Pathology

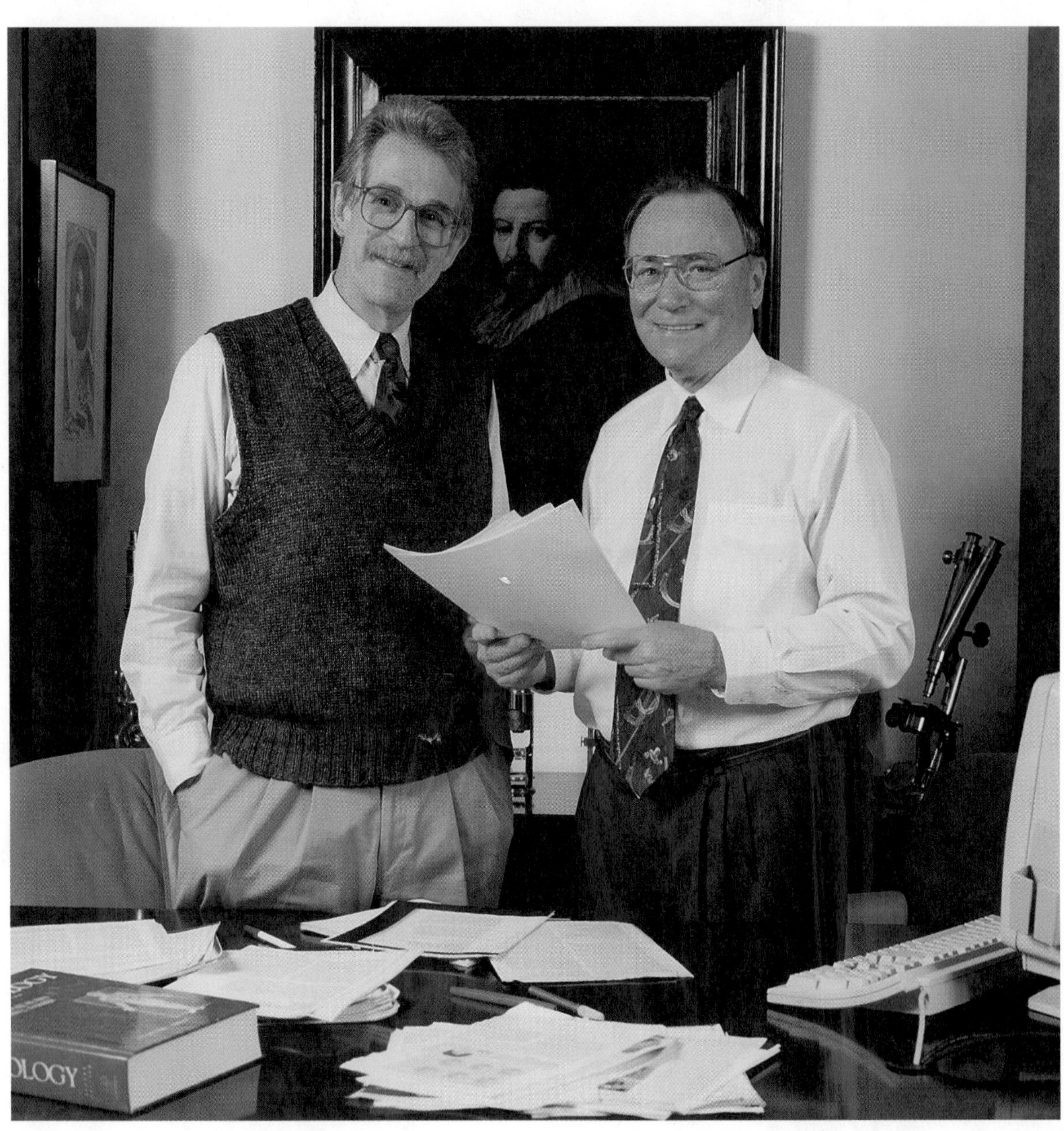

John L. Farber (*left*), Emanuel Rubin (*right*).

Pathology

THIRD EDITION

EDITED BY

Emanuel Rubin, M.D.

Gonzalo E. Aponte Professor and Chairman
Department of Pathology, Anatomy and Cell Biology
Jefferson Medical College
Thomas Jefferson University
Philadelphia, Pennsylania

John L. Farber, M.D.

Professor of Pathology, Anatomy and Cell Biology
Jefferson Medical College
Thomas Jefferson University
Philadelphia, Pennsylania

WITH 47 CONTRIBUTORS

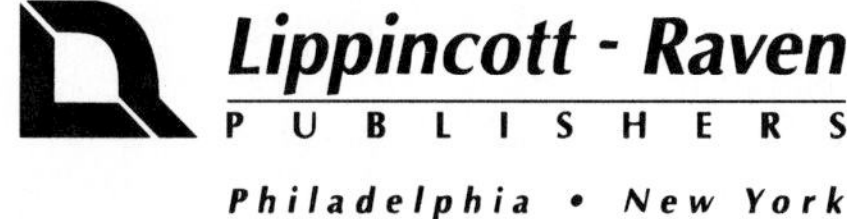

Philadelphia • New York

To our parents:
Jacob and Sophie Rubin
Lionel and Freda Farber

and our wives:
Linda Anne and Susan

Acquisitions Editor: Richard Winters
Developmental Editor: Mary Beth Murphy
Manufacturing Manager: Dennis Teston
Production Manager: Cassie Moore
Production Editor: Kimberly Monroe
Indexer: Maria Coughlin
Compositor: Maryland Composition
Printer: R. R. Donnelly

Printed in the United States of America

9 8 7 6 5 4 3 2 1

Library of Congress Cataloging-in-Publication Data

Pathology/edited by Emanuel Rubin, John L. Farber. — 3rd ed.
p. cm.
Includes bibliographical references and index.
ISBN 0-397-58422-9
1. Pathology. I. Rubin, Emanuel, 1928– . II. Farber, John L, 1941– .
[DNLM: 1. Pathology. QZ 4 P29854 1998]
RB111.P29 1998
616.07—dc21
DNLM/DLC
for Library of Congress 98-3831
CIP

Contributors

Vernon W. Armbrustmacher, M.D.
Medical Examiner, Neuropathologist
Office of the Chief Medical Examiner
New York, New York

Adam Bagg, M.D.
Associate Professor of Pathology and Medicine
Georgetown University Medical Center
Director of Hematopathology and Clinical Hematology
Georgetown University School of Medicine
Washington, D.C.

Károly Balogh, M.D.
Associate Professor of Pathology
Harvard Medical School;
Pathologist
New England Deaconess Hospital
Boston, Massachusetts

Sue A. Bartow, M.D.
Associate Professor of Laboratory Medicine and Pathology
University of Minnesota Medical School
Minneapolis, Minesota

Earl P. Benditt, M.D.*
Professor of Pathology Emeritus
University of Washington School of Medicine;
Distinguished Physician
Veterans Administration Medical Center
Seattle, Washington

Hugh Bonner, M.D.
Adjunct Associate Professor of Pathology
University of Pennsylvania School of Medicine
Philadelphia, Pennsylvania;
Director of Anatomic Pathology
The Chester County Hospital
West Chester, Pennsylvania

Thomas W. Bouldin, M.D.
Professor of Pathology and Ophthalmology
University of North Carolina School of Medicine;
Attending Pathologist
University of North Carolina Hospitals
Chapel Hill, North Carolina

Stephen W. Chensue, M.D. Ph.D.
Assistant Professor of Pathology
University of Michigan Medical School;
Staff Pathologist
Veterans Affairs Medical Center
Ann Arbor, Michigan

Wallace H. Clark, M.D.*
Visiting Professor of Pathology
Harvard Medical School;
Senior Pathologist
Beth Israel Hospital
Boston, Massachusetts

Daniel H. Connor, M.D.
Visiting Professor of Pathology
Georgetown University School of Medicine;
Rockville, Maryland

Jeffrey Cossman, M.D.
Oscar Benwood Hunter Professor of Pathology
Georgetown University School of Medicine
Washington, D.C.

John E. Craighead, M.D.
Professor of Pathology Emeritus
University of Vermont College of Medicine;
Attending Pathologist
Fletcher Allen Health Care
Burlington, Vermont

Maire A. Duggan, M.B., B.C.H., F.R.C.P.
Professor of Pathology
University of Calgary;
Consultant Pathologist
Calgary Laboratory Services
Calgary, Alberta, Canada

Hormoz Ehya, M.D.
Senior Member and Director of Cytopathology
Fox Chase Cancer Center
Clinical Professor of Pathology
MCP-Hahnemann School of Medicine;
Adjunct Clinical Professor of Pathology, Anatomy and Cell Biology
Jefferson Medical College
Philadelphia, Pennsylvania

**Deceased*

Joseph C. Fantone, M.D.
Professor of Pathology
University of Michigan Medical School;
Pathologist
University of Michigan Medical Center
Ann Arbor, Michigan

John L. Farber, M.D.
Professor of Pathology, Anatomy and Cell Biology
Jefferson Medical College
Thomas Jefferson University
Philadelphia, Pennsylvania

Gregory N. Fuller, M.D.
Assistant Professor of Pathology
MD Anderson Cancer Center
Houston, Texas

Robert M. Genta, M.D.
Professor of Pathology, Medicine,
Microbiology and Immunology
Baylor Medical College
Chief of Pathology and Laboratory Medicine
Veterans Administration Medical Center
Houston, Texas

Avrum I. Gotlieb, M.D.
Professor and Chairman
Department of Laboratory Medicine and Pathobiology
Faculty of Medicine
University of Toronto
Director of Vascular Research Laboratories
Toronto Hospital
Toronto, Ontario, Canada

Stanley R. Hamilton, M.D.
Head
Division of Pathology/Laboratory Medicine
University of Texas
MD Anderson Cancer Center
Houston, Texas

Terence J. Harrist, M.D.
Clinical Assistant Professor of Pathology
Harvard Medical School
Senior Pathologist
Beth Israel Hospital
Boston, Massachusetts

Arthur P. Hays, M.D.
Associate Professor of Pathology
College of Physicians and Surgeons
Columbia University
New York, New York

J. Charles Jennette, M.D.
Professor of Pathology and Laboratory
Medicine
University of North Carolina School
of Medicine
Chapel Hill, North Carolina

Robert B. Jennings, M.D.
James B. Duke Professor of Pathology
Duke University Medical Center
Durham, North Carolina

Kent J. Johnson, M.D.
Professor of Pathology
University of Michigan Medical School;
Pathologist
University of Michigan Medical Center
Ann Arbor, Michigan

Robert Kisilevsky, M.D., Ph.D., F.R.C.P.
Professor of Pathology and Biochemistry
Queen's University;
Attending Pathologist
Kingston General Hospital
Kingston, Ontario, Canada

Gordon K. Klintworth, M.D., Ph.D.
Professor of Pathology
Joseph A. C. Wadsworth Research
Professor of Ophthalmology
Duke University Medical Center
Durham, North Carolina

Robert J. Kurman, M.D.
Professor of Pathology and Obstetrics
and Gynecology
Johns Hopkins University School
of Medicine
Director of Gynecologic Pathology
Johns Hopkins Hospital
Baltimore, Maryland

Ernest A. Lack, M.D.
Professor of Pathology
Georgetown University School of Medicine
Director of Anatomic Pathology
Georgetown University Medical Center
Washington, D.C.

Antonio Martinez-Hernandez, M.D.
Professor of Pathology
University of Tennessee College of Medicine;
Chief of Pathology and Laboratory Medicine
Veterans Administration Medical Center
Memphis, Tennessee

Wolfgang J. Mergner, M.D., Ph.D.
Professor of Pathology
University of Maryland School of Medicine;
Director of Anatomic Pathology
University of Maryland Medical Center
Baltimore, Maryland

Robert O. Petersen, M.D., Ph.D.
Professor of Pathology, Anatomy and Cell Biology
Jefferson Medical College
Thomas Jefferson University;
Attending Pathologist
Thomas Jefferson University Hospital
Philadelphia, Pennsylvania

Timothy R. Quinn, M.D.
Instructor in Pathology
Harvard Medical School;
Pathologist
Beth Israel Hospital
Boston, Massachusetts

Stanley J. Robboy, M.D.
Professor of Pathology and Obstetrics and Gynecology
Duke University Medical School;
Vice-Chairman of Pathology
Duke University Medical Center
Durham, North Carolina

Emanuel Rubin, M.D.
Gonzalo E. Aponte Professor and Chairman
Department of Pathology, Anatomy and Cell Biology
Jefferson Medical College
Thomas Jefferson University
Philadelphia, Pennsylvania

Dante G. Scarpelli, M.D., Ph.D.
Earnest J. and Hattie H. Magerstadt
Professor of Pathology
Northwestern University Medical School
Chicago, Illinois

Brian Schapiro, M.D.
Instructor in Pathology
Harvard Medical School;
Pathologist
Beth Israel Hospital
Boston, Massachusetts

Alan L. Schiller, M.D.
Irene Heinz Given and John LaPorte Given
Professor and Chairman of Pathology
Mount Sinai School of Medicine;
Director of Pathology
The Mount Sinai Hospital
New York, New York

Stephen M. Schwartz, M.D., Ph.D.
Professor of Pathology
University of Washington School of Medicine
Seattle, Washington

Benjamin H. Spargo, M.D.
Professor of Pathology Emeritus
University of Chicago School of Medicine;
Emeritus Director of Renal Pathology
University of Chicago Medical Center
Chicago, Illinois

Charles Steenbergen, Jr., M.D., Ph.D.
Assistant Professor of Pathology
Duke University Medical Center
Durham, North Carolina

Steven L. Teitelbaum, M.D.
Messing Professor of Pathology
Washington University Medical Center
St. Louis, Missouri

William D. Travis, M.D.
Co-Chairman Department of Pulmonary
and Mediastinal Pathology
Armed Forces Institute of Pathology
Washington, D.C.

Benjamin F. Trump, M.D.
Professor and Chairman
Department of Pathology
University of Maryland School of Medicine
Baltimore, Maryland

F. Stephen Vogel, M.D.
Clinical Professor of Pathology
Medical College of Georgia;
Secretary-Treasurer and Executive Director
United States and Canadian Academy of Pathology
Augusta, Georgia

Peter A. Ward, M.D.
Godfrey D. Stobbe Professor and Chairman
Department of Pathology
University of Michigan Medical School
Ann Arbor, Michigan

Preface

An honest tale speeds best being plainly told.
(Shakespeare, Richard III)

As we stated in the Preface to the previous editions of *Pathology*, this third edition continues to view pathology as the medical science that deals with all aspects of disease, but with special reference to the essential nature, the causes, and the development of abnormal conditions. In this sense, literacy in pathology is the bedrock of practice and research for the student of medical science.

As in the earlier editions, *Pathology* maintains the traditional custom of dividing the subject matter into general (Chapters 1–9) and systemic (Chapters 10–30) pathology. General pathology emphasizes the towering achievements in the study of cell and molecular biology, biochemistry, and immunology, all of which are related to the contemporary understanding of the pathogenesis of disease. Although systemic pathology is concerned principally with the description of specific maladies, the concepts detailed in general pathology are utilized to explain their underlying causes. Particular attention continues to be paid throughout to the impact of molecular genetics on our insights into the causes and manifestations of disease, including the correlations between genotype and phenotypic expression. For reference purposes, wherever possible we have identified the relevant gene mutations and their chromosomal locations.

Our original decision to present separate chapters on two systemic diseases, namely diabetes and amyloidosis, has been amply justified by the striking accumulation of new knowledge in these areas. We also recognize the increasing importance of cytopathology as a diagnostic modality by retaining a chapter on this subject.

In his treatise *On the Natural Faculties*, Galen wrote, "the chief merit of language is clearness, and we know that nothing detracts from this as do unfamiliar terms." As in the first two editions, we have always kept this admonition in mind in editing the text and the graphic material. To enhance the clarity of presentation, the third edition features definitions of all disease in the form of initial italicized statements. We continue with the format of designating for every disease separate sections of pathogenesis, pathology, and clinical features. Attention is often directed to the key points by the use of bulleted lists and boldface type.

To aid the student in understanding and retaining complex and detailed information, we have retained the emphasis on graphic representations of the pathogenesis of disease, the complications of various disorders, and the sequences of pathological alterations. Because graphic images utilize pattern recognition, one of the most fundamental characteristics of the human brain, they powerfully communicate abstract and complex material, as any lecturer who has referred to a graph will attest. At the same time, we have been guided by Einstein's admonition that "everything should be made as simple as possible, but not simpler." For the third edition, we have added many new drawings and have revised virtually all of the previous ones. In particular, all the artwork is now presented in full color, taking maximum advantage of contemporary computer graphics. The number of color photographs has also been increased.

We mourn the passing of three of our most distinguished original authors, namely Earl Benditt, Wally Clark, and Don Hackel. At the same time, we welcome the participation of many new authors in the chapters on hemodymanic disorders, infectious diseases, blood vessels, respiratory system, gastrointestinal tract, kidney, blood, endocrine system, skin, bones, skeletal muscle, and the nervous system.

Sadly, attempting to edit a comprehensive textbook of pathology without missing any errors is like trying to live without sin—worth the effort, but probably impossible. However, the inevitability of human mistakes has not deterred us from including new and still controversial concepts. Some of these will stand the test of time; the others will be corrected in the next edition.

Emanuel Rubin
John L. Farber

Contents

Pathology

CHAPTER 1

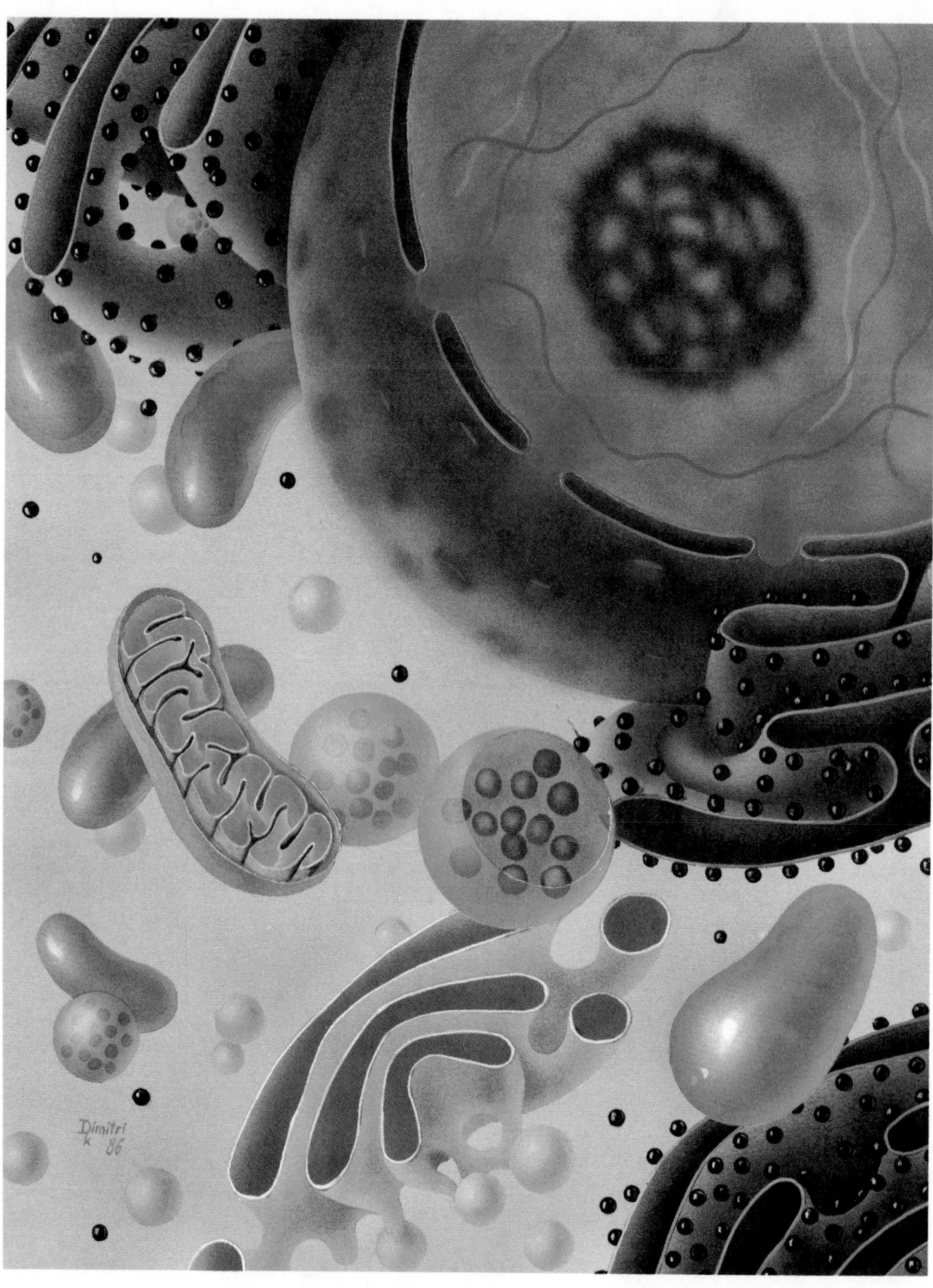

Cell Injury

Emanuel Rubin
John L. Farber

FIGURE **1-1** *(see opposite page)*
Interior of an idealized cell.

Pathology in its simplest sense is the study of structural and functional abnormalities that are expressed as diseases of organs and systems. Classic theories of disease attributed all disorders to systemic imbalances or to noxious effects of humors on specific organs. In the 19th century, Rudolf Virchow, often referred to as the father of modern pathology, broke sharply with such traditional concepts by proposing that the basis of all disease is injury to the smallest living unit of the body, namely, the cell. A century and a half later, both clinical and experimental pathology remain rooted in Virchow's cellular pathology.

To appreciate the mechanisms of injury to the cell, it is useful to consider its global needs in a philosophical sense. In the reaction against mystical or vitalistic theories of biology, teleology—the study of design or purpose in nature—was discredited as a means of scientific investigation. Nevertheless, although facts can be established only by observations, teleological thinking can be important in framing questions. As an analogy, without an understanding of the goals of chess and prior knowledge that a particular computer is programmed to play it, no analysis of the machine would be likely to uncover its method of operation. Moreover, it would be futile to search for the sources of defects in the specific program or overall operating system while lacking an appreciation of the goals of the device. In this sense, it is helpful to understand the problems with which the cell is confronted and the strategies that have evolved to cope with them.

A living cell must maintain an organization capable of producing energy. Thus, the most pressing need for a free living cell, whether prokaryotic or eukaryotic, is to establish a structural and functional barrier between its internal milieu and a hostile environment. The plasma membrane serves this purpose in three ways:

- It maintains a constant internal ionic composition against very large chemical gradients between the interior and exterior compartments.
- It selectively admits some molecules while excluding or extruding others.
- It provides a structural envelope to contain the informational, synthetic, and catabolic constituents of the cell.
- It provides an environment to house signal transduction molecules that mediate communication between the external and internal milieus.

At the same time, to survive, the cell must be able to adapt to adverse environmental conditions, such as changes in temperature, solute concentrations, or oxygen supply; the presence of noxious agents; and so on. The evolution of multicellular organisms eased the hazardous lot of individual cells by establishing a controlled extracellular environment in which temperature, oxygenation, ionic content, and nutrient supply are relatively constant. It also permitted the luxury of differentiation of cells for such widely divergent functions as nutrient storage (liver cell glycogen and adipocytes), communication (neurons), contractile activity (heart muscle), synthesis of proteins or peptides for export (liver, pancreas, and endocrine cells), absorption (intestine), and defense against foreign invaders (polymorphonuclear leukocytes, lymphocytes, and macrophages).

Cells encounter many stresses as a result of changes in their internal and external environments. **The patterns of response to this stress constitute the cellular bases of disease.** If an injury exceeds the adaptive capacity of the cell, it dies. A cell exposed to persistent sublethal injury has a limited repertoire of responses, the expression of which we interpret as evidence of cell injury. In general, the mammalian cell adapts to injury by conserving its resources; it decreases or ceases its differentiated functions and reverts to its ancestral, unicellular character, which is concerned with functions exclusively dedicated to its own survival. **In this perspective, pathology is the study of cell injury and the expression of a preexisting capacity to adapt to such injury, on the part of either injured or intact cells.** Such an orientation leaves little room for the concept of parallel—normal and pathological—biologies.

CELLULAR PATTERNS OF RESPONSE TO STRESS

All cells have efficient mechanisms to deal with shifts in environmental conditions. Thus, ion channels open or close, harmful chemicals are detoxified, metabolic stores such as fat or glycogen may be mobilized, and catabolic processes lead to the segregation of internal particulate materials. It is when environmental changes exceed the capacity of the cell to maintain normal homeostasis that we recognize acute cell injury. If the stress is removed in time, or if the cell is able to withstand the assault, cell injury is reversible, and complete structural and functional integrity is restored. For example, when circulation to the heart is interrupted for less than 30 minutes, all structural and functional alterations prove to be reversible. The cell can also be exposed to persistent sublethal stress, as in mechanical irritation of the skin or exposure of the bronchial mucosa to tobacco smoke. In such instances, the cell has time to adapt to reversible injury in a number of ways, each of which has its morphological counterpart.

On the other hand, if the stress is severe, irreversible injury leads to death of the cell. The precise moment at which reversible injury gives way to irreversible injury, the "point of no return," cannot at present be identified. The morphological pattern of cell death occasioned by disparate exogenous environmental stresses is **coagulative necrosis**. This type of necrosis is common to almost all forms of cell death and precedes the other varieties to be described.

REVERSIBLE CELL INJURY

Hydropic Swelling

Hydropic swelling is an increase in cell volume characterized by a large, pale cytoplasm and a normally located nucleus (Fig. 1-2). The greater volume reflects an increased water content. Hydropic swelling is a reflection of acute, reversible cell injury and may result from such varied causes as chemical and biological toxins, viral or bacterial infections, ischemia, excessive heat or cold, and so on. The archaic description "cloudy swelling" refers to the gross appearance of injured tissue that contains hydropically swollen cells.

By electron microscopy, the number of organelles is unchanged, although they appear dispersed in a larger volume. The excess fluid seems to accumulate preferentially in the cisternae of the endoplasmic reticulum, which are conspicuously dilated, presumably because of ionic shifts into this compartment (Fig. 1-3). It deserves emphasis that hydropic swelling is entirely reversible when the cause is removed.

Hydropic swelling results from impairment of cellular volume regulation, a process that controls ionic concentrations in the cytoplasm. This regulation, particularly for sodium, operates at three levels: (1) the plasma membrane itself, (2) the plasma membrane sodium pump, and (3) the supply of adenosine triphosphate (ATP). The plasma membrane imposes a barrier to the flow of sodium down a concentration gradient into the cell and prevents a similar efflux of potassium from the cell. The barrier to sodium is imperfect, and the relative leakiness to that ion permits the passive entry of sodium into the cell. To compensate for this intrusion, the energy-dependent plasma membrane sodium pump (Na^+-K^+ ATPase), which is fueled by ATP, extrudes sodium. Injurious agents may interfere with this membrane-regulated process by (1) increasing the permeability of the plasma membrane to sodium, thereby exceeding the capacity of the pump to extrude sodium; (2) damaging the pump directly; or (3) interfering with the synthesis of ATP and depriving the pump of its fuel. In any event, the accumulation of sodium in the cell leads to an increase in water content to maintain isosmotic conditions, and the cell then swells.

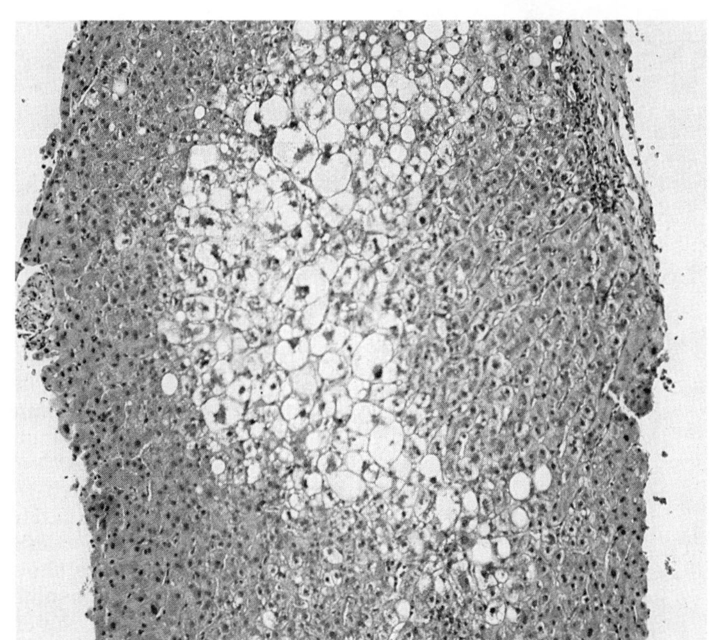

FIGURE *1-2*
Hydropic swelling. A needle biopsy of the liver in a patient with toxic hepatic injury shows severe hydropic swelling in the centrilobular zone. The affected hepatocytes exhibit central nuclei and cytoplasm distended (ballooned) by excess fluid.

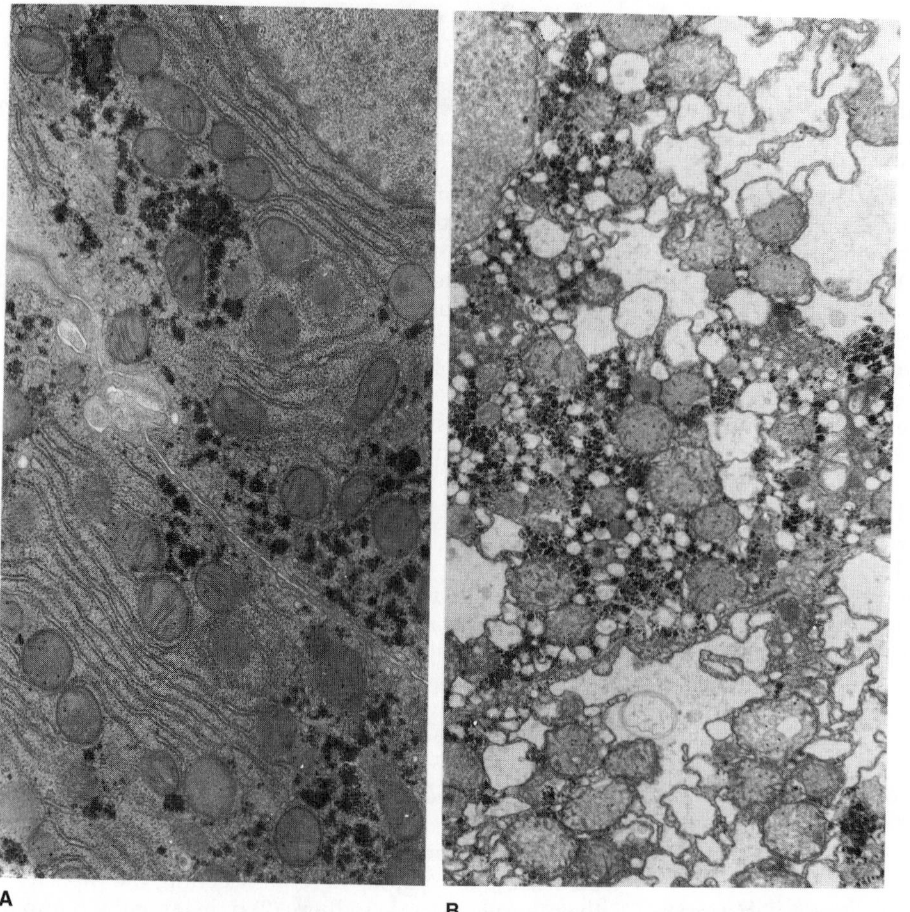

FIGURE *1-3*
Ultrastructure of hydropic swelling of a liver cell. (*A*) Two apposed normal hepatocytes with tightly organized, parallel arrays of rough endoplasmic reticulum. (*B*) Swollen hepatocyte in which the cisternae of the endoplasmic reticulum are dilated by excess fluid.

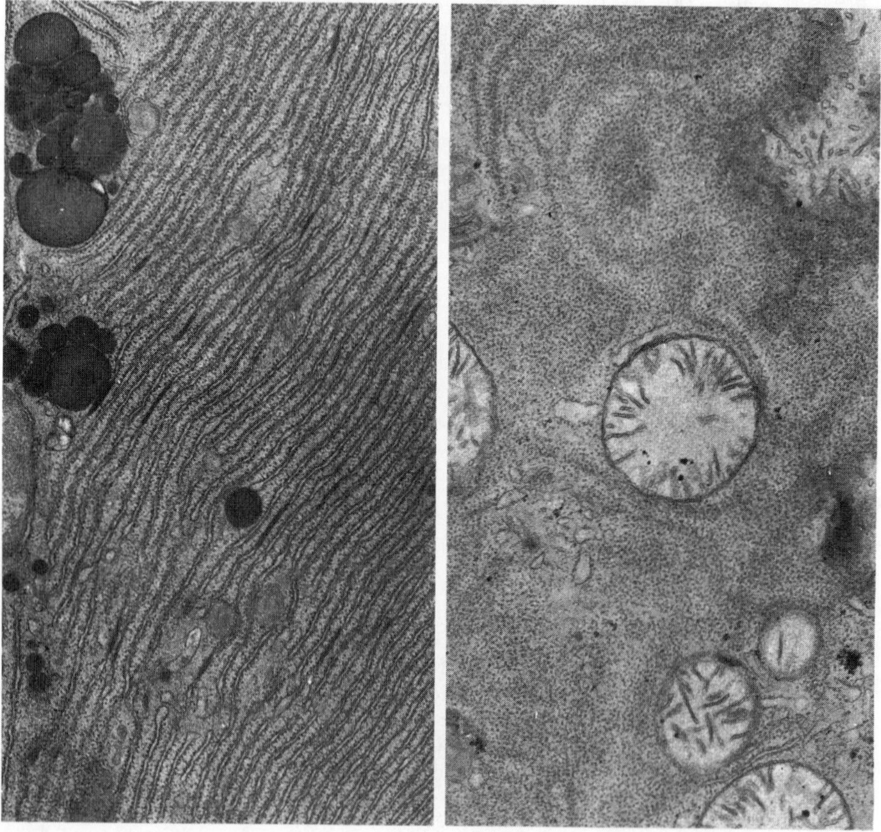

FIGURE *1-4*
Disaggregation of membrane-bound polyribosomes in acute, reversible liver injury. (*A*) Normal hepactocyte, in which the profiles of endoplasmic reticulum are studded with ribosomes. (*B*) An injured hepatocyte, showing detachment of ribosomes from the membranes of the endoplasmic reticulum and the accumulation of free ribosomes in the cytoplasm.

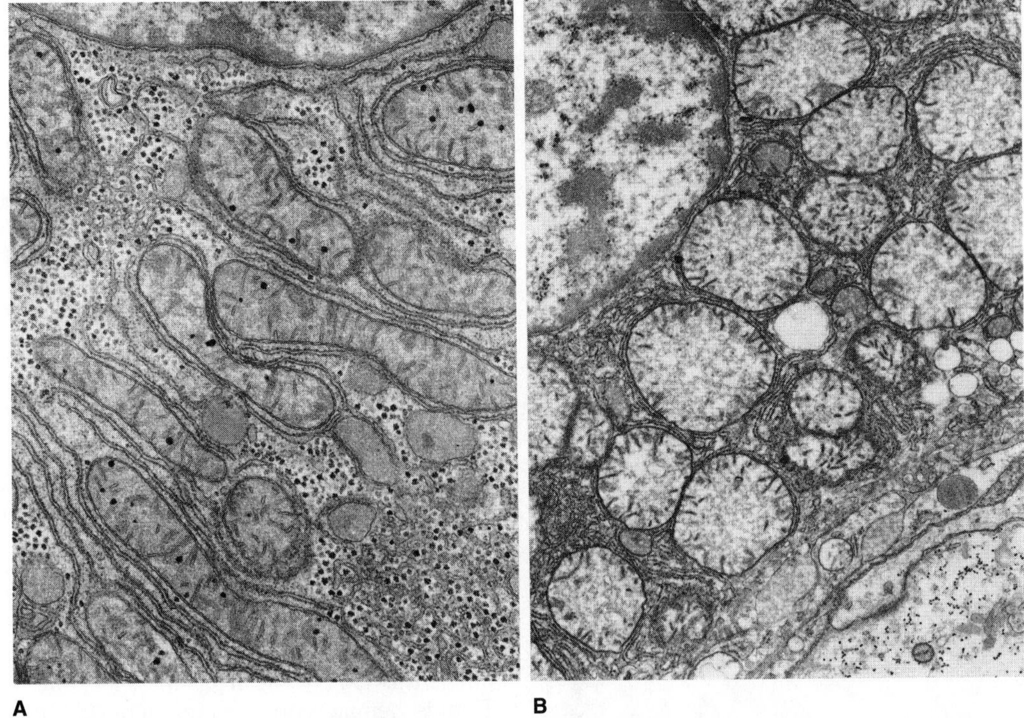

FIGURE 1-5
Mitochondrial swelling in acute ischemic cell injury. (*A*) Normal mitochondria are elongated and display prominent cristae, which traverse the mitochondrial matrix. (*B*) Mitochondria from an ischemic cell are swollen and round and exhibit a decreased matrix density. The cristae are less prominent than in the normal organelle.

Ultrastructural Changes

Changes in the ultrastructure of intracellular organelles occur in reversibly injured cells.

- **Endoplasmic reticulum:** The cisternae of the endoplasmic reticulum are distended by fluid in hydropic swelling (see Fig. 1-3). In other forms of acute, reversible cell injury, membrane-bound polysomes may undergo disaggregation and detach from the surface of the rough endoplasmic reticulum (Fig. 1-4).
- **Mitochondria:** In some forms of acute injury, particularly ischemia, mitochondria swell (Fig. 1-5). This enlargement is probably caused by the dissipation of the energy gradient and consequent impairment of mitochondrial volume control. Amorphous densities rich in phospholipid may appear, but these effects are fully reversible on recovery.
- **Plasma membrane:** Blebs of the plasma membrane—that is, focal extrusions of the cytoplasm—are occasionally noted. These can detach from the membrane into the external environment without the loss of cell viability.
- **Nucleolus:** In the nucleus, reversible injury is reflected principally in nucleolar change. The fibrillar and granular components of the nucleolus may segregate. Alternatively, the granular component may be diminished, leaving only a fibrillar core. These morphological changes are accompanied by reduced synthesis of ribosomal RNA species.

It is important to recognize that after withdrawal of an acute stress that has led to reversible cell injury, by definition, the cell returns to its normal state.

MORPHOLOGICAL REACTIONS TO PERSISTENT STRESS

Persistent stress is often described as leading to chronic cell injury. Yet few if any of the morphological changes at the cellular level reflect the type of persistent damage seen in chronically injured organs. Similar responses to insults at the cellular level can produce different gross appearances in injured organs. For example, chronic ischemia of the brain leads to permanent injury and shrinkage of that organ. Chronic liver injury produces irreversible damage in the form of a diffuse scarring, called cirrhosis. **In general, permanent organ injury is associated with the death of individual cells. By contrast, the cellular response to persistent sublethal injury, whether chemical or physical, reflects adaptation of the cell to a hostile environment.** Again, these changes are, for the most part, reversible on discontinuation of the stress. In response to

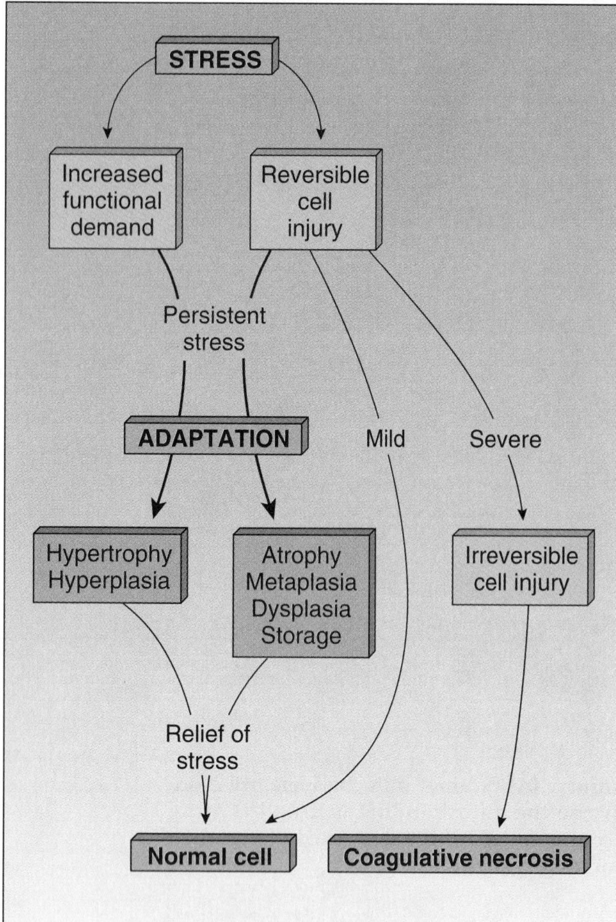

FIGURE **1-6**
Reactions of cells to stress.

persistent stress, a cell dies or adapts. Cells experiencing persistent stress manifest few if any of the characteristic alterations described for acute cell injury. It is thus our view that at the cellular level it is more appropriate to speak of chronic adaptation than of chronic injury (Fig. 1-6). The major adaptive responses are atrophy, hypertrophy, hyperplasia, metaplasia, dysplasia, and intracellular storage. According to some theories, certain forms of neoplasia may also result from adaptive responses.

Atrophy

Atrophy is a decrease in the size and function of a cell. Clinically, it is often recognized as a diminution in the size or function of an organ (Fig. 1-7). Atrophy is often seen in areas of vascular insufficiency or chronic inflammation and may result from disuse of skeletal muscle. Atrophy may be thought of as an adaptive response to stress, in which the cell shrinks in volume and shuts down its differentiated functions, thereby reducing its need for energy to a minimum. In general, the genes expressed in all cells fall into two broad categories, namely the "housekeeping" genes necessary for the maintenance and survival of any cell and those that determine the differentiated phenotype of any particular cell. With atrophy the expression of differentiation genes is repressed, without significant effects on the expression of housekeeping genes. On restoration of normal conditions, atrophic cells are fully capable of resuming their differentiated functions; size increases to normal, and specialized functions, such as protein synthesis or contractile force, return to their original levels. Atrophy occurs under a variety of conditions outlined below.

Reduced Functional Demand

The most common form of atrophy follows reduced functional demand. For example, after immobilization of a limb in a cast as treatment for a bone fracture, or after prolonged bed rest, muscle cells atrophy and muscular strength is reduced. With resumption of normal activity, normal size and function are restored.

Inadequate Supply of Oxygen

Interference with blood supply to tissues is known as ischemia. Total ischemia, with cessation of oxygen perfusion of tissues, results in cell death. Partial ischemia occurs after incomplete occlusion of a blood vessel or in areas of inadequate collateral circulation following a complete vascular occlusion. This results in a chronically reduced oxygen supply, a condition often compatible with cell viability. Under such circumstances, cell atrophy is common. It is frequently seen around the inadequately perfused margins of ischemic necrosis (infarcts) in the heart, brain, and kidneys following vascular occlusion in these organs.

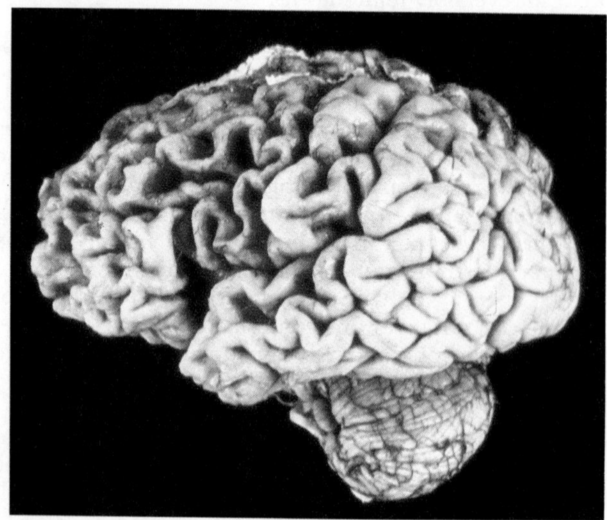

FIGURE *1-7*
Atrophy of the brain. Marked atrophy of the frontal lobe is noted in this photograph of the brain. The gyri are thinned and the sulci conspicuously widened.

Insufficient Nutrients

Starvation or inadequate nutrition associated with chronic disease leads to cell atrophy, particularly in skeletal muscle. From a teleological point of view, it is striking that reduction in mass is particularly prominent in cells that are not vital to the survival of the organism. One cannot dismiss the possibility that a portion of the cell atrophy caused by partial ischemia reflects a lack of nutrients.

Interruption of Trophic Signals

The functions of many cells depend on signals transmitted by chemical mediators. The endocrine system and neuromuscular transmission are the best examples. The demands placed on the cell by the actions of hormones or, in the case of skeletal muscle, by synaptic transmission, can be eliminated by removing the source of the signal. This can be accomplished through, for example, ablation of an endocrine gland or denervation. If the anterior pituitary is surgically resected, the loss of thyroid-stimulating hormone (TSH), adrenocorticotropic hormone, and follicle-stimulating hormone (FSH) results in atrophy of the thyroid, adrenal cortex, and ovaries, respectively. Atrophy secondary to endocrine insufficiency is not restricted to pathological conditions—witness the atrophy of the endometrium caused by decreased estrogen levels following menopause (Fig. 1-8). Moreover, even cancer cells can be induced to undergo atrophy, to some extent, by hormonal deprivation. Androgen-dependent cancer of the prostate partially regresses after the administration of testosterone antagonists. The growth of certain types of thyroid cancer is halted by inhibiting pituitary TSH secretion with thyroxine. Neurological conditions resulting in denervation of muscle, and thus in loss of the neuromuscular transmission necessary for muscle tone, cause atrophy of the affected muscles. The wasting caused by poliomyelitis or traumatic paraplegia falls into this category.

Persistent Cell Injury

Persistent cell injury is most commonly caused by chronic inflammation associated with prolonged viral or bacterial infections. Chronic inflammation may be seen in a variety of other circumstances, including immunological and granulomatous disorders. Whether cell injury results from the inciting agent, the inflammatory process itself, or both is not always clear. In any event, cells in areas of chronic inflammation are often atrophic. A good example is the profound atrophy of the gastric mucosa that occurs in association with chronic gastritis (see Chapter 13). Similarly, villous atrophy of the small intestinal mucosa follows the chronic inflammation characteristic of celiac dis-

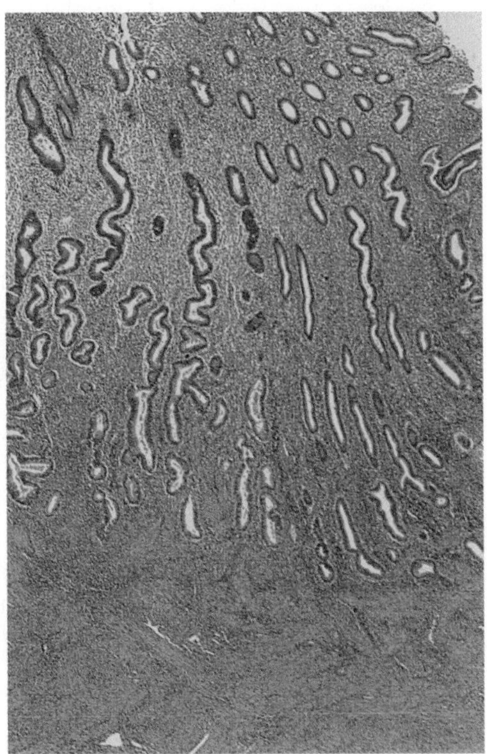

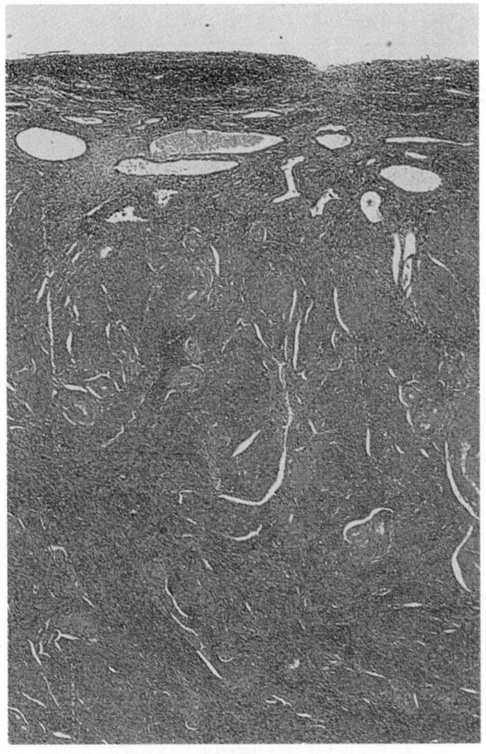

FIGURE *1-8*
Proliferative endometrium. ***(A)*** **A section of the uterus from a woman of reproductive age reveals a thick endometrium composed of proliferative glands in an abundant stroma.** ***(B)*** **The endometrium of a 75-year-old woman (shown at the same magnification as A) is thin and contains only a few atrophic and cystic glands.**

ease. Even physical injury, such as prolonged pressure in inappropriate locations, produces atrophy. Heart failure leads to increased pressure in sinusoids of the liver because the heart cannot efficiently pump the venous return from that organ. Accordingly, the cells exposed to the greatest pressure—those in the center of the liver lobule—become atrophic.

Aging

One of the hallmarks of aging, particularly in nonreplicating cells such as those of the brain and heart, is cell atrophy. The size of all the parenchymal organs of the body decreases with age. The size of the brain is invariably decreased, while in the very old the size of the heart may be so diminished that the term **senile atrophy** has been used.

Hypertrophy

Hypertrophy is an increase in the size of a cell accompanied by an augmented functional capacity. Unlike hydropic swelling, the hypertrophied cell does not contain excess water or electrolytes. Hypertrophy is a response to trophic signals or increased functional demands and is commonly a normal process. Hypertrophy can be thought to represent the opposite of atrophy, with increased expression of differentiation genes.

Physiological (Hormonal) Hypertrophy

Physiological hypertrophy occurs during maturation under the influence of a variety of hormones. An increased production of sex hormones at puberty leads to hypertrophy of the juvenile sex organs and organs associated with secondary sex characteristics. The lactating woman, under the influence of prolactin and estrogen, exhibits hypertrophy of breast tissue.

Although hypertrophy results from certain normal hormonal signals, it is also a response to abnormal levels of hormones. Exogenous anabolic steroids are taken by athletes precisely for their capacity to induce muscle hypertrophy. Endogenous overproduction of TSH by the pituitary is responsible for the thyroid enlargement (goiter) that occurs with nutritional iodine deficiency. In the absence of sufficient iodine, thyroid hormone is not produced. Consequently, there is no feedback inhibition of TSH secretion, and the unopposed TSH, acting as a trophic hormone, induces hypertrophy of thyroid follicular cells. Increased hormone levels can also result from abnormal hormone production by tumors. For example, secretion of corticotropic hormone by pituitary tumors results in hypertrophy of the adrenal cortex.

Increased Functional Demand

Hypertrophy caused by an increased functional demand is exemplified by greater muscle size and strength following repeated exercise. In an analogous fashion, an exogenous metabolic demand is placed on the liver cell by the administration of drugs that are detoxified by the mixed-function oxidase system. Cytochrome P_{450} and other enzymes of this drug-metabolizing system reside in the smooth endoplasmic reticulum. The liver cell responds to the metabolic demand of detoxification by increasing the amount of smooth endoplasmic reticulum, with consequent hypertrophy of the cell (Fig. 1-9).

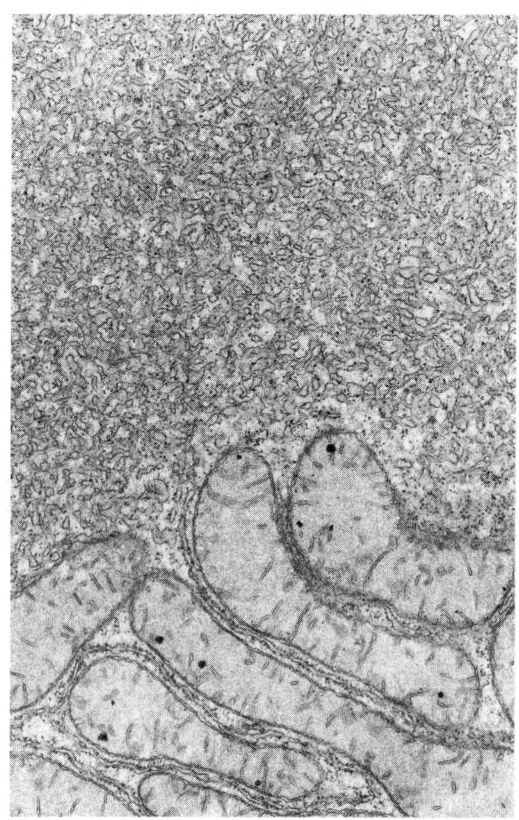

FIGURE *1-9*
Proliferation of smooth endoplasmic reticulum in a liver cell in response to phenobarbital administration.

Increased demand occurs under pathological conditions as well. The heart may be called on to increase its contractile force because of mechanical interference with the aortic outflow or because of systemic hypertension, both conditions requiring the heart to eject blood under higher pressure (Fig. 1-10). As in exercise-induced hypertrophy of skeletal muscle, the myocardial cells enlarge, and the heart may more than double in weight. Increased demand also results from the loss of functional mass. If one kidney is surgically removed or rendered inoperative because of vascular occlusion, the contralateral kidney hypertrophies to accommodate the increased demand.

Cellular Mechanisms of Hypertrophy

The elucidation of the cellular and molecular mechanisms underlying the hypertrophic response is still actively investigated, although it is clear that the final steps must include increases in messenger and ribosomal RNA and

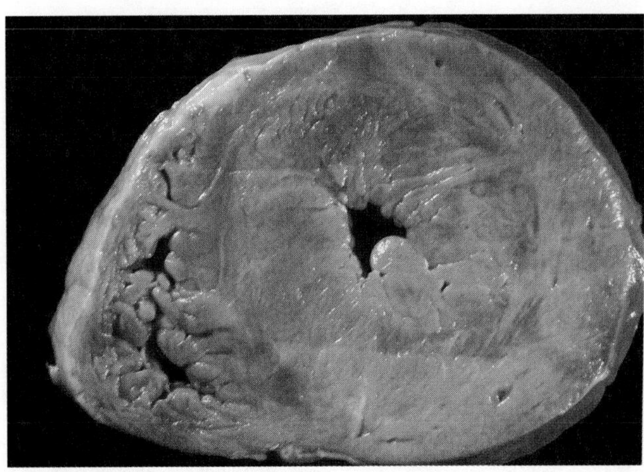

FIGURE *1-10*
Myocardial hypertrophy. Cross-section of the heart of a patient with long-standing hypertension shows pronounced, concentric left ventricular hypertrophy.

protein. Thus, cell hypertrophy in some way results from transcriptional regulation. The growth in the size of a cell and DNA replication can be independently regulated by different growth factors. Experimental cardiac hypertrophy is the best-studied model at this time and is discussed in Chapter 11.

The molecular basis of hypertrophy has also been studied in the kidney. After experimental extirpation of one kidney, the remaining kidney exhibits little change in cell number but rather a striking increase in the size of the tubular cells. As in the heart, this compensatory hypertrophic response is accompanied by an increased expression of growth-promoting genes (protooncogenes), such as *myc*, *fos*, and *ras*. When renal tubular cells in culture are exposed to mitogens, they enter into DNA synthesis and divide. However, when the mitogens are added in the presence of inhibitors of DNA synthesis, the cells do not replicate but rather undergo hypertrophy. Thus, the same stimulus can lead to hypertrophy or hyperplasia, depending on the presence of other growth factors or inhibitors.

Hyperplasia

Hyperplasia is an increase in the number of cells in an organ or tissue. Hypertrophy and hyperplasia are not mutually exclusive and are often seen concurrently.

Hormonal Stimulation

Hormonal signals can induce a physiological hyperplastic effect. For example, the normal increase in estrogen levels at puberty and during the early phase of the menstrual cycle leads to an increased number of both endometrial and uterine stromal cells. A similar hyperplastic response is commonly produced by the administration of exogenous estrogen in postmenopausal women. Estrogens also produce hyperplasia in men. Gynecomastia, an enlargement of the male breast characterized by hyperplasia of the epithelial cells lining the ducts, occurs after the treatment of prostatic carcinoma with exogenous estrogens. Similarly, gynecomastia is seen in patients with chronic liver disease, a malady in which circulating estrogen levels are raised because of diminished hepatic inactivation. Hormones produced by tumors can also lead to hyperplasia. For example, secretion of erythropoietin by cancer of the kidney leads to an increase in the number of erythrocyte precursors in the bone marrow.

Increased Functional Demand

Hyperplasia, like hypertrophy, may also follow increased physiological demand. Residence at high altitude, where the oxygen content of the air is relatively low, leads to compensatory hyperplasia of erythrocyte precursors in the bone marrow and an increased number of circulating erythrocytes (secondary polycythemia). The decrease in the amount of oxygen carried in each erythrocyte is balanced by an increase in the number of cells. On return to sea level, the number of erythrocytes promptly falls to normal. Similarly, chronic blood loss, as in abnormal uterine bleeding, causes hyperplasia of erythrocytic elements. The immune system's response to many antigens—a vital mechanism for protection from foreign invaders—constitutes another example of demand-induced hyperplasia. Morphologically, lymphocyte hyperplasia is conspicuous in chronic inflammation caused by conditions such as bacterial infection or transplant rejection. An increased demand for parathyroid hormone results in hyperplasia of the parathyroid glands, a sequence found in some cases of chronic renal disease. In such cases, decreased calcium absorption from the small intestine results in mobilization of calcium from the bones to maintain appropriate blood calcium levels. This demand is mediated by parathyroid hormone, and the gland responds with an increase in the number of cells.

Persistent Cell Injury

Persistent cell injury may lead to hyperplasia. Whether such hyperplasia should be viewed as a compensatory response to decreased function or simply as a manifestation of mitotic signals generated by injury is not clear in most instances. The point is that, especially in the skin and the lining epithelium of some viscera, chronic inflammation or chronic exposure to physical or chemical injury results in a hyperplastic response. For instance, pressure from ill-fitting shoes causes hyperplasia of the skin of the foot, so-called corns or calluses. It is not too fanciful to consider the primary function of the skin as protection of underlying structures. In this perspective, such hyperplasia, with resultant thickening of the skin, serves to enhance functional capacity. Chronic inflammation of the bladder (chronic cystitis) commonly causes hyperplasia of the bladder epithelium, a condition easily viewed grossly by endoscopy as whitish plaques of the bladder lining. Inappropriate hyperplasia can itself be harmful—witness the unpleasant consequences of psoriasis, a malady of un-

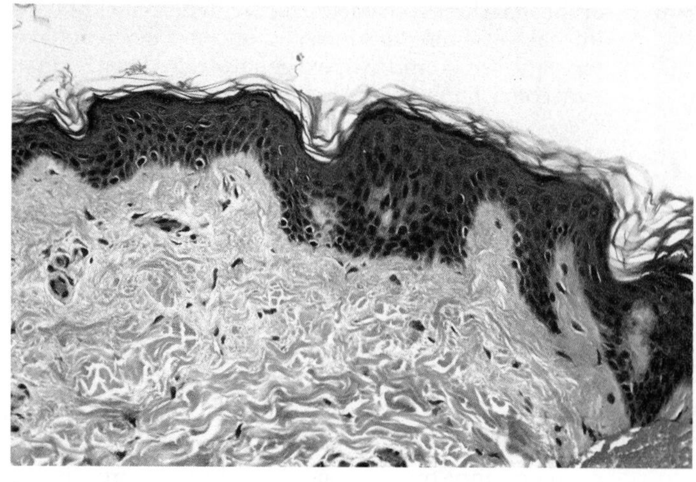

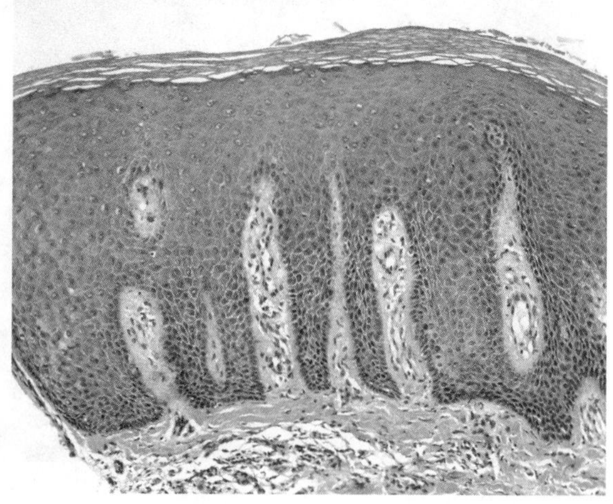

FIGURE 1-11
Epidermal hyperplasia. (*A*) Normal epidermis. (*B*) Epidermal hyperplasia in psoriasis, shown at the same magnification as in *A*. The epidermis is thickened, owing to an increase in the number of squamous cells.

known etiology characterized by conspicuous hyperplasia of the skin (Fig. 1-11).

The cellular and molecular mechanisms that are responsible for the hyperplastic response clearly relate to the control of cell proliferation. This topic is so broad that it is beyond the scope of this discussion, and the student is referred to the reading list at the end of the chapter.

Metaplasia

Metaplasia is the conversion of one differentiated cell type to another. The most common sequence is the replacement of a glandular epithelium by a squamous one. It is almost invariably a response to persistent injury and can be thought of as an adaptive mechanism. Columnar or cuboidal lining cells committed to differentiated functions, such as mucus production, assume a simpler form, providing more protection against a pernicious chemical action or the effects of chronic inflammation. Prolonged exposure of the bronchi to tobacco smoke leads to squamous metaplasia of the bronchial epithelium. A comparable response, associated with chronic infection, occurs in the endocervix (Fig. 1-12). In molecular terms, metaplasia represents the substitution of the expression of one set of differentiation genes for another.

Metaplasia is not restricted to squamous differentiation. In cases of chronic reflux of highly acidic gastric contents into the lower esophagus, the squamous epithelium is occasionally replaced by a gastric-like glandular mucosa (Barrett epithelium). This can be thought of as an adaptive response that protects the esophagus from the injurious effects of gastric acid and pepsin, to which the normal gastric mucosa is resistant. Metaplasia may also consist of replacement of one glandular epithelium by another. In chronic gastritis, a disorder of the stomach characterized by chronic inflammation, atrophic gastric glands are replaced by cells resembling those of the small intestine. The adaptive value of this condition, known as intestinal metaplasia, is not apparent. One also sees metaplasia of transitional epithelium to glandular epithelium in chronic inflammation of the bladder (cystitis glandularis).

It should be emphasized that metaplasia is not necessarily a harmless process, even though this response may be thought of as adaptive. Squamous metaplasia can impair bronchial function and predispose a person to recurrent pneumonia. Furthermore, neoplastic transformation may occur in metaplastic epithelium; cancers of the lung, cervix, stomach, and bladder have their origins in such areas. It is unlikely that the metaplastic epithelium itself is responsible for cancer formation. More probably, the nox-

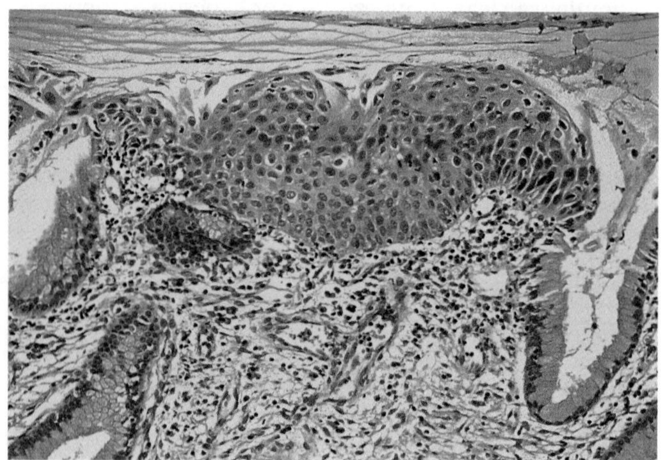

FIGURE 1-12
Squamous metaplasia. A section of endocervix shows the normal columnar epithelium at both margins and a focus of squamous metaplasia in the center.

ious stimuli leading to metaplasia are also carcinogenic to metaplastic cells.

Metaplasia is usually fully reversible. If the stimulus is removed (for example, when one stops smoking), the metaplastic epithelium eventually returns to normal.

Dysplasia

Cellular dysplasia refers to an alteration in the size, shape, and organization of the cellular components of a tissue. The cells comprising an epithelium normally exhibit uniformity of size, shape, and nucleus. Moreover, they are arranged in a regular fashion, as in the progression from plump basal cells to flat superficial cells in a squamous epithelium. When we speak of dysplasia, we mean that this monotonous appearance is disturbed by (1) variations in the size and shape of the cells; (2) enlargement, irregularity, and hyperchromatism of the nuclei; and (3) disorderly arrangement of the cells within the epithelium (Fig. 1-13). Dysplasia occurs most commonly in hyperplastic squamous epithelium, as seen in epidermal actinic keratosis (caused by sunlight), and in areas of squamous metaplasia, such as in the bronchus or the cervix. It is not, however, exclusive to squamous epithelium. Ulcerative colitis, an inflammatory disease of the large intestine, is often complicated by dysplastic changes in the mucosal cells.

Like metaplasia, dysplasia reflects the persistence of injurious influences and will customarily regress, for example, on cessation of smoking or cure of chronic cervicitis. However, dysplasia shares many cytological features with cancer, and the line between the two may be very fine indeed. For example, a common diagnostic problem for the pathologist is the distinction between severe dysplasia and early cancer of the cervix. **It is established that dysplasia is a preneoplastic lesion, in the sense that it is a necessary stage in the multistep cellular evolution to cancer.** In fact, dysplasia is today included in the morphological classifications of the stages of intraepithelial neoplasia in a variety of organs (e.g., cervix, prostate, bladder). Accordingly, severe dysplasia is considered an indication for aggressive preventive therapy to cure the underlying cause, eliminate the noxious agent, or surgically remove the offending tissue.

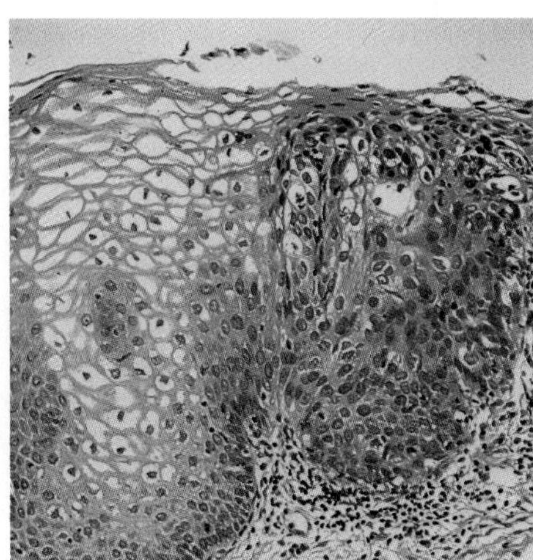

FIGURE *1-13*
Dysplasia. A section of the cervix shows an area of epithelial dysplasia (*right*) adjacent to an area of normal squamous epithelium. The dysplastic epithelium lacks the normal polarity, and the individual cells show hyperchromatic nuclei, a larger nucleus-to-cytoplasm ratio, and a disorderly arrangement.

Dysplasia as a process is not easy to reconcile with adaptation. Yet in a teleological sense, it can be included in this category. The dysplastic cell is less differentiated than its hyperplastic or metaplastic neighbors and is likely to be more resistant to injury. Although not autonomous in its growth, its replication is clearly not as well regulated as that of the hyperplastic or metaplastic cell. Thus, in terms of its own survival, the dysplastic cell has found ways to cope with a dangerous environment. Such adaptation could be considered beneficial. It not only enhances the survival of the individual cell but also protects the integrity of the tissue. It would not do to have a gaping hole in the bronchus because the epithelial cells were destroyed by cigarette smoke. Unfortunately, the system is not so finely tuned that adaptation stops with dysplasia, and it can overshoot its adaptive mark. The ultimate adaptation is transformation to a cancer cell—a return to the conditions of the free living cell—free of endogenous growth restraints and free to wander, perhaps to a more hospitable environment. Here the needs of the cell clash with those of the organism, since no case can be made for an advantage to the person of metastatic cancer. Yet cancer has little if any evolutionary impact, since most cancers occur well after the reproductive period.

Intracellular Storage

Intracellular storage is a normal function of the tissues of multicellular organisms. Cells store nutritional constituents that are used at a later time, including fat, glycogen, vitamins, and minerals. They also store the products of the turnover of endogenous membranes, principally in the form of degraded phospholipids. Furthermore, storage is also the mechanism by which certain cells deal with substances that cannot be eliminated by intracellular digestion. For example, carbon particles inhaled in the form of soot cannot be metabolized or dissolved. They would accumulate indefinitely in the alveoli if they were not engulfed by macrophages. Finally, many inborn errors of metabolism lead to the accumulation of intermediate metabolites or an abnormal material. A variety of human diseases are characterized by an exaggeration of the normal storage functions of specialized cells.

Fat

Bacteria and other unicellular organisms continuously ingest nutrients. By contrast, mammals are freed from the necessity of continuous eating. They can eat periodically and can survive a prolonged fast because they store nutrients in specialized cells for later use—fat in adipocytes and glycogen in the liver, heart, and muscle. Yet the excess storage of fat is not beneficial. Overeating leads to the storage of excess calories as fat (i.e., obesity).

The abnormal accumulation of fat is most conspicuous in the liver, a subject treated in detail in Chapter 14. Briefly, liver cells always contain some fat, because free fatty acids released from adipose tissue are taken up by the liver, where they are either oxidized or converted to triglycerides. Most of the newly synthesized triglycerides are secreted as lipoproteins by the liver. When the delivery of free fatty acids to the liver is increased, as in diabetes, or when the intrahepatic metabolism of lipids is disturbed, as in alcoholism, triglycerides accumulate in the liver cell. Fatty liver is identified morphologically by the presence of lipid globules in the cytoplasm. Other organs, including the heart, kidney, and skeletal muscle, also store fat. It is important to recognize that fat storage is always reversible, and there is no evidence that the presence of excess fat in the cytoplasm interferes with the function of the cell.

Glycogen

Glycogen is a long-chain polymer of glucose formed and largely stored in the liver and to a lesser extent in muscles. It is depolymerized to glucose and liberated as needed. The degradation of glycogen is accomplished in steps by a series of enzymes, each of which may be deficient as a result of an inborn error of metabolism. Regardless of the specific enzyme deficiency, the result is a glycogen storage disease (see Chapter 6). These inherited disorders affect the liver, heart, and skeletal muscle and range from mild and asymptomatic conditions to inexorably progressive and fatal diseases (see Chapters 11, 14, and 27).

The amount of glycogen stored in cells is regulated by the blood glucose concentration, and hyperglycemic states are associated with increased glycogen stores. Thus, in uncontrolled diabetes, hepatocytes and epithelial cells of the renal proximal tubules are enlarged by excess glycogen.

Inherited Lysosomal Storage Diseases

Similar to the metabolism of glycogen, the breakdown of certain complex lipids and mucopolysaccharides (glycosaminoglycans) is accomplished by a sequence of enzymatic steps. Since these enzymes are located in the lysosomes, their absence results in the lysosomal storage of incompletely degraded lipids, such as cerebrosides (e.g., Gaucher disease) and gangliosides (e.g., Tay-Sachs disease), or products of the catabolism of mucopolysaccharides (e.g., Hurler and Hunter syndromes). These disorders are all progressive but vary from asymptomatic organomegaly to rapidly fatal brain disease. See Chapter 6 for the metabolic bases of these disorders and Chapters 26 and 28 for specific organ pathology.

Iron

About 25% of the body's total iron content is in an intracellular storage pool composed of the iron-storage proteins ferritin and hemosiderin. The liver and bone marrow are particularly rich in ferritin, although it is present in virtually all cells. Hemosiderin is a partially denatured form of ferritin that easily aggregates and is recognized microscopically as yellow-brown granules in the cytoplasm. Normally, hemosiderin is found mainly in the spleen, bone marrow, and Kupffer cells of the liver.

Total body iron may be increased by enhanced intestinal iron absorption, as in some anemias, or by parenteral administration of iron-containing erythrocytes in a transfusion. In either case, the excess iron is stored intracellularly as both ferritin and hemosiderin. Increasing the body's total iron content results in a progressive accumulation of hemosiderin, a condition termed **hemosiderosis**. In this condition, iron is present not only in the organs in which it is normally found but also throughout the body, in such places as the skin, pancreas, heart, kidneys, and endocrine organs. The intracellular accumulation of iron in hemosiderosis does not injure the cells. However, there are a number of situations in which the increase in total body iron is extreme; we then speak of **iron overload syndromes** (see Chapter 14), disorders in which iron deposition is so severe that it damages vital organs—the heart, liver, and pancreas. Severe iron overload can result from a genetic abnormality in iron absorption, termed **hereditary hemochromatosis** (Fig. 1-14). Alternatively, severe iron overload may occur after multiple blood transfusions, such as those required in treating hemophilia or certain hereditary anemias.

Excessive iron storage in some organs is also associated with an increased risk of cancer. The pulmonary siderosis encountered among certain metal polishers is accompanied by an increased risk of lung cancer. Hemochromatosis leads to a higher incidence of liver cancer. The storage of other metals also presents dangers. In Wilson disease, a hereditary disorder of copper metabolism, storage of excess copper in the liver and brain leads to severe chronic disease of those organs.

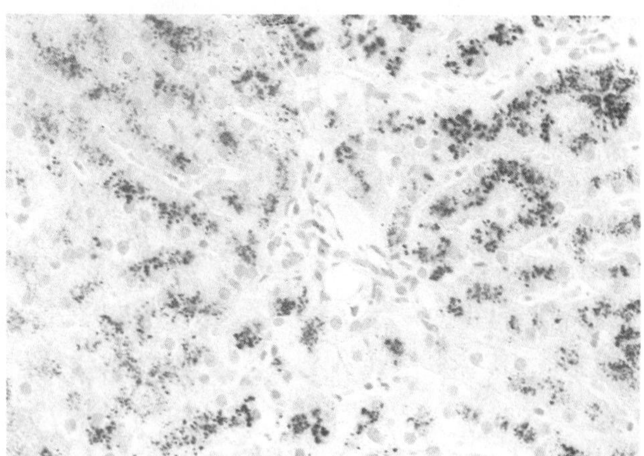

FIGURE *1-14*
Iron storage in hereditary hemochromatosis. A Prussian blue stain of the liver reveals large deposits of iron within hepatocellular lysosomes.

Lipofuscin

Lipofuscin, classically known as the "wear-and-tear" pigment, is composed of golden-brown granules found predominantly in cells that either are terminally differentiated (neurons and cardiac myocytes) or cycle only infrequently (hepatocytes) (Fig. 1-15). This material is a normal constituent of many cells and increases with age. It is often more conspicuous in conditions associated with atrophy of an organ.

Lipofuscin derives from the normal turnover of membrane constituents of the cell. Fragments of subcellular organelles are continuously being segregated within autophagic vacuoles in which the lipids and proteins are degraded. Peroxidation of the unsaturated lipids, and the formation of heterogeneous lipid–protein complexes, render these materials resistant to further digestion. The insoluble products are stored indefinitely as lysosome-derived residual bodies. Despite the occasional prominence of intracellular lipofuscin, there is no reason to believe that this pigment interferes in any way with the function of the cell.

Melanin

Melanin is an insoluble, brown-black pigment found almost exclusively in the epidermal cells of the skin. It is located in intracellular organelles known as melanosomes and results from the polymerization of certain oxidation products of tyrosine. The amount of melanin is responsible for the differences in skin color among the various races, as well as the color of the eyes. It serves a protective function owing to its ability to absorb ultraviolet light. In white persons, exposure to sunlight increases melanin formation (tanning). The hereditary inability to produce melanin results in the disorder known as albinism. The presence of melanin is also a marker of the cancer that arises from melanocytes (melanoma). Melanin is discussed in detail in Chapter 24.

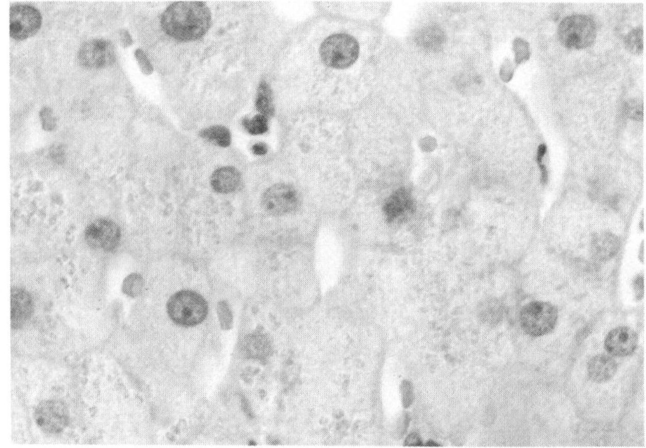

FIGURE *1-15*
Lipofuscin. A photomicrograph of the liver from an 80-year-old man shows golden cytoplasmic granules, which represent lysosomal storage of lipofuscin.

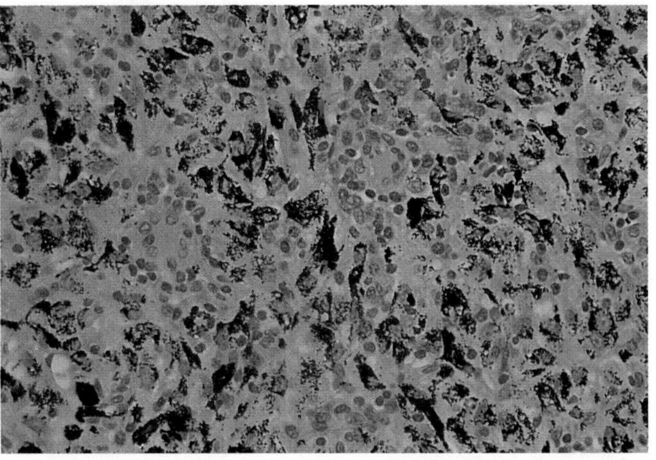

FIGURE *1-16*
Carbon pigment storage. A mediastinal lymph node, which drains the lungs, exhibits numerous macrophages that contain black anthracotic (carbon) pigment. This material was inhaled and originally deposited in the lungs.

Exogenous Pigments

Anthracosis refers to the storage of carbon particles in the lung and regional lymph nodes (Fig. 1-16). Virtually all urban dwellers inhale particulates of organic carbon generated by the burning of fossil fuels. These particles accumulate in alveolar macrophages and are also transported to hilar and mediastinal lymph nodes, where the indigestible material is stored indefinitely within macrophages. Although the gross appearance of the lungs of persons with anthracosis may be alarming, the condition is entirely innocuous.

Tattoos are the result of the introduction of insoluble metallic and vegetable pigments into the skin where they are engulfed by dermal macrophages and persist for a lifetime.

IRREVERSIBLE CELL INJURY

If the acute stress to which a cell must react exceeds its ability to adapt, the resulting changes in structure and function lead to the death of the cell. Among the more common causes of cell death are viruses, reduction in blood supply (ischemia), and physical agents such as ionizing radiation, extreme temperatures, or toxic chemicals. Cell death is classified into two types according to the presumed underlying mechanisms responsible for the loss of viability, namely **necrosis and apoptosis**. The latter is generally held to result from the expression of a genetically determined cell death program, which can be activated by a variety of physiological signals or cellular injuries (see later). By contrast, necrosis is the consequence of a catastrophic injury to the mechanisms that maintain the integrity of the cell. Although these two types of cell death can often be distinguished ultrastructurally, at the level of light microscopy they tend to be indistinguishable and have the appearance of **coagulative necrosis**. In a few specific circumstances, cell death can be dissociated from coagulative necrosis—for example, in the killing of a cell in tissue culture or by fixation of a biopsy specimen. **It should be emphasized, however, that when a tissue is examined for morphological evidence of irreversible injury, coagulative necrosis remains the criterion by which cell death (necrosis or apoptosis) is identified.** This is not to deny that there is a definable point prior to the appearance of coagulative necrosis when cell injury is irreversible—the point of no return. Such a point, however, cannot be appreciated in any morphological alteration of the injured cell.

The Morphology of Necrosis

Coagulative Necrosis

Coagulative necrosis refers to light microscopic alterations in a dead or dying cell. The term includes changes in both the cytoplasm and the nucleus (Figs. 1-17 and 1-18). When stained with the usual combination of hematoxylin and eosin, the cytoplasm is more eosinophilic than usual, owing both to a loss of basophilia and to an increased affinity of the cytoplasmic proteins for eosin. The nucleus displays an initial clumping of the chromatin followed by a redistribution along the nuclear membrane. Three morphological changes typically follow:

1. **Pyknosis:** The nucleus becomes smaller and stains deeply basophilic as chromatin clumping continues.
2. **Karyorrhexis:** The pyknotic nucleus breaks up into many smaller fragments scattered about the cytoplasm.
3. **Karyolysis:** The pyknotic nucleus may be extruded from the cell, or it may manifest progressive loss of chromatin staining.

There are a few instances in which the specific circumstances responsible for cell killing modify the morphological manifestations of the resulting coagulative necrosis. These changes result in a number of historically well-recognized variants, including liquefactive, fat, caseous, and fibrinoid necrosis. In most cases, necrotic tissue is eventually removed by an inflammatory reaction. However, when the areas of coagulative necrosis are particularly large, as in the occlusion of a coronary artery and the death (infarction) of a substantial area of the myocardium, the central region may be inaccessible to the inflammatory process. The necrotic tissue will then persist in place, sometimes for years.

Liquefactive Necrosis

There are two circumstances in which the rate of dissolution of the necrotic cells is considerably faster than the rate of repair. The polymorphonuclear leukocytes of the acute inflammatory reaction are endowed with potent hydrolases capable of completely digesting dead cells. A sharply localized collection of these acute inflammatory cells, generally in response to a bacterial infection, produces the rapid death and dissolution of tissue, so-called **liquefactive necrosis**. The result is often an **abscess** (Fig. 1-19).

Coagulative necrosis of the brain as a result of cerebral artery occlusion is frequently followed by rapid dissolution—liquefactive necrosis—of the dead tissue by a mechanism that cannot be attributed to the action of an acute inflammatory response. It is not clear why coagulative necrosis in the brain, and not elsewhere, is followed

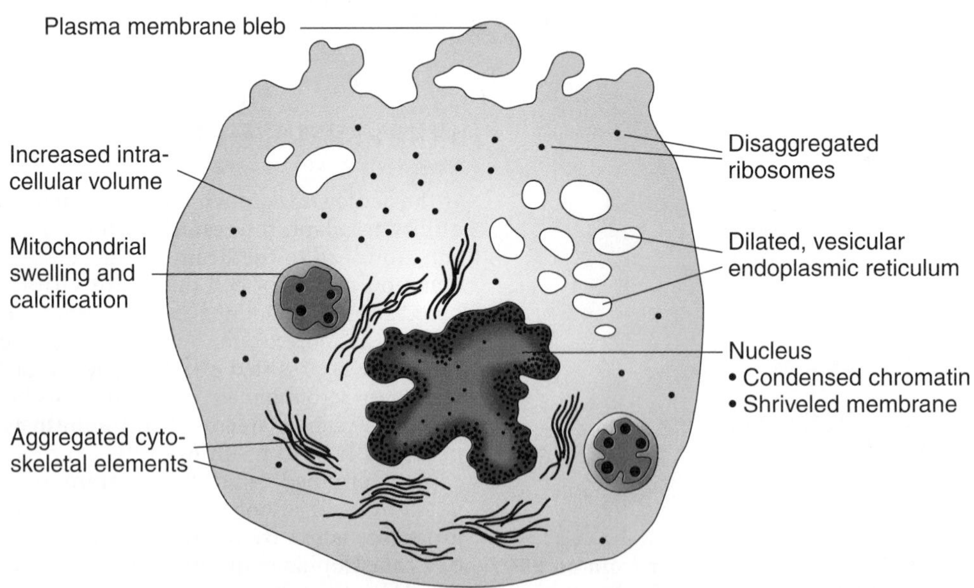

FIGURE *1-17*
Ultrastructural features of coagulative necrosis.

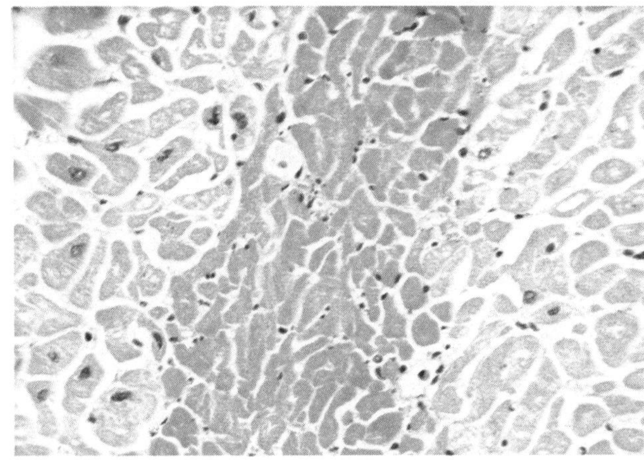

FIGURE *1-18*
Coagulative necrosis. A photomicrograph of the heart in a patient with an acute myocardial infarction. In the center, the deeply eosinophilic necrotic cells have lost their nuclei. The necrotic focus is surrounded by paler-staining, viable cardiac myocytes.

by the dissolution of the necrotic cells, but the phenomenon may be related to the presence of more abundant lysosomal enzymes or different hydrolases specific to the cells of the central nervous system. The liquefactive necrosis of large areas of the central nervous system can result in the formation of an actual cavity or cyst that will persist for the life of the person.

Fat Necrosis

Fat necrosis specifically affects adipose tissue and most commonly results from pancreatitis or trauma (Fig. 1-20). The unique feature determining this type of necrosis is the presence of triglycerides in adipose tissue. The process is begun when digestive enzymes, normally found only in the pancreatic duct and small intestine, are released from

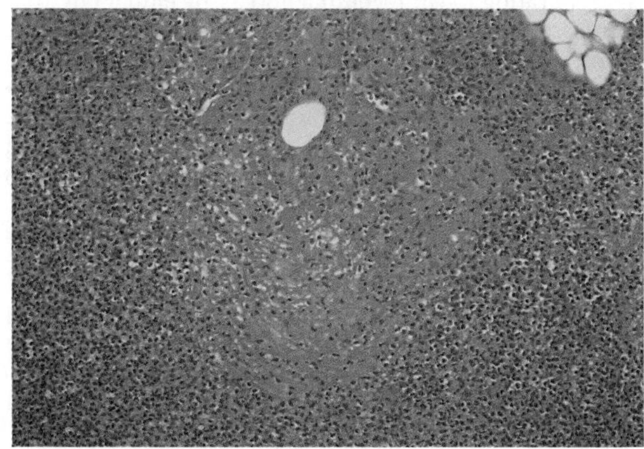

FIGURE *1-19*
Liquefactive necrosis in an abscess of the skin. The abscess cavity is filled with polymorphonuclear leukocytes.

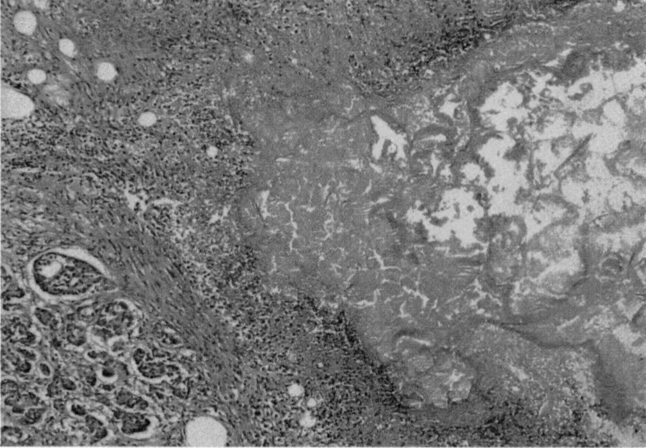

FIGURE *1-20*
Fat necrosis. A photomicrograph of peripancreatic adipose tissue from a case of acute pancreatitis shows an island of necrotic adipocytes (*on the right*) adjacent to an acutely inflamed area. Fatty acids are precipitated as calcium soaps, which accumulate as amorphous, basophilic deposits at the periphery of the irregular island of necrotic adipocytes.

injured pancreatic acinar cells and ducts into the extracellular spaces. On extracellular activation, these enzymes digest the pancreas itself as well as the surrounding tissues, including adipose cells, as follows.

1. Phospholipases and proteases attack the plasma membrane of the fat cells, releasing their stored triglycerides.
2. Pancreatic lipase then hydrolyzes the triglycerides, a process that produces free fatty acids.
3. The fatty acids are precipitated as calcium soaps, which accumulate microscopically as amorphous, basophilic deposits at the periphery of the irregular islands of necrotic adipocytes.

On gross examination, fat necrosis appears as an irregular, chalky white area embedded in otherwise normal adipose tissue. In the case of traumatic fat necrosis, we presume that triglycerides and lipases are released from the injured adipocytes.

Caseous Necrosis

Caseous necrosis is a lesion characteristic of tuberculosis (Fig. 1-21). The lesions of tuberculosis are the tuberculous granulomas, or tubercles. In the center of such a granuloma, the accumulated mononuclear cells mediating the chronic inflammatory reaction to the offending mycobacteria are killed. In caseous necrosis, unlike coagulative necrosis, the necrotic cells fail to retain their cellular outlines. They do not, however, disappear by lysis, as in liquefactive necrosis. Rather, the dead cells persist indefinitely as amorphous, coarsely granular, eosinophilic debris. Grossly, this debris appears grayish white and is soft and friable. It resembles clumpy cheese, hence the name *caseous necrosis*. This distinctive type of necrosis is

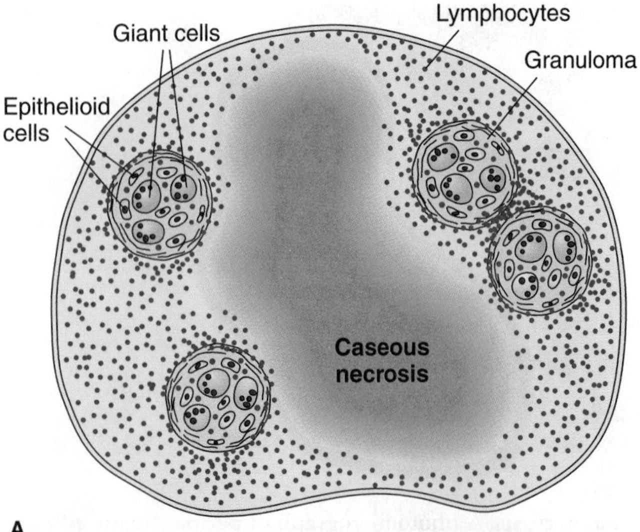

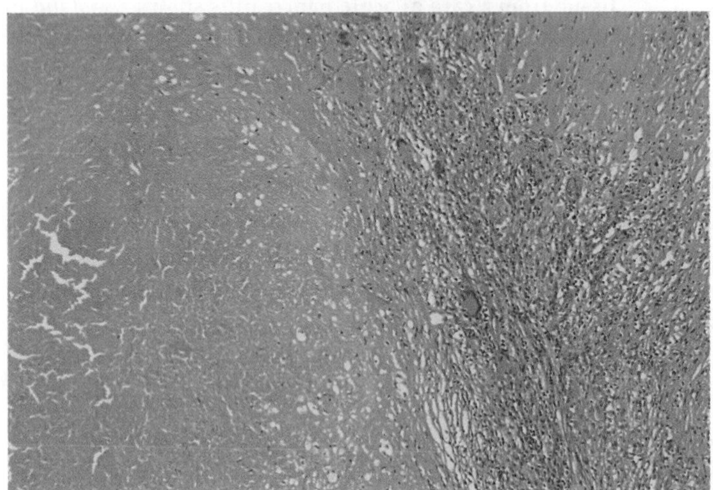

FIGURE 1-21
Caseous necrosis in a tuberculous lymph node. (*A*) The typical amorphous, granular, eosinophilic, necrotic center is surrounded by granulomatous inflammation. (*B*) A photomicrograph shows a tuberculous granuloma with central caseous necrosis.

generally attributed to the toxic effects of the unusual cell wall of the mycobacterium, which contains complex waxes (peptidoglycolipids) that exert potent biological effects.

Fibrinoid Necrosis

Fibrinoid necrosis refers to an alteration of injured blood vessels, in which the insudation and accumulation of plasma proteins cause the wall to stain intensely with eosin (Fig. 1-22). The term is something of a misnomer, however, because the eosinophilia of the accumulated plasma proteins obscures the underlying alterations in the blood vessel, making it difficult, if not impossible, to determine whether there truly is necrosis in the vascular wall.

The Pathogenesis of Coagulative Necrosis

The cellular alterations constituting coagulative necrosis are not specific for a particular insult. The morphological manifestation of cell death—coagulative necrosis—is the same regardless of whether the cells have been killed by a virus, by ionizing radiation, or by an interruption in blood supply.

Living cells exist in striking disequilibrium with their external environment. The plasma membrane is the barrier separating the intracellular and extracellular environments. By both passive and active mechanisms, the plasma membrane maintains the numerous concentration gradients that characterize the difference between the intracellular and extracellular milieu. With cell death, these gradients are dissipated. The largest gradient in all living cells is that of calcium. The concentration of calcium ions in extracellular fluids is in the millimolar range (10^{-3} M). By contrast, the concentration in the cytosol is some 10,000-fold lower, on the order of 10^{-7} M. This large concentration gradient is maintained by both the passive impermeability of the plasma membrane to calcium ions and by the active extrusion of calcium from the cell. It is not surprising, therefore, that coagulative necrosis is accompanied by the accumulation of calcium ions in the dead cells.

Calcium ions are biologically very active, and their accumulation in dead or dying cells may actually contribute to the morphological transformations that characterize coagulative necrosis. The influx and accumulation of calcium ions, and the resultant morphological changes

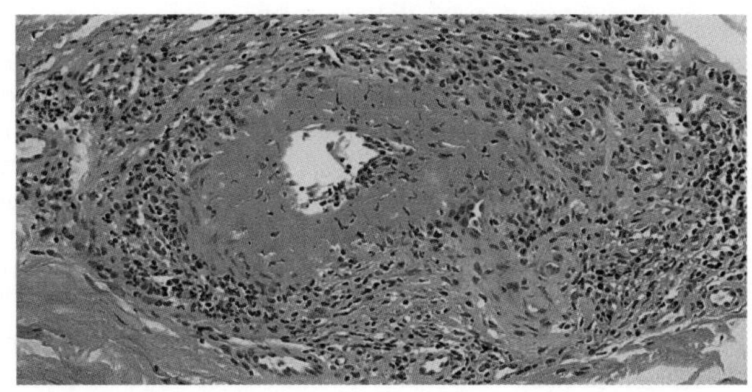

FIGURE *1-22*
Fibrinoid necrosis. An inflamed muscular artery in a case of systemic arteritis shows a sharply demarcated, homogeneous, deeply eosinophilic zone of necrosis.

of coagulative necrosis, can account for the common morphology of cell death. The sequence of events leading to coagulative necrosis may then be described as (1) irreversible injury and cell death, (2) loss of the plasma membrane's ability to maintain a gradient of calcium ions, (3) an influx and accumulation of calcium ions in the cell, and (4) the morphological appearance of coagulative necrosis. Under such a scheme, coagulative necrosis occurs after the point of no return—that is, after irreversible injury and "death" of the cell.

Alternatively, cell injury may lead to potentially reversible plasma membrane damage. In such a scheme, the large gradient of calcium ions can no longer be maintained by the plasma membrane. Excess calcium ions then accumulate in the injured cells and cause coagulative necrosis. This scenario has two specific implications. First, it does not define a stage of cell death distinct from coagulative necrosis. Second, it envisions the accumulation of calcium ions as the point at which potentially reversible cell injury becomes irreversible. There are some experimental data to support such a hypothesis. Agents that block calcium fluxes across biological membranes have been shown to prevent the coagulative necrosis that usually follows reperfusion of liver cells otherwise irreversibly injured by ischemia. Such experiments are difficult to interpret, however, because we cannot specifically implicate the inhibition of calcium accumulation as the mechanism by which the drug prevents coagulative necrosis. Any alternative action of the drug that results in cytoprotection would similarly prevent the accompanying accumulation of calcium.

The preceding discussion is summarized as follows: **Whatever the role of calcium, the disruption of the permeability barrier of the plasma membrane seems to be a critical event in lethal cell injury.** Loss of the plasma membrane's barrier function results in an equilibration of the concentration gradients that characterize living cells. As these gradients are dissipated, the cells are transformed into necrotic debris.

Ischemic Cell Injury

The interruption of blood flow—ischemia—is probably the most important cause of coagulative necrosis in human disease. The complications of atherosclerosis, for example, are generally the result of ischemic cell injury in the brain, heart, small intestine, kidneys, and lower extremities. Highly differentiated cells, such as the proximal tubular cells of the kidney, cardiac myocytes, and the neurons of the central nervous system, depend on aerobic respiration to produce ATP for the performance of their specialized functions. When ischemia limits the supply of oxygen and ATP is depleted, these cells rapidly manifest many changes in structure and function.

The effects of ischemic injury are all reversible if the duration of ischemia is short. For example, changes in myocardial contractility, membrane potential, metabolism, and ultrastructure are short lived if the circulation is rapidly restored. However, when ischemia persists, the affected cells become irreversibly injured—that is, the cells continue to deteriorate and become necrotic despite reperfusion with arterial blood. By definition, all metabolic alterations associated with reversible ischemic cell injury are either quantitatively or qualitatively insufficient to produce irreversible injury. With longer periods of ischemia, some biochemical alteration develops that causes irreversible injury.

Two phenomena illustrate the difference between irreversibly and reversibly injured ischemic cells. An inability to reverse mitochondrial dysfunction on reperfusion or reoxygenation correlates with a similar inability to reverse the cell injury in general. This finding was originally interpreted as indicating that ischemic cell death is a consequence of irreversible mitochondrial injury, particularly since mitochondria develop a series of structural and functional abnormalities with ischemia. However, it has been shown that the environment to which reperfusion exposes irreversibly injured cells does not allow mitochondria to recover from injury that would otherwise be reversible. In particular, it has been demonstrated that during reperfusion of irreversibly injured cells a large influx of Ca^{2+} ions occurs. An excess of Ca^{2+} ions is known to induce loss of mitochondrial function, and it may be that the inability to reverse mitochondrial dysfunction reflects the flooding of the cells with Ca^{2+}, rather than being a consequence of the mitochondrial abnormalities themselves.

Recent evidence has renewed interest in mitochondrial injury as a key element in the pathogenesis of irreversible cell injury. Under ischemic conditions, mitochondria exhibit a nonspecific increase in the permeability of the inner membrane. This effect is attributed to the opening of a proteinaceous pore in the membrane (mitochondrial permeability transition). Agents that inhibit this transition protect against irreversible ischemic cell injury, both *in vitro* and in the intact animal. Thus, mitochondria are now again identified as potentially critical in the development of ischemic cell death.

A disturbance in membrane function in general, and in the plasma membrane in particular, is the second characteristic of the loss of reversibility in ischemic injury. Some have therefore maintained that defective cell membrane function is the primary event in the genesis of irreversible cell injury in ischemia. Indeed, the results of morphological, functional, and biochemical studies clearly suggest that defects in cell membranes are an early feature of irreversible ischemic cell injury. Yet a definitive understanding of the mechanism underlying membrane damage in irreversible ischemic injury remains elusive. There are, however, potential candidates for this mechanism.

Reperfusion Injury and Activated Oxygen

A popular theory postulates a role for partially reduced, and thus activated, oxygen species in the genesis of membrane damage in irreversible ischemia. The general problem of how activated oxygen species may injure cells is discussed later in this chapter; here, we consider the mechanisms by which activated oxygen (superoxide, H_2O_2, hydroxyl radicals) is formed in ischemia and the evidence that it injures ischemic cells.

It might seem paradoxical that oxygen species cause cell injury when that injury is attributed to an insufficient oxygen supply. This dilemma is more apparent than real. Toxic oxygen species are generated not during the period of ischemia itself but rather on restoration of blood flow, or reperfusion, hence the term **reperfusion injury**.

Some event occurs during the period of ischemia that results in an overproduction of toxic oxygen species on the later restoration of the oxygen supply. Two sources of activated oxygen species have been proposed, namely, production by intracellular xanthine oxidase and extracellular release by activated neutrophils.

In some circumstances, for example as originally described with experimental intestinal ischemia, xanthine dehydrogenase may be converted by proteolysis during the period of ischemia into xanthine oxidase. On return of the oxygen supply with reperfusion, the abundant purines derived from the catabolism of ATP during ischemia provide substrates for the activity of xanthine oxidase. This enzyme requires oxygen in catalyzing the formation of uric acid, and activated oxygen species are byproducts of this reaction.

A second source of activated oxygen species during reperfusion may be the neutrophil. It is thought that alterations in the cell surface that occur during ischemia and on reperfusion induce the adhesion and activation of circulating neutrophils. These cells release large quantities of activated oxygen species and hydrolytic enzymes, both of which may injure the previously ischemic cells. This concept is supported by the protection afforded by reperfusing ischemic tissue with blood depleted of neutrophils. In addition to the generation of toxic oxygen species in reperfusion injury, other agents, such as cytokines, nitric oxide, platelet activating factor (PAF), and other molecules, have been proposed as mediators or modulators of tissue damage.

The specific role that reperfusion injury plays in the genesis of irreversible ischemic injury in human disease remains to be defined. We can put reperfusion injury in perspective by emphasizing that there are three different degrees of cell injury, depending on the duration of the ischemia:

1. With short periods of ischemia, reperfusion (and, therefore, the resupply of oxygen) completely restores the structural and functional integrity of the cell. Cell injury in this case is completely reversible.
2. With longer periods of ischemia, reperfusion is not associated with restoration of cell structure and function but rather with deterioration and death of the cells. As we have seen, this seemingly paradoxical response to reoxygenation is a consequence of the formation of reduced oxygen species on reperfusion, and it is these activated oxygen species that injure the cells. It is important to emphasize that, in this case, lethal cell injury occurs during the period of reperfusion.
3. Lethal cell injury may develop during the period of ischemia itself, in which case reperfusion is not a factor. A longer period of ischemia is needed to produce this third type of cell injury. In this case, cell damage is not dependent on the formation of activated oxygen species. When cells are reperfused after periods of ischemia that produce this type of injury, there is an explosive accumulation of sodium and calcium ions in the cells. This accumulation is a result of plasma membrane damage that developed during the period of ischemia—not during reperfusion.

The damage to the plasma membrane directly associated with irreversible ischemic injury, and not dependent on reperfusion, has been attributed to two mechanisms. One of these mechanisms relates to changes in the metabolism of the phospholipid bilayer, whereas the other emphasizes alterations in cytoskeletal structures.

Altered Phospholipid Metabolism

Plasma membrane damage in irreversible ischemia has been attributed, at least in part, to accelerated degradation of membrane phospholipids. Evidence for this hypothesis has been derived in a number of experimental systems, including liver, heart, brain, and kidney ischemia.

Experimental ischemia has been shown to result in a loss of phospholipids from cell membranes, accompanied by a release of their fatty acids. Structural alterations in cellular membranes accompany this increased hydrolysis of phospholipids. Microsomes and plasma membranes display aggregations of intramembranous particles, a finding suggestive of phase separations in the lipid bilayer. Interfaces between lipid domains of differing molecular order are believed to be sites of increased permeability. Indeed, microsomal membranes prepared from ischemic livers exhibit a 25- to 50-fold increase in their passive permeability to calcium.

The mechanism responsible for the accelerated degradation of membrane phospholipids in ischemia is not fully understood. It has been proposed that membrane-associated phospholipases are activated by increases in cytosolic free calcium during ischemia. According to this hypothesis, energy depletion dissipates the mitochondrial gradient that permits the retention of calcium in that organelle. With ischemia, the release of mitochondrial calcium elevates the cytosolic calcium concentration and activates phospholipases. Support for this hypothesis comes from studies of cardiac myocytes, in which cytosolic calcium has been reported to increase at the same time that fatty acids are released from the phospholipids of cellular membranes. By contrast, phospholipid degradation in anoxic liver cells can proceed in the absence of an elevated cytosolic free calcium. Thus, the role of phospholipase activation by calcium in ischemic injury remains to be defined.

Cytoskeletal Alterations

The intimate association of cytoskeletal elements with the plasma membrane of many cells suggests that the cytoskeleton plays a role in the regulation of the structure of the cell membrane. Thus, it has been postulated that alterations in the cytoskeleton provide another mechanism by which ischemia damages the plasma membrane. Evidence has been forthcoming that anoxia may lead to activation of phospholipases by interfering with the intimate relationship between the cytoskeleton and the plasma membrane. In a number of experimental systems, both ischemia and anoxia lead to the formation of prominent blebs of the plasma membrane, which have been attributed to cytoskeletal changes. These fluid-containing blebs are not seen in reversibly injured cells. The biochemical basis for the formation of plasma membrane blebs, or for the postulated participation of the cytoskeleton, remains to be elucidated.

It is of interest that although the participation of the cytoskeleton in ischemic injury is not entirely defined, direct modification of the cytoskeleton can have profound effects on the viability of the cell. The best example is the liver injury produced by phalloidin, one of the active agents of the toxic mushroom *Amanita phalloides*. Phalloidin binds to actin filaments, thereby preventing their depolymerization. The resulting accumulation of microfilaments in immediate association with the plasma membrane produces numerous invaginations of that structure

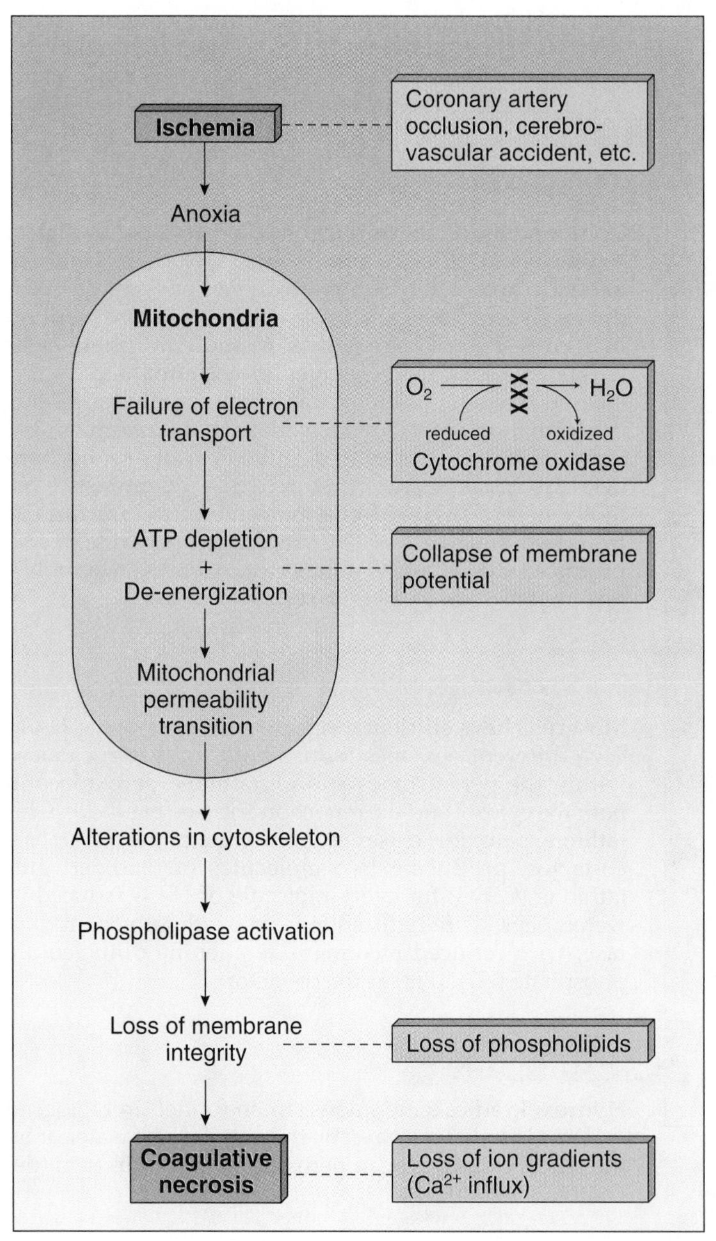

FIGURE 1-23
Possible sequence of events in the pathogenesis of irreversible cell injury caused by anoxia/ischemia.

and eventually lethal injury to the cell. The fungal metabolite cytochalasin B enhances the depolymerization of actin and prevents the toxicity of phalloidin.

The events leading to irreversible ischemic cell injury are summarized in Figure 1-23.

Cell Injury Caused by Oxygen Free Radicals

Partially reduced oxygen species have been identified as the likely cause of cell injury in an increasing number of diseases (Fig. 1-24). We referred earlier to reperfusion injury when discussing the mechanism of cell injury in ischemia. The inflammatory process, whether acute or chronic, can cause considerable tissue destruction. Partially reduced oxygen species produced by phagocytic cells are important mediators of cell injury in such circumstances. Damage to cells resulting from oxygen radicals formed by inflammatory cells has been implicated in diseases of the joints and of many organs, including the kidney, lungs, and heart. The toxicity of many chemicals may reflect the formation of toxic oxygen species. The killing of cells by ionizing radiation is most likely the result of the direct formation of hydroxyl radicals from the radiolysis of water. There is also evidence of a role for oxygen species in chemical carcinogenesis, during either initiation or promotion. Finally, oxidative damage has been implicated in biological aging (see later).

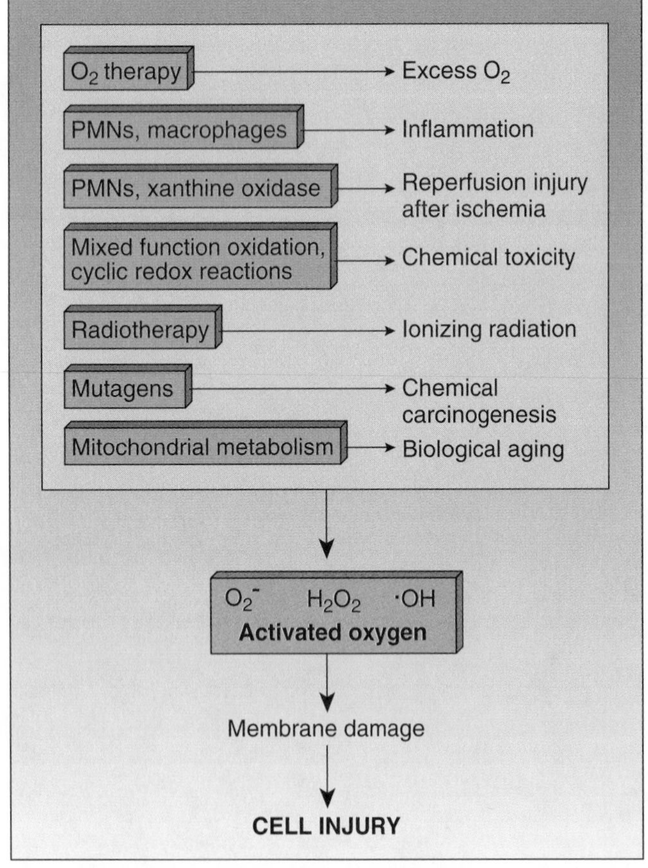

FIGURE *1-24*
The role of activated oxygen species in human disease.

Cells also may be injured when oxygen is present at concentrations greater than normal. In the past, this occurred largely in those therapeutic circumstances in which oxygen was given to patients at concentrations greater than the normal 20% of inspired air. The lungs of adults and the eyes of premature newborns were the major targets of such oxygen toxicity.

Oxygen has a major metabolic role as the terminal acceptor for mitochondrial electron transport. Cytochrome oxidase catalyzes the four-electron reduction of O_2 to water. The resultant energy is harnessed as an electrochemical potential across the mitochondrial inner membrane.

There are three partially reduced species that are intermediate between O_2 and H_2O, representing transfers of varying numbers of electrons. They are O_2^-, superoxide (one electron); H_2O_2, hydrogen peroxide (two electrons); and $\cdot OH$, the hydroxyl radical (three electrons). These partially reduced oxygen species are not produced by cytochrome oxidase but are derived from other enzymatic and nonenzymatic reactions (Fig. 1-25).

Superoxide

Components of the mitochondrial electron transport chain may be directly auto-oxidized by O_2 to yield superoxide anions (O_2^-). Superoxide anions are also produced by enzymes such as xanthine oxidase and cytochrome P_{450}. Phagocytosis by polymorphonuclear leukocytes and macrophages is accompanied by increased oxygen consumption, which largely represents the formation of O_2^- by an oxidase in the plasma membrane. O_2^- anions produced in the cytosol or mitochondria are catabolized by superoxide dismutase. One molecule of H_2O_2 and one molecule of O_2 are formed from two molecules of O_2^-. Hydrogen peroxide is also produced directly by a number of oxidases in cytoplasmic peroxisomes (see Fig. 1-25).

Hydrogen Peroxide

Most cells have efficient mechanisms for removing H_2O_2. Two different enzymes reduce H_2O_2 to water: catalase within the peroxisomes and glutathione peroxidase in both the cytosol and the mitochondria (see Fig. 1-25). Glutathione peroxidase uses reduced glutathione (GSH) as a co-factor, producing two molecules of oxidized glutathione (GSSG) for every molecule of H_2O_2 reduced to water. GSSG is re-reduced to GSH by glutathione reductase, with reduced nicotinamide adenine dinucleotide phosphate (NADPH) as the co-factor.

Hydroxyl Radical

Hydroxyl radicals are known to be formed in biological systems in only two ways: by the radiolysis of water or by the reaction of hydrogen peroxide with ferrous iron (the Fenton reaction).

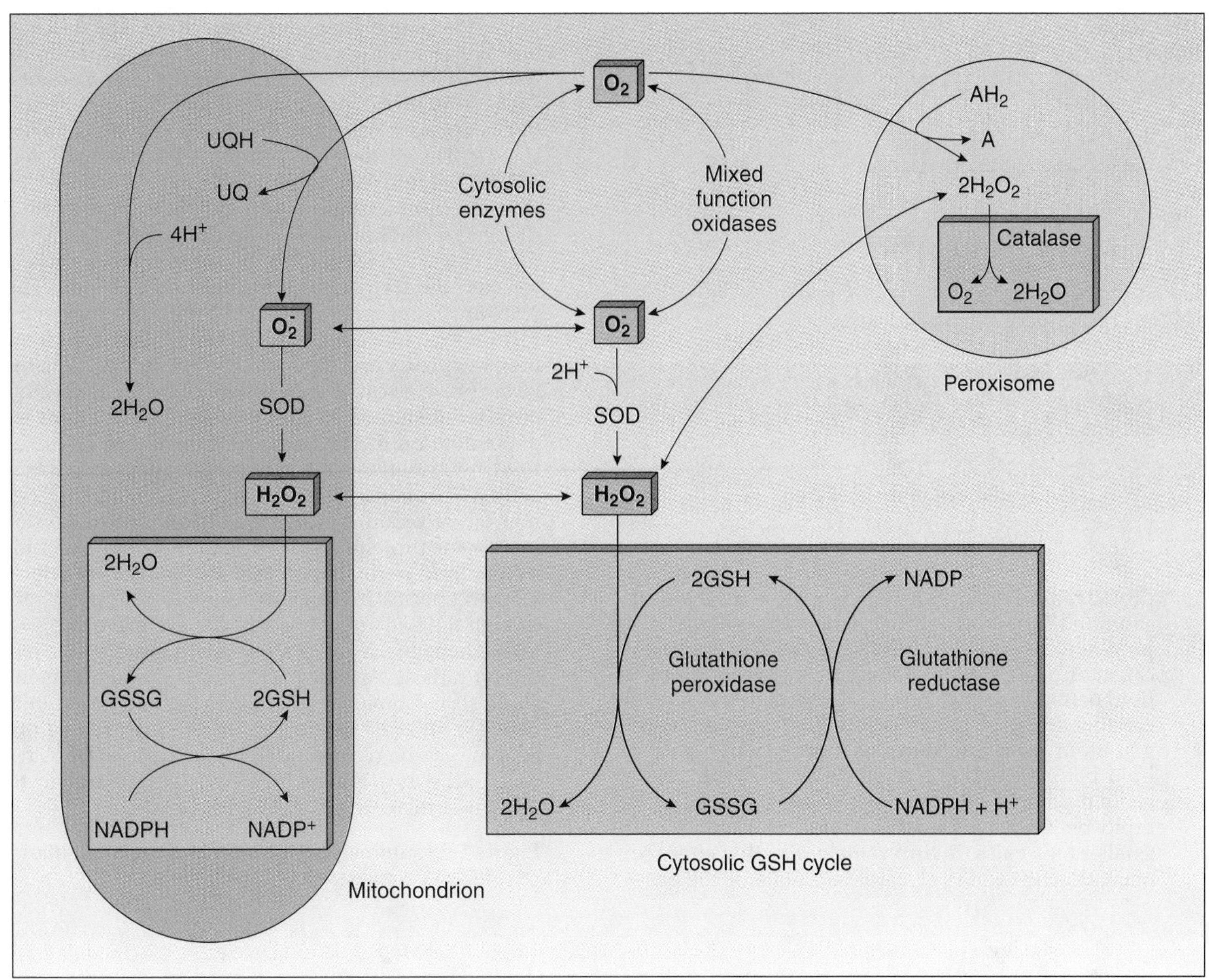

FIGURE *1-25*
Cellular metabolism of oxygen and the accompanying antioxidant defense mechanisms.

The Role of Iron

All respiring cells require iron; it is used, for example, to form cytochromes for electron transport in the mitochondria. Cells obtain iron from the plasma as ferric iron bound to transferrin. Transferrin binds to specific receptors on the cell surface and is delivered to the cytoplasm within an endosome, where an acidic environment releases free ferric iron. Free iron first is used for the synthesis of hemoproteins and then is stored as ferritin; it is subsequently returned to newly synthesized or recycled transferrin and is then secreted by the cell. Cellular iron stores may be mobilized by the autophagocytosis of ferritin. Following the fusion of autophagosomes with lysosomes, the acid proteases activated by the low pH release free ferric iron. Figure 1-26 summarizes these events, emphasizing the presence of a **pool of free ferric iron formed as a result of both the uptake and the release of iron from cells**.

It is this pool of free ferric iron that seems to be required for partially reduced oxygen species to injure cells. Free ferric iron can be reduced by superoxide anions to ferrous iron. Hydrogen peroxide, formed either directly or (more commonly) by the dismutation of superoxide anions, then reacts with the ferrous iron by the Fenton reaction to produce hydroxyl radicals. This sequence, starting with superoxide anions and ferric iron and leading to the generation of hydroxyl radicals without the consumption of ferric iron, is called an iron-catalyzed Haber-Weiss reaction.

Hydroxyl Radicals and Macromolecules

The hydroxyl radical (·OH) is an extremely reactive species, and there are several mechanisms by which it might damage membranes.

- **Lipid peroxidation:** The best known effect of hydroxyl radicals on membranes relates to ·OH as an initiator of lipid peroxidation (Fig. 1-27). The hy-

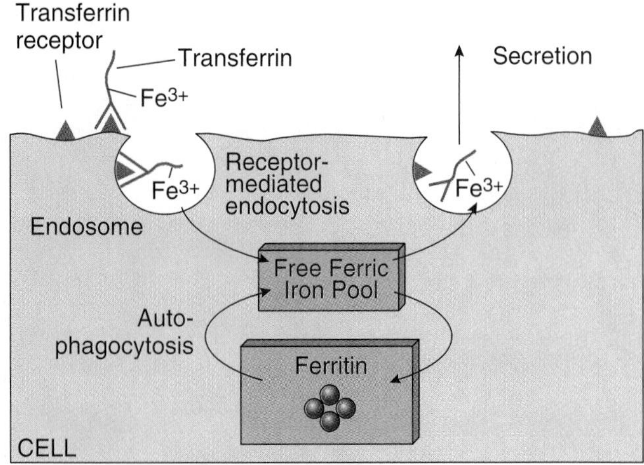

FIGURE 1-26
Cellular metabolism of iron.

droxyl radical removes a hydrogen atom from the unsaturated fatty acids of membrane phospholipids, a process that forms a free lipid radical. The lipid radical, in turn, reacts with molecular oxygen and forms a lipid peroxide radical. Like ·OH, this peroxide radical can function as an initiator, removing another hydrogen atom from a second unsaturated fatty acid. A lipid peroxide and a new lipid radical result, and a chain reaction is initiated.
Lipid peroxides are unstable and break down into smaller molecules (hydroxyaldehydes) that either remain attached to the glycerol backbone of the phospholipid or are released into the cytosol. The destruction of the unsaturated fatty acids of phospholipids results in a loss of membrane integrity. Antioxidants, such as vitamin E, prevent the injury that usually follows exposure of cells to partially reduced oxygen species. This protection is attributed to the inhibition of lipid peroxidation by antioxidants.

- **Protein interactions:** Hydroxyl radicals may also damage membranes by altering their proteins. They may cause cross-linking of membrane proteins through the formation of disulfide (S-S) bonds. The resulting aggregation of membrane proteins may form ion channels or may otherwise disrupt membrane structure and function. The SH groups of membrane proteins can also be modified by the formation of mixed disulfides in a reaction with GSH, a process dependent on the hydroxyl radical. The products of lipid peroxidation form carbonyl adducts with intracellular proteins, thereby providing a convenient marker of oxidative damage. The modification of membrane proteins has been suggested as an alternative to lipid peroxidation as a mechanism by which oxygen species produce irreversible cell injury, although the two are not necessarily exclusive.
- **DNA damage:** DNA is an important target of the hydroxyl radical. A variety of structural alterations include strand breaks, modified bases, and cross-links between strands. In most cases, the integrity of the genome can be reconstituted by the various DNA repair pathways. However, if oxidative damage to DNA is sufficiently extensive, the cell dies.

Figure 1-28 summarizes the mechanisms of cell injury by activated oxygen species.

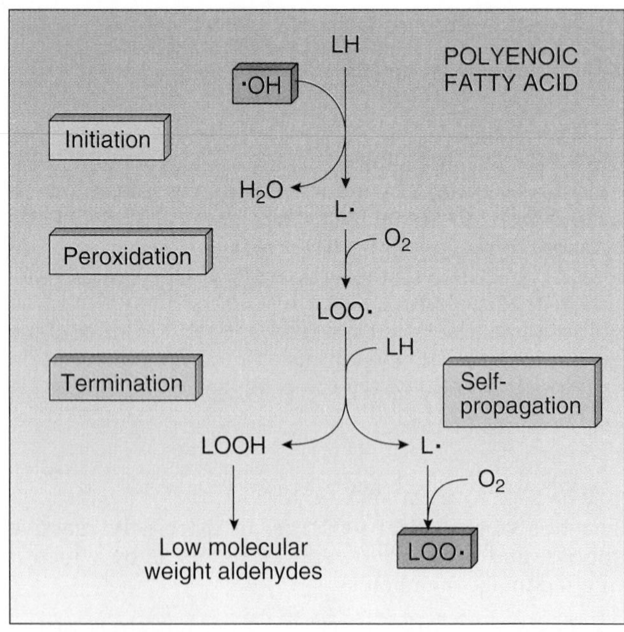

FIGURE 1-27
Lipid peroxidation initiated by the hydroxyl radical.

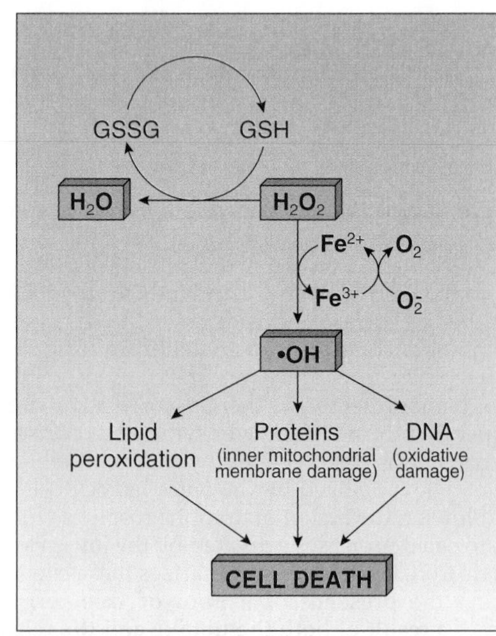

FIGURE 1-28
The mechanisms of cell injury by activated oxygen species.

How Ionizing Radiation Kills Cells

The discussion of activated oxygen species can be extended to include the mechanism by which ionizing radiation injures cells. The adjective "ionizing" in reference to electromagnetic radiation connotes an ability to effect the radiolysis of water, thereby directly forming hydroxyl radicals. These hydroxyl radicals then produce membrane injury by the mechanisms already discussed.

As noted previously, hydroxyl radicals can also interact with DNA. An important functional consequence of such damage is the inhibition of DNA replication. For a nonproliferating cell, such as a hepatocyte or a neuron, the inability to replicate DNA is of little consequence. For a proliferating cell, however, the inability to replicate DNA represents a catastrophic loss of function. Once a proliferating cell is prevented from replicating, a mechanism (apoptosis, see later) is set in motion that leads to its demise. Induction of cell death or inhibition of cell replication would clearly serve to rid the body of those cells that had lost their prime function. If the dose of ionizing radiation is sufficiently large, the resulting DNA damage may kill the cell directly. In this case, the extensive single-strand breaks exaggerate the DNA repair process, thereby depleting the cells of energy and initiating a cascade of events that leads to cell death. Figure 1-29 summarizes the mechanisms of cell killing by ionizing radiation.

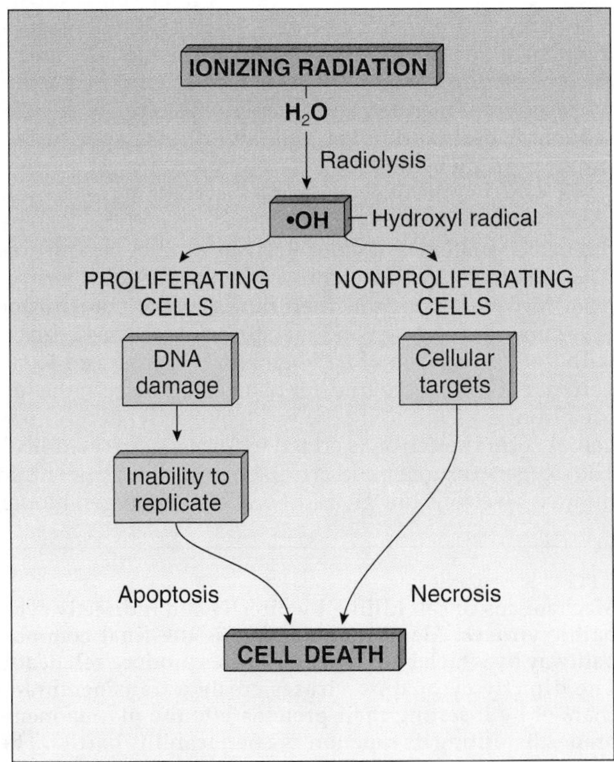

FIGURE *1-29*
Mechanisms of cell injury by ionizing radiation.

How Viruses Kill Cells

Viruses kill cells in two distinct ways. The infection of a cell by a **directly cytopathic** virus leads to lethal injury without invoking the host immune system. **Indirectly cytopathic viruses**, on the other hand, require the participation of the immune system.

Poliovirus is typical of the group of viruses that are directly cytopathic. It consists of a single strand of RNA surrounded by a protein capsule. After binding to specific receptors on the surface of the target cell, the virus is internalized by endocytosis. The endosome fuses with a cellular lysosome to form a phagolysosome, after which the protein capsule is removed by proteolysis. The viral genome is released into the cytosol and is recognized by the protein synthetic apparatus as just another messenger RNA molecule. As a result, the viral genome is translated by the host cell into capsular proteins and a specific RNA polymerase. The polymerase, in turn, leads to replication of the viral genome. Virally coded proteins insert into the host cell plasma membrane and form a pore, or channel, that disrupts the permeability barrier, allowing equilibration of ionic gradients. Potassium ions leave, and sodium and calcium ions enter. The cell is dead.

Hepatitis B virus is an example of an indirectly cytopathic virus. This agent consists of a double-stranded DNA genome enclosed in a protein capsule. Like poliovirus, hepatitis B virus binds to specific receptors on the target cell surface, is internalized, and has its capsule removed by acidic proteases after the phagosome fuses with a lysosome. Unlike poliovirus, however, the viral DNA genome cannot be directly translated by the protein synthetic machinery. It must first be transcribed into viral messenger RNA before it can be translated into viral proteins. The transcription of the viral DNA genome is accomplished in the nucleus by the host cell's DNA-dependent RNA polymerase. The resulting viral RNAs are transported to the cytoplasm, where they are translated into proteins. The viral proteins include a DNA polymerase that replicates the viral genome and the capsular proteins. Progeny viruses are assembled and released from the host cell without lethal cell injury. Yet all is not well.

The process of viral assembly or release exposes viral proteins on the external surface of the plasma membrane. These proteins are recognized by the immune system as nonself, or foreign, antigens. A cellular and humoral immune response develops in reaction to the viral proteins on the surface of the infected host cells. **It is this immune response that seems to be responsible for the lethal injury of the virus-infected cell.** T cells recognize and bind to the viral antigen(s) on the target cell surface, a process that results in the death of the infected cell by two mechanisms. The T cells may release a protein (perforin) that interacts with the target cell plasma membrane. Disruption of the membrane's functional integrity and cell death proceed in a manner similar to that seen with the directly cytopathic viruses. The action of perforin is similar to that of complement, a group of plasma proteins that on activation form a membrane attack complex. Once formed, this complex is inserted into the plasma membrane of a target cell to form a pore that disrupts its permeability. Al-

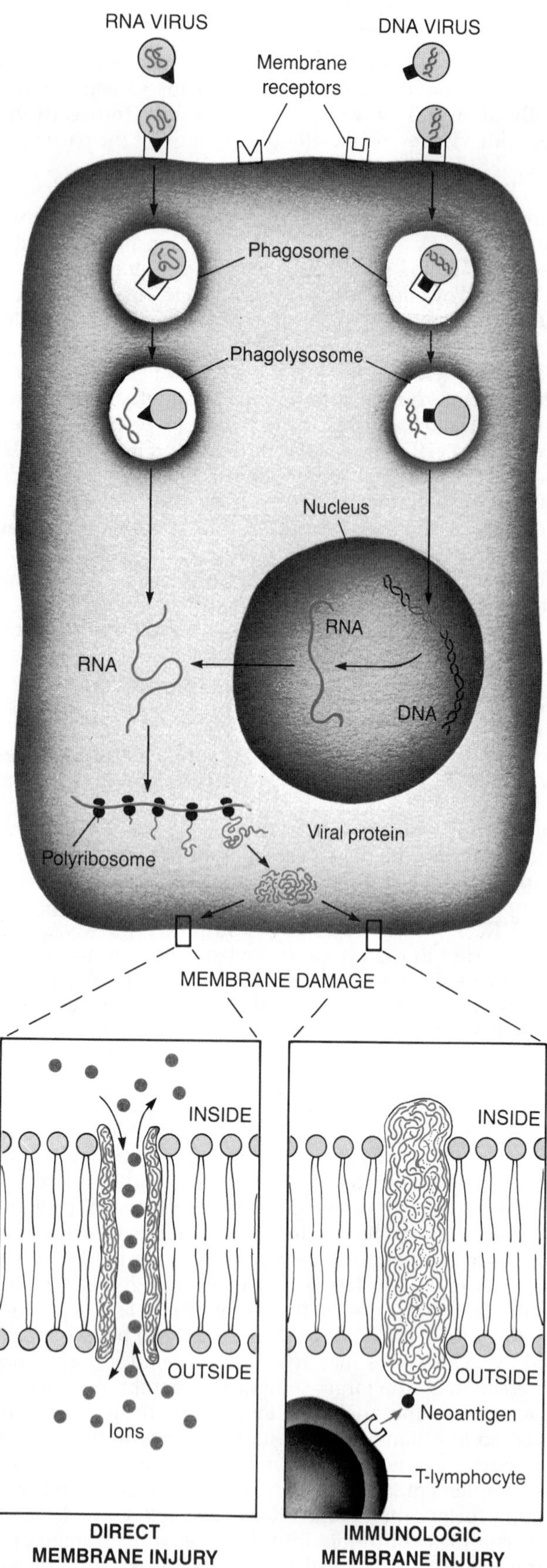

ternatively, the binding of the T cell to the virus-infected cell leads to the interaction of a T-cell ligand (Fas ligand) with its specific receptor (Fas receptor) on the surface of the target cell, thereby initiating a sequence of events that results in cell death by apoptosis (see later).

Figure 1-30 summarizes the mechanisms of cell killing by directly and indirectly cytopathic viruses.

How Chemicals Kill Cells

There are innumerable chemicals that can damage almost any cell in the body. The science of toxicology attempts to define the mechanisms that determine both the target cell specificity and the mechanism of action of such chemicals. Toxic chemicals are divided into two general classes: (1) those that interact directly with cellular constituents without requiring metabolic activation and (2) those that are themselves not toxic but are metabolized to yield an ultimate toxin that interacts with the target cell. This target cell need not be the same cell that metabolizes the toxin.

Liver Necrosis Caused by the Metabolism of Chemicals

Studies of a few compounds that produce liver cell necrosis in rodents have enhanced our understanding of how chemicals injure cells. These studies have focused principally on those compounds that are converted to toxic metabolites.

Carbon tetrachloride, acetaminophen, and bromobenzene are well-studied hepatotoxins. Each is metabolized by the mixed-function oxidase system of the endoplasmic reticulum, and each causes liver cell necrosis. How does this metabolic process relate to the damage of the plasma membrane that results in irreversible injury? Each of the three hepatotoxins is metabolized in a somewhat different manner, and it is possible to relate the subsequent evolution of lethal cell injury to the specific features of this metabolism.

The active site of cytochrome P_{450} contains ferric iron. During substrate binding, NADPH–cytochrome P_{450} reductase transfers a single electron to the cytochrome P_{450}–substrate complex, thus reducing ferric to ferrous iron. Molecular oxygen then binds to the cytochrome P_{450}–substrate complex in much the same way as it reacts with the ferrous iron of hemoglobin. O_2 is reduced to superoxide (O_2^-) by the transfer of an electron from the ferrous iron, thus initiating the reductive activation of oxygen. A second electron is added to form a peroxyl radical. The oxygen–oxygen bond is broken in such a manner that the two electrons are given to one of the oxygen atoms,

FIGURE *1-30*
Mechanisms of cell killing by directly and indirectly cytopathic viruses. Membrane damage is the final common pathway by which both types of viruses produce cell death. The directly cytopathic viruses create a transmembrane channel by inserting their proteins into the plasma membrane, disrupting its function as a permeability barrier. The indirectly cytopathic viruses also insert their proteins into the plasma membrane and create an antigenic target for cytotoxic T lymphocytes.

thus reducing it to water. The remaining activated oxygen atom bound to the cytochrome–substrate complex is highly reactive. Through a mechanism still poorly understood, the substrate is oxidized by reaction with this activated oxygen atom. The final products are native ferric cytochrome P_{450}, one molecule of oxidized substrate, and one molecule of water. The equation for the oxidation of a given substrate (RH) can then be summarized as follows:

$$RH + 2e^- + O_2 + 2H^+ \rightarrow ROH + H_2O$$

CARBON TETRACHLORIDE: The metabolism of carbon tetrachloride (CCl_4), a model compound for toxicological studies, is a variation on the mechanism described earlier. Again, when most chemicals bind to the ferric cytochrome P_{450}, an electron is added to the complex. With CCl_4, however, the addition of an electron immediately results in the reductive cleavage of a carbon–chlorine bond rather than in the reduction of iron. The products are a chlorine atom and a highly reactive trichloromethyl free radical. Oxygen is not involved in the metabolic activation of CCl_4.

Thus, the toxicity of CCl_4 depends on its metabolism and relates to the formation of the trichloromethyl free radical. Like the hydroxyl radical, the trichloromethyl radical is a potent initiator of lipid peroxidation. It abstracts a hydrogen atom from unsaturated fatty acids of the membrane phospholipids of the endoplasmic reticulum. Chloroform is produced, and a lipid radical is formed. The reaction of the lipid radical with O_2 then initiates the peroxidative decomposition of the phospholipids of the endoplasmic reticulum. However, the liver cells do not die because of damage to the endoplasmic reticulum alone. Peroxidizing lipids release soluble products that can diffuse over significant distances and produce further membrane injury at other cellular loci, such as the plasma membrane.

ACETAMINOPHEN AND BROMOBENZENE: It has been suggested that the hepatotoxicity of the two model hepatotoxins bromobenzene and the analgesic acetaminophen might reflect covalent binding of electrophilic metabolites to critical cellular macromolecules. Bromobenzene is metabolized to a reactive, electrophilic epoxide, which can react with reduced glutathione. If glutathione is depleted, the epoxide is free to react with cellular macromolecules. Acetaminophen is also metabolized to an electrophilic intermediate that can react with both GSH and cellular macromolecules. However, studies of the mechanisms by which bromobenzene and acetaminophen kill liver cells have suggested an alternative to the covalent binding of electrophilic metabolites. It has been possible to dissociate covalent binding from cell killing, and it is possible that liver necrosis is actually related to the toxicity of activated oxygen species. How are these species formed?

Acetaminophen is oxidized to the metabolite N-acetylimidoquinone without the addition of oxygen. Like CCl_4, acetaminophen is metabolized by a modification of the normal cytochrome P_{450} cycle, in which a number of electron transfer reactions result in the formation of superoxide and hydrogen peroxide. The liver cells may then be lethally injured by these activated oxygen species through mechanisms similar to those discussed earlier.

The metabolism of bromobenzene to produce an epoxide is a standard mixed-function oxidation, without the kinds of modifications characterizing the metabolism of CCl_4 and acetaminophen. How then are the liver cells injured by activated oxygen species? There are two possible mechanisms. On the one hand, the mixed-function oxidation of many substrates produces superoxide anions because the intermediate complex of cytochrome P_{450}, substrate, and reduced oxygen is inherently unstable; it may dissociate spontaneously to yield native cytochrome P_{450}, the original substrate, and superoxide. On the other hand, it is possible that, as a result of GSH depletion from the reaction with the bromobenzene epoxide, the antioxidant defenses of the cells are so weakened that they become sensitive to endogenous activated oxygen species.

To summarize, the metabolism of hepatotoxic chemicals by mixed-function oxidation leads to irreversible cell injury through mechanisms that may be unrelated, at least in part, to the covalent binding of reactive metabolites. What is emerging is a common theme of membrane damage as a result of the peroxidation of the constituent phospholipids. Lipid peroxidation is initiated by (1) a metabolite of the original compound (as with CCl_4) or (2) by activated oxygen species formed during the metabolism of the toxin (as with acetaminophen), the latter augmented by weakened antioxidant defenses.

Chemicals that Are Not Metabolized:

Directly cytotoxic chemicals do not have to be metabolized to injure the target cell and interact directly with cellular constituents. The critical cellular targets are diverse and include, for example, mitochondria (heavy metals), cytoskeleton (phalloidin, taxol), and DNA (chemotherapeutic alkylating agents). In addition, the interaction of directly cytotoxic chemicals with glutathione (alkylating agents) may weaken the antioxidant defenses of the cell.

Apoptosis (Programmed Cell Death)

Apoptosis refers to a genetically determined, internal, self-destruct mechanism of cell death, which is activated under a variety of circumstances. These include the following situations:

- Developmental morphogenesis
- The physiological turnover of cells in renewable tissues
- Immune regulation, as exemplified by the deletion of self-reactive T cells in the thymus during development and of B cells in the germinal centers of peripheral lymph nodes
- Deprivation of hormones and other trophic factors in some tissues
- Environmental hazards, including certain viral infections, ultraviolet exposure, ionizing radiation, and toxic cell injury
- Cancers, in which the vast majority of neoplastic cells undergo apoptosis, a feature that accounts for the slow growth of many malignant tumors

Multicellular organisms must control the elimination of damaged or surplus cells as strictly as they regulate the formation of new ones. Just as billions of hemopoietic elements, mucosal cells of the gastrointestinal tract, and epidermal cells of the skin are created daily, an equal number of cells in the same tissues are simultaneously lost by apoptosis. Programmed cell death is particularly important during development. For example, the formation of discrete digits of the hands and toes requires the elimination of interdigital webs of tissue. Similarly, half or more of many types of newly formed neurons are actually surplus and normally die soon after they form synaptic connections with their target cells. Another instance is the regression of the mesonephric precursor of the adult kidney in the development of the genitourinary system.

Many examples of apoptosis are relevant to the biology of adult tissues. For example, removal of the normal androgen stimulus to the prostate results in substantial shrinkage of the gland, partly by apoptosis and partly by atrophy of the epithelial cells. In women, the involution of the lactating breast is mediated by a reduction in prolactin secretion by the pituitary. These examples emphasize the positive roles of trophic factors in the maintenance of cell viability. Conversely, upon deprivation of such factors, many types of cells (neurons, hemopoietic precursors, endocrine cells, etc.) are programmed to die by apoptosis.

The ability of chemicals to trigger apoptosis is the basis for the effectiveness of many chemotherapeutic agents in the treatment of cancer. During normal development, glucocorticoids are produced within the thymus, in which location they may remove thymocytes that have escaped other selective pressures. This effect is, in turn, reflected in the capacity of high doses of adrenal steroids (glucocorticoids) to induce apoptosis in adult T lymphocytes, thereby contributing to the anti-inflammatory and immunosuppressive actions of these hormones.

THE MORPHOLOGY OF APOPTOSIS: However, apoptosis is typically seen in individual cells against a background of viable ones, in contrast to necrosis, which characteristically affects a mass of dying cells. The individual apoptotic cell tends to be shrunken and detached from its neighbors and is often engulfed by macrophages. Moreover, the inflammatory response elicited by necrotic cells is ordinarily absent or attenuated during apoptosis. By electron microscopy, apoptosis features (1) nuclear condensation and fragmentation, (2) segregation of cytoplasmic organelles into distinct regions, (3) surface membrane blebs, and (4) fragmentation of the dead or dying cell into membrane-bound bodies, which may or may not contain nuclear components.

The fragmentation of the nucleus characteristic of apoptosis (Fig. 1-31) has its counterpart in the electrophoretic pattern of DNA isolated from the dying cells. Since the internucleosomal distance in chromatin corresponds to approximately 200 base pairs, the cleavage of DNA by the activated endonuclease produces fragments that are multiples of this value. Upon electrophoresis of the cleaved DNA, a characteristic "ladder" of bands is typical of apoptosis (Fig. 1-32). Moreover, a nuclease that cleaves chromatin, which is activated in apoptosis, has been identified. Apoptotic cells can be detected in tissue sections after labeling fragmented DNA by means of the so-called TUNEL (terminal deoxynucleotidyl transferase dUTP nick end labeling) assay.

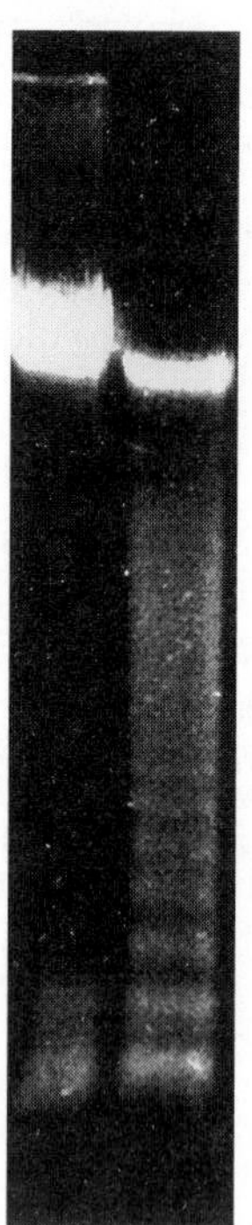

FIGURE *1-32*
DNA fragmentation in apoptosis. Agarose gel electrophoresis of DNA isolated from control (*left*) and apoptotic cells (*right*). In the control preparation, fragmented high-molecular-weight DNA is retained at the top of the gel. By contrast, internucleosomal cleavage of DNA in apoptosis is reflected in multiple fragments of varying molecular weight.

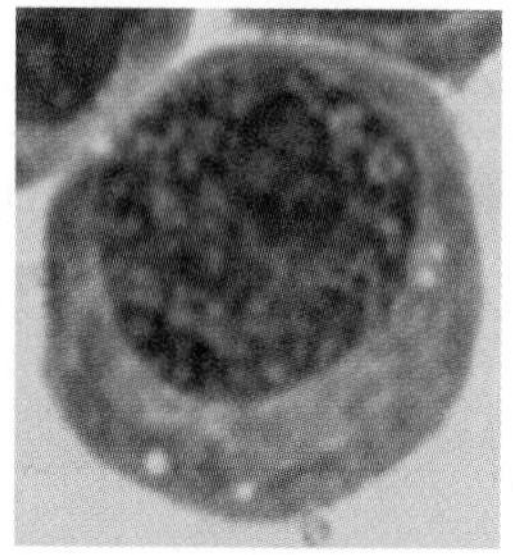

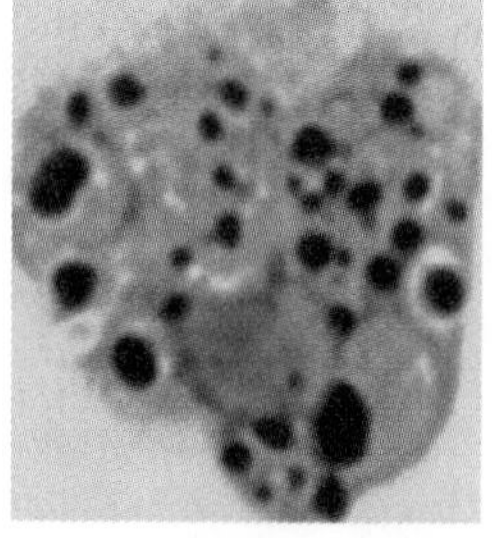

FIGURE *1-31*
Apoptosis. A viable leukemic cell (*left*) contrasts with an apoptotic cell (*right*) in which the nucleus has undergone condensation and fragmentation.

The Mechanisms of Apoptosis

The programmatic nature of apoptosis is well illustrated by studying lineage-dependent death of cells in the nematode worm *Caenorhabditis elegans*. In this model, specific cells die sequentially, and genes that control their programmed death have been identified and collectively termed **ced** (cell death) genes. Importantly, homologues of the ced genes are present in mammalian cells, one of which (ced-3) encodes a protein termed interleukin converting enzyme (ICE), which belongs to a family of cysteine proteases collectively labeled caspases. Loss of ced-3 function in the worm and caspase inhibitors in mammalian cells protect against apoptosis. A variety of other genes that participate in programmed cell death has been found in *C. elegans*, *Drosophila*, and other models.

Programmed cell death has become the subject of intense study, and numerous phenomena that contribute to apoptotic cell death have been described. It is beyond the scope of this discussion to enter deeply into the controversies in this field, but a few examples of proposed mechanisms in apoptosis merit review. At present, the two best-characterized models of programmed cell death are those that involve the activation of the Fas-receptor (e.g., cell killing by T lymphocytes) and apoptosis following DNA damage (Fig. 1-33).

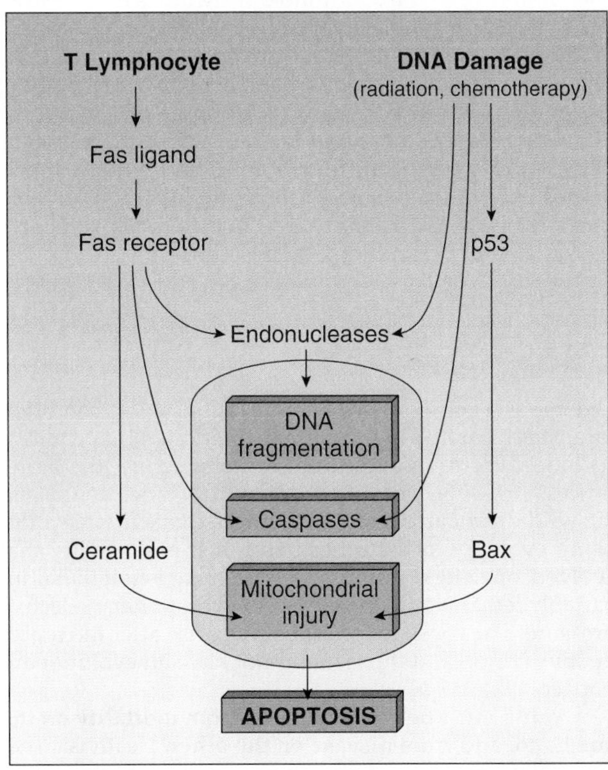

FIGURE 1-33
Mechanisms of apoptosis. Two major pathways that mediate cell death in apoptosis are illustrated. Cytotoxic T cells bear the Fas ligand, which binds and activates the Fas receptor on the surface of target cells. As a result, three biochemical consequences that collectively mediate apoptosis ensue: (1) activation of an endonuclease causes DNA fragmentation; (2) activation of caspases leads to the proteolysis of a variety of substrates; and (3) the generation of ceramide injures mitochondria. The same three events characterize the apoptosis induced by DNA damage. In this case, however, the upregulation of p53 induces Bax synthesis, which leads to mitochondrial injury.

FAS RECEPTOR ACTIVATION: Cytotoxic (CD8+) T cells bear a Fas ligand protein on the surface. Upon interaction of the T cell receptor with a target cell, the Fas ligand binds to and activates the Fas receptor on the surface membrane of the latter. Activation of the Fas receptor leads to a series of reactions that culminates in the activation of caspases (ICE-like proteases) and subsequent proteolytic cleavage of their substrates. At the same time, other events that are consequences of Fas receptor activation lead to the generation of ceramide (a product of the hydrolysis of the plasma membrane phospholipid sphingomyelin). This lipid messenger is thought to mediate mitochondrial injury. In a still undefined manner, the combined effects of increased caspase activity and mitochondrial damage eventuate in the death of the cell, a process that is accompanied by endonuclease activation and the internucleosomal fragmentation of DNA.

DNA DAMAGE: Diverse agents that damage DNA (e.g., ionizing radiation, chemotherapeutic compounds, and activated oxygen species) may induce apoptosis. Despite the differences in the nature of the injurious agents, the pathway toward apoptosis appears to be uniform. DNA damage upregulates the nuclear protein p53, which, in general, controls the reactions of cells to the compromise of genome integrity (see Chapter 5). The p53 protein is a transcriptional activator that results in the expression of several genes involved in the regulation of the cell cycle and in apoptosis. In particular, p53 induces the synthesis of Bax, a death-promoting protein that is thought to injure mitochondria. Caspases also contribute to cell death initiated by DNA damage, although the mechanisms underlying their activation and functions remain to be identified.

REGULATORS OF APOPTOSIS: In *C. elegans*, genes that inhibit apoptosis have also been identified. The best known of these is ced-9, whose human homologue is the oncogene *Bcl*-2, a protein that is present in certain B cell malignancies and that also inhibits apoptosis (see Chapters 5 and 20). The inappropriate expression of *Bcl*-2 allows the persistence of cells ordinarily destined to be removed by apoptosis and results in the abnormal accumulation of neoplastic cells, which describes the clinical presentation of follicular lymphoma. Viruses (adenovirus, papillomavirus, vaccinia virus, hepatitis B virus) can also thwart apoptotic cell death by virtue of gene sequences that code for products that can bind to and inhibit proteins in death-promoting pathways, including p53, caspases, and possibly Bax.

CALCIFICATION

The deposition of mineral salts of calcium is, of course, a normal process in the formation of bone from cartilage.

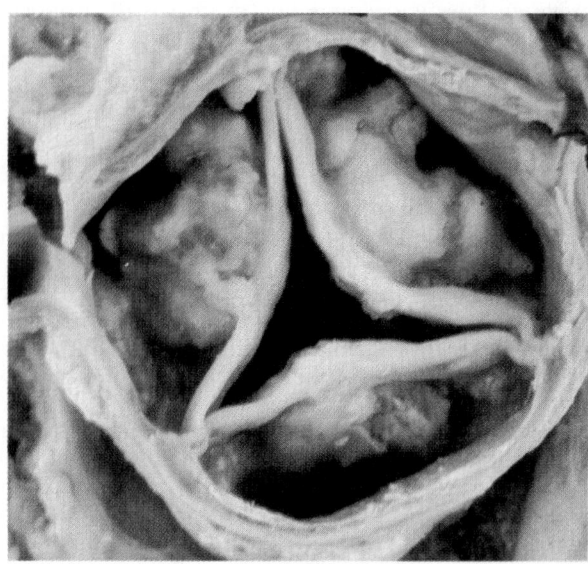

FIGURE *1-34*
Calcific aortic stenosis. Large deposits of calcium salts are evident in the cusps and the free margins of the thickened aortic valve, as viewed from above.

As we have learned, calcium entry into dead or dying cells is usual, owing to the inability of such cells to maintain a steep calcium gradient. This cellular calcification is not ordinarily visible except as inclusions within mitochondria (see Fig. 1-18).

Dystrophic calcification *refers to the macroscopic deposition of calcium salts in injured tissues.* This type of calcification does not simply reflect an accumulation of calcium derived from the bodies of dead cells but rather represents an extracellular deposition of calcium from the circulation or interstitial fluid. Dystrophic calcification apparently requires the persistence of necrotic tissue; it is often visible to the naked eye and ranges from gritty, sandlike grains to firm, rock-hard material. In many locations, such as in cases of tuberculous caseous necrosis in the lung or lymph nodes, calcification has no functional consequences. However, dystrophic calcification may also occur in crucial locations, such as in the mitral or aortic valves (Fig. 1-34). In such instances, calcification leads to impeded blood flow because it produces inflexible valve leaflets and narrowed valve orifices (mitral and aortic stenosis). Dystrophic calcification in atherosclerotic coronary arteries contributes to narrowing of those vessels.

Dystrophic calcification also plays a role in diagnostic radiography. Mammography is based principally on the detection of calcifications in breast cancers; congenital toxoplasmosis, an infection involving the central nervous system, is suggested by the visualization of calcification in the infant brain.

Metastatic calcification *reflects deranged calcium metabolism in contrast to dystrophic calcification, which has its origin in cell injury.* Metastatic calcification is associated with an increased serum calcium concentration (hypercalcemia). In general, almost any disorder that increases the serum calcium level can lead to calcification in such inappropriate locations as the alveolar septa of the lung, renal tubules, and blood vessels. Calcification is seen in various disorders, including chronic renal failure, vitamin D intoxication, and hyperparathyroidism.

The formation of stones containing calcium carbonate in sites such as the gallbladder, renal pelvis, bladder, and pancreatic duct is another form of pathological calcification. Under certain circumstances, the mineral salts precipitate from solution and crystallize about foci of organic material. Those who have suffered the agony of gallbladder or renal colic will attest to the unpleasant consequences of this type of calcification.

HYALINE

The word "hyaline" simply refers to any material that exhibits a reddish, homogeneous appearance when routinely stained with hematoxylin and eosin. The student will encounter the term hyaline in classic descriptions of diverse and unrelated lesions. Standard terminology includes hyaline arteriolosclerosis, alcoholic hyaline in the liver, hyaline membranes in the lung, and hyaline droplets in various cells. The various lesions called hyaline actually have nothing in common. Alcoholic hyaline is composed of cytoskeletal filaments; the hyaline found in arterioles of the kidney is derived from basement membranes; and hyaline membranes consist of plasma proteins deposited in alveoli. The term is anachronistic and of questionable value, except as a handy morphological descriptor.

CELLULAR AGING

Old age is a consequence of civilization; it is a condition rarely encountered in the animal kingdom or in primitive societies. From an evolutionary perspective, the aging process presents conceptual difficulties. Since animals in the wild do not attain their maximum longevity, how did aging evolve? On the other hand, if it is longevity that evolved, one might intuitively expect that a trait that is invariably lethal would be subject to evolutionary selective pressure. The consequences of aging arise after the reproductive period and thus should not have an evolutionary impact.

Aging must be distinguished from mortality on the one hand, and from disease on the other. Death is an accidental event; an aged person who does not succumb to the most common cause of death will die from the second, third, or tenth most common cause. Although the increased vulnerability to disease among the elderly is an interesting problem, disease itself is entirely distinct from aging.

Life Span

Millennia ago the psalmist sang of a natural life span of 70 years, which with vigor may extend to 80. On an evolutionary scale, biblical figures lived in our era of literate

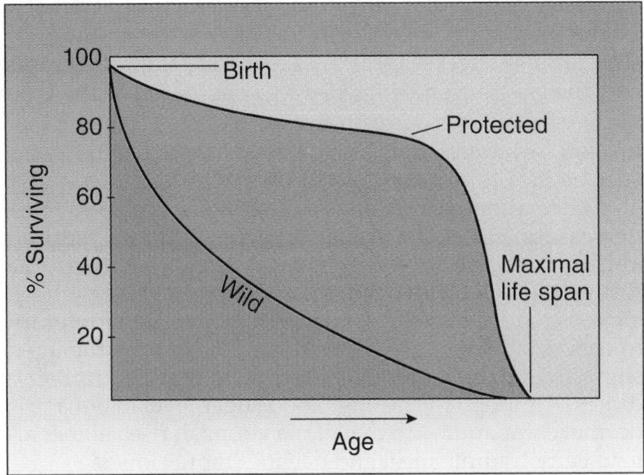

FIGURE 1-35
Life span of animals in their natural environment compared with a protected habitat. Note that both curves reach the same maximal life span.

civilization. By contrast, it is estimated that the usual age at death of neolithic humans was 20 to 25 years, and the average life span in many primitive cultures today is often barely 10 years more.

The difference between humans in primitive and in civilized environments is analogous to that observed between animals in their natural habitat and those in a zoo (Fig. 1-35). For animals in the wild, after an initial high mortality during maturation, a progressive linear decline in survival is noted, ending at the maximum life span of the species. This steady decrease in the number of mature animals reflects not aging but random events, such as encounters with beasts of prey, accidental trauma, infections, starvation, and so on. On the other hand, survival in the protected environment of a zoo is characterized by slow attrition until senescence, at which time the steep decline in numbers is attributable to aging. Of interest is the fact that the maximum life span attained is not significantly altered by a protected environment. An analogous situation is seen in studies of human mortality (Fig. 1-36). Less than a century ago, the steep linear slope of mortality in the adult principally reflected random accidents and infections. With greater attention to safety and sanitation, the development of antibiotics and other specific drugs, safer blood transfusions, and improved diagnostic and therapeutic methods, mortality through the middle years has substantially decreased. Yet mortality during old age remains steep, and the maximum human life span has remained constant at about 110 years. What would happen if diseases associated with old age, such as coronary artery disease and cancer, were eliminated? Such triumphs might lead to an **ideal survival curve** (see Fig. 1-36) but to only a modest increase in average life expectancy. A long period of good health and low mortality would inevitably be followed by a precipitously increased mortality owing to aging itself; the life span would, for practical purposes, remain on the lower side of 100. Given the current mean life expectancy, which in women is approaching 80, the prevention or cure of the causes of premature death would have little impact on mean longevity.

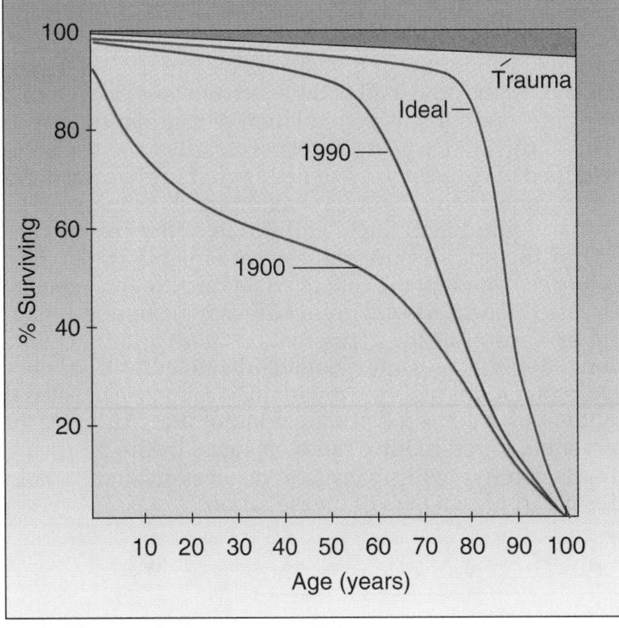

FIGURE 1-36
Ideal human life span contrasted with those seen in 1900 and 1980. Note again that the same maximal life span is reached in all cases.

Why do women live longer than men? From 1900 to 1980, the male-to-female mortality ratio in the United States rose continuously, but in the last two decades this ratio has stabilized. Although as many as 170 male zygotes are conceived for every 100 female, the male-to-female ratio declines during pregnancy and is only 106:100 at birth. From that time on, more women than men survive at every age, and at age 75 the male-to-female ratio is 2:3. Interestingly, a greater female longevity is almost universal in the animal kingdom.

At the cellular level, somatic cells with the female phenotype are no hardier than those with the male pattern. A major cause of the difference in average longevity is clearly the greater male mortality rate from violent causes and a greater susceptibility to cardiovascular disease, cancer, respiratory illness, and cirrhosis in middle and old age.

The historical differences between the sexes in cigarette smoking and alcohol consumption are important in the gender gap in longevity. Indeed, smoking alone has been estimated to account for 4 of the 7 years of sex differential in longevity at birth. Thus, if men escape from the hazards noted earlier, the gap in longevity between the sexes is progressively reduced with advancing age to just over 1 year beyond age 85.

Functional and Structural Changes

The insidious effects of aging can be detected in otherwise healthy persons. The great leaps of imagination by theoretical physicists and mathematicians are almost exclu-

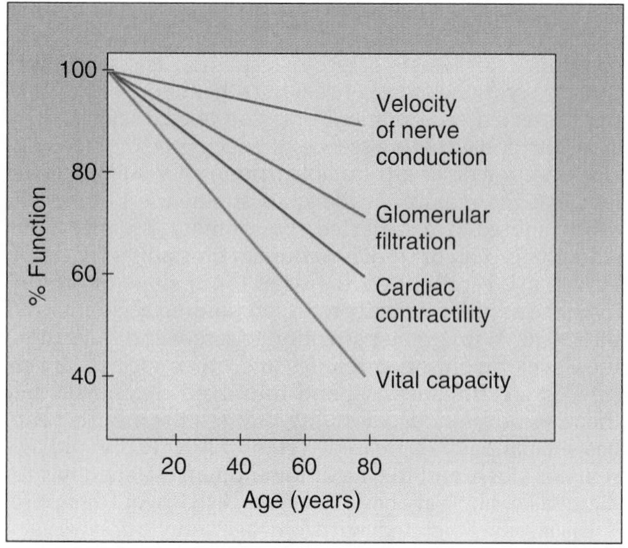

FIGURE 1-37
Decrease in human physiological capacities as a function of age.

sively the province of the young, and an athlete in his or her 30s may be referred to as "aged." Even in the absence of specific diseases or vascular abnormalities, beginning in the fourth decade of life there is a progressive decline in many physiological functions (Fig. 1-37), including such easily measurable parameters as muscular strength, cardiac reserve, nerve conduction time, pulmonary vital capacity, glomerular filtration, and vascular elasticity. These functional deteriorations are accompanied by structural changes (Fig. 1-38). Lean body mass decreases and the proportion of fat rises. Constituents of the connective tissue matrix are progressively cross-linked. Lipofuscin ("wear and tear") pigment accumulates in organs such as the brain, heart, and liver.

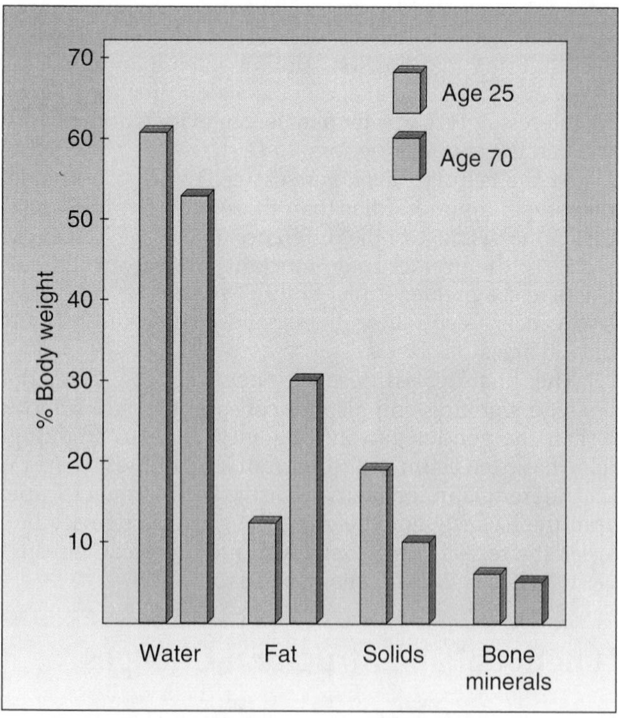

FIGURE 1-38
Structural changes with age in the human body.

The salient characteristic of aging is not so much a decrease in basal functional capacity as it is a reduced ability to adapt to environmental stress. Although the resting pulse is unchanged, the maximal increase with exercise is reduced with age, and the time required for return to a normal heart rate is prolonged. Similarly, the aged show an impaired adaptive response to ingested carbohydrates. Although the fasting blood sugar level in old age is normal compared with that of the young, it rises higher after a carbohydrate meal and declines more slowly.

The Cellular Basis of Aging

Although the biological basis for aging is obscure, there is general agreement that its elucidation, as in all pathological conditions, should be sought at the cellular level. Various theories of cellular aging have been proposed, but the evidence adduced for each is at best indirect and is often derived from data obtained in cultured cells. An adequate theory should be parsimonious, compatible with the species-specific differences in life spans, and consistent with the fact that most noncycling cells, such as neurons and myocytes, undergo a linear, relatively uniform functional decline with age. Most findings to date can be considered the result of aging as easily as the cause.

There is no shortage of speculation regarding cellular aging, but the fundamental information necessary for a coherent theory is lacking. Current opinions of the mechanisms underlying aging encompass a broad spectrum. At one extreme is the concept of a species-specific, predetermined genetic program that sets the life span of the organism. At the other end of the spectrum, are theories that attribute aging to an accumulation of random defects in cellular function, which are not necessarily genetically determined. Evidence for a genetic program has been derived from (1) studies of the "senescence" of animal cells in tissue culture, (2) the identification of the genetic control of life span in invertebrate organisms (*C. elegans*, *Drosophila*), and (3) the characterization of human genetic diseases associated with premature aging. Support for aging as a result of the accumulation of a variety of functional deficits has come from the identification of phenotypic alterations associated with increasing age in several models, as well as the prolongation of life span after interventions that modify these changes. In the following discussion, we will review the major considerations in this controversial field of investigation.

Aging as a Genetic Program

Cellular Senescence *in vitro*

Support for the concept of a genetically programmed life span comes from studies of replicating cells in tissue culture. Unlike cancer cells, normal cells in tissue culture do

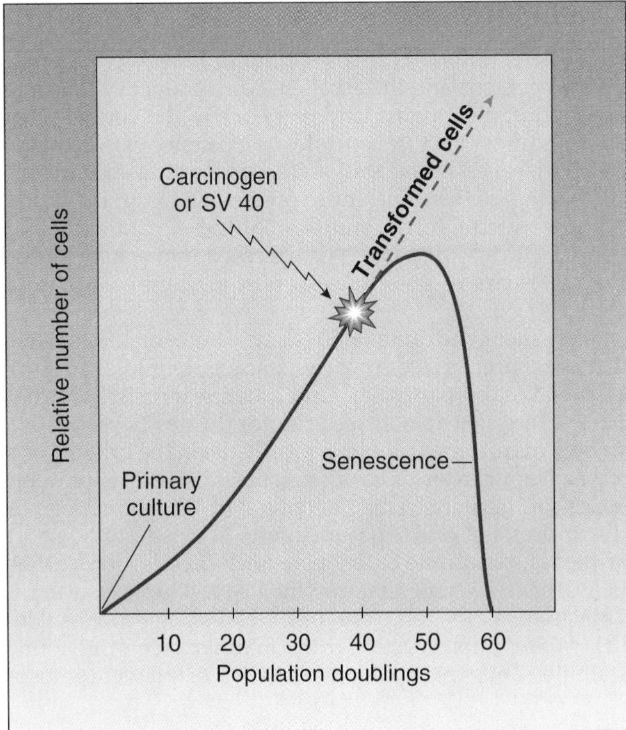

FIGURE *1-39*
Cellular senescence in cultured human fibroblasts. The number of cultured cells is a function of the number of population doublings. After about 50 population doublings, the cells no longer divide and the culture dies out. However, if the cells are transformed with a virus or chemical, cellular senescence is not seen; the cells are "immortalized" and continue to divide indefinitely.

not exhibit an unrestrained capacity to replicate. Cultured human fibroblasts undergo about 50 population doublings, after which they no longer divide and the culture dies out (Fig. 1-39). If the cells are transformed into cancer cells, by exposure to an oncogenic virus (SV40) or a chemical carcinogen, they continue to replicate; in a sense, they become immortal. A rough correlation between the number of population doublings in fibroblasts and life span has been reported in several species. As an example, rat fibroblasts exhibit considerably fewer doublings than do human ones. Moreover, cells obtained from patients with precocious aging, such as those with progeria (see later), also display a conspicuously reduced number of population doublings *in vitro*.

There is no demonstrable age-related change *in vivo* in the replicative capacity of rapidly cycling cells, such as epithelial cells of the intestine. Therefore, one is left with the apparent paradox that replicating cells in culture have a limited life span but aging *in vivo* seems principally to affect the functional capacity of postmitotic cells. In other words, persons do not age because the cells of the intestinal tract fail to replicate. However, if one considers that the function of cells *in vitro* is to proliferate, then they indeed display a major failure in functional capacity. Thus, cells in culture do represent a model for the study of aging.

Studies have demonstrated that cellular senescence *in vitro* is apparently a dominant genetic trait. The evidence for this concept is the demonstration that hybrids between normal human cells *in vitro*, which exhibit a finite life span, and immortal cells with an indefinite life span undergo senescence. This finding shows that senescence is dominant over immortality. Interestingly, such hybrid cells that escape senescence have either lost chromosome 1 or exhibit specific deletions in the long arm (1q). The introduction of chromosome 1 from a normal human cell with a limited life span into an otherwise immortalized hybrid cell induces senescence (Fig. 1-40). Cell senes-

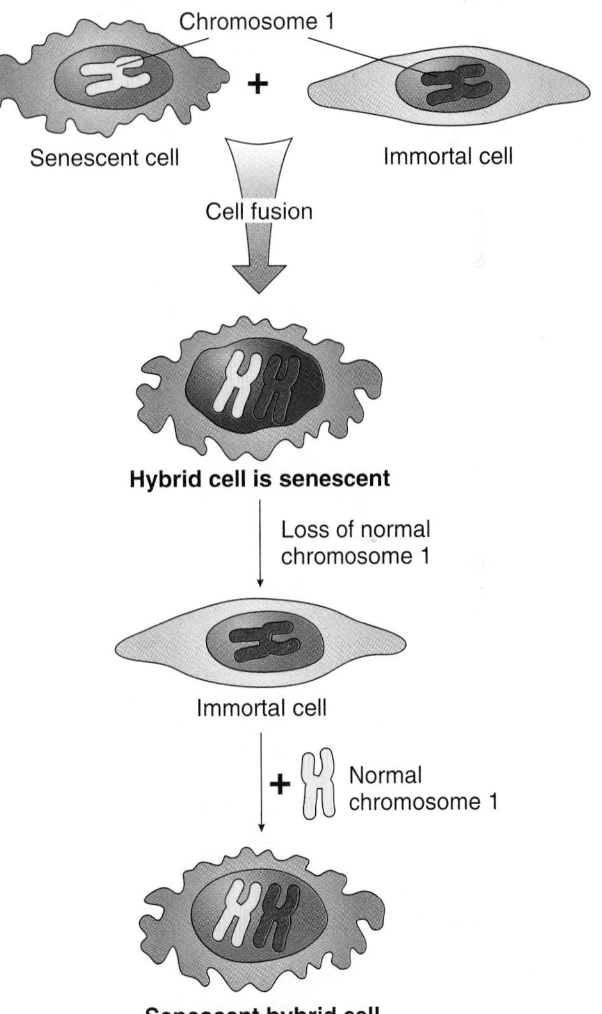

FIGURE *1-40*
The role of human chromosome 1 in cellular senescence *in vitro*. When a normal human fibroblast with a limited life span is fused with a transformed hamster cell, the resulting hybrid cell undergoes senescence, demonstrating that senescence is dominant over immortality. The loss of the human chromosome 1 from the hybrid cell restores immortality, whereas the reintroduction of a normal human chromosome 1 again leads to senescence.

cence–related genes have also been identified on other human chromosomes, but the function(s) coded for by any of the senescence genes have not been identified.

An alternative explanation for cell senescence *in vitro* centers on the genetic elements at the tips of chromosomes termed telomeres. These are composed of short repetitive nucleotide sequences (TTAGGG in vertebrates), which vary in size from 70 in *Tetrahymena* to 2000 in human chromosomes. Since DNA polymerase is unable to copy the linear chromosomes all the way to the tip, the telomeres would tend to shorten with each cell division until a critical diminution in size would interfere with cell viability. To overcome this "end-replication" problem, most eukaryotic cells utilize a ribonucleoprotein enzyme termed telomerase, which is capable of extending chromosome ends. However, many somatic mammalian cells lack telomerase activity, and progressive telomere shortening occurs over the replicative life span of such cells in tissue culture. It has, therefore, been proposed that telomere shortening acts as a molecular clock that produces senescence after a defined number of cell divisions *in vitro*. Indeed, declining telomere length is currently the best molecular correlate of the capacity of cultured mammalian cells to replicate. Interestingly, after immortalization of cells *in vitro*, telomerase activity can be demonstrated. However, it has recently been observed that telomeres do not always shorten significantly with age, and cancer cells (immortalized) do not always have telomeres of a constant length. Thus, the relevance of telomere shortening to aging remains to be established.

Genetic Control of Life Span in Invertebrates

C. elegans is the only metazoan in which single-gene mutations that extend life span have been identified. A variety of such mutations (Age mutations) increase the life span of the nematode up to fivefold, a greater increase than has been reported for any other model. In addition to prolonging the life span, Age mutations in *C. elegans* also confer a complex array of other phenotypes. For example, the so-called clock (clk) mutations slow most functions that relate to the overall metabolic rate (cell cycle progression, swimming, food pumping, etc.). Age mutations also confer resistance to both environmental (extrinsic) and intrinsic stresses, including oxygen free radicals, heat shock, and ultraviolet radiation. Thus, genes that prolong life in *C. elegans* apparently act to reduce the accumulation of cellular "injuries" that impair homeostatic mechanisms and, thereby, shorten life span.

In experiments with *Drosophila*, strains of long-lived flies can be readily created by using the oldest flies for breeding. In such studies, the better health of the aged flies is associated with a "trade-off" of decreased fitness in the young flies, as evidenced by lesser activity and fertility compared to wild-type flies. Thus, the original population must have had a set of alleles that determines greater fitness at a young age and decreased fitness at an older one, a phenomenon termed "antagonistic pleiotropy." Similar to the situation in *C. elegans*, long-lived fruit flies, depending on the strain, also exhibit resistance to oxidative stress, desiccation, food deprivation, and heat.

Diseases of Premature Aging

In humans, the modest correlation in longevity between related persons and the excellent concordance of life span among identical twins lend credence to the concept that aging is under genetic control. The existence of human genetic diseases associated with accelerated aging buttresses this notion. The entire process of aging, including features such as male-pattern baldness, cataracts, and coronary artery disease, is compressed into a span of less than 10 years in a heritable syndrome termed **progeria** (Fig. 1-41).

Werner syndrome (WS) is a rare autosomal recessive disease characterized by early cataracts, hair loss, atrophy of the skin, osteoporosis, and atherosclerosis. Affected persons are also at increased risk for the development of a variety of cancers. Patients typically die in the fifth decade either from cancer or cardiovascular disease, as do their older counterparts. This phenotype of WS patients gives the impression of premature aging. Located on the short arm of chromosome 8, the gene for WS codes for a DNA helicase, an enzyme that unwinds DNA duplexes to provide access of the template to DNA-binding proteins. Helicases are, thus, crucial for the maintenance of genomic stability. Cells from patients with WS display chromoso-

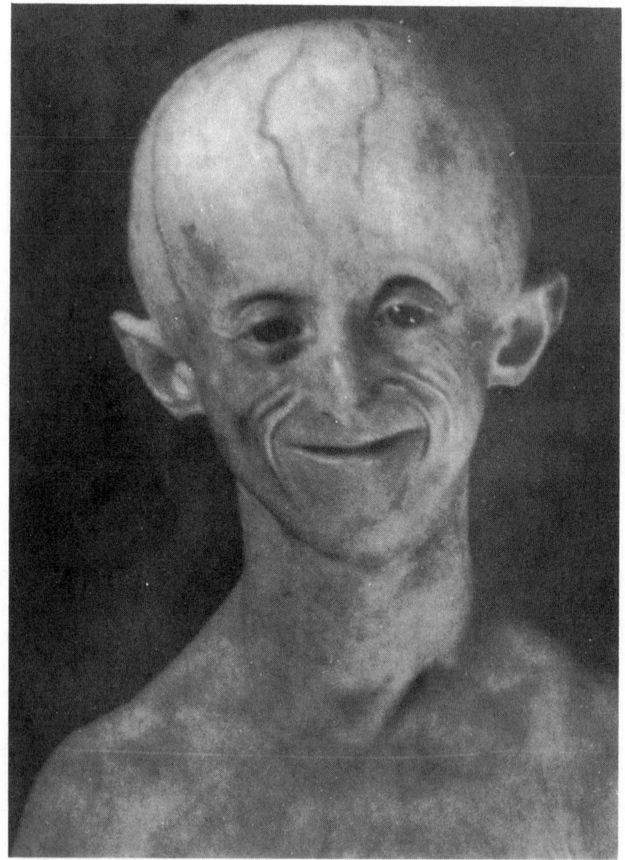

FIGURE *1-41*
Progeria. A 14-year-old boy shows the signs of accelerated aging.

mal deletions, inversions, and reciprocal translocations (see Chapter 6). It is presumed that the premature aging in this disorder results from the progressive accumulation of genetic damage and consequent functional derangements.

Aging as Accumulated Somatic Damage

Cells may sustain a variety of injuries during a lifetime, and the precise catalogue of molecular lesions responsible for aging remains to be defined. Currently, most attention of investigators in this area is directed toward the molecular consequences of persistent oxidative stress. The oxidative stress hypothesis holds that the loss of function characteristic of aging is caused by the progressive and irreversible accrual of molecular oxidative damage. Such lesions would be manifested as peroxidation of membrane lipids, DNA modification (strand breaks, base alterations, DNA-protein cross-linking), and protein oxidation (loss of sulfhydryl groups, carbonylation). Oxidative stress in normal cells is hardly trivial, with as much as 3% of total oxygen consumption being converted to the generation of superoxide anions and hydrogen peroxide. It has been estimated that a single rodent cell undergoes some 100,000 attacks on DNA a day by oxygen free radicals and that at any one time 10% of protein molecules are modified by carbonyl adducts. Thus, antioxidant defenses are not fully efficient, and progressive oxidative damage to the cell may be responsible, at least in part, for the aging process.

The rate of generation of reactive oxygen species correlates with the overall metabolic rate of an organism. The theory that aging is related to oxidative stress is based to some extent on several observations: (1) larger animals usually have longer life spans than smaller ones; (2) the metabolic rate is inversely related to body size (the larger the animal, the lower the metabolic rate); and (3) the generation of activated oxygen species is directly related to body size.

The role of oxidative stress in aging has been emphasized by experiments in *Drosophila*, in which the overexpression of genes for superoxide dismutase or catalase, significantly prolongs the life span of the fly. Furthermore, as discussed above, virtually all long-lived worms and flies display increased antioxidant defenses. Superoxide dismutase activity in the livers of different primates has also been reported to be proportional to the maximal life span.

The correlation of oxidative damage with aging is further exemplified by supporting biochemical data: (1) In mammalian and insect tissues, the ratios of redox couples (GSH-GSSG, NADPH-NADP$^+$, NADH-NAD$^+$) is shifted toward more prooxidant values during aging; (2) the exhalation of products of lipid peroxidation (ethane, pentane) is augmented with age; (3) a threefold increase in the concentration of oxidatively damaged proteins is present in older tissues; and (4) DNA oxidative damage (measured as the concentration of 8-hydroxydeoxyguanosine) increases with age in various tissues.

Additional evidence for progressive oxidative damage with aging is the deposition of lipofuscin pigment, principally in postmitotic cells of organs such as the brain, heart, and liver. This brown pigment is located in lysosomes and contains products of the peroxidation of unsaturated fatty acids. Although no functional derangements are directly attributed to the accumulation of lipofuscin, it has been proposed that the presence of this pigment reflects continuing lipid peroxidation of cellular membranes as a result of inadequate defenses against the stress of activated oxygen.

Recently, oxidative damage to mitochondria has been proposed to play a major role in aging. Aerobic respiration in mitochondria is the richest source of reactive oxygen species in the cell. More than a dozen large deletions in mitochondrial DNA of postmitotic cells have been identified in the tissues of older persons and are interpreted as evidence of oxidative damage. In turn, these DNA defects may lead to further increases in the mitochondrial generation of toxic oxygen species, thereby establishing a vicious circle.

Caloric restriction in rodents has been known for more than half a century to increase longevity. This phenomenon has also been reported in lower species, such as fish, spiders, and other nonrodent species. Conversely, food consumption above an optimal level progressively shortens longevity. However, a prolongation of the life span by caloric restriction has not been demonstrated in primates or humans. There is evidence to indicate that the extension of the life span by caloric restriction in rodents is associated with a hypometabolic state, analogous to the effect of the "clock" mutations in *C. elegans*. Animals subjected to caloric restriction show attenuation of age-related increases in the rates of mitochondrial generation of reactive oxygen species, slower accrual of oxidative damage, and decreased evidence of lipid peroxidation and oxidative alterations of proteins.

Summary Hypothesis of Aging

In establishing a theory of aging, it is necessary to maintain an evolutionary perspective. In this context, aging should be thought of as a spectrum of phenotypes that have escaped the force of natural selection. After the reproductive period, evolution loses interest in a species and abandons the organism to events against which nature confers no protection. As reviewed above, the doctrine of antagonistic pleiotropy posits the existence of genes that are beneficial during development and the reproductive period but exert baleful influences later in life. The alternative hypothesis of mutation accumulation holds that the evolutionary suppression of genes that are harmful to young individuals of a species creates pressure favoring alleles that defer the attainment of a deleterious phenotype until the postreproductive period. Finally, the major nongenetic theories hold that simple accumulation of various cell injuries eventuate in senescence. It is our view that current evidence supports the notion that these hypotheses are not mutually contradictory and that all may contribute to aging (Fig. 1-42). According to this concept, although aging is under genetic control, it is unlikely that a predetermined genetic program for aging exists. It is likely that the combined effects of a number of genes eventually lead to the accumulation of somatic mutations,

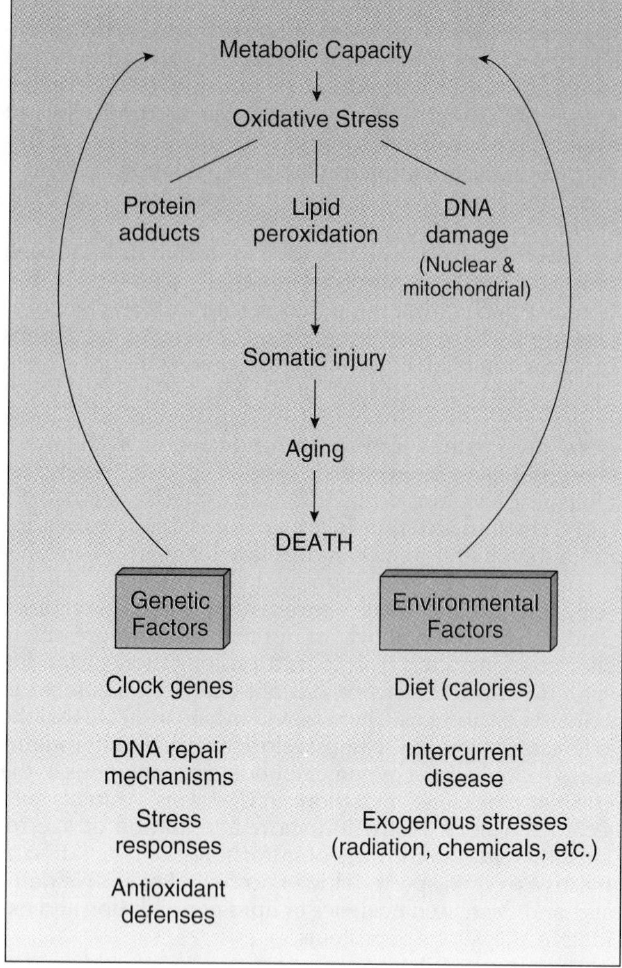

FIGURE *1-42*
Summary hypothesis of the mechanisms responsible for biological aging. It is likely that aging represents the progressive accumulation of a variety of somatic injuries, including damage to proteins, membrane lipids, and nuclear and mitochondrial DNA. The extent of these injuries has been linked to the oxidative stress produced by cellular metabolism. In turn, both genetic and environmental factors have been invoked as determining the metabolic capacity and the antioxidant and other defenses of a cell.

deficiencies in DNA repair, the accretion of oxidative damage to macromolecules, and a variety of other defects in cell function, all culminating in the progressive failure of homeostatic mechanisms characteristic of aging. As Maimonides said, "The same forces that operate in the birth and temporal existence of man also operate in his destruction and death."

SUGGESTED READING

Epstein CJ, Motulusky AG: Werner syndrome: Entering the helicase era. *BioEssays* 18:1025–1027, 1996.

Farber JL: Mechanisms of cell injury by activated oxygen species. *Environ Health Perspect* 102:17–24, 1994.

Grace PA: Ischaemia-reperfusion injury. *Br J Surg* 81:637–647, 1994.

Greider CW, Blackburn EH: Telomeres, telomerase and cancer. *Sci Am* 274:92–97, 1996.

Karlsson C, Stenman G, Vojta PJ, Bongcam-Rudloff E, Barrett C, Westermark B, Lithgow GJ: Invertebrate gerontology: The age mutations of *Caenorhabditis elegans*. *BioEssays* 18:809–815, 1996.

Martin GM: The genetics of aging. *Hosp Pract* 32:47–75, 1997.

Nakae D, Yamamoto K, Yoshiji H, et al: Liposome-encapsulated superoxide dismutase prevents liver necrosis induced by acetaminophen. *Am J Pathol* 136:787–795, 1990.

Neyses L, Pelzer T: The biological cascade leading to cardiac hypertrophy. *Eur Heart J* 16:8–11, 1995.

Osborne BA, Schwartz LM: Essential genes that regulate apoptosis. *Trends Cell Biol* 4:394–397, 1994.

Paulsson Y: Escape from senescence in hybrid cell clones involves deletions of two regions located on human chromosome 1q. *Cancer Res* 56:241–245, 1996.

Rattan SIS: Gerontogenes: Real or virtual? *FASEB J* 9:284–286, 1995.

Sanders EJ, Wride MA: Programmed cell death in development. *Int Rev Cytol* 163:105–173, 1995.

Sohal RS, Weindruch R: Oxidative stress, caloric restriction, and aging. *Science* 273:59–63, 1996.

Tower J: Aging mechanisms in fruit flies. *BioEssays* 18:799–807, 1996.

White K, Grether ME, Abrams JM, Young L, Farrell K, Steller H: Genetic control of programmed cell death in *Drosophila*. *Science* 264:677–683, 1994.

CHAPTER 2

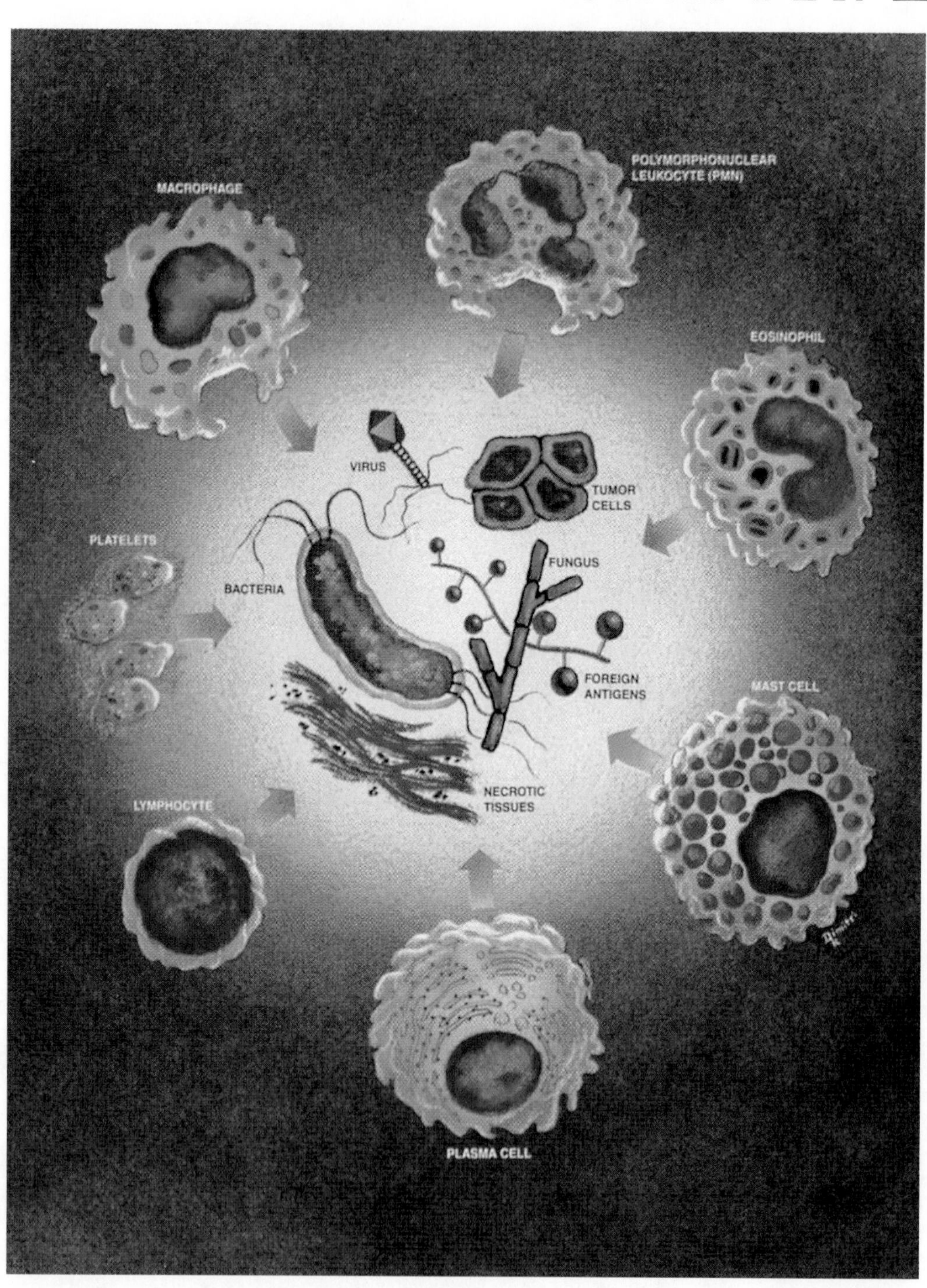

MACROPHAGE
POLYMORPHONUCLEAR LEUKOCYTE (PMN)
EOSINOPHIL
VIRUS
TUMOR CELLS
PLATELETS
FUNGUS
BACTERIA
FOREIGN ANTIGENS
MAST CELL
NECROTIC TISSUES
LYMPHOCYTE
PLASMA CELL

Inflammation

Joseph C. Fantone
Peter A. Ward

FIGURE **2-1** (*see opposite page*)
Participants in acute and chronic inflammatory reactions.

Inflammation is the reaction of a tissue and its microcirculation to a pathogenic insult. It is characterized by the generation of inflammatory mediators and movement of fluid and leukocytes from the blood into extravascular tissues. This is frequently an expression of the host's attempt to localize and eliminate metabolically altered cells, foreign particles, microorganisms, or antigens.

The clinical signs of inflammation, termed *phlogosis* by the Greeks and *inflammatio* in Latin, were described in classical times. In the second century AD, the Roman encyclopedist Aulus Celsus described the four cardinal signs of inflammation, namely, **rubor** (redness), **calor** (heat), **tumor** (swelling), and **dolor** (pain). According to medieval concepts, inflammation represented an imbalance of various "humors," including blood, mucus, and bile. The modern understanding of the vascular basis of inflammation began in the 18th century with the observations of John Hunter, who noted dilatation of blood vessels and appreciated that pus represented an accumulation of material derived from the blood. That inflammation is usually a reaction to prior tissue injury was described by Rudolf Virchow, whose pupil Julius Cohnheim was then the first to associate inflammation with the emigration of leukocytes through the walls of the microvasculature. At the turn of the 19th century, the role of phagocytosis in the inflammatory process was emphasized by the great Russian zoologist Eli Metchnikoff. Finally, the importance of chemical mediators in the inflammatory response was described in 1927 by Thomas Lewis, who demonstrated that histamine and other substances produced an increase in vascular permeability and the migration of leukocytes into the extravascular spaces.

GENERAL CONSIDERATIONS

The primary purpose of the inflammatory response is to eliminate the pathogenic insult and remove injured tissue components. This process accomplishes either regeneration of the normal tissue architecture and return of physiological function or the formation of scar tissue to replace what cannot be repaired. Further extension of injury or the effects of the inflammatory response itself may lead to loss of function of the organ or tissue. Inflammation can be thought to proceed as follows:

1. **Initiation** of the mechanisms responsible for the localization and clearance of foreign substances and injured tissues is stimulated by the recognition that injury to tissues has occurred.
2. **Amplification** of the inflammatory response, in which both soluble mediators and cellular inflammatory systems are activated, follows recognition of injury.
3. **Termination** of the inflammatory response, after generation of inflammatory agents and elimination of the foreign agent, is accomplished by specific inhibitors of the mediators.

Under certain conditions, the ability to clear injured tissue and foreign agents is impaired, or the regulatory mechanisms of the inflammatory response are altered. In these circumstances, inflammation is harmful to the host and leads to excessive tissue destruction and injury. In other instances, an immune response to residual microbial products or to altered tissue components also triggers a persistent inflammatory reaction.

Initiation of the inflammatory response begins as the result of direct injury or stimulation of the cellular or structural components of a tissue including the following:

- Parenchymal cells
- Microvasculature
- Tissue macrophages and mast cells
- Mesenchymal cells (e.g., fibroblasts)
- Extracellular matrix

One of the earliest responses following tissue injury occurs within the microvasculature at the level of the capillary and postcapillary venule. Within this vascular network are the major components of the inflammatory response, including plasma, platelets, erythrocytes, and circulating leukocytes (Figs. 2-1 and 2-2). These components are normally confined within the intravascular compartment by a continuous layer of endothelial cells, which are connected to each other by tight junctions and separated from the tissue by a limiting basement membrane. Following injury to a tissue, changes in the struc-

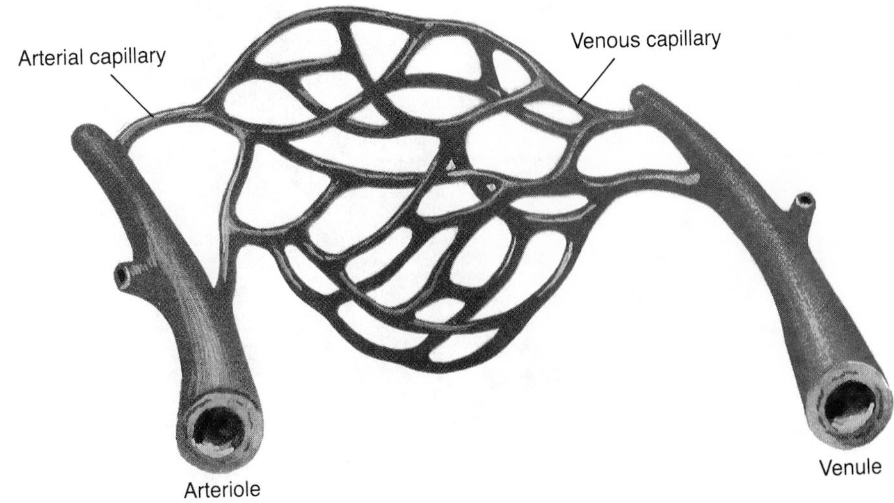

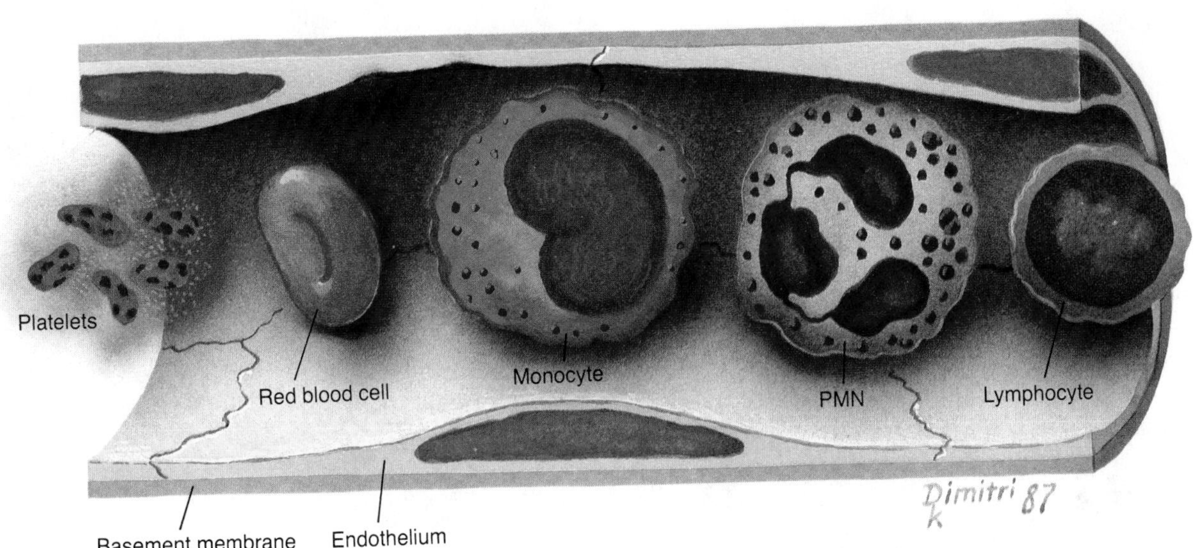

FIGURE 2-2
The microcirculation and cellular components of the blood.

ture of the vascular wall lead to the following:

- Loss of endothelial cell integrity
- Leakage of fluid and plasma components from the intravascular compartment
- Emigration of both erythrocytes and leukocytes from the intraluminal space into the extravascular tissue

Specific inflammatory mediators produced at the sites of injury regulate this response of the vasculature to injury (Fig. 2-3). Among these mediators are vasoactive molecules that act directly on the vasculature to increase vascular permeability. In addition, chemotactic factors are generated that recruit leukocytes from the vascular compartment into the injured tissue. Once present in tissues, recruited leukocytes secrete additional inflammatory mediators that either enhance or inhibit the inflammatory response.

Acute Inflammation versus Chronic Inflammation

Historically, inflammation has been referred to as either **acute** or **chronic** inflammation, depending on the persistence of the injury, clinical symptoms, and the nature of the inflammatory response. **The hallmarks of acute inflammation include (1) accumulation of fluid and plasma components in the affected tissue, (2) intravas-**

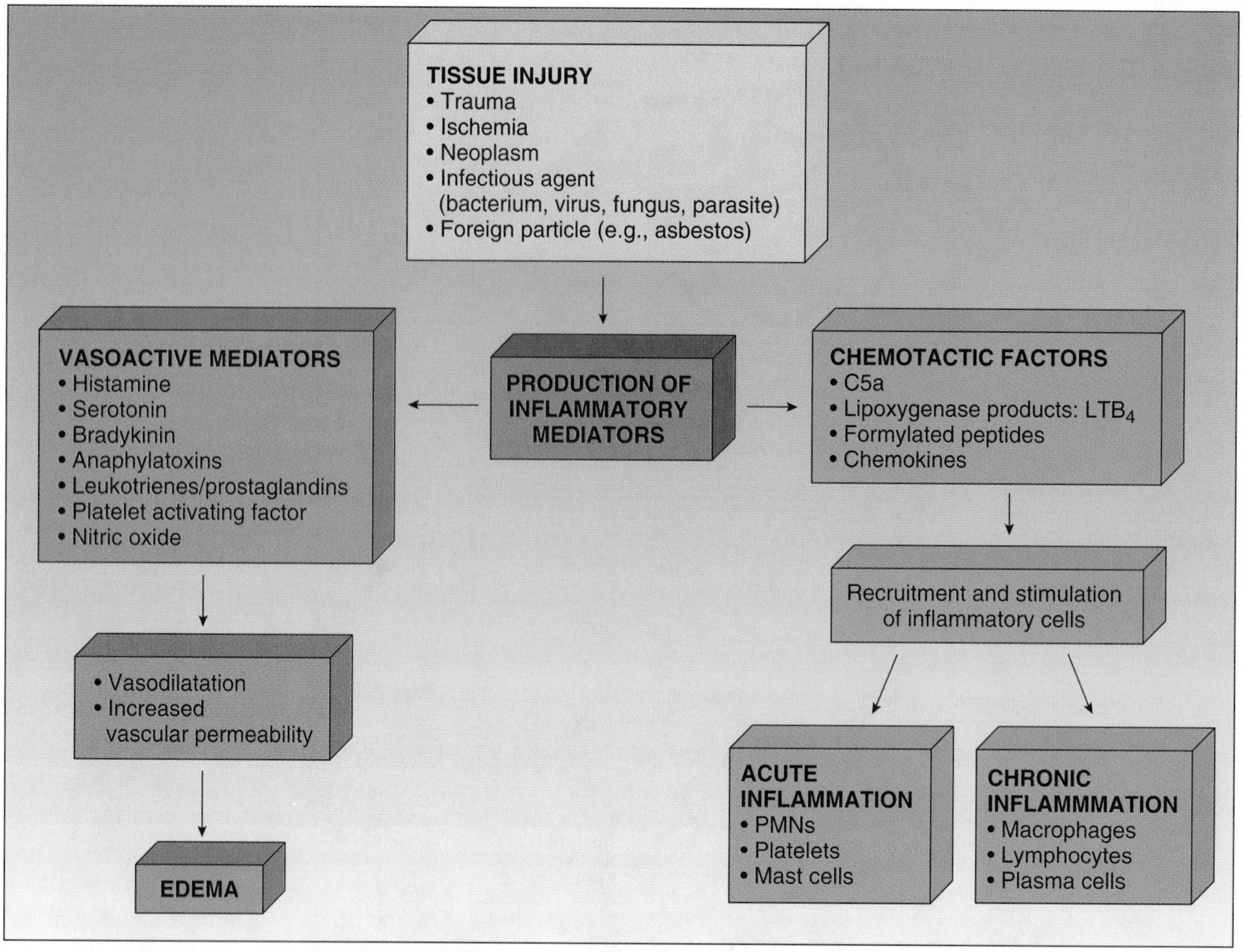

TISSUE INJURY
- Trauma
- Ischemia
- Neoplasm
- Infectious agent (bacterium, virus, fungus, parasite)
- Foreign particle (e.g., asbestos)

PRODUCTION OF INFLAMMATORY MEDIATORS

VASOACTIVE MEDIATORS
- Histamine
- Serotonin
- Bradykinin
- Anaphylatoxins
- Leukotrienes/prostaglandins
- Platelet activating factor
- Nitric oxide

- Vasodilatation
- Increased vascular permeability

EDEMA

CHEMOTACTIC FACTORS
- C5a
- Lipoxygenase products: LTB_4
- Formylated peptides
- Chemokines

Recruitment and stimulation of inflammatory cells

ACUTE INFLAMMATION
- PMNs
- Platelets
- Mast cells

CHRONIC INFLAMMMATION
- Macrophages
- Lymphocytes
- Plasma cells

FIGURE *2-3*
Mediators of the inflammatory response.

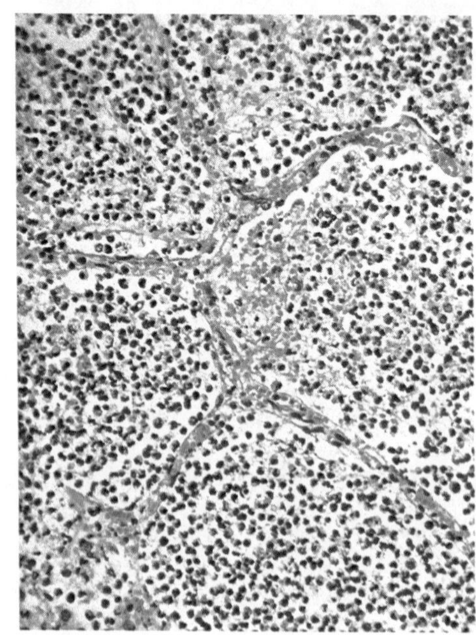

FIGURE *2-4*
Acute inflammation. A photomicrograph of the lung from a patient with pneumonia shows densely packed polymorphonuclear leukocytes in the alveoli.

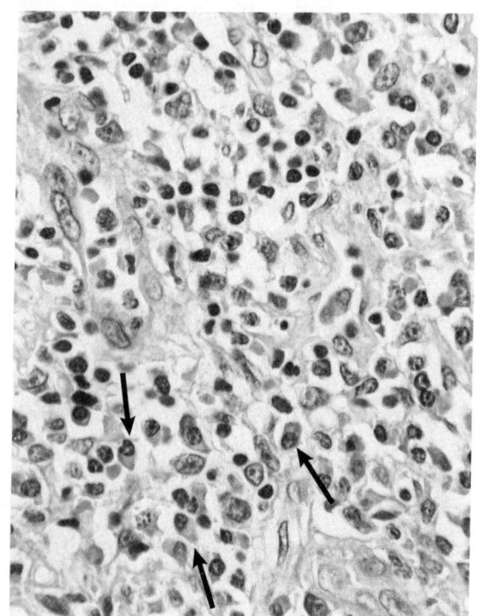

FIGURE *2-5*
Chronic inflammation. Lymphocytes, plasma cells *(arrows),* and a few macrophages are present.

cular stimulation of platelets, and (3) the presence of polymorphonuclear leukocytes (Fig. 2-4). **By contrast, the characteristic cell components of chronic inflammation are lymphocytes, plasma cells, and macrophages** (Fig. 2-5).

Activation of the inflammatory response results in a number of distinct outcomes:

- **Resolution:** Under ideal conditions the source of the tissue injury is eliminated, the inflammatory response resolves, and normal tissue architecture and physiological function are restored.
- **Abscess:** If the area of acute inflammation is walled off by the collection of inflammatory cells, destruction of the tissue by products of the polymorphonuclear leukocytes (also known as neutrophils) takes place. This is the mechanism by which an abscess is formed.
- **Scar:** If the tissue is irreversibly injured, the normal architecture is often replaced by a scar, despite elimination of the initial pathological insult.
- **Persistent inflammation:** When inflammatory cells fail to eliminate the pathological insult, the inflammatory reaction persists and may be associated with a cell-mediated immune reaction. The area of chronic inflammation often expands, leading to fibrosis and scar formation.

ACUTE INFLAMMATION

An understanding of the acute inflammatory response requires a discussion of the mechanisms that regulate vascular permeability, leukocyte recruitment, and the effects of specific mediators and inflammatory cell products on tissues.

Vascular Permeability and Edema

Normal Regulation of Fluid Transport

Under normal physiological conditions, there is a continual movement of fluid from the intravascular compartment to the extravascular space. Fluid that accumulates in the extravascular space is normally cleared through lymphatics and returned to the circulation. The regulation of transport of fluid across the vascular wall is in part described by **Starling's law**. This principle recognizes that the pressure gradient across the vascular wall depends on both the hydrostatic and the oncotic pressure differentials between the intravascular and extravascular compartments (Fig. 2-6). Thus, either an increase in intravascular hydrostatic pressure (e.g., venous obstruction) or a decrease in intravascular oncotic pressure (e.g., protein depletion) promotes the extravasation of fluid across the vessel wall.

Noninflammatory Edema

In certain conditions, the movement of fluid into the extravascular space exceeds the clearance ability of the lymphatics. The resulting increase in extravascular fluid is called **edema**, and its clinical manifestation is swelling. Examples of clinical conditions in which edema occurs include (1) pulmonary edema resulting from increased hydrostatic pressure in the pulmonary vasculature, secondary to left ventricular cardiac failure; (2) soft tissue edema in the leg as a consequence of increased hydrostatic pressure caused by thrombosis of the femoral vein; and (3) diffuse soft tissue edema secondary to decreased intravascular oncotic pressure in a patient with nephrotic syndrome. Obstruction of lymphatic flow can also cause fluid to accumulate in tissues, in which case it is referred to as **lymphedema**. Lymphedema may follow surgery or be secondary to tumor metastasis.

Inflammatory Edema

Alterations in the anatomy and function of the microvasculature are among the earliest responses to tissue injury and may promote fluid accumulation in tissues (see Figs. 2-6 and 2-7). These pathological changes are characteristic of the classic "triple response" first described by Sir Thomas Lewis. In the original experiments, a dull red line developed at the site of mild trauma to skin, followed by the development of a red halo (flare) and then swelling (wheal). Lewis postulated the presence of a vasoactive mediator that causes vasodilatation and increased vascular permeability at the site of injury. The triple response can be explained as follows:

1. **Transient vasoconstriction of arterioles** at the site of injury is the earliest vascular response to mild injury of the skin. This process is mediated by both neurogenic and chemical mediator systems and usually resolves within seconds to minutes.
2. **Vasodilatation of precapillary arterioles** then increases blood flow to the tissue, a condition known as **hyperemia**. Vasodilatation is caused by the release of specific mediators and is responsible, in part, for the redness and warmth at sites of tissue injury.
3. **An increase in the permeability of the endothelial cell barrier** results in leakage of fluid from the intravascular compartment into extravascular spaces, termed **edema**. The loss of fluid from the intravascular compartments as blood passes through the capillary venules leads to local stasis and plugging of dilated small vessels with erythrocytes. These changes are reversible following mild injury, and within several minutes to hours the extravascular fluid is cleared through lymphatics.

Injury to the vasculature is a dynamic event and frequently involves sequential physiological and pathological changes. **Vasoactive mediators**, originating from both plasma and cellular sources, are generated at sites of tissue injury by a variety of mechanisms (see Fig. 2-7). These mediators bind to specific receptors on vascular endothelial and smooth muscle cells, causing vasoconstriction or vasodilatation. Vasodilatation of arterioles increases blood flow and can exacerbate fluid leakage into the tissue. At the same time, vasoconstriction of postcapillary

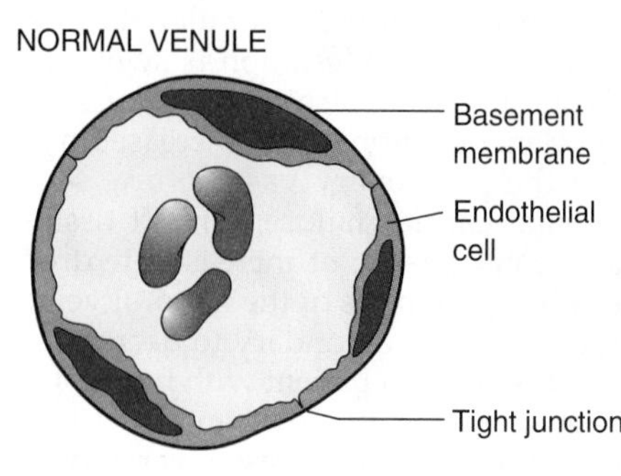

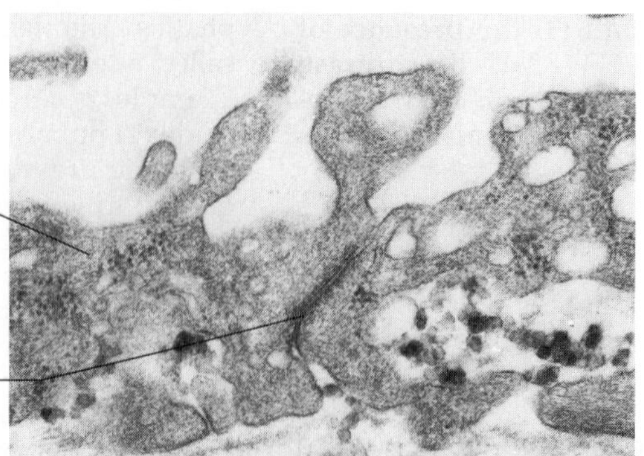

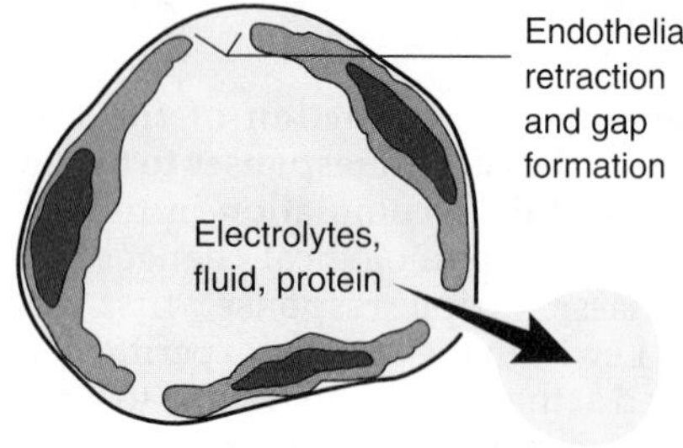

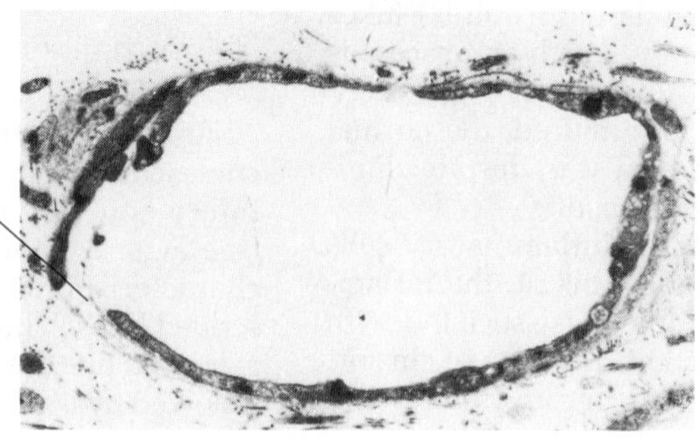

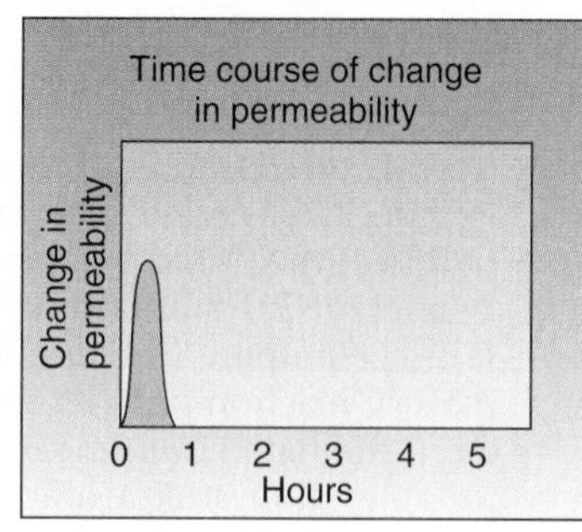

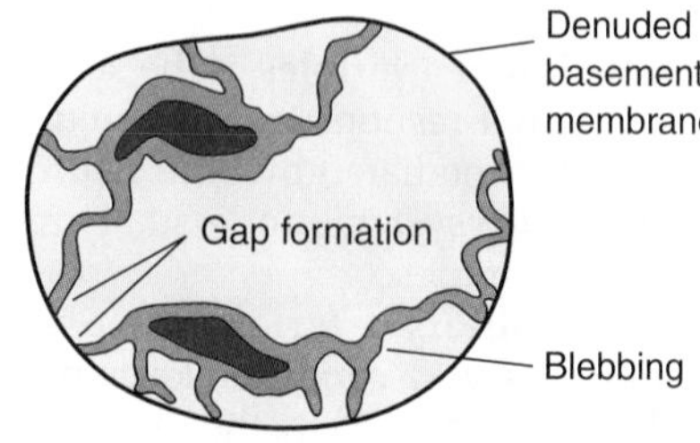

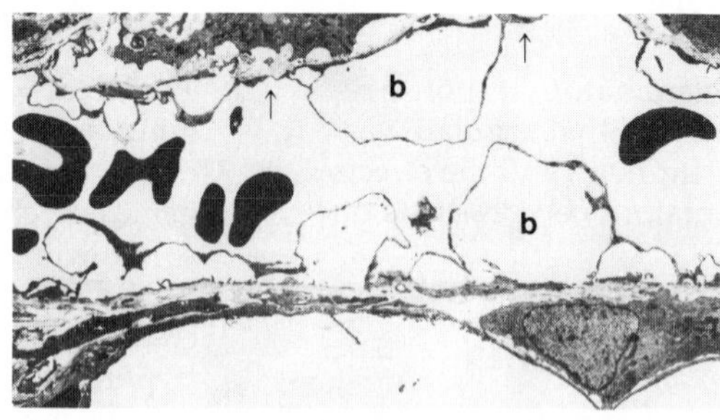

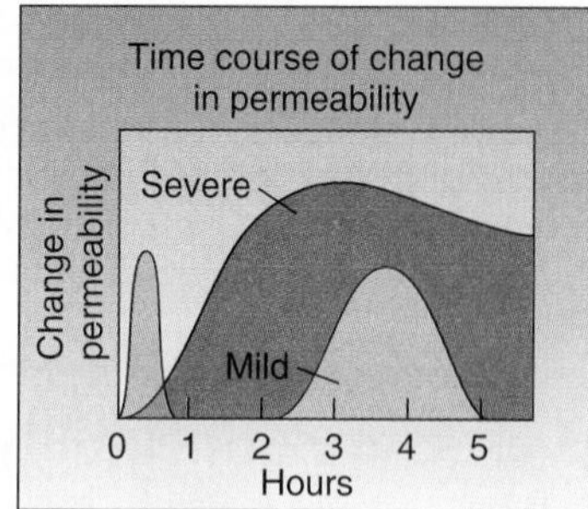

FIGURE 2-6
Responses of the microvasculature to injury. The wall of the normal venule is sealed by tight junctions between adjacent endothelial cells. During mild vasoactive mediator–induced injury, the endothelial cells separate and permit the passage of the fluid constituents of the blood. With severe direct injury, the endothelial cells form blebs (b) and separate from the underlying basement membrane. Areas of denuded basement membrane *(arrows)* allow a prolonged escape of fluid elements from the microvasculature.

venules increases the hydrostatic pressure in the capillary bed, potentiating edema formation. Vasodilatation of venules decreases capillary hydrostatic pressure and inhibits the movement of fluid into the extravascular spaces. Therefore, when the role of a particular vasoactive mediator in the development of inflammatory response is being examined, the effects of this mediator on specific tissues and components of the vasculature must be identified.

The postcapillary venule is the primary site at which vasoactive mediators induce endothelial changes. Binding of vasoactive mediators to specific receptors on endothelial cells results in cell activation, causing endothelial cell contraction and gap formation. This break in the endothelial barrier leads to the extravasation (leakage) of intravascular fluids into the extravascular space. Endothelial retraction with gap formation is a reversible process. Local injection of classic vasoactive mediators into the skin results in an acute change in vascular permeability that peaks between 15 and 20 minutes after injection but is corrected within 1 hour.

In contrast to this action of vasoactive mediators, direct injury to the endothelium, such as that caused by burns or caustic chemicals, may result in irreversible damage. In such cases, the endothelium is separated from the basement membrane. This effect leads to cell blebbing

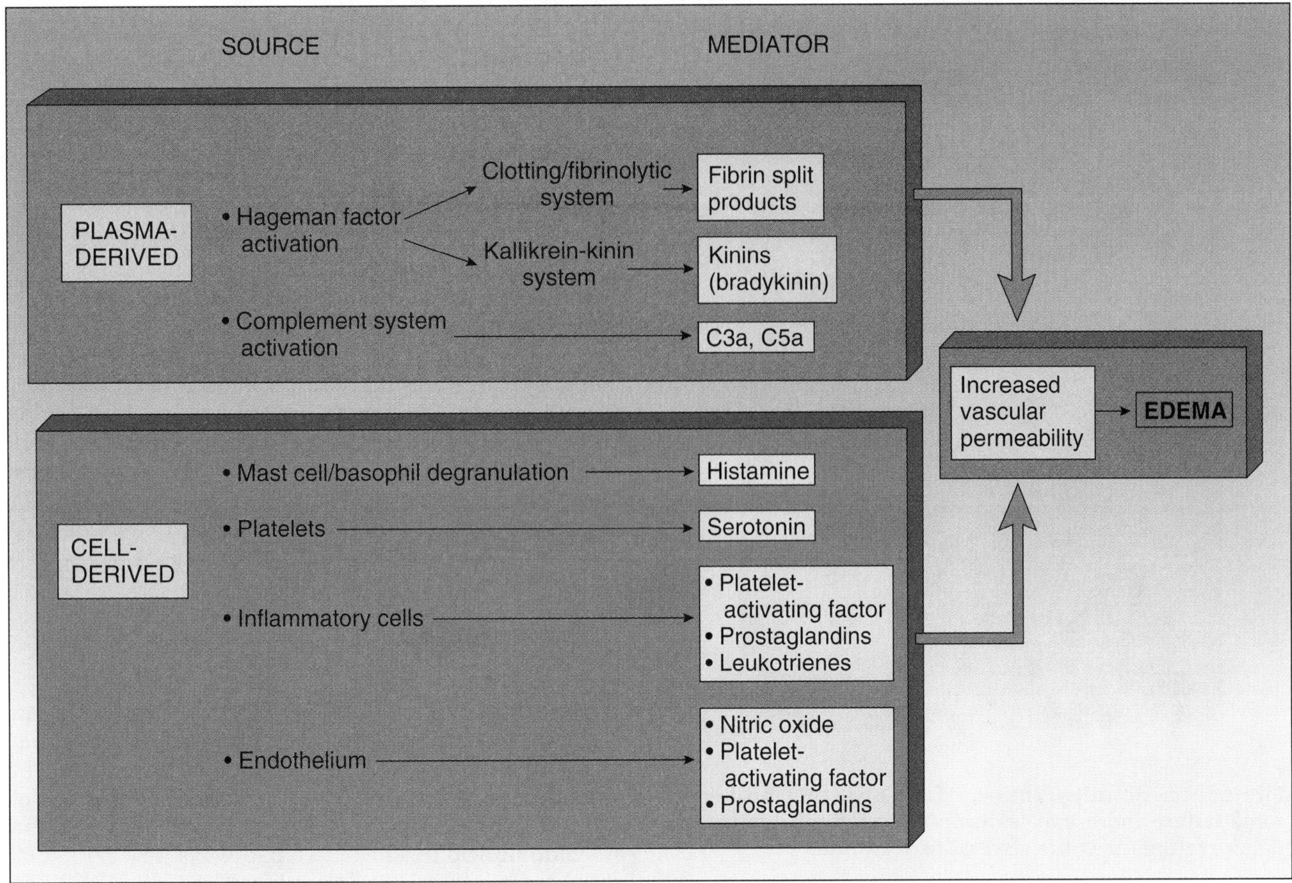

FIGURE 2-7
Vasoactive mediators of increased vascular permeability.

(the appearance of blisters or bubbles between the endothelium and the basement membrane) and areas of denuded basement membrane. Mild direct injury to the endothelium results in a biphasic response: an early change in permeability occurs 15 to 30 minutes after the injury, followed by a second increase in vascular permeability after 3 to 5 hours. When damage is severe, the exudation of intravascular fluid into the extravascular compartment increases progressively, reaching a peak between 3 and 4 hours after injury.

Several definitions are important for understanding the consequences of inflammation:

- **Edema** refers to the accumulation of fluid within the extravascular compartment and interstitial tissues.
- **An effusion** is excess fluid in the cavities of the body, for instance the peritoneum or pleura.
- **A transudate** describes edema fluid with a low protein content (specific gravity <1.015).
- **An exudate** is edema fluid with a high protein concentration (specific gravity >1.015), which frequently contains inflammatory cells. Exudates are observed early in acute inflammatory reactions and are produced by mild injuries, such as sunburn or traumatic blisters.
- **A serous exudate or effusion** is characterized by the absence of a prominent cellular response and has a yellow, strawlike color.
- **Serosanguineous** refers to a serous exudate or effusion that contains erythrocytes and has a red tinge.
- **A fibrinous exudate** contains large amounts of fibrin as a result of activation of the coagulation system. When a fibrinous exudate occurs on a serosal surface, such as the pleura or pericardium, it is referred to as fibrinous pleuritis or fibrinous pericarditis (Fig. 2-8).
- **A purulent exudate or effusion** is one that contains prominent cellular components. Purulent exudates and effusions are frequently identified with pathological conditions such as pyogenic bacterial infections (Fig. 2-9), in which the predominant cell type is the polymorphonuclear leukocyte (see Fig. 2-4).
- **Suppurative inflammation** describes a condition in which a purulent exudate is accompanied by significant liquefactive necrosis; it is the equivalent of pus.

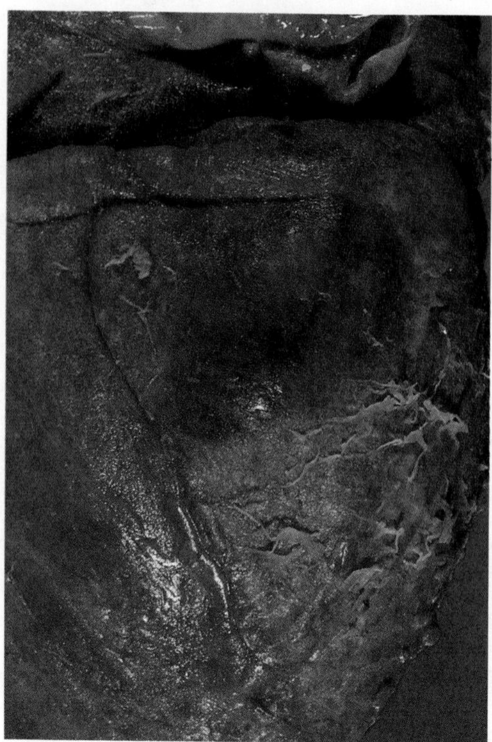

FIGURE *2-8*
Fibrinous pericarditis. The heart from a patient who died in renal failure and uremia exhibits a shaggy, fibrinous exudate covering the entire visceral pericardium.

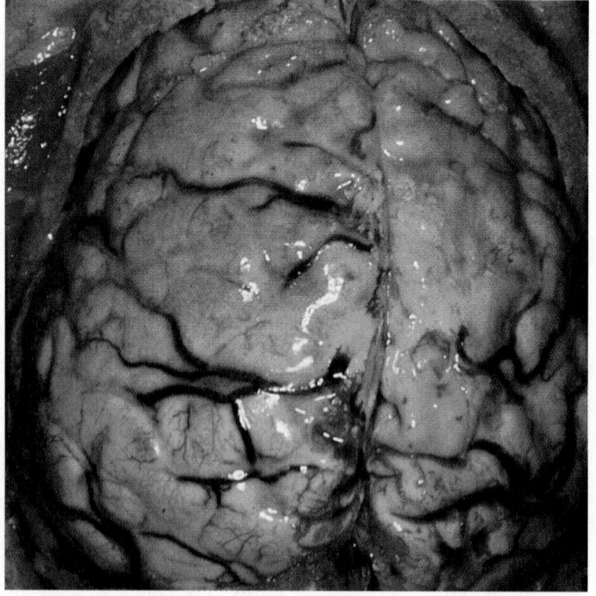

FIGURE *2-9*
Purulent exudate. In this case of bacterial meningitis, a viscid, cream-colored, acute inflammatory exudate is present within the subarachnoid space.

Mediators of Increased Permeability in Inflammatory Edema

The primary sources of vasoactive mediators are cells and plasma.

Cell-Derived Vasoactive Mediators

Circulating platelets, tissue mast cells, basophils, polymorphonuclear leukocytes, endothelial cells, monocyte/macrophages, and the injured tissue itself are all potent cellular sources of vasoactive mediators. In general, these mediators are (1) preformed and stored in cytoplasmic granules (e.g., histamine, serotonin, lysosomal hydrolases), (2) derived from the metabolism of phospholipids and arachidonic acid (e.g., prostaglandins, leukotrienes, thromboxanes, platelet activating factor), or (3) represent altered production of normal regulators of vascular function (e.g., nitric oxide and neurotransmitters).

Phospholipid Metabolism and Arachidonic Acid Metabolites

GENERATION OF ARACHIDONIC ACID: Certain derivatives of phospholipids and fatty acids are among the mediators generated by inflammatory cells and injured tissues. Depending on the specific inflammatory cell and the nature of the stimulus, activated cells generate arachidonic acid by one of two pathways (Fig. 2-10). One pathway involves stimulus-induced activation of phospholipase A_2, an enzyme that cleaves arachidonic acid from the glycerol backbone of membrane phospholipids. Phosphatidylcholine, an important substrate of phospholipase A_2, is the major source of arachidonic acid in inflammatory cells. The other mechanism for the generation of arachidonic acid is the metabolism of phosphatidylinositol phosphates to diacylglycerol and inositol phosphates by phospholipase C. Diacylglycerol lipase then cleaves arachidonic acid from diacylglycerol. Once generated, arachidonic acid, a polyunsaturated (20:4) fatty acid is metabolized through two pathways, (1) cyclooxygenation, with the subsequent production of prostaglandins and thromboxanes, and (2) lipoxygenation, to form monohydroxyeicosatetranoic (HETEs) and dihydroxyeicosatetranoic acids (diHETEs) and leukotrienes.

CYCLOOXYGENASE: Inflammatory cells contain specific cyclooxygenase enzymes that generate endoperoxide derivatives of arachidonic acid, including prostaglandin G_2, (PGG_2) and prostaglandin H_2 (PGH_2). The endoperoxides are unstable and, depending on the specific inflammatory cell or tissue, are further metabolized to more stable prostaglandins. The latter include PGI_2 (also known as prostacyclin), $PGF_{2\alpha}$, PGE_2, PGD_2, and thromboxane A_2 (TxA_2). The primary cyclooxygenase metabolite in platelets is TxA_2; endothelial cells secrete principally PGI_2. Monocyte/macrophages, depending on their state of activation, produce any or all of these derivative products.

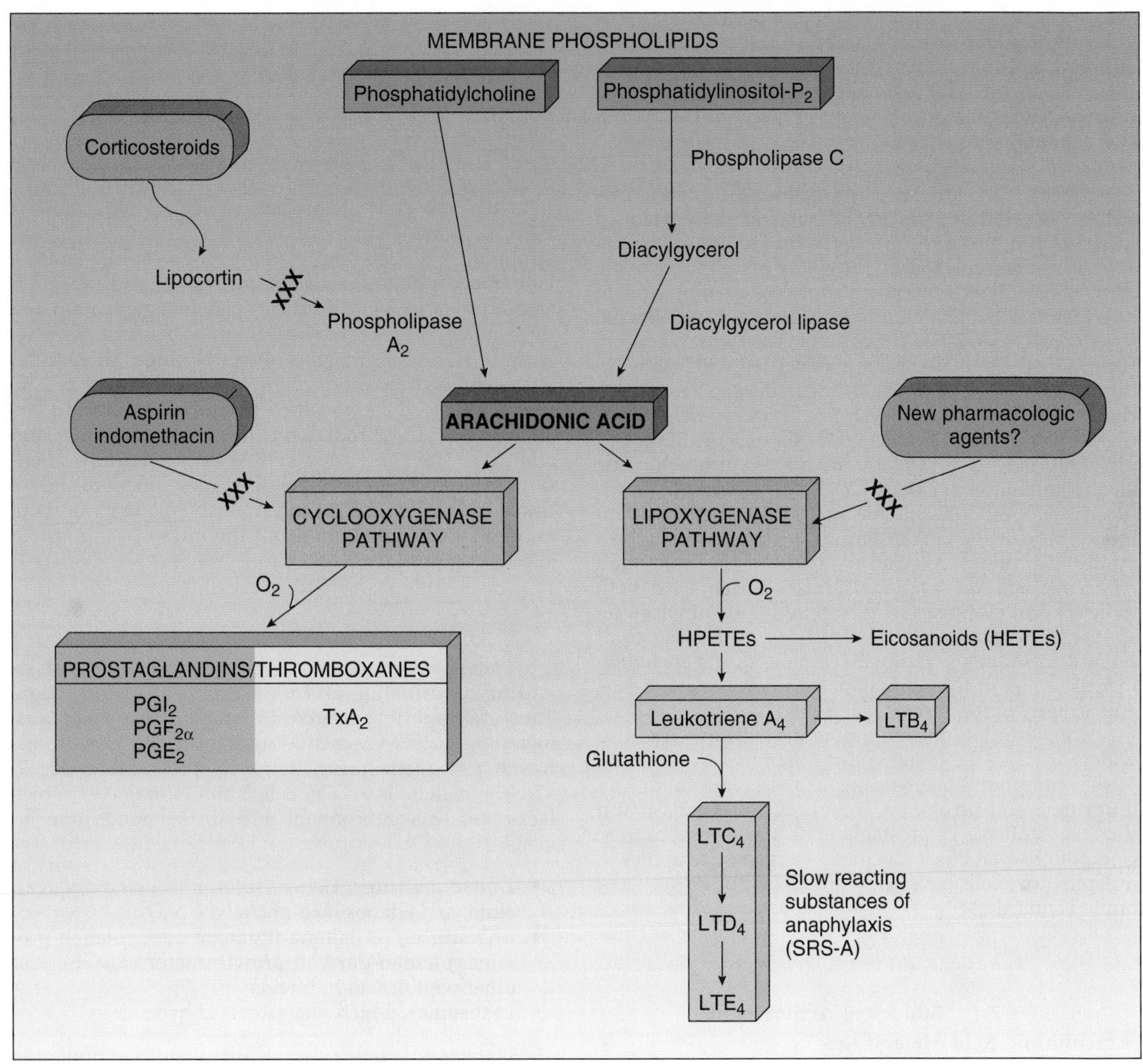

FIGURE *2-10*
Arachidonic acid metabolism.

PGI_2 and PGE_2, owing to their vasodilating effects, have been used clinically to enhance tissue perfusion and in the lung to improve blood oxygenation. However, vasodilatation can enhance vascular permeability at sites of inflammation. TxA_2 is a potent vasoconstrictor and plays an important role in the mediation of the "second wave" of platelet aggregation. PGI_2 and PGE_2 bind to specific receptors on inflammatory cells, thereby activating adenylyl cyclase and increasing intracellular cyclic adenosine monophosphate (cAMP) levels. These effects inhibit the functional responses of these cells to other inflammatory stimuli.

LIPOXYGENASE: A second pathway by which arachidonic acid is metabolized in inflammatory cells and tissues is lipoxygenation, with the formation of hydroperoxyeicosatetranoic acid compounds (HPETEs). Hydroperoxy compounds may be metabolized to hydroxyeicosatetranoic acids (HETEs) or to leukotriene A_4; the latter contains three conjugated double bonds and serves as a precursor for other leukotriene molecules. In the neutrophil and in certain macrophage populations, leukotriene A_4 is metabolized to leukotriene B_4, a compound with potent chemotactic activity for neutrophils, monocytes, and macrophages. In other cell types, especially mast cells, basophils, and macrophages, the addition of glutathione to leukotriene A_4 results in the formation of leukotriene C_4. Leukotrienes D_4 and E_4 are formed following sequential removal of the amino acids glycine and glutamine, respectively. Leukotrienes C_4, D_4, and E_4 are collectively known as slow-reacting substances of anaphylaxis (SRS-As). They stimulate the contraction of smooth muscle and enhance vascular permeability. The generation of leukotriene B_4 at sites of tissue injury plays an important role in the recruitment of polymorphonuclear leukocytes, whereas leukotrienes C_4, D_4, and E_4 are responsible for the development of much of the clinical symptomatology associated with allergic-type reactions.

INHIBITORS OF ARACHIDONIC ACID METABOLITES: Arachidonic acid metabolites are important in mediating many of the effects of the inflammatory response, as demonstrated by the ability of inhibitors of the enzymes involved in the production of these molecules to attenuate both the pathological changes and clinical symptoms (Table 2-1). Corticosteroids are widely used to suppress the tissue destruction associated with many inflammatory diseases, including allergic responses, rheumatoid arthritis, and systemic lupus erythematosus. Corticosteroids induce the synthesis of an inhibitor of phospholipase A_2 and block the release of arachidonic acid in inflammatory cells. Originally described as two proteins, lipomodulin and macrocortin, the regulatory inhibitor induced by corticosteroids is now known to be a family of proteins, referred to as lipocortins. Although corticosteroids such as prednisone are widely used, both topically and systemically, to suppress inflammatory responses, the prolonged administration of these compounds can have significant deleterious effects, including increased risk of infection, damage to connective tissue, and atrophy of the adrenal glands.

Nonsteroidal anti-inflammatory drugs are also widely used in the treatment of inflammatory diseases. These compounds, including aspirin, indomethacin, ibuprofen, and piroxicam, inhibit cyclooxygenase and thus the synthesis of prostaglandins and thromboxanes. Compounds that block specific lipoxygenase activities in inflammatory cells have been developed but are as yet of limited clinical use.

TABLE *2-1* **Biological Activities of Arachidonic Acid Metabolites**

Metabolite	Biological Activity
PGE_2, PDG_2	Induce vasodilatation, bronchodilation; inhibit inflamatory cell function
PGI_2	Induces vasodilatation, bronchodilation; inhibits inflamatory cell function
$PGF_{2\alpha}$	Induces vasodilatation, bronchoconstriction
TxA_2	Induces vasoconstriction, bronchoconstriction; enhances inflammatory cell functions (esp. platelets)
LTB_4	Chemotactic for phagocytic cells; stimulates phagocytic cell adherence; enhances microvascular permeability
LTC_4, LTD_4, LTE_4	Induce smooth muscle contraction; constrict pulmonary airways; increase microvascular permeability

Platelet Activating Factor

Platelet activating factor (PAF) is a class of vasoactive mediators with the structure of an acetylated lysophospholipid. It is not preformed but is generated by the stimulation of virtually all activated inflammatory cells, endothelial cells, and injured tissue cells. PAF is produced by the deacylation of phospholipids by phospholipase A_2, followed by acetylation mediated by an acetyltransferase. PAF has a wide range of activities, among which are stimulatory effects on platelets, neutrophils, monocyte/macrophages, endothelial cells, and vascular smooth muscle cells. It induces platelet aggregation and degranulation at sites of tissue injury and enhances the release of serotonin, thereby causing changes in vascular permeability. In addition, exposure of phagocytic cells to PAF "primes" them, resulting in enhanced functional responses (e.g., O_2^- production, degranulation) to a second stimulus. The expression of PAF on the surface of endothelial cells augments leukocyte recruitment to sites of tissue injury. PAF is also an extremely potent vasodilator and enhances permeability of the microvasculature at sites of tissue injury.

Platelets

Platelets play a primary role in normal homeostasis and in the initiation and regulation of clot formation. They are important sources of inflammatory mediators, including potent vasoactive substances and growth factors that modulate mesenchymal cell proliferation (Fig. 2-11). The platelet is a small cell, 2 mm in diameter, which lacks a nucleus and contains three distinct kinds of inclusions:

- **Dense granules,** rich in serotonin, histamine, calcium, and adenosine diphosphate (ADP)
- **α-Granules,** containing fibrinogen, coagulation proteins, platelet-derived growth factor (PDGF), and other peptides and proteins
- **Lysosomes,** which sequester acid hydrolases

Platelet adherence, aggregation, and degranulation occur when platelets come in contact with (1) fibrillar collagen (following vascular injury that exposes the interstitial matrix proteins) or (2) thrombin (after activation of the coagulation system). Degranulation is associated with the release of **serotonin** (5-hydroxytryptamine), which directly induces changes in vascular permeability. In addition, the arachidonic acid metabolite TxA_2 is produced by platelets. TxA_2 not only plays a key role in the second wave of platelet aggregation but also mediates smooth muscle constriction. On activation, platelets, as well as phagocytic cells, secrete cationic proteins that neutralize the negative charges on endothelium and promote increased permeability.

Mast Cells and Basophils

Mast cells and basophils both contain receptors for immunoglobulin E (IgE) on their cell surface and are ad-

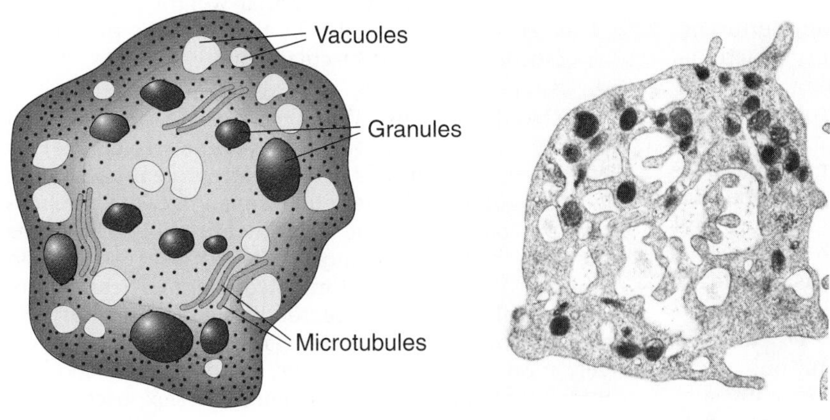

CHARACTERISTICS AND FUNCTIONS
- Thrombosis; promotes clot formation
- Regulates permeability
- Regulates proliferative response of mesenchymal cells

PRIMARY INFLAMMATORY MEDIATORS
- Dense granules
  - -Serotonin
  - -Ca^{2+}
  - -ADP
- α-granules
  - -Cationic proteins
  - -Fibrinogen and coagulation proteins
  - -Platelet-derived growth factor (PDGF)
- Lysosomes
  - -Acid hydrolases
- Thromboxane A_2

FIGURE *2-11*
Platelets: morphology and functions.

ditional cellular sources of vasoactive mediators. Mast cells are localized within the connective tissue of the body, whereas basophils are present in low numbers in the circulation. Mast cells are especially prevalent along mucosal surfaces of the lung and gastrointestinal tract, the dermis of the skin, and the microvasculature. This distribution places the mast cell at the interface between environmental antigens and the host for participation in a variety of allergic and inflammatory conditions.

When an IgE-sensitized mast cell or basophil is stimulated by antigen, a variety of inflammatory mediators contained in dense cytoplasmic granules are secreted into extracellular tissues (Fig. 2-12). These granules contain histamine, acid mucopolysaccharides (including heparin), serine proteases, and chemotactic mediators for neutrophils and eosinophils. Because of their ability to secrete specific mediators following stimulation, both mast cells and basophils play an important role in the regulation of vascular permeability and bronchial smooth muscle tone, especially in many forms of allergic hypersensitivity reactions (see Chapter 4).

Histamine is also released from the dense granules when mast cells are stimulated with anaphylatoxins derived from the third and fifth components of the complement system (C3a and C5a). When injected into the skin, both histamine and serotonin induce reversible en-

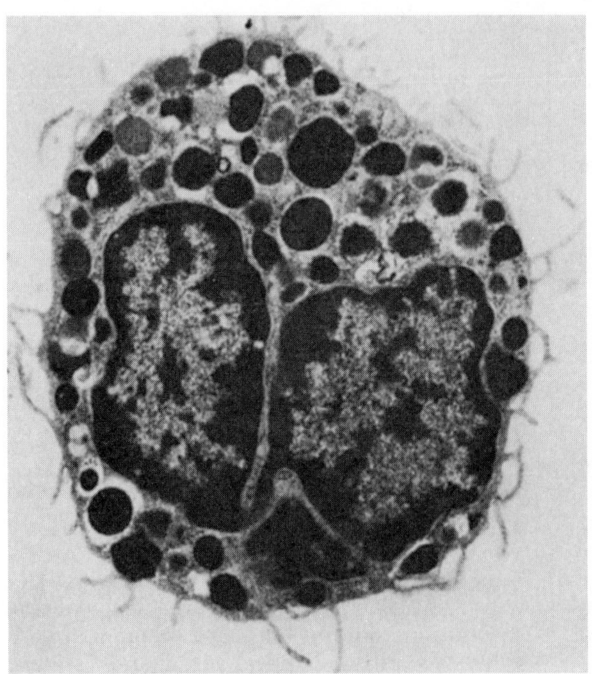

Mast Cell (Basophils)

CHARACTERISTICS AND FUNCTIONS
- Binds IgE molecules
- Contains electron-dense granules

PRIMARY INFLAMMATORY MEDIATORS
- Histamine
- Leukotrienes (LTC_4, LTD_4, LTE_4)
- Platelet activating factor
- Eosinophil chemotactic factors
- Cytokines (e.g., TNF-α IL-4)

FIGURE *2-12*
Mast cells: morphology and functions.

dothelial cell contraction, gap formation, and edema. **The most important effects of histamine (and serotonin) occur early in the evolution of inflammatory reactions.** Histamine acts on the vasculature by binding to specific H_1 receptors in the vascular wall, an effect that can be inhibited pharmacologically by H_1-receptor antagonists. Degranulation of mast cells and basophils may also be induced by physical agonists, such as cold and trauma, and by cationic proteins derived from platelets and neutrophil lysosomal granules.

Stimulation of mast cells and basophils also leads to the release of products of arachidonic acid metabolism, including leukotrienes C_4, D_4, and E_4. These lipoxygenase products of arachidonic acid metabolism, previously referred to as slow-reacting substances of anaphylaxis (SRS-As), induce smooth muscle contraction and increase vascular permeability in the skin. They produce their effects by binding to specific receptors on cell membranes and are important in delayed changes in vascular permeability at sites of inflammation.

It has recently been recognized that several distinct populations of mast cells are also important sources of cytokines (e.g., tumor necrosis factor-alpha [TNF-α], interleukin-4 [IL-4]). In addition to their role in the regulation of vascular permeability and the inflammatory response, mast cell–derived mediators participate in immediate hypersensitivity reactions (Chapter 4), neovascularization, wound healing, and tumorigenesis.

Endothelial Cells

One of the important functions of endothelial cells is the regulation of tissue perfusion under physiological and pathological conditions (Fig. 2-13). This regulation is mediated by the secretion of both vasoconstrictor and vasodilator substances, as well as by the influence of platelet aggregation and the coagulation pathways. In inflammatory conditions, the altered production of vasoregulatory mediators, or the modulation of platelet aggregation and thrombus formation, profoundly affects the functions of organs and tissues and the recruitment and accumulation of inflammatory cells.

The most important vasoactive mediators produced by endothelial cells include PGI_2, nitric oxide, and endothelin.

- **PGI_2**, a metabolite of arachidonic acid, has potent vasodilator and antiaggregatory effects.
- **Nitric oxide (NO)**, originally identified as endothelium-derived relaxing factor (EDRF), is a low-molecular-weight vasodilator that inhibits platelet aggregation and regulates vascular tone by stimulating smooth muscle relaxation. NO is synthesized *in vivo* from L-arginine and is the active compound produced from several vasodilator drugs that are used clinically. Specific mediators, including acetylcholine and bradykinin, induce NO· release from venous and arterial endothelial cells. NO stimulates relaxation of vascular smooth muscle cells by activating guanylyl cyclase and increasing intracellular cyclic guanosine monophosphate (cGMP).
- **Endothelin** is a low-molecular-weight peptide produced by endothelial cells that induces prolonged vasoconstriction of vascular smooth muscle.

COAGULATION: When exposed to bacterial lipopolysaccharide or specific cytokines (e.g., IL-1 or TNF-α), endothelial cells play a central role in regulating blood coagulation. These cells secrete increased amounts of the procoagulant tissue factor that promotes thrombus formation through activation of the extrinsic coagulation pathway. When they are stimulated, mononuclear phagocytic cells also express increased tissue factor activity. By contrast, smooth muscle cells and fibroblasts constitutively express tissue factor. Thus, an injury to a blood vessel wall that alters the endothelial barrier exposes a local procoagulant signal, whereas bacterial infection and cytokine production lead to the expression of a procoagulant signal distant from the site of injury.

FIBRINOLYSIS: Endothelial cells also mediate the patency of blood vessels and tissue perfusion by regulating fibrinolysis. Endothelial cells secrete both plasminogen activators and plasminogen activator inhibitors (see Chapter 10). Thus, the action of an endothelial cell depends on the pathological insult and the mediators generated at sites of inflammation. The cell has the capacity either to promote or to inhibit tissue perfusion through multiple mechanisms, thereby modulating tissue function and the development of the inflammatory response.

Monocyte/Macrophages

Circulating monocytes are derived from the bone marrow and exit the circulation to accumulate at sites of acute inflammation. Both circulating and tissue momonuclear cells are now included in the term **monocyte/macrophage system**.

As previously noted, monocyte/macrophages are a direct source of potent vasoactive mediators, including the products of arachidonic acid metabolism (prostaglandins, leukotrienes) and PAF. Moreover, these cells act indirectly to modify vascular integrity by releasing cytokines (e.g., IL-1 and TNF-α) that activate endothelial cells (see later).

Plasma-Derived Vasoactive Mediators

The plasma contains three major enzyme cascades in an inactive state, each of which is composed of a series of sequentially activated proteases. These interrelated systems include (1) the coagulation cascade, (2) kinin generation, and (3) complement.

Hageman Factor and the Kinins

Hageman factor (clotting factor XII), generated within the plasma, provides an additional source of vasoactive mediators (Fig. 2-14). Hageman factor is activated by exposure to negatively charged surfaces, such as basement membranes, proteolytic enzymes, bacterial lipopolysaccharide, and foreign materials (including

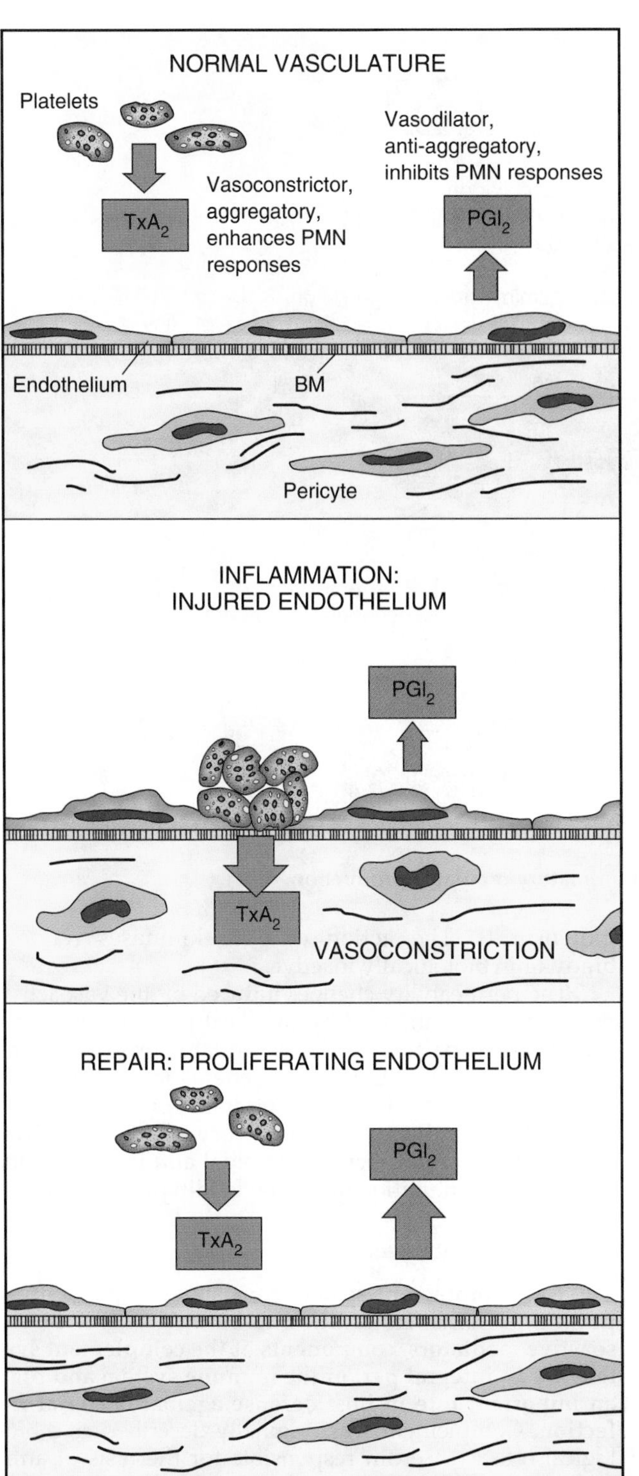

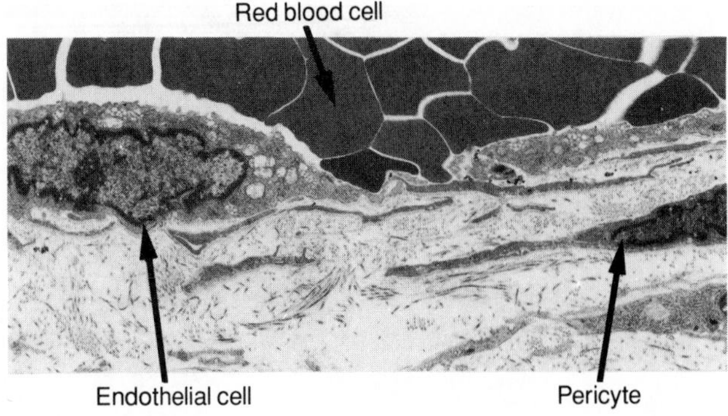

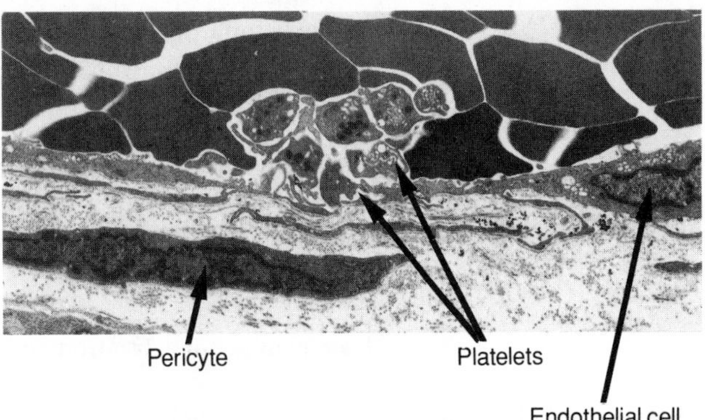

FIGURE *2-13*

Regulation of platelet and endothelial cell interactions by thromboxane A_2 and prostaglandin I_2. During inflammation, the normal balance is shifted to vasoconstriction, platelet aggregation, and polymorphonuclear leukocyte responses. During repair, the prostaglandin effects predominate.

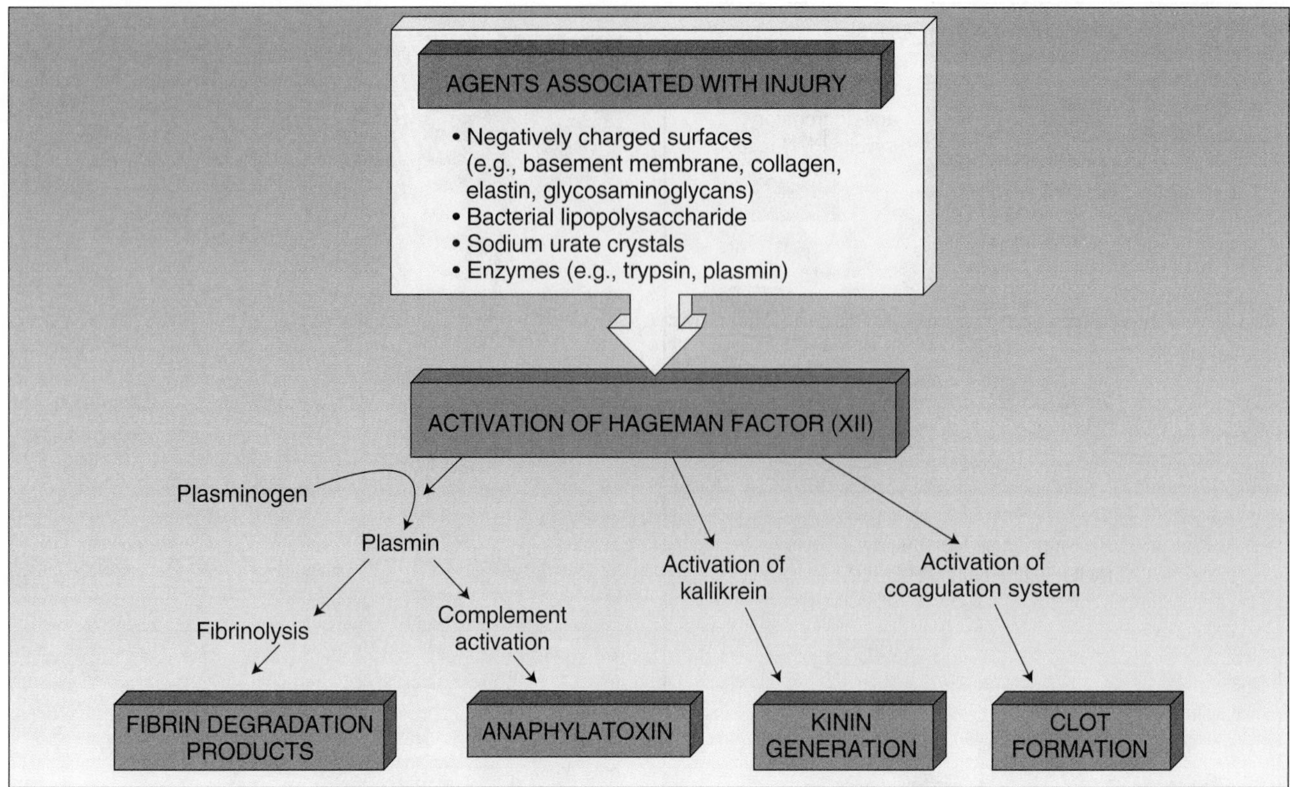

FIGURE *2-14*
Hageman factor activation and inflammatory mediator production.

urate crystals in gout). In turn, this process results in the activation of several additional plasma proteases, which lead to the following:

- Conversion of plasminogen to plasmin
- Conversion of prekallikrein to kallikrein
- Activation of the alternative complement pathway

Plasmin generated by activated Hageman factor induces fibrinolysis. In turn, the products of fibrin degradation (fibrin-split products) augment vascular permeability in both the skin and the lung. Plasmin also cleaves components of the complement system, thereby generating biologically active products, including the anaphylatoxins C3a and C5a. These molecules increase vascular permeability in the skin both directly and indirectly (e.g., by a mast cell–dependent mechanism).

Plasma kallikrein, generated by activated Hageman factor, cleaves high-molecular-weight kininogen, thereby producing several vasoactive peptides of low molecular weight, collectively referred to as **kinins** (Fig. 2-15). **Bradykinin** is the best characterized of these vasoactive kinins. When injected into skin, bradykinin elicits reversible changes of the endothelium that lead to edema. Many kinins are under the tight regulatory control of specific inactivating enzymes. For instance, plasma carboxypeptidase N (kininase I) selectively cleaves the carboxyterminal peptide of bradykinin. A dipeptidase known as kininase II cleaves the dipeptides of bradykinin. Kininase II is also termed **angiotensin-converting enzyme** (ACE), because it converts angiotensin I to angiotensin II. The action of both kininases renders bradykinin biologically inactive.

The permeability changes induced by the vasoactive mediators are enhanced by the local production of vasodilators. In particular, the vasodilator prostaglandins (PGI_2, PGE_2, and PGD_2) increase edema formation when injected locally at sites of tissue injury. One proposed mechanism for the anti-inflammatory effects of aspirin, indomethacin, and other nonsteroidal anti-inflammatory drugs is their inhibition of prostaglandin production.

Complement System

The complement system consists of a group of 20 plasma proteins. In addition to being a source of vasoactive mediators, components of the complement system are an integral part of the immune system and play an important role in host defense against bacterial infection. Complement was originally described as a biological effect of serum responsible for the lysis of antibody-coated cells. It is now known that this activity is present in an inactive form in plasma and that the proteins involved in the activation are sequentially activated by three convergent pathways, termed **classical, alternative, and lectin binding** (Fig. 2-16).

The functional roles of the complement system are as follows:

- A source of vasoactive mediators: anaphylatoxins
- The production of leukocyte chemoattractants
- Enhanced leukocyte phagocytosis
- Cell lysis

CLASSICAL PATHWAY: Activators of the classical pathway (Table 2-2) include antigen–antibody (Ag-Ab) immune complexes and products of bacteria and viruses. The cascade that leads from activation to the formation of the membrane attack complex proceeds as follows:

1. The activation of the classical pathway requires recognition of the inflammatory agent by the first component of complement, C1, which consists of three separate proteins, C1q, C1r, and C1s. When IgM immunoglobulins, or molecules of specific IgG subclasses, are bound to antigens on target cells or tissue substrates, alterations in the conformation of the immunoglobulin Fc component initiate the binding of C1q. This results in sequential enzymatic activation of the other two components of C1, namely, C1r and C1s.

2. Two additional components of the complement system, C4 and C2, serve as the substrates for the enzymatically active C1s. The action of C1s on C4 and C2 is responsible for the release of the first soluble anaphylatoxin, C4a, and the generation of the complex C4b,2b. The formation of C4b exposes a highly reactive thioester group within the molecule, which reacts with proteins on the surface of cells to form a covalent bond (Fig. 2-17). This reaction localizes both the C4b,2b complex and the subsequent activation of the complement cascade at specific tissue sites. If a covalent bond is not formed, the thioester group reacts with water and is inactivated. This process prevents the diffusion of C4b and the activation of the complement cascade in normal host cells and tissues. The C4b,2b complex has proteolytic activity for the C3 molecule and has been defined as the classical pathway C3 convertase.

3. C3 convertase cleaves C3, generating a second soluble anaphylatoxin molecule, C3a, and a residual C3 product, C3b. The C3 convertase cleaves multiple C3 molecules within its vicinity and, thereby, amplifies the activation of the complement cascade, locally generating large amounts of C3a and C3b. C3b also expresses a reactive thioester bond that can react with surface proteins, thereby localizing it to the cell surface. The "fixation" of C3b and its degradation products (e.g., iC3b) on surfaces of a pathogen plays a critical role in the clearance of pathogens by phagocytic cells. When C3b fixation occurs on pathogens, phagocytosis is enhanced by the binding of C3b and its degradation products to specific phagocytic

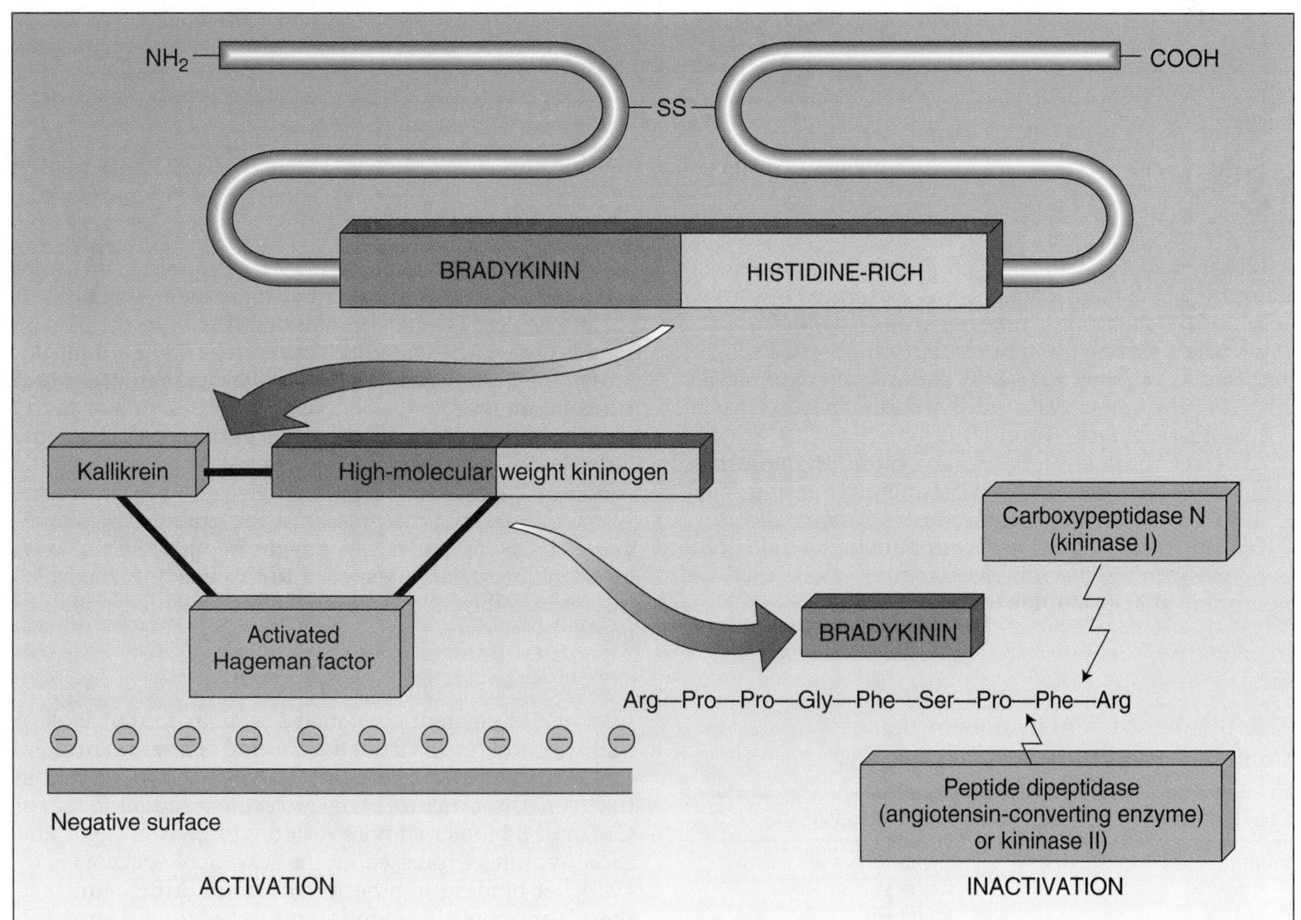

FIGURE *2-15*
The bradykinin precursor kininogen interacts with kallikrein and activated Hageman factor to form a trimolecular complex. Kallikrein releases bradykinin from kininogen. Bradykinin is, in turn, inactivated by kininases.

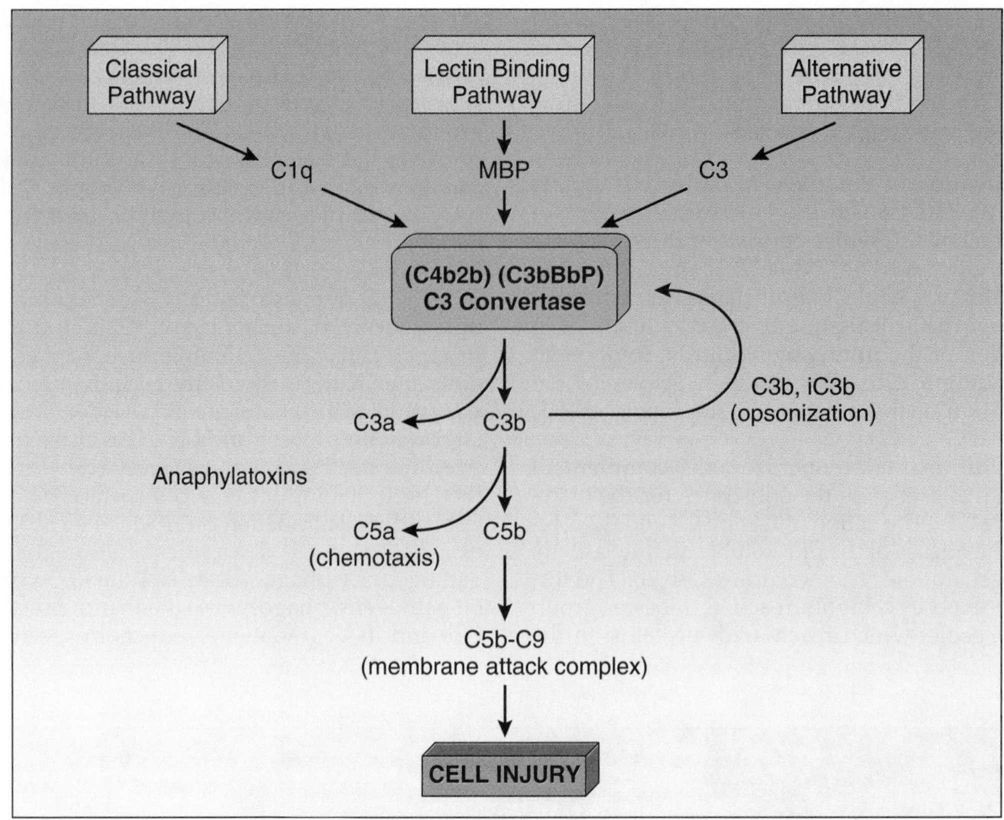

FIGURE *2-16*
The complement system and its biologically active products.

cell receptors. The coating of the pathogen with a molecule that enhances phagocytosis is termed **opsonization**, and the molecule is referred to as an **opsonin**.

4. The resulting multimolecular complex (C4b,2b,3b) functions as a C5 convertase. By binding and cleaving C5, this complex generates a third soluble anaphylatoxin, C5a, and a residual C5 product, C5b.

5. The C5b molecule serves as a nidus on the surface membranes of target cells for the sequential binding of C6, C7, and C8 and the polymerization of C9 molecules.

6. This cascade leads to the formation of a lipid-soluble, pore-forming, macromolecular complex, termed the **membrane attack complex (MAC)**.

TABLE 2-2 **Activators of the Complement System**

Classical Pathway	Alternative Pathway
Immune complexes (IgM, IgG)	Zymosan (yeast cell wall)
Aggregated antibody	Cobra venom factor
Proteases	Endotoxin
Urate crystals	Polysaccharides
Polyanions (polynucleotides)	Radiographic contrast media; dialysis membranes; parasites, fungi, viruses

The assembly of the highly lipophilic MAC on target cell surfaces occurs through hydrophobic interactions of the molecules. The insertion of the MAC into the plasma membrane creates a cylindrical hole, an effect that destroys the barrier function of the plasma membrane and leads to cell lysis.

Complement also participates in the lysis of bacteria. Gram-negative bacteria are protected from the cytolytic action of the MAC by a peptidylglycan layer. However, lysozyme, an enzyme present in the granules of phagocytic cells, is capable of cleaving the peptidylglycan layer. Once the bacteria are exposed to this enzyme, the MAC inserts into the cell membrane, after which lysis is initiated.

LECTIN-BINDING PATHWAY: This second pathway of complement activation is similar to the classical pathway and results from the binding of a serum protein, mannose-binding protein (MBP), which is synthesized in the liver. The structure of the molecule is similar to that of C1q, and it binds mannose residues of glycoproteins and carbohydrates expressed on the surface of specific bacteria. After binding to a bacterial surface, MBP, similar to the C1qrs complex, binds and activates C4 and C2, thereby forming C4b,2b,C3 convertase. Host cells are protected from the indiscriminate binding of MBP because the mannose residues of vertebrate cells are not exposed on their external surfaces. C-reactive protein, which is

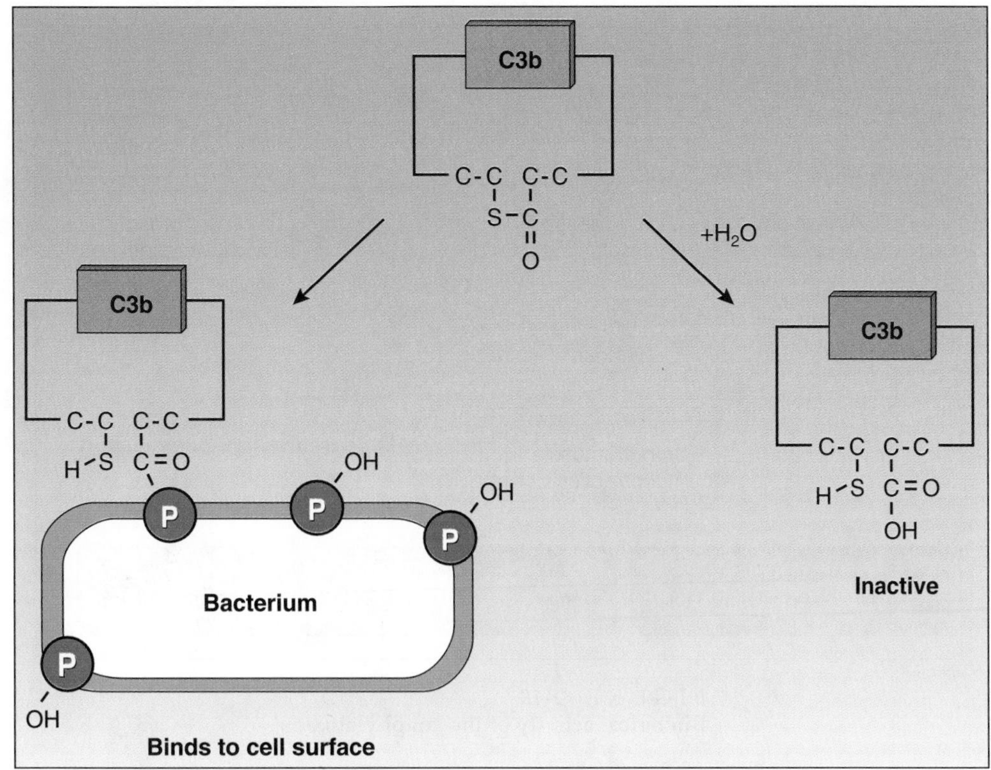

FIGURE *2-17*
Covalent binding of complement to cell surfaces.

synthesized by the liver and is present in serum, binds phosphorylcholine of specific bacteria and fungi. Macrophages possess receptors for both MBP and C-reactive protein, molecules that also function as opsonins to enhance phagocytosis of bacteria.

ALTERNATIVE PATHWAY: Activation of the alternative pathway of the complement system is initiated by derivative products of infectious organisms and by foreign materials through a cascade-like interaction of specific plasma proteins (see Table 2-1). Although they functioned in the classical pathway, C1, C4, and C2 are not involved in the alternative pathway. Activation of the alternative pathway proceeds as follows:

1. The binding of C3 with two plasma proteins, factor B and factor D, results in the formation of an enzymatically active derivative of factor B.
2. The larger fragment, Bb, catalyzes the conversion of C3, forming C3b and C3a.
3. When C3b is bound to Bb, a C3 convertase (C3bBb) is generated, greatly amplifying the subsequent conversion of C3 and generating additional C3b and C3a.
4. The binding of a second C3b molecule to C3b,Bb forms a C5 convertase, which in turn generates C5b and C5a, with subsequent assembly of the MAC.

Thus, whether the alternative, classical, or lectin-binding complement pathways are activated, the end-results are the same: (1) the generation of biologically active anaphylatoxins (C4a,C3a,C5a), (2) the fixation of opsonins (C3b) on cell surfaces, and (3) the formation of the MAC capable of inducing cell lysis.

ANAPHYLATOXINS: The anaphylatoxins C3a, C4a, and C5a are important products of complement activation through the classical pathway. Each of these molecules has potent effects on smooth muscle and the vasculature, including enhancement of smooth muscle contraction and an increase in vascular permeability (Fig. 2-18). The relative potencies of these effects are C3a>C5a>>C4a. Both C3a and C5a also induce degranulation of mast cell and basophils, and the consequent release of histamine further potentiates the increase in vascular permeability. In addition to their effects on vascular smooth muscle, the anaphylatoxins stimulate contraction of bronchial smooth muscle and cause airway narrowing by two mechanisms. One is dependent on arachidonic acid metabolism in the lung, whereas the other is mediated by the release of mast cell products.

C5a is also a potent chemotactic factor for neutrophils, monocytes, eosinophils, and basophils. Additional effects of C5a-induced stimulation of neutrophils include the following:

- Increased expression of cell adhesion molecules and complement receptors.
- Induction of low levels of neutrophil degranulation and superoxide anion production.
- Enhancement of the phagocytic response and (in response to a second stimulus) degranulation and superoxide anion production. This enhancement is referred to as cell priming and is similar to that observed with PAF and cytokines such as TNF-α.

C3a and C5a also modulate certain immune responses. Whereas C3a inhibits T-lymphocyte prolifera-

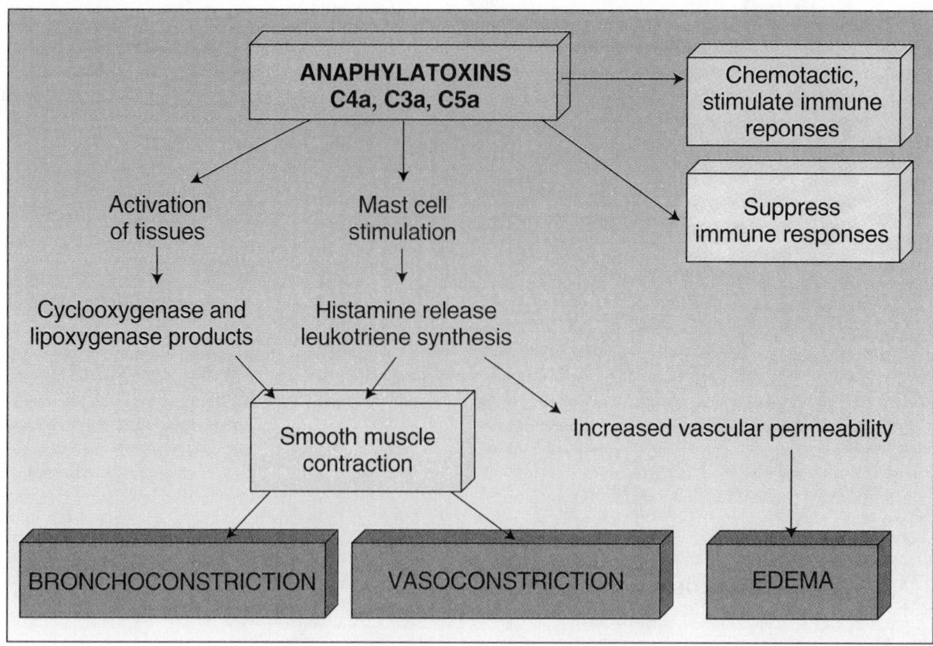

FIGURE *2-18*
Biological activity of the anaphylatoxins.

tion, C5a promotes immune reactions. These immune-regulatory properties of C3a and C5a are discussed in greater detail in Chapter 4.

REGULATION OF THE COMPLEMENT SYSTEM: Proteins in the serum and on cell surfaces protect the host from indiscriminate injury from complement. Deficiencies of several of these regulatory proteins are associated with specific clinical syndromes. Activation of the complement system is regulated by four mechanisms:

- **Spontaneous decay** of the enzymatically active complexes C4b2a and C3bBb and their cleavage products C3b and C4b.
- **Proteolytic inactivation** of specific components by plasma inhibitors. These inhibitors include factor I (an inhibitor of C3b and C4b) and serum carboxypeptidase N (SCPN). SCPN cleaves the carboxyterminal arginine from the anaphylatoxins C4a, C3a, and C5a in a manner similar to that of bradykinin. Removal of this single amino acid markedly decreases the biological activity of each of these molecules.
- **Binding of active components** by specific proteins in the plasma. C1 esterase inhibitor (C1 INA) binds C1r and C1s, forming an irreversibly inactive complex. Additional binding proteins in the plasma include factor H and C4b binding protein. These proteins form complexes with C3b and C4b, respectively, and enhance their susceptibility to proteolytic cleavage by factor I.
- **Cell membrane–associated molecules** also have potent regulatory effects on complement activation. They protect host cells from injury through spontaneous activation of C3 on their surface. Membrane cofactor protein (protectin, CD59) binds membrane-associated C4b and C3b and promotes its inactivation by factor I. Two proteins that are linked to the cell membrane by glycophosphoinositol (GPI) anchors play key roles in protecting cells from complement-mediated injury. Decay accelerating factor (DAF) breaks down the alternative pathway C3 convertase, and protectin prevents the formation of the MAC. Patients with defects in enzymes that generate protein–GPI linkages suffer from **paroxysmal nocturnal hemoglobinuria**, a disease characterized by episodes of spontaneous, intravascular, complement-mediated hemolysis (see Chapter 20).

The complement system is important in many forms of immunological tissue injury (see Chapter 4) and is a vital defense mechanism against bacterial infection. Bacterial activation of the complement system may occur either by direct activation of the alternative pathway or as an outcome of antibody or MBP binding to the surface of the organism and activation of the classical and lectin-binding pathways. Once the complement system is activated, bacteriolysis may follow, either by means of the assembled MAC or by enhanced bacterial clearance following opsonization. **Bacterial opsonization** is the process by which a specific molecule (e.g., IgG or C3b) binds to the surface of the bacterium. The process enhances phagocytosis by enabling receptors on the phagocytic cell membrane (e.g., the Fc receptor or the C3b receptor) to recognize and bind to the opsonized bacterium. Viruses, parasites, and transformed cells also activate the complement system by similar mechanisms, an effect that leads to their inactivation or death.

Receptors for complement components, especially C3b and its degradation products, are not only crucial for bacterial phagocytosis but also for the clearance of soluble Ag-Ab immune complexes (see Chapter 4). Complement receptors on erythrocytes bind and "scavenge" circulating immune complexes that have bound C4b or C3b. In the spleen and liver, mononuclear phagocytic cells bind and degrade the erythrocyte-bound complexes, returning the cells to the circulation. In certain autoimmune diseases, such as systemic lupus erythematosus, this clearance pathway is thought to be saturated, owing to excess Ag-Ab complex formation, with consequent tissue deposition and injury.

COMPLEMENT DEFICIENCY:The importance of an intact and appropriately regulated complement system is exemplified in persons who have deficiencies of either specific complement components or regulatory proteins. Deficiencies of complement components may be either acquired or congenital. The most common congenital defect is a C2 deficiency, which is inherited as an autosomal codominant trait, with a gene frequency of approximately 1%. Acquired deficiencies of early complement components occur in patients with certain autoimmune diseases, especially those associated with circulating immune complexes. These include certain forms of membranous glomerulonephritis and systemic lupus erythematosus.

Persons with congenital deficiencies in the early components of the complement system have recurrent symptoms resembling those of systemic lupus erythematosus. Patients with deficiencies of the middle (C3, C5) components are at particular risk of pyogenic bacterial infections, whereas those who lack terminal (C6, C7, or C8) complement components are vulnerable to infections with *Neisseria* species. Such a difference in susceptibility emphasizes the importance of individual components of the complement system in host surveillance against bacterial infection. Congenital defects have been reported in regulatory proteins of the complement system, including C1 INA and SCPN. Deficiency of C1 INA is associated with the syndrome of **hereditary angioedema**, characterized by episodic, painless, nonpitting edema of soft tissues. This disorder is the result of chronic complement activation, with the generation of a vasoactive peptide from C2, and may be life-threatening because of the occurrence of laryngeal edema.

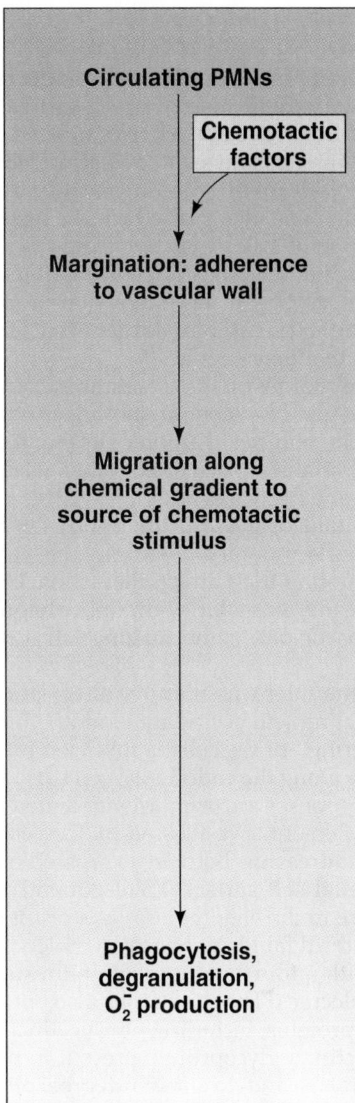

FIGURE *2-19*
Leukocyte exudation and phagocytosis.

Cell Recruitment

The second phase of the acute inflammatory response involves the accumulation of leukocytes, especially polymorphonuclear leukocytes (PMNs), at sites of tissue injury (Fig. 2-19). Beginning within minutes and continuing throughout the first 24 hours after the initiation of injury, many PMNs accumulate. This attraction of neutrophils to the inflammatory site involves a dynamic interaction between circulating leukocytes, endothelium, and the extracellular matrix. The primary mediators responsible for the recruitment of leukocytes are low-molecular-weight soluble compounds that are collectively referred to as **chemotactic factors**. They are generated in high concentrations at sites of tissue injury, with a decreasing gradient away from the injured tissue. In some cases, chemotactic factors are expressed on cell surfaces or bind to extracellular matrix, thereby creating a fixed chemotactic gradient.

The physiological responses of circulating leukocytes exposed to chemotactic factors include the following:

- **Margination** of the cells along the vascular wall
- **Adherence** of the leukocytes to the endothelium or vascular basement membrane
- **Emigration** through the vascular wall
- **Chemotaxis**, the unidirectional migration toward increasing concentrations of a soluble chemotactic agent
- **Haptotaxis**, chemotaxis along a fixed (insoluble) chemotactic gradient

Margination

Under normal circumstances, blood flow in the venules is characterized by a central stream of formed elements and a clear peripheral zone of plasma. On vasodilatation following injury, the blood flow slows and leukocytes appear in the peripheral region, which was previously acellular. This process is termed **margination**.

Adherence

The adherence of inflammatory cells to the endothelium or vascular basement membrane is critical for the recruitment of these circulating cells to sites of tissue injury. The adherence between circulating leukocytes and the vascular wall involves both physical and receptor-specific interactions, many of which are mediated by the local generation of inflammatory mediators. Importantly, the processes that mediate adherence within the vasculature are also critical for the interaction of inflammatory cells with the extravascular targets (bacteria, necrotic cells, debris) that they engulf.

Negative charges on the membranes of inflammatory cells and vascular basement membrane mutually repulse each other. The number of anionic sites (and hence, negative charges) on the surface of endothelial cells and basement membrane decreases after injury. This defect results in a concomitant decrease in the repulsion between the circulating inflammatory cells and the vascular wall, thereby promoting their direct interaction. Other components of plasma, vascular wall, and phagocytic membranes also participate in modulating cell adherence reactions.

Within the microvasculature, direct interactions between circulating leukocytes and endothelium occur. An initial "tethering" of the cells is followed by "rolling" of the leukocyte along the endothelial cell surface (Fig. 2-20). These two responses are primarily mediated by two families of complementary adhesion molecules, namely **selectins and addressins**. Both are expressed on leukocytes and endothelial cell surfaces. Subsequently, leukocytes tightly adhere to the endothelium as a result of the direct binding of a third family of adhesion molecule, termed **β-integrins**, with a fourth immunoglobulin superfamily of adhesion molecules. The β-integrins also bind to extracellular matrix proteins, including fibronectin and laminin.

Fibronectin, a glycoprotein present in plasma, basement membranes, and, to a lesser degree, phagocytic cell membranes, is important in modulating the attachment of phagocytic cells to vascular walls. Following injury to the vascular wall or tissues, increased amounts of fibronectin are deposited at the injury site. Fibronectin is also a potent opsonin, and as such it enhances phagocytosis of bacteria and phagocytic cell adherence. **Laminin**, another glycoprotein, is a structural component of basement membranes and modulates inflammatory cell function, secondary to its binding to specific receptors.

Cell Adhesion Molecules

Cell adhesion molecules are membrane glycoproteins that promote adherence and are among the factors that enhance phagocytic cell attachment to vascular walls and phagocytic particles. Four distinct families of cell adhesion molecules participate in the regulation of leukocyte recruitment and platelet localization at sites of inflammation (Fig. 2-21). These include selectins, addressins, integrins, and the immunoglobulin superfamily adhesion molecules.

SELECTINS: Selectins are a family of adhesion molecules of similar structure with an extracellular lectin-like binding domain. They are expressed on the surface of leukocytes, platelets, and endothelial cells and have been named for the cell in which they were first characterized: L-selectin, P-selectin, and E-selectin, respectively. The distinguishing lectin-binding region of the molecule recognizes specific carbohydrates on cell surface glycoproteins, known as vascular addressins. One of the important carbohydrate moieties recognized by selectins is sulfated sialyl Lewis X. Together, the three selectin molecules promote the initial localization and rolling of leukocytes along endothelium at sites of tissue injury. Patients with inherited deficiencies in fucosyl transferase activity and selectin-dependent binding (leukocyte adhesion deficiency-2 [LAD-2]) experience recurrent bacterial infections.

P-selectin is preformed and is stored within Weibel-Palade bodies of endothelial cells and the α-granules of platelets. On stimulation with histamine, thrombin, or specific inflammatory cytokines, endothelial cells trans-

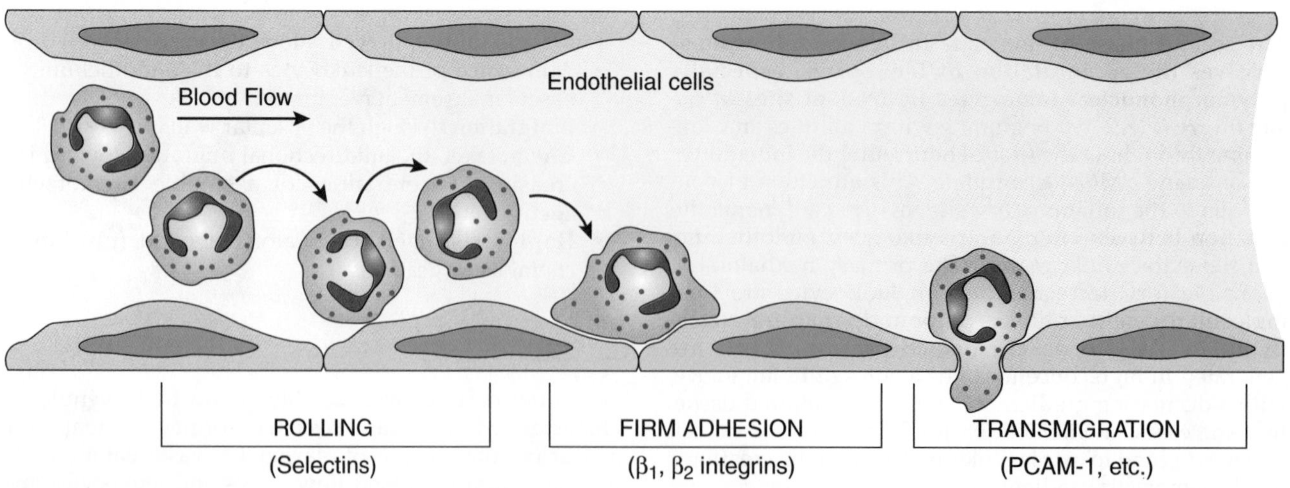

FIGURE 2-20
Mechanisms of leukocyte adherence.

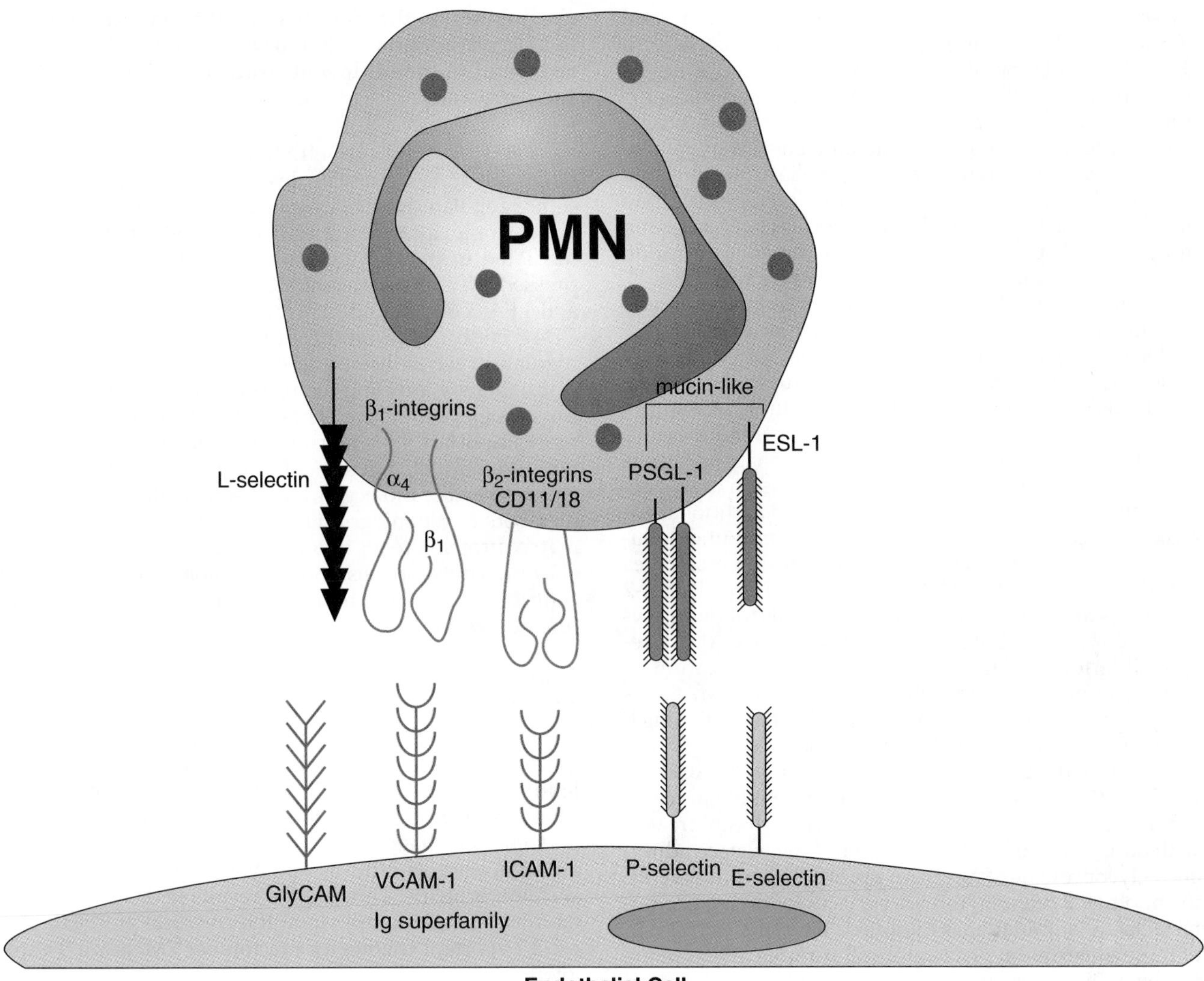

FIGURE *2-21*
Leukocyte and endothelial cell adhesion molecules.

port these protein molecules to the surface within minutes. P-selectin, which can also be rapidly expressed on the surface of stimulated platelets, binds to a glycoprotein on leukocyte surfaces (PSGL-1) and participates in the interactions between neutrophils and endothelial cells and those between platelets and neutrophils.

E-selectin is synthesized by cytokine-activated endothelial cells and requires several hours for its expression following stimulation with specific cytokines (IL-1, TNF-α) or bacterial lipopolysaccharide. Its natural ligand is a protein expressed on the cell surface of leukocytes, which contains sialic acid and fucosyl carbohydrate residues. Thus, it appears that P-selectin promotes the initial localization of leukocytes and platelets at sites of inflammation, whereas E-selectin enhances the recruitment of leukocytes.

L-selectin (also referred to as Leu-8 differentiation antigen) was originally defined as the "homing receptor" on lymphocytes. This molecule regulates lymphocyte binding to high endothelial lymph node venules and regulates their trafficking through lymphoid tissue. This molecule is (1) constitutively expressed on the surfaces of lymphocytes and neutrophils, (2) binds several addressin molecules expressed on endothelium (e.g., GlyCam-1), and (3) helps localize leukocytes to sites of tissue injury. On stimulation by chemotactic factors, L-selectin is released from the surface of neutrophils. L-selectin is a significant factor in lymphocyte activation (see Chapter 4).

ADDRESSINS: Vascular addressins are mucin-like molecules that possess carbohydrate regions that bind the lectin domain of selectins. Addressins are expressed on the surface of leukocytes and specific tissue endothelium and regulate the localization of subpopulations of leukocytes. These molecules also have a role to play in the activation of lymphocytes (see Chapter 4).

INTEGRINS: Integrins make up another class of adhesion molecules that are crucial for the recruitment of leukocytes and their migration to inflammatory sites.

These transmembrane adhesive molecules are composed of α and β subunits, arranged as heterodimers. Integrins act in the regulation of cell–matrix and cell–cell adhesive interactions. The β_1-integrins bind specific regions of extracellular matrix and endothelial cell surface proteins. The β_1-integrin VLA-4 (very late antigen-4) is expressed on leukocytes and binds the endothelial cell adhesion molecule VCAM-1 (vascular cell adhesion molecule-1), a member of the immunoglobulin superfamily of adhesion molecules. The β_1-integrins promote cell migration through the vasculature and extracellular matrix.

Several of the best-studied molecules of this family are the β_2-integrins (also referred to as CD11/CD18 molecules). The β_2-integrins represent three distinct molecules, designated MAC-1, leukocyte function antigen-1 (LFA-1), and gp150,95. In each of these molecules, the β-chain is conserved, and the specificity for adherence is conferred by the β-chain. Activation of phagocytic cells by chemotactic stimuli increases the expression of β_2-integrins on their cell surface. β_2-integrins bind additional adhesion molecules that are members of the immunoglobulin superfamily, termed **intercellular adhesion molecules 1 and 2 (ICAM-1, ICAM-2)**. Both ICAM-1 and ICAM-2 molecules are expressed on endothelial cells following cytokine stimulation. Binding of β_2-integrins to ICAMs is responsible for the "tight adhesion" and localization of leukocytes at sites of tissue injury. In addition, MAC-1 is the receptor for the inactivated form of C3b (iC3b), which functions as an important bacterial opsonin.

As noted above, persons deficient in MAC-1 or gp150,95 (i.e., those with LAD-1) are susceptible to recurrent bacterial infection. When phagocytic cells are treated with antibodies to block expression of the surface adherence glycoproteins MAC-1 and gp150,95, their adherence to endothelial cells and foreign surfaces following chemotactic factor stimulation is inhibited. Thus, the expression of these integrins on phagocytic cell surfaces assists in the localization of circulating cells at sites of tissue injury and in the host defense against bacterial infection.

IMMUNOGLOBULIN SUPERFAMILY ADHESION MOLECULES: Certain intercellular adhesion molecules (e.g., ICAM-1, -2) are members of the immunoglobulin superfamily and help localize leukocytes to areas of tissue injury. They are expressed on the cell surface of cytokine-stimulated endothelial cells and leukocytes and bind to LFA-1 (CD11a/CD18) and MAC-1 (CD11b/CD18), surface molecules of neutrophils and macrophages. ICAM-1 is also an important receptor for rhinovirus, whereas LFA-1 functions in cell killing by T cells and natural killer (NK) cells (see Chapter 4). A second intercellular adhesion molecule, VCAM-1, is expressed on endothelial cell surfaces and binds to the leukocyte β_1-integrin VLA-4.

Endothelial cells at sites of tissue injury also express on their surface increased numbers of specific adhesion molecules and PAF, which bind circulating leukocytes and platelets. The expression of P-selectin and PAF is induced by histamine and thrombin early in the inflammatory response. Subsequently, the levels of additional adhesion molecules (e.g., E-selectin, ICAM-1, and ICAM-2) on the endothelial surface are increased in response to cytokines, including TNF-α. **Together, the local coordinated expressions of PAF, adhesion molecules, and chemokines on the endothelial cell surface result in the local accumulation of leukocytes and platelets, which can result in blood flow obstruction and decreased tissue perfusion.**

OTHER CELL ADHESION MOLECULES: Additional cell adhesion molecules distinct from the T-cell receptor regulate lymphocyte interactions with other cells. For example, the binding of T lymphocytes to host cells is mediated in part by the interaction of two proteins expressed on cell surfaces, CD2 (a T-cell surface protein) and LFA-3 on antigen-presenting cells. Another protein, CD44, is expressed on the surface of T lymphocytes and regulates their adhesion to endothelial cells and monocytes, thereby affecting the recruitment of T lymphocytes to sites of inflammation. These represent only a few of the most important mechanisms by which cell–cell interactions are regulated at sites of inflammation. Other leukocyte cell surface molecules have been identified, including members of the integrin family that bind to extracellular matrix proteins (e.g., fibronectin, laminin, collagen, and elastin). The synthesis and expression of these proteins contribute to the regulation of leukocyte migration and function within tissues.

Chemotaxis

Chemotaxis refers to the process of directed cell migration, which is a dynamic and energy-dependent activity. The cell extends a pseudopod in the direction of the increasing chemotactic gradient. At the leading front of the pseudopod, marked changes in the levels of intracellular calcium are associated with the assembly and contraction of cytoskeleton proteins. This process results in drawing the remaining tail of the cell along the chemical gradient. The most important chemotactic factors for PMNs are the following:

- **C5a,** derived from complement
- **Bacterial and mitochondrial products,** particularly low-molecular-weight *N*-formylated peptides (such as *N*-formyl-methionyl-leucyl-phenylalanine [FMLP])
- **Products of arachidonic acid metabolism,** especially leukotriene B_4
- **Chemokines,** notably IL-8

***Cytokines** is a term that refers to a group of low-molecular-weight proteins that are secreted by cells.* These include the following:

- Interleukins
- Growth factors and colony-stimulating factors
- TNF-α
- Interferons
- Chemokines

Many of these cytokines are produced at sites of inflammation, and those with chemotactic activity are referred to as **chemokines**. Two families of chemokines (α- and β-chemokines) are defined by the molecular relationship of specific cysteine residues within the molecule. The α-chemokines include IL-8 and are potent chemoattractants for neutrophils. The β-chemokines (e.g., macrophage chemotactic peptide-1 [MCP-1]) are preferentially chemotactic for monocytes. Both α- and β-chemokines are produced by a variety of cell types, including tissue macrophages, endothelial cells, keratinocytes, fibroblasts, and smooth muscle cells. Thus, they represent one of the most important mechanisms of leukocyte recruitment. One of the mechanisms by which chemokines generate a chemotactic gradient is the binding to proteoglycans of the extracellular matrix. As a result, high concentrations of the chemokines persist at sites of tissue injury. In turn, specific receptors on the surface of the migrating leukocytes bind to the matrix-bound chemokines and associated adhesion molecules, a process that tends to move the cells along the chemotactic gradient to the site of injury. This process of responding to a matrix-bound chemoattractant is termed **haptotaxis**. Interestingly, chemokines and other chemoattractants all bind to receptors of similar structure. Each is an integral membrane protein with seven membrane-spanning regions, which binds a G protein within the cell and is associated with a specific tyrosine kinase.

Chemotactic factors for cell types other than neutrophils and monocytes, including lymphocytes, basophils, and eosinophils, are also produced at sites of tissue injury. In addition to the agents listed earlier, chemotactic factors may be generated from plasma components or the extracellular matrix (C5a, degradation products of fibrin, fibronectin, and collagen). They may also be secreted by activated endothelial cells, tissue parenchymal cells, or other inflammatory cells and include PAF, transforming growth factor-beta (TGF-β), neutrophilic cationic proteins, and lymphokines.

Cytokine Networks in Inflammation

The production of cytokines at sites of tissue injury regulates the inflammatory response (Fig. 2-22), ranging from initial changes in vascular permeability to resolution. These molecules function as inflammatory hormones that exhibit autocrine, paracrine, and endocrine functions (Fig. 2-23). Through its production of cytokines, the macrophage is the pivotal cell in the orchestration of the inflammatory response within tissues. Lipopolysaccharide (LPS), a molecule derived from the outer cell membrane of gram-negative bacteria, is one of the most potent stimuli of macrophages. LPS can either directly, or after binding with a serum protein (LPS-binding protein [LBP]), activate macrophages through specific receptors. It is a potent stimulus for the production of several cytokines, including TNF-α and IL-1, -6, -8, and -12. As a result, macrophage-derived mediators modulate endothelial cell–leukocyte adhesion (TNF-α), leukocyte recruit ment (IL-8), the acute phase response (IL-6, IL-1), and immune functions (IL-1, IL-6, IL-12). LPS can also directly affect endothelial cell function and activate PMNs.

A second potent stimulus of macrophage activation and cytokine production is interferon-gamma (IFN-γ). Although IFN-γ is produced by a subset of T lymphocytes as part of the immune response (see Chapter 4), it is also synthesized by NK cells as a primary host response to intracellular pathogens (e.g., *Listeria monocytogenes*) and certain viral infections. NK cells are lymphocytes that possess large cytoplasmic granules, which contain proteins that cause cell lysis. They are present in the circula-

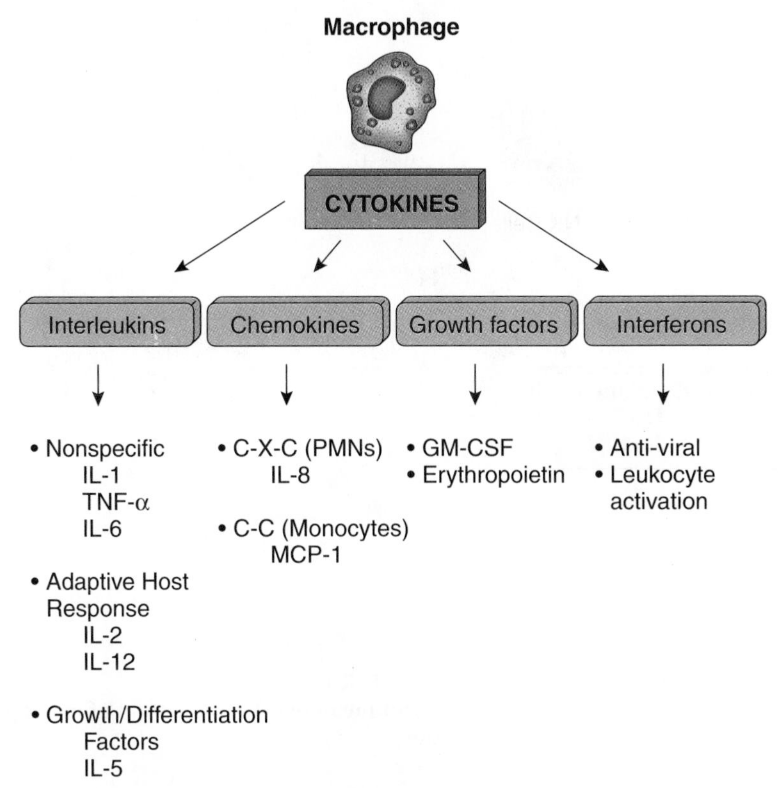

FIGURE 2-22
Cytokine activities.

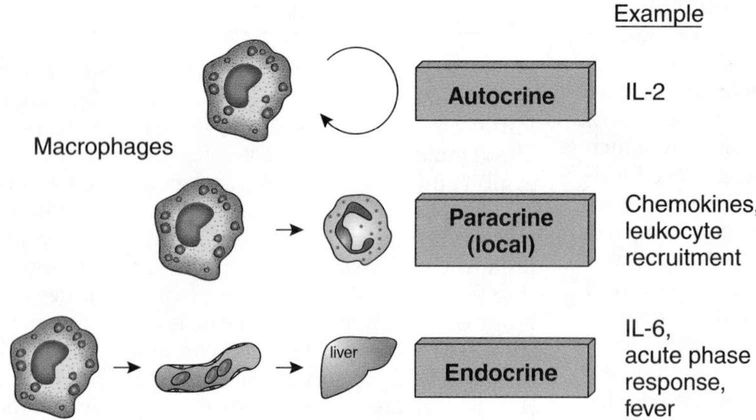

FIGURE 2-23
Functional roles of cytokines.

tion and migrate into tissues at sites of injury. When exposed to IL-12 and TNF-α, NK cells are activated to produce IFN-γ. Thus, an amplification pathway exists by which activated tissue macrophages produce TNF-α and IL-12 and thereby stimulate IFN-γ production by NK cells, with subsequent stimulation of additional macrophages (Fig. 2-24).

The recruitment of inflammatory cells to sites of tissue injury involves cell-cell communication networks (Fig. 2-25). This communication is effected both by direct cell contact, mediated in part by specific adherence proteins, and by the production, secretion, and receptor-specific binding of cytokines to target cells. In addition, the cellular expression of certain adherence proteins is regulated by cytokines that are produced at inflammatory sites. The recruitment of neutrophils to sites of bacterial infection is an example of this interrelationship between adherence proteins, cytokines, and inflammatory cells. During the initial stages of bacterial infection, formylated chemotactic peptides are produced, and C5a is generated in response to activation of the complement system by the organisms. Each of these compounds is a potent chemotactic factor for neutrophils. In addition, other products of the bacteria, such as endotoxin (LPS), activate tissue macrophages to produce (1) IL-8, (2) MCPs, and (3) other cytokines, such as TNF-α and IL-1.

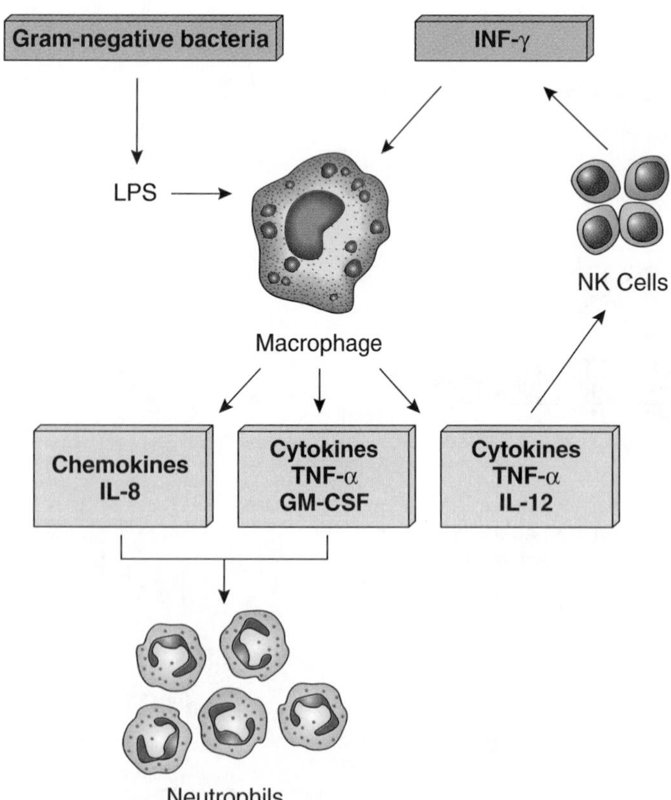

FIGURE 2-24
Cytokine networks: regulation of macrophage activation.

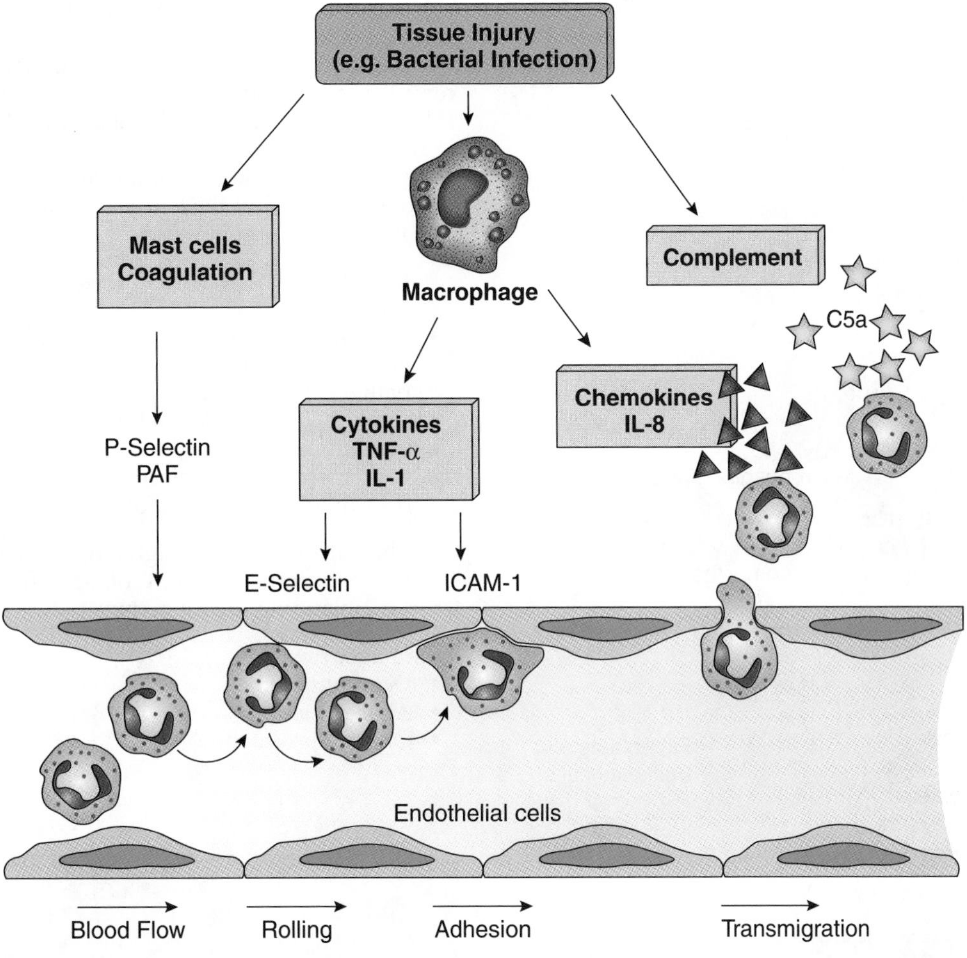

FIGURE 2-25
Regulation of leukocyte recruitment.

IL-1 and TNF-α stimulate a variety of cell types, including endothelial cells, and induce the expression of adherence glycoproteins (e.g., endothelial leukocyte adhesion molecule [ELAM-1], ICAM-1) and the production of chemotactic cytokines (e.g., IL-8 and MCPs). Furthermore, TNF-α acts in an autocrine manner to activate macrophages, thereby further enhancing the production of IL-8 and MCPs. IL-1 and TNF-α also induce the synthesis of similar chemokines in fibroblasts and epithelial cells (Fig. 2-26). Maximum secretion of these chemotactic peptides requires several hours, in contrast to the rapid activation of complement, generation of C5a, and production of PAF and leukotriene B_4 by neutrophils.

Thus, the initial recruitment of neutrophils to sites of tissue injury is largely dependent on C5a and the generation of lipid mediators, whereas following injury the prolonged recruitment from 6 to 48 hours is mediated by the production of chemotactic cytokines. Additional cytokines may be secreted that are chemotactic for lymphocytes, initiate wound healing and repair (see Chapter 3), or promote systemic responses (e.g., IL-6). Once the inflammatory cells are recruited to sites of injury and remove the initiating insult (e.g., bacteria or products of tissue injury), the production of inflammatory mediators decreases with resolution of the inflammatory response.

Inflammatory Cell Activation

Polymorphonuclear leukocytes, mast cells, mononuclear phagocytes cells, and platelets are important cellular components of the inflammatory reaction. Once stimulated, these cells release inflammatory mediators that can cause tissue injury.

The PMN is activated in response to phagocytic stimuli, cytokines, chemotactic mediators, or Ab–Ag complexes that bind to specific receptors on their cell membrane. Neutrophil receptors react with the following:

- Fc portion of IgG and IgM molecules
- Complement system components C5a, C3b, and iC3b
- Arachidonic acid metabolites (e.g., leukotriene B_4)
- Chemotactic factors (e.g., FMLP, IL-8)
- Cytokines (e.g., TNF-α)

Mast cells, platelets, and mononuclear phagocytic cells are also activated in a receptor-specific manner.

The process by which diverse stimuli lead to the functional responses of inflammatory cells (e.g., degranulation or aggregation) is referred to as stimulus–response coupling. Common intracellular pathways associated with inflammatory cell activation include the following (Fig. 2-27):

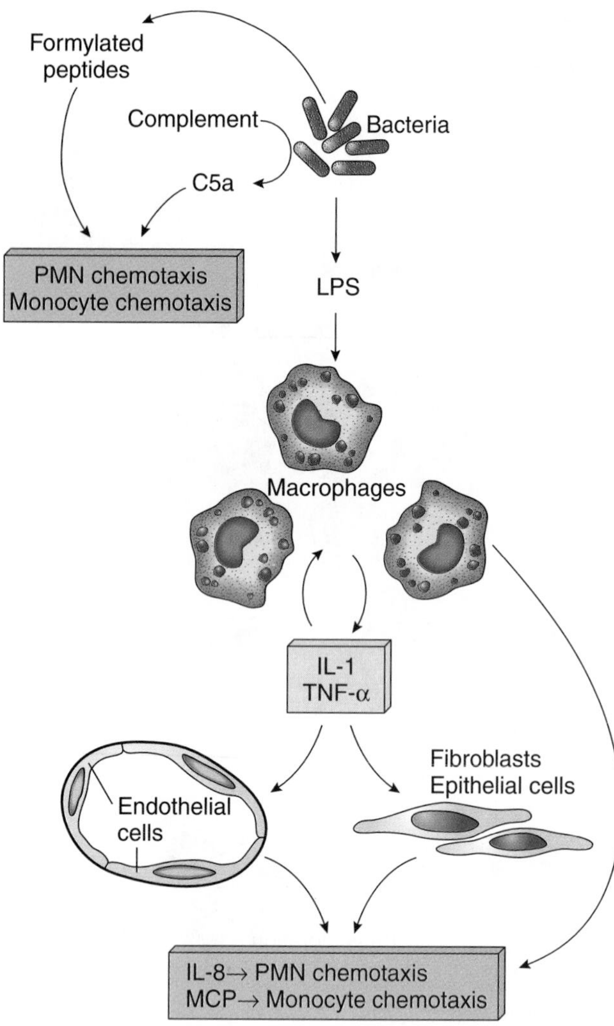

FIGURE 2-26
Cytokine networks in acute inflammation.

- Stimulus-induced increases in phospholipi metabolism of cell membranes (e.g., the phosphoinositide or arachidonic acid systems)
- Elevated cytosolic free calcium
- Protein phosphorylation and dephosphorylation
- Protein kinase C
- Tyrosine kinases
- Protein phosphatases

For example, the binding of a chemotactic factor to a specific receptor on the cell membrane results in the formation of a ligand–receptor complex (Fig. 2-28). A guanine nucleotide regulatory protein (G protein) couples the ligand–receptor complex to the activation of specific enzymes associated with the leukocyte plasma membrane, including phospholipase C. In turn, phospholipase C hydrolyzes a phosphoinositide in the plasma membrane (phosphatidylinositol bisphosphate [PIP_2]), thereby forming two potent metabolites, diacylglycerol and inositol trisphosphate. **Inositol trisphosphate releases calcium stored in the endoplasmic reticulum.** The release of intracellular calcium, in conjunction with an influx of calcium ions from the extracellular environment, increases cytosolic free calcium, a critical event for the activation of most inflammatory cells.

In addition, specific tyrosine kinases bind the ligand–receptor complex and initiate a series of protein phosphorylations. The precise mechanisms by which an increase in free calcium and tyrosine kinase initiate protein phosphorylations and mediate inflammatory cell activation remain undefined, but they appear to be critical for a number of events:

- Potentiation of phospholipase A_2 and phospholipase D activity
- Activation of protein kinase C and other protein kinases, which activate other intracellular signaling pathways, including gene transcription
- Assembly of cytoskeletal elements: the microtubular system and actin–myosin complexes are crucial for the secretion of cytoplasmic granules and for chemotaxis of neutrophils and other inflammatory cells

The outcome of these signaling mechanisms involves induction or enhancement of specific functional responses, including the following:

- Phagocytosis
- Degranulation
- Aggregation
- Oxidant production

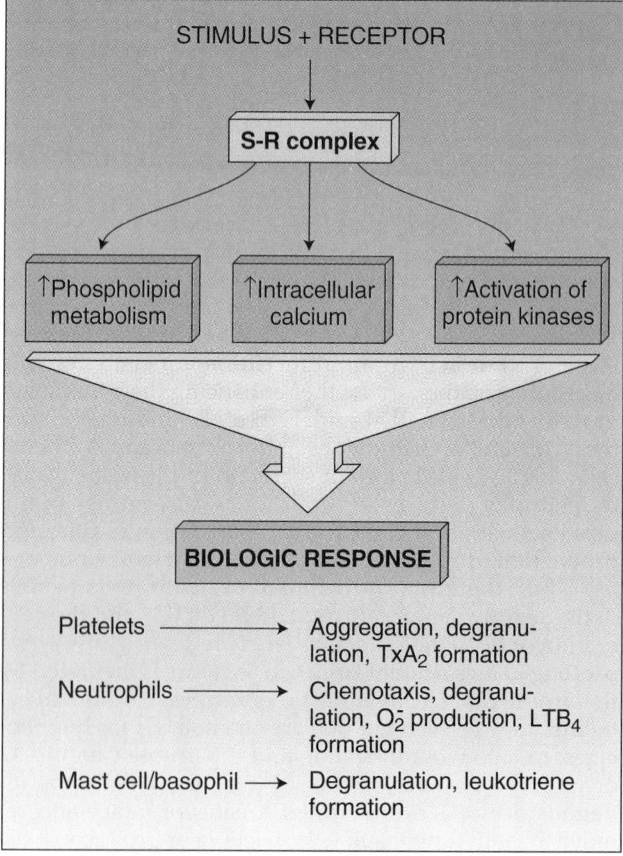

FIGURE 2-27
Mechanisms of inflammatory cell activation.

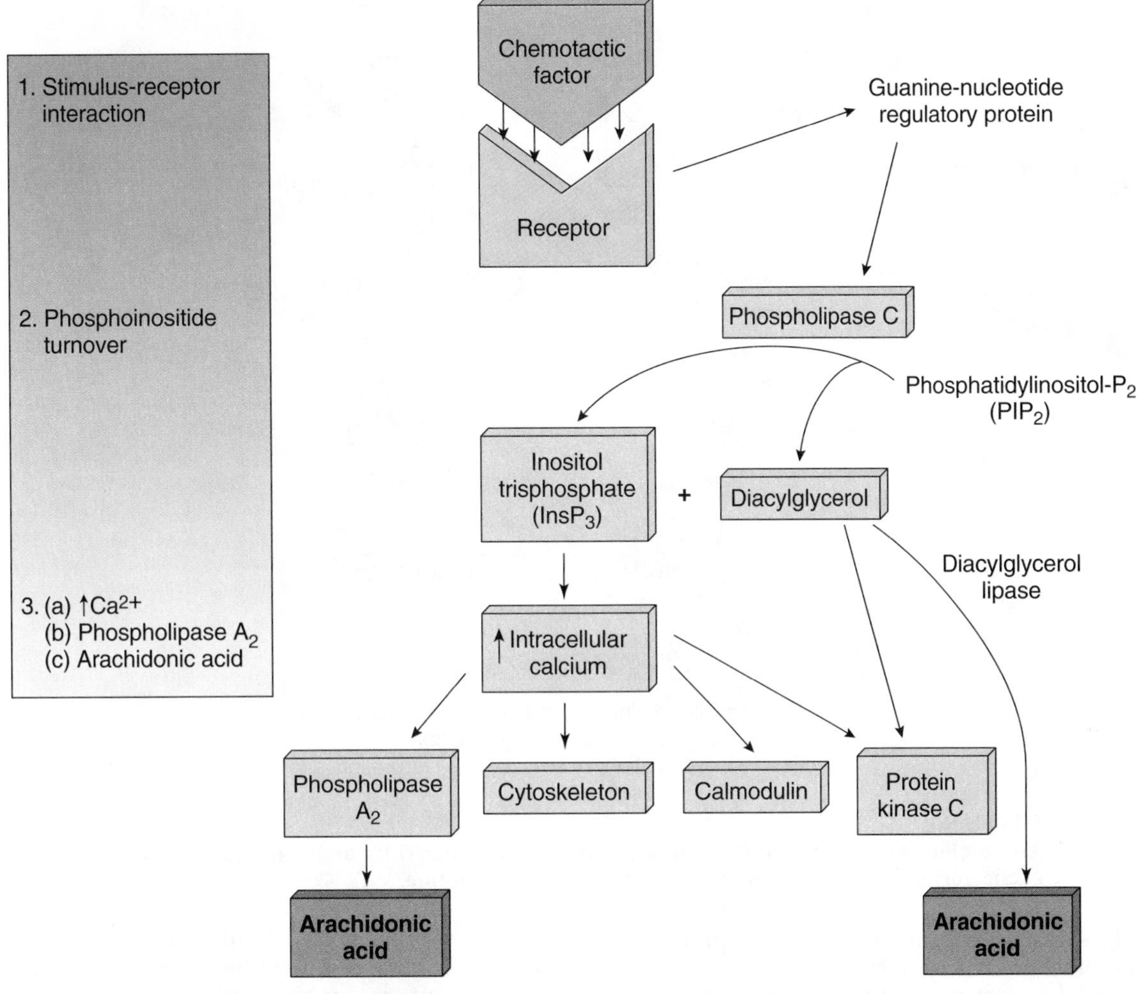

FIGURE 2-28
Initial events in polymorphonuclear leukocyte activation.

- Adhesion molecule receptor expression
- Gene transcription and cytokine production

An understanding of inflammatory cell stimulation provides the basis for new strategies for therapeutic modulation of inflammation in human disease. For instance, specific lipoxygenase or phospholipase inhibitors could be developed to inhibit the early activation processes of inflammatory cells, suppressing in this way the tissue injury associated with certain diseases.

Modulation of Inflammatory Cell Function

A variety of pharmacological agents are used clinically to modulate inflammatory cell function. Nonsteroidal anti-inflammatory drugs (NSAIDs) represent the largest group of compounds and include several classes of structurally distinct compounds: salicylates (e.g., aspirin), indolacetic acids (e.g., indomethacin), phenylacetic acids (e.g., ibuprofen), as well as others. One of the primary effects of NSAIDs is inhibition of cyclooxygenase activity and the synthesis of prostaglandins and thromboxane. Corticosteroids, including hydrocortisone and prednisone, have multiple suppressive effects on inflammatory cell function, for example, diminished cell adhesion, phagocytosis, and cytokine production. One mechanism postulated for the action of corticosteroids is the induction of a cytosolic protein, lipocortin, that inhibits phospholipase A_2 activity and arachidonic acid generation.

CYCLIC NUCLEOTIDES: The activation of inflammatory cells can be inhibited by pharmacological modulation, exemplified by the effects of E-series prostaglandins and PGI_2 on mast cells, neutrophils, macrophages, and platelets. These compounds inhibit inflammatory cell function by increasing intracellular cAMP levels, secondary to their activation of adenylyl cyclase (Fig. 2-29). Adenylyl cyclase is also stimulated by β-adrenergic agonists and adenosine (and experimentally by cholera toxin), all of which inhibit the function of inflammatory cells. Furthermore, treatment with an inhibitor (e.g., theophylline) of cAMP phosphodiesterase, the enzyme that hydrolyzes cAMP, leads to an increase in the level of cAMP, an effect that potentiates the inhibitory effects of adenylyl cyclase agonists. By contrast, mediators that activate guanylyl cyclase and increase the level

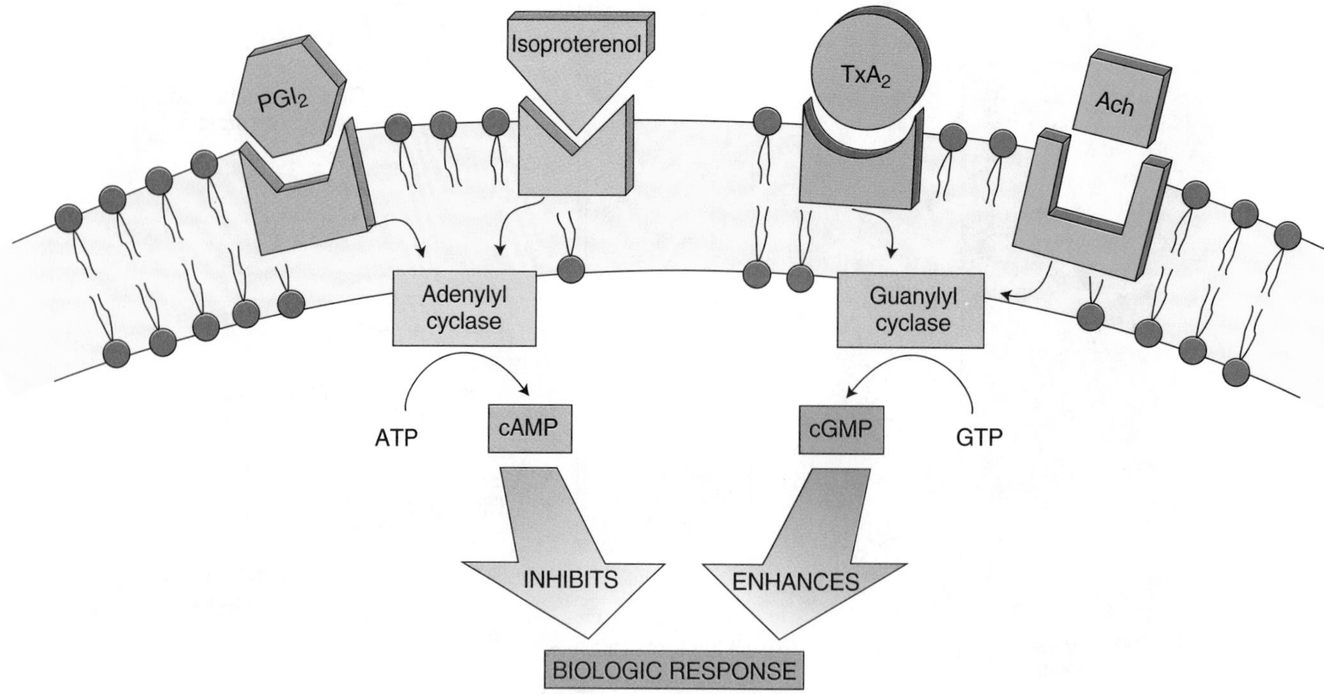

FIGURE 2-29
The biological response of inflammatory cells is modulated by activating and inhibitory cyclic nucleotides. TxA_2, thromboxane A_2; Ach, acetylcholine.

of cGMP, such as TxA_2 and acetylcholine, promote the functions of inflammatory cells.

Adenylyl cyclase agonists and phosphodiesterase inhibitors also affect tissues other than inflammatory cells. For instance, an increased level of cAMP in smooth muscle causes bronchiolar relaxation and blocks the effects of mediators that stimulate bronchoconstriction. For this reason, phosphodiesterase inhibitors are used to prevent mast cell degranulation and to treat symptoms associated with certain allergic reactions.

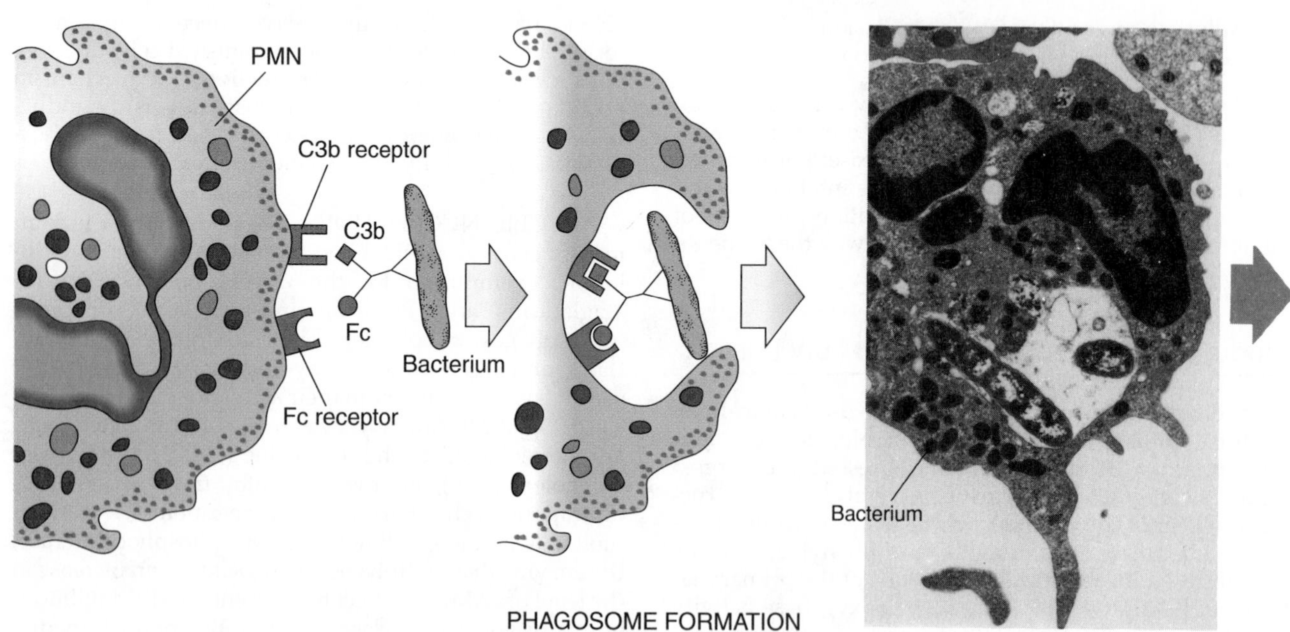

FIGURE 2-30
Mechanisms of polymorphonuclear leukocyte bacterial phagocytosis and cell killing.

In summary, the response of both inflammatory cells and target tissues to specific inflammatory mediators is modulated by intracellular cyclic nucleotides and is subject to pharmacological modulation of the inflammatory response.

PROSTAGLANDIN I_2: PGI_2, a secretory product of endothelial cells, exerts a number of effects (see Fig. 2-29):

- Inhibition of the activation of neutrophils and platelets
- Maintenance of vascular integrity
- Modulation of the recruitment of neutrophils to sites of inflammation

Under normal conditions, PGI_2 increases the amount of cAMP, thereby suppressing the activation of platelets and PMNs within the vascular compartment. A variety of injuries promote the activation of these cells by (1) decreasing the endothelial production of PGI_2, (2) increasing the sensitivity of platelets and PMNs to PGI_2, or (3) presenting an overwhelming inflammatory stimulus (e.g., high levels of C5a or thrombin). Alterations in the homeostatic balance between the activation of platelets and the suppression of this process by PGI_2 have been postulated as important in the development of vascular thrombi and the pathogenesis of atherosclerosis. Similarly, a decline in the inhibitory effect of PGI_2 on the activation of PMNs caused by endothelial injury probably participates in the initiation of acute inflammatory reactions.

Mechanisms of Inflammatory Cell Functions

Phagocytosis

Many inflammatory cells, including PMNs, monocytes, and tissue macrophages, function by recognizing, internalizing, and digesting foreign material or the debris of injured cells. This process is termed **phagocytosis**, and the effector cells are known as **phagocytes**. In general terms, the critical events of phagocytosis proceed as follows (Fig. 2-30):

1. **Recognition:** The incubation of phagocytic cells with an inert material (e.g., glass beads or carbon particles) results in the internalization of the foreign substance. Under these circumstances, the mechanism by which the phagocyte "recognizes" the particle as foreign is poorly understood. Since both the phagocyte and biological materials such as bacteria and cell membranes carry net negative charges, they would be expected to repel each other. Therefore, the phagocytosis of most biological agents is substantially enhanced, if not dependent on, their coating (opsonization) with plasma components (opsonins), particularly immunoglobulins or the C3b fragment of complement. Phagocytic cells possess specific receptors for C3b, iC3b, and the Fc fragment of immunoglobulin molecules, and the binding of opsonized particles to these receptors greatly facilitates the recognition process, thereby overcoming any electrostatic repulsion.

2. **Internalization:** The attachment of a particle to the surface of a phagocytic cell triggers its internalization. In some cases, binding to a receptor is sufficient to initiate the engulfment of a foreign agent by the cell membrane, whereas in other circumstances activation of phagocytosis also requires the concurrent binding of extracellular matrix components (fibronectin, laminin) or cytokines secreted by macrophages or T cells. Internalization is accomplished by an invagination of the plasma membrane that encloses the foreign material in a cytoplasmic vacuole, termed a **phagosome**.

3. **Digestion:** The phagosome fuses with cytoplasmic lysosomal granules to form a phagolysosome, into which the lysosomal enzymes are released. These hydrolytic enzymes are activated by the acid pH within the phagolysosome, after which they degrade the phagocytosed material.

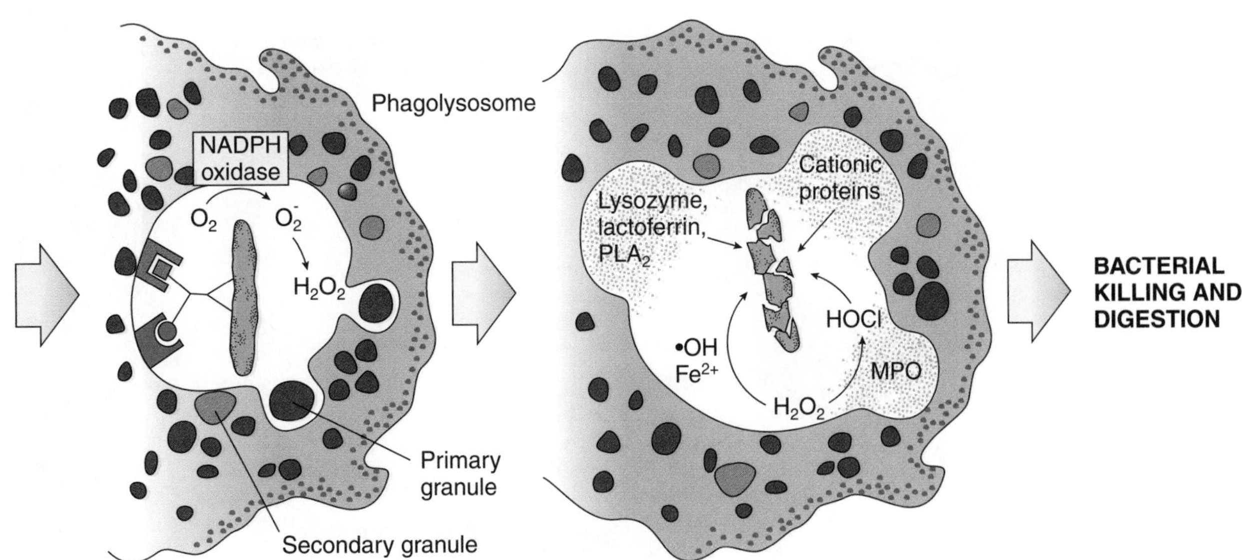

Neutrophil Granules

Three distinct granules in the cytoplasm of PMNs are designated as primary, secondary, and tertiary granules, which can be differentiated morphologically and biochemically (Fig. 2-31). Each granule displays a unique spectrum of enzymes.

- **Primary granules:** These cytoplasmic inclusions, also known as azurophilic granules, contain potent acid hydrolases capable of digesting a wide variety of biological materials. They enclose elastase and cathepsin G, which are serine proteases capable of digesting structural proteins of tissues, including elastin and collagen. Also present in these granules are cationic proteins that enhance the adherence of neutrophils to targets and initiate the killing of certain cell types. Both of these functions of the cationic proteins are important in killing bacteria. Other primary granule enzymes with known bactericidal activity are lysozyme and phospholipase A_2, which degrade bacterial cell walls and biological membranes, respectively. Myeloperoxidase, an enzyme also present in these granules, enhances cytotoxicity by metabolizing hydrogen peroxide in the presence of halide ions (e.g., Cl^- or I^-) to form hypohalous acid (see later).
- **Secondary granules:** These structures, similar to primary granules, also contain phospholipase A_2 and lysozyme. In addition, their contents include the cationic protein lactoferrin, a vitamin B_{12}–binding protein, and a collagenase specific for type IV collagen.
- **Tertiary granules:** These granules are also referred to as C particles. They contain cathepsins and gelatinase, the latter a metalloproteinase that digests basement membranes and denatured collagen. Tertiary granules are released at the leading front of neutrophils during chemotaxis and are believed to be the source of enzymes that promote the migration of cells through basement membranes and tissues. Similar granules are present in monocytes and macrophages.

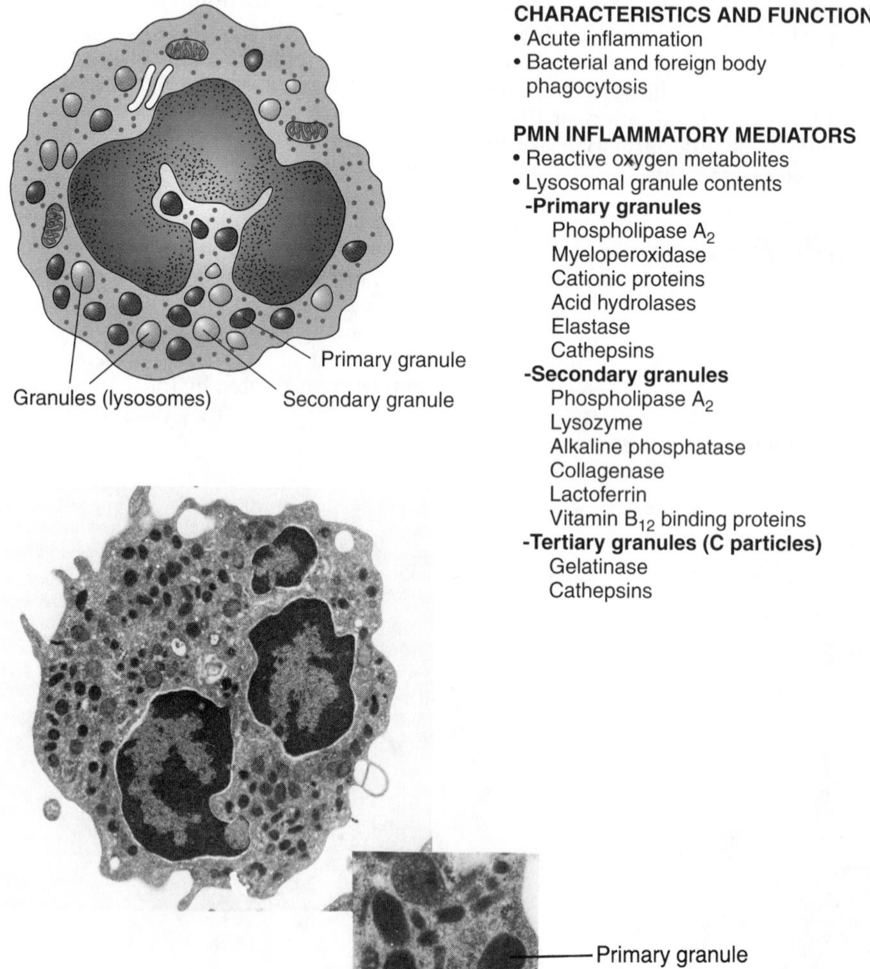

FIGURE *2-31*
Polymorphonuclear leukocyte: morphology and function.

Bactericidal Activity of Inflammatory Cells

The bactericidal activity of PMNs and macrophages is mediated in part by the production of reactive oxygen species and in part by oxygen-independent mechanisms.

Bacterial Killing by Activated Oxygen Species

Phagocytosis is accompanied by metabolic reactions within inflammatory cells that lead to the production of a number of oxygen metabolites. These products are more reactive than oxygen itself and contribute to the killing of ingested bacteria.

- **Superoxide anion (O_2^-):** In addition to releasing granular enzymes into the phagolysosome, phagocytosis activates a nicotinamide adenine dinucleotide phosphate (NADPH) oxidase in the cell membrane of PMNs (see Fig. 2-31). NADPH oxidase is a multicomponent electron transport complex that reduces molecular oxygen to the superoxide anion, O_2^-. The activation of NADPH oxidase is enhanced by prior exposure of the cells to small amounts of a chemotactic stimulus or bacterial lipopolysaccharide. NADPH oxidase activation is associated with an increase in oxygen consumption and the stimulation of the hexose–monophosphate shunt. Together, these cell responses are referred to as the **respiratory burst**. Almost all the oxygen consumed during the initiation of the respiratory burst can be accounted for by the generation of O_2^-.
- **Hydrogen peroxide (H_2O_2):** O_2^- is reduced to H_2O_2 by the superoxide dismutase reaction at the cell surface and within phagolysosomes. H_2O_2 is stable and serves as a substrate for the generation of additional reactive oxidants.
- **Hypochlorous acid:** H_2O_2 can react with myeloperoxidase in the presence of a halide to form hypohalous acid (Table 2-3). The most prominent halogen in biological systems is chlorine, and thus hypochlorous acid (HOCl) is produced following neutrophil stimulation. This acid (the primary component of household bleach) is a more potent oxidant than hydrogen peroxide itself and appears to be a major bactericidal agent produced by phagocytic cells. In addition to its bactericidal action, HOCl also participates (together with granular proteases) in the activation of neutrophil-derived collagenase and gelatinase, both of which are secreted as latent enzymes.
- **Hydroxyl radical ($\cdot OH$):** Further reduction of H_2O_2 occurs through Haber-Weiss reaction, which forms the highly reactive hydroxyl radical ($\cdot OH$) (see Chapter 1). Although this reaction occurs slowly at physiological pH, it is facilitated by reduced transition metals, particularly ferrous iron. In the presence of Fe^{2+}, a Fenton-type reaction converts H_2O_2 to $\cdot OH$, a radical with potent bactericidal activity. Further reduction of $\cdot OH$ leads to the formation of H_2O.

Monocytes, macrophages, and eosinophils also produce superoxide anion and hydrogen peroxide, depending on their state of activation and the stimulus to which they are exposed. The production of reactive oxygen metabolites by these cells has been implicated in their bactericidal and fungicidal activity, as well as in their ability to kill certain parasites. Phagocytic cells from several animal species have been shown to produce NO, which serves as an important bactericidal agent. However, in contrast to its important role in human endothelial cell function, the effect of NO on human phagocytic cells remains to be demonstrated.

The importance of oxygen-dependent mechanisms in the bacterial killing by phagocytic cells is exemplified in **chronic granulomatous disease of childhood**. Children with this disease suffer from a hereditary deficiency of NADPH oxidase. This defect results in a failure to produce the superoxide anion and hydrogen peroxide during phagocytosis. Persons with this disorder are susceptible to recurrent infections, especially with gram-positive cocci (Table 2-4). Similarly, patients deficient in myeloperoxidase are unable to produce HOCl and experience an increased incidence of infections with the fungal pathogen *Candida*.

TABLE 2-3 Reactions Involving Reactive Oxygen Metabolites Produced by Phagocytic Cells

Reaction	Product
Reduction of molecular oxygen	
$O_2 + e^- \rightarrow O_2^-$	Superoxide anion
Dismutation of O_2^-	
$O_2^- + O_2^- + 2H^- \rightarrow O_2 + H_2O_2$	Hydrogen peroxide
Haber-Weiss Reaction	
$H_2O_2 + O_2^- \rightarrow OH^- + \cdot OH$	Hydroxyl radical
Fenton reaction (iron-catalyzed)	
$H_2O_2 + Fe^{2+} \rightarrow Fe^{3+} + OH^- + \cdot OH$	Hydroxyl radical
Myeloperoxidase reaction	
$H_2O_2 + Cl^- + H^- \rightleftharpoons + HOCl$	Hypochlorous acid

TABLE 2-4 Congenital Diseases of Defective Phagocytic Cell Function Characterized by Recurrent Bacterial Infections

Disease	Defect
Leukocyte adhesion deficiency	LAD-1 (CD11/CD18) LAD-2 (defective fucosylation, selectin binding)
Hyper-IgE-recurrent infection (Job) syndrome	Poor chemotaxis
Chédiak-Higashi syndrome	Defective lysosomal granules, poor chemotaxis
Neutrophil-specific granule deficiency	Absent neutrophil granules
Chronic granulomatous disease	Deficient NADPH oxidase, with absent H_2O_2 production
Myeloperoxidase deficiency	Deficient HOCl production

Nonoxidative Bacterial Killing

Phagocytic cells, particularly PMNs and monocyte/macrophages, exhibit substantial antimicrobial activity that is oxygen independent. This activity relies principally on a number of bactericidal proteins that are preformed constituents of cytoplasmic granules. These include many lysosomal acid hydrolases and specialized noncatalytic proteins with microbicidal activity that are unique to inflammatory cells.

- **Lysosomal hydrolases:** The primary and secondary granules of neutrophils and the lysosomes of mononuclear phagocytes contain various hydrolases that possess antimicrobial activity, including proteases, lipases, hydrolases active against polysaccharides and DNA, and other enzymes such as sulfatases and phosphatases. Cathepsin G is a neutral protease in the primary granules of neutrophils that demonstrates antimicrobial properties. Interestingly, the bactericidal activity of cathepsin G is independent of its catalytic properties, since it kills microorganisms even after heat inactivation of its protease activity.
- **Bactericidal/permeability-increasing protein (BPI):** This cationic protein has been isolated from the primary granules of PMNs and is potently bactericidal toward many gram-negative bacteria, but it is not toxic to gram-positive bacteria or to eukaryotic cells. BPI has the following effects on susceptible bacteria: (1) insertion into the outer membrane of the bacterial envelope, (2) an increase in the permeability of the outer membrane, and (3) an activation of certain phospholipases and enzymes that degrade bacterial peptidylglycans.
- **Defensins:** Primary granules of PMNs and the lysosomes of some mononuclear phagocytes contain a family of cationic proteins, termed **defensins**, that kill a wide variety of gram-positive and gram-negative bacteria, fungi, and some enveloped viruses. These polypeptides are distinct from BPI, and on a molar basis they exert far less potent bactericidal activity. However, defensins are so abundant (30% to 50% of the granule protein) that their overall activity is probably significant. Some of these polypeptides also can kill host cells in a manner that is dependent on the active metabolism of the target tissue. One defensin is strongly and specifically chemotactic for monocytes, suggesting that the release of defensin by neutrophils facilitates the local accumulation of monocytes during acute inflammatory reactions. The precise mechanisms by which defensins exert microbicidal activity are unclear, but they have been shown to permeabilize *E. coli*, presumably by inserting into the cell membranes.
- **Lactoferrin:** Lactoferrin is an iron-binding glycoprotein contained in the secondary granules of neutrophils. It is also present in most secretory fluids in the body. Its antimicrobial properties are related to its iron-chelating capacity, which allows it to compete with bacteria for iron. In addition, lactoferrin may also participate in oxidative killing of bacteria by enhancing ·OH formation.
- **Lysozyme:** Lysozyme occurs in many tissues and fluids in the body and is contained in primary and secondary granules of neutrophils and in the lysosomes of mononuclear phagocytes. The peptidoglycans of gram-positive bacterial cell walls are exquisitely sensitive to degradation by lysozyme, whereas gram-negative bacteria are as a rule resistant to its action.
- **Bactericidal proteins of eosinophils:** Eosinophils contain several granule-bound cationic proteins, the most important of which are major basic protein (MBP) and eosinophilic cationic protein. MBP accounts for about half of the total protein of the eosinophil granule. Both proteins are ineffective against bacteria but are potent cytotoxic agents for a large number of parasites.

Tissue Injury by Inflammatory Cells

Inflammatory cells, whose functions evolved to combat microorganisms and other foreign agents, are also capable of damaging the host tissue by the extracellular release of enzymes and activated oxygen.

Lysosomal Enzymes

Lysosomal enzymes involved in the intracellular degradation of phagocytosed material are released into the extracellular environment by three processes:

- Escape of granule contents from the cell interior during fusion of the granule with a developing phagosome that is still open to the exterior
- Release of lysosomal enzymes on the death and dissolution of the phagocyte (the life span of a circulating neutrophil is only 6 hours)
- Uncommon situations in which the plasma membrane of a neutrophil cannot surround a particle attached to a flat surface (e.g., the glomerular basement membrane), in which case the contents of the granules that have fused with the invaginated membrane are released to the exterior

It deserves emphasis that the same enzymes that are beneficial when active intracellularly during phagocytosis are harmful to the tissues when released to the extracellular environment.

The biological activities of extracellular proteases, such as elastase and cathepsin G, are regulated by inhibitors in plasma and tissue fluids. For example, α_1-antitrypsin is synthesized by hepatocytes and is the primary inhibitor of neutrophil elastase. The importance of this inhibitory activity is evident in persons with a genetic deficiency of α1-antiprotease. Such persons develop pulmonary emphysema, presumably as a result of the lack of elastase inhibitory activity. Another antiprotease in plasma is α2-macroglobulin, a protein that also inhibits elastase and cathepsin G activities. Additionally, both α1-antiprotease and α2-macroglobulin inhibit the activities of plasmin, trypsin, and chymotrypsin. **Thus, circulating serum inhibitors not only block protease activity derived from phagocytic cells but also inhibit protease activity generated within the plasma and tissues.**

Another class of protease inhibitors secreted by macrophages and mesenchymal cells (e.g., fibroblasts) plays an important role in regulating the activity of metalloproteinases, including phagocytic cell collagenases and gelatinase. Collectively referred to as tissue inhibitors of metalloproteinases (TIMPs), these proteins bind metalloproteinases and block the degradation of extracellular matrix. Changes in the relative secretion of metalloproteinases and TIMPs are critical for the regulation of extracellular matrix turnover and the modulation of tissue injury and repair (see Chapter 3).

Activated Oxygen

Similar to lysosomal enzymes, the activated oxygen species that mediate the bactericidal activity of phagocytes and endothelial cell–derived NO· can produce tissue injury in extracellular sites. Unlike granular enzymes, specific oxygen metabolites diffuse through the plasma membrane. Reactive oxygen metabolites injure cells and tissues by the following mechanisms:

- Lipid peroxidation
- DNA damage
- Oxidation of the sulfhydryl groups in proteins
- Degradation of extracellular matrix components

Phagocytic Cell Adherence

The adherence of phagocytic cells to their targets is associated with increased cytotoxicity and the degradation of substrates. The ability of phagocytic cells to recognize and adhere to a target serves to "focus" the functional responses of the cell along the adherent surface. For instance, when stimulated phagocytic cells cling to basement membranes, the production of reactive oxygen metabolites is greatest at the point of attachment. Moreover, this is also the site of greatest lysosomal degranulation. In addition, close approximation of the phagocytic cell to its target also serves to exclude macromolecular inhibitors (e.g., α_1-antitrypsin) from the interface between the cell and the substrate.

In summary, tissue injury produced by inflammatory cells is related to the pathogenesis of several diseases, for instance pulmonary emphysema, rheumatoid arthritis, certain immune complex diseases, gout, and the adult respiratory distress syndrome. Phagocytic cell adherence, the escape of reactive oxygen metabolites, and the release of lysosomal enzymes function in a synergistic manner to enhance cytotoxicity and tissue degradation.

Diseases Associated with Defects in Phagocytosis

The importance of the protection afforded by acute inflammatory cells is emphasized by the frequency and severity of infections in persons with defective phagocytic cells. **The most common defect is actually iatrogenic neutropenia secondary to cancer chemotherapy.** Functional impairment of phagocytic cells may occur almost anywhere in the sequence that includes adherence, emigration, chemotaxis, and phagocytosis. These disorders may be acquired or congenital. Acquired diseases such as leukemia, diabetes mellitus, malnutrition, viral infections, and sepsis are often accompanied by defects in inflammatory cell function (Table 2-5). Representative examples of congenital diseases linked to defective phagocytic function are shown in Table 2-4.

TABLE 2-5 Causes of Acquired Defects in Phagocytic Cell Locomotion

Overwhelming infections
Severe trauma or burn
Diabetes mellitus
Chronic debilitating disease

CHRONIC INFLAMMATION

Chronic inflammation may be a sequel to acute inflammation or an immune response to a foreign antigen. The process may become chronic if the inflammatory response is unable to eliminate the injurious agent or restore injured tissue to its normal state. **Chronic inflammation primarily serves to contain and remove a pathological agent or process within a tissue.**

The cellular components of the chronic inflammatory response are (1) macrophages, (2) plasma cells, (3) lymphocytes, and, in certain conditions, (4) eosinophils. Chronic inflammation is mediated by both immunological and nonimmunological mechanisms and is frequently observed in conjunction with reparative responses, namely, granulation tissue and fibrosis (see Chapter 3).

The macrophage is the pivotal cell in regulating the reactions that lead to chronic inflammation. It functions as a source of both inflammatory and immunological mediators (Fig. 2-32). The accumulation of macrophages mainly reflects the recruitment of circulating monocytes by chemotactic stimuli and their differentiation in tissues (Fig. 2-33). The local proliferation of resident tissue macrophages may also contribute, albeit to a lesser degree, to the local increase in mononuclear phagocytes. In addition to generating inflammatory mediators, macrophages regulate lymphocyte responses to antigens and secrete other mediators that modulate the proliferation and function of fibroblasts and endothelial cells (see Chapter 4).

Plasma cells also participate in the chronic inflammatory response (Fig. 2-34). These lymphoid cells, which are rich in rough endoplasmic reticulum, are the primary source of antibodies. The production of antibody to specific antigens at sites of chronic inflammation is important in antigen neutralization, clearance of foreign antigens and particles, and antibody-dependent cell-mediated cytotoxicity.

Lymphocytes are a prominent feature of chronic inflammatory reactions (Fig. 2-35) and perform vital functions in both humoral and cell-mediated immune responses. T lymphocytes not only function in the regulation of macrophage activation and recruitment through the secretion of specific mediators (lymphokines) but also modulate antibody production and cell-mediated cytotoxicity. Recently, NK cells and specialized forms of lymphocytes (e.g., T cells, CD5 B cells) have been implicated as participants in the defense against viral and bacterial

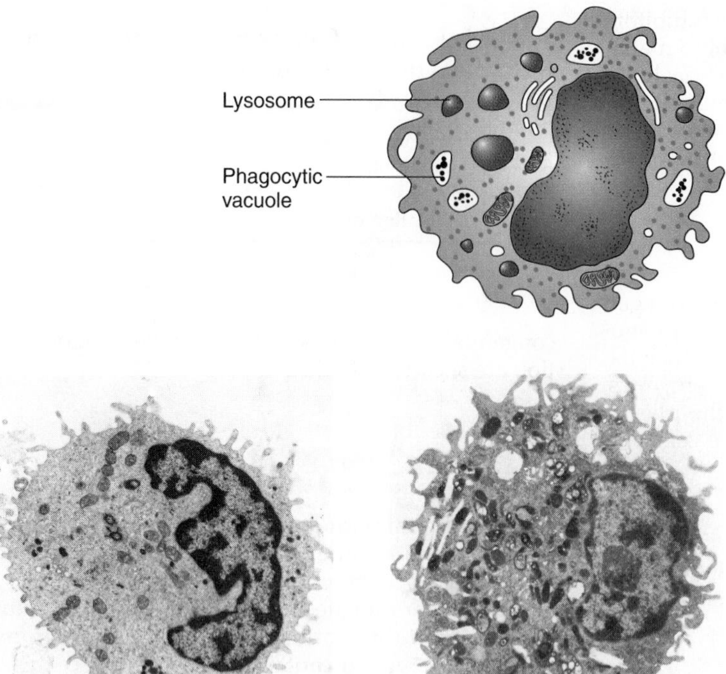

CHARACTERISTICS AND FUNCTIONS
- Regulates inflammatory response
- Regulates coagulation/fibrinolytic pathway
- Regulates immune response (see Chapt. 4)

PRIMARY INFLAMMATORY MEDIATORS
- cytokines
  - -IL-1
  - -TNF-α
  - -IL-6
  - -Chemokines (e.g. IL-8, MCP-1)
- lysosomal enzymes
  - -acid hydrolases
  - -serine proteases
  - -metalloproteases (e.g. collagenase)
- cationic proteins
- prostaglandins/leukotrienes
- plasminogen activator
- procoagulant activity
- oxygen metabolite formation

FIGURE 2-32
Monocyte/macrophage: morphology and function.

infections. Their activity does not require previous sensitization to foreign antigens.

Eosinophils are occasionally a conspicuous component of the chronic inflammatory response. They are particularly evident during allergic-type reactions and parasitic infestations. Eosinophils share many functional features with the neutrophil. Their rhomboid, crystalloid granules are rich in acid phosphatase and have a specific peroxidase activity (Fig. 2-36). As previously noted, the granules also contain unique basic proteins that are toxic to certain parasites and normal host cells. The precise role of eosinophils in chronic inflammatory reactions is less clear.

Polymorphonuclear leukocytes, although characteristic of acute inflammation, may also be observed at sites of chronic inflammation.

Acute inflammation and chronic inflammation represent ends of a dynamic continuum, in which the morphological features of these inflammatory responses frequently overlap.

Chronic Inflammation as a Primary Response

The presence of cells characteristic of chronic inflammation does not necessarily imply the existence of persistent inflammation. A chronic inflammatory infiltrate is the primary response to viral infections, certain autoimmune diseases, parasitic infestations, and malignant tumors. Cell killing by cytotoxic T lymphocytes or by antibody-dependent mechanisms is often associated with chronic inflammation in many viral diseases, including influenza A pneumonia, viral hepatitis, and viral myocarditis. Similarly, a chronic inflammatory response may be observed in association with certain cancers. In this circumstance, the presence of chronic inflammatory cells, especially macrophages and T lymphocytes, may be the morphological expression of an immune response to the cancer. Many autoimmune diseases, including rheumatoid arthritis, chronic thyroiditis, and primary biliary cirrhosis, are characterized by a chronic inflammatory response in the affected tissues, which may be associated with the activation of both antibody-dependent and cell-mediated immune mechanisms. It is thought that the autoimmune response accounts for cellular injury in the affected organs. Varying degrees of fibrosis may also be present, depending on the extent of tissue injury and the persistence of the pathological stimulus and inflammatory response.

Lymphadenitis

Localized acute inflammation and chronic inflammation both lead to a reaction in the lymphatics and lymph nodes that drain the affected tissue. Inflammatory mediators generated at sites of injury, as well as necrotic debris, drain into the lymphatic system and flow to the regional lymph nodes. Severe injury thus causes secondary inflammation of the lymphatic channels (lymphangitis) and lymph nodes (lymphadenitis). This response represents either a nonspecific reaction to mediators released from the injured tissue or an immunological response to a specific foreign antigen.

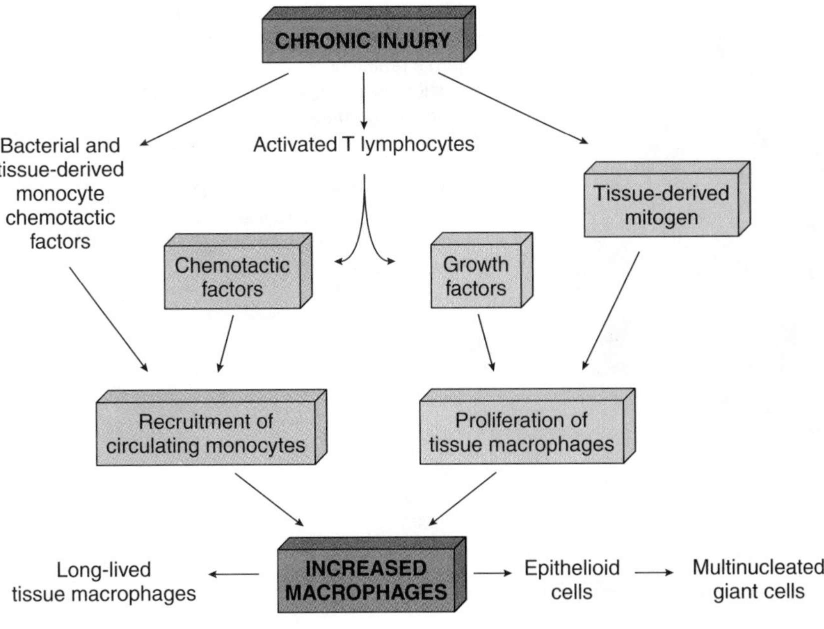

FIGURE 2-33
The accumulation of macrophages in chronic inflammation.

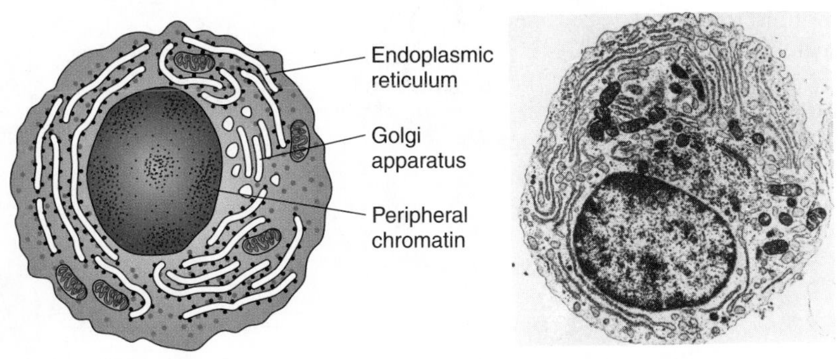

CHARACTERISTICS AND FUNCTIONS

- Associated with:
  - -antibody synthesis and secretion
  - -chronic inflammation
- Derived from B lymphocytes

FIGURE 2-34
Plasma cell: morphology and function.

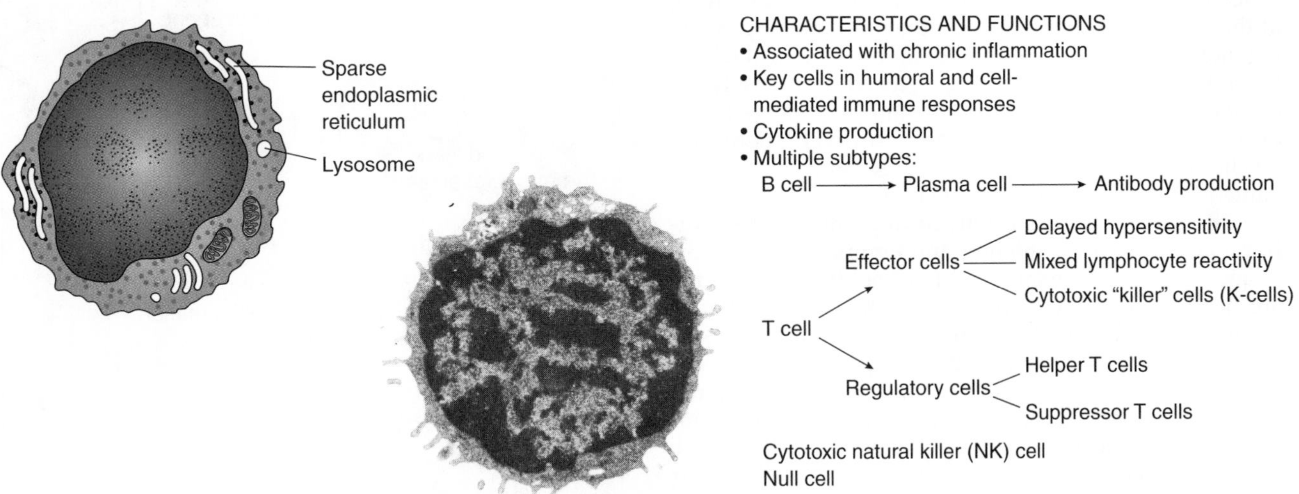

FIGURE 2-35
Lymphocyte: morphology and function.

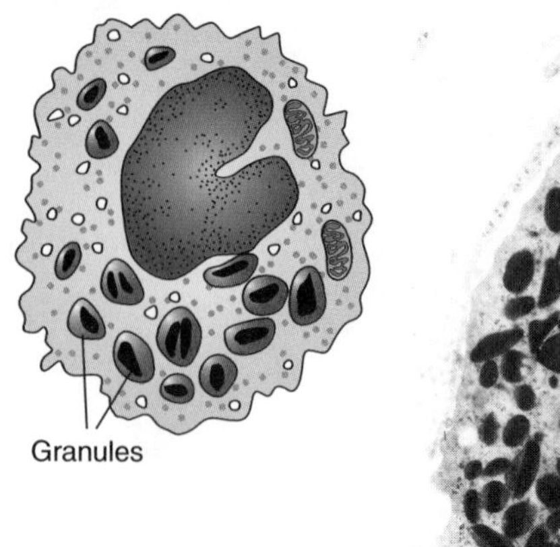

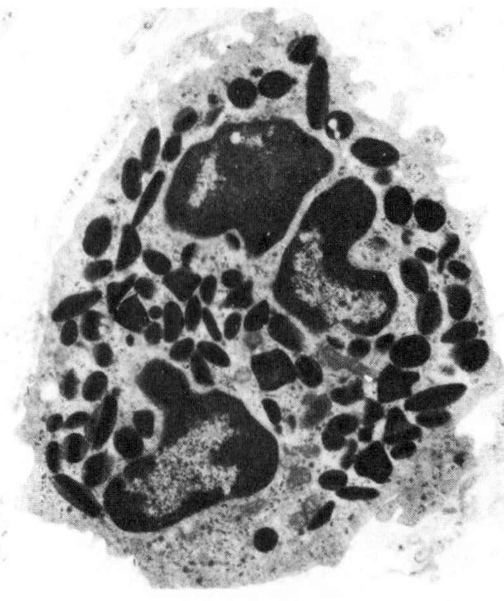

CHARACTERISTICS AND FUNCTIONS
- Associated with:
  - -Allergic reactions
  - -Parasite-associated inflammatory reactions
  - -Chronic inflammation
- Modulates mast cell-mediated reactions

PRIMARY INFLAMMATORY MEDIATORS
- Reactive oxygen metabolites
- Lysosomal granule enzymes (primary crystalloid granules)
  - -Major basic protein
  - -Eosinophil cationic protein
  - -Eosinophil peroxidase
  - -Acid phosphatase
  - -β-glucuronidase
  - -Arylsulfatase B
  - -Histaminase
- Phospholipase D
- Prostaglandins of E series
- Cytokines

FIGURE *2-36*
Eosinophil: morphology and function.

Clinically, the inflamed lymphatic channels in the skin manifest as red streaks, and the lymph nodes themselves are enlarged and painful. Microscopically, the lymph nodes exhibit hyperplasia of the lymphoid follicles and proliferation of mononuclear phagocytes in the sinuses (sinus histiocytosis). The presence of painful palpable lymph nodes is more commonly associated with inflammatory processes, whereas firm nonpainful lymph nodes are characteristic of neoplasms.

GRANULOMATOUS INFLAMMATION

Neutrophils ordinarily remove agents that incite an acute inflammatory response by phagocytosis and digestion. However, there are circumstances in which the substances that provoke the acute inflammatory reaction cannot be digested by the reacting neutrophils. Such a situation is potentially dangerous, because it might lead to a vicious circle of phagocytosis, failure of digestion, death of the neutrophil, and release of the undigested, provoking agent. The offending material, once free of the neutrophil, would again be phagocytosed by a newly recruited neutrophil. The result would be persistent and destructive acute inflammation. However, there is a mechanism for dealing with indigestible substances, namely, granulomatous inflammation (Fig. 2-37).

The principal cells involved in granulomatous inflammation are macrophages and lymphocytes. Macrophages are much longer lived than neutrophils. If they are not killed by the noxious agent that incites the inflammatory reaction, they can sequester it in their cytoplasm for indefinite periods, thereby preventing it from continuing to provoke an acute inflammatory reaction.

Macrophages are mobile cells that continuously migrate through the extravascular connective tissues of the body. Their recruitment to sites of injury, as well as their activation, is regulated by the local generation of chemotactic factors: bacterial products (e.g., LPS) and cytokines secreted by activated T lymphocytes. Several cytokines

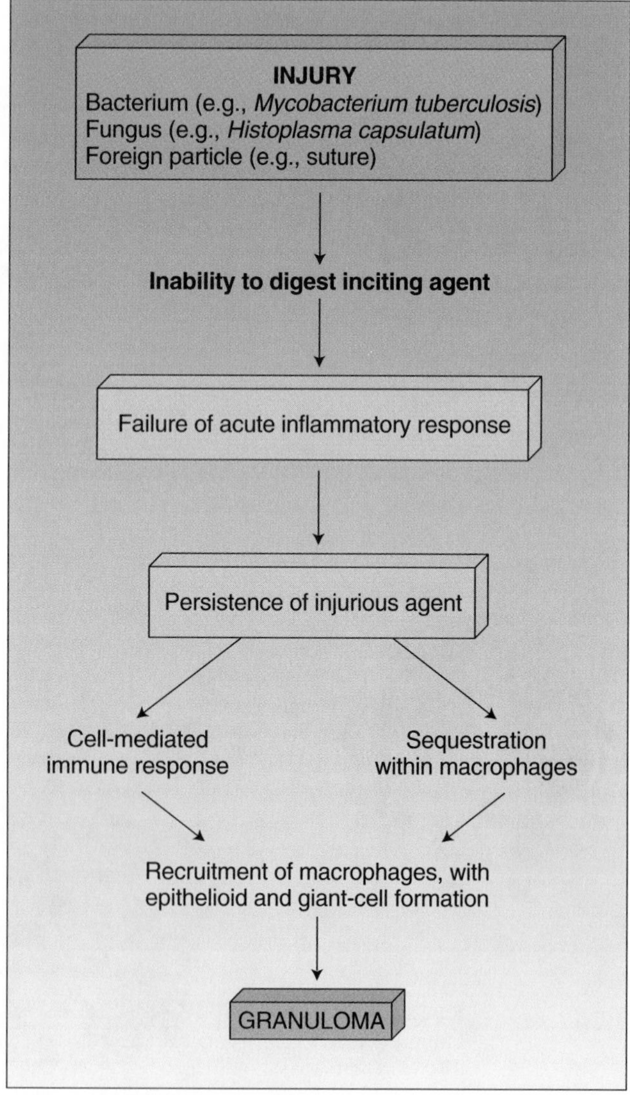

FIGURE 2-37
Mechanism of granuloma formation.

stimulate macrophage function (e.g., IFN-γ), whereas others inhibit macrophage activation (e.g., IL-4, IL-10). Thus, lymphocytes are vital for regulating the development and resolution of inflammatory responses.

After amassing substances that they cannot digest, the macrophages lose their motility and accumulate at the site of injury. Macrophages then undergo a characteristic change in their structure that transforms them into **epithelioid cells**. The latter have considerably more pale cytoplasm than monocytes and tissue macrophages and are so-named because of their resemblance to epithelial cells. **Nodular collections of epithelioid cells form granulomas, which are the morphological hallmark of granulomatous inflammation.**

Granulomas are small (<2 mm) collections of epithelioid cells, which are frequently surrounded by a rim of lymphocytes (Fig. 2-38). Unlike circulating monocytes, epithelioid cells have vacuoles and numerous lysosomal granules. In addition, granulomas are populated by multinucleated giant cells, which are formed by the cytoplasmic fusion of macrophages. Such cells may contain up to 50 separate nuclei. When the nuclei are arranged around the periphery of the cell in a horseshoe pattern, the cell is termed a **Langhans giant cell** (Fig. 2-39). Frequently, a foreign pathogenic agent (e.g., silica or a *Histoplasma* spore) or other indigestible material is identified within the cytoplasm of a multinucleated giant cell, in which case the term **foreign body giant cell** is used (Fig. 2-40). Giant cells are functionally inactive. All the other cell types characteristic of chronic inflammation, including lymphocytes, eosinophils, and fibroblasts, may also be associated with granulomas.

Despite the long life of macrophages in granulomatous reactions, these cells do turn over, albeit slowly. On the death of the macrophage, the offending indigestible agent is released and may continue to provoke an acute inflammatory reaction in granulomas that have been present for months or years. Thus, many granulomatous reactions display variable numbers of PMNs. The turnover of epithelioid cells is also influenced by the toxicity of the inciting agent. The more inert the agent, the slower the turnover of the cells.

The fate of a granulomatous reaction is influenced not only by the cytotoxicity of the inciting agent but also by its immunogenicity. Immunological sensitivity may develop to a noxious agent that is slowly released from macrophages and epithelioid cells. In particular, cell-mediated immune responses to the inciting agent may modify the granulomatous reaction by recruiting and activating more macrophages and lymphocytes.

Figure 2-37 summarizes the mechanisms in the generation of granulomatous inflammation. Granulomatous inflammation is typical of the tissue response elicited by fungal infections, tuberculosis, leprosy, schistosomiasis, and the presence of foreign material (e.g., suture or talc). It is characteristically associated with areas of caseous necrosis produced by infectious agents, particularly *Mycobacterium tuberculosis*. Some diseases of unknown etiology, especially sarcoidosis, are distinguished by florid granulomatous inflammation, although the inciting agent is not apparent.

SYSTEMIC MANIFESTATIONS OF INFLAMMATION

The objective of the inflammatory response is to (1) confine the area of injury, (2) clear the inciting pathological agent and damaged tissue, and (3) restore function to the tissue. However, under certain conditions, local injury may result in prominent systemic effects that can themselves be debilitating. Many times, these effects are the result of a pathogen entering the bloodstream, a condition known as sepsis. This event can result in systemic activation of mediator systems in the plasma and inflammatory cells. Alternatively, the local injury may be severe and lead to the release of inflammatory mediators, especially cytokines, into the circulation, thereby causing systemic effects. The most prominent systemic manifestations of

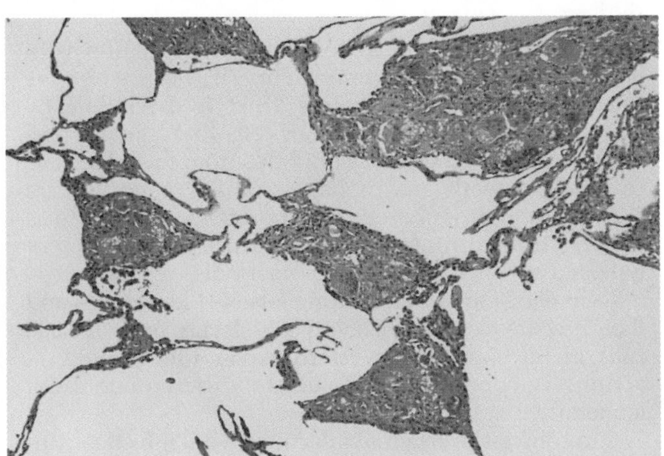

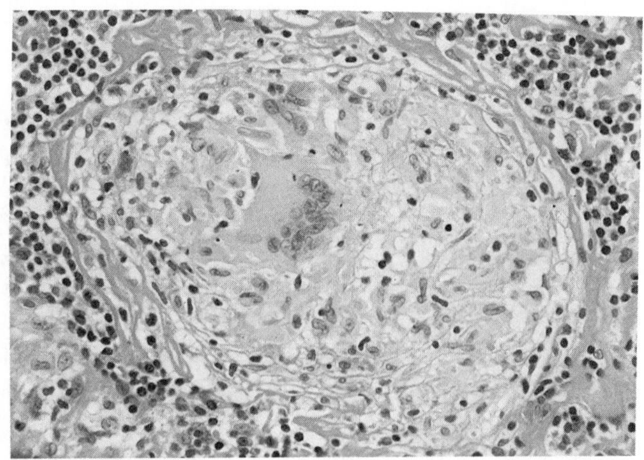

FIGURE 2-38
Granulomatous inflammation. *(A)* Section of lung from a patient with sarcoidosis reveals numerous discrete granulomas. *(B)* A higher-power photomicrograph of a single graunuloma in a lymph node from the same patient depicts a multinucleated giant cell amid numerous pale epithelioid cells. A thin rim of fibrosis separates the granuloma from the lymphoid cells of the node.

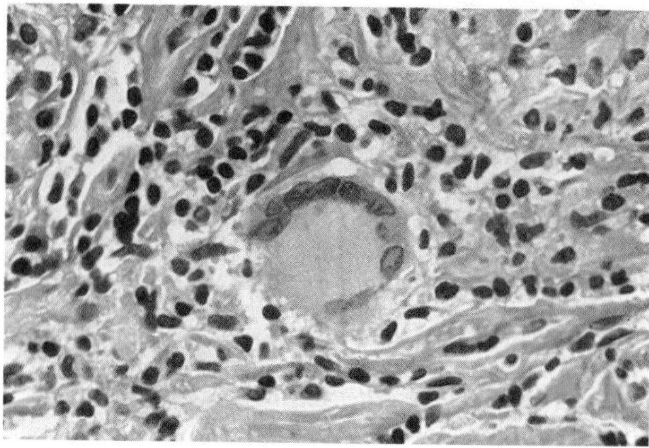

FIGURE 2-39
A Langhans giant cell shows nuclei arranged on the periphery of an abundant cytoplasm.

inflammation are as follows:

- Fever
- Shock
- Leukocytosis
- Leukopenia
- Acute phase response

Fever

Fever is a clinical hallmark of inflammation. There is scant evidence that the release of exogenous pyrogens (molecules that cause fever) by bacteria, viruses, or injured cells directly affect the hypothalamic thermoregulatory center. Rather, they stimulate the production of endogenous pyrogens, namely IL-1, IL-6, and TNF-α. IL-1 is a 15-kd protein that is released by macrophages following exposure to bacterial endotoxin, viruses, or lymphocyte products. IL-1 stimulates prostaglandin synthesis in the hypothalamic thermoregulatory centers, thereby altering the "thermostat" that controls body temperature. Inhibitors of cyclooxygenase (e.g., aspirin) block the fever response by inhibiting IL-1-stimulated PGE_2 synthesis in the hypothalamus. TNF-α and IL-6 also increase body temperature by a direct action on the hypothalamus. In addition, TNF-α promotes the release of IL-1 from macrophages, and both IL-1 and TNF-α induce IL-6 synthesis in the liver.

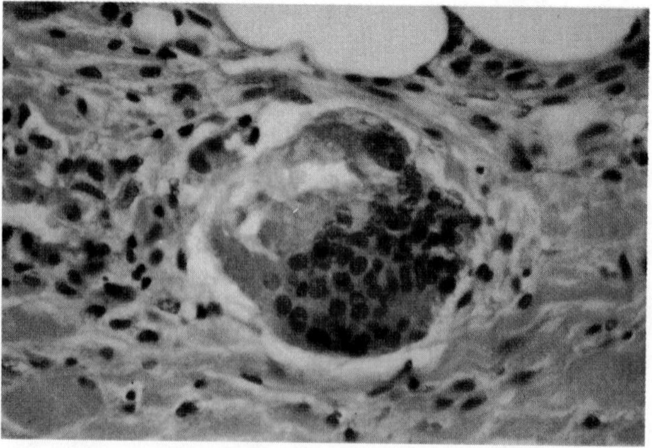

FIGURE 2-40
Foreign body giant cell. The numerous nuclei are randomly arranged in the cytoplasm.

Shock

As discussed previously, TNF-α is one of the primary cytokine mediators associated with the inflammatory response, protecting the host against bacterial infection. However, under conditions of massive tissue injury or infection that spreads to the blood (sepsis), significant amounts of TNF-α may be generated in the circulation. Under those circumstances, even small quantities of this cytokine can have deleterious effects on the patient. Systemic vasodilatation, with increased vascular permeability and intravascular volume loss, may lead to hypotension and shock (see Chapter 6). In severe cases, systemic activation of the coagulation pathways may also occur, generating microthrombi throughout the body with consumption of clotting components and subsequent predisposition to bleeding. This condition is defined as disseminated intravascular coagulation and can result in multisystem organ failure and death (see Chapter 20).

Leukocytosis

Leukocytosis is defined as an increase in the number of circulating leukocytes and commonly accompanies acute inflammation. Leukocytosis presents as a twofold to threefold increase in the number of leukocytes; the predominant cells are usually PMNs **(neutrophilia)**. An increase in the number of immature PMNs ("band" forms) may also be seen in the peripheral blood.

Neutrophilia is most common in association with bacterial infections and tissue injury. It is caused by the release of specific mediators (IL-1 and TNF-α) by macrophages and perhaps other cells that initially promote an accelerated release of PMNs from the bone marrow. Subsequently, macrophages and T lymphocytes are stimulated to produce a group of proteins, referred to as **colony-stimulating factors**, that induce proliferation of bone marrow hemopoietic precursor cells.

On occasion, the circulating levels of leukocytes and their precursors may reach very high levels, up to 100,000 cells/μl. Such a situation, referred to as a **leukemoid reaction**, is sometimes difficult to differentiate from leukemia.

In contrast to bacterial infections, viral infections (including infectious mononucleosis) are characterized by an absolute increase in the number of circulating lymphocytes **(lymphocytosis)**. Parasitic infestations and certain allergic reactions cause an increase in the number of eosinophils in the peripheral blood **(eosinophilia)**. Eosinophils, which normally constitute 1% to 3% of pe-

TABLE 2-6 **Acute Phase Proteins**

Protein	Function
Mannose binding protein	Opsonization/complement activation
C-reactive protein	Opsonization
α_1-Antitrypsin	Serine protease inhibitor
Haptoglobin	Binds hemoglobin
Ceruloplasmin	Antioxidant, binds copper
Fibrinogen	Coagulation
Serum amyloid A protein	Apolipoprotein
α_2-Macroglobulin	Antiprotease
Cysteine protease inhibitor	Antiprotease

ripheral leukocytes, can reach levels as high as 90% in some parasitic infections, particularly trichinosis.

Leukopenia

Leukopenia is defined as an absolute decrease in the circulating white cell count. It is occasionally encountered under conditions of chronic inflammation, especially in patients who are malnourished or who suffer from a chronic debilitating disease such as disseminated cancer. Leukopenia may also be caused by typhoid fever and certain viral and rickettsial infections. The mechanisms responsible for the suppression of leukopoiesis are not well understood.

Acute Phase Response

The acute phase response is a regulated physiological reaction that occurs in inflammatory conditions. It is characterized clinically by fever, leukocytosis, decreased appetite and altered sleep patterns, and chemically by changes in the plasma levels of **acute phase proteins.** These proteins are a group of molecules (Table 2-6) synthesized primarily by hepatocytes and released in large numbers into the circulation in response to an acute inflammatory challenge. Changes in the plasma levels of acute phase proteins are mediated primarily by IL-1, IL-6, and TNF-α. These cytokines bind to specific receptors on hepatocytes, thereby inducing the synthesis of acute phase proteins. Several of these proteins, for example, the opsonins MBP and C-reactive protein, participate directly in host defense mechanisms. Increased plasma levels of some acute phase proteins are reflected in an accelerated **erythrocyte sedimentation rate**, which is a qualitative index used clinically to monitor the activity of many inflammatory diseases.

SUGGESTED READING

BOOKS

Gallin JI, Goldstein IM, Snyderman R (eds): *Inflammation: Basic principles and clinical correlates,* 2nd ed. New York: Raven Press, 1992.

Janeway CA, Travers P: *Immunobiology,* 2nd ed. New York: Garland, 1996.

Kelley WN, Harris ED, Ruddy S, Sledge CB (eds): *Textbook of rheumatology,* 4th ed. Philadelphia: WB Saunders, 1993.

REVIEW ARTICLES

Albeda SM, Buck CA: Integrins and other cell adhesion molecules. *FASEB J* 4:2868–2880, 1990.

Arai KI, Lee F, Miyajima A, Miyatake S, Arai N, Yokota T: Cytokines: Coordinators of immune and inflammatory responses. *Ann Rev Biochem* 59:783–836, 1990.

Ben-Baruch A, Michiel DF, Oppenheim JJ: Signals and receptors involved in the recruitment of inflammatory cells. *J Biol Chem* 270:11703–11706, 1995.

Gura T: Chemokines take center stage in inflammatory ills. *Science* 272:954–956, 1996.

Ley K, Tedder TF: Leukocyte interactions with vascular endothelium: New insights into selectin-mediated attachment and rolling. *J Immunol* 155:525–528, 1995.

Springer TA: Traffic signals for lymphocyte recirculation and leukocyte emigration: The multistep paradigm. *Cell* 76:301–314, 1994.

Stossel TP: On the crawling of animal cells. *Science* 260:1086–1094, 1993.

Tracey KJ, Cerami A: Tumor necrosis factor, cytokines and disease. *Ann Rev Cell Biol* 9:317–343, 1993.

CHAPTER 3

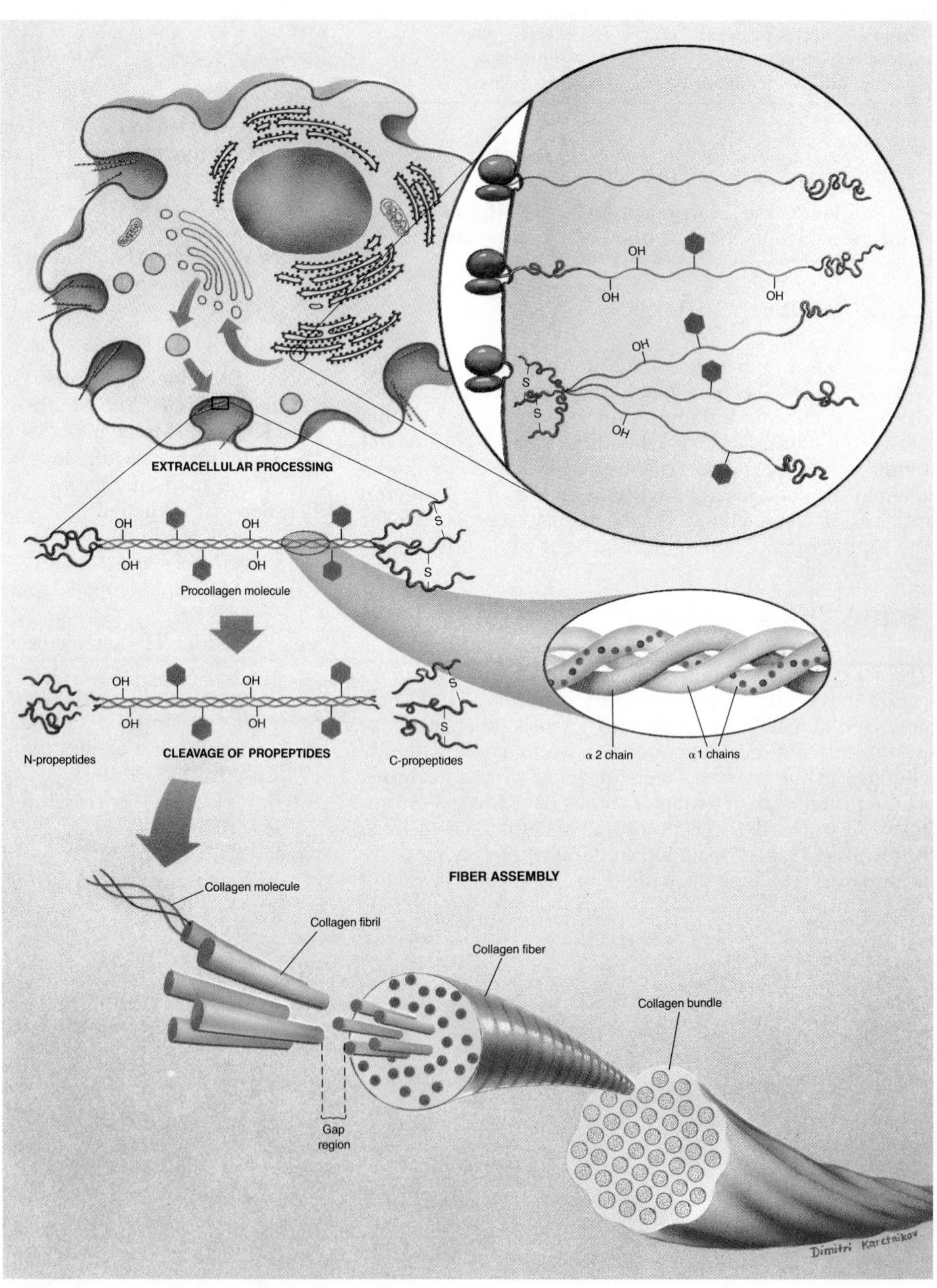

OH
OH
OH
S
S
OH
OH
EXTRACELLULAR PROCESSING
OH
OH
S
OH
OH
S
Procollagen molecule
OH
OH
S
OH
OH
S
N-propeptides
CLEAVAGE OF PROPEPTIDES
C-propeptides
α 2 chain
α 1 chains
FIBER ASSEMBLY
Collagen molecule
Collagen fibril
Collagen fiber
Collagen bundle
Gap
region
Dimitri Karetnikov

Repair, Regeneration, and Fibrosis

Antonio Martinez-Hernandez

FIGURE 3-1 *(see opposite page)*
Collagen synthesis, secretion, and assembly. The initial steps of collagen synthesis, that is, translation by membrane-bound ribosomes and passage of the nascent chains into the rough endoplasmic reticulum (RER), follow pathways common to all proteins destined for secretion. (1) In the cisternae of the RER, the pre-propeptide sequences are removed, (2) proline and lysine residues become hydroxylated, (3) the propeptides are glycosylated, (4) individual α chains associate by disulfide bonds, and (5) triple helices are formed. After all these post-translational modifications have taken place, individual procollagen molecules are secreted into the extracellular space. In the case of type I collagen, at least, the propeptides must be cleaved before fiber assembly can occur. Several collagen molecules associate in a quarter-staggered manner to form collagen fibrils, and fibrils associate to form collagen fibers with the characteristic cross-banding. In turn, collagen fibers associate to form bundles recognizable by light microscopy.

Humans are constantly subjected to injuries that result in cell death and tissue destruction. Healing is part of the response to this injury and represents an attempt to maintain normal structure and function. It overlaps the inflammatory process, and it is only for didactic purposes that the two are separated. Some primitive organisms can replace almost any cell or tissue with a new one, a process called regeneration. Invertebrates and amphibians can actually regenerate lost parts: lobsters regrow lost claws, salamanders develop a new lens from the iris, and newts replace lost extremities.

When a newt's limb is amputated, the epidermal cells adjacent to the wound divide and rapidly cover the stump. As epithelial cell proliferation continues, the cells pile up at the apex, forming an apical cap. The connective tissue cells in the stump—fibroblasts, myocytes, and osteocytes—then divide. The daughter cells lack some of the differentiated properties of the parent cells as a result of a process termed dedifferentiation. The original dense extracellular matrix in the stump is catabolized and replaced by a loose, edematous stroma resembling embryonic mesenchyme (blastema). The blastemal cells multiply rapidly, endothelial cells proliferate and vascularize the blastema, and orderly differentiation into bone, muscle, tendon, and blood vessels follows. The end result is the accurate replacement of the lost part (epigenetic regeneration).

In mammals, the granulation tissue formed during wound healing is reminiscent of the amphibian blastema. However, rather than forming a limb, granulation tissue matures only into dense connective tissue and eventuates in a scar. The replacement of lost tissue by scar tissue is termed repair. The major components of the repair reaction are the extracellular matrix and the cells.

THE EXTRACELLULAR MATRIX

The extracellular matrix is a stable complex of macromolecules that underlies epithelial cells and surrounds connective tissue cells. **A matrix must contain molecular information in order to direct cellular migration, attachment, differentiation, and organization.** The information contained in the extracellular matrix is as important for development as it is for wound healing. The importance of various components of the extracellular matrix for a multicellular organism is underscored by the fact that the production of collagen, laminin, and fibronectin occurs as early as the cleavage stage of the fertilized ovum.

The extracellular matrix not only provides tissues with structural support but also exchanges information with cells, thereby modulating a host of processes, including development, cell migration, attachment, differentiation, and repair. It plays a crucial role in wound healing through its chemotactic, opsonic, and attachment properties. The strength of the healed wound and the properties of the scar ultimately depend on the deposition of an adequate extracellular matrix.

The extracellular matrix has five major components: collagens, basement membranes, elastic fibers, structural glycoproteins, and proteoglycans.

The Collagens

The collagens are a family of closely related proteins that have common properties. In spite of the differences in tertiary structure, physical properties, and biological context, the collagens of invertebrates, fish, reptiles, birds, and mammals share the same plan. A third of their amino acid content is glycine, and they are rich in the amino acids serine, proline, threonine, and alanine. These four amino acids are encoded in nucleotide triplets that differ from each other only in the first nucleotide of the code; the second and third bases, namely cytosine and uracil are common. Fibrillar proteins with great apparent disparities—for example, the invertebrate fibroin, silk, and resilin, as well as human collagens and elastin—share this common plan. It is likely that the present collagen polymorphism reflects evolution from a single primordial gene.

Collagens contain repeating triplet sequences of amino acids (Gly-X-Y) and are rich in two hydroxylated amino acids, hydroxyproline and hydroxylysine. A glycine in every third position imparts a right-handed helicity to each polypeptide chain. The collagen molecule itself is formed by three polypeptide chains, which intertwine in a left-handed supercoil to form a triple helical rope. The individual polypeptide chains, encoded in separate genes, are designated by the Greek letter α. An Arabic numeral after the α designates the constituent chains of the trimer. For example, type I collagen consists of two $\alpha 1$ chains and one $\alpha 2$ chain. The different trimers are designated by Roman numerals and represent the collagen

TABLE 3-1 Genetically Distinct Vertebrate Collagen Types

Type	Chains	Macromolecular Association	Aggregate Form	Localization
I	α1(I), α2(I)			Most abundant collagen: Ubiquitous—skin, bone, etc.
II	α1(II)			Major cartilage collagen: Cartilage, vitreous humor
III	α1(III)			Abundant in pliable tissues: Blood vessels, uterus, skin, etc.
IV	α1(IV), α2(IV)			All basement membranes
V	α1(V), α2(V), α3(V)	???		Minor component of most interstitial tissues
VI	α1(VI), α2(VI)			Abundant in most interstitial tissues
VII	α1(VII)			? Anchoring fibrils
VIII	α1(VIII)	???		Produced by some endothelia
IX	α1(IX), α2(IX), α3(IX)	???		Cartilage
X	α1(X)	???		Mineralizing cartilage

types. The different types of collagen are distinguished by placing the appropriate Roman numeral in parentheses after the Arabic numeral, for example, α1(I) and α1(III). A heteropolymer is a collagen molecule composed of at least two different α chains, whereas in a homopolymer the three chains are identical. At least 19 genetically distinct collagen types have been described, representing the products of some 33 genes. The composition and distribution of 10 collagen types are summarized in Table 3-1.

- **Type I collagen: This is the major collagen of bone, skin, and tendon and the predominant collagen in mature scars.** It is a heteropolymer that consists of two α1(I) chains and one α2(I) chain $[\alpha1(I)]_2\ \alpha2(I)$. By electron microscopy, type I collagen appears as cross-banded fibers with 67-nm periodicity (Figs. 3-1 and 3-2). A homopolymer of this collagen type $[\alpha1(I)]_3$, consisting of three α1(I) chains, is found in some chronic inflammatory conditions.

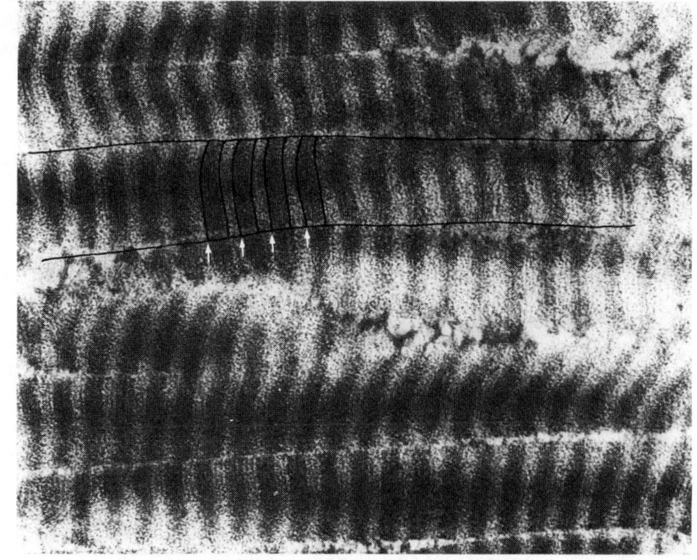
A

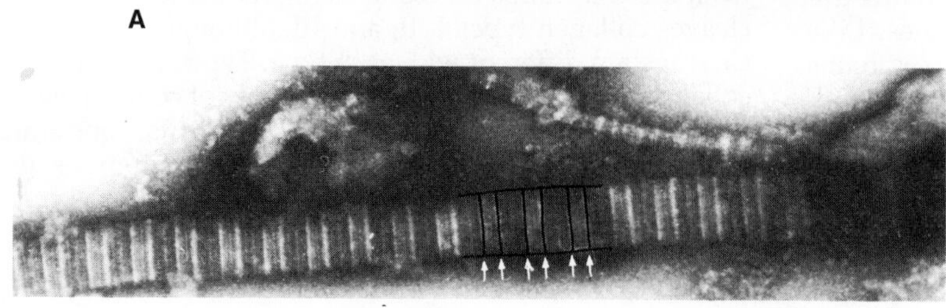
B

FIGURE 3-2
Collagen fibers viewed by electron microscopy. (*A*) Groups of parallel collagen fibers form a collagen bundle. The characteristic cross-banding (repeating bands at 67 nm) is distinct (*arrows*). (*B*) Isolated collagen fibers were negatively stained. The conspicuous cross-banding is due to penetration of the metallic stain at the gap regions (see Fig. 3-1).

- **Type II collagen: This is the major collagen in cartilage and has also been found in the vitreous humor and the nucleus pulposus.** It contains three identical $[\alpha1(II)]_3$ chains. Type II collagen fibers are thinner than those of type I and exhibit a barely discernible periodicity.
- **Type III collagen: This collagen is abundant in embryonic tissues, and in the adult it predominates in pliable organs, such as blood vessels, the uterus, and the gastrointestinal tract.** It is a homopolymer, $[\alpha1(III)]_3$, that appears as thin, beaded filaments, often associated with type I fibers. Type III is the first collagen deposited in wound healing.

Collagen types I, II, and II are rich in alanine, contain fewer hydroxylated residues than the other collagen types, and are resistant to nonspecific proteases.

- **Type IV collagen: This component of the extracellular matrix is found exclusively in basement membranes.** Type IV collagen does not form individual fibers but associates with laminin and other matrix components to constitute basement membranes. Six distinct chains have been identified in this collagen, namely $\alpha1$(IV) to $\alpha6$(IV). Their exact ratio in any basement membrane is not established, but it is likely that both homopolymers and heteropolymers exist. Whereas other collagens are subjected to cleavage of propeptides to form definitive molecules, type IV collagen is incorporated into aggregates without such cleavage. The collagenous triple helix of type IV collagen is interrupted at several sites by globular domains that are susceptible to nonspecific proteases.
- **Type V collagen:** This protein is widely distributed in most tissues, but never as a major component. Three constituent chains of type V collagen have been identified—$\alpha1$(V), $\alpha2$(V), and $\alpha3$(V). Several homopolymers and heteropolymers have been reported. Type V collagen forms thin, delicate, nonbanded filaments, often connecting type I fibers to each other and to other structures.
- **Type VI collagen: This collagen is prevalent in most connective tissues.** The triple helical domain makes up only one third of the polypeptide chain in this collagen type; the globular domains at both ends contribute the remainder. Type VI collagen forms delicate filaments resembling those of type V collagen.

Collagen Biosynthesis

The steps in the synthesis, secretion, and assembly of collagen into extracellular structures are summarized in Figure 3-1.

1. **Synthesis:** The individual polypeptide chains are synthesized on membrane-bound ribosomes. Like other export proteins, these pre-procollagen chains contain signal sequences at the amino-terminal end, which are cleaved shortly after translation. The resulting procollagen chains display extension peptides (propeptides) at both ends of the molecule. The pro-α chains therefore have three major domains: the α-chain, the amino-terminal peptide, and the carboxy-terminal p]eptide.
2. **Formation of procollagen:** In the cisternae of the rough endoplasmic reticulum, three pro-chains interact to form a procollagen molecule.
3. **Intracellular processing:** Hydroxylation of proline and lysine residues, glycosylation, chain association, disulfide bonding, and triple helix formation take place before the secretion of collagen. **Hydroxylation of the collagen polypeptide requires vitamin C, a need that explains the inadequate wound healing characteristic of vitamin C deficiency (scurvy).** All collagens are glycoproteins and are glycosylated in the Golgi complex before secretion. The degree of glycosylation varies among the different genetic types.
4. **Secretion:** The modified procollagen molecules are packaged into granules and secreted into the extracellular space.
5. **Extracellular processing:** Collagen types I, II, III, and V must be processed in the extracellular space before the definitive structures can be assembled. The extension peptides are cleaved by aminoproteases and carboxyproteases. Failure of the aminoprotease to cleave the molecule leads to the retention of the N-terminal propeptide and defective fiber formation, as in the case of the hereditary condition Ehler-Danlos disease, type VII.
6. **Formation of collagen fibers:** After removal of the extension propeptides, collagen molecules aggregate to form collagen fibers (see Figs. 3-1 and 3-2). However, the full tensile strength of these fibers is not achieved until a series of intramolecular and intermolecular bonds forms. Some of these bonds result from the action of specific enzymes, such as lysyl oxidase, a metalloenzyme that requires copper as cofactor. Experimental chelation of copper by nitriles causes a toxic disorder called **lathyrism**. Certain inherited diseases of copper metabolism result in reduced lysyl oxidase activity and consequently poorly cross-linked collagen fibers that lack tensile strength.

Collagen Catabolism and Collagenase

Collagen has a slow turnover (months) in adult tissues. In fact, for a long time it was thought that collagen was inert and remained unchanged in the tissues for life. Native collagen is resistant to most nonspecific proteases. The collagenases are a family of enzymes with diverse cellular origins and substrate specificities. These enzymes digest native triple-helical collagen at physiological temperature, ionic concentration, and pH. Most vertebrate collagenases cleave a single peptide bond at the same locus in the three constituent chains of collagen, one fourth of the distance from the C-terminal end. In general, the same collagenase cleaves collagen types I, II, and III, although the rates of cleavage are different with each type. Type IV and type V collagen are degraded by another family of collagenases.

Collagenases release two large fragments, consisting of three fourths and one fourth of the collagen molecule. There is no further action by collagenases on these fragments, and final degradation is accomplished by nonspecific extracellular proteases or by lysosomal enzymes after phagocytosis of the fragments.

Fibroblasts are the main source of collagenases, although they are also produced by other cells, including macrophages, epithelial cells, and endothelial cells. Collagenases are secreted in an inactive form, that is, as a proenzyme. In turn, the proenzyme is converted to an active form by other proteases, for example trypsin and plasmin. Several collagenase inhibitors are present in plasma, including α_2-macroglobulin, α_1-antitrypsin, and β_1-globulin. Fibronectin, a protein that is present in plasma and tissues, has a specific binding site for collagen, which is adjacent to the collagenase-susceptible bond. It is likely that fibronectin bound to collagen fibers protects them from the action of collagenases. Thus, control of collagenase activity is exerted at several levels, from the intracellular steps regulating protein synthesis to the extracellular activators and inhibitors that influence collagen remodeling.

Morphology and Functions of Collagen

Collagen molecules self-assemble nonenzymatically to form a number of structures.

- **Collagen fibrils** are the smallest collagen structures recognizable by conventional electron microscopy. Fibrils appear as thin (4 nm in diameter) filaments consisting of four or five quarter-staggered collagen molecules.
- **Collagen fibers** consist of several fibrils that are aligned in parallel. The characteristic cross-banding of fibers at 67-nm intervals reflects the staggered array of the collagen molecules.
- **Collagen bundles** are groups of collagen fibers that are oriented along the same axis (see Fig. 3-1).

A single collagen bundle may be composed of several collagen types. Type I fibers form the backbone, to which types III, V, and VI collagen are attached. Collagen bundles have various sizes and orientations, depending on the organ and function. For example, tendons consist of dense, parallel bundles composed almost exclusively of type I collagen. By contrast, the cornea is formed by sheets of type I collagen orthogonal to each other, with some filaments of collagen types V and VI.

The formation of collagen bundles is influenced by (1) the cell surface, (2) proteoglycans, (3) structural glycoproteins, and (4) interactions among different collagen types. Collagen fibers are beyond the resolving power of the light microscope, and only large bundles can be identified. The reticulin stain (a silver impregnation) demonstrates the fine connective tissue network of many organs by binding silver to various glycoproteins, including fibronectin and several collagen types. Thus, there is no structure that can properly be called a "reticulin fiber." The reticulin stain simply allows the visualization of argyrophilic extracellular matrix components.

The best-known function of the collagens is physical support. Type I collagen predominates in organs in which tensile strength is needed, such as tendon and bone. By contrast, type III collagen is found in organs with some plasticity, such as blood vessels, uterus, gastrointestinal tract, and dermis. Nevertheless, collagens should not be regarded as merely inert scaffolds. They bind to cell surfaces and modulate morphogenesis, chemotaxis, platelet adhesion and aggregation, cell attachment, and cell phenotype.

Basement Membranes

Morphology

Basement membranes are delicate structures at the interface between cells and stroma. They contain type IV collagen, laminin, and other matrix components. By light microscopy, basement membranes appear as pale, amorphous bands that react with histochemical stains for carbohydrate groups (e.g., periodic acid–Schiff [PAS]). By electron microscopy, the appearance of basement membranes is variable. Most basement membranes have two layers with distinct electron densities (Fig. 3-3). The layer of lower electron density, the lamina rara or lamina lucida, abuts the plasma membrane. The lamina densa, the layer of higher electron density, is adjacent to the stroma. In most tissues, both laminae are of equal thickness—40 to 60 nm. However, some basement membranes, for example, lens capsule and Descemet membrane, have only a lamina densa. By contrast, the mature glomerular basement membrane is trilaminar, with a central lamina densa of double thickness, sandwiched between two outer 40-nm laminae rarae. This trilaminar appearance results from the fusion

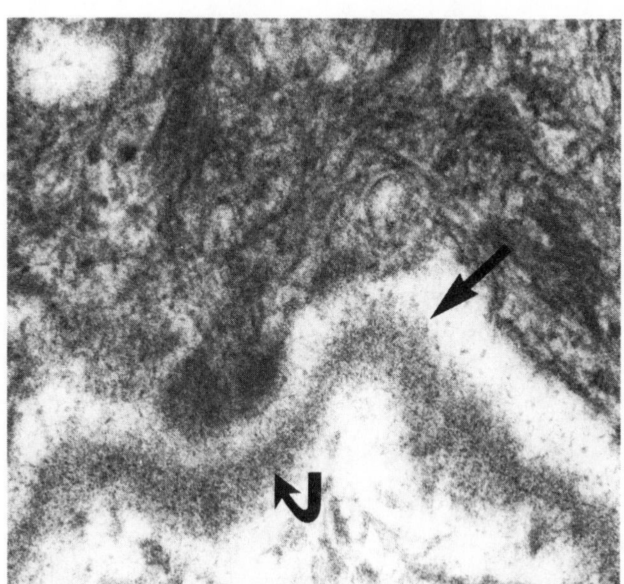

FIGURE *3-3*
Basement membrane of the epidermis viewed by electron microscopy. The layer of lower electron density (*straight arrow*), the lamina rara, abuts against the plasma membrane of a keratinocyte. The lamina densa (*curved arrow*) is adjacent to the stroma.

of the developmentally distinct endothelial and epithelial basement membranes. Segments of the alveolar basement membrane in the lung are also trilaminar.

All epithelia (epidermal, endocrine, genitourinary, respiratory, gastrointestinal) are separated from the stroma by continuous basement membranes. The liver is an exception, since hepatocytes lack a basement membrane. The central nervous system has only vascular basement membranes. In the peripheral nervous system, Schwann cells are surrounded by a basement membrane. **All vascular endothelial cells are separated from the underlying stroma by a basement membrane, except for the sinusoidal endothelium of the bone marrow, lymphoid organs, and liver.** Adipocytes and cardiac, skeletal, and smooth muscle cells are individually surrounded by basement membranes. All other cells of mesodermal origin, that is, fibroblasts, macrophages, synovial cells, lymphoid cells, and other blood cells lack basement membranes.

Composition

Basement membranes are complex structures that result from the interaction of several macromolecules with type IV collagen (Table 3-2). The recently described types XV and XIX collagen seem to be present in some basement membranes.

- **Laminin:** This molecule of the basement membrane is an 800-kd glycoprotein that is composed of three chains, one large and two smaller chains. The large chain can be either A or M; one of the small chains is always B2, whereas the other is either S or B1. These three chains are assembled into a crosslike structure. Laminin (1) is found in both basement membrane laminae, (2) is susceptible to several proteases, including pepsin and trypsin, and (3) plays a role in cell adhesion and attachment. A specific laminin-binding protein (integrin) is present on many cell surfaces.
- **Entactin:** This protein is a highly sulfated, 150-kd glycoprotein that is found only in basement membranes. It interacts with laminin, binds calcium, and may participate in basement membrane assembly.
- **Heparan sulfate proteoglycan (perlecan):** This molecule consists of several polysaccharide (glycosaminoglycan) chains covalently bound to a core protein. The protein core is specific for basement membrane and is located in clusters, preferentially within the lamina rara. Because of its high charge density, perlecan is important in glomerular filtration.

Basement membranes are synthesized by the cells resting on them. The actual assembly of the various basement membrane components into a distinct entity is poorly understood, but it seems to occur extracellularly. Basement membranes are stable structures, which normally have a slow turnover. However, in certain situations, such as embryonic development, organ remodeling, invasion by cancer cells, and wound healing, basement membranes are rapidly degraded. There are specific metalloproteinases that degrade type IV collagen, but the globular domains of type IV collagen are also susceptible to nonspecific proteases, such as trypsin and plasmin. Laminin, entactin, and perlecan are also digested by these nonspecific proteases.

TABLE 3-2 Basement Membrane Components

Component	Constituent Chains	Molecular Composition	Supramolecular Aggregate	Function
Collagen type IV	α1 (IV) α2 (IV) α3 (IV) α4 (IV) α5 (IV) α6 (IV)	3 α-chains		Structural
Laminin	A, M, S, B1, B2	3 chains: Either A or M, either S or B1, and B2		Cell attachment Growth promoter
Entactin	Single polypeptide chain	Single polypeptide chain		Ca^{2+} binding
Heparan sulfate, proteoglycan	Polypeptide chain Glycosaminoglycan side chains	Protein core Glycosaminoglycan side chains		Electrostatic charge

Function

Basement membranes have substantial tensile strength and provide physical support to structures resting on them. They also function as a site for cell attachment. Many cells overlying basement membranes express a membrane protein (integrin) that specifically binds to laminin. Basement membranes also serve as filters. This function is more obvious in capillaries and has been extensively studied in the renal glomerulus. Initially, it was assumed that basement membranes filtered molecules on the basis of their size and shape. It is now recognized that the high anionic charge of the basement membrane also is critical for selective filtration. By a combination of these functions, basement membranes allow cells to create and maintain their own special microenvironment.

Elastic Fibers

Tissues such as the uterus, blood vessels, skin, and lung require elasticity in addition to tensile strength for their function. **Whereas tensile strength is provided by members of the collagen family, the ability to recoil after transient stretching is provided by elastic fibers.** By electron microscopy, elastic fibers have two distinct components, a central amorphous core and a peripheral rim of microfibrils. Elastic fibers vary in size, from large sheets visible by light microscopy (elastic lamellae of large arteries) to delicate fibers demonstrable only by electron microscopy.

Elastin, a 70-kd glycoprotein, constitutes the central core of elastic fibers. Similar to collagen, elastin is rich in glycine and proline, but unlike collagen, it contains almost no hydroxylated amino acids. Elastin molecules are cross-linked to form an extensive network. Unlike most other proteins, elastin does not form definitive folds but rather oscillates between different states to form random coils. It is this cross-linked, random-coiled structure of elastin that determines the capacity of the elastic network to stretch and recoil. The interwoven and inelastic collagen fibers limit elasticity and maintain tissue integrity. The exact composition and function of the peripheral microfibrils associated with elastic fibers are unknown, but a glycoprotein (fibrillin) unique to microfibrils associated with elastic fibers has been identified. Defects in microfibrils are the basis for Marfan syndrome, a genetic disease of connective tissue.

Structural Glycoproteins

In addition to collagens and elastin, the extracellular matrix contains several other glycoproteins.

Fibronectin

The fibronectins (*nectere,* to bind) comprise a family of glycoproteins with almost identical amino acid compositions and similar properties. All forms of fibronectin are derived from a single gene. Minor variations in splicing determine the differences in amino acid composition, which, in turn, are responsible for the slight variations in biological properties within the family. Fibronectin exists in two major forms, plasma fibronectin and tissue fibronectin.

Fibronectins have two nearly identical 200-kd polypeptide chains, held together by disulfide bridges. Plasma fibronectin is a dimer, which is soluble under physiological conditions. By contrast, tissue fibronectin is a mixture of dimers and larger polymers, which are soluble only at alkaline pH. **Specific binding sites in specialized domains of the fibronectin molecule allow it to bind avidly to collagens, proteoglycans, glycosaminoglycans, fibrinogen, fibrin, cell surfaces, bacteria, and DNA.** The varied binding properties of fibronectin permit it to connect cells with other components of the extracellular matrix, thereby integrating the tissue into a functional unit. Through the action of transglutaminases (one of them being factor XIII of the clotting cascade), fibronectin is covalently cross-linked with itself, fibrinogen, fibrin, or collagen. This cross-linking is probably of great importance in the early phases of wound healing.

Plasma fibronectin is synthesized and secreted by hepatocytes, as are other plasma proteins. Most mesenchymal cells, including fibroblasts and endothelial cells, secrete tissue fibronectin. Fibronectin is ubiquitous in the extracellular matrix, where it is found (1) as delicate filaments, (2) as small aggregates, (3) attached to collagen fibers, and (4) on cell surfaces. Plasma fibronectin is occasionally trapped in basement membranes that have prominent filtering functions, such as those in the renal glomerulus.

Tissue fibronectin is one of the first structural macromolecules to be deposited during embryonic development. It forms a "primitive" matrix that allows the initial organization to be replaced by the definitive, organ-specific matrix. This role of tissue fibronectin as the initial, "undifferentiated" matrix is recapitulated in the early phases of wound healing.

Osteonectin

Osteonectin is a 32-kd, bone-associated, structural glycoprotein that binds to collagen type I and to hydroxyapatite. The name reflects the ability of this protein to bind both the mineral and collagenous components of bone. Osteonectin is also found in dentin, but not in tooth enamel or calcified cartilage. In the bone, osteonectin lies immediately subjacent to the zone of calcified cartilage on new bone surfaces and on mineralized metaphyseal and subperiosteal trabeculae of long and membranous bones. It seems that this glycoprotein contributes to the initiation of mineralization. However, osteonectin is also present in nonosseous tissues that contain basement membranes. Interestingly, the amino acid sequence of osteonectin is over 90% homologous with that of SPARC (secreted protein rich in cysteine), another component of some basement membranes. Osteopontin and osteocalcin are other structural glycoproteins present in osseous tissues.

Tenascin

Tenascin (*tenere,* to hold; *nasci,* to be born) consists of six, 240-kd, disulfide-linked subunits. This protein is found in perichondrium, developing and mature tendons, and myotendinous junctions, and in association with chondroitin sulfate proteoglycan in cultures of skeletal muscle cells. Tenascin also appears to participate in chondrogenesis and osteogenesis. Of note is the persistence of tenascin on the perichondrium and periosteum, tissues that contain stem cells capable of chondrogenic or osteogenic differentiation. This distribution is consistent with a modulatory function for tenascin in limb development. This protein is also found in the dense extracellular matrix adjacent to developing tooth buds, hair follicles, and mammary glands, suggesting a role in mesenchymal condensation and epithelial growth. Tenascin interacts with other matrix components, including fibronectin and laminin.

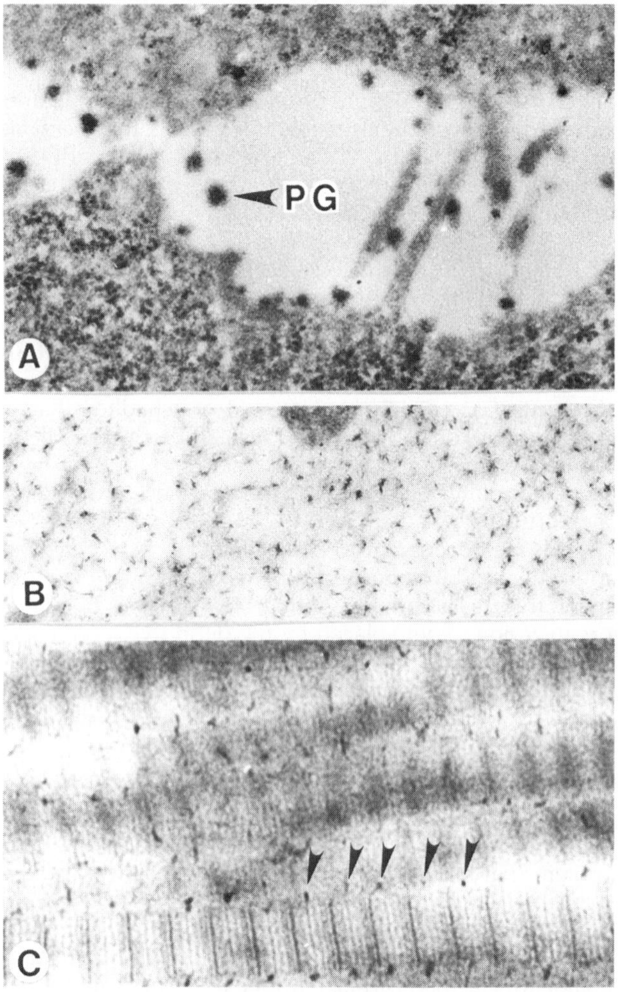

FIGURE 3-4
Proteoglycans viewed by electron microscopy. (*A*) Proteoglycan granules (PG) are associated with the plasma membrane or its microvilli and interact with a number of ligands. The proteoglycans appear as electron-dense particles after exposure to the cationic dye ruthenium red. By virtue of their polyanionic nature, the glycosaminoglycan side chains bind the cationic dye and collapse into electron-dense particles when reacted with osmium tetroxide. (*B*) Proteoglycans, stained here with cuprolinic blue, are also intrinsic constituents of basement membranes and influence the passage of molecules through them. (*C*) Proteoglycans associated with collagen are demonstrated by staining with cuprolinic blue. A small proteoglycan, termed decorin for its ability to decorate collagen type I, is visualized in (*C*). Notice the periodic association of decorin with the "d" band of collagen (*arrowheads*).

Proteoglycans

Proteoglycans are molecules of the extracellular matrix formed by long, unbranched polysaccharide chains, which are covalently bound to a protein core. Proteoglycans are widely distributed in all extracellular matrices, and they are also found in cell surfaces and in most biological fluids. The carbohydrate polymers were formerly termed **mucopolysaccharides**, but they are more properly referred to as **glycosaminoglycans**, because one of the sugar residues in the repeating disaccharide unit is always an amino sugar. Up to 95% of the dry weight of proteoglycans consists of carbohydrate. Glycosaminoglycans are negatively charged, extended molecules that occupy large volumes. They are also highly hydrophilic and form hydrated gels, even at low concentrations.

The distribution of proteoglycans and glycosaminoglycans is tissue specific. For example, cartilage contains abundant chondroitin-4-sulfate, keratan sulfate, and hyaluronic acid but no heparan sulfate or dermatan sulfate. Basement membranes contain heparan sulfate, whereas the dermis contains hyaluronic acid, chondroitin sulfate, and dermatan sulfate. Proteoglycan-containing hydrated gels help maintain tissue turgor. Their high charge density also allows them to act as selective filters. Perlecan seems to provide most of the charge selectivity of basement membranes. Proteoglycans participate in the organization of the extracellular matrix by binding to collagen fibers (Fig. 3-4), elastic fibers, and fibronectin. In cartilage, where they are particularly abundant, proteoglycans regulate the size of type II collagen fibers. As organizers of the extracellular matrix, these molecules are deposited in the early phases of wound healing, before collagen deposition becomes prominent.

CELL PROLIFERATION

Tissues periodically renew their cell populations, except for organs composed of nondividing (permanent) cells. This orderly renewal is under rigorous control as expressed in the cell cycle. Interactions with the extracellular matrix also influence the maintenance of the differentiated state. For example, chondrocytes remain differentiated only as long as they are in contact with type II collagen and cartilage-specific proteoglycans. Basal cells of the epidermis retain their stem cell character provided that they are attached to the basement membrane. Finally, interactions among cells also contribute to tissue maintenance. For example, a skin wound promotes the proliferation and migration of epidermal cells, to cover the defect. As soon as contact is established between the cells approaching from the apposed edges, migration stops and differentiation into squamous cells begins.

The Cell Cycle

The maintenance of the structure of tissues composed of short-lived cells (e.g., gastrointestinal epithelium, epidermis, neutrophils) and the regeneration of injured tissues require rigorously controlled cell proliferation to maintain an appropriate cell number. The cell cycle, that is, the period of time between two successive cell divisions, is divided into four phases of unequal duration (Fig. 3-5):

- **M phase** (M, mitosis): This phase describes the interval between the onset of the mitotic prophase and the conclusion of the telophase, at which time the cell has divided.
- **G_1 phase** (G, gap): Following mitosis, the cell enters the G_1 phase, during which it is devoted to its own specialized activities. The main difference between rapidly dividing and slowly dividing cells is in the length of the G_1 phase.
- **S phase** (S, synthesis): After the G_1 phase, a doubling of DNA takes place in the S phase.
- **G_2 phase**: Upon completion of nuclear DNA duplication, the cells enter the G_2 phase, which is followed by the next mitosis, or M phase.

Thus, interphase is composed of successive G_1, S, and G_2 phases, which constitute 90% or more of the time required for the total cell cycle.

- **G_0 phase**: Some cells remain quiescent after an M phase and do not divide unless stimulated. After an appropriate stimulus, they may reenter the cycle at G_1 and continue through the cycle to mitosis.

Classification of Cells by their Proliferative Potential

The cells of the body divide at different rates. Some mature cells do not divide at all, whereas others complete a cycle every 16 to 24 hours.

- **Labile cells** are found in tissues that are in a constant state of renewal, for example, the epithelial lining of the gastrointestinal tract or the hemopoietic system.
- **Stable cells** are found in tissues that normally are renewed very slowly but are capable of more rapid renewal after tissue loss. The liver and the proximal renal tubules are examples of stable cell populations.
- **Permanent cells** are terminally differentiated and have lost all capacity for regeneration. Neurons are representative of permanent cells.

Labile Cells

Tissues in which more than 1.5% of the cells are in mitosis at any one time are composed of labile cells. Such tissues include the epidermis; the mucosa of the gastrointestinal, respiratory, urinary, and genital tracts; the bone marrow;

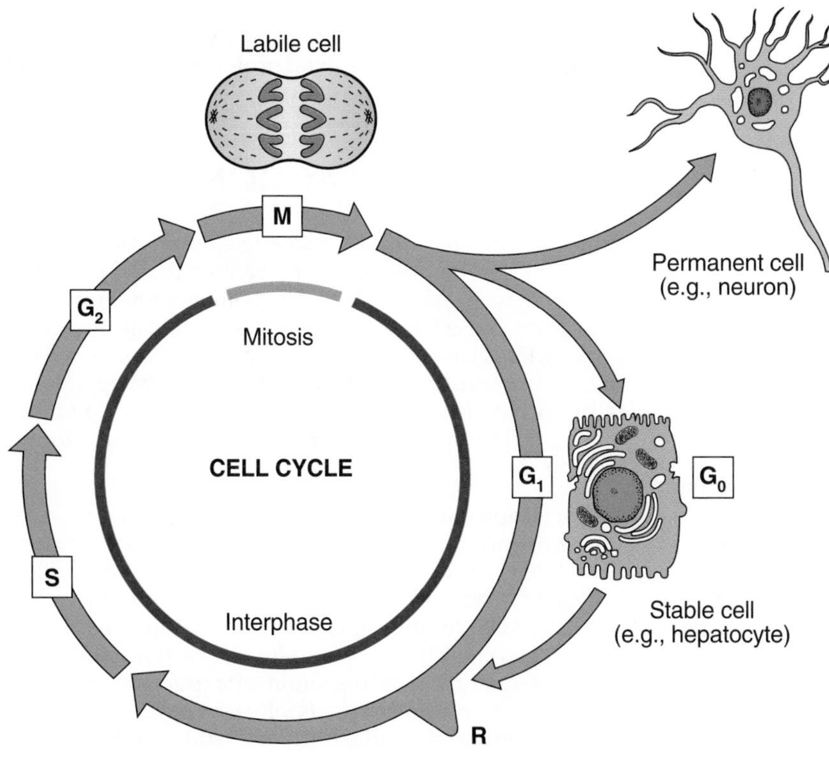

FIGURE 3-5
The cell cycle. Labile cells (e.g., intestinal crypt cells) undergo continuous replication, and the interval between two consecutive mitoses is designated the cell cycle. After division, the cells enter a gap phase (G_1), in which they pursue their own specialized activities. If they continue in the cycle, after passing the restriction point (R) they are committed to a new round of division. The G_1 phase is followed by a period of nuclear DNA synthesis (S) in which all chromosomes are replicated. The S phase is followed by a short gap phase (G_2) and then by mitosis. After each cycle, one daughter cell will become committed to differentiation and the other will continue cycling. Other cell types, such as hepatocytes, are stable; that is, after mitosis the cells take up their specialized functions (G_0). They do not reenter the cycle unless stimulated by the loss of other cells. Permanent cells (e.g., neurons) become terminally differentiated after mitosis and cannot reenter the cell cycle.

and the lymphoid organs. However, not all the cells in these tissues are continuously cycling.

Stem cells are constituents of labile tissues that are programmed to divide continuously. One daughter cell of each division becomes another stem cell, whereas the other follows an irreversible path to terminal differentiation. The basal cells of the epidermis and of the gastrointestinal crypts are examples of stem cells.

Unipotent stem cells give rise to progeny that differentiate into only one type of cell. For instance, the daughter cells of a basal epidermal cell mature only into keratinized cells, which eventually desquamate.

Pluripotent stem cells generate more than one cell type. Hemocytoblasts of the bone marrow yield erythrocytes, neutrophils, eosinophils, basophils, monocytes, lymphocytes, and megakaryocytes.

Tissues composed of labile cells regenerate after injury, provided that enough stem cells remain.

Stable Cells

Stable cells populate tissues in which fewer than 1.5% of the cells are in mitosis. Stable tissues, for example, endocrine glands, endothelium, and liver, do not have conspicuous stem cells. Rather, their cells require an appropriate stimulus to divide. **It is the potential to replicate and not the actual number of steady state mitoses that determines the ability of an organ to regenerate.** For example, the liver, a stable tissue with less than one mitosis for every 15,000 cells, regenerates rapidly after a loss of as much as 75% of its mass.

Permanent Cells

Permanent cells are terminally differentiated and do not enter the cell cycle. Neurons, cardiac myocytes, and cells of the lens are permanent cells. **If lost, permanent cells cannot be replaced.** Although permanent cells do not divide, most of them do renew their organelles. The extreme example of permanent cells is the lens. Every lens cell generated during embryonic development and postnatal life is preserved in the adult without turnover of its constituents.

CELL–MATRIX INTERACTIONS

The structure of normal mature tissues is dependent on a close relationship between cells and their surrounding connective tissue matrix, as exemplified by the relationship between epithelial, endothelial, and muscle cells and their basement membranes. In addition, close interactions between cells and matrix components are crucial for cell migration and differentiation during embryogenesis and wound healing.

Cell Migration

Embryonic development and wound healing require the orderly movement of both cells and extracellular matrix. For example, during the repair of a wound, the interactions between the extracellular matrix and cells are critical for the "directed" migration of the respective cell types into the area of injury. Whereas soluble factors attract inflammatory and fibrogenic cells to the wound site (chemotaxis), the distribution, organization, and orientation of these cells is determined by information contained in the insoluble matrix.

Haptotaxis *is defined as the migration of cells along an adhesion gradient on a substrate.* During haptotaxis, cells randomly extend processes in all directions. When they contact a proper substrate, they adhere to it and spread, preventing other processes from attaching to that site. The binding of the plasma membrane to specific extracellular matrix components creates an anchorage point on which cells can advance. The unattached portions of the membrane form new processes and contribute to the formation of a new advancing edge. Depending on the cell type, different components of the extracellular matrix, such as fibronectin and laminin, enhance directed cell migration.

Integrins

Integrins comprise a family of cell surface receptors that bind components of the extracellular matrix, including collagen, laminin, and fibronectin (see Chapter 2). By interacting with integrins, the extracellular matrix can modify cell behavior. In turn, the matrix is reciprocally modified by the cells with which it is in contact. Many of the adhesive extracellular matrix proteins contain a specific tripeptide known as the RGD sequence (arginine-glycine-aspartate), which binds to the integrins on the cell surface. Integrins transduce signals from the extracellular matrix by interacting with cytoskeletal proteins, such as talin and actin.

CELL–CELL INTERACTIONS

In addition to the influence exerted by physical contact between cells themselves and between cells and the extracellular matrix, many cells secrete soluble proteins termed cytokines. These factors (1) bind to specific cell surface receptors, (2) act as growth factors, and (3) modulate cell behavior. The programmed elaboration of many cytokines is important in embryogenesis, normal tissue maintenance, inflammation, immune responses, and wound healing.

- **Macrophage-derived growth factor (MDGF):** Under appropriate circumstances, macrophages produce MDGF, which stimulates the proliferation of quiescent fibroblasts, endothelial cells, and smooth muscle cells. Depletion of circulating monocyte/macrophages inhibits the proliferation of fibroblasts and consequently the deposition of extracellular matrix. Fibronectin and products of gram-negative bacteria (endotoxin) stimulate the secretion of MDGF by macrophages.
- **Platelet-derived growth factor (PDGF):** This polypeptide is a potent mitogen for mesodermal-derived

cells, including smooth muscle cells, fibroblasts, and microglia. PDGF is stored in the α-granules of platelets and is released after platelet aggregation during hemostasis. Several other cells, including macrophages, endothelial cells, smooth muscle cells, and transformed fibroblasts, produce PDGF-like molecules.

Platelet-derived growth factor contains two disulfide-bonded polypeptide chains. The activity of the molecule is mediated by the PDGF receptor on the surface of target cells. This transmembrane protein has tyrosine kinase activity in its cytoplasmic domain, a property that is probably associated with its mitogenic activity. PDGF is also a potent chemotactic signal for inflammatory cells, including monocyte/macrophages and neutrophils. The chemotactic and mitogenic activities of PDGF can be dissociated, since inflammatory cells that respond to its chemotactic property seem to have a receptor different from that on cells that react to its mitogenic activity (e.g., smooth muscle cells and fibroblasts).

The chemotactic and mitogenic properties of PDGF may be important for processes such as (1) the recruitment of inflammatory cells, fibroblasts, endothelial cells, and smooth muscle cells to a wound site, (2) the activation of neutrophils and monocytes, and (3) the proliferation of connective tissue cells.

- **Epidermal growth factor (EGF):** This small polypeptide exhibits a wide range of physiological effects. EGF binds to a glycosylated transmembrane receptor that is present in most mammalian cell types but is most abundant on epithelial cells. The binding of EGF activates a tyrosine kinase in the cytoplasmic domain of the EGF receptor, thereby phosphorylating the receptor itself and other intracellular proteins. As a result, the cell assumes a less differentiated appearance and begins to proliferate. EGF accelerates the healing of corneal and skin wounds and gastrointestinal ulcers. It also stimulates collagen deposition during wound healing by stimulating the proliferation of fibroblasts and other cells.
- **Fibroblast growth factor (FGF):** FGF is a single-chain, nonglycosylated protein that stimulates the growth of capillaries and is mitogenic for fibroblasts, endothelial cells, smooth muscle cells, and several other mesenchymal cells. This cytokine leads to an increase in collagen, protein, and DNA content and thereby accelerates wound healing. FGF exists in two forms, basic and acidic, the basic type being 10 times more active than the acidic one. Both isoforms are products of a single gene on chromosome 4.
- **Transforming growth factor-beta (TGF-β):** The name of this cytokine is derived from its secretion by transformed cells in culture. Platelets have high concentrations of TGF-β in their α-granules, and activation of lymphocytes induces transcription of the TGF-β gene. TGF-β is involved in terminating cellular proliferation in the regenerating liver and inhibits the growth of many cell types in culture. By contrast, it is mitogenic for fibroblasts and increases the amount of collagen and other proteins during wound healing. TGF-β also induces the formation of granulation tissue (see later) when injected subcutaneously. In fact, there is an increasing body of evidence that points to TGF-β as a key cytokine whose sustained production underlies the development of tissue fibrosis during wound healing. TGF-β, a 25-kd dimer composed of two identical subunits held together by disulfide bonds, binds to specific receptors present on the surface of virtually all cells.

The complex functions and interaction of cytokines imply that they are the conductors of the repair orchestra. This point is illustrated by recent experiments in which the application of a single dose of a cytokine (TGF-β, PDGF, or FGF) at the time of injury changed the rate of healing, the type of matrix deposited, and the cell types present in the wound. PDGF accelerates the deposition of a provisional matrix, and TGF-β hastens the deposition and maturation of collagen. By contrast, FGF induces a florid angiogenic response, which delays wound maturation.

WOUND HEALING

Healing is the restoration of integrity to an injured tissue. Following the creation of a wound, an initial inflammatory phase leads to the formation of an exudate rich in fibrin and fibronectin. Before necrotic tissue can be replaced by regeneration or scarring, phagocytic cells of the inflammatory response remove the dead cells and other debris that accumulate after the injury.

After the inflammatory phase, wound healing is accomplished by three mechanisms: contraction, repair, and regeneration. In most instances, all three mechanisms are operative simultaneously. Thus, in a skin wound, part of the defect is closed by wound contraction, part by repair and part by regeneration of epithelial cells. Figure 3-6 summarizes the events in the healing of a skin wound.

Wound Contraction

Contraction is a reduction in the size of a wound mediated principally by myofibroblasts. This process is most prominent in the skin, but it also contributes to the healing of wounds in the gastrointestinal and genitourinary tracts. The decrease in wound size is achieved by the inward migration of surrounding mesenchymal cells. Under some circumstances, contraction reduces the size of an open defect by as much as 70%. **Wound contraction results in faster healing, since only one third to one half of the original defect has to be repaired.** If contraction is prevented, large, unsightly scars result.

MYOFIBROBLASTS: Myofibroblasts migrate into the wound 2 or 3 days after injury, and their active contraction decreases the size of the defect (Fig. 3-7). These cells have features intermediate between those of fibroblasts (Fig. 3-8) and those of smooth muscle cells. The nuclei are irregular and indented. The cytoplasm contains actin and myosin bundles and occasional dense bodies resembling those of smooth muscle cells. The rough endoplasmic reticulum and the Golgi complex are prominent. Myofibroblasts have cell junctions and are occasionally

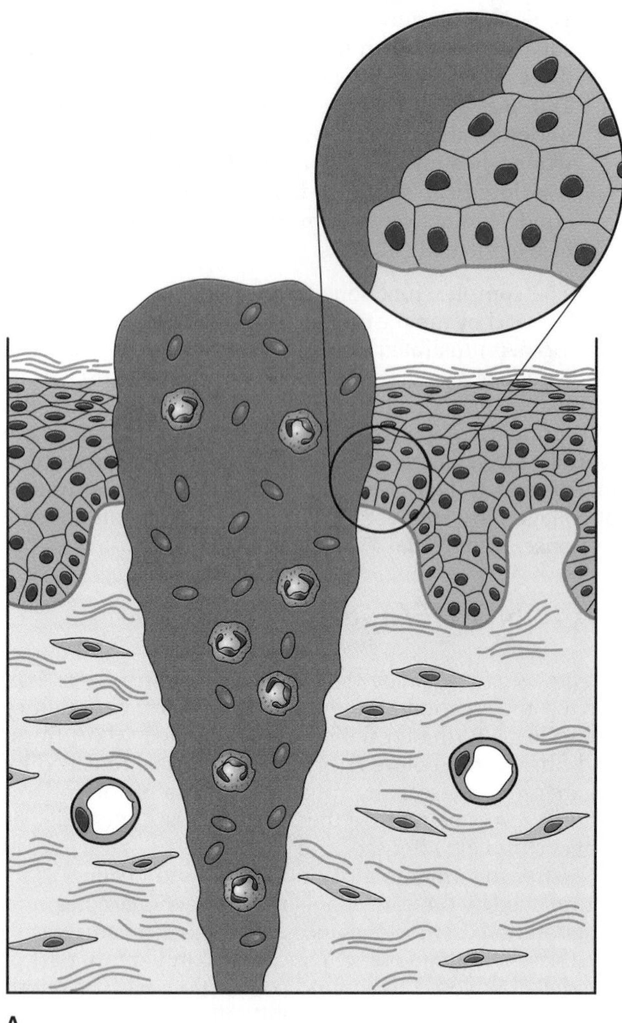

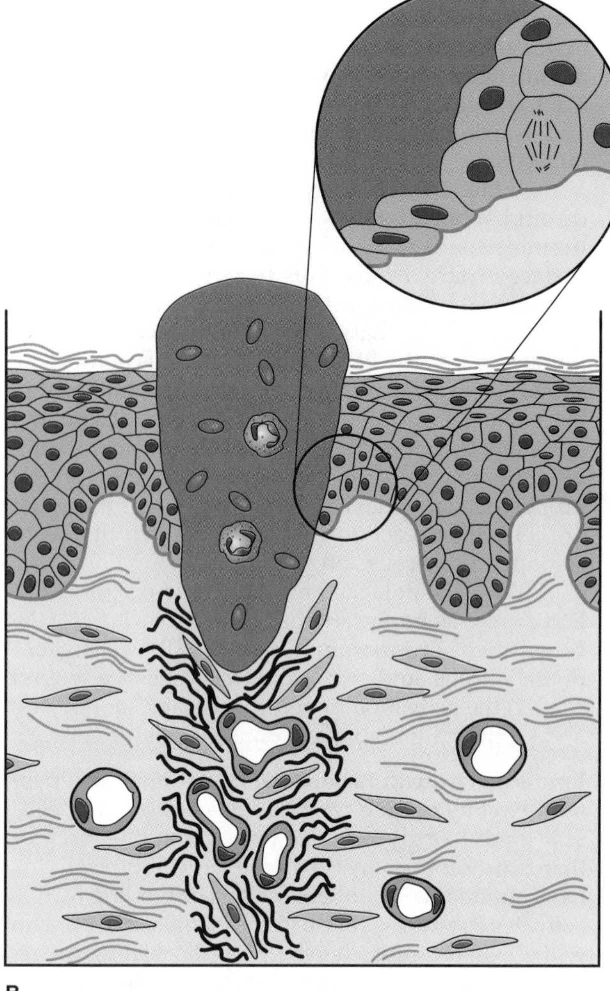

FIGURE *3-6*
Skin healing. (*A*) In any wound, the initial gap is filled by blood that upon clotting (formation of fibrin polymers) provides the initial stability to the wound. Plasma fibronectin, present in the clot, can be cross-linked with extracellular matrix components and fibrin to bridge the clot and tissues. (*B*) The epidermal cells at the edges of the wound lose contact with other epithelial cells and with their basement membranes. At the same time, this loss of contact probably acts as a signal to trigger migration of the cells. Concurrently, basal epidermal cells adjacent to the migrating cells undergo division. The result of this coordinated migration and cell division is the gradual covering of the epidermal defect. The breakdown products from the injured cells, fibronectin, and lysosomal enzymes from leukocytes act as chemoattractants, resulting in an influx of macrophages, myofibroblasts, and fibroblasts. Simultaneously, endothelial cells proliferate and neovascularization begins. The phagocytic cells attracted to the wound remove part of the clot, while fibroblasts and myofibroblasts begin to deposit a new extracellular matrix.

surrounded by a basement membrane. The origin of myofibroblasts is not entirely clear, but they probably derive either from perivascular cells (pericytes) or from mesenchymal stem cells.

Repair

Repair is the orderly process by which a wound is eventually replaced by a scar. Wounds in which only the lining epithelium is affected are termed erosions and heal exclusively by regeneration. Proliferation of the epithelial cells surrounding the erosion covers the defect, without the formation of a scar. By contrast, wounds that extend through the basement membrane to the connective tissue, for example, the dermis in the skin or the submucosa in the gastrointestinal tract, lead to the formation of granulation tissue and eventual scarring.

Granulation Tissue

Granulation tissue is the initial response to a wound and consists of a richly vascular connective tissue, which contains new

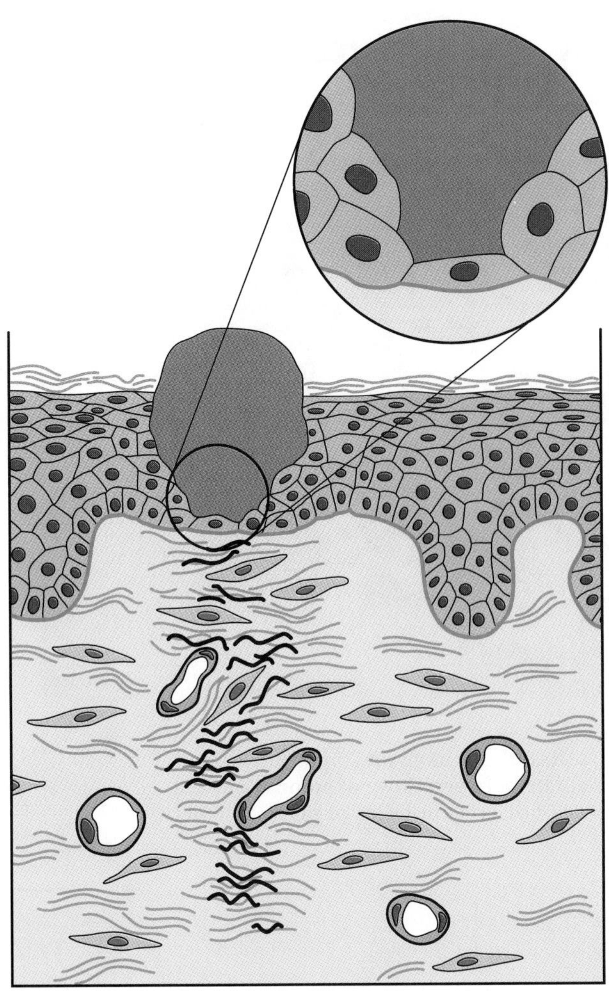

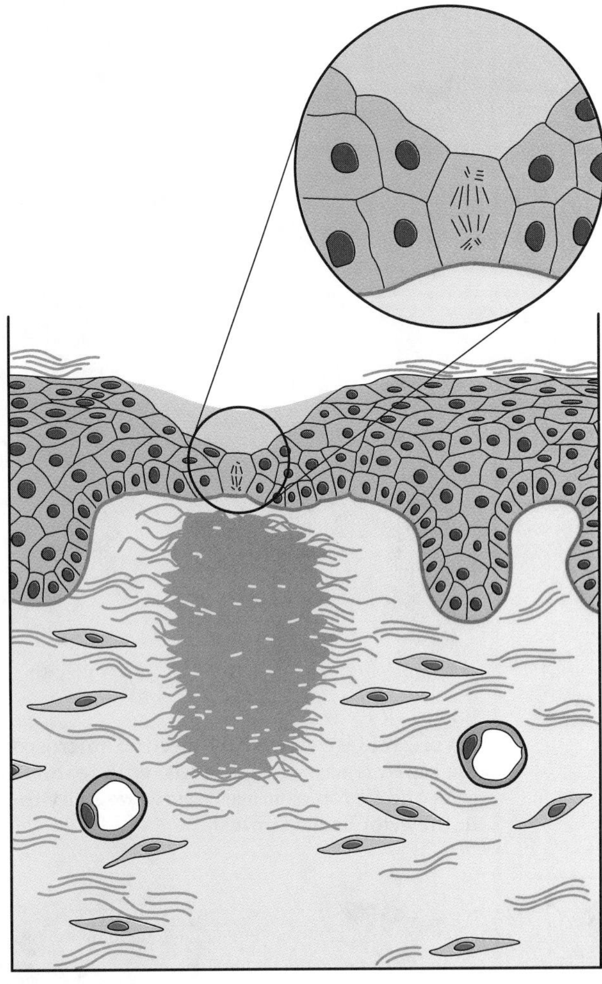

FIGURE 3-6 *(continued)*
(*C*) The concentric migration of epidermal cells, sustained by the mitotic activity of the trailing cells, fills the wound gap and displaces the remnants of the original clot (scab) toward the surface. Contact with other epidermal cells is the signal that stops migration. The trailing cells not only divide but also secrete basement membrane components. In this manner, the continuity of the epidermal basement membrane is restored. In a similar fashion, the concerted activity of fibroblasts, myofibroblasts, macrophages, and endothelial cells fills the dermal gap. At this point, the number of macrophages and myofibroblasts declines. Those capillaries that failed to establish a definitive flow pattern begin to be obliterated, and accumulation of the definitive extracellular matrix is initiated. (*D*) The gap created by the wound has been repaired. The mitotic activity of the epidermal cells will restore the epidermal thickness. Most capillaries of the initial granulation tissue have been reabsorbed, and the dermal gap has been filled with a dense, almost avascular, extracellular matrix, composed predominantly of type I collagen.

capillaries, abundant fibroblasts, and variable numbers of inflammatory cells (Fig. 3-9). The formation of granulation tissue is a regulated process, which involves a number of events, including the growth of new capillaries, fibrogenesis, and involution during maturation of the scar.

Angiogenesis

A striking vascular proliferation starts 48 to 72 hours after a wound injury and lasts for several days. Endothelial cells near the wound divide and form solid sprouts extending from preexisting vessels (see Fig. 3-9). Intracytoplasmic vacuoles form, and the fusion of several vacuoles produces a lumen. Subsequently, vascular sprouts arborize and anastomose to form a new capillary bed. At its peak, granulation tissue has more capillaries per unit volume than any other tissue type. These sprouting capillaries tend to protrude from the surface of the wound as minute red granules, imparting the name "granulation" tissue (see Fig. 3-9). Eventually, portions of the new capillary bed differentiate into arterioles and venules. Many of the new capillaries do not develop a definitive blood flow and are reabsorbed.

The cellular sources of angiogenesis factor(s) in

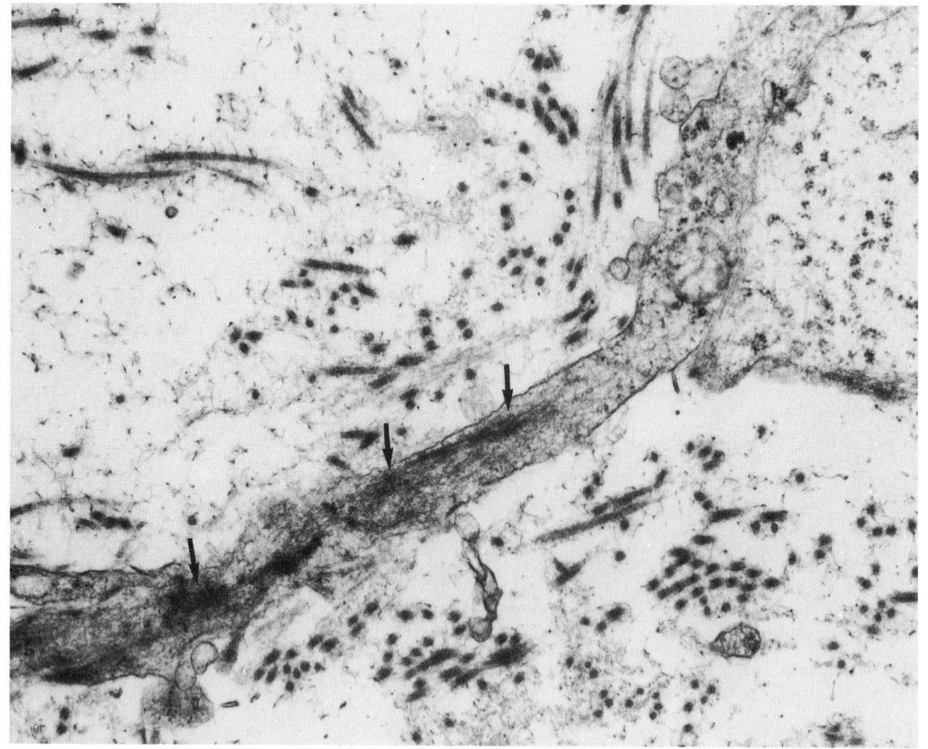

FIGURE 3-7
Myofibroblast viewed by electron microscopy. Myofibroblasts have an important role in the repair reaction. These cells, with features intermediate between those of smooth muscle cells and fibroblasts, are characterized by the presence of discrete bundles of myofilaments in the cytoplasm (*arrows*).

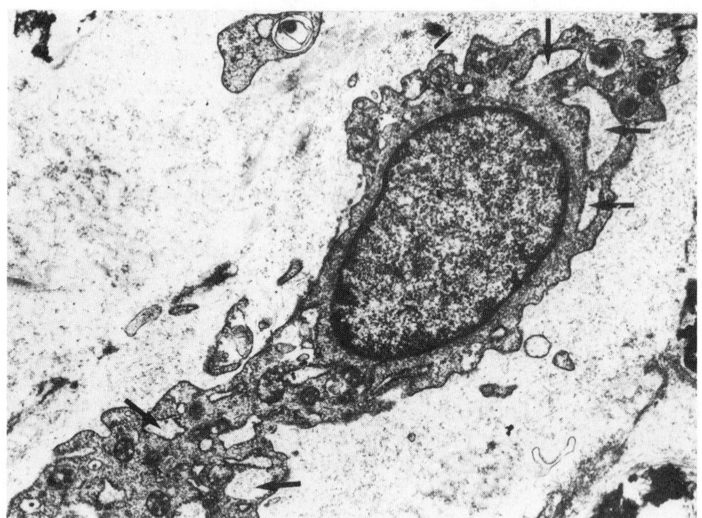

FIGURE 3-8
Fibroblast viewed by electron microscopy. This elongated cell, with multiple, delicate cell processes and an oval nucleus, is an active fibroblast. During the repair reaction, fibroblasts secrete extracellular matrix components. This activity is manifested by the distended cisternae of the rough endoplasmic reticulum (*arrows*).

FIGURE 3-9
Granulation tissue. (*A*) Granulation tissue has two major components: cells and proliferating capillaries. The cells are mostly fibroblasts, myofibroblasts, and macrophages. The macrophages are derived from monocytes and macrophages. The fibroblasts and myofibroblasts derive from mesenchymal stem cells, and the capillaries arise from adjacent vessels by division of the lining endothelial cells (*detail*), in a process termed *angiogenesis*. Endothelial cells put out cell extensions, called *pseudopodia*, that grow toward the wound site. Cytoplasmic growth enlarges the pseudopodia, and eventually the cells divide. Vacuoles formed in the daughter cells eventually fuse to create a new lumen. The entire process continues until the sprout encounters another capillary, with which it will connect. At its peak, granulation tissue is the most richly vascularized tissue in the body. (*B*) Once repair has been achieved, most of the newly formed capillaries are obliterated and then reabsorbed, leaving a pale avascular scar. (*C*) A photomicrograph of granulation tissue shows thin-walled vessels embedded in a loose connective tissue matrix containing mesenchymal cells and occasional inflammatory cells.

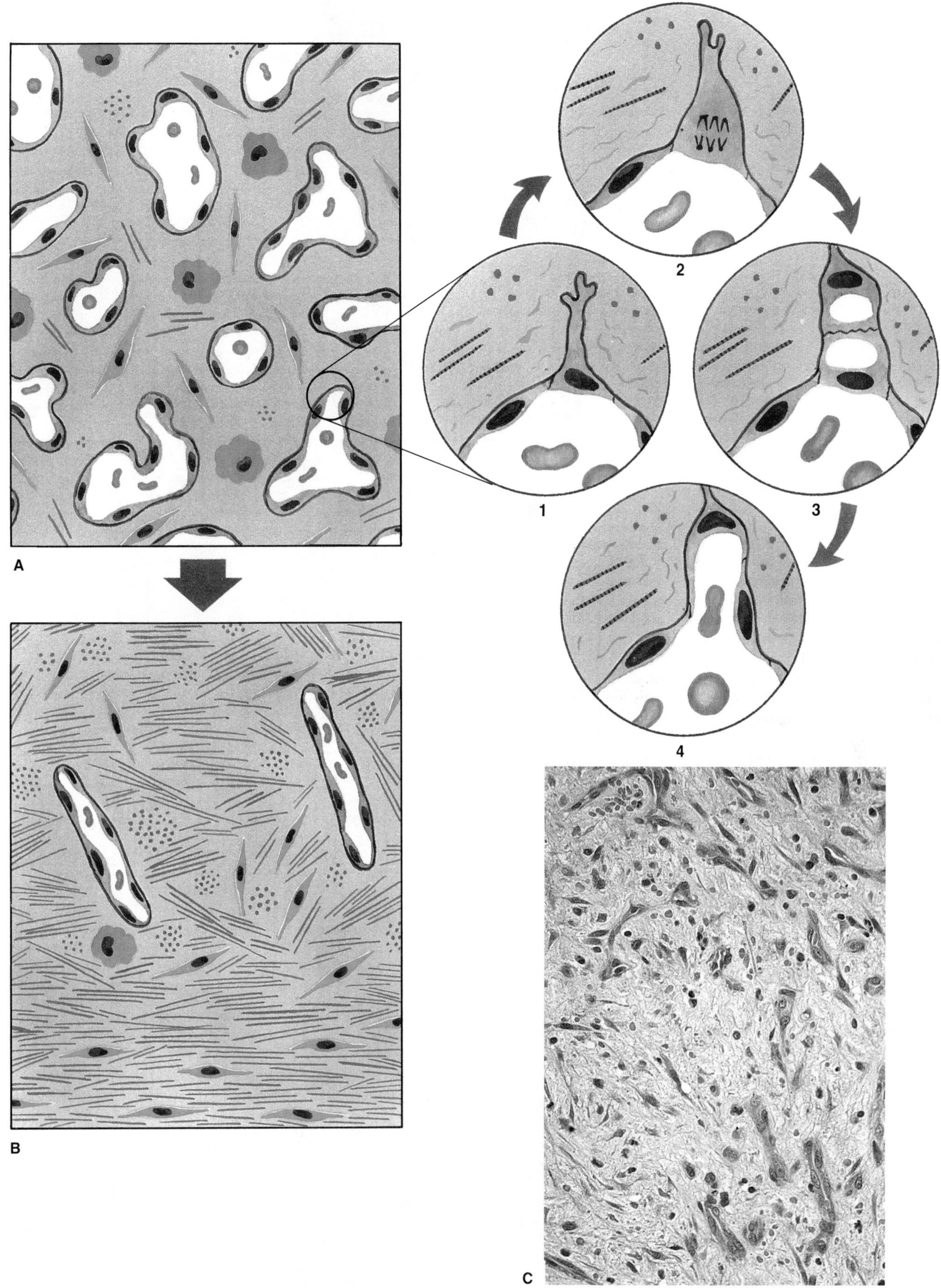

FIGURE *3-9*

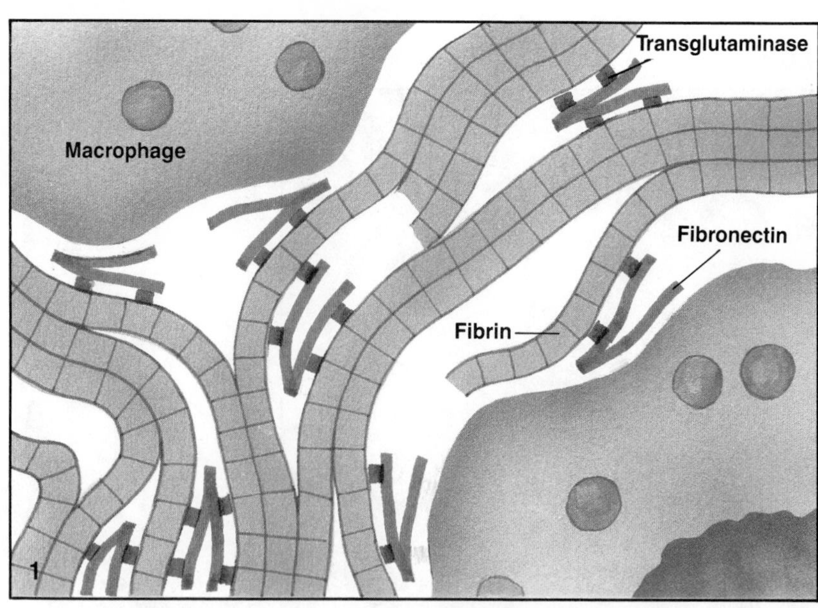

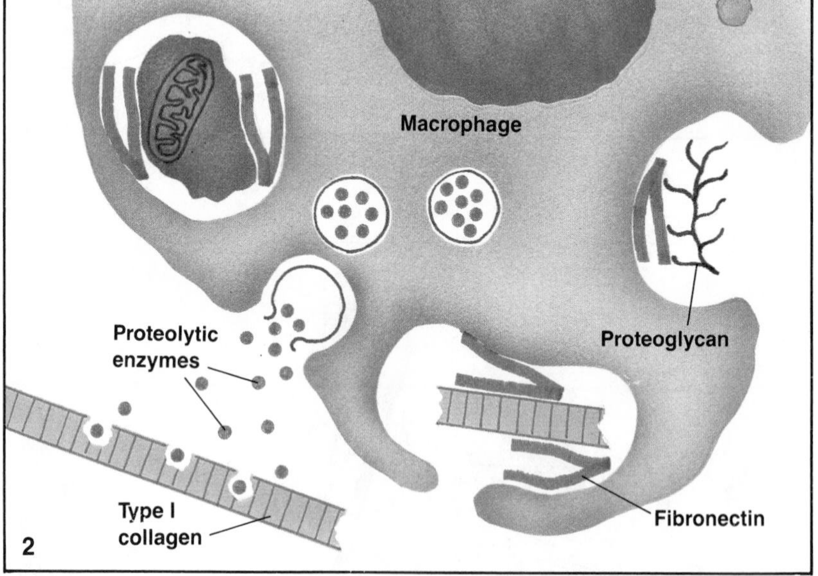

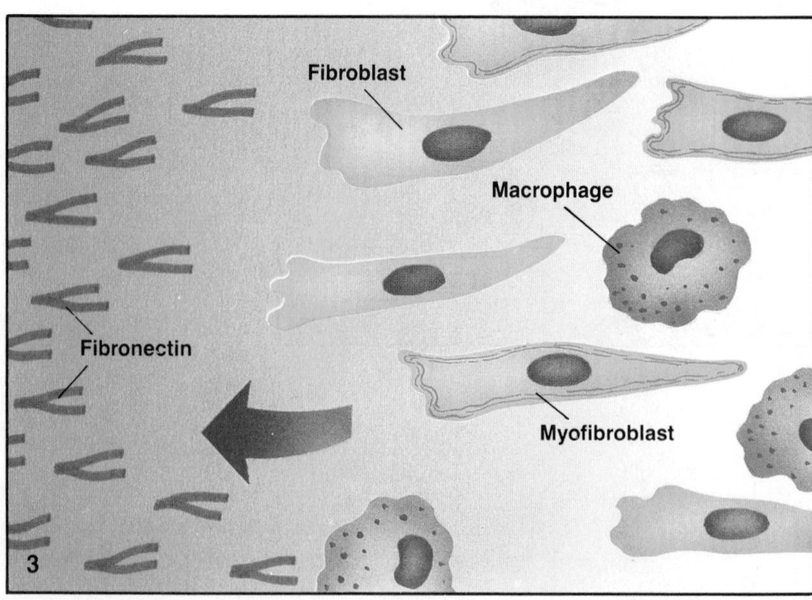

FIGURE *3-10*
Summary of the healing process. ***This page:*** **The initial phase of the repair reaction, which typically begins with hemorrhage into the tissues. *(1)* A fibrin clot forms and fills the gap created by the wound. Fibronectin in the extravasated plasma is cross-linked to fibrin, collagen, and other extracellular matrix components by the action of transglutaminases. This cross-linking provides a provisional mechanical stabilization of the wound. (2) Macrophages recruited to the wound area process cell remnants and damaged extracellular matrix. The binding of fibronectin to cell membranes, collagens, proteoglycans, DNA, and bacteria (opsonization) facilitates phagocytosis of these elements; collagenases and other proteases secreted by leukocytes and macrophages contribute to the removal of debris. (3) Fibronectin, cell debris, and bacterial products are chemoattractants for a variety of cells that are recruited to the wound site.** ***Next page:*** **Intermediate phase of the repair reaction. *(1)* As a new extracellular matrix is deposited at the wound site, the initial fibrin clot is lysed by a combination of extracellular proteolytic enzymes and phagocytosis. (2) Concurrent with fibrin removal there is deposition of a temporary matrix formed by proteoglycans, glycoproteins, and type III collagen. (3) Final phase of the repair reaction. Eventually the temporary matrix is removed by a combination of extracellular and intracellular digestion, and the definitive matrix, rich in type I collagen, is deposited.**

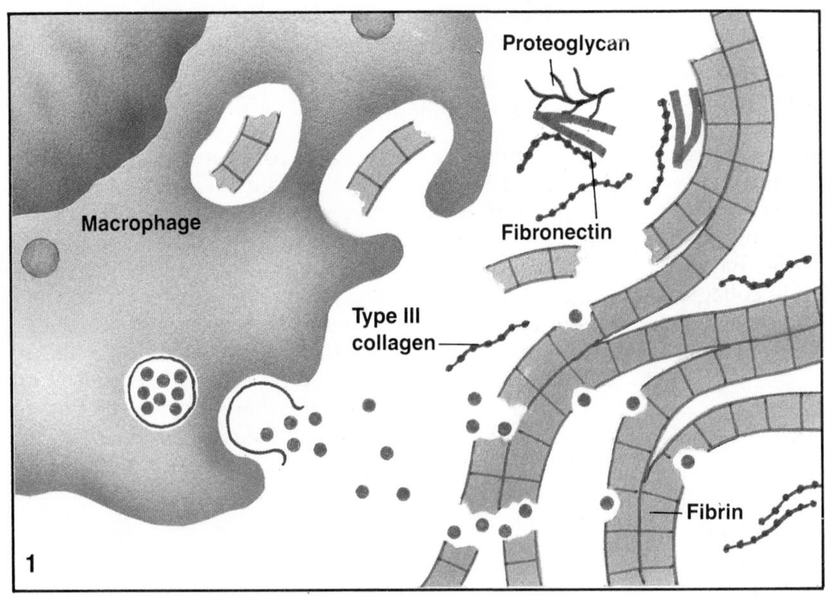
Proteoglycan
Macrophage
Fibronectin
Type III collagen
Fibrin
1

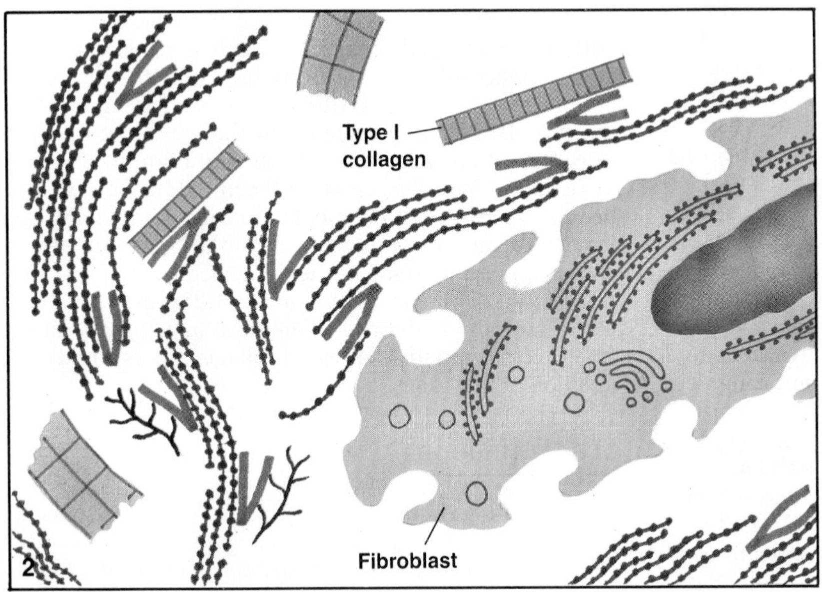
Type I collagen
Fibroblast
2

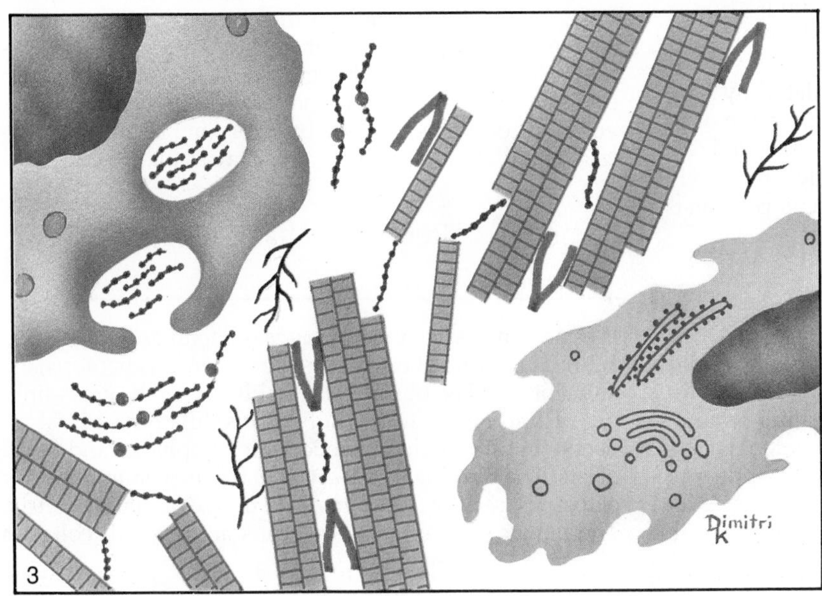
Dimitri K
3

wound healing have not been conclusively identified. Macrophages produce angiogenesis factors *in vitro*, although they probably are not the only cells responsible for endothelial proliferation. Basic FGF is a potent angiogenesis factor, although its precise cell of origin is still debated. Interestingly, malignant tumors depend on neovascularization for their continuous growth, and many cancers secrete factors that induce the growth of endothelial cells (see Chapter 5). Angiogenesis is probably also modulated by inhibitory factors, such molecules having been identified in tissues such as cartilage and in collagen VI. Thus, it is likely that angiogenesis, like the overall regulation of cell proliferation, is controlled by combinations of signals rather than by a single factor.

Cell Proliferation

Early wound healing features not only debris, inflammatory cells, and capillaries but also abundant fibroblasts. Following the initial influx of inflammatory cells from the blood into a wound site, fibroblasts move into the injured area. By light microscopy, inactive fibroblasts are oval cells with an indistinct cytoplasm and an elongated, homogeneous nucleus. Cells with this appearance comprise at least three functionally distinct mesenchymal cell types: (1) stem cells of connective tissues; (2) cells with Fc receptors and phagocytic capacities (macrophages); (3) cells specialized in the synthesis of extracellular matrix components (fibrocytes).

The activation and proliferation of mesenchymal or stem cells give rise to **activated fibroblasts** (see Fig. 3-8). These are oval cells with distinct cytoplasm, an intensely basophilic nucleus, and frequent mitoses. They are detected 2 to 3 days after injury. After 4 to 5 days, activated fibroblasts become bipolar and show abundant rough endoplasmic reticulum and a prominent Golgi complex. They secrete extracellular matrix components, including fibronectin, proteoglycans, and collagen types I and III.

The precise regulation of fibroblast proliferation has not been elucidated, but FGF, TGF-β, and PDGF are likely to be important. In addition, plasma fibronectin, extravasated as a consequence of an injury, is chemotactic for mesenchymal cells. Fibroblast proliferation is also dependent on the presence of macrophages, which presumably secrete specific growth factors. In turn, the synthetic activities of macrophages are in part modulated by lymphokines, particularly interferons. The proliferation of fibroblasts and the growth of capillaries are related. Fibroblasts align themselves at right angles to newly formed vascular arches, and inadequate vascularization is associated with poor fibroblast proliferation.

Deposition of Noncollagenous Extracellular Matrix

Fibroblasts secrete components of the extracellular matrix. Fibronectin and hyaluronic acid are the first fibroblast products to be deposited in the healing wound. Sulfated proteoglycans appear later. Since proteoglycans are very hydrophilic, their accumulation contributes to the edematous appearance of wounds. The concentrations of proteoglycans and fibronectin in the wound peak 4 to 6 days after injury and then decline, falling to normal levels by day 12.

Collagen Synthesis

Although the synthesis of collagen by fibroblasts begins within 24 hours of wound injury, significant collagen deposition in the wound is not apparent until 4 days. Initially, type III collagen predominates, but after a week, type I is abundant and eventually becomes the major collagen of mature scar tissue. A similar sequence takes place during organogenesis. In embryonic development, proteoglycans and glycoproteins are deposited first in the extracellular matrix. Collagen type III and later type I are then laid down. To some extent, therefore, wound healing recapitulates development and has similarities to amphibian regeneration. The main difference is the inability of higher vertebrates to form a pluripotential blastema that regenerates the missing parts.

Collagen Turnover

Collagen also rapidly turns over at the healing site. Although many cell types are capable of producing collagenase, macrophages and fibroblasts play the major role in collagen degradation during wound healing. Most of the type III collagen secreted in the early phases is removed, perhaps because of its susceptibility to digestion by nonspecific proteases. After the initial stages of wound healing and the establishment of tensile strength, the capillaries of the newly formed granulation tissue are resorbed and remodeling of the tissue begins. As part of the remodeling, collagen fibers and bundles are reoriented along new lines of stress. This process involves the removal of the initially deposited collagen fibers and the deposition of new ones.

Scar Formation

As the healing of the wound progresses, the rate of collagen synthesis exceeds that of its degradation. As a result, collagen accumulates at a steady rate during scar formation, usually reaching a maximum in 2 to 3 months. **However, the tensile strength of the wound continues to increase many months after the collagen content has peaked.** This physical change is related to an increase in collagen cross-linking. As the scar matures, vascular involution continues, thereby transforming richly vascularized granulation tissue into a pale, avascular scar.

Summary of Repair Mechanisms During Wound Healing

We can summarize the processes of repair as follows (Fig. 3-10): The initial event at the site of injury is hemorrhage and clotting. The fibrin clot is stabilized by the cross-linking of fibronectin to fibrin by transglutaminases. Fibronectin, in turn, is chemotactic for macrophages and fibroblasts. The fibroblasts attracted to the area, stimulated by cytokines, secrete components of the extracellular matrix. The newly secreted proteoglycans and type III collagen bind specifically to fibronectin and provide tensile strength to the wound while the fibrin clot is being lysed. Eventually, most of the proteoglycans, fibronectin, and type III collagen are removed and replaced by type I collagen to form a permanent scar. Each one of these molecules has different cell and matrix interactions and participates in feedback loops that modulate cellular functions. As a result, the cells secrete various products that, in turn, convey new information that modulates other cells. The repair process can be viewed as a cascade of events (similar to the clotting cascade but without the multiplication characteristic of coagulation). Each stage completes the previous one and initiates the subsequent one (Fig. 3-11). Thus, a continuous cell–cell, cell–matrix, and matrix–matrix exchange of information permits healing to take place. These interactions are summarized in Figure 3-12.

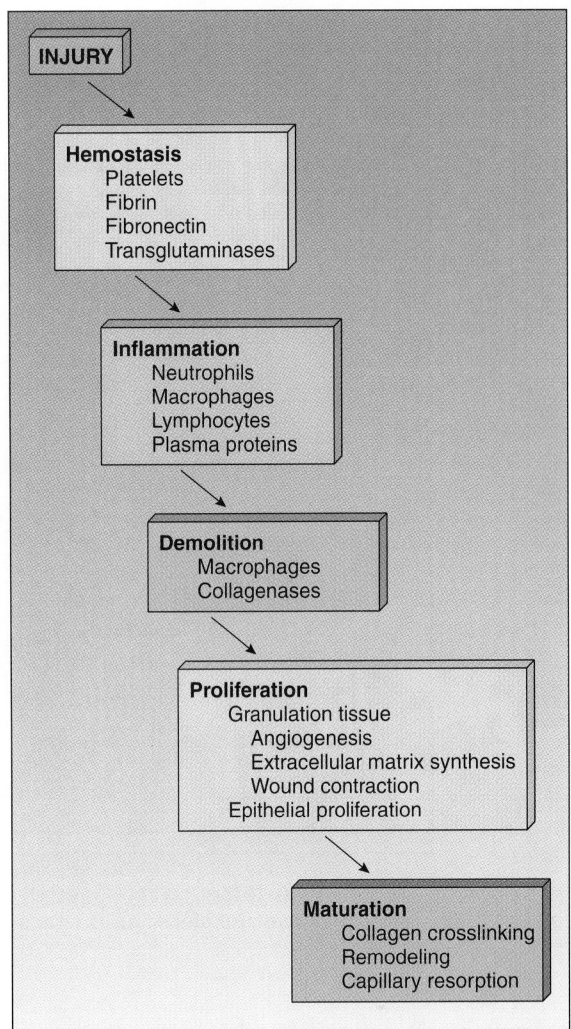

FIGURE *3-11*
The repair cascade. Repair can be viewed as a chain of events, each stage completing the previous one and initiating the subsequent one.

Regeneration

Regeneration (generare, to bring to life) is the renewal of a lost tissue or part in which the lost cells are replaced by identical ones. Strictly speaking, regeneration represents compensatory hyperplasia of the remaining cells. This process has been well studied in the skin. As long as the basement membrane beneath the epidermis is not breached, damage to the epidermis is easily repaired by the proliferation of epithelial cells at the wound margin. Epidermal reserve cells detach from the underlying basement membrane and increase their surface area by flattening, although they still retain their contacts with other cells. Thus, simply by changing their shape, the epithelial cells at the margins of the wound cover part of the denuded area without cell division. Mitosis occurs in cells that are slightly behind the advancing edge, and the epithelium advances across the wound. Migration also requires dissolution of the complex system that anchors the epithelial cells to the basement membrane. Epithelial cells secrete collagenases and probably additional enzymes that digest other extracellular matrix components.

As long as the migrating cells do not make contact with other epithelial cells, the advancing front is only one or two cells thick. However, when the wound surface is completely covered, and the migrating cells are in contact with each other, the cells recover their usual shape and attach themselves to the basement membrane. Squamous differentiation proceeds, and the normal thickness of the epithelium is restored. Although there are variations, depending on the cell type and the organ, most tissues that are capable of regeneration show a similar pattern, namely (1) change in cell shape, (2) dissolution of attachments to the extracellular matrix, and (3) proliferation of the cells behind the advancing front.

Much of what has been said previously about cell proliferation and tissue maintenance also applies to regeneration. A number of growth factors, including EGF, FGF, PDGF, TGF-β, and nerve growth factor (NGF), have been implicated in regeneration of various tissues. Insulin, glucagon, and thyroid hormones, and even the extracellular matrix components fibronectin and laminin, also play a role. The complexity of the problem is illustrated by liver regeneration. Liver regeneration is regulated by insulin, glucagon, calcitonin, thyroid hormone, parathormone, glucocorticoids, EGF, hepatocyte growth factor (HGF), several amino acids, and probably laminin. What is the stimulus that triggers regeneration? Again there is no clear answer. In endocrine organs, a decrease in the number of functional cells results in decreased hormone secretion. The target organs respond by producing substances that stimulate regeneration of the endocrine organ. In the case of covering epithelia, the loss of contact between epithelial cells (contact inhibition) may be a major factor.

Whatever the stimulus, the magnitude of the response in some organs is remarkable. The mammalian liver regenerates after a loss of 70% of the original mass. In the rat, more than 40% of the removed mass is replaced by 48 hours after partial hepatectomy, and in 6 days, regeneration is complete. This rate of growth is higher than that of the normal embryo or of most cancers. In fact, no other tissue, normal or abnormal, grows faster than the regenerating liver.

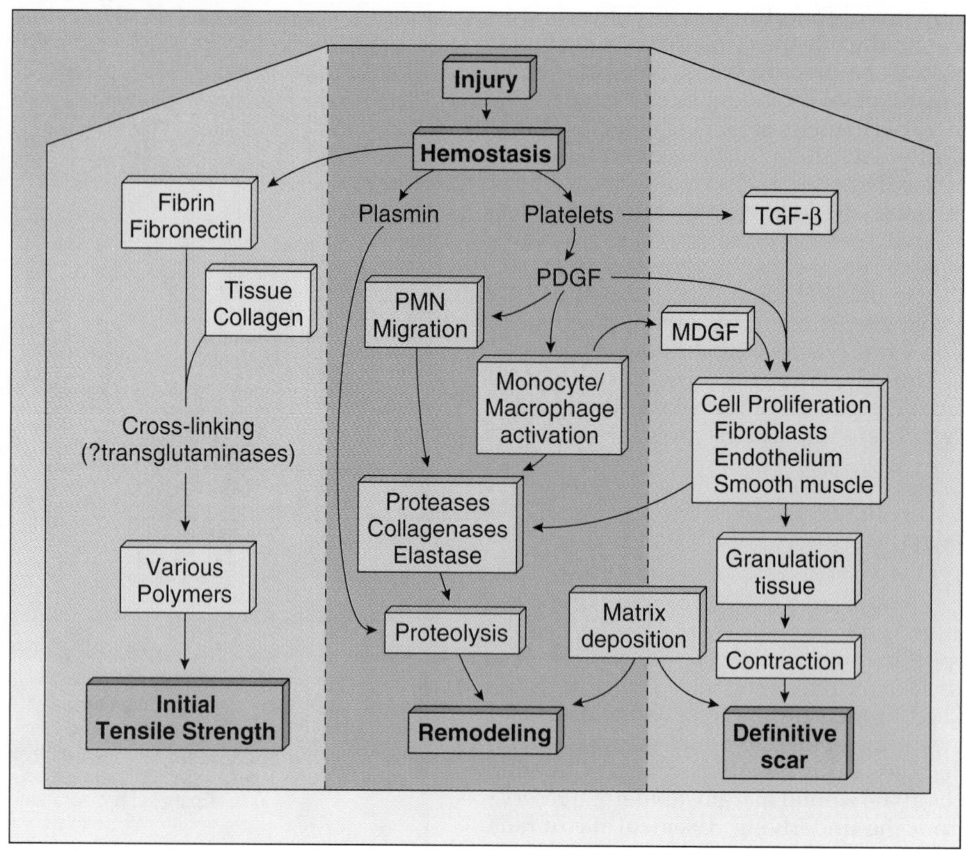

FIGURE *3-12*
The major steps and interactions in three phases of wound healing.

Healing by Primary and Secondary Intention

It is traditional to make a distinction between the healing of the apposed edges of a clean incised wound (healing by primary intention) and the separated edges of a gouged wound (healing by secondary intention). Although the end results—minimal and prominent scarring, respectively (Fig. 3-13)—are clearly different, the basic mechanisms are the same for both. In other words, the differences between healing by primary and healing by secondary intention are quantitative and not qualitative.

Healing of Wounds with Apposed Edges (Primary Intention)

Immediately after an incision, a hematoma rich in fibrin and fibronectin forms. Acute inflammation and dissolution of the clot rapidly follow the hematoma. Within 48 hours in a well-approximated wound, a continuous layer of epithelial cells covers the site of injury. By the third or fourth day, granulation tissue invades the wound, and collagen deposition begins. For the first month, tensile strength closely parallels the collagen content of the wound. Granulation tissue prevents epithelial migration deep into the wound. The epithelial cells on the surface divide and differentiate, thereby restoring a multilayered

FIGURE *3-13*
Healing by primary intention. (*A*) A wound with closely apposed edges and minimal tissue loss. (*B*) Such a wound requires only minimal cell proliferation and neovascularization to heal. (*C*) The result is a small scar.
Healing by secondary intention. (*A*) A gouged wound, in which the edges are far apart and in which there is substantial tissue loss. (*B*) This wound requires wound contraction, extensive cell proliferation, and neovascularization (granulation tissue) to heal. (*C*) The wound is reepithelialized from the margins, and collagen fibers are deposited in the granulation tissue. (*D*) Granulation tissue is eventually resorbed and replaced by a large scar that is functionally and esthetically unsatisfactory.

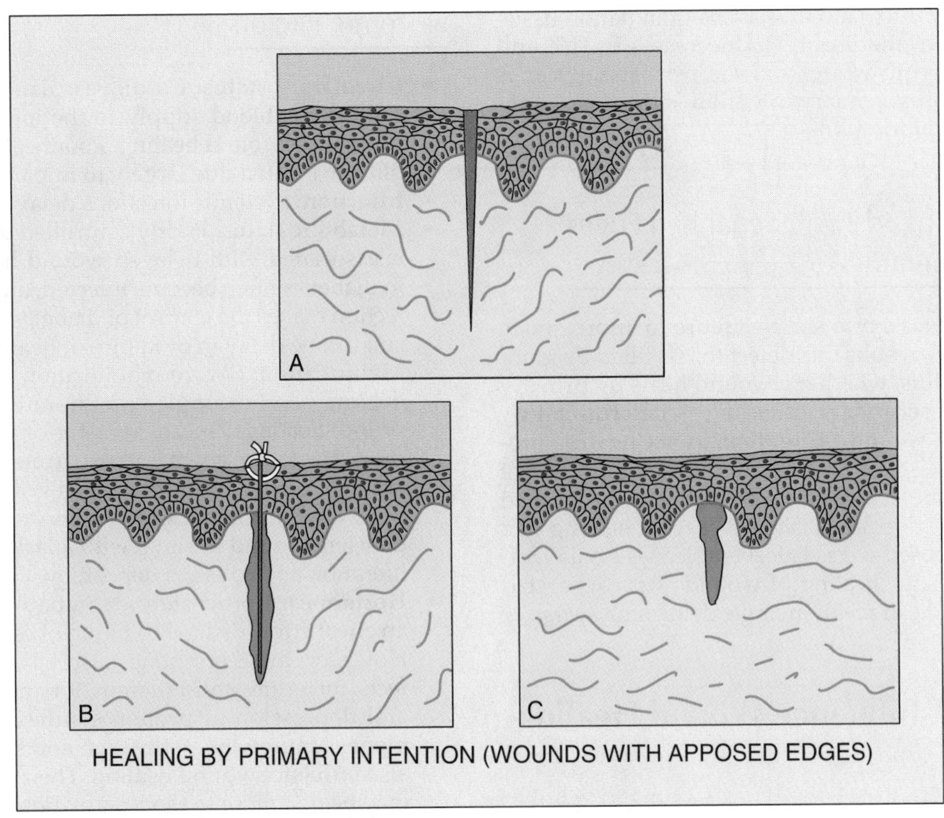
A
B
C
HEALING BY PRIMARY INTENTION (WOUNDS WITH APPOSED EDGES)

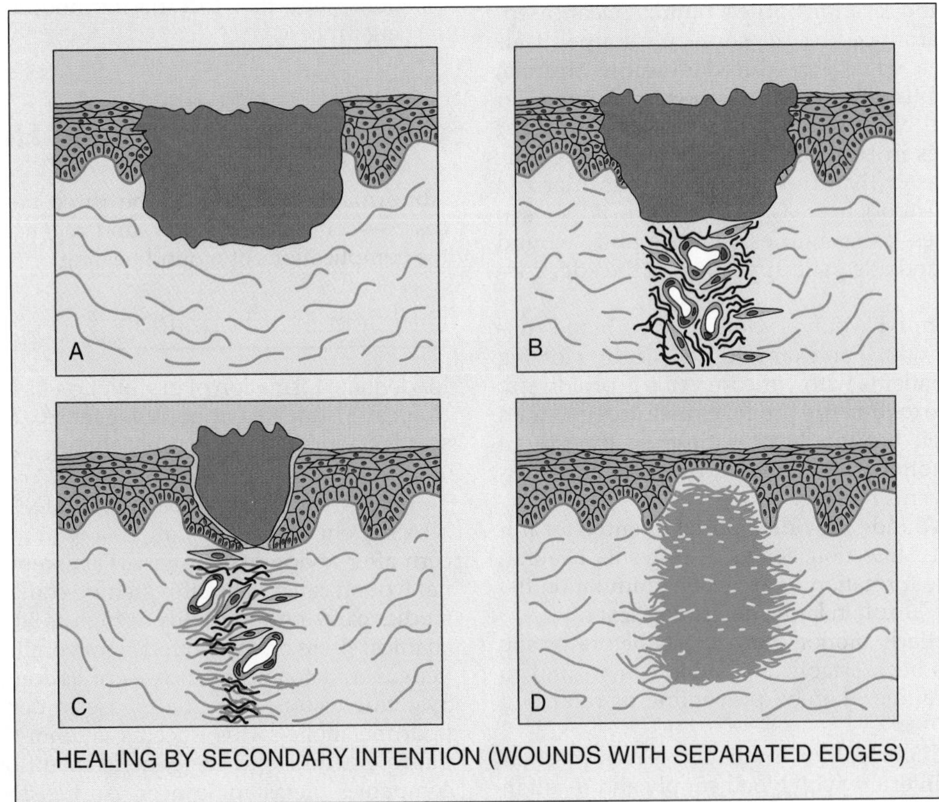
A
B
C
D
HEALING BY SECONDARY INTENTION (WOUNDS WITH SEPARATED EDGES)

FIGURE *3-13*

epithelium. After 1 to 3 months, as the granulation tissue is devascularized, the linear scar decreases in size and changes from red to white, and the permanent scar is formed. **Healing by primary intention is the desired result in all surgical incisions.**

Healing of Wounds with Separated Edges (Secondary Intention)

Extensive tissue loss, or a simple failure to approximate the wound edges, results in a defect that is filled by granulation tissue. **Thus, whether a wound heals by primary intention or by secondary intention is determined by the nature of the wound, rather than by the healing process itself.** The degree of inflammation and the amount of granulation tissue are considerably greater in gouged wounds than in surgical incisions. Whereas healing of a wound with apposed edges is fast and leaves a small, often unapparent scar, healing of wounds with separated edges is slow and can result in large, deforming scars.

Factors that Influence Wound Healing

Local Factors

- **Type, size, and location of the wound:** A clean, aseptic wound produced by the surgeon's scalpel heals faster than a wound produced by blunt trauma, which exhibits abundant necrosis and irregular edges. Small blunt wounds heal faster than larger ones. Injuries in richly vascularized areas (e.g., the face) heal faster than those in poorly vascularized ones (e.g., the foot). In areas where the skin adheres to bony surfaces, as in injuries over the tibia, wound contraction and adequate apposition of the edges are difficult.
- **Vascular supply:** Wounds with impaired blood supply heal slowly. For example, the healing of leg wounds in patients with varicose veins is prolonged. Ischemia due to pressure produces bedsores and then prevents their healing. Ischemia caused by arterial obstruction, often in the lower extremities of diabetics, also prevents healing.
- **Infection:** Wounds provide a portal of entry for microorganisms. Infection delays or prevents healing, promotes the formation of excessive granulation tissue, and may result in large, deforming scars.
- **Movement:** Early motion, particularly before tensile strength has been established, subjects a wound to persistent trauma, thereby preventing or retarding healing.
- **Ionizing radiation:** Prior irradiation leaves vascular lesions that interfere with blood supply and result in slow wound healing. Acutely, irradiation of a wound blocks cell proliferation, inhibits contraction, and retards the formation of granulation tissue.
- **Ultraviolet light:** Exposure of wounds to ultraviolet light accelerates the rate of healing.

Systemic Factors

- **Circulatory status:** Cardiovascular status, by determining the blood supply to the injured area, is important for wound healing. Poor healing attributed to old age is often due largely to impaired circulation.
- **Infection:** Systemic infections delay wound healing.
- **Metabolic status:** Poorly controlled diabetes mellitus is associated with delayed wound healing. Wounds in diabetics often become infected, and, in turn, an infection makes the control of diabetes difficult. The result can be delay in or failure of healing.
- **Malnutrition:** Severe malnutrition impedes wound healing. For example, methionine is needed for proper healing. Zinc, a co-factor of several enzymes, promotes faster healing in experimental animals. Vitamin C is required for collagen synthesis and secretion. Vitamin C deficiency (scurvy) results in grossly deficient wound healing, with a lack of vascular proliferation and collagen deposition.
- **Hormones:** Corticosteroids impair wound healing, an effect attributed to inhibition of collagen synthesis. However, these hormones also have many other effects, including anti-inflammatory actions and a general depression of protein synthesis. Thyroid hormones, androgens, estrogens, and growth hormone also influence wound healing. Their effects, however, may be due more to their regulation of general metabolic status than to a specific modification of the healing process.

Complications of Wound Healing

Abnormalities in any of the three basic healing processes—contraction, repair, and regeneration—result in the complications of wound healing.

Deficient Scar Formation

Inadequate formation of granulation tissue or an inability to form a suitable extracellular matrix leads to deficient scar formation and its complications.

WOUND DEHISCENCE AND INCISIONAL HERNIAS: Dehiscence (bursting of a wound) is of most concern after abdominal surgery. Dehiscence of an abdominal wound can be a life-threatening complication, in some studies carrying a mortality as high as 30%. Increased mechanical stress on the wound from vomiting, coughing, or ileus is a factor in most cases of abdominal dehiscence. Systemic factors that predispose to dehiscence include poor metabolic status, such as vitamin C deficiency, hypoproteinemia, and the general inanition that often accompanies metastatic cancer. An incisional hernia, usually of the abdominal wall, refers to a defect caused by prior surgery into which the intestines protrude. Such hernias from weak scars are often the consequence of insufficient deposition of extracellular matrix or inadequate cross-linking of the matrix.

ULCERATION: Wounds ulcerate because of an inadequate intrinsic blood supply or insufficient vascularization during healing. For example, leg wounds in persons with varicose veins or severe atherosclerosis typically ulcerate. Nonhealing wounds also develop in areas devoid of sensation because of persistent trauma. Such **trophic or neuropathic ulcers** are occasionally seen in patients with spinal involvement from tertiary syphilis (tabes dorsalis), in leprosy, and in diabetic peripheral neuropathy.

Excessive Scar Formation

An excessive deposition of extracellular matrix at the wound site results in a **hypertrophic scar** (an excessively large scar localized to the site of initial injury) or a **keloid** (an exuberant scar that tends to progress beyond the site of initial injury and recurs after excision) (Fig. 3-14). Histologically, both of these types of scars exhibit abundant, broad, and irregular collagen bundles, with more capillaries and fibroblasts than expected for a scar of the same age. The rate of collagen synthesis, the ratio of type III to type I collagen, and the number of reducible cross-links remain high, a situation that indicates a "maturation arrest," or block, in the healing process.

Excessive Contraction

A decrease in the size of a wound depends on the presence of myofibroblasts, development of cell–cell contacts, and sustained cell contraction. An exaggeration of these processes is termed **contracture** and results in severe deformity of the wound and surrounding tissues. Interestingly, the regions that normally show minimal wound contraction (such as the palms, the soles, and the anterior aspect of the thorax) are the ones prone to contractures. Contractures are particularly conspicuous in the healing of serious burns. Contractures of the skin and underlying connective tissue can be sufficiently severe to compromise the movement of joints. In the alimentary tract, a contracture (stricture) can result in obstruction to the passage of food in the esophagus or a block in the flow of intestinal contents.

Several diseases are characterized by contracture and irreversible fibrosis of the superficial fascia, including **Dupuytren contracture (palmar contracture), plantar contracture (Lederhosen disease), and Peyronie disease (contracture of the cavernous tissues of the penis)**. In these diseases, there is no known precipitating injury, even though the basic process is similar to contracture in wound healing.

HEALING IN SPECIFIC TISSUES

The general principles of wound healing apply to all tissues. Each organ, however, contains specialized cells and distinctive extracellular matrices, imparting some organ specificity to the healing response (Fig. 3-15).

Liver

Liver injury is followed by complete parenchymal regeneration, the formation of scars, or a combination of both.

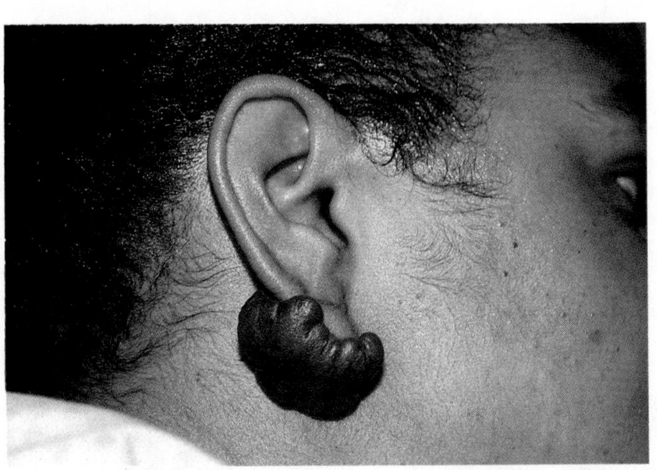

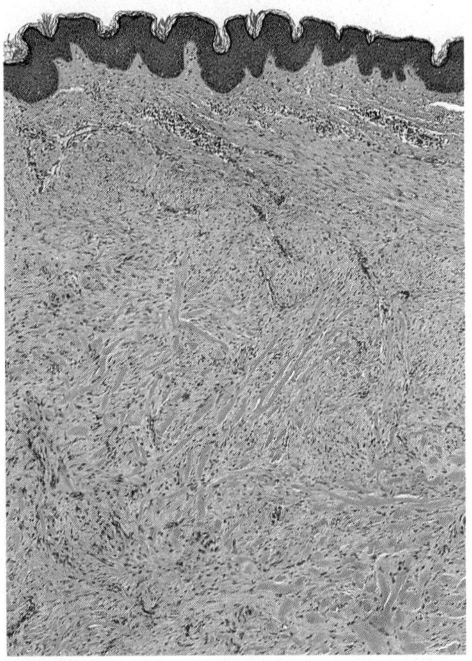

FIGURE *3-14*
Keloid. (*A*) A light-skinned black woman developed a keloid as a reaction to having her earlobe pierced. (*B*) Microscopically, the dermis is markedly thickened by the presence of collagen bundles with random orientation and abundant cells.

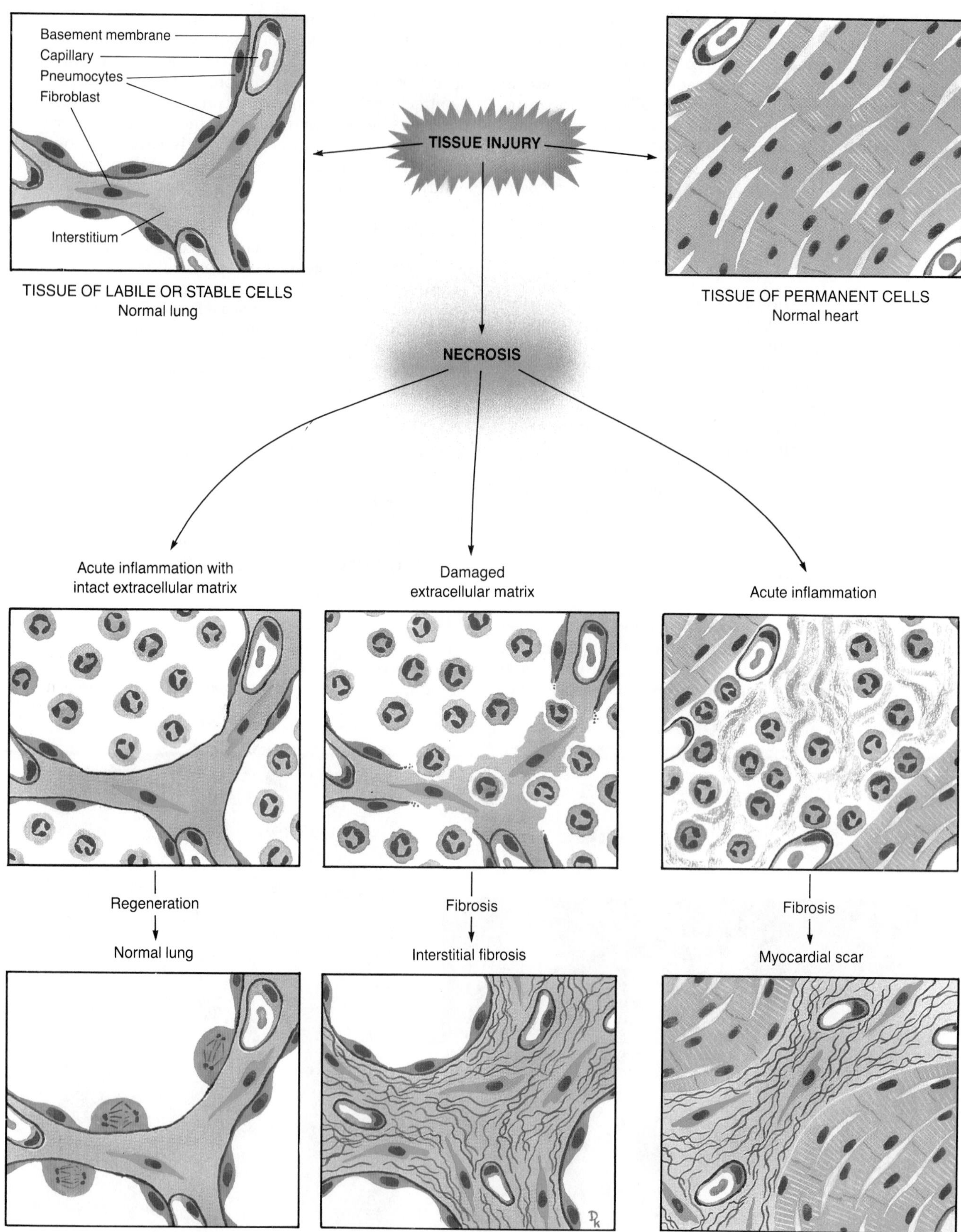
Basement membrane
Capillary
Pneumocytes
Fibroblast
Interstitium
TISSUE OF LABILE OR STABLE CELLS
Normal lung
TISSUE INJURY
TISSUE OF PERMANENT CELLS
Normal heart
NECROSIS
Acute inflammation with
intact extracellular matrix
Damaged
extracellular matrix
Acute inflammation
Regeneration
Normal lung
Fibrosis
Interstitial fibrosis
Fibrosis
Myocardial scar

FIGURE 3-15

The outcome depends on the extent and chronicity of the insult.

The hepatocytes lost after focal or zonal necrosis of the liver are restored by regeneration. The normal architecture is reestablished, and no fibrosis occurs because the framework provided by the extracellular matrix is not affected. In massive hepatic necrosis, death from liver failure often ensues within a few days, although some patients survive the acute episode. In the latter situation, the surviving hepatocytes regenerate. However, because the extracellular matrix framework is destroyed, regeneration of hepatocytes forms irregular parenchymal nodules that are separated by broad scars. Forms of chronic hepatic injury that destroy the extracellular matrix framework (e.g., chronic viral hepatitis, alcoholic liver injury) elicit a combination of regeneration and fibrosis, an appearance that is termed cirrhosis (Fig. 3-16).

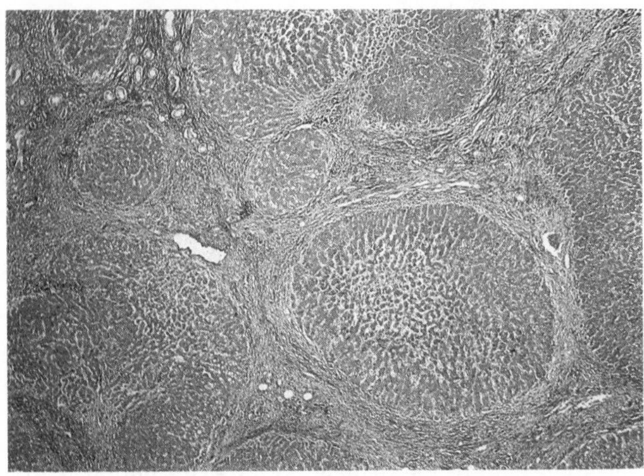

FIGURE *3-16*
Cirrhosis of the liver. The consequence of chronic hepatic injury is the formation of regenerating nodules separated by bands of fibrous connective tissue (*blue*).

Kidney

The kidney has a limited regenerative capacity and usually responds to injury with a combination of hypertrophy and hyperplasia. If the injury is not extensive and the extracellular matrix framework is not destroyed, the tubular epithelium regenerates. In most clinically relevant lesions, however, there is some destruction of the extracellular matrix framework. Regeneration is incomplete, and repair with scar formation is the usual outcome. The regenerative capacity of renal tissue is maximal in cortical tubules, less in medullary tubules, and nonexistent in glomeruli.

- **Cortical renal tubules:** Normally, there is some turnover of tubular epithelium, leading to desquamation of cells in the urine. No reserve cell has been identified, and simple division accomplishes replacement. The outcome of injury depends on whether the tubular basement membrane is ruptured. If the injury does not produce discontinuities in the tubular basement membrane, the surviving tubular cells in the vicinity of the wound flatten, acquire a squamous appearance, and migrate into the necrotic area along the basement membrane. Mitoses are frequent and occasional clusters of epithelial cells project into the lumen. Within 1 week, the flattened cells are more cuboidal, and differentiated cytoplasmic elements appear. Changes in the interstitium are usually minimal. Tubular morphology and function are normal by 3 to 4 weeks.
- **Tubulorrhexis:** Tubulorrhexis refers to the rupture of the tubular basement membrane. The sequence of events resembles that for tubular damage in which the basement membrane is intact, except that interstitial changes are more prominent. Proliferation of fibroblasts, increased deposition of extracellular matrix, and collapse of the tubular lumen are seen. The final result is regeneration of some tubules and fibrosis of others, usually with a loss of functional nephrons in the latter.
- **Medullary renal tubules:** Medullary diseases are often associated with extensive necrosis, which involves tubules, interstitium, and blood vessels. If the lesion is not fatal, the necrotic tissue sloughs off into the urine. The surviving stump heals, and extensive fibrosis produces urinary obstruction within the kidney. Although there is some epithelial proliferation, there is no significant regeneration.
- **Glomeruli:** Unlike tubules, glomeruli do not regenerate. Injuries that produce necrosis of glomerular endothelial or epithelial cells, whether focal, segmental,

FIGURE *3-15*
Possible outcomes of the healing response. A crucial factor in determining the outcome of any injury is the constituent cells of the injured tissue. In this figure, the lung represents tissues composed of labile or stable cells and the heart represents tissues of permanent cells. If the injury to the lung produces cell necrosis, but the framework of the organ is left intact, the surviving cells will proliferate. They migrate along the intact basement membrane and reconstruct the normal organ structure. On the other hand, if the injury destroys not only cells but also the basement membrane, when the surviving cells proliferate they lack the master plan provided by the extracellular matrix. As a consequence, the repair reaction fails to duplicate the normal structure, and scarring of the lung ensues with varying degrees of functional impairment. In tissues composed of permanent cells, as exemplified by the heart, lost parenchymal cells cannot be restored. Therefore, cell necrosis invariably results in permanent loss of parenchymal cells, in fibrosis, and, if extensive enough, in functional impairment.

or diffuse, heal by scarring (glomerulosclerosis). Mesangial cells seem to have some capacity for regeneration.

Lung

The epithelium lining the respiratory tract has an excellent regenerative capacity, provided that the underlying extracellular matrix framework is not destroyed. Superficial injuries to tracheal and bronchial epithelia heal by regeneration from the adjacent epithelium. The outcome of alveolar injury ranges from complete regeneration of structure and function to incapacitating fibrosis. The determining factors are, again, the degree of cell necrosis and the extent of the damage to the extracellular matrix framework (see Fig. 3-15).

- **Alveolar injury with intact basement membranes:** Alveolar injury occurs in many pulmonary diseases and with acute exposures to toxic fumes. Following injury there is a variable degree of alveolar cell necrosis. The alveoli are flooded with an inflammatory exudate particularly rich in plasma proteins. **As long as the alveolar basement membrane remains intact, healing is by regeneration, and neutrophils and macrophages clear the alveolar exudate.** If these cells fail to lyse the alveolar exudate, it is organized by granulation tissue, and intra-alveolar fibrosis results. Alveolar type II pneumocytes are the alveolar reserve cells. After injury, they migrate to denuded areas and undergo mitosis to generate cells with features intermediate between those of type I and type II pneumocytes. As these cells cover the alveolar surface, they establish contact with other epithelial cells. Mitosis then stops and the cells differentiate into type I pneumocytes.
- **Alveolar injury with ruptured basement membranes**: Extensive damage to the alveolar basement membrane elicits a repair reaction that results in scarring and fibrosis. Mesenchymal cells from the alveolar septa proliferate and differentiate into fibroblasts and myofibroblasts. The role of macrophage products in inducing fibroblast proliferation in the lung is well documented. The myofibroblasts and fibroblasts migrate into the alveolar spaces, where they secrete extracellular matrix components, mainly type I collagen and proteoglycans. Scarring (pulmonary fibrosis) is the end result.

Heart

Myocardial cells have no significant regenerative capacity. Myocardial necrosis, from whatever cause, heals by the formation of granulation tissue and eventual scarring (Fig. 3-17). Not only does myocardial scarring result in the loss of contractile elements, but the fibrous tissue also decreases the effectiveness of contraction in the surviving myocardium.

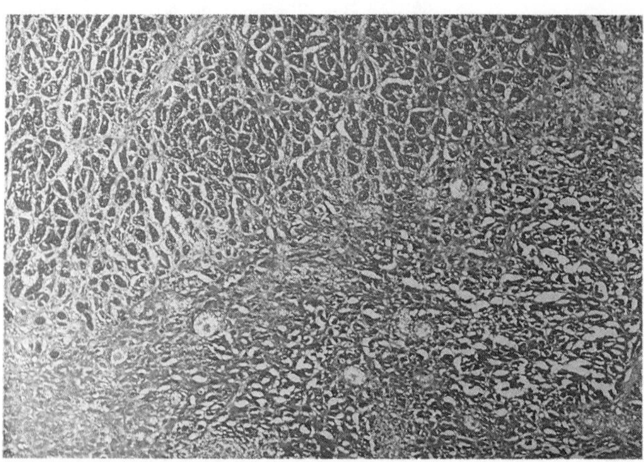

FIGURE *3-17*
Healed myocardial infarct. Tissues with permanent cells can replace dead cells with scar tissue only. After a myocardial infarct, the lost cardiac myocytes are replaced with dense connective tissue (*blue*).

Nervous System

Mature neurons are permanent postmitotic cells and cannot divide. Following trauma, only regrowth and reorganization of the surviving neuronal cell processes can reestablish neural connections. Whereas the peripheral nervous system has the capacity for axonal regeneration, the central nervous system lacks this property.

CENTRAL NERVOUS SYSTEM: Any damage to the brain or spinal cord is followed by capillary growth and gliosis (i.e., astrocytic and microglial proliferation). Gliosis in the central nervous system is the equivalent of scar formation elsewhere; once established, it remains permanently. In spinal cord injuries, axonal regeneration can be seen up to 2 weeks after injury. After 2 weeks, gliosis has taken place and attempts at axonal regeneration end. In the central nervous system, axonal regeneration occurs only in the hypothalamic–hypophyseal region, where glial and capillary barriers do not interfere with axonal regeneration. Axonal regeneration seems to require contact with extracellular fluid containing plasma proteins.

PERIPHERAL NERVOUS SYSTEM: Neurons in the peripheral nervous system can regenerate their axons, and under ideal circumstances section of a peripheral nerve results in complete functional recovery. However, if the cut ends are not in perfect alignment or are prevented from establishing continuity by inflammation or a scar, a traumatic neuroma results. This bulbous lesion consists of disorganized axons and proliferating Schwann cells and fibroblasts (Fig. 3-18). The regenerative capacity of the peripheral nervous system can be ascribed to (1) the fact that the blood–nerve barrier, which insulates peripheral axons from extracellular fluids, is not restored for 2 to 3 months and (2) the presence of Schwann cells with basement membranes. Laminin, a basement membrane component, and nerve growth factor stimulate neurite growth.

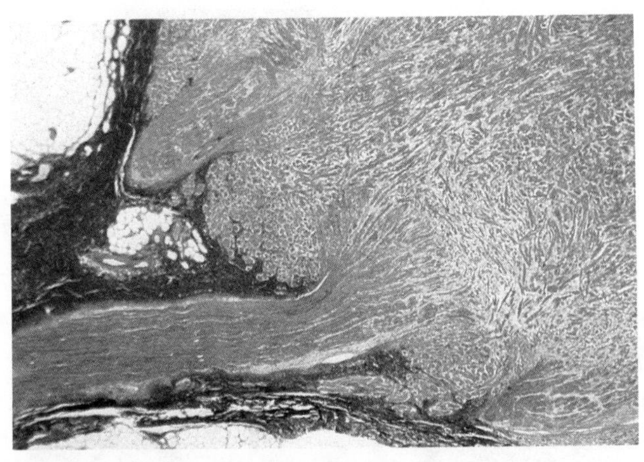

FIGURE *3-18*
Traumatic neuroma. In this photomicrograph, the original nerve (*lower left*) enters the neuroma. The nerve is surrounded by dense collagenous tissue, which appears dark blue with this trichrome stain.

SUGGESTED READING

BOOKS

Alberts B, Bray D, Lewis J, et al: *Molecular biology of the cell.* New York: Garland, 1995.

Cohen I, Diegelman RF, Lindblad WJ: *Wound healing.* Philadelphia: WB Saunders, 1992.

Hay ED (ed): *Cell biology of extracellular matrix.* Mt. Kisco, NY: Plenum Press, 1981.

Majno G, Joris I: *Cells, tissues, and disease.* Cambridge: Blackwell, 1994.

Perez-Tamayo R: *Mechanisms of disease,* 2nd ed. Chicago: Year Book Medical, 1985.

Piez KA, Reddi AH: *Extracellular matrix biochemistry.* New York: Elsevier, 1984.

REVIEW ARTICLES

Majno G: The story of the myofibroblasts. *Am J Surg Pathol* 3:535–542, 1979.

Martinez-Hernandez A, Amenta PS: The basement membrane in pathology. *Lab Invest* 48:656–677, 1983.

Martin P: Wound healing—aiming for perfect skin regeneration. *Science* 276:75–81, 1997.

Martinez-Hernandez A, Amenta PS: The extracellular matrix in hepatic regeneration. *FASEB J* 9:1401–1410, 1995.

Perez-Tamayo R: Pathology of collagen degradation. *Am J Pathol* 92:509–566, 1978.

Shosham S: Wound healing. *Int Rev Connect Tissue Res* 9:1–24, 1981.

CHAPTER 4

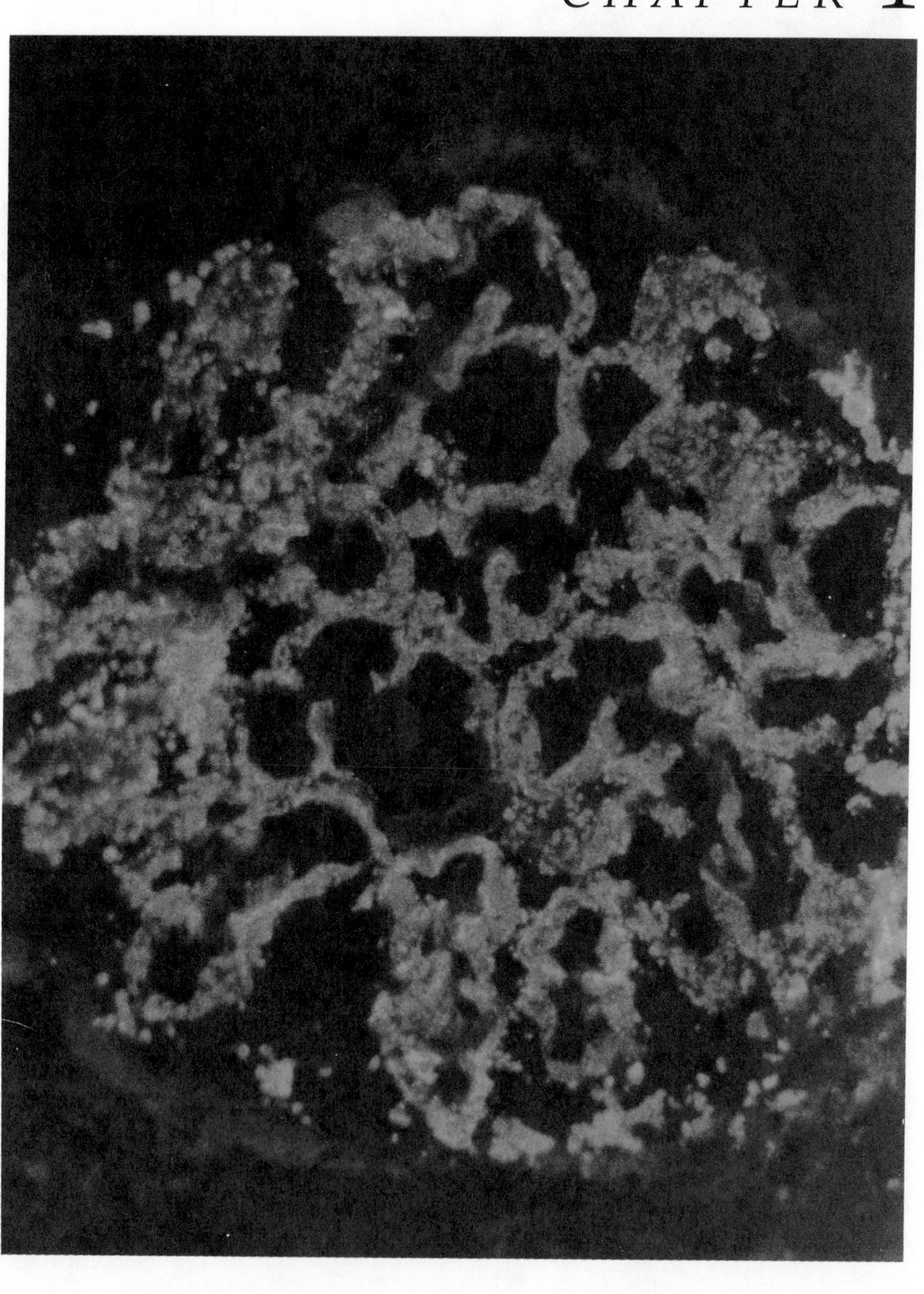

Immunopathology

Kent J. Johnson
Steven W. Chensue
Peter A. Ward

FIGURE *4-1* (*see opposite page*)
Demonstration by immunofluorescence of an extensive deposition of IgG in a renal glomerulus from a patient with systemic lupus erythematosus.

During evolution, plants and animals have acquired a variety of mechanisms to defend themselves from invasion by a vast spectrum of microorganisms, ranging from viruses to multicellular parasites. These defenses extend from simple phagocytosis and digestion in protozoa to the exquisitely complex network of cellular and humoral elements of the mammalian immune system. The importance of immune defenses is dramatically illustrated by the consequences of inherited or acquired defects in the immune system. For example, patients with the acquired immunodeficiency syndrome (AIDS) almost invariably succumb to infectious diseases caused by a bewildering variety of microorganisms, including viruses, bacteria, fungi, and parasites. The sad fate of persons infected with the human immunodeficiency virus (HIV) attests to the silent and unremitting battle that the body constantly wages against foreign invaders.

The body's defense against microorganisms consists of two interrelated but conceptually distinct systems: **natural immunity** and the more specific **acquired immunity**. Natural immunity is mediated principally by the cells involved in the inflammatory response discussed in Chapter 2. Natural immunity does not require prior exposure to the offending agent, nor is it enhanced by such exposure. Moreover, natural immunity is nonspecific; that is, it does not discriminate among various foreign materials. By contrast, acquired immunity is specific. The functions of the cells that participate in acquired immune responses require a sensitizing exposure to the offending agent, and their response is magnified by subsequent exposures to the same macromolecule (antigen).

Although both natural (inflammatory) and acquired (immunological) defense mechanisms are crucial for survival, they are also capable of damaging host tissues. Tissue injury mediated by inflammatory reactions has been described in Chapter 2. Here we discuss the cells that orchestrate immune responses, and we describe the immunopathological manifestations of exaggerated or dysfunctional immune reactions, mediated by both antibodies and immune effector cells.

CELLULAR COMPONENTS OF THE IMMUNE RESPONSE

Lymphocytes

Lymphocytes, because they have the capacity to recognize and react with specific foreign molecules, are the primary directors of antigen-specific immune responses. In the traditional model of lymphocyte development, all cells follow one of two major pathways of development (Fig. 4-2). Lymphocytes originate from primitive yolk sac progenitor cells that become either T cells (thymus-derived) or B cells (bone marrow–derived), depending on subsequent migration and molecular signals. In addition, a third class of lymphocytes (null cells) lacks the defining characteristics of T and B cells. The ontogeny of null cells is unclear. The natural killer (NK) cells, which are described later, belong in this category. T lymphocytes and B lymphocytes are defined on the basis of several functional and phenotypic characteristics acquired during their development.

T Lymphocytes

The development of T cells in the thymus is summarized in Figure 4-3. The stem cell precursors interact with thymic epithelium via surface glycoproteins or adhesion molecules. The latter provide the molecular signals that cause the sequential expression of genes that confer the functional and phenotypic characteristics of T cells. Within the thymus, two differentiation pathways result in T cells that display either of two classes of antigen receptors. The first pathway involves the pro–T cell stage, in which rearrangements of variable (V), diversity (D), and joining (J) regions of the gamma chain gene occur. These code for the antigen-binding receptor of gamma/delta T cells. Pro–T cells that fail to create a stable gamma chain can then initiate beta chain rearrangements. This process is followed by alpha chain rearrangements at the pre–T cell stage, ultimately leading to the mature alpha/beta T cells. A spectrum of functionally related T-cell membrane antigens has been defined with monoclonal antibody reagents, thereby enabling the maturational stages of the T cell to be identified.

Various names have been given to similar target membrane antigens because of differing antibody sources. In order to standardize the nomenclature, cluster designation (CD) numbers have been assigned to distinguish lymphocyte subsets. **T cells at different stages of maturation are characterized by their expression of specific surface markers.**

T-cell development begins with the proliferation of antigen-specific clones in the cortical regions of thymic lobes. The differentiation of T lymphocytes proceeds as follows:

- **Early cortical T cells:** The early, or least mature, cortical thymocytes comprise 10% of the lymphocytes. As illustrated in Figure 4-3, immature T lymphocytes express the membrane antigens designated CD38, CD44, and CD71. The early-stage markers, CD44 and CD71, are lost in the late cortical stage. By contrast, CD38 antigen persists throughout subsequent maturation within the thymus. CD71 and CD38 are markers of activation, that is, they are associated with proliferating or metabolically stimulated T cells. The CD71 antigen is the receptor for transferrin and provides a means to acquire iron during active metabolic states. It should be noted that these markers are not always exclusively expressed by immature T cells; some can be reexpressed during antigen-elicited activation and maturation.
- **Late cortical T cells:** Late cortical thymocytes account for 80% of the thymic population and express new antigens, designated CD1, CD4, CD5, and CD8. These cells lose the early CD71 antigen. Whereas the CD5 and CD7 antigens persist on all T cells, the CD1 antigen is transient and disappears by the time thymocytes migrate to medullary areas of the thymus.
- **Medullary T cells:** In the thymic medulla, the CD4 and CD8 antigens are distributed among two separate cell populations, which display helper (CD4) and cytotoxic/suppressor (CD8) functions. The medullary T cells also acquire the CD3 membrane complex, which is associated with the antigen receptor and persists for the life of the cell. The expression of antigen-specific receptors on T lymphocytes does not require the presence of antigen but, as noted above, is the result of programmed gene expression and rearrangement.
- **Peripheral T cells:** The final stages of T-cell development occur with the migration of T cells to the blood and the lymphatic system, where the CD38 antigen is lost. **In the blood and peripheral lymphoid organs, CD4+ (helper) cells comprise 65% of all T cells, and CD8+ (cytotoxic/suppressor) cells account for 35%.**

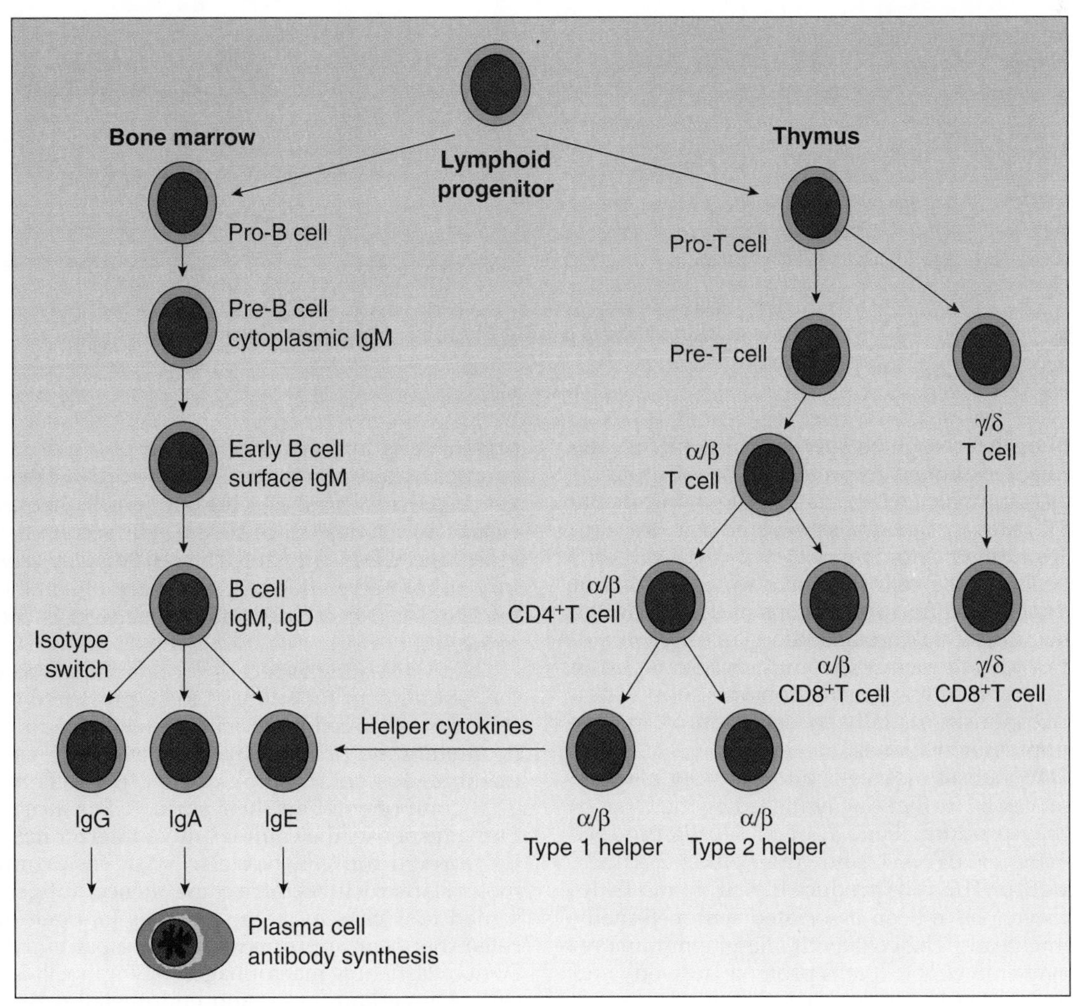

FIGURE 4-2
Major maturational stages of lymphocytes.

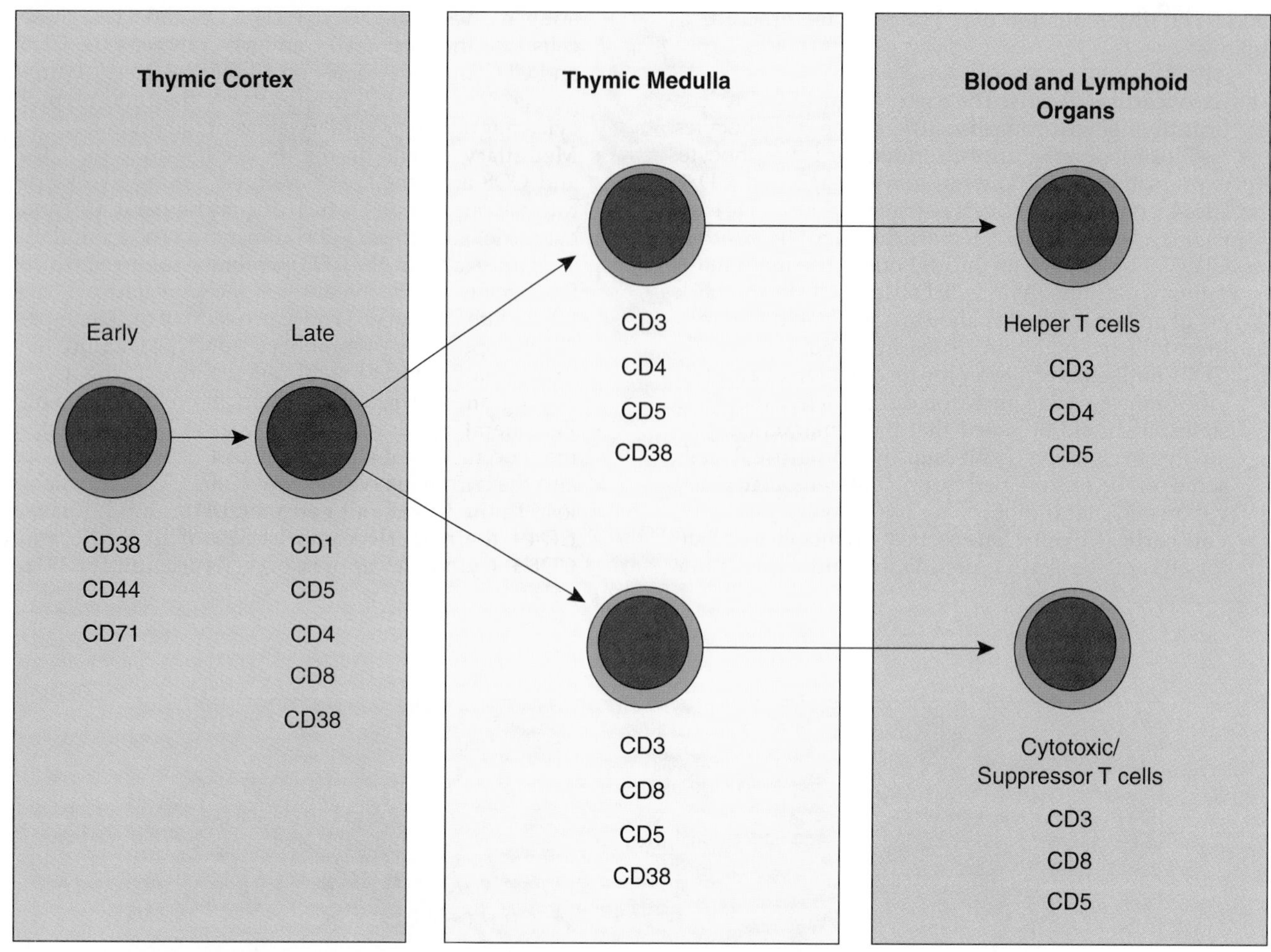

FIGURE 4-3
Membrane marker changes during thymic T-cell maturation.

T lymphocytes recognize specific antigens, usually proteins or haptens bound to proteins. They respond as directed by (1) intrinsic factors that dictate maturational events, and (2) exogenous signals delivered by extracellular molecules termed cytokines. CD4+ and CD8+ cells are, in fact, subsets of T cells that have varied effector or regulatory functions. Effector functions include secretion of proinflammatory cytokines and killing of cells containing foreign or altered membrane antigens. Examples of regulatory functions are augmentation and suppression of immune responses, usually by secretion of specific helper or suppressor cytokines.

The CD4+ subset of T cells and possibly also the CD8+ subset can be further distinguished by the types of cytokines they produce. Type 1, or Th1, cells produce interferon-gamma (IFN-γ) and interleukin-2 (IL-2), whereas type 2, or Th2, cells produce IL-4, IL-5, and IL-10. Th1 lymphocytes have been associated with cell-mediated phenomena and Th2 cells with allergic immune responses. In general, CD4+ T cells promote antibody and inflammatory responses. By contrast, CD8+ cells for the most part exert suppressor and cytotoxic functions. Suppressor cells inhibit the activation phase of immune responses, whereas cytotoxic cells are capable of killing target cells that express specific antigens. However, there is clearly an overlap, since CD8+ cells secrete helper cytokines, and CD4+ Th1 and Th2 cells display cross-regulatory suppressive effects. A summary of some of the important T-cell cytokines and their effects is provided in Table 4-1.

An interesting aspect of T-cell antigen recognition is the requirement for antigens to be presented on the surface of another cell in association with a histocompatibility membrane protein. In other words, T cells have a membrane receptor complex (the α/β T-cell receptor plus CD3 components) on their surface. For a maximal immune response, the complex must interact not only with the foreign antigen but also with histocompatibility molecular structures. As a consequence, antigens are presented to T cells by accessory cells (antigen-presenting cells) that bear appropriate histocompatibility antigens. Such cells include macrophages, B lymphocytes, dendritic cells, Langerhans cells, and endothelial cells. Antigens may also be presented to certain T cells by a variety of

TABLE *4-1* **Polypeptide Cytokines Produced by Lymphocytes**

Cytokine	Molecular Weight	Major Activities
Interferon-γ	20–24 kD	Antiviral, activates phagocytes; induces class I and II MHC antigens and IgG2a synthesis.
Interleukin-2	15–18 kD	Promotes lymphocyte growth, NK-cell activity, and phagocyte activation.
Interleukin-3	14–15 kD	Stimulates myeloid and erythroid differentiation.
Interleukin-4	15–19 kD	Promotes lymphocyte growth, IgE and IgG1 synthesis, FcRϵ expression, and adhesion molecule expression.
Interleukin-5	20 kD	Promotes B-cell differentiation, eosinophil growth, and IgE synthesis.
Interleukin-6	21–28 kD	Produced by macrophages, endothelial cells, fibroblasts, and epithelial cells; promotes lymphocyte growth, acute phase synthesis, and thrombopoiesis.
Interleukin-9	32–39 kD	Promotes T-cell growth.
Interleukin-10	35–40 kD	Promotes B- and mast-cell growth; inhibits IL-12, IFN-γ, TNF, and IL-1 synthesis; also produced by nonlymphoid cells.
Interleukin-12	65–75 kD (dimer)	Promotes IFN-γ production, NK-cell activity, and growth of cytotoxic T cells; opposes IL-10 actions; also produced by macrophages.
Interleukin-13	16–19 kD	Promotes lymphocyte growth and IgE synthesis; many functions similar to IL-4.
Interleukin-14	53 kD	Promotes B-cell growth.
Interleukin-15	14–15 kD	Can replace IL-2 functions, but much of its amino acid sequence differs from IL-2.
Tumor necrosis factor α and β	17 kD	Cytotoxic for some tumor cells; promotes expression of adhesion molecules; stimulates fibroblast growth, synthesis of acute phase proteins; causes fever, cachexia; TNF-α is also a major product of activated macrophages.

cells that are not normally antigen-presenting cells, when they express on their surface a foreign or altered self-protein in association with a histocompatibility molecule.

The relevant histocompatibility antigens are derived from genes in the major histocompatibility complex (MHC). This region codes for human leukocyte antigen (HLA) class I and class II membrane proteins, a subject that will be discussed in greater detail later. In general, CD8+ cells (cytotoxic T cells) recognize antigens in conjunction with class I molecules, whereas CD4+ cells (helper T cells) recognize antigens together with class II molecules. The membrane CD4 and CD8 molecules of α/β T cells help to stabilize binding interactions. γ/δ T cells may also acquire CD8 extrathymically and thereby utilize class I antigens for binding target cells. It should be noted that foreign class I and class II molecules, which are not histocompatible with the host (e.g., transplanted histocompatibility antigens), are themselves potent immunogens and are recognized by host T cells. In addition to the binding of foreign peptides presented by MHC molecules to the T cell receptor complex, a number of other receptor-ligand interactions must occur in order to activate maximally lymphocytes. Figure 4-4 shows schematics of some of the interactions that occur between CD4+ T helper cells and antigen-presenting cells. The CD4+ T cell becomes an activated effector cell when stimulated via the T cell receptor complex and receptors (CD28 and CTLL-4) that recognize co-stimulatory molecules (e.g., B7 and B7.2). In turn, the activated T helper cell recognizes an antigen-specific B cell via its receptor. The T helper cell then provides co-stimulatory and regulatory signals, such as the CD40 ligand and helper cytokines (e.g., IL-4 and IL-5).

B Lymphocytes

B lymphocytes are cells that bear membrane immunoglobulins. Under appropriate conditions they differentiate into antibody-secreting cells as follows:

- **Pre-B cells:** Following development in the embryonic yolk sac, precursor B cells (pro-B cells) migrate to the fetal liver and later to the bone marrow (see Fig. 4-2). These cells interact with stromal cells at those sites and become a proliferating population of pre-B cells. In a manner analogous to that of T cells, they undergo rearrangements of VDJ genes.

  The pre-B cells contain cytoplasmic heavy-chain μ immunoglobulins but neither light-chain nor surface immunoglobulins. However, receptors for complement fragment C3b and HLA class II proteins are present on the plasma membrane. In the fetal liver and bone marrow, pre-B cells multiply and diversify into a vast number of clones.
- **Early B cells:** Immature B cells are recognized by the presence of surface monomeric immunoglobulin M (IgM), which appears once light chain genes have undergone rearrangements and transcription. Upon leaving the bone marrow, B cells express surface IgD. Other membrane markers are also acquired, for example, receptors for IgG-Fc component, complement fragment C3d, and Epstein-Barr virus.
- **Mature B cells:** Mature B lymphocytes are primarily in a resting state, awaiting activation by foreign antigens. Activation involves cross-linking of membrane immunoglobulin receptors by antigens that are presented on accessory cells, as well as interactions with membrane molecules of helper T cells. This initial

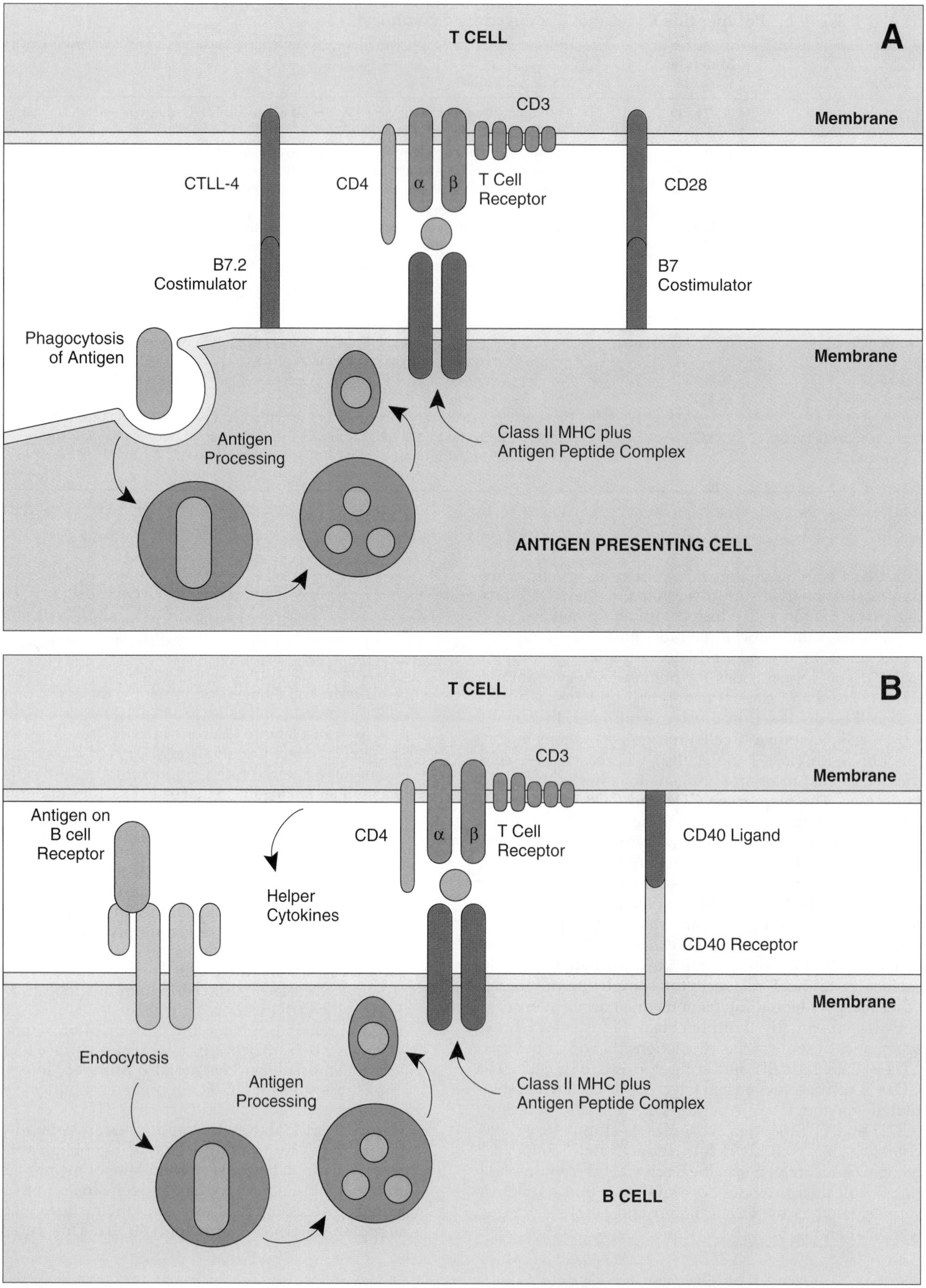

T CELL

A

CD3

Membrane

CTLL-4

CD4

α β

T Cell
Receptor

CD28

B7.2
Costimulator

B7
Costimulator

Phagocytosis
of Antigen

Membrane

Antigen
Processing

Class II MHC plus
Antigen Peptide Complex

ANTIGEN PRESENTING CELL

T CELL

B

CD3

Membrane

Antigen on
B cell
Receptor

CD4

α β

T Cell
Receptor

CD40 Ligand

Helper
Cytokines

CD40 Receptor

Membrane

Endocytosis

Antigen
Processing

Class II MHC plus
Antigen Peptide Complex

B CELL

FIGURE *4-4*

stimulus leads to the proliferation and clonal expansion of B cells, which are amplified by cytokines derived from accessory cells and T cells, such as IL-1 and IL-4. If no further signal is provided, the proliferating B cells return to the resting state and enter the memory cell pool. These events largely occur in lymphoid tissues and are observed as cellular aggregates called germinal centers. Within these centers, B-cells undergo further somatic gene rearrangements, leading to isotype switching.

- **Isotype switching:** The term **isotype** refers to the class of the defining heavy chain of an immunoglobulin molecule. In the absence of antigenic stimulation, a proportion of the B-cell clones proceed to express other heavy-chain isotypes: IgG ($\gamma 1$, $\gamma 2$, $\gamma 3$), IgA (1 or 2), or IgE (ϵ). T cells are also involved in the differentiation of B cells. In the presence of antigen, T cells produce helper cytokines that either stimulate B-cell isotype switching or induce the proliferation of particular committed isotype populations. For example, IL-4 induces switching to the IgE isotype.
- **Plasma cells:** The final stage of B-cell differentiation into antibody-synthesizing plasma cells generally requires exposure to additional T-cell products (e.g., IL-5, IL-6). This is the case for responses to most protein antigens. However, some polyvalent agents directly induce proliferation of B cells and their differentiation into plasma cells, bypassing the requirements for B-cell growth and differentiation factors. Such agents are called **polyclonal B-cell activators** because they do not interact with antigen-binding sites and hence are not specific antigens. Examples of polyclonal B-cell activators are bacterial products (lipopolysaccharide, protein A) and certain viruses (Epstein-Barr virus, cytomegalovirus).

It is noteworthy that the spectrum of immunoglobulins produced during immune responses changes with age. Newborns tend to produce predominantly IgM. By contrast, older children and adults initially produce IgM following antigenic challenge but then rapidly shift toward IgG synthesis.

Natural Killer Cells

Natural killer cells comprise a population of lymphocytes that have the capacity to recognize and kill various tumor cells and virus-infected cells *in vitro*. These large lymphocytes, which contain cytoplasmic granules, cannot be precisely classified as T, B, or myelomonocytic cells. **Thus, NK cells represent a subset of so-called null cells.** These cells possibly have several receptors for various structures in the target cell membrane.

Natural killer cells are affected by several molecular mediators. For example, IL-2 and IL-12 support their growth, and interferon promotes their killing activity. By contrast, prostaglandin E_2 is highly suppressive of NK cell activity. NK cells also have Fc receptors and thus can kill target cells by antibody-dependent cell-mediated cytotoxicity. So called lymphokine-activated killer (LAK) cells are NK cells that have been activated *in vitro* by high concentrations of the lymphokine IL-2 to kill tumor cells and virally infected targets. The role of LAK cells in physiological immune responses is obscure. They have been used in attempts to treat cancer patients but with only limited success.

Mononuclear Phagocytes

Mononuclear phagocyte is a general term applied to populations of phagocytic cells found in virtually all organs and connective tissues. Among these cells are macrophages, monocytes, and Kupffer cells of the liver. The older term histiocyte is today synonymous with macrophage, either a circulating or a fixed tissue macrophage. Mononuclear phagocytes are identified by their nonsegmented nuclei, abundant cytoplasm, and phagocytic function.

There may be subpopulations of macrophages with different functional and phenotypic characteristics. Precursor cells (monoblasts and promonocytes) arise in the bone marrow, enter the circulation as monocytes, and then migrate to tissues, where they take up residence as tissue macrophages (i.e., histiocytes). In the lung, liver, and spleen, numerous macrophages populate sinuses and capillaries to form an effective filtering system that removes effete cells and foreign particulate material from the blood. This system was formerly known as the "reticuloendothelial system," but it is now termed the **mononuclear phagocytic system**. In addition to their housekeeping functions, macrophages play a critical role in the induction of immune responses and in the maintenance and resolution of inflammatory reactions.

Macrophages are important accessory cells by virtue of their expression of class II histocompatibility antigens. They actively ingest and process antigens for presentation to T cells in conjunction with class II antigens. The subsequent T-cell responses are further amplified by macrophage-derived cytokines. One of the best characterized of these is IL-1, which promotes the expression of the IL-2 receptor by T cells. As a result, T-cell proliferation that is driven by IL-2 is augmented. IL-1 also has a broad spectrum of effects on other tissues and, in general, prepares the body to combat infection: for example, it induces fever and promotes catabolic metabolism.

Macrophages are dominant participants in subacute and chronic inflammatory reactions. During persistent inflammation, increased numbers of monocytes are recruited from the bone marrow. Under chemotactic influences, they migrate to sites of inflammation, where they mature into macrophages. Both recruited and local tissue macrophages proliferate at these foci. Table 4-2 summarizes some of the many secretory products of macrophages that can function at sites of inflammation. Among

FIGURE *4-4*
Interactions of T cells with antigen-presenting cells (APCs) and B cells. (*A*) CD4 T cells are activated by APCs via the T-cell receptor and CD28 or CTLL-4. (*B*) Antigen-specific B cells are activated via interaction with the T-cell receptor and CD40.

TABLE 4-2 Major Macrophage Products

Proteins
Enzymes
- Neutral proteinases (e.g., plasminogen activator, elastase, collagenases)
- Lysozyme
- Arginase
- Lipoprotein lipase
- Angiotensin-converting enzyme
- Acid hydrolases

Plasma proteins
- Coagulation proteins
- Complement components
- α_2-Macroglobulin
- Fibronectin

Cytokines
- IL-1, 10, 12
- Tumor necrosis factor
- Interferon α/β
- Angiogenesis factor

Reactive Oxygen Species
- Superoxide anion
- Hydrogen peroxide
- Oxygen radicals
- Nitric oxide

Bioactive Lipids
- Prostaglandin E_2
- Prostacyclin I_2
- Thromboxane B_2
- Leukotriene B_4, C_4, D_4, E_4
- Hydroxyeicosatetraenoic acids (HETEs)

Nucleotides
- Thymidine, uracil
- cAMP
- Uric acid

these are proteins, lipids, nucleotides, and reactive oxygen metabolites. Functionally, these molecules are (1) digestive, (2) opsonic, (3) cytotoxic, (4) growth promoting, or (5) growth inhibiting. Thus, macrophages are ideal cells to direct inflammatory events, locally and systemically.

The functional activity of macrophages and the spectrum of molecules that they produce are regulated by external factors, such as T cell–derived cytokines. Macrophages exposed to such factors become "activated"; that is, they acquire a greater capacity to release oxygen metabolites and kill tumor cells and intracellular microorganisms.

If the agent that incites an inflammatory process is poorly digestible, a **granulomatous reaction** may ensue. Under such conditions, macrophages show additional maturation and become epithelioid cells and multinucleated giant cells. Epithelioid cells are macrophages with abundant eosinophilic cytoplasm, which appear to be predominantly secretory. Giant cells result from macrophage fusion, resulting in syncytia containing multiple nuclei. Depending upon the inciting agent, different types of giant cells may form. For example, granulomas elicited by mycobacteria often contain Langhans-type giant cells, which have a circular arrangement of nuclei. Giant cells of foreign body granulomas have a random distribution of nuclei. Both epithelioid cells and giant cells are poorly phagocytic; they mainly sequester and digest foreign material.

Human Major Histocompatibility Complex

The discovery that the sera of multiparous women and multiply transfused patients contain antibodies against foreign blood leukocytes led to the definition of an intricate system of membrane proteins known as the **major histocompatibility complex**. Individual MHC antigens are referred to as *human leukocyte antigens*. **MHC proteins, which are highly polymorphous within the human population, are the main target antigens during rejection of transplanted organs.** Such antigens allow for self-recognition during cell–cell interactions, especially in immune responses.

The MHC genes are located on the short arm of chromosome 6 (Fig. 4-5), where they code for three major classes of molecules, designated I, II, and III. Class III antigens represent certain complement components and are not histocompatibility antigens.

CLASS I HISTOCOMPATIBILITY MOLECULES: Class I molecules were originally defined using the sera of multiparous women. They are coded for by genes in the A, B, and C regions of the MHC. These loci code for molecules of similar structure and are expressed in virtually all tissues. Class I histocompatibility antigens are heterodimeric structures consisting of two chains, a 44-kD polymorphic transmembrane glycoprotein and a 12-kD nonpolymorphic molecule called β_2-microglobulin. The latter is a superficial surface protein lacking a membrane component and is in noncovalent association with the larger heavy chain. It is coded for by a gene on chromosome 15. The heavy α-chain, encoded by the MHC complex, contains the polymorphic antigenic determinants that define the many alleles of the A, B, and C loci. Antigenic polymorphism occurs primarily in the extracellular regions of the α-chain. Since the alleles are expressed codominantly, tissues bear class I antigens from both parents. These antigens are recognized by cytotoxic T cells during graft rejection or during killing of virus-infected cells.

CLASS II HISTOCOMPATIBILITY MOLECULES: Class II molecules are coded for by multiple loci in the D region: DP, DN, DM, DO, DQ, and DR. The D region loci code for molecules of similar structure, which are expressed primarily on accessory cells involved in antigen presentation, such as monocytes, macrophages, dendritic cells, Kupffer cells, and B cells. Class II antigens are also referred to as Ia (immunity-associated) antigens. They are analogous to the mouse MHC genes of that name, which are associated with the immune response. Class II molecules are heterodimers consisting of two noncovalently linked glycoprotein chains. The 34-kD β-chain has a sin-

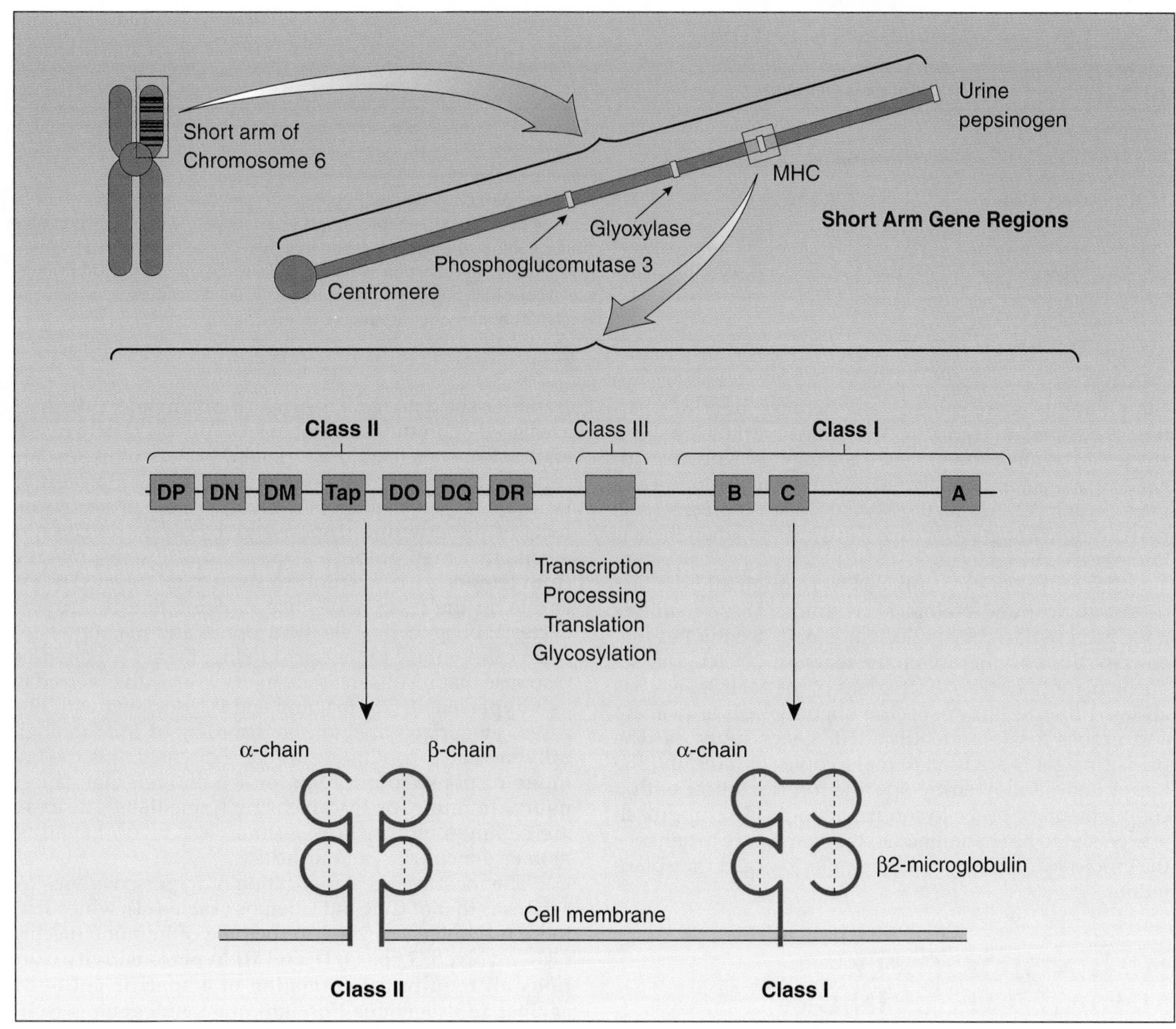

FIGURE 4-5
The genes of the human major histocompatibility complex (MHC) and their protein products.

gle disulfide bond; its extracellular domain is the major site of class II antigenic variability. The 29-kD α-chain has two disulfide bonds. Both are transmembrane proteins. As in the case of class I antigens, the alleles are expressed co-dominantly, and tissues bear antigens from both parents.

SIGNIFICANCE OF MHC MOLECULES: The histocompatibility molecules are important for interactions between immune cells, particularly in antigen presentation to T cells. X-ray crystallographic studies of classes I and II molecules indicate that processed foreign peptides are bound to a groove formed by their tertiary structures. The two classes of MHC molecules allow for presentation of antigen derived from different cellular compartments, namely the cytosol and endosomes.

Intracellular pathogens such as viruses generate cytosolic peptides, which are transported to the endoplasmic reticulum by transporter-associated processing (TAP) molecules. There the peptides join with class I molecules to form a stable complex that migrates to the cell surface, where they can be recognized by CD8+ T cells. Unlike class I molecules, class II molecules do not associate with peptides during their assembly in the endoplasmic reticulum. They are, rather, transported to phagolysosomes, where under acid proteolytic conditions they acquire peptides and protein fragments derived from endocytosed proteins or microorganisms. The resulting complexes are then fused to the surface membrane, where they are recognized by CD4+ T cells.

DETECTION OF MHC MOLECULES: Table 4-3 summarizes the methods used to define class I and class II antigens for tissue typing prior to organ transplantation.

TABLE 4-3 **Methods of Tissue Typing**

Assay	Antigens Detected	Principle
Microcytotoxicity assay	Class I	Defined antibodies directed against specific MHC antigens are mixed with patient's cells in the presence of complement. Cells bearing the target antigens are lysed.
Mixed leukocyte assay	Class II (DR and DQ)	Mitomycin-treated, HLA-defined typing cells are mixed with patient's cells. The patient's cells will not proliferate in response to cells with compatible antigens. (Note: this assay is being largely replaced by DNA allotyping.)
DNA allotyping assay	Class I (B locus) and class II (DR, DQ, DP)	The polymerase chain reaction is performed using oligonucleotide primers and probes that detect polymorphisms in DNA sequences, which can be related to allotypic differences in MHC antigens.

Class I antigens are serologically defined. Briefly, a battery of defined antisera directed against various antigens are tested against the patient's leukocytes. Known antigens are named and numbered according to the loci of origin (e.g., A1, A2, A3, B4, B6, C1, C2). Tissue typing reveals two different antigens for each locus, except when there is homozygosity at a locus.

Class II membrane antigens were originally defined by serological and biological methods. These methods have been replaced by molecular genetic techniques that employ the **polymerase chain reaction (PCR)**. The sequencing of hypervariable regions of the MHC genes has allowed the design of specific oligonucleotide primers and probes that can identify MHC genes subtypes. The primer reagents are used to make copies of (amplify) the target gene, followed by specific hybridization with a complementary probe to confirm identity. This approach is expected to be streamlined in the near future to enhance the efficiency of tissue matching prior to organ transplantation.

IMMUNOLOGICALLY MEDIATED TISSUE INJURY

Immune responses constitute a protective mechanism to combat invasion by foreign organisms, but they also often lead to tissue damage. Thus, many inflammatory diseases are based on immune mechanisms. A wide variety of foreign substances (e.g., dust, pollen, bacteria, viruses) are capable of acting as antigens and provoking a protective immune response. In certain situations, the protective effects of the immune response give way to deleterious events that may produce a spectrum of lesions, ranging from temporary discomfort to substantial injury. For example, in the process of phagocytizing and destroying bacteria, phagocytic cells (neutrophils and macrophages) often cause injury to the surrounding tissue. An immune response that results in tissue injury is broadly referred to as a **hypersensitivity reaction** and is associated with diseases categorized as immune disorders or immunologically mediated conditions. In these diseases, it is the immune response to a foreign or self-antigen that causes injury. Immune, or hypersensitivity-mediated, diseases are common and include asthma, hay fever, hepatitis, glomerulonephritis, and arthritis.

The most useful classification of hypersensitivity reactions is that of Gell and Coombs (Table 4-4), which lists these reactions according to the type of immune mechanism involved. **Types I, II, and III hypersensitivity reactions all require the formation of a specific antibody against an exogenous (foreign) or an endogenous (self) antigen. However, the antibody class, which is variable, is a critical determinant in the mechanism by which tissue injury occurs.**

TABLE 4-4 **Classification of Hypersensitivity Reactions**

Type	Immunological Mechanism	Examples
Type I (anaphylactic type): Immediate hypersensitivity	IgE antibody–mediated—mast cell activation and degranulation	"Hay fever," asthma, anaphylaxis
Type II (cytotoxic type): Cytotoxic antibodies	Cytotoxic (IgG, IgM) antibodies formed against cell surface antigens. Complement is usually involved.	Autoimmune hemolytic anemias, antibody-dependent cellular cytotoxicity (ADCC), Goodpasture disease
Type III (immune complex type): Immune complex disease	Antibodies (IgG, IgM, IgA) formed against exogenous or endogenous antigens. Complement and leukocytes (neutrophils, macrophages) are often involved.	Autoimmune diseases (SLE, rheumatoid arthritis), most types of glomerulonephritis
Type IV (cell-mediated type): Delayed-type hypersensitivity	Mononuclear cells (T lymphocytes, macrophages) with interleukin and lymphokine production	Granulomatous diseases (tuberculosis, sarcoidosis)

- **Type I hypersensitivity:** In type I, or immediate-type, hypersensitivity reactions, IgE antibody is formed and binds to receptors on mast cells and basophils. The binding of antigen that reacts with the IgE releases products from these cells and results in the characteristic symptoms of diseases such as asthma or anaphylaxis.
- **Type II hypersensitivity:** In type II hypersensitivity reactions, IgG or IgM antibody is formed against an antigen, usually a protein on a cell surface or (less commonly) a component of the extracellular matrix, such as basement membranes. This antigen–antibody coupling leads to complement activation, which in turn is responsible for the lysis of the cell (cytotoxicity) or damage to the extracellular matrix.
- **Type III hypersensitivity:** In type III hypersensitivity reactions, the antibody responsible for tissue injury is also IgM or IgG, but the mechanism of tissue injury differs. The antigen is not fixed to the cell surface but circulates in the vascular compartment and is eventually deposited in tissues. Complement activation at sites of antigen localization leads to the recruitment of leukocytes, which are responsible for the subsequent tissue injury.
- **Type IV hypersensitivity:** Type IV reactions, also known as cell-mediated or delayed hypersensitivity reactions, do not require the formation of an antibody. Rather, antigenic activation of T lymphocytes, usually with the help of macrophages, causes the release of products by these cells, thereby leading to tissue injury.

Although the Gell and Coombs classification is useful in categorizing immunologically mediated tissue injury, it is important to remember that it is oversimplified. Many immunological diseases are mediated by more than one type of hypersensitivity reaction. A good example is hypersensitivity pneumonitis, a condition in which lung injury results from hypersensitivity to an inhaled fungal antigen. Types I, III, and IV hypersensitivity reactions are all involved in the events that culminate in this disease. We will briefly describe the immunological mechanisms involved in the various hypersensitivity reactions.

Type I Hypersensitivity (Immediate Type or Anaphylaxis)

Immediate-type hypersensitivity, or anaphylaxis (Greek ana, excessive; phylaxis, protection), is manifested by a localized or generalized reaction that occurs immediately (within minutes) after exposure to an antigen to which the person has previously become sensitized. The reactions depend on the site of antigen exposure. For example, when the reactions involve the skin, the characteristic local reaction is swelling and edema (**hives**). When the localized manifestations of immediate hypersensitivity involve the upper respiratory tract and conjunctiva, causing sneezing and conjunctivitis, we speak of **hay fever**. In its generalized, most severe form, an immediate hypersensitivity reaction is associated with bronchial constriction, airway obstruction, and circulatory collapse, as seen in the **anaphylactic syndrome**. Fortunately, severe anaphylactic reactions are rare, even though immediate-type hypersensitivity reactions, particularly of the localized variety, are common (e.g., millions of persons every year have allergic rhinitis).

Pathogenesis

The mechanism involved in all immediate hypersensitivity reactions is related to the formation of IgE antibody. IgE antibodies are formed by a CD4+, Th2 T-cell-dependent mechanism and bind avidly to Fc receptors on mast cells and basophils. The specific binding of IgE accounts for the term **cytotropic** antibody. Once exposed to a specific allergen that has resulted in the formation of IgE, a person is **sensitized**; subsequent responses to the allergen induce an immediate hypersensitivity reaction. After IgE antibody is formed, reexposure to the antigen often results in the production of additional IgE antibodies, rather than the formation of other antibody classes, such as IgG or IgM ("class switching"). For example, a person who has responded with IgM antibody to an antigenic challenge will produce IgG after subsequent exposure to the same antigen. This response is induced by IL-4.

It should also be stressed that IgE bound to receptors on mast cells and basophils persists for long periods of time (weeks), a feature unique to IgE. Upon subsequent reexposure, the soluble antigen binds to the IgE coupled to its surface receptor. This event activates mast cells and basophils, an effect that releases the potent inflammatory mediators that are responsible for the development of the hypersensitivity reactions. As shown in Figure 4-6, the antigen (allergen) binds to IgE antibody through its Fab sites. Cross-linking of the antigen to more than one IgE antibody molecule, attached to receptors on mast cells and basophils, is required to activate the cells. Cells can also be activated by agents other than antibodies. As also shown in Figure 4-6, the complement anaphylatoxin peptides, C3a and C5a, directly stimulate mast cells by a different receptor-mediated process. This event causes the release of granule constituents or the rapid synthesis and release of other mediators. Other compounds, including mellitin (from bee venom) and drugs (e.g., morphine), also directly activate mast cells and cause the release of granule constituents. Many anaphylactic deaths from bee stings in sensitized persons occur in the United States every year.

CALCIUM: No matter how the mast cell activation sequence is initiated, calcium influx into the cell cytoplasm is required. The rise in cytosolic free calcium is associated with (1) increases in cyclic adenosine monophosphate (cAMP), (2) activation of several metabolic pathways within the mast cell, and (3) subsequent secretion of preformed and newly synthesized products.

PREFORMED PRODUCTS: Potent mediators are rapidly released from granules. Because they are preformed and stored in granules, they exert immediate biological effects on their release. Of the granule constituents listed in Figure 4-6, the biogenic amine histamine is perhaps the most important.

Histamine induces constriction of vascular and nonvascular smooth muscle and causes microvascular

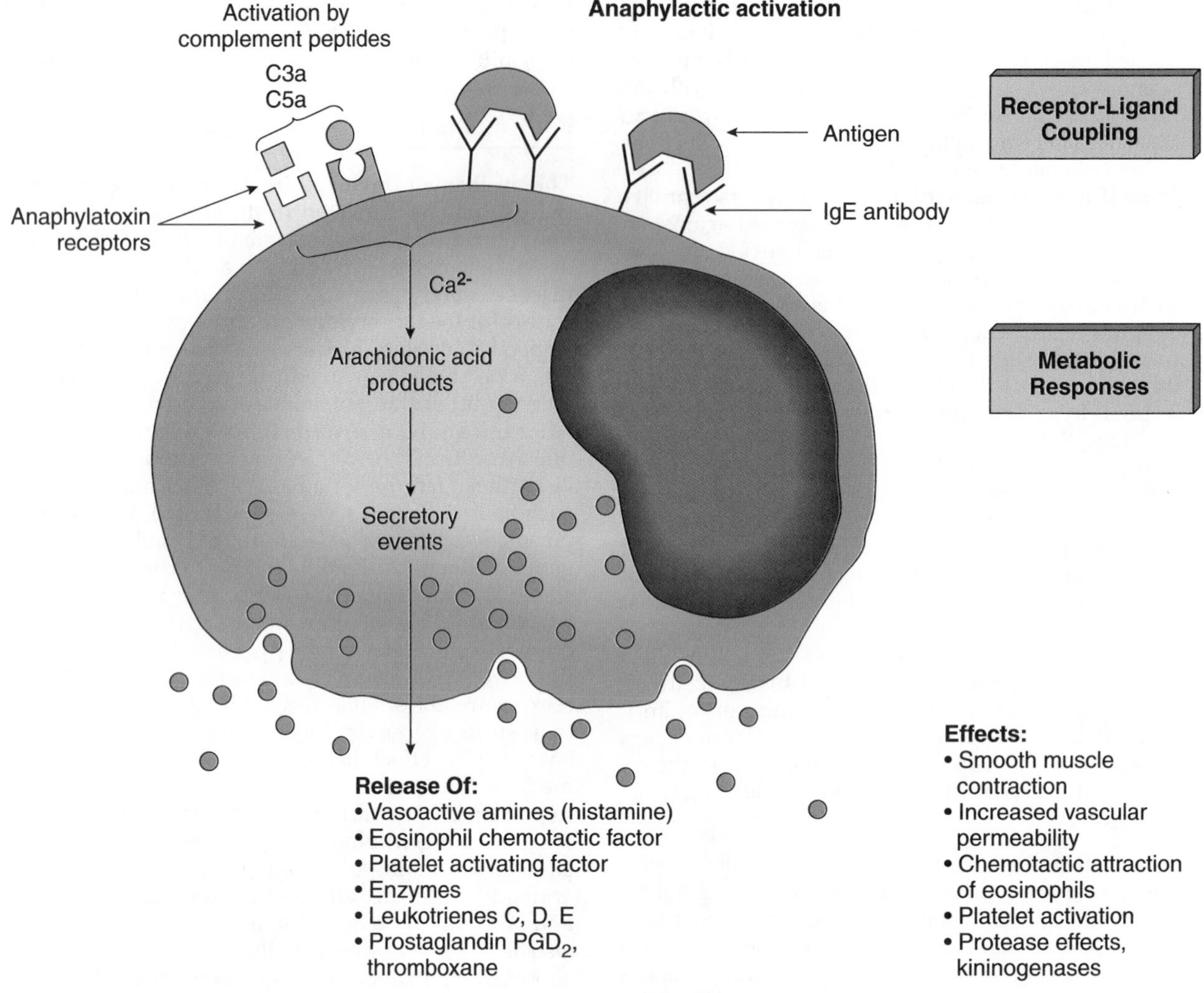

FIGURE *4-6*
Type I hypersensitivity. Activation of the mast cell and the potent inflammatory mediators released or synthesized by the cell.

dilatation and increased permeability of the venules. These biological effects are largely mediated by H_1 histamine receptors. Histamine also increases gastric acid secretion through H_2 histamine receptors. In the skin, histamine provokes the "wheal and flare" reaction. In the lung, it is responsible for the classic early manifestations of immediate hypersensitivity, namely, bronchospasm, vascular congestion, and edema.

Other preformed products released from mast cell granules include heparin, neutral proteases (trypsin, chymotrypsin, carboxypepidase, acid hydrolases), and at least two chemotactic factors: a neutrophil chemotactic factor and an eosinophil chemotactic factor. The last is responsible for the accumulation of eosinophils, an effect characteristic of immediate hypersensitivity.

MEDIATORS DERIVED FROM ARACHIDONIC ACID: Upon activation of mast cells, the synthesis of potent inflammatory mediators is also initiated. Foremost among these mediators are the various products of the arachidonic acid pathway, which are formed following the activation of phospholipase A_2 (see Chapter 2). Products derived from the activities of cyclooxygenase (prostaglandins D_2, E_2, F_2, and thromboxane) and lipoxygenase (leukotrienes B_4, C_4, D_4, E_4) are formed. These arachidonic acid products, which are also generated by a variety of other cells, induce effects such as smooth muscle contraction, vasodilatation, and edema. Of particular interest is the finding that leukotrienes C_4, D_4, and E_4 are the **slow-reacting substances of anaphylaxis** (SRS-As), molecules that are important in the delayed bronchoconstriction phase of anaphylaxis. Leukotriene B_4, a potent chemotactic factor for neutrophils, macrophages, and eosinophils, is formed during anaphylaxis and may be involved in attracting inflammatory cells into tissues.

PLATELET ACTIVATING FACTOR: Another inflammatory mediator synthesized by the mast cell is platelet activating factor (PAF), a lipid derived from membrane phospholipids (see Chapter 2). As the name implies, platelet activating factor is a powerful stimulant for platelet aggregation and the release of vasoactive amines from platelets. It has a broad range of biological activity and is able to activate all types of phagocytic cells.

CYTOKINE MEDIATORS: As mentioned earlier, there is good evidence that activated T cells, specifically those with a Th2-type response, produce several cytokines that have important effects on the allergic response. These activated Th2 T-cell subsets produce IL-4, IL-5, and IL-6 in the mouse, leading to IgE production and increased numbers of mast cells and eosinophils. In man, this response also occurs with T-cell clones that produce IL-4 in allergic persons. IL-6 and IL-2 levels are also increased in allergic individuals. These patients also have lowered levels of IFN-γ, which has been shown to suppress the development of Th2 clones and the subsequent production of IgE.

Summary

The type I (immediate) hypersensitivity reaction is characterized by a specific cytotropic antibody (IgE), which binds to receptors on basophils and mast cells and reacts with a specific antigen. This process results in the activation of mast cells and basophils, which then release preformed (granule) products and synthesize mediators that cause the classic manifestations of immediate hypersensitivity.

Type II Hypersensitivity (Cytotoxic Type)

Type II hypersensitivity is also caused by an antigen–antibody reaction. However, as the name implies, the antibodies are often cytotoxic and are directed against antigens on cell surfaces or in connective tissues. IgG and IgM are the classes of antibody usually involved in these reactions. The most important characteristic of these antibodies is their ability to activate the complement system through Fc receptors. There are several antibody-dependent mechanisms of cytotoxicity.

Complement-Mediated Cytotoxicity

The classic model of antibody-mediated cytotoxicity directed against erythrocytes is illustrated in Figure 4-7.

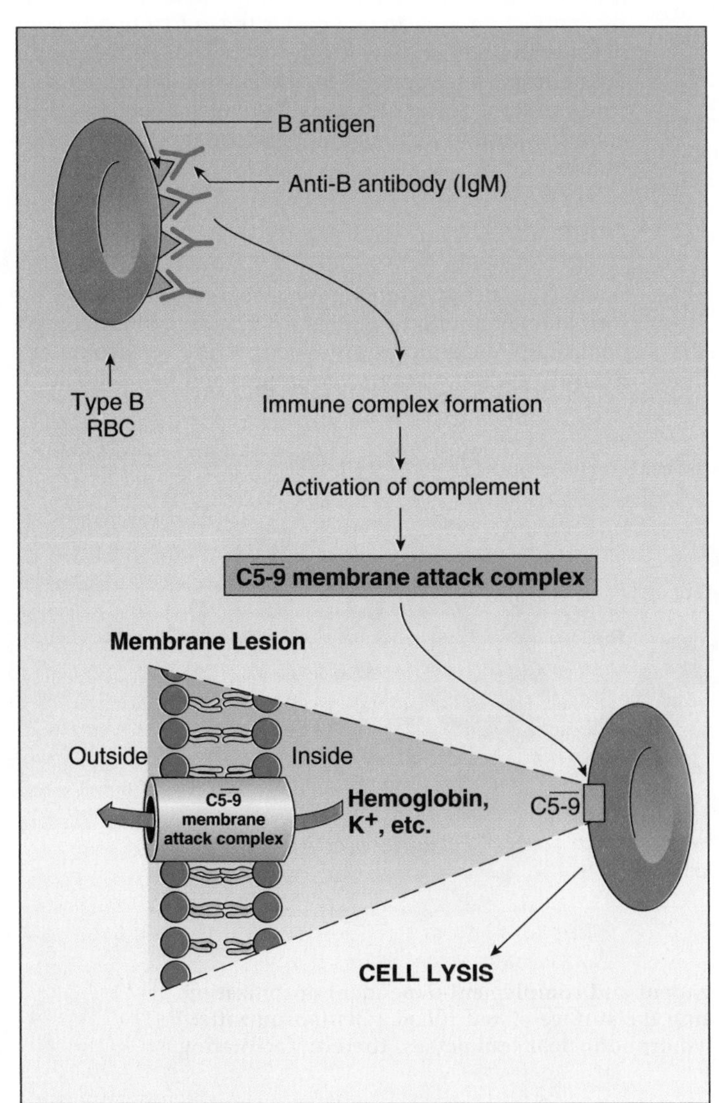

FIGURE 4-7
Type II hypersensitivity. Antibody- and complement-mediated red blood cell lysis due to complement activation and the formation of the C5b–9 membrane attack complex (MAC).

IgM or IgG antibody binds to an antigen on the surface of the erythrocyte membrane. This antibody binding induces activation of the complement system through the classic pathway, via interaction with C1q (see Chapter 2). Once activated, complement leads to the destruction of the target cell by two distinct mechanisms.

DIRECT LYSIS: Complement products directly lyse the target cells by the formation of a complex of C5b–9 complement components (see Fig. 4-7). This complex is referred to as the **membrane attack complex** because of its ability to insert into the plasma membrane and form "holes" or ionic channels, thereby destroying the permeability barrier and inducing lysis of the cell. This type of complement-mediated cell lysis is exemplified by certain types of autoimmune hemolytic anemias that involve the formation of cold-reactive antibodies against blood group antigens on erythrocytes. In transfusion reactions that result from major blood group incompatibilities, hemolysis occurs because the activation of complement leads to the destruction of erythrocytes.

OPSONIZATION: Complement also indirectly enhances the destruction of a target cell by opsonization, in which complement interaction on the target cell surface leads to the formation of C3b (Fig. 4-8). Many phagocytic cells, including neutrophils and macrophages, express receptors for C3b on their cell membranes. By binding to its receptor, C3b bridges the target cell and the effector (phagocytic) cell, thereby enhancing phagocytosis and the intracellular destruction of the complement-coated cell. Certain types of autoimmune hemolytic anemias and some drug reactions are mediated by this type of complement-associated opsonization.

ANTIBODY-DEPENDENT, CELL-MEDIATED CYTOTOXICITY: There is another type of antibody-mediated cytotoxicity that does not require participation of the complement system. Antibody-dependent, cell-mediated cytotoxicity (ADCC) involves cell-destroying leukocytes that attack antibody-coated target cells through Fc receptors. Phagocytic cells and null or killer lymphocytes are the effector cells in ADCC. The mechanism by which the target cell is destroyed in these reactions is not clear. It appears that the effector cells synthesize homologues of terminal complement proteins, which may be related to the cytotoxic events. Only rarely is antibody alone directly cytotoxic. In those cases involving primarily lymphoid cells, apoptotic mechanisms are activated. ADCC may be involved in the pathogenesis of some autoimmune diseases, for example autoimmune thyroiditis.

Antibody-Mediated Functional Changes

In some type II reactions, antibody binding to a specific target cell receptor does not lead to death of the cell but rather to physiological changes. The autoimmune diseases myasthenia gravis and Graves disease (hyperthyroidism) feature autoantibodies against hormone receptors (Fig. 4-9). In Graves disease, the autoantibody against the thyroid-stimulating hormone (TSH) receptor mimics the effect of TSH, thereby stimulating thyroid acinar cells. By contrast, in myasthenia gravis the autoantibody competes with acetylcholine for the acetylcholine receptor in the neuromuscular endplate, thereby inhibiting synaptic transmission. Autoantibodies have also been described against receptors for insulin, prolactin, and growth hormone.

Antibody-Mediated Connective Tissue Injury

Some type II hypersensitivity reactions result from the formation of antibody against a connective tissue component. Classic examples are Goodpasture syndrome and the bullous skin diseases pemphigus and pemphigoid. In

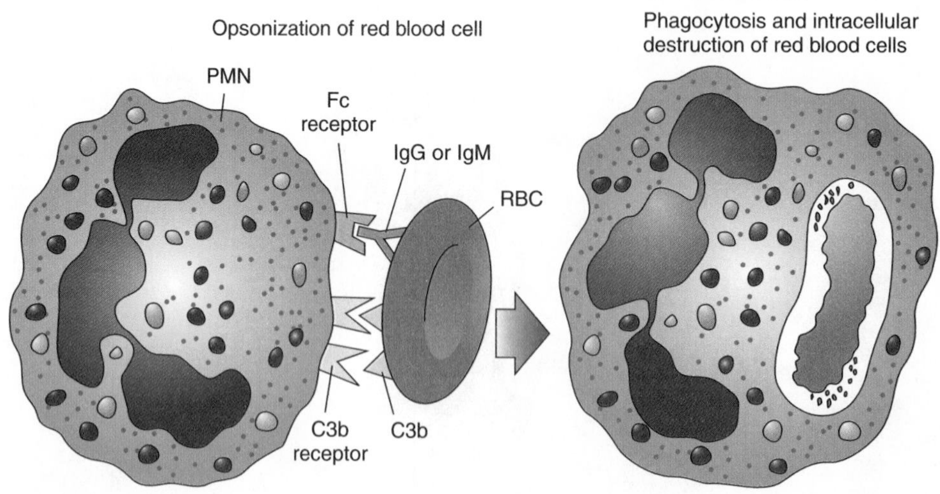

FIGURE 4-8
Type II hypersensitivity. Antibody-dependent and complement-dependent opsonization. Immunoglobulins and complement coating the surface of red blood cells (opsonization) bind to receptors on the surface of polymorphonuclear leukocytes, thereby facilitating phagocytosis.

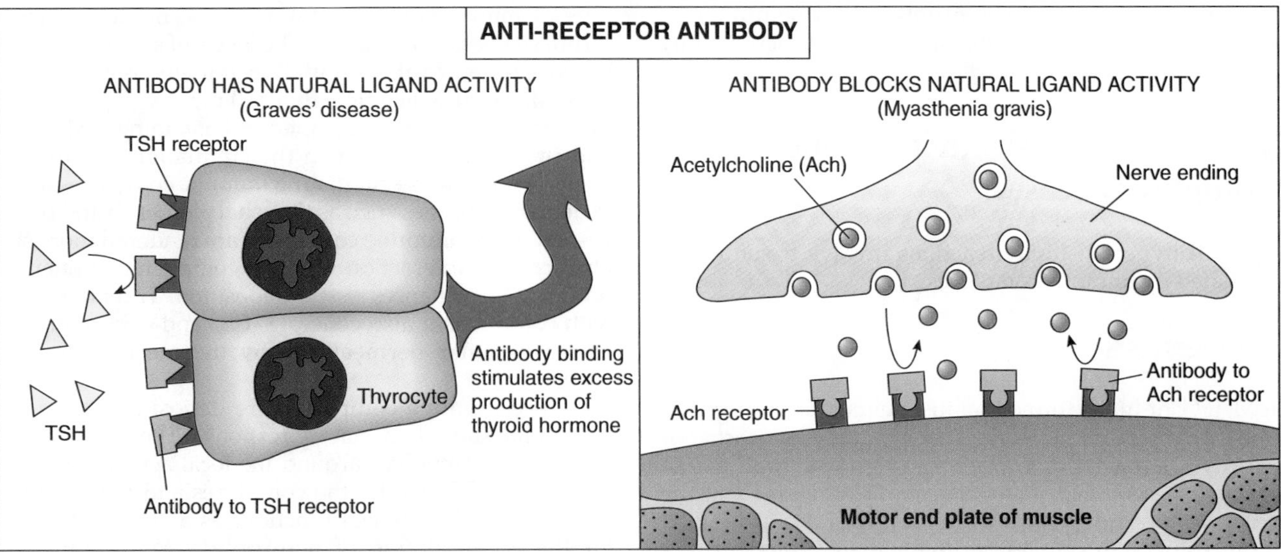

FIGURE 4-9
Type II hypersensitivity. Noncytotoxic antireceptor antibodies in Graves disease and myasthenia gravis. The binding of the antibody to the TSH receptor in Graves disease results in hyperthyroidism, whereas the inhibition of synaptic transmission in myasthenia gravis leads to profound muscle weakness.

these diseases, circulating antibody binds to a fixed connective tissue antigen and evokes a local inflammatory response. In the case of Goodpasture disease (Fig. 4-10), an autoantibody binds to an antigen or antigens in pulmonary and glomerular basement membranes. Local complement activation recruits neutrophils into the site, resulting in pulmonary hemorrhage and glomerulonephritis. Direct complement-mediated damage to the basement membranes of the lung and kidney through formation of the membrane attack complex may also be involved.

Summary

Type II hypersensitivity reactions are directly or indirectly cytotoxic and involve the formation of antibodies against antigens on cell surfaces or in connective tissues. Complement is required for many of these cytotoxic events. Lysis is mediated directly by complement or indirectly by opsonization or the chemotactic attraction of phagocytic cells. Complement-independent reactions, such as ADCC, also fall into this category. Many human diseases, including the autoimmune hemolytic anemias,

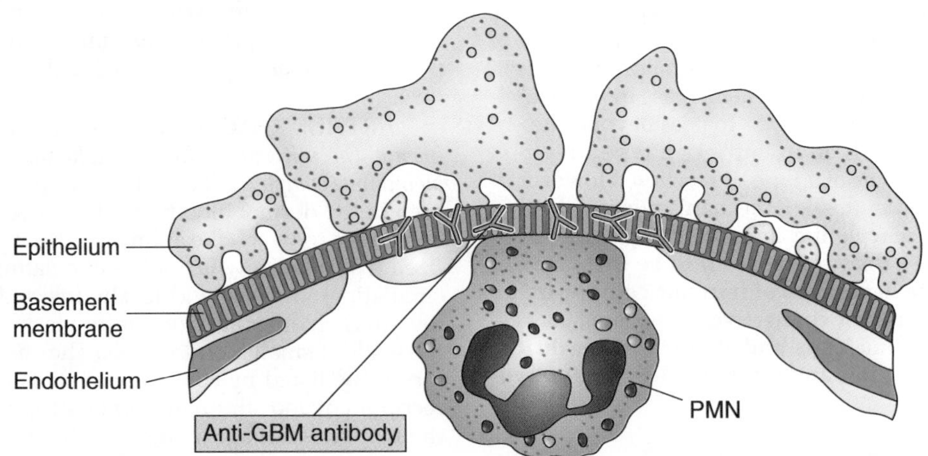

FIGURE 4-10
Type II hypersensitivity. Antibody against glomerular basement membrane antigens in Goodpasture disease. The binding of antibody to antigens of basement membrane activates complement, thereby recruiting polymorphonuclear leukocytes and provoking tissue injury.

Goodpasture syndrome, pemphigus and pemphigoid, Graves disease, and myasthenia gravis, are mediated by type II hypersensitivity reactions.

Type III Hypersensitivity: Immune Complex Diseases

Type III hypersensitivity reactions involve tissue injury mediated by immune complexes.

Pathogenesis

IgM, IgG, or IgA is formed against a circulating antigen or one that is present in tissues. Based on the physicochemical characteristics of the immune complexes, such as size and charge, antigen–antibody complexes formed in the circulation are deposited in tissues, including the renal glomerulus, skin venules, choroid plexus, lung, and synovium. Once deposited, immune complexes elicit an inflammatory response by activating complement, thereby leading to chemotactic recruitment of neutrophils and macrophages to the site. These cells are then activated and release their tissue-damaging mediators, such as proteases and oxygen radicals.

Immune complexes have been implicated in the pathogenesis of many human diseases. The most compelling case is one in which the demonstration of immune complexes in the injured tissue correlates with the development of the injury. A convincing example of this is periarteritis nodosa associated with hepatitis B, in which medium-size arteries contain immune complexes of IgG and the hepatitis B surface antigen (HBsAg) in the vessel wall. In many diseases, immune complexes are detected in the plasma without concomitant evidence of tissue injury. The physicochemical properties of these circulating complexes differ from those of complexes deposited in tissues, the presence of which correlates with tissue injury. In some cases, vasopermeability factors may play a key role in the localization of circulating immune complexes. In this regard, immune complex deposition in the renal glomerulus may be facilitated by the interaction of antigen with IgE-coated basophils. This binding results in the release of histamine and a local increase in permeability, thereby permitting complexes to pass beyond the endothelial barrier. This is an example of a type I reaction that affects the outcome of a type III reaction. However, it is not known whether this IgE mechanism is involved in the deposition of circulating immune complexes in human disease. **The diseases that seem to be most clearly attributable to the deposition of immune complexes are autoimmune diseases of connective tissue, such as systemic lupus erythematosus and rheumatoid arthritis, some types of vasculitis, and most varieties of glomerulonephritis.**

SERUM SICKNESS: *Serum sickness is an acute, self-limited disease that occurs 6 to 8 days after the injection of a foreign protein (bovine albumin) and is characterized by fever, arthralgias, vasculitis, and an acute glomerulonephritis.* Several experimental models of immune complex injury allow a precise definition of the mediator involved in this type of injury. Foremost among these models is acute serum sickness in the rabbit. The levels of exogenously injected antigen in the circulation remain constant until about day 6, at which time they fall rapidly (Fig. 4-11). At the same time, immune complexes (containing IgM or IgG and the antigen) appear in the circulation. Simultaneously, some of these circulating immune complexes begin to deposit in tissues such as the renal glomeruli and blood vessels. These immune complexes are rendered more soluble by their interaction with the complement system, a process that enhances tissue deposition. The interaction with complement also generates C3a and C5a, which increase vascular permeability by the mechanisms described.

Once immune complexes are deposited in tissues, they induce an inflammatory response. The mediation of this response revolves around the local activation of the complement system by the complexes and the resulting formation of C5a, which functions as a chemoattractant for the accumulation of neutrophils. Many adhesion molecules and cytokines are critical in the neutrophil recruitment and activation. The actual recruitment of these cells is mediated by chemotactive peptides such as C5a, leukotriene B_4 (LTB_4), and IL-8. The adherence and migration of neutrophils into the sites of immune complex deposition are mediated by several adhesive interactions (see Chapter 2). Many cytokines have been implicated in modulating this neutrophilic response. The early production of IL-1 and tumor necrosis factor-alpha (TNF-α) mediates the upregulation of adhesion molecules and other cytokines. These include platelet-derived growth factor (PDGF), transforming growth factor-beta (TGF-β), and the interleukins IL-4, IL-6, and IL-10, which serve to modulate the activation of leukocytes and fibroblasts. Not all cytokines are proinflammatory. IL-10, in particular, appears to downregulate the inflammatory response. Once neutrophils arrive, they are activated through contact with and ingestion of immune complexes. As a result, they release many inflammatory mediators, including proteases, oxygen radicals, and arachidonic acid products, which collectively produce tissue injury. Experimental injury associated with serum sickness, such as that seen in the renal glomerulus, mimics the histological appearance of many types of human glomerulonephritis.

ARTHUS REACTION: *The Arthus reaction is an experimental vasculitis model in which a localized injury is induced by immune complexes* (Fig. 4-12). This reaction is classically seen in the dermal blood vessels by the local injection of an antigen to which the animal has been previously sensitized (i.e., against which it has circulating antibody). The circulating antibody and locally injected antigen diffuse toward each other and form immune complex deposits in the walls of small blood vessels. The ensuing vascular injury is mediated by complement activation, followed by recruitment and stimulation of neutrophils, which release their tissue-damaging factors. Because the injury is caused by recruited neutrophils and their products, 2 to 6 hours are required for evidence of tissue injury, in marked contrast to type I (immediate) hypersensitivity reactions. Histologically, the affected vessels show large numbers of neutrophils and evidence of damage to the vessel, with edema and hemorrhage into the surrounding tissue (see

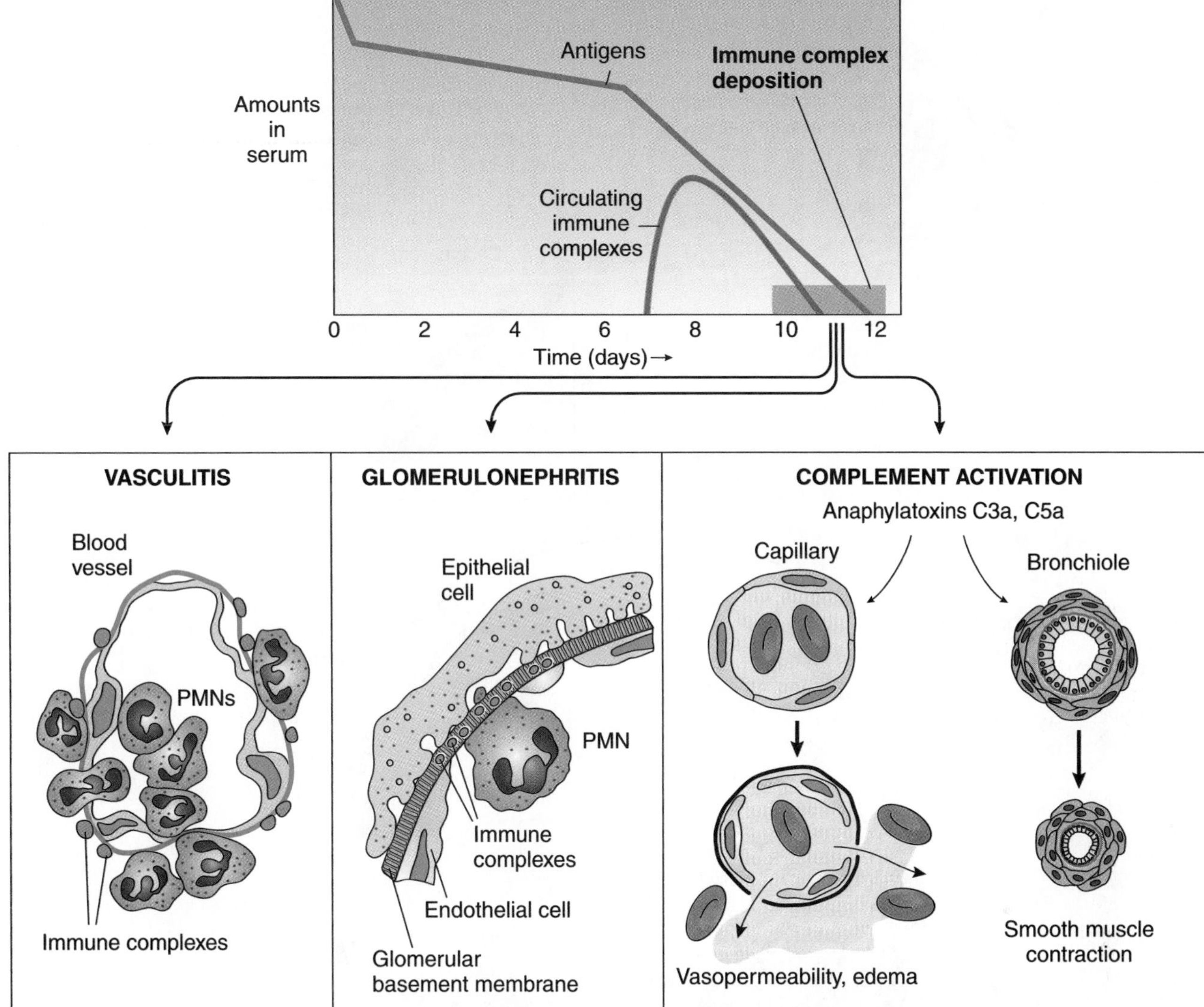

FIGURE *4-11*
Type III hypersensitivity. In the serum sickness model of immune complex tissue injury, antibody is produced against a circulating antigen, and immune complexes form in the blood. These complexes deposit in tissues such as blood vessels and glomeruli and, augmented by complement activation, induce tissue injury or dysfunctional responses.

Fig. 4-12). In addition, the presence of fibrin creates the classic appearance of an immune complex–induced vasculitis, referred to as **fibrinoid necrosis**. This experimental model of localized vasculitis is the prototype for many forms of vasculitis seen in man, for example, the various types of cutaneous vasculitides that characterize certain drug reactions.

Summary

Type III hypersensitivity reactions represent the classic example of immune complex–mediated injury, in which antigen–antibody complexes, which are usually not organ specific, are formed in the circulation and deposited in the tissues. These complexes then induce a localized inflammatory response by activating the complement system, consequently attracting neutrophils and macrophages. Activation of these cells by the immune complexes, with the release of potent inflammatory mediators, is directly responsible for the injury. **Many human diseases, including auto-immune diseases such as systemic lupus erythematosus and most types of glomerulonephritis, are mediated by type III hypersensitivity reactions.**

Type IV Hypersensitivity: Cell-Mediated Immunity

Cell-mediated hypersensitivity is an antigen-elicited cellular immune reaction that results in tissue damage and does not

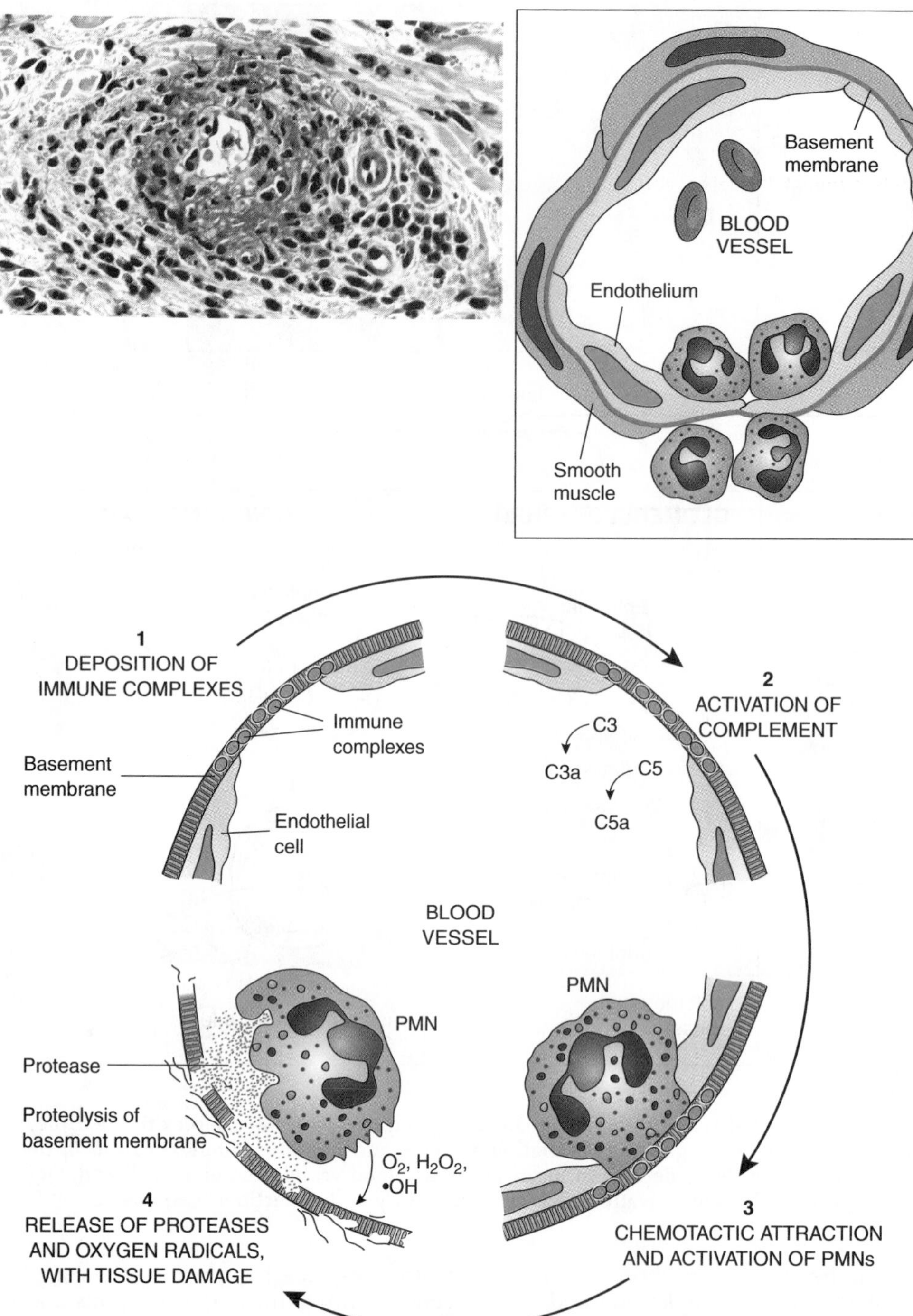

FIGURE *4-12*

Type III hypersensitivity. Localized immune complex-induced vasculitis in the Arthus reaction is depicted. The deposition of immune complexes in the vessel wall leads to localized complement activation and the recruitment of polymorphonuclear leukocytes, as shown in the photomicrograph. The leukocytes produce injury to the vessel wall, with edema and fibrin deposition.

require the participation of antibodies. Included among these reactions are delayed-type cellular inflammatory responses and cell-mediated cytotoxic effects. These reactions often occur together with superimposed antibody reactions, which makes it difficult to define these processes under natural circumstances. Studies with several experimental models suggest that the type of tissue response is largely determined by the nature of the inciting agent.

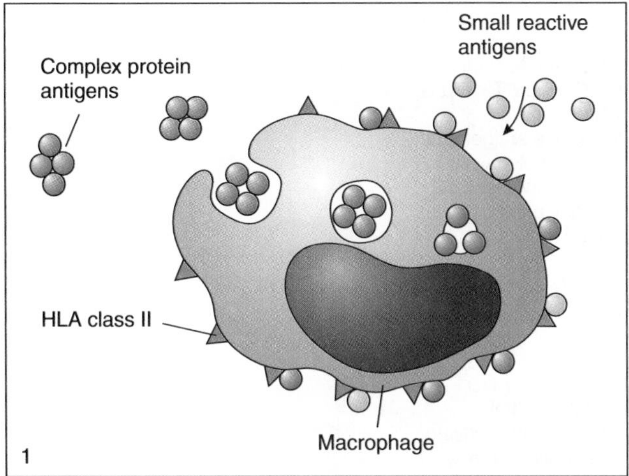

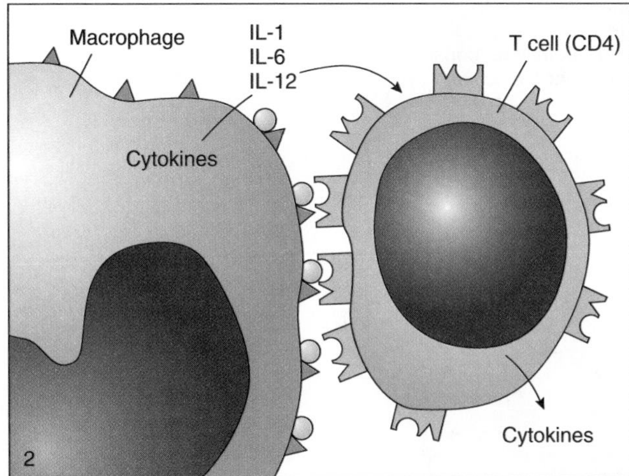

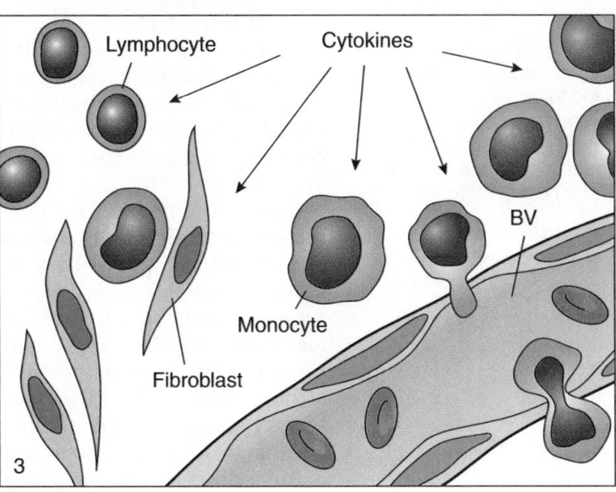

Delayed-Type Hypersensitivity

Classically, delayed-type hypersensitivity is defined as a tissue reaction, primarily involving lymphocytes and mononuclear phagocytes, that occurs in response to the subcutaneous injection of a soluble protein antigen and reaches greatest intensity 24 to 48 hours after injection. A naturally occurring example of this reaction is the contact sensitivity response to poison ivy. Although the chemical ligands in poison ivy are not proteins, they bind covalently to cell proteins, after which the altered molecules are recognized by antigen-specific lymphocytes.

Figure 4-13 summarizes the main stages of the delayed-type hypersensitivity reaction. In the initial phase, foreign protein antigens or chemical ligands interact with accessory cells (macrophages) bearing class II HLA-D molecules. The protein antigens are actively processed into short peptides within phagolysosomes of macrophages and then presented on the cell surface in conjunction with the class II HLA-D molecules (see previous discussion of MHC molecules). The latter are recognized by CD4+ T cells, which become activated and begin the synthesis of a spectrum of cytokines (see Table 4-1). In turn, the cytokines recruit and activate lymphocytes, monocytes, fibroblasts, and other inflammatory cells. If the antigenic stimulus is eliminated, the reaction spontaneously resolves after 48 hours, possibly with only a scar remaining as the result of fibroblast activity. If the stimulus persists, an attempt to sequester the inciting agent results in a granulomatous reaction.

T Cell–Mediated Cytotoxicity

Another mechanism by which T cells effect tissue damage is direct cytolysis of target cells. This immune mechanism is important for the destruction and elimination of cells infected by viruses and possibly tumor cells that express neoantigens. Cytotoxic T cells also play an important role in graft or transplant rejection.

Figure 4-14 summarizes the events in T cell–mediated cytotoxicity. In contrast to the situation in delayed hypersensitivity reactions, cytotoxic CD8+ T cells must simultaneously interact with target antigens joined with class I MHC antigens, HLA-A, HLA-B, or HLA-C. In the case of virus-infected cells and tumor cells, foreign antigens are actively presented together with self-MHC antigens. In

FIGURE *4-13*
Delayed-type hypersensitivity reaction. (*Panel 1*) Complex antigens are phagocytosed and "processed" by macrophages and then presented on the membrane complexed with class II (Ia) antigens. By contrast, chemically reactive ligands bind directly to membrane proteins. (*Panel 2*) Antigen-specific T cells recognize the membrane protein–antigen complexes and receive growth-promoting signals (monokines), such as interleukin-1, from macrophages. T cells then become activated and begin the synthesis and secretion of molecular mediators (lymphokines). (*Panel 3*) The lymphokines and monokines recruit additional inflammatory cells and initiate local cellular proliferation and activation. BV, blood vessel.

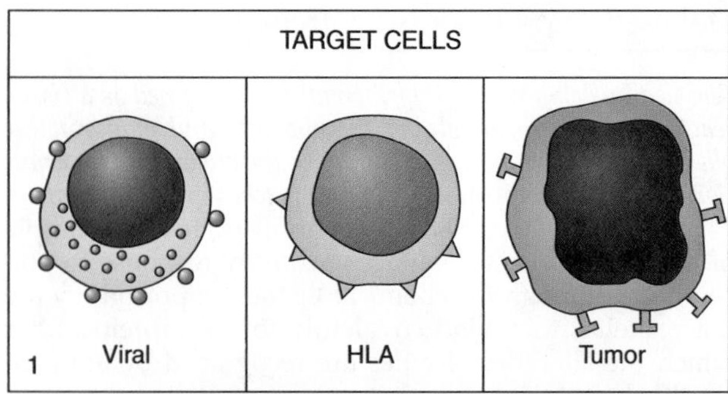

TARGET ANTIGENS
- Virally-coded membrane antigen
- Foreign or modified histocompatibility antigen
- Tumor-specific membrane antigens

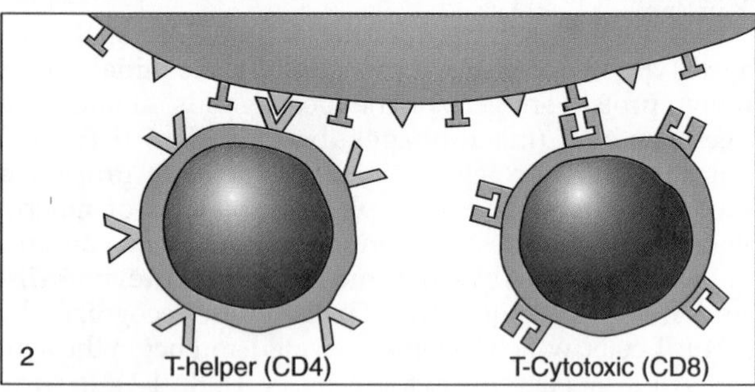

RECOGNITION OF ANTIGEN BY T CELLS
- T-helper cells recognize antigen plus class II molecules
- T-cytotoxic/killer cells recognize antigen plus class I molecules

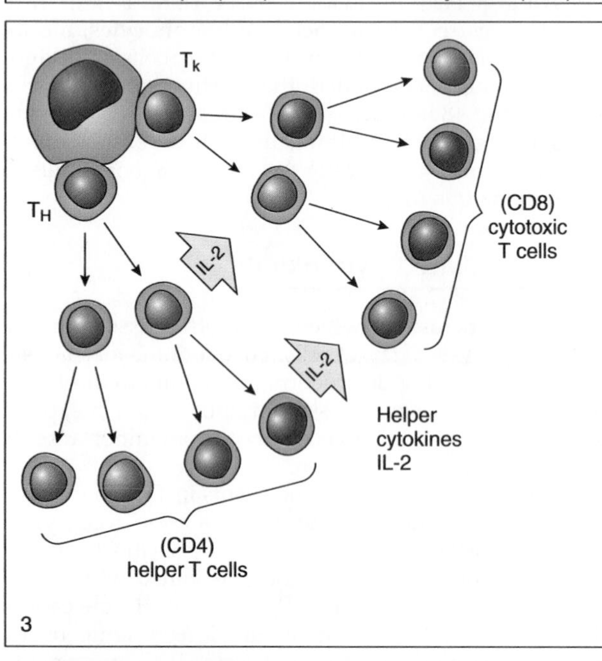

ACTIVATION AND AMPLIFICATION
- T-helper cells activate and proliferate, releasing helper molecules (e.g., IL-2)
- T-cytotoxic/killer cells proliferate in response to helper molecules

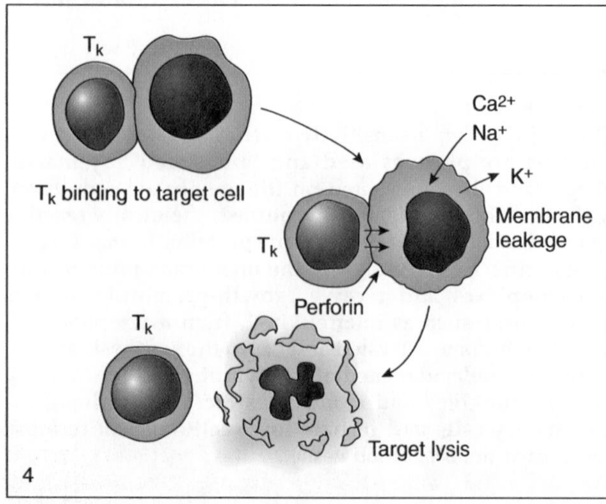

TARGET CELL KILLING
- T-cytotoxic/killer cells bind to target cell
- Killing signals perforin release and target cell loses membrane integrity
- Target cell undergoes lysis

FIGURE *4-14*
T cell–mediated cytotoxicity. (*Panel 1*) Potential target cells of T cells include virally infected cells, histoincompatible cells (e.g., transplanted organ), and tumor cells expressing neoantigens. (*Panel 2*) T cells recognize foreign antigens and class I histocompatibility antigens. (*Panel 3*) T cells become activated and begin to proliferate. T helper cells release lymphokines that amplify proliferation. (*Panel 4*) T killer cell binds to target cell and delivers a signal, resulting in disruption of the sodium–potassium pump. The target cell is then lysed.

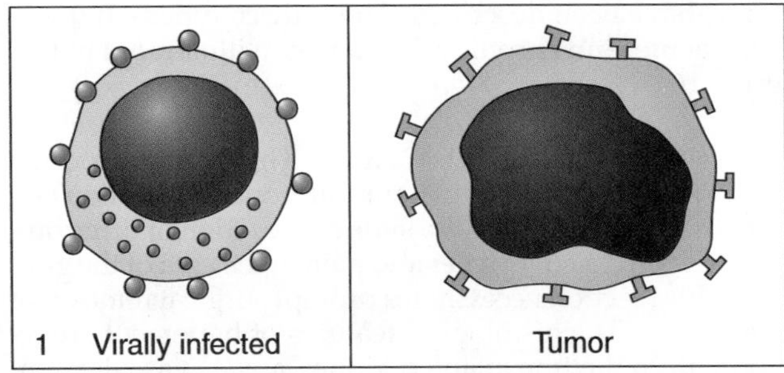

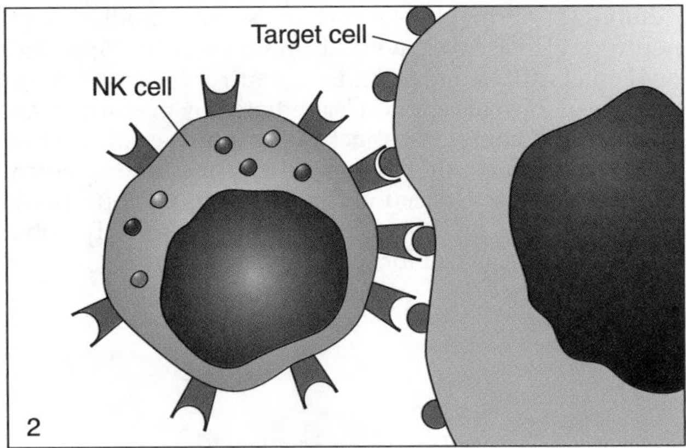

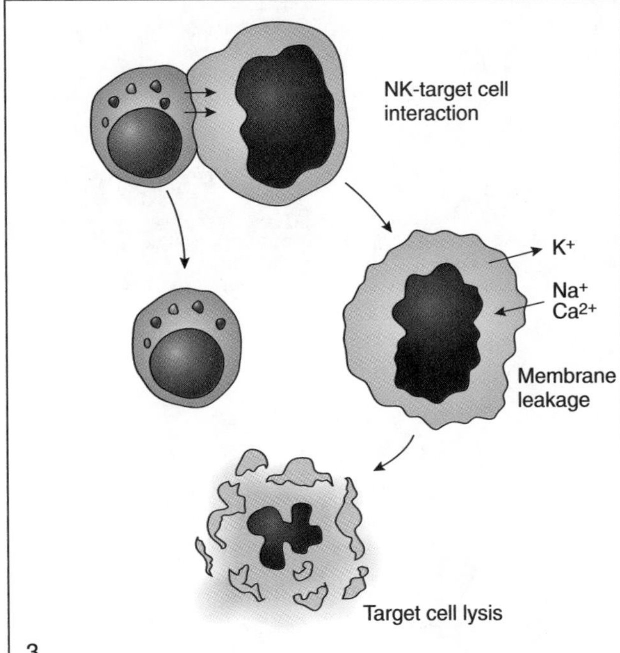

FIGURE *4-15*
Natural killer (NK) cell–mediated cytotoxicity. (*Panel 1*) Potential targets of NK cells include virally infected cells and tumor cells. (*Panel 2*) Recognition of antigen. NK cells bear receptors for a variety of membrane glycoproteins, allowing for cell–cell binding. (*Panel 3*) Following binding, the NK cell delivers the killer signal. The target-cell sodium–potassium pump is disrupted, and the target cell is lysed.

graft rejection, foreign MHC antigens are themselves potent activators of CD8+ T cells. Once activated by the antigenic stimulus, the proliferation of the cytotoxic cells is promoted by helper or amplifier cells and is mediated by soluble growth factors such as IL-2. An expanded population of antigen-specific killer cells is thus generated for attacking target cells. The actual killing event requires energy-dependent binding of the killer cell to the target cell. The killer cell next delivers the molecular signal perforin, which disrupts the membrane permeability of the target, causing an influx of sodium, calcium, and water, and ultimately lysis. Once the cytotoxic signal is delivered, the subsequent lytic events are energy independent and irreversible.

Natural Killer Cell–Mediated Cytotoxicity

The defining characteristics of NK cells have been described, but the extent to which such cells participate in tissue-damaging immune reactions is unclear. Mounting evidence indicates that NK cells exert both effector and immunoregulatory functions.

Figure 4-15 summarizes the events of target-cell killing by NK cells. Unlike killer T cells, NK cells recognize a variety of target cells. They bear receptors that bind either several different antigenic structures or similar antigens on different target cells. The target antigens are membrane glycoproteins that are expressed by certain virus-infected cells or tumor cells. In a series of events similar to that described for killer T cells, NK cells bind to the target cell through their membrane receptors and then deliver a molecular signal that results in its lysis. NK cells also have membrane Fc receptors. Thus, they acquire antibodies that allow for the binding and killing of target cells by an antibody-directed mechanism (i.e., ADCC). NK cell activity is influenced by a variety of cytokines. For example, NK cell activity is increased by IL-2, IL-12, and IFN-γ, and decreased by prostaglandins.

Summary

The type IV hypersensitivity reaction, unlike the other types of hypersensitivity reactions, is not an antibody-mediated response. Rather, antigens are processed by macrophages and presented to antigen-specific T lymphocytes. These lymphocytes become activated and release a variety of mediators, or cytokines, that recruit and activate lymphocytes, macrophages, and fibroblasts. The resulting injury is caused by the T lymphocytes themselves or the macrophages or both. The chronic inflammation characteristic of a wide variety of autoimmune diseases, such as chronic thyroiditis, Sjögren syndrome, and primary biliary cirrhosis, is an example of type IV hypersensitivity reactions.

IMMUNE REACTIONS TO TRANSPLANTED ORGANS AND TISSUES

It is now clear that histocompatibility antigens are the critical immunogenic molecules that stimulate rejection of transplanted organs. The optimal survival of a graft occurs when the recipient and donor are closely matched with regard to these histocompatibility antigens, especially in the case of renal transplantation. In practice, an exact HLA match is rarely obtained, except in the case of transplantation between monozygotic twins. As a result, vigilant monitoring of the status of the graft and immunosuppressive therapy are required after transplantation. In recent years, such therapies have greatly improved transplant success rates, even when there is documented histoincompatibility. When rejection does occur, any combination of immune responses may destroy the graft.

Host-versus-Graft Reactions

The histopathological features of graft rejection are well demonstrated in rejected renal allografts. Three major types of rejection, based on the time of onset of the rejection episode and the corresponding histological features, have been described. These three types—hyperacute, acute, and chronic rejection—are illustrated in Figure 4-16.

HYPERACUTE REJECTION: This reaction occurs within the first minutes to hours after transplantation and is manifested clinically as a sudden cessation of urine output, accompanied by fever and pain in the area of the graft site. This reaction necessitates prompt surgical removal of the kidney. The histological features of hyperacute rejection within the transplanted kidney are (1) vascular congestion, (2) fibrin–platelet thrombi within capillaries, (3) neutrophilic vasculitis with fibrinoid necrosis, (4) prominent interstitial edema, and (5) neutrophilic infiltrates. This rapid form of rejection is mediated by **preformed** antibodies and complement activation products, including chemotactic and other inflammatory mediators. Fortunately, hyperacute rejection is not common if appropriate antibody screening is performed, using recipient lymphocytes as the target cell for the antibody assay.

A
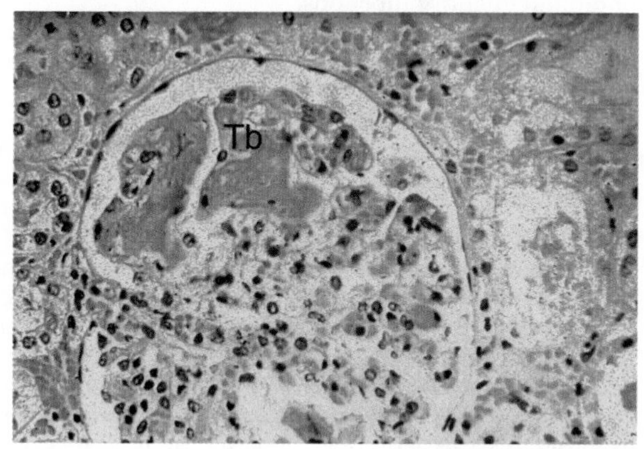

B
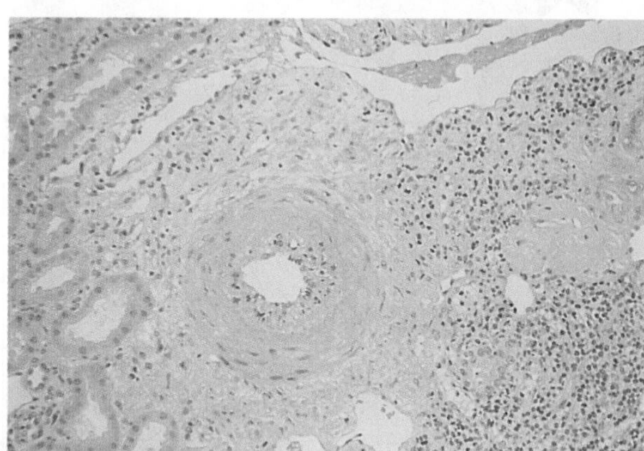

C
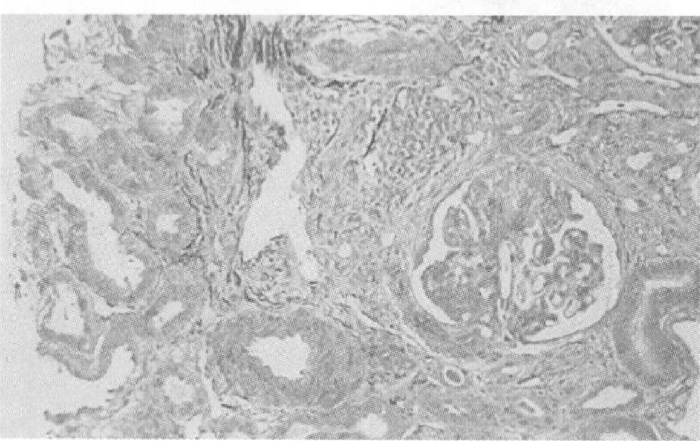

FIGURE *4-16*
Histological features of major forms of renal transplant rejection. (*A*) Hyperacute rejection occurs in minutes to hours after transplant. This glomerulus shows intravascular fibrin–platelet thrombi and infiltrates of polymorphonuclear leukocytes. There is interstitial edema of surrounding tissue. (*B*) Acute cellular rejection occurs within weeks to months after transplant. There is infiltration by mononuclear leukocytes with associated tubular damage. The small artery in the middle of the photo is also infiltrated, indicating vasculitis. (*C*) Chronic rejection is observed months to years after transplant. There is extensive deposition of fibrous tissue (stained blue) between tubules and around glomeruli. Tubules show atrophy and there are patchy interstitial infiltrates of mononuclear cells. Glomerular capillary walls are focally thickened. Tb, thrombi.

ACUTE REJECTION: Acute rejection occurs in the first few weeks or months after transplantation. Clinically, there is sudden onset of azotemia and oliguria, which may be associated with fever and graft tenderness. A needle biopsy is often performed to differentiate between a rejection episode and acute tubular necrosis or toxicity from immunosuppressive agents. The microscopic findings of acute graft rejection include (1) interstitial infiltrates of lymphocytes and macrophages, (2) edema, (3) lymphocytic tubulitis, and (4) tubular necrosis. The most severe form also shows vascular damage, manifested as arteritis, fibrinoid necrosis, and thrombosis. Vascular involvement is an ominous sign because it usually means the rejection episode will be refractory to therapy. Acute rejection likely involves both cell-mediated and humoral mechanisms of tissue damage. If detected in its early stages, acute rejection can be reversed with immunosuppressive therapy.

CHRONIC REJECTION: The transplanted kidney may undergo rejection several months to years after transplantation. Clinically, the patient develops progressive azotemia, oliguria, hypertension, and weight gain. The dominant histological features of chronic rejection are (1) arterial and arteriolar intimal thickening, causing stenosis or obstruction, (2) thick glomerular capillary walls, (3) tubular atrophy, and (4) interstitial fibrosis. The interstitium often has scattered mononuclear infiltrates and tubules containing proteinaceous casts. Chronic rejection may be the end-result of repeated episodes of cellular rejection, either asymptomatic or clinically apparent. This advanced state of damage is not responsive to therapy.

It should be noted that the histological features of acute and chronic rejection described earlier may overlap and vary in degree, so that a clear distinction may not be apparent on renal biopsy. Moreover, treatment with immunosuppressive drugs, such as cyclosporine, complicate the histological diagnosis by modifying immune responses, as well as by exerting direct toxic effects on renal tubular cells.

Graft-versus-Host Reactions

The discussion of graft rejection describes reactions to a transplanted organ in a recipient with an intact immune system. The advent of bone marrow transplantation to bone marrow–depleted or immunodeficient patients has resulted in the complication of graft-versus-host disease. Immunocompetent lymphocytes in the grafted marrow tend to reject the host tissues. Graft-versus-host disease also occurs when severely immunodeficient patients are transfused with blood products containing HLA-incompatible lymphocytes.

The skin and intestine reveal mononuclear cell infiltrates and epithelial cell necrosis in graft-versus-host disease. The liver shows periportal inflammation, damaged bile ducts, and liver cell injury. Clinically, graft-versus-host disease manifests as rash, diarrhea, abdominal cramps, anemia, and liver dysfunction. A chronic form of graft-versus-host disease is characterized by dermal sclerosis, sicca syndrome (dry eyes and dry mouth secondary to chronic inflammation of the lacrimal and salivary glands), and immunodeficiency. Treatment of graft-versus-host disease requires immunosuppressive therapy.

ASSESSMENT OF IMMUNE STATUS

Immunodeficiency is usually suspected in an infant or adult with chronic, recurrent, or unusual infections. The specific type of immunodeficiency is suggested by the kinds of infections and other clinical features. However, diagnosis and confirmation usually require laboratory studies. A number of laboratory methods are used to assess the various components of the immune system: antibody-mediated immunity (B cells), cell-mediated immunity (T cells), phagocytosis, and complement.

IMMUNOGLOBULIN LEVELS: The total concentrations of various immunoglobulins are crudely measured by serum protein electrophoresis. In this technique, serum proteins are separated electrophoretically, stained, and then quantitated by densitometry. Figure 4-17A shows the characteristic electrophoretic patterns of a normal person and a person with hypogammaglobulinemia, and their corresponding densitometric tracings. The immunoglobulins comprise the gamma globulin fraction, which migrates to the cathode and is significantly reduced in a patient with hypogammaglobulinemia.

Immunoglobulins are more precisely measured by quantitation of individual subclasses. Various methods can be used, but automated nephelometry is the most common. All of the methods employ specific antibodies directed against the different heavy-chain isotypes. Quantitation allows the detection of selective deficiencies of immunoglobulin subclasses and provides a measure of total available immunoglobulins. A number of conditions have been described in which there is a specific deficiency of IgA, IgM, or IgG.

ANTIBODY-DEPENDENT IMMUNITY: Subtle immune deficiencies are evaluated by serological methods that measure the levels of circulating antibodies to specific antigens to which persons are commonly exposed through vaccination or the environment (e.g., tetanus, diphtheria, typhoid, rubella, and major blood groups). These methods uncover more elusive deficiencies, even when total immunoglobulin levels are normal.

CELL-MEDIATED IMMUNITY: Since most blood lymphocytes are T cells, the total lymphocyte count is a crude indication of cell-mediated immunity. Functional screening of delayed hypersensitivity is done by **skin testing**. Subjects are given intradermal injections of antigens to which most of the population should be sensitive (e.g., *Candida albicans*, tetanus toxoid, streptokinase). A normal response is notable swelling, redness, and induration (>5 mm) at the skin injection site.

T-LYMPHOCYTE FUNCTION: Figure 4-17B diagrams a commonly employed assay in which lymphoid

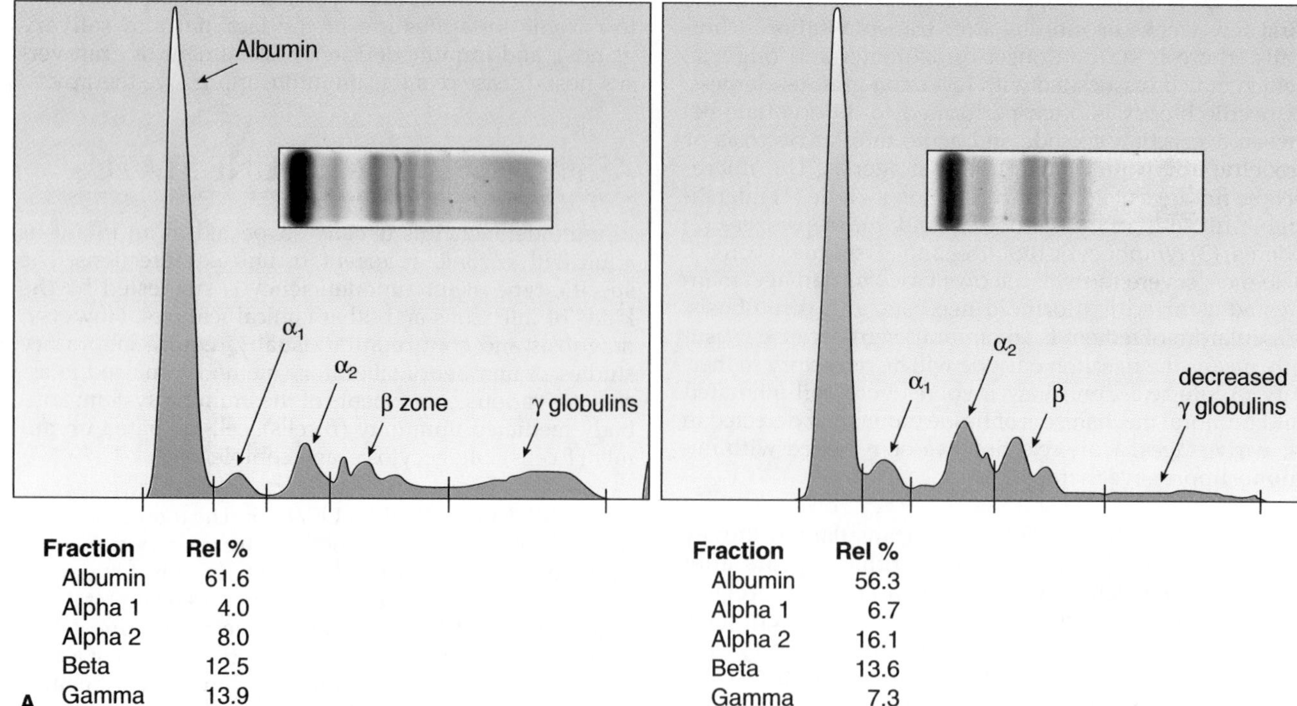

Fraction	Rel %
Albumin	61.6
Alpha 1	4.0
Alpha 2	8.0
Beta	12.5
Gamma	13.9

Fraction	Rel %
Albumin	56.3
Alpha 1	6.7
Alpha 2	16.1
Beta	13.6
Gamma	7.3

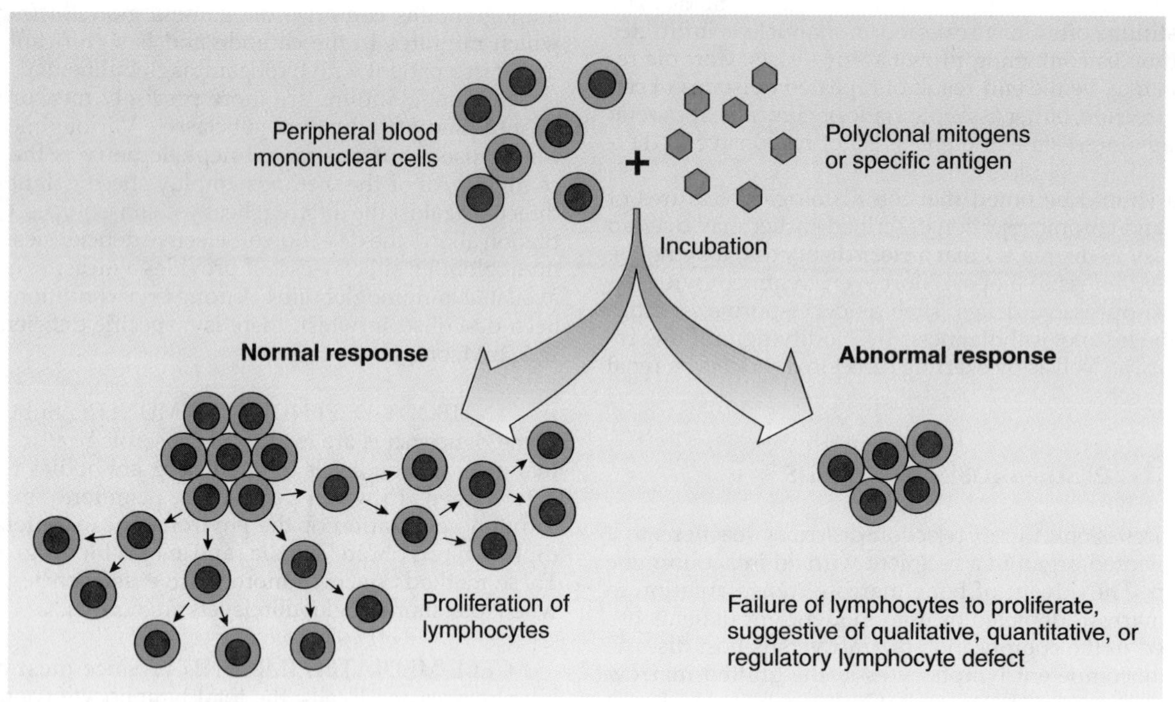

FIGURE 4-17
(*A*) Normal and hypogammaglobulinemic serum protein electrophoresis (SPEP). SPEP provides a rapid means to evaluate the major protein components of serum. (*B*) T-cell mitogenic or blastogenic response assay. This assay tests the capacity of peripheral blood T cells to respond to mitogenic or antigenic stimuli.

cells are isolated from a blood sample and then incubated with a polyclonal T-cell mitogen (i.e., phytohemagglutinin), a common microbial antigen (e.g., *Candida*, streptokinase), or histoincompatible cells. Normal T cells proliferate in response to such stimuli. A poor or absent response suggests a qualitative, quantitative, or regulatory lymphocyte defect.

LYMPHOCYTE QUANTITATION: Both antibody-mediated immunity and cell-mediated immunity can be evaluated by quantitation of peripheral blood T- and B-lymphocyte populations. Historically, T cells were measured by their ability to bind sheep erythrocytes spontaneously and form rosettes *in vitro*. B cells were identified with fluorochrome-labeled rabbit or goat antibodies directed against human immunoglobulins. These antibodies bind to B cells, which are then identified by fluorescence microscopy.

Flow cytometry, a method dependent on laser technology and monoclonal antibodies with specificities for lymphocyte subpopulations, has enabled more detailed analyses of lymphoid cells and other leukocytes. Briefly, cell preparations are stained with a fluorochrome-labeled monoclonal antibody specific for the target populations (e.g., CD3, CD4, CD8). The cells are then passed individually through a narrow beam of laser light of appropriate wavelength. Diffracted light is analyzed by a forward light scatter detector. Various blood cell types (e.g., lymphocytes, neutrophils, monocytes) are recognized by their characteristic forward light scatter pattern. A second detector positioned at 90° to the incident beam monitors cells for fluorescence intensity. The information from both detectors is subjected to computer analysis, which yields total counts of specific populations as well as their intensity of marker expression.

IMMUNODEFICIENCY DISEASES

Immunodeficiency disorders involving lymphocytes may be classified as antibody (B-cell), cellular (T-cell), and combined T-cell and B-cell deficiencies. In addition, immunodeficiency can result from defects in other cells that participate in immune reactions, such as phagocytic cells. The latter conditions were discussed in Chapter 2. Lymphoid functional defects may be localized to particular maturational stages in the ontogeny of the immune system or due to interruptions of immune activation events (Fig. 4-18). The defects can be **primary** (congenital) or **secondary** (acquired). Molecular biological studies have begun to define the specific functional and genetic abnormalities in immunodeficient individuals (Table 4-5).

Deficiencies of Antibody (B-Cell) Immunity

CONGENITAL X-LINKED INFANTILE HYPOGAMMAGLOBULINEMIA: Congenital (Bruton) X-linked infantile hypogammaglobulinemia is observed in male infants at 5 to 6 months of age, the time when maternal antibody levels begin to decline. The infant usually presents with recurrent pyogenic infections and severe hypogammaglobulinemia involving all immunoglobulin isotypes. There is an absence both of mature B cells in the peripheral blood and of plasma cells in the lymphoid tissues. Pre-B cells, however, can be detected. The gene defect is located on the long arm of the X chromosome and is an inactivating mutation of the gene for B-cell tyrosine kinase (agammaglobulinemia tyrosine kinase [ATK]), an enzyme critical to maturation beyond the pre-B cell stage.

TABLE 4-5 **Major Immunodeficiency Diseases**

Condition	Inheritance Pattern	Chromosome Defect Site	Pathogenesis
X-linked agammaglobulinema	XL	Xq21.3–22	Mutation of ATK gene
Immunoglobulin deficiency with hyper-IgM	XL, AR	Xq26–27	Mutation of CD40 ligand gene in XL form
Common variable immunodeficiency	Variable, AD, AR, or unknown	Unknown	Variable, likely represents several types of defects
IgA deficiency	Variable, AR, or unknown	Unknown	Failure of differentiation to IgA-producing B cells
DiGeorge syndrome	Hemizygous deletions	22q11	Polytypic embryonic field defects involving thymus
Severe combined immunodeficiency	XL and AR forms	Xq13.1–13.3 (AR unknown)	Mutation of gamma chain or receptors for T-cell growth cytokines in XL form Mutation in nonreceptor JAK-3 protein kinase in AR form
Adenosine deaminase deficiency	AR	20q13-ter	Lymphocyte dysfunction due to accumulation of toxic adenosyl metabolites
Purine nucleoside phosphorylase deficiency	AR	14q13.1	Lymphocyte dysfunction due to metabolites
Wiskott-Aldrich syndrome	XL	Xp11.22–11.23	Defective function of a rho-type GTPase due to deficiency of Wiskott-Aldrich syndrome protein (WASP)

XL, X-linked; AR, autosomal recessive; AD, autosomal dominant; q, long arm; p, short arm.

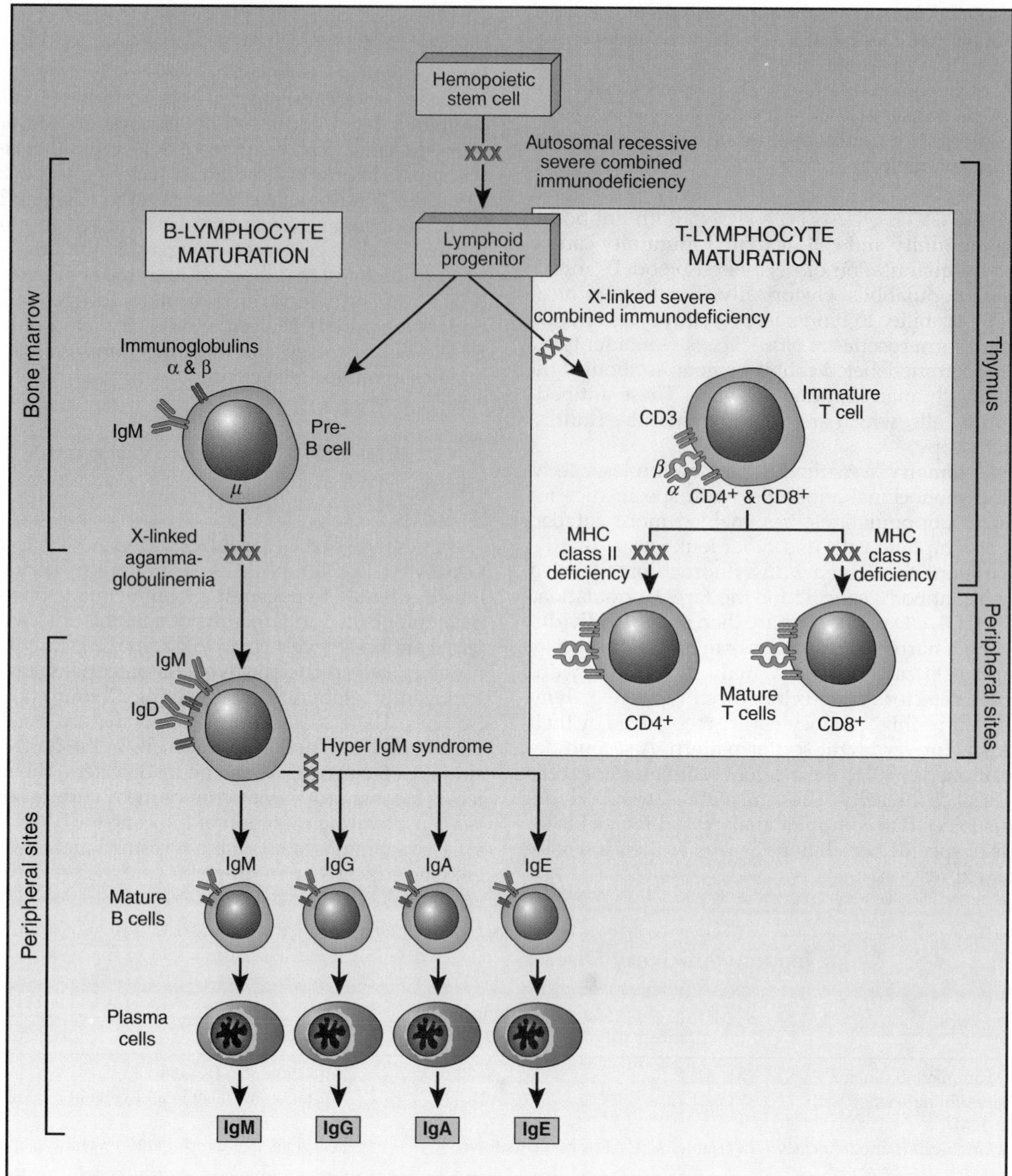

FIGURE *4-18*

Maturation of B and T lymphocytes. After hemopoietic stem cells give rise to progenitor cells, the latter enter either the B-cell (bone marrow) or T-cell (thymus) developmental pathway. In the thymus, CD4 and CD8 are transiently expressed on immature T cells. Maturation to CD4+ or CD8+ T cells is determined by the interaction of CD4 with MHC class II or of CD8 with MHC class I molecules on thymic stromal cells. In the bone marrow, the interaction of progenitor B cells with stromal cells yields pre-B cells, which initially express cytoplasmic μ heavy chains and subsequently an IgM-receptor complex and the transmembrane Ig α and β signal-transduction unit. After leaving the bone marrow, pre-B cells express surface IgD and then differentiate into mature, Ig-specific B cells and eventually Ig-secreting plasma cells. The location in these developmental sequences of heritable immunodeficiency disorders are indicated by *red xxx* in the directional arrows.

TRANSIENT HYPOGAMMAGLOBULINEMIA OF INFANCY: This condition is characterized by prolonged hypogammaglobulinemia after maternal antibodies have reached a nadir. Some affected infants develop recurrent infections and require therapy, but all eventually produce immunoglobulins. **Infants with transient hypogammaglobulinemia have mature B cells that are temporarily unable to produce antibodies.** The defect is thought to represent a delay in helper T-cell signals.

IMMUNOGLOBULIN DEFICIENCY WITH NORMAL OR INCREASED IgM: This syndrome represents a group of distinct entities, of which 70% are X-linked and the remaining are of autosomal inheritance. Infants with the X-linked form of the disease exhibit pyogenic and opportunistic infections, especially with *Pneumocystis carinii*. They also tend to develop autoimmune diseases involving the formed elements of the blood, namely autoimmune hemolytic anemia, thrombocytopenic purpura, and recurrent, severe neutropenia. The levels of IgG and IgA are low, but those of IgM are high normal or conspicuously elevated. Circulating B cells bear only IgM and IgD. The defect appears to be at the level of the "switch" to other heavy-chain isotopes. In the X-linked form, the genetic defect appears to be a mutation of the gene for the CD40 ligand (Xq26), which is normally expressed by T cells. Interaction of the CD40 receptor on the surface of the B cell with this ligand is required for isotype switching.

COMMON VARIABLE IMMUNODEFICIENCY: Common variable immunodeficiency represents a group of diseases characterized by pronounced hypogammaglobulinemia, in which patients present with recurrent severe pyogenic infections, especially pneumonia, and diarrhea, the latter often due to *Giardia lamblia*. Recurrent attacks of herpes simplex are common, and herpes zoster develops in one fifth of the patients. The disease appears years to decades after birth, with a mean age at onset of 30 years. The incidence is estimated to be 1:50,000 to 1:200,000. The inheritance pattern is variable, and the disease probably reflects a variety of maturational and regulatory defects of the immune system.

A remarkable incidence of malignant disease is seen in common variable immunodeficiency, including a 50-fold increase in stomach cancer. Interestingly, lymphoma is 300 times more frequent in women with this immunodeficiency than in affected men. Malabsorption secondary to lymphoid hyperplasia and inflammatory bowel diseases are more frequent. The patients are also susceptible to other autoimmune disorders, including hemolytic anemia, neutropenia, thrombocytopenia, and pernicious anemia.

SELECTIVE IgA DEFICIENCY: An inadequate amount of IgA is the most common immunodeficiency syndrome, with an incidence of 1:700 among Europeans and 1:18,000 in the Japanese. Persons with IgA deficiency are often asymptomatic but sometimes present with respiratory or gastrointestinal infections of varying severity. There is also a strong predilection for allergies and collagen vascular diseases. Patients with IgA deficiency have normal numbers of IgA-bearing B cells, and their defect seems to be an inability to synthesize and secrete IgA subclasses.

OTHER ANTIBODY-RELATED DEFICIENCIES: There are a variety of other deficiency states involving antibodies. These include selective deletions of immunoglobulin heavy chains or selective loss of light-chain expression. In addition, there are persons who have normal levels and structure of immunoglobulins but fail to produce antibodies that react with specific antigens, usually polysaccharides. This condition is known to result in recurrent sinusitis and pulmonary infections.

Deficiencies of Cell-Mediated (T-Cell) Immunity

DiGEORGE SYNDROME: In its complete form, DiGeorge syndrome is one of the most severe forms of deficient T-cell immunity. The disease usually presents in an infant with congenital heart defects and severe hypocalcemia (due to hypoparathyroidism) and is recognized shortly after birth. Infants who survive the neonatal period are subject to recurrent or chronic viral, bacterial, fungal, and protozoal infections. DiGeorge syndrome is caused by defective embryological development of the third and fourth pharyngeal pouches, which become the thymus and parathyroid glands. Most patients have a point deletion in the long arm of chromosome 22. In the absence of a thymus, T-cell maturation is interrupted at the pre-T cell stage. The disease can be corrected by transplanting thymic tissue. The majority of patients have a partial DiGeorge syndrome, in which a small remnant of thymus is present. With time, these persons recover T-cell function without treatment.

CHRONIC MUCOCUTANEOUS CANDIDIASIS: Another congenital defect in T-cell function is characterized by susceptibility to candidal infections and is associated with an endocrinopathy (hypoparathyroidism, Addison disease, diabetes mellitus). Although most T-cell functions are intact, there is a defective response to *Candida* antigens. The precise cause of the defect in chronic mucocutaneous candidiasis is unknown, but it could occur at any of several points during T-cell development. Recent studies suggest that persons with this disorder react to *Candida* antigens in a manner different from that of normal individuals. In particular, they mount a type 2 (IL-4/IL-6) helper T-cell response, which is ineffective in resisting the organism. By contrast, the normal response features type 1 (IL-2/IFN-γ) T cells, which effectively resist *Candida* infection.

Combined T-Cell and B-Cell Deficiencies

SEVERE COMBINED IMMUNODEFICIENCY: Severe combined immunodeficiency (SCID), a disease of T and B lymphocytes, is characterized by recurrent viral, bacterial, fungal, and protozoal infections. A virtually complete absence of T cells is associated with severe hypogammaglobulinemia. Many of these infants have severely reduced lymphoid tissue and an immature thymus that lacks lymphocytes. In some patients, lymphocytes fail to develop beyond pre-B cells and pre-T cells.

The disease occurs in X-linked and autosomal recessive (Swiss type) forms and typically appears at about 6 months of age. In some patients with the autosomal recessive form, B lymphocytes are present but do not function, possibly because of a lack of helper cell activity. In the X-linked form, the defect is due to a mutation of the γ-chain of the IL-2 receptor, which is also used by receptors for other cytokines, namely IL-4, IL-7, IL-9, and IL-15. Patients with the autosomal recessive form of SCID have demonstrated mutations of the Jak-3 gene, a protein kinase that associates with the γ-chain of the cytokine receptors. Thus, abnormalities in the Jak/STAT signaling pathway may account for both forms of SCID.

ADENOSINE DEAMINASE DEFICIENCY: This disease is an autosomal recessive form of combined immunodeficiency due to mutations of the adenosine deaminase gene on chromosome 20q13. Adenosine deaminase participates in the catabolism of purine nucleotides, converting adenosine to inosine or deoxyadenosine to deoxyinosine. If the enzyme is defective or absent, deoxyadenosine and deoxyadenosine triphosphate accumulate. Deoxyadenosine triphosphate inhibits ribonucleotide reductase, thereby causing depletion of deoxyribonucleoside triphosphates and defective lymphocyte function. The clinical manifestations of adenosine deaminase deficiency range from mild to severe dysfunction of T cells and B cells.

PURINE NUCLEOSIDE PHOSPHORYLASE DEFICIENCY: This condition is another congenital immunodeficiency syndrome involving an enzyme of purine metabolism. It is characterized by immune defects attributed to a paucity of circulating T cells, but, unlike adenosine deaminase deficiency, B-cell function is preserved.

OTHER COMBINED IMMUNODEFICIENCIES: Combined immunodeficiencies have been observed in persons with stem cell dysgenesis, impaired expression of MHC class II molecules, defective T-cell receptors (CD3), and mutations in receptor-associated signal transduction enzymes. All are autosomal recessive conditions and illustrate that appropriate immune function can be undermined at many stages.

Wiskott-Aldrich Syndrome

Wiskott-Aldrich syndrome is a rare X-linked immunodeficiency disorder clinically characterized by (1) recurrent infections, (2) hemorrhages secondary to thrombocytopenia, and (3) eczema. It typically presents in boys within the first few months of life as petechiae and infections (e.g., otitis media).

The Wiskott-Aldrich syndrome is caused by numerous distinct mutations in a gene on the X chromosome (Xp11.23) that encodes WASP (Wiskott-Aldrich syndrome protein). WASP is an effector for one member (CDC42Hs) of the Rho family of GTPases, which control diverse biological processes, including cell morphology and mitogenesis. The loss of this effector function of WASP is thought to result in a disturbance of the actin cytoskeleton, which may, in turn, account for the varied functional abnormalities of the Wiskott-Aldrich syndrome. A characteristic feature of the disorder is impaired CD43 glycoprotein expression on lymphocytes. No mutations have been found in the CD43 gene located on chromosome 16, and the loss of WASP function may be responsible for the altered expression of CD43.

Immunological Abnormalities

Both cellular and humoral immunities are impaired in Wiskott-Aldrich syndrome. Whereas the levels of most immunoglobulins are normal or elevated, IgM levels are characteristically reduced by half. Interestingly, the antibody response to many antigens is normal, whereas it is completely absent for others. In particular, Wiskott-Aldrich syndrome is the only immunological disorder characterized by a complete failure to produce antibodies to an entire class of antigens, namely polysaccharides. Thus, patients with this condition have low or absent isohemagglutinins and are highly vulnerable to infection with encapsulated organisms such as *Streptococcus pneumoniae*.

Similar to the situation that prevails with humoral immunity, boys with Wiskott-Aldrich syndrome have selective deficiencies of cell-mediated immunity. Despite adequate numbers of T lymphocytes and a normal CD4:CD8 ratio, patients with Wiskott-Aldrich syndrome are for the most part anergic for cutaneous delayed hypersensitivity and exhibit prolonged survival of skin allografts. Although the lymphocytes respond normally to exogenous mitogens (e.g., phytohemagglutinin) *in vitro*, they proliferate poorly in response to antigens or allogeneic cells. Moreover, they do not exhibit virus-specific cytotoxic T cells, even though they may produce antibodies against the same virus.

Clinical Features

Patients with Wiskott-Aldrich syndrome typically have infections with *Streptococcus pneumoniae*, *Haemophilus influenzae*, and opportunistic organisms, such as *Pneumocystis carinii* and *Candida albicans*. They also contract infections with cytomegalovirus, and some have died of disseminated herpes simplex and varicella infections. Not only is thrombocytopenia severe (platelet counts $<30{,}000/\mu L$), but Wiskott-Aldrich syndrome is the only disorder characterized by small platelets. In one third of these patients, bleeding is the cause of death.

A variety of autoimmune diseases often complicate Wiskott-Aldrich syndrome. Such disorders include autoimmune hemolytic anemia and thrombocytopenia, a severe polyarthritis, and vasculitis of the coronary or cerebral arteries. In addition, a high incidence of cancer is noted in these patients, principally malignant lymphoma.

Bone marrow transplantation has been reported to be

more successful in Wiskott-Aldrich syndrome than in any other condition, with the cure rate exceeding 90%. The major form of thrombocytopenia (nonimmune) is almost always cured by splenectomy alone.

Acquired Immunodeficiency Syndrome

Acquired immunodeficiency syndrome (AIDS) is a widespread fatal disease that is caused by human immunodeficiency viruses 1 and 2 (HIV-1 and -2). The vast majority of cases of AIDS represent infection with HIV-1. Persons infected with this virus exhibit a variety of immunological defects, the most devastating of which is the complete loss of cellular immunity. As a result, catastrophic opportunistic infections are virtually inevitable. The relentless progression of HIV infection is now recognized as a continuum that extends from an initial asymptomatic state to the immune exhaustion that characterizes the patient with overt AIDS. **The fundamental lesion in AIDS is infection of CD4+ (helper) T lymphocytes by HIV, leading to the depletion of this cell population and consequent impaired immune function.** As a result, rather than dying of HIV infection itself, patients with AIDS usually die of opportunistic infections. There is also a high incidence of malignant tumors associated with AIDS, principally **B-cell lymphomas** and **Kaposi sarcoma**. Finally, infection of the central nervous system with HIV often leads to a form of encephalopathy termed **AIDS dementia complex**.

☐ **Epidemiology:** AIDS was first recognized in 1981 with the description of *Pneumocystis carinii* pneumonia in five homosexual men who had been diagnosed over an 8-month period in Los Angeles. However, antibodies to HIV have been found in stored blood samples from Zaire dating to 1959, although newer PCR-based analyses have questioned this finding. In any event, sporadic cases of diseases that can retrospectively be attributed to AIDS occurred in Africa during the 1960s. In the late 1970s, there were clusters of strange infectious diseases in New York and Miami among homosexual men, intravenous drug users, and Haitians; these are now recognized as having been secondary to AIDS. By 1982, the unusual infections and the occurrence of Kaposi sarcoma were found to reflect an underlying immune deficiency, and the acronym AIDS was coined. At the same time, it became clear that AIDS was spread by contact with the blood of persons suspected to bear an infectious agent. In addition to homosexual men and intravenous drug abusers who shared needles, transfusion recipients, heterosexual contacts, and infants born to female drug abusers were at risk. In 1983, the AIDS virus, now termed **HIV-1**, was identified. The development of a serological test for antibodies to HIV-1 in 1985 permitted accurate diagnosis of the infection and public health surveillance.

Although AIDS is believed to have originated in sub-Saharan Africa, the disease has now become a worldwide pandemic. The spread of HIV is attributable to the ease of international travel and enhanced population mobility, which in many societies have coincided with a rapid increase in sexual promiscuity and sexually transmitted diseases. By 1996, the World Health Organization (WHO) estimated that a cumulative total of 6 million cases of AIDS had occurred worldwide in adults and children. In addition, 20 million adults are alive and infected with HIV. WHO projects a cumulative total of 40 million HIV infections by the year 2000.

UNITED STATES: More cases of AIDS have been reported from the United States than from any other country, with a prevalence by 1994 of 1 million HIV-positive persons. Originally, homosexual men represented two thirds of these cases, and 30% were accounted for by intravenous drug users and their sexual partners. However, because of behavioral changes, the prevalence of infection among homosexuals has recently decreased. Men account for 95% of AIDS cases in the United States, although the prevalence in women has been increasing. Contaminated blood and blood products were the source of infection in 4%. In fact, 70% of patients with hemophilia A and 35% with hemophilia B who received blood products before 1985 were infected with HIV-1. Fortunately, since 1985 donations of blood and plasma have been screened for HIV-1 antibodies, and clotting factor concentrates used in the treatment of hemophilia are heat-treated to inactivate the AIDS virus. Children who have acquired HIV from their mothers comprise 2% of all AIDS cases. Currently, only 4% of cases occur through heterosexual contact with an HIV-infected person.

AFRICA: Inhabitants of sub-Saharan Africa suffer more from the ravages of AIDS than persons in other regions. Although accurate statistics from this area are not as readily available as in the industrialized countries, in parts of sub-Saharan Africa it is estimated that nearly 25% of the population is HIV positive. The epidemiological pattern is different from that in the United States, as African patients rarely report homosexuality or intravenous drug use, and the sex ratio for AIDS shows only a slight male predominance. These data are interpreted as evidence for the predominant heterosexual spread of the infection in Africa.

The spread of AIDS was from central Africa to East Africa, probably along truck routes where the drivers often have sexual contact with prostitutes who congregate at truck stops, thereby creating an "ecological corridor" for the spread of the disease. The explosive dissemination of HIV in East Africa is illustrated by the increase of HIV-1 in prostitutes in Nairobi, Kenya, from 4% in 1981 to 88% in 1988. Although initially spared, West Africa has now experienced the emergence of AIDS in epidemic form. Risk factors for HIV infection in Africa include frequent sexual congress with prostitutes, lack of circumcision, and genital ulcers from sexually transmitted diseases.

OTHER REGIONS: Many cases of AIDS have been reported in countries of western Europe. As in the United States, most have occurred in homosexual men, intravenous drug users and their sexual partners, and prostitutes. Many cases of AIDS have now been reported from Asia, and some countries in that region (Thailand, India) describe an exponential increase in HIV infection.

Transmission of Human Immunodeficiency Virus

It is now clear that with the exception of direct transmission of HIV through blood or blood products, as in intravenous drug abusers and transfusion recipients, AIDS is transmitted principally as a venereal disease, both homosexually and heterosexually. Significant amounts of HIV have been isolated not only from blood, but also from semen, vaginal secretions, breast milk, and cerebrospinal fluid. Except for cerebrospinal fluid, the occurrence of HIV in these fluids reflects the presence of both lymphocytes and free virus.

Among homosexual men, the receptive partner in anal intercourse is at particularly high risk of becoming infected with HIV. The virus is transmitted from semen through tears in the rectal mucosa. It is also possible that HIV can infect the epithelial cells of the rectum directly. In heterosexual contact, transmission from male to female is more likely than the reverse, perhaps reflecting the greater concentration of HIV in semen than in vaginal fluids. The risk of infecting a woman with HIV is evidenced by the demonstration that 8% to 50% of women artificially inseminated with semen from donors later shown to be HIV positive became infected with the AIDS virus. Additionally, genital lesions, usually caused by other sexually transmitted diseases, facilitate entry of the virus and lead to a particularly high risk of contracting AIDS.

AIDS is not transmissible by nonsexual, casual exposure to infected persons. A particular concern of health care workers is the possibility of HIV infection from accidental exposure to the virus. In prospective studies of hundreds of health care workers who sustained needle sticks or other accidental exposures to blood from AIDS patients, fewer than 1% developed antibodies to HIV. Immediate treatment with zidovudine is beneficial.

☐ **Pathogenesis:** **The etiological agent of AIDS is HIV-1, an enveloped RNA retrovirus that contains a reverse transcriptase (RNA-dependent DNA polymerase).** HIV-1 is a member of the retrovirus family and specifically the subfamily of lentiviruses. Animal lentiviruses have been recognized for a century, but human lentiviruses have been identified for less than two decades.

The HIV-1 genome consists of two identical 9.7-kD single strands of RNA enclosed within a core of viral proteins. The core is in turn enveloped by a phospholipid bilayer derived from the host cell membrane, in which are found virally encoded glycoproteins (gp120 and gp41). In addition to the *gag*, *pol*, and *env* genes characteristic of all replication-competent RNA viruses, HIV-1 contains six other genes coding for proteins that regulate viral replication. **The specific target cells for HIV-1 are CD4+ helper T lymphocytes and mononuclear phagocytes, although infection of other cells, such as B lymphocytes, glial cells, and intestinal epithelial cells, occurs.**

THE LIFE CYCLE: The replicative life cycle of HIV-1 proceeds as follows (Fig. 4-19):

1. **Binding:** Free HIV or an infected lymphocyte can transmit the virus to an uninfected cell. The HIV envelope glycoprotein gp120, either on the free virus or on the surface of an infected cell, binds to the CD4 molecule on the surface of helper T lymphocytes.
2. **Internalization:** The binding of gp120 to CD4 allows gp41 to insert into the cell membrane of the lymphocyte, thereby promoting fusion of the viral envelope with that of the lymphocyte, with consequent internalization of the virus. The entry of HIV-1 into the target cell *in vivo* requires viral binding to a co-receptor, namely the β-chemokine receptor 5 (CCR-5). The chemokine ligands for this receptor are RANTES, MIP-1α, and MIP-1β. About 1% of Caucasians are homozygous for major deletions in the CCR-5 gene and remain uninfected with HIV despite extensive exposure to the agent. There is evidence that even heterozygosity for the mutant CCR-5 allele provides partial protection against HIV infection. Interestingly, the mutant allele is found in up to 20% of Caucasians but is absent in blacks and Asians. Some persons who are multiply exposed to HIV-1 and who do not seroconvert, and possibly some long-term HIV-infected individuals who do not progress to AIDS, have high levels of chemokines, which may block the co-receptors for HIV.
3. **DNA synthesis:** In the cytoplasm of the T lymphocyte, the virus is uncoated and its RNA is copied into double-stranded DNA by retroviral reverse transcriptase.
4. **Viral integration:** The DNA derived from the virus is integrated into the host genome by the viral integrase protein, thereby producing the latent proviral form of HIV-1. Viral genes are replicated along with host chromosomes and, therefore, persist for the life of the cell.
5. **Viral replication:** Viral RNA is reproduced by transcriptional activation of the integrated HIV provirus, a process that requires "activation" of the T cell and the presence of certain inducible host transcription factors.
6. **Viral dissemination:** To complete the life cycle, nascent virus is assembled in the cytoplasm and disseminated to other target cells. This is accomplished either by fusion of an infected cell with an uninfected one or by the budding of virions from the plasma membrane of the infected cell (Fig. 4-20).

The mechanism by which HIV kills infected T lymphocytes is still poorly understood. Among the potential mechanisms for the depletion of CD4+ lymphocytes are direct viral cytotoxicity, immune clearance of infected cells, and the actions of secondary mediators such as cytokines. Whatever the mechanism, there is a clear association between increasing amounts of viral burden and the decline in CD4+ lymphocyte counts.

VIRAL LATENCY AND ACTIVATION: The long interval between HIV-1 infection and the appearance of the clinical symptoms of AIDS is related to the small number of infected T lymphocytes and the latency of the virus. Only 1/100,000 to 1/10,000 circulating mononuclear cells displays detectable viral mRNA, although about 1% of circulating T cells contain proviral DNA. Although many

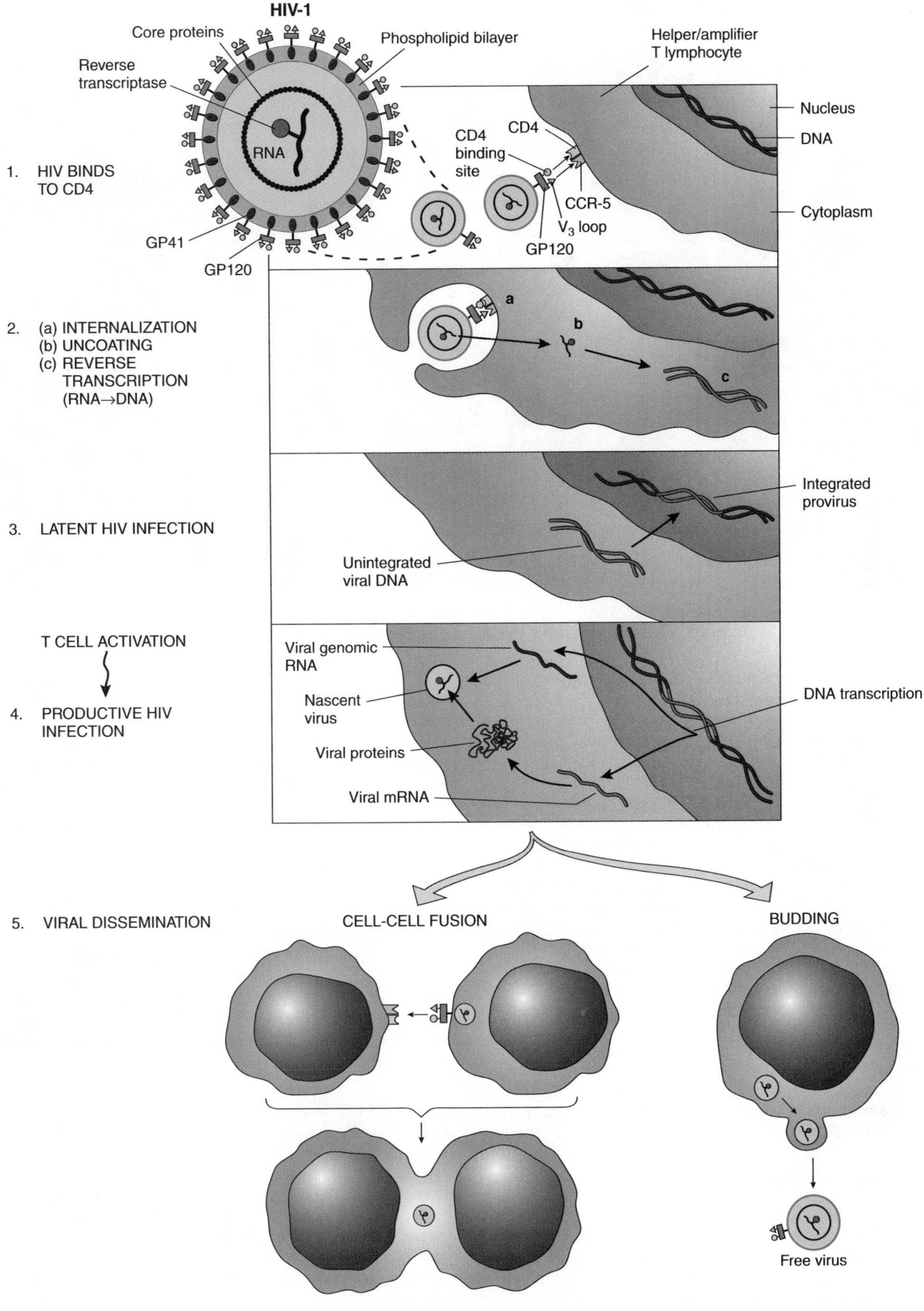

FIGURE *4-19*
The life cycle of HIV-1.

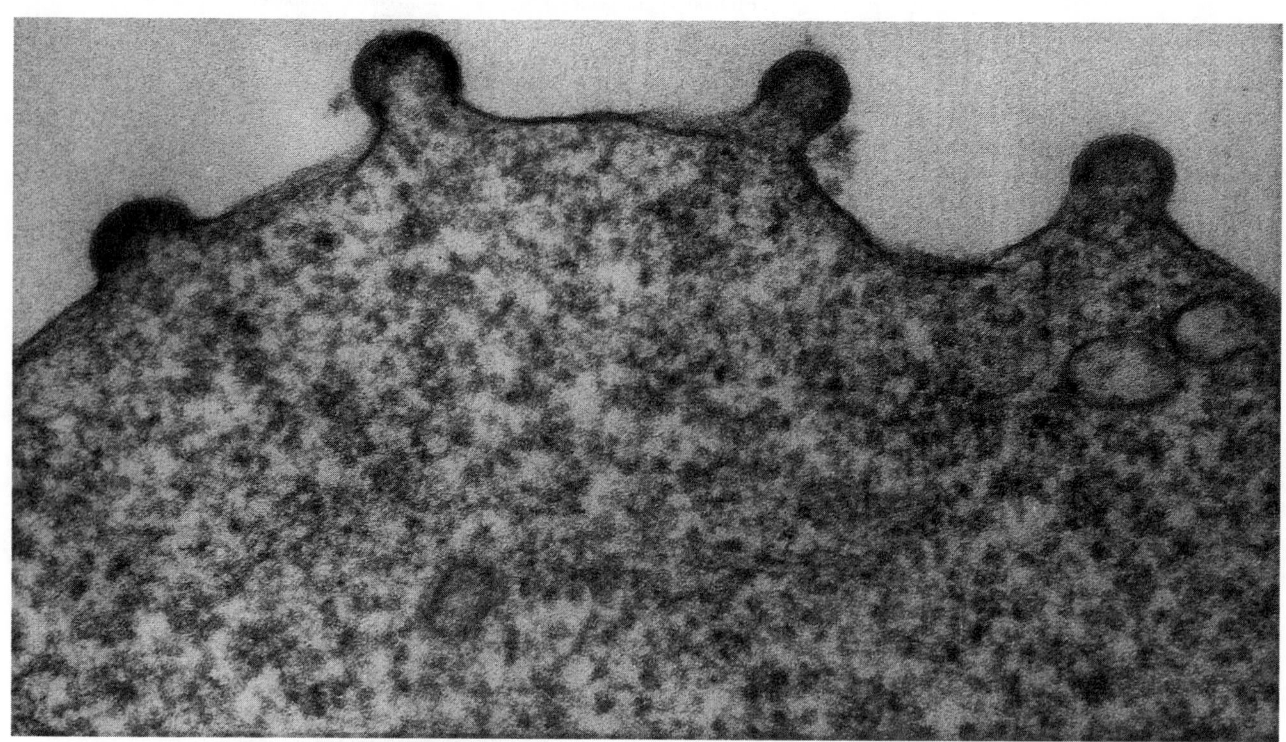

FIGURE *4-20*
Budding of virions from the plasma membrane of an HIV-infected cell.

infected cells do not replicate the virus, but rather harbor latent HIV-1, recent data indicate that many cells contain actively replicating virus. During latent infection, the virus can exist in three forms: (1) untranscribed viral RNA may exist in the cytoplasm of resting T cells; (2) unintegrated, and thus untranscribed, viral DNA may be present in the cell; and (3) in a resting T cell, integrated proviral DNA may remain untranscribed. The mechanisms underlying latency and the conversion to a lytic infection are poorly understood.

The initiation of viral replication in latent HIV-1 infection is critically dependent on the induction of host proteins during T-cell activation. The regulation of viral transcription involves the long terminal repeats (LTRs) that flank both ends of the viral genome. The LTRs are activated by many T-cell mitogens and by various cytokines produced by monocyte/macrophages, including TNF-α and IL-1. Moreover, the LTRs can also be activated by proteins produced by other viruses known to infect patients with AIDS, such as herpesvirus, Epstein-Barr virus, adenovirus, and cytomegalovirus. Thus, activation of the immune system by a variety of infectious agents may promote HIV replication.

Immunology of AIDS

The destruction of CD4+ T cells by HIV-1 constitutes an attack on the Achilles heel of the entire immune system, because this subset of lymphocytes exerts critical regulatory and effector functions that involve both cellular and humoral immunity. **Thus, in the typical AIDS patient, all the elements of the immune system are eventually perturbed, including T cells, B cells, NK cells, and monocyte/macrophages.**

T CELLS: CD4+ lymphocytes include two functional types: helper and amplifier (or inducer) cells. The first population affected in HIV infection is the amplifier subset. Eventually, total CD4 counts fall to less than 500 cells/μL, and the helper-to-suppressor T-cell ratio declines from a normal of 2.0 to as little as 0.50. The number of CD8+ (cytotoxic/suppressor) cells is variable, although in AIDS most of these cells seem to be of the cytotoxic variety.

The defects in T-cell function are manifested by defective responses to skin testing with a variety of antigens (delayed hypersensitivity) and by impaired proliferative responses to mitogens and antigens *in vitro*. Moreover, the deficiency of CD4+ cells reduces the levels of IL-2, the cytokine produced in response to antigens that stimulate cytotoxic T-cell killing. **Thus, the patient with AIDS cannot generate the antigen-specific cytotoxic T cells that are required for the clearance of viruses and other infectious agents.**

B CELLS: In persons infected with HIV, humoral immunity is also abnormal. The production of antibodies in response to specific antigenic stimulation is markedly decreased, often to less than 10% of normal. B cells also demonstrate a decreased proliferative response *in vitro* to mitogens and antigens. Yet, the serum of patients with AIDS usually shows high levels of polyclonal immunoglobulins, autoantibodies, and immune complexes. This apparent paradox is explained by the fact that concurrent infection with polyclonal B cell–activating viruses (e.g., Epstein-Barr virus or cytomegalovirus) constantly stimulates B cells to produce nonspecific immunoglobulins. The lack of CD4+ lymphocytes impairs the proliferation of cytotoxic T cells that normally would eliminate the Epstein-Barr virus–infected B cells.

NATURAL KILLER CELLS: NK cell activity is severely decreased in AIDS. Since these cells kill both virus-infected cells and tumor cells, this defect may contribute to the appearance of malignant tumors and the viral infections that plague these patients. The suppression of NK cell activity has been related both to a decrease in the number of NK cells and to a reduction in IL-2 levels owing to the loss of CD4+ cells.

MONOCYTE/MACROPHAGES: Lentiviruses tend to target monocyte/macrophages, and it is therefore not surprising that macrophages are infected by HIV-1 and may serve as a reservoir for dissemination of the virus. Interestingly, some macrophages express CD4 on their surfaces. Unlike T lymphocytes, which are killed by HIV, infected macrophages display little if any cytotoxicity. Macrophages from patients with AIDS show impaired phagocytosis of immune complexes and opsonized particles, decreased chemotaxis, and impaired responses to antigenic challenges.

☐ **Pathology and Clinical Features:** Persons infected with HIV exhibit a spectrum of clinical manifestations, beginning with an acute, self-limited illness, and months to years later culminating in fulminant immunodeficiency and its fatal complications (Table 4-6 and Fig. 4-21).

ACUTE HIV INFECTION: Two to 3 weeks after exposure to HIV, before the appearance of antibodies against the virus, infected persons often present with an acute illness that resembles infectious mononucleosis.

TABLE **4-6** **Classification of HIV Infections**

Group	Type	Description
Group I	Acute infection	Mononucleosis-like syndrome with associated seroconversion for HIV antibody.
Group II	Asymptomatic infection	No signs or symptoms of HIV. There may or may not be laboratory evidence of disease.
Group III	Persistent generalized lymphadenopathy	Lymphadenopathy (≥1 cm) at two or more extrainguinal sites persisting for more than 3 months in the absence of a condition other than HIV infection to explain the findings. There may or may not be laboratory evidence of disease.
Group IV	Other disease	*Subgroup A.* Constitutional disease, fever (>1 month), weight loss (>10% of baseline), or diarrhea (>1 month), in the absence of a condition other than HIV infection to explain the findings.
		Subgroup B. Neurological disease such as dementia, myelopathy, or peripheral neuropathy in the absence of a condition other than HIV infection to explain the findings.
		Subgroup C. Diagnosis of an infectious disease associated with HIV infection or at least moderately indicative of a defect in cell-mediated immunity.
		Category C-1. Disease due to at least one of the following:
		Pneumocystis carinii
		Toxoplasma
		Stronglyoides (extraintestinal)
		Cryptococcus
		Atypical mycobacteria (*avium* complex or *kansasii*)
		Progressive multifocal leukoencephalopathy
		Cytomegalovirus
		Cryptosporidia
		Isosporidia
		Candida (esophageal, pulmonary or bronchial)
		Candida (chronic mucocutaneous)
		Histoplasma
		Herpes simplex (disseminated)
		Category C-2. Disease due to one of the following:
		Oral hairy leukoplakia
		Nocardia
		Tuberculosis
		Oral candidiasis
		Multidermatomal herpes zoster
		Salmonella bacteremia (recurrent)
		Subgroup D. Secondary cancers known to be associated with HIV infection; Kaposi sarcoma, lymphoma, or primary lymphoma of the brain.
		Subgroup E. Clinical conditions not defined above that may be due to HIV infection or indicative of defective cell-mediated immunity. Also included are patients with signs and symptoms that may be due to HIV or other clinical illness.

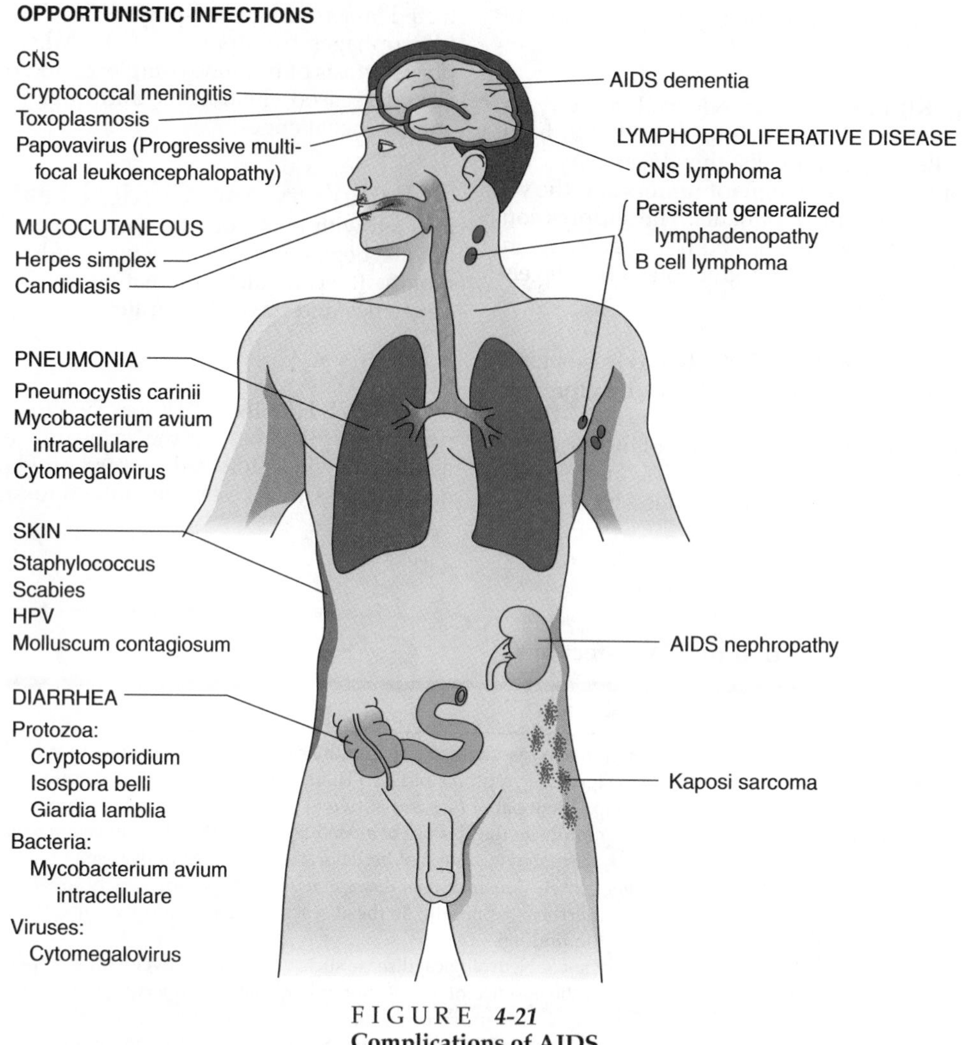

FIGURE *4-21*
Complications of AIDS.

Less commonly, they manifest neurological symptoms that suggest encephalitis or some form of neuropathy. Fever, myalgia, lymphadenopathy, sore throat, and a macular rash are common. Most of these symptoms resolve within 2 to 3 weeks, although lymphadenopathy, fever, and myalgia may persist for a few months. Seroconversion occurs 1 to 10 weeks after the onset of this acute illness. The proportion of patients in whom seroconversion occurs without the development of acute symptoms is unknown.

PERSISTENT GENERALIZED LYMPHADENOPATHY: This condition is defined as palpable lymphadenopathy at two or more extrainguinal sites, persisting for more than 3 months in persons infected with HIV. The disorder develops either as part of the acute HIV syndrome or within a few months of seroconversion. The most common sites of involvement are the axillary, inguinal, and posterior cervical nodes, although almost any group of lymph nodes may be affected. Many cells within the affected lymph nodes, especially follicular dendritic cells, harbor actively replicating virus. Biopsies of the lymph nodes are nondiagnostic and reveal reactive changes with follicular hyperplasia (see Chapter 20). Persistent generalized lymphadenopathy does not have any prognostic significance with respect to the progression of HIV infection to AIDS.

PROGRESSION TO AIDS: Most persons infected with HIV exhibit viral antigens and antibodies within 6 months. **Viral replication remains at minimal levels for variable times (up to 10 or more years), during which time the infected person is asymptomatic.** However, as discussed earlier, viral replication virtually always resumes at some time, and the number of helper T cells begins to decrease. Patients generally remain asymptomatic until the total number of CD4+ lymphocytes falls below 500/μL. At that time, nonspecific constitutional symptoms may appear, together with opportunistic infections. Below 150 CD4+ cells/μL and CD4:CD8 ratios less than 0.8, the disease progresses rapidly. A wide variety of bacteria, viruses, fungi, and protozoa attack the immunocompromised patient, Kaposi sarcoma and lymphoproliferative disorders may appear, and neurological disease is common. Thus far, AIDS has been uniformly fatal.

OPPORTUNISTIC INFECTIONS: The diversity of infectious agents that ravage patients with AIDS reads like a textbook of microbiology. It is beyond the scope of this discussion to treat this subject in any detail, and only a few representative examples will be mentioned.

- **Lungs:** The large majority of AIDS patients suffer from opportunistic pulmonary infections. ***Pneumocystis carinii* pneumonia occurs at some time in more than two thirds of the patients,** and pulmonary infection with cytomegalovirus and *Mycobacterium avium-intracellulare* are common. Patients with AIDS are also susceptible to tuberculosis and *Legionella* infections.
- **Central nervous system:** Cryptococcal meningitis is a devastating and usually fatal complication, representing 5% to 8% of all opportunistic infections in patients with AIDS. Toxoplasmosis of the brain is the most common cause of intracerebral mass lesions. Herpes encephalitis occasionally complicates AIDS.
- **Gastrointestinal tract:** Diarrhea is the single most common gastrointestinal symptom in AIDS, occurring in more than 75% of patients. Simultaneous infections with more than one organism are common. The most frequent pathogens are protozoans, including *Cryptosporidium*, *Isospora belli*, and *Giardia*. *Mycobacterium avium-intracellulare* and *Salmonella* species are the most common bacterial causes of diarrhea in patients with AIDS. Cytomegalovirus infection of the gastrointestinal tract can manifest as a colitis associated with watery diarrhea.
- **Skin:** Virtually all patients with AIDS develop some form of skin disease, with infections being prominent causes. *Staphylococcus aureus* is the most common cutaneous bacterial offender, causing bullous impetigo, deeper purulent lesions (ecthyma), and folliculitis. Chronic mucocutaneous herpes simplex infection is so characteristic of AIDS that it is considered an index infection in establishing the diagnosis. Skin lesions produced by *Molluscum contagiosum* and human papillomavirus are common, as are scabies and infections with *Candida* species.

NEUROLOGICAL MANIFESTATIONS OF AIDS: Postmortem studies of patients who died of AIDS have disclosed pathological findings in more than three fourths of the cases, and clinically neurological symptoms occur in 30% to 40% of the patients. Direct infection of the brain with HIV leads to a subacute encephalopathy, also termed the **AIDS dementia complex**. Progressive multifocal leukoencephalopathy, presumably reflecting infection with a papovavirus, is also a lethal complication.

AIDS-ASSOCIATED CANCERS: **Kaposi sarcoma** (KS) is an otherwise rare, multicentric, malignant neoplasm. It is characterized by cutaneous and, less commonly, visceral nodules, in which endothelium-lined channels and vascular spaces are admixed with spindle-shaped cells. The disease was classically described in elderly men but was also associated with immunosuppressive therapy prior to the AIDS pandemic. Treatment with corticosteroids and azathioprine therapy for renal transplantation and autoimmune diseases were found to be associated with some cases of KS. Similarly, patients with AIDS, particularly homosexual men rather than intravenous drug abusers, are at very high risk of developing KS. **In fact, the occurrence of KS in an otherwise healthy person younger than 60 years is considered strong evidence for the diagnosis of AIDS.** Unlike the classic indolent variety of KS, the cutaneous tumor in AIDS is commonly aggressive, often involving the gastrointestinal tract or lungs. Lung involvement frequently leads to death.

Recent studies have incriminated a new strain of herpesvirus (HHV8) in all forms of KS, including AIDS-associated KS, the classic European variety in elderly men, and KS in immunosuppressed recipients of organ transplants. HHV8 is also thought to be the cause of a peculiar lymphoma associated with AIDS (primary effusion lymphoma) and of AIDS-associated Castleman disease (see Chapter 20). The virus has been detected in both the spindle cells and the flat endothelial cells of KS lesions (see Chapter 10). The presence of HHV8 in the blood is strongly predictive of the later development of KS. In fact, 75% of HIV-infected persons with HHV8 in the blood developed KS within 5 years. It is thought that HHV8 is sexually transmitted, since almost all homosexual HIV carriers are infected, whereas only a quarter of heterosexual drug abusers with HIV infection harbor HHV8.

Congenital and acquired immunodeficiency states are associated with B-cell hyperplasia, commonly manifested as generalized lymphadenopathy. This lymphoproliferative syndrome may be followed by the appearance of high-grade B-cell lymphomas. In fact, patients who have been subjected to immunosuppressive therapy for renal transplants are at a 35-times-greater risk of developing lymphoma, and in one third of these cases the disease is confined to the central nervous system. The lymphomas in chronically immunodeficient patients may present as an invasive polyclonal B-cell proliferation or as a monoclonal B-cell lymphoma. Many of these patients exhibit serological evidence of infection with Epstein-Barr virus, and the genome of this virus has been demonstrated in the neoplastic cells.

Patients with AIDS are similarly at substantial risk for the development of B-cell proliferative diseases. As discussed earlier, B-cell hyperplasia and generalized lymphadenopathy are common in HIV-infected persons and precede the appearance of malignant lymphoproliferative disease. HIV-associated lymphomas usually present as the large cell variety, typically noted in other immunodeficient conditions, although a few small cell lymphomas are encountered. A conspicuous feature of lymphomas associated with AIDS is the predilection for extranodal disease, particularly primary lymphomas of the brain. In addition, lymphomas of the gastrointestinal tract, liver, and bone marrow are frequent. The Epstein-Barr virus genome has also been demonstrated in many of the lymphomas occurring with AIDS.

Treatment

Pharmacological antiretroviral therapy for HIV infection is not curative, but it has greatly impaired progression of the disease. The first approved inhibitor of HIV replication was zidovudine (formerly azidothymidine [AZT]), a drug that prolonged the lives of many patients with CD4+ cell counts less than 500/μL. Since zidovudine, a number of new reverse transcriptase inhibitors have been developed. In addition, virus-targeted protease inhibitors are likewise available. Recently, combination therapy using two or three different agents has shown the most beneficial effects. Disease monitoring has improved significantly through the development of assays that directly measure viral RNA levels in the blood. Considerable efforts continue to be directed toward the development of an AIDS vaccine, but the task has proved to be difficult and many problems remain to be solved.

HIV-2

In 1985, otherwise healthy prostitutes in Senegal were discovered to harbor antibodies that cross-reacted with a monkey retrovirus, now termed **simian immunodeficiency virus (SIV)**. A year later, a retrovirus similar to HIV-1 was isolated from West African patients with AIDS who were negative for antibodies against HIV-1. Antibodies to this new retrovirus, now termed **HIV-2**, also cross-reacted with SIV antigens. Frozen sera from West Africa dating to the 1960s have been shown to contain antibodies to HIV-2. In Guinea-Bissau, infection with HIV-2 has been shown in 8% of pregnant women, 10% of male blood donors, and more than one third of prostitutes. The infection has now also been reported from other parts of Africa, Europe, and the United States.

HIV-2 is morphologically similar to HIV-1, and the immunodeficiency state associated with HIV-2 infection is indistinguishable from AIDS caused by HIV-1. The risk factors for infection in both diseases seem to be similar. However, HIV-2 is far more difficult to transmit than HIV-1, and persons infected with the former are less likely to progress to AIDS.

Other Acquired Immunodeficiencies

Acquired immunodeficiency states can be secondary to a large number of conditions, including infections (viral, bacterial, and fungal), malnutrition, autoimmune diseases (systemic lupus erythematosus, rheumatoid arthritis), nephrotic syndrome, uremia, sarcoidosis, cancer, lymphomas, and treatment with immunosuppressive agents (e.g., radiation, corticosteroids, chemotherapy, cyclosporin A). **The widespread use of immunosuppressive agents is today the main cause of immunodeficiency and the resulting increased risk for opportunistic infections.**

AUTOIMMUNITY

Autoimmunity implies that an immune response has been generated against self-antigens (autoantigens). Central to the concept of autoimmunity is a breakdown in the ability of the immune system to differentiate between self- and non–self-antigens. Autoimmunity was classically interpreted as an abnormal immune response that invariably caused disease. However, it is now clear that autoimmune responses are common and are necessary for the regulation of the immune system. The normal development of anti-idiotype antibodies (antibodies against immunoglobulins), which serve as important regulatory proteins for the immune response, is by definition an autoimmune response. **Thus, the regulated production of autoantibodies is a normal event.** When these regulatory mechanisms are in some way deflected, the uncontrolled production of autoantibodies, or the appearance of abnormal cell–cell recognition, produces disease. The presence of specific autoantibodies, as shown in Table 4-7, is useful in the diagnosis of autoimmune diseases, but it is not sufficient for a designation of autoimmune disease. It is necessary to demonstrate a cause-and-effect relationship in which the autoimmune reaction (whether cellular or humoral) is directly related to the disease process. At present, only a few diseases (e.g., lupus erythematosus and thyroiditis) fit this criterion.

An abnormal autoimmune response to self-antigens implies that there is a loss of immune tolerance. The term **tolerance** traditionally denotes a condition in which there is no measurable immune response to specific (usually self) antigens. The reasons for the loss of tol-

TABLE 4-7 **Characteristic Autoantibodies in Autoimmune Diseases**

Disease	Nature of Antigen	Autoantibody
Systemic lupus erythematosus (SLE)	DNA	Anti-double–stranded DNA
	Sm (ribonuclear protein)	Anti-Sm
	Histone	Anti-histone
Drug-induced SLE	Histone	Anti-histone
Sjögren syndrome	Ribonucleoproteins	Anti-SS-A, Anti-SS-B
	SS-A (Ro)	SS-B (La)
Scleroderma (systemic)	Nucleolar RNA polymerase	Anti-nucleolar
	Topoisomerase I (SCL-70)	Anti-SCL-70
Scleroderma (limited—CREST)	Centromere proteins	Anti-centromere
Dermatomyositis	Histidyl-tRNA synthetase	Anti-Jo-1
	Nuclear proteins	Anti-Mi-2
Polymyositis	Histidyl-tRNA synthetase	Anti-Jo-1
	Cytoplasmic RNA–protein complex	Anti-SRP
Mixed connective tissue disease	U1-Ribonucleoprotein	Anti-U1-RNP

erance in autoimmune diseases are not understood. Experimental studies suggest that normal tolerance to self-antigens is an active process, requiring contact between self-antigens and immune cells. In the fetus, tolerance is readily established to antigens that in the adult cause vigorous immune responses. In contrast to the classic theory of Burnet, which postulated that tolerance is caused by "clonal deletion" of antigen-reactive T cells, there is extensive evidence that induction of tolerance is an active immune response that can be produced in a variety of ways. **Thus, tolerance is best looked on as an active state in which the immune response is blocked by inhibitory products.** Induction of tolerance to an antigen is partly related to the dose of antigen to which cells of the intact organism are exposed. Both T cells and B cells are rendered tolerant, helper T cells after exposure to low doses of the antigen and B cells after large doses.

Theories of Autoimmunity

The most popular theories explaining the loss of tolerance in autoimmune disease are listed in Table 4-7.

SEQUESTERED ANTIGENS: The simplest hypothesis states that an immune reaction develops to a self-antigen not normally present in the circulation. Tissue antigens are usually contained within cells and are not exposed or released until some type of tissue injury occurs. When these antigens are released into the circulation, an immune response develops. Examples of this type of response are antibody formation against spermatozoa, lens tissue, and myelin. Whether these autoantibodies are capable of directly inducing injury is another matter. In the case of antisperm antibodies, aside from a localized orchitis there is no evidence that they induce generalized injury. **Thus, although autoantibodies may form against normally "sequestered" antigens, there is little evidence that they are pathogenic.**

ABNORMAL T-CELL FUNCTION: Autoimmune reactions have been claimed to develop as a result of abnormalities in the T-lymphocyte system. Most immune responses require T-cell participation to activate antigen-specific B cells. Thus, alterations in the number or functional activities of helper or suppressor T cells would be expected to influence the ability of the host to mount an immune response. In fact, defects in T cells, particularly suppressor T cells, have been described in many autoimmune diseases. For example, there are reports of defective suppressor cell activity in human and experimental systemic lupus erythematosus. Lymphocytotropic antibodies have also been described in patients with the disease. Abnormalities in suppressor cell function characterize other autoimmune diseases, including primary biliary cirrhosis, thyroiditis, multiple sclerosis, myasthenia gravis, rheumatoid arthritis, and scleroderma. However, the critical question is whether these alterations in suppressor cell function are the primary cause of these diseases or merely a secondary response. In this regard, defects in suppressor cell function have also been described in persons with no evidence of autoimmune disease.

There has also been interest in abnormalities in helper T-cell function in autoimmune disease. Helper T cells are defined by their role in antigen-specific B-cell activation. It is believed that these cells maintain the helper T-cell tolerance induced by low doses of antigen. Recent evidence has found that these cells become autoreactive in many autoimmune diseases. One key mechanism in this T-cell autoimmunity is that of DNA hypomethylation caused by drugs and other agents. This leads to upregulation of leukocyte function antigen 1 (LFA-1) and B-cell activation independent of antigen. An example of this T-cell autoreactivity and loss of antigen specificity is drug-induced lupus. Experimentally, it is also possible to "break" this type of tolerance by altering the antigen in such a way that the helper T-cell is activated and triggers the B cell. Examples are antigen modification by partial degradation and complexing of antigen to a carrier protein. Some rheumatic diseases display autoantibodies to partially degraded connective tissue proteins, such as collagen or elastin. In some drug-induced hemolytic anemias, the binding of the drug to the erythrocyte membrane induces hemolysis.

A third mechanism by which the helper T-cell tolerance is overcome involves antibodies against foreign antigens that cross-react with self-antigens. Here helper T cells function correctly and do not induce autoantibody formation. Rather, the efferent limb of the immune response is abnormal. An example is rheumatic heart disease, in which antibodies formed against streptococcal bacterial antigens cross-react with antigens from cardiac muscle (a phenomenon known as **biological mimicry**).

POLYCLONAL B-CELL ACTIVATION: Another postulated mechanism to explain the loss of tolerance involves polyclonal B-cell activation, in which B lymphocytes are directly activated by complex substances that contain many antigenic sites (e.g., bacterial cell walls and viruses). **There is some evidence that polyclonal B-cell activation may be involved in the formation of autoantibodies.** The development of rheumatoid factor in rheumatoid arthritis, anti-DNA antibodies in lupus erythematosus, and other autoantibodies has been described after bacterial, viral, and parasitic infections.

Mediation of Tissue Injury in Autoimmune Diseases

Autoimmune diseases have traditionally been considered to be prototypes of immune complex disease, the immune complexes forming in either the circulation or the tissues. Thus, type II (cytotoxic) and type III (immune complex) hypersensitivity reactions are implicated as the cause of tissue injury in most types of autoimmune diseases. Although it is probably true that these hypersensitivity reactions explain most of the autoimmune tissue injury, the story is actually more complicated. In some types of autoimmune diseases, T cells sensitized to self-antigens (such as thyroglobulin) may directly cause tissue injury (type IV reaction), but it is not clear to what extent.

Examples of autoimmune diseases presumably mediated by type II hypersensitivity reactions are listed in

TABLE 4-8 **Types of Hypersensitivity Reactions Involved in Autoimmune Disease**

Reaction Type	Disease
Type II	Autoimmune hemolytic anemias, neutropenias, lymphopenias, thrombocytopenias
	Goodpasture disease
	Antireceptor antibody diseases
	Myasthenia gravis
	Graves disease
	Anti-insulin receptor antibody
	Bullous skin diseases
	Pemphigus
	Pemphigoid
Type III	Systemic lupus erythematosus
	Rheumatoid arthritis
	Sjögren syndrome
	Scleroderma
	Polymyositis/dermatomyositis

Table 4-8. In these disorders, an antibody is formed against either a cell surface antigen or components of connective tissue. Local complement activation by the antibody causes most of the injury, either by direct complement-mediated lysis or, in the case of phagocytic cells, by opsonization.

Another mechanism of tissue injury is antibody-directed cellular cytotoxicity. However, not all autoantibodies cause injury by cytotoxic reactions. In the antireceptor antibody diseases, such as Graves disease and myasthenia gravis, the autoantibody binds to the receptor but has no cytotoxic effect itself. In Graves disease, the autoantibody against the TSH receptor acts as an agonist to stimulate the production of thyroid hormone, whereas in myasthenia gravis the autoantibody blocks the binding of acetylcholine to its receptor, thereby leading to muscle weakness. Anti-insulin receptor antibodies have also been described in diseases such as acanthosis nigricans and ataxia telangiectasia, in which some patients exhibit a form of diabetes characterized by extreme insulin resistance.

Type III hypersensitivity reactions (immune complex disease) explain tissue injury in some types of autoimmune diseases. As shown in Table 4-8, the prototypical disease in this category is systemic lupus erythematosus. In this disorder, DNA–anti-DNA complexes are formed in the circulation and are deposited in tissues, where they induce various diseases, such as vasculitis, glomerulonephritis, and arthritis. Other examples are rheumatoid arthritis, scleroderma, polymyositis/dermatomyositis, and Sjögren disease. All of these disorders are characterized by the deposition of circulating immune complexes in tissue and are classified under the rubric "collagen vascular" diseases. **Because the pathogenesis of these maladies largely involves circulating immune complexes, the clinical manifestations are systemic, and many organs and systems are involved. By contrast, cytotoxic or type II–mediated autoimmune reactions are, for the most part, organ specific.**

Systemic Lupus Erythematosus

Systemic lupus erythematosus (SLE) is a chronic, autoimmune, multisystemic, inflammatory disease that may involve almost any organ but characteristically affects the kidneys, joints, serous membranes, and skin (Table 4-9). It is the prototype of a systemic autoimmune disease in which autoantibodies are formed against a variety of self-antigens, including (1) plasma proteins (complement components and clotting factors), (2) cell surface antigens (lymphocytes, neutrophils, platelets, erythrocytes), (3) intracellular cytoplasmic components (microfilaments, microtubules, lysosomes, ribosomes, RNA), and (4) nuclear DNA, ribonucleoproteins, and histones. The most important diagnostic autoantibodies are those against nuclear antigens—in particular, antibody to double-stranded DNA and to the soluble nuclear antigen termed Sm antigen. High titers of these two autoantibodies (called antinuclear antibodies) are pathognomonic of SLE (see Table 4-7). These antinuclear antibodies are usually not directly cytotoxic. Antigen–antibody complexes form in the circulation and deposit in tissues, creating the characteristic injury of **vasculitis, synovitis, and glomerulonephritis.** It is for this reason that SLE is considered the prototype of type III hypersensitivity reactions. Occasionally in this disease, some directly cytotoxic antibodies are present—particularly antibodies formed against cell surface antigens of leukocytes and erythrocytes.

The prevalence of SLE varies worldwide, being 40/100,000 in North America and northern Europe. In the United States, the disease appears to be more severe in blacks and Hispanics, although socioeconomic factors may in part be responsible. More than 80% of the cases are seen in women of childbearing age, and SLE may strike as many as many as 1 in 1000 women in this age group.

☐ **Pathogenesis:** The etiology of SLE is unknown. The characteristic feature of the disease—the presence of numerous autoantibodies, particularly antinuclear antibodies—suggests that there is a breakdown in the normal immune surveillance mechanisms. Presumably this is the defect that leads to a loss of normal self-tolerance. Many of symptoms of SLE result from tissue injury caused by

TABLE 4-9 **Primary Organ System Involvement in Systematic Lupus Erythematosus**

Organ System	Percentage	Characteristic Pathology
Joints	90	Nonerosive synovitis with neutrophils and mononuclear cells
Kidney	75	Immune complex glomerulonephritis, interstitial nephritis
Serosal membranes	35	Pleuritis, pericarditis, peritonitis secondary to immune complex deposition
Heart	45–50	Pericarditis, myocarditis, endocarditis

vascular disease mediated by immune complexes. Other clinical manifestations, for example thrombocytopenia or the antiphospholipid syndrome, are caused by autoantibodies directed against molecules on cell membranes or serum components. In this context, it deserves emphasis that the diagnostic antinuclear antibodies are not incriminated in the pathogenesis of SLE. There appear to be many factors that predispose to the development of SLE (Fig. 4-22).

VIRUSES: Although there was earlier widespread interest in C-type virus particles in experimental murine models of SLE, recent evidence mitigates against a viral etiology for human SLE.

HORMONAL FACTORS: The clear female predisposition for SLE is true for all autoimmune diseases, and sex hormones may in part be the explanation. The immune response in animals is strongly influenced by sex hormones. In mouse models of SLE, estrogens accelerate the progression of the disease, whereas androgens have a retarding effect. However, it is controversial whether the course of human SLE can be manipulated in the same manner. Experimentally, estrogens have been described as increasing the likelihood of overcoming immune tolerance.

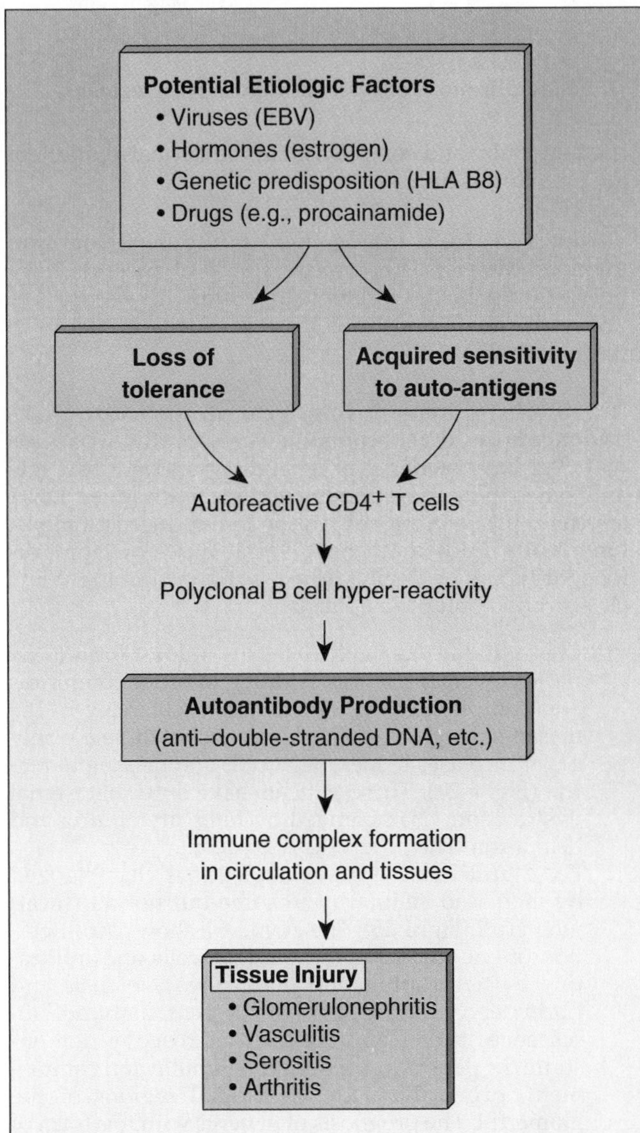

FIGURE 4-22
Pathogenesis of systemic lupus erythematosus.

GENETIC FACTORS: There appears to be some genetic predisposition to lupus, and a higher incidence is described in families. Monozygotic twins show a concordance of 30% to 50%, indicating that both genetic and environmental factors play a role. With respect to the latter, it has been noted that pet dogs whose masters suffer from SLE have a higher prevalence of anti-DNA antibodies than do those that belong to disease-free owners.

The incidence of lupus (and the other autoimmune diseases) is higher among persons who express certain class II antigens belonging to the DR and DQ loci of the major histocompatibility complex. These genes participate in two unlinked functions, namely, immunoregulation and the effector limb of the immune response. Thus, the HLA-B8 haplotype, which is often found in association with autoimmune diseases, is also associated with the DR antigens in certain immunoregulatory abnormalities. These disorders include abnormal lymphocyte responses to antigens, decreased numbers of circulating suppressor cells, and increased numbers of B cells in the blood. Among the effector functions associated with these HLA haplotypes is a decrease in C3b receptors on cells that clear circulating immune complexes. A critical role for the D/DR region in the pathogenesis of SLE is supported by the observation that inherited deficiencies of certain complement components, particularly C2 and C4, are associated with an increased incidence of the disease. The genes that code for these early complement components are within the HLA region, close to the D/DR site.

IMMUNOLOGICAL ABNORMALITIES: The production of autoantibodies against a large variety of antigens is characteristic of SLE. The precise mechanisms underlying this B-cell hyperreactivity are unknown. Two general hypotheses have been advanced. One attributes the disease to a nonspecific, polyclonal B-cell activation, although the nature of the stimulus is speculative. The second hypothesis holds that the antibodies formed in SLE represent a response to specific antigenic stimulation. Support for the latter hypothesis comes from the observation that with time the antibodies of SLE demonstrate gene rearrangements and mutations that are typical of an antigen-driven response. Moreover, a patient with SLE often has antibodies to more than one epitope on a single antigen, further suggesting a primary role for antigens. With respect to the antigen-driven hypothesis, the inciting antigens have not been identified. However, a number of factors render normal body constituents more immunogenic, including infection, ultraviolet exposure, or other environmental agents that damage cells. Foreign antigens that might induce molecular mimicry are most likely to be viral proteins, although direct evidence for this conjecture is lacking.

Whether or not the autoimmune response in SLE is primarily driven by antigens, the variety of autoantibodies strongly suggests a general disturbance of immune tolerance, which is a phenomenon that is dependent on T lymphocytes. Recent evidence suggests that CD4+ T cells are important in this process. In SLE, these cells become autoreactive secondary to DNA hypomethylation. These autoreactive CD4+ T cells overexpress the cell adhesion molecule LFA-1 (CD11a), which stabilizes the interaction between the T cells and the antigen-presenting cells such as macrophages. These autoreactive CD4+ T cells are also capable of activating B cells in the absence of antigen. Various abnormalities in CD8+ suppressor T cells have also been described, most completely in the mouse models. However, in humans no consistent defect in the T suppressor cell population has been found. Other immunological abnormalities described in SLE include increased circulating levels of IL-6, which in these patients is associated with B-cell differentiation.

TYPE III HYPERSENSITIVITY: The evidence for the hypothesis that SLE is predominantly mediated by immune complexes is as follows:

- Circulating immune complexes, which contain nuclear antigens, are often detected during the active stages of lupus.
- Immune complexes in injured tissues are identified by immunofluorescence in lupus-induced tissue injury—for example, vasculitis or glomerulonephritis.
- Immune complexes extracted from the tissues contain nuclear antigens.

Thus, there is good reason to believe that the bulk of the injury in lupus is due to the deposition of immune complexes formed against self-antigens, particularly against DNA.

Although most of this multisystemic involvement in SLE can be traced to the deposition of circulating preformed immune complexes in the tissues, recent evidence suggests that under certain conditions the formation of immune complexes occurs *in situ*—that is, in the tissues rather than in the circulation. Examples include antibody formed against connective tissue components and perhaps the membranous form of lupus glomerulonephritis. Type II hypersensitivity reactions may also participate in lupus, since cytotoxic antibodies against leukocytes, erythrocytes, and platelets have been described.

□ Pathology and Clinical Features:

Because circulating immune complexes deposit in almost all tissues, virtually every organ in the body can be involved. The organs with the most serious involvement by SLE are shown in Figure 4-23 and Table 4-9.

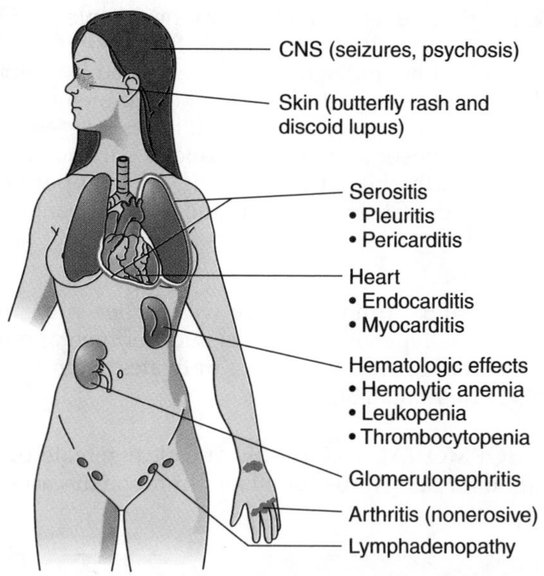

FIGURE *4-23*
Complications of systemic lupus erythematosus.

SKIN: Skin involvement is common and is manifested by an erythematous rash in sun-exposed sites, a "butterfly" malar rash being the most characteristic. Microscopically, the skin exhibits a perivascular lymphoid infiltrate and liquefactive degeneration of the basal cells. Immunofluorescence studies reveal the deposition of immunoglobulin and complement at the dermal–epidermal junction (lupus band).

JOINTS: **Joint involvement is the most common manifestation of SLE, and over 90% of patients have polyarthralgias.** An inflammatory synovitis occurs, but unlike rheumatoid arthritis there is usually no injury to the joint itself.

KIDNEYS: **Renal involvement, in particular glomerulonephritis, is very common.** Three fourths of patients with SLE have evidence of renal disease at autopsy. IgG antibodies to double-stranded and single-stranded DNA appear to play a prominent role in SLE-induced glomerulonephritis. Four main histological types of glomerulonephritis can be distinguished, as defined in the WHO classification of lupus nephritis.

1. **Mesangial lupus nephritis** is the mildest form of renal involvement. In this disorder, immune complexes and complement deposit almost exclusively in the mesangial regions of the glomeruli, but there are only slight increases in mesangial cells and mesangial matrix (Fig. 4-24). These patients have only slight renal dysfunction, characterized by mild proteinuria and hematuria. The prognosis is excellent.
2. **Focal proliferative lupus nephritis** is characterized by increased cellularity in some but not all (focal) glomeruli (Fig. 4-25). The glomeruli show a proliferation of endothelial and mesangial cells and infiltration by neutrophils and monocytes. Necrosis and fibrin deposition are also often present. Immunofluorescence studies and electron microscopy demonstrate the deposition of immunoglobulin and complement, primarily in the mesangial regions of the glomeruli. The prognosis of patients with this form of lupus nephritis is mixed. Some remain with only mild disease, whereas others progress to renal failure.

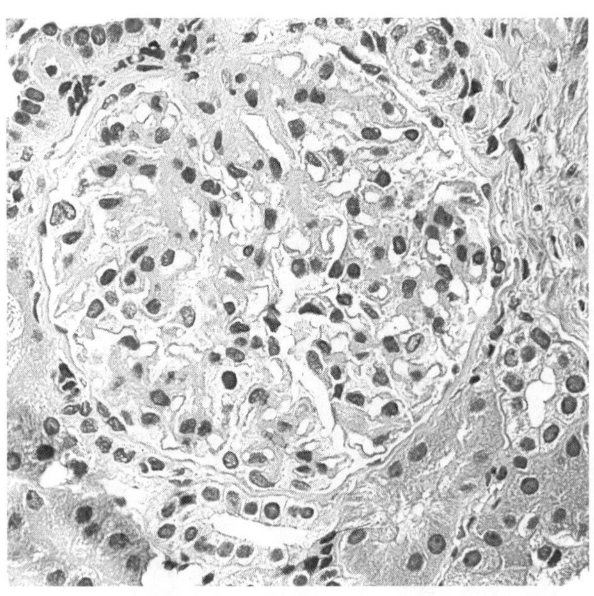

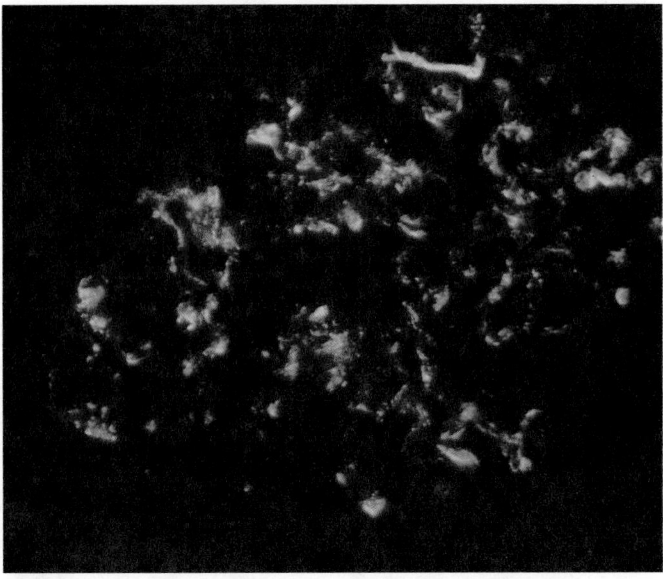

A B

FIGURE 4-24
Mesangial form of lupus nephritis. (*A*) The mesangial component of the glomerulus is more prominent because of an increase in both cells and matrix. (*B*) Immunofluorescent staining with an antibody to immunoglobulin demonstrates the deposition of immunoglobulin in the mesangium. The deposition of complement in the same location is also demonstrated by this technique.

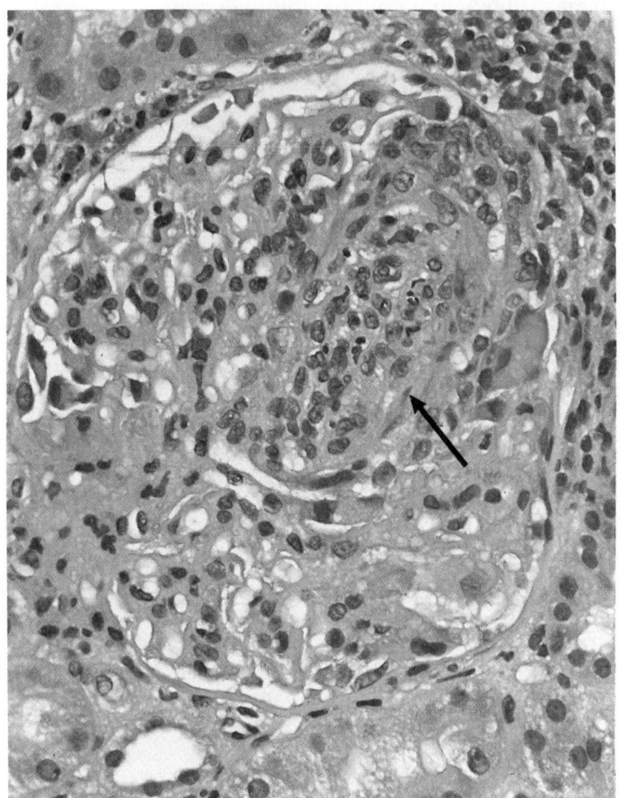

FIGURE 4-25
Focal proliferative lupus nephritis with segmental proliferation (*arrow*) in the glomerulus.

3. **Diffuse proliferative lupus nephritis** is the most serious type of renal disease. It occurs in as many as 50% of patients who suffer lupus with renal involvement and is associated with conspicuous increases in glomerular cellularity, fibrin deposition, and necrosis (Fig. 4-26). Epithelial crescents are also commonly seen. By immunofluorescence and electron microscopy, widespread deposition of immune complexes is seen throughout the glomeruli, primarily in the mesangium and underneath the glomerular basement membrane (subendothelial). Many patients with this form of lupus nephritis progress to renal failure.
4. **Membranous lupus nephritis** resembles other forms of membranous glomerulonephritis that are associated with massive proteinuria and the nephrotic syndrome. There is often minimal hypercellularity. Instead, diffusely thickened glomerular capillary loops, caused by the deposition of immunoglobulin and complement on the epithelial surface of the glomerular basement membrane (subepithelial), are present. This pattern of lupus involvement is usually not associated with renal failure.

Although glomerulonephritis is the most common renal manifestation of SLE, occasionally an interstitial nephritis or (rarely) a vasculitis is associated with the disease. In many of these cases, immunoglobulins and complement are present in the interstitium and blood vessels of the kidney. A fuller discussion of lupus nephritis is found in Chapter 16.

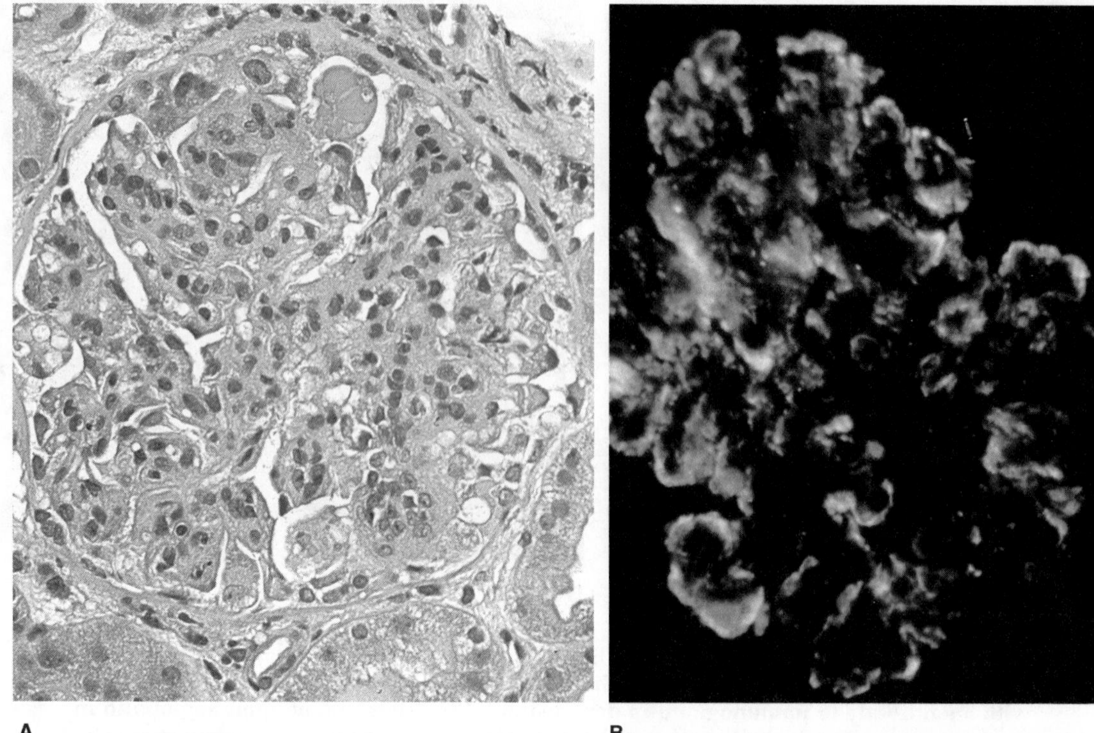

FIGURE 4-26
Diffuse proliferative lupus nephritis. (*A*) There is a diffuse increase in the cellularity of the glomerulus. (*B*) Immunofluorescent staining with an antibody to immunoglobulin demonstrates a conspicuous deposition of immunoglobulin in the mesangium and capillary walls. Similar deposition of complement in the same locations is also demonstrated by this technique.

SEROUS MEMBRANES: Involvement of serous membranes is common in SLE. More than one third of patients have pleuritis and a pleural effusion. Pericarditis and peritonitis occur less frequently.

LUNG: The involvement of the respiratory system in SLE is frequent, and the clinical manifestations are diverse, ranging from pleural disease to upper airway involvement and parenchymal disease of the lungs. Pneumonitis is thought to be caused by the deposition of immune complexes in the alveolar septa and is associated with patchy acute inflammation. Progressive interstitial fibrosis develops in some patients. An increased incidence of pulmonary hypertension has also been reported.

HEART: Cardiac involvement is common in SLE, although congestive heart failure is rare and is usually associated with a myocarditis. All layers of the heart may be involved, with pericarditis being the most common finding. Endocarditis, which is usually not clinically significant, is characterized by small nonbacterial vegetations on the valve leaflets termed **Libman-Sacks endocarditis**. These lesions should be differentiated from the larger, more bulky vegetations of bacterial endocarditis or the small vegetations of rheumatic endocarditis, which are confined to the lines of valve closure.

BRAIN: **Involvement of the central nervous system is a life-threatening complication of lupus.** Vasculitis is the common underlying lesion leading to hemorrhage and infarction of the brain, which are often lethal. In addition, patients with diffuse central nervous system involvement often have antineuronal and anti-ribonucleoprotein (anti-RNP) autoantibodies.

THROMBOEMBOLIC COMPLICATIONS: One third of the patients with SLE display antiphospholipid antibodies. This autoimmune reaction results in thromboembolic complications, including stroke, pulmonary embolism, deep venous thrombosis, and portal vein thrombosis.

Other organ involvement occurs less frequently and is often due to a vasculitis, which is also characteristic of lupus. Thus, lesions in the spleen are characterized by thickening and concentric fibrosis of the penicillary arteries—the so-called onion-skin pattern.

Course and Prognosis

The clinical course of SLE is highly variable and typically exhibits exacerbations and remissions. Before the advent of corticosteroids and other immunosuppressive therapies, SLE was considered a rapidly fatal disease. However, with the recognition of mild forms of the disease, improved antihypertensive medications, and the use of immunosuppressive agents, the overall 10-year survival approaches 90%. The worst prognosis is found in patients with severe disease of the kidneys and brain and those with systolic hypertension.

Summary

The dominant abnormality in SLE is polyclonal B-cell hyperactivity, which is associated with a loss of normal self-tolerance and autoantibody formation to a variety of self-antigens, the most important of which is DNA. The reason for this B-cell hyperactivity is not clear, but emerging evidence suggests a critical role for autoreactive CD4+ helper cells. The systemic injury seen in SLE is caused by the deposition of immune complexes in tissues.

Other Forms of Lupus Erythematosus

Drug-Induced Lupus

The administration of certain drugs, including procainamide (arrhythmias), hydralazine (hypertension), and isoniazid (tuberculosis), is occasionally complicated by the development of a syndrome similar to SLE. Unlike SLE, drug-induced lupus shows no sex predominance, and most patients are older than 50 years. Factors that predispose to the development of this syndrome include (1) large daily doses of the drug, (2) slow drug-acetylator status, and (3), in hydralazine-induced lupus, the presence of the HLA-DR4 genotype. As in SLE, the deposition of immune complexes is a feature of drug-induced lupus.

Patients with drug-induced lupus suffer from polyarthritis, pleuritis, and pericarditis and exhibit antinuclear antibodies. In addition, they may develop rheumatoid factor, a false-positive test for syphilis (Venereal Diseases Research Laboratory, VDRL), and a positive Coombs test. However, renal and central nervous system involvement rarely occurs, and antibodies to double-stranded DNA, antibodies to Sm antigen, and low serum complement levels are unusual. On the other hand, autoantibodies to histones are typical in drug-induced lupus. As in idiopathic SLE, autoreactive CD4+ T cells have been implicated in the polyclonal B-cell activation. Discontinuation of the offending drug is ordinarily curative.

Chronic Discoid Lupus

This cutaneous disorder is the most common variety of localized lupus erythematosus, although it may also occur in some cases of SLE (see Chapter 24). Erythematous, depigmented, and telangiectatic plaques are found most commonly on the face and scalp. The deposition of immunoglobulins and complement at the dermal–epidermal interface is similar to that observed in SLE, but the uninvolved skin in patients with discoid lupus, unlike SLE, shows no immune deposits. Although antinuclear antibodies develop in about one third of the patients, antibodies to double-stranded DNA and Sm antigen are not encountered. The large majority of patients with discoid lupus are not otherwise ill, but up to 10% eventually manifest the features of SLE.

Subacute Cutaneous Lupus

This generalized form of cutaneous lupus is characterized by papular and annular lesions, principally on the trunk. The disorder is aggravated by exposure to ultraviolet light (sunlight), although the lesions eventually resolve without scarring. Antibodies to ribonucleoprotein (SS-A) and an association with the HLA-DR3 genotype are characteristic of subacute cutaneous lupus.

Sjögren Syndrome

Sjögren syndrome (SS) is an autoimmune disorder characterized by keratoconjunctivitis sicca (dry eyes) and xerostomia (dry mouth) in the absence of other connective tissue diseases. This definition is used to separate primary SS from secondary types that are occasionally associated with other disorders of connective tissue, such as SLE, rheumatoid arthritis, scleroderma, and polymyositis. Although the main targets in SS are the salivary and the lacrimal glands, the primary type is also frequently associated with involvement of other organs, including the thyroid gland, the lung, and the kidney.

Primary SS is the second most common connective tissue disorder after SLE and affects up to 3% of the population. Like most autoimmune diseases, it occurs mostly in women (30 to 65 years old). There are strong associations between primary SS and certain MHC types, notably HLA-B8, Dw3, HLA-DR3, DRW-52, HLA-Dw2, and MT2, the last a B-cell alloantigen. Familial clustering occurs, and in these families there is also a high incidence of other autoimmune diseases.

☐ **Pathogenesis:** The cause of SS is unknown. The production of autoantibodies, particularly antinuclear antibodies, typically occurs in patients with SS. These autoantibodies may be directed against DNA, histones, or nonhistone proteins in the nucleus. Autoantibodies to soluble nuclear nonhistone proteins characterize primary SS, particularly the antigens SS-A (RO) and SS-B (La) (see Table 4-7). Antibodies to these autoantigens are found in half of the patients with SS and are associated with more severe glandular and extraglandular manifestations. Autoantibodies to DNA or histones are rare, and their presence suggests secondary SS due to lupus. Rheumatoid factor is also commonly found in saliva, tears, and the circulation. Organ-specific autoantibodies, such as those directed against salivary gland antigens, are distinctly uncommon. As in SLE, it remains controversial whether the production of autoantibodies in SS primarily reflects polyclonal activation of B cells or is essentially antigen-driven, although these processes are not mutually exclusive.

Sjögren syndrome has become the prototype for the

investigation of a viral etiology for autoimmune disease. Particular attention has been paid to the possible roles of Epstein-Barr virus (EBV) and the retrovirus human T-cell leukemia virus-1 (HTLV-1). Although it is still difficult to assign a role for EBV in the pathogenesis of SS, there is evidence that reactivation of this virus may be involved in the perpetuation of SS, polyclonal B-cell activation, and the development of lymphoma. In Japan, the seroprevalence of HTLV-1 among patients with SS is 23%, compared to 3.4% among blood donors. Conversely, among HTLV-1 seropositive persons, more than three quarters demonstrated evidence of SS. Mice infected with or transgenic for retroviruses develop SS-like pathogenic changes and are currently being studied as animal models of the disease. The evidence to date suggests that persistent viral infection of the salivary epithelium mediates upregulation of class II MHC and Ro and La antigens, leading to immune activation and the formation of autoantibodies to Ro and La.

□ Pathology and Clinical Features:

Sjögren syndrome is characterized by an intense lymphocytic infiltrate in the salivary and lacrimal glands (Fig. 4-27). Focal lymphocytic infiltrates in these glands are initially observed in a periductal location. The majority of lobules, especially the centers of the lobules, are affected. Well-defined germinal centers are rare. The lymphoid infiltrates destroy acini and ducts, and the latter often become dilated and filled with cellular debris. The stroma of the gland is preserved, an appearance that helps to differentiate this disorder from a lymphoma. The lymphocytic infiltrates in the glands are predominantly CD4+ T cells, but a few B cells are also present. In the late stage of the disease, the glands atrophy and may be replaced by hyalinized tissue and fibrosis. Owing to the absence of tears, the cornea becomes dry and fissured and may ulcerate. The lack of saliva causes atrophy, inflammation, and cracking of the oral mucosa. The pathology of the salivary and lacrimal glands is described in greater detail in Chapter 25.

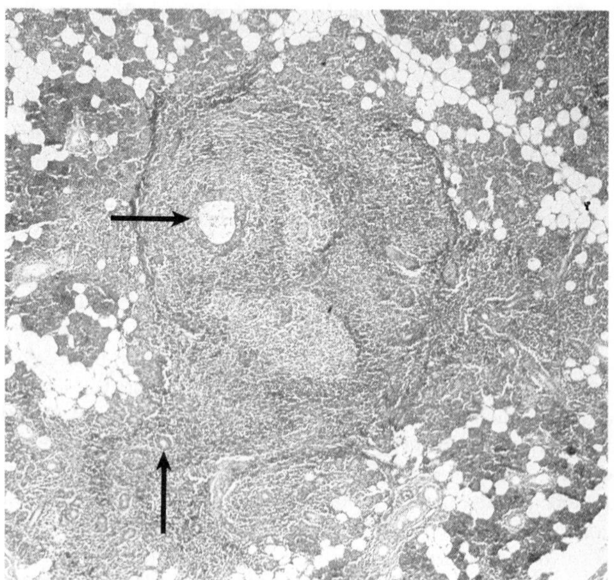

FIGURE 4-27
Sjögren syndrome involving a major salivary gland. An intense lymphoid infiltrate destroys the gland's acini but spares the ducts (*arrows*).

Involvement of extraglandular sites is also common in SS:

- **Pulmonary disease** occurs in most patients, and bronchial glands atrophy following lymphoid infiltration. This causes thick tenacious secretions, focal atelectasis, recurrent infections, and bronchiectasis.
- **The gastrointestinal tract is also affected**, and many patients have difficulty in swallowing (dysphagia). The submucosal glands of the esophagus are infiltrated by lymphocytes. In addition, atrophic gastritis occurs secondary to lymphoid infiltration of the gastric mucosa.
- **Liver disease**, especially primary biliary cirrhosis, is present in 5% to 10% of patients with SS and is associated with the destruction of intrahepatic bile ducts and nodular lymphoid infiltrates.
- **Interstitial nephritis and chronic thyroiditis** occasionally accompany SS.

Sjögren syndrome is associated with a 40-fold increased risk of malignant lymphoma. There is reason to believe that B-cell clonal expansion plays an integral role in the pathophysiology of the lymphoid infiltrates and may explain the increased incidence of malignant lymphoma associated with this disorder. In the proliferating B cells, both heavy-chain and light-chain immunoglobulin genes are rearranged.

Scleroderma (Progressive Systemic Sclerosis)

Scleroderma, or the more contemporary term progressive systemic sclerosis, is an autoimmune disease of connective tissue characterized by excessive collagen deposition in the skin and internal organs such as the lung, gastrointestinal tract, heart, and kidney. The disease occurs four times as often in women as in men, mostly in persons between 25 and 50 years of age. Familial incidence has been reported. There is an association between HLA-DQB1 and the formation of the characteristic autoantibodies in this disease.

□ Pathogenesis:

IMMUNOLOGICAL ABNORMALITIES: Patients with scleroderma exhibit abnormalities of the humoral and cellular immune systems. The number of circulating B lymphocytes is normal, but there is evidence of hyperactivity, as manifested by hypergammaglobulinemia and cryoglobulinemia. Antinuclear antibodies are common but are usually in a lower titer than in SLE. **Antibodies virtually specific for scleroderma include (1) nucleolar autoantibodies (primarily against RNA polymerase), (2) antibodies to Scl-70, a nonhistone nuclear protein topoisomerase, and (3) anticentromere antibodies, which are associated with the CREST variant of the dis-**

ease (see later). The Scl-70 autoantibody is the most common and specific for the diffuse form of scleroderma and is seen in 70% of these patients. However, there is no correlation between the titer of antinuclear antibodies and the severity of the disease process. Rheumatoid factor is commonly present in scleroderma, and autoantibodies are occasionally directed against other tissues, such as smooth muscle, thyroid gland, and salivary glands. Antibodies against types I and IV collagen have also been described and may be relevant to the pathogenesis of this disease.

There are several cellular immune derangements in patients with progressive systemic sclerosis. Reductions in CD8+ T-suppressor cells in the circulation are found, and there is evidence of T-cell activation, with alterations in functions mediated by IL-1 and elevations in IL-2 and the soluble IL-2 receptor in active disease. The levels of IL-4 and IL-6 have also been described as being increased. The tissues exhibit active mononuclear inflammation, which precedes the development of the vasculopathy and the fibrosis characteristic of this disease. In this infiltrate, increased numbers of CD4+ and YS+ T cells (which adhere to fibroblasts) are present, as well as macrophages. Mast cells (degranulated) are also present in the skin of these patients. The incidence of other autoimmune disorders, such as thyroiditis and primary biliary cirrhosis, is increased in patients with progressive systemic sclerosis. Circulating male fetal cells have been demonstrated in the blood of many women with scleroderma who bore male children many years before the onset of the disease. It has been suggested that scleroderma in these patients is similar to graft-versus-host reaction.

FIBROSIS: Progressive systemic sclerosis is characterized by excessive collagen deposition in many tissues. Although the cause remains unclear, there is emerging evidence that there is expansion and activation of fibrogenic clones of fibroblasts in the active disease. These clones of fibroblasts behave autonomously and display augmented procollagen synthesis, including increased circulating levels of type III collagen aminopropeptide. Several factors may be responsible for this fibroblast activation. The YS+ T cells adhere to fibroblasts and may induce activation via cytokine generation. Cytokines implicated in this process include TGF-β, which is elevated in the tissues of these patients, as well as IL-1 and IL-4, all of which stimulate fibroblast proliferation and collagen biosynthesis. There is also an increased level of IL-6, which is involved in the upregulation of matrix metalloproteinase and is important in the modulation of collagen metabolism. Activated fibroblasts themselves produce cytokines and growth factors, such as IL-1, prostaglandin E (PGE), TGF-β, and PDGF, which may in turn serve to activate other fibroblasts. Finally, activated fibroblasts also express adhesion molecule ICAM-1 on their surface, which may be important in the adherence of T cells and macrophages and their subsequent activation.

☐ **Pathology:** The skin in scleroderma displays early edema and then induration, with the latter characterized by the following:

- A striking increase in collagen fibers in the reticular dermis
- Thinning of the epidermis with loss of rete pegs
- Atrophy of dermal appendages
- Hyalinization and obliteration of arterioles
- Variable mononuclear infiltrates, consisting primarily of T cells

The stage of induration may progress to atrophy or revert to normal. Similar histological alterations occur in the synovium, lungs, gastrointestinal tract, heart, and kidneys.

BLOOD VESSELS: Lesions in the arteries, arterioles, and capillaries are typical, and in some cases may be the first effect of the disease. Initial subintimal edema with fibrin deposition is followed by thickening and fibrosis of the vessel and reduplication or fraying of the internal elastic lamina (Fig. 4-28). The involved vessels are usually severely restricted in terms of blood flow and may actually be thrombosed.

KIDNEYS: The kidneys are involved in more than half of patients with scleroderma. They show marked vascular changes, often with focal hemorrhage and cortical infarcts. Among the most severely affected vessels are the interlobular arteries and afferent arterioles. Early fibromuscular thickening of the subintima causes luminal narrowing, which is followed by fibrosis (see Fig. 4-28). "Fibrinoid" necrosis is commonly seen in afferent arterioles. The glomerular alterations are nonspecific, and focal changes range from necrosis extending from the afferent arterioles to fibrosis. There is diffuse deposition of immunoglobulin, complement, and fibrin in affected vessels early in the disease, probably because of increased vascular permeability.

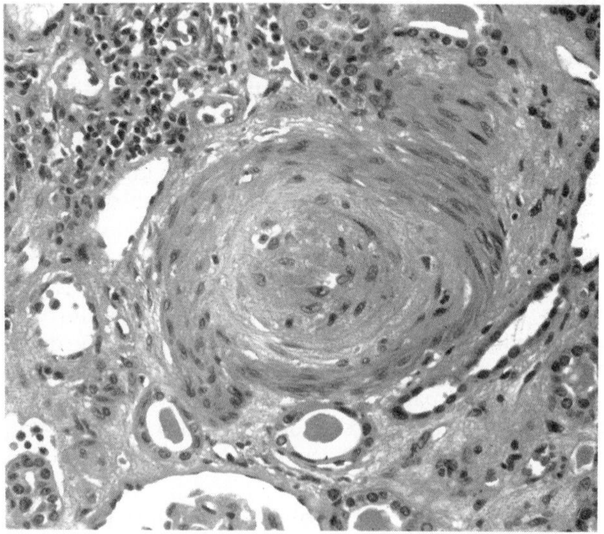

FIGURE *4-28*
Scleroderma with characteristic renal vascular involvement. The interlobular artery shows marked intimal thickening, with virtual obliteration of the lumen.

LUNGS: Diffuse interstitial fibrosis is the primary abnormality in the lungs. The disease progresses to end-stage pulmonary fibrosis, eventuating in a "honeycomb" lung.

HEART: The large majority of patients with scleroderma have patchy myocardial fibrosis, and in about one fourth of cases, more than 10% of the myocardium is involved. These lesions result from focal myocardial necrosis, which may reflect focal ischemia secondary to a Raynaud-like reactivity of the coronary microvasculature.

GASTROINTESTINAL TRACT: Progressive systemic sclerosis can involve any portion of the gastrointestinal tract. Esophageal dysfunction is the most common and troublesome gastrointestinal complication. Atrophy of the smooth muscle and fibrous replacement are seen in the lower esophagus. The small bowel is often involved with patchy fibrosis, principally of the muscular layers.

□ **Clinical Features:** Scleroderma presents as two distinct clinical entities, the generalized form and the CREST variant.

GENERALIZED SCLERODERMA: This disorder is characterized by severe and progressive disease of the skin and the early onset of all or most of the associated abnormalities of visceral organs. The symptoms usually begin with Raynaud phenomenon (intermittent episodes of ischemia of the fingers, marked by pallor, paresthesias, and pain), accompanied or followed by edema of the fingers and hands, tightening and thickening of the skin, polyarthralgia, and complaints referable to involvement of specific internal organs.

The typical patient with generalized scleroderma has a "stone facies" owing to tightening of the facial skin and restricted motion of the mouth. The progression of vascular lesions in the fingers is reflected in the appearance of ischemic ulcerations of the fingertips in many patients, with subsequent shortening and atrophy of the digits. Many patients suffer from painful tendinitis, and joint pain is common. Involvement of the esophagus leads to hypomotility and dysphagia, and fibrosis in the small bowel interferes with intestinal motility, with consequent overgrowth of bacteria and secondary malabsorption.

Dyspnea on exertion is the initial symptom of pulmonary fibrosis in scleroderma, occurring is more than half of the patients. The pulmonary disease progresses to dyspnea at rest and eventually to respiratory failure. Patients with long-standing disease are at risk for the development of pulmonary hypertension and cor pulmonale. Although most patients with scleroderma have some degree of myocardial fibrosis, congestive heart failure is uncommon. However, ventricular arrhythmias are a cause of sudden death.

The vascular involvement of the kidneys in generalized scleroderma is responsible for the so-called scleroderma renal crisis, characterized by (1) the sudden onset of malignant hypertension, (2) progressive renal insufficiency, and (3) frequently, microangiopathic hemolytic anemia. The syndrome, which reflects ischemic injury to the kidneys, usually occurs in the first few years of the disease and is marked by conspicuously elevated levels of circulating renin.

CREST VARIANT: This form of scleroderma is a milder disease than generalized scleroderma; it is characterized by calcinosis (C), Raynaud phenomenon (R), esophageal dysfunction (E), sclerodactyly (S), and telangiectasia (T). The CREST variant usually does not display severe systemic involvement, but it does exhibit anticentromere antibodies.

Polymyositis/Dermatomyositis

Polymyositis and dermatomyositis are chronic inflammatory myopathies that, together with inclusion body myositis (IBM), comprise a group of autoimmune diseases of muscle. These inflammatory myopathies are rare (1/100,000) and occur in children as well as adults, juvenile dermatomyositis being the most common. There is an increased incidence in certain families and racial groups; in blacks the incidence is three times that in whites. A strong association is present with HLA-DR3, HLA-DRw52, and HLA-DQ, as well as with the gene encoding the constant region of the immunoglobulin molecule (the Gm phenotype). Women are affected twice as frequently as men. In many patients, particularly adult men, there is an association between myositis and cancer. Finally, myositis may also be seen in syndromes that overlap with other autoimmune diseases such as SLE, scleroderma, mixed connective tissue disease, and SS.

□ **Pathogenesis:** As for other systemic autoimmune diseases, the etiology of these inflammatory myopathies remains to be fully elucidated. Viral agents, such as picornavirus and retroviruses (including HIV), have been implicated. In fact, HIV can initially present as a myositis. However, selective molecular techniques have not detected viral particles in human myositis.

In polymyositis and IBM, injury seems to be mediated by activated T cells and macrophages. Muscle damage is associated with CD8+ cytotoxic T cells surrounding muscle fibers that express MHC class I antigens. *In vitro,* these T cells are directly cytotoxic to autologous muscle fibers. Macrophages are also activated, as assessed by their production of cytokines.

In dermatomyositis, CD4+ T cells are also present in the muscle, but there is evidence that humoral immune mechanism play the dominant role. B cells occur in the muscle, and the production of antibodies directed against intramuscular capillaries and endothelial cells appears to be primary to the disease process. Immunoglobulin and complement are deposited in the walls of the intramuscular capillaries. Complement, in particular C5b–9, has been implicated in the pathogenesis of the vascular injury.

Various autoantibodies are present in 60% to 80% of patients with inflammatory myopathies, including antibodies against muscle antigens such as myosin, as well as various antinuclear antibodies. The most specific autoantibodies are called myositis-specific antibodies (MSAs), a category that includes autoantibodies directed against rRNA synthetases, of which anti-Jo-1 is the most common. These antibodies are found both in polymyositis and dermatomyositis. Other specific but less common MSAs include those directed against a cytoplasmic RNA–protein complex (anti-SRP) found in polymyositis and anti-Mi-2 antibodies directed against nuclear proteins in dermatomyositis. The anti-PM-scl autoantibody directed against nucleolar proteins is specific for the common scleroderma-myositis overlap syndrome. There is no evidence that these specific autoantibodies are directly pathogenic.

☐ **Pathology:** The histological features of the three types of myositis are distinctive, reflecting their different pathogenetic mechanisms. Dermatomyositis features a humorally mediated microangiopathy, with early deposition of immune complexes and complement. The inflammatory infiltrate consists primarily of CD4+ T cells, B lymphocytes, and macrophages. The end-result of chronic dermatomyositis is a reduction in the number of capillaries in the muscle fibers, with atrophy and fibrosis reflecting secondary ischemia.

Polymyositis and IBM display no evidence of an angiopathy. Rather, there are infiltrates of CD8+ cytotoxic T cells and activated macrophages, which surround normal-appearing muscle fibers that express MHC class I molecules. Thus, in these diseases, cytotoxic T cells are thought to be primarily responsible for injury to the myocytes. IBM also exhibits pathognomonic vacuolar inclusion bodies in the myocytes.

SKIN: In 40% of patients with inflammatory myopathies, skin involvement is manifested by an erythematous rash on the face (and elsewhere), resembling that seen in SLE. If it involves the eyelids (heliotropic rash), it is considered specific for dermatomyositis. As in SLE, the skin changes involve a perivascular lymphoid infiltrate and liquefactive degeneration of the basal epithelial cells. Immunofluorescence studies of skin are helpful to differentiate between these two entities. In SLE, the deposition of granular immunoglobulin and complement at the dermal–epidermal junction occurs in uninvolved and involved skin and is virtually pathognomonic for that disease. By contrast, dermatomyositis is not associated with the deposition of immune components at the dermal–epidermal junction.

OTHER ORGAN SYSTEMS: Other organ systems are also affected, including joints, kidneys, lungs, and gastrointestinal tract. In the childhood form of polymyositis/dermatomyositis, a vasculitis may also be present. Renal involvement was initially believed to be rare, but newer reports suggest that a small proportion of patients (5% to 10%) indeed have immune complex renal disease.

☐ **Clinical Features:** The diagnosis of these acquired inflammatory myopathies rests not only on the histological appearance of the involved muscles but also on (1) the location of the involved muscles, (2) electromyographic alterations, and (3) elevated activities of muscle enzymes in the blood, namely, the MM isoenzyme of creatine phosphokinase and aldolase.

The proportion of patients with polymyositis/dermatomyositis who have an associated malignancy is disputed and varies from less than 10% to as many as 50%. In any event, the frequency of cancer is many-fold higher than that in the general population. **The association with malignancy is particularly evident in men older than 50 years, among whom three fourths have a cancer already diagnosed or will be shown to have one within 1 year.** Thus, polymyositis/dermatomyositis is often a paraneoplastic syndrome, and a careful search for an underlying malignancy is justified. Most of the cancers are in the lung, colon, and stomach, although in affected women, tumors of the breast, ovaries, and uterus are also encountered.

Dermatomyositis usually responds to treatment with adrenocortical steroids, and the prognosis is generally considered good. Some patients, however, develop classic scleroderma, and others have significant pulmonary and brain involvement.

The inflammatory myopathies are discussed in further detail in Chapter 27.

Mixed Connective Tissue Disease

Mixed connective tissue disease combines features of systemic lupus erythematosus, scleroderma, and dermatomyositis. The symptoms characteristic of SLE include rash, Raynaud phenomenon, arthritis, and arthralgias, whereas those of scleroderma are swollen hands, esophageal hypomotility, and pulmonary interstitial disease. Some patients also develop symptoms suggestive of rheumatoid arthritis. The incidence of mixed connective tissue disease is unknown. Between 80% and 90% of patients are female, and most are adults (mean age, 37 years). Patients with mixed connective tissue disease have been reported to respond well to corticosteroid therapy, although some studies have challenged this assertion.

☐ **Pathogenesis:** The etiology and pathogenesis of mixed connective tissue disease are unknown. Patients often have substantial evidence of B-cell activation with hypergammaglobulinemia and a positive rheumatoid factor. Antinuclear antibodies are present but, unlike in SLE, are usually not against double-stranded DNA. The most distinctive antinuclear antibody is directed against an extractable nuclear antigen. Specifically, patients with mixed connective tissue disease have high titers of antibody to uridine-rich ribonucleoprotein (anti-UI-RNP) in the absence of other extractable nuclear antigens, including PM-1 and Jo-1. Anti-RNP antibodies are also occasionally seen in SLE but usually in lower titer than in mixed connective tissue disease.

The cause for the formation and maintenance of the high titer of anti-RNP antibody is unclear. However, there is an association with HLA-DR4 and HLA-DR2 genotypes, suggesting a role for T cells in the autoantibody production. There is no direct evidence that these antibodies induce the characteristic involvement of the various organ systems. There is also controversy over whether mixed connective tissue disease is a separate disease entity or represents a heterogeneous collection of patients with SLE, scleroderma, or polymyositis who do not present initially with the classic manifestations of these diseases. For example, in some patients, mixed connective tissue disease seems to have evolved into typical scleroderma. Other patients develop evidence of renal disease, a finding consistent with SLE. Still others differentiate into rheumatoid arthritis. Thus, mixed connective tissue disease in many patients seems to be an intermediate stage in a genetically determined progression to a recognized autoimmune disease. Persons whose disease remains undifferentiated may comprise a distinct subset.

At this time, whether mixed connective tissue disease represents a distinct entity or simply an overlap of symptoms in patients with other types of collagen vascular diseases remains an open question.

SUGGESTED READING

BOOKS

Abbas AK, Lichtman AH, Pober JS: *Cellular and molecular immunology,* 2nd ed. Philadelphia: WB Saunders, 1994.

Ioachim HL: *Pathology of AIDS.* Philadelphia: JB Lippincott, 1989.

Janeway C, Travers P: *Immunobiology: The immune system in health and disease.* London: Current Biology Limited, 1996.

Kunkel SL, Remick DG: *Cytokines in health and disease.* New York: Marcel Dekker, 1992.

Lachmann PJ, Peters K, Rosen F: *Clinical aspects of immunology.* Boston: Blackwell Scientific, 1993.

Roitt I, Brosoff J, Male D: *Immunology,* 4th ed. St. Louis: CV Mosby, 1996.

REVIEW ARTICLES

Arnett FC, Edworthy SM, Block DA, et al: The American Rheumatism Association 1987 revised criteria for the classification of rheumatoid arthritis. *Arthritis Rheum* 31:315–324, 1988.

Barnaba V: Viruses, hidden self-epitopes and autoimmunity. *Immunol Rev* 152:47–66, 1996.

Boumpas DT, Austin HA, Fessler BJ, Balow JE: Systemic lupus erythematosus: Emerging concepts. Part 1: Renal, neuropsychiatric, cardiovascular, pulmonary, and hematologic disease. *Ann Intern Med* 122: 940–950, 1995.

Boumpas DT, Fessler BJ, Austin HA, Balow JE, Klippel JH, Lockshin MD: Systemic lupus erythematosus: Emerging concepts. Part 2: Dermatologic and joint disease, the antiphospholipid antibody syndrome, pregnancy and hormonal therapy, morbidity and mortality, and pathogenesis. *Ann Intern Med* 123: 42–53, 1995.

Campbell RD, Trowsdale J: Map of the human MHC. *Immunol Today* 14:349–352, 1993.

Davies JM: Molecular mimicry: Can epitope mimicry induce autoimmune disease? *Immunol Cell Biol* 75: 113–126, 1997.

Fox RI: Sjögren's syndrome: Controversies and progress. *Clin Lab Med* 17:431–444, 1997.

Frederick M, Grimm E, Krohn E, Smid C, Yu TK: Cytokine-induced cytotoxic function expressed by lymphocytes of the innate immune system: Distinguishing characteristics of NK and LAK based on functional and molecular markers. *Interferon Cytokine Res* 17:435–447, 1997.

Germain RN: MHC-dependent antigen processing and peptide presentation: Providing ligands for T lymphocyte activation. *Cell* 76:287–299, 1994.

Goodnow CC: Balancing immunity, autoimmunity, and self-tolerance. *New York Acad Sci* 815:55–66, 1997.

Hentges F: B lymphocyte ontogeny and immunoglobulin production. *Clin Exp Immunol* 97(suppl 1):3–9, 1994.

Jiminez SA, Hitraya E, Varga J: Pathogenesis of scleroderma: Collagen. *Rheum Dis Clin North Am* 22: 647–674, 1996.

Kunkel SL, Lukacs NW, Strieter RM, Chensue SW: Th1 and Th2 responses regulate experimental lung granuloma development. *Sarcoidosis Vasc Diffuse Lung Dis* 13:120–128, 1996.

Lukacs NW, Ward PA: Inflammatory mediators, cytokines and adhesion molecules in pulmonary inflammation and repair. *Adv Immunol* 62:257–304, 1996.

Mach B: Genetics of histocompatibility. *Curr Opinion Hematol* 1:4–11, 1994.

Mastaglia FL, Phillips BA, Zilko P: Treatment of inflammatory myopathies. *Muscle Nerve* 20:651–664, 1997.

Mills JA: Systemic lupus erythematosus. *N Engl J Med* 330:1871–1879, 1994.

Mitchell H, Bolster MB, LeRoy EC: Scleroderma and related conditions. *Med Clin North Am* 81:129–149, 1997.

Morris A, Hewitt C, Young S: The major histocompatibility complex: Its genes and their roles in antigen presentation. *Mol Aspects Med* 15:377–403, 1994.

Oddis CV, Medsger TA Jr: Inflammatory myopathies. *Baillere's Clin Rheumatol* 9:497–514, 1995.

Pantaleo G, Fauci AS: Immunopathogenesis of HIV infection. *Annu Rev Microbiol* 50:825–854, 1996.

Plotz PH: NIH conference. Myositis: Immunologic contributions to understanding cause, pathogenesis, and therapy. *Ann Intern Med* 122:715, 1995.

Report of a WHO Scientific Group: Primary immunodeficiency diseases. *Clin Exp Immunol* 99(suppl 1):1–24, 1995.

Rigg KM: Renal transplantation: Current status, complications and prevention. *J Antimicrob Chemotherap* 36(suppl B):51–57, 1995.

Saadi S, Platt JL: Immunology of xenotransplantation. *Life Sci* 62:365–387, 1998.

Smart BA, Och HD: The molecular basis and treatment of primary immunodeficiency disorders. *Curr Opinion Pediat* 9:570–576, 1997.

Sunthanthiran M, Strom TB: Immunobiology and immunopharmacology of organ allograft rejection. *J Clin Immunol* 15:161–171, 1995.

Swanson PC, Yung RL, Blatt NB, et al: New concepts in the pathogenesis of drug-induced lupus. *Lab Invest* 73:746–759, 1995.

Tan EM, Cohen AS, Fries JF et al: The 1982 revised criteria for the classification of systemic lupus erythematosus. *Arthritis Rheum* 25:1271–1277, 1982.

Theofilopoulos AN: The basis of autoimmunity: Part 1. Mechanisms of aberrant self-recognition. *Immunol Today* 16:90–98, 1995.

Trentham DE: Rheumatologic therapy for the 1990's: Evolution or revolution? *Rheum Dis Clin North Am* 15:407–412, 1989.

White B: Immunologic aspects of scleroderma. *Curr Opin Rheumatol* 7:541–545, 1995.

Yung RL, Johnson KJ, Richardson BC: New concepts in the pathogenesis of drug-induced lupus. *Lab Invest* 73:746–759, 1995.

CHAPTER 5

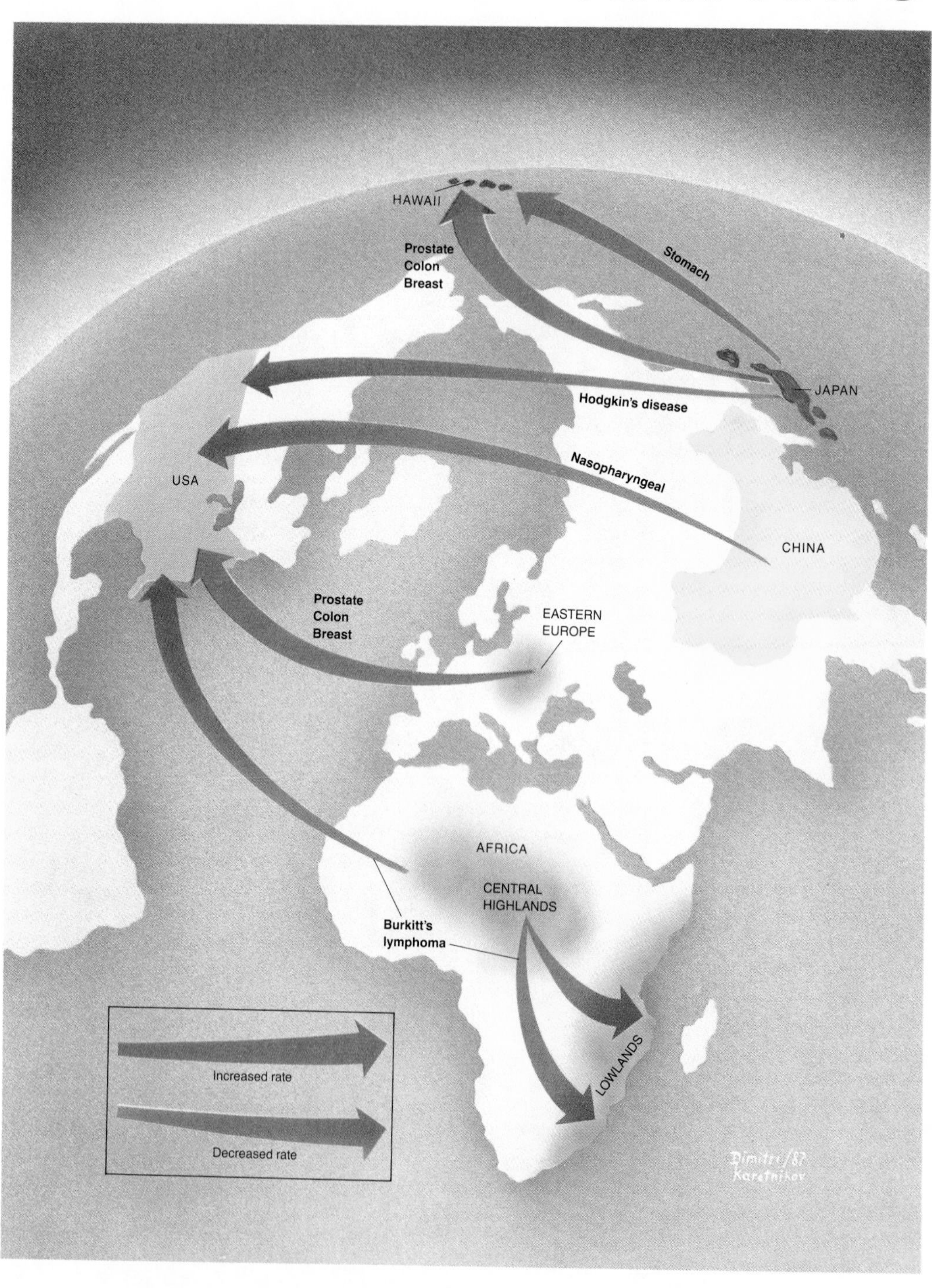
HAWAII
Prostate
Colon
Breast
Stomach
JAPAN
Hodgkin's disease
Nasopharyngeal
USA
CHINA
Prostate
Colon
Breast
EASTERN
EUROPE
AFRICA
CENTRAL
HIGHLANDS
Burkitt's
lymphoma
LOWLANDS
Increased rate
Decreased rate
Dimitri/87
Karetnikov

Neoplasia

Emanuel Rubin
John L. Farber

FIGURE *5-1* (*see opposite page*)
Cancer epidemiology. The influence of environmental factors on the incidence of cancer is illustrated by the results of several classic epidemiological studies of migrant populations. Offspring of Japanese immigrants to Hawaii exhibited (1) a decreased incidence of stomach cancer; (2) an increased incidence of cancers of the breast, colon, and prostate; and (3) an increased incidence of Hodgkin disease. The incidence of nasopharyngeal carcinoma decreased in the offspring of immigrants to the United States from China. Eastern Europeans who immigrated to the United States showed an increased incidence of carcinoma of the breast, colon, and prostate. Finally, the incidence of Burkitt lymphoma changed in Africans who immigrated from the central highlands to coastal lowlands or to the United States.

Cancer, for the most part, represents an uncontrolled proliferation of cells that express varying degrees of fidelity to their precursors. However, in some instances, for example follicular lymphoma (see Chapter 20), the accumulation of neoplastic cells reflects an aberration in programmed cell death (apoptosis). The structural resemblance of the cancer cell to its cell of origin enables specific diagnoses as to the source and potential behavior of the neoplasm. Although the causes of most cancers are not identified, and the mechanisms of carcinogenesis remain obscure, considerable information on the biological attributes of neoplasia has been generated. A wide variety of human and experimental data suggest that the neoplastic process entails not only cellular proliferation but also a modification of the differentiation of the involved cell types. Thus, in a sense, cancer may be viewed as a burlesque of normal development.

Cancer is not a new disease. Evidence of bone tumors has been found in prehistoric remains, and the disease is mentioned in ancient writings from India, Egypt, Babylonia, and Greece. Hippocrates is actually reported to have distinguished benign from malignant growths. He also introduced the term **karkinos**, from which our term **carcinoma** is derived. In particular, Hippocrates described cancer of the breast, and Paul of Aegina in the 7th century A.D. commented on its frequency.

The incidence of neoplastic disease increases with age, and the greater longevity in modern times necessarily enlarges the population at risk. Hence, for this reason alone, the overall incidence of cancer is increasing. In previous generations, on average, humans did not live long enough to develop many cancers that are particularly common in middle and old age, such as those of the prostate, colon, pancreas, and kidney. Despite assertions that contemporary society is or will be subject to an "epidemic" of cancer, the epidemiological data do not support such a concept. If all deaths from cancers caused by tobacco smoke are removed from the statistics, there has been no increase in the overall age-adjusted cancer death rate in men in the past half-century, and there has been a continually decreasing rate in women.

In general, neoplasms are irreversible, and their growth is, for the most part, autonomous and persists after the stimulus that produced it has been removed. Several observations are important at this point:

- Neoplasms are derived from cells that normally maintain a proliferative capacity. Thus, mature neurons and cardiac myocytes do not give rise to tumors.
- A tumor may express varying degrees of differentiation, from relatively mature structures that mimic normal tissues to a collection of cells so primitive that the cell of origin cannot be identified.
- The stimulus responsible for the uncontrolled proliferation may not be identifiable; in fact, it is not known for most human neoplasms.

BENIGN VERSUS MALIGNANT TUMORS

By definition, benign tumors do not penetrate (invade) adjacent tissue borders, nor do they spread (metastasize) to distant sites. They remain as localized overgrowths in the area in which they arise. As a rule, benign tumors are more differentiated than malignant ones—that is, they more closely resemble their tissue of origin. *By contrast, malignant tumors, or cancers, have the added property of invading contiguous tissues and metastasizing to distant sites, where subpopulations of malignant cells take up residence, grow anew, and again invade.*

In common usage, the terms benign and malignant refer to the overall biological behavior of a tumor rather than to its morphological characteristics. In most circumstances, malignant tumors kill, whereas benign ones spare the host. However, so-called benign tumors in critical locations can be deadly. For example, a benign intracranial tumor of the meninges (meningioma) can kill by exerting pressure on the brain. A minute benign tumor of the ependymal cells of the third ventricle (ependymoma) can block the circulation of cerebrospinal fluid, and the resulting hydrocephalus is lethal. A benign mesenchymal tumor of the left atrium (myxoma) may kill suddenly by blocking the orifice of the mitral valve. In certain locations, the erosion of a benign tumor of smooth muscle can lead to serious hemorrhage—witness the peptic ulceration of a gastric leiomyoma. On rare occasions, a functioning, benign endocrine adenoma can be life-threatening, as in the case of the sudden hypoglycemia associated with an insulinoma of the pancreas or the hypertensive crisis produced by a pheochromocytoma of the adrenal medulla. Conversely, certain types of malignant tumors are so indolent that many are curable by surgical resection. In this category are a considerable proportion of cancers of the breast and some malignant tumors of connective tissue, such as fibrosarcoma.

There are a number of tumors that are difficult to classify because they do not fit all the criteria for either benign or malignant neoplasms. The best-known example is basal cell carcinoma of the skin, which is histologically malignant (i.e., it invades aggressively) but does not metastasize to distant sites. Similarly, the local growth of a pleomorphic adenoma of a salivary gland, which is classified as benign, may be so aggressive that it defies surgical cure.

CLASSIFICATION OF NEOPLASMS

In any language, the classification of objects and concepts is pragmatic and useful only insofar as its general acceptance permits effective communication. Similarly, the nosology of tumors reflects historical concepts, technical jargon, location, origin, descriptive modifiers, and predictors of biological behavior. Although the language of tumor classification is neither rigidly logical nor consistent, it still serves as a reasonable mode of communication.

Benign Tumors

The primary descriptor of any tumor, benign or malignant, is its cell or tissue of origin. The classification of benign tumors is the basis for the names of their malignant variants. **Benign tumors are identified by the suffix "oma," which is preceded by reference to the cell or tissue of origin.** For instance, a benign tumor that resembles chondrocytes is called *chondroma* (Fig. 5-2). If the tumor resembles the precursor of the chondrocyte, it is labeled *chondroblastoma*. When a chondroma is located entirely within the bone, it is designated *enchondroma*. Tumors of epithelial origin are given a variety of names based on what is believed to be their outstanding characteristic.

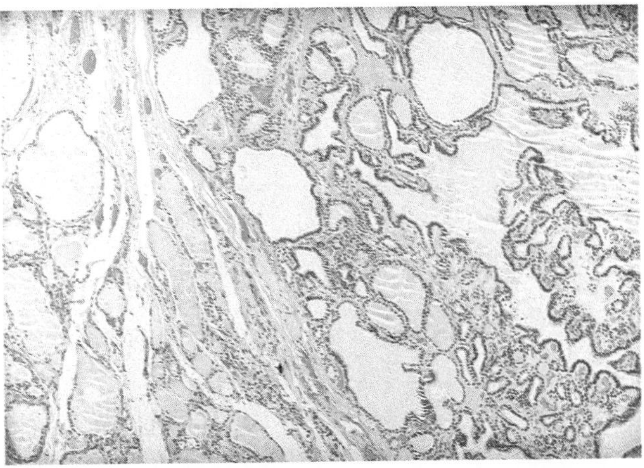

FIGURE 5-3
Benign thyroid adenoma. The follicles of a thyroid adenoma (*right*) contain colloid and resemble those of the normal thyroid tissue (*left*).

Thus, a benign tumor of the squamous epithelium may be called simply *epithelioma* or, when branched and exophytic, may be termed *papilloma*. Benign tumors arising from glandular epithelium, such as in the colon or the endocrine glands, are named *adenoma*. Accordingly, we refer to a thyroid adenoma (Fig. 5-3) or an islet cell adenoma. In some instances, the predominating feature is the gross appearance, in which case we speak, for example, of an *adenomatous polyp* of the colon or of the endometrium.

Benign tumors that arise from germ cells and contain derivatives of different germ layers are labeled *teratoma*. These tumors occur principally in the gonads and occasionally in the mediastinum and may contain a variety of structures, such as skin, neurons and glial cells, thyroid, intestinal epithelium, and cartilage. Localized, disordered differentiation during embryonic development results in a *hamartoma*, a disorganized caricature of normal tissue

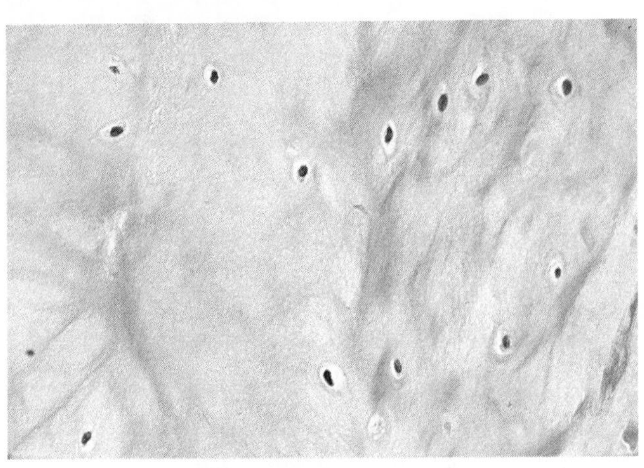

A

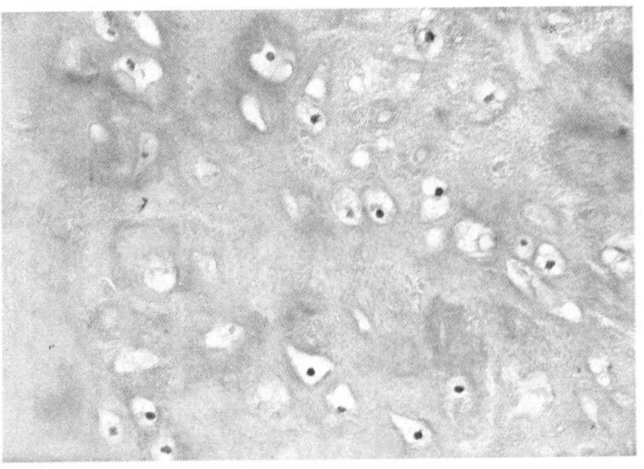

B

FIGURE 5-2
Benign chondroma. (*A*) Normal cartilage. (*B*) A benign chondroma closely resembles normal cartilage.

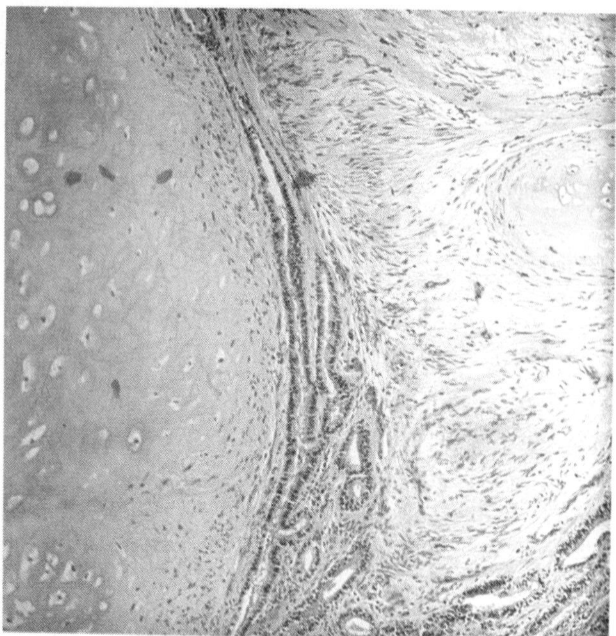

FIGURE 5-4
Hamartoma of the lung. The tumor contains islands of hyaline cartilage and clefts lined by cuboidal epithelium embedded in a fibromuscular stroma.

components (Fig. 5-4). Such tumors, which are not strictly neoplasms, contain varying combinations of cartilage, ducts or bronchi, connective tissue, blood vessels, and lymphoid tissue. Ectopic islands of normal tissue, called *choristoma*, may also be mistaken for true neoplasms. These small lesions are represented by pancreatic tissue in the wall of the stomach or intestine, adrenal rests under the renal capsule, and nodules of splenic tissue in the peritoneal cavity. Certain benign growths, recognized clinically as tumors, are not truly neoplastic but rather represent overgrowth of normal tissue elements. Examples are vocal cord polyps, skin tags, and hyperplastic polyps of the colon.

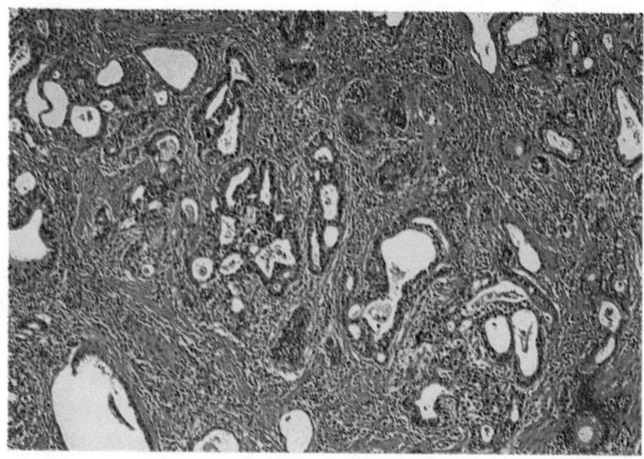

FIGURE 5-5
Adenocarcinoma of the stomach. Irregular neoplastic glands infiltrate the gastric wall.

Malignant Tumors

In general, the malignant counterparts of benign tumors usually carry the same name, except that the suffix "carcinoma" is applied to epithelial cancers and "sarcoma" to those of mesenchymal origin. For instance, a malignant tumor of the stomach is a *gastric adenocarcinoma* or *adenocarcinoma of the stomach. Squamous cell carcinoma* is an invasive tumor of the skin (Fig. 5-5) or a neoplasm that arises in the metaplastic squamous epithelium of the bronchus or endocervix. *Transitional cell carcinoma* is a malignant neoplasm of the bladder. By contrast, we speak of *chondrosarcoma* (Fig. 5-6) or *fibrosarcoma.* Sometimes the name of the tumor suggests the tissue type of origin, as in *osteogenic sarcoma* or *bronchogenic carcinoma.* Some tumors display neoplastic elements of different cell types but are not germ cell tumors. For example, *fibroadenoma* of the breast, composed of epithelial and stromal elements, is benign, whereas, as the name implies, *adenosquamous carcinoma* of the uterus or the lung is malignant. A rare malignant tumor that contains intermingled carcinomatous and sarcomatous elements is known as *carcinosarcoma.*

The persistence of certain historical terms adds a note of confusion. *Hepatoma* of the liver, *melanoma* of the skin, *seminoma* of the testis, and the lymphoproliferative tumor, *lymphoma*, are all highly malignant. Tumors of the hemopoietic system are a special case in which the relationship to the blood is indicated by the suffix "emia." Thus, *leukemia* refers to a malignant proliferation of leukocytes.

Secondary descriptors (again, with some inconsistencies) refer to a tumor's morphological and functional characteristics. For example, the term *papillary* describes a frondlike structure (Fig. 5-7). *Medullary* signifies a soft, cellular tumor with little connective tissue stroma, whereas *scirrhous* or *desmoplastic* implies a dense fibrous stroma (Fig. 5-8). *Colloid* carcinomas secrete abundant mucus, in which float islands of tumor cells. *Comedocarcinoma* is an intraductal neoplasm in which necrotic mate-

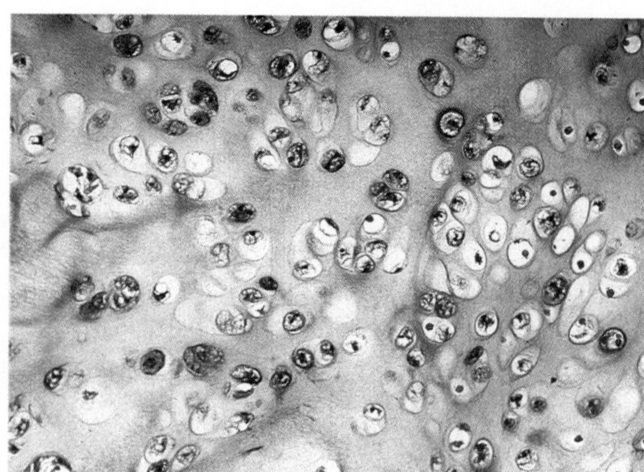

FIGURE 5-6
Chondrosarcoma of bone. The tumor is composed of malignant chondrocytes, which have bizarre shapes and irregular hyperchromatic nuclei, embedded in a cartilaginous matrix. Compare with Figure 5-2.

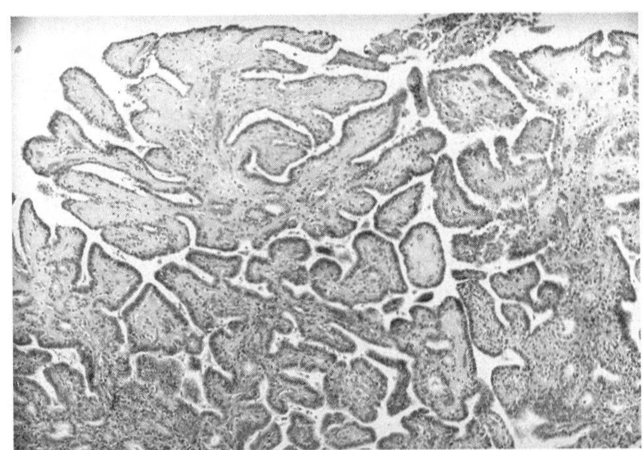

FIGURE 5-7
Papillary adenocarcinoma of the thyroid. The tumor exhibits numerous fronds lined by malignant epithelial cells.

rial can be expressed from the ducts. Certain visible secretions of the tumor cells lend their characteristics to the classification—for example, production of mucin or serous fluid. A further designation describes the gross appearance of a cystic mass. From all these considerations we derive such common terms as *papillary serous cystadenocarcinoma* of the ovary, *comedocarcinoma* of the breast, *adenoid cystic carcinoma* of the salivary glands, *polypoid adenocarcinoma* of the stomach, and *medullary carcinoma* of the thyroid. Finally, tumors in which the histogenesis is poorly understood are often given an eponym—as in, for example, Hodgkin disease, Ewing sarcoma of bone, or Brenner tumor of the ovary.

HISTOLOGICAL DIAGNOSIS OF MALIGNANCY

The distinction between benign and malignant tumors is, from a practical point of view, the most important diagnostic challenge faced by the pathologist. In most cases, the differentiation poses few problems, whereas in a few, careful study is required before an accurate diagnosis is secure. However, there remain tumors that defy the diagnostic skills and experience of any pathologist; in these cases, the correct diagnosis must await the clinical outcome. In effect, the criteria used to assess the true biological nature of any tumor are based not on scientific principles but rather on a historical correlation of histological and cytological patterns with clinical outcomes. Although general criteria for malignancy are recognized, they must be used with caution in specific cases. For instance, a reactive proliferation of connective cells termed *nodular fasciitis* (Fig. 5-9) has a more alarming histological appearance than many fibrosarcomas, and misdiagnosis can lead to unnecessary surgery. Conversely, many well-differentiated endocrine adenocarcinomas are histologically indistinguishable from benign adenomas.

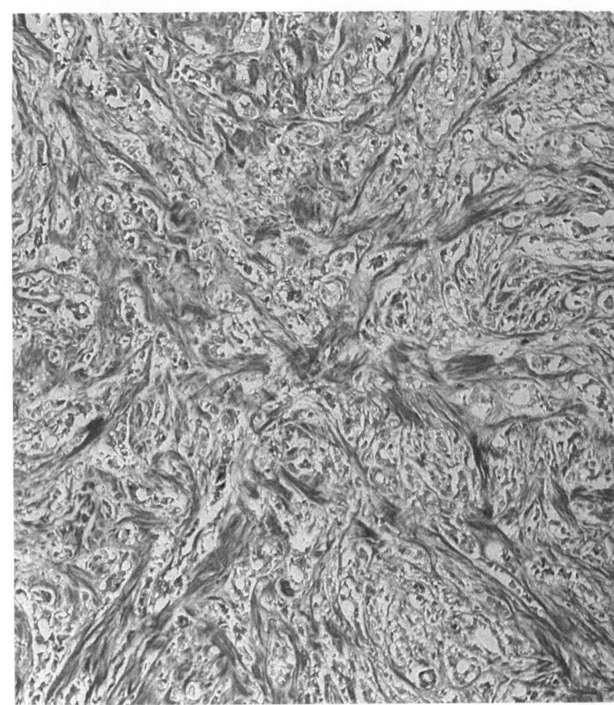

FIGURE 5-8
Scirrhous adenocarcinoma of the breast. A trichrome stain shows nests of cancer cells *(red)* embedded in a dense fibrous stroma *(blue)*.

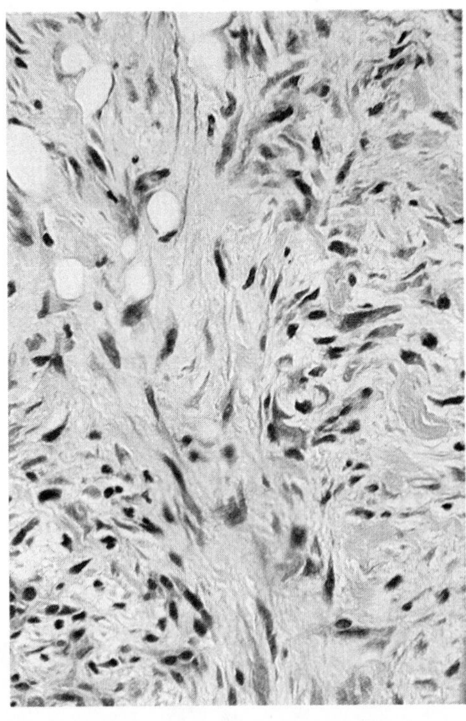

FIGURE 5-9
Nodular fasciitis. This cellular reactive lesion contains atypical and bizarre fibroblasts, which may be mistaken for a fibrosarcoma.

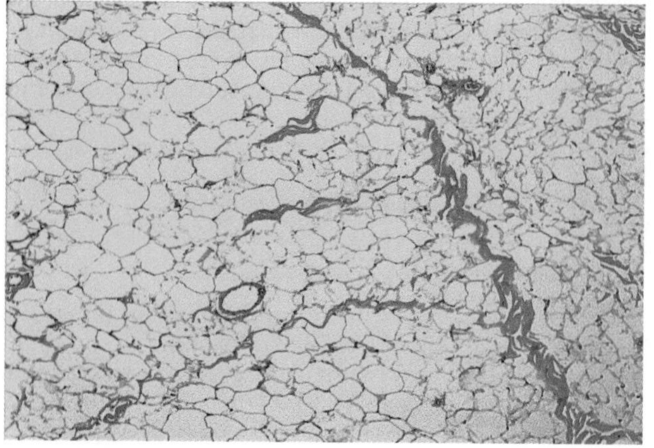

FIGURE 5-10
Lipoma. This subcutaneous, nodular tumor of adipocytes is grossly and microscopically indistinguishable from normal fat.

Benign Tumors

Benign tumors in general resemble their parent tissues, both histologically and cytologically. For example, lipomas, despite their often lobulated gross appearance, seem to be composed of normal adipocytes (Fig. 5-10). Fibromas are composed of mature fibroblasts and a collagenous stroma. Chondromas exhibit chondrocytes dispersed in a cartilaginous matrix. Thyroid adenomas form acini and produce thyroglobulin. The gross structure of a benign tumor may depart from the normal and assume papillary or polypoid configurations, as in papillomas of the bladder and skin and adenomatous polyps of the colon. **However, the lining epithelium of a benign tumor resembles that of the normal tissue.** Although many benign tumors are circumscribed by a connective tissue capsule, many equally benign neoplasms are not encapsulated. Unencapsulated benign tumors include papillomas and polyps of the visceral organs, hepatic adenomas, many endocrine adenomas, and hemangiomas. **It bears repetition that the definition of a benign tumor resides above all in an inability to invade adjacent tissue and to metastasize.**

Malignant Tumors

Malignant tumors depart from the parent tissue morphologically and functionally, although an accurate diagnosis of their origin depends not only on the location but also on a histological and cytological resemblance to a normal tissue. Some of the histological features that favor malignancy include the following:

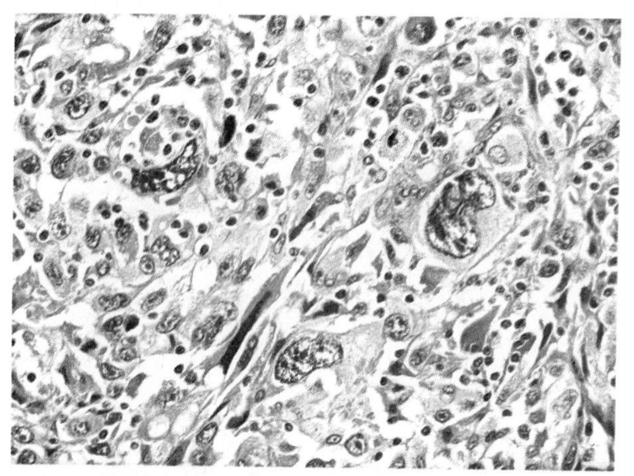

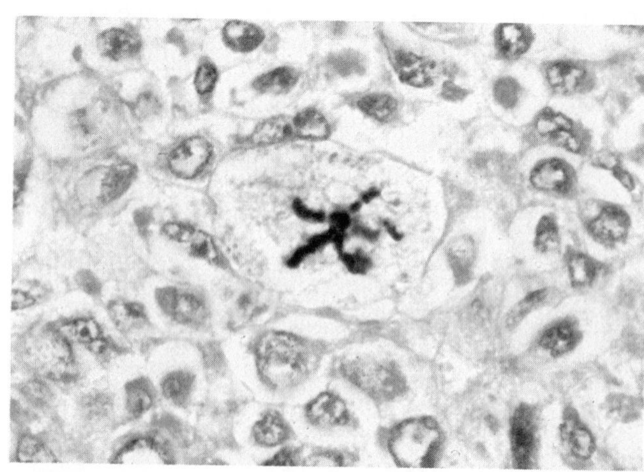

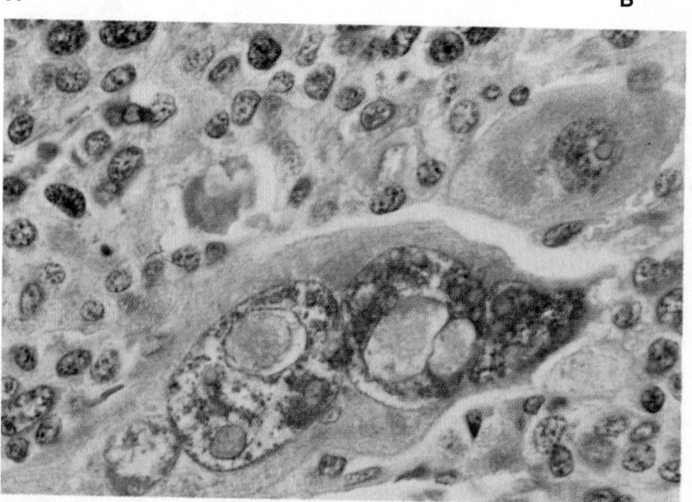

FIGURE 5-11
Anaplastic features of malignant tumors. (*A*) The cells of this anaplastic carcinoma are highly pleomorphic (i.e., they vary in size and shape). The nuclei are hyperchromatic and are large relative to the cytoplasm. (*B*) A malignant cell in metaphase exhibits an abnormal mitotic figure. (*C*) Multinucleated tumor giant cell.

- **Anaplasia or cellular atypia:** These terms refer to the lack of differentiated features in a cancer cell. In general, the degree of anaplasia correlates with the aggressiveness of the tumor. Cytological evidence of anaplasia includes (1) variation in the size and shape of cells and cell nuclei (**pleomorphism**), (2) enlarged and hyperchromatic nuclei with coarsely clumped chromatin and prominent nucleoli, (3) atypical mitoses, and (4) bizarre cells, including tumor giant cells (Fig. 5-11).
- **Mitotic activity:** Abundant mitoses are characteristic of many malignant tumors but are not a necessary criterion. However, in some cases (e.g., leiomyosarcomas), the diagnosis of malignancy is based on the finding of even a few mitoses.
- **Invasion:** Malignancy is proved by the demonstration of invasion, particularly of blood vessels and lymphatics. In some circumstances, such as squamous carcinoma of the cervix or carcinoma arising in an adenomatous polyp, the diagnosis of malignant transformation is made on the basis of local invasion.
- **Metastases:** It is intuitively obvious that the presence of metastases identifies a tumor as malignant, but occasionally it reveals the true character of a tumor previously considered benign. In metastatic disease that was not preceded by a clinically diagnosed primary tumor, the site of origin is often not readily apparent from the morphological characteristics of the tumor. In such cases, electron microscopic examination and the demonstration of a specific tumor marker may establish the correct diagnosis.

Electron Microscopy of Tumors

The study of the ultrastructure of malignant tumors has failed to enhance our understanding of the pathogenesis of cancer. It is clear that in general the organization of the cytoplasm becomes simpler with increasing anaplasia. Thus, anaplastic tumors from highly differentiated tissues often do not show the rich cytoplasmic complexity of the parent tissue, in terms of organelles and specialized cytoplasmic components. **However, there are no specific determinants of malignancy or even of neoplasia itself that can be detected by electron microscopy.** On the other hand, electron microscopy has proved of significant value in the diagnosis of poorly differentiated cancers, whose classification is problematic by routine light microscopy. For example, it is often difficult to decide by light microscopy whether a poorly differentiated tumor is a carcinoma, a sarcoma, or a lymphoma. However, by electron microscopy, carcinomas often exhibit desmosomes and specialized junctional complexes, structures that are not typical of mesenchymal tumors and are absent in lymphomas.

Characteristically, the microvilli of carcinomas are short and blunt and are associated with a terminal web, whereas those of mesotheliomas are long and slender. By contrast, the microvilli of lymphoid and mesenchymal tumors do not show a terminal web. Cells of ectodermal origin often have many cilia, as opposed to the solitary cilia occasionally found in other cell types. The presence of bundles of tonofilaments is highly suggestive of an epithelial tumor, whereas slender microfilaments are more common in mesenchymal tumors. A metastatic tumor can often be correctly identified by visualizing cytoplasmic granules and identifying their nature. For example, the presence of melanosomes signifies a melanoma, whereas small, membrane-bound granules with a dense core are features of endocrine neoplasms (Fig. 5-12). Another example of a diagnostically useful granule is the characteristic crystal-containing granule of an insulinoma derived from the pancreatic islets.

Tumor Markers

Tumor markers are products of malignant neoplasms that can be detected in the cells themselves or in body fluids. The ultimate tumor marker would be one that allows the unequivocal distinction between benign and malignant cells, but unfortunately no such marker is in sight. Nevertheless, markers do exist that are often useful in identifying the cell of origin of a metastatic or poorly differentiated primary tumor. Metastatic tumors may be so undifferentiated microscopically as to preclude even the distinction between an epithelial and a mesenchymal origin. Tumor markers rely on the preservation of characteristics of the progenitor cell or the synthesis of specialized proteins by the neoplastic cell to make this distinction. The determination of the cell lineage of undifferentiated tumors is more than an academic exercise, because thera-

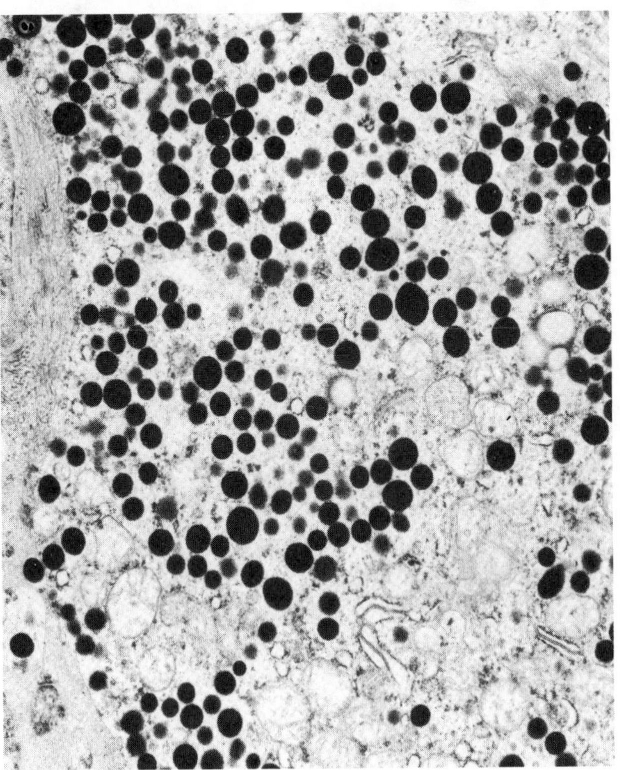

FIGURE *5-12*
Electron micrograph of a metastatic cancer of the adrenal medulla (pheochromocytoma). The neuroendocrine origin of this poorly differentiated tumor was identified by the presence of characteristic cytoplasmic secretory granules.

peutic decisions may be based on the appropriate identification. For instance, the treatment of carcinomas usually involves surgery, whereas malignant lymphomas are treated with radiation therapy and chemotherapy. Among these diagnostically useful markers are such diverse products as immunoglobulins, fetal proteins, enzymes, hormones, and cytoskeletal and junctional proteins.

Carcinomas uniformly express cytokeratins, which are intermediate filaments belonging to a multigene family of proteins. Insoluble proteins of desmosomal junctions, termed desmoplakins, are frequently associated with cytokeratins and are also markers for epithelial differentiation.

Lineage-associated markers are often useful in establishing the origin of a poorly differentiated carcinoma. For example, prostatic carcinomas consistently express a glycoprotein named prostate-specific antigen (PSA) and are also positive for prostate-specific acid phosphatase (PSAP). By contrast, colon cancers are consistently negative for these markers, but most of them express carcinoembryonic antigen (CEA). Some thyroid carcinomas demonstrate thyroglobulin, and breast cancers frequently show nuclear receptors for estrogen and progesterone. Expression of the sialated form of the Lewis a antigen (CA 19-9) has been associated with pancreatic and gastrointestinal cancers, whereas CA 125 is a sensitive marker for ovarian cancers.

Neuroendocrine tumors share the positivity for cytokeratins with other carcinomas. However, they can be identified by their content of chromogranins, a family of proteins found in neurosecretory granules. Neuron-specific enolase is another, albeit less specific, marker for neuroendocrine cells. Other markers for neuroendocrine differentiation are synaptophysin and Leu-7 (CD57). Specific antibodies exist for a number of peptide hormones, such as gastrin, bombesin, corticotropic hormone (ACTH), insulin, glucagon, somatostatin, and serotonin.

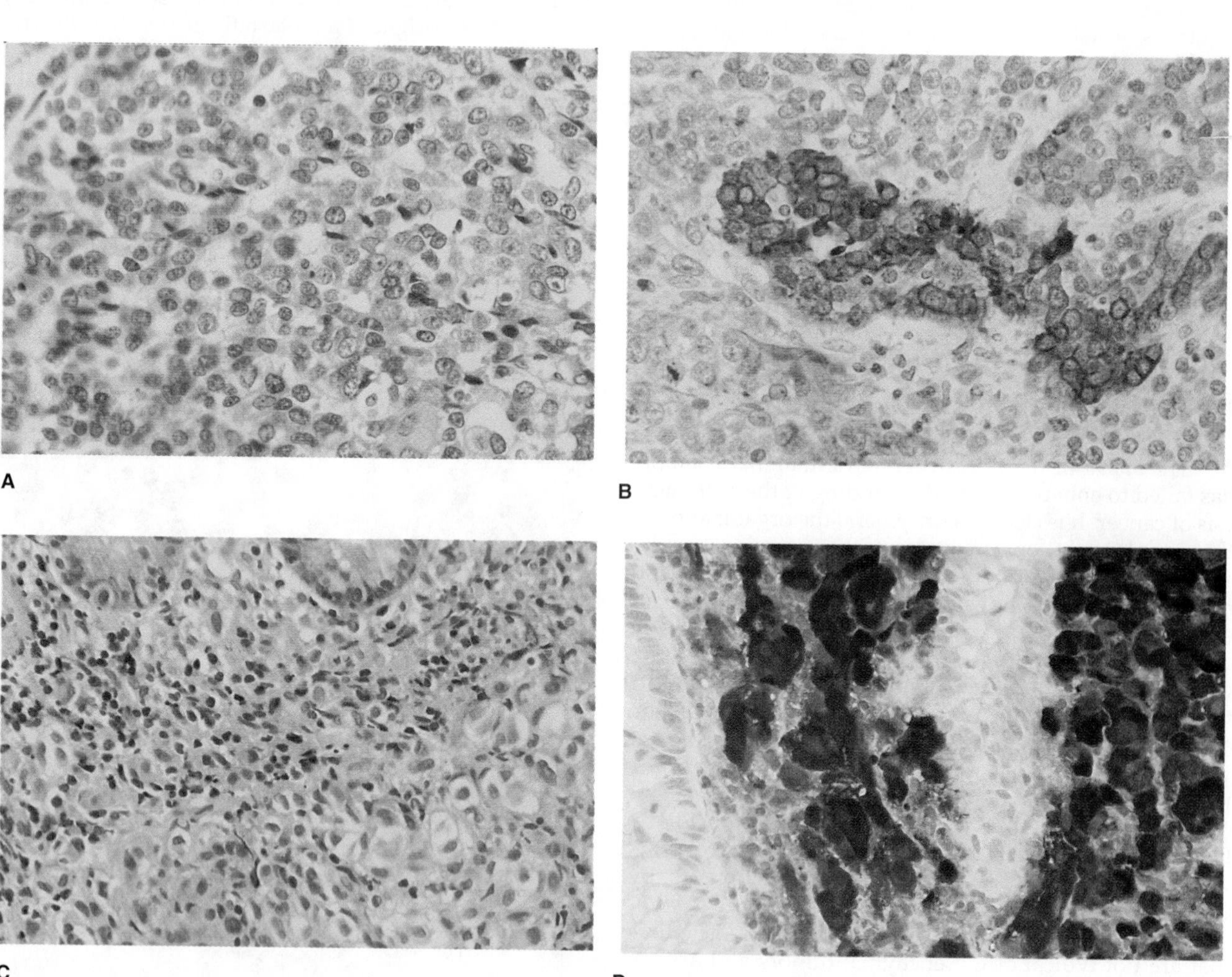

FIGURE *5-13*
Tumor markers in the identification of undifferentiated neoplasms. (*A*) A poorly differentiated metastatic bladder cancer is difficult to identify as a carcinoma with the hematoxylin and eosin stain. (*B*) A section of the tumor depicted in *A* is positive for cytokeratin with an immunoperoxidase stain and is identified as carcinoma. (*C*) A metastasis to the colon of an undifferentiated malignant melanoma is not pigmented, and its origin is unclear. (*D*) An immunoperoxidase stain of the tumor shown in *C* reveals numerous cells positive for S-100 protein, a commonly used marker for cells of melanocytic origin.

TABLE 5-1 Frequently Used Markers to Identify Tumors

Marker	Target Cell
Epithelial Cells	
Cytokeratins	Carcinomas, mesothelioma
CK7	Many adenocarcinomas
CK20	Gastrointestinal carcinomas, Merkel cell tumor
Epithelial membrane antigen (EMA)	Carcinomas, some large cell lymphomas
Mesothelial Cells	
Cytokeratins	Mesothelioma
Vimentin	Mesothelioma
Ber-Ep4	Most carcinomas, but not in mesothelioma
HBME	Mesothelioma and some carcinomas
B72.3 (tumor-associated)	Many adenocarcinomas, but not in mesothelioma
CEA	Many adenocarcinomas, but not in mesothelioma
CD15	Many adenocarcinomas, but not in mesothelioma
Melanocytes	
HMB-45	Malignant melanoma
S-100 protein	Malignant melanoma
Neuroendocrine and Neural Cells	
Chromogranins	Neuroendocrine carcinoma, carcinoid tumor
Synaptophysin	Neuroendocrine carcinoma, carcinoid tumor
Neuron-specific enolase	Neuroendocrine carcinoma, carcinoid tumor, and ganglion cells
CD57	Neuroendocrine carcinoma
Neurofilament proteins	Neuroblastoma
Glial Cells	
Glial fibrillary acidic protein (GFAP)	Astrocytoma and other glial tumors
Mesenchymal Cells	
Vimentin	Most sarcomas
Desmin	Muscle tumors (myosarcomas)
Muscle-specific actin	Muscle tumors (myocsarcomas)
CD99	Ewing sarcoma, peripheral neuroectodermal tumors (PNET)
Specific Organs	
Prostate-specific antigen (PSA)	Prostatic cancer
Prostate-specific alkaline phosphatase (PSAP)	Prostatic cancer
Thyroglobulin	Thyroid cancer
α-Fetoprotein (AFP)	Hepatocellular carcinomas, yolk sac tumor
Carcinoembryonic antigen (CEA)	Gastrointestinal cancers
Placental alkaline phosphatase (PLAP)	Seminoma
Human chorionic gonadotropin (hCG)	Trophoblastic tumors
CA19.9	Pancreatic and gastrointestinal carcinomas
CA125	Ovarian carcinoma
CD-Markers	
CD1	Thymocytes, dendritic cells, some T-cell leukemias
CD2	T cells, T-cell malignancies
CD3	T cells, T-cell malignancies
CD4	T-helper cells, T-cell malignancies
CD5	T cells, B-cell chronic lymphocytic leukemia
CD8	Cytotoxic/suppressor T cells
CD10 (common ALL antigen, CALLA)	Some acute lymphocytic leukemias
CD13	Myeloid leukemias
CD19	B cells, B-cell malignancies
CD20	B cells, B-cell malignancies
CD30	Large cell lymphomas, Hodgkin disease
CD33	Myeloid leukemias
CD34	Leukemias
CD45 (leucocyte common antigen)	Leukemias and lymphomas
Immunoglobulins	
κ-Light chain	B-cell malignancies
λ-Light chain	B-cell malignancies
Endothelial Markers	
von Willebrand Factor (vWF)	Vascular neoplasms
CD31	Vascular neoplasms
CD34	Vascular neoplasms
Lectins	Vascular neoplasms

Malignant melanomas may be unpigmented and appear similar to other poorly differentiated carcinomas. They can be distinguished by immunohistochemical studies (Fig. 5-13). Melanomas express vimentin, melanoma-associated antigen, and S-100 protein, but unlike most carcinomas, they are not positive for cytokeratins.

Soft tissue sarcomas express the intermediate filament vimentin. Since this marker is also present in numerous nonmesenchymal tumors, its expression is meaningful only in concert with other markers and morphological criteria. Desmin, another useful intermediate filament, is present in all benign and malignant neoplasms originating from either smooth or striated muscle fibers. Muscle-specific actin is another marker for muscle tissue with comparable sensitivity and specificity. Neurofilament proteins are excellent markers for tumors originating from neurons, including neuroblastomas and ganglioneuroma. Neuron-specific enolase also shows a strong association with neurogenic tissue and is found in almost all neuroblastomas. Glial fibrillary acidic protein (GFAP), the first intermediate filament discovered, is strongly expressed on astrocytes and in most glial cell neoplasms.

Malignant lymphomas are generally positive for leukocyte common antigen (LCA, CD45). Markers for lymphomas and leukemias are grouped by so-called cluster designations (CD), at present numbering about 130. Markers for CD antigens help to discriminate between T and B lymphocytes, monocytes, and granulocytes and the mature and immature variants of these cells. B-cell malignancies, including plasmacytomas, manifest immunoglobulin light-chain restriction. A single B cell expresses κ- or λ-light chains. The presence of both κ- and λ-positive B cells argues against malignancy, whereas the demonstration of only one type of light chain on the lymphocytes strongly suggests a monoclonal B-cell lymphoma.

Vascular tumors derived from endothelial cells, including hemangiomas and hemangiosarcomas, are identified by antibodies against factor VIII–related antigen or by the binding of certain lectins.

Proliferating cells display Ki-67 and the proliferating cell nuclear antigen (PCNA). Although the presence of proliferating cells alone does not establish a diagnosis of malignancy, the presence of cycling cells at sites in which cell growth is normally absent frequently suggests a cancer.

Serum tumor markers are not disease-specific but allow for the monitoring of tumor recurrence after surgery. For example, high serum levels of CEA are associated with carcinomas of the gastrointestinal tract and the breast. Increased serum α-fetoprotein (AFP) suggests liver cancer or a yolk sac tumor. Human chorionic gonadotropin (hCG) is used for monitoring the recurrence of malignant trophoblastic tumors. Elevated CA 19-9 serum titers are found in patients with pancreatic or gastrointestinal cancers, and high CA 125 levels are associated with ovarian carcinomas. Increased serum levels of PSA accompany prostatic cancers. Elevated titers of human placental alkaline phosphatase (HPAP) occur with seminomas.

Table 5-1 lists many of the commonly used tumor markers.

INVASION AND METASTASIS

The two properties that are unique to cancer cells are the ability to invade locally and the capacity to metastasize to distant sites. It is these characteristics that are responsible for the vast majority of deaths from cancer; the primary tumor itself is generally amenable to surgical extirpation.

Direct Extension

Most carcinomas begin as localized growths confined to the epithelium in which they arise. As long as these early cancers do not penetrate the basement membrane on which the epithelium rests, such tumors are termed carcinoma *in situ* (Fig. 5-14). In this stage, it is unfortunate that they are asymptomatic, because they are invariably curable. When the *in situ* tumor acquires invasive potential and extends directly through the underlying basement membrane, it is in a position to compromise neighboring tissues and to metastasize. In those situations in which cancer arises from cells that are not confined by a basement membrane, such as connective tissue cells, lymphoid elements, and hepatocytes, an *in situ* stage is not defined.

Malignant tumors characteristically grow within the tissue of origin, where they enlarge and infiltrate normal structures. They may also extend directly beyond the confines of that organ to involve adjacent tissues. In some cases, the growth of the cancer may be so extensive that

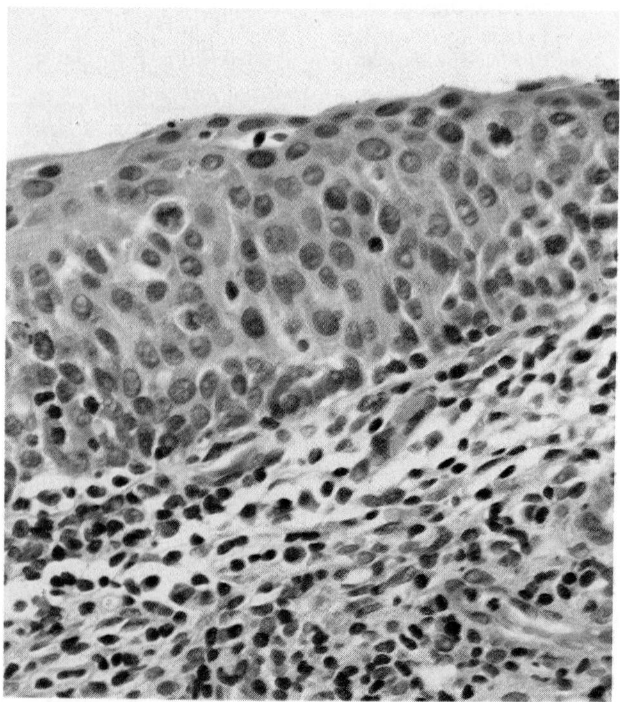

FIGURE *5-14*
Carcinoma *in situ*. A section of the uterine cervix shows neoplastic squamous cells occupying the full thickness of the epithelium and confined to the mucosa by the underlying basement membrane.

replacement of the normal tissue results in functional insufficiency of the organ. Such a situation is not uncommon in primary cancer of the liver. Tumors of the brain, such as astrocytomas, infiltrate the brain until they compromise vital regions. The direct extension of malignant tumors within an organ may also be life-threatening because of their location. A common example is the intestinal obstruction produced by cancer of the colon (Fig. 5-15).

The invasive growth pattern of malignant tumors often leads to their direct extension outside the tissue of origin, in which case the tumor may secondarily impair the function of an adjacent organ. Squamous carcinoma of the cervix often grows beyond the genital tract to produce vesicovaginal fistulas and obstruction of the ureters. Neglected cases of breast cancer are often complicated by extensive ulceration of the skin. Even small tumors can produce severe consequences when they invade vital structures. A small cancer of the lung can cause a bronchopleural fistula when it penetrates the bronchus, or exsanguinating hemorrhage when it erodes a blood vessel. The agonizing pain of pancreatic carcinoma results from direct extension of the tumor to the celiac nerve plexus. Tumor cells that reach serous cavities (e.g., those of the peritoneum or pleura) spread easily by direct extension or can be carried by the fluid to new locations on the serous membranes. The most common example is the seeding of the peritoneal cavity by certain types of ovarian cancer (Fig. 5-16). Although malignant brain tumors do not customarily metastasize extracranially, cells that reach the cerebrospinal fluid may be transported to other sites within the central nervous system.

Metastatic Spread

Metastasis refers to the transfer of malignant cells from one site to another not directly connected with it. The invasive properties of malignant tumors bring them into contact with

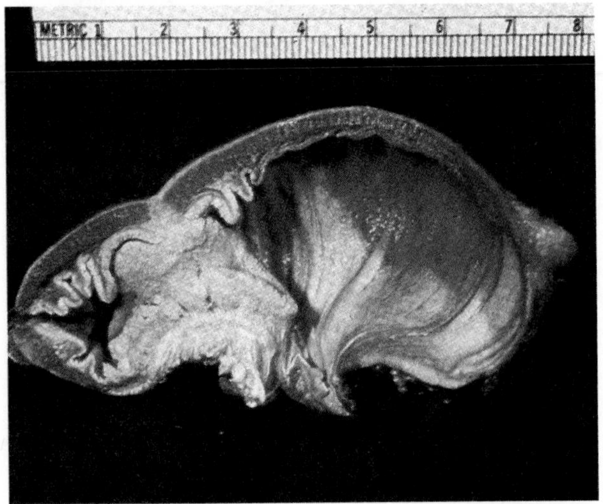

FIGURE *5-15*
Adenocarcinoma of the colon with intestinal obstruction. The lumen of the colon at the site of the cancer is narrow. The colon above the obstruction is dilated.

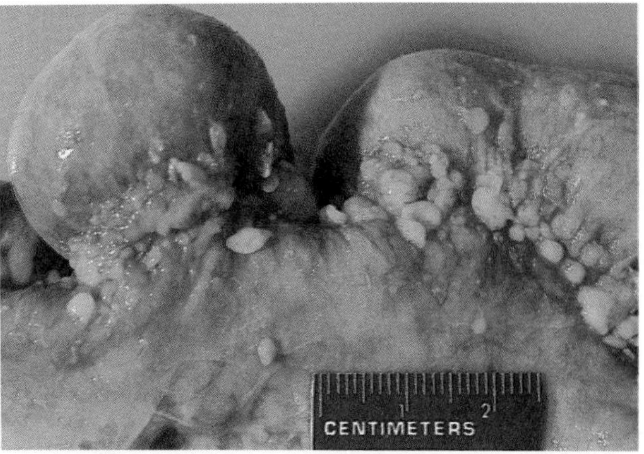

FIGURE *5-16*
Peritoneal carcinomatosis. The mesentery attached to a loop of small bowel is studded with small nodules of metastatic ovarian carcinoma.

blood and lymphatic vessels. **In the same way that they can invade parenchymal tissue, neoplastic cells can also penetrate vascular and lymphatic channels, through which they are disseminated to distant sites.** In general, metastases resemble the primary tumor histologically, although they are occasionally so anaplastic that their cell of origin is obscure.

Hematogenous Metastases

Cancer cells commonly invade capillaries and venules, whereas the thicker-walled arterioles and arteries are relatively resistant. The appearance of malignant cells in the blood should not be construed as synonymous with metastasis, because most of these cells are destroyed in the circulation. Nevertheless, it is likely that the probability of viable metastases correlates directly with the number of malignant cells released into the circulation. Before they can form viable metastases, circulating tumor cells must lodge in the vascular bed of the metastatic site (Fig. 5-17). Here they presumably attach to the walls of blood vessels, either to endothelial cells or to naked basement membranes, although the mechanisms remain a matter of study. For many but not all tumors, this sequence of events explains why the liver and the lung are so frequently the sites of metastases. Because abdominal tumors seed the portal system, they lead to hepatic metastases, whereas other tumors penetrate systemic veins that eventually drain into the vena cava and hence to the lungs. In this respect, it should be noted that some tumor cells released into the venous system survive passage through the microcirculation and are thus transported to more distant organs. For instance, tumor cells may traverse the liver and produce pulmonary metastases, and neoplastic cells may also survive passage through the pulmonary microcirculation to reach the brain, bones (Fig. 5-18), and other organs through arterial dissemination. Neoplastic cells arrested in the microcirculation are believed to penetrate the vessel walls at the site of metastasis using the same mechanisms by which the primary tumor invades.

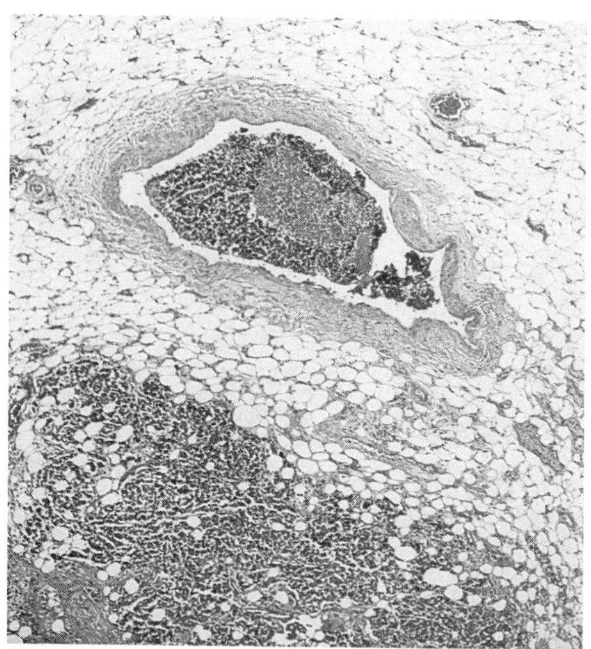

FIGURE 5-17
Hematogenous spread of cancer. A malignant tumor (*bottom*) has invaded adipose tissue and penetrated into a small vein.

Lymphatic Metastases

An historical dogma of metastatic spread held that epithelial tumors (carcinomas) preferentially metastasize through lymphatic channels, whereas mesenchymal neoplasms (sarcomas) are distributed hematogenously. This distinction is no longer considered valid, because of clinical observations of metastatic patterns and the demonstration of numerous connections between the lymphatic and vascular systems. Tumors arising in tissues that have a rich lymphatic network (e.g., the breast) often metastasize by this route, although the particular properties of specific neoplasms may play a role in the route of spread.

Basement membranes envelop only the large lymphatic channels; they are lacking in the lymphatic capillaries. Thus, there is reason to believe that invasive tumor cells may penetrate lymphatic channels more readily than blood vessels. Once in the lymphatic vessels, the cells are carried to the regional draining lymph nodes, where they initially lodge in the marginal sinus and then extend throughout the node. Lymph nodes bearing metastatic deposits may be enlarged to many times their normal size, often exceeding the diameter of the primary lesion. The cut surface of the lymph node usually resembles that of the primary tumor in color and consistency and may also exhibit the necrosis and hemorrhage commonly seen in primary cancers (Fig. 5-19).

The regional lymphatic pattern of metastatic spread is most prominently exemplified by cancer of the breast. In breast cancer, the initial metastases are almost always lymphatic, and these regional lymphatic metastases have considerable prognostic significance. Cancers that arise in the lateral aspect of the breast characteristically spread to the lymph nodes of the axilla, whereas those arising in the medial portion drain to the internal mammary lymph nodes in the thorax.

Lymphatic metastases are occasionally found in lymph nodes distant from the site of the primary tumor; these are termed skip metastases. For example, abdominal cancers may initially be signaled by the appearance of an enlarged supraclavicular node, the so-called "sentinel node." A graphic example of the relationship of lymphatic anatomy to the spread of malignant tumors is afforded by cancers of the testis. Rather than metastasizing to the regional nodes, as do other tumors of the male external genitalia, testicular cancers typically involve the draining abdominal periaortic nodes. The explanation lies in the descent of the testis from an intra-abdominal site to

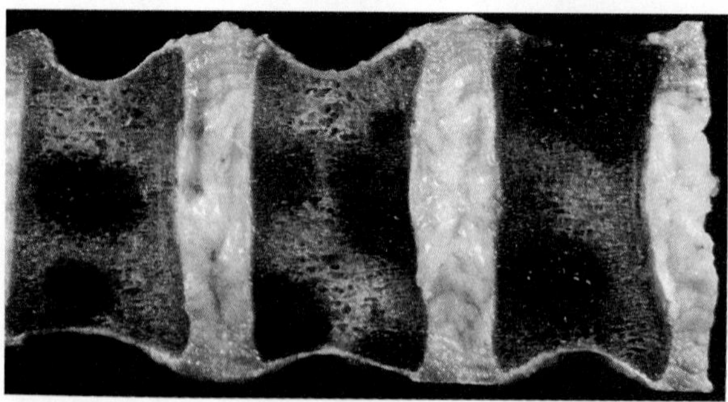

FIGURE 5-18
Multiple pigmented metastases in the vertebral bodies in a patient who died of malignant melanoma.

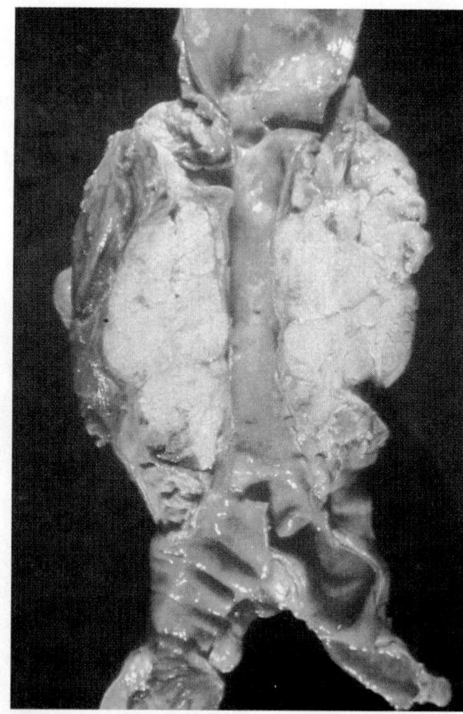

FIGURE 5-19
Metastatic carcinoma in periaortic lymph nodes. The aorta has been opened and the nodes bisected.

the scrotum, during which it is accompanied by its own lymphatic supply.

Lymph nodes that drain a tumor may be enlarged not only by the presence of metastases but also by reactive hyperplasia, which is presumably a response to the released antigens from viable or necrotic tumor cells and the phagocytosis of cell debris. Thus, the clinical presence of an enlarged lymph node is not necessarily synonymous with a metastasis. Conversely, the absence of tumor cells in a resected lymph node does not guarantee that there is no underlying cancer.

Biology of Invasion and Metastasis

A number of steps are required for malignant cells to establish a metastasis (Fig. 5-20):

1. Invasion of the basement membrane underlying the tumor
2. Movement through the extracellular matrix
3. Penetration of vascular or lymphatic channels
4. Survival and arrest within the circulating blood or lymph
5. Exit from the circulation into a new tissue site
6. Survival and growth as a metastasis, a process that involves angiogenesis

Most cancers originate from the malignant transformation of a single cell (monoclonal origin of tumors). Nevertheless, the inherent genetic instability of the malignant phenotype leads to the appearance of subpopulations with diverse biological characteristics and profound variations in their metastatic potential (**tumor heterogeneity**). An important demonstration of tumor heterogeneity has come from experiments in which a variety of tumors were cloned *in vitro*, after which each clone was individually injected into a host animal. If the tumor cells were originally homogeneous, then a comparable number of metastases would be expected in each animal. In fact, the clones displayed widely varying metastatic activity. The demonstration of tumor heterogeneity has led to the concept that at each step of the metastatic cascade, only the fittest cells survive. Thus, the metastatic process can be viewed as a competition in which a subpopulation of cells within the primary cancer ultimately prevails as a metastasis. The notion of tumor heterogeneity extends beyond metastatic potential to include the expression of hormone receptors and, of great importance, sensitivity to chemotherapeutic agents.

Invasion

Inherent in the definition of a malignant cell is the capacity to invade the surrounding tissue. In epithelial tumors, invasion requires disruption of and penetration through the underlying basement membrane and passage through the extracellular matrix. Similarly, circulating cells destined to establish metastases must reproduce these same events in order to exit from the vascular or lymphatic compartment and establish residence in the distant extracellular matrix site.

Adhesion Molecules

The entire metastatic sequence, from the initial binding of the tumor cell to the underlying extracellular matrix to the growth in a distant location, depends on the expression of numerous adhesion molecules by the malignant cells. The display of such surface molecules varies with (1) the type of tumor, (2) the individual clone (tumor heterogeneity), and (3) the stage of the metastatic process.

INTEGRINS: Integrins comprise a family of transmembrane receptors that mediate the adhesive interactions between cells themselves and between cells and the extracellular matrix. The binding of integrins to their substrates also stimulates intracellular signaling and gene expression that play a role in cell migration, proliferation, differentiation, and survival. In addition, the expression of integrins affects the cell surface localization of metalloproteinases and promotes angiogenesis.

Much has been learned about the role of integrins and other adhesion molecules in invasion and metastasis by studying excised human melanoma cells, which exhibit considerable phenotypic heterogeneity with respect to their metastatic potential. In general, a clear correlation exists between the metastatic capacity of different malignant clones and the expression of integrins on the cell surface. Transfection of an integrin gene into integrin-deficient, nontumorigenic cancer cells confers a metastatic potential.

IMMUNOGLOBULIN SUPERGENE FAMILY: A number of intercellular adhesion molecules belong to this superfamily, including intercellular adhesion molecule-1 (ICAM-1), MUC18, vascular cell adhesion molecule-1 (VCAM-1), and CD44. The expression of ICAM-1, MUC18, and CD44 correlates positively with the aggressiveness of a variety of tumor cell types. By contrast, VCAM-1, which promotes the interaction of cancer cells with endothelium, is downregulated in highly metastatic clones. Presumably, the loss of adhesive properties caused by decreased expression of VCAM-1 allows detachment of individual tumor cells from the parent tumor.

CADHERINS AND CATENINS: Cadherins are a family of cell–cell adhesion molecules, which are Ca^{2+}-dependent, transmembrane glycoproteins. The best-characterized of the cadherins, E-cadherin, is expressed on the surface of all epithelia and mediates cell–cell adhesion by mutual zipper interactions. Catenins (α, β, and ξ) are proteins that interact with the intracellular domain of E-cadherin and create a mechanical linkage between the latter and the cytoskeleton, which is essential for effective epithelial cell interactions. Overall, cadherins and catenins suppress invasion and metastasis. The expression of both E-cadherin and catenins is reduced or lost in most carcinomas, an effect that permits individual malignant cells to leave the main tumor mass and thereby metastasize. Interestingly, β-catenin also binds to the adenomatous polyposis coli (APC) gene product, an effect that is independent of its interaction with E-cadherin and α-catenin. Mutations in either the APC or β-catenin gene are implicated in the development of colon cancer (see later and Chapter 13).

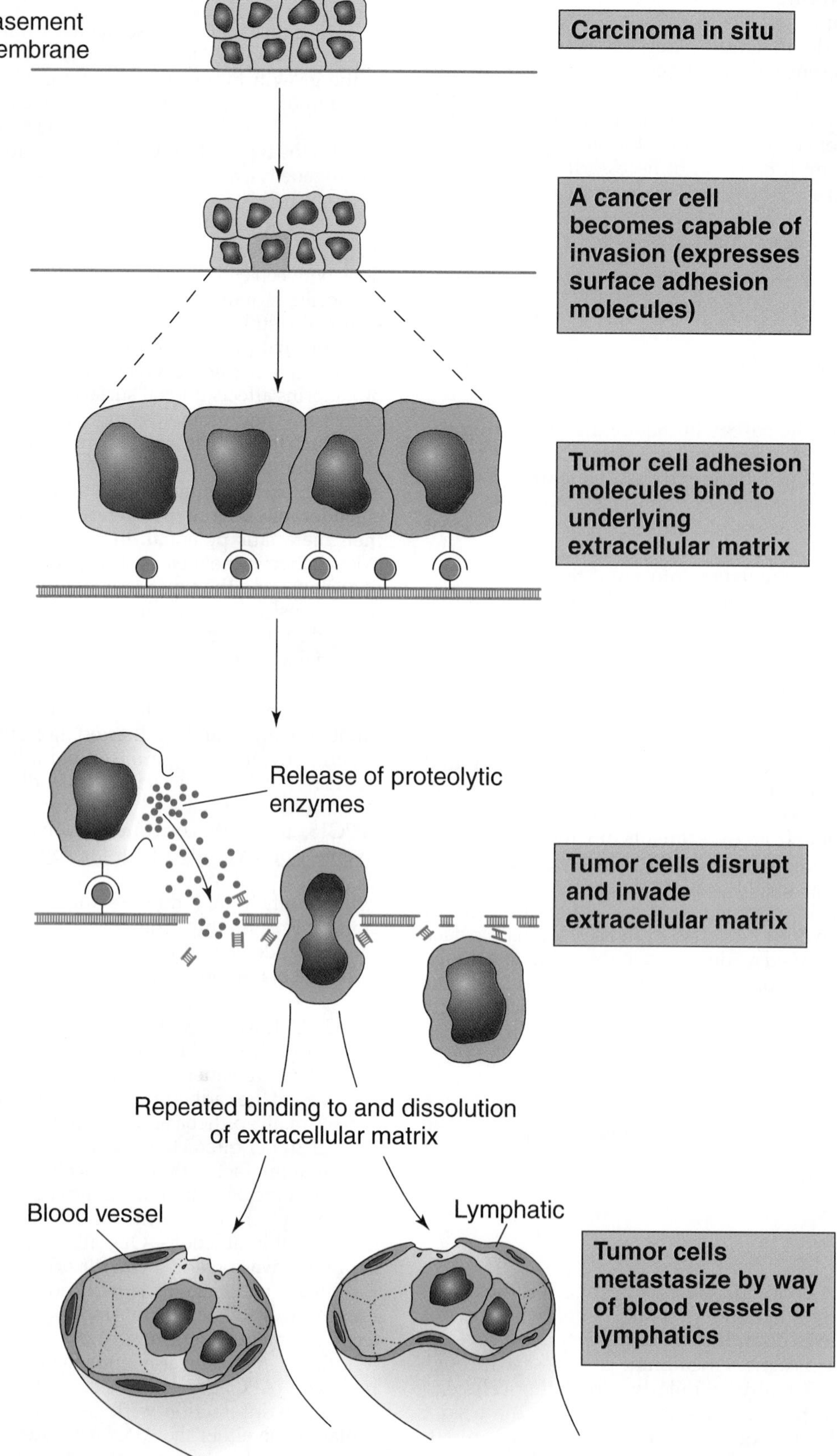
Basement membrane
Carcinoma in situ
A cancer cell becomes capable of invasion (expresses surface adhesion molecules)
Tumor cell adhesion molecules bind to underlying extracellular matrix
Release of proteolytic enzymes
Tumor cells disrupt and invade extracellular matrix
Repeated binding to and dissolution of extracellular matrix
Blood vessel
Lymphatic
Tumor cells metastasize by way of blood vessels or lymphatics

FIGURE 5-20

Autocrine Motility Factor

Autocrine motility factor (AMF) belongs to a family of tumor cell cytokines that stimulate motility via a receptor-mediated signaling pathway. AMF not only regulates motility but also modulates the expression of cell surface integrins. The expression of the AMF receptor (gp78) in normal cells is regulated by cell contact, whereas in many cancer cells it is constitutively expressed. Binding of AMF (which has been identified as a phosphohexose isomerase) to gp78 initiates a signal transduction pathway involving 12-lipoxygenase and protein kinase C, resulting in enhanced tumor cell adhesion to the matrix, lysosomal enzyme release, and cell migration.

Proteolytic Enzymes

The breach of the basement membrane separating epithelia from the mesenchymal compartment is the first event in tumor cell invasion. The basement membrane is composed of a number of extracellular matrix components, including type IV collagen, laminin, and proteoglycans (see Chapter 3). Malignant cells and stromal cells associated with cancers elaborate a variety of proteases that degrade one or more of the basement membrane components. Such enzymes include the urokinase-type plasminogen activator (u-PA) and matrix metalloproteinases (MMP) of the collagenase family.

Plasmin is a serine protease that degrades laminin and activates type IV procollagenase. Experimentally, antibodies to u-PA attenuate the metastatic capacity of cancer cells, whereas overexpression of the enzyme by these cells enhances their ability to metastasize. The activity of u-PA is balanced by its inhibitor PAI (plasminogen activator inhibitor), and changes in this activity have also been reported in some cancers.

The MMPs comprise a family of zinc-dependent endopeptidases, which are susceptible to tissue inhibitors of metalloproteinases (TIMPs). To date, four types of MMPs are recognized, namely interstitial collagenases, stromelysins, gelatinases, and membrane-type MMPs. Three distinct TIMPs have also been identified. The MMPs are synthesized and secreted by normal cells under conditions associated with physiological tissue remodeling, such as wound healing and placental implantation. Under these circumstances, a balance between MMPs and TIMPs is strictly regulated. By contrast, the invasive and metastatic phenotypes of cancer cells are characterized by a dysregulation of this balance.

A direct correlation between increased expression of MMPs and augmented invasive capacity or metastatic potential of tumor cells has been observed in many cancers. In addition, many of these same tumors exhibit decreases in TIMP expression. MMPs are present in either the tumor cells or the surrounding stromal cells, or both, depending on the particular neoplasm. In some instances, MMPs secreted by stromal cells are bound to integrins on the surface of the tumor cells, thereby providing a particularly high local concentration of protease activity at the site of tumor invasion. Dysregulated MMP activity permits entry of cancer cells into and their passage through the extracellular matrix.

Metastasis

Following the invasion of surrounding tissue, malignant cells may spread to distant sites by a process that includes a number of steps:

1. **Invasion of the circulation**: After invading the interstitial tissue, malignant cells penetrate lymphatic or vascular channels. In the lymph nodes, communications between lymphatics and venous tributaries allow the cells access to the systemic circulation. The vast majority of tumor cells do not survive their journey in the bloodstream, and less than 0.1% remain to establish a new colony.
2. **Escape from the circulation**: Circulating tumor cells may arrest mechanically in capillaries and venules, where they attach to endothelial cells. This adherence causes the retraction of the endothelium, thereby exposing the underlying basement membrane to which the tumor cells now bind. Clumps of tumor cells may also arrest in arterioles, where they grow within the vascular lumen. In both situations, the tumor cells eventually extravasate by mechanisms similar to those responsible for local invasion.
3. **Local growth**: In a hospitable site, the extravasated cancer cells grow in response to autocrine and possibly local growth factors produced by the host tissue. However, a new vascular supply is necessary for the tumor to grow to a diameter greater than 0.5 mm. Thus, many tumors secrete polypeptides (e.g., platelet-derived growth factor [PDGF], fibroblast growth factor [FGF], and transforming growth factor-beta [TGF-β]) that stimulate the growth of new vessels in the host tissue, a process termed **angiogenesis** (see later). The newly established metastatic colony must also escape detection and destruction by the host immune defenses (see later). The metastasis can also metastasize, either within the same organ or to distant sites.

FIGURE *5-20*
Mechanisms of tumor invasion and metastasis. The mechanism by which a malignant tumor initially penetrates a confining basement membrane and then invades the surrounding extracellular environment involves several steps. The tumor first acquires the ability to bind components of the extracellular matrix. These interactions are mediated by the expression of a number of adhesion molecules. Proteolytic enzymes are then released from the tumor cells, and the extracellular matrix is degraded. After moving through the extracellular environment, the invading cancer penetrates blood vessels and lymphatics by the same mechanisms.

The establishment of a metastatic colony does not mean that it inevitably enlarges. It is well known clinically that tumors may recur locally or at metastatic sites many years after the primary cancer has been surgically removed. For example, patients treated for breast cancer or malignant melanoma may be apparently cured for 20 or more years, only to have the tumor suddenly recur. The mechanism of such tumor dormancy is not well understood. It has been proposed that cancer cells may lie dormant because of immunological suppression, a lack of host growth factors, or inadequate vascularity.

Target Organs in Metastatic Disease

It was recognized more than 100 years ago that the distribution of metastases in breast cancer is not due to chance. Rather, it was concluded that the spread of tumor cells (the seed) cannot be explained simply by anatomical considerations but requires the favorable environment of specific organs (the soil). By contrast, others have argued that metastatic spread depends solely on the blood flow to an organ. Today, there is evidence that both mechanisms operate, depending on the tumor. For example, cancers of the breast, prostate, and thyroid metastasize to bone, a tropism that suggests a favored soil. Conversely, despite their size and abundant blood flow, neither the spleen nor skeletal muscle is a common site of metastases. Yet for many cancers the vascular anatomy unquestionably influences the pattern of metastatic spread. Malignant tumors of the gastrointestinal tract commonly metastasize to the first capillary bed they encounter, namely the liver. Similarly, lung cancers often spread to the brain.

The need for a hospitable host environment has been elegantly demonstrated experimentally. Grafts of various organs were transplanted into the skeletal muscle of inbred mice, after which the animals were injected with mouse tumor cells. Metastases appeared only in grafts from organs that normally are the locale of secondary tumors. The mechanism underlying such preferential "homing" of neoplastic cells to specific organs is not well understood, but there is experimental evidence to suggest that the surface properties of the cells (such as integrins) are involved. For example, breast cancers preferentially metastasize to bone, a characteristic that may be related to the expression of several bone matrix proteins by the tumor cells. In addition, a specific integrin ($\alpha v\beta 3$) is overexpressed by breast cancer metastases to bone, compared to the cells of the primary tumor. Deficient expression of certain HLA antigens has been correlated with lymph node metastases, and selective expression of certain adhesion molecules (e.g., E-selectin) has been found in specific organ metastases of breast and colon cancers.

THE GRADING AND STAGING OF CANCERS

In an attempt to predict the clinical behavior of a malignant tumor and to establish criteria for therapy, many cancers are classified according to cytological and histological grading schemes or by staging protocols that describe the extent of spread.

Cancer Grading

Cytological/histological grading, which is necessarily subjective and at best semiquantitative, is based on the degree of anaplasia and on the number of proliferating cells. The degree of anaplasia is determined from the shape and regularity of the cells, and from the presence of distinct differentiated features, such as functioning gland-like structures in adenocarcinomas or epithelial pearls in squamous carcinomas. Evidence of rapid or abnormal growth is provided by large numbers of mitoses, the pres-

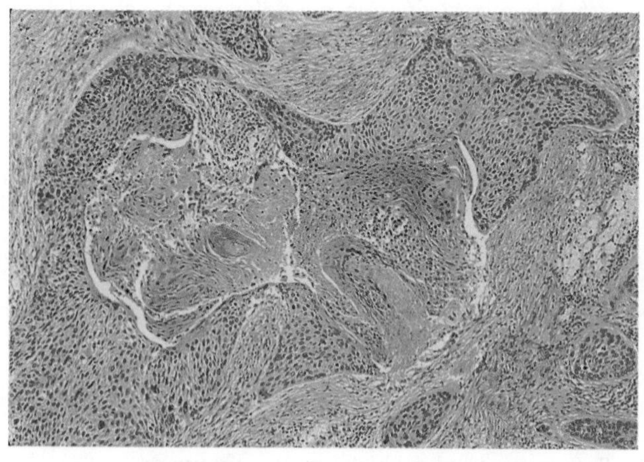

A

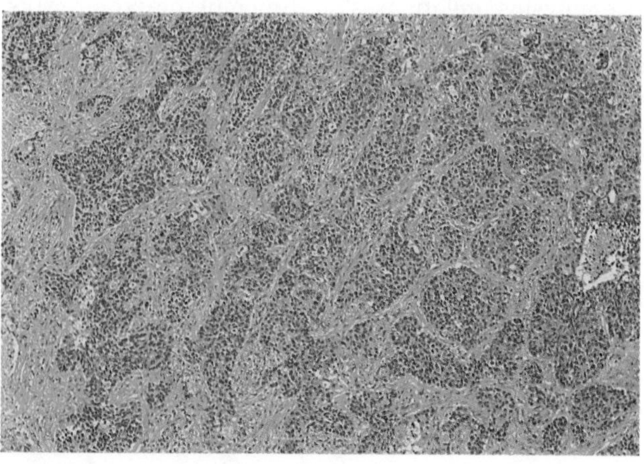

B

FIGURE *5-21*
Cytological grading of squamous cell carcinoma of the lung. (*A*) Well-differentiated (grade 1) squamous cell carcinoma. The tumor cells bear a strong resemblance to normal squamous cells and synthesize keratin, as evidenced by epithelial pearls. (*B*) Poorly differentiated (grade 3) squamous cell carcinoma. The malignant cells are difficult to identify as being of squamous origin.

ence of atypical mitoses, nuclear pleomorphism, and tumor giant cells. Most grading schemes classify tumors into three or four grades of increasing degrees of malignancy (Fig. 5-21). The general correlation between the cytological grade and the biological behavior of a neoplasm is not invariable: There are many examples of tumors of low cytological grades that express substantial malignant properties.

Cancer Staging

The choice of surgical approach or the selection of treatment modalities is influenced more by the stage of a cancer, which refers to the extent of spread, than by its cytological grade. Moreover, most statistical data related to cancer survival are based on the stage rather than the cytological grade of the tumor. Clinical staging is independent of cytological grading. The significant criteria used for staging vary with different organs. Commonly used criteria include (1) tumor size, (2) the extent of local growth, whether within or without the organ, (3) the presence of lymph node metastases, and (4) the presence of distant metastases. These criteria have been codified in the international **TNM cancer staging** system, in which T refers to the size of the primary tumor, N to the number and distribution of lymph node metastases, and M to the presence and extent of distant metastases.

In some cases, the distinction between benign and malignant tumors is based solely on size. For example, on the basis of clinical experience with renal cancers, tumors smaller than 2 cm in diameter are considered benign adenomas, whereas those of larger size are labeled renal carcinomas. The choice of surgical therapy is often influenced by size alone. For instance, a primary breast cancer smaller than 2 cm in diameter can be treated with local excision and radiation therapy, whereas larger masses often necessitate mastectomy. Local extension can also be used to estimate prognosis, as in the Dukes classification of colorectal cancer. Penetration of the tumor into the muscularis and serosa of the bowel is associated with a poorer prognosis than that of a more superficial tumor. Clearly, the presence of lymph node metastases mandates more aggressive treatment than does their absence, whereas the presence of distant metastases is generally a contraindication to surgical intervention other than for palliation.

THE BIOCHEMISTRY OF THE CANCER CELL

Despite more than a half century of intensive investigation of the biochemical basis of neoplasia, no alterations unique to cancer cells or crucial to carcinogenesis have emerged. Among the earliest studies, the most prominent were those of Warburg, who proposed that the biochemical basis of neoplasia was the dependence of tumor cells on anaerobic glycolysis rather than aerobic respiration. According to Warburg's theory, the neoplastic stimulus is an irreversible injury to aerobic respiration, followed by a compensatory increase in anaerobic fermentation and the production of a neoplastic cell. However, although it is true that most cancers do exhibit high rates of glycolysis, many display normal rates. An increase in glycolysis seems, therefore, to be a characteristic of only some tumors and to be an effect rather than a cause of neoplastic transformation. Later investigations found an association between neoplasia and numerous enzyme deficits, lowered protein levels, the appearance of unusual isozymes, and the production of fetal proteins. However, detailed studies of tumors with varying degrees of differentiation have clearly shown that this phenotypic heterogeneity of tumor cells simply reflects a variable degree of differentiation. **The search for a common qualitative biochemical defect to explain neoplasia has to date been unsuccessful.**

THE GROWTH OF CANCERS

Cell Cycle Kinetics

Historically, cancer was considered to result from a totally unregulated growth of cells, and a logical corollary was that neoplastic cells proliferate at a faster rate than normal ones. When tritiated thymidine became available, accurate measurements of growth kinetics were made possible. The observation that the cell cycle time of intestinal cells was shorter than that of very rapidly growing tumors cast doubt on the validity of these basic assumptions. **It is now clear that tumor cells do not necessarily proliferate at a faster rate than their normal counterparts.** Tumor growth depends on other factors, such as the growth fraction (proportion of cycling cells) and the rate of cell death. In normal proliferating tissues, such as the intestine and the bone marrow, an exquisite balance between cell renewal and cell death is strictly maintained. **By contrast, the major determinant of tumor growth is clearly the fact that more cells are produced than die in a given time.**

Doubling Time

The growth of a tumor may be expressed in terms of the doubling time—that is, the time taken for the number of cells in the mass to double. Internal cancers are not usually detected before they attain a size of about 1 cm^3 (1 g), which corresponds to 10^8 to 10^9 cells. The origin of most tumors from a single cell implies that the mass has doubled at least 30 times to reach this size. If the cancer is neglected and enlarges to the impressive size of 1 kg, it now contains 10^{12} cells. Yet, the growth from 1 g to 1 kg (assuming no cell death) can be achieved by only 10 population doublings. Thus, when cancers are initially detected clinically, they are already far advanced in their natural history. Because of the variable death rate of tumor cells and differences in cell cycle kinetics, the actual doubling time of human tumors is highly unpredictable.

The doubling time is not necessarily correlated with the growth fraction. Since the duration of mitosis in cancer cells is often prolonged, the number of mitoses in a histological section can be misleading as an indicator of overall growth. For example, a doubling in the time required for mitosis results in twice as many visible mitoses without any real increase in the rate of growth. In most cases, the theoretical tumor doubling time, calculated from the growth fraction and the cell cycle time, bears little relation to the actual clinical situation. For example, if a tumor weighing 1 g (often the smallest size clinically detectable) produces 2 new cells per 1000 cells in each mitotic cycle, the theoretical net increase would be a staggering 10^6 cells per hour, a figure totally at variance with the experience with most solid tumors. **Because of this difference between the theoretical and observed growth of tumors, it has been estimated that in human skin tumors as many as 97% of proliferated cells die spontaneously.** The causes of tumor cell death are not precisely defined but probably include such factors as programmed cell death (apoptosis); inadequate blood supply, with consequent ischemia; a paucity of nutrients; and vulnerability to specific and nonspecific host defenses.

Tumor Angiogenesis

Angiogenesis refers to the sprouting of new capillaries from preexisting blood vessels and is a requirement for the continued growth of cancers, whether primary or metastatic. In the absence of new vessels to supply the nutrients and remove waste products, malignant tumors do not grow larger than 1 to 2 mm in diameter. In this context, the density of capillaries within the primary tumor (e.g., cancers of the breast, prostate, and colon) predicts metastases and decreased survival. Moreover, inhibitors of angiogenesis have been shown experimentally to suppress the growth and spread of malignant tumors. Importantly, the process of tumor angiogenesis occurs in non-neoplastic host tissue and is comparable to that in wound healing and other physiological circumstances (see Chapter 3). Neovascularization of the evolving cancer may appear at various stages of tumor development and probably is related to phenotypic and genetic changes in the tumors. However, it is still unclear whether tumor angiogenesis is fundamentally a response to tissue hypoxia or to a distinct angiogenic tumor phenotype.

A number of factors are capable of stimulating an angiogenic response; some act directly on endothelial cells and others stimulate inflammatory cells to promote the formation of new blood vessels. Among these factors are aFGF and bFGF , TGF-α and TGF-β, tumor necrosis factor-alpha (TNF-α), vascular endothelial growth factor (VEGF), PDGF, angiogenin, and epidermal growth factor (EGF). The role of such angiogenic factors is underscored by the ability of antiangiogenesis molecules to suppress tumor growth. These include antibodies to VEGF, a dominant negative mutant of a VEGF receptor (Flk-1), and antisense oligonucleotides to bFGF. In fact, two new angiogenesis inhibitors (angiostatin and endostatin) have recently been reported to eliminate widespread tumors in mice. Tumor angiogenesis may also be influenced by variations in the production of angiogenic inhibitors, such as thrombospondin, TIMPs, platelet factor 4, and interferons α and β.

Tumor Dormancy

It is often the clinical situation that metastatic disease is not detectable at the time of the removal of a primary cancer. With some tumors, notably breast cancer and melanoma, metastases may remain dormant for many years, only to become apparent without any obvious cause. It is not clear whether tumor dormancy represents a balance between cell growth and cell death or whether the tumor cells are in cell cycle arrest. In the absence of tumor angiogenesis, it is likely that cell proliferation is balanced by apoptosis. On the other hand, in a mouse lymphoma model, dormancy can be induced by anti-idiotype antibodies. In this situation, restraint of cell proliferation is achieved by exposure of the malignant cells to a ligand whose binding to its receptor initiates a growth inhibitory signal. Hence, such a signal can reverse the malignant phenotype of the cells without affecting the genetic lesion responsible for their tumorigenic potential. The development of ligands that induce or maintain tumor dormancy may be clinically beneficial in the management of cancers that are not controlled by available chemotherapeutic regimens.

THE MOLECULAR GENETICS OF CANCER

The belief that cancer has a genetic basis, embodied in the concept of "cancer genes," was prevalent for most of this century and was rooted in the recognition of four factors: (1) hereditary predisposition, (2) the presence of chromosomal abnormalities in neoplastic cells, (3) a correlation between impaired DNA repair and the occurrence of cancer, and (4) the close association between carcinogenesis and mutagenesis. **It is now recognized that the unregulated growth of cancer cells results from the sequential acquisition of somatic mutations in genes that control cell growth and differentiation or that maintain the integrity of the genome**. Similar mutations may also be present in the germline of persons with hereditary predispositions to a variety of cancers. Mutations can be produced by environmental mutagens such as chemical carcinogens or radiation (see later). Mutagens can also arise during normal cellular metabolism, particularly the formation of activated oxygen species (see Chapter 1). It is, however, likely that the most common mechanism of mutagenesis relates to spontaneous errors in DNA replication and repair. Considering that 10^{17} mitoses occur during an average human lifetime, corresponding to incorporation of the more than 10^{26} nucleotides into nascent DNA, it is impossible for this extent of DNA replication to occur without the introduction of unrepaired errors (mutations). Since the body is composed of 10^{14} cells and the mutation rate is roughly 10^{-6} per gene per generation, it is inevitable that everyone is a somatic mosaic at many genetic loci. The vast majority of such mutations are of no consequence, because they either do not affect the function of the cell or are lost as a result of the death of the cell. However, if the mutation involves genes that control growth or that protect the stability of the genome, it may give rise to a clone of cells that possess a growth advantage with respect to their normal neighbors. Successive mutations in similar genes result in increasingly aberrant clones until a malignant phenotype eventually emerges.

The genes involved in the pathogenesis of cancer can be conveniently grouped into three categories:

- **Oncogenes** are altered versions of normal genes, termed protooncogenes, that regulate normal cell growth and differentiation. Gain-of-function (dominant) mutations activate protooncogenes to become oncogenes and are positive effectors of the neoplastic phenotype.
- **Tumor suppressor genes** are normal genes whose products inhibit cellular proliferation. Loss-of-function (recessive) mutations inactivate the inhibitory activities of tumor suppressor genes, thereby permitting unregulated cell growth.
- **Mutator genes** normally maintain the integrity of the genome and the fidelity of DNA replication. Inactivating mutations of these genes allow the successive accumulation of further mutations.

Oncogenes

The concept of oncogenes was originally derived from studies of animal tumor viruses. The role of such viruses in the spontaneous and experimental induction of cancer is thoroughly established. A historical overview of the oncogenic animal viruses provides an appropriate background for understanding the role of oncogenes in carcinogenesis.

- **Chicken leukemias and lymphomas:** These avian malignancies were at one time not uncommon and appeared in epidemic form. The transmissibility of avian erythroblastosis by cell-free extracts from diseased chickens was recognized shortly after the turn of the century, but the successful transfer of chicken lymphomatosis by cell extracts was not accomplished until 1941. Ten years later, a vaccine against chicken lymphomatosis, the first anticancer vaccine, successfully eradicated this economic hazard from poultry flocks.
- **Rous sarcoma virus:** This RNA virus was originally derived in 1910 from a cell-free extract of a breast sarcoma in a chicken. When injected into young chickens, sarcomas developed at the site of injection and metastasized to many other organs.
- **Shope papillomavirus:** This DNA poxvirus was isolated from warty growths in wild cottontail rabbits in the early 1930s. Shope demonstrated for the first time that cell-free extracts from naturally occurring tumors could transmit the disease.
- **Bittner virus:** Formerly known as the Bittner milk factor, this RNA virus was shown in 1936 to be the agent that transmits mammary cancer in mice. It had long been known that certain strains of mice have a high incidence of mammary tumors, whereas other strains have virtually none. Although the susceptibility to mammary cancer clearly seemed to be hereditary, it did not follow mendelian laws. When the mother was from a tumor-susceptible strain, the daughters were susceptible. On the other hand, when the father was from a susceptible strain and the mother from a resistant strain, the daughters of the cross did not develop mammary tumors. The solution to the problem lay in the mother's milk, rather than in her genes. Bittner showed that if the offspring are delivered by cesarean section and suckled by dams from a tumor-free strain, the daughters did not develop cancer. Conversely, when young newborn mice from a tumor-free strain were suckled by dams of a susceptible strain, they developed mammary cancer. The responsible virus was subsequently isolated.
- **Polyoma virus:** Discovered in the 1950s, this DNA virus produces an astonishing variety of carcinomas and sarcomas in mice, rats, rabbits, and hamsters, the last being especially sensitive.
- **SV-40 virus:** This DNA virus, a member of the polyomavirus group, was isolated from monkey cells (simian virus [SV]) and was shown to be a potent transforming agent *in vitro*.

Many other oncogenic DNA viruses have now been found to produce solid tumors and lymphoproliferative disorders in a variety of species, including frogs, birds, rodents, and monkeys. Similarly, other oncogenic RNA viruses were also found to produce similar neoplasms in comparably diverse species. These include the Gross, Friend, Moloney, Kirsten, and Rauscher leukemia viruses. In 1970, the discovery of reverse transcriptase revolutionized the study of oncogenic RNA viruses and led to their being renamed retroviruses.

Retroviral Oncogenes

The discovery of DNA as the basis of heredity was entirely consistent with the transforming capability of DNA-containing viruses. It was argued that the induction of the permanent, heritable characteristics of the transformed cell reflects the incorporation of viral DNA into the cellular genome. However, the transforming properties of RNA-containing viruses posed a dilemma: the central dogma of molecular biology held that information flowed in a unidirectional manner, from DNA to RNA to protein. How then, could the genetic information encoded in RNA be communicated to subsequent generations of stable lines of transformed cells? In the mid 1960s, a revolutionary hypothesis was put forward to the effect that the genome of RNA-containing oncogenic viruses is transcribed into DNA by a reversal of the usual direction of information flow. This hypothesis implied that (1) the DNA segment in the host genome (now called a provirus) is derived from viral RNA and (2) that the virally derived DNA functions as a gene from which viral mRNA is, in turn, transcribed. Moreover, the theory implied that the mRNA transcribed from the integrated segment of DNA becomes the genome of nascent viral progeny. This hypothesis was validated in 1970 by the demonstration of **reverse transcriptase**, the viral enzyme that synthesizes DNA from the viral RNA genome. This discovery opened a new era of research into the molecular biology of cancer.

The oncogenic retroviruses can be divided into two general groups, based on the interval between viral infection and the development of a tumor (Fig. 5-22):

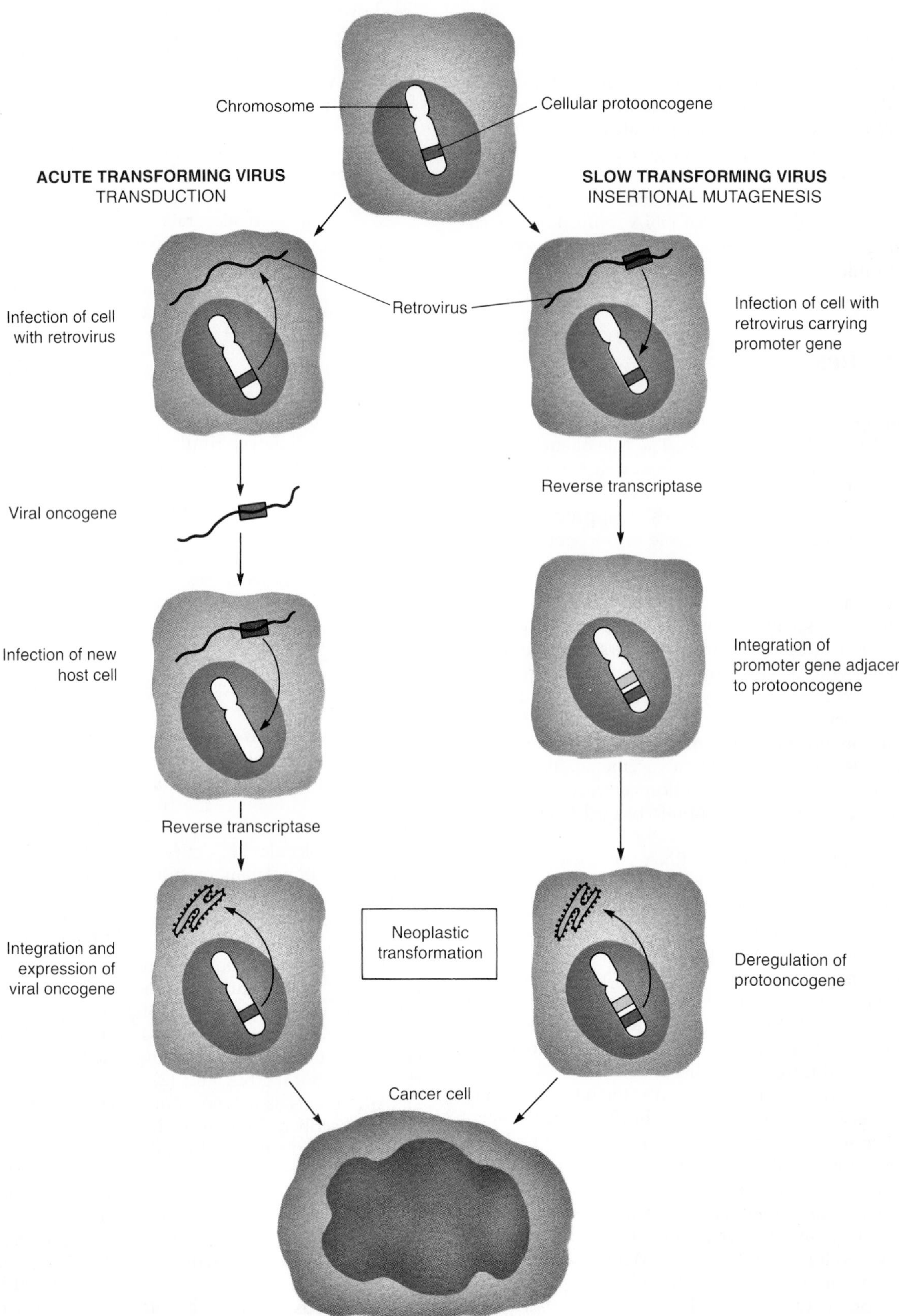
Chromosome
Cellular protooncogene
ACUTE TRANSFORMING VIRUS
TRANSDUCTION
SLOW TRANSFORMING VIRUS
INSERTIONAL MUTAGENESIS
Retrovirus
Infection of cell with retrovirus
Infection of cell with retrovirus carrying promoter gene
Reverse transcriptase
Viral oncogene
Infection of new host cell
Integration of promoter gene adjacent to protooncogene
Reverse transcriptase
Integration and expression of viral oncogene
Neoplastic transformation
Deregulation of protooncogene
Cancer cell

FIGURE 5-22

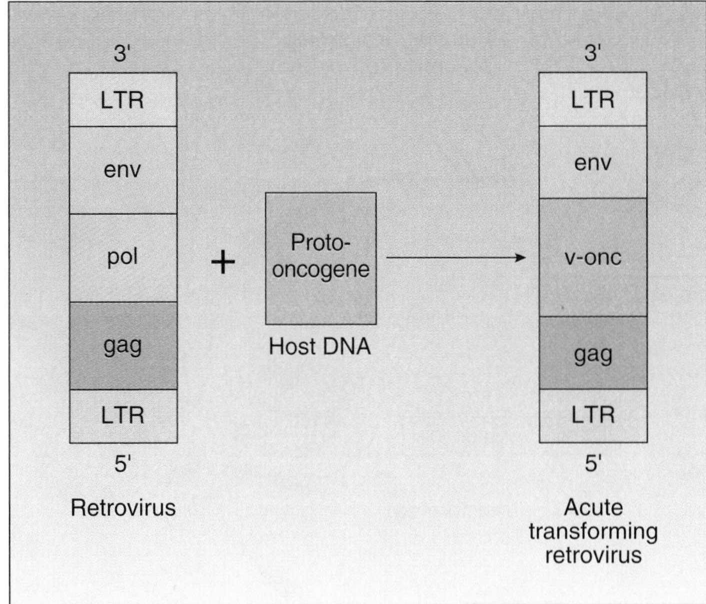

FIGURE 5-23
Conversion by transduction of a replication-competent retrovirus into a replication-incompetent acute transforming virus. The genome of a retrovirus contains three gene regions *gag*—the core protein; *pol*—polymerase (in this case reverse transcriptase); and *env*—envelope protein. These regions are flanked by long terminal repeats (LTR). An acute transforming virus has replaced the *pol* region with sequences derived from a cellular protooncogene by a process termed transduction. As a result, the acute transforming virus has no reverse transcriptase activity and can no longer replicate.

- **Acute transforming viruses** produce tumors in a few weeks.
- **Slow transforming viruses** require months before cancers are evident.

The difference in the latency period between the acute and the slow transforming viruses reflects differences in their genetic composition. Acute transforming viruses have acquired, by a process known as **transduction**, portions of cellular genes, whose expression in cells leads to the rapid development of tumors. Such transduced viral genes are termed **viral oncogenes (v-onc)**, and the cellular genes from which they are derived are known as **cellular oncogenes (c-onc)** or **protooncogenes**. Infection with an acute transforming retrovirus leads to the incorporation of a viral oncogene into the host DNA, where it is expressed as a transforming factor. To date, close to two dozen retroviral oncogenes have been identified, and in almost half of these corresponding cellular oncogenes have been recognized.

Slow transforming viruses do not possess viral oncogenes. Rather, they produce tumors by integrating the provirus (the DNA copy of the viral RNA genome) at critical sites in the cell genome, thereby deregulating a neighboring cellular oncogene. This integration of the provirus into host DNA and the resulting activation of a cellular oncogene is termed **insertional mutagenesis**.

The difference in latency between acute transforming and slow transforming retroviruses is a function of the probability that a viral oncogene or a cellular oncogene will be expressed. Both types of retroviruses contain promoter and enhancer sequences in the long terminal repeats (LTR) at both ends of their genomes. Insertion of a provirus into the host genome occurs randomly. In the case of an acute transforming virus, transcription of the viral oncogene is controlled by its own LTR. **Thus, the expression of a viral oncogene does not depend on the site of viral insertion.**

In contrast to an acute transforming virus, the growth-promoting activity of a slow transforming virus resides in the capacity of the viral promoter and enhancer sequencers to augment the transcription of an immediately adjacent cellular oncogene. Since the provirus inserts into the host DNA at random, there is only a low probability that it will come to rest adjacent to a cellular oncogene. **Therefore, the long latency for transformation by a slow transforming virus reflects the time required for a rare event to occur.**

The complete viral genome is necessary for the replication of a retrovirus. In most cases, acute transforming retroviruses cannot replicate, because the viral oncogene has replaced the polymerase (reverse transcriptase) gene (Fig. 5-23). By contrast, slow transforming retroviruses can replicate, because they contain an intact viral genome.

FIGURE 5-22
Mechanisms of tumorigenesis by RNA retroviruses. Acute transforming RNA viruses contain a viral oncogene formed by transduction of a cellular protooncogene. Infection of a cell by such a virus results in the integration and expression of the viral oncogene, presumably leading to neoplastic transformation. By contrast, slow transforming viruses do not contain a viral oncogene but rather a promoter gene. The integration of this promoter gene deregulates the expression of cellular protooncogene (a process called insertional mutagenesis), again presumably leading to neoplastic transformation.

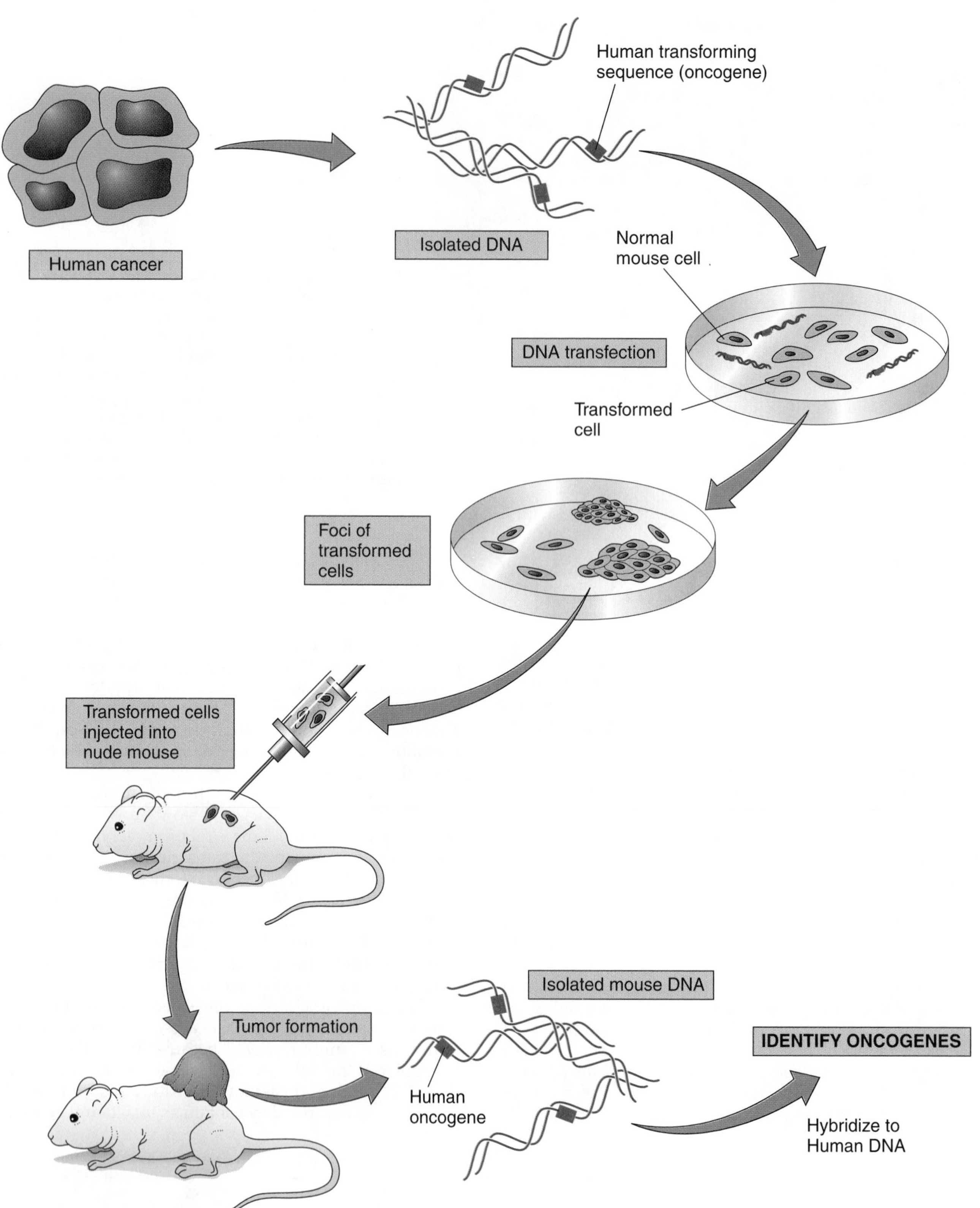

FIGURE *5-24*
Identification of human oncogenes by DNA transfection. DNA from a human cancer transforms cultured mouse cells. When injected into a nude mouse, the transformed cells form tumors. DNA from the nude mouse tumor contains the human oncogene, which is identified by hybridization with human DNA.

Identification of Human Oncogenes

After the discovery that v-onc genes represent mutated alleles of normal genes (c-onc or protooncogenes), it was predicted that sporadic (nonviral) human cancers would harbor similar mutations in the same genes. This expectation was realized and served to identify the genetic alterations that underlie many cancers. Most of these oncogenes have been identified by three methods.

Gene Transfer *in vitro* (DNA Transfection)

After the demonstration of the existence of retroviral oncogenes, similar oncogenes were identified in chemically induced rodent tumors and spontaneously occurring human cancers. It was shown that the DNA extracted from a malignant tumor has the ability to transform cells in culture, a process known as **transfection** (Fig. 5-24). **Importantly, the transforming oncogenes in human tumors that have been identified by the technique of gene transfer are somatic mutants of normal protooncogenes.**

Although DNA transfection is historically important, it has resulted in the identification of only a limited number of oncogenes, primarily those of the ras family. For example, the transforming genes of human lung and bladder cancers, neuroblastoma, and promyelocytic leukemia are homologous with the v-ras oncogenes of certain acute transforming retroviruses. In fact, 15% of biopsy specimens from unselected human cancers have activated *ras* oncogenes, as detected by DNA transfection. This figure is even higher in selected tumors, such as colorectal cancer, in which activated ras genes may be present in more than half the cases. The oncogenes identified by transfection of DNA from human tumors are not restricted to homologues of viral oncogenes, and novel transforming genes have also been found (*neu*, *met*, *trk*, *mas*, *HST*, and *KS3*).

Chromosomal Alterations

Human cancers commonly exhibit nonrandom chromosomal abnormalities, such as certain translocations (see Chapter 6) and homogeneously staining regions (pale chromosomal segments that do not exhibit a banding pattern). Importantly, specific chromosomal alterations are consistently observed in particular cancers, indicating that the lineage from which the cancer originated is especially susceptible to the oncogenic effects of the gene involved in the chromosomal lesion. In this context, activated protooncogenes have been demonstrated at the sites of translocation breakpoints by *in situ* hybridization with DNA probes of known oncogenes. For example , *c-myc* has been localized to the translocation in Burkitt lymphoma and *c-abl* has been found at the breakpoint in the Philadelphia chromosome of chronic myelogenous leukemia (see later). Homogeneously staining regions in chromosomes of a number of human cancers contain amplified protooncogenes, that is, an increased number of gene copies. A case in point is the 700-fold amplification in human neuroblastomas of N-*myc*, a protooncogene normally expressed during development.

Mechanisms of Activation of Cellular Oncogenes

The similarity of oncogenes (both viral and tumor) to normal genes that code for proteins involved in growth and development poses the question as to how these normal genes become oncogenes, or are "activated." There are two general mechanisms by which this activation is accomplished:

- An alteration in the structure of the protooncogene itself results in an abnormal gene product. A change in nucleic acid sequence, by point mutation, deletion, or chromosomal translocation, leads to the synthesis of a mutant protein that functions abnormally.
- An increase in the expression of the protooncogene causes overproduction of a normal gene product. Increased transcription of a normal protooncogene occurs in situations such as insertional mutagenesis, chromosomal translocation, and gene amplification. Additional mechanisms for increased transcription include deletion in noncoding sequences, altered promotion of RNA polymerase, and hypomethylation of the protooncogene.

Activation by Mutation

Historically, retroviral oncogenes served as the prototype for the study of oncogene activation. It was demonstrated in a number of systems that v-onc sequences contain mutations when compared with their cellular counterparts. These include both point mutations and deletions. As a result of such changes, mutant proteins are synthesized and the regulation of transcriptional and post-transcriptional events is altered. **It is now well documented that mutations of v-onc sequences increase the tumorigenic potential of acute transforming retroviruses.**

The first oncogene identified in a human tumor was activated *c-ras* from a bladder cancer. This gene was found to have a remarkably subtle alteration, namely a point mutation in codon 12, a change that results in the substitution of valine for glycine in the ras protein. Subsequent studies of other cancers have revealed point mutations involving other codons of the *ras* gene, suggesting that these positions are critical for the normal function of the ras protein.

The possible importance of point mutations in protooncogenes is well illustrated in an animal model. The *erb B* oncogene, which encodes a protein that closely resembles the EGF receptor, was identified by transfection studies using DNA from a chemically induced rat glioblastoma. In the mutated gene, a glutamic acid is substituted for valine in the transmembrane domain. When placed in transgenic mice, mutant *erb B* stimulated the development of adenocarcinomas of the breast in 100% of female and male animals that expressed the transgene. Further evidence for the tumorigenic role of this transgenic oncogene was the observation that these adenocarcinomas were polyclonal and that the malignant process involved the entire epithelium of each gland.

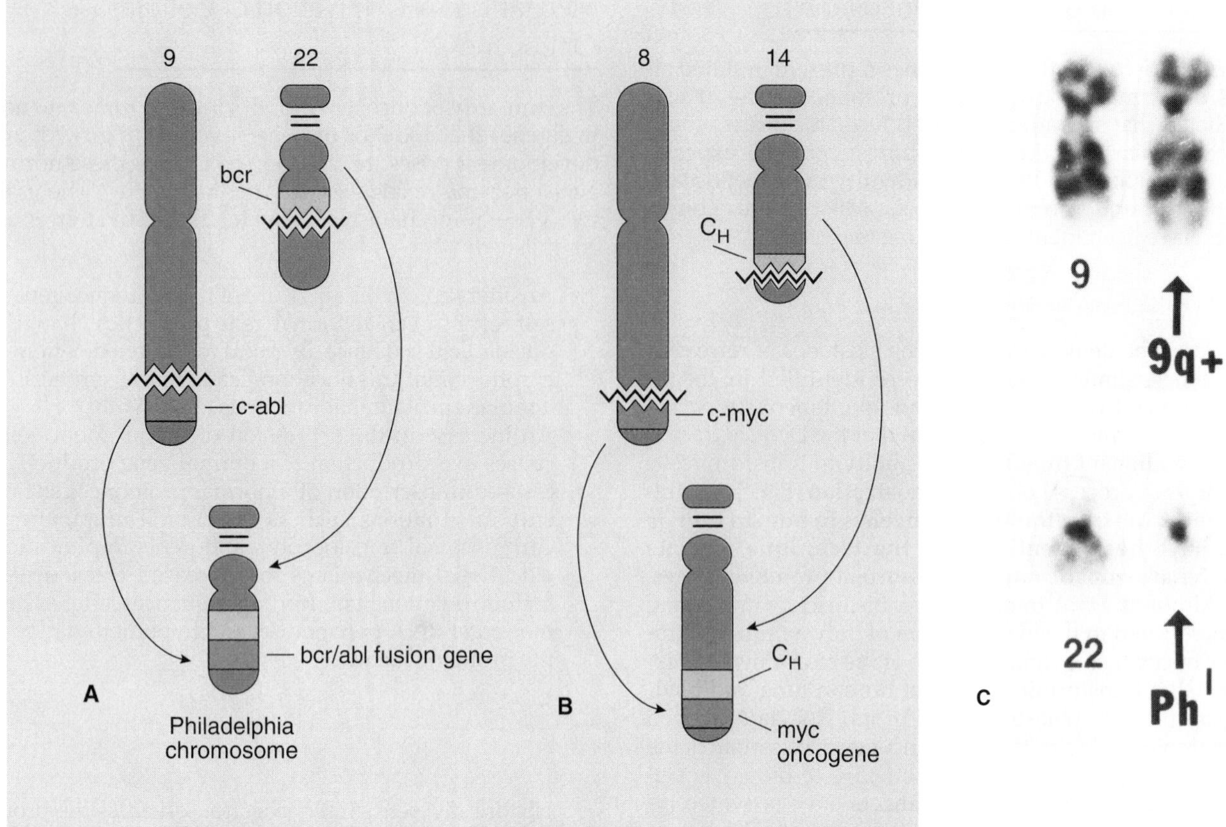

FIGURE 5-25
Oncogene activation by chromosomal translocation. (*A*) Chronic myelogenous leukemia. Breaks at the ends of the long arms of chromosomes 9 and 22 allow reciprocal translocations to occur. The c-*abl* protooncogene on chromosome 9 is translocated to the breakpoint region (bcr) of chromosome 22. The result is the Philadelphia chromosome, which contains a new fusion gene coding for a hybrid oncogenic protein (bcr-abl), presumably involved in the pathogenesis of chronic myelogenous leukemia. (*B*) Burkitt lymphoma. In this disorder, chromosomal breaks involve the long arms of chromosomes 8 and 14. The c-*myc* gene on chromosome 8 is translocated to a region on chromosome 14 adjacent to the gene coding for the constant region of an immunoglobulin heavy chain (C_H). The expression of c-*myc* is enhanced by its association with the promoter/enhancer regions of the actively transcribed immunoglobulin genes. (*C*) Karyotypes of a patient with chronic myelogenous leukemia showing the results of reciprocal translocations between chromosomes 9 and 22. The Philadelphia chromosome is recognized by a smaller-than-normal chromosome 22 (22q−). One chromosome 9 (9q+) is larger than its normal counterpart.

Activating, or gain-of-function, mutations in protooncogenes are almost always somatic rather than germline alterations. It is likely that germline mutations in protooncogenes, which are known to be important regulators of growth during development, are lethal *in utero*. The only known exception to this rule is *c-ret*, a gene that in its mutated (activated) form is incriminated in the pathogenesis of familial thyroid cancers and multiple endocrine neoplasia, type II. Since the function of the *c-ret* product (a receptor tyrosine kinase) is unknown, it remains to be seen whether *ret* may not eventually be classified as some other type of cancer-promoting gene.

Activation by Chromosomal Translocation

Chromosomal translocations, that is, the transfer of a portion of one chromosome to another, have been implicated in the pathogenesis of several human leukemias and lymphomas. The first and still the best-known example of an acquired chromosomal translocation in a human cancer is the **Philadelphia chromosome**, which is found in 95% of patients with chronic myelogenous leukemia (Fig. 5-25). The *c-abl* protooncogene on chromosome 9 is translocated to chromosome 22, where it is placed in juxtaposition to a site known as the breakpoint cluster region (bcr). The *c-abl* gene and bcr region unite to produce a hybrid oncogene that codes for an aberrant protein with very high tyrosine kinase activity. Tyrosine kinases are important in the normal regulation of cellular proliferation, but the precise involvement of this abnormal protein in the pathogenesis of myelogenous leukemia is not known. The chromosomal translocation that produces the Philadelphia chromosome is an example of activation of an oncogene by the formation of a chimeric (fusion) protein.

In 75% of patients with Burkitt lymphoma (a type of B-cell lymphoma, see Chapter 20), there is a translocation of the *c-myc* protooncogene from its site on chromosome 8 to a position on chromosome 14 (see Fig. 5-25). This translocation places *c-myc* adjacent to the genes that control the transcription of the immunoglobulin heavy chains. As a result, the *c-myc* protooncogene is activated by the promoter/enhancer sequences of these immunoglobulin genes and is consequently expressed constitutively rather than in a regulated manner. In 25% of patients with Burkitt lymphoma, the *c-myc* protooncogene remains on chromosome 8 but is activated by the translocation of Ig light-chain genes from chromosome 2 or 22 to the 3′ end of the *c-myc* gene. In either case, a chromosomal translocation does not create a novel chimeric protein, but rather stimulates the overproduction of a normal gene product. In Burkitt lymphoma, the excessive amount of the normal *c-myc* product, probably in association with other genetic alterations, leads to the emergence of a dominant clone of B cells, driven relentlessly to proliferate as a monoclonal neoplasm.

Activation by Gene Amplification

Chromosomal alterations that result in an increase in the number of copies of a gene (i.e., gene amplification) have been found primarily in human solid tumors. Such aberrations are recognized as (1) **homogeneous staining regions (HSRs)** (Fig. 5-26); (2) **abnormal banding regions** on chromosomes; or (3) **double minutes**, which are visualized as multiple, small, paired, cytoplasmic bodies (Fig. 5-27). In some cases, gene amplification has been shown to involve protooncogenes. For example, HSRs may be seen in neuroblastomas and are all derived from the N-*myc* protooncogene. The presence of N-*myc* HSRs is associated with up to a 700-fold amplification of this gene and is a marker of advanced disease with a poor prognosis. Activation of *myc*-family protooncogenes by means of gene amplification has also been demonstrated in small cell carcinoma of the lung, Wilms tumor, and hepatoblastoma.

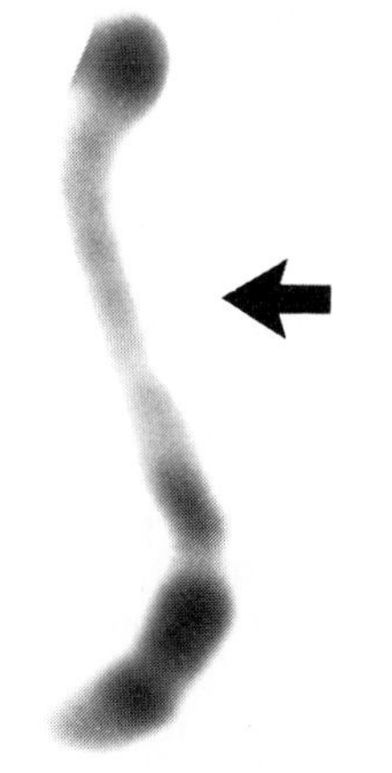

FIGURE 5-26
Homogeneously staining region (HSR, *arrow*) in a chromosome from an ovarian carcinoma.

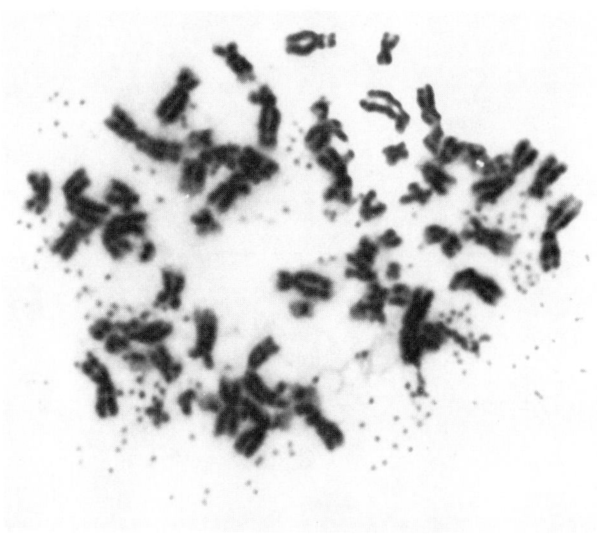

FIGURE 5-27
Double minutes in a karyotype of a soft tissue sarcoma appear as multiple small bodies.

The *erb B* protooncogene is amplified in as many as a third of breast and ovarian cancers. The *erb B* gene codes for a receptor-type tyrosine kinase that shows close structural similarity to the EGF receptor. It has been reported in some studies (but not in others) that amplification of *erb B* in breast and ovarian cancer is associated with poor overall survival and decreased time to relapse.

Mechanisms of Action of Oncogenes

Oncogenes can be classified according to the roles of their normal counterparts (protooncogenes) in the biochemical pathways that regulate growth and differentiation. These include the following (Fig. 5-28):

- Extracellular growth factors
- Cell surface receptors
- Intracellular signal transduction pathways
- DNA-binding nuclear proteins (transcription factors)
- Cell cycle proteins (cyclins and cyclin-dependent protein kinases)
- Inhibitors of apoptosis (bcl-2)

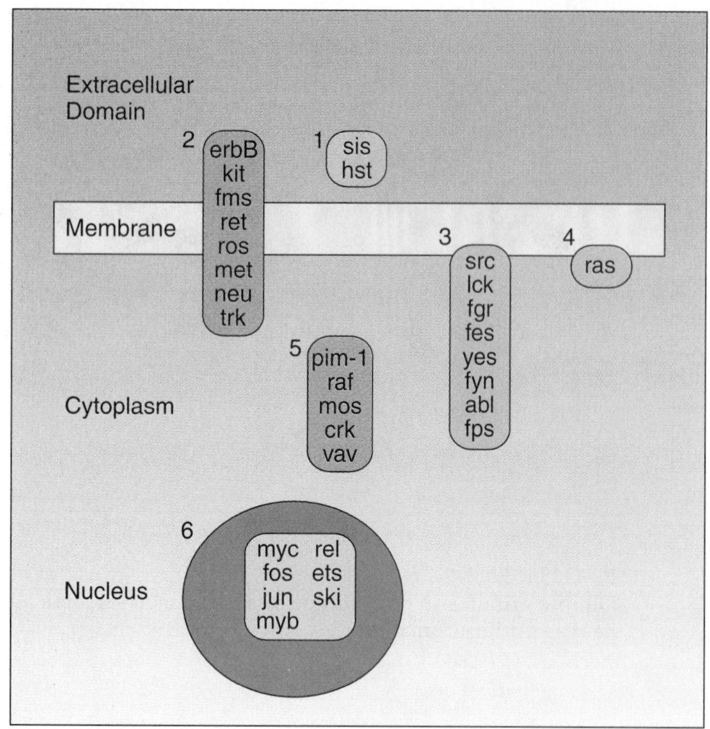

FIGURE 5-28
Cellular compartments in which oncogene or protooncogene products reside. (1) Growth factors, (2) transmembrane growth factor receptors (tyrosine kinase), (3) integral membrane receptors, (4) *ras* GTPase family, (5) cytoplasmic oncogenes, (6) nuclear oncogenes.

Oncogenes and Growth Factors

The first oncogene shown to code for a growth factor was v-*sis*, a retroviral oncogene that encodes a protein with striking sequence similarity to the B-chain of PDGF. PDGF is the protein product of the c-*sis* protooncogene and is a potent mitogen for fibroblasts, smooth muscle cells, and glial cells. Cells derived from human sarcomas and glioblastomas (a malignant glial cell tumor) produce PDGF-like polypeptides, whereas their normal counterparts do not. Transfection of c-*sis* into cultured mouse fibroblasts results in their transformation. Thus, a normal human gene (c-*sis*) that encodes a growth factor (PDGF) acquires transforming capacity when it is constitutively expressed in a cell that responds to this signal. **The synthesis of a PDGF-like growth factor by neoplastic cells that express a receptor for this activity is an example of autocrine growth stimulation, which is a mechanism implicated in oncogenesis.**

An oncogene (*HST* or *KS3*) that codes for a protein with homology to FGF has been identified in human stomach cancer and Kaposi sarcoma. Moreover, neoplastic cells often express TGF in rodent models . TGF-α binds to the EGF receptor, and TGF-β has its own receptor. Further evidence that autocrine stimulation secondary to inappropriate synthesis of growth factors may contribute to malignant transformation comes from the demonstration that a novel oncogene can be constructed from sequences that encode EGF.

Despite these examples, mutational activation of growth factor genes is not well characterized in human cancers. Nevertheless, whether caused by genetic or epigenetic mechanisms, cancer cells generally produce a mixture of growth factors with autocrine or paracrine activity, including PDGF, TGF-α, FGF, colony-stimulating factor-1 (CSF-1), and hepatocyte growth factor (HGF).

Oncogenes and Growth Factor Receptors

Many growth factors stimulate cellular proliferation by interacting with a family of cell surface receptors that are integral membrane proteins with tyrosine kinase activity. Binding of a ligand to the extracellular domain of such a receptor stimulates an intrinsic kinase activity in the cytoplasmic domain of the molecule that phosphorylates tyrosine residues in other proteins. For example, the phosphorylation of a specific phospholipase C by "receptor type" tyrosine kinase links the binding of a growth factor to the phosphoinositide signaling pathway, which activates protein kinase C and elevates cytosolic free calcium. **Thus, because growth factor receptors can generate potent mitogenic signals, they harbor a latent oncogenic potential, which when activated overrides the normal controls of signaling pathways.**

A number of retroviral oncogenes code for mutant versions of normal growth factor receptors (Fig. 5-29). Among these are receptors for well-characterized growth factors, including EGF receptor (v-erbB), hepatocyte growth factor receptor (met), stem cell factor receptor (kit), nerve growth factor receptor (trk), and colony-stimulating factor-1 receptor (fms). Mutations in putative receptors whose ligands have not been identified have also been found in human cancers, for example ros and ret. In some cases, the truncation of an N-terminal domain of the receptor is thought to eliminate the conformational constraints that necessitate ligand binding for activation of the tyrosine kinase domain. In other instances, deletions or mutations in the C-terminal portion of the receptor abolish domains that inhibit tyrosine kinase activity. In both of these examples (and other mutations as well), the altered receptor provides a constitutive, ligand-independent, growth signal.

Although mutations of growth factor receptors have been demonstrated in retroviral oncogenesis and in a subset of human neoplasms, their role in human cancer appears to be limited. In some human malignancies (e.g., breast, ovarian, and stomach cancers), amplification of *her-2/neu* results in autocrine activation mediated by the overexpression of this growth factor receptor. Of greater importance in human cancers are epigenetic changes that cause increased synthesis of growth factors and receptors.

Oncogenes and Membrane-Associated and Cytoplasmic Protein Kinases

A number of protein kinases are loosely associated with the inner aspect of the plasma membrane and possess tyrosine kinase activity but are neither integral membrane proteins nor growth factor receptors. The prototype of an oncogene that codes for mutant forms of these protein kinases is v-*src* (see Fig. 5-29), although a number of other oncogenes (*abl, lck, yes, fgr, fps, fes*) belong to the src family. The homologous c-*src* protooncogene product is highly expressed in platelets and some neurons, and to a lesser extent in most cells. Although the functions of the src family of tyrosine kinases are not fully understood, they are thought to bind to the cytoplasmic domains of a variety of cell surface receptors. As a result, they act as the catalytic subunit for the receptor and, in turn, phosphorylate cellular proteins. Oncogenic activation of members of the c-*src* family of tyrosine kinases leads to unregulated delivery of growth-promoting signals.

In human cancer, the best studied example of an oncogene that codes for a src-type of tyrosine kinase is activated *abl*. As previously discussed, in chronic myelogenous leukemia this protooncogene, which codes for a cytoplasmic tyrosine kinase, is translocated from chromosome 9 to the breakpoint cluster region (bcr) of chromosome 22. The bcr-abl fusion gene encodes a mutant protein with conspicuously elevated tyrosine kinase activity, which is necessary for the oncogenic action of the chimeric protein.

Soluble cytoplasmic oncoproteins (*raf, mos, pim*-1) that phosphorylate serine/threonine residues have also been described. These enzyme activities are similar to those of protein kinase C, the protein stimulated by the phosphoinositide signal transduction system. Interestingly, overexpression of a cloned protein kinase C in cultured cells leads to their partial transformation, and a mutant form of PKC acts as an oncoprotein. The best-studied of the soluble cytoplasmic oncoproteins, *raf*, plays a role in the signal transduction cascade that converts ligand binding by cell surface receptors into nuclear transcriptional activation.

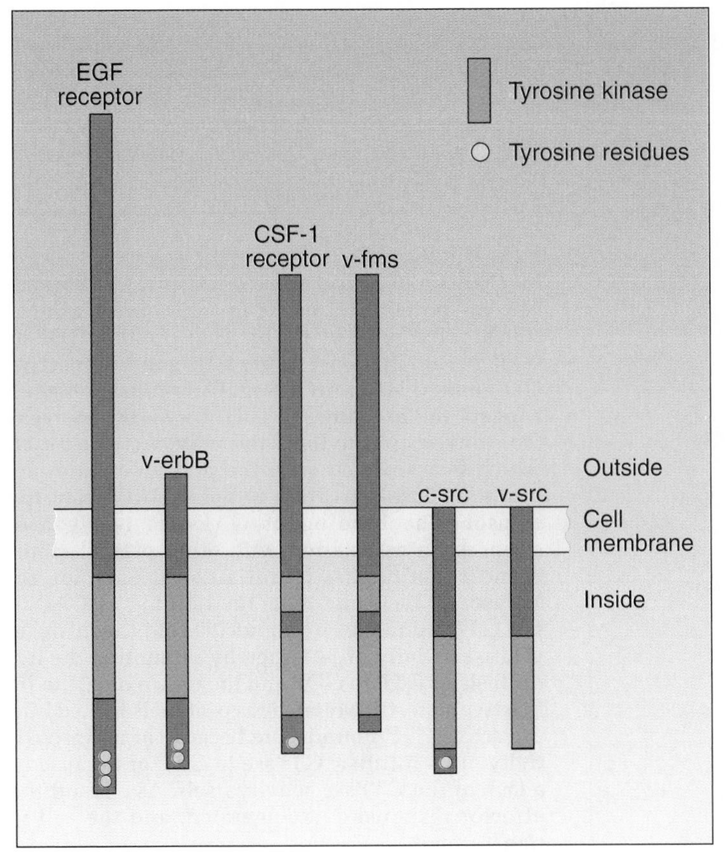

FIGURE 5-29
Cell surface receptors and oncogene products with tyrosine kinase activities. The product of the v-*erb*B oncogene is homologous to the EGF receptor, with the difference that a large portion of the extracellular domain and a smaller portion of the intracellular domain are absent. The v-*fms* oncogene product closely resembles the CSF-1 receptor, except that a short peptide consequence containing a terminal tyrosine residue is deleted. A similar deletion characterizes the difference between the v-*src* oncogene and the c-*src* protooncogene.

Ras Oncogenes

The *ras* protooncogene codes for a product, p21, that belongs to a family of small cytoplasmic proteins (G proteins) that bind guanosine triphosphate (GTP) and guanosine diphosphate (GDP). The ras protein, p21, is distinct from the integral membrane G proteins that are involved in receptor-mediated signal transduction (Fig. 5-30). The protein p21 is active when it binds GTP and is inactive when it binds GDP. Bound GTP is converted to GDP by the intrinsic GTPase activity of p21. This enzyme activity is normally very low but is stimulated more than 100-fold by a GTPase-activating protein (GAP). Thus, the inactivating switch for the ras protein is the p21 GTPase.

The discovery of an activated version of the *ras* protooncogene in bladder cancer cells was the first demonstration of a human oncogene. Furthermore, the point mutation in which valine was substituted for glycine at position 12 in p21 was the first mutation characterized in a human oncogene. It is now evident that activation of *ras* genes (Ha-*ras*, Ki-*ras*, or N-*ras*) is the most frequent dominant mutation in human cancers.

The mutant forms of p21 are characterized by persistence of GTP binding, which maintains the protein in its active conformation. Point mutations in the *ras* protooncogene interfere with the hydrolysis of GTP to GDP by rendering p21 resistant to the action of GAP. In addition, some mutations decrease the intrinsic ATPase activity of the ras protein. The persistence of the GTP-bound state results in uncontrolled stimulation of ras-related functions, because p21 is locked in the "on" position. Ras is an effector molecule in the signal transduction cascade that couples the activation of growth factor receptors to changes in gene transcription in the nucleus. Figure 5-31 illustrates the pathway by which Ras couples the binding of growth factors to a receptor with changes in nuclear transcription. It deserves emphasis that mutations in the genes coding for many of the components of this pathway result in the synthesis of oncoproteins.

Oncogenes and Nuclear Regulatory Proteins

There is a group of nuclear proteins encoded by protooncogenes that are intimately involved in the sequential expression of genes that regulate cellular proliferation and differentiation. Many of these proteins have the capacity to bind to DNA and are believed to regulate the expression of other genes. In models of stimulated cellular proliferation, the transitory expression of several protooncogenes is necessary for the cells to pass through specific points in the cell cycle. As an example, the binding of PDGF to cultured fibroblasts causes the cells to leave G_0 and enter the G_1 phase of the cell cycle. Shortly thereafter, several genes, including c-*myc*, c-*fos*, and c-*jun*, are expressed. However, the cells are not yet fully programmed to divide by the expression of these genes and will enter S phase and mitosis only after further stimulation by other

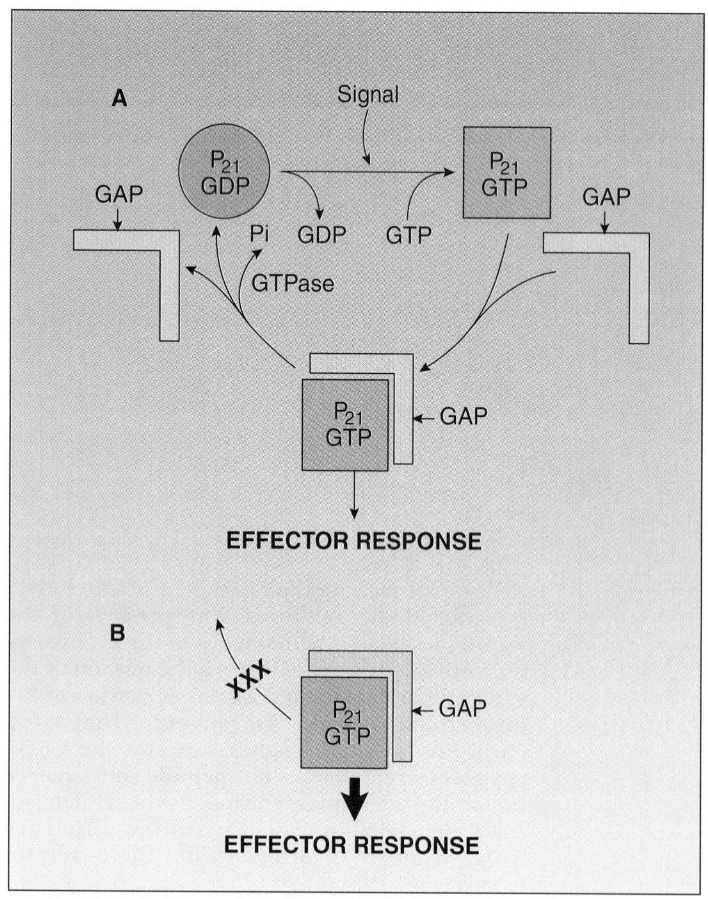

FIGURE 5-30
Mechanism of action of *ras* oncogene. (*A*) Normal. The *ras* protein p21 exists in two conformational states, determined by the binding of either GDP or GTP. Normally, most of the p21 is in the inactive GDP-bound state. An external stimulus, or signal, triggers the exchange of GTP for GDP, an event that converts p21 to the active state. Activated p21, which is associated with the plasma membrane, binds GTPase-activating protein (GAP) from the cytosol. The binding of GAP has two consequences. In association with other plasma membrane constituents, it initiates the effector response. At the same time, the binding of GAP to p21 GTP stimulates by about 100-fold the intrinsic GTPase activity of p21, thereby promoting the hydrolysis of GTP to GDP and the return of p21 to its inactive state. (*B*) Mutated ras protein is locked into the active GTP-bound state because of an insensitivity of its intrinsic GTPase to GAP or because of a lack of the GTPase activity itself. As a result the effector response is exaggerated, and the cell is transformed.

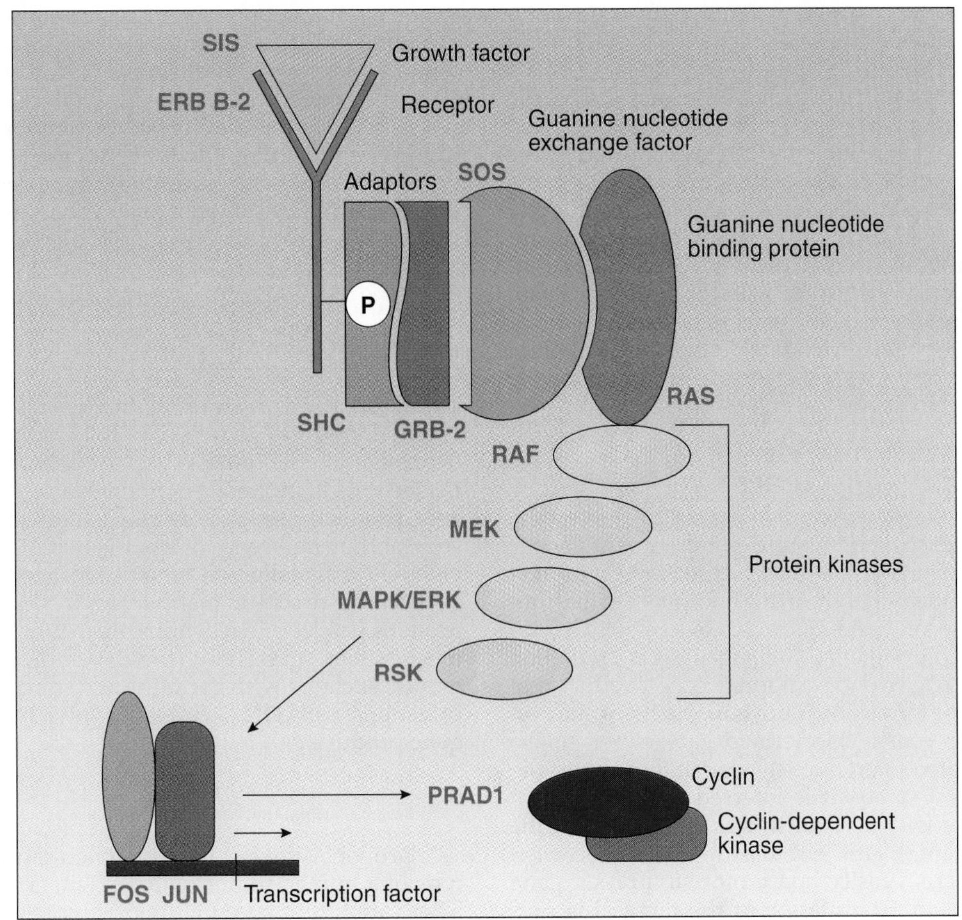

FIGURE 5-31
The ras cascade. Examples shown in *red* are oncogenic or induce cell transformation when activated or overexpressed.

factors, such as EGF or insulin-like growth factor (IGF). Protooncogenes that are expressed early in the cell cycle, such as *myc* and *fos*, render the cells competent to receive the final signals for mitosis and are, therefore, termed **competence genes**. In general, competence genes play a role in (1) progression from G_1 to S phase in the cell cycle, (2) stability of the genome, (3) apoptosis, and (4) positive or negative effects in cellular maturation.

The proteins encoded by c-*fos* and c-*jun* are components of AP-1, a transcription factor that activates the expression of a variety of genes. Jun is one target for the downstream signaling cascade that depends on ras activation. Mutations of the jun protein eliminate a negative regulatory domain, thereby prolonging the half-life of the protein. Few mutations of c-*jun* are described in human tumors, but overexpression of the protein has been described in lung and colorectal cancers.

Although nuclear proteins encoded by protooncogenes have the capacity to promote cellular proliferation, in some circumstances, they stimulate differentiation. A rapid increase in c-*fos* expression follows the induction of differentiation in a variety of cells *in vitro*, including several hemopoietic cell lines and teratocarcinomas.

c-*Myc* is a nuclear protein that binds to a variety of other proteins to regulate gene transcription. Among other proteins, such targets include p53 and ornithine decarboxylase. Activation of c-*myc* in cultured cells that have been arrested in the cell cycle by deprivation of growth factors results in their reentry into the cell cycle. As previously discussed, the translocation characteristic of Burkitt lymphoma (t8:14) constitutively activates *myc* expression.

Bcl-2 and Apoptosis

Follicular B-cell lymphomas (see Chapter 20) display a characteristic chromosomal translocation, t(14;18), in which the *bcl*-2 gene on chromosome 18 is brought under the transcriptional control of the immunoglobulin light-chain gene promoter, thereby causing overexpression of *bcl*-2. Rather than stimulating cell proliferation, *bcl*-2 is a unique oncogene that inhibits the programmed cell death (apoptosis) of the malignant B cells. As a result, the neoplastic clone accumulates in the affected lymph nodes. Since its demonstration in follicular lymphomas, *bcl*-2 expression has been observed in a variety of other human cancers and non-neoplastic conditions, although the contribution of *bcl*-2 to the disease process in these cases is not defined. Another oncogene that has anti-apoptotic properties and that has been implicated in human tumorigenesis is *lyt*10, a member of the *rel* family that codes for a protein homologous to the p50 component of the transcriptional factor NF-κB.

Mice in which the *bcl*-2 gene has been knocked out die *in utero* with prominent apoptosis of the hemopoietic and neuronal lineages, suggesting that *bcl*-2 is important in the normal development of these systems. Although the mechanism by which *bcl*-2 prevents apoptosis is not fully understood, it appears to involve its interaction with another *blc*-2 family member, namely *bax* (see Chapter 1). The expression of *bax* correlates with the apoptotic death of a variety of cell types, and *bax* is regarded as a major mediator of programmed cell death. Thus, prevention of the lethal effect of *bax* by *bcl*-2 readily accounts for the anti-apoptotic action of the latter.

Tumor Suppressor Genes

The concept of oncogenes postulates a dominant genetic alteration that results in the overproduction of a normal gene product or the synthesis of an abnormally active mutant protein. A second general mechanism by which a genetic alteration contributes to carcinogenesis is a mutation that creates a deficiency of a normal gene product that suppresses tumor formation. Since both alleles of such tumor suppressor genes (also termed gatekeeper genes) must be inactivated to produce the deficit that allows the development of a tumor, it is inferred that the normal suppressor gene is dominant. In this circumstance, the heterozygous state is sufficient to protect against cancer. **The loss of heterozygosity in a tumor suppressor gene by deletion or somatic mutation of the remaining normal allele predisposes to tumor development.**

Evidence for Tumor Suppressor Genes

The evidence for the existence of tumor suppressor genes is derived from experiments in tissue culture, studies of intact organisms, and analyses of human hereditary tumors. In tissue culture, it is possible to fuse two cells to form a single hybrid cell (heterokaryon), which contains all the chromosomes of both cells in a single nucleus. When a tumor cell is fused with a normal one, the resulting hybrid cell is not tumorigenic. It is thought that the genes from the normal cell provide a tumor suppressor function that is absent in the malignant cells.

The existence of tumor suppressor genes has been demonstrated in *Drosophila* fruit flies, in which at least 24 such genes have been identified. When two flies that are heterozygous for one of these tumor suppressor genes are mated, those offspring that are homozygous for the defective allele invariably develop tumors. Moreover, the specific gene defect determines the type of the tumor. When the cloned normal gene is introduced into mutant flies, no tumors develop. It deserves emphasis that, in a manner similar to that of protooncogenes, whose products control normal cellular functions, the tumor suppressor genes of *Drosophila* code for proteins that are crucial for normal growth and differentiation.

Studies of human hereditary cancers, of which at least 50 have been identified, provide compelling evidence for the importance of tumor suppressor genes. It has emerged that in some of these, notably retinoblastoma, Wilms tumor, and familial APC, homozygous deletions or mutations at specific genetic loci are frequent and possibly invariable features of the tumor cells. Moreover, in some tumors that are not considered hereditary (e.g., cancers of the breast and lung), there is increasing evidence that the loss of both alleles at a specific genetic locus is a regular feature.

The Role of Tumor Suppressor Genes in Carcinogenesis

Tumor suppressor genes are increasingly being incriminated in the pathogenesis of both hereditary and spontaneous cancers in humans. Two such genes have been particularly well studied. The retinoblastoma (Rb) and p53 gene products serve to restrain cell division in many tissues, and their absence or inactivation is linked to the development of malignant tumors. Oncogenic DNA viruses also encode products that interact with these suppressor proteins, thereby inactivating their functions. **Thus, the mechanisms underlying the development of some tumors associated with germline and somatic mutations or infections with DNA viruses involve the same cellular gene products.**

The Retinoblastoma Gene

Retinoblastoma, a rare childhood cancer, is the prototype of a human tumor whose origin is attributed to the inactivation of a specific tumor suppressor gene. About 40% of cases are associated with a germline mutation, whereas the remainder are not hereditary. In patients with hereditary retinoblastoma, all somatic cells carry one missing or defective allele of a gene (the Rb gene) located on the long arm of chromosome 13. By contrast, both alleles of the Rb gene are inactive in all the retinoblastoma cells. Thus, the Rb gene is assumed to have a tumor suppressor function, and the development of hereditary retinoblastoma has been attributed to two genetic events (the "two-hit" hypothesis) (Fig. 5-32).

An affected child inherits one defective Rb allele, together with one normal gene. This heterozygous state is not associated with any observable changes in the retina, presumably because 50% of the Rb gene product is sufficient to prevent the development of retinoblastoma. If the remaining normal Rb allele is inactivated by deletion or mutation, the loss of its suppressor function leads to the appearance of a retinoblastoma. Thus, the susceptibility to retinoblastoma is inherited in a dominant fashion, that is, the heterozygote develops the disease. Paradoxically, the genetic defect in the tumor itself is recessive. In sporadic cases of retinoblastoma, the child begins life with two normal Rb alleles in all somatic cells, but both are inactivated by postzygotic mutations in the retina. Since somatic mutations in the Rb gene are uncommon, the incidence of sporadic retinoblastoma is very low (1/30,000).

The Rb gene encodes a nuclear protein (p105Rb) that is crucial in the control of cell proliferation. The Rb protein interacts with a family of transcription factors (E2F) that promote the progression of the cell cycle. p105Rb exists in

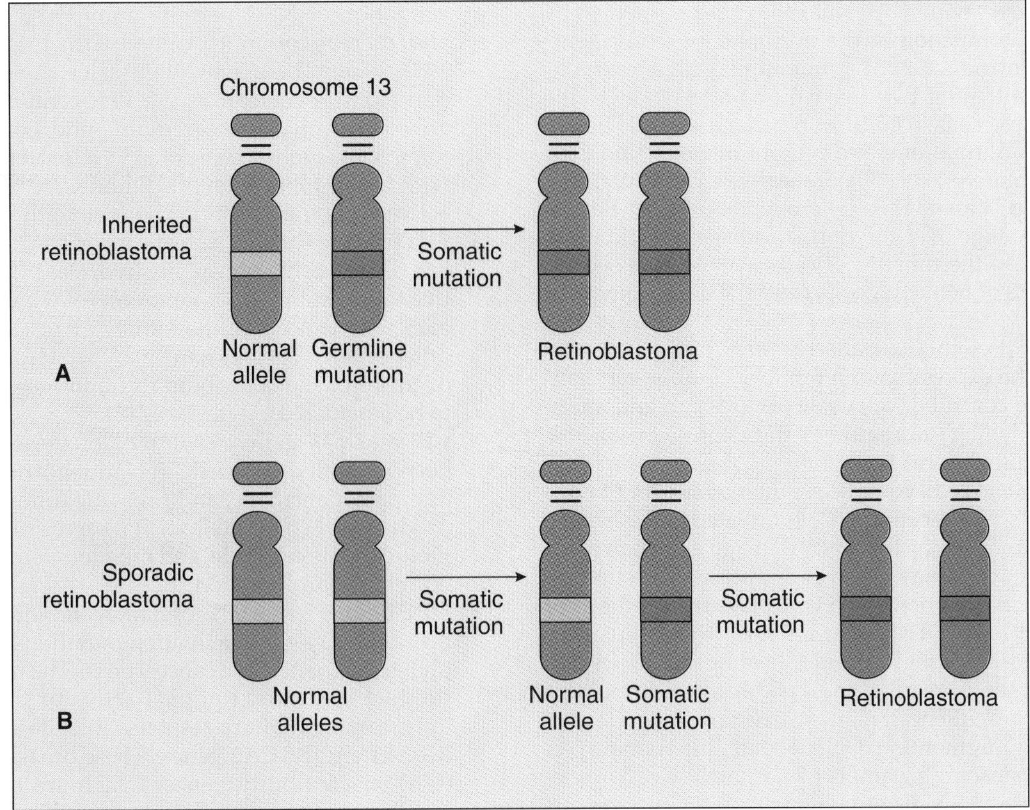

FIGURE 5-32
The "two-hit" origin of retinoblastoma. (*A*) A child with the inherited form of retinoblastoma is born with a germline mutation in one allele of the retinoblastoma gene located on the long arm of chromosome 13. A second somatic mutation in the retina leads to the inactivation of the functioning Rb allele and the subsequent development of a retinoblastoma. (*B*) In sporadic cases of retinoblastoma, the child is born with two normal Rb alleles. It requires two independent somatic mutations to inactivate Rb gene function and allow the appearance of a neoplastic clone.

two phosphorylation states; phosphorylation creates a switch between the active (hypophosphorylated) and inactive (hyperphosphorylated) forms. Shortly before entry of a cell into S phase of the cell cycle, p105Rb is phosphorylated, an effect that frees E2F from the inhibitory action of Rb, thereby permitting the cell to proceed through the S phase. This phosphorylation is dependent on cyclins, cyclin-dependent kinases (cdk), and cdk inhibitors. **It is thought that the function of Rb represents the most critical checkpoint in the cell cycle, and inactivating mutations of Rb permit unregulated cell proliferation.**

Children who inherit a mutant Rb gene also suffer a 200-fold increased risk of developing mesenchymal tumors in early adult life. More than 20 different cancers have been described, with osteosarcoma being by far the most common. Chromosomal analysis has demonstrated abnormalities of the Rb locus in 70% of cases of osteosarcoma and in some instances of small cell lung cancer, carcinoma of the breast, and other human tumors.

The p53 Gene

The p53 gene is located on the small arm of chromosome 17, and its protein product is present in virtually all normal tissues. This gene is deleted or mutated in 70% to 80% of cases of colorectal cancer and frequently in breast cancer, small cell carcinoma of the lung, hepatocellular carcinoma, astrocytoma, and numerous other tumors. **In fact, mutations of p53 seem to be the most common genetic change in human cancer.** In normal cells, p53 is a negative regulator of cell division. In response to DNA damage, p53 levels rise and prevent cells from entering the S phase of the cell cycle, thereby allowing time for DNA repair to take place. In this way, p53 acts as a guardian of the genome by restricting uncontrolled cellular proliferation under circumstances in which cells with abnormal DNA might propagate. Mutations of p53 allow cells with damaged DNA to progress through the cell cycle.

Many human cancers exhibit deletion of both p53 alleles, in which case the cell contains no p53 gene product. For instance, 80% of colon cancers carry abnormalities in both p53 alleles, usually deletion of the gene in one allele and point mutations in the other. By contrast, in some cancers, the malignant cells express one normal p53 allele and one mutant version. In these cases, the mutant p53 protein forms complexes with the normal p53 protein and thereby inactivates the function of the normal suppressor gene. Indeed, the introduction of a mutant p53 allele into normal cells (containing two normal p53 alleles) alters the growth of these cells in culture. When a mutant allele inactivates the normal one, the mutant allele is said be a dominant negative gene. Theoretically, a cell containing one mutant p53 allele (i.e., heterozygous) might have a growth advantage over the normal cells, a situation that would increase the number of cells at risk for a second mutation (loss of heterozygosity) and the development of cancer.

The p53 protein is a transcriptional factor that promotes both the expression of a number of other genes involved in the control of cell cycle progression and apoptosis. DNA damage upregulates the expression of p53, which in turn enhances the synthesis of CIP1. The latter inactivates cyclin/cdk complexes, thereby leading to cell arrest at the G_1/S checkpoint. Cells arrested at this checkpoint may either repair the DNA damage and then reenter the cycle or they may undergo apoptosis. The stimulation of gene transcription by p53 results in the synthesis of proteins (CIP1, GADD45) that enhance DNA repair by binding to proliferating cell nuclear antigen (PCNA). In this manner, the upregulation of p53 has two important and related consequences, namely arresting cell cycle progression and augmenting DNA repair. Interestingly, a gene on chromosome 1, namely p73, resembles p53 in several regions and may also function as tumor suppressor. Another gene (ING-1) codes for p33, protein that binds to p53 and promotes its activity.

Li-Fraumeni syndrome *refers to an inherited predisposition to develop cancers in many organs.* Persons with this condition carry germline mutations in one p53 allele, whereas their tumors display mutations at both alleles. This situation is similar to that determining inherited retinoblastoma and is another example of Knudson's two-hit hypothesis.

Other Tumor Suppressor Genes

A number of unrelated syndromes have now been shown to harbor germline mutations in other tumor suppressor genes.

- **APC gene:** This gene is implicated in the pathogenesis of familial adenomatous polyposis coli and some sporadic colorectal cancers. The APC gene product binds to and inhibits the function of β-catenin, a protein that interacts with Tcf and Lef transcription factors. Constitutive activation of the target genes of these transcription factors secondary to the loss of APC function may contribute to unregulated cell proliferation.
- **WT-1 gene:** The tumor suppressor gene WT-1 is mutated or deleted in hereditary Wilms tumor (WT) and is essential for the normal development of the urogenital tract. It encodes a nuclear DNA binding protein that represses transcription and also binds p53.
- **NF-1 gene:** Neurofibromatosis (NF) type 1 is related to germline alterations of the NF-1 gene, which encodes neurofibromin, a negative regulator of *ras*. Inactivation of NF-1 permits unopposed *ras* function and, thereby, promotes cell growth.
- **VHL gene:** The inactivation of the von Hippel-Lindau (VHL) gene causes the VHL syndrome, associated with renal cell carcinoma and hemangioblastoma of the brain. The normal VHL protein complexes with and inhibits elongins B and C, two factors that activate the transcription factor elongin A.
- **FHIT gene:** The fragile histidine triad (FHIT) protein is a dinucleoside phosphate hydrolase that is a putative tumor suppressor, mutations of which are associated with cancers of the kidney, digestive tract, and other organs. The mechanism by which abnormalities of this enzyme contribute to tumorigenesis remains to be elucidated.
- **p15 and p16 genes:** Deletions of these genes have been identified primarily in bladder cancers, but also in breast, pancreatic, and prostatic tumors. The gene products are cdk inhibitors that serve as negative regulators of the cell cycle, and their loss removes a brake on cellular proliferation.
- **DPC4 gene:** Some 90% of pancreatic carcinomas feature allelic loss or inactivating mutations in the DPC4 (deleted in pancreatic cancer) gene. The normal DPC4 product is a transcriptional activator that mediates the growth inhibitory response to TGF-β.
- **BRCA1 and BRCA2 genes:** These breast (BR) cancer (CA) susceptibility genes, which are also incriminated in some ovarian cancers, are tumor suppressors that are thought to be involved in checkpoint functions of the cell cycle in response to DNA damage. There is evidence that BRCA1 inhibits cell cycle progression into S phase by inducing the CDK inhibitor p21.
- **PTEN gene:** Termed the phosphatase and tensin homologue deleted on chromosome 10, this gene is mutated in many prostate cancers and gliomas, as well as other tumors. The gene product may suppress tumor cell growth by antagonizing tyrosine kinases and may regulate invasion and metastasis through interactions at focal adhesions.

Tumor Suppressor Genes and Oncogenic DNA Viruses

For many years, the mechanism of tumorigenesis by DNA viruses was puzzling. Unlike RNA tumor viruses, whose oncogenes have normal cellular counterparts, the transforming genes of DNA viruses are not homologous with any cellular genes. This conundrum was resolved with the discoveries that linked the gene products of oncogenic DNA viruses to the inactivation of tumor suppressor proteins. This phenomenon is analogous to the ability of mutant tumor suppressor proteins to inhibit their normal counterparts. Furthermore, the binding of a human papillomavirus protein to p53 accelerates the degradation of this suppressor protein. It is now recognized that the transforming proteins of polyomaviruses (including SV40), adenoviruses, and human papillomaviruses inactivate both the Rb and p53 proteins by binding to these tumor suppressors. These observations indicate that oncogenic DNA viruses use a common mechanism for altering growth regulation and, thereby, transforming cells.

Mutator Genes

The third class of genes in which mutations contribute to the pathogenesis of cancer is so-called mutator genes. In general, the normal versions of these genes (also termed caretaker genes) exercise surveillance over the integrity of genetic information by participating in the cellular response to DNA damage. The loss of these gene functions renders the DNA susceptible to the progressive accumulation of mutations; when these affect protooncogenes or tumor suppressor genes, cancer may result. The study of two hereditary syndromes associated with an increased risk of cancer, namely hereditary nonpolyposis colon cancer and ataxia telangectasia, have shed light on the roles of mutator genes.

HEREDITARY NONPOLYPOSIS COLON CANCER (HNPCC): *Also known as Lynch syndrome, HNPCC is a familial predisposition to the development of colorectal cancers in persons who do not suffer from APC.* It is estimated that some 5% of all colorectal cancers fall into this category. Patients with HNPCC display heterozygous germline mutations in at least one of four genes involved in the DNA mismatch repair system, whereas the tumors have lost the function of both alleles in the affected gene. After DNA replication is complete, this system leads to the excision and replacement of mismatched nucleotides. Mutations in these error correction genes are associated with up to a 1000-fold general increase in the rate of mutation. The incidence of cancers of the stomach and small bowel is increased in patients with HNPCC, and women with this syndrome display an increased risk for endometrial and ovarian cancers.

ATAXIA TELANGIECTASIA: *Ataxia telangiectasia (AT) is a rare hereditary syndrome that features cerebellar degeneration, immunological abnormalities, oculocutaneous telangiectasia, and a predisposition to cancer, including lymphomas, leukemias, stomach cancer, and breast cancer.* About 15% of patients with this syndrome eventually die from a malignant disease. The gene responsible for AT (AT mutated [ATM]), located on chromosome 11q22-q23, codes for a nuclear phosphoprotein that participates in multiple responses to DNA damage, including control of checkpoints in the cell cycle, activation of DNA repair enzymes, and regulation of apoptosis. There is evidence that heterozygous mutations in ATM increase the risk of breast cancer in women. In view of a carrier rate of 1% in the general population, it has been suggested that ATM mutations may contribute to a significant number of sporadic breast cancers.

Telomerase and Cancer

As cells in tissue culture continue to divide, the tips of the chromosomes, termed telomeres, progressively shorten (see Chapter 1). These structures are thought to protect the integrity of the DNA at the ends of the chromosomes, possibly by preventing exonuclease attack on these regions. Somatic cells do not normally express telomerase, an enzyme that recognizes the end of a chromosome and adds repetitive telomeric sequences to maintain the length of the telomere. Thus, with each round of cell repli-

TABLE 5-2 **Genes Implicated in the Pathogenesis of Human Cancers**

Gene	Human Cancer
Growth Factor Receptor Tyrosine Kinases	
ERB-B/HER	Squamous carcinoma, glioblastoma
ERB-B2/NEU/HER-2	Cancers of breast, ovary, stomach
RET	Thyroid cancers (papillary and medullary), MEN 2A, 2B
PDGF Receptor	Chronic myelomonocytic leukemia
TGF-β Receptor	Colon cancer
ABL (nonreceptor)	Chronic myelogenous leukemia
Cell Surface Molecules	
APC	Colon cancer
E-cadherin	Breast cancer
PTC/NBCCS	Nevoid basal cell cancer syndrome
TAN-1	T-cell acute lymphocytic leukemia
Signaling Molecules	
BCL-2	B-cell follicular lymphoma
DPC-4	Pancreatic cancer
Guanine Nucleotide Binding and Exchanger Proteins	
BCR	Chronic myelogenous leukemia
NF-1	Neurofibromatosis, type 1
RAS	Many cancers
Nuclear Proteins and Transcription Factors	
BRCA-1	Cancers of breast and ovary
BRCA-2	Breast cancer
EVII	Acute myelogenous leukemia
GLI	Glioma
MLL	Acute myelogenous leukemia
MYC	Burkitt lymphoma
N-MYC	Neuroblastoma
L-MYC	Lung cancer
VHL	Renal cancer
WT-1	Wilms tumor
Cell Cycle and DNA Damage	
ATM	Many cancers
FACC	Leukemia
FHIT	Lung cancer
MUT-L/MUT-S	Hereditary nonpolyposis colon cancer
MDM-2	Sarcomas
p53	More than 50% of all cancers
PRAD-1/BCL-1	Parathyroid adenoma, B-cell chronic lymphocytic leukemia
RB	Retinoblastoma, osteosarcomas, other cancers

TABLE 5-3 **Inherited Neoplasia Syndromes**

Disease	Associated Neoplasms	Inheritance[a]
Chromosomal Instability Syndromes		
Bloom syndrome	Leukemia, gastrointestinal cancer	R
Fanconi anemia	Leukemia, squamous cell carcinoma, hepatoma	R
Werner syndrome	Sarcomas	R
Hereditary Skin Diseases		
Nevi	Malignant melanoma	D
Giant hairy nevi	Malignant melanoma	D
Xeroderma pigmentosum	Skin cancers	R
Multiple trichoepitheliomas	Basal and squamous cell carcinomas	D
Epidermodysplasia verruciformis	Basal cell carcinoma, Bowen disease, squamous carcinoma	R
Familial atypical nevi	Malignant melanoma	D
Nevoid basal carcinoma syndrome	Basal cell carcinoma, medulloblastoma, ovarian carcinoma	D
Tylosis	Esophageal cancer	D
Endocrine System		
Multiple endocrine neoplasia syndromes	Adenomas of endocrine glands	D
Nervous System		
Retinoblastoma	Retinoblastoma	D
Neuroblastoma	Neuroblastoma	R
Phacomatoses		
Neurofibromatosis (von Recklinghausen disease)	Fibrosarcoma, schwannoma, meningioma, optic glioma	D
Tuberous sclerosis	Glial tumors, rhabdomyoma of heart, angiomyolipoma of kidney	D
von Hippel-Lindau syndrome	Cerebellar hemangioblastoma, retinal angioma, other hemangiomas	D and R
Sturge-Weber syndrome	Multiple angiomas	D
Gastrointestinal System		
Familial polyposis coli	Intestinal polyps and carcinomas	D
Gardener syndrome	Intestinal polyps and cancers, osteomas, fibromas	D
Peutz-Jegher syndrome	Intestinal polyps and cancers	D
Vascular Syndromes		
Osler-Weber-Rendu syndrome	Angiomas	D
Multiple angiolipomas	Angiolipomas	D
Ataxia telangiectasia	Lymphoma, leukemia, gastric cancer, brain tumors	R
Urogenital System		
Gonadal dysgenesis	Gonadoblastoma, dysgerminoma	R
Wilms tumor		R and D
Immunological Syndromes		
Agammaglobulinemia (Swiss type)	Lymphoma, leukemia	R
X-linked agammaglobulinemia	Lymphoma, leukemia	XR
DiGeorge syndrome	Squamous carcinoma of upper respiratory tract	D
Wiscott-Aldrich syndrome	Lymphoma	XR
Severe combined immunodeficiency	Lymphoma, leukemia, sarcoma	XR
Familial Cancer Syndrome	Carcinomas of colon, breast, endometrium, lung	D

[a] D, autosomal dominant; R, autosomal recessive; XR, X-linked recessive.

cation, the telomere progressively shortens. It has been proposed that the length of the telomeres acts as a molecular clock that governs the life span of replicating cells. Since cancer cells have been found to express telomerase, the reactivation of this enzyme is said to be necessary for the immortalization of cancer cells. Interestingly, spontaneous regression of childhood neuroblastoma is associated with a failure to upregulate telomerase. However, the subject is controversial and requires further study.

Table 5-2 lists genes that have been implicated in the pathogenesis of human cancers.

Inherited Cancer Syndromes

The etiology of cancer, as of most diseases, is intertwined with both hereditary and environmental factors. As an example, although smoking is unquestionably an environmental cause of cancer, only a minority of smokers develop any of the cancers associated with it. A parallel can be drawn with the effects of radiation. The incidence of leukemia was considerably increased in the Japanese survivors of the atom bomb explosions, but only a small proportion of these victims developed leukemia or any other cancer. In both of these examples, "constitutional" or hereditary factors presumably influence the development of cancer. In as genetically diverse a population as humans, it is unlikely that many cancers have either a purely environmental or an unequivocally hereditary etiology. In all probability, they constitute a continuum in which both these components contribute to a greater or lesser extent. Compounding this uncertainty is our ignorance of most of the environmental and hereditary factors that may be involved. Heritable cancer syndromes attributed to germline mutations comprise only 1% of all cancers.

The hereditary tumors can be arbitrarily divided into three categories: (1) inherited malignant tumors (e.g., retinoblastoma, Wilms tumor, and many endocrine tumors); (2) benign inherited tumors that remain benign or have a malignant potential (e.g., APC); and (3) inherited syndromes associated with a high risk of malignant tumors (e.g., Bloom syndrome and AT). Most of these are discussed in detail in the chapters dealing with specific organs, and selected examples are given in Table 5-3. In many cases, the underlying genetic defect responsible for the tumor development has been identified. Some disorders that are difficult to classify, called **phacomatoses**, have both developmental and neoplastic features. The tumors associated with these syndromes mostly involve the nervous system.

Although only a small proportion of all cancers show a mendelian pattern of inheritance, certain cancers exhibit an undeniable tendency to run in families. It is estimated that for many tumors other members of the family of an affected person have a twofold to threefold increase in the risk of developing the same cancer. This predisposition is particularly marked for cancer of the breast and colon. The interplay of heredity and environment is exemplified by the case of lung cancer. Smokers who are closely related to a person with lung cancer have a higher risk of developing lung cancer themselves than smokers without this familial background.

THE CLONAL ORIGIN OF CANCER

Studies of human and experimental tumors have provided strong evidence that most cancers arise from a single transformed cell. This theory has been most thoroughly examined in connection with proliferative disorders of the hemopoietic system. The most common piece of clinical evidence in its favor is the production by neoplastic plasma cells of a single immunoglobulin unique to an individual patient with multiple myeloma. Indeed, such a "monoclonal spike" in the serum electrophoresis from a patient with suspected myeloma is regarded as conclusive evidence of the disease. Similarly, cell surface markers have been used to establish a monoclonal origin for many other hemopoietic malignant disorders. For example, B-cell lymphomas are composed of cells that exclusively display either κ- or λ-light chains on

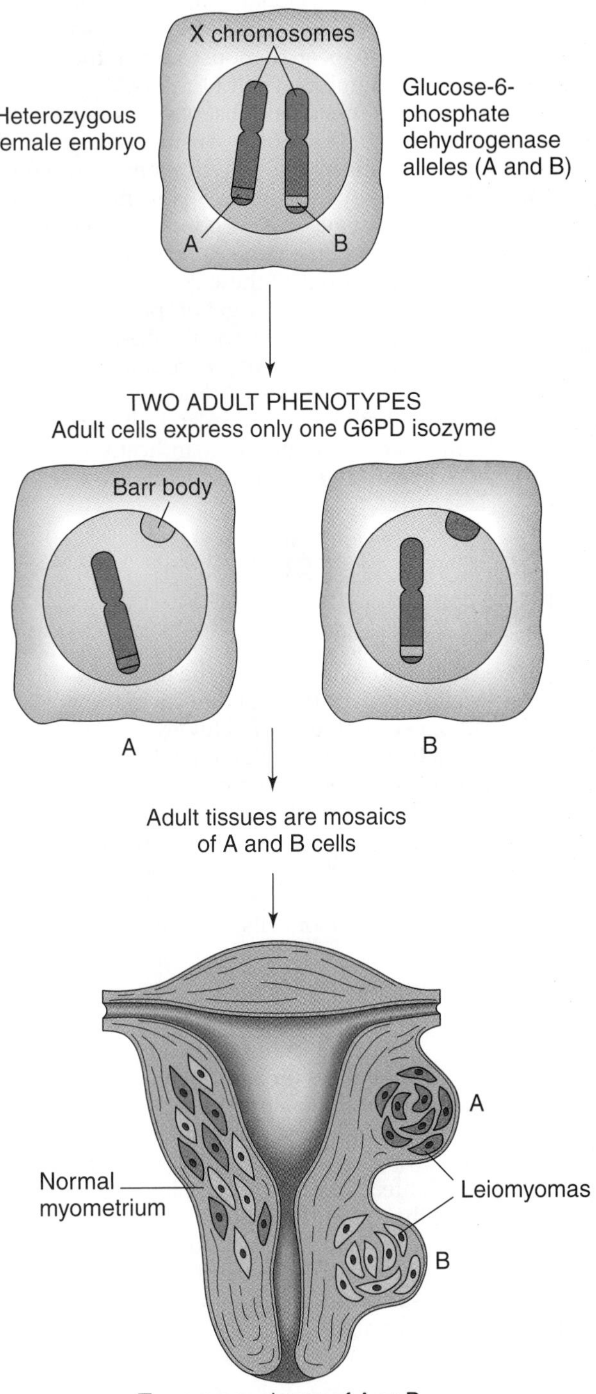

FIGURE 5-33
Monoclonal origin of human tumors. Some females are heterozygous for the two alleles of glucose-6-phosphate dehydrogenase (G6PD) on the long arm of the X chromosome. Early in embryogenesis, one of the X chromosomes is randomly inactivated in every somatic cell and appears cytologically as a Barr body attached to the nuclear membrane. As a result, the tissues are a mosaic of cells that express either the A or the B isozyme of G6PD. Leiomyomas of the uterus have been shown to contain one or the other isozyme (A or B) but not both, a finding that demonstrates the monoclonal origin of the tumors.

their surface, whereas polyclonal lymphoid proliferations are characterized by the presence of both types of cells. Monoclonality has also been demonstrated in the individual metastases of a number of solid tumors.

One of the most important observations in regard to the monoclonal origin of cancer was derived from the study of glucose-6-phosphate dehydrogenase in women who were heterozygous for its two isozymes, A and B (Fig. 5-33). These isozymes are encoded by genes located on the X chromosome. Since one X chromosome is randomly inactivated, only one of these genes is expressed in any given cell. Thus, whereas the genotypes of all cells are the same, their phenotypes vary with regard to the expression of isozyme A or B. An examination of benign uterine smooth muscle tumors (leiomyomas, or "fibroids") revealed that all the cells in an individual tumor expressed either A or B, but not both, indicating that each tumor was derived from a single progenitor cell.

CANCER AS ALTERED DIFFERENTIATION

We have seen that in many cancers the malignant phenotype results, at least in part, from defects in the normally strict control of cell proliferation. However, in some cancers, it is thought that the malignant cells result from a maturation arrest in the sequence of development from a stem cell to a fully differentiated cell. According to this theory, tumor cells accumulate because the mechanisms that control the total number of cells in the fully differentiated compartment of some tissues do not apply when less differentiated precursor cells fail to mature.

SQUAMOUS CELL CARCINOMA: In many tumors, most of the neoplastic cells are outside the cell cycle and, thus, do not contribute to the malignancy of the tumor. For example, as previously noted, fewer than 3% of the cells in a squamous carcinoma maintain the malignant potential of the tumor, and most differentiate and die spontaneously. When such terminally differentiated tumor cells are transplanted into appropriate hosts, they do not grow, whereas their undifferentiated counterparts from the same tumor form typical squamous carcinomas. Such observations support the theory that the initial step in the development of some cancers is a failure of the stem cell to differentiate normally.

TERATOCARCINOMA: Further evidence to support the concept of cancer as a failure of differentiation has come from the study of experimental malignant germ cell tumors (teratocarcinomas). A single embryonal carcinoma cell, the stem cell of a teratocarcinoma, when transplanted into a mouse, gives rise to a tumor that contains cells derived from all three germ layers. Clearly, the progeny of the original transplanted tumor cell differentiate into more mature cells, which express recognizable phenotypes of more fully differentiated tissues. When these differentiated tissues of the teratocarcinoma are separated from the malignant embryonal cells and transplanted into compatible hosts, they not only survive but also function with no detriment to the host. These cells are clearly benign, and the dogma "once a cancer cell, always a cancer cell" does not hold in this case.

A further refinement of this approach involves the transplantation of a single teratocarcinoma stem cell from a mouse into an early mouse embryo. At term, the entirely normal pup is a mosaic composed of cells derived from both the embryo proper and the teratocarcinoma. The progeny of the malignant cell, under the influence of normal developmental controls, has differentiated into mature tissue elements. Thus, at least in the experimental situation, the altered expression of genetic information inherent in the definition of a cancer may be redirected into modes of expression that are normal for that particular cell.

Clinical analogies to the experimental situation do exist. The best known is illustrated by the rare spontaneous conversion of a malignant neuroblastoma to its better-differentiated, benign counterpart, ganglioneuroma.

LEUKEMIAS AND LYMPHOMAS: The most comprehensive systematic analysis of human neoplasia from the perspective of developmental biology has come from the study of leukemias and lymphomas. During normal B- and T-lymphocyte maturation, there are well-documented sequential changes of membrane antigens and rearrangements of immunoglobulin and T-cell receptor genes. In acute lymphoblastic leukemia of childhood, the neoplastic cells exhibit only partial assembly of the cell surface receptor molecules that characterize mature lymphocytes. In other words, the leukemic cell phenotype bears a strong resemblance to lymphocytes that appear transiently during the developmental sequence of the normal lymphocyte. Thus, the leukemic cells appear to be "frozen" in the act of receptor gene assembly and expression.

Acute myeloid leukemia is similar to acute lymphoblastic leukemia in that the malignant cells express phenotypes of transient, immature myeloid populations. Likewise, studies of chronic lymphocytic leukemias and lymphomas have revealed that these malignant disorders represent clonal expansions of lymphocyte populations corresponding to subsets found in normal lymphoid tissue.

In normal hemopoietic maturation, differentiation is tightly coupled to proliferation—that is, terminally differentiated cells are continually lost, to be replaced by newly proliferated and differentiated cells. By contrast, the data reviewed earlier suggest that certain leukemias and lymphomas are not truly proliferative disorders but rather reflect an uncoupling of differentiation from proliferation, with the resulting accumulation of cells that have not attained terminal differentiation. According to this theory, leukemia and lymphoma may represent the stabilization of a phenotype that is also expressed, though only transiently, in developing normal cells. It has been said that the cell phenotypes in a leukemia or lymphoma can be compared with the phenotype of the ostrich, which is believed to be "primitive and conserved rather than degenerate."

RETINOIDS: The view that certain cancers may reflect impaired differentiation has led to a search for maturation-enhancing drugs. The interest in the retinoids derives from experiments showing that administration of excess vitamin A or its derivatives inhibits chemically induced carcinogenesis in the skin, lung, bladder, colon, and mammary gland.

A dramatic response to all-*trans*-retinoic acid is generated in acute promyelocytic leukemia, in which the administration of this agent induces a complete remission in the majority of patients. In this disease, the reciprocal translocation between chromosomes 15 and 17 results in a fusion gene consisting of the retinoic acid receptor and the PML gene. The chimeric protein blocks myeloid differentiation at the promyelocyte stage, a process that is reversed by retinoic acid. Other forms of retinoic acid have shown limited activity against mycosis fungoides (cutaneous T-cell lymphoma) and certain low-grade skin cancers.

VIRUSES AND HUMAN CANCER

Despite the existence of viral oncogenes in acute transforming viruses and transforming genes in oncogenic DNA viruses, the number of human cancers definitely associated with viral infections is limited. Nevertheless, it is estimated that viral infections are responsible for 15% of all human cancers. The strongest associations between the presence of viruses and the development of cancer in humans are (1) the RNA retrovirus human T-cell leukemia virus type I and T-cell leukemia/lymphoma, (2) human papillomavirus (DNA) and squamous carcinoma of the cervix, (3) hepatitis B virus (DNA) and primary hepatocellular carcinoma, (4) Epstein-Barr virus and certain forms of lymphoma and nasopharyngeal carcinoma, and (5) human herpesvirus 8 (DNA) and Kaposi sarcoma. Worldwide, infections with hepatitis B virus and human papillomaviruses alone account for 80% of all virus-associated cancers

Human T-Cell Leukemia Viruses (HTLV-I and -II)

The one human cancer that has been firmly linked to infection with an RNA retrovirus is the rare adult T-cell leukemia, which is endemic to parts of Japan, Africa, the Caribbean basin, and the southeastern United States. The etiological agent, human T-cell leukemia virus (HTLV-I), is tropic for CD4+ T lymphocytes and has also been incriminated in the pathogenesis of a number of neurological disorders. It is estimated that leukemia develops in 1% to 4% of persons infected with HTLV-I. A closely related virus, HTLV-II, has been associated with a few cases of a T-cell variant of hairy cell leukemia, but firm evidence for its oncogenic potential is still lacking.

HTLV-I differs from other oncogenic retroviruses in two important respects: (1) the genome of the virus contains no known oncogene, and (2) it does not integrate at specific sites within the host genome. Thus, it is inappropriate to group HTLV-I with either the acute or slow transforming retroviruses. On structural grounds, HTLV is analogous to a number of other retroviruses, including simian T-cell leukemia virus type I, bovine leukemia virus, and human immunodeficiency viruses (HIV-1 and HIV-2). To understand these similarities, it is helpful to compare the viral genomes of these retroviruses.

In general, replication-competent transforming retroviruses have three sequential open reading frames, which code for (1) the core protein (gag), (2) the DNA polymerase (pol), and (3) the envelope protein (env). Promoter and enhancer sequences are present in the form of the LTRs at each end of the genome. These regulatory sequences act in a *cis* fashion, that is they promote the transcription of adjacent regions, in this instance the *gag*, *pol*, and *env* genes.

By contrast, HTLV-I (and the analogous viruses mentioned earlier) contains not only the components of the usual retroviral genome but also a novel region at the 3′ end that encodes regulatory proteins. These proteins, termed **Tax** and **Rex** in HTLV-I, are *trans*-regulatory, that is, they act at a distance from the site of their transcription. Tax and Rex are nuclear proteins that are essential for viral replication. Tax protein increases the transcription from its own viral LTR and promotes the activity of other genes involved in cell proliferation. These include genes that code for interleukin-2 (IL-2) and its receptor, granulocyte macrophage colony-stimulating factor (GM-CSF), and the protooncogenes c-*fos* and c-*sis*. Although the precise roles of Tax and Rex in HTLV-induced transformation of T cells have not been elucidated, it is likely that they participate in the early transformational events. Since lymphocyte transformation *in vitro* by HTLV-I is initially polyclonal and only later monoclonal, it is thought that Tax and Rex may initiate the transformation process, but that additional genetic events are required for the appearance of the complete malignant phenotype. In this respect, the multistep process hypothesized for HTLV-I-induced oncogenesis is similar to that proposed for most human cancers.

DNA Viruses

Almost all groups of DNA viruses contain at least one representative virus that produces or is closely associated with an animal tumor. Four DNA viruses (human papillomavirus, Epstein-Barr virus, hepatitis B virus, herpesvirus 8) are incriminated in the development of human cancers.

Infection of cultured cells with oncogenic DNA viruses almost always leads to the appearance of clones that express viral genes, and the expressed viral proteins are required for the maintenance of the transformed state. The transforming genes of oncogenic DNA viruses exhibit virtually no homology with cellular genes, whereas the transforming genes of retroviruses (oncogenes) are derived from and are homologous with their cellular counterparts (protooncogenes). As discussed earlier, oncogenic DNA viruses have genes that encode protein products that bind to specific host proteins (the products of tumor suppressor genes) involved in the regulation of cell proliferation. Thus, they decouple cell proliferation from inhibitory control and play a role in the creation of the transformed phenotype of a cancer cell.

Human Papillomaviruses

Human papillomaviruses (HPVs) induce lesions in humans that progress to squamous cell carcinoma. Papillomaviruses manifest a pronounced tropism for epithelial tissues, unlike other tumor viruses, which are associated principally with sarcomas and hemopoietic neoplasms. The full productive life cycle of HPV occurs only in squamous cells. In animals, papillomaviruses produce benign papillomas of squamous epithelia (e.g., the skin and esophagus), adenomas of the glandular epithelium of the intestine, and papillomas of the bladder. A significant proportion of these benign animal tumors progress to frank malignancy. A similar situation is seen in humans. As in animals, HPV definitely causes benign lesions of squamous epithelium, including warts, laryngeal papillomas, and condylomata acuminata (genital warts) of the vulva, penis, and perianal region. Occasionally condylomata acuminata and laryngeal papillomas undergo malignant transformation to squamous cell carcinoma. Although warts of the skin invariably remain benign, in a rare hereditary disease, termed **epidermodysplasia verruciformis**, HPV produces flat warts that commonly progress to squamous carcinoma. It is noteworthy that all of these malignant transformations of benign squamous lesions in animals and humans exemplify the multistep nature of cancer development, proceeding through dysplasia and carcinoma *in situ*, to frank invasion.

Human papillomavirus contains circular double-stranded DNA, 8000 base pairs in length. More than 75 different types of HPV have been identified. Since the virus cannot be typed by serological methods, it is classified by DNA hybridization; viruses that differ by more than 50% DNA homology are categorized as different types. Each of the various types of HPV has been associated with a particular clinical syndrome, including plantar warts, verruca vulgaris, laryngeal papillomas, genital warts, and Bowen disease. Certain strains of HPV (particularly types 16 and 18) are associated with the development of epithelial dysplasia of the uterine cervix, which can progress to carcinoma *in situ* and eventually to invasive squamous cell carcinoma. Importantly, it is clear that HPV infection by itself is not sufficient for progression from dysplasia to carcinoma. This multistep sequence requires other factors, probably additional mutations. The role of HPV in the pathogenesis of squamous cancers of the female genital tract is discussed in detail in Chapter 18. HPV, particularly type 16, is also incriminated in the development of penile cancer.

The major oncoproteins encoded by HPV are E6 and E7. E6 binds to p53 and targets it for degradation. Interestingly, E6 also activates telomerase. E7 binds to Rb, thereby releasing its inhibitory effect on cell cycle progression. The transforming genes of HPV are similar to those of polyomaviruses (T antigen) and adenoviruses (E1A and E1B) in binding to tumor suppressor proteins.

Epstein-Barr Virus

Epstein-Barr virus (EBV), a well-defined human herpesvirus, is composed of linear double-stranded DNA, about 170,000 base pairs in length. This virus is so widely disseminated that 95% of adults in the world have antibodies to it. EBV infects B lymphocytes in humans and other primates, a situation similar to the tropism of other herpesviruses of nonhuman primates. The binding of EBV to CD21, a glycoprotein on the surface of B lymphocytes, initiates the transformation of these cells into lymphoblasts with an indefinite life span. In a small proportion of primary infections with EBV, this lymphoblastoid transformation is manifested as infectious mononucleosis (see Chapter 9), a short-lived lymphoproliferative disease. However, EBV is also intimately associated with the development of certain human cancers.

When B lymphocytes are infected with EBV, they acquire the ability to proliferate indefinitely *in vitro*. A number of EBV genes are implicated in this lymphocyte immortalization, including Epstein-Barr nuclear antigens (EBNAs) and latent-infection-associated membrane proteins (LMPs). The EBNAs maintain the EBV genome in its episomal state and activate the transcription of viral and cellular genes. LMP1 interacts with cellular proteins that normally transduce signals from the TNF receptor, a critical pathway in lymphocyte activation and proliferation. Both EBNAs and LMPs can be demonstrated in most EBV-associated cancers.

BURKITT LYMPHOMA: EBV was the first virus to be unequivocally linked to the development of a human tumor. In 1958, Burkitt described a form of childhood lymphoma in a geographic belt across equatorial Africa, which he suggested might have a viral etiology. A few years later, Epstein and Barr discovered viral particles in cell lines cultured from patients with Burkitt lymphoma.

African Burkitt lymphoma is a B-cell tumor, in which the neoplastic lymphocytes invariably contain EBV in their DNA and manifest EBV-related antigens. The tumor has also been recognized in non-African populations, but in those cases only about 20% contain the EBV genome. The localization of Burkitt lymphoma to equatorial Africa is not understood, but it has been suggested that prolonged stimulation of the immune system by endemic malaria may be important. Under normal circumstances, the EBV-stimulated B-lymphocyte proliferation is controlled by suppressor T cells. The lack of an adequate T-cell response often reported in chronic malarial infections might result in uncontrolled B-cell proliferation, thereby providing the background for further genetic events that lead to the development of lymphoma. One of these is known to be a chromosomal translocation, in which the c-*myc* protooncogene is deregulated by being brought into proximity with an immunoglobulin promoter region. In 75% of the cases, the c-*myc* protooncogene on chromosome 8 is translocated to chromosome 14 at the site of the immunoglobulin promoter. In 25% of the cases, the c-*myc* protooncogene remains in its normal location on chromosome 8, but an immunoglobulin promoter from either chromosome 2 or chromosome 22 is translocated to chromosome 8. A role for the deregulation of c-*myc* in the pathogenesis of Burkitt lymphoma is supported by the demonstration that the introduction of an activated c-*myc* gene into EBV-infected human B lymphocytes renders the cells tumorigenic. Thus, a postulated sequence in the multistep pathogenesis of African Burkitt lymphoma is as follows:

1. Infection and polyclonal lymphoblastoid transformation of B lymphocytes by EBV
2. Proliferation of B cells and inhibition of suppressor T cells induced by malaria

3. Deregulation of the c-*myc* protooncogene by chromosomal translocation in a single transformed B lymphocyte
4. Uncontrolled proliferation of a malignant clone of B lymphocytes

Burkitt lymphoma is further discussed in Chapter 20.

POLYCLONAL LYMPHOPROLIFERATION IN IMMUNODEFICIENT STATES: Congenital or acquired immunodeficiency states can be complicated by the development of EBV-induced B-cell proliferative disorders. These lesions may be clinically and pathologically indistinguishable from true malignant lymphomas, but they differ in that most of them are polyclonal. The incidence of lymphoid neoplasia in immunosuppressed renal transplant recipients is 30 to 50 times that of the general population. In virtually all cases of lymphoproliferations associated with organ transplantation, EBNA or EBV genomic material is present in the neoplastic tissue. Similar B-cell lymphoproliferative disorders are seen in a number of other acquired immunodeficiencies, notably, acquired immunodeficiency syndrome (AIDS). Occasionally, a true monoclonal lymphoma may develop in the background of an EBV-induced lymphoproliferative disorder.

Congenital immunodeficiency states, including X-linked lymphoproliferative syndrome (XLP), Wiskott-Aldrich syndrome, and AT, are associated with EBV infections and aggressive lymphoproliferations. The best studied of these conditions is XLP. In this familial disorder, clinical immunodeficiency is commonly inapparent until the onset of a particularly severe, and often fatal, form of infectious mononucleosis. In many of these patients who survive infectious mononucleosis, lymphoproliferative disorders and lymphomas ensue. Patients with XLP lack EBV-specific immune responses, including the formation of cytotoxic T cells that normally eliminate EBV-infected B cells.

NASOPHARYNGEAL CARCINOMA: Nasopharyngeal carcinoma is a variant of squamous cell carcinoma that has a worldwide distribution and is particularly common in certain parts of Africa and Asia. EBV DNA and EBNA are present in virtually all of these cancers. EBV gains access to the squamous epithelial cells of the nasopharynx by forming an IgA-EBV complex, which is then taken up by endocytosis. It has been suggested that the pathogenesis of nasopharyngeal carcinoma is related to infection with EBV in early childhood, with reactivation at 40 to 50 years of age and the appearance of tumors 1 to 2 years thereafter. Fortunately, 70% of patients with this disease are cured by radiation therapy alone.

Hepatitis B Virus

Hepatitis B virus (HBV), a partially double-stranded DNA virus, infects only humans, although separate, closely related hepadnaviruses infect woodchucks, ground squirrels, and domestic ducks. **Epidemiological studies have clearly established an association between chronic infection with HBV (chronic hepatitis and cirrhosis) and the development of primary hepatocellular carcinoma.**

The geographic incidence of hepatocellular carcinoma correlates well with the prevalence of chronic carriers of HBV. Moreover, prospective studies in Asia, where HBV infection is endemic, have shown that the risk for hepatocellular carcinoma in carriers is more than 200 times greater than that in noncarriers (see Chapter 14). Animals chronically infected with hepadnaviruses also exhibit a high incidence of primary hepatocellular carcinoma.

Two mechanisms have been invoked to explain the mechanism of carcinogenesis in HBV-related liver cancer. One theory holds that the continued liver cell proliferation that accompanies chronic liver injury eventually leads to malignant transformation. Transgenic mice expressing the gene for the surface antigen of HBV (HBsAg) have consistently demonstrated a prolonged interval of chronic liver injury and inflammation, culminating in the appearance of hepatocellular carcinoma. In addition, chronic infection with a hepatotropic RNA virus (hepatitis C virus [HCV]) also carries a high risk for the development of hepatocellular carcinoma. Thus, chronic liver cell injury and regeneration may be sufficient to cause hepatocellular carcinoma, and HBV may be oncogenic in humans by virtue of its ability to induce chronic liver disease.

A second theory implicates a virally encoded protein in the pathogenesis of HBV-induced liver cancer. Transgenic mice expressing the HBx gene, a small viral regulatory protein, also developed liver cancer, but without evident preexisting liver cell injury and inflammation. The HBx gene product has been shown *in vitro* to upregulate a number of cellular genes. In addition, similar to other DNA viral oncoproteins, HBx binds to and inactivates p53. The underlying mechanisms in HBV-induced carcinogenesis are still controversial and require further investigation.

Human Herpesvirus 8 and Kaposi Sarcoma

Kaposi sarcoma is a vascular neoplasm that was originally described in eastern European elderly men and later in central African blacks (see Chapter 10). Kaposi sarcoma is today the most common neoplasm associated with AIDS. The neoplastic cells have recently been shown to contain sequences of a novel virus known as human herpesvirus 8 (HHV 8) or Kaposi sarcoma–associated herpesvirus (KSHV). Interestingly, HHV 8 has also been demonstrated in specimens of Kaposi sarcoma from HIV-negative patients. In addition to infecting the spindle cells of Kaposi sarcoma, HHV 8 is lymphotropic and has been implicated in two uncommon B-cell lymphoid malignancies, namely body cavity–based lymphoma and multicentric Castleman disease.

CHEMICAL CARCINOGENESIS

A brief historical overview of chemical carcinogenesis is not only of inherent interest but also points the way to the details that require amplification. The entire field of chemical carcinogenesis originated some two centuries ago in descriptions of an occupational disease. (This was not the first recognition of an occupation-related cancer, since a peculiar predisposition of nuns to breast cancer was appreciated even earlier.) To the English physician Sir Percival Pott goes the credit for relating cancer of the scrotum in chimney sweeps to a specific chemical exposure, namely soot. Interestingly, the great German pathologist Rudolf Virchow attributed these scrotal tumors to irritation rather than to chemicals. He persisted in this mistaken notion even though at about the same time the high incidence of skin cancer in some German workers had been ascribed to an exposure to coal tar, whose ingredients were known to be remarkably similar to soot. Almost a century elapsed between those observations and the realization that other products of the combustion of organic materials are responsible for a man-made epidemic of cancer, namely, cancer of the lung in cigarette smokers.

The experimental production of cancer by chemicals dates to 1915, when Japanese investigators produced skin cancers in rabbits with coal tar. Since that time, the list of organic and inorganic carcinogens has grown exponentially. Yet a curious paradox existed for many years. Many compounds known to be potent carcinogens are relatively inert in terms of chemical reactivity. **The solution to this riddle became apparent in the early 1960s, when it was shown that most, although not all, chemical carcinogens require metabolic activation before they can react with cell constituents.** On the basis of those observations and the close correlation between mutagenicity and carcinogenicity, an *in vitro* assay utilizing *Salmonella* organisms for screening potential chemical carcinogens—the Ames test—was developed a decade later. Subsequently, a variety of assays for genotoxicity were developed and are still used to screen chemicals and new drugs for potential carcinogenicity.

Chemical Carcinogens as Mutagens

Associations between exposure to a specific chemical and human cancers have historically been established on the basis of epidemiological studies. These studies have numerous inherent disadvantages, including uncertainties in estimated doses, variability of the population, long and variable latency, and dependence on clinical and public health records of questionable accuracy. Moreover, a negative result—that is, a lack of association between the chemical and cancer—often does not necessarily exclude a weak carcinogenic effect. As an alternative to epidemiological studies, investigators turned to the use of studies involving animals. Indeed, such studies are legally required before the introduction of a new drug. Yet the logarithmic increase in the number of chemicals synthesized every year makes even this method prohibitively cumbersome and expensive. The search for rapid, reproducible, and reliable screening assays for potential carcinogenic activity has centered on the relationship between carcinogenicity and mutagenicity.

A mutagen is an agent that can permanently alter the genetic constitution of a cell. The most widely used screening test, the Ames test, uses the appearance of frameshift mutations and base-pair substitutions in a culture of bacteria of the *Salmonella* species. Mutations and unscheduled DNA synthesis (DNA repair) are also detected in rat hepatocytes, mouse lymphoma cells, and Chinese hamster ovary cells. Cultured human cells are now increasingly used for assays of mutagenicity. About 90% of known carcinogens are mutagenic in these systems. Moreover, most, but not all, mutagens are carcinogenic. This close correlation between carcinogenicity and mutagenicity presumably occurs because both reflect damage to DNA. Although not infallible, the *in vitro* mutagenicity assay has proved to be a valuable tool in screening for the carcinogenic potential of chemicals.

Chemical Carcinogenesis as a Multistep Process

We have previously mentioned that carcinogenesis is a multistep process. Studies of chemical carcinogenesis in experimental animals have shed light on the individual stages in the progression of normal cells to cancer. Early studies of chemical carcinogenesis demonstrated that a single application of a carcinogen to the skin of a mouse was not, by itself, sufficient to produce cancer (Fig. 5-34). However, when a proliferative stimulus was then applied locally, in the form of a second, noncarcinogenic, irritating chemical (e.g., a phorbol ester), tumors appeared. The first effect was termed **initiation**. The action of the second, noncarcinogenic chemical was called **promotion**. Subsequently, further experiments in rodent models of a variety of organ-specific cancers (liver, skin, lung, pancreas, colon, etc.) expanded the concept of a two-stage mechanism to our present understanding of carcinogenesis as a multistep process.

From these studies, one can abstract four stages of chemical carcinogenesis:

1. **Initiation** is the first stage and likely represents mutations in a single cell. The phenotype of the initiated cells is influenced by its tissue of origin, and it encompasses resistance to the toxicity of the initiating agent, maturation abnormalities, and changes in response to hormones and growth factors.

FIGURE *5-34*
The concept of initiation and promotion. (*A*) The single application of an initiator to the skin of a mouse produces initiated cells, but no papillomas form. (*B*) Likewise, the application of a promoter alone to the skin produces no papillomas. (*C*) If the promoter is applied to the skin before the application of the initiator, no papillomas form, although initiated cells are present. (*D*) When the skin is first exposed to the initiator, the subsequent application of the promoter results in papillomas. If the promoter is withdrawn, the papillomas regress, leaving initiated cells in their place. When the promoter is applied to mouse skin bearing papillomas, invasive squamous cell carcinomas are produced.

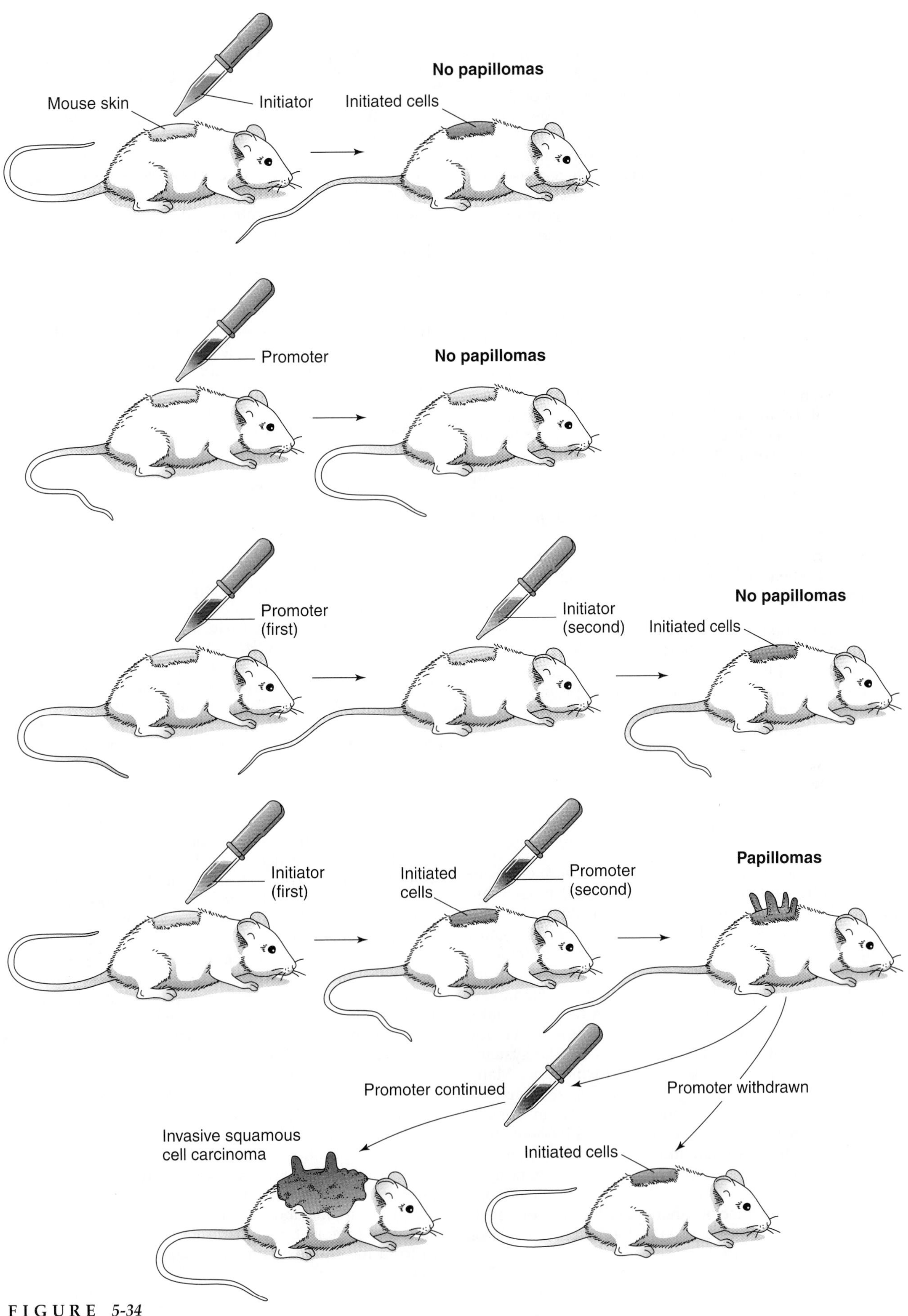
No papillomas
Mouse skin
Initiator
Initiated cells
Promoter
No papillomas
Promoter
(first)
Initiator
(second)
No papillomas
Initiated cells
Initiator
(first)
Initiated
cells
Promoter
(second)
Papillomas
Promoter continued
Promoter withdrawn
Invasive squamous
cell carcinoma
Initiated cells

FIGURE *5-34*

2. **Promotion** is the stage that follows initiation and is characterized by clonal expansion of the initiated cell. During this second stage, the altered cells do not exhibit autonomous growth but remain dependent on the continued presence of the promoting stimulus. This stimulus may be an exogenous chemical or physical agent, or it may reflect an endogenous mechanism (e.g., hormonal stimulation [breast, prostate] or the effect of bile salts [colon]). In this context, persons carrying a germline oncogenic mutation may develop cancer in a particular organ that is sensitive to a tissue-specific promoter, for instance the effect of estrogen on the endometrium or the breast.
3. **Progression** is the third stage, in which growth becomes autonomous. At this stage, the progression to cancer is independent of the carcinogen or the promoter. The mechanism underlying spontaneous progression is thought to relate to constitutive genomic instability and is characterized by nonrandom, sequential genetic events (e.g., deletions, activating [oncogenes] or inactivating [tumor suppressor genes] mutations, or gene amplifications). These genomic changes in individual cells presumably endow them with a relative growth advantage, which in turn results in their further clonal expansion.
4. **Cancer**, the end result of the entire sequence, is established when the cells acquire the capacity to invade and metastasize.

The morphological changes that reflect multistep carcinogenesis in humans is best exemplified in epithelia, such as those of the skin, cervix, and colon. Although initiation has no morphological counterpart, promotion and progression are represented by the sequence of hyperplasia, dysplasia, and carcinoma *in situ*.

Chemical Carcinogens and their Metabolism

Chemicals cause cancer either directly or, more often, after metabolic activation. The direct-acting carcinogens are inherently sufficiently reactive to bind covalently to cellular macromolecules. In addition to a number of organic compounds, such as nitrogen mustard, *bis*(chloromethyl)ether, and benzyl chloride, certain metals are included in this category. The great majority of organic carcinogens, however, require conversion to an ultimate, more reactive compound. This conversion is enzymatic and, for the most part, is effected by the cellular systems involved in drug metabolism and detoxification. Many cells in the body, particularly liver cells, possess enzyme systems that are capable of converting procarcinogens to their active forms. Yet each carcinogen has its own spectrum of target tissues, often limited to a single organ. The basis for organ specificity in chemical carcinogenesis is not well understood, but there is experimental evidence to suggest that other factors are required for tumor development in certain tissues, such as the suspected role of cystitis in bladder cancer.

POLYCYCLIC AROMATIC HYDROCARBONS: The polycyclic aromatic hydrocarbons, originally derived from coal tar, are among the most extensively studied carcinogens. In this class are such model compounds as benzo(a)pyrene, 3-methylcholanthrene, and dibenzanthracene. These compounds have a broad range of target organs and generally produce cancers at the site of application. The specific type of cancer produced varies with the route of administration and includes tumors of the skin, soft tissues, and breast. Since polycyclic hydrocarbons have been identified in cigarette smoke, it has been suggested that they may be involved in the production of lung cancer.

Polycyclic hydrocarbons are metabolized by cytochrome P_{450}-dependent mixed-function oxidases to electrophilic epoxides, which in turn react with proteins and nucleic acids. The formation of the epoxide depends on the presence of an unsaturated carbon–carbon bond. For example, vinyl chloride, the simple two-carbon molecule from which the widely used plastic polyvinyl chloride is synthesized, is metabolized to an epoxide, which is responsible for its carcinogenic properties. Workers exposed to the vinyl chloride monomer in the ambient atmosphere later developed angiosarcomas of the liver.

AFLATOXIN: In contrast to the polycyclic hydrocarbons, which are for the most part formed either by the combustion of organic material or synthetically, a heterocyclic hydrocarbon, aflatoxin B_1, is a natural product of the fungus *Aspergillus flavus*. Like the polycyclic aromatic hydrocarbons, aflatoxin B_1 is metabolized to an epoxide, which either is detoxified or binds covalently to DNA (Fig. 5-35). Aflatoxin B_1 is among the most potent liver carcinogens recognized, producing tumors in fish, birds, rodents, and primates. Since *Aspergillus* species are ubiquitous, contamination of vegetable foods, particularly peanuts and grains exposed to the warm moist conditions that favor the growth of this mold, may result in the formation of significant amounts of aflatoxin B_1. It has been suggested that aflatoxin-rich foods may contribute to the high incidence of cancer of the liver in parts of Africa and Asia. In rodents exposed to aflatoxin B_1, the resulting liver tumors exhibit a specific inactivating mutation in the p53 gene (G:C → T:A transversion at codon 249). Interestingly, human liver cancers in areas of high dietary concentrations of aflatoxin carry the same p53 mutation. However, the relationship between aflatoxin consumption and the development of hepatocellular carcinoma must be viewed with caution, since hepatitis B and C are also endemic in these areas and have been incriminated as causes of hepatocellular carcinoma.

AROMATIC AMINES AND AZO DYES: Aromatic amines and azo dyes, in contrast to the polycyclic aromatic hydrocarbons, are not ordinarily carcinogenic at the point of application. However, they commonly produce bladder and liver tumors, respectively, when fed to experimental animals. Both aromatic amines and azo dyes are primarily metabolized in the liver. The activation reaction undergone by aromatic amines is *N*-hydroxylation to form the hydroxylamino derivatives, which are then

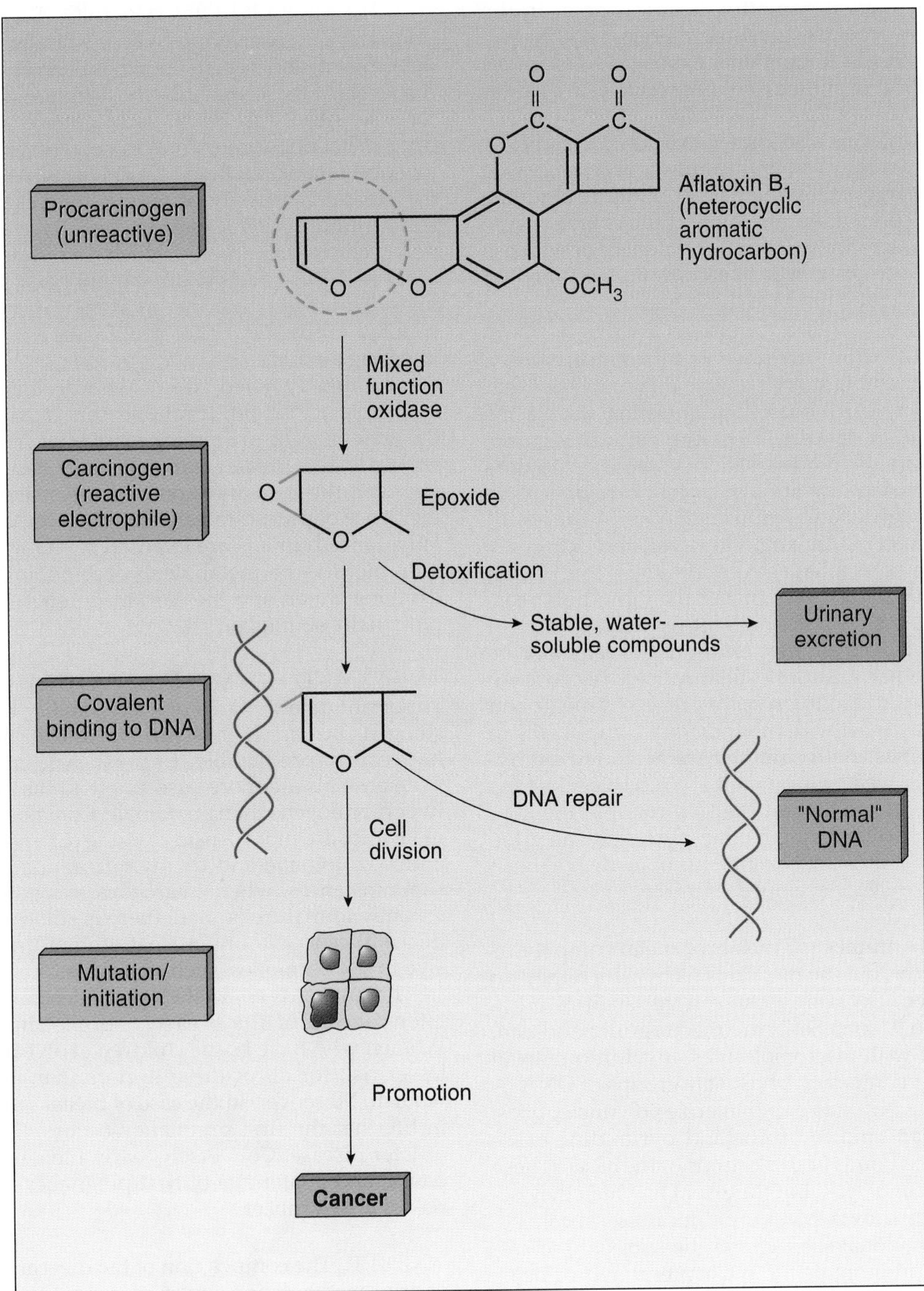

FIGURE 5-35
Metabolic activation of aflatoxin B_1. The unreactive procarcinogen aflatoxin B_1 is metabolized by the mixed-function oxidase of the hepatic endoplasmic reticulum to yield an epoxide. This electrophilic metabolite can be detoxified by conjugation with glutathione (GSH) and excreted in the urine. Alternatively, the epoxide of aflatoxin B_1 can covalently bind to liver cell macromolecules and, in particular, can bind to DNA. The resulting DNA damage can be repaired, a process that restores the integrity of the DNA. If the hepatocyte divides before DNA repair is complete, initiated liver cells result. With the appropriate regimen, these initiated hepatocytes can be promoted to a hepatocellular carcinoma.

detoxified by conjugation with glucuronic acid. In the bladder, hydrolysis of the glucuronide releases the reactive hydroxylamine. Occupational exposure to aromatic amines in the form of aniline dyes has resulted in bladder cancer.

Aminoazo dyes are also known to be carcinogenic. At one time, butter yellow (dimethylaminoazobenzene) was used to color margarine or pale winter butter to simulate the richness of summer butter. Maraschino cherries were tinted with scarlet red, a structural component of which is *o*-aminoazotoluene. However, there are no documented cases of cancer in humans from these agents.

NITROSAMINES: Carcinogenic nitrosamines are a subject of considerable study because it is suspected that they may play a role in human gastrointestinal neoplasms and possibly other cancers. The simplest nitrosamine, dimethylnitrosamine, produces kidney and liver tumors in rodents. Nitrosamines are also potent carcinogens in primates, although unambiguous evidence of cancer induction in humans is lacking. However, the extremely high incidence of esophageal carcinoma in the Hunan province of China (100 times higher than in other areas) has been correlated with the high nitrosamine content of the diet. There is concern that nitrosamines may also be implicated in other gastrointestinal cancers because nitrites, commonly added to preserve processed meats and other foods, may react with other dietary components to form nitrosamines. Nitrosamines are activated by hydroxylation, followed by formation of a reactive alkyl carbonium ion. A carbonium ion is also formed in the liver by the metabolism of carcinogenic pyrrolizidine alkaloids, which are important constituents of medicinal bush and herbal teas in less developed countries.

METALS: A number of metals or metal compounds can induce cancer, but the mechanisms by which they do so are unknown. Divalent metal cations, such as Ni^{2+}, Pb^{2+}, Cd^{2+}, Co^{2+}, and Be^{2+}, are electrophilic and can, therefore, react with macromolecules. In addition, metal ions react with guanine and phosphate groups of DNA. A metal ion such as Ni^{2+} can depolymerize polynucleotides. Some metals can bind to purine and pyrimidine bases through covalent bonds or pi electrons of the bases. These reactions all occur *in vitro*, but the extent to which they occur *in vivo* is not known. Most metal-induced cancers occur in an occupational setting, and the subject is, therefore, discussed in more detail in Chapter 9, which deals with environmental pathology.

Factors Influencing Chemical Carcinogenesis

Chemical carcinogenesis in experimental animals is influenced by a variety of factors, including species and strain, age and sex of the animal, hormonal status, diet, and the presence or absence of inducers of drug-metabolizing systems and tumor promoters. A similar role for such factors in humans has been postulated on the basis of epidemiological studies.

METABOLISM OF CARCINOGENS: Mixed function oxidases are enzymes whose activities are genetically determined, and a correlation has been observed between the levels of these enzymes in various strains of mice and their sensitivity to chemical carcinogens. The levels of drug-metabolizing enzymes in newborn animals are very low and take some time to reach adult levels. Therefore, the greater sensitivity of young animals to induction of some tumors seems paradoxical. By way of example, polycyclic hydrocarbons, which do not produce liver tumors in adult rodents, are carcinogenic for young animals. However, this inconsistency can be readily accounted for by the higher proliferative activity of tissues in young animals.

As already noted, most chemical carcinogens require metabolic activation. It follows that agents that enhance the activation of procarcinogens to ultimate carcinogens should lead to greater carcinogenicity, whereas those that augment the detoxification pathways should reduce the incidence of cancer. In general, this is the case experimentally. Since humans are exposed to many chemicals that may modify the metabolism of xenobiotics in the diet, drinking water, and the workplace, such interactions are potentially significant.

SEX AND HORMONAL STATUS: These factors are important determinants of susceptibility to chemical carcinogens but are highly variable and in many instances not readily predictable. In most experimental species, male animals are more susceptible to the aromatic amine liver carcinogens than are female animals. By contrast, female mice are more sensitive to the carcinogenic effects of aminoazotoluene and diethylnitrosamine. Moreover, in some instances, when a carcinogen is administered to a sexually immature animal, there is still a sex-linked incidence of cancer in organs that are not primarily responsive to sex hormones, such as the liver.

Pregnancy is associated with a decreased incidence of later cancers of the breast, endometrium, and ovary. Women who have borne children at an early age are at a lesser risk for all of these tumors than are nulliparous women. Moreover, in the case of breast cancer, the earlier in life that the first pregnancy occurs, the less the risk of later disease. Conversely, early menarche, late menopause, and a later age of first pregnancy all increase the risk of breast cancer.

DIET: The composition of the diet can affect the level of drug-metabolizing enzymes. A low-protein diet, which reduces the hepatic activity of mixed-function oxidases, is associated with a decreased sensitivity to hepatocarcinogens. In the case of dimethylnitrosamine, the decreased incidence of liver tumors is accompanied by an increased incidence of kidney tumors, an observation that emphasizes the fact that the metabolism of carcinogens may be regulated differently in different tissues.

There is both experimental and epidemiological evidence that obesity is associated with an increased number of tumors. However, the mechanisms by which caloric intake influences carcinogenesis are complex and poorly understood. Much attention has recently been focused on an alleged association between fat in the diet and the incidence of breast and colon cancers. Indeed it has been clearly shown experimentally that a diet high in fat increases susceptibility to chemically produced breast cancer in rodents. There is a very large (greater than fivefold) variation internationally in the incidence of breast cancer and in the consumption of fat, and an excellent correlation has been demonstrated for these parameters. However, the results of case-control studies that have examined this association within individual populations, in which the amount of dietary fat varies far less than between different populations, have been inconclusive. Thus, the relationship between breast cancer and fat consumption in humans remains controversial.

Dietary fiber has also been suggested as an influence on the occurrence of colorectal cancer. In this case, a plausible explanation lies in the effect of fiber on increasing the motility of the gut and thereby hastening the elimination of potentially harmful chemicals in the fecal stream. However, despite the recommendations of health officials and the claims of manufacturers of certain foods, there is no clinical or epidemiological evidence that the introduction of more fiber into the Western diet reduces the risk of colorectal cancer.

PHYSICAL CARCINOGENESIS

The physical agents of carcinogenesis discussed here are ultraviolet light, asbestos, and foreign bodies. Because of the significant implications for public health stemming from the diagnostic and therapeutic use of x-rays and radioisotopes in medicine, and because of the widespread concern about the safety of nuclear reactors and the dangers of atomic war, radiation carcinogenesis is discussed in Chapter 9, which is concerned with environmental pathology.

Ultraviolet Radiation

Among fair-skinned persons, a glowing tan is commonly considered the mark of a successful holiday. However, this overt manifestation of the alleged healthful effects of the sun conceals underlying tissue damage. The harmful effects of solar radiation were recognized by ladies of a bygone era, who shielded themselves from the sun with parasols to maintain a "roses-and-milk" complexion and to prevent wrinkles. The current fad for a tanned complexion has been accompanied not only by cosmetic deterioration of facial skin but also by an increase in the incidence of the major skin cancers.

Cancers attributed to sun exposure, namely, basal cell carcinoma, squamous carcinoma, and melanoma, occur predominantly in persons of the white race. The skin of persons of the darker races is protected by the increased concentration of melanin pigment, which absorbs ultraviolet radiation. In fair-skinned people, the areas exposed to the sun are most prone to develop skin cancer. Moreover, there is a direct correlation between total exposure to sunlight and the incidence of skin cancer.

Ultraviolet (UV) radiation is the short-wavelength portion of the electromagnetic spectrum adjacent to the violet region of visible light. The earth is shielded from much of the UV radiation from the sun by the ozone layer. Unfortunately, there is reason to believe that this layer is being depleted by industrial gases, and the long-term consequences are possibly hazardous. The first evidence of cell damage produced by UV radiation dates to a century ago, when it was reported that this form of energy rendered bacteria inactive. Subsequently it was found that the effectiveness of energy of different wavelengths in killing bacteria paralleled the absorption spectrum of nucleic acids. It appears that only certain portions of the UV spectrum are associated with tissue damage, and a carcinogenic effect occurs at wavelengths between 290 and 320 nm. However, in experimental models of melanoma, wavelengths greater than 320 nm also are effective in producing tumors. **The effects of UV radiation on cells include enzyme inactivation, inhibition of cell division, mutagenesis, cell death, and cancer.**

The most important biochemical effect of UV radiation is the formation of **pyrimidine dimers in DNA**, a type of DNA damage that is not seen with any other carcinogen. Pyrimidine dimers may form between thymine and thymine, between thymine and cytosine, or between cytosine pairs alone. Dimer formation leads to a cyclobutane ring, which distorts the phosphodiester backbone of the double helix in the region of each dimer. The central role of pyrimidine dimers in the tissue injury caused by UV radiation is evidenced by the demonstration that restoring these dimers to their original monomeric state by photoreactivation protects against UV-induced damage. Unless efficiently eliminated by the nucleotide excision repair pathway, genomic injury produced by UV radiation is mutagenic and carcinogenic.

Xeroderma pigmentosum, an autosomal recessive disease, exemplifies the importance of DNA repair in protecting against the harmful effects of UV radiation. In this rare disorder, a sensitivity to sunlight is accompanied by a high incidence of skin cancers, including basal cell carcinoma, squamous cell carcinoma, and melanoma. Both the neoplastic and non-neoplastic disorders of the skin in xeroderma pigmentosum are attributed to an impairment in the excision of UV-damaged DNA.

Asbestos

Pulmonary asbestosis and asbestosis-associated neoplasms are discussed in Chapter 12, which deals with diseases of the lungs. Here we will review possible mechanisms of carcinogenesis attributed to asbestos. In this context, it is not conclusively established whether the cancers related to asbestos exposure should be considered as examples of chemical carcinogenesis or of physically induced tumors.

Asbestos, a material widely used in construction, insulation, and manufacturing, is a family of related fibrous silicates, which are classed as "serpentines" or "amphiboles." Serpentines, of which chrysotile is the only example of commercial importance, occur as flexible fibers, whereas the amphiboles, represented principally by crocidolite and amosite, are firm narrow rods.

The sources of inhaled asbestos fibers include (1)

mining and manufacturing of asbestos, (2) the installation of asbestos insulation, (3) air in the vicinity of asbestos plants, (4) contaminated air in buildings undergoing repair or demolition, and (5) the clothing of asbestos workers. The deposition of asbestos fibers in the lung relates more to their diameter than to their length. The thick fibers lodge in the upper respiratory tract, but thin ones are deposited in the terminal airways and alveoli. Asbestos fibers can be coated with complexes of iron and protein and are then visualized particularly well with iron stains, which reveal so-called **ferruginous bodies (asbestos bodies)**. However, most asbestos fibers remain uncoated and are, therefore, not visible by light microscopy.

The characteristic tumor associated with asbestos exposure is malignant mesothelioma of the pleural and peritoneal cavities. This cancer, which is exceedingly rare in the general population, has been reported to occur in 2% to 3% (in some studies even more) of heavily exposed workers. The latent period—that is, the interval between exposure and the appearance of a tumor—is usually about 20 years but may be twice that figure. Fibrotic pleural lesions (pleural plaques) are often found in those exposed to asbestos but are not related to the development of malignant mesothelioma. It is reasonable to surmise that mesotheliomas of both the pleura and the peritoneum reflect the close contact of these membranes with asbestos fibers transported to them by lymphatic channels.

The pathogenesis of asbestos-associated mesotheliomas is obscure. In rats, the dimensions of the fiber, rather than its chemical composition, were reported to be crucial. Long, thin fibers deposited in the pleural space produced tumors, whereas short, thick fibers did not. This finding is compatible with the clinical observation that the long, thin crocidolite fibers are associated with a considerably greater risk of mesothelioma than the shorter and thicker amosite fibers or the flexible chrysotile fibers. However, the distinction between these fibers in the causation of human disease should not be taken as absolute, particularly since mixtures of these fibers are characteristically found in human lungs.

A role for a simian virus, SV40, in the pathogenesis of asbestos-induced mesotheliomas has been postulated because genomic sequences of this monkey virus have been identified in many cases of mesothelioma. Moreover, placement of SV40 into the pleural space of hamsters resulted in a 100% incidence of pleural mesotheliomas. However, the contribution of SV40 to the development of mesothelioma, if any, requires further study.

An association between cancer of the lung and asbestos exposure is clearly established in smokers. A small increase in the prevalence of lung cancer has been reported in nonsmokers exposed to asbestos, but this association remains controversial. An increased incidence of cancer of the larynx has also been reported among asbestos workers who smoke. Claims that exposure to asbestos increases the risk of gastrointestinal cancer have not withstood statistical analysis of the collected data.

Foreign Body Carcinogenesis

A number of different sarcomas have been induced in rodents by the implantation of inert materials, such as plastic and metal films, various fibers (including fiberglass), plastic sponges, glass spheres, and dextran polymers. The chemical nature of these implants does not seem to be the critical feature, since disks made of pure carbon also produce sarcomas. Rather, the size, smoothness, and durability of the implanted surface are important. Foreign body carcinogenesis is highly species specific. For example, rats and mice are highly susceptible to foreign body carcinogenesis, but guinea pigs are resistant. **Humans are certainly highly resistant to foreign body carcinogenesis, as evidenced by the lack of cancers following the implantation of prostheses constructed of plastics and metals.** A few reports of cancer developing in the vicinity of foreign bodies in humans probably reflect scar formation, which in some organs seems to be associated with an increased incidence of cancers. As an aside, it deserves mention that despite numerous contrary claims in lawsuits, there is no evidence that a single traumatic injury can lead to any form of cancer.

A special case of possible foreign body carcinogenesis is represented by the tumors associated with certain parasitic infestations. Squamous cell carcinoma of the bladder in persons harboring *Schistosoma haematobium* in that organ has long been recognized and probably reflects the presence of squamous metaplasia. Cancer of the bile ducts occasionally follows infection with the liver fluke *Clonorchis sinensis*, which takes up residence in the biliary passages. It is not clear whether the development of cancer in these circumstances reflects the foreign body reaction itself or the release of carcinogens from the parasites.

TUMOR IMMUNOLOGY

It has long been recognized that malignant tumors elicit a chronic inflammatory response that is unrelated to necrosis or infection of the tumor. This observation led early investigators to postulate a host immune reaction to the neoplastic cells, but a refined understanding awaited the development of modern immunology. The inflammatory reaction is correlated with a better prognosis in some tumors, such as medullary carcinoma of the breast and seminoma, but in general no clear correlation exists. Although the infiltrate is composed principally of T cells and macrophages, suggesting a cell-mediated immune response, the antigens to which the cells respond have not been identified. Despite the paucity of direct evidence in human cancers, it is clear from animal experiments that immune defenses against malignant tumors exist.

Immunological Defenses Against Cancer in Experimental Animals

To invoke a role for an immune defense against cancer, it is necessary to postulate that tumor cells express antigens that are different from normal cells and that are recognized as foreign by the host. Such a condition has been indirectly demonstrated in experiments with inbred mice (Fig. 5-36). When cells from a chemically induced or virally induced tumor are transplanted into a syngeneic mouse, the cells form a tumor. When cells from this tumor are passed into a second mouse, they again form a tumor. On the other hand, if the first transplanted tumor is removed before it metastasizes (i.e., the mouse is cured of its tumor), reinjection of the tumor cells back into the cured mouse will not produce a tumor. **The transplanted tumor is rejected because of immunity acquired as a result of the first tumor transplant.** Moreover, irradiated tumor cells or preparations of tumor cell membranes, when injected experimentally, augment resistance to tumor growth.

An important observation is that tumors induced by the same chemical in different mice are antigenically distinct, whereas those induced by the same virus express the same virally determined antigens. Accordingly, mice sensitized to one chemically induced tumor accept a second tumor induced by the same chemical, whereas mice that have received a virus-induced tumor reject another similar tumor. These experiments provide compelling evidence that immunological mechanisms can play a role in host defenses against tumors, at least against experimental tumors in animals.

Further evidence for the existence of immune mechanisms in the defense against cancer comes from studies in nude mice. These animals are devoid of T cell–mediated immunity and thus accept grafts from different species. Similarly, tumors from different species grow in an unrestrained fashion when transplanted into nude mice.

The effectiveness of immune mechanisms to limit the growth of malignant cells can be demonstrated by mixing mouse tumor cells with immune effector cells from a syngeneic mouse that has been sensitized to the tumor. The mixture is then injected into a normal (unsensitized) syngeneic recipient. In many instances, the growth of the tumor cells in the recipient is inhibited, compared with that of tumor cells mixed with unsensitized lymphoid cells.

Tumor Antigens

The immune response to experimental tumors must necessarily be directed against tumor antigens on the surface of the malignant cells. Such antigens can be tumor specific; that is, they are novel antigens that are expressed only by the cancer cells. Conversely, other tumor antigens represent proteins that are not present on adult cells but are normal cellular constituents during embryonic development. Such antigens are tumor-associated, rather than tumor-specific.

In experimental animals, tumors produced by chemicals and viruses display tumor-specific antigens. As previously noted, each chemically induced cancer expresses unique tumor antigens, that is, no two tumors are antigenically alike. The precise nature of these antigens is obscure, although some may be altered histocompatibility antigens. By contrast, all tumors induced by the same virus express the same tumor-specific antigens, presumably because they are products encoded by the viral genome. Interestingly, tumor-specific antigens are expressed weakly or not at all in the neoplasms that appear spontaneously in rodents.

It is much more difficult to document the presence of tumor-specific antigens in human cancers, because patients cannot be subjected to an immunization challenge with tumor cells, as is used in experimental animals (see Fig. 5-36). As a result, the search for tumor-specific antigens in human cancers has relied principally on *in vitro* assays for humoral or cellular immune responses. Such studies have reported cell-mediated recognition of antigens on human cancer cells, although the precise antigens in most cases have not been identified. An exception is the case of melanoma, in which a number of HLA-associated, specific antigens have been described. The development of immunotherapies against human cancers is based on the concept of tumor-specific antigens and includes studies of tumor infiltrating lymphocytes, immune response modifiers (interferon, interleukins, etc.), and potential vaccines.

Cancers that arise in both experimental animals and humans may display tumor-associated antigens. These are generally proteins that may be present in small amounts in the adult but are abundant during development. These oncodevelopmental antigens are not specific for a given tumor but are shared by cancers of varying histological type and even of different species. There is no reason to believe that immune responses to these fetal antigens play any role in the host defense against cancer. However, as previously noted, their presence in the blood or the tumor (e.g., carcinoembryonic antigen, α-fetoprotein) is useful in clinical diagnosis and treatment.

Mechanisms of Immunological Cytotoxicity

The contribution of any specific immunological mechanism to tumor cell destruction *in vivo* has not been clearly defined. A number of possible mechanisms are recognized (Fig. 5-37):

- **T cell–mediated cytotoxicity:** The capacity of cytotoxic T cells to mediate the specific rejection of transplanted tumors is evidenced by the demonstration that lymphocytes from tumor-bearing hosts can transfer tumor immunity when injected into normal animals. Moreover, the transferred immunity is eliminated by the administration of antibodies directed against T-cell antigens. The mechanisms of T cell–mediated immunological cell killing have been discussed in Chapter 4.
- **Natural killer cell–mediated cytotoxicity:** Another set of lymphocytes, the natural killer (NK) cells, have tumoricidal activity that is not dependent on prior sensitization. These lymphocytes are generally more effective than untransformed cells in killing tumor cells. Tumor cells that are resistant to the action of NK cells may be lysed by NK cells that have been activated by interleukin (IL)-2. Such activated NK cells are referred to as lymphokine-activated killer (LAK) cells.
- **Macrophage-mediated cytotoxicity:** Macrophages are capable of killing tumor cells in a nonspecific manner. However, their role in the control of malignant tumors is far from clear, since under some circumstances *in vitro* factors derived from macrophages can actually stimulate the proliferation of tumor cells.
- **Antibody-dependent cell-mediated cytotoxicity (ADCC):** Tumor-associated antigens are capable of eliciting a humoral antibody response, but these immunoglobulins by themselves do not kill tumor cells.

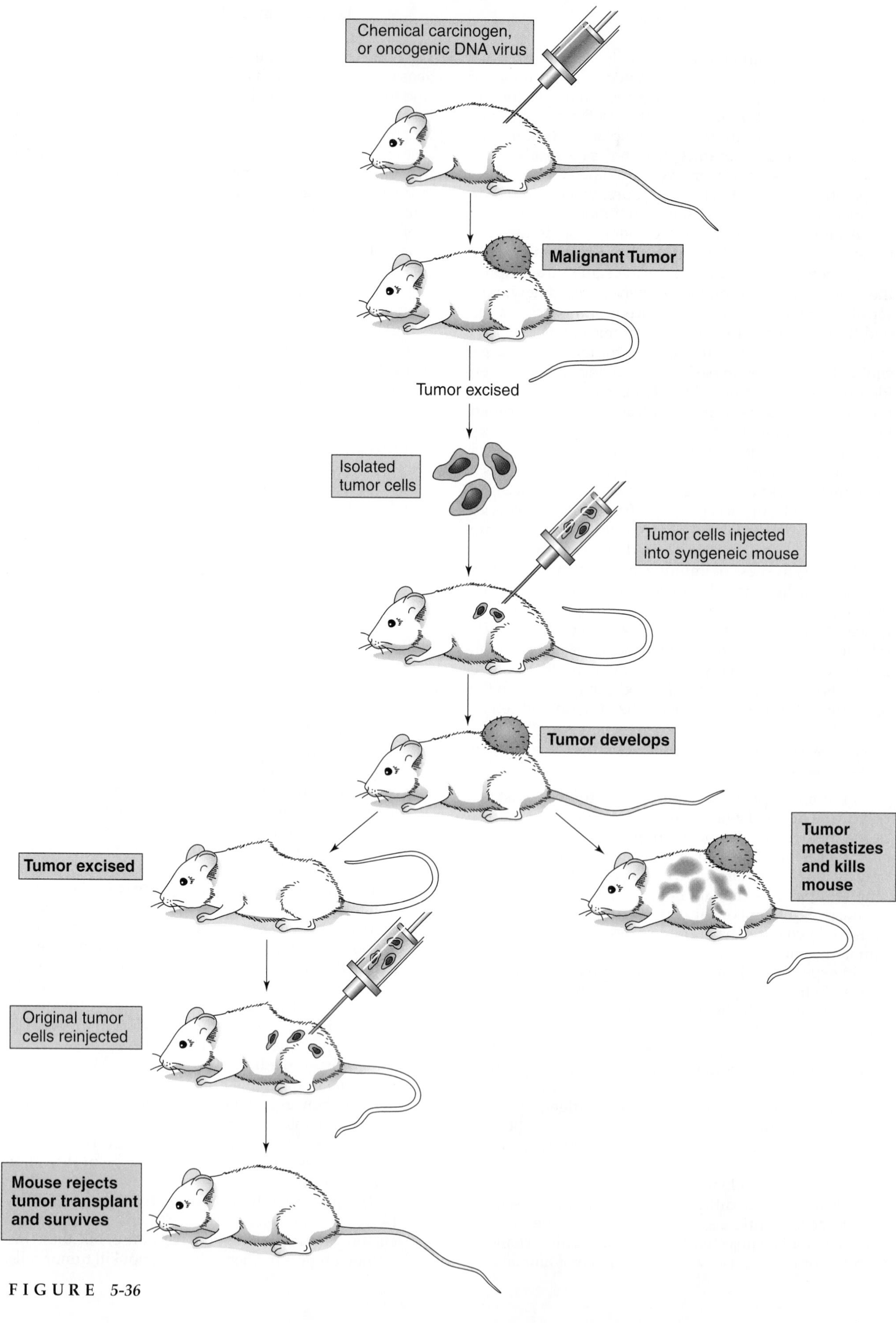
Chemical carcinogen, or oncogenic DNA virus
Malignant Tumor
Tumor excised
Isolated tumor cells
Tumor cells injected into syngeneic mouse
Tumor develops
Tumor excised
Tumor metastizes and kills mouse
Original tumor cells reinjected
Mouse rejects tumor transplant and survives

FIGURE 5-36

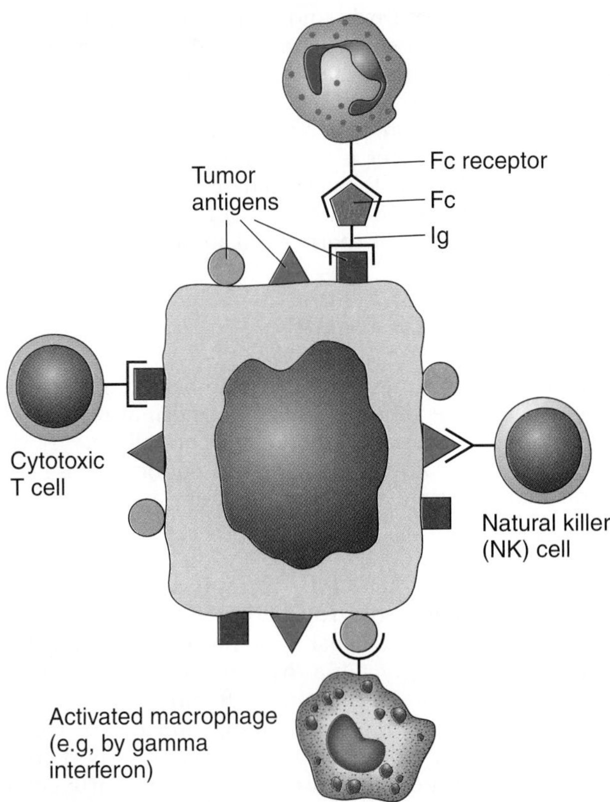

FIGURE 5-37
Possible mechanisms of immunological tumor cytotoxicity in animal studies.

However, as discussed in Chapter 4, such antibodies can participate in ADCC. The antibody binds both to the tumor antigen and to the Fc receptor of the effector cell, thereby bringing the effector cell into direct contact with its target. Depending on the conditions, the effector cells may be a lymphocyte killer cell (null cell), macrophage, or neutrophil.

- **Complement-mediated cytotoxicity:** Tumor cells that have been coated with specific antibodies may be lysed by the activation of complement. This mechanism operates only on cells in suspension (e.g., leukemic cells) and has not been demonstrated to occur with solid tumors.

Immune Surveillance

Considering the enormous number of chemical, viral, and physical agents that are carcinogenic, it seems remarkable that the incidence of cancer is not far greater than current statistics indicate. The theory of immune surveillance holds that mutant clones with neoplastic potential frequently arise but are recognized and expunged by cell-mediated immune responses. However, the evidence for this concept is highly controversial, and the subject deserves further study.

Immunological Defenses Against Cancer in Humans

Although some circumstantial evidence exists for the participation of immunological defenses in the resistance to cancer in humans, it deserves emphasis that conclusive proof for their clinical importance is lacking. Perhaps the strongest argument for immunological tumor rejection in humans is the observation that immunodeficiency, whether acquired or congenital, is associated with an increased incidence of cancers, almost all of which are B-cell lymphomas. There are three prominent examples that are widely cited, namely XLP, AIDS, and patients who receive immunosuppressive therapy following organ transplantation. In XLP and AIDS, the enormously increased risk can be attributed to a polyclonal lymphoid hyperplasia induced by infection with EBV, coupled with a lack of cytotoxic T cells that normally limit the proliferation of virus-infected B cells. In immunosuppressed transplant patients, who manifest a 75-fold increased incidence of lymphomas, it remains unclear whether a direct effect of immunosuppressive agents on the regulation of lymphocyte proliferation and maturation or a nonspecific depression of immune defenses is responsible.

Additional arguments for the effectiveness of immunological defenses against cancer in humans are also far from definitive. Rare instances of the regression of primary and metastatic tumors have been attributed to immunological mechanisms, but many other factors may have been responsible (e.g., hormonal, nutritional, vascular). Similarly, as previously noted, the phenomenon of tumor dormancy may be related to comparable nonimmunological circumstances. The presence of lymphoid cells and macrophages in the stroma of many cancers may represent a reaction to tumor antigens, but their effectiveness in limiting growth is problematic.

Evasion of Immunological Cytotoxicity

The fact that cancer is alive and well despite the presence of potential immunological defenses implies that such mechanisms are either ineffective or that tumor cells have the capacity to evade immunological cytotoxicity. A number of factors have been proposed to account for the failure of immune responses to limit tumor growth. It deserves emphasis that these explanations remain theoretical, and even controversial.

FIGURE 5-36
Immunogenicity of tumors. Cancer cells injected into a syngeneic mouse form tumors, which metastasize and kill the animal. Excision of the tumor before it has metastasized allows the rejection of a second tumor implant, presumably as a consequence of immunity acquired from exposure to the original tumor.

It is intuitively clear that an absence of tumor-specific antigens, or a lack of immunogenicity by such antigens, will permit unhampered growth of the neoplasm. **In this respect, tumor-specific antigens have not been found in the large majority of human tumors.** Moreover, substantial variations in immunological responses, presumably of genetic origin, have been demonstrated in many clinical situations.

The concept of tumor heterogeneity predicts that even in strongly antigenic tumors, clones will arise that do not express tumor antigens or histocompatibility antigens and thus will be selected for survival. In this way, a tumor might develop resistance to immunological defenses in a manner analogous to that of bacterial resistance to antibiotics.

THE SYSTEMIC EFFECTS OF CANCER ON THE HOST

The symptoms of cancer are, for the most part, referable to the local effects of either the primary tumor or its metastases. However, in a minority of patients, cancer produces remote effects that are not attributable to tumor invasion or to metastasis, which are collectively termed **paraneoplastic syndromes**. Although such effects are rarely lethal, in some cases they dominate the clinical course. It is important to recognize these syndromes for several reasons. First, the signs and symptoms of the paraneoplastic syndrome may be the first clinical manifestation of a malignant tumor. When they are recognized, the cancer may be detected early enough to permit a cure. Second, the syndromes may be mistaken for those produced by advanced metastatic disease and may, therefore, lead to inappropriate therapy. Third, when the paraneoplastic syndrome itself is disabling, treatment directed toward alleviating those symptoms may have important palliative effects. Finally, certain tumor products that result in paraneoplastic syndromes provide a means of monitoring recurrence of the cancer in patients who have had surgical resections or are undergoing chemotherapy or radiation therapy.

Fever

It is not uncommon for cancer patients to present initially with fever of unknown origin that cannot be explained by an infectious disease. Fever attributed to cancer correlates with tumor growth, disappears after treatment, and reappears on recurrence. The cancers in which this most commonly occurs are Hodgkin disease, renal cell carcinoma, and osteogenic sarcoma, although many other tumors are occasionally complicated by fever. Tumor cells may themselves release pyrogens, or the inflammatory cells in the tumor stroma can produce IL-1.

Anorexia and Weight Loss

A paraneoplastic syndrome of anorexia, weight loss, and cachexia is very common in patients with cancer, often appearing before its malignant cause becomes apparent. Although cancer patients often have a decreased caloric intake because of anorexia and abnormalities of taste, restricted food intake does not explain the profound wasting so common among them; in fact, the mechanisms responsible are poorly understood. It is known, however, that unlike starvation, which is associated with a lowered metabolic rate, cancer is often accompanied by an elevated metabolic rate. It has been demonstrated that TNF-α and other cytokines (interferons, IL-6) can produce a wasting syndrome in experimental animals.

Endocrine Syndromes

Malignant tumors may produce a number of peptide hormones whose secretion is not under normal regulatory control. Most of these hormones are normally present in the brain, gastrointestinal tract, or endocrine organs. Their inappropriate secretion can cause a variety of effects.

CUSHING SYNDROME: Ectopic secretion of corticotropin (adrenocorticotropic hormone, ACTH) by a tumor leads to features of Cushing syndrome, including hypokalemia, hyperglycemia, hypertension, and muscle weakness. The other prominent features of this syndrome, such as obesity, buffalo hump, and a moon facies, are less common. Corticotropin production is most commonly seen with cancers of the lung, particularly small cell (oat cell) carcinoma. It also complicates carcinoid tumors and other neuroendocrine tumors, such as pheochromocytoma, neuroblastoma, and medullary carcinoma of the thyroid.

INAPPROPRIATE ANTIDIURESIS: The production of arginine vasopressin (antidiuretic hormone, ADH) by a tumor may cause sodium and water retention to such an extent that it is manifested as water intoxication, resulting in altered mental status, seizures, coma, and sometimes death. The tumor that most often produces this syndrome is small cell carcinoma of the lung. It is also reported with carcinomas of the prostate, gastrointestinal tract, and pancreas and with thymomas, lymphomas, and Hodgkin's disease.

HYPERCALCEMIA: Hypercalcemia, a paraneoplastic complication that afflicts 10% of all cancer patients, is usually caused by metastatic disease of bone. However, in about one tenth of cases it occurs in the absence of bony metastases. The most common cause of paraneoplastic hypercalcemia is the secretion of a parathormone-like peptide by an epithelial tumor, usually squamous cell carcinoma of the lung or adenocarcinoma of the breast. In multiple myeloma and lymphomas, hypercalcemia is attributed to the secretion of osteoclast activating factor. Other mechanisms of hypercalcemia involve the production of prostaglandins, active metabolites of vitamin D, TGF-α, and TGF-β.

HYPOCALCEMIA: Cancer-induced hypocalcemia is actually more common than hypercalcemia and complicates osteoblastic metastases from cancers of the lung, breast, and prostate. The cause of hypocalcemia is not known, but low calcium levels have been reported in association with calcitonin-secreting medullary carcinoma of the thyroid.

HYPOPHOSPHATEMIC OSTEOMALACIA: Certain benign mesenchymal tumors are complicated by a vitamin D–resistant osteomalacia, characterized by phosphaturia, low serum phosphate levels, and normal serum calcium levels. This syndrome is usually associated with neoplasms such as giant cell tumors of bone and large hemangiomas. The cause is obscure but may involve a vitamin D antagonist, abnormal metabolism of vitamin D, or a direct effect on the renal tubule to inhibit reabsorption of phosphate.

GONADOTROPIC SYNDROMES: Gonadotropins may be secreted by germ cell tumors, gestational trophoblastic tumors (choriocarcinoma, hydatidiform mole), and pituitary tumors. Less commonly, gonadotropin secretion is observed with hepatoblastomas in children and cancers of the lung, colon, breast, and pancreas in adults. High gonadotropin levels lead to precocious puberty in children, gynecomastia in men, and oligomenorrhea in premenopausal women.

HYPOGLYCEMIA: The best-understood cause of hypoglycemia associated with tumors is excessive insulin production by islet cell tumors of the pancreas. Other tumors, especially large mesotheliomas and fibrosarcomas and primary hepatocellular carcinoma, are associated with hypoglycemia. The cause of hypoglycemia in nonendocrine tumors is not established, but the most likely candidate is production of somatomedins (insulin-like growth factors), a family of peptides normally produced by the liver under regulation by growth hormone.

Neurological Syndromes

Neurological disorders are common in cancer patients, usually resulting from metastases or from endocrine or electrolyte disturbances. Vascular, hemorrhagic, and infectious conditions affecting the nervous system are also common. However, there remains a small group of cancer patients who suffer from a variety of neurological complaints without any demonstrable cause. Such disorders are thought to reflect remote effects of cancer on the nervous system. Cerebral complications include dementia, subacute cerebellar degeneration, limbic encephalitis, and optic neuritis.

Spinal Cord

Subacute motor neuropathy, a disorder of the spinal cord, is characterized by slowly developing lower motor neuron weakness without sensory changes. It is so strongly associated with cancer that an intensive search for an occult neoplasm, often a lymphoma, should be made in patients who present with these symptoms.

Amyotrophic lateral sclerosis is well described among cancer patients. Conversely, as many as 10% of patients with this disease are found to have cancer. A rapidly ascending motor and sensory paralysis to the thoracic level, with severe destruction of gray and white matter, has been described.

Peripheral Nerves

Sensorimotor peripheral neuropathy, characterized by distal weakness and wasting and sensory loss, is common in cancer patients and when not associated with an overt neoplasm suggests the possibility of an occult tumor. Interestingly, the removal of the primary tumor usually does not reverse the neuropathy.

Purely sensory neuropathy, resulting from degenerative changes in the dorsal root ganglia, may also develop in persons with cancer.

Autonomic and gastrointestinal neuropathies, manifested as orthostatic hypotension, neurogenic bladder, and intestinal pseudo-obstruction, are associated with small cell carcinoma of the lung.

Skeletal Muscle Syndromes

Patients with dermatomyositis or polymyositis have an incidence of cancer 5 to 7 times higher than that in the general population. The association is most striking in affected men older than 50 years: in this group more than 70% have cancer. In most cases, the muscle disorder and cancer present within a year of each other.

Eaton-Lambert syndrome is an uncommon myasthenic disorder that is strongly associated with small cell carcinoma of the lung. Although the symptoms superficially resemble those of true myasthenia gravis, muscle strength improves with exercise and there is a poor response to an anticholinesterase (edrophonium [Tensilon]). The association of true myasthenia gravis with thymoma is well recognized, although a wide variety of other tumors have on occasion been linked to this disorder of the neuromuscular junction.

Hematological Syndromes

The most common hematological complications of neoplastic disease result either from direct infiltration of the marrow or from treatment. However, hematological paraneoplastic syndromes, which antedate the modern era of chemotherapy and radiation therapy, are well described.

Erythrocytosis

Cancer-associated erythrocytosis is a complication of some tumors, particularly renal cell carcinoma, hepatocellular carcinoma, and cerebellar hemangioblastoma. Interestingly, benign kidney disease, such as cystic disease or hydronephrosis, and uterine myomas can lead to erythrocytosis. Elevated erythropoietin levels are found in the tumor and in the serum in about half of the patients with erythrocytosis. The diagnosis of erythrocytosis is made when there is an increased erythrocyte mass.

Anemia

One of the most common findings in patients with cancer is anemia, but the mechanism for this disorder is not clear. The anemia is usually normocytic and normochromic, although iron deficiency anemia is common in cancers that bleed into the gastrointestinal tract, such as colorectal cancers. **Pure red cell aplasia**, often associated with thymomas, and megaloblastic anemia are sometimes encountered. **Autoimmune hemolytic anemia** may be associated with B-cell neoplasms and with solid tumors, particularly in the elderly. In fact, autoimmune hemolytic anemia in an older person suggests the possibility of an underlying neoplasm. **Microangiopathic hemolytic anemia** is occasionally seen, often in association with disseminated intravascular coagulation and thrombotic thrombocytopenic purpura.

Leukocytes and Platelets

Paraneoplastic granulocytosis, characterized by a peripheral granulocyte count over 20,000/μL, is a finding that may lead to an erroneous diagnosis of leukemia. This condition is usually caused by the secretion of a colony-stimulating factor by the tumor.

Eosinophilia is occasionally noted in association with cancer, particularly in Hodgkin disease, in which it may occur in one fifth of cases.

Thrombocytosis, with platelet counts above 400,000/μL, occurs in one third of cancer patients. The platelet count usually returns to normal with successful treatment of the malignant disease.

Thrombocytopenia, similar to that of idiopathic thrombocytopenic purpura, occurs in rare instances of cancer. However, an immune mechanism has not been demonstrated.

The Hypercoagulable State

The association between cancer and venous thrombosis was noted more than a century ago. Since then, other abnormalities resulting from a hypercoagulable state (e.g., disseminated intravascular coagulation and nonbacterial thrombotic endocarditis) have been recognized. The cause of this hypercoagulable state is still debated.

VENOUS THROMBOSIS: This condition is most distinctly associated with carcinoma of the pancreas, in which there is a 50-fold increased incidence of this complication compared with cases of chronic pancreatitis. Venous thrombosis, commonly in the deep veins of the legs, is also particularly frequent in association with other mucin-secreting adenocarcinomas of the gastrointestinal tract and with lung cancer. Tumors of the breast, ovary, prostate, and other organs are occasionally complicated by venous thrombosis.

DISSEMINATED INTRAVASCULAR COAGULATION: The widespread appearance of thrombi in small vessels in association with cancer may come to attention because of the chronic occurrence of thrombotic phenomena or an acute hemorrhagic diathesis. Sometimes a coagulation disorder is detected by laboratory tests alone. This complication is most commonly found with acute promyelocytic leukemia and adenocarcinomas.

NONBACTERIAL THROMBOTIC ENDOCARDITIS: The presence of noninfected verrucous deposits of fibrin and platelets on the left-sided heart valves occurs in cancer patients, particularly in debilitated persons. This form of endocarditis (also called marantic endocarditis) develops with or without disseminated intravascular coagulation. Although the effects on the heart are not of clinical importance, emboli to the brain present a great danger. Paraneoplastic endocarditis may develop early in the course of a cancer and signal its presence long before the tumor would otherwise become symptomatic. This cardiac complication is most common with solid tumors but may occasionally be noted with leukemias and lymphomas.

Gastrointestinal Syndromes

Malabsorption of a variety of dietary components is an occasional paraneoplastic symptom, and half of cancer patients develop some histological abnormalities of the small intestine. The classic tumor associated with malabsorption is lymphoma of the small intestine. However, such changes can occur even with tumors that do not directly involve the bowel.

Hypoalbuminemia may result from a paraneoplastic depression of albumin synthesis by the liver. In rare cases, hypoalbuminemia is attributable to a protein-losing enteropathy. In this paraneoplastic disorder, there is an exudative loss of proteins into the bowel lumen, sometimes associated with mucosal inflammation and occasionally occurring without recognizable morphological abnormalities.

Renal Syndromes

Nephrotic syndrome, as a consequence of renal vein thrombosis or amyloidosis, is a well-known complication of cancer. The nephrotic syndrome may also represent a paraneoplastic complication in the form of minimal-change disease (lipoid nephrosis) or a glomerulonephritis produced by the deposition of immune complexes. Although the antigens in glomerulonephritis of this kind are not generally identified, tumor-specific antibodies and carcinoembryonic antigen–antibody complexes have been eluted from the kidneys in a few cases.

Cutaneous Syndromes

Pigmented lesions and keratoses are well-recognized paraneoplastic effects.

Acanthosis nigricans is a cutaneous disorder marked by hyperkeratosis and pigmentation of the axilla, neck, flexures, and anogenital region. **It is of particular interest because more than half of patients with acanthosis nigricans have cancer**. The development of the disease may precede, accompany, or follow the detection of the cancer. Over 90% of the cases occur in association with gastrointestinal carcinomas, with tumors of the stomach accounting for one half to two thirds. Regression of the skin lesions after removal of the cancer has been recorded in a few cases.

Seborrheic keratoses, which develop suddenly or rapidly increase in size, may herald the presence of a malignant tumor, albeit rarely.

Exfoliative dermatitis occasionally complicates certain lymphomas and Hodgkin disease, without any cutaneous involvement by tumor.

Erythema gyratum repens is an unusual skin disorder, which presents with scaling and itching and is seen almost exclusively in cancer patients.

Amyloidosis

About 15% of cases of amyloidosis occur in association with cancers, particularly with multiple myeloma and renal cell carcinoma but also with other solid tumors and lymphomas. The presence of amyloidosis implies a poor prognosis; in patients with myeloma, amyloidosis is associated with a median survival of 14 months or less.

THE EPIDEMIOLOGY OF CANCER

The causes of most cancers in humans remain obscure, but there is ample reason to believe that, at least in some cases, chemical, viral, physical, and genetic factors are involved. This is not to deny the possibility that other agents or mechanisms, as yet unknown, may also be important in the pathogenesis of many human cancers. Experimental studies require exposure of animals to specific agents, and obviously this approach cannot be used for the study of human neoplasia. In attempts to identify the etiologies of human cancers, epidemiological studies have been very useful. Such studies correlate the occurrence of cancers in defined human populations, residing in specified geographic locations, with genetic and environmental factors. In the following discussion, we will not deal with occupational epidemiology or exposure to specific agents, such as tobacco smoke or alcohol, since these are treated in Chapter 8.

The mere compilation of raw epidemiological data is of little use unless they are subjected to careful analysis. In evaluating the relevance of epidemiological observations to cancer causation, the following criteria are germane:

- Strength of the association
- Consistency under different circumstances
- Specificity
- Temporality (i.e., the cause must precede the effect)
- Biological gradient (i.e., there is a dose–response relationship)
- Plausibility
- Coherence (i.e., a cause-and-effect relationship does not violate basic biological principles)
- Analogy to other known associations

It is not mandatory that a valid epidemiological study satisfy all these criteria, nor does adherence to them guarantee that the hypothesis derived from the data is necessarily true. However, as a guideline they remain useful.

The Incidence of Cancer in the United States

Cancer accounts for one fifth of the total mortality in the United States and is the second leading cause of death after cardiovascular diseases and stroke. For most cancers, death rates in the United States have largely remained flat for more than half a century, with some notable exceptions (Fig. 5-38). The death rate from cancer of the lung among men has risen dramatically from 1930, when it was an uncommon tumor, to the present, when it is by far the most common cause of death from cancer in men. As discussed in Chapter 8, the entire epidemic of lung cancer deaths is attributable to smoking. Among women, smoking did not become fashionable until World War II. Considering the time lag needed between starting to smoke and the development of cancer of the lung, it is not surprising that the increased death rate from cancer of the lung in women did not become significant until after 1965. In the United States, the death rate from lung cancer in women now exceeds that for breast cancer, and it is now, as in men, the most common fatal cancer. By contrast, for reasons difficult to fathom, cancer of the stomach, which in 1930 was by far the most common cancer in men and was only slightly less common than breast cancer in women, has shown a remarkable and sustained decline in frequency. Similarly, there has been an unexplained decline in the death rate from cancer of the uterus, although better screening, diagnostic, and therapeutic methods may account for some of this reduction. Overall, after decades of steady increases, the age-adjusted mortality due to all cancers has now reached a plateau. The ranking of the incidence of tumors in men and women in the United States is shown in Table 5-4.

Individual cancers have their own age-related profiles, but for most, increased age is associated with an increased incidence. The most striking example of the dependency on age is carcinoma of the prostate, in which the incidence increases 30-fold between age 50 and 85 years. Certain neoplastic diseases, such as acute lymphoblastic leukemia in children and testicular cancer in young adults, show different age-related peaks of incidence (Fig. 5-39).

Geographic and Ethnic Differences in Cancer Incidence

NASOPHARYNGEAL CANCER: Nasopharyngeal cancer is rare in most of the world except for certain regions of China, Hong Kong, and Singapore. Nasopharyngeal carcinoma has been associated with infection by the EBV.

ESOPHAGEAL CARCINOMA: The range in incidence of esophageal carcinoma varies from extremely low in Mormon women in Utah to a value some 300 times

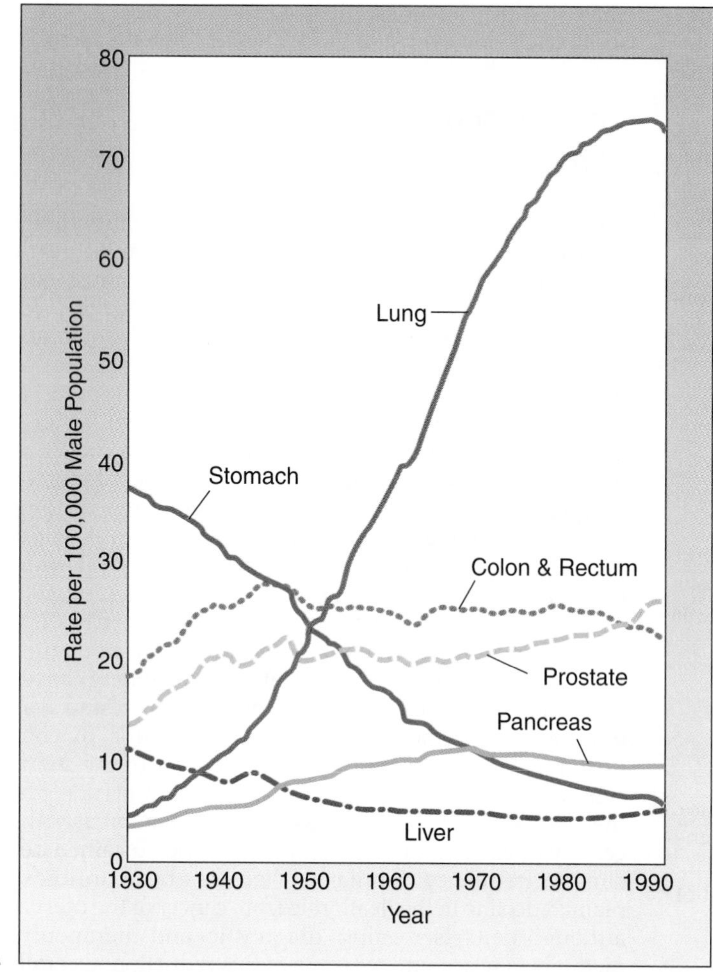

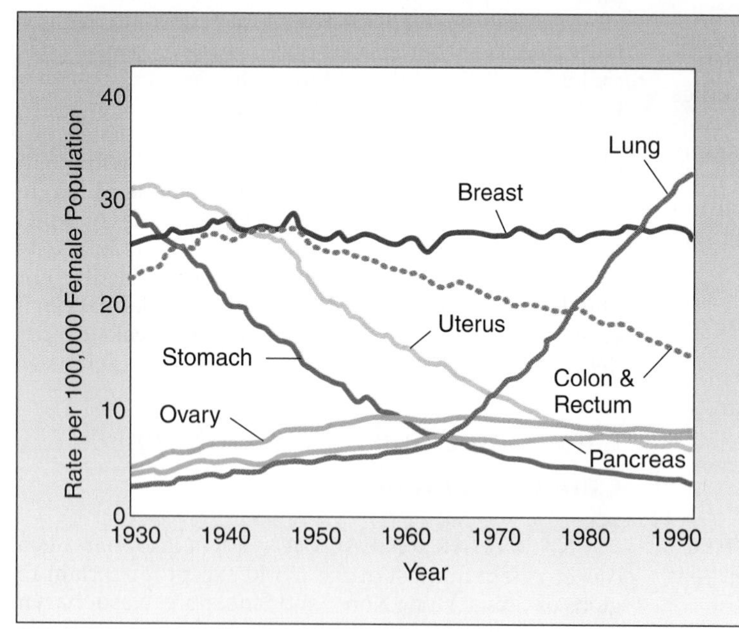

FIGURE 5-38
Cancer death rates in the United States, 1930 to 1990, among men (*A*) and women (*B*).

TABLE 5-4 Most Common Tumor Types in Men and Women

Men	
Type	**%**
Lung	20
Prostate	20
Colon and rectum	14
Urinary	10
Leukemia and lymphoma	8
Oral	4
Skin	3
Pancreas	3
All others	18

Women	
Type	**%**
Breast	27
Colon and rectum	16
Lung	11
Uterus	10
Leukemia and lymphoma	7
Ovary	4
Urinary	4
Pancreas	3
Skin	3
Oral	2
All others	13

higher in the female population of northern Iran. Particularly high rates of esophageal cancer are noted in a so-called Asian esophageal cancer belt, which includes the great land mass stretching from European Russia to eastern China. Interestingly, throughout this region, as the incidence rises the proportional excess in males decreases; in some of the areas of highest incidence there is even a female excess. The disease is also more common in certain regions of Africa inhabited predominantly by blacks and among blacks in the United States. The causes of esophageal cancer are obscure, but it is known that it disproportionately affects the poor in many areas of the world, and the combination of alcohol abuse and smoking is associated with a particularly high risk.

STOMACH CANCER: The highest incidence of stomach cancer occurs in Japan, where the disease is almost 10 times as frequent as it is among American whites. A high incidence has also been observed in Latin American countries, particularly Chile. Stomach cancer is also common in Iceland and eastern Europe.

COLORECTAL CANCER: The highest incidence of colorectal cancer is found in the United States, where it is 3 or 4 times more common than in Japan, India, Africa, and Latin America. It has been theorized that the high fiber content of the diet in low-risk areas and the high fat content in the United States are related to this difference, although this concept has been seriously questioned.

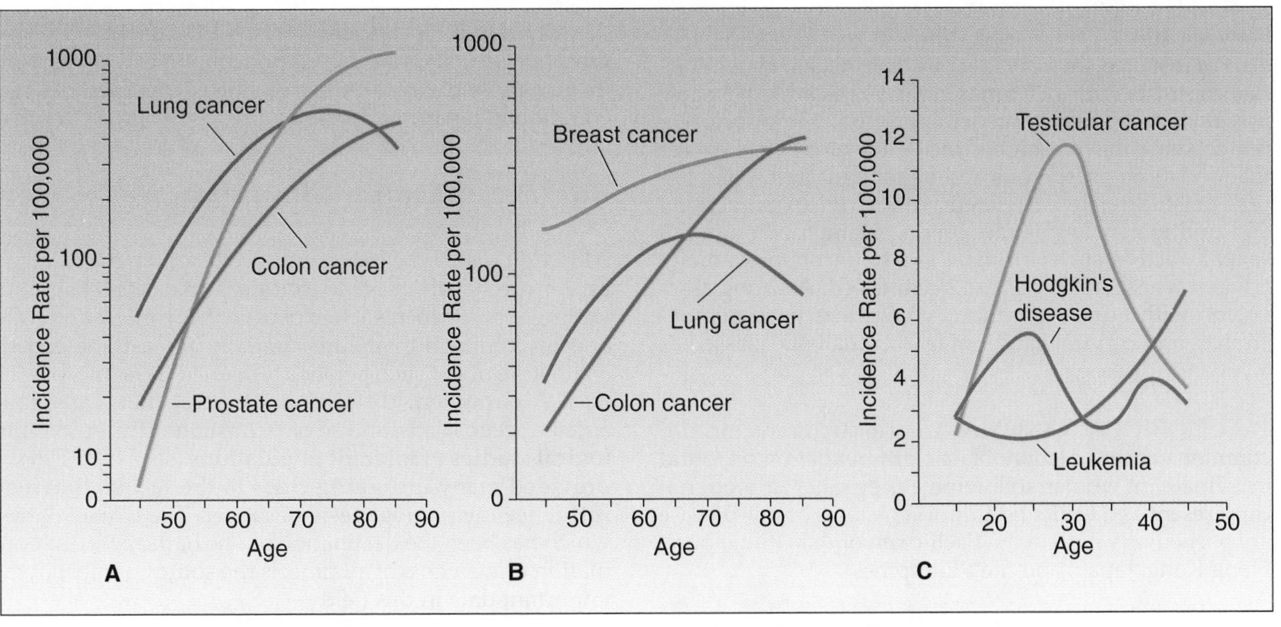

FIGURE 5-39
Incidence of specific cancers as a function of age. (*A*) Men. (*B*) Women. (*C*) Testicular cancer in men and Hodgkin disease and leukemia in both sexes. The incidence of these cancers in *C* peaks at younger ages than do those in *A* and *B*.

LIVER CANCER: There is a strong correlation between the incidence of primary hepatocellular carcinoma and the prevalence of hepatitis B and C. Endemic regions for both diseases include large parts of sub-Saharan Africa and most of the Orient, Indonesia, and the Philippines. It must be remembered, too, that levels of aflatoxin B_1 are high in the staple diets of many of the high-risk areas.

SKIN CANCER: As previously noted, the rates for skin cancers vary with skin color and exposure to the sun. Thus, particularly high rates have been reported in northern Australia, where the population is principally of Celtic origin and sun exposure is intense. Increased rates of skin cancer have also been noted among the white population of the American Southwest. The lowest rates are found among persons with pigmented skin (e.g., Japanese, Chinese, and Indians). The rates for African blacks, despite their heavily pigmented skin, are occasionally higher than those for Asians because of the higher incidence of melanomas of the soles and palms in blacks.

BREAST CANCER: Adenocarcinoma of the breast, the most common female cancer in many parts of Europe and North America, shows considerable geographic variation. The rates in African and Asian populations are only one fifth to one sixth of those prevailing in Europe and the United States. Epidemiological studies have contributed little to our understanding of the etiology of breast cancer. Although hormonal factors are clearly involved, except for a good correlation with age at first pregnancy, few confirmed hormonal correlations have surfaced. The role of dietary fat in the pathogenesis of breast cancer is still debated.

CANCER OF THE CERVIX: Striking differences in the incidence of squamous carcinoma of the cervix exist between ethnic groups and different socioeconomic levels. For instance, the very low rate in Ashkenazi Jews of Israel contrasts with a 25 times greater rate in the Hispanic population of Texas. In general, groups of low socioeconomic status have a higher incidence of cervical cancer than the more prosperous and better educated. This cancer is also directly correlated with early sexual activity and multiparity and is rare among women who are not sexually active, such as nuns. It is also uncommon among women whose husbands are circumcised. A strong association with human papillomaviruses has been demonstrated, and cervical cancer may eventually be classed as a venereal disease.

CHORIOCARCINOMA: Choriocarcinoma, an uncommon cancer of trophoblastic differentiation, is found principally in women following a pregnancy, although it can present as a testicular tumor. The rates of this disease are particularly high in the Pacific rim of Asia (Singapore, Hong Kong, Japan, and the Philippines).

PROSTATIC CANCER: Very low incidences of prostatic cancer are reported for Asian populations, particularly Japanese, whereas the highest rates described are in American blacks, in whom the disease occurs some 25 times more often. The incidence in American and European whites is intermediate.

TESTICULAR CANCER: An unusual aspect of testicular cancer is its universal rarity among black populations. Interestingly, although the rate in American blacks is only about one fourth that in whites, it is still considerably higher than the rate among African blacks.

CANCER OF THE PENIS: This squamous carcinoma is virtually nonexistent among circumcised men of any race but is common in many parts of Africa and Asia. Interestingly, in the highlands of New Guinea, where both circumcision and washing are rarely practiced, this tumor is also rare, a finding that is contrary to expectation.

CANCER OF THE URINARY BLADDER: The rates for transitional cell carcinoma of the bladder are fairly uniform. Squamous carcinoma of the bladder, however, is a special case. Ordinarily far less common than transitional cell carcinoma, it has a high incidence in areas where schistosomal infestation of the bladder (bilharziasis) is endemic.

BURKITT LYMPHOMA: Burkitt lymphoma, a disease of children, was first described in Uganda, where it accounts for half of all childhood tumors. Since then, a high frequency has been observed in other African countries, particularly in hot, humid lowlands. It has been noted that these are areas where malaria is also endemic. High rates have been recorded in other tropical areas, such as Malaysia and New Guinea, but European and American cases are encountered only sporadically.

MULTIPLE MYELOMA: This malignant tumor of plasma cells is uncommon among American whites but displays a three to four times higher incidence in American and South African blacks.

CHRONIC LYMPHOCYTIC LEUKEMIA: Chronic lymphocytic leukemia is common among elderly persons in Europe and North America but is considerably less common in Japan.

Studies of Migrant Populations

Although planned experiments on the etiology of human cancer are hardly feasible, certain populations have unwittingly performed such experiments by migrating from one environment to another. Initially at least, the genetic characteristics of such persons remained the same, but the new environment differed in climate, diet, infectious agents, occupations, and so on. **Consequently, epidemiological studies of migrant populations** (see Fig. 5-1) **have provided many intriguing clues to the factors that may influence the pathogenesis of cancer.** The United States, which has been the destination of one of the greatest population movements of all time, is the source of most of the important data in this field.

CANCER OF THE STOMACH: A study of Japanese residents of Hawaii found that emigrants from Japanese regions with the highest risk of stomach cancer continued to exhibit an excess risk in Hawaii. By contrast, their offspring who were born in Hawaii had the same incidence of this cancer as American whites. Although dietary factors, such as pickled vegetables and salted fish, have been postulated to account for the higher incidence in Japan and the lower incidence in Hawaii, no firm evidence has been adduced to support this contention. More recently it has been shown in Japan that the population in regions at high risk for stomach cancer also display a high prevalence of chronic atrophic gastritis with intestinal metaplasia, lesions that are considered precursors of gastric cancer. Interestingly, when persons from these regions move to low-risk areas, they carry the high prevalence of intestinal metaplasia with them. Thus, the environmental factors associated with stomach cancer may not be directly carcinogenic but rather may be related to atrophic gastritis and intestinal metaplasia.

COLORECTAL, BREAST, ENDOMETRIAL, OVARIAN, AND PROSTATIC CANCERS: Emigrant studies of the incidence of colorectal cancer show opposite trends to those of stomach cancer. Emigrants from low-risk areas in Europe and Japan exhibit an increased risk of colorectal cancer in the United States. Moreover, their offspring continue at higher risk and reach the incidence levels of the general American population. This rule for colorectal cancer also prevails for cancers of the breast, endometrium, ovary, and prostate.

CANCER OF THE LIVER: As previously noted, primary hepatocellular carcinoma is common in Asia and Africa, where it has been associated with hepatitis B. In American blacks and Asians, however, the neoplasm is no more common than in American whites, a situation that presumably reflects the low prevalence of hepatitis B in the United States.

BURKITT LYMPHOMA: In Central Africa, emigrants from highland regions to lowland areas, where Burkitt lymphoma is rare, develop tumors at an older age than do those born in endemic areas. This presumably reflects a later age of exposure to EBV or a more potent stimulation of the antigenic response by malaria. Moreover, the incidence of Burkitt lymphoma is higher among emigrants to high-risk areas than among the same group who stay in the low-risk areas. Indeed, the risk of Burkitt lymphoma is higher in emigrants to high-risk areas than among adults who were born in the high-risk area. It is probable that many adults in the high-risk areas who have escaped Burkitt lymphoma in their youth are immune to the disease.

HODGKIN DISEASE: In general, in poorly developed countries the childhood form of Hodgkin's disease is the one reported most often. In developed Western countries, by contrast, the disease is most common among young adults. Such a pattern is characteristic of certain viral infections, although there is no evidence for an infectious etiology of Hodgkin disease. An exception to this generalization is noted in Japan, a developed country where young adult disease is distinctly uncommon. Further evidence for an environmental influence is the increased incidence of Hodgkin disease in Americans of Japanese descent, compared with that in Japan.

SUGGESTED READING

BOOKS

DeVita VT Jr, Hellman S, Rosenberg SA: *Cancer: Principles and practice of oncology*, 5th ed. Philadelphia: Lippincott–Raven, 1997.

Sherbet, Lakshmi: *Genetics of cancer*. San Diego, CA: Academic Press, 1997.

Vogelstein B, Kinzler KW: *Genetics of cancer*. New York: McGraw-Hill, 1997.

REVIEWS

Battegay EJ: Angiogenesis: Mechanistic insights, neovascular diseases, and therapeutic prospects. *J Mol Med* 73:333–346, 1995.

Boyd D: Invasion and metastasis. *Cancer Metastasis Rev* 15:77–89, 1996.

Dunlop MG: Mutator genes and mosaicism in colorectal cancer. *Curr Opin Genet Dev* 6:767–781, 1996.

Hartwell LH, Kastan MB: Cell cycle control and cancer. *Science* 266:1821–1828, 1994.

zur Hausen H: Papillomavirus infections: A major cause of human cancers. *Biochim Biophys Acta* 1288:F55–F78, 1996.

de The G: Viruses and human cancers: Challenges for preventive strategies. *Environ Health Perspect* 103(suppl 8):169–173, 199.

Jiang WG: E-cadherin and its associated protein catenins, cancer invasion and metastasis. *Br J Surg* 83:437–446, 1996.

Lavin MF, Shiloh Y: Ataxia-telangiectasia: A multifaceted genetic disorder associated with defective signal transduction. *Curr Opin Immunol* 8:459–464, 1996.

Modrich P, Lahue R: Mismatch repair in replication fidelity, genetic recombination, and cancer biology. *Annu Rev Biochem* 65:101–133, 1996.

Pines J: Cyclins, CDKs and cancer. *Semin Cancer Biol* 6:63–72, 1995.

Pitot HC, Dragan YP: The multistage nature of chemically induced hepatocarcinogenesis in the rat. *Drug Metab Rev* 26:209–220, 1994.

Rowley JD. Molecular cytogenetics: Rosetta stone for understanding cancer. *Cancer Res* 50:3816–3825, 1990.

Stetler-Stevenson WG, Hewitt R, Corcoran M: Matrix metallproteinases and tumor invasion: From correlation and causality to the clinic. *Semin Cancer Biol* 7:147–154, 1996.

Uhr JW, Marches R, Racila E, et al: Role of antibody signaling in inducing tumor dormancy. *Adv Exp Med Biol* 406:69–74, 1996.

Varmus HE: Retroviruses and oncogenes. *Biosci Rep* 10:413–430, 1990.

Varner JA, Cheresh DA: Integrins and cancer. *Curr Opin Cell Biol* 8:724–730, 1996.

Vogelstein B, Kinzler KW: The multistep nature of cancer. *Trends Genet* 9:138–141, 1993.

CHAPTER 6

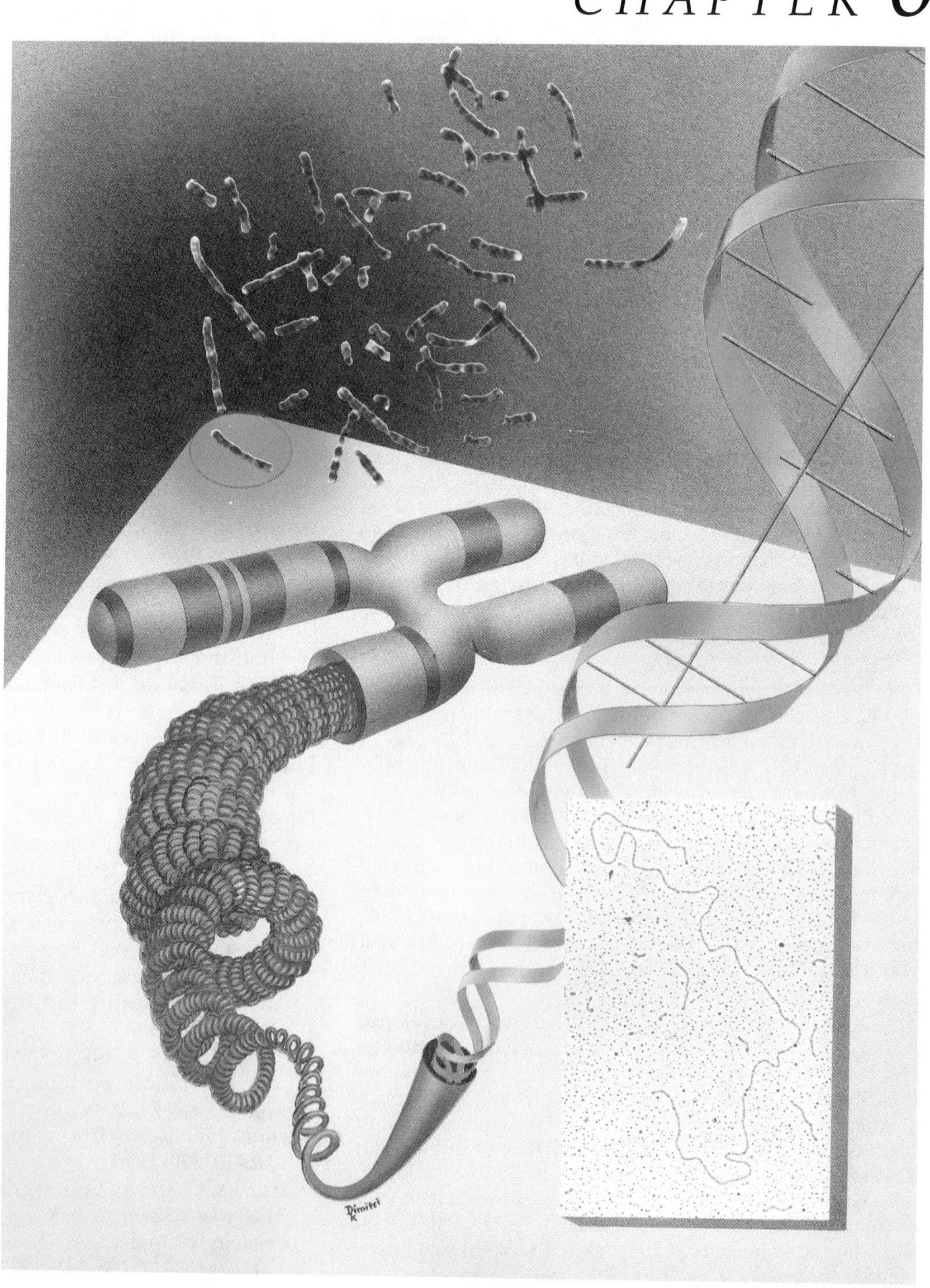

Developmental and Genetic Diseases

Emanuel Rubin
John L. Farber

FIGURE *6-1* (*see opposite page*)
Squash preparation of human chromosomes stained by the Giemsa banding technique. The X chromosome is enlarged and depicted schematically.

It has been known since biblical times that certain disorders are inherited or related to disturbances in intrauterine development. The earliest sanitary codices contain guidelines on how to choose a healthy spouse, how to conceive healthy children, and what to do or not do during pregnancy. Nevertheless, most of our present scientific knowledge about developmental and genetic disorders has been gathered only within the past three decades, and the exponential growth of molecular genetics has provided the tools for unraveling the etiology and pathogenesis of these disorders. In fact, the molecular basis of most inherited disorders caused by single gene mutations are either known today or likely to be described within the next few years.

Diseases that originate during prenatal development range from conditions caused solely by factors in the fetal environment to those that are exclusively determined by genomic abnormalities. There are also diseases that exemplify the interaction between genetic defects and environmental influences. An example is phenylketonuria, in which a genetic deficiency of phenylalanine hydroxylase causes mental retardation only if the infant is exposed to dietary phenylalanine.

Developmental and genetic disorders are classified as follows:

- Errors of morphogenesis
- Chromosomal abnormalities
- Single gene defects
- Polygenic inherited diseases

The fetus may also be injured by adverse transplacental influences or by deformities and injuries caused by intrauterine trauma or during parturition. After birth, acquired diseases of infancy and childhood are also important causes of morbidity and mortality.

MAGNITUDE OF THE PROBLEM

Each year, about one quarter of a million babies are born in the United States with a birth defect. Worldwide, at least 1 in 50 newborns has a major congenital anomaly, 1 in 100 has a single gene abnormality, and 1 in 200 has a major chromosomal abnormality.

In more than two thirds of all birth defects, the cause is not apparent (Fig. 6-2). No more than 6% of total birth defects can be attributed to uterine factors, maternal disorders such as metabolic imbalances or infections during pregnancy, and other environmental hazards, including exposure to drugs, chemicals, and radiation. Most of the remaining conditions are accounted for by genomic defects, either hereditary traits or spontaneous mutations, and a smaller number of chromosomal abnormalities.

Although chromosomal abnormalities account for only a small fraction of birth defects in newborns, cytogenetic analysis of fetuses spontaneously aborted in early pregnancy indicates that two thirds show chromosomal abnormalities. **The incidence of specific numerical chromosomal abnormalities in the abortuses is several times higher than in term infants, indicating that most inborn chromosomal defects are lethal.** The conceptus dies in early pregnancy, and only a small number of children with cytogenetic abnormalities are born alive.

In advanced Western countries, developmental and genetic birth defects account for half of the total mortality in infancy and childhood. This contrasts with the situation in less-developed countries, where 95% of infant mortality is attributable to environmental causes such as infectious diseases and malnutrition. In industrialized societies, genetic counseling, early prenatal diagnosis, identification of high-risk pregnancies, and avoidance of possible exogenous teratogens are the only practical approaches that can reduce the incidence of birth anomalies. In this context, it deserves mention that prenatal dietary supplementation with folic acid has been shown to reduce the incidence of congenital neural tube defects.

PRINCIPLES OF TERATOLOGY

Teratology is the discipline concerned with the study of developmental anomalies (Gk. *teraton*, monster). **Teratogens** are chemical, physical, and biological agents that cause developmental anomalies. There are few proven teratogens in humans, but many drugs and chemicals are teratogenic in animals and should, therefore, be considered as potentially dangerous for humans.

Malformation *refers to a morphological defect or abnormality of an organ, part of an organ, or anatomical region that results from perturbed morphogenesis.* Exposure to a teratogen may result in a malformation, but this is not invariably the case. Such observations have led to the formulation of general principles of teratology:

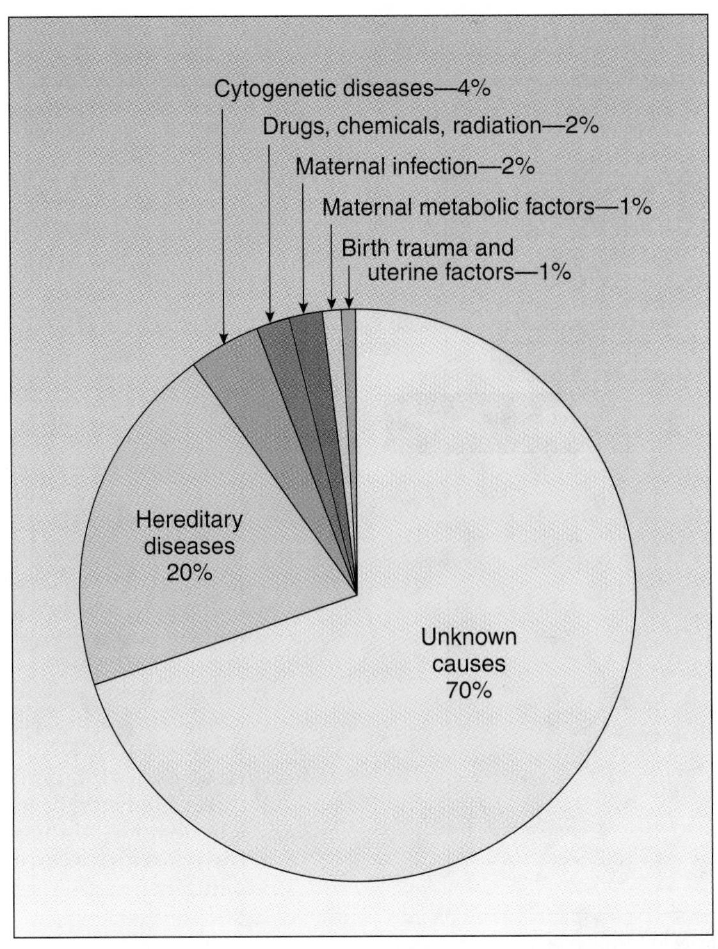

FIGURE 6-2
Causes of birth defects in humans. Most birth defects have unknown causes.

- **Susceptibility to teratogens is variable.** Presumably the principal determinants of this variability are the genotypes of the fetus and the mother. Experimental evidence for this concept comes from the demonstration that certain strains of inbred mice are susceptible to some teratogens whereas others are not. An example of human variability in the vulnerability to teratogens is the fetal alcohol syndrome, which affects some children of alcoholic mothers whereas others are resistant.
- **Susceptibility to teratogens is specific for each developmental stage.** Most agents are teratogenic only during critical stages of development (Fig. 6-3). For example, maternal rubella infection causes abnormalities in the fetus only during the first 3 months of pregnancy.
- **The mechanism of teratogenesis is specific for each teratogen.** Teratogenic drugs inhibit the activity of crucial enzymes or receptors, interfere with the formation of the mitotic spindle, or block energy production, and thus inhibit metabolic steps critical for normal morphogenesis. Many drugs and viruses affect specific tissues (e.g., neurotropism, cardiotropism) and thereby damage some developing organs more than others.
- **Teratogenesis is dose-dependent.** Theoretically, this means that each teratogen should have a "safe" dose, below which no teratogenesis occurs. In practice, however, because of the multiple determinants of teratogenesis, all established teratogens should be avoided during pregnancy; an absolutely safe dose cannot be predicted for every woman.
- **Teratogens produce death, growth retardation, malformation, or functional impairment.** The outcome depends on the interaction between the teratogenic influences, the maternal organism, and the fetal-placental unit.

The search for human teratogens requires (1) population surveys, (2) prospective and retrospective studies of single malformations, and (3) the investigation of reported adverse effects of drugs or other chemicals. The list of proven teratogens is long and includes most cytotoxic drugs, alcohol, some antiepileptic drugs, heavy metals, and thalidomide. On the other hand, many drugs and chemicals have been declared as safe for use during pregnancy because of negative teratogenic studies in laboratory animals. However, there is species specificity for every drug, and the fact that a drug is not teratogenic for mice and rabbits is not necessarily evidence that it is innocuous for humans. In fact, the best known drug-related teratogenic incident—complex malformations related to the ingestion of the hypnotic drug thalidomide—occurred after the drug was found not to be teratogenic in mice and rats. Interestingly, long after the drug was found

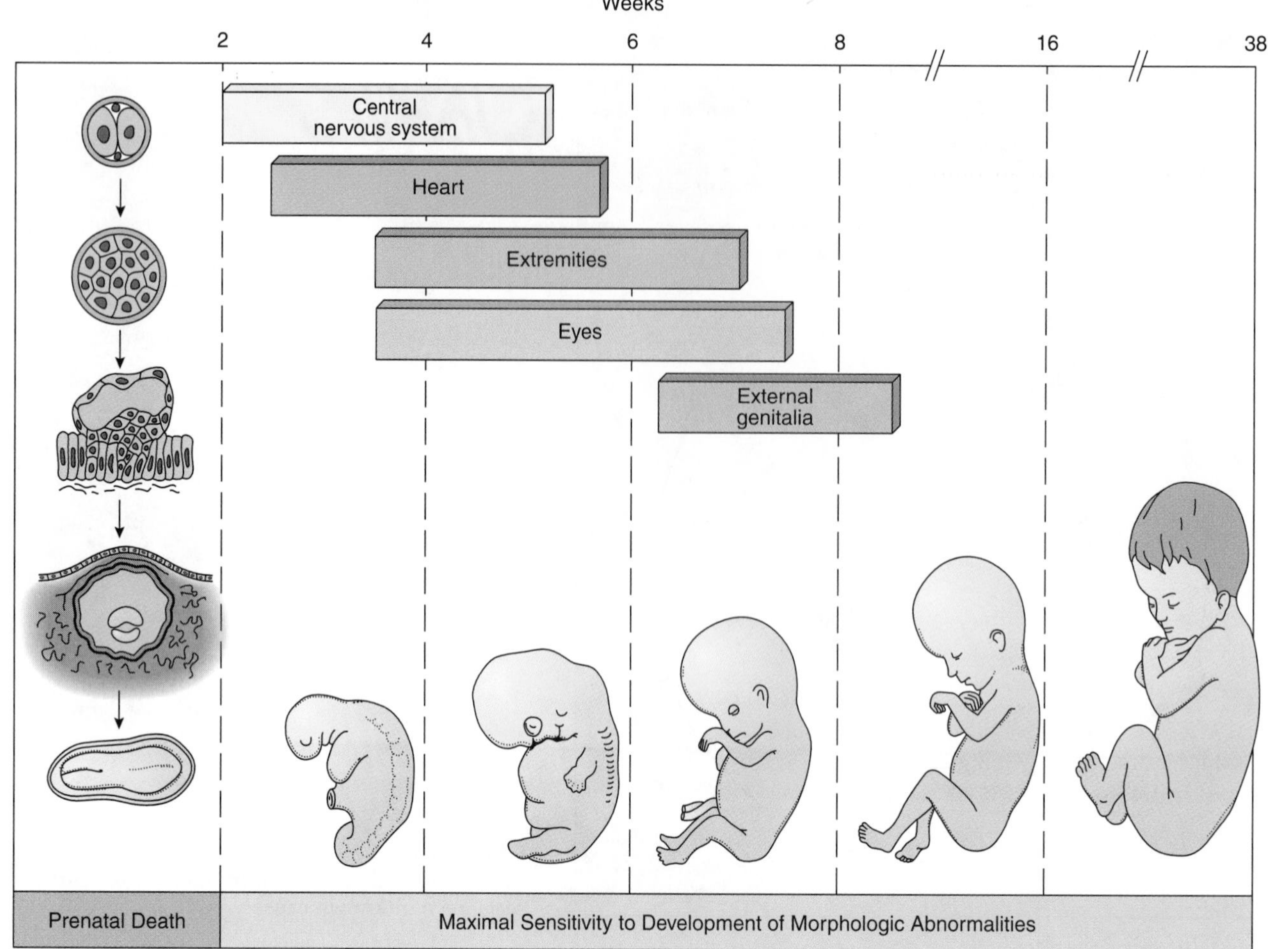

FIGURE *6-3*
Sensitivity of specific organs to teratogenic agents at critical stages of human embryogenesis. Exposure to adverse influences in the preimplantation and early postimplantation stages of development (*far left*) leads to prenatal death. Periods of maximal sensitivity to teratogens (*horizontal red bars*) vary for different organ systems but overall are limited to the first 8 weeks of pregnancy.

to be teratogenic in humans, its teratogenicity was also demonstrated in rabbits and monkeys.

ERRORS OF MORPHOGENESIS

Normal intrauterine and postnatal development depends on sequential activation and repression of genes inherited from the parents. Although the fertilized ovum (zygote) has all the genes found in the adult organism, most of them are inactive. As the zygote enters cleavage stages of development, individual genes or sets of genes are activated in a stage-specific manner. Initially, activation involves only genes essential for cellular replication and growth, cell-to-cell interaction, and the regulation of important morphogenetic movements. **Abnormally activated or structurally abnormal genes in the zygote and early embryonic cells result in early death.**

The cells that form the two-cell and four-cell embryos (blastomeres) are developmentally equipotent, and each can give rise to an adult organism. Separation of the embryonic cells at this stage results in identical twins or quadruplets. Since the blastomeres are equipotent and interchangeable, loss of a single blastomere at this stage of development may pass without any serious consequences. On the other hand, since the blastomeres are identical, if one blastomere contains a set of lethal genes it is likely that other blastomeres contain the same genes. Thus, their activation invariably leads to the death of the conceptus. Furthermore, if the conceptus is exposed to untoward exogenous influences, the noxious agent exerts the same effect on all blastomeres and also causes death. **We conclude that adverse environmental influences on preimplantation-stage embryos exert an all-or-nothing effect: either the conceptus dies or development proceeds uninterrupted, since the interchangeable blastomeres replace the loss.** As a rule, exogenous toxins acting on preimplantation-stage embryos do not produce errors of morphogenesis and do not result in malformations (see Fig. 6-3). **The most common consequence of toxic exposure at the preimplantation stage is embryonic death, which often passes unnoticed or is perceived as heavy, albeit delayed, menstrual bleeding.**

Injury during the first 8 to 10 days after fertilization usually results in an incomplete separation of blastomeres, an effect that leads to the formation of double monsters. Symmetric double monsters represent incompletely separated twins ("Siamese twins") joined at various anatomical sites, such as the head (craniopagus), thorax (thoracopagus), or rump (ischiopagus). Asymmetric double monsters have one well-developed and one rudimentary or hypoplastic twin. The rudimentary twin is always abnormal and is either externally attached to or internally included in the body of the better-developed sibling (fetus in fetu). Some of the congenital teratomas, especially those in the sacrococcygeal area, are actually asymmetric monsters.

Most complex developmental abnormalities affecting several organ systems are due to injuries inflicted from the time of implantation of the blastocyst through early organogenesis. In addition to rapid cell division, this period is characterized by differentiation of cells and formation of so-called **developmental fields**, in which cells interact and determine each other's developmental fate. This process leads to irreversible differentiation of groups of cells. Complex morphological movements form organ primordia (anlage), and organs are then interconnected in functionally active systems. **The formation of primordial organ systems is the stage of embryonic development most susceptible to teratogenesis, and many major developmental abnormalities are probably due to faulty gene activity or the deleterious effects of exogenous toxins on the embryo at this time** (see Fig. 6-3). Disorganized or disrupted morphogenesis may have minor or major consequences at the level of (1) cells and tissues, (2) organs or organ systems, and (3) anatomical regions.

Agenesis *is the complete absence of an organ primordium.* It may present as (1) complete absence of an organ, as in unilateral or bilateral agenesis of kidneys; (2) the absence of part of an organ, as in agenesis of the corpus callosum of the brain; or (3) the absence of tissue or cells within an organ, as in the absence of testicular germ cells in congenital infertility ("Sertoli cell only" syndrome).

Aplasia *is the absence of an organ coupled with persistence of the organ anlage or a rudiment that never developed completely.* Thus, aplasia of the lung refers to a condition in which the main bronchus ends blindly in nondescript tissue composed of rudimentary ducts and connective tissue.

Hypoplasia *refers to reduced size owing to the incomplete development of all or part of an organ.* Examples include microphthalmia (small eyes), micrognathia (small jaw), and microcephaly (small brain and head).

Dysraphic anomalies *are defects caused by the failure of apposed structures to fuse.* Spina bifida is an anomaly in which the spinal canal has not closed completely and the overlying bone and skin have not fused, thus leaving a midline defect.

Involution failures *reflect the persistence of embryonic or fetal structures that should involute at certain stages of development.* A persistent thyroglossal duct is the result of incomplete involution of the tract that connects the base of the tongue with the developing thyroid.

Division failures *are caused by the incomplete cleavage of embryonic tissues, when that process depends on the programmed death of cells.* Fingers and toes are formed at the distal end of the limb bud through the loss of cells located between the primordia that contain the cartilage. If these cells do not die in a programmed manner, the fingers will be conjoined or incompletely separated (syndactyly).

Atresia *refers to defects caused by the incomplete formation of a lumen.* Many hollow organs originate as strands and cords of cells, the centers of which are programmed to die, thus forming a central cavity or lumen. Atresia of the esophagus is characterized by partial occlusion of the lumen, which was not fully established in embryogenesis.

Dysplasia *is caused by abnormal organization of cells into tissues, a situation that results in abnormal histogenesis.* (Dysplasia has a different meaning here from that used in characterizing the precancerous lesion epithelial dysplasia [see Chapter 1].) Tuberous sclerosis is a striking example of dysplasia, being characterized by abnormal development of the brain, which contains aggregates of normally developed cells arranged into grossly visible "tubers."

Ectopia or heterotopia *is an anomaly in which an organ is outside its normal anatomical site.* Thus, an ectopic heart is located outside the thorax. Heterotopic parathyroid glands can be located within the thymus in the anterior mediastinum.

Dystopia *refers to the retention of an organ at a site where it is located during development.* For example, the kidneys are initially in the pelvis and then move into a more craniad lumbar position. Dystopic kidneys are those that remain in the pelvis. Dystopic testes are retained in the inguinal canal, not having completed their descent into the scrotum (cryptorchidism).

Developmental anomalies caused by interference with morphogenesis are often multiple:

- ***A polytopic effect*** *refers to a situation in which the noxious stimulus affects several organs that are simultaneously in critical stages of development.*
- ***A monotopic effect*** *denotes a single localized anomaly that results in a cascade of pathogenetic events.*
- ***A developmental sequence anomaly*** *(anomalad or complex anomaly) is a pattern of defects that is related to a single anomaly or pathogenetic mechanism.* In a developmental sequence anomaly, different factors lead to the same consequences through a common pathway. Such a situation, which represents the result of a monotopic effect, is well illustrated by Potter complex (Fig. 6-4), in which pulmonary hypoplasia, external signs of intrauterine fetal compression, and morphological changes of the amnion, are all related to oligohydramnios (a severely reduced amount of amniotic fluid). A fetus enclosed in an amniotic sac with insufficient fluid develops the distinctive features of Potter complex irrespective of the cause of the oligohydramnios.

A developmental syndrome *refers to multiple anomalies that are pathogenetically related.* The term *syndrome* implies a single cause for anomalies in diverse organs that have been damaged by the same polytopic effect during a critical developmental period. Many of the developmental syndromes are related to chromosomal abnormalities or single-gene defects. By contrast, ***developmental association or syntropy*** refers to multiple anomalies that are associated statistically but do not necessarily share the same pathogenetic mechanisms. Many of the anomalies that now seem unrelated may one day prove to have the same cause. However, until such associations are proved, it is important to note that not all multiple congenital defects are interrelated. In practical terms, the birth of a child with multiple anomalies does not prove that the mother was exposed to an exogenous teratogen or that all the diverse anomalies are caused by the same genetic defect. The recognition of specific syndromes, and their distinction from random associations, is essential for the estimation of the risk of recurrence of similar anomalies in subsequent children in the same family.

After the third month of pregnancy, exposure of the human fetus to teratogenic influences rarely results in major errors of morphogenesis. However, morphological and, especially, functional consequences are still found in children exposed to exogenous teratogens during the second and third trimesters. Although organs have already been formed by the end of the third month of pregnancy, most still undergo the restructuring and maturation required for extrauterine life. Functional maturation proceeds at different rates in different organs. For example, the central nervous system does not attain functional maturity until several years after birth and is, thus, susceptible to adverse exogenous influences not only during pregnancy but for some time after birth.

*A **deformation** is defined as an abnormality of form, shape, or position of a part of the body caused by mechanical forces.* Most anatomical defects caused by adverse influences in the latter two trimesters of pregnancy fall into this category. The responsible forces may be external (e.g., amniotic bands in the uterus) or intrinsic (e.g., fetal hypomobility caused by central nervous system injury). Thus, a deformity known as equinovarus foot can be due to the compression of the extremities by the uterine wall in oligohydramnios or to spinal cord abnormalities that lead to defective innervation and movement of the foot.

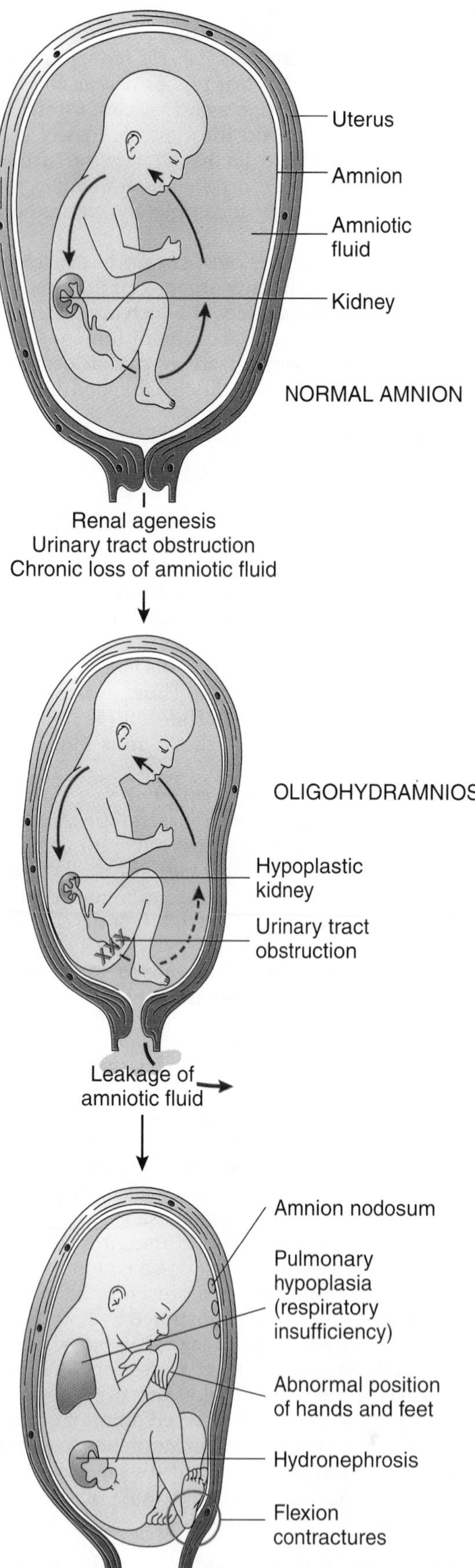

FIGURE *6-4*
Potter complex. The fetus normally swallows amniotic fluid and, in turn, excretes urine, thereby maintaining its normal volume of amniotic fluid. In the face of urinary tract disease, such as renal agenesis or urinary tract obstruction, or leakage of amniotic fluid, the volume of amniotic fluid decreases, a situation termed *oligohydramnios*. Oligohydramnios results in a number of congenital abnormalities termed *Potter complex*, which includes pulmonary hypoplasia and contractures of the limbs. The amnion has a nodular appearance. In cases of urinary tract obstruction, congenital hydronephrosis is also seen although this abnormality is not considered part of Potter complex.

Clinically Important Malformations

Anencephaly and Other Neural Tube Defects

Anencephaly

Anencephaly refers to the congenital absence of the cranial vault, with cerebral hemispheres completely missing or reduced to small masses attached to the base of the skull.

□ Epidemiology: Anencephaly is a typical multifactorial birth defect that exhibits a worldwide geographic variation in incidence. In the United States, the frequency of this anomaly is 0.3 per 1000 live births and stillbirths, whereas in Ireland and Wales, the frequency is 20-fold greater (5 to 6 per 1000 conceptuses). Interestingly, Irish immigrants to North America have the highest incidence of anencephaly on the continent, although it is lower (2 to 3 per 1000) than that in Ireland. A high frequency of anencephaly has also been reported in Iran. The incidence of this disorder is particularly low in blacks.

□ Pathogenesis and Pathology: Anencephaly is a dysraphic defect of neural tube closure. During fetal development the neural plate invaginates and is transformed into the neural tube by fusion of the posterior surfaces (Fig. 6-5). The mesenchymal tissue overlying the primitive neural tube then molds the skull and the vertebral arches posterior to the spinal cord. Failure of the neural tube to close results in the lack of closure of the overlying bony structures of the cranium and an absence of the calvarium, skin, and subcutaneous tissues of this region. The exposed brain is incompletely formed or even entirely absent. In most cases, the base of the skull contains only fragments of neural and ependymal tissue and residues of the meninges. **Acrania** (complete or partial absence of the cranium) results from an injury to the fetus between the 23rd and 26th days of gestation.

Genetic factors seem to play a role in the pathogenesis of anencephaly. The anomaly is twice as common in females as in males, and it occurs with higher frequency in certain families. The risk of a second anencephalic fetus is 2% to 5%, and after two anencephalic fetuses the risk rises to 25% for each subsequent pregnancy.

Folic acid supplied in the periconceptional period lowers the incidence of neural tube defects (NTDs). In this context, mild elevations of blood homocysteine levels (homocysteinemia) in pregnant women carry an increased risk of NTDs. Women with a common polymorphism (677C $\rightarrow$ T) of the enzyme 5,10-methylenetetrahydrofolate reductase (MTHFR) have (1) reduced enzyme activity, (2) decreased function of the folate methylation cycle, (3) increased plasma homocysteine levels, and (4) a sevenfold increased risk of bearing an infant with an NTD. Experimental data indicate that homocysteine is a teratogen for the central nervous system and the heart. Pharmacological doses of folic acid lower plasma homocysteine levels, a finding that is thought to explain the protective effect of folate for NTDs. As a consequence, the Food and Drug Administration has approved the supplementation of flour with folate as a means to prevent these anomalies.

□ Clinical Features: Two thirds of anencephalic fetuses die *in utero*, and those that are alive at birth rarely survive for more than a week. Screening of pregnant women for serum α-fetoprotein and examination by ultrasonography allow detection of virtually all anencephalic fetuses. The use of organs from anencephalic infants for transplantation remains a thorny ethical problem.

Other Neural Tube Defects

The neural tube closes sequentially in a craniocaudad direction, and a defect in this process results in abnormalities of the vertebral column.

- ***Craniorachischisis*** *occurs when defective closure extends from the cranium into the spinal cord and vertebral column.*
- ***Spina bifida*** *refers to the incomplete closure of the spinal cord and vertebral column.* This anomaly is usually localized to the lumbar region and represents the mildest dysraphic abnormality of the central nervous system. Spina bifida results from an insult between the 25th and 30th days of gestation, reflecting the sequential closure of the neural tube.
- ***Meningocele*** *is a hernial protrusion of the meninges through a defect in the vertebral column.*
- ***Myelomeningocele*** *refers to the same condition as meningocele, but it is complicated by hernial protrusion of the spinal cord itself.*

Neural tube defects are illustrated in Figure 6-5 and discussed in greater detail in Chapter 29.

Thalidomide-Induced Malformations

Limb-reduction deformities, involving one or up to all four extremities, are rare congenital defects of unknown origin that affect 1 in 5000 liveborn infants. These defects have been known for ages: a Goya depiction of a typical example is in the Louvre Museum in Paris. In the 1960s, a sudden increase in the incidence of limb-reduction deformities in Germany and England was linked to maternal intake of a sedative during the early stages of pregnancy. Known under the generic name of thalidomide, this derivative of glutamic acid is teratogenic between the 28th and 50th days of pregnancy. Many of the children born to mothers exposed to thalidomide presented with skeletal deformities and pleomorphic defects in other organs, most commonly the ears (**microtia** and **anotia**) and the heart. Typically, the arms of the affected children were short and malformed (Fig. 6-6) and resembled the flippers of the seal (**phocomelia**). Sometimes limbs were completely missing (**amelia**). The central nervous system was not involved, and the children had normal intelligence. After it was recognized that the defects were causally linked to thalidomide, the drug was banned from the

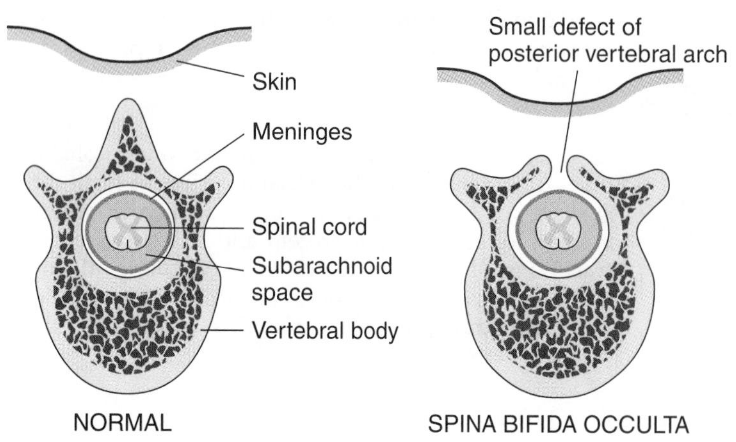

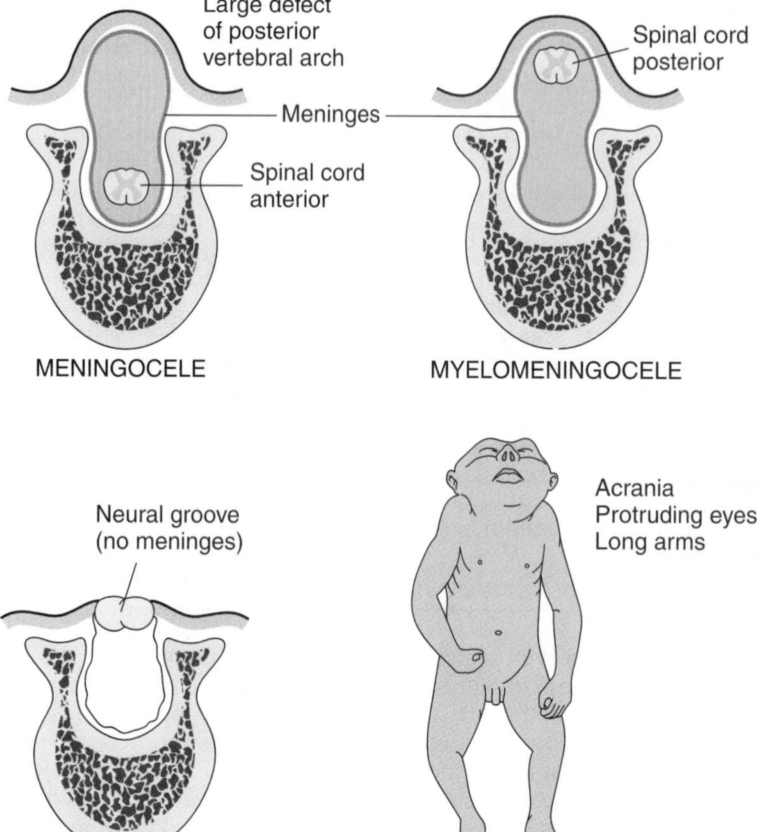

FIGURE *6-5*
Dysraphic defects of the neural tube. Incomplete fusion of the neural tube and overlying bone, soft tissues, or skin leads to several defects, varying from mild anomalies, such as spina bifida occulta, to severe anomalies, such as anencephaly.

market, but not before an estimated 3000 malformed children were born.

Fetal Hydantoin Syndrome

Approximately 10% of children born to epileptic mothers treated during pregnancy with antiepileptic drugs such as hydantoin show characteristic facial features, hypoplasia of nails and digits, and various congenital heart defects. Since this syndrome occurs only two to three times more often in treated epileptics than in untreated ones, it is uncertain whether the defects are entirely due to the adverse effects of the drug. Nevertheless, it appears that fetal susceptibility to this disorder correlates with the fetal level of the microsomal detoxifying enzyme epoxide hydrolase. Presumably,

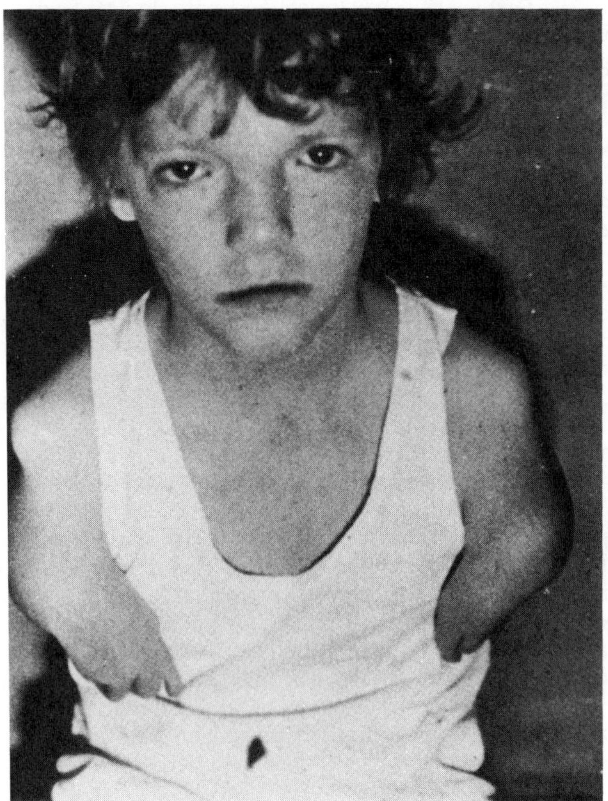

FIGURE 6-6
Thalidomide-induced deformity of the arms.

the accumulation of poorly detoxified reactive intermediates of hydantoin metabolism promotes teratogenesis.

Fetal Alcohol Syndrome

Fetal alcohol syndrome refers to a complex of abnormalities induced by the maternal consumption of alcoholic beverages that includes (1) growth retardation, (2) dysfunction of the central nervous system, and (3) characteristic facial dysmorphology. Since not all children adversely affected by maternal alcohol abuse exhibit the entire spectrum of abnormalities, the term **fetal alcohol effect** is also used.

☐ Epidemiology and Pathogenesis: An injurious effect of intrauterine exposure to alcohol was noted in biblical times and was reported during the historic London gin epidemic (1720 to 1750). However, it was not until 1968 that a specific syndrome was identified. The prevalence of fetal alcohol syndrome in the United States and Europe is 1 to 3 per 1000 live births. However, in populations with extremely high rates of alcoholism, such as some tribes of Native Americans, the incidence may be astounding (20 to 150 per 1000). **It is thought that abnormalities related to fetal alcohol effect, particularly mild degrees of mental deficiency and emotional disorders, are far more common than the full-blown fetal alcohol syndrome.**

The minimum amount of alcohol that results in fetal injury is not well established, but children with the entire spectrum of fetal alcohol syndrome are usually born to mothers who are chronic alcoholics. Heavy alcohol consumption during the first trimester of pregnancy is particularly dangerous. The mechanism by which alcohol damages the developing fetus remains unknown despite a large body of research.

☐ Pathology and Clinical Features: Infants born to alcoholic mothers often exhibit prenatal growth retardation, which continues after birth. The facial dysmorphology of fetal alcohol syndrome includes microcephaly, epicanthal folds, short palpebral fissures, maxillary hypoplasia, a thin upper lip, a small jaw (micrognathia), and a poorly developed philtrum. Septal defects of the heart are described in as many as one third of the patients, although many of these close spontaneously. Minor abnormalities of the joints and limbs may occur.

Fetal alcohol syndrome is a common cause of mental retardation. In a major study, one fifth of children with fetal alcohol syndrome had IQs less than 70, and 40% of the IQs were between 70 and 85. Even with a normal IQ, these children tend to have short memory spans, impulsiveness, and emotional instability.

TORCH Complex

The acronym TORCH refers to a complex of similar signs and symptoms produced by fetal or neonatal infection with a variety of microorganisms, including Toxoplasma (T), rubella (R), cytomegalovirus (C), and herpes simplex virus (H). In the acronym TORCH, the letter "O" represents "others." The term was coined to alert pediatricians to the fact that the infections in the fetus and newborn by TORCH agents are usually indistinguishable from each other and that testing for one of the four major TORCH agents should include testing for the other three and for some possible others as well (Fig. 6-7). As noted by the original authors, other infections include syphilis, tuberculosis, listeriosis, leptospirosis, varicella-zoster virus infection, and Epstein-Barr virus infection. Human immunodeficiency virus and human parvovirus (B19) have been suggested as additions to the list.

Infections with TORCH agents occur in 1% to 5% of all liveborn infants in the United States and are among the major causes of neonatal morbidity and mortality. Severe damage inflicted by these organisms is mostly irreparable, and prevention (when possible) is the only alternative. Unfortunately, the titers of serum antibodies against TORCH agents in the newborn or the mother is usually not diagnostic and the precise etiology of the condition often remains obscure.

- **Toxoplasmosis:** Asymptomatic toxoplasmosis is common, and 25% of women in their reproductive years exhibit antibodies to this organism. On the other hand, intrauterine Toxoplasma infection occurs in only 0.1% of all pregnancies.

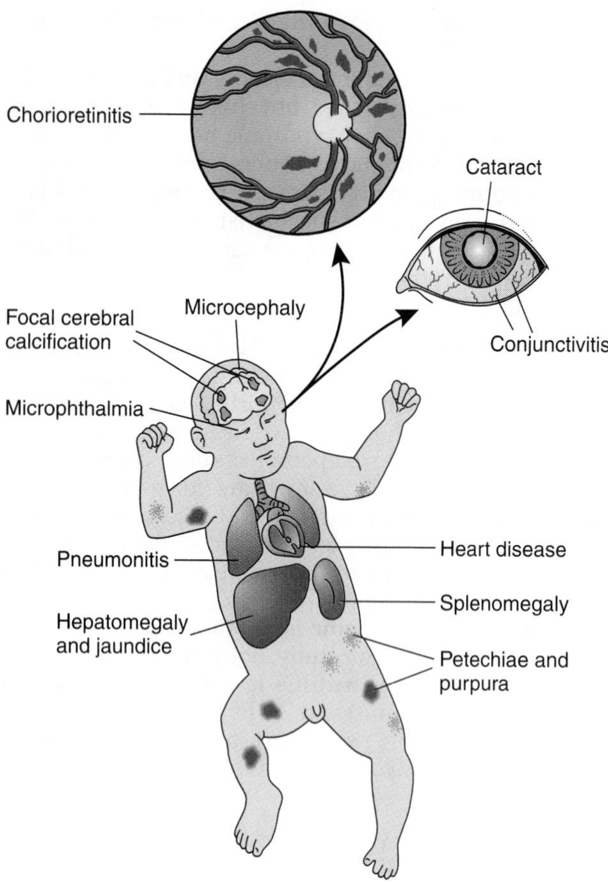

FIGURE *6-7*
TORCH complex. Children infected *in utero* with Toxoplasma, rubella virus, cytomegalovirus, or herpes simplex virus show remarkably similar symptoms.

- **Rubella:** The introduction of the rubella vaccine in the United States has virtually eliminated congenital rubella, and fewer than 10 cases are reported each year.
- **Cytomegalovirus:** Two thirds of women of child-bearing age test positive for cytomegalovirus immunoglobulin G (IgG), and up to 2% of newborns in the United States are congenitally infected with this virus. Since most normal infants carry maternally transmitted antibodies, the "gold standard" for the diagnosis of cytomegalovirus is a urine culture.
- **Herpesvirus:** Intrauterine infection with herpes simplex virus type 2 is uncommon, and infection is most often acquired during passage through the birth canal of a mother with active genital herpes. The diagnosis is established by clinical examination of the mother, the appearance of typical skin lesions in the newborn, and serological testing and culture for herpes simplex virus type 2. Congenital herpes infection can be prevented by cesarean section of mothers who exhibit active genital lesions.

The specific organisms of the TORCH complex are discussed in greater detail in Chapter 9.

☐ Pathology: The clinical and pathological findings in the symptomatic newborn vary, and only a minority present with a multisystem disease and the entire spectrum of abnormalities (Table 6-1). Growth retardation and abnormalities of the brain, eyes, liver, hemopoietic system, and heart are common.

Lesions of the brain represent the most serious pathological changes in TORCH-infected children. Acute encephalitis is associated with foci of necrosis, which are initially surrounded by inflammatory cells. Later the lesions become calcified and are visualized radiologically, most prominently in congenital toxoplasmosis. Microcephaly, hydrocephalus, and abnormally shaped gyri and sulci (microgyria) are frequent. Radiologically, defects of cerebral matter (porencephaly), missing olfactory bulbs, and other major brain defects may be identified. Severe brain damage is reflected in psychomotor retardation, neurological defects, and seizures.

Ocular defects are prominent in the TORCH complex, particularly in rubella embryopathy, in which more than two thirds of patients present with cataracts and microphthalmos. Glaucoma and malformations of the retina (coloboma) may occur. Choroidoretinitis, which is common in infections with rubella, Toxoplasma, and cytomegalovirus, is usually bilateral, and on funduscopy presents as pale, mottled areas surrounded by a pigmented rim. Keratoconjunctivitis is the most common ocular lesion in newborns afflicted with herpes simplex.

TABLE *6-1* **Pathological Findings in the Fetus and Newborn Infected with TORCH Agents**

General	Prematurity, intrauterine retardation	
Central nervous system	Encephalitis	
	Microcephaly	
	Hydrocephaly	
	Intracranial calcifications	
	Psychomotor retardation	
Ear	Inner ear damage with hearing loss	
Eye	Chorioretinitis	(TCH)
	Pigmented retina	(R)
	Keratoconjunctivitis	(H)
	Cataracts	(RH)
	Glaucoma	(R)
	Visual impairment	(TRCH)
Liver	Hepatomegaly	
	Liver calcifications	(R)
	Jaundice	
Hemopoietic system	Hemolytic and other anemias	
	Thrombocytopenia	
	Splenomegaly	
Skin and mucosae	Vesicular or ulcerative lesions (H)	
	Petechiae and ecchymoses	
Cardiopulmonary system	Pneumonitis	
	Myocarditis	
	Congenital heart disease	
Skeleton	Various bone lesions	

T, Toxoplasma; R, rubella virus; C, cytomegalovirus; H, herpesvirus.

Cardiac anomalies occur in many children with the TORCH complex, most commonly in congenital rubella. Patent ductus arteriosus and various septal defects are the most frequent abnormalities, although occasionally stenosis of the pulmonary artery and complex cardiac anomalies are encountered.

Congenital Syphilis

The organism that causes syphilis, *Treponema pallidum*, is transmitted to the fetus by a mother who has acquired syphilis during pregnancy. There is a possibility that the fetus will develop syphilis if the mother became infected in the 2 years preceding the pregnancy, although the actual risk cannot be accurately assessed. It has been estimated that congenital syphilis affects 1 in 2000 liveborn infants in the United States. In pregnant syphilitic women, stillbirth occurs in one third, and of the infants carried to term, two thirds manifest congenital syphilis.

T. pallidum invades the fetus at any point during pregnancy. Early infections most likely induce abortions, and the grossly visible signs of congenital syphilis appear only in fetuses infected after the 16th week of pregnancy. The spirochetes grow in all fetal tissues, and the clinical presentation is thus characterized by protean manifestations.

Children born with congenital syphilis are initially normal or show changes indistinguishable from those of the TORCH complex. The early lesions in various organs teem with spirochetes and are characterized by infiltrates of lymphocytes and plasma cells, particularly around blood vessels and granuloma-like lesions termed **gummas**. Many infants are asymptomatic, only to develop the typical stigmata of congenital syphilis in the first few years of life. Late symptoms of congenital syphilis become apparent many years later and reflect slowly evolving tissue destruction and repair:

- **Rhinitis:** A conspicuous mucopurulent nasal discharge, colloquially known as "snuffles," is almost always present as an early sign of congenital syphilis. The nasal mucosa is edematous and tends to ulcerate, leading to nosebleeds. Destruction of the nasal bridge eventually results in flattening of the nose, so-called **saddle nose**.
- **Skin:** A maculopapular rash is a common early finding in congenital syphilis. The palms and soles are usually affected (similar to secondary syphilis of the adult), although it may involve the entire body or any part. Cracks and fissures (**rhagades**) around the mouth, anus, and vulva occur. Flat raised plaques (**condylomata lata**) around the anus and female genitalia may develop early or after a few years.
- **Visceral organs:** A distinctive pneumonitis, characterized by pale hypocrepitant lungs (**pneumonia alba**), may develop in the neonatal period. Hepatosplenomegaly, anemia, and lymphadenopathy may also be observed in early congenital syphilis.
- **Teeth:** The buds of the incisor teeth and the 6th-year molars develop early in postnatal life, the time when congenital syphilis is particularly aggressive. Thus, the permanent incisors may be notched (**Hutchinson teeth**) and the molars malformed (**mulberry molars**).
- **Bones:** The most common osseous lesion is an inflammation of the periosteum together with new bone formation (periostitis). This complication is particularly evident in the anterior tibia, resulting in a distinctive outward curving called **saber shin**.
- **Eye:** A progressive vascularization of the cornea (**interstitial keratitis**) is an especially vexing complication of congenital syphilis, occurring as early as 4 years of age and as late as 20 years. The cornea eventually scars and becomes opaque.
- **Nervous system:** The nervous system is commonly involved in congenital syphilis, with symptoms beginning in infancy or after 1 year of age. **Meningitis** predominates in early congenital syphilis, resulting in convulsions, mild hydrocephalus, and mental retardation. **Meningovascular syphilis** is a common lesion in later syphilis, which may result in deafness, mental retardation, paresis, and other manifestations of neurosyphilis. **Hutchinson triad** refers to the combination of deafness, interstitial keratitis, and notched incisor teeth.

The diagnosis of congenital syphilis is suggested by clinical findings and a history of maternal infection. Serological confirmation of syphilitic infection may be difficult in the newborn because the transplacental transfer of maternal IgG gives false-positive results. If the infant presents with skin lesions, the diagnosis is established by demonstrating *T. pallidum* in swabs from tissue. In children born to syphilitic mothers who do not have clinically detectable disease, one should perform monthly quantitative reagin tests in an attempt to detect the infant's own immune response to *T. pallidum*. If the transfer of maternal antibodies accounts for a positive test, the titer in the infants's serum should slowly decrease over 2 to 3 months. However, if the infant itself is infected with *T. pallidum*, the titers of reaginic antibodies will remain high or even increase. Penicillin is still the drug of choice for both intrauterine and postnatal syphilis. If penicillin is given during intrauterine life or during the first 2 years of postnatal life, the prognosis is excellent, and most symptoms of early and late congenital syphilis will be prevented.

CHROMOSOMAL ABNORMALITIES

During cell division, the nuclear material condenses to form the **chromosomes**, distinct threadlike particles composed of nucleic acids and proteins. All somatic cells in the human body contain 46 chromosomes: 44 autosomes and 2 sex chromosomes. **Cytogenetics** is the discipline concerned with the study of chromosomes and chromosomal abnormalities. The classification system now in use is the International System for Human Cytogenetic Nomenclature (ISCN).

Normal Chromosomes

Cytogenetic analysis can be performed on any spontaneously dividing cell. However, in most instances the analysis is performed on circulating lymphocytes, which are easily stimulated to undergo mitosis. Mitotic cells are treated with colchicine to arrest them in metaphase, after which they are spread on glass slides to disperse the chromosomes. The chromosomes are stained with standard hematological techniques that enable more precise identification of chromosomes on the basis of distinct bands.

Chromosome Structure

Using hematological stains such as Giemsa, the chromosomes are classified according to their **length** and the positioning of the constriction, or **centromere**. The centromere is the point at which the two identical double helices of the chromosomal DNA, called **sister chromatids**, attach to each other during mitosis. The location of the centromere is used to classify the chromosomes as **metacentric, submetacentric, or acrocentric**. In metacentric chromosomes (numbers 1, 3, 19, and 20), the centromere is exactly in the middle. In submetacentric chromosomes, the centromere divides the chromosome into a short arm (p, from French *petit*) and a long arm (q, the next letter in the alphabet). Acrocentric chromosomes (numbers 13, 14, 15, 21, 22, and Y) have very short arms or stalks and satellites attached to an eccentrically located centromere. Chromosomes of many animal species have terminally located centromeres, but these **telocentric** chromosomes are not found in humans.

Hematological stains are used to classify chromosomes into seven groups, conveniently labeled with letters from A to G. Thus, group A contains two large metacentric and a large submetacentric chromosome, group B contains two distinct large submetacentric chromosomes, group C contains six submetacentric chromosomes, and so forth.

Chromosomal Banding

To identify each chromosome individually, special stains delineate specific bands of different staining intensity on each chromosome. **The pattern of bands is unique to each chromosome and makes possible (1) the pairing of two homologous chromosomes, (2) the recognition of each chromosome, and (3) the identification of defects on each segment of a chromosome.**

Chromosome bands are labeled as follows:

- **G bands:** These chromosomal segments stain with Giemsa (hence G).
- **Q bands:** These bands stain with Giemsa and also fluoresce when stained with quinacrine (hence Q).
- **R bands:** On appropriate staining, R bands present as the reverse (hence R) image of G and Q bands, that is, dark G bands are light R bands, and vice versa.
- **C banding:** This is a method for staining centromeres (hence C) and other portions of chromosomes containing constitutive heterochromatin. By contrast, facultative heterochromatin forms the inactive X chromosome (Barr body).
- **Nucleolar organizing region (NOR) staining:** Secondary constrictions (stalks) of chromosomes with satellites are demonstrated by NOR staining.
- **T banding:** This technique stains the terminal (hence T) ends of chromosomes.

Structural Chromosomal Abnormalities

Structural abnormalities of chromosomes may arise during somatic cell division (mitosis) or during gametogenesis (meiosis). In the case of somatic cell division (most common in rapidly proliferating tissues, e.g., intestines or skin), the structurally abnormal chromosome that arises during mitosis may still code for all of the essential functions of the cell, thereby permitting survival for the normal (usually short) life span of the cell. Alternatively, structural or metabolic deficiencies resulting from a structurally abnormal chromosome may be lethal, in which case only a single cell dies. In both of these instances, structural chromosomal abnormalities that occur during somatic cell division are of no consequence. However, under some circumstances, structural abnormalities may involve protooncogenes and contribute to the pathogenesis of certain cancers (see Chapter 5).

The structural chromosomal abnormalities that originate during gametogenesis are important in a different context, because they are transmitted to all somatic cells of the offspring and may result in heritable diseases. During normal meiosis, homologous chromosomes (e.g., two chromosomes 1) form pairs, termed **bivalents**. By a normal process known as crossing-over, parts of these chromosomes are exchanged, thereby rearranging the genetic constituents of each chromosome. Such an exchange of genetic material may also take place between nonhomologous chromosomes (e.g., between chromosomes 3 and 21), by an abnormal process termed **translocation**. Two major forms of chromosomal translocations are recognized, namely reciprocal and robertsonian.

Reciprocal Translocations

A reciprocal translocation refers to the exchange of acentric chromosomal segments between two different (nonhomologous) chromosomes (Fig. 6-8). A reciprocal translocation is said to be **balanced** when there is no loss of genetic material, that is, when each chromosomal segment is translocated in its entirety. When such translocations are present in the gametes (sperm or ova), the progeny maintain the abnormal chromosomal structure in all somatic cells. **Since balanced translocations are not associated with the loss of genes or the disruption of vital gene loci, most carriers of such balanced translocations are phenotypically normal.** Balanced reciprocal translocations can be inherited for many generations. Reciprocal translocations are particularly well demonstrated by current banding techniques.

Carriers of balanced translocations, however, are at risk for producing offspring with unbalanced karyotypes and severe phenotypic abnormalities (Fig. 6-9).The

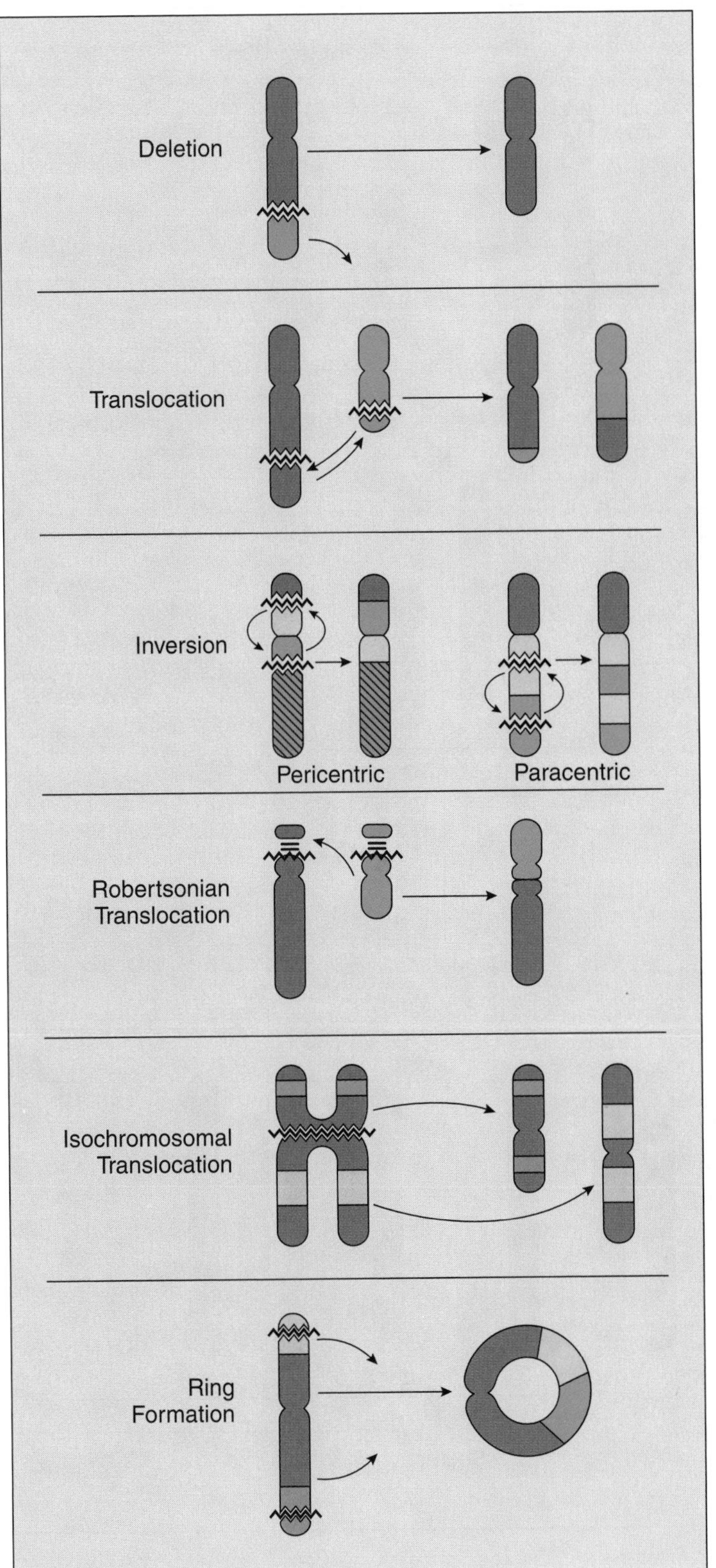

FIGURE *6-8*
Structural abnormalities of human chromosomes. The deletion of a portion of a chromosome leads to the loss of genetic material and a shortened chromosome. A reciprocal translocation involves breaks on two nonhomologous chromosomes, with exchange of the acentric segments. An inversion requires two breaks in a single chromosome. If the breaks are on opposite sides of the centromere, the inversion is "pericentric," whereas it is "paracentric" if the breaks are on the same arm. A robertsonian translocation occurs when two nonhomologous acrocentric chromosomes break near their centromeres, after which the long arms fuse to form one large metacentric chromosome. Isochromosomes arise from faulty centromere division, which leads to duplication of the long arm (iso q) and deletion of the short arm, or the reverse (iso p). Ring chromosomes involve breaks of both telomeric portions of a chromosome, deletion of the acentric fragments, and fusion of the remaining centric portion.

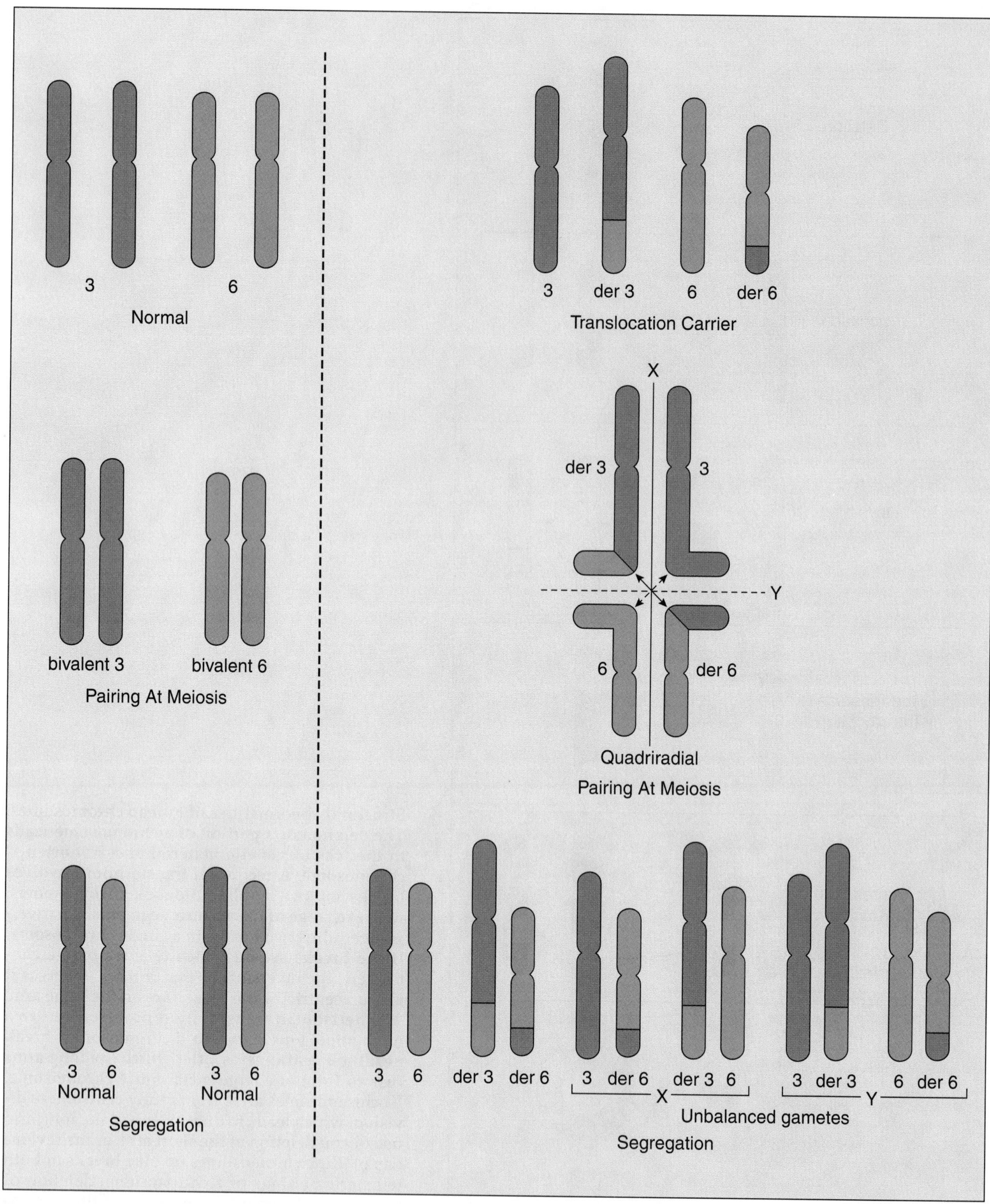
3
6
Normal
3
der 3
6
der 6
Translocation Carrier
X
der 3
3
Y
6
der 6
Quadriradial
Pairing At Meiosis
bivalent 3
bivalent 6
Pairing At Meiosis
3 6
Normal
3 6
Normal
Segregation
3 6
der 3 der 6
3 der 6
der 3 6
X
3 der 3
6 der 6
Y
Unbalanced gametes
Segregation

FIGURE 6-9

abnormal positions of the exchanged chromosomal segments may result in a disturbance of meiosis and lead to abnormal segregation of chromosomes. In a translocation carrier, the formation of bivalents may be disturbed. To achieve complete pairing of the translocated segments, a complex cross-like structure (quadriradial), which consists of two chromosomes bearing the translocations and their two normal homologues, is formed. Unlike the normal bivalent, which typically resolves by an orderly migration of the two chromosomes to the opposite poles, the quadriradial can divide along several different planes. Some of the resulting gametes carry unbalanced chromosomes and on fertilization result in zygotes with various combinations of partial trisomy and monosomy for segments of the translocated chromosomes.

Robertsonian Translocations

Robertsonian translocation (centric fusion) involves the centromere of acrocentric chromosomes. When two nonhomologous chromosomes are broken near the centromere, they may exchange two arms to form one large metacentric chromosome and a small chromosomal fragment. The fragment is devoid of a centromere and is usually lost during subsequent divisions. As in a reciprocal translocation, a robertsonian translocation is balanced if there is no significant loss of genetic material. The carrier is also usually phenotypically normal, although he or she may suffer from infertility. **When fertile, however, carriers of balanced robertsonian translocations are at risk of producing unbalanced translocations in their gametes, in which case the offspring may be born with congenital malformations** (see Fig. 6-9).

Chromosomal Deletions

A deletion is the loss of a portion of a chromosome and involves either a terminal or an intercalary (middle) segment. Disturbances during meiosis in germ cells, or breaks of chromatids during mitosis in somatic cells, may result in the formation of chromosomal fragments that are not incorporated into any of the chromosomes and are thus lost in subsequent cell divisions.

The shortening of the chromosome because of a deletion may be apparent in routinely stained chromosome preparations. Banding techniques are applied to determine whether the arm of the chromosome is shortened because of a deletion of the terminal portion or because of a double break in the more central portions. The latter event leads to intercalary deletion and subsequent fusion of adjoining residual fragments.

Gametic deletion can be associated with either normal or abnormal development. An example of the latter is the **cri du chat syndrome**, which is associated with the deletion of part of the short arm of chromosome 5. Deletion is related to several cancers in humans, including some hereditary forms of cancer. For example, some familial **retinoblastomas** are associated with deletions in the long arm of chromosome 13. **Wilms tumor aniridia syndrome** is associated with deletions in the short arm of chromosome 11.

Chromosomal Inversions

Chromosomal inversion refers to (1) the break of a chromosome at two points, (2) the inversion of the segment between the breaks, and (3) the rejoining of the two broken ends. **Pericentric inversions** result from breaks on opposite sides of the centromere, whereas **paracentric inversions** involve breaks on the same arm of the chromosome (see Fig. 6-8). During meiosis, homologous chromosomes that carry inversions do not exchange segments of chromatids by crossing over as readily as normal chromosomes, because of an interference with pairing. Although this is of little consequence for the phenotype of the offspring, it may be important in evolutionary terms, since it may lead to clustering of certain hereditary features.

Ring Chromosomes

Ring chromosomes are formed by a break involving both telomeric ends of a chromosome, followed by the deletion of the acentric fragments and end-to-end fusion of the remaining centric portion of the chromosome (see Fig. 6-8). The consequences depend primarily on the amount of genetic material lost because of the break. The abnormally shaped chromosome may impede normal meiotic division, but in most instances this chromosomal abnormality is of no consequence.

FIGURE *6-9*
Meiotic segregation in a reciprocal balanced translocation involving chromosomes 3 and 6. (*A*) The pairing of homologous chromosomes 3 and 6 in normal meiosis forms bivalents, which then segregate uniformly to create two gametes, each of which bears a single chromosome 3 and chromosome 6. (*B*) The translocation carrier is depicted as carrying a balanced exchange of portions of the long arms of chromosomes 3 and 6. The chromosomes that carry the translocated genetic material are termed *derivative chromosomes* (der 3 and der 6). Diploid germ cells contain pairs of homologous chromosomes 3 and 6, each of which consists of one normal chromosome and one that carries a translocation. During meiosis, instead of the normal pairing into two bivalents, a quadriradial structure, containing all four chromosomes, is formed. In this circumstance, the chromosomes can segregate along several different planes of cleavage, shown as X and Y. In addition, the chromosomes can segregate diagonally (*arrows*). As a result, six different gametes can be produced, four of which are unbalanced and can result in congenital abnormalities.

Isochromosomes

Isochromosomes are formed by the faulty division of the centromere. Normally, centromere division occurs in a plane parallel to the long axis of the chromosome, leading to the formation of two identical hemichromosomes. If the centromere divides in a plane transverse to the long axis, pairs of isochromosomes are formed. One pair corresponds to the short arms attached to the upper portion of the centromere and the other to the long arms attached to the lower segment (see Fig. 6-8).

The most important clinical condition involving isochromosomes is **Turner syndrome**, in which 15% of those affected have an isochromosome of the X chromosome. Thus, a woman with a normal X chromosome and an isochromosome composed of long arms of the X chromosome is monosomic for all the genes located on the missing short arm (i.e., the other isochromosome, which is lost during the meiotic division). She has three sets of the genes located on the long arm. The absence of the genes from the short arm accounts for the abnormal development in these persons.

Numerical Chromosomal Abnormalities

A number of terms are important for the understanding of developmental defects associated with aberrations in the number of chromosomes.

- **Haploid:** A single set of each of the chromosomes characteristic of a species (23 in humans). Only germ cells have a haploid number (n) of chromosomes.
- **Diploid:** A double set (2n) of each of the chromosomes (46 in humans). Most somatic cells are diploid.
- **Euploid:** Any multiple (from n to 8n) of the haploid number of chromosomes. For example, many normal liver cells contain twice (4n) the DNA of diploid somatic cells and are, therefore, euploid, or more specifically tetraploid. When the multiple is greater than 2 (i.e., greater than diploid), the karyotype is said to be **polyploid**.
- **Aneuploid:** Karyotypes that are not exact multiples of the haploid number. Many cancer cells are aneuploid, a characteristic often associated with an aggressive biological behavior.
- **Monosomy:** The absence in a somatic cell of one chromosome of a homologous pair. For example, Turner syndrome is characterized by the presence of a single X chromosome.
- **Trisomy:** The presence in a somatic cell of an extra copy of a normally paired chromosome. For example, Down syndrome is caused by the presence of three chromosomes 21.

Nondisjunction

Nondisjunction is a failure of paired chromosomes or chromatids to separate and move to opposite poles of the spindle at anaphase, either during mitosis or meiosis. ***Numerical chromosomal abnormalities arise primarily from nondisjunction.*** Nondisjunction leads to aneuploidy if only one pair of chromosomes fails to separate. It results in polyploidy if the entire set does not divide and all the chromosomes are segregated into a single daughter cell. In somatic cells, aneuploidy secondary to nondisjunction leads to one daughter cell that exhibits trisomy ($2n + 1$) and the other monosomy ($2n - 1$) for the affected chromosome pair. Aneuploid germ cells have two copies of the same chromosome ($n + 1$) or lack the affected chromosome entirely ($n - 1$).

Anaphase lag is a special form of nondisjunction in which a single chromosome or chromatid fails to pair with its homologue during anaphase. It lags behind the others on the spindle and is, therefore, not incorporated into the nucleus of the daughter cell. As a result of anaphase lag and the loss of a single chromosome, one daughter cell is monosomic for the missing chromosome, whereas the other remains euploid.

Pathogenesis of Numerical Aberrations

The causes of chromosomal aberrations are obscure. Putative exogenous factors, such as radiation, viruses, and chemicals, affect the mitotic spindle or DNA synthesis and produce mitotic and meiotic disturbances in experimental animals. However, the role of these factors in the production of human chromosomal abnormalities remains conjectural. Immune factors have been invoked, in view of the correlation between autoantibodies and chromosomal anomalies in families with autoimmune thyroid disorders. The familial occurrence of meiotic failure and chromosomal anomalies provides some evidence for the existence of human genes that predispose to faulty cell division. However, these explanations are hypothetical and there are only two documented phenomena known to be of importance in the genesis of numerical aberrations.

- **Nondisjunction during meiosis occurs more commonly in persons with structurally abnormal chromosomes.** This is probably related to the fact that such chromosomes do not pair or segregate during gametogenesis as readily as normal ones.
- **Children born to older women have more frequent numerical chromosomal abnormalities than those born to younger mothers.**

Effects of Chromosomal Aberrations

Most major chromosomal abnormalities are incompatible with life. The defects are usually lethal to the developing conceptus, leading to early death and spontaneous abortion. The loss of genetic material, for example, autosomal monosomies, results in embryos that generally do not survive pregnancy. By contrast, monosomy of the X chromosome (45,X) may be compatible with life, although some 90% of such embryos are lost during pregnancy. The absence of an X chromosome (i.e., the karyotype 45,Y) invariably results in early abortion.

Autosomal trisomies are associated with several developmental abnormalities, and the affected fetus usually dies during pregnancy or shortly after birth. Trisomy 21, which defines Down syndrome, is an exception, and such

TABLE 6-2 **Chromosomal Nomenclature**

Numerical designation of autosomes	1–22
Sex chromosomes	X, Y
Addition of a whole or part of a chromosome	+
Loss of a whole or part of a chromosome	−
Numerical mosaicism (e.g., 46/47)	/
Short arm of chromosome (petite)	p
Long arm of chromosome	q
Isochromosome	i
Ring chromosome	r
Deletion	del
Insertion	ins
Translocation	t
Derivative chromosome (carrying translocation)	der
Terminal	ter
Representative karyotypes	
Male with trisomy 21 (Down syndrome)	47, XY, +21
Female carrier of fusion-type translocation between chromosomes 14 and 21	45,XX,−14,−21, +t(14q21q)
Cri du chat syndrome (male) with deletion of a portion of the short arm of chromosome 5	46,XY,del(5p)
Male with ring chromosome 19	46,XY,r(19)
Turner syndrome with monosomy X	45,X
Mosaic Klinefelter syndrome	46,XY/47,XXY

persons survive for years. Trisomy of the X chromosome may result in abnormal development but is not lethal.

Mitotic nondisjunction may involve embryonic cells during early stages of development and result in chromosomal aberrations. These are transmitted selectively through some cell lineages but not through others. *The condition in which the body contains two or more karyotypically different cell lines is called* ***mosaicism***. Like all chromosomal abnormalities related to nondisjunction, mosaicism may involve autosomes or sex chromosomes. The phenotype of a mosaic person depends on the chromosome involved and the extent of mosaicism. Autosomal mosaicism is rare, most likely because this condition is usually lethal. On the other hand, mosaicism involving sex chromosomes is common and is found in patients with gonadal dysgenesis who present with Turner or Klinefelter syndrome.

Nomenclature of Chromosomal Aberrations

Structural and numerical chromosomal abnormalities are classified according to (1) the total number of chromosomes, (2) the designation (number) of the affected chromosomes, and (3) the nature and location of the defect on the chromosome (Table 6-2). The karyotype is described sequentially in the following order: (1) the total number of chromosomes, (2) the sex chromosome complement, and (3) any abnormality. The short arm of a chromosome is designated **p**, and the long arm is designated **q**. The addition of chromosomal material, whether an entire chromosome or a part of one, is indicated by a plus sign **(+)** before the number of the affected chromosome, and the loss of chromosomal material by a minus sign **(−)**. Alternatively, the loss (deletion) of part of a chromosome may be designated by the symbol **del** followed by the location of the deleted material on the affected chromosome. A translocation is written as a **t**, followed by brackets containing the involved chromosomes.

Structural or numerical chromosomal aberrations are found in 5 to 7 per 1000 liveborn infants, although most are balanced translocations and asymptomatic.

Syndromes of the Autosomal Chromosomes

Clinical syndromes that reflect disorders of the autosomal chromosomes may arise from numerical or structural abnormalities (Table 6-3). Numerical autosomal aberrations in liveborn infants are virtually all trisomies. Structural aberrations that may result in clinical disorders include translocations, deletions, and chromosomal breakage.

TABLE 6-3 **Clinical Features of the Autosomal Chromosomal Syndromes**

Syndromes	Features
Trisomic Syndromes	
Chromosome 21 (Down syndrome 47,XX or XY, +21:1/800)	Epicanthic folds, speckled irides, flat nasal bridge, congenital heart disease, simian crease of palms, Hirschsprung disease, increased risk of leukemia
Chromosome 18 (47,XX or XY, +18: 1/8000)	Female preponderance, micrognathia, congenital heart disease, horseshoe kidney, deformed fingers
Chromosome 13 (47,XX or XY, +13: 1/20,000)	Persistent fetal hemoglobin, microcephaly, congenital heart disease, polycystic kidneys, polydactyly, simian crease
Deletion Syndromes	
5p− syndrome (Cri du chat 46,XX or XY,5p−)	Catlike cry, low birth weight, microcephaly, epicanthic folds, congenital heart disease, short hands and feet, simian crease
11p− syndrome (46,XX or XY, 11p−)	Aniridia, Wilms tumor, gonadoblastoma, male genital ambiguity
13q− syndrome (46,XX or XY,13q−)	Low birth weight, microcephaly, retinoblastoma, congenital heart disease

All of these syndromes are associated with mental retardation.

Trisomy 21 (Down Syndrome)

Trisomy 21 is the single most common cause of mental retardation. Furthermore, liveborn infants represent only a fraction of all conceptuses with this chromosomal defect. Two thirds are aborted spontaneously or die *in utero*. Life expectancy is also reduced. Recent advances in the therapy for infections, operations for congenital heart defects, and chemotherapy for leukemia—the leading causes of death in patients with Down syndrome—are increasing life expectancy.

☐ Pathogenesis: There are three mechanisms by which three copies of the genes on chromosome 21 that are responsible for Down syndrome may be present in somatic cells:

- **Nondisjunction** during the first meiotic division of gametogenesis accounts for the large majority (92% to 95%) of patients with Down syndrome that have trisomy 21 (Fig. 6-10). DNA polymorphism analysis has shown that the extra chromosome 21 is of maternal origin in about 95% of Down syndrome children. Interestingly, virtually all maternal nondisjunction seems to result from events occurring in the first meiotic division (meiosis I).
- **Translocation** of an extra long arm of chromosome 21 to another acrocentric chromosome causes about 5% of cases of Down syndrome.
- **Mosaicism** for trisomy 21 is caused by nondisjunction during mitosis of a somatic cell in the early stages of embryogenesis and is responsible for 2% of children born with Down syndrome.

The incidence of trisomy 21 correlates strongly with increasing maternal age, that is, older mothers are at a substantially greater risk of giving birth to an infant with Down syndrome (Fig. 6-11). Up to their mid 30s, women have a constant risk of giving birth to a trisomic child of about 1 per 1000 liveborn infants. The risk then increases dramatically and reaches an incidence of 1 in 30 at age 45 years. The risk of recurrence of Down syndrome in subsequent children born to the same mother is 1% irrespective of maternal age, unless the syndrome is associated with translocation of chromosome 21.

The mechanism by which increasing maternal age is associated with a greater risk of bearing a child with trisomy 21 is not known. The "older egg" hypothesis holds that meiotic nondisjunction is more frequent with advanced maternal age. Alternatively, the "relaxed selection" model predicts no maternal age effect on gametic nondisjunction and argues that older women are less able than younger ones to abort a trisomic embryo. Conclusive evidence to resolve this controversy has not yet been derived. Clearly, Down syndrome associated with a translocation or mosaicism is not related to maternal age.

Down syndrome caused by translocation of an extra portion of chromosome 21 occurs in two situations. Either

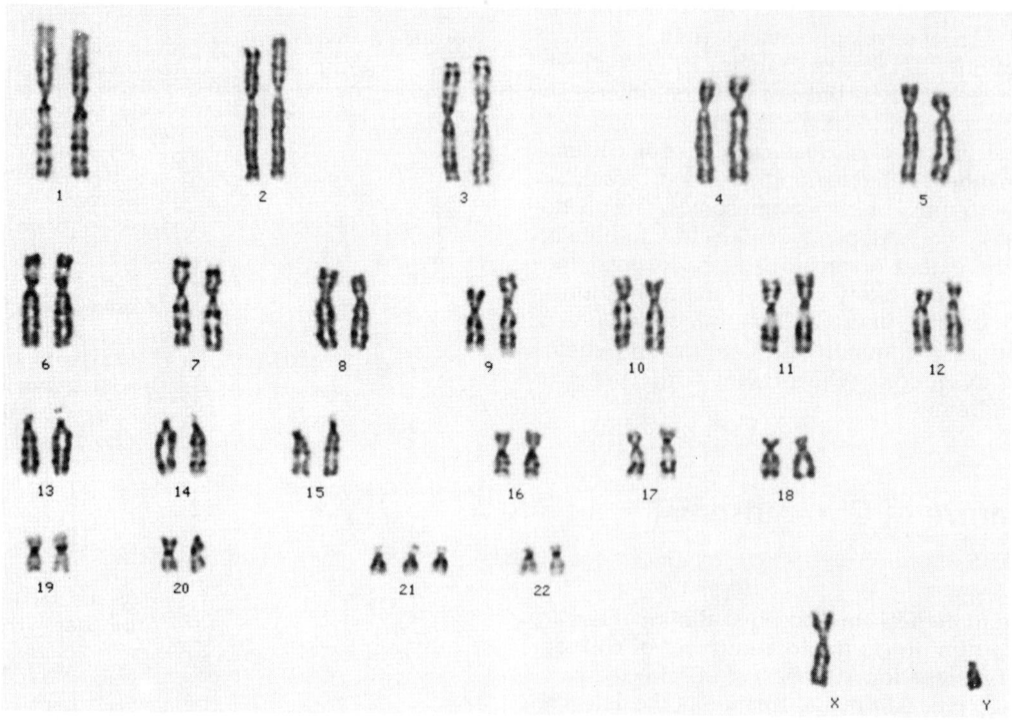

FIGURE 6-10
Trisomy 21 in the karyotype of a child with Down syndrome. All other chromosomes are normal.

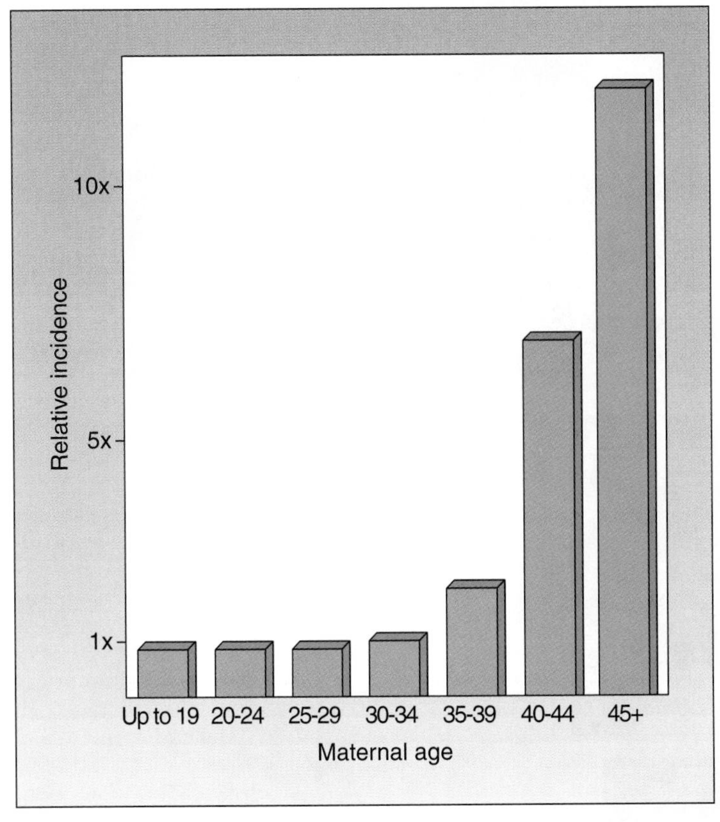

FIGURE *6-11*
Incidence of Down syndrome in relation to maternal age. A conspicuous increase in the frequency of this disorder is seen over the age of 35 years.

parent may be a phenotypically normal carrier of a balanced translocation or the translocation may arise *de novo* during gametogenesis. These translocations are typically robertsonian, tending to involve only acrocentric chromosomes, with short arms consisting of a satellite and stalk (chromosomes 13, 14, 15, 21, and 22). Translocations between these chromosomes are particularly common because they cluster during meiosis and are, therefore, subjected more frequently than other chromosomes to breakage and recombination. The most common translocation in Down syndrome (50%) is fusion of the long arms of chromosomes 21 and 14, t(14q;21q), followed in frequency (40%) by similar fusion involving two chromosomes 21, t(21q;21q).

If the translocation is inherited from a parent, a balanced translocation has been converted to an unbalanced one, as illustrated in Figure 6-9. According to this scheme, one would expect a one in three chance of Down syndrome among the offspring of a carrier of a balanced robertsonian translocation. However, when the mother carries the translocation, the actual incidence is only 10% to 15%, and, for unknown reasons, it is less than 5% when the father is the carrier. This reduced incidence probably relates to the early loss of the majority of embryos with trisomy 21.

Molecular Genetics of Down Syndrome

Chromosome 21 is the smallest human autosome, comprising less than 2% of the human genome. It has an acrocentric structure, and all genes of known function (other than for ribosomal RNA) are located on the long arm (21q). Based on studies of inherited translocations, in which only a portion of chromosome 21 is duplicated, the region on chromosome 21 responsible for the full Down syndrome phenotype has been restricted to band 21q22.2, a 4-Mb region of DNA termed the **Down syndrome critical region**. The gene(s) responsible for Down syndrome remains undetermined. Interesting speculation centers on a recently identified homologue of the *Drosophila* gene "minibrain" in this region. Transgenic mice that overexpress the human gene exhibit defects in learning and memory.

☐ Pathology and Clinical Features: The diagnosis of Down syndrome is ordinarily made at the time of birth by observing the flaccid state and characteristic physical appearance of the infant. The diagnosis is then confirmed by cytogenetic analysis. As the child develops, a typical constellation of abnormalities appears (Fig. 6-12).

- **Mental status:** Children with Down syndrome invariably suffer severe mental retardation, with a relentless and progressive decline in the IQ with age. Beginning with a mean IQ of 70 below the age of 1 year, intelligence deteriorates during the first decade of life to a mean of 30. The major defect seems to be an inability to develop more advanced cognitive strategies and processes, problems that become more apparent as the child grows older. Although these children have traditionally been described as particularly

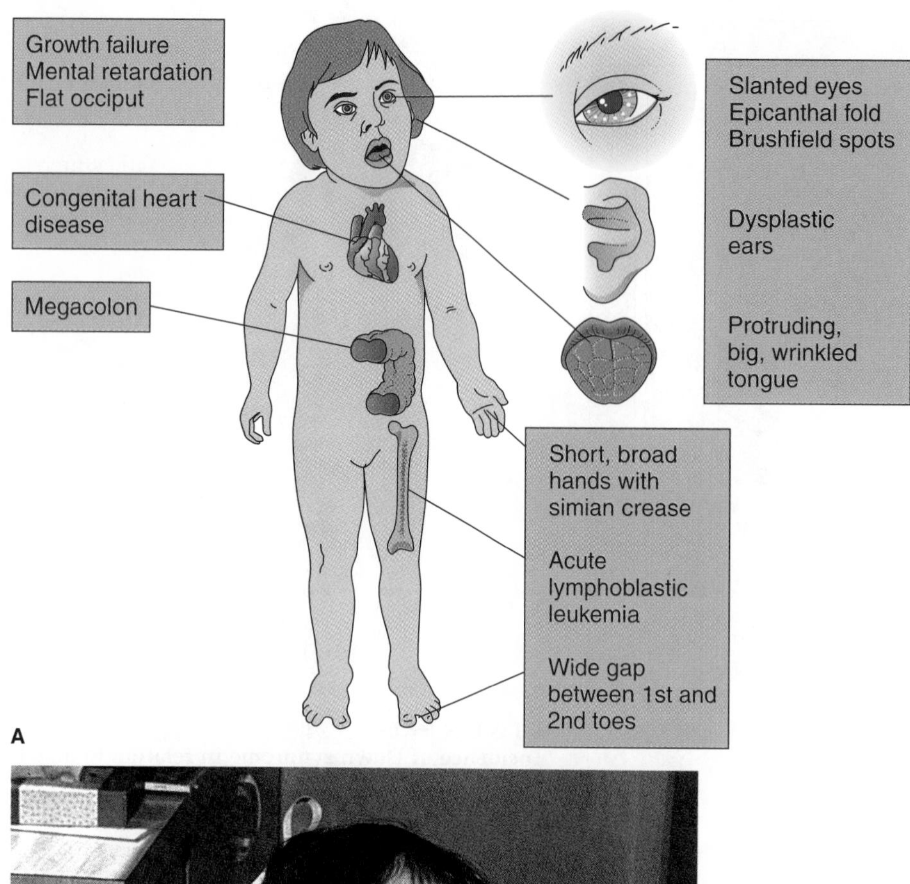

B

FIGURE *6-12*
(*A*) Clinical features of Down syndrome. (*B*) A young girl exhibits the facial features of Down syndrome.

gentle and affectionate, newer studies have cast serious doubt on the validity of these personality stereotypes.

- **Craniofacial features:** The face and occiput tend to be flat, with a low-bridged nose, reduced interpupillary distance, and oblique palpebral fissures. Epicanthal folds of the eyes impart an Oriental appearance, a feature that accounts for the obsolete term **mongolism**. A speckled appearance of the iris is referred to as **Brushfield spots**. The ears are enlarged and malformed. A prominent tongue, which typically lacks a central fissure, protrudes through an open mouth.
- **Heart:** One third of children born with Down syndrome suffer from congenital cardiac disease, and the incidence is even higher in aborted fetuses. The anomalies take the form of atrioventricular canal, ventricular and atrial septal defects, tetralogy of Fallot, and patent ductus arteriosus. Most of the cardiac defects seem to be variations of a common problem in the formation of the venous inflow tract of the heart.
- **Skeleton:** These children tend to be small, owing to shorter than normal bones of the ribs, pelvis, and extremities. The hands are broad and short and exhibit a "simian crease," that is, a single transverse crease

across the palm. The middle phalanx of the fifth finger is hypoplastic, an abnormality that leads to inward curvature of this digit.

- **Gastrointestinal tract:** Duodenal stenosis or atresia, imperforate anus, and Hirschsprung disease (megacolon) occur in 2% to 3% of children with Down syndrome.
- **Reproductive system:** Men with trisomy 21 are invariably sterile, owing to arrested spermatogenesis. A few women with Down syndrome have given birth to children, of which 40% had trisomy 21.
- **Immune system:** Although the immune system in Down syndrome has been the subject of numerous studies, no clear pattern of specific defects has emerged. Nevertheless, affected children are unusually susceptible to respiratory and other infections. Prior to the antibiotic era, most of these children died in infancy from infectious diseases.
- **Hematological disorders:** It has been known for many years that persons with Down syndrome are at a particularly high risk of developing leukemia at all ages. **The risk of leukemia in Down syndrome children younger than the age of 15 years is about 15-fold greater than normal.** In children younger than the age of 3 years, acute nonlymphocytic leukemia predominates. After that age, when most of the leukemias in Down syndrome occur, the majority of cases are acute lymphoblastic leukemias. The basis for the high incidence of leukemia is unknown, but leukemoid reactions (transient pronounced neutrophilia) are frequent in the newborn with Down syndrome. Interestingly, in mosaic Down syndrome, the proliferating leukocytes are invariably trisomic for chromosome 21.
- **Neurological disorders:** The search for specific neuropathological alterations in the brain associated with Down syndrome has proved futile, and no clear pattern of abnormal "wiring" has emerged. Furthermore, there are no characteristic changes in the electroencephalogram. Nevertheless, it is possible that the nerve cells in trisomy 21 are indeed different from normal. Virtually all electrical parameters and a number of physiological ones are altered in cultured neurons from infants with Down syndrome.

  One of the most intriguing neurological features of Down syndrome is its association with Alzheimer disease, a relationship that has been appreciated for more than half a century. The morphological lesions characteristic of Alzheimer disease progress in all patients with Down syndrome and are universally demonstrable by age 35. These changes in the brain include (1) granulovacuolar degeneration, (2) neurofibrillary tangles, (3) senile plaques, and (4) loss of neurons. The senile plaques and cerebral blood vessels of both Alzheimer disease and Down syndrome always contain an amyloid composed of the same fibrillar protein (β-amyloid protein). The similarity between the neuropathological features of Down syndrome and those of Alzheimer disease is also reflected in the appearance of dementia in one fourth to one half of older Down syndrome patients and the progressive loss of many intellectual functions that cannot be attributed to mental retardation alone.
- **Life expectancy:** During the first decade of life, the major determinant of survival in Down syndrome is the presence or absence of congenital heart disease. In those who have a normal heart, only about 5% succumb before age 10, whereas about 25% with heart disease die by that time. After age 10, the estimated life expectancy (the age at death) is 55 years, a life span some 20 years or more less than that of the general population. By age 70, only 10% are still alive.

Trisomies of Chromosomes 18, 13, and 22

Trisomy 18 is the second most common autosomal syndrome, occurring about once in 8000 live births, an order of magnitude less frequent than Down syndrome. The disorder results in mental retardation and affects females four times as often as males. Virtually all infants with trisomy 18 suffer from congenital heart disease and succumb within the first 3 months of life.

Trisomies 13 and 22 are rare, and both are associated with mental retardation, congenital heart disease, and other abnormalities. Syndromes associated with trisomies of chromosomes 8 and 9 have also been described.

Translocation Syndromes

The prototypical translocation that results in partial trisomy is Down syndrome. Many other partial trisomies have been documented, the best documented of which is the 9p− trisomy syndrome. In this disorder, the short arm of chromosome 9 may be translocated to a number of different autosomes, and many kindreds in which this syndrome occurs have been described. Importantly, as in Down syndrome, the carriers of a balanced chromosome 9 translocation are asymptomatic but may transmit an unbalanced translocation to their offspring. The clinical disorder is characterized by mental retardation, microcephaly, and other craniofacial abnormalities. A reciprocal translocation between the long arms of chromosomes 22 and 11 is also well known. The children of carriers may have an extra chromosome containing portions of both 11 and 22, in which case they have partial trisomy of both chromosomes, resulting in microcephaly and a variety of other anomalies.

Chromosomal Deletion Syndromes

The deletion of an entire autosomal chromosome, namely monosomy, is usually not compatible with life. However, several syndromes arise from the deletions of parts of several chromosomes. In most cases, the congenital syndromes are sporadic, but in a few instances, reciprocal translocations have been demonstrated in the parents. Virtually all of these deletion syndromes are characterized by low birth weight, mental retardation, microcephaly, and craniofacial and skeletal abnormalities. Congenital heart disease and urogenital abnormalities are common.

- **5p− syndrome (cri du chat syndrome):** This is the best-known deletion syndrome, because the high-pitched cry of the infant is similar to that of a kitten and calls attention to the disorder. The majority of cases are sporadic, but reciprocal translocations have been reported in some parents.
- **11p− syndrome:** Deletion of the short arm of chromosome 11, specifically band 11p13, results in congenital absence of the iris (aniridia) and is often accompanied by Wilms tumor.
- **13q− syndrome:** A deletion of the long arm of chromosome 13 is associated with retinoblastoma, owing to the loss of the Rb tumor suppressor gene (see Chapter 5).
- **Other deletion syndromes:** Deletions of both the short and the long arms of chromosome 18 are documented, leading to varying patterns of mental retardation and craniofacial anomalies. The loss of material for chromosomes 19, 20, 21, and 22 is usually associated with the formation of ring chromosomes. Syndromes associated with 21q− and 22q− are the most common and often resemble Down syndrome.

Chromosomal Breakage Syndromes

A number of recessive syndromes associated with frequent chromosomal breakage and rearrangements are accompanied by a significant risk of leukemia and other cancers. These disorders include xeroderma pigmentosum, Bloom syndrome (congenital telangiectatic erythema with dwarfism), Fanconi anemia (constitutional aplastic pancytopenia), and ataxia telangiectasia. Acquired chromosomal breaks and rearrangements (translocations) are associated with leukemias and lymphomas, the best documented of which are chronic myelogenous leukemia, t(9;22), and Burkitt lymphoma, mostly t(8;14) (see Chapters 5 and 20).

Syndromes of the Sex Chromosomes

Numerical aberrations of sex chromosomes (Fig. 6-13) are considerably more common than those of the autosomes. The reasons are not entirely clear, but it is possible that additional sex chromosomes produce less genetic imbalance than extra autosomes and therefore do not disturb critical stages of development.

The contrast between the X and Y chromosomes is striking. Whereas the X chromosome is one of the larger chromosomes, containing 6% of the total DNA, the Y chromosome is distinctly small. More than 50 genes in the X chromosome have been identified, but it is expected that several thousand will eventually be recognized. By contrast, there are relatively few genes on the Y chromosome; one of these is the testis-determining gene.

The Y Chromosome

Historically, the sex of a person was believed to be determined by the number of X chromosomes, the situation that was observed in genetic studies of *Drosophila*. However, with the discoveries that the XXY phenotype (Klinefelter syndrome) is male and that the XO phenotype (Turner syndrome) is female, the role of the Y chromosome in conferring the male phenotype was recognized.

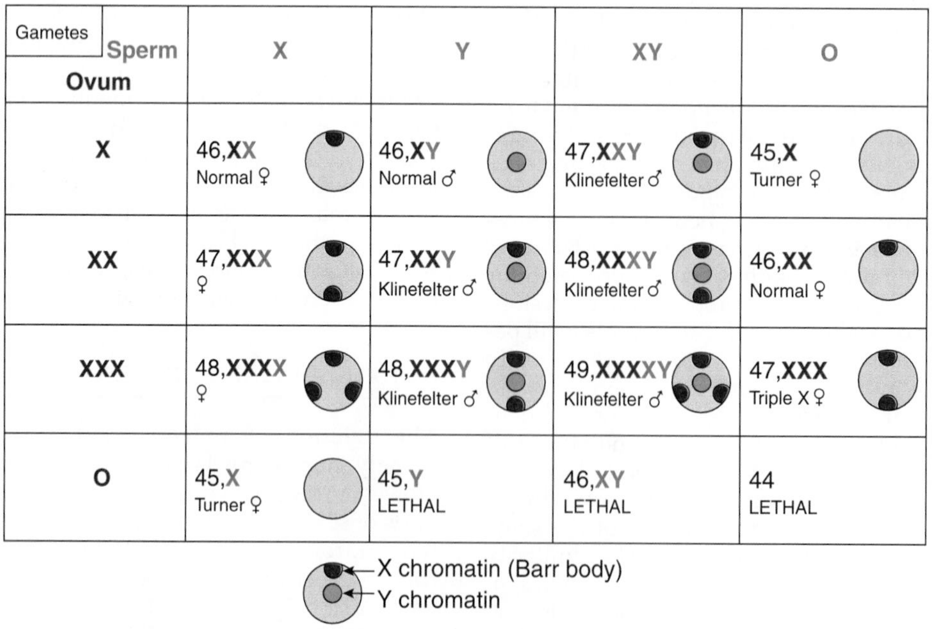

Gametes: Sperm / Ovum	X	Y	XY	O
X	46,XX Normal ♀	46,XY Normal ♂	47,XXY Klinefelter ♂	45,X Turner ♀
XX	47,XXX ♀	47,XXY Klinefelter ♂	48,XXXY Klinefelter ♂	46,XX Normal ♀
XXX	48,XXXX ♀	48,XXXY Klinefelter ♂	49,XXXXY Klinefelter ♂	47,XXX Triple X ♀
O	45,X Turner ♀	45,Y LETHAL	46,XY LETHAL	44 LETHAL

X chromatin (Barr body)
Y chromatin

FIGURE 6-13
Numerical aberrations of sex chromosomes. Nondisjunction in either the male or female gamete is the principal cause of these abnormalities.

The testis-determining gene (SRY, sex-determining region,Y) is a single exon near the end of the short arm of the Y chromosome. The SRY gene encodes a small nuclear protein with a DNA binding domain. This protein binds to another protein (SIP-1) to form a complex that functions as a transcriptional activator of autosomal genes whose expression controls the development of the male phenotype.

A small proportion of infertile men with azoospermia or severe oligospermia have small deletions in regions of the Y chromosome. However, the size and location of the deletions are variable and do not correlate with the severity of spermatogenic failure.

The X Chromosome

Although males carry only one X chromosome, both males and females produce the same amounts of gene products encoded by the X chromosome. This seeming discrepancy has been explained by the **Lyon effect**, on which the following principles are based:

- One X chromosome is irreversibly inactivated early in embryogenesis. The inactivated X chromosome is detectable in interphase nuclei as a heterochromatic clump of chromatin attached to the inner nuclear membrane, termed the **Barr body**. The inactive X chromosome is extensively methylated at gene control regions and transcriptionally repressed. Nevertheless, a significant minority of X-linked genes escape inactivation and continue to be expressed by both X chromosomes. The probability that an X chromosome is rendered inactive seems to correlate with the level of expression of another X-linked gene, namely XIST, which is expressed only by the inactive partner.
- Either the paternal or maternal X chromosome is inactivated randomly.
- The inactivation of the X chromosome is virtually complete.
- The inactivation of the X chromosome is permanent and transmitted to progeny cells. In other words, paternally or maternally derived X chromosomes are clonally propagated. **Thus, all females are mosaic for paternally and maternally derived X chromosomes.** Mosaicism for glucose-6-phosphate dehydrogenase in females was important in the demonstration of the monoclonal origin of neoplasms (see Chapter 5).

The inactivation of the X chromosome poses a problem in understanding the phenotypes of several disorders characterized by an abnormal complement of X chromosomes. If one X chromosome is rendered entirely nonfunctional, persons with XXY (Klinefelter) or XO (Turner) karyotypes should be phenotypically normal. The fact that such persons show a variety of phenotypic abnormalities indicates that the inactivated X chromosome retains some functioning genes. Indeed, at least two genes on the short arm of the X chromosome (Xga blood group antigen and steroid sulfatase) have been demonstrated to retain their activity. **Furthermore, in both phenotypically male and female children with extra X chromosomes, the degree of mental retardation shows a rough correlation with the number of X chromosomes.**

Klinefelter Syndrome (47,XXY)

Klinefelter syndrome, or testicular dysgenesis, is related to the presence of one or more X chromosomes in excess of the normal male XY complement. It is the most important clinical condition associated with trisomy of sex chromosomes (Fig. 6-14). This syndrome is a prominent cause of male hypogonadism and infertility.

☐ Pathogenesis: The large majority (80%) of persons with Klinefelter syndrome have one extra X chromosome, that is, a 47,XXY karyotype. A minority are mosaics (e.g., 46,XY/47,XXY) or have more than two X chromosomes (e.g., 48,XXXY). **Interestingly, regardless of the number of supernumerary X chromosomes (even up to four), the presence of a Y chromosome ensures a male phenotype.** Nevertheless, additional X chromosomes correlate with a more abnormal phenotype, despite the inactivation of the extra X chromosomes. Presumably, the

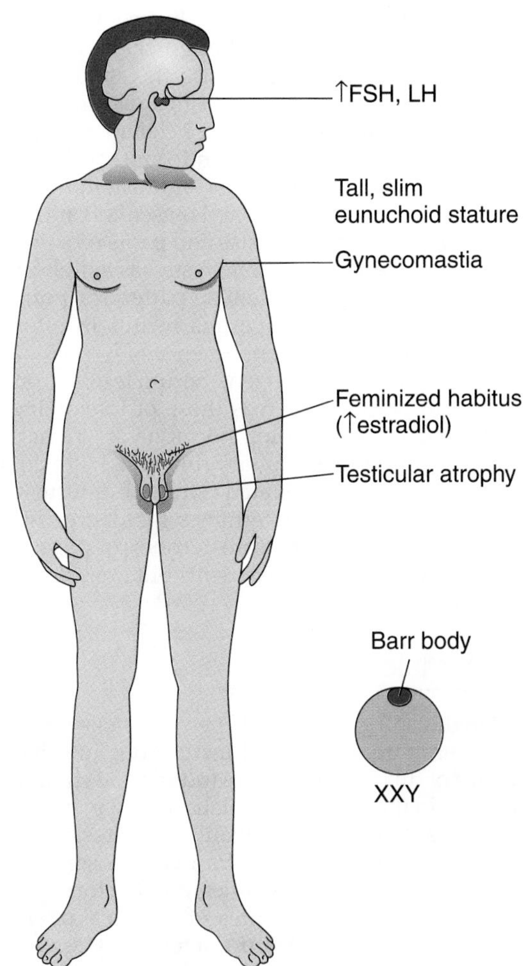

FIGURE 6-14
Clinical features of Klinefelter syndrome.

same genes that escape inactivation in the normal female remain functional in Klinefelter syndrome.

Klinefelter syndrome occurs in 1 per 1000 male newborns, roughly comparable to the incidence of Down syndrome. Interestingly, half of all 47,XXY conceptuses are lost as spontaneous abortions. The additional X chromosome(s) arises as a result of meiotic nondisjunction during gametogenesis, and the extra X chromosome is of maternal origin in two thirds of the case.

☐ Pathology: After puberty, the intrinsically abnormal testes do not respond to stimulation by gonadotropins and show sequentially regressive alterations. The seminiferous tubules display atrophy, hyalinization, and peritubular fibrosis. Germ cells and Sertoli cells are characteristically absent, and eventually the tubules are represented by dense cords of collagen. Although Leydig cells usually appear to be increased in number, their function is impaired, as evidenced by low testosterone levels in the face of elevated luteinizing hormone levels.

☐ Clinical Features: The diagnosis of Klinefelter syndrome is usually not made until after puberty, because the principal manifestations of the disorder during childhood are behavioral and psychiatric. Gross mental retardation is uncommon, although the average IQ is probably somewhat reduced. Since the syndrome is so common, it should be suspected in all boys with some degree of mental deficiency or severe behavioral problems.

Children with Klinefelter syndrome tend to be tall and thin, with relatively long legs (eunuchoid body habitus). Normal testicular growth and masculinization at puberty do not occur, and the testes and penis remain small. Feminine characteristics are manifested as a high-pitched voice, gynecomastia, and a female pattern of pubic hair (female escutcheon). Azoospermia results in infertility. All of these changes are a consequence of hypogonadism and a resulting lack of androgens. Serum testosterone levels are low to normal, whereas those of luteinizing hormone and follicle-stimulating hormone are remarkably high, indicating normal pituitary function. High circulating estradiol creates an elevated estradiol-to-testosterone ratio, the level of which determines the degree of feminization. Treatment with testosterone preparations is successful in virilizing these patients but does not restore fertility.

The XYY Male

Interest in the XYY phenotype (1 per 1000 male newborns) derives from studies in penal institutions in which the prevalence of this karyotype was found to be significantly greater than in the general population. However, the concept that these "supermales" manifest aggressive antisocial behavior as a result of an extra Y chromosome has not been substantiated in other studies, and the topic remains controversial. The only features of the XYY phenotype that are agreed on are tall stature, a tendency toward cystic acne, and some problems in motor and language development. Aneuploidy of the Y chromosome is a consequence of meiotic nondisjunction in the father.

Turner Syndrome (45,X)

Turner syndrome refers to the spectrum of abnormalities that results from the presence of complete or partial monosomy of the X chromosome in a phenotypic female. It is less common than Klinefelter syndrome, occurring in about 1 per 5000 female liveborn infants. In three fourths of the cases, the single X chromosome of Turner syndrome is of maternal origin, suggesting that the meiotic error tends to be paternal. The incidence of the syndrome does not correlate with maternal age, and the risk of producing a second affected female infant is not increased.

The 45,X karyotype is actually one of the most common aneuploid abnormalities in human conceptuses, but 99% are aborted spontaneously. In fact, up to 2% of all abortuses manifest this aberration. Since patients with Turner syndrome survive normally after birth, why is the missing X chromosome lethal during fetal development? Moreover, the presence of only one chromosome implies that the inactivated X chromosome in normal females (or the Y chromosome in males) protects against early demise of the embryo. It is suspected that homologues of Y genes on the X chromosome (e.g., ribosomal protein gene, RPS4) normally escape inactivation and are critical to the survival of a female conceptus.

Only about half of women with Turner syndrome lack an entire X chromosome (monosomy X). The remainder are mosaics or display structural aberrations of the X chromosome, such as isochromosome of the long arm, translocations, and deletions. Mosaics characterized by a 45,X/46,XX karyotype (15%) tend to have milder phenotypic manifestations of Turner syndrome and may even be fertile. In about 5% of patients, the mosaic karyotype is 45,X/46,XY, in which case an original male zygote was subsequently modified by a mitotic nondisjunction. Such mosaic persons are at a 20% risk of developing a germ cell cancer and should have prophylactic removal of the abnormal gonads.

☐ Pathology and Clinical Features: The clinical hallmark of Turner syndrome is sexual infantilism with primary amenorrhea and sterility (Fig. 6-15). In most cases, the disorder is not discovered until the absence of menarche brings the child to medical attention. Virtually all of these women are less than 5 ft (152 cm) tall. Other clinical features include a short, webbed neck (pterygium coli), a low posterior hairline, a wide carrying angle of the arms (cubitus valgus), a broad chest with widely spaced nipples, and hyperconvex fingernails. Half of the patients have abnormal urograms, the most common anomalies being horseshoe kidney and malrotation. Many have facial abnormalities, among which are a small mandible, prominent ears, and epicanthal folds. Defective hearing and vision are common, and as many as one fifth are reported to be mentally defective. Pigmented nevi become prominent as the patient ages. For unknown reasons, women with Turner syndrome are at a greater risk for chronic autoimmune thyroiditis and goiter.

Cardiovascular anomalies are common in Turner syndrome, occurring in almost half the patients. Coarctation of the aorta is seen in 15%, and a bicuspid aortic valve is detected by echocardiography in as many as a third. Essential hypertension occurs in some cases, and dissecting aneurysm of the aorta is occasionally a cause of death.

The pathological alterations in the ovary of women with Turner syndrome represent a curious acceleration of the normal aging of this organ. The ovary of a female fetus initially contains 7 million oocytes, of which fewer than half survive to the time of birth. A relentless loss of oocytes continues, so that at menarche only about 5% (400,000) of the original total remain and at menopause a mere 0.1% have survived. Although the ovaries of fetuses with Turner syndrome initially contain oocytes, they are rapidly degraded, and none remain by 2 years of age. The ovaries are converted to fibrous streaks, whereas the uterus, fallopian tubes, and vagina develop normally. It may be said that the child with Turner syndrome has undergone menopause long before reaching menarche.

Interestingly, families are known in which several women have premature menopause and exhibit deletions of portions of the long arm of one X chromosome. Such data, together with observations of Turner syndrome, further support the concept that the genes controlling ovarian development and function in the inactivated X chromosome continue to be expressed in the normal female.

Children with Turner syndrome are treated with growth hormone and estrogens and enjoy an excellent prognosis for a normal life.

Syndromes in Females with Multiple X Chromosomes

One extra X chromosome in a phenotypic female, that is, a 47,XXX karyotype, is the most frequent abnormality of sex chromosomes in women, occurring at about the same rate as Klinefelter syndrome. Most of these women are of normal intelligence, although they are reported to display some difficulty in speech, learning, and emotional responses. Minor physical anomalies are encountered, including epicanthal folds and clinodactyly (inward curvature of the fifth finger). Fertility is the rule, but an increased incidence of congenital defects may be found in the children of 47,XXX women.

Women with four and five X chromosomes have been documented, virtually all of whom have been mentally retarded. These women superficially resemble women with Down syndrome and do not mature sexually. It is noteworthy that women with supernumerary X chromosomes have additional Barr bodies, indicating inactivation of all but one X chromosome. Clearly, some genes on the inactivated X chromosomes continue to be expressed.

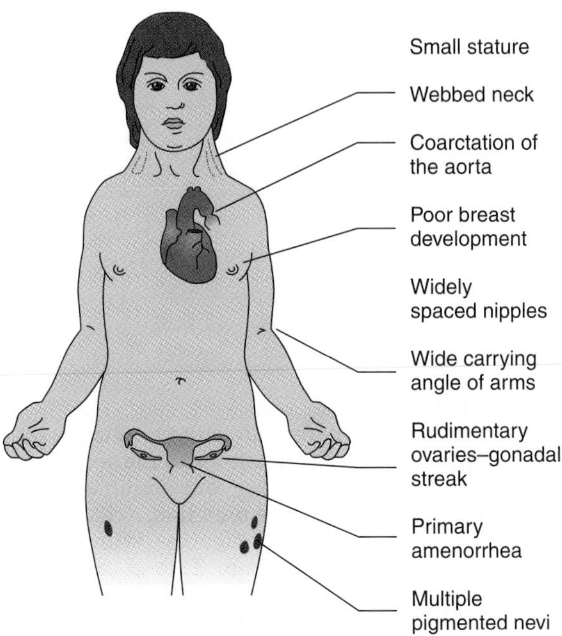

FIGURE *6-15*
Clinical features of Turner syndrome.

SINGLE GENE ABNORMALITIES

The classic laws of mendelian inheritance, named in honor of Gregor Mendel, imply that single genes encode identifiable traits that segregate sharply within families.

- **A mendelian trait** is determined by two copies of the same gene, called alleles, which are located at the same locus on two homologous chromosomes.
- **Autosomal genes** refer to those located on one of the 22 autosomes.
- **Sex-linked genes** are important in the pathogenesis of heritable diseases and reside on the X chromosome.
- **A dominant phenotypic trait** requires the expression of only one allele of a homologous gene pair. In other words, the dominant phenotype is present whether the allelic genes are homozygous or heterozygous.
- **A recessive phenotypic trait** demands that both alleles be identical, that is homozygous.
- **Co-dominance** refers to a situation in which both alleles in a heterozygous gene pair are fully expressed, for example the AB blood group genes.

Mendelian traits are classified as (1) autosomal dominant, (2) autosomal recessive, (3) sex-linked dominant, or (4) sex-linked recessive. Diseases associated with the expression of sex-linked dominant genes are rare and of little practical significance.

Biochemical Basis

Mutations

The central dogma of molecular biology holds that DNA is transcribed into RNA, after which the latter is processed into mRNA, which in turn is translated into proteins. Thus, a change in DNA can be reflected in either a corresponding change in the amino acid sequence of a specific protein or an interference with its synthesis.

A mutation is a stable heritable change in DNA. The consequences of mutations are highly variable. Some have no functional consequences, whereas others are lethal and cannot be transmitted from one generation to another. Between these extremes is a broad range of mutations that account for the profound genetic polymorphisms of any species. **On the basis of many studies, it appears that 1 in 250 base pairs is polymorphic in the human genome.** Indeed, evolution is based on the occurrence over time of nonlethal mutations that alter the adaptability of a species to its environment. From the viewpoint of human disease, we are interested principally in mutations that result in perceptible alterations in the structure or function of proteins. The major types of mutations encountered in the study of human genetic disorders are as follows:

- **Point mutations:** *The replacement of one base by another is termed a point mutation.* In the coding region, a point mutation has three consequences.

  A **synonymous mutation** is one in which the new codon containing the mutation still codes for the same amino acid. For example, UUU and UUC both code for phenylalanine.

  A **missense mutation** (three fourths of base substitutions in the coding region) refers to a situation in which the new codon codes for a different amino acid. In sickle anemia, an adenine to thymine substitution results in the replacement of glutamic acid (GAG) by valine (GUG) in the β-globin chain of hemoglobin.

  A **nonsense mutation** (4%) is one in which the base substitution changes the normal codon to a termination codon, so that translation is halted at the site of the mutation. For example, UAU codes for tyrosine, but UAA is a stop codon.
- **Frameshift mutations:** *Insertions or deletions of one or more bases into the coding region of DNA changes the reading frame of the genetic code.* In this situation, every codon in the same gene downstream from the mutation has a new sequence and codes for a different amino acid or a termination signal (Fig. 6-16). Frameshift mutations can also alter the transcription, splicing, or processing of mRNA.
- **Large deletions:** When an extensive segment of DNA is deleted, the coding region of a gene may be entirely removed, in which case the protein product is absent. On the other hand, a large deletion may result in the approximation of neighboring genes, thereby producing a fused gene that codes for a hybrid protein, that is, one in which the initial sequence of one protein is followed by the terminal sequence of another.

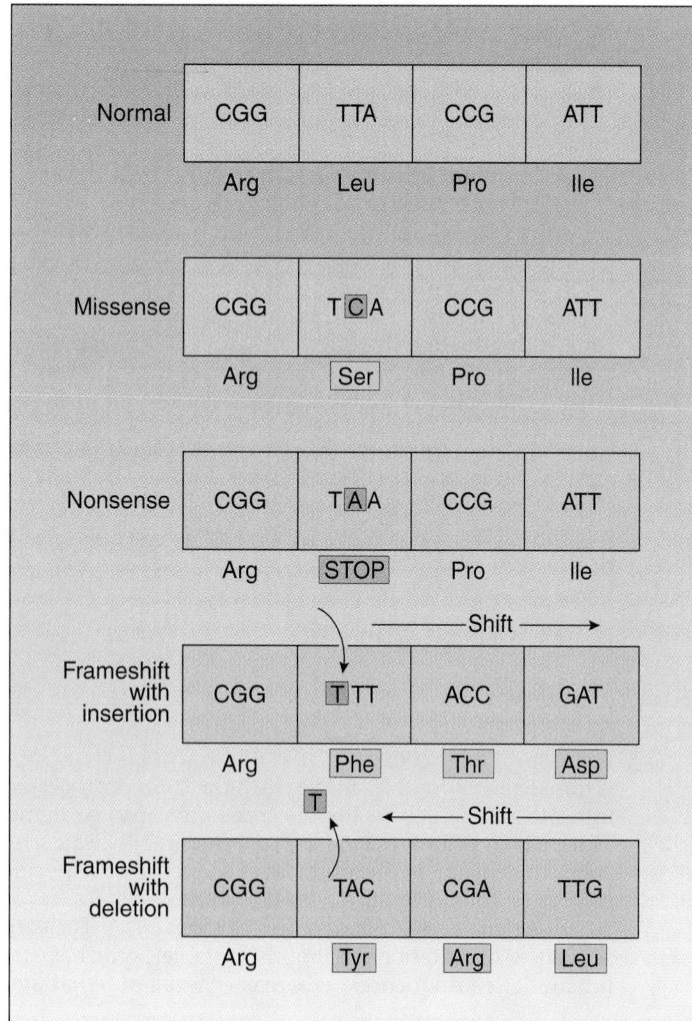

FIGURE 6-16
Point mutations that alter the reading frame of DNA. A variety of mutations in the second codon of a normal sequence of four amino acids is depicted. With a missense mutation, a change from T to C substitutes serine for leucine. With a nonsense mutation, a change from T to A converts the leucine codon to a stop codon. A shift in the reading frame to the right results from an insertion of a T, hereby changing the sequence of all subsequent amino acids. Conversely, a deletion of a T shifts the reading frame one base to the left and also changes the sequence of subsequent amino acids.

- **Expansion of unstable trinucleotide repeat sequences:** The human genome contains frequent tandem trinucleotide repeat sequences, of which there are 10 different combinations. The length of the repeat segment varies among individuals, thereby representing allelic polymorphism of the genes in which they are found. In general, the number of repeats below a particular threshold does not change during mitosis or meiosis, whereas above this threshold the number of repeats can expand or contract, the former being far more common. A number of distinct trinucleotide expansions have been identified in human disease (Table 6-4):

  Huntington disease (HD): HD is an inherited neurodegenerative disease caused by the expansion of a **CAG** repeat within the coding sequence of the gene that codes for the protein huntingtin. In HD, the stable alleles contain 10 to 30 repeats, whereas persons affected by the disease exhibit 40 to 100 repeats. CAG codes for glutamine, and the abnormal expansion of the polyglutamine tract in HD confers a toxic gain-of-function to huntingtin. Although the precise mechanism by which mutant huntingtin causes selective neuronal loss is not understood, there is evidence to suggest altered protein–protein interactions as the basis for this effect. In addition to HD, expanded CAG repeats have been identified as the cause of four other neurodegenerative disorders (see Table 6-4).

  Fragile X syndrome: This genetic disorder, the most common cause of inherited mental retardation (see later), is caused by the expansion of a **CGG** repeat in a noncoding region immediately adjacent to the FMR1 gene on the X chromosome. In a poorly understood manner, the expanded CGG repeat silences the FMR1 gene by methylation of its promoter. The abnormal repeat is also associated with an inducible "fragile site" on the X chromosome, defined as a nonstaining gap or a chromosomal break.

  Myotonic dystrophy (MD): MD, the most frequent autosomal muscular dystrophy (see Chapter 27), is caused by expansion of a **CTG** repeat in the 3′-untranslated region of the myotonic dystrophy gene. Normal persons bear up to 35 CTG repeats, whereas MD patients display up to 2000 repeats. Interestingly, the structure of the protein product of the MD gene, a protein kinase, is unaffected by the mutation. It is suspected that the abnormal expansion renders other nearby genes dysfunctional.

  Friedreich ataxia (FA): FA is an autosomal recessive degenerative disease affecting the central nervous system and the heart that is associated with expansion of a GAA repeat in the frataxin gene (see Chapter 28), which apparently codes for a mitochondrial protein. Affected persons have 120 to 1700 repeats in the first intron (noncoding) of the frataxin gene.

Functional Consequences of Mutations

A biochemical pathway represents the sequential actions of a series of enzymes, which are coded for by specific genes. A typical pathway can be represented by the conversion of a substrate (A) through intermediate metabolites (B and C) to the final product (D).

A	→ B → C	→ D
initial substrate	intermediary metabolites	end-products

A single gene defect can have several consequences:

- **Failure to complete a metabolic pathway:** In this situation, the end-product (D) is not formed because an enzyme that is essential for the completion of a metabolic sequence is missing:

  $$A \rightarrow B \rightarrow C \rightarrow (D)$$

  An example of the failure to complete a metabolic pathway is albinism, a pigment disorder caused by a deficiency of tyrosinase. This enzyme catalyzes the conversion of tyrosine to melanin (through the intermediate formation of dihydroxyphenylalanine, or DOPA). In the absence of tyrosinase, the end-product, namely melanin, is not formed, and the affected person (an "albino") is devoid of pigment in all organs that normally contain it, primarily the eyes and the skin.
- **Accumulation of unmetabolized substrate:** The enzyme that converts the initial substrate into the first intermediary metabolite may be missing, a situation that results in an excessive accumulation of the initial substrate.

  $$A\,(\uparrow) \rightarrow \underset{x}{\overset{x}{x}}\, B\,(\downarrow)\; C\,(\downarrow)\; D\,(\downarrow)$$

  An example of this situation is phenylketonuria, a disease in which dietary phenylalanine accumulates owing to an inborn deficiency of phenylalanine hydroxylase. The resulting toxic concentration of

TABLE 6-4 **Representative Diseases Associated with Trinucleotide Repeats**

Disease	Location	Sequence	Normal Length	Premutation	Full Mutation
Huntington disease	4p16.3	CAG	10–35	—	40–100
Kennedy disease	Xq21	CAG	15–25	—	40–55
Spinocerebellar ataxia	6p23	CAG	20–35	—	45–80
Fragile X syndrome	Xq27.3	CGG	5–55	50–200	200–>1000
Myotonic dystrophy	19q13	CTG	5–35	37–50	50–4000
Friedreich ataxia	9q13	GAA	7–30	—	120–1700

phenylalanine interferes with the postnatal development of the brain and causes severe mental retardation.

- **Storage of an intermediary metabolite:** An intermediary metabolite, which is readily processed into the final product and is normally present only in minute amounts, accumulates in large quantities if the enzyme responsible for its metabolism is deficient.

$$A \rightarrow B\,(\uparrow) \overset{X}{\underset{X}{x}} C\,(\downarrow)\, D\,(\downarrow)$$

This type of genetic disorder is exemplified by von Gierke disease, a glycogen storage disease that results from a deficiency of glucose-6-phosphatase. The inability to convert glucose-6-phosphate to glucose leads to the alternative conversion of this substrate to glycogen.

- **Formation of an abnormal end-product:** In this situation, a mutant gene codes for an abnormal protein. Sickle cell anemia results from the substitution of a valine for a glutamic acid in the β-chain of hemoglobin.

Autosomal Dominant Disorders

Autosomal dominant inheritance refers to traits that are expressed in heterozygotes. In other words, a dominant disease occurs when only one defective gene (i.e., a mutant allele) is present, whereas its paired allele on the homologous chromosome is normal. The salient features of autosomal dominant traits are as follows (Fig. 6-17):

- Males and females are equally affected since, by definition, the mutant gene resides on one of the 22 autosomal chromosomes.
- The trait encoded by the mutant gene can be transmitted to successive generations (unless the disease interferes with reproductive capacity).
- Unaffected members of the family do not transmit the trait to their offspring. As a corollary, every person with the disease has an affected parent, assuming that the disorder does not represent a new mutation.
- The proportions of normal and diseased offspring of patients with the disorder are on average equal, because most affected persons are heterozygous, whereas their normal mates do not harbor the defective gene.

New Mutations versus Inherited Mutations

As noted previously, an autosomal dominant disease may result from a new mutation rather than transmission from an affected parent. Nevertheless, the offspring of persons with a new dominant mutation are at a 50% risk of developing the disease. **The ratio of new mutations to transmitted ones among persons with dominant autosomal disorders varies with the effect of the disease on reproductive capacity.** The greater the damage to reproductive capacity, the greater the proportion of new mutations. At one end of the spectrum, a dominant mutation that leads to complete infertility would invariably be a new mutation. When reproductive capacity is only partially impaired, the proportion of new mutations is correspondingly less. Such a situation occurs with tuberous sclerosis, an autosomal dominant condition in which mental retardation limits reproductive potential and in which new mutations account for 80% of cases. Finally, in a dominant disease that has little effect on reproductive activity (e.g., familial hypercholesterolemia), virtually all affected persons exhibit pedigrees showing classic vertical transmission of the disorder.

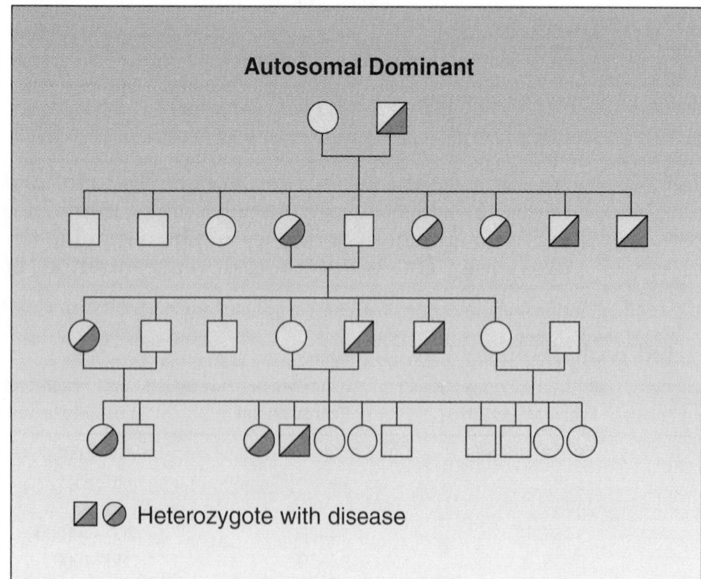

FIGURE *6-17*
Autosomal dominant inheritance. Only symptomatic persons transmit the trait to the next generation, and heterozygotes are symptomatic. Both males and females are affected.

TABLE 6-5 **Representative Autosomal Dominant Disorders**

Disease	Frequency	Chromosome
Familial hypercholesterolemia	1/500	19p
von Willebrand disease	1/8000	12p
Hereditary spherocytosis (major forms)	1/5000	14,8
Hereditary elliptocytosis (all forms)	1/2500	1,1p,2q,14
Osteogenesis imperfecta (types I–IV)	1/10,000	17q,7q
Ehlers-Danlos syndrome, type III	1/5000	?
Marfan syndrome	1/10,000	15q
Neurofibromatosis type 1	1/3500	17q
Huntington chorea	1/15,000	4p
Retinoblastoma	1/14,000	13q
Wilms tumor	1/10,000	11p
Familial adenomatous polyposis	1/10,000	5q
Acute intermittent porphyria	1/15,000	11q
Hereditary amyloidosis	1/100,000	18q
Adult polycystic kidney disease	1/1000	16p

Biochemical Basis of Autosomal Dominant Disorders

There are two major mechanisms by which the presence of one mutant allele and one normal allele is responsible for clinical disease. When the gene product is a rate-limiting component of a complex metabolic network (e.g., a receptor or an enzyme), half of the normal amount of gene product may be insufficient to maintain the normal state. Examples of this mechanism include von Willebrand disease and familial hypercholesterolemia. Alternatively, mutations in genes that encode structural proteins (e.g., collagens and cytoskeletal constituents) result in abnormal molecular interactions and the disruption of normal morphological patterns. Such a situation is exemplified by osteogenesis imperfecta and hereditary spherocytosis.

More than 1000 human diseases are inherited as autosomal dominant traits, although most of them are rare. Examples of human autosomal dominant diseases are given in Table 6-5.

Heritable Diseases of Connective Tissue

The numerous autosomal dominant genetic disorders of collagen are heterogeneous and, in many instances, difficult to classify. This discussion will be limited to three of the most common and best studied entities: Marfan syndrome, Ehlers-Danlos syndrome, and osteogenesis imperfecta. Even in these well-delineated disorders, the clinical symptomatology often overlaps. For instance, some patients exhibit the joint dislocations typical of the Ehlers-Danlos syndrome, whereas other members of the same family suffer from multiple fractures characteristic of osteogenesis imperfecta. Yet other persons in the family, with the same genetic defect, may be totally without symptoms. It is clear, therefore, that the current classifications, which are based on clinical criteria, will eventually be replaced by references to specific gene defects, in a manner analogous to the hemoglobinopathies.

Marfan Syndrome

Marfan syndrome is an autosomal dominant, inherited disorder of connective tissue characterized by a variety of abnormalities in many organs, including the heart, aorta, skeleton, eyes, and skin. Although the condition is inherited as an autosomal dominant trait, one third of the cases represent sporadic mutations. The incidence in the United States is 1 per 10,000.

☐ Pathogenesis: The cause of Marfan syndrome has been established as private missense mutations in the gene coding for **fibrillin-1** (FBN1), which has been mapped to the long arm of chromosome 15 (15q21.1). Fibrillin is a family of connective tissue proteins analogous to the collagens, of which there are now about a dozen genetically distinct forms. Fibrillin is widely distributed in many tissues in the form of a fiber system termed **microfibrils**. By electron microscopy, microfibrils are threadlike filaments that form larger fibers organized into rods, sheets, and interlaced networks. **Microfibrillar fibers** are believed to serve as a scaffold for the deposition of elastin during embryonic development, and these fibers then constitute part of elastic tissues. For example, the deposition of elastin on lamellae of microfibrillar fibers produces the concentric rings of elastin in the aortic wall. With the use of immunofluorescent microscopy, microfibrillar fibers have been visualized in all the tissues affected in Marfan syndrome.

Fibrillin-1 is a large, cysteine-rich glycoprotein that forms 10-nm microfibrils in the extracellular matrix. Fibrillin has been localized to them in many tissues. Interestingly, the ciliary zonules that suspend the lens of the eye are devoid of elastin but consist almost exclusively of microfibrillar fibers (fibrillin). Dislocation of the lens is a characteristic feature of Marfan syndrome. Furthermore, using monoclonal antibodies against fibrillin, deficiencies in the amount and distribution of microfibrillar fibers have been demonstrated in the skin and fibroblast cultures of patients with Marfan syndrome. The consistent finding of fragmented elastic fibers in many affected tissues suggests that a lack of normal microfibrillar fibers renders the elastic fibers incompetent to resist normal stress.

☐ Pathology and Clinical Features: Persons with Marfan syndrome are usually (but not invariably) tall, and the lower body segment (pubis-to-sole) is longer than the upper body. A slender habitus, which reflects a paucity of subcutaneous fat, is complemented by long, thin extremities and fingers, which accounts for the term **arachnodactyly** (spider fingers) (Fig. 6-18). Overall,

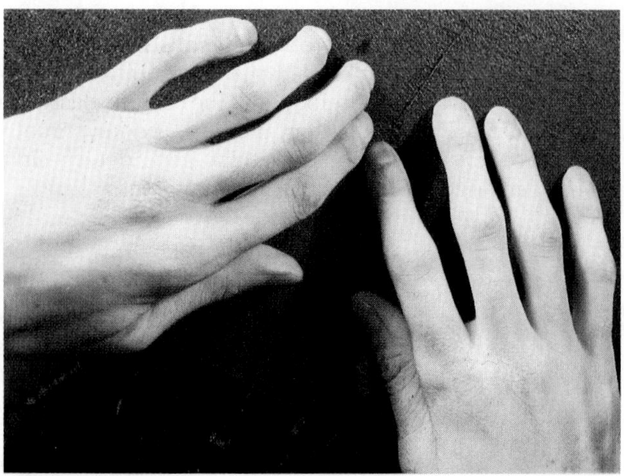

FIGURE 6-18
Long, slender fingers (arachnodactyly) in a patient with Marfan syndrome.

the affected persons resemble figures in a painting by El Greco.

- **Skeletal system:** The skull in Marfan syndrome is characteristically long (dolichocephalic), with prominent frontal eminences. Disorders of the ribs are conspicuous and produce pectus excavatum (concave sternum) and pectus carinatum (pigeon breast). The tendons, ligaments, and joint capsules are weak, a condition that leads to hyperextensibility of the joints (double-jointedness), dislocations, hernias, and kyphoscoliosis; the last is often severe.
- **Cardiovascular system: The most important cardiovascular defect resides in the aorta, in which the principal lesion is a faulty media.** Weakness of the media leads to variable dilatation of the ascending aorta and to a high incidence of dissecting aneurysms. The dissecting aneurysm, usually of the ascending aorta, may rupture into the pericardial cavity or make its way down the aorta and rupture into the retroperitoneal space. Dilatation of the aortic ring results in aortic regurgitation, which may be so severe as to produce angina pectoris and congestive heart failure. The mitral valve may exhibit redundant valve leaflets and chordae tendineae—changes that result in the mitral valve prolapse syndrome. Cardiovascular disorders are the most common causes of death in Marfan syndrome.

  Microscopic examination of the aorta reveals a conspicuous fragmentation and loss of elastic fibers, accompanied by an increase in metachromatic mucopolysaccharide. Focally, the defect in the elastic tissue results in discrete pools of amorphous metachromatic material, reminiscent of that seen in Erdheim idiopathic cystic medial necrosis of the aorta. Smooth muscle cells are enlarged and lose their orderly circumferential arrangement.
- **Eyes:** Ocular changes are common in Marfan syndrome and reflect the intrinsic lesion in connective tissue. These include dislocation of the lens (ectopia lentis), severe myopia owing to elongation of the eye, and retinal detachment.

Untreated men with Marfan syndrome usually die in their 30s, and women who are untreated often die in their 40s. However, with the use of drugs that reduce blood pressure and replacement of the aorta with prosthetic grafts, life expectancy approaches normal.

Ehlers-Danlos Syndromes

The Ehlers-Danlos syndromes (EDS) comprise a group of rare, autosomal dominant inherited disorders of connective tissue that feature remarkable hyperelasticity and fragility of the skin, joint hypermobility, and often a bleeding diathesis. The disorder is clinically and genetically heterogeneous (Table 6-6).

TABLE 6-6 **Ehlers-Danlos Syndromes**

Type	Inheritance	Frequency	Biochemical Lesion	Clinical Features
I	AD	1/30,000	Type V collagen	Hyperextensible skin; hypermobile joints
II	AD	1/30,000	Type V collagen	Similar to, but less severe than, type I
III	AD	1/5000	Unknown	Hypermobile joints
IV	AD	1/100,000	Type III collagen	Thin skin, easy bruising, rupture of arteries, intestine and gravid uterus
V	XLR	Rare	Unknown	Similar to type II
VI	AR	Rare	Lysyl hydoxylase	Ocular lesions and blindness, hyperextensible, hypermobile joints
VII	AD	Rare	Type I collagen	Congenital hip dislocation, hypermobile joints
VIII	AD	Rare	Unknown	Periodontal disease, hyperextensible skin
IX	XLR	Rare	Lysyl oxidase (copper metabolism)	Lax skin, bladder diverticula and rupture, skeletal deformities
X	AR	Rare	Fibronectin	Similar to type II

AD, autosomal dominant; AR, autosomal recessive; XLR, X-linked recessive.

More than 10 varieties of EDS have been distinguished, and the molecular lesions have been identified in several.

☐ Pathogenesis: The genetic and biochemical lesions in 7 of the 10 types of EDS have been established. **The common feature of all is a generalized defect in collagen, including abnormalities of the biochemical structure, synthesis, secretion, and degradation of collagen.** In EDS I through IV, VI, and X, electron microscopic studies of the skin have shown an increased size of collagen fibrils, with unusually small bundles, features that are consistent with the presence of abnormal collagen. Such changes involve type III collagen in EDS IV and type I collagen in EDS VII. EDS VII arises from mutations that alter the amino-terminal cleavage sites of either the 1 or 2 procollagen chains of type I collagen. Deficiencies of specific collagen processing enzymes, including lysyl hydroxylase and lysyl oxidase, have been identified in EDS VI and IX, respectively. Whatever the underlying biochemical defect may be, the end result is deficient or defective collagen. Depending on the type of EDS, these molecular lesions are associated with conspicuous weakness of the supporting structures of the skin, joints, arteries, and visceral organs.

☐ Pathology and Clinical Features: All types of EDS are characterized by a soft, fragile, and hyperextensible skin. Patients are typically able to stretch the skin many centimeters, and trivial injuries can lead to serious wounds. Because sutures do not hold well, dehiscence of surgical incisions is common. Hypermobility of the joints allows unusual extension and flexion, a situation that accounted for the "human pretzel" and other contortionists in the freak shows of an earlier age. EDS IV is the most dangerous variety, owing to a tendency to spontaneous rupture of large arteries, the bowel, and the gravid uterus. Death from such complications is common in the third and fourth decades of life.

Ehlers-Danlos syndrome VI also has major complications, including severe kyphoscoliosis, blindness from retinal hemorrhage or rupture of the globe, and death from aortic rupture. Severe periodontal disease, with loss of teeth by the third decade, characterizes EDS VIII. EDS IX features the development of bladder diverticula during childhood, with a danger of bladder rupture, and skeletal deformities.

Many persons who exhibit clinical abnormalities suggestive of EDS do not conform to any of the documented types of this disorder. Further genetic and biochemical characterization of such cases is likely to expand the classification of EDS.

Osteogenesis Imperfecta

Osteogenesis imperfecta (OI), or brittle bone disease, comprises a group of inherited disorders in which a generalized abnormality of connective tissue is expressed principally as fragility of bone. OI is inherited in an autosomal dominant pattern, although there are rare cases that are autosomal recessive.

☐ Pathogenesis: The genetic defects in all of the four types of OI are heterogeneous, but all affect the synthesis of type I collagen. In 90% of the cases, mutations in the pro-α1(I) and pro-α2(I) collagen genes are present, most of them resulting in the substitution of other amino acids for the obligate glycine at every third residue.

☐ Pathology and Clinical Features: **Type I** OI is characterized by a normal appearance at birth, but fractures of many bones occur during infancy and at the time the child learns to walk. Such patients have been described as being as "fragile as a china doll." Children with type I OI typically have blue sclerae as a result of the deficiency in collagen fibers, which imparts translucence to the sclera. A high incidence of hearing loss occurs because fractures and fusion of the bones of the middle ear restrict their mobility.

Type II OI is usually fatal *in utero* or shortly after birth. The infants have a characteristic facial appearance and skeletal abnormalities. Those who are born alive usually die of respiratory failure within the first month of life.

Type III OI is the progressively deforming variant, which is ordinarily detected at birth by the presence of short stature and deformities caused by fractures *in utero*. Dental defects and hearing loss are common. Unlike the other types of OI, type III is often inherited as an autosomal recessive trait.

Type IV OI is similar to type I, except that the sclerae are normal and the phenotype is more variable.

Osteogenesis imperfecta is discussed in further detail in Chapter 26.

Neurofibromatosis

The neurofibromatoses include two distinct autosomal dominant disorders characterized by the development of multiple neurofibromas, which are benign tumors of peripheral nerves of Schwann cell origin.

Neurofibromatosis Type I (von Recklinghausen Disease)

Neurofibromatosis type I (NF1) is characterized by (1) disfiguring neurofibromas, (2) areas of dark pigmentation of the skin (café-au-lait spots), and (3) pigmented lesions of the iris (Lisch nodules). It is one of the more common autosomal dominant disorders, affecting 1 in 3500 persons of all races. The NF1 gene has an unusually high rate of mutation, and half of the cases are sporadic rather than familial. The condition was first described in 1882 by von Recklinghausen, but references to this disorder can be found as early as the 13th century. Public interest in the disease was stimulated by the disturbing account in a play and film of a severely disfigured man, the so-called Elephant Man. Interestingly, Joseph Merrick, the original patient, is now thought actually to have suffered from a different malady, namely, Proteus syndrome.

☐ Pathogenesis: Germline mutations in the NF1 gene, located on the long arm of chromosome 17

(17q11.2), include deletions, missense mutations, and nonsense mutations. The protein product of the NF1 gene, termed **neurofibromin**, is expressed in many tissues and belongs to a family of GTPase-activating proteins (GAP), which inactivate the ras protein (see Chapter 5). In this sense, NF1 is a classic tumor suppressor gene. The loss of GAP activity permits uncontrolled ras activation, an effect that presumably predisposes to the formation of neurofibromas.

☐ Clinical Features: The clinical manifestations of NF1 are highly variable and difficult to explain entirely on the basis of a single gene defect. The typical features of NF1 include the following:

- **Neurofibromas:** More than 90% of patients with NF1 develop cutaneous and subcutaneous neurofibromas in late childhood or adolescence. These cutaneous tumors, which may total more than 500, appear as soft, pedunculated masses, usually about 1 cm in diameter (Fig. 6-19). However, on occasion they may reach alarming proportions and dominate the physical appearance of the patient, with lesions up to 25 cm in largest dimension. Subcutaneous neurofibromas present as soft nodules along the course of peripheral nerves. **Plexiform neurofibromas** occur only within the context of NF1 and are diagnostic of that condition. These tumors usually involve the larger peripheral nerves but on occasion may arise from cranial or intraspinal nerves. Plexiform neurofibromas are often large, infiltrative tumors that cause severe disfigurement of the face or an extremity. The microscopic appearance of neurofibromas is discussed in Chapter 28. **One of the major complications of NF1, occurring in 3% to 5% of patients, is the appearance of a neurofibrosarcoma in a neurofibroma, usually a larger one of the plexiform type.** NF1 is also associated with an increased incidence of other neurogenic tumors, including meningioma, optic glioma, and pheochromocytomas.
- ***Café-au-lait* spots:** Although normal persons may exhibit occasional light brown patches on the skin, more than 95% of persons affected by NF1 display six or more such lesions. These are over 5 mm before puberty and greater than 1.5 cm thereafter. *Café-au-lait* spots tend to be ovoid, with the longer axis oriented in the direction of a cutaneous nerve. Numerous freckles, particularly in the axilla, are also common.
- **Lisch nodules:** More than 90% of persons with NF1 display pigmented nodules of the iris, which consist of masses of melanocytes. These raised lesions are believed to be hamartomas.
- **Skeletal lesions:** A number of bone lesions occur frequently in NF1. These include malformations of the sphenoid bone and thinning of the cortex of the long bones, with bowing and pseudarthrosis of the tibia, bone cysts, and scoliosis.
- **Mental status:** Mild intellectual impairment is frequent in patients with NF1, but severe retardation is not part of the syndrome.
- **Leukemia:** The risk of malignant myeloid disorders in children with NF1 is 200 to 500 times the normal risk. In some patients, both alleles of the NF1 gene are inactivated in the leukemic cells.

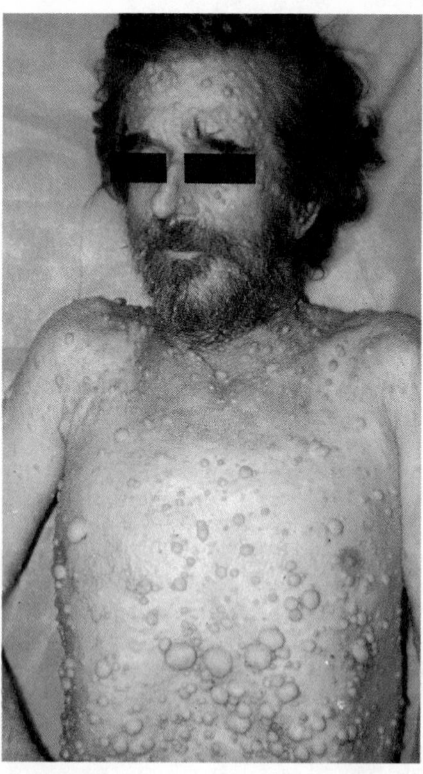

FIGURE *6-19*
Neurofibromatosis, type I. Multiple cutaneous neurofibromas are noted on the face and trunk.

Neurofibromatosis Type II (Central Neurofibromatosis)

Neurofibromatosis type II (NF2) refers to a syndrome defined by bilateral tumors of the eighth cranial nerve (acoustic neuromas) and, commonly, by meningiomas and gliomas. The disorder is considerably less common than NF1, occurring in 1 in 50,000 persons. Most patients suffer from bilateral acoustic neuromas, but the condition can be diagnosed in the presence of a unilateral eighth nerve tumor if two of the following are present: neurofibroma, meningioma, glioma, schwannoma, or juvenile posterior lenticular opacity.

Despite the superficial similarities between NF1 and NF2, they are not variants of the same disease and, indeed, have separate genetic origins. The NF2 gene resides in the middle of the long arm of chromosome 22 (22q, 11.1-13.1). In contrast to NF1, the tumors in NF2 frequently show deletions or loss of heterozygous DNA markers in the affected chromosome. The NF2 gene encodes a tumor suppressor protein termed merlin or schwannomin, which is a member of a superfamily of proteins that link the cytoskeleton to the cell membrane. Other members of this family include ezrin, moesin, radixin, talin, and protein 4.1. Merlin is detectable in most differentiated tissues, including Schwann cells.

Achondroplastic Dwarfism

Achondroplastic dwarfism is an autosomal dominant, hereditary disturbance of epiphyseal chondroblastic development that leads to inadequate enchondral bone formation. This abnormality causes a distinctive form of dwarfism characterized by short limbs with a normal head and trunk. The affected person has a small face, a bulging forehead, and a deeply indented bridge of the nose. Achondroplastic dwarfism is not infrequent, occurring in 1 per 3000 live births. Achondroplasia is discussed in Chapter 26.

Familial Hypercholesterolemia

Familial hypercholesterolemia is an autosomal dominant disorder characterized by high levels of low-density lipoproteins (LDL) in the blood, accompanied by the deposition of cholesterol in arteries, tendons, and skin. It is one of the most common autosomal dominant disorders, and in its heterozygous form it affects at least one in 500 adults in the United States. Only 1 in 1 million persons is homozygous for the disease. **The interest in this disease stems from the striking acceleration of atherosclerosis and its complications.** This subject is discussed in detail in Chapter 10.

☐ Pathogenesis: Familial hypercholesterolemia results from abnormalities in the gene that codes for the cell surface receptor that removes LDL from the blood. The gene for the LDL receptor is located on the short arm of chromosome 19. More than 150 different mutations in the LDL receptor gene have been described, including insertions, deletions, and nonsense and missense point mutations.

The LDL receptor is (1) synthesized in the endoplasmic reticulum, (2) transferred to the Golgi complex, (3) transported to the cell surface, and (4) internalized by receptor-mediated endocytosis in coated pits after binding LDL. Classes of genetic defects in each of these steps have been described:

- **Class 1:** The most common class of defect leads to failure of the synthesis of nascent LDL receptor protein in the endoplasmic reticulum. Most class 1 defects reflect large deletions in the gene (null alleles).
- **Class 2:** These mutations prevent the transfer of the nascent receptor from the endoplasmic reticulum to the Golgi apparatus (transport-defective alleles). Thus, the mutant receptor never appears on the cell surface.
- **Class 3:** The LDL receptors of class 3 mutations are expressed on the cell surface but are defective in the ligand-binding domain (binding-defective alleles).
- **Class 4:** In this rare class of mutations, LDL binding to the receptor is normal, but the genetic defect prevents the clustering of the receptors in coated pits, thereby blocking their internalization by endocytosis (internalization-defective alleles).
- **Class 5:** In this situation, the internalized LDL–receptor complex is not discharged from the endosome, and recycling of the receptor to the plasma membrane is defective (recycling-defective alleles).

The LDL receptor resides on the surface of hepatocytes and to some extent on other cells. After binding to the receptor, LDL is internalized and degraded in lysosomes, thereby freeing cholesterol for further metabolism. A deficiency in LDL receptors leads to an increase in plasma LDL because the rate of LDL clearance is inversely proportional to the number of LDL receptors. As a result, LDL cholesterol is taken up by tissue macrophages and accumulates to form occlusive arterial plaques (atheromas) and papules or nodules of lipid-laden macrophages (xanthomas). The central role of the liver in the pathogenesis of familial hypercholesterolemia is confirmed by the successful treatment of this disorder by liver transplantation.

☐ Clinical Features: Heterozygous and homozygous familial hypercholesterolemia constitute two distinct clinical syndromes, reflecting a clear gene dosage effect. In heterozygotes, elevated blood cholesterol levels (mean, 350 mg/dL; normal, <200 mg/dL) are noted at birth. Tendon xanthomas develop in half the patients before the age of 30 years, and symptoms of coronary heart disease often occur before the age of 40. In homozygotes, the blood cholesterol content reaches astronomic levels (600 to 1200 mg/dL), and virtually all patients exhibit tendon xanthomas and generalized atherosclerosis in childhood. Untreated homozygotes typically die of myocardial infarction before 30 years of age.

Autosomal Recessive Disorders

Autosomal recessive diseases are associated with clinical symptoms only when both alleles at a given locus on homologous chromosomes are defective. In other words, the affected person is homozygous for the recessive trait (Fig. 6-20). **The large majority of genetic metabolic diseases exhibit an autosomal recessive mode of inheritance** (Table 6-7). The fact that recessive genes are uncommon and the need for two mutant alleles for the expression of clinical disease determine the important characteristics of autosomal recessive inheritance. Some of the salient features of autosomal recessive disorders are as follows:

- The more infrequent the mutant gene is in the general population, the less is the probability that unrelated parents are heterozygous for the trait. **Thus, rare autosomal recessive disorders are often the product of consanguineous marriages.**
- Both parents are usually heterozygous for the trait and are clinically normal.
- Symptoms appear on average in one fourth of the offspring. One half of all offspring are heterozygous for the trait and are therefore asymptomatic.
- As in autosomal dominant disorders, autosomal recessive traits are transmitted equally to males and females, since by definition the mutant gene resides on one of the 22 different autosomal chromosomes.
- The symptomatology of autosomal recessive disorders is ordinarily less variable than that of dominant diseases. As a result, recessive traits are more commonly evident in childhood, whereas dominant disorders may initially appear in adults.

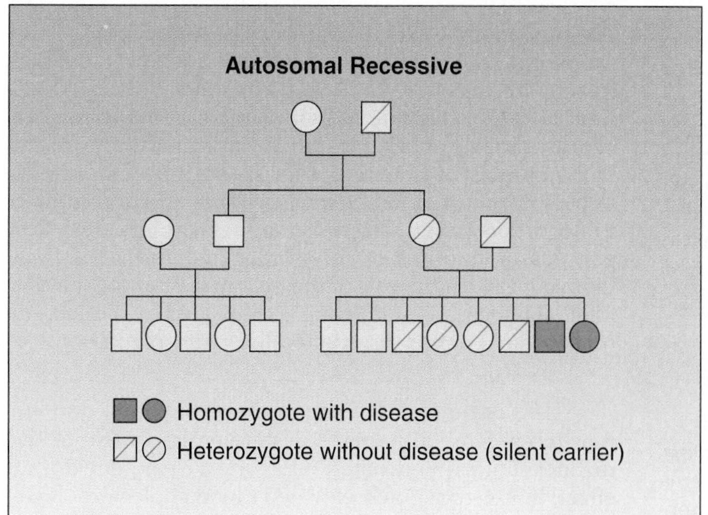

FIGURE 6-20
Autosomal recessive inheritance. Symptoms of the disease appear only in homozygotes, male or female. Heterozygotes are asymptomatic carriers. Symptomatic homozygotes result from the mating of asymptomatic heterozygotes.

- The variability in the clinical expression of many autosomal recessive diseases is determined by the residual activity of the affected enzyme. This variability is manifested in (1) different degrees of clinical severity, (2) age at onset, or (3) the existence of acute and chronic forms of the specific disease.

Most mutant genes responsible for autosomal recessive disorders are rare in the general population, because the homozygotes for the trait tend to die before reaching reproductive age. Paradoxically, a few lethal autosomal recessive diseases are common. In the case of sickle cell anemia, it has been suggested that the resistance of the heterozygote to malarial parasitization of the erythrocyte confers a biological advantage that compensates for the loss of homozygotes. Almost all patients afflicted with cystic fibrosis are sterile, and any enhanced biological fitness of the heterozygote remains obscure.

TABLE 6-7 **Representative Autosomal Recessive Disorders**

Disease	Frequency	Chromosome
Cystic fibrosis	1/2500	7q
α-Thalassemia	High	16p
β-Thalassemia	High	11p
Sickle cell anemia	High	11p
Myeloperoxidase deficiency	1/2000	17q
Phenylketonuria	1/10,000	12q
Gaucher disease	1/1000	1q
Tay-Sachs disease	1/4000	15q
Hurler syndrome	1/100,000	22p
Glycogen storage disease Ia (von Gierke disease)	1/100,000	17
Wilson disease	1/50,000	13q
Hereditary hemochromatosis	1/1000	6p
α_1-Antitrypsin deficiency	1/7000	14q
Oculocutaneous albinism	1/20,000	11q
Alkaptonuria	<1/100,000	3q
Metachromatic leukodystrophy	1/100,000	22q

New mutations for recessive diseases are difficult to identify clinically because the resulting heterozygotes are asymptomatic. Nonconsanguineous mating of two such heterozygotes would occur by chance only many generations later, if at all.

Biochemical Basis of Autosomal Recessive Disorders

Autosomal recessive diseases characteristically are caused by deficiencies in enzymes rather than abnormalities in structural proteins. A mutation that results in the inactivation of an enzyme does not ordinarily produce an abnormal phenotype, because compensatory mechanisms readily correct the functional defect. For instance, since most cellular enzymes operate at substrate concentrations significantly below saturation, an enzyme deficiency is easily corrected simply by increasing the amount of substrate. By contrast, the loss of both alleles in a homozygote results in the complete loss of enzyme activity, a situation that is not amenable to correction by regulatory mechanisms. It follows that diseases caused by the impairment of catabolic pathways that involve the accumulation of dietary substances (e.g., phenylketonuria, galactosemia) or cellular constituents (e.g., Tay-Sachs, Hurler) are autosomal recessive, since the accumulation of substrate overcomes any partial enzymatic defect in the heterozygote.

Cystic Fibrosis

Cystic fibrosis (CF) is an autosomal recessive disorder affecting children, which is characterized by (1) chronic pulmonary disease, (2) deficient exocrine pancreatic function, and (3) other complications of inspissated mucus in a number of organs, including the small intestine, the liver, and the reproductive tract. The disease results from abnormal electrolyte transport caused by impaired function of the chloride channel of epithelial cells.

Cystic fibrosis is the most common lethal autosomal recessive disorder in the white population, with an inci-

dence of 1 in 2500 newborns. More than 95% of cases have been reported in whites, and the disease is found only exceptionally in blacks, and almost never in Asians. It is estimated that 1 in 25 whites is a heterozygous carrier of the CF gene. The high prevalence of CF mutations in white populations has raised the question of a possible selective advantage for heterozygotes. Although this topic has been a source of lively speculation, a selective advantage for the CF gene has yet to be demonstrated.

☐ Pathogenesis: The gene responsible for CF is located on the long arm of chromosome 7 (7q31.2) and encodes a protein of 1480 amino acids termed the **cystic fibrosis transmembrane conductance regulator (CFTR).** CFTR is a member of the adenosine triphosphate (ATP)-binding family of membrane transporter proteins that constitutes a chloride channel present in most epithelia. The protein has two membrane-spanning domains, two domains that bind ATP, and an "R" domain that contains phosphorylation sites. The activity of the channel is regulated by the balance between kinase and phosphatase activities (i.e., phosphorylation and dephosphorylation). Phosphorylation of the R domain stimulates chloride channel activity by enhancing the binding of ATP. Activation by phosphorylation is principally effected by cyclic adenosine monophosphate (cAMP)–dependent protein kinase A, although other kinases may also contribute. The secretion of chloride anions by mucus-secreting epithelial cells controls the parallel secretion of fluid and, consequently, the viscosity of the mucus. In normal mucus-secreting epithelia, cAMP activates protein kinase A, which in turn phosphorylates the regulatory domain of CFTR and permits channel opening. The binding of ATP to CFTR also contributes to the regulation of channel function.

In CF, the mutations in the gene encoding CFTR that disturb chloride channel function can be classified as follows (Fig. 6-21):

- **Failure of CFTR synthesis:** Mutations of the CFTR gene that result in premature termination signals lead to interference with the synthesis of the full-length CFTR protein. As a result there is a complete loss of CFTR-mediated chloride secretion in the involved epithelia.
- **Failure of CFTR transport to the plasma membrane:** Certain mutations prevent the proper folding of the nascent protein, which is then targeted for degradation rather than for transport to the plasma membrane. The mutation responsible for 70% of all cases of CF in the United States, namely the loss of a phenylalanine residue at position 508, ΔF_{508}, is of this class. However, the contribution of the ΔF_{508} mutation to CF shows significant geographic and ethnic variability. In Denmark, this mutation accounts for almost 90% of all CF cases, whereas among Ashkenazi Jews the figure is only 30%. An analysis of haplotypes suggested that the ΔF_{508} mutation originated 50,000 years ago in the Middle East, from where it progressively spread throughout the European land mass.
- **Defective ATP binding to CFTR:** Certain mutations in CFTR proteins that reach the plasma membrane affect the ATP-binding domains, thereby interfering with the regulation of the channel and decreasing, but not abolishing, chloride secretion.
- **Defective chloride secretion by mutant CFTR:** Mutations in the channel pore inhibit chloride secretion.

The relationship between the these genotypes (more than 400 allelic variations are known) and the clinical severity of CF is complicated and not always consistent. The best correlation seems to be between children with or without pancreatic insufficiency. Severe symptoms are generally found in those with pancreatic insufficiency (85% of all cases of CF), whereas milder cases are associated with preservation of pancreatic function. Class I and class II mutations are generally found among severely affected patients. By contrast, milder forms of CF feature class III and class IV mutations.

All of the pathological consequences of CF can be attributed to the presence of the abnormally thick mucus, which obstructs the lumina of airways, pancreatic and biliary ducts, and the fetal intestine and impairs mucociliary function in the airways. In fact, an older term for CF was **mucoviscidosis**. The normal CFTR has

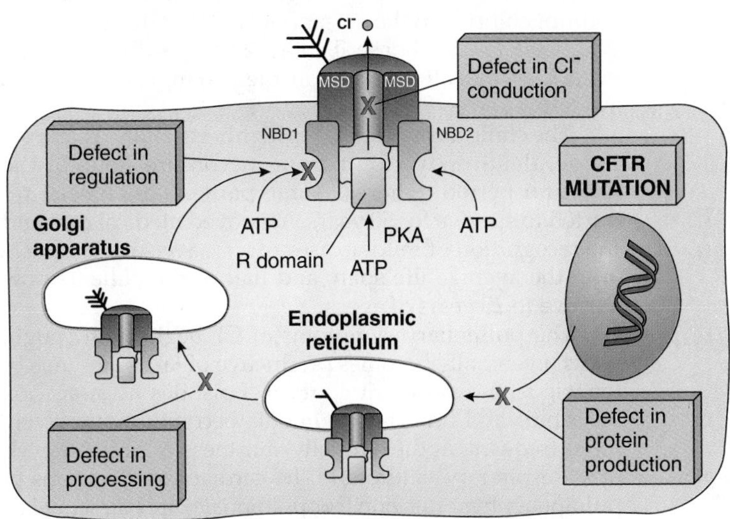

FIGURE 6-21
Cellular sites of the disruptions in the synthesis and function of cystic fibrosis transmembrane conductance regulator (CFTR) in CF.

been shown to correct the deficiency in chloride secretion in cultured cells from patients with CF.

□ Pathology

RESPIRATORY TRACT: **Pulmonary disease is responsible for most of the morbidity and mortality associated with CF.** The earliest lesion is obstruction of bronchioles by mucus, with secondary infection and inflammation of the bronchiolar walls. Recurrent cycles of obstruction and infection result in **chronic bronchiolitis and bronchitis**, which increase in severity as the disease progresses. The mucous glands in the bronchi undergo hypertrophy and hyperplasia, and the airways are distended by thick and tenacious secretions. Widespread **bronchiectasis** becomes apparent by age 10, and often earlier. In the late stages of the disease, large bronchiectatic cysts and lung abscesses are common. Vascular changes of secondary pulmonary hypertension complicate the chronic bronchitis.

PANCREAS: As noted, the large majority (85%) of patients with CF have a form of **chronic pancreatitis**, and in long-standing cases, little or no functional exocrine pancreas remains. The inspissated secretions in the pancreatic ducts produce secondary dilatation and cystic change of the distal ducts (Fig. 6-22). Recurrent pancreatitis leads to the loss of acinar cells and extensive fibrosis. At autopsy, the pancreas is often represented simply by cystic fibroadipose tissue containing islets of Langerhans, hence the original designation of this disease as cystic fibrosis of the pancreas.

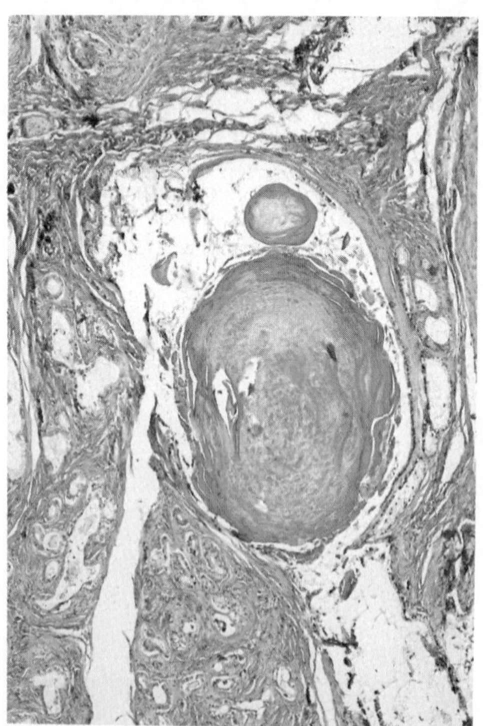

FIGURE 6-22
Intraductal concretion and atrophy of the acini in the pancreas of a patient with cystic fibrosis.

LIVER: Inspissated mucous secretions in the intrahepatic biliary system obstruct the flow of bile in the drainage areas of the affected ducts and are responsible for the development of focal **secondary biliary cirrhosis**, seen in one fourth of patients at autopsy. Microscopically, the liver exhibits inspissated concretions in bile ducts and ductules, chronic portal inflammation, and septal fibrosis. On occasion (2% to 5%), the hepatic lesions are sufficiently widespread to lead to the clinical manifestations of biliary cirrhosis.

GASTROINTESTINAL TRACT: Shortly after birth, the normal newborn passes the intestinal contents that have accumulated *in utero* (meconium). The most important lesion of the gastrointestinal tract in CF is small bowel obstruction in the newborn, termed **meconium ileus**, which is caused by the failure to pass meconium in the immediate postpartum period. This complication, which occurs in 5% to 10% of newborns with CF, has been attributed to the failure of pancreatic secretions to digest meconium, possibly augmented by the greater viscosity of small bowel secretions.

REPRODUCTIVE TRACT: Almost all boys with CF exhibit atrophy or fibrosis of the reproductive duct system, including the vas deferens, epididymis, and seminal vesicles. The pathogenesis of these lesions relates to obstruction of the lumen by inspissated secretions early in life and even *in utero*. As a result, only 2% to 3% of males become fertile, the large majority demonstrating an absence of spermatozoa in the semen.

Only a minority of women with CF are fertile, many of them suffering from anovulatory cycles as a result of poor nutrition and chronic infections. Moreover, the cervical mucous plug is abnormally thick and tenacious.

□ Clinical Features:

The diagnosis of CF is most reliably made by the demonstration of increased concentrations of electrolytes in the sweat. The decreased chloride conductance characteristic of CF results in a failure of chloride reabsorption by the cells of the sweat gland ducts, and hence to the accumulation of sodium chloride in the sweat (Fig. 6-23). Indeed, children with CF have been described as "tasting salty" and may even display salt crystals on their skin after vigorous sweating.

The clinical course of CF is highly variable. At one extreme, death may result from meconium ileus in the neonatal period, whereas some patients have been reported to survive for 50 years. Improved medical care and the recognition of milder cases of CF have served to prolong the average life span, and half of the patients now survive to 25 years of age.

The pulmonary symptoms of CF begin with cough, which eventually becomes productive of large amounts of tenacious and purulent sputum. Episodes of infectious bronchitis and bronchopneumonia become progressively more frequent, and eventually shortness of breath develops. Respiratory failure and the cardiac complications of pulmonary hypertension (cor pulmonale) are late sequelae.

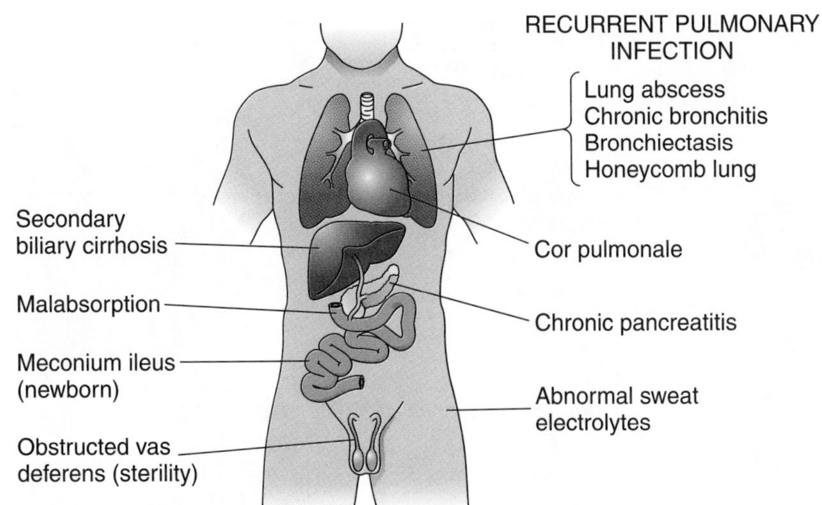

FIGURE 6-23
Clinical features of cystic fibrosis.

The most common organisms that infect the respiratory tract in CF are *Staphylococcus* and *Pseudomonas* species. As the disease advances, *Pseudomonas* may be the only organism cultured from the lung. **In fact, the recovery of *Pseudomonas* species, particularly the mucoid variety, from the lungs of a child with chronic pulmonary disease is virtually diagnostic of CF.**

The failure of pancreatic exocrine secretion leads to the malabsorption of fat and protein, an effect that is reflected in bulky, foul-smelling stools (steatorrhea), nutritional deficiencies, and growth retardation.

Postural drainage of the airways, antibiotic therapy, and pancreatic enzyme supplementation are the mainstays of the treatment of CF. The molecular prenatal diagnosis of CF in specimens obtained by amniocentesis or chorionic villus sampling is now accurate in 95% of cases.

Lysosomal Storage Diseases

Lysosomal storage diseases, inherited as autosomal recessive traits, are characterized by the accumulation (or "storage") of unmetabolized normal substrates in the lysosomes, owing to deficiencies of specific acid hydrolases. Lysosomes are membranous bags of hydrolytic enzymes used for the controlled intracellular digestion of macromolecules. Lysosomal digestive enzymes are referred to as "acid hydrolases" because they function optimally in the acidic range (pH 3.5 to 5.5), an environment maintained by an ATP-dependent proton pump in the lysosomal membrane. These enzymes degrade virtually all types of biological macromolecules. Extracellular macromolecules that are incorporated by endocytosis or phagocytosis, and intracellular constituents that are subjected to autophagy, are digested in the lysosomes to their basic components. The end-products may be transported across the lysosomal membrane into the cytosol, where they are reutilized in the synthesis of new macromolecules.

Virtually all lysosomal storage diseases result from mutations in genes that encode lysosomal hydrolases. A deficiency in one of the more than 40 acid hydrolases can result in an inability to catabolize the normal macromolecular substrate of that enzyme. As a result, the undigested substrate accumulates in the lysosomes, thereby leading to engorgement of these organelles and expansion of the lysosomal compartment of the cell. The resulting distention of the lysosomes is often at the expense of other critical cellular components, particularly in the brain and the heart, and can lead to a failure of cell function.

Lysosomal storage diseases are classified according to the material retained within the lysosomes. Thus, when the substrates that accumulate are sphingolipids, we speak of the sphingolipidoses. Similarly, the storage of mucopolysaccharides (glycosaminoglycans) leads to the mucopolysaccharidoses. More than 30 distinct lysosomal storage diseases have been described, but we will restrict our discussion to the more important examples.

Sphingolipidoses are lysosomal storage diseases characterized by the accumulation of certain lipids derived from the turnover of obsolete cell membranes. Cerebrosides, gangliosides, sphingomyelin, and sulfatides are sphingolipid components of the membranes of a variety of cells. These substances are degraded within lysosomes by complex metabolic pathways to sphingosine and fatty acids (Fig. 6-24). Deficiencies of many of the acid hydrolases that mediate specific steps in these pathways result in the accumulation of undigested intermediate substrates in the lysosomes.

Gaucher Disease

Gaucher disease is characterized by the accumulation of glucosylceramide, primarily in the lysosomes of macrophages. The disorder was first described in 1882 in a doctoral thesis by Gaucher, but the familial occurrence was not recognized for some 20 years.

☐ Pathogenesis: The underlying abnormality in Gaucher disease is a deficiency in glucocerebrosidase, a type of lysosomal acid β-glucosidase. The enzyme deficiency can be traced to a variety of single base mutations in the β-glucosidase gene, which resides on the long arm of chromosome 1 (1q21). Each of the three clinical types of

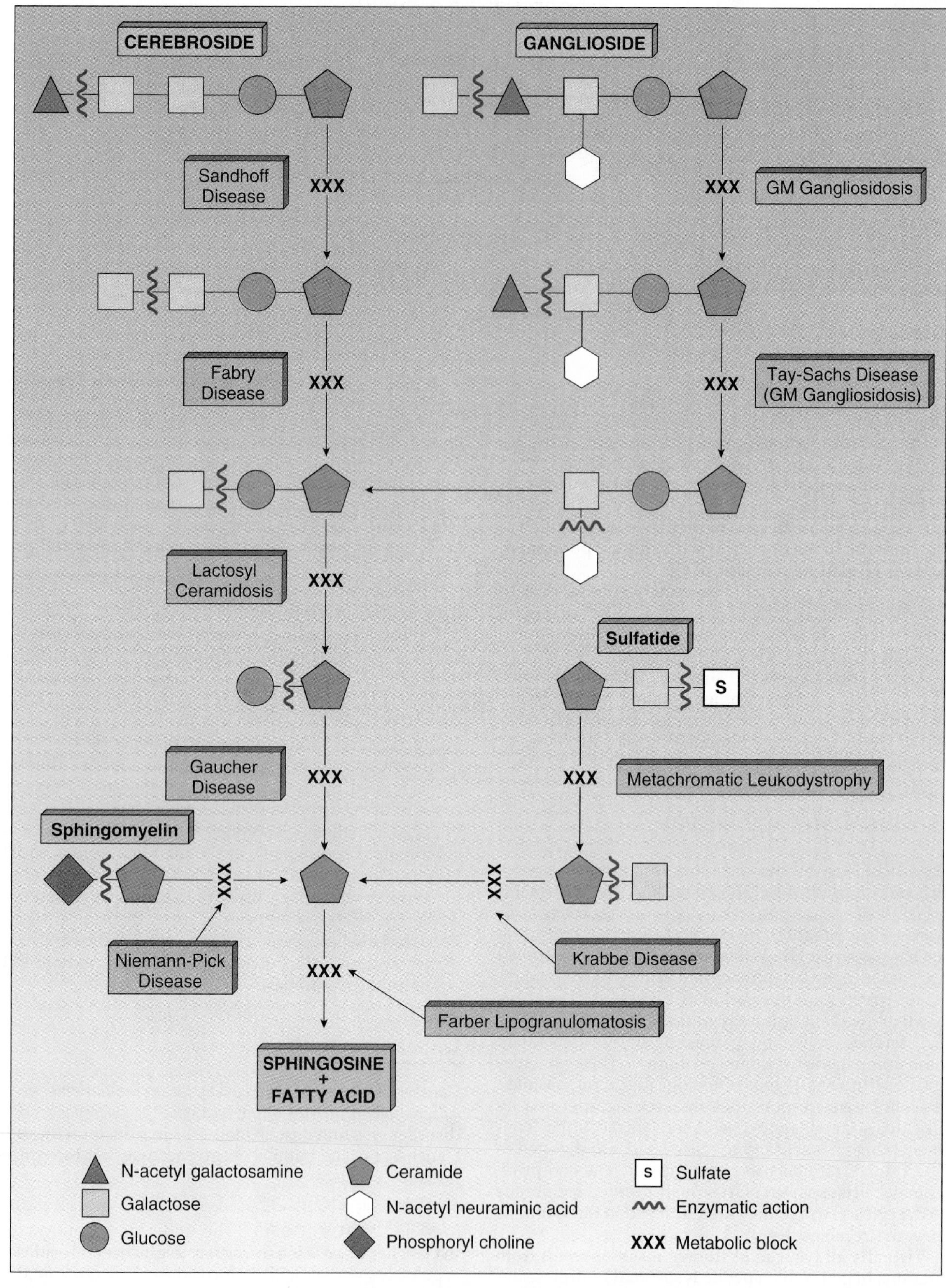

FIGURE 6-24
Disturbances of lipid metabolism in various sphingolipidoses.

the disease (see later) exhibits heterogeneous mutations in the β-glucosidase gene, although the molecular basis for the phenotypic differences remains to be firmly established.

The glucosylceramide that accumulates in the Gaucher cells in the spleen, liver, bone marrow, and lymph nodes derives principally from the catabolism of senescent leukocytes. The membranes of these cells are rich in the cerebrosides, and when their degradation is blocked by the deficiency of glucocerebrosidase, the intermediate metabolite, glucosylceramide, accumulates. The glucosylceramide of Gaucher cells in the brain is believed to originate from the turnover of plasma membrane gangliosides of cells in the central nervous system.

☐ Pathology: The hallmark of this disorder is the presence of **Gaucher cells**, which are lipid-laden macrophages that are characteristically present in the red pulp of the spleen, liver sinusoids, lymph nodes, lungs, and bone marrow, although they may be found in virtually any organ of the body. These cells are derived from the resident macrophages in the respective organs, for example, the Kupffer cells in the liver and the alveolar macrophages in the lung. In the uncommon variants of Gaucher disease with involvement of the central nervous system, the Gaucher cells originate from periadventitial cells in the Virchow-Robin spaces.

The Gaucher cell is large (20 to 100 μm in diameter) and has a clear cytoplasm and an eccentric nucleus (Fig. 6-25). By light microscopy, the cytoplasm has a characteristic fibrillar appearance, which has been likened to "wrinkled tissue paper" and is intensely positive with the periodic acid–Schiff (PAS) stain. By electron microscopy, the storage material is found within enlarged lysosomes and appears as parallel layers of tubular structures.

Enlargement of the spleen is virtually universal in Gaucher disease. In the adult form of the disorder, splenomegaly may be massive, with spleen weights up to 10 kg. The cut surface of the enlarged spleen is firm and pale and often contains sharply demarcated infarcts. Microscopically, the red pulp shows nodular and diffuse infiltrates of Gaucher cells, together with moderate fibrosis.

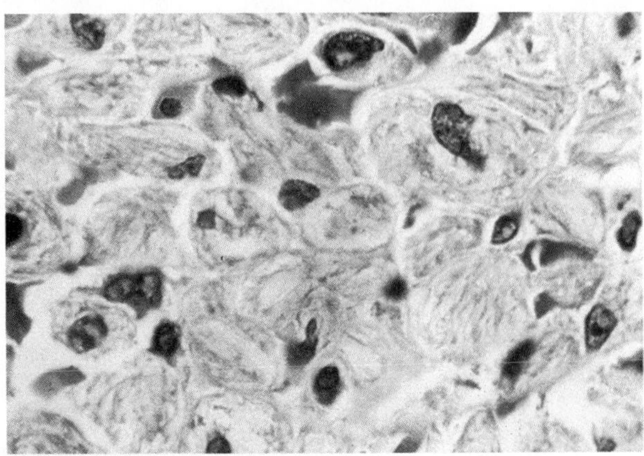

FIGURE *6-25*
The spleen in Gaucher disease. Typical Gaucher cells have foamy cytoplasm and eccentrically located nuclei.

The liver is usually enlarged by the presence of Gaucher cells within the sinusoids, but the hepatocytes are unaffected. In severe cases, hepatic fibrosis, and even cirrhosis, may ensue. The extent of bone marrow involvement is variable but leads to some radiological abnormalities in 50% to 75% of cases (see Chapter 26).

Gaucher cells may also be found in many other organs, including the lymph nodes, lungs, endocrine glands, skin, gastrointestinal tract, and kidneys, although symptoms referable to these organs are uncommon.

When the brain is affected, Gaucher cells are present in the Virchow-Robin spaces around blood vessels. In the infantile (neuronopathic) form of Gaucher disease, these cells have also been found in the parenchyma, where they may stimulate gliosis and the formation of microglial nodules.

☐ Clinical Features: Gaucher disease is classified into three distinct forms, based on the age at onset and degree of neurological involvement.

- **Type 1 (chronic non-neuronopathic):** This variant of Gaucher disease is the most common of all lysosomal storage diseases and is found principally in adult Ashkenazi Jews, among whom the incidence is between 1 in 600 and 1 in 2500. The age at onset is highly variable, with some cases being diagnosed in infants and others in persons 70 years of age. Similarly, the severity of clinical manifestations varies widely. The majority of cases are not diagnosed until adulthood and present initially as painless splenomegaly and the complications of hypersplenism (i.e., anemia, leukopenia, and thrombocytopenia). Whereas hepatomegaly is common, clinical liver disease is infrequent. Bone involvement, in the form of pain and pathological fractures, is the leading cause of disability and may be severe enough to confine the patient to a wheelchair. The life expectancy of most persons with type 1 Gaucher disease is normal. This type of Gaucher disease is now successfully treated by the intravenous administration of modified acid glucose cerebrosidase, although the extremely high cost limits its use. Marrow transplantation is also effective but is little used because of the risks associated with this therapy. Prenatal diagnosis, based on β-glucosidase activity in amniotic fluid or chorionic villi or on DNA technology, is now routinely available.
- **Type 2 (acute neuronopathic):** Type 2 Gaucher disease is rare and distinctly different from type 1 in the age at onset and the clinical presentation. It usually presents by age 3 months with hepatosplenomegaly and has no ethnic predilection. Within a few months, the infant exhibits neurological signs, with the classic triad of trismus, strabismus, and backward flexion of the neck. Further neurological deterioration rapidly follows, and most patients die before the age of 1 year.
- **Type 3 (subacute neuronopathic):** This form of Gaucher disease is also rare and combines features of type 1 and type 2 disease. Neurological deterioration presents at an older age than in patients with type 2 and is more slowly progressive.

Tay-Sachs Disease (GM_2 Gangliosidosis, Type 1)

Tay-Sachs disease is the catastrophic infantile variant of a class of lysosomal storage diseases, known as the GM_2 gangliosidoses, in which this ganglioside is deposited in neurons of the central nervous system, owing to a failure of lysosomal degradation. The association of a "cherry-red spot" in the retina and profound mental and physical retardation was first pointed out in 1881 by Warren Tay, a British ophthalmologist. Fifteen years later, Bernard Sachs, an American neurologist, described the histological features of the disorder and coined the term "amaurotic (blind) family idiocy." Tay-Sachs disease is inherited as an autosomal recessive trait and is predominantly a disorder of Ashkenazi Jews, in whom the carrier rate is 1 in 30, and the natural incidence of homozygotes is 1 in 4000 live newborns. By contrast, the incidence of Tay-Sachs disease in non-Jewish American populations is less than 1 in 100,000 live births. Screening programs for heterozygotes among Ashkenazi Jews have now reduced the disease incidence by 90%. The other GM_2 gangliosidoses are exceedingly rare.

□ Pathogenesis: Gangliosides are glycosphingolipids consisting of a ceramide and an oligosaccharide chain that contains N-acetylneuraminic acid (see Fig. 6-24). They are present in the outer leaflet of the plasma membrane of animal cells, particularly in brain neurons.

The lysosomal catabolism of 1 of the 12 known gangliosides in the brain, namely ganglioside GM_2, is accomplished through the activity of the β-hexosaminidases (A and B), which are composed of α- and β-subunits and require the participation of the GM_2 activator protein. A deficiency in any of these components results in clinical disease.

Tay-Sachs disease (also known as hexosaminidase α-subunit deficiency) results from about 50 different mutations in the gene on chromosome 15q23-24 that codes for the α-subunit of hexosaminidase A, with a resulting defect in the synthesis of this enzyme. An insertion of four nucleotides in exon 11 is the most common mutation among Ashkenazi Jews, accounting for over two thirds of the carriers, or about 2% of that population. The β-subunits are synthesized normally and associate to form the dimer known as hexosaminidase B, the levels of which are normal or even increased in Tay-Sachs disease.

Sandhoff disease is the result of a mutation in the gene on chromosome 5 that encodes the β-subunit and leads to deficiencies of both hexosaminidase A and B.

A third rare variant is the result of a defect in the synthesis of the GM_2 activator protein (chromosome 5), in the face of normal activities of the hexosaminidases.

□ Pathology: GM_2 ganglioside accumulates in the lysosomes of all organs in Tay-Sachs disease, but it is most prominent in brain neurons and cells of the retina. The size of the brain varies with the length of survival of the affected infant. Early cases are marked by brain atrophy, whereas the brain may be as much as doubled in weight in those who survive beyond a year. Microscopic examination reveals neurons markedly distended with storage material that stains positively for lipids. By electron microscopy, the neurons are stuffed with "membranous cytoplasmic bodies," which are composed of concentric whorls of lamellar structures (Fig. 6-26). As the disease progresses, neurons are lost and numerous lipid-laden macrophages are conspicuous in the gray matter of the cerebral cortex. Eventually, gliosis becomes prominent, and myelin and axons in the white matter are lost. The pathological changes in the other forms of GM_2 gangliosidosis are similar to those of Tay-Sachs disease, although usually less severe.

□ Clinical Features: The symptomatology of Tay-Sachs disease appears between 6 and 10 months of age and is characterized by progressive weakness, hypotonia, and decreased attentiveness. Progressive motor and mental deterioration, often with generalized seizures, follow rapidly. Vision is seriously impaired, and blindness (Gk. *amaurosis*) is the feature that was responsible for the original designation of the disease as familial amaurotic idiocy. Involvement of the retinal ganglion cells is detected by ophthalmoscopy as a **cherry-red spot** in the macula. This feature reflects the pallor of the affected cells, which enhances the prominence of the vessels underlying the central fovea. Most children with Tay-Sachs disease die before 4 years of age.

Niemann-Pick Disease

Niemann-Pick disease (NPD) refers to lipidoses that are characterized by the lysosomal storage of sphingomyelin in macrophages of many organs, in hepatocytes, and in the brain. These disorders are classified into two categories, termed types A and B. Type A NPD appears in infancy and is

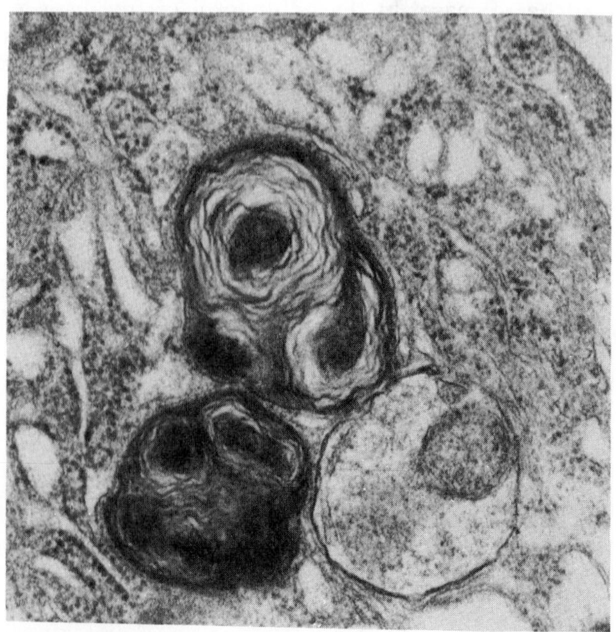

FIGURE *6-26*
Tay-Sachs disease. The cytoplasm of the nerve cell contains lysosomes filled with whorled membranes.

characterized by hepatosplenomegaly and progressive neurodegeneration, with death occurring by 3 years of age. Type B NPD is more variable and features principally hepatosplenomegaly and minimal neurological symptomatology, with survival to adulthood. A particularly high frequency of NPD is observed among Ashkenazi Jews, but the disorder is present in other ethnic groups. Among the former, the incidence of type A NPD is 1 in 40,000 and of type B 1 in 80,000, with a combined heterozygote prevalence of 1 in 100.

☐ Pathogenesis: Sphingomyelin is a membrane phospholipid, composed of phosphorylcholine, sphingosine (a long-chain amino alcohol), and a fatty acid, that accounts for up to 14% of the total phospholipids of the liver, spleen, and brain. The metabolic defect in NPD reflects 12 different mutations in the gene (11p15.1-15.4) that encodes **sphingomyelinase**, the lysosomal enzyme that hydrolyzes sphingomyelin to ceramide and phosphorylcholine. Type A NPD reflects the complete absence of sphingomyelinase activity, whereas in type B patients up to 10% of normal activity can be detected.

☐ Pathology: The characteristic storage cell in NPD is a foam cell, that is, an enlarged (20 to 90 μm) macrophage in which the cytoplasm is distended by the presence of uniform vacuoles that contain sphingomyelin and cholesterol. By electron microscopy, whorls of concentrically arranged lamellar structures distend the lysosomes.

Foam cells are particularly numerous in the spleen, lymph nodes, and bone marrow but are also found in the liver, lungs, and gastrointestinal tract. The spleen is enlarged, often to massive proportions, and, microscopically, foam cells are diffusely distributed throughout the red pulp. Lymph nodes enlarged by foam cells are seen in many locations. The hemopoietic tissues in the bone marrow may be displaced by aggregates of foam cells. The liver is enlarged by the presence of stored sphingomyelin and cholesterol in the lysosomes of both Kupffer cells and hepatocytes.

The brain is the most important organ involved in type A NPD, and neurological damage is the usual cause of death. At autopsy, the brain is atrophic and in severe cases may be reduced to as little as half the normal weight. Neurons are distended by the presence of vacuoles containing the same stored lipids found elsewhere in the body. Advanced cases are characterized by a severe loss of neurons and sometimes by demyelination. Foam cells are noted in many locations. Half of the children affected by type A disease demonstrate a cherry-red spot in the retina, similar to that seen in Tay-Sachs disease.

☐ Clinical Features: Type A NPD presents in early infancy with conspicuous enlargement of the spleen and liver, and psychomotor retardation. There is a progressive loss of motor and intellectual function, and the child typically dies between the of ages of 2 and 3 years. Most type B patients are identified in childhood because of conspicuous hepatosplenomegaly. Pulmonary infiltration with sphingomyelin-laden macrophages eventually leads to compromised respiratory function in many patients with type B disease. However, these patients have little in the way of neurological symptoms and may survive for many years.

Mucopolysaccharidoses

The mucopolysaccharidoses (MPS) comprise an assortment of lysosomal storage diseases characterized by the accumulation of glycosaminoglycans (mucopolysaccharides) in many organs. All types of MPS are inherited as autosomal recessive traits, with the exception of Hunter syndrome, which is X-linked recessive. These rare diseases are caused by deficiencies in any one of the 10 lysosomal enzymes involved in the sequential degradation of glycosaminoglycans (Fig. 6-27). Six abnormal phenotypes are described, each varying with the specific enzyme deficiency (Table 6-8).

☐ Pathogenesis: Glycosaminoglycans (GAGs) are large polymers composed of repeating disaccharide units containing N-acetylhexosamine and a hexose or a hexuronic acid. Either of the disaccharide components may by sulfated. The accumulated GAGs (dermatan sulfate, heparan sulfate, keratan sulfate, and chondroitin sulfates) in MPS are all derived from the cleavage of proteoglycans, which are important constituents of the extracellular matrix. GAGs are degraded in a stepwise fashion by removing sugar residues or sulfate groups. Thus, a deficiency in any one of the glycosidases or sulfatases results in the accumulation of undegraded GAGs. A special case is a deficiency of an N-acetyltransferase, which leads to the deposition of heparan sulfate in Sanfilippo C disease.

☐ Pathology: Although the severity and location of the lesions in MPS vary with the specific enzyme deficiency, certain features are common to most of these syndromes. The undegraded GAGs tend to accumulate in connective tissue cells, mononuclear phagocytes (including Kupffer cells), endothelial cells, neurons, and hepatocytes. The affected cells are swollen and clear, and stains for metachromasia confirm the presence of GAGs. By electron microscopy, numerous enlarged lysosomes containing granular or striped material are noted.

The most important lesions of the MPS involve the central nervous system, the skeleton, and the heart, although hepatosplenomegaly and corneal clouding are common.

The central nervous system initially demonstrates only the accumulation of GAGs, but with advancing disease there is an extensive loss of neurons and increasing gliosis, changes that are reflected in cortical atrophy. Communicating hydrocephalus, owing to meningeal involvement, is often reported.

The skeletal deformities are a consequence of the accumulation of GAGs in chondrocytes, a process that eventually interferes with the normal endochondral sequence of ossification. Abnormal foci of osteoid and woven bone are common in the deformed skeleton.

Cardiac lesions are often severe and are characterized by thickening and distortion of the valves, chordae tendineae, and endocardium. The coronary arteries are

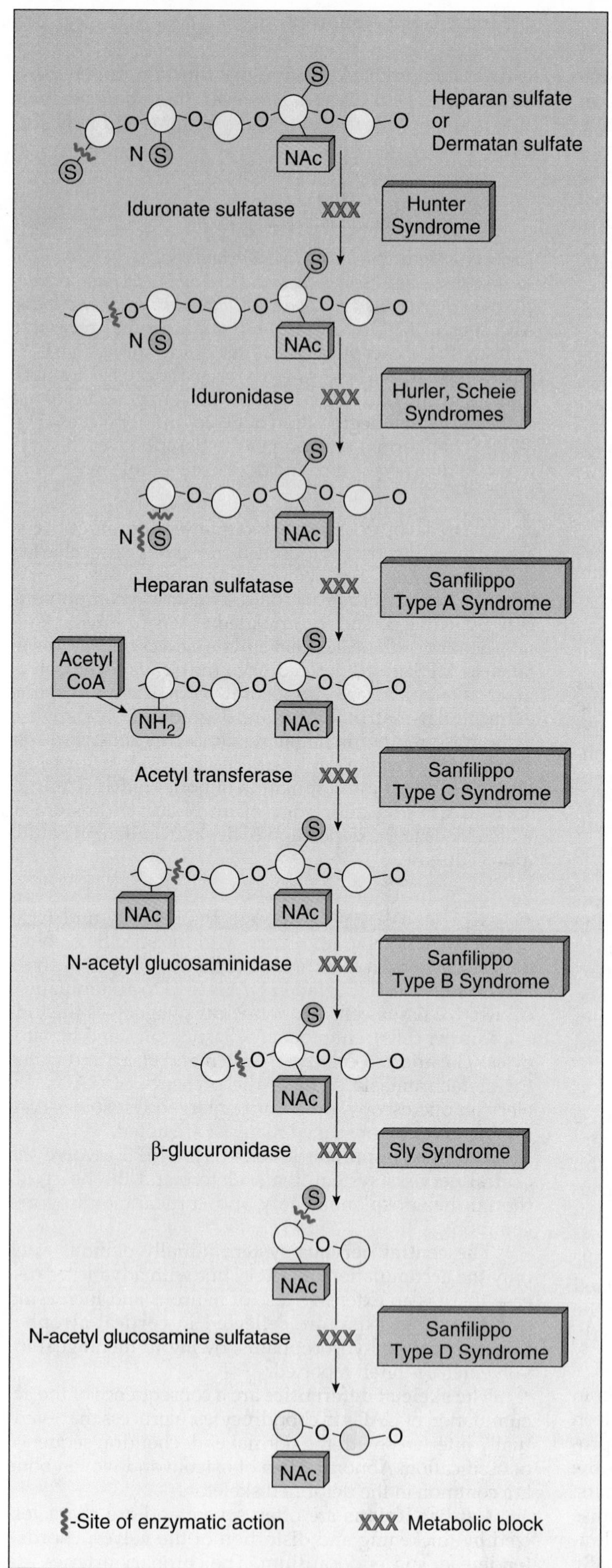

FIGURE 6-27
Metabolic blocks in various mucopolysaccharidoses that affect the degradation of heparan sulfate and dermatan sulfate.

TABLE 6-8 **Mucopolysaccharidoses**

Type	Eponym	Location of Gene	Clinical Features
I H	Hurler	4p16.3	Organomegaly, cardiac lesions, dysostosis multiplex, corneal clouding, death in childhood
I S	Scheie	4p16.3	Stiff joints, corneal clouding, normal intelligence, longevity
II	Hunter	X	Organomegaly, dysostosis multiplex, mental retardation, death earlier than 15 years of age
III	Sanfillipo	12q14	Mental retardation
IV	Morquio	16q24	Skeletal deformities, corneal clouding
V	Obsolete	—	—
VI	Maroteaux Lamy	5q13–14	Dysostosis multiplex, corneal clouding, death in second decade
VII	Sly	7q21.1–22	Hepatosplenomegaly, dysostosis multiplex

frequently narrowed by intimal thickening caused by GAG deposits in smooth muscle cells.

Hepatosplenomegaly is secondary to the distention of Kupffer cells and hepatocytes in the liver and the accumulation of macrophages filled with GAGs in the spleen.

☐ Clinical Features: Hurler syndrome (MPS IH), the most severe clinical form of the mucopolysaccharidoses, remains the prototype of these syndromes. The clinical features of the other varieties of MPS are summarized in Table 6-8. The symptoms of Hurler syndrome become apparent between the ages of 6 months and 2 years. These children typically exhibit skeletal deformities, an enlarged liver and spleen, a characteristic facies, and joint stiffness. The combination of coarse facial features and dwarfism is reminiscent of the gargoyle figures decorating Gothic cathedrals and accounts for the term **gargoylism** previously appended to this syndrome.

Children with Hurler syndrome suffer developmental delay, hearing loss, clouding of the cornea, and progressive mental deterioration. Increased intracranial pressure, owing to communicating hydrocephalus, can be troublesome. Most patients die before the age of 10 years from recurrent pulmonary infections and cardiac complications.

The detection of heterozygotes is difficult, because of the overlap in enzyme activity of cultured cells with the normal population. Prenatal diagnosis is possible for all the mucopolysaccharidoses and is routine for Hurler and Hunter syndromes.

Glycogenoses (Glycogen Storage Diseases)

The glycogenoses are a group at least 10 distinct inherited disorders characterized by the accumulation of glycogen, principally in the liver, skeletal muscle, and heart. Each entity reflects a deficiency of one of the specific enzymes involved in the metabolism of glycogen (Fig. 6-28). With one rare exception (X-linked phosphorylase kinase deficiency), all types of glycogen storage disease represent autosomal recessive traits. The glycogenoses are rare diseases, varying in frequency from 1 in 100,000 to 1 in 1 million.

Glycogen is a large glucose polymer (20,000 to 30,000 glucose units per molecule) that is stored in most cells to provide a ready source of energy during the fasting state. The liver and muscle are particularly rich in glycogen, although its function is different in each organ. The liver stores glycogen not for its own use but rather for the rapid supply of glucose to the blood, particularly for the benefit of the brain. By contrast, glycogen in skeletal muscle is utilized as a local fuel when the supply of oxygen or glucose falls. Glycogen is synthesized and degraded sequentially by the action of a number of enzymes, a deficiency in any of which leads to the accumulation of glycogen.

Although each of the glycogen storage diseases involves an accumulation of glycogen, the significant organ involvement varies with the specific enzyme defect. Some predominantly affect the liver, whereas others are principally manifested by cardiac or skeletal muscle dysfunction. **Importantly, the symptoms of a glycogenosis can reflect either the accumulation of glycogen itself (Pompe disease, Andersen disease) or the lack of the glucose that is normally derived from glycogen degradation (von Gierke disease, McArdle disease).** We will discuss only several representative examples of the known glycogenoses.

VON GIERKE DISEASE (TYPE IA GLYCOGENOSIS): *von Gierke disease is characterized by the accumulation of glycogen in the liver as a result of a deficiency in glucose-6-phosphatase.* The symptoms reflect the inability of the liver to convert glycogen to glucose, a defect that results in hepatomegaly and hypoglycemia. The disorder is usually evident in infancy or early childhood. Although growth is commonly stunted, with modern treatment the prognosis for normal mental development and longevity is generally good.

POMPE DISEASE (TYPE II GLYCOGENOSIS): *Pompe disease is a lysosomal storage disease that involves virtually all organs and results in death from heart failure before the age of 2 years.* The juvenile and adult variants are less common and have a better prognosis. Normally, a small proportion of cytoplasmic glycogen is degraded within lysosomes following an autophagic sequence. Type II glycogenosis is caused by a deficiency in the lysosomal enzyme acid α-glucosidase (17q23), which leads to the inexorable accumulation of undegraded glycogen in the lysosomes of many different cells. Interestingly, the patients do not suffer from hypoglycemia, because the major metabolic pathways of glycogen synthesis and degradation in the cytoplasm remain normal.

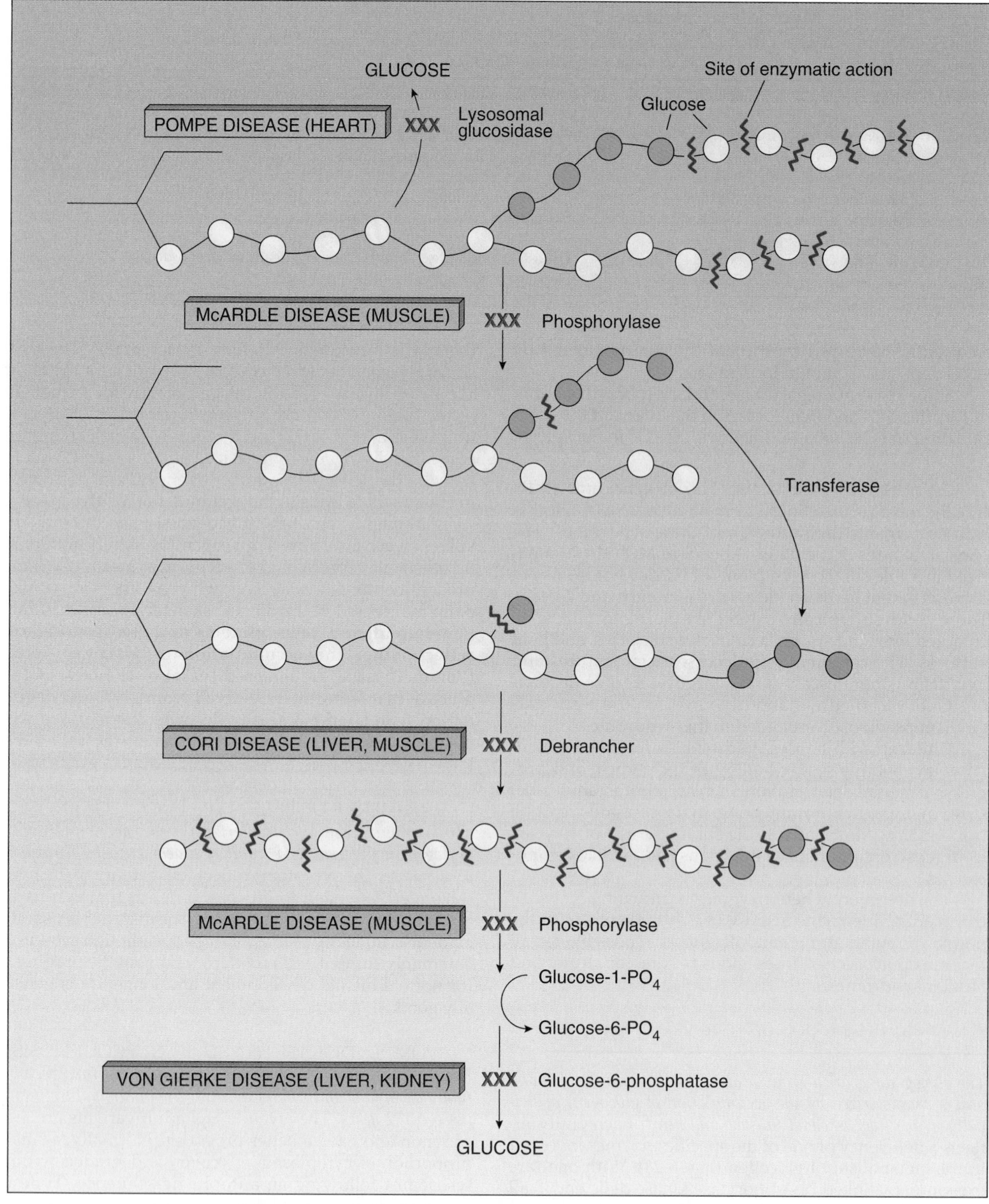
GLUCOSE
Site of enzymatic action
Glucose
POMPE DISEASE (HEART)
XXX
Lysosomal glucosidase
McARDLE DISEASE (MUSCLE)
XXX
Phosphorylase
Transferase
CORI DISEASE (LIVER, MUSCLE)
XXX
Debrancher
McARDLE DISEASE (MUSCLE)
XXX
Phosphorylase
Glucose-1-PO4
Glucose-6-PO4
VON GIERKE DISEASE (LIVER, KIDNEY)
XXX
Glucose-6-phosphatase
GLUCOSE

FIGURE 6-28

ANDERSEN DISEASE (TYPE IV GLYCOGENOSIS): *Andersen disease is a very rare condition in which an abnormal form of glycogen, termed amylopectin, is deposited principally in the liver, but also in the heart, muscles, and nervous system.* Children with type IV glycogenosis typically die between the ages of 2 and 4 years from **cirrhosis of the liver**. The disorder results from a deficiency in the branching enzyme (amyloglucantransferase) (3p12) responsible for creating the branch points in the normal glycogen molecule. The absence of brancher enzyme leads to the formation and accumulation of an insoluble and toxic form of glycogen that is normally not present in animal cells and resembles plant starch. Liver transplantation cures Andersen disease. Remarkably, the deposits of amylopectin in the heart and other extrahepatic tissues are significantly reduced following liver transplantation, although the mechanism for this paradoxical effect is obscure.

McARDLE DISEASE (TYPE V GLYCOGENOSIS): *McArdle disease is characterized by the accumulation of glycogen in skeletal muscles, owing to a deficiency of muscle phosphorylase (11q13), the enzyme responsible for the release of glucose-1-phosphate from glycogen.* Symptoms usually appear in adolescence or early adulthood and consist of muscle cramps and spasms during exercise and sometimes myocytolysis and resulting myoglobinuria. Avoidance of exercise prevents the symptoms.

Inborn Errors of Amino Acid Metabolism

Heritable disorders involving the metabolism of many amino acids have been described (Table 6-9). Some are lethal in early childhood, whereas others are asymptomatic biochemical defects that have no clinical significance. Some of these are treated in chapters dealing with specific organs. Here we restrict our discussion to the examples provided by defects in the metabolism of phenylalanine and tyrosine (Fig. 6-29).

Phenylketonuria

Phenylketonuria (PKU, hyperphenylalaninemia) is an autosomal recessive disorder characterized by progressive mental deterioration in the first few years of life owing to high levels of circulating phenylalanine secondary to a deficiency of the hepatic enzyme phenylalanine hydroxylase. The overall incidence of PKU is 1 per 10,000 in white and Asian populations, but it varies widely across different geographic areas. The frequency of the disease is highest (1 in 5000) in Ireland and western Scotland and among Yemenite Jews.

TABLE *6-9* **Representative Inherited Disorders of Amino Acid Metabolism**

Phenylketonuria (hyperphenylalaninemia)
Tyrosinemia
Histidinemia
Ornithine transcarbamylase deficiency (ammonia intoxication)
Carbamyl phosphate synthetase deficiency (ammonia intoxication)
Maple syrup urine disease (branched chain ketoacidemia)
Arginase deficiency
Arginosuccinic acid synthetase deficiency (citrulline accumulation)

☐ Pathogenesis: Phenylalanine is an essential amino acid that is derived exclusively from the diet and is oxidized in the liver to tyrosine by phenylalanine hydroxylase (PAH). A deficiency in PAH results in both hyperphenylalaninemia and the formation of phenylketones from the transamination of phenylalanine. The excretion in the urine of phenylpyruvic acid and its derivatives accounts for the original name of phenylketonuria. However, it is now established that phenylalanine itself, rather than its metabolites, is responsible for the neurological damage central to this disease. **Thus, the term hyperphenylalaninemia is actually a more appropriate designation than PKU.**

A variety of point mutations in the PAH gene, located on the long arm of chromosome 12 (12q22-24.1), are responsible for the deficiency in PAH in most patients of European origin. By contrast, PKU among Yemenite Jews has been ascribed to a single deletion in the PAH gene. An analysis of family histories of the Yemenite Jewish community has traced the origin of this defect to a common ancestor who lived in Sanà, the capital of Yemen, before the 18th century. A different deletion in the PAH gene has been identified in the affected Scottish population.

FIGURE *6-28*
The sequential catabolism of glycogen and the enzymes that are deficient in various glycogenoses. Glycogen is a long-chain branched polymer of glucose residues, which are connected by α-1,4 linkages, except at branch points, where an α-1,6 linkage is present. Phosphorylase hydrolyzes α-1,4 linkages to a point three glucose residues distal to an α-1,6-linked sugar. These three glucose residues are transferred to the chain linked by α-1,4 bonds, by the bifunctional debrancher enzyme amylo-1,6-glucosidase. Subsequently the same enzyme removes the α-1,6 linked sugar at the original branch point. This creates a linear α-1,4 chain, which is degraded by phosphorylase to glucose-1-phosphate. Following the conversion to glucose-6-phosphate, glucose is released by the action of glucose-6-phosphatase. A small proportion of glycogen is totally degraded within lysosomes by acid α-glucosidase.

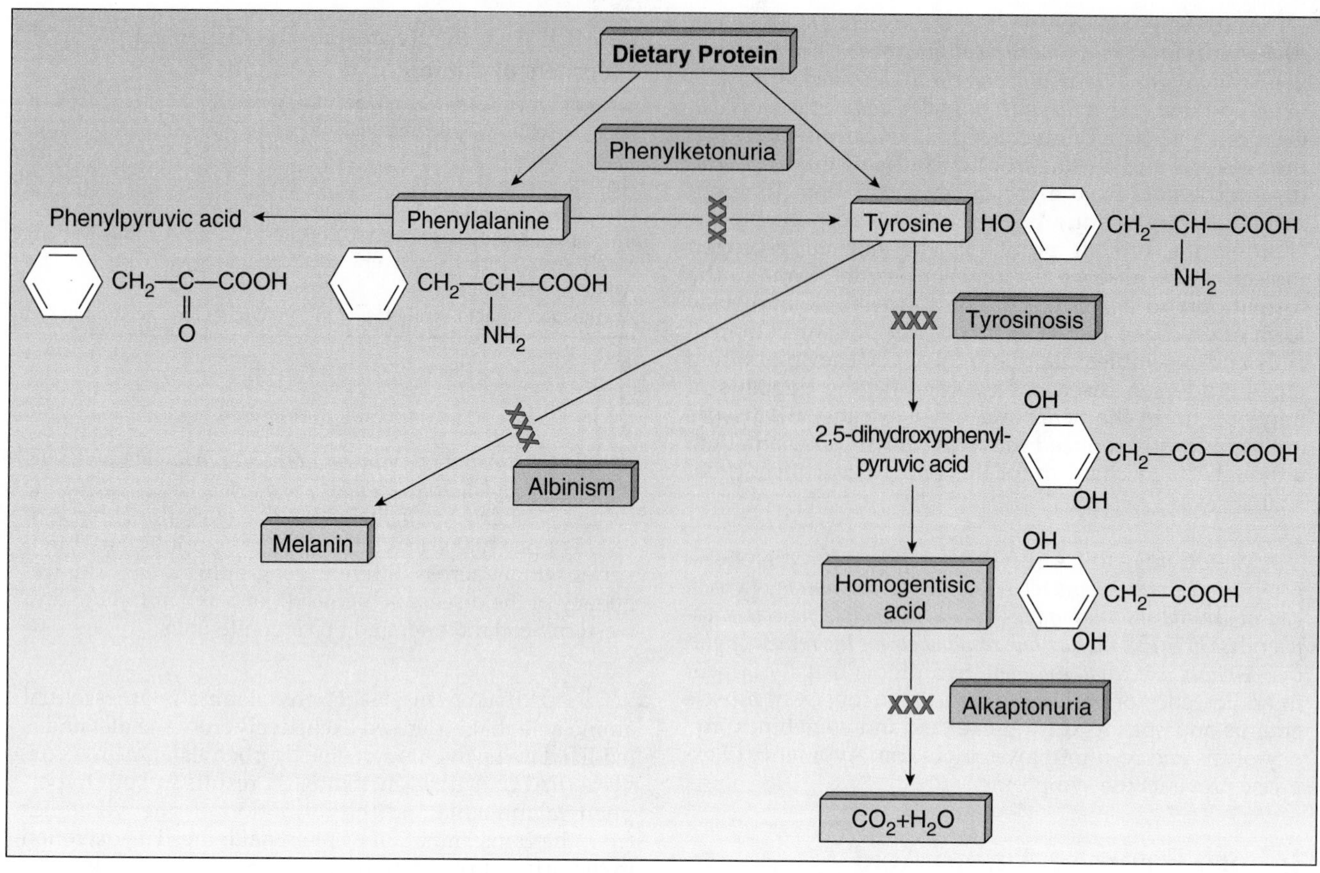

FIGURE 6-29
Diseases caused by disturbances of phenylalanine and tyrosine metabolism.

The mechanism of the neurotoxicity associated with hyperphenylalaninemia during infancy has not been precisely established, but several processes have been implicated: (1) competitive interference with amino acid transport systems in the brain, (2) inhibition of the synthesis of neurotransmitters, and (3) disturbance of other metabolic processes. These effects presumably lead to inadequate development of neurons and defective synthesis of myelin.

The deficiency in PAH activity is not necessarily absolute, and milder degrees of hyperphenylalaninemia than occur in classic PKU are described. In such cases, phenylpyruvic acid is not excreted in the urine. Patients with less than 1% of the normal activity of PAH generally have a PKU phenotype, whereas those with more than 5% are considered to exhibit non-PKU hyperphenylalaninemia. Importantly, the latter do not suffer neurological damage and develop normally. It is presumed that non-PKU hyperphenylalaninemia is caused by mutations different from those in classic PKU.

Malignant hyperphenylalaninemia occurs in a few (<5%) infants with hyperphenylalaninemia. In this condition, dietary restriction of phenylalanine fails to arrest neurological deterioration. These patients have a deficiency in tetrahydrobiopterin (BH_4), a co-factor required for the hydroxylation of phenylalanine by PAH. In some instances, this defect results from a failure to regenerate BH_4, owing to an inherited lack of dihydropteridine reductase (DHPR), the enzyme that reduces dihydrobiopterin (BH_2) to the tetrahydro form (BH_4). The mutant DHPR gene is distinct from the PAH gene, being located on the short arm of chromosome 4. Alternatively, in some cases the synthesis of BH_4 is impaired. Although these infants with malignant hyperphenylalaninemia are initially indistinguishable phenotypically from those with classic PKU, BH_4 deficiency also interferes with the synthesis of the neurotransmitters dopamine (tyrosine hydroxylase-dependent) and serotonin (tryptophan hydroxylase-dependent). Thus, the mechanism underlying the brain damage in malignant hyperphenylalaninemia likely involves more than a simple elevation in the levels of phenylalanine.

□ Clinical Features: Phenylketonuria illustrates the interaction between "nature and nurture" in the pathogenesis of disease. The disorder is based on a genetic defect, but its expression depends on the provision of a dietary constituent. **The affected infant appears normal at birth, but mental retardation is evident within a**

few months. By the age of 12 months, the untreated infant has lost about 50 IQ points, which means that a child with normal intelligence has been reduced to an imbecile who requires institutionalization. Infants with PKU tend to have fair skin, blond hair, and blue eyes, because the inability to convert phenylalanine to tyrosine leads to reduced melanin synthesis. These patients exude a "mousy" odor, owing to the formation of phenylacetic acid.

The treatment of PKU involves the restriction of phenylalanine in the diet to between 250 and 500 mg/day, which usually requires a semisynthetic formula. The required duration of such dietary therapy is controversial. Although at one time it was believed that the dietary regimen could be relaxed by 6 years of age, that is, after the brain has in large part matured, newer evidence suggests that many older patients suffer some deleterious effect on the reintroduction of phenylalanine into the diet. Thus, it is recommended that some degree of phenylalanine restriction be maintained indefinitely.

In developed countries, the clinical phenotype of classical PKU is now more of historical interest than of significant public health concern. About 10 million newborns worldwide are screened annually for hyperphenylalaninemia by a simple blood test, and most of the estimated 1000 new cases are promptly treated.

Tyrosinemia

Hereditary tyrosinemia (hepatorenal tyrosinemia, tyrosinemia type I) is a rare (1 in 100,000) autosomal recessive inborn error of tyrosine catabolism that presents as acute liver disease in early infancy or as a more chronic disease of the liver, kidneys, and brain in children. Elevated levels of tyrosine and its metabolites are found in the blood. Both forms of the disease are caused by a deficiency of fumarylacetoacetate hydrolase (15q23-25), the last enzyme in the catabolic pathway that converts tyrosine to fumarate and acetoacetate. The acute form is characterized by a complete lack of enzyme activity, whereas children with chronic disease exhibit variable amounts of residual activity. Cell injury in hereditary tyrosinemia is attributed to the formation of abnormal toxic metabolites, namely succinylacetone and succinylacetoacetate.

Acute tyrosinemia presents during the first few months of life as hepatomegaly, edema, failure to thrive, and a cabbage-like odor. Within a few months, the infant dies of hepatic failure.

Chronic tyrosinemia is characterized by cirrhosis of the liver, renal tubular dysfunction (Fanconi syndrome), and neurological abnormalities. **Hepatocellular carcinoma supervenes in more than a third of the patients.** Most children die before the age of 10 years. Liver transplantation corrects the hepatic metabolic abnormalities and prevents the neurological crises. Combined liver–kidney transplants have also been performed in the treatment of chronic tyrosinemia. Prenatal diagnosis is accomplished by demonstrating succinylacetone in amniotic fluid or fumarylacetoacetate hydrolase deficiency in cells obtained by amniocentesis or chorionic villus sampling.

Alkaptonuria (Ochronosis)

Alkaptonuria is a rare autosomal recessive disease characterized by the excretion of homogentisic acid in the urine, generalized pigmentation, and arthritis. A deficiency in hepatic and renal homogentisic acid oxidase prevents the catabolism of homogentisic acid, an intermediate product in the metabolism of phenylalanine and tyrosine. Alkaptonuria is of greater historical significance than of clinical importance. Studies almost a century ago by Garrod and others described the mode of inheritance of alkaptonuria and were among the first to define the concept of hereditary inborn errors of metabolism.

Patients with alkaptonuria excrete urine that darkens rapidly on standing, reflecting the formation of a pigment on the nonenzymatic oxidation of homogentisic acid (Fig. 6-30). In long-standing alkaptonuria, a similar pigment is deposited in numerous tissues, particularly the sclera, cartilage in many areas (ribs, larynx, trachea), tendons, and synovial membranes. Although the pigment appears bluish black on gross examination, it is brown under the microscope, accounting for the term **ochronosis** (color of ocher) coined by Virchow. A degenerative and frequently disabling arthropathy ("ochronotic arthritis") often develops after years of alkaptonuria. It is tempting to ascribe the joint disease to the pigment deposition, but this has not been proved. Despite the involvement of many organs, alkaptonuria does not reduce the longevity of affected persons.

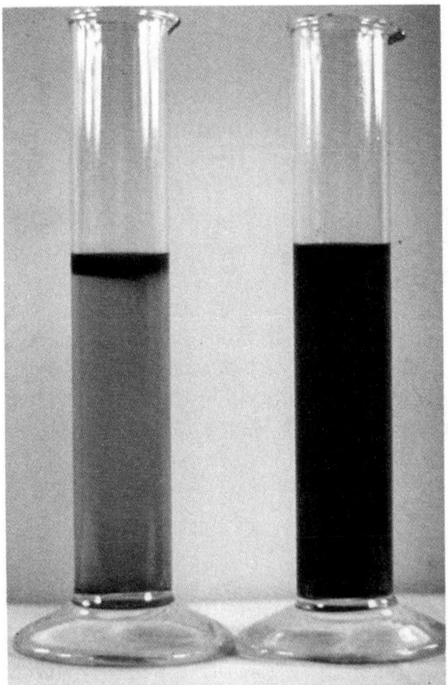

FIGURE *6-30*
Urine from a patient with alkaptonuria. The specimen on the *left*, which has been standing for 15 minutes, shows some darkening at the surface, owing to the oxidation of homogentisic acid. After 2 hours (*right*), the urine is entirely black.

Albinism

Albinism refers to a heterogeneous group of at least 10 inherited disorders characterized by hypopigmentation as a result of absent or reduced biosynthesis of melanin. This condition is found throughout the animal kingdom (from insects to humans). The most common type is oculocutaneous albinism (OCA), a family of closely related diseases that (with a single rare exception) represent autosomal recessive traits. OCA is characterized by a deficiency or complete absence of melanin pigment in the skin, hair follicles, and eyes. The frequency of OCA in whites varies from 1 per 18,000 in the United States to 1 per 10,000 in Ireland. American blacks have the same high frequency of OCA as the Irish.

The two major forms of oculocutaneous albinism are distinguished by the presence or absence of tyrosinase, the first enzyme in the biosynthetic pathway that converts tyrosine to melanin.

Tyrosinase-positive OCA is the most common type of albinism in both whites and blacks. These patients typically begin life with complete albinism, but with age a small amount of clinically detectable pigment accumulates. The defect responsible for the impairment in melanin synthesis in tyrosinase-positive OCA is attributed to mutations in the P gene (15q11.2-13), which is homologous with the mouse pink-eyed (p) gene. The P gene has been postulated to code for a tyrosine transport protein.

Tyrosinase-negative OCA is the second most common type of albinism and is characterized by a complete absence of tyrosinase (11q14-21) and melanin, although melanocytes are present and contain unpigmented melanosomes. The affected person has snow-white hair, pale pink skin, blue irides, and prominent red pupils, owing to an absence of retinal pigment. Persons with OCA typically have severe ophthalmic problems, including photophobia, strabismus, nystagmus, and decreased visual acuity. The skin of all types of albinos exhibits a striking sensitivity to sunlight and requires the application of sunscreen lotions to exposed areas. These patients are at a greatly increased risk for the development of squamous cell carcinoma of the skin in sun-exposed sites. In fact, among a group of more than 500 albinos in equatorial Africa, not one survived beyond the age of 40 years, nearly all having succumbed to their cancer. Interestingly, albinos seem to have a lower than normal frequency of malignant melanoma.

X-Linked Disorders

An X-linked disorder is one in which the gene responsible for the disease resides on the X chromosome (Fig. 6-31). As a result, the expression of the disorder is different in males and females. Females, having two X chromosomes, may be homozygous or heterozygous for a given trait. It follows that the clinical expression of the trait in a female is variable, depending on whether it is dominant or recessive. By contrast, males have only one X chromosome and are said to be *hemizygous* for the same trait. **Thus, regardless of whether the trait is dominant or recessive, it is invariably expressed in the male.**

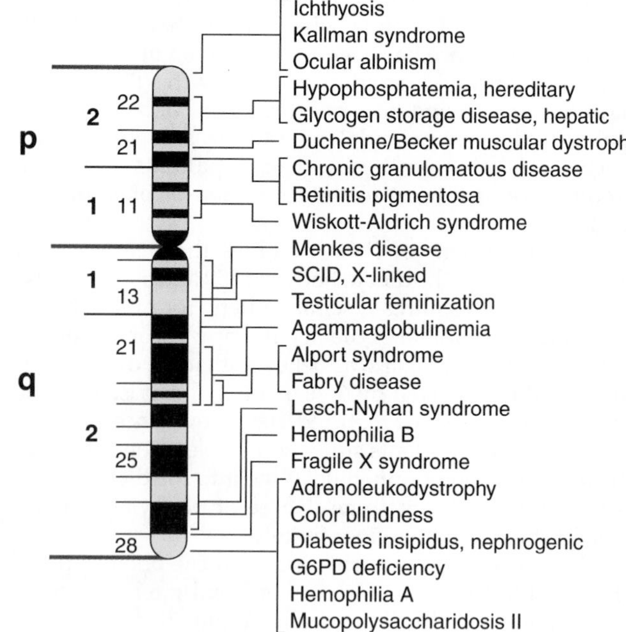

FIGURE *6-31*
The localization of representative inherited diseases on the X chromosome.

A cardinal attribute of X-linked inheritance, whether dominant or recessive, is the lack of transmission from father to son. This reflects the fact that the symptomatic father donates only his normal Y chromosome to his male offspring. By contrast, he always donates his X chromosome to his daughters, who are therefore obligate carriers of the trait. As a consequence, the disease classically skips a generation in the male, the female carrier transmitting the trait to the grandsons of the original symptomatic male.

X-Linked Dominant Traits

X-linked dominance refers to the expression of a trait only in the female, since the hemizygous state in the male precludes a distinction between dominant and recessive inheritance (Fig. 6-32). The distinctive features of X-linked dominant disorders are as follows:

- Females are affected twice as frequently as males.
- A heterozygous woman transmits the disorder to half her children, whether male or female.
- A man with a dominant X-linked disorder transmits the disease only to his daughters.
- The clinical expression of the disease tends to be less severe and more variable in heterozygous females than in hemizygous males.

Only a few X-linked dominant disorders are described, among which are familial hypophosphatemic rickets and ornithine transcarbamylase deficiency. In such diseases, the variations in the phenotypic expression of the trait in the female may be explained, at least in part, by the Lyon effect, that is, the inactivation of one X chro-

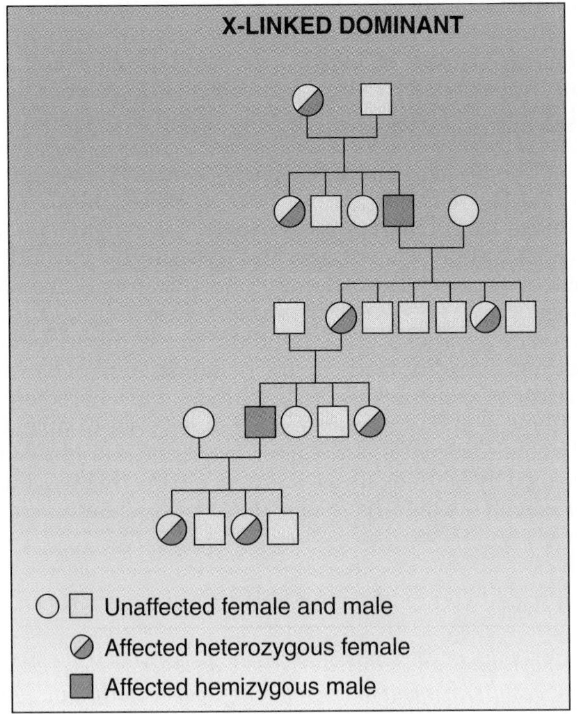

FIGURE 6-32
X-linked dominant inheritance. A heterozygous woman transmits the trait equally to males and females, whereas men transmit the trait only to their daughters. Asymptomatic males and females do not carry the trait.

mosome. This random inactivation results in mosaicism for the mutant allele, a condition that may be associated with inconstant expression of the trait.

X-Linked Recessive Traits

Most X-linked traits are recessive, that is, heterozygous females do not exhibit clinical disease (Fig. 6-33). The characteristics of this mode of inheritance are as follows:

- Sons of women who are carriers of the trait have a 50% chance of inheriting the disease, whereas the daughters are not symptomatic.
- All daughters of affected men are asymptomatic carriers, but the sons of these men are free of the trait and, thus, cannot transmit the disease to their children.
- Symptomatic homozygous females result only from the rare mating of an affected man and an asymptomatic, heterozygous woman.
- The trait tends to occur in maternal uncles and in male cousins descended from the mother's sisters.

Table 6-10 presents a list of representative X-linked recessive disorders.

X-Linked Muscular Dystrophies (Duchenne and Becker Muscular Dystrophies)

The muscular dystrophies comprise a number of devastating muscle diseases, most of which are X-linked, although a few are autosomal recessive. The X-linked muscular dystrophies are among the most frequent human genetic diseases, occurring in 1 per 3500 boys, an incidence approaching that of CF.

Duchenne muscular dystrophy (DMD), the most common variant, is a fatal progressive degeneration of muscle that appears before the age of 4 years (Fig. 6-34).

Becker muscular dystrophy (BMD) is allelic with DMD but is a less frequent and milder disorder.

□ Pathogenesis: **Both DMD and BMD are caused by a deficiency of dystrophin, a member of the family of membrane cytoskeletal proteins, which includes α-actinin and spectrin.** The protein is located on the cytoplasmic face of the plasma membrane of muscle cells and is linked to it by integral membrane glycoproteins (dystrophin-associated glycoprotein complex), which in turn are bound to extracellular laminin (Fig. 6-35). Thus, dystrophin molecules form a network connecting actin fibers to the extracellular matrix, a function that

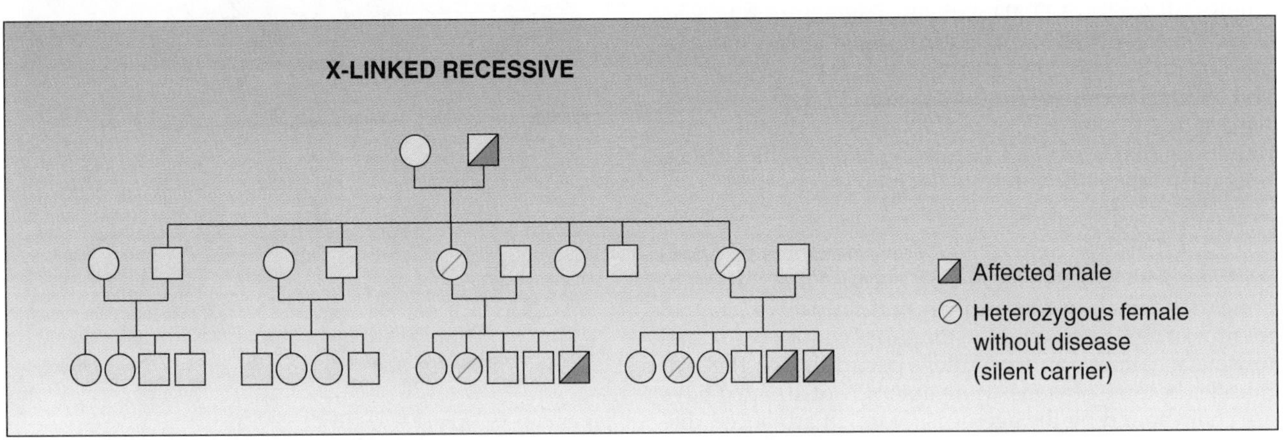

FIGURE 6-33
X-linked recessive inheritance. Only males are affected, whereas daughters of affected men are all asymptomatic carriers. Asymptomatic men do not transmit the trait. Clinical expression of the disease skips a generation.

TABLE *6-10* **Representative X-Linked Recessive Diseases**

Disease	Frequency in Males
Fragile X syndrome	1/2000
Hemophilia A (factor VIII deficiency)	1/10,000
Hemophilia B (factor IX deficiency)	1/70,000
Duchenne-Becker muscular dystrophy	1/3500
Glucose-6-phosphate dehydrogenase deficiency	Up to 30%
Lesch-Nyhan syndrome (HPRT deficiency)	1/10,000
Chronic granulomatous disease	Not rare
X-linked agammaglobulinemia	Not rare
X-linked severe combined immunodeficiency	Rare
Fabry disease	1/40,000
Hunter syndrome	1/70,000
Adrenoleukodystrophy	1/100,000
Menke disease	1/100,000

probably maintains the mechanical properties of the muscle cell and the flexibility that is needed during the contraction and relaxation of muscle fibers. It has been proposed that the absence of dystrophin leads to a defective membrane that is damaged during contraction, an effect that predisposes to necrosis of the myocyte.

The DMD gene, which encodes dystrophin, is one of the largest known human genes (about 2×10^6 base pairs) and is located on the short arm of the X chromosome (Xp21). Deletions in the DMD gene are responsible for the defects in more that 60% of the cases of muscular dystrophy, with most of the remaining cases representing point mutations. The more severely affected Duchenne patients have no detectable dystrophin, whereas patients with the Becker variant have a smaller than normal dystrophin molecule. One third of patients with DMD represent new mutations, one third mutations in the mother, and only one third mutations that have been in the family for more than one generation.

In most cases, the differences between DMD and BMD reflect the nature of the mutation in the DMD gene. Almost all (96%) of DMD patients have frameshift deletions that result either in the complete absence of detectable dystrophin or in a protein that is reduced in size and exhibits abnormalities or deletions of the C-terminal region. By contrast, 85% of BMD patients harbor in-frame mutations that lead to a truncated version of the protein, but one in which the C-terminal region is conserved.

□ Clinical Features: The symptoms of DMD progress with age. During the first year of life, the infant appears normal, but more than half fail to walk by 18 months of age. Subsequently, the gait is clumsy. Proximal muscle weakness and pseudohypertrophy of the calf muscles become obvious. More than 90% of afflicted boys are chair-bound by the age of 11 years. In advanced disease, cardiac symptoms are almost universal and cardiomyopathy is a common cause of death. There is an overall decrease in intelligence, and one fifth of patients are significantly retarded. The demonstrated presence of dystrophin in the cerebral cortex presumably accounts for this association of DMD with mental deficiency. The mean age at death in boys with DMD is 17 years, a figure that is only 2 years greater than that reported a century ago.

The Becker variant of muscular dystrophy is similar to the Duchenne form, but later in onset and milder in clinical symptomatology. Virtually all patients are still walking at 12 years of age, and 95% survive beyond the age of 21. Mental retardation is not a feature of the BMD phenotype.

The diagnosis of DMD/BMD in the proper clinical setting is readily made by the demonstration of elevated creatine kinase levels in the blood and characteristic pathological findings in a muscle biopsy (see Chapter 27). Prenatal diagnosis and carrier detection can be accomplished by DNA analysis. It is noteworthy that two thirds of carrier women have elevated serum creatine kinase levels.

Hemophilia A (Factor VIII Deficiency)

Hemophilia is an X-linked recessive disorder of blood clotting that results in spontaneous bleeding, particularly into joints, muscles, and internal organs. It is now clear that classic hemophilia is actually two distinct diseases, one resulting from mutations in the gene encoding factor VIII (hemophilia A) and the other caused by defects in the

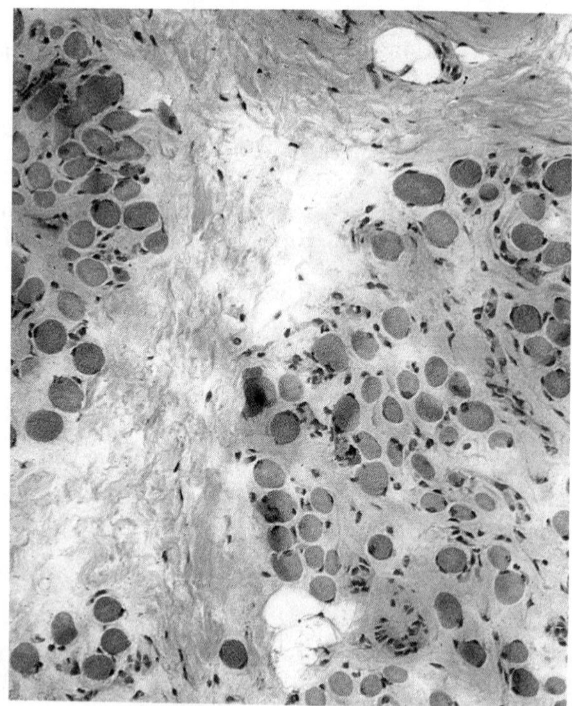

FIGURE *6-34*
Dystrophic skeletal muscle in Duchenne muscular dystrophy. The muscle cells are atrophic and embedded in intrafascicular fibrosis. A few inflammatory cells are present.

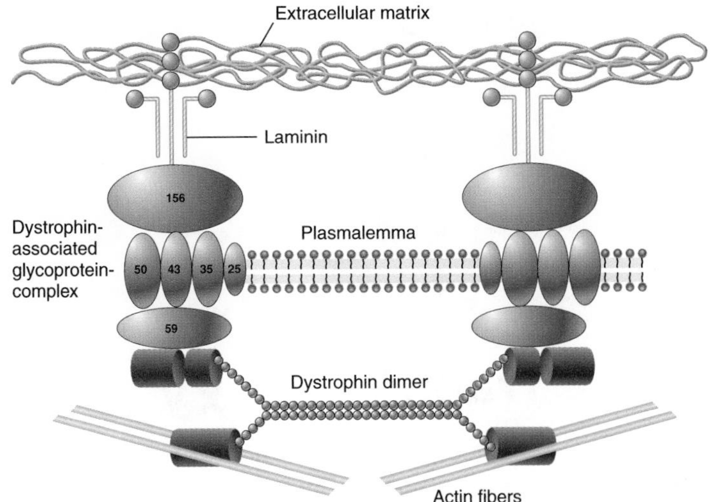

FIGURE 6-35
The correlation of alterations in dystrophin domains with the severity of muscular dystrophy. Small deletions in the N-terminal domain and in both the first 13 and last 8 repeats result in the mild Becker variant, whereas deletions of the cysteine-rich and adjacent C-terminal domains lead to the severe Duchenne type of muscular dystrophy. The numbers refer to the domains in the dystrophin.

gene for factor IX (hemophilia B). Since hemophilia A is the most frequently encountered, sex-linked inherited bleeding disorder (1 per 5000 to 10,000 males), our discussion will be limited to that variant.

Hemophilia is one of the oldest human genetic diseases recorded, having been described in the Talmud almost 2000 years ago. Male infants of Jewish families with a history of fatal bleeding after circumcision were accordingly excused from this ritual. The transmission of a bleeding tendency to boys from their unaffected mothers has been known for 200 years. Subsequently, the disorder became a subject of public interest following the dissemination of hemophilia throughout the royal families of Europe by the daughters of Queen Victoria. Finally, the gene for factor VIII was cloned in 1984, allowing investigation of the molecular basis of hemophilia A.

☐ Pathogenesis: The mutations in the very large factor VIII gene at the tip of the long arm of the X chromosome (Xq28) include deletions, point mutations, and insertions. Each family with hemophilia in its history actually harbors a different mutation (private mutant allele). In half of the cases of hemophilia A, the disease can be traced through many generations, but in the other half, *de novo* mutations occurring within two generations are the cause of this bleeding diathesis. In most of these *de novo* mutations, an origin in the mother, maternal grandfather, or maternal grandmother has been identified.

☐ Pathology and Clinical Features: Patients with hemophilia A exhibit a mild, moderate, or severe bleeding tendency. In most of these patients, the severity of the illness parallels the amount of factor VIII activity in the blood. Half of the patients have virtually no factor VIII activity and often suffer spontaneous bleeding. A third of the patients, who have up to 10 units of factor VIII per deciliter, have spontaneous bleeding only occasionally, but hemorrhages are common after minor trauma. One fifth of hemophiliacs have greater than 10 U/dL and bleed only after significant trauma or surgery.

The most frequent complication of hemophilia A is a deforming arthritis caused by repeated bleeding into many joints. Although uncommon, bleeding into the brain was formerly the most frequent cause of death in hemophiliacs. Hematuria, intestinal obstruction, and respiratory obstruction may all occur with bleeding into the respective organs.

Treatment with factor VIII transfusions to maintain the levels of this clotting factor generally control the bleeding diathesis. Unfortunately, many of these patients have developed the acquired immunodeficiency syndrome (AIDS) and viral hepatitis as a result of contamination of pooled factor VIII preparations. These complications have been virtually eliminated by screening blood donors and heat treatment to inactivate the human immunodeficiency virus (HIV) in the purified factor VIII product. The availability of human recombinant factor VIII should now avoid all infectious complications. Screening of women to detect carriers and prenatal diagnosis of affected fetuses by the use of DNA markers are highly accurate.

Fragile X Syndrome

Fragile X syndrome is the most common form of inherited mental retardation and is caused by expansion of a CGG repeat at the Xq27 fragile site. It is second only to Down syndrome as an identifiable cause of retardation. The disease afflicts 1 in 1250 males and 1 in 2500 females.

☐ Pathogenesis: The well-known fact that more males than females are institutionalized for mental retardation was traditionally ascribed to societal factors. However, it was recognized in the early 1970s that X-linked inheritance of mental retardation accounted for most of this excess of males. Whereas fully 20% of all cases of heritable mental retardation are X-linked disorders, one fifth of these are associated with a single genetic defect, namely an inducible fragile site on the X chromosome (Xq27).

A fragile site represents a specific locus, or band, on a chromosome that breaks easily, after which it is usually detected in cytogenetic preparations as a nonstaining gap or constriction (Fig. 6-36). Less commonly, a complete break occurs, with a resulting acentric fragment. Importantly, under the routine conditions of preparing cells for karyotypic analysis, most fragile sites are not detected. However, when the same cells in culture are subjected to treatment that impairs DNA synthesis (e.g., methotrexate, floxuridine), fragile sites are revealed. At least 11, and possibly as many as 50, fragile sites occur in the genomes of most persons, both on autosomes and on the X chromosome. **However, only the locus at Xq27 is associated with mental retardation or other clinical disorders**. As discussed, the fragile site at the Xq27 locus represents a distinct kind of mutation characterized by amplification of a CGG repeat.

Within fragile X families, the probability of being affected with the disorder is related to the position in the pedigree, that is, latter generations are more likely to be affected than earlier ones (Sherman paradox, or genetic anticipation). This phenomenon relates to the progressive nature of the triplet repeat expansion. Early expansions enlarge the abnormal segment up to 200 repeats, the threshold for the clinical phenotype of mental retardation, which are referred to as premutations. Expansions greater than 200 repeats are associated with mental retardation and represent full mutations. Expansion of a premutation to a full mutation during gametogenesis takes place only in females. Thus, the daughters of men with premutations (carriers) are never clinically symptomatic, whereas the sisters of the transmitting males occasionally produce affected daughters. However, the daughters of carrier males always harbor the premutation. The frequency of conversion of a premutation to a full mutation in such women (that is, the probability of their sons suffering fragile X syndrome) varies with the length of the expanded tract. Premutations with more than 90 repeats are almost always converted to full mutations. In view of the recessive nature of fragile X syndrome, most of the daughters of carrier males transmit mental retardation to 50% of their sons. These considerations explain the greater risk of the disorder in succeeding generations of fragile X families.

☐ Clinical Features: The male newborn afflicted with the fragile X syndrome appears normal, but during childhood, characteristic features appear, including an increased head circumference, facial coarsening, joint hyperextensibility, enlarged testes, and abnormalities of the cardiac valves. Mental retardation is profound, with IQ scores varying from 20 to 60. **Interestingly, a significant proportion of autistic male children carry a fragile X chromosome**. Among female carriers who are mentally handicapped, the severity of the impairment varies from a learning disability with normal IQ to serious retardation.

Only 80% of males who exhibit the Xq27 fragile site are mentally retarded, whereas the remaining 20% are clinically normal but can transmit the trait. Among females who are known to bear a fragile X chromosome (obligate carriers), two thirds are intellectually normal, and the fragile site on the X chromosome cannot be demonstrated. By contrast, of the one third of female carriers who are mentally retarded, virtually all display a fragile Xq27 locus. Although the evidence is contradictory, it has been suggested that this variability in phenotypic expression in females relates to the pattern of X-inactivation.

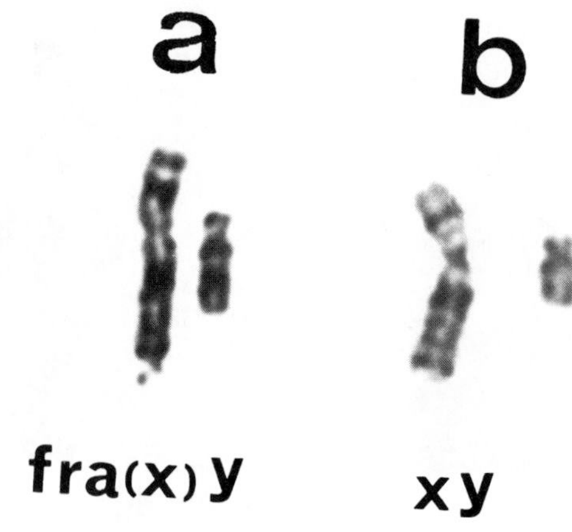

FIGURE 6-36
Fragile X chromosome.

MITOCHONDRIAL DISEASES

Mitochondrial proteins are encoded by both the nuclear and mitochondrial genomes. In particular, the majority of respiratory chain proteins are encoded by nuclear genes, whereas several are the products of the mitochondrial genome. A few rare, autosomal recessive (mendelian) disorders that represent defects in nuclear encoded mitochondrial proteins have been described. However, most inherited defects in mitochondrial function result from mutations in the mitochondrial genome itself. An appreciation of these conditions requires an understanding of the unique genetics of the mitochondria. These features include the following:

- **Maternal inheritance:** All vertebrate mitochondria are inherited from the mother via the ovum, which possesses up to 300,000 copies of mitochondrial DNA (mtDNA).
- **Variability of mtDNA copies:** The number of mitochondria and the number of copies of mtDNA per mitochondrion vary in different tissues. Each mitochondrion contains 2 to 10 mtDNA copies, and the need of various cell types for ATP correlates with the DNA content per mitochondrion.
- **Threshold effect:** Since any given cell contains numerous mitochondria and, therefore, hundreds or thousands of mtDNA copies, mutations in mtDNA lead to mixed populations of mutant and normal mitochondrial genomes. The phenotype associated with

mtDNA mutations reflects the severity of the mutation, the proportion of mutant genomes, and the demand of the tissue for ATP. In this context, different tissues require different minimum rates (or thresholds) of ATP production to sustain their characteristic metabolic activity, the brain, heart, and skeletal muscle having particularly great energy demands.

- **High mutation rate:** The rate of mutation of mtDNA is considerably higher than that of nuclear DNA, owing (at least in part) to a lesser DNA repair capacity.

Diseases caused by mutations in the mitochondrial genome principally affect the nervous system, heart, and skeletal muscle. The functional deficits in all of these disorders can be traced to inadequate oxidative phosphorylation (OXPHOS). **OXPHOS diseases** have been divided into the following classes: I, nuclear mutations; II, mtDNA point mutations; III, mtDNA deletions; and IV, as yet undefined defects. All inherited mitochondrial diseases are rare and have variable clinical presentations based on the considerations discussed above. The first human disease caused by an mtDNA point mutation was **Leber hereditary optic neuropathy**, a condition characterized by progressive loss of vision. Since that time, various mitochondrial myopathies and encephalomyopathies have been described; they are discussed in Chapter 27. Hypertrophic cardiomyopathy (see Chapter 11) is also a common manifestation of OXPHOS diseases.

GENETIC IMPRINTING

Genetic imprinting refers to the observation that the phenotype associated with some genes differs depending on whether the allele is inherited from the mother or the father. This phenomenon implies that in the case of imprinted genes, either the maternal or paternal allele is consistently inactivated. In the extreme case, it has been demonstrated experimentally that mammalian embryos in which both sets of chromosomes are derived exclusively from one parent, either the mother or the father, never survive to term. A less severe manifestation of genetic imprinting is *uniparental disomy*, in which both members of a single chromosome pair have been inherited from the same parent. In this instance, the offspring may manifest an autosomal recessive disease when only one parent carries the trait, as has been observed in a few cases of CF and hemophilia A. Loss of a chromosome from a trisomy or duplication of a chromosome in the case of a monosomy can lead to uniparental disomy. Interestingly, as many as 1% of viable pregnancies carry uniparental disomy for at least one chromosome.

The existence of genetic imprinting is well illustrated by certain hereditary diseases whose phenotype is determined by the parental source of the mutant allele. Deletion of the 15q11-13 chromosomal locus results in **Prader-Willi syndrome** when the affected chromosome is inherited paternally and in **Angelman syndrome** when it is of maternal origin. The phenotypes of these disorders are remarkably different. Prader-Willi syndrome features hypotonia, obesity, hypogonadism, mental retardation, and a specific facies. By contrast, Angelman syndrome patients are hyperactive, display inappropriate laughter, have a facies different from that of Prader-Willi syndrome, and suffer from seizures. Clearly, there exists a gene or group of genes in the 15q11-13 region that is expressed only on the chromosome derived from the father, the deletion of which results in Prader-Willi syndrome. Conversely, a gene in the same region is active only on the maternal autosome, and its loss leads to Angelman syndrome.

Genetic imprinting is implicated in a number of other situations relevant to human disease. For example, in some childhood cancers, including Wilms tumor, osteosarcoma, bilateral retinoblastoma, and embryonal rhabdomyosarcoma, the maternal allele of a putative tumor suppressor gene is lost, and the remaining allele is on a chromosome of paternal origin. In the case of familial glomus tumor, an adult neoplasm, both males and females may carry the trait, but it is transmitted only through the male. Thus, the responsible gene is active only when it is located on the paternal autosome. Finally, as previously noted, the premutation of fragile X syndrome is expanded to the full mutation only during female gametogenesis, implying that the trinucleotide repeat is treated differently on passage through the female versus the male.

Genetic imprinting is thought to occur during meiosis, but the mechanism is poorly understood. Differential methylation of genes may play a role, since all imprinted genes that have been identified have domains in which the maternal and paternal DNA copies are methylated differently at cytosine–guanine base pairs. It is likely that the influence of genetic imprinting on human biology will assume greater importance as more information becomes available.

MULTIFACTORIAL INHERITANCE

Multifactorial inheritance is a term that describes a process by which a disease is the consequence of the additive effects of a number of abnormal genes and environmental factors. Most normal human traits are inherited neither as dominant nor as recessive mendelian attributes but rather in a more complex manner. For example, multifactorial inheritance determines intelligence, height, skin color, body habitus, and even emotional disposition. Similarly, most of the common chronic disorders of adults represent multifactorial genetic diseases and are well known to "run in families." Such maladies include diabetes, atherosclerosis, many forms of cancer and arthritis, and hypertension. The inheritance of a number of birth defects is also multifactorial (e.g., cleft lip and palate, pyloric stenosis, and congenital heart disease) (Table 6-11).

The concept of multifactorial inheritance is based on the notion that multiple genes interact with various environmental factors to produce disease in an individual patient. Such inheritance leads to familial aggregation that does not obey simple mendelian rules. As a consequence, the inheritance of polygenic diseases is studied by the methods of population genetics, rather than by the analysis of individual family pedigrees.

TABLE 6-11 Representative Diseases Associated with Multifactorial Inheritance

Adults	Children
Hypertension	Pyloric stenosis
Atherosclerosis	Cleft lip and palate
Diabetes, type II	Congenital heart disease
Allergic diathesis	Meningomyelocele
Psoriasis	Anencephaly
Schizophrenia	Hypospadias
Ankylosing spondylitis	Congenital hip dislocation
Gout	Hirschprung disease

The number of involved genes is not known for any polygenic disease. Thus, it is not possible to ascertain accurately the risk of a particular disorder in an individual case. The probability of disease can only be predicted from the number of relatives affected and the severity of their disease, supplemented by statistical projections based on population analyses. Whereas monogenic inheritance implies a specific risk of disease (e.g., 25% or 50%), the probability of symptoms in first-degree relatives of a person affected with a polygenic disease is usually on the order of 5% to 10%.

The biological basis of polygenic inheritance rests on the evidence that more than one fourth of all genetic loci in normal humans contain polymorphic alleles. Such genetic heterogeneity provides a background for the wide variability in the susceptibility to many diseases, which is compounded by a multiplicity of interactions with environmental factors.

- **The expression of symptoms is proportional to the number of mutant genes.** Close relatives of an affected person have more mutant genes than the population at large and have a greater chance of expressing clinical disease. The probability of expressing the same number of mutant genes is highest in identical twins.
- **Environmental factors influence the expression of the trait.** Thus, concordance of disease occurs in only one third of monozygotic twins.
- **The risk in all first-degree relatives (parents, siblings, children) is the same (5% to 10%).** The probability of disease is considerably lower in second-degree relatives.
- **The probability of expression in later offspring is influenced by expression of the trait in earlier siblings.** If one or more children are born with a multifactorial defect, the chance for recurrence in subsequent offspring is doubled. This contrasts with mendelian traits, in which the probability is independent of the number of affected siblings.
- **The more severe the defect, the greater is the risk of transmitting it to offspring.** Patients with more severe polygenic defects presumably have more mutant genes, and their children thus have a greater chance of inheriting the abnormal genes than the offspring of less severely affected persons.
- **Some abnormalities characterized by multifactorial inheritance show a sex predilection.** For example, pyloric stenosis is more common in male infants, whereas congenital dislocation of the hip is more common in females. Such a differential susceptibility is believed to represent a difference in the threshold for the expression of mutant genes in the two sexes. For example, if the number of mutant genes required to produce pyloric stenosis in males is X, it may require 4X in the female. In such a circumstance, a woman who had pyloric stenosis as an infant has more mutant genes than a similarly afflicted man to transmit to her children. Indeed, the son of such a woman actually has a 25% chance of being born with pyloric stenosis, compared with a 4% risk for the son of an affected man. **As a general rule, if there is an altered sex ratio in the incidence of a polygenic defect, the less affected sex has a much greater probability of transmitting the defect.**

Cleft Lip and Cleft Palate

Cleft lip and cleft palate are excellent paradigms to illustrate the principles of multifactorial inheritance. At the 35th day of gestation, the frontal prominence fuses with the maxillary process to form the upper lip. This process is under the control of many genes, and disturbances in gene expression (hereditary or environmental) at this time lead to interference with proper fusion and result in cleft lip, with or without cleft palate (Fig. 6-37). This anomaly may also be part of a systemic malformation syndrome caused by teratogens (rubella, anticonvulsants) and is often encountered in children with chromosomal abnormalities.

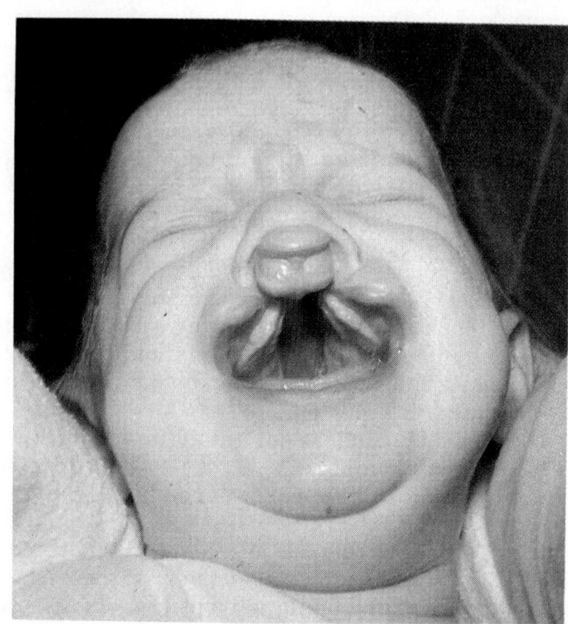

FIGURE 6-37
Cleft lip and palate in an infant.

The incidence of cleft lip, with or without cleft palate, is 1 in 1000, and the incidence of cleft palate alone is 1 in 2500. If one child is born with a cleft lip, the chances are 4% that the second child will also exhibit the same defect. If the first two children are affected, the risk of cleft lip increases to 9% for the third child. The more severe the anatomical defect, the greater the probability of transmitting cleft lip will be. Whereas 75% of cases of cleft lip occur in boys, the sons of women with cleft lip have a four times higher risk of acquiring the defect than the sons of affected fathers.

PRENATAL DIAGNOSIS OF GENETIC DISORDERS

Amniocentesis and chorionic villus biopsy are the most important methods for diagnosis of a developmental or genetic disorder. Both procedures are safe, reliable, and easily performed. The indications for chorionic villus biopsy or amniocentesis in pregnant women are as follows:

- **Age 35 years old and over:** The risk of having a child with Down syndrome is about 1 in 300 for the 40-year-old woman, compared with 1 in 1200 at age 25. This risk rises even higher with advanced maternal age.
- **Previous chromosomal abnormality:** The overall risk of recurrence of Down syndrome in a succeeding child of a woman who has already borne an infant with trisomy 21 is 1%.
- **Translocation carrier:** Estimates of risks to the offspring of translocation carriers vary from 3% to 15%. Carriers of balanced translocations are at increased risk for producing children with unbalanced karyotypes and resulting phenotypic abnormalities.
- **History of familial inborn error of metabolism:** The recessive inborn errors of metabolism have a risk of 25% for each child. Prenatal diagnosis should be considered in all of these disorders for which a definitive biochemical diagnosis can be made.
- **Identified heterozygotes:** Carrier detection programs, such as the Tay-Sachs Disease Prevention Program, detect couples in which both spouses are carriers of the same recessive gene. Each pregnancy in such couples has a 25% risk of an affected child, and prenatal diagnosis should be routinely made.
- **Family history of X-linked disorders:** Fetal sex determination, using amniotic cells, should be offered to women known to be carriers of X-linked disorders. The diagnosis of some of these conditions can be established biochemically by amniotic fluid analysis.

New molecular techniques for carrier detection and early prenatal diagnosis are of ever-increasing utility. Gene-specific DNA probes have been developed for many genetic diseases, including hemophilia A and B, the hemoglobinopathies, phenylketonuria, and α_1-antitrypsin deficiency. The large majority of heterozygous carriers for Duchenne and Becker muscular dystrophies, Huntington chorea, and cystic fibrosis can be identified.

DISEASES OF INFANCY AND CHILDHOOD

The period from birth to puberty has been traditionally subdivided into several stages.

- Neonatal age (the first 4 weeks)
- Infancy (the first year)
- Early childhood (1 to 4 years)
- Late childhood (5 to 14 years)

Each of these periods has its own distinct anatomical, physiological, and immunological characteristics, which determine the nature and form of various pathological processes. Morbidity and mortality rates in the neonatal period differ considerably from those in infancy and childhood. Infants and children are not simply "small adults," and they may be afflicted by diseases unique to their particular age group.

PREMATURITY AND INTRAUTERINE GROWTH RETARDATION

The duration of human pregnancy is normally 40 ± 2 weeks, and most newborns weigh 3300 ± 600 g. Prematurity has been defined by the World Health Organization as a gestational age of less than 37 weeks (from the first day of the last menstrual period). The traditional definition of prematurity was a birthweight of less than 2500 g regardless of gestational age. However, it is now appreciated that full-term infants may weigh less than 2500 g because of intrauterine growth retardation rather than premature birth. **Thus, low-birth-weight infants (less than 2500 g) are classed as (1) appropriate for gestational age (AGA) or (2) small for gestational age (SGA).**

In the United States, the frequency of low-birth-weight infants is less than 6% among whites, and two thirds of these infants are premature (AGA). By contrast, when the frequency of low-birth-weight infants exceeds 10%, as it does for blacks (>12%), the majority suffer from intrauterine growth retardation and are considered SGA.

About 1% of all infants born in the United States weigh less than 1500 g and are referred to as **very low-birth-weight infants**. Such infants account for half of all neonatal deaths, and their survival is determined by their birth weight. Historically, newborns weighing more than 1250 g had a 90% survival rate, whereas 2% of those weighing between 500 g and 600 g could be expected to live. Today, in advanced societies in which premature newborns are cared for in neonatal intensive care units, 90% of infants over 750 g survive. Between 500 g and 750 g, 45% survive, of whom more than half develop normally.

☐ Etiology: The factors that predispose to the premature birth of an infant (AGA) are (1) maternal illness, (2) uterine incompetence, (3) fetal disorders, and (4) placental abnormalities. When the life of a fetus is threatened by such conditions, it may be necessary to induce premature delivery to salvage the infant. In a substantial proportion of AGA infants, the cause of premature birth is unknown. Intrauterine growth retardation and the resulting birth of SGA infants are associated with disorders that (1) impair maternal health and nutrition, (2) interfere with placental circulation or function, or (3) disturb the growth or development of the fetus.

☐ Clinical Features: It deserves emphasis that there is a substantial overlap between the complications of prematurity itself (AGA) and intrauterine growth retardation (SGA). However, certain general principles apply. Prematurity is often associated with severe respiratory distress, metabolic disturbances (e.g., hyperbilirubinemia, hypoglycemia, hypocalcemia), circulatory problems (anemia, hypothermia, hypotension), and bacterial sepsis. By contrast, SGA infants comprise a much more heterogeneous group, including many infants with congenital anomalies and infections acquired *in utero*. Even when these causes of intrauterine growth retardation are excluded, the neonatal complications of SGA infants reflect gestational age more than birth weight. In addition to many of the problems associated with prematurity, SGA infants often suffer from perinatal asphyxia, meconium aspiration, necrotizing enterocolitis, pulmonary hemorrhage, and disorders related to birth defects or inherited metabolic diseases.

Organ Immaturity

The maturity of the newborn can be defined in both anatomical and physiological terms. The maturing organs differ morphologically from those in term infants, although complete morphological and physiological maturity of many organs is not achieved for periods of time varying from days (lungs) to years (brain).

THE LUNGS: Immaturity of the lungs poses one of the most common and immediate threats to the viability of the low-birth-weight infant. The lining cells of the fetal alveoli do not differentiate into type I and type II pneumocytes until late pregnancy. The amniotic fluid, which fills the fetal alveoli, drains from the lungs at birth, after which air expands the respiratory spaces. Often the sluggish respiratory movements of the immature infant do not suffice to evacuate the amniotic fluid from the lungs. As a result, such newborns die of respiratory failure with incompletely expanded lungs. On gross examination, the lungs are not crepitant, and microscopically the alveoli are variably expanded. The air passages contain desquamated squamous cells (squames) and lanugo hair from the fetal skin and protein-rich amniotic fluid (Fig. 6-38). Although this appearance is often termed **amniotic fluid aspiration**, it actually represents retained amniotic fluid.

Alveoli are maintained in the expanded state not only by connective tissue but also by the reduction in surface tension achieved by the presence of **pulmonary surfactant**. This material, which is produced by type II pneumocytes, is a complex mixture of several phospholipids, 75% phosphatidylcholine (lecithin) and 10% phosphatidylglycerol. The composition of lung surfactant changes as the fetus matures: (1) The concentration of lecithin increases rapidly at the beginning of the third trimester and thereafter rises rapidly to reach a peak near term (Fig. 6-39). (2) Whereas most of the lecithin in the mature lung is dipalmitate, in the immature lung it is the less surface-active α-palmitate, β-myristate species. (3) Phosphatidylglycerol is not present in the lungs before the 36th week of pregnancy. (4) Before the 35th week, the immature surfactant contains a higher proportion of sphingomyelin than adult surfactant.

Pulmonary surfactant is released into the amniotic fluid, which can be sampled by amniocentesis to assess the maturity of the fetal lung. A lecithin-to-sphingomyelin ratio above 2:1 implies that the fetus will survive without developing the respiratory distress syndrome. After the 35th week, the appearance of phosphatidylglycerol in the amniotic fluid is the best proof of the maturity of the fetal lungs.

THE LIVER: The liver of premature infants is morphologically similar to that of the adult organ, with the exception of conspicuous extramedullary hemopoiesis. However, the hepatocytes tend to be functionally immature. The fetal liver is deficient in glucuronyl transferase and the resulting inability of the organ to conjugate bilirubin often leads to neonatal jaundice. This enzyme deficiency is aggravated by the rapid destruction of fetal

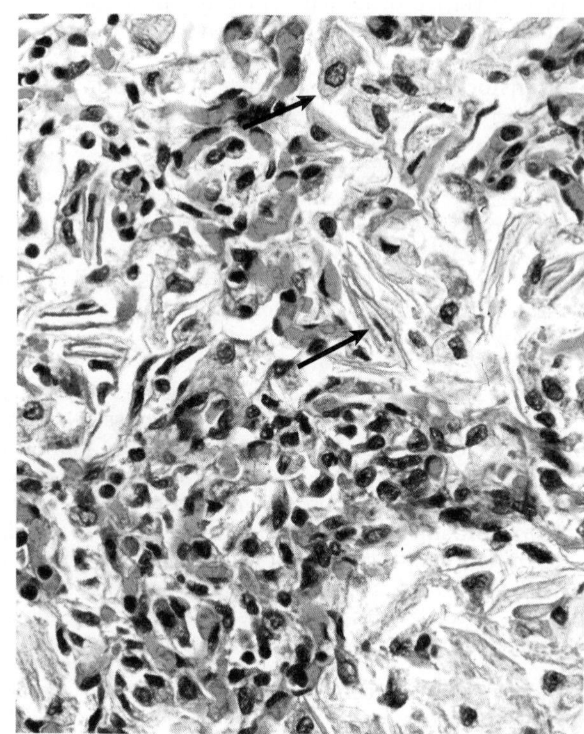

FIGURE 6-38
Retention of amniotic fluid in the lung of a premature newborn. The incompletely expanded lung contains squames (*arrows*), consisting of squamous epithelial cells shed into the amniotic fluid from the fetal skin.

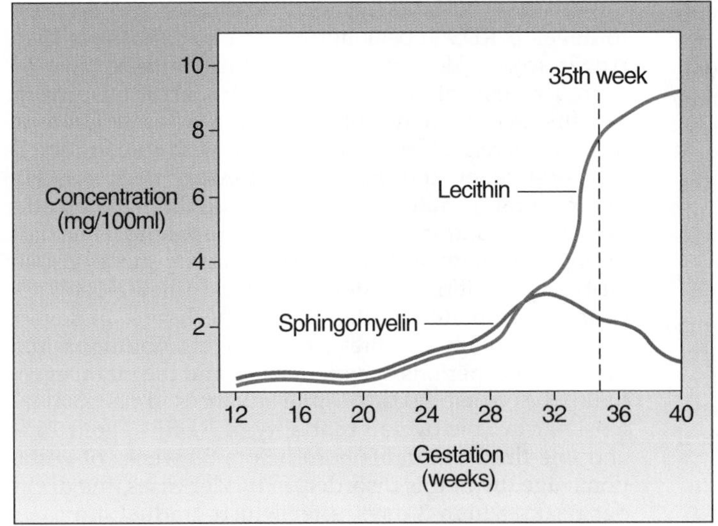

FIGURE 6-39
Changes in amniotic fluid composition during pregnancy.

erythrocytes, a process that results in an increased supply of bilirubin.

THE BRAIN: Although the brain of the immature newborn differs from that of the adult, both morphologically and functionally, this difference is rarely fatal. On the other hand, the incomplete development of the central nervous system is often reflected in poor vasomotor control, hypothermia, feeding difficulties, and recurrent apnea.

The Apgar Score

A clinical assessment of neonatal maturity is usually performed at 1 minute and 5 minutes after delivery, and certain parameters are scored according to the criteria recommended by Virginia Apgar (Table 6-12). In general, the higher the Apgar score, the better is the clinical condition of the infant. The score taken at 1 minute is an index of asphyxia and of the need for assisted ventilation. The 5-minute score is a more accurate indication of impending death or the likelihood of persistent neurological damage. For example, in newborns weighing less than 2000 g who have a 5-minute Apgar score of 9 or 10, the mortality during the first month is less than 5%, whereas it is almost 80% when the Apgar score is reduced to 3 or less.

Respiratory Distress Syndrome of the Newborn (Hyaline Membrane Disease)

The respiratory distress syndrome (RDS) of the newborn is an acquired, life-threatening disorder of the lungs caused by a deficiency of surfactant. RDS is principally associated with prematurity. It is the leading cause of morbidity and mortality among premature infants and accounts for half of all neonatal deaths in the United States. The incidence of RDS varies inversely with gestational age and birth weight. Thus, more than half of newborns younger than 28 weeks gestational age are afflicted with RDS, whereas only one fifth of infants between 32 and 36 weeks are affected. In addition to prematurity, other risk factors for RDS include (1) neonatal asphyxia, (2) maternal diabetes, (3) delivery by cesarean section, (4) precipitous delivery, and (5) twin pregnancies.

☐ Pathogenesis: **The pathogenesis of RDS of the newborn is intimately linked to a deficiency of surfactant** (Fig. 6-40). In the normal newborn, the onset of breathing is associated with a massive release of stored surfactant. This material lowers the surface tension of the alveoli at low lung volumes and thereby prevents collapse (atelectasis) of the alveoli during expiration. As

TABLE *6-12* **Apgar Score**

Sign	0	1	2
Heart rate	Not detectable	Below 100/min	Over 100/min
Respiratory effort	None	Slow, irregular	Good, crying
Muscle tone	Poor	Some flexion of extremities	Active motion
Response to catheter in nostril	No response	Grimace	Cough or sneeze
Color	Blue, pale	Body pink, extremities blue	Completely pink

Sixty seconds after the completion of birth, these five objective signs are evaluated, and each is given a score of 0, 1, or 2. A maximum score of 10 is assigned to infants in the best possible condition.

noted previously, the immature lung is deficient in both the amount and composition of surfactant. Moreover, any damage to type II pneumocytes (e.g., from asphyxia) will interfere with the synthesis and secretion of surfactant. Atelectasis secondary to surfactant deficiency results in perfused but not ventilated alveoli, a situation that leads to hypoxia and acidosis, with further compromise in the ability of type II pneumocytes to produce surfactant. Moreover, hypoxia produces pulmonary arterial vasoconstriction, thereby increasing right-to-left shunting through the ductus arteriosus and foramen ovale and within the lung itself. The resulting pulmonary ischemia further aggravates alveolar epithelial damage and injures the endothelium of the pulmonary capillaries. The leak of protein-rich fluid into the alveoli from the injured vascular bed contributes to the typical clinical and pathological features of RDS.

☐ Pathology: On gross examination, the lungs are dark red and airless. Microscopically, the alveoli are collapsed, and the alveolar ducts and respiratory bronchioles are dilated. Within these expanded spaces, cellular debris, proteinaceous edema fluid, and erythrocytes are evident. The alveolar ducts are lined by conspicuous, eosinophilic, fibrin-rich, amorphous structures, termed **hyaline membranes**, which accounts for the original designation of RDS as **hyaline membrane disease** (Fig. 6-41). The walls of the collapsed alveoli are thick, the capillaries are congested, and the lymphatics are filled with proteinaceous material.

☐ Clinical Features: Most newborns destined to develop RDS appear normal at birth and have high Apgar scores. However, some of these infants have required resuscitation because of intrapartum asphyxia. The first symptom, usually appearing within an hour of birth, is increased respiratory effort, with forceful intercostal retraction and the use of accessory neck muscles. The respiratory rate increases to more than 100 breaths per minute, and cyanosis becomes apparent. The chest radiograph shows a characteristic "ground-glass" granularity, and in terminal stages the fluid-filled alveoli appear as complete "white out" of the lungs. In severe cases, the infant becomes progressively obtunded and flaccid. Long periods of apnea ensue, and the infant eventually dies of asphyxia. Despite advances in neonatal intensive care, the overall mortality of RDS is about 15%, and one third of infants born before 30 weeks of gestational age die of this disorder. In milder cases, the disorder peaks within 3 days, after which gradual improvement takes place.

The major complications of RDS relate to anoxia and acidosis and include the following:

- **Intraventricular cerebral hemorrhage:** The periventricular germinal matrix in the newborn brain is particularly vulnerable to hemorrhage, because the dilated, thin-walled veins in this area rupture easily (Fig. 6-42). The pathogenesis of this complication is not fully understood but is believed to reflect anoxic injury to the periventricular capillaries, venous sludging and thrombosis, and impaired vascular autoregulation.

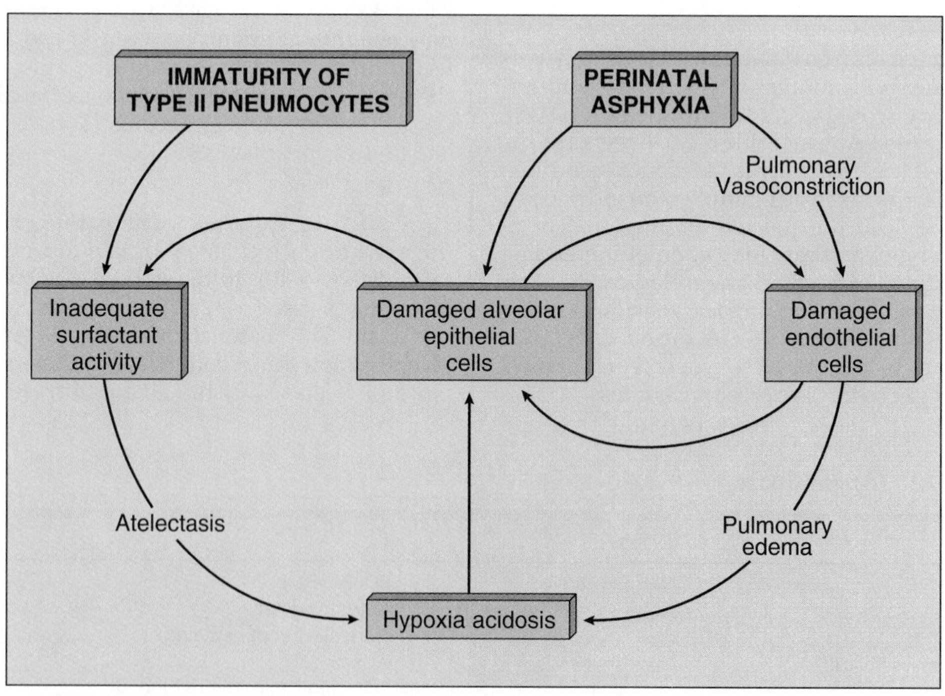

FIGURE *6-40*
Pathogenesis of the respiratory distress syndrome of the neonate. Immaturity of the lungs and perinatal asphyxia are the major pathogenetic factors.

- **Persistence of the patent ductus arteriosus:** In almost one third of newborns who survive RDS, the ductus arteriosus remains patent. With recovery from the pulmonary disease, the pressure in the pulmonary circulation declines, and the higher pressure in the aorta reverses the direction of blood flow in the ductus, thereby creating a persistent left-to-right shunt. Congestive heart failure often ensues and requires correction of the patent ductus.
- **Necrotizing enterocolitis:** This intestinal complication of RDS is the most common acquired gastrointestinal emergency in newborns. Although the pathogenesis is not completely understood, it is believed to be related principally to ischemia of the intestinal mucosa. This injury is followed by bacterial colonization, usually with *Clostridium difficile*. The lesions vary from those of typical pseudomembranous enterocolitis to gangrene and perforation of the bowel.
- **Bronchopulmonary dysplasia:** This late complication of RDS usually occurs in infants who weigh less than 1500 g and were maintained on a positive-pressure respirator with high oxygen tensions. It is thought that the disorder results from oxygen toxicity superimposed on RDS. In such patients, respiratory distress persists after the third or fourth day and is reflected in hypoxia, acidosis, oxygen dependency, and the onset of right-sided heart failure. Radiographs of the lungs change from almost complete opacification to a spongelike appearance, characterized by small lucent areas alternating with denser foci. Microscopic examination of the lungs reveals hyperplasia of the bronchiolar epithelium and squamous metaplasia in the bronchi and bronchioles. Atelectasis, interstitial edema, and thickening of the alveolar basement membranes are noted. Most surviving infants eventually recover normal pulmonary function, but right-sided heart failure and viral necrotizing bronchiolitis pose threats to a favorable outcome.

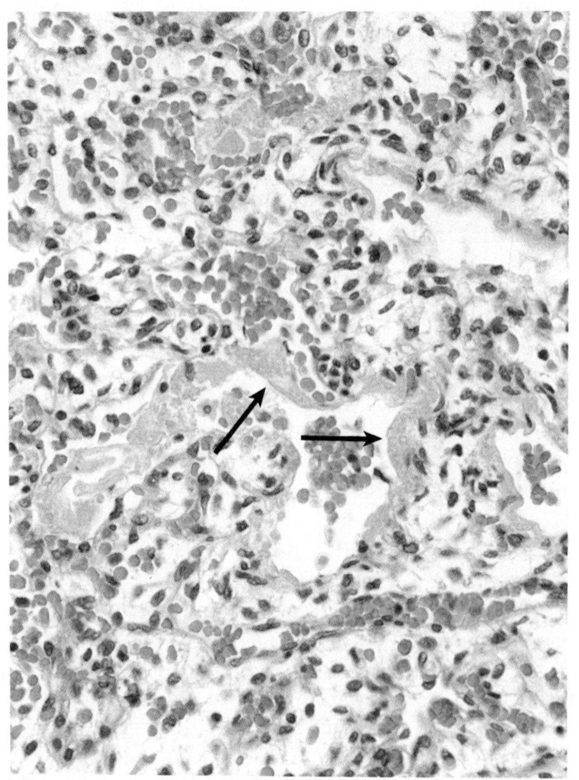

FIGURE 6-41
The lung in the respiratory distress syndrome of the neonate. The alveoli are atelectatic, and a dilated alveolar duct is lined by a fibrin-rich hyaline membrane (*arrows*).

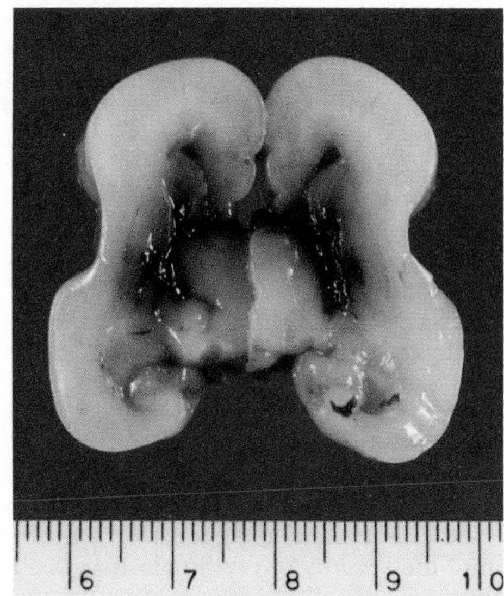

FIGURE 6-42
Intraventricular hemorrhage in a premature infant suffering from respiratory distress syndrome of the neonate.

Erythroblastosis Fetalis and Neonatal Hemolytic Anemia

Erythroblastosis fetalis is a hemolytic disease of the fetus or newborn caused by the transplacental passage of maternal antibodies against fetal erythrocytes. The disorder was first recognized by Hippocrates but was not fully understood until 1940, when the Rh (Rhesus) antigen on erythrocytes was identified. More than 60 antigens on the surface of erythrocytes can elicit an antibody response, but only the D antigen of the Rh group and the ABO system are associated with a significant incidence of hemolytic disease.

Rh Incompatibility

The distribution of Rh antigens among ethnic groups is variable. In American whites, 15% are Rh negative (Rh-d), whereas only 8% of blacks are Rh negative. Japanese, Chinese, and Native American Indian populations contain essentially no Rh-negative persons. By contrast, in the Basque population, among whom the mutation that causes the Rh-d phenotype may have arisen, the prevalence of Rh-negative persons is 35%.

☐ Pathogenesis: The Rh blood group system consists of some 25 components, of which only the alleles cde/CDE need to be considered in this discussion. Among infants with erythroblastosis fetalis caused by Rh incompatibility, 90% are due to antibodies against D, with the remaining cases involving C or E. The introduction of Rh-positive fetal erythrocytes (>1 mL) into the circulation of an Rh-negative mother at the time of delivery sensitizes her to the D antigen (Fig. 6-43). Erythroblastosis fetalis does not ordinarily occur during the first pregnancy, because the quantity of fetal blood necessary to sensitize the mother is introduced into her circulation only at the time of delivery, too late to affect the fetus. However, when the sensitized mother again bears an Rh-positive fetus, much smaller quantities of fetal D antigen elicit an increase in antibody titer. In contrast to IgM, IgG antibodies are small enough to cross the placenta and thus produce hemolysis in the fetus. This cycle is exaggerated in multiparous women, and the severity of erythroblastosis tends to increase progressively with each succeeding pregnancy.

Since 15% of white women are Rh negative, and since they have an 85% chance of marrying an Rh-positive man, 13% of all marriages are theoretically at risk for maternal–fetal Rh incompatibility. The actual incidence of erythroblastosis fetalis is, however, much less. This apparent discrepancy is explained by several factors: (1) More than half of Rh-positive men are heterozygous (D/d), and thus only half of their offspring express the D antigen. (2) Only half of all pregnancies have large enough fetal-to-maternal transfusions to sensitize the mother. (3) Even in those Rh-negative women who are exposed to significant amounts of fetal Rh-positive blood, many do not mount a substantial immune response. Even after multiple pregnancies, only 5% of Rh-negative women are ever delivered of infants with erythroblastosis fetalis.

☐ Pathology and Clinical Features: The severity of erythroblastosis fetalis varies from a mild hemolysis to fatal anemia, and the pathological findings are determined by the extent of the hemolytic disease.

- ***Death in utero*** occurs in the most extreme form of the disease, in which case severe maceration is evident on delivery. Numerous erythroblasts are demonstrable in visceral organs that are not extensively autolyzed.
- ***Hydrops fetalis*** *refers to the most serious form of erythroblastosis fetalis* (Fig. 6-44) *in liveborn infants and is characterized by severe edema secondary to congestive heart failure caused by the severe anemia.* The infant generally dies, unless adequate exchange transfusions with Rh-negative cells correct the anemia and ameliorate the hemolytic disease. Although the infant is not jaundiced at birth, progressive hyperbilirubinemia develops rapidly. In infants who die, autopsy reveals conspicuous hepatosplenomegaly and bile-stained organs. Microscopically, erythroblastic hyperplasia of the bone marrow and extramedullary hemopoiesis in the liver, spleen, lymph nodes, and other sites are prominent.
- ***Kernicterus****, also termed* ***bilirubin encephalopathy****, is defined as a neurological condition associated with severe jaundice and characterized by bile staining of the brain, particularly of the basal ganglia, pontine nuclei, and dentate nuclei in the cerebellum.* Although brain damage in jaundiced newborns was first mentioned in the 15th century, the association of kernicterus with high levels of unconjugated bilirubin was not appreciated until 1952. Kernicterus (Ger. *kern*, nucleus) is essentially confined to newborns with severe unconjugated hyperbilirubinemia, usually related to erythroblastosis. The bilirubin derived from the destruction of erythrocytes and the catabolism of the released heme is not easily conjugated by the immature liver, which is deficient in glucuronyl transferase.

  The development of kernicterus is directly related to the level of unconjugated bilirubin and in term infants is rare, with serum bilirubin levels less than 20 mg/dL. Premature infants are more vulnerable to hyperbilirubinemia and may develop kernicterus at levels as low as 12 mg/dL. The mechanism by which bilirubin injures the cells of the brain is obscure but is believed to relate to interference with mitochondrial function. Immaturity of the blood–brain barrier in the newborn was traditionally considered to be an important contributing factor to kernicterus. However, in light of newer data, there is little reason to believe that an exaggerated permeability of the blood–brain barrier to free bilirubin plays any role.

  Severe kernicterus leads initially to loss of the startle reflex and athetoid movements, which in 75% progresses to lethargy and death. Most surviving infants have severe choreoathetosis and mental retardation, whereas a minority have varying degrees of intellectual and motor retardation.

PREVENTION AND TREATMENT: Exchange transfusions may keep the maximum serum bilirubin at an acceptable level. However, phototherapy, which converts the toxic unconjugated bilirubin into isomers that are nontoxic and excreted in the urine, has greatly reduced the need for exchange transfusions.

The incidence of erythroblastosis fetalis secondary to Rh incompatibility has been greatly reduced (to <1% of women at risk) by the use of human anti-D globulin (RhoGAM) within 72 hours of delivery. The quantity of RhoGAM administered is sufficient to neutralize 10 mL of antigenic fetal cells that may have entered the maternal circulation during delivery.

ABO Incompatibility

Since the availability of RhoGAM prophylaxis of Rh-negative mothers, the incidence of Rh-incompatible erythroblastosis has drastically decreased, and today ABO incompatibility is the principal cause of hemolytic disease of the newborn. Despite the fact that 25% of pregnancies result in ABO incompatibility between mother and offspring, hemolytic disease develops in only 10% of the children, usually in infants with type A blood. The low antigenicity of the ABO factors in the fetus accounts for the mildness of ABO hemolytic disease. The natural anti-A and anti-B antibodies are IgM, which does not cross the placenta.

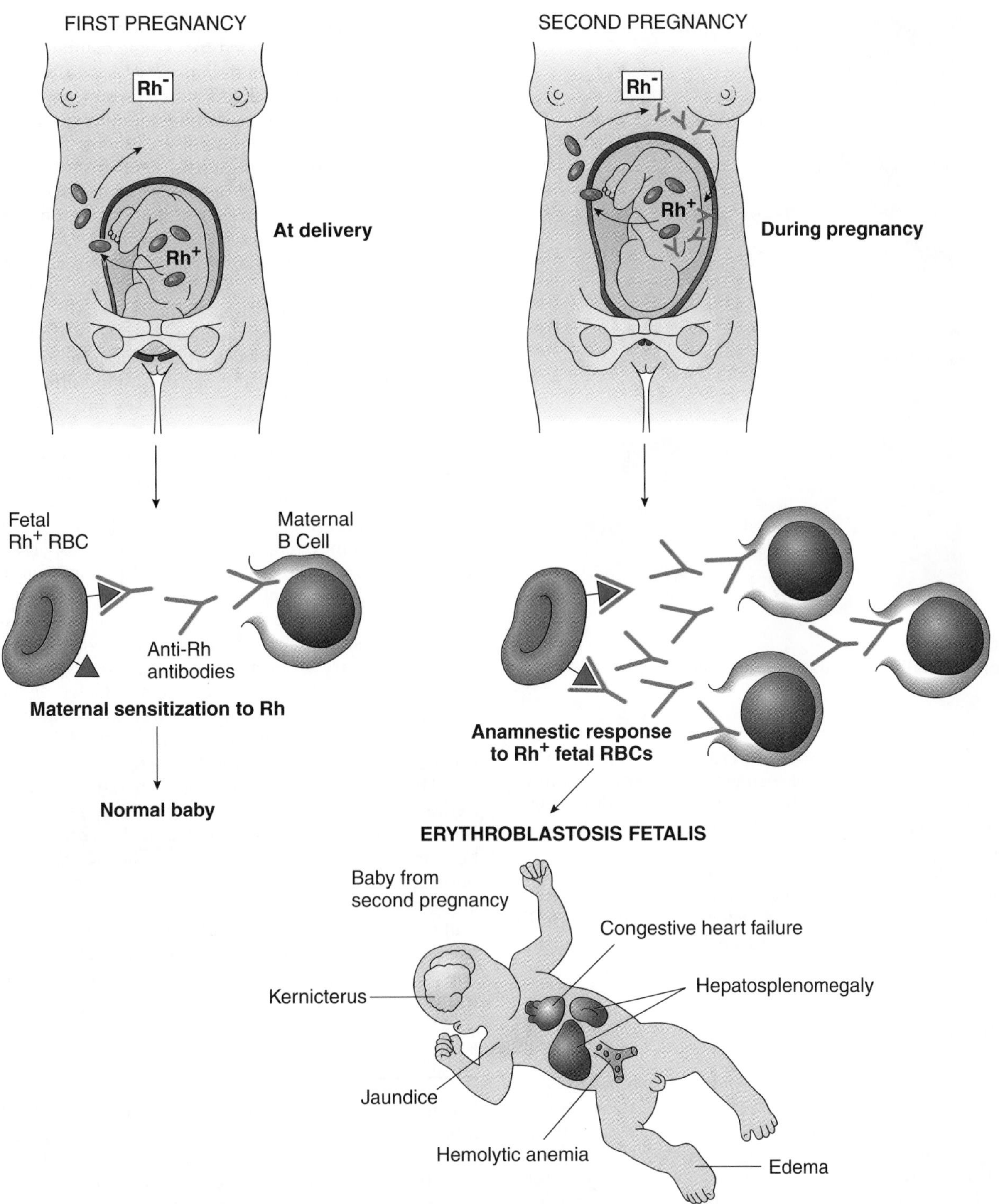

FIGURE *6-43*
Pathogenesis of erythroblastosis fetalis due to maternal–fetal Rh incompatibility. Immunization of the Rh-negative mother with Rh-positive erythrocytes in the first pregnancy leads to the formation of anti-Rh antibodies of the IgG type. These antibodies cross the placenta and damage the Rh-positive fetus in subsequent pregnancies.

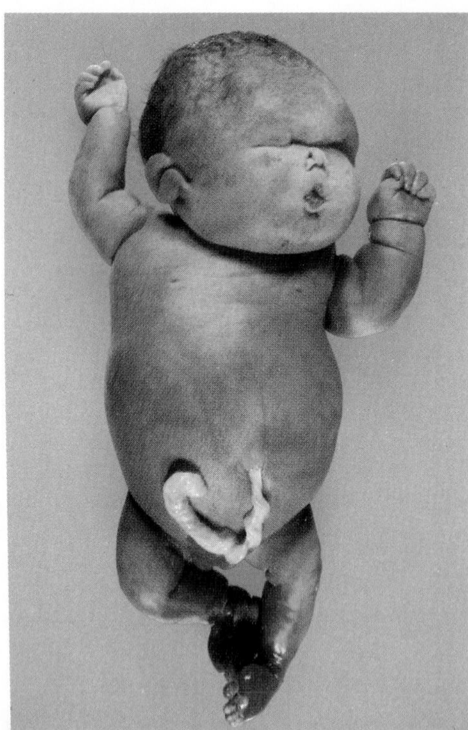

FIGURE 6-44
Hydrops fetalis. The infant shows severe anasarca.

However, certain incomplete antibodies to A antigen may be IgG, which does cross the placenta. Therefore, ABO isoimmune disease may be seen in firstborn infants. However, most cases of hemolytic anemia from ABO incompatibility are seen after a previous incompatible pregnancy.

The majority of infants with ABO incompatibility suffer mild disease, and jaundice is the only clinical feature. The complications of erythroblastosis associated with Rh incompatibility are unusual with ABO disease. Nevertheless, kernicterus has occasionally been reported.

Birth Injury

Birth injury is a broad term that spans the spectrum of mechanical trauma to anoxic damage. Some of these injuries relate to poor obstetric manipulation, whereas many are unavoidable sequelae of routine delivery. Birth injuries occur in about 5 per 1000 live births. Factors that predispose to birth injury include cephalopelvic disproportion, dystocia (difficult labor), prematurity, and breech presentation.

Cranial Injury

Caput succedaneum refers to edema of the scalp caused by trauma to the head incurred during the passage through the birth canal. The swelling rapidly disappears and is more a source of parental anxiety than of clinical concern.

Cephalohematoma is defined as a subperiosteal hemorrhage that is confined to a single cranial bone and becomes apparent within the first few hours after birth. It may or may not be associated with a linear fracture of the underlying bone. Most cephalohematomas resolve without complications and require no treatment.

Skull fractures during birth result from the impact of the head on the pelvic bones or pressure from obstetric forceps. Linear fractures, the most common variety, are asymptomatic and do not require any treatment. Depressed fractures are usually caused by trauma from forceps. Although many depressed fractures do not initially produce symptoms, they usually require mechanical elevation because of the risk of underlying cranial trauma from persistent pressure. In contrast to most fractures, those of the occipital bone often extend through the underlying venous sinuses and produce fatal hemorrhage.

Intracranial hemorrhage is one of the most dangerous birth injuries and may be traumatic or secondary to asphyxia. Rarely, such hemorrhage may be the presenting symptom of an underlying bleeding diathesis. Traumatic intracranial hemorrhage occurs in the setting of (1) significant cephalopelvic disproportion, (2) precipitous delivery, (3) breech presentation, (4) prolonged labor, or (5) the inappropriate use of forceps. These traumas can result in **subdural or subarachnoid hemorrhage**, which are commonly secondary to lacerations of the falx cerebri or tentorium cerebelli that involve the vein of Galen or the venous sinuses. As previously noted, anoxic injury from asphyxia, particularly in the premature infant, is often associated with intraventricular hemorrhage.

The prognosis for the newborn with intracranial hemorrhage varies with its extent. Massive hemorrhage is often rapidly fatal. If the infant survives, recovery may be complete, or the child may be afflicted with chronic neurological residuals, usually in the form of cerebral palsy or hydrocephalus. It deserves emphasis, however, that many cases of cerebral palsy have been shown by ultrasound studies to relate to brain damage acquired at least 2 weeks prior to birth rather than from birth trauma.

Peripheral Nerve Injury

Brachial palsy, with varying degrees of paralysis of the upper extremity, is caused by excessive traction on the head and neck or shoulders during delivery. The injury may be permanent if the nerves are severed. Function may return within a few months if the palsy results from edema and hemorrhage.

Phrenic nerve paralysis, and associated paralysis of a hemidiaphragm, may be associated with brachial palsy and results in breathing difficulties. The condition generally resolves spontaneously within a few months.

Facial nerve palsy usually presents as a unilateral flaccid paralysis of the face caused by injury to the seventh cranial nerve during labor or delivery, especially with forceps. When severe, the entire affected side of the face is paralyzed and even the eyelid cannot be closed.

The prognosis again depends on whether the nerve was lacerated or simply injured by pressure.

Fractures

The clavicle is more vulnerable to fracture during delivery than any other bone and may be associated with fracture of **the humerus**. Immobilization of the arm and shoulder are almost invariably the only treatment required for complete healing. Fractures of other long bones and the nose occasionally occur during birth but again heal easily.

Rupture of the Liver

The only internal organ other than the brain that is injured with any frequency during labor and delivery is the liver. This organ is injured by mechanical pressure during difficult or premature births. Rupture of the liver may lead to the formation of a hematoma large enough to cause a palpable abdominal mass and anemia, and surgical repair of the laceration may be required.

Sudden Infant Death Syndrome

The sudden infant death syndrome (SIDS), also known as "crib death," is defined as "the sudden death of an infant or young child which is unexpected by history and in which a thorough postmortem examination fails to demonstrate an adequate cause of death." Although the diagnosis of SIDS is arrived at solely by excluding other specific causes of sudden death, this catastrophe is nevertheless considered a distinct clinicopathological entity. SIDS actually was first described in the American colonies in 1686, but modern attention to the disorder dates only a few decades.

Typically, the victim of SIDS is an apparently healthy young infant who has been asleep without any hint of impending calamity. The infant does not awake spontaneously at the usual time, and when it cannot be aroused, the parent realizes that it has died. Postmortem examination does not disclose a cause of death, such as pneumonia, food aspiration, sepsis, or cerebral hemorrhage. This tragic sequence has aroused great public concern, because it must be separated from homicide, which has been demonstrated in a number of cases to be the true cause of mysterious death in children.

☐ Epidemiology: Beyond the neonatal period, SIDS is the leading cause of death during the first year of life, accounting for more than one third of all deaths in this period. The incidence in the United States is 2 per 1000 live births. The large majority (90%) of cases occur before 6 months of age. Most deaths from SIDS occur during the winter months, but no association between particular respiratory infections and infant death has been established. The large majority of deaths occur at night or during periods associated with sleep, but the position in which the infants are found in bed varies and is probably unrelated to the fatal event. It has been proposed that infants who sleep in the prone position are at greater risk of SIDS.

The risk factors for SIDS have been difficult to ascertain and are based principally on retrospective studies. **The strongest maternal risk factors** appear to be the following:

- Low socioeconomic status (limited education, unmarried mother, poor prenatal care)
- Age younger than 20 years at first pregnancy
- Cigarette smoking during pregnancy
- Use of illicit drugs during pregnancy

The risk factors for the infant are controversial. The consensus includes the following:

- Low birth weight
- Prematurity
- An illness, often gastrointestinal, within the last 2 weeks before death
- Subsequent siblings of SIDS victims
- Survivors of an apparent life-threatening event, defined as an episode characterized by some combination of apnea, color change, marked alteration in muscle tone, and choking or gagging. A definite cause, such as seizures or aspiration after vomiting, is established in only half the cases of an apparent life-threatening event.

☐ Pathogenesis: The pathogenesis of SIDS remains elusive and controversial, and no clear answers are forthcoming at this time. It is also unclear whether SIDS is a single entity or whether it represents the common endpoint of several different conditions. The most popular hypothesis relates SIDS to a prolonged spell of apnea, followed by a cardiac arrhythmia or shock, in a susceptible, sleeping infant who cannot arouse himself and prevent the process from progressing to a fatal outcome. However, it deserves emphasis that fewer than 10% of parents of SIDS victims report an episode of apnea or an apparent life-threatening event at any time prior to the fatal event. **Thus, while it is possible that sleep apnea contributes to the sequence of events leading to SIDS, available data do not support a strong and predictable relationship between the two conditions.**

Numerous other causes for SIDS have found various champions, but the evidence for any one of these is indeed weak. They include cardiovascular abnormalities triggering fatal arrhythmias, abnormal brain stem sensitivity to respiratory stimuli, gastroesophageal reflux, various types of infections, inborn errors of metabolism, and bronchopulmonary dysplasia.

☐ Pathology: At autopsy, a number of morphological alterations have been described in victims of SIDS, but their relevance to the etiology and pathogenesis of this disorder remains unclear. Chronic hypoxia is said to be evidenced by gliosis of the brain stem, medial hypertrophy of small pulmonary arteries, persistence of extramedullary hematopoiesis in the liver, retention of periadrenal brown fat, and right ventricular hypertrophy. However, with the exception of brain stem gliosis, none of these changes occur with any regularity. Petechiae on the surfaces of the lungs, heart, pleura, and thymus, which have been reported in most infants dying of SIDS, are probably terminal events and have been attributed to negative intrathoracic pressure produced by respiratory efforts.

NEOPLASMS OF INFANCY AND CHILDHOOD

Malignant tumors between the ages of 1 and 15 years are distinctly uncommon, but cancer remains the leading cause of death from disease in this age group. In children, 10% of all deaths are due to malignancies, and only accidental trauma kills a larger number. **Unlike adults, in whom the large majority of cancers are of epithelial origin (e.g., carcinomas of the lung, breast, and gastrointestinal tract), most malignant tumors in children arise from hemopoietic, nervous, and soft tissues** (Fig. 6-45). Another feature that distinguishes childhood tumors from those of adults is the fact that many of the former are part of developmental complexes. Examples include Wilms tumor associated with aniridia, genitourinary malformations, and mental retardation (WAGR complex); hemihypertrophy of the body associated with Wilms tumor, hepatoblastoma, and adrenal carcinoma; and tuberous sclerosis in association with renal tumors and rhabdomyomas of the heart. Some tumors are apparent at birth and are obviously developmental tumors that have evolved *in utero*. In addition, abnormally developed organs, persistent organ primordia, and displaced organ rests are all vulnerable to neoplastic transformation.

The individual cancers of childhood, including disorders such as the leukemias, neuroblastoma, Wilms tumor, various sarcomas, and germ cell neoplasms, are discussed in detail in the chapters dealing with the respective organs. The basic principles of neoplasia and carcinogenesis, including those applicable to pediatric cancers, are discussed in Chapter 5.

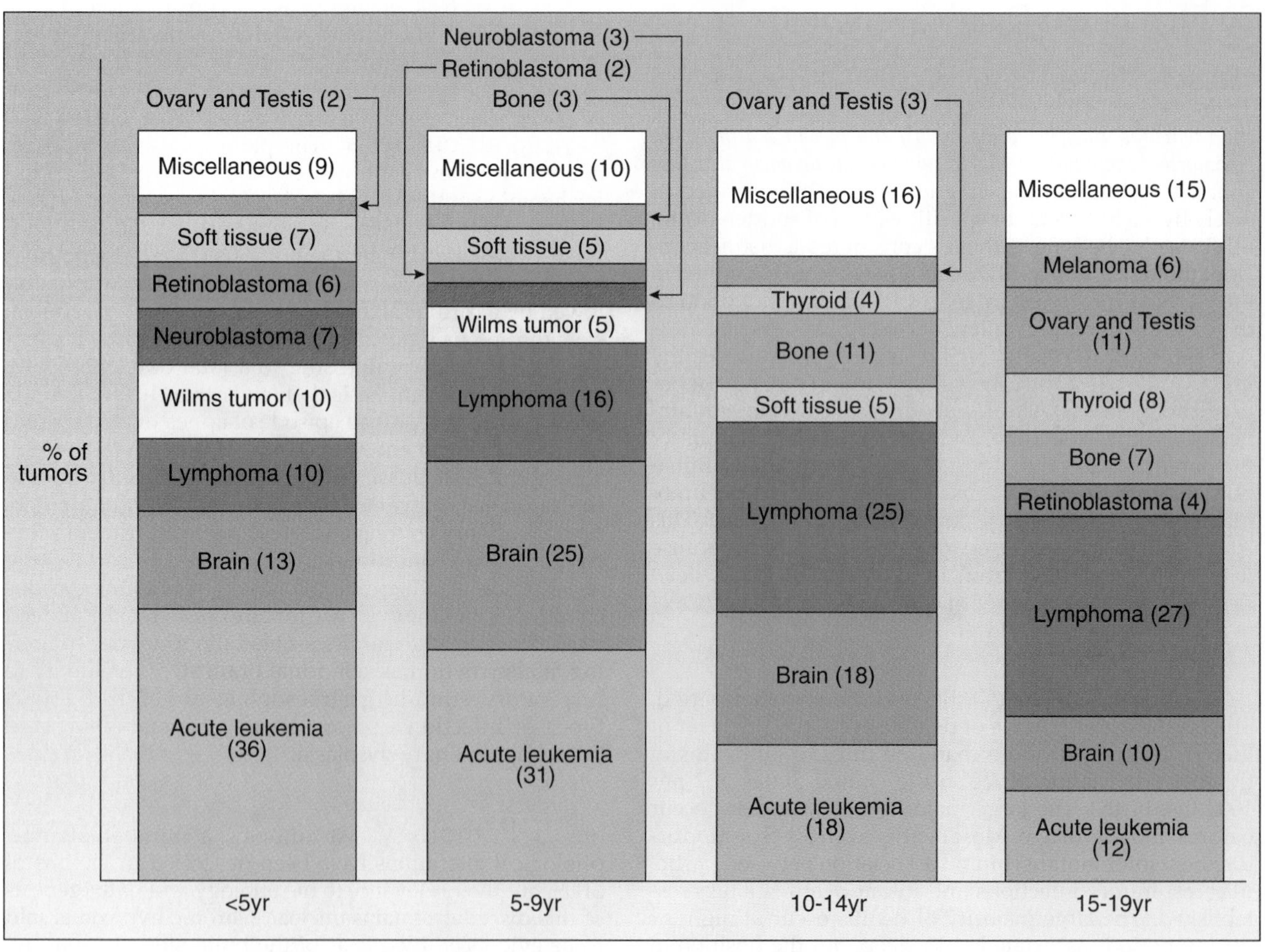

FIGURE *6-45*
Distribution of childhood tumors according to age and primary site.

Benign Tumors and Tumor-Like Conditions

HAMARTOMAS: These lesions represent focal, benign overgrowths of one or more of the mature cellular elements of a normal tissue, often with one element predominating. Although the cells of a hamartoma are often arranged in a highly irregular fashion, the distinction between this developmental abnormality and a true benign neoplasm is often conjectural.

CHORISTOMAS: Also called heterotopias, choristomas are similar to hamartomas but are minute or microscopic aggregates of normal tissue components in aberrant locations. Choristomas are represented by rests of pancreatic tissue in the wall of the gastrointestinal tract or of adrenal tissue in the renal cortex.

HEMANGIOMAS: These lesions, of varying size and in diverse locations, are the most frequently encountered tumors in childhood. Whether hemangiomas are true neoplasms or hamartomas is unclear, although half are present at birth and most regress with age. Occasionally, large rapidly growing hemangiomas can be serious lesions, especially when they occur on the head or neck. **A port wine stain** is a congenital capillary hemangioma that involves the skin of the face and scalp and is often large enough to be disfiguring, imparting a dark purple color to the affected area. Unlike many small hemangiomas, they persist for life and are not easily treated.

LYMPHANGIOMAS: Also termed **cystic hygromas**, lymphangiomas are poorly demarcated swellings that are usually present at birth and thereafter rapidly increase in size. Most lymphangiomas occur on the head and neck, but the floor of the mouth, mediastinum, and buttocks are not uncommon sites. The classification of these tumors is imprecise, with some researchers considering them developmental malformations or hamartomas and others calling them neoplasms. Lymphangiomas appear as unilocular or multilocular cysts with thin, transparent walls and straw-colored fluid. Microscopically, myriad dilated lymphatic channels are separated by fibrous septa. Unlike hemangiomas, these lesions do not regress spontaneously and should be resected, although their tendency to infiltrate soft tissue may require extensive dissection.

SACROCOCCYGEAL TERATOMAS: Although rare, these germ cell neoplasms are the most common solid tumors in the newborn, with an incidence of 1 in 40,000 live births. At least 75% of sacrococcygeal teratomas occur in girls, and a substantial number have been encountered in twins. The tumors are usually noticed at birth as a mass in the region of the sacrum and buttocks. They are commonly large, lobulated masses, often as large as the infant's head. One half of the tumors grow externally and may be connected to the body by a small stalk. Some have both external and intrapelvic components, whereas a small minority grow entirely in the pelvis. Microscopically, sacrococcygeal teratomas are composed of numerous tissues, particularly of neural origin. The large majority (90%) of sacrococcygeal teratomas detected before the age of 2 months are benign, but up to half of those diagnosed later in life are malignant. Associated congenital anomalies of the vertebrae, genitourinary system, and anorectum are common. The lesion should be resected promptly, although extension within the pelvis and surrounding bony structures may present surgical problems.

Malignant Tumors

Cancers in the pediatric age group are uncommon, with an incidence of 1.3 per 10,000 per year in children younger than the age of 15 years. The mortality clearly varies with the intrinsic behavior of the tumor and the response to therapy, but as an overall figure the death rate for childhood cancer is only about one third the incidence. Almost half of all malignant diseases in patients younger than 15 years of age are acute leukemias and lymphomas. Leukemias alone, particularly acute lymphoblastic leukemia, account for one third of all cases of childhood cancer. Most of the other malignant neoplasms are neuroblastomas, brain tumors, Wilms tumors, retinoblastomas, bone cancers, and various soft tissue sarcomas.

The genetic influences in the development of childhood tumors have been particularly well studied in the case of retinoblastoma, Wilms tumor, and osteosarcoma. The issues relating to the interaction of inherited mutations and environmental influences in the pathogenesis of malignant tumors in both children and adults are discussed in Chapter 5.

SUGGESTED READING

BOOKS

Behrman RE, Kliegman RM, Arvin AM: *Nelson's textbook of pediatrics,* 15th ed. Philadelphia: WB Saunders, 1996.

Gelehrter TD, Collins FS: *Principles of medical genetics*, 2nd ed. Baltimore: Williams & Wilkins, 1997.

Scriver CR, Beaudet AL, Sly WS, Valle D: *The metabolic basis of inherited disease,* 7th ed. New York: McGraw-Hill, 1995.

Strachen T, Read AP: *Human molecular genetics.* New York: Wiley-Liss, 1996.

REVIEW ARTICLES

Antomarakis SE, Kazazian HH Jr: The molecular basis of hemophilia A in man. *Trends Genet* 4:233, 1988.

Goyco PG, Beckerman RC: Sudden infant death syndrome. *Curr Probl Pediatr* 20:297–346, 1990.

Graeter LJ, Mortensen ME: Kids are different: Develomental variability in toxicology. *Toxicology* 111:15–20, 1996.

Greger R, Mall M, Bleich M, Ecke D, Warth R, Riedemann N, Kunzelmann K: Regulation of epithelial ion channels by the cystic fibrosis transmembrane conductance regulator. *J Mol Med* 74:527–534, 1996.

Harris S, Moncrieff C, Johnson K: Myotonic dystrophy:

Will the real gene please step forward? *Hum Mol Genet* 5(spec. no.):1417–1423, 1996.

Hendrickx J, Willems PJ: Genetic deficiencies of the glycogen phosphorylase system. *Hum Genet* 97:551–556, 1996.

Hernandez D, Fisher EM: Down syndrome genetics: Unravelling a multifactorial disorder. *Hum Mol Genet* 5:1411–1416, 1996.

Horowitz M, Zimran A: Mutations causing Gaucher disease. *Hum Mutat* 3:1–11, 1994.

Koch R, Fishler K, Azen C, Guldberg P, Guttler F: The relationship of genotype to phenotype in phenylalanine hydroxylase deficiency. *Biochem Mol Med* 60:92–101, 1997.

Ogata T, Matsuo N: Turner syndrome and female sex chromosome aberrations: Deduction of the principal factors involved in the development of clinical features. *Hum Genet* 95:607–629, 1995.

Ozawa E, Yoshida M, Suzuki A, Mizuno Y, Hagiwara Y: Dystrophin-associated proteins in muscular dystrophy. *Hum Mol Genet* 4(spec. no.):1711–1716, 1995.

Paulson HL, Fischbeck KH: Trinucleotide repeats in neurogenetic disorders. *Annu Rev Neurosci* 19:79–107, 1996.

Pope FM, Burrows NP: Ehlers-Danlos syndrome has varied molecular mechanisms. *J Med Genet* 34:400–410, 1997.

Swain RA, St Clair L: The role of folic acid in deficiency states and prevention of disease. *J Fam Pract* 44:138–144, 1997.

Timchenko LT, Caskey CT: Trinucleotide repeat disorders in humans: Discussion of mechanisms and medical issues. *FASEB J* 10:1589–1597, 1996.

West JR, Chen WJ, Pantazis NJ: Fetal alcohol syndrome: The vulnerability of the developing brain and possible mechanism of damage. *Metab Brain Dis* 9:291–322, 1994.

Wraith JE: The mucopolysaccharidoses: A clinical review and guide to management. *Arch Dis Child* 72:263–267, 1995.

Zwarthoff EC: Neurofibromatosis and associated tumour-suppressor genes. *Pathol Res Pract* 192:647–657, 1996.

CHAPTER 7

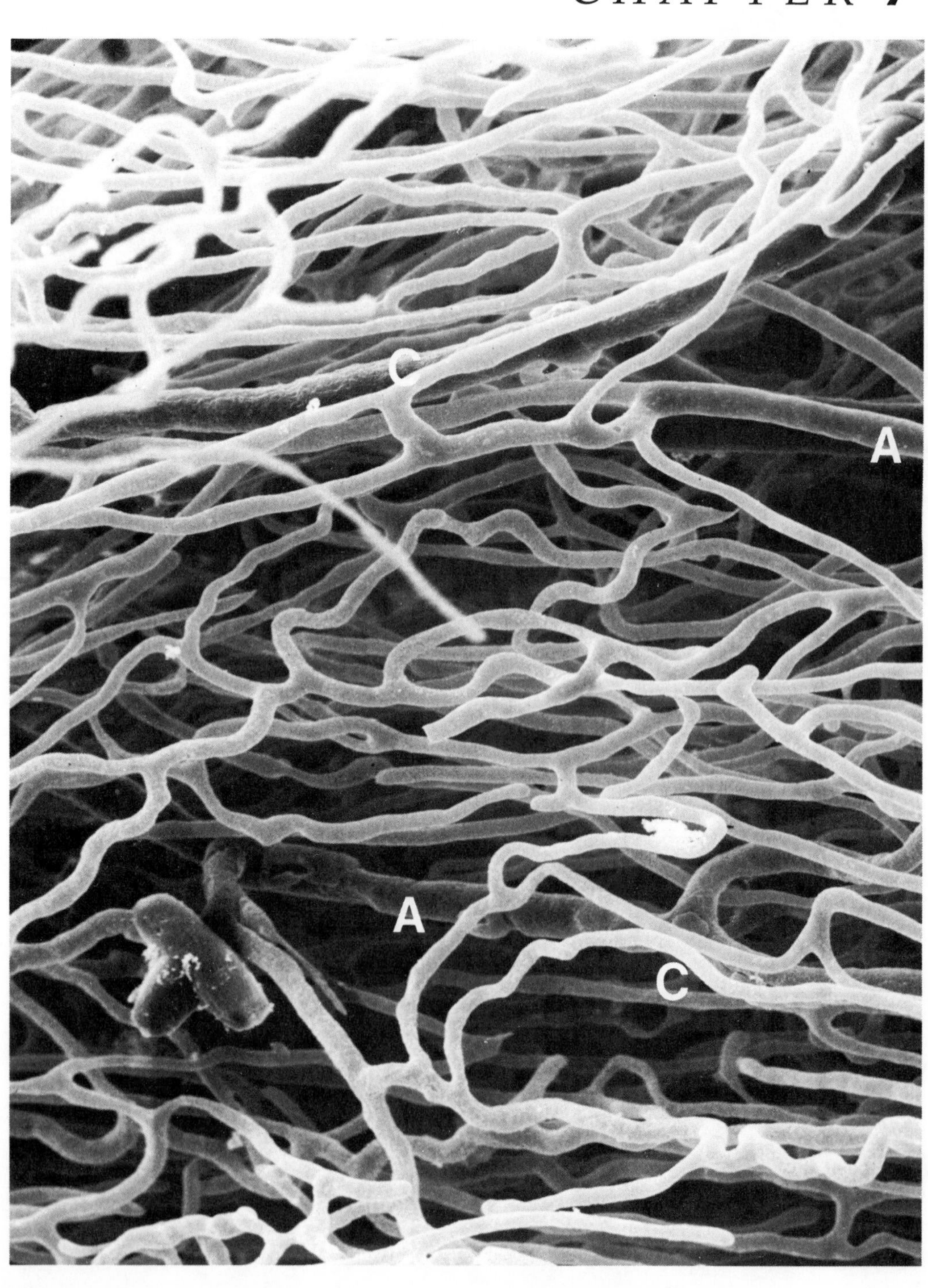

Hemodynamic Disorders

Wolfgang J. Mergner
Benjamin F. Trump

FIGURE 7-1 *(see opposite page)*
Capillary system of the heart. The coronary arteries were washed with Ringer's solution and filled with a low-viscosity plastic. Subsequently, the heart tissue was digested with concentrated potassium hydroxide. The cast of the capillaries was then observed under low-magnification scanning electron microscopy. C, capillary; A, arteriole.

THE NORMAL CIRCULATION

The metabolism of organs and cells depends on an intact circulation for the continuous delivery of oxygen, nutrients, hormones, electrolytes, and water and for the removal of metabolic waste and carbon dioxide. **Delivery and elimination at the cellular level are controlled by exchanges between the intravascular space, interstitial space, cellular space, and lymphatic space.**

The Heart

The heart is a two-sided pump, with the two vascular circuits placed in series. The amount of blood pumped by the right ventricle must, over time, exactly equal the amount of blood pumped by the left ventricle. The hemodynamically important parameters are (1) cardiac output, (2) perfusion pressure, and (3) peripheral resistance.

- **Cardiac output** is the volume of blood pumped by each ventricle per minute and represents the total blood flow in the pulmonary and systemic circulations.
- **Perfusion pressure** (also called driving pressure) is the difference in the dynamic pressure between two points along a tube or vessel. Blood flow to any segment of the circulation is ultimately dependent on the arterial driving pressure. However, each organ can autoregulate flow and thereby determine the amount of blood that it receives from the circulation.
- **Peripheral vascular resistance** refers to the sum of the factors that determine the regional blood flow in each organ. Two thirds of the resistance in the systemic vasculature is determined by the arterioles.

The sum of all regional flows equals the venous return, which in turn determines the cardiac output.

The Aorta and Arteries

The aorta and major arteries are "conducting vessels" whose major functions are the transport of blood to the organs and the conversion of pulsatile flow into sustained regular flow. The latter function derives from the elastic properties of the aorta and the resistance produced by the arteriolar sphincters.

The Microcirculation

The velocity of the blood in the microcirculation (Fig. 7-1) is 1 mm/s. The average length of a capillary is 1 mm. Blood from an arteriole enters the capillaries, which freely anastomose with each other either directly or through metarterioles. Entry into the capillary system is guarded by **precapillary sphincters**, except in the case of **thoroughfare channels**, which bypass capillaries and are always open. Since not all capillaries are open at all times, blood flow can be increased by recruiting capillaries. The sum of the flow through the capillary bed, the thoroughfare channels, and the arteriovenous anastomoses determines the regional blood flow. The exact means by which an organ regulates blood flow according to its metabolic needs is still debated, but there is a link between oxygen demand and blood flow. In the heart, blood flow is adjusted on a second-to-second basis. Factors that mediate and link metabolic vasodilatation to cellular metabolism include adenosine, other nucleotides, nitric oxide, certain prostaglandins, carbon dioxide, and pH. The microcirculation is an important contributor to all forms of hyperemia and edema and is a target in septic shock (see later).

Veins and Venules

Blood from the capillaries enters the venules and eventually the veins on its route back to the heart. The veins not only serve as a conduit for blood, but also act as a blood reservoir, 64% of the total blood volume residing in the venous system.

The Interstitium

The spaces between cells, collectively termed "interstitium," comprises 15% of the total body volume. The interstitial fluid provides a means for the delivery of nutrients and the elimination of waste. Most of the interstitial water is bound to a dense network of glycosaminoglycans.

The Lymphatics

Interstitial fluid is reabsorbed into the circulation at the venous end of the capillary, and a small portion is drained through lymphatics. Lymphatic capillaries conduct the lymph from the periphery to the central venous system via the thoracic duct. Lymph is a solvent for large molecules that cannot return to the circulation through the blood capillaries.

DISORDERS OF PERFUSION

Hemodynamic disorders are characterized by disturbed perfusion that results in organ and cellular injury.

Hyperemia

Hyperemia is defined as an excess amount of blood in an organ. It may be caused either by an increased supply of blood from the arterial system (active hyperemia) or by an impediment to the exit of blood through venous pathways (passive hyperemia or congestion).

Active Hyperemia

Active hyperemia is an augmented supply of blood to an organ, usually as a physiological response to an increased functional demand, as in the case of the heart and skeletal muscle during exercise. Neurogenic and hormonal influences play a role in active hyperemia, exemplified at both extremes of the female reproductive span—namely, in the form of the blushing bride and the menopausal flush. Although these examples do not appear to promote any useful function, hyperemia of the skin in febrile states serves to dissipate heat. In addition, skeletal muscle may increase its blood flow (and thus oxygen delivery) 20-fold during exercise. The increased blood supply is brought about by arteriolar dilatation and recruitment of inactive or latent capillaries.

The most striking active hyperemia occurs in association with inflammation. Vasoactive materials released by inflammatory cells (see Chapter 2) cause dilatation of blood vessels; in the skin this results in the classic "tumor, rubor, and calor" of inflammation. In pneumonia, the alveolar capillaries are engorged with erythrocytes as a hyperemic response to inflammation. Since inflammation can also damage endothelial cells and increase capillary permeability, the hyperemia of inflammation is often accompanied by edema and local extravasation of erythrocytes.

Reactive hyperemia occurs after temporary interruption of blood supply. The release of the obstruction is followed by active hyperemia, which repays the oxygen deficit accrued during the period of ischemia.

Passive Hyperemia (Congestion)

Passive hyperemia, or congestion, refers to the engorgement of an organ with venous blood. Acute passive congestion is clinically a consequence of acute failure of the left ventricle. The resulting venous engorgement of the lung leads to the accumulation of a transudate in the alveoli, a condition termed **pulmonary edema**.

A generalized increase in venous pressure, typically from chronic heart failure, results in slower blood flow, and a consequent increase in the volume of blood in many organs, including the liver, spleen, and kidneys. In the past, heart failure from rheumatic mitral stenosis was a common cause of generalized venous congestion, but with the decline in the prevalence of rheumatic fever and the advent of surgical valve replacement, such cases are unusual. Congestive heart failure secondary to coronary artery disease and right-sided failure because of pulmonary disease are now more common causes.

Passive congestion may also be confined to a limb or an organ as a result of more localized obstruction to the venous drainage. Examples include thrombophlebitis of the leg veins, with resulting edema of the lower extremity, and thrombosis of the hepatic veins (Budd-Chiari syndrome), with secondary chronic passive congestion of the liver.

THE LUNG: Chronic failure of the left ventricle constitutes an impediment to the exit of blood from the lungs and leads to chronic passive congestion of the lungs. As a result, the pressure in the alveolar capillaries is increased, and these vessels become engorged with blood. The increased pressure in the alveolar capillaries has four major consequences:

1. Microhemorrhages release erythrocytes into the alveolar spaces, where they are phagocytosed and degraded by alveolar macrophages. The released iron, in the form of hemosiderin, remains in the macrophages, which are then called "heart failure cells."
2. The increased hydrostatic pressure forces fluid from the blood into the alveolar spaces, resulting in pulmonary edema, a dangerous condition that interferes with gas exchange in the lung.
3. The increased pressure, together with other poorly understood factors, stimulates fibrosis in the interstitial spaces of the lung. The presence of fibrosis and iron is viewed grossly as a firm, brown lung ("brown induration").
4. The increased capillary pressure is transmitted to the pulmonary arterial system, a condition labeled **pulmonary hypertension**. This disorder may lead to right-sided heart failure and consequent generalized venous congestion.

Chapter 12 discusses the morphological changes associated with chronic passive congestion of the lungs.

THE LIVER: The liver, with the hepatic veins emptying into the vena cava immediately inferior to the heart, is particularly vulnerable to chronic passive congestion. The central veins of the hepatic lobule become dilated. The increased venous pressure is transferred to the sinusoids, where it leads to dilatation of the sinusoids with blood and pressure atrophy of the centrilobular hepatocytes (Fig. 7-2).

In extreme cases, frank hemorrhagic necrosis of the hepatocytes in the centrilobular zones is conspicuous. Grossly, the cut surface of the chronically congested liver exhibits dark foci of centrilobular congestion surrounded by paler zones composed of unaffected peripheral portions of the lobules. The result is a curious reticulated appearance, resembling a cross-section of a nutmeg, and is

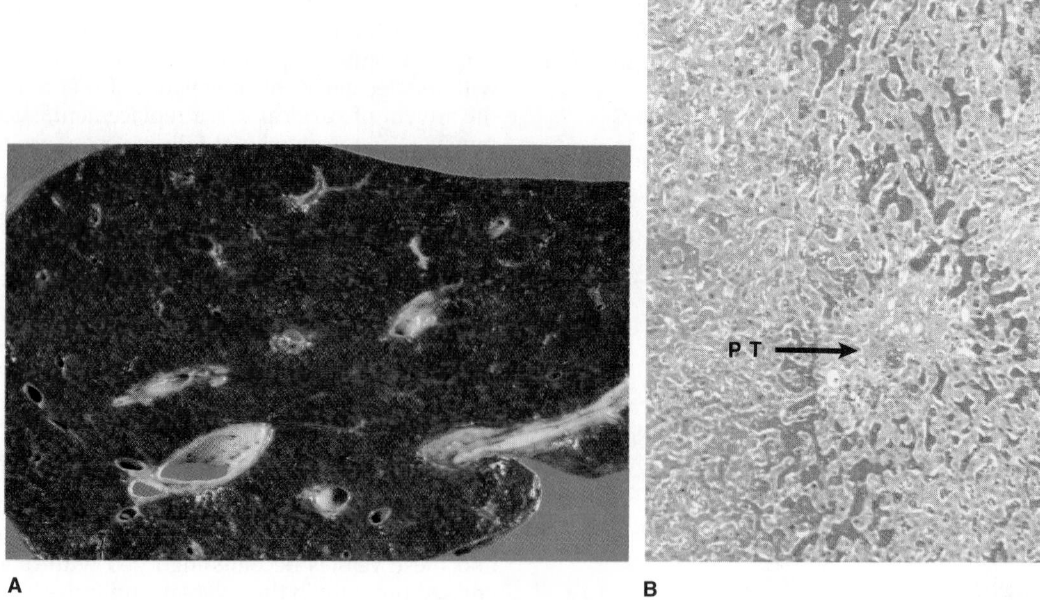

FIGURE 7-2
Passive congestion of the liver. (*A*) A gross photograph shows the pattern of chronic passive congestion, in which lighter-appearing tissue segments form an interlacing pattern with dark-staining centrilobular blood spaces. (*B*) A photomicrograph of the liver shows centrilobular sinusoids dilated with blood. The intervening plates of hepatocytes show pressure atrophy. PT, portal tract.

appropriately called "nutmeg liver" (see Fig. 7-2). Prolonged venous congestion of the liver eventually leads to thickening of the central veins and centrilobular fibrosis. Only in the most extreme cases of venous congestion (e.g., constrictive pericarditis or tricuspid stenosis) is the fibrosis sufficiently generalized and severe to justify the label "cardiac cirrhosis."

THE SPLEEN: Increased pressure in the liver, from cardiac failure or an intrahepatic obstruction to the flow of blood (e.g., cirrhosis), results in higher splenic vein pressure and congestion of the spleen. The organ becomes enlarged and tense, and the cut section oozes dark blood. In long-standing congestion, diffuse fibrosis of the spleen is seen, together with iron-containing, fibrotic, and calcified foci of old hemorrhage (Gamna-Gandy bodies). Fibrocongestive splenomegaly may result in an organ that weighs 250 to 750 g, compared with a normal weight of 150 g. The enlarged spleen sometimes displays excessive functional activity—a condition termed hypersplenism—which leads to hematological abnormalities.

EDEMA AND ASCITES: Venous congestion impedes the flow of blood in the capillaries, thereby increasing hydrostatic pressure and promoting edema formation. The accumulation of edema fluid in heart failure is particularly noticeable in dependent tissues: the legs and feet in ambulatory patients and the back in bedridden persons. Ascites, the accumulation of fluid in the peritoneal space, reflects (among other factors) the lack of tissue rigor, a condition in which there is no countervailing external pressure to oppose hydrostatic pressure.

Hemorrhage

Hemorrhage (i.e., bleeding) is a discharge of blood from the vascular compartment to the exterior of the body or into nonvascular body spaces. The most common and obvious cause is trauma—usually accidental, but often by the surgeon's scalpel. An artery may be ruptured in ways other than laceration. For instance, severe atherosclerosis may so weaken the wall of the abdominal aorta that it balloons to form an aneurysm, which then ruptures and bleeds into the retroperitoneal space. By the same token, an aneurysm may complicate a congenitally weak cerebral artery (berry aneurysm) and lead to subarachnoid hemorrhage. Certain infections (e.g., pulmonary tuberculosis) erode blood vessels; a similar vascular injury is caused by invasive tumors.

Hemorrhage also results from damage at the level of the capillaries. For instance, the rupture of capillaries by blunt trauma is evidenced by the appearance of a bruise. Increased venous pressure also causes extravasation of blood from capillaries in the lung. Vitamin C deficiency is associated with capillary fragility and bleeding, owing to a defect in the supporting structures. It is important to recognize that the capillary barrier by itself is not sufficient to contain the blood within the intravascular space. The minor trauma imposed on small vessels and capillaries by normal movement requires an intact coagulation system to prevent hemorrhage. Thus, a severe decrease in the number of platelets (thrombocytopenia) or a deficiency of a coagulation factor (e.g., factor VIII in hemophilia) is associated with spontaneous hemorrhages unrelated to any apparent trauma.

A person may exsanguinate into an internal cavity, as in the case of gastrointestinal hemorrhage from a peptic ulcer (arterial hemorrhage) or esophageal varices (venous hemorrhage). In such cases, large amounts of fresh blood fill the entire gastrointestinal tract. Bleeding into a serous cavity can result in the accumulation of a large amount of blood, even to the point of exsanguination. A few definitions are in order:

- **Hematoma:** Hemorrhage into the soft tissues. Such collections of blood can be merely painful, as in a muscle bruise, or fatal, if located in the brain.
- **Hemothorax:** Hemorrhage into the pleural cavity.
- **Hemopericardium:** Hemorrhage into the pericardial space.
- **Hemoperitoneum:** Bleeding into the peritoneal cavity.
- **Hemarthrosis:** Bleeding into a joint space.
- **Purpura:** Diffuse superficial hemorrhages in the skin, up to 1 cm in diameter.
- **Ecchymosis:** A larger superficial hemorrhage. Following a bruise or in association with a coagulation defect, an initially purple discoloration of the skin turns green and then yellow before resolving. This sequence reflects the progressive oxidation of bilirubin released from the hemoglobin of degraded erythrocytes. A good example of an ecchymosis is a "black eye."
- **Petechia:** A pinpoint hemorrhage, usually in the skin or conjunctiva. This lesion represents the rupture of a capillary or arteriole and occurs in conjunction with coagulopathies or vasculitis, the latter classically associated with infections of the heart valves (bacterial endocarditis).

THROMBOSIS

Thrombosis refers to the formation within a vascular lumen of a thrombus, defined as an aggregate of coagulated blood containing platelets, fibrin, and entrapped cellular elements. ***A thrombus*** is by definition adherent to the vascular endothelium and should be distinguished from a simple blood clot, which reflects only the activation of the coagulation cascade and can form *in vitro* or *in situ* in the postmortem state. Similarly, a thrombus is different from a hematoma, which results from hemorrhage and subsequent clotting outside the vascular system. The details of thrombus formation and the coagulation cascade are discussed in more detail in Chapters 10 and 20. Here we present the causes and consequences of thrombosis in different sites.

Thrombosis in the Arterial System

☐ **Pathogenesis:** The most common cause of arterial thrombosis is atherosclerosis, and the most important vessels involved are the coronary, cerebral, mesenteric, and renal arteries and the arteries of the lower extremities. Uncommonly, arterial thrombosis occurs in other disorders, including inflammation of the arteries (arteritis), trauma, and diseases of the blood. Thrombi are common in aneurysms (localized dilatations of the lumen) of the aorta and its major branches, in which the distortion of blood flow, combined with intrinsic vascular disease, promotes thrombosis.

The pathogenesis of arterial thrombosis involves principally three factors:

- **Damage to the endothelium,** usually by atherosclerosis, disturbs the anticoagulant properties of the vessel wall and serves as the nidus for platelet aggregation and fibrin formation.
- **Alterations in blood flow,** whether from turbulence in an aneurysm or at the sites of arterial bifurcation, or slowing in narrowed arteries, tend to favor thrombosis.
- **Increased coagulability of the blood,** as seen in polycythemia vera, or after the use of oral contraceptives, is associated with an increased risk of thrombosis.

☐ **Pathology:** Initially, an arterial thrombus, which is attached to the vessel wall, is soft, friable, and dark red, with fine alternating bands of yellowish platelets and fibrin, the so-called **lines of Zahn**. Once formed, arterial thrombi have several outcomes.

- **Lysis** of an arterial thrombus may occur, owing to the potent thrombolytic activity of the blood.
- **Propagation** of a thrombus (i.e., an increase in its size) may occur, because the thrombus serves as the focus for further thrombosis.
- **Organization** refers to the eventual invasion of connective tissue elements, which causes a thrombus to become firm and grayish white.
- **Canalization** is the process by which new lumina lined by endothelial cells form in an organized thrombus. The functional significance of this change is often questionable.

The organized structure of a thrombus reflects a tight interaction between platelets and fibrin and differs in appearance from a postmortem clot or one formed in a test tube. The lines of Zahn stabilize the thrombus formed during life, whereas the **postmortem clot** has a more gelatinous structure. Postmortem clots occur in stagnant blood in which gravity fractionates the erythrocytes. The part of the clot that contains many red blood cells is called **currant jelly**. The overlying clot, which represents coagulated plasma without red blood cells, is called **chicken fat** because of its color and consistency. The determination of whether or not a clot formed during life (antemortem clot) or after death (postmortem clot) is often important in a medical autopsy and in forensic pathology.

☐ **Clinical Features:** **Arterial thrombosis is the most common cause of death in Western industrialized countries**. Since most arterial thrombi occlude the vessel, they often lead to ischemic necrosis of the tissue supplied by the artery—that is, an **infarct**. Thus, thrombosis of a coronary or cerebral artery results in a **myocardial infarct** (heart attack) or **cerebral infarct** (stroke). Other end-arteries that are affected by atherosclerosis and often suffer thrombosis include the mesenteric arteries (intestinal infarction), renal arteries (kidney infarcts), and arteries of the leg (gangrene).

Thrombosis in the Heart

As in the arterial system, endocardial injury and changes in blood flow in the heart are associated with mural thrombosis. The disorders in which mural thrombosis occurs include the following:

- **Myocardial infarction:** Adherent mural thrombi form in the cavity of the left ventricle over areas of myocardial infarction, owing to damaged endocardium and alterations in blood flow associated with an adynamic segment of the myocardium.
- **Atrial fibrillation:** A disorder of atrial rhythm (atrial fibrillation) leads to slower blood flow in the left atrium, a situation that predisposes to the formation of mural thrombi in that location.
- **Cardiomyopathy:** Primary diseases of the myocardium are associated with mural thrombi in the left ventricle. The reasons are poorly understood but presumably relate to endocardial injury and altered hemodynamics associated with poor myocardial contractility.
- **Endocarditis:** Small thrombi, termed **vegetations**, may also develop on cardiac valves, usually mitral or aortic, that are damaged by a bacterial infection (bacterial endocarditis). Occasionally, in the absence of valve infection, vegetations form on a mitral or tricuspid valve injured by systemic lupus erythematosus (Libman-Sacks endocarditis). In chronic wasting states, such as occur with terminal cancer, large, friable vegetations may appear on cardiac valves (marantic endocarditis), possibly reflecting a hypercoagulable state.

The major complication of thrombi in any location in the heart is the detachment of fragments and their transport to distant sites (embolization), where they lodge and occlude arterial vessels.

Thrombosis in the Venous System

At one time, venous thrombosis was widely referred to as *thrombophlebitis*, implying that an inflammatory or infectious process had injured the vein, thereby causing thrombosis. However, with the recognition that in most cases there is no evidence of inflammation, the term *phlebothrombosis* is more accurate. Nevertheless, both terms have been replaced for the most part by the expression *deep venous thrombosis*. This term is particularly appropriate for the most common manifestation of the disorder, namely, thrombosis of the deep venous system of the legs.

☐ **Pathogenesis:** Deep venous thrombosis is caused in general by the same factors that dispose toward arterial and cardiac thrombosis, namely endothelial injury, stasis, and a hypercoagulable state. Conditions that favor the development of deep venous thrombosis include the following:

- **Stasis** (heart failure, chronic venous insufficiency, postoperative immobilization, prolonged bed rest)
- **Injury** (trauma, surgery, childbirth)
- **Hypercoagulability** (oral contraceptives, late pregnancy, cancer)
- **Advanced age**
- **Sickle cell disease**

☐ **Pathology:** The large majority (>90%) of venous thromboses occur in the deep veins of the legs, with the remainder usually involving veins in the pelvis. Most venous thrombi begin in the calf veins, frequently in the sinuses above the venous valves. In this location, venous thrombi have several potential fates:

- **Lysis:** Venous thrombi generally remain small and are eventually lysed, posing no further threat to health.
- **Organization:** Many thrombi undergo organization similar to thrombi of arterial origin. Small organized venous thrombi may be incorporated into the wall of the vessel, whereas larger ones may undergo canalization, with partial restoration of venous drainage.
- **Propagation:** It is not uncommon for venous thrombi to serve as a nidus for further thrombosis and thereby propagate proximally to involve the larger iliofemoral veins (Fig. 7-3).
- **Embolization:** Large venous thrombi or those that have propagated proximally represent a significant hazard to life, since they may dislodge and be carried to the lungs as pulmonary emboli.

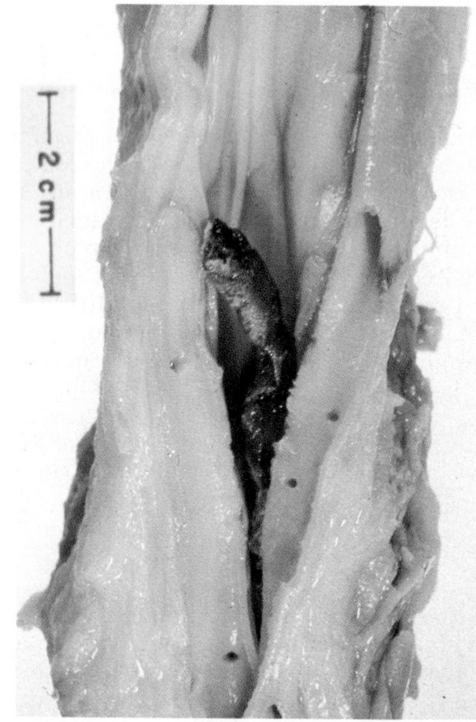

FIGURE 7-3
Venous thrombosis. The femoral vein has been opened to reveal a large thrombus within the lumen.

☐ **Clinical Features:** Small thrombi in the calf veins are ordinarily asymptomatic, and even larger thrombi in the iliofemoral system may cause no symptoms. Some patients have tenderness in the calf, often associated with forced dorsiflexion of the foot (Homans sign). Occlusive thrombosis of the femoral or iliac veins leads to severe congestion, edema, and cyanosis of the lower extremity. Symptomatic deep venous thrombosis is treated with systemic anticoagulants, and thrombolytic therapy has been useful in selected cases.

The function of the venous valves is always impaired in a vein subjected to thrombosis, organization, and canalization. As a result, chronic deep venous insufficiency (i.e., a failure of venous drainage) is virtually inevitable. If the lesion is restricted to a small segment of the deep venous system, the condition may remain asymptomatic. However, more extensive involvement results in pigmentation, edema, and induration of the skin of the leg. Ulceration above the medial malleolus is often troublesome and difficult to treat.

EMBOLISM

Embolism is the passage through the venous or arterial circulations of any material capable of lodging in a blood vessel and thereby obstructing the lumen. The usual embolus is a thromboembolus—that is, a blood clot formed in one location that detaches from the vessel wall and travels to a distant site.

Pulmonary Embolism

For the clinician, pulmonary embolism remains an important diagnostic and therapeutic challenge. In fact, pulmonary thromboemboli are reported in more than half of all autopsies. Furthermore, this complication occurs in 1% to 2% of postoperative patients over the age of 40 years. The risk increases with advancing age, obesity, length of the operative procedure, postoperative infection, the presence of cancer, and preexisting venous disease.

The large majority of pulmonary emboli (90%) arise from the deep veins of the lower extremities; most of the fatal ones arise from the iliofemoral veins (Fig. 7-4). Only half of patients with pulmonary thromboembolism have signs of deep vein thrombosis. Some thromboemboli arise from the pelvic venous plexus and others from the right side of the heart. Emboli are also derived from thrombi around indwelling lines in the systemic venous system or the pulmonary artery. The upper extremities are a rare source of thromboemboli.

Depending on the size of the embolus, the health of the patient, and his circulatory status, the clinical features of acute pulmonary embolism vary, but they can be divided into the following syndromes:

- Asymptomatic small pulmonary emboli
- Transient dyspnea and tachypnea without other symptoms
- Pulmonary infarction, with pleuritic chest pain, hemoptysis, and pleural effusion
- Cardiovascular collapse with sudden death

Massive Pulmonary Embolism

One of the most dramatic and tragic calamities typically complicating hospitalization is the sudden collapse and death of a patient who appeared to be well on the way to an uneventful recovery. The cause of this catastrophe is often massive pulmonary embolism as a consequence of the release of a large deep venous thrombus from a lower extremity. Classically, a postoperative patient succumbs immediately on getting out of bed for the first time. The muscular activity dislodges a thrombus that formed as a result of the stasis associated with prolonged bed rest. Excluding deaths related to surgery itself, massive pulmonary embolism is the most common cause of death after major orthopedic surgery and is the most frequent nonobstetric cause of postpartum death. It also is an especially common cause of death in patients who suffer from chronic heart and lung diseases and in those who are subjected to prolonged immobilization for any reason.

A large pulmonary embolus often lodges at the bifurcation of the main pulmonary artery (saddle embolus), thereby obstructing the blood flow to both lungs (Fig. 7-5). Somewhat smaller lethal emboli may be found in the right or left pulmonary arteries or in multiple primary and secondary branches. With acute obstruction of more than half of the pulmonary arterial tree, the patient often goes into shock immediately and may die within minutes.

The hemodynamic consequences of such massive pulmonary embolism are the result of acute right ventricular failure, because of sudden obstruction to outflow, and a pronounced reduction in left ventricular cardiac output, secondary to the loss of right ventricular function. The low cardiac output is responsible for the sudden appearance of cardiogenic shock.

Pulmonary Infarction

Small pulmonary emboli are not ordinarily lethal. They tend to lodge in peripheral pulmonary arteries and in some patients (15% to 20% of all pulmonary emboli) they produce infarcts of the lung. Clinically, pulmonary infarction is usually seen in the context of congestive heart failure or chronic lung disease, because the normal dual circulation of the lung ordinarily protects against ischemic necrosis. Pulmonary infarcts are typically hemorrhagic, because the bronchial artery pumps blood into the necrotic area. They tend to be pyramidal, with the base of the pyramid on the pleural surface. Patients experience cough, stabbing pleuritic pain, shortness of breath, and occasional hemoptysis. Pleural effusion is common and often bloody. With the passage of time, the blood in the infarct is resorbed and the center of the infarct becomes pale. Granulation tissue forms on the edge of the infarct, after which it is organized to form a fibrous scar.

Pulmonary Embolism Without Infarction

Since the lung has a dual circulation, supplied by both the bronchial arteries and the pulmonary artery, the large majority (75%) of small pulmonary emboli do not produce infarcts. Although most small emboli do not attract clinical

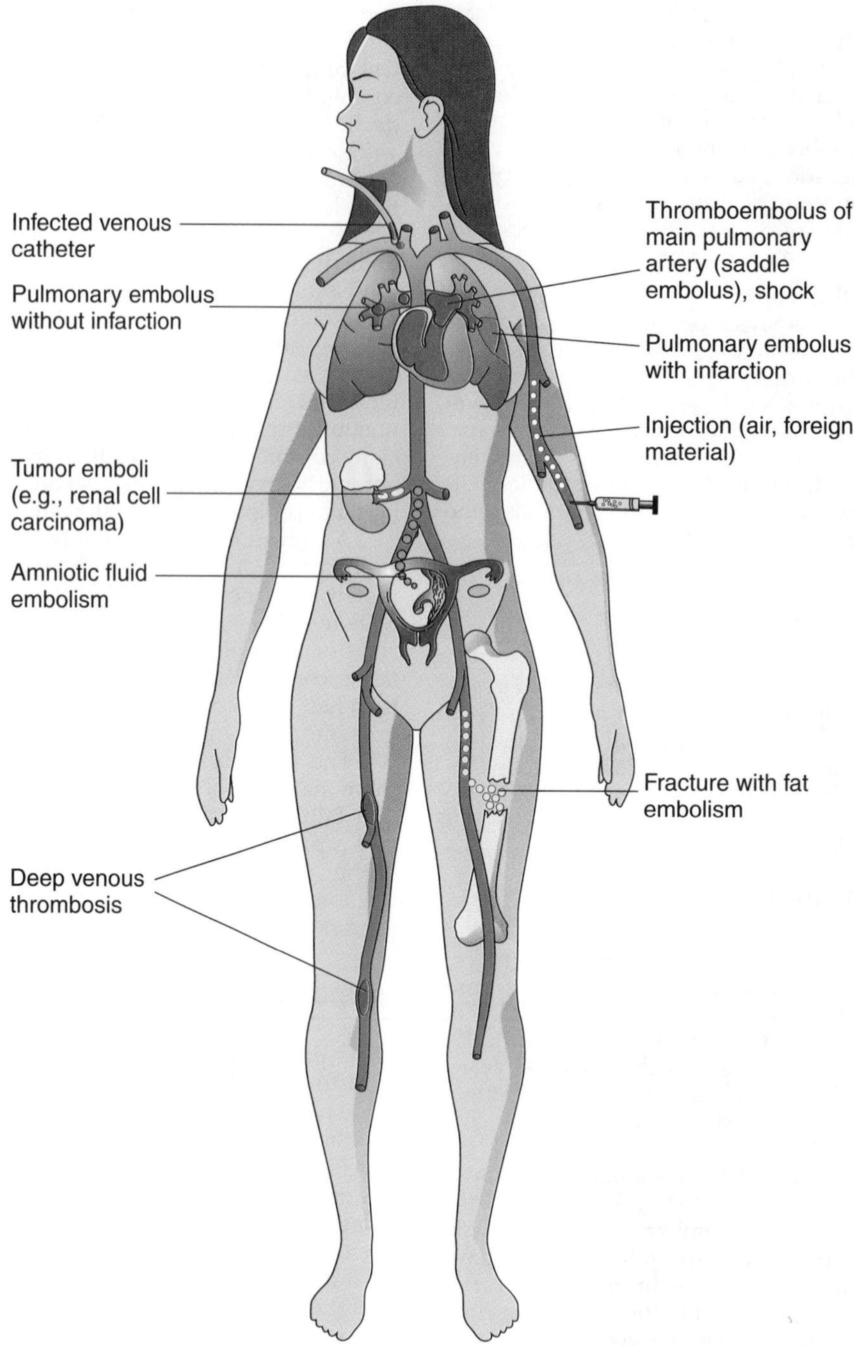

FIGURE *7-4*
Sources and effects of venous emboli.

attention, a few lead to a syndrome characterized by dyspnea, cough, chest pain, and hypotension, with attacks of shortness of breath. Rarely (3%) recurrent pulmonary emboli produce pulmonary hypertension by mechanical blockage of the arterial bed. In this circumstance, reflex vasoconstriction and bronchial constriction, owing to release of vasoactive substances, may contribute to a reduction in the size of the functional pulmonary vascular bed.

In the clinical syndrome of "partial infarction," patients have the clinical and radiological findings of pulmonary infarction due to thromboembolism. However, the lesion resolves instead of contracting to leave a scar. In such cases, hemorrhage and necrosis of the lung tissue in the affected area occur, but the tissue framework remains. Collateral circulation maintains the viability of the tissue and enables its regeneration.

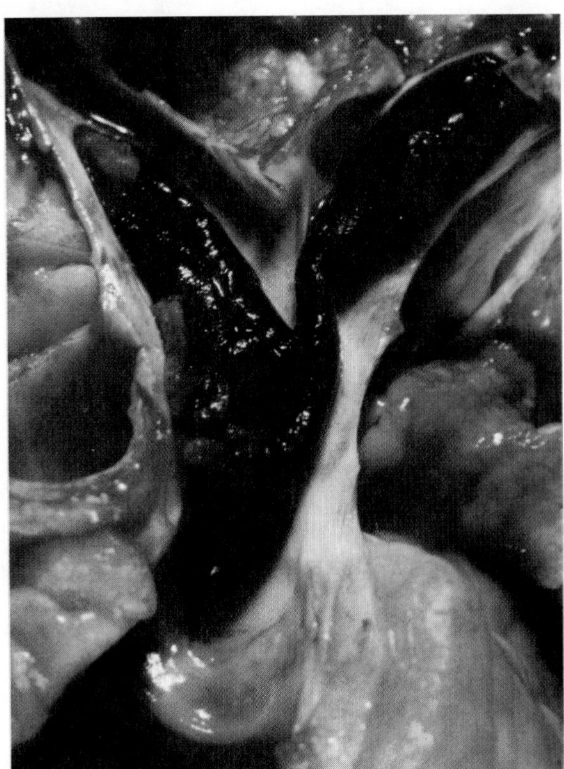

FIGURE 7-5
Pulmonary embolism. The main pulmonary artery and its bifurcation have been opened to reveal a large saddle embolus.

Fate of Pulmonary Thromboemboli

Small pulmonary emboli may completely resolve, depending on (1) the embolic load, (2) the adequacy of the pulmonary vascular reserve, (3) the state of the bronchial collateral circulation, and (4) the activity of the thrombolytic process. Alternatively, thromboemboli may become organized and leave strings of fibrous tissue attached to the vessel wall in the lumen of pulmonary arteries. Radiological studies have indicated that half of all pulmonary thromboemboli are resorbed and organized within 8 weeks, with little narrowing of the vessels.

Paradoxical Embolism

Paradoxical embolism refers to emboli that arise in the venous circulation and bypass the lungs by traveling through an incompletely closed foramen ovale, subsequently entering the left side of the heart and blocking flow in systemic arteries.

Arterial Embolism

The heart is the most common source of arterial emboli (Fig. 7-6), which usually arise from mural thrombi (Fig. 7-7) or diseased valves. Emboli tend to lodge at points where the vessel lumen narrows abruptly, for example, at bifurcations or in the area of an atherosclerotic plaque. The viability of the tissue supplied by the vessel depends on the availability of collateral circulation and on the fate of the embolus. The embolus may propagate locally and lead to a more severe obstruction, or it may fragment and lyse. The organs that suffer the most from arterial embolism include the following:

- **Brain:** Arterial emboli to the brain cause strokes.
- **Intestine:** In the mesenteric circulation, emboli cause infarction of the bowel, a complication that presents as an acute abdomen and requires immediate surgery.
- **Lower extremity:** Embolism of an artery of the leg leads to sudden pain, absence of pulses, and a cold limb. In some cases, the limb must be amputated.
- **Kidney:** Renal artery embolism may infarct the entire kidney but more commonly results in small peripheral infarcts.
- **Heart:** Coronary artery embolism and resulting myocardial infarcts are reported but are rare.

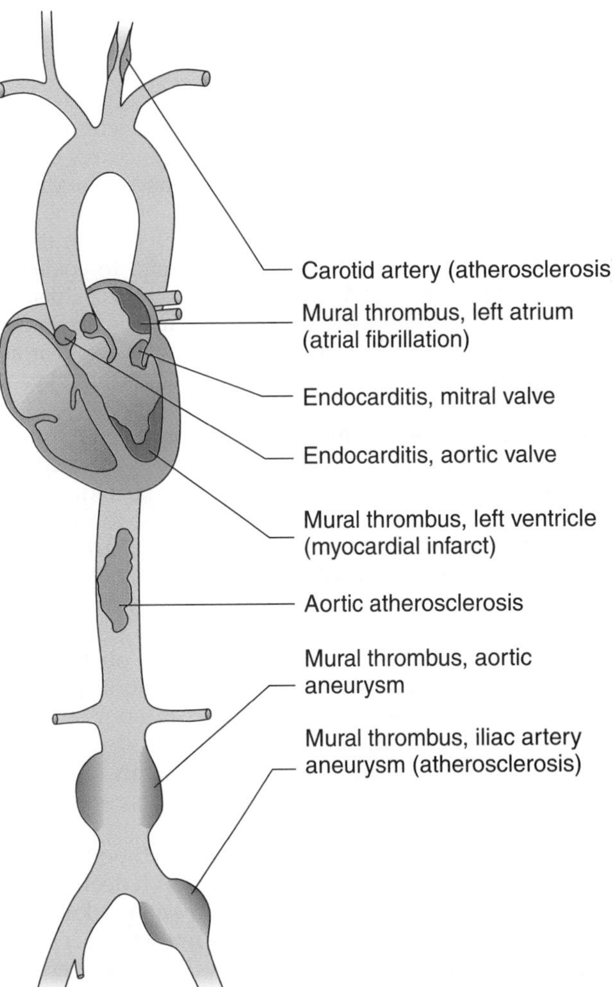

FIGURE 7-6
Sources of arterial emboli.

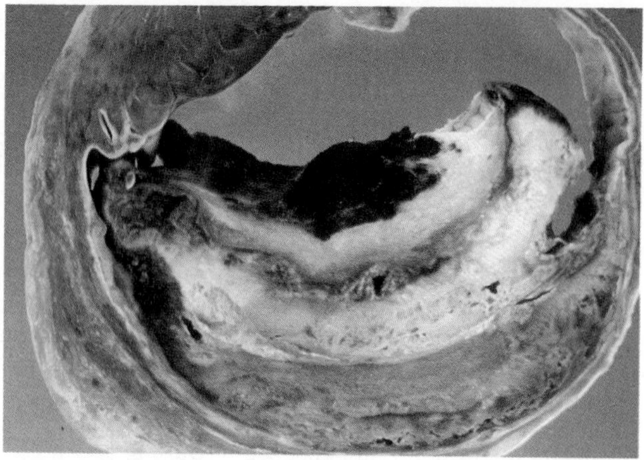

FIGURE 7-7
Mural thrombus of the left ventricle. A laminated thrombus adheres to the endocardium overlying a healed aneurysmal myocardial infarct.

The more common sites of infarction from arterial emboli are summarized in Figure 7-8.

Air Embolism

Air may be introduced into the venous circulation through neck wounds, thoracocentesis, punctures of the great veins during invasive procedures, and hemodialysis. Small amounts of circulating air in the form of bubbles are of little consequence, but quantities of 100 mL or more can lead to sudden death. Air bubbles tend to coalesce and physically obstruct the flow of blood in the right side of the heart, the pulmonary circulation, and the brain. On histological examination, bubbles of air, which appear as empty spaces, can be seen in the capillaries and small vessels of the lung.

Persons exposed to increased atmospheric pressure, such as scuba divers and workers in underwater occupations (e.g., tunnels, drilling platform construction) are subject to **decompression sickness**, a unique form of gas embolism. During descent, large amounts of inert gas (nitrogen or helium) are dissolved in body fluids. When the diver ascends, the gas is released from solution and exhaled. However, if the ascent is too rapid, gas bubbles form in the circulation and within tissues, obstructing blood flow and directly injuring cells. Air embolism is the second most common cause of death in sport diving (drowning being the first).

Acute decompression sickness, commonly known as "**the bends**," is characterized by temporary muscular and joint pain, owing to small vessel obstruction in these tissues. However, involvement of the cerebral blood vessels may be severe enough to cause coma or even death.

Caisson disease refers to decompression sickness in which the vascular obstruction causes multiple foci of ischemic (avascular) necrosis of bone, particularly affecting the head of the femur, tibia, and humerus. This complication was originally described in construction workers in diving bells (caissons).

Amniotic Fluid Embolism

Amniotic fluid embolism refers to the entry of amniotic fluid containing fetal cells and debris into the maternal circulation through the open uterine and cervical veins. It is a rare maternal complication of childbirth, but when it occurs it is often catastrophic. This disorder usually occurs at the end of labor when the pulmonary emboli are composed of the solid epithelial constituents (squames) contained in the

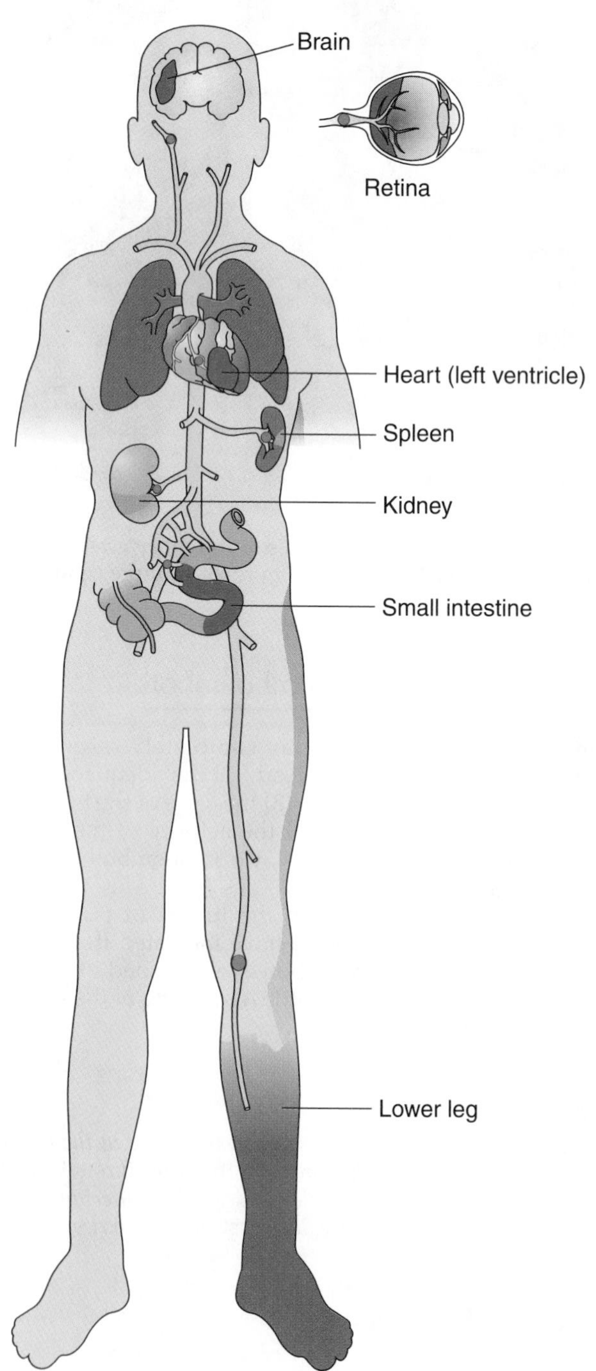

FIGURE 7-8
Common sites of infarction from arterial emboli.

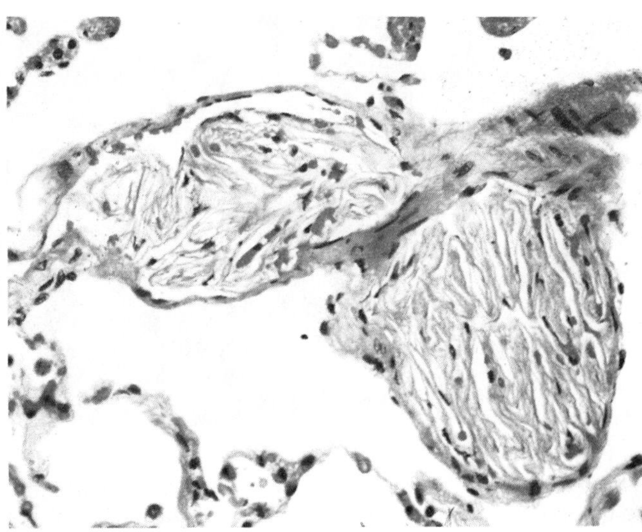

FIGURE 7-9
Amniotic fluid embolism. A section of lung shows pulmonary capillaries distended by epithelial squames.

amniotic fluid (Fig. 7-9). Of greater importance is the initiation of a potentially fatal consumptive coagulopathy caused by the high thromboplastin activity of amniotic fluid.

The clinical presentation of amniotic fluid embolism can be dramatic, with the sudden onset of cyanosis and shock, followed by coma and death. If the mother survives this acute episode, she may die of disseminated intravascular coagulation. Should she overcome this complication, she is at substantial risk of acute respiratory distress syndrome. Minor amniotic fluid embolism is probably a common asymptomatic event, since autopsies of mothers dying of other causes in the perinatal period frequently present evidence of this complication.

Fat Embolism

Fat embolism describes the release of emboli of fatty marrow (Fig. 7-10A) into damaged blood vessels following severe trauma to fat-containing tissue, particularly accompanying bone fractures. In most instances, fat embolism is clinically inapparent. However, cases of severe fat embolism are marked by the development of a **fat embolism syndrome**, which appears 1 to 3 days after the injury. In its most severe form, which may be fatal, this syndrome is characterized by respiratory failure, mental changes, thrombocytopenia, and widespread petechiae. A chest radiograph reveals a diffuse opacity, which may progress to a "white-out" typical of the adult respiratory distress syndrome. In such cases, at autopsy innumerable fat globules are seen in the microvasculature of the lungs (see Fig. 7-10B) and brain, and sometimes other organs. The lungs typically exhibit the changes of the adult respiratory distress syndrome (see Chapter 12). The lesions in the brain include cerebral edema, small hemorrhages, and occasionally microinfarcts.

Fat embolism is usually considered a direct consequence of trauma, with fat entering ruptured capillaries at the site of the fracture. However, this explanation may be too simplistic. It has been suggested that hemorrhage into the marrow cavity, and perhaps also into the subcutaneous fat, increases the interstitial pressure above capillary pressure, so that fat is forced into the circulation. Moreover, the amount of fat in the pulmonary vascular system is larger

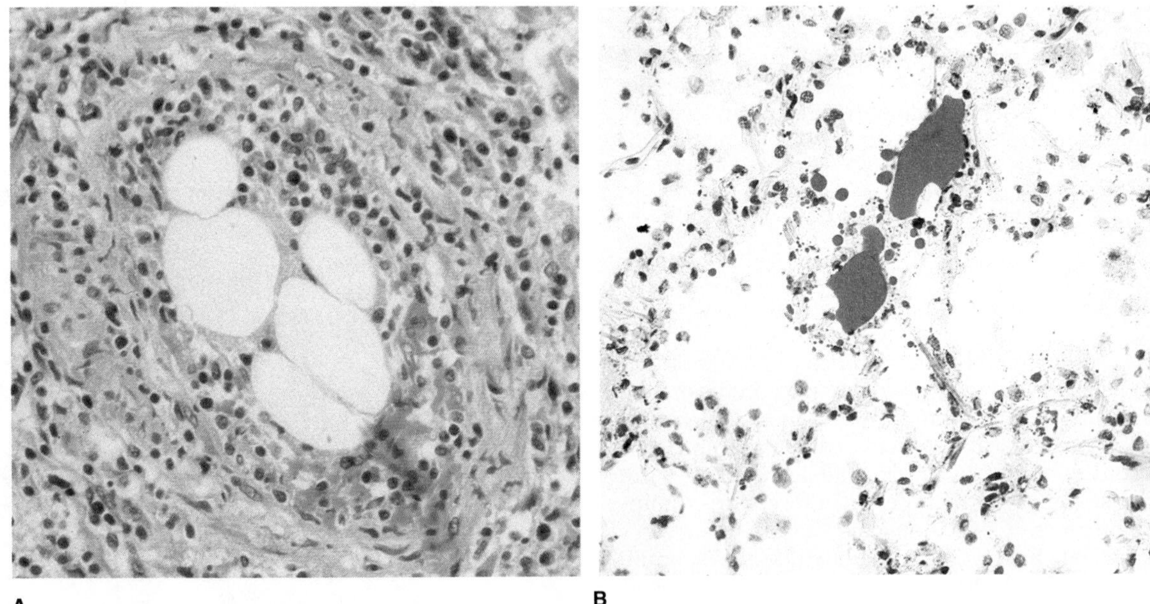

FIGURE 7-10
Fat embolism. (*A*) The lumen of a small pulmonary artery is occluded by a fragment of bone marrow consisting of fat cells and hemopoietic elements. (*B*) A frozen section of lung stained with sudan red shows capillaries occluded by red-staining fat emboli.

than can be accounted for by the simple transfer of fat from peripheral depots. In addition, the chemical composition of the fat in the lung is different from that in tissue. Finally, there is a discrepancy between the frequency of fat embolism and bone marrow embolism.

Bone Marrow Embolism

Bone marrow emboli, complete with hemopoietic cells and fat, are often seen in the lung at autopsy. They are usually encountered after cardiac resuscitation, a procedure in which fractures of the bones of the thorax, sternum, and ribs are common. No symptoms are attributed to bone marrow embolism.

Miscellaneous Pulmonary Emboli

Intravenous drug abusers who use talc as a carrier for illicit drugs may introduce it into the lung via the blood stream. These emboli produce a granulomatous response in the lungs. **Cotton emboli** are surprisingly common and are due to cleansing of the skin prior to venipuncture. **Schistosomiasis** may be associated with the embolization of ova to the lungs from the bladder or the gut, in which case they incite a foreign body granulomatous reaction. **Tumor emboli** are occasionally seen in the lung during hematogenous dissemination of cancer.

INFARCTION

Infarction is defined as the process by which coagulative necrosis develops in an area distal to the occlusion of an end-artery. The necrotic zone is termed an **infarct**. Infarcts of vital organs such as the heart, brain, and intestine are serioius medical conditions and are major causes of morbidity and mortality. If the victim survives, the infarct heals with a scar. Partial arterial occlusion (i.e., stenosis) occasionally causes necrosis, but more commonly it results in a variety of atrophic changes associated with chronic ischemia. For example, in the heart these changes include vacuolization of cardiac myocytes, atrophy, loss of muscle cell myofibrils, and interstitial fibrosis.

Pathology

The gross and microscopic appearance of an infarct depends on its location and age. On vascular occlusion, the area supplied by the vessel rapidly becomes swollen and deep red. Microscopically, vascular dilatation and congestion, and occasionally interstitial hemorrhage, are noted. Subsequently, two types of infarcts are distinguishable by gross examination: pale and red infarcts.

Pale infarcts are typical in the heart, kidneys, brain, and spleen (Fig. 7-11). Dry gangrene of the leg as a result of arterial occlusion, often noted in diabetes, is actually a large pale infarct. On gross examination, 1 or 2 days after the initial hyperemia, the infarct becomes soft, sharply delineated, and light yellow (Fig. 7-12). The border tends to be dark red, reflecting hemorrhage into the surrounding viable tissue. Microscopically, a pale infarct exhibits uniform coagulative necrosis.

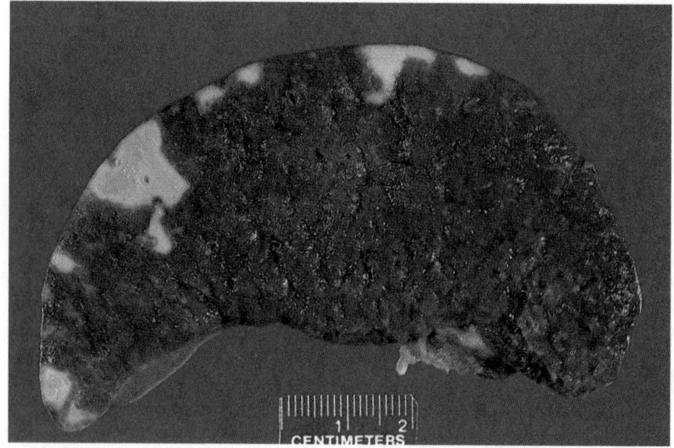

FIGURE 7-11
Spleen infarcts. A cut section of spleen shows multiple pale, wedge-shaped infarcts beneath the capsule.

Red infarcts, which may result from either arterial or venous occlusion, are also characterized by coagulative necrosis but are distinguished by bleeding into the necrotic area from adjacent arteries and veins. This occurs principally in organs with a dual blood supply, such as the lung, or those with extensive collateral circulation, such as the small intestine and brain. Grossly, red infarcts are sharply circumscribed, firm, and dark red to purple (Fig. 7-13).

Over a period of several days, acute inflammatory cells infiltrate the necrotic area from the viable border. The cellular debris is phagocytized and digested by polymorphonuclear leukocytes, and later by macrophages. Granulation tissue eventually forms, to be ultimately replaced by a scar. In a large infarct of an organ such as the heart or kidney, the necrotic center remains inaccessible to the inflammatory exudate and may persist for months. In the brain, an infarct typically undergoes liquefactive necrosis and may become a fluid-filled cyst.

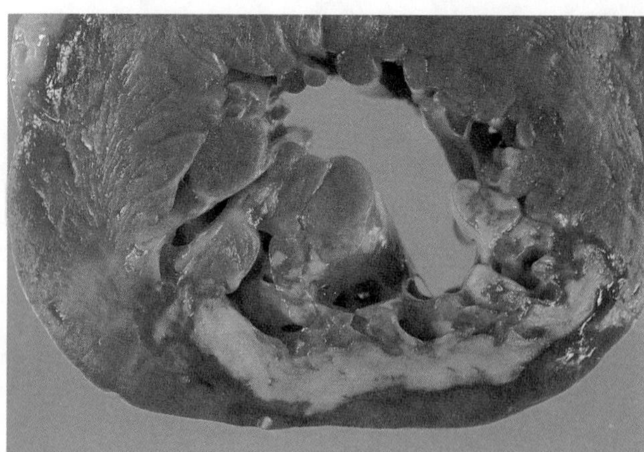

FIGURE 7-12
Acute myocardial infarct. A cross-section of the left ventricle reveals a sharply circumscribed, soft, yellow area of necrosis in the posterior wall.

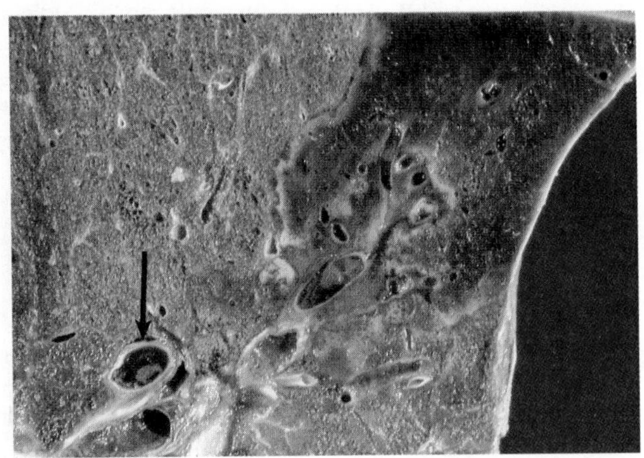

FIGURE 7-13
Pulmonary infarct. A section of lung shows a well-demarcated subpleural red infarct. An embolus (*arrow*) occludes the lumen of a small pulmonary artery at the apex of the infarct.

A septic infarct results when the necrotic tissue of an infarct is seeded by pyogenic bacteria and becomes infected. Pulmonary infarcts are not uncommonly infected, presumably because the necrotic tissue offers little resistance to inhaled bacteria. In the case of bacterial endocarditis, the emboli themselves are infected and the resulting infarcts are often septic. A septic infarct may became a frank abscess.

Infarction in Specific Locations

Myocardial Infarcts

Myocardial infarcts are transmural (through the entire wall) or subendocardial. A transmural infarct results from complete occlusion of a major extramural coronary artery. Subendocardial infarction reflects prolonged ischemia caused by partially occluding, atherosclerotic, stenotic lesions of the coronary arteries when the requirement for oxygen exceeds the supply. Such a situation prevails in disorders such as shock, anoxia, or severe tachycardia (rapid pulse). A myocardial infarct is initially pale, but hemorrhage occurs with reflow into the injured vascular bed.

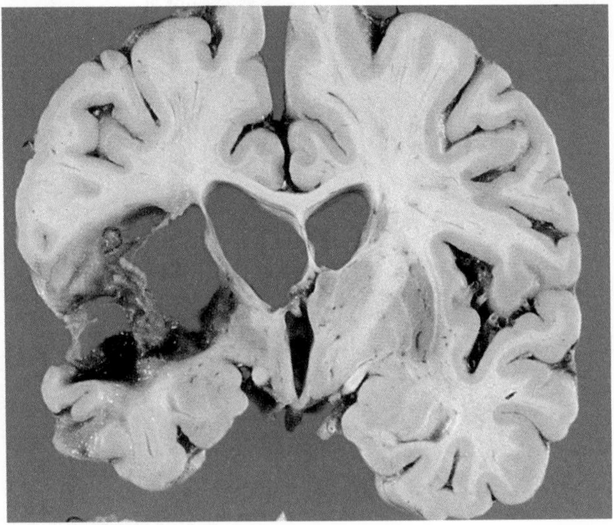

FIGURE 7-14
Cystic infarct of the brain. A section of the brain shows cystic transformation of an old infarct.

Pulmonary Infarcts

Only about 10% of pulmonary emboli elicit clinical symptoms referable to pulmonary infarction, usually after occlusion of a middle-sized pulmonary artery. Infarction occurs only if the circulation from the bronchial arteries inadequately compensates for the loss of supply from the pulmonary arteries. This circumstance is often found in congestive heart failure, although stasis in the pulmonary circulation may contribute. Hemorrhage into the alveolar spaces of the necrotic lining tissue occurs within 48 hours.

Cerebral Infarcts

Infarction of the brain may be the result of local ischemia or of a generalized reduction in blood flow. A generalized reduction in blood flow resulting from systemic hypotension, as in shock, produces infarction in the border zones between the distributions of the major cerebral arteries (watershed infarct). If prolonged, severe hypotension can cause widespread brain necrosis. The occlusion of a single vessel in the brain (e.g., after an embolus has lodged) causes ischemia and necrosis in a well-defined area. This type of cerebral infarct may be pale or red, the latter being common with embolic occlusions. The occlusion of a large artery produces a wide area of necrosis, which may ultimately resolve as a large fluid-filled cavity in the brain (Fig. 7-14).

Intestinal Infarcts

The earliest tissue changes in intestinal ischemia are necrosis of the tips of the villi in the small intestine and necrosis of the superficial mucosa in the large intestine. In either case, more severe ischemia leads to hemorrhagic necrosis of the submucosa and muscularis, but not the serosa. Small mucosal infarcts heal in a few days, but more severe injury leads to ulceration. These ulcers can eventually reepithelialize. However, if the ulcers are large, they are repaired by scar tissue, a process that may lead to strictures. Severe transmural necrosis is associated with massive bleeding or perforation, complications that often result in irreversible shock, sepsis, and death.

EDEMA

Edema refers to the presence of excess fluid in the interstitial spaces of the body. Edema may be local or generalized.

Local edema in most instances occurs with inflammation, the tumor of "tumor, rubor, and calor." Local edema of a limb, usually the leg, results from venous or lymphatic obstruction. Burns cause prominent local edema by disrupting the permeability of the local vasculature. Local edema may be a prominent component of an immune reaction, for example, urticaria (hives) or edema of the epiglottis or larynx (angioneurotic edema).

Generalized edema, affecting the visceral organs and the skin of the trunk and lower extremities (Fig. 7-15), reflects a global disorder of fluid and electrolyte metabolism, most often occasioned by heart failure. Generalized edema is also seen in certain renal diseases associated with loss of serum proteins to the urine (nephrotic syndrome), and in cirrhosis of the liver. **Anasarca** refers to extreme generalized edema, a condition evidenced by conspicuous fluid accumulation in the subcutaneous tissues, visceral organs, and body cavities. Edema fluid may accumulate in body spaces, such as the pleural cavity (hydrothorax), peritoneal cavity (ascites), or pericardial cavity (hydropericardium).

Mechanisms of Edema Formation

Normal Capillary Filtration

The normal formation and retention of interstitial fluid depends on filtration and reabsorption at the level of the capillaries (Starling forces). In the arteriolar segment of the capillary, the internal or hydrostatic pressure is 32 mm Hg, and at the middle of the capillary it is 20 mm. Since the interstitial hydrostatic pressure is only 3 mm Hg, there is an outward fluid filtration of 14 mL/min. The hydrostatic pressure is opposed by the oncotic pressure of the plasma (26 mm Hg), which results in an osmotic reabsorption of 12 mL/min at the venous end of the capillary. Thus, interstitial fluid is formed at the rate of 2 mL/min and is reabsorbed by the lymphatics, so that in equilibrium there is no net fluid gain or loss in the interstitium.

Sodium and Water Metabolism

Water represents 50% to 70% of body weight and comprises two major compartments—the extracellular and the intracellular fluid spaces. Extracellular fluid is further divided into interstitial and vascular compartments. Interstitial fluid constitutes roughly 75% of the extracellular compartment.

Total body sodium is the principal determinant of extracellular fluid volume, because sodium is the major cation that determines the osmolality of the extracellular fluid. In other words, an increase in total body sodium must be balanced by more extracellular water to maintain constant osmolality. The control of extracellular fluid volume depends to a large extent on the regulation of renal sodium excretion, which is influenced by (1) atrial natriuretic factor, (2) the renin–angiotensin system of the juxtaglomerular apparatus, and (3) sympathetic nervous system activity.

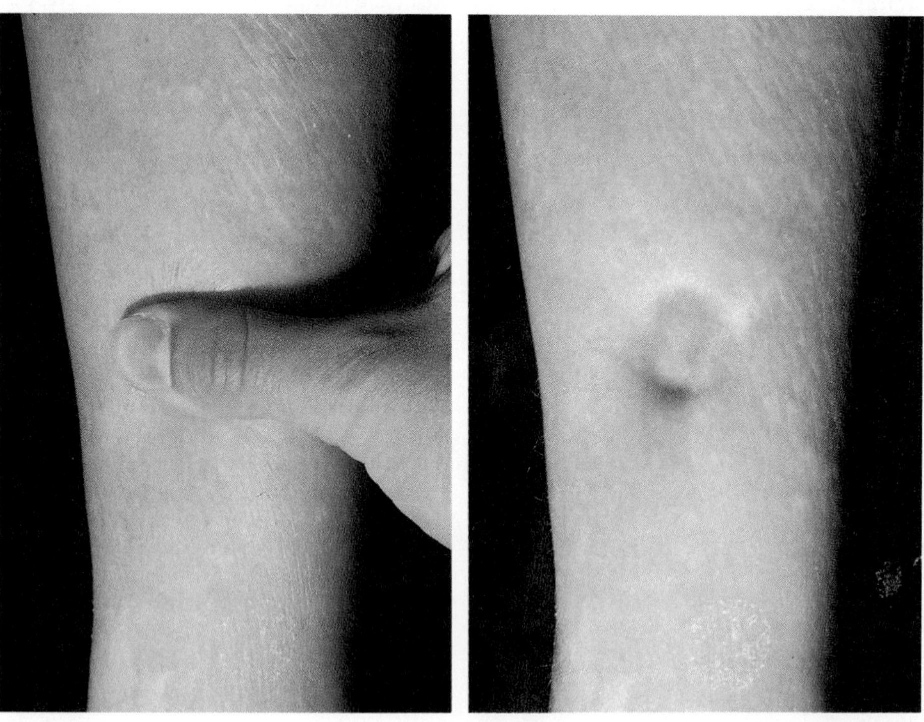

FIGURE 7-15
Pitting edema of the leg. (*A*) In a patient with congestive heart failure, severe edema of the leg is demonstrated by applying pressure with a finger. (*B*) The resulting "pitting" reflects the inelasticity of the fluid-filled tissue.

Edema Caused by Increased Hydrostatic Pressure

It is intuitively clear that an unopposed increase in hydrostatic pressure will result in greater filtration of fluid into the interstitial space and its retention as edema. Such a situation is particularly prominent in the case of decompensated heart disease, in which back-pressure in the lungs secondary to failure of the left ventricle leads to acute pulmonary edema, and failure of the right side of the heart contributes to systemic edema. Similarly, back-pressure caused by venous obstruction in the lower extremity causes edema of the leg. Obstruction to portal blood flow in cirrhosis of the liver contributes to the formation of abdominal fluid (ascites).

Edema Caused by Decreased Oncotic Pressure

The difference in pressure between the intravascular and interstitial compartments is largely determined by the concentration of plasma proteins, especially that of albumin. Any condition that lowers plasma albumin levels, whether it be albuminuria in the nephrotic syndrome or reduced albumin synthesis in chronic liver disease, tends to promote generalized edema.

Edema Caused by Lymphatic Obstruction

Under normal circumstances, more fluid is filtered into the interstitial spaces than is reabsorbed into the vascular bed. This excess interstitial fluid is removed by the lymphatics. Thus, obstruction to the lymphatic flow leads to localized edema formation. Lymphatic channels can be obstructed by (1) malignant tumors, (2) fibrosis resulting from inflammation or irradiation, and (3) surgical ablation. For instance, the inflammatory response to filarial worms (Bancroftian and Malayan filariasis) can result in lymphatic obstruction that produces massive lymphedema of the scrotum and lower extremities (elephantiasis) (Fig. 7-16). Lymphedema of the upper extremity often complicates radical mastectomies for cancer of the breast, owing to the removal of the axillary lymph nodes and lymphatics.

Lymphatic edema difers from other forms of edema in its high protein content, since lymph is the vehicle by which proteins and interstitial cells are returned to the circulation. The increased protein concentration may be a fibrogenic stimulus in the formation of dermal fibrosis in chronic edema (indurated edema).

The Role of Sodium Retention in Edema

Generalized edema and ascites invariably reflect an increased total body sodium content, as a consequence of sodium retention by the kidneys. When peripheral edema is first clinically detectable, the extracellular fluid volume has already expanded by at least 5 L. The most common conditions in which generalized edema is found include congestive heart failure, cirrhosis of the liver,

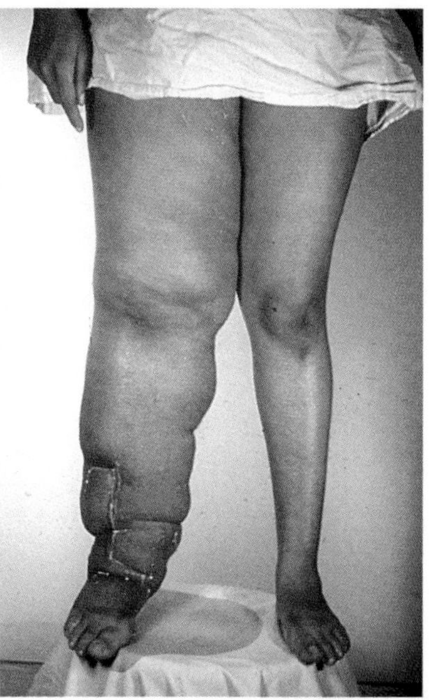

FIGURE *7-16*
Edema secondary to lymphatic obstruction. Massive edema of the right lower extremity (elephantiasis) in a patient with obstruction of the lymphatic drainage.

nephrotic syndrome, and some cases of chronic renal insufficiency.

The mechanisms of edema formation and representative disorders associated with them are summarized in Figure 7-17 and Table 7-1.

Congestive Heart Failure

Congestive heart failure describes the consequences of inadequate cardiac output relative to the needs of the body. It is estimated that two to three million people in the United States have congestive heart failure, and 15% die annually. In fact, half of all patients with congestive heart failure who require admission to the hospital will die within 1 year. In the United States, this disorder is most commonly associated with ischemic heart disease, although virtually any chronic cardiac disorder may eventuate in congestive heart failure (see Chapter 11).

☐ **Pathogenesis:** The argument regarding the relative contributions of "forward failure" (low cardiac output) versus "backward failure" (venous congestion) in the pathogenesis of the edema of congestive heart failure is no longer a burning issue. It is now recognized that both systolic and diastolic dysfunction contribute to the low cardiac output and high ventricular filling pressure characteristic of congestive heart failure, although systolic dysfunction is more important in the majority of patients.

The inadequacy of the cardiac output in congestive heart failure leads to a decreased glomerular filtration rate and and an increased secretion of renin. The latter activates angiotensin, leading to the release of aldosterone,

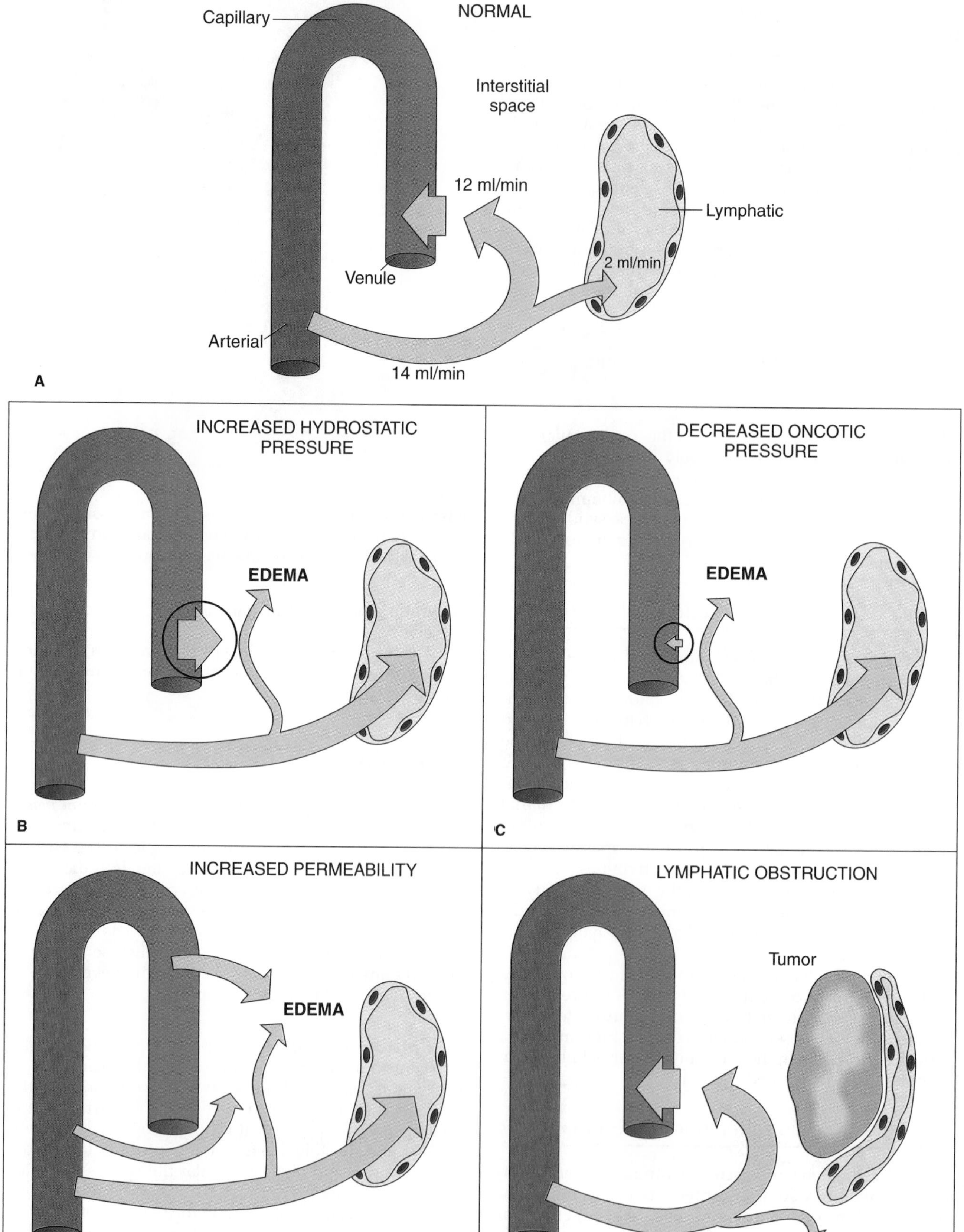

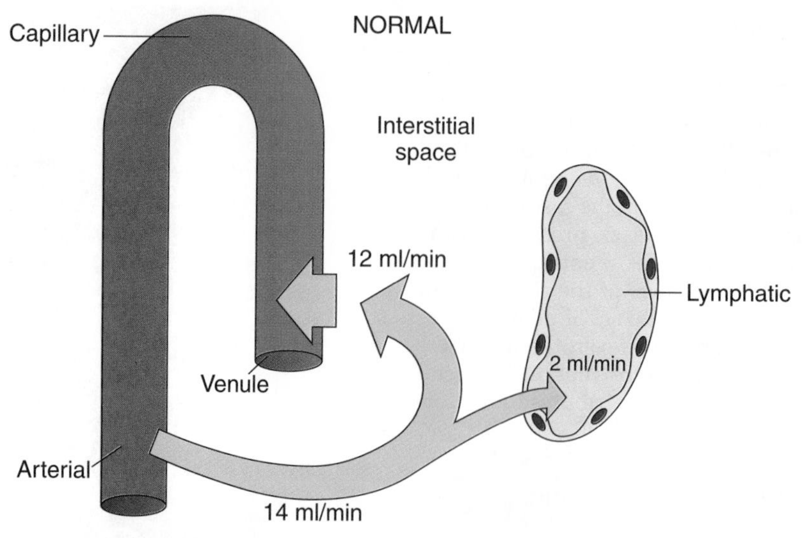
NORMAL
Capillary
Interstitial space
12 ml/min
Lymphatic
2 ml/min
Venule
Arterial
14 ml/min
A

INCREASED HYDROSTATIC PRESSURE
EDEMA
B
DECREASED ONCOTIC PRESSURE
EDEMA
C
INCREASED PERMEABILITY
EDEMA
D
LYMPHATIC OBSTRUCTION
Tumor
EDEMA
E

FIGURE 7-17

TABLE 7-1 **Disorders Associated with Edema**

Increased hydrostatic pressure	
Arteriolar dilatation	Inflammation Heat
Increased venous pressure	Venous thrombosis Congestive heart failure Cirrhosis (ascites) Postural inactivity (e.g., prolonged standing)
Hypervolemia	Sodium retention (e.g., decreased renal function)
Decreased oncotic pressure	
Hypoproteinemia	Nephrotic syndrome Cirrhosis Protein-losing gastroenteropathy Malnutrition
Increased capillary permeability	Inflammation Burns Adult respiratory distress syndrome
Lymphatic obstruction	Cancer Postsurgical lymphedema Inflammation

subsequent sodium reabsorption, and fluid retention. Furthermore, reduced blood flow to the liver impairs the catabolism of aldosterone, thereby further raising its concentration in the blood. The increased fluid volume is a compensatory mechanism that preserves an adequate intracardiac pressure. In addition, increased sympathetic discharge and the augmented levels of catecholamines stimulate cardiac contractility, thereby further counteracting the impairment in cardiac performance. At the same time, distention of the atria by the increased blood volume promotes the release of atrial natriuretic peptide, which stimulates sodium excretion by the kidney.

After longstanding heart failure, these compensatory mechanisms fail, in which case renal sodium retention again becomes important. The further expansion of plasma volume leads to an increase in pulmonary and systemic venous pressure, which produces increased hydrostatic pressure in the respective capillary beds. The increased capillary pressure, together with decreased plasma oncotic pressure, results in the edema of congestive heart failure.

☐ **Pathology:** Failure of the left ventricle is associated principally with passive congestion of the lungs and pulmonary edema (Fig. 7-18). In turn, chronic passive congestion leads to pulmonary hypertension and eventual failure of the right ventricle. Right ventricular failure is characterized by generalized subcutaneous edema, most prominent in the dependent portions of the body, ascites, and pleural effusions. The liver, spleen, and other splanchnic organs are typically congested. At autopsy, the heart is enlarged and its chambers dilated.

☐ **Clinical Features:** Patients in congestive heart failure complain of shortness of breath (dyspnea) on exertion and when recumbent (orthopnea). They may be awakened from sleep by sudden episodes of shortness of breath (paroxysmal nocturnal dyspnea). Physical examination usually reveals distended jugular veins and pitting edema of the lower extremities. The liver is enlarged and tender; when ascites is present, the abdomen is distended. Patients in congestive heart failure with pulmonary edema have crackling breath sounds (rales) caused by the expansion of fluid-filled alveoli.

Pulmonary Edema

Pulmonary edema refers to increased fluid in the alveolar spaces and interstitium of the lung. This condition leads to decreased gas exchange in the lung, causing hypoxia and retention of carbon dioxide (hypercapnia).

☐ **Pathogenesis and Pathology:** The lung is a loose tissue without much connective tissue support and, therefore, requires certain conditions to prevent the development of edema. Among these protective devices are the following:

- Low perfusion pressure in the lung capillaries owing to low right ventricular pressure

FIGURE 7-17
The capillary system and mechanisms of edema formation. (*A*) *Normal.* The differential between the hydrostatic and oncotic pressures at the arterial end of the capillary system is responsible for the filtration into the interstitial space of approximately 14 mL of fluid per minute. This fluid is reabsorbed at the venous end at the rate of 12 mL/min. It is also drained through the lymphatic capillaries at a rate of 2 mL/min. Proteins are removed by the lymphatics from the interstitial space. (*B*) *Hydrostatic edema.* If the hydrostatic pressure at the venous end of the capillary system is elevated, reabsorption is decreased. As long as the lymphatics are able to drain the surplus fluid, no edema results. If their capacity is exceeded, however, edema fluid accumulates. (*C*) *Oncotic edema.* Edema fluid also accumulates if reabsorption is diminished by a decrease in the oncotic pressure of the vascular bed, owing to a loss of albumin. (*D*) *Inflammatory and traumatic edema.* Edema, either local or systemic, results if the vascular bed becomes leaky following injury to the endothelium. (*E*) *Lymphedema.* Lymphatic obstruction causes the accumulation of interstitial fluid because of insufficient reabsorption and deficient removal of proteins, the latter increasing the oncotic pressure of the fluid in the interstitial space.

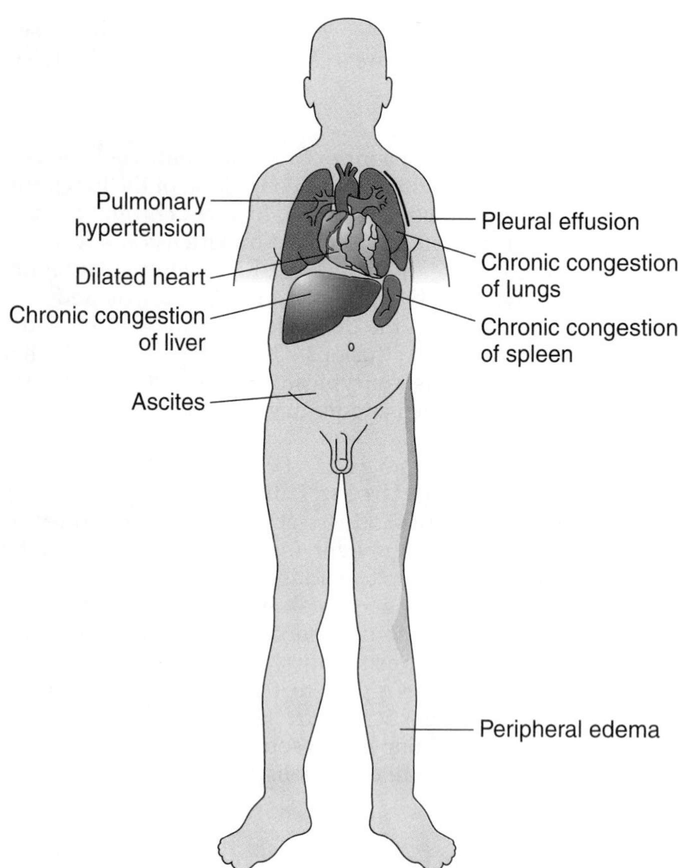

FIGURE *7-18*
Pathological consequences of chronic congestive heart failure.

- Effective drainage of the interstitial space of the lung by lymphatics, which are under a slightly negative pressure and can accommodate up to 10 times the regular lymph flow
- Tight cellular junctions between endothelial cells, which control capillary permeability

If these protective mechanisms are perturbed, pulmonary edema results. The most common causes of pulmonary edema relate to hemodynamic alterations in the heart that increase the perfusion pressure in the pulmonary capillaries and block effective lymphatic drainage. These include left ventricular failure (the most common cause), mitral stenosis, and mitral insufficiency. Disruption of capillary permeability is the cause of pulmonary edema in acute lung injury associated with the adult respiratory distress syndrome, inhalation of toxic gases, aspiration of gastric contents, viral infections, and uremia. Acute lung injury is reflected in destruction of endothelial cells or disruption of their tight junctions.

Pulmonary edema may be interstitial or alveolar. Interstitial edema represents the earliest phase and is an exaggeration of the normal process of fluid filtration. Lymphatics become distended and fluid accumulates in the interstitium of the lobular septa and around veins and the bronchovascular bundles. Radiological examination reveals a reticulonodular pattern, more marked in the bases of the lung. Lobular septa become edematous and produce linear shadows (Kerley B lines). Edema results in the shunting of blood flow from the bases to the upper lobes of the lungs, and increased airflow resistance occurs because of edema of the bronchovascular tree. Patients are often asymptomatic in this early stage.

When the fluid can no longer be contained in the interstitial space, it spills into the alveoli, a condition termed **alveolar edema**. At this stage, a radiological alveolar pattern is seen, usually worse in the central portions of the lung and in the lower zones. The patient becomes acutely short of breath and bubbly rales are heard. In extreme cases, frothy fluid is coughed up or wells up out of the trachea.

Sections of the edematous lung reveal severely congested alveolar capillaries and alveoli filled with a homogeneous, pink-staining fluid permeated by air bubbles (Fig. 7-19). In cases of pulmonary edema caused by alveolar damage, cell debris, fibrin, and proteins form films of proteinaceous material, called hyaline membranes, in the alveoli.

☐ **Clinical Features:** Pulmonary fluid accumulation may go unnoticed initially, but eventually dyspnea and coughing become prominent. If the edema is severe, large amounts of frothy sputum, which is often pink, are expectorated. Hypoxemia is manifested as cyanosis.

Pulmonary function is restricted in severe congestion and in interstitial pulmonary edema because the accumulation of fluid in the interstitial space causes reduced compliance—that is, a stiffening of the lung tissue. Thus, increased respiratory work is required to maintain

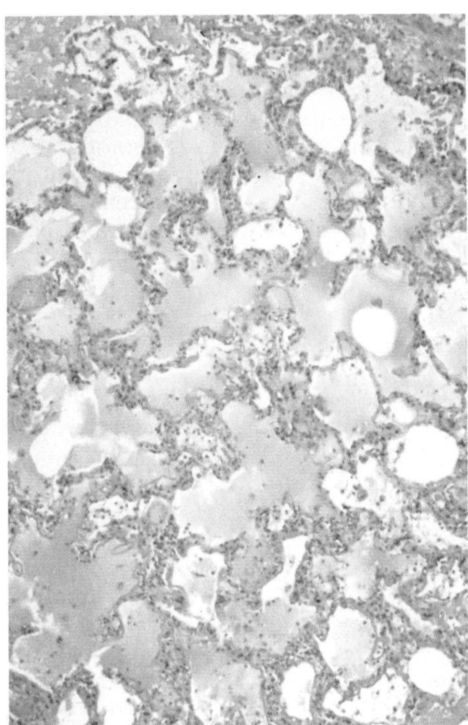

FIGURE 7-19
Pulmonary edema. A photomicrograph of the lung from a patient in acute left-sided heart failure shows pink-staining fluid filling the alveoli.

ventilation. Since the alveolar walls are thickened, there is a greater barrier to the exchange of oxygen and carbon dioxide. The exchange of carbon dioxide is less affected than that of oxygen, a situation that results in hypoxia with near-normal carbon dioxide levels.

Edema in Cirrhosis of the Liver

Cirrhosis of the liver is often accompanied by ascites and peripheral edema. Scarring of the liver obstructs the portal blood flow and leads to portal hypertension, a condition that increases the hydrostatic pressure in the splanchnic circulation. This situation is compounded by a decreased hepatic synthesis of albumin as a result of liver dysfunction. The consequent accumulation of peritoneal fluid leads to a decreased effective blood volume, which results in renal retention of sodium by mechanisms similar to those that are operative in congestive heart failure. Alternatively, chronic liver disease itself causes renal retention of sodium. The subsequent expansion of extracellular fluid volume further promotes ascites and edema, thus establishing a vicious circle. In addition, the increased transudation of lymph from the liver capsule adds to the accumulation of fluid in the abdomen.

The Nephrotic Syndrome

The nephrotic syndrome is caused by a massive loss of protein to the urine, the magnitude of which exceeds the rate at which it is replaced by the liver. The resulting decline in the concentration of plasma proteins, particularly albumin, reduces the oncotic pressure of the plasma and promotes edema. The ensuing decrease in blood volume stimulates the renin–angiotensin–aldosterone mechanism, leading to sodium retention. The edema is generalized but appears preferentially in soft connective tissues, the eyes, the eyelids, and subcutaneous tissue. Ascites and pleural effusions also occur.

Cerebral Edema

Edema of the brain is dangerous because the confined space of the cranium allows little room for expansion. Increased intracranial pressure from edema compromises the blood supply, distorts the gross structure of the brain, and interferes with the function of the central nervous system (see Chapter 28). Cerebral edema is divided into vasogenic, cytotoxic, and interstitial forms.

Vasogenic edema, the most common variety of edema, refers to excess fluid in the extracellular space of the brain. It results from increased vascular permeability, principally in the white matter. The tight endothelial junctions of the blood-brain barrier are disrupted, and fluid filters into the interstitial space. Clinical disorders associated with cerebral vasogenic edema include trauma, tumors, encephalitis, abscesses, infarcts, hemorrhage, and toxic brain injury (e.g., lead poisoning).

Cytotoxic edema is equivalent to hydropic cell swelling (i.e., the accumulation of intracellular water). It is usually a response to cell injury, such as that produced by ischemia. Cytotoxic cerebral edema preferentially affects the gray matter.

Interstitial edema is a consequence of hydrocephalus, in which fluid accumulates in the cerebral ventricles and periventricular white matter.

At autopsy, the edematous brain is soft and heavy. The gyri are flattened and the sulci narrowed. Because of alterations in brain function, patients with cerebral edema suffer vomiting, disorientation, and convulsions. Severe cerebral edema leads to herniation of the cerebral tonsils, ordinarily a lethal event.

Fluid Accumulation in Body Cavities

The body cavities, such as the pericardium and the pleural and peritoneal spaces, are extensions of the interstitial space.

The Pleural Space

Pleural effusion (i.e., fluid in the pleural space) is a straw-colored transudate of low specific gravity that contains few cells (mainly exfoliated mesothelial cells). Fluid commonly accumulates as an expression of a generalized tendency to form edema in diseases such as the nephrotic syndrome, cirrhosis of the liver, and congestive heart failure. Pleural effusion is also a frequent response to an inflammatory process or tumor in the lung or on the pleural surface.

The Pericardium

Fluid in the pericardial cavity may result from either hemorrhage (hemopericardium) or injury to the pericardium (pericardial effusion). Pericardial effusions occur with pericardial infections, metastatic tumors to the pericardium, uremia, and systemic lupus erythematosus. They are also occasionally encountered after cardiac operations (postpericardiotomy syndrome) or after radiation therapy for cancer.

Pericardial fluid may accumulate rapidly, particularly with hemorrhage caused by a ruptured myocardial infarct, dissecting aortic aneurysm, or trauma. In this circumstance, the pressure in the pericardial cavity rises to exceed the filling pressure of the heart, a condition termed **cardiac tamponade** (Fig. 7-20). The resulting precipitous decline in cardiac output is often fatal. When fluid in the pericardium accumulates rapidly, the tolerable limit may be only 90 to 120 mL, but a liter or more of fluid can be accommodated when the process is gradual.

The Peritoneum

Peritoneal effusion, also called ascites, is caused mainly by cirrhosis of the liver, abdominal tumors, pancreatitis, cardiac failure, the nephrotic syndrome, and hepatic venous obstruction (Budd-Chiari syndrome). Obstruction of the thoracic duct by cancer may lead to chylous ascites, in which the fluid has a milky appearance and a high fat content. The pathogenesis of ascites in cirrhosis of the liver was discussed earlier.

Patients with severe ascites accumulate many liters of fluid and have a conspicuously distended abdomen. The complications of ascites derive from increased abdominal pressure and include anorexia and vomiting, reflux esophagitis, dyspnea, ventral hernia, and leakage of fluid into the pleural space.

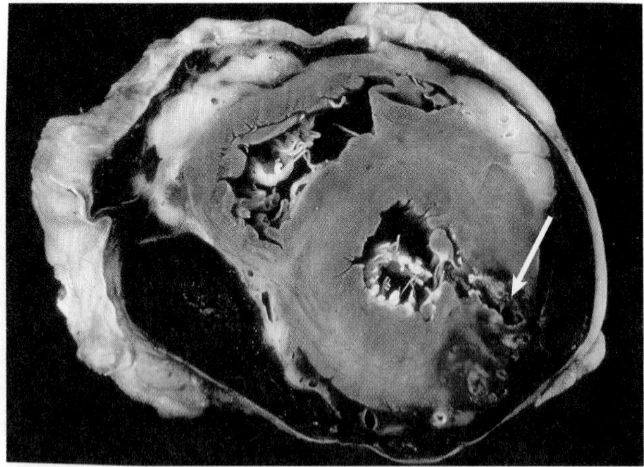

FIGURE *7-20*
Cardiac tamponade. A cross-section of the heart shows rupture of a myocardial infarct (*arrow*) with the accumulation of a large quantity of blood in the pericardial cavity.

FLUID LOSS AND OVERLOAD

Excessive fluid loss (dehydration) and fluid overload are clinical situations that have potentially grave consequences. Fluid imbalance causes hemodynamic disorders; alterations in the osmolality and quantity of the fluid in the intravascular, interstitial, and cellular spaces may affect perfusion or the delivery of substrates, electrolytes, or fluids.

Dehydration

Dehydration refers to a condition in which there is inadequate fluid to fill the fluid compartments of the body. Such a condition results from insufficient fluid intake or excessive fluid loss or both. Water loss may exceed intake in cases of vomiting, diarrhea, burns, excessive sweating, and diabetes insipidus. When excessive fluid loss occurs, fluid is recruited from the interstitial space to the plasma space. The fluids in the cell and within the interstitial and vascular compartments become more concentrated, particularly if there is a preferential loss of water, such as during inappropriate secretion of antidiuretic hormone in diabetes insipidus. When patients suffer from burns, vomiting, excessive sweating, or diarrhea, they not only lose fluid but also suffer electrolyte disturbances.

Clinically, only dryness of the skin and mucous membranes is noted initially, but as dehydration progresses the turgor of the skin is lost. If dehydration persists, oliguria (reduced urine output) occurs as a compensation for the fluid loss. More severe degrees of fluid loss are accompanied by a shift of water from the intracellular space to the extracellular space, a process that causes severe cell dysfunction, particularly in the brain. Shrinkage of brain tissue may result in the rupture of small vessels and subsequent bleeding. Systemic blood pressure falls with continuous dehydration, and declining perfusion eventually leads to death.

Overhydration

Excessive hydration occurs when fluid intake exceeds the compensatory capacity of the kidney to excrete a fluid overload. This is ordinarily a rare situation, unless renal injury limits the excretory function of the kidney, or unless the kidney is prevented from proper counter-regulation (e.g., through excessive secretion of antidiuretic hormone).

Fluid overload today is mostly iatrogenic, caused by the administration of excessive amounts of intravenous fluids. The most serious effect of this type of fluid overload is the induction of cerebral edema or congestive heart failure in patients with cardiac dysfunction.

SHOCK

Shock is a condition of profound hemodynamic and metabolic disturbance characterized by failure of the circulatory system to maintain an appropriate blood supply to the microcirculation, with consequent inadequate perfusion of vital organs. In this often catastrophic circumstance, tissue perfusion and oxygen delivery fall below the levels required to meet normal demands, including a failure to remove metabolites adequately. The term **shock** encompasses all the reactions that occur in response to such disturbances. In the course of uncompensated shock, a rapid circulatory collapse leads to impaired cellular metabolism and death. However, in many cases, compensatory mechanisms sustain the patient, at least for a while. When these adaptations fail, shock becomes irreversible.

Shock is not synonymous with low blood pressure, although hypotension is commonly a part of the shock syndrome. Hypotension is actually a late sign in shock and indicates a failure of compensation. At the same time that peripheral blood flow falls below critical levels, extreme vasoconstriction can maintain arterial blood pressure. This distinction between shock and hypotension is important clinically because the rapid restoration of systemic blood flow is the primary goal in treating shock. When blood pressure alone is raised with vasopressive drugs, systemic blood flow may actually be diminished.

Pathogenesis

Decreased perfusion in shock is generally the result of a decreased cardiac output, resulting either from the inability of the heart to pump the normal venous return or from a decreased volume of blood secondary to a decreased venous return. These two mechanisms, which lead to a decreased cardiac output, define the two major types of shock: cardiogenic and hypovolemic shock (Fig. 7-21).

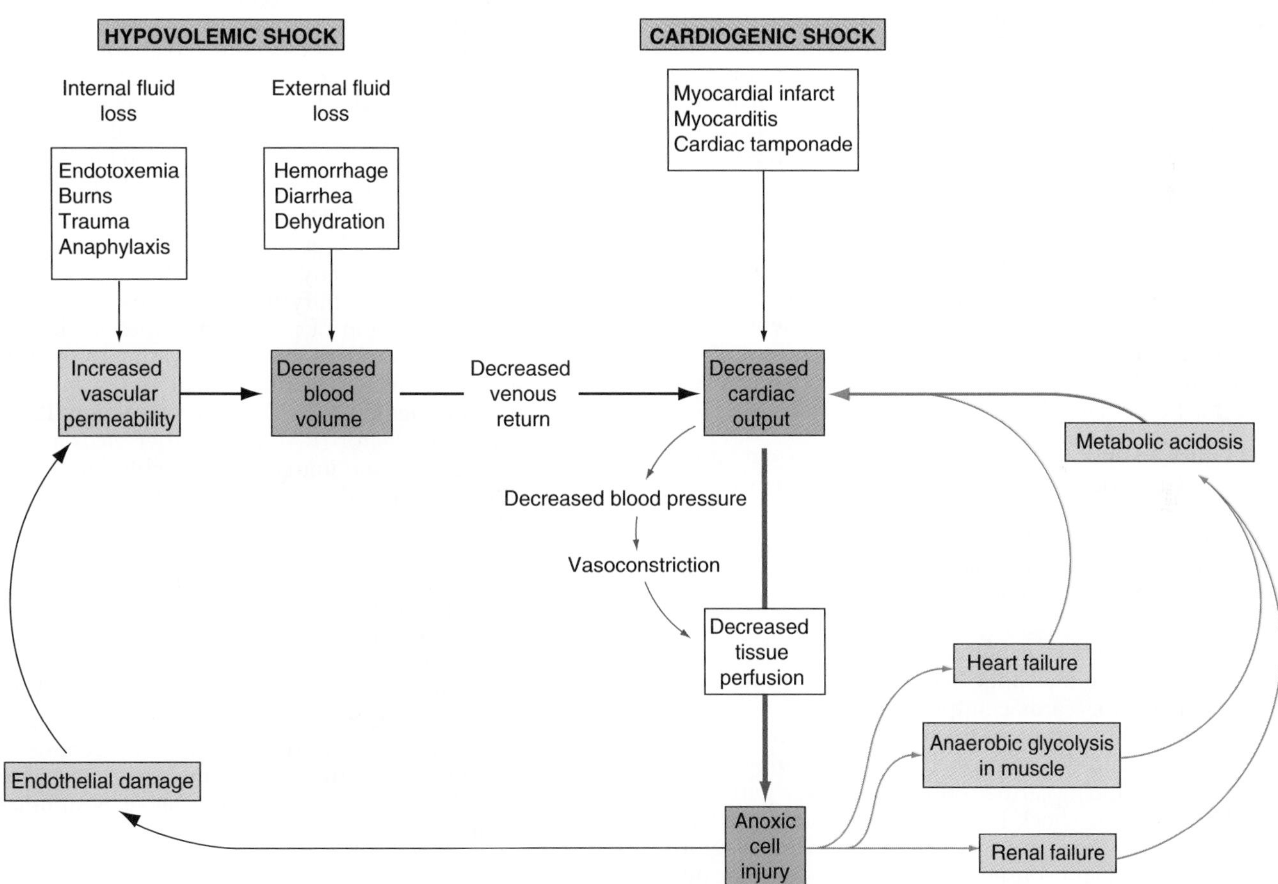

FIGURE *7-21*
The pathogenesis of shock. This drawing shows the integration of many factors in the progression of shock. Shock is initiated by one of two principal events: pump failure, or "cardiogenic shock," and loss of circulatory volume, also called "hypovolemic shock." Hypovolemic shock follows internal fluid loss, such as that in endotoxemia, burns, trauma, or anaphylaxis, or external fluid loss, such as that caused by hemorrhage, diarrhea, and dehydration. The effect of both events is decreased cardiac output and decreased tissue perfusion. The resulting anoxic cell injury sets into motion several vicious circles. Metabolic acidosis (renal failure, increased anaerobic glycolysis) and heart failure lead to a further decline in cardiac output. Endothelial damage increases vascular permeability and decreases effective blood volume, reducing venous return and decreasing cardiac output.

Cardiogenic shock is usually caused by myocardial infarction, and less commonly by myocarditis. In these conditions, depressed systolic cardiac function (ejection fraction <20%) is responsible for the decreased cardiac output. Events that prevent left or right heart filling reduce cardiac output, resulting in "obstructive" shock. Such conditions include pulmonary embolism, cardiac tamponade, and rarely atrial myxoma.

Hypovolemic shock is secondary to a pronounced decrease in blood volume, caused by the loss of fluid from the vascular compartment. Hemorrhage, diarrhea, excessive urine formation, and perspiration are the major mechanisms of external fluid loss. Internal fluid loss usually results from an increase in the permeability of the microvasculature caused by endotoxemia, burns, trauma, or anaphylaxis. In the case of burns or trauma, direct damage to the microcirculation increases vascular permeability. Immunological mechanisms, coupled to the activation of complement and the release of anaphylotoxins, enhance vascular permeability in anaphylaxis. Neurogenic shock can follow acute injury to the brain or spinal cord, which impairs the neural control of vasomotor tone, thereby leading to generalized vasodilatation. The subsequent redistribution of blood to the periphery reduces the effective circulating volume and causes a type of hypovolemic shock (distributive shock).

In both hypovolemic and cardiogenic shock, a decreased cardiac output and resultant decreased tissue perfusion comprise the essential pathogenetic mechanisms in the progression from reversible to irreversible shock. Anoxic injury is the common cellular consequence of the initial decrease in tissue perfusion (see Fig. 7-21). A vicious circle of decreasing tissue perfusion and further cell injury is perpetuated by several mechanisms:

- Injury to endothelial cells, secondary to the anoxia caused by decreased tissue perfusion, increases vascular permeability.
- The increased exudation of fluid from the circulation reduces (1) blood volume, (2) venous return, and (3) cardiac output, thereby aggravating anoxic cell injury.
- Decreased perfusion of the kidneys and skeletal muscles results in metabolic acidosis, which in turn further decreases cardiac output and tissue perfusion.
- Decreased perfusion of the heart injures the myocardial cells and decreases their ability to pump blood, further reducing cardiac output and tissue perfusion.
- Hypovolemic shock is caused by a pronounced decrease in blood volume, which reduces venous return to the heart and consequently decreases cardiac output.

Septic Shock (Endotoxic Shock)

Septicemia with gram-negative organisms is the most common cause of septic shock. The invading bacteria are responsible for the release of **endotoxin**, a term historically used to describe the cell-associated toxin found in gram-negative bacteria. Endotoxin is now known to be a lipopolysaccharide (LPS), the toxic activity of which resides in the lipid A component. On entry of LPS into the circulation, it binds to a specific protein, after which the complex binds to the CD14 receptor on the surface of monocytes/macrophages. The latter binding causes these cells to secrete large quantities of tumor necrosis factor (TNF), a cytokine that mediates the overwhelming cardiovascular collapse characteristic of septic shock. TNF may also be involved in the pathogenesis of shock unassociated with endotoxemia. Although LPS may be the most potent stimulus for the release of TNF, other antigens also stimulate its biosynthesis and secretion. These include toxin-1 of the toxic shock syndrome, enterotoxin, antigens of mycobacteria, fungi, parasites, and viruses, and products of complement activation.

Tumor necrosis factor exerts beneficial effects by enhancing remodeling, wound healing, and the defense against local infections. However, in septic shock this protein is suddenly released in great excess by exposure of macrophages to bacterial endotoxin, resulting in effects that are often lethal. The infusion of large amounts of TNF to animals precipitates a syndrome strikingly similar to that of human septic shock. The administration of anti-TNF antibody before exposure of the animal to endotoxin or to the gram-negative bacteria completely protects against the development of septic shock. Unfortunately, clinical trials of agents that block TNF or its receptor have thus far not been successful in ameliorating septic shock in humans.

The mechanisms by which TNF precipitates shock are not fully elucidated. TNF appears to have a direct toxic effect on endothelial cells, although the reason is unclear. TNF also acts indirectly by (1) initiating a cascade of other mediators that amplify its deleterious effects, (2) promoting the adhesion of polymorphonuclear leukocytes to endothelial surfaces, and (3) activating the extrinsic coagulation pathway. The presence of TNF stimulates the release of interleukin-1 (IL-1) and interleukin-6 (IL-6), platelet activating factor (PAF), and other eicosanoids that may mediate tissue injury. Interestingly, nonlethal doses of TNF become lethal when administered together with small amounts of IL-1. TNF also increases the expression of intercellular adhesion molecules (ICAMs) and endothelial-leukocyte adhesion molecules (ELAMs) on endothelial surfaces, thereby promoting leukostasis. This mechanism presumably plays a role in the respiratory distress syndrome induced by the infusion of TNF, in which leukocytes aggregate in the pulmonary vasculature. Activated neutrophils sequestered in the pulmonary circulation are believed to be important in the pathogenesis of the adult respiratory distress syndrome associated with septic shock. The pathogenesis of septic shock is summarized in Figure 7-22.

SYSTEMIC INFLAMMATORY RESPONSE SYNDROME (SIRS)/MULTIPLE ORGAN DYSFUNCTION SYNDROME (MODS): Improvements in the early treatment of shock and sepsis have allowd patients to survive long enough to manifest a new problem, namely progressive deterioration of organ function. Almost all septic patients suffer from dysfunction of at least one organ, and MODS is seen in one third of the cases. MODS also develops in one third of patients afflicted by trauma or burns and in a quarter of those with acute pancreatitis. Whatever the cause, the clinical deterioration of MODS is held to be the result of common mechanisms of tissue injury subsumed under the rubric of SIRS. The latter syndrome

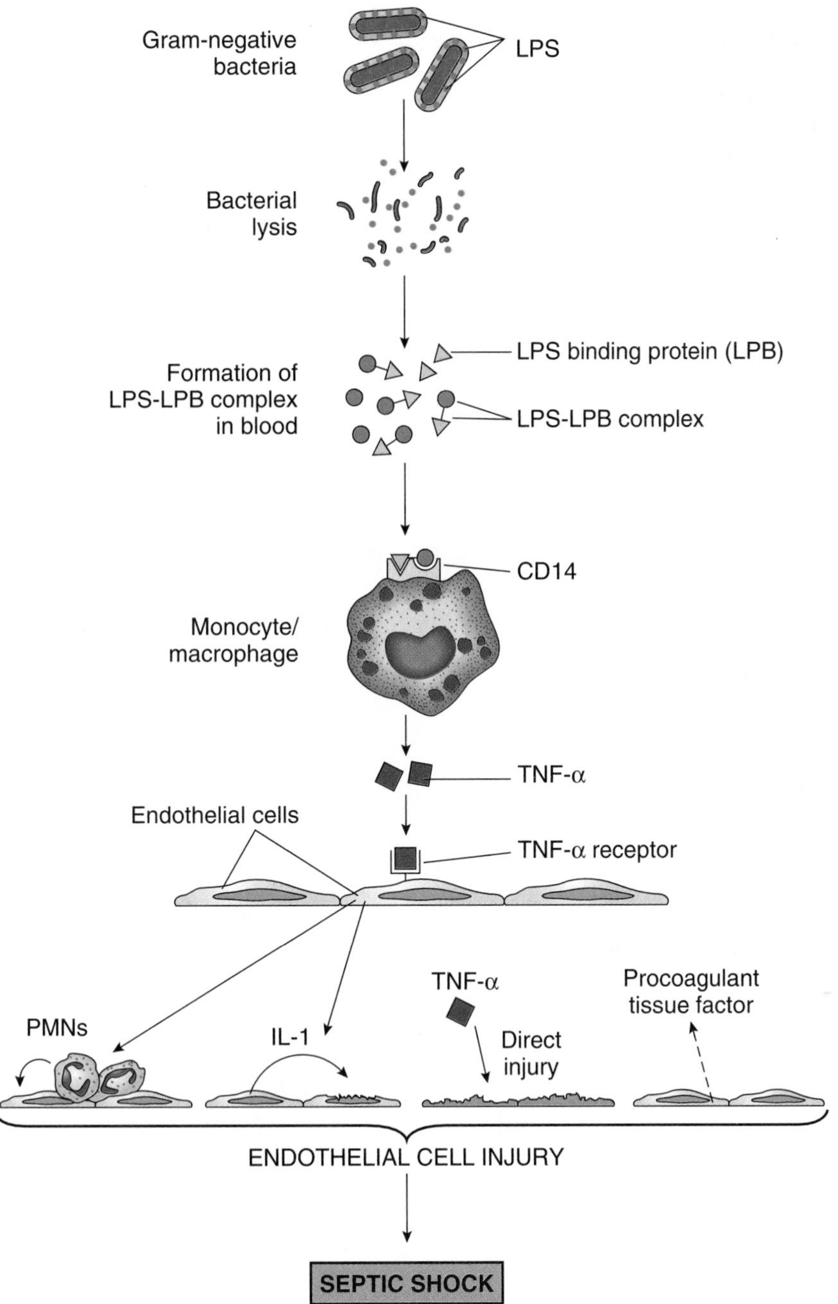

FIGURE 7-22
Pathogenesis of endothelial cell injury in endotoxic shock. In sepsis caused by gram-negative bacteria, the lysis of the organisms releases endotoxin (lipopolysaccharide [LPS]) into the circulation, where it binds to the LPS-binding protein (LBP). The LPS-LBP complex binds to CD14 on the surface of monocytes/macrophages, which are stimulated to secrete substantial quantities of tumor necrosis factor-alpha (TNF-*α*). TNF-*α* mediates septic shock by causing endothelial cell injury by a number of mechanisms: (1) direct cytotoxicity; (2) enhancing the adherence of polymorphonuclear leukocytes; (3) stimulating the release of interleukin-1 (IL-1), a cytokine that injures endothelial cells; and (4) promoting the expression of procoagulant tissue factor, thereby leading to thrombosis and local ischemia.

is a hypermetabolic state and is defined as two or more signs of systemic inflammation, such as fever, tachycardia, tachypnea, leukocytosis, or leukopenia, in the setting of a known cause of inflammation. Such a cause may be shock, infection, ischemia, trauma, or other catastrophic events. SIRS/MODS now accounts for most deaths in noncoronary intensive care units in the United States, with mortality rates well in excess of 50%.

It is thought that the massive inflammatory reaction defined by SIRS is the consequence of a systemic release of cytokines, TNF, IL-1, IL-6, and PAF being the most important. Actually, over 30 endogenous mediators have been described in this condition, and their collective interactions may be important in the pathogenesis of MODS. Importantly, there are no differences between the response of patients with MODS in the presence or absence of sepsis. Even when infection is present, the type of microorganism makes no difference in the response. Thus, the mechanisms underlying SIRS/MODS are not fully understood and are the subjects of continuing research.

Vascular Compensatory Mechanisms

Compensatory mechanisms in shock maintain blood flow to the heart and the brain, shifting it away from the periphery, skeletal muscle, skin, splanchnic bed, adipose tissue, limbs, and some parenchymal organs. These responses involve the sympathetic nervous system, the release of endogenous vasoconstrictors and hormonal substances, and local vasoregulation. The result is an increase in cardiac output achieved by a faster heart rate and augmented myocardial contractility in the presence of enhanced arterial and arteriolar vasoconstriction.

Increased sympathetic discharge increases the release of catecholamines by the adrenal medulla. The skeletal muscle, splanchnic bed, and skin arterioles respond to increased sympathetic discharge, whereas the cardiac and cerebral arterioles are less reactive. In this manner, the increased sympathetic tone tends to shift blood flow from the periphery to the heart and brain. The marked arteriolar vasoconstriction results in reduced capillary hydrostatic pressure and in less fluid shifted into the interstitium, thereby permitting an osmotic fluid shift from the interstitium to the vascular system. The sympathetic–adrenal response can completely compensate for a blood loss of 10% of intravascular volume. With a greater volume deficit, cardiac output and blood pressure can no longer be properly maintained and blood flow to the tissues is reduced.

The renin–angiotensin–aldosterone system also contributes a compensatory mechanism by stimulating sodium and water reabsorption, thereby helping to maintain intravascular volume. A similar water-preserving action is provided by pituitary antidiuretic hormone.

Vascular autoregulation preserves regional blood flow to vital organs, particularly the heart and the brain, by vasodilatation of the coronary and cerebral circulations in response to hypoxia and acidosis. The peripheral circulation of organs such as the skin and skeletal muscles, which are less sensitive to hypoxia, do not display such a tightly controlled autoregulation.

Pathology

Shock is associated with specific changes in a number of organs (Fig. 7-23), including acute tubular necrosis of the kidney, acute respiratory distress syndrome, liver failure, depression of host defense mechanisms, and heart failure.

The Heart

The heart shows petechial hemorrhages of the epicardium and endocardium. Microscopically, necrotic foci in the myocardium range from the loss of single fibers to large areas of necrosis. Prominent contraction bands are visible by light microscopy but are better seen by electron mi-

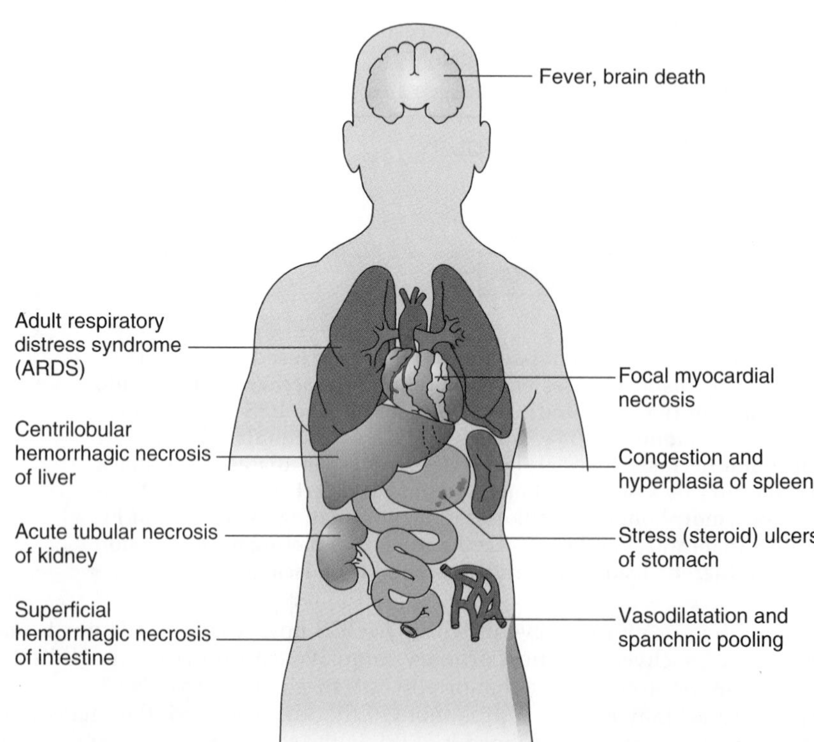

FIGURE 7-23
Complications of shock.

croscopy. Ultrastructurally, flattened areas of the intercalated disk are a sign of cell swelling and invagination of adjacent cells is considered a catecholamine-induced lesion.

The Kidney

Acute tubular necrosis (acute renal failure), a major complication of shock, has been divided into three phases: (1) **the initiation phase**, from the onset of injury to the beginning of renal failure; (2) **the maintenance phase**, from the onset of renal failure to a stable, reduced renal function; and (3) **the recovery phase**. In those who survive an episode of shock, the recovery phase begins about 10 days after its onset and lasts up to 8 weeks.

Renal blood flow is restricted to one third of normal following the acute ischemic phase, an effect that is even more severe in the outer cortex. The constriction of arterioles reduces the filtration pressure, thereby reducing the amount of filtrate and contributing to oliguria. Interstitial edema occurs, possibly through a process termed **backflow**. Excessive vasoconstriction is also believed to be related to stimulation of the renin–angiotensin system.

During acute renal failure, the kidney is large, swollen, and congested, although the cortex may be pale. Cross-section reveals blood pooling in the outer stripe of the medulla. Microscopically, fully developed acute tubular necrosis is evidenced by dilatation of the proximal tubules and focal necrosis of cells. Frequently, pigmented casts in the tubular lumina indicate leakage of hemoglobin or myoglobin. Coarse, "ropy" casts are seen in the distal nephron and distal convoluted tubules. Interstitial edema is prominent in the cortex, and mononuclear cells accumulate within the tubules and surrounding interstitium. Acute tubular necrosis is discussed in greater detail in Chapter 16.

The Lung

Following the onset of severe and prolonged shock, injury to the alveolar wall results in focal or generalized interstitial pneumonitis. This condition goes under the name of **shock lung** and is considered a cause of the adult respiratory distress syndrome. The sequence of changes is mediated by polymorphonuclear leukocytes and includes interstitial edema, necrosis of endothelial cells, microthrombi, and necrosis of the alveolar epithelium.

The lung is firm and congested, and frothy fluid exudes from the cut surface. Interstitial edema is first seen around the peribronchial connective tissue and lymphatics, subsequently filling the interstitial connective tissue. In this initial period, a large fluid volume drains into the pulmonary lymphatics. If removal of this fluid becomes insufficient, or if the balance of forces that keep the fluid in the interstitial space is disturbed, alveolar edema develops.

Shock-induced lung injury leads to the appearance of hyaline membranes in the alveoli, which are frequently expelled into the alveolar ducts and terminal bronchioles. These lung changes may heal entirely, but in half of patients, the repair processes continue and cause a thickening of the alveolar wall. Type II pneumocytes proliferate to line the alveoli, interfering with gas exchange. Fibrous tissue proliferation also leads to organization of the alveolar exudate. These chronic changes may lead to persistent respiratory distress and even death. Shock lung and the adult respiratory distress syndrome are more fully discussed in Chapter 12.

The Gastrointestinal Tract

Shock often results in diffuse gastrointestinal hemorrhage. Erosions of the gastric mucosa and superficial ischemic necrosis in the intestines are the usual sources of this bleeding. Interruption of the barrier function of the intestine may be related to the development of septicemia. More severe necrotizing lesions contribute to the deterioration in the final phase of shock.

The Liver

In patients who die in shock, the liver is enlarged and has a mottled cut surface that reflects marked centrilobular pooling of blood. The most prominent histological lesion is centrilobular congestion and necrosis. The cells in the center of the lobule are the most distant from the blood supply that comes from the portal tracts and are, therefore, presumably more vulnerable to circulatory disturbances. Hypoxia of the liver leads to the development of cytoplasmic vacuoles, which represent dilated cisternae of the endoplasmic reticulum. An increase in intracellular fat is consistently noted in persons who have survived shock.

The Pancreas

The splanchnic vascular bed, which supplies the pancreas, is particularly affected by impaired circulation during shock. The resulting ischemic damage to the exocrine pancreas unleashes activated catalytic enzymes and causes acute pancreatitis, a complication that further promotes shock.

The Brain

Brain lesions are rare in shock. Occasionally, microscopic hemorrhages are seen, but patients who recover do not display neurological deficits. In severe cases, particularly in persons with cerebral atherosclerosis, hemorrhage and necrosis may appear in the overlapping region between the terminal distributions of major arteries, so-called **watershed infarcts**.

The Adrenals

In severe shock, the adrenal glands exhibit conspicuous hemorrhage in the inner cortex. Frequently, this hemorrhage is only focal. However, it can be massive and accompanied by hemorrhagic necrosis of the entire gland, as seen in the Waterhouse-Friderichsen syndrome (Fig. 7-24), typically associated with overwhelming meningococcal septicemia.

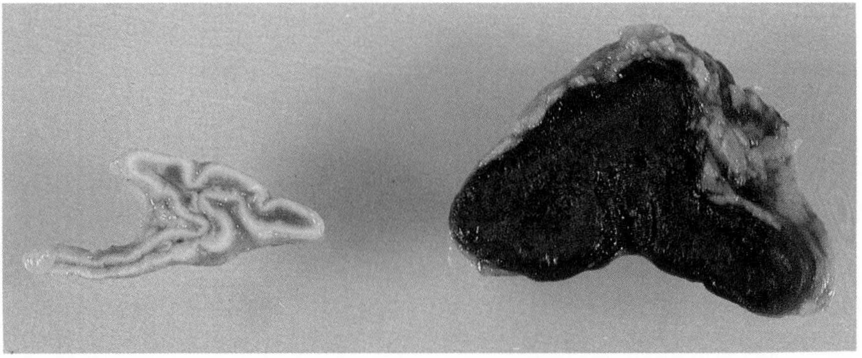

FIGURE 7-24
Waterhouse-Friderichsen syndrome. A normal adrenal gland (*left*) is contrasted with an adrenal gland enlarged by extensive hemorrhage obtained from a patient who died of meningococcemic shock.

Host Defenses

The alterations of the immunological system and host defenses in shock are not well defined, although it is common for patients who survive the acute phase to succumb to subsequent overwhelming infection. It may well be that several factors interact, namely ischemic colitis, tissue trauma, suppression of the immune system, and metabolic suppression of host defenses. Humoral immunity and phagocytic activity by leukocytes and mononuclear macrophages are both depressed, but the mechanisms underlying these effects are not clear.

SUGGESTED READING

BOOKS

Braunwald E: *Heart disease: A textbook of cardiovascular medicine*, 5th ed. Philadelphia: WB Saunders, 1997.

Gravanis MB: *Cardiovascular disorders: Pathogenesis and pathophysiology*. St. Louis: CV. Mosby, 1993.

Kelley WN: *Textbook of internal medicine*, 3rd ed. Philadelphia: Lippincott–Raven, 1997.

Virmani R, Burke A, and Farb A: *Atlas of cardiovascular pathology*. Philadelphia: WB Saunders, 1996.

REVIEW ARTICLES

Beal AL, Cerra FB: Multiple organ failure syndrome in the 1990s. Systemic inflammatory response and organ dysfunction. *JAMA* 271:226–233, 1994.

Beutler B, Cerami A: The biology of cachectin/TNF-α: a primary mediator of the host response. *Annu Rev Immunol* 7:625–655, 1989.

Bone RC: Toward a theory regarding the pathogenesis of the systemic inflammatory response syndrome: What we do and do not know about cytokine regulation. *Crit Care Med* 24:163–172, 1996.

Parrillo JE: Pathogenetic mechanisms of septic shock. *N Engl J Med* 3328:1471–1477, 1993.

Rink L, Kirchner H: Recent progress in the tumor necrosis factor-alpha field. *Int Arch Allergy Immunol* 111: 199–209, 1996.

Schlag G, Reddl H: Mediators of injury and inflammation. *World J Surg* 20:406–410, 1996.

Tracey KJ, Cerami A: Tumor necrosis factor: a pleiotropic cytokine and therapeutic target. *Annu Rev Med* 45: 491–503, 1994.

CHAPTER 8

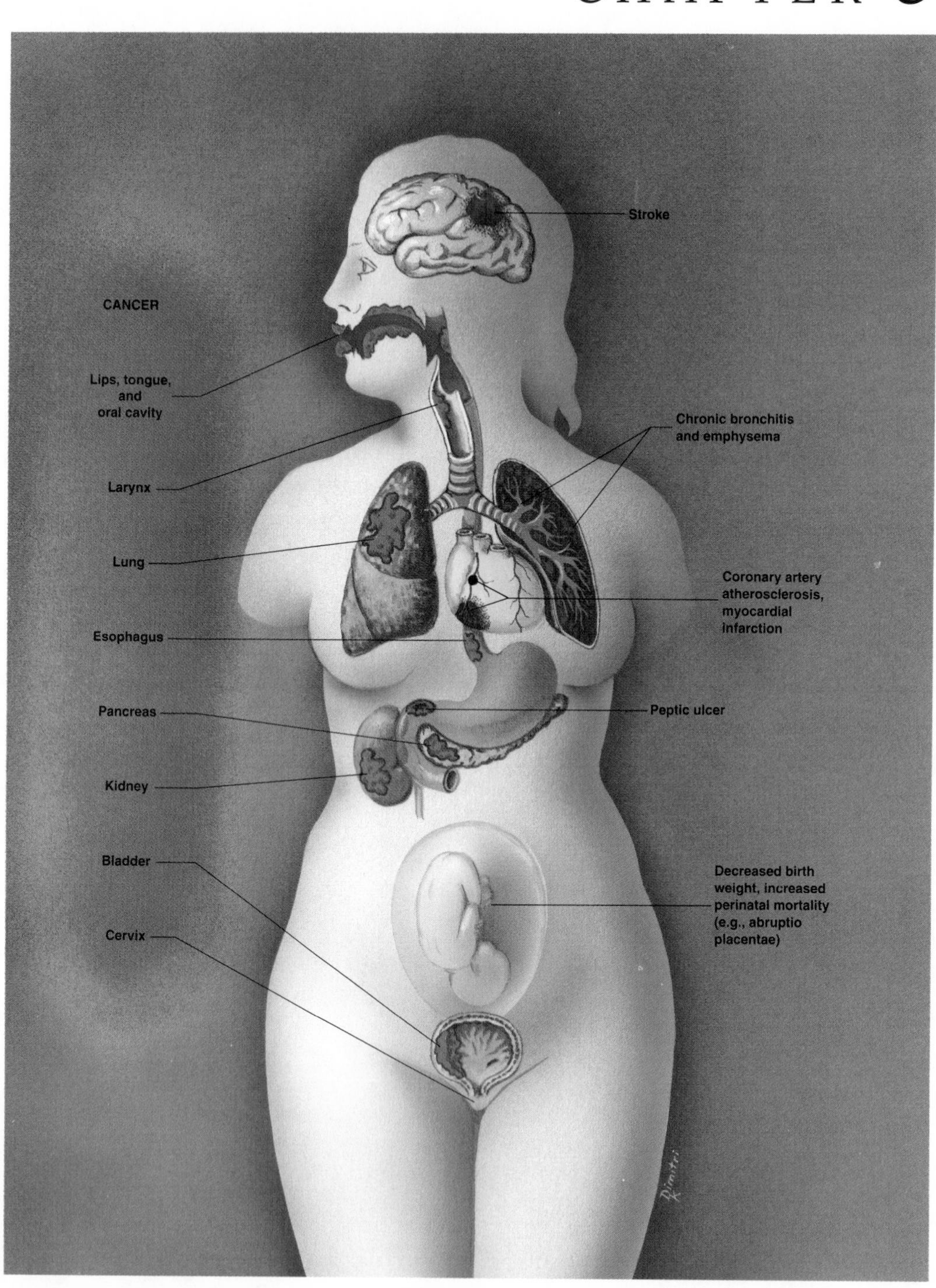

Stroke
CANCER
Lips, tongue, and oral cavity
Larynx
Lung
Esophagus
Pancreas
Kidney
Bladder
Cervix
Chronic bronchitis and emphysema
Coronary artery atherosclerosis, myocardial infarction
Peptic ulcer
Decreased birth weight, increased perinatal mortality (e.g., abruptio placentae)

Environmental and Nutritional Pathology

Emanuel Rubin
John L. Farber

FIGURE *8-1 (see opposite page)*
Diseases associated with cigarette smoking. The cancers whose incidences are known to be increased in cigarette smokers are shown on the *left*. The non-neoplastic diseases associated with cigarette smoking are shown on the *right*.

Environmental pathology is the field that deals with the diseases caused by exposure to harmful external agents and deficiencies of vital substances; in a sense it encompasses all nutritional, infectious, chemical, and physical causes of illness. A half century ago a few physicians cultivated an interest in diseases that seemed to have strict geographic boundaries. "Geographic pathology" was concerned with diseases endemic to certain areas of the world, notably parasitic and infectious diseases that seemed unique to those locales. A minor component dealt with nutritional disease, and a separate discipline covered forensic medicine. With the discovery that chemical agents are mediators of a variety of tissue changes, and with the recognition that many of these causative agents are environmental contaminants, a component called "occupational disease" was added to the roster. Finally, disease due to all environmental factors in the broadest sense was included to constitute the field of "environmental pathology."

The mortality and morbidity from the voluntary intake of tobacco smoke, alcohol, and illicit psychoactive drugs dwarfs those from all other environmental hazards combined. In fact, it is estimated that one quarter of all adult deaths in the United States are attributable to these three agents. Were tobacco or alcohol to be introduced at this time, it is inconceivable that either would be approved by the Food and Drug Administration. Because of ingrained cultural habits throughout the world, a simple prohibition of these substances is clearly not effective. The experiment with the legal prohibition of alcoholic beverages in the United States and the current inability to control the distribution and intake of illicit drugs attest to the difficulty of persuading people that exposure to culturally acceptable agents is indeed dangerous. Radiation, air pollution, and industrial exposures are relatively minor dangers compared with the problems that people willingly bring on themselves.

SMOKING

Smoking tobacco is the single largest preventable cause of death in the United States, with direct health costs to the economy of tens of billions of dollars a year. **Over 400,000 deaths a year—about one sixth of the total mortality in the United States—occur prematurely because of smoking.** Recent estimates have incriminated tobacco in 11% to 30% of cancer deaths (Fig. 8-1), 17% to 30% of cardiovascular deaths, 30% of deaths from lung diseases, and 20% to 30% of the incidence of low-birth-weight infants. Life expectancy is shortened, and overall mortality is proportional to the amount and duration of cigarette smoking, commonly quantitated as "pack-years." (Fig. 8-2). For example, a person who smokes two packs of cigarettes a day at the age of 30 years will live an average of 8 years less than a nonsmoker. One of the less desirable fallouts from the feminist movement has been the assumption of the smoking habit by many women. As a result, the epidemic of smoking-related disease that assaulted men more than a generation ago has now reached the female population. Women whose smoking characteristics are similar to those of men exhibit mortality rates similar to those of men. In fact, the mortality from cancer of the lung, almost all of which is related to cigarette smoking, exceeds that from cancer of the breast as the most common cause of death from malignant neoplasms in women in the United States. The excess mortality associated with cigarette

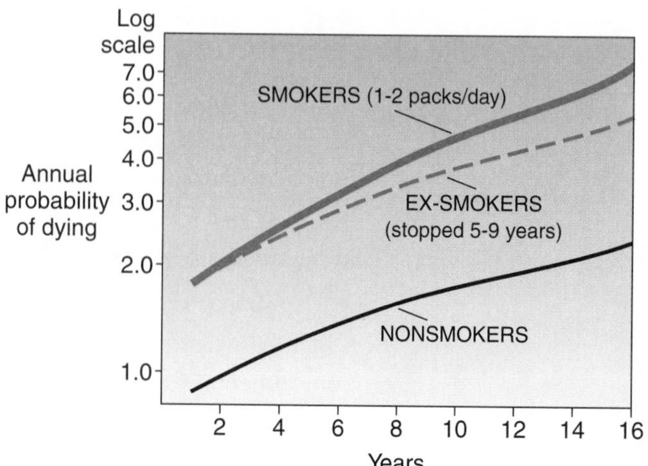

FIGURE *8-2*
The risk of dying in smokers and nonsmokers. Note that the annual probability of an individual dying, indicated on the ordinate, is a log scale. Individuals who have smoked for 1 year have a twofold greater probability of dying than a nonsmoker, whereas those who have smoked for more than 15 years have more than a threefold greater probability of dying.

smoking declines after cessation of the habit, and after 15 years of abstinence from cigarettes the mortality of ex-smokers is similar to that of those who have never smoked at all. Overall mortality among those who smoke only cigars or pipes is only slightly higher than that in the nonsmoking population.

The major diseases responsible for the excess mortality reported in cigarette smokers are, in order of frequency, coronary heart disease, cancer of the lung, and chronic obstructive pulmonary disease (see Fig. 8-1). Smokers also suffer an increased incidence of cancer of the oral cavity, larynx, esophagus, pancreas, bladder, kidney, colon, and cervix. In addition, smokers exhibit excess mortality from atherosclerotic aortic aneurysms and peptic ulcer disease.

Cardiovascular Disease

A relationship between tobacco use and ischemic heart disease was reported more than half a century ago. **Today, cigarette smoking is recognized as a major independent risk factor for myocardial infarction and acts synergistically with other risk factors, such as high blood pressure and elevated blood cholesterol levels** (Fig. 8-3). It not only serves to precipitate initial myocardial infarction but also increases the risk for second heart attacks and diminishes survival after a heart attack among those who continue to smoke. Importantly, the proportion of heart attacks caused by tobacco is about 80% for persons in their 30s or 40s, 65% in those in their 50s, and 50% for those in their 60s and 70s. Smoking also increases the incidence of sudden cardiac death, possibly by exacerbating regional ischemia, an effect that may promote electrical instability of the heart.

Cigarette smoking has recently emerged as an independent risk factor for ischemic stroke. The risk correlates with the number of cigarettes smoked and is reduced after cessation of smoking. Tobacco use also increases the risk of certain forms of intracranial hemorrhage. The combination of smoking and oral contraceptive use in women older than 35 years of age increases the risk of myocardial infarction. Similarly, the use of cigarettes by women who are using oral contraceptives significantly augments their risk of stroke.

Atherosclerosis of the coronary arteries and the aorta is more severe and extensive among cigarette smokers than among nonsmokers, and the effect is dose related. As a consequence, cigarette smoking is a strong risk factor for atherosclerotic aortic aneurysms. The incidence and severity of atherosclerotic peripheral vascular disease are also remarkably increased by smoking. It should be noted that the increase in the severity of coronary atherosclerosis is not enough to account entirely for the greater risk of coronary heart disease in smokers, and other factors are assumed to play a role. In particular, smoking is a major risk factor for coronary vasospasm, disturbs regional coronary blood flow in patients with coronary artery disease, and lowers the threshold for ventricular fibrillation and cardiac arrest in patients with established ischemic heart disease. Other effects of smoking that may predispose to myocardial infarction include pharmacological actions of nicotine itself, the inhalation of carbon monoxide, a reduction in plasma high-density lipoprotein levels, increased plasma fibrinogen levels, and a higher leukocyte count.

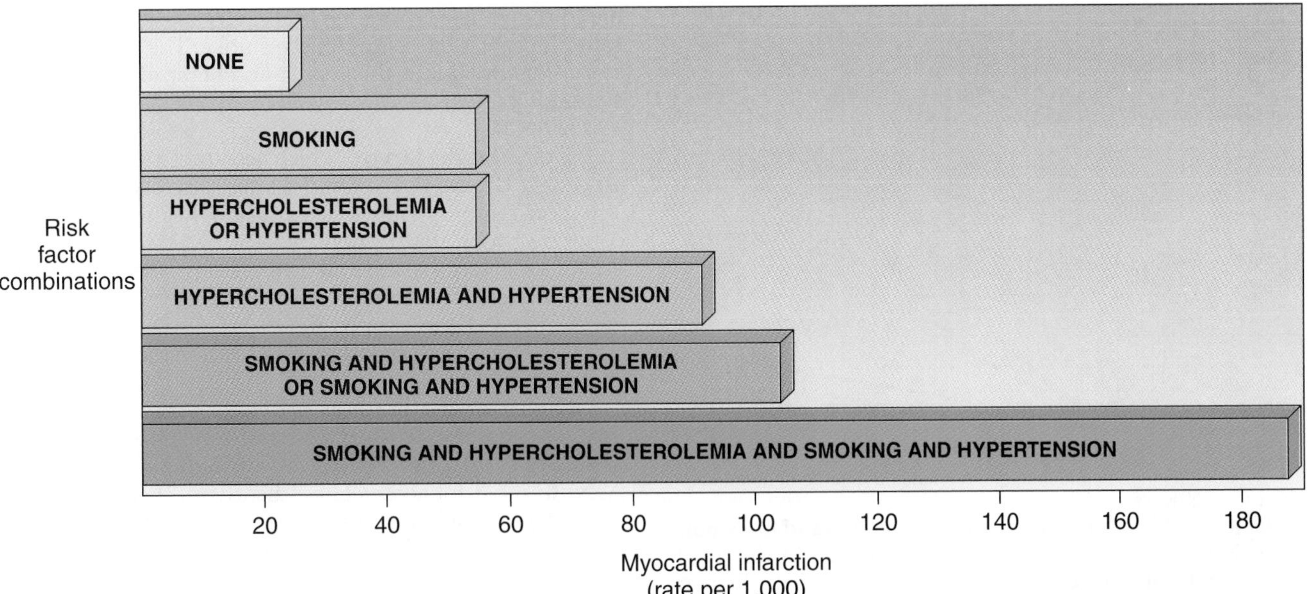

FIGURE *8-3*
The risk of myocardial infarction in cigarette smokers. Smoking is an independent risk factor and increases the risk of a myocardial infarction to about the same extent as does hypertension of hypercholesterolemia alone. The effects of smoking are additive to those of these other two risk factors.

In the earlier part of this century, a peculiar inflammatory and occlusive disease of the vasculature of the lower leg was described in a patient population consisting principally of Eastern European Jews, almost all of whom were heavy smokers. This disorder, termed **Buerger disease**, was characterized by inflammation, fibrosis, and thrombosis of both the artery and its accompanying vein, leading to gangrene and amputation of the lower extremities. Although Buerger disease is unquestionably related to smoking, it is rarely reported today.

Cancer

Death from cancer of the lung, more than 85% of which is attributed to cigarette smoking, is today the single most common cancer death in both men and women in the United States (Fig. 8-4). Although the precise offenders in cigarette smoke have not been identified, it is clear that cigarette smoke is toxic and carcinogenic to the bronchial mucosa. When cigarette smoke is passed through a filter, it is separated into gas and particulate phases. Cigarette tar, the material that is deposited on the filter, contains more than 2000 compounds, many of which have been identified as carcinogens, tumor promoters, and ciliotoxic agents. Compounds with similar toxic properties are found in the gas phase, but they are fewer.

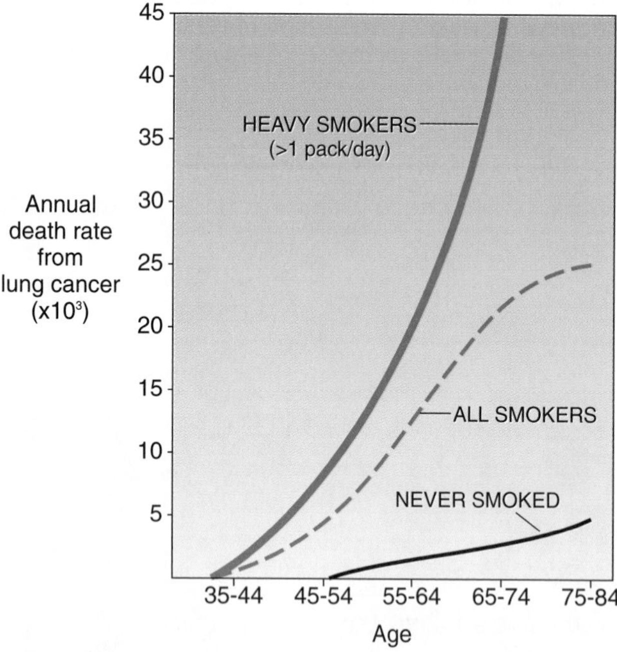

FIGURE *8-4*
Death rate from lung cancer among smokers and nonsmokers. Nonsmokers exhibit a small, linear rise in the death rate from lung cancer from the age of 50 onwards. By contrast, those who smoke more than one pack per day show an exponential rise in the annual death rate from lung cancer starting at about age 35. By age 70, heavy smokers have about a 20-fold greater death rate from lung cancer than nonsmokers.

The initial change in the morphological sequence leading to cancer of the lung is squamous metaplasia of the bronchial mucosa. As is often the case in a squamous mucosa (e.g., the cervix), the metaplastic epithelium becomes dysplastic and eventually neoplastic. In time, carcinoma *in situ* of the bronchial mucosa invades the basement membrane of the epithelium and metastasizes to regional nodes and distant sites. The risk of developing lung cancer is directly related to the number of cigarettes smoked (Fig. 8-5).

Cigarette smoking is also an important factor in the induction of lung cancer that is associated with certain occupational exposures. In general, it is difficult to separate damage due to smoking from that due to certain types of occupational exposures, but in some cases they appear to be additive. For instance, uranium miners have an increased rate of lung cancer, presumably because of the inhalation of radon daughters. However, the rate of lung cancer among miners who smoke is considerably greater than that among nonminers with similar smoking habits.

Another example is the case of asbestos workers. Whereas heavy smokers in the general population have a risk of lung cancer some 20 times greater than nonsmokers, asbestos workers who smoke heavily have a risk that is more than 60 times that of nonsmokers. Thus, in this group, the risk is not simply additive but seems to reflect a synergism. The subject is interesting from a legal point of view, since it is difficult to say whether asbestos exposure is particularly dangerous in smokers or smoking is more dangerous in asbestos workers; the relative contribution of each to the extraordinary incidence of cancer of the lung is uncertain.

Cancers of the lip, tongue, and buccal mucosa occur principally (>90%) in tobacco users. All forms of tobacco use—cigarette, cigar, and pipe smoking, as well as tobacco chewing—expose the oral cavity to the compounds found in raw tobacco or tobacco smoke. The precursor lesion—leukoplakia, a thickening and keratinization of the squamous mucosa—is followed by dysplasia and eventually neoplasia.

Cancer of the larynx, which accounts for about 1% of all cancer deaths in the United States, involves a similar situation. Among white male smokers the mortality ratio, compared with that in nonsmokers, varies from 6 to 13, and in some large studies all deaths from cancer of the larynx occurred in smokers.

Cancer of the esophagus in the United States and Great Britain is estimated to result from smoking in 80% of the cases.

Cancer of the bladder is twice as great a cause of death in cigarette smokers as in nonsmokers. In fact, 30% to 40% of all bladder cancers are attributable to smoking. As with most tobacco-related disorders, there is a clear dose-response relationship between the incidence of bladder cancer, the number of cigarettes smoked per day, and the duration of cigarette smoking.

Adenocarcinoma of the kidney is increased 50% to 100% among smokers. A modest increase in cancer of the renal pelvis has also been documented.

Cancer of the pancreas has shown a steady increase in incidence, which is, at least in part, related to cigarette

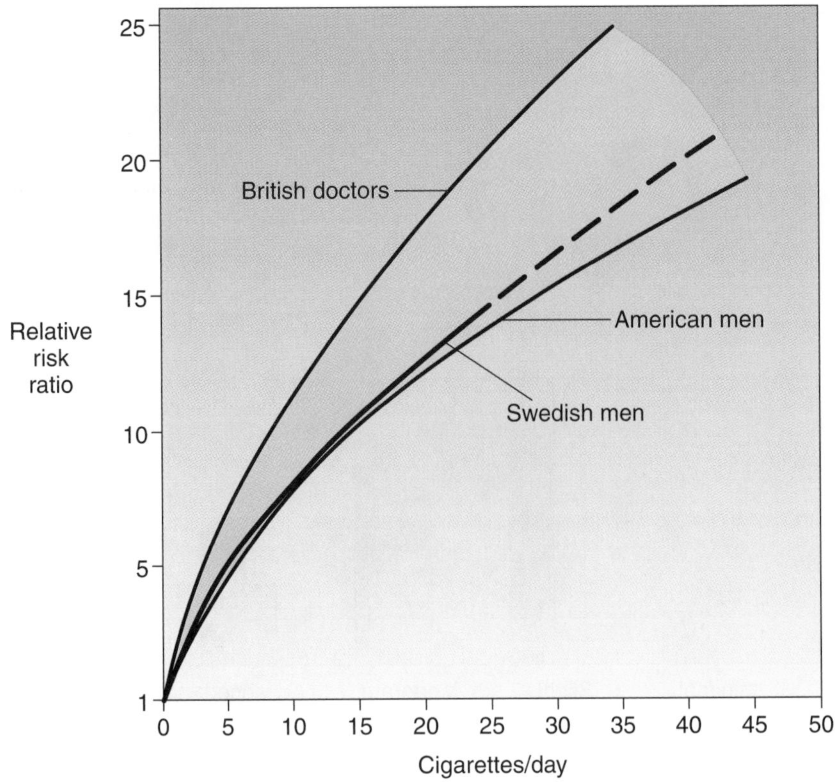

FIGURE *8-5*
Dose-dependent relationship between cigarette smoking and the risk of lung cancer. Prospective studies of three different populations of smokers found a dependence of the risk of lung cancer on the number of cigarettes smoked per day. For example, there is about a threefold greater risk of developing lung cancer in those who smoke 15 cigarettes a day as opposed to those who smoke 5. The *dashed line* is an extrapolation of the data for Swedish men who smoke from 25 to 50 cigarettes a day.

smoking. The risk ratio in male smokers for adenocarcinoma of the pancreas is 2 to 3, and a dose-response relationship exists (Fig. 8-6). In fact, men who smoke more than two packs a day have a five times greater risk of the development of pancreatic cancer than nonsmokers.

Cancer of the uterine cervix is significantly increased in women smokers, and it has been estimated that about 30% of cervical cancer mortality is attributable to this habit.

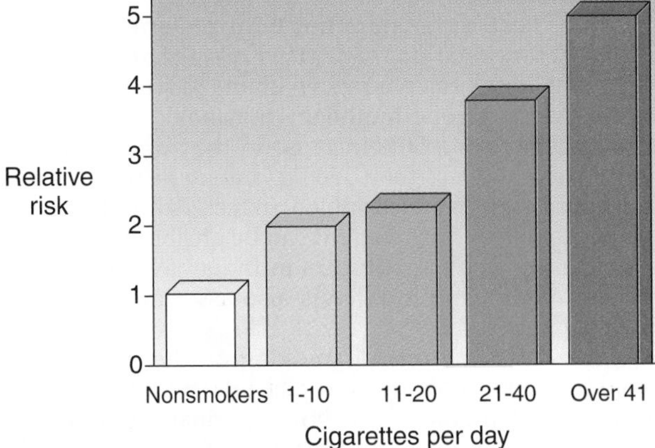

FIGURE *8-6*
Dose-dependent relationship between smoking and the risk of pancreatic cancer. The relative risk of pancreatic cancer increases with the number of cigarettes smoked per day.

Other Non-Neoplastic Diseases in Smokers

Chronic bronchitis and emphysema are primarily diseases of smokers (Fig. 8-7) (see Chapter 12). Not only is this relationship established by pulmonary function studies and symptomatic histories, but cigarette smokers also demonstrate more frequent abnormalities in macroscopic and microscopic lung sections at autopsy than do nonsmokers. Furthermore, there is a dose-response relationship between these changes and the intensity of smoking.

Peptic ulcer disease has a 70% greater prevalence in male cigarette smokers than in nonsmokers. The converse has also been shown: the proportion of smokers is higher among patients with peptic ulcer disease than among controls. Moreover, it now appears that smoking retards the healing of peptic ulcers of the stomach and duodenum.

Osteoporosis in women is exacerbated by tobacco use. Women who smoke one pack of cigarettes a day during their reproductive period will at the time of menopause exhibit a 5% to 10% deficit in bone density, which is enough to increase the risk of bone fractures. In this regard, smoking is a risk factor for vertebral, forearm, and hip fractures.

Thyroid diseases are linked to cigarette smoking. The most conspicuous association is with Graves disease, especially when the hyperthyroidism is complicated by exophthalmos. Tobacco use also increases the severity of established hypothyroidism, presumably by decreasing hormone secretion and antagonizing peripheral thyroid action in these patients.

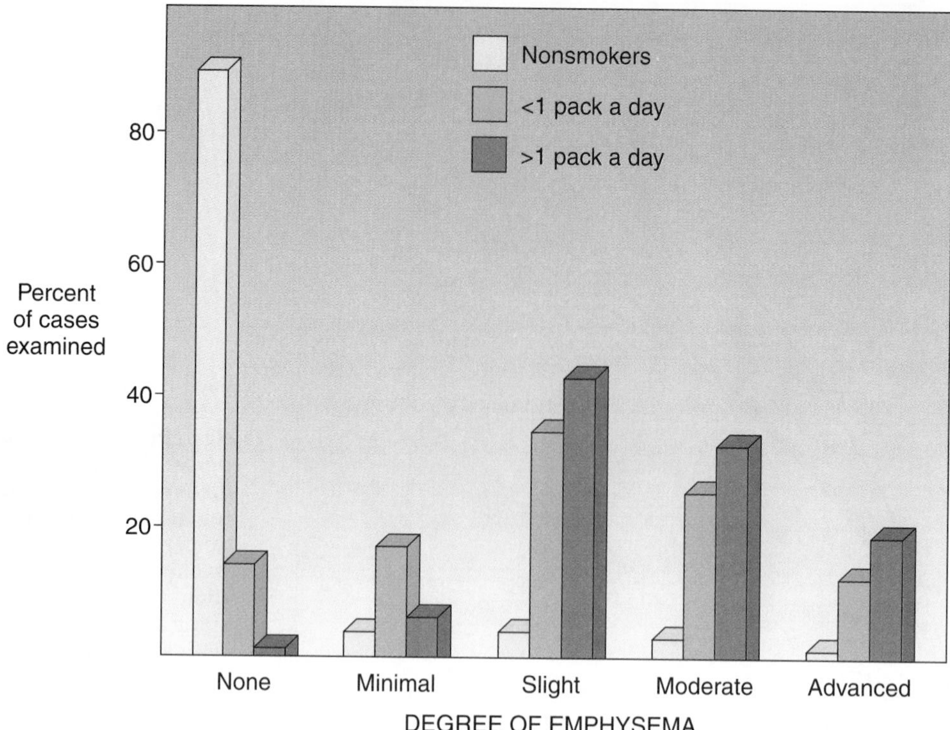

FIGURE 8-7
The association between cigarette smoking and pulmonary emphysema. Ninety percent of nonsmokers have no detectable emphysema at autopsy. In contrast, virtually all those who smoke more than one pack per day have morphological evidence of emphysema at autopsy. Emphysema shows a slight dose dependence on the number of cigarettes smoked. Those who smoke less than one pack per day tend to have less severe emphysema, but 85% to 90% of such smokers have some emphysema at autopsy.

Smoking and Female Reproductive Function

Reproductive function in women is affected by cigarette smoking in a number of ways. It is now clear that women who smoke experience an **earlier menopause** than nonsmokers, possibly because of the effects of tobacco on estrogen metabolism.

In the liver, estradiol is hydroxylated to estrone, which then enters one of two irreversible metabolic pathways. In one, 16-hydroxylation leads to the production of estriol, a compound with potent estrogenic activity. In the other, which involves 2-hydroxylation, the end product is methoxyestrone, a compound that has no estrogenic activity. **In women smokers, the pathway leading to the inactive metabolite is stimulated and, as a result, circulating levels of the active estrogen, estriol, are reduced.** As well as earlier menopause, an increased incidence of postmenopausal osteoporosis in smoking women has been attributed to decreased estriol levels. In view of the alarming increase in smoking among teenage girls, it might be useful to make this information widely known.

Fetal Tobacco Syndrome

Fetal tobacco syndrome refers to the deleterious effects of maternal cigarette smoking on the development of the fetus. Infants born to women who smoke during pregnancy are, on average, 200 g lighter than infants born to comparable women who do not smoke. This decrease in birth weight is independent of other determinants of birth weight, since there is a downward shift of the entire set of weights of smokers' infants (Fig. 8-8). Thus, this effect of smoking is not idiosyncratic but reflects a direct retardation of fetal growth. **These infants are not born preterm but rather are small for gestational age at every stage of pregnancy.** The prevalence of newborns weighing less than 2500 g is much greater among mothers who smoke. Among light smokers, there is a 50% increase in the number of newborns weighing less than 2500 g; among heavy smokers, this figure is more than doubled. In fact, 20% to 40% of the incidence of low birth weight can be attributed to maternal cigarette smoking. Studies in India have shown that the use of chewing tobacco is also associated with low birth weight.

The noxious effect of smoking on the fetus is mirrored by its effect on the uteroplacental unit. Every major well-controlled study has shown perinatal mortality to be increased among the offspring of smokers, the increase ranging from 20% among the progeny of women who smoke less than a pack per day to almost 40% among the offspring of those who smoke more than a pack per day. It is important to recognize that this excess mortality does not reflect specific abnormalities of the fetus but rather problems related to the uteroplacental sys-

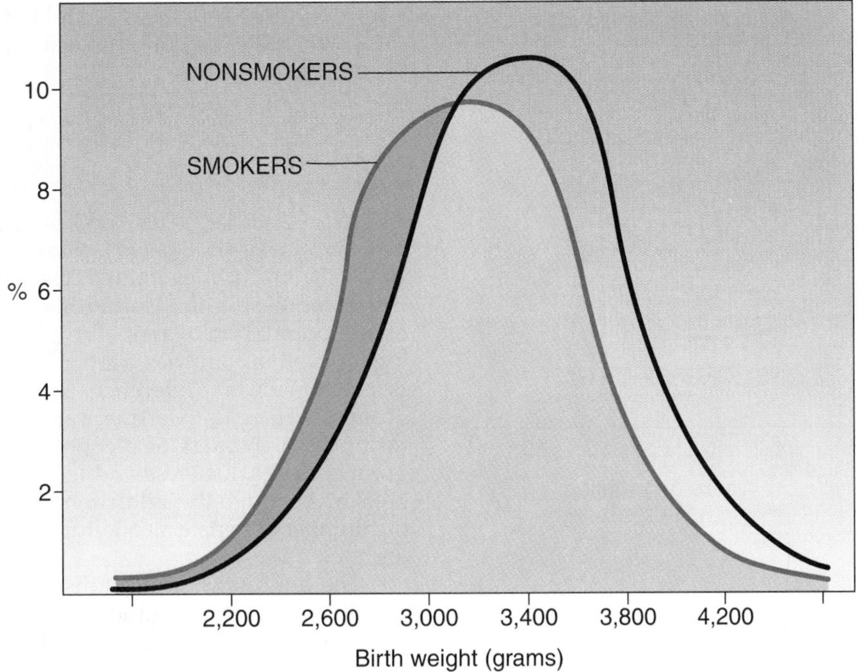

FIGURE *8-8*
Effect of smoking on birth weight. Mothers who smoke give birth to smaller infants. In particular, the incidence of babies weighing less than 3000 g is significantly increased by smoking.

tem. **The incidences of abruptio placentae, placenta previa, uterine bleeding, and premature rupture of the membranes are all increased** (Fig. 8-9). These complications of smoking tend to occur at times when the fetus is not viable or is at great risk, namely, from 20 to 32 weeks of gestation.

There is substantial evidence that the injurious effects of maternal cigarette smoking are not limited to the fetus and the newborn but extend to the physical, cognitive, and emotional development of the children at older ages. Thus, in a number of studies the children of mothers who smoke have exhibited measurable deficiencies in physical growth, intellectual maturation, and emotional development that are independent of other known predisposing factors. In the most comprehensive study to date, 17,000 children born during one week in Great Britain were studied at ages 7 and 11 years. The children of mothers who smoked 10 or more cigarettes a day during pregnancy were, on average, 1.0 cm shorter than children of nonsmoking mothers and were 3 to 5 months retarded in reading, mathematics, and general intellectual ability. Moreover, the deficits increased with the number of cigarettes smoked during pregnancy. These studies were carefully controlled for associated social and biological factors. A number of other studies have come to the same conclusions, and although the studies of performance on psychological tests have not shown statistically significant differences, the direction of differences is always in favor of the nonsmoker's child. Thus, it appears that the children of women who smoke, on average, do not catch up with the fetal retardation induced by smoking. Although more data are needed, it is also possible that deficits in growth and development may occur in children of normal birth weight whose mothers were habituated to smoking.

Passive Smoking

Involuntary exposure to tobacco smoke in the environment has been seriously considered as a risk factor for disease in nonsmokers for about two decades. As a result, knowledge of the effects of passive exposure to cigarette smoke is far more limited than that for active smoking, and there remains considerable controversy concerning the association of environmental tobacco smoke with certain diseases.

Passive exposure to cigarette smoke in nonsmokers is an order of magnitude less than that in smokers. Nevertheless, an increased incidence of respiratory illnesses and hospitalizations has been reported among infants whose parents smoke. Furthermore, several studies have shown a mild impairment of pulmonary function among children of smokers. Although passive smoking does not appear to cause asthmatic attacks in children, it tends to exacerbate preexisting asthma. The risk of lung cancer in adults exposed to environmental tobacco smoke is not precisely known but is probably in the range of 1.2 to 2.0. Smoke-exposed persons also tend to show an increase in resting pulse rate and in the level of blood carboxyhemoglobin. Interestingly, nonsmoking married men or women whose spouses smoke may have an increased risk of death from coronary heart disease. Thus, even if the increased risk of death attributable to passive smoking is

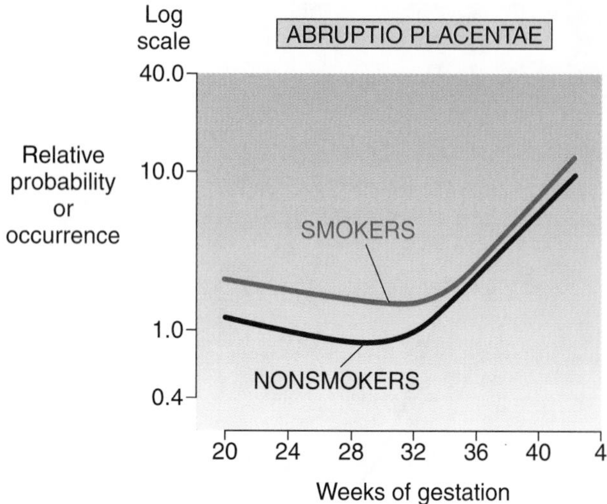

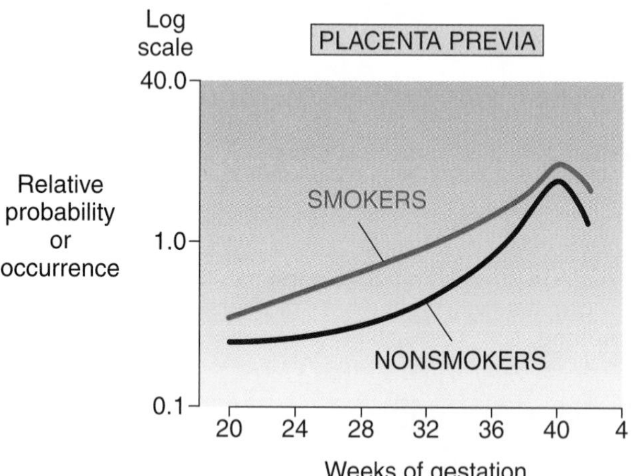

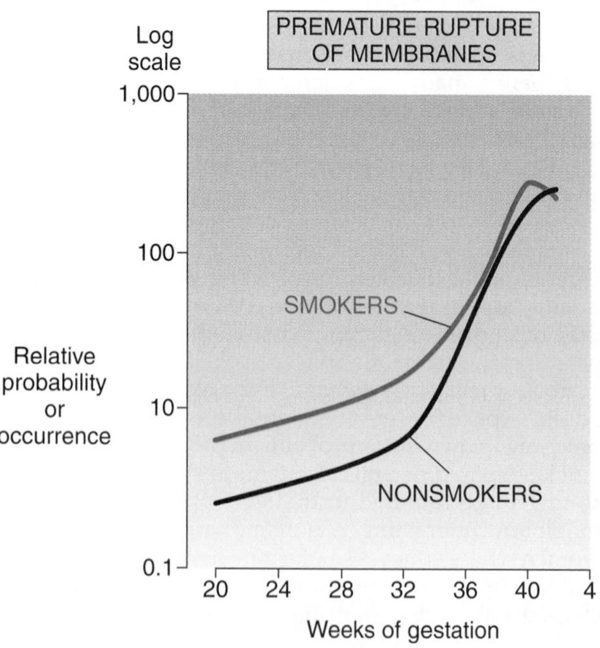

only 1% of that from active smoking, it is estimated that there will be 3000 premature deaths per year in passively exposed nonsmokers.

ALCOHOLISM

Alcoholism is an addiction to ethanol that features dependence, withdrawal symptoms, and the acute and chronic toxic effects of alcohol the body. **It is estimated that there are about 12 million alcoholics in the United States, or about one tenth of the population at risk.** The proportion may be even higher in other countries, particularly those in which wine is consumed in preference to water. Certain ethnic groups, such as Native Americans and Eskimos, have notoriously high rates of alcoholism. By contrast, other groups, such as Chinese and Jews, experience little alcoholism. Although this addiction is more common in men, the number of female alcoholics has been rapidly increasing.

The definition of alcoholism is difficult and varies widely with different authors. In view of the large differences in individual susceptibility both to the acute intoxicating effects of alcohol and to the development of alcohol-related disease, it is difficult to derive a simple number for the consumption of ethanol above which a diagnosis of alcoholism can be made. It is sufficient that chronic alcoholism be defined as the regular intake of a quantity of alcohol that is enough to injure a person socially, psychologically, or physically. Although there are no firm rules for most persons, a daily consumption of more than 40 g alcohol should probably be discouraged. Intakes of 100 g or more a day may be dangerous (10 g alcohol = 1 oz, or 30 mL, of 86 proof [43%] spirits).

The acute effects of alcohol on the brain need no elaboration since they are familiar to most people, either through personal experience or through the observation of acute alcoholic intoxication. Although the mechanism of inebriation is not understood, alcohol, like other anesthetic agents, acts as a central nervous system depressant. However, it is such a weak anesthetic that it must be drunk by the glassful to exert any significant effect. In the normal person, characteristic behavioral changes can be detected at low alcohol concentrations (below 50 mg/dL). Levels above 100 mg/dL are usually associated with gross incoordination and in most American jurisdictions are considered legal evidence of intoxication while driving a motor vehicle. At levels above 300 mg/dL, most people become comatose, and at concentrations above 400 mg/dL death from respiratory failure is common. In hu-

FIGURE *8-9*
Effect of smoking on the incidence of abruptio placentae, placenta previa, and the premature rupture of amniotic membranes. In each, the ordinate shows the probability of one of three complications of the third trimester of pregnancy. Note that it is a log scale. Smoking increases the probability of abruptio placentae and premature rupture of the amniotic membranes prior to 34 weeks of gestation, at which time the fetus is still premature. Smoking increases the risk of placenta previa up to 40 weeks of gestation.

mans, the LD_{50} is about 5 g alcohol per kilogram of body weight.

The situation is somewhat different in chronic alcoholics, who develop central nervous system tolerance to alcohol. Such persons often easily tolerate blood alcohol levels of 100 to 200 mg/dL, and in fatal automobile accidents, blood levels of 500 to 600 mg/dL or more have been found by medical examiners. The mechanism underlying tolerance has not been established for alcohol or any other drug.

Acute alcohol intoxication is hardly a benign condition. About half of all fatalities from motor vehicle accidents involve alcohol—20,000 to 25,000 deaths a year in the United States. Alcoholism is also a major contributor to fatal home accidents, death in fires, and suicide.

Many of the chronic diseases associated with alcoholism were, at one time, attributed to malnutrition, and it is true that some alcoholics suffer from nutritional deficiencies, such as thiamine deficiency (Wernicke encephalopathy) or folic acid deficiency (megaloblastic anemia). **However, most alcoholics have adequate diets, and the great majority of alcohol-related disorders should be attributed to the toxic effects of alcohol.** The diseases associated with alcoholism are discussed in detail in chapters dealing with individual organs, and we shall restrict this discussion to the spectrum of disease (Fig. 8-10).

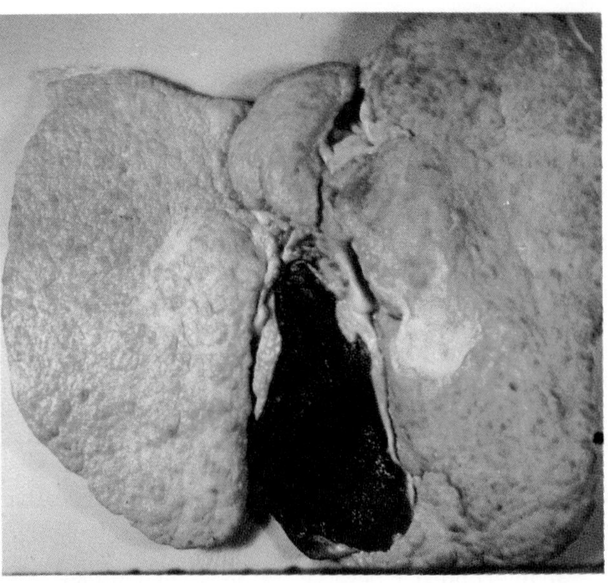

FIGURE 8-11
Cirrhosis of the liver in a chronic alcoholic. The surface displays innumerable small nodules of hepatocytes, separated by interconnecting bands of fibrous tissue. The dark structure is the gallbladder.

Effects of Alcohol Ingestion on Organs and Tissues

Liver

Liver disease associated with the excess consumption of alcoholic beverages has been recognized for several thousand years, having been implied in the Ayur Veda, the ancient medical text of India. Almost 300 years ago, the noted English clinician Thomas Heberden wrote about the increase in "scirrhous" livers in those who consume large quantities of "spirituous liquors." **Alcoholic liver disease, the most common medical complication of alcoholism, accounts for a majority of the cases of cirrhosis of the liver in the industrialized countries.** The nature of the alcoholic beverage is largely irrelevant; consumed in excess, beer, wine, whiskey, hard cider, and so on all produce cirrhosis. Only the total daily dose of alcohol itself is relevant. Alcoholic liver disease is conventionally divided into three major phases: (1) a reversible fatty liver, which has few functional consequences; (2) alcoholic hepatitis, an inflammatory and necrotizing disease of the liver, which has a significant mortality; and (3) cirrhosis, an irreversible scarring of the liver (Fig. 8-11). The last leads to liver failure or the consequences of portal hypertension, particularly gastrointestinal hemorrhage.

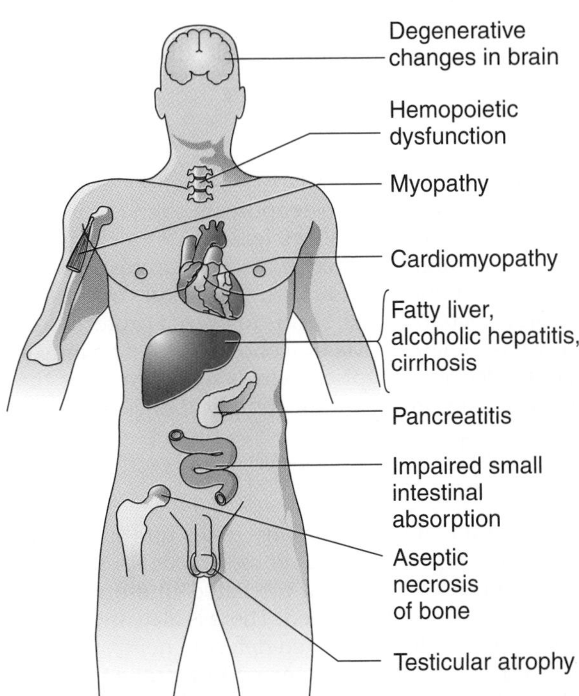

FIGURE 8-10
Complications of chronic alcohol abuse.

Pancreas

The relationship of acute pancreatitis to alcoholism is unclear, but such episodes occur with sufficient frequency to suggest that it is a complication of alcoholism. **Chronic calcifying pancreatitis, on the other hand, is an unquestioned result of alcoholism and is an important cause of incapacitating pain, pancreatic insufficiency, and pancreatic stones.** Among men in industrialized countries, alcoholism may be the cause of the majority of cases of chronic pancreatitis.

Heart

Alcohol-related heart disease was recognized over a century ago in Germany, where it was referred to as the "beer-drinker's heart." This degenerative disease of the myocardium is a form of dilated cardiomyopathy, termed **alcoholic cardiomyopathy**, and leads to low-output congestive heart failure. Although the pathogenesis is obscure, it is widely accepted as a toxic effect of ethanol. This cardiomyopathy is clearly different from the heart disease associated with thiamine deficiency (beri-beri), a disorder characterized by high-output failure. Cardiac changes in alcoholics are far more common than are usually appreciated, and the strength of the myocardium (as measured by the ejection fraction) has been negatively correlated with the total lifetime dose of ethanol. Interestingly, the vulnerability of the heart to the deleterious effects of alcohol abuse on the heart is considerably greater in women than in men. The alcoholic heart seems also to be more susceptible to arrhythmias, and the occurrence of abnormal cardiac rhythms after an alcoholic binge has been called the "holiday heart." Many cases of sudden death in alcoholics are probably caused by sudden, fatal arrhythmias.

In this context, it deserves emphasis that moderate alcohol comsumption or "social drinking" (1 to 2 drinks a day) provides a measure of protection against coronary arterty disease (atherosclerosis) and its consequence, myocardial infarction. Similarly, compared to abstainers, social drinkers have a lesser incidence of ischemic stroke.

Skeletal Muscle

Muscle weakness is extremely common in alcoholics and is often attributed to general debility or nutritional deficiency. However, when carefully tested clinically, even well-nourished alcoholics usually show some weakness, particularly of the proximal muscles. A wide range of changes in skeletal muscle occurs in chronic alcoholics, varying from mild alterations in muscle fibers evident only by electron microscopy to a severe, debilitating chronic myopathy, with degeneration of muscle fibers and diffuse fibrosis. On rare occasions, **acute alcoholic rhabdomyolysis**—acute necrosis of muscle fibers and release of myoglobin to the circulation—occurs. This sudden event can be fatal because of renal failure secondary to myoglobinuria.

Endocrine System

The principal endocrine effect of alcoholism in men is on the testes, which are reduced in size. Feminization of chronic alcoholics, together with loss of libido and potency, is common. The distribution of fat may change, giving the alcoholic male a female habitus. The breasts become enlarged (gynecomastia), body hair is lost, and a female distribution of pubic hair (female escutcheon) develops. Some of these changes can be attributed to an impaired metabolism of estrogens due to chronic liver disease, but many of the changes—particularly atrophy of the testes—occur in the absence of any liver disease. Chronic alcoholism leads to lower levels of circulating testosterone because of a complex interference with the pituitary-gonadal axis, possibly complicated by an accelerated metabolism of testosterone by the liver. Alcohol has been shown to have a direct toxic effect on the testes; thus, sexual impairment in the male is one of the prices exacted by alcoholism.

Gastrointestinal Tract

Since the esophagus and stomach may be exposed to 10 molar ethanol, it is not surprising that a direct toxic effect on the mucosa of these organs is common. Injury to the mucosa of both organs is potentiated by the hypersecretion of gastric hydrochloric acid stimulated by ethanol. **Reflux esophagitis** may be particularly painful, and peptic ulcers are also more common in the alcoholic. Violent retching may lead to tears at the esophageal-gastric junction (**Mallory-Weiss syndrome**), sometimes so severe as to result in exsanguinating hemorrhage. The mucosal cells of the small intestine are also exposed to circulating alcohol, and a variety of absorptive abnormalities and ultrastructural changes have been demonstrated. Alcohol inhibits the active transport of amino acids, thiamine, and vitamin B_{12}.

Blood

Megaloblastic anemia secondary to a deficiency of folic acid is not uncommon in malnourished alcoholics. A nutritional deficiency of folic acid is the most important factor, but alcohol is itself considered a weak folic acid antagonist in humans. Moreover, absorption of folate in the small intestine may be decreased in alcoholics. In addition, chronic ethanol intoxication leads directly to an **increase in erythrocyte volume**. In the presence of alcoholic cirrhosis, the spleen is often enlarged by portal hypertension; in such cases, **hypersplenism** often causes **hemolytic anemia**. Acute transient **thrombocytopenia** is common after acute alcohol intoxication and may result in bleeding. Alcohol also interferes with the aggregation of platelets, thereby contributing to bleeding.

Bone

Chronic alcoholics, particularly postmenopausal women, are at increased risk for **osteoporosis**. Although it is well established that alcohol, at least *in vitro*, inhibits osteoblast function, the precise mechanism responsible for accelerated bone loss is not understood. Interestingly, moderate alcohol intake seems to exert a protective effect against osteoporosis. Male alcoholics exhibit an unusually high incidence of **aseptic necrosis of the head of the femur**. The mechanism for this complication is also obscure.

Immune System

Despite tantalizing clinical anecdotes and a substantial number of serious investigations, no consistent effect of alcohol on humoral or cell-mediated immunity has yet been conclusively established. There is also no convincing evidence of an alcohol-related defect in neutrophils. Clinically, however, **alcoholics seem to be prone to many infections** (particularly pneumonias) with organisms that are unusual in the general population, such as *Haemophilus influenzae*.

Nervous System

A general cortical atrophy of the brain is common in alcoholics and may reflect a toxic effect of alcohol. By contrast, most of the characteristic brain diseases in alcoholics are probably a result of nutritional deficiency.

Wernicke encephalopathy is caused by thiamine deficiency and is characterized by mental confusion, ataxia, abnormal ocular motility, and polyneuropathy. The pathological changes involve the diencephalon and brain stem. Lesions are always present in the mamillary bodies and are frequently observed in the walls of the third ventrical and the periaqueductal gray matter. Necrosis of nerve cells and myelinated fibers, together with glial responses, is noted.

Korsakoff psychosis is characterized by retrograde amnesia and confabulatory symptoms. The condition was once believed to be pathognomonic of chronic alcoholism but has now been identified in a number of organic mental syndromes and is considered nonspecific. However, it is mostly associated with Wernicke encephalopathy, which may be a precursor lesion.

Alcoholic cerebellar degeneration is differentiated from other forms of acquired or familial cerebellar degeneration by the uniformity of its manifestations. Progressive unsteadiness of gait, ataxia, incoordination, and reduced deep tendon reflex activity are present. The cerebellar vermis displays varying degrees of shrinkage of the folia and widening of the sulci. At the microscopic level, the Purkinje cells in the cerebellum are the neuronal elements primarily destroyed, but in advanced cases, the molecular and granular cell layers are also affected.

Central pontine myelinolysis is another characteristic change in the brain of alcoholics, apparently caused by electrolyte imbalance—usually after electrolyte therapy, after an alcoholic binge, or during withdrawal. In this complication, a progressive weakness of bulbar muscles causes dysphagia and dysarthria and may be rapidly succeeded by an inability to swallow. Quadriparesis and coma eventually terminate in respiratory paralysis. Microscopic examination reveals foci of demyelination in the pons.

Amblyopia (impaired vision) is occasionally seen in alcoholics and may result from an alcohol-related decrease in tissue vitamin A, although other vitamin deficiencies may also be involved.

Polyneuropathy is common in chronic alcoholics. This condition is usually associated with deficiencies of thiamine and other B vitamins, but a direct neurotoxic effect of ethanol may play a role. The most common complaints include numbness, paresthesias, pain, weakness, and ataxia.

Fetal Alcohol Syndrome

Infants born to mothers who consume excess alcohol during pregnancy may show a cluster of abnormalities that together constitute the fetal alcohol syndrome. These include growth retardation, microcephaly, facial dysmorphology, neurological dysfunction, and other congenital anomalies. About 6% of the offspring of alcoholic mothers are afflicted by the full syndrome. More often, the exposure of the fetus to high concentrations of ethanol leads to less severe abnormalities, prominent among which are mental retardation, intrauterine growth retardation, and minor dysmorphic features. The fetal alcohol syndrome is discussed in greater detail in Chapter 6.

Cancer

The incidence of cancer of the oral cavity and esophagus is unquestionably greater in alcoholics than in the general population, but the precise relationship of cancer to alcohol consumption is confused by the fact that most alcoholics are also smokers.

Mechanisms of Alcohol-Induced Tissue Injury

The mechanism by which alcohol injures any organ or tissue is not understood. In the liver, the change in the redox potential occasioned by the metabolism of ethanol has been proposed as a major factor. During the oxidation of ethanol to acetaldehyde, NAD is reduced to NADH, thereby greatly increasing the reducing power of the cell. However, although certain metabolic abnormalities may be attributed to this change in the NAD/NADH ratio, no tissue injury has been directly shown to be caused by it. Moreover, other organs that also exhibit alcohol-induced injury, such as the heart and the pancreas, do not metabolize ethanol to any appreciable extent.

Acetaldehyde is the highly toxic product of alcohol metabolism. In the liver, acetaldehyde is rapidly converted by aldehyde dehydrogenase to acetate, but measurable levels of acetaldehyde (usually $<50\ \mu M$) can be found in the liver. However, circulating levels of acetaldehyde are extremely low, and it is difficult to attribute all of the changes associated with alcoholism to this metabolite. Other metabolites that have been proposed as causes of tissue injury include fatty acid ethyl esters, phosphatidyl ethanol, and hydroxyethanol.

An effect of ethanol common to all cells, regardless of their origin or location, is disordering of cell membranes. Like all anesthetics, ethanol intercalates within the lipid bilayer and decreases the molecular order of the acyl chains of phospholipids (a process known as fluidization). As an adaptive response, the composition of the membranes is changed, so that they become resistant to this fluidizing effect of ethanol. Such a mechanism may be important for central nervous system tolerance to alcohol, but its relationship to cell injury requires further study.

DRUG ABUSE

Drug abuse has been defined as "the use of any substance in a manner that deviates from the accepted medical, social, or legal patterns within a given society." For the most part, drug abuse involves agents that affect the higher functions of the brain and that are used to alter mood and perception. These chemicals include (1) derivatives of opium (heroin, morphine); (2) depressants (barbiturates, tranquilizers, alcohol); (3) stimulants (cocaine, amphetamines), marijuana, psychedelic drugs (LSD); and (4) inhalants (amyl nitrite, organic solvents such as those in glue). The use of psychotropic chemicals to produce euphoric states has a long history and a worldwide distribution. In addition to alcoholic beverages, examples are hashish in the Middle East, opium in the Far East, coca leaves in South America, and mescaline among Native Americans of the Southwest. However, the current epidemic of drug abuse in western industrialized countries is of recent origin. A notable difference in the pattern of drug intake, namely, the intravenous injection of illicit drugs, reflects the easy availability of syringes and hypodermic needles in industrialized societies. This change in the pattern of drug intake and the development of newer and more potent drugs have led to a profound change in the nature of the diseases related to drug abuse. The social and emotional consequences of drug abuse are beyond the scope of this chapter, but it should be noted that suicide, homicide, and accidents are responsible for one fourth to one half of deaths related to narcotic abuse. The use of illicit drugs is estimated to cause about 20,000 deaths a year in the United States.

Heroin

Heroin, the potent diacetyl derivative of morphine, is the preferred illicit opiate in use today. It is ordinarily administered subcutaneously or intravenously and in the usual dosage is effective for about 5 hours. The drug produces euphoria and drowsiness, but overdoses are characterized by hypothermia, bradycardia, and respiratory depression. Naloxone is a specific opiate antagonist that rapidly reverses the respiratory depression produced by heroin. Withdrawal symptoms are extremely uncomfortable but rarely fatal.

Stimulants

Cocaine

Cocaine is an alkaloid derived from South American coca leaves. At one time, it was a drug of the affluent, but its current wide availability has led to an epidemic of use. The traditional route of intake among South American Indians was the chewing of raw coca leaves. However, the processing of pure forms of cocaine allowed nasal and intravenous administration. The more potent freebase form of cocaine is hard and is "cracked" into smaller pieces that are smoked ("crack"). The half-life of cocaine in the blood is about 1 hour.

Cocaine users report extreme euphoria and a sense of heightened sensitivity to a variety of stimuli. However, with addiction, paranoid states and conspicuous emotional lability occur. The mechanism of action of cocaine is related to its interference with the reuptake of the neurotransmitter dopamine.

Cocaine overdose leads to anxiety and delirium and occasionally to seizures. Cardiac arrhythmias and other effects on the heart may cause sudden death in otherwise apparently healthy persons. Chronic abuse of cocaine is associated with the occasional development of a characteristic dilated cardiomyopathy, which may be fatal. Abstinence from cocaine does not produce a well-defined withdrawal syndrome.

Amphetamines

Amphetamines were initially used as nasal decongestants and are still widely employed in this manner. However, their ability to disguise fatigue and decrease appetite has led to widespread abuse. This family of drugs, which are relatively easy to synthesize, are sympathomimetic and resemble cocaine in their effects, although they exhibit a longer duration of action.

The most serious complications of the abuse of amphetamines are seizures, cardiac arrhythmias, and hyperthermia. Amphetamine use has been reported to lead to vasculitis of the central nervous system, and both subarachnoid and intracerebral hemorrhages have been described. Physical dependence on amphetamines has not been demonstrated. Numerous analogues of amphetamine have been synthesized, but they differ little in their effects, except that some also have psychedelic properties.

Hallucinogens

Hallucinogens comprise a group of chemically unrelated drugs that alter perception and sensory experience.

Phencyclidine (PCP) is an anesthetic agent that has psychedelic or hallucinogenic effects. As a recreational drug, it is known as "angel dust" and is taken orally, intranasally, or by smoking. Because the half-life of PCP varies from 12 to 90 hours, its effects are often difficult to control. The anesthetic properties of phencyclidine lead to a diminished capacity to perceive pain and, therefore, to self-injury and trauma. Other than the behavioral effects, PCP commonly produces tachycardia and hypertension, and high doses result in deep coma, seizures, and even decerebrate posturing.

Lysergic acid diethylamide (LSD) is a hallucinogenic drug whose popularity peaked in the late 1960s, and it is little used today. The drug causes a perceptual distortion of the senses, an interference with logical thought, an alteration of time perception, and a sense of depersonalization. "Bad trips" are characterized by anxiety and panic and objectively by sympathomimetic effects that include tachycardia, hypertension, and hyperthermia. Large overdoses cause coma, convulsions, and respiratory arrest. No chronic neurological sequelae have been documented.

Organic Solvents

The recreational inhalation of organic solvents is widespread, particularly among adolescents. Various commercial preparations such as fingernail polish, glues, plastic cements, and lighter fluid are all sniffed. Among the active ingredients are benzene, carbon tetrachloride, acetone, and toluene. Acute intoxication with organic solvents is similar to inebriation with alcohol. Large doses produce nausea and vomiting, hallucinations, and even-

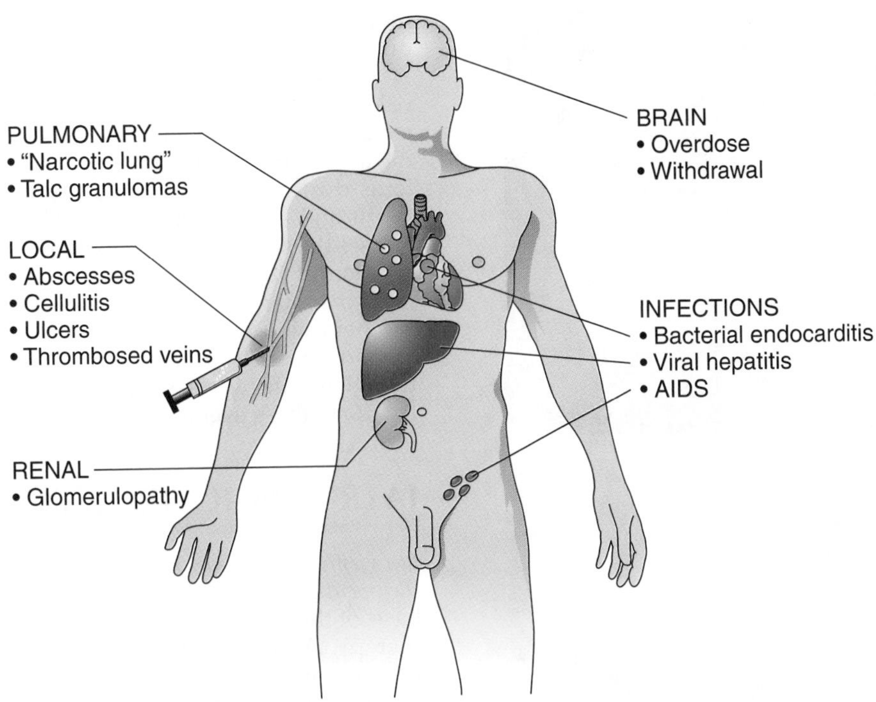

FIGURE 8-12
Complications of intravenous drug abuse.

tually coma. Chronic abuse of organic solvents may result in disease of the brain, kidneys, liver, lungs, and hematopoietic system.

Complications of Intravenous Drug Abuse

Apart from reactions related to the pharmacological or physiological effects of substance abuse, the most common complications (15% of directly drug-related deaths) are caused by the introduction of infectious organisms by a parenteral route. The most common infections are local at the site of injection. Among these are cutaneous abscesses, cellulitis, and ulcers (Fig. 8-12). When these heal, "track marks" persist, and these areas may also exhibit hypopigmentation or hyperpigmentation. Thrombophlebitis of the veins draining the sites of injection is common. Self-administration of street drugs is a major cause of tetanus, particularly when the injection is subcutaneous or intramuscular. The intravenous introduction of bacteria also leads to septic complications in many organs. Bacterial endocarditis, often involving *Staphylococcus aureus*, occurs on both sides of the heart (Fig. 8-13). Other complications of bacteremia are pulmonary, renal, and intracranial abscesses, meningitis, osteomyelitis, and mycotic aneurysms (Fig. 8-14).

Perhaps the most feared infectious complications today are of viral etiology. Addicts who exchange needles constitute one of the highest risk groups for acquired immunodeficiency syndrome (AIDS) and viral hepatitis. Addicts also suffer from the complications of viral hepatitis, such as chronic active hepatitis, necrotizing angiitis, and glomerulonephritis. A focal glomerulosclerosis ("heroin nephropathy") is characterized by the presence of immune complexes in the absence of a known antigen and has been ascribed to an immune reaction to impurities contaminating illicit drugs. The prognosis in this form of glomerulonephritis is poor, and progression to uremia is common.

The intravenous injection of talc, a material used to dilute the pure drug, is associated with the appearance of foreign body granulomas in the lung (Fig. 8-15). These may be severe enough to lead to interstitial pulmonary fibrosis. In some cases, talc-induced thrombosis of pul-

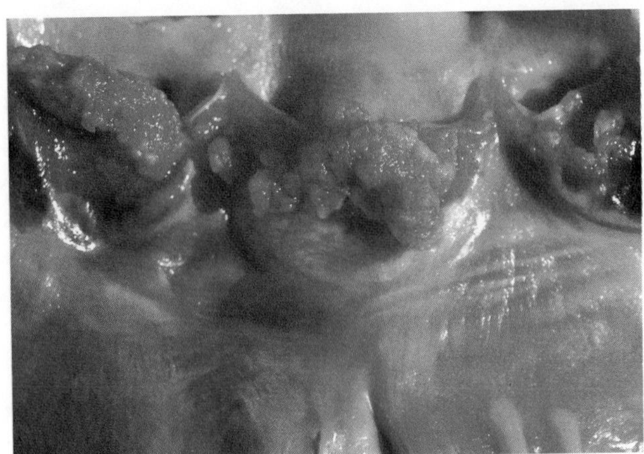

FIGURE 8-13
Bacterial endocarditis. The aortic valve of an intravenous drug abuser displays adherent vegetations.

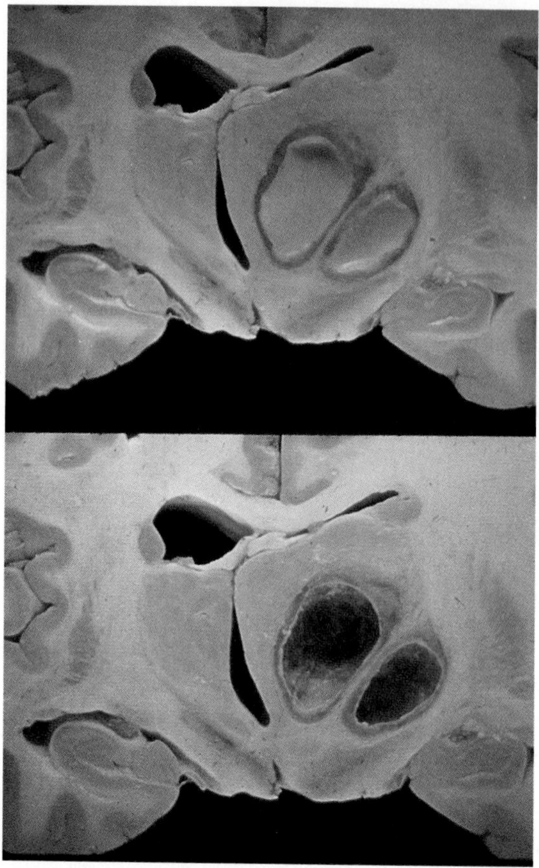

FIGURE 8-14
Brain abscess. Cross-section of the brain from an intravenous drug abuser shows two encapsulated cavities containing pus (*top*) and the same abscesses after removal of their contents (*bottom*).

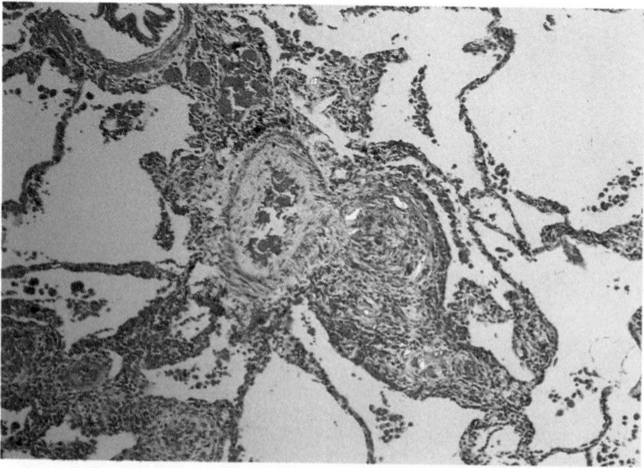

FIGURE 8-15
Talc granulomas in the lung. A section of lung from an intravenous, drug abuser viewed under polarized light reveals a granuloma adjacent to a pulmonary artery. The refractile material is talc that was used to dilute the drug prior to its intravenous injection.

monary vessels results in pulmonary hypertension or cor pulmonale.

Drug addiction in pregnant women poses substantial risks for the fetus. Infants of drug-dependent mothers often exhibit a full-blown withdrawal syndrome. Moreover, the appearance of the drug withdrawal syndrome in the fetus during labor may result in excessive fetal movements and increased oxygen demand, a situation that increases the risk of intrapartum hypoxia and meconium aspiration. If labor occurs when maternal drug levels are high, the infant is often born with respiratory depression. Mothers who are addicted to drugs experience higher rates of toxemia of pregnancy and premature labor, although it is unclear to what extent smoking may also contribute to these events.

IATROGENIC DRUG INJURY

Iatrogenic drug injury refers to the unintended side effects of therapeutic or diagnostic drugs prescribed by physicians. The basis of the scientific practice of medicine is rational drug therapy. Although few agents act as specifically and effectively as antibiotics, when properly used, drugs constitute the foundation of patient management. However, the administration of therapeutic agents exacts a price. Adverse reactions are surprisingly common, being found in 2% to 5% of patients hospitalized on medical services; of these reactions, 2% to 12% are fatal. The typical hospitalized patient is given about 10 different medications, and some receive five times as many. The risk of an adverse reaction increases proportionately with the number of different drugs; for example, the risk of injury is at least 40% when more than 15 drugs are administered. Because they are so ubiquitously prescribed, drugs represent a significant environmental hazard. Untoward effects of drugs result from (1) overdose, (2) an exaggerated physiological response, (3) a genetic predisposition, (4) hypersensitivity mechanisms, (5) interactions with other drugs, and (6) other unknown factors. It is beyond the scope of this chapter to describe in detail adverse reactions to individual drugs; the characteristic pathological changes associated with these reactions are treated in chapters dealing with specific organs. Some general principles are discussed here.

An overdose implies an excessive pharmacological effect of the drug. The intake of an inordinate amount of a drug can be a deliberate suicide attempt or can be accidental, as often happens in children or in those who are addicted to illicit drugs. The lethal physiological effect may be different from the desired effect at lower doses—for example, depression of the respiratory centers in barbiturate poisoning. A minor physiological effect may be dangerous in a susceptible person, as with lethal cardiac arrhythmias in some cocaine users. A dose considered safe for the general population may be excessive in someone who has a genetically slow metabolizing apparatus. Others may show an exaggerated reactivity (e.g., neurological or cardiovascular) to the pharmacological action of specific drugs. Drugs that have a wide therapeutic window—that is, a substantial distance between therapeutic and toxic levels—are less likely to produce these side effects than those with a steep dose-response curve. It is of-

TABLE *8-1* **Differential Sensitivity of Various Tissues to Acute Ionizing Radiation**

Very sensitive	Hemopoietic cells
	Lymphoid tissue
	Spermatogonia
	Ovarian follicles
Sensitive	Gastrointestinal mucosa
	Endothelial cells
	Hair follicles
	Breast
	Pancreas
	Bladder
	Heart and lungs
Least sensitive	Bone and cartilage
	Skeletal muscle
	Nervous tissue

ten not appreciated that drug reactions can produce a bewildering variety of disorders in virtually all organs. An example of a drug reaction is illustrated in Figure 8-16.

Oral Contraceptives

The most important contemporary drugs with important gynecologic effects are the oral contraceptives. These hormonal preparations, barely known a generation ago, are now the most commonly used method of contraception in industrialized countries. Almost all current formulations are combinations of synthetic estrogens and steroids with progesterone-like activity.

Hormonal Actions

The oral contraceptives act by either inhibiting the surge of gonadotropins at mid cycle, thereby preventing ovulation, or preventing implantation by altering the phase of the endometrium. Most of the complications are produced by the estrogenic component, but some may be related to the progestin component or to a combination of the two (Fig. 8-17). The current preparations contain only one fifth as much estrogen as earlier ones, and the incidence of side effects has progressively decreased as the amount of the hormone in the proprietary oral contraceptives has been reduced.

Ethinyl estradiol, the synthetic estrogen in many oral contraceptives, augments the liver's synthesis of several globulins of the coagulation system and may thus cause a hypercoagulable state and thrombosis. An increased production of angiotensinogen may cause an increase in the level of angiotensin II, thereby raising blood pressure. Estrogen's stimulation of tryptophan metabolism in the liver may result in a decrease in the level of tryptophan in the blood; it may also lead to low levels of serotonin, the end-product of tryptophan metabolism. Presumably, this effect can produce depression and behavioral changes.

The progestational agents, or gestagens, are related structurally to androgenic steroids and therefore exert certain virilizing effects, including weight gain, acne, and

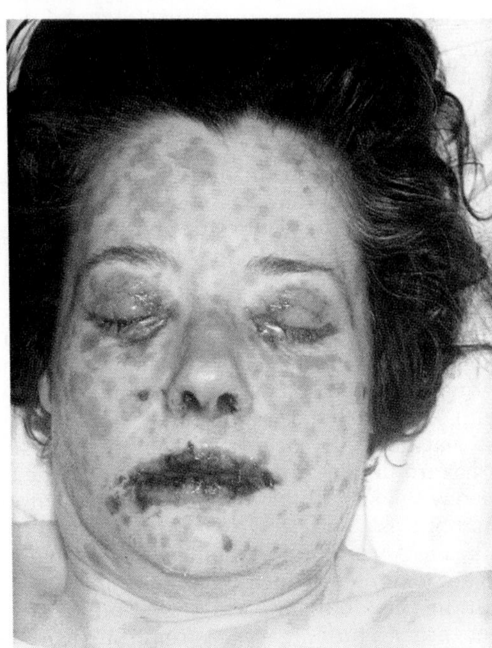

FIGURE *8-16*
Erythema multiforme secondary to sulfonamide therapy.

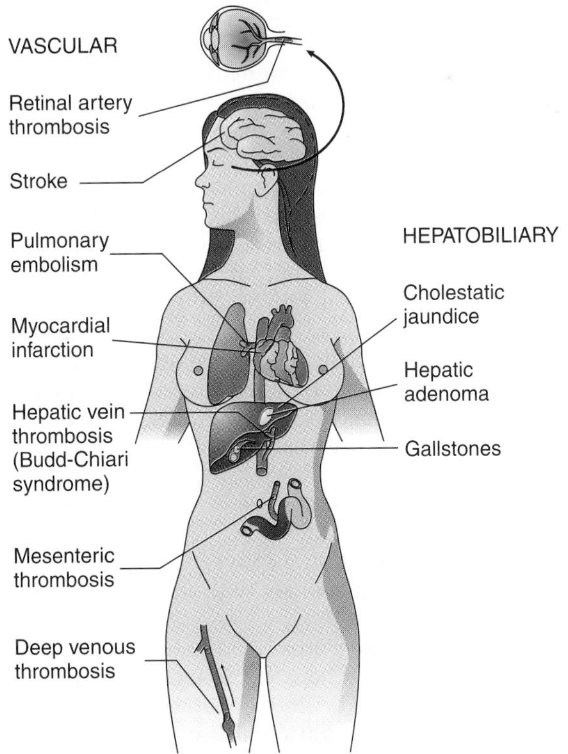

FIGURE *8-17*
Complications of oral contraceptives.

amenorrhea. The weight gain is presumed to be an anabolic effect of the progestin component. The progestins decrease the number of estrogen receptors in the endometrium, and endometrial growth is therefore decreased, leading to amenorrhea.

Vascular Complications

Deep vein thrombosis is a recognized complication of oral contraceptive use, the risk being increased three to four times. As a consequence, the risk of thromboembolism is correspondingly increased.

The incidence of stroke was increased in women who used oral contraceptives, but newer formulations do not carry this risk.

Myocardial infarction is a possible complication of the use of oral contraceptives, which occurs principally in women older than 35, in women who smoke, or in those who have another associated risk factor, such as hypertension or hypercholesterolemia. Nevertheless, the incidence of myocardial infarction is low—about 1 in 5000 a year.

It should be emphasized that most of the epidemiological evidence linking the use of oral contraceptives with cardiovascular diseases is derived from experience with earlier formulations containing higher doses of estrogens than are used today. Thus, the current risk associated with oral contraceptives will require further study.

Neoplastic Complications

Cancers of the female reproductive organs, namely the ovary, endometrium, and breast, are strongly linked to hormonal influences. Thus, there has been substantial concern that the use of oral contraceptive might increase the risk of such tumors. Fortunately, the available epidemiological data suggest that the use of oral contraceptives actually decreases the risk of ovarian and endometrial cancers by about half, presumably because of suppression of the production of pituitary gonadotropins.

With respect to breast cancer, oral contraceptives have not produced an increase in the overall incidence of breast cancer. However, they seem to increase the risk of breast cancer to a small degree in women under the age of 45 years who have used this method of birth control for many years.

Benign liver adenomas are rare hepatic neoplasms that are significantly increased in incidence among women who use oral contraceptives. The risk of these tumors increases conspicuously with the duration of use, particularly after 5 years.

Several small case-control studies in developed countries with low rates of hepatitis B and C infection have suggested an increased risk of **hepatocellular carcinoma** among women using oral contraceptives. Fortunately, this cancer is distinctly uncommen in young women without chronic viral hepatitis, and no more than 1 case in 100,000 long-term users can be expected.

Other Complications

For reasons unknown, oral contraceptives may induce an increased pigmentation of the malar eminences, called **chloasma**, which is accentuated by sunlight and persists for a long time after the contraceptives are discontinued.

Cholelithiasis is more frequent (twofold increase) in women who have used oral contraceptives for 4 years or less but decreases to lower than normal after that period of time. Thus, oral contraceptives accelerate the process of cholelithiasis but do not increase its overall incidence.

Benefits of Oral Contraceptives

In considering the potential side effects of the use of oral contraceptive agents, it is important to recognize that certain benefits accrue. In addition to a signficant reduction in the risk of ovarian and endometrial cancers, the use of these agents decreases the risk of pelvic inflammatory disease, uterine leiomyomas, endometriosis, and fibrocystic disease of the breast.

ENVIRONMENTAL CHEMICALS

An awareness of the potential hazards posed by the presence of harmful chemicals in the environment is not new. As the following quote from Maimonides shows, concerns about air pollution existed even in the 12th century.

> Comparing the air of cities to the air of deserts is like comparing waters that are befouled and turbid to waters that are fine and pure. In the city, because of the height of its buildings, the narrowness of its streets, and all that pours forth from its inhabitants, the air becomes stagnant, turbid, thick, misty, and foggy. If there is no choice in this matter, if we have grown up in the cities and become accustomed to them, we should endeavor at least to dwell out at the outskirts of the city. Wherever the air is altered ever so slightly, you will find men develop dullness of understanding, failure of intelligence, and defects of memory.

Humans inhale, bathe in, and eat a variety of chemical materials that are found as contaminants in foods and in the food chain, the water supply, and the general ecosystem in which they live. In the past 2 decades, man-made contamination and the effects of these chemicals have caused considerable alarm. However, predictions of widespread destruction of flora and fauna and an epidemic of human cancer have yet to materialize. In fact, efforts to quantitate the potency of environmental contaminants and to estimate past and present human exposure suggest that **naturally occurring chemicals pose a far greater hazard than man-made products**, and the former have been with us for millennia. Our natural environment is not without risk, and even oxygen can be harmful.

There are several important mechanisms that govern the effect of toxic agents, including the toxin's absorption, distribution, metabolism, and excretion. Absorption (whether through pulmonary, gastrointestinal, or dermal routes) depends in part on the chemical structure of the agent. For example, because of their solubility in lipids, the insecticides chlordane and heptachlor are rapidly absorbed and stored in body fat. By contrast, the water-soluble herbicide paraquat is readily eliminated.

The effects of many chemicals are exerted by their metabolic products rather than by the parent compound. The capacity of the xenobiotic systems to modify these materials varies among tissues. Moreover, these detoxifying systems may produce different metabolites in different sites, which may vary in their capacity to produce disease. The cellular content of these enzyme systems varies with age, sex, hormonal and nutritional status, and previous drug intake.

The storage, distribution, and excretion of these materials control their concentrations in the organism at any given time. It follows that agents stored in adipose tissue exert a prolonged low-level effect, whereas the more water-soluble materials that are easily excreted by the kidney have a shorter duration of action.

It is worth pointing out that the fact that a toxic agent can be detected in the workplace does not mean that it necessarily produces disease. For example, carbon tetrachloride, a recognized species-dependent hepatotoxin, is used frequently in the machining of steel. Yet liver disease derived from this haloalkane is not an occupational hazard in the steel fabricating industry. Thus, although there is little question that chemicals can and do produce human disease, in many cases, our information is far from conclusive.

Among the most important chemical hazards to which humans are exposed are environmental dusts and carcinogens. Inhalation of mineral and organic dusts occurs primarily in occupational settings (e.g., mining, industrial manufacturing, farming) and occasionally as a result of unusual situations (e.g., bird fanciers, pituitary snuff inhalation). The inhalation of mineral dusts leads to the pulmonary diseases known as pneumoconioses, whereas organic dusts produce hypersensitivity pneumonitis. Pneumoconioses were formerly common, but control of dust exposure in the workplace through modification of manufacturing techniques, improvements in air handling, and the use of facial masks has substantially reduced the incidence of these diseases. Because of their importance, pneumoconioses and hypersensitivity pneumonitis are discussed in detail in Chapter 12.

Chemical carcinogens are ubiquitous in the environment, and their potential for causing human disease has elicited widespread concern. In particular, exposure to carcinogens in the workplace has been associated epidemiologically with a number of cancers (Table 8-2). Chemical carcinogenesis is reviewed in Chapter 5.

TABLE 8-2 **Cancers Associated with Exposure to Occupational Carcinogens**

Agent or Occupation	Site of Cancer
Arsenic	Lung cancer
Asbestos	Mesothelioma (pleura and peritoneum)
	Lung cancer (in smokers)
Aromatic amines	Bladder cancer
Benzene	Leukemia, multiple myeloma
bis-(Chloromethyl)ether	Lung cancer
Chromium	Lung cancer
Furniture and shoe manufacturing	Nasal carcinoma
Hematite mining	Lung cancer
Isopropyl alcohol	Paranasal sinus cancer
Nickel	Lung cancer, paranasal sinus cancer
Tars and oils	Cancers of lung, gastrointestinal tract, bladder, and skin
Vinyl chloride	Angiosarcoma of liver

Toxic versus Hypersensitivity Responses

Many substances elicit disease in a variety of animal species in a dose-dependent manner, with a regular time delay and a predictable target organ response. Furthermore, the morphological changes in the injured tissues are constant and reproducible. By contrast, other agents show great variability in the production of disease, an irregular lag before any manifestation of injury, no dose dependency, and a lack of reproducibility. It has been assumed that the predictable dose-response reactions reflect a direct action of the compound or its metabolite on a tissue—that is, a "toxic" effect. The second, unpredictable type of reaction is believed to reflect "hypersensitivity," or an immunological response. Yet despite the wealth of information that has been accumulated about the mechanisms of cell injury, such a separation with respect to mechanisms of action has not been conclusively established. There are, clearly, immunological responses, but the mechanisms by which delayed, irregular responses to toxic agents occur have yet to be explained.

Responses to Chemical Substances

Our current fund of information does not permit an easy cataloging of responses to the variety of man-made and natural products. For the purposes of this discussion, we will mention certain chemicals as illustrations or because of the importance of the pathological changes they induce.

Beginning with the industrial revolution, there has been an exponential rise in the number of chemicals manufactured and a corresponding increase in the risk of human exposure. This potential problem has elicited widespread public concern and has particularly attracted the attention of journalists and attorneys. In any consideration of this topic, it is crucial to differentiate between the problems of acute poisoning and chronic toxicity. One must also distinguish industrial and accidental exposure from that which is likely to occur in the general environment. The lack of adequate quantitative data in humans and the obvious problems involved in obtaining such information have led to the extrapolation to humans of experimental data derived from animal studies. Such projections can be hazardous because of (1) species differences in sensitivity, (2) differing routes of administration, and (3) the use of unrealistically high concentrations of the test agent. Yet the doctrine is enshrined in American law that any agent that produces malignant tumors in any species, and at any dose, is unfit for human use. For example, large doses of the artificial sweeteners saccharin and the cyclamates were reported to be associated with the development of bladder tumors in experimental animals. As a result, the cyclamates have been withdrawn from use and saccharin has been subjected to strong criticism. Yet there are no adequate epidemiological data in humans that suggest a similar harmful effect among those who have regularly consumed these substances.

Except for certain hypersensitivity reactions in susceptible persons, acute poisoning by environmental chemicals does not pose a significant threat to the general population. The concentrations necessary to cause acute functional disorders or structural damage are ordinarily encountered only in the workplace or as a consequence of uncommon accidents. The latter category includes the exposure to the largest amount of tetrachloro-dibenzodioxin (TCDD) ever to contaminate the environment, which followed an explosion in a chemical plant in Seveso, Italy, in 1976. This compound, a potent herbicide, is a byproduct of the synthesis of 2,4,5-trichlorphenoxyacetic acid (2,4,5-T), a defoliant used by the U.S. Army in Vietnam under the name "Agent Orange." As expected, some exposed persons developed acute symptoms, although none died. It is noteworthy that more than 20 years later, with the exception of chloracne, there have been no confirmed chronic effects in the persons exposed at Seveso. Moreover, after 20 years, Air Force veterans exposed to Agent Orange in Vietnam experienced no increased incidence of cancer or other diseases compared to comparable veterans not so exposed.

Although accidental mass poisonings with the pesticides endrin and parathion have led to as many as 100 deaths in a single event, no chronic sequelae among the survivors have been documented. Despite claims of an association between progressive chronic disease and exposure to pesticides, the small number of cases, coupled with the nonspecific nature of the complaints, does not permit such a conclusion. It should be stressed that the action of most environmental toxins is specific and that a causal relationship to disease implies damage to a specific organ or organ system, with specific alterations of these tissues. As a corollary, multisystem involvement, particularly when the symptoms are vague, should be viewed with skepticism. The experimental literature dealing with the acute and chronic toxicity of industrial chemicals is voluminous and complicated and often contradictory. It is for this reason that we shall largely restrict the following discussion to documented effects in humans.

Volatile Organic Solvents and Vapors

Volatile organic solvents and vapors are widely used in industry to dissolve other compounds (degreasers) and as fuels. With few exceptions the exposures are industrial or accidental and represent acute dangers rather than chronic toxicity. However, chronic exposure to organic solvents has been linked to the development of anti–basement membrane glomerulonephritis, with an estimated threefold to ninefold increased risk for this disorder. For the most part, exposure to solvents is by inhalation rather than by ingestion.

- **Chloroform ($CHCl_3$) and carbon tetrachloride (CCl_4):** These solvents exert anesthetic effects on the central nervous system but are better known as hepatotoxins. With both, large doses lead to acute hepatic necrosis, fatty liver, and liver failure. Whereas chronic administration of carbon tetrachloride to rats invariably produces cirrhosis, such a situation does not pertain to humans, because each exposure to the toxin results in recognizable clinical liver injury. Unlike the rat, a person who suffers a bout of jaundice after exposure to carbon tetrachloride will not be permitted another episode of poisoning.
- **Trichloroethylene (C_2HCl_3):** A ubiquitous industrial solvent, trichloroethylene in high concentrations depresses the central nervous system, but hepatotoxicity is minimal. There is no evidence for chronic sequelae in humans following ordinary long-term industrial exposure.
- **Methanol (CH_3OH):** This compound was originally called "wood alcohol," because it was derived from the distillation of wood. The odor and taste of methanol are similar to those of ethanol, and methanol does not carry the burden of a tax. It is, therefore, used by some impoverished chronic alcoholics as a substitute for ethanol or by unscrupulous merchants as an adulterant of alcoholic beverages. In methanol poisoning, inebriation similar to that produced by ethanol is succeeded by gastrointestinal symptoms, visual dysfunction, coma, and death. The major toxicity of methanol is believed to arise from its metabolism to formaldehyde, principally by alcohol dehydrogenase, followed by its oxidation to formic acid by aldehyde dehydrogenase.

  The most characteristic lesion of methanol toxicity is necrosis of retinal ganglion cells and subsequent degeneration of the optic nerve, a process presumably mediated by the metabolites of methanol oxidation. Interestingly, methanol-induced blindness occurs only in primates. It is not clear whether the metabolic acidosis seen in cases of methanol poisoning results from a direct effect of formate or from an inhibition of glucose oxidation.
- **Ethylene glycol ($HOCH_2CH_2OH$):** Commonly used as an antifreeze, ethylene glycol has been ingested by chronic alcoholics as a substitute for ethanol for many years. Poisoning with this compound has come into prominence because it has been used to adulterate wines in Austria and Italy, owing to its sweet taste and solubility. Like methanol, ethylene glycol is much more toxic in humans than in animals. The major toxicity relates to acute tubular necrosis in the kidney. Oxalate crystals in the tubules and oxaluria are often noted.
- **Gasoline and kerosene:** These fuels are mixtures of aliphatic hydrocarbons and branched, unsaturated, and aromatic hydrocarbons. Despite prolonged exposure to gasoline, gas station attendants, auto mechanics, and so on do not manifest any evidence of toxicity. The increased use of kerosene as a home heating fuel has led to accidental poisoning of children.
- **Benzene (C_6H_6):** The prototypic aromatic hydrocarbon is benzene, which must be distinguished from benzine, a mixture of aliphatic hydrocarbons. Ben-

zene is one of the most widely used chemicals in industrial processes, being employed as the starting point for innumerable syntheses and as a solvent. It is also a constituent of fuels, accounting for as much as 3% of gasoline. Virtually all cases of acute and chronic benzene toxicity have occurred against the background of industrial exposure. Many instances have been reported in shoemakers and workers in shoe manufacturing, occupations that at one time were associated with heavy exposure to benzene-based glues.

Acute benzene poisoning primarily affects the central nervous system, and death results from respiratory failure. However, it is the chronic effects of benzene exposure that have attracted the most attention. The bone marrow is the principal target in chronic benzene intoxication. Those patients who develop hematological abnormalities characteristically exhibit **hypoplasia or aplasia of the bone marrow and pancytopenia**. Aplastic anemia usually is seen while the workers are still exposed to high concentrations of benzene. In a substantial proportion of cases of benzene-induced anemias, **acute myeloblastic leukemia, erythroleukemia, or multiple myeloma** develops during continuing exposure to benzene, or after a variable latent period following removal of the worker from the hazardous environment. Some cases of acute leukemia have occurred without a prior history of aplastic anemia. Although instances of chronic myeloid and chronic lymphocytic leukemia have been reported, a cause-and-effect relationship with benzene exposure is less convincing than with cases of acute leukemia. Overall, the risk of leukemia is increased 60-fold in workers exposed to the highest atmospheric concentrations of benzene. The closely related compound toluene, also widely used for its solvent properties, has not been incriminated as a cause of hematological abnormalities.

Agricultural Chemicals

Pesticides, fungicides, herbicides, and organic fertilizers are crucial to the success of modern agriculture. Without the use of pesticides, it is estimated that agricultural production would fall by about half, and it is possible that epidemic and endemic famine would again become commonplace. However, the realization that many of these chemicals persist in soil and water and pose a potential long-term hazard has caused substantial concern. The problem of acute poisoning with very large concentrations of any of these chemicals has already been alluded to, and it is clear that exposure to industrial concentrations or inadvertently contaminated food can cause severe acute illness. A particularly common acute poisoning occurs in children who ingest home gardening preparations.

The symptoms of acute toxicity are often related to the mode of action of the toxin. For example, the organophosphate insecticides exert their effect by inhibiting acetylcholinesterase, and thus acute toxicity in humans is principally reflected in symptoms referable to the nervous system. In the United States, 30 to 40 persons die annually of acute pesticide poisoning. However, in underdeveloped countries, where the use of safety equipment is unusual, many more fatalities occur. If the acute incident is not fatal, in most cases there are no chronic sequelae. However, delayed neurotoxicity has been reported with a few compounds, the most notorious of which is triorthocresyl phosphate (TOCP). Acute poisoning with this compound leads to a peripheral neuropathy that progresses to motor weakness of limbs, which in some cases is only partially reversible. Contamination of illicit ginger liquor with TOCP in the United States during the 1930s led to an epidemic of "ginger jake paralysis." In Morocco, the adulteration of cooking oil with lubricating oil containing TOCP produced an outbreak of a similar peripheral neuropathy.

The problem of widespread chronic human exposure to low levels of agricultural chemicals has profound health, economic, and legal implications. From a practical point of view, these chemicals cannot be eliminated from our environment, but because they produce a variety of disorders in experimental animals, it is appropriate to search for evidence of disease in humans. Potential effects that have elicited public concern include cancer, chronic degenerative diseases, congenital abnormalities, and a host of nonspecific complaints ranging from asthenia to impotence. However, no persuasive data have emerged to substantiate these fears, with the possible exception of certain types of hemopoietic malignancies in farmers who employ large amounts of herbicides, particularly 2,4-dichlorophenoxyacetic acid (2,4-D). In this respect, several studies have linked occupational exposure to herbicides with an increased incidence of soft tissue sarcomas, lymphomas, and Hodgkin disease.

The current state of our knowledge can be summarized with the simple recognition that although chronic toxicity and reproductive failure have been clearly established in predatory birds and fish, there are no reliable data to support a similar link in humans. Until such a connection has been validated, the burden of proof will remain on those who postulate a cause-and-effect relationship.

Aromatic Halogenated Hydrocarbons

The halogenated aromatic hydrocarbons that have received considerable attention include (1) the polychlorinated biphenyls (PCBs), (2) chlorophenols (pentachlorophenol, used as a wood preservative), (3) hexachlorophene, employed as an antibacterial agent in soaps), and (4) the dioxin TCDD, a byproduct of the synthesis of herbicides and hexachlorophene and, therefore, a contaminant of these preparations. The lack of chronic effects after acute TCDD poisoning has been discussed earlier. Serious questions have been raised regarding the danger of chronic exposure to dioxin, and there is now a consensus that at the very least this compound is far more carcinogenic in rodents than in humans. The problem of the presence of PCBs in the environment resembles that of agricultural chemicals: chronic animal toxicity is well documented, but the most recent data indicate that there are no significant increases in the incidence of cancer or other diseases in workers exposed to PCBs. The same situation pertains to hexachlorophene and pentachlorophenol.

Cyanide

Prussic acid (HCN) is the classic murderer's tool in detective fiction, where the smell of bitter almonds (*Amygdalus prunus*) betrays the crime. A more contemporary homicidal application of cyanide is its surreptitious addition to a number of commercially available medicinal capsules. Amygdalin, a glycoside found in the pits of several fruits (including apricots, peaches, and wild cherries) and in the seeds of almonds and hydrangeas, is a combination of glucose, benzaldehyde, and cyanide. Although humans do not possess the β-glucosidase needed to liberate the cyanide, intestinal flora are capable of effecting this release, thereby leading to cyanide intoxication. Amygdalin is, therefore, far more toxic when ingested than when injected intravenously. These considerations may appear esoteric, except for the fact that extracts of apricot pits are used in the formulation of fraudulent anticancer nostrums and have resulted in cases of cyanide poisoning.

Cyanide blocks cellular respiration, reversibly binding to mitochondrial cytochrome oxidase, the terminal acceptor in the electron transport chain, which is responsible for reducing molecular oxygen to water. The pathological consequences are similar to those produced by any acute global anoxia.

Air Pollutants

A precise definition of air pollution is elusive, since the meaning of "pure air" is not established. In the absence of man-made pollutants, the atmosphere has always been dirtied by natural contaminants. These include the products of vegetation (spores, pollens, airborne molds), emissions from decaying plants (carbon dioxide, hydrogen sulfide), volcanic gases and dusts, and aerosolized bacteria and viruses. However, for the purposes of this discussion, the most important pollutants are those generated by the combustion of fossil fuels for the production of heat and energy.

The most important air pollutants that are implicated as factors in human disease are the irritants sulfur dioxide, nitrogen dioxide, and ozone, in addition to suspended particulates and acid aerosols. Particulate air pollution refers to the presence in the atmosphere of solid particles and liquid droplets, which are of variable size, composition, and origin. Fine particles (2.5 μm or less in aerodynamic diameter) are a mixture of soot, sulfate and nitrate particles, and acid condensates. Because of their small size, they can be inhaled more deeply into the lungs. Owing to their composition, they are also more toxic than larger particles.

Epidemiological studies of the relationship between urban air pollution and adverse respiratory and cardiovascular effects are difficult to interpret because of the confounding effects of cigarette smoking, social class, occupation, age, and so on. However, it is indisputable that episodes of unusually severe air pollution, such as those that occurred in the Meuse valley in Belgium (1930), Donora, Pennsylvania (1948), and London (1952), were associated with striking increases in mortality. During each of these occurrences, the concentrations of sulfur dioxide and particulates are believed to have been remarkably increased.

A substantial body of contemporary epidemiological literature describes adverse health effects from lower levels of particulate air pollution. In studies that adjust for cigarette smoking, the overall mortality in highly polluted cities is still some 25% greater than that in the least polluted areas. The excess mortality is largely attributable to increases in the incidence of lung cancer and cardiopulmonary disease.

Sulfur dioxide results from the combustion of sulfur-containing petroleum and coal in power plants, oil refineries, and industries such as paper mills and smelters. Ozone and nitrogen oxides do not derive principally from industrial activities but rather result from the action of sunlight on the products of vehicular internal combustion engines. Automobiles and trucks emit unburnt hydrocarbons and nitrogen dioxide, after which ultraviolet irradiation leads to complex chemical reactions that produce ozone, various nitrates, and other organic and inorganic compounds in both gas and particulate phases. This mixture of pollutants comprises the "smog" that is characteristic of areas with numerous vehicles and abundant sunlight. Prolonged exposure to gas phase pollutants (SO_2, NO_2, and O_3) is associated with an increase in the frequency of chronic bronchitis and asthmatic attacks and a decrease in pulmonary function.

A number of studies have established an association between these atmospheric contaminants and both chronic respiratory symptoms and mortality. The adverse effects of this type of air pollution principally involve those persons with existing respiratory ailments (asthma, chronic bronchitis, and emphysema) and cardiovascular disease. By contrast, the evidence to incriminate sulfur oxides and particulates in the pathogenesis of chronic respiratory disease remains equivocal.

Carbon Monoxide

Carbon monoxide is an odorless and nonirritating gas that results from the incomplete combustion of organic substances. It combines with hemoglobin with an affinity 240 times greater than that of oxygen to form carboxyhemoglobin. In addition, the binding of carbon monoxide to hemoglobin increases the affinity of the remaining heme moieties for oxygen. As a consequence, oxygen does not readily dissociate from such hemoglobin in the tissues and the hypoxia that results from carbon monoxide poisoning is far greater than can be attributed to the loss of oxygen-carrying capacity alone.

Environmental carbon monoxide is derived principally from automobile exhaust emissions, fires, and in some areas, home heating systems. A concentration of carboxyhemoglobin less than 10% is commonly found in smokers and ordinarily does not produce symptoms. Concentrations up to 30% usually cause only headache and mild exertional dyspnea. Higher levels of carboxyhemoglobin lead to confusion and lethargy; and at concentrations greater than 50%, coma and convulsions ensue. Levels greater than 60% are usually fatal. In fatal cases of carbon monoxide poisoning, a characteristic cherry-red color is imparted to the skin by the carboxyhemoglobin in the superficial capillaries. Recovery from severe carbon monoxide poisoning may be associated with brain damage, which may be manifested as subtle intellectual deficits, memory loss, or extrapyramidal symptoms (e.g., parkinsonism). Treatment of acute carbon monoxide poisoning, as in persons who attempt suicide or are trapped in fires, consists principally of the administration of 100% oxygen.

Deleterious effects of chronic exposure to low levels of carbon monoxide have been difficult to substantiate. However, concentrations of carboxyhemoglobin less than 5% to 8% (often found in smokers) have accelerated the onset of exertional angina and changed the electrocardiograms in patients with ischemic heart disease. Thus, carboxyhemoglobin saturation levels even as low as 2.5% are held to be undesirable in such patients.

Metals

Metals are an important group of environmental chemicals that have caused disease in humans from ancient times to the present. Although for centuries lead and mercury were known to cause disease, the industrial revolution was accompanied by a proliferation of occupational exposures to these and other toxic metals. In our own time, attention has increasingly turned to the ominous threat of the pollution of environment by toxic metals.

Lead

Lead is a ubiquitous heavy metal that is common in the environment of industrialized countries. The concentrations of lead in air, water, food, and soil have sharply increased since the onset of the industrial revolution, and a further increase was related to the introduction of leaded gasoline in the earlier part of this century.

Prior to the widespread awareness of chronic exposure to lead in the 1950s and 1960s, the classic symptoms of lead poisoning were commonly encountered in children and adults. In the United States, lead poisoning was primarily a pediatric problem related to pica, the habit of chewing on cribs, toys, furniture, and woodwork and the eating of painted plaster and fallen paint flakes. Most dwellings built before 1940 were decorated on the interior and exterior with paint that contained lead (up to 40% of dry weight). Children living in dilapidated older homes heavily coated with flaking paint were at significant risk of developing chronic lead poisoning. To these sources of lead was added a heavy burden of atmospheric lead in the form of dust derived from the combustion of lead-containing gasoline. Children and adults living near point sources of environmental lead contamination, such as smelters, were exposed to even higher levels of lead.

In adults, occupational exposure to lead occurred primarily among those engaged in the smelting of lead, a process that releases metal fumes and deposits lead oxide dust in the industrial environment. Lead oxide is a constituent of battery grids, and an occupational exposure to lead is a hazard in the manufacture and recycling of automobile batteries. Accidental poisonings occasionally occurred from the use of pottery that had been improperly fired with a lead glaze, the renovation of an old residence heavily coated with lead paint, the consumption of "moonshine" whiskey made in lead stills, or the "sniffing" of lead-containing gasoline.

METABOLISM: Lead is absorbed through either the lungs or the gastrointestinal tract. Once in the blood, it rapidly equilibrates with the plasma and erythrocytes and is excreted by the kidneys. A portion of blood lead remains freely diffusible and enters either of two types of tissues. Bones, teeth, nails, and hair represent a tightly bound pool of lead that is not generally regarded as harmful. By contrast, the amount of lead in the brain, liver, kidneys, and bone marrow is directly related to its toxic effects. With chronic exposure, 90% of the total body lead burden is in the bones. During metaphyseal bone formation in children, lead and calcium are deposited to produce the increased bone densities ("lead lines") seen radiographically at the metaphysis, thereby providing a simple method of detecting increased body stores of lead in children (Fig. 8-18).

TOXICITY: Classic lead toxicity, which is rarely encountered in the United States today, is manifested in the dysfunction of three important organ systems: (1) the nervous system, (2) the kidneys, and (3) the hemopoietic system (see Fig. 8-20).

The brain is the target of lead toxicity in children; adults usually present with manifestation of peripheral neuropathy. Children with lead encephalopathy are typically irritable and ataxic. They may convulse or display altered states of consciousness, from drowsiness to frank coma. Children with blood lead levels above 80 μg/mL, but with concentrations lower than those in children with frank encephalopathy (120 μg/mL), exhibit mild central nervous system symptoms such as clumsiness, irritability, and hyperactivity.

Lead encephalopathy is a condition in which the brain is edematous and displays flattened gyri and compressed ventricles. There may be herniation of the uncus and cerebellar tonsils. Microscopically, congestion, petechial hemorrhages, and foci of neuronal necrosis are seen. A diffuse astrocytic proliferation in both the gray and white matter may accompany these changes. Vascular lesions in the brain are particularly prominent, with dilatation and proliferation of capillaries.

Peripheral motor neuropathy is the most common manifestation of lead neurotoxicity in the adult, typically affecting the radial and peroneal nerves and resulting in **wristdrop** and **footdrop**, respectively. Lead-induced neuropathy is probably also the basis of the paroxysms of gastrointestinal pain known as **lead colic**.

Anemia is a cardinal sign of lead intoxication. Lead disrupts heme synthesis in bone marrow erythroblasts through inhibition of δ-aminolevulinic acid dehydratase, the second enzyme in the *de novo* synthesis of heme. It also inhibits ferrochelatase, the enzyme that catalyzes the incorporation of ferrous iron into the porphyrin ring. The resulting inability to produce heme adequately is expressed as a microcytic and hypochromic anemia resembling that seen in iron deficiency, in which heme synthesis is also impaired. The anemia of lead intoxication is also

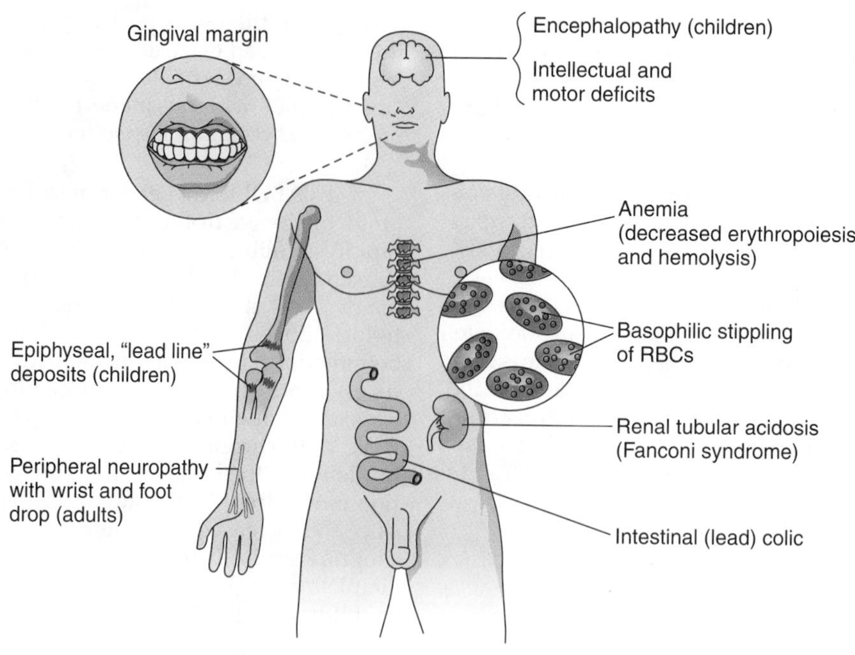

FIGURE *8-18*
Complications of lead intoxication.

characterized by prominent basophilic stippling of the erythrocytes, related to the clustering of ribosomes. The life span of the erythrocytes is decreased; thus, the anemia of lead intoxication is due to both ineffective hemopoiesis and accelerated erythrocyte turnover.

Lead nephropathy reflects the toxic effect of the metal on the proximal tubular cells of the kidney. The resulting dysfunction is characterized by aminoaciduria, glycosuria, and hyperphosphaturia (Fanconi syndrome). Such functional alterations are accompanied by the formation of inclusion bodies in the nuclei of the proximal tubular cells. These inclusions are characteristic of lead nephropathy and are composed of a lead-protein complex containing more than 100 times the concentration of lead in the whole kidney.

Lead poisoning is treated with chelating agents such as calcium ethylene diamine tetraacetic acid (EDTA), either alone or in combination with dimercaprol (BAL). Both the hematological and renal manifestations of lead intoxication are usually reversible, whereas the alterations in the central nervous system are generally irreversible.

The laboratory diagnosis of an increased lead burden is made by demonstrating high levels of lead in the blood and increased free erythrocyte protoporphyrin. Elevated urinary excretion of δ-aminolevulinic acid and decreased levels of aminolevulinic acid dehydratase in erythrocytes are confirmatory.

EFFECTS OF CHRONIC EXPOSURE TO LOW LEAD LEVELS: As a result of the increased use of unleaded gasoline, improvements in housing, substitution of titanium for lead in paints, and the control of industrial point sources, ambient levels of lead have fallen significantly in the past three decades. In fact, blood levels in the general population of the United States decreased from an average of 16 μg/dL of blood in 1976 to less than 10 μg/dL in 1980. The dramatic fall in mean blood lead levels has been accompanied by the near elimination of lead-related childhood fatalities and encephalopathy. At the same time, the safe threshold for blood levels of lead in children was progressively reduced from 60 to 25 μg/dL and is now thought to be lower than 10 μg/dL.

The effects of chronic exposure of children who appear to be in good health to low levels of environmental lead has been extensively studied. The evidence is compelling that low lead exposure in children, while not producing recognizable symptoms, consistently decreases cognitive performance. Moreover, the deficits in intellectual and motor functions persist into adult life. During the last 15 years, efforts to reduce environmental lead exposure have led to a decrease in the percentage of children in the United States with blood levels of 10 μg lead or greater from 89% to 9%. However, elevated blood lead concentrations remain a problem among poor, mainly black children, and more vigorous campaigns to ameliorate this situation are justified.

The margin of safety between "safe" levels of lead and those producing adverse health effects is extremely small. This is particularly important in view of the kinetics of lead metabolism, since a high body burden of lead may not be evident at the time of blood sampling. Even if it were certain that 20 μg/dL is harmless (probably not the case), an increase of only 50% would place the concentration in the range of suspected toxicity. No other environmental pollutant has such a narrow margin between safety and risk.

Mercury

Mercury has been used since prehistoric times and has been known to be an occupation-related hazard at least since the Middle Ages. As the use of mercury has changed, so have the populations at risk. At first, mercurialism was mainly a disease of mercury miners. In the 16th and 17th centuries, mercury poisoning was an occupational disease among gilders of gold, silver, or copper, who used mercury in the process of preparing a surface to be decorated. Mercury was subsequently introduced into the manufacture of fur felt, and mercurialism became an occupational hazard of the hatting industry. The neurological syndrome of tremor ("hatter's shakes") and mental symptoms ("mad as a hatter") was well known in the 19th century.

Although mercury poisoning still occurs in some occupations, there has been increasing concern over the potential health hazards brought about by the contamination of many ecosystems following several well-known outbreaks of methylmercury poisoning. The most widely publicized episodes occurred in Japan, first in Minamata Bay in the 1950s and then in Niigata. In both cases, local inhabitants developed severe, chronic organic mercury intoxication. This poisoning was traced to the consumption of fish contaminated with mercury that had been discharged into the environment in the effluents from a fertilizer and a plastics factory. To date, over 1000 cases of methylmercury poisoning have been reported from Japan. In the early 1970s, there was a more extensive outbreak of mercury poisoning in Iraq resulting from the consumption of bread made from cereal grains that had been treated with organic mercury fungicides. Six thousand persons were affected, 500 of whom died. Interestingly, in prenatally exposed children, later studies showed delayed achievement of developmental milestones and abnormal reflexes, despite the fact that fetal exposure was estimated to be 5 to 10 times lower than that for adults.

In the past two decades, it has become ominously clear that mercury released into the environment may be bioconcentrated and enter the food chain. Bacteria in the bottoms of bays and oceans can convert mercury compounds released from industrial wastes into highly neurotoxic organomercurials. These compounds are then transferred up the food chain and are eventually concentrated in the large predatory fish that make up a substantial part of the diet in many countries.

Although inorganic mercury is not efficiently absorbed in the gastrointestinal tract, organic mercurial compounds are readily absorbed because of their lipid solubility. Both inorganic and organic mercury are preferentially concentrated in the kidney, and methylmercury also distributes to the brain. **Although the kidney is the principal target of the toxicity of inorganic mercury, the brain is damaged by organic mercurials.**

NEPHROTOXICITY: At one time, mercuric chloride was widely used as an antiseptic, and acute mercuric chloride poisoning was much more common; the compound was ingested by accident or for suicidal purposes. Under such circumstances, **proximal tubular necrosis** was accompanied by oliguric renal failure. Mercurial diuretics were also widely prescribed in the past, and chronic mercury nephrotoxicity was a not uncommon complication of their chronic use. Today, chronic mercurial nephrotoxicity is almost always a consequence of a chronic industrial exposure. Proteinuria is common in chronic mercurial nephrotoxicity, and there may be a nephrotic syndrome with more severe intoxication. Pathologically, there is a membranous glomerulonephritis with subepithelial electron-dense deposits, suggesting immune complex deposition.

NEUROTOXICITY: The neurological effects of mercury, now known as **Minamata disease**, are manifested as a constriction of visual fields, paresthesias, ataxia, dysarthria, and hearing loss. Pathologically, there is cerebral and cerebellar atrophy. Microscopically, the cerebellum exhibits atrophy of the granular layer, without loss of Purkinje cells, and spongy softenings in the visual cortex and other cortical regions.

Arsenic

The toxic properties of arsenic have been known for centuries. Arsenic-containing compounds are toxic to a broad spectrum of living systems and, therefore, have been widely used as insecticides, weed killers, and wood preservatives. In the past, the medicinal uses of arsenic ranged from the treatment of a variety of cancers to its use as a "tonic." In the United States, the use of arsenicals in human medicine has declined, although they remain in common use in veterinary medicine and in agriculture. Arsenic compounds contaminate the soil and drinking water as a result of coal burning and the use of arsenical pesticides. As with mercury, there is evidence for the bioaccumulation of arsenic along the food chain.

Acute arsenic poisoning is almost always the result of accidental or homicidal ingestion, and death is due to **central nervous system toxicity**. Chronic arsenic intoxication is characterized initially by such nonspecific symptoms as malaise and fatigue. Eventually, gastrointestinal disturbances develop, along with changes in the skin and a peripheral neuropathy. The latter is characterized by paresthesias, motor palsies, and painful neuritis. On epidemiological grounds, **cancers of the skin and respiratory tract** have been attributed to industrial and agricultural exposure to arsenic. Arsenic in the drinking water has also been related to local increases in the incidence of skin cancer.

Cadmium

Cadmium is used in the manufacture of alloys, in the production of alkali storage batteries, in electroplating of other metals (such as automobile parts and musical instruments), and as a pigment. Fumes of cadmium oxide are released in the course of welding steel parts previously plated with a cadmium anticorrosive.

Acute cadmium inhalation irritates the respiratory tract, with pulmonary edema the most dangerous result. The lungs and the kidneys are the principal target organs of chronic cadmium intoxication. Emphysema has been the major finding in the fatal cases of chronic cadmium pneumonitis that have been studied. Proteinuria, which reflects tubular rather than glomerular damage, has been the most consistent finding in cadmium workers with renal damage.

Nickel

Nickel is a widely used metal in electronics, coins, steel alloys, batteries, and food processing. Dermatitis ("nickel itch"), the most frequent effect of exposure to nickel, may occur from direct contact with metals containing nickel, such as coins and costume jewelry. The dermatitis is a sensitization reaction; the body reacts to nickel-conjugated proteins formed following the penetration of the epidermis by nickel ions. Exposure to nickel, as to arsenic, increases the risk of development of specific types of cancer. Epidemiological studies have demonstrated that workers who were occupationally exposed to nickel compounds have an increased incidence of **lung cancer and cancer of the nasal cavities**.

Iron

Iron deficiency anemia is a common disease, particularly in women. Oral iron preparations contain largely ferrous sulfate, the form absorbed by the gastrointestinal mucosa and then converted to the trivalent form. Acute poisoning from the accidental ingestion of ferrous sulfate tablets occurs chiefly in children, particularly those between the ages of 1 and 2 years. As little as 1 to 2 g of ferrous sulfate may be lethal, but most fatal cases follow ingestion of 3 to 10 g. Hemorrhagic gastritis and acute liver necrosis have been the most prominent findings at autopsy.

A chronic, excessive dietary intake of iron does not lead to abnormal iron accumulation in the body, except in the Bantus of South Africa, among whom it is common. These persons have a high iron content in their diet. Although some of it is derived from iron cooking pots, the major source is the iron drums used for the preparation of fermented alcoholic beverages. The acidic pH of these brews readily solubilizes the iron, and their low alcohol content allows large volumes to be consumed. Whether this high dietary iron intake is solely responsible for the iron overload in these persons is still debated. In any case, a large proportion of the excess iron is in the liver, and there is a correlation between the degree of siderosis and the presence of cirrhosis. There is also a high incidence of diabetes and heart disease in this "Bantu siderosis."

Miscellaneous Metals

COBALT: In the 1960s, an epidemic of an unusual cardiomyopathy, clinically characterized by fulminant congestive heart failure, appeared in drinkers of a particular brand of beer, first in the Canadian province of Quebec and subsequently in the United States and Europe. The heart disease was traced to an excessive intake of cobalt, which had been added to the beer to enhance foaming qualities. When the cobalt was removed from the beer, no further cases of heart disease were reported.

ALUMINUM: In 1972, a new syndrome, called "dialysis encephalopathy," was first reported in patients with uremia undergoing chronic renal dialysis. The subsequent finding of high concentrations of aluminum in the gray matter of the brains of patients who died led to the suggestion that the **encephalopathy resulted from aluminum intoxication**. Epidemiological studies implicated the aluminum in the tap water used to prepare the dialysates, and the disease could be eliminated by removing aluminum from the water. Aluminum intoxication with encephalopathy and osteomalacia can occur in patients (generally children) with uremia who are not dialyzed but who are given oral phosphate-binding gels that contain aluminum.

THERMAL REGULATORY DYSFUNCTION

Body temperature is regulated by the thermal regulatory center of the hypothalamus, which modifies heat loss from the body, and by heat production, primarily from muscular activity. The hypothalamic center is sensitive to thermal, neural, and humoral stimulation. There is also evidence that it responds to changes in the perfusing blood temperature of as little as 0.5°C. A lowering of skin temperature below 32.8°C (91°F) causes a neural discharge of this center. Fever is produced by a short polypeptide, interleukin-1, which is released from macrophages. There is also a diurnal variation in body temperature of about 0.5°C.

Body heat is produced as a result of cellular metabolic activity and muscular work. Cold stress produces an increase in heat production of 50% to 100% by increasing muscle tone, a modification not associated with significant physical movement. Increased heat production beyond this level requires actual muscular contraction, often in the form of shivering, which can further increase the heat yield considerably.

Heat loss accounts for 50% of the heat produced by the body; the remainder of the heat energy provides for the 37°C ± 1°C body temperature. In large part, heat loss is regulated by the volume of blood. Two major factors are involved in the dermal regulatory system: (1) blood flow to the skin and (2) the use of the thermal energy to warm the portion of the skin surface that is wet with perspiration. Dilatation of these arcades to bring the blood nearer the skin surface facilitates the transfer of the heat, a process that underlies the flushed appearance during strenuous exercise or hot weather. The means for heat dissipation from the body are conduction, convection, and radiation of thermal energy, as well as the evaporation of sensible and insensible perspiration from the surface of the skin. Under basal conditions, roughly 5% of the cardiac output goes to the skin, but when vasodilatation is called on to increase heat loss, this value may reach roughly half of the normal cardiac output. In the reverse process, environmental cold leads to vasoconstriction and a reduction in blood flow to the skin, an effect seen as blanching.

Although the skin surface is the major avenue of heat loss, smaller quantities of heat energy are lost through the warming of inspired air and through sweating. The skin has abundant sweat glands whose orifices deposit perspiration on the surface. The evaporation of this fluid contributes to the loss of heat energy by extracting the heat of vaporization. At rest, a person normally loses about 1 liter of insensible perspiration a day. During strenuous physical activity or in a hot environment, the production of sweat serves as an important additional source of cooling.

The dermis is also provided with a fatty layer that

serves as an effective insulator. Humans appear to use body fat as an adaptive device for cold climates. Persons living near and above the Arctic Circle frequently have thicker dermal fat layers than their southern counterparts.

Hypothermia

Hypothermia refers to a decrease in body temperature below 35°C (95°F). It can result in systemic or focal injury, the latter exemplified by **trenchfoot** or **immersion foot**. In localized hypothermia of these types, actual tissue freezing does not occur. **Frostbite**, by contrast, involves the crystallization of tissue water. It should not be forgotten that the hospitalized patient, especially if sedated, is often placed in a thermal environment that is cooler than optimal and that can exert a stressful effect. Heat loss during a surgical procedure can be remarkable, and the administration of muscle relaxants further compromises the ability to generate heat.

Generalized Hypothermia

Acute immersion in water at 4°C to 10°C leads to a reduction in central blood flow, coupled with a decreased core body temperature and cooling of the blood perfusing the brain, which results in mental confusion. Muscle tetany makes swimming impossible. Furthermore, an increased vagal discharge leads to premature ventricular contractions, ventricular arrhythmias, and even fibrillation.

In an attempt to increase heat production, the immersed body immediately responds by increasing muscle activity and oxygen consumption. However, there are limits to the sources of energy available for sustained warming. Within 30 minutes, heat loss exceeds heat production because of the combination of high direct conduction of heat from the whole skin surface and the altered muscle tone caused by decreased arterial carbon dioxide and exhaustion. Core temperature then begins to fall. Peripheral vasoconstriction is another response to conserve heat. In addition, there is an increased sympathetic neural discharge, resulting in increased heart and basal metabolic rates and shivering. When the core temperature approaches 35°C, this activity may be three to six times above normal. Below this temperature, declines in respiratory rate, heart rate, and blood pressure ensue because of the reduction in functional reserve.

With prolonged cooling, a "cold-induced" diuresis results in an increased blood viscosity. As a result, blood flow decreases and oxygen-hemoglobin association is less effective. Cardiac stroke volume decreases and peripheral vascular resistance increases as a direct result of both blood "sludging" and loss of plasma. The most important factor in causing death is cardiac arrhythmia or sudden cardiac arrest. These observations have been confirmed and extended in the past several decades, largely because of the need to induce hypothermia in patients undergoing open-heart surgery. In fact, with careful pharmacological control, prolonged periods of decreased body temperature can be achieved with no residual harm.

During prolonged hypothermia—for example, after an accident to a mountain climber—several of the consequences of decreased body temperature are related to altered cerebrovascular function. When the body core temperature reaches 32°C (89.6°F), the exposed person becomes lethargic, apathetic, and withdrawn. A characteristic response is inappropriate behavior, including disrobing, even when cold. A further decline in temperature increases the lethargy to intermittent "stupor" and eventually coma. A core temperature below 28°C (82.4°F) results in a weak pulse, feeble respiration, and coma.

Although there are no specific morphological changes in those who have succumbed to hypothermia, the skin exhibits red and purple discolorations, swelling of the ears and hands, and irregular vasoconstriction and vasodilatation. Areas of myocytolysis are seen within the heart. The lung may display pulmonary edema and intraalveolar, intrabronchial, and interstitial hemorrhage.

Focal Thermal Alterations

As discussed previously, local reduction in tissue temperature, particularly in the skin, is associated with local vasoconstriction. Tissue water crystallizes if blood circulation is insufficient to counter persistent thermal loss. When freezing occurs slowly, ice crystals form within tissue cells and in the interstitial space. Concomitantly, electrolyte-rich gels are excluded. Injury to the cellular organelles reflects the drastic changes in ionic concentrations in the excluded volume. Denaturation of macromolecules follows, as well as physical disruption of cellular membranes by the ice. When freezing is rapid, a gel-like structure forms within the cell that lacks the crystalloids of water. This water-solid reduces the extent of mechanical and chemical injury. The most significant cellular damage apparently occurs on thawing, when mechanical disruption of membrane structures occurs. This may be the result of a transformation from the gel to the crystal state.

The most biologically significant cell injury appears in the endothelial lining of the capillaries and venules, an effect that alters small vessel permeability. This injury initiates extravasation of plasma, formation of localized edema and blisters, and an inflammatory reaction. Whereas frostbite results from the actual freezing of water, immersion foot (trenchfoot) is caused by a prolonged reduction in tissue temperature to a point not low enough to freeze tissue. This cooling causes cellular disruption and vascular changes that resemble those observed during the healing phase of local tissue freezing. The target, again, seems to be the endothelial cell. Local thrombosis and changes caused by altered permeability are prominent. Vascular occlusion often leads to gangrene.

Hyperthermia

Tissue responses to hyperthermia are similar in some respects to those caused by freezing injuries. In both instances, injury to the vascular endothelium results in altered vascular permeability, edema, and blisters. The degree of injury is dependent on both the extent of temperature elevation and the rapidity with which it is reached. Clearly, increased temperature of any living system increases its metabolic rate. However, above a certain thermal limit, denaturation of enzymes and precipitation of other proteins occur. In addition, "melting" of the lipid bilayers of cell membranes takes place.

Systemic Hyperthermia

Systemic hyperthermia is an elevation of body core temperature. It occurs because of (1) increased heat production, (2) decreased elimination of heat from the body (reflecting an aberrant response of the thermal regulatory center), or (3) a disturbance of the thermal regulatory center itself. It can also occur because heat is conducted into the body faster than the system can clear the additional "thermal load."

A body temperature higher than 42.5°C (108.5°F) leads to profound functional disturbances, including general vasodilatation, inefficient cardiac function, and altered respiration. Isolated heart-lung preparations fail at about the same temperature, suggesting an inherent temperature limitation in the cardiovascular system and perhaps in the myocardial cells themselves. **In general, systemic temperature elevations above 41°C to 42°C are not compatible with life.**

Systemic temperature elevations are commonly designated "fever." During infectious processes and inflammatory responses, interleukin-1 and tumor necrosis factor, derived from macrophages, apparently reset the body's "thermostat" to permit a higher body core temperature level. However, this may not be the sole thermal factor.

There are few, if any, defined pathological changes that are associated with fever alone. Physical findings include increased heart and respiratory rates, peripheral vasodilatation, and diaphoresis, all recognized mechanisms for thermal regulation. The central nervous system responds with irritability, restlessness, and, particularly in children, convulsions. Nocturnal temperature elevations with "night sweats" are a feature of pulmonary granulomatous infection (especially tuberculosis) and are also observed in lymphoproliferative diseases. Prolonged temperature elevation can produce wasting, principally because of an increased metabolic rate.

Malignant hyperthermia is a peculiar thermal alteration that occurs during surgery in susceptible persons. The cause of this prolonged temperature elevation is not known, but it may be a hypersensitivity response to anesthetic agents.

Heat stroke is a form of hyperthermia that is not mediated by endogenous pyrogens. It appears under conditions of very high ambient temperatures and reflects impaired cooling responses of the thermal regulatory systems. Heat stroke characteristically occurs in infants and young children and in the very aged. Often the disorder is associated with an underlying chronic illness and the intake of diuretics, tranquilizers that may affect the hypothalamic thermal regulatory center, or drugs that inhibit perspiration. Another form of heat stroke is seen in healthy men during unusually vigorous exercise. Lactic acidosis, hypocalcemia, and rhabdomyolysis may be severe problems, and almost one third of patients with exertional heat stroke develop myoglobinuric acute renal failure. Heat stroke is not amenable to treatment with standard antipyretics, and only external cooling and fluid and electrolyte replacement are effective therapy.

Cutaneous Burns

Cutaneous burns are the most frequent form of localized hyperthermia. Both the elevated temperature and the rate of temperature change are important in determining the pattern of the tissue response. A temperature of 70°C or higher for several seconds causes necrosis of the entire dermal epithelium, whereas a temperature of 50°C may be sustained for 10 minutes or more without killing the cells.

Cutaneous burns have been separated into three categories of severity: first-, second-, and third-degree burns (Fig. 8-19). A more contemporary classification refers to full-thickness (third-degree) and partial thickness (first- and second-degree) burns.

FIRST DEGREE

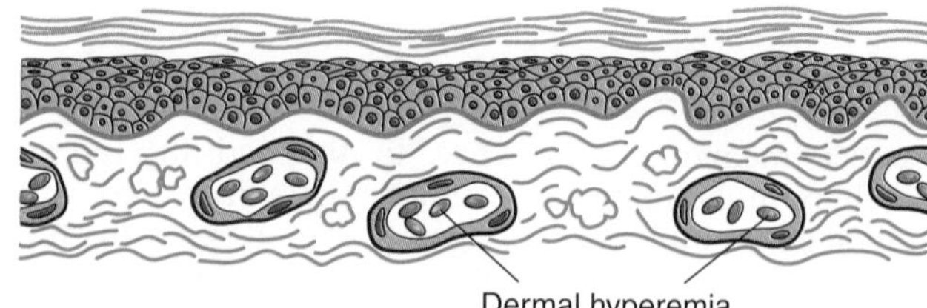

SECOND DEGREE

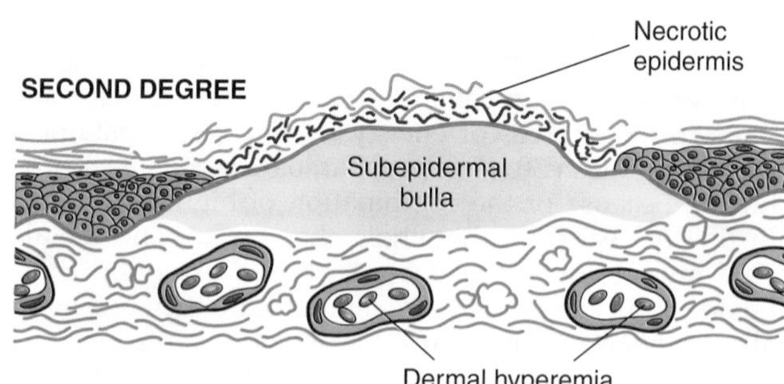

THIRD DEGREE

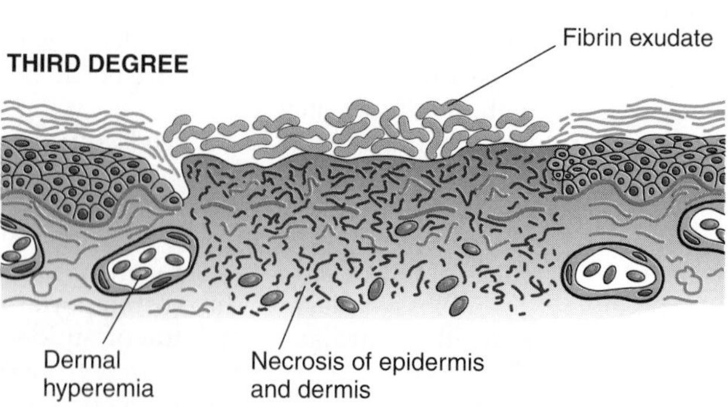

FIGURE *8-19*
The pathology of cutaneous burns. A first-degree skin burn exhibits only dilatation of the dermal blood vessels. In a second-degree burn, there is necrosis of the epidermis, and subepidermal edema collects under the necrotic epidermis to form a bulla. In a third-degree burn, both the epidermis and dermis are necrotic.

- **First-degree burns**, such as a mild sunburn, are recognized by congestion and pain but are not associated with necrosis. Mild endothelial injury produces vasodilatation, increased vascular permeability, and slight edema.
- **Second-degree burns** cause necrosis of the epithelium but spare the dermis. Clinically, these burns are recognized by blisters, in which the epithelium is separated from the dermis.
- **Third-degree burns** char both the epithelium and the underlying dermis. Histologically, the epidermis and the dermis are carbonized and the cellular structure is lost.

One of the most serious systemic disturbances caused by extensive cutaneous burns arises from the fact that the denuded skin surfaces "weep" plasma. Persons with third-degree burns can lose about 0.3 mL body water per square centimeter of burned area a day. The resulting hemoconcentration and poor vascular perfusion of the skin and other viscera complicate the recovery of these patients. Many severely burned persons, particularly with more than 70% of their body surface involved with third-degree burns, develop shock and acute tubular necrosis, in which circumstance the mortality is very high. Severely burned patients who survive longer are at great risk of lethal surface infections and sepsis.

The healing of cutaneous burns is related to the extent of the tissue destruction. First-degree burns, by definition, display little if any cell loss, and healing requires only repair or replacement of the injured endothelial cells. Second-degree burns also heal without a scar because the basal cells of the epidermis are not destroyed and serve as a source of regenerating cells for the epithelium. Third-degree burns, in which there is destruction of the entire thickness of the epidermis, pose a separate set of problems. If the destruction spares the skin appendages, reepithelialization can arise from these foci. Initially, islands of proliferation at the orifices of these glands grow and coalesce to cover the surface. Saprophytic infection of the charred tissue is common and poses another difficulty for healing. Deeper burns that destroy the skin appendages require new epidermis to be grafted to the debrided area to establish a functional covering. Burned skin that is not replaced by a graft heals with the formation of a dense scar. Since this connective tissue lacks the elasticity of normal skin, contractures that limit motion may be the eventual result. In severe burns, epithelial layers have been produced *in vitro* from cultured keratinocytes derived from the patient's own surviving skin. The application of these layers of squamous epithelium to the burned areas has permitted the survival of severely injured patients who previously would have surely died.

Inhalation Burns

Persons trapped in burning buildings and vehicles are exposed to air and aerosolized flammable materials that have been heated to very high temperatures. The inhalation of these noxious fumes injures or destroys the respiratory tract epithelium from the oral cavity to the alveoli. If the patient survives the acute episode, the end-result of such a burn is the development of the adult respiratory distress syndrome (ARDS), which itself may be fatal.

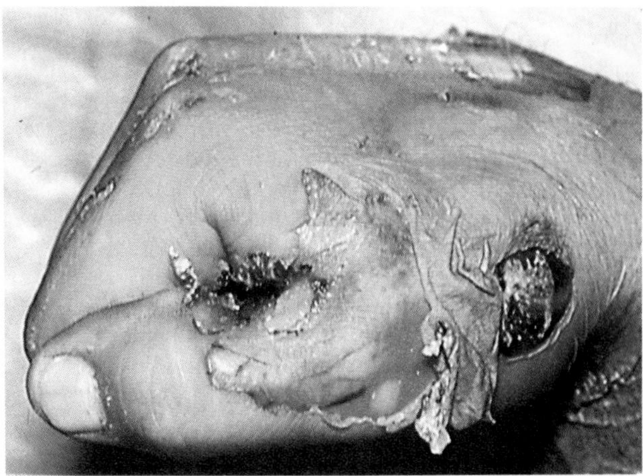

FIGURE *8-20*
Electrical burn of the skin. The victim was electrocuted after attempting to stop a fall from a ladder by grasping a high-voltage electrical line.

Electrical Burns

Electrical injury produces damage through two modalities: (1) through an electrical dysfunction of the cardiovascular conduction system and the nervous system, and (2) through the conversion of electrical energy to heat energy when the current encounters the resistance of the tissues. **Because electrical energy has the potential to disrupt the electrical system within the heart, it frequently causes death through ventricular fibrillation.** The amount of current necessary to produce such a disruption depends in part on its pathway through the body and its ease in penetrating the skin. Someone who inadvertently touches a 120-V line in a living room may suffer burns on the hand because of the electrical resistance of the skin that contacts the wire. A person inadvertently touching the same line in a bathtub may have no cutaneous manifestations but may be killed by disordered electrical activity in the heart. In the latter instance, the wet skin provides a low-resistance entry for the current, thereby permitting greater current flow to the entire body.

Electrical burns of the skin reflect the voltage, the area of electrical conductance, and the duration of current flow (Fig. 8-20). Very high-voltage current chars the tissue and produces a third-degree burn. On the other hand, broad, moist surfaces exposed to the same flow exhibit less severe change. With very high-voltage currents, the force may be almost "explosive," in which case vaporization of tissue water produces extensive damage.

ALTITUDE-RELATED ILLNESSES

High-altitude illness is rare, in large part because of the acclimation of mountain climbers before extreme altitudes are achieved. However, there is an altitude limit beyond which human life cannot be sustained for prolonged periods. Communities in the Andes succeed at 4000 to 4300 meters. The inhabitants adapt to the decreased pressure and availability of oxygen by developing elevated hematocrits and large "barrel" chests with increased lung volume. Even those who live in this zone do not survive at elevations above 5500 to 6000 meters. Prolonged stays at this altitude result in weight loss, difficulty in sleeping, and lethargy, perhaps because of the redirection of cellular energy simply for survival. For example, 75% to 90% of the oxygen obtained per inspiration at 6000 meters is used for the effort of inspiration alone.

The modifications induced by high altitude are related to a decreased atmospheric pressure and, therefore, to decreased oxygen availability. It has been suggested that the decreased oxygen tension and the limited ability of the lungs to extract oxygen at lower pressures produce the hypoxia that is probably the most important factor in causing high-altitude illness. The narrow reserve is illustrated by the observation that physical activity at these elevations leads to a decrease in the partial pressure of arterial oxygen, whereas comparable physical activity at sea level does not change oxygen saturation. At sea level, cardiac output limits exercise, whereas at high altitudes the diffusing capacity of the lung for oxygen seems to be the determinant.

Acclimation to chronic hypoxia at high altitudes results in a reduced ventilatory drive. Acclimated persons exhibit increases in (1) the number of capillaries per unit of brain, muscle, and myocardium; (2) the amount of myoglobin within tissues; (3) the number of mitochondria per cell; and (4) the hematocrit. An increase in erythrocyte levels of 2′3′-diphosphoglycerate, which enhances oxygen delivery to tissues, occurs within hours, but the induction of polycythemia requires months. Some of the minor effects of high altitude are systemic edema, retinal hemorrhages, and flatus expulsion. The more serious nonfatal diseases are acute and chronic mountain sickness and high-altitude deterioration. Fatal disease can develop in the form of **high-altitude pulmonary edema and high-altitude encephalopathy**.

- **High-altitude systemic edema:** This condition results from an asymptomatic modification of vascular permeability, particularly in the hands, face, and feet and most often occurs at elevations over 3000 meters. It is reflected only in weight gain; on return to lower altitude, a diuresis causes the edema to disappear. This disorder is twice as common in women as in men. The cause of this peculiar condition is not known, and an endothelial response to hypoxia provides only a partial explanation.
- **High-altitude retinal hemorrhage:** A critical analysis by funduscopic examination revealed that 30% to 60% of those sleeping above 5000 meters had retinal hemorrhages. The initial effect includes retinal vascular engorgement and tortuousness. Optic disc hyperemia is also noted, and multiple flame-shaped hemorrhages subsequently occur. These changes are reversible.
- **High-altitude flatus:** Changes in external pressure and the production of intestinal gas provide for the expansion of the luminal contents of the intestine and increased flatus at altitudes above 3500 meters. No specific physical disease has been associated with these changes, although social problems have been encountered.
- **Acute mountain sickness:** This condition is rare below 2500 meters but is present to some degree in nearly everyone at 3000 to 3600 meters. The initial presentation includes headache, lassitude, anorexia, weakness, and difficulty in sleeping. The pathophysiological mechanism that underlies this disease is in part related to hypoxia and a shift in plasma fluid to the interstitial space. Adaptation through a modification of pulmonary function (increased respiratory rate) causes some amelioration of the disease. Descent to lower altitudes is certainly indicated. Chronic or subacute exacerbation of this disease also occurs, frequently at lower altitudes, and the symptoms may be severe. The basis of the disease is not known.
- **High-altitude deterioration:** Generally occurring at higher elevations (5500 meters or more), high-altitude deterioration presents as a decrease in physical and mental performance. The combination of chronic hypoxia, inadequate fluid intake, and inadequate nutrition, together with decreased plasma volume and hemoconcentration, are aggravating factors.
- **High-altitude pulmonary edema and cerebral edema:** Serious high-altitude problems, including pulmonary edema and cerebral edema, can occur with a rapid ascent to heights over 2500 meters, particularly in susceptible persons who have difficulty tolerating sleeping at higher altitudes. Tachycardia, right ventricular overload, and a marked reduction in arterial oxygen pressure occur, but there is no change in pH or carbon dioxide retention. A characteristic patchy pulmonary infiltrate is noted radiographically. Pulmonary hypertension is common in patients with high-altitude pulmonary edema. Hypoxic vasoconstriction and intravascular thrombosis have been proposed as causes of pulmonary hypertension. Eventually, cardiac output is decreased and systemic blood pressure falls. The precapillary arterioles become dilated, increasing capillary bed pressure and inducing interstitial and alveolar edema. Autopsy findings include severe confluent pulmonary edema, proteinaceous alveolar exudates, and hyaline membrane formation. Capillary obstruction by thrombi has been noted. A dilated heart and enlarged pulmonary arteries are commonly found.
- **High-altitude encephalopathy** is characterized by confusion, stupor, and coma. Autopsies have consistently revealed cerebral edema and vascular congestion. A proposed mechanism is severe cerebral hypoxia, with inhibition of the sodium pump and resultant intracellular edema.

PHYSICAL INJURIES

The effect of mechanical trauma is related to the force transmitted to the tissue, the rate at which the transfer occurs, the surface area to which the force is transferred, and the area of the body that is injured. The disruption of the continuity of the tissue results in a wound. It should be remembered, however, that the transmission of the energy absorbed can produce alterations elsewhere in the body.

- **Force expended:** The amount of energy released is related to the velocity and mass of the object that strikes the person, or to that of the person who collides with a stationary object. In addition to the lateral displacement, many objects that strike people—from bullets to car wheels—have rotational forces. Prolongation of the period of impact dissipates some of the energy, as when a boxer "rolls with a punch."

- **Transfer area:** The area over which transfer of force occurs is particularly important. The intensity—that is, the force exerted per unit area—decreases with the increasing area. A protective helmet does not lessen the force of a blow or projectile but diffuses it over a larger area.
- **Body area:** The area of the body that is affected by physical trauma plays an important role. The compressibility of the tissue adjacent to the transmitted force in part determines its effect. A blow over a large muscle mass, such as the thigh or upper arm, is often less injurious than a direct blow to a poorly shielded bone, such as the anterior tibia. Furthermore, the distribution of the force is important. Blows over a hollow viscus can rupture the organ because of compression of the fluid or gas it contains; organs nestled beneath the skin, such as the liver, can be easily ruptured. An impact directly over the heart can even disturb its electrical systems.

Contusions

A contusion is a localized area of mechanical injury with focal hemorrhage. A force with sufficient energy may disrupt capillaries and venules within an organ by physical means alone. If this occurs in the skin, a loss of blood into the tissue space occurs, with consequent altered coloration. The change may be so limited that the only histological change is hemorrhage in tissue spaces outside the vascular compartment. The presence of a discrete blood pool within the tissue is termed a **hematoma**. Initially, the deoxygenated blood renders the area blue to blue-black, as in the classic "black eye." Macrophages ingest the erythrocytes and convert the hemoglobin to bilirubin, thereby changing the color from blue to yellow. Both mobilization of the pigment by macrophages and further metabolism of bilirubin cause the yellow to fade to yellowish green and then to disappear.

Abrasions

An abrasion is a skin defect caused by a direct or tangential impact that crushes or scrapes the epithelial surface. The disruptive force may destroy some of the cells by crushing them, and thus may provide a portal of entry for microorganisms. There may be disruption of the epidermis itself, and there may also be vascular distortion of the cells within the dermis. The impact of the agent and its configuration are frequently seen in these wounds and are of special interest to the forensic pathologist.

Lacerations

A laceration is a split or tear of the skin that results from an impact stronger than that causing an abrasion. Lacerations are usually the result of unidirectional displacement, but they may have crushed margins, in which case they are termed abraded lacerations.

Incisions and Wounds

An incision is the deliberate opening of the skin by a cutting instrument, usually the surgeon's scalpel. Incisions have particularly sharp edges and, importantly, spare no tissue to the depth of the wound. **Deep penetrating wounds** produced by high-velocity projectiles, such as bullets, are often deceptive, because the energy of the missile as it passes through the body may be released at sites distant from the entrance itself. Bullets, because they rotate, produce a well-defined and usually round entrance wound (Fig. 8-21). Once the projectile enters the flesh, however, it may fragment, tumble, or actually explode, resulting in a

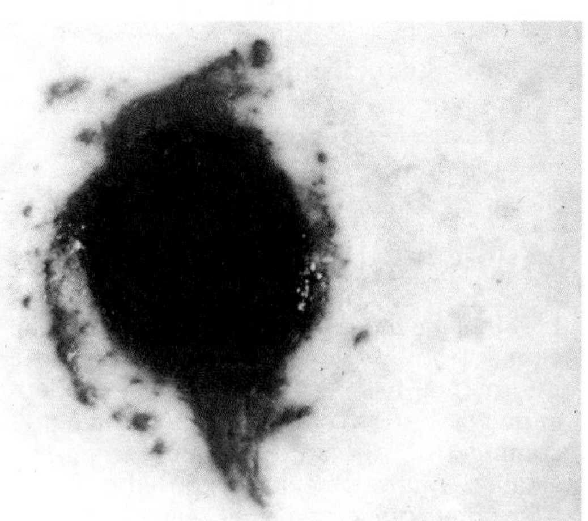
A

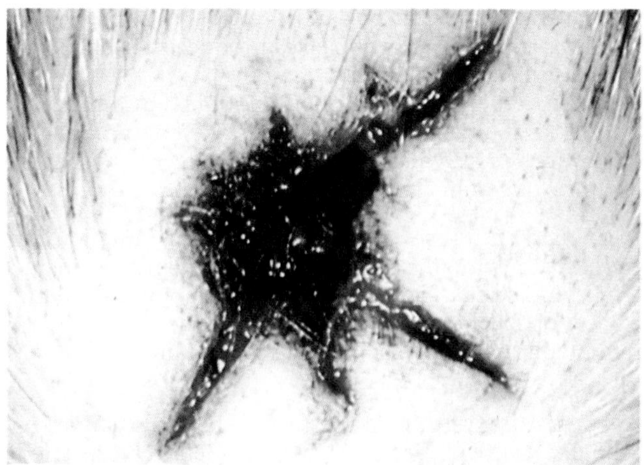
B

FIGURE *8-21*
Bullet wounds. (*A*) The entrance wound is sharply punched out. (*B*) The exit wound is irregular with the characteristic stellate lacerations.

remarkable degree of tissue damage and a large, ragged exit wound. The interested student may refer to the reading list at the end of the chapter for further information in this area of forensic pathology.

RADIATION

We can define radiation simply as the emission of energy by one body, its transmission through an intervening medium, and its absorption by another body. By this definition, radiation encompasses the entire electromagnetic spectrum and certain charged particles emitted by radioactive elements. However, since the latter also have wave characteristics, this distinction is to some extent arbitrary. Alpha particles such as the radiation emitted by ^{32}P and the beta particles of elements such as tritium (^{3}H) and ^{14}C are of immense use scientifically and diagnostically but pose few hazards for humans. High-energy radiation, in the form of gamma or x-rays, is the mediator of most of the biological effects discussed here. We do not consider the effects of ultraviolet radiation here, since they are discussed in Chapters 5 and 24.

Medical practice is inconceivable today without the use of diagnostic and therapeutic radioisotopes, clinical radiographs, and radiation therapy. On the other hand, nuclear explosions and accidental exposure to radiation in nuclear power plants have caused injury and death. Here, we focus on the pathological consequences of radiation exposure. Radiation is quantitated in a number of ways:

- **A roentgen** is a measure of the emission of radiant energy from a source. This unit refers to the amount of ionization produced in air.
- **A rad** measures the absorption of radiant energy, which is biologically the more important parameter. A rad defines the energy, expressed as ergs, absorbed by a tissue. One rad equals 100 ergs per gram of tissue.
- **A gray** is a unit that corresponds to 100 rads (1 joule/kg tissue)
- **The rem** unit was introduced to describe the biological effect produced by a rad of high-energy radiation, because low-energy particles produce more biological damage than gamma or x-rays.
- **A sievert** is the dose in grays multiplied by an appropriate quality factor Q, so that 1 sievert of radiation is roughly equivalent in biological effectiveness to 1 gray of gamma rays.

For the purposes of this discussion of radiation-induced pathology, the roentgen, rad, and rem are considered comparable. The details of radiation biology are the subject of a voluminous literature, and the student may refer to this chapter's list of suggested reading.

☐ **Pathogenesis:** At the cellular level, radiation essentially has two effects: (1) a somatic effect, associated with acute cell killing, and (2) the induction of genetic damage. Radiation-induced cell death is believed to be caused by the acute effects of the radiolysis of water (see Chapter 1). The production of activated oxygen species may result in lipid peroxidation, membrane injury, and possibly an interaction with macromolecules of the cell. Genetic damage to the cell, whether caused by direct absorption of energy by DNA (the target theory) or caused indirectly by a reaction of DNA with oxygen radicals, is expressed either as a mutation or as reproductive failure. Both mutation and reproductive failure may lead to delayed cell death, and mutation is incriminated in the development of radiation-induced neoplasia.

The differential sensitivity of tissues to radiation has been recognized since the beginning of the century (see Table 8-2 on page 323). For example, the intestine and the hemopoietic bone marrow are far more vulnerable to radiation than tissues such as bone and brain. These differences should not be construed as a reflection of variable sensitivity to acute cell killing, even though there may be slight differences in the acute somatic response of cells to radiation based on antioxidant and other metabolic defenses. The important consideration is that the vulnerability of a tissue to radiation-induced damage depends on its proliferative rate, which in turn correlates with the natural life span of the constituent cells. Damage to the DNA of a long-lived, nonproliferating cell does not necessarily pose a threat to its function or viability because the reproductive and metabolic functions of the cell are separate properties. By contrast, a short-lived, proliferating cell, such as an intestinal crypt cell or a hemopoietic precursor, must be rapidly replaced by the division of stem cells and committed precursor. When radiation-induced DNA damage precludes mitosis of these cells, the mature elements are not replaced and the tissue can no longer function.

Before discussing the structural and functional injury produced by radiation, it is important to distinguish between whole-body irradiation and localized irradiation. Except for unusual circumstances, as in the high-dose irradiation that precedes bone marrow transplantation, significant levels of whole-body irradiation result only from industrial accidents or from the explosion of nuclear weapons. By contrast, localized irradiation is an inevitable byproduct of any diagnostic radiological procedure, and it is the intended result of radiation therapy. Rapid somatic cell death occurs only with extremely high doses of radiation, well in excess of 1000 rads. It is morphologically indistinguishable from the coagulative necrosis produced by other causes (see Chapter 1). By contrast, irreversible damage to the replicative capacity of cells requires far lower doses, possibly as little as 50 rads.

Whole-Body Irradiation

Fortunately, there have been few instances of human disease caused by whole-body irradiation, and most of our information has been derived from studies of Japanese atom bomb survivors. Further information may be forthcoming from the study of the survivors of the much smaller sample of persons exposed in the accident at the Chernobyl nuclear power plant in the former Soviet Union in 1986.

Since comparable doses of radiant energy are transmitted to all organs in whole-body irradiation, the development of the different acute radiation syndromes re-

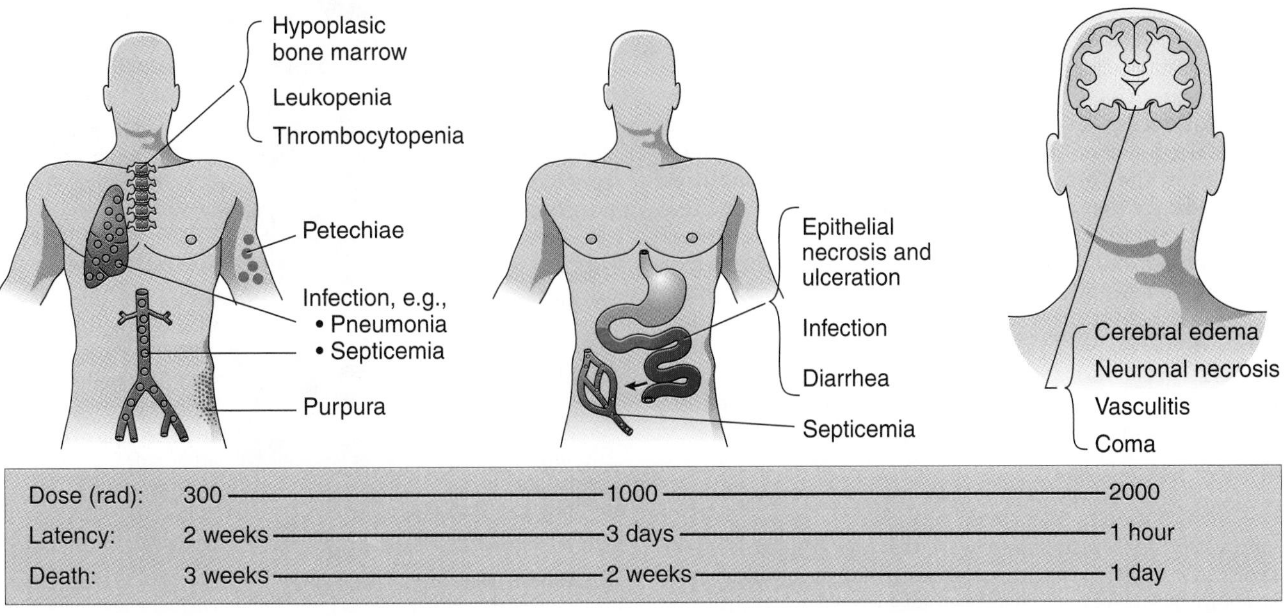

FIGURE 8-22
Acute radiation syndromes. At a dose of approximately 300 rads of whole body radiation, a syndrome characterized by hemopoietic failure develops within 2 weeks. In the vicinity of 1000 rads, a gastrointestinal syndrome with a latency of only 3 days is seen. With doses of 2000 rads or greater, disease of the central nervous system appears within 1 hour, and death ensues rapidly.

flects the dissimilarities in vulnerability of the target tissues (Fig. 8-22).

300 RADS: At a dose of approximately 300 rads, a syndrome characterized by **hemopoietic failure** develops within 2 weeks. Since all hemopoietic precursor elements are highly sensitive to radiant energy, a pancytopenia typically characterizes the hemopoietic whole-body irradiation syndrome. Following an initial depletion of circulating lymphocytes, a progressive decrease in formed elements of the blood eventually leads to bleeding, anemia, and infection. The last is often the cause of death.

1000 RADS: With more intense radiation, in the vicinity of 1000 rads, the principal cause of death is related to the **gastrointestinal system**. Although gastrointestinal symptoms characterize the entire dose range of whole-body exposure, at higher levels severe destruction of the entire epithelium of the gastrointestinal tract occurs within 3 days, the time that corresponds to the normal life span of the villous and crypt cells. As a result, the fluid homeostasis of the bowel is disrupted and severe diarrhea and dehydration ensue. Moreover, the epithelial barrier to intestinal bacteria is breached, and organisms invade and disseminate throughout the body. Septicemia and shock kill the victim.

2000 RADS: With exposure to whole-body doses of 2000 rads and greater, central nervous system damage causes death within hours. In most cases, cerebral edema and loss of the integrity of the blood-brain barrier, owing to endothelial injury, predominates. With extreme doses, radiation necrosis of neurons can be expected. Convulsions, coma, and death follow.

FETAL EFFECTS: The effects of whole-body irradiation on the human fetus have been documented in studies of the survivors of the atom bomb explosions in Japan. Pregnant women exposed to doses of 25 rads or greater gave birth to infants with reduced head size, diminished overall growth, and mental retardation.[1] In studies of the clinical status of children who were exposed to therapeutic doses of radiation *in utero*, the most likely time for the production of growth retardation and microcephaly was between the 3rd and 20th week of gestation. Other effects of irradiation *in utero* include hydrocephaly, microphthalmia, chorioretinitis, blindness, spina bifida, cleft palate, clubfeet, and genital abnormalities. Data derived from experimental and human studies strongly support the conclusion that major congenital malformations are highly unlikely with doses of less than 20 rads after day 14 of pregnancy. However, lower doses may produce more subtle effects, such as a decrease in mental capacity. **To protect against such a possibility, the established maximum permissible dose to the fetus from exposure of the expectant mother is far below the known teratogenic dose.**

[1] Intrauterine exposure to radiation at Nagasaki was significantly less teratogenic than at Hiroshima. This disparity has been attributed to a difference in the quality of the radiation in the two cities. The bomb dropped on Hiroshima produced far greater fast-neutron radiation (20% as opposed to 1% of the total energy released), which is lower in energy than comparable doses of gamma rays and, therefore, produces greater biological damage.

GENETIC EFFECTS: The potential genetic effects of radiation have been the source of considerable public alarm. Again, there is a dearth of evidence, and most of the data on which predictions of human genetic effects are based are derived from experimental data. **After long-term follow-up, even the survivors of Hiroshima and Nagasaki have failed to manifest evidence of genetic damage in the form of either congenital abnormalities or hereditary diseases in subsequent offspring or their descendants.** In experimental animals, the risk of induced mutation per rad is at most only 0.5% to 5% of the risk of spontaneous mutation (estimated to be 10% of live births in humans). In other words, the experimental radiation exposure necessary to double the spontaneous mutation rate is 20 to 200 rads. Thus, even with the most pessimistic estimates, the risk of genetic damage to future generations from radiation appears vanishingly small.

AGING: The finding that rodents exposed to whole-body irradiation have a shortened life span has led to the suggestion that radiation accelerates the aging process. A mortality study of the survivors of the atom bomb explosions in Japan has not disclosed any excess mortality not attributable to neoplasia. Nor is there any evidence of acceleration in disease among the survivors in any part of the age range. **Thus, the effects of ionizing radiation on mortality are specific and focal, and there is no reason to believe that premature aging in humans or radiation-induced carcinogenesis is due to a general acceleration of aging.**

Localized Radiation Injury Associated with Radiation Therapy

In the course of radiation therapy for malignant neoplasms, some normal tissue is inevitably included in the radiation field. Although almost any organ can be damaged by radiation, the clinically important tissues are the skin, lungs, heart, kidney, bladder, and intestine—organs that are difficult to shield (Fig. 8-23). Localized damage to the bone marrow is clearly of little functional consequence because of the immense reserve capacity of the hemopoietic system.

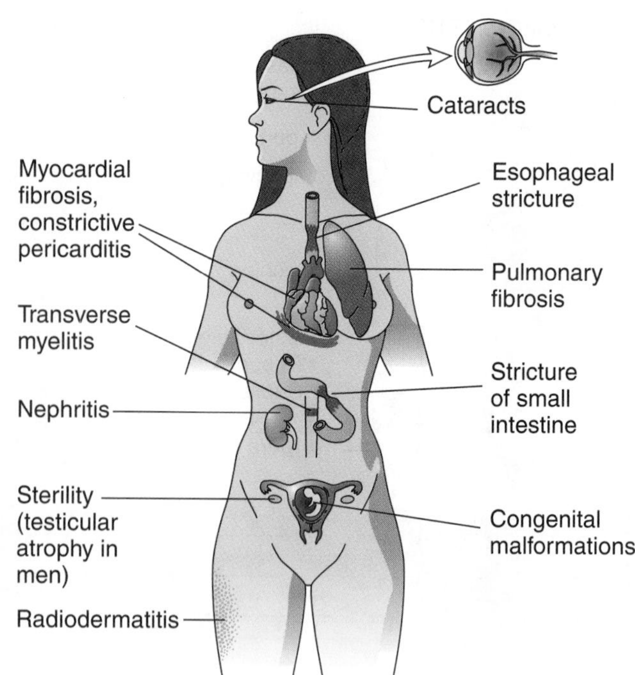

FIGURE 8-23
The non-neoplastic complications of radiation.

☐ **Pathology:** Persistent damage to radiation-exposed tissue can be attributed to two major factors: (1) compromise of the vascular supply and (2) a fibrotic repair reaction to acute necrosis and chronic ischemia. Radiation-induced tissue injury predominantly affects small arteries and arterioles. The endothelial cells are the most sensitive elements in the blood vessels and acutely exhibit swelling and necrosis. Chronically the walls become thickened by endothelial cell proliferation and subintimal deposition of collagen and other connective tissue elements. Striking vacuolization of intimal cells, the so-called foam cells, is typical. Fragmentation of the internal elastic lamina, loss of smooth muscle cells and scarring in the media, and fibrosis of the adventitia are seen in the small arteries. The fibroblastic repair reaction is nonspecific but may be exaggerated, possibly owing to altered epithelial–mesenchymal interactions consequent on impaired regeneration. Bizarre fibroblasts with large, hyperchromatic nuclei are common and, again, probably reflect radiation-induced DNA damage.

☐ **Clinical Features:** Acute necrosis from radiation is represented by such disorders as **radiation pneumonitis, cystitis, dermatitis** and diarrhea from **enteritis**. Chronic disease is characterized by **interstitial fibrosis** in the heart and lungs, strictures in the esophagus and small intestine, and **constrictive pericarditis**. Chronic **radiation nephritis**, which simulates malignant nephrosclerosis, is primarily a vascular disease that leads to severe hypertension and progressive renal insufficiency.

Since radiation therapy inevitably traverses the skin, it often leads to **radiation dermatitis**. The initial damage is evidenced by dilatation of blood vessels, recognized as **erythema**. Necrosis of the skin may follow and linger as **indolent ulcers** that do not heal because the epithelium is unable to regenerate. A further consequence of this poor regenerative capacity is the difficulty faced by the surgeon, for whom the impairment of wound healing in irradiated areas poses a serious problem. **Poorly healed** or **dehisced wounds** or **persistent ulcers** often require full-thickness skin grafts. **Chronic radiation dermatitis** results from the repair and revascularization of the skin and is characterized by atrophy, hyperkeratosis, telangiectasia, and hyperpigmentation (Fig. 8-24).

The gonads, both testes and ovaries, are similar to other tissues in their dependence on continuous cell cycling and are exquisitely radiosensitive. The acute inhibition of mitosis in the testis results in necrosis of the germinal stem cells, the spermatogonia. The combination of radiation-induced vascular injury and direct damage to

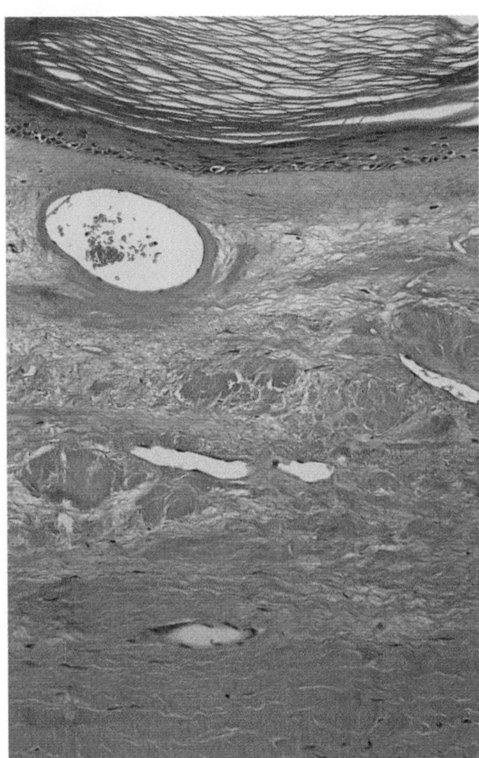

FIGURE 8-24
Chronic radiation dermatitis. The epidermis is atrophic. The dermis is densely fibrotic and contains dilated superficial blood vessels.

the germ cells leads to progressive atrophy of the seminiferous tubules, peritubular fibrosis, and loss of reproductive function. However, since the interstitial and Sertoli cells do not cycle rapidly, they are more resistant than the germ cells and so persist, thereby preserving the normal hormonal status. Comparable injury is seen in the irradiated ovary; the follicles become atretic, and the organ eventually becomes fibrous and atrophic.

Cataracts (lenticular opacities) may be produced if the eye lies in the path of the radiation beam. **Transverse myelitis** and paraplegia occur when the spinal cord is unavoidably irradiated during treatment of certain thoracic or abdominal tumors. **Vascular damage in the cord** may bring about localized ischemia.

Radiation and Cancer

High doses of radiation cause cancer. The evidence is incontrovertible and comes both from animal experiments and from studies of the effects of occupational exposure, radiation therapy for nonneoplastic conditions, the diagnostic use of certain radioisotopes, and the atom bomb explosions (Fig. 8-25). In the early part of this century, scientists and radiologists tested their equipment by placing their hands in the path of the beam. As a result, they developed basal and squamous cell carcinomas of the exposed skin. In addition, early instruments were not properly shielded and the hazards associated with fluoroscopy were not appreciated. The radiologists of that era suffered an unusually high incidence of leukemia, a situation that has disappeared with the use of modern shielding and protective equipment.

An unusual occupational exposure to radiation occurred among workers who painted radium-containing material onto watches to create luminous dials. These workers were in the habit of licking their paint brushes to produce a point, which led to the ingestion of the radioactive element and its subsequent localization in their bones. As a consequence, they were exposed to a long-lived isotope that persisted in their bones indefinitely. They later experienced a high incidence of cancer of the bone and of the paranasal sinuses. Another example of occupational exposure to a radioactive element is the high rate of lung cancer in uranium miners who have inhaled radioactive dusts. Since most of these workers also smoke, it is difficult to distinguish the independent effects from the synergistic effects of radiation in the induction of their cancers, but the evidence strongly favors a synergistic effect.

At one time, thymic irradiation of infants for a mysterious "ailment" known as "status thymicolymphaticus" was popular. Although the irradiation produced no perceptible improvement in the overall health of these infants, as adults they did develop cancer of the thyroid. An explosive increase in the incidence of thyroid cancer among children in geographic areas contaminated by the nuclear catastrophe at Chernobyl in Ukraine in 1986 has been linked to the release of radioactive iodine isotopes.

The risk of solid tumors, especially breast cancer, is particularly high among adult women who were treated with radiation for Hodgkin disease as children. Long-term survivors of childhood Hodgkin disease, who were treated with radiation therapy, are at an almost 20-fold increased risk of developing a second neoplasm. Another example of iatrogenic cancer resulted in Great Britain from the widespread use of low-dose spinal irradiation as a treatment for ankylosing spondylitis. A beneficial effect on the course of this disease was claimed, but the penalty was the later development of aplastic anemia, myelogenous leukemia, and other tumors. An increase in brain tumors was found in persons who had received cranial irradiation for tinea capitis infection of the scalp in childhood. Radiation delivered by long-lived radioactive isotopes used for diagnostic purposes was also not without danger. Thorium dioxide (Thorotrast), a material avidly ingested by phagocytic cells, was at one time used for radionuclide imaging. The persistence in the liver of a long-lived radioisotope resulted in the development of a number of tumors, particularly angiosarcomas of the liver.

The survivors of the atom bomb explosions suffered from a number of cancers. These persons exhibited a more than 10-fold increase in the incidence of leukemia, which reached its zenith from 5 to 10 years after exposure and subsequently declined to background rates.[2] Two thirds were acute leukemia; the remainder were of the chronic

[2] An increased incidence of leukemia was evident in those exposed to doses as low as 50 rads in Hiroshima, but required more than 100 rads in Nagasaki. As previously suggested, this difference in sensitivity may reflect the greater neutron component of the radiation in Hiroshima.

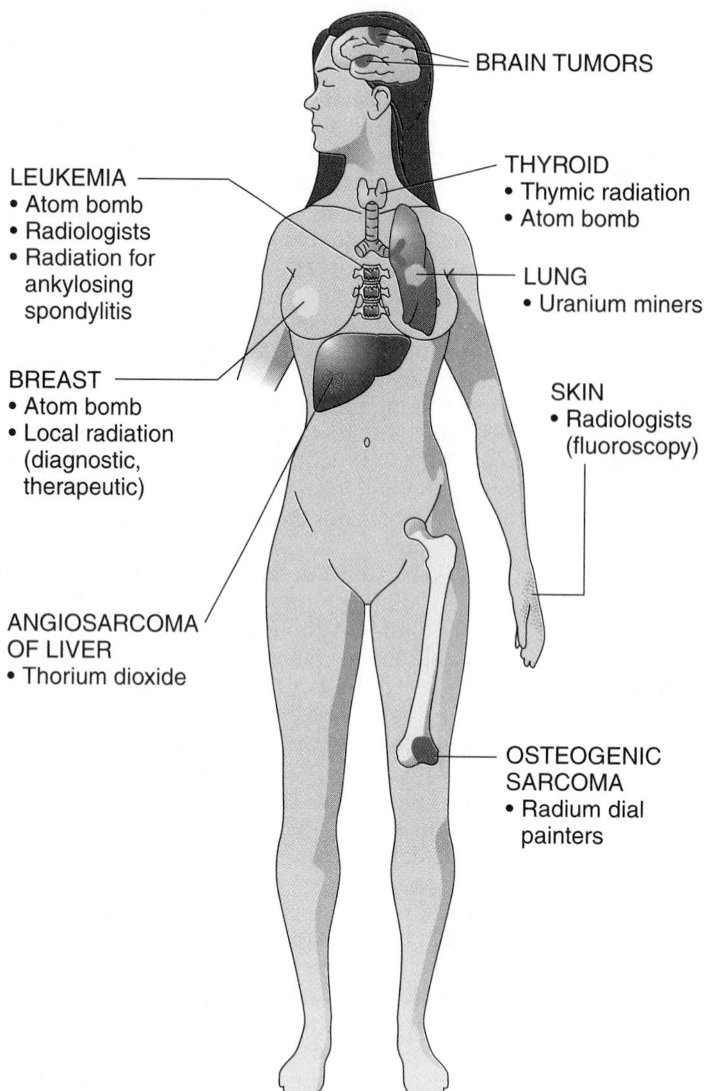

FIGURE *8-25*
Radiation-induced cancers.

myelogenous variety. Chronic lymphocytic leukemia, an uncommon disease in Japan, showed no increase in incidence. The risk of multiple myeloma increased fivefold, and there was a small increment in the incidence of lymphoma. The frequency of solid tumors, although not as great as that for leukemia, was clearly increased for the breast, lung, thyroid, gastrointestinal tract, and urinary tract. The development of malignant tumors, including leukemia, showed a dose-response relationship.

LOW-LEVEL RADIATION AND CANCER: Few debates have engendered as much heat and as little light as that concerning the potential carcinogenic effect of low levels of radiation. All assumptions are based on extrapolations to zero of the risk of cancer at higher doses or from epidemiological studies to which valid exception may be taken. **The key question that needs to be answered is whether there is a threshold dose of radiation below which there is no increase in the incidence of cancer or whether any exposure carries a significant risk.**

The "no threshold hypothesis"—that is, the theory that postulates no safe dose—is based on a linear (proportional to dose) projection of low doses of radiation to zero. However, as is the case with many drugs, there is no *a priori* reason to accept such an assumption; an alternative analysis of the same data uses a quadratic (proportional to dose squared) dependence of risk on dose. With this analysis, the curve is steep at higher doses but is appreciably flattened at the lowest ones. A more sophisticated approach is the linear-quadratic analysis, in which the quadratic dependence gives way to a linear dependence at the lowest doses. At low doses, the linear-quadratic model is intermediate between the highest level of risk of radiogenic cancer projected by the linear analysis and the lowest risk indicated by the quadratic projection.

For instance, based on data from the Nagasaki survivors, the risk of leukemia from a 1-rad dose, expressed as excess cases per million per year, ranges from 2.5 for the linear model to 0.016 for the quadratic model—a 156-fold difference in risk. Comparable differences can be derived from other epidemiological studies of cancer incidence.

Human epidemiological studies do not provide data precise enough to permit an accurate estimate of cancer risk from low-level radiation, except to suggest that it lies between zero and some projected upper limit. However, experiments involving the effects of radiation on cells in culture and in other mammals suggest a dose relation that is less than linear for x- and gamma irradiation. Such a conclusion implies that the established permissible exposures to radiation (which are based on a linear relation) are highly conservative and may exaggerate the risks.

A discussion of the effects of low-level radiation must include consideration of naturally occurring background radiation—that is, the radiation derived from cosmic and terrestrial radiation and the inhalation and ingestion of natural and man-made radioactive isotopes. This background radiation is estimated at about 100 millirads per year at sea level and somewhat greater at higher altitudes. Since exposure to this radiation is universal, it is clearly impossible to determine directly whether this level of exposure contributes to the spontaneous incidence of cancer in humans. However, using the linear hypothesis to estimate the risk from the low levels of background radiation, it has been estimated that the leukemia rate in 20- to 30-year-old women in the United States that can be attributed to this radiation is between 3 and 4 per million per year. The actual leukemia rate in this group is 18 per million per year; thus, background radiation can only account for about one fifth of the cases. However, other attempts to estimate cancer incidence from the linear hypothesis have yielded conflicting conclusions. For example, a linear extension back from the observed cancer incidence and radiation exposure among uranium miners predicts a cancer rate that is four times higher than the rate actually observed in a population of nonsmokers. Cancer mortality has been recorded in two regions of China that have different levels of background radiation. In the low-background region, persons were exposed to 72 millirads per year, while in the high-background region, the exposure was almost three times greater. Despite this difference, no difference in cancer mortality existed. Moreover, pilots and cabin crews of commercial airlines, who are exposed to significantly higher doses of background radiation at high altitude, have not manifested any increased cancer incidence. These and other studies suggest that the contribution of background radiation to the occurrence of human cancer may not be as significant as many believe.

The arguments for a risk of radiogenic cancer from low-level radiation (between 1 and 10 rads) has been buttressed by a number of epidemiological studies. It has been reported that children exposed to radioactive fallout from atmospheric testing of nuclear weapons had a higher incidence of leukemia than similar children not so exposed. However, close inspection of the data reveals that, oddly enough, this apparent increase is explained not by an increased incidence of leukemia relative to the general population but rather by an unusually low leukemia rate in the controls. Interestingly, the incidence of other types of cancer was decreased in the high-fallout areas by a factor of two compared with immediately adjacent low-fallout areas, and this observed reduction is as significant statistically as the apparent increase in leukemia.

Another epidemiological study of radiation associated with nuclear bomb tests involved military personnel engaged in exercises during and after the detonation of a nuclear device named "Smokey" in Nevada in 1957. An unusual feature of this study was the availability of film badges that measured the dose of external radiation. After a 20-year follow-up, 7 cases of myelocytic leukemia were found, with a mean whole-body dose of 1 rad, compared with 1.8 cases expected from the spontaneous incidence of this disease. If these cases were induced by radiation, the risk can be calculated as 80 times greater than the risk established by all other major studies. Moreover, the unusually long latent period of 11 to 19 years for the occurrence of myelocytic leukemia is also at variance with the experience from the study of atom bomb survivors. Thus, the data from the "Smokey" episode should be interpreted with caution and with the recognition that other unrelated factors may have played a role. Equally compelling arguments can be raised against many other studies of the carcinogenic effect of low-level radiation, and there are also studies that failed to show such an effect. For example, analyses of cancer mortality among British radiologists, x-ray technicians trained during World War II, and women given radiation therapy for cervical cancer did not establish a higher risk of leukemia than the expected spontaneous rate.

In summary, the data currently available from radiation studies of cancer induction in animals, chromosomal damage in human cell cultures, malignant transformation of mammalian cells *in vitro*, and populations exposed to radiation show that the estimates of risk at low doses derived from a linear extrapolation from risk at high doses exaggerate the risk, perhaps by an order of magnitude. On the other hand, the data do not by any means show that the risk of radiogenic cancer from low-level radiation is zero. **When the data from atomic bomb survivors are subjected to a linear-quadratic analysis, the lifetime risk from 1 rad of whole-body x- or gamma irradiation is 1 excess cancer death per 10,000 persons.**

RADON: The recent finding that some homes in the United States are contaminated with radon has elicited considerable public concern. Radon is a gas formed as a result of the decay chain of the uranium–radium series of elements. The daughter products of radon emit alpha particles that bind to dust in the home and may be inhaled and deposited in the lungs.

It has been estimated that 4% to 5% of homes in the United States have levels of radon at least five times the average value, and in up to 2% the concentrations are increased eightfold. Based on extrapolations from the incidence of lung cancer in uranium miners, who are exposed to far greater doses of radiation, it was feared that environmental radon exposure might result in as many as 16 excess lung cancer deaths per 100,000 population. Indeed, case-control studies of persons living in homes with substantial radon contamination have indicated an excess lifetime risk of lung cancer in nonsmokers of 1 in 200. The risk in smokers seems to be even higher, and the combination of tobacco use and radon exposure may be synergistic. However, more recent studies in Canada, Finland, Missouri, and China have all found no connection between residential radon exposure and lung cancer risk, and the subject remains controversial.

Microwave Radiation, Electromagnetic Fields, and Ultrasound

Microwaves, produced by ovens, radar, and diathermy, are electromagnetic waves that penetrate tissue but do not produce ionization. Unlike x- and gamma radiation, the absorption of microwave energy produces only heat. The activation energy of radiofrequency and microwave radiation is too low to modify chemical bonds or alter DNA below levels that produce thermal effects. Thus, exposure to microwave radiation under ordinary circumstances is highly unlikely to produce any injury. Moreover, an epidemiological study of 20,000 radar technicians in the Navy who were chronically exposed to high levels of microwave radiation failed to detect any increased incidence of cancer.

Considerable controversy also surrounds the possible carcinogenic effects of exposure to nonionizing electromagnetic fields, such as those encountered in the vicinity of high-voltage electric lines. Particular concern has been expressed regarding the risk of leukemia. However, the epidemiological evidence to date does not support a conclusion that exposure to electromagnetic fields raises the incidence of leukemia or other cancers.

Ultrasound, the vibrational waves in air above the audible range, produces mechanical compression but, again, no ionization. Highly focused and energetic ultrasound devices are used to disrupt tissue *in vitro* for chemical analysis and to clean various surfaces, including teeth. However, there is no reason to believe that diagnostic ultrasound or accidental exposure to any industrial device results in any measurable damage.

NUTRITIONAL DISORDERS

Obesity

Obesity is an increase in adipose tissue beyond the physical requirements of the body. Obesity is the most common nutritional disorder in the industrialized countries, where it is far more common than all the nutritional deficiencies combined. There is no single ratio of increased weight to height or body area at which an increased morbidity and mortality can be said to begin. Thus, as in the case of anemia or hypertension, arbitrary standards are employed. **If one defines obesity as beginning at 20% above the mean adiposity, then 20% to 30% of middle-aged American men and 30% to 40% of women are obese.** Although the prevalence of obesity declines in the elderly, it is possible that this reflects, in part, the increased mortality associated with obesity. Socioeconomic and cultural factors are important because they influence not only the type and amount of food but also the social acceptability of obesity. Genetic factors may also play a role in some ethnic and racial groups. For instance, blacks, particularly women, have a considerably higher prevalence of obesity than do whites in the United States.

It is indisputable that obesity results from a chronic excess of caloric intake relative to the expenditure of energy. The ability to store energy in the form of fat during plentiful times clearly confers an evolutionary advantage in an environment in which periods of food scarcity may occur. Presumably, evolution has been unable to anticipate the advances in societal organization and food production that have converted this evolutionary advantage into a leading cause of morbidity and mortality.

☐ **Pathogenesis:** Whatever the underlying cause of obesity, it clearly results from the excess storage of triglycerides derived from the dietary calories in adipose tissue depots, owing either to excessive caloric intake, insufficient expenditure of energy, or both. The controversies regarding the pathogenesis of obesity are mostly centered on the relative contributions of nature versus nurture, that is, hereditary factors as opposed to environmental ones.

The environmental influence on obesity is clearly demonstrated by the conspicuous increase in the prevalence of obesity among Asians and Indians in the United States, compared with their counterparts in their native lands. By contrast, studies of identical twins reared apart document a striking concordance in adiposity, indicating a heritablity of 80% to 90%. It is fair to say that both genetic and environmental factors are important in the pathogenesis of obesity, but the contributions of each or their interactions vary significantly throughout the population.

Only a minor imbalance between caloric intake and expenditure is sufficient to produce significant obesity. For example, an excess consumption of only 100 calories per day, the amount contained in a slice of bread, will result in a weight gain of almost 5 kg over the course of a year. The fine balance between caloric intake and energy utilization necessary to maintain constant body weight implies that each person has an internal set point, or *lipostat*, that regulates these processes.

Insights into the mechanisms that mediate the operation of this lipostat have come from the analysis of genetically obese mice, which are homozygous for the ob gene (ob/ob). The Lep gene encodes a protein, termed **leptin** (leptos: Greek, thin), that is produced only by adipocytes and informs the brain of the amount of adipose tissue present in the body. Leptin acts by binding to its receptor in the hypothalamus, which then transmits signals that cause a decrease in appetite and an increase in energy use. In addition, leptin directly increases glucose metabolism. In the obese mice, two separate mutations (termed ob) in the Lep gene result in either a premature stop codon or the total absence of leptin mRNA. As a result, in the absence of functional leptin, the afferent loop of the lipostat is defective and incapable of regulating caloric intake and utilization. The administration of recombinant leptin to these mice restores a normal body phenotype.

The human gene encoding the leptin gene (LEP) has been identified, but unlike its counterpart in the mouse, mutations have to date not been found in obese subjects. In addition, the amount of leptin mRNA in adipocytes correlated with body weight, and the plasma concentration of leptin varied directly with the amount of adipose tissue. Thus, it seems that human obesity is more likely to be due to central mechanisms regulating food intake and energy expenditure than simply to defective signaling by adipocytes to the hypothalamus through leptin. In this respect, only few mutations have to date been found in the human genes encoding leptin or the leptin receptor. However, a heritable mutation in the LEP gene was found in a consanguineous family and resulted in severe early-onset obesity in the children.

Other mechanisms that have been incriminated in the regulation of body adiposity include the β_3 adrenergic receptor, which is expressed predominantly in fat and adipocytes lining the gastrointestinal tract and, at least in rodents, regulates thermogenesis and lipolysis. Persons bearing mutations in the gene encoding the β_3 adrenergic receptor tend to gain weight more rapidly than those with the wild-type alleles. Pharmacological studies also suggest a possible role for central serotonergic systems in the regulation of body weight.

An interesting animal model for maturity-onset obesity is the *tubby* mouse, in which an autosomal recessive mutation of the *tub* gene results in slowly developing obesity and a doubling of body weight in the adult. The *tub* gene has been cloned and sequenced and may code for a cytoplasmic phosphodiesterase.

☐ **Pathology and Clinical Features:** The distribution of excess body fat in obesity shows two major patterns. Some overweight persons accumlate fat on the upper trunk, shoulders, and arms, whereas others exhibit pelvic girdle obesity. Persons with upper truncal obesity can usually reduce body fat by diet, whereas those who deposit fat in the buttocks, hip, and lower abdomen retain their obese configuation despite rigorous control of food consumption.

Obesity leads to an increase in overall mortality. **The most important consequence of obesity** (Fig. 8-26) **is maturity-onset (type II) diabetes, which is associated with normal or high levels of circulating insulin and peripheral resistance to insulin's action.** This complication is

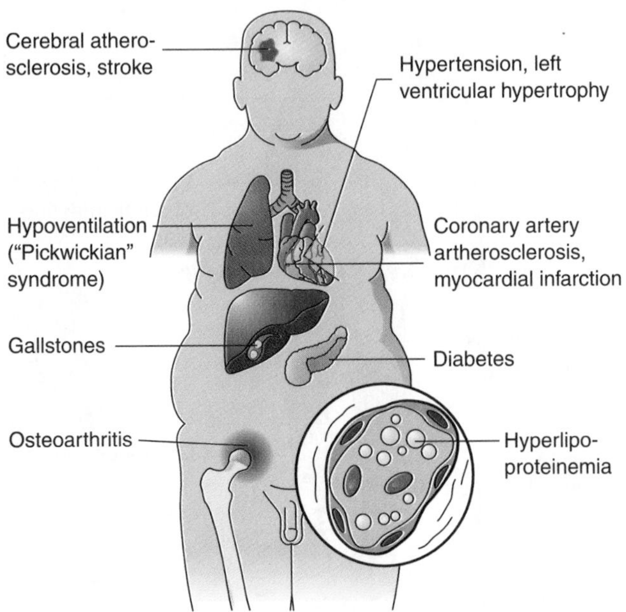

FIGURE *8-26*
Complications of obesity.

more frequent in persons with upper truncal obesity than those with pelvic girdle adiposity. In the United States, more than 80% of type II diabetes occurs in obese persons. The precise mechanism is not understood, but in experimental animals, it has been found that weight gain directly stimulates insulin secretion by the beta cells of the pancreas. Higher levels of circulating insulin decrease the number of insulin receptors on the surfaces of muscle and adipose cells—a form of negative feedback inhibition. This observation has led to the theory that this peripheral resistance to the action of insulin stimulates insulin production, leading to a further decrease in the number of receptors. Eventually, the beta cell is unable to secrete enough insulin to overcome the peripheral resistance to its effect. In an analogy to the heart, the final result is "high output failure" of the beta cells of the pancreas. Weight reduction usually ameliorates the glucose intolerance of type II diabetes, presumably owing to a decrease in the stimulus for insulin secretion by the pancreatic beta cells. This subject is more fully discussed in Chapter 22.

Obesity is also linked to atherosclerosis and myocardial infarction. Even mild-to-moderate obesity increases this risk. It is noteworthy that obesity is associated with all the major risk factors for myocardial infarction, including hypercholesterolemia, low levels of high-density lipoproteins, diabetes, and hypertension. The relationship of hypertension to obesity is not understood, but it may involve an increase in circulating blood volume and dietary salt intake. In addition to its deleterious effect on the heart, hypertension is also responsible for the greater incidence of stroke and vascular disease of the kidneys prevalent in obese persons. Atherosclerosis seems to be linked to the disordered lipid metabolism associated with obesity.

Obesity and hypercholesterolemia are also linked to an increased incidence of gallstones, particularly in women. Severe degrees of obesity result in the deposition of fat in the liver and minor functional changes, but these are generally of little clinical significance. For reasons that are not clear, blood uric acid levels are increased in obese persons, as is the incidence of gout.

A number of complications can be traced simply to the physical effect of an increase in body weight and skin fold thickness. Osteoarthritis, or degenerative joint disease, is common in weight-bearing joints, such as those of the hip, knee, and spine. Excessive subcutaneous fat, particularly beneath the breasts and in the crural areas in women, often is responsible for an intertriginous dermatitis, owing to an accumulation of moisture and maceration of the epidermis. The moisture in the intertriginous areas may predispose to fungal infections of the skin. Hernias of the ventral abdominal wall and of the diaphragm are not uncommon. Because the fat deposits place greater pressure on the veins, and possibly because tissue turgor is decreased, varicose veins of the lower extremities are more common in obese persons and the incidence of deep venous thrombosis is increased correspondingly.

Obesity also poses a physical impediment to surgery, which is made more difficult technically. Because of the longer time needed for surgery, the risks of anesthesia, pulmonary complications, and infection are increased, and the overall surgical mortality for the obese is probably twice as great as that for persons of normal weight.

Obesity also has an important effect on the female reproductive system. **Oligomenorrhea and amenorrhea are common in premenopausal obese women.** Pregnant obese women have a higher incidence of toxemia of pregnancy. Postmenopausal obese women have higher rates of endometrial carcinoma and uterine fibroids. It has been postulated that the increased body fat provides a larger storage space for estrogens and that the conversion of adrenal androgens to compounds with estrogenic activity is increased. Such mechanisms might lead to greater hormonal stimulation of the endometrium and myometrium.

The treatment of obesity is difficult, especially in those who have been overweight since childhood. Despite the commercial success of innumerable fad diets that purport to enhance weight loss, there is no evidence that any particular form of caloric restriction is more effective than any other. Simply put, any caloric intake that is less than energy expenditure will result in weight loss. Since some unusual diets (e.g., protein hydrolysates) may actually pose health risks, such as cardiac arrhythmias, the most reasonable regimen for most obese persons is a balanced diet containing less than 1000 calories a day. The use of diuretics to achieve weight loss borders on the fraudulent, and administration of thyroid hormone has a greater effect on lean body mass than on adipose tissue.

Protein-Calorie Malnutrition

Protein-calorie malnutrition is a direct result of inadequate dietary protein coupled with a deficient intake of the carbohydrates and lipids necessary to provide an adequate energy source. A secondary form of this condition arises when disease prevents absorption of nutrients from the intestine or provokes an increased nutritional demand. It should be recalled that a lack of carbohydrates and lipids results in the oxidation of endogenous protein, a complication that leads to wasting. These states are found not only in children and adults in endemic areas of restricted food supply but also in as many as 25% of hospitalized adult patients, because of the increased nutritional needs associated with the underlying disease. The manifestations of protein-energy deficiency vary depending on the person and his state of development. Infants and children are particularly susceptible because of their requirements for growth.

There are two ends of the spectrum of protein-calorie malnutrition, reflecting the relative imbalance between the components of the diet. **Marasmus** refers to a deficiency of calories from all sources. **Kwashiorkor** is a form of malnutrition in children caused by a diet deficient in protein alone.

Actually, the classic manifestations of either of these conditions are uncommon when compared with the high prevalence of intermediate states of undernutrition. Moreover, both marasmus and kwashiorkor, as well as their intermediate states, are often complicated by deficiencies in vitamins and minerals.

Marasmus

Global starvation—that is, a deficiency of all elements of the diet—leads to marasmus. The condition is common throughout the nonindustrialized world, particularly when breast feeding is stopped and a child must subsist on a calorically inadequate diet. The pathological changes are similar to those in starving adults, and consist of decreased body weight, diminished subcutaneous fat, a protuberant abdomen, muscle wasting, and a wrinkled face. In general, the child is a "shrunken old person." Wasting and increased lipofuscin pigment are seen in most visceral organs, especially the heart and the liver. No edema is present. The pulse, blood pressure, and temperature are low, and diarrhea is common. Because immune responses are impaired, the child suffers from numerous infections. An important consequence of marasmus is growth failure. If these children are not provided with an adequate diet during childhood, they will not reach their full potential stature as adults. The effects on ultimate intelligence are controversial.

Kwashiorkor

Kwashiorkor (Fig. 8-27) *is a syndrome that results from a deficiency of protein in a diet relatively high in carbohydrates.* It is one of the most common diseases of infancy and childhood in the nonindustrialized world. As in the case of marasmus, the disorder usually occurs after the in-

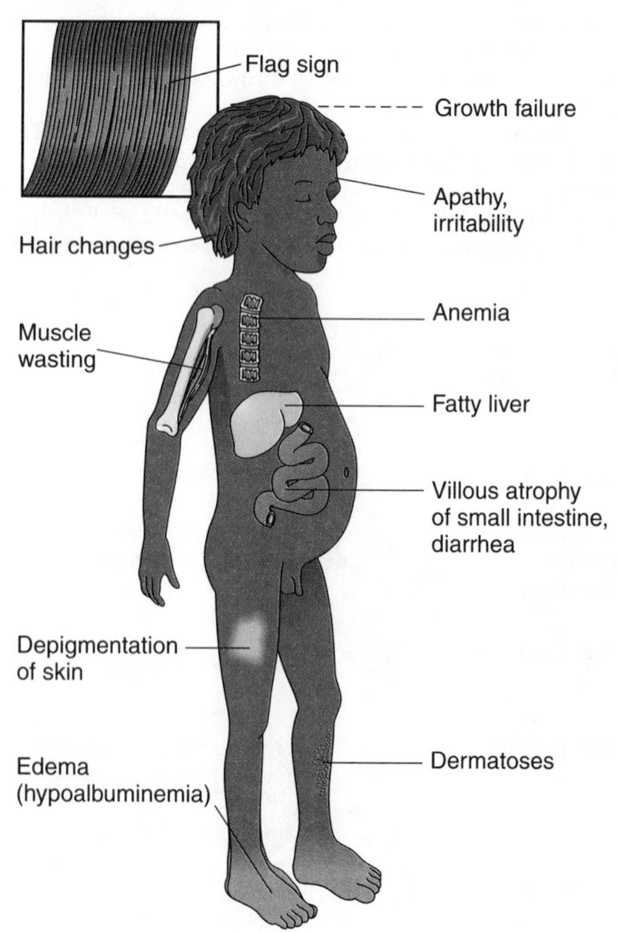

FIGURE 8-27
Complications of kwashiorkor.

fant is weaned, at which time a protein-poor diet, consisting principally of staple carbohydrates, replaces the mother's milk. Although there is generalized growth failure and muscle wasting, as in marasmus, the subcutaneous fat is normal, owing to an adequate caloric intake. Extreme apathy is a notable feature, in contrast to children with marasmus, who may be alert. Also in contrast to marasmus, severe edema, hepatomegaly, depigmentation of the skin, and dermatoses are usual. "Flaky paint" lesions of the skin, located on the face, extremities, and perineum, are dry and hyperkeratotic. The hair becomes a sandy or reddish color; a characteristic linear depigmentation of the hair ("flag sign") provides evidence of particularly severe periods of protein deficiency. The abdomen is distended because of flaccid abdominal muscles, hepatomegaly, and ascites. Along with generalized atrophy of the viscera, villous atrophy of the intestine may interfere with nutrient absorption, and diarrhea is common. Anemia is a usual feature, although it is not generally life-threatening. The nonspecific effects on growth, pulse, temperature, and the immune system are similar to those in marasmus. Although it has been claimed that kwashiorkor not only impairs physical development but also stunts later intellectual growth, the subject requires further study.

Microscopically, the liver in kwashiorkor is conspicuously fatty, and the accumulation of lipid within the cytoplasm of the hepatocyte displaces the nucleus to the periphery of the cell. The adequacy of dietary carbohydrate provides the lipid to the hepatocyte, but the inadequate protein stores do not permit the synthesis of enough apoprotein carrier to transport the lipid from the liver cell. The changes, with the possible exception of mental retardation, are fully reversible when sufficient protein is made available. In fact, the fatty liver reverts to normal after early childhood, even when the diet remains deficient. In any event, the hepatic changes are not progressive and are not associated with the development of chronic liver disease.

Vitamins

"Vitamin" is a general term for a number of unrelated organic catalysts that are not endogenously synthesized but are necessary in trace amounts for normal metabolic functions. **The body is, therefore, totally dependent on dietary sources for these crucial substances.** Critical to the definition of a vitamin is the demonstration that a lack of this compound results in a clearly definable disease. Thus, vitamins in one species are not necessarily vitamins in another. For example, whereas humans are unable to synthesize ascorbic acid (vitamin C) and therefore require dietary ascorbate to prevent scurvy, most lower animals are fully capable of producing their own ascorbic acid and do not require it as a vitamin. By contrast, the importance of the antioxidant vitamin E in rats is clear; however, its precise role in human nutrition has not been well elucidated, and a deficiency state is only poorly characterized. Another example is choline, a deficiency of which produces fatty liver and cirrhosis in rats. Thus, although not a vitamin, choline may be considered an essential nutrient for that species. However, no lesions attributable to choline deficiency have been demonstrated in humans. Vitamins A, D, and K are fat soluble, a property that allows for their storage in the liver and that also accounts for their malabsorption in diseases that interfere with lipid absorption, such as pancreatic disease, biliary obstruction, and primary disease of the small bowel (sprue). Because the water-soluble vitamins—vitamin B complex and vitamin C—are not stored as efficiently as the fat-soluble vitamins, deficiency states occur more rapidly after deprivation of dietary sources.

Vitamin A

Vitamin A, a fat-soluble substance, is important for the maintenance of a number of specialized epithelial linings, skeletal maturation, and the structure of the cell membranes. In addition, it is an important constituent of the photosensitive pigments in the retina. Vitamin A occurs naturally as retinoids or as a precursor, β-carotene. The source of the precursor, carotene, is in plants, principally leafy, green vegetables. Fish livers are a particularly rich source of vitamin A itself.

Metabolism

Both forms of vitamin A are absorbed from the intestinal mucosa, vitamin A as 80% to 90% of the available food load, and β-carotene as only 40% to 50%. β-Carotene is cleaved in the intestinal mucosa to the aldehyde and then reduced to retinoids. The retinoids are bound to palmitic acid, absorbed to chylomicrons, and transported by the lymph to the general circulation. Lipoprotein lipase releases the retinoid, after which it is stored in the liver, where 90% of the body's vitamin A is located. Retinol is bound to a retinol-binding protein, transported with albumin, and extracted by cell surfaces throughout the body. Usually, rapid transit of food through the small intestine, or modification of available lipid by the addition of nonabsorbable lipid carriers (e.g., mineral oil) decreases the absorption of vitamin A.

Vitamin A Deficiency

Although vitamin A deficiency is distinctly uncommon in the developed countries, it remains a significant health problem in poorer regions of the world, including much of Africa, China, and Southeast Asia. **The lack of vitamin A results principally in squamous metaplasia, especially in glandular epithelium** (Fig. 8-28). One effect of this change is the formation of an epithelium whose structure is not adapted to functional needs. Stratified squamous epithelium keratinizes, and the keratin debris blocks sweat and tear glands. Squamous metaplasia is common in the trachea and the bronchi, and bronchopneumonia is a frequent cause of death. The lining epithelia of the renal pelvis, pancreatic ducts, uterus, and salivary glands are also commonly affected. Epithelial changes in the renal pelvis are occasionally associated with kidney stones. With further diminution of vitamin A stores, squamous metaplasia of the epithelial cells of the conjunctiva and tear ducts occurs, which leads to **xerophthalmia**, a dryness of the cornea and conjunctiva. The

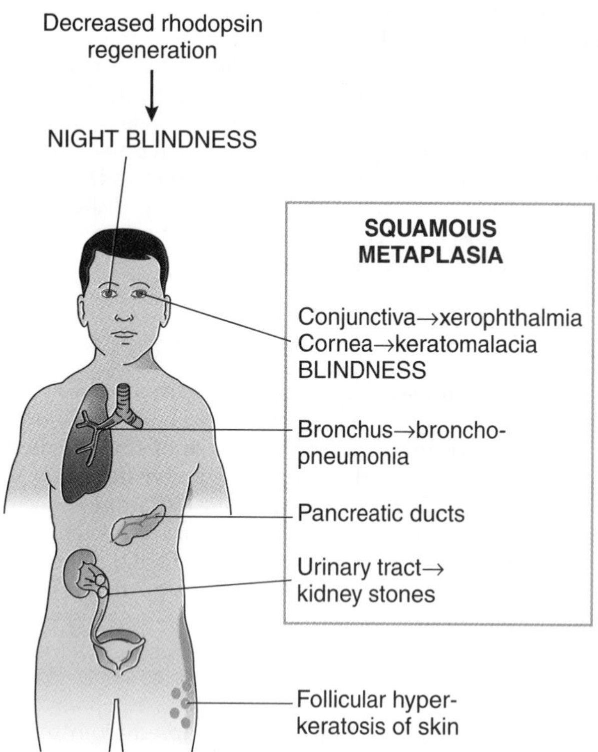

FIGURE *8-28*
Complications of vitamin A deficiency.

cornea becomes softened (**keratomalacia**) and is vulnerable to ulceration and bacterial infection, complications that may lead to blindness. Follicular hyperkeratosis, a skin disorder that results from occluded sebaceous glands, is also a feature of this disease.

The earliest sign of vitamin A deficiency often is diminished vision in dim light. Vitamin A is a necessary component in the pigment of the retinal rods and is active in light transduction. Since the aldehyde of vitamin A, retinal, is constantly being degraded during the generation of the light signal, a continuous supply of vitamin A is necessary for night vision.

Vitamin A Toxicity

Poisoning by excessive doses of vitamin A is usually caused by overenthusiastic administration of vitamin supplements to children. Early Arctic explorers were said to have experienced vitamin A toxicity because they ate polar bear livers, which are particularly rich in the vitamin. Enlargement of the liver and spleen are common, and microscopically these organs show lipid-laden macrophages. In the liver, vitamin A is also present in hepatocytes, and prolonged vitamin A toxicity has been incriminated in the production of cirrhosis. Bone pain and neurological symptoms, such as hyperexcitability and headache, may be the presenting symptoms. Discontinuation of excess vitamin A consumption reverses all or most of the lesions. Excessive carotene intake is benign and simply stains the skin yellow, an appearance that may be mistaken for jaundice.

Synthetic derivatives of retinoic acid are now increasingly used for their pharmacological effects in alleviating severe acne. The dosage of these compounds, which display potent vitamin A activity, is limited by vitamin A toxicity. Both retinoic acid and a high dietary intake of preformed vitamin A are particularly dangerous in pregnancy because of their potent teratogenic actions. Retinoids are also effective in the treatment of certain experimental tumors and may find a place in the treatment of human cancer.

Vitamin B Complex

Vitamins in the B group of water-soluble vitamins are numbered 1 through 12, but most are not distinct vitamins. The members of the complex currently recognized as true vitamins are vitamins B_1 (thiamine), niacin, B_2 (riboflavin), B_6 (pyridoxine), and B_{12} (cyanocobalamin). With the exception of vitamin B_{12}, which is derived only from animal sources, the vitamins of the B complex, although chemically distinct, are found principally in leafy green vegetables, milk, and liver.

Thiamine

Thiamine was the active ingredient in the original description of vitamin B, which was defined as a watersoluble extract in rice polishings that cured beri-beri (clinical thiamine deficiency). This disease was classically seen in the Orient, where the staple food was polished rice that had been deprived of its thiamine content by processing. With increased awareness of the disease and improved nutrition in some areas, the disorder is less common now than in previous generations. In Western countries, the disease occurs in alcoholics, neglected persons with poor overall nutrition, and food faddists. **The cardinal symptoms of thiamine deficiency are polyneuropathy, edema, and cardiac failure** (Fig. 8-29). The deficiency syndrome is classically divided into **dry beri-beri**, with symptoms referable to the neuromuscular system, and **wet beri-beri**, in which the manifestations of cardiac failure predominate.

□ **Pathogenesis:** Patients with dry beri-beri present with paresthesias, depressed reflexes, and weakness and atrophy of the muscles of the extremities. Wet beri-beri is characterized by generalized edema, a reflection of severe congestive failure. The basic lesion is an uncontrolled, generalized vasodilatation and significant peripheral arteriovenous shunting. This combination leads to a compensatory increase in cardiac output and eventually to a large dilated heart and congestive heart failure. In the absence of a documented metabolic disease (e.g., hyperthyroidism), high output failure and generalized edema are strongly suggestive of thiamine deficiency.

The biochemical basis for the symptoms of thiamine deficiency is not understood. As a result of the defect in oxidative decarboxylation, pyruvate accumulates. However, experimental pyruvate administration does not produce the same lesions. Moreover, it is difficult to attribute the symptomatology to a generalized defect in energy metabolism.

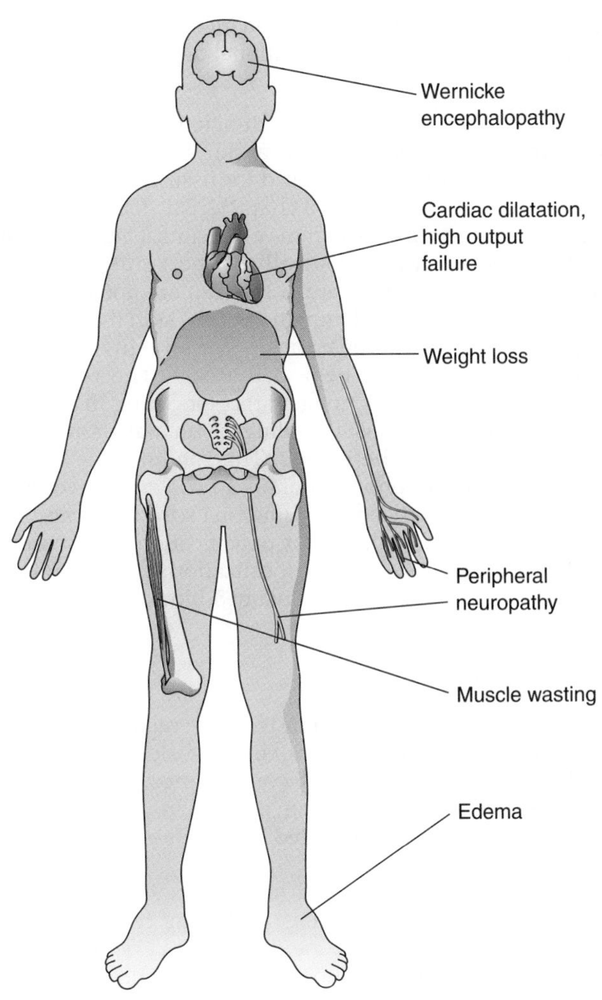

FIGURE *8-29*
Complications of thiamine deficiency (beri-beri).

☐ **Pathology:** Thiamine deficiency in chronic alcoholics may be manifested by involvement of the brain in the form of **Wernicke syndrome**, in which progressive **dementia**, **ataxia**, and **ophthalmoplegia** (paralysis of the extraocular muscles) are prominent. **Korsakoff syndrome**, in which a thought disorder is conspicuous, at one time was attributed solely to thiamine deficiency, but it now appears to be a finding both in chronic alcoholics and in patients with other organic mental syndromes.

Pathological examination of the nervous system in cases of thiamine deficiency has not defined a pathognomonic change in the peripheral nerves, since similar or identical changes can be seen in a variety of other diseases characterized by peripheral neuropathy. A characteristic alteration is degeneration of myelin sheaths, often beginning in the sciatic nerve and then involving other peripheral nerves, and sometimes the spinal cord itself. In the few advanced cases that have been studied, fragmentation of the axons has been noted. In Wernicke encephalopathy, the most striking lesions are found in the mamillary bodies and surrounding areas that abut on the third ventricle. Indeed, atrophy of the mamillary bodies can be visualized in alcoholics by computed tomography and magnetic resonance imaging. Microscopically, degeneration and loss of ganglion cells, rupture of small blood vessels, and ring hemorrhages are seen in the brain.

The changes in the heart are also nonspecific. Grossly, the heart is flabby, dilated, and increased in weight. The process may affect either the right or the left side of the heart or both. The microscopic changes are nondescript and include edema, inconsistent fiber hypertrophy, and occasional foci of fiber degeneration. At one time, all primary myocardial diseases in the alcoholic were considered to reflect thiamine deficiency, but it is now recognized that the large majority are unrelated to thiamine and are caused by a direct toxic effect of alcohol (alcoholic cardiomyopathy).

The most reliable diagnostic test for thiamine deficiency is an immediate and dramatic response to parenteral administration of thiamine. Measurements of levels of thiamine in the blood and erythrocyte transketolase activity are also useful.

Niacin

Niacin refers to two chemically distinct compounds: nicotinic acid and nicotinamide. These biologically active components are derived from dietary niacin or are biosynthesized from available tryptophan. Niacin plays a major role in the formation of nicotinamide adenine dinucleotide (NAD) and its phosphate (NADP), compounds important in intermediary metabolism and a wide variety of oxidation-reduction reactions. Animal protein, as found in meat, eggs, and milk, is high in tryptophan and is therefore a good source of endogenously synthesized niacin. Niacin itself is available in many types of grain.

PELLAGRA: Pellagra refers to clinical niacin deficiency and is uncommon today. It is seen principally in patients who have been weakened by other diseases and in malnourished alcoholics. Food faddists who do not eat sufficient protein may suffer a deficiency of tryptophan, which in combination with a lack of exogenous niacin may result in mild pellagra. Malabsorption of tryptophan, as in Hartnup disease, or excessive utilization of tryptophan for the synthesis of serotonin in the carcinoid syndrome, may also lead to mild symptoms of pellagra. Deficiencies of pyridoxine and riboflavin increase the requirement for dietary niacin because both of these cofactors are required for the biosynthesis of niacin from tryptophan. Pellagra is particularly prevalent in areas where corn (maize) is the staple food because the niacin in corn is chemically bound and thus poorly available. Corn is also a poor source of tryptophan.

☐ **Pathology:** Pellagra (Ital., "rough skin") is characterized by the three D's of niacin deficiency: dermatitis, diarrhea, and dementia (Fig. 8-30). Those areas exposed to light, such as the face and the hands, and those subjected to pressure, such as the knees and the elbows, exhibit a rough, scaly dermatitis. The involvement of the hands leads to so-called "glove dermatitis." The lesions are discrete and show areas of pigmentation and of depigmentation. Microscopically, hyperkeratosis, vascularization, and chronic inflammation of the skin are characteristic. Subcutaneous fibrosis and scarring may be seen in late

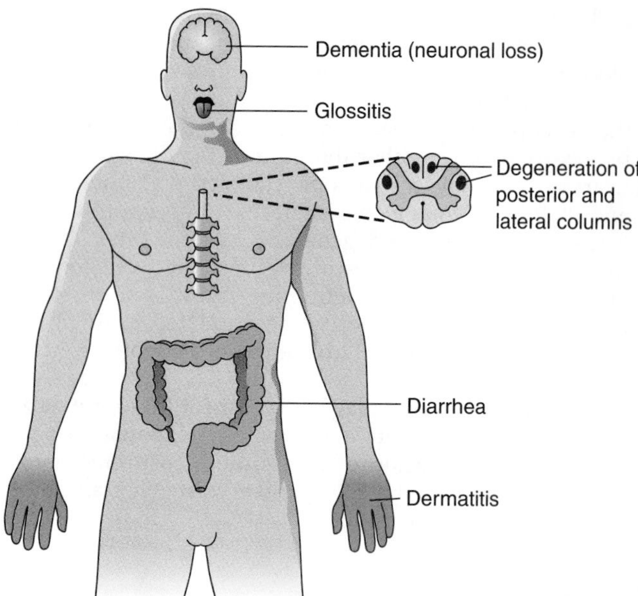

FIGURE *8-30*
Complications of niacin deficiency (pellagra).

stages. Similar lesions are found in the mucous membranes of the mouth and vagina. In the mouth, inflammation and edema lead to a large, red tongue, which in the chronic stage is fissured and is likened to raw meat. A chronic, watery diarrhea is a typical feature of the disease, presumably caused by mucosal atrophy and ulceration in the entire gastrointestinal tract, particularly in the colon. The dementia, characterized by aberrant ideation bordering on psychosis, is represented in the brain by degeneration of ganglion cells in the cortex. Myelin degeneration of tracts in the spinal cord resembles the subacute combined degeneration of vitamin B_{12} deficiency. Severe longstanding pellagra adds another D, namely death.

Riboflavin

Riboflavin, a vitamin derived from many plant and animal sources, is important for the synthesis of flavin nucleotides, which play an important role in electron transport and other reactions in which the transfer of energy is crucial. Riboflavin is converted within the body to flavin mononucleotides and dinucleotides. Riboflavin itself and flavin mononucleotides are absorbed from the proximal small bowel, whereas flavin adenine dinucleotide (FAD) must be degraded to flavin mononucleotide prior to absorption. The conjugated and unconjugated forms circulate bound to serum proteins, but storage sites have not been clearly defined. Clinical symptoms of riboflavin deficiency are uncommon; they are usually seen only in debilitated patients with a variety of diseases and in poorly nourished alcoholics.

Deficiencies of thiamine, riboflavin, and niacin are unusual in the industrialized countries because bread and cereals are fortified with these vitamins. Occasionally, a mild deficiency of riboflavin is seen during pregnancy and lactation or during the period of rapid growth of childhood and adolescence, when increased demands are combined with moderate nutritional deprivation.

☐ **Pathology:** Riboflavin deficiency is manifested principally by lesions of the facial skin and the corneal epithelium. **Cheilosis**, a term used for fissures in the skin at the angles of the mouth, is a characteristic feature (Fig. 8-31). These cracks in the skin may be painful and often become infected. Microscopically, hyperkeratosis and a mild mononuclear infiltrate of the skin are noted. **Seborrheic dermatitis**, an inflammation of the skin that exhibits a greasy, scaling appearance, typically involves the cheeks and the areas behind the ears. The tongue is smooth and a purplish (magenta) color owing to atrophy of the mucosa. The most troubling lesion may be an **interstitial keratitis of the cornea**. The conjunctivae are injected, and severe photophobia is a problem. The cornea is initially vascularized by numerous sprouting capillaries. This process is followed by opacification of the cornea and eventual ulceration. The localization of the lesions in riboflavin deficiency is not explained biochemically.

Pyridoxine

Vitamin B_6 activity is found in three related, naturally occurring compounds: pyridoxine, pyridoxal, and pyridoxamine. For the sake of convenience, they are all grouped under the heading pyridoxine. These compounds are widely distributed in vegetable and animal foods.

Pyridoxine is converted to pyridoxal phosphate, a coenzyme for many enzymes, including transaminases and carboxylases. Pyridoxine deficiency is rarely caused by an inadequate diet, although infants who have been fed a poorly prepared powdered formula in which the pyridoxine has been destroyed during preparation have suffered convulsions. A higher demand for the vitamin,

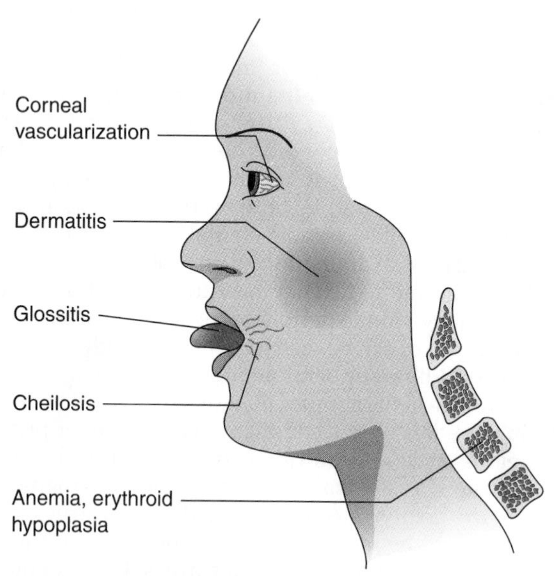

FIGURE *8-31*
Complications of riboflavin deficiency.

such as may occur in pregnancy, may lead to a secondary deficiency state. Of particular concern is the deficiency of pyridoxine that follows prolonged medication with a number of drugs, particularly isoniazid, cycloserine, and penicillamine. A deficiency state is also occasionally reported in alcoholics.

There are no clinical manifestations of pyridoxine deficiency that can be considered characteristic or pathognomonic. The usual dermatological complications of other B vitamin deficiencies occur with pyridoxine deficiency. **The primary expression of the disease is in the central nervous system, a feature consistent with the role of this vitamin in the formation of pyridoxal-dependent decarboxylase of the neurotransmitter γ-aminobutyric acid (GABA).** In infants and children, diarrhea, anemia, and seizures have occurred.

Conditions are encountered in which there is no clinical or biochemical evidence of pyridoxine deficiency, yet large (pharmacological) doses of the vitamin are useful in treating the disorder. Such diseases are termed **pyridoxine-dependency syndromes** and include anemia, convulsions, and homocystinuria caused by cystathionine synthetase deficiency.

Pyridoxine-responsive anemia is hypochromic and microcytic and therefore can be confused with iron deficiency anemia. Unlike iron-deficiency anemia, however, pyridoxine-responsive anemia is characterized by saturation of iron stores and an increased saturation of transferrin. Thus, administration of iron may simply make pyridoxine-responsive anemia worse. By definition, the anemia responds well to massive doses of pyridoxine.

Vitamin B_{12} and Folic Acid Deficiencies

Deficiencies of vitamin B_{12} are almost always seen in cases of pernicious anemia and result from the lack of secretion of intrinsic factor in the stomach, which prevents absorption of the vitamin in the ileum. Since vitamin B_{12} is found in almost all animal protein, including meat, milk, and eggs, dietary deficiency is seen only in rare cases of extreme vegetarianism, and that only after many years of a restricted diet. Parasitization of the small intestine by the fish tapeworm, *Diphyllobothrium latum*, may lead to vitamin B_{12} deficiency because the parasite absorbs the vitamin in the lumen of the gut.

Deficiency of folic acid, the trivial name for pteroylmonoglutamic acid, is commonly of dietary origin. Leafy vegetables, liver, kidney, and yeast are rich sources of folic acid. However, excessive cooking destroys much of the folic acid in foods. Dietary folic acid deficiency is usually accompanied by multiple vitamin deficiencies. Pregnancy increases the requirement for folic acid 5-fold to 10-fold. **It has been estimated that two thirds of anemic pregnant women are folate deficient**, although this may be combined with iron deficiency. Folic acid is absorbed principally in the upper third of the small intestine, and therefore folate deficiency is common in certain diseases of malabsorption, notably nontropical and tropical sprue. The latter condition is responsive to treatment with folic acid.

Deficiencies of both vitamin B_{12} and folic acid are associated with **megaloblastic anemia**. In addition, pernicious anemia is complicated by a neurological condition called **subacute combined degeneration of the spinal cord**. Comprehensive discussions of vitamin B_{12} and folic acid deficiencies are found in Chapters 20 and 28.

Vitamin C (Ascorbic Acid)

Ascorbic acid is a powerful biological reducing agent that is involved in numerous oxidation-reduction reactions and the transfer of protons. This vitamin is important in the synthesis of chondroitin sulfate and in the hydroxylation of proline to form the hydroxyproline of collagen. It serves many other important functions, such as preventing the oxidation of tetrahydrofolate and augmenting the absorption of iron from the gut. Without vitamin C, the biosynthesis of certain neurotransmitters is impaired because of a reduction in the activity of dopamine β-hydroxylase. Wound healing and immune functions are also under the influence of ascorbic acid. The best dietary sources of vitamin C are citrus fruits, green vegetables, and tomatoes. Humans and the guinea pig lack the ability to make ascorbic acid, an incapacity that can be explained only as an evolutionary quirk.

Scurvy

The term scurvy refers to the clinical vitamin C deficiency state. The first demonstration of the need for this vitamin was the remarkable effect of lime in preventing scurvy among 18th century British sailors. The distribution of limes in the British navy led to the name "limey" for the seamen. Scurvy is uncommon in the western world, but is often noted in nonindustrialized countries in which other forms of malnutrition are prevalent. In the industrialized countries, scurvy is now a disease of persons afflicted with chronic diseases who do not eat well, the neglected aged, and malnourished alcoholics. Elderly persons who consume a "tea and toast" diet are particularly vulnerable to ascorbic acid deficiency because of an inadequate intake of the vitamin. The stress of cold, heat, fever, or trauma (accidental or surgical) leads to an increased requirement for vitamin C. Children who are fed only milk for the first year of life develop scurvy, as do alcoholics. Mild depression of ascorbic acid levels also occurs in other conditions, including cigarette smoking, tuberculosis, rheumatic fever, and many debilitating disorders. Some women who use oral contraceptives may have a mild decrease in serum vitamin C levels. The rate of catabolism of ascorbic acid is about 3% of the body pool a day, a value that is consistent with the fact that on a diet lacking in vitamin C the symptoms of scurvy take some months to develop.

☐ **Pathology:** **Most of the events associated with vitamin C deficiency are caused by the formation of abnormal collagen that lacks tensile strength** (Fig. 8-32). Within 1 to 3 months, subperiosteal hemorrhages lead to pain in the bones and joints. Petechial hemorrhages, ecchymoses, and purpura are common, particularly after mild trauma or at pressure points. Perifollicular hemorrhages in the skin are particularly typical of scurvy. In advanced cases, swollen, bleeding gums are a classic finding. Alveolar bone resorption results in the loss of teeth.

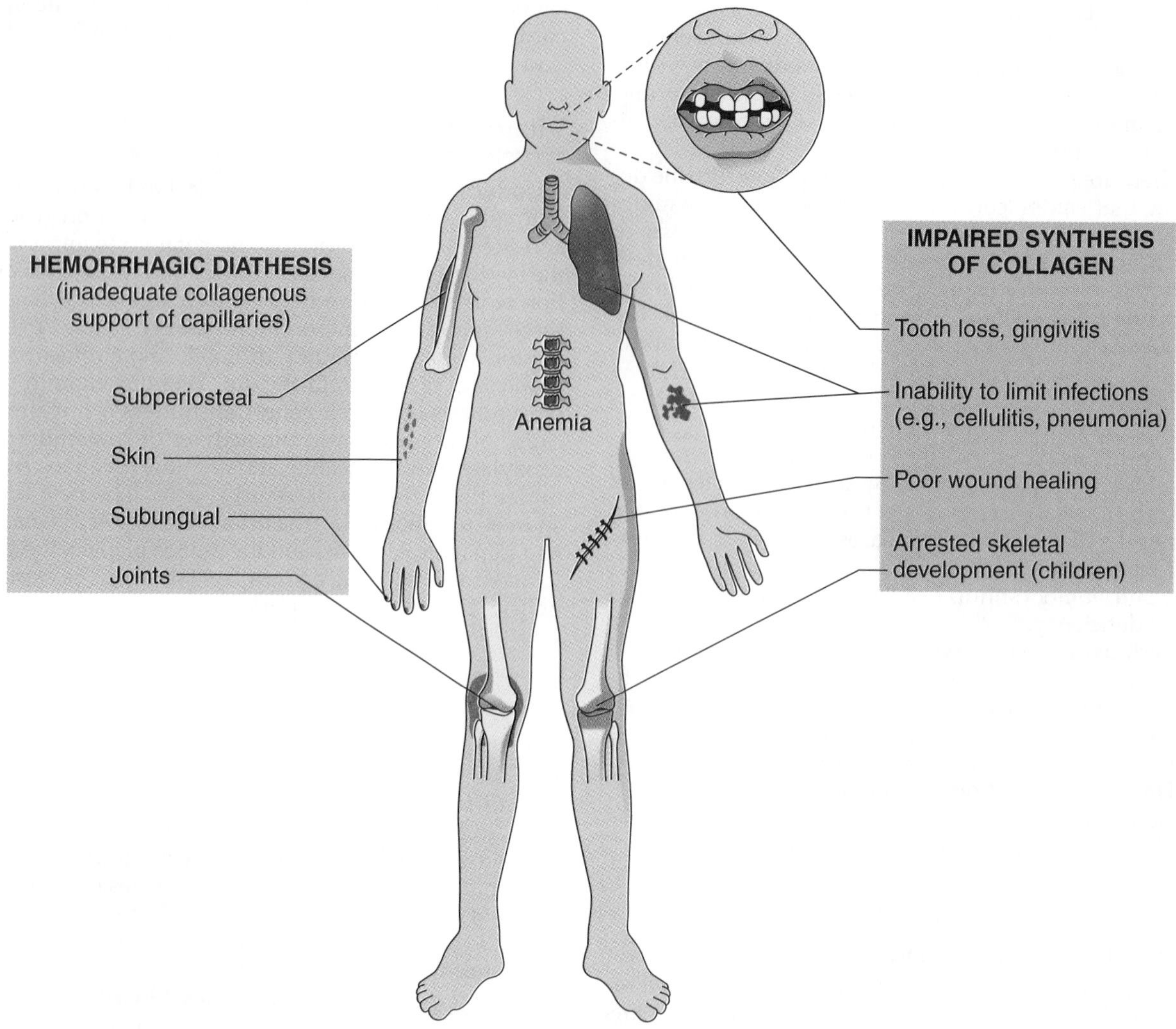

FIGURE *8-32*
Complications of vitamin C deficiency (scurvy).

Wound healing is poor, and dehiscence of previously healed wounds occurs. Anemia may result from prolonged bleeding, impaired iron absorption, or an associated folic acid deficiency.

In children, vitamin C deficiency leads to growth failure, and collagen-rich structures such as the teeth, bones, and blood vessels develop abnormally. The effects on developing bone are conspicuous and relate principally to impaired function of osteoblasts. The effects of scurvy on bone are discussed in greater detail in Chapter 26. In addition to poor wound healing, scorbutic patients have difficulty in walling off an infection to form an abscess, and infections therefore spread more easily. The diagnosis of scurvy is confirmed by finding low levels of ascorbic acid in the serum.

Widespread publicity has attended claims that very large doses of ascorbic acid are useful in the prevention of the common cold and in the treatment of metastatic cancer. There is no credible evidence to support either contention.

Vitamin D

Vitamin D is a fat-soluble steroid hormone found in two forms: vitamin D_3 (cholecalciferol) and vitamin D_2 (ergocalciferol), both of which have equal biological potency in humans. Vitamin D_3 is produced in the skin, and vitamin D_2 is derived from plant ergosterol. The vitamin is absorbed in the jejunum along with fats and is transported in the blood bound to an α-globulin (vitamin D–binding protein). **To achieve biological potency, vitamin D must be hydroxylated to active metabolites in the liver and kidney. The active form of the vitamin promotes calcium and phosphate absorption from the small intestine** and may directly influence mineralization of bone, although the latter effect is not well delineated.

Vitamin D Deficiency

Vitamin D deficiency results from (1) insufficient vitamin D in the diet, (2) insufficient production of vitamin

D in the skin because of limited sunlight exposure as a result of occupation or dress, (3) inadequate absorption of vitamin D from the diet (as in the fat malabsorption syndromes), or (4) abnormal conversion of vitamin D to its bioactive metabolites. The last occurs in liver disease and chronic renal failure. **In children, vitamin D deficiency causes rickets; in adults, osteomalacia occurs.**

The bone lesions of vitamin D deficiency in children (rickets) have been recognized for centuries and were common in the western industrialized world until recently. It was a disease that affected the urban poor to a much greater extent than their rural counterparts. A partial explanation for this difference lies in the greater exposure of rural residents to sunlight. The addition of vitamin D to milk and many processed foods, the administration of vitamin preparations to young children, and generally improved levels of nutrition have made rickets a curiosity in industrialized countries. A full discussion of the metabolism of vitamin D and its relationship to rickets and osteomalacia is found in Chapter 26.

Hypervitaminosis D

The most common cause of excess vitamin D is the inordinate consumption of vitamin preparations. Abnormal conversion of vitamin D to biologically active metabolites is occasionally seen in granulomatous diseases such as sarcoidosis. In cases of calcium malabsorption, when the underlying disease is corrected the sensitivity of target tissues to vitamin D may be increased.

The initial response to excess vitamin D is **hypercalcemia**, which leads to nonspecific symptoms such as weakness and headaches. The increased excretion of calcium by the kidneys results in **nephrolithiasis** or **nephrocalcinosis**. **Ectopic calcification** in other organs, such as blood vessels, the heart, and lungs, may be seen. Infants are particularly susceptible to excess vitamin D, and if the condition is not corrected they may develop premature arteriosclerosis, supravalvular aortic stenosis, and renal acidosis.

Vitamin E

Vitamin E is an antioxidant that, experimentally at least, protects membrane phospholipids against lipid peroxidation by free radicals formed by cellular metabolism. The activity of this fat-soluble vitamin is found in a number of dietary constituents, principally in α-tocopherol. Corn and soy beans are particularly rich in vitamin E. No specific carrier protein in the blood has been identified for vitamin E, nor is it stored in any specific organ.

A dietary deficiency of vitamin E is rare, except among patients receiving total parenteral nutrition. Low vitamin E levels have also been found in patients with disorders of fat absorption from the intestine. A clearly definable syndrome associated with vitamin E deficiency has not been identified in adults. Inconsistent reports of abnormalities of the posterior columns of the spinal cord, together with functional disturbances of gait, proprioception, and vibration have been recorded. Although the lifespan of the erythrocyte may be shortened, clinical anemia is not attributable to vitamin E deficiency alone.

In premature infants, hemolytic anemia, thrombocytosis, and edema have been associated with a deficiency of vitamin E. Food faddists and enterprising entrepreneurs have endorsed vitamin E as an antiaging vitamin and an enhancer of sexual potency. There is no objective evidence to support these claims. On the other hand, vitamin E therapy has been reported to improve hemolytic anemia in premature newborns and may reduce the severity but not the incidence of retrolental fibroplasia. Vitamin E is reported to retard the development of cirrhosis in infants with congenital biliary atresia. A number of interesting experimental effects are produced by vitamin E, such as inhibition of (1) platelet aggregation, (2) the conversion of dietary nitrites to carcinogenic nitrosamines, and (3) prostaglandin synthesis. Protection against toxins that exert their activity through the production of free radical oxygen species has also been shown. The applicability of these results to humans requires further study.

Vitamin K

Vitamin K, a fat-soluble material, occurs in two forms: vitamin K_1, from plants, and vitamin K_2, which is principally synthesized by the normal intestinal bacteria. Green leafy vegetables are rich in vitamin K, and liver and dairy products contain smaller amounts. Dietary deficiency is very uncommon in the United States; most cases are associated with other disorders. However, inadequate dietary intake of vitamin K does occasionally occur in conjunction with chronic illness associated with anorexia.

Vitamin K deficiency is common in severe fat malabsorption, as seen in sprue and biliary tract obstruction. The destruction of intestinal flora by antibiotics may also result in vitamin K deficiency. Newborn infants frequently exhibit vitamin K deficiency because the vitamin is not transported well across the placenta, and the sterile gut of the newborn does not have bacteria to produce it. Vitamin K, which confers calcium-binding properties to certain proteins, is important for the activity of four clotting factors: prothrombin, factor VII, factor IX, and factor X. Deficiency of vitamin K can be serious, because it can lead to catastrophic bleeding. Parenteral vitamin K therapy is rapidly effective.

Minerals

The essential trace minerals are, for the most part, components of enzymes and co-factors necessary for metabolic functions. These include iron, copper, iodine, zinc, cobalt, selenium, manganese, nickel, chromium, tin, molybdenum, vanadium, silicon, and fluorine. Dietary deficiencies of these minerals are clinically important in the case of iron and iodine, and these are discussed in Chapters 20 and 21, which deal with blood diseases and endocrinologic pathology, respectively.

Chronic zinc deficiency has been reported in Iran and Egypt to result in hypogonadal dwarfism in boys. The children usually are those who eat clay, a substance that may bind zinc, but a deficiency in dietary protein is usually also present. An inherited disorder of zinc metabolism, acrodermatitis enteropathica, which is a chronic form of zinc deficiency, is characterized by diarrhea, rash, hair loss, muscle wasting, and mental irritability. Similar symptoms are seen in acute zinc deficiency associated with total parenteral nutrition. Zinc deficiency is also seen in diseases that cause malabsorption, such as Crohn disease, sprue, cirrhosis, and alcoholism.

Dietary copper deficiency is rare but may occur in certain inherited disorders, malabsorption syndromes, and during total parenteral nutrition. The most common result is a microcytic anemia, although megaloblastic changes have also been described.

Manganese deficiency has been described and causes poor growth, skeletal abnormalities, reproductive impairment, ataxia, and convulsions. Industrial exposure to manganese causes symptoms closely related to those of parkinsonism.

CONCLUSION

The dawn of life was marked by an incredibly hostile environment. The earth revolved on its axis more than 10^{12} times before a creature evolved who could consciously manipulate the environment. In the process, the 18-year average life span of Cro-Magnon man has risen for industrialized humans to surpass the biblical 3 score and 10. This remarkable success should not lead us to complacency in our efforts to improve the quality and extent of life, but it is important to maintain a realistic perspective on the impact of civilization on the environment.

SUGGESTED READING

BOOKS

Alcohol, Drug Abuse, and Mental Health Administration: The Sixth Special Report to the US Congress on Alcohol and Health from the Secretary of Health and Human Services. Item No. 498-C-6. Rockville, MD, US Department of Health and Human Services, 1987.

Abel EL: *Fetal alcohol syndrome.* Oradell, NJ: Medical Economics, 1990.

Amdur MO, Doull J, Klaassen CD: *Casarett and Doull's toxicology*, 4th ed. New York: Pergamon Press, 1991.

Committee on the Biological Effects of Ionizing Radiations (BEIR III): The Effects on Populations of Exposure to Low Levels of Ionizing Radiation. Washington, DC, National Academy of Sciences, 1980.

Craighead JE: *Pathology of environmental and occupational disease.* St. Louis: Mosby, 1995.

Hall EJ: *Radiobiology for the radiologist*, 3rd ed. Philadelphia: JB Lippincott, 1988.

Karch SB: *The pathology of drug abuse.* Boca Raton, FL: CRC Press, 1993.

Office on Smoking and Health: The Health Consequences of Smoking: Cancer and Chronic Lung Disease in the Workplace: A Report of the Surgeon General. Item No. 85-50207. Rockville, MD, US Department of Health and Human Services, 1985.

Rubin E (ed): *Alcohol and the cell.* Ann NY Acad Sci. New York: NY Academy of Sciences, 1987.

Strickland GT (ed): Nutritional deficiencies and heat-associated illnesses. In: *Hunter's tropical medicine*, 6th ed. Philadelphia: WB Saunders, 1984.

Tedeschi CG, Eckert WG, Tedeschi LG: *Forensic medicine: A study in trauma and environmental hazards.* Philadelphia: WB Saunders, 1977.

REVIEW ARTICLES

Baghurst PA, McMichael AJ, Wigg NR: Environmental exposure to lead and children's intelligence at age of seven years. The Port Pirie cohort study. *New Engl J Med* 327:1279–1284, 1992.

Blair A, Zahm S: Cancer among farmers. *Occup Med* 6:335–354, 1991.

Brent RL: The effects of ionizing radiation, microwaves, and ultrasound on the developing embryo: Clinical interpretations and applications of the data. *Curr Probl Pediatr* 14:1–87, 1984.

Cantor K, Blair A, Everett G: Pesticides and other agricultural risk factors for non-Hodgkin's lymphoma among men in Iowa and Minnesota. *Cancer Res* 52:2447–2455, 1992.

Department of Energy: Health and environmental consequences of the Chernobyl nuclear power plant accident. Publication No. DOE/ER-0332. National Technical Information Service, Washington, DC, 1987.

Goldfrank LR, Hoffman RS: The cardiovascular effects of cocaine: update 1992. In: *Acute cocaine intoxication: Current methods of treatment.* NIDA Research Monograph No. 123. National Institute of Drug Abuse, Rockville, MD, 1993.

Karch SB: Introduction to the forsenic pathology of cocaine. *Am J Forensic Med Pathol* 12:126–131, 1991.

McBride PE: The health consequences of smoking: cardiovascular diseases. *Med Clin N Am* 76:333–353, 1992.

National Council on Radiation Protection and Measurements: The relative biological effectiveness of radiations of different quality. Report No. 104, Bethesda, MD, 1990.

Newcomb PA, Carbone PP: The health consequences of smoking. *Med Clin N Am* 76:305–331, 1992.

Webster EW: Garland lecture: On the question of cancer induction by small x-ray doses. *Am J Roentgenol* 137:647–666, 1981.

CHAPTER 9

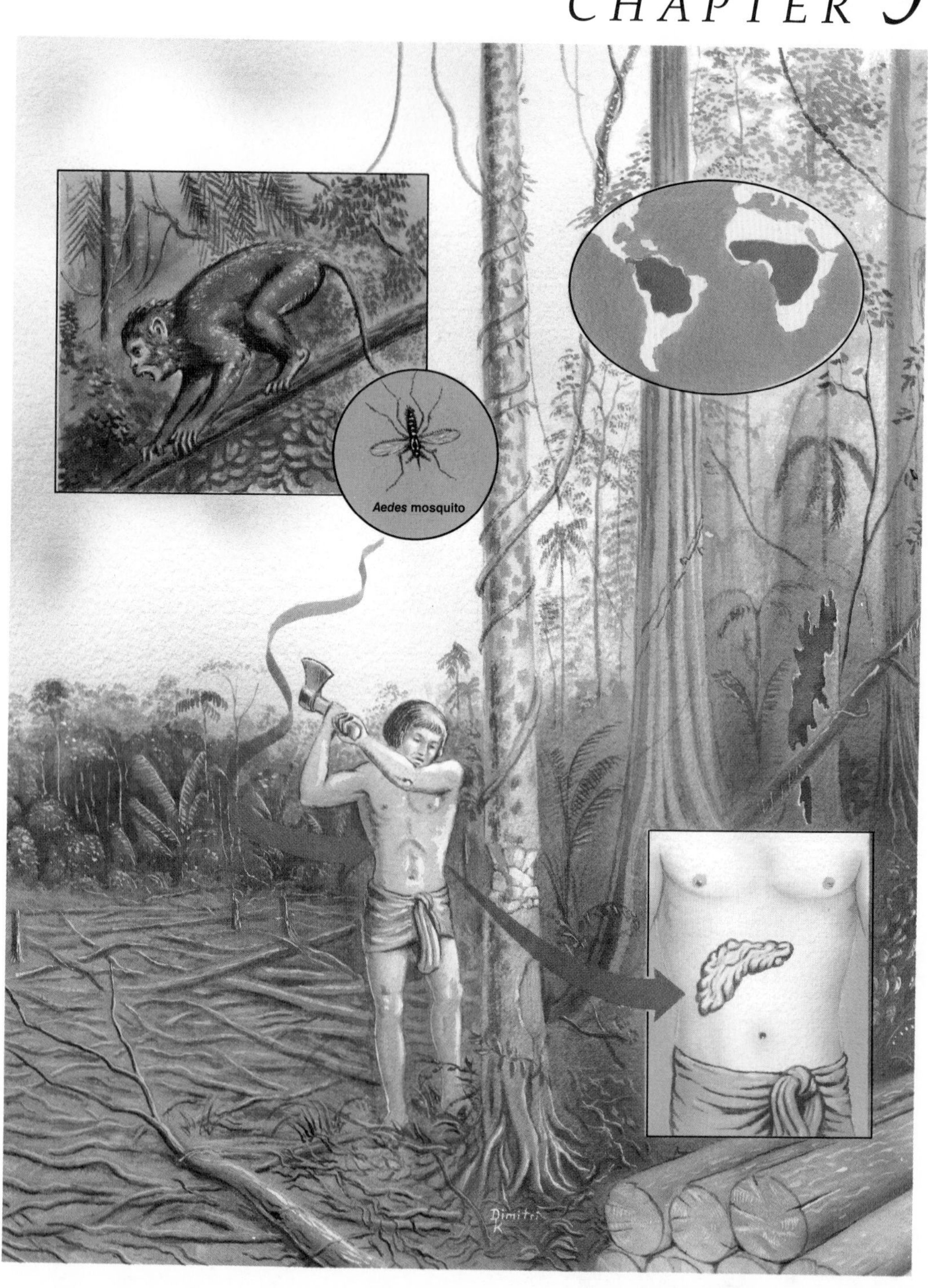

Infectious and Parasitic Diseases

Robert M. Genta
Daniel H. Connor

(continued)

FIGURE 9-1 *(see opposite page)*
Epidemiology of yellow fever. The usual reservoir for the yellow fever virus is the tree-dwelling monkey. The virus is passed from monkey to monkey in the forest canopy by mosquitoes of the genus *Aedes*. Felling a tree brings mosquitoes down with the tree, increasing the chance of being bitten and inoculated with the virus.

Fungal Infections

Candida

Aspergillosis

Mucormycosis (Zygomycosis)

Cryptococcosis

Histoplasmosis

Coccidioidomycosis

Blastomycosis

Paracoccidioidomycosis (South American Blastomycosis)

Sporotrichosis

Chromomycosis

Dermatophyte Infections

Mycetoma

Protozoa

Malaria

Babesiosis

Toxoplasmosis

Pneumocystis carinii Pneumonia

Amebiasis

Balantidiasis

Cryptosporidiosis

Giardiasis

Leishmaniasis

Chagas Disease (American Trypanosomiasis)

African Trypanosomiasis

Primary Amebic Meningoencephalitis

Helminthic Infection

Filarial Nematodes

Intestinal Nematodes

Hookworms

Strongyloidiasis

Pinworm Infection (Enterobiasis)

Tissue Nematodes

Trematodes (Flukes)

Cestodes

Infectious diseases are the most frequent afflictions of mankind worldwide, the most common reasons that people seek medical care, and the leading causes of death from disease. Bacterial and viral diarrheas, bacterial pneumonias, tuberculosis, measles, malaria, hepatitis B, pertussis, and tetanus kill more people each year than all cancers and cardiovascular diseases (Table 9-1). The impact of infectious diseases is greatest in less-developed countries, where millions of people, mostly children younger than 5 years of age, die of treatable or preventable infectious diseases. Even in the developed countries of Europe and North America, the mortality, morbidity, and loss of economic productivity from infectious diseases is enormous. In the United States each year, infectious diseases cause over 200,000 deaths, more than 50 million days of hospitalization, and almost 2 billion days lost from work or school.

The significance of infectious diseases should not be surprising. We share this world with a myriad of organisms small enough to live on or in the human body, using it as a source of energy and material for their own survival and propagation. Although humans possess diverse protective mechanisms, some organisms may overcome or circumvent these defenses.

Infectious diseases are disorders in which tissue damage or dysfunction is produced by a microorganism. Many of these diseases, such as influenza, syphilis, and tuberculosis, are contagious, that is, transmissible from person to person. Yet many infectious diseases, such as legionellosis, histoplasmosis, and toxoplasmosis, are not contagious. Humans acquire infecting organisms not only from other humans but also from diverse sources, including animals, insects, soil, air, inanimate objects, and the endogenous microbial flora of the human body.

INFECTIVITY AND VIRULENCE

Virulence refers to the complex of properties that allows an organism to achieve infection and cause disease of different degrees of severity. The organism must (1) gain access to the body, (2) avoid multiple host defenses, (3) accommodate to growth in the human milieu, and (4) parasitize human resources.

HOST DEFENSE MECHANISMS

The means by which the body prevents or contains infections are known as defense mechanisms (Table 9-2). There are major anatomical barriers to infection—the skin and the aerodynamic filtration system of the upper airway—that prevent most organisms from ever penetrating the body. The mucociliary blanket of the airways is also an essential defense, providing a means of expelling organisms that gain access to the respiratory system. The microbial flora normally resident in the gastrointestinal tract and in various body orifices compete with outside organisms, preventing them from gaining sufficient nutrients or binding sites in the host. The body's orifices are also protected by secretions that possess antimicrobial properties,

TABLE 9-1 **Sources of Global Deaths**

Illness	Annual Deaths
Cardiovascular disease	12 × 10^6
Diarrheal diseases (Rotavirus, Norwalk-like viruses, *Salmonella, Shigella,* diarrheogenic *E. coli*)	5 × 10^6
Cancer	4.8 × 10^6
Pneumonia	4.8 × 10^6
Tuberculosis	3 × 10^6
Chronic obstructive lung disease	2.7 × 10^6
Measles	1.5 × 10^6
Malaria	1–2 × 10^6
Hepatitis B	1–2 × 10^6
Tetanus (neonatal)	775 × 10^3
Pertussis (whooping cough)	500 × 10^3
Maternal mortality	500 × 10^3
AIDS	200 × 10^3
Schistosomiasis	200 × 10^3
Amebiasis	40–110 × 10^3
Hookworm	50–60 × 10^3
Rabies	35 × 10^3
Typhoid	25 × 10^3
Yellow fever	25 × 10^3
African trypanosomiasis (sleeping sickness)	20 × 10^3
Ascariasis	20 × 10^3

(Modified from the World Health Organization, 1990.)

both nonspecific (e.g., lysozyme and interferon) and specific (usually IgA immunoglobulins). In addition, gastric acid and bile chemically destroy many ingested organisms.

HOST FACTORS IN INFECTIONS

In the historical investigations of infectious diseases, there was a simple notion of "one organism, one disease"; a concept that a single microorganism produces the same outcome in all infected hosts. Actually, this is rarely true, and a single infecting microorganism often causes a wide range of effects in exposed persons. An infectious agent, for instance, the influenza virus, may (1) fail to infect some persons, (2) produce asymptomatic infections in others, (3) cause modest symptomatic disease in some, and (4) produce lethal infections in still others. In infectious diseases, variability in outcomes of exposure is the rule, rather than the exception. This is due to diverse host factors, heritable variability, age, integrity of host defenses, and behavior.

TABLE 9-2 **Host Defenses Against Infection**

Skin
Tears
Normal bacterial flora
Gastric acid
Bile
Salivary and pancreatic secretions
Filtration system of nasopharynx
Mucociliary blanket
Bronchial, cervical, urethral, and prostatic secretions
Neutrophils
Monocytes
Complement
Stationary mononuclear phagocyte system
Immunoglobulins
Cell-mediated immunity

Heritable Differences in Response to Infecting Agents

The first step in infection is often a highly specific interaction of a binding molecule on the infecting organism with a receptor molecule on the host. If the host lacks the appropriate receptor molecule, then the attachment of the organism to the target cannot occur. An example is *Plasmodium vivax*, one of the organisms that causes human malaria. It infects human erythrocytes by using the Duffy blood group determinants on the cell surface as receptor molecules. These determinants, however, are not conserved in all human populations. Many persons, particularly blacks, lack them and are not susceptible to infection with *P. vivax*. As a result, *P. vivax* malaria is absent from much of Africa.

The containment or elimination of an infecting organism also depends on specific molecular interactions between the host and the organism. This is illustrated by the racial variations in the response to *Coccidioides immitis* infection. This fungus is present in the environment in restricted geographic regions. In most persons infected with *C. immitis*, cell-mediated immunity rapidly controls the infection, and the disease is usually mild and self-limited. By contrast, some otherwise healthy persons do not contain the infection, because their immune system fails to respond to the organism. In these persons, infection spreads throughout the body and becomes potentially lethal. Whereas disseminated coccidioidomycosis is rare in healthy whites, it is 14 times more common in blacks and 175 times more frequent in persons of Filipino ancestry, a pattern that reflects heritable differences in the ability to contain the organism.

Effect of Age on Response to Infection

The age of the host affects the outcome of exposure to many infectious agents. This is well illustrated in the case of fetal infections. Some organisms produce more severe disease *in utero* than in children or adults. Infections of the fetus with cytomegalovirus, rubellavirus, human parvovirus B19, and *Toxoplasma gondii* interfere with fetal development. Depending on the organism and time of exposure, fetal infection can produce minimal damage, major congenital abnormalities, or death. By contrast, when these organisms infect children or adults, they usually produce asymptomatic or minimally symptomatic diseases.

Age also has an effect on the course of common illnesses, such as the diverse viral and bacterial diarrheas. In older children and adults, these infections cause discomfort, inconvenience, and sometimes embarrassment, but rarely severe injury. The outcome can be different in children younger than 3 years of age, who lack the capacity to compensate for the rapid volume loss that results from profuse diarrhea. Thus, if intense fluid replacement is not provided, the fluid and electrolyte disturbances resulting from diarrheal disease can rapidly kill small children.

There are numerous other examples of how age influences the outcome of exposure to an infectious agent. Infection with *Mycobacterium tuberculosis* often produces severe, disseminated tuberculosis in children younger than the age of 3 years, probably because of the immaturity of the cell-mediated immune system. By contrast, older persons fare much better. Maturity, however, is not always an advantage in infections. Epstein-Barr virus is more likely to cause symptomatic infections in adolescents and adults than in younger children. Varicella-zoster virus, the cause of chickenpox, produces more severe disease in adults, who are more likely to develop viral pneumonia.

The elderly fare more poorly with almost all infections than younger persons. Common respiratory illnesses such as influenza and pneumococcal pneumonia are more often fatal in those older than 65 years of age.

Effect of Behavior on Infection

Behavior is another host factor that influences infections. The link between behavior and infection is probably most obvious for the sexually transmitted diseases. Syphilis, gonorrhea, urogenital chlamydial infections, acquired immune deficiency syndrome (AIDS), and a number of other infectious diseases are transmitted primarily by sexual contact. The type and number of sexual encounters profoundly influence the risk of acquiring sexually transmitted diseases.

Other aspects of behavior also influence the risk of acquiring infections. Humans contract brucellosis and Q fever, which are primarily bacterial diseases of domesticated farm animals, by close contact with infected animals or their secretions. These infections occur in farmers, herders, meat processors, and, in the case of brucellosis, in persons who drink unpasteurized milk. The transmission of a number of parasitic diseases is strongly affected by behavior. Schistosomiasis, acquired when water-borne infective parasite larvae penetrate the skin of a susceptible host, is primarily a disease of farmers who work in fields irrigated by infected water. In addition, children who swim in lakes and ponds containing these organisms organisms become infected. The larvae of hookworm and *Strongylodes stercoralis* live in humid soil and penetrate the skin of the lower extremities in people who walk barefoot. The introduction of shoes has probably been the single most important factor in reducing the prevalence of infection with soil-transmitted nematodes. Anisakiasis and diphyllobothriasis are two helminthic diseases acquired by eating incompletely cooked fish. Toxoplasmosis is a protozoan infection transmitted from animals to humans by ingestion of incompletely cooked, infected meat or by exposure to infected cat feces. Botulism, a food poisoning caused by a bacterial toxin, is contracted by ingestion of improperly canned food.

As humans change their behavior, they open up new possibilities for infectious diseases. The introduction of hyperabsorbent tampons in the late 1970s led to an epidemic of toxic shock syndrome, a previously unrecognized disease caused by *Staphylococcus aureus*. The novel tampons provided an excellent vehicle for the production and delivery of a staphylococcal toxin. Although the agent of legionnaires disease is common in the environment, aerosols generated by cooling plants, faucets, and humidifiers now have provided the means for causing human infections. Traditional behaviors are not necessarily health promoting. Hundreds of thousands of cases of neonatal tetanus in less-developed countries are linked to coating umbilical stumps with dirt, dung, or even homemade cheese to stop the bleeding. These materials stop the bleeding but often contain the spores of *Clostridium tetani*, which germinate and release the toxin that causes tetanus. In parts of Africa, numerous cases of cysticercosis are caused by the ingestion of locally prepared potions containing, among other ingredients, the stools of persons infected with *Taenia solium*.

Effect of Compromised Host Defenses on Infection

The state of host defense mechanisms affects both susceptibility and response to infection. A disruption or absence of any of the complex host defenses results in increased numbers and severity of infections. Disruption of the skin surface by trauma or burns frequently leads to invasive bacterial or fungal infections. Injury to the mucociliary apparatus of the airways, as occurs in smoking or influenza, impairs the clearing of inhaled microorganisms and results in an increased incidence of bacterial pneumonias. Congenital absence of complement components C5, C6, C7, and C8 prevents formation of a fully functional membrane attack complex and permits disseminated *Neisseria* infections. Diseases and drugs that interfere with neutrophil production or function increase the likelihood of bacterial infection.

The technological capacity to prolong the lives of debilitated persons, the broad use of cytotoxic and immunosuppressive therapies, and the rapid expansion of the AIDS epidemic have led to an exponential increase in the number of patients with severe defects in host defenses. Burn and trauma units, transplantation centers, and medical and surgical intensive care facilities are filled with patients who lack the normal capacity to ward off infections. Many are immunocompromised, meaning that their defects affect their capacity to mount inflammatory or immunological responses. Not only do compromised hosts become infected more easily, but they are often attacked by organisms that are innocuous to normal persons. For example, patients deficient in neutrophils frequently develop life-threatening bloodstream infections with commensal microorganisms that normally populate the skin and gastrointestinal tract.

Organisms that cause disease predominantly in hosts with impaired immunity are known as **opportunistic pathogens**. This term implies that such organisms, most of which are part of the normal endogenous human or environmental microbial flora, take advantage of the host's inadequate defense mechanisms to stage a more violent attack. In fact, so called opportunistic organisms are as much victims as the compromised host. As a result of an opportunistic infection, both host and organism usually perish, when in fact it is an evolutionary advantage for an infectious agent to have little or no pathogenicity. Nevertheless, the term "opportunistic pathogen" is firmly established in the medical vocabulary, and we will, therefore, use this term.

The organisms to be discussed in this chapter vary in their virulence. The opportunistic pathogens are organisms of low virulence. On their own they produce little, if any, damage in the human host with intact defenses. At the opposite extreme are the "classic" human pathogens, such as *Yersinia pestis, Corynebacterium diphtheriae, Plasmodium falciparum*, or *Mycobacterium leprae*. These microorganisms are highly virulent and cause destructive infections in persons with intact defenses.

Viral Infections

Viruses, the smallest human pathogens, range in size from 20 to 300 nm and consist of RNA or DNA, contained in a protein shell. Some viruses are enveloped in a lipid membrane. **Viruses are incapable of independent metabolism or reproduction and thus are obligate intracellular parasites, requiring living cells in which to replicate.** After invading cells, these microorganisms divert their biosynthetic and metabolic capacities to the synthesis of viral-encoded nucleic acids and proteins.

Viruses often cause disease by killing the infected cells. Many viruses, however, produce disease without killing infected cells. For example, rotavirus, a common cause of diarrhea, interferes with the function of infected enterocytes without immediately killing these cells. The virus prevents enterocytes from synthesizing proteins that transport molecules from the intestinal lumen and thereby causes diarrhea.

Viruses also produce disease by promoting the release of chemical mediators that incite inflammatory or immunological responses. The symptoms of the common cold are due to the release of bradykinin from infected cells. Some viruses produce disease by causing cells to proliferate and form tumors. Human papillomaviruses, for instance, cause squamous cell proliferative lesions, which include common warts and anogenital warts.

Some viruses infect and persist in cells without interfering with normal cellular functions, a process known as latency. Viruses that establish latent infections can emerge to produce disease or transmit infection long after the primary infection. Opportunistic infections are frequently caused by viruses that have established latent infections. Cytomegalovirus and herpes simplex viruses are among the most frequent opportunistic pathogens because they are commonly present as latent agents, which emerge in persons with impaired cell-mediated immunity.

RESPIRATORY VIRUS INFECTIONS

The Common Cold

Common colds are acute, self-limited, upper respiratory tract infections caused by a variety of RNA viruses, including over 100 distinct rhinoviruses and several coronaviruses. Colds are frequent and worldwide in distribution, spreading from person to person by contact with infected secretions. Infection is more likely during the winter months in temperate areas and during the rainy seasons in the tropics, when spread is facilitated by indoor crowding. In the United States, children usually suffer six to eight colds per year and adults suffer two to three.

☐ **Pathogenesis and Pathology:** Virus-containing secretions are carried to the nose, by means of infectious aerosols or direct contact such as contaminated hands. The viruses parasitize nasal respiratory epithelial cells, causing increased mucus production and tissue swelling. The rhinoviruses and coronaviruses have a tropism for respiratory epithelium and optimally reproduce at temperatures well below 37°C. Thus, infection remains confined to the cooler passages of the upper airway. The parasitized cells release chemical mediators, such as bradykinin, which produce most of the symptoms associated with the common cold. Increased mucus production, together with nasal congestion and Eustachian tube obstruction, predispose to secondary bacterial infections, resulting in bacterial sinusitis and otitis media. Rhinoviruses and coronaviruses do not destroy the infected respiratory epithelium and produce no alterations visible by routine light microscopy. Clinically, the common cold (coryza) is characterized by rhinorrhea, pharyngitis, cough, and low-grade fever. Symptoms last about a week.

Influenza

Influenza is an acute, self-limited, infection of the upper and lower airways, caused by strains of influenza virus. These viruses are enveloped and contain single-stranded RNA. Although three distinct types of influenza virus—types A, B, and C—cause human disease, influenza A is by far the most common pathogen and causes the most severe disease. Ten to 40 million cases of influenza occur annually in the United States. Influenza is highly contagious, and epidemics often spread from an original focus around the world. The virus periodically alters its surface antigens, so that the host immunity that develops in one epidemic often does not protect against the next one.

☐ **Pathogenesis and Pathology:** Influenza spreads from person to person by virus-containing respiratory droplets and secretions. Sneezing, coughing, and even talking spread the virus. Once the influenza virus has contacted the respiratory epithelial cell surface, it binds and enters the cell by fusion with the cell membrane. This process is mediated by a viral glycoprotein, referred to as a hemagglutinin, which binds to sialic acid residues on human respiratory epithelium. This interaction is highly specific and can be blocked by antibody directed at the particular hemagglutinin. Once inside the cell, the virus directs it to produce progeny viruses and causes cell death. The infection usually involves both the upper and the lower airways. Symptoms may represent disease at both sites or may be primarily those of an upper respiratory infection or those of tracheitis, bronchitis and pneumonia. Destruction of the ciliated epithelium cripples the mucociliary blanket, predisposing to bacterial pneumonia.

In the airways, influenza virus causes necrosis and desquamation of the ciliated respiratory tract epithelium, associated with a predominantly lymphocytic inflammatory infiltrate. Extension of the infection to the lungs leads to necrosis and sloughing of alveolar lining cells and the histological appearance of viral pneumonitis.

☐ **Clinical Features:** Influenza presents as a rapid onset of fever, chills, myalgia, headaches, weakness, and nonproductive cough. The illness can be incapacitating for 3 to 5 days and is followed by gradual improvement. Influenza is especially injurious to the elderly or persons with underlying cardiopulmonary disease, who cannot tolerate further impaired respiratory function. Epidemics are accompanied by deaths from both the disease and its complications. Killed viral vaccines specific to epidemic strains are 75% effective in preventing influenza.

Parainfluenza Virus Infection

The parainfluenza viruses cause acute upper and lower respiratory tract infections, which can be particularly severe in young children. These enveloped, single-stranded RNA viruses are the most common cause of croup (laryngotracheobronchitis). This condition is common in children younger than the age of 3 years and is characterized by subglottic swelling, airway compression, and respiratory distress.

There are four antigenically distinct parainfluenza viruses. These viruses spread from person to person through infectious respiratory aerosols and secretions. Infection is highly contagious, and disease is present worldwide. The parainfluenza viruses are isolated from 10% of young children with acute respiratory tract illnesses.

☐ **Pathogenesis and Pathology:** Parainfluenza viruses infect and kill ciliated respiratory epithelial cells, thereby inciting an inflammatory response. In very young children, this process frequently extends into the lower respiratory tract, causing bronchiolitis and pneumonitis. This pattern is most common for parainfluenza type 3. In young children, the trachea is narrow, and its cartilaginous rings are pliable. Moreover, the larynx is small. When laryngotracheitis occurs, the local tissue swelling compresses the upper airway sufficiently to obstruct breathing and cause croup. Parainfluenza virus infection causes necrosis and sloughing of the respiratory tract epithelium, associated with a predominantly lymphocytic inflammatory infiltrate.

☐ **Clinical Features:** Parainfluenza infection is associated with fever, hoarseness, and cough. Croup is evidenced by a characteristic barking cough and inspiratory stridor. Treatment is largely supportive. If hypoxemia or hypercapnia develops, the child with croup may require intubation and assisted respiration. When parainfluenza virus infects older children or adults, the symptoms are usually mild.

Respiratory Syncytial Virus Infection

Respiratory syncytial virus (RSV) is an enveloped, single-stranded RNA virus and is the major cause of bronchiolitis and pneumonia in children younger than 1 year of age. RSV spreads from child to child in respiratory aerosols and secretions. The virus, which is present worldwide, is highly contagious, and most children have been infected with RSV by school age. The spread of RSV is particularly rapid in confined susceptible populations, such as young children on a hospital ward.

☐ **Pathogenesis and Pathology:** RSV infects and kills respiratory epithelium. Viral surface proteins interact with specific receptors on host respiratory epithelium to cause viral binding and fusion. RSV produces necrosis and sloughing of bronchial, bronchiolar, and alveolar epithelium, associated with a predominantly lymphocytic inflammatory infiltrate. The virus can cause fusion of infected cells, and multinucleated syncytial cells are sometimes seen in infected tissues.

☐ **Clinical Features:** Infants and young children with RSV bronchiolitis or pneumonitis present with wheezing, cough, and respiratory distress, sometimes accompanied by fever. The illness is usually self-limited, resolving in 1 to 2 weeks. Antiviral therapy with ribavirin may be of value in some cases. In older children and adults, RSV produces much milder disease. Among otherwise healthy young children, the mortality from RSV infection is very low, but it rises dramatically (to 20% to 40%) among hospitalized children compromised by congenital heart disease or immunosuppression.

Adenovirus Infection

Adenoviruses are nonenveloped DNA viruses that are isolated from the respiratory and intestinal tract of humans and animals. Certain serotypes are common causes of acute respiratory disease and adenovirus pneumonia in military recruits coming together for the first time for basic training. Some adenoviruses are important causes of chronic pulmonary disease in infants and young children.

Pathological changes include necrotizing bronchitis and bronchiolitis, in which the sloughed epithelial cells and inflammatory infiltrate may fill the damaged bronchioles. Interstitial pneumonitis is characterized by areas of consolidation with extensive necrosis, hemorrhage, and a mononuclear inflammatory infiltrate. Two distinctive types of intranuclear inclusions—smudge cells and

Cowdry type A inclusions—involve bronchiolar epithelial cells and alveolar lining cells.

Adenoviruses types 40 and 41 infect colonic and small intestinal epithelial cells and may cause diarrhea in immunocompetent as well as in immunocompromised hosts. AIDS patients are particularly susceptible to urinary tract infections caused by adenovirus type 35.

VIRAL EXANTHEMS

Measles (Rubeola)

Measles virus is an enveloped, single-stranded RNA virus that causes an acute, highly contagious, self-limited illness, characterized by upper respiratory tract symptoms, fever, and a rash.

☐ **Epidemiology:** Humans are the only reservoir for measles virus. Measles is transmitted in respiratory aerosols and secretions. Since infected persons shed large amounts of virus, even before the onset of characteristic symptoms, there is little warning of impending infection. In nonimmunized populations, measles is primarily a disease of children.

Currently available live, attenuated measles vaccines are highly effective in preventing measles and in eliminating the spread of the virus. Recent efforts at nationwide immunization have made measles uncommon in the United States. Similar efforts are underway worldwide to immunize all children.

Measles is a particularly severe disease when it affects the very young, the sick, or the malnourished. In impoverished countries, the disease has a high mortality rate (10% to 25%). In recent years, measles has been estimated to kill 1.5 million children each year and remains a major vaccine-preventable cause of death worldwide. When measles was first introduced to previously unexposed populations (e.g., Native Americans, Pacific Islanders), the resulting widespread infections had devastatingly high mortality rates.

☐ **Pathogenesis:** The initial site of infection in measles is the mucous membranes of the nasopharynx and bronchi. Rubeola virus possesses two surface glycoproteins, designated the "H" and "F" proteins, which mediate viral attachment and fusion with respiratory epithelium. From these cells, the virus extends to the regional lymph nodes and then to the bloodstream, leading to widespread dissemination. Virus then infects various tissues, with prominent involvement of the skin and lymphoid tissues. The rash is thought to result from the action of T lymphocytes on virally infected vascular endothelium.

☐ **Pathology:** Measles virus produces necrosis of infected respiratory epithelium, associated with a predominantly lymphocytic inflammatory infiltrate. In the skin, the virus produces a vasculitis of small blood vessels. The affected vessels are edematous and rimmed by a lymphocytic infiltrate. Lymphoid hyperplasia is often prominent in the cervical and mesenteric lymph nodes, spleen, and appendix. In the lymphoid tissues, the virus sometimes causes fusion of infected cells, producing multinucleated giant cells containing up to 100 nuclei, with both intracytoplasmic and intranuclear inclusions. These cells, named **Warthin-Finkeldey giant cells** (Fig. 9-2), are pathognomonic for measles.

☐ **Clinical Features:** After an incubation period of 10 to 21 days, measles first presents with fever, rhinorrhea, cough, and conjunctivitis and progresses to the characteristic mucosal and skin lesions. The mucosal lesions, known as "Koplik spots," appear on the posterior buccal mucosa and consist of minute gray-white dots on a red base. The skin lesions begin on the face as an erythematous maculopapular rash, which usually spreads to involve the trunk and extremities. The rash fades in 3 to 5 days, and the symptoms gradually resolve. The clinical course of measles may be much more severe in very young children, malnourished persons, or immunocompromised patients. Measles often leads to secondary bacterial infections, especially otitis media and pneumonia.

Rubella

Rubellavirus is an enveloped, single-stranded RNA virus, that causes a mild, self-limited systemic disease, usually associated with a rash. Many infections are so mild that they go unnoticed. However, in pregnant women, rubella is a destructive fetal pathogen. Infection early in gestation can produce fetal death, premature delivery, and congenital anomalies, including deafness, cataracts, glaucoma, heart defects, and mental retardation.

☐ **Epidemiology:** Humans are the only host of rubellavirus. The agent spreads from person to person primarily by the respiratory route. Infection occurs worldwide, except in vaccinated populations. Rubella is

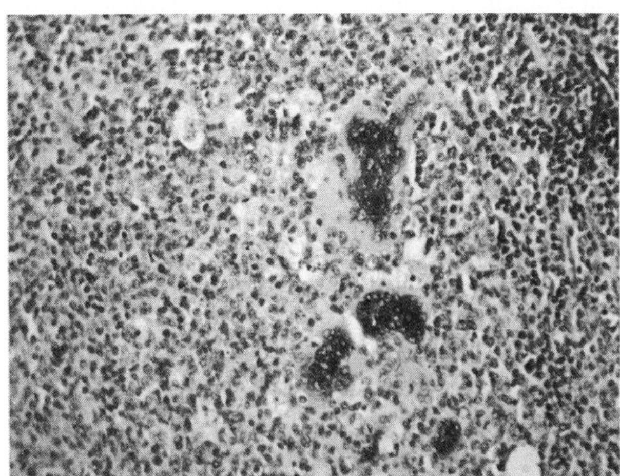

FIGURE 9-2
Warthin-Finkeldey giant cells in measles. A photomicrograph of a hyperplastic lymph node from a patient with measles shows several multinucleated giant cells.

not highly contagious, and in unvaccinated populations, 10% to 15% of young women remain susceptible to infection into their reproductive years.

The live attenuated viral vaccine that is currently available prevents rubella, and vaccination programs have largely eliminated the disease from developed countries. This disease is now uncommon in the United States.

□ **Pathogenesis:** Rubella infects the respiratory epithelium and then disseminates to various organs through the bloodstream and lymphatics. As in measles, the rubella rash is believed to result from an immunological response to the disseminated virus. Fetal infection occurs through the placenta during the viremic phase of maternal illness. A congenitally infected fetus remains persistently infected and sheds large amounts of virus in body fluids, even after birth. Maternal infection after 20 weeks' gestation usually does not cause significant fetal disease.

□ **Pathology:** The pathology of congenital rubella is variable. The heart, eye, and brain are the organs most frequently affected. Cardiac lesions include pulmonary valvular stenosis, pulmonary artery hypoplasia, ventricular septal defects, and patent ductus arteriosus. Ocular abnormalities are characterized by cataracts, glaucoma, and retinal defects. Deafness is a common complication of fetal rubella. Severe brain involvement can produce microcephaly and mental retardation.

□ **Clinical Features:** Rubella is a mild, acute febrile illness, with rhinorrhea, conjunctivitis, postauricular lymphadenopathy, and a rash that spreads from face to trunk and extremities. The rash resolves within 3 days, and complications are rare. As many as 30% of infections are completely asymptomatic.

Human Parvovirus B19 Infection

Human parvovirus B19 is a single-stranded DNA virus that causes systemic infections, characterized by rash, arthralgias, and transient interruption in erythrocyte production. Most persons suffer a mild exanthematous illness, known as **erythema infectiosum** ("fifth disease"), accompanied by an asymptomatic interruption in erythropoiesis. In persons with chronic hemolytic anemias, however, the interruption in erythrocyte production causes profound, potentially fatal anemia, known as **transient aplastic crisis**. When the fetus is infected by human parvovirus B19, a transient cessation of erythropoiesis can lead to severe anemia, hydrops fetalis, and death *in utero*, an outcome that occurs in as many of 10% of maternal infections.

Human parvovirus B19 spreads from person to person by the respiratory route. Infection is common and occurs in outbreaks, mostly among children. It is not known which cells, other than erythroid precursors, support parvovirus B19 replication, but replication at some respiratory site prior to dissemination to erythropoietic cells seems likely.

Human parvovirus B19 produces characteristic cytopathic effects in erythroid precursor cells. The nucleus of an affected cell is enlarged, and the chromatin is displaced peripherally by central glassy eosinophilic material.

Smallpox (Variola)

Before its eradication, smallpox was an acute highly contagious exanthematous viral infection caused by a double-stranded DNA virus. The virus produces a typical plaque, or "pock," when cultured on the chorioallantoic membrane of embryonated chicken eggs. Since Jenner's pioneering work in 1796, a similar virus—vaccinia, the causative agent of cowpox—has been used for "vaccination" to protect against smallpox.

Smallpox is evidently an ancient disease; a rash resembling smallpox was found in the mummified remains of the Egyptian pharaoh Ramses V, who died in 1160 BC. The disease once had a worldwide distribution, afflicting persons of both sexes and all ages, but particularly children.

In 1967, the World Health Organization began its uniquely successful campaign to eradicate smallpox. At that time, the disease had already been controlled in developed countries but was still endemic in the less-developed world. Remarkably, in 10 years, the vaccination campaign eliminated the disease. The successful eradication of smallpox depended on several factors, including (1) the permanence of immunity following vaccination, (2) the stability of the smallpox virus (in contrast to the instability of influenza viruses and many others), and (3) the lack of an animal reservoir for the virus.

Smallpox was transmitted in respiratory droplets and almost always involved face-to-face contact. The infection led to the development of vesicles and pustules over much of the body (Fig. 9-3). The pustules umbilicated and desiccated to form scabs, which contained the smallpox virus. The scabs sloughed from the skin, thereby creating pitted scars or "pock marking." The most severe form, known as "hemorrhagic smallpox," was characterized by bleeding into the vesicles and was almost always fatal.

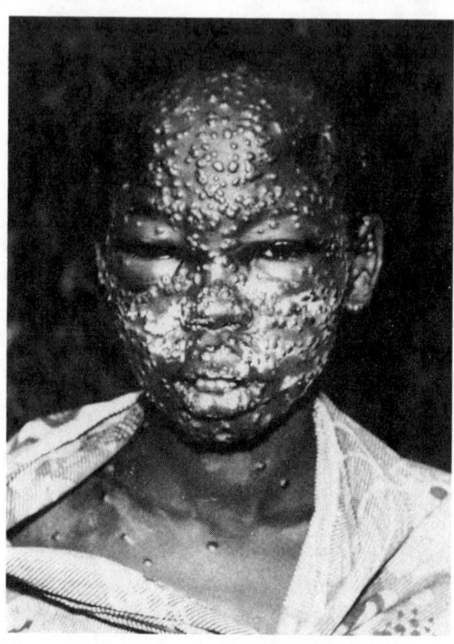

FIGURE *9-3*
Smallpox, eastern Zaire, 1968.

MUMPS

Mumps virus is an enveloped, single-stranded RNA virus that causes an acute, self-limited systemic illness, characterized by parotid gland swelling and meningoencephalitis.

☐ **Epidemiology:** Humans are the only reservoir for mumps virus, and the disease spreads from person to person through the respiratory route. Infection is highly contagious, and 90% of exposed, susceptible persons become infected, although only 60% to 70% develop symptoms. Mumps is present worldwide, except in immunized populations, and is primarily a disease of childhood.

A live attenuated mumps vaccine prevents mumps, and the disease has been largely eliminated from most developed countries.

☐ **Pathogenesis:** Mumps infection begins with viral infection of respiratory tract epithelium. The virus then disseminates through the blood and lymphatic systems to infect other sites, most commonly the salivary glands (especially parotids), central nervous system, pancreas, and testes. The central nervous system is involved in more than half of cases, producing symptomatic disease in 10%. Epididymo-orchitis occurs in 30% of males infected after puberty.

☐ **Pathology:** Mumps virus causes necrosis of infected cells, which is associated with a predominantly lymphocytic inflammatory infiltrate. The affected salivary glands are swollen, the ducts lined by necrotic epithelium, and the interstitium infiltrated with lymphocytes. In mumps epididymo-orchitis, the testis can be swollen to three times the normal size. The swelling of testicular parenchyma, confined within the tunica albuginea, produces focal ischemic infarctions. Mumps orchitis is usually unilateral and, thus, rarely causes sterility.

☐ **Clinical Features:** After an incubation period of 2 to 3 weeks, mumps begins with fever and malaise, followed by painful swelling of the salivary glands, usually one or both parotids. Symptomatic meningeal involvement most often presents as headache, stiff neck, and vomiting. Meningitis is the most common extra-salivary manifestation of mumps. Prior to widespread vaccination, mumps was a leading cause of viral meningitis and encephalitis in the United States. Although severe disease of the pancreas is rare in mumps, most patients exhibit elevated serum amylase activity.

INTESTINAL VIRUS INFECTIONS

Rotavirus Infection

Rotavirus is the most common cause of severe diarrhea worldwide, producing a profuse watery diarrhea that can lead to dehydration and death if untreated. This double-stranded RNA virus usually infects young children.

☐ **Epidemiology:** Rotavirus infection spreads from person to person by the oral-fecal route. Infection is most common among children, who shed huge amounts of virus in the stool. Siblings, playmates, parents, food, water, and environmental surfaces are readily contaminated with the virus. The peak age of infection is 6 months to 2 years, and virtually all children have been infected by the age of 4 years. In the United States, rotavirus causes more than 3 million infections annually, resulting in about 100 deaths in young children. Worldwide rotavirus causes 140 million infections annually, and over 1 million deaths.

☐ **Pathogenesis and Pathology:** Rotavirus infects the enterocytes of the upper small intestine, disrupting the absorption of sugars, fats, and various ions. The resulting osmotic load causes a net loss of fluid into the bowel lumen, producing diarrhea and dehydration. Infected cells are shed from the intestinal villi, and the regenerating epithelium initially lacks full absorptive capabilities.

Pathological changes in rotavirus infection are largely confined to the duodenum and jejunum, where there is shortening of the intestinal villi, associated with a mild infiltrate of neutrophils and lymphocytes. There is no alteration in the gross appearance of the infected intestine.

☐ **Clinical Features:** Rotavirus infection presents as vomiting, fever, abdominal pain, and profuse, watery diarrhea. The vomiting usually persists for 2 to 3 days, while the diarrhea continues for 5 to 8 days. Without adequate fluid replacement, the diarrhea can produce rapidly fatal dehydration in young children.

Norwalk Virus Infection and Other Viral Diarrheas

In addition to rotavirus, there are numerous other viral causes of diarrhea, including adenoviruses, caliciviruses, and astroviruses. The best understood are the Norwalk family of nonenveloped RNA viruses, a group of caliciviruses which carry a host of individual names (e.g., Norwalk virus, Snow Mountain virus, Sapporo virus) associated with the locations of particular outbreaks. Norwalk viruses are responsible for one third of all outbreaks of diarrheal disease. They produce gastroenteritis in children and adults, with self-limited vomiting and diarrhea, similar to that caused by rotavirus. The Norwalk viruses infect cells of the upper small bowel and produce changes similar to those that occur with rotavirus.

VIRAL HEMORRHAGIC FEVERS

Viral hemorrhagic fevers are a group of at least 13 distinct viral infections that cause varying degrees of hemorrhage and shock, and sometimes death. There are many similar viral hemorrhagic fevers in different parts of the world, for the most part named for the area where they were first described.

On the basis of differences in routes of transmission, vectors, and other epidemiological characteristics, the viral hemorrhagic fevers have been divided into four groups (Table 9-3): mosquito-borne, tick-borne, zoonotic, and the filoviruses, Marborg and Ebola virus, in which the route of transmission is unknown. The agents in the last group have emerged as human pathogens only in the past three decades, presumably because humans have encroached on wild indigenous reservoirs of infection previously isolated from human contact. In 1996, an epidemic of Ebola virus infection broke out in sub-saharan Africa, killing 200 to 300 persons. Of the viral hemorrhagic fevers, only yellow fever will be discussed in detail.

Yellow Fever

Yellow fever is an acute hemorrhagic fever, sometimes associated with extensive hepatic necrosis and jaundice. The illness is caused by an insect-borne flavivirus, an enveloped, single-stranded RNA virus.

☐ **Epidemiology:** First described in the Caribbean, yellow fever is the oldest known viral hemorrhagic fever. It was first recognized as a nosological entity in the New World in the 17th century, but its origins probably were in Africa. Today, the virus is restricted to certain regions of Africa and South America, including both jungle and urban settings. The usual reservoir for the virus is tree-dwelling monkeys, the agent being passed among them in the forest canopy by mosquitoes. These monkeys serve as a reservoir because the virus neither kills them nor makes them ill. Humans acquire jungle yellow fever by entering the forest and being bitten by infected *Aedes* mosquitoes (see Fig. 9-1). Felling trees increases the risk of infection, because mosquitoes are brought down with the tree. On returning to the village or city, the human victim becomes the reservoir for epidemic yellow fever in the urban setting, where *Aedes aegyptii* is the vector.

☐ **Pathogenesis:** On inoculation by the mosquito, the virus multiplies within tissue and vascular endothelium and then disseminates through the bloodstream. The virus has a tropism for liver cells, where it sometimes produces extensive acute hepatocellular destruction. Extensive damage to the endothelium of small blood vessels may lead to the loss of vascular integrity and consequent hemorrhages and shock.

TABLE **9-3** **Viral Hemorrhagic Fevers**

Vector	Viral Fever
Mosquitoes	Yellow fever Rift valley fever Dengue hemorrhagic fever Chikungunya hemorrhagic fever
Ticks	Omsk hemorrhagic fever Crimean hemorrhagic fever Kyasanur forest disease
Rodents	Lassa fever Bolivian hemorrhagic fever Argentine hemorrhagic fever Korean hemorrhagic fever
Undefined	Ebola virus disease Marburg virus disease

☐ **Pathology:** Yellow fever virus causes coagulative necrosis of hepatocytes, which begins among cells in the middle of hepatic lobules and spreads toward the central veins and portal tracts. The infection sometimes produces confluent areas of necrosis in the middle of the hepatic lobules (i.e., midzonal necrosis). In the most severe cases, the entire lobule may be necrotic. Some necrotic hepatocytes lose their nuclei and become intensely eosinophilic. They often dislodge from adjacent hepatocytes, in which case they are known as **Councilman bodies** (recognized today as apoptotic bodies). Hepatocytes also show microvesicular fatty change.

☐ **Clinical Features:** Yellow fever usually begins with the abrupt onset of fever, chills, headache, myalgias, nausea, and vomiting. After 3 to 5 days, some patients develop manifestations of hepatic failure, with jaundice (hence the term **yellow fever**), deficiencies of clotting factors, and diffuse hemorrhages. Vomiting clotted blood ("black vomit") is a classic feature of severe cases of yellow fever. Patients with massive hepatic failure lapse into coma and die, usually within 10 days of onset of illness. The overall mortality of yellow fever is 5%, but among those with jaundice, it rises to 30%.

HERPESVIRUS INFECTIONS

The virus family Herpesviridae includes a large number of enveloped, DNA viruses, many of which infect humans. Almost all herpesviruses express some common antigenic determinants, and many produce type A nuclear inclusions (acidophilic bodies surrounded by a halo). The most important human pathogens among the herpesviruses are varicella-zoster, herpes simplex, Epstein-Barr virus, human herpervirus 6 (HHV6, the cause of roseola), and cytomegalovirus. Recently, human herpesvirus 8 (HHV8) was implicated in the pathogenesis of Kaposi sarcoma in human immunodeficiency virus (HIV)–infected patients. Herpesviruses are also distinguished by their capacity to remain latent for long periods of time.

Varicella-Zoster Infection

Varicella-zoster virus causes two distinct diseases, chickenpox and herpes zoster (Fig. 9-4). The first exposure to varicella-zoster virus produces chickenpox, an acute systemic illness whose dominant feature is a generalized vesicular skin eruption. The virus then becomes latent, and its reactivation causes herpes zoster ("shingles"), a localized vesicular skin eruption.

☐ **Epidemiology:** Varicella-zoster virus is restricted to human hosts and spreads from person to per-

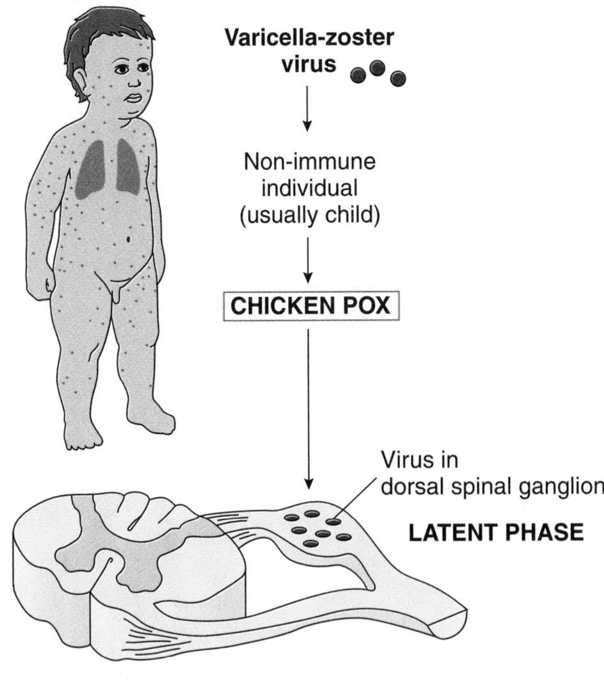

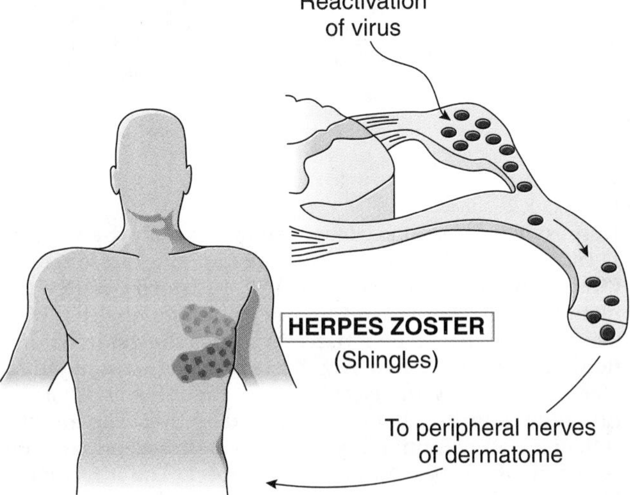

FIGURE 9-4
Varicella (chickenpox) and herpes zoster (shingles). Varicella-zoster virus (VZV) in droplets is inhaled by a nonimmune person (usually a child) and initially causes a "silent" infection of the nasopharynx. This progresses to viremia, seeding of fixed macrophages, and dissemination of VZV to skin (chickenpox) and viscera. VZV resides in a dorsal spinal ganglion, where it remains dormant for many years. Latent VZV is reactivated and spreads from ganglia along the sensory nerves to the peripheral nerves of sensory dermatomes, causing shingles.

son primarily by the respiratory route. It can also be spread by contact with secretions from the skin lesions. The virus is present worldwide and is highly contagious. Most children in the United States are infected by early school age.

☐ **Pathogenesis:** Varicella-zoster virus is believed initially to infect cells of the respiratory tract or possibly the conjunctival epithelium. There it reproduces and spreads throughout the body through the bloodstream and lymphatic systems. Many organs are infected during this viremic stage, but skin involvement usually dominates the clinical picture. The virus spreads from the capillary endothelium to the epidermis, where viral replication destroys the basal cells. As a result, the upper layers of the epidermis separate from the basal layer to form vesicles.

During primary infection with varicella-zoster virus, the agent establishes latent infection in perineuronal satellite cells of the dorsal nerve root ganglia. Transcription of viral genes continues during latency, but complete viral replication cycles do not occur, and the virus cannot be cultured from ganglion tissue. However, viral DNA can be demonstrated by *in situ* hybridization for many years after the initial infection.

Shingles occurs when full replication of the virus occurs in ganglion cells, and the agent travels down the sensory nerve serving a dermatome. It infects the epidermis of that dermatome, producing a localized, painful vesicular eruption. The risk of shingles in an infected person increases with age, and most cases occur among the elderly. Impaired cell-mediated immunity also increases the risk of herpes zoster reactivation.

☐ **Pathology:** The skin lesions of chickenpox and shingles are indistinguishable from each other and also from the lesions produced by herpes simplex virus. The vesicle fills with neutrophils and soon erodes to become a shallow ulcer. In infected cells, varicella-zoster virus produces a characteristic cytopathic effect, consisting of nuclear homogenization, intranuclear inclusions (Cowdry type A), and formation of multinucleated cells (Fig. 9-5). The inclusion occupies more than one half of the nuclear diameter, is separated from the nuclear membrane by a clear zone (halo), and is eosinophilic. Over several days,

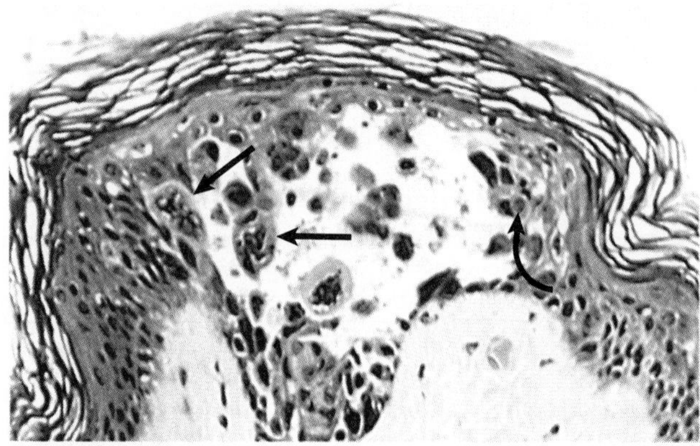

FIGURE 9-5
Varicella. Photomicrograph of the skin from a patient with chickenpox shows an intraepidermal vesicle. Multinucleated giant cells (*straight arrows*) and nuclear inclusions (*curved arrow*) are present.

the vesicles become pustules, after which they rupture and heal.

☐ **Clinical Features:** After an incubation period of 11 to 21 days, chickenpox presents as fever, malaise, and a distinctive pruritic rash, beginning on the head and spreading to the trunk and extremities. The skin lesions begin as maculopapules that rapidly evolve into vesicles. The latter become pustules, which soon ulcerate and crust. Lesions appear in crops, and any one area contains lesions in various stages of evolution. Vesicles may also appear on the mucous membranes, especially the mouth. The fever and systemic symptoms resolve in 3 to 5 days, whereas the skin lesions heal in several weeks.

Shingles presents with a unilateral, painful, vesicular eruption, similar in appearance to chickenpox, but in a dermatomal pattern, usually localized to a single dermatome. Although shingles can appear anytime after chickenpox, most cases do not occur until after age 50. Pain can persist for months after the resolution of the skin lesions.

Herpes Simplex Virus Infection

Herpes simplex viruses (HSV) are common human viral pathogens, producing necrotizing infections at diverse body sites (Table 9-4). HSV most frequently produces recurrent painful vesicular eruptions of the skin and mucous membranes. Two antigenically and epidemiologically distinct herpes simplex viruses, HSV-1 and HSV-2, cause human disease (Fig. 9-6):

- **HSV-1** is transmitted in oral secretions and typically causes disease "above the waist," including oral, facial, and ocular lesions.
- **HSV-2** is transmitted in genital secretions and typically produces disease "below the waist," including genital ulcers and neonatal herpes infection.

Both HSV-1 and HSV-2 can cause severe protracted and disseminated disease in immunocompromised persons.

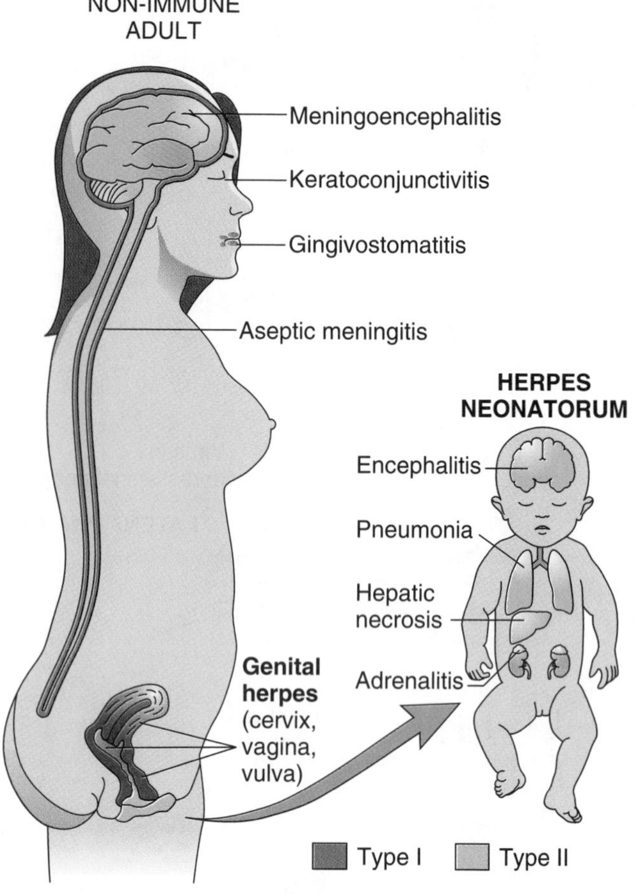

FIGURE *9-6*
Herpesvirus infections. Herpes simplex virus type 1 (HSV-1) infects a nonimmune adult, causing gingivostomatitis ("fever blister" or "cold sore"), keratoconjunctivitis, meningoencephalitis, and aseptic spinal meningitis. Herpes simplex virus type 2 (HSV-2) infects the genitalia of a nonimmune adult, involving the cervix, vagina, and vulva. Herpes simplex virus type 2 infects the fetus as it passes through the birth canal of an infected mother. The infant's lack of a mature immune system results in disseminated infection with herpes simplex virus type 1. The infection is often fatal, involving lung, liver, adrenal glands, and central nervous system.

TABLE *9-4* **Herpes Simplex Viral Diseases**

Viral Type	Common Presentations	Infrequent Presentations
HSV-1	Oral-labial herpes	Conjunctivitis, keratitis Encephalitis Herpetic whitlow Esophagitis[a] Pneumonia[a] Disseminated infection[a]
HSV-2	Genital herpes	Perinatal infection Disseminated infection[a]

[a] These conditions usually occur in immunocompromised hosts.

☐ **Epidemiology:** HSV spreads from person to person, primarily through direct contact with infected secretions or open lesions. HSV-1 spreads in oral secretions, and infection frequently occurs in childhood, most persons (50% to 90%) being infected by adulthood. HSV-2 spreads by contact with genital lesions and is primarily a venereally transmitted pathogen. Neonatal herpes is acquired during passage of the newborn through an infected birth canal.

☐ **Pathogenesis:** Primary HSV disease occurs at a site of initial viral inoculation, such as the oropharynx, genital mucosa, or skin. There the virus infects epithelial cells, producing progeny viruses and destroying the infected cells. Destruction of basal cells in the squamous epithelium disrupts the epithelium and leads to vesicle formation. Cell necrosis also incites an inflammatory response, initially dominated by neutrophils and then followed by lymphocytes. Primary infection resolves with the development of humoral and cell-mediated immunity to the virus.

Latent infection is established in a manner analogous to that of varicella-zoster virus. The virus invades sensory nerve endings in the oral or genital mucosa, ascends within axons, and establishes a latent infection in sensory neurons within the corresponding ganglia. From time to time, the latent infection is reactivated, and HSV travels back down the nerve to the epithelial site served by the ganglion, where it again infects epithelial cells. Sometimes this secondary infection produces ulcerating vesicular lesions. At other times, the secondary infection does not cause visible tissue destruction, but contagious progeny viruses are shed from the site of infection. Various factors, usually typical for a given person, can induce the reactivation of latent HSV infection. These include intense sunlight, emotional stress, febrile illness, and menstruation.

Herpes encephalitis is a rare (1 in 100,000 HSV infections), but devastating, manifestation of HSV-1 infection. In some instances, it occurs when the virus, latent in the trigeminal ganglion, is reactivated and travels retrograde to the brain. However, herpes encephalitis also occurs in persons who have no history of "cold sores," and the pathogenesis of the encephalitis in these cases is poorly understood (see Chapter 28).

Neonatal herpes is a serious complication of maternal genital herpes. The virus is transmitted to the fetus from the infected birth canal, often the uterine cervix, and readily disseminates in the unprotected newborn child.

Humoral and cell-mediated immunity are crucial to the control of HSV infections, and immunocompromised persons are at risk of severe HSV disease. In those with impaired cell-mediated immunity, primary and secondary HSV infections are more protracted and often spread from the initial site of infection to other body sites.

☐ **Pathology:** The skin and mucous membranes are the usual sites of HSV infection, but the disease sometimes involves the brain, eye, liver, lungs, and other organs. In any location, both HSV-1 and HSV-2 cause necrosis of infected cells, which is accompanied by a vigorous inflammatory response. Clusters of painful ulcerating vesicular lesions on the skin or mucous membranes are the most frequent manifestation of HSV infection (Fig. 9-7A). These lesions persist for 1 to 2 weeks and then resolve. The cellular alterations include (1) nuclear homogenization, (2) Cowdry type A intranuclear inclusions, and (3) the formation of multinucleated giant cells (see Fig. 9-7B).

☐ **Clinical Features:** The clinical features of HSV infections vary according to host susceptibility (e.g., neonate, normal host, compromised host), viral type, and site of infection. A prodromal "tingling" sensation at the site often precedes the appearance of lesions. Recurrent lesions appear weeks, months, or years later, at the initial site or at a site subserved by the same nerve ganglion. Recurrent herpetic lesions in the mouth or on the lip are commonly called "cold sores" or "fever blisters" and frequently appear following sun exposure, trauma, or a febrile illness.

Patients with AIDS and other immunocompromised persons are prone to develop herpes esophagitis. The presentation features the acute onset of severely painful and difficult swallowing and constant retrosternal pain. Early lesions consist of rounded 1- to 3-mm vesicles located predominantly in the mid to distal esophagus. As the HSV-infected squamous cells slough from the lesions, sharply demarcated ulcers with elevated margins form and coalesce. This process may result in denudation of the esophageal mucosa. Superimposed Candida infection is common at this stage. In immunocompromised patients,

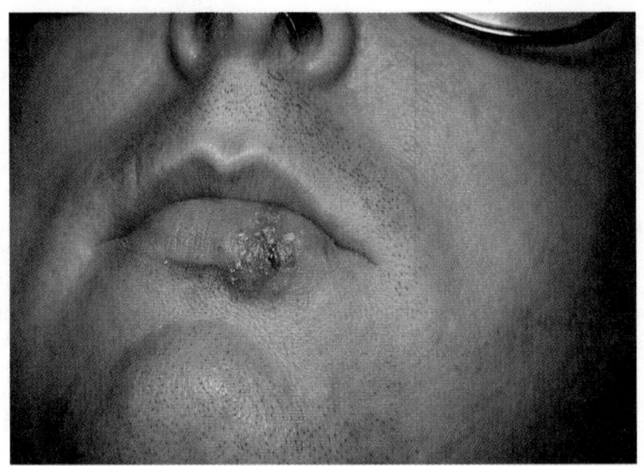
A

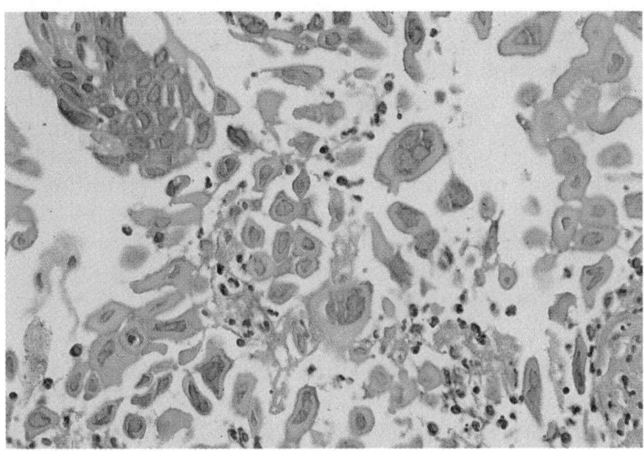
B

FIGURE *9-7*
Herpes simplex, type 1. (*A*) Herpetic vesicles are seen on the surface of the lower lip. (*B*) Epithelial cells infected with herpes simplex virus type 1 demonstrate Cowdry type A intranuclear inclusions and multinucleated giant cells.

HSV may also infect the anal mucosa, where it causes painful blisters and ulcers.

Neonatal herpes begins 5 to 7 days after delivery, with irritability, lethargy, and a mucocutaneous vesicular eruption. The infection rapidly spreads to involve multiple organs, including the brain. The infected newborn develops jaundice, bleeding problems, respiratory distress, seizures, and coma. Treatment of severe herpes simplex infections with acyclovir is often effective, but neonatal herpes still carries a high mortality.

Epstein-Barr Virus Infection (Infectious Mononucleosis)

Infectious mononucleosis is a viral disease characterized by fever, pharyngitis, lymphadenopathy, and increased circulating lymphocytes. By the time of adulthood, most persons have been infected with Epstein-Barr virus (EBV). In most instances, the infection is asymptomatic, but in some persons, EBV causes infectious mononucleosis. EBV infection also has been associated with several cancers, including African Burkitt lymphoma, B-cell lymphoma in immunosuppressed persons, and nasopharyngeal carcinoma. These neoplastic complications are discussed in Chapters 20 and 25.

☐ **Epidemiology:** In impoverished areas of the world, where children often live in crowded conditions, infection with EBV usually occurs at a young age. For example, in central Africa, virtually all children are infected with EBV before the age of 3 years, and infectious mononucleosis is not encountered. In developed countries, where there is less crowding of children, many persons remain uninfected into adolescence or early adulthood. In such instances, two thirds of those newly infected develop clinically evident infectious mononucleosis.

Epstein-Barr virus spreads from person to person primarily through contact with infected oral secretions (Fig. 9-8). Once infected with the virus, persons remain asymptomatically infected for life and a few (10% to 20%) intermittently shed EBV. This lifelong latent infection with EBV is analogous to latent infections characteristic of the other herpesviruses. Transmission of the virus requires close contact with infected persons. Thus, EBV spreads readily among young children in crowded conditions, where there is considerable "sharing" of oral secretions. Spread proceeds more slowly among older persons who are usually less generous with saliva, although kissing can be an effective mode of transmission.

☐ **Pathogenesis:** The virus first binds to and infects nasopharyngeal cells and then B lymphocytes. Infection with the virus is initiated by the binding of a viral glycoprotein to a cell membrane protein, which also serves as the receptor for the complement fragment C3d. There is evidence that EBV binds IgA before being internalized in epithelial cells. Circulating B lymphocytes carry the virus throughout the body, producing a generalized infection of lymphoid tissues.

Epstein-Barr virus induces a polyclonal activation of B cells. In turn, the activated B cells stimulate the proliferation of specific killer T lymphocytes and suppressor T cells. The former destroy virally infected B cells, whereas the suppressor cells inhibit the production of immunoglobulins by the B cells.

Although EBV is clearly implicated in the pathogenesis of African Burkitt lymphoma (Fig. 9-9), B-cell lymphomas in immunosuppressed persons, and nasopharyngeal carcinoma, its precise role remains uncertain. The viral genome can be demonstrated within tumor cells, and EBV is known to immortalize and induce proliferation of infected cells. It is thought that EBV is an initiator in the process of carcinogenesis and that other proliferative stimuli (e.g., malaria in African Burkitt lymphoma) act as promotors. The oncogenic properties of EBV are discussed in Chapter 5.

☐ **Pathology:** The pathological changes of infectious mononucleosis are prominent in the lymph nodes and spleen. In most patients, the lymphadenopathy is symmetric and most striking in the neck. The nodes are movable, discrete, and tender. Microscopically, the general architecture is preserved. The germinal centers are enlarged and have indistinct margins, because of a proliferation of immunoblasts. They contain frequent mitoses and scattered nuclear debris, presumably from degenerated B cells. The nodes contain occasional large hyperchromatic cells with polylobated nuclei that resemble Reed-Sternberg cells. The appearance of the nodes may present diagnostic problems because of the morphological similarity to Hodgkin disease or lymphomas.

The spleen is large and soft, owing to hyperplasia of the red pulp, and is susceptible to rupture. Many immunoblasts are present throughout the pulp and infiltrate the walls of vessels, the trabeculae, and the capsule. The liver is almost always involved, and the sinusoids and portal tracts contain atypical lymphocytes.

One of the features of infectious mononucleosis is a lymphocytosis with atypical lymphocytes. The increased lymphocytes are activated T lymphocytes, which are involved in the suppression and killing of EBV-infected B lymphocytes. "Atypical" lymphocytes are enlarged cells with lobulated, eccentric nuclei and vacuolated cytoplasm.

Another distinguishing feature of infectious mononucleosis is the development of a specific heterophile antibody, known as the Paul Bunnell antibody. A heterophile antibody is an immunoglobulin produced in one species that reacts with antigens of another species. Paul Bunnell antibodies are raised in persons with infectious mononucleosis and are recognized by their affinity for sheep erythrocytes. This heterophile reaction is a standard diagnostic test for infectious mononucleosis. Specific serological tests for the presence of antibodies against EBV and for the presence of EBV antigens are also available.

☐ **Clinical Features:** Infectious mononucleosis presents as fever, malaise, lymphadenopathy, pharyngitis, and splenomegaly. Patients usually have an elevated leukocyte count, with a predominance of lymphocytes

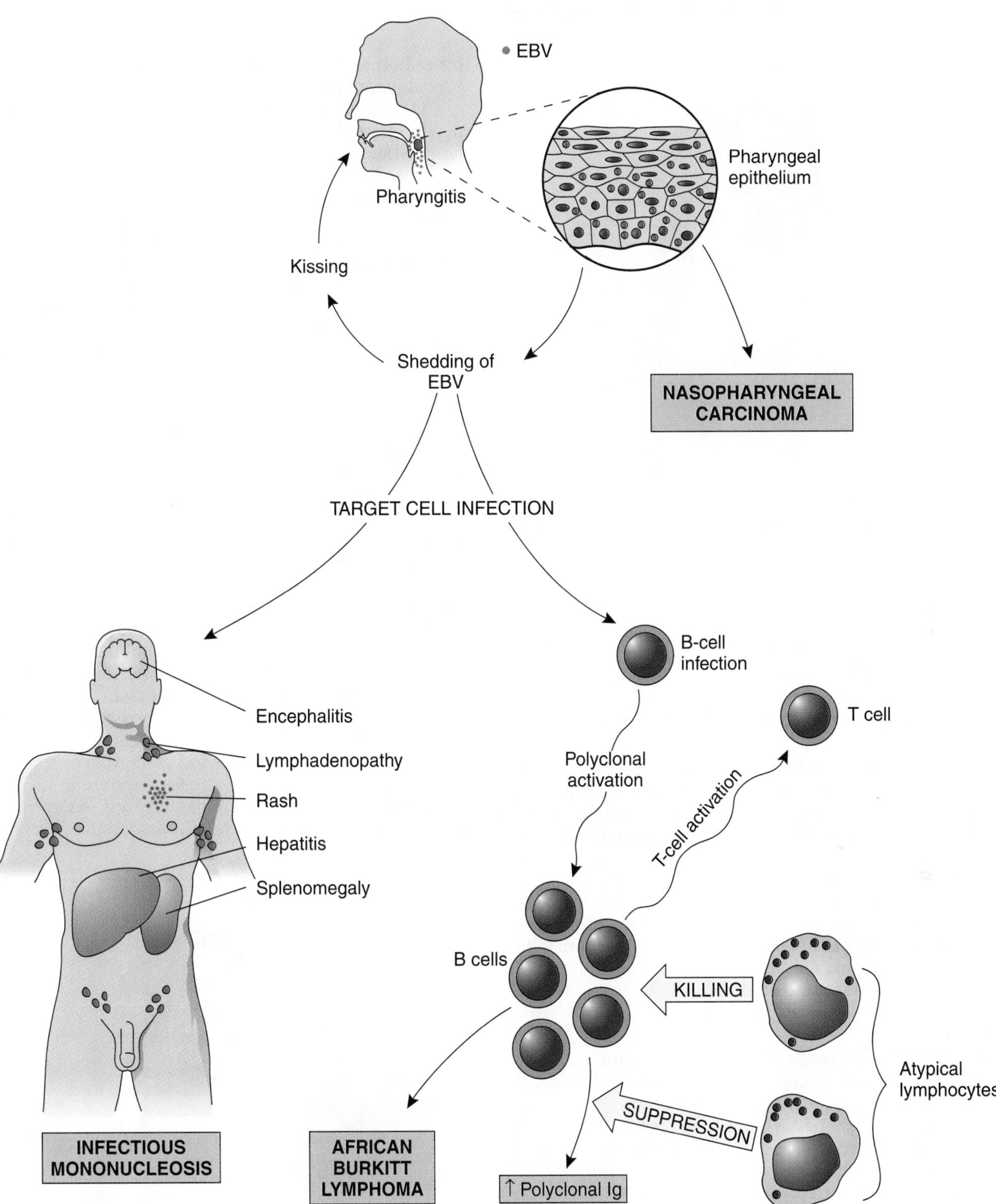

FIGURE *9-8*
Role of Epstein-Barr virus (EBV) in infectious mononucleosis, nasopharyngeal carcinoma, and Burkitt lymphoma. EBV invades and replicates within the salivary glands or pharyngeal epithelium, and is shed into the saliva and respiratory secretions. In some people, the virus transforms pharyngeal epithelial cells, leading to nasopharyngeal carcinoma. In people who are not immune from childhood exposure, EBV causes infectious mononucleosis. EBV infects B lymphocytes, which undergo polyclonal activation. These B cells stimulate the production of atypical lymphocytes, which kill virally infected B cells and suppress the production of immunoglobulins. Some infected B cells are transformed into immature malignant lymphocytes of Burkitt lymphoma.

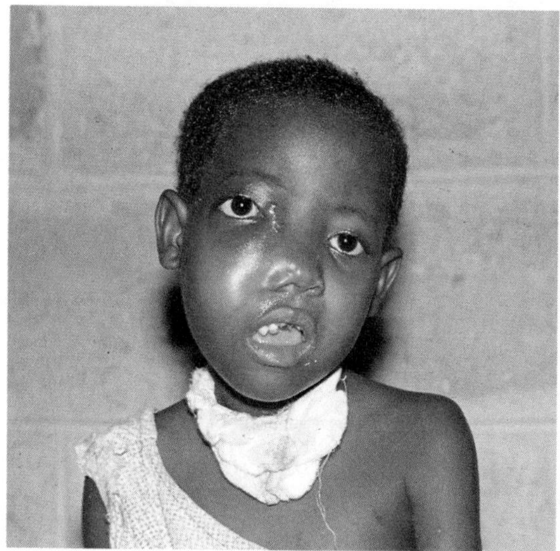

FIGURE 9-9
African Burkitt lymphoma. A tumor of the jaw distorts the child's face.

and monocytes. Treatment is supportive, and symptoms usually resolve in 3 to 4 weeks. The clinical features of tumors associated with EBV infections are discussed in Chapters 20 and 25.

Cytomegalovirus Infection

Cytomegalovirus (CMV) is a congenital and opportunistic pathogen that infects many persons worldwide but produces disease only uncommonly. The fetus and immunocompromised persons are particularly vulnerable to the destructive effects of the virus. CMV infects 0.5% to 2.0% of all fetuses and injures 10% to 20% of these, making it the most common congenital pathogen. Affected children show predominantly neurological defects, which range from subtle learning disabilities to profound retardation. In the immunocompromised patient, CMV infection causes necrotizing lesions, particularly in the gastrointestinal tract, eye, brain, adrenals, and lung.

☐ **Epidemiology:** CMV spreads from person to person by contact with infected secretions and fluids, including saliva, blood, urine, semen, breast milk, and cervical secretions. The virus is transmitted to the fetus across the placenta. Children spread the virus to each other in saliva or urine, while among adolescents and adults, transmission occurs primarily through sexual contact. Infection is present worldwide, and although there is considerable geographic variation, most persons become infected by adulthood.

☐ **Pathogenesis:** CMV infects various human cells, including epithelial cells, lymphocytes, and monocytes and establishes latency in leukocytes. The normal immune response rapidly controls CMV infection, and infected persons usually show no ill effects, although they shed virus periodically in body secretions. Similar to other herpesviruses, CMV can remain latent for years, probably for life.

Destructive CMV infections of the fetus occur when a newly infected pregnant woman passes the virus to her fetus. In such primary maternal infections, the fetus is not protected by maternally derived antibodies, and the virus invades fetal cells with little initial immunological response. This infection produces widespread cellular necrosis and inflammation. A similar situation occurs in persons with profound suppression of cell-mediated immunity. In such patients, the virus spreads to susceptible cells, causing widespread cellular necrosis and inflammation. In most immunosuppressed persons, disseminated CMV infection derives from reactivation of endogenous latent infection, although the virus can also come from exogenous sources.

☐ **Pathology:** In the fetus with CMV disease, the most common sites of involvement are the brain, inner ears, eyes, liver, and bone marrow. The most severely affected fetuses may have microcephaly, hydrocephalus, cerebral calcifications, hepatosplenomegaly, and jaundice. Microscopically, the lesions of fetal CMV disease show cellular necrosis and a characteristic cytopathic effect, consisting of marked cellular and nuclear enlargement, with nuclear and cytoplasmic inclusions. The giant nucleus, which is usually solitary, contains a large central inclusion surrounded by a clear zone (Fig. 9-10). The cytoplasmic inclusions are less prominent.

In persons with depressed cell-mediated immunity, CMV produces localized or disseminated necrotizing lesions. In patients with AIDS and in immunosuppressed transplant recipients, CMV causes chorioretinitis, gastrointestinal ulcers, pneumonitis, hepatitis, encephalitis, and adrenal insufficiency. The CMV cytopathic effect occurs in affected tissues.

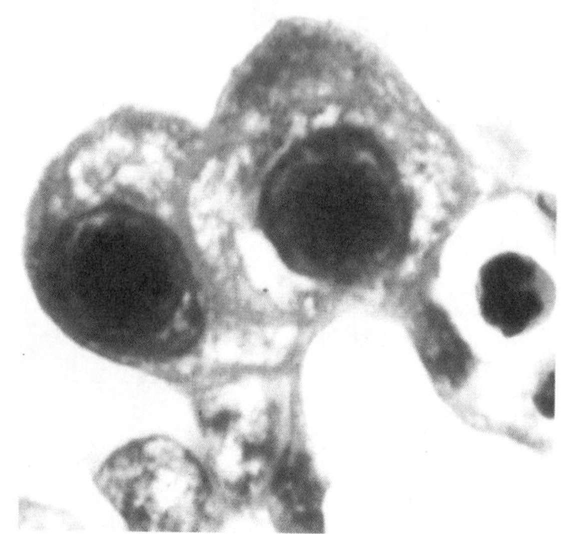

FIGURE 9-10
Cytomegalovirus pneumonitis. Type II pneumocytes display enlarged nuclei containing solitary inclusions surrounded by a clear zone.

☐ **Clinical Features:** Congenitally acquired CMV has a wide range of clinical presentations. Severe disease causes fetal death *in utero*, conspicuous lesions of the central nervous system, liver disease, and bleeding problems. However, most congenital CMV infections do not produce gross abnormalities but present as subtle learning or hearing defects, which are not detected until later in life.

Cytomegalovirus disease in immunosuppressed patients has diverse clinical manifestations, depending on the site of involvement and the degree of suppression of cell-mediated immunity. CMV disease can present as decreased visual acuity (chorioretinitis), diarrhea or gastrointestinal hemorrhage (colonic ulcerations), change in mental status (encephalitis), shortness of breath (pneumonitis), or a wide range of other symptoms. Recently developed antiviral agents, such as gancyclovir, have been effective in arresting some cases of CMV disease in immunosuppressed persons.

HUMAN PAPILLOMAVIRUS INFECTIONS

Human papillomaviruses (HPV) cause proliferative lesions of squamous epithelium, including common warts, flat warts, plantar warts, anogenital warts (condyloma acuminatum), and laryngeal papillomatosis. HPV infection also contributes to the development of squamous cell dysplasias and squamous cell carcinomas of the genital tract.

The agents are nonenveloped, double-stranded DNA viruses, which are members of the papovavirus group. Over 60 distinct types of HPV are identified, and different viral types are associated with different lesions. For instance, HPV types 1, 2, and 4 produce common warts and plantar warts. Types 6, 10, 11, and 40 through 45 cause anogenital warts. Types 16, 18, and 31 are associated with squamous cell dysplasias and squamous cell carcinoma of the female genital tract.

Human papillomavirus infection is widespread and is transmitted from person to person by direct contact. Most children develop common warts. The viruses that cause anogenital warts and genital flat warts are transmitted sexually, and these lesions are now the most prevalent sexually transmitted disease in the United States.

☐ **Pathogenesis:** HPV infection begins with viral inoculation into a stratified squamous epithelium, where the virus enters the nuclei of basal cells. Infection stimulates the replication of the squamous epithelium, producing the various HPV-associated proliferative lesions. Some HPV types produce raised (exophytic) lesions; other HPV types cause flat (endophytic) lesions, which are less readily visible to the naked eye.

The rapidly growing squamous epithelium replicates innumerable progeny viruses, which are shed in the degenerating superficial cells. Many HPV lesions resolve spontaneously. Depressed cell-mediated immunity is associated with the persistence and spread of HPV lesions. The mechanism by which HPV infections participate in malignant change is discussed in Chapter 5.

☐ **Pathology:** HPV infection produces squamous proliferative lesions, which vary in appearance and biological behavior. The individual lesions are discussed in detail in chapters dealing with specific organs. Most lesions show a thickening of the affected epithelium, owing to enhanced squamous cell proliferation. Some HPV-infected cells display a characteristic cytopathic effect, termed **koilocytosis**. Koilocytes are large squamous cells with shrunken nuclei enveloped in large cytoplasmic vacuoles.

☐ **Clinical Features:** **Common warts** (verruca vulgaris) are firm, circumscribed, raised, rough-surfaced lesions, which usually appear on surfaces subject to trauma, especially the hands. They are common in children but rare in the elderly. **Plantar warts** are similar squamous proliferative lesions on the soles of the feet but are compressed inward by standing and walking. Common plantar warts persist for months, even years, but eventually resolve spontaneously. They can be treated with various local destructive therapies, including salicylic acid application.

Anogenital warts (condyloma acuminatum) are soft, raised, fleshy lesions found on the penis, vulva, vaginal wall, cervix, or perianal region. They are usually treated by local application of caustics, cauterization, or surgical excision.

Flat warts in the genital area are now recognized to be more common than typical raised anogenital warts. Flat warts are difficult to detect on routine examination, but they can be made to stand out against uninvolved skin or mucosa by the application of acetic acid. When caused by certain HPV types, these flat warts can develop into malignant squamous cell proliferations.

The relationship between HPV, cervical intraepithelial neoplasia (CIN), and invasive squamous carcinoma is discussed in Chapter 18.

Bacterial Infections

Bacteria are the smallest living cells, ranging in size from 0.1 to 10 μm in greatest dimension. They have three basic structural components: nuclear body, cytosol, and envelope. The nuclear body consists of a single, coiled circular molecule of double-stranded DNA with associated RNA and proteins. The nuclear body is not separated from the cytoplasm by a nuclear membrane, a key feature that distinguishes bacteria, which are prokaryotes, from eukaryotes. The cytosol is densely packed with ribosomes, proteins, and carbohydrates and lacks the structured organelles of eukaryotic cells, such as mitochondria and Golgi apparatus. The nuclear body and cytosol together are surrounded by an envelope, which serves as a permeability barrier but is also actively involved in transport, protein synthesis, energy generation, DNA synthesis, and cell division.

Bacteria are classified according to the structural features of the bacterial envelope. The simplest bacterial envelope consists of only a cell membrane composed of a phospholipid-protein bilayer. For example, the mycoplasmas, which are discussed later, have such a simple envelope. Most bacteria, however, have a rigid cell wall, which surrounds the cell membrane. Two basic types of bacterial cell walls are identified by their tinctorial properties with the Gram stain.

- **Gram-positive bacteria** retain iodine-crystal violet complexes when decolorized and appear dark blue. Their cell walls contain teichoic acids and a thick peptidoglycan layer.
- **Gram-negative bacteria** lose the iodine-crystal violet stain when decolorized and appear red with a counterstain. The outer membrane of gram-negative bacteria contains a lipopolysaccharide component, known as endotoxin, which is a potent mediator of the shock that complicates infections with these organisms.

Both gram-positive and gram-negative cell walls may be surrounded by an additional layer of polysaccharide or protein gel. When this gel is condensed about the cell wall, it is called a capsule. The capsule aids in bacterial attachment and colonization and may prevent phagocytosis by leukocytes. Bacteria are often described as "encapsulated" or "unencapsulated" because of the importance of the capsule in some infections.

The cell wall confers rigidity to bacteria and allows them to be distinguished on the basis of shape and pattern of growth. Round or oval bacteria are called "cocci," and those that grow in typical pairs are called "diplococci." Elongate bacteria are known as **rods** or **bacilli**, and curved ones are termed **vibrios**. Some spiral-shaped bacteria are called **spirochetes**.

Most bacteria can be grown *in vitro* on artificial media devoid of living cells, and they are frequently described according to their growth requirements on these media. Bacteria that require high levels of oxygen are called **aerobic**; those that grow best in the absence of oxygen are termed **anaerobic**; those that thrive with limited amounts of oxygen are designated **microaerophilic**. Bacteria that grow well both in the presence and absence of oxygen are referred to as **facultative anaerobes**.

BACTERIAL EXOTOXINS: Many bacteria secrete toxins, known as exotoxins, which damage human cells either at the site of bacterial growth or at a distant site. These toxins are often named for the site or mechanism of their activity. Thus, those that act on the nervous system are called **neurotoxins** and those that affect intestinal cells are termed **enterotoxins**. Some toxins, such as diphtheria toxin or some of the *Clostridium perfringens* toxins, kill target cells and are referred to as **cytotoxins**. Other toxins, such as the diarrheogenic toxin of *Vibrio cholerae* or the potent neurotoxin of *Clostridium botulinum*, disturb the normal functions of their target cells without causing structural damage or death of these targets. Some bacteria, such as *V. cholerae*, produce a single toxin that causes profound, often rapidly fatal disease. Other organisms, such as *C. perfringens*, produce over 20 different toxins that damage the human body in diverse ways.

BACTERIAL ENDOTOXINS: As mentioned earlier, gram-negative bacteria contain in their outer membranes a structural element called lipopolysaccharide. Also known as endotoxin, lipopolysaccharide activates the complement, coagulation, fibrinolysis, and bradykinin systems. It also causes the release of primary mediators of inflammation, including tumor necrosis factor and interleukin-1, and various colony-stimulating factors. The actions of endotoxin produce shock, complement depletion, and disseminated intravascular coagulation.

Many bacteria damage tissues through the inflammatory or immune responses that they elicit. *Streptococcus pneumoniae* is an excellent example. It does not produce toxins but possesses a capsule that protects the organism from phagocytosis while activating the inflammatory response. Within the lung, the encapsulated organism causes an exudation of fluid and cells that fills the alveoli. This inflammatory response impairs breathing but does not, at least initially, limit the proliferation of the organism. Syphilis is another disease in which the pathology is largely due to the inflammatory and immune response to the organism. *Treponema pallidum*, the spirochete that causes syphilis, persists in the body for years and elicits inflammatory and immune responses that continuously damage host tissues.

We often think incorrectly of bacteria as simply causing pyogenic infections. Although it is true that many common bacterial infections (e.g., *Staphylococcus aureus* skin infections) are characterized by purulent exudates, the tissue response in bacterial disease is highly variable. In some bacterial diseases, such as cholera, botulism, and tetanus, there is no inflammatory response at the critical site of cellular injury. Other bacterial infections, including syphilis and Lyme disease, lead to a predominantly lymphocytic and plasma cellular response. Still others (e.g., brucellosis) are characterized by granuloma formation.

Many bacterial diseases are due to organisms that normally inhabit the human body. There is an extensive endogenous bacterial flora of the gastrointestinal tract, upper respiratory tract, skin, and vagina. Under normal circumstances, these microorganisms are commensal and cause no harm. However, when they gain access to usually sterile sites, or when host defenses are impaired, these bacteria can cause extensive destruction. *Staphylococcus aureus*, *Streptococcus pneumoniae*, and *Escherichia coli* are examples of the normal human flora that are also major human pathogens.

PYOGENIC GRAM-POSITIVE COCCI

Staphylococcus aureus

Staphylococcus aureus is a gram-positive coccus that typically grows in clusters and is one of the most common bacterial pathogens. The organism normally resides on the skin and is readily inoculated into deeper tissues, where it causes suppurative infections. **In fact, it is the most common cause of suppurative infections involving the skin, joints, and bones, and it is a leading cause of infective endocarditis.** *S. aureus* is commonly distinguished from other, less virulent staphylococci by the coagulase test. *S. aureus* is coagulase positive whereas the other staphylococci are coagulase negative.

S. aureus spreads by direct contact with colonized surfaces or persons. Most children and adults are intermittently colonized with *S. aureus*, carrying the organism on the skin, in the nares, or on clothing. The organism also survives on inanimate surfaces for long periods of time.

☐ **Pathogenesis:** *S. aureus* cannot invade through intact skin or mucous membranes, and infection usually begins with traumatic inoculation of the organism. Once inside the body, the organism is a virulent pathogen, secreting a number of enzymes and toxins that harm host tissues. *S. aureus* elaborates at least five different membrane-damaging toxins, which are capable of destroying erythrocytes, leukocytes, platelets, fibroblasts, and other human cells. It also possesses a surface protein, designated protein A, that binds the Fc receptor of IgG, thereby blocking complement activation by the classical pathway.

Many *S. aureus* infections begin as localized infections of the skin and skin appendages. Equipped with its armamentarium of destructive enzymes and toxins, the organism sometimes invades beyond the initial site, spreading by the bloodstream or lymphatic system to almost any location in the body. The bones, joints, and heart valves are the most common sites of metastatic *S. aureus* infections.

S. aureus also causes several distinct diseases, such as scalded skin syndrome, toxic shock syndrome, and staphylococcal food poisoning, by the elaboration of toxins that are carried to distant sites. Certain *S. aureus* strains produce toxins that cause skin exfoliation in infants. Other strains secrete a toxin that mediates toxic shock syndrome. There is evidence that this toxin acts by inducing the release of interleukin-1 by macrophages.

Many *S. aureus* strains elaborate enterotoxins that cause food poisoning when ingested. When food that supports rapid bacterial growth is contaminated with one of these strains and allowed to sit at room temperature, the organism proliferates and produces large amounts of enterotoxin. The enterotoxins survive heating at temperatures that kill the organisms and produce nausea and vomiting within a few hours of ingestion.

☐ **Pathology:** When *S. aureus* is inoculated into a previously sterile site, the infection usually produces suppuration and abscess formation. The abscesses range in size from microscopic foci to lesions several centimeters in diameter. They are filled with pus and bacteria, which can usually be identified on Gram stain.

☐ **Clinical Features:** The clinical manifestations of *S. aureus* disease vary enormously according to the sites and types of infection.

- **Furuncles (boils) and styes:** Boils are deep-seated infections with *S. aureus* in and around hair follicles, often in a nasal carrier. They occur on hairy surfaces, such as the neck, thighs, and buttocks of men and the axillae, pubic area, and eyelids of both sexes. The boil begins as a nodule at the base of a hair follicle, followed by a pimple that remains painful and red for a few days. A yellow apex forms, and the central core becomes necrotic and fluctuant. Rupture or incision of the boil relieves the pain. Several boils may occur in close proximity, and they often recur. Styes are boils that involve the sebaceous glands around the eyelid. **Paronychia** refers to staphylococcal infection of the nail bed, and **felons** are the same infections on the palmar side of the fingertips.
- **Carbuncles:** These lesions result from coalescing infections with *S. aureus* around hair follicles and produce draining sinuses (Fig. 9-11). Most carbuncles are on the neck, but they also occur on the limbs, trunk, face, and scalp. Necrosis spreads deeply into the skin, and some patients develop bacteremia, with a risk to life.
- **Scalded skin syndrome:** This disease affects infants and children younger than the age of 3 years who present with a sunburn-like rash, which begins on the face and spreads over the body. Bullae then begin to form, and even gentle rubbing causes the skin to desquamate. The disease begins to resolve in 1 to 2 weeks, as the epithelium regenerates. The desquamation is due to the systemic effects of a specific exotoxin, and the site of *S. aureus* proliferation is often occult.
- **Osteomyelitis:** Acute staphylococcal osteomyelitis, usually in the bones of the legs, most commonly afflicts boys between 3 and 10 years of age, most of whom have a history of infection or trauma. Many patients have had a previous bacteremia. Osteomyelitis may become chronic if not properly treate. Adults older than 50 years of age are more frequently afflicted with osteomyelitis of the vertebrae. It may follow staphylococcal infections of the skin or urinary tract, prostatic surgery, or pinning of a fracture.
- **Infections of burns or surgical wounds:** These sites often become infected with *S. aureus* from the patient's own nasal carriage or from medical personnel. Newborns and elderly, malnourished, diabetic, and obese persons all have increased susceptibility.

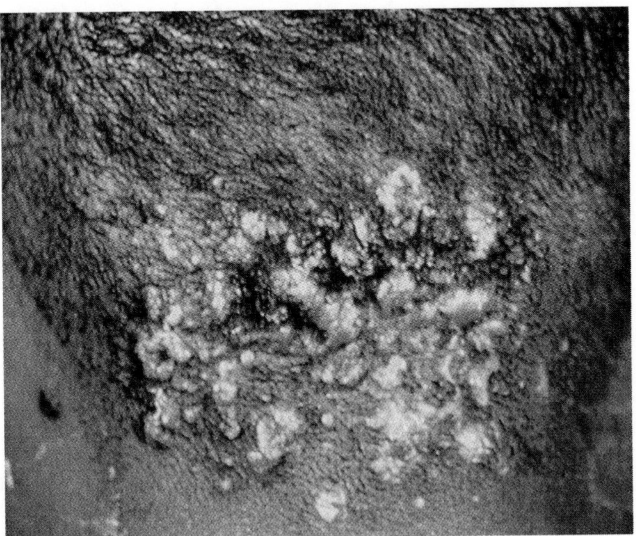

FIGURE *9-11*
Staphylococcal carbuncle. The posterior neck is indurated and shows multiple follicular abscesses discharging purulent material.

- **Respiratory tract infections:** Staphylococcal infections of the respiratory tract are most common in infants younger than 2 years of age, and especially in those younger than 2 months of age. The child often has an underlying skin infection and may be suffering from a viral respiratory disease. The infection is characterized by ulcers of the upper airway, scattered foci of pneumonia, pleural effusion, empyema, and pneumothorax. In adults, staphylococcal pneumonia may follow viral influenza, a disease that destroys the ciliated surface epithelium and leaves the bronchial surface vulnerable to secondary infections. Patients with chronic lung disease are also at increased risk for staphylococcal pneumonia.
- **Bacterial arthritis:** S. aureus is the causative organism in half of all cases of septic arthritis, mostly in patients 50 to 70 years old. Rheumatoid arthritis and corticosteroid therapy are common predisposing conditions.
- **Septicemia:** Septicemia with *S. aureus* afflicts patients with lowered resistance who are in the hospital for other diseases. Some have underlying staphylococcal infections (e.g., osteomyelitis, septic arthritis), some have had surgery, such as transurethral resection of the prostate, and some have infections from an indwelling intravenous catheter. Miliary abscesses and endocarditis are serious complications.
- **Bacterial endocarditis:** Bacterial endocarditis is a common complication of *S. aureus* septicemia. It may develop spontaneously on normal valves, valves damaged by rheumatic fever, or prosthetic valves. Intravenous drug abuse is a predisposing factor to staphylococcal endocarditis.
- **Toxic shock syndrome:** This disorder most commonly afflicts menstruating women, who present with high fever, nausea, vomiting, diarrhea, and myalgias. Subsequently, they develop shock, and within several days a sunburn-like rash. The disease has been associated with the use of tampons, particularly hyperabsorbent tampons, which provide a site for *S. aureus* replication and toxin elaboration. Toxic shock syndrome occurs rarely in children and men and is then usually associated with an occult *S. aureus* infection.
- **Staphylococcal food poisoning:** Staphylococcal food poisoning typically begins less than 6 hours after a meal. Nausea and vomiting begin abruptly and usually resolve within 12 hours.

Coagulase-Negative Staphylococci

Coagulase-negative staphylococci are the major cause of infections associated with the introduction of medical devices, including intravenous catheters, prosthetic heart valves, heart pacemakers, orthopedic prostheses, cerebrospinal fluid shunts, and peritoneal catheters.

Disease due to coagulase-negative staphylococci usually derives from the normal bacterial flora. Of the over 20 known species of coagulase-negative staphylococci, 10 are normal residents of human skin and mucosal surfaces. ***Staphylococcus epidermidis* is the most frequent cause of infections associated with medical devices.** Another species, *Staphylococcus saprophyticus*, causes 10% to 20% of acute urinary tract infections in young women.

☐ **Pathogenesis:** Because of their ubiquitous presence on human surfaces, coagulase-negative staphylococci readily contaminate foreign bodies. The organisms slowly proliferate on implanted devices, inducing an inflammatory response that damages adjacent tissue. If the bacteria are present on an intravascular surface, such as the tip of an intravascular catheter, they can spread through the bloodstream to cause metastatic infections. Coagulase-negative staphylococci lack the enzymes and toxins that permit *S. aureus* to cause extensive local tissue destruction. Some strains of coagulase-negative staphylococci produce a polysaccharide gel, called "slime," which facilitates the growth of the organisms on implanted medical devices. The slime enhances adherence of the bacteria to foreign objects and protects them from host antimicrobial defenses.

☐ **Pathology:** Medical devices infected with coagulase-negative staphylococci are usually thinly coated with tan, fibrinous material. In contrast to infections caused by *S. aureus*, coagulase-negative staphylococcal infections usually do not produce extensive local tissue necrosis or large quantities of pus. However, tissue adjacent to infected devices is acutely inflamed. Microscopic examination of infected devices shows clusters of gram-positive bacteria embedded in fibrin and cellular debris, with an associated acute inflammatory infiltrate.

☐ **Clinical Features:** Coagulase-negative staphylococcal infections usually have subtle clinical presentations. Often the only symptom of infection is persistent low-grade fever. Infection of orthopedic prostheses frequently causes progressive loosening and dysfunction of the devices. In most persons, these infections are indolent, but in neutropenic or otherwise severely compromised persons, the infections can be fatal. Treatment usually requires replacement of any infected foreign object and appropriate antibiotic therapy.

Streptococcus pyogenes Infection

Streptococcus pyogenes, also known as group A Streptococcus, is one of the most frequent bacterial pathogens of humans, causing many diseases of diverse organ systems, which range from acute self-limited pharyngitis to major illnesses such as rheumatic fever (Fig. 9-12). *S. pyogenes* is a gram-positive coccus, which is frequently part of the endogenous flora that colonizes the skin and oropharynx.

The diseases caused by *S. pyogenes* may be considered in two categories: suppurative and nonsuppurative. Suppurative diseases occur at sites where the bacteria invade and cause tissue necrosis, usually inducing an acute inflammatory response. Suppurative *S. pyogenes* infections include pharyngitis, impetigo, cellulitis, myositis, pneumonia, and puerperal sepsis. By contrast, nonsuppurative diseases occur at sites remote from the site of bacterial in-

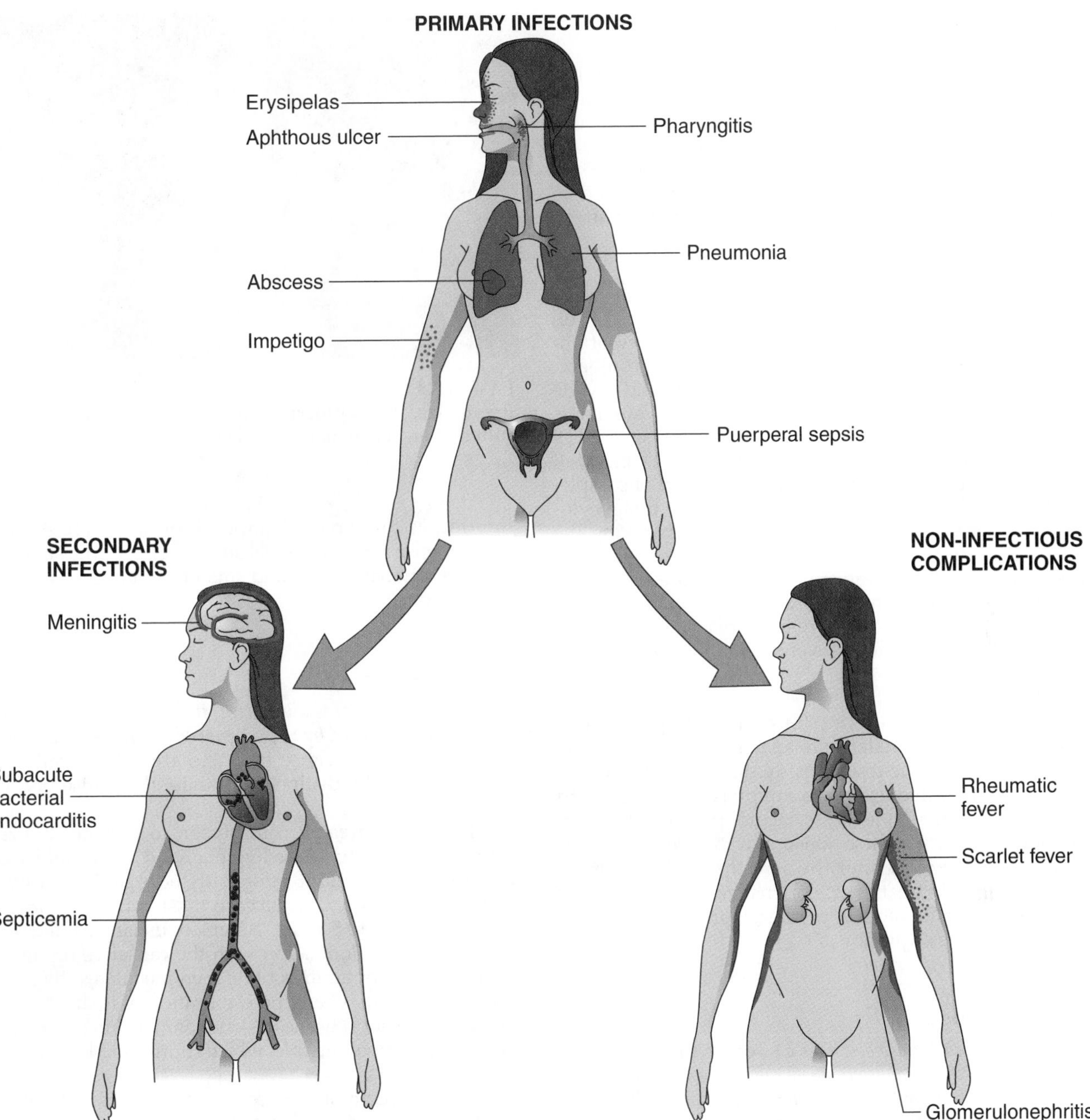

FIGURE *9-12*
Streptococcal diseases.

vasion. *S. pyogenes* causes two major nonsuppurative complications: rheumatic fever and acute poststreptococcal glomerulonephritis. These (1) involve organ systems far from the sites of streptococcal invasion, (2) usually occur some time after the acute infection, and (3) are probably caused by an immunological response. Rheumatic fever is discussed in Chapter 11 and poststreptococcal glomerulonephritis is described in Chapter 16.

STREPTOCOCCAL EXOTOXINS: *S. pyogenes* elaborates several exotoxins, including erythrogenic toxins and cytolytic toxins (streptolysins S and O). Erythrogenic toxins are responsible for the rash of scarlet fever. Most, but not all, strains of *S. pyogenes* produce both streptolysin S and streptolysin O. These toxins are not only hemolysins but also are cytolytic. Hemolysis on blood agar plates is largely caused by streptolysin S, which also lyses bacterial protoplasts (L-forms) and probably destroys neutrophils after they ingest *S. pyogenes*. Because streptolysin S is not immunogenic, its effects may be unimpeded even after repeated infections. By contrast, streptolysin O induces a persistently high antibody titer, an effect that provides a useful marker for the diagnosis of *S. pyogenes* infections and their nonsuppurative complications.

Streptococcal Pharyngitis ("Strep Throat")

S. pyogenes is the common bacterial cause of pharyngitis. The organism spreads from person to person by direct contact with oral or respiratory secretions, and spread is enhanced by crowding. Persons remain infected with the organism for weeks after symptomatic resolution of the pharyngitis and thus serve as a reservoir for infection. "Strep throat" occurs worldwide, predominantly affecting children and adolescents.

☐ **Pathogenesis and Pathology:** *S. pyogenes* attaches to epithelial cells by binding to fibronectin on their surface. The bacterium produces a battery of enzymes, including hemolysins, DNAase, hyaluronidase, and streptokinase, which allow it to damage and invade human tissues. *S. pyogenes* also has cell wall components that protect it from the inflammatory response. One of these, designated M protein, protrudes from the cell wall of virulent strains and prevents the deposition of complement, thereby protecting the bacterium from phagocytosis. Another surface protein destroys C5a, blocking the opsonizing effect of complement and inhibiting phagocytosis. The invading organism elicits an acute inflammatory response, often producing an exudate of neutrophils in the tonsillar fossae. Reactive hyperplasia of the tonsils and the cervical lymph nodes are common responses.

☐ **Clinical Features:** "Strep throat" presents as sore throat, fever, malaise, headache, and an elevated leukocyte count. The disease is self-limited, usually lasting 3 to 5 days. In a few cases, streptococcal pharyngitis leads to rheumatic fever or acute poststreptococcal glomerulonephritis. These nonsuppurative complications usually occur weeks after the sore throat itself has resolved. Penicillin treatment shortens the clinical course of "strep throat" and, more importantly, prevents the major nonsuppurative sequelae.

Scarlet Fever

Scarlet fever (scarlatina) describes a punctate red rash that appears on the skin and mucous membranes in some suppurative S. pyogenes infections, most commonly pharyngitis. The rash usually begins on the chest and spreads to the extremities. The tongue may develop a yellow-white coating, which sheds to reveal a "beefy-red" surface. Scarlet fever is caused by an erythrogenic toxin elaborated by certain streptococcal strains.

Erysipelas

Erysipelas is an erythematous swelling of the skin caused chiefly by S. pyogenes (Fig. 9-13). It is the classic cutaneous streptococcal infection, usually beginning on the face and spreading rapidly. Erysipelas is common in warm climates but is not often seen before the age of 20 years. The map-like area of brawny erythema has a sharp, well demarcated, serpiginous border. A diffuse, edematous, acute inflammatory reaction in the epidermis and dermis extends into the subcutaneous tissues. The inflammatory infiltrate is principally composed of neutrophils and is most intense around vessels and adnexae of the skin. Cutaneous microabscesses and small foci of necrosis are not uncommon.

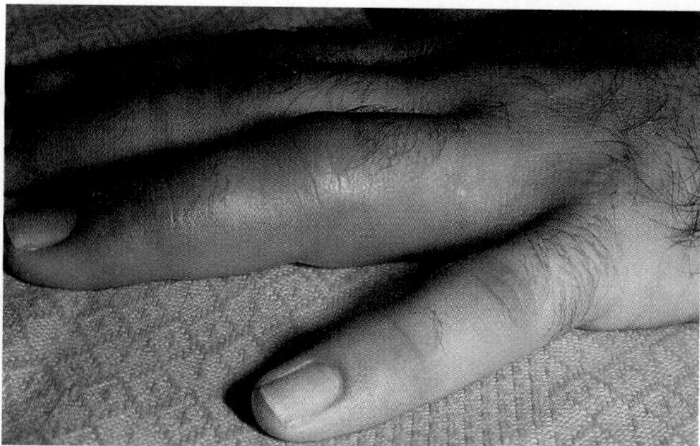

FIGURE *9-13*
Erysipelas. A streptoccocal infection of the skin has resulted in an erythematous and swollen finger.

Impetigo

Impetigo (pyoderma) is a localized, intraepidermal infection of the skin that is caused by S. pyogenes or S. aureus. The strains of *S. pyogenes* that cause impetigo are antigenically and epidemiologically distinct from those that cause pharyngitis.

Impetigo spreads from person to person by direct contact. Crowding, poor hygiene, and warm moist climates favor skin colonization with the organisms responsible for impetigo. The disease most commonly affects children aged 2 to 5 years. A person, usually a child, first develops skin colonization with the causative organism. Minor trauma or an insect bite then inoculates the bacteria into the skin, where the elaboration of toxins and enzymes allows local tissue destruction. The infection forms an intraepidermal pustule, which ruptures to leak a purulent exudate.

Lesions begin on exposed body surfaces as localized erythematous papules (Fig. 9-14). These become pustules, which erode within a few days to form a thick honey-colored crust. The skin lesions are rarely accompanied by systemic symptoms. Impetigo sometimes leads to poststreptococcal glomerulonephritis but not to rheumatic fever.

Streptococcal Cellulitis

S. pyogenes is one of the most common causes of cellulitis, an acute spreading infection of the loose connective tissue of the deeper layers of the dermis. This suppurative infection results from traumatic inoculation of microorganisms into the skin and frequently occurs on the extremities in the context of impaired lymphatic drainage. Cellulitis usually begins at sites of unnoticed injury and appears as spreading areas of redness, warmth, and swelling.

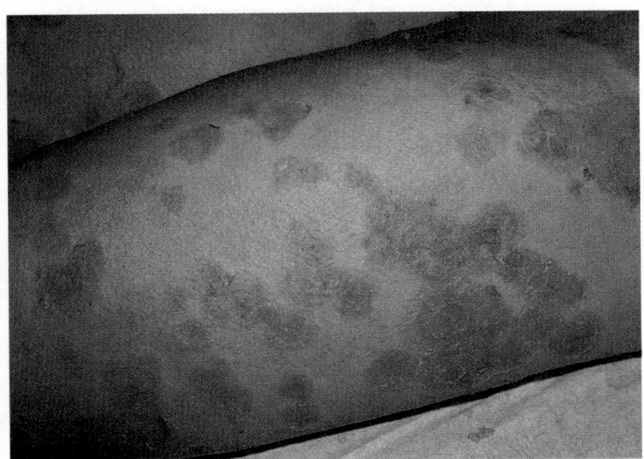

FIGURE *9-14*
Streptococcal impetigo. The lower extremities exhibit numerous erythematous papules, with central ulceration and the formation of crusts.

Puerperal Sepsis

Puerperal sepsis refers to pospartum infection of the uterine cavity by S. pyogenes. The disease was formerly common but is now rare in developed countries. The infection originates from the contaminated hands of attendants at delivery, an association first established by the historic observations of Semmelweiss.

Streptococcus pneumoniae Infection

Streptococcus pneumoniae, often simply called pneumococcus, causes pyogenic infections, primarily involving the lungs (pneumonia), middle ear (otitis media), sinuses (sinusitis), and meninges (meningitis). **It is one of the most common bacterial pathogens of humans, and by age 5, most children in the world have suffered at least one episode of pneumococcal disease (usually otitis media).** After *Hemophilus influenzae*, pneumococcus is the second leading cause of bacterial meningitis.

S. pneumoniae is an aerobic, encapsulated, gram-positive diplococcus. The capsule is often not visible on tissue stains, and individual cocci are bullet or lancet shaped. There are over 80 antigenically distinct serotypes of pneumococcus; antibody to one serotype does not protect against infection with another. Pneumococcal disease arises from organisms normally resident in the oropharynx. *S. pneumoniae* is a commensal organism in the oropharynx, and virtually all persons are colonized at some time.

□ **Pathogenesis and Pathology:** Pneumococcal disease begins when the organism gains access to sterile sites, usually those in proximity to its normal residence in the oropharynx. Pneumococcal sinusitis and otitis media are usually preceded by a viral illness, such as the common cold, which injures the protective ciliated epithelium and fills the affected air spaces with fluid. Pneumococci then thrive in the nutrient-rich tissue fluid. Infection of the sinuses or middle ear can spread to the adjacent meninges.

Pneumococcal pneumonia arises in a similar fashion. The lower respiratory tract is protected by the mucociliary blanket and cough response, which normally expel organisms that are inhaled into the lower airway. Insults that interfere with the function of these defenses, including influenza, other viral respiratory illness, smoking, and alcoholism, allow access to *S. pneumoniae*. Once in the alveoli, the organisms proliferate and elicit an acute inflammatory response.

The polysaccharide capsule is the major determinant of virulence of *S. pneumoniae*. The capsule prevents activation of the alternate complement pathway, thereby blocking the production of the opsonin C3b. Thus, before a specific IgG antibody is produced, the organism can proliferate and spread unimpeded by phagocytes.

In the lungs, *S. pneumoniae* spreads rapidly to involve an entire lobe or several lobes (lobar pneumonia). Alveoli fill with proteinaceous fluid, neutrophils, and bacteria. When the pneumonia resolves, there is usually no residual damage to the pulmonary parenchyma.

□ **Clinical Features:** **Pneumococcal pneumonia** presents with the abrupt onset of high fever, shaking chills, and cough, often producing bloody or rust-colored sputum. In younger persons who acquire the disease outside the hospital, a chest radiograph shows a lobar pattern of consolidation. Hospital-acquired infections, particularly in the elderly, more often appear as diffuse bronchopneumonia. Pneumococcus is so frequently a cause of pneumonia that empirical antibiotic therapy always includes antipneumococcal coverage. In young adults treated for pneumococcal pneumonia, death is today uncommon. However, in hospitalized patients older than 70 years of age, the death rate exceeds 50%. Antipneumococcal vaccines are effective in the prophylaxis of pneumonia in the elderly.

Pneumococcal otitis media primarily affects young children and presents as fever, irritability, and pain. The symptoms and the appearance of the ear drums are not specific for a particular etiology, and antibiotic therapy is empirically directed to cover all common causes. Acute pneumococcal sinusitis presents as tenderness over the affected sinus, headache, and fever.

Acute pneumococcal meningitis affects all age groups and presents as fever, headache, and stiff neck. Meningitis progresses rapidly, and patients are often desperately ill within 12 to 24 hours, with changes in consciousness rapidly progressing to coma. Antibiotic therapy is often begun before a specific etiology for the meningitis has been defined. The mortality of pneumococcal meningitis is highest in infants and the aged.

Group B *Streptococcus* Infection

Group B Streptococcus (S. agalactiae) is the leading cause of neonatal pneumonia, meningitis, and sepsis. The organism is also an infrequent cause of pyogenic infections in adults. Group B *Streptococcus* is a gram-positive bacterium that grows in short chains.

Several thousand neonatal infections with group B streptococci occur in the United States each year, and about 30% of infected infants die. Group B *Streptococcus* is part of the normal vaginal flora and is found in 30% of women. Most newborns born to colonized women acquire the organism as they pass through the birth canal, but less than 1% of these infants develop group B streptococcal infections.

☐ **Pathogenesis and Pathology:** Particular risk factors have been associated with the development of neonatal group B streptococcal infections. These include delivery before 37 weeks' gestation and low levels of maternally derived IgG antibodies specifically directed against the organism. Newborns have little functional reserve for granulocyte production, and once established, the bacterial infection rapidly overwhelms the body's defense capacity.

Group B streptococcal infection may be limited to the lungs or central nervous system or may be widely disseminated. Histopathologically, the involved tissues show a pyogenic response, often with overwhelming numbers of gram-positive cocci.

☐ **Clinical Features:** Symptoms of severe infection in the newborn are not specific, and group B streptococcal infection typically presents as lethargy, poor feeding, and respiratory distress. In the first few days of life, fever may not be present, but if infection occurs several weeks after birth, fever is usually prominent.

BACTERIAL INFECTIONS OF CHILDHOOD

Diphtheria

Diphtheria is a necrotizing upper respiratory tract infection sometimes associated with cardiac and neurological disturbances. Corynebacterium diphtheriae is an aerobic, pleomorphic, gram-positive rod. The organism uncommonly produces cutaneous disease, although this rarely results in systemic complications. Diphtheria is preventable by vaccination with inactivated *C. diphtheriae* toxin (toxoid).

☐ **Epidemiology:** Humans are the only significant reservoir for *C. diphtheriae*, and most persons are asymptomatic carriers. The organism spreads from person to person in respiratory droplets or oral secretions. Infection of the pharynx is more common in children, whereas cutaneous infections are more frequent in adults living in the tropics.

At one time, diphtheria was a leading cause of death in children 2 to 15 years of age. In developed countries, immunization programs have largely eliminated the disease. However, diphtheria persists as a major health problem in less-developed countries.

☐ **Pathogenesis:** Diphtheria begins with the entry of *C. diphtheriae* into the pharynx, where the organisms proliferate, commonly on the tonsils. The pathogenicity of the strain depends on the presence of a toxin-producing, lysogenic bacteriophage and a critical concentration of iron in the environment. Diphtheria toxin is absorbed systemically and acts on tissues throughout the body, with the heart, nerves, and kidneys being most susceptible to damage. Diphtheria toxin is composed of two subunits, designated A and B. The B subunit binds to glycolipid receptors on target cells, and the A subunit acts within the cytoplasm on elongation factor 2 to interrupt protein synthesis. The toxin is one of the most potent known, and only one molecule is sufficient to kill the cell.

☐ **Pathology:** The characteristic lesions of diphtheria are the thick, gray, leathery membranes that line the affected respiratory passages (Gk. *diphtheria*, "leather"). These membranes are composed of sloughed epithelium, necrotic debris, neutrophils, fibrin, and bacteria. The epithelial surface beneath the membranes is denuded, and the submucosa is acutely inflamed and hemorrhagic. Sometimes the membrane is so extensive that it forms a cast of the entire upper airway, and aspiration of the membrane can be fatal. The inflammatory process often produces swelling in the surrounding soft tissues, which can be sufficiently severe as to cause respiratory compromise. When the heart is affected, the myocardium displays fat droplets in the myocytes and focal necrosis (Fig. 9-15). In the case of neural involvement, the affected peripheral nerves exhibit demyelination.

☐ **Clinical Features:** Diphtheria begins with fever, sore throat, and malaise. The dirty gray membrane usually develops first on the tonsils and may spread throughout the posterior oropharynx. The membrane is firmly adherent, and an attempt to strip it from the underlying mucosa produces bleeding. Cardiac and neurological symptoms develop in a minority of infected persons, usually those with the most severe local disease. Cardiac involvement presents as conduction abnormalities, dysrhythmias, or congestive heart failure. Neurological disease is evidenced by motor weakness in the affected cranial and peripheral nerves.

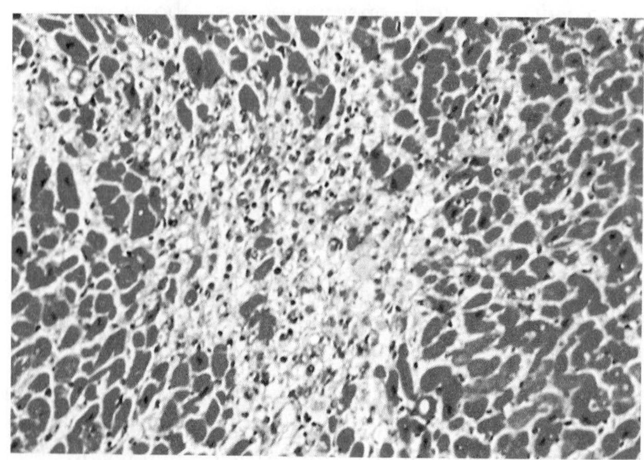

FIGURE *9-15*
Diphtheric myocarditis. Focal degeneration of cardiac myocytes is evident.

Cutaneous diphtheria, which results from inoculation of the organism into a break in the skin, presents as a pustule or ulcer. Cutaneous disease is only rarely associated with cardiac or neurological complications. Diphtheria is treated by prompt administration of antitoxin and antibiotics.

Pertussis

Pertussis, commonly called whooping cough, is a prolonged upper respiratory tract infection, characterized by debilitating coughing paroxysms. The paroxysm is followed by a long, high-pitched inspiration, the "whoop," which gives the disease its name. The causative organism is *Bordetella pertussis*, a small, gram-negative coccobacillus, similar in appearance to *Hemophilus* species.

☐ **Epidemiology:** *B. pertussis* is highly contagious and spreads from person to person, primarily by infected respiratory aerosols. Humans are the only reservoir of infection. In susceptible populations, pertussis is primarily a disease of children younger than the age of 5 years, and many cases occur in children younger than 1 year of age. Vaccination protects against *B. pertussis*. Because the disease frequently affects infants, vaccination must begin as early as possible, usually at the age of 6 to 8 weeks. In the United States, where vaccination is not rigorously pursued among the whole population, there are thousands of cases of pertussis per year, but death is uncommon. Worldwide, there are estimated to be 50 million cases of pertussis each year, resulting in almost 1 million deaths, particularly in infants.

☐ **Pathogenesis and Pathology:** *B. pertussis* initiates infection by attaching to the cilia of respiratory epithelial cells. The organism then reproduces and elaborates a cytotoxin, which kills the ciliated cells but spares the nonciliated ones. The progressive destruction of ciliated respiratory epithelium and the ensuing inflammatory response cause the local respiratory symptoms. Several other toxins are produced. "Pertussis toxin" is an agent that causes the pronounced lymphocytosis often associated with whooping cough. Another toxin inhibits adenylyl cyclase, an effect that blocks bacterial phagocytosis.

B. pertussis causes an extensive tracheobronchitis, with necrosis of the ciliated respiratory epithelium and an acute inflammatory response. With the loss of the protective mucociliary blanket, there is an increased risk of pneumonia from aspirated oral bacteria. Coughing paroxysms and vomiting make aspiration all the more likely, and secondary bacterial pneumonias are a common cause of death in pertussis.

☐ **Clinical Features:** Whooping cough is a prolonged upper respiratory tract illness, lasting 4 to 5 weeks and passing through three stages:

1. **Catarrhal stage:** The first stage of whooping cough resembles a common viral upper respiratory tract illness, with low-grade fever, runny nose, conjunctivitis, and cough.
2. **Paroxysmal stage:** One week into the illness, the cough worsens and becomes paroxysmal, with 5 to 15 consecutive coughs, often followed by an inspiratory whoop. The paroxysms are exhausting and often accompanied by vomiting. During this phase of the illness, the patient is afebrile but develops a marked lymphocytosis, with the total leukocyte count often exceeding 40,000 cells/μL. The paroxysms persist for 2 to 3 weeks.
3. **Convalescent phase:** As the paroxysms gradually subside, the patient enters the convalescent phase of the illness, which usually lasts for several weeks.

Hemophilus influenzae Infection

Hemophilus influenzae causes pyogenic infections, primarily in young children, involving the middle ear, sinuses, facial skin, epiglottis, meninges, lungs, and joints. The organism is a major pediatric bacterial pathogen and the leading cause of bacterial meningitis worldwide. *H. influenzae* is an aerobic, pleomorphic gram-negative coccobacillus, which exists in both encapsulated and nonencapsulated strains. Nonencapsulated strains usually produce localized infections, including otitis media, acute sinusitis, conjunctivitis, and pneumonia. The unencapsulated strain, designated *H. influenzae* type b, is more virulent and causes over 95% of the invasive bacteremic infections, including meningitis, facial cellulitis, epiglottitis, and septic arthritis.

☐ **Epidemiology:** *H. influenzae* is a strict parasite of humans and spreads from person to person, primarily in respiratory droplets and secretions. The organism is normally resident in the human nasopharynx, colonizing 20% to 50% of healthy adults. Most colonizing strains are nonencapsulated, but 3% to 5% are *H. influenzae* type b.

Most severe *H. influenzae* type b infections occur in children younger than the age of 6 years. The incidence of serious disease peaks at 6 to 18 months of age, corresponding to the period between the loss of maternally acquired immunity and the acquisition of native immunity. *H. influenzae* type b causes over 20,000 severe infections in the United States annually, resulting in over 1,000 deaths. It is estimated that 15,000 of these infections and over 700 deaths could be prevented by inoculating infants with available *H. influenzae* type b vaccine.

☐ **Pathogenesis:** Unencapsulated *H. influenzae* strains and the encapsulated *H. influenzae* type b differ significantly in their pathogenicity. Unencapsulated strains produce disease by spreading locally from their normal sites of residence to adjoining sterile locations, such as the sinuses or middle ear. This is facilitated by injury to the normal defense mechanisms, as occurs with a viral upper respiratory tract illness. Within these previously sterile sites, unencapsulated organisms proliferate and elicit an acute inflammatory response, which injures the local tissue but eventually contains the infection. Under most circumstances, the unencapsulated strains do not invade to produce a bacteremia.

The situation is different for *H. influenzae* type b, which is capable of tissue invasion. The capsular polysaccharide of type b organisms allows them to evade phagocytosis, and bacteremic infections are common. Epiglottitis, facial cellulitis, septic arthritis, and meningitis result from invasive bacteremic infections. *H. influenzae* type b also elaborates an IgA protease, which facilitates local survival of the organism in the respiratory tract.

□ **Pathology:** *H. influenzae* elicits a pronounced acute inflammatory response, and specific pathological features vary according to the sites affected. *H. influenzae* meningitis resembles other acute bacterial meningitides, with a predominantly neutrophilic infiltrate in the leptomeninges, sometimes extending into the subarachnoid space.

H. influenzae pneumonia usually complicates chronic lung disease, and in half the patients it follows a viral infection of the respiratory tract. The alveoli are filled with neutrophils, macrophages containing bacilli, and fibrin. The bronchiolar epithelium is necrotic and infiltrated by macrophages.

Epiglottitis consists of swelling and acute inflammation of the epiglottis, aryepiglottic folds, and pyriform sinuses, which sometimes completely obstruct the upper airway. In facial cellulitis, the site of infection and inflammation is the dermis, usually of the cheek or periorbital region.

□ **Clinical Features:** Most bacteremic *H. influenzae* infections afflict young children. ***H. influenzae* is the most common cause of meningitis in children younger than the age of 2 years.** The onset is insidious and may follow an otherwise unremarkable upper respiratory tract infection or otitis media.

Bronchopneumonia or lobar pneumonia produced by *H. influenzae* is characterized by fever, cough, purulent sputum, and dyspnea.

Epiglottitis resulting from *H. influenzae* infection affects primarily children aged 2 to 7 years but also occurs in adults. The onset is usually abrupt, with sore throat, fever, dysphagia, and pooling of oral secretions. Death may occur from obstruction of the upper respiratory tract.

Septic arthritis caused by *H. influenzae* is secondary to bacteremic seeding of large weight-bearing joints. Symptoms include fever, heat, erythema, swelling, and pain on movement. The diagnosis is made by culturing the organism from the joint fluid.

Facial cellulitis or periorbital cellulitis is another severe bacteremic infection affecting primarily young children. Patients present with fever, profound malaise, and a raised, hot, red-blue discolored area of the face, usually involving the cheek or an area about the eye. There is often concomitant meningitis or septic arthritis.

Neisseria meningitidis

Neisseria meningitidis, commonly termed meningococcus, causes pyogenic meningitis and disseminated blood-borne infections, often accompanied by shock and profound disturbances in coagulation (Fig. 9-16). The organism is aerobic and appears as paired, bean-shaped, gram-negative cocci. There are eight major serogroups, three of which (A, B, C) cause most infections.

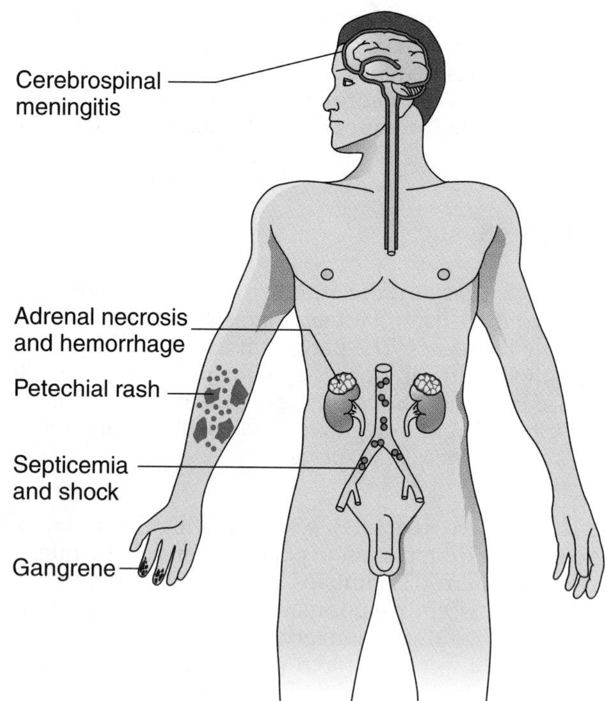

FIGURE *9-16*
Meningococcemia. Meningococcal infections have a variety of clinical manifestations including meningitis, septicemia, shock, and associated complications.

□ **Epidemiology:** Meningococci spread from person to person, primarily by respiratory droplets; close contact facilitates dissemination. At any given time, a small proportion (5% to 15%) of the population carries the organism in the nasopharynx as a commensal. Carriers develop antibodies to the particular colonizing strain of *N. meningitidis* and are immune to meningococcal disease caused by that strain.

Meningococcal diseases appear as sporadic cases, clusters of cases, and epidemics. Most infections in industrialized countries are sporadic and afflict children younger than the age of 5 years. In these countries, epidemic disease occurs most frequently in crowded quarters, such as among military recruits in barracks. There are over 6000 cases of meningococcal meningitis each year in the United States, resulting in over 600 deaths. Fatalities from meningococcal disease are more common in less developed countries. In a belt across the northern savanna of sub-Saharan Africa, from Gambia to Ethiopia, major epidemics occur, principally in children 5 to 14 years of age.

□ **Pathogenesis:** On colonizing the upper respiratory tract, *N. meningitidis* attaches to nonciliated respiratory epithelium by means of its pili. Most exposed persons then develop protective bactericidal antibodies over the following weeks, and some become carriers. If the organism spreads to the bloodstream before the development of protective immunity, it can proliferate rapidly in unprotected human tissue, resulting in fulminant meningococcal disease.

Many of the systemic effects of meningococcal disease are due to the endotoxin of the outer membrane lipopolysaccharide of the bacterium. Endotoxin promotes a conspicuous increase in the production of tumor necrosis factor and the simultaneous activation of the complement cascade, coagulation cascade, Hageman factor, and prekallikrein. Disseminated intravascular coagulation, fibrinolysis, and shock follow.

☐ **Pathology:** Meningococcal disease can be confined to the central nervous system or may be disseminated throughout the body in the form of septicemia. In the case of menigococcal meningitis, the leptomeninges and subarachnoid space are infiltrated with neutrophils, and the underlying brain parenchyma is swollen and congested. Meningococcal septicemia is characterized by diffuse damage to the endothelium of small blood vessels, thereby resulting in widespread petechiae and purpura in the skin and viscera.

Affected blood vessels initially show dilatation, with hemorrhage into adjacent perivascular tissue. This is soon followed by an intense neutrophilic infiltrate of the vessel walls. Small vessels throughout the body are also occluded by fibrin clots. Rarely (3% to 4% of all cases), the vasculitis and thrombosis produce hemorrhagic necrosis of both adrenals, a phenomenon known as the **Waterhouse-Friderichsen syndrome.**

Some patients who survive the early phase of meningococcemia develop late allergic complications, such as polyarthritis, cutaneous vasculitis, and pericarditis. Occasionally, severe vasculitis is associated with extensive cutaneous ulceration and sometimes even gangrene of the distal extremities.

☐ **Clinical Features:** Meningococcal diseases, both meningitis and sepsis, most often present as fulminant illnesses. Meningitis begins with the rapid onset of fever, stiff neck, and headache. In the case of meningococcal sepsis, fever, shock, and mucocutaneous hemorrhages appear abruptly. Patients can progress to shock in minutes, and treatment requires rapid support of blood pressure and antibiotics. In the preantibiotic era, meningococcal disease was almost invariably fatal, but modern treatment has reduced the fatality rate to less than 15%.

SEXUALLY TRANSMITTED BACTERIAL DISEASES

Gonorrhea

Neisseria gonorrhoeae, also termed gonococcus, causes gonorrhea, an acute suppurative infection of the genital tract, which is reflected in urethritis in men and endocervicitis in women. It is one of the oldest and still one of the most common sexually transmitted diseases. *N. gonorrhoeae* is an aerobic, bean-shaped, gram-negative diplococcus, which is morphologically indistinguishable from *N. meningitidis.*

Male homosexuals are at risk for gonococcal pharyngitis and proctitis. In women, infection often ascends the genital tract, producing endometritis, salpingitis, and pelvic inflammatory disease. Ascending spread in men is less common, but when it does occur epididymitis results. Rarely, gonococcal infection becomes bacteremic, in which circumstance septic arthritis and skin lesions develop.

Neonatal infections derived from the birth canal of a mother with gonorrhea usually present as conjunctivitis, although disseminated infections are occasionally encountered. Neonatal gonococcal conjunctivitis has been largely eliminated in developed countries by the routine instillation of antibiotics into the conjunctiva at birth, but it is still a major cause of blindness in much of Africa and Asia.

☐ **Epidemiology:** Infection is spread directly from person to person, and except for perinatal transmission, spread is almost always by sexual intercourse. Infected persons who are asymptomatic serve as a significant reservoir of infection. Although effective antibiotic therapy has been available for almost 50 years, the disease remains rampant throughout the world. Over 2 million cases of gonorrhea occur in the United States annually.

☐ **Pathogenesis:** Gonorrhea begins as an infection of the mucous membranes of the urogenital tract (Fig. 9-17). The bacteria attach to the surface cells, after which they invade superficially and provoke acute inflammation. Gonococcus lacks a true polysaccharide capsule, but hairlike extensions, termed **pili**, project from the cell wall. The pili contain a protease that digests IgA on the mucous membrane, thereby facilitating the attachment of the bacterium to the columnar and transitional epithelium of the urogenital tract.

☐ **Pathology:** Gonorrhea is a suppurative infection, characterized by a vigorous acute inflammatory response, producing copious pus and often forming submucosal abscesses. Stained smears of pus reveal numerous neutrophils, often containing phagocytosed bacteria. If untreated, the inflammatory response becomes chronic, with macrophages and lymphocytes predominant.

☐ **Clinical Features:** After an incubation period of 3 to 5 days, men exposed to *N. gonorrhoeae* present with a purulent urethral discharge (Fig. 9-18) and dysuria. With prompt antibiotic treatment, the infection is arrested and the organism remains confined to the mucosa of the anterior urethra. However, if treatment is not instituted promptly, urethral stricture is a common complication. The organisms may also extend to the prostate, epididymis, and accessory glands, where they cause epididymitis and orchitis, and may result in infertility.

In about one half of infected women, gonorrhea remains asymptomatic. The other infected women initially manifest endocervicitis, with a vaginal discharge or bleeding. Urethritis presents as dysuria, rather than as a urethral discharge. The infection often extends to the fal-

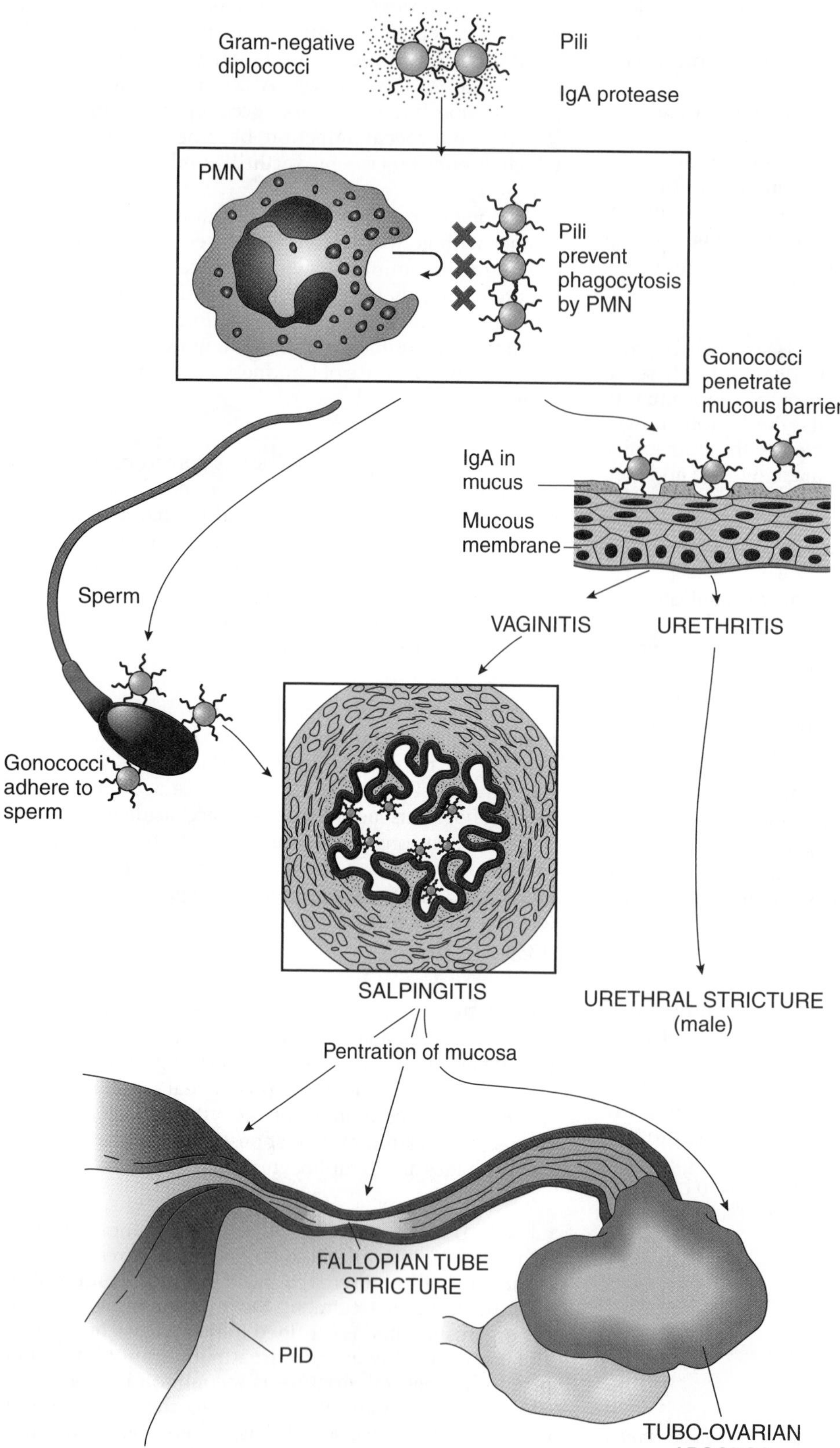

FIGURE *9-17*
Pathogenesis of gonococcal infections. *Neisseria gonorrhoea* is a gram-negative diplococcus whose surface pili form a barrier against phagocytosis by neutrophils. The pili contain an IgA protease that digests IgA on the luminal surface of the mucous membranes of the urethra, endocervix, and fallopian tube, thereby facilitating attachment of gonococci. Gonococci cause endocervicitis, vaginitis, and salpingitis. In men, gonococci attached to the mucous membrane of the urethra cause urethritis and, sometimes, urethral stricture. Gonococci may also attach to sperm heads and be carried into the fallopian tube. Penetration of the mucous membrane by gonococci leads to stricture of the fallopian tube, pelvic inflammatory disease (PID), or tubo-ovarian abscess.

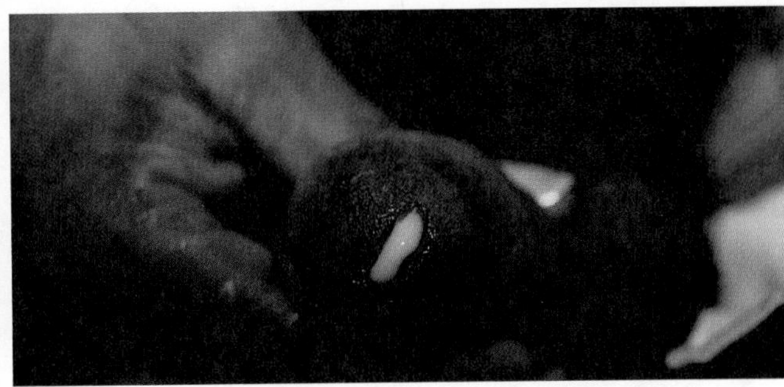

FIGURE 9-18
Acute gonorrhea. A purulent discharge emanates from the penile urethra.

lopian tubes, where it produces acute and chronic salpingitis and eventually pelvic inflammatory disease. The fallopian tubes swell with pus (Fig. 9-19), causing acute abdominal pain. Infertility occurs when inflammatory adhesions block the tubes.

From the fallopian tubes, gonorrhea spreads to the peritoneum, healing as fine ("violin string") adhesions between the liver and the parietal peritoneum. Chronic endometritis is a persistent complication of gonococcal infection and is usually the consequence of chronic gonococcal salpingitis.

Gonorrhea is readily cured with effective antibiotic regimens, especially penicillin. However, susceptibility to penicillin can no longer be routinely assumed, because penicillinase-producing strains are increasingly being encountered, initially in Africa and Asia and recently also in North America and Europe.

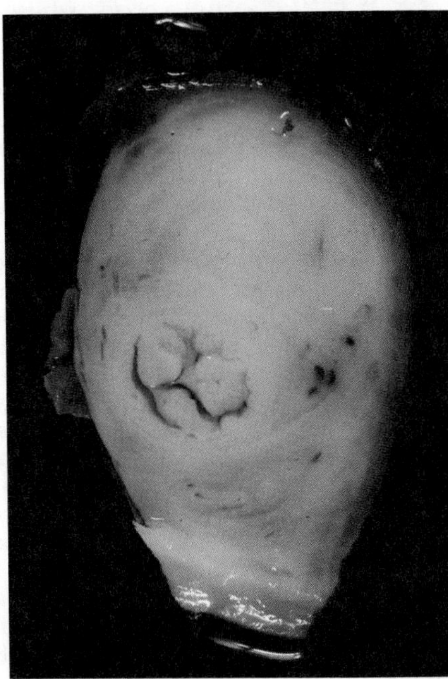

FIGURE 9-19
Gonorrhea of the fallopian tube. Cross-section of a "pus tube" shows thickening of the wall and a lumen swollen with pus.

Chancroid

Chancroid, sometimes called "the third venereal disease" (after syphilis and gonorrhea), is an acute sexually transmitted infection caused by Hemophilus ducreyi. The organism is a small, gram-negative bacillus, which appears in tissue as clusters of parallel bacilli and as chains, resembling schools of fish. Chancroid is characterized by painful genital ulcerations and associated lymphadenopathy.

☐ **Epidemiology:** Chancroid is most common in tropical and subtropical regions, especially in Africa and parts of Asia. The infection is more frequent in men than in women and is associated with promiscuity and poor personal hygiene. *H. ducreyi* is transmitted from person to person by sexual contact. Chancroid is the leading cause of genital ulcers in many less-developed countries. Because the infection is widespread in African countries that have high rates of heterosexual transmission of AIDS, it has been suggested that the genital ulcers facilitate the spread of HIV. Although chancroid remains uncommon in developed countries, the incidence in the United States has risen during the past decade, and there are now about 5000 cases annually.

☐ **Pathogenesis and Pathology:** *H. ducreyi* enters through unnoticed breaks in the skin, where it multiplies and produces a raised lesion, which then ulcerates. Organisms are carried within macrophages to regional lymph nodes, which may suppurate. *H. ducreyi* does not spread to distant sites or cause systemic symptoms.

The ulcers of chancroid are located on the skin and mucous membranes of the genitalia. A papule develops 1 to 14 days after sexual contact, becomes pustular, and then ulcerates. The ulcers vary from 0.1 to 2 cm in diameter, although large and mutilating lesions have been described. Seven to 10 days after the appearance of the primary lesion, half of the patients develop unilateral, painful, suppurative, inguinal lymphadenitis (bubo). The overlying skin becomes inflamed, breaks down, and drains pus from the underlying node.

Microscopically, the typical ulcer exhibits three zones. The superficial zone contains neutrophils, fibrin, erythrocytes, and debris. The broad middle zone is composed of granulation tissue, and the deep zone exhibits plasma cells and lymphocytes concentrated around blood vessels.

The diagnosis is made by identifying the bacillus in tissue sections or gram-stained smears prepared from the ulcers. Treatment of chancroid with erythromycin is usually effective.

Granuloma Inguinale

Granuloma inguinale is a sexually transmitted, chronic, superficial ulceration of the genitalia and the inguinal and perianal regions. It is caused by *Calymmatobacterium granulomatis*, a small, encapsulated, nonmotile, gram-negative bacillus.

☐ **Epidemiology:** Humans are the only hosts of *C. granulomatis.* Granuloma inguinale is rare in temperate climates but is common in tropical and subtropical areas. New Guinea, central Australia, and India have the highest incidence. The highly variable susceptibility to infection and the low level of infectivity have sparked controversy about sexual transmission. For instance, spouses of infected persons often remain uninfected. However, epidemiological data still favor sexual transmission. Most patients are 15 to 40 years of age, the period of greatest sexual activity. Because male homosexuals who take the passive role have only anal lesions, and because *C. granulomatis* has been isolated from the feces, the organism is believed to inhabit the intestinal tract. It causes granuloma inguinale through autoinoculation, anal intercourse, or vaginal intercourse if the vagina is colonized by enteric bacteria.

☐ **Pathology:** The characteristic lesion of granuloma inguinale is a raised, soft, beefy-red, superficial ulcer. The exuberant granulation tissue resembles a fleshy mass herniating through the skin. Microscopically, the epithelium of the ulcer margin is hyperplastic. The dermis and subcutis are infiltrated by numerous macrophages and plasma cells and by fewer neutrophils and lymphocytes. The neutrophils in the ulcer bed are clustered into poorly defined microabscesses. Interspersed macrophages contain many bacteria, which are termed **Donovan bodies** (Fig. 9-20). The bacteria are difficult to see in routinely stained sections but are clearly revealed by silver impregnation.

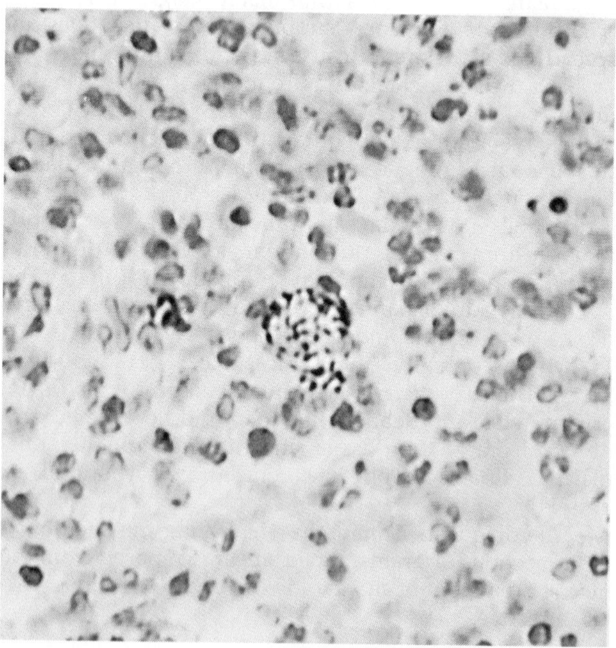

FIGURE *9-20*
Granuloma inguinale. A photomicrograph of a skin lesion shows *C. granulomatis* (Donovan bodies) clustered in a large macrophage. Intense silvering by Warthin-Starry technique makes the organisms large, black, and easily seen.

☐ **Clinical Features:** The incubation period of granuloma inguinale varies from 1 week to 6 months, with 2 to 4 weeks being average. The initial lesion may be a papule, a subcutaneous nodule, or an ulcer. In heterosexual men, early ulceration of the penile and scrotal skin commonly extends to the adjacent inguinal areas. In women, ulcerations spread to the perineal and perianal skin. Homosexual men display anal and perianal lesions. Although regional lymphadenopathy is not a feature, subcutaneous inflammation in the inguinal areas may occasionally be confused with the bubo of lymphogranuloma venereum. Sometimes infection of the vagina and cervix mimics carcinoma. Extragenital lesions have also been reported.

Untreated granuloma inguinale follows an indolent, relapsing course, often healing with an atrophic scar. Secondary fusospirochetal infection may cause ulceration, with mutilation or amputation of the genitalia. Massive scarring of the dermis and subcutis causes genital elephantiasis by lymphatic obstruction. It is uncertain whether there is an association between granuloma inguinale and squamous cell carcinoma, because both diseases share common risk factors, such as poor hygiene, fusospirochetal flora, and a large number of sexual partners. Antibiotic therapy is effective in early cases.

ENTEROPATHOGENIC BACTERIAL INFECTIONS

Escherichia coli

Escherichia coli is among the most frequent and important bacterial pathogens of humans, causing more than 90% of all urinary tract infections and many cases of diarrheal illness worldwide. It is also a major opportunistic pathogen, frequently producing pneumonia and sepsis in immunocompromised hosts and meningitis and sepsis in newborns.

E. coli organisms comprise a group of antigenically and biologically diverse, aerobic (facultatively anaerobic), gram-negative bacteria. Most strains are intestinal commensals, well adapted to growth within the human colon without causing harm to the host. However, *E. coli* can be aggressive when it gains access to usually sterile body sites, such as the urinary tract, meninges, or peritoneum. Strains of *E. coli* that produce diarrhea possess specialized virulence properties, usually plasmid-borne, which confer the capacity to cause intestinal disease.

E. coli Diarrhea

There are four distinct strains of *E. coli* that cause diarrhea. These diarrheogenic strains are known as enterotoxigenic, enteroinvasive, enteropathogenic, and enterohemorrhagic *E. coli.*

ENTEROTOXIGENIC E. COLI: *Enterotoxigenic E. coli is a major cause of diarrhea in poor tropical areas and probably causes most "traveler's diarrhea" among visitors to such regions.* Enterotoxigenic *E. coli* is acquired from contaminated water and food. Many persons in Latin America, Africa, and Asia carry this strain asymptomatically in their intestine, providing an enormous reservoir of infection. Nonimmune persons, either local children or travelers from abroad, develop diarrhea when they encounter the organism. Enterotoxigenic strains produce diarrhea by adhering to the intestinal mucosa and elaborating one or more of at least three enterotoxins that cause secretory dysfunction of the small bowel. The organisms neither invade nor destroy the epithelium. One of the enterotoxins is structurally and functionally similar to cholera toxin, and another acts on guanylyl cyclase. Enterotoxigenic *E. coli* produces no distinctive macroscopic or light-microscopic alterations in the intestine.

Enterotoxigenic *E. coli* causes an acute, self-limited diarrheal illness with watery stools lacking neutrophils and erythrocytes. The fluid and electrolyte loss can cause severe dehydration and even death.

ENTEROPATHOGENIC *E. COLI*: *Historically, enteropathogenic E. coli was the first group of this genus to be identified as a casual agent of diarrhea.* The organism is a major cause of diarrheal illness in poor tropical areas, especially in infants and young children. Although it has virtually disappeared from developed countries, it still causes sporadic outbreaks of diarrhea, particularly among hospitalized infants younger than 2 years of age. Enteropathogenic *E. coli* is acquired by the ingestion of contaminated food or water. The organism lacks invasive properties and causes disease by adhering to and deforming the microvilli of the intestinal epithelial cells (Fig. 9-21A). Enteropathogenic *E. coli* produces diarrhea, vomiting, fever, and malaise. Diarrhea tends to persist longer than in other childhood diarrheal illnesses.

ENTEROHEMORRHAGIC *E. COLI*: *Enterohemorrhagic E. coli (serotype 0157:H7) causes a bloody diarrhea, which occasionally is followed by the hemolytic-uremic syndrome* (see Chapter 16). In the cases studied, the source of infection has been the ingestion of contaminated meat and milk. Enterohemorrhagic *E. coli* adheres to the colonic mucosa and elaborates an enterotoxin that destroys the epithelial cells. The enterotoxin is virtually identical to Shiga toxin. Unlike *Shigella* species, enterohemorrhagic *E. coli* lacks the capacity to invade the mucosa. Patients infected with *E. coli* 0157:H7 present with cramping abdominal pain, low-grade fever, and sometimes frankly bloody diarrhea. Microscopic examination of the stool shows both leukocytes and erythrocytes.

ENTEROINVASIVE *E. COLI*: *Enteroinvasive E. coli causes dysentery that is clinically and pathologically indistinguishable from that caused by Shigella.* The disease, a food-borne enteric infection, is less common than that due to other pathogenic strains of *E. coli*. Enteroinvasive *E. coli* shares extensive DNA homology and antigenic and biochemical characteristics with *Shigella*. It invades and destroys mucosal cells of the distal ileum and colon (see Fig. 9-21B). As in shigellosis, the mucosa of the distal ileum and colon are acutely inflamed and focally eroded, and are sometimes covered by an inflammatory pseudomembrane.

Patients present with cramping abdominal pain, fever, tenesmus, and bloody diarrhea. Symptoms persist for about a week. Antibiotic treatment is similar to that for shigellosis.

E. coli Urinary Tract Infection

☐ Epidemiology: Urinary tract infections are most common in sexually active women and in persons of both sexes who have structural or functional abnormalities of the urinary tract. Such infections are extremely common, afflicting more than 10% of the human population, often repeatedly. *E. coli* in the urinary tract usually derives from the resident flora of the perineum and periurethral areas, reflecting fecal contamination of these regions.

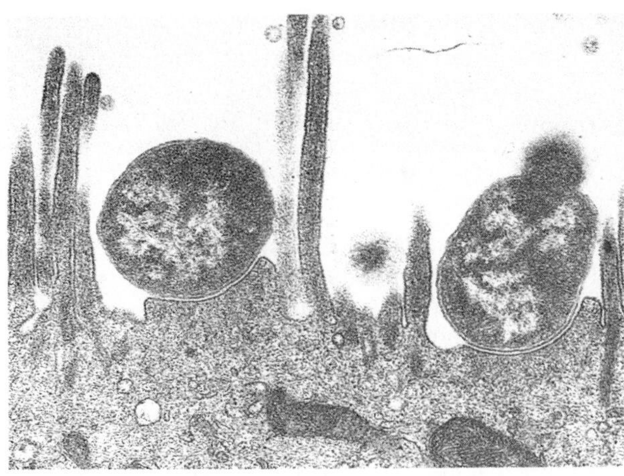

A

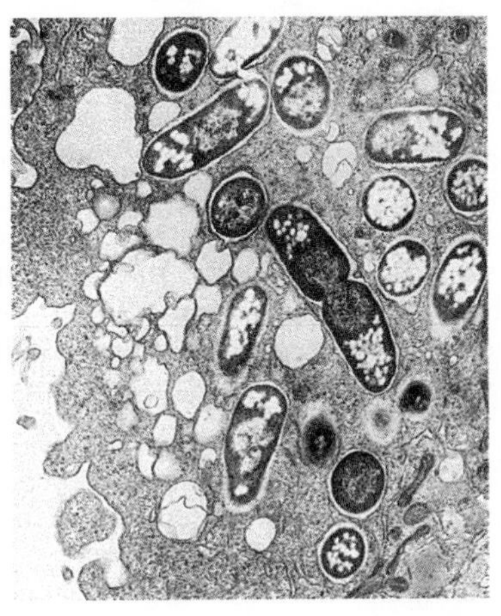

B

FIGURE 9-21
(*A*) Enteropathogenic *E. coli* infection. An electron micrograph shows adherence of the bacteria to the intestinal mucosal cells and localized destruction of microvilli. (*B*) Enteroinvasive *E. coli* infection. An electron micrograph shows organisms within a cell.

□ **Pathogenesis:** *E. coli* gains access to the sterile proximal urinary tract by ascending from the distal urethra. The mechanical flushing of urination, the length of the urethra, and the pH and osmolality of urine defend against such ascending infections. Because the shorter female urethra provides a less effective mechanical barrier to infection, women are much more prone to urinary tract infections. Sexual intercourse can be sufficient to propel organisms into the female urethra. Urinary tract infections can then ascend to the bladder and eventually to the kidneys.

Certain strains of *E. coli* are more frequently associated with urinary tract infections. These uropathogenic *E. coli* organisms have specialized adherence factors (Gal-Gal) on the pili, which enable them to bind to galactopyranosyl-galactopyranoside residues on the uroepithelium. Such adherence permits the organisms to resist the flushing of urination.

Structural abnormalities of the urinary tract (e.g., congenital deformities, prostatic hyperplasia, strictures) and instrumentation (catheterization) overwhelm normal host defenses and facilitate the establishment of urinary tract infections. These conditions account for most urinary tract infections in men.

□ **Pathology:** *E. coli* urinary tract infections initially produce an acute inflammatory infiltrate at the site of infection, usually the bladder mucosa. An infiltrate of neutrophils spills from the mucosa into the urine, and the blood vessels of the submucosa are dilated and congested. If the infection becomes chronic, the inflammatory infiltrate becomes a mixture of neutrophils and mononuclear cells.

□ **Clinical Features:** Urinary tract infections involving the bladder or urethra present as urinary urgency, burning on urination (dysuria), and leukocytes in the urine. If the infection ascends to involve the kidney (pyelonephritis), the patient develops acute flank pain, fever, and an elevated leukocyte count. Chronic infection of the kidneys with *E. coli* may lead to chronic pyelonephritis and renal failure (see Chapter 16).

E. coli Pneumonia

Pneumonias due to enteric gram-negative bacteria are opportunistic infections, often occurring in debilitated persons. *E. coli* is the most common cause, but other normal bowel flora, such as *Klebsiella*, *Serratia*, and *Enterobacter* species, produce similar disease, and the following discussion applies to all opportunistic gram-negative pneumonias.

□ **Epidemiology:** *E. coli* pneumonia occurs in persons weakened by alcoholism, chronic lung disease, and diabetes, as well as in almost any severely ill, hospitalized patient. The pneumonia derives from endogenous *E. coli*, which may colonize the oropharynx in debilitated persons.

□ **Pathogenesis and Pathology:** Enteric gram-negative bacteria are transiently introduced into the oral cavity of healthy persons, but they cannot compete successfully with the predominant gram-positive flora, which adhere to the fibronectin that coats the surface of mucosal cells. Chronically ill or severely stressed persons elaborate a salivary protease that degrades fibronectin, allowing gram-negative enteric bacteria to compete successfully with the normal gram-positive flora and colonize the oropharynx.

Inevitably, droplets of the resident oral flora are aspirated into the respiratory tract. Debilitated persons often have markedly diminished respiratory tract defenses and are incapable of destroying these organisms. Decreased gag and cough reflexes, abnormal neutrophil chemotaxis, injured respiratory epithelium, and the presence of foreign bodies, such as endotracheal tubes, all facilitate entry and survival of the aspirated organisms.

E. coli pneumonia results from the proliferation of aspirated organisms in the terminal airways, usually at multiple sites in the lung. Multifocal areas of consolidation result, and the terminal airways and alveoli are filled with proteinaceous fluid, fibrin, neutrophils, and macrophages.

□ **Clinical Features:** Because pneumonia caused by *E. coli* and other enteric gram-negative organisms afflicts patients who are often already severely ill, the symptoms of pneumonia may be less obvious than in healthy persons. Increased malaise, fever, and labored breathing are often the first signs of pneumonia. If *E. coli* pneumonia remains untreated, the organisms may invade the bloodstream to produce a fatal septicemia. Treatment requires parenteral antibiotics.

E. coli Sepsis (Gram-Negative Sepsis)

E. coli is the most common cause of enteric gram-negative sepsis, but various other gram-negative rods, including *Pseudomonas*, *Klebsiella*, and *Enterobacter*, produce identical disease. The following discussion pertains to gram-negative sepsis in general.

□ **Epidemiology:** *E. coli* sepsis is acquired from the normal enteric bacterial flora. It is usually an opportunistic infection, occurring in persons with predisposing conditions, such as neutropenia, pyelonephritis, or cirrhosis. Because of its association with severe illness, *E. coli* sepsis frequently occurs in hospitalized patients.

□ **Pathogenesis:** *E. coli* and the other enteric gram-negative rods that normally reside in the human colon occasionally seed the bloodstream. In healthy persons, mononuclear macrophages and circulating neutrophils phagocytose and kill these bacteria, which are usually opsonized by complement. Patients with neutropenia or cirrhosis develop *E. coli* sepsis because of an impaired capacity to eliminate even low-level bacteremias. Persons with ruptured abdominal organs or acute pyelonephritis suffer gram-negative sepsis because the large numbers of organisms that gain access to the circulation overwhelm the normal defenses.

The presence of *E. coli* in the bloodstream causes septic shock through the effects of tumor necrosis factor, whose release from macrophages is stimulated by bacterial endotoxin. The pathogenesis and pathology of septic shock are discussed in Chapter 7.

Neonatal *E. coli* Meningitis and Sepsis

E. coli and group B *Streptococcus* are the primary causes of meningitis and sepsis in the first month after birth. Both organisms colonize the vagina, and the newborn acquires the organisms on passage through the birth canal. *E. coli* then colonizes the infant's gastrointestinal tract. It is postulated that the organisms spread to the bloodstream from the gastrointestinal tract and then seed the meninges, but the factors that permit this spread are not understood.

The pathology of *E. coli* meningitis is identical to that of other bacterial meningitides. The leptomeninges are clouded by an acute inflammatory infiltrate, and there may be collections of pus in the subarachnoid space and ventricles. The symptoms are nonspecific and include lethargy, poor feeding, and respiratory distress. Fever is only variably present. Although antibiotic treatment for neonatal *E. coli* meningitis and sepsis is often effective, the mortality rate still ranges from 15% to 50%. Almost half of the survivors suffer neurological sequelae.

Salmonella Enterocolitis and Typhoid Fever

The bacterial genus *Salmonella* comprises over 1500 antigenically distinct but biochemically and genetically related gram-negative rods, which cause two important human diseases, namely, *Salmonella* enterocolitis and typhoid fever. *Salmonella* enterocolitis is an acute, self-limited diarrheal illness produced by *Salmonella* infection confined to the intestinal epithelium. Several hundred different *Salmonella* strains, often designated simply the nontyphoidal *Salmonella*, cause *Salmonella* enterocolitis. Typhoid fever, on the other hand, is a severe, prolonged systemic illness produced by particular typhoidal strains of *Salmonella*, usually *Salmonella typhi*.

Salmonella Enterocolitis

Salmonella enterocolitis is an acute self-limited (1 to 3 days) gastrointestinal illness, which presents as nausea, vomiting, diarrhea, and fever. The infection is typically acquired by ingestion of food contaminated with nontyphoidal *Salmonella* strains and is commonly called "*Salmonella food poisoning.*"

☐ **Epidemiology:** The nontyphoidal *Salmonella* infect diverse animal species, including amphibians, reptiles, birds, and mammals. They also readily contaminate foodstuffs derived from infected animals (e.g., meat, poultry, eggs, or dairy products). If these foods are not cooked, pasteurized, or irradiated, the bacteria persist and, particularly at warm temperatures, proliferate. Since only a small portion of ingested bacteria survive gastric acidity, a large inoculum is usually needed to produce enterocolitis. Once a person is infected, the organism can spread from person to person by fecal-oral contamination. Such spread is infrequent among adults but occurs readily among small children in day-care settings or within families.

There are estimated to be 2 million cases of *Salmonella* food poisoning in the United States each year. *Salmonella* enterocolitis remains a major cause of childhood mortality in less developed countries.

☐ **Pathogenesis and Pathology:** If the *Salmonella* organisms survive exposure to gastric acidity, they then proliferate in the small intestine and invade enterocytes in the distal small bowel and colon. Achlorhydria, antacid use, prior gastric surgery, and other processes that interfere with gastric acidity or speed gastric transit all promote *Salmonella* infections. The nontyphoidal *Salmonella* species do not invade beyond the superficial enterocytes but elaborate several toxins that may contribute to the dysfunction of intestinal cells. In *Salmonella* enterocolitis, the mucosa of the ileum and colon is acutely inflamed and sometimes superficially ulcerated.

☐ **Clinical Features:** *Salmonella* enterocolitis characteristically presents as diarrhea, beginning 12 to 48 hours after the ingestion of contaminated food. This stands in contrast to staphylococcal food poisoning, which is caused by a preformed toxin and begins 1 to 6 hours after the ingestion of contaminated food. The diarrhea of *Salmonella* food poisoning is self-limited, lasting from 1 to 3 days, and is often accompanied by nausea, vomiting, cramping abdominal pain, and fever. Treatment is supportive, and antibiotics rarely improve the clinical course.

Typhoid Fever

Typhoid fever is an acute systemic illness caused by infection with S. typhi. Paratyphoid fever is a clinically similar but milder disease that results from infection with other species of Salmonella, including *S. paratyphi.* The term **enteric fever** includes both typhoid and paratyphoid fever.

☐ **Epidemiology:** Humans are the only natural reservoir for *S. typhi*, and typhoid fever is acquired from convalescing patients or from chronic carriers. The latter tend to be older women with gallstones or biliary scarring, in whom *S. typhi* colonizes the gallbladder or biliary tree. Typhoid fever is spread primarily through the ingestion of contaminated water and food, especially dairy products and shellfish. Less commonly, the organisms are disseminated by direct finger-to-mouth contact with feces, urine, or other secretions. Infected food handlers with poor personal hygiene are a notorious source of infection.

Although concentrations of *S. typhi* in water and food may be too low to cause infection, the organisms proliferate when environmental conditions are favorable. Shellfish in contaminated water filter large volumes and concentrate the bacteria, a process that may deliver enormous doses of *S. typhi* in raw shellfish. Urine from patients with typhoidal pyelonephritis can be a significant source of in-

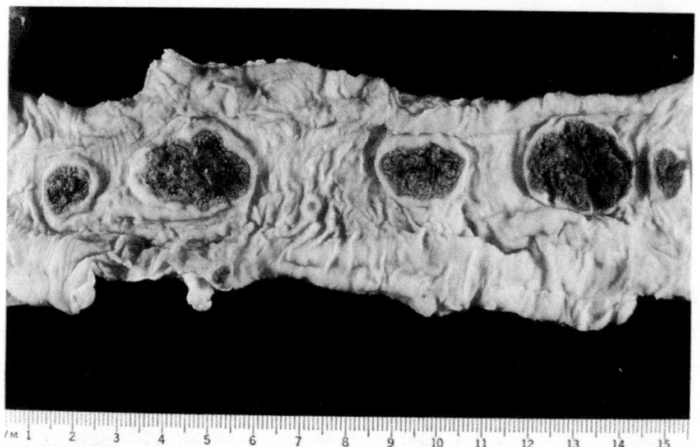

FIGURE 9-22
Ulcers of the terminal ileum in fatal typhoid fever. The ulcers have a longitudinal orientation because they are over hyperplastic and necrotic Peyer patches.

fection. Throughout history armies and refugees have been especially susceptible to typhoid fever. The disease has become rare in countries with modern control of sewage and of water and milk supplies.

Typhoid fever is one of the leading preventable global causes of death due to infectious disease, accounting for over 25,000 annual deaths worldwide. The disease has become uncommon in the United States, where only 500 cases are reported each year, two thirds of which occur in new immigrants or those returning from travel abroad.

□ **Pathogenesis:** *S. typhi* attaches to and invades the small bowel mucosa without causing clinical enterocolitis. Invasion tends to be most prominent in the ileum in areas overlying Peyers patches, where the organisms are engulfed by macrophages. The organisms block the respiratory burst of the phagocytes and multiply within these cells. They spread first to regional lymph nodes and then throughout the body through the lymphatics and bloodstream, infecting mononuclear macrophages in lymph nodes, bone marrow, liver, and spleen. The infection of macrophages stimulates the production of interleukin-1 and tumor necrosis factor, thereby causing the prolonged fever, malaise, and wasting characteristic of typhoid fever.

□ **Pathology:** The earliest pathological change in typhoid fever is the degeneration of the brush border of the intestinal epithelium, as a result of bacterial attachment and penetration. As the bacteria invade, Peyer patches become hypertrophic. In some cases, lymphoid hyperplasia in the intestine progresses to capillary thrombosis, causing necrosis of the overlying mucosa and the characteristic ulcers oriented along the long axis of the bowel (Fig. 9-22). These gastrointestinal ulcerations frequently bleed and occasionally perforate, producing infectious peritonitis. Systemic dissemination of the organisms leads to focal granulomas in the liver, spleen, and other organs, termed **typhoid nodules**. These are composed of aggregates of macrophages ("typhoid cells") containing ingested bacteria, erythrocytes, and degenerated lymphocytes.

□ **Clinical Features:** Prior to the antibiotic era, untreated typhoid fever was classically divided into five stages (Fig. 9-23):

1. **Incubation:** After infection with *S. typhi*, the patient remains asymptomatic for 10 to 14 days.
2. **Active invasion/bacteremia:** For a period of about a week, the patient suffers a variety of nonspecific symptoms, including daily stepwise elevation in temperature (up to 105°F), malaise, headache, arthralgias, and abdominal pain.
3. **Fastigium:** Fever and malaise increase over several days until the infected person is bedridden. In severe cases, patients become toxic (delirious, stuporous, or comatose) as a consequence of the release of endotoxins from dead bacteria. Hepatomegaly is accompanied by derangements in liver function tests. The spleen is conspicuously enlarged.
4. **Lysis:** After about a week of sustained fever (fastigium), patients destined to survive exhibit a gradual reduction in fever, and the toxic symptoms recede. Although gastrointestinal tract bleeding and perforation of the intestine at the site of ulceration may occur in any stage, it is most common during lysis, which commonly lasts a week.
5. **Convalescence:** After about 4 weeks of symptomatic disease, the fever abates, and with the exception of patients who relapse or have metastatic foci of infection, patients gradually regain strength and recover over a period of several weeks to months.

FIGURE 9-23
Stages of typhoid fever.

Incubation (10–14 days). Water or food contaminated with *S. typhi* is ingested. Bacilli attach to the villi in the small intestine, invade the mucosa, and pass to the intestinal lymphoid follicles and draining mesenteric lymph nodes. The organisms proliferate further within mononuclear phagocytic cells of the lymphoid follicles, lymph nodes, liver, and spleen. Bacilli are sequestered intracellularly in the intestinal and mesenteric lymphatic system.

Active invasion/bacteremia (1 week). Organisms are released and produce a transient bacteremia. The intestinal mucosa becomes enlarged and necrotic, forming characteristic mucosal lesions. The intestinal lymphoid tissues become hyperplastic and contain "typhoid nodules"—aggregates of macrophages ("typhoid cells") that phagocytose bacteria, erythrocytes, and degenerated lymphocytes. Bacilli proliferate in several organs, reappear in the intestine, are excreted in stool, and may invade through the intestinal wall. Fastigium (1 week). Dying bacilli release endotoxins that cause systemic toxemia.

Lysis (1 week). Necrotic intestinal mucosa sloughs, producing ulcers, which hemorrhage or perforate into the peritoneal cavity.

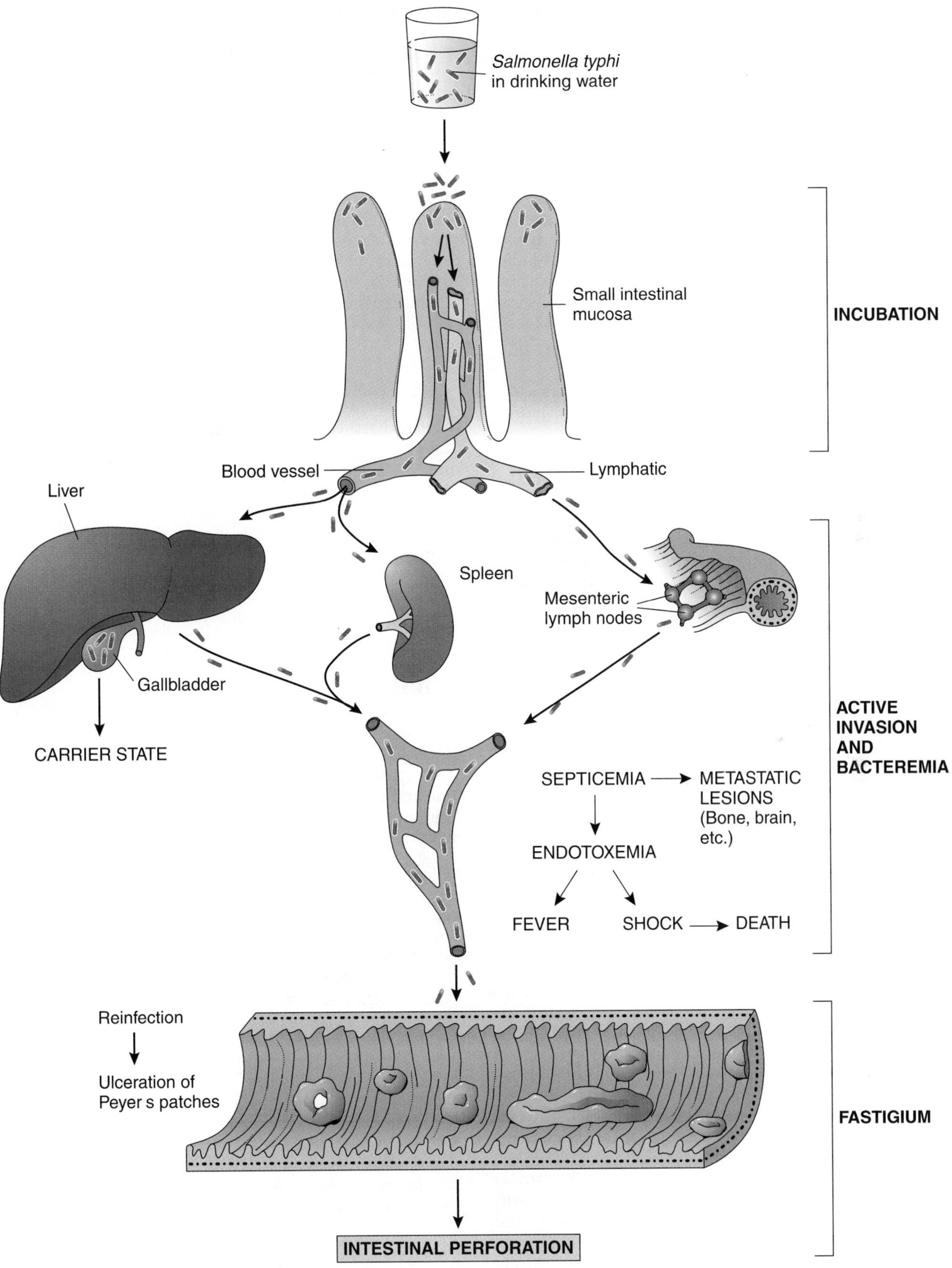
Salmonella typhi in drinking water
Small intestinal mucosa
INCUBATION
Blood vessel
Lymphatic
Liver
Spleen
Mesenteric lymph nodes
Gallbladder
CARRIER STATE
ACTIVE INVASION AND BACTEREMIA
SEPTICEMIA
METASTATIC LESIONS (Bone, brain, etc.)
ENDOTOXEMIA
FEVER
SHOCK
DEATH
Reinfection
Ulceration of Peyer s patches
FASTIGIUM
INTESTINAL PERFORATION

FIGURE 9-23

The treatment of typhoid fever entails antibiotics and supportive care. If untreated, 10% to 20% of patients die, usually of secondary complications, such as pneumonia. However, treatment within 3 days of the onset of fever is generally curative.

Shigellosis

Shigellosis is an acute bacterial dysentery characterized by a necrotizing infection of the distal small bowel and colon. It is caused by any of the four species of *Shigella* (*S. boydii*, *S. dysenteriae*, *S. flexneri*, and *S. sonnei*), which are aerobic, gram-negative rods. Of the various species, *S. dysenteriae* is the most virulent. Shigellosis is a self-limited disease, which typically presents as abdominal pain and bloody, mucoid stools.

☐ **Epidemiology:** *Shigella* organisms are spread from person to person by the fecal-oral route. Unlike salmonellae, shigellae have no animal reservoir, and they do not survive well outside the stool. Therefore, infection usually occurs through ingestion of fecally contaminated food or water, but it can be acquired by oral contact with any contaminated surface (e.g., clothing, towels, or skin surfaces). As a result, endemic shigellosis is more common in populations with poor standards of hygiene and sanitation. Shigellosis is also spread in closed communities, such as hospitals, barracks, and households. In developed countries, *S. flexneri* and *S. sonnei* are more common and infection tends to be sporadic.

Shigella are among the most virulent enteropathogens known. Disease is produced by the ingestion of as few as 10 to 100 organisms, and there are few asymptomatic carriers. *S. dysenteriae* caused a 1968 pandemic in Central and North America, in which mortality rates reached 20% to 50%.

In the United States, there are estimated to be 300,000 cases of shigellosis annually, but the incidence of the disease is much greater in countries lacking sanitary systems for human waste disposal. Like the other diarrheal illnesses, shigellosis is a significant cause of childhood mortality in developing countries.

☐ **Pathogenesis:** In contrast to salmonellae, shigellae are more capable of surviving the host defenses of the upper gastrointestinal tract, and small numbers of organisms are sufficient to produce disease. Shigellae proliferate rapidly in the small bowel and attach to enterocytes. The organisms are then engulfed by endocytosis and replicate within the cytoplasm of infected cells. Endocytosis is essential to the virulence of the organism, and the factor that induces it is encoded on a plasmid. The replicating shigellae kill infected cells and spread to adjacent cells and into the lamina propria.

Shigellae also produce a potent exotoxin, known as Shiga toxin. It appears that the severity of diarrhea and the degree of bleeding in shigellosis are related to the amount of toxin produced by different *Shigella* strains. Shiga toxin has two major effects. It attaches to the 60S ribosomal subunits and thereby inhibits protein synthesis. It also causes watery diarrhea, probably by inducing a failure of fluid absorption in the colon. Although shigellae extensively damage the epithelium of the ileum and colon, they rarely invade beyond the intestinal lamina propria, and bacteremia is uncommon.

☐ **Pathology:** In shigellosis, the distal colon is almost always affected, although the entire colon and distal ileum can be involved. The affected mucosa is edematous, acutely inflamed, and focally eroded. Ulcers appear first on the edges of mucosal folds, perpendicular to the long axis of the colon. A patchy inflammatory pseudomembrane, composed of neutrophils, fibrin, and necrotic epithelium, is commonly found on the most severely affected areas. Regeneration of infected colonic epithelium occurs rapidly, and healing is usually complete within 10 to 14 days.

☐ **Clinical Features:** Shigellosis often begins with watery diarrhea, which changes in character within 1 to 2 days to the classic dysenteric stools. These are small-volume stools that contain gross blood, sloughed pseudomembranes, and mucus. Cramping abdominal pain, tenesmus, and urgency at stool typically accompany the diarrhea. Fever is present in only about half of the patients. Symptoms persist for 3 to 8 days, if the disease is untreated. The course of disease is usually more severe in children younger than 2 years of age. Treatment with antibiotics shortens the course of the illness.

Cholera

Cholera is a severe diarrheal illness caused by the enterotoxin of Vibrio cholerae, an aerobic, curved gram-negative rod. The organism proliferates in the lumen of the small intestine and causes profuse watery diarrhea, rapid dehydration, and (if fluids are not restored) shock and death within 24 hours of the onset of symptoms.

☐ **Epidemiology:** In the 19th century, cholera was common in most parts of the world, but it periodically "disappeared" spontaneously. A major pandemic occurred between 1961 and 1974, extending throughout Asia, the Middle East, southern Russia, the Mediterranean basin, and parts of Africa. A more recent epidemic of cholera in Peru and contiguous regions of South America was responsible for numerous deaths. The disease remains endemic in the river deltas of India and Bangladesh, where it may cause up to 500,000 deaths annually.

Cholera is acquired by ingesting *V. cholerae*, primarily in contaminated food or water. Cholera epidemics spread readily in areas where human feces pollute the water supply. Shellfish and plankton may serve as a natural reservoir for the organism, and shellfish ingestion accounts for most of the sporadic cases seen in the United States.

☐ **Pathogenesis and Pathology:** A large number of organisms must be ingested to survive normal gastric acidity. Bacteria that survive passage through the stomach thrive and multiply in the mucus layer of the small bowel. **They do not themselves invade the mucosa but cause diarrhea by the elaboration of a potent exotoxin, known as cholera toxin.** The toxin is composed of A and B subunits. The B subunit binds the toxin to GM_1 ganglioside in the cell membrane of the enterocyte. The A subunit then enters the cell, where it activates adenylyl cyclase. The consequent increase in the content of cyclic adenosine monophosphate (cAMP) results in the massive secretion of sodium and water from the enterocyte into the intestinal lumen (Fig. 9-24). The greatest fluid secretion occurs in the small bowel, where there is a net loss of water, potassium, and bicarbonate into the bowel lumen. *V. cholerae* causes little visible alteration in the affected intestine, which appears grossly normal or only slightly hyperemic. Microscopically, the intestinal epithelium is intact but depleted of mucus.

☐ **Clinical Features:** Cholera begins with a few loose stools, usually evolving within hours into severe watery diarrhea. The stools are often flecked with mucus, imparting a "rice water" appearance. The volume of diarrhea is highly variable, but the rapidity and volume loss of severe cases can be truly staggering. With adequate volume replacement, infected adults can lose up to 20

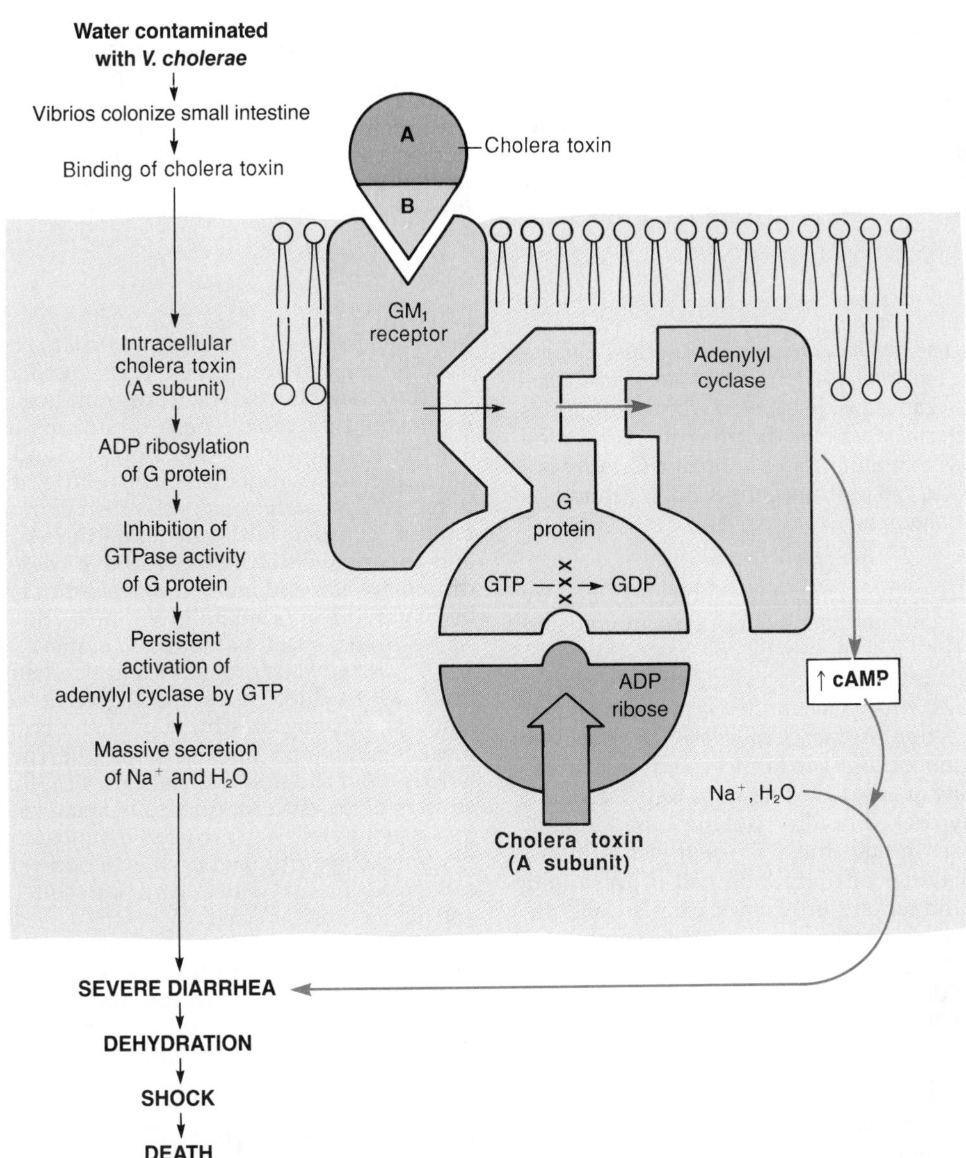

FIGURE *9-24*
Cholera. Infection comes from water contaminated with *Vibrio cholerae* or food prepared with contaminated water. The vibrios traverse the stomach, enter the small intestine, and propagate. Although they do not invade the intestinal mucosa, the vibrios elaborate a potent toxin that induces a massive outpouring of water and electrolytes. Severe diarrhea ("rice-water stool") leads to dehydration and hypovolemic shock.

liters of fluid in a single day. Fluid and electrolyte loss initially causes thirst, oliguria, and muscle cramping. This can advance to shock and death within hours if fluid volume is not replaced. Untreated cholera has a 50% mortality rate. Replacement of lost salts and water is a simple, effective treatment, which can often be accomplished by oral rehydration with preparations of salt, glucose, and water. The illness subsides spontaneously in 3 to 6 days. Antibiotic therapy shortens the duration of the illness. Infection with *V. cholerae* confers long-term immunity to the development of recurrent illness, and vaccines are now being developed.

VIBRIO PARAHEMOLYTICUS: There are a number of so-called noncholera vibrios, of which *V. parahemolyticus* is the most common. This organism is a gram-negative bacillus that causes acute gastroenteritis. It is found in marine life and coastal waters around the world in temperate climates, causing outbreaks in the summer. Gastroenteritis is associated with the consumption of inadequately cooked or poorly refrigerated seafood. The clinical syndrome resembles that produced by *Salmonella* enteritis, and no deaths have been reported.

Campylobacter jejuni

C. jejuni is the major human pathogen in the genus Campylobacter and causes an acute, self-limited inflammatory diarrheal illness. The organism is distributed worldwide and is the leading bacterial agent of diarrhea in the United States, causing over 2 million cases annually. *C. jejuni* is a microaerophilic, curved gram-negative rod, morphologically similar to the vibrios.

☐ **Epidemiology:** *C. jejuni* infection is acquired by the ingestion of organisms, usually through contaminated food or water. The bacteria inhabit the gastrointestinal tracts of diverse animal species, including cows, sheep, chickens, and dogs, which constitute a significant animal reservoir for infection. In fact, *Campylobacter* infections cause serious economic losses to farmers because of abortions and infertility of infected cattle and sheep. Raw milk and inadequately cooked poultry and meat are frequent sources of disease. In one study, *C. jejuni* was cultured from the body cavities of more than half of fresh and frozen chickens and turkeys in 10 major cities around the world. *C. jejuni* can also spread from person to person by fecal-oral contact. The organism is a major cause of childhood mortality in developing countries and is responsible for many cases of "travelers' diarrhea."

☐ **Pathogenesis:** Ingested *C. jejuni* organisms that survive gastric acidity multiply in the alkaline environment of the upper small intestine. When they reach the distal ileum and colon, they cause superficial necrosis of the intestinal epithelium and elicit an acute inflammatory response. *C. jejuni* elaborates several proteins that are toxins *in vitro*. Although their role in causing disease is still unclear, the severity of the symptoms has been correlated with toxin production.

☐ **Pathology:** *C. jejuni* causes a superficial enterocolitis, primarily involving the terminal ileum and colon, with focal necrosis of the intestinal epithelium, accompanied by an acute inflammatory infiltrate. In severe cases, this progresses to small ulcers and patchy inflammatory exudates (pseudomembranes) composed of necrotic cells, neutrophils, fibrin, and debris. The crypts of the colonic epithelium often fill with neutrophils, forming so-called crypt abscesses. These pathological changes resolve in 7 to 14 days. The inflammation resolves and the intestinal epithelium regenerates in 7 to 14 days.

☐ **Clinical Features:** The acute enterocolitis associated with *C. jejuni* infection resembles *Shigella* dysentery and begins with fever, headache, malaise, cramping abdominal pain, and diarrhea. Patients usually produce more than 10 stools per day, varying from profuse watery stools to small-volume stools containing gross blood and mucus. The symptoms tend to resolve in 5 to 7 days. Treatment with antibiotics is probably of marginal benefit in most cases. A few patients develop a more severe, protracted illness resembling acute ulcerative colitis, including toxic megacolon and extraintestinal complications.

Yersinia Infection

Yersinia infections of the gastrointestinal tract produce painful diarrhea. They are caused by *Y. enterocolitica* and *Y. pseudotuberculosis*, both of which are gram-negative coccoid or rod-shaped bacteria. These organisms are facultative anaerobes found in the feces of wild and domestic animals, including rodents, sheep, cattle, dogs, cats, and horses. *Y. pseudotuberculosis* is also commonly encountered in domestic birds, including turkeys, ducks, geese, and canaries. Both organisms have been isolated from drinking water and milk. *Y. enterocolitica* is more likely to be acquired from contaminated meat and *Y. pseudotuberculosis* from contact with infected animals.

Y. enterocolitica proliferates in the ileum, invades the mucosa, produces ulceration and necrosis of Peyer patches, and migrates by way of the lymphatics to the mesenteric lymph nodes. Fever, diarrhea (sometimes bloody), and abdominal pain begin 4 to 10 days after penetration of the mucosa. Abdominal pain in the right lower quadrant has led to an incorrect diagnosis of appendicitis. Arthralgia, arthritis, and erythema nodosum are complications. Septicemia is an uncommon sequel but kills about one half of those affected.

Y. pseudotuberculosis penetrates the ileal mucosa, localizes in ileal-cecal lymph nodes, and produces abscesses and granulomas in the lymph nodes, spleen, and liver. Fever, diarrhea, and abdominal pain may also lead to an erroneous diagnosis of appendicitis.

PULMONARY INFECTIONS WITH GRAM-NEGATIVE BACTERIA

Klebsiella and Enterobacter

Klebsiella and Enterobacter species are short, encapsulated, gram-negative bacilli that cause a necrotizing lobar pneumonia.

☐ **Epidemiology:** These organisms cause 10% of all infections acquired in the hospital, including pneumonia and infections of the urinary tract, biliary tract, and surgical wounds. Person-to-person transmission by hospital personnel is a special hazard. Predisposing factors are indwelling catheters and endotracheal tubes, a variety of debilitating conditions, immunosuppression, and obstructive pulmonary disease. Secondary pneumonias caused by these bacteria may complicate influenza or other viral infections of the respiratory tract, especially in immunocompromised persons and patients taking glucocorticosteroids.

☐ **Pathology:** *Klebsiella* and *Enterobacter* species are inhaled and multiply within the alveolar spaces. The pulmonary parenchyma becomes consolidated, and the mucoid exudate that fills the alveoli is dominated by macrophages, fibrin, and edema fluid. Neutrophils are inhibited by a neutral polysaccharide in the capsule of the bacterium and are not a significant part of the early exudate. Numerous encapsulated, gram-negative bacilli appear free in the exudate and in alveolar macrophages. As the exudate accumulates, the alveolar walls become compressed and then necrotic. Numerous small abscesses may coalesce and lead to cavitation.

☐ **Clinical Features:** Pneumonia caused by these organisms is most commonly nosocomial. When it occurs in the hospital, the onset is sudden, with fever, pleuritic pain, cough, and **a characteristic thick mucoid sputum**. When infection is severe, these symptoms progress to dyspnea, cyanosis, and death in 2 to 3 days. The pneumonia, or other infections with *Klebsiella* and *Enterobacter* species may be complicated by a fulminating, often fatal, septicemia, even without disseminated lesions in other tissues. Aggressive antibiotic therapy is required.

Legionnaires Disease (Legionellosis)

Legionella species cause pneumonia that ranges from a relatively mild disease to a severe, life-threatening necrotizing pneumonia, known as Legionnaires disease. Six months after an outbreak of a severe respiratory disease of unknown cause at the 1976 state convention of the American Legion in Philadelphia, *L. pneumophila* was first identified by the Centers for Disease Control. Subsequently, retrospective studies demonstrated antibodies in sera from previously unexplained epidemics. The first epidemic so recognized occurred in 1957 in a Minnesota meat-packing plant. *L. pneumophila* was also responsible for a "flulike" illness known as Pontiac fever.

L. pneumophila is a minute aerobic bacillus that has the cell wall structure of a gram-negative organism but reacts poorly with Gram stains and can rarely be visualized by the routine study of clinical material.

☐ **Epidemiology:** *Legionella* is present in small numbers in natural bodies of fresh water. It survives chlorination and proliferates in man-made devices, such as cooling towers, water heaters, humidifiers, and evaporative condensers. Infection occurs when persons inhale aerosols from contaminated sources. Legionnaires disease is not contagious, and the organism is not part of the normal human oropharyngeal flora. There are an estimated 75,000 cases of *Legionella* infection in the United States annually.

☐ **Pathogenesis:** *Legionella* causes two distinct diseases: pneumonia and Pontiac fever. The pathogenesis of *Legionella* pneumonia (Legionnaires disease) is understood in some detail, whereas that of Pontiac fever remains largely a mystery. *Legionella* pneumonia begins with the arrival of the organisms in the terminal bronchioles or alveoli, where they are phagocytosed by alveolar macrophages. The bacteria are not killed by these cells but survive and replicate within their phagosomes. They protect themselves by blocking the fusion of lysosomes with the phagosomes. Although neutrophils and monocytes are recruited to the site of infection, they initially do not kill the organisms. Rather, the multiplying *Legionella* are released from their host cells and infect freshly arriving phagocytes. Replication of *Legionella* and recruitment of inflammatory cells continues, involving more of the pulmonary parenchyma, until checked by a specific cell-mediated immune response. With the development of this immunity, macrophages become activated and cease to support intracellular growth of the organisms.

The native respiratory tract defenses, such as the mucociliary blanket of the airway, provide a first line of defense against lower respiratory tract *Legionella* infection. Factors such as smoking, alcoholism, and chronic lung diseases, which interfere with normal functions of the respiratory defenses, increase the risks of developing *Legionella* pneumonia.

☐ **Pathology:** Legionnaires disease is an acute bronchopneumonia. The process is usually patchy but sometimes produces a lobar pattern of infiltration. Affected alveoli and bronchioles are filled with an exudate composed of proteinaceous fluid, fibrin, macrophages, and neutrophils (Fig. 9-25), and microabscesses are frequently found. The alveolar walls become necrotic and are destroyed. Many macrophages show eccentric nuclei, pushed aside by cytoplasmic vacuoles containing *L. pneumophila*. Silver impregnation stains, such as the Dieterle stain, increase the size of the organisms and better demonstrate their presence. With resolution of the pneumonia, the lungs heal with little permanent damage.

☐ **Clinical Features:** In its severe form, Legionnaires disease presents as a rapidly progressive pneumonia, accompanied by fever, a nonproductive cough, and myalgia. After an incubation of 2 to 10 days, the clinical onset is abrupt. Patients rapidly develop a persistent high fever and respiratory rales. Chest radiographs reveal unilateral, diffuse, patchy consolidation, progressing to widespread nodular consolidation, usually without cavitation. Toxic symptoms, hypoxia, and obtundation may be prominent, and death may follow within a few days. In those who survive, convalescence is prolonged. Erythromycin is the antibiotic of choice. The mortality rate

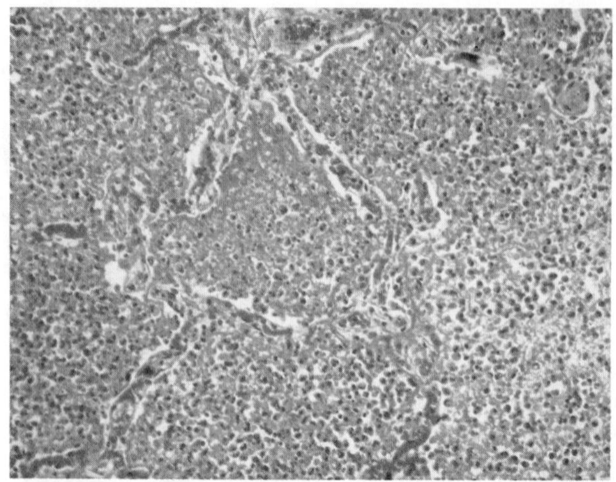

FIGURE 9-25
Legionnaires pneumonia. The alveoli are packed with an exudate composed of fibrin, macrophages, and neutrophils.

among hospitalized patients averages 15%, although there is a much greater risk of death among persons with serious underlying illness.

Pontiac fever is a self-limited, flulike illness with fever, malaise, myalgias, and headache. It differs from Legionnaires disease in showing no evidence of pulmonary consolidation. The disease resolves spontaneously in 3 to 5 days.

Pseudomonas aeruginosa

Pseudomonas aeruginosa is a major opportunistic pathogen and one of the most frequent hospital-acquired pathogens. The organism only infrequently infects humans, but it can cause disease, particularly in the hospital environment, where it is associated with pneumonia, wound infections, urinary tract disease, and sepsis in debilitated persons. Burns, urinary catheterization, cystic fibrosis, diabetes, and neutropenia all predispose to infection with *P. aeruginosa.*

P. aeruginosa is a ubiquitous aerobic, gram-negative rod, which requires moisture and only minimal nutrients. It thrives in soil and water, on animals, and on moist environmental surfaces. **Antibiotic use tends to select for *P. aeruginosa* infection, since the organism is among the most antibiotic-resistant bacteria.**

☐ **Pathogenesis:** *P. aeruginosa* elaborates an array of proteins, which allow it to attach to, invade, and destroy host tissues, while avoiding host inflammatory and immune defenses. Injury to epithelial cells uncovers surface molecules that serve as binding sites for the pili of *P. aeruginosa.* Many strains of *P. aeruginosa* produce a proteoglycan that surrounds the bacteria, protecting them from mucociliary action, complement, and phagocytes. The organism releases extracellular enzymes, including an elastase, an alkaline protease, and a cytotoxin, which facilitate tissue invasion and are partially responsible for the necrotizing lesions of *Pseudomonas* infections. The elastase is probably responsible for the distinctive ability of *P. aeruginosa* to invade blood vessel walls. The organism also produces systemic pathological effects through endotoxin and several systemically active exotoxins.

☐ **Pathology:** If the host has the capacity to respond to the invading bacteria with neutrophils, *Pseudomonas* infection will produce an acute inflammatory response. The organism often invades small arteries and veins, producing vascular thrombosis and hemorrhagic necrosis, particularly in the lungs and skin. Blood vessel invasion, of course, predisposes to bacteremia, dissemination, and sepsis. Vascular invasion often leads to the rapid development of multiple metastatic nodular lesions in the lungs. Gram stains of necrotic tissue infected with *Pseudomonas* commonly show blood vessel walls densely infiltrated with organisms. Sometimes disseminated infections are marked by the development of typical skin lesions called **ecthyma gangrenosum**. These nodular, necrotic lesions represent sites where the organism has disseminated to the skin, invaded blood vessels, and produced localized hemorrhagic infarctions.

☐ **Clinical Features:** Signs and symptoms of *Pseudomonas* infections vary with the site of infection and the state of host defenses. These infections are among the most aggressive human bacterial diseases, often progressing rapidly to sepsis. They require immediate medical intervention and are associated with a high mortality.

Melioidosis

Melioidosis (Rangoon beggars disease) is an uncommon infectious disease caused by Pseudomonas pseudomallei, a small gram-negative bacillus in the soil and surface water of Southeast Asia and other tropical areas. During the conflict in Vietnam, several hundred servicemen acquired melioidosis. The organism flourishes in wet environments, such as rice paddies and marshes. The skin is the usual portal of entry, and organisms enter through preexisting lesions, including penetrating wounds and burns. Humans may also be infected by inhaling contaminated dust or aerosolized droplets. The incubation period varies up to months, and possibly years, and the clinical course is variable.

***Acute melioidosis** is a pulmonary infection, ranging from a mild tracheobronchitis to an overwhelming cavitary pneumonia* (Fig. 9-26). Patients with severe cases present with the sudden onset of high fever, constitutional symptoms, and a cough that may produce blood-stained sputum. Splenomegaly, hepatomegaly, and jaundice are sometimes present. Diarrhea may be as severe as that in cholera. Fulminating septicemia, shock, coma, and death may develop in spite of antibiotic therapy. Acute septicemic melioidosis causes discrete abscesses throughout the body, especially in the lungs, liver, spleen, and lymph nodes.

***Chronic melioidosis** is a persistent localized infection involving the lungs, skin, bones, or other organs.* The lesions are suppurative or granulomatous abscesses and in the lung may be mistaken for tuberculosis. Chronic melioidosis

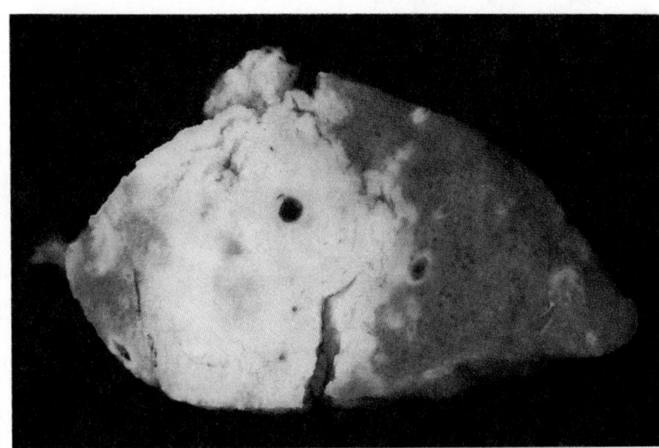

FIGURE 9-26
Acute melioidosis. The lung is consolidated and necrotic.

may lie dormant for months or years, only to appear suddenly—hence the colloquial name "Vietnamese time bomb."

CLOSTRIDIAL DISEASES

Clostridia are gram-positive, spore-forming bacilli that are obligate anaerobes. The vegetative bacilli are found in the gastrointestinal tract of herbivorous animals and humans. Anaerobic conditions promote vegetative division, whereas aerobic ones lead to sporulation. Spores pass in animal feces and contaminate soil and plants, where they are able to survive unfavorable environmental circumstances. Under anaerobic conditions, the spores revert to vegetative cells, thereby completing the cycle. During sporulation, vegetative cells degenerate and their plasmids produce a variety of specific toxins that cause widely differing diseases, depending on the species (Fig. 9-27).

- **Food poisoning and necrotizing enteritis** (pigbel) are caused by the enterotoxins of *Clostridium perfringens*.
- **Gas gangrene** is produced by the myotoxins of *C. perfringens*, *C. novyi*, *C. septicum*, and other species.
- **Tetanus** is related to the neurotoxin of *C. tetani*.
- **Botulism** results from the action of the neurotoxin of *C. botulinum*.
- **Pseudomembranous enterocolitis** is the consequence of the action of the exotoxins of *C. difficile*.

Clostridial Food Poisoning

Clostridium perfringens is one of the most common causes of bacterial food poisoning in the world, characterized by an acute, generally benign, diarrheal disease, usually lasting less than 24 hours. This organism is the most widely disseminated of all pathogenic bacteria, being 10 to 100 times more numerous than *E. coli* in the stool. It is also omnipresent in the environment, contaminating soil, water, air samples, clothing, dust, and meat.

☐ **Pathogenesis:** Spores of *C. perfringens* survive cooking temperatures and germinate to yield vegetative forms, which proliferate when food is allowed to stand without refrigeration. Cooking drives out enough air to make the food anaerobic, a condition that is conducive to growth but not to sporulation. As a result, the contaminated food contains the vegetative clostridia but little preformed enterotoxin. (This contrasts with the situation in botulism, in which preformed neurotoxin is ingested.) Clostridial food poisoning results from the ingestion of food containing large numbers ($>10^5/g$) of these vegetative bacteria. Certain types of food, including meats, gravies, and sauces, are ideal substrates for *C. perfringens*. Clostridial food poisoning is prevented by prompt refrigeration of food after cooking.

Sufficient numbers of *C. perfringens* must be ingested so that some survive upper gastrointestinal tract defenses. The vegetative bacteria sporulate in the small bowel. The pathogenicity of the organism (types A, C, and D) resides in its ability to elaborate a variety of exotoxins, which are cytotoxic to enterocytes. Damage to these cells leads to the loss of intracellular ions and fluid.

☐ **Clinical Features:** Clostridial food poisoning presents as abdominal cramping and watery diarrhea. Symptoms begin 8 to 24 hours after the ingestion of contaminated food and usually resolve within 24 hours.

Necrotizing Enteritis

Clostridium perfringens type C also produces an enterotoxin that causes a necrotizing enterocolitis. The illness may date back to accounts of enteric disease described by Hippocrates, but is seldom encountered in the industrialized world. However, the necrotizing enteritis caused by C. perfringens is still endemic in the highlands of New Guinea, especially in children who have participated in pig feasts (hence the pidgin term pigbel).

☐ **Pathogenesis:** Spit roasting of pig carcasses encourages the growth of *C. perfringens*. Adults tend not to develop pigbel, because they have circulating antibodies. The normal diet of the children is derived principally from sweet potatoes. The combination of protein malnutrition and the presence of a trypsin inhibitor in sweet potatoes renders the children deficient in intestinal proteases, to which the enterotoxin of *C. perfringens* is very sensitive.

☐ **Pathology:** Necrotizing enteritis is a segmental disease that may be restricted to a few centimeters or may involve the entire small intestine. Green, necrotic pseudomembranes are seen in segmental areas of necrosis and peritonitis. More advanced lesions perforate the bowel wall. Histological sections reveal infarction of the intestinal mucosa, with edema, hemorrhage, and a suppurative transmural infiltrate. The pseudomembrane is composed of necrotic epithelium containing *C. perfringens*.

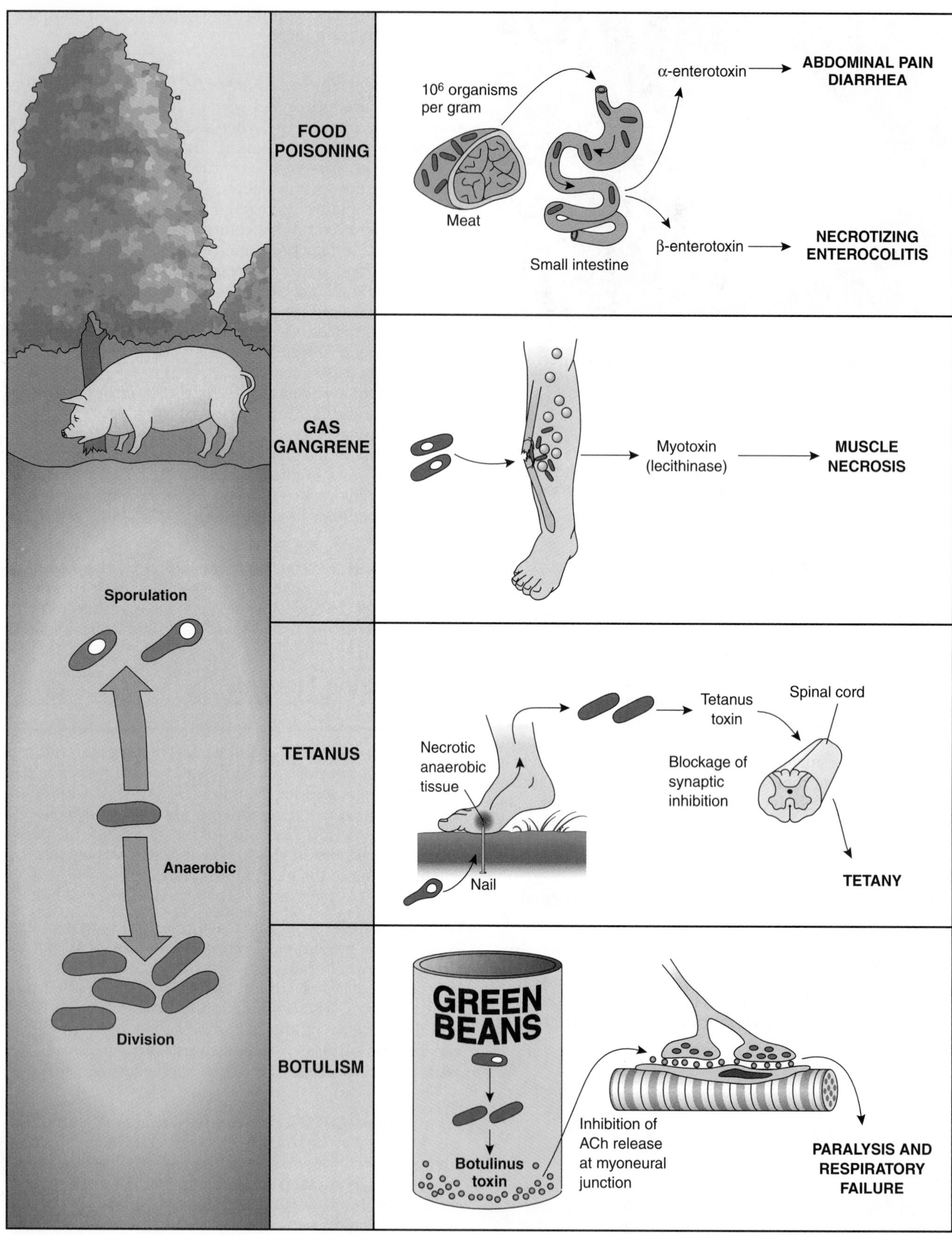

FOOD POISONING
10^6 organisms per gram
Meat
Small intestine
α-enterotoxin
ABDOMINAL PAIN DIARRHEA
β-enterotoxin
NECROTIZING ENTEROCOLITIS
GAS GANGRENE
Myotoxin (lecithinase)
MUSCLE NECROSIS
Sporulation
Anaerobic
Division
TETANUS
Necrotic anaerobic tissue
Nail
Tetanus toxin
Spinal cord
Blockage of synaptic inhibition
TETANY
BOTULISM
GREEN BEANS
Botulinus toxin
Inhibition of ACh release at myoneural junction
PARALYSIS AND RESPIRATORY FAILURE

FIGURE 9-27

☐ **Clinical Features:** The incubation period of pigbel is 48 hours after the ingestion of contaminated meat. The presenting symptoms include severe abdominal pain and distention, vomiting, and passage of bloody or black stools. Patients with fulminating pigbel die within 24 hours of onset. Others have mild pigbel, which resembles gastroenteritis. Half of the patients require segmental resection of the bowel. Passive immunization with specific antitoxin and active immunization with a pigbel toxoid vaccine reduce morbidity and mortality.

Gas Gangrene (Clostridial Myonecrosis)

Gas gangrene is a necrotizing, gas-forming infection that begins in contaminated wounds and spreads rapidly to adjacent tissues. The disease can be fatal within hours of onset. *C. perfringens* is the most common cause of gas gangrene, but other Clostridial species occasionally produce the disease.

☐ **Pathogenesis:** Gas gangrene follows the deposition of *C. perfringens* into tissue under anaerobic conditions. Since the organisms are present throughout the environment, they readily contaminate wounds. The anaerobic conditions necessary to foster clostridial growth are fortunately uncommon in human tissues and are usually produced only in the presence of extensive devitalized tissue, such as occurs with severe trauma, wartime injuries, and septic abortions. However, only a small proportion of wounds contaminated with clostridia develop gas gangrene. Contributing factors include hypoxia from injury to blood vessels near the wound site, pressure dressings, tourniquets, local injection of vasoconstrictors, foreign bodies, damaged tissues from earlier injury, and concurrent microbial infections. Clostridial myonecrosis is rare when wounds are subjected to prompt and thorough debridement of traumatized tissue.

The necrosis of previously healthy muscle is caused by myotoxins elaborated by a few species of clostridia. *C. perfringens* type A is the most common source of myotoxin (80% to 90% of cases), but myotoxin may also be produced by *C. novyi* and *C. septicum*. Clostridial myotoxin is a phospholipase that destroys the membranes of muscle cells and of leukocytes and erythrocytes.

☐ **Pathology:** Initially, affected tissues are pale and edematous, but they rapidly become mottled and then frankly necrotic. Tissues such as muscle may even liquefy. The overlying skin becomes tense, as edema and gas expand the underlying soft tissues. Microscopic examination shows extensive tissue necrosis with dissolution of the normal cellular architecture. A striking feature is the paucity of neutrophils, which are apparently destroyed by the myotoxin. Gram stain of affected tissues often shows typical, lozenge-shaped, gram-positive rods.

☐ **Clinical Features:** The incubation period of gas gangrene is commonly 2 to 4 days after injury. Sudden, severe pain occurs at the site of the wound, which is tender and edematous. The skin darkens, because of hemorrhage and cutaneous necrosis. The lesion develops a thick, serosanguineous discharge, which has a fragrant odor and may contain gas bubbles. Sweating, low-grade fever, and disproportionate tachycardia rapidly give way to hemolytic anemia, hypotension, and renal failure. In the terminal stages, coma, jaundice, and shock supervene.

FIGURE 9-27

Clostridial diseases. Clostridia in the vegetative form (bacilli) inhabit the gastrointestinal tract of humans and animals. Spores pass in the feces, contaminate soil and plant materials, and are ingested or enter sites of penetrating wounds. Under anaerobic conditions they revert to vegetative forms. Plasmids in the vegetative forms elaborate toxins that cause several clostridial diseases.

Food poisoning and necrotizing enteritis. Meat dishes left to cool at room temperature grow large numbers of clostridia (> 10^6 organisms per gram). When contaminated meat is ingested, *C. perfringens* types A and C produce alpha-enterotoxin in the small intestine during sporulation, causing abdominal pain and diarrhea. Type C also produces beta-enterotoxin.

Gas gangrene. Clostridia are widespread and may contaminate a traumatic wound or surgical operation. *C. perfringens* type A elaborates a myotoxin (alpha-toxin), a lecithinase that destroys cell membranes, alters capillary permeability, and causes severe hemolysis following intravenous injection. The toxin causes necrosis of previously healthy skeletal muscle.

Tetanus. Spores of *C. tetani* are in soil, and enter the site of an accidental wound. Necrotic tissue at the wound site causes spores to revert to the vegetative form (bacilli). Autolysis of vegetative forms releases tetanus toxin. The toxin is transported in peripheral nerves and (retrograde) through axons to the anterior horn cells of the spinal cord. The toxin blocks synaptic inhibition, and the accumulation of acetylcholine in damaged synapses leads to rigidity and spasms of the skeletal musculature (tetany).

Botulism. Improperly canned food is contaminated by the vegetative form of *C. botulinum*, which proliferates under aerobic conditions and elaborates a neurotoxin. After the food is ingested, the neurotoxin is absorbed from the small intestine and eventually reaches the myoneural junction, where it inhibits the release of acetylcholine. The result is a symmetric descending paralysis of cranial nerves, trunk, and limbs, with eventual respiratory paralysis and death.

Tetanus

Tetanus is a severe, acute neurological syndrome of humans and other mammals caused by tetanus toxin, an extremely potent neurotoxin elaborated by plasmids of C. tetani. The disease is characterized by spastical contractions of skeletal muscles. It is also known as "lockjaw" because of early involvement of the muscles of mastication.

☐ **Epidemiology:** *C. tetani* is a common environmental organism, present in the soil and the lower intestine of many animals. Tetanus occurs when the organism contaminates wounds and proliferates in tissue, releasing its exotoxin. A vaccine composed of inactivated tetanus toxin is highly effective in preventing tetanus, and immunization programs have largely eliminated the disease from developed countries. Nonetheless, tetanus remains a frequent and lethal disease in developing countries. In the United States, fewer than 150 cases of tetanus occur annually, resulting in fewer than 50 deaths. On the other hand, more than 1 million cases occur annually worldwide, most of which are fatal. Contributing factors include the presence of herbivorous animals (especially horses and cattle), frequency of tetanus-prone wounds, abortion practices, and the immune status of the population. Many deaths occur in newborns, owing to the custom of coating the umbilical stump with dirt or dung to prevent bleeding. In developed countries, tetanus is frequently associated with drug addiction.

☐ **Pathogenesis:** At the site of injury, necrotic tissue and suppuration contribute to the creation of an anaerobic environment, a condition that causes spores to revert to vegetative cells. Tetanus toxin is released from autolyzed vegetative cells. Although the clostridial infection remains localized, the potent neurotoxin (tetanospasmin) undergoes retrograde transport through the ventral roots of peripheral nerves to the anterior horn cells of the spinal cord. The toxin crosses the synapse and binds to ganglioside receptors on presynaptic terminals of motor neurons in the ventral horns. Following internalization, the endopeptidase activity of the toxin selectively cleaves a protein responsible for the exocytosis of synaptic vesicles. As a result, the release of inhibitory neurotransmitters is blocked, thereby permitting unopposed neural stimulation and sustained contraction of skeletal muscles (tetany). The block to the release of inhibitory neurotransmitters also induces acceleration of the heart rate, hypertension, and cardiovascular instability. Tetanospasmin produces no specific histopathology.

☐ **Clinical Features:** The incubation period of tetanus is 1 to 3 weeks. The disease begins subtly with fatigue, weakness, and muscle cramping, which progresses to muscle rigidity. Spastic rigidity often begins in the muscles of the face, giving rise to "lockjaw" or spastic rigidity of several facial muscles, causing a fixed grin (risus sardonicus). Rigidity of the muscles of the back produces a backward arching (opisthotonos) (Fig. 9-28). Abrupt stimuli, including noise, light, or touch, can precipitate painful generalized muscle spasms. Swallowing and breathing may be impaired by involvement of associated muscles. Prolonged spasm of the respiratory and laryngeal musculature may lead to death.

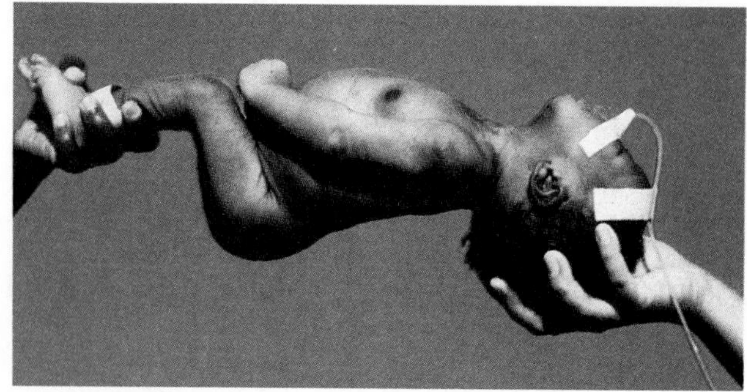

FIGURE *9-28*
Tetanus. Opisthotonus (backward arching) in an infant due to intense contraction of the paravertebral muscles.

The outcome of tetanus depends on the age of the patient, the inoculum of toxin, and the availability of medical support. Administration of antibody to bind unabsorbed toxin, antibiotics to eliminate infection, and supportive care, including respiratory support, are the mainstays of therapy. Infants and persons older than 50 years of age have the highest mortality.

Botulism

Botulism is a paralyzing illness that follows the ingestion of food containing the preformed neurotoxins of C. botulinum. The disease is characterized by a symmetric descending paralysis of cranial nerves, limbs, and trunk.

☐ **Epidemiology:** The spores of *C. botulinum* are widely distributed in soil and animals and contaminate many foods . The spores survive unfavorable conditions and are especially resistant to drying and boiling. **In the United States, the toxin is most commonly present in vegetables or other foods that have been improperly home-canned and stored without refrigeration. These circumstances provide suitable anaerobic conditions for the growth of the vegetative cells that elaborate the neurotoxins (A-G).** There is no overt clue to the fact that the food is tainted, since toxin production does not alter the appearance or taste of the food.

Botulism can also be contracted from home-cured ham and other meats that have been left unrefrigerated for several days and from raw, smoked, and fermented fish products. The disease is also caused by the absorption of toxin from organisms proliferating in the intestine of infants (infantile botulism) or rarely by the absorption of toxin from organisms growing in contaminated wounds (wound botulism).

☐ **Pathogenesis:** After food containing botulinum neurotoxin is ingested, the toxin resists gastric digestion and is readily absorbed into the blood from the proximal small intestine. Circulating toxin reaches the cholinergic nerve endings at the myoneural junction and binds to gangliosides of the presynaptic nerve terminals. In this location, it inhibits the release of acetylcholine by a mechanism similar to that of tetanus toxin and produces a flaccid paralysis. The toxin is present in extraordinarily minute quantities, and its action at the neuromuscular junction produces no distinctive pathological changes.

☐ **Clinical Features:** Botulism causes a descending paralysis, first affecting the cranial nerves and beginning with blurred vision, photophobia, dry mouth, and dysarthria. Weakness progresses to involve the neck muscles, extremities, diaphragm, and accessory muscles of breathing. Respiratory weakness can progress rapidly to complete respiratory arrest and death. Nonfatal, flaccid paralysis can also produce significant secondary effects, including severe wasting, bedsores, and aspiration pneumonia.

Prompt administration of antitoxin prevents the action of botulinum toxin that has not been bound to the presynaptic membrane. Supportive care includes assisted respiration. Untreated botulism food poisoning is usually lethal, but treatment reduces the mortality to 25%.

Clostridium difficile Colitis

C. difficile colitis is an acute necrotizing infection of the terminal small bowel and colon. C. difficile colitis is responsible for a large fraction (25% to 50%) of the antibiotic-associated diarrheas and is potentially lethal.

☐ **Epidemiology:** *C. difficile* resides in the colon in some healthy persons. A change in intestinal flora, usually precipitated by antibiotic administration, allows the organism to flourish, produce toxin, and damage the colonic mucosa.

Because of its association with antibiotic administration, *C. difficile* colitis is frequently called "antibiotic-associated colitis." Such colitis, however, can also be precipitated by other insults to the colonic flora, such as bowel surgery, dietary changes, and antineoplastic chemotherapeutic agents. In hospitals where many patients receive antibiotics, *C. difficile* colitis is usually a leading cause of diarrhea, and fecal shedding of the organism leads to person to person spread.

☐ **Pathology:** The colonic flora ordinarily prevent the pathogenic action of *C. difficile.* Alterations in the normal flora permit *C. difficile* to proliferate, elaborate toxins, and destroy mucosal cells. The bacterium does not invade the colonic mucosa but rather produces two exotoxins. Toxin A causes fluid secretion, whereas toxin B is directly cytopathic.

C. difficile destroys colonic mucosal cells and incites an acute inflammatory infiltrate. Lesions range from focal colitis limited to a few crypts and only detectable on biopsy, to massive confluent mucosal ulceration. The inflammatory infiltrate initially involves only the mucosa, but if the disease progresses, it can extend into the submucosa and muscularis propria. An inflammatory exudate, called a "pseudomembrane," often forms over affected areas of the colon. This membrane is composed of cellular debris, neutrophils, and fibrin. *C. difficile* colitis is often called pseudomembranous colitis, even though this organism is only one of several causes of pseudomembranous colitis.

☐ **Clinical Features:** *C. difficile* colitis may present with very mild symptoms or with diarrhea, fever and abdominal pain. Stools may be profuse and often contain neutrophils. The symptoms and signs are not specific and do not distinguish *C. difficile* colitis from other acute inflammatory diarrheal illnesses. Mild cases of *C. difficile* diarrhea can often be treated simply by discontinuing the precipitating antibiotic. More severe cases require treatment with an antibiotic effective against *C. difficile.*

BACTERIAL INFECTION WITH ANIMAL RESERVOIRS OR INSECT VECTORS

Brucellosis

Brucellosis is a zoonotic disease caused by one of four Brucella species. Human brucellosis may present as an acute systemic disease or as a chronic infection characterized by waxing and waning febrile episodes, weight loss, and fatigue. Brucella species are small, aerobic, gram-negative rods, which in humans primarily infect monocytes/macrophages.

☐ **Epidemiology:** Each species of *Brucella* has its own animal reservoir:

- *B. melitensis*: sheep and goats
- *B. abortus*: cattle
- *B. suis*: swine
- *B. canis*: dogs

Brucellosis is encountered worldwide and in all climates. Virtually every type of domesticated animal and many wild ones are affected. The prevalence of human disease relates to occupational exposure, cultural or socioeconomic conditions that lead to close contact with animals, and consumption of contaminated milk or milk products.

The organisms reside in the genitourinary systems of these animals, and infection is often endemic in animal herds. Humans acquire the bacteria by several mechanisms, including (1) contact with infected blood or tissue, (2) ingestion of contaminated meat or milk, or (3) inhalation of contaminated aerosols. Brucellosis is an occupational hazard among ranchers, herders, veterinarians, and slaughterhouse workers.

Elimination of infected animals and vaccination of herds have reduced the incidence of brucellosis in many countries, including the United States, where only about 200 cases are reported to the Centers for Disease Control annually. Yet, the disease remains prevalent throughout Central and South America, Africa, Asia, and Southern Europe. Unpasteurized milk and cheese remain a major source of infection in these areas. In the arctic and subarctic regions, humans acquire brucellosis by eating raw bone marrow of infected reindeer.

☐ **Pathology:** Bacteria enter the circulation through skin abrasions, the conjunctiva, oropharynx, or lungs. They then spread in the bloodstream to the liver, spleen, lymph nodes, and bone marrow, where they multiply in macrophages. A generalized hyperplasia of these cells may ensue, causing lymphadenopathy and hepatosplenomegaly in 10% to 20% of patients infected with *B. melitensis* and in 40% of those infected with *B. abortus*. Patients infected with *B. abortus* develop conspicuous noncaseating granulomas in the liver, spleen, lymph nodes, and bone marrow. By contrast, classic granulomas are not present in patients infected with *B. melitensis*, who may have only small aggregates of mononuclear inflammatory cells scattered throughout the liver. *B. suis* infection may cause suppurative liver abscesses rather than granulomas. The organisms usually cannot be demonstrated histologically. Periodic release of organisms from infected phagocytic cells may be responsible for the febrile episodes of the illness.

☐ **Clinical Features:** Brucellosis is a systemic infection that can involve any organ or organ system of the body. Symptoms are nonspecific, generally occurring within 2 to 3 weeks of inoculation. The onset of disease is insidious in half of the cases. The disease is characterized by a multitude of somatic complaints, such as fever, sweats, anorexia, fatigue, weight loss, and depression. By contrast, there can be a paucity of abnormal physical findings, of which the most notable are fever, mild lymphadenopathy, and occasionally hepatosplenomegaly. Fever occurs in all patients at some time during the illness, but it can wax and wane (hence the term *undulant fever*) over a period of weeks to months when untreated. Occasionally symptoms related to a single organ predominate, in which case the disease is termed localized. Not unexpectedly, localization usually involves an organ rich in elements of the mononuclear phagocyte system. The mortality rate from brucellosis is less than 1%; death is usually caused by endocarditis.

The most common complications of brucellosis involve the bones and joints and include spondylitis of the lumbar spine and suppuration in large joints. Peripheral neuritis, meningitis, orchitis, endocarditis, myocarditis, and pulmonary lesions are described. Prolonged treatment with tetracycline is usually effective; the relapse rate is dramatically reduced if rifampin or an aminoglycoside is added.

Plague

Yersinia pestis causes plague, a bacteremic infection that is usually accompanied by enlarged, painful regional lymph nodes (bubos) and is often fatal. Historically, devastating epidemics made this disease the scourge of the civilized world. *Y. pestis* is a short gram-negative rod, which tends to stain more heavily at the ends (i.e., bipolar staining), particularly with Giemsa stains.

☐ **Epidemiology:** *Y. pestis* infection is an endemic zoonosis in many parts of the world, including the Americas, Africa, and Asia. The organisms are found in wild rodents, such as rats, squirrels, and prairie dogs. Fleas transmit the bacterium from animal to animal, and most human infections result from the bites of infected fleas. Some infected humans develop plague pneumonia, shedding large numbers of organisms in aerosolized respiratory secretions. Infection can be transmitted from person to person in these respiratory aerosols.

Major plague epidemics have occurred when *Y. pestis* was introduced into large urban rat populations in crowded, squalid cities. Infection spreads first among the rats; as the rats die, large numbers of infected fleas begin feeding on the human population, causing widespread disease. Spread from rats to persons, the "black death" of the mid-14th century killed over one fourth of the European population.

Plague still occurs, almost always as sporadic cases, throughout endemic areas. In the United States, 30 to 40 cases of plague occur annually, most in the desert southwest.

☐ **Pathology:** After inoculation into the skin, *Y. pestis* is phagocytosed by neutrophils and macrophages. Organisms ingested by neutrophils are killed, but those engulfed by macrophages survive and replicate intracellularly. The bacteria are carried to regional lymph nodes, where they continue to multiply, producing extensive hemorrhagic necrosis. From the regional lymph nodes, they disseminate throughout the body through the bloodstream and lymphatics. In the lungs, *Y. pestis* produces a necrotizing pneumonitis that releases organisms into the alveoli and airways. These are expelled by coughing, enabling pneumonic spread of the disease.

Affected lymph nodes, known as "bubos," are frequently enlarged and fluctuant, owing to extensive hemorrhagic necrosis. Microscopic examination shows irregular zones of cytolysis with large numbers of bacteria in cellular debris. In plague pneumonia, the consolidation can be patchy or diffuse. Microscopically, the affected portions of the lung show hemorrhagic necrosis of alveolar walls and large numbers of bacteria are apparent within the alveoli. Infected patients often develop necrotic, hemorrhagic skin lesions, hence the name "black death" for this disease.

☐ **Clinical Features:** There are three clinical presentations of *Y. pestis* infection, although they often overlap.

Bubonic plague begins within 2 to 8 days of the flea bite, with headache, fever, and myalgias, accompanied by painful enlargement of regional lymph nodes, most commonly those of the groin, because flea bites usually occur in the lower extremities. The disease progresses to septic shock within hours to days after the appearance of the bubo.

Septicemic plague (10% of cases) occurs when bacteria are inoculated directly into the blood and do not produce bubos. Patients die of the overwhelming growth of the bacteria in the bloodstream. Fever, prostration, and meningitis occur suddenly, and death ensues within 48 hours. All blood vessels contain bacilli, and fibrin casts surround the organisms in renal glomeruli and dermal vessels.

Pneumonic plague results from the inhalation of airborne particles from the carcasses of animals or the cough of infected persons. Within 2 to 5 days after infection, there is a sudden onset of high fever, cough, and dyspnea. The sputum teems with bacilli. Respiratory insufficiency and endotoxic shock kill the patient within 1 to 2 days.

All types of plague carry a high mortality rate (50% to 75%) if untreated. Tetracycline combined with streptomycin is the recommended therapy.

Tularemia

Tularemia is an acute, febrile, granulomatous disease caused by Francisella tularensis, a small, gram-negative coccobacillus.

☐ **Epidemiology:** Tularemia is a zoonosis whose most important reservoirs are rabbits and rodents, although other wild and domestic animals may harbor the organisms. Human infection with *F. tularensis* results from contact with infected animals or from the bites of infected insects, including ticks, deerflies, and mosquitoes. Ticks and rabbits are responsible for most human infections. The blood-sucking insect inoculates the organism into the skin on feeding. The bacteria may also be inoculated into unnoticed breaks in the skin by direct contact with an infected animal. In addition, tularemia can result from the inhalation of infected aerosols, ingestion of contaminated food and water, or inoculation into the eye. Tularemia is found in temperate zones of the Northern Hemisphere. The incidence of the infection has fallen dramatically in the United States in the past five decades, to about 250 cases annually, presumably related to a decline in hunting and trapping.

☐ **Pathogenesis:** *F. tularensis* multiplies at the site of inoculation, where it produces a focal ulceration. The bacteria then spread to regional lymph nodes. Dissemination in the bloodstream leads to metastatic infections that involve the monocyte/macrophage system and sometimes the lungs, heart, and kidneys. *F. tularensis* survives within macrophages, until these cells are activated by a cell-mediated immune response to the infection.

☐ **Pathology:** Lesions of tularemia occur at the inoculation site and in lymph nodes, spleen, liver, bone marrow, lungs (Fig. 9-29), heart, and kidneys. The initial skin lesion is an exudative, pyogenic ulcer. Later, disseminated lesions undergo central necrosis and are surrounded by a perimeter of granulomatous reaction resembling the lesions of tuberculosis. Hyperemia and the presence of numerous macrophages in the sinuses make lymph nodes large and firm; they subsequently soften as necrosis and suppuration develop. The spleen tends to be enlarged but shows only nonspecific changes. The pulmonary lesions resemble those of primary tuberculosis.

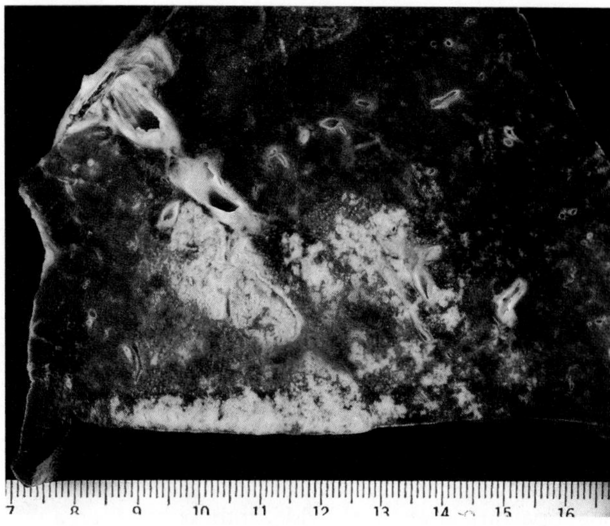

FIGURE *9-29*
Tularemia. The lung shows firm, consolidated, and necrotic areas.

☐ **Clinical Features:** The incubation period of tularemia ranges from 1 to 14 days, depending on the dose and route of transmission, with a mean of 3 to 4 days. There are four distinct clinical presentations.

- **Ulceroglandular tularemia** is the most common form of the disease (80% to 90% of the cases) and begins as a tender, erythematous papule at the site of inoculation, usually on a limb. This develops into a pustule, which then ulcerates. The regional lymph nodes become large and tender and may suppurate and drain through sinus tracts. In some instances, generalized lymphadenopathy (glandular tularemia) is the first manifestation of the infection.
  The initial bacteremia is accompanied by fever, headache, myalgias, and occasionally prostration. Within a week, generalized lymphadenopathy and splenomegaly become evident. The most serious infections are complicated by secondary pneumonia and endotoxic shock, in which case the prognosis is grave. Some patients develop meningitis, endocarditis, pericarditis, or osteomyelitis.
- **Oculoglandular tularemia** is rare (<2% of the cases) and is characterized by a primary papule in the conjunctiva, which forms a pustule and ulcerates. Lymphadenopathy of the head and neck become prominent. Severe ulceration may cause blindness, owing to penetration of the sclera and infection of the optic nerve.
- **Typhoidal tularemia** is diagnosed when fever, hepatosplenomegaly, and toxemia are the presenting signs and symptoms.
- **Pneumonic tularemia**, in which pneumonia is a major feature, may complicate any of the other types.

The duration of illness is 1 week to 3 months, but this may be shortened by prompt treatment with streptomycin.

Anthrax

Anthrax is a necrotizing disease caused by Bacillus anthracis, which is rapidly fatal when it disseminates from localized sites of infection. The cause of anthrax is a large spore-forming, gram-positive rod.

☐ **Epidemiology:** Anthrax is a zoonosis in which the major reservoirs are goats, sheep, cattle, horses, pigs, and dogs. Spores form in the soil and dead animals, resisting heat, desiccation, and chemical disinfection for years. Humans are infected when spores enter the body through breaks in the skin, by inhalation, or by ingestion. Human disease may also result from exposure to contaminated animal byproducts, such as hides, wool, brushes, or bone meal.

Although there are foci of *B. anthracis* in contaminated pasture lands worldwide, anthrax has been a persistent problem in Iran, Turkey, Pakistan, and the Sudan. An epidemic of inhalation anthrax with a large number of deaths occurred in 1979 in the former Soviet Union as a result of the accidental explosion of a biological weapons plant located in an urban area. The disaster was revealed only after the collapse of the Soviet Union, years after it occurred. In North America, human infection is extremely rare (one case per year for the past few years) and usually results from exposure to imported animal products.

☐ **Pathology:** The spores of *B. anthracis* germinate in the human body to yield vegetative bacteria, which multiply and release a potent necrotizing toxin. In 80% of cases of cutaneous anthrax, the infection remains localized, and the host immunological response eventually eliminates the organism. If the infection disseminates, as occurs when the organisms are inhaled or ingested, the resulting widespread tissue destruction is usually fatal.

B. anthracis produces extensive tissue necrosis at the sites of infection, associated with only a mild infiltrate of neutrophils. Cutaneous lesions are ulcerated, contain numerous organisms and are covered by a black scab. Pulmonary infection produces a necrotizing, hemorrhagic pneumonia, associated with hemorrhagic necrosis of mediastinal lymph nodes and widespread dissemination of the organism.

☐ **Clinical Features:** There are four presentations of anthrax, depending on the site of inoculation.

- **Malignant pustule**, which accounts for 95% of all anthrax, is the cutaneous form of the disease. The infected person presents with an elevated cutaneous papule that enlarges and erodes into an ulcer. Bloody purulent exudate accumulates and gradually darkens to purple or black. The ulcer is often surrounded by a zone of brawny edema, which seems disproportionately large relative to the size of the ulcer. Regional lymphadenitis portends a poor prognosis, because invasion of lymphatics precedes septicemia. If the infection does not disseminate, the cutaneous lesions heal without sequelae.
- **Pulmonary anthrax**, sometimes called "woolsorters' disease," is a hazard of handling raw wool and develops after the inhalation of the spores of *B. anthracis*. Pulmonary anthrax presents as a flu-like illness that rapidly progresses to respiratory failure, shock, and death. The only hope is early antibiotic therapy.
- **Septicemic anthrax** more commonly follows pulmonary anthrax than malignant pustule. Disseminated intravascular coagulation is a common complication. Moreover, a bacterial toxin depresses the respiratory center, which explains the fact that death can occur even when antibiotic therapy has cured the infection.
- **Gastrointestinal anthrax** is rare and is acquired by eating contaminated meat. Ulceration of the stomach or bowel and invasion of the regional lymphatics are common. Death is caused by fulminant diarrhea and massive ascites.

Listeriosis

Listeriosis is a systemic multiorgan infection caused by Listeria monocytogenes, a small, motile, gram-positive coccobacillus.

☐ **Epidemiology:** Listeriosis is usually sporadic but may also be epidemic. The organism has been isolated worldwide from surface water, soil, vegetation, the feces of healthy persons, many species of wild and domestic mammals, and several species of birds. In spite of this wide distribution, the spread of infection from animals to humans is rare. Most human infections are in urban rather than rural environments, and in the Northern Hemisphere, occur during July and August. The peak months of infection in animals are January through May. Some infections have been traced to unpasteurized milk. *L. monocytogenes* grows at refrigerator temperatures, and outbreaks of listeriosis have been traced to contaminated cheese and other dairy products.

☐ **Pathogenesis:** *L. monocytogenes* has an unusual life cycle, which accounts for its ability to evade intracellular and extracellular antibacterial defense mechanisms. After phagocytosis by host cells, the organism enters a phagolysosome, where the acidic pH activates **lysteriolysin O**, an exotoxin that disrupts the vesicular membrane and permits escape of the bacterium into the cytoplasm. After replicating, the bacteria usurp the contractile elements of the host cytoskeleton to form elongated protrusions that are ingested by adjacent cells. Thus, *Listeria* spread from one cell to another without exposure to the extracellular environment.

☐ **Pathology and Clinical Features:** Most *Listeria* infections fall into one of two groups. **Listeriosis of pregnancy includes prenatal and postnatal infections.** Listeriosis of the adult population is most commonly characterized by **meningoencephalitis and septicemia**, but may be localized to skin, eyes, lymph nodes, endocardium or bones.

Maternal infection early in pregnancy leads to abortion or premature delivery. Infected premature infants develop symptoms of infection within a few hours of birth, including respiratory distress, hepatosplenomegaly, cutaneous and mucosal papules, leukopenia, and thrombocytopenia. Neonatal listeriosis may also be acquired during delivery, in which case the onset of clinical disease is 3 days to 2 weeks after birth. Intrauterine infections involve many organs and tissues, including the amniotic fluid, placenta, and the umbilical cord. Widespread abscesses are found in many organs. Microscopically, foci of necrosis and suppuration contain many bacteria. Older lesions tend to be granulomatous. Neurological sequelae are common, and the mortality is high even with prompt antibiotic therapy.

Chronic alcoholics, patients with cancer, and those receiving immunosuppressive therapy are all susceptible to listeriosis. Patients with AIDS are 100 to 300 times more susceptible to infection than the general population. Meningitis is the most common form of the disease in adults and resembles other bacterial meningitides. Microscopically, the leptomeninges are infiltrated with lymphocytes, plasma cells, macrophages, and neutrophils.

Septicemic listeriosis is most common in immunodeficient patients. It is a severe febrile illness that may lead to shock and disseminated intravascular coagulation, a situation that may be erroneously diagnosed as gram-negative sepsis. A suppurative leptomeningitis can occur, and the brain may be seeded with miliary abscesses. Prolonged treatment with antimicrobials is usually required in cases of listeriosis because patients tend to experience relapse if therapy is administered for less than 3 weeks. Despite such aggressive therapy, the overall mortality from systemic listeriosis remains at 25%.

Cat-Scratch Disease

Cat-scratch disease is a self-limited infection usually caused by Bartonella henselae, and more rarely by B. quintana. The bacteria are small (0.2 to 0.6 μm) gram-negative rods. These organisms are difficult to culture but are easily seen in tissue sections of the skin, lymph nodes, and conjunctiva, when stained with a silver impregnation technique (Fig. 9-30).

☐ **Epidemiology:** The reservoir is thought to be cats; various surveys have shown that up to 30% of cats are bacteremic. Infection begins when the bacillus is inoculated into the skin by the claws of cats (and rarely other animals) or by thorns or splinters. Sometimes the conjunctiva is contaminated by close contact with a cat, possibly by licking around the eye. In fact, cat-scratch disease is the most common cause of the **oculoglandular syndrome**, characterized by swelling of the eye, jaw, and cervical lymph nodes. Infections are more common in children (80%) than in adults, and there may be clustering of cases when a stray cat joins a family.

☐ **Pathology:** At the site of inoculation, the bacteria multiply in the walls of small vessels and about collagen fibers. The organisms are then carried to regional lymph nodes, where they produce a **suppurative and granulomatous lymphadenitis**. In early lesions, clusters of bacteria fill and expand the lumina of small blood vessels. Bacteria are rare in late lesions.

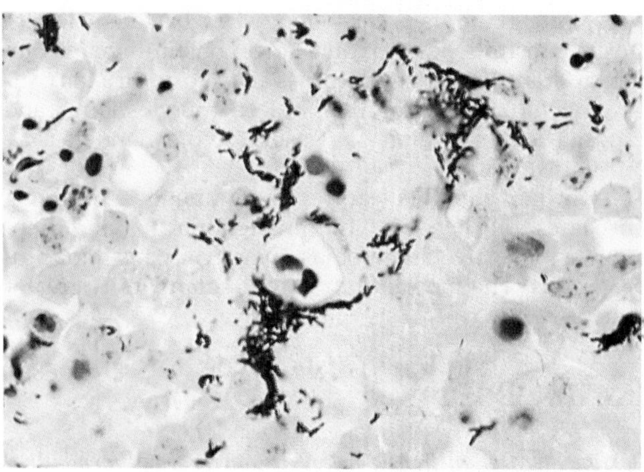

FIGURE *9-30*
Cat-scratch disease. Section of a lymph node shows the bacilli, which are gram-negative but difficult to visualize with tissue gram stains. They are blackened by the Warthin-Starry silver impregnation technique.

☐ **Clinical Features:** Most patients develop a papule at the site of inoculation, although it may be small and overlooked. The papule begins 3 to 14 days after the scratch and may persist for 2 months. Tenderness and enlargement of regional lymph nodes ensue. The nodes remain enlarged for 3 to 4 months and may drain through the skin. About half of the patients have other symptoms, including fever and malaise, rash, a brief encephalitis, and erythema nodosum. Parinaud oculoglandular syndrome (preauricular adenopathy secondary to conjunctival infection) is common.

Without biopsy and the visualization of the characteristic bacteria, the diagnosis of cat-scratch disease is supported when three criteria are met: (1) contact with a cat, a cat scratch, or a primary lesion of the skin or conjunctiva; (2) a positive serological test for antibodies against *B. henselae* antigen; and (3) negative results from laboratory studies for other causes of lymphadenopathy. No antibiotic has been accepted as beneficial.

Glanders

Glanders is an infection of equine species (horses, mules, donkeys) that is only rarely transmitted to humans, in whom it causes acute or chronic granulomatous disease. The cause is *Pseudomonas mallei*, a small gram-negative, nonmotile bacillus. Although uncommon, the infection remains endemic in South America, Asia, and Africa. Humans acquire the disease by contact with infected equines through broken skin or by inhalation of contaminated aerosols. The clinical course of glanders may be acute and severe or protracted and wasting.

Acute glanders is characterized by bacteremia, with severe prostration, fever, and other constitutional symptoms. Granulomatous abscesses may form in many organs, including the lung, liver, spleen, muscles, joints, and especially the subcutaneous tissues. Acute glanders is almost always fatal.

Chronic glanders features low-grade fever, draining abscesses of the skin, lymphadenopathy, and hepatosplenomegaly. Granulomas in many organs mimic tuberculosis. The mortality in chronic glanders is greater than 50%.

Bartonellosis

Bartonellosis is an infection by Bartonella bacilliformis that causes acute anemia (Oroya fever) and a chronic skin disease (verruga peruana). The organism is a small, multiflagellated, gram-negative coccobacillus.

☐ **Epidemiology:** Bartonellosis occurs only in Peru, Ecuador, and Colombia in river valleys of the Andes. Interestingly, deformities that appear to represent verruga peruana are depicted in the pottery of the pre-Incan inhabitants of Peru, and the disease was noted by the Spanish conquistadors almost five centuries ago.

Bartonellosis is transmitted by sandflies. Humans provide the only reservoir and acquire the infection at sunrise and sunset, when sandflies are most active. In endemic areas, 10% to 15% of the population have latent infections. Newcomers are susceptible, whereas the indigenous population tends to be resistant.

☐ **Pathology and Clinical Features:** Bartonellosis presents a biphasic pattern, with acute hemolytic anemia first, followed some months later by a chronic dermal phase. Either phase may occur by itself.

The most severe consequence of bartonellosis is hemolyic anemia. After *B. bacilliformis* has been inoculated into the skin by a sandfly, the bacteria proliferate in the vascular endothelium and then invade erythrocytes. The growth of the organisms within the erythrocytes results in profound hemolysis.

The acute anemic phase follows an incubation period of 3 weeks and is characterized by an abrupt onset of fever, skeletal pains, and a severe, often macrocytic, hemolytic anemia. The erythrocyte count may fall in a few days to less than 500,000/μL. Secondary *Salmonella* septicemia is frequent and contributes to the high mortality. In untreated bartonellosis, 40% of patients in the anemic phase die. If the patient does not succumb, the bacilli in the erythrocytes gradually decline in number, and hemolysis ceases.

The dermal eruptive phase of bartonellosis may coexist with the anemic phase, but is usually separated by an interval of 3 to 6 months. Many small hemangioma-like lesions stud the dermis, and bacteria may be identified in endothelial cells. Nodular lesions may be prominent on the extensor surfaces of the arms and legs. Large deep-seated lesions, which tend to ulcerate, develop near joints and limit motion. Clinically and microscopically, the lesions of chronic cutaneous bartonellosis must be distinguished from Kaposi sarcoma and pyogenic granuloma. The dermal eruptive phase is often prolonged but eventually heals spontaneously. The mortality in this phase is less than 5%.

A number of antibiotics are effective against *B. bacilliformis*, but the chronic phase does not respond well.

INFECTIONS CAUSED BY BRANCHING FILAMENTOUS ORGANISMS

Actinomycosis

Actinomycosis is a slowly progressive, suppurative, fibrosing infection involving the jaw, thorax, or abdomen. The disease is caused by a number of anaerobic and microaerophilic bacteria termed *Actinomyces.* These organisms are branching, filamentous, gram-positive rods, which grow slowly only under conditions of reduced oxygen and normally reside in the human oropharynx, gastrointestinal tract, and vagina. Although *Actinomyces* organisms are now recognized as bacteria, they were long considered fungi because of their filamentous morphology. Several *Actinomyces* species cause human disease, the most common being *Actinomyces israelii.*

Actinomyces organisms inhabit the anaerobic crevices of the mouth, including the tonsillar crypts, gingival crevices, and areas covered by dental plaque. Actinomycosis is acquired from the endogenous flora and is not transmitted from person to person.

☐ **Pathology:** *Actinomyces* is not ordinarily virulent, and the organisms reside as saprophytes in the body without producing disease. Two uncommon conditions must occur for *Actinomyces* to establish disease First, the organism must be inoculated into deeper tissues, since it cannot invade. Second, an anaerobic atmosphere is necessary for the bacteria to proliferate. Trauma can produce tissue necrosis, providing an excellent anaerobic medium for growth of *Actinomyces*, and can inoculate the organism into normally sterile tissue. Actinomycosis occurs at four distinct sites:

- **Cervicofacial actinomycosis** results from jaw injury, dental extraction, or dental manipulation.
- **Thoracic actinomycosis** is caused by the aspiration of organisms contaminating dental debris.
- **Abdominal actinomycosis** follows traumatic or surgical disruption of the bowel, especially the appendix.
- **Pelvic actinomycosis** is associated with the prolonged use of intrauterine devices (IUD). Women with neglected IUDs have increased actinomycotic flora of the vagina and cervix, and the attached string becomes a nidus for the growth of the organisms. Moreover, the endometrium about the IUD becomes sufficiently necrotic that colonizing bacteria may thrive and spread, with a risk of tubal or ovarian actinomycosis.

Actinomycosis begins as a nidus of proliferating organisms, which attracts an acute inflammatory infiltrate. The small abscess grows slowly, becoming a series of abscesses connected by sinus tracts. Tracts burrow across normal tissue boundaries and into adjacent organs. Eventually, a tract may penetrate onto an external surface or mucosal membrane, producing a draining sinus. The walls of the abscess and tracts are composed of granulation tissue, often thick, densely fibrotic, and chronically inflamed. Within the abscesses and sinuses are pus and colonies of organisms. The slowly expanding fibrotic mass tends to invade across tissue boundaries and contains multiple areas of necrosis, often resembling a malignant tumor.

The colonies of *Actinomyces* within these lesions can grow to several millimeters in diameter and be visible to the naked eye. They appear as hard, yellow grains known as **sulfur granules**, because of their resemblance to elemental sulfur. Sulfur granules consist of tangled masses of narrow, branching filaments, embedded in a polysaccharide—protein matrix (Splendore-Hoeppli material). Histologically, the colonies appear as rounded, purple (with hematoxylin) grains with scalloped eosinophilic borders (Fig. 9-31A). The individual filaments of *Actinomyces* cannot be discerned with the hematoxylin and eosin stain but are readily visible on Gram staining or silver impregnation (see Fig. 9-31B).

☐ **Clinical Features:** Actinomycosis is an indolent, slowly progressive infection. Fever is variably present and often low grade. Constitutional symptoms of fatigue and weight loss commonly appear late in the course of infection. The eruption of a draining sinus tract may be the first evidence of disease. Untreated actinomycosis may destroy vital structures.

The signs and symptoms of actinomycosis vary according to the site of infection. Actinomycosis originating in a tooth socket or the tonsils is characterized by swelling of the jaw ("lumpy jaw"), face, and neck, at first painless and fluctuant but later painful. In pulmonary infections, sinus tracts may penetrate from lobe to lobe, through the pleura, and into ribs and vertebrae. Abdominal or pelvic disease may be encountered as an expanding mass, suggesting a locally spreading tumor. Actinomycosis responds to prolonged antibiotic therapy, and penicillin is a highly effective drug.

Nocardiosis

Nocardiosis is a suppurative infection of the lung that may spread to the brain and skin, and, less commonly, to the thyroid, liver, and other organs, frequently in immunocompromised persons. Nocardia are aerobic, gram-positive filamentous, branching bacteria. They are weakly acid-fast, a characteristic used to distinguish them from the morphologically similar actinomycetes.

☐ **Epidemiology:** *Nocardia* species are widely distributed in soil, and human disease is caused by inhalation or inoculation of soil-borne organisms. Nocardiosis is not transmitted from person to person. *Nocardia asteroides* is the species that most frequently produces human disease.

Nocardiosis affects both normal and immunocompromised hosts, but disease is more common in persons with impaired immunity, particularly cell-mediated immunity. Organ transplantation, long-term corticosteroid therapy, lymphomas, leukemias, and various other debilitating diseases predispose to *Nocardia* infections.

Two other pathogenic species of *Nocardia*, namely *N. brasiliensis* and *N. caviae*, deserve mention. Either of these may cause pulmonary nocardiosis resembling that produced by *N. asteroides*, but more characteristically they are encountered in underdeveloped countries as a cause of mycetomas. Such lesions must be distinguished from the mycetomas caused by fungi and nonfilamentous bacteria.

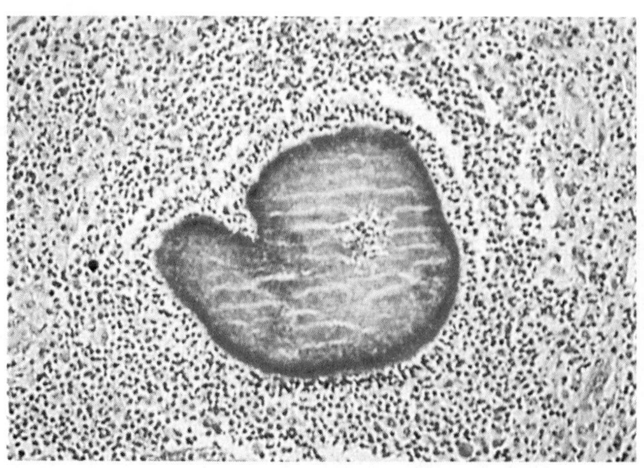
A

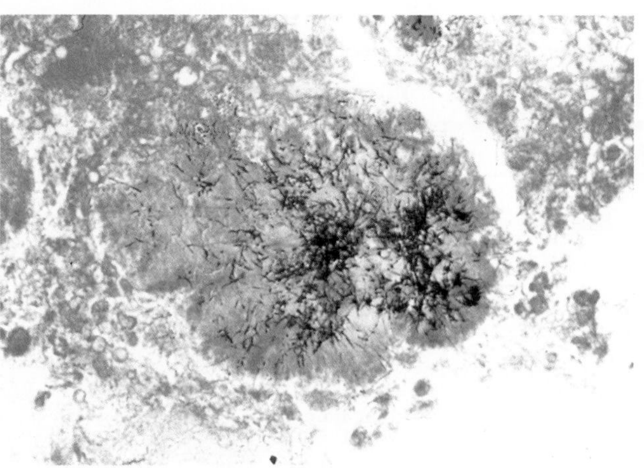
B

FIGURE *9-31*
Actinomycosis. (*A*) A typical sulfur granule lies within an abscess. (*B*) The individual filaments of *A. israeli* are readily visible with the silver impregnation technique.

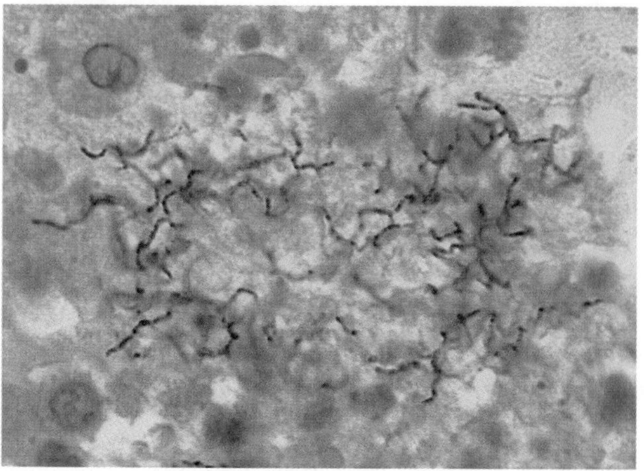

FIGURE 9-32
Nocardiosis. A silver stain of a necrotic exudate reveals the branching, filamentous rods of *N. asteroides*.

☐ Pathology: The respiratory tract is the usual portal of entry for *Nocardia*. The organism elicits a brisk infiltrate of neutrophils, and disease begins as a slowly progressive, pyogenic pneumonia. If the infected person mounts a vigorous cell-mediated immune response, the infection may be eliminated. In immunocompromised persons, however, *Nocardia* produces pulmonary abscesses, which are frequently multiple and confluent. The brain is secondarily involved in one third of infected persons. Nocardial abscesses are filled with neutrophils, necrotic debris, and scattered organisms. Bacteria are not visible on hematoxylin and eosin stains but can be demonstrated by silver impregnation (Fig. 9-32). With the Gram stain, they appear as beaded, filamentous, gram-positive rods.

☐ Clinical Features: Nonspecific, constitutional symptoms of nocardiosis include fever, fatigue, and weight loss. Invasion of the lung causes bronchopneumonia, which may extend to become lobar. Direct extension to the pleura, trachea, and heart and metastases to the brain or skin through the circulation carry a grave prognosis. Untreated nocardiosis is usually fatal. Sulfonamides or related antibiotics for several months are often effective therapy.

Spirochetal Infections

Spirochetes are long, slender, helical bacteria with specialized cell envelopes that permit them to move by flexion and rotation. Spirochetes are 0.10 to 0.30 μm in width and 10 to 30 μm in length. The thinner organisms are below the resolving power of routine light microscopy, and specialized techniques, such as darkfield microscopy or silver impregnation, are needed for their demonstration. Although spirochetes have the basic cell wall structure of gram-negative bacteria, they stain poorly with the Gram stain.

Three genera of spirochetes, *Treponema*, *Borrelia*, and *Leptospira*, cause human disease. Although the diseases and their organisms are highly diverse (Table 9-5), they share some general features. They are all inoculated locally, and disease produced at the inoculation site may disseminate through the bloodstream. Spirochetes are adept at evading host inflammatory and immunological defenses, and diseases caused by these organisms are all chronic or relapsing. Many spirochetal infections persist for years with progressive manifestations in diverse organ systems.

SYPHILIS

Syphilis (lues) is a chronic, sexually transmitted, systemic infection caused by Treponema pallidum. The disease was first recognized in Europe in the 1490s and has been related to the return of Christopher Columbus and his seamen from

TABLE 9-5 **Spirochete Infections**

Disease	Organism	Clinical Manifestation	Distribution	Mode of Transmission
	Treponemes			
Syphilis	*T. pallidum*	See text	Common worldwide	Sexual contact, congenital
Bejel	*T. endenicum (T. Pallidum,* subspecies *en denicum)*	Mucosal, skin, and bone lesions	Middle East	Mouth-to-mouth contact
Yaws	*T. pertenue (T. pallidum* subspecies *pertenue)*	Skin and bone	Tropics	Skin-to-skin contact
Pinta	*T. carateum*	Skin lesions	Latin America	Skin-to-skin contact
	Borrelia			
Lyme disease	*B. burgdorferi*	See text	North America, Europe, Russia, Asia, Africa, Australia	Tick bite
Relapsing fever	*B. recurrentis* and related species	Relapsing flulike illness	Worldwide	Tick bite, louse bite
	Leptospira			
Leptospirosis	*L. interrogans*	Flulike illness, meningitis	Worldwide	Contact with animal urine

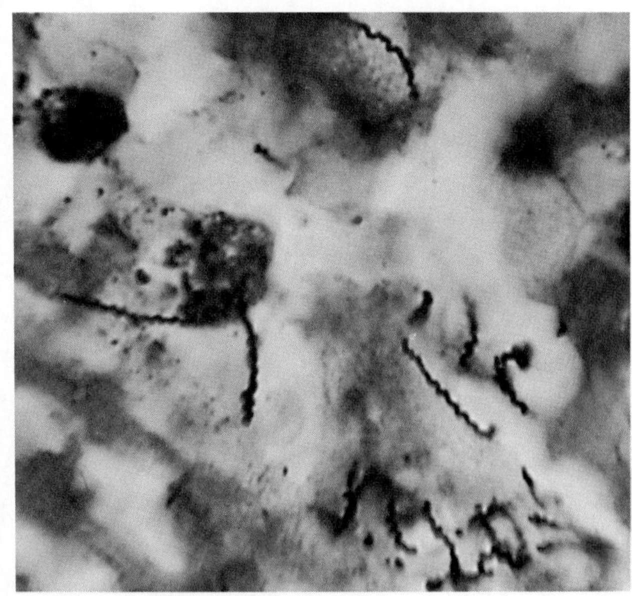

FIGURE 9-33
Syphilis. Spirochetes of *T. pallidum*, visualized by silver impregnation, in the eye of a child with congenital syphilis.

the New World. Urbanization and mass movements of people caused by war contributed to its rapid spread. Originally, syphilis was an acute disease that caused destructive skin lesions and early death, but it has become milder, with a more protracted and insidious clinical course.

T. pallidum is a thin, long spirochete (Fig. 9-33), which cannot be grown in artificial media. The organism is too thin to be seen by routine light microscopy, and techniques that amplify the width of the organism (e.g., darkfield microscopy, silver impregnation stains) must be employed to demonstrate the organism in tissue or fluids.

☐ **Epidemiology:** Syphilis is a worldwide disease, which is transmitted almost exclusively by sexual contact. The infection is also spread from an infected mother to her fetus (congenital syphilis). Blood transfusions, direct inoculation, and nonsexual contact are only rare causes of syphilis. In the United States, the incidence of primary and secondary syphilis had declined steadily since the introduction of penicillin therapy at the end of World War II. Beginning in the early 1960s, however, the incidence has increased again. Since 1990, it has again declined steadily, falling from 20 to 6 cases per 100,000 population per year.

☐ **Pathogenesis:** *T. pallidum* is very fragile and is killed by soap, antiseptics, drying, and cold. Person-to-person transmission requires direct contact between a rich source of spirochetes (e.g., an open lesion) and mucous membranes or abraded skin of the genital organs, rectum, mouth, fingers, or nipples. The organisms reproduce at the site of inoculation, pass to regional lymph nodes, gain access to the systemic circulation, and are disseminated throughout the body. Although *T. pallidum* induces an inflammatory response and is taken up by phagocytic cells, it persists and proliferates. Chronic infection and inflammation cause tissue destruction, sometimes for decades.

The course of syphilis is classically divided into three stages (Fig. 9-34):

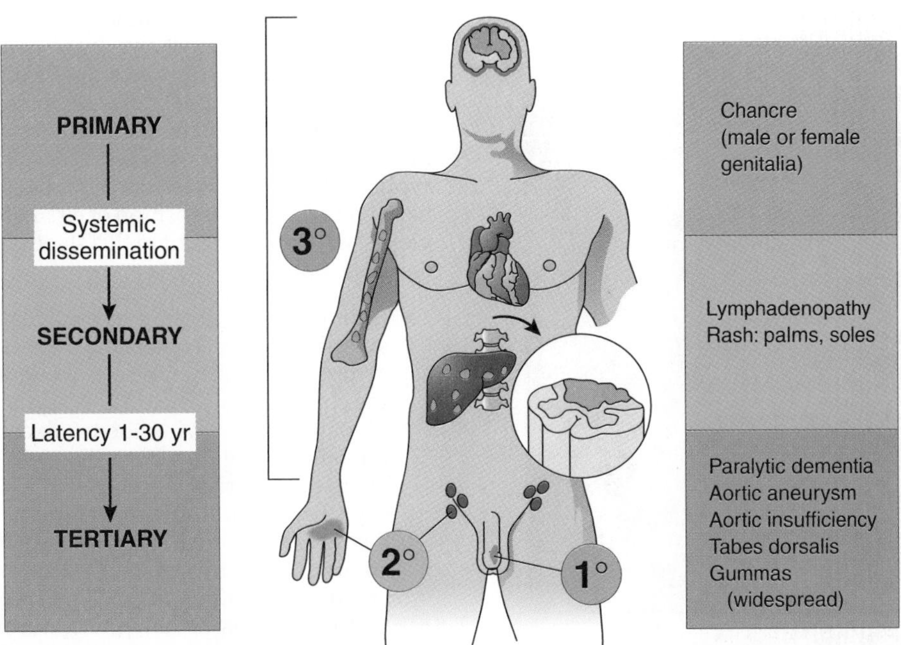

FIGURE 9-34
Clinical characteristics of the various stages of syphilis.

1. **Primary syphilis:** The first lesion (a chancre) appears within several weeks of exposure at the site of inoculation.
2. **Secondary syphilis:** From the primary lesion, the spirochetes are disseminated throughout the body, producing systemic manifestations and widespread lesions.
3. **Tertiary syphilis:** The continued presence of spirochetes at some sites and the associated immunological response produce chronic destructive lesions, which often manifest years after primary and secondary disease.

Primary Syphilis

The classic lesion of primary syphilis is the chancre (Fig. 9-35), a characteristic ulcer located at the site of *T. pallidum* inoculation, usually the penis, vulva, anus, or mouth. It appears 1 week to 3 months after exposure, with an average incubation period of 3 weeks. The chancre tends to be solitary and has a firm, raised border. Unless secondarily infected, the chancre lacks a purulent exudate. Microscopically, spirochetes may be anywhere in the chancre but tend to be concentrated in the walls of vessels and in the epidermis around the ulcer. **Chancres, as well as the lesions of the other stages of syphilis, display a characteristic "luetic vasculitis," in which endothelial cells proliferate and swell and the walls of the vessels become thickened by lymphocytes and fibrous tissue.**

The chancre begins as a papule that quickly erodes to a characteristic ulcer. Chancres are painless and can go unnoticed in some locations, such as the uterine cervix, anal canal, and mouth. The chancre lasts from 3 to 12 weeks and is frequently accompanied by inguinal lymphadenopathy. It heals without scarring. Penicillin remains effective therapy.

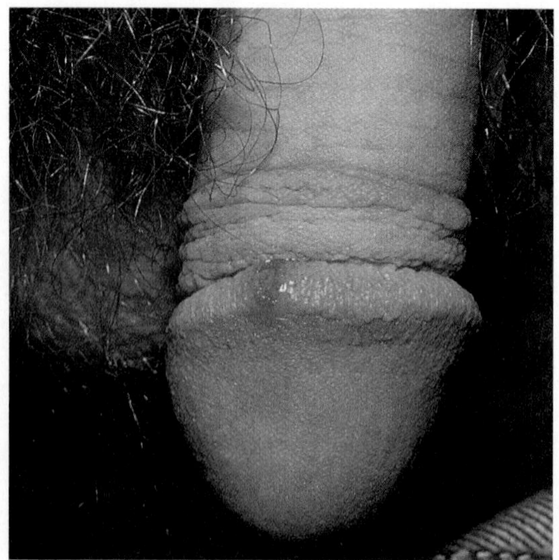

FIGURE *9-35*
Syphilitic chancre. A patient with primary syphilis displays a raised, erythematous penile lesion.

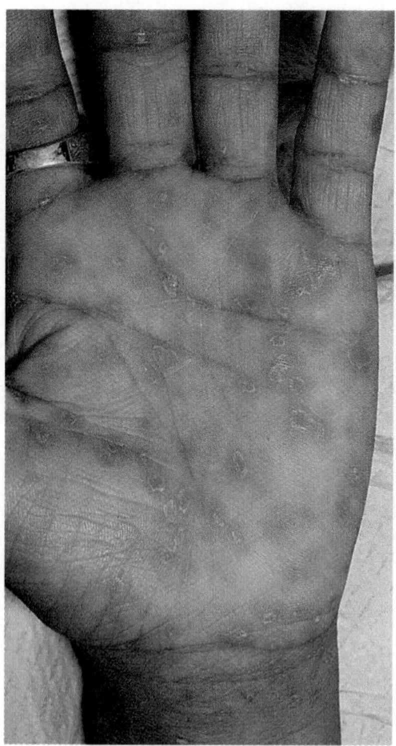

FIGURE *9-36*
Secondary syphilis. A maculopapular rash is present on the palm.

Secondary Syphilis

Secondary syphilis is characterized by lesions in a variety of organs, especially the skin, mucous membranes, lymph nodes, meninges, stomach, and liver. This stage is the result of the systemic dissemination and proliferation of *T. pallidum*. Because almost any organ or combination of organs can be involved in secondary syphilis, this stage of the disease is enormously diverse in its clinical presentation, earning syphilis its nickname as "The Great Imitator." Histopathologically, the lesions of secondary syphilis show a perivascular lymphocytic infiltrate, perhaps related to the deposition of circulating immune complexes, which are present in this stage of infection, and endarteritis obliterans.

- **Skin:** The most common presentation of secondary syphilis is a rash, accompanied by constitutional symptoms, which appear 2 weeks to 3 months after the chancre heals. The rash is erythematous and maculopapular, involving the trunk and extremities and often including the palms (Fig. 9-36) and soles.
  There are a variety of other skin lesions in secondary syphilis, including **condylomata lata** (exudative plaques in the perineum, vulva, or scrotum, which abound in spirochetes) (Fig. 9-37); **follicular syphilids** (small papular lesions around hair follicles that cause loss of hair); and **nummular syphilids** (coinlike lesions involving the face and perineum).
- **Mucous membranes:** Lesions on mucosal surfaces of the mouth and genital organs, called "mucous

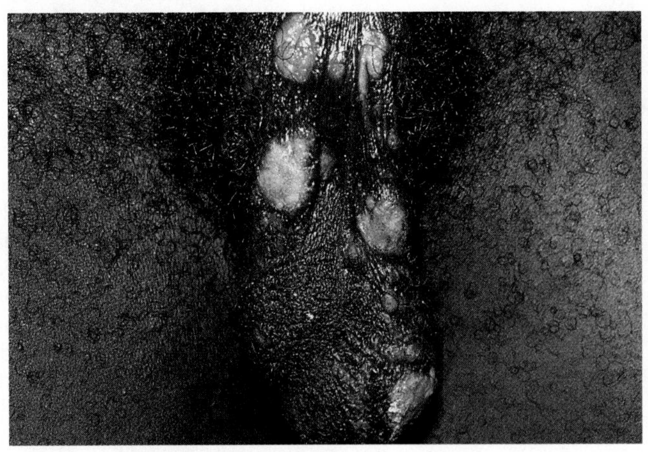

A

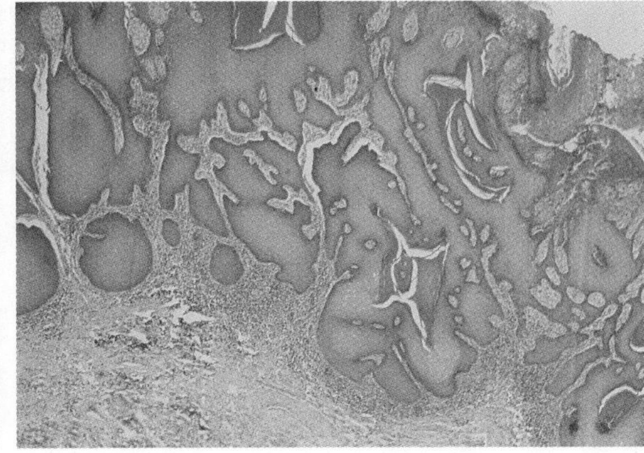

B

FIGURE *9-37*
Condylomata lata in secondary syphillis. (*A*) Whitish plaques are seen on the vulva and perineum. (*B*) A photomicrograph shows papillomatous hyperplasia of the epidermis with underlying chronic inflammation.

patches," teem with organisms and are highly infectious. The mucocutaneous lesions are accompanied by fever, malaise, pharyngitis, weight loss, and lymphadenopathy.

- **Lymph nodes:** Characteristic changes in lymph nodes include a thickened capsule, follicular hyperplasia, increased numbers of plasma cells and macrophages, and luetic vasculitis. Numerous spirochetes are present in the lymph nodes of secondary syphilis. Swelling of the epitrochlear lymph nodes, uncommon in other diseases, has long been associated with syphilis.
- **Meninges:** Although the meninges are commonly seeded with *T. pallidum*, this involvement is frequently asymptomatic. Occasionally, patients complain of headache and stiff neck.

The symptoms of secondary syphilis may begin before the chancre of primary syphilis has resolved and persist for varying periods of time, ranging from a few days to many months. If untreated, secondary syphilis can relapse.

Tertiary Syphilis

After the lesions of secondary syphilis have subsided, an asymptomatic period lasts for years or decades. However, during this latent period, spirochetes continue to multiply, and the deep-seated lesions of tertiary syphilis gradually develop and expand. During this stage of apparent well-being, spirochetes may be passed in blood transfusions or across the placenta to the fetus.

One third of untreated patients with syphilis develop tertiary lesions. **Focal ischemic necrosis secondary to obliterative endarteritis is the underlying mechanism for many of the processes associated with tertiary syphilis.** *T. pallidum* induces a mononuclear inflammatory infiltrate predominantly composed of lymphocytes and plasma cells. These cells infiltrate small arteries and arterioles, producing a characteristic obstructive vascular lesion (endarteritis obliterans). The small arteries are inflamed and their endothelial cells are swollen. They are surrounded by concentric layers of proliferating fibroblasts, which confer an "onion skin" appearance to the vascular lesions.

- **Syphilitic aortitis:** This lesion results from a slowly progressive endarteritis obliterans of the vasa vasorum that eventually leads to necrosis of the aortic media, a gradual weakening and stretching of the aortic wall, and the formation of an aortic aneurysm. The syphilitic aneurysm is saccular and involves the ascending aorta, an unusual site for the much more common atherosclerotic aneurysms. On gross examination, the intima of the aorta appears rough and pitted (tree-bark appearance) (Fig. 9-38). The specialized arrangement of the aortic media, which includes a delicate and intimate weave elastica, smooth muscle, and collagen, is gradually replaced by scar tissue. It is the specialized tissues of the media that gives the aorta its strength and resilience. When these are replaced by scar tissue, the aorta gradually stretches, becoming progressively thinner to the point of rupture, massive hemorrhage, and sudden death.
  Damage to and scarring of the ascending aorta also commonly lead to dilatation of the aortic ring, separation of the valve cusps, and regurgitation of blood through the aortic valve (aortic insufficiency). Luetic vasculitis of the coronary arteries may narrow or occlude these vessels and cause myocardial infarction.
- **Neurosyphilis:** The slowly progressive infection damages the meninges, cerebral cortex, spinal cord, cranial nerves, or eyes. Tertiary syphilis involving the central nervous system is subclassified according to the predominant tissue affected. Thus, there are references to **meningovascular syphilis** (meninges), **tabes dorsalis** (spinal cord), and **general paresis**

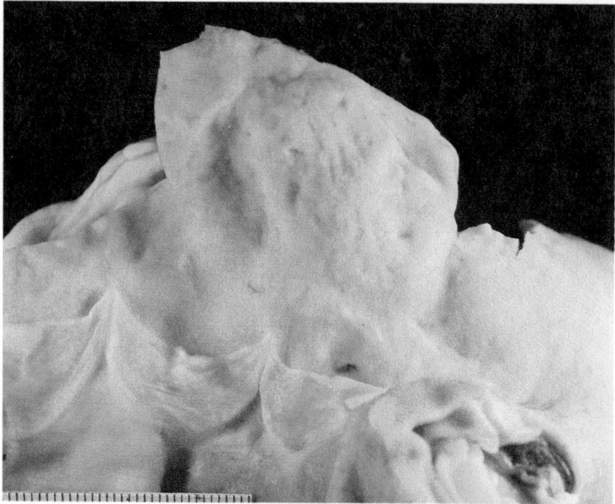

FIGURE 9-38
Syphilic aortitis. The ascending aorta exhibits a roughened intima ("tree bark" appearance), owing to destruction of the media.

(cerebral cortex). The lesions of neurosyphilis are discussed in detail in Chapter 28.

- **Benign tertiary syphilis:** The appearance of a gumma (Fig. 9-39) in any organ or tissue is the hallmark of benign tertiary syphilis. Gummas are most commonly found in the skin, bone, and joints, although lesions can occur at any body site. These granulomatous lesions are composed of a central area of coagulative necrosis, epithelioid macrophages, occasional giant cells, and peripheral fibrous tissue. Gummas are usually localized lesions, which do not significantly damage the patient.

Congenital Syphilis

Syphilis may be acquired *in utero*. When *T. pallidum* is transmitted from an infected mother to the fetus, the organism disseminates in fetal tissues, which are injured by the proliferating organisms and accompanying inflammatory response. Fetal infection produces stillbirth, neonatal illness or death, or progressive postnatal disease.

Histopathologically, the lesions of congenital syphilis are identical to those of adult disease. Infected tissues show a chronic inflammatory infiltrate, composed of lymphocytes and plasma cells, and endarteritis obliterans. Virtually any tissue can be affected, but skin, bones, teeth, joints, liver, and central nervous systems are characteristically involved (see Chapter 6).

The clinical features of congenital syphilis are highly variable, and infected newborns are often completely asymptomatic. Early signs of infection include a rhinitis (**snuffles**) and a desquamative rash. Infection of periosteum, bone, cartilage, and dental pulp produce deformities of bones and teeth, including **saddle nose**, anterior bowing of the legs (**saber shins**), and peg-shaped upper incisor teeth (**Hutchinsons teeth**). Progression of congenital syphilis can be arrested by penicillin, and serological testing of newborns readily detects asymptomatic disease.

Laboratory Diagnosis of Syphillis

The laboratory test that is most specific and sensitive for verifying a clinical diagnosis of primary syphilis is the finding of treponemes by darkfield microscopic examination of fluid obtained from the surface of the chancre. Patients with syphilis produce two classes of antibodies that can be detected by appropriate serological tests and that are important as diagnostic tools: (1) Antibody to cardiolipin, as measured in so-called nontreponemal antibody tests such as the RPR (rapid plasma reagin) or the VDRL (Venereal Disease Research Laboratory) test; and (2) antibody to outer membrane proteins of *T. pallidum*, as measured by the *T. pallidum* hemagglutination assay (TPHA or NMA-TP). Cardiolipin is a component of mammalian cells that is incorporated and, presumably, modified by *T. pallidum* so that the infected host generates antibody to it. Thus, in a manner of speaking, anticardiolipin antibody is an autoantibody.

The RPR test is positive, often at a relatively low level, in about 80% of patients at the time they come to medical attention for primary syphilis. It is positive in high titer in all persons with secondary syphilis. Within 1 to 2 years of treatment, this reactivity generally disappears. A number of nonsyphilitic infections including Lyme disease, chickenpox, infectious mononucleosis, and kala-azar cause a reactive RPR. The TPHA or N1HA-TP test is positive in 90% of patients at the time they seek medical attention for a chancre. It is always positive in secondary syphilis. Once positive, the NMA-TP remains so for life. No other disease renders this test positive. Thus, despite its remarkable sensitivity and specificity, a positive result does not establish a diagnosis of primary syphilis, since antibody may be present as a result of some earlier infection. Conversely, 10% of patients with primary syphilis have a negative test result. The major use of the test for antibody to treponemal proteins is to exclude the diagnosis of

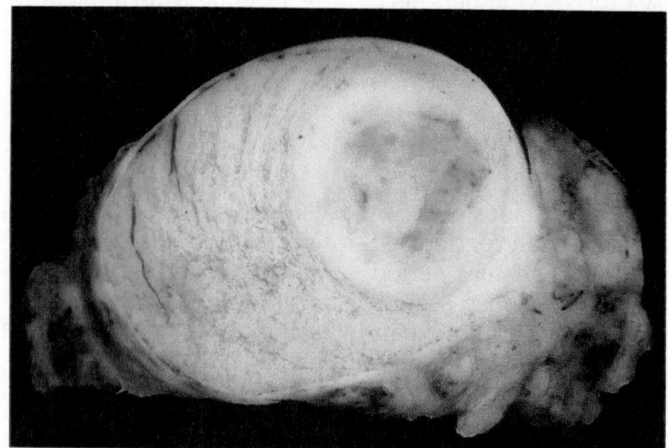

FIGURE 9-39
Syphilitic gumma. A patient with tertiary syphilis shows sharply circumscribed gumma in the testis, characterized by a fibrogranulomatous wall and a necrotic center.

syphilis in someone who has a rash that might represent secondary syphilis or a neurological or cardiological syndrome that might reflect neurosyphilis.

T. pallidum can be demonstrated in tissue by silver impregnation stains, such as the Warthin-Starry or Steiner stains, and by immunofluorescent antibody staining.

Nonvenereal Treponematoses

In tropical and subtropical countries, there is a group of nonvenereal, chronic diseases that are caused by treponemes indistinguishable from *T. pallidum*. Similar to syphilis, they result from the inoculation of the organism into mucocutaneous surfaces. They also pass through clearly defined clinical and pathological stages, including a primary lesion at the site of inoculation, secondary skin eruptions, a latent period, and a tertiary, late stage. Although the nonvenereal treponematoses (yaws, bejel, pinta) are distinct clinical entities, the responsible spirochetes cannot be distinguished from each other or from *T. pallidum* by molecular analyses.

Yaws

Yaws is a systemic treponematosis that produces chronic lesions of the bone and skin. The disease is caused by *T. pertenue* and occurs among poor rural populations in warm, humid areas of tropical Africa, South America, Southeast Asia, and Oceania. Importantly, *T. pertenue* does not cause disease of the cardiovascular or central nervous systems. Children and adolescents living in deprived tropical regions are at risk. Transmission is by skin-to-skin contact and is facilitated by breaks or abrasions.

☐ **Pathology and Clinical Features:** Two to 5 weeks after exposure, a single "mother yaw" appears at the site of inoculation, usually on an exposed part. The lesion begins as a papule and becomes a 2- to 5-cm "raspberry-like" papilloma. The secondary or disseminated stage begins with the eruption of a similar, but smaller, yaw on other parts of the skin. Microscopically, the mother yaw and the disseminated lesions show hyperkeratosis, papillary acanthosis, and an intense neutrophilic infiltrate of the epidermis. The epidermis at the apex of the papilloma lyses to form a shallow ulcer. Plasma cells invade the upper dermis. Spirochetes are numerous in the dermal papillae, particularly in foci of neutrophils and in the superficial exudate. Unlike the causative organism of syphilis, *T. pertenue* does not involve blood vessels.

Painful papillomas on the soles of the feet lead the patient to walk on the sides of the feet like a crab, a condition called "crab yaw." The treponemes are borne by the blood to bones, lymph nodes, and skin. There they grow during a latent period of 5 or more years. The lesions in the late stage include gummas of the skin, which are destructive to the face and upper airway. Periostitis of the tibia causes "saber shins" or "boomerang legs." A single dose of long-acting penicillin cures yaws.

Bejel

Bejel (also known as "endemic syphilis") is a treponemal disease characterized by gummas of the skin, airway mucosa, and bone. It has a focal distribution in Africa, western Asia, and Australia. Poor children who live in rural, arid areas under unsanitary conditions are affected. Bejel is transmitted by nonvenereal routes, such as from an infected infant to the breast of the mother, from mouth to mouth, or from utensils to the mouth, and is caused by *T. pallidum* subspecies *endemicum*. Other than on the nursing breast, primary lesions are rare. Secondary lesions in the mouth are identical to the mucosal lesions of syphilis and may spread from the upper airway to the larynx. Lesions of the perineum and bone are encountered, and gummas of the breast occur. However, cardiovascular and neurological lesions are rare.

Pinta

Pinta (Sp., "painted" or "blemish") is a treponematosis characterized by variably colored spots on the skin. It is caused by *T. carateum* and prevails in remote, arid, inland regions and river valleys of the American tropics. The lesions of the three stages of pinta are limited to the skin and tend to merge. Transmission is by skin-to-skin inoculation, usually after long intimate contact with an infected person.

Ten days after inoculation, a small papule appears, most often on the leg. The lesion enlarges and in 1 to 3 months may involve a 10-cm patch of skin. The papule flattens and displays irregular margins and a scaly and pigmented surface. The lesion initially appears slate blue in dark-skinned persons, but after several years it leaves an area of hypopigmentation. In secondary pinta (5 to 18 months later), generalized pale, pink macules (pintids) appear on exposed surfaces. These lesions later become depigmented and hyperkeratotic. Treponemes abound in the primary and secondary lesions but not the late ones. The latter are characterized by acanthosis and hyperkeratosis of the epidermis, follicular plugging, elongation of rete ridges, intraepidermal microabscesses, and an absence of pigment in the basal layer. The inflammatory infiltrate is diminished in the tertiary stage. A single dose of long-acting penicillin is curative.

LYME DISEASE

Lyme disease is a chronic systemic infection, which begins with a characteristic skin lesion and later manifests as cardiac, neurological, or joint disturbances. The causative agent is *Borrelia burgdorferi*, a large (11 × 39 μm), microaerophilic spirochete.

☐ **Epidemiology:** Lyme disease was first described in patients from Lyme, Connecticut, but was later recognized in many other areas. *B. burgdorferi* is transmitted from its animal reservoir to humans by the bite of the minute *Ixodes* tick. The insect is found in wooded areas, where it usually feeds on mice and deer. Transmission to humans is most likely to occur from May through July, when nymph forms of the tick feed.

Lyme disease is a growing problem in the United States, where the disease has become the most common tick-borne illness, causing an estimated 15,000 to 20,000 cases annually. Disease is concentrated mainly in three areas, along the eastern seaboard from Maryland to Massachusetts, in the Midwest in Minnesota and Wisconsin, and in the West in California and Oregon. The disease is also present in Europe, Australia, countries of the former Soviet Union, Japan, and China.

□ **Pathology and Clinical Features:** *B. burgdorferi* reproduces locally at the site of inoculation, spreads to regional lymph nodes, and is disseminated throughout the body in the bloodstream. Like other spirochetal diseases, Lyme disease is chronic, occurring in stages, with remissions and exacerbations. The histopathological features of Lyme disease have not been well defined since tissue, other than skin, is rarely available for pathological examination. Studies of skin and synovium have shown that *B. burgdorferi* elicits a chronic inflammatory infiltrate, composed of lymphocytes and plasma cells. In patients who died of the disease, organisms have been seen at autopsy in sections from virtually every organ affected, including skin, myocardium, liver, central nervous system, and the musculoskeletal system.

Lyme disease is a prolonged illness with features that change over time. Although three clinical stages are described, they are rarely well defined in an individual patient:

- **Stage 1:** A distinctive feature of the first stage of Lyme disease is the characteristic skin lesion, **erythema chronicum migrans**, which appears at the site of the tick bite. This begins 3 to 35 days after the bite as an erythematous macule or papule, which grows to become an erythematous patch 3 to 7 cm in diameter. It often is intensely red at its periphery and shows some degree of central clearing, imparting an annular appearance to the lesion. Erythema chronicum migrans is accompanied by fever, fatigue, headache, arthralgias, and regional lymphadenopathy. Secondary annular skin lesions develop in about half of the patients and tend to appear and fade at different times, in some cases, persisting for long periods. During this phase, patients experience constant malaise and fatigue, headache, and fever. Intermittent manifestations may also include meningeal irritation, migratory myalgia, cough, generalized lymphadenopathy, and testicular swelling.
- **Stage 2:** The first stage merges indistinctly into the second stage and begins within several weeks to months of the appearance of the skin lesion. This stage is characterized by exacerbation of migratory musculoskeletal pains and the development of cardiac and neurological abnormalities. The migratory pains may involve joints, bursae, muscles, and tendons and usually have no associated swelling. Cardiac abnormalities occur in 10% of infected persons. These are usually conduction abnormalities, particularly atrioventricular block, which result from a myocarditis. Neurological abnormalities, most commonly meningitis and facial nerve palsies, occur in 15% of patients.
- **Stage 3:** The third stage of Lyme disease begins months to years after the tick bite and is manifested by joint, skin, and neurological abnormalities. Joint abnormalities develop in over half of infected persons and include severe arthritis of the large joints, especially the knee. The histopathological changes in affected joints are virtually indistinguishable from those of rheumathoid arthritis, with villous hypertrophy and a conspicuous mononuclear infiltrate in the subsynovial lining area. The white cell count of the joint fluid ranges from 1000 to 100,000 cells/mm^3 and polymorphonuclear neutrophils predominate.

It is now recognized that neurological manifestations may begin months to years after the onset of the disease. They range from intermittent tingling paresthesias without demonstrable neurological deficits to slowly progressive encephalomyelitis, transverse myelitis, organic brain syndromes, and dementia. There is a distinctive late skin manifestation of Lyme disease, **acrodermatitis chronica atrophicans**, which occurs years after erythema chronicum migrans and presents as patchy atrophy and sclerosis of the skin.

The diagnosis of Lyme disease is established by culturing *B. burgdorferi* from infected patients, but the yield is low. Therefore, the determination of antibody titers (initially IgM and later IgG) against the organism remains the most practical way to establish the diagnosis. Treatment with tetracycline or erythromycin is effective in eliminating early Lyme disease. In later stages and when there are extensive extracutaneous manifestations, high doses of intravenous penicillin G and other combinations of antibiotic regimens for long periods are necessary.

LEPTOSPIROSIS

Leptospirosis is an infection with spirochetes of the genus Leptospira, which is for the most part (90% of patients) a mild, self-limited, febrile disease. In persons with more severe infections, hepatic and renal failure may prove fatal. The leptospires are 0.1 μm wide and 6 to 12 μm long, with 18 or more coils.

□ **Epidemiology:** Leptospirosis is a zoonosis of worldwide distribution. Although about 180 serovars of *Leptospira interrogans* have been identified, virtually all are capable of causing leptospirosis, and there is no correlation between the serotype and the clinical syndromes. Thus, it is currently preferred to refer to the illness caused by all serotypes of *Leptospira* as leptospirosis.

Leptospires penetrate abraded skin or mucous membranes following contact with infected rats, contaminated water, or mud. Since warm, moist environments favor survival of the spirochetes, the incidence is greater in the tropics. Between 30 and 100 cases of leptospirosis are reported annually in the United States, some of them in slaughterhouse workers and trappers, but recently some cases were reported to occur among destitute persons in urban areas. Soldiers engaged in jungle warfare during the Vietnam war were at particular risk. Intrauterine infection causes fetal death.

□ **Pathology and Clinical Features:** The symptoms of leptospirosis begin 4 days to 3 weeks after exposure to *L. interrogans*. In most cases, the disease resolves within a week without sequelae. In more severe infections, leptospirosis is a biphasic disease.

- **The leptospiremic phase** is characterized by the presence of leptospires in the blood and cerebrospinal fluid. There is an abrupt onset of fever, shaking chills, headache, and myalgias. After 1 to 2 weeks, the symptoms abate as the leptospires disappear from the blood and body fluids.
- **The immune phase**, which begins within 3 days of the end of the leptospiremic phase, is accompanied by the production of IgM antibodies. The earlier symptoms recur, and signs of meningeal irritation become apparent. At this time, the cerebrospinal fluid shows a prominent pleocytosis. In severe cases, jaundice precedes the onset of hepatic and renal failure and the appearance of widespread hemorrhages and shock. This severe form of leptospirosis has historically been referred to as **Weil disease**.

At autopsy, the tissues are bile stained and hemorrhages are observed in many organs. Microscopically, the principal lesion is a diffuse vasculitis with capillary injury. The liver shows dissociation of the liver cell plates, erythrophagocytosis by Kupffer cells, minimal necrosis of hepatocytes, neutrophils in the sinusoids, and a mixed inflammatory cell infiltrate in the portal tracts. Kidneys display swollen and necrotic tubules. Spirochetes are numerous in the lumina of the tubules and particularly in bile-stained casts (Fig. 9-40).

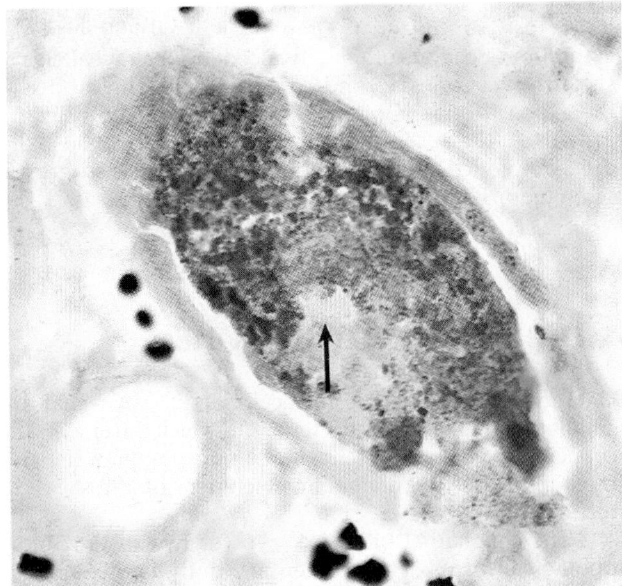

FIGURE *9-40*
Leptospirosis. A distal renal tubule is obstructed by a bile-stained mass of hemoglobin and cellular debris. A leptospire (*arrow*) is in the center of this mass.

Culture of the blood and cerebrospinal fluid is an effective means of confirming the diagnosis in the first phase. Leptospires grow from the urine after the second week, and serological tests are useful during the immune phase. Untreated Weil disease carries a mortality rate of 5% to 30%. Large doses of penicillin and tetracyclines are effective if administered within 4 days of the onset of symptoms.

RELAPSING FEVER

Relapsing fever is an acute, febrile, septicemic illness caused by spirochetes of the genus Borrelia. The organisms are 0.2 to 0.5 μm wide and 3 to 20 μm long, with 310 coarse, irregular coils. There are two main types of relapsing fever:

- **Epidemic relapsing fever** is caused by *B. recurrentis* and is transmitted by the bite of an infected louse. Humans are the only reservoir.
- **Endemic relapsing fever** is caused by a number of *Borrelia* species and is transmitted from rodents and other animals by the bite of an infected tick.

□ **Epidemiology:** The human body louse, *Pediculus humanus humanus*, becomes infected with *B. recurrentis* when it feeds on an infected person. The spirochetes cross the gut wall of the louse into the hemolymph, where they multiply. Here they remain, unless the louse is crushed when feeding. If this occurs, the borrelliae escape and penetrate at the site of the bite or even through the intact skin. War, crowded migrant worker camps, and heavy clothing during cold weather all favor mobilization of lice and the spread of relapsing fever. Furthermore, lice dislike the higher temperatures of the feverish victims and seek new hosts, another factor in the rapid spread of relapsing fever during epidemics. Louse-borne relapsing fever is currently encountered in a number of African countries, especially Ethiopia and Sudan, and is also seen in the South American Andes.

In endemic, tick-borne relapsing fever, ticks are infected while biting rats and other hosts. The borelliae grow in the hemocoelom of the tick and invade other tissues, including the salivary glands. Humans are infected by the saliva or coxal fluid of the tick. Ticks have a considerably longer life span than lice and may harbor spirochetes for 12 to 15 years without a blood meal. Tick-borne relapsing fever occurs sporadically worldwide.

□ **Pathology and Clinical Features:** Following the bite of an infected arthropod, fever, headache, myalgias, arthralgias, and lethargy appear within 1 to 2 weeks. The liver and spleen enlarge, and there are petechiae of the skin, conjunctival hemorrhages, and abdominal tenderness. Within 3 to 9 days after the onset of symptoms, the fever ends abruptly, only to begin 7 to 10 days later. During the afebrile period, the spirochetes disappear from the blood and change their antigenic coats. With each relapse, the symptoms are milder and the duration of illness is shorter. In severe cases, the initial episode may be characterized by a rash, meningitis, myocarditis, liver failure, and coma.

In fatal infections, the spleen is enlarged and contains miliary microabscesses. Spirochetes form tangled aggregates around the necrotic centers. Lymphocytes and neutrophils infiltrate central and midzonal areas of the liver, where spirochetes lie free in the sinusoids. Focal hemorrhages involve many organs. Tetracycline is an effective treatment for both types of relapsing fever.

FUSOSPIROCHETAL INFECTIONS

Tropical Phagedenic Ulcer

Tropical phagedenic (rapidly spreading and sloughing) ulcer, also known as **tropical foot,** *is a painful, necrotizing lesion of the skin and subcutaneous tissues of the leg that afflicts persons in tropical climates.* Although the flora in the ulcers are often mixed, bacteriological studies indicate *Bacillus fusiformis* and *Treponema vincentii* to be the cause. Malnutrition may predispose the patient to infection.

The lesion usually starts on the skin at a point of trauma and develops rapidly. The surface sloughs to form an ulcer with raised borders and a cup-shaped crater, which contains a gray, putrid exudate (Fig. 9-41). The ulcer may be so deep that the underlying bone and tendons are exposed. The margin becomes fibrotic, but complete healing may be delayed for years. In addition to secondary infection, tibial osteomyelitis and squamous cell carcinoma may be late complications. Antibiotics may be effective, but reconstructive plastic surgery is often necessary to close the defect.

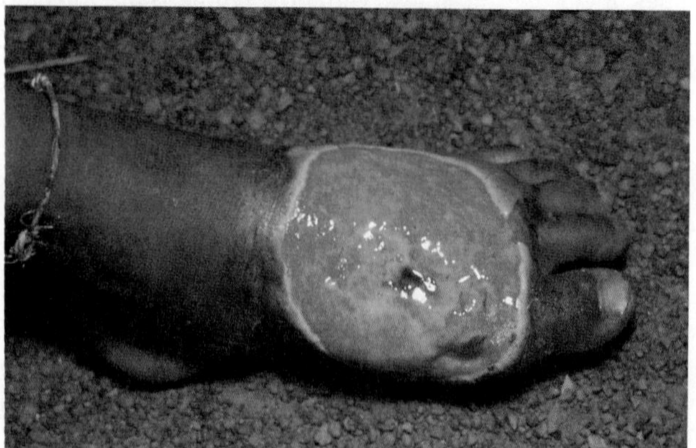

FIGURE 9-41
Tropical phagedenic ulcer caused by infection by fusospirochetal organisms, following penetrating trauma.

Noma

Noma, or gangrenous stomatitis or cancrum oris, is a rapidly progressive necrosis of soft tissues and bones of the mouth and face, and less commonly of other sites, such as the chest, limbs, and genitalia. It afflicts malnourished children in the tropics, many of whom are further debilitated by recent infections (e.g., measles, malaria, or leishmaniasis). A variety of bacteria may be recovered from these lesions, but *Treponema vincentii, Bacillus fusiformis, Bacteroides,* and *Corynebacterium* tend to predominate. The ulceration is destructive and disfiguring and usually unilateral (Fig. 9-42). The initial lesion is a small papule, often on the cheek opposite the molars or premolars. From this early lesion, large malodorous defects quickly develop. The lesions are painful and accompanied by variable systemic symptoms. Sections of the advanced lesions reveal necrosis of the skin, muscle, and adipose tissue. The surface of the exposed bone is often covered by a mixed bacterial growth. In the absence of treatment, the patients usually die. Antibiotics are helpful, but reconstructive surgery is often required to correct the deformity.

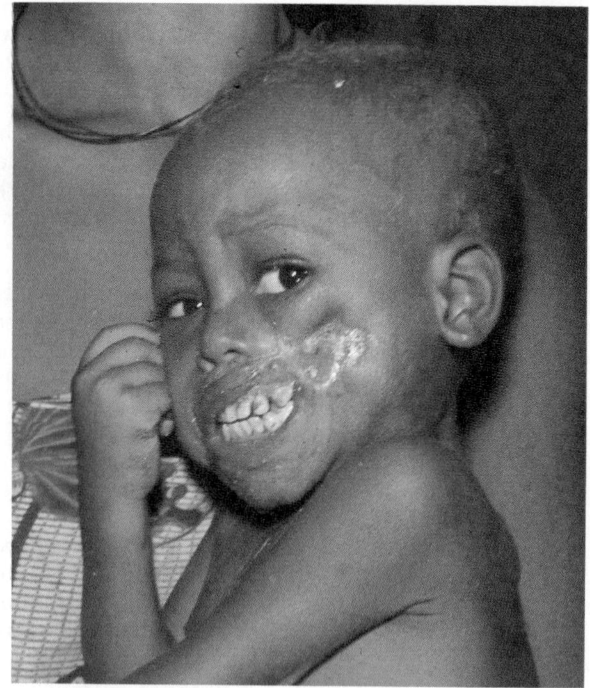

FIGURE 9-42
Noma. There is massive destruction of the soft tissues and bones of the mouth and cheek.

Chlamydial Infections

Chlamydiae are obligate intracellular parasites that are smaller than most other bacteria. They lack the enzymatic capacity to generate adenosine triphosphate (ATP) and must parasitize the metabolic machinery of a host cell to reproduce.

The chlamydial life cycle involves two distinct morphological forms. **The elementary body** is the smaller, metabolically inactive form, which survives extracellularly. It attaches to the appropriate host cell and induces endocytosis, forming a vacuole. It then transforms into the larger, metabolically active form, **the reticulate body**, which commandeers host cell metabolism to fuel chlamydial replication. The reticulate body divides repeatedly, forming daughter elementary bodies and destroying the host cell. Necrotic debris elicits inflammatory and immunological responses that further damage infected tissue.

Chlamydial infections are widespread among birds and mammals, and as many as 20% of humans are infected. Three species of chlamydiae (*C. trachomatis*, *C. psittaci*, and *C. pneumoniae*) cause human infection.

CHLAMYDIA TRACHOMATIS INFECTION

The species *C. trachomatis* contains a variety of strains (serovars), which cause three distinct types of disease, namely (1) genital and neonatal disease, (2) lymphogranuloma venereum, and (3) trachoma.

Genital and Neonatal Diseases

C. trachomatis serovars D through K cause a genital epithelial infection, which is now among the most common sexually transmitted diseases in developed countries. In fact, chlamydial infection of the genital tract has surpassed gonorrhea as the leading cause of sexually contracted disease in North America. In men, this infection produces urethritis and sometimes epididymitis or proctitis. In women, the infection usually begins with cervicitis, which can progress to endometritis, salpingitis, and generalized infection of the pelvic adnexal organs (pelvic inflammatory disease). Repeated infections of the fallopian tubes are particularly associated with scarring, which may interfere with passage of sperm or fertilized ova and result in infertility or ectopic pregnancy. Perinatal transmission of *C. trachomatis* causes neonatal conjunctivitis and pneumonia.

☐ **Epidemiology:** The organism spreads from person to person in infected genital secretions. Infection is chronic and frequently asymptomatic, providing an enormous reservoir for transmission. As with all sexually transmitted diseases, persons with the largest number of sexual partners are at greatest risk of infection. There are estimated to be 3 million cases of genital *C. trachomatis* infection in the United States annually.

Newborns acquire the organism by contact with infected endocervical secretions on passage through an infected birth canal. Sixty to 70% of exposed newborns develop *C. trachomatis* conjunctivitis.

☐ **Pathology:** Regardless of the site, chlamydial infection elicits an inflammatory infiltrate of neutrophils and lymphocytes. Lymphoid aggregates, with or without germinal centers, may appear at the site of infection. In newborns, the conjunctival epithelium often contains characteristic vacuolar cytoplasmic inclusions, and the disease is frequently called **inclusion conjunctivitis**.

☐ **Clinical Features:** Most genital *C. trachomatis* infections are completely asymptomatic. In men, clinically apparent infection presents as a purulent penile discharge, associated with dysuria and urinary urgency. Chlamydial cervicitis causes a mucopurulent drainage from the cervical os. Treatment in adults is with tetracycline.

Chlamydial disease in the newborn presents as reddened conjunctivae with a watery or purulent discharge. Untreated neonatal conjunctivitis is potentially serious, although it may resolve without sequelae. Chlamydial pneumonia presents in the second or third month with tachypnea and paroxysmal cough, usually without fever. Inclusion conjunctivitis is treated with systemic or topical antibiotics.

Lymphogranuloma Venereum

Lymphogranuloma venereum is a sexually transmitted disease, which begins as a genital ulcer, progresses to a local necrotizing lymphadenitis (Fig. 9-43A), *and may eventuate in local scar-*

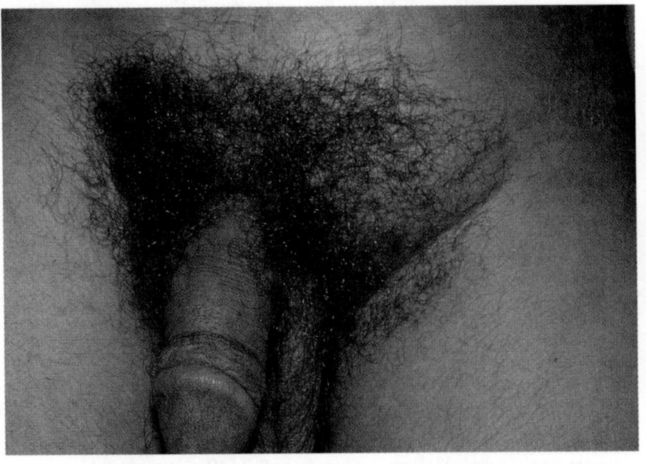

A

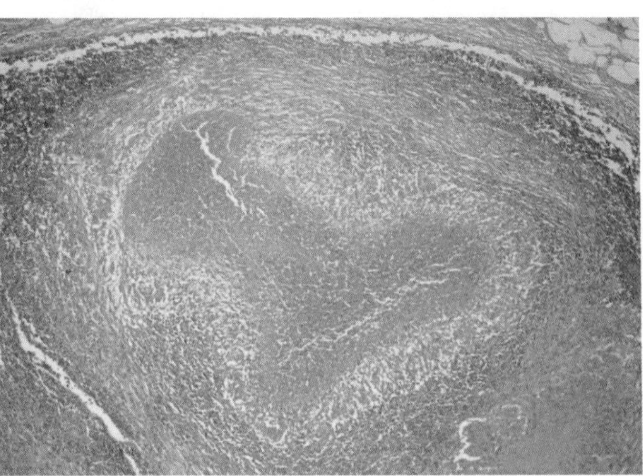

B

FIGURE 9-43
Lymphogranuloma venereum. (*A*) Painful inguinal lymphadenopathy in a man infected with *C. trachomatis.* (*B*) Microscopic section of a lymph node shows a necrotic central area surrounded by a granulomatous zone.

ring. The disease is caused by *C. trachomatis* serovars L1 through L3. Lymphogranuloma venereum is uncommon in developed countries, but it is endemic in the tropics and subtropics. It accounts for 5% of sexually transmitted disease in Africa, India, parts of southeast Asia, South America, and the Caribbean. In North America, where fewer than 250 cases were reported in 1994, and Europe, lymphogranuloma venereum is now primarily a disease of homosexual men.

☐ **Pathology:** The organism is introduced through a break in the skin. After an incubation period of 4 to 21 days, an ulcer appears, usually on the penis, vagina, or cervix, although lips, tongue, and fingers may also be primary sites. The organisms are transported by lymphatics to regional lymph nodes, where a necrotizing lymphadenitis erupts 1 to 3 weeks after the primary lesion. Abscesses develop within involved lymph nodes, often extending to adjacent lymph nodes. Over the next few weeks, the nodes become tender and fluctuant, and frequently ulcerate and discharge pus. The intense inflammatory process can result in severe scarring, which may produce chronic lymphatic obstruction, ischemic necrosis of overlying structures, or strictures and adhesions. The necrotizing process produces enlarged and matted lymph nodes, containing multiple, coalescing abscesses, which often develop a stellate shape (see Fig. 9-43B). The abscesses have a granulomatous appearance, containing neutrophils and necrotic debris in the center, surrounded by palisading epithelioid cells, macrophages, and occasional giant cells. The abscesses are rimmed by lymphocytes, plasma cells, and fibrous tissue. The nodal architecture is eventually effaced by fibrosis.

☐ **Clinical Features:** Patients with lymphogranuloma venereum present with lymphadenopathy, with or without systemic signs and symptoms, such as fever, myalgia, arthralgia, headache, and meningismus. Most infections resolve completely even without antimicrobial therapy. However, progressive ulceration of the penis, urethra, or scrotum, with fistulas and urethral stricture, develop in 5% of men. Women and homosexual men often present with hemorrhagic proctitis, and the large majority of late complications, such as rectal stricture, rectovaginal fistulas, and genital elephantiasis, occur in women. Chronic ulcers of the vulva (esthiomene) and smooth pedunculated, perianal growths (lymphorrhoids) are also occasional complications in women. Tetracycline is recommended for the treatment of acute lymphogranuloma venereum.

Trachoma

Trachoma is a chronic infection of the conjunctiva that progressively scars the conjunctiva and cornea and is a leading cause of blindness in many developing countries. C. trachomatis serovars A, B, Ba, and C cause the disease.

☐ **Epidemiology:** Trachoma is worldwide, associated with poverty, and most prevalent in dry or sandy regions. Only humans are naturally infected, and poor personal hygiene and inadequate public sanitation are common factors. Endemic regions have been reduced in size since World War II, but trachoma remains a major problem in parts of Africa, India, and the Middle East. In the United States, Native Americans are most susceptible. The infection is spread mostly by direct contact, but it may also be transmitted by fomites, contaminated water, and probably flies. Subclinical infections are an important reservoir. In endemic areas, infection is acquired early in childhood, becomes chronic, and eventually progresses to blindness.

☐ **Pathology:** When *C. trachomatis* is inoculated into the eye, it reproduces within the conjunctival epithelium, thereby inciting a mixed acute and chronic inflammatory infiltrate. Aggregates of lymphocytes and macrophages form beneath the conjunctiva. With reinfections these follicles expand, focally scarring the conjunctiva, and resulting in a chronic follicular keratoconjunctivitis. Progressive scarring distorts the eyelids so that they abrade the cornea, and the distorted eye is subject to secondary bacterial infections. If not interrupted, this process of chronic inflammation, scarring, mechanical distortion, abrasion, and secondary bacterial infection eventuates in blindness.

Histological examination of the early lesions shows chronic inflammation, lymphoid aggregates, focal degeneration of the conjunctiva, and chlamydial inclusions within the conjunctival epithelium. As trachoma progresses, the lymphoid aggregates enlarge, and the conjunctiva becomes scarred and focally hypertrophic. The cornea is invaded by blood vessels and fibroblasts, forming a scar reminiscent of a cloth ("pannus" in Latin), and is eventually opacified.

☐ **Clinical Features:** Early trachoma is characterized by the abrupt onset of palpebral and conjunctival inflammation, which leads to tearing, purulent conjunctivitis, and photophobia. **The lymphoid aggregates can be seen as small yellow grains beneath the palpebral conjunctivae within 3 to 4 weeks of infection.** Chronic inflammation, progressing over months and years, leads to scarring of the eyelids and inflammation of the cornea (keratitis), with the formation of a vascular pannus. Deformities of the eyelids eventually interfere with normal ocular function, and secondary bacterial infections and corneal ulcerations are common. Tetracycline eye ointments are effective therapy, but reinfections are common in endemic areas. Deformities of the eyelids must be treated surgically.

PSITTACOSIS (ORNITHOSIS)

Psittacosis is a self-limited pneumonia transmitted to humans from birds. The causative agent, *Chlamydia psittaci*, is spread by infected birds, and the resulting disease is known as both psittacosis (because of its association with parrots) or ornithosis (because of the association with birds in general).

☐ **Epidemiology:** *C. psittaci* is present in the blood, tissues, excreta, and feathers of infected birds. Humans inhale infectious excreta or dust from feathers. Although infection is endemic in tropical birds, *C. psittaci* can infect almost any species. Human disease has resulted from exposure to various bird species, including parrots, parakeets, canaries, pigeons, sea gulls, ducks, chickens, and turkeys. Use of tetracycline-containing bird feeds and quarantine of imported tropical birds limits the spread of disease, and fewer than 50 cases of psittacosis are reported annually in the United States.

☐ **Pathology:** *C. psittaci* first infects pulmonary macrophages, which carry the organism to the phagocytic cells of the liver and spleen, where it reproduces. The organism is then distributed from the liver and spleen by the bloodstream, producing systemic infection, particularly diffuse involvement of the lungs. *C. psittaci* infects and reproduces in alveolar lining cells. These cells are destroyed, and an inflammatory response is elicited.

The pneumonia is predominantly interstitial, and the inflammatory infiltrate within alveolar septa is composed largely of lymphocytes. Type II pneumocytes are hyperplastic and may show characteristic chlamydial cytoplasmic inclusions. In severe pulmonary disease, hemorrhage and fibrin fill the alveoli and bacterial superinfection may produce multiple abscesses. Dissemination of the infection, which may be fatal, is characterized by foci of necrosis in the liver and spleen and diffuse mononuclear cell infiltrates in the heart, kidneys, and brain.

☐ **Clinical Features:** The spectrum of clinical illness varies widely. There is usually a persistent dry cough, accompanied by constitutional symptoms of high fever, headache, malaise, myalgias, and arthralgias. If untreated, the fever persists for 2 to 3 weeks and then subsides as the pulmonary disease regresses. The mortality rate in the preantibiotic era exceeded 20%, but with tetracycline therapy the disease is only rarely fatal.

Chlamydia pneumoniae (TWAR) Infection

Chlamydia pneumoniae is a newly discovered chlamydial pathogen, which causes acute, self-limited, usually mild respiratory tract infections, including pneumonia. Before 1989, *C. pneumoniae* was known as the TWAR agent (its working laboratory designation), because of uncertainty about its relationship to other chlamydial species. It is now clear that *C. pneumoniae* is a distinct species of chlamydia.

C. pneumoniae is transmitted from person to person, and infection appears to be very common (5 to 10 times more frequent than *C. trachomatis* infection). In those parts of the developed world where *C. pneumoniae* has been investigated, half of all of adults show evidence of past infection.

C. pneumoniae infections vary widely in severity but are usually mild, and only 10% of infections result in clinically apparent pneumonia. Symptomatic persons complain of fever, sore throat, and cough. Severe pneumonia occurs only in those with an underlying pulmonary condition. In most cases, untreated disease resolves in 2 to 4 weeks.

Rickettsial Infections

The rickettsiae are small, gram-negative coccobacillary bacteria that are obligate intracellular pathogens. These organisms are no larger than 0.2 to 0.5 μm by 1 to 2 μm. Similar to chlamydiae, they cannot replicate outside a host. Rickettsiae have a proton motive force and can synthesize their own ATP via proton-translocating ATPase. They can also obtain ATP from the host via the ATP/ADP translocase. It has not yet been established why they are unable to replicate outside the host cell. Rickettsiae induce endocytosis by target cells and replicate within the cytoplasm of the host cell. They have the cell wall structure of gram-negative bacteria but, unlike chlamydiae, replicate by binary fission. Although structurally gram-negative, the rickettsiae do not stain well with the Gram stain and are best demonstrated by the Gimenez method or with acridine orange.

Humans are accidental hosts for most species of *Rickettsia*. The organisms reside in animals and insects and do not require humans for perpetuation. Human rickettsial infection results from insect bites. Several species of *Rickettsia* cause different human diseases (Table 9-6), but rickettsial infections have many features in common. **The hu-**

TABLE *9-6* **Rickettsial Infections**

Disease	Organism	Distribution	Transmission
	Spotted-fever group		
Rocky Mountain spotted fever	*R. rickettsii*	Americas	Ticks
Queensland tick fever	*R. australis*	Australia	Ticks
Boutonneuse fever, Kenya tick fever	*R. conorii*	Mediterranean, Africa, India	Ticks
Siberian tick fever	*R. sibirica*	Siberia, Mongolia	Ticks
Rickettsialpox	*R. akari*	United States, Russia, Central Asia, Korea, Africa	Mites
	Typhus group		
Louse-borne typhus (epidemic typhus)	*R. prowazekii*	Latin America, Africa, Asia	Lice
Murine typhus (endemic typhus)	*R. typhi*	Worldwide	Fleas
Scrub typhus	*R. tsutsugamushi*	South Pacific, Asia	Mites
Q fever	*Coxiella burnetti*	Worldwide	Inhalation

man target cell for all rickettsiae is the endothelial cell of capillaries and other small blood vessels. The organisms reproduce within these cells, killing them in the process and producing a necrotizing vasculitis.

Human rickettsial infections present as systemic symptoms of headache, myalgias, and fever, followed by a rash. They are traditionally divided into the "spotted fever group" and the "typhus group."

ROCKY MOUNTAIN SPOTTED FEVER

Rocky Mountain spotted fever is an acute, potentially fatal, systemic vasculitis, usually manifested by headache, fever, and rash. The causative organism, *Rickettsia rickettsii*, is transmitted to humans by tick bites.

☐ **Epidemiology:** Rocky Mountain spotted fever is acquired by bites of infected ticks, which are the vectors and major reservoirs for *R. rickettsii*. The organism passes from mother to progeny ticks without killing them, thereby maintaining a natural reservoir for human infection.

Rocky Mountain spotted fever occurs in various areas throughout North, Central, and South America. In the United States, most cases occur in a large cluster of states extending from the eastern seaboard (Georgia to New York) westward to Texas, Oklahoma, and Kansas. Cases in the Rocky Mountain region are uncommon. The name of the disease is misleading, deriving from its discovery in Idaho, rather than its area of greatest prevalence. Some 500 cases occur annually in the United States.

☐ **Pathogenesis:** *R. rickettsii* in the salivary glands of the tick is introduced into the skin while the tick is feeding. The organisms apparently spread via lymphatics and small blood vessels to the systemic and pulmonary circulation. Here they attach to vascular endothelial cells, are engulfed, and reproduce within the cytoplasm. They are then shed into the vascular and lymphatic systems. Further infection and destruction of vascular endothelium causes a systemic vasculitis. The rash, produced by inflammatory damage to cutaneous vessels, is the most visible manifestation of the generalized phenomenon of vascular injury. Whereas other rickettsiae infect only capillary endothelial cells, *R. rickettsii* spreads to vascular smooth muscle and endothelium of larger vessels. Extensive damage to blood vessel walls causes loss of vascular integrity, exudation of fluid, and disseminated intravascular coagulation. Fluid loss can be so extensive that it leads to shock. Damage to pulmonary capillaries can produce pulmonary edema and acute alveolar injury.

☐ **Pathology:** The vascular lesions of Rocky Mountain spotted fever are found throughout the body, affecting capillaries, venules, arterioles, and sometimes larger vessels. There is necrosis and reactive hyperplasia of vascular endothelium, often associated with thrombosis of the smaller-caliber vessels. Vessel walls are infiltrated, initially with neutrophils and macrophages and later with lymphocytes and plasma cells. Vascular inflammation and thrombosis is associated with microscopic infarctions and extravasation of blood into surrounding tissues. The orientation of the intracellular bacilli in parallel rows and in an end-to-end pattern gives them the appearance of a "flotilla at anchor facing the wind."

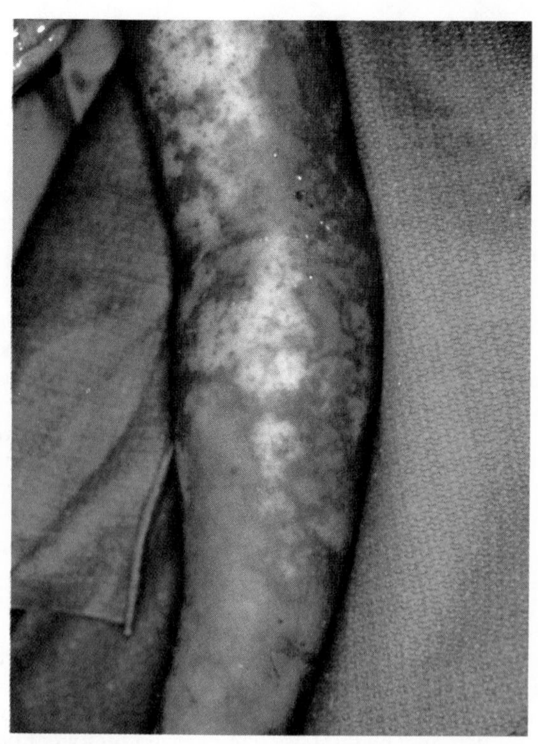

FIGURE *9-44*
Rocky mountain spotted fever. A severe petechial and purpuric eruption is noted on the arm in this fatal case.

☐ **Clinical Features:** The incubation period varies from 2 to 14 days. Rocky Mountain spotted fever presents with fever, headache, and myalgias, followed by a rash. The rash begins as a maculopapular eruption but rapidly becomes petechial, spreading centripetally from the distal extremities to the trunk (Fig. 9-44). Cutaneous lesions usually appear on the palms and soles, a distinctive feature of the disease. If untreated, more than 20% to 50% of infected persons die within 8 to 15 days. Prompt diagnosis and antibiotic treatment (chloramphenicol and tetracycline) is lifesaving, and in the United States, mortality has been reduced to less that 5%.

EPIDEMIC (LOUSE-BORNE) TYPHUS

Epidemic typhus is a severe systemic vasculitis transmitted by the bite of infected lice. The disease is caused by *Rickettsia prowazekii*, an organism that has a human-louse-human life cycle (Fig. 9-45).

☐ **Epidemiology:** *R. prowazekii* is transmitted from one infected person to another by the bite of an infected body louse. The disease is widely distributed in some re-

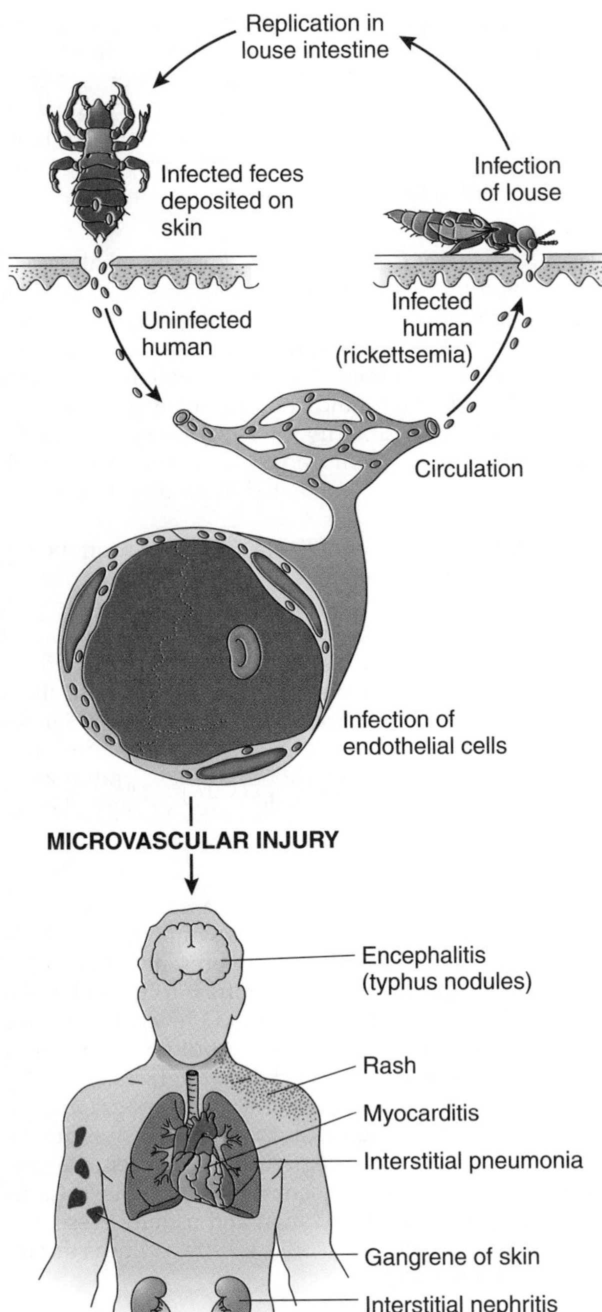

FIGURE *9-45*
Epidemic typhus (louse-borne typhus). *R. prowazekii* has a man-louse-man life cycle. The organism multiplies in endothelial cells, which detach, rupture, and release organisms into the circulation (rickettsemia). A louse taking a blood meal becomes infected with rickettsiae, which enter the epithelial cells of its midgut, multiply, and rupture the cells, thereby releasing rickettsiae into the lumen of the louse intestine. Contaminated feces are deposited on the skin or clothing of a second host and penetrate an abrasion or are inhaled. The rickettsiae then enter endothelial cells, multiply, and rupture the cells, thus completing the cycle.

gions of Africa, Asia, Europe, and the Western Hemisphere. Devastating epidemics of typhus were associated with cold climates, poor sanitation, and crowding during natural disasters, famine, or war. Infrequent bathing and lack of changes of clothing lead to louse infestation of human populations and consequently epidemics of typhus. With the mass displacements of populations in Eastern Europe in World War I, epidemic typhus affected over 30 million persons, killing over 3 million. Epidemic louse-borne typhus last occurred in the United States in 1921, but rare sporadic cases have been reported in persons who have been in contact with flying squirrels (*Glaucomys volans*), the only known nonhuman reservoir of *R. prowazekii*.

After a louse takes a blood meal from a person infected with *R. prowazekii*, the organisms enter the epithelial cells of the midgut, multiply, and rupture the cells within 3 to 5 days. Large numbers of rickettsiae are released into the lumen of the louse intestine. The louse deposits its contaminated feces on the skin or clothing of a second host, where they may remain infectious for more than 3 months. A person becomes infected when the contaminated louse feces penetrate an abrasion or scratch or when the person inhales airborne rickettsiae from clothing containing louse feces.

□ Pathology:

Epidemic typhus begins with localized infection of capillary endothelium and progresses to a systemic vasculitis. Louse-borne typhus differs from the other rickettsial diseases in that *R. prowazekii* can establish latent infection and produce recrudescent disease **(Brill-Zinsser disease)** many years after primary infection.

The pathological changes produced by *R. prowazekii* are similar to those of Rocky Mountain spotted fever and the other rickettsial diseases. At autopsy, there are few gross findings except for splenomegaly and occasional areas of necrosis. Microscopically, collections of mononuclear cells are found in various organs (e.g., skin, brain, and heart). The infiltrate includes mast cells, lymphocytes, plasma cells, and macrophages, which are frequently arranged as **typhus nodules** around arterioles and capillaries. Throughout the body, the endothelium of small blood vessels is focally necrotic and hyperplastic, and the walls are infiltrated by neutrophils, macrophages, lymphocytes, and plasma cells. Rickettsiae can be demonstrated within the endothelial cells.

□ Clinical Features:

After an incubation period of 7 to 14 days, louse-borne typhus presents as fever, headache, and myalgias, followed by a rash. Macular lesions, which become petechial, appear on the upper trunk and axillary folds and spread centrifugally to the extremities. In fatal cases, the rash commonly becomes confluent and purpuric. Mild rickettsial pneumonia is followed by a superimposed bacterial pneumonia. Dying patients may exhibit the symptoms of encephalitis, myocarditis, interstitial pneumonia, interstitial nephritis, and shock. In patients who recover, the symptoms abate after about 3 weeks, and fatalities usually occur during the second or third week of illness.

Epidemic typhus can be controlled by large-scale delousing of the population, by steam sterilization of clothing, and the use of insecticides. Typhus is treated with tetracycline or chloramphenicol.

ENDEMIC (MURINE) TYPHUS

Endemic typhus is similar to epidemic typhus but tends to be a milder disease. Humans are infected with *R. typhi* by interrupting the rat-flea-rat cycle of transmission. When the flea defecates on the surface of the skin, the feces contaminate the small wound made by the bite. The rickettsiae also contaminate clothes and become airborne. When they are inhaled, they cause pulmonary infection. Outbreaks of murine typhus are associated with an exploding population of rats, although sporadic infections occur in the southwestern United States. These are associated with rat-infested dwellings and with occupations that bring humans into contact with rats, such as the handling and storage of grain.

SCRUB TYPHUS

Scrub typhus ***(tsutsugamushi fever)*** *is an acute, febrile illness of humans that is caused by Rickettsia tsutsugamushi.* Rodents are the natural mammalian reservoir. From rats, the organism is passed to trombiculid mites known as chiggers. These insects transmit the infection to their larvae, which crawl to the tips of vegetation and attach to passers-by. While feeding, mites inoculate the organisms into the skin. Rickettsemia and lymphadenopathy follow shortly. Scrub typhus is widely distributed in eastern and southern Asia, and the islands of the southern and western Pacific, including Japan. Endemic infection is unknown in the western world.

A multiloculated vesicle forms at the inoculation site and ulcerates, after which an eschar forms. As the lesion heals, there is a sudden onset of headache and fever, followed by pneumonia, a macular rash, lymphadenopathy, and hepatosplenomegaly. Severe infections are complicated by meningoencephalitis, myocarditis, and shock. The mortality rates in untreated patients have ranged up to 30%.

Q FEVER

Q fever is a self-limited, systemic infection, usually presenting as headache, fever, and myalgias. The disease is caused by *Coxiella burnetii*, a small (0.3 × 1μm) pleomorphic coccobaciluus with a gram-negative cell wall. Unlike true rickettsiae, *C. burnetii* enter cells by a passive mechanism, being phagocytized by macrophages. Also unlike true rickettsial infections, *C. burnetii* infection does not produce a vasculitis, and thus there is no associated rash.

☐ **Epidemiology:** Humans acquire *C. burnetii* infection by exposure to infected animals or animal products. Infection is endemic in many wild and domesticated animals, but cattle, sheep, and goats are the usual sources of human infection. These animals shed large numbers of organisms in urine, feces, milk, body fluids, and birth products. Humans acquire the infection by inhaling organisms aerosolized from these materials. Q fever is most often seen in herders, slaughterhouse workers, veterinarians, dairy workers, and other persons with occupational exposure to infected domesticated animals. Aerosol droplets may spread the infection from person to person. Q fever is rare in the United States.

☐ **Pathology:** Q fever begins with the inhalation of organisms, after which they are phagocytosed by alveolar macrophages. *C. burnetii* replicates in phagolysosomes. Recruitment of neutrophils and macrophages produces a focal bronchopneumonia. The nonactivated phagocytes fail to kill *C. burnetii*, and the organism disseminates through the body, primarily infecting cells of the monocyte/macrophage system. Most infections resolve with the onset of specific cell-mediated immunity. Occasional cases persist as chronic infections.

The lungs and liver are the organs most prominently involved in Q fever. The lungs demonstrate single or multiple irregular areas of consolidation, in which the pulmonary parenchyma is infiltrated by neutrophils and macrophages. Organisms may be demonstrated in macrophages by the Giemsa stain. Hepatic involvement in Q fever is usually characterized by multiple microscopic granulomas, which have a distinctive "fibrin ring" or "doughnut ring" configuration. In these granulomas, epithelioid macrophages encircle a ring of fibrin, sometimes containing a lipid vacuole.

☐ **Clinical Features:** In most cases in endemic areas, Q fever is a self-limited mildly symptomatic febrile disease. More severe cases typically present as headache, fever, fatigue, and myalgias. In contrast to the rickettsial diseases, there is usually no rash in Q fever. Pulmonary infection is virtually always present, but it may manifest as an atypical pneumonia with dry cough, as a rapidly progressive pneumonia, or as chest roentgenographic abnormalities without significant respiratory symptoms. Many patients have some degree of hepatosplenomegaly. The disease resolves spontaneously in 2 to 14 days. Cases of chronic Q fever are uncommon and usually present as persistent fever of unknown origin. Tetracycline is the antibiotic of choice for Q fever.

Mycoplasmal Infections

The mycoplasmas, formerly known as pleuropneumonia-like organisms, are the smallest free-living prokaryotes, measuring less than 0.3 μm in greatest dimension. They lack the rigid cell walls of the more complex bacteria. Mycoplasmas are widespread, both geographically and ecologically, as saprophytes and as parasites of a broad range of animals and plants. Numerous *Mycoplasma* species are known to inhabit the human body, but only three are pathogenic, namely, *M. pneumoniae*, *M. hominis*, and *Ureaplasma urealyticum*. The diseases associated with these organisms are shown in Table 9-7.

TABLE 9-7 **Mycoplasmal Infections**

Organism	Disease
Mycoplasma pneumoniae	Tracheobronchitis Pneumonia Pharyngitis Otitis media
Ureaplasma urealyticum	Urethritis Chorioamnionitis Postpartum fever
Mycoplasma hominis	Postpartum fever

MYCOPLASMA PNEUMONIAE INFECTION

M. pneumoniae causes acute, self-limited lower respiratory tract infections (tracheobronchitis and pneumonia), affecting mostly children and young adults. M. pneumoniae can also cause pharyngitis and otitis media.

☐ **Epidemiology:** Most infections occur in small groups of persons who have frequent close contact, for example, families, college fraternities, military units, and residents of closed institutions. The organism is spread by aerosol transmission from person to person over a period of several months, with an attack rate of greater than 50% within the group. *M. pneumoniae* infection occurs worldwide, and in developed countries the organism causes 15% to 20% of all pneumonias.

☐ **Pathogenesis:** *M. pneumoniae* initiates infection by attaching to a glycolipid on the surface of the respiratory epithelium. The organism remains outside the cells, where it reproduces and causes progressive dysfunction and eventual death of the host cells. Because *M. pneumoniae* infection rarely produces symptomatic disease in children younger than the age of 5 years, it is thought that the host immune response plays a role in tissue injury.

☐ **Pathology:** Pneumonia caused by *M. pneumoniae* usually shows patchy consolidation of a single segment of a lower lung lobe, although the process can be more widespread. The mucosa of the affected airways is edematous and infiltrated by a predominantly mononuclear inflammatory infiltrate. The alveoli display a largely interstitial process, with reactive alveolar lining cells and infiltration by mononuclear cells. The pulmonary changes are often complicated by bacterial superinfection. The organism itself is too small to be detected in infected tissue by routine light microscopy.

☐ **Clinical Features:** Pneumonia or tracheobronchitis produced by *M. pneumoniae* presents as fever, headache, and malaise, followed by the onset of a nonproductive cough. The pneumonia tends to be milder than other bacterial pneumonias, a fact that has earned the disease the appellation "walking pneumonia." Fever ordinarily persists for no more than 2 weeks, although the cough may linger for 6 weeks or more. Death from *M. pneumoniae* infection is rare. The infection is treated with tetracycline or erythromycin.

Mycobacterial Infections

The Mycobacteria are distinctive organisms, 2 to 10 μm in length, which share the cell wall architecture of gram-positive bacteria, but also contain large amounts of lipid. The high lipid content interferes with staining by aniline dyes, including crystal violet used in the Gram stain. Thus, although the Mycobacteria are gram-positive on a structural basis, this property is difficult to demonstrate by routine staining. The waxy lipids of the cell wall make the Mycobacteria "acid fast," that is, they retain carbolfuchsin after rinsing with acid alcohol.

The Mycobacteria grow more slowly than other pathogenic bacteria, and mycobacterial diseases are all chronic, slowly progressive illnesses. The Mycobacteria produce no known toxins, and they damage human tissues by inducing inflammatory and immunological responses. Most mycobacterial pathogens are able to replicate within cells of the monocyte-macrophage lineage and elicit granulomatous inflammation. The outcome of mycobacterial infection is largely determined by the host's capacity to contain the organism through delayed-type hypersensitivity mechanisms and cell-mediated immune responses.

The two primary mycobacterial pathogens, *M. tuberculosis* and *M. leprae*, exclusively infect humans and enjoy no environmental reservoir. The remaining pathogenic Mycobacteria are environmental organisms, which only occasionally cause human disease.

TUBERCULOSIS

Tuberculosis is a chronic, communicable disease, in which the lungs are the prime target, but in which any organ may be infected. The disease is caused principally by M. tuberculosis hominis (Koch bacillus), but also occasionally by M. tuberculosis bovis. The lungs are the prime target, but any organ may be infected. **The characteristic lesion is a spherical granuloma with central caseous necrosis.**

M. tuberculosis is a slender, beaded, nonmotile, acid-fast bacillus (Fig. 9-46), which is an obligate aerobe. The organism grows slowly in culture, with a doubling time of 24 hours, and 3 to 6 weeks are commonly required to produce visible growth in culture.

☐ **Epidemiology:** Distributed throughout the world, tuberculosis is clearly one of the most important bacterial diseases in humans. Although the risk of infection has been significantly reduced in developed countries, it remains high for HIV-infected persons, homeless, and malnourished persons in impoverished areas, and immigrants from regions where the disease is endemic. In the United States, for example, the annual incidence of tuberculosis is 12 per 100,000, and the mortality is 1 to 2 per

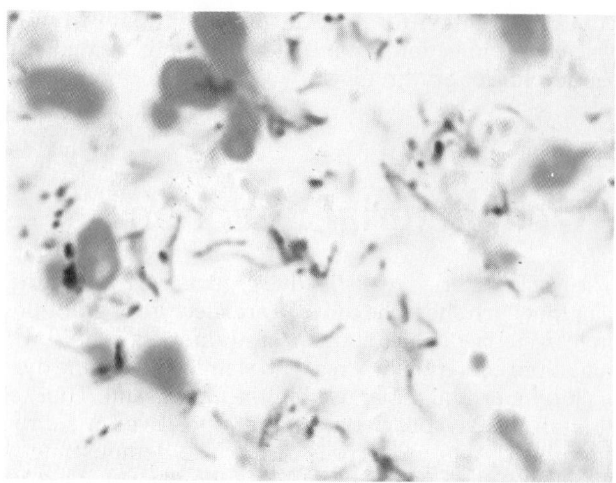

FIGURE 9-46
Mycobacterium tuberculosis. **A smear of a pulmonary lesion shows slender, beaded, acid-fast bacilli.**

100,000. By contrast, in some developing countries, the incidence reaches 450 per 100,000, and many of these persons die of the disease. There are also racial and ethnic differences. Jews, other whites, and Mongolians have greater natural resistance than Africans, Native Americans, and Eskimos. Age may also be a factor. In the United States, tuberculosis is highest among the elderly, possibly reflecting reactivation of infections acquired earlier in life before the decline in the prevalence of the disease.

M. tuberculosis is transmitted from person to person by aerosolized droplets. Coughing, sneezing, and talking all create aerosolized respiratory droplets; usually, the droplets evaporate, leaving an organism ("droplet nucleus") that is readily carried in the air. Crowding of urbanization and industrialization fueled the tuberculosis epidemics that devastated Europe in the 18th and 19th centuries, accounting for as many as one third of all deaths.

Tuberculosis can also be caused by *M. tuberculosis bovis*, an animal pathogen closely related to *M. tuberculosis hominis*. Humans acquire this form of tuberculosis by the ingestion of infected milk. It has ceased to be a significant public health problem in countries where milk is pasteurized or milk-producing animals are inspected.

☐ **Pathogenesis:** Depending on the age and immunological status of the infected person, as well as the total burden of organisms, tuberculosis can pursue radically different courses. Some patients exhibit only an indolent, completely asymptomatic infection, whereas in others, tuberculosis progresses to disseminated destructive disease. Many more persons are infected with *M. tuberculosis* than develop clinical symptoms, and a distinction is made between tuberculous infection and active tuberculosis. **Tuberculous infection** refers to growth of the organism in a person, whether the infection produces symptomatic disease or not. **Active tuberculosis** is the term for the subset of tuberculous infections manifested by destructive, symptomatic disease.

Primary tuberculosis occurs on first exposure to the organism and can pursue either an indolent or an aggressive course (Fig. 9-47). **Secondary tuberculosis** refers to disease that develops long after the primary infection, most commonly as a result of the reactivation of the primary infection. Secondary tuberculosis can also be produced by exposure to exogenous organisms and is always an active disease.

Primary Infection

Primary tuberculosis is an infection of persons who have not had prior contact with the tubercle bacillus.

☐ **Pathogenesis:** Inhaled *M. tuberculosis* are deposited in the alveoli, usually in the lower segments of the lower and middle lobes and anterior segments of the upper lobes. The organisms are phagocytosed by alveolar macrophages but resist killing; the cell wall lipids of *M. tuberculosis* apparently block the fusion of phagosomes and lysosomes and allow the bacilli to proliferate within the macrophages.

As the tubercle bacilli multiply, macrophages degrade some mycobacteria and present antigen to T lymphocytes. Some macrophages carry organisms from the lung to regional (hilar and mediastinal) lymph nodes, from which sites they may be disseminated by the bloodstream to other areas in the body. The bacilli continue to proliferate at the primary site of deposition in the lungs, as well as at other hospitable sites, including lymph nodes, kidneys, meninges, epiphyseal plates of long bones and vertebrae, and apical areas of the lungs.

Although the macrophages that first ingest *M. tuberculosis* cannot kill these organisms, they initiate hypersensitivity and cell-mediated immunologic responses, which eventually contain the infection. Infected macrophages present tuberculous antigens to T lymphocytes. A clone of sensitized cells proliferates, produces interferon γ, and activates macrophages, thereby increasing their concentrations of lytic enzymes and augmenting their capacity to kill mycobacteria. When released, the lytic enzymes in these activated macrophages, which include epitheloid macrophages and Langhans giant cells, also damage host tissues.

The development of a population of activated lymphocytes responsive to *M. tuberculosis* antigen constitutes the hypersensitivity response to the organism. The related development of activated macrophages capable of ingesting and destroying the bacilli comprises the cell-mediated immune response. The hypersensitivity and cell-mediated immune responses work in concert to combat the proliferating organisms, a process that requires 3 to 6 weeks to come into play.

If the infected person is immunologically competent and the burden of organisms is small, a vigorous granulomatous reaction is produced. Tubercle bacilli are ingested and killed by activated macrophages, surrounded by fibrous tissue, and successfully contained. When the number of organisms is high, the hypersensitivity reaction produces significant tissue necrosis, which has a characteristic cheese-like (caseous) consistency. Although not invariably caused by *M. tuberculosis*, caseous necrosis is so strongly

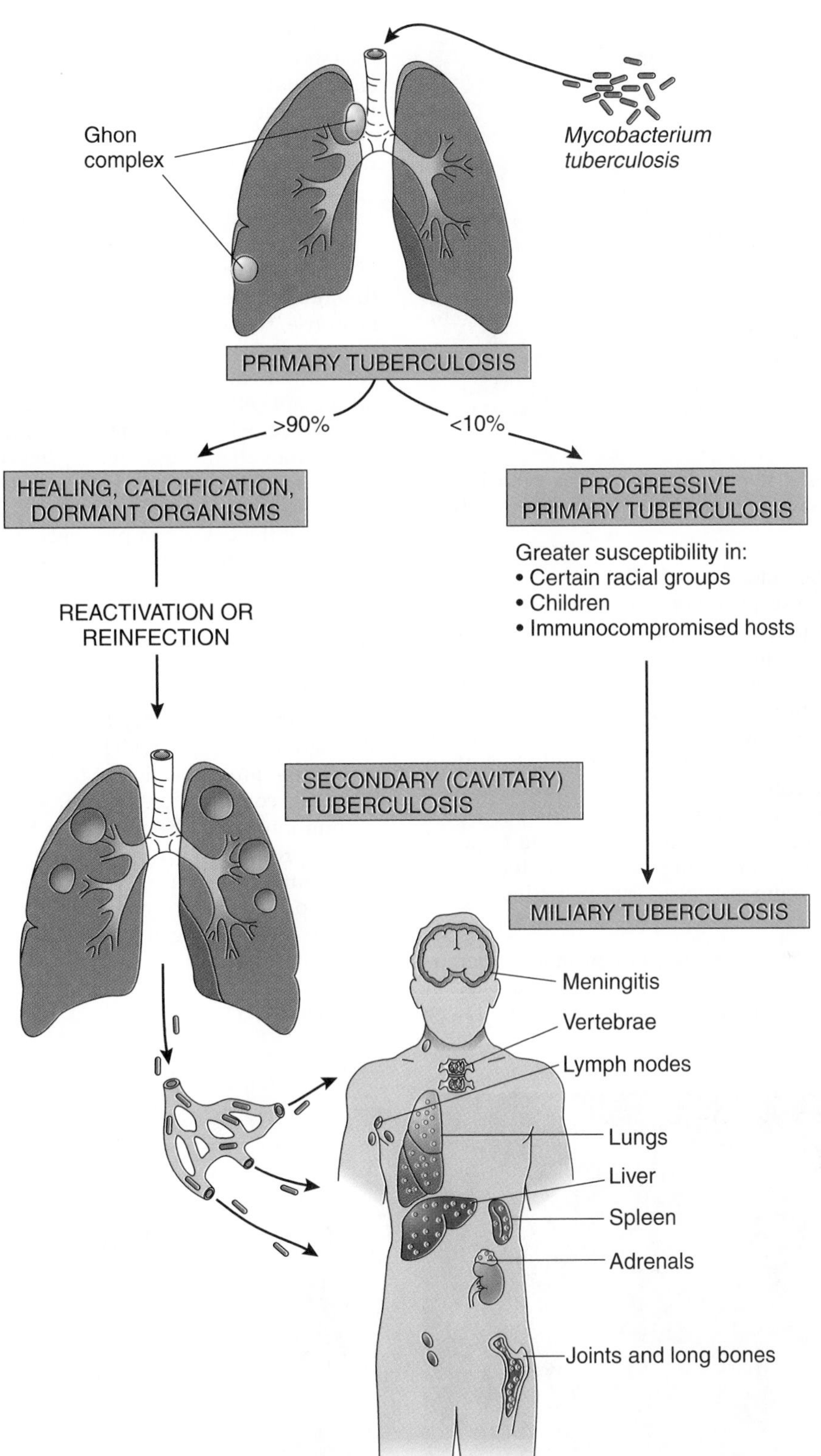

FIGURE 9-47
Stages of the tuberculosis. Primary tuberculosis (in a person lacking previous contact or immune responsiveness). Progressive primary tuberculosis develops in less than 10% of infected normal adults, but more frequently in children and immunosuppressed patients.

Secondary (cavitary) tuberculosis results from reactivation of dormant endogenous bacilli or reinfection with exogenous bacilli. Miliary tuberculosis is caused by dissemination of tubercle bacilli to produce numerous, minute, yellow-white lesions (resembling millet seeds) in distant organs.

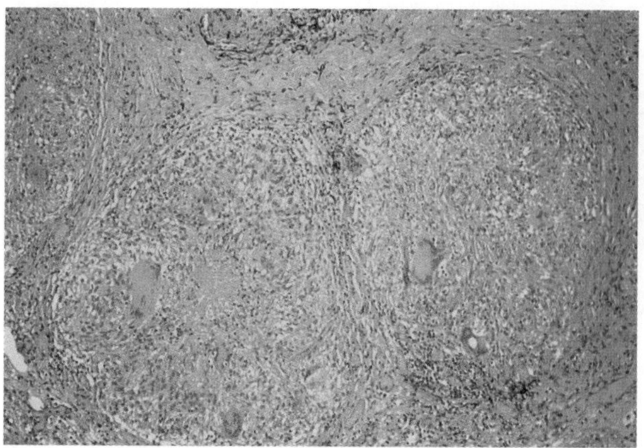

FIGURE 9-48
Primary tuberculosis. Photomicrograph of a hilar lymph node shows a tuberculous granuloma with central caseation.

associated with tuberculosis, that its discovery in tissue almost always raises a suspicion of this disease.

If the infected person is immunologically immature, as in a young child, or immunosuppressed as in a patient with AIDS, the course of this primary tuberculous infection is often quite different. Such persons lack the capacity to coordinate integrated hypersensitivity and cell-mediated immune responses to the organism and, thus, often lack the capacity to contain the infection. Granulomas are poorly formed, or not formed at all, and infection progresses at the primary site in the lung, in the regional lymph nodes, or in multiple sites of dissemination. This process produces progressive primary tuberculosis.

☐ **Pathology:** The lung lesion of primary tuberculous infection is known as the **Ghon focus**. It is located in the subpleural area of the upper segments of the lower lobes or in the lower segments of the upper lobes. Initially, the Ghon focus is a small ill-defined area of inflammatory consolidation. The infection then drains to the hilar lymph nodes. The combination of the peripheral Ghon focus and the involved mediastinal or hilar lymph nodes is referred to as the **Ghon complex**.

Microscopically, the classic lesion of tuberculosis is a caseous granuloma (Fig. 9-48), which has a soft, semisolid core surrounded by epithelioid macrophages, Langhans giant cells, lymphocytes, and peripheral fibrous tissue. If the infected person lacks an appropriate immunological response, the granuloma formed in response to *M. tuberculosis* is less organized and may consist of only an aggregate of macrophages, lacking the architecture and Langhans giant cells of the classic granuloma.

In over 90% of normal adults, tuberculous infection follows a self-limited course, because the cellular immune response is sufficient to control the multiplication of the bacilli. In both the lungs and the lymph nodes, the lesions of the Ghon complex heal, undergoing shrinkage, fibrous scarring, and calcification, the last visible radiographically. Most of the organisms die, but a small proportion may remain viable for years. Later, if immune mechanisms wane or fail, the resting bacilli may proliferate and break out, causing serious tuberculous infection (secondary tuberculosis).

Progressive primary tuberculosis is a less common alternative course, in which the immune response fails to control the multiplication of the tubercle bacilli. Infection takes this course in less than 10% of normal adults, but it is common in children younger than 5 years of age. In adults, progressive primary tuberculosis is most common in patients with suppressed or defective immunity.

In progressive primary tuberculosis, the Ghon focus in the lung enlarges and may even erode into the bronchial tree. The affected hilar and mediastinal lymph nodes also enlarge, sometimes compressing the bronchi to produce atelectasis of the distal lung; collapse of the mid-

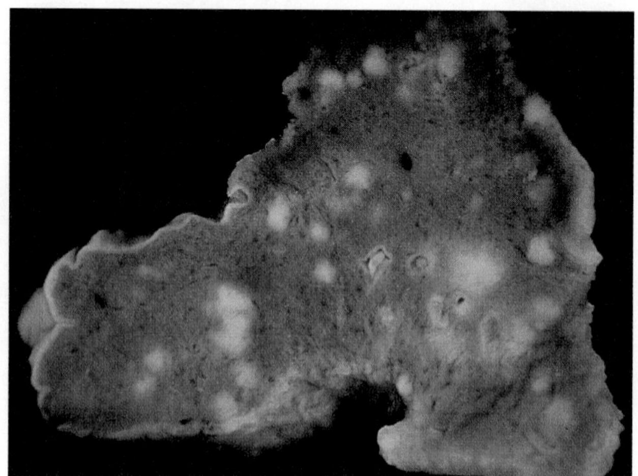

A

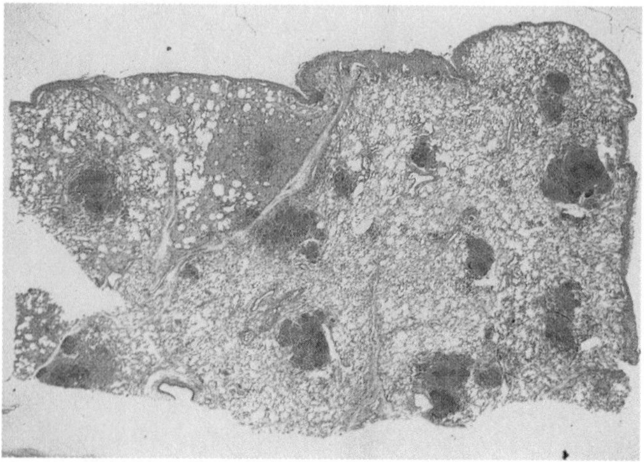

B

FIGURE 9-49
Miliary tuberculosis. (*A*) The cut surface of the lung reveals numerous uniform, white, nodules. (*B*) A low-power photomicrograph discloses many foci of granulomatous inflammation.

dle lobe ("middle lobe syndrome") is a common result of this compression. In some instances, the infected lymph nodes erode into an airway to spread organisms throughout the lungs.

Miliary tuberculosis *refers to infection at disseminated sites that produces multiple, small, yellow, nodular lesions in several organs* (Fig. 9-49). The term **miliary** was coined to emphasize the resemblance of the disseminated lesions to millet seeds. The lungs, lymph nodes, kidneys, adrenals, bone marrow, spleen, and liver are common sites of miliary lesions. Progressive disease may involve the meninges and cause tuberculous meningitis.

□ **Clinical Features:** The vast majority of persons successfully contain the primary infection, and primary tuberculosis is generally asymptomatic. In those who develop progressive primary disease, the symptoms are usually insidious and nonspecific. Constitutional symptoms of fever, weight loss, fatigue, and night sweats are often the first clinical manifestations of disease. Sometimes the onset of symptoms is abrupt, and the disease presents as high fever, pleurisy, a pleural effusion, and lymphadenitis. Cough and hemoptysis develop only when active pulmonary disease is well established. With disseminated (miliary) tuberculosis, specific symptoms vary according to the organs affected and tend to occur late in the course of disease.

Secondary (Cavitary) Tuberculosis

Secondary tuberculosis results from the proliferation of M. tuberculosis in a person who has been previously infected and has mounted an immunological response. The source of the bacteria in secondary tuberculosis may be either dormant organisms from old granulomas (which is usually the case) or newly acquired bacilli. Various conditions predispose to the reemergence of endogenous (dormant) *M. tuberculosis*, including cancer, antineoplastic chemotherapy, immunosuppressive therapy, AIDS, and old age. Secondary tuberculosis may develop any time after the primary infection, even decades later.

□ **Pathology:** The lungs are by far the most common site for secondary tuberculosis, although any locale of previous dissemination may manifest secondary disease. In the lungs, secondary tuberculosis usually begins in the apical-posterior segments of the upper lobes, where organisms are commonly seeded during the primary infection. The bacilli proliferate at these sites and elicit an inflammatory response, which results in a localized area of consolidation. **The ensuing T cell–mediated immune responses to the now familiar tuberculous antigens lead to tissue necrosis and the production of tuberculous cavities** (Fig. 9-50). Apical cavities are optimal sites for the multiplication of *M. tuberculosis*, and large numbers of organisms are produced in this environment. Cavities are typically 2 to 4 cm in diameter when first detected clinically but can range to well over 10 cm. Tuberculous cavities contain caseous material teeming with mycobacteria and are surrounded by a granulomatous response.

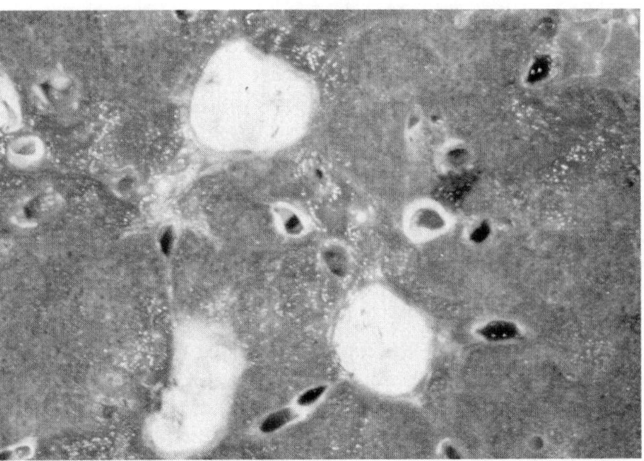

FIGURE *9-50*
Secondary pulmonary tuberculosis. A cross-section of lung shows several tuberculous cavities filled with necrotic, caseous material.

The pulmonary lesions of secondary tuberculosis may be complicated by a variety of secondary effects. These include (1) scarring and calcification; (2) spread to other areas; (3) pleural fibrosis and adhesions; (4) rupture of a caseous lesion, spilling bacilli into the pleural cavity; (5) erosion into a bronchus, which seeds the bronchioles, bronchi, and trachea; and (6) implantation of bacilli in the larynx, causing hoarseness and pain on swallowing. Tubercle bacilli may also spread throughout the body through the lymphatics and bloodstream to cause miliary tuberculosis.

□ **Clinical Features:** The symptoms of secondary tuberculosis begin with cough, which may be erroneously attributed to smoking or to a cold. Low-grade fever develops, with general malaise, fatigue, anorexia, weight loss, and often night sweats. Cavitary disease may be accompanied by brisk hemoptysis, on occasion severe enough to cause exsanguination. Chest radiographs showing unilateral or bilateral apical cavities suggest the diagnosis of secondary tuberculosis. If the disease is disseminated, the signs and symptoms reflect the particular organs involved.

Untreated secondary tuberculosis is a wasting disease, which is eventually fatal. Prior to the antibiotic era, chronic cavitary tuberculosis was one of the most common causes of secondary amyloidosis. Tuberculosis is treated with prolonged courses of antituberculous antibiotics, including isoniazid, pyrizinamide, rifampin, and ethambutol. Strains of *M. tuberculosis* that are resistant to these antibiotics have recently emerged, usually as a result of failure to take prescribed medications consistently and for the full time-period.

LEPROSY

Leprosy (Hansen disease) is a chronic, slowly progressive, destructive process involving peripheral nerves, skin, and mucous membranes caused by Mycobacterium leprae. This agent is a slender, weakly acid-fast rod, which cannot be cultured on artificial media or in cell culture.

☐ **Epidemiology:** Leprosy is one of the oldest recognized human diseases. Lepers were isolated from the community in the Old Testament, although some of those segregated persons may have suffered from psoriasis and other skin conditions. For centuries, leprosy was widespread in Europe, including England. In 1873, Hansen documented the first human bacterial pathogen when he described the lepra bacillus in fresh mounts of scrapings from a skin lesion of a Norwegian patient.

Lepra bacilli multiply in experimental animals at sites with temperatures below that of the internal organs, such as the foot pads of mice and the ear lobes of hamsters, rats, and other rodents. Naturally acquired leprosy has been recognized in armadillos (Louisiana and Texas), in a chimpanzee trapped in Sierra Leone, and in a mangabey captured in Nigeria. Lepra bacilli have been experimentally transmitted to armadillos, whose susceptibility is related, at least in part, to their low body temperature (32°C to 35°C).

Leprosy is transmitted from person to person, usually as a result of years of intimate contact. *M. leprae* is shed in nasal secretions or from ulcerated lesions of an infected person. The mode of infection is unclear, but it probably involves inoculation of bacilli into the respiratory tract or into open wounds. Although leprosy is now rare in developed countries, 15 million persons are infected worldwide, primarily in tropical areas, including India, Papua-New Guinea, Southeast Asia, and tropical Africa. Fewer than 400 cases are diagnosed annually in the United States, the vast majority in immigrants from endemic areas.

☐ **Pathogenesis:** *M. leprae* multiplies best at temperatures cooler than core human body temperature, and lesions tend to occur in cooler parts of the body (e.g., the hands and face). Leprosy exhibits a bewildering variety of clinical and pathological features. The lesions vary from the small, insignificant, and self-healing macules of tuberculoid leprosy to the diffuse, disfiguring, and sometimes fatal lesions of lepromatous leprosy (Fig. 9-51). This extreme variation in the presentation of the disease is probably related to differences in immune reactivity.

The large majority (95%) of all persons have a natural protective immunity to *M. leprae* and are not infected even through intimate and prolonged exposure. In the susceptible population (5%) who may develop symptomatic infections, a broad immunological spectrum ranges from anergy to hyperergy. **Anergic patients (i.e., those with little or no resistance) have lepromatous leprosy, whereas hyperergic patients (i.e., those with high resistance) develop tuberculoid leprosy.** Borderline leprosy is the term applied to the broad middle ground into which most symptomatic patients fall.

Tuberculoid Leprosy

Tuberculoid leprosy occurs in infected persons who mount an effective granulomatous response that limits the proliferation of the bacillus and the extent of the disease.

☐ **Pathology:** Tuberculoid leprosy is characterized by a single lesion or very few lesions of the skin. These usually appear on the face, extremities, or trunk. Microscopically the lesions show well-formed, circumscribed dermal granulomas, composed of epithelioid granulomas, Langhans giant cells, and lymphocytes. Nerve fibers are almost invariably swollen and infiltrated with lymphocytes. The destruction of small dermal nerve twigs accounts for the sensory deficit associated with tuberculoid leprosy. Bacilli are rare and often not found with acid-fast stains. The condition is termed tuberculoid leprosy because the granulomas vaguely resemble the lesions of tuberculosis. However, the granulomas of leprosy lack caseous necrosis.

☐ **Clinical Features:** The skin lesions of tuberculoid leprosy appear as well-demarcated, hypopigmented or erythematous, dry, hairless patches, with raised outer edges. Nerve involvement causes diminished sensation or numbness within the patch. As the lesion expands at its periphery, it often heals centrally. In contrast to lepromatous leprosy, the lesions of tuberculoid leprosy cause minimal disfigurement and are not infectious.

FIGURE *9-51*
(*A, top*) Lepromatous leprosy. There is diffuse involvement, including a leonine face, loss of eyebrows and eyelashes, and nodular distortions, especially on the face, ears, forearms, and hands—the exposed (cool) parts of the body. (*A, bottom*) The nodular skin lesions of advanced lepromatous leprosy. Swelling has flattened the epidermis (loss of Rete ridges). A characteristic "clear zone" of uninvolved dermis separates the epidermis from tumor-like accumulations of macrophages, each containing numerous lepra bacilli (*Mycobacterium leprae*). (*B, top*) Tuberculoid leprosy on the cheek, showing a hypopigmented macule with a raised, infiltrated border. The central portion may be hypesthetic or anesthetic. (*B, bottom*) Macular skin lesion of tuberculoid leprosy. Skin from the raised "infiltrated" margin of the plaque contains discrete granulomas that extend to the basal layer of the epidermis (without a clear zone). The granulomas are composed of epithelioid cells and Langhans giant cells, and are associated with lymphocytes and plasma cells. Lepra bacilli are rare. (*C*) Distribution of leprosy. Prevalence is greatest in tropical regions of Africa, Asia, and Latin America.

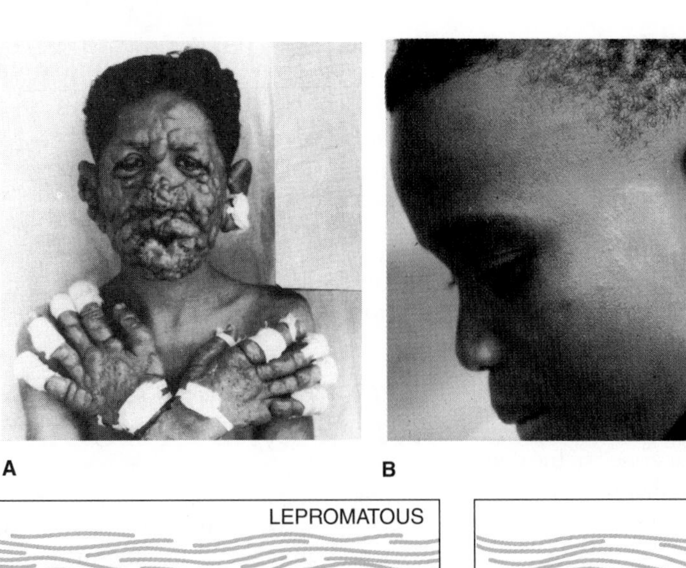
A
B

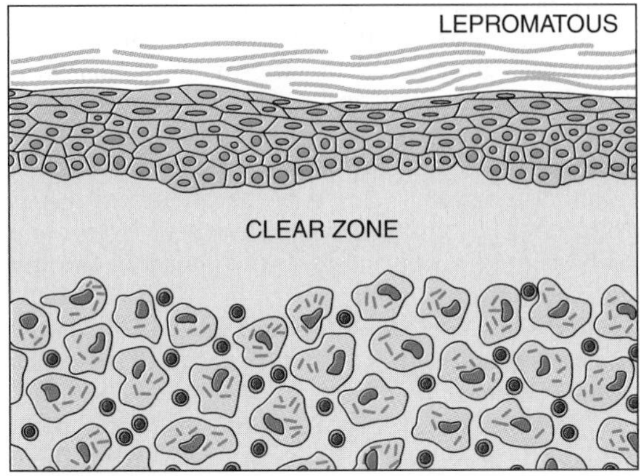
LEPROMATOUS
CLEAR ZONE

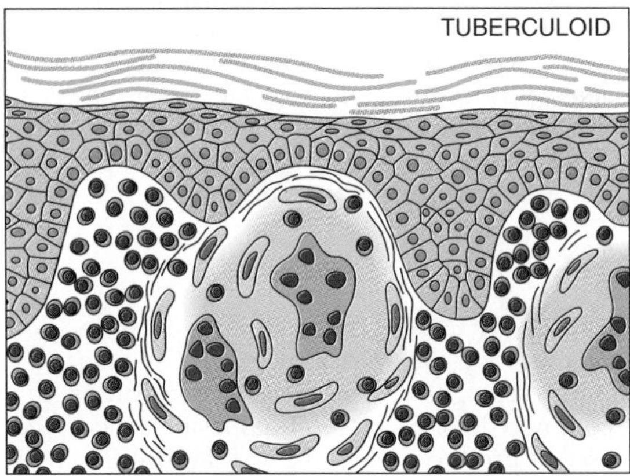
TUBERCULOID

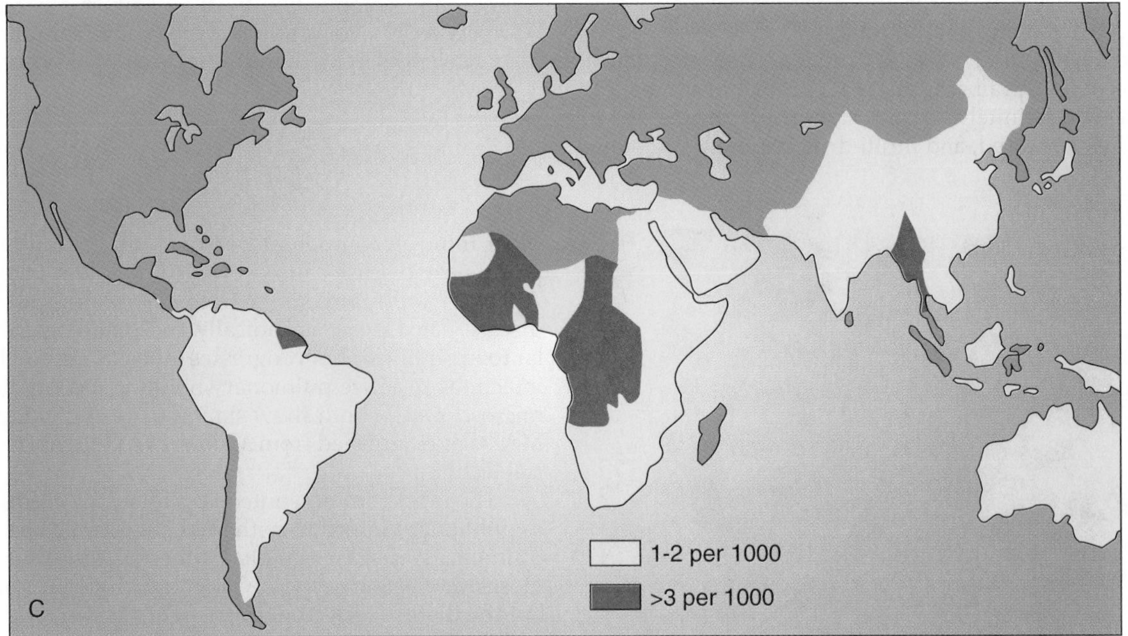
1-2 per 1000
>3 per 1000
C

FIGURE ***9-51***

Lepromatous Leprosy

Lepromatous leprosy occurs in persons who fail to develop an adequate immune response to the lepra bacillus. These patients cannot retard the proliferation of the organisms and suffer progressive destructive lesions filled with mycobacteria.

□ **Pathology:** Lepromatous leprosy exhibits multiple, tumor-like lesions of the skin, eyes, testes, nerves, lymph nodes, and spleen. Nodular or diffuse infiltrates of foamy macrophages contain myriads of bacilli (Fig. 9-52). The epidermis is stretched thinly over the nodules, and beneath it is a narrow, uninvolved "clear zone" of the dermis. Rather than destroying the bacilli, the macrophages appear to act as microincubators. When stained with acid-fast stains, the numerous organisms within the foamy macrophages appear as aggregates of acid-fast material, called **globi**. The dermal infiltrates expand slowly to distort and disfigure the face, ears, and upper airway and to destroy the eyes, eyebrows and eyelashes, nerves, and testes.

□ **Clinical Features:** The nodular skin lesions of lepromatous leprosy sometimes ulcerate. Claw-shaped hands, hammertoes, saddle-nose, and pendulous ear lobes are common deformities. Nodular lesions of the face may coalesce to produce a lion-like appearance (**leonine facies**). Involvement of the upper respiratory tract leads to a chronic nasal discharge and voice change, and infection of the eyes may cause blindness.

The most commonly used drug, dapsone, effectively eliminates the lepra bacilli in 4 to 5 years, but it must be continued indefinitely. Dapsone-resistant strains of *M. leprae* have appeared, and multi-drug regimens are often now used.

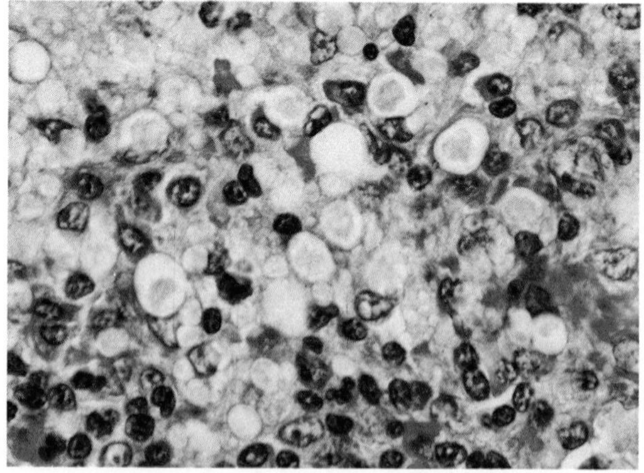

FIGURE 9-52
Lepromatous leprosy. A section of skin shows a tumor-like mass of foamy macrophages. The faint masses within the vacuolated macrophages are enormous numbers of lepra bacilli.

Borderline Leprosy

Patients with borderline leprosy have a highly variable combination of features of both lepromatous and tuberculoid leprosy. The term **indeterminate leprosy** is used when the biopsy sample is taken from a lesion that is so early in the course of the disease that the cellular response does not reveal the type of leprosy. Indeterminate lesions may heal spontaneously or progress to either lepromatous or tuberculoid forms.

MYCOBACTERIUM AVIUM-INTRACELLULARE COMPLEX

Mycobacterium avium and *Mycobacterium intracellulare* are similar mycobacterial species, which cause identical diseases and are classed together as *M. avium-intracellulare* (MAI) complex, or simply MAI. MAI causes two types of disease: (1) a rare, slowly progressive granulomatous pulmonary disease in immunocompetent persons and (2) a progressive systemic disease in patients with AIDS. Prior to the AIDS epidemic, infection with MAI was so rare as to be a medical curiosity, but today it is the third most common opportunistic infection in AIDS patients in the United States. In fact, it is thought that *M. avium complex* may eventually infect most, if not all, HIV-positive persons.

MAI is found in soil, water, and foodstuffs worldwide. Humans probably acquire MAI from the environment by inhalation of aerosols from infected water sources, and colonization by the organisms is common. As many as 70% of healthy persons show immunological responsiveness to MAI, indicating a prior exposure.

Granulomatous Pulmonary Disease in Immunocompetent Persons

Most immunocompetent persons with granulomatous pulmonary disease caused by MAI are older (aged 50 to 70 years) and many suffer from preexisting pulmonary disease. The disease is clinically and pathologically similar to tuberculosis but progresses much more slowly. Both infections produce pulmonary nodules and cavities, and microscopically both show similar caseating granulomas. MAI is distinguished from *M. tuberculosis* by microbiological techniques.

The most common antecedent illnesses predisposing to pulmonary infection with MAI are chronic obstructive pulmonary disease, treated tuberculosis, pneumoconioses, and bronchiectasis. Cough is a frequent symptom, but the disease lacks the fever, night sweats, fatigue, and weight loss that characterize tuberculosis. MAI pulmonary disease is indolent or only slowly progressive, producing a gradual decline in pulmonary function over years or decades. MAI is invariably resistant *in vitro* to all first-line antituberculous drugs. Combinations of these drugs are used in treatment, but the results are often disappointing.

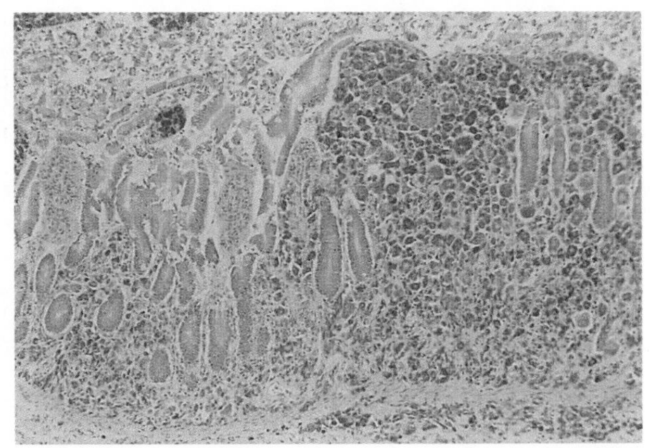

FIGURE 9-53
Mycobacterium avium-intracellulare **(MAI). A section of small bowel from a patient with AIDS reveals the presence of numerous macrophages stuffed with acid-fast bacilli in lamina propria.**

M. avium-intracellulare Infections in Patients with AIDS

One third of AIDS patients in the United States develop overt MAI infections, and as many as one half have evidence of infection at autopsy. In AIDS patients, progressive depletion of helper T cells cripples the immune responses that normally prevent MAI disease. Although macrophages phagocytose the organisms, they are unable to kill them. The bacilli replicate, fill the cells, spread to other macrophages, and are disseminated throughout the body by the lymphatics and bloodstream.

Infected macrophages are found in various organs, particularly the bowel, lymph nodes, spleen, liver, bone marrow, and lungs. Proliferation of organisms and recruitment of additional macrophages produce expanding nodular lesions. Depending on the residual state of cell-mediated immunity, this response leads to a wide spectrum of lesions. These range from structured epithelioid granulomas containing few organisms to loose aggregates of foamy macrophages packed with acid-fast bacilli (Fig. 9-53). This spectrum is reminiscent of the variety of lesions seen in leprosy. With progressive immune depletion, the loose aggregates of MAI-laden macrophages expand. Lymph nodes, spleen, and bone marrow may be almost completely replaced by aggregates of macrophages, and lesions in the bowel eventually erode into the lumen of the gut. As the organisms progressively supplant normal tissues, the body burden of mycobacteria becomes staggering.

The early, constitutional symptoms of MAI disease in AIDS resemble those of tuberculosis and include fever, night sweats, fatigue, and weight loss. Progressive involvement of the small bowel produces malabsorption and diarrhea, often accompanied by abdominal pain. Although the lungs are commonly involved, pulmonary disease is usually clinically insignificant. Combinations of as many as five or more different antibiotics, usually including clarithromycin, may control but rarely cure disseminated MAI infection in AIDS patients.

ATYPICAL MYCOBACTERIA

Several other species of environmental mycobacteria occasionally produce human disease. These organisms are also present in surface waters, dust, and dirt, and people

TABLE 9-8 **Atypical Mycobacterial Infections**

Organism	Disease	Ages Affected	Pathology	Source	Distribution
M. kansasii	Chronic granulomatous pulmonary disease (similar to that caused by *M. avium-intracellulare*)	50–70	Granulomatous inflammation	Inhaled organisms from soil, dust, or water	Worldwide
M. scrofulaceum	Cervical lymphadenitis	1–5	Granulomatous inflammation	Probably ingested organisms from soil or dust	Worldwide
M. marinum	Localized skin lesions	All	Granulomatous inflammation	Direct inoculation of organisms from fish or underwater surfaces (swimming pools, fish tanks)	Worldwide
M. ulcerans	Large, solitary, severe ulcer of skin and subcutaneous tissue	Usually 5–25	Coagulative necrosis	Probably inoculation of environmental organisms	Australia, Africa
M. fortuitum-chelonei	Infections associated with traumatic or iatrogenic inoculations	All	Pyogenic inflammation	Inoculation of environmental organisms	Worldwide

acquire infection by inhalation, inoculation, or ingestion of environmental material.

These bacteria, including MAI, are often lumped together as the "atypical mycobacteria" (in contrast to *M. tuberculosis*, regarded as the "typical" mycobacterium). The atypical mycobacteria are biologically diverse, and the uncommon diseases that they produce in humans differ in circumstances of acquisition, pathology, clinical presentations, and therapies. The features of these diseases are compared in Table 9-8.

M. kansasii causes a chronic, slowly progressive granulomatous pulmonary disease in older persons (over age 50 years), similar to that produced by MAI in immunocompetent patients.

M. scrofulaceum, a common soil inhabitant, causes a draining, granulomatous, cervical lymphadenitis in young children (aged 1 to 5 years). The infection affects the submandibular lymph nodes and probably results from inoculation or ingestion of organisms by toddlers playing in soil. The disease is localized, and surgical excision of the affected lymph nodes is curative.

M. marinum, commonly found on underwater surfaces, produces a localized nodular skin lesion ("swimming pool granuloma"), sometimes with lymphatic involvement. Infection is acquired by traumatic inoculation, such as abrading an elbow on a swimming pool ladder or cutting a finger on a fish spine. The tissue reaction can be pyogenic or granulomatous.

M. ulcerans leads to a severe ulcerating skin disease in Australia, Africa, and New Guinea. The infection presents as a solitary, undermining, deep ulcer of the skin and subcutaneous fat of the extremities. The ulcers show extensive necrosis, with large clusters of acid-fast organisms in the ulcer bed. The natural habitat of the organism and the mode of human acquisition are unknown.

M. chelonae* and *M. fortuitum are closely related organisms that are present throughout the environment. Infection is associated with traumatic or iatrogenic inoculation of material contaminated with organisms. Painless, fluctuant abscesses appear at the site of inoculation, ulcerate, and gradually heal spontaneously. The tissue reaction can be pyogenic or granulomatous.

Fungal Infections

Of more than 100,000 known fungi, only a few invade and destroy human tissue. Of these, most are "opportunists"—that is, they infect only persons with impaired immune mechanisms. Why are fungi, although abundant in nature, so poorly represented among the infectious agents of mankind? The reasons may be found in the hostile environment these organisms encounter in the body. The elevated temperature arrests their growth, and cell-mediated immune mechanisms destroy them. Even the thermally dimorphic fungi (i.e., those that grow in living tissues as well as in soil) do not usually survive phagocytosis by neutrophils and macrophages. Most invading fungi thus fail to establish infection, and of those that do, the majority infect only when cellular immunity fails. Although cell-mediated systems effectively protect against fungi, humoral antibodies play little or no role. Defective neutrophils, or inhibition of the function of neutrophils or macrophages, invites infection. **Thus, corticosteroid administration, antineoplastic therapy, and congenital or acquired T-cell deficiencies all predispose to mycotic infections.** The fungi that cause opportunistic infections are environmental organisms or part of the endogenous human flora. Only the dermatophytes are primary pathogens, producing disease on routine exposures.

Fungi are larger and more complex organisms than bacteria, ranging in size from 2 to 100 μm. They sometimes form multicellular, functionally differentiated structures. Fungi are eukaryotes, having nuclear membranes and cytoplasmic organelles, such as mitochondria and endoplasmic reticulum.

There are two basic morphological types of fungi: yeasts and molds.

- **Yeasts** are the unicellular form of fungi. They are round or oval cells that reproduce by budding, a process in which the daughter organism pinches off from the parent. Some yeasts produce buds that do not detach but instead produce a chain of elongated yeast cells that resemble hyphae and are termed **pseudohyphae**.
- **Molds** are multicellular filamentous fungal colonies that consist of branching tubules, 2 to 10 μm in diameter, termed **hyphae**. The mass of tangled hyphae in the mold form is called a **mycelium**. Some hyphae are separated by septa that are located at regular intervals, whereas others are nonseptate.
- **Dimorphic fungi** can grow as either yeasts or molds, depending on the environmental circumstances.

Most fungi are visible on tissue sections stained with hematoxylin and eosin. The periodic acid–Schiff (PAS) reaction and Gomori methenamine silver stain outline fungal cell walls and are commonly used to detect fungal infection in tissues.

CANDIDA

The genus *Candida*, comprising over 20 species of yeasts, includes the most common opportunistic pathogens. Many *Candida* species are endogenous human flora, well adapted to life on or in the human body. However, they are capable of causing disease when host defenses are compromised. Although the various forms of candidiasis vary in clinical severity, most are localized, superficial diseases, limited to a particular mucocutaneous site, including the following:

- **Intertrigo:** infection of opposed skin surfaces
- **Paronychia:** infection of the nail bed
- **Diaper rash**
- **Vulvovaginitis**
- **Thrush:** oral infection
- **Esophagitis**

Candidal infections of deep tissues are much less common than superficial infections but can be life-threatening. The most common deep sites affected are the brain, eye, kidney, and heart. Deep infections, with candidal sepsis and disseminated candidiasis, occur only in immunologically compromised persons and are often fatal.

Most candidal infections derive from endogenous flora. *C. albicans* resides in small numbers in the oropharynx, gastrointestinal tract, and vagina and is the most frequent candidal pathogen, being responsible for more than 95% of these infections.

☐ **Pathogenesis:** Mechanical barriers, inflammatory cells, humoral immunity, and cell-mediated immunity relegate *Candida* to superficial, nonsterile sites. In turn, the resident bacterial flora normally limit the number of fungal organisms. Bacteria (1) block candidal attachment to epithelial cells, (2) compete with the organisms for nutrients, and (3) prevent conversion of the fungus to its tissue-invasive forms. When any of the above defenses is compromised, candidal infections can occur (Table 9-9). **Antibiotic use results in the suppression of the competing bacterial flora and is the most common precipitating factor for candidiasis.** Under conditions of unopposed growth, the yeast converts to its invasive form (hyphae or pseudohyphae), invades superficially, and elicits an inflammatory or immunological response.

Intact dry skin is an effective barrier to candidal infection. Even though the organism inhabits the skin surface, it does not produce cutaneous disease without some predisposing skin lesion. The most common precipitating factor is maceration, a softening and destruction of the skin. Chronically warm and moist areas, such as those between fingers and toes, between skin folds, and under diapers, are prone to maceration and thus superficial candidal disease.

The incidence of severe candidal infections has increased in recent years, in part owing to increased numbers of neutropenic and immunodeficient patients. Other aspects of contemporary medical care also exacerbate the problem. Frequent use of potent broad-spectrum antibiotics leads to extensive candidal colonization in debilitated patients. Expanded use of medical devices, such as intravascular catheters, monitoring devices, endotracheal tubes, and urinary catheters, provides access to sterile sites. Intravenous drug users also develop deep candidal infections because of inoculation of the fungi into the bloodstream.

TABLE *9-9* **Candidal Infections**

Disease	Predisposing Conditions
Superficial Infections	
Intertrigo (opposed skin surfaces)	Maceration
Paronychia (nail beds)	Maceration
Diaper rash	Maceration
Vulvovaginitis	Alteration in normal flora
Thrush (oral)	Decreased cell-mediated immunity
Esophagitis	Decreased cell-mediated immunity
Deep Infections	
Urinary tract infections	Indwelling urinary catheters
Sepsis and disseminated infection	Neutropenia, indwelling vascular catheters, and change in normal flora

☐ **Pathology:** The pathology of candidal infections varies according to the site of infection. Superficial infections of the skin, oropharynx (Fig. 9-54A), and esophagus show invasive organisms in the most superficial layers of the epithelium and are associated with acute inflammatory infiltrates. Yeasts, pseudohyphae, and hyphae are present (see Fig. 9-54). The yeast cells are round and 3 to 4 μm in diameter, and the hyphae are septate. Candidal vaginitis is characterized by superficial invasion of the squamous epithelium, but the inflammatory infiltrate is usually sparse. Deep candidal infections consist of multiple microscopic abscesses composed of yeasts and hyphae, necrotic debris, and neutrophils. Rarely, a granulomatous response to the organism occurs.

The various superficial cutaneous infections present as tender, erythematous papules, which expand to form confluent erythematous areas. Cutaneous candidal infections are treated topically.

- **Thrush:** This distinctive candidal lesion involves the tongue and mucous membranes of the mouth. Early in life, oral thrush is the most common form of mucocutaneous candidiasis, and candidal vaginitis during pregnancy predisposes the newborn to infection. Thrush consists of friable, white, curdlike membranes adherent to the affected surfaces. These patches are composed of fungi, necrotic debris, neutrophils, and bacteria and can be dislodged by scraping. Removal of the membranes leaves a painful, bleeding surface.
- **Candidal vulvovaginitis:** This condition presents as vaginal and vulvar itching, associated with a thick, white vaginal discharge. Involved areas of the vulva are erythematous and tender. Candidal vaginitis is most intense when the vaginal pH is low. Antibacterial antibiotics, pregnancy, diabetes mellitus, and corticosteroids predispose to the development of this common form of vaginitis.
- **Candidal sepsis and disseminated candidiasis:** Systemic candidiasis is rare, and it is ordinarily a terminal event of an underlying disorder associated with an altered immune system. In addition to *C. albicans*, other candidal species are capable of producing invasive candidiasis. The organisms may enter through an ulcerative lesion of the skin or mucous membrane, or may be introduced by iatrogenic means (e.g., peritoneal dialysis, intravenous lines, or urinary catheters). The urinary tract is most commonly involved, and the incidence in women is four times greater than in men. Renal lesions may be bloodborne or may arise from an ascending pyelonephritis.
- **Candidal endocarditis:** This infection is characterized by large vegetations on the valves and a high incidence of embolization to large arteries. In most patients with candidal endocarditis, the cause is not immunosuppression but unusual vulnerability. Drug addicts who use unsterilized needles and persons with preexisting valvular disease who have had prolonged antibacterial therapy or indwelling vascular catheters are at risk for endocarditis. One of the most

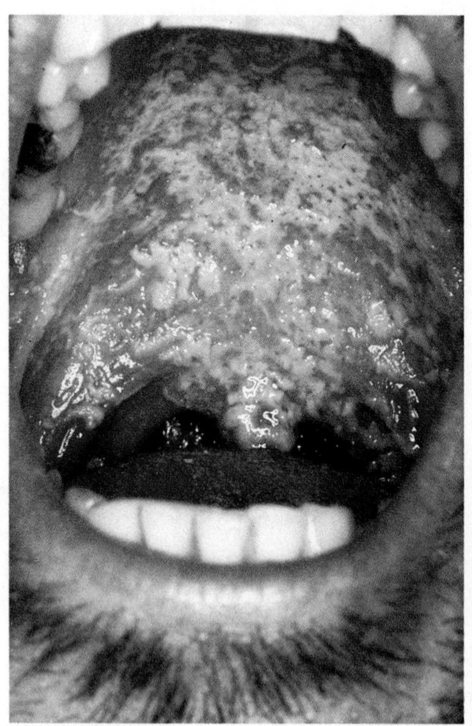

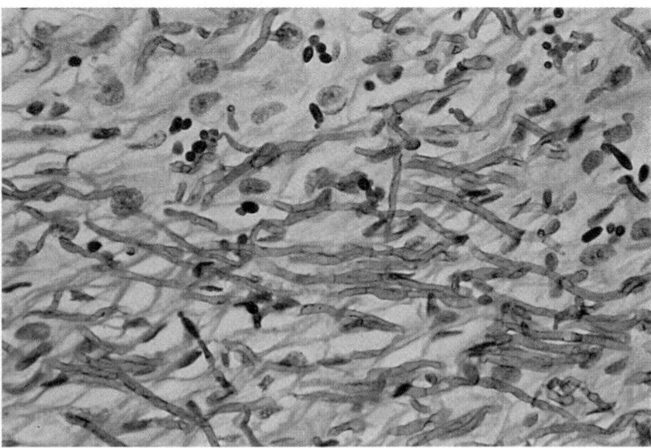

A B

FIGURE 9-54
Candidiasis. (*A*) The oral cavity of a patient with AIDS is covered by a white, curdlike exudate containing numerous fungal organisms. (*B*) A periodic acid–Schiff (PAS) stain shows numerous septate hyphae and yeast forms.

serious complications of invasive candidiasis is septic embolism to the brain.

The symptoms of disseminated candidiasis vary according to the organ involvement. There are no characteristic clinical features, and illness is often masked by other major medical problems. The diagnosis is suggested by clinical deterioration or persistent fever in a neutropenic or immunocompromised person or one who has had an indwelling vascular catheter. Disseminated candidiasis is treated with amphotericin B.

ASPERGILLOSIS

Aspergillus species are common environmental fungi that produce opportunistic infections, usually involving the lungs. There are three distinct types of pulmonary aspergillosis: (1) allergic bronchopulmonary aspergillosis; (2) colonization of a preexisting pulmonary cavity (aspergilloma or fungus ball); and (3) invasive aspergillosis. Of the over 200 identified species of *Aspergillus*, approximately 20 have been associated with human disease. One species, *A. fumigatus*, is by far the most frequent human pathogen.

☐ **Epidemiology:** *Aspergillus* is present throughout the world, growing as saprophytes in soil, decaying plant matter, and dung. Pulmonary aspergillosis is acquired by inhalation of environmental organisms. The fungus reproduces by releasing numerous small (2 to 3 μm) spores, known as conidia, which are carried in the air into almost every human environment. The spores are small enough to reach the alveoli when inhaled. Exposure to *Aspergillus* is greatest when its native habitat is disturbed, as during soil excavations or handling of decaying organic matter.

Aspergillus has a characteristic appearance in tissue. Septate hyphae, 2 to 7 μm in diameter and branching progressively at acute angles, are seen. The multiple dichotomous branching is responsible for the name *Aspergillus* (from the Latin *aspergere*, "to sprinkle"). It derived from a fancied resemblance to the aspergillum, a device used to sprinkle holy water during religious ceremonies of the Catholic church.

Allergic Bronchopulmonary Aspergillosis

The inhalation of *Aspergillus* spores exposes the airways and the alveoli to *Aspergillus* antigens; subsequent contact initiates an allergic response in susceptible persons. The situation is aggravated if the spores germinate and grow in the airways, thereby producing a chronic exposure to the antigen. Allergic bronchopulmonary aspergillosis is virtually restricted to asthmatics, 20% of whom eventually develop this disorder.

Bronchi and bronchioles in allergic bronchopulmonary aspergillosis are inflamed, with an infiltrate of lymphocytes, plasma cells, and variable numbers of eosinophils. Sometimes the airways are impacted with mucus and fungal hyphae. Patients experience exacerbations of asthma, often accompanied by pulmonary infiltrates and eosinophilia.

Aspergilloma

Aspergilloma, also termed ***fungus ball****, occurs in persons with pulmonary cavities or bronchiectasis.* Inhaled spores germinate in the warm humid atmosphere provided by these hollows and fill them with masses of hyphae. The organisms do not invade, being confined to the air spaces by neutrophils and macrophages.

☐ Pathology: An aspergilloma consists of a dense, round or lobulated mass of tangled hyphae, 1 to 7 cm in diameter, within a fibrous cavity. The fungal mass may fill the cavity, although it is rarely attached to it. The wall of the cavity is composed of collagenous connective tissue, infiltrated by lymphocytes and plasma cells. The hyphae do not invade the adjacent pulmonary parenchyma.

☐ Clinical Features: Aspergillomas occur in persons with underlying lung disease, most commonly old cavitary tuberculosis, and the symptoms correspond to the underlying disease. The radiological appearance of a dense round ball in a cavity is characteristic. For the most part, aspergillomas are best left untreated, but surgical excision may be indicated in some cases.

Invasive Aspergillosis

Any condition that profoundly diminishes the number or activity of neutrophils predisposes to invasive aspergillosis. The most common circumstances are acute leukemias and high-dose cytotoxic therapy, both of which are accompanied by depletion of bone marrow elements. In profoundly neutropenic patients, inhaled spores germinate to produce hyphae, which invade through the bronchi into the pulmonary parenchyma, from where the fungi may spread widely.

☐ Pathology: *Aspergillus* readily invades blood vessels and produces thrombosis (Fig. 9-55). As a result, multiple nodular infarcts are found throughout both lungs. Involvement of larger pulmonary arteries results in large, wedge-shaped, pleural-based infarcts. Vascular invasion by the fungi also leads to widespread dissemination of the infection to the brain, heart, kidney, and other organs. Microscopically, *Aspergillus* hyphae are arranged radially around blood vessels and extend through their walls from the surrounding pulmonary parenchyma. Acute aspergillosis may also start in a nasal sinus and spread to the face, orbit, and brain.

☐ Clinical Features: Invasive aspergillosis presents as fever and multifocal pulmonary infiltrates in a patient with profound neutropenia. Nothing in the clinical presentation clearly distinguishes invasive aspergillosis from other opportunistic pneumonias, and the diagnosis requires demonstration of the organism on tissue biopsy. Because of the frequent thrombosis and bloodstream dissemination, invasive aspergillosis is often fatal. Antifungal therapy with amphotericin B may be successful but must be initiated early and given in high doses.

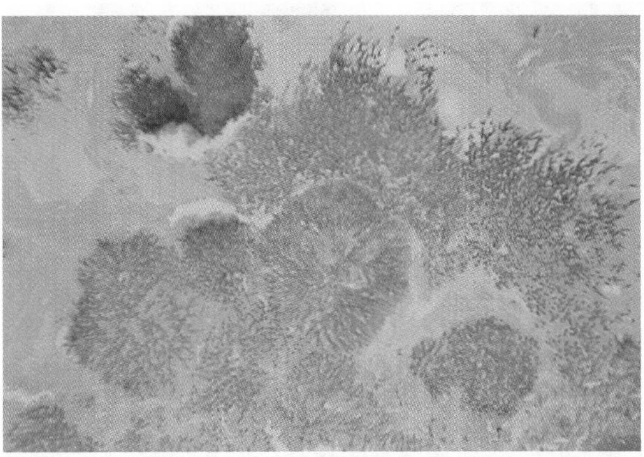

FIGURE *9-55*
Invasive aspergillosis. A section of lung impregnated with silver shows branching fungal hyphae surrounding blood vessels and invading the adjacent parenchyma.

MUCORMYCOSIS (ZYGOMYCOSIS)

Several related environmental fungi, namely *Rhizopus*, *Mucor*, and *Absidia* species, produce severe, necrotizing, invasive, opportunistic infections, which begin in the nasal sinuses or lungs. These organisms are members of the class Zygomycetes, order Mucormorales, and the infections that they produce are usually called mucormycosis or zygomycosis.

Zygomycetes have a characteristic appearance in tissue sections and can be readily distinguished from other pathogenic fungi. They are large (8 to 15 μm across), branch at right angles, have thin walls, and lack septa. In sections, they appear as hollow tubes. Lacking cross walls, their liquid contents flow, leaving long empty segments. Zygomycetes also may resemble "twisted ribbons," which represent collapsed hyphae.

☐ Epidemiology: *Rhizopus*, *Mucor*, and *Absidia* are ubiquitous in the environment, inhabiting soil, food, and decaying vegetable matter. They often cause the "mold" seen on bread or fruit. These fungi grow rapidly and release numerous spores, which circulate in the air to expose humans on a constant basis. The small spores are inhaled, and in susceptible persons disease begins in the lungs. Mucormycosis occurs almost exclusively in the context of an underlying illness, particularly severe diabetes or profound neutropenia. In uncontrolled diabetics, neutrophils and macrophages fail to kill the fungi. Furthermore, whereas normal serum inhibits the growth of zygomycetes, serum from diabetics in ketoacidosis actually stimulates fungal growth.

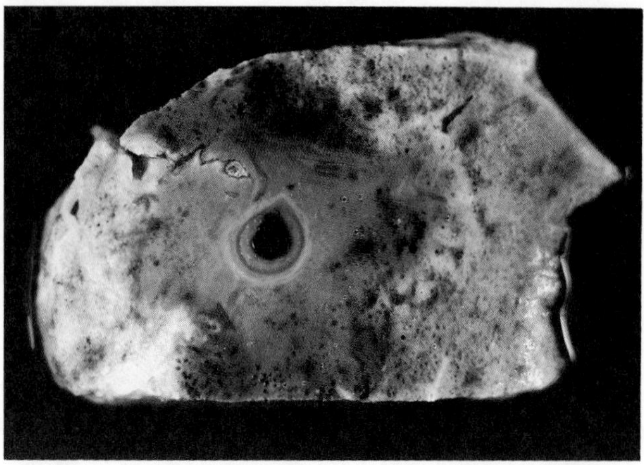

FIGURE 9-56
Pulmonary mucormycosis. A cross-section of the lung shows the vessel in the center of the field to be invaded by mucormycetes and occluded by a septic thrombus. The surrounding tissue is infarcted.

☐ **Pathology:** The three predominant forms of mucormycosis are rhinocerebral, pulmonary, and subcutaneous.

- **Rhinocerebral mucormycosis:** In this disease, fungi proliferate in the nasal sinuses and invade surrounding tissues, extending into the facial soft tissues, nerves, blood vessels, and brain. The palate or nasal turbinates are covered by a black crust, and the underlying tissue is friable and hemorrhagic.

  Rhinocerebral mucormycosis presents as facial pain, headache, cranial nerve dysfunction, or a persistent change in mental status. Often a blood-tinged nasal discharge is followed by orbital pain; a bulging, discolored eye; and a fixed pupil. The fungal hyphae grow into the arteries and cause a devastating, rapidly progressive, septic infarction of the affected tissues. Extension into the brain leads to a fatal, necrotizing, hemorrhagic encephalitis. Therapy requires the surgical excision of involved tissues, administration of amphotericin B, and correction of the predisposing abnormality.
- **Pulmonary mucormycosis:** This infection occurs primarily in neutropenic persons and resembles invasive pulmonary aspergillosis, with vascular invasion and multiple areas of septic infarction throughout the lungs (Fig. 9-56).

  Pulmonary mucormycosis manifests as fever and progressive pneumonia in a severely neutropenic patient. Therapy is similar to that for rhinocerebral disease. Unfortunately, despite heroic efforts, both rhinocerebral and pulmonary mucormycosis are usually fatal.
- **Subcutaneous zygomycosis:** This infection is limited to the tropics and is caused by *Basidiobolus haptosporus*. The fungus grows slowly in the panniculus, producing a gradually enlarging, hard inflammatory mass, usually on the shoulder, trunk, buttock, or thigh. These lesions respond to orally administered potassium iodide.

CRYPTOCOCCOSIS

Cryptococcosis is a systemic mycosis caused by Cryptococcus neoformans, which principally affects the meninges and the lungs (Fig. 9-57). *C. neoformans* has a worldwide distribution. The main reservoir for the fungus is pigeon droppings, which are alkaline and hyperosmolar. These conditions keep the cryptococci small, thereby allowing the inhaled organisms to penetrate to the terminal bronchioles. *C. neoformans* is unique among pathogenic fungi in having a proteoglycan capsule, which is essential for their pathogenicity. The organisms appear as faintly stained, basophilic yeasts that vary from 4 to μm in diameter and have a clear 3 to 5 μm thick mucinous capsule.

***Cryptococcus* almost exclusively affects persons with impaired cell-mediated immunity.** Although the organism is ubiquitous, and exposure is common, cryptococcosis remains a rare disease in the absence of a predisposing illness. Because some immune defect is necessary for infection to occur, disease is rare even among persons such as pigeon fanciers, who are exposed to large inoculums of the organism. Cryptococcosis occurs in patients with AIDS, lymphomas, particularly Hodgkin disease, leukemias, and sarcoidosis and in those treated with high doses of corticosteroids.

☐ **Pathogenesis:** With few exceptions, in the immunologically intact person, neutrophils and alveolar macrophages kill *C. neoformans,* and no clinical disease develops. By contrast, in a patient with defective cell-mediated immunity, the cryptococci survive, reproduce locally, and then disseminate. Even though the lung is the

FIGURE 9-57
Pulmonary and disseminated fungal infection. Fungi grow in soil, air, and the feces of birds and bats, and produce spores, some of which are infectious. When inhaled, spores cause primary pulmonary infection. In a few patients, the infection disseminates.

Histoplasmosis. Primary infection is in the lung. In susceptible patients, the fungus disseminates to target organs, namely the monocyte/macrophage system (liver, spleen, lymph nodes, and bone marrow), and the tongue, mucous membranes of mouth, and the adrenals.

Cryptococcosis. Primary infection of the lung disseminates to the meninges.

Blastomycosis. Primary infection of the lung disseminates widely. The principal targets are the brain, meninges, skin, spleen, bone and kidney.

Coccidioidomycosis. Primary infection of the lung may disseminate widely. The skin, meninges, and bone are common targets.

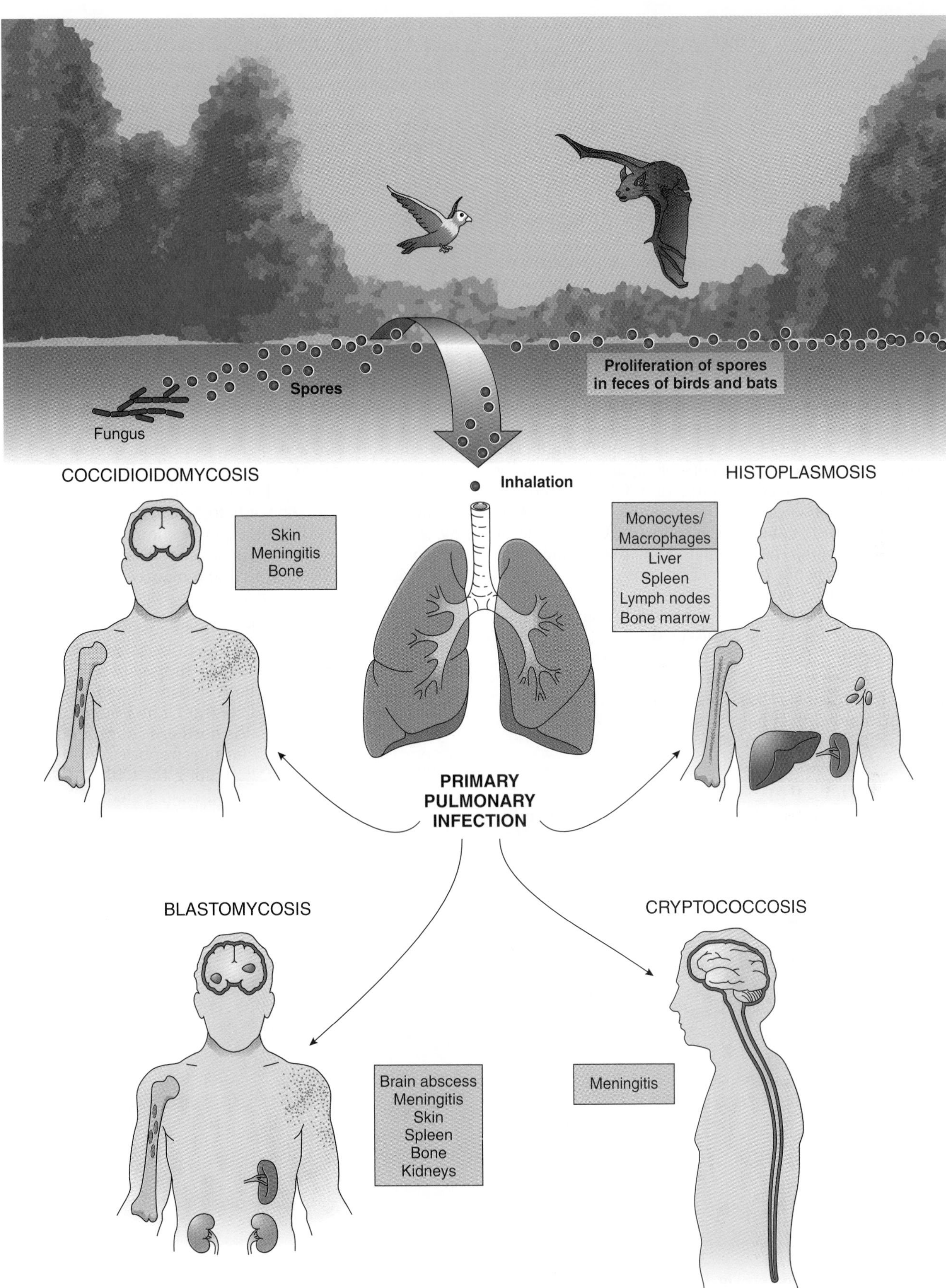
Spores
Fungus
Proliferation of spores in feces of birds and bats
Inhalation
COCCIDIOIDOMYCOSIS
Skin
Meningitis
Bone
HISTOPLASMOSIS
Monocytes/ Macrophages
Liver
Spleen
Lymph nodes
Bone marrow
PRIMARY PULMONARY INFECTION
BLASTOMYCOSIS
Brain abscess
Meningitis
Skin
Spleen
Bone
Kidneys
CRYPTOCOCCOSIS
Meningitis

FIGURE 9-57

site of entry of the organism, the central nervous system is the most common site of disease, owing to the excellent environment provided by the cerebrospinal fluid. It is speculated that dopamine in the central nervous system promotes the growth of virulent cryptococci.

□ **Pathology:** Over 95% of cryptococcal infections involve the meninges and the brain. Lesions in the lungs can be demonstrated in half of the patients, and a small minority have involvement of the skin, liver, spleen, adrenals, and bones.

In cryptococcal meningoencephalitis, the entire brain is swollen and soft, and the leptomeninges are thickened and gelatinous, owing to infiltration by the thickly encapsulated organisms. The inflammatory response is highly variable, but is often minimal, with large numbers of cryptococci infiltrating tissue that is devoid of inflammatory cells. When present, the inflammatory response is neutrophilic, lymphocytic, or granulomatous.

Cryptococcosis in the lung may present as diffuse disease or as isolated areas of consolidation. The affected alveoli are distended by clusters of organisms, usually with minimal associated inflammation. Old granulomas containing cryptococci are occasionally found in immunocompetent persons. These represent the residue of old exposure that has been contained by the immune system, rather than active pulmonary disease.

Because of its thick capsule, *C. neoformans* stains poorly with the routine hematoxylin and eosin stain and appears as bubbles or holes in tissue sections (Fig. 9-58A). The routine fungal stains (PAS and Gomori methenamine silver) demonstrate the yeasts well but fail to stain the polysaccharide capsule. As a result, the organism appears to be surrounded by a halo. The capsule can be demonstrated with a mucicarmine stain (see Fig. 9-58B).

□ **Clinical Features:** Cryptococcal disease of the central nervous system often begins insidiously with nonfocal symptoms, including headache, dizziness, sleepiness, and loss of coordination. Defects in mental status are often present but are frequently overlooked by the patient because of their subtle onset. There is usually little or no fever or nuchal rigidity. Untreated cryptococcal meningitis is invariably fatal, and therapy requires the prolonged systemic administration of antifungal medication. Cryptococcal pneumonia presents as diffuse progressive pulmonary disease, which is not clinically distinct from other opportunistic pulmonary infections.

HISTOPLASMOSIS

Histoplasmosis is a mycosis caused by Histoplasma capsulatum, which is usually self-limited, but may lead to a systemic grannulomatous disease. Although most cases of histoplasmosis are asymptomatic, progressive, disseminated infections occur in persons with impaired cell-mediated immunity. *H. capsulatum* is a dimorphic fungus of worldwide distribution, which grows as a mold at ambient temperatures and always as a yeast in the body (37°C). The yeast cell is round and has a central basophilic body surrounded by a clear zone or halo, which in turn is encircled by a rigid cell wall 2 to 4 μm in diameter. In caseous lesions, where the yeasts are degenerating, silver impregnation is needed to identify the remains of the yeasts.

□ **Epidemiology:** Histoplasmosis is acquired by the inhalation of infectious spores of *H. capsulatum* (see Fig. 9-57). The reservoir for the fungus is in bird droppings and in the soil. In the Americas, hyperendemic areas are in the eastern and central United States, western Mexico, Central America, the northern countries of South America, and Argentina. Starlings imported from Europe in 1890 became concentrated along the Ohio-Mississippi valley in the United States and contributed to the establishment of this midwestern area as a major endemic fo-

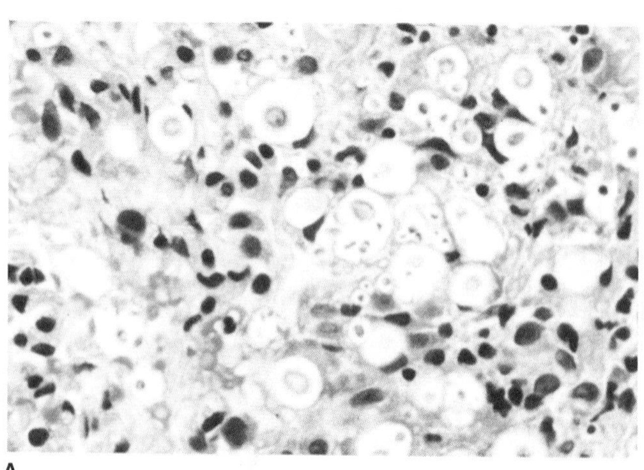

A

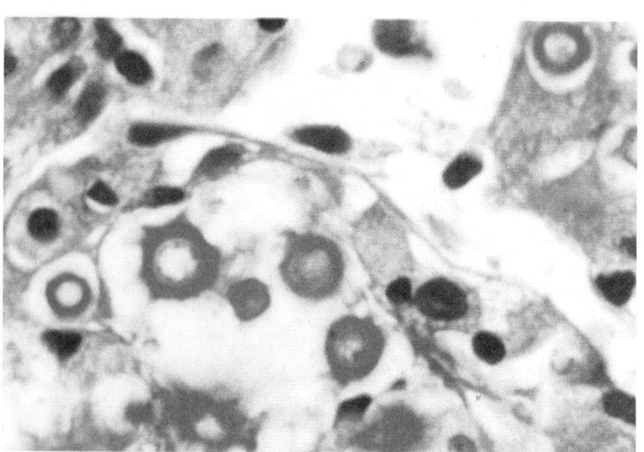

B

FIGURE 9-58
Cryptococcosis. (*A*) In a section of the lung stained with hematoxylin and eosin, *C. neoformans* appears as holes or bubbles. (*B*) The same section stained with mucicarmine illustrates the capsule of the organism.

cus. As a result, the population in this area displays a high prevalence of positive histoplasmin skin test results. In the tropics, bat nests, caves, and soil beneath trees are foci of exposure. In the soil, *H. capsulatum* produces characteristic macroconidia (8 to 16 μm in diameter) and microconidia (2 to 5 μm in diameter). Because they are smaller, the microconidia reach the alveolar spaces, where they are transformed into yeasts.

□ **Pathogenesis:** Histoplasmosis resembles tuberculosis in many ways. Primary infection begins with phagocytosis by alveolar macrophages. Like *M. tuberculosis*, *H. capsulatum* survives and reproduces in immunologically naive macrophages. As the organisms grow, additional macrophages are recruited to the site of infection, producing an area of pulmonary consolidation. A few macrophages carry organisms first to hilar and mediastinal lymph nodes, and then throughout the body, where the fungi infect cells of the monocyte/macrophage system. The organisms proliferate within parasitized macrophages, until the host mounts hypersensitivity and cell-mediated immune responses, usually within 1 to 3 weeks. The normal immunological response contains the organisms in most infected persons. Activated macrophages destroy the phagocytosed yeasts, forming necrotizing granulomas at the sites of infection. The granulomas undergo caseation, develop progressively thicker fibrous capsules, and often eventually calcify.

The course of the infection varies with the size of the infecting inoculum and the immunological competence of the host. Most infections (95%) involve small inoculums of organisms in immunologically competent persons. They affect small areas of the lung and regional lymph nodes and remain completely unnoticed. On the other hand, inhalation of a large inoculum, as occurs in an excavated bird roost, may lead to a rapidly evolving pulmonary histoplasmosis, with large areas of consolidation, prominent mediastinal and hilar nodal involvement, and extension of the infection to the liver, spleen, and bone marrow. Nevertheless, even such extensive disease is usually brought under control by immune responses.

Disseminated histoplasmosis develops in persons who fail to mount an effective immune response to *H. capsulatum*. Infants, persons with AIDS, and patients treated with corticosteroids are at particular risk. In addition, some persons with no known underlying illness also develop disseminated histoplasmosis; they are thought to have a specific defect of host responsiveness to *H. capsulatum*. Similar to secondary tuberculosis, disseminated histoplasmosis may be caused by a new exposure to environmental organisms or by reactivation of fungi that have remained viable in old *Histoplasma* granulomas.

□ **Pathology:** **Acute self-limited histoplasmosis** is characterized by the development of necrotizing, caseous granulomas in the lung, mediastinal and hilar lymph nodes, spleen, and liver. Early in the course of infection, the caseous material is surrounded by macrophages, Langhans giant cells, lymphocytes, and plasma cells. Yeast forms of *H. capsulatum* can be demonstrated both within macrophages and in the caseous material. Eventually, the cellular components of the granuloma largely disappear and the caseous material calcifies, forming a "fibrocaseous nodule" (Fig. 9-59A).

Disseminated histoplasmosis is characterized by progressive organ infiltration with macrophages containing *H. capsulatum* (see Fig. 9-59B). The course and pathology of the infection depends on the degree of host immunodeficiency. In mild cases, the immunological response is sufficient to inhibit, but not eliminate, the infection. For long periods of time, the disease remains largely confined to the macrophages in the lymph nodes, bone marrow, liver, and spleen, although there may be oropharyngeal involvement. Aggregates of macrophages contain a few *H. capsulatum* yeasts. In the mildest cases, tuberculoid granulomas sometimes form.

In cases of profound immunodeficiency, there is little, if any restraint on the proliferation of the fungus, and

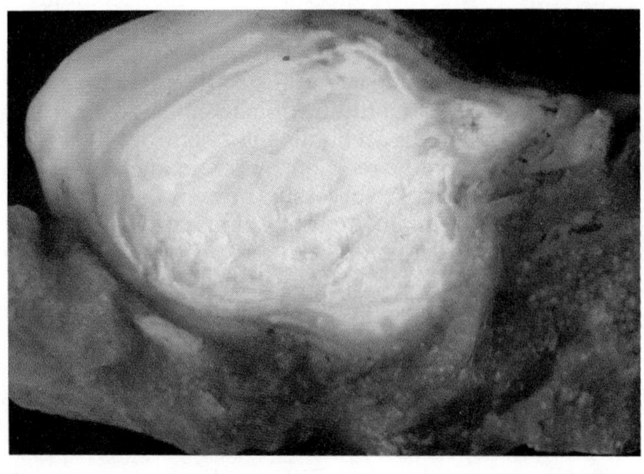

A

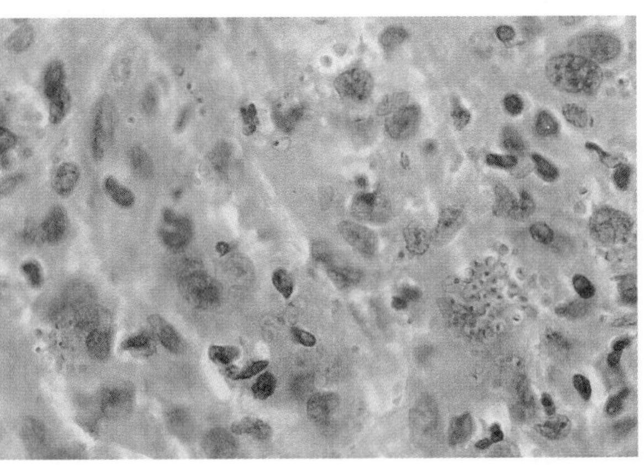

B

FIGURE *9-59*
Histoplasmosis. (*A*) A section of lung shows an encapsulated, subpleural, fibrocaseous nodule. (*B*) A section of liver from a patient with disseminated histoplasmosis reveals Kupffer cells containing numerous yeasts of *H. capsulatum* (PAS stain).

eventually large clusters of macrophages filled with *H. capsulatum* infiltrate the liver, spleen, lungs, intestine, adrenals, and meninges. The accumulation of infected macrophages displaces and destroys the affected tissues.

☐ **Clinical Features:** The course of acute, self-limited histoplasmosis is highly variable. The large majority of infections are asymptomatic, but with extensive disease, patients present with fever, headache, and cough. In such cases, the chest radiograph shows small, scattered infiltrates and hilar lymphadenopathy, an appearance that may be confused with pulmonary tuberculosis. The symptoms persist from a few days to a few weeks, but the disease requires no therapy.

In disseminated histoplasmosis, patients present with weight loss, intermittent fever, and weakness. In cases of subtle immunodeficiency, usually adults with no obvious underlying illness, the disease may persist and progress for years, even decades. With more profound immunodeficiency, disseminated histoplasmosis progresses rapidly, often causing high fever, cough, pancytopenia, and changes in mental status. Disseminated histoplasmosis is treated with systemic antifungal agents.

COCCIDIOIDOMYCOSIS

Coccidioidomycosis is a chronic, necrotizing mycotic infection that clinically and pathologically resembles tuberculosis. The disease, caused by *Coccidioides immitis*, includes a spectrum of infections that begin as focal pneumonitis. Most are mild and asymptomatic and are limited to the lungs and regional lymph nodes. Occasionally, *C. immitis* infections spread outside the lungs to produce life-threatening disease.

☐ **Epidemiology:** *C. immitis* is a dimorphic fungus that grows as a mold in the soil, where it reproduces by segmentation of hyphae to form spores, called arthroconidia. The spores are inhaled into the alveoli and terminal bronchioles (see Fig. 9-57), enlarge into spherules, and then mature to form sporangia, which are structures that are 30 to 60 μm across. The sporangia gradually fill with endospores, 1 to 5 μm across, which accumulate by endosporulation, a process unique among the pathogenic fungi. The sporangia eventually rupture and release endospores, which then repeat the cycle.

C. immitis is present in the soil in restricted climatic regions, particularly the Lower Sonoran life zones of the Western hemisphere. These are areas with sparse rainfall, hot summers, and mild winters. In the United States, large portions of California, Arizona, New Mexico, and Texas are a natural habitat for *C. immitis*, and most exposures occur in these states. The disease is particularly common in the San Joaquin Valley of California, where it is called "valley fever." Coccidioidomycosis also occurs in Mexico and parts of South America.

Long-term residents of endemic regions are almost invariably infected with *C. immitis*, and even brief visits to these areas can produce infection (usually asymptomatic). Dry, windy weather, which lifts arthrospores into the air, favors infection. The forms of *C. immitis* that grow in the human body are not transmitted from person to person, and coccidioidomycosis is not contagious.

☐ **Pathogenesis:** Coccidioidomycosis begins with focal bronchopneumonia at the site where the arthrospores are deposited. These elicit a mixed inflammatory infiltrate, composed of neutrophils and macrophages, but the spores survive the onslaught of the immunologically naive inflammatory cells. The host is unable to control the infection until inflammatory cells become activated. With the onset of specific hypersensitivity and cell-mediated immune responses, necrotizing granulomas form, killing or containing the fungi.

Similar to tuberculosis and histoplasmosis, the course of coccidioidomycosis varies according to the size of the infecting inoculum and the immunological status of the host. A broad spectrum of illness ranges from acute self-limited disease to disseminated infections. **The large majority of infections are produced by small inoculums of organisms in immunologically competent hosts and are acute and self-limited.** Extensive pulmonary involvement and fulminant disease may occur in persons from a nonendemic region exposed to large numbers of organisms (e.g., New Yorkers who participate in an archaeological dig in southern Arizona). Even such persons usually recover from the infection.

Disseminated coccidioidomycosis occurs in immunocompromised persons, either from a primary infection or from reactivation of old disease. Patients with lymphomas, leukemias, or AIDS and those receiving immunosuppressive therapy are at risk of dissemination. Certain racial groups, including Filipinos, other Asians, and blacks, are particularly susceptible to dissemination of coccidioidomycosis, probably because of a specific immunological defect. The risk of dissemination in Filipinos is actually 175 times greater than in whites. Pregnant women are also unusually susceptible to spread of the disease if they develop primary infection during the latter half of pregnancy.

☐ **Pathology:** Acute self-limited coccidioidomycosis produces a solitary lesion or patchy areas of pulmonary consolidation, in which the affected alveoli are infiltrated by neutrophils and macrophages (Fig. 9-60). *C. immitis* spherules elicit an infiltrate of macrophages, whereas the endospores attract predominantly neutrophils. With the onset of an immune reaction, a necrotizing, caseous granuloma develops. A successful immunological response causes the granuloma to heal, sometimes leaving a fibrocaseous nodule composed of caseous material and rimmed by residual macrophages and a thin capsule. In contrast to histoplasmosis, the old granulomas of coccidioidomycosis rarely calcify.

The spherules and endospores of *C. immitis* both stain with hematoxylin and eosin. Spherules in various stages of development appear as basophilic rings. Mature spherules (sporangia) contain endospores that appear as smaller basophilic rings. PAS and Gomori methenamine silver stains can be used to enhance the staining of *C. immitis*.

Disseminated coccidioidomycosis may involve almost any body site and may manifest as a single ex-

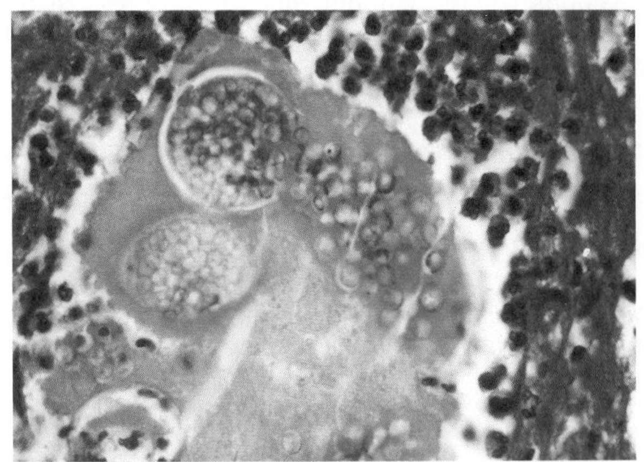

FIGURE 9-60
Coccidioidomycosis. A photomicrograph of the lung from a patient with acute coccidioidal pneumonia shows an acute inflammatory infiltrate surrounding spherules and endospores of *C. immitis.*

trathoracic site or as widespread disease, including lesions of the skin (Fig. 9-61), bones, meninges, liver, spleen, and genitourinary tract. The inflammatory response at the sites of dissemination is highly variable, ranging from an infiltrate of neutrophils to a granulomatous response. Deficiencies of cell-mediated immunity usually prevent the formation of necrotizing granulomas.

☐ **Clinical Features:** Coccidioidomycosis is a disease of protean manifestations, which vary from a subclinical respiratory infection to one that disseminates and is rapidly fatal. Physicians in endemic areas who are most experienced in diagnosing coccidioidomycosis state that almost any complaint or syndrome may be a manifestation of this infection. It thus joins syphilis and typhoid fever as a "great imitator."

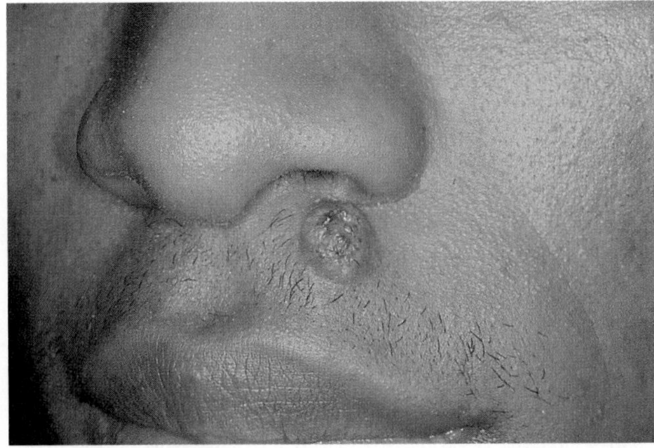

FIGURE 9-61
Disseminated coccidioidomycosis. A single raised, central ulcerated lesion is present on the face.

Most persons with coccidioidomycosis (>60%) are asymptomatic. The remaining ones develop a flu-like syndrome, characterized by fever, cough, chest pain, and malaise. Infection usually resolves spontaneously. Cavitation is the most frequent complication of pulmonary coccidioidomycosis, although it fortunately occurs in only few patients (<5%). The cavity, which may be mistaken for tuberculosis, is usually solitary and may persist for years. Progression or reactivation may lead to destructive lesions in the lungs, or more seriously, to disseminated lesions.

The signs and symptoms of disseminated coccidioidomycosis vary according to the site affected. Coccidioidal meningitis presents with headache, fever, alteration in mental status, or seizures and is fatal if untreated. Skin lesions of disseminated coccidioidomycosis frequently have a warty appearance (see Fig. 9-61). Even with prolonged amphotericin B therapy, the prognosis is poor in acute disseminated coccidioidomycosis, especially if there is meningitis.

BLASTOMYCOSIS

Blastomycosis is a chronic granulomatous and suppurative disease of the lungs, which is often followed by dissemination to other body sites, principally the skin and bone. The causative organism is *Blastomyces dermatitidis,* a dimorphic fungus that grows as a mold in warm moist soil, rich in decaying vegetable matter. It reproduces by releasing spores, and in mammals it grows as a thick-walled yeast that reproduces by broad-based budding.

☐ **Epidemiology:** Blastomycosis is acquired by the inhalation of infectious spores from the soil (see Fig. 9-57). Symptomatic blastomycosis is a less common disease (100 cases annually in the United States) than histoplasmosis or coccidioidomycosis. The infection occurs within restricted geographic regions of North America, Central and South America, Africa, and possibly the Middle East. In North America, the fungus is endemic along the distributions of the Mississippi and Ohio Rivers, the Great Lakes, and the St. Lawrence River. The full extent of *B. dermatitidis* infection is unknown, because the skin tests for the detection of asymptomatic infected persons are unreliable.

In endemic areas, blastomycosis tends to occur in restricted geographic locations, where the organism grows in nature. Disturbance of the soil, either by construction or by leisure activities such as hunting or camping, leads to the formation of aerosols containing fungal spores. In turn, inhalation of such aerosols causes human and canine illness.

☐ **Pathogenesis:** The inhaled spores of *B. dermatitidis* germinate to form yeasts, which reproduce by budding. The host responds to the proliferating organisms with neutrophils and macrophages, producing a focal bronchopneumonia. Despite the inflammatory response, the organisms persist until the onset of specific hypersensitivity and cell-mediated immunity, when activated neutrophils and macrophages kill them. Although asymptomatic infections certainly occur, their frequency is unknown.

☐ **Pathology:** Blastomycosis is usually confined to the lungs, where the infection most frequently produces small areas of pulmonary consolidation. *B. dermatitidis* incites a mixed suppurative and granulomatous inflammatory response, and even in the same patient, lesions may range from neutrophilic abscesses to epithelioid granulomas. Although the pulmonary disease usually resolves by scarring, some patients develop progressive miliary lesions or cavities. When the infection spreads outside the lungs, the skin (>50%), bones (>10%), and less commonly, the prostate are common sites of involvement. Skin infection often elicits a marked pseudoepitheliomatous hyperplasia, imparting a warty appearance to the lesions.

The infected areas contain numerous yeasts of *B. dermatitidis*, which are spherical and 8 to 14 μm across, with broad-based buds and multiple nuclei in a central body (Fig. 9-62). With the hematoxylin and eosin stain, the yeasts appear as rings with thick, sharply defined cell walls. The yeasts may be found in epithelioid cells, macrophages, or giant cells, or they may lie free in microabscesses.

☐ **Clinical Features:** Pulmonary blastomycosis is self-limited in one third of the cases. Symptomatic acute infection presents as a flu-like illness, with fever, arthralgias, and myalgias. Progressive pulmonary disease manifests as low-grade fever, weight loss, cough, and predominantly upper lobe infiltrates on the chest radiograph. Skin lesions, which often resemble squamous cell carcinomas of the skin, are the most common manifestation of extrapulmonary dissemination. Although the pulmonary infection may apparently resolve completely, in some patients, blastomycosis may appear at distant sites months to years later. Acute self-limited infections resolve without therapy. Progressive pulmonary or disseminated disease requires treatment with systemic antifungal agents.

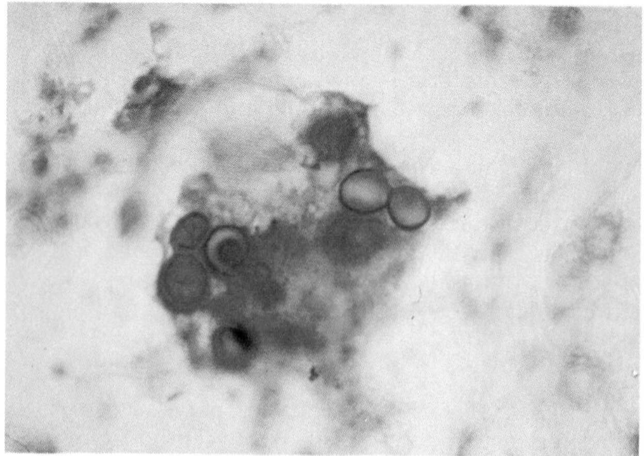

FIGURE 9-62
Blastomycosis. The yeasts of *B. dermatitidis* have a doubly contoured wall and nuclei in the central body. The buds have broad-based attachments.

PARACOCCIDIOIDOMYCOSIS (SOUTH AMERICAN BLASTOMYCOSIS)

Paracoccidioidomycosis, also known as South American blastomycosis, is a chronic granulomatous infection that begins with pulmonary involvement and disseminates to involve the skin, oropharynx, adrenals, and the macrophages of the liver, spleen, and lymph nodes. The causative organism is *Paracoccidioides brasiliensis*, a dimorphic fungus, whose mold form is thought to reside in the soil, but whose natural habitat has not been defined.

☐ **Epidemiology:** Paracoccidioidomycosis is acquired by the inhalation of spores from the environment in restricted regions of Central and South America. The endemic regions have relatively constant moderate temperatures and high humidity. The infection is the predominant dimorphic fungal disease in Latin America, and Brazilians living in rural areas constitute the largest affected group. The large majority of infections with *P. brasiliensis* are asymptomatic. Reactivation of latent infection occurs, and persons can develop active disease many years after moving from an endemic region. Interestingly, men develop symptomatic infections 15 times more often than women, presumably because of hormonal influences on the conversion of the organism to its yeast phase.

☐ **Pathology:** Infection with *P. brasiliensis* is initiated by the inhalation of its spores, which convert to a distinct replicative yeast form at body temperature. Paracoccidioidomycosis can involve the lungs alone or multiple extrapulmonary sites, most commonly skin, mucosal surfaces, and lymph nodes. *P. brasiliensis* elicits a mixed suppurative and granulomatous response, producing lesions similar to those seen in blastomycosis and coccidioidomycosis.

The fungus has a characteristic appearance on microscopic examination. The yeast reproduces by generating multiple, narrow-based buds arising circumferentially from the mother organism, giving the appearance of a ship's pilot wheel (Fig. 9-63). The mother organism is large, ranging up to 60 μm in diameter, and the associated progeny are considerably smaller, 5 to 10 μm in diameter.

☐ **Clinical Features:** Paracoccidioidomycosis is usually an acute, self-limited, and minimally symptomatic disease. In patients with progressive disease, symptoms vary according to the sites affected. The symptoms of progressive pulmonary involvement resemble those of tuberculosis. Chronic mucocutaneous ulcers are a frequent manifestation of extrapulmonary disease. Later, the lesions become proliferative and form vegetations.

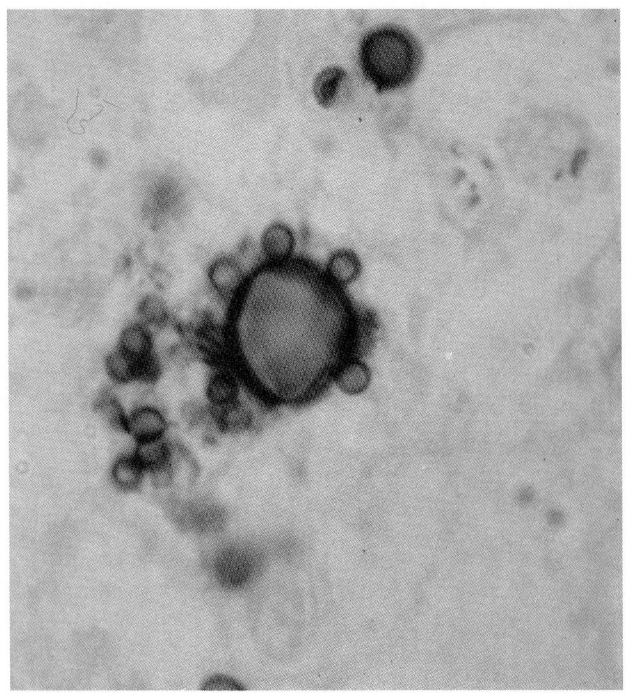

FIGURE 9-63
Paracoccidioidomycosis. The lung contains *P. braziliensis*, which displays many external buds arising circumferentially from the mother organism.

Progressive pulmonary and extrapulmonary disease requires systemic antifungal therapy.

SPOROTRICHOSIS

Sporotrichosis is a chronic infection of the skin, subcutaneous tissues, and regional lymph nodes caused by Sporothrix schenkii. This dimorphic fungus grows as a mold in soil and decaying plant matter and as a yeast in the body. Sporotrichosis is endemic in parts of the Americas and southern Africa. Most cases are cutaneous, resulting from the accidental inoculation of the fungus from thorns or splinters or by handling reeds or grasses. Cutaneous sporotrichosis is particularly common among gardeners (especially rose gardeners), nursery workers, and other persons who suffer abrasions while working with soil, moss, hay, or timbers. However, the disease can also be transmitted by infected animals, particularly cats.

□ **Pathology:** On inoculation into the skin, *S. schenkii* proliferates locally, inducing an inflammatory response that produces an ulceronodular lesion. The infection frequently spreads along subcutaneous lymphatic channels, resulting in a chain of similar nodular skin lesions (Fig. 9-64A). Extracutaneous disease is much less common than skin disease. Joint and bone involvement is the most frequent form of extracutaneous disease, and infections of the wrist, elbow, ankle, or knee account for most (80%) of the cases. Although the origin of bone and joint infection is uncertain, the locations on the extremities suggest direct traumatic inoculation.

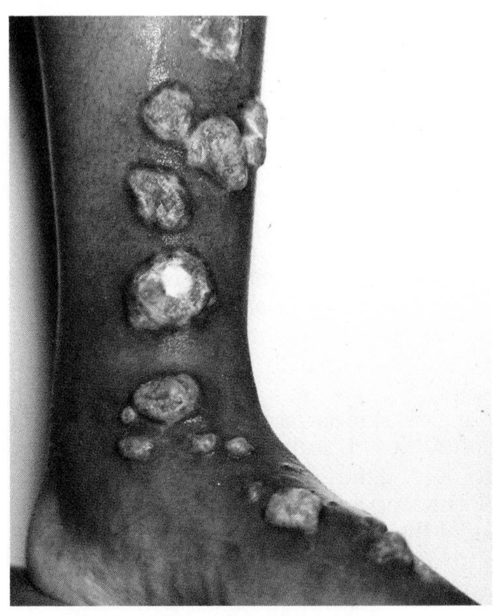

A

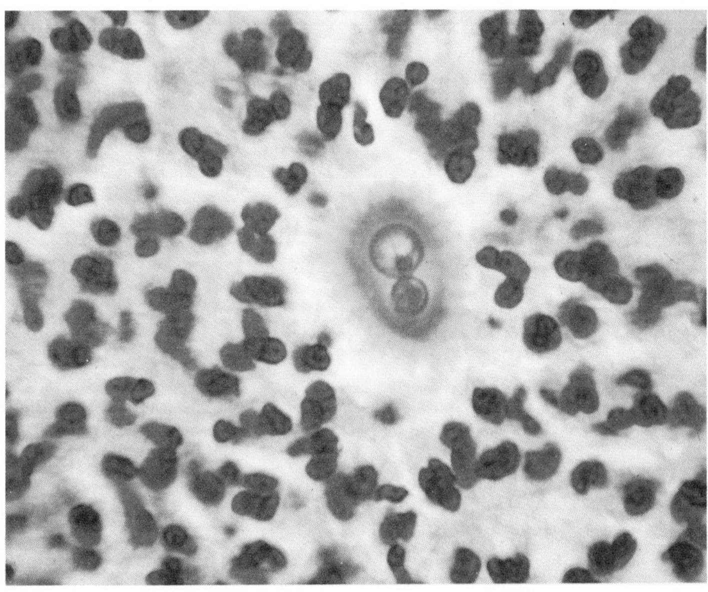

B

FIGURE 9-64
Sporotrichosis. (*A*) The leg shows typical lymphocutaneous spread. (*B*) A section of the lesion in (*A*) shows an asteroid body, composed of a pair of budding yeasts of *S. schenckii* surrounded by a layer of Splendore-Hoeppli substance, with radiating projections.

The lesions of cutaneous sporotrichosis are usually centered in the dermis or subcutaneous tissue. The periphery of the nodules is granulomatous, and the center is suppurative. The surrounding skin displays exuberant pseudoepitheliomatous hyperplasia. The lesions contain only few organisms, which are difficult to find on microscopic examination because they stain poorly with hematoxylin and eosin. The yeasts appear as round or elongated (cigar-shaped) cells. They are best demonstrated with routine fungal stains (Gomori methenamine silver and PAS) and are 2 to 3 μm in diameter; the cigar-shaped bodies are 1 to 2 μm thick and 4 to 5 μm long. Some of the yeasts are surrounded by an eosinophilic, spiculated zone and are termed **asteroid bodies** (see Fig. 9-64B). The material surrounding the yeasts (Splendore-Hoeppli substance) probably consists of antigen-antibody complexes.

☐ **Clinical Features:** Cutaneous sporotrichosis begins as a solitary nodular lesion at the site of inoculation, typically on a hand, arm, or leg. Weeks after the appearance of the first lesion, additional nodules may appear along the lymphatic drainage of the primary lesion. The nodules frequently ulcerate and drain serosanguineous fluid. Joint involvement presents as pain and swelling of the affected joint, without involvement of the overlying skin. If untreated, cutaneous sporotrichosis continues to spread along the skin. The skin infection responds to systemic iodine therapy, but extracutaneous sporotrichosis requires systemic antifungal therapy.

CHROMOMYCOSIS

Chromomycosis is a chronic infection of the skin caused by several species of fungi that live as saprophytes in soil and decaying vegetable matter. The fungi are brown, round, thick walled, and 8 μm across and have been likened to "copper pennies" (Fig. 9-65). The infection is most common in barefooted agricultural workers in the tropics, in whom the fungus is implanted by trauma, usually below the knee. The lesions begin as papules and over the years become verrucous, crusted, and sometimes ulcerated. The infection spreads by contiguous growth and through lymphatics and eventually may involve an entire limb.

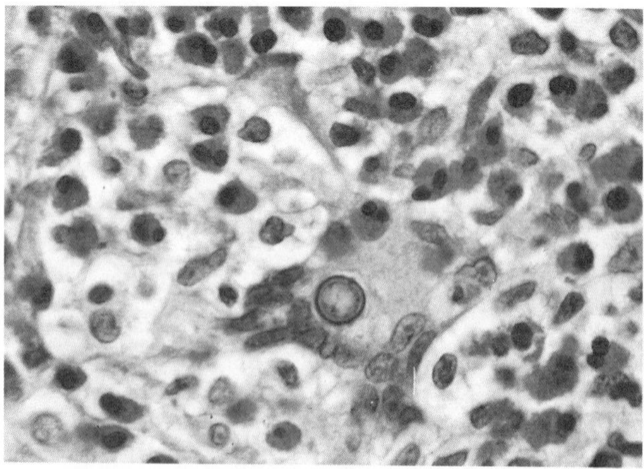

FIGURE 9-65
Chromomycosis. A section of skin shows a giant cell in the center, which contains a thick-walled, brown, sclerotic body (copper penny) representing the fungus.

DERMATOPHYTE INFECTIONS

Dermatophytes are fungi that cause localized superficial infections of keratinized tissues, including skin, hair, and nails. There are about 40 species of dermatophytes within three genera: *Trichophyton*, *Microsporum*, and *Epidermophyton*. Although dermatophyte infections are minor illnesses, they are among the most common skin diseases for which persons seek medical care.

Dermatophytes are resident in the soil, on animals, and on other humans. Most dermatophyte infections in temperate countries are acquired by direct contact with persons who have infected hairs or skin scales. Infection can also be transmitted by unclean hair cutting equipment or by shared bathing facilities.

☐ **Pathology:** Dermatophytes proliferate within the superficial keratinized tissues, which are no longer viable. In skin, they spread centrifugally from the inoculation site, producing round, expanding lesions with sharply defined margins. The clinical appearance once suggested that a worm is responsible for the disease, thus the names "ringworm" and "tinea" (from the Latin *tinea*, "worm"). If infection occurs at sites where keratinized cells are eliminated rapidly, it is often self-limited. On the other hand, if infection occurs at a site where turnover of keratinized cells is slow, such as the soles of the feet, it is likely to become chronic.

Dermatophyte infections produce a thickening of the squamous epithelium, with increased numbers of keratinized cells. Lesions severe enough to be biopsied show a mild lymphocytic inflammatory infiltrate in the dermis. Hyphae and spores of the infecting dermatophytes are confined to the nonviable portions of skin, hair, and nails.

☐ **Clinical Features:** Dermatophyte infections are named according to the sites of involvement (e.g., scalp—tinea capitis; feet—tinea pedis, "athlete's foot"; nails—tinea unguium; and intertriginous areas of the groin—tinea cruris, "jock itch"). These infections range from asymptomatic disease to chronic, fiercely pruritic eruptions. On most skin surfaces, dermatophyte infections begin as slightly raised, scaling papules that spread centrifugally, conferring the "ringworm" appearance. Foot infection (athlete's foot) is characterized by pruritus, scaling, and splitting of the intertriginous skin. Dermatophyte infections are treated with topical antifungal agents.

MYCETOMA

A mycetoma is a slowly progressive, localized, and often disfiguring infection of the skin, soft tissues, and bone produced by inoculation of various soil-dwelling fungi and filamentous bacteria. The foot is the most common site of infection, and

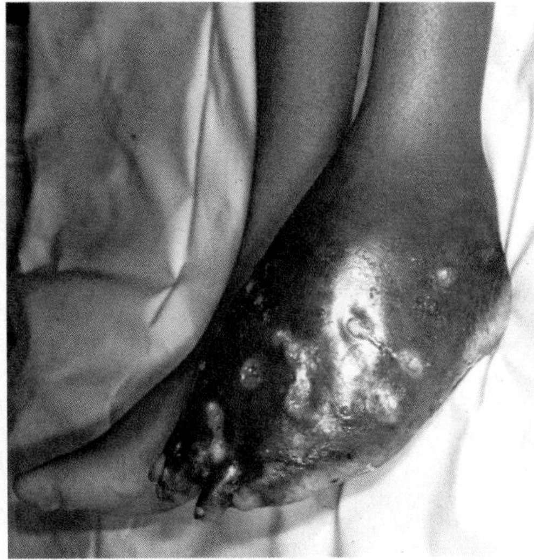
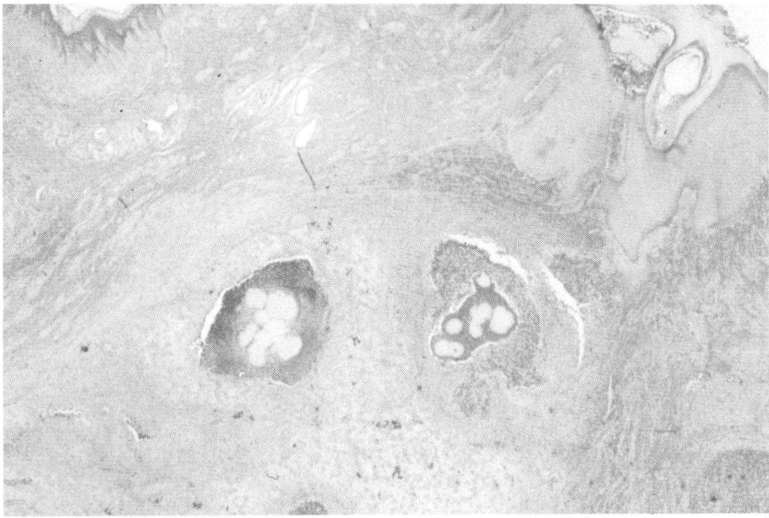

A B

FIGURE 9-66
Mycetoma of the foot. (*A*) The foot is swollen and painful and drains through the skin. The extremity was amputated. (*B*) A photomicrograph of (*A*) demonstrates mycotic grains in the dermis. These are clusters of fungi *(P. boydii)* surrounded by an abscess with a granulomatous perimeter. The grains are erupting through the surface and are in a tunnel of keratin.

the disease is also known as "Madura foot." Responsible organisms include *Madurella mycetomatis, Petrilidium boydii, Actinomadura madurae,* and *Nocardia brasiliensis.*

Mycetoma usually occurs in the tropics among farmers and outdoor laborers whose skin is exposed to trauma. The foot is a common site of infection in locales where people walk barefoot on soggy ground. Frequent immersion of the foot macerates the skin, facilitating deep inoculation with soil organisms.

□ **Pathology:** Within the subcutaneous tissue, the inoculated organisms proliferate and spread to adjacent tissues, including bone. The infection incites a mixed suppurative and granulomatous inflammatory infiltrate, which fails to eliminate the infecting organism. Surrounding granulation tissue and scarring produce progressive disfigurement of the affected sites.

A mycetoma begins as a solitary subcutaneous abscess, which slowly expands to form multiple abscesses interconnected by sinus tracts (Fig. 9-66A). The sinus tracts eventually drain to the skin surface. The abscesses contain colonies of compact bacteria or fungi surrounded by neutrophils and an outer layer of granulomatous inflammation. The colonies of organisms, called "grains," resemble the "sulfur granules" at actinomycosis (see Fig. 9-66B).

□ **Clinical Features:** A mycetoma initially presents as a painless, localized swelling at the site of a penetrating injury. The lesion slowly expands, eventually producing sinus tracts, which tend to follow fascial planes in their lateral and deep spread through connective tissue, muscle, and bone. The treatment is radical excision of the affected area, although meticulous microbiological studies of the causal organisms followed by specific therapy has been effective.

Protozoa

The protozoa are a diverse group of single-celled eukaryotes, classified on the basis of their modes of locomotion and reproduction. The protozoa that cause human disease fall into three general classes: amebae, flagellates, and sporozoites. Amebae move by projection of cytoplasmic extensions termed pseudopods. Flagellates move through threadlike structures, known as flagella, which extend out from the cell membrane. Sporozoites do not possess organelles of locomotion and also differ from the amebae and flagellates in their mode of replication.

Protozoa cause human disease by diverse mechanisms. Some, such as *Entamoeba histolytica*, are extracellular parasites capable of digesting and invading human tissues. Others, such as the plasmodia, are obligate intracellular parasites, which replicate within human cells, thereby killing them. Still others, such as the trypanosomes, damage human tissue largely through the inflammatory and immunological responses that they elicit. Some of the protozoa, for example, *Toxoplasma gondii*, have the capacity to establish latent infections and produce reactivation disease in immunocompromised hosts.

MALARIA

Malaria is a mosquito-borne, hemolytic, febrile illness. The World Health Organization recognizes malaria as causing

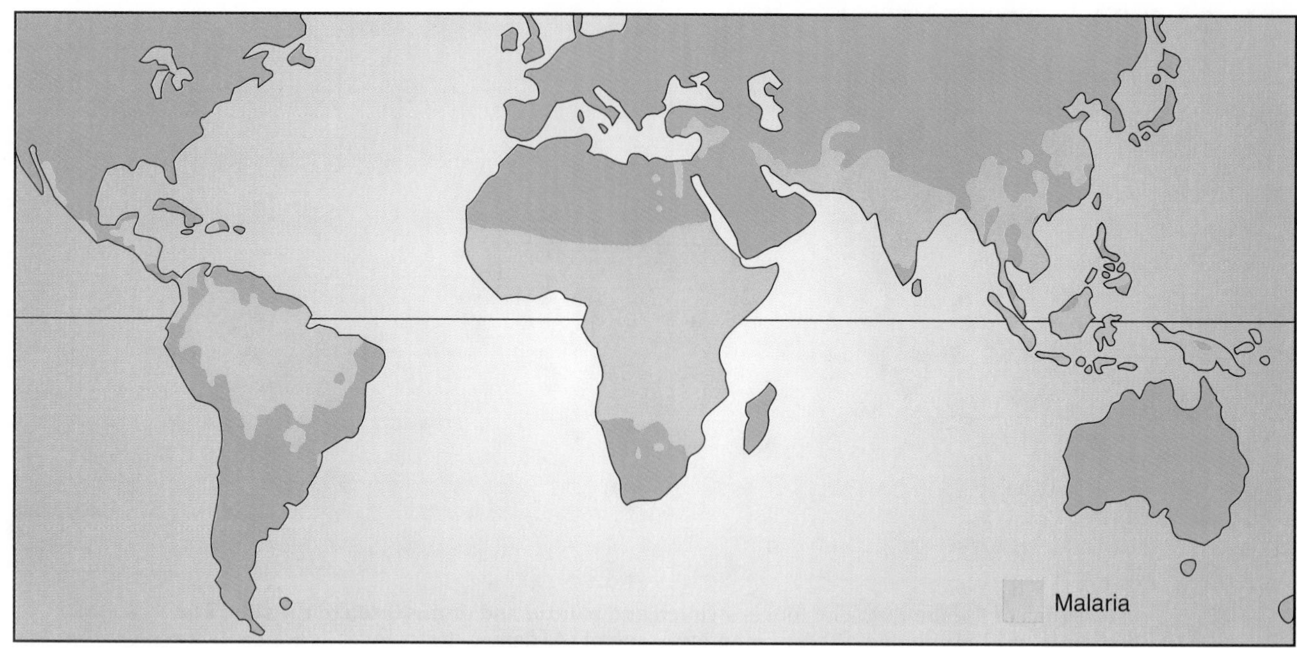

FIGURE *9-67*
The geographic distribution of malaria.

more morbidity than any other disease. Malaria infects over 200 million persons and yearly kills more than 1 million. Four species of *Plasmodium* cause malaria: *P. falciparum*, *P. vivax*, *P. ovale*, and *P. malariae*. All of these plasmodia infect and destroy human erythrocytes, producing chills, fever, anemia, and splenomegaly. *P. falciparum* causes more severe disease than the other plasmodial species and accounts for most malarial deaths.

☐ **Epidemiology:** Malaria has been eradicated in North America, Europe, Australia, Japan, and other developed countries but continues to be a scourge in tropical and subtropical areas, especially tropical Africa, parts of South and Central America, India, and Southeast Asia (Fig. 9-67). The rural poor, infants, children, malnourished persons, and pregnant women are all especially susceptible to infection. All inhabitants of hyperendemic regions are presumed to harbor malarial parasites, even though they may have no clinical symptoms.

Malaria is transmitted from person to person by the bite of the female *Anopheles* mosquito. Although *P. falciparum and P. vivax* are the most common pathogens, there is considerable geographic variation in species distribution. *P. vivax* is rare in Africa, where much of the black population lacks the erythrocyte cell surface receptors required for infection. *P. falciparum* and *P. ovale* are the predominant species in Africa. *P. malariae* is the least common and mildest form of malaria, although it enjoys a broad geographic distribution.

FIGURE *9-68*
Life cycle of malaria. An *Anopheles* mosquito bites an infected person, taking blood that contains micro- and macrogametocytes (sexual forms). In the mosquito, sexual multiplication ("sporogony") produces infective sporozoites in the salivary glands. (1) During the mosquito bite, sporozoites are inoculated into the bloodstream of the vertebrate host. Some sporozoites leave the blood and enter the hepatocytes, where they multiply asexually (exoerythrocytic schizogony), and form thousands of uninucleated merozoites. (2) Rupture of hepatocytes releases merozoites, which penetrate erythrocytes and become trophozoites, which then divide to form numerous schizonts (intraerythrocytic schizogony). Schizonts divide to form more merozoites, which are released on the rupture of erythrocytes and reenter other erythrocytes to begin a new cycle. After several cycles, subpopulations of merozoites develop into micro- and macrogametocytes, which are taken up by another mosquito to complete the cycle. (3) Parasitized erythrocytes obstruct capillaries of the brain, heart, kidney, and other deep organs. Adherence of parasitized erythrocytes to capillary endothelial cells causes fibrin thrombi, which produce microinfarcts. These result in encephalopathy, congestive heart failure, pulmonary edema, and frequently death. Ruptured erythrocytes release hemoglobin, erythrocyte debris, and malarial pigment. (4) Phagocytosis leads to monocyte/macrophage hyperplasia and hepatosplenomegaly. (5) Released hemoglobin produces hemoglobinuric nephrosis, which may be fatal.

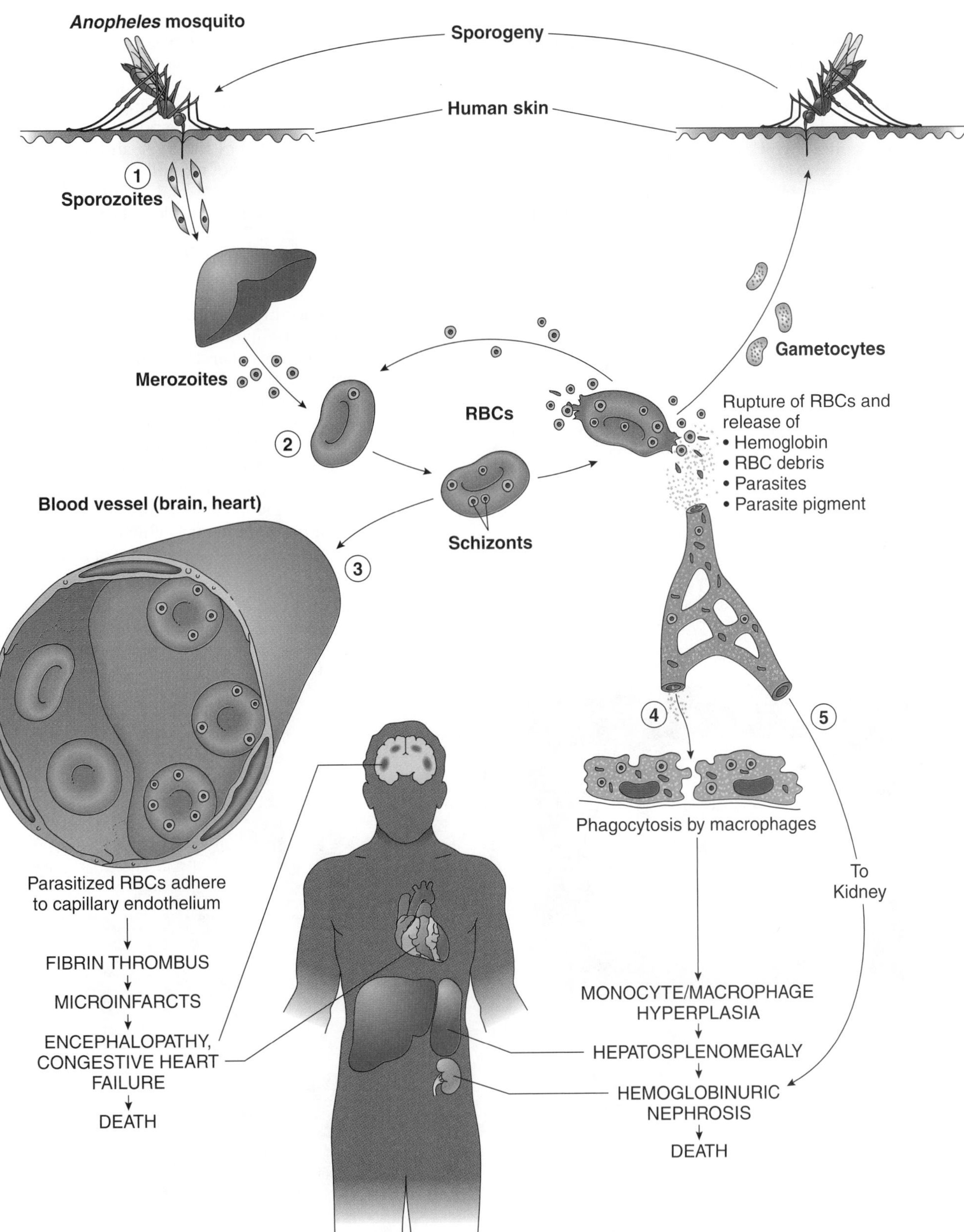
Anopheles mosquito
Sporogeny
Human skin
1
Sporozoites
Merozoites
2
RBCs
Schizonts
Gametocytes
Rupture of RBCs and release of
• Hemoglobin
• RBC debris
• Parasites
• Parasite pigment
Blood vessel (brain, heart)
3
4
5
Phagocytosis by macrophages
To Kidney
Parasitized RBCs adhere to capillary endothelium
FIBRIN THROMBUS
MICROINFARCTS
ENCEPHALOPATHY, CONGESTIVE HEART FAILURE
DEATH
MONOCYTE/MACROPHAGE HYPERPLASIA
HEPATOSPLENOMEGALY
HEMOGLOBINURIC NEPHROSIS
DEATH

FIGURE *9-68*

Pathogenesis: The life cycle of the *Plasmodium* species responsible for human malaria requires both human and mosquito hosts (Fig. 9-68). Infected humans produce forms of the organism (gametocytes) that mosquitoes acquire on feeding. Within these insects, the organism reproduces sexually, producing plasmodial forms (sporozoites), which the mosquito transmits to humans when it feeds.

The anopheline mosquito inoculates malarial sporozoites into the human bloodstream, where they undergo asexual division (schizogony). Circulating sporozoites rapidly invade hepatocytes and reproduce in the liver, yielding numerous daughter organisms, known as merozoites (exoerythrocytic phase). Within 2 to 3 weeks of hepatic infection, merozoites exit into the bloodstream by rupturing their host hepatocytes and invade erythrocytes, establishing the erythrocytic phase of malarial infection.

The merozoites feed on hemoglobin, grow, and reproduce within the erythrocytes. Within 2 to 4 days, depending on the species of *Plasmodium*, mature progeny merozoites are produced. These burst from infected erythrocytes and invade previously uninfected red cells, initiating another cycle of erythrocytic parasitism.

The erythrocytic cycle is repeated many times. Eventually, subpopulations of merozoites differentiate into sexual forms known as gametocytes. A mosquito feeding on an infected host ingests gametocytes, thereby completing the life cycle of the malarial parasite.

The rupture of infected erythrocytes causes the chills and fever of malaria through the release of as yet unidentified pyrogenic material. Anemia results both from the rupture of circulating infected erythrocytes and from sequestration of cells in the enlarging spleen. Hepatosplenomegaly reflects the response of the fixed mononuclear phagocytes of the liver and spleen to the parasitism and destruction of red cells.

P. falciparum, the cause of malignant malaria, produces much more aggressive and lethal disease than the other human malarias. This organism is distinguished from other malarial parasites in four respects:

- It has no secondary exoerythrocytic (hepatic) stage.
- It parasitizes erythrocytes of any age, causing marked parasitemia and anemia. In other types of malaria, only subpopulations of erythrocytes (e.g., only young or old forms) are parasitized, and thus low-level parasitemias and more modest anemias occur.
- There may be several parasites in a single red cell.
- *P. falciparum* alters the flow characteristics and adhesive properties of infected erythrocytes, so that they adhere to the endothelial cells of small blood vessels. The obstruction of small blood vessels frequently produces severe tissue ischemia, which is probably the most important factor in the virulence of *P. falciparum*.

Pathology: In all forms of malaria, the spleen and liver enlarge as erythrocytes are sequestered by the fixed

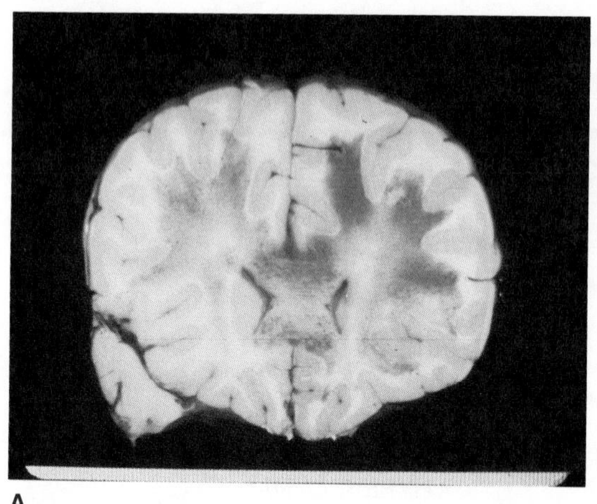
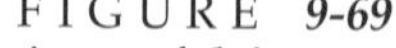

A

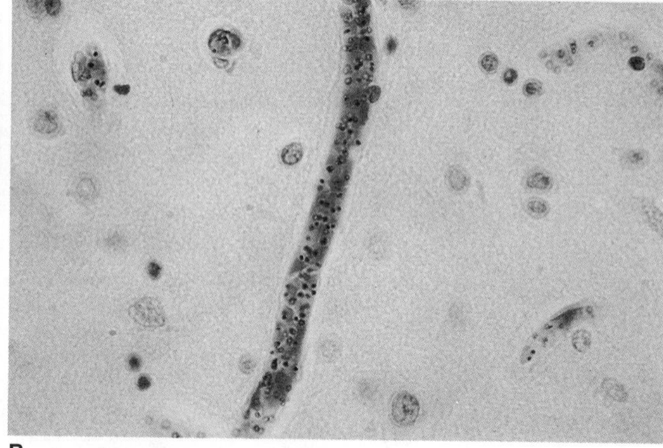

B

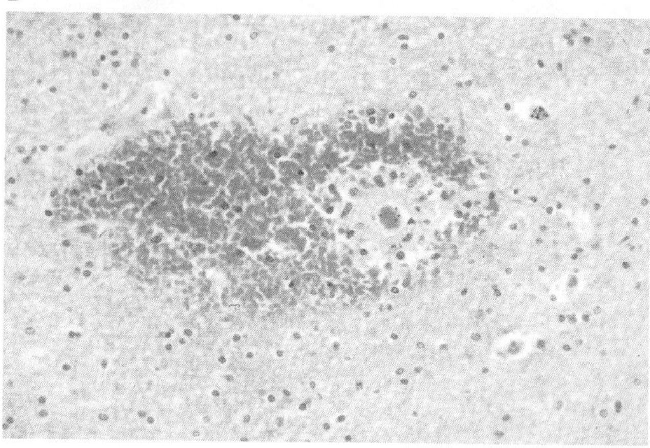

C

FIGURE 9-69
Acute falciparum malaria of the brain. (*A*) There is severe diffuse congestion of the white matter and focal hemorrhages. (*B*) A section of (*A*) shows a capillary packed with parasitized erythrocytes. (C) Another section of (*A*) displays a ring hemorrhage around a thrombosed capillary, which contains parasitized erythrocytes in a fibrin thrombus.

mononuclear phagocyte system. The organs of this system (liver, spleen, lymph nodes) are darkened ("slate gray") by macrophages filled with hemosiderin and malarial pigment, the end-product of parasitic digestion of hemoglobin.

The adherence of infected red cells to the microvascular endothelium in falciparum malaria has two consequences. First, parasitized erythrocytes attached to endothelial cells do not circulate, so patients with severe falciparum malaria have few circulating parasites. Second, capillaries of deep organs, especially the brain, become obstructed, leading to ischemia of the brain, kidneys, and lungs. The brains of persons who die of cerebral malaria show congestion and thrombosis of small blood vessels in the white matter, which are rimmed with edema and hemorrhage ("ring hemorrhages") (Fig. 9-69). Obstruction of blood flow in the kidney produces acute renal failure, while intravascular hemolysis leads to hemoglobinuric nephrosis ("blackwater fever"). In the lung, damage to alveolar capillaries produces pulmonary edema and acute alveolar damage.

□ **Clinical Features:** Recurrent bouts of chills and high fever, known as paroxysms, are characteristic of malaria. The paroxysm begins with chills and sometimes headache. This "cold phase" of the paroxysm is then followed by a "hot phase" of high, spiking fever and tachycardia, often accompanied by nausea, vomiting, and abdominal pain. The high fever produces a marked vasodilatation and often an associated orthostatic hypotension. When the fever defervesces after several hours, the patient is usually exhausted and drenched in sweat, the "wet phase" of the paroxysm.

A period of 2 to 3 days then follows during which the patient feels well, only to be followed by a new paroxysm. The paroxysms recur for weeks, eventually subsiding as the infected person mounts an immunological response. Each paroxysm corresponds to the rupture of infected erythrocytes and the release of daughter merozoites. As the mononuclear macrophage system responds to the infection, patients develop hepatosplenomegaly. Splenic enlargement can be dramatic (some of the largest spleens on record represent the effects of chronic malaria). Hypersplenism can exacerbate the anemia of malarial infection.

As mentioned earlier, *P. falciparum* infection frequently produces much graver disease than the other forms of malaria. As the level of parasitemia grows, fever can become virtually continuous. Ischemic injury to the brain causes symptoms ranging from somnolence, hallucinations, and behavioral changes to seizures and coma. Central nervous system disease is dangerous, with a mortality of 20% to 50%. Malaria is diagnosed by the demonstration of the organisms on Giemsa-stained smears of peripheral blood, and the different species of *Plasmodium* are distinguished by their appearance in infected erythrocytes. Malarias other than falciparum malaria are treated with oral chloroquine, sometimes with the addition of primaquine. Therapy for falciparum malaria varies, as new treatments are constantly being developed to meet the challenge of widespread chloroquine resistance.

BABESIOSIS

Babesiosis is a malaria-like infection caused by protozoa of the genus Babesia, which is transmitted by hard-bodied ticks. *Babesia* infections are common in animals and in some locations are responsible for serious economic losses to the livestock industry. By contrast, human babesiosis is almost a medical curiosity, with the parasites infecting humans only when they intrude into the zoonotic cycle between the tick vector and its vertebrate host. Human babesiosis has been reported only in Europe and North America. Infections in the United States have been concentrated in islands off the New England coast.

The causative organisms, which resemble those of malaria, invade and destroy erythrocytes. However, they differ from malarial parasites in several important ways: they (1) are transmitted by ticks; (2) make no pigment; (3) produce no sexual forms; and (4) have no exoerythrocytic stage. *Babesias* infect a variety of mammals, including cattle, horses, and dogs. The parasites are ingested by ticks when they feed on infected animals, after which the organisms are transmitted in the saliva when the tick feeds again. *Babesia* invade red cells, where the organisms assume an ameboid, round, rod-shaped, or irregular appearance. They are 1 to 5 μm in diameter; with the Giemsa stain, they have a blue cytoplasm and a mass of red chromatin.

Splenectomy and diabetes are predisposing factors for babesiosis. After an incubation period of 2 to 6 weeks, the patient experiences the sudden onset of chills and fever, sometimes with muscle aches and pains, prostration, jaundice, dark urine, and diarrhea. The progressive invasion and destruction of erythrocytes causes hemoglobinemia, hemoglobinuria, and renal failure. The disease is usually self-limited, but uncontrolled infections can be fatal. *Babesia* species are resistant to most antiprotozoal drugs used in human medicine.

TOXOPLASMOSIS

Toxoplasmosis is a worldwide infectious disease caused by Toxoplasma gondii, a protozoan that may produce the most common human infection. Most infections are asymptomatic, but when they occur in the fetus or an immunocompromised host, devastating necrotizing disease may result.

□ **Epidemiology and Pathogenesis:** In some areas (e.g., Paris), the prevalence of *T. gondii* infection exceeds 80% of adults, whereas in other regions (e.g., the southwestern part of the United States), only a small portion of the population is infected.

T. gondii infects a wide variety of mammals and birds as intermediate hosts. The only final host is the cat, which becomes infected by ingesting cysts of the organism in the tissues of an infected mouse or other intermediate host. Within the cat's intestinal epithelium, five multiplicative stages end with the shedding of oocysts. The oocysts sporulate in feces and soil and differentiate into sporocysts, which contain sporozoites. The sporocysts are ingested by intermediate hosts, such as birds, mice, or humans. The sporozoites develop in the intermediate host to complete the life cycle. *T. gondii* has two stages in tissue: tachyzoites and bradyzoites, both crescent-shaped and measuring 2 × 6 μm. During acute infection, tachyzoites multiply rapidly to form "groups" within intracellular vacuoles of the parasitized cells, a process that eventually causes the rupture of the cells. Tachyzoites spread from the gut through the lymphatics to regional lymph nodes and through the blood to the liver, lungs, heart, brain, and other organs.

During chronic infection, the organisms, now called bradyzoites, multiply slowly. The bradyzoites store PAS-positive material, and hundreds of organisms are tightly packed in "cysts." The cysts originate in intracellular vacuoles, enlarge beyond the usual size of the cell, and push the nucleus to the periphery.

Except for congenital infection, toxoplasmosis is acquired by the ingestion of infectious forms of the organism. In the tropics, where children are predominantly infected, oocysts in contaminated soil are the principal source of infection. By contrast, in developed countries, the ingestion of incompletely cooked meat (lamb and pork) that contains *Toxoplasma* tissue cysts is the major mechanism of infection. Another source of infection is cat feces. The oocysts contaminate the hands and food of persons who live in close association with cats. Congenital infection is acquired by transplacental transmission of infectious forms from an acutely infected (usually asymptomatic) mother to the fetus.

The active infection is usually terminated by cell-mediated immunological responses. **In most *T. gondii* infections, little significant tissue destruction occurs before the immunological response brings the active phase of the infection under control, and infected persons suffer few clinical effects.** *T. gondii* establishes latent infection, however, by forming the dormant tissue cysts in some infected cells. These survive for decades in host cells. If the infected person loses cell-mediated immunity, the organism can emerge from its encysted form and reestablish a destructive infection.

Toxoplasma Lymphadenopathy Syndrome

The most frequent manifestation of *T. gondii* infection in the immunocompetent host is lymphadenopathy. Virtually any lymph node group may be involved, but enlarged cervical nodes are most readily apparent. The histological appearance of affected lymph nodes is distinctive, with numerous epithelioid macrophages surrounding and encroaching on reactive germinal centers.

In *Toxoplasma* lymphadenitis (Fig. 9-70A), patients present with nontender regional lymph node enlargement, sometimes accompanied by fever, sore throat, hepatosplenomegaly, and circulating atypical lymphocytes. Hepatitis, myocarditis (see Fig. 9-70B), and myositis have been documented. Lymphadenopathy usually resolves spontaneously in several weeks to several months, and therapy is seldom required.

Congenital Toxoplasma Infections

T. gondii infection in the fetus is much more destructive than in the child or adult. The developing brain and eye are readily infected, and the fetus lacks the immunological capacity to contain the infection. Central nervous system infection produces a necrotizing meningoencephalitis, which in the most severe cases results in the loss of brain parenchyma, cerebral calcifications, and marked hydrocephalus (Fig. 9-71). Ocular infection causes chorioretinitis (i.e., necrosis and inflammation of the choroid and retina).

The most severe fetal disease is produced by infection early in pregnancy. The earliest infections probably produce spontaneous abortion. In infants born with congenital toxoplasmosis, the effects of brain involvement range from severe mental retardation and seizures to subtle psychomotor defects. Ocular involvement may cause congenital visual impairment. Latent ocular infection estab-

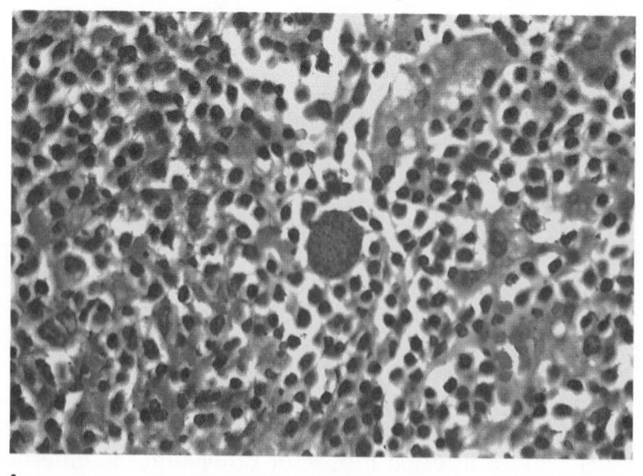

A

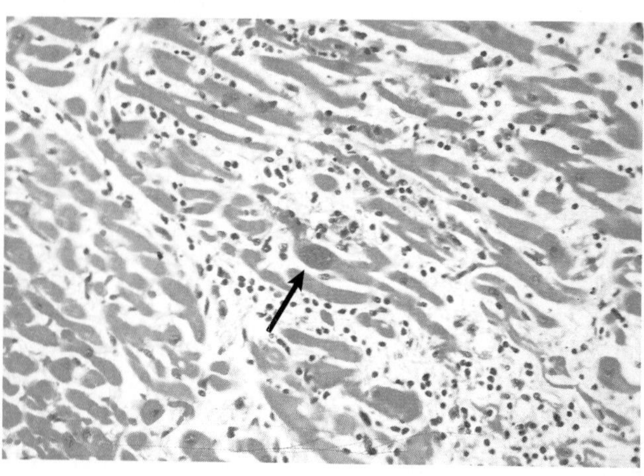

B

FIGURE 9-70
Toxoplasmosis. (*A*) A photomicrograph of an enlarged lymph node reveals bradyzoites of *T. gondii* within a cyst. (*B*) A section of heart shows a cyst of bradyzoites of *T. gondii* within a myofiber (*arrow*), with edema and inflammatory cells in the adjacent tissue.

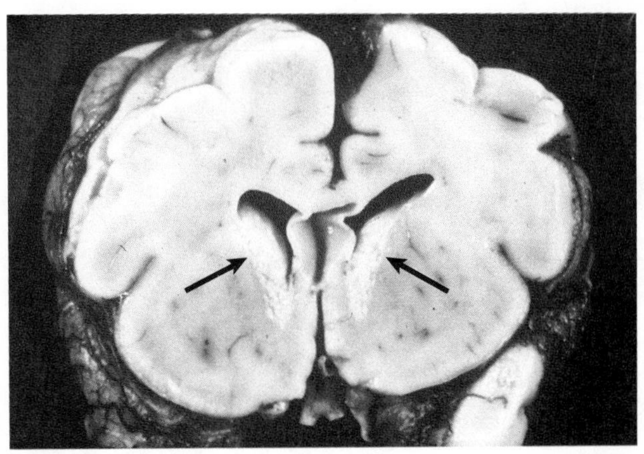

FIGURE *9-71*
Congenital toxoplasmosis. The brain of a premature infant reveals subependymal necrosis with calcification appearing as bilaterally symmetric areas of whitish discoloration (*arrows*).

lished *in utero* may also recrudesce later in life to produce visual loss. Some newborns have *Toxoplasma* hepatitis, with large areas of necrosis and giant cells. Adrenal necrosis is also occasionally observed. Congenital toxoplasmosis requires therapy with antiprotozoal agents.

Toxoplasmosis in Immunocompromised Hosts

Devastating *T. gondii* infections occur in persons with decreased cell-mediated immunity (e.g., patients with AIDS or those receiving immunosuppressive therapy for transplantation). In most cases, the disease represents a reactivation of a latent infection. The brain is the most commonly affected organ, where infection with *T. gondii* produces a multifocal necrotizing encephalitis.

Patients with encephalitis present with paresis, seizures, alterations in visual acuity, and changes in mentation. *Toxoplasma* encephalitis in the immunocompromised patient is fatal if not treated with effective antiprotozoal agents.

PNEUMOCYSTIS CARINII PNEUMONIA

Pneumocystis carinii causes progressive, often fatal, pneumonia in persons with severely impaired cell-mediated immunity and is the one of the most common, serious opportunistic pathogens in persons with AIDS. Although previously considered a protozoan, the taxonomy of *P. carinii* has been called into question by recent nucleic acid studies, and the organism may be more closely related to the fungi than to the protozoa.

☐ **Epidemiology:** *P. carinii* is distributed worldwide, and since 75% of the population have acquired antibodies by 5 years of age, it is reasonable to assume that the organisms are inhaled regularly by all. Whether *P. carinii* is acquired from the environment, from infected humans, or from animals is unknown. In persons with intact cell-mediated immunity, *P. carinii* infection is rapidly contained without producing symptoms.

In the 1960s and 1970s, between 100 to 200 cases of active *Pneumocystis* disease were reported annually in the United States. These cases occurred primarily among persons with hematological malignancies, transplant recipients, or patients with autoimmune diseases who were treated with corticosteroids or cytotoxic therapy. The situation changed dramatically in the 1980s with the AIDS pandemic. **Eighty percent of all AIDS patients develop *Pneumocystis carinii* pneumonia during the course of their illness.**

☐ **Pathogenesis:** *P. carinii* reproduces in intimate association with alveolar type 1 lining cells, and active disease is confined to the lungs. Infection begins with the attachment of the *Pneumocystis* trophozoite to the alveolar lining cell. The trophozoite feeds on the host cell, enlarges, and transforms into the cyst form, which contains daughter organisms. The cyst ruptures to release new trophozoites, which attach to additional alveolar lining cells. If the process is not checked by the host immune system or antibiotic therapy, the infected alveoli eventually fill with organisms and proteinaceous fluid. The progressive filling of alveoli prevents adequate gas exchange, and the patient slowly suffocates.

It is assumed, but not proven, that most cases of pneumocystosis derive from latent endogenous infection. Outbreaks of *Pneumocystis* pneumonia have also occurred among severely malnourished (and thus immunosuppressed) infants in nurseries; these uncommon cases are believed to represent primary infection with the organism.

☐ **Pathology:** *P. carinii* causes a progressive consolidation of the lungs. Microscopically, the alveoli contain a frothy eosinophilic material, which is composed of alveolar macrophages and cysts and trophozoites of *P. carinii* (Fig. 9-72). There are hyaline membranes and prominent type 2 lining cells. In newborns, the alveolar septa are thickened by lymphoid cells and macrophages. The prominence of plasma cells in the infantile disease led to the term **plasma cell pneumonia**.

The various forms of *P. carinii* are difficult to discern with hematoxylin and eosin stains. Methenamine silver stains the cyst form of *P. carinii*, which measures 58 μm in diameter (see Fig. 9-72B). Giemsa does not stain the cyst but rather the extracellular trophozoites and intracystic forms of the organism. These appear as irregularly shaped cells, 1 to 3 μm across, with punctate violet nuclei.

☐ **Clinical Features:** *P. carinii* pneumonia presents as fever and progressive shortness of breath, often exacerbated by exertion and accompanied by a nonproductive cough. The dyspnea may be subtle in onset and slowly progressive over many weeks. Chest radiographs show a diffuse pulmonary process. The diagnosis requires recovery of alveolar material (by bronchoscopy, endobronchial washing, or sputum induction) for staining. *P. carinii* is fa-

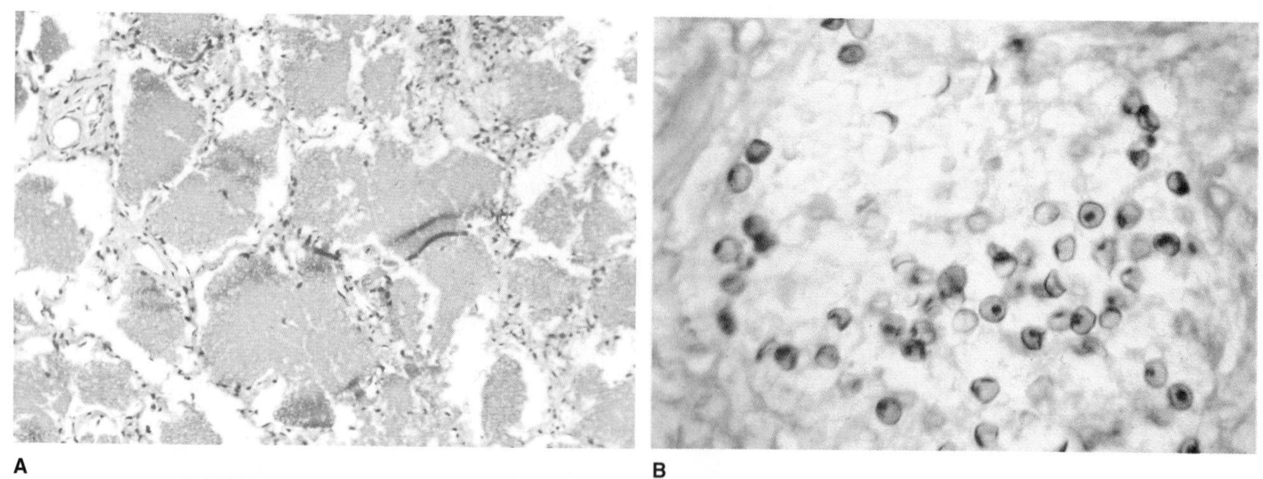

FIGURE 9-72
***Pneumocystis carinii* pneumonia. (*A*) The alveoli contain a frothy eosinophilic material, which is composed of alveolar macrophages and cysts and trophozoites of *P. carinii*. (*B*) A silver stain shows crescent-shaped organisms, which are collapsed and degenerated. Some have a characteristic dark spot in their walls.**

tal if untreated. Treatment consists of the administration of trimethoprim-sulfamethoxazole or pentamidine.

AMEBIASIS

Amebiasis refers to an infection with Entamoeba histolytica, which principally involves the colon and occasionally the liver. *E. histolytica* is named for its lytic actions on tissue. Intestinal infection ranges from asymptomatic colonization to severe invasive infections with bloody diarrhea. On occasion, the parasites spread beyond the colon to involve other organs. The most common site of extraintestinal disease is the liver, where *E. histolytica* causes slowly expanding, necrotizing abscesses.

☐ **Epidemiology:** Humans are the only known reservoir for *E. histolytica,* which reproduces in the colon and passes in the feces. Although amebiasis is worldwide, it is more common and more severe in tropical and subtropical areas, where poor sanitation prevails. **Amebiasis is acquired by ingestion of materials contaminated with human feces.**

☐ **Pathogenesis:** *E. histolytica* has three distinct stages: the trophozoite (the ameboid form), the precyst, and the cyst.

Amebic trophozoites, 15 to 20 μm across, are found in the stools of patients with acute symptoms. They are spherical or oval and have a thin cell membrane, a single nucleus, condensed chromatin on the interior of the nuclear membrane, and a central karyosome. The trophozoites sometimes contain phagocytosed erythrocytes. PAS stains the cytoplasm of the trophozoites and makes them stand out in tissue sections.

Amebic cysts are found only in the stools, since they do not invade tissue. They are spherical, have thick walls, measure 5 to 25 μm across, and usually have four nuclei.

The cysts are found in contaminated water or food and constitute the infective stage (Fig. 9-73). On ingestion, the cysts traverse the stomach and excyst in the lower ileum. A metacystic ameba containing four nuclei divides to form four small, immature trophozoites, which then grow to full size. The trophozoites thrive in the colon and feed on bacteria and human cells. Trophozoites may colonize any portion of the large bowel, but the area of maximum disease is usually the cecum. Precysts and cysts form when the passage of feces through the bowel is slow. Precysts form a cyst wall and develop into a mature quadrinucleate cyst—the transmission stage to the next host. The cysts contaminate water, food, or fingers, thereby completing the cycle. Patients with symptomatic amebic colitis pass both cysts and trophozoites, but the latter survive only briefly outside the body and are also destroyed by gastric secretions. Strains of *E. histolytica* capable of invading human colonic epithelium cause human disease, whereas others merely colonize the colon. Host factors, such as nutritional status, coexistent colonic flora, and immunological status, also contribute to the course of *E. histolytica* infection.

FIGURE 9-73
Amebic colitis and its complications. Amebiasis results from the ingestion of food or water contaminated with amebic cysts. In the colon, the amebae penetrate the mucosa and produce flask-shaped ulcers of the mucosa and submucosa. The organisms may invade submucosal venules, thereby disseminating the infection to the liver and other organs. The liver abscess can expand to involve adjacent structures.

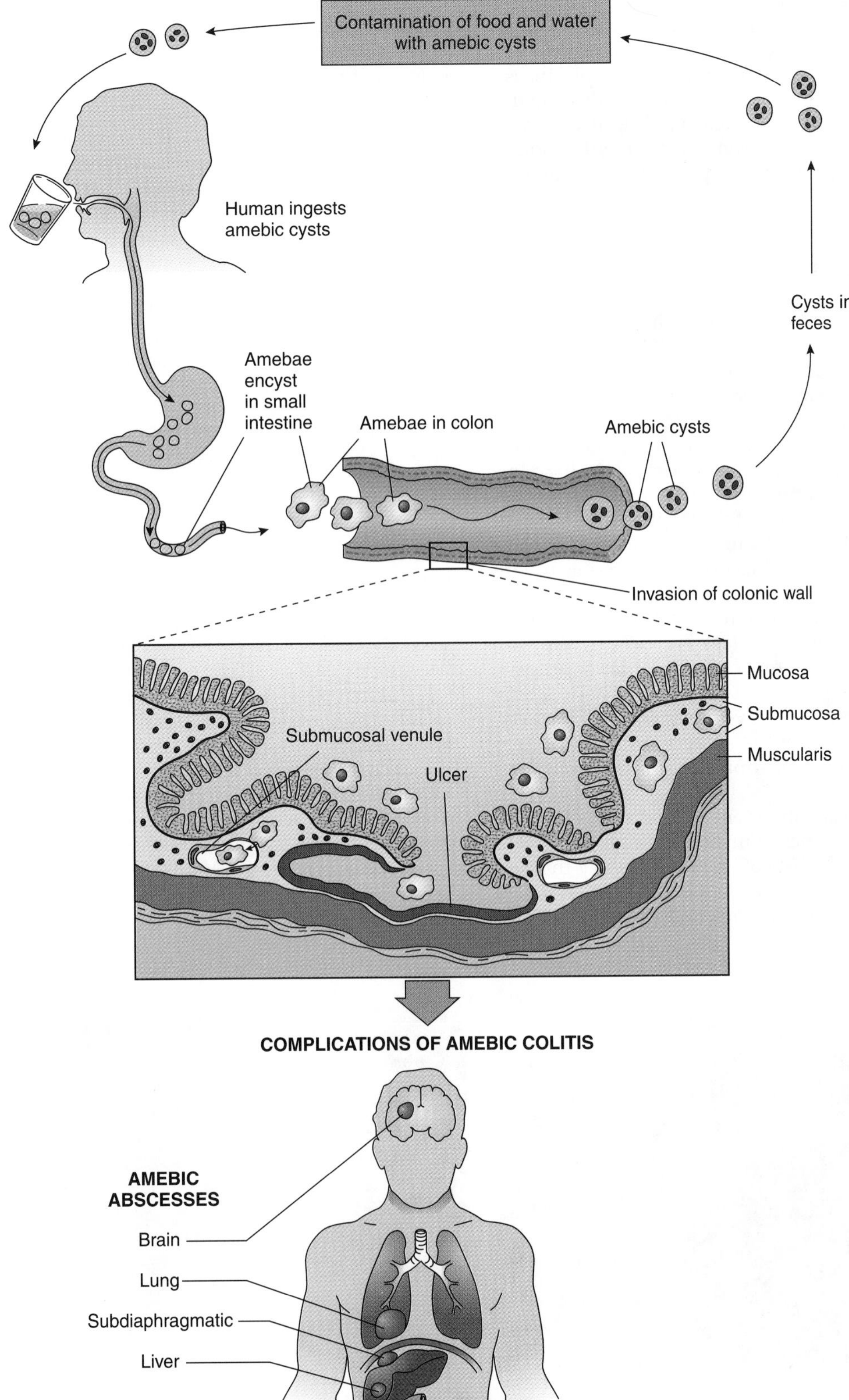
Contamination of food and water with amebic cysts
Human ingests amebic cysts
Cysts in feces
Amebae encyst in small intestine
Amebae in colon
Amebic cysts
Invasion of colonic wall
Mucosa
Submucosa
Muscularis
Submucosal venule
Ulcer
COMPLICATIONS OF AMEBIC COLITIS
AMEBIC ABSCESSES
Brain
Lung
Subdiaphragmatic
Liver
Amebic ulcers
Ameboma

FIGURE *9-73*

Invasion begins with the attachment of a trophozoite to a colonic epithelial cell. The organism kills the target cell by elaborating a lytic protein that breaches the cell membrane. Progressive death of mucosal cells produces a superficial ulcer. The disease may arrest with this superficial ulceration or proceed to extensive deep invasion. In the latter case, trophozoites sometimes invade submucosal blood vessels and are carried to distant extraintestinal sites.

Intestinal Amebiasis

☐ **Pathology:** Amebic lesions begin as small foci of necrosis that progress to ulcers (Fig. 9-74A). Some remain small and discrete, but others expand. Undermining of the ulcer margin and confluence of the expanding ulcers lead to sloughing of the mucosa in broad, irregular, geographic patterns. The bed of the ulcer is gray and necrotic, being composed of fibrin and cellular debris. A sharp line divides the viable and necrotic mucosa, a feature that demonstrates the lytic action of the trophozoite. The exudate raises the undermined mucosa, producing chronic amebic ulcers whose shape has been described as resembling a flask or a bottle neck.

Trophozoites are found on the surface of the ulcer, in the exudate, and in the crater (see Fig. 9-74B). They are also frequent in the submucosa, muscularis propria, serosa, and small veins of the submucosa. There is little inflammatory response in early amebic ulcers. However, as the ulcer enlarges, there is an accumulation of neutrophils, lymphocytes, macrophages, plasma cells, and sometimes eosinophils.

An ameboma is an infrequent complication of amebiasis, occurring when amebae invade through the intestinal wall. The lesion consists of an inflammatory thickening of the wall of the bowel that resembles carcinoma of the colon in location, symptoms, and gross and radiographic appearance. The ameboma tends to form a "napkin-ring constriction." Histological sections reveal granulation tissue, fibrosis, chronic inflammatory cells, and clusters of trophozoites.

☐ **Clinical Features:** Intestinal amebiasis ranges from a completely asymptomatic infection to a severe dysenteric disease. The incubation period for acute amebic colitis is 8 to 10 days. Gradually increasing abdominal discomfort, tenderness, and cramps are accompanied by chills and fever. Nausea, vomiting, malodorous flatus, and intermittent constipation are typical features. Liquid stools (up to 25 a day) contain bloody mucus, but the diarrhea is rarely so prolonged as to result in dehydration. Amebic colitis often persists for months or years, and the patients may become emaciated and anemic. The clinical features are occasionally bizarre, and sometimes must be differentiated from those of appendicitis, cholecystitis, intestinal obstruction, or diverticulitis. In severe amebic colitis, massive destruction of the colonic mucosa may lead to fatal hemorrhage, perforation, or peritonitis. Therapy for intestinal amebiasis includes metronidazole, which acts against trophozoites, and diloxanide, which is effective against cysts.

Extraintestinal Amebiasis

☐ **Pathology:** **Liver abscess** is a major complication of intestinal amebiasis. *E. histolytica* trophozoites that have invaded into submucosal veins of the colon enter the portal circulation and reach the liver. Here the organisms kill hepatocytes, producing a slowly expanding necrotic cavity, filled with a dark brown, odorless semisolid material, reported to resemble "anchovy paste" in color and consistency (Fig. 9-75). Neutrophils are rare within the cavity, which is not a proper abscess, and trophozoites are found along the edges adjacent to hepatocytes.

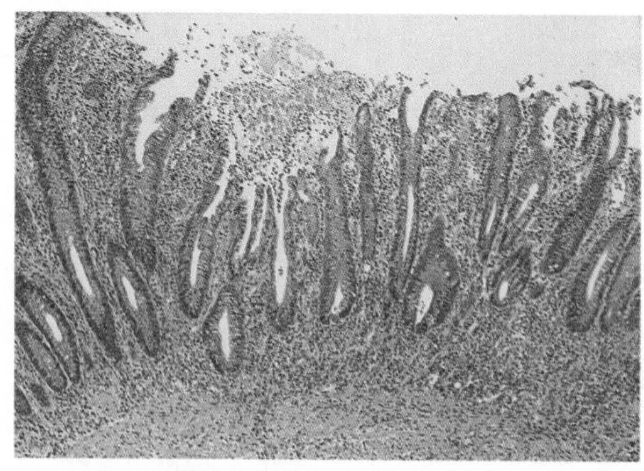

A

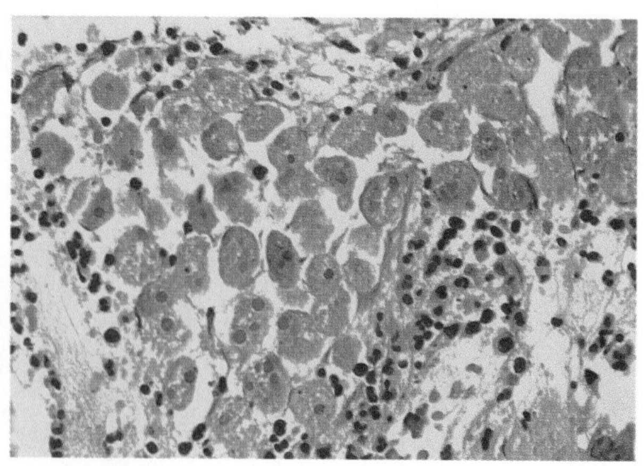

B

FIGURE *9-74*
Intestinal amebiasis. (*A*) The colonic mucosa shows superficial ulceration beneath a cluster of trophozoites of *E. histolytica*. The lamina propria contains excess acute and chronic inflammatory cells, including eosinophils. (*B*) Higher-power view shows numerous trophozoites in the luminal exudate.

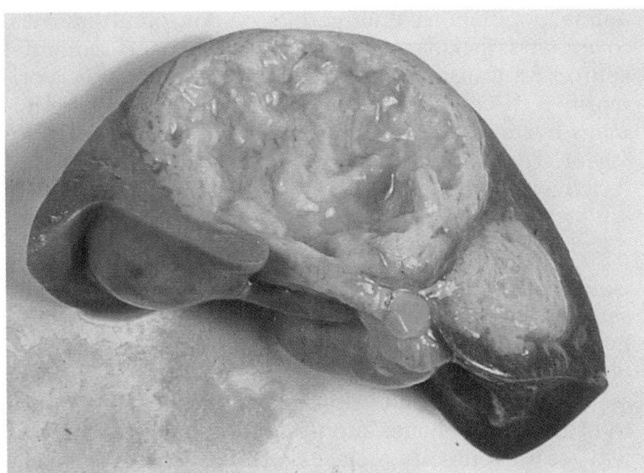

FIGURE 9-75
Amebic abscesses of the liver. The cut surface of the liver shows multiple abscesses containing "anchovy paste" material.

An amebic liver abscess may expand and rupture through the capsule, extending into the peritoneum, diaphragm, pleural cavity, lungs, or pericardium. Rarely, a liver abscess, or even a lesion in the colon, may spread amebae to the brain by a hematogenous route to form large necrotic lesions. Cutaneous amebiasis results from extension of rectal amebiasis to the anus, perianal skin, and vulva, or from infection of the penile skin acquired during anal intercourse. Trophozoites are concentrated over ulcerations in the epidermis. Ulcers of the abdominal wall and penis, which may extend rapidly, are acutely tender, have a putrid odor, and exhibit a gray-white necrotic base.

☐ **Clinical Features:** Patients with amebic liver abscess present with severe right upper quadrant pain, low-grade fever, and weight loss. Only a minority of patients give a history of an antecedent diarrheal illness, and *E. histolytica* is demonstrated in the feces of less than one third of patients with extraintestinal disease. The diagnosis is usually made by radiological or ultrasound demonstration of the abscess, in conjunction with serological testing for antibodies to *E. histolytica*. Extraintestinal amebiasis is treated with metronidazole and diloxanide.

BALANTIDIASIS

Infection with the large, ciliated, ameba-like protozoan *Balantidium coli* is encountered worldwide but is more common in warm climates. *B. coli* infects many animals, but pigs and rats are the source of most human infections. Humans become infected by ingesting cysts of *B. coli* in water or food, after which the trophozoites live in the large intestine. Most balantidial infections are asymptomatic, but severe ones may resemble intestinal amebiasis.

CRYPTOSPORIDIOSIS

Cryptosporidiosis refers to an enteric infection with a protozoan of the genus Cryptosporidium that causes diarrheal disease in persons with compromised immunity. Cryptosporidium causes an enteric infection of animals and is of particular concern in patients with AIDS. Cryptosporidiosis varies from a self-limited gastrointestinal infection to a potentially life-threatening diarrheal illness.

Cryptosporidiosis is acquired by the ingestion of *Cryptosporidium* oocysts, which are shed in the feces of infected humans and animals. Most infections probably result from person-to-person transmission, but many domesticated animals harbor the parasite, providing a large reservoir for human infection.

☐ **Pathogenesis and Pathology:** The *Cryptosporidium* oocyst survives passage through the stomach and releases forms that attach to the microvillous surface of the small bowel. Unlike *Toxoplasma* and other coccidia, *Cryptosporidium* remains an extracellular parasite. The organisms reproduce on the luminal surface of the gastrointestinal tract, from the stomach to the rectum, forming progeny that also attach to the epithelium. The mechanism by which these organisms cause diarrhea is unknown.

In immunologically competent persons, the infection is terminated by unknown immune responses. Patients with AIDS and some congenital immunodeficiencies cannot contain the parasite and develop chronic infections, which sometimes spread from the bowel to involve the gallbladder and intrahepatic bile ducts.

Cryptosporidiosis produces no grossly visible alterations. The organisms are visible microscopically as round, 2- to 4-μm blebs attached to the luminal surface of the epithelium. The stomach is only rarely infected. In the small intestine, there may be moderate or severe chronic inflammation in the lamina propria and a degree of villous atrophy that is directly related to the density of the parasites. The colon exhibits a chronic active colitis with minimal architectural disruption.

☐ **Clinical Features:** Cryptosporidiosis presents as an acute, profuse, watery diarrhea, sometimes accompanied by cramping abdominal pain or low-grade fever. Extraordinary volumes of fluid can be lost as diarrhea, and intensive fluid replacement is required. In immunologically competent persons, the diarrheal illness resolves spontaneously in 1 to 2 weeks. In the immunocompromised, diarrhea persists indefinitely and may contribute to death. Treatment is supportive.

GIARDIASIS

Giardiasis is an infection of the small intestine caused by the flagellated protozoan Giardia lamblia (G. intestinalis) and characterized by abdominal cramping and diarrhea.

☐ **Epidemiology:** *G. lamblia* has a worldwide distribution, with a prevalence of infection from less that 1%

to more than 25% in some areas with warmer climates and crowded, unsanitary environments. Children are more susceptible than adults. Giardiasis is acquired by the ingestion of infectious cyst forms of the organism, which are shed in the feces of infected humans and animals. Infection spreads directly from person to person and also in contaminated water or food. *Giardia* can be acquired from wilderness water sources, where infected animals, such as beavers and bears, serve as the reservoir of infection. The infection may be epidemic, and outbreaks have occurred in orphanages and institutions for the mentally retarded.

☐ **Pathogenesis and Pathology:** *G. lamblia* has two stages: trophozoites and cysts. The trophozoites are flat, pear-shaped, binucleate organisms, with four pairs of flagella. They are most numerous in the duodenum and proximal small intestine. A curved, disk-like "sucker plate" on the ventral surface aids mucosal attachment. The ingested cysts contain two or four nuclei and revert to trophozoites on reaching the intestine. The stools usually contain only cysts, but trophozoites may also be present in patients with diarrhea.

Giardia cysts survive gastric acidity and rupture within the duodenum and jejunum to release trophozoites. The latter attach to the microvilli of the small bowel epithelium and reproduce. The mechanism by which *Giardia* causes diarrhea is unknown, although the infection leads to the malabsorption of fats and carbohydrates.

Giardiasis produces no grossly visible alterations. Microscopic examination shows *Giardia* trophozoites on the surface of villi and within crypts, with minimal associated mucosal changes. Occasionally, the villi are shortened and flattened.

☐ **Clinical Features:** Although *G. lamblia* is a harmless commensal in most persons, it can cause acute or chronic symptoms. Acute giardiasis presents with the abrupt onset of abdominal cramping and frequent, foul-smelling stools. The course of infection is highly variable. In some patients, the symptoms resolve spontaneously in 1 to 4 weeks. Others complain of persistent abdominal cramping and poorly formed stools for months. In children, chronic giardiasis may cause malabsorption, weight loss, and retarded growth. The infection is effectively treated with various antibiotics, including metronidazole.

LEISHMANIASIS

Leishmaniae are protozoans that are transmitted to humans by insect bites and cause a spectrum of clinical syndromes, ranging from indolent, self-resolving cutaneous ulcers to fatal disseminated disease. There are numerous species of *Leishmania*, which differ in their natural habitats and the types of disease that they produce.

☐ **Epidemiology:** Leishmaniasis is transmitted by the bites of the *Phlebotomus* sandflies, which acquire infection from feeding on infected animals. In many subtropical and tropical areas, leishmanial infection is endemic in animal populations; thus, gerbils, dogs, ground squirrels, foxes, and jackals serve as reservoirs and potential sources for transmission to humans. Leishmaniasis is primarily a disease of less-developed countries, where humans live in close proximity to animal hosts and the fly vector. There are estimated to be 20 million persons infected worldwide.

☐ **Pathogenesis:** Infection begins when the organisms are inoculated into human skin by the bite of the sandfly. Shortly thereafter, *Leishmaniae* are phagocytosed by mononuclear phagocytes and transform into amastigotes, which reproduce within the macrophage. Daughter amastigotes eventually rupture from the cell and spread to other macrophages. Reproduction continues in this way, and eventually a cluster of infected macrophages forms at the site of inoculation.

From this initial local infection, the disease may take widely divergent courses depending on two factors: the immunological capabilities of the host and the infecting species of *Leishmania*. Three distinct clinical entities are recognized: (1) localized cutaneous leishmaniasis, (2) mucocutaneous leishmaniasis, and (3) visceral leishmaniasis.

Localized Cutaneous Leishmaniasis

Several *Leishmania* species in Central and South America, Northern Africa, the Middle East, India, and China produce localized cutaneous disease, also known as "oriental sore" or "tropical sore."

☐ **Pathology:** Localized cutaneous leishmaniasis begins as a collection of amastigote-filled macrophages that ulcerates the overlying epidermis. In tissue sections, the oval amastigotes measure 2 μm and contain two internal structures, a nucleus and a kinetoplast. When examined under low power, the amastigotes in macrophages appear as multiple regular cytoplasmic dots, known as Leishman-Donovan bodies.

With the progressive development of cell-mediated immunity to the parasite, macrophages become activated and kill the intracellular parasites. As a result, the number of amastigote-filled macrophages in the ulcer declines. The lesion slowly assumes a more mature granulomatous appearance, with epithelioid macrophages, Langhans giant cells, plasma cells, and lymphocytes. Over the course of months, the cutaneous ulcer heals spontaneously.

☐ **Clinical Features:** Cutaneous leishmaniasis begins as an itching, solitary papule, which erodes to form a shallow ulcer with a sharp, raised border. This ulcer can grow to 6 to 8 cm in diameter. Satellite lesions develop along draining lymphatics. The ulcers begin to resolve at 3 to 6 months, but healing may take a year or longer.

Diffuse cutaneous leishmaniasis develops in some patients who lack specific cell-mediated immune responses to leishmania. The disease begins as a single nodule, but adjacent satellite nodules slowly form, eventually involving much of the skin. These lesions so closely resemble lepromatous leprosy that some patients have been cared for in leprosaria. The nodule of anergic leishmaniasis is caused by enormous numbers of macrophages replete with leishmaniae.

Mucocutaneous Leishmaniasis

Mucocutaneous leishmaniasis is a late complication of cutaneous leishmaniasis caused by infection with *L. braziliensis*. Most cases occur in Central and South America, where rodents and sloths are reservoirs for *L. braziliensis*.

☐ **Pathology and Clinical Features:** The early course and pathologic changes of mucocutaneous leishmaniasis are similar to those of localized cutaneous leishmaniasis. A solitary ulcer appears, expands, and resolves spontaneously. Years after the primary lesion has healed, an ulcer develops at a mucocutaneous junction, such as the larynx, nasal septum, anus, or vulva. The mucosal lesion is slowly progressive, highly destructive, and disfiguring, eroding mucosal surfaces and cartilage. Destruction of the nasal septum sometimes produces a "tapir nose" deformity. The ulcers may also kill the patient by obstructing the airways. Mucocutaneous leishmaniasis requires treatment with systemic antiprotozoal agents.

Visceral Leishmaniasis (Kala-azar)

Visceral leishmaniasis, or kala-azar, is a potentially fatal, disseminated infection of the monocyte/macrophage system produced by several subspecies of L. donovani.

☐ **Epidemiology:** The reservoirs of *L. donovani*, and the susceptible age groups, vary in different parts of the world. Humans are the reservoir in India, and foxes in southern France, central Italy, and some parts of South America. Jackals are the source of infection for sporadic cases in rural areas of the Middle East and Central Asia. Dogs harbor the organism in the Mediterranean basin, China, and some parts of South America. The reservoirs in Africa are incompletely known but may include humans, domestic dogs, rats, and other rodents.

☐ **Pathology:** As in the other forms of leishmaniasis, infection with *L. donovani* begins with a localized collection of infected macrophages at the site of a sandfly bite (Fig. 9-76); however, unlike the other leishmanial infections, infected macrophages spread the organisms throughout the mononuclear phagocyte system. Most infected persons destroy *L. donovani* by a cell-mediated immune response, but 5% cannot contain the organisms and develop disseminated disease. Young children and malnourished persons are especially prone to develop visceral leishmaniasis, probably because of a failure to mount an adequate cell-mediated immune response.

In kala-azar, the liver (Fig. 9-77A), spleen, and lymph node become massively enlarged, as the mononuclear phagocytes in these organs fill with proliferating leishmanial amastigotes (see Fig. 9-77). The normal architecture of these organs and the bone marrow is progressively supplanted by sheets of parasitized macrophages (see Fig. 9-77B). Eventually, these cells accumulate in other organs, including the heart and kidney.

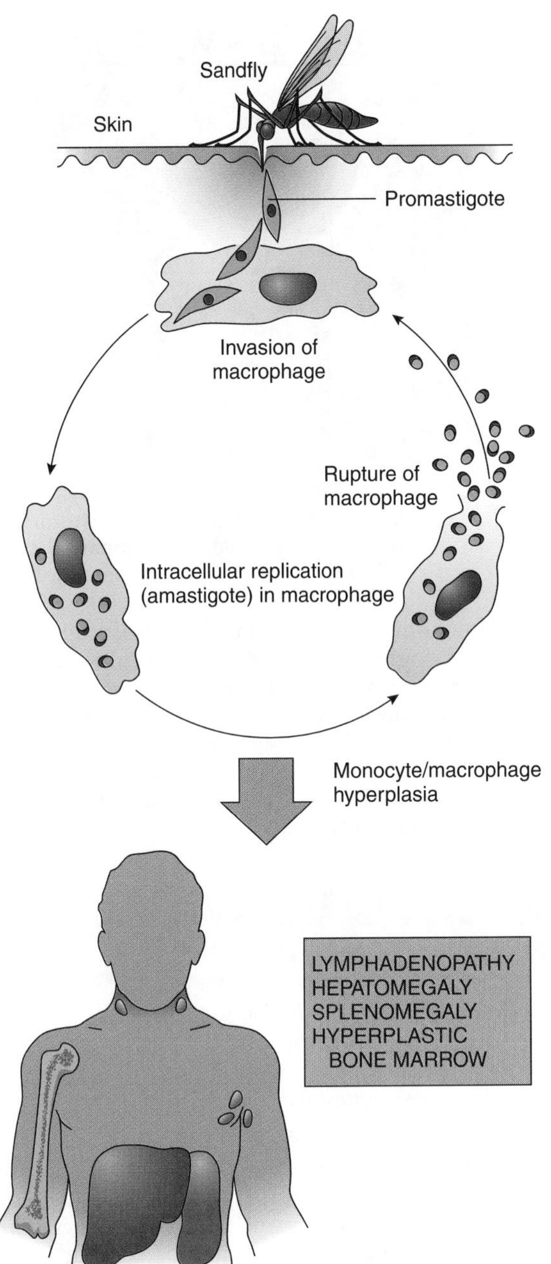

FIGURE *9-76*
Leishmaniasis. Blood-sucking sandflies ingest amastigotes from an infected host. These are transformed in the sandfly gut into promastigotes, which multiply and are injected into the next vertebrate host. There they invade macrophages, revert to the amastigote form, and multiply, eventually rupturing the cell. They then invade other macrophages, thus completing the cycle.

☐ **Clinical Features:** Visceral leishmaniasis manifests as persistent fever, with progressive weight loss,

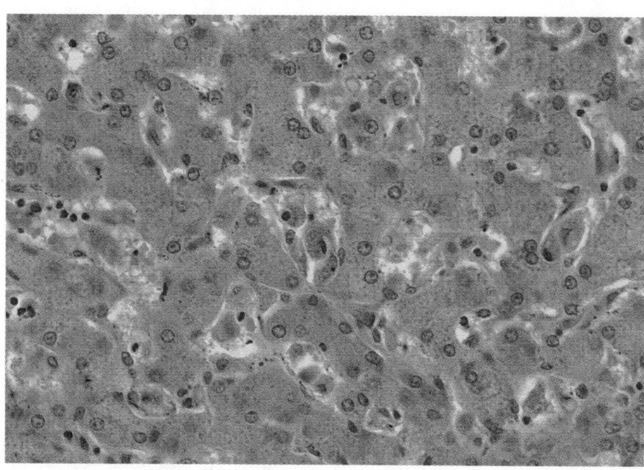

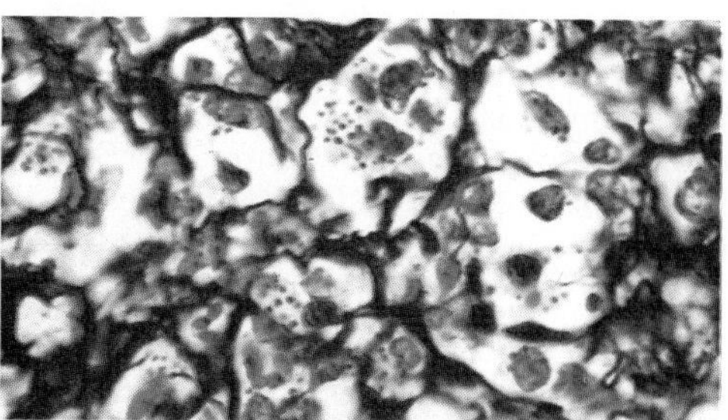

FIGURE 9-77
Visceral leishmaniasis. (*A*) *A* photomicrograph of an enlarged liver shows prominent Kupffer cells distended by leishmanial amastigotes. (*B*) A section of bone marrow subjected to silver impregnation shows macrophages filled with proliferating leishmanial amastigotes.

hepatosplenomegaly, anemia, thrombocytopenia, and leukopenia. Light-skinned persons develop a darkening of the skin; the Hindi name for leishmaniasis, *kala-azar*, literally means "black sickness." Over the course of months, the patient with visceral leishmaniasis becomes profoundly cachectic, and the spleen enlarges massively. If untreated, the disease is invariably fatal. Treatment entails systemic antiprotozoal therapy.

CHAGAS DISEASE (AMERICAN TRYPANOSOMIASIS)

Chagas disease is an insect-borne, zoonotic infection by the protozoan Trypanosoma cruzi, which causes a systemic infection of humans with acute manifestations and long-term sequelae in the heart and gastrointestinal tract.

☐ **Epidemiology:** *T. cruzi* infection is endemic in wild and domesticated animals (e.g., rats, dogs, goats, cats, armadillos) in Central and South America, where the parasite is transmitted by the reduviid ("kissing") bug. Infection with *T. cruzi* is promoted by contact between humans and infected bugs, usually in mud or thatched dwellings of the rural and suburban poor. The bugs hide in cracks of rickety houses and in vegetal roofing, emerge at night, and feed on sleeping victims. Congenital infection occurs upon passage of the parasite from mother to fetus. It is estimated that some 20 million persons in Latin America are infected with *T. cruzi*, more than half of whom live in Brazil. An annual total of 50,000 deaths are attributable to the Chagas disease.

☐ **Pathogenesis:** Metacyclic trypomastigotes of *T. cruzi* are discharged in the feces of the reduviid bug while it takes its blood meal. Itching and scratching promote contamination of the wound by the insect feces. The trypomastigotes penetrate through the site of the bite or other abrasions, or may penetrate the mucosa of the eyes or lips. Once in the body, trypomastigotes lose their flagella and undulating membranes, round up to become amastigotes, and enter macrophages, where they undergo repeated divisions. Importantly, amastigotes also invade other sites, including cardiac myofibers and brain. Within the host cells, amastigotes differentiate into trypomastigotes, which break out and enter the bloodstream (Fig. 9-78). Ingested in a subsequent bite of a reduviid bug, trypomastigotes multiply in the alimentary tract of the insect and differentiate into metacyclic trypo-

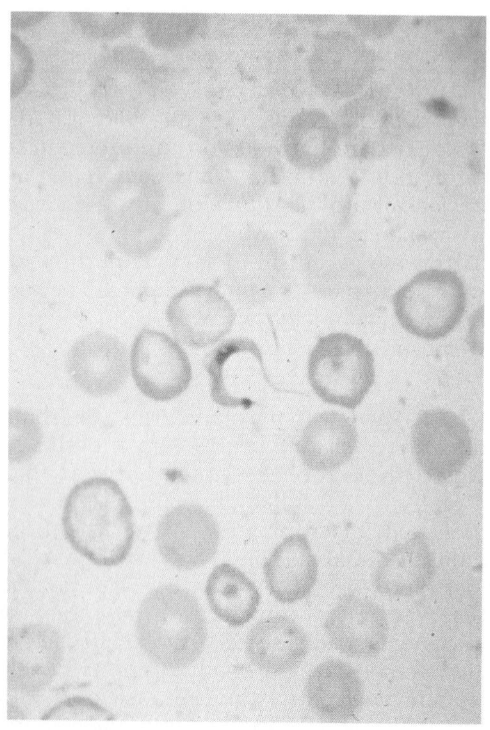

FIGURE 9-78
Chagas disease. A blood smear demonstrates a trypomastigote of *T. cruzi*, with its characteristic "C" shape, flagellum, nucleus, and terminal kinetoplast.

mastigotes, which congregate in the rectum of the bug and are discharged in the feces.

T. cruzi infects cells at the site of inoculation, reproducing within them to form a localized nodular inflammatory lesion, known as a **chagoma**. The organism then disseminates in the bloodstream, infecting cells throughout the body. Strains of *T. cruzi* differ in their predominant target cells; infections of cardiac myocytes, gastrointestinal ganglion cells, and meninges produce the most significant disease. The parasitemia and widespread cellular infection are responsible for the systemic symptoms of acute Chagas disease. The onset of cell-mediated immunity eliminates the acute manifestations, but chronic tissue damage may continue. The progressive destruction of cells at sites of *T. cruzi* infection, particularly the heart, esophagus, and colon, causes dysfunction of these organs, manifested decades after the acute infection.

Acute Chagas Disease

Acute symptoms develop after an incubation period of 1 to 2 weeks following inoculation with *T. cruzi*. A subcutaneous, inflammatory nodule, the chagoma, develops at the site. Parasitemia appears 2 to 3 weeks after inoculation and is usually associated with a mild illness characterized by fever, malaise, lymphadenopathy, and hepatosplenomegaly. However, the disease can be lethal when there is extensive myocardial or meningeal involvement.

☐ **Pathology:** *T. cruzi* circulates in the blood as a 20-μm long, curved, flagellate that is easily recognized on blood films. Within infected cells it reproduces as a nonflagellated amastigote, 2 to 4 μm in diameter. In fatal cases, the heart is enlarged and dilated, with a pale, focally hemorrhagic myocardium. Microscopically, numerous parasites are seen in the heart, and amastigotes are evident within pseudocysts in myofibers (Fig. 9-79). There is extensive chronic inflammation with lymphocytes, plasma cells, and macrophages. Phagocytosis of parasites is conspicuous. Myofibers are destroyed, and the heart shows interstitial edema, endocarditis, pericarditis, and inflammatory and parasitization of the sinus node and atrioventricular node.

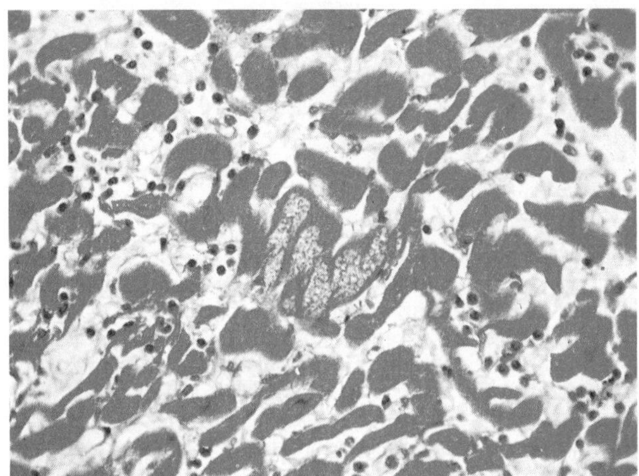

FIGURE *9-79*
Acute Chagas myocarditis. The myofibers in the center contain numerous amastigotes of *T. cruzi* and are surrounded by edema and chronic inflammation.

Chronic Chagas Disease

The most frequent and most serious consequences of infection with *T. cruzi* develop years or decades after the acute infection. It is estimated that 10% to 40% of acutely infected persons eventually develop chronic disease. In this phase of the illness, *T. cruzi* is no longer present in the blood or tissue. Infected organs have been damaged, however, by a chronic, progressive inflammatory process.

☐ **Pathology and Clinical Features:** Chronic myocarditis is characterized by a dilated heart, prominent right ventricular outflow tract, and dilatation of the valve rings. The interventricular septum is often deviated to the right and may immobilize the adjacent tricuspid leaflet. Microscopically, there is extensive interstitial fibrosis, hypertrophied myofibers, and focal lymphocytic inflammation, often involving the cardiac conduction system. Progressive cardiac fibrosis causes dysrhythmias or congestive heart failure. In endemic regions, chronic Chagas disease is a leading cause of heart failure in young adults.

Megaesophagus, that is, dilatation of the esophagus caused by failure of the lower esophageal sphincter (achalasia), is a common complication of chronic Chagas disease. It results from the destruction of parasympathetic ganglion cells in the wall of the lower esophagus and leads to difficulty in swallowing, which may be so severe that the patient can consume only liquids.

Megacolon, massive dilatation of the large bowel, is similar to megaesophagus in that the myenteric plexus of the colon is destroyed. The progressive aganglionosis of the colon causes severe constipation.

Congenital Chagas disease occurs in some pregnant women with parasitemia. Infection of the placenta and fetus leads to spontaneous abortion. In the infrequent live births, the infants die of encephalitis within a few days or weeks.

Antiprotozoal chemotherapy is effective for acute Chagas disease but is of no value for its the chronic sequelae. Cardiac transplanation has been effective in a number of patients.

AFRICAN TRYPANOSOMIASIS

African trypanosomiasis, popularly termed sleeping sickness, is an infection with Trypanosoma brucei gambiense or T. brucei rhodesiense, which produces a life-threatening meningoencephalitis. Gambian trypanosomiasis is a chronic infection often lasting more than a year. By contrast, East African (Rhodesian) trypanosomiasis is a rapidly progressive infection that kills the patient in 3 to 6 months. The organisms are curved flagellates, 15 to 30 μm in length. Although they can be demonstrated in blood or cerebrospinal fluid, they are difficult to find in infected tissues.

☐ **Epidemiology:** *T. brucei gambiense* and *T. brucei rhodesiense* are hemoflagellate protozoa, which are transmitted by several species of blood-sucking tsetse flies of the genus *Glossina*. The patchy distribution of African trypanosomiasis is related to the habitats of the tsetse flies. In Gambian trypanosomiasis, *T. brucei gambiense* is transmitted by tsetse flies of the riverine bush, mainly in endemic pockets of West and Central Africa. **Humans are the only important reservoir for this trypanosome.**

In East African trypanosomiasis, *T. brucei rhodesiense* is spread by tsetse flies of the woodland savanna of East Africa. Antelope, other game animals, and domestic cattle are natural reservoirs of *T. brucei rhodesiense.* **Infection of humans is an occupational hazard of game wardens, fisherman, and cattle herders.**

☐ **Pathogenesis:** While biting an infected animal or human, the tsetse fly ingests trypomastigotes with the blood (Fig. 9-80). These forms (1) lose their coat of surface antigen; (2) multiply in the midgut of the fly; (3) migrate to the salivary gland; (4) develop over a 3-week period through the epimastigote stage; and (5) multiply in the fly's saliva as infective metacyclic trypomastigotes. During another bite, the metacyclic trypomastigotes are injected into the lymphatics and blood vessels of a new host. The organisms disseminate to the bone marrow and tissue fluids, and some eventually invade the central nervous system. After replicating by binary fission in blood, lymph, and spinal fluid, trypomastigotes are ingested by another fly, to complete the cycle.

The pathogenesis of African trypanosomiasis involves the formation of immune complexes by variable trypanosomal antigens and antibodies. In addition, the production of autoantibodies to antigenic components of erythrocytes, brain, and heart may participate in the production of disease. The trypanosome evades immune attack in the mammalian host by periodically altering its glycoprotein antigenic coat. The alterations take place in a genetically determined pattern, not by mutation. Thus, each wave of circulating trypomastigotes includes immunologically distinct antigenic variants that are a step ahead of the immune response.

☐ **Pathology:** *T. brucei* multiplies at the site of inoculation, occasionally producing a localized nodular lesion termed a **primary chancre**. Early in the course of the disease, there is prominent generalized involvement of lymph nodes and spleen. Microscopic changes in the affected nodes and spleen include foci of lymphocyte and macrophage hyperplasia. Infection eventually localizes to the small blood vessels of the central nervous system, where the replicating organisms elicit a destructive vasculitis. The vasculitis of the brain and meninges produces the progressive decrease in mentation characteristic of sleeping sickness. In *T. brucei rhodesiense* infection, the organisms also localize to blood vessels in the heart, sometimes producing a fulminant myocarditis. On microscopic

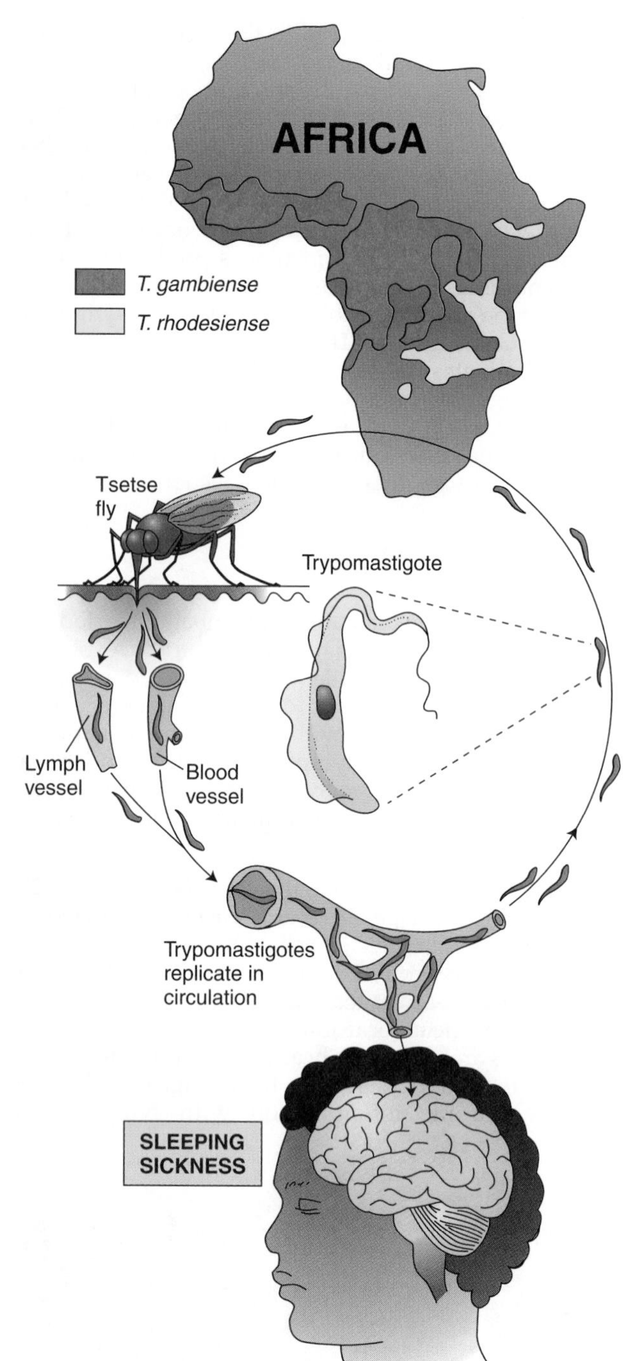

FIGURE 9-80
African trypanosomiasis (sleeping sickness). The distribution of Gambian and Rhodesian trypanosomiasis is related to the habitats of the vector tsetse flies (*Glossina* sp.). A tsetse fly bites an infected animal or human and ingests trypomastigotes, which multiply into infective, metacyclic trypomastigotes. During another fly bite, these are injected into lymphatic and blood vessels of a new host. A primary chancre develops at the site of the bite (stage 1a). Trypomastigotes replicate further in the blood and lymph, causing a systemic infection (stage 1b). Another fly ingests hypomastigotes to complete the cycle. In stage 2, invasion of the central nervous system by trypomastigotes leads to meningoencephalomyelitis and associated symptoms, including lethargy and daytime somnolence. Patients with Rhodesian trypanosomiasis may die within a few months.

examination, the interstitial and perivascular spaces of the endocardium, myocardium, and epicardium are infiltrated by mononuclear inflammatory cells (pancarditis).

Lesions in the lymph nodes, brain, heart, and various other sites (including the inoculation site) show vasculitis of small blood vessels, with endothelial cell hyperplasia and dense perivascular infiltrates of lymphocytes, macrophages, and plasma cells. Vasculitis of the meninges and brain causes destruction of neurons, demyelination, and gliosis. There is a perivascular mononuclear infiltrate that thickens the leptomeninges and involves the Virchow-Robin spaces (Fig. 9-81).

□ **Clinical Features:** In general, African trypanosomiasis can be divided into three clinical stages:

1. **Primary chancre:** After an incubation period of 5 to 15 days, a 3- to 4-cm papillary swelling topped by a central red spot appears at the dermal inoculation site. The chancre subsides spontaneously within 3 weeks.
2. **Systemic infection:** Shortly after the appearance of the chancre (if any), and within 3 weeks of the bite, invasion of the bloodstream is marked by intermittent fever, which lasts up to a week and is often accompanied by splenomegaly and local and generalized lymphadenopathy. **Winterbottom sign** refers to enlargement of the posterior cervical lymph nodes and is characteristic of Gambian trypanosomiasis. The evolving illness is marked by remitting irregular fevers, headache, joint pains, lethargy, and muscle wasting. Myocarditis may be a complication and is more common and severe in Rhodesian trypanosomiasis. Dysfunction of the lungs, kidneys, liver, and endocrine system are frequently observed in both forms of the disease.
3. **Brain invasion:** Differences between the forms of sleeping sickness are primarily a matter of time scale, especially with regard to invasion of the brain. This feature develops early (weeks or months) in Rhodesian trypanosomiasis and late (months or years) in the Gambian form. Brain invasion is marked by apathy, daytime somnolence, and sometimes coma. A diffuse meningoencephalitis is characterized by tremors of the tongue and fingers; fasciculations of the muscles of the limbs, face, lips, and tongue; oscillatory movements of the arms, head, neck, and trunk; indistinct speech; and cerebellar ataxia, leading to problems in walking.

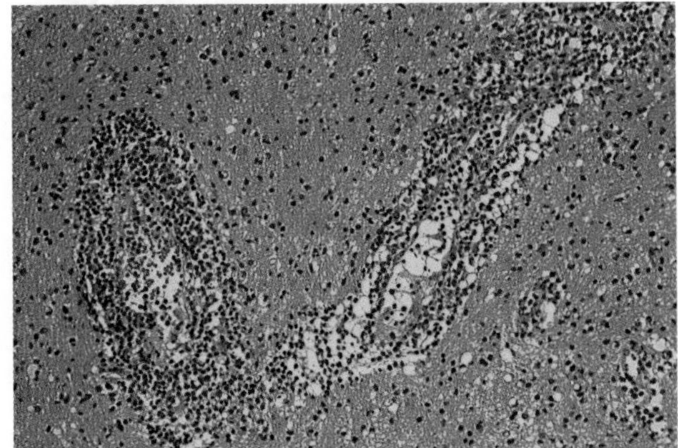

FIGURE *9-81*
African trypanosomiasis. A section of brain from a patient who died from infection with *T. brucei rhodesiense* shows a perivascular mononuclear cell infiltrate.

PRIMARY AMEBIC MENINGOENCEPHALITIS

Amebic meningoencephalitis, caused by Naegleria fowleri, is a fatal, acute suppurative inflammation of the brain and meninges.

□ **Epidemiology:** *N. fowleri* is a free-living, soil ameba that inhabits ponds and lakes throughout tropical and subtropical regions, but has occasionally been found in temperate areas. Primary amebic meningoencephalitis is a rare disease (fewer than 300 reported cases) affecting persons who swim or bathe in these waters. The disease has been recognized in many parts of the world, including the United States, Europe, Australia, New Zealand, South America, and Africa. It has been diagnosed principally on histological evidence, with only a few cases confirmed by culture.

□ **Pathogenesis and Pathology:** *N. fowleri* is inoculated into the nasal mucosa near the cribriform plate when a person swims in or dives into water containing high concentrations of the organism. The amebae subsequently invade the olfactory nerves, migrate through the cribriform plate to the olfactory bulbs, and then proliferate in the meninges and brain.

In tissue sections, trophozoites of *Naegleria* measure 8 to 15 μm across. The cytoplasm is not distinctive, but the nuclei are sharply outlined and stain deeply with hematoxylin. Cysts of *Naegleria* have not been seen in tissue sections.

On gross examination, the brain is swollen and soft, with vascular congestion and a purulent exudate on the meningeal surface, most prominent over the lateral and basal areas. There is massive destruction of the brain by amebae, which invade the brain along the Virchow-Robin spaces. Thrombosis and destruction of blood vessels are associated with extensive hemorrhage in the affected areas. The olfactory tract and bulbs are enveloped and destroyed, and there is an exudate between the bulb and the inferior surface of the temporal lobe. Extensive proliferation of *Naegleria* in the brain often leads to the formation of solid masses of amebae (amebomas). Meningitis can extend the full length of the cord.

□ **Clinical Features:** Primary amebic meningoencephalitis due to *N. fowleri* begins suddenly with fever, nausea, vomiting, and headache. The disease progresses rapidly, and within hours the patient suffers a profound deterioration in mental status. The cerebrospinal fluid contains numerous neutrophils, blood, and amebae. The disease is rapidly fatal.

Helminthic Infection

Helminths, or worms, are among the most common human pathogens. At any given time, 25% to 50% of the world's population is infected with at least one helminth species. Although the large majority of helminthic infections cause little harm, some produce significant disease. Schistosomiasis, for instance, ranks among the leading global causes of morbidity and mortality.

Helminths are the largest and most complex organisms capable of living within the human body. Their adult forms range from 0.5 mm to greater than 1 m in length, and most are readily visible to the naked eye. Helminths are multicellular animals with differentiated tissues, including specialized nervous tissues, digestive tissues, and reproductive systems. Their maturation from eggs or larvae to adult worms is complex, often involving multiple morphological transformations (molts). Some helminths undergo these metamorphoses in different hosts before attaining adulthood, and the human host may be only one in a series of hosts that support this maturation process. Within the human body, the helminths frequently migrate from the port of entry through several organs to a site of final infection.

The majority of helminth infections are minimally symptomatic. Most helminths that infect humans are well adapted to human parasitism, producing limited or no damage to host tissues. Their life cycles are long and complex, and significant damage to the host would impair the parasite's own life cycle. Moreover, the number of infecting helminths in the body, the so-called worm burden, is low in most hosts. Helminth infections are acquired by ingestion, direct skin penetration, or insect bites, and the number of infecting organisms is determined by the number or frequency of these inoculations. Unlike viruses, bacteria, and fungi, the helminths (with two exceptions) cannot multiply within the human body; thus the inoculation of a single organism cannot be amplified into an overwhelming infection. The exceptions are *Strongyloides stercoralis* and *Capillaria philippinensis*, which are capable of completing their life cycle and multiplying within the human body.

Helminths cause disease in various ways. A few compete with their human host for limited nutrients. Some grow to block vital structures, producing disease by mass effect. Most, however, cause dysfunction through the destructive inflammatory and immunological responses that they elicit. For example, morbidity and mortality in schistosomiasis, the most destructive helminth infection, result from the granulomatous response to the schistosome eggs deposited in tissue.

Eosinophils contain basic proteins toxic to some helminths and are a major component of the inflammatory responses to these organisms. These cells are present in acute infiltrates induced by helminths and in the chronic infiltrates and granulomas that form in response to helminth eggs, larvae, or adult forms. However, these responses are usually not effective in protecting the host from the parasite.

In schistosomiasis, the eggs, not the viable adult worms, are the target of the destructive inflammatory reaction. This is true in many other helminth infections in which adult or larval forms persist for years without eliciting an inflammatory response. Some helminths avoid inflammatory and immunological surveillance by coating themselves with host material. When the helminths die, however, their antigens leak into the surrounding tissue and cause a vigorous inflammatory response.

Parasitic helminths are divided into three broad categories based on overall morphology and the structure of digestive tissues.

- **Roundworms (nematodes)** are elongate cylindrical organisms with tubular digestive tracts.
- **Flatworms (trematodes)** are dorsoventrally flattened organisms with digestive tracts that end in blind loops.
- **Tapeworms (cestodes)** are segmented organisms with separate head and body parts; they lack a digestive tract and absorb nutrients through their outer walls.

FILARIAL NEMATODES

Lymphatic Filariasis (Bancroftian and Malayan Filariasis)

Lymphatic filariasis is an inflammatory parasitic infection of lymphatic vessels caused by the filarial roundworms Wuchereria bancrofti and Brugia malay, which results in massive lymphedema (elephantiasis) of the affected tissuesi. The adult worms inhabit the lymphatics, most frequently those in the inguinal, epitrochlear, and axillary lymph nodes, testis, and epididymis. There they elicit an inflammatory response that causes acute lymphangitis and, in a minority of infected subjects, eventual lymphatic obstruction, leading to severe lymphedema (Fig. 9-82). These and other similar organisms are known as filarial worms, because of their threadlike appearance (from the Latin *filum*, meaning thread). Adult females release live-born progeny called microfilariae.

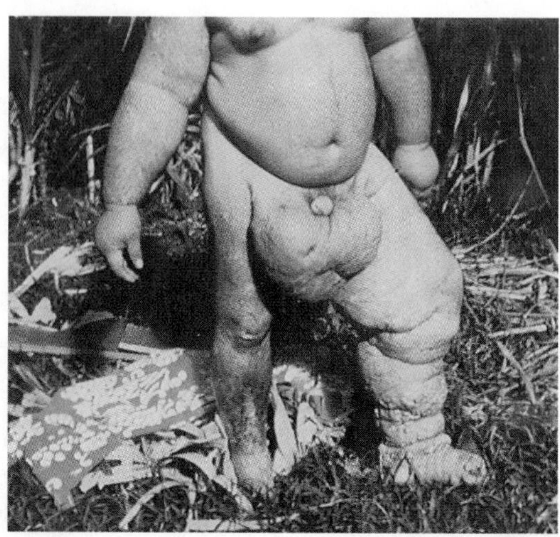

FIGURE *9-82*
Bancroftian filariasis. Massive lymphedema (elephantiasis) of the scrotum and left lower extremity are present.

☐ **Epidemiology:** The elephantiasis characteristic of lymphatic filariasis was familiar to Hindi and Persian physicians as early as 600 BC. Humans, the only definitive host of these filarial nematodes, acquire infection from the bites of at least 80 species of mosquitoes of the genera *Culex, Aedes, Anopheles,* and *Mansonia*. *W. bancrofti* infection is widespread in southern Asia, the Pacific, Africa, and portions of South America. *B. malayi* is localized to coastal southern Asia and western Pacific islands. Worldwide, between 100 and 200 million persons are estimated to be infected.

☐ **Pathogenesis:** Mosquito bites transmit infectious larvae that migrate to lymphatics and lymph nodes. After maturing into adult forms over several months, the worms mate and the female releases microfilariae into lymphatics and the bloodstream. The manifestations of filariasis result from the inflammatory response to degenerating adult worms in the lymphatics.

The initial inflammatory response is an acute lymphangitis, which resolves in 1 to 2 weeks. Repeated filarial infections are common in endemic regions and produce repeated bouts of lymphangitis (filarial fevers), which eventually (over years) may cause extensive scarring and obstruction of lymphatics. The lymphatic obstruction causes localized dependent edema, most commonly affecting the legs, arms, genitalia, and breasts. In its most severe form, which occurs in less than 5% of the infected population, this edematous distortion of body parts is known as elephantiasis.

☐ **Pathology:** The adult nematode is a white, threadlike worm that is much convoluted within the lymph nodes where they reside. The female is twice the size of the male and measures 80 to 100 mm in length and 0.20 to 0.3 mm in width. In blood films stained with Giemsa, the microfilariae appear as gracefully curved worms, measuring about 300 μm in length.

The lymphatic vessels harboring the adult worms are dilated and the endothelial lining is thickened. In the adjacent tissue, a chronic inflammatory infiltrate, consisting of lymphocytes, macrophages, plasma cells, and eosinophils, surrounds the worms. A granulomatous reaction may develop, and degenerating worms can provoke acute inflammation. Microfilariae are seen in blood vessels and lymphatics, and degenerating microfilariae also provoke a chronic inflammatory reaction. After repeated bouts of lymphangitis, the lymph nodes and lymphatics become densely fibrotic, often containing calcified remnants of the worms.

☐ **Clinical Features:** Filariasis is a disease with a wide spectrum of manifestations. In endemic areas, most of the infected population displays either antifilarial antibodies with no detectable infection or asymptomatic microfilaremia. A smaller number of the infected persons develop recurrent episodes of filarial fevers, with malaise, lymphadenopathy, and lymphangitis, which persist for 1 to 2 weeks and then resolve spontaneously. In most of these patients, the fevers decrease in frequency over a period of years and eventually cease. In a small subset of these patients, the late manifestations of disease may appear after two to three decades of recurrent bouts of filarial fevers. Lymphatic obstruction produces chronic edema of dependent tissues, and the overlying skin becomes thickened and warty. The diagnosis is made by identifying the microfilariae in blood samples. Those should be obtained at night because during the day microfilariae tend to congregate in the pulmonary circulation. This phenomenon is called periodic microfilaremia and is reversed in areas of the world where mosquitoes bite preferentially during the day. Diethylcarbamazine and ivermectin are the chemotherapeutic agents effective against lymphatic filariasis.

Occult filariasis, a condition characterized by indirect evidence of filarial infection (circulating anti-filarial antibodies), is the cause of **tropical pulmonary eosinophilia**. This manifestation of filariasis is virtually restricted to southern India and some Pacific Islands. Patients present with cough, wheezing, diffuse pulmonary infiltrates, and peripheral eosinophilia. Its severity is variable, ranging from mild asthma-like manifestations to severe fatal pneumonia. In some of these patients, filariae have been found at autopsy.

Onchocerciasis

Onchocerciasis ("river blindness") is a chronic inflammatory disease of the skin, eyes, and lymphatics caused by the filarial nematode Onchocerca volvulus. **Blindness is the most severe consequence of onchocerciasis.**

☐ **Epidemiology:** Onchocerciasis is one of the world's major endemic diseases, afflicting an estimated 40 million persons, of whom 2 million are blind. Humans are the only definitive host. *Simulium damnosum* blackflies transmit infectious larvae to humans on biting. These insects require rapidly running water for breeding, and onchocerciasis is therefore endemic along rivers and streams (hence the name "river blindness") in parts of tropical Africa, southern Mexico, Central America, and South America.

☐ **Pathogenesis:** Adult worms live as coiled tangled masses in the deep fasciae and subcutaneous tissues. They do not cause tissue damage and do not elicit inflammatory responses, but the gravid females release millions of microfilariae, which migrate into the skin, eyes, lymph nodes, and deep organs, thereby producing corresponding onchocercal lesions. Ocular onchocerciasis results from the migration of microfilariae into all regions of the eye, from the cornea to the optic nerve head.

When microfilariae die, they incite a vigorous inflammatory and immunological response. Inflammatory damage to the cornea, choroid, or retina leads to partial or total loss of vision. The inflammatory response in the skin results in microabscess formation and chronic degenerative changes in the epidermis and dermis. In the lymph nodes and lymphatics, the response to dying microfilariae causes chronic lymphatic obstruction and resulting localized dependent edema.

☐ **Pathology:** *Onchocerca volvulus* is a thin and very long nematode, the female measuring 400 × 0.3 mm and the male 30 × 0.2 mm. Masses of adult worms become encapsulated by a fibrous scar, forming discrete, 1- to 3-cm, onchocercal nodules in the deep dermis and subcutaneous tissues. Nodules form over bony prominences of the skull, scapula, ribs, iliac crest, trochanter, sacrum, and knee. Microscopically, the subcutaneous nodules contain coiled adult worms and have an outer fibrous layer and a central inflammatory infiltrate, which varies from suppurative to granulomatous. Arborization of capillaries around adult worms provides them with nutrition. Dermatitis begins when microfilariae degenerate in the dermis, an event that is accompanied by degranulation of eosinophils and the deposition of major basic protein on the cuticle.

The active lesions in the eyes and lymphatics all show degenerating microfilariae surrounded by a dense inflammatory infiltrate of eosinophils, macrophages, lymphocytes, and plasma cells. Involvement of the eye leads to sclerosing keratitis, iridocyclitis, chorioretinitis, and optic atrophy. The femoral or inguinal nodes become enlarged and then fibrotic.

☐ **Clinical Features:** The nodules harboring adult worms are asymptomatic. Symptoms of onchocerciasis result from the inflammatory response to degenerating microfilariae. Skin manifestations begin with generalized pruritus that becomes so intense that it often interferes with sleeping. Continuing damage produces areas of depigmentation, hypertrophy, or atrophy of the skin. Progressive destruction of the cornea, choroid, or uvea leads to loss of vision. Chronic lymphadenitis results in localized edema that may cause chronic swelling (elephantiasis) of the legs, scrotum, or other dependent portion of the body. Systemic antihelmintic therapy, particularly with ivermectin, is effective in treating onchocerciasis.

Loiasis

Loiasis is infection by the filarial nematode Loa loa, the African "eyeworm." It is prevalent in the rain forests of Central and West Africa. Humans and baboons are the definitive hosts, and infection is transmitted by mango flies. Adult worms (4 cm long) migrate in the skin and occasionally cross the eye beneath the conjunctiva, making the patient acutely aware of this infection (Fig. 9-83). Gravid worms discharge microfilariae, which circulate in the bloodstream during the day but reside in capillaries of the skin, lungs, and other organs at night.

Migrating worms cause no inflammation, but static worms are surrounded by plasma cells, lymphocytes, eosinophils, neutrophils, and a foreign body giant cell reaction. Rarely, infected subjects may develop acute generalized loiasis. At autopsy, these patients have obstructive fibrin thrombi in small vessels of most organs, which contain degenerating microfilariae. When the brain is involved, obstruction of vessels by filarial thrombi kills the patient through sudden and diffuse ischemia.

Most infections are asymptomatic but persist for years. Some patients have pruritic, red, subcutaneous

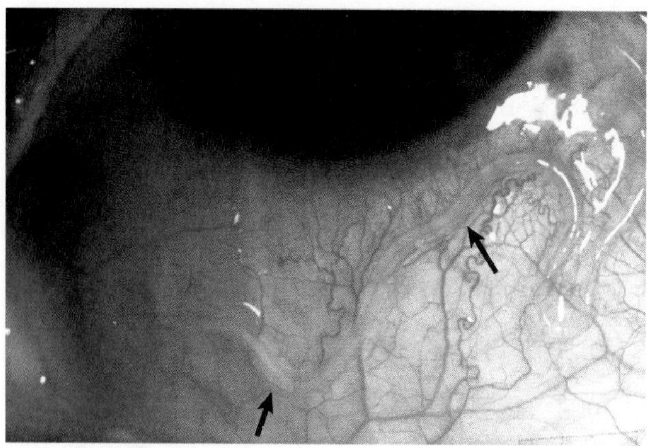

FIGURE *9-83*
Loiasis. A threadlike *L. loa* (*arrows*) is migrating in the subconjunctival tissues.

"Calabar" swellings, which may be a reaction to migrating adult worms or to microfilariae in the skin. Ocular symptoms include swelling of the eyelids, itching, and pain. Worms may be extracted during their migration beneath the conjunctiva. Systemic reactions include fever, pain, itching, urticaria, and eosinophilia. Dead worms in or near major nerves may cause paresthesias or paralyses. Treatment with microfilariacides may cause massive death of microfilariae and provoke fever, meningoencephalitis, and death.

Dirofilariasis

Several filarial nematodes belonging to the genus *Dirofilaria* are transmitted to humans by mosquitoes. *D. immitis* is the heartworm of dogs and other mammals found in Japan, Australia, and the southern United States. In humans, microfilariae do not reach maturity; the immature worms are carried by the venous circulation into the lungs, where they obstruct small pulmonary arteries and cause subpleural infarcts, which resolve as granulomas. Most of these lesions are clinically silent and are discovered incidentally during radiological examination of the chest.

D. tenuis is a parasite of raccoons in the United States, and *D. repens* infects dogs and cats in Europe, Asia, and Africa. These organisms cause subcutaneous dirofilariasis in humans. Humans are abnormal hosts, and no microfilariae are seen in the circulation. A coiled, degenerating worm provokes a subcutaneous abscess, which later becomes granulomatous. The most common site is the subcutaneous tissue of the trunk, but the conjunctiva, eyelid, scrotum, and breast can also be affected.

INTESTINAL NEMATODES

The adult forms of a number of nematode species (Table 9-10) reside in the human bowel. They are all well adapted to human parasitism, commonly infecting hu-

TABLE *9-10* **Intestinal Nematodes**

Species	Common Name	Site of Adult Worm	Clinical Manifestations
Ascaris lumbricoides	Roundworm	Small bowel	Allergic reactions to lung migration; intestinal obstruction
Ancylostoma duodenale	Hookworm	Small bowel	Allergic reactions to cutaneous inoculation and lung migration; intestinal blood loss
Necator americanus	Hookworm	Small bowel	Allergic reactions to cutaneous inoculation and lung migration; intestinal blood loss
Trichuris trichiura	Whipworm	Large bowel	Abdominal pain and diarrhea; rectal prolapse (rare)
Strongyloides stercoralis	Threadworm	Small bowel	Abdominal pain and diarrhea; dissemination to extraintestinal sites in immunocompromised persons
Enterobius vermicularis	Pinworm	Cecum, appendix	Perianal and perineal itching

mans but only rarely causing symptomatic disease. In fact, severe symptomatic illness occurs almost exclusively in persons who are infected with large numbers of worms or in those who are immunocompromised. Humans are the exclusive or primary host for all of the intestinal nematodes, and infection spreads from person to person through eggs or larvae passed in the stool or deposited in the perianal region. Infection is most prevalent in locations where hand washing and hygienic disposal of human feces are lacking (e.g., less-developed countries, day-care centers). Warm, moist climates are required for environmental survival of the infectious forms of many of the intestinal nematodes, and these worms are therefore endemic in most tropical and subtropical environments.

Ascariasis

Ascariasis refers to infection of the small intestine by the large roundworm Ascaris lumbricoides. It is the most common helminth infection of humans, affecting one fourth of the world's population, usually without causing symptoms.

□ **Epidemiology:** Ascariasis is found worldwide, but infection is most common in areas with warm climates and poor sanitation. Nevertheless, it is estimated that over 4 million persons in the United States harbor the parasite. Adult worms live in the small intestine, where gravid females discharge eggs that pass in the feces. The eggs develop in warm moist soil to become infective in 3 to 4 weeks. Humans acquire the infection by ingesting eggs in contaminated soil, food, or water.

□ **Pathogenesis:** The eggs hatch when ingested, and the *Ascaris* larvae emerge in the small intestine, penetrate the bowel wall, and, while maturing, reach the lungs through the venous circulation. From the pulmonary capillaries they enter the alveolar spaces and migrate up the trachea to the glottis, where they are swallowed and again reach the small bowel. They mature in the small bowel and live as adult worms within the lumen for 1 to 2 years.

□ **Pathology and Clinical Features:** Adult worms (15 to 35 cm long) usually cause no pathological changes, and the patients are entirely asymptomatic. Heavy infections may cause vomiting, malnutrition, and sometimes intestinal obstruction (Fig. 9-84). On rare occasions, worms migrate into the ampulla of Vater or the pancreatic or biliary ducts, where they may cause biliary obstruction, acute pancreatitis, suppurative cholangitis, and liver abscesses. Eggs deposited in the liver or other tissues may produce necrosis, granulomatous inflammation, and fibrosis. *Ascaris* pneumonia, which may be fatal, develops when large numbers of larvae migrate within the air spaces.

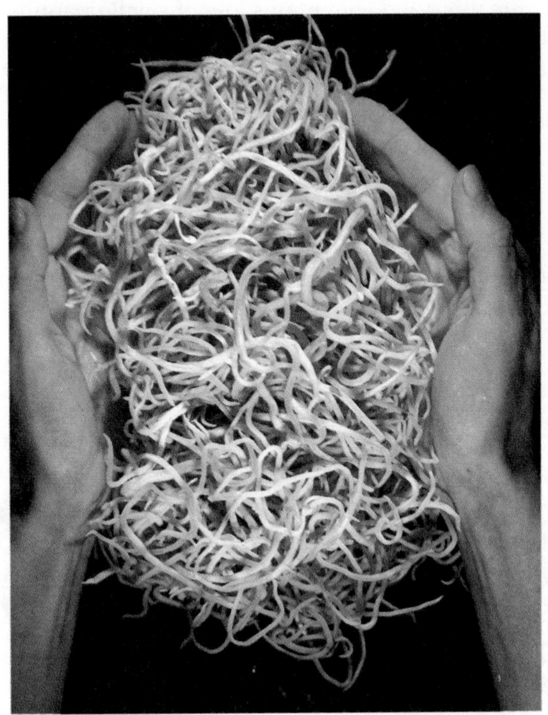

FIGURE *9-84*
Ascariasis. This mass of over 800 worms of *A. lumbricoides* obstructed and infarcted the ileum of a 2-year-old girl in South Africa.

The diagnosis of ascariasis is made by identifying eggs in the feces. Occasionally, adult worms may pass with the stools or even emerge from the nose or mouth. Ascaricidal drugs are effective.

Trichuriasis

Trichuriasis is a superficially invasive infection of the large bowel by the intestinal nematode Trichuris trichiura ("whipworm").

☐ **Epidemiology:** Whipworm infection is found worldwide with over 800 million persons infected. Although parasitism is most common in areas with warm, moist climates and poor sanitation, it is estimated that over 2 million persons in the United States are infected. Children are especially susceptible.

Adult worms live in the cecum and upper colon, where they attach to the intestinal wall by burying their head just under the epithelial layer (Fig. 9-85). Female worms produce eggs that pass in the feces. Eggs embryonate in moist soil and become infective in 3 weeks. Humans are infected by ingesting eggs in contaminated soil, food, or drink.

☐ **Pathogenesis and Pathology:** Larvae emerge from the ingested eggs in the small bowel and, while maturing, migrate to the cecum and colon. There the adult worms burrow their anterior portions into the superficial mucosa. This invasion causes small erosions, focal active inflammation, and continuous loss of small quantities of blood.

T. trichiura measures 3 to 5 cm in length, with a long, slender anterior portion and a short, blunt posterior. The gross appearance of the whip-shaped worms attached to the large bowel mucosa is striking.

☐ **Clinical Features:** The large majority of *T. trichiura* infections are asymptomatic. Infections with large numbers of worms may produce cramping abdominal pain, bloody diarrhea, weight loss, and anemia. The diagnosis is made by finding the characteristic eggs in the stool. Mebendazole is effective therapy.

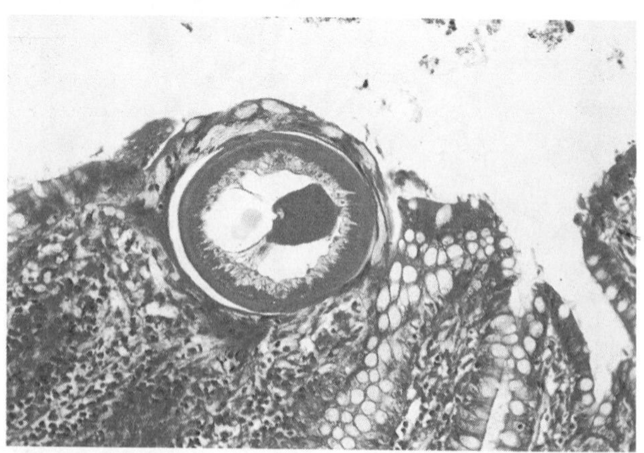

FIGURE 9-85
Trichuriasis. The anterior "whip" end of *T. trichiura* is threaded into the mucosa of the colon.

HOOKWORMS

Necator americanus and Ancylostoma duodenale ("hookworms") are intestinal nematodes that infect the human small bowel. These worms lacerate the bowel mucosa, causing intestinal blood loss, which can produce symptomatic disease in heavy infestations.

☐ **Epidemiology:** Hookworm infections are encountered in moist warm temperate and tropical areas and cause serious public health problems across large areas of the globe. In fact, both *A. duodenale* ("Old World" hookworm) and *N. americanus* ("American" hookworm) prevail on most continents and have overlapping epidemiological boundaries. In general, *A. duodenale* is less common in the Western Hemisphere, Australia, and Africa, where *N. americanus* is more common. Likewise, *A. duodenale* is frequent in the Mediterranean basin, where there is no infection by *N. americanus*. Both species are common in Southeast Asia. Worldwide over 700 million persons are infected with hookworms, and it is estimated that 700,000 persons in the United States harbor the parasite.

Tropical areas with poor sanitation are ideal for transmission. Warm, moist, sandy soil with adequate shade from direct sunlight favors the survival of the soil-borne infective larvae. Hookworm infection is commonly found among persons who walk barefoot in endemic areas.

☐ **Pathogenesis and Pathology:** On contact with human skin, filariform larvae directly penetrate the epidermis and enter the venous circulation. They travel to the lungs, where they lodge in alveolar capillaries. After rupturing into the alveoli, the larvae migrate up the trachea to the glottis and are then swallowed. They molt in the duodenum, attach to the mucosal wall with toothlike buckle plates, clamp off a section of the villus, and ingest it (Fig. 9-86). The resulting intestinal blood loss varies according to the number and the species of hookworm. *A. duodenale* causes a greater blood loss (~0.3 mL/day per adult worm) than does *N. americanus* (~0.02 mL/day per worm). With extensive worm infestations, particularly with *A. duodenale*, the blood loss can be considerable, resulting in anemia and hypoalbuminemia.

Hookworms are anteriorly bent and measure about 1 cm in length. The worms are grossly visible attached to the mucosal surface of the small bowel, alongside punctate areas of hemorrhages. There is essentially no associated inflammation.

☐ **Clinical Features:** **Although the majority of persons with hookworm infection are not symptomatic, infestation with this parasite is the most important cause of chronic anemia worldwide**. The balance between the dietary iron intake and the blood loss caused by the intestinal worms determines whether an infected in-

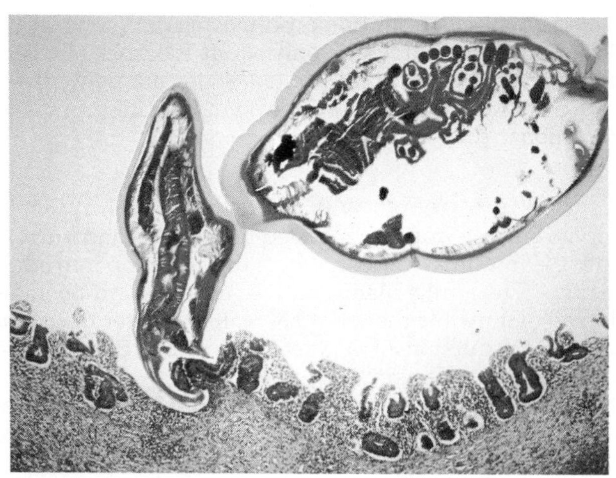

FIGURE 9-86
Ancylostomiasis. Section of the ileum shows two portions of a single adult worm, *A. duodenale*. A plug of mucosa is in the buccal cavity of the hookworm.

dividual will develop anemia. Thus, in persons with heavy worm burdens (particularly women who consume a diet low in iron) and in populations with inadequate iron intake, chronic intestinal blood loss can produce severe iron deficiency anemia.

Skin penetration is sometimes associated with a pruritic eruption ("ground itch"), and the phase of larval migration through the lungs occasionally causes asthma-like symptoms.

STRONGYLOIDIASIS

Strongyloidiasis refers to a small intestinal infection with the nematode Strongyloides stercoralis ("threadworm"). Although most cases of strongyloidiasis are asymptomatic, the infection can progress to lethal disseminated disease in immunocompromised hosts. The worldwide prevalence of *S. stercoralis* is unknown, but this parasite is believed to be much less common than hookworm or *A. lumbricoides*. Infection is most frequent in areas with warm, moist climates and poor sanitation. However, endemic pockets of strongyloidiasis still exist in the United States, particularly in the Appalachian region and in institutions where personal hygiene is poor, such as hospitals for the mentally ill. It is also endemic in several countries of central and southern Europe.

☐ **Pathogenesis and Pathology:** *S. stercoralis* is the smallest of the intestinal nematodes, measuring 0.2 to 0.3 cm in length. The adult females are buried in the crypts of the duodenum or jejunum but produce no visible alterations. Microscopic examination shows the coiled females, along with eggs and developing larvae, within the mucosa, usually with no associated inflammation (Fig. 9-87).

Parasitic females live within the mucosa of the small intestine, where they lay eggs that quickly hatch and release rhabditiform larvae. The larvae are passed in the feces, and in the soil become filariform, the infective stage able to penetrate human skin. On entering the skin, *S. stercoralis* larvae pass in the bloodstream to the lungs and then to the small bowel, in a manner similar to that of hookworms. The worms mature in the small bowel. In contrast to other intestinal nematodes, *S. stercoralis* may reproduce within the human host by a mechanism known as **autoinfection**. This process occurs when rhabditiform larvae become infective (filariform) within the host's intestine and repenetrate either the intestinal wall or the perianal skin, thereby starting a new parasitic cycle within a single host. Some degree of autoinfection occurs in all infected hosts, but a balance seems to be reached whereby a small parasitic population that does no harm to the host is maintained indefinitely.

☐ **Clinical Features:** The large majority of infected persons are completely asymptomatic. Moderate peripheral eosinophilia is common in patients with chronic strongyloidiasis. **Disseminated strongyloidiasis or hyperinfection syndrome** occurs in patients with suppressed immunity, particularly those receiving corticosteroids. In such patients, the rate of internal autoinfection is greatly increased, and extraordinary numbers of filariform larvae penetrate the intestinal walls and disseminate to distant organs. In disseminated strongyloidiasis, the gut may exhibit ulceration, edema, and severe inflamma-

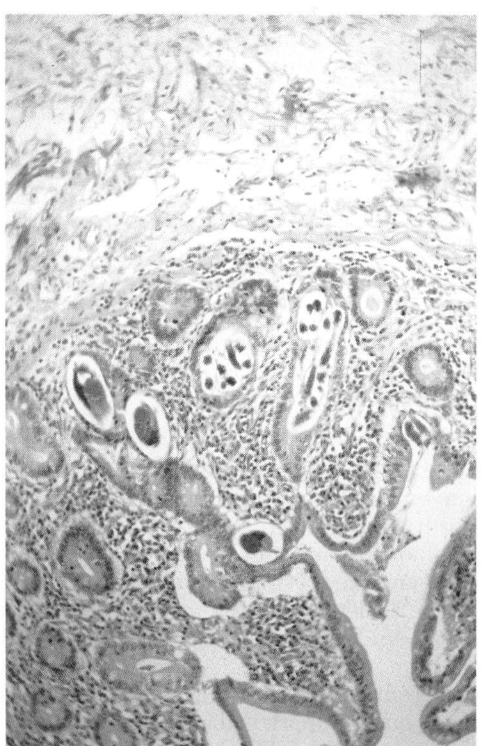

FIGURE 9-87
Stronglyoidiasis. A section of jejunum shows adult worms, larvae, and eggs of *S. stercoralis* in the mucosal crypts. The lamina propria is infiltrated with lymphocytes, plasma cells, and eosinophils. The patient had a hyperinfected syndrome and presented with malabsorption.

tion. Sepsis, usually with gram-negative organisms, and infection of parenchymal organs occur almost invariably in these patients. If untreated, disseminated strongyloidiasis is universally fatal; even with prompt treatment with thiabendazole or ivermectin, the survival rate remains in the range of 30% to 40%.

PINWORM INFECTION (ENTEROBIASIS)

Enterobius vermicularis ("pinworm") is an intestinal nematode that causes intense perianal itching. The organism is encountered worldwide but is more frequent in temperate zones. Although people can be infected at any age, parasitism is most common among young children. It is estimated that more than 200 million persons are infected with *E. vermicularis* worldwide and that 4 to 5 million school-age children harbor the worm in the United States.

The adult female worm resides in the cecum and appendix but migrates to the perianal and perineal skin to deposit eggs. The eggs stick to fingers, bed linens, towels, and clothing and are readily transmitted from person to person. Ingested eggs hatch in the small bowel to yield larvae that mature into adult worms. The adult female (1 cm × 0.5 mm) is occasionally seen incidentally in a surgically removed appendix, but its presence rarely causes tissue damage.

Some infected persons are asymptomatic, but most complain of anal or perineal pruritus, caused by the migrating worms depositing eggs. Scratching may cause perianal dermatitis, which may become secondarily infected. Several agents, including mebendazole, are effective against pinworms.

TISSUE NEMATODES

Trichinosis

Trichinosis is a myositis produced by the roundworm Trichinella spiralis, which humans acquire from eating the muscles of domestic pigs or wild animals.

☐ **Epidemiology:** Infection with *T. spiralis* is cosmopolitan but is most common in eastern and central Europe, North America, and South America. Humans acquire trichinosis by ingesting inadequately cooked meat containing encysted *T. spiralis* larvae. The larvae are found in the skeletal muscles of various carnivorous or omnivorous wild and domesticated animals, including pigs, rats, bears, and walruses. Although human infection can result from eating incompletely cooked meat from any of these animals, pork is the most common source of human trichinosis (Fig. 9-88).

Animals acquire trichinosis by feeding on the flesh of other infected animals. Infection is common among some wild animal populations and can be readily introduced into domesticated animals, such as pigs, when they feed on garbage or uncooked meat. Meat inspection programs and restriction of feeding practices have largely eliminated *T. spiralis* from domesticated pigs in many developed countries. Although only about 100 cases of trichinosis are reported in the United States annually, these represent only the most severely symptomatic cases, and infection is probably much more common.

☐ **Pathogenesis:** Within the small bowel, *T. spiralis* larvae emerge from the ingested tissue cysts and burrow into the intestinal mucosa, where they develop into adult worms. The adults mate, and the female worm liberates larvae that invade the intestinal wall and enter the circulation. Production of larvae may continue for 1 to 4 months, until the worms are finally expelled from the intestine. The larvae are capable of invading nearly any tissue but can survive only in striated skeletal muscle, where they encyst and remain viable for years. The resulting myositis is especially prominent in the diaphragm, extrinsic ocular muscles, tongue, intercostal muscles, gastrocnemius, and deltoids. Sometimes the central nervous system or heart is also involved in the inflammatory response, producing a meningoencephalitis or myocarditis.

☐ **Pathology:** In *T. spiralis* infections, the small bowel is grossly unremarkable. In heavy infestations, adult worms may be found on microscopic examination at the base of villi and may be associated with an inflammatory infiltrate of neutrophils, eosinophils, lymphocytes, and plasma cells.

The skeletal muscles are the major sites of tissue damage in trichinosis. When a larva infects a myocyte, the cell undergoes basophilic degeneration, swelling, and loss of its cross-striations. Early myocyte infection incites an intense inflammatory infiltrate of neutrophils, eosinophils, macrophages, and lymphocytes. The larva grows to 10 times its initial size, folds on itself, and develops a capsule. With encapsulation, the inflammatory infiltrate subsides. Several years later, the larva dies and the cyst calcifies.

☐ **Clinical Features:** Most human infections with *T. spiralis* involve small numbers of cysts and are totally asymptomatic. Symptomatic trichinosis is usually a self-limited disease from which patients recover in a few months. When large numbers of cysts are eaten, abdominal pain and diarrhea may result from small bowel invasion by the worms. The major clinical manifestations develop several days later with the onset of skeletal muscle invasion. Patients suffer severe pain and tenderness of affected skeletal muscles, together with fever and weakness. Eosinophilia is the rule and may be extreme (over 50% of all leukocytes). Involvement of the extraocular muscles produces periorbital edema. Infection of the brain or myocardium can be fatal. Severe cases of trichinosis are treated with corticosteroids to attenuate the inflammatory response. Antihelminthic drugs are required to remove adult worms from the intestine.

Visceral Larva Migrans (Toxocariasis)

Visceral larva migrans is an infection of deep organs by helminthic larvae migrating in aberrant hosts. It is a sporadic

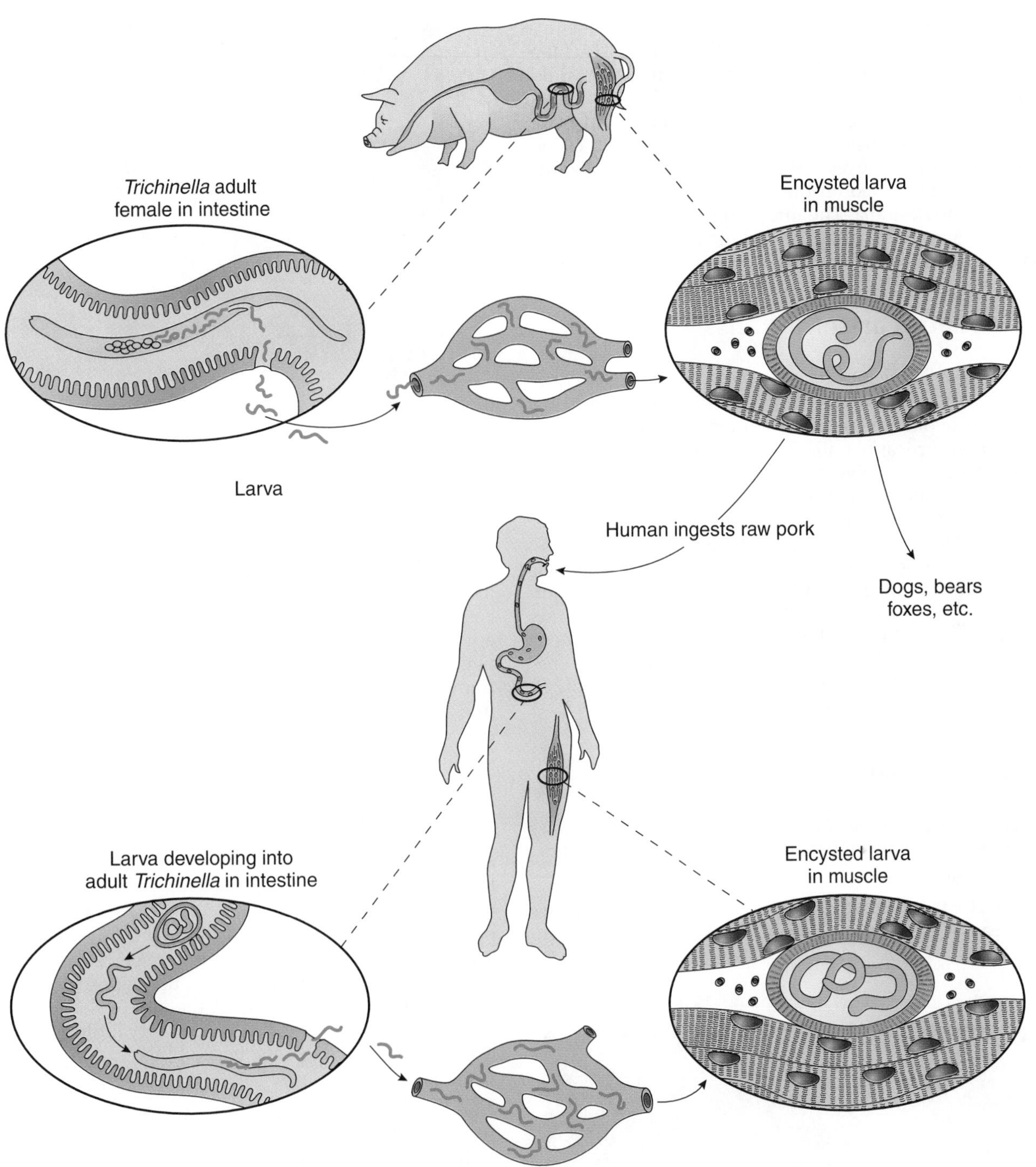

FIGURE 9-88
Trichinosis. After being ingested by the pig, cysts of *Trichinella* are digested in the gastrointestinal tract, liberating larvae that mature to adult worms. Female worms release larvae that penetrate the intestinal wall, enter the circulation, and lodge in striated muscle, where they encyst. When humans ingest inadequately cooked pork, the cycle is repeated, resulting in the muscle disease characteristic of trichinosis.

disease, primarily of young children, which characteristically occurs in areas where there are overcrowded dwellings, dogs, and cats. The most common causes of visceral larva migrans are *Toxocara* species, especially *T. canis* and *T. cati*. These roundworms live in the intestine of dogs and cats, and infection is transmitted to humans by the ingestion of embryonated ova. Ingested eggs hatch, and the larvae invade the intestinal wall. They are carried to the liver, from where a few emerge to reach the systemic circulation and may be carried to any part of the body. In tissues, larvae die and stimulate the formation of small granulomas, which eventually heal by scarring.

Many cases of visceral larva migrans are asymptomatic, but any infection is potentially capable of causing severe disease. The typical symptomatic patient is a child with hypereosinophilia, pneumonitis, and hypergammaglobulinemia. In these patients, ocular manifestations are common and the chief complaint is often the loss of vision in one eye. In fact, eyes with toxocaral endophthalmitis have been enucleated on the supposition that the lesion was a retinoblastoma. The infection is generally self-limited, and symptoms disappear within a year. The disease is treated with diethylcarbamazine and thiabendazole.

Cutaneous Larva Migrans

Cutaneous larva migrans is caused by the migration of a variety of larval nematodes through the skin. The migrating worms provoke severe inflammation, which appears as serpiginous urticarial trails (Fig. 9-89). The names applied to cutaneous larva migrans are as varied as the organisms that cause it and include creeping eruptions, sand worm, plumber's itch, duck hunter's itch, and epidermis linearis migrans. The more common larval nematodes include *S. stercoralis*, *Ancylostoma braziliensis*, and *Necator americanus*. Dogs and cats infected with hookworms are the major source of the disease. Outbreaks of cutaneous larva migrans occur at subtropical and tropical beaches. Plumbers who crawl under houses and animal caretakers are frequently infected. Thiabendazole is the treatment of choice.

Dracunculiasis

Dracunculiasis is an infection of the connective and subcutaneous tissues with the guinea worm, Dracunculus medinensis.

☐ **Epidemiology:** Dracunculiasis is common in rural areas of sub-Saharan Africa, the Middle East, India, and Pakistan, where it is estimated that 10 million persons are infected. The disease is transmitted in drinking water contaminated with the intermediate host, a microscopic aquatic crustacean of the genus *Cyclops*. The adult female nematode resides in subcutaneous tissues and releases numerous larvae through an ulcerated blister. When the infected part is immersed in water, the larvae are ingested by the *Cyclops* crustaceans, which are in turn ingested by humans.

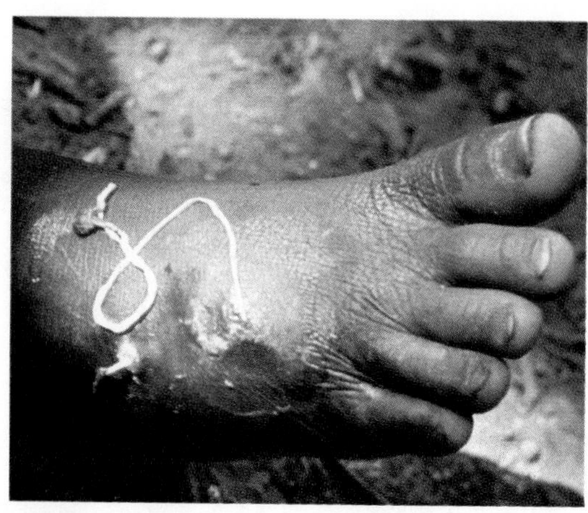

FIGURE *9-90*
Dracunculiasis. A female guinea worm is seen emerging from the foot, which is swollen because of secondary bacterial infection.

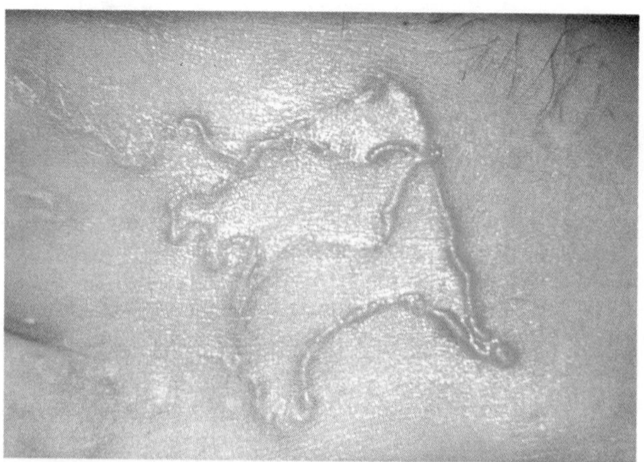

FIGURE *9-89*
Cutaneous larva migrans. The skin shows a creeping eruption with the characteristic serpiginous, raised lesion.

☐ **Pathogenesis and Pathology:** Ingested crustaceans are destroyed by gastric secretions, releasing *D. medinensis* larvae, which penetrate the stomach or small bowel. The larvae mature as they migrate through human tissues. The male dies, but the female continues to grow, passing through connective tissue toward the lower legs. As it nears the surface, the adult female releases a substance that produces painful local tissue destruction and eventual blistering of skin. At the site of the ulcer, the worm is surrounded by an inflammatory infiltrate of neutrophils, macrophages, and eosinophils.

☐ **Clinical Features:** About a year after infection, systemic allergic symptoms, including a pruritic urticarial rash, appear. A few hours later, a reddish papule, often around the ankles, develops and vesiculates. Beneath this sterile blister is the anterior end of the female worm. The blister bursts when it comes into contact with water, and the female worm, now measuring up to 120 cm in length and containing 3 million larvae, partially emerges (Fig. 9-90). The worm then spews myriad larvae into the water. Secondary infection of the blister, often with spreading cellulitis, is common. Dead worms provoke an intense inflammatory response, accounting for the debilitation seen in many cases of dracunculosis. The worm is often extracted by local practitioners by progressively twisting it onto a small stick. Treatment also includes anthelmintic drugs.

TREMATODES (FLUKES)

Schistosomiasis

Schistosomiasis (bilharziasis) is the most important helminthic disease of humans, in which intense inflammatory and immunological responses damage the liver, intestine, or urinary bladder. Three species of schistosomes, namely, *Schistosoma mansoni*, *S. haematobium*, and *S. japonicum*, are responsible for the disease.

☐ **Epidemiology:** Schistosomiasis is as old as civilization. Pharonic temple murals of the 19th dynasty in ancient Egypt (ca. 1500 BC) depict men with ascites and scrotal edema, generally accepted as evidence of hepatic schistosomiasis. Schistosome eggs have also been identified in mummies of the 20th dynasty (1200–1090 BC). In more recent times, Napoleonic memoirs recall the "menstruating males of Egypt," persons probably suffering from urogenital schistosomiasis.

Today, schistosomiasis causes greater morbidity and mortality than all other worm infestations. The disease is increasing in prevalence, affecting about 10% of the world's population and ranking second only to malaria as a cause of disabling disease. The three schistosomal pathogens inhabit distinct geographic regions, dictated by the distribution of their specific host snail species (Fig. 9-91). *S. mansoni* is found in much of tropical Africa, parts of southwest Asia, South America, and the Caribbean Islands. *S. haematobium* is endemic in large regions of tropical Africa and parts of the Middle East. *S. japonicum* occurs in parts of China, the Philippines, southeast Asia, and India.

The schistosomes have complicated life cycles, alternating between asexual generations in the invertebrate host (snail) and sexual generations in the vertebrate host (Fig. 9-92). A schistosome egg hatches in fresh water, liberating a motile form (miracidium) that penetrates a snail, where it develops into the final larval stage, the cercaria. The cercaria escapes from the snail into the water and penetrates the skin of the human host, during which process it loses its forked tail and becomes a schistosomule. The schistosomule migrates through tissues, penetrates a blood vessel, and is carried to the lung and subsequently to the liver. In the intestinal venules of the portal drainage, the schistosomules mature, forming pairs of male and female worms. The female worms of *S. mansoni* and *S. japonicum* deposit immature eggs in the intestinal venules, whereas *S. haematobium* lays eggs in those of the urinary bladder. Embryos develop during the passage of eggs through the tissues, and the larvae are mature when the eggs pass through the wall of the intestine or the urinary bladder and are discharged in the feces or urine. The eggs hatch in fresh water, liberating miracidia and completing the life cycle.

☐ **Pathogenesis and Pathology:** The immunological and inflammatory reactions to the schistosomal eggs in tissue cause the manifestations of schistosomiasis. **The basic lesion is a circumscribed granuloma or a cel-**

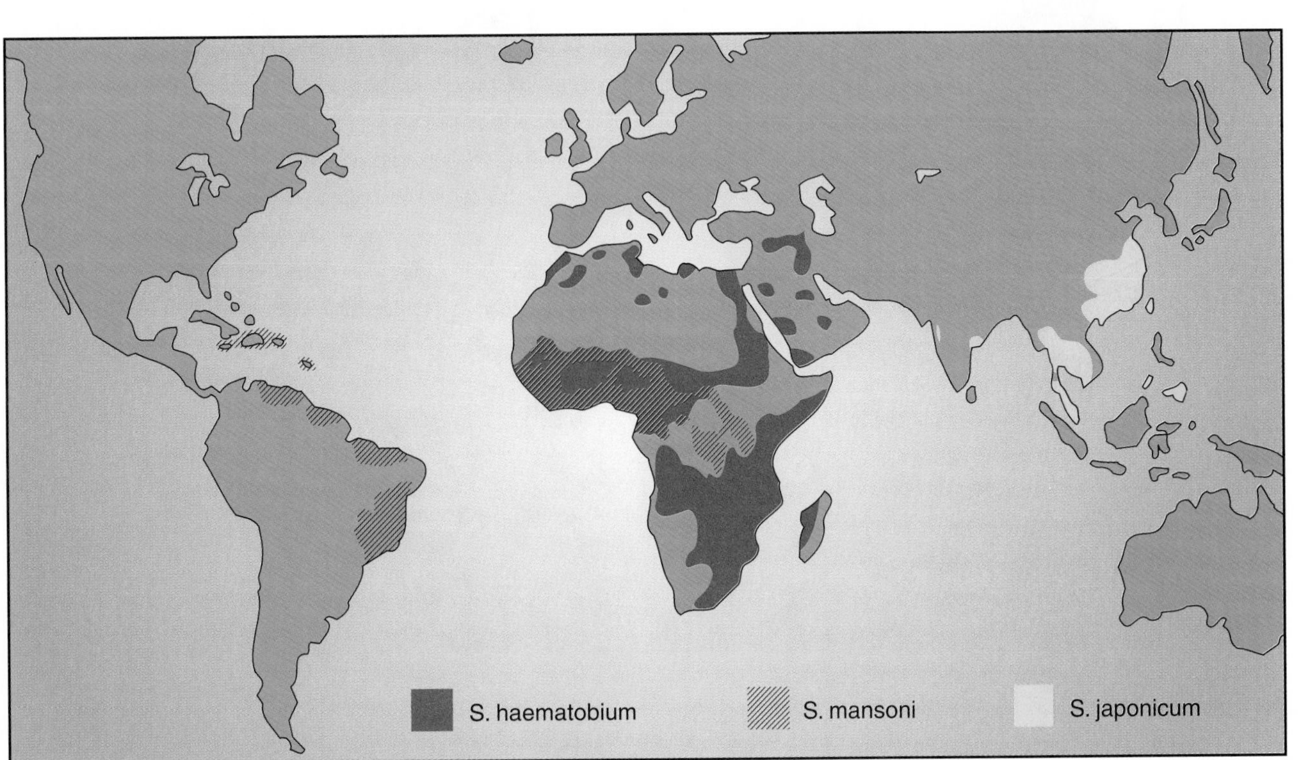

FIGURE *9-91*
Distribution of schistosomiasis caused by *Schistosoma mansoni, S. haematobium,* and *S. japonicum.*

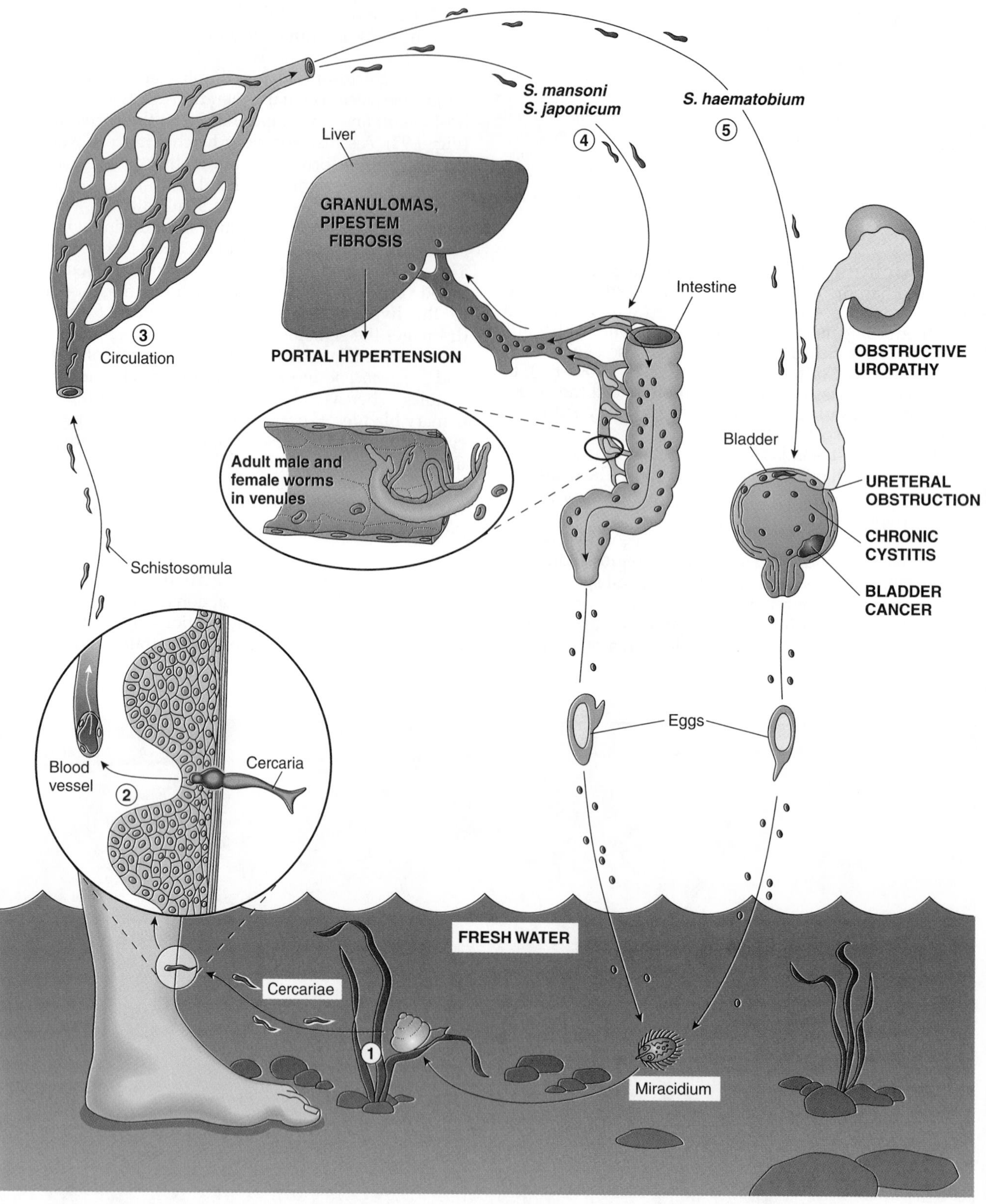
S. mansoni
S. japonicum
S. haematobium
④
⑤
Liver
GRANULOMAS, PIPESTEM FIBROSIS
PORTAL HYPERTENSION
③
Circulation
Intestine
OBSTRUCTIVE UROPATHY
Adult male and female worms in venules
Bladder
URETERAL OBSTRUCTION
CHRONIC CYSTITIS
BLADDER CANCER
Schistosomula
Eggs
Blood vessel
②
Cercaria
FRESH WATER
Cercariae
①
Miracidium

FIGURE 9-92

lular infiltrate of eosinophils and neutrophils around an egg. Adult schistosomes provoke no inflammation while alive in the veins. Granulomas that form about the eggs also obstruct the microvascular blood supply and produce ischemic damage to adjacent tissue. The result is progressive scarring and dysfunction in the affected organs.

The female worm deposits hundreds or thousands of eggs daily for 5 to 35 years. Fortunately, most infected persons harbor fewer than 10 adult females. However, when the worm burden is large, the granulomatous response to the enormous number of eggs poses significant problems. The site of involvement is determined by the tropism of the particular schistosome species.

- *S. mansoni* inhabits the branches of the inferior mesenteric vein, thereby affecting the distal colon and liver.
- *S. haematobium* winds its way to the veins serving the rectum, bladder, and pelvic organs.
- *S. japonicum* deposits eggs predominantly in the branches of the superior mesenteric vein, thereby damaging the small bowel, ascending colon, and liver.

Liver disease caused by *S. mansoni* or *S. japonicum* begins as periportal granulomatous inflammation (Fig. 9-93) and progresses to dense periportal fibrosis (pipestem fibrosis) (Fig. 9-94). In severe cases of hepatic schistosomiasis, this results in obstruction of portal blood flow and portal hypertension. *S. mansoni* and *S. japonicum* also damage the intestine, where the granulomatous response produces inflammatory polyps and foci of mucosal and submucosal fibrosis.

Urogenital schistosomiasis, caused by *S. haematobium*, features eggs that are most numerous in the bladder, ureter, and seminal vesicles, although they may also reach lungs, colon, and appendix. Eggs in the urinary bladder and ureters lead to a granulomatous reaction, inflammatory protuberances, and patches of mucosal and mural fibrosis. These can obstruct urine flow, producing secondary inflammatory damage to the bladder, ureters, and kidneys. **The bladder disease produced by *S. haematobium* is related to the development of squamous cell carcinoma of the bladder.**

The granulomas of schistosomiasis surround schistosome eggs. Eosinophils often predominate in early granulomas. In older granulomas, epithelioid macrophages and giant cells are conspicuous, and the oldest granulomas are densely fibrotic. The eggs of the various schistosomal species are identified on the basis of their size and shape.

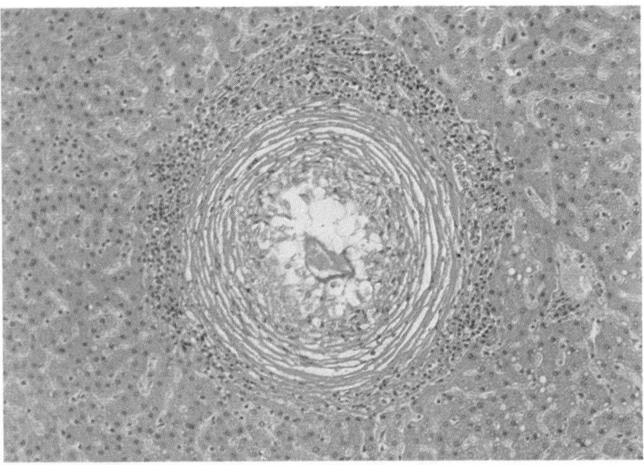

FIGURE 9-93
Hepatic schistosomiasis. A hepatic granuloma surrounds a degenerating egg of *S. mansoni*.

☐ **Clinical Features:** Skin penetration by the schistosome larvae is sometimes associated with a self-limited, intensely pruritic rash. Early in the infection, some cases of schistosomiasis present as an illness similar to serum sickness, characterized by fever, arthralgias, and myalgias. However, most cases are dominated by the manifestations of chronic granulomatous tissue damage. Hepatic involvement leads to portal hypertension, with splenomegaly, ascites, and bleeding esophageal varices. Although intestinal disease is usually only minimally symptomatic, some patients experience abdominal pain and blood in the stools. Schistosomiasis of the bladder causes hematuria, recurrent urinary tract infections, and sometimes progressive obstructive damage leading to renal failure. The diagnosis is made by identifying schistosome eggs in the urine or feces. Although schistosomes are effectively killed by systemic anthelminthic agents, the structural changes resulting from extensive fibrosis and scarring are irreversible.

FIGURE 9-92
Life cycle of *Schistosoma* and clinical features of schistosomiasis. The schistosome egg hatches in water, liberates a miracidium that penetrates a snail, and develops through two stages to a sporocyst to form the final larval stage, the cercaria. (1) The cercaria escapes from the snail into water, "swims," and penetrates the skin of a human host. (2) The cercaria loses its forked tail to become a schistosomule, which migrates through tissues, penetrates a blood vessel, and (3) is carried to the lung and later to the liver. In hepatic portal venules, the schistosomule becomes sexually mature and forms pairs, each with a male and a female worm, the female worm lying in the gynecophoral canal of the male worm. The organism causes lesions in the liver, including granulomas, portal ("pipestem") fibrosis, and portal hypertension. (4) The female worm deposits immature eggs in small venules of the intestine and rectum (*S. mansoni* and *S. japonicum*) or (5) of the urinary bladder (*S. haematobium*). The bladder infestation leads to obstructive uropathy, ureteral obstruction, chronic cystitis, and bladder cancer. Embryos develop during passage of the eggs through tissues, and larvae are mature when eggs pass through the wall of the intestine or urinary bladder. Eggs hatch in water and liberate miracidia to complete the cycle.

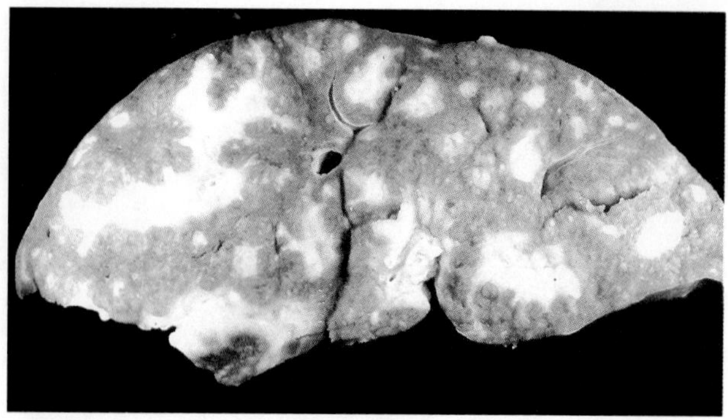

FIGURE 9-94
Hepatic schistosomiasis. Chronic infection of the liver with *S. japonicum* has led to the characteristic "pipestem" fibrosis.

Clonorchiasis

Clonorchiasis is an infection of the hepatic biliary system by the Chinese liver fluke, Clonorchis sinensis. Although the presence of the fluke usually causes only mild symptoms, it is sometimes associated with bile duct stones, cholangitis, and bile duct cancer.

□ **Epidemiology:** Clonorchiasis is endemic in east Asia, from Vietnam to Korea, where uncooked freshwater fish is common fare. In parts of Vietnam, China, and Japan, over 50% of the adult population is infected. The infection persists for years and is seen among Asian immigrants in North America and Europe. Human infection is acquired by the ingestion of inadequately cooked freshwater fish containing *C. sinensis* larvae.

Adult worms are flat and transparent, live in human bile ducts, and pass eggs to the intestine and feces. After ingestion by a specific snail, the egg hatches into a miracidium. Cercariae escape from the snail and seek out certain fish, which they penetrate and in which they encyst. When humans eat the fish, the cercariae emerge in the duodenum, enter the common bile duct through the ampulla of Vater, and mature in the distal bile ducts to an adult fluke.

□ **Pathogenesis and Pathology:** The presence of *Clonorchis* in the bile ducts elicits an inflammatory response, which fails to eliminate the worm but which causes dilatation and fibrosis of the ducts. Sometimes the worms cause calculus formation within the hepatic bile ducts, leading to ductal obstruction. The adult *Clonorchis* persists in the ducts for decades, and long-standing infection is associated with an increased incidence of carcinoma of the bile duct epithelium (cholangiocarcinoma).

In heavy *Clonorchis* infections, the liver may be up to three times the normal size. Dilated bile ducts are seen through the capsule, and the cut surface is punctuated with thick-walled dilated bile ducts (Fig. 9-95). The flukes (up to 2.5 cm in length), sometimes in the thousands, can be expressed from the bile ducts. Microscopically, the epithelial lining of the ducts is initially hyperplastic and then becomes metaplastic. The surrounding stroma is fibrotic. Secondary bacterial infection is common and may be associated with suppurative cholangitis. Eggs deposited in the hepatic parenchyma are surrounded by a fibrous and granulomatous reaction. Masses of eggs may become lodged in the bile ducts and cause cholangitis. The pancreatic ducts may also be invaded and become dilated, thickened, lined by metaplastic epithelium, and eventually surrounded by scar tissue.

□ **Clinical Features:** The migration of *C. sinensis* into the bile ducts results in transient fever and chills, although most infected persons remain completely asymptomatic. Patients with clonorchiasis may die of a variety of complications, including biliary obstruction, bacterial cholangitis, pancreatitis, and cholangiocarcinoma. The diagnosis of clonorchiasis is made by identifying the eggs of *C. sinensis* in stools or duodenal aspirates. The infestation is effectively treated with systemic antihelminthic agents.

Paragonimiasis

Paragonimiasis refers to a pulmonary infection by several species of the genus Paragonimus, the oriental lung fluke. The most common human pathogen is *P. westermani.*

□ **Epidemiology:** *Paragonimus* is the only helminthic parasite of humans that in the form of the adult worm naturally infects the lungs. Paragonimiasis is common in Asian countries (Korea, the Philippines, Taiwan, and China), where uncooked, lightly salted or wine-soaked fresh crabs are considered delicacies. The use of raw crab juices as medicinal beverages or seasonings also has been associated with the infection. Paragonimiasis is acquired by eating inadequately cooked freshwater crabs or crayfish infected with larval forms of *Paragonimus.*

Paragonimus eggs are coughed up from the lungs, swallowed, and passed in the stool. Miracidia emerge in water and infect a mollusk, which becomes an intermedi-

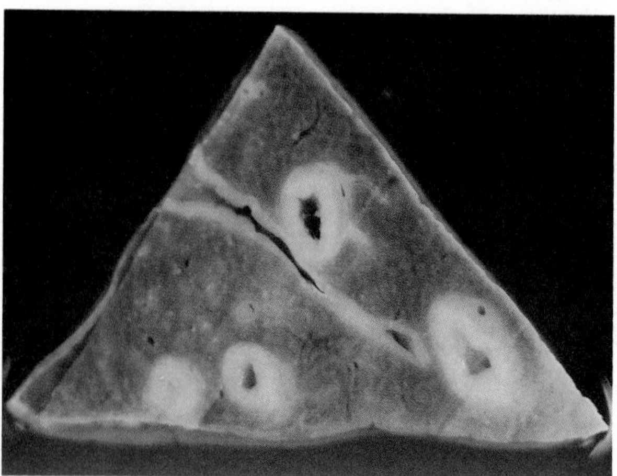

FIGURE 9-95
Clonorchiasis of the liver. The bile ducts are greatly thickened and dilated because of the presence of adult flukes (*C. sinensis*).

ate host and eventually releases infective cercariae. The latter penetrate the gills of a crustacean, migrate to soft tissue, and encyst. After humans ingest the cyst, a metacercaria emerges and penetrates the wall of the stomach, migrates to the diaphragm, bores through the pleura, and settles in the lung. There it matures into an adult worm, which survives for 20 years.

☐ **Pathogenesis and Pathology:** In the lungs, the worms incite a vigorous inflammatory response that walls them off from the surrounding pulmonary parenchyma. Sometimes the inflammatory response erodes into an adjacent airway, producing hemoptysis and releasing *Paragonimus* eggs to be coughed up in the sputum. Although the adult worms cause pulmonary disease, they occasionally produce lesions at ectopic sites, including brain, liver, gut, skeletal muscle, testes, and lymph nodes.

The pulmonary lesions of paragonimiasis are abscesses, measuring 2 to 5 cm in diameter. Early lesions contain adult worms (red, plump, measuring ~1 cm in maximum length), eggs, neutrophils, eosinophils, and macrophages. The older lesions have dense fibrous capsules and often contain only necrotic debris. *Paragonimus* eggs are usually present in the adjacent pulmonary tissue, where they elicit a granulomatous and eosinophilic inflammatory infiltrate.

☐ **Clinical Features:** Pulmonary paragonimiasis is frequently misdiagnosed as tuberculosis. The disease presents as fever, malaise, night sweats, chest pain, and cough. However, unlike tuberculosis, peripheral eosinophilia is common. The sputum is sometimes blood-tinged, and chest radiographs reveal transient diffuse pulmonary infiltrates. The prognosis in pulmonary paragonimiasis is good, but ectopic lesions of the brain may be fatal. Eggs in the sputum or stools provide the definitive diagnosis. Treatment is with systemic antihelminthic agents.

Fascioliasis

Fascioliasis is an infection of the liver by the sheep liver fluke, Fasciola hepatica.

☐ **Pathogenesis:** Humans may acquire the infection wherever sheep are raised. The eggs, passed by the sheep in their feces, require 2 weeks in fresh water before a miracidium emerges. Miracidia infect specific snails, after which infective cercariae emerge and encyst on submerged vegetation. Humans become infected by eating vegetation, such as watercress, that is contaminated with the cysts. Metacercariae excyst in the duodenum, pass through the wall into the peritoneal cavity, penetrate the liver, and migrate through the hepatic parenchyma into the bile ducts. The larvae mature to adults and live in both the intrahepatic and extrahepatic bile ducts. Later, the adult flukes penetrate the wall of the bile ducts and wander back into the liver parenchyma, where they feed on liver cells and deposit their eggs.

☐ **Pathology and Clinical Features:** The eggs of *F. hepatica* lead to hepatic abscesses and granulomas. The worms induce hyperplasia of the lining epithelium of the bile ducts, portal and periductal fibrosis, proliferation of bile ductules, and varying degrees of biliary obstruction. Eosinophilia, vomiting, and acute gastric pain are characteristic features. Severe untreated infections may be fatal. The diagnosis is made by recovering eggs from the stools or biliary tract. Early diagnosis and aggressive treatment with an anthelmintic agent prevent irreparable damage to the liver.

Fasciolopsiasis

Fasciolopsiasis is an infestation of the small intestine with the giant intestinal fluke, Fasciolopsis buski. The disease prevails throughout most of the Orient. Humans acquire the infection by eating aquatic vegetables contaminated with the encysted cercariae. The worm is large (3 × 7 cm) and attaches to the duodenal or jejunal wall. The point of attachment may ulcerate and become infected, causing pain similar to that of a peptic ulcer. Acute symptoms may also be caused by intestinal obstruction or by toxins released by large numbers of worms. The diagnosis is made by identifying the eggs of *F. buski* in the stool. Treatment is with systemic antihelminthic agents.

CESTODES

Intestinal Tapeworms

Taenia saginata, Taenia solium, and *Diphyllobothrium latum* are tapeworms that infect humans, growing to their adult forms within the intestine (Table 9-11). The presence of these adult worms rarely damages the human host.

☐ **Epidemiology:** The intestinal tapeworm infections are acquired by eating inadequately cooked beef (*T. saginata*), pork (*T. solium*), or fish (*D. latum*), which contain the larval forms of the organisms. The life cycles of these tapeworms involve cystic larval stages in animals and worm stages in the human. The life cycles of the beef and pork tapeworms require that the animals ingest material tainted with infected human feces. The cystic larval forms of the worms develop in the muscles of the animals. Mod-

TABLE **9-11** **Tapeworm Infections**

Species	Human Disease	Source of Human Infection
Taenia saginata	Adult tapeworm in intestine	Beef
Taenia solium	Adult tapeworm in intestine; cysticercosis	Pork; human feces
Diphyllobothrium latum	Adult tapeworm in intestine	Fish
Echinococcus granulosus	Hydatid cyst disease	Dog feces

ern cattle and pig farming practices, together with meat inspection, have largely eliminated beef and pork tapeworms in industrialized countries, but infection remains common throughout the underdeveloped world. Fish tapeworm infection is prevalent in regions where raw, pickled, or partly cooked freshwater fish are common fare.

☐ **Pathogenesis:** The larval form ingested in the meat or fish develops into the adult tapeworm in the human small intestine. The adult attaches to the intestinal mucosa by muscular sucking disks or grooves, where it feeds and grows within the rich intestinal stream, usually for years. Intestinal tapeworm infection rarely harms the human host. The fish tapeworm (*D. latum*) competes for vitamin B_{12}, and a small number (<2%) of infected persons develop a deficiency of this nutrient.

☐ **Clinical Features:** Adult tapeworm infection is usually asymptomatic, and the presence of the adult worms in the human intestine is only rarely of pathological consequence. Often the most significant concern is the distress produced when the infected person passes portions of the worm in the stool. Adult tapeworm infections can be eliminated with niclosamide.

Cysticercosis

Cysticercosis is a systemic infection by the cystic larval stage (cysticercus) of Taenia solium, the pork tapeworm. The adult *T. solium* is acquired by eating undercooked pork infected with cysticerci (measly pork). Pigs acquire cysticerci by ingesting eggs of *T. solium* shed in human feces. This cycle, although a public health concern, is essentially benign for both humans and pigs. **However, when humans accidentally ingest the eggs from human feces and become infected with cysticerci, the consequences may be catastrophic.** The eggs release oncospheres, which penetrate the wall of the gut, enter the bloodstream, lodge in tissue, encyst, and differentiate to cysticerci.

The cysticercus is a spherical, milky white cyst about 1 cm in diameter that contains fluid and an invaginated scolex (head of the worm) with birefringent hooklets. Viable cysts can be shelled out from the infected tissue. The cysticerci remain viable for an indefinite period and provoke no inflammation; rather, as they grow they compress adjacent tissues. Degenerating cysts, the ones usually responsible for symptoms, are attached to the tissue and are densely inflamed with neutrophils, eosinophils, lymphocytes, and plasma cells. Multiple cysticerci in the brain sometimes impart a "Swiss cheese" appearance to the tissue (Fig. 9-96).

Cysticercosis of the brain presents as headaches or seizures, and symptoms vary according to the sites affected. Massive cysticercosis of the brain causes convulsions and death. Cysticerci in the retina blind the patient. In the heart, cysticerci may cause arrhythmias and sudden death. Depending on the site of involvement, cysticercosis is treated with surgery or anthelmintic therapy.

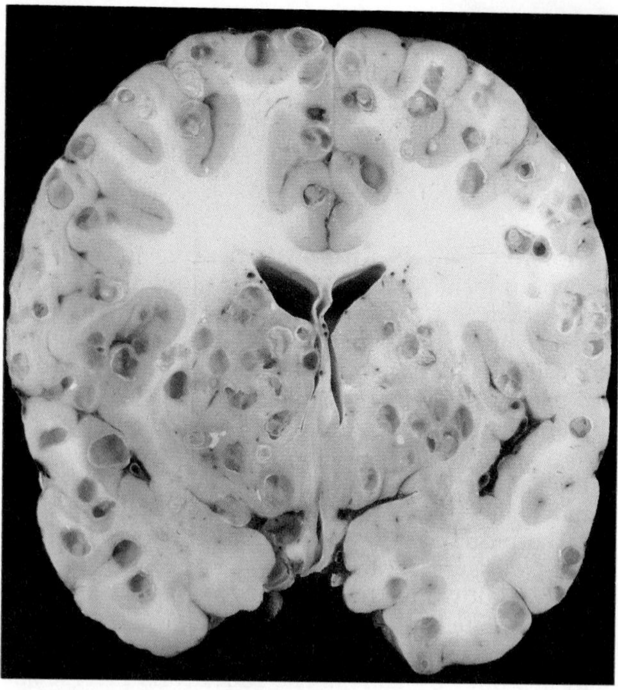

FIGURE *9-96*
Cysticercosis. A cross-section of the brain from a patient infected with the larvae of *T. solium* shows many cysticerci in the gray matter, imparting a "Swiss cheese" appearance.

Echinococcosis (Hydatid Disease)

Echinococcosis is a zoonotic infection caused by larval cestodes of the genus Echinococcus, which result in space occupying cysts, principally in the liver and lungs. The most common offender is *E. granulosus*, which causes cystic hydatid disease. Rarely, *E. multilocularis* and *E. vogeli* infect humans.

☐ **Epidemiology:** Infestation with the tapeworm *E. granulosus* is endemic in sheep, goats, and cattle and their attendant dogs. These animals, particularly dogs, contaminate their habitats (and their human keepers) with infectious eggs. Humans become infected when they inadvertently ingest the tapeworm eggs. The resulting hydatid disease is present worldwide among herding populations who live in close proximity to dogs and herd animals. Disease is especially common in Australia, New Zealand, Argentina, Greece, and herding countries of Africa and the Middle East. In the United States, hydatid cyst disease is seen among immigrants and among the indigenous sheep-herding populations of the southwest.

The adult tapeworms (2 to 6 mm long) live in the small intestine of a carnivorous host, such as the wolf, fox, coyote, jackal, or dog (Fig. 9-97). *E. granulosus* has a scolex with suckers and numerous hooklets for attachment to the intestinal mucosa. A short neck is followed by three segments (proglottids). The terminal gravid proglottid breaks off and releases eggs, which are eliminated in the feces of the carnivore. Contaminated herbage is then

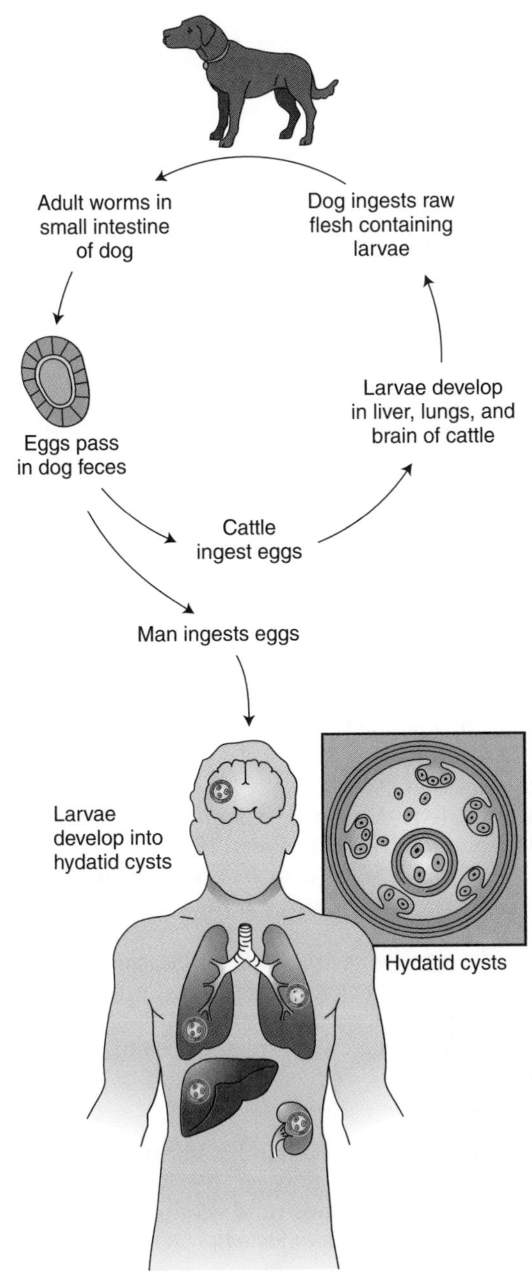

FIGURE 9-97
Life cycle of *Echinococcus granulosus* and cystic hydatid disease. The adult cestode lives in the small intestine of a dog (the definitive host). A gravid proglottid ruptures, releasing cestode eggs into the dog's feces. Cestode eggs are ingested by cattle or sheep (the intermediate hosts), hatch in the intestine, and release oncospheres that penetrate the wall of the gut, enter the bloodstream, disseminate to various deep organs, and grow to form hydatid cysts, containing brood capsules and scolices. When another dog ingests raw flesh from the cattle or sheep, the scolices are ingested and develop into mature worms in the dog's intestine to complete the cycle. A person who ingests cestode eggs in contaminated plant material becomes an accidental intermediate host. The larvae increase in size, but the parasite reaches a "dead end" without developing into an adult tapeworm. Hydatid cysts in humans occur predominantly in the liver but may also involve lung, kidney, brain and other organs.

eaten by herbivorous intermediate hosts, including deer, moose, antelopes, cattle, and sheep. Humans are also infected by ingesting plant material contaminated by the cestode eggs. Larvae released from the eggs penetrate the wall of the gut, enter the bloodstream, and disseminate to deep organs, where they grow to form large cysts containing brood capsules and scolices. When the flesh of the herbivore is eaten by a carnivore, the scolices develop into sexually mature worms in the latter, thereby completing the cycle.

E. multilocularis causes alveolar hydatid disease in humans. The wild definitive hosts are the wolf, fox, and coyote, which are carnivores that are predators of the intermediate hosts, the field mouse, mole, shrew, and lemming. Dogs and cats are domestic definitive hosts, and the domestic intermediate host is the house mouse. Rare infections by *E. multilocularis* have been reported in Germany, Switzerland, China and the republics of the former Soviet Union.

Dogs are definitive hosts for *E. vogeli*. Humans may become accidental intermediate hosts for *E. vogeli* by ingesting eggs shed by domestic dogs. Polycystic hydatid disease caused by *E. vogeli* has been reported in Central and South America.

☐ **Pathogenesis and Pathology:** After the larvae of *E. granulosus* penetrate the bowel wall, most are carried to the liver, but some reach the lungs, skeletal muscles, and other body sites. The larvae develop into hydatid cysts, which expand by 1 to 5 cm per year and remain asymptomatic until their size or location interferes with normal organ function. The most common sites of hydatid cysts are the liver (75%), lungs (10%), and skeletal muscle (5%).

On gross examination, unilocular hydatid cysts are fluid-filled structures varying from a few millimeters to as many as 20 cm in diameter (Fig. 9-98A). Cysts are lined by daughter cysts, which bud from the internal cyst wall. Microscopically, the thin cyst wall is composed of an outer laminated layer and an internal germinal membrane, from which brood capsules and scolices develop (see Fig. 9-98B). Fluid aspirated from the cyst often contains "hydatid sand" consisting of free daughter cysts and scolices.

Multilocular cysts of *E. multilocularis* involve only the liver. The cysts spread by budding infiltrative growth, creating an "alveolar" pattern. The multilocular cysts grow very slowly, and an infected person may remain asymptomatic for decades.

Polycystic hydatid cysts of *E. vogeli* have been found in the liver, lung, heart, skeletal muscles, stomach, and omentum. Individual cysts are about 1 cm in diameter, and aggregates of several centimeters across may form. The cysts may be so extensive that they replace most of the liver.

☐ **Clinical Features:** The slowly growing hydatid cyst is found by chance or becomes obvious when its size and position interferes with normal bodily functions. A hepatic cyst often presents as a palpable mass in the right upper quadrant. Compression of intrahepatic bile ducts by the cyst may lead to obstructive jaundice. Pulmonary

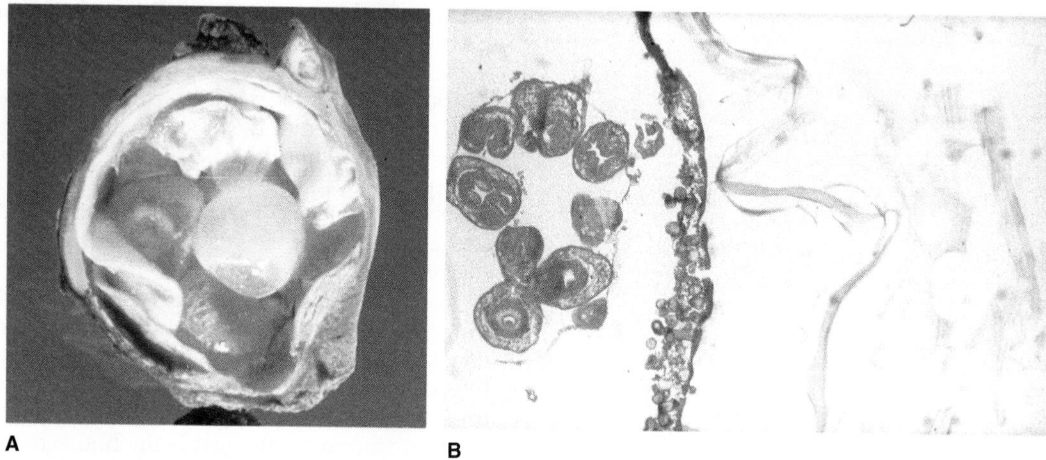

FIGURE 9-98
Echinococcal cyst. (*A*) An echinococcal cyst showing daughter cysts was resected from the liver of a patient infected with *E. granulosus.* (*B*) A photomicrograph of the cyst wall shows (*from right to left*) a laminated, non-nuclear layer, a nucleated germinal layer with brood capsules attached, and numerous scolices in the cyst cavity.

cysts are often asymptomatic and discovered incidentally on a chest radiograph.

A major complication of cyst rupture is the seeding of adjacent tissues with brood capsules and scolices. When these "seeds" germinate, they produce many additional cysts, each with the growth potential of the original cyst. Traumatic rupture of a hydatid cyst of the liver or other abdominal organ results in severe diffuse pain, resembling that of peritonitis. The rupture of a cyst in the lung may cause pneumothorax and empyema. Moreover, when a hydatid cyst ruptures into a body cavity, the release of cyst contents can cause fatal allergic reactions. Treatment of echinococcal cysts frequently requires careful surgical removal. Cysts must be sterilized with formalin before drainage or extirpation to prevent intraoperative anaphylactic shock.

SUGGESTED READING

BOOKS

Baron S (ed): *Medical micobiology.* 4th ed. New York: Churchill Livingstone, 1996.

Cook M: *Manson's tropical disease.* 20th ed. Philadelphia: WB Saunders, 1995.

Gutierrez Y: *Diagnostic pathology of parasitic infections with clinical correlations.* Philadelphia: Lea & Febiger, 1990.

Gorbach SL, Bartlett JG, Blacklow NR (eds): *Infectious diseases in medicine and surgery*, 2nd ed., Philadelphia: WB Sauders, 1997.

Holmes KK, Mardh P, Sparling PF, et al (eds): *Sexually transmitted diseases*, 3rd ed. New York: McGraw-Hill, 1997.

Mandell GL, Bennett JE, Dolin E (eds): *Principles and practice of infectious diseases*, 3rd ed. New York: Churchill Livingstone, 1995.

Murray PR (ed): *Manual of clinical microbiology.* 6th ed. Washington DC: ASM Press, 1995.

Remington JS, Klein JO (eds): *Infectious diseases of the fetus and newborn infant*, 4th ed. Philadelphia: WB Saunders, 1994.

Rippon JW: *Medical mycology: the pathogenic fungi and the pathogenic actinomycetes*, 3rd ed. Philadelphia: WB Saunders, 1988.

Rom WN, Garay (ed): *Tuberculosis.* Boston: Little Brown, 1996.

REVIEWS

Genta RM: Diarrhea in helminthic infections. *Clin Inf Dis* 19:S122–S129, 1993.

Meslin FX: Surveillance and control of emerging zoonoses. *World Health Statistics Quarterly* 45:200–207, 1992.

Steere AC: Lyme disease. *N Engl J Med* 321:586–596, 1989.

Walker DH, Barbour AG, Olivier JH, et al: Emerging bacterial zoonotic and vector-borne diseases. Ecological and epidemiological factors. *JAMA* 275:463–469, 1996.

Walker DH, Yamolska O, Grinberg LM: Death at Sverdlovsk: what have we learned? *Am J Pathol* 144:1135–1141, 1994.

CHAPTER 10

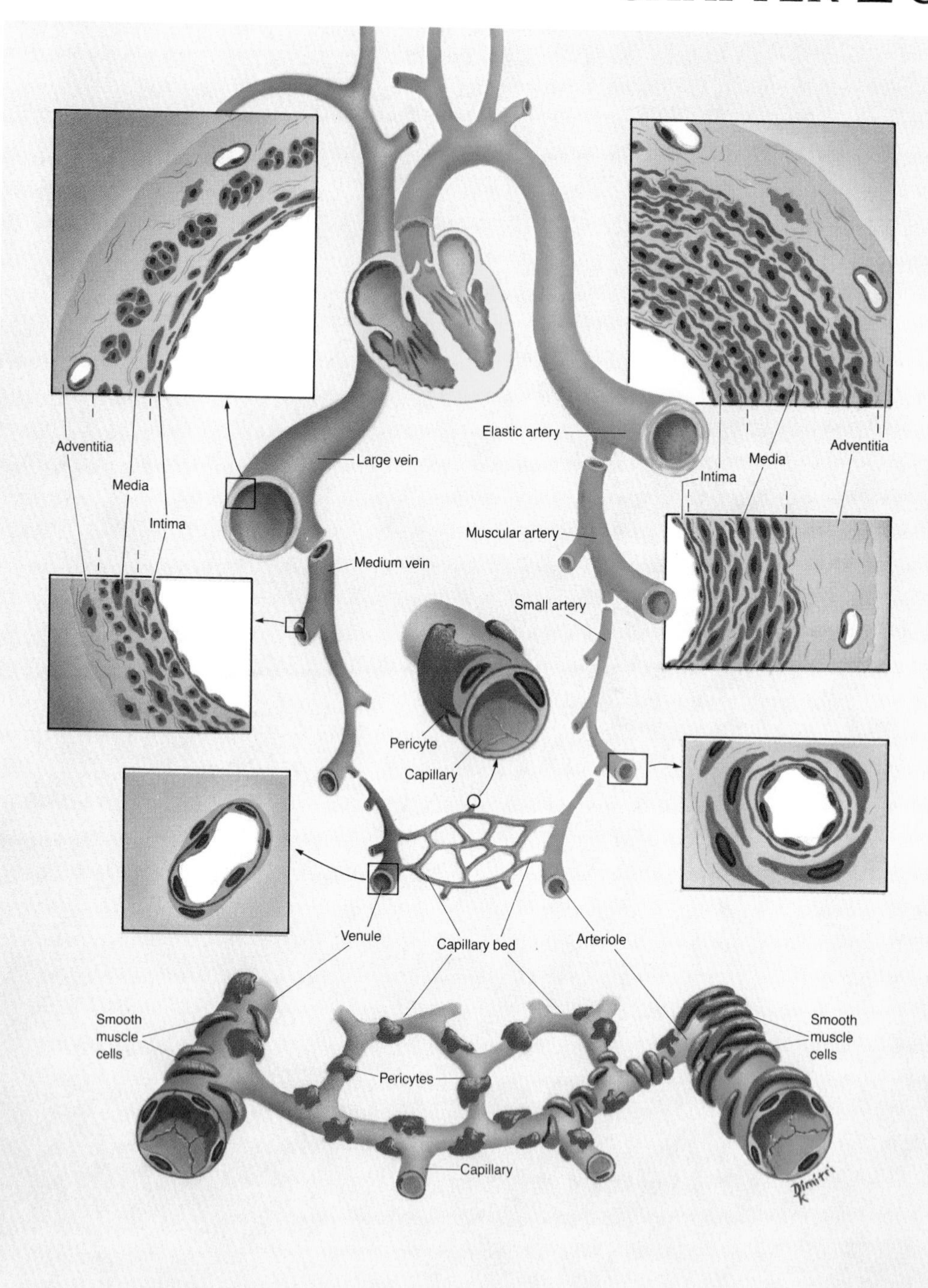

Adventitia
Media
Intima
Large vein
Medium vein
Elastic artery
Intima
Media
Adventitia
Muscular artery
Small artery
Pericyte
Capillary
Venule
Capillary bed
Arteriole
Smooth muscle cells
Pericytes
Capillary
Smooth muscle cells
Dimitri K

Blood Vessels

Avrum I. Gotlieb
Earl P. Benditt
Stephen M. Schwartz

(continued)

FIGURE *10-1 (see opposite page)*
Subdivisions and histological structure of the vascular system. Each subdivision is subject to a set of pathological changes conditioned by the structure–function relationship of that part of the system. For example, the aorta, an elastic artery subject to great pressure, frequently shows a pathological dilatation (aneurysm) if the supporting elastic media is damaged. Muscular arteries are the most significant sites of atherosclerosis. Small arteries, particularly arterioles, are sites of hypertensive changes. Capillary beds, venules, and veins each display their own types of pathological changes.

Syphilic Aneurysms

Mycotic (Infectious) Aneurysms

Veins

Varicose Veins of the Legs

Varicose Veins at Other Sites

Deep Venous Thrombosis

Saphenous Vein Bypass Grafts

Lymphatic Vessels

Lymphangitis

Lymphatic Obstruction

Benign Tumors of Blood Vessels

Hemangiomas

Glomus Tumor (Glomangioma)

Hemangioendothelioma

Malignant Tumors of Blood Vessels

Angiosarcoma

Hemangiopericytoma

Kaposi Sarcoma

Tumors of the Lymphatic System

Capillary Lymphangioma

Cystic Lymphangioma (Cystic Hygroma, Cavernous Lymphangioma)

Lymphangiosarcoma

EMBRYONIC DEVELOPMENT OF BLOOD VESSELS

Endothelial Cells

The earliest embryonic vascular primordia are clusters of endothelial cells that arise on the yolk sac between the splanchnic mesoderm and endoderm. Blood vessels then develop through a programmed sequence:

1. The early structures, called **blood islands** (Fig. 10-2), soon separate into peripheral cells, which become endothelium and more centrally located cells, which produce a short-lived line of primitive blood cells.
2. The vascular primordia arising on the yolk sac consolidate into a plexus, which eventually connects with a system of endothelial tubes originating independently within the body of the embryo. Recent studies suggest that tube formation is dependent on cell adhesion molecules and on the extracellular matrix.
3. The original capillaries, represented by bare endothelial tubes, recruit the mesenchymal cells that become the smooth muscle cells of the media and the fibroblasts of the adventitia.
4. Mesenchymal cells differentiate into phenotypes appropriate for their locations in the vessel wall and secrete extracellular matrix. In the fourth fetal month, the three coats of the arterial wall become clearly evident.

Once the embryonic vascular system is firmly established, it extends by forming new branches from preexisting vessels. The signals controlling this process are known as angiogenic factors, and the process is termed **angiogenesis**. For example, basic fibroblast growth factor (FGF-2) and vascular endothelial growth factor (VEGF) are both angiogenic factors. Angiogenesis is likely mediated by a balance between several inducers and inhibitors of angiogenesis. For example, the angiogenesis inhibitor platelet factor 4 suppresses the proliferation of blood vessels in the chicken chorioallantoic membrane, a commonly used test system to evaluate angiogenesis. The angiostatic effect is due to specific inhibition of endothelial cell proliferation stimulated by growth factors. Angiogenesis is important in wound healing and tumor growth, as well as in embryonic development.

The stability of the single cell layer of endothelial cells in the intima depends on several types of adhesion complexes. These junctions are essential for the maintenance of proper endothelial function and the permeation of solutes across this barrier. Moreover, the interaction of endothelial cells with circulating blood cells is also governed, in part, by the expression of adhesive molecules. The receptors for those molecules and their ligands fall into three functional categories:

- **Cell-substrate adhesion molecules**, which provide for the attachment of endothelial cells to their substrate (e.g., basal lamina). For example, endothelial cell integrins act as receptors for the binding of endothelial cells to adhesive glycoproteins, including laminin, fibronectin, and thrombospondin.
- **Cell-cell adhesion molecules** act to attach one endothelial cell to another. For instance, cadherin is located at intercellular adhesion junctions, and occludin at intercellular tight junctions.
- **Leukocyte adhesion molecules**, located at the cell surface, are available for the adherence of different kinds of leukocytes. For example, members of the selectin and the immunoglobulin family of adhesion molecules are involved in leukocyte adhesion. E-selectin and P-selectin, which are present on the endothelial surface, bind ligands on leukocytes as do vascular cell adhesion molecule 1 (VCAM-1) and intercellular adhesion molecule 1 (ICAM-1) of the immunoglobulin superfamily.

The cell–substrate and cell–cell adhesion molecules are linked to the actin cytoskeleton of the cell, which regulates, in part, the structural integrity of the endothelium.

Smooth Muscle Cells

Smooth muscle cells are derived from the local mesoderm after the endothelial tubes are formed. There may actually

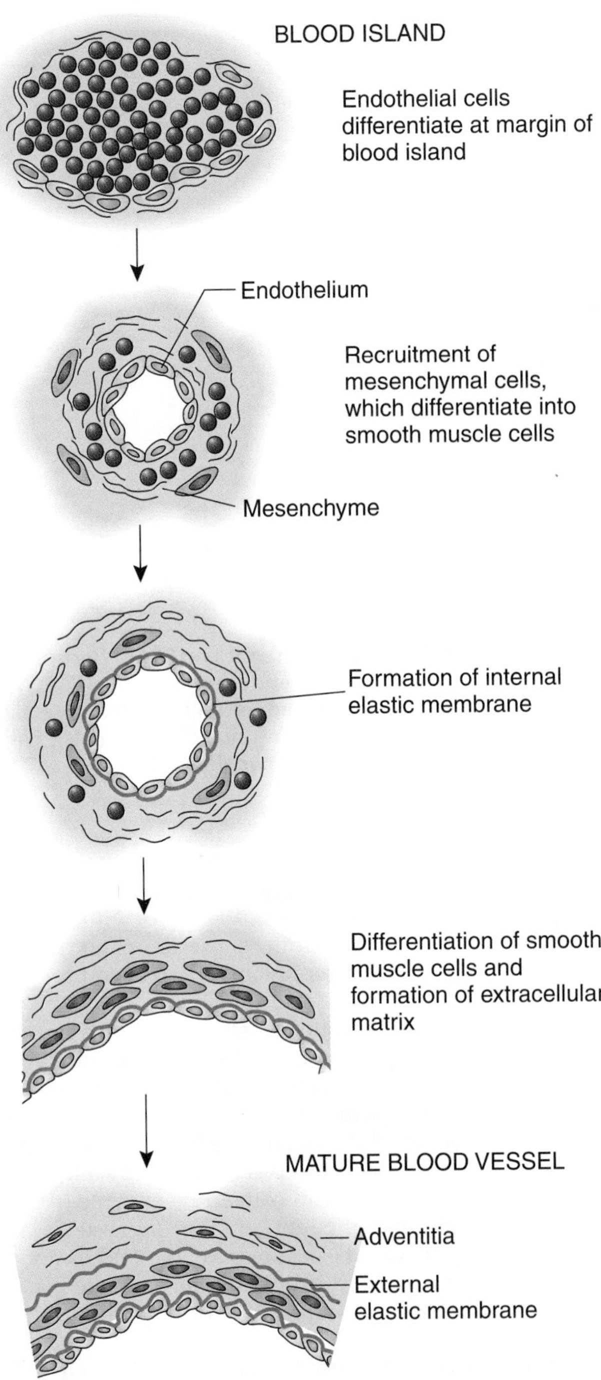

FIGURE 10-2
Differentiation of vessels in early embryos. The course of events from the development of blood islands on the chorioallantoic membrane starts with differentiation of endothelium and proceeds to fully developed arteries or veins.

be two distinct embryological origins for smooth muscle. The smooth muscle cells that populate the major arteries in the upper part of the body are thought to represent "mesectoderm," derived from neural crest cells. Thus, despite the fact that smooth muscle cells of the media appear monotonously uniform, they exhibit significant heterogeneity. This has important implications in relation to the development of lesions in the vascular system. The contractile properties of smooth muscle cells also vary according to the location of the blood vessel, some being more reactive to various stimuli than others.

STRUCTURE OF BLOOD VESSELS

Cells of the Vessel Wall

Blood vessels are among the simplest tissue structures in the body (see Fig. 10-1). The vessel wall is composed of only two cell types, namely endothelial cells and smooth muscle cells. In turn, most vascular diseases result from the malfunction of these cell types, or they arise from the interaction of leukocytes with them. The cells surrounding the vessel wall, namely, those of the connective tissue of the adventitia and the pericytes of capillaries and venules, ordinarily do not play a leading role in the pathogenesis of most vascular disease processes. Pericytes, however, influence endothelial cell function, and the cells of the adventitia react to medial disruption, as occurs after angioplasty and in vasculitis.

A single row of endothelium lines the tunica intima, the innermost layer of the vessel wall (Fig. 10-3). A layer of connective tissue is interposed between the endothelium and the underlying smooth muscle of the tunica media. At one time, the endothelium was considered to be an uncomplicated structural barrier that simply modulates permeation through the vessel wall by providing pores of appropriate size. The endothelial cells do not normally proliferate, unlike other cell types, such as epithelial cells of the skin and gut, which are also exposed to hostile environments. However, in the face of vascular injury and loss of endothelium, the cells have the capacity to proliferate rapidly to reestablish the integrity of the endothelium. We now recognize that endothelial cells actually accomplish a large variety of metabolic functions (Table 10-1). In fact, endothelial dysfunction, is an important feature in the pathogenesis of vascular disease. In some diseases, endothelial dysfunction is associated with the subendothelial accumulation of blood-borne materials. For example, the accretion of lipid beneath the endothelium in atherosclerotic lesions reflects the failure of the endothelium to serve as an effective barrier between tissue and plasma. Thus, a modern view of endothelium holds that the metabolic and endocrine functions of its cells play a critical role in both health and disease by synthesizing a number of biologically active factors:

- **Autacoids**: The term autacoid refers to potent bioactive compounds that are released locally, act at short distances, and are rapidly inactivated. Endothelial cells release autacoids and thereby exert effects on vascular tone and platelet activity. For example, **prostacyclin**, the first autacoid observed, relaxes smooth muscle and inhibits the aggregation of platelets. One of the functionally most important autacoids is **nitric oxide (NO)**. NO is produced by the action of NO synthase (NOS) which oxidizes L-arginine to form citrulline and NO. Although endothelial NOS is constitutively expressed, it can be regulated. NO inhibits the adhesion and aggregation of

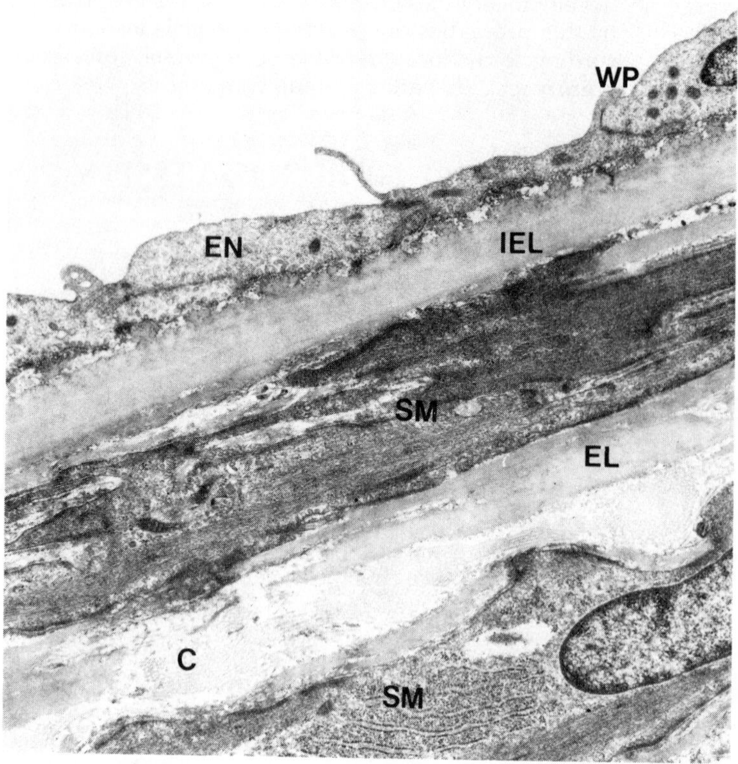

FIGURE 10-3
Luminal side of the rat aorta. An electron micrograph shows endothelial cells *(EN)* with Weibel-Palade bodies *(WP)*, internal elastic lamina *(IEL)*, smooth muscle cells *(SM)*, collagen *(C)*, and elastic lamellae *(EL)*.

platelets and the proliferation of vascular smooth muscle by attenuating the rise in intracellular free calcium induced by a variety of agonists. In addition, NO likely has a physiological role in the control of the vascular tone of large arteries and resistance vessels. Inhibition of NO synthesis in experimental animals leads to a chronic elevation of blood pressure. Both prostacyclin and NO are released following stimulation of endothelial receptors by agonists and act together to inhibit platelet aggregation. Compounds that promote the release of NO include acetylcholine, bradykinin, and adenosine diphosphate (ADP). NO is more labile than even prostacyclin, with a half-life of 6 seconds.

- **Peptides:** Vascular tone is also affected by a number of bioactive peptides. **Endothelin** is a potent vasoconstrictive protein synthesized by the endothelium. **Angiotensin II**, which is also a potent vasoconstrictor, is an octapeptide that results from a series of proteolytic steps. The last step is mediated by a terminal dipeptidase (angiotensin-converting enzyme [ACE]), located in the endothelium. Another suggested mediator, 13-hydroxy-9,11-octadecadienoic acid, is not released, but acts from inside the cell to make the endothelial surface nonadhesive for circulating blood cells.
- **Immunoactive factors**: Endothelial cell-derived factors are also important in the control of the immune response. Similar to macrophages, endothelial cells express class II histocompatibility antigens when they are stimulated. In this way, they are able to participate with monocytes—or even to replace them—in activating lymphocytes. Immune responses to endothelial cells are a major part of organ rejection following transplantation. Endothelial cells also synthesize interleukin-1 (IL-1) and several factors involved in coagulation and thrombosis.

Less is known about the metabolic functions of the smooth muscle cells of the vessel wall. These cells maintain the integrity of the vessel, providing support for the

TABLE 10-1 **Functions of Endothelial Cells of the Blood Vessels**

Permeability barrier
Vasoactive factors: Nitric oxide (EDRF) endothelin
Antithrombic agent production: Prostacyclin (PGI_2), adenine metabolites
Prothrombic agent production: Factor VIIIa (von Willebrand factor)
Anticoagulant production: Thrombomodulin, other proteins
Fibrinolytic agent production: Tissue plasminogen activator, urokinase-like factor
Procoagulant production: Tissue factor, plasminogen activator/inhibitor, factor V
Inflammatory mediator production: Interleukin-1, cell adhesion molecules
Receptors for factor IX, factor X, low-density lipoproteins, modified low-density lipoproteins, thrombin
Growth factor production: Blood cell colony-stimulating factor, insulin-like growth factors, fibroblast growth factor, platelet-derived growth factor
Growth inhibitor: Heparin
Replication

endothelium. They also control blood flow by contracting or dilating in response to specific stimuli. In addition, smooth muscle cells synthesize the connective tissue matrix of the vessel wall, which includes elastin, collagen, and proteoglycans. Adult smooth muscle cells, like endothelial cells, show very low levels of proliferation in the normal artery, but both have the capacity to undergo prominent proliferation in response to injury of the vessel.

Arteries

The simple two-cell structure of blood vessels is made more complex by the organization of the wall into layers called "tunicae" (see Fig. 10-1).

Elastic Arteries

The largest blood vessels in the body, including the aorta, are the elastic arteries. They function as conduits to smaller arterial branches for blood from the heart and are composed of three layers:

- **Tunica intima**: This layer consists of the endothelium and the connective tissue on the luminal side of the internal elastic lamina. Many of the pathological changes in elastic arteries (e.g., atherosclerosis) develop in this layer. The tunica intima of the aorta is thick and contains a matrix of collagen, proteoglycans, and small amounts of elastin. In addition to the endothelial cells, the normal intima also contains smooth muscle cells. Occasional resident lymphocytes, macrophages, and other inflammatory cells derived from the blood are also present.
- **Tunica media**: The next layer outward, the tunica media, displays layers of smooth muscle cells. In the elastic arteries, elastic fibers interposed between smooth muscle cells provide a means of minimizing energy loss during the pressure changes between systole and diastole. A breakdown of the media, particularly of its elastic layers, leads a dilatation of the artery, called an **aneurysm**. Much of the disease that occurs in arteries (e.g., atherosclerosis) involves proliferation of medial smooth muscle cells. Alternatively, during normal aging and in hypertension, smooth muscle cells undergo "endoreplication," that is, they replicate their DNA without cell division. As a result, they become tetraploid, octaploid, or even of higher ploidy. This phenomenon is accelerated in the aorta, at least in the hypertensive rat.

  Medial smooth muscle cells may also undergo degenerative changes, even leading to cell death, because they do not receive adequate nutrients or cannot effectively exchange wastes with the circulating blood. In smaller vessels, particularly those with fewer than 30 layers of smooth muscle cells, nutrition for the media is provided only from the lumen of the blood vessel, through the endothelium and the layers of smooth muscle. However, in larger blood vessels, such as the aorta, this pathway is apparently inadequate. This problem is resolved in blood vessels that have more than 28 layers of smooth muscle cells by the provision of a vasculature of their own, namely, the **vasa vasorum**. The vasa vasorum penetrate the exterior of the vessel wall and provide blood for the tunica media. The rich blood supply that develops in atherosclerotic plaques is derived from the vasa vasorum. In addition to this external vascular supply, the tunica media also contains autonomic nerve fibers that influence vascular contractility.
- **Tunica adventitia**: This coat is the most external layer of the vessel wall. The tunica adventitia is a connective tissue sheath composed of fibroblasts, small vessels that give rise to the vasa vasorum, and nerves.

Muscular Arteries

The blood conducted by the elastic arteries is distributed to individual organs through large muscular arteries (Fig. 10-4). The tunica media of a muscular artery consists of layers of smooth muscle cells without prominent bands of elastin. Nevertheless, the wall does have a prominent internal elastic lamina and usually an external elastic lamina. The continuity of the internal elastic lamina is interrupted by fenestrae, which permit the migration of smooth muscle cells from the media into the intima. The absence of the heavy elastin layers allows for better contraction of the muscular arteries. The intima of the muscular arteries, like that of the aorta, also contains smooth muscle cells, connective tissue, and occasional inflammatory cells. Vasa vasorum penetrate the walls of the thicker muscular arteries, but are not seen in the smaller ones. As the vascular tree branches further, the tunica media becomes thinner, and except for the endothelium the tunica intima disappears.

The small muscular arteries play an important role in the regulation of blood flow. The narrow lumen of these vessels produces an increased resistance, thereby reducing blood pressure to levels appropriate for the exchange of water and plasma constituents across the thin-walled capillaries. In addition to reducing pressure to capillary levels, the small muscular arteries, sometimes called "resistance vessels," maintain systemic pressure by regulating total peripheral resistance.

Arterioles

The arterioles are the smallest elements of the arterial vascular tree and consist of an endothelial lining surrounded by one or two layers of smooth muscle cells. No elastic layers are evident. The smallest arterioles provide a dynamic regulation of blood flow by controlling the distribution of blood in the capillary tree. The minute size of these vessels makes them susceptible to mechanical damage and rupture.

Capillaries

The smallest blood vessels, the capillaries, consist of endothelium supported only by sparse smooth muscle cells. The capillary endothelium provides for the interchange of solutes and cells between the blood and the extracellular fluid. A necessary feature of this exchange is a marked reduction in pressure, compared with that prevailing in the

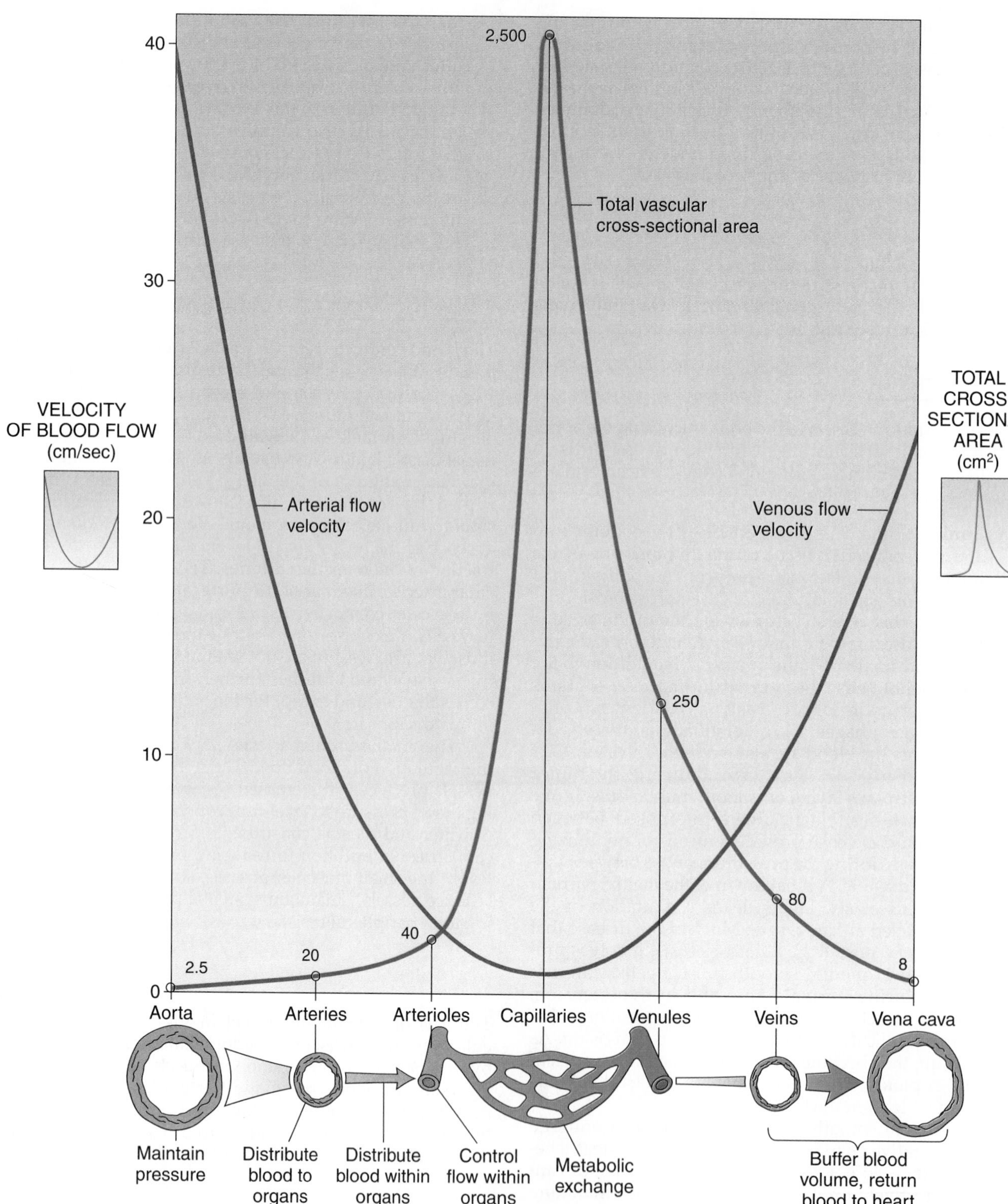

FIGURE *10-4*

Relationship between velocity of blood flow and cross-sectional area in the vasculature. The vascular tree is a circuit that conducts blood from the heart through large-diameter, low-resistance conducting vessels to small arteries and arterioles, which lower blood pressure and protect the capillaries. The capillaries are thin-walled and allow the exchange of nutrients and waste products between tissue and blood, a process that requires a very large surface area. The circuit back to the heart is completed by the veins, which are distensible and provide a volume buffer that acts as a capacitance for the vascular circuit.

feeding arteries and arterioles. Without this change, the filtration pressure across the capillaries would be so high that all of the vascular fluid would be quickly shifted into the extracellular space. On the other hand, if the capillary wall had a thick tunica media, no exchange would occur, because the distance between the exchange surface of the endothelium and the extravascular tissue would be excessive. **The compromise is a low-pressure capillary adapted to exchange across the endothelium by filtration and diffusion.**

The capillary endothelium acts as a semipermeable membrane, in which the exchange of plasma solutes with extracellular fluid is controlled by molecular size and charge. The endothelium also plays an active metabolic role as follows:

- It synthesizes factors that influence the surrounding cells.
- It modifies molecules in transit across the endothelium.
- It participates in the inflammatory response by synthesizing inflammatory mediators.

Pericytes are modified smooth muscle cells that surround the capillaries and share a basement membrane that envelopes the endothelial cells and the pericyte, thereby bringing the two cells into close contact (see Fig. 10-1). The functions of pericytes are largely unknown. The adventitia of the capillary merges with the surrounding connective tissue and cannot be distinguished from it.

The permeability of capillaries depends on the ultrastructure of their endothelial cells. Brain capillaries are highly impermeable. Their endothelium has tightly sealed junctions between individual cells, which prevent the exchange of proteins across the vessel wall. Transport in other capillary beds is mediated either by the passage of molecules through incomplete cell junctions or by micropinocytosis, a process by which molecules traverse the cytoplasm through vesicular transport in a "bucket brigade" fashion.

Some researchers believe that little transport occurs by way of micropinocytosis. Rather, they contend, vesicles are connected with each other, thereby providing a channel for direct transport of plasma proteins across the cytoplasm. In some locations, the endothelium itself may be fenestrated. It may have permanent channels across the endothelium, or it may exhibit discontinuous gaps between endothelial cells. Fenestrated capillaries in the renal glomerulus are specifically adapted to filter plasma. The liver sinusoids, which are not true capillaries, also show a fenestrated endothelium, which permits free access of the plasma to the liver cell. Pathological changes in the structure of the capillary and venular endothelium result in the accumulation of excess fluid in the interstitial space, that is, edema (see Chapter 7).

Veins

The venous system comprises the vessels that return blood from the capillaries to the heart. The venules are the first vessels that collect blood from the capillaries. The thin media of the venule is appropriate for a vessel that is not required to withstand a high luminal pressure. Only few pericytes are associated with the venules.

Venules merge into **small and medium-sized veins,** which in turn converge into **large veins**. The walls of large veins do not display the characteristic elastic lamellae of elastic arteries, and even the internal elastic lamina is well developed only in the largest veins. The media tends to thin and is virtually absent in the smaller tributaries. Many veins, particularly those in the extremities, have valves formed by endothelial-lined folds of the tunica intima. These structures prevent backflow and assist in the transport of blood under the low-pressure conditions of the venous circulation.

Lymphatics

The lymphatic vessels are composed essentially of endothelium. This set of channels drains interstitial fluid that has filtered through the capillaries and venules endothelium from the plasma. The lymphatics act as a pathway to the regional lymph nodes for cells, foreign material, and microorganisms. Lymph is returned to the circulation by the pumping action of lymphatic vessels containing smooth muscle cells in the wall.

HEMOSTASIS AND THROMBOSIS

Hemostasis *is defined as the arrest of hemorrhage and is a response to vascular injury.* This process involves vasoconstriction, tissue swelling, coagulation, and thrombosis.

Thrombosis *refers to the formation of a blood clot in the circulation.* A thrombus is an aggregate of coagulated blood that contains platelets, fibrin, leukocytes, and red blood cells.

The hemostatic system is an exquisitely controlled mechanism whose main function is to prevent blood loss following injury. The complex system that controls hemostasis is (1) a network of activating and inactivating enzymes, and (2) co-factors derived from different cells and tissues, some circulating and some locally produced. Some coagulation factors were originally named for the first patient found with a deficiency of the factor or for the discoverer of the disease. Current nomenclature, for the most part, uses number designations for the factors in the cascade (Table 10-2). The disorders of hemostasis are discussed in detail in Chapter 20.

The hemostatic complex can be divided into several functional areas that combine coagulation of blood proteins and aggregation of platelets to form a hemostatic "plug." Contact activation of factors required for coagulation include:

- Blood coagulation
- Platelet aggregation
- Endothelial cell interactions

It is important to understand the difference between coagulation and thrombosis. Coagulation can occur *in vitro*, for example, in a test tube, solely as a result of the activation of the clotting cascade. By contrast, thrombosis is the formation of a blood clot *in situ*. Thrombosis also in-

TABLE 10-2 **Coagulation Factor Designations**

Factor	Standard Name	Alternative Designations
I	Fibrinogen	
II	Prothrombin	
III	Tissue factor	Thromboplastin
IV	Calcium ions	
V	Proaccelerin	Labile factor, accelerator globulin (AcG), thrombogen
(VI)		No longer considered in the scheme of hemostasis
VII	Proconvertin	Stable factor, serum prothrombin conversion accelerator (SPCA)
VIII	Antihemophilic factor (AHF)	Antihemophilic globulin (AHG), antihemophilic factor A, platelet co-factor 1, thromboplastinogen
IX	Plasma thromboplastin (PTC)	Christmas factor, antihemophilic factor B, autoprothrombin II, platelet co-factor 2
X	Stuart factor	Prower factor, autoprothrombin III, thrombokinase
XI	Plasma thromboplastin antecedent (PTA)	Antihemophilic factor C
XII	Hageman factor	Glass factor, contact factor
XIII	Fibrin stabilizing factor (FSF)	Laki-Lorand factor (LLF), fibrinase, plasma transglutaminase, fibrinoligase
—	Prekallikrein	Fletcher factor
—	HMW kininogen	High-molecular-weight kininogen, contact activation cofactor, Fitzgerald factor, Williams factor, Flaujeac factor, Reid factor, Washington factor

volves (1) the adherence and aggregation of platelets, (2) the participation of cellular elements of the monocyte-macrophage system, and (3) active paraticipation of endothelial cells.

Blood Coagulation

Coagulation of blood entails the conversion of soluble plasma fibrinogen to an insoluble fibrillar polymer, fibrin, a reaction catalyzed by the proteolytic enzyme thrombin. It is intuitively evident that this event cannot represent a sudden process, since the entire circulation might be converted into a massive clot. Instead, a series of finely tuned steps mediated by a number of coagulation factors (Table 10-2), many of which are restricted by specific inhibitors, amplifies the initial signal into the eventual generation of thrombin. **The production of thrombin is probably the most important factor in the progression and stabilization of the thrombus.**

Historically, the coagulation cascade was divided into two arms, termed the "intrinsic" and "extrinsic" pathways. The intrinsic pathway was so-named because blood clotting could be initiated without the addition of an extrinsic trigger and required only contact of factor XII with a thrombogenic surface. By contrast, the extrinsic pathway depended on the fact that *in vivo* coagulation requires the exposure of blood to an extravascular (subendothelial) "tissue factor" (TF). However, it is today recognized that this partition of the coagulation cascade into

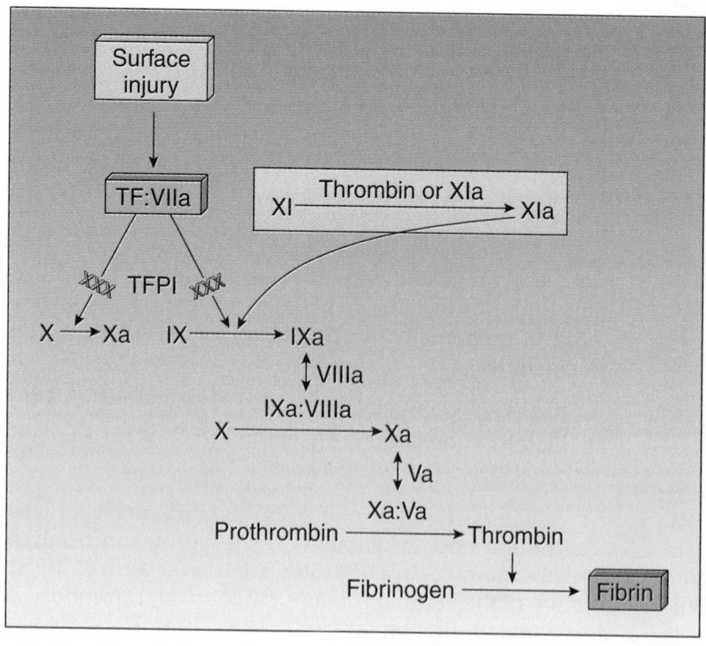

FIGURE 10-5
Coagulation cascade. The coagulation cascade is initiated by endothelial injury, which releases tissue factor. The latter combines with activated factor VII (VIIa) to form a complex that activates small amounts of X to Xa and IX to IXa. The complex of IXa with VIIIa further activates X. The complex of Xa with Va then catalyzes the conversion of prothrombin to thrombin, after which fibrin is formed from fibrinogen.

two distinct arms is arbitrary and does not accurately reflect the underlying mechanisms of clotting.

The current view of the coagulation cascade (Fig. 10-5) holds that the association of factor VIIa-TF complexes with TF pathway inhibitor (TFPI) is crucial to the generation of a thrombus. The initiation of hemostasis takes place when factor VII, or activated factor VII (VIIa), in the blood encounters TF at the site of injury. As a result, small amounts of factors X and IX are activated to form Xa and IXa. The activation of larger amounts of X to Xa is promoted by factor VIIIa and IXa. Traces of thrombin catalyze the activation of factor XI, which in turn augments the conversion of factor IX to IXa. The complex of IXa and VIII converts larger amounts of factor X to Xa. Xa then binds Va to form a complex that converts prothrombin to thrombin. Besides its important role in the coagulation cascade and in platelet aggregation, thrombin modulates numerous endothelial cell functions, including the production of fibrinolytic molecules and the regulation of growth factors and leukocyte adhesion molecules. Thrombin also increases endothelial permeability through alterations in cell shape.

Platelet Adhesion and Aggregation

The circulating cellular element most intimately involved with injury to the blood vessel is the platelet. When vessels are injured, platelets interact with one another to form a platelet thrombus, that is, an aggregate of activated platelets (Fig. 10-6). These platelet aggregates occlude injured small vessels and prevent the leakage of blood.

Once platelets are stimulated to adhere to the vessel wall, their granular contents are released. In turn, these contents promote aggregation with new platelets. **Adhesion** is enhanced by the release of von Willebrand factor; this substance is adhesive for Gp1b platelet membrane protein and for fibrinogen. Activated platelets also release ADP and thromboxane A_2, which recruit additional platelets, thereby causing changes in platelet shape, release of granule contents, and more aggregation. The platelet membrane protein complex GpIIb-IIIa adheres to fibrinogen, a process that tends to enhance aggregation and stabilize the forming thrombus. Activated platelets, in turn, release factors that initiate clotting, resulting in the formation of a complex thrombus on the vessel wall. Thrombin itself is sufficient to stimulate further release of platelet granules and the subsequent recruitment of new platelets.

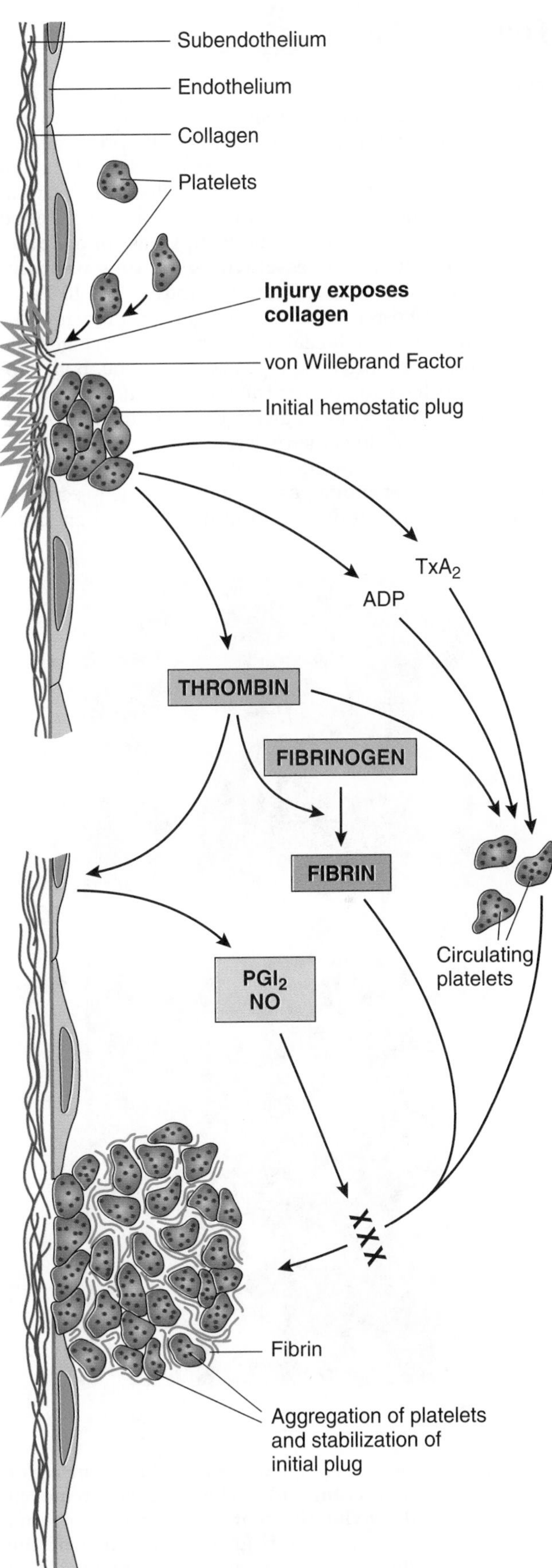

FIGURE *10-6*
The role of platelets in thrombosis. Following vessel wall injury and alteration in flow, platelets adhere and then aggregate. Adenosine diphosphate and thromboxane A_2 are released and, along with locally generated thrombin, recruit additional platelets, causing the mass to enlarge. The growing platelet thrombus is stabilized by fibrin. Other elements, including leukocytes and red blood cells, are also incorporated into the thrombus. The release of prostacyclin (PGI_2) and nitric oxide (NO) by endothelial cells regulates the process by inhibiting platelet aggregation.

Endothelial Factors

The major initiating event for most coagulation and thrombosis is some form of injury to the endothelium (see Fig. 10-6). Thrombus formation is normally prevented by blood flow and the antithrombotic properties of the endothelium. Thrombi form when endothelial function is altered, when endothelial continuity is lost, or when blood flow is altered or becomes static. **Simple loss of endothelial cells or injury to a vessel with good flow produces platelet pavementing, but not thrombosis** (Fig. 10-7).

For thrombosis to occur, endothelial continuity must be disrupted or the endothelial cell surface must change from an anticoagulant surface to a procoagulant one. Both processes are believed to occur. The most common denuding endothelial injury is the progressive disruption of endothelium by an advancing atherosclerotic lesion. Denuding endothelial injury has also been described in other conditions (e.g., in homocysteinuria), as a response to the injection of radiological contrast dyes, and in hypoxia and endotoxemia. Endothelial injury and denudation also occur during various therapies for atherosclerotic disease, including the construction of saphenous vein bypass grafts, angioplasty and atherectomy, and the insertion of stents. In addition, the interactions of a thrombus with the underlying endothelium may cause a further disturbance of endothelial integrity. For example, fibrin applied to the superficial surface of an endothelial cell in culture causes a marked change in cell shape. **Thrombin also initiates endothelial shape changes and promotes disruption of endothelial integrity.** Finally, inflammatory agents, including cytokines released from monocytes, activate procoagulant activities on the surface of an intact endothelium.

Why are blood vessels not normally thrombogenic? The simplest view is that subendothelial thrombogenic molecules are covered by a nonthrombogenic cell layer—the endothelium. According to this view, in the same way that platelets do not aggregate with other blood elements, they also do not aggregate with endothelial cells; there is thus no need for a specific inhibitory mechanism.

It is now apparent, however, that the endothelium plays an active rather than a passive role in the control of thrombosis (Table 10-3). It has been suggested that the major antithrombotic mechanism of the endothelium is the secretion of prostaglandin I_2, also known as prostacyclin. This molecule may actually have a minor role, and several other features of the endothelium support its antithrombotic activity. Endothelial cells metabolize ADP, which is a strong promoter of thrombogenesis, although its metabolites are antithrombogenic. The luminal

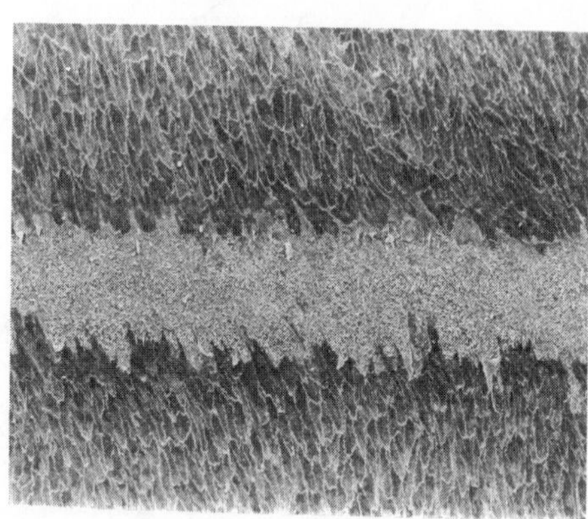

A

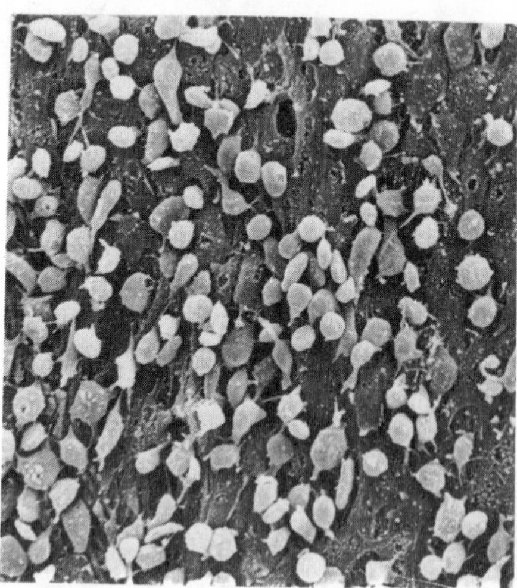

B

FIGURE *10-7*
Scanning electron micrograph of the endothelial surface of a rat aorta 1 hour after the endothelial cells were removed by scraping with a nylon filament. (*A*) Intact endothelium and scratched portion. (*B*) Higher-power view of the scratched area showing a pavement of intact platelets that adheres to the underlying connective tissue in the high-velocity arterial stream.

TABLE *10-3* **Regulation of Coagulation at the Endothelial Cell Surface**

Down-Regulation

1. Thrombin inactivators
   a. Antithrombin III
   b. Thrombomodulin
2. Activated protein C pathway
   a. Synthesis and expression of thrombomodulin
   b. Synthesis and expression of protein S
   c. Thrombomodulin-mediated activation of protein C
   d. Inactivation of factor V_a and factor VIII_a by APC-protein S complex
3. Tissue factor pathway inhibition
4. Fibrinolysis
   a. Synthesis of tissue plasminogen activator, urokinase plasminogen activator, and plasminogen activator inhibitor 1
   b. Conversion of GLU-plasminogen to LYS-plasminogen
   c. APC-mediated potentiation
5. Synthesis of unsaturated fatty acid metabolites
   a. Lipoxygenase metabolites-13-HODE
   b. Cyclo-oxygenase metabolites-PGI_2 and PGE_2

Procoagulant Pathways

1. Synthesis and expression of:
   a. Tissue factor (thromboplastin)
   b. Factor V
   c. Platelet activating factor (PAF)
2. Binding of clotting factors IX/IX_a, X (prothrombinase complex)
3. Down-regulation of APC pathway
4. Increased synthesis of plasminogen activator inhibitor
5. Synthesis of 15-HPETE

surface of the endothelium is coated with heparan sulfate. There is no direct evidence that this substance participates directly in the inhibition of blood clotting, as does exogenous heparin, but heparan sulfate does bind a number of clotting factors, including the antiprotease α_2-macroglobulin. Endothelial cells may also lyse some clots as they form. In addition, they may take up vasoactive amines released from platelets at the site of thrombosis. Similarly, endothelial cells may limit coagulation by consuming thrombin created during the procoagulant process.

There are several other more specific endothelial anticoagulant mechanisms. A co-factor on the endothelial cell surface inactivates thrombin by forming a complex with it and antithrombin 3, a plasma antiprotease. Thrombin itself activates protein C through an interaction with its receptor, called thrombomodulin, which is located on the surface of endothelial cells. Both protein C and thrombomodulin are synthesized by endothelial cells. Activated protein C destroys coagulation factors V and VIII. Tissue factor pathway inhibitor is thought to be bound to endothelium, where it is generated during coagulation and inhibits the tissue factor: VIIa complex.

Thus, the formation of a thrombus is a dynamic process within the vascular system that involves a "tug of war" between factors that promote thrombosis, and those that inhibit it. The presence of these antithrombotic mechanisms on the endothelial surface has raised the intriguing possibility that endothelial dysfunction alone might lead to thrombosis. There is also evidence that endothelial cells have prothrombotic functions. At least in culture, endothelial cells synthesize von Willebrand factor, which promotes platelet adherence and activates clotting factor V. Cultured endothelial cells also bind factors IX and X, a process that favors coagulation on the endothelial surface *in vivo*. Finally, endothelial cells treated with IL-1 or tumor necrosis factor (TNF) present thromboplastin to the plasma, thereby potentially initiating coagulation through the extrinsic pathway. Thus, one can envision that procoagulant injuries at the surface of blood vessels are produced either by the loss of a normal endothelial function or by the stimulation of an abnormal one.

Clot Lysis

A thrombus may undergo several fates, including (1) lysis, (2) growth and propagation, (3) embolization, or (4) organization and canalization. The combination of aggregated platelets and clotted blood is made unstable by the activation of the fibrinolytic enzyme plasmin (Fig. 10-8). During clot formation, plasminogen is bound to fibrin and, therefore, is an integral part of the forming platelet mass. Endothelial cells synthesize plasminogen activator, but in larger thrombi circulating plasminogen may also be converted to plasmin by products of the coagulation cascade. Plasminogen activator bound to fibrin activates plasmin. In turn, by digesting fibrin, plasmin lyses the clots and disrupts the thrombus. The synthesis of plasminogen activator represents still another antithrombotic mechanism of the endothelial cell. Endothelial cells also synthesize an inhibitor of plasminogen activator. Thus, this cell again displays both procoagulant and anticoagulant properties. The ultimate defense against clot lysis is the inhibition of plasmin itself by α2-antiplasmin.

ATHEROSCLEROSIS

Atherosclerosis is a disease of large and medium-sized arteries that results in the progressive accumulation within the intima of smooth muscle cells, lipids, and connective tissue. The con-

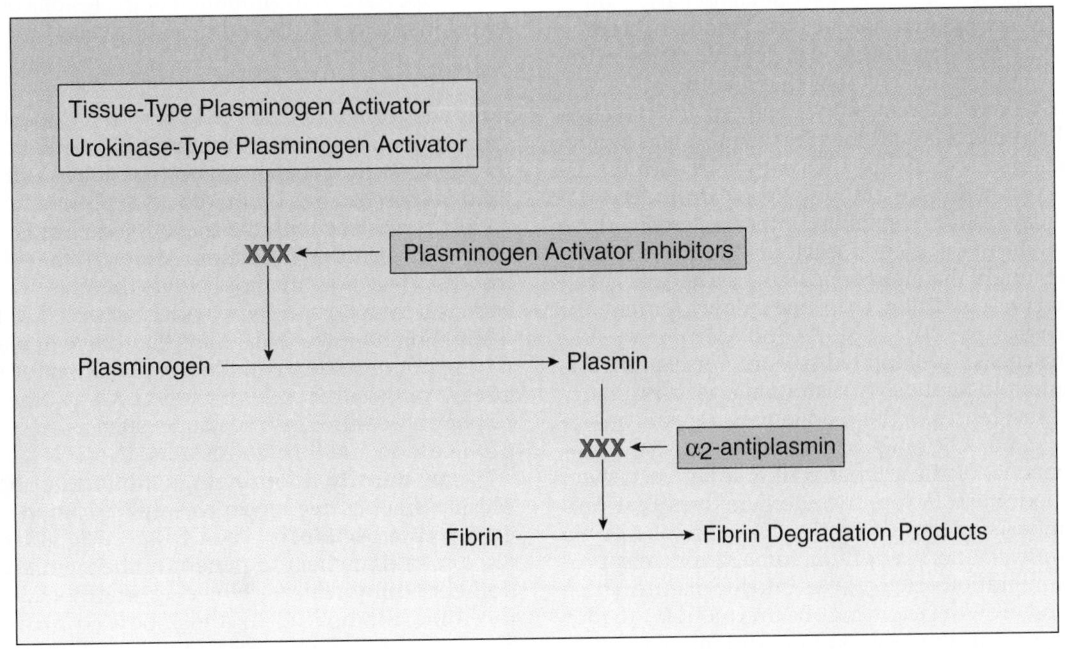

FIGURE *10-8*
Mechanisms of fibrinolysis. Plasmin formed from plasminogen lyses fibrin. The conversion of plasminogen to plasmin and the activity of plasmin itself are suppressed by specific inhibitors.

tinued growth of the lesions encroaches on other layers of the arterial wall and narrows the lumen of the vessel. **The major complications of atherosclerosis, including ischemic heart disease, myocardial infarction, stroke, and gangrene of the extremities, account for more than half of the annual mortality in the United States.** In fact, ischemic heart disease is by itself the leading cause of death. The incidence of ischemic heart disease in the United States and other Western countries rose progressively from the turn of the century to a peak in the late 1960s, but subsequently it has fallen by more than 30%. There are wide geographic and racial variations in the incidence of ischemic heart disease. For example, the mortality from ischemic heart disease is eightfold higher in Sweden than it is in Japan.

□ Pathogenesis and Pathology:

Atherosclerotic lesions, referred to as atherosclerotic plaques, atheromas, fibrous plaques or fibrofatty lesions, develop in the tunica intima of elastic and muscular arteries as a result of two critical processes: the proliferation of intimal smooth muscle cells and the accumulation of lipid. As the lesion forms, the intima comes to contain smooth muscle cells, macrophages, lymphocytes, and connective tissue. Later, as the lesion advances, the endothelium breaks down and platelets are deposited. In a more advanced stage, small capillaries penetrate the vessel wall, vascularizing the plaque with endothelialized channels. The expansion of this lesion, together with thrombosis, produces the final clinical result, namely, occlusion of a distributing artery. Thus, the pathogenesis of the atherosclerotic plaque is a dynamic process that usually occurs over several decades.

No current theory adequately accounts for the fact that blood vessels in some persons conduct blood for a lifetime with little or no evidence of arterial disease, whereas in others vascular lesions develop early, sometimes with catastrophic consequences. Another puzzling problem is the fact that lesions develop much more frequently in some anatomic regions than in others.

An early (and oversimplified) view of the development of atherosclerosis held that the disorder was simply the deposition of excess lipid from the circulation. Although animals fed large amounts of fat do indeed develop vascular lesions resembling atherosclerosis, these lesions contain many elements other than lipids. Currently, it is thought that lipid deposition is a necessary but not sufficient condition for the development of atherosclerosis.

The presence of proliferated smooth muscle cells has called attention to peptides that stimulate their proliferation. Other substances in the plaque may also act as signals that trigger a wide range of responses among the resident components of the arterial wall and between them and the blood. Such factors include cytokines that promote thrombosis or that cause the death of cells in the atherosclerotic plaque. In addition, some factors may promote the immigration of leukocytes into the plaque. These cytokines and growth factors may be produced by all four cell types found in the lesions. In addition, growth inhibitors for smooth muscle cells may be produced. Both genetic and hemodynamic factors could modify these responses, and we need at this point to consider the main elements that are involved in the production of an atherosclerotic plaque.

- **The vascular endothelium** interacts with macromolecules and formed elements of the blood and plays a role in the transport of plasma proteins.
- **The arterial smooth muscle cell** is important in (1) the control of artery wall tone, (2) maintenance and repair of the vessel wall, (3) the metabolism of various blood-borne substances, including lipids, and (4) the secretion of various cytokines.
- **The mononuclear phagocyte** (macrophage) has many functions, including the uptake of low-density lipoproteins (LDL) and the secretion of various hydrolases and cytokines.
- **Lymphocytes** may participate in autoimmune reactions, such as may occur with viral infections in vessels of transplanted organs. Neutrophils are involved in the response to tissue injury.

Recent studies have shown that proliferative activity in macrophages and smooth muscle cells occurs in the atherosclerotic plaque. Smooth muscle replication is at a very low level, suggesting that the proliferation of these cells may be only an early part of lesion formation or may be episodic.

Atherogenic Processes

At least six hypotheses have been proposed to explain the origins of atherosclerotic plaques. It deserves emphasis that these hypotheses are not mutually exclusive, and numerous experimental and clinical observations have shown how the processes highlighted in one theory are linked with those of another. Viewed in this light, most of the controversy lies in opinions as to which process is most important in the initiation of the lesions or their progression into clinically significant disease.

INSUDATION HYPOTHESIS: Conventional wisdom has for some years held that the critical events in atherosclerosis center on the focal accumulation of fat in the vessel wall. The insudation hypothesis states that the lipid in these lesions is derived from plasma lipoproteins, a view consistent with the role of blood lipids as risk factors for myocardial infarction. Although there is still controversy over how the lipid enters the vessel wall, the insudation hypothesis is now widely accepted. Whereas the insudation hypothesis explains the source of plaque lipid, it does not provide a complete explanation for the pathogenesis of the atherosclerotic lesion. Many other clinically important features of the plaque, such as smooth muscle proliferation and thrombosis, remain unexplained.

Low-density lipoprotein is the form of lipid in the plasma that has been most closely associated with accelerated atherosclerosis. The LDL particle is far too large (20 nm in diameter) to penetrate the tightly closed endothelial cell junctions. However, endothelial cells have receptors for both LDL and modified forms of LDL. Transport can occur across an intact endothelium either by receptor-mediated uptake of lipoprotein or by nonspecific uptake into micropinocytic channels. Alternatively, lipid may be engulfed by macrophages in the blood and then transported into the vascular wall inside these cells.

ENCRUSTATION HYPOTHESIS: A theory first suggested in the 19th century asserted that material from the blood is deposited on the inner surface of arteries and leads to thickening of the inner lining. At the time that this suggestion was made, the details of the clotting mechanisms and the functions of platelets in thrombosis were unknown. A modern version of this idea holds that small mural thrombi represent the initial event in atherosclerosis. Organization of these thrombi leads to the formation of plaques, and the expansion of these lesions reflects repeated episodes of thrombosis and organization.

We now know from experimental studies of hyperlipidemic animals, and from autopsy studies of children, that the mural thrombus is not the initial event in atherogenesis. However, mural thrombosis is a critical part of the later progression of the atherosclerotic lesion and is the major event leading to vascular occlusion, especially in coronary arteries.

REACTION TO INJURY HYPOTHESIS: This theory attempts to explain the accumulation of smooth muscle cells in atherosclerotic lesions. It is held that smooth muscle proliferation depends on the release of polypeptide growth factors by endothelial cells and monocytes, and by smooth muscle cells themselves, that accumulate at sites of injury. This theory has been broadened to focus on the role of the cells found in the artery wall in the initiation and growth of an atherosclerotic lesion. Thus, endothelial dysfunction is considered to be an important event. It results in loss of the integrity of the endothelial barrier to macromolecules and in the activation of leukocyte adhesion molecules to promote macrophage deposition in the subendothelium.

The "reaction to injury" hypothesis evolved from the discovery that the growth of smooth muscle cells in culture requires one or more platelet-derived polypeptides. The best known of these is platelet-derived growth factor (PDGF), which is secreted by both macrophages and vascular wall cells. This factor is not only mitogenic for smooth muscle cells *in vitro*, but is also chemotactic for them. Thus, in addition to stimulating the proliferation of cells already located in the intima, PDGF may recruit smooth muscle cells from the media. The number of growth factors that can potentially induce proliferation of cells in culture has multiplied. These include FGF, PDGF, transforming growth factor-beta (TGF-β), thrombin, LDL, endothelin, and others. There are also growth inhibitors, such as heparin and NO.

The "reaction to injury" hypothesis points to a mechanism for smooth muscle proliferation. It has recently been modified to suggest that the cellular responses that occur during the pathogenesis of the fibrofatty lesion constitute an inflammatory and fibroproliferative response to injury.

MONOCLONAL HYPOTHESIS: The monoclonal concept is also focused on smooth muscle proliferation and was originally derived from the observation that the fibrous caps of atherosclerotic plaques (see later) are composed of smooth muscle cells. Furthermore, these cells appear to migrate from the underlying media and then proliferate. Can the lesion, therefore, arise as an aberration of growth control in one, or at most a few cells, in a manner analogous to the process in a benign smooth muscle tumor such as a leiomyoma? On the other hand, might it not arise from the polyclonal proliferation of many cells, as would be expected in a healing wound?

Based on studies of women who are mosaic for X-linked markers, it has been established that many plaques are monoclonal, that is, they originate from one or very few smooth muscle cells. This interpretation has been criticized on the grounds that the marker may be linked to another gene that provides the smooth muscle cells with a selective growth advantage, without the atherosclerotic lesion being monoclonal in origin. The monoclonality of the fibrous cap suggests that some unknown etiological factor, perhaps circulating mutagens or viruses, might induce cap formation by altering growth control in the smooth muscle cells of the arterial wall. Although research has been done on the possible role of viruses in the pathogenesis of atherosclerosis, particularly herpesvirus and cytomegalovirus, a cause and effect relationship has yet to be established.

INTIMAL CELL MASS AND NEOINTIMA FORMATION HYPOTHESIS: The location of atherosclerotic lesions has been related to the focal accumulation of smooth muscle cells in the normal intima at branch points and other sites in certain vessels, particularly the coronary arteries. Intimal cell masses or neointimal thickening are found in infancy and are more pronounced in male infants. They occur in the vessels of persons of varying ethnicity and geographic location, irrespective of the incidence of atherosclerosis. The distribution of intimal cell masses in children resembles the distribution of atherosclerotic lesions in adults. Intimal cell masses in animals fed high-fat diets develop into lesions that display many of the characteristics of fully developed human atherosclerotic lesions. These observations suggest that the intimal cell mass is either the early lesion of atherosclerosis or a precursor of it.

Little is known about the development of the intimal cell mass, its growth potential, or its clonality. If the intimal cell mass is indeed the precursor of atherosclerosis, it is probable that all humans are susceptible to this disease. In that case, we would view other factors, such as hyperlipidemia or hypertension, as critical for the progression of the disease to a clinically significant state.

HEMODYNAMIC HYPOTHESIS: The role of hemodynamics in the origin of atherosclerosis is frequently mentioned, and certain observations are compatible with the concept that elevated blood pressure enhances the process. The distribution of atherosclerotic lesions in large vessels, and the differences in location and frequency of lesions in different vascular beds, has encouraged a belief in the role of hemodynamic factors. In humans, atherosclerotic lesions tend to occur at sites where shear stresses are low but rapidly fluctuating, whereas in rabbit models of hypercholesterolemia, areas exposed to high shear are at risk for lesion formation. The fact that hypertension enhances the severity of atherosclerotic lesions in various systems, and that low blood pressure is generally associated with increased longevity, further encourages the idea that hemodynamic factors somehow play a role in the development of sclerotic vascular disease.

An example of the role of hypertension in large arteries is seen in the pulmonary artery, which rarely exhibits atherosclerosis. In cases of pulmonary hypertension, typical fibrous atheromatous plaques can be found in the pulmonary artery and its major branches. The demonstration that shear-stress affects endothelial cell structure and function adds support to the concept that hemodynamic factors may promote endothelial cell dysfunction and accelerate the development of atherosclerotic lesions. For example, hemodynamic forces have been shown to induce gene expression of several factors in endothelial cells that are likely to promote atherosclerosis, including FGF-2, tissue factor, plasminogen activator, and endothelin. Shear stress also induces gene expression of agents that may be antiatherogenic, including nitric oxide synthase (NOS) and plasminogen activator inhibitor-1 (PAI-1).

A Unifying Hypothesis

To tie the foregoing concepts together, we can construct a hypothetical sequence divided into three stages, namely, formation, adaptation, and the clinical stage (Fig. 10-9):

1. The intimal lesion initially occurs at sites that are predisposed to lesion formation, owing to endothelial dysfunction or the accumulation of subendothelial smooth muscle cells, such as occurs in an intimal cell mass or an intimal thickening at branch points. In persons at increased risk of atherosclerosis, lesions also occur in nonpredisposed areas.
2. Lipid accumulation in these foci depends on disruption of the integrity of the endothelial barrier or the properties of intimal smooth muscle cells. The types of connective tissue synthesized by the cells in the intima render these sites prone to lipid accumulation. Lipid insudation in these accumulations of intimal cells produces cell injury, thereby leading to the accumulation of macrophages by upregulation of leukocyte adhesion molecules and disruption of the tight integrity of the endothelial barrier.
3. In turn, the macrophages release growth factors, as proposed in the "reaction to injury" hypothesis. Mononuclear macrophages may play a central role by participating in lipid accumulation and releasing growth factors, thereby stimulating further accumulation of smooth muscle cells. Oxidized lipoproteins promote tissue damage and further macrophage accumulation.

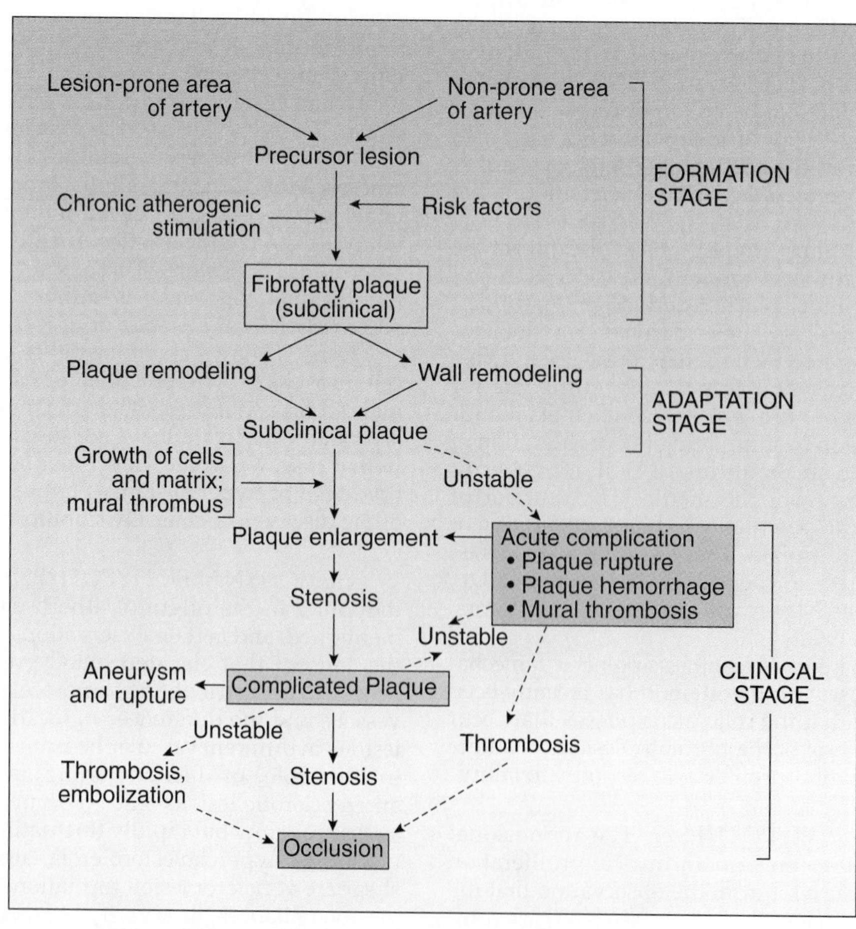

FIGURE 10-9
A unifying hypothesis for the pathogenesis of atherosclerosis.

4. As the lesion progresses, endothelial injury leads to the loss of the anticoagulant properties of the normal wall. The resulting mural thrombosis stimulates the release of PDGF and further accelerates smooth muscle proliferation and the secretion of matrix components. The thrombus becomes organized and is incorporated into the plaque.

   The intima is thickened so that its deeper parts are poorly nourished and undergo necrosis, an event augmented by proteolytic enzymes released by macrophages and tissue damage caused by oxidized LDL and other agents.

   The fibrofatty plaque is formed, angiogenesis promotes vascularization of the plaque, and the plaque becomes heterogeneous with respect to inflammatory cell infiltration and matrix organization.
5. The artery adapts to the atherosclerotic plaque. As the lumen is encroached upon by the plaque (e.g., in coronary arteries), the wall of the artery undergoes remodeling to maintain the lumen size. Once a plaque encroaches upon half of the lumen, compensatory remodeling can no longer maintain the normal size of the lumen, which becomes narrowed (stenosis). Hemodynamic shear stress is an important regulator of vessel wall remodeling. It is likely that cell proliferation, apoptosis, and matrix synthesis and degradation are also important processes that modulate vascular remodeling in the face of atherosclerosis. It is also possible that the plaque itself undergoes remodeling.
6. Plaque progression continues as a dynamic process involving the smooth muscle cells, macrophages, lymphocytes, and matrix synthesis and degradation. Surface thrombi may be incorporated into the plaque. Hemorrhage into a plaque without rupture may increase its size.
7. Plaque complications develop, including surface ulceration, fissure formation, calcification, and aneurysm formation. Continued plaque growth leads to occlusion of the lumen. The catastrophic events of plaque rupture and ensuing thrombosis and occlusion occur in advanced plaques. However, recent angiographic studies suggest that plaques with even 50% stenosis may rupture. Factors that promote rupture of a plaque have been proposed to include (1) hemodynamic shear stress on the shoulder of the plaque, (2) inflammatory activity at the interface between an area of lipid deposition and fibrous tissue, and (3) the presence of metalloproteinases that digest connective tissue matrix.

Whether or not this theoretical scenario is entirely correct, some aspects of these hypotheses probably do operate as distinct processes during different phases of the development of an atherosclerotic plaque. Figure 10-9 shows how these hypotheses might interact over the course of early lesion development.

The Initial Lesion of Atherosclerosis

Two distinct lesions have been proposed as the initial structural abnormality of atherosclerosis.

FATTY STREAK: Fatty streaks are flat or slightly elevated lesions that contain accumulations of intracellular and extracellular lipid in the intima. Fatty streaks are found in young children, as well as in adults. In these simple focal lesions, cells filled with lipid droplets ("foam cells") accumulate (Fig. 10-10). A balanced view holds that the cells with the greatest amount of lipid are indeed macrophages, but that smooth muscle cells also contain fat.

In children who die accidentally, significant numbers of fatty streaks are usually evident in many parts of the arterial tree. However, these do not correspond to the distribution of atherosclerotic lesions in adults. For example, fatty spots are common in the thoracic aorta in children, but atherosclerosis in adults is typically prominent in the abdominal aorta. Nonetheless, many believe that fatty infiltration represents the initial lesion of atherosclerosis and that other factors control the distribution of the later and more clinically significant lesions.

INTIMAL CELL MASS: As we have already proposed (see Fig. 10-9), the intimal cell mass is an alternative candidate for the initial lesion of atherosclerosis. Intimal cell masses are white, thickened areas at branch points in the arterial tree. Microscopically, they contain smooth muscle cells and connective tissue but no lipid. The location of these lesions, also known as "cushions," at arterial branch sites correlates well with the location of later atherosclerotic lesions.

The concept of the intimal cell mass as the initial lesion is controversial. First, if it is indeed the initial lesion of atherosclerosis, then the very early stages of lesion development should be common to everyone, regardless of age. However, a gradual increase in the thickness of the intima occurs diffusely throughout large arteries as a normal part of aging, and for this reason many prefer to distinguish intimal thickening from atherosclerosis.

The Characteristic Lesion of Atherosclerosis

The characteristic lesion of atherosclerosis is the fibrofatty plaque (Fig. 10-11). On gross examination, simple plaques are elevated, pale yellow, smooth-surfaced lesions. They are focal in distribution and irregular in shape, but have well-defined borders. Fibrofatty plaques tend to be oval, with the larger diameter being 8 to 12 cm. In smaller vessels, such as the coronary or cerebral arteries, a plaque is often eccentric, that is, it occupies only part of the circumference of the lumen. In advanced stages, the fusion of plaques in muscular arteries can give rise to larger lesions, which occupy several square centimeters.

Microscopically, the plaque is initially covered by endothelium and tends to involve the intima and only very little of the upper media. The area between the lumen and the necrotic core, termed the **fibrous cap**, contains smooth muscle cells, monocytes, lymphocytes, lipid-laden cells (foam cells), and connective tissue components. The central core contains necrotic debris. Cholesterol crystals and foreign body giant cells may be present within the fibrous tissue and the necrotic areas. Foam cells are noted in this area and as focal groups within the tissue matrix. They consist of both macrophages (derived from blood mono-

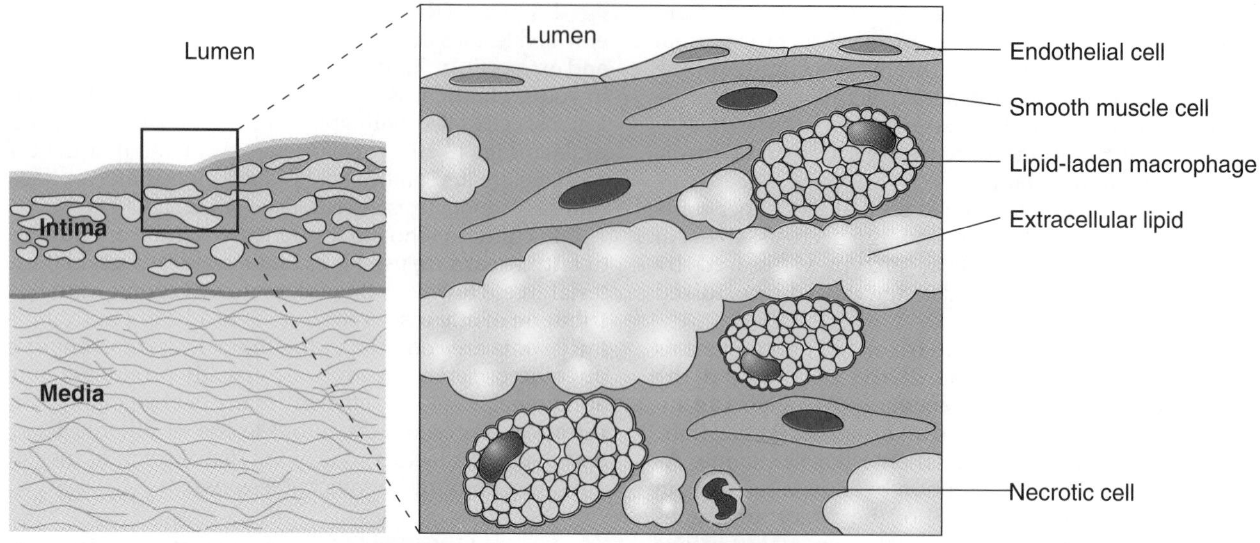

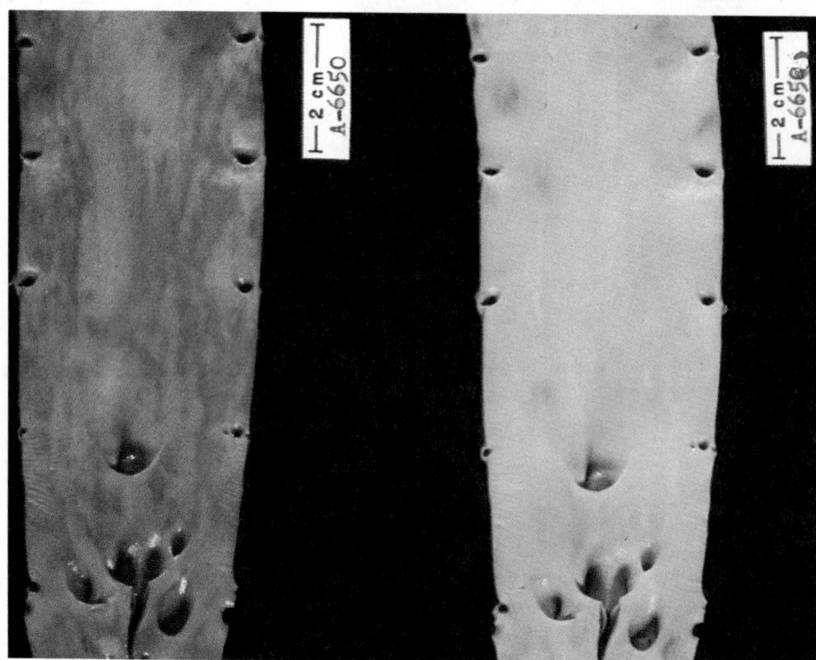

FIGURE 10-10
Fatty streak of atherosclerosis. (*A*) The fatty streak, composed largely of foamy macrophages, is presumed to be an early stage in the formation of atherosclerotic lesions. Note the intimal thickening in the left panel and the infiltrating cells in the enlargement on the right. (*B*) The aorta of a young man shows numerous fatty streaks on the luminal surface when stained with Sudan red. The unstained specimen is shown on the right.

cytes) and smooth muscle cells that have taken up lipids. Smooth muscle cells are also present throughout the plaque matrix. Numerous inflammatory and immune cells, especially T cells, are present within a plaque.

Neovascularization is an important contributor to plaque growth and the subsequent complications. It is postulated that vessels grow in from the vasa vasorum. They are rare in healthy coronary arteries, but plentiful in atherosclerotic plaques. Newly formed vessels are fragile and may rupture, resulting in an acute expansion of the plaque from intraplaque hemorrhage. Foci of hemosiderin-laden macrophages are often present in the plaque, indicating a remote plaque hemorrhage.

Complicated Plaques

The term complicated plaque describes several conditions: erosion, ulceration or fissuring of the surface of the plaque, plaque hemorrhage, mural thrombosis, calcification, and aneurysm (Fig. 10-12). Erosion, ulceration, and fissuring follow focal denudation of the surface endothelium.

Calcification occurs both in areas of necrosis and elsewhere in the plaque. The calcium compounds in the aortic tissue are hydroxyapatite-like and consist of calcium, phosphate, and carbonate. The crystals are often deposited on collagen fibrils and tend to be oriented in the same direction as the fibril.

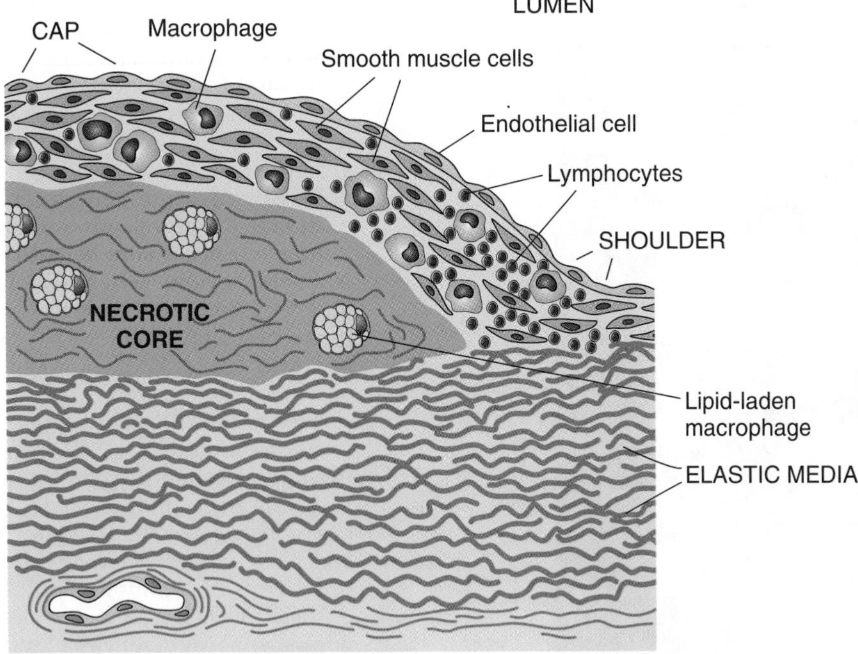

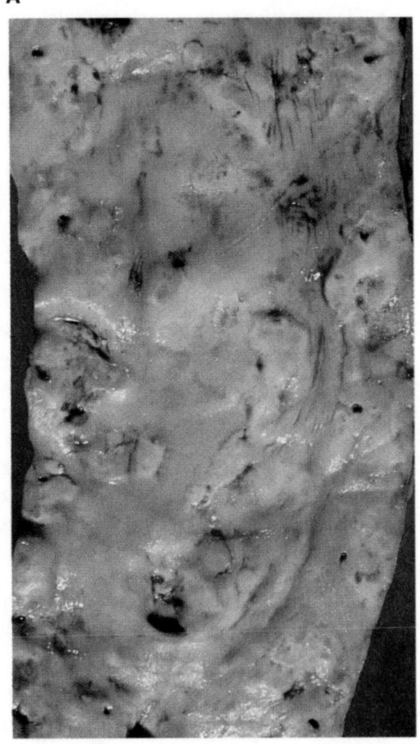

FIGURE *10-11*
Fibrofatty plaque of atherosclerosis. (*A*) In this fully developed fibrous plaque, the core contains lipid-filled macrophages and necrotic smooth muscle cell debris. The "fibrous" cap is composed largely of smooth muscle cells, which produce collagen, small amounts of elastin, and glycosaminoglycans. Also shown are infiltrating macrophages and lymphocytes. Note that the endothelium over the surface of the fibrous cap frequently appears intact. (*B*) The aorta shows discrete, raised, tan plaques. Focal plaque ulcerations are also evident.

Mural thrombosis results from disrupted blood flow around the plaque, at the site of its protrusion into the lumen. The disturbance in flow also causes damage to the endothelial lining, which may become locally denuded, no longer forming a thromboresistant surface. Mural thrombi in the proximal region of a coronary artery may embolize to more distal sites.

Plaque hemorrhage may result from tearing of the fibrous cap at the shoulder of the plaque or rupture of thin, newly formed vessels within the plaque. Plaque rupture has been associated with hemodynamic shear stress and with proteolytic enzymes found in the fibrous cap in areas of inflammation. Once the plaque ruptures, the thrombogenic material in the plaque promotes thrombosis in the lumen, resulting in the formation of an occlusive thrombus.

Progression from a simple fibrofatty atherosclerotic plaque to a complicated lesion may occur in some persons

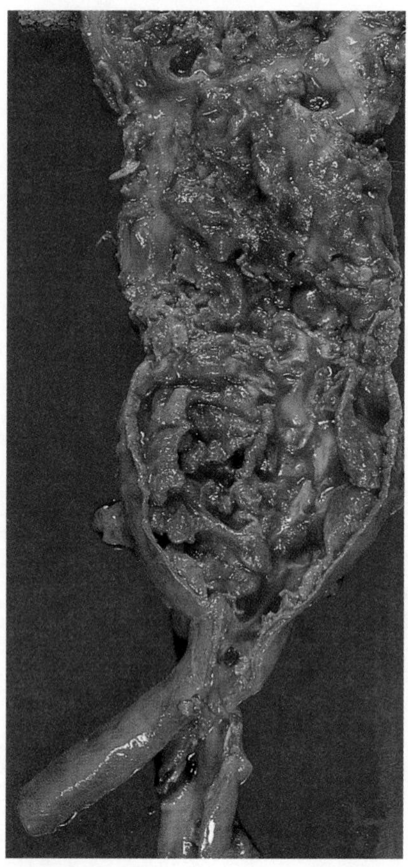

FIGURE 10-12
Complicated lesions of atherosclerosis. The luminal surface of the abdominal aorta and the common iliac arteries shows numerous fibrous plaques and raised, ulcerated lesions containing friable, atheromatous debris. The distal portion of the aorta displays a small aneurysmal dilatation.

while they are still in their 20s and in most people by 50 or 60 years of age. Although the simple lesions are clinically insignificant, they may progress to severe stenosis or occlusion in a short time, after which they are associated with angina pectoris or acute myocardial infarction.

The Mechanisms of Lesion Progression in Atherosclerosis

The sequence of events in the development of atherosclerosis may begin as early as the fetal stage, with the formation of intimal cell masses, or perhaps shortly after birth, when fatty streaks begin to evolve. However, the characteristic lesion, which is not clinically significant, requires as long as 20 to 30 years to form. Moreover, the clinically important complicated lesions emerge after several more decades of development (Fig. 10-13). Some of the factors and cellular processes that may contribute to the progression of the simple lesions to complicated ones are as follows (Fig. 10-14):

- **Cytokines:** A prominent factor in lesion progression is the macrophage, a cell that may participate even in the earliest events. In this context, a large part of the lipid that accumulates in lesions of fat-fed animals is found in the mononuclear macrophage. Once the macrophages are in the lesion, progression may depend on the inflammatory functions of the monocytes. For example, the monocyte synthesizes PDGF, FGF, TNF, IL-1, interferon-α, and TGF-β. Each of these can modulate the growth of smooth muscle or endothelial cells, either positively or negatively. Interferon and TGF-β inhibit cell proliferation and could account for the failure of endothelial cells to maintain continuity over the lesion. Alternatively, such growth inhibitors could exert a negative feedback effect in the presence of large amounts of growth-stimulatory peptides.

  Mediators secreted by monocytes and macrophages are also thought to change the functions of overlying endothelial cells in ways that may be important for lesion progression. Of particular interest is the discovery that IL-1 and TNF stimulate the expressions of platelet-activating factor, tissue factor, and plasminogen activator inhibitor by endothelial cells. Thus, the combination of monocytes and endothelial cells may be capable of transforming the normal anticoagulant vascular surface to a procoagulant one.
- **T lymphocytes**: Atherosclerotic plaques also contain T lymphocytes. The expression of HLA-DR antigens on both endothelial cells and smooth muscle cells in plaques implies that these cells have undergone some kind of immunological activation, perhaps in response to interferon-γ released by activated T cells in the plaque. It is possible that the presence of T cells reflects an autoimmune response that is important for the progression of atherosclerotic lesions.
- **Endothelium:** A loss of endothelial continuity on the luminal surface is another potential antecedent of plaque progression. Such damage would (1) increase the permeability of the wall to lipoproteins and, therefore, accelerate lipoprotein accumulation; (2) permit platelet interaction with the vessel wall and the subsequent release of growth factors, resulting in more rapid lesion progression; and (3) allow the formation of a thrombus on the surface of an atherosclerotic lesion.

  Endothelial-lined channels are found in many advanced plaques, and some fully developed vessels may be encountered within the muscular media, mainly in the shoulders of fibrous caps. The vessels in the plaque itself may derive from the vasa vasorum, but a large number appear to come from the proliferation of luminal endothelial cells. These vascular channels are a potential source of hemorrhage into plaques. Alternatively, blood may enter the plaque from the circulation through tears in its surface. The rupture of the fibrous cap of the plaque and the exposure of plaque contents to the circulation lead to the formation of a thrombus, which is most often occlusive.
- **Thrombosis:** The formation of a thrombus (Fig. 10-15) is the most common clinical event that leads to myocardial infarction, and an intervention aimed at dissolving such a thrombus can prevent or limit the size of an evolving myocardial infarction. Many

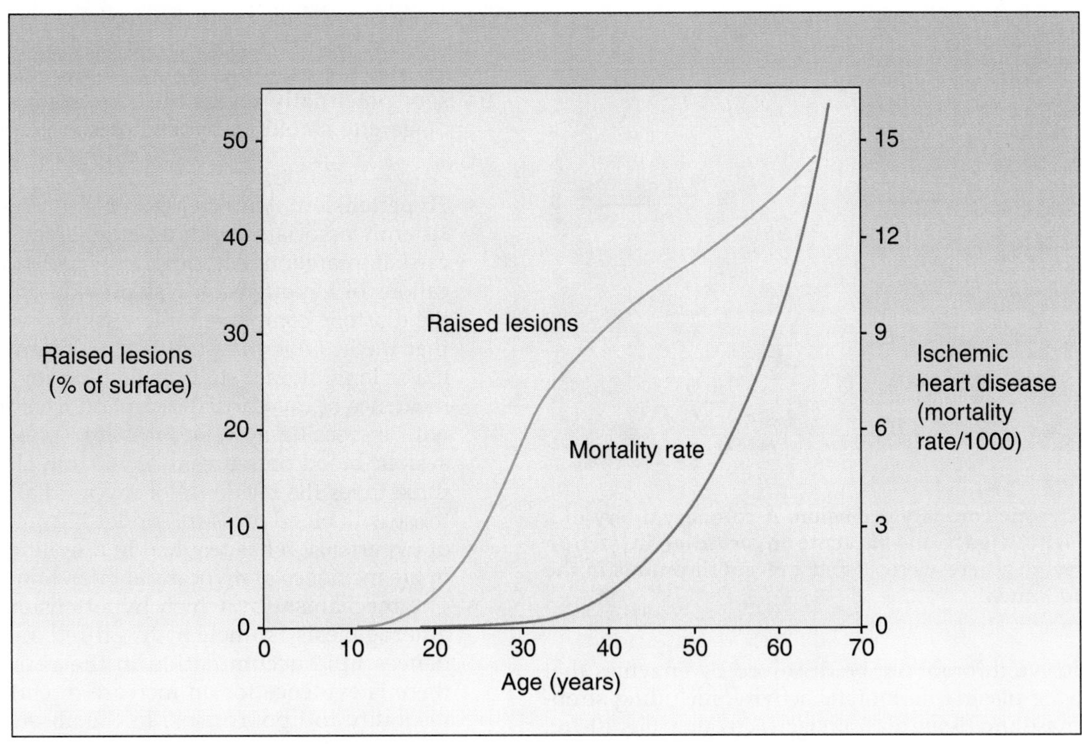

FIGURE 10-13
Raised lesions in coronary arteries and the mortality rate from ischemic heart disease as a function of age. There is a protracted incubation period of about 25 years between the appearance of raised lesions in the coronary vessels and their lethal complications.

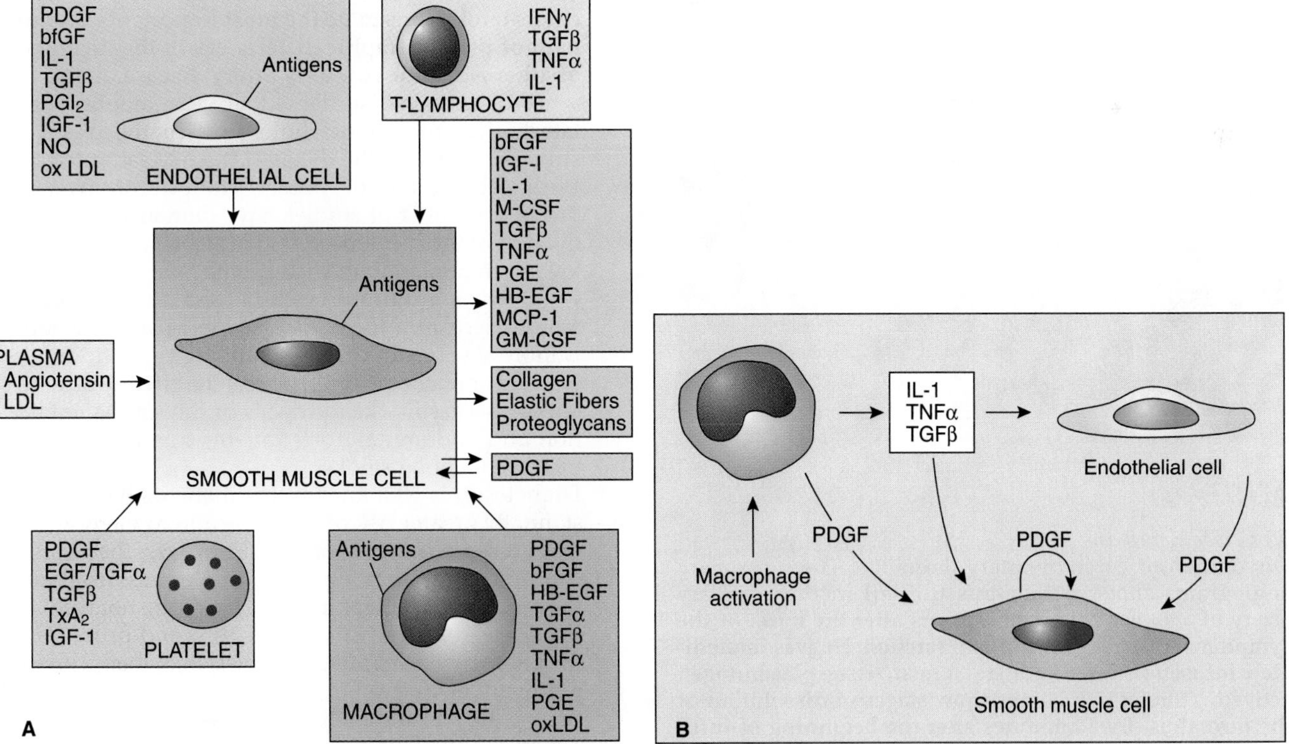

FIGURE 10-14
Cellular interactions in the progression of the atherosclerotic plaque. (*A*) Endothelium, platelets, macrophages, T lymphocytes, and smooth muscle cells elaborate a variety of cytokines, growth factors, and other substances. The scheme illustrated here emphasizes their influence on smooth muscle cells. (*B*) The cellular interactions that promote the proliferation of smooth cells.

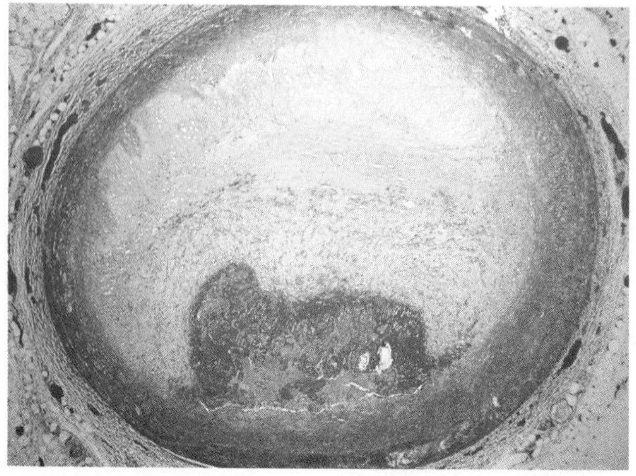

FIGURE 10-15
Atherosclerotic coronary occlusion. A coronary artery of a patient who died from an acute myocardial infarction shows severe atherosclerosis and a recent thrombus in the narrowed lumen.

occlusive thrombi can be dissolved by enzymes that activate plasma fibrinolytic activity, including streptokinase and tissue plasminogen activator (Fig. 10-16).

Risk Factors

The concept of risk factors for atherosclerosis has emerged from studies of ischemic heart disease in human populations. Any factor associated with a doubling in the incidence of ischemic heart disease has been defined as a "risk factor." A risk factor can be regarded as either **not reversible**, for example, aging, male gender, genetic traits, or **potentially reversible**—for example, hypertension, cigarette smoking, hypercholesterolemia, and obesity.

- **Hypertension:** An increase in blood pressure is consistently associated with an augmented risk of myocardial infarction. Although the incidence of complications of hypertension was previously attributed to the diastolic component, there is increasing evidence that the systolic pressure is equally important. In a major longitudinal study extending for 24 years, the incidence of myocardial infarction rose progressively with increasing systolic pressure. In fact, men with systolic blood pressures over 160 mm Hg had almost three times the incidence of myocardial infarction as those with blood pressures under 120 mm Hg. Control of hypertension has resulted in a significant decrease in the incidence of myocardial infarction and stroke.
- The mechanism by which hypertension accelerates atherogenesis is unclear. In fat-fed animals, it enhances lipid accumulation in the vessel wall, and there is evidence for an increase in endothelial permeability to lipoproteins. In the absence of a fatty diet, hypertension has also been shown to augment the rate of intimal thickening.
- **Blood cholesterol level:** In cross-sectional population studies, the levels of serum cholesterol have been directly correlated with the incidence of ischemic heart disease. **Indeed, of all the known risk factors, serum cholesterol seems to be the most important determinant of the geographic differences in the incidence of atherosclerotic coronary artery disease.** In the absence of genetic disorders of lipid metabolism (see later), the amount of cholesterol in the blood is strongly related to the dietary intake of saturated fat. With the advent of potent cholesterol-lowering drugs, a number of studies have demonstrated a reduction in the incidence of myocardial infarction following treatment with such agents
- **Cigarette smoking:** As discussed in Chapter 8, atherosclerosis of the coronary arteries and the aorta is more severe and extensive among cigarette smokers than among nonsmokers, and the effect is dose-related. As a result, the incidence of myocardial infarction and abdominal aortic aneurysms is markedly increased among smokers.
- **Diabetes:** It is well known that diabetics have a substantially greater risk of occlusive atherosclerotic vascular disease in many organs. However, the relative contributions of carbohydrate intolerance itself and the secondary changes in blood lipids are not well defined. The role of advanced glycation end-products in the pathogenesis of atherosclerosis in diabetics is currently under study.
- **Increasing age and male sex:** These factors are strong determinants of the risk for myocardial infarction, but both are probably secondary to the accumulated effects of other risk factors.
- **Physical inactivity and stressful life patterns:** Both of these factors have been correlated with an increased risk of ischemic heart disease, although their

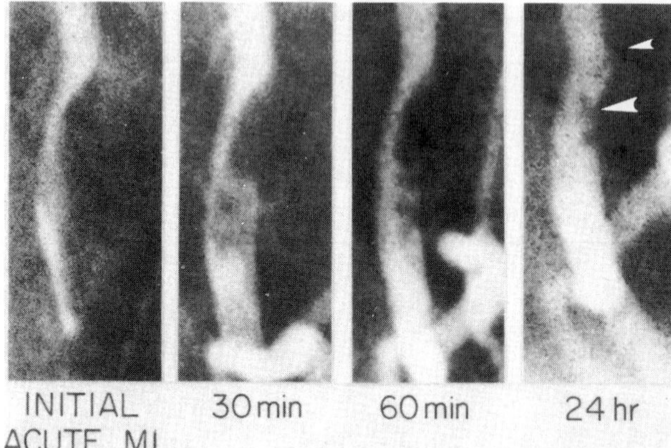

FIGURE 10-16
Dissolution of coronary artery thrombus. These coronary angiograms show a thrombus (initial) in the coronary artery of a 48-year-old man, 3 hours after the onset of the symptoms of acute myocardial infarction. He was immediately infused with recombinant human tissue plasminogen activator. Successive frames show stages of dissolution of the thrombus. By 60 minutes after the beginning of infusion, the thrombus is distinctly smaller. The infusion was continued for 6 hours, and at 24 hours the thrombus is almost completely lysed. The *lower arrow* indicates a small remaining portion of plaque or thrombus; the apparent bulge indicated by the *upper arrow* is interpreted as an ulceration of the plaque.

precise relationship to the evolution of atherosclerosis is not established.

Viruses and Atherosclerosis

A number of studies have implicated viral infection as a possible factor in the pathogenesis of atherosclerosis. In chickens, an avian herpesvirus that causes a neurolymphomatous neoplasm (Marek disease) also produces a fatty proliferative lesion in muscular arteries. In tissue culture, infection of chicken cells by the virus of Marek disease and infection of human smooth muscle cells by herpes simplex virus alter the metabolism of lipid and cholesterol in these cells. Genomic sequences of herpesviruses and cytomegalovirus have also been found in human lesions.

Although a role for viruses in the pathogenesis of atherosclerosis has not been conclusively demonstrated, viral infection is compatible with the importance of cell proliferation in the formation of atheromatous plaques. It could also explain several puzzling features of atherosclerosis, namely, (1) intimal cell proliferation in the absence of certain common risk factors and (2) the monoclonal nature of cell populations found in many human atherosclerotic lesions. In addition, infection of endothelial cells by herpes simplex virus infection may enhance their procoagulant properties and reduce their anticoagulant activities, the net result being increased platelet adherence.

Lipid Metabolism and Atherosclerosis

In the 19th century, Virchow identified cholesterol crystals in atherosclerotic lesions. Since that time, there has evolved a large body of information on lipoproteins and their role in lipid transport and metabolism.

The insolubility of cholesterol and other lipids (mainly triglycerides), which are important as structural elements in cell membranes and as energy sources, necessitates a special transport system. This function is subserved by a system of lipoprotein particles (Table 10-4; Fig. 10-17). The lipoproteins have been divided into

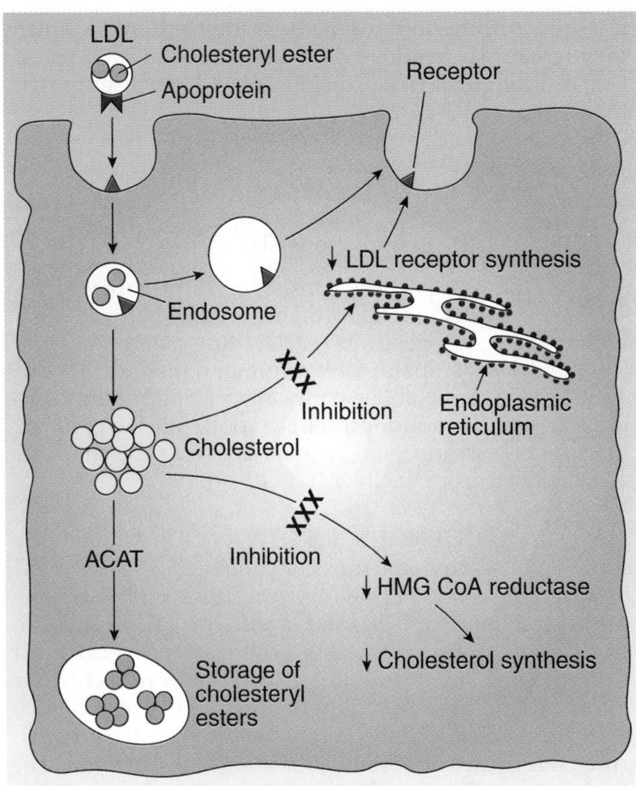

FIGURE *10-17*
The relationship between circulating low-density lipoprotein-cholesterol, low-density lipoprotein receptors, and the synthesis of cholesterol. The low-density lipoprotein, which contains cholesteryl esters, is taken up by cells into vesicles by a receptor-mediated pathway to form an endosome. The receptor and lipids are dissociated, and the receptor is returned to the cell surface. The exogenous cholesterol, now in the cytoplasm, causes a reduction in receptor synthesis in the endoplasmic reticulum and inhibits the activity of HMG CoA reductase in the cholesterol synthesizing pathway. Excess cholesterol in the cell is esterified to cholesteryl esters and stored in vacuoles.

TABLE *10-4* **The Apolipoproteins**

Apolipoprotein	Approximate Molecular Weight	Major Density Class	Major Sites of Synthesis in Humans	Major Function in Lipoprotein Metabolism
AI	28,000	HDL	Liver, intestine	Activates lecithin: cholesterol acyltransferase
AII	18,000	HDL	Liver, intestine	
AIV	45,000	Chylomicrons	Intestine	
B-100	250,000	VLDL IDL LDL	Liver	Binds to LDL receptor
B-48	125,000	Chylomicrons VLDL IDL	Intestine	
CI	6500	Chylomicrons VLDL HDL	Liver	Activates lecithin: cholesterol acyltransferase
CII	10,000	Chylomicrons VLDL HDL	Liver	Activates lipoprotein lipase
CIII	10,000	Chylomicrons	Liver	Inhibits lipoprotein uptake by the liver
D	20,000	HDL		Cholesteryl ester exchange protein
E	40,000	Chylomicrons VLDL HDL	Liver, macrophage	Binds to E receptor system

classes according to the density of the medium in which they remain suspended when centrifuged at high speed (100,000*g* or greater). The major classes of particles are the following:

- Chylomicrons
- Very-low-density lipoproteins (VLDL)
- Low-density lipoproteins (LDL)
- High-density lipoproteins (HDL)

Each of these particles consists of a lipid core with associated proteins (apolipoproteins). A number of the latter have been described, and each is designated by a letter (frequently accompanied by a number), as indicated in Table 10-4. The metabolic pathways for lipoproteins containing the B apolipoproteins (apoB) are two major lipoprotein cascades, one originating from the intestine and the other from the liver (Fig. 10-18).

THE EXOGENOUS PATHWAY: This metabolic route involves chylomicrons containing apoB-48 secreted by the intestine. Following secretion, chylomicrons rapidly acquire apoCII and apoE from HDL. These triglyceride-rich lipoproteins primarily transport lipid from the intestine to the liver. The triglycerides in chylomicrons are hydrolyzed by lipoprotein lipase, which is attached to the endothelial cells of the capillary walls. ApoCII activates lipoprotein lipase and causes removal of triglycerides. Thus, chylomicrons are converted to "remnants" and finally to intermediate-density lipoproteins (IDL). The chylomicron remnants are removed by the hepatocytes through an apoE-mediated (remnant) receptor process.

THE ENDOGENOUS PATHWAY: This network of reactions involves triglyceride-rich lipoproteins containing apoB-100 secreted by the liver. As with the chylomicrons, the liver VLDL particles acquire apoCII and apoE from HDL shortly after their secretion. The triglycerides on VLDL undergo hydrolysis by lipoprotein lipase. The lipoproteins containing apoB-100 are initially converted to IDLs and finally to LDLs. With the conversion of IDL to LDL, most apoCII and apoE dissociates from the particles and reassociates with HDL. The conversion of IDL to LDL may, in part, be mediated by hepatic lipase. This enzyme functions both as a triglyceride hydrolase and, more importantly, as a phospholipase. LDL, which contains apoB-100, interacts with high-affinity receptors on hepatocytes and on peripheral cells, including smooth muscle cells, fibroblasts, and adrenal cells (see Fig. 10-17). The interaction of LDL with its receptor initiates receptor-mediated endocytosis, which is followed by the catabolism of LDL.

HIGH-DENSITY LIPOPROTEIN: HDL containing apoAI and apoAII is synthesized by several pathways. These include direct secretion of HDL by the intestine and liver and transfer of the lipid and apolipoprotein constituents released during the lipolysis of lipoproteins that contain apoB. Two major functions have been proposed for HDL: (1) a reservoir for apolipoproteins, particularly apoCII and apoE, and (2) an interaction with cells in the transport system to carry extrahepatic cholesterol to the liver for ultimate removal from the body. The latter function has been termed **reverse cholesterol transport**. A receptor for HDL has been identified in the liver and steroid-producing endocrine glands of mice. The cholesterol removed from the cells is principally free cholesterol, which rapidly undergoes esterification to cholesteryl esters. Cholesteryl esters are transferred to the core of the lipoprotein particle or are exchanged to VLDL and LDL. The transfer of cholesteryl esters between lipoprotein particles is mediated by specific transfer proteins. Defects in cholesteryl ester transfer and exchange lead to dyslipoproteinemias, increased intracellular cholesteryl esters, and premature atherosclerosis.

OXIDIZED LOW-DENSITY LIPOPROTEIN: As noted earlier, macrophage-derived foam cells constitute a significant component of atherosclerotic lesions. Early studies of the uptake of LDL by macrophages *in vitro*

FIGURE ***10-18***
Exogenous and endogenous cholesterol transport pathway. In the exogenous pathway, cholesterol and fatty acids from food are absorbed through the intestinal mucosa. Fatty acid chains are linked to glycerol to form triglycerides. Triglycerides and cholesterol are packaged into chylomicrons that are returned via the lymph to the blood. The lipids are coupled to proteins by enzymes such as the microsomal transfer protein complex. In the capillaries (mainly of fat tissue and muscle, but also other tissues), the ester bonds holding the fatty acids in triglycerides are split by lipoprotein lipase. Fatty acids are removed, leaving cholesterol-rich lipoprotein remnants. These bind to special remnant receptors and are taken up by liver cells. The cholesterol of the remnant is either secreted into the intestine, largely as bile acids, or packaged as very low-density lipoprotein particles (VLDL), which are then secreted into the circulation. This is the first step in the endogenous cycle. In fat or muscle tissue the triglyceride is removed from the VLDL with the aid of lipoprotein lipase. The intermediate-density lipoprotein particles (IDL [*not shown*]) remain in the circulation. Some IDL is immediately taken up by the liver via the mediation of low-density lipoprotein (LDL) receptors for ApoB/E. The remaining IDL in the circulation is either taken up by nonliver cells or converted to LDL. Most of the LDL in the circulation bind to hepatocytes or other cells and are removed from the circulation. High-density lipoproteins (HDL) take up cholesterol from cells. This cholesterol is esterified by the enzyme lecithin: cholesterol acyltransferase (LCAT), after which the esters are transferred to LDL and taken up by cells.

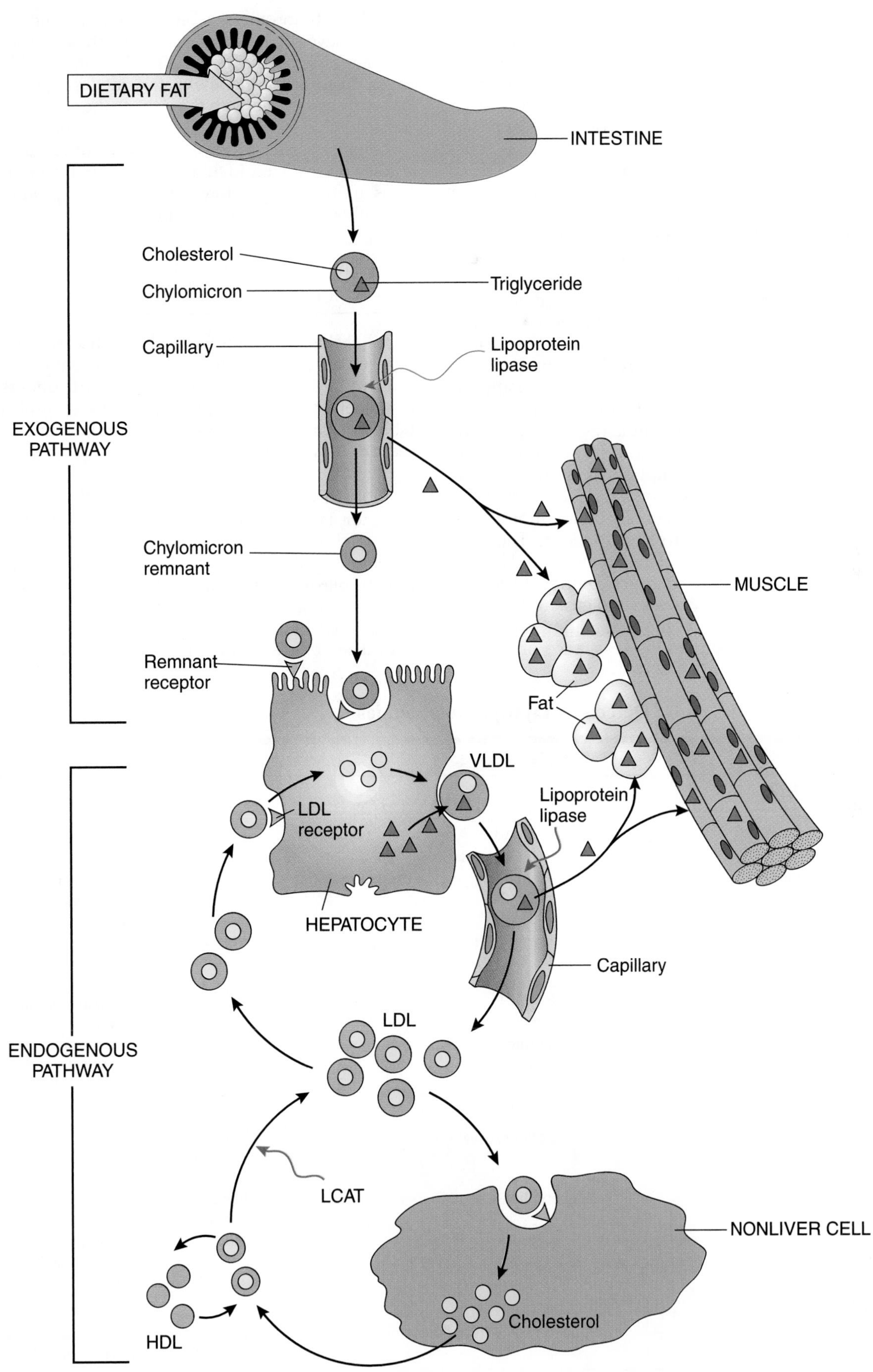

DIETARY FAT
INTESTINE
EXOGENOUS PATHWAY
Cholesterol
Chylomicron
Triglyceride
Capillary
Lipoprotein lipase
Chylomicron remnant
MUSCLE
Remnant receptor
Fat
VLDL
LDL receptor
Lipoprotein lipase
HEPATOCYTE
Capillary
ENDOGENOUS PATHWAY
LDL
LCAT
NONLIVER CELL
Cholesterol
HDL

FIGURE *10-18*

showed that foam cells did not form under these conditions. However, when the LDL was modified by acetylation or oxidation, the macrophages readily recognized, ingested, and retained LDL cholesterol. **Subsequent studies established that oxidized LDL is present in atherosclerotic plaques** and that each of the cell types in atherosclerotic lesions (macrophages, endothelial cells, smooth muscle cells) is capable of oxidizing LDL, a change that facilitates recognition by the macrophage scavenger receptor. Unlike the uptake of native LDL by the LDL receptors on macrophages, the uptake of oxidized LDL by these cells is not subject to negative-feedback regulation and thus results in the massive uptake of cholesterol by macrophages. In addition, oxidized LDL products are present in the macrophages of human atherosclerotic lesions. Evidence is now emerging, especially from *in vitro* systems, that oxidized lipoproteins also affect other processes that may contribute to atherogenesis, including the regulation of vascular tone, the activation of inflammatory and immune responses, and coagulation. Oxidized LDL is toxic to cells of the vascular wall and may lead to the disruption of endothelial integrity and to the accumulation of cell debris within the atheroma. Oxidized LDL is chemotactic for monocytes and promotes the accumulation of macrophages. These effects promote the accumulation of macrophages and inhibit endothelial repair by suppressing cell migration. Oxidized LDL has variable effects on cytokines and growth factors in atherosclerotic lesions and on the coagulation and fibrinolytic processes that regulate the resistance of the endothelium to thrombosis. Studies in hypercholesterolemic animals have suggested that chronic antioxidant therapy retards the atherogenic process. In this context, epidemiological studies suggest that the dietary intake of antioxidants is inversely associated with the risk of atherosclerosis, further implying that oxidized LDL may be an important mediator of human vascular disease. Although the results of these studies on oxidized LDL are intriguing, further investigations are necessary before a role for these products in human atherosclerosis can be confirmed.

Hereditary Disorders of Lipid Metabolism and Atherosclerosis

Familial clustering of ischemic heart disease has been recognized for decades, but it is only in recent years that significant strides have been made toward understanding the genetic basis for this predisposition. A number of heritable defects that produce dyslipoproteinemias are now recognized (Table 10-5).

FAMILIAL HYPERCHOLESTEROLEMIA: The LDL receptor is a cell surface glycoprotein that regulates plasma cholesterol by mediating the endocytosis and recycling of apoE, the major cholesterol transport protein in human plasma. Mutations in the LDL receptor gene, located on the short arm of chromosome 19, are responsible for familial hypercholesterolemia, an autosomal dominant disease in which the prevalence of heterozygotes is

TABLE *10-5* **Molecular Defects in Dyslipoproteinemias**

Disease	Genetic Defect	Clinical Features
Apolipoprotein Defects		
ApoA1 deficiency	ApoA1 truncations or rearrangements (11q23)	Absent HDL, severe atherosclerosis
ApoA1 variants	ApoA1 point mutations (11q23)	Reduced HDL, variable atherosclerosis
Abetalipoproteinemia (absence of both ApoB-100 and ApoB-48)	Microsomal triglyceride protein mutation (4q22–24)	Ataxia, malabsorption, hemolytic anemia, visual defects, absence of atherosclerosis
ApoB-100 absence	Unknown (2p24)	Mild ataxia, malabsorption, absence of atherosclerosis
ApoCII deficiency	ApoCII mutations (19q13.2)	Type I hyperlipidemia: severe hypertriglyceridemia, variable atherosclerosis
ApoE variants	ApoE mutations (19q13.2)	Type III hyperlipidemia: elevated triglycerides, premature atherosclerosis
Enzyme Defects		
Lipoprotein lipase deficiency	Lipoprotein lipase mutations (8p22)	Type I hyperlipidemia: hypertriglyceridemia; minimal atherosclerosis
Hepatic lipase deficiency	Hepatic lipase mutations (15q21–23)	Elevations of IDL and HDL; severe atherosclerosis
Lecithin:cholesterol acyltransferase deficiency	LCAT mutations (16q22.1)	Mild hypertriglyceridemia; reduced HDL corneal opacities; variable atherosclerosis
Receptor Defect		
Familial hypercholesterolemia	LDL receptor mutations (19p13.2)	Type II hyperlipidemia: severe elevation of LDL; premature atherosclerosis

about 1 in 500 persons. However, among persons who have had myocardial infarctions associated with hyperlipidemia, the prevalence of familial hypercholesterolemia is much higher, reaching 6% in some populations.

The LDL receptor gene is located on chromosome 19. More than 400 mutant alleles for familial hypercholesterolemia have been described, including point mutations, insertions, and deletions. The mutations fall into five main classes, based on their effects on the functions of the receptor protein (Fig. 10-19). The genetic considerations of familial hypercholesterolemia are discussed more fully in Chapter 6.

The early onset and malignant course of ischemic heart disease in patients with homozygous familial hypercholesterolemia is arguably the most compelling argument for a relationship between circulating cholesterol and the development of atherosclerosis. Homozygotes exhibit plasma cholesterol levels between 600 and 1000 mg/dL, a value fourfold to sixfold higher than the mean value in most whites. Most untreated homozygotes die from coronary artery disease before the age of 20 years. In heterozygotes, LDL cholesterol levels vary from 250 to 500 mg/dL, roughly twice the normal range. These patients suffer from premature myocardial infarction, but at a later mean age than do the homozygotes (40 to 45 years in men). Pathologically, the atherosclerotic lesions in per-

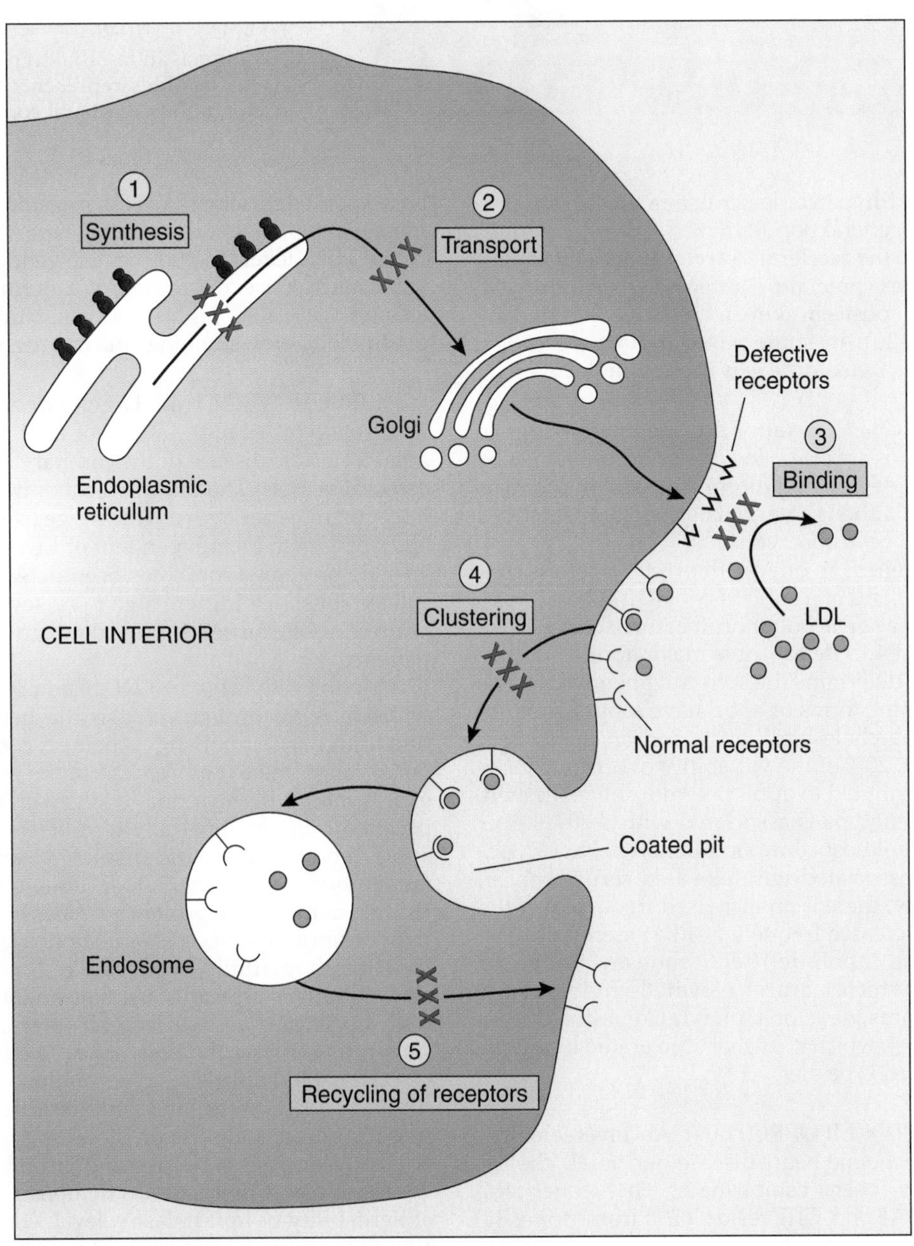

FIGURE *10-19*
Mutations of the low-density lipoprotein receptor in familial hypercholesterolemia.

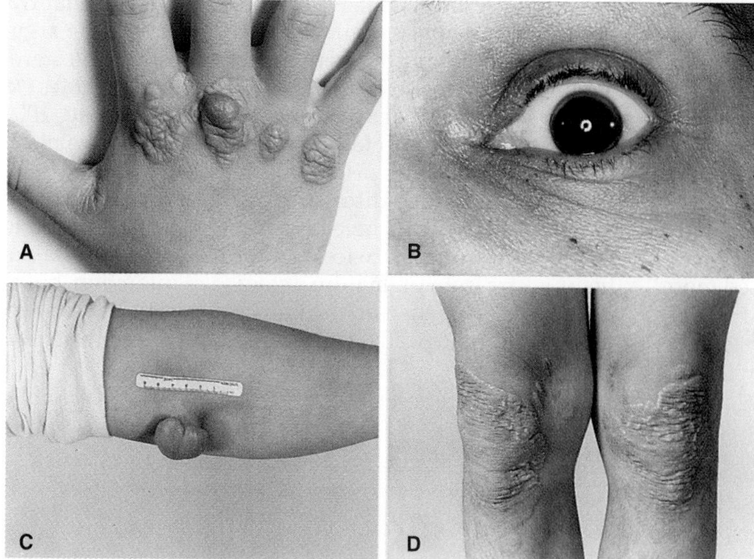

FIGURE *10-20*
Xanthomas in familial hypercholesterolemia. Arcus lipoides represents the deposition of lipids in the peripheral cornea.

sons with familial hypercholesterolemia are identical to those seen in the general population.

In addition to the accelerated accumulation of cholesterol in the arteries (premature atherosclerosis), the LDL cholesterol also deposits in skin and tendons to form xanthomas (Fig. 10-20). In some cases (before age 10 in homozygotes), an arcus corneae is present in the eye.

APOLIPOPROTEIN E (apoE): Genetic variations in various apoproteins are also known to be accompanied by alterations in LDL levels. Polymorphisms are present particularly in apoE, although variants of apolipoprotein AI and AII have also been observed.

Apolipoprotein E is one of the main protein constituents of VLDL and of a subclass of HDL. The gene locus that codes for apoE is polymorphic; three common alleles, E2, E3, and E4, code for three major apoE isoforms, respectively, and determine the six apoE phenotypes. The several polymorphic forms of apoE have a significant influence on plasma cholesterol levels and on lipoprotein variations. In fact, 20% of the variability of serum cholesterol has been attributed to apoE polymorphism. In men, the apoE 3/2 phenotype is associated with a 20% lower LDL level than the most common phenotype, apoE 3/3. The E4 allele is associated with elevated serum cholesterol. Interestingly, there is an increased frequency of the E2 allele and a decreased frequency of E4 among male octogenarians. The apoE-deficient mouse model of atherosclerosis, which features elevated chylomicrons and VLDL remnants, develops human-like lesions on an ordinary chow diet, which is further accelerated by a typical human Western-type diet.

HIGH-DENSITY LIPOPROTEIN: An inverse correlation between ischemic heart disease and HDL cholesterol levels has been established. The genes for apolipoproteins AI and CIII reside on chromosome 11 and are physically linked, whereas the gene for A-II is on chromosome 1. Polymorphisms of apoAI are associated with premature atherosclerosis, as are rare cases of hereditary apoAI deficiency. Antiatherogenic effects are seen in transgenic mice that overexpress apoA1. Factors that increase HDL levels include female gender, estrogens, and vigorous exercise. Decreased HDL occurs with low-fat diets and with diets high in polyunsaturated fats, truncal obesity, diabetes, smoking, and androgen administration.

LIPOPROTEIN (a): High circulating levels of lipoprotein (a)—Lp(a)—are associated with a high risk of atherosclerotic disease of the coronary arteries and larger cerebral vessels. The plasma level of this cholesterol-rich lipoprotein varies over a wide range (<1 to >140 mg/dL) and appears to be independent of LDL levels. The Lp(a)-specific protein, apo(a), has been detected in atherosclerotic lesions. In addition, high Lp(a) levels have been correlated with target organ damage in hypertensive patients.

Lipoprotein (a) is an LDL-like lipoprotein particle to which the glycoprotein apo(a) is attached through a disulfide bridge with apoB-100. Apo(a) is coded for by a gene on chromosome 6 (6q2.7), close to the gene for plasminogen. Apo(a) is highly homologous with plasminogen, the precursor of the fibrinolytic molecule plasmin. Both apo(a) and plasminogen display a variable number of tandemly repeated, triple-loop units termed "kringles." Kringle domains are protein modules found in a wide variety of fibrinolytic and coagulation-related proteins that show binding affinity for lysine residues and for fibrin. These domains appear to mediate an interaction of Lp(a) with fibrin and cell surface receptors. Lp(a) has been shown to enhance the delivery of cholesterol to injured blood vessels, suppress the generation of plasmin on fibrin and cell surfaces, and promote the proliferation of smooth muscle cells. Thus, Lp(a) may be an important link between atherosclerosis and thrombosis.

Family and twin studies demonstrate a high degree of heritability of Lp(a) plasma levels. Lp(a) levels are not altered by the usual cholesterol-lowering drugs but are reduced by nicotinic acid therapy. Taken together, this information distinguishes a risk factor that appears to be related to serum cholesterol, but the effect of which may actually be linked to an alteration in clot lysis.

HOMOCYSTEINE: The observation that homocysteinuria, a rare autosomal recessive disease caused by mutations in the gene encoding cystathionine synthase, results in premature and severe atherosclerosis. This observation stimulated studies of the relationship between homocysteine concentrations in the blood and the occurrence of occlusive vascular disease. **It is now recognized that milder elevations of plasma homocysteine are common and represent an independent risk factor for atherosclerosis of the coronary arteries and other large vessels.** The increased risk of vascular disease associated with high levels of plasma homocysteine is comparable to that of smoking or hyperlipidemia and increases the risk conferred by smoking and hypertension. Homocysteine is toxic to endothelial cells, and it has been demonstrated that several different anticoagulant mechanisms mediated by the vascular endothelium are inhibited by this amino acid. In this regard, homocysteine inhibits thrombomodulin on the endothelial cell surface; the antithrombin III binding activity of heparan sulfate proteoglycan; the binding of tissue plasminogen activator; and the ecto-ADPase activity on the endothelial cell surface, which promotes the aggregation of platelets. In addition, oxidative interactions between homocysteine, lipoproteins, and cholesterol have been shown.

The precise cause of mild hyperhomocysteinemia has not been determined, but it may reflect heterozygosity for cystathionine synthase deficiency or an inherited thermolability of the enzyme that remethylates homocysteine into methionine. In addition, a low dietary intake of folic acid, found exclusively in fruits and vegetables, may aggravate an underlying genetic predisposition to hyperhomocysteinemia. Treatment with folic acid, sometimes supplemented with pyridoxine, vitamin B_{12}, or choline, reduces plasma homosysteine levels, but it has not been established that this dietary intervention actually protects against atherosclerotic vascular disease.

C-REACTIVE PROTEIN: The plasma level of this protein is a marker for systemic inflammation. Elevated concentrations of C-reactive protein have been associated with an increased risk of myocardial infarction and ischemic stroke. It has therefore been suggested that systemic inflammation may contribute to atherogenesis.

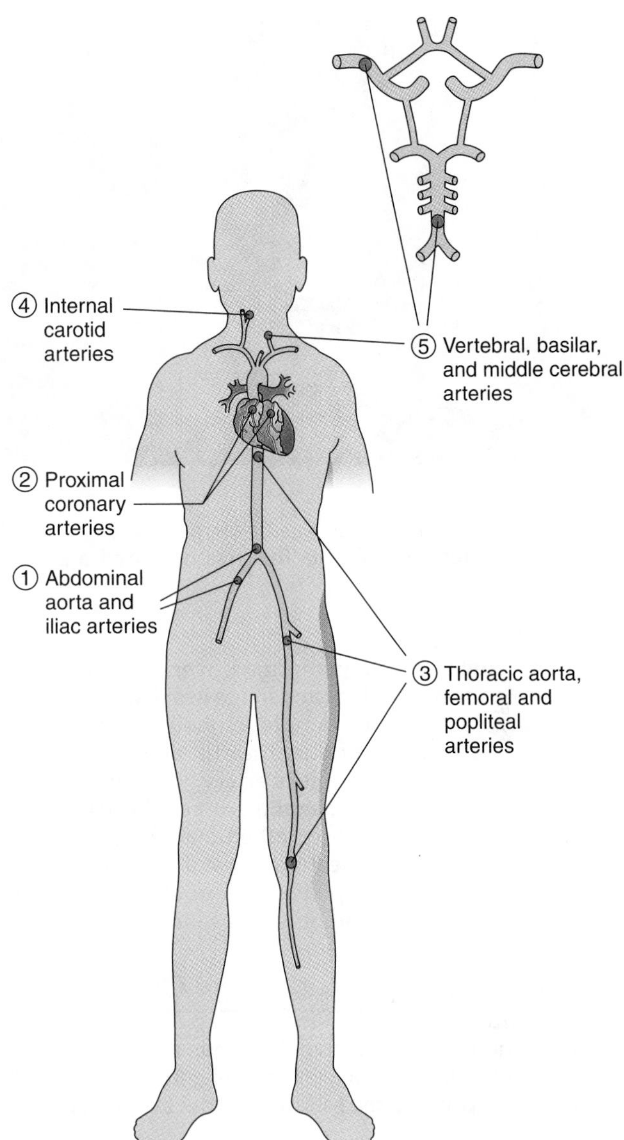

FIGURE ***10-21***
Sites of severe atherosclerosis in order of frequency.

Complications of Atherosclerosis

The complications of atherosclerosis vary with the location and the size of the affected vessel and the chronicity of the process (Fig. 10-21).

- **Acute occlusion:** Thrombosis on an atherosclerotic plaque, often in association with plaque rupture (with or without plaque hemorrhage), may abruptly occlude the lumen of a muscular artery. The result is ischemic necrosis (infarction) of the tissue supplied by that vessel, manifested clinically as myocardial infarction, stroke, or gangrene of the intestine or lower extremities.
- **Chronic narrowing of the vessel lumen:** As an atherosclerotic plaque grows, it often impinges on the lumen, thereby progressively reducing the blood flow to the distribution of the artery. Chronic ischemia of the affected tissue is evidenced by atrophy of the organ, as exemplified by (1) unilateral renal artery stenosis with atrophy of a kidney, (2) intestinal stricture in mesenteric artery atherosclerosis, or (3) ischemic atrophy of the skin in a diabetic with severe peripheral vascular disease.
- **Aneurysm formation:** The complicated lesions of atherosclerosis may extend into the media of an elastic artery and sufficiently weaken the wall to allow the formation of an aneurysm, typically in the abdominal aorta. These aneurysms may develop small leaks or may suddenly rupture and precipitate a vascular catastrophe.

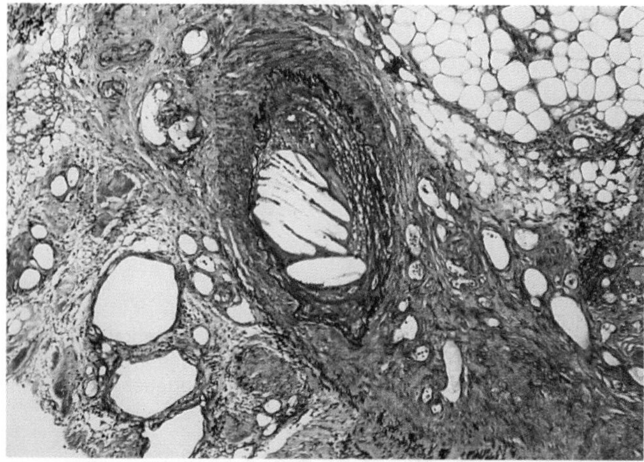

FIGURE *10-22*
Cholesterol crystal embolus. Needle-shaped clefts are seen in an atherosclerotic embolus that has occluded a small artery.

- **Embolism:** A thrombus formed over an atherosclerotic plaque may detach and lodge in a distal vessel as an embolus. As an example, embolization from a thrombus in an abdominal aortic aneurysm may acutely occlude the popliteal artery, with subsequent gangrene of the leg. Ulceration of an atherosclerotic plaque may also dislodge atheromatous debris and lead to so-called **cholesterol crystal emboli**, which appear as needle-shaped spaces in affected tissues (Fig. 10-22), most commonly in the kidney.

Thrombosis and Coronary Artery Occlusion

The formation of an occlusive thrombus in the lumen of an atherosclerotic coronary artery (Fig. 10-23) typically proceeds according to the following sequence of events:

1. The primary process involves a coronary artery wall that is distorted by a plaque. Narrowing and changes in local elasticity cause some alteration in blood flow. At this point, the surface may not be thrombogenic, and the endothelium is intact.
2. **Some change occurs in the lesion to make it thrombogenic.** Endothelial dysfunction may favor anticoagulation or antifibrinolysis. For example, activated macrophages in the lesion may secrete TNF or IL-1, causing endothelial cells to secrete tissue factor. Perhaps the lesion ulcerates. Possibly, toxic products released by macrophages alter endothelial cell viability, so that the cells are sloughed. Vasa vasorum may hemorrhage into the plaque. Any of these circumstances will lead to exposure of the connective tissue of the vessel wall to the circulating blood.
3. In any event, platelets are stimulated to interact with collagen, fibronectin, or fibrin on the injured surface, after which they adhere and become activated. The activated platelets stimulate platelet aggregation by releasing thromboxane A_2 and ADP. Von Willebrand factor is liberated from platelet α-granules and possibly from injured endothelial cells, a process that further accelerates platelet aggregation. The α-granules contribute to the stabilization of the forming aggregate by liberating fibrinogen and fibronectin. Platelet granules also release ADP and vasoactive elements, including histamine, epinephrine, and serotonin. Calcium discharged by the platelets helps to stimulate the coagulation sequence.
4. Activation of the platelet surface also promotes coagulation by the intrinsic pathway, because it leads to the binding of factor X, factor V, and calcium. In addition to stimulating platelet aggregation, thromboxane A_2 also provokes constriction of the surrounding vessels, thereby aggravating the occlusion of the lumen. The initiation of the intrinsic clotting cascade results in the release of thrombin. In addition to stimulating the formation of fibrin, thrombin itself is a powerful promoter of platelet aggregation. Thus, the initial aggregate of platelets becomes converted to a mixture of platelets and thrombus. Injury to surrounding smooth muscle and endothelial cells results in the release of tissue factor, which then initiates the extrinsic coagulation pathway. The resulting thrombus may occlude the lumen and precipitate a myocardial infarction or may remain nonocclusive and undergo several possible fates. Fibrinolytic processes may lyse the thrombus, especially if it is small. Alternatively, the thrombus may detach and embolize downstream, or it may propagate and eventually occlude the lumen.
5. The mural thrombus overlying an atherosclerotic plaque is a rich source of chemotactic factors and mitogens. These agents stimulate the growth of smooth muscle cells in the plaque and the secretion of collagen, thereby converting a labile structure into a more permanent one. An organized thrombus is a permanent structure formed when the thrombus is invaded by smooth muscle cells and connective tissue. New vessels may invade the organized thrombus (i.e., canalization [see Chapter 7]) and provide some blood flow across it. Unfortunately, these new vessels are almost always too small to maintain a clinically significant level of blood flow. Occasionally, the organized thrombus becomes incorporated into the plaque.
6. **A thrombus over an atherosclerotic plaque may form following the rupture of its fibrous cap.** The

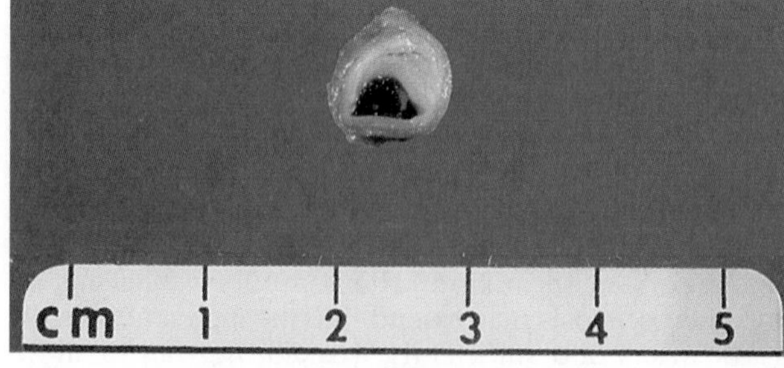

FIGURE *10-23*
Coronary artery thrombosis. A cross-section of a coronary artery shows a fresh thrombus overlying an atherosclerotic plaque and occluding the lumen.

rupture is thought to be due to physical forces exerted on the shoulder of the plaque, proteolytic enzyme digestion of plaque matrix, or sudden intraplaque hemorrhage after the rupture of plaque vessels. The liberated plaque contents then initiate thrombosis. This mechanism is probably the most common cause of occlusion of the coronary arteries and is especially important because the recent introduction of thrombolytic therapy has in many cases permitted the reestablishment of the lumen. It is now possible to dissolve an early thrombus and reduce the extent of myocardial infarction by injecting enzymes that activate plasmin, for example, streptokinase or plasminogen activating factor.

Nonatherosclerotic Intimal Proliferation

An interesting example of mural thrombus formation has been documented in a number of deaths following the intravenous or intranasal use of cocaine. These deaths have been associated with acute myocardial infarction or with arrhythmias. In these case reports, coronary lesions fall into three categories: (1) fresh mural platelet thrombi; (2) lesions involving proliferation of smooth muscle cells in the intima; and (3) organized, canalized thrombi. These lesions occur in young persons (21 to 44 years of age) who frequently show no evidence of atherosclerosis or vasculitis elsewhere. The older lesions have been described as "nonatherosclerotic intimal proliferations." It is possible that coronary spasm leads to an alteration in blood flow, with endothelial injury being followed by thrombus formation.

Angioplasty and Restenosis

Angioplasty has become an important form of interventional therapy for occlusive vascular disease, especially that of the epicardial coronary arteries. A balloon catheter is manipulated into the coronary arteries, similar to an angiogram catheter, and the balloon is inflated to dilate the stenotic artery. The balloon causes endothelial damage and tears in the atherosclerotic plaque and the media. In 30% to 40% of the cases in which the vessel lumen is satisfactorily dilated, restenosis of the vessel takes place over a period 3 to 6 months.

The pathogenesis of restenosis is likely multifactorial. Intimal hyperplasia due to smooth muscle proliferation and matrix deposition, with or without an organized mural thrombus on the luminal surface, leads to restenosis. In addition, the dynamic process of vascular wall remodeling, induced in part by the trauma to the vessel wall, also results in luminal narrowing.

HYPERTENSIVE VASCULAR DISEASE

Hypertension affects up to 20% of the population in industrial countries throughout the world, and is responsible for many cases of myocardial infarction, stroke, and chronic renal disease. Blacks particularly suffer from the ravages of hypertension, and are more likely than whites to experience severe complications. More than half of the patients with angina pectoris, sudden death, stroke, and atherothrombotic occlusion of the abdominal aorta or its branches have hypertension. Three fourths of patients with dissecting aortic aneurysm, intracerebral hemorrhage, or rupture of the myocardial wall also have an elevated blood pressure.

In recent years, it has become clear that the treatment of hypertension prolongs life. The etiology of most hypertension remains unknown, 95% of patients having no clearly identifiable cause. Thus, the large majority of hypertensive persons are described as having "essential" or "primary" hypertension.

The definition of hypertension depends on a statistical estimate of the distribution of systolic and diastolic blood pressures in the general population. Over the course of the day, blood pressure varies widely, depending on exertion, emotional state, and other poorly understood factors. Blood pressure also varies with age. The mean systolic blood pressure in 20-year-old men is about 130 mm Hg, but the 95% confidence limits include a range from 105 to 150 mm Hg. With age, the average systolic blood pressure increases, so that in 80-year-olds, it reaches 170 mm Hg, with the 95% confidence limits extending from 125 to 220. Against this background, the "diagnostic level" of blood pressure that defines hypertension remains controversial. **The World Health Organization has defined hypertension as a systolic pressure greater than 160 mm Hg, a diastolic pressure greater than 90, or both.**

☐ **Pathogenesis:** It is intuitively evident that blood pressure is simply the product of cardiac output and the systemic vascular resistance to blood flow. However, both of these functions are critically influenced by renal function and sodium homeostasis. **The most widespread hypothesis holds that primary hypertension results from an imbalance in the interactions between these mechanisms** (Fig. 10-24).

A complex endocrine axis centers on the renin–angiotensin system. Renal artery occlusion or dietary salt restriction leads to an increased secretion of renin by the kidney. Renin is a protease that splits angiotensinogen to a decapeptide, termed angiotensin I. In turn, angiotensin I is converted to angiotensin II by angiotensin-converting enzyme (ACE), a protein found on the surface of the endothelial cell. Angiotensin II was originally believed to be primarily a vasoconstrictor. However, it is now recognized that it also has major effects on centers in the central nervous system that control sympathetic outflow and stimulate aldosterone release from the adrenal gland. Aldosterone acts on renal tubules to increase sodium reabsorption. The net effect of all these actions is an increase in total body fluid volume. Thus, the **renin–angiotensin** system elevates blood pressure by three mechanisms:

- Increased sympathetic output
- Increased mineralocorticoid secretion
- Direct vasoconstriction

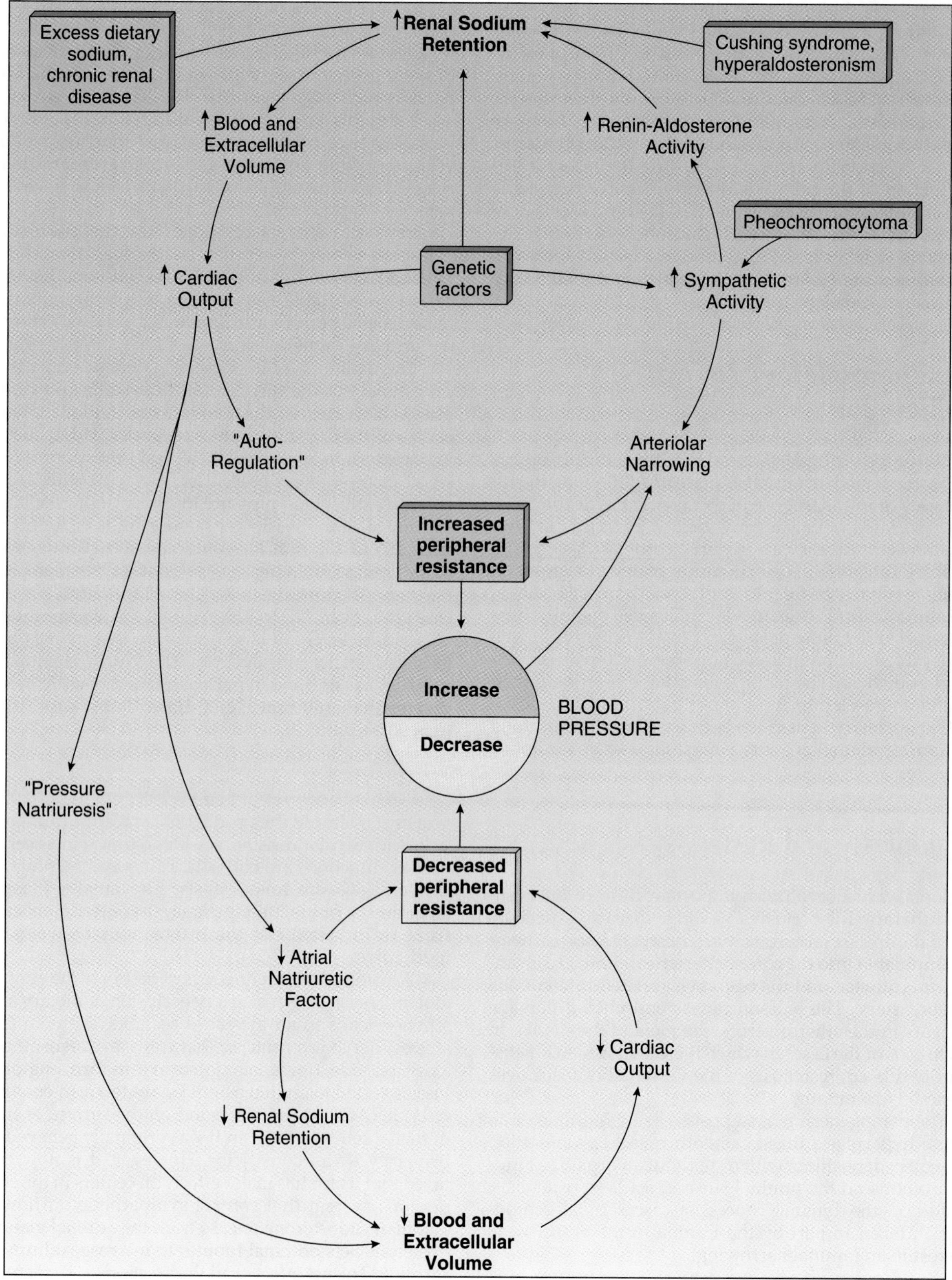

FIGURE *10-24*
Factors contributing to hypertension and the counter-regulatory factors that lower blood pressure. An imbalance in these factors results in the increased peripheral resistance that is responsible for most cases of essential (primary) hypertension. Note the central role of peripheral resistance.

The renin–angiotensin–aldosterone axis is antagonized by **atrial natriuretic factor (ANF)**, a hormone secreted by specialized cells in the cardiac atria. ANF binds to specific receptors in the kidney and increases the urinary excretion of sodium, thereby opposing the vasoconstrictor effects of angiotensin II. Secretion of ANF may be controlled by atrial distention, a consequence of increased volume, or by as yet undefined endocrine interactions.

The importance of this axis of hormones in regulating blood pressure in hypertension is demonstrated by the therapeutic success of sympathetic antagonists (β-adrenergic blockers), diuretics, and inhibitors of ACE. **Nonetheless, there is no clear evidence that a specific defect in the renin–angiotensin axis is the crucial lesion in essential hypertension.** It has proved difficult to identify a central defect in this system, because the vasculature responds quickly to hemodynamic changes in the tissues by autoregulation (Fig. 10-25).

In the case of hypertension, the end-result of autoregulation is always increased peripheral resistance. For example, hypertension can be induced in dogs by surgical resection of large amounts of renal tissue, followed by the administration of excess sodium and water. Cardiac output, and therefore blood pressure, is rapidly increased as a result of the rapid change in blood volume. However, within a few days, pressure-induced diuresis results in a return to near-normal cardiac output and plasma volume. At this point, blood pressure is maintained by increased peripheral resistance. **Even though the elevation in blood pressure was initially due to increased volume, compensatory mechanisms have successfully masked the volume changes and caused apparent essential hypertension.** It is possible that many cases of human hypertension also represent the end-stage of a process that begins with alterations in cardiac output, salt metabolism, or ANF release.

Molecular Genetics of Hypertension

We know from family and twin studies that genetic factors are likely to be important in the pathogenesis of essential hypertension. For example, there is a familial association of hypertension with alterations in the membrane transport of sodium (measured as lithium transport). Interestingly, spontaneous hypertension can be produced in rats in as few as six generations of inbreeding for elevated blood pressure. However, no specific genetic defect has been shown to be causal in rats or humans, and the inheritance of essential hypertension is most likely polygenic.

Although it is clear that essential hypertension likely involves the interactions of a number of gene products, the study of rare mendelian forms of hypertension has provided a novel opportunity to identify candidate genes that may contribute to the control of blood pressure. Three hereditary forms of human hypertension have been well defined in which a single gene mutation results in high blood pressure:

- **Glucocorticoid-remediable aldosteronism (GRA):** GRA is an autosomal dominant trait in which congenital hypertension is mediated by the mineralocorticoid receptor in the kidney. In this condition, the excess production of aldosterone is prompted by corticotropin (ACTH) rather than by the normal secretegogue for aldosterone, angiotensin II. The aldosterone synthase gene on chromosome 8 is normally expressed in the adrenal glomerulosa, where its product catalyzes the biosynthesis of aldosterone. This gene is 95% homologous to the steroid 11β-hydroxylase gene, which regulates the biosynthesis of cortisol in the adrenal fasiculata. Being located in close proximity on the same chromosome, mutations in the aldosterone synthase and 11β-hydroxylase genes cre-

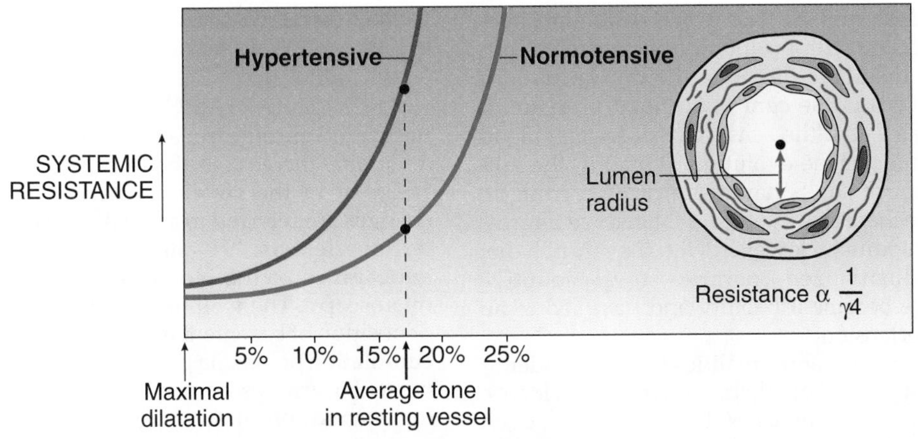

FIGURE *10-25*
Structural autoregulation of blood pressure. Hypertension, regardless of its primary etiology, increases the ability of the resistance vessel walls to respond to vasoactive stimuli. Resistance is increased even in maximally dilated vessels because the lumen size is decreased in the hypertensive vascular bed. As the smooth muscle cells contract, the increase in vessel wall thickness increases the resistance, which is inversely proportional to the fourth power of the radius of the lumen. Note that at the average resting muscular tone, the resistance in hypertensives is considerably higher than normal.

ate a hybrid gene, with ectopic production of aldosterone in the zona fasiculata under the control of corticotropin. In turn, the unrestrained secretion of mineralocorticoids leads to prolonged volume expansion and hypertension.

- **Syndrome of apparent mineralocorticoid excess (AME):** In this autosomal recessive form of early-onset hypertension, stimulation of the mineralocorticoid receptor is present in the face of very low levels of aldosterone. Under normal circumstances, the mineralocorticoid receptor responds not only to aldosterone but also to cortisol, albeit much more weakly. The aldosterone-like activity of cortisol is suppressed through its conversion to cortisone by 11β-hydroxysteroid dehydrogenase in the renal tubular epithelial cells. In AME, inactivating mutations in the gene for this enzyme allow cortisol to accumulate and constitutively stimulate the mineralocorticoid receptor. Interestingly, the consumption of large quantities of licorice can produce a syndrome similar to AME, and a substance in licorice (glycyrrhetinic acid) inhibits 11β-hydroxysteroid dehydrogenase.
- **Liddle syndrome**: Patients with this autosomal dominant form of hypertension exhibit low levels of mineralocorticoids but have a constitutively activated sodium channel in the renal tubule. The defect represents a "gain-of-function" mutation in the gene on chromosome 16 that codes for the amiloride-sensitive epithelial sodium channel. Sustained activation of the channel results in excessive renal reabsorption of salt and water independent of the action of mineralocorticoids, thereby leading to volume expansion and hypertension.

The mutations that cause hereditary hypertension all result in constitutively increased renal sodium reabsorption. Conversely, mutations that result in sodium wastage (pseudohypoaldosteronism type I and Gitelman syndrome) are associated with profound hypotension. Thus, these mendelial disorders illustrate the central role for sodium homeostasis in the control of blood pressure. It has been speculated that the sensitivity of human blood pressure to salt reflects the evolution of man in the salt-poor environment of sub-Saharan Africa. According to this scenario, mechanisms evolved to conserve aggressively total body sodium. However, with the salt-rich diet prevalent in industrialized countries, these adaptive mechanisms have become a liability and have led to an epidemic of hypertension.

Although no genetic abnormalities have been identified in essential hypertension, there is increasing evidence that common polymorphisms of the angiotensinogen gene contribute to the disease. Three findings buttress the potential importance of angiotensinogen variants: (1) the angiotensinogen locus shows linkage to elevated blood pressure in sibling pairs; (2) specific angiotensinogen variants have been linked to hypertension in case-control studies; and (3) the same variants are linked to increased levels of plasma angiotensinogen. Interestingly, in transgenic mice that overexpress the angiotensinogen gene, the degree of blood pressure elevation parallels the number of angiotensinogen copies. However, the identity of angiotensinogen variants and their mode of action remain to be clarified.

Acquired Causes of Hypertension

In a small proportion of all cases of hypertension, acquired causes are identifiable. These include renal artery stenosis, most forms of chronic renal disease, primary elevation of aldosterone levels (Conn syndrome), Cushing syndrome, pheochromocytoma, hyperthyroidism, coarctation of the aorta, and renin-secreting tumors. In addition, persons with severe atherosclerosis may have a high systolic pressure, because the sclerotic aorta cannot properly absorb the kinetic energy of the pulse wave.

☐ **Pathology: The central lesion in most cases of hypertension is a decrease in the caliber of the lumen of small muscular arteries and arterioles**. These resistance vessels control the flow of blood through the capillary bed (see Fig. 10-25). The lumen may be restricted by active contraction of the vessel wall, an increase in the structural mass of the vessel wall, or both. Structural changes in hypertension have been demonstrated by morphometric analysis of the arterial walls. Constriction of a structurally thicker vessel wall would be expected to produce an even more marked narrowing of the lumen than would occur with a normal thinner wall. The rapid drop in blood pressure after the treatment of hypertensive animals or persons with smooth muscle relaxants suggests that active constriction is very important.

Arteriosclerosis

Chronic hypertension leads to reactive changes in the smaller arteries and arterioles throughout the body, collectively referred to as arteriosclerosis. In the arterioles, the alterations are termed arteriolosclerosis.

BENIGN ARTERIOSCLEROSIS: This condition reflects mild chronic hypertension, and the major change is a variable increase in the thickness of arterial walls (Fig. 10-26A). In the smallest arteries and arterioles, these changes are referred to as **hyaline arteriosclerosis and arteriolosclerosis**. "Hyaline" refers to the glassy, scarred appearance of the blood vessel walls as seen by light microscopy. The wall of the arteriole is thickened by the deposition of basement membrane material and by the accumulation of plasma proteins (see Fig. 10-26B). The small muscular arteries display new layers of elastin, presenting as a reduplication of the intimal elastic lamina, and increased connective tissue. The vascular lesions of benign arteriosclerosis are particularly evident in the kidney, where they result in a loss of renal parenchyma, termed **benign nephrosclerosis** (see Chapter 17).

The finding of benign arteriosclerosis is not diagnostic of hypertension, since comparable morphological alterations commonly occur as part of the aging process. However, hyaline arteriosclerosis is accelerated in diabetes and in hypertension, diseases that are also associated with accelerated atherosclerosis.

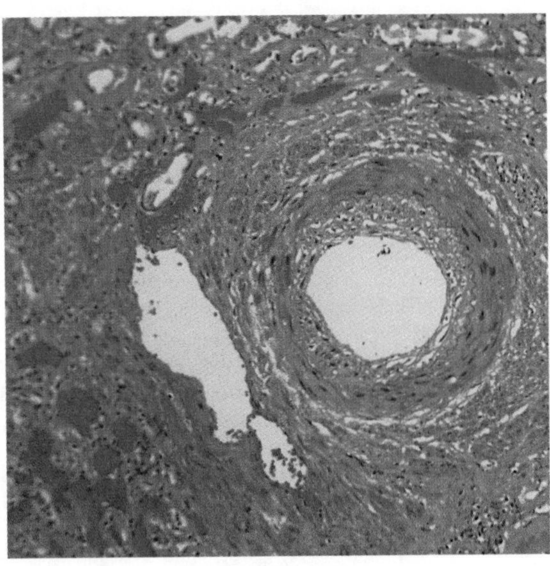

A

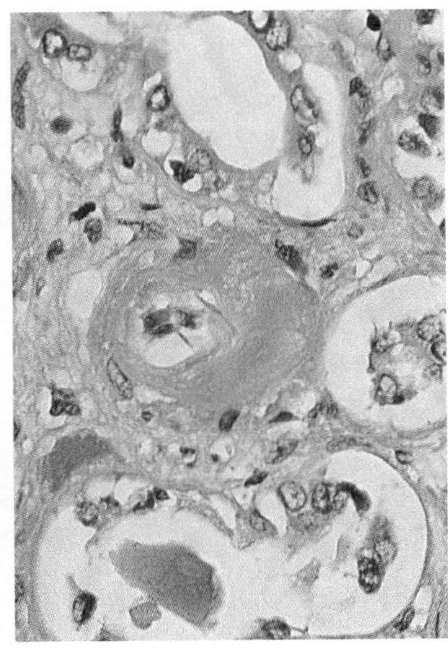

B

FIGURE *10-26*
Benign arteriosclerosis. (*A*) A cross-section of a renal intralobular shows irregular thickening of the intima. (*B*) A renal arteriole exhibts hyalin arteriolosclerosis.

MALIGNANT (ACCELERATED) HYPERTENSION: This term refers to a situation in which an elevated blood pressure results in rapidly progressive vascular compromise, with the onset of symptomatic disease of the brain, heart, or kidney. Although malignant hypertension cannot be defined strictly by the degree of blood pressure elevation, it is ordinarily not evident with pressures below 160/110 mm Hg. Modern antihypertensive therapy has made malignant hypertension a rare disorder.

The morphological changes associated with moderate elevations of blood pressure are often too subtle to be detected by simple histological studies. On the other hand, severe or malignant hypertension produces dramatic changes, particularly at the microvascular level. Segmental constriction and dilatation of the retinal arterioles in severely hypertensive persons are sufficiently prominent to allow the diagnosis of hypertension by ophthalmoscopy. If the blood pressure rises rapidly, the retinal arterioles are unable to resist the increased pressure, and microaneurysms, focal hemorrhages, and scarring of the retina result. Ischemic necrosis and edema of the retina are visible with the ophthalmoscope as "cotton wool spots" (see Chapter 29). These retinal changes are typical of those in other resistance vessels when the pressure rises rapidly.

In malignant hypertension, small muscular arteries show segmental dilatation as a result of necrosis of smooth muscle cells. Endothelial integrity is lost in these regions, and the increase in vascular permeability leads to the entry of plasma proteins into the vessel wall, the deposition of fibrin, and an appearance termed **fibrinoid necrosis**. The period of acute injury is rapidly followed by smooth muscle proliferation and a striking concentric increase in the number of layers of smooth muscle cells, which yields the so-called "onion-skin" appearance (Fig. 10-27). This form of smooth muscle proliferation may be a response to the release of growth factors derived from platelets and other cells at the sites of vascular injury. Taken together, these changes are labeled **malignant arteriosclerosis** or **arteriolosclerosis**, depending on the size of the vessels affected. In the kidney, the lesions of malignant hypertension are known as **malignant nephrosclerosis**.

MONCKEBERG MEDIAL SCLEROSIS

Monckeberg medial sclerosis refers to degenerative calcification of the media of large- and medium-sized muscular arteries. The disorder occurs principally in older persons. The arteries of the upper and lower extremities are most often involved. On gross examination, the involved arteries are hard and dilated. Microscopically, the smooth muscle of the media is focally replaced by pale-staining, acellular, hyalinized fibrous tissue, which exhibits concentric dystrophic calcification. Osseous metaplasia in calcified areas is occasionally observed. **Monckenberg medial sclerosis is distinct from atherosclerosis and ordinarily does not lead to any clinical disorder.**

RAYNAUD PHENOMENON

Raynaud phenomenon refers to intermittent, bilateral attacks of ischemia of the fingers or toes, and sometimes of the ears or nose. It is characterized by severe pallor (Fig. 10-28) and is often accompanied by paresthesias and pain. The symptoms are precipitated by cold or emotional stimuli and relieved by heat.

Raynaud phenomenon may occur as an isolated disorder or as a prominent feature of a number of systemic diseases of connective tissue (collagen vascular disorders), particularly scleroderma. The entity includes primary and secondary cold sensitivity, livedo reticularis,

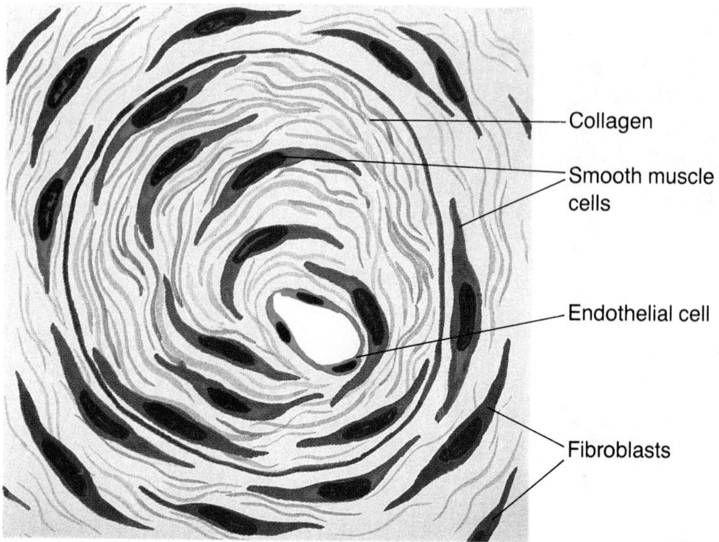

FIGURE *10-27*
Arteriolosclerosis. In cases of hypertension, the arterioles exhibit smooth muscle cell proliferation and increased amounts of intercellular collagen and glycosaminoglycans, resulting in an "onion-skin" appearance. The mass of smooth muscle and associated elements tends to fix the size of the lumen and restrict the arteriole's capacity to dilate.

and acrocyanosis. **Whatever the cause, Raynaud phenomenon represents arterial vasospasm in the skin.**

Primary cold sensitivity of the Raynaud type is more common in women, often starting in the late teens. It is bilateral and symmetric, and on rare occasions may lead to ulcers or gangrene of the tips of the digits. The hands are more commonly affected than the feet.

FIBROMUSCULAR DYSPLASIA

Fibromuscular dysplasia is a rare, noninflammatory thickening of large and medium-sized muscular arteries, which is distinct from atherosclerosis and arteriosclerosis. The cause is unknown. In the renal arteries, the stenosis produced by this condition is an important cause of renovascular hypertension, although the disorder may affect almost any other vessel, including the carotid, vertebral, and splanchnic arteries. Fibromuscular dysplasia is typically a disease of women during their reproductive years, but it can appear at any age, even in childhood. In the majority of cases, the distal two thirds of the renal artery and its primary branches display several segmental stenoses, which represent fibrous and muscular ridges that project into the lumen. Microscopically, these segments exhibit a disorderly arrangement and proliferation of the cellular elements of the vessel wall, without necrosis or inflammation. Smooth muscle is replaced by fibrous tissue and myofibroblasts. In some cases, intimal fibroplasia predominates, and in unusual instances, connective tissue encircles the adventitia. Other than renal hypertension, the major complication of fibromuscular dysplasia is dissecting aneurysm of the affected arteries.

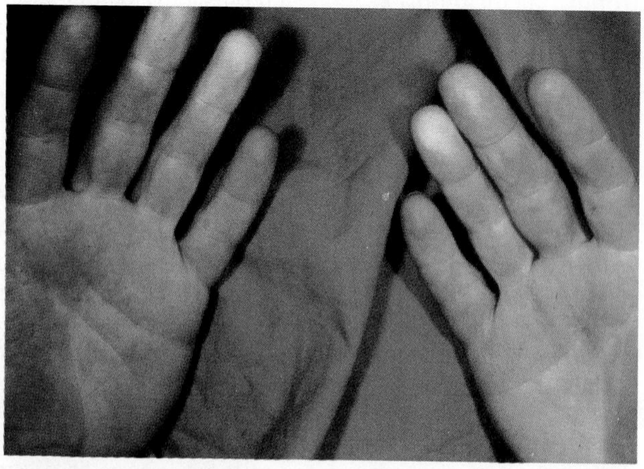

FIGURE *10-28*
Raynaud phenomenon. The tips of the fingers show marked pallor.

VASCULITIS

Vasculitis refers to inflammation and necrosis of blood vessels, including arteries, veins, and capillaries (Table 10-6). Arteries

TABLE *10-6* **Inflammatory Disorders of Blood Vessels**

Polyarteritis nodosa group of systemic necrotizing vasculitis
- Classic polyarteritis nodosa
- Allergic angiitis and granulomatosis (Churg-Strauss variant)
- "Overlap syndrome" of systemic angiitis

Hypersensitivity vasculitis
- Serum sickness and similar reactions
- Henoch-Schönlein purpura
- Vasculitis associated with connective tissue disorders
- Vasculitis in cases of essential mixed cryoglobulinemia
- Vasculitis associated with other primary disorders

Wegener granulomatosis

Lymphomatoid granulomatosis

Giant cell arteritis
- Temporal arteritis
- Takayasu arteritis

Central nervous system vasculitis

Vasculitis associated with cancer

Mucocutaneous lymph node syndrome (Kawasaki disease)

Thromboangiitis obliterans (Buerger disease)

Behçet disease

Miscellaneous vasculitis syndromes

or veins may be damaged by infectious agents, mechanical trauma, radiation, or toxins. However, in many cases of vasculitis, no specific etiology is determined.

☐ **Pathogenesis:** Vasculitic syndromes are thought to involve immune mechanisms, including (1) the deposition of immune complexes, (2) a direct attack on the vessels by circulating antibodies, and (3) various forms of cell-mediated immunity. Although the agents responsible for inciting the immune reaction are largely unknown, there is evidence that in some instances vasculitis is associated with a viral infection.

Serum sickness was one of the first human immunological disorders associated with vasculitis. In animal models of serum sickness, immune complexes and complement are found in the local tissue reaction (see Chapter 4). However, in most cases of human vasculitis, the search for immune complexes has yielded variable results, and firm evidence for immune complexes in the pathogenesis of most cases of vasculitis is lacking.

Viral antigens have been suspected as a cause of vasculitis in experimental animals and in humans. A case in point is chronic infection with hepatitis B virus, which is associated with some cases of polyarteritis nodosa. In this circumstance, circulating viral antigen-antibody complexes, as well as the deposition of these immune complexes in the vascular lesions, have been demonstrated. Human vasculitis has also been associated with a variety of other viral infections, including herpes simplex, cytomegalovirus, and parvovirus. In addition, several bacterial antigens have been identified in the lesions of some cases of vasculitis.

Small vessel vasculitides, for example, Wegener granulomatosis and microscopic polyarteritis (see later), are associated with anti-neutrophil cytoplasmic antibodies (ANCA), but the contribution of these autoantibodies to the vasculitis is not understood. ANCA may cause endothelial damage by activating neutrophils, and antibody titers correlate with disease activity. ANCA is detected by indirect immunofluorescence assays using the patient's serum and ethanol-fixed neutrophils. Common patterns include a perinuclear immunofluorescence (P-ANCA, mainly against myeloperoxidase) and a more general cytoplasmic immunofluorescence (C-ANCA, mainly against proteinase 3).

Polyarteritis Nodosa

Polyarteritis nodosa is an acute, necrotizing vasculitis that affects medium-sized and smaller muscular arteries, and occasionally larger arteries. It occurs primarily in whites and is somewhat more common in men than in women. Polyarteritis was regarded as a rarity until the 1940s, when there was a striking rise in its incidence. The greater frequency of polyarteritis nodosa at that time seemed to be associated with the widespread use of antisera to bacteria and toxins produced in animals and with the administration of sulfonamides. The incidence of polyarteritis nodosa now seems to be subsiding.

☐ **Pathology:** The characteristic lesions of polyarteritis nodosa affect the small to medium-sized muscular arteries and are distributed in a patchy manner. However, on occasion they extend into larger-sized arteries, such as the renal, splenic, or coronary arteries. Each lesion is no more than a millimeter in length and may involve the entire circumference of the vessel or only a part of it. The most prominent morphological feature of the affected artery is an area of fibrinoid necrosis, in which the medial muscle and adjacent tissues are fused into a structureless eosinophilic mass that stains for fibrin. A vigorous acute inflammatory response envelops the area of necrosis, usually involving the entire adventitia (periarteritis), and extends through the other coats of the vessel (Fig. 10-29). Neutrophils, lymphocytes, plasma cells, and macrophages are present in varying proportions, and eosinophils are often conspicuous. Polyarteritis nodosa affecting small vessels is frequently associated with the presence of P-ANCA.

As a result of thrombosis in the lumen of an affected segment, infarcts are commonly found in the involved organs. Injury to larger arteries results in the formation of small aneurysms (<0.5 cm in diameter), particularly in branches of the renal, coronary, and cerebral arteries. An aneurysm may rupture and, if located in a critical area, may be the source of fatal hemorrhage.

If the patient survives for some months, many of the vascular lesions will show evidence of healing, especially if corticosteroids have been administered. The necrotic tissue and inflammatory exudate are resorbed, and the vessel is left with fibrosis of the media and conspicuous gaps in the elastic laminae.

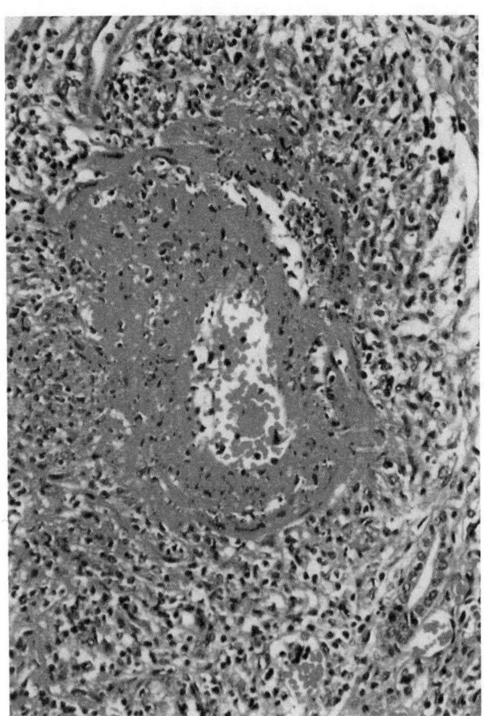

FIGURE *10-29*
Polyarteritis nodosa. The intense inflammatory cell infiltrate in the arterial wall and surrounding connective tissue is associated with fibrinoid necrosis and disruption of the vessel wall.

☐ **Clinical Features:** The clinical manifestations of polyarteritis nodosa are highly variable, depending on the chance occurrence of lesions in different organs. The kidneys, heart, skeletal muscle, skin, and mesentery are most frequently involved, but lesions may also occur in almost any organ of the body, including the bowel, pancreas, lungs, liver, and brain. Constitutional symptoms such as fever and weight loss are common.

Without treatment polyarteritis nodosa is usually fatal, but antiinflammatory and immunosuppressive therapy, in the form of corticosteroids and cyclophosphamide, leads to remissions or cures in the large majority of patients.

Hypersensitivity Angiitis

Hypersensitivity angiitis refers to a broad category of inflammatory vascular lesions that are thought to represent a response to exogenous substances such as bacterial products or drugs. In the case of vascular lesions confined predominantly to the skin, the terms **leukocytoclastic vasculitis** (referring to the nuclear debris from disintegrating neutrophils), **cutaneous vasculitis**, or **cutaneous necrotizing venulitis** (emphasizing the predominant involvement of the venules) are applied. Systemic hypersensitivity angiitis, also referred to as **microscopic polyarteritis**, affects many of the same organs as polyarteritis nodosa but is restricted to the smallest arteries and arterioles.

Cutaneous vasculitis typically follows the administration of a wide variety of drugs, including aspirin, penicillin, and thiazide diuretics. It is also commonly related to disparate infections, such as streptococcal and staphylococcal illnesses, viral hepatitis, tuberculosis, and bacterial endocarditis. The disease typically presents as palpable purpura, principally on the lower extremities. Microscopically, the superficial cutaneous venules display fibrinoid necrosis and an acute inflammatory reaction. Cutaneous vasculitis is generally self-limited. A detailed description of cutaneous necrotizing venulitis is found in Chapter 24.

Systemic hypersensitivity angiitis may be an isolated entity or a feature of other conditions, including collagen vascular diseases (lupus erythematosus, rheumatoid arthritis, Sjögren syndrome), Henoch-Schönlein purpura, dysproteinemias, and a variety of malignant neoplasms. Patients with systemic hypersensitivity angiitis may also present with purpuric lesions in the skin. The most feared complication of microscopic polyarteritis is renal involvement, characterized by **rapidly progressive glomerulonephritis** and **renal failure** (see Chapter 16). Microscopic polyarteritis is strongly associated with the presence of ANCA (60% P-ANCA and 40% C-ANCA).

Allergic Granulomatosis and Angiitis (Churg-Strauss Syndrome)

Churg-Strauss syndrome is a systemic vasculitis with prominent eosinophilia that occurs in young persons with asthma. C-ANCA or P-ANCA is demonstrated in two thirds of the patients. Widespread necrotizing vascular lesions of the small and medium-sized arteries (Fig. 10-30), arterioles, and veins are found in the lungs, spleen, kidney, heart, liver, central nervous system, and other organs. The lesions are characterized by granulomas and an intense eosinophilic infiltrate in and around blood vessels. The resulting fibrinoid necrosis, thrombosis, and aneurysm formation may simulate polyarteritis nodosa, although Churg-Strauss syndrome seems to be a distinct entity. The disease must also be distinguished from other eosinophilic syndromes, such as parasitic and fungal infestations, Wegener granulomatosis, eosinophilic pneumonia (Loeffler syndrome), and drug vasculitis. Untreated persons with allergic granulomatosis and angiitis have a poor prognosis, but corticosteroids are now almost always successful in the treatment of the disease.

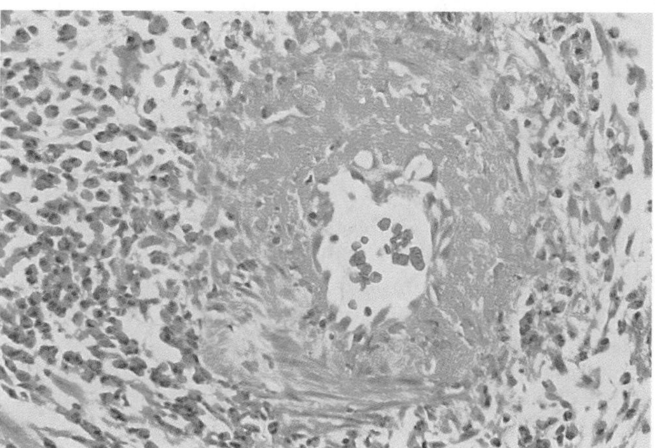

FIGURE *10-30*
Churg-Strauss syndrome. A medium-sized artery shows fibrinoid necrosis and a surrounding eosinophilic infiltrate.

Giant Cell Arteritis (Temporal Arteritis, Granulomatous Arteritis)

Giant cell arteritis describes a focal, chronic, granulomatous inflammation of the temporal arteries. **It is today the most common form of vasculitis.** Although the disease most often affects the temporal artery, it can also involve additional cranial arteries, the aorta (giant cell aortitis) and its branches, and occasionally other arteries. The average age at onset is 70 years, and the disease rarely occurs in those younger than 50. The incidence rises with age and may reach 1% by 80 years of age. Women are affected slightly more often than men. The age at onset helps differentiate this entity from other vasculitides that may affect the same vessels, such as Takayasu disease, which occurs in much younger persons.

The etiology of giant cell arteritis is obscure. The association of this disease with HLA-DR4 and its occurrence in first-degree relatives support a genetic component in its pathogenesis. The morphological alterations, including the presence of activated CD4+ T-helper cells, suggest an immunological reaction, and a cell-mediated response to arterial antigens has been reported in some cases. The generalized muscle aching and widespread distribution of its manifestations are consistent with a relationship to rheumatoid diseases.

☐ **Pathology:** In giant cell arteries, the affected vessels is cordlike and exhibits nodular thickening. The lumen is reduced to a slit or may be obliterated by a thrombus. **Microscopic examination reveals granulomatous inflammation of the media and intima consisting of aggregates of macrophages, lymphocytes, and plasma cells, with varying admixtures of eosinophils and neutrophils** (Fig. 10-31A). Giant cells, which tend to be distributed at the site of the internal elastic lamina (see Fig. 10-31B), are usually conspicuous, but vary widely in number. Both foreign-body giant cells and Langhans giant cells may be found. Foci of necrosis are characterized by changes in the internal elastica, which becomes swollen, irregular, and fragmented, and in advanced lesions may completely disappear. Fragments of the elastica occasionally appear in the giant cells. In the late stages, the intima is conspicuously thickened and the media is fibrotic. Thrombosis may obliterate the lumen, after which organization and canalization occur.

☐ **Clinical Features:** Giant cell arteritis tends to be benign and self-limited, with the symptoms subsiding in 6 to 12 months. Patients present with headache and throbbing temporal pain. In some instances, there are early constitutional symptoms, including malaise, fever, and weight loss, accompanied by generalized muscular aching or stiffness in the shoulders and hips (polymyalgia rheumatica). The throbbing and pain over the temporal artery are accompanied by swelling, tenderness, and redness in the skin overlying the vessel. Visual symptoms occur in almost half of the patients and may proceed from transient to permanent blindness in one or both eyes. In an occasional patient, the disease gives rise to infarcts in the myocardium, brain, or gastrointestinal tract, which may be fatal.

Biopsy of the temporal artery may not disclose the disease in as many as 40% of patients with otherwise classic manifestations. The response to corticosteroid therapy is usually dramatic, with symptoms subsiding in a matter of days.

Wegener Granulomatosis

Wegener granulomatosis is a systemic necrotizing vasculitis of unknown etiology characterized by granulomatous lesions of the respiratory tract (the nose, sinuses, and lungs) and renal glomerular disease. Men are affected more often than women, usually in the fifth and sixth decades of life. The etiology of the disease is unknown, and no infectious agent has been uncovered. More than 90% of patients with Wegener granulomatosis exhibit ANCA in the blood, of whom 75% have C-ANCA. It has been suggested that these antibodies activate circulating neutrophils to attack blood vessels. The response to immunosuppressive therapy supports an immunological basis for the disease.

☐ **Pathology:** The lesions of Wegener granulomatosis feature parenchymal necrosis, vasculitis, and a granulomatous inflammation composed of neutrophils, lymphocytes, plasma cells, macrophages, and eosinophils. The individual lesions in the lung may be as large as 5 cm across and must be distinguished from those of tuberculosis. **Vasculitis involving small arteries and veins** may

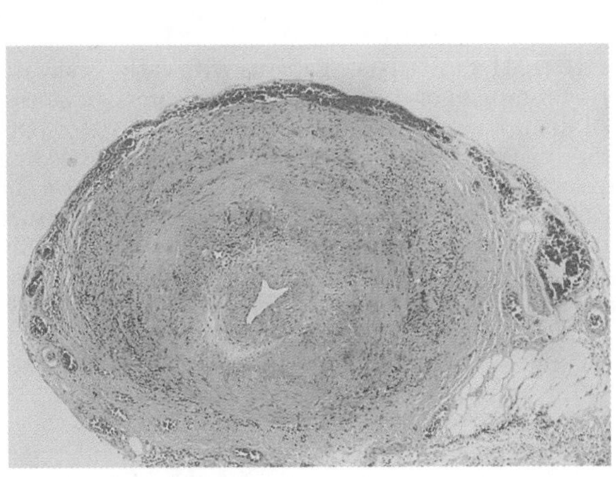

A

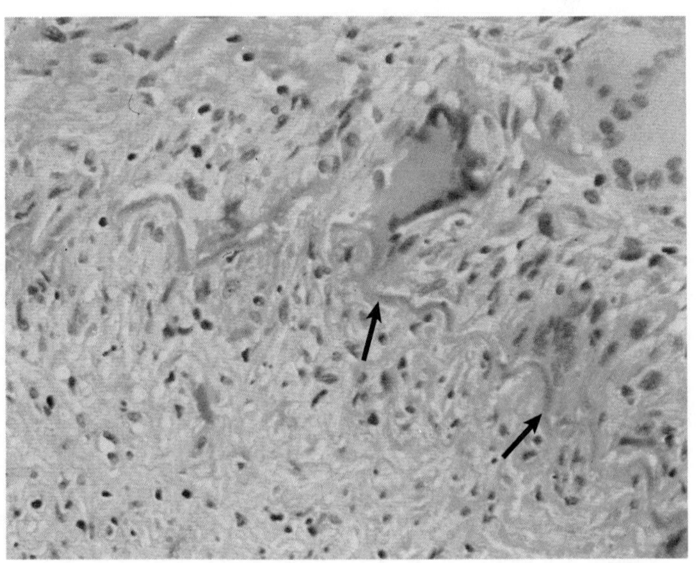

B

FIGURE *10-31*
Temporal arteritis. ***(A)*** **A photomicrograph of a temporal artery shows chronic inflammation throughout the wall, giant cells, and a lumen severely narrowed by intimal thickening.** ***(B)*** **A high-power view shows giant cells adjacent to the fragmented internal elastic lamina (*arrows*).**

be found anywhere, but occurs most frequently in the respiratory tract (Fig. 10-32), kidney, and spleen. The arteritis is characterized principally by chronic inflammation, although acute inflammation, necrotizing and non-necrotizing granulomatous inflammation, and fibrinoid necrosis are frequently present. Medial thickening and intimal proliferation are common and often result in narrowing or obliteration of the lumen.

The most prominent pulmonary feature is a persistent bilateral pneumonitis, with nodular infiltrates that undergo cavitation in a manner similar to that of tuberculous lesions (although the mechanisms are clearly different). The kidney initially exhibits focal necrotizing glomerulonephritis, which progresses to crescentic glomerulonephritis (see Chapter 17). Chronic sinusitis and ulcerations of the nasopharyngeal mucosa are common.

☐ **Clinical Features:** The large majority of patients with Wegener granulomatosis present with symptoms referable to the respiratory tract, particularly pneumonitis and sinusitis. In fact, the lung is eventually involved in over 90% of patients. Radiologically, multiple pulmonary infiltrates, which are often cavitary, are prominent. Hematuria and proteinuria are common, and the glomerular disease can progress to renal failure. Rashes, muscular pains, joint involvement, and neurological symptoms occur. In untreated Wegener granulomatosis, most persons (80%) die within a year of onset, with a mean survival of 5 to 6 months. Treatment with cyclophosphamide produces a striking improvement in the prognosis, and both complete remissions and substantial disease-free intervals are induced in most patients. Interestingly, the administration of antimircobialsulfa drugs significantly reduces the incidence of remissions, suggesting a relationship of the disease to bacterial infections.

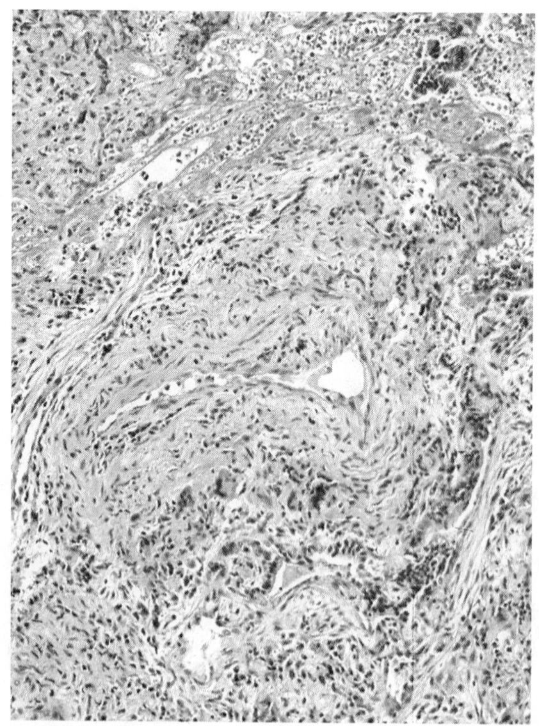

FIGURE *10-32*
Wegener granulomatosis. A photomicrograph of the lung shows vasculitis of a pulmonary artery. There are chronic inflammatory cells and Langhans giant cells in the wall and thickening of the intima.

Takayasu Arteritis

Takayasu arteritis refers to an inflammatory disorder of large arteries, classically the aortic arch and its major branches. The malady has a worldwide distribution and primarily affects young women (90%), the large majority of whom are younger than 30 years of age. The cause of Takayasu arteritis is unknown, but an autoimmune basis has been proposed.

☐ **Pathology:** Takayasu arteritis is classified according to the extent of aortic involvement: (1) disease restricted to the aortic arch and its branches, (2) arteritis involving only the descending thoracic and abdominal aorta and its branches, and (3) combined involvement of the arch and descending aorta. The pulmonary artery is also occasionally affected, and involvement of the retinal vasculature is often a prominent feature.

On gross examination, the aorta is thickened and the intima exhibits focal, raised plaques. The branches of the aorta often display localized stenosis or occlusion, which interferes with blood flow and accounts for the synonym "pulseless disease" when the subclavian arteries are affected. The aorta, particularly the distal thoracic and abdominal segments, commonly shows variably sized aneurysms. The early lesions of the aorta and its main branches consist of an acute panarteritis, with infiltrates of neutrophils, mononuclear cells, and occasional Langhans giant cells. Inflammation of the vasa vasorum in Takayasu arteritis requires differentiation from syphilitic aortitis. Late lesions display fibrosis and severe intimal proliferation, and secondary atherosclerotic changes may obscure the basic disease.

☐ **Clinical Features:** Patients with early Takayasu arteritis complain of constitutional symptoms, dizziness, visual disturbances, dyspnea, and occasionally syncope. As the disease progresses, cardiac symptoms become more severe and intermittent claudication of the arms or legs appears. Asymmetric differences in blood pressure may develop, and the pulse in one extremity may actually disappear. Hypertension may reflect coarctation of the aorta or renal artery stenosis. The majority of patients eventually manifest congestive heart failure or loss of visual acuity, ranging from field defects to total blindness. Early Takayasu arteritis responds to corticosteroids, but the later lesions require surgical reconstruction.

Kawasaki Disease (Mucocutaneous Lymph Node Syndrome)

Kawasaki disease is an acute necrotizing vasculitis of infancy and early childhood characterized by high fever, rash, conjunctival and oral lesions, and lymphadenitis. In 70% of the

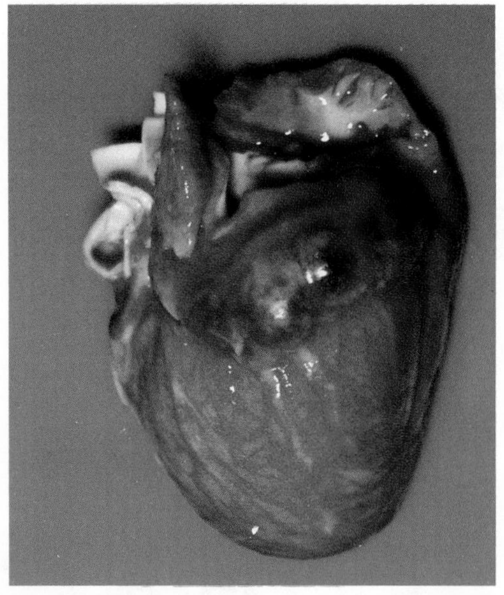

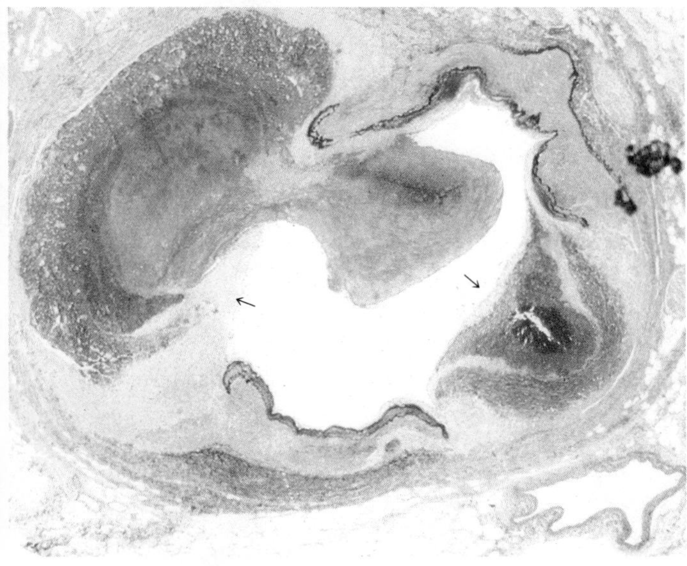

A B

FIGURE *10-33*
Kawasaki disease. (*A*) The heart of a child who died from Kawasaki disease shows conspicuous coronary artery aneurysms. (*B*) A microscopic section of a coronary artery from the same patient shows two large defects (*arrows*) in the internal elastic lamina with two small aneurysms filled with thrombus.

patients, the vasculitis affects the coronary arteries and leads to the formation of coronary artery aneurysms (Fig. 10-33). Such lesions are the cause of death in 1% to 2% of cases.

Kawasaki disease is usually self-limited, and although an infectious cause has been sought, none has been conclusively proved. Infection with parvovirus B19 has been implicated in some cases, and there is evidence for various bacterial infections in others. The common theme seems to be viral or bacterial production of superantigens, molecules that bind to major histocompatibility complex (MHC) class II receptors and the V-beta region of the T cell receptor, thereby overstimulating the immune system.

Thromboangiitis Obliterans (Buerger Disease)

Thromboangiitis obliterans defines an occlusive, inflammatory disease of the medium and small arteries in the distal arms and legs. Buerger disease occurs almost exclusively in young and middle-aged men who smoke heavily.

☐ **Pathogenesis:** The etiological role of smoking in Buerger disease is emphasized by the observation that cessation of smoking can be followed by a remission, and resumption of smoking by an exacerbation. Yet the mechanism of action of tobacco smoke is obscure. Although carbon monoxide has been postulated as a cause, there is no evidence to support such a notion. Interestingly, certain polyphenols from tobacco elicit antibodies and can induce inflammation. Smokers show a higher incidence of such sensitivity to tobacco than do nonsmokers. Cell-mediated hypersensitivity to collagen types II and III has also been observed.

Although at one time the disorder was common in Jewish men in Eastern Europe and their immigrant counterparts in the United States, Buerger disease is now rare in both locations. Its greater frequency in Japan, Israel, and India suggests possible predisposing genetic factors. An increased prevalence of the HLA-A9 and HLA-B5 haplotypes among victims of the disease lends further credence to the idea that a genetically controlled hypersensitivity to tobacco is involved in the pathogenesis of disease.

☐ **Pathology:** The earliest change in Buerger disease is an acute inflammation of medium-sized and small arteries. The neutrophilic infiltrate extends to involve neighboring veins and nerves. The involvement of the endothelium in the inflamed areas leads to thrombosis and obliteration of the lumen (Fig. 10-34A). Small microabscesses of the vessel wall, featuring a central area of neutrophils surrounded by fibroblasts and Langhans giant cells, distinguish the process from thrombosis associated with atherosclerosis. The early lesions often become severe enough to result in gangrene of the extremity, for which the only treatment is amputation. Late in the course of the disease, the thrombi are completely organized and partly canalized.

☐ **Clinical Features:** The symptoms of Buerger disease usually start between the ages of 25 and 40 years and take the form of intermittent claudication (cramping

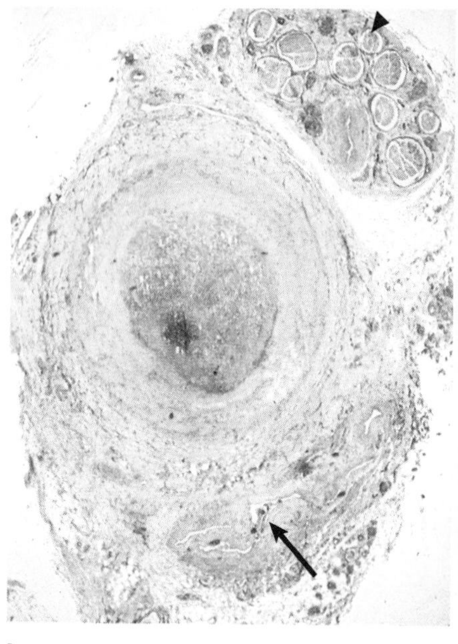
A

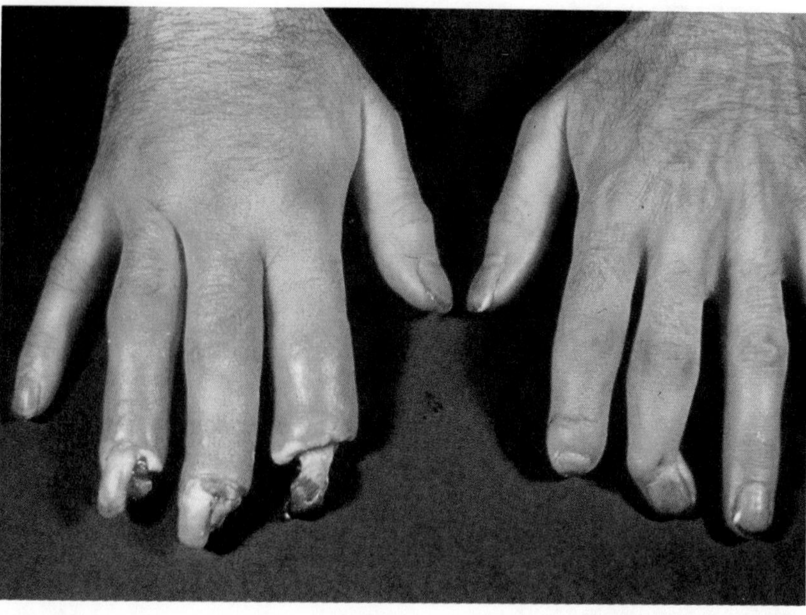
B

FIGURE *10-34*
Buerger disease. (*A*) Section of the upper extremity shows an organized arterial thrombus, which has occluded the lumen. Some inflammatory cells are evident in the adventitial fat. In this instance, the vein (*arrow*) and the adjacent nerve (*arrowhead*) show foci of chronic inflammation. (*B*) The hand shows necrosis of the tips of the fingers.

pains in muscles following exercise, which are quickly relieved by rest). Patients often present with painful ulceration of a digit, which can progresses to destruction of the tips of the involved digits (see Fig. 10-34B). Persons with Buerger disease who continue to smoke may slowly lose both hands and feet.

Behçet Disease

Behçet disease is a systemic vasculitis characterized by oral aphthous ulcers, genital ulceration, and ocular inflammation, and occasionally lesions in the central nervous system, the gastrointestinal tract, and the cardiovascular system. Both large and small vessels display a vasculitis. The mucocutaneous lesions show a nonspecific vasculitis of arterioles, capillaries, and venules, characterized by infiltration of the walls and perivascular tissue by lymphocytes and plasma cells. Occasional endothelial cells are proliferated and swollen. Medium- and large-sized arteries disclose a destructive arteritis, with fibrinoid necrosis, mononuclear infiltration, thrombosis, aneurysms, and hemorrhage. The cause of Behçet syndrome is unknown, but an association with specific HLA subtypes suggests an immune basis. The disease is often responsive to corticosteroids.

Rickettsial Vasculitis

Rickettsiae are obligate intracellular parasites, which produce a characteristic vasculitis. The vasculitis in each of the different rickettsial diseases affects different types of small vessels, and its extent and severity varies. In general, the organisms disseminate from the entry site into the bloodstream and invade endothelial cells, smooth muscle cells of the media of small vessels, and capillaries. These infections are discussed in detail in Chapter 9.

ANEURYSMS

Arterial aneurysms are localized dilatations of blood vessels caused by a congenital or acquired weakness in the media. They are not rare, and their incidence tends to rise with age. In fact, aneurysms of the aorta and other arteries are found in as many as 10% of autopsies. The wall of an aneurysm is formed by the stretched remnants of the arterial wall.

Aneurysms are classified by location, configuration, and etiology (Fig. 10-35). The location refers to the type of vessel involved—artery or vein—and the specific vessel affected, such as the aorta or popliteal artery.

- **A fusiform aneurysm** is an ovoid swelling parallel to the long axis of the vessel.
- **A saccular aneurysm** is a bubble-like outpouching of the arterial wall at the site of a weakened media.
- **A dissecting aneurysm** is actually a dissecting hematoma, in which hemorrhage into the media separates the layers of the vascular wall by a column of blood.
- **An arteriovenous aneurysm** is a direct communication between an artery and a vein.

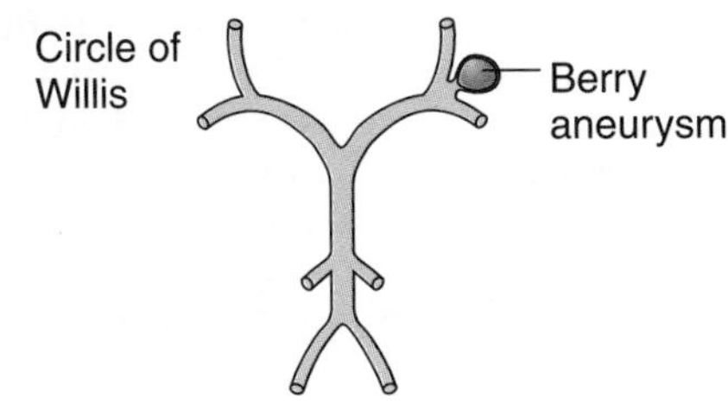

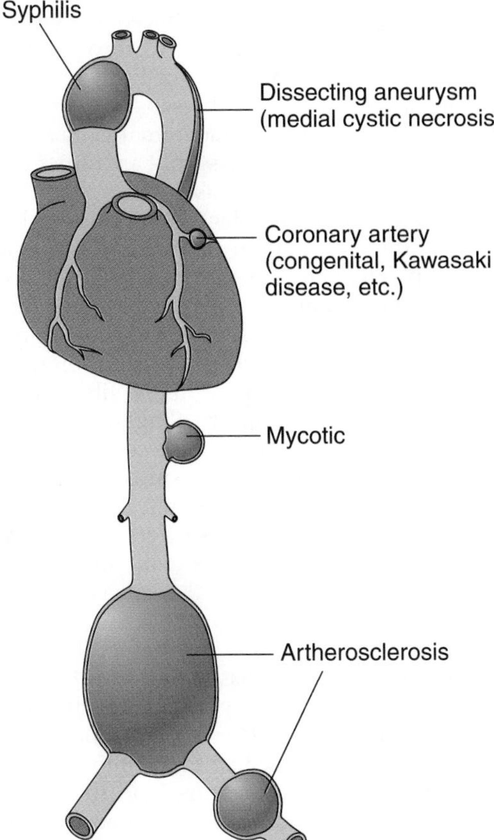

FIGURE 10-35
The locations of aneurysms. Syphilitic aneurysms are the common variety in the ascending aorta, which is usually spared by the atherosclerotic process. Atherosclerotic aneurysms can occur in the abdominal aorta or muscular arteries, including the coronary and popliteal arteries and other vessels. Berry aneurysms are seen in the circle of Willis, mainly at branch points; their rupture leads to subarachnoid hemorrhage. Mycotic aneurysms occur almost anywhere that bacteria can deposit on vessel walls.

Abdominal Aortic Aneurysms

An aneurysm of the abdominal aorta is defined as a dilatation of the vessel in which its diameter is increased at least 50% They are the most frequent aneurysms, usually developing after the age of 50 years, and are associated with severe atherosclerosis of the artery, with a prevalence rising to 6% after the age of 80 years. Aortic aneurysms occur much more often in men than in women, and half of the patients are hypertensive. Occasionally, aneurysms are found in the ascending arch and descending parts of the thoracic aorta, and they also can occur in the iliac and popliteal arteries.

Although abdominal aortic aneurysms invariably occur in the context of atherosclerosis, it is thought that the disease is actually multifactorial. Familial clustering suggests a role for genetic predisposition. A variety of changes in the extracellular matrix of the aortic wall has been described and hemodynamic factors have also been implicated, particularly with regard to hypertension.

☐ **Pathology:** Most abdominal aneurysms of the aorta are distal to the renal arteries and proximal to the bifurcation (Fig. 10-36). The aneurysms are usually fusiform, although saccular varieties are occasionally encountered. The lesions may be of almost any size, but the majority of the symptomatic ones are more than 5 to 6 cm in diameter. Some of these aneurysms extend into the iliac arteries, which may also exhibit distinct aneurysms distal to the one in the aorta. Aneurysms that extend above the renal arteries may occlude the origin of the superior mesenteric artery and the celiac axis.

The large majority of abdominal aortic aneurysms are lined by raised, ulcerated, and calcified (complicated) atherosclerotic lesions. Most contain a mural thrombus of

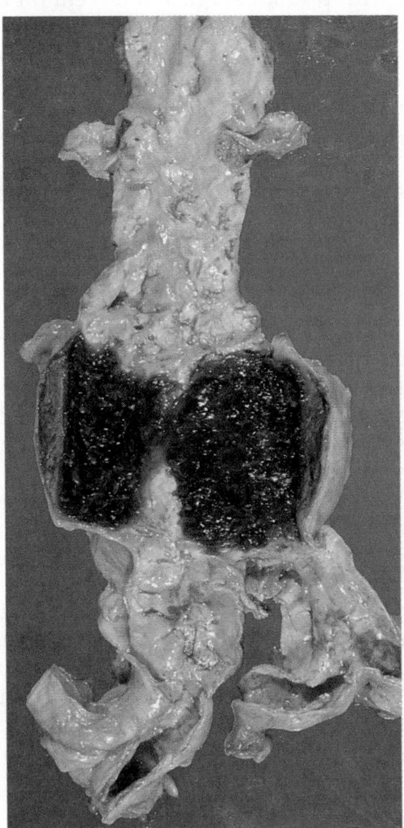

FIGURE 10-36
Atherosclerotic aneurysm of the abdominal aorta. The aneurysm has been opened longitudinally to reveal a large mural thrombus in the lumen. The aorta and common iliac arteries display complicated lesions of atherosclerosis.

varying degrees of organization. Portions of the thrombus may dislodge and be carried in the bloodstream as emboli to peripheral arteries. Infrequently, the thrombus itself may enlarge sufficiently to compromise the lumen of the aorta.

Microscopic examination reveals complicated atherosclerotic lesions, with destruction of the normal arterial wall and its replacement by fibrous tissue. Remnants of normal media are seen focally, and atheromatous lesions extend to variable depths. The adventitia is thickened and focally inflamed. The inflammation is considered to be part of the response to the severe atherosclerosis and does not represent a specific atherosclerotic entity.

☐ **Clinical Features:** Many abdominal aortic aneurysms are asymptomatic and are discovered only by the palpation of a mass in the abdomen or during radiological examination for some other reason. In some cases, the condition is brought to medical attention by the onset of abdominal pain, which often reflects the expansion of the aneurysm. Abrupt occlusion of a peripheral artery by an embolus from the mural thrombus presents as sudden ischemia of a lower limb. The most dreaded complication of aortic aneurysms is rupture and exsanguinating retroperitoneal (or thoracic) hemorrhage, in which case the patient presents with pain, shock, and a pulsatile mass in the abdomen. Such a situation is an acute emergency, and even with prompt surgical intervention half the patients die. Therefore, large aneurysms, even if entirely asymptomatic, are often replaced by or bypassed with prosthetic grafts.

The risk of rupture of an abdominal aortic aneurysm relates to the size of the lesion. Aneurysms less than 4 cm in diameter rarely rupture (2%), whereas 25% to 40% of those larger than 5 cm in diameter rupture within 5 years of their discovery.

Aneurysms of Cerebral Arteries

Aneurysms of cerebral arteries are particularly important because they lead to fatal subarachnoid hemorrhage. The most common type is saccular and is called a berry aneurysm, because it resembles a berry attached to a twig of the arterial tree. The aneurysm results from a congenital defect in a branch point of the arterial wall. Berry aneurysms tend to arise at one of the branching angles of the circle of Willis or in one of the arterial branches. The most common sites are (1) between the anterior cerebral artery and the anterior communicating artery, (2) between the internal carotid artery and the posterior communicating artery, and (3) between the first main divisions of the middle cerebral artery and the bifurcation of the internal carotid artery. Berry aneurysms are discussed in detail in Chapter 28.

Dissecting Aneurysms

Dissecting aneurysm refers to the entry of blood into the arterial wall and its extension along the length of the vessel (Fig. 10-37). In effect, the blood is encompassed by a false lumen within the wall of the artery. Although this lesion is conventionally termed an aneurysm, it is actually a form of hematoma. Dissecting aneurysm most often affects the aorta and its major branches. The frequency of occurrence has been estimated to be as high as 1 in 400 autopsies, with men being affected three times as frequently as women. A dissecting aneurysm may occur at almost any age, but is most common in the sixth and seventh decades of life. **The large majority of patients have a history of hypertension.**

☐ **Pathogenesis:** The pathogenesis of dissecting aneurysm in most instances can be traced to a weakening of the aortic media. The changes were originally described as **cystic medial necrosis** (of Erdheim), because focal loss of elastic and muscle fibers in the media leads to "cystic" spaces filled with a metachromatic myxoid material. These spaces are not true cysts but are rather pools of matrix collected between the cells and tissues of the media. The cause of the medial degeneration is not known. Some cases of dissecting aneurysm represent a complication of Marfan syndrome, an autosomal dominant disorder in which there is a mutation in the gene encoding fibrillin-1 on chromosome 15 (see Chapter 6). Aging also results in mild degenerative changes in the aorta, characterized by focal elastin loss and medial fibrosis. In animals, defective cross-linking of collagen induced by a copper-deficient diet (lysyl oxidase is a copper-dependent enzyme) causes dissecting aneurysm of the aorta. The same lesion is produced by feeding β-aminoproprionitrile, an inhibitor of lysyl oxidase. Persons with Wilson disease who are treated with penicillamine, a copper chelator, also may develop medial necrosis of the aorta. **Taken together, these data suggest that the common factor in these several situations is a defect that leads to weakness of the connective tissue of the aorta.**

The initial event that triggers medial dissection is controversial. More than 95% of cases of dissecting aneurysm show a transverse tear in the intima and internal media, and many investigators hold that a spontaneous laceration of the intima allows blood from the lumen to enter and dissect the media. Alternatively, it has been proposed that hemorrhage from the vasa vasorum into the media weakened by cystic medial necrosis initiates stress on the intima, which in turn leads to the ubiquitous intimal tear.

☐ **Pathology:** The gross appearance of a dissecting aneurysm is striking. The majority of intimal tears are found in the ascending aorta 1 or 2 cm above the aortic ring. The dissection in the media, which occurs within seconds, separates the inner two thirds of the aorta from the outer third. It can also involve the coronary arteries, great vessels of the neck, or the renal, mesenteric, or iliac arteries. Since the outer wall of the false channel of the dissecting aneurysm is thin, hemorrhage into the extravascular space, including the pericardium, mediastinum, pleural space, and the retroperitoneum, is a frequent cause of death. In 5% to 10% of the cases, the blood within the dissecting aneurysm reenters the lumen through a second distal tear to form a "double-barreled aorta." In a comparable proportion, a reentry site leads to communication of the aorta with a major artery, most often the iliac artery.

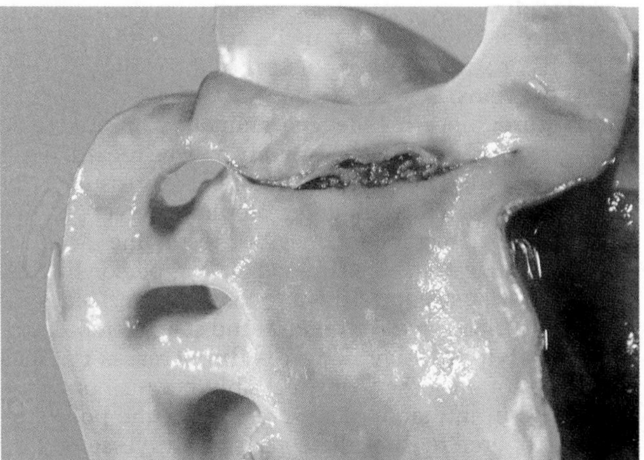

A

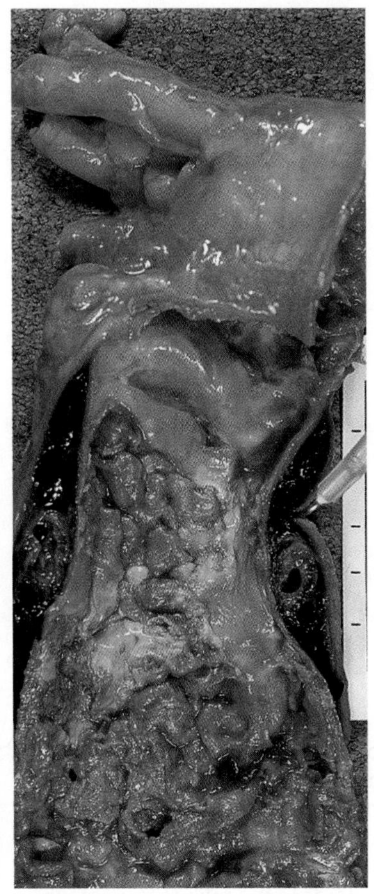

B

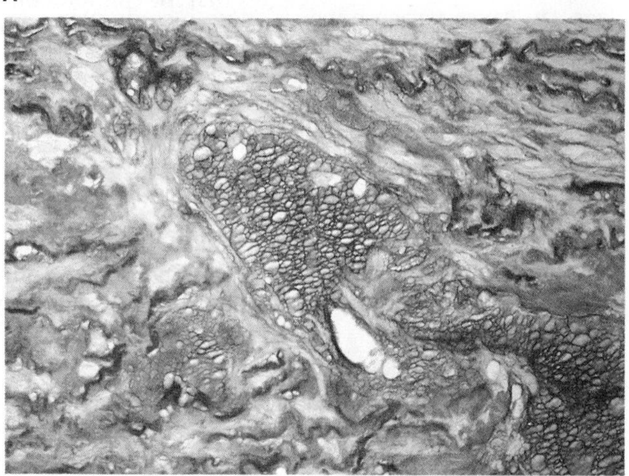

C

FIGURE *10-37*
Dissecting aneurysm of the aorta. (*A*) A transverse tear is present in the aortic arch. The orifices of the great vessels are on the left. (*B*) The thoracic aorta has been open longitudinally and reveals clotted blood dissecting the media of the vessel. The luminal surface shows extensive complicated lesions of atherosclerosis. (*C*) A section of the aortic wall stained with aldehyde fuchsin shows pools of metachromatic material characteristic of the degenerative process known as cystic medial necrosis.

□ **Clinical Features:** The typical patient with an aortic dissection presents with the acute onset of severe, "tearing" pain in the anterior chest, which is sometimes misdiagnosed as myocardial infarction. A loss of one or more arterial pulses is common, and a murmur of aortic regurgitation is often present. Whereas hypertension is a frequent finding, hypotension is an ominous sign, suggesting aortic rupture. Cardiac tamponade or congestive heart failure is diagnosed by the usual criteria.

Before antihypertensive and surgical treatment became available, more than a third of patients with aortic dissection died within 24 hours, and 80% succumbed by 2 weeks. Of the survivors, half died within 3 months. Surgical intervention and control of hypertension have now reduced the overall mortality to less than 20%.

Syphilitic Aneurysms

Syphilitic (luetic) aneurysms were once the most common form of aortic aneurysm, but the decline in the prevalence of syphilis has led to a marked decrease in syphilitic vas-

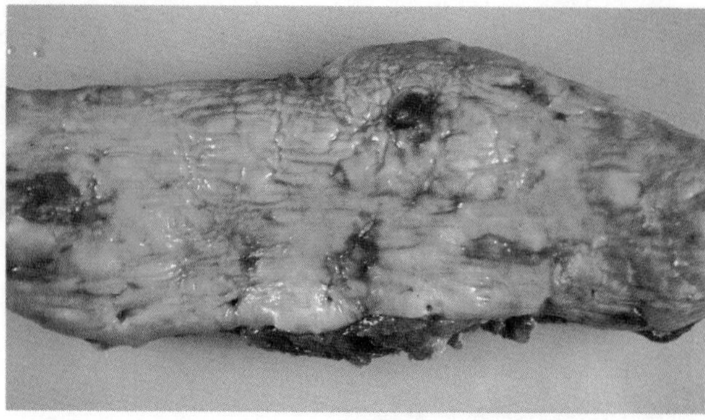

FIGURE 10-38
Syphilitic aortitis. The thoracic aorta is dilated, and its inner surface shows the typical "tree bark" appearance.

cular disease, including aortitis and aneurysms. These aneurysms preferentially affect the ascending aorta, where microscopic examination shows endarteritis and periarteritis of the vasa vasorum. These vessels ramify in the adventitia and penetrate the outer and middle thirds of the aorta, where they become encircled by lymphocytes, plasma cells, and macrophages. Obliterative changes in the vasa vasorum cause focal necrosis and scarring of the media, with disruption and disorganization of the elastic lamellae. The depressed medial scars lead to a roughened intimal surface, which imparts a "tree bark" appearance (Fig. 10-38). The weakened wall of the ascending aorta and aortic arch eventually yields to the relentless pressure of the blood and balloons to form a fusiform aneurysm.

Mycotic (Infectious) Aneurysms

Mycotic aneurysms result from the weakening of the vessel wall by a microbial infection and have a tendency to rupture and hemorrhage. They may develop in the aortic wall or in cerebral vessels during the course of a septicemia, most commonly secondary to bacterial endocarditis. Mesenteric, splenic, or renal arteries are also common sites of involvement. In addition, mycotic aneurysms may occur adjacent to a tuberculous infection or a bacterial abscess.

VEINS

Varicose Veins of the Legs

A varicose vein is an enlarged and tortuous blood vessel. Superficial varicosities of the leg veins, usually in the saphenous system, are among the most common ailments of humans. They vary from a trivial knot of dilated veins to disabling distention of the whole venous system of the leg, with secondary trophic disturbances. It has been estimated that as much as 10% to 20% of the population has some varicosities in the leg veins, but only a fraction of these persons develop symptoms.

☐ **Pathogenesis:** There are a number of risk factor for varicose veins:

- **Age:** The incidence of varicose veins rises with age and may reach 50% in persons older than the age of 50 years. The increase in the frequency of varicose veins with age may reflect degenerative changes of the connective tissues in the vein walls, together with loss of the supporting fat and connective tissues, a more flaccid muscle tone, and inactivity.
- **Sex:** In the 30- to 50-year-old age group, women are affected by varicose veins more often than men, particularly women who have experienced the increased venous pressure associated with the weight of the pregnant uterus on the iliac veins.
- **Heredity:** There is a strong familial predisposition to varicose veins, possibly owing to inherited configurations or structural weaknesses of the walls or valves of the veins.
- **Posture:** Since four-legged animals do not develop varicose veins, this abnormality may be regarded as a price exacted by the erect posture. The pressure in the leg veins is 5 to 10 times greater in the erect position than in the recumbent one. As a result, the incidence of varicose veins is increased among persons whose occupations require them to stand in one place for long periods, such as dentists and sales clerks.
- **Obesity:** Excessive body weight increases the incidence of varicose veins, possibly because of an increase in intraabdominal pressure or the poor support offered by subcutaneous fat to the vessel walls.

Other factors that augment venous pressure in the legs can cause varicose veins. These include pelvic tumors, congestive heart failure, and thrombotic obstruction of the main venous trunks of the thigh or pelvis.

In the pathogenesis of varicose veins, it is not clear whether incompetence of the valves or dilatation of the vessels comes first. Whatever the case, the two reinforce each other. The vein increases both in length and diameter, so that tortuosities develop. Once the process has begun, the varicosity extends progressively throughout the length of the affected vein. As each valve becomes incompetent, a progressively increasing strain is thrown on the vessel and valve below.

☐ **Pathology:** Microscopically, varicose veins exhibit variations in the thickness of the wall. Thinning due to dilatation is present in some areas, whereas others are thickened by muscle hypertrophy, subintimal fibrosis, and the incorporation of mural thrombi into the wall. Patchy calcification is frequently seen. Valvular deformities consist of thickening, shortening, and rolling of the cusps.

☐ **Clinical Features:** The diagnosis of varicose veins of the leg is easily made by inspection. Except for their cosmetic impact, most varicose veins are without clinical effects and require no treatment. The principal symptoms are aching in the legs, aggravated by standing and relieved by elevation. Severe varicosities (Fig. 10-39) may lead to trophic alterations in the skin drained by the

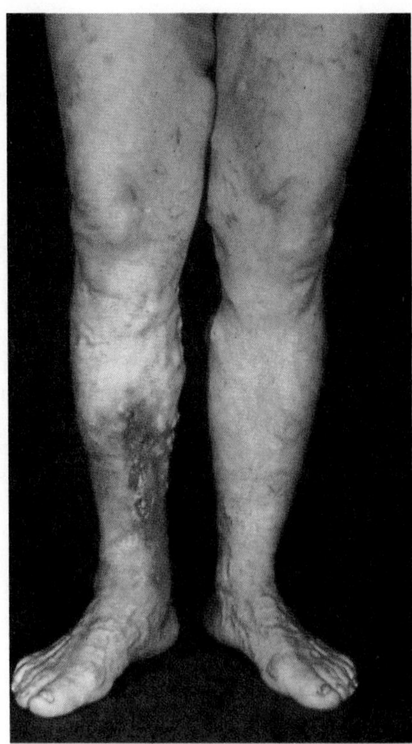

FIGURE *10-39*
Varicose veins of the legs. Severe varicosities of the superficial leg veins have led to stasis dermatitis and secondary ulcerations.

affected veins, termed stasis dermatitis. Surgical intervention is mandated in the presence of ulceration of the overlying skin, spontaneous bleeding, or extensive thrombosis (which may lead to pulmonary embolism).

Varicose Veins at Other Sites

HEMORRHOIDS: These dilatations of the veins of the rectum and anal canal may occur inside or outside the anal sphincter (see Chapter 13). Although there may be a hereditary predisposition, the condition is aggravated by constipation and pregnancy. It may also result from venous obstruction by rectal tumors. Hemorrhoids often bleed, a sign that can cause confusion with bleeding rectal cancers. Thrombosed hemorrhoids are exquisitely painful.

ESOPHAGEAL VARICES: This complication of portal hypertension is caused mainly by cirrhosis of the liver (see Chapter 14). High portal pressure leads to distention of the anastomoses between the portal system and the systemic veins at the lower end of the esophagus. Although they may be prominent radiologically, esophageal varices are usually unimpressive at autopsy. After their collapse at death, often all that is evident on gross examination are bluish streaks in the esophageal mucosa. Hemorrhage from esophageal varices is one of the most common causes of death in cirrhosis.

VARICOCELE: A varicocele is a palpable mass in the scrotum formed by varicosities of the pampiniform plexus (see Chapter 17).

Deep Venous Thrombosis

Thrombophlebitis describes inflammation and secondary thrombosis of small veins, and sometimes larger ones, commonly as part of a local reaction to bacterial infection. **Phlebothrombosis** is the term for venous thrombosis that occurs in the absence of an initiating infection or inflammation. Since the majority of cases of venous thrombosis are not associated with inflammation or infection, the term **deep venous thrombosis** now refers to both phlebothrombosis and thrombophlebitis. The condition is associated with prolonged bed rest or reduced cardiac output and frequently affects the deep leg veins. Such thrombi can be a major threat to life because of embolization to the lung (witness the well-known phenomenon of sudden death occurring on ambulation after surgery). Deep venous thrombosis is discussed more fully in Chapter 7.

Saphenous Vein Bypass Grafts

Autopsy studies have shown that the transplanted saphenous veins used as autografts in coronary artery bypass operations undergo a series of adaptive and reparative changes. These include (1) intimal thickening associated with phlebosclerosis, (2) occasional foci of medial calcification, (3) focal muscle cell hypertrophy, and (4) eventually, scarring of the adventitia. Venous grafts in place for a few years have atherosclerotic plaques indistinguishable from those found in native coronary arteries.

Endothelial cells are frequently lost during the handling of the autografts, and transient adhesion of platelets and inflammatory cells, microthrombi, and edema are found in the intima and inner media. Intimal cells proliferate over the first 4 to 6 weeks, reaching a maximum by 4 to 6 months after insertion of the saphenous graft. Condensation of intimal tissue occurs over the next 6 months, so that by 1 year the graft has a thickened wall adapted to the increased arterial pressure.

Complications, including thrombosis and exuberant proliferation of intimal cells, occurred often in the early years of bypass surgery. Acute thrombosis occurs as a result of turbulent flow and vessel wall injury, especially at the site of the distal anastomosis. However, with gentler methods of handling the grafts and a better understanding of the hemodynamics at anastomosis sites, this problem has become much less frequent. In the long term, half of the grafts occlude within 5 to 10 years, owing to neointimal hyperplasia and atherosclerosis.

LYMPHATIC VESSELS

The lymphatic vessels provide drainage of plasma filtrates, cells, and foreign material from the interstitial spaces. In this way, they also serve as pathways for the spread of two major pathological processes, namely, inflammation and neoplasia. Congenital malformations and primary neoplasms may occur in lymphatics.

Lymphangitis

Lymphangitis, that is, inflammation of the lymphatic vessels, is caused by the entrance of bacteria and inflammatory cells from the sites of drainage. These elements are then conveyed to the regional lymph nodes, where they incite a lymphadenitis. The periphery of a focus of inflammation reveals dilated lymphatics filled with fluid exudate, cells, cellular debris, and bacteria. Lymphatic dilatation depends on a system of fine fibers attached to the surrounding tissues. When the tissues are expanded by exudate, there is a comparable distention of the lymphatic channels.

Almost any virulent pathogen can cause acute lymphangitis, but group β-hemolytic streptococci (Streptococcus pyogenes) are particularly notorious offenders. The process may extend beyond the lymphatic channels into the surrounding tissues. The draining lymph nodes are regularly enlarged and inflamed. Clinically, painful subcutaneous red streaks, often accompanied by painful regional lymph nodes, are characteristic of acute lymphangitis.

Lymphatic Obstruction

Lymphatics may be obstructed by scar tissue, intraluminal tumor cells, pressure from surrounding tumor tissue, or plugging with parasites. Since collateral lymphatic routes are abundant, lymphedema (distention of tissue by lymph) usually occurs only when major trunks are obstructed, especially in the axilla or groin. For example, when radical mastectomy for breast cancer was routine, dissection of the axillary lymph nodes frequently disrupted lymphatic channels and led to lymphedema of the arm. Prolonged lymphatic obstruction causes progressive dilatation of lymphatic vessels, called **lymphangiectasia**, and overgrowth of fibrous tissue. The term **elephantiasis** describes a lymphedematous limb that has become grossly enlarged. An important cause of elephantiasis in the tropics is filariasis, in which a parasitic worm invades the lymphatics (see Chapter 9).

Milroy disease is *an inherited type of lymphedema that is present at birth.* It usually affects only one limb, but it may be more extensive and involve the eyelids and lips. The affected tissues show enormously dilated lymphatic channels, and the entire area appears honeycombed or spongy. This lesion is more properly considered a lymphangiectasia rather than simply lymphedema.

BENIGN TUMORS OF BLOOD VESSELS

Tumors of the vascular system are common, and many are not true neoplasms but rather hamartomas, that is, masses of mature but disorganized cells and tissues characteristic of the particular organ.

Hemangiomas

Hemangiomas are common benign tumors composed of vascular channels. They usually occur in the skin but may also be found in internal organs. Although they are clearly benign, their true origin is uncertain, and they represent either true neoplasms or hamartomas. The evidence in favor of a hamartoma, that is, a malformation, includes the following: (1) the lesion is present at birth; (2) it grows only with the growth of the rest of the body and remains limited in size; and (3) following cessation of growth, it usually remains unchanged indefinitely, unless accidents such as trauma, thrombosis, or hemorrhage supervene.

The development of these vascular malformations recalls the embryology of the vascular system. A network of endothelial channels undergoes remodeling, acquiring a muscular coat and adventitia. In this view, vascular malformations reflect the persistence of the original or modified channels and mixtures of connective tissue elements derived from the mesenchyme.

Hemangiomas are classified by histological type and location.

CAPILLARY HEMANGIOMA: *This lesion is composed of vascular channels that have the size and structure of normal capillaries.* Capillary hemangiomas may be located in any tissue. The most common sites are the skin, subcutaneous tissues, mucous membranes of the lips and the mouth, and internal viscera, including the spleen, kidneys, and liver. Capillary hemangiomas vary from a few millimeters to several centimeters in diameter. Their color is bright red to blue, depending on the degree of oxygenation of the blood. In the skin, capillary hemangiomas are known as "birthmarks" or "ruby spots." The only disability is cosmetic disfiguration.

JUVENILE HEMANGIOMA: Also called **strawberry hemangiomas**, these lesions are found on the skin of newborns. They grow rapidly in the first few months of life, begin to fade at 1 to 3 years of age, and completely regress in the majority of cases (80%) by 5 years of age. Histologically, juvenile hemangioma is composed of packed masses of capillaries separated by a connective tissue stroma. The endothelium-lined channels are usually filled with blood. Thromboses, sometimes organized, are seen. Occasionally, the vascular channels rupture, causing scarring and the accumulation of hemosiderin pigment. Juvenile hemangiomas are usually well demarcated despite the lack of a capsule, although finger-like projections of the vascular tissue may give the impression of invasion. However, the growths are not malignant and they do not invade or metastasize.

CAVERNOUS HEMANGIOMA: *This designation is reserved for lesions consisting of large vascular channels, frequently interspersed with small, capillary-type vessels.* Cavernous hemangiomas occur in the skin (Fig. 10-40), where they are termed **port wine stains**. They also appear on mucosal surfaces and visceral organs, including the spleen, liver, and pancreas. Occasionally, they are found in the brain, where after long quiescent periods they may slowly enlarge and cause neurological symptoms.

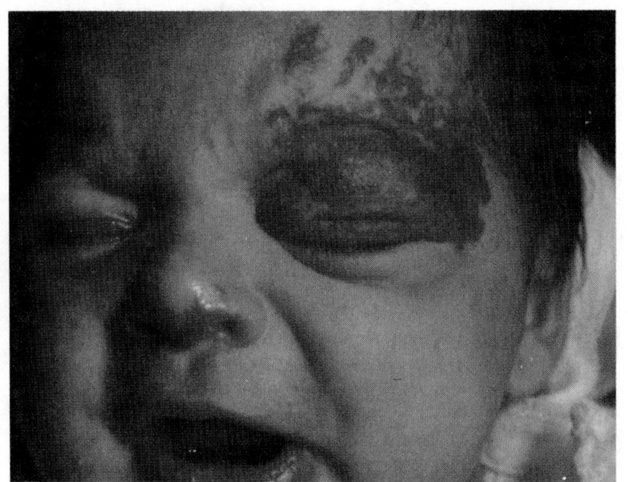

FIGURE 10-40
Congenital cavernous hemangioma of the skin.

A cavernous hemangioma appears as a red-blue, soft, spongy mass, with a diameter of up to several centimeters. Unlike the capillary hemangioma, a cavernous hemangioma does not regress spontaneously. Although the lesion is demarcated by a sharp border, it is not encapsulated. Large endothelial-lined, blood-containing spaces are separated by sparse connective tissue. Cavernous hemangiomas can undergo a variety of changes, including thrombosis and fibrosis, cystic cavitation, and intracystic hemorrhages.

MULTIPLE HEMANGIOMATOUS SYNDROMES: A number of hemangiomas may be found in a single tissue. Two or more tissues may be involved, such as the skin and the nervous system or the spleen and the liver. Eponym enthusiasts have defined various combinations of sites. For example, **von Hippel-Lindau syndrome** is a rare entity in which cavernous hemangiomas occur within the cerebellum or brain stem and the retina. **Sturge-Weber syndrome** is characterized by a developmental disturbance of blood vessels in the brain and skin. Other closely related lesions are plexiform or racemose angiomas, cirsoid aneurysms, and angiomatous dilatation of vessels of the central nervous system and elsewhere.

Glomus Tumor (Glomangioma)

A glomus tumor is a benign, exquisitely painful neoplasm of the glomus body, a convoluted arteriolar-venous anastomosis. Glomus bodies are normal neuromyoarterial receptors that are sensitive to temperature and regulate arteriolar flow. They are widely distributed in the skin, but are most frequent in the distal regions of the fingers and toes. This pattern is reflected in the location of glomus tumors at these sites, typically in a subungual location.

The lesions are small, usually less than 1 cm in diameter, and many are smaller than a few millimeters. In the skin, they are slightly elevated, rounded, red-blue, and firm (Fig. 10-41). The two main histological components are branching vascular channels in a connective tissue stroma and aggregates or nests of the specialized glomus cells. The latter are regular, round to cuboidal cells, which by electron microscopy reveal typical smooth muscle cell features.

Hemangioendothelioma

Hemangioendothelioma refers to a vascular tumor of endothelial cells that is intermediate between benign hemangiomas and frankly malignant angiosarcomas. **The epithelioid, or histiocytoid, variant** displays endothelial cells with considerable eosinophilic, often vacuolated, cytoplasm. Vascular lumina are evident, and there is a paucity of mitoses. These tumors occur in almost all locations. Surgical removal is generally curative, but about one fifth of the patients develop metastases.

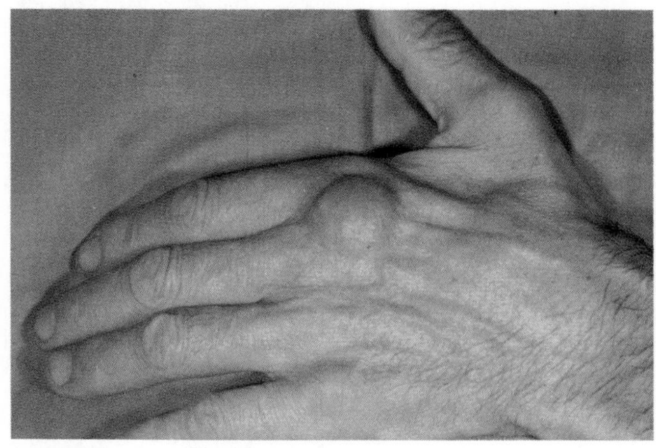

A

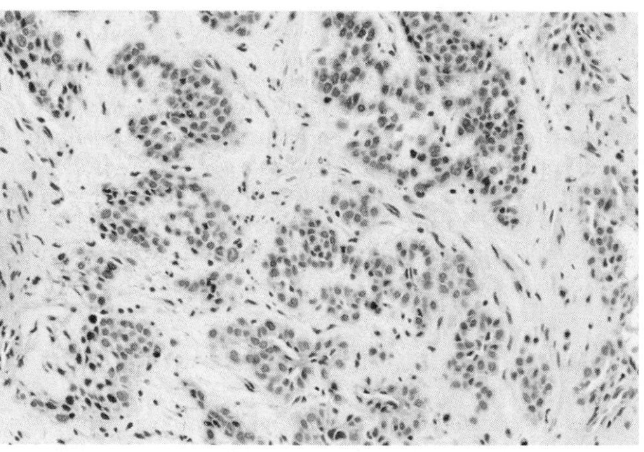

B

FIGURE 10-41
Glomus tumor. *(A)* **The dorsal surface of the hand displays a prominent tumor nodule on the proximal third finger.** *(B)* **A photomicrograph of** *A* **reveals nests of glomus tumor cells embedded in a fibrovascular stroma.**

Spindle cell hemangioendothelioma occurs principally in males of any age, usually in the dermis and subcutaneous tissue of the distal extremities. The tumor features vascular, endothelial-lined spaces into which papillary projections extend. Although the lesion may recur locally after excision, this variant of hemangioendothelioma rarely metastasizes.

MALIGNANT TUMORS OF BLOOD VESSELS

Malignant vascular neoplasms are rare, and only a few arise in preexisting benign tumors.

Angiosarcoma

Angiosarcoma is a rare, highly malignant tumor composed of single or multiple masses of neoplastic endothelial cells. The lesions occur in either sex and at any age and begin as small, painless, sharply demarcated, red nodules. The most common locations are skin, soft tissue, breast, bone, liver, and spleen. Eventually, most angiosarcomas enlarge to become pale gray, fleshy masses without a capsule. Often these tumors undergo central necrosis, with softening and hemorrhage.

Angiosarcomas exhibit varying degrees of differentiation, ranging from those composed mainly of distinct vascular elements to undifferentiated tumors with few recognizable blood channels. The latter display frequent mitoses, pleomorphism, and giant cells and tend to be more malignant. Almost half of all patients with an angiosarcoma will die of the disease.

Angiosarcoma of the liver is of special interest because of its association with environmental carcinogens. Arsenic is a component of pesticides, and vinyl chloride is used in the production of plastics. Hepatic angiosarcoma has also been associated with the administration of thorium dioxide (Thorotrast), a material used by radiologists prior to 1950. This radioactive contrast medium is engulfed by the macrophages of the liver sinusoids, where it remains for life.

There is a long latent period between exposure to the chemicals or radionuclide and the development of angiosarcoma of the liver. The earliest detectable changes are atypism and diffuse hyperplasia of the cells lining the hepatic sinusoids. The tumors are frequently multicentric and may arise in the spleen as well as the liver. Hepatic angiosarcomas are highly malignant and exhibit both local invasion and metastatic spread.

Hemangiopericytoma

Hemangiopericytoma is a rare malignant neoplasm that presumably arises from pericytes, the modified smooth muscle cells that are external to the walls of capillaries and arterioles. Hemangiopericytomas present as small masses and consist of capillary-like channels surrounded by, and frequently enclosed within, nests and masses of round to spindle-shaped cells. The tumor cell type is identified by a characteristic investment of basement membrane, similar to that of its normal counterpart.

Hemangiopericytomas can occur anywhere, but are most frequently encountered in the retroperitoneum and lower extremities. The majority of hemangiopericytomas are removed surgically without having invaded or metastasized. The reported metastatic rate varies from 10% to 50%, depending on the series. Malignant hemangiopericytomas metastasize to lungs, bone, liver, and lymph nodes.

Kaposi Sarcoma

Kaposi sarcoma is a malignant tumor derived from endothelial cells. It was originally described in the 19th century by Moritz Kaposi (née Kohn) as a sporadic tumor in the sixth and seventh decades of life, with an incidence 10 times higher in men than in women. However, this picture has changed dramatically, and Kaposi sarcoma has now appeared in epidemic form in association with acquired immune deficiency syndrome (AIDS). In this respect, it is interesting that for some years before AIDS appeared, Kaposi sarcoma was known to be common in parts of Central Africa (where AIDS is now rampant) and to afflict younger men. The etiology of this formerly rare disease is now clearer. Its association with the current AIDS epidemic as a widespread, multifocal lesion suggests that it is related to the loss of immunity. A virus of the herpes family (HHV8) is a newly detected agent in endothelial and spindle cells of Kaposi sarcoma and is thought to contribute to the genesis of the tumor (see Chapter 4).

Kaposi sarcoma begins as painful purple or brown nodules in the skin, varying from 1 mm to 1 cm in diameter. They occur most often on the hands or feet but may appear anywhere. The histological appearance of Kaposi sarcoma is highly variable. One form resembles a simple hemangioma and is characterized by tightly packed clusters of capillaries and scattered hemosiderin-laden

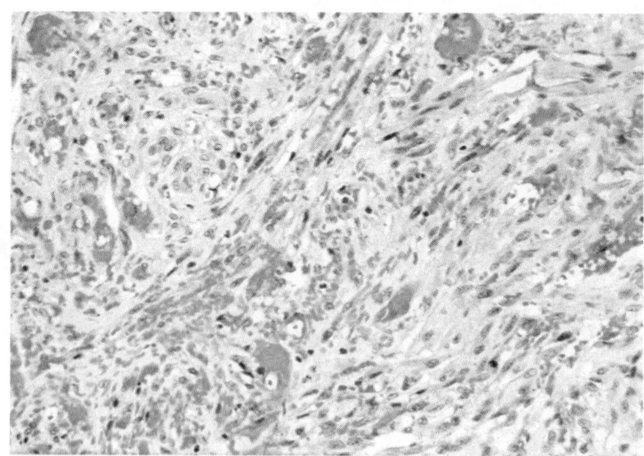

FIGURE *10-42*
Kaposi sarcoma. A photomicrograph of a vascular lesion from a patient with acquired immune deficiency syndrome shows numerous poorly differentiated, spindle-shaped neoplastic cells and a vascular lesion filled with red blood cells.

macrophages. In other forms of the tumor, the lesions are highly cellular and the vascular spaces are less prominent (Fig. 10-42). These lesions may be difficult to distinguish from fibrosarcomas, but the characteristic features of endothelial cells can be demonstrated immunochemically and by electron microscopy. Although Kaposi sarcoma is considered to be a malignant lesion and may be widely disseminated in the body, it is only exceptionally a cause of death.

TUMORS OF THE LYMPHATIC SYSTEM

Many histological and clinical variants of local enlargements of the lymphatics have been described. It is difficult to distinguish among anomalies, proliferations due to stasis, and true neoplasms. In general, lymphatic tumors are distinguished by their size and location. The spaces may be small, as in capillary lymphangiomas, or large and dilated, as in cystic or cavernous lesions. Lymphangiomatous lesions can arise at almost any site, including the skin, mediastinum, retroperitoneum, spleen, and other locations.

Capillary Lymphangioma

Sometimes called "simple lymphangiomas," these benign tumors are small, circumscribed, grayish pink, fleshy nodules, which can be single or multiple. They are subcutaneous and found in the skin of the face, lips, chest, genitalia, or extremities. Capillary lymphangiomas are composed of variably sized, thin-walled spaces that are lined by endothelial cells and contain lymph and occasional leukocytes.

Cystic Lymphangioma (Cystic Hygroma, Cavernous Lymphangioma)

These benign lesions occur most often in the neck and axilla, less commonly in the mediastinum, and occasionally in the retroperitoneum. They may reach a size of 10 to 15 cm in diameter or more and fill the axilla or distort structures of the neck.

Cystic lymphangiomas are soft, spongy, and pink, and watery fluid exudes from their cut surface. Microscopically, they are composed of endothelial-lined spaces that contain a protein-rich fluid. These spaces are distinguished from blood vessels by their lack of erythrocytes and leukocytes. An abundance of irregularly distributed smooth muscle and connective tissue cells may be present.

Lymphangiosarcoma

A rare malignant tumor develops in 0.1% to 0.5% of patients with lymphedema of the arm following radical mastectomy. A distinction between this tumor and angiosarcoma is difficult, and some authors equate the two cancers. Lymphangiosarcoma may also occur in other regions, for example, in the leg following radiation therapy for uterine cervical carcinoma.

Lymphangiosarcomas present as purplish, frequently multiple nodules in the edematous skin. Histologically, the nodules are composed of cells that resemble capillary epithelial cells, with a few pinocytotic vesicles and microfilaments. There are zonulae adherentes between the cells, similar to those in endothelial cells. The walls of the tumor vessels have a rudimentary form of basal basement membrane. Lymphangiosarcomas are highly malignant and, despite radical surgery, carry a poor prognosis.

SUGGESTED READING

BOOKS

Bloom S: *Diagnostic criteria for cardiovascular pathology*. Philadelphia: Lippincott–Raven, 1997.

Fuster V, Ross R, Topol EJ: *Atherosclerosis and coronary artery disease*. Philadelphia: Lippincott–Raven, 1996.

Numano F, Ross R (eds): Atherosclerosis IV: Recent advances in atherosclerosis research. The Fourth Saratoga International Conference on Atherosclerosis. *Ann New York Acad Sci*, p. 811, 1997.

Tilson D, Boyd CD (eds): The abdominal aortic aneurysm: Genetics, pathophysiology, and molecular biology. *Ann New York Acad Sci*, p. 800, 1996.

REVIEW ARTICLES

Alexander RW: Hypertension and the pathogenesis of atherosclerosis. Oxidative stress and the mediation of arterial inflammatory response: A new perspective. *Hypertension* 25:155–161, 1995.

Dammerman M, Breslow JL: Genetic basis for lipoprotein disorders. *Circulation* 91:505–512, 1995.

Demers LL, Watson KE, Bostrom K: Mechanism of calcification in atherosclerosis. *Trends Cardiovasc Med* 4:45–49, 1994.

Ettenson DA, Gotlieb AI: Role of endothelial cells in vascular integrity and repair in atherosclerosis. *Adv Pathol Lab Med* 6:285–309, 1993.

Frid MG, Dempsey EC, Durmowicz AG, Stenmark KR: Smooth muscle heterogeneity in pulmonary and systemic vessels. *Arterioscler Thromb Vasc Biol* 17: 1203–1209, 1997.

Fuster V, Badimon L, Badimon JJ, Chesebro JH: The pathogenesis of coronary artery disease and the acute coronary syndromes. *N Engl J Med* 326:242–250 and 326:310–318, 1992.

Garlanda C, Dejana E: Heterogeneity of endothelial cells: Specific markers. *Arterioscler Thromb Vasc Biol* 17: 1193–1202, 1997.

Glagov S: Intimal hyperplasia, vascular remodeling and the restenosis problem. *Circulation* 89:2888–2891, 1994.

Hurt–Camejo E, Olsson U, Wiklund O, Bondjers G, Camejo G: Cellular consequences of the association of ApoB lipoproteins with proteoglycans. *Arterioscler Thromb Vasc Biol* 17:1011–1017, 1997.

Introna M, Mantovani A: Early activation signals in endothelial cells: Stimulation by cytokines. *Arterioscler Thromb Vasc Biol* 17:423–428, 1997.

Lahav J, Vermylen J (eds): 1995: State of the art. *Thrombosis and Haemostasis* 74:1–579, 1995.

Lee RT, Libby P: The unstable atheroma. *Arterioscler Thromb Vasc Biol* 17:1859–1867, 1997.

Nicholson AC, Hajjar DP: Herpesviruses in atherosclerosis and thrombosis: Etiologic agents or ubiquitous bystanders? *Arterioscler Thromb Vasc Biol* 18:339–348, 1998.

Pepper MS: Manipulating angiogenesis: From basic science to the bedside. *Arterioscler Thromb Vasc Biol* 17: 605–619, 1997.

Schoen FJ, Libby P: Cardiac transplant graft arteriosclerosis. *Trends Cardiovasc Med* 1:216–223, 1991.

Schwartz SM, de Blois D, O'Brien ERM: The intima: Soil for atherosclerosis and restenosis. *Circ Res* 77: 445–465, 1995.

Stary HC, Blankenhorn DH, Chandler AB, et al: A definition of the intima of human arteries and of its atherosclerosis-prone regions: A report from the Committee on Vascular Lesions of the Council on Arteriosclerosis, American Heart Association. *Circulation* 85:391–405, 1992.

Stary HC, Chandler AB, Glagov S, et al: A definition of initial, fatty streak, and intermediate lesions of atherosclerosis: A report from the Committee on Vascular Lesions of the Council on Arteriosclerosis, American Heart Association. *Arterioscler Thromb* 14:840–856, 1994.

Stary HC, Chandler AB, Dinsmore RE, et al: A definition of advanced types of atherosclerotic lesions and a histological classification of atherosclerosis: A report from the Committee on Vascular Lesions of the Council on Arteriosclerosis, American Heart Association. *Arterioscler Thromb Vas Biol* 15:1512–1531, 1995.

Sundy JS, Haynes BF: Pathogenic mechanisms of vessel damage in vasculitis syndromes. *Rheum Dis Clin North Am* 21:861–881, 1995.

Waller BF, Orr CM, Pinkerton CA, et al: Morphologic observations late after coronary balloon angioplasty: Mechanisms of acute injury and relationship to restenosis. *Radiology* 174:961–967, 1990.

CHAPTER 11

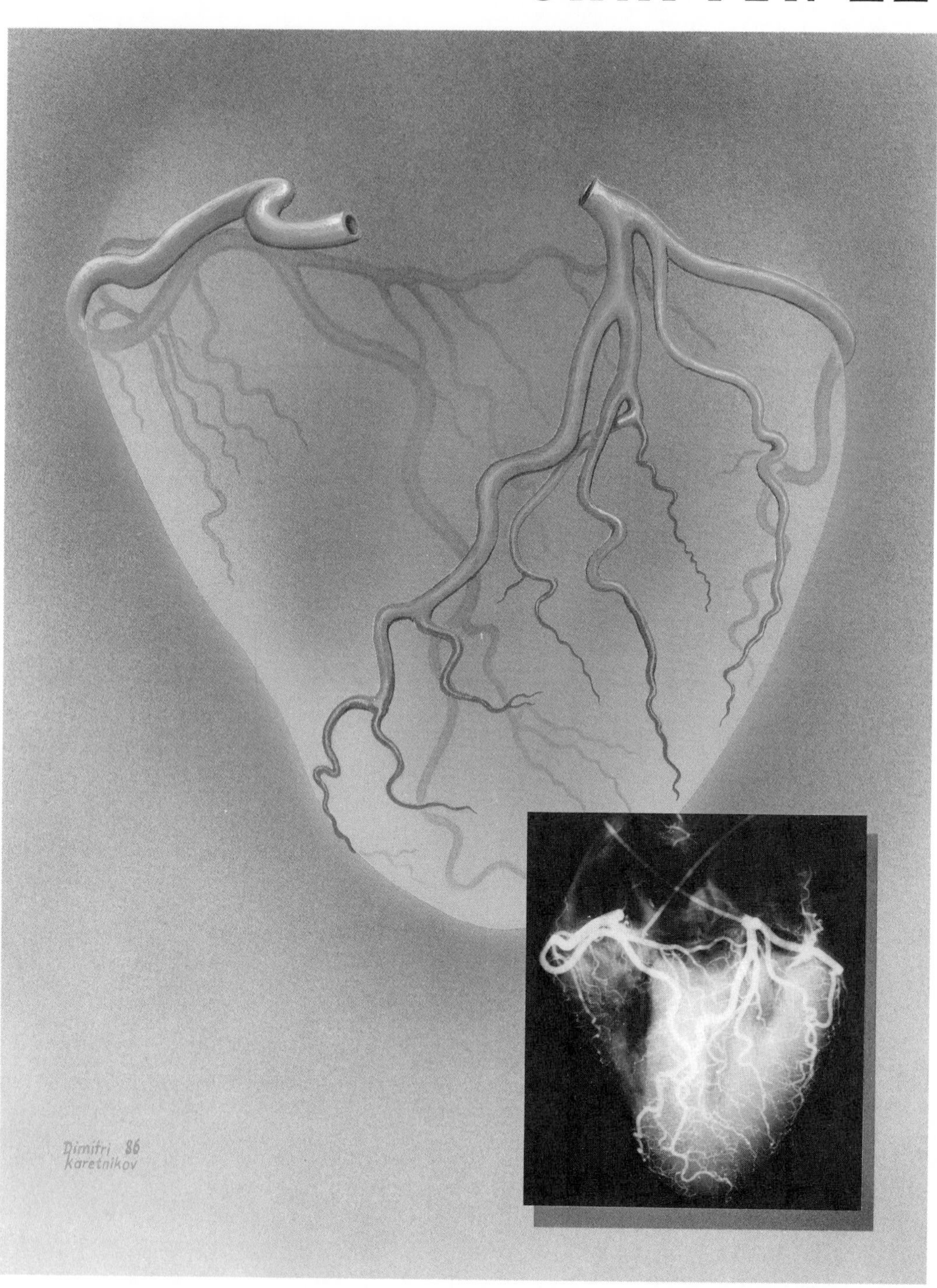

The Heart

Robert B. Jennings
Charles Steenbergen, Jr.

(continued)

FIGURE *11-1 (see opposite page)*
The coronary circulation. The right coronary artery *(green)* supplies the back of the left ventricle and gives rise to the posterior descending artery. The left main coronary artery divides into the anterior descending *(red)* and the circumflex *(orange)* branches. *(Inset)* Postmortem coronary arteriogram.

Nonbacterial Thrombotic Endocarditis (Marantic Endocarditis)

Calcific Aortic Stenosis

Calcification of the Mitral Valve Annulus

Mitral Valve Prolapse

Papillary Muscle Dysfunction

Carcinoid Heart Disease

Primary Myocardial Diseases

Myocarditis

Metabolic Diseases of the Heart

Hyperthyroid Heart Disease

Hypothyroid Heart Disease

Thiamine Deficiency (Beriberi) Heart Disease

Cardiomyopathy

Idiopathic Dilated Cardiomyopathy

Secondary Dilated Cardiomyopathy

Hypertrophic Cardiomyopathy

Restrictive Cardiomyopathy

Cardiac Tumors

Cardiac Myxoma

Rhabdomyoma

Papillary Fibroelastoma

Other Tumors

Diseases of the Pericardium

Pericardial Effusion

Acute Pericarditis

Constrictive Pericarditis

Pathology of Interventional Therapies

Coronary Angioplasty

Coronary Bypass Grafts

Prosthetic Valves

Heart Transplantation

The heart is a fist-sized muscular pump that has a remarkable capacity to work unceasingly for the 70 to 80 years of a human lifetime. As demand requires, it can increase its output manyfold, in part because the coronary circulation can augment its blood flow to a rate more than 10 times normal. The ventricles also respond to an acute increase in their workload by dilating, in accordance with Starling's law of the heart. When an increased workload is imposed for a longer period, for example in cases of essential hypertension, the left ventricle hypertrophies, an adaptation that increases its work capacity. However, when this compensatory mechanism reaches its limits, the heart no longer provides an adequate supply of blood to the peripheral tissues, with the result being congestive heart failure. Damage to the myocardium, caused mostly by ischemic heart disease, also limits the capacity of the left ventricle to pump blood, and similarly results in heart failure.

ANATOMY OF THE HEART

The heart of a normal adult man weighs 280 to 340 g, and that of a woman, 230 to 280 g. The organ is a two-sided pump, with blood entering each side through a thin-walled atrium, from which it is propelled forward by thicker muscular ventricles. Owing to the low venous pressure and the relatively low afterload on the right side, the right ventricle is considerably thinner (<0.5 cm) than the left ventricle (1.3 to 1.5 cm). Blood enters the ventricles across the atrioventricular valves, the mitral valve on the left and the tricuspid valve on the right. The leaflets of these valves are held in place by the chordae tendineae, which are strong fibrous cords attached to the inner surface of the ventricular wall. The aorta and pulmonary arteries are guarded by the aortic and pulmonary valves, respectively, each consisting of three semilunar cusps. The wall of the heart is composed of three layers: an outer epicardium, a middle myocardium, and an inner endocardium. The heart is surrounded and enclosed by the visceral and parietal pericardia, separated by the pericardial cavity.

The Cardiac Myocyte

The myocardium is composed of a syncytial network of myocytes, each of which has a single nucleus and is separated from adjacent cells by intercalated disks. Electron microscopy shows the sarcolemma, the sarcoplasmic reticulum (SR), the T system of tubules, the nucleus, and numerous mitochondria (Fig. 11-2). The contractile elements of the myocyte, the myofilaments, are arranged in bundles, referred to as myofibrils, which are separated by mitochondria and SR. The myofibrils are organized into repeating units termed sarcomeres.

The sarcomere is the basic functional unit of the contractile apparatus. It consists of a Z line on each end and interdigitated thick and thin filaments, which are oriented perpendicular to the Z line (see Fig. 11-2). The thick filaments contain myosin and are limited to the A band.

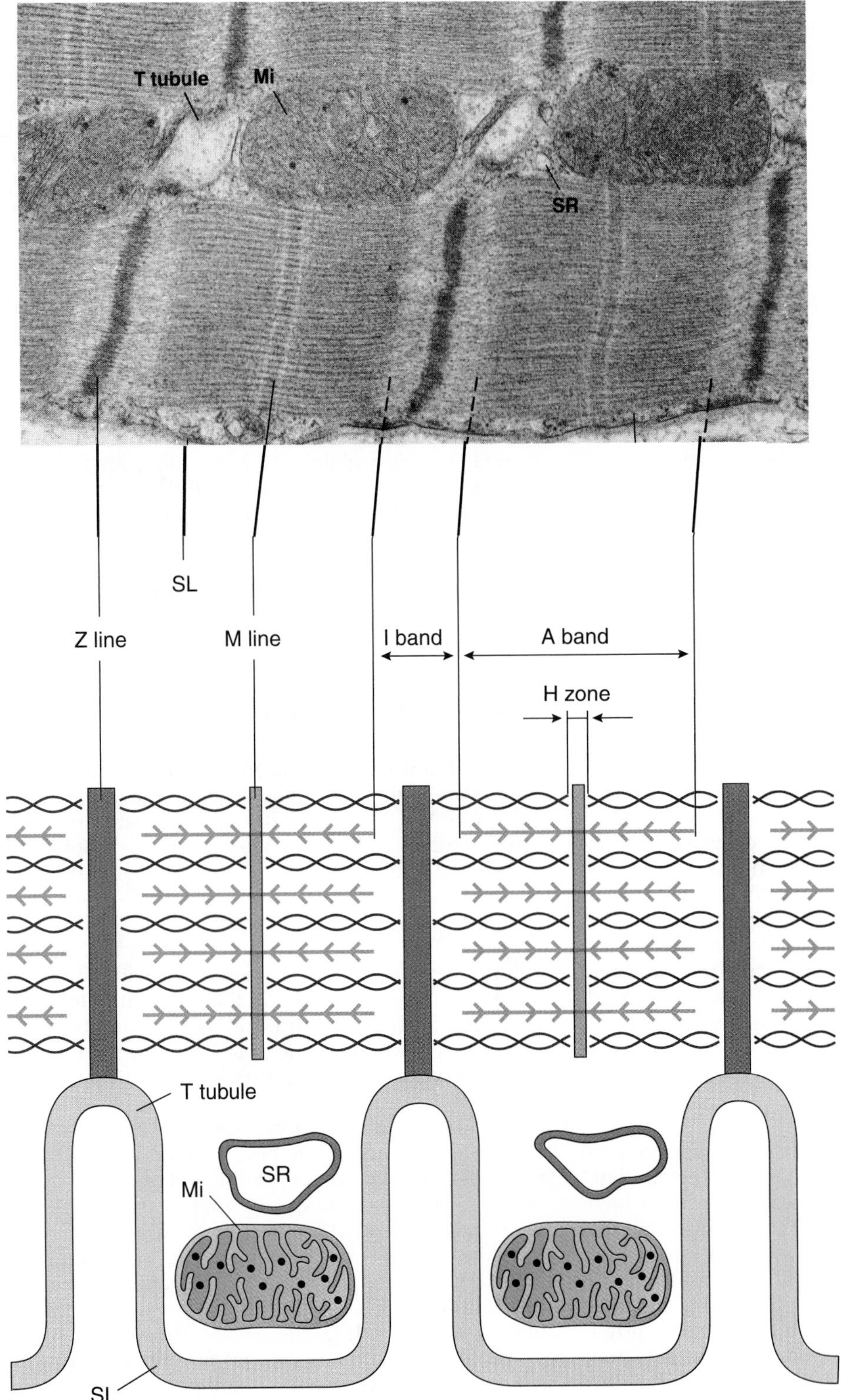

FIGURE 11-2
Ultrastructure of the myocardium. *(Top)* Electron micrograph of left ventricle in the longitudinal plane, showing the sarcolemma (SL); the sarcomeres of the myofibrils, which are delimited by Z lines; A bands; I bands; H zones; and M lines. Also present are mitochondria (Mi), sarcoplasmic reticulum (SR), and T tubules. The I bands and H zones are absent when the myofibrils are shortened. *(Bottom)* The structural basis for the banding shown in the electron micrograph. The fine threads that extend at right angles to the thick (myosin) filaments are the cross bridges that form the force-generating cross-links with actin. The amount of force that can be generated is proportional to the length of the adjoining myofilaments and is at a maximum when the sarcomeres are between 2 μm and 2.2 μm in length. When the sarcomeres are less than 2 μm in length, the thin filaments slide across each other and overlap, decreasing the potential for force-generating cross-links; similarly, when the sarcomeres are stretched beyond 2.2 μm, there is a decrease in force that is proportional to the widening of the H zone. It is apparent that this mechanism can be invoked as the basis for Starling's law of the heart.

The actin filaments (thin filaments), with their associated regulatory proteins tropomyosin and troponin, extend from the Z line through the I band and into the A band. The interaction of these myofilaments generates the force for contraction. The amount of force that can be generated is proportional to the extent of overlap between adjoining thick and thin filaments and is at a maximum when the sarcomeres are 2.0 to 2.2 μm in length.

When the sarcomere length is less than 2 μm, the thin filaments slide across each other and overlap, decreasing the potential for force-generating cross-links. When the sarcomere is stretched beyond 2.2 μm, there is a decrease in force that is proportional to the widening H zone. **This mechanism is the basis for Starling's law of the heart, which states that the contractile force of the heart is a function of diastolic fiber length.** The average sarcomere length is about 2.2 μm when the end-diastolic pressure in the left ventricle is at the upper limit of normal.

The contraction of cardiac muscle is initiated by an increase in cytosolic free calcium. In the normal myocyte, the action potential triggers the entry of calcium into the myocyte through slow calcium channels in the sarcolemma. In turn, calcium penetrating into the cell stimulates the release of calcium sequestered in the SR (Ca^{2+}-induced Ca^{2+}-release). The increase in cytosolic free calcium produces a conformational change in the regulatory proteins of the myofilaments, in particular troponin, which permits the cross-bridges between actin and myosin to break and reform repetitively. As a result, the filaments slide over one another, causing contraction of the myocardium. **The number of contractile sites activated and the resulting force that is generated are directly proportional to the concentration of calcium in the vicinity of the myofibrils.**

The myocardium relaxes when the cytosolic calcium returns to its normal low concentration of 10^{-7} M. This process is dependent on the calcium adenosine triphosphatase (ATPase) of the SR, which pumps Ca^{2+} from the cytosol into the SR. Cytosolic Ca^{2+} also is lowered by its outward transport through sodium–calcium exchange and the sarcolemmal calcium pumps. **Thus, myocardial relaxation is an active, energy-requiring event.**

The Conducting System

The cardiac conducting system consists of specialized myocytes that have two major functions: (1) they initiate the heartbeat through their automatic rhythmicity, which is more rapid in the sinoatrial node than in the more distal parts of the system; and (2) they conduct at a faster rate than the contractile fibers, with the exception of the myocytes in the atrioventricular node, which delay the passage of the impulse. Thus, the heartbeat normally originates in the sinoatrial node. If the sinoatrial node is prevented from functioning as the pacemaker for the heartbeat, more distal parts of the system become the pacemaker. As a rule, the slower the heart rate, the more distal is the pacemaker site.

On leaving the sinoatrial node, the electrical impulse continues through the atrioventricular node, passing through the common bundle (bundle of His) and along the left and right bundle branches to the apex of the ventricles, which is the region that is first stimulated to contract. In the normal adult heart, the common bundle is the only electrical connection between the atria and the ventricles. Occasionally, however, additional bypass pathways are present, including lateral accessory atrioventricular pathways (bundles of Kent), nodoventricular and fasciculoventricular pathways (Mahaim fibers), and intranodal and atriofascicular pathways (James fibers). Bypass fibers often are found in patients with certain arrhythmias. They probably permit preexcitation of the ventricles and also establish a circus movement that results in tachycardia. Bypass pathways also have been postulated to cause the Wolff–Parkinson–White syndrome, in which preexcitation is manifested in the electrocardiogram by the delta wave and a short PR interval.

It is often possible to identify at autopsy specific abnormalities of the conducting fibers that explain the arrhythmias that were present during life. Such lesions may cause irregularity of the cardiac rhythm (slowing or accelerating of the heart rate) or partial or complete heart block. These functional defects may be transient or permanent, depending on the conditions of the injury. For example, acute myocardial infarction or surgical trauma may injure the conducting fibers in a way that results in heart block. Normal sinus rhythm often returns when the local inflammatory and hemorrhagic changes subside.

The Coronary Arteries

The right and left main coronary arteries originate in or immediately above the sinuses of Valsalva of the aortic valve (see Fig. 11-1). The left main coronary artery bifurcates within 1 cm of its origin into the left anterior descending (LAD) and left circumflex coronary arteries. The left circumflex coronary artery rests in the left atrioventricular groove and supplies the lateral wall of the left ventricle (Fig. 11-3). The LAD coronary artery lies in the anterior interventricular groove and provides blood to (1) the anterior left ventricle, (2) the adjacent anterior right ventricle, and (3) the anterior two thirds of the interventricular septum. In the apical region, the LAD coronary artery supplies the ventricles circumferentially (see Fig. 11-3).

The right coronary artery occupies the right atrioventricular groove and nourishes the remainder of the right ventricle and the posteroseptal region of the left ventricle (see Fig. 11-3), including the posterior third of the interventricular septum at the base of the heart (also referred to as the "inferior" or "diaphragmatic" wall). From these distributions, one can predict the location of the infarct that follows occlusion of any of the three coronary artery branches (see Fig. 11-3).

Epicardial coronary arteries usually are arranged in the so-called right coronary–dominant distribution. Dominance is determined by the coronary artery that contributes most of the blood to the posterior descending coronary artery (see Fig. 11-1). In 10% of human hearts, there is a left-dominant pattern, with the left circumflex coronary artery supplying the posterior descending coronary artery.

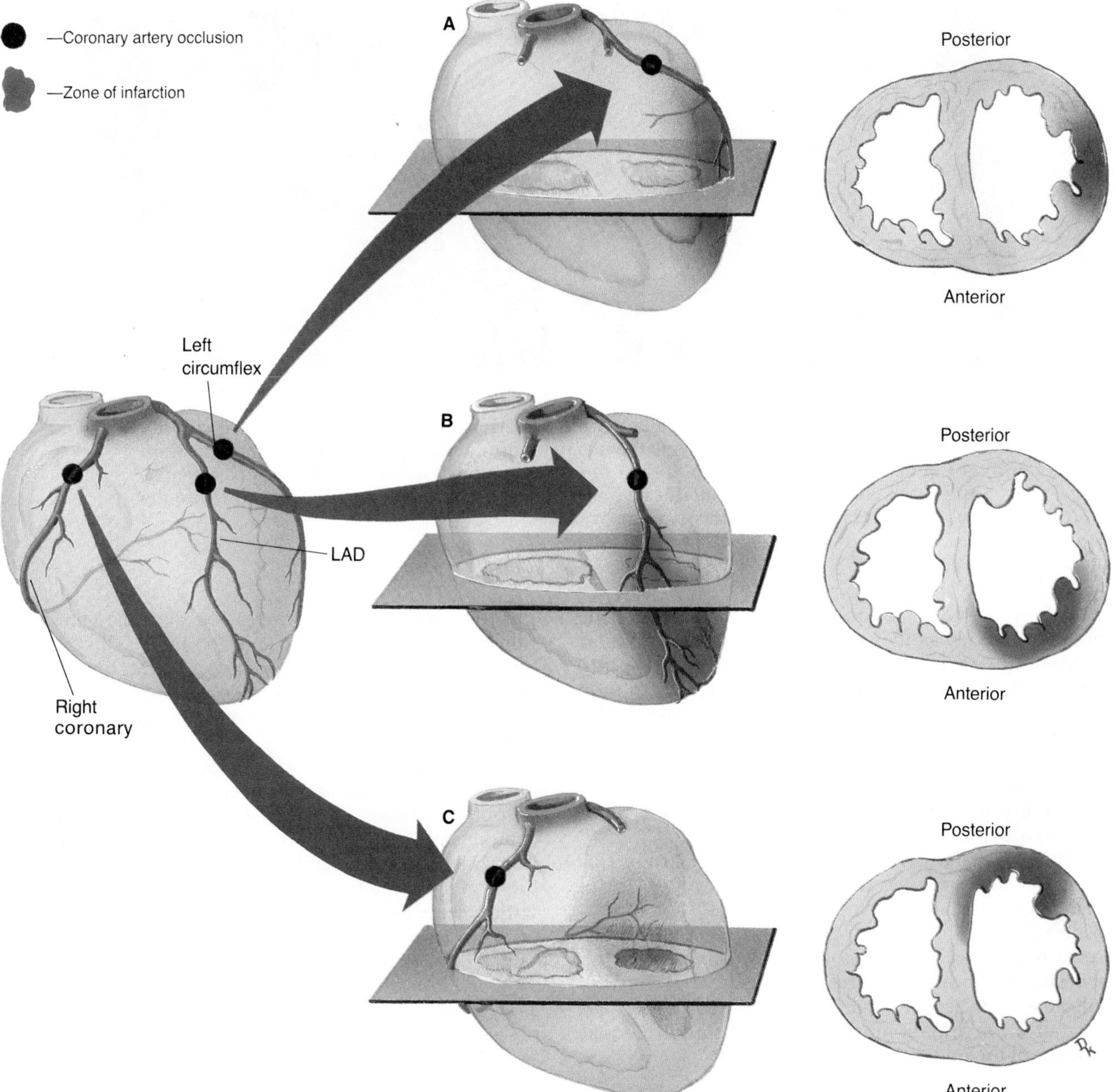

FIGURE *11-3*
Position of left ventricular infarcts resulting from occlusion of each of the three main coronary arteries. *(A)* Posterolateral infarct, which follows an occlusion of the left circumflex artery and is present in the posterolateral wall. *(B)* Anterior infarct, which follows occlusion of the anterior descending branch *(LAD)* of the left coronary artery. The infarct is located in the anterior wall and adjacent two thirds of the septum, in the apical three fourths of the left ventricle. It involves the entire circumference of the wall near the apex. *(C)* A posterior ("inferior" or "diaphragmatic") infarct results from occlusion of the right coronary artery and involves the posterior wall, including the posterior third of the interventricular septum and the posterior papillary muscle in the basal half of the ventricle. Note the lateral displacement of the posterior papillary muscle caused by the expansion (i.e., stretching) of the infarct region of the left ventricle.

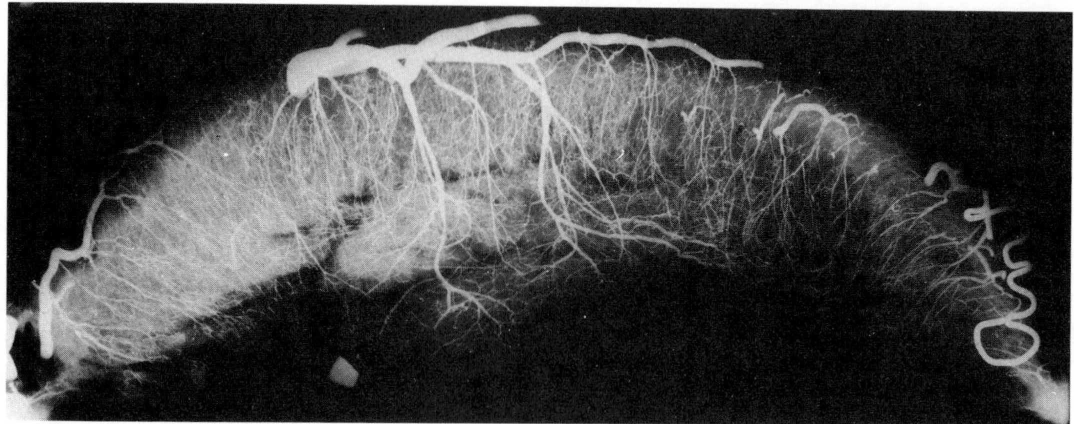

FIGURE *11-4*
Arteriogram of a longitudinal segment of the posterior wall of the left ventricle, including the posterior papillary muscle. Note the two types of branches passing into the myocardium at right angles to the epicardial artery *(top)*: class A, which quickly divides into a fine network; and class B, which maintains a large diameter and pass with little branching into the subendocardial region and the papillary muscle.

It is enlightening to look at the arrangement of the coronary arteries as they pass through the ventricular walls at right angles to the epicardial vessels (Fig. 11-4). Some of these small coronary arteries branch as they course through the ventricular wall, whereas others maintain a large diameter and pass to the endocardial surface without branching. Because the capillary networks arising from these penetrating arteries do not interconnect, distinct borders between viable and infarcted myocardium occur after coronary artery occlusion.

The epicardial portion of each coronary artery fills and expands during systole and empties and narrows during diastole. The intramyocardial arteries have the opposite action and are narrowed by the systolic muscular pressure. As a result, blood flow within the myocardium, especially in the subendocardial regions of the ventricle, is decreased or absent during systole. Nevertheless, because of autoregulation, blood flow is roughly equal throughout the myocardium.

MYOCARDIAL HYPERTROPHY AND HEART FAILURE

In the normal heart, the ventricles are compliant, and diastolic filling occurs at low atrial pressures. During systole, the ventricles contract vigorously and eject about 65% of the blood present in the ventricle at the end of diastole (ejection fraction). When the heart is injured, cardiac function is impaired. Regardless of the precise cause of cardiac dysfunction, the clinical consequences are similar. **If the initial impairment is severe, cardiac output is not maintained despite compensatory changes, and the result is acute, life-threatening, cardiogenic shock.** When the functional impairment is less extensive, compensatory mechanisms (see later) allow the cardiac output to be maintained by increasing diastolic ventricular filling pressure and end-diastolic volume. This situation results in the characteristic signs and symptoms of congestive heart failure. Because of the heart's capacity to compensate, congestive heart failure is often tolerated for many years.

The ability of the heart to compensate after cardiac injury is based on the same mechanisms that allow cardiac output to increase in response to stress. **The fundamental compensatory mechanism is based on the Frank–Starling mechanism, which states that the stroke volume of the heart is a function of diastolic fiber length and that, within certain limits, the normal heart will pump whatever volume is brought to it by the venous circulation** (Fig. 11-5). Stroke volume is a measure of ventricular function. It is enhanced by increasing ventricular end-diastolic volume secondary to an increase in atrial filling pressure.

The increase in contractile force that occurs in response to ventricular dilatation is a consequence of myofibrillar organization. Stretching of the sarcomeres results in a greater potential for overlap of thick and thin filaments during contraction, which allows enhanced force generation as long as the sarcomere is not stretched beyond 2.2 μm. When there is a sudden need to increase cardiac output in a normal heart, such as during exercise, catecholamine stimulation causes an increase in contractility. As a result, the normal relationship between end-diastolic volume and stroke volume is shifted upward (from curve A to curve X in Fig. 11-5). End-diastolic volume also may increase, resulting in a large increase in cardiac output.

In the presence of cardiac injury, overall cardiac function tends to be is depressed in the basal state. Under these circumstances, higher than normal filling pressures are required to maintain cardiac output (curve Y in Fig. 11-5). Moreover, during cardiac failure, catecholamine

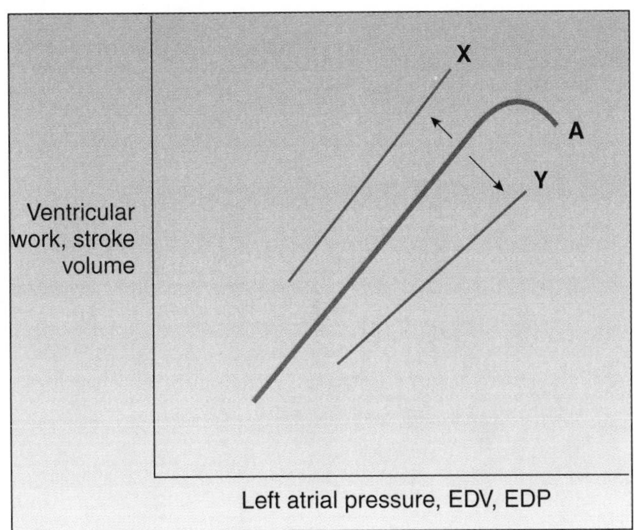

FIGURE 11-5
The relation of the work of the heart (or stroke volume) to the level of venous inflow, as measured by atrial pressure, or by ventricular end-diastolic volume or end-diastolic pressure. Curve *A* indicates that as the ventricular end-diastolic volume *(EDV)*, end-diastolic pressure *(EDP)*, or left atrial pressure increases, the amount of work done by the heart increases linearly up to a point. Beyond this point, there is a decrease in the work done, and the heart fails. However, the downslope of this curve is reached only at very high left atrial pressures. The curve may shift up to position *X* or down to position *Y*, depending on whether the heart is more contractile (e.g., because of the action of norepinephrine) or is less contractile (i.e., in failure), respectively. The failing heart usually functions on the ascending limb of a depressed curve.

stimulation is often present in the basal state, so that a comparable increase in cardiac output requires a larger increase in atrial pressure in the failing heart than in the normal heart. **The most prominent feature of heart failure is the abnormally high atrial filling pressure relative to stroke volume.** The absolute values of stroke volume and cardiac output are generally well maintained.

Myocardial hypertrophy provides another compensatory mechanism that requires time to develop. It is an adaptive process by the failing heart that permits compensation for overloading and plays a significant role in augmenting the contractile strength of the myocytes. However, it is important to realize that the hypertrophied myocyte is not a normal cell.

Pathogenesis of Myocardial Hypertrophy and Congestive Heart Failure

Cardiac hypertrophy is an adaptive response to hemodynamic overload, which occurs in association with chronic hypertension (pressure overload), myocardial injury, valvular insufficiency (volume overload), and other stresses that increase the workload of the heart. The importance of this adaptive mechanism was noted more than a century ago by Austin Flint, who suggested that, similar to the enlargement of skeletal muscle in athletes, cardiac hypertrophy compensates for hemodynamic overloading of the heart. The hypertrophic response features enlargement of cardiac myocytes and an accumulation of sarcomeric proteins, without an increase in the number of cells. Initially, hypertrophy reflects a compensatory and potentially reversible mechanism, but with persistent stress on the heart, the myocardium becomes irreversibly enlarged and dilated. The factors that mediate both the reversible and irreversible phases of myocardial hypertrophy and heart failure remain poorly understood, although much has been learned in the last few years (Fig. 11-6).

ANGIOTENSIN II (ANG II): It is known that contractile cells respond to mechanical stimuli such as stretching in response to an external load. In this context, muscle cells are intrinsically able to sense such a load, even in the absence of neuronal or hormonal factors. However, the mechanism by which muscle cells sense a stretch stimulus and convert it into growth-regulating intracellular signals is not clear. All components of the renin–angiotensin system (renin, angiotensinogen, angiotensin-converting enzyme [ACE], and Ang II receptor) are present in cardiac myocytes. Recent studies suggest that locally produced Ang II triggers the hypertrophic response of the myocardium. In experimental hypertensive animals, a drug-induced decrease in blood pressure did not lead to regression oFf cardiac hypertrophy, whereas treatment with an ACE inhibitor normalized the heart size. ACE inhibitors prevented cardiac hypertrophy induced by experimental coarctation of the aorta, without changing the increased arterial pressure. Postnatal growth of the heart, which is due exclusively to hypertrophy, was prevented by treatment of newborn pigs with an ACE inhibitor. Finally, mechanical stretch of cultured cardiac myocytes caused the release of Ang II from the cells and induced biochemical changes characteristic of cardiac hypertrophy. Binding of Ang II to its receptor activates an intracellular signal-transduction mechanism, which increases the activity of the mitogen-activated protein (MAP) kinase cascade and eventuates in enhanced gene expression and protein synthesis. Thus, a local renin–angiotensin system in the heart is believed to be critical in mediating cardiac hypertrophy.

ENDOTHELIN-1 (ET-1): ET-1 is a vasoconstrictor produced by a variety of cells, including endothelial cells and cardiac myocytes. This peptide is also a potent growth factor for cardiac myocytes. Similar to Ang II, ET-1 activates the MAP kinase cascade on binding to its specific receptor to cause cardiac hypertrophy *in vivo* and *in vitro*. Interestingly, ET-1 also is released by cardiac myocytes as a response to mechanical stretching and is constitutively elaborated by neonatal heart tissue. Thus, in

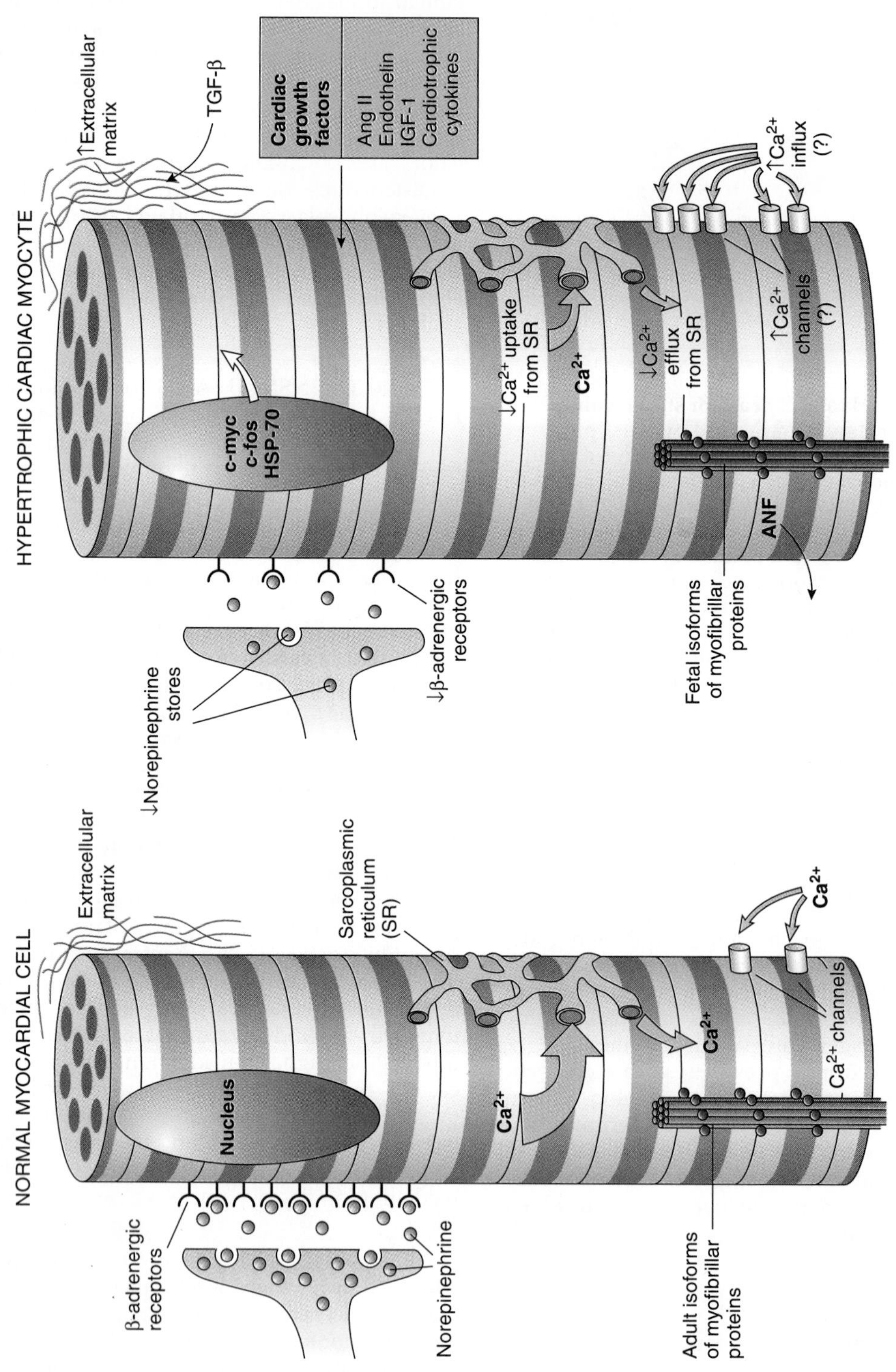

FIGURE 11-6
Biochemical characteristics of myocardial hypertrophy and congestive heart failure.

addition to Ang II, ET-1 is thought to be an important mediator of cardiac hypertrophy.

INSULIN-LIKE GROWTH FACTOR-1 (IGF-1): IGF-1 is a growth-promoting peptide that mediates the activity of pituitary growth hormone and is produced principally in the liver. However, most tissues synthesize IGF-1 locally, and this molecule also has been shown to be a growth factor for cardiac myocytes. In experimental models, there is substantial evidence that IGF-1 participates in the pathogenesis of cardiac hypertrophy.

CARDIOTROPHIN-1: A family of cytokines (leukemia inhibitory factor, interleukin-11 [IL-11], oncostatin M, and others) mediates pleiotropic actions on a variety of cell types, including hepatocytes, megakaryocytes, osteoclasts, and neuronal cells. The most recent addition to this family is cardiotrophin-1, a cytokine that shares many properties with other similar molecules, including the induction of cardiac myocyte hypertrophy *in vitro*.

EXPRESSION OF FETAL GENES: A number of contractile protein isoforms are expressed in the fetal heart but not after birth. In cardiac hypertrophy induced by hemodynamic overload, many of these genes are reexpressed. For example, atrial natriuretic factor (ANF) is expressed in both the ventricle and atrium in the fetus, but after birth, the expression of ANF is restricted to the atrium. In the hypertrophic ventricle, however, ANF is abundantly reexpressed and serves to reduce the hemodynamic overload through its effect on salt and water metabolism.

Cardiac hypertrophy also is accompanied by the reexpression of fetal isoforms of several contractile proteins. In the rat, α-myosin heavy chain, the normal adult isoform, has a high ATPase activity and a rapid shortening velocity. By contrast, the β-myosin heavy chain, the fetal isoform, has a lower ATPase activity and a slower shortening velocity. In experimental cardiac hypertrophy, "fast" α-myosin is replaced by "slow" β-myosin, thereby leading to impaired myocardial contractility. However, this change in myosin gene expression also has adaptive features, insofar as it increases the tension generated during each systole and improves the efficiency of contraction, thereby conserving energy. Hypertrophied human hearts exhibit similar, but not identical, changes in myosin isoforms. The human ventricle contains only slow myosin, and the hypertrophic heart exhibits a change from fast to slow myosin only in the atrium. However, other fetal isoforms of myofibrillar proteins appear in the human ventricular myocardium. Thus, a feature of the hypertrophic response is induction of a program of fetal gene expression. The hypertrophied heart also exhibits changes in other protein isoforms, including fetal forms of actin and tropomyosin, and abnormal varieties of lactic dehydrogenase (LDH), creatine kinase (CK), and the sarcolemmal sodium pump. The changes in protein isoforms documented to date are likely to be only a small portion of the molecular adaptations in cardiac hypertrophy, and their functional consequences remain to be elucidated.

ALTERATIONS IN CALCIUM HOMEOSTASIS: A variety of defects in calcium homeostasis have been reported to occur in hypertrophy and heart failure. The density of both ryanodine-sensitive and IP_3-sensitive calcium-release channels in the SR is decreased. The ryanodine-sensitive calcium-release channel is responsible for calcium-induced calcium release during the action potential, and a decrease in the number of these channels impairs contractile function by reducing the rate of release of Ca^{2+} from the SR. A decreased rate of Ca^{2+} uptake by the SR also has been observed and appears to be mediated by a decrease in the amount of SR Ca^{2+}-ATPase. This change interferes with Ca^{2+} sequestration during diastole and leads to impaired relaxation. Although it is not yet clear whether these changes are primary or secondary, they likely contribute to the systolic and diastolic dysfunction seen in heart failure.

β-ADRENERGIC DESENSITIZATION: The chronically failing heart has a markedly depressed response to catecholamines, presumably as an adaptive response to the increased secretion of autonomic neurotransmitters. In patients with heart failure, receptor desensitization may contribute to the sluggish response of the heart to exercise. Chronic overstimulation of the β-adrenergic receptors of the myocytes by endogenous catecholamines leads to a decrease in the number of receptors and to a depressed responsiveness of the remaining receptors, presumably as a result of receptor desensitization. In addition, there appears to be a defect in the coupling of β-adrenergic receptor to adenylyl cyclase through G proteins. In this respect, the ratio of the alpha subunit of the G protein that inhibits adenylyl cyclase (G_i) to the alpha subunit of the stimulatory G protein (G_s) is increased. There also is evidence that the failing heart contains less norepinephrine stored in the autonomic nerve endings.

PROTOONCOGENES AND MYOCARDIAL HYPERTROPHY: Within an hour of the stress produced by an acute pressure overload, myocardial cells respond by inducing the expression of the protooncogenes c-*myc* and c-*fos* and heat shock protein 70 (HSP 70). It is suspected that the transcription of protooncogenes may underlie the reexpression of fetal protein isoforms in the hypertrophic heart.

EXTRACELLULAR MATRIX: An acute overload of the heart leads to a prompt increase in the synthesis of collagen. Fibrosis also occurs in heart failure, at least in part, as a result of stimulation of cardiac fibroblasts by transforming growth factor-beta (TGF-β) and possibly Ang II. This response is adaptive in the sense that it may protect against excessive dilatation of the ventricle, thereby maintaining mechanical efficiency. After a myocardial infarction, fibrosis also is important in replacing necrotic myocytes and in preventing cardiac rupture. On the other hand, as with many of the acute adaptive responses of the heart, myocardial fibrosis eventually interferes with diastolic relaxation and may impair the diffusion of oxygen and nutrients to the myocytes.

Pathology of Heart Failure

Anything that causes the heart to increase its workload for a prolonged period or produces anatomical damage that makes it more difficult for the heart to function may eventuate in myocardial failure. **Ischemic heart disease is by far the most common condition responsible for cardiac failure, accounting for more than 80% of deaths from heart disease.** Between 1% and 3% of cardiac deaths are due to hypertensive heart disease, 1% are caused by rheumatic heart disease, and the remaining types account for less than 1% each. Virtually all of the organs of the body suffer the effects of heart failure. The subject is discussed in detail in Chapter 7, and only the salient features are reviewed here.

Other than the changes characteristic of specific disease entities, for instance, ischemic heart disease or cardiac amyloidosis, the morphological changes in the failing heart are nonspecific. The ventricles are conspicuously dilated and, in cases of chronic failure, tend to be hypertrophied. Although the weight of the hypertrophied heart is invariably increased, both ventricles often appear to be of normal thickness, owing to dilatation that masks the hypertrophy. The distribution of organ involvement depends on whether the heart failure is predominantly left-sided or right-sided.

Left-sided heart failure is the more common type of heart failure, because the most frequent causes of cardiac injury (e.g., ischemic heart disease, hypertension) primarily affect the left ventricle. As a compensatory response to left ventricular failure, left atrial pressure and pulmonary venous pressure both increase, resulting in passive pulmonary congestion. The capillaries in the alveolar septa fill with blood, and small ruptures allow the escape of erythrocytes. As a result, the alveoli contain many hemosiderin-laden macrophages. Moreover, if capillary hydrostatic pressure exceeds plasma osmotic pressure, fluid leaks from the capillaries into the alveoli. The resultant pulmonary edema may be massive, with alveoli being drowned in a transudate. Interstitial pulmonary fibrosis results when congestion is present over an extended period.

Right-sided heart failure commonly complicates left-sided failure, or it can develop independently secondary to intrinsic pulmonary disease and pulmonary hypertension, which create resistance to the flow of blood through the lungs. As a consequence, right atrial pressure and systemic venous pressure both increase, resulting in jugular venous distention, edema of the lower extremities, and congestion of the liver and spleen.

Hepatic congestion in heart failure is characterized by distended central veins, which stand out as dark red foci against the yellow of the cells in the periphery of the lobule. This imparts to the liver a gross appearance that has been compared with the cut surface of a nutmeg (hence the term **nutmeg liver**; see Chapter 14).

Clinical Features of Heart Failure

The clinical symptoms of left-sided failure include dyspnea on exertion, orthopnea (dyspnea when lying down), and paroxysmal nocturnal dyspnea. Dyspnea on exertion reflects the increasing pulmonary congestion that accompanies a higher end-diastolic pressure in the left atrium and ventricle. Orthopnea and paroxysmal nocturnal dyspnea result when thoracic blood volume increases, owing to reduced blood volume in the lower extremities while the patient is recumbent.

Although much of the clinical presentation of heart failure can be explained by venous congestion (backward failure), two aspects of congestive failure involve inadequate arterial perfusion of vital organs (forward failure). Most patients with left-sided heart failure retain sodium and water (edema), owing to decreased renal perfusion, a decreased glomerular filtration rate, and activation of the renin–angiotensin–aldosterone system (see Chapter 7). Inadequate cerebral perfusion can result in confusion, memory loss, and disorientation, whereas reduced perfusion of skeletal muscle leads to fatigue and weakness.

CONGENITAL HEART DISEASE

Congenital heart disease (CHD) results from faulty embryonic development, expressed either as misplaced structures (e.g., transposition of the great vessels) or an arrest in the progression of a normal structure from an early stage to a more advanced one (e.g., atrial septal defect).

The incidence of CHD is cited as almost 1% of all live births. This figure does not include certain common defects that are not functionally significant, such as an anatomically patent foramen ovale that is functionally closed by the right atrial flap that covers it. In this circumstance, the foramen ovale remains closed as long as the left atrial pressure is higher than that in the right atrium. A bicuspid aortic valve is also common and usually is asymptomatic until adulthood. The figures for the incidence of particular cardiovascular anomalies vary depending on many factors, and a range derived from several sources is shown in Table 11-1.

Pathogenesis

The cause of CHD is usually not ascertained. However, it is worthwhile to determine whether the defect in any one

TABLE *11-1* Relative Incidence of Specific Anomalies in Patients with Congenital Heart Disease

Ventricular septal defects—25% to 30%
Atrial septal defects—10% to 15%
Patent ductus arteriosus—10% to 20%
Tetralogy of Fallot—6% to 15%
Pulmonary stenosis—5% to 7%
Coarctation of the aorta—5% to 7%
Aortic stenosis—4% to 6%
Complete transposition of the great arteries—4% to 10%
Truncus arteriosus—2%
Tricuspid atresia—1%

case can be recognized as being mainly of genetic origin or primarily acquired, because this consideration is important to the parents with respect to planning future pregnancies.

Most congenital defects of the heart reflect a combination of multifactorial genetic factors and environmental influences. As in other diseases with multifactorial inheritance (see Chapter 6), there is an increased risk of recurrence among the siblings of an affected child. Whereas the incidence of CHD in the general population is roughly 1%, it increases up to 6% for a second pregnancy after the birth of a child with a heart defect. The risk for a third affected child may be as high as 30%. Moreover, an infant born to a mother with CHD also has an increased risk of cardiac lesions.

Single-gene syndromes are only rare causes of CHD. A number of chromosomal abnormalities are associated with an increased incidence of congenital anomalies of the heart, most prominently Down syndrome (trisomy 21), but also other trisomies and Turner syndrome. However, these account for no more than 5% of all cases of CHD.

The best evidence for an intrauterine influence on the occurrence of congenital cardiac defects relates to maternal infection with rubella virus during the first trimester, especially during the first 4 weeks of gestation. An association with other viral infections is suspected but is not as well documented. The maternal use of drugs in early pregnancy also is associated with an increased number of cardiac defects in the offspring. For example, the thalidomide syndrome (phocomelia) was associated with a 10% incidence of CHD. Other drugs implicated in the pathogenesis of CHD include alcohol, phenytoin, amphetamines, lithium, and estrogenic steroids.

Classification of Congenital Heart Disease

There are several ways to categorize hearts with congenital defects. One of the earliest clinically useful schemes was proposed by Maude Abbott, who grouped cases in three categories according to the presence or absence of cyanosis, as follows:

- **The acyanotic group** does not have an abnormal communication between the two circulations. Examples of the acyanotic group described by Abbott include coarctation of the aorta, right-sided aortic arch, Ebstein malformation, and congenital tricuspid insufficiency.
- **The cyanose tardive** group is defined as an initial left-to-right shunt with late reversal of flow. Abbott illustrated this group with cases of patent ductus arteriosus (PDA), patent foramen ovale, and ventricular septal defect. In patients with these anomalies, cyanosis supervenes later (i.e., tardive). The shunt is initially from left to right but later becomes a right-to-left shunt (Eisenmenger complex), because pulmonary vascular changes develop and increase pulmonary vascular resistance. (In a protective surgical procedure, the pulmonary artery is banded, thereby decreasing the pulmonary blood flow.)
- **The cyanotic group** describes a permanent right-to-left shunt. In this category of CHD, Abbott included tetralogy of Fallot, truncus arteriosus, and complete transposition of the great vessels.

Since Abbott's grouping, numerous classification schemes have been developed to provide the detail necessary to meet clinical requirements, especially those of the cardiac surgeon. A more contemporary classification divides the cases into the groups shown in Table 11-2.

TABLE *11-2* **Classification of Congenital Heart Disease**

Initial Left-to-Right Shunt
Ventricular septal defect
Atrial septal defect
Patent ductus arteriosus
Persistent truncus arteriosus
Anomalous pulmonary venous drainage
Right-to-Left Shunt
Tetralogy of Fallot
No Shunt
Complete transposition of the great vessels
Coarctation of the aorta
Pulmonary stenosis
Aortic stenosis
Coronary artery origin from pulmonary artery
Ebstein malformation
Complete heart block
Endocardial fibroelastosis

Initial Left-to-Right Shunt

Ventricular Septal Defect (Roger Disease)

Ventricular septal defects are the most common of all congenital heart lesions (see Table 11-2) and occur as isolated lesions or in combination with other malformations.

☐ **Pathogenesis:** The fetal heart consists of a single chamber until the fifth week of gestation, after which it is divided by the development of the interatrial and interventricular septa and by the formation of the atrioventricular valves from the endocardial cushions. A muscular interventricular septum grows upward from the apex toward the base of the heart (Fig. 11-7). The muscular septum is joined by the down-growing membranous septum, thereby separating the right and left ventricles. **The most common ventricular septal defect is related to the failure of the membranous portion of the septum to form in whole or in part.**

☐ **Pathology:** Defects in the muscular portion of the ventricular septum are more common anteriorly but can occur anywhere in the muscular septum. Ventricular septal defects vary in size. They occur as (1) a small hole in the membranous septum, (2) a large defect involving more than the membranous region (perimembranous defects), or (3) a complete absence of the muscular septum (leaving a single ventricle).

Ventricular septal defects occur most commonly in the superior portion of the septum below the outflow tract of the pulmonary artery (below the crista supraventricularis, i.e., infracristal) and behind the septal leaflet of the tricuspid valve. The common bundle (bundle of His) is located immediately below the defect (inlet type). Less commonly, the defect occurs above the crista supraventricularis (supracristal) and just below the pulmonary valve (infraarterial). The supracristal variety of septal defect is often associated with other defects, such as an overriding pulmonary artery (the Taussig–Bing type of double-outlet right ventricle), transposition of the great vessels, or persistent truncus arteriosus.

☐ **Clinical Features:** **A small septal defect may have little functional significance and may actually close spontaneously as the child matures.** Closure is accomplished by either hypertrophy of the adjacent muscle or adherence of the tricuspid valve leaflets to the margins of the defect. In infants with large septal defects, the higher pressure in the left ventricle creates initially a left-to-right shunt. Left ventricular hypertrophy and congestive heart failure are common complications of such shunts. If the defect is small enough to permit prolonged survival in the face of a significant left-to-right shunt, the augmented pulmonary blood flow caused by the higher left ventricular pressure eventually results in thickening of the pulmonary arteries and increased pulmonary vascular resistance. This increased vascular resistance may be so great that the direction of the shunt is reversed and goes from right to left (**Eisenmenger complex**). A patient with this condition displays a late onset of cyanosis (i.e., tardive cyanosis). These children develop right ventricular hypertrophy and right-sided congestive heart failure.

Additional complications of ventricular septal defects include infective endocarditis at the site of the lesion, paradoxical emboli, and prolapse of an aortic valve cusp (with resulting aortic valve insufficiency). Large ventricular septal defects are repaired surgically.

Atrial Septal Defects

Atrial septal defects range in severity from clinically insignificant and asymptomatic anomalies to chronic, life-threatening conditions.

☐ **Pathogenesis:** The embryological development of the atrial septum occurs in a sequence that permits the continued passage of oxygenated placental blood from the right to the left atrium through the valve of the inferior vena cava (eustachian valve). The developing atrial septum is programmed to permit this right-to-left shunt to continue until birth. Beginning at the fifth week of intrauterine life, the septum primum extends downward from the roof of the atrium to join with the endocardial cushions, thereby closing the incomplete segment, or "ostium primum" (see Fig. 11-7). Before this closure is complete, the midportion of the septum primum develops a defect, or "ostium secundum," so that right-to-left flow continues. During the sixth week, a second septum (septum secundum) develops to the right of the septum primum, passing from the roof of the atrium toward the endocardial cushions. This process leaves a patent foramen at about the midpoint of the septum, known as the **foramen ovale**. The defect persists after birth until it is sealed off by the fusion of the septum primum and septum secundum, after which it is termed the **fossa ovalis**.

☐ **Pathology:** The atrial septum may be defective at a number of sites (see Fig. 11-7).

- **Patent foramen ovale:** Tissue derived from the septum primum situated on the left side of the foramen ovale functions as a flap valve that normally fuses with the margins of the foramen ovale, thereby sealing the opening. An incomplete seal of the foramen ovale, which can be detected with a probe (probe patent foramen ovale), is found in 25% of normal adults and is not normally functional. However, it may become a true shunt if circumstances increase

FIGURE *11-7*
Pathogenesis of ventricular and atrial septal defects. ***(A)*** **The common atrial chamber is being separated into the right and left atria (RA and LA) by the septum primum. Because the septum primum has not yet joined the endocardial cushion material, there is an open ostium primum. The ventricular cavity is being divided by a muscular interventricular septum into right and left chambers (RV and LV). SVC, superior vena cava; IVC, inferior vena cava.** ***(B)*** **The septum primum has joined the endocardial cushions, but at the same time has developed an opening in its midportion (the ostium secundum). This opening is partly overlaid by the septum secundum, which has now grown down to cover the foramen ovale in part. Simultaneously, the membranous septum joins the muscular interventricular septum to the base of the heart, completely separating the ventricles.** ***(C)*** **The sinus venosus type of atrial septal defect is located in the most cephalad region and is adjacent to the inflow of the right pulmonary veins, which thus tend to open into the right atrium.** ***(D)*** **The ostium primum defect occurs just above the valve ring, sometimes in the presence of an intact valve ring. It may also, in conjunction with a defect of the valve ring and ventricular septum, form an atrioventricular canal, as shown in** ***(E)*****. This common opening allows free communication between atria and ventricles.**

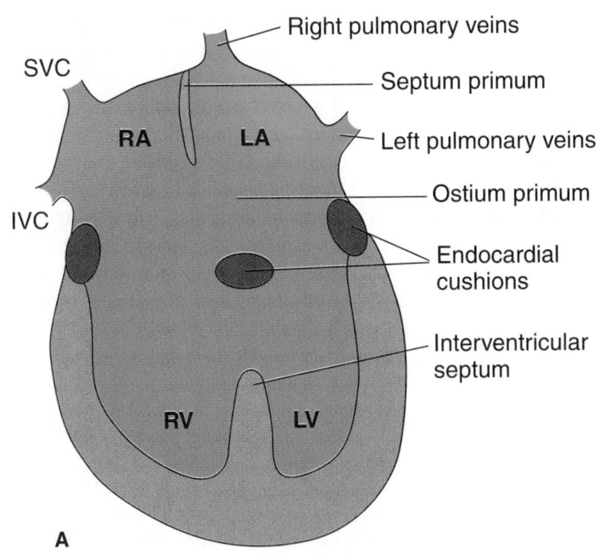
Right pulmonary veins
SVC
Septum primum
RA
LA
Left pulmonary veins
Ostium primum
IVC
Endocardial cushions
Interventricular septum
RV
LV
A

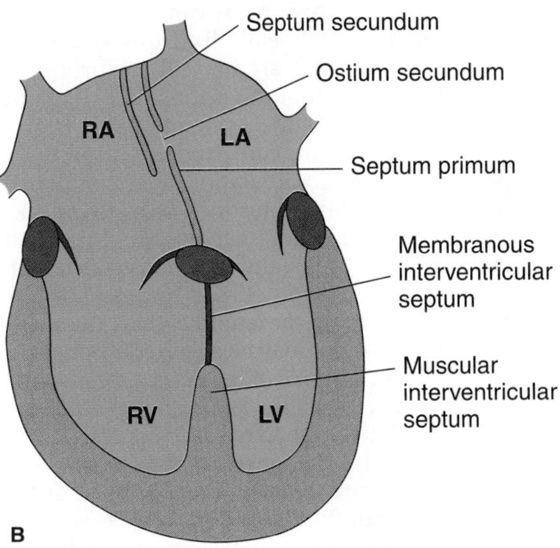
Septum secundum
Ostium secundum
RA
LA
Septum primum
Membranous interventricular septum
Muscular interventricular septum
RV
LV
B

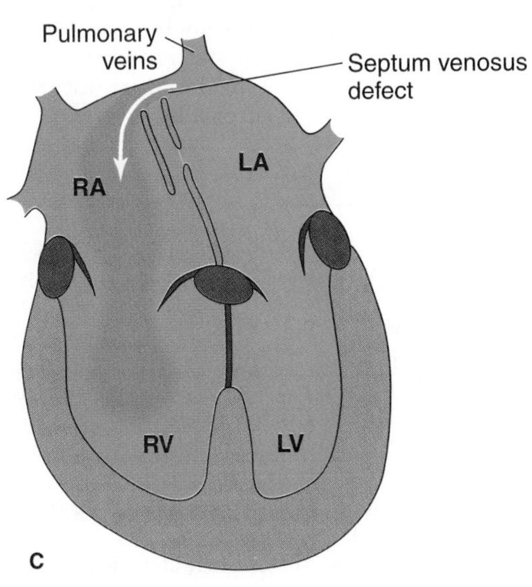
Pulmonary veins
Septum venosus defect
RA
LA
RV
LV
C

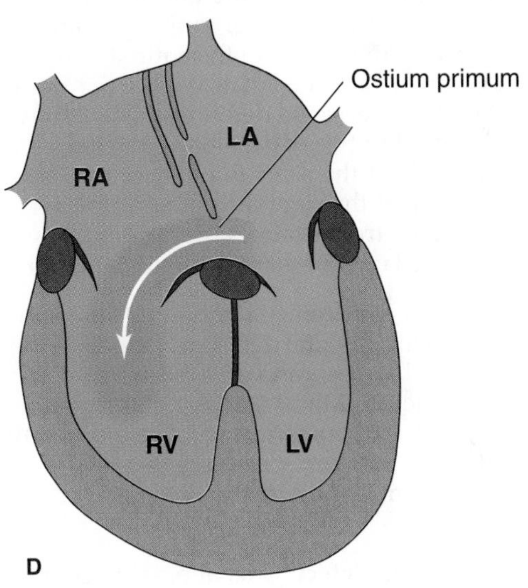
Ostium primum
LA
RA
RV
LV
D

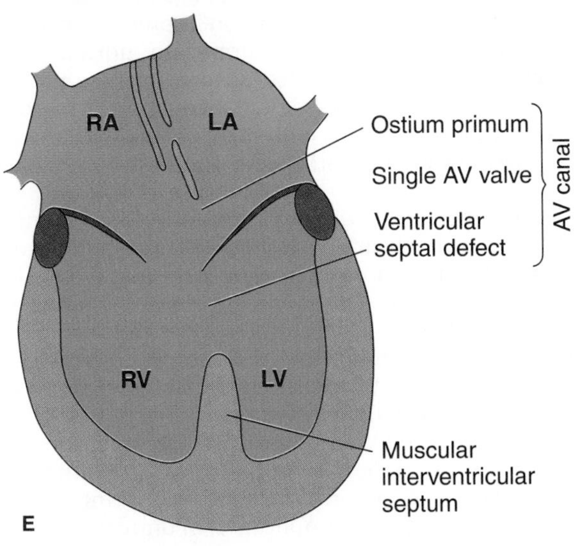
RA
LA
Ostium primum
Single AV valve
Ventricular septal defect
AV canal
RV
LV
Muscular interventricular septum
E

FIGURE *11-7*

the right atrial pressure, as can occur with recurrent pulmonary thromboemboli. If this situation develops, a right-to-left shunt will be produced, and thromboemboli from the right-sided circulation will pass directly into the systemic circulation. These paradoxical emboli can produce infarcts in many parts of the arterial circulation, most commonly in the brain, heart, spleen, intestines, kidneys, and legs.

A widely patent foramen ovale is occasionally encountered and is actually an acquired atrial septal defect caused by a disproportion between the size of the foramen ovale and the length of the valve covering it. The foramen ovale may be enlarged by obstructive lesions on the right side of the heart. On the other hand, conditions in which the left atrium is dilated may result in a relatively short valve.

- **Atrial septal defect, ostium secundum type:** This lesion is by far the most common of the atrial septal defects, accounting for 90% of the cases. It reflects a true deficiency of the atrial septum and should not be confused with a patent foramen ovale. An ostium secundum defect occurs in the middle portion of the septum and varies in size, ranging from a trivial opening to a large defect of the entire fossa ovalis region. When the defect is small, it is not normally functional. If the atrial septal defect is larger, it may result in sufficient shunting of the blood from the left side to the right side of the heart to produce dilatation and hypertrophy of the right atrium and right ventricle. Under these circumstances, the pulmonary artery may become larger in diameter than the aorta.

Lutembacher syndrome, a variant of the ostium secundum type of atrial septal defect, is defined as the combination of mitral stenosis and an ostium secundum type of atrial septal defect. Mitral stenosis may be either congenital or a result of rheumatic fever. It is thought that increased left atrial pressure secondary to the mitral valve obstruction influences the continued patency of the atrial septum.

- **Sinus venosus defect:** This anomaly occurs in the upper portion of the atrial septum above the fossa ovalis near the entry of the superior vena cava. It is usually accompanied by drainage of the right pulmonary veins into the right atrium. This is an uncommon defect, occurring in only 5% of atrial septal defects.
- **Atrial septal defect, ostium primum type:** This condition involves the region adjacent to the endocardial cushion and is also rare, accounting for 7% of all atrial septal defects. There are usually clefts in the anterior leaflet of the mitral valve and the septal leaflet of the tricuspid valve, which may be accompanied by an associated defect in the adjacent interventricular septum.
- **Persistent common atrioventricular canal:** This anomaly represents the fully developed combined atrial and ventricular septal defects. Although ordinarily rare, this defect is common in patients with Down syndrome.

  Complete atrioventricular canal is the consequence of a failure of the atrioventricular endocardial cushions to fuse. As a result, the lesion includes (1) an enlarged ostium primum atrial septal defect, (2) a ventricular septal defect, and (3) clefts in the septal leaflets of the tricuspid and mitral valves.

  Incomplete (partial) atrioventricular canal is a situation in which an ostium primum atrial septal defect is adjacent to the atrioventricular valves, which are often abnormal.
- **Coronary sinus atrial septal defect:** This abnormality is the rarest of the atrial septal defects. It is situated in the posteroinferior part of the interatrial septum at the site of the coronary sinus ostium and is associated with a persistent left superior vena cava, which drains into the roof of the left atrium.

□ **Clinical Features:** Young children with atrial septal defects are ordinarily asymptomatic, although they may complain of easy fatigability and dyspnea on exertion. Later in life, usually in adolescence, changes in the pulmonary vasculature may reverse the flow of blood through the defect and create a right-to-left shunt. In such cases, cyanosis and clubbing of the fingers ensue. Complications of atrial septal defects include pulmonary hypertension, right ventricular hypertrophy, heart failure, paradoxical emboli, and bacterial endocarditis. Symptomatic cases are treated surgically.

Patent Ductus Arteriosus

Early in its development, the embryo supposedly recapitulates an ancestral evolutionary stage, with six aortic arches connecting the ventral and dorsal aortas as part of the branchial cleft system (Fig. 11-8). The left sixth aortic arch is partly preserved as the pulmonary arteries, and the arterial continuation on the left to the descending thoracic aorta is retained as the **ductus arteriosus**. The ductus conveys most of the pulmonary outflow into the aorta. After birth, the ductus contracts in response to the increased arterial oxygen content and becomes occluded by fibrosis (ligamentum arteriosus).

Persistent PDA is one of the most common congenital cardiac defects and is especially frequent in infants whose mothers were infected with rubellavirus early in pregnancy. PDA is not uncommon in premature infants, in whom this structure is anatomically normal but in whom prematurity precludes closure. In these patients, the ductus usually closes spontaneously. On the other hand, in full-term infants with PDA, the ductus has an abnormal endothelium and media and only rarely closes spontaneously.

The lumen of a PDA varies greatly. A small shunt has little effect on the heart. By contrast, a large shunt leads to considerable diversion of blood from the aorta to the low-pressure pulmonary artery. In severe cases, more than half of the left ventricular output may be shunted into the pulmonary circulation. As a result of the increased demand for cardiac output, left ventricular hypertrophy and failure ensue. In patients with a smaller but functional PDA, the increased volume and pressure of blood in the pulmonary circulation eventually lead to pulmonary hypertension and its cardiac complications. Infective endarteritis is a frequent complication in untreated patients with PDA.

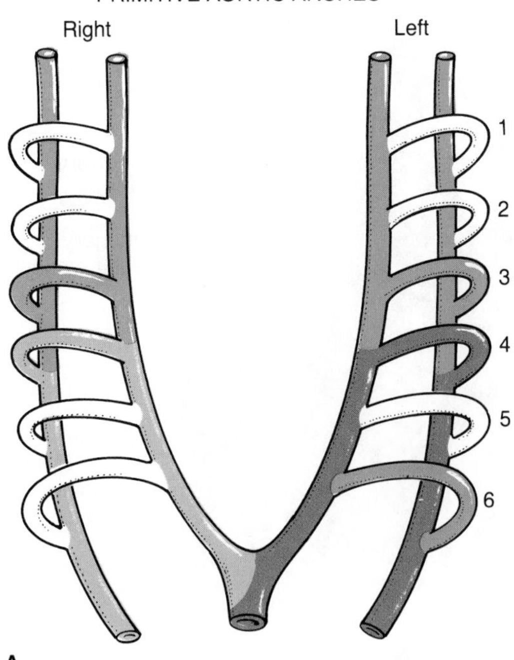

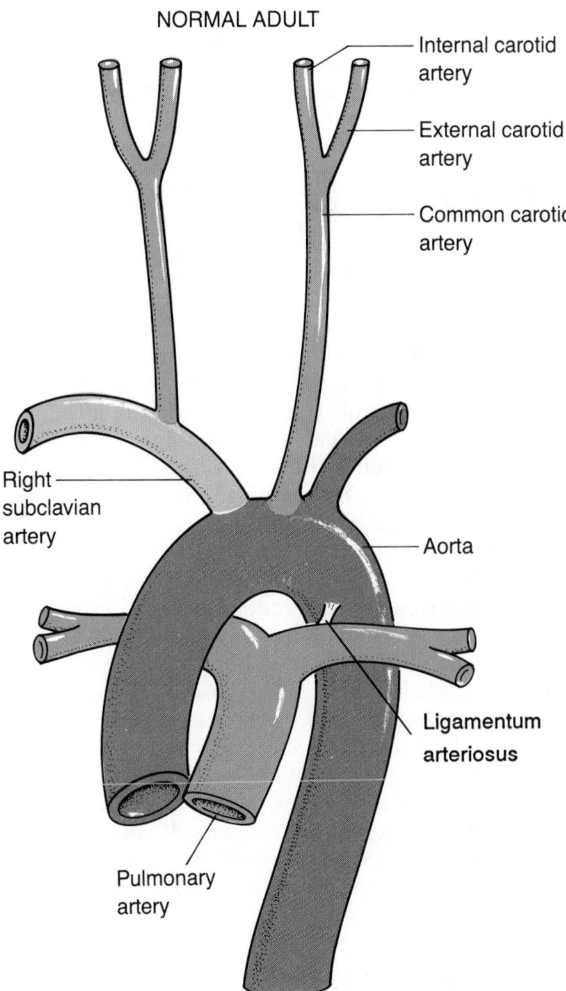

Patent ductus arteriosus can be corrected surgically, usually with complete success. Much of the treatment of PDA changed from surgical to medical when it was discovered that the ductus arteriosus can be kept open after birth by the administration of prostaglandins (PGE_2). This effect is used in treating patients born with a cardiac defect that requires the presence of a left-to-right shunt to survive. Examples include patients with isolated pulmonary stenosis and those with complete transposition of the great vessels. Conversely, in patients with PDA, the ductus can be caused to contract and then close by inhibitors of prostaglandin synthesis (e.g., indomethacin).

Aortopulmonary window is a defect between the base of the aorta and the pulmonary artery. It is a rare condition that is functionally similar to PDA and is clinically difficult to differentiate from it.

Other abnormalities of the aortic arch system can be predicted by visualizing the variations that could occur in the development of the complete aortic arch system (see Fig. 11-8). For example, the right side of the aortic arch system rather than the left may be retained, resulting in the condition known as a **right aortic arch**. This variant is seen in about 25% of patients with tetralogy of Fallot and in 50% of patients with truncus arteriosus. A right aortic arch is innocuous, unless it comes as a surprise to the cardiac surgeon.

Truncus Arteriosus

Persistent truncus arteriosus refers to a common trunk for the origin of the aorta, pulmonary arteries, and coronary arteries. It results from an absent or incomplete partitioning of the truncus arteriosus by the spiral septum. There are several variants of truncus arteriosus:

- **Type 1** is the most common variant and consists of a single trunk that gives rise to a common pulmonary artery and ascending aorta.
- **Type 2** displays right and left pulmonary arteries that originate from a common site in the posterior midline of the truncus.
- **Type 3** has separate pulmonary arteries that originate laterally from a common trunk.
- **Type 4** consists of other rare variants in which there is no pulmonary trunk at all and in which the pulmonary circulation is supplied from the aorta by enlarged bronchial arteries. This type is difficult to differentiate from tetralogy of Fallot with pulmonary artery atresia.

Truncus arteriosus always overrides a ventricular septal defect and receives blood from both ventricles. The valve of the truncus usually has three semilunar cusps but may have as few as two or as many as six. The coronary arteries arise from the base of the valve.

FIGURE *11-8*
Derivatives of the aortic arches. *(A)* Complete primitive aortic arch system. *(B)* In the normal adult, the left fourth aortic arch is preserved as the arch of the adult aorta, and the left sixth arch is represented by the pulmonary artery and ligamentum arteriosus.

☐ **Clinical Features:** Most infants with truncus arteriosus have a torrential pulmonary blood flow and have heart failure and recurrent respiratory tract infections, often resulting in an early death. There is little or no cyanosis. In children with prolonged survival, pulmonary vascular disease develops, in which case cyanosis, polycythemia, and clubbing of the fingers appear. Open-heart surgery has proven to be an effective treatment.

Anomalous Pulmonary Vein Drainage

The pulmonary veins form a network in the dorsal mesoderm. A bud from the region of the atrium joins the pulmonary venous confluence, and eventually all four pulmonary veins drain into the left atrium. Failure of these tissues to join correctly results in various venous anomalies.

Total anomalous pulmonary vein drainage may occur as an isolated defect, or it may be part of the asplenia syndrome (splenic agenesis, congenital heart defects, and situs inversus of abdominal organs). Most commonly, the pulmonary veins drain into a common pulmonary venous chamber, and then through a persistent left superior vena cava (the persistent left pericardial vein) into the innominate vein or into the right superior vena cava. A second route for the common pulmonary vein drainage leads into the coronary sinus. A third drainage route consists of persistent posterior and subcardinal veins, which form a mid-dorsal trunk that crosses the diaphragm and enters the portal vein or the ductus venosus. The third type of drainage is often associated with some pulmonary venous obstruction.

In total anomalous pulmonary drainage, there is no direct venous return to the left side of the heart, and life is sustained only in the presence of an atrial septal defect or a patent foramen ovale. Heart failure, severe anoxemia, and pulmonary venous obstruction result from total anomalous pulmonary vein drainage. The results of surgical correction have been good.

Partial anomalous pulmonary venous drainage may result from less severe circulatory impairment. This anomaly may involve one or two pulmonary veins, especially in association with a sinus venosus type of atrial septal defect. The prognosis here is excellent, similar to that of atrial septal defects.

Tetralogy of Fallot (Dominant Right-to-Left Shunt)

Tetralogy of Fallot is the most common cyanotic CHD in older children and adults, representing 10% of all cases of CHD. The four anatomicalal changes that define the tetralogy of Fallot are as follows (Fig. 11-9):

- **Pulmonary stenosis**
- **Ventricular septal defect**
- **Dextroposition of the aorta so that it overrides the ventricular septal defect**
- **Right ventricular hypertrophy**

The ventricular septal defect, which may be as large as the aortic orifice, is the result of incomplete closure of the membranous septum and involves both the muscular septum and the endocardial cushions. In addition, the development of the spiral septum, which normally divides the common truncus region into an aorta and pulmonary artery, is probably abnormal. As a result, the aorta is displaced into a more dextral position overlying the septal defect. The ventricular septal defect is immediately below the overriding aorta. Pulmonary stenosis is usually due to subpulmonary muscular hypertrophy, with an enlarged infundibular muscle obstructing blood flow into the pulmonary artery. However, in about one third of these hearts, the valve itself is the main cause of the stenosis; in such cases, the valve is usually funnel shaped, with the narrow part being more distal.

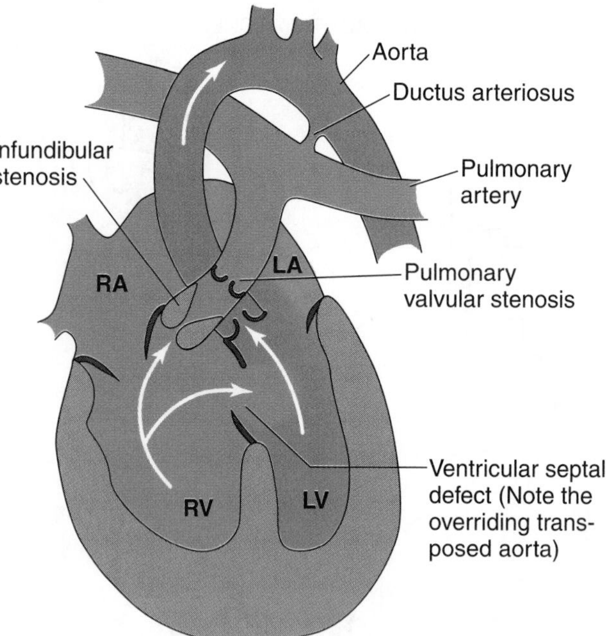

FIGURE *11-9*
Tetralogy of Fallot. Note the pulmonary stenosis, which is due to infundibular hypertrophy as well as to pulmonary valvular stenosis. The ventricular septal defect involves the membranous septum region. Dextroposition of the aorta and right ventricular hypertrophy are shown. Because of the pulmonary obstruction, the shunt is from right to left, and the patient is cyanotic.

The heart is hypertrophied in such a way as to give it a boot shape. Almost half of the patients with tetralogy of Fallot display other cardiac anomalies, including ostium secundum atrial septal defects, PDA, left superior vena cava, and endocardial cushion defects. The aortic arch is on the right side in about 25% of cases of tetralogy of Fallot, an incidence that is of importance to the surgeon. In addition to the hazard of being surprised by a right aortic arch, the surgeon must remember that a large branch of the right coronary artery may cross the pulmonary conus region, which is the cardiotomy site. It should be noted that patency of the ductus arteriosus is protective, because it provides a source of blood to the otherwise deprived pulmonary vascular bed.

☐ **Clinical Features:** In the face of severe pulmonary stenosis, right ventricular blood is shunted through the ventricular septal defect into the aorta, resulting in arterial desaturation and cyanosis. Dyspnea on exertion is particularly noticeable, and the affected child often assumes a squatting position to relieve the shortness of breath. Physical development is characteristically retarded. Owing to marked polycythemia, cerebral thromboses may complicate the course of the disease. The patients are also at risk for bacterial endocarditis and brain abscesses. Increasing cyanosis and shortness of breath may indicate that a beneficial patent ductus has closed spontaneously. Heart failure is not a common complication.

In the absence of surgical intervention, tetralogy of Fallot carries a dismal prognosis. However, total correction is now possible with open-heart surgery, which carries less than a 10% mortality. After successful surgery, the patients are asymptomatic and have an excellent long-term prognosis.

Congenital Heart Diseases without Shunts

Transposition of the Great Arteries

Transposition of the great arteries (TGA) refers to a situation in which the aorta arises from the right ventricle and the pulmonary artery from the left ventricle. The condition shows a male predominance and is more common in the offspring of mothers with diabetes. TGA is responsible for more than half of the deaths in infants with cyanotic heart disease younger than 1 year.

☐ **Pathogenesis:** The normal division of the embryonic truncus arteriosus into the aorta and pulmonary artery is dependent on the spiral septum. Its abnormal development can produce an aberrant positioning of the great arteries, such that the aorta is anterior to the pulmonary artery and connects with the right ventricle. In this circumstance, the pulmonary artery receives the outflow of the left ventricle (Fig. 11-10). Because the venous blood from the right side of the heart flows to the aorta, and the oxygenated blood from the lungs returns to the pulmonary artery, there are in effect two independent and parallel blood circuits for the systemic and pulmonary circulations. Thus, survival is possible only in the presence of a communication between the circuits. Virtually all infants with TGA have an atrial septal defect, one half have a ventricular septal defect, and two thirds have a PDA.

☐ **Pathology:** The aorta normally arises posterior to and to the left of the pulmonary artery, and in its ascending portion, courses behind and to the right of the pulmonary artery. In TGA, the aorta is anterior to the pulmonary artery and to its right ("d" transposition) all the way from its origin.

☐ **Clinical Features:** Before the advent of cardiac surgery, the outlook for infants born with TGA was hopeless, with 90% dying within the first year. However, it is now possible to correct the malformation within the first 2 weeks of life by means of an arterial-switch operation, with an overall survival rate of 90%.

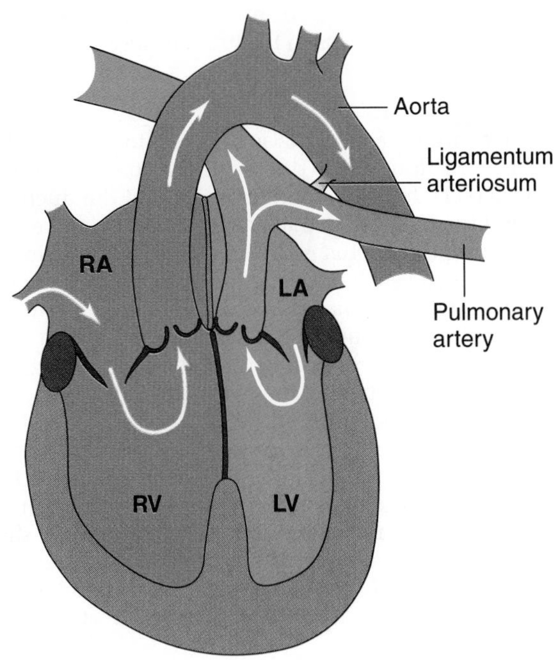

FIGURE *11-10*
Complete transposition of great arteries, regular type. The aorta is anterior to, and to the right of, the pulmonary artery ("D-transposition") and arises from the right ventricle. Because there are no interatrial or interventricular connections and no patent ductus arteriosus, this anomaly is incompatible with life.

Congenitally corrected transposition is a condition in which the aorta is anterior to, but passes to the left of, the pulmonary artery ("l" transposition). Although the great arteries are thus abnormally related to each other, they nevertheless arise from anatomically correct ventricles. Patients in whom corrected TGA is the only malformation are clinically entirely normal. Unfortunately, many cases are complicated by other cardiac anomalies, which require their own specific interventions.

The Taussig–Bing malformation is a double-outlet right ventricle, in which a ventricular septal defect is above the crista supraventricularis and directly beneath an overriding pulmonary artery. This condition functionally and clinically is similar to TGA with a ventricular septal defect and pulmonary hypertension.

Coarctation of the Aorta

Coarctation of the aorta is a local constriction of this vessel that almost always is seen immediately below the origin of the left subclavian artery at the site of the ductus arteriosus. Rare cases occur at any point from the aortic arch to the abdominal bifurcation. The condition is two to five times more frequent in males than in females and is associated with a bicuspid aortic valve in two thirds of the patients. Malformations of the mitral valve, ventricular septal defects, and subaortic stenosis also may accompany coarctation of the aorta. There is a particular association of this condition with Turner syndrome, and an increased incidence of berry aneurysms in the brain is observed.

☐ Pathogenesis and Pathology: The pathogenesis of coarctation of the aorta is believed to be related to the pattern of flow in the ductus arteriosus during fetal life (Fig. 11-11). *In utero* blood flow through the ductus is considerably greater than that across the aortic valve. The blood leaving the ductus is diverted into two streams by a posterior aortic shelf opposite the orifice of the ductus. One stream passes cephalad into the relatively hypoplastic aortic isthmus to supply the head and upper extremities, whereas the other stream enters the descending thoracic aorta. In late fetal life, the increasing left ventricular output dilates the isthmus, and the increased blood flow bypasses the obstruction (represented by the posterior shelf) through the wide ductal orifice. After birth, the ductal orifice is obliterated, and the posterior shelf normally involutes, thereby removing the obstruction. The shelf may not involute because of an inadequate antegrade flow in the aortic arch *in utero* secondary to anomalies that limit left ventricular output (e.g., bicuspid aortic valve). Alternatively, in many instances, the obstructing shelf does not involute for unknown reasons. In any event, the result is the most common type of coarctation of the aorta, a **juxtaductal constriction**.

The infantile (preductal) type of coarctation results when the aortic isthmus remains narrow (hypoplastic) into late fetal life and after birth. This lesion is usually accompanied by a patent ductus arteriosus and a right-to-left shunt through a ventricular septal defect.

☐ Clinical Features: The clinical hallmark of coarctation of the aorta is a discrepancy between the blood pressure in the upper extremities and that in the lower ones. The pressure gradient produced by the coarctation causes hypertension proximal to the narrowed segment and, occasionally, dilatation of that portion of the aorta. In children older than 1 year, the mean systolic blood pressure measured in the arm is 145 mm Hg compared with 70 mm Hg in the leg.

Hypertension in the upper part of the body results in left ventricular hypertrophy and may produce dizziness, headaches, and nosebleeds. The increased pressure also

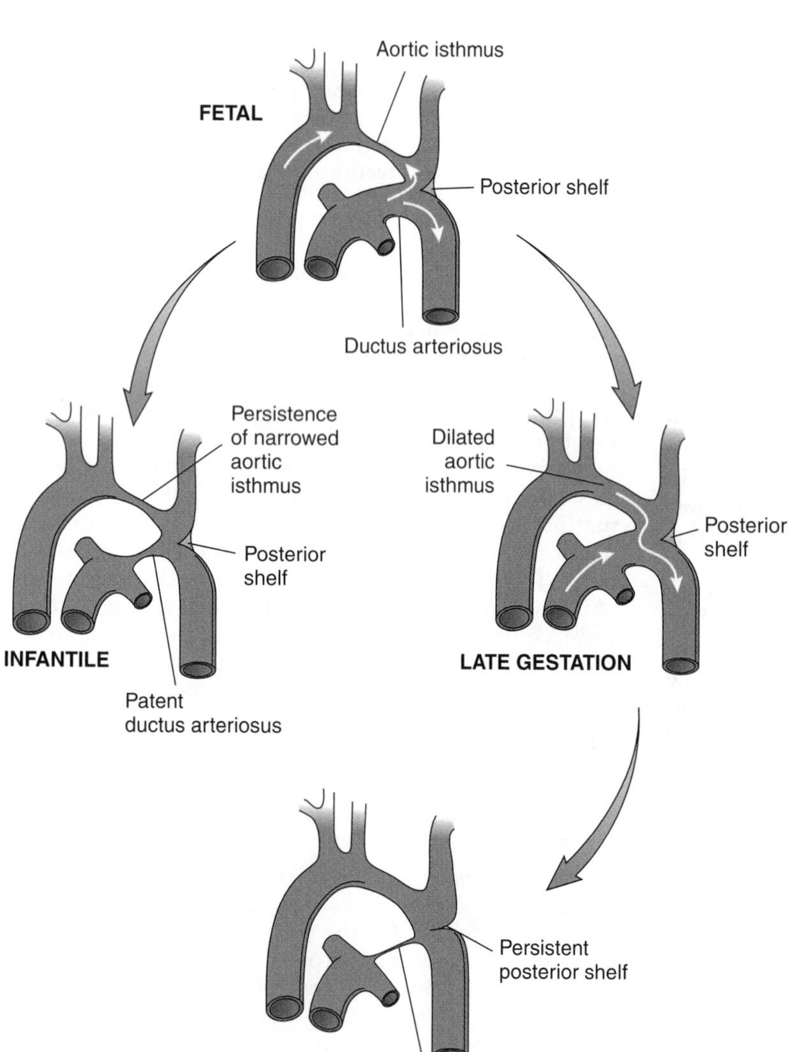

FIGURE *11-11*
Pathogenesis of coarctation of the aorta. In the fetus, the ductal blood is diverted into cephalad and descending streams by the posterior aortic shelf. In late fetal life, the isthmus dilates, and the increased descending blood flow is accommodated by the ductal orifice. After birth, if the shelf does not undergo the normal involution, obliteration of the ductal orifice does not permit free flow around the persistent posterior shelf, thereby creating a juxtaductal obstruction to the flow of blood to the distal aorta. If the aortic isthmus does not dilate during late fetal life, it remains narrow, resulting in an infantile or preductal coarctation. In this circumstance, the ductus arteriosus usually remains patent.

may cause the rupture of a berry aneurysm and consequent subarachnoid hemorrhage. Hypotension below the coarctation leads to weakness, pallor, and coldness of the lower extremities. In an attempt to bridge the obstruction between the upper and lower aortic segments, collateral vessels enlarge. Radiological examination of the chest shows **notching of the inner surfaces of the ribs**, owing to pressure from the markedly dilated intercostal arteries.

Most patients with coarctation of the aorta who remain untreated die by age 40 years. Complications include (1) heart failure, (2) rupture of a dissecting aneurysm (secondary to cystic medial necrosis of the aorta), (3) infective endarteritis at the point of narrowing or at the site of jet-stream impingement on the wall immediately distal to the coarctation, (4) cerebral hemorrhage, and (5) stenosis or infective endocarditis of a bicuspid aortic valve. Coarctation of the aorta is successfully treated by surgical excision of the narrowed segment, preferably between 2 and 4 years of age.

Pulmonary Stenosis

Pulmonary stenosis results from (1) developmental deformities arising from the endocardial cushion region of the heart (with involvement of the pulmonary valves), (2) an abnormality of the right ventricular infundibular muscle (subvalvular or infundibular stenosis, especially as part of tetralogy of Fallot), or (3) abnormal development of the more distal parts of the pulmonary artery tree (peripheral pulmonary stenosis). Peripheral pulmonary stenosis, which is a much less common condition than the other two, may produce "coarctation" of the pulmonary arteries at one or several sites.

Isolated pulmonary stenosis ordinarily involves the valve cusps, which are fused to form an inverted cone or funnel type of constriction. The artery distal to the valve may develop poststenotic dilatation after several years. In severe cases, the infants exhibit hypertrophy of the right ventricle and atrium. In the presence of a patent foramen ovale, there is a right-to-left shunt with cyanosis, secondary polycythemia, and clubbing of the fingers. Good results have been obtained with balloon dilatation of the stenotic valve.

Congenital Aortic Stenosis

Three types of congenital aortic stenosis are recognized: valvular, subvalvular, and supravalvular.

VALVULAR AORTIC STENOSIS: This is the most common type of congenital aortic stenosis and reflects abnormal development of the endocardial cushions. It is considerably more frequent (4:1) in males than in females and is associated with other cardiac anomalies (e.g., coarctation of the aorta) in 20% of the cases. Congenital valvular aortic stenosis usually features fusion of two of the three semilunar cusps (the right coronary cusp with one of the adjacent two cusps). Over the years, the resulting bicuspid valve tends to become thickened and calcified.

Hypoplastic left heart syndrome is characterized by hypoplasia of the left ventricle, ascending aorta, and mitral valve. It is a condition in which severe aortic valvular stenosis or atresia is often the main defect. If the mitral valve is atretic rather than hypoplastic, the left ventricle may consist of only a thin slit.

Many children with valvular aortic stenosis are asymptomatic, but in severe cases, exertional dyspnea and angina pectoris may be prominent features. Sudden death poses a distinct threat to patients with severe obstruction, principally owing to ventricular arrhythmias. Bacterial endocarditis sometimes complicates the course of the disease. In symptomatic cases, aortic valvulotomy has had a high degree of success, although valve replacement is occasionally indicated. No treatment other than cardiac transplantation is available for the hypoplastic left heart syndrome.

SUBVALVULAR AORTIC STENOSIS: This type accounts for 10% of all cases of congenital aortic stenosis and is caused by the abnormal development of a band of subvalvular fibroelastic tissue or a muscular ridge. The stenosis results from a membranous diaphragm or fibrous ring that surrounds the left ventricular outflow tract immediately below the aortic valve. It is twice as common in male as in female patients.

In many persons with subvalvular aortic stenosis, thickening and immobility of the aortic cusps develops, with mild aortic regurgitation. Bacterial endocarditis carries its own risks and may also aggravate the regurgitation. Surgical treatment of subvalvular aortic stenosis is accomplished by excising the membrane or fibrous ridge.

SUPRAVALVULAR AORTIC STENOSIS: This type of stenosis is much less common than the other two forms and is often associated with idiopathic infantile hypercalcemia (Williams syndrome), characterized by mental retardation and multiple system disorders.

Origin of a Coronary Artery from the Pulmonary Artery

A coronary artery, or rarely both, may originate from the pulmonary artery rather than from the aorta. When one coronary artery has an anomalous origin (most commonly the left coronary), anastomoses usually develop between the right and left coronary arteries. This process produces an arteriovenous shunt through which blood flows from the artery originating from the aorta to that arising from the pulmonary artery. As a result, the myocardium supplied by the anomalous artery tends to become chronically ischemic. The result may be myocardial infarction, fibrosis, and calcification, and endocardial fibroelastosis.

Ebstein Malformation

Ebstein malformation is a downward displacement of an abnormal tricuspid valve into an underdeveloped right ventricle. One or more of the tricuspid valve leaflets is plastered to the right ventricular wall for a variable distance below the right atrioventricular annulus.

The septal and posterior leaflets of the tricuspid valve are usually involved in Ebstein malformation. They are irregularly elongated and adherent to the right ventricular wall, so that the upper part of the right ventricular cavity (inflow region) functions separately from the distal chamber. The anterior leaflet is usually the least involved of the three and may be normal. The valve ring may or may not be displaced downward from its usual position. In any event, the effective tricuspid valve orifice is displaced downward into the ventricle, thereby dividing it into two separate parts: the "atrialized" ventricle (proximal ventricle) and the functional right ventricle (distal ventricle). In two thirds of such cases, conspicuous dilatation of the functional ventricle hinders its ability to pump the blood efficiently through the pulmonary arteries. The degree of insufficiency of the tricuspid valve depends on the severity and configuration of the defect in the leaflets.

Ebstein malformation leads to heart failure, massive right ventricular dilatation, arrhythmias with palpitations and tachycardia, and sudden death. Surgical treatment of Ebstein malformation has met with variable success.

Congenital Heart Block

Congenital complete heart block usually occurs in association with other cardiac anomalies. The disruption in the continuity of the conducting system is probably caused by the accompanying cardiac abnormality. However, in cases of isolated complete heart block, failure of the atrioventricular conduction system is believed to result from the lack of regression of the sulcus tissue, which entirely encloses the conducting tissue during early development.

The hearts of patients with congenital heart block tend to show a lack of continuity between the atrial myocardium and the atrioventricular node. Alternatively, the defect may consist of a fibrous separation of the atrioventricular node from the ventricular conducting tissue. Interestingly, infants whose mothers have systemic lupus erythematosus have a high incidence of congenital heart block.

Although their heart rate is abnormally slow, patients with isolated heart block often have little functional difficulty. Later in life, cardiac hypertrophy, attacks of Stokes–Adams syncope (dizziness and unexpected fainting), arrhythmias, and heart failure may develop.

Endocardial Fibroelastosis

Endocardial fibroelastosis (EFE) is characterized by a fibroelastic thickening of the endocardium of the left ventricle, which also may affect the valves. The disorder is classified as primary or secondary, the latter being far more common.

SECONDARY ENDOCARDIAL FIBROELASTOSIS: This disorder occurs in association with underlying cardiovascular anomalies that lead to left ventricular hypertrophy in the face of an inability to meet the increased oxygen demands of the myocardium. Thus secondary EFE is a frequent complication of congenital aortic stenosis (including hypoplastic left ventricle syndrome) and coarctation of the aorta. On gross examination, the endocardium of the left ventricle displays irregular, white, opaque, thickened patches, which also may be present on the cardiac valves. Microscopically, these plaques correspond to fibroelastic thickening, frequently accompanied by degeneration of the subendocardial myocytes. The valves may show collagenous thickening.

PRIMARY ENDOCARDIAL FIBROELASTOSIS: Defined as the presence of fibroelastosis in the absence of any associated lesion, this disorder is of unknown etiology and afflicts infants, usually between 4 and 10 months of age. Although the disease has occurred in siblings, no specific mode of inheritance has been established.

The left ventricle is usually conspicuously dilated but occasionally contracted and hypertrophic. Diffuse endocardial thickening involves most of the left ventricle (Fig. 11-12) and the aortic and mitral valve leaflets. The thickened endocardium tends to obscure the trabecular pattern of the underlying myocardium, and the papillary muscles and chordae tendineae are thick and short. Mural thrombi may complicate the situation.

Infants with primary EFE develop progressive heart failure, and the prognosis is dismal. Cardiac transplantation offers the only hope for a cure.

Dextrocardia

Dextrocardia refers to an inverted position of the heart, which represents a mirror image of the normal left-sided location and configuration. The position of the heart chambers is determined by the direction of the embryonic cardiac loop. If the loop protrudes to the right, the future right ventricle develops on the right and the left ventricle comes to occupy its proper position. If the loop protrudes to the left, the opposite obtains.

When dextrocardia occurs without abnormal positioning of the visceral organs (situs inversus), the condition is invariably associated with severe cardiovascular anomalies. These include transposition of the great arter-

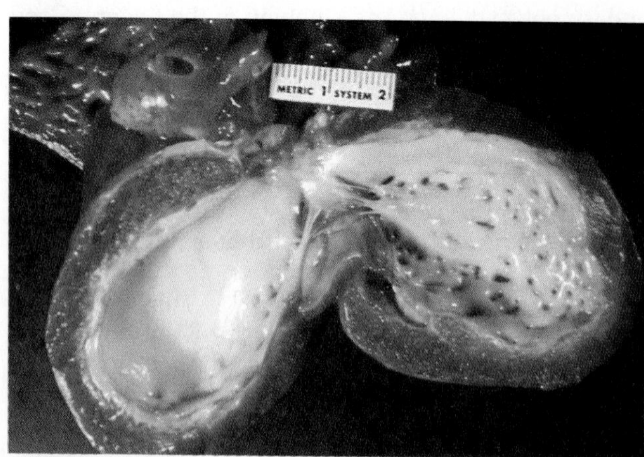

FIGURE *11-12*
Endocardial fibroelastosis. The left ventricle of an infant who died of endocardial fibroelastosis has been opened to reveal a thickened endocardium lining most of the cavity, which virtually obliterates the trabeculae carneae.

ies, a variety of atrial and ventricular septal defects, anomalous pulmonary venous drainage, and many others. In dextrocardia that occurs in combination with situs inversus, the heart is functionally normal, although minor anomalies are not uncommon.

ISCHEMIC HEART DISEASE

Ischemic heart disease is, in the vast majority of cases, a consequence of atherosclerosis of the coronary arteries and develops when blood flow is inadequate to provide for the oxygen demands of the heart. **Ischemic heart disease is by far the most common type of heart disease in the United States and other industrialized lands (e.g., Scandinavia, England, Germany), where it remains the leading cause of death and is responsible for at least 80% of all deaths of heart disease.** By contrast, atherosclerotic heart disease is far less frequent in underdeveloped countries, such as those of Africa and many parts of Asia. The pathogenesis of ischemic cell injury is discussed in detail in Chapter 1. The principal effects of ischemic heart disease are angina pectoris, myocardial infarction, and sudden death.

ANGINA PECTORIS: *This term refers to pain in the chest and is the most common symptom of ischemic heart disease.* Coronary atherosclerosis usually becomes symptomatic only when the luminal cross-sectional area of the affected vessel is reduced by more than 75%. A patient with typical angina pectoris exhibits recurrent episodes of chest pain, usually brought on by increased physical activity or emotional excitement. The pain is of limited duration (1 to 15 minutes) and is relieved by reducing physical activity or by treatment with sublingual nitroglycerin (a potent vasodilator). The chest pain typically is substernal but may radiate from the chest to involve the left arm, the jaw, and the upper abdomen.

Although the most common cause of angina pectoris is severe coronary atherosclerosis, decreased coronary blood flow can result from other conditions, including coronary vasospasm, aortic stenosis, or aortic insufficiency. Angina pectoris is not associated with any characteristic anatomical change in the myocardium as long as the duration and severity of the ischemic episode are insufficient to cause myocardial necrosis.

Prinzmetal angina (variant angina) *is an atypical form of angina that occurs at rest and is secondary to coronary artery spasm.* The cause is unknown, but the spasm often develops in a portion of the coronary artery adjacent to an atherosclerotic plaque. Whereas coronary artery spasm may contribute to the pathogenesis of an acute myocardial infarction or to the size of the infarct, it is generally not the principal cause of infarction.

Unstable angina, *a variety of chest pain that has a less predictable relationship to exercise than does stable angina and may occur during rest or sleep, is associated with the development of nonocclusive thrombi over atherosclerotic plaques.* In some cases of unstable angina, the patient complains of pain that develops with progressively increasing frequency and duration over a 3- to 4-day period. The electrocardiographic changes are not characteristic of infarction, and the serum levels of CK and LDH (evidence of myocardial necrosis) do not become elevated. **Unstable angina also is termed preinfarction angina, accelerated angina, "crescendo" angina, or coronary insufficiency.** Most of these patients ultimately progress to frank myocardial infarction, although in some cases, the symptoms may regress.

MYOCARDIAL INFARCTION: *A myocardial infarct refers to a discrete focus of ischemic necrosis in the heart.* This definition excludes patchy foci of necrosis that are caused by drugs and toxins (e.g., epinephrine, isoproterenol, alcohol) or by viruses. The development of an infarct is related to the duration of ischemia and the metabolic rate of the ischemic tissue. In experimental coronary artery ligation, foci of necrosis will result from as little as 20 minutes of ischemia and become more extensive as the period of ischemia is extended.

SUDDEN DEATH: The initial manifestation of ischemic heart disease may be unexpected ventricular fibrillation, an arrhythmia that results in sudden death. Provided that treatment is given immediately, this irregularity can often be converted to a normal rhythm by controlled electric shock.

Some authorities consider death to be sudden only if it occurs within 1 hour of the onset of symptoms. Others view death within 24 hours after the onset of symptoms to be sudden or require that sudden death be diagnosed only if it is unexpected. **In any event, coronary atherosclerosis underlies most cases of cardiac death occurring during the first hour after the onset of symptoms.**

Experimental animals subjected to acute coronary occlusion show a high incidence of ventricular fibrillation during the first hour of ischemia. It is clear that sudden cardiac death due to ventricular fibrillation also occurs in humans as a result of acute thrombosis of a coronary artery. On the other hand, this arrhythmia also appears in patients with marked coronary artery disease and no detectable thrombosis. If cardiopulmonary resuscitation is initiated promptly in persons who have suddenly lost consciousness because of ventricular fibrillation, more than half of the patients successfully resuscitated exhibit no myocardial infarction.

Many other less common conditions are associated with sudden cardiac death, including calcific aortic stenosis, dissecting aneurysm, conduction system abnormalities, myxomatous degeneration of the mitral valve, hypertrophic cardiomyopathy, anomalous coronary artery origin, certain drugs such as the phenothiazine antidepressants, and alcoholism.

Epidemiology

The major elements that predispose a person to coronary artery disease are an elevated blood cholesterol level, hypertension, and cigarette smoking. Any one of these factors significantly increases the risk of myocardial infarction (heart attack), and the presence of all three augments the risk more than sevenfold (see Chapter 8).

In the United States, there has been a reversal in the trend to progressively increasing mortality from ischemic heart disease. Beginning some 3 decades ago, the mortality rate from ischemic disease has steadily declined by more than half. In 1950, the age-adjusted death rate from myocardial infarction was 226 per 100,000 cases, whereas 40 years later it was only 108. This shift may be due, at least in part, to a reduction in smoking, to consumption of less saturated fat in the average diet, to the effective control of hypertension, and to the more recent use of cholesterol-reducing agents. For example, a man between 30 and 40 years of age with a blood cholesterol level of less than 175 mg/dL has less than half the risk of having a myocardial infarct than one with a level more than 240 mg/dL. An increase in serum low-density lipoproteins (LDLs) indicates an increased risk of heart disease. By contrast, persons with high levels of serum high-density lipoproteins (HDLs) are less likely to develop severe atherosclerosis and myocardial infarction. The total cholesterol-to-HDL cholesterol ratio appears to be a better predictor of coronary artery disease than is the serum cholesterol level alone.

Most populations in which men have high mean serum cholesterol values exhibit a high rate of coronary artery disease; the usual diet of these persons is high in saturated fat. Correspondingly, the diet is low in saturated fat in most countries whose inhabitants have low serum cholesterol levels and low rates of coronary artery disease. Moreover, the fat consumed by these populations is derived mainly from unsaturated fish and vegetable oils. Large prospective studies of groups at high risk of coronary events in which the dietary intake of saturated fat was decreased demonstrated a moderate reduction in the incidence of myocardial infarction, although overall mortality was unchanged. A study comparing Japanese men in Japan with Japanese immigrants in Hawaii and in San Francisco found that the risk of heart attack increased progressively from Japan to Hawaii to the mainland United States. It is thought that this trend probably relates to dietary differences among these groups.

In addition to factors related to cholesterol metabolism, high nonfasting triglyceride levels appear to be an independent predictor of the risk for myocardial infarction. This association is particularly strong when the total level of cholesterol is also increased. In recent years, substantial evidence has accumulated suggesting that the level of plasma fibrinogen is also directly correlates with the risk of ischemic heart disease, presumably because of the role of fibrinogen in atherogenesis and coronary artery thrombosis. Other factors that are involved in atherogenesis (see Chapter 10) have been reported to contribute to an increased risk of myocardial infarction, including levels of factor VII, plasminogen activator inhibitor-1, homocysteine, and decreased fibrinolytic activity.

The risk of ischemic heart disease also increases with increasing blood pressure. A person with a blood pressure of 160/95 mm Hg has twice the risk of ischemic heart disease compared with one whose blood pressure is 140/75 mm Hg or less. **Cigarette smoking is considered to be the major modifiable cause of coronary artery disease, and the risk of ischemic heart disease is increased in proportion to the number of cigarettes smoked.** Passive exposure to environmental tobacco smoke may also increase the risk of coronary atherosclerosis, albeit only slightly. Smoking is synergistic with other risk factors and has been estimated to be responsible for 20% of all death from cardiovascular disease in the United States.

Other risk factors for ischemic heart disease include the following:

- **Diabetes mellitus:** Ischemic heart disease is a major consequence of both type I and type II diabetes, the risk being twofold to threefold greater than that in the nondiabetic population. Conversely, atherosclerotic cardiovascular disease (myocardial infarction, stroke, peripheral vascular disease) accounts for 80% of all deaths in patients with diabetes.
- **Obesity:** In a major, longitudinal study of one population (Framingham Heart Study), obesity was an independent risk factor for cardiovascular disease, with an increased risk for obese persons compared with lean ones of 2 to 2.5.
- **Age:** The risk of infarction is greater with increasing age, up to age 80 years.
- **Sex:** Men remain at increased risk of ischemic heart disease, with 60% of coronary events occurring in men. Angina pectoris is considerably more frequent in men than in women; the ratio at ages younger than 50 years is 4:1 and that at age 60 years is 2:1.
- **Family history:** In one study that controlled for other risk factors, relatives of patients with ischemic heart disease had a twofold to fourfold increased risk for coronary artery disease. The genetic basis for this familial risk may interact with the other risk factors discussed here.
- **Use of oral contraceptives:** Women older than 35 years who smoke cigarettes and use oral contraceptives have an increased incidence of myocardial infarction.
- **Sedentary life habits:** Regular exercise seems to reduce the risk of myocardial infarction, perhaps by increasing HDL levels. In one study, the least-fit quartile of persons subjected to exercise testing had a risk of myocardial infarction 6.5 times greater than that of persons in the fittest quartile.
- **Personality features:** Early studies indicated that hard-driving, aggressive, time-conscious, executive-type persons ("type A" personality) have a higher incidence of heart disease than do more easygoing, relaxed persons ("type B" personality). "Coronary-prone" persons, those of the type A behavior pattern, tend to differ from those of type B, having higher plasma triglyceride and cholesterol levels and greater urinary catecholamine excretion. However, there is some controversy as to the relationship between coronary artery disease and the presence of the type A personality, and more recent studies failed to show the strong association previously reported.

Conditions that Limit the Supply of Blood to the Heart

The heart is an aerobic organ, requiring oxidative phosphorylation to provide energy for contraction. The anaerobic glycolysis of skeletal muscle is an insufficient source of energy for cardiac contraction. Ischemic heart disease is caused by an imbalance between the oxygen demands of

TABLE *11-3* **Causes of Ischemic Heart Disease**

Decreased Supply of Oxygen

Conditions that Influence the Supply of Blood

Atherosclerosis and thrombosis
Thromboemboli
Coronary artery spasm
Collateral blood vessels
Blood pressure, cardiac output, and heart rate
Miscellaneous: arteritis (e.g., periarteritis nodosa), dissecting aneurysm, luetic aortitis, anomalous origin of coronary artery, muscular bridging of coronary artery

Conditions that Influence the Availability of Oxygen in the Blood

Anemia
Shift in the hemoglobin–oxygen dissociation curve
Carbon monoxide
Cyanide

Increased Oxygen Demand (i.e., Increased Cardiac Work)

Hypertension
Valvular stenosis or insufficiency
Hyperthyroidism
Fever
Thiamine deficiency
Catecholamines

the myocardium and the supply of oxygenated blood (Table 11-3).

Atherosclerosis and Thrombosis

The pathogenesis of atherosclerosis is described in detail in Chapter 10. Here we only briefly discuss the features that are of special importance in relation to the coronary arteries. These vessels are small muscular arteries with a prominent internal elastic lamina. In a healthy person, they can dilate to accommodate four to eight times the resting blood flow. In the normal heart, the large coronary arteries provide almost no resistance to blood flow, and the myocardial circulation is controlled mainly by constriction and dilatation of small, intramyocardial branches less than 400 μm in diameter. In advanced atherosclerosis of the main coronary arteries (Fig. 11-13), stenosis develops and causes a decrease in blood pressure distal to the narrowed zone. To compensate for the consequent reduction in perfusion pressure, the microvessels dilate, thereby maintaining normal resting blood flow. As a result, most patients with coronary atherosclerosis do not have ischemia or angina at rest. However, with exercise, the capacity of the microcirculation to dilate further becomes limiting, and the demand for oxygen on the part of the myocardium exceeds the blood supply. The result is ischemia and angina.

Maximal blood flow to the myocardium is not impaired until 75% of the cross-sectional area of coronary artery (50% of the diameter) is compromised by atherosclerosis. However, resting blood flow is not reduced until more than 90% of the lumen is occluded. In patients with long-standing angina pectoris, the extent of collateral circulation exerts an important influence on the risk of acute myocardial infarction. There are conditions, such as hypotension or tachycardia, in which the demand for oxygen and the perfusion pressure may be in such imbalance that myocardial infarction ensues even when the narrowing of a coronary artery is not ordinarily sufficient to produce ischemia.

The angiographic demonstration of thrombotic obstruction plus the results of studies of experimental coronary occlusion establish that coronary artery thrombosis is the event that usually precipitates an acute myocardial infarction. More than 80% of patients who were studied by coronary angiography within 4 hours of the clinical onset of an acute myocardial infarction showed thrombotic occlusion of a coronary artery, whereas only half of patients examined between 12 and 24 hours had a thrombus. This discrepancy is explained by the dissolution of the thrombus through local and systemic thrombolytic mechanisms. In many cases, the thrombus occluding the vessel can be lysed and the ischemia relieved by the infusion of thrombolytic enzymes, such as streptokinase or tissue plasminogen activator.

Thromboemboli

Thromboembolism is a rare cause of myocardial infarction, and the coronary embolus is usually traced to the heart itself. The most common source is valvular vegetations, caused either by infectious or nonbacterial endocarditis. Coronary emboli occur in patients with atrial fibrillation and old rheumatic mitral valve disease who have mural thrombi in the left atrial appendage (Fig. 11-14). Thromboembolic occlusion of a coronary artery also is seen in patients with mural thrombi in the left ventricle secondary to infarction, aneurysm, or dilated cardiomyopathy.

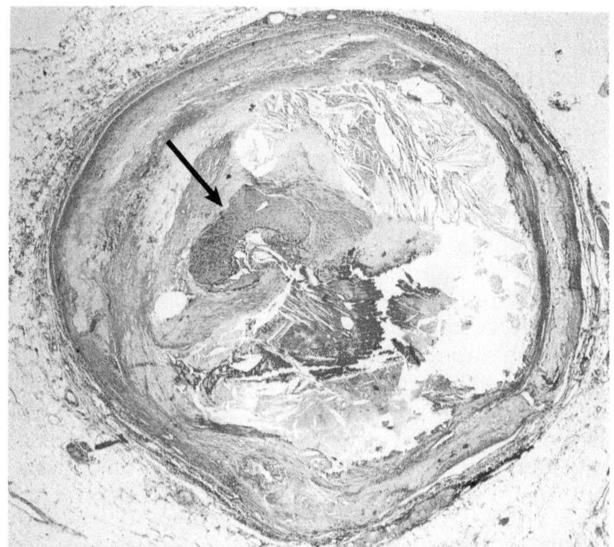

FIGURE *11-13*
Coronary atherosclerosis. Cross-section of an epicardial coronary artery shows severe atherosclerosis. The wall is thickened, and the lumen *(arrow)* is narrowed by an accumulation of atheromatous debris, including cholesterol crystals (needle-like spaces).

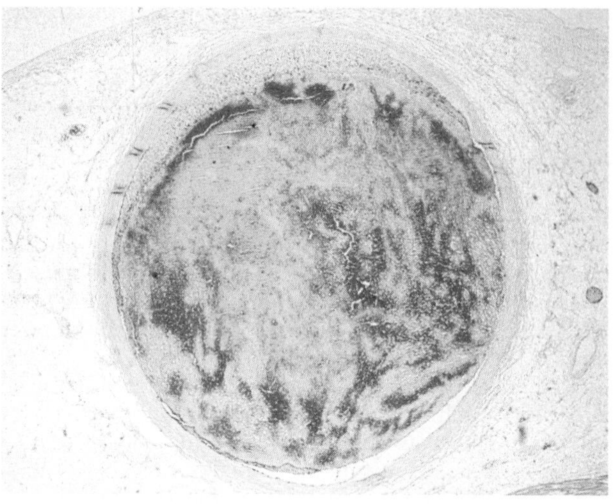

FIGURE *11-14*
Thromboembolus in the left anterior descending coronary artery of a man who had old rheumatic heart disease, mitral stenosis, and a mural thrombus in the left atrial appendage.

Coronary Collateral Circulation

Normal coronary arteries function as end-arteries, although most normal hearts have some anastomoses between coronary vessels 20 to 200 μm in diameter. These collateral vessels do not function under normal circumstances, because there is no pressure gradient between the arteries that they connect. However, after abrupt occlusion of a coronary artery, the pressure at one end of the anastomosis decreases precipitately, allowing blood to flow from the patent coronary artery to the ischemic area. More extensive collateral connections develop in hearts that are chronically ischemic because of coronary atherosclerosis. These collaterals may actually provide sufficient arterial flow to the area of myocardium supplied by an occluded coronary artery to prevent infarction completely or to limit its size.

The presence of coronary collaterals can explain certain unusual situations, such as an anterior infarct after recent thrombotic occlusion of the right coronary artery. This circumstance reflects the presence of coronary collaterals that develop between the LAD and right coronary arteries in response to gradual atherosclerotic narrowing of the LAD coronary artery. As a result, the myocardium previously supplied by the LAD coronary artery distal to the occlusion becomes dependent on the blood flow from the right coronary artery through the collaterals. Under these conditions, an acute thrombosis of the right coronary artery results in the paradoxical infarction of the anterior left ventricle ("infarction at a distance").

Other Conditions that Limit Coronary Blood Flow

- **Coronary arteritis,** a disorder usually caused by periarteritis nodosa, may be the basis of coronary artery obstruction.
- **Dissecting aneurysm of the aorta** on rare occasions obstructs the coronary arteries. Occasionally, medial necrosis and dissecting aneurysm are confined to the coronary artery.
- **Syphilitic aortitis** may extend to a coronary artery orifice and obliterate it.
- **Congenital anomalous origin of a coronary artery** has been associated with sudden death.
- **An intramural course of the LAD coronary artery** may cause myocardial ischemia and sudden death. This artery normally runs in the epicardial fat, but in some hearts, it dips into the myocardium for a short distance. The muscular bridge over the LAD coronary artery may result in compression of the vessel during systole or may predispose to coronary spasm.

Conditions that Limit Oxygen Availability

Anemia is a common cause of decreased oxygen supply to the myocardium. Although a heart with normal circulation can survive severe anemia, in the presence of coronary atherosclerosis, the capacity of the vessel to carry increased coronary blood flow may be limited, and cardiac necrosis may result. Furthermore, anemia increases the workload of the heart because an increased cardiac output is needed to supply the other organs with adequate oxygen.

Carbon monoxide poisoning results in decreased oxygen delivery to the tissues. The high affinity of hemoglobin for carbon monoxide displaces oxygen, and high carbon monoxide levels therefore lead to oxygen deprivation of the tissues. Cigarette smoking has been shown to produce a significant carbon monoxide level in the smoker's blood.

Increased Oxygen Demand

Any increase in the workload of the heart augments its need for oxygen. Conditions that increase the blood pressure or the cardiac output, such as exercise or pregnancy, result in an increased oxygen demand by the myocardium and may contribute to angina pectoris or myocardial infarction. Disorders in this category include valvular disease (mitral or aortic insufficiency, aortic stenosis), infection, and conditions such as hypertension, coarctation of the aorta, and hypertrophic cardiomyopathy. The increased metabolic rate and tachycardia in patients with hyperthyroidism is accompanied by an increase in oxygen demand as well as an increase in the workload of the heart. This is especially important to recognize clinically because treatment of the underlying thyroid disease is the most effective therapy for a hyperthyroid patient with symptoms of ischemic heart disease. Fever also increases the basal metabolic rate, cardiac output, and heart rate.

Pathology of Myocardial Infarction

Location of Infarcts

Transmural infarcts conform to the distribution of one of the three major coronary arteries (see Fig. 11-2).

- **Right coronary artery:** An occlusion of the proximal portion of this vessel results in an infarct of the posterior basal region of the left ventricle and the posterior third of the interventricular septum ("inferior" infarct).
- **Left anterior descending coronary artery:** Blockage of the LAD coronary artery produces an infarct of the apical, anterior, and anteroseptal walls of the left ventricle.
- **Left circumflex coronary artery:** Obstruction of this vessel is the least common cause of a myocardial infarct and leads to an infarct of the lateral wall of the left ventricle.

Infarcts may involve predominantly the subendocardial portion of the myocardium, or they may be transmural. There are important differences between these two types of infarctions (Table 11-4). A subendocardial infarct affects the inner one third to one half of the left ventricle; it is commonly circumferential, so that it is not necessarily in the distribution of any one coronary artery. Subendocardial infarction generally occurs as a consequence of hypoperfusion of the heart in disorders such as aortic stenosis or hemorrhagic shock or as a result of hypoperfusion during the course of cardiopulmonary bypass. Because the necrosis is limited to the inner layers of the heart, the fibrinous epicarditis seen in transmural infarcts is not present. Coronary artery thrombosis is not usually a cause of circumferential subendocardial infarcts, and coronary artery stenosis need not be present.

Occlusion of a coronary artery often results in a transmural infarct. **The volume of arterial collateral flow is the chief factor affecting the transmural progression of the infarct.** With chronic cardiac ischemia, the presence of extensive collateral vessels that preferentially supply the outer or subepicardial layer limits the infarct to the subendocardial portion of the myocardium. Whereas the subendocardial myocardium is involved in virtually all infarcts, ischemic lesions of the deeper myocardium and subepicardial region are variable. In fatal cases of acute myocardial infarction, transmural infarcts are more common than those restricted to the subendocardium.

Infarcts involve the left ventricle much more commonly and extensively than they do the right ventricle. This difference may be partly due to the greater workload imposed on the left ventricle and the greater thickness of the left ventricular wall. In the presence of right ventricular hypertrophy (e.g., in cases of pulmonary hypertension), the incidence of right ventricular infarcts is increased. Infarction of the right ventricle in posterior myocardial infarcts is actually not uncommon, occurring in about a third of such cases. However, most of these are extensions of a transmural left ventricular infarct, and lesions limited to the right ventricle are rare.

TABLE ***11-4*** **Differences Between Subendocardial and Transmural Infarcts**

Subendocardial Infarcts	Transmural Infarcts
Multifocal	Unifocal
Patchy	Solid
Circumferential	In distribution of a specific coronary artery
Coronary thrombosis rare	Coronary thrombosis common
Often **result** from hypotension or shock	Often **cause** shock
No epicarditis	Epicarditis common
Do not form aneurysms	May result in aneurysm

Macroscopic Characteristics of Myocardial Infarcts

The early stages in the evolution of a myocardial infarct can be observed experimentally. About 10 seconds after the ligation of a coronary artery, the affected myocardium becomes cyanotic and, rather than contracting, bulges outward during systole. If the obstruction is promptly relieved, myocardial contractions resume, and no anatomical damage ensues, although contractility may be depressed in the postischemic tissue for many hours (stunned myocardium). This reversible stage continues for 20 to 30 minutes of total ischemia, beyond which time damaged myocytes progressively die.

On gross examination, an acute myocardial infarct is not identifiable within the first 12 hours after the onset. By 24 hours, the infarct can be recognized on the cut surface of the involved ventricle by its pallor. After 3 to 5 days, the infarct is mottled and more sharply outlined, with a central pale, yellowish, necrotic region bordered by a hyperemic zone (Fig. 11-15). Occasionally, the infarcted region is hemorrhagic, especially when thrombolytic drugs have been administered and the infarct has been reperfused with arterial blood. By 2 to 3 weeks, the infarcted region is depressed and soft, with a refractile, gelatinous appearance. Older, healed infarcts are firm and contracted and have the pale gray appearance of scar tissue (Fig. 11-16).

Microscopic Characteristics of Myocardial Infarcts

THE FIRST 24 HOURS: Electron microscopy provides the earliest morphological evidence of ischemia (Fig. 11-17). Reversibly injured myocytes show sarcoplasmic edema, mild mitochondrial swelling, and loss of glycogen. After 30 to 60 minutes of ischemia, when myocyte injury has become irreversible, the mitochondria are greatly swollen and exhibit disorganized cristae and amorphous matrix densities. The nucleus shows clumping and margination of chromatin, and the sarcolemma is focally disrupted.

The loss of sarcolemmal integrity leads to the release of intracellular proteins, such as myoglobin, lactic dehydrogenase (LDH), and creatine kinase (CK), from the myocytes to the extracellular space. Ion gradients also are dissipated, and tissue potassium decreases as the sodium and chloride increase.

The noncontractile ischemic myocytes are stretched with each systole and become "wavy fibers." In longitudinal sections, the periphery of the infarct exhibits contraction bands. By 24 hours, the myocytes are deeply eosinophilic (Fig. 11-18) and show the characteristic changes of coagulation necrosis. However, it takes several

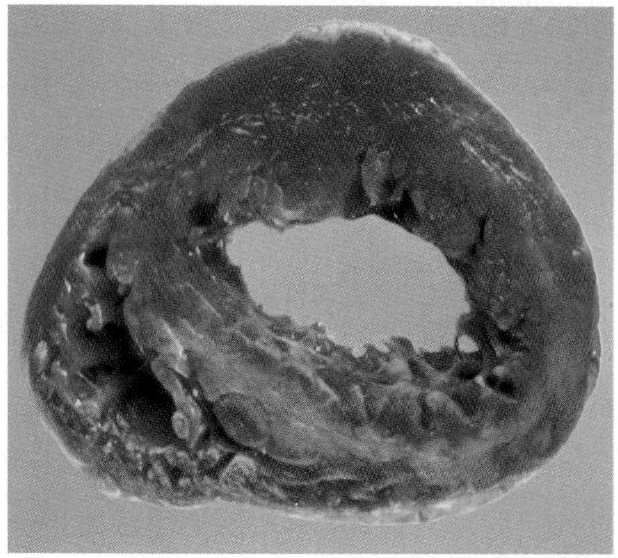

FIGURE *11-15*
Acute myocardial infarct. A cross-section of the ventricles of a man who died a few days after the onset of severe chest pain shows a transmural infarct in the posterior and septal regions of the left ventricle. The necrotic myocardium is soft, yellowish, and sharply demarcated.

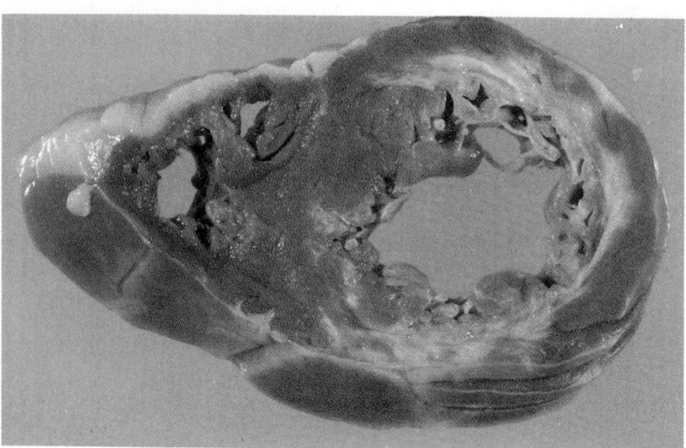

FIGURE *11-16*
Healed myocardial infarct. A cross-section of the heart from a man who died after a long history of angina pectoris and several myocardial infarctions shows circumferential scarring of the left ventricle.

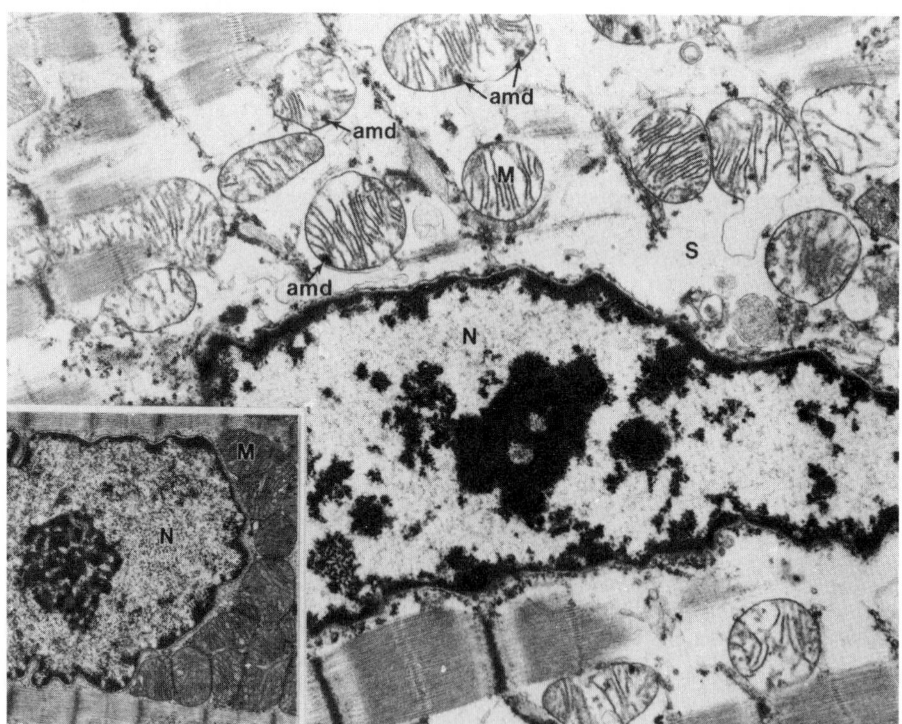

FIGURE *11-17*
Ultrastructure of myocardial ischemia. Electron micrograph of an irreversibly injured myocyte from a canine heart subjected to 40 minutes of low-flow ischemia, induced by proximal occlusion of the circumflex branch of the left coronary artery. A nonischemic control myocyte from the same heart is shown in the inset. The affected myocyte is swollen and has abundant clear sarcoplasm *(S)*. The mitochondria *(M)* also are swollen and contain amorphous matrix densities *(amd)*, which are characteristic of lethal cell injury. The sarcolemma of this myocyte *(not shown)* exhibited small areas of disruption. The chromatin of the nucleus *(N)* is aggregated peripherally, in contrast to the uniformly distributed chromatin in normal tissue.

days for the myocyte nucleus to disappear totally. Myocytes also show an increase in periodic acid–Schiff (PAS)-positive material, which is resistant to diastase and thus is not glycogen.

TWO TO 3 DAYS: Polymorphonuclear leukocytes are attracted to the necrotic myocytes and reach their maximal concentration in infarcts after 2 days (Figs. 11-18 and 11-19). Interstitial edema and areas of hemorrhage commonly appear. By 2 to 3 days, the muscle cells are more clearly necrotic, nuclei disappear, and striations become less prominent. Some of the polymorphonuclear leukocytes that were attracted to the area begin to undergo karyorrhexis.

FIVE TO 7 DAYS: By this time, the acute inflammatory leukocytic response has abated, so that few, if any, polymorphonuclear leukocytes are present. The periphery of the infarcted region shows phagocytosis of the dead muscle by macrophages. Fibroblasts begin to proliferate, and new collagen formation is evident. Lymphocytes and pigment-laden macrophages are prominent. The process of repair is initiated at about 5 days, beginning at the periphery of the infarct and gradually extending toward the center.

ONE TO 3 WEEKS: Collagen deposition proceeds, the inflammatory infiltrate gradually recedes, and the newly sprouted capillaries are progressively obliterated.

MORE THAN 4 WEEKS: Considerable dense fibrous tissue is present. The debris is progressively removed, and the scar becomes more solid and less cellular as it matures (Fig. 11-20).

This timetable of events after a coronary artery occlusion can be altered by local or systemic events. For example, the immediate extension of an infarct into a region that previously displayed patchy necrosis may not show the expected changes. A large infarct tends not to mature in its center as rapidly as a smaller infarct. In estimating the age of a large infarct, it is more accurate to base the interpretation on the outer border where repair begins, rather than on changes in the central region. In fact, in some large infarcts, rather than being removed, the dead myocytes remain in a "mummified" form indefinitely.

Contraction band necrosis refers to the presence of thick, irregular, transverse bands across necrotic myocytes as a result of hypercontraction (Fig. 11-21). By electron microscopy, these irreversible bands consist of small groups of hypercontracted disorganized sarcomeres with thickened Z lines. The architecture of the myocyte is disrupted, and there are breaks in the sarcolemma. The mitochondria, located between the contraction bands, are swollen and may contain deposits of calcium phosphate in the matrix, as well as amorphous matrix densities. The pathogenesis of hypercontraction involves an uncontrolled increase in calcium concentration in the SR of myocytes that are sufficiently intact to generate the high-energy phosphates necessary for hypercontraction.

Contraction band necrosis is prominent in regions where blood flow persists, such as at the margins of an acute infarct. It is also seen in situations in which reflow occurs, for example, in patients who have had emergency coronary artery bypass grafts, who have been treated with thrombolytic drugs or angioplasty to clear an obstructed coronary artery, or who spontaneously lyse an occluding thrombus. In cases of restored flow, contraction band necrosis is seen in the territory supplied by the grafted or dilated artery.

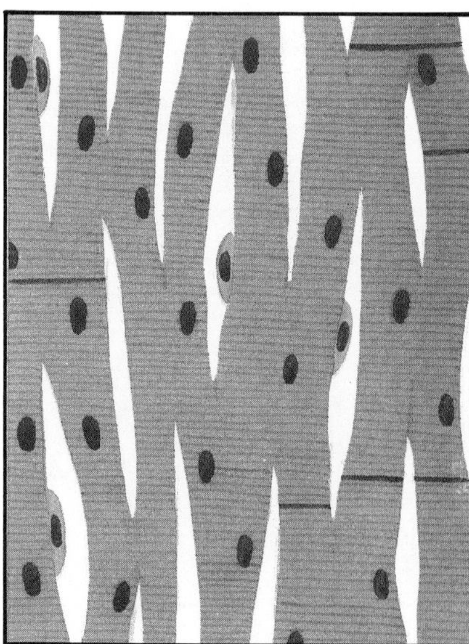
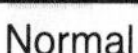
Normal

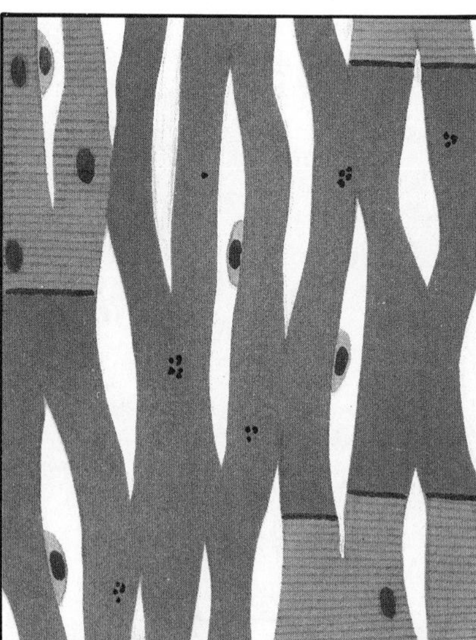
12-18 hours

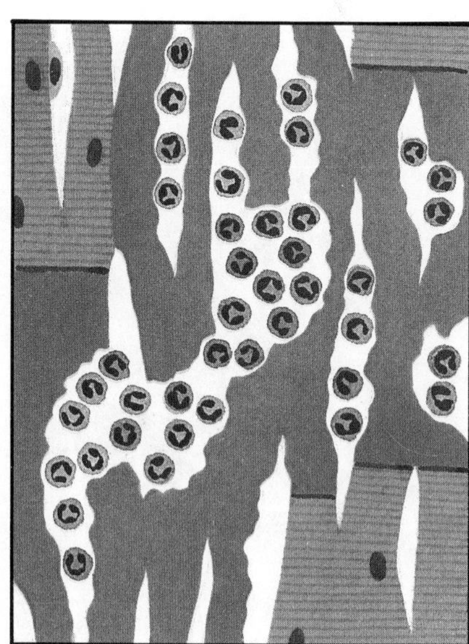
1 day

FIGURE *11-18*
Development of a myocardial infarct. (*A*) Normal myocardium. (*B*) After about 12 to 18 hours, the infarcted myocardium shows eosinophilia (red staining) in sections of the heart stained with hematoxylin and eosin. (*C*) About 24 hours after the onset of the infarct, polymorphonuclear neutrophils infiltrate around the necrotic myocytes.

Clinical Diagnosis of Acute Myocardial Infarction

The onset of acute myocardial infarction is often sudden, with severe substernal or precordial crushing pain. The pain may be an epigastric burning (simulating indigestion) or may extend into the jaw or down the inside of either arm. It is often accompanied by sweating, nausea, vomiting, and shortness of breath. In some cases, an acute myocardial infarction is preceded by unstable angina of several days duration. **One fourth to one half of all nonfatal myocardial infarctions occur without any symptoms, and the infarcts are identified only later by electrocardiographic changes or at autopsy.**

The diagnosis of acute myocardial infarction is confirmed by electrocardiography and the appearance of increased levels of certain enzymes or proteins in the serum. The electrocardiogram exhibits new Q waves and changes in the ST segment and the conformation of the T wave. Serum enzyme changes, particularly in the isoenzymes of LDH and CK, are detectable after significant myocardial necrosis has occurred. There are five isoenzymes of LDH, with LDH-1 in the highest concentration in the heart. After the death of myocytes, the normally low serum level of LDH-1 is increased within 6 to 12 hours as a result of leakage of the enzyme from the dead cells and remains increased for many days. Because the level of LDH-2 is not proportionally increased, the ratio of LDH-1 to LDH-2 is reversed.

A more reliable diagnostic criterion for acute myocardial infarction is the MB isoenzyme of CK, which is found almost exclusively in the myocardium. The serum level of CK-MB enzyme is increased 7 to 48 hours after the onset of symptoms, reaching its peak in 20 hours.

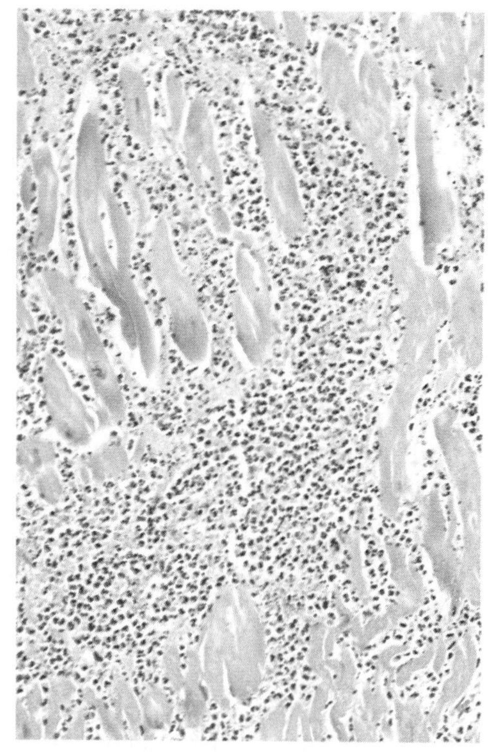

FIGURE *11-19*
Acute myocardial infarct. The necrotic myocardial fibers, which are eosinophilic and devoid of cross striations and nuclei, are immersed in a sea of acute inflammatory cells.

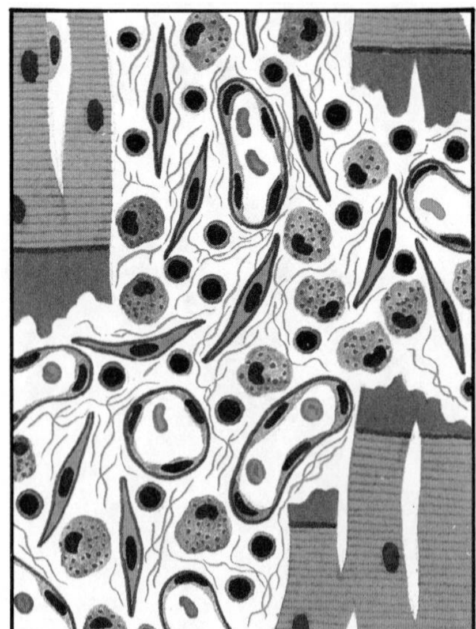

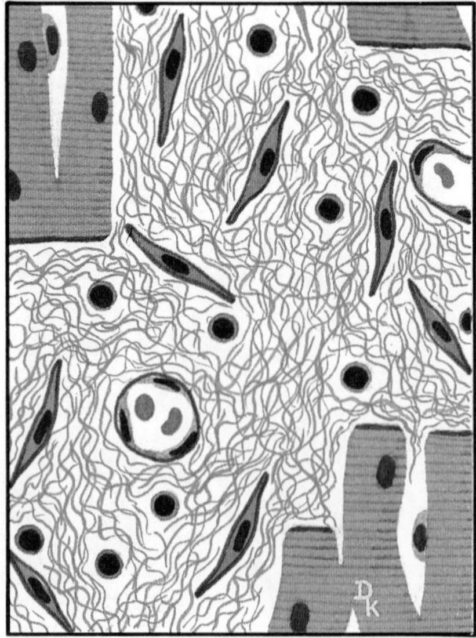

FIGURE *11-18 (continued)*
***(D)* After about 3 weeks, the infarct contains granulation tissue with prominent capillaries, fibroblasts, lymphoid cells, and macrophages. The necrotic debris has been largely removed, and a small amount of collagen has been laid down. *(E)* After 3 months or more, the infarcted region has been replaced by scar tissue.**

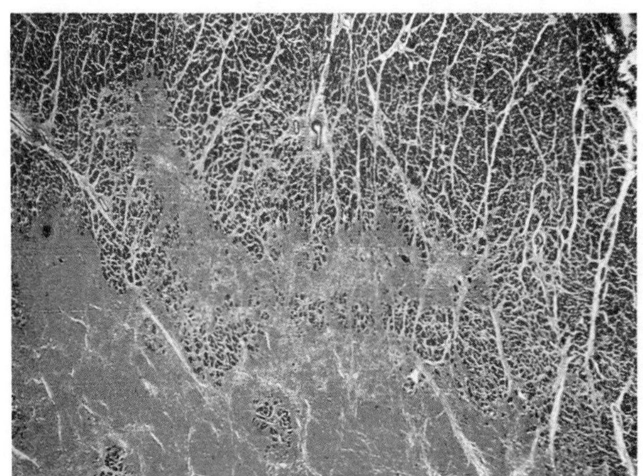

FIGURE 11-20
Healed myocardial infarct. A section of the scarred myocardium stained for collagen shows dense, acellular fibrosis sharply demarcated from the adjacent viable myocardium.

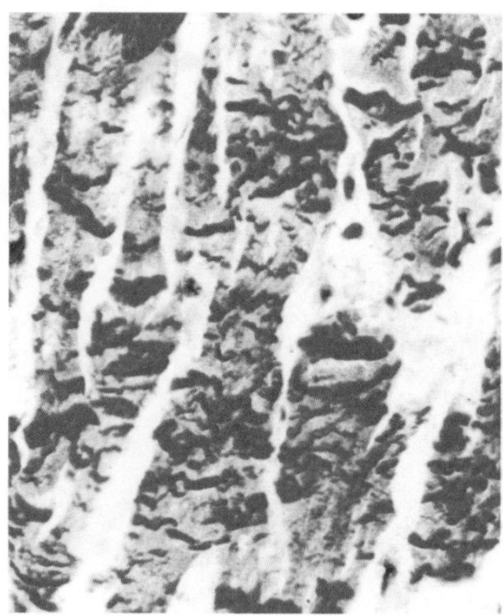

FIGURE 11-21
Contraction band necrosis. A section of infarcted myocardium shows prominent, thick, wavy, transverse bands in the myofibers.

Recently, increased levels of cardiac troponin T (cTnT) in the serum were found to be a useful index of myocardial necrosis. The cTnT remains increased longer than CK-MB and appears to be a more predictive marker of mortality than is MB-CK.

Complications of Myocardial Infarction

In some cases of acute myocardial infarction, the patient succumbs to pump failure (cardiogenic shock). However, in the majority of cases, the clinical course is dominated by a variety of other functional or mechanical complications of the infarct.

ARRHYTHMIAS: Virtually all patients who have a myocardial infarct have some abnormality of cardiac rhythm at some time during the course of their illness. In fact, arrhythmias account for half of the deaths caused by ischemic heart disease. Premature ventricular beats, sinus bradycardia, ventricular tachycardia, ventricular fibrillation, paroxysmal atrial tachycardia, and partial or complete heart block can occur. The causes of the arrhythmias are often obscure, but many are believed to reflect enhanced sympathetic activity mediated by increased levels of local or circulating catecholamines.

LEFT VENTRICULAR FAILURE AND CARDIOGENIC SHOCK: Now that ventricular fibrillation can be treated effectively by electric-shock resuscitation, the most feared complication in acute myocardial infarction is cardiogenic shock. The incidence of this complication is now only about 7%, owing to the development of techniques that assist the damaged myocardium (intraaortic balloon pump) or that increase perfusion through the obstructed coronary artery (thrombolytic therapy, angioplasty). Cardiogenic shock is most likely to occur early in the course of the illness when the infarct involves more than 40% of the left ventricle; the mortality rate in these cases is as high as 90%. The hemodynamic consequences of cardiogenic shock are discussed in Chapter 7.

At autopsy, in patients who have succumbed to cardiogenic shock, the heart exhibits marginal extension of the original infarct and foci of necrosis in remote areas of the left and right ventricles. These changes are most likely secondary to shock, rather than to the original ischemic episode. In more than two thirds of cases of cardiogenic shock, the luminal cross-section of all three coronary arteries is reduced by more than 90%, a situation that limits the perfusion of the heart.

EXTENSION OF THE INFARCT: Clinically recognizable extension of an acute myocardial infarct occurs in the first 1 to 2 weeks in up to 10% of patients. In careful echocardiographic studies, half of all patients with anterior myocardial infarction showed some extension of the infarct during the first 2 weeks, indicating that many episodes of infarct extension are not recognized. Clinically significant infarct extension is associated with a twofold increased mortality.

RUPTURE OF THE FREE WALL OF THE MYOCARDIUM: Myocardial rupture (Fig. 11-22) may occur at almost any time within the first 3 weeks of an acute myocardial infarction but is most common between the first and fourth days, when the infarcted wall is weakest. After this time, the scar becomes progressively stronger, so that rupture becomes less likely. Rupture of the free wall is generally a complication of large transmural infarcts that involve at least 20% of the left ventricle. It usually occurs at the junction of the infarct and the normal muscle.

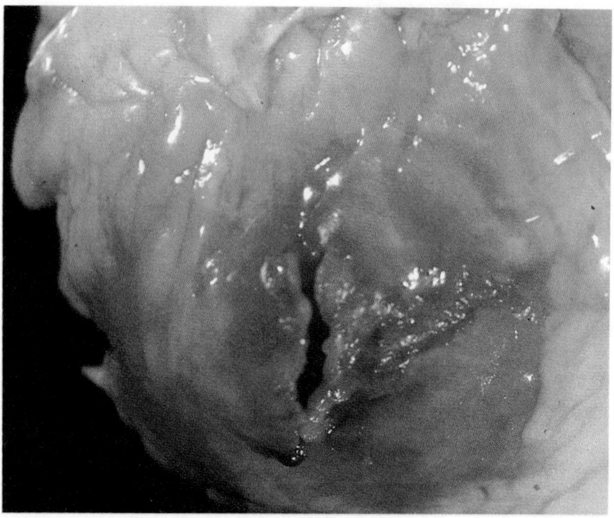

FIGURE *11-22*
Rupture of an acute myocardial infarct. An elderly woman with a recent myocardial infarct died of cardiac tamponade. The pericardium was filled with blood, and the external surface of the left ventricle shows a linear rupture of the necrotic myocardium.

Rupture of the infarcted myocardium most often results in hemopericardium and death of pericardial tamponade. Myocardial rupture accounts for 10% of the deaths of acute myocardial infarction in hospitalized patients. This complication is more common in the elderly, and possibly, in women and in patients with hypertension. In rare instances, a ruptured ventricle may be walled off, and the patient survives with a false aneurysm (Fig. 11-23).

OTHER FORMS OF MYOCARDIAL RUPTURE: A few patients in whom a myocardial infarct involves the interventricular septum develop a **septal perforation**, varying in length from 1 cm or more. The magnitude of the resulting left-to-right shunt, and therefore the prognosis, varies with the size of the rupture.

Rupture of a portion of a papillary muscle occurs and results in mitral regurgitation. In unusual cases, an entire papillary muscle is transected, in which case, massive mitral valve incompetence is fatal.

ANEURYSMS: Left ventricular aneurysms complicate 10% to 15% of healed transmural myocardial infarcts. After an acute transmural myocardial infarct, the affected ventricular wall tends to bulge outward during systole in one third of patients. As the infarct matures, the collagenous scar tissue is susceptible to further stretching. Localized thinning and stretching of the ventricular wall in the region of a healing myocardial infarct is termed **infarct expansion** and is actually an early aneurysm. Such an aneurysm is composed of a thin layer of necrotic myocardium and collagenous tissue, which expands with each contraction of the heart. As the evolving aneurysm becomes more fibrotic, its tensile strength increases. However, the aneurysm continues to dilate with each beat, thereby "stealing" some of the left ventricular output and contributing to the workload of the heart. Patients with left ventricular aneurysms are at increased risk of myocardial rupture and have a poorer prognosis. Mural thrombi develop within the aneurysm in half of these cases and are a source of systemic emboli.

A distinction should be made between "true" and "false" aneurysms (see Fig. 11-23). True aneurysms are much more common than false aneurysms and are caused by bulging of the weakened, but intact, left ventricular

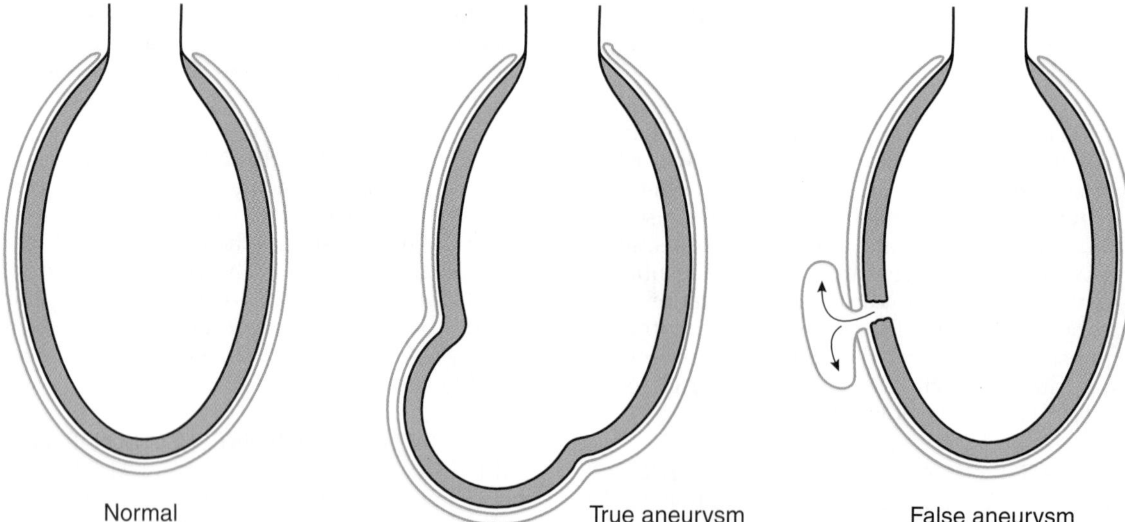

FIGURE *11-23*
True and false aneurysms of the left ventricle. *(Left)* Normal heart. The left ventricular wall *(shaded)* is enclosed by a pericardial sac. *(Center)* True aneurysm shows an intact wall *(black)*, which bulges outward. *(Right)* False aneurysm shows a ruptured infarct, which is walled off externally by adherent pericardium. Note that the mouth of the true aneurysm is wider than that of the false aneurysm.

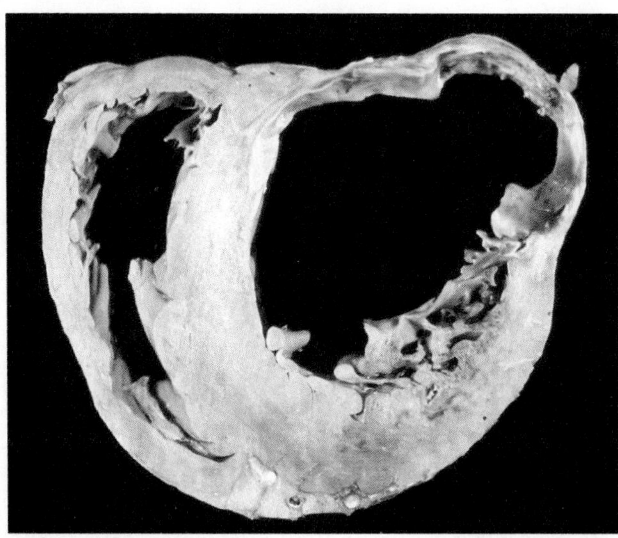

FIGURE *11-24*
Ventricular aneurysm. A cross-section through the ventricles of a heart obtained at autopsy from a patient with a history of a posterior wall myocardial infarction shows thinning and aneurysmal dilatation of the left ventricular wall in the region of the healed infarct.

wall (Fig. 11-24). By contrast, false aneurysms result from the rupture of a portion of the left ventricle that has been walled off by pericardial scar tissue. Thus, the wall of a false aneurysm is composed of pericardium and scar tissue and not left ventricular myocardium.

MURAL THROMBOSIS AND EMBOLISM: Almost half of all patients who die after myocardial infarction are discovered at autopsy to have mural thrombi overlying the infarct (Fig. 11-25), particularly when it involves the apex of the heart. In turn, half of these patients have some evidence of systemic embolization.

Involvement of the endocardium over an infarct predisposes to the adhesion of platelets and to the deposition of fibrin. Moreover, the poor contractile function of the underlying myocardium allows the fibrin–platelet mural thrombus to grow. Pieces of the thrombus can detach and be swept along with the arterial blood. Therefore, the presence of a mural thrombus justifies anticoagulant therapy and antiplatelet medications.

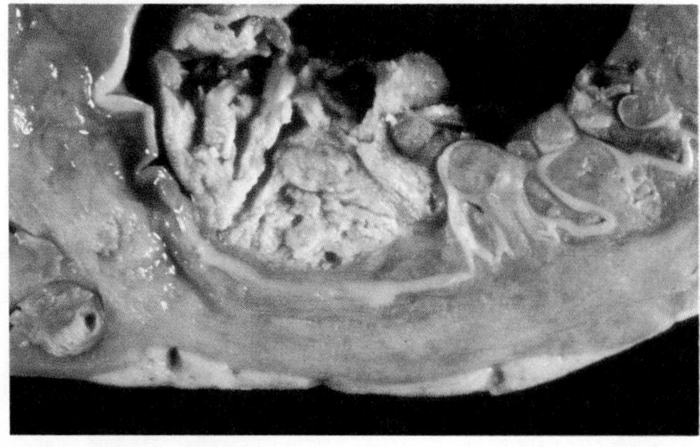

FIGURE *11-25*
Mural thrombus overlying a healed myocardial infarct. In this cross-section of a fixed heart, an organized, friable, grayish-white mural thrombus overlies a thickened endocardium situated over a scarred myocardium.

PERICARDITIS: A transmural myocardial infarct involves the epicardium and leads to inflammation of the pericardium in 10% to 20% of patients. This pericarditis is manifested clinically as chest pain and a pericardial friction rub. A fourth of the patients with acute myocardial infarction, particularly those with larger infarcts and congestive heart failure, develop a pericardial effusion, with or without pericarditis. Less frequently, anticoagulant therapy has been associated with the appearance of a hemorrhagic pericardial effusion and even with cardiac tamponade.

Postmyocardial infarction syndrome (Dressler syndrome) refers to a delayed pericarditis, which develops 2 to 10 weeks after infarction. A similar disorder may occur after cardiac surgery. The fact that antibodies to heart muscle appear in patients with Dressler syndrome and the observation that the condition is ameliorated by corticosteroid therapy suggest that this condition has an immunological basis.

Therapeutic Interventions that Limit Infarct Size

Because the dimensions of an infarct are an important predictor of morbidity and mortality, any therapy that limits its size should be beneficial. By definition, such therapy is directed at preventing the death of reversibly injured, ischemic myocytes and limiting infarct extension. For some time after the onset of ischemia, damaged myocytes can be salvaged if the tissue is reperfused successfully with arterial blood. As the period of ischemia is extended, increasing numbers of myocytes die. Reperfusion of areas of acute myocardial ischemia results in a mixture of living myocytes damaged by ischemia and dead myocytes exhibiting contraction band necrosis.

Restoration of arterial blood flow remains the only way to salvage ischemic myocytes permanently, although a number of interventions can delay ischemic injury. The most notable is hypothermia, which is used during cardiac surgery to minimize myocardial injury. There are several methods to restore blood flow to the area of myocardium supplied by an obstructed coronary artery.

Thrombolytic enzymes, such as tissue plasminogen activator or streptokinase, can be infused intravenously or directly into an obstructed coronary artery to dissolve the clot causing the obstruction.

Percutaneous transluminal coronary angioplasty (PTCA) refers to dilatation of a narrowed coronary artery by the inflation of a balloon catheter. This procedure can be performed quickly after the onset of ischemia and, together with thrombolytics, restores arterial blood flow. PTCA also allows the placement of a stent in the coronary artery to maintain the patency of the lumen.

Coronary artery bypass grafting can restore blood flow to the distal segment of a coronary artery with a proximal occlusion.

Procedures that restore blood flow must be performed as quickly as possible, preferably in the first few hours after the onset of symptoms. After 6 hours, it is unlikely that any salvageable ischemic myocardium remains. Moreover, after this interval, reperfusion frequently produces hemorrhage in the center of the infarct because of microvascular damage in this region.

On the basis of animal experiments, it has been suggested that some myocytes, alive but injured at the time of reperfusion, may be further injured or even killed after restoration of blood flow. Such reperfusion injury (see Chapter 1) appears to be related to the generation of toxic oxygen radicals and to the accumulation of excess calcium in the damaged myocytes. It is further suggested that reperfusion injury may result in a temporary but reversible impairment of myocardial contractility, referred to as "myocardial stunning." However, the clinical significance of stunned myocardium after an infarction remains controversial.

Chronic Ischemic Heart Disease

Patients with severe coronary atherosclerosis follow a pattern of increasingly frequent episodes of angina pectoris, reflecting progressive narrowing of one or more coronary arteries. In many cases, a diseased artery is eventually occluded by a thrombus, which has formed on a ruptured atherosclerotic plaque. During the interval between the onset of intermittent angina and the development of an infarct, the patient may be incapacitated by anginal pain, although cardiac function need not be impaired. If the infarct is small, it may be difficult to detect any functional deficit, but if it is large, regional contractility may be absent (akinesis) or defective (dyskinesis). Under these conditions, overall cardiac function, which is often evaluated by measurement of the ejection fraction, declines in proportion to the amount of infarcted myocardium. **Thus, in most patients with chronic ischemic heart disease, persistently depressed cardiac function reflects the presence of infarcts.**

ISCHEMIC CARDIOMYOPATHY: In a minority of patients with severe coronary atherosclerosis, myocardial contractility is impaired globally in the absence of discrete infarcts, a situation that mimics dilated cardiomyopathy. In many cases, this situation reflects a combination of ischemic myocardial dysfunction, diffuse fibrosis, and multiple small healed infarcts. However, there remains a group of patients with left ventricular failure in whom cardiac dysfunction occurs without obvious infarction. These patients are said to have **ischemic cardiomyopathy**. In some patients, the dysfunctional myocardium is persistently ischemic, with oxygen delivery inadequate to sustain normal contraction but sufficient to maintain viability, a circumstance referred to as hibernating myocardium. The contractile function of hibernating myocardium is restored when the affected tissue is revascularized. Thus, to the extent that hibernation plays a role in ischemic cardiomyopathy, surgical revascularization is potentially beneficial.

HYPERTENSIVE HEART DISEASE

Hypertension has been defined by the World Health Organization as a persistent increase of blood pressure to levels greater than 160 mm Hg systolic or 90 mm Hg diastolic, or both (see Chapter 10). Chronic hypertension leads to pressure overload, compensatory left ventricular hypertrophy, and eventually, cardiac failure. The term *hypertensive heart disease* is used when the heart is enlarged in the absence of a cause other than hypertension.

Effects of Hypertension on the Heart

Hypertension causes compensatory left ventricular hypertrophy as a result of the increased workload imposed on the heart. The left ventricle is thickened (Fig. 11-26), and the overall weight of the heart is increased, exceeding 375 g in men and 350 g in women. Microscopically, the hypertrophic myocardial cells have an increased diameter, with enlarged, hyperchromatic, and rectangular nuclei (boxcar nuclei) (Fig. 11-27).

Myocardial hypertrophy clearly adds to the ability of the heart to handle an increased workload up to a point, beyond which additional hypertrophy is damaging. This upper limit to useful hypertrophy may reflect the increasing diffusion distance between the interstitium and the center of each myofiber; if the distance becomes too great, the supply of oxygen to the myofiber will be deficient.

Diastolic dysfunction is the most common functional abnormality caused by hypertension and by itself can lead to congestive heart failure. **Hypertension also is associated with an increased severity of atherosclerosis of the coronary arteries.** The combination of increased cardiac workload (systolic dysfunction), diastolic dysfunction, and narrowed coronary arteries leads to a greater risk of myocardial ischemia, infarction, and heart failure.

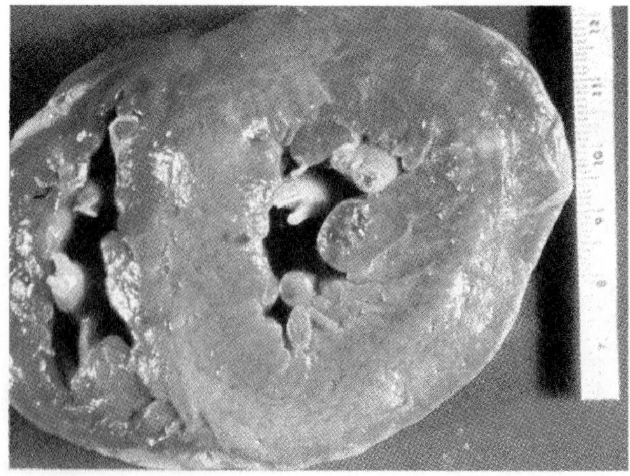

FIGURE *11-26*
Hypertensive heart disease. A cross-section of the heart shows prominent hypertrophy of the left ventricular myocardium.

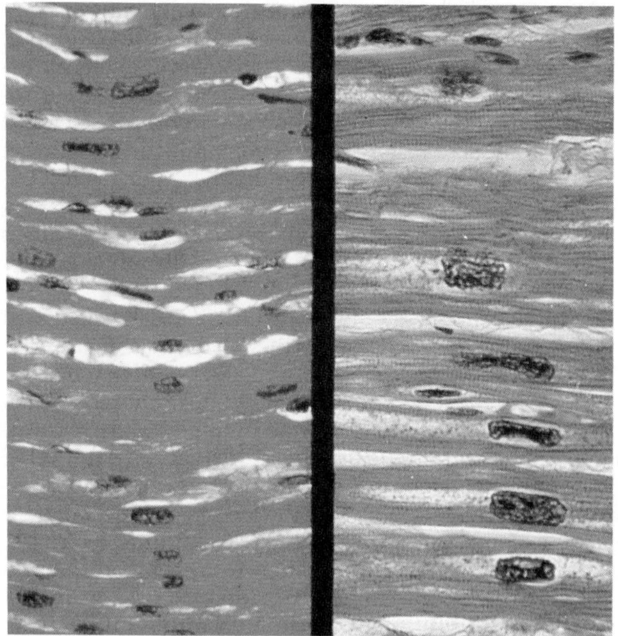

FIGURE 11-27
Hypertensive heart disease with myocardial hypertrophy. Compared with a normal myocardium *(left)*, the hypertrophic myocardium *(right)* shows thicker fibers and enlarged, hyperchromatic, and rectangular nuclei.

Cause of Death in Patients with Hypertension

Congestive heart failure is the most common cause of death in hypertensive patients, accounting for 40% of all deaths caused by hypertension. Intracerebral hemorrhage is also a frequent fatal complication. In addition, death may occur as a result of coronary atherosclerosis and myocardial infarction, dissecting aneurysm of the aorta, or ruptured berry aneurysm of the cerebral circulation. Finally, death in renal failure may supervene when nephrosclerosis induced by hypertension becomes severe.

COR PULMONALE

Cor pulmonale is defined as right ventricular hypertrophy and dilatation secondary to pulmonary hypertension. Increased pressure in the lesser circulation may reflect a disorder of the pulmonary parenchyma, or more rarely, a primary disease of the vasculature (e.g., primary pulmonary hypertension, recurrent small pulmonary emboli).

Acute cor pulmonale refers to the sudden occurrence of pulmonary hypertension, most commonly as a result of sudden, massive pulmonary embolization. This condition causes acute right-sided heart failure and is a medical emergency. At autopsy, the only cardiac findings are severe dilatation of the right ventricle and sometimes of the right atrium.

Chronic Cor Pulmonale

Chronic cor pulmonale is a common heart disease, accounting for 30% to 40% of all cases of heart failure in an English study and 10% to 30% in a series in the United States. This frequency reflects the prevalence of chronic pulmonary disease in these countries, especially chronic bronchitis and emphysema. In many cases of chronic disease of the lung, the severity of pulmonary hypertension correlates more closely with survival than does any other variable. In fact, fewer than 10% of patients with a pulmonary artery pressure greater than 45 mm Hg survive 5 years.

☐ **Pathogenesis:** Chronic cor pulmonale may be caused by any pulmonary disease that interferes with ventilatory mechanics or gas exchange or obstructs the pulmonary vasculature (Table 11-5). **The most common causes of chronic cor pulmonale are chronic obstructive pulmonary disease and pulmonary fibrosis.** Severe kyphoscoliosis may deform the chest wall and interfere with its function as a bellows, resulting in hypoxemia and pulmonary vasoconstriction. A small number of cases of cor pulmonale is attributed to primary pulmonary hypertension, a disorder of unknown etiology. As discussed earlier, some congenital heart diseases associated with increased pulmonary blood flow are complicated by pulmonary hypertension and cor pulmonale.

The pathogenesis of pulmonary hypertension secondary to recurrent pulmonary emboli is clearly progressive mechanical obstruction to blood flow. However, the situation in chronic parenchymal diseases of the lungs is more complicated. In addition to the obliteration of blood vessels in the lung, these disorders also lead to pulmonary arteriolar vasoconstriction, which reduces the effective

TABLE 11-5 Causes of Cor Pulmonale

Parenchymal Diseases of the Lung
Chronic bronchitis and emphysema
Pulmonary fibrosis (from any cause)
Cystic fibrosis
Pulmonary Vascular Diseases
Recurrent pulmonary emboli
Primary pulmonary hypertension
Peripheral pulmonary stenosis
Intravenous drug abuse
Residence at high altitude
Schistosomiasis
Congenital Heart Diseases
Impaired Movement of the Thoracic Cage
Kyphoscoliosis
Pickwickian syndrome
Pleural fibrosis
Neuromuscular disorders
Idiopathic hypoventilation

cross-sectional area of the pulmonary vascular bed without destruction of the vessels. Hypoxia, acidosis, and hypercapnia directly cause pulmonary vasoconstriction. Hypoxia also acts indirectly by leading to polycythemia. In turn, the latter results in hyperviscosity of the blood, an effect that increases pulmonary vascular resistance. Persons living at very high altitude, for instance, natives of the South American Andes mountain range, often develop cor pulmonary secondary to the effects of chronic hypoxemia.

☐ **Pathology:** Chronic cor pulmonale is characterized by conspicuous hypertrophy of the right ventricle (Fig. 11-28), which measures more than 1.0 cm in thickness (normal range, 0.3 to 0.5 cm). Hypertrophy of the trabeculae carneae and papillary muscles is also readily evident.

ACQUIRED VALVULAR AND ENDOCARDIAL DISEASES

A variety of inflammatory, infectious, and degenerative diseases damage the cardiac valves and impair their function. The valves normally consist of thin flexible membranes, which close tightly to prevent backward blood flow. When the valves become damaged, the leaflets or cusps may be so thickened as to narrow the aperture and result in obstruction to blood flow, a condition termed **valvular stenosis**. Diseases that destroy valve tissue also may allow retrograde blood flow, termed **valvular regurgitation or insufficiency**. In many instances, diseases involving the cardiac valves produce both stenosis and insufficiency, but generally one or the other predominates.

Stenosis of a cardiac valve results in hypertrophy of the myocardium proximal (in terms of blood flow) to the obstruction. **Pressure overload** eventually causes myocardial failure and dilatation of the chamber proximal to the valve after compensatory mechanisms have been exhausted. Thus, mitral stenosis leads to left atrial hypertrophy and dilatation. As the left atrium decompensates and is no longer able to force the venous return through the stenotic mitral valve, signs of pulmonary congestion develop and are followed by right ventricular hypertrophy and even cor pulmonale. Similarly, aortic stenosis causes left ventricular hypertrophy and eventually left heart failure.

Valvular regurgitation or insufficiency also results in hypertrophy and dilatation of the cardiac chamber proximal to the valve, owing to **volume overload**. In aortic insufficiency, the left ventricle first hypertrophies and then dilates when it can no longer accommodate the regurgitant volume and provide adequate cardiac output. On the other hand, an incompetent mitral valve leads to hypertrophy and dilatation of both the left atrium and left ventricle, because both are subjected to volume overload. Marked left ventricular dilatation from any condition in which cardiac contractility is inadequate, for example, congestive failure after a large myocardial infarct, also may widen the mitral valve ring. This effect may be so severe that the valve leaflets cannot close properly, thereby causing mitral regurgitation.

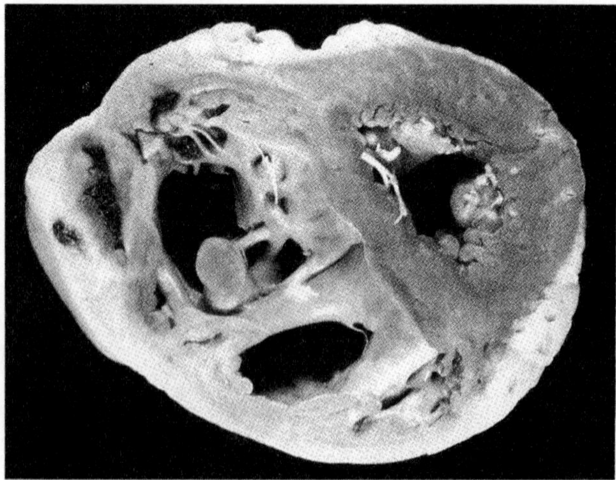

FIGURE 11-28
Cor pulmonale. A cross-section of the heart from a patient with severe pulmonary fibrosis and pulmonary hypertension shows a hypertrophied right ventricle. The right ventricular cavity is dilated in comparison with the much smaller cavity of the left ventricle.

Rheumatic Heart Disease

Rheumatic heart disease encompasses myocarditis during acute rheumatic fever and residual chronic valvular deformities.

Acute Rheumatic Fever

Rheumatic fever (RF) is a multisystem childhood disease that follows a streptococcal infection and is characterized by an inflammatory reaction involving the heart, joints, and central nervous system. A century ago, RF had an incidence of more than 100 per 100,000 population in the United States, compared with less than 2 per 100,000 at the present time.

☐ **Epidemiology:** RF is a complication of an acute streptococcal infection, almost always a pharyngitis (see Chapter 9). The offending agent is *Streptococcus pyogenes*, also known as group A, β-hemolytic *Streptococcus*. In some epidemics of streptococcal pharyngitis, the incidence of RF has been as high as 3%. RF is principally a disease of childhood, the median age being 9 to 11 years, although it can occur in adults. No differences in susceptibility related to sex, race, or ethnicity have been documented.

In the first half of the 20th century, RF reached almost epidemic proportions in the United States, but the incidence of this disease has decreased dramatically. In the period from 1950 to 1972, the death rate decreased from 14.5 to 6.8 per 100,000, and it has further decreased since that time. Although this decline may have been partly the result of widespread antibiotic treatment, such therapy cannot account for the entire decline, because the death rate had begun to decline well before antibiotics were generally available. It is probable that improved socioeconomic conditions, in particular less crowded living circumstances, contributed to the decrease. **Despite its declining importance in the industrialized countries, RF remains the leading cause of death of heart disease in persons between the ages of 5 and 25 years in less developed regions.**

☐ **Pathogenesis:** The pathogenesis of RF remains unclear, and with the exception of the link to streptococcal infection, no theory is generally accepted. Most hypotheses relate rheumatic carditis to immunological phenomena. Among other conjectures, it has been proposed that antibodies raised against streptococcal antigens cross-react with heart antigens, an observation that raises the possibility of an autoimmune etiology related to so-called molecular mimicry (Fig. 11-29).

Streptococcal antigens structurally similar to those in the heart include hyaluronate in the bacterial capsule, cell wall polysaccharides similar to the carbohydrate moiety of heart valve glycoproteins, and bacterial membrane antigens that share epitopes with sarcolemma and smooth muscle. Although antibodies to these antigens are found in patients with RF, it has not been proved that they are cytotoxic or that they are involved in the pathogenesis of the disease. It deserves emphasis that a direct toxic effect of some streptococcal product on the myocardium has not yet been excluded.

☐ **Pathology:** Acute rheumatic heart disease is a pancarditis, involving all three layers of the heart.

MYOCARDITIS: In severe cases of RF, the heart tends to be dilated, and a few patients die in the acute stage of the disease. At autopsy, the heart exhibits a nonspecific myocarditis, in which lymphocytes and macrophages predominate, although a few neutrophils and eosinophils may be evident. Fibrinoid degeneration of collagen, in which the fibers become swollen and eosinophilic, is characteristic.

The Aschoff body is the typical lesion of rheumatic myocarditis (Fig. 11-30), developing several weeks after the onset of symptoms. This structure initially consists of a perivascular focus of swollen eosinophilic collagen surrounded by lymphocytes, plasma cells, and macrophages. With time, the Aschoff body assumes a granulomatous appearance, with a central fibrinoid focus associated with a perimeter of lymphocytes, plasma cells, macrophages, and giant cells. Eventually, the Aschoff body is replaced by a nodule of scar tissue.

Anitschkow cells are unusual cells within the Aschoff body, whose nuclei contain a central band of chromatin. In cross-section, these nuclei have an "owl eye" appearance and when cut longitudinally, they resemble a caterpillar. Anitschkow cells may become multinucleated, in which case they are termed **Aschoff myocytes**.

PERICARDITIS: Tenacious irregular deposits of fibrin are found on both the visceral and parietal surfaces of the pericardium. These deposits resemble the shaggy surfaces of two slices of buttered bread that have been pulled apart ("bread-and-butter pericarditis"). The pericarditis may be recognized clinically by a friction rub, but it has little functional effect and ordinarily does not lead to constrictive pericarditis.

ENDOCARDITIS: During the acute stage of rheumatic carditis, an endocarditis involves mainly the mitral and aortic valves, which show a finely nodular "verrucous" appearance at the line of closure. Areas of focal collagen degeneration in the valve are surrounded by inflammation, and ulceration of the valve surface and the deposition of fibrin lead to the verrucous lesions.

☐ **Clinical Features:** There is no specific test for RF, and the clinical diagnosis of RF is made when two major—or one major and two minor—criteria (the Jones criteria) are met. If this diagnosis is supported by evidence of a recent streptococcal infection, the probability of RF is high.

The major criteria of acute RF include carditis (murmurs, cardiomegaly, pericarditis, and congestive heart failure), polyarthritis, chorea, erythema marginatum, and subcutaneous nodules.

The minor criteria are a previous history of RF, arthralgia, fever, certain laboratory tests indicative of an inflammatory process (e.g., increased sedimentation rate, positive test for C-reactive protein, leukocytosis), and electrocardiographic changes.

The symptoms of RF occur 2 to 3 weeks after an infection with *S. pyogenes*. By this time, the throat culture is usually negative. Increasing titers of serum antibodies to group A streptococcal antigens, such as antistreptolysin O, anti-DNAase B, and anti-hyaluronidase, provide concrete evidence that there has been a recent infection with group A *Streptococcus*. The acute symptoms of RF usually subside within 3 months, but in the presence of severe carditis, clinical activity may continue for 6 months or more. The mortality from acute rheumatic carditis is low, and the main cause of death is heart failure caused by myocarditis, although valvular dysfunction may also play a role.

Recurrent attacks of RF are associated with types of group A β-hemolytic streptococci to which the patient has not been previously exposed and, therefore, to which immunity has not developed. The rate of recurrence of RF is related to the elapsed interval between the initial episode and a subsequent streptococcal infection. In patients with a history of a recent attack of RF, the recurrence rate is as high as 65%, whereas after 10 years, a streptococcal infection is followed by an acute relapse in only 5%.

Prompt treatment of streptococcal pharyngitis with penicillin prevents an initial attack of RF and, less often, a recurrence of the disease. There is no specific treatment for acute RF, but corticosteroids and salicylates are helpful in the management of the symptoms.

Chronic Rheumatic Heart Disease

Severe valvular scarring may develop over a period of months or years after a single bout of acute RF. On the other hand, recurrent episodes of acute RF are common and result in repeated and progressively increasing

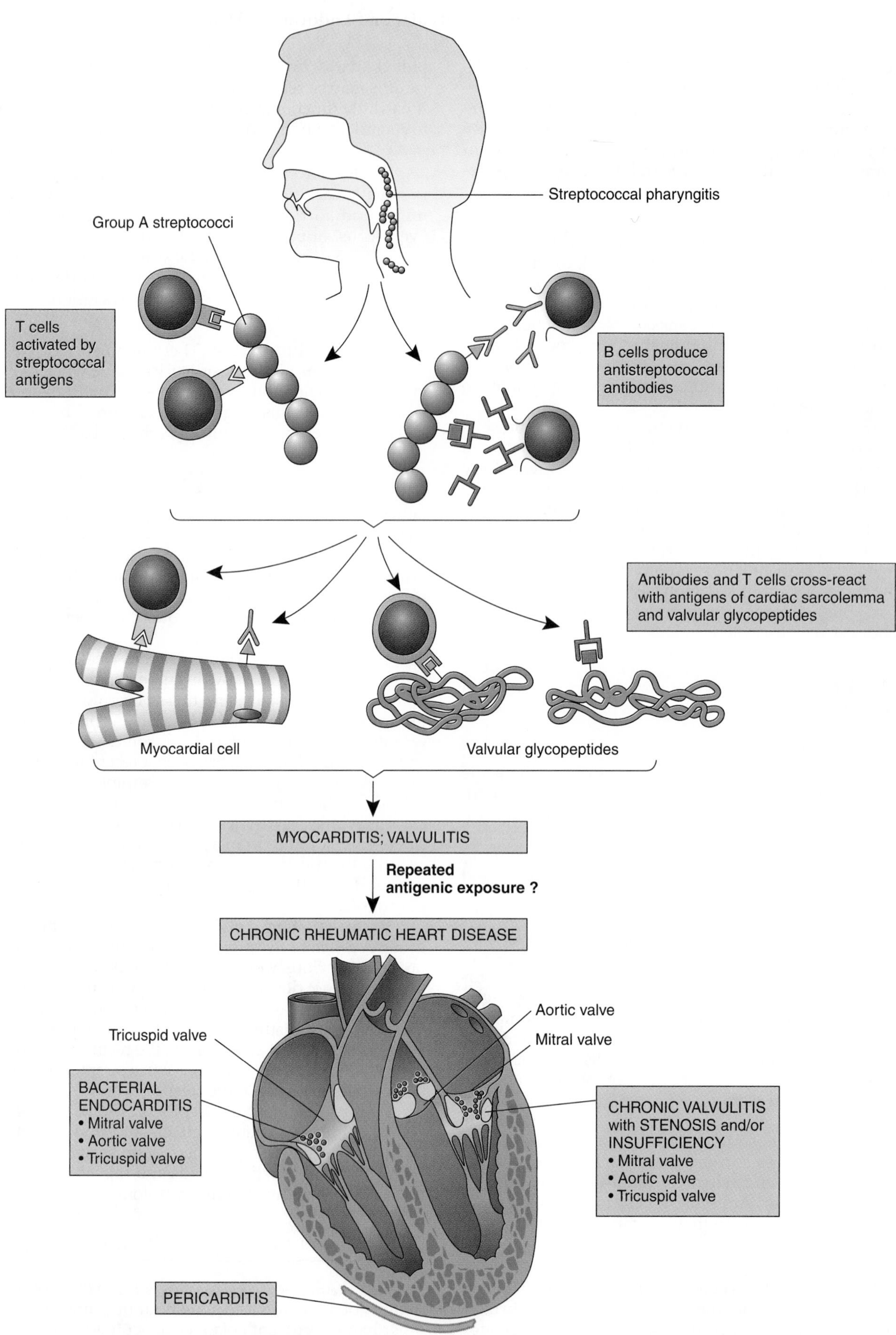
Streptococcal pharyngitis
Group A streptococci
T cells activated by streptococcal antigens
B cells produce antistreptococcal antibodies
Antibodies and T cells cross-react with antigens of cardiac sarcolemma and valvular glycopeptides
Myocardial cell
Valvular glycopeptides
MYOCARDITIS; VALVULITIS
Repeated antigenic exposure ?
CHRONIC RHEUMATIC HEART DISEASE
Aortic valve
Mitral valve
Tricuspid valve
BACTERIAL ENDOCARDITIS
• Mitral valve
• Aortic valve
• Tricuspid valve
CHRONIC VALVULITIS with STENOSIS and/or INSUFFICIENCY
• Mitral valve
• Aortic valve
• Tricuspid valve
PERICARDITIS

FIGURE ***11-29***

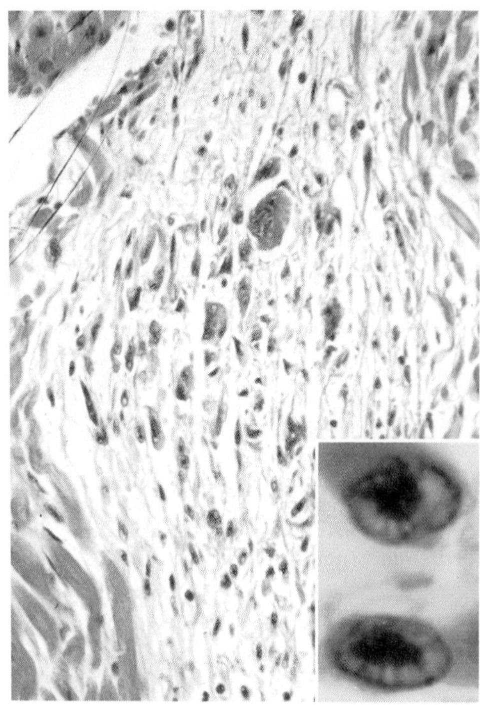

FIGURE 11-30
Acute rheumatic heart disease. A spindle-shaped Aschoff body is located interstitially in the myocardium. Collagen degeneration, lymphocytes, and a multinucleated giant cell (Aschoff myocytes) are noted. *(Inset)* Nuclei of Anitschkow myocytes, showing "owl-eyed" appearance in cross-section and "caterpillar" shape longitudinally.

damage to the heart valves. **The mitral valve is the most commonly and severely affected valve in chronic rheumatic disease.** Chronic mitral valvulitis is characterized by conspicuous, irregular thickening and calcification of the leaflets, often with fusion of the commissures and the chordae tendineae (Fig. 11-31). As a result, the valve cannot close properly, and mitral regurgitation results. Varying degrees of mitral stenosis may also be present and when severe may be the predominant functional lesion. When viewed from the atrial aspect, a severely stenotic mitral valve has a narrowed orifice that has the appearance of a "fish mouth" (Fig. 11-32). A focus of rough, wrinkled endocardium in the posterior aspect of the left atrium, referred to as **MacCallum patch**, may be present and serve as a clue to previous rheumatic involvement.

The aortic valve is the second most commonly involved valve in rheumatic heart disease and shows fused commissures and pronounced thickening of the cusps. This valve often becomes calcified as the patient ages, resulting in stenosis and insufficiency, although either lesion may predominate. The tricuspid valve is deformed in 10% of patients with chronic rheumatic heart disease, virtually always in association with mitral and aortic lesions. The pulmonic valve is rarely affected.

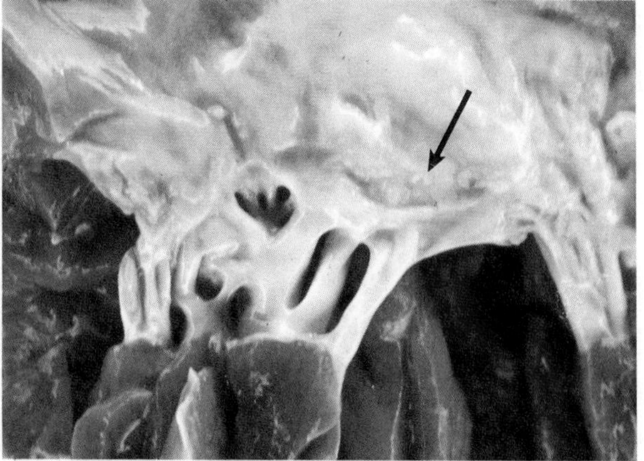

FIGURE 11-31
Chronic rheumatic valvulitis. The mitral valve leaflet is thickened and focally calcified *(arrow)*. The chordae tendineae are short, thick, and fused.

Complications of Chronic Rheumatic Heart Disease

- **Bacterial endocarditis** follows episodes of bacteremia, such as those that occur during dental procedures. The scarred valves of rheumatic heart disease provide an attractive environment for bacteria that would ordinarily bypass a normal valve.
- **Mural thrombi** form in the atrial or ventricular chambers in 40% of patients with rheumatic valvular disease. They give rise to thromboemboli, which produce infarcts in various organs. Rarely, a large thrombus in the left atrial appendage develops a stalk and acts as a ball valve that obstructs the mitral valve orifice.
- **Congestive heart failure** is associated with rheumatic disease of both the mitral and aortic valves.
- **Cor pulmonale** may develop as a result of secondary pulmonary hypertension.
- **Adhesive pericarditis** commonly follows the fibrinous pericarditis of the acute attack, but almost never results in constrictive pericarditis.

FIGURE 11-29
Biological factors in rheumatic heart disease. The upper portion illustrates the initiating β-hemolytic streptococcal infection of the throat, which introduces the streptococcal antigens into the body and may also activate cytotoxic T cells. These antigens lead to the production of antibodies to various antigenic components of the streptococcus, which can cross-react with certain cardiac antigens, including those from the myocyte sarcolemma and from the glycoproteins of the valves. This may be the mechanism for the production of the acute inflammation of the heart in acute rheumatic fever that involves all cardiac layers (endocarditis, myocarditis, and pericarditis). This inflammation becomes apparent after a latent period of 2 to 3 weeks. The insult may progress to chronic stenosis or insufficiency of the valves. These lesions involve the mitral, aortic, tricuspid, and pulmonary valves, in that order of frequency.

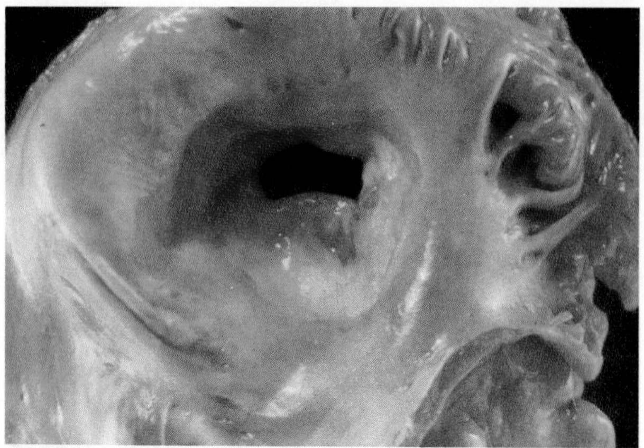

FIGURE 11-32
Chronic rheumatic valvulitis. A view of the mitral valve from the left atrium shows rigid, thickened, and fused leaflets with a narrow orifice, creating the characteristic "fish mouth" appearance of rheumatic mitral stenosis.

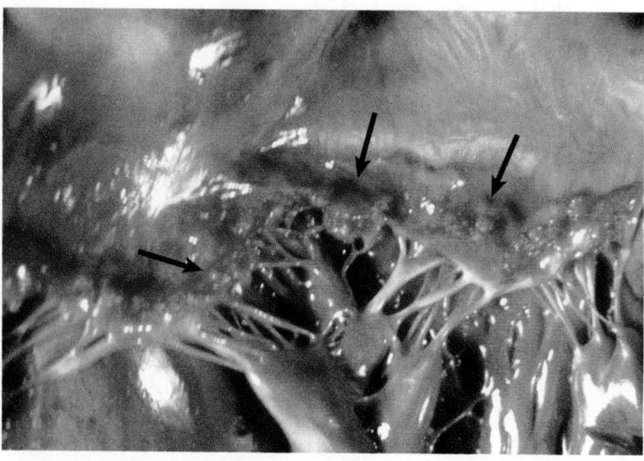

FIGURE 11-33
Libman–Sacks endocarditis. The heart of a patient who died of complications of systemic lupus erythematosus displays verrucous vegetations on the leaflets of the mitral valve.

The Heart in Collagen Vascular Diseases

Systemic Lupus Erythematosus

The heart is often involved in systemic lupus erythematosus (SLE), but the cardiac symptoms are usually less prominent than other manifestations of the disease. The most common cardiac lesion is a fibrinous pericarditis, usually with an effusion. Myocarditis in SLE, at least in the form of subclinical left ventricular dysfunction, is also common and reflects the severity of the disease in other organs. Microscopically, fibrinoid necrosis of small vessels and focal degeneration of interstitial tissue are seen.

Endocarditis is the most striking cardiac lesion of SLE. Verrucous vegetations, measuring up to 4 mm across, occur on the endocardial surfaces and are termed **Libman–Sacks endocarditis**. They are most common on the surfaces of the mitral valve (Fig. 11-33), characteristically the undersurface, close to the origin of the leaflets from the valve ring. Rare aortic valve involvement has been described, and the verrucae may extend onto the chordae tendineae and the papillary muscles. The lesions may contain **hematoxylin bodies** (basophilic nuclear fragments), but otherwise this lesion is indistinguishable from acute rheumatic mitral valvulitis. Libman–Sacks endocarditis ordinarily does not produce a functional deficit and heals without scarring.

Rheumatoid Arthritis

On rare occasions, the heart is involved in patients with rheumatoid arthritis. Characteristic rheumatoid granulomatous inflammation, with fibrinoid necrosis and palisaded lymphocytes and macrophages, may occur in the pericardium, myocardium, or valves. Involvement of the heart in rheumatoid arthritis does not compromise function.

Ankylosing Spondylitis

A characteristic aortic valve lesion develops in as many as 10% of patients with long-standing ankylosing spondylitis. The aortic valve ring is dilated, and the valve cusps are scarred and shortened. Focal inflammatory lesions occur in all layers of the aortic wall, particularly near the valve ring. The principal functional consequence is aortic regurgitation.

Scleroderma (Progressive Systemic Sclerosis)

Involvement of the heart in patients with scleroderma is second only to renal disease as a cause of death in this illness. The myocardium exhibits intimal sclerosis of small arteries, which leads to small infarctions and patchy fibrosis. As a result, congestive heart failure and arrhythmias are common. In fact, electrocardiographic studies have revealed some ventricular irritability in two thirds of patients with scleroderma and serious arrhythmias in one fourth. Cor pulmonale secondary to interstitial fibrosis of the lungs and hypertensive heart disease (caused by renal involvement) also are seen.

Polyarteritis Nodosa

The heart is involved in up to 75% of cases of polyarteritis nodosa. The necrotizing lesions of branches of the coronary arteries result in myocardial infarction, arrhythmias, or heart block. Cardiac hypertrophy and failure secondary to renal vascular hypertension often occur.

Bacterial Endocarditis

Bacterial endocarditis refers to colonization of the cardiac valves by bacteria. Fungi, chlamydia, and rickettsiae may also produce an infective endocarditis, but such cases are distinctly uncommon. Before the antibiotic era, bacterial endocarditis was untreatable and almost invariably fatal. The infection was classified according to its clinical

TABLE 11-6 Etiological Factors in Bacterial Endocarditis

	Children (%)		Adults (%)	
	Newborns	<15 years	15–60 years	>60 years
Underlying Disease				
Congenital heart disease	30	80	10	2
Rheumatic heart disease	—	5	25	8
Mitral valve prolapse	—	10	10	10
Valvular calcification	—	—	5	30
Intravenous drug abuse	—	—	15	10
Other	—	—	10	10
None	70	5	25	30
Microorganisms[a]				
Staphylococcus aureus	45	25	35	30
Coagulase-negative staphylococci	10	5	5	10
Streptococci	15	45	45	35
Enterococci	—	5	5	15
Gram-negative bacteria	10	5	5	5
Fungi	10	Rare	Rare	Rare
Negative culture	5	10	5	5

[a] About 5% of neonatal infections are polymicrobial.

course as either acute or subacute endocarditis (Table 11-6).

Acute endocarditis was described as an infection of a normal cardiac valve by suppurative organisms, typically *Staphylococcus aureus* and *S. pyogenes*. The affected valve was rapidly destroyed, and the patient died within 6 weeks in acute heart failure or of overwhelming infection.

Subacute endocarditis was a less fulminant disease in which less-virulent organisms, for example, *Staphylococcus viridans* or *Staphylococcus epidermidis*, colonized deformed valves, which had usually been damaged by rheumatic heart disease. In these cases, the patients typically survived for 6 months or more, and infectious complications were uncommon.

The introduction of antimicrobial therapy has changed the clinical patterns of bacterial endocarditis, and the classical presentations described earlier are today unusual. The disease is now classified according to the anatomical location and the offending organism.

☐ **Epidemiology:** The large majority of children with bacterial endocarditis have an underlying cardiac lesion. In the past, rheumatic heart disease accounted for a third of such cases. However, with the declining incidence of rheumatic fever, fewer than 10% of cases of bacterial endocarditis in children are today attributable to this disease. **The most common predisposing condition for bacterial endocarditis in children is now CHD.**

The epidemiology of bacterial endocarditis also has changed in adults. Whereas rheumatic heart disease accounted for as many as three fourths of the cases in the past, it now underlies only one fourth, and 25% to 50% have no predisposing cardiac lesion. **Mitral valve prolapse and CHD are today the most frequent basis for bacterial endocarditis in adults.**

Intravenous drug abusers inject pathogenic organisms along with their illicit drugs, and bacterial endocarditis is a notorious complication. In such patients, 80% have no underlying cardiac lesion, and the tricuspid valve is infected in fully half of the cases. The most common source of bacteria in intravenous drug abusers is the skin, with *S. aureus* causing more than half of the infections.

Prosthetic valves are the site of infection in 10% of all cases of endocarditis in adults, and up to 4% of patients with prosthetic valves have this complication. Staphylococci are again responsible for half of these infections, with most of the remainder being caused by gram-negative aerobic organisms, streptococci and enterococci, and fungi. Another iatrogenic form of endocarditis results from the bacterial colonization of indwelling vascular catheters.

Transient bacteremia from any procedure may lead to infective endocarditis. Examples include dental procedures, urinary catheterization, gastrointestinal endoscopy, and obstetric procedures. Antibiotic prophylaxis is recommended for such maneuvers if the physician has reason to believe that the patient is at increased risk for bacterial endocarditis (e.g., a history of rheumatic fever or the presence of a cardiac murmur).

The elderly also show an increasing trend to develop endocarditis independent of cardiac-valve replacement. A number of degenerative changes in the cardiac valves predispose to endocarditis, including calcific aortic stenosis and calcification of the mitral annulus. Diabetes and pregnancy also are associated with an increased incidence of bacterial endocarditis.

☐ **Pathogenesis:** Virulent organisms, such as *S. aureus*, can infect apparently normal valves, but the mechanism of such bacterial colonization is poorly understood. The pathogenesis of the infection of a damaged valve by less-virulent organisms has been related to (1) hemodynamic factors, (2) the formation of an initially sterile platelet and fibrin thrombus, and (3) the adherence properties of the microorganisms.

A high-velocity jet stream and a pressure gradient across a narrow orifice (valve or congenital defect) tend to denude endothelial surfaces, thereby allowing the deposition of platelets and fibrin. These small sterile vegetations are, in turn, hospitable sites for bacterial colonization and growth. In fact, in this protected environment, colony counts may indicate 10^{10} organisms per gram of tissue.

Factors that promote the adherence of bacteria to the sterile vegetations are believed to be important in the pathogenesis of endocarditis. Cell-associated and circulating fibronectin bind to surface molecules of the bacteria, thereby facilitating adhesion of fibrin, collagen, and cells. Some microorganisms produce extracellular polysaccharides, which also function as adhesion factors.

☐ **Pathology:** Bacterial endocarditis most commonly involves the mitral or aortic valve, or both. In rheumatic heart disease, the mitral valve is affected in more than 85% of cases of bacterial endocarditis, and the aortic valve is infected in 50%. Involvement of a single valve occurs more often in women (2:1) in the case of mitral valve disease, whereas the male-to-female ratio in isolated aortic endocarditis is 4:1. The most frequent congenital heart lesions that underlie bacterial endocarditis are PDA, tetralogy of Fallot, and ventricular septal defect. Bicuspid aortic valve is an increasingly recognized risk factor, especially in men older than 60 years.

The vegetations, composed of platelets, fibrin, cell debris, and masses of organisms, form on the valve surface at the point of closure of the leaflets or cusps (Fig. 11-34). The underlying valve is edematous and inflamed and may eventually be so damaged that it becomes insufficient. The lesions vary from a small superficial deposit to exuberant vegetations. The infective process may spread locally to involve the valve ring or the adjacent mural endocardium and chordae tendineae.

Infected thromboemboli travel to multiple systemic sites, causing infarcts or abscesses in many organs, including the brain, kidneys, intestine, and spleen.

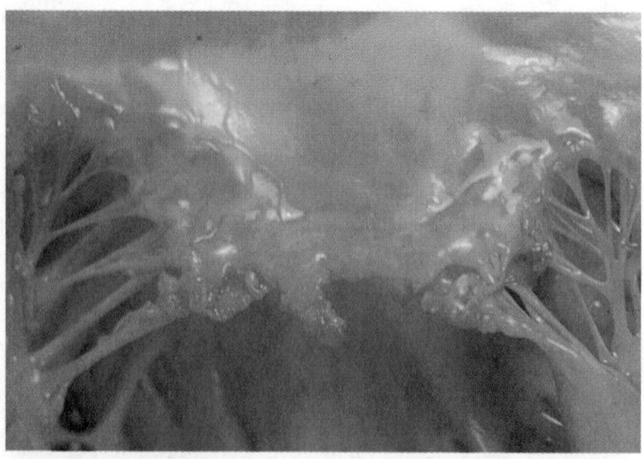

FIGURE *11-34*
Bacterial endocarditis. The mitral valve shows destructive vegetations, which have eroded through the free margins of the valve leaflets.

Focal embolic glomerulonephritis is another complication of infective endocarditis (see Chapter 16). The term embolic is a misnomer, because the disease is the result of immune-complex deposition in the glomeruli. The patchy hemorrhagic appearance of the kidneys at autopsy accounts for the term **flea-bitten kidneys**.

☐ **Clinical Features:** Many patients manifest the early symptoms of bacterial endocarditis within a week of the bacteremic episode, and almost all are symptomatic within 2 weeks. The disease begins with nonspecific symptoms of low-grade fever, fatigue, anorexia, and weight loss. Heart murmurs develop almost invariably, often with a changing pattern, during the course of the disease. In cases of more than 6 weeks' duration, splenomegaly, petechiae, and clubbing of the fingers are frequent. In a third of the patients, systemic emboli are recognized at some time during the illness, and pulmonary emboli are characteristic of tricuspid valve endocarditis in drug addicts. One third of the victims of bacterial endocarditis manifest some evidence of neurological dysfunction, owing to the frequency of embolization to the brain. Mycotic aneurysms of cerebral vessels, brain abscesses, and intracerebral bleeding are observed.

The most common serious complication of bacterial endocarditis is congestive heart failure, usually as a result of the destruction of a valve. Myocardial abscesses and infarction secondary to coronary artery emboli occasionally contribute to heart failure. Renal insufficiency may result from glomerulonephritis or embolic renal infarction.

Antibacterial therapy is effective in limiting the morbidity and mortality of bacterial endocarditis, and most patients defervesce within a week of instituting such therapy. However, the prognosis depends to some extent on the offending organism and the stage at which the infection is treated. **As many as 25% to 40% of cases of endocarditis caused by *S. aureus* are still fatal.** Cardiac surgery with valve replacement is necessary in some cases in which the bacteria have been eliminated, but in which structural damage remains.

Nonbacterial Thrombotic Endocarditis (Marantic Endocarditis)

Nonbacterial thrombotic endocarditis (NBTE) refers to the presence of sterile vegetations on apparently normal cardiac valves, almost always in association with cancer or some other wasting disease. NBTE affects the mitral (Fig. 11-35) and aortic valves equally and is similar in gross appearance to infective endocarditis. However, it does not destroy the affected valve, and on microscopic examination, neither inflammation nor microorganisms can be demonstrated.

The cause of NBTE is poorly understood, and it has been attributed to increased blood coagulability or immune-complex deposition. It is commonly a paraneoplastic condition, usually complicating adenocarcinomas (particularly of the pancreas and lung) and hematological malignancies. It may be part of the disseminated intravascular coagulation syndrome and also may accompany a variety of debilitating non-neoplastic diseases,

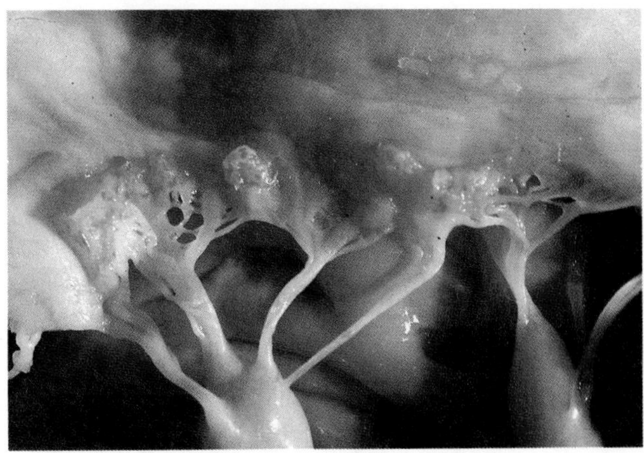

FIGURE 11-35
Marantic endocarditis. Sterile vegetations are seen on the leaflets of an apparently normal mitral valve.

hence the synonym "marantic endocarditis" (Gr., *marantikos*, "wasting away"). The principal danger posed by NBTE is embolization to distant organs, clinically manifested as infarcts of the brain, kidneys, spleen, intestines, or extremities.

Calcific Aortic Stenosis

Calcific aortic stenosis refers to a narrowing of the aortic valve lumen as a result of the deposition of calcium in the cusps and valve ring. It occurs in a number of situations.

- Calcific stenosis develops in elderly patients as a degenerative process involving a symmetric tricuspid aortic valve, which shows none of the stigmata of rheumatic disease, such as commissural fusion. Almost all patients (90%) older than 65 years with calcific aortic stenosis have no evidence of other valvular disease (see later).

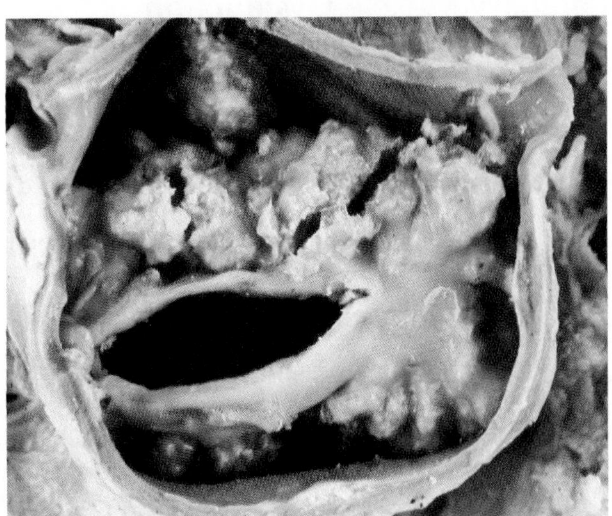

FIGURE 11-36
Calcific aortic stenosis of a congenitally bicuspid aortic semilunar valve.

- Calcification may develop in an aortic valve scarred as a result of rheumatic fever.
- A congenital bicuspid aortic valve often becomes calcified with age (Fig. 11-36).
- Severe atherosclerosis of the aorta (e.g., in familial hypercholesterolemia) may be associated with calcific aortic stenosis.

Isolated calcific aortic stenosis in both congenitally malformed valves and normal ones is thought to be caused by the cumulative effect of years of trauma, owing to turbulent blood flow around the valve. Dystrophic calcification produces nodules restricted to the base and lower half of the cusps, rarely involving the free margins. In the absence of rheumatic scarring, the commissures are not fused, and three distinct cusps are evident.

Severe aortic stenosis results in striking concentric left ventricular hypertrophy, with the heart achieving a weight as great as 1000 g (cor bovinum). Eventually, the heart dilates and fails. The disease is treated with great success (5-year survival rate of 85%) with surgical valve replacement, after which the hypertrophic left ventricle is restored to a normal size.

Calcification of the Mitral Valve Annulus

Calcification of the mitral valve annulus occurs commonly in the elderly and is usually without functional significance, although it often produces a murmur. However, if it is severe enough to interfere with closure of the mitral leaflets during systole, mitral regurgitation occurs. Calcification of the mitral valve annulus in the elderly differs from the calcification that occurs in rheumatic mitral valve disease in location and degree of deformation of the valve leaflets. In rheumatic mitral valve disease, the valve leaflets become thickened, particularly along their free edges. The commissures become fused, and the calcium deposits occur primarily in the valve leaflets. In calcification of the mitral valve annulus, there is little or no deformation of the valve leaflets, and the calcification is most prominent in the annulus. In contrast to rheumatic disease, degenerative calcification of the mitral valve annulus is more common in women than in men. About 40% of women older than 90 years exhibit this lesion, whereas in men, the incidence is only 15%. Calcification of the mitral valve annulus is aggravated by the presence of aortic stenosis, hypertension, and diabetes.

Calcific deposits transform the mitral ring into a rigid, curved bar up to 2 cm in diameter, which is evident radiologically. The posterior mitral leaflet is often distorted and displaced upward. Microscopically, amorphous masses of calcified material are first seen in the connective tissue of the valve ring. However, with time, the calcification extends into the base of the leaflets and eventually to the ventricular septum.

Mitral Valve Prolapse

Mitral valve prolapse (MVP) refers to a situation in which redundant mitral valve leaflets fail to approximate during systole, resulting in mitral regurgitation. This abnormality is caused

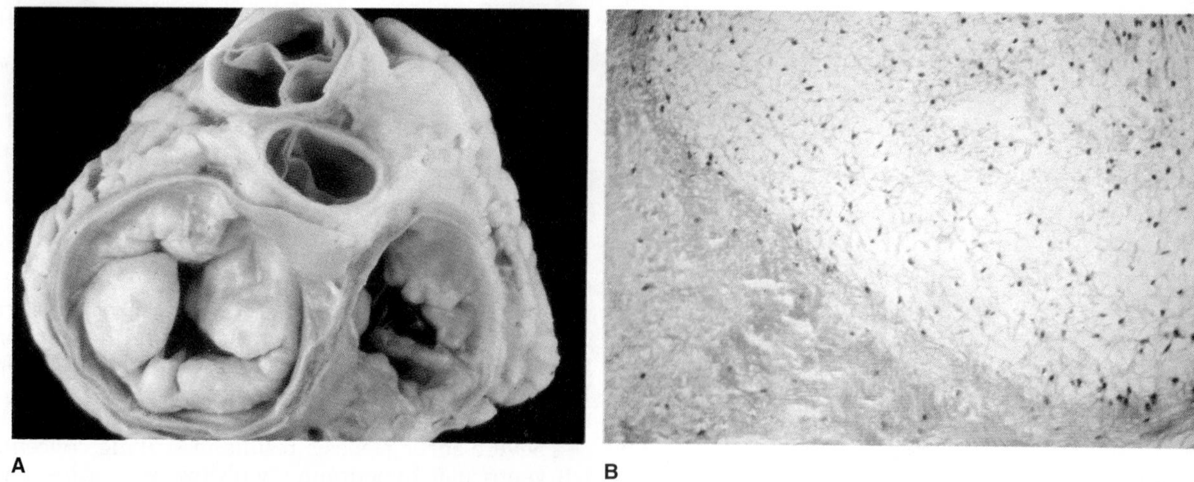

FIGURE 11-37
Mitral valve prolapse. ***(A)*** **A view of the mitral valve** ***(left)*** **from the left atrium shows redundant and deformed leaflets, which billow into the left atrial cavity.** ***(B)*** **A microscopic section of one of the mitral valve leaflets reveals conspicuous myxomatous connective tissue in the center of the leaflet.**

by a variety of conditions, all of which have in common excessive mobility of the mitral valve leaflets (Fig. 11-37A), which allows them to billow or prolapse into the left atrium during systole. The condition is one of the most prevalent cardiac abnormalities, affecting 5% to 10% of the adult population. In fact, MVP is today the most frequent cause of mitral regurgitation that requires surgical replacement of the valve.

☐ **Pathogenesis:** MVP has an important hereditary component, and many cases appear to be transmitted as an autosomal dominant trait. Patients with primary MVP exhibit a striking accumulation of myxomatous connective tissue in the center of the valve leaflet (see Fig. 11-37B). This abnormality is believed to be related to an as-yet-undefined defect in the metabolism of the extracellular matrix. The amount of proteoglycans in the mitral valve is increased, and by electron microscopy, the collagen fibrils are fragmented. MVP is usually an isolated finding, although it may occur in the context of a variety of other conditions, including Marfan syndrome, inherited disorders of collagen metabolism, and myotonic muscular dystrophy. It is also seen in association with hyperthyroidism, certain congenital heart lesions, and von Willebrand disease. There seems to be an unusually high incidence of MVP in persons with an asthenic habitus and a number of congenital thoracic deformities.

☐ **Pathology:** On gross examination, the mitral valve leaflets are redundant and deformed, and on cross-section, they have a gelatinous appearance. Myxomatous proliferation may involve not only the mitral valve leaflets but also the annulus and the chordae tendineae. Owing to these changes, mitral valve regurgitation may be aggravated by dilatation and calcification of the annulus and lengthening of the chordae. The damage to the chordae is often so severe that chordal rupture occurs, with a consequent flail valve that is totally incompetent. Myxomatous proliferation also has been described in the other cardiac valves, especially in patients with Marfan syndrome, 90% of whom have some clinical evidence of MVP.

☐ **Clinical Features:** The large majority of patients with MVP are entirely asymptomatic. Clinical recognition of the abnormality is based on the auscultatory findings of mid to late systolic clicks and a late systolic murmur if mitral regurgitation is significant. Endocarditis, both infective and nonbacterial, is sometimes a serious complication, and cerebral emboli are common. In 15% of patients with MVP, significant mitral regurgitation develops in 10 to 15 years and often requires mitral valve replacement.

Papillary Muscle Dysfunction

Dysfunction of the left ventricular papillary muscles is an important cause of acute mitral regurgitation and is most often caused by ischemia. The papillary muscles are especially vulnerable to ischemic injury because they are supplied by the terminal branches of the intramyocardial coronary arteries. Thus, any reduction in coronary blood flow may preferentially interfere with the function of the papillary muscles. Brief periods of ischemia (e.g., during episodes of angina pectoris) result in transient papillary muscle dysfunction and temporary mitral regurgitation. By contrast, severe, prolonged ischemia (e.g., after a myocardial infarction in the region of the papillary muscles) results in the scarring of these structures and permanent mitral regurgitation. In fact, one third of all patients being evaluated for coronary artery bypass surgery have some evidence of mitral regurgitation. Papillary muscle dysfunction also may be associated with a healed myocardial infarct, in which abnormal contractility of the myocardium at the base of the papillary muscle interferes with its function. Rarely, patients may die quickly of rupture of an acutely infarcted papillary muscle, which causes acute mitral regurgitation in an already compromised heart.

Carcinoid Heart Disease

Carcinoid heart disease refers to the changes in the right side of the heart in patients with carcinoid tumors that have metastasized to the liver. The cardiac lesions consist of deposits of pearly gray, uniform, fibrous tissue on the tricuspid (Fig. 11-38) and pulmonary valves and on the endocardial surface of the right ventricle. Microscopically, these patches appear "tacked on" to the endocardium and are without elastic fibers.

Carcinoid involvement of the endocardium can result in tricuspid insufficiency or stenosis and in pulmonary valve stenosis. It is thought that the endocardial lesions are caused by high concentrations of tumor-produced serotonin or other tumor products, which are metabolized in the lung. As a result, the carcinoid secretions affect almost exclusively the right side of the heart, whereas the left side tends to be spared.

PRIMARY MYOCARDIAL DISEASES

Primary myocardial diseases can be divided into inflammatory diseases (myocarditis), metabolic diseases, and cardiomyopathies. These disorders result in diffuse damage to individual cardiac myocytes and affect overall cardiac function.

Myocarditis

Myocarditis refers to generalized inflammation of the myocardium associated with necrosis and degeneration of myocytes. This definition specifically excludes ischemic heart disease. The true incidence of myocarditis is difficult to establish because many cases are asymptomatic. Myocarditis can occur at any age and is one of the few heart diseases that can produce acute heart failure in previously healthy adolescents or young adults. Although unusual, it can occur with the sudden onset of arrhythmias and even sudden cardiac death. Numerous infectious agents can cause myocarditis, as can hypersensitivity reactions and some toxic injuries.

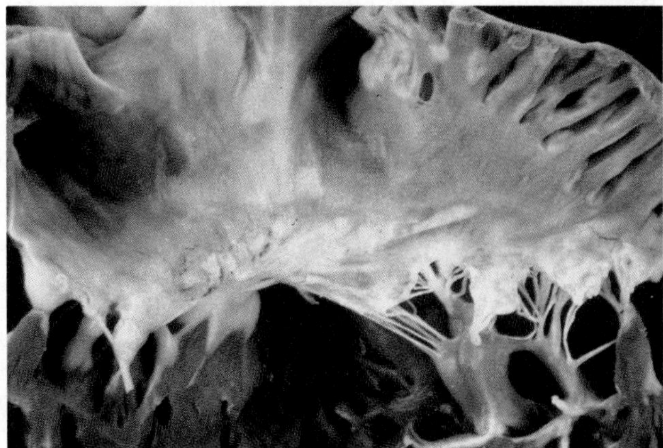

FIGURE 11-38
Carcinoid heart disease. Pearly white deposits are seen on the tricuspid valve leaflets and the adjacent endocardium.

Viral Myocarditis

Most cases of myocarditis in North America occur without a demonstrable etiology. The majority, however, are believed to be viral, although the evidence is largely circumstantial. A viral etiology is suggested by the histological similarity of human myocarditis to that produced experimentally by the inoculation of cardiotropic viruses into animals. Patients with a presumptive diagnosis of viral myocarditis may give a history of a recent upper respiratory tract viral syndrome, with a positive throat culture for a specific virus and increased serum antibody titers to the same agent. However, viruses usually cannot be cultured from the heart, even when endomyocardial biopsy or autopsy tissue is studied during the most active phase of the inflammatory process. Even in the case of a severely inflamed myocardium, electron microscopic study only rarely reveals viral particles. Viral genes have been detected by *in situ* hybridization or gene amplification by polymerase chain reaction (PCR) in some cases of myocarditis. The most common viruses that cause myocarditis are listed in Table 11-7.

☐ **Pathogenesis:** The pathogenesis of viral myocarditis is believed to involve direct viral cytotoxicity or cell-mediated immune reactions directed against infected myocytes. In animal models, the inoculation of a cardiotropic virus is followed shortly by replication of the organism in the myocardium. Microscopically, only small isolated foci of acute myocyte necrosis, with little if any inflammatory cell infiltration, are seen, and there is little evidence of functional impairment. Over the next few days, the virus can no longer be cultured from the blood,

TABLE 11-7 **Causes of Myocarditis**

Idiopathic

Infectious

- Viral: Coxsackievirus, echovirus, influenza virus, human immunodeficiency virus, and many others
- Rickettsial: Typhus, Rocky Mountain spotted fever
- Bacterial: Diphtheria, staphylococcal, streptococcal, meningococcal, and leptospiral infection
- Fungi and protozoan parasites: Chagas disease, toxoplasmosis, aspergillosis, cryptococcal, and candidal infection
- Metazoan parasites: *Echinococcus, Trichina*

Noninfectious

- Hypersensitivity and immunologically related diseases: Rheumatic fever, systemic lupus erythematosus, scleroderma, drug reaction (e.g., to penicillin or sulfonamide), and rheumatoid arthritis
- Radiation
- Miscellaneous: Sarcoidosis, uremia

and a few days later, virus can no longer be isolated from the heart. At the same time, mononuclear cells, principally T lymphocytes and macrophages, extensively infiltrate the myocardium. At the point of maximum inflammation, the animals show signs of heart failure, although viral cultures of both blood and myocardium are negative. This finding is consistent with the observation that patients with symptomatic myocarditis generally have negative viral cultures. In experimental viral myocarditis, it is clear that T lymphocytes cause much or all of the myocyte injury. The stimulus for the immune attack on the myocyte has not been established but appears to involve the major histocompatibility antigens. Animals depleted of T lymphocytes exhibit much less myocardial injury in response to the inoculation of a cardiotropic virus than do those with intact immune systems. Myocytes in biopsy specimens from patients with myocarditis exhibit a significant increase in the expression of major histocompatibility antigens.

□ **Pathology:** The hearts of symptomatic patients with myocarditis during the active inflammatory phase show biventricular dilatation and generalized hypokinesis of the myocardium. At autopsy, the heart of patients dying of acute illness is flabby and dilated, whereas chronic myocarditis is associated with myocardial hypertrophy. The histological changes of viral myocarditis vary with the clinical severity of the disease. Most cases show a patchy or a diffuse interstitial infiltrate composed principally of T lymphocytes and macrophages (Fig. 11-39). Multinucleated giant cells may be present in the predominantly mononuclear inflammatory cell infiltrate. The inflammatory cells often surround individual myocytes, and there is focal or patchy acute myocyte necrosis associated with the inflammatory cell infiltrate. In the early stages, necrosis and accumulation of interstitial proteinaceous material are prominent, whereas during the resolving phase, fibroblast proliferation and interstitial collagen deposition predominate. When necrosis is extensive, the histological features are similar to those seen in an infarct—a neutrophilic infiltrate being followed by organization and repair. Most viruses that cause myocarditis also cause pericarditis.

□ **Clinical Features:** The symptoms of viral myocarditis usually begin a few weeks after the infection. Despite extensive inflammation, most patients recover from acute myocarditis, although a few die of congestive heart failure or arrhythmias. The disease may be unusually severe in infants and in pregnant women. During the resolving phase of viral myocarditis, subtle functional impairment may persist for years, and progression to overt cardiomyopathy has been observed in a few cases. There is no specific treatment for viral myocarditis, and supportive measures are the rule.

MYOCARDITIS IN AIDS: Up to one half of all patients with acquired immunodeficiency syndrome (AIDS) have some clinical or pathological evidence of cardiac disease (pericardial effusions, myocarditis, endocarditis, or cardiomyopathy). Opportunistic infections account for many of these disorders, but a significant number are not associated with any other known cause and may represent infection of the heart with human immunodeficiency virus. Only a small minority of cases of AIDS-related heart disease are symptomatic.

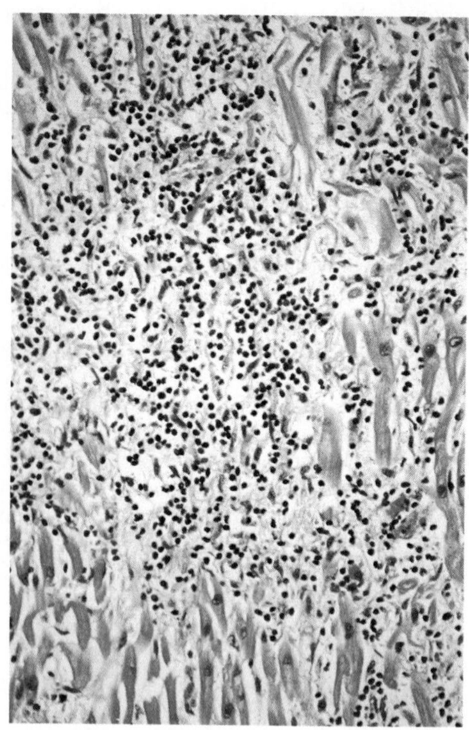

FIGURE *11-39*
Viral myocarditis. The myocardial fibers are disrupted by a prominent interstitial infiltrate of lymphocytes and macrophages.

Other Forms of Infectious Myocarditis

In addition to viruses, other infectious agents that gain access to the bloodstream can colonize the heart. For example, brucellosis, meningococcemia, and psittacosis are often associated with an infectious myocarditis. Moreover, some bacteria (e.g., diphtheria organisms) produce cardiotoxins, which may produce a fatal myocarditis. The most common cause of myocarditis in South America is infection with the protozoan *Trypanosoma cruzi*, the agent of Chagas disease (see Chapter 9).

Bacterial infection of the myocardium is characterized by multiple foci of a mixed inflammatory cell infiltrate, with neutrophils as the major component. Organisms can often be identified by special stains. Microabscesses can occur when septic emboli lodge in the coronary circulation, often as a consequence of infective endocarditis.

Rickettsial diseases commonly cause widespread vasculitis, which affects small coronary blood vessels.

Fungal colonization of the myocardium can occur in generalized fungal infections, particularly in immunocompromised patients.

Toxoplasmosis can involve the myocardium in immunosuppressed patients; the intracellular parasites proliferate within cardiac myocytes and elicit a focal mixed inflammatory response, with neutrophils and eosinophils.

Chagas disease likewise is associated with the proliferation of parasites within cardiac myocytes and a mixed inflammatory cell infiltrate, composed primarily of lymphocytes, plasma cells, and macrophages.

Hypersensitivity Myocarditis

Hypersensitivity reactions to drugs, such as methyldopa, certain antibiotics and sulfonamides, anticonvulsants, diuretics, and anti-inflammatory agents, can affect the heart. The hypersensitivity reaction is often confined to the myocardium and may not affect other organs. The composition of the inflammatory cell infiltrate in hypersensitivity myocarditis differs from that in infectious myocarditis, but the inflammation is otherwise similar. In hypersensitivity myocarditis, the inflammatory infiltrate is predominantly interstitial and perivascular and includes many eosinophils, as well as lymphocytes and plasma cells. The degree of myocyte necrosis is often slight in comparison with the intensity of the inflammation. Involvement of the conduction system is not infrequent and can be responsible for fatal ventricular arrhythmias.

Hypersensitivity myocarditis is often asymptomatic and is discovered only incidentally at autopsy. When the disease causes symptoms, treatment consists of discontinuation of the offending drug and the administration of corticosteroids or immunosuppressive agents.

Giant Cell Myocarditis

Giant cell myocarditis refers to an uncommon inflammatory disease of the heart, in which a granulomatous reaction, replete with multinucleated giant cells, accompanies necrosis of myocytes. The cause of the disorder is unknown, but it is sometimes encountered in association with systemic lupus erythematosus, hyperthyroidism, and thymoma. Although an autoimmune etiology has been suggested, no persuasive evidence for this theory has been presented.

Giant cell myocarditis is usually a rapidly fatal disease of adults in their third to fifth decades of life, and, aside from cardiac transplantation, there is no effective therapy. Patients die of congestive heart failure or sudden death from arrhythmias. At autopsy, the heart is flabby and dilated and may contain mural thrombi. Microscopically, prominent giant cells, together with lymphoid cells and macrophages, are seen at the margins of serpiginous areas of myocardial necrosis.

The only effective treatment for giant cell myocarditis is cardiac transplantation. However, the disease recurs in the transplanted heart in one fourth of the cases.

METABOLIC DISEASES OF THE HEART

Hyperthyroid Heart Disease

Hyperthyroidism causes conspicuous tachycardia and an increased cardiac workload, owing to decreased peripheral resistance and increased cardiac output. The disorder may eventually lead to angina pectoris and high-output failure. In addition to its multiple effects in the body, thyroid hormone has direct inotropic and chronotropic effects on the heart. Thyroid hormone (1) increases the activity of the sarcolemmal sodium pump, (2) enhances the synthesis of a myosin isoform with rapid ATPase activity, (3) reduces the production of a slower isoform, and (4) upregulates the expression of slow calcium channels in the sarcolemma, thereby facilitating contractility.

Hypothyroid Heart Disease

Patients with severe hypothyroidism (myxedema) have a decreased cardiac output, reduced heart rate, and impaired myocardial contractility, changes that are the reverse of those seen in hyperthyroidism. There may be a pericardial effusion, owing to increased capillary permeability and leakage of fluid and protein into the pericardial cavity. The pulse pressure is decreased because of increased peripheral resistance and decreased blood volume.

The hearts of patients with myxedema are flabby and dilated. The myocardium exhibits myofiber swelling, and basophilic (mucinous) degeneration is common. Interstitial fibrosis also may be present. Despite these changes, myxedema does not produce congestive heart failure in the absence of other cardiac disorders.

Thiamine Deficiency (Beriberi) Heart Disease

Beriberi heart disease has been seen in the Orient in patients who consume a diet inadequate in vitamin B_1 (thiamine) for at least 3 months (see Chapter 8). Persons who partake of foods composed largely of shelled rice and white bread are at particular risk. In the United States, thiamine deficiency is seen occasionally in alcoholic or neglected persons. Beriberi heart disease results in decreased peripheral vascular resistance and increased cardiac output, a combination similar to that produced by hyperthyroidism. The result is again high-output failure. Interestingly, heart failure may develop so suddenly that the patient dies within 2 days of the onset of symptoms. At autopsy, the heart is dilated and shows only nonspecific microscopic changes.

CARDIOMYOPATHY

Cardiomyopathy refers to primary disease of the myocardium and in this sense excludes myocardial disease caused by ischemia, hypertension, valvular dysfunction, congenital anomalies, or inflammatory disorders. The cardiomyopathies are divided into three categories: dilated (congestive), hypertrophic, and restrictive (infiltrative). Dilated cardiomyopathy (DCM) is the most common type of cardiomyopathy and is characterized by biventricular dilatation, impaired contractility, and eventually congestive heart failure. DCM can be secondary to a large number of cardiac insults, or it may be idiopathic (primary). In addition, inherited metabolic and structural disorders of skeletal muscle (e.g., mitochondrial myopathies or muscular dystrophies) also can result in cardiomyopathy.

Idiopathic Dilated Cardiomyopathy

Idiopathic DCM is a primary myocardial disease characterized by left ventricular or biventricular dilatation and impaired contractility.

☐ **Pathogenesis:** Numerous theories regarding the etiology of idiopathic DCM have been proposed, but none has been established.

Genetic factors now appear to be more important than previously believed. Among patients with idiopathic DCM, 20% have at least one first-degree relative with evidence of a similar heart disease. Although most familial cases seem to be transmitted as an autosomal dominant trait, autosomal recessive, X-linked recessive, and mitochondrial inheritance also have been described. In the case of X-linked idiopathic DCM, mutations at the Xp21 locus of the dystrophin gene (see Chapters 6 and 27) have been reported. There is an increased frequency of the DD genotype of angiotensin-converting enzyme (ACE) among patients with idiopathic DCM. In addition, certain human leukocyte antigen (HLA) class II antigens (DR4 and DQw4) are almost 3 times as common among patients with idiopathic DCM as in the general population.

Viral myocarditis has been suggested to precipitate an autoimmune attack on the myocardium that eventuates in DCM. However, this attractive hypothesis is weakened by the observation that only 15% of patients with known myocarditis evolve into DCM. Moreover, gene amplification by PCR has failed to detect viral genomic sequences. Thus viral myocarditis, at most, appears to be responsible for only few cases of idiopathic DCM.

Immunological abnormalities involving both cellular and humoral effects have been recognized in both myocarditis and idiopathic DCM. Autoantibodies to cardiac antigens that have been identified include those directed against a variety of mitochondrial antigens, cardiac myosin, and β-adrenergic receptors. However, as in many cases of autoimmune disease, a pathogenic role for immune mechanisms remains to be proved, and circulating autoantibodies may simply reflect long-standing myocardial injury.

☐ **Pathology:** The pathological changes in patients with DCM are for the most part similar whether the disorder is idiopathic or secondary. At autopsy, the heart is enlarged, owing to both hypertrophy and dilatation. The weight of the heart may be as much as tripled (900 g). All chambers of the heart are dilated, although the ventricles are more severely affected than the atria (Fig. 11-40). The myocardium is flabby and pale, and small subendocardial scars are occasionally evident. The endocardium of the left ventricle, especially at the apex, tends to be thickened, and adherent mural thrombi are often present in this area.

Microscopically, DCM is characterized by both atrophic and hypertrophic myocardial fibers. Interstitial and perivascular fibrosis of the myocardium is evident, especially in the subendocardial zone. Although scattered chronic inflammatory cells may be present, they are not prominent. By electron microscopy, myofilaments are decreased, and the number of mitochondria is increased.

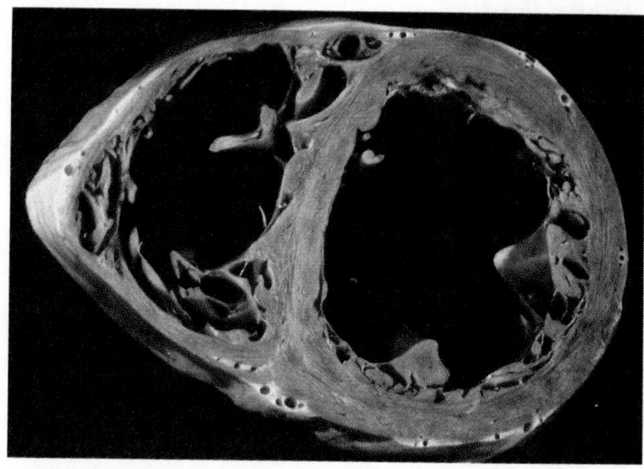

FIGURE *11-40*
Idiopathic dilated cardiomyopathy. A cross-section of the enlarged heart reveals conspicuous dilatation of both ventricles.

☐ **Clinical Features:** The clinical courses of idiopathic and secondary DCM are comparable. The disease begins insidiously with asymptomatic left ventricular dilatation. Commonly, exercise intolerance progresses relentlessly to frank congestive heart failure, and 75% of the patients die within 5 years. Although supportive treatment is useful, cardiac transplantation offers the only hope of cure. In fact, DCM is the principal indication for heart transplantation in adults and children.

Secondary Dilated Cardiomyopathy

Almost 100 distinct myocardial diseases can result in the clinical features of DCM. Thus secondary DCM is best viewed as a final common pathway for the effects of virtually any toxic, metabolic, or infectious disorder that causes widespread degenerative changes in the myocardium. In this context, alcohol abuse, hypertension, pregnancy, and viral myocarditis are thought to predispose to secondary DCM. Cigarette smoking also has been linked to an increased incidence of this disorder.

Toxic Cardiomyopathy

Numerous chemicals and drugs cause myocardial injury, but only a few of the more important chemicals that cause DCM are discussed here.

ETHANOL: Alcoholic cardiomyopathy is the single most common identifiable cause of DCM in the United States and Europe, probably accounting for more than half of all the cases. Ethanol abuse can lead to chronic, progressive cardiac dysfunction, which may be fatal. Both men and women alcoholics are equally susceptible to ethanol-induced cardiomyopathy, but the disorder is more common in men, because alcoholism is more frequent in men than in women. The typical patient is between 30 and 55 years of age and has been drinking heavily for at least 10 years.

The mechanism by which alcohol injures the heart remains obscure, but the degree of myocardial damage has been correlated with the total lifetime dose of ethanol. It is clear that ethanol exerts an immediate negative inotropic effect. However, the immediate action of alcohol on the cardiac myocyte is entirely reversible, and the reason for the conversion to irreversible cell injury after long-standing alcohol abuse is unknown. In the early stages of alcoholic cardiomyopathy, abstinence ameliorates or even reverses the disorder, but such behavior may be too late in advanced stages.

COBALT: Cobalt cardiomyopathy was originally misdiagnosed as alcoholic cardiomyopathy in the mid 1960s, because persons who drank large amounts of a certain type of beer developed DCM. It was subsequently shown that the cardiac manifestations were caused by cobalt that had been added as a foam stabilizer rather than by ethanol itself. Interestingly, cobalt cardiomyopathy has been reported almost exclusively in alcohol abusers rather than in moderate drinkers.

CATECHOLAMINES: In high concentrations, catecholamines can cause focal myocyte necrosis. Toxic myocarditis may occur in patients with pheochromocytomas, in persons who require inotropic drugs to maintain blood pressure, and in accident victims who sustain massive head trauma. The mechanisms of myocardial injury may involve platelet aggregation, increased intracellular calcium levels, focal ischemia, or the toxicity of catecholamine oxidation products.

ANTHRACYCLINES: Drugs such as doxorubicin (Adriamycin) and daunorubicin are potent chemotherapeutic agents whose usefulness is limited by a cumulative, dose-dependent cardiac toxicity. The major effect is a chronic, irreversible degeneration of cardiac myocytes, characterized pathologically by vacuolization and loss of myofibrils and functionally by depressed contractility. Myocyte necrosis is rare, but once severe degeneration occurs, intractable congestive heart failure develops, and the prognosis is grim.

Dilated cardiomyopathy begins to appear in patients who receive a cumulative dose of more than 500 mg doxorubicin per m^2, and those who are treated with more than 550 mg/m^2 have a 35% incidence of cardiomyopathy. The mechanism by which anthracyclines damage the heart is not understood.

CYCLOPHOSPHAMIDE: This potent chemotherapeutic drug is often used in high doses before bone marrow transplantation. Although it is not responsible for classical DCM, it can cause pericarditis and occasionally massive hemorrhagic myocarditis. The latter is believed to be due to endothelial injury and thrombocytopenia.

COCAINE: The use of this illicit drug is frequently associated with chest pain and palpitations. Although true DCM is not a usual complication of cocaine abuse, myocarditis, focal necrosis, and thickening of intramyocardial coronary arteries have been reported in some cases. A few instances of myocardial ischemia or infarction associated with cocaine use have been attributed to coronary vasoconstriction in the presence of an increased myocardial oxygen demand. Sudden death caused by ventricular arrhythmias has received a great deal of public attention. The mechanisms underlying these effects of cocaine are unclear; they include vasoconstriction, sympathomimetic activity, hypersensitivity responses, and direct toxicity.

Cardiomyopathy of Pregnancy

A unique form of DCM develops during the last trimester of pregnancy or during the first 6 months after delivery. The disorder is uncommon in the United States, but in some regions of Africa, it is encountered in as many as 1% of pregnant women. The risk for cardiomyopathy of pregnancy is greatest in black, multiparous women older than 30 years. The cause of this form of DCM is unknown, but there is increasing evidence of an underlying myocarditis in many patients.

Unlike most other varieties of DCM, half of the women with cardiomyopathy of pregnancy spontaneously recover normal cardiac function. The other half are left with persistent left ventricular dysfunction or proceed to congestive heart failure and early death. In patients who survive, subsequent pregnancies pose a high risk of recurrence and maternal mortality.

Hypertrophic Cardiomyopathy

Hypertrophic cardiomyopathy (HCM) refers to an uncommon condition in which cardiac hypertrophy is out of proportion to the hemodynamic load on the heart. The disorder is identified as a genetically transmitted autosomal trait in half of the patients, whereas the cause is unknown in the remainder. Moreover, one fourth of asymptomatic first-degree relatives of patients with HCM display morphological and echocardiographic changes similar to those of the fully developed disease. HCM is actually more frequent than previously appreciated, with a prevalence in the United States of about 1 in 500.

☐ **Pathogenesis:** Four separate disease loci have been identified in HCM, and it is suspected that there will be more, because not all families with HCM are linked to one of the known defects. The most common abnormalities, accounting for one third to one half of cases, are missense mutations in the cardiac β-myosin heavy chain gene on chromosome 14. Less commonly, missense or splice-site mutations in the cardiac troponin T gene on chromosome 1 (~15%) or in the β-tropomyosin gene on chromosome 15 (<5%) are responsible for the disease. More recently, mutations in the myosin-binding protein C gene on chromosome 11 have been identified, and another as-yet-unidentified locus appears to be on chromosome 7. Within each gene, a number of different mutations, usually missense, have been found and, despite similar clinical manifestations, specific mutations can be associated with differences in prognosis. Although troponin T mutations are associated with less hypertrophy than are those that involve the β-myosin heavy chain, the former have a high risk of sudden death and markedly reduced life expectancy. All of the defects involve sarcomeric proteins, and it is thought that changes in protein conformation may affect sarcomere assembly and turnover. Interestingly, the mutations in the β-myosin heavy chain are not located in the nucleotide sequences encoding myosin ATPase or the binding sites for actin and for myosin light chains. Perhaps mutations in these critical domains are lethal. It also appears that some sporadic cases of hypertrophic cardiomyopathy are due to *de novo* mutations in the same genes that are responsible for the familial form of the disease; in some cases, *de novo* mutations can be passed on to offspring.

☐ **Pathology:** The heart in HCM is always enlarged, with an average weight of about 500 g. The wall of the left ventricle is thick, and its cavity is small, sometimes being reduced to a slit. The papillary muscles and trabeculae carneae are prominent and encroach on the ventricular lumen. More than half of the cases exhibit asymmetric hypertrophy of the interventricular septum, with a ratio of the thickness of the septum to that of the left ventricular free wall greater than 1.5 (Fig. 11-41A). The hypertrophy is uniformly concentric (symmetric) in only 5% of the cases. Hypertrophy of the interventricular septum may also encroach on the right ventricular outflow tract. An endocardial mural plaque is often present in the left ventricular outflow tract, corresponding to the contact point where the anterior mitral valve leaflet impinges on the septal wall of the outflow tract during systole. Both atria are commonly dilated.

The most notable histological feature of HCM is myofiber disarray, which is most extensive in the interventricular septum. Instead of the usual parallel arrangement of myocytes into muscle bundles, myofiber disarray is characterized by an oblique and often perpendicular orientation of adjacent hypertrophic myocytes (see Fig. 11-41). By electron microscopy, the myofibrils and myofilaments within the individual myocytes also are disorganized. Myofiber and myofibrillar disarray is not entirely pathognomonic for HCM. These structures are frequently present in infants with congenital heart defects and can be observed under a wide variety of circumstances. However, they are always extensive in HCM and are not widespread in other situations.

☐ **Clinical Features:** Most patients with HCM have few if any symptoms, and the diagnosis is commonly made on the screening of the family of a patient with symptomatic HCM. Despite the absence of symptoms, such persons are at risk for sudden death, particu-

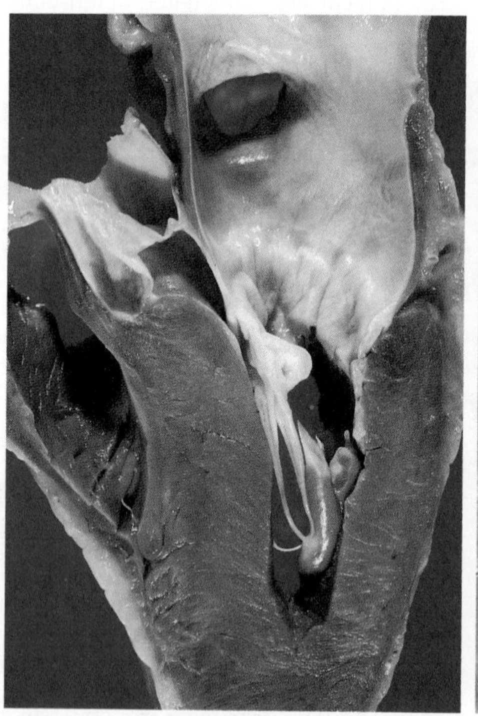

A

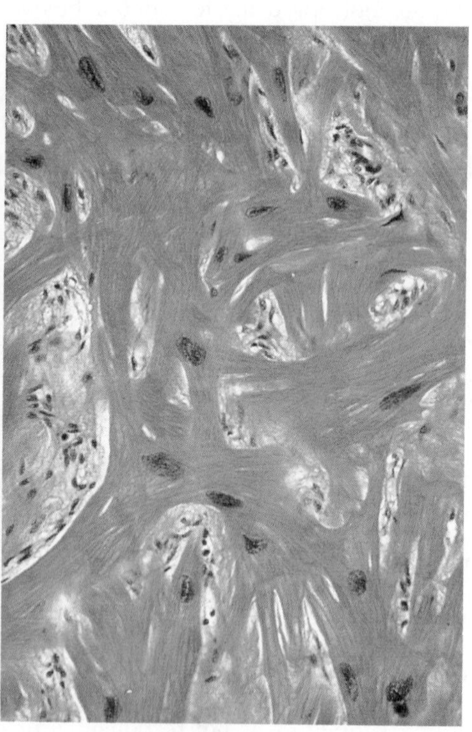

B

FIGURE *11-41*
Hypertrophic cardiomyopathy. ***(A)*** **The heart has been opened to show striking asymmetric left ventricular hypertrophy. The interventricular septum is thicker than the free wall of the left ventricle and impinges on the outflow tract.** ***(B)*** **A section of the myocardium shows myofiber disarray characterized by an oblique and often perpendicular orientation of adjacent hypertrophic myocytes.**

larly during severe exertion. In fact, unsuspected HCM is the most common abnormality found at autopsy in young competitive athletes who die suddenly. Clinical recognition of HCM can occur at any age, often in the third, fourth, or fifth decade of life, but the disorder also is encountered in the elderly.

Death is usually sudden and commonly precedes functional cardiac deterioration. However, some patients with HCM become incapacitated by cardiac symptoms, although the severity of the clinical disease and the risk of sudden death bear little relation to the degree of cardiac hypertrophy. Dyspnea, angina pectoris, and syncope are the most common symptoms. The clinical course tends to remain stable for many years, although eventually the disease can progress to congestive heart failure. In 10% of the patients, DCM supervenes.

The most prominent dysfunctional aspect of HCM is decreased left ventricular compliance (diastolic dysfunction), which results in increased end-diastolic pressure. In one fourth of the patients, functional obstruction of the left ventricular outflow tract occurs near the end of systole, resulting in a pressure gradient between the apex and the subvalvular region of the left ventricle.

Hypertrophic cardiomyopathy responds paradoxically to pharmacological interventions. Heart failure from other causes is typically treated with cardiac glycosides to increase myocardial contractility and with diuretics to reduce intravascular volume. By contrast, in HCM these drugs aggravate the symptoms. The most efficacious drugs for the treatment of HCM are β-adrenergic blockers and calcium channel blockers. These agents reduce contractility, decrease outflow-tract obstruction, and may improve left ventricular relaxation during diastole. Surgical removal of a portion of the hypertrophic septum has been successful in many patients.

Restrictive Cardiomyopathy

Restrictive cardiomyopathy refers to a group of diseases in which myocardial or endocardial abnormalities limit diastolic filling, while allowing contractile function to remain relatively normal. It is the least common category of cardiomyopathy in Western countries, although in some less developed regions (e.g., parts of equatorial Africa, South America, and Asia), endomyocardial disease (EMD) leads to many cases of restrictive cardiomyopathy.

Restrictive cardiomyopathy is caused by (1) interstitial infiltration of amyloid, metastatic carcinoma, or sarcoid granulomas; (2) EMD; (3) storage diseases, including hemochromatosis; and (4) a marked increase in interstitial fibrous tissue. The consequences of the impaired diastolic compliance are restricted ventricular filling, increased end-diastolic pressure, atrial dilatation, and venous congestion. In many respects, these hemodynamic changes are similar to the consequences of constrictive pericarditis. Although a variety of specific causes of restrictive cardiomyopathy have been identified, many cases are classified as idiopathic, with interstitial fibrosis as the only histological abnormality.

Restrictive cardiomyopathy almost invariably progresses to congestive heart failure, and only 10% of the patients survive for 10 years. There is no specific treatment for the condition.

Amyloidosis

The heart is affected in most of the generalized forms of amyloidosis (see Chapter 23). In fact, restrictive cardiomyopathy is the most common cause of death in the AL amyloidosis of plasma cell dyscrasias.

☐ **Pathology:** Amyloid infiltration of the heart results in cardiac enlargement without significant ventricular dilatation. The ventricular walls are thickened, firm, and rubbery. Microscopically, amyloid deposits are interstitial, perivascular, or endocardial (Fig. 11-42). Endocardial involvement is particularly common in the atria, where nodular endocardial deposits often impart a granular appearance to the endocardial surface. Amyloid deposits also can cause thickening of cardiac valves. In rare cases, amyloid deposition in the intramural coronary arteries narrows the lumina and causes ischemic injury.

☐ **Clinical Features:** Cardiac amyloidosis most often is seen as a restrictive cardiomyopathy, with symptoms predominantly referable to the right side of the heart, particularly peripheral edema. Infiltration of the conduction system can result in arrhythmias, and sudden

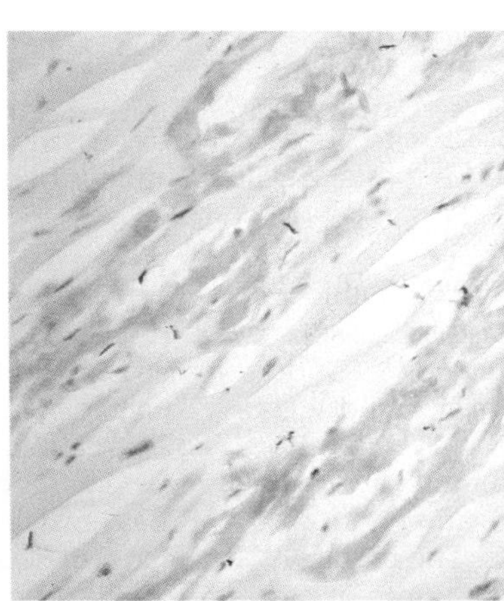

A

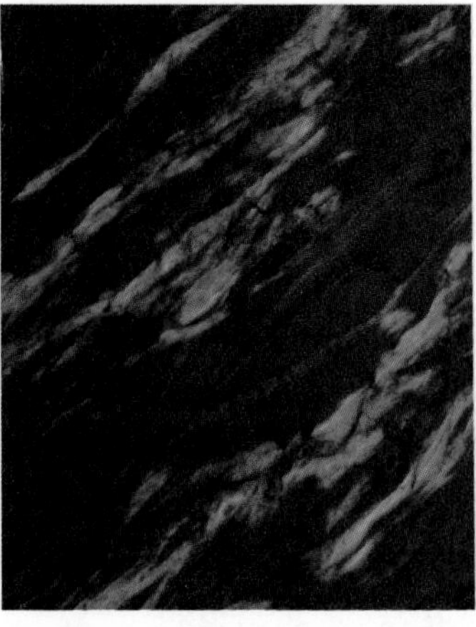

B

FIGURE *11-42*
Cardiac amyloidosis. A section of myocardium stained with Congo red *(A)* shows interstitial, pink-staining deposits of amyloid. Under polarized light *(B)*, the same section displays the characteristic green birefringence of amyloid fibrils.

cardiac death is not unusual. Cardiomegaly is characteristically prominent; echocardiography shows marked wall thickening and decreased wall motion.

Many patients with cardiac amyloidosis initially are seen with congestive heart failure secondary to impairment of systolic or contractile function. In these patients, the diastolic dysfunction is often inconspicuous. As in patients with a restrictive presentation, the prognosis is grim.

Senile Cardiac Amyloidosis

Senile cardiac amyloidosis refers to the deposition of a protein closely related to prealbumin (transthyretin) in the hearts of elderly persons (see Chapter 23). The disorder has been reported to be present in 25% of patients who are 80 years old or older. It not only involves the heart (atria and ventricles) but, in many cases, the lungs and rectum as well. Amyloid deposits also may be found in blood vessel walls in many organs, but virtually never in the renal glomeruli. The functional significance of senile cardiac amyloidosis is often minimal. Even when the amyloid deposition is extensive and is associated with symptoms of congestive heart failure, the progression of the disease is much slower than that in AL amyloidosis.

Two additional forms of isolated cardiovascular amyloidosis are common in the elderly: senile aortic amyloidosis and isolated atrial amyloidosis. Neither of these forms of amyloid contains prealbumin or closely related proteins.

Endomyocardial Disease

Endomyocardial disease comprises two geographically separate disorders.

ENDOMYOCARDIAL FIBROSIS: This disorder is particularly common in equatorial Africa, where it accounts for 10% to 20% of all deaths attributed to heart disease. The malady also is occasionally encountered in other tropical and subtropical regions of the world. It is most common is children and young adults but has been reported to occur up to age 70 years. Endomyocardial fibrosis leads to progressive myocardial failure and has a poor prognosis, although survival for as long as 12 years has been reported.

EOSINOPHILIC ENDOMYOCARDIAL DISEASE (LÖFFLER ENDOCARDITIS): This is a cardiac disorder of temperate regions characterized by hypereosinophilia. The disease is usually encountered in men in the fifth decade and is often accompanied by a rash. Peripheral eosinophil counts may attain levels as high as 50,000/μL. Löffler endocarditis typically progresses to congestive heart failure and death, although corticosteroids may improve the survival rate.

☐ **Pathogenesis:** Whereas endomyocardial fibrosis and Löffler endocarditis have in the past been considered to be distinct entities, there is a growing consensus that they represent variants of the same underlying disease. EMD is suspected to result from myocardial injury produced by eosinophils, possibly mediated by cardiotoxic constituents of the granules. In the tropics, transient high blood eosinophil counts often result from parasitic infestations, whereas in temperate climates, idiopathic hypereosinophilia is often persistent. In the latter case, it is much easier to document the relationship between the hypereosinophilia and endomyocardial injury. EMD can be divided into three stages.

1. The necrotic stage occurs within the first few months of the illness and is characterized by an intense eosinophilic infiltrate involving the inner layers of the myocardium, usually of both ventricles. The infiltrate is perivascular and interstitial, and there is evidence of vascular injury and myocyte necrosis. The necrotic stage lasts for several months, but significant functional impairment is infrequent. In Löffler endocarditis, the necrotic stage is often detected, but it is infrequently seen in endomyocardial fibrosis.
2. The thrombotic stage develops about a year later and features mural thrombi attached to the injured endocardium. At this time, the myocardium is no longer inflamed but shows early hypertrophy. The endocardium displays early thickening, and embolization is a common complication.
3. The fibrotic stage is the chronic phase of EMD and features conspicuous fibrotic thickening of the endocardium. Marked endocardial fibrosis results in decreased compliance and abnormal diastolic function. Adherence of the posterior mitral valve leaflet to the endocardium results in mitral regurgitation, or, in the case of the right side, in tricuspid regurgitation.

☐ **Pathology:** At autopsy, a grayish-white layer of thickened endocardium extends from the apex of the left ventricle over the posterior papillary muscles to the posterior leaflet of the mitral valve and a short distance into the left outflow tract. On cut section of the ventricle, endocardial fibrosis spreads into the inner one third to one half of the wall. Mural thrombi in various stages of organization may be present. When the right ventricle is involved, the entire cavity may exhibit endocardial thickening, which may penetrate as far as the epicardium. Microscopically, the fibrotic endocardium contains only a few elastic fibers. Myofibers trapped within the collagenous tissue display a variety of degenerative changes.

Storage Diseases

The various lysosomal storage diseases are discussed in detail in Chapter 6, and only the cardiac manifestations are reviewed here.

GLYCOGEN STORAGE DISEASES: Of the various forms of glycogen storage disease, types II (Pompe disease), III (Cori disease), and IV (Andersen disease) affect the heart. The most common and severe cardiac involvement occurs with type II glycogen storage disease. In infants with this condition, the heart is markedly enlarged (up to 7 times normal), and endocardial fibroelastosis is seen in 20% of patients. The myocytes are vacuolated as a result of the large amounts of stored glycogen. The functional changes are those of a restrictive type of cardiomyopathy, and the usual cause of death is cardiac failure.

MUCOPOLYSACCHARIDOSES: Several of the numerous mucopolysaccharidoses involve the heart. Cardiac disease results from the lysosomal accumulation of mucopolysaccharides (glycosaminoglycans) in various cells. In general, pseudohypertrophy of the ventricles develops, and contractility gradually diminishes. The coronary arteries may be narrowed by thickening of the intima and media, and in Hurler and Hunter syndromes, myocardial infarction is common. The valve leaflets may be thickened, thereby producing progressive valvular dysfunction, manifested as aortic stenosis (Scheie syndrome) or mitral regurgitation (Hurler and Morquio syndromes). Cor pulmonale may result from the pulmonary hypertension related to narrowing of the airways.

SPHINGOLIPIDOSES: **Fabry disease** may result in the accumulation of glycosphingolipids in the heart, with functional and pathological changes similar to those that complicate the mucopolysaccharidoses. **Gaucher disease**, which only rarely involves the heart, may feature interstitial infiltration of the left ventricle by cerebroside-laden macrophages, leading to impairment of left ventricular compliance and cardiac output.

HEMOCHROMATOSIS: This multiorgan disease is associated with excessive iron deposition in many tissues and is caused by a genetic defect in iron metabolism (see Chapter 14). The degree of iron deposition in the heart is variable and only roughly correlates with that in other organs. Involvement of the heart creates features of both dilated and restrictive cardiomyopathy, with systolic and diastolic impairment. **Congestive heart failure occurs in as many as one third of patients with hemochromatosis.**

At autopsy, the heart is dilated, and the ventricular walls are thickened. The brown color seen on gross examination correlates with the deposition of iron in cardiac myocytes. Interstitial fibrosis is invariable, but its extent does not correlate well with the degree of iron accumulation. The severity of myocardial dysfunction seems to be proportional to the quantity of iron deposited.

Sarcoidosis

Sarcoidosis is a generalized granulomatous disease that can involve the heart (see Chapter 12). Whereas one fourth of sarcoidosis cases that come to autopsy show some granulomas in the heart, fewer than 5% of patients with this condition have clinical symptoms. Sarcoid heart disease is seen as a mixed pattern of dilated and restrictive cardiomyopathy. Sudden death from an arrhythmia is common, owing to involvement of the conducting system. In a few patients, myocardial disease is severe enough to result in a ventricular aneurysm. Microscopic examination of the heart in severe cases of sarcoid heart disease reveals infiltration of the myocardium by noncaseating granulomas, destruction of myocytes, and replacement by interstitial fibrosis (Fig. 11-43).

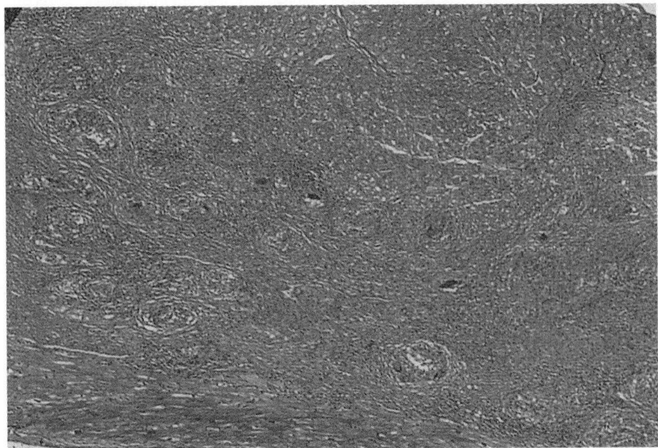

FIGURE *11-43*
Cardiac sarcoidosis. The myocardium is infiltrated by noncaseating granulomas, with prominent giant cells.

CARDIAC TUMORS

Primary cardiac tumors are rare, but when they occur, they can result in serious problems.

Cardiac Myxoma

The most common primary tumor of the heart is myxoma, accounting for 35% to 50% of all primary cardiac tumors. The tumor is usually sporadic, but it is occasionally associated with familial autosomal dominant syndromes. Most myxomas (75%) arise in the left atrium, although they can occur in any cardiac chamber or on a valve. The tumor appears as a glistening, gelatinous, polypoid mass, usually 5 to 6 cm in diameter, with a short stalk (Fig. 11-44). Sometimes the tumor is sufficiently mobile as to obstruct the mitral valve orifice. Microscopically, cardiac myxoma has a loose myxoid matrix containing abundant proteoglycans. Polygonal, stellate cells are found within the matrix, occurring singly or in small clusters.

More than half of the patients with left atrial myxoma have clinical evidence of mitral valve dysfunction. One third of those with a myxoma of the left atrium or left ventricle die of embolization of the tumor to the brain. Surgical removal of the tumor is successful in most cases.

Rhabdomyoma

This tumor is the most common primary cardiac tumor in infants and children and forms nodular masses in the myocardium. There is reason to believe that cardiac rhabdomyoma may actually be a hamartoma rather than a true neoplasm, although the issue is still debated. Almost all rhabdomyomas are multiple and involve both the left and right ventricles and, in one third of the cases, the atria as well. In half of the cases, the tumor mass projects into the cardiac chamber and obstructs the lumen or the valve orifices.

On gross examination, cardiac rhabdomyomas are

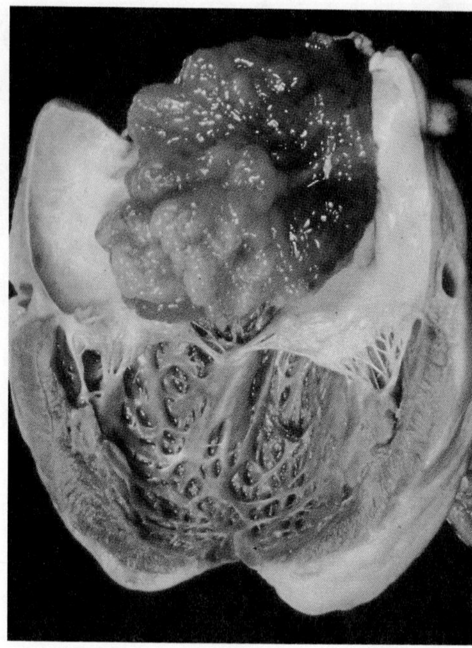

FIGURE 11-44
Cardiac myxoma. The left atrium contains a large, polypoid tumor, which protrudes into the mitral valve orifice.

pale masses varying from 1 mm to several centimeters in diameter. Microscopically, the cells show small central nuclei and abundant glycogen-containing, clear cytoplasm in which fibrillar processes radiate to the margin of the cell ("spider cell"). Rhabdomyomas often occur in association with tuberous sclerosis (one third to one half of the cases). A few cardiac rhabdomyomas have been successfully excised.

Papillary Fibroelastoma

Papillary fronds, measuring up to 3 to 4 cm in diameter, may grow on the heart valves. These tumors are not neoplasms and are more appropriately termed hamartomas.

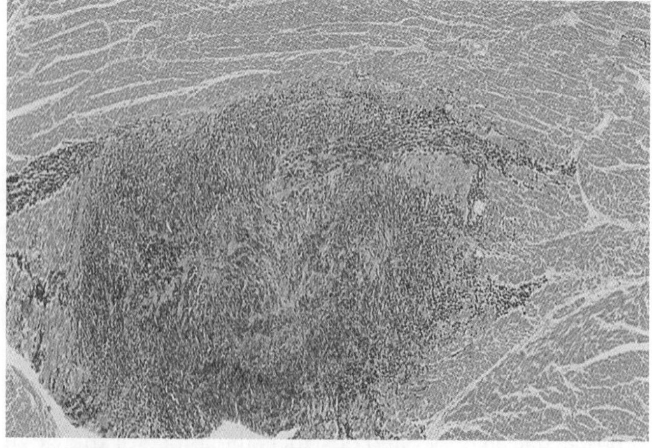

FIGURE 11-45
Malignant melanoma metastatic to the heart. The myocardium contains a heavily pigmented tumor.

The fronds have a central dense core of collagen and elastic fibers surrounded by looser connective tissue. They are covered by a continuation of the endothelial cells of the valve on which the tumor originates. In most instances, papillary fibroelastomas pose no clinical problem, but they have the potential to fragment and embolize to other organs, or they may occlude a coronary artery orifice and produce myocardial ischemia.

Other Tumors

Other primary tumors of the heart are even rarer than those described earlier. These include angiomas, fibromas, lymphangiomas, neurofibromas, and the sarcomatous counterparts of these tumors. Lipomatous hypertrophy of the interatrial septum and encapsulated lipomas have been reported.

Metastatic tumors of the heart derive from cancer of the lung, breast, and gastrointestinal tract. Lymphomas and leukemia also may involve the heart. For unknown reasons, many malignant melanomas metastasize to the heart (Fig. 11-45). Metastatic cancer of the myocardium can result in the manifestations of restrictive cardiomyopathy.

DISEASES OF THE PERICARDIUM

The pericardium serves a number of functions. It (1) maintains the heart in its normal anatomical orientation despite changes in body position, (2) prevents excessive friction between the heart and adjacent organs, (3) protects against the spread of intrathoracic infection to the heart, and (4) may subserve a circulatory function related to cardiac volume. Diseases of the pericardium, although they may cause chest pain, are most important for their effects on the heart.

Pericardial Effusion

Pericardial effusion refers to the accumulation of excess fluid, in the form of either a transudate or an exudate, within the pericardial cavity. The pericardial sac normally contains no more than 50 mL of lubricating fluid. If the pericardium is slowly distended, it can stretch to accommodate as much as 2 L of fluid without notable hemodynamic consequences. However, the rapid appearance of as little as 150 to 200 mL of pericardial fluid or blood may significantly increase intrapericardial pressure and thereby restrict diastolic filling.

Serous pericardial effusion is often a complication of an increase in extracellular fluid volume, as occurs in congestive heart failure or the nephrotic syndrome. The fluid has a low protein content and few cellular elements.

Chylous effusion (fluid containing chylomicrons) results from a communication of the thoracic duct with the pericardial space secondary to lymphatic obstruction by tumor or infection.

Serosanguineous pericardial effusion may be present after chest trauma, either accidental or after cardiopulmonary resuscitation.

Hemopericardium refers to bleeding directly into the pericardial cavity (Fig. 11-46). The most common cause is

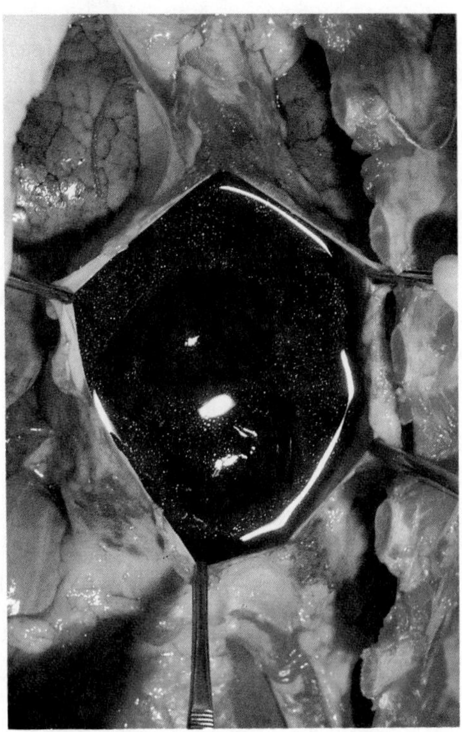

FIGURE 11-46
Hemopericardium. The parietal pericardium has been opened to reveal the pericardial cavity distended with fresh blood. The patient had sustained a rupture of a myocardial infarct.

rupture of a myocardial infarct, although penetrating cardiac trauma, dissecting aneurysm of the aorta, rupture of a vessel by infiltrating tumor, or a bleeding diathesis may be responsible.

Cardiac tamponade *is the syndrome produced by the rapid accumulation of pericardial fluid, which restricts the filling of the heart.* The hemodynamic consequences range from a minimally symptomatic condition to abrupt cardiovascular collapse and death. As the pericardial pressure increases, it reaches and then exceeds the central venous pressure, thereby limiting the return of blood to the heart. Cardiac output and blood pressure decrease, and **pulsus paradoxicus** (an abnormal decrease in systolic pressure with inspiration) occurs in almost all patients. Acute cardiac tamponade is almost invariably fatal, unless the pressure is relieved by removal of the pericardial fluid, either by needle pericardiocentesis or by a number of surgical procedures.

Acute Pericarditis

Pericarditis refers to inflammation of the visceral or parietal pericardium. The causes of pericarditis are similar to those for myocarditis (see Table 11-7). In most cases, the etiology of acute pericarditis is obscure and (as in myocarditis) is attributed to undiagnosed viral infection. At one time, pneumococcal pericarditis secondary to lobar pneumonia was not uncommon, but today all forms of bacterial pericarditis are unusual. Metastatic neoplasms also may induce a serofibrinous or hemorrhagic exudate and inflammatory reaction when they involve the pericardium. Pericarditis associated with myocardial infarction and rheumatic fever was discussed earlier.

Acute pericarditis can be classified according to its gross morphologic characteristics. For example, it can be described as being **fibrinous**, **purulent**, or **hemorrhagic**. Uremia is frequently the cause of a fibrinous pericarditis (Fig. 11-47). Viral infection also produces a fibrinous pericarditis, as do myocardial infarcts. Bacterial infection leads to a purulent pericarditis.

The initial manifestation of acute pericarditis is sudden, severe, substernal chest pain, sometimes referred to the back, shoulder, or neck. It is distinguished from the pain of angina pectoris or myocardial infarction by its failure to radiate down the left arm. A characteristic pericardial friction rub is easily heard. Electrocardiographic changes reflect repolarization abnormalities of the myocardium.

Idiopathic or viral pericarditis is a self-limited disorder, although it may infrequently lead to constrictive pericarditis. Corticosteroids are the treatment of choice. The therapy for other specific forms of acute pericarditis varies with the etiology.

Constrictive Pericarditis

Constrictive pericarditis is a chronic fibrosing disease of the pericardium that compresses the heart and restricts inflow. The condition is today infrequent, and in developed countries, it is predominantly idiopathic. Previous radiation therapy to the mediastinum and cardiac surgery account for more than one third of the cases, whereas in others, constrictive

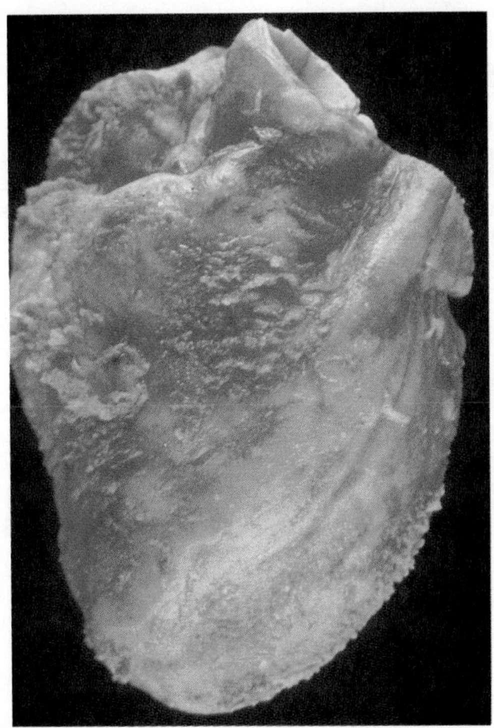

FIGURE 11-47
Fibrinous pericarditis. The heart of a patient who died in uremia displays a shaggy, fibrinous exudate covering the visceral pericardium.

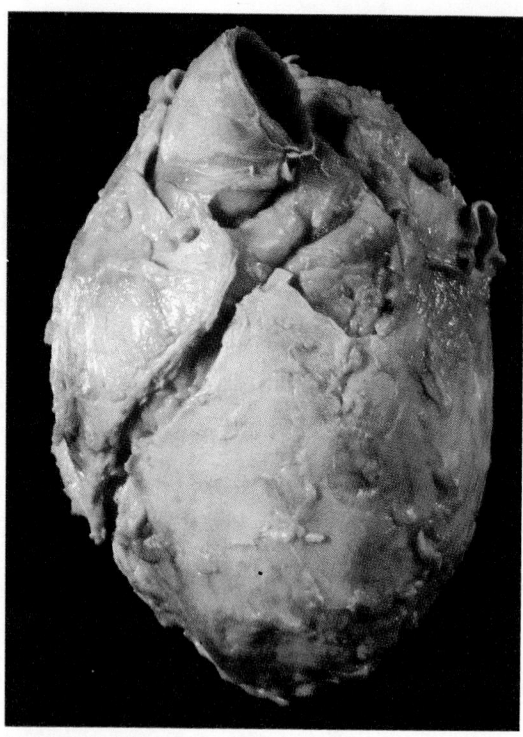

FIGURE 11-48
Constrictive pericarditis. The heart is encased in a fibrotic, thickened, and adherent pericardium.

pericarditis follows a purulent or tuberculous infection. Although tuberculosis today accounts for fewer than 15% of cases of constrictive pericarditis in persons in industrialized countries, it is still the major cause of this condition in underdeveloped regions.

The scarred pericardium may be so thick (up to 3 cm) that it obliterates the pericardial space and is seen as a rigid mass of fibrous tissue, which narrows the orifices of the venae cavae (Fig. 11-48). The fibrous envelope may contain deposits of calcium. Adhesive pericarditis is commonly an incidental finding at autopsy; it is the sequel of many different types of pericarditis that have healed and left only minor fibrous adhesions.

Patients with constrictive pericarditis have a small, quiet heart, in which venous inflow is restricted, and the rigid pericardium determines the diastolic volume of the heart. These patients have high venous pressure, low cardiac output, small pulse pressure, and fluid retention, with ascites and peripheral edema. Total pericardiectomy is the treatment of choice.

PATHOLOGY OF INTERVENTIONAL THERAPIES

Coronary Angioplasty

Percutaneous transluminal coronary angioplasty is used to dilate an artery narrowed by an atherosclerotic plaque. A balloon catheter is advanced through the stenotic segment, and its inflation fractures the plaque and stretches the underlying vessel wall. Major complications of PTCA occur in up to 10% of patients. In some cases, blood dissects into the media, thereby compressing the lumen and obstructing the vessel. Moreover, the initial luminal expansion may be followed by thrombus formation, owing to endothelial damage and the exposure of thrombogenic plaque elements. Perforation of an artery is a rare occurrence.

In addition to acute complications, progressive re-stenosis can occur, usually developing within 4 to 6 months. This complication is the result of a repair process of the arterial wall, which results in variable amounts of intimal hyperplasia. The extent of re-stenosis appears to be inversely proportional to the rate of blood flow; intimal hyperplasia is less marked in arteries with high rates of blood flow after angioplasty than in arteries that exhibit distal stenosis and poor blood flow.

Coronary Bypass Grafts

Coronary bypass grafting, by using either a saphenous vein or the left internal mammary artery, is a commonly performed procedure for the treatment of proximal coronary stenosis. Although the operative mortality is low and early symptomatic relief occurs in most patients, improvement in myocardial perfusion can be transient, owing to several complications in the grafts. These include (1) early thrombosis, (2) intimal hyperplasia, and (3) atherosclerosis of vein grafts. Moreover, progressive atherosclerosis of the native coronary arteries is not affected by the grafting procedure.

Internal mammary artery grafts develop fewer pathological changes than vein grafts, an effect that is most likely due to multiple factors. The excised saphenous veins segments used as grafts have a period of ischemia before their anastomosis, which results in endothelial cell injury. A portion of the adventitia is stripped away, thereby disrupting the vasa vasorum. Once the vein is grafted and arterial blood begins to flow, the vein is exposed to blood pressures that are much greater than those in its previous location. Finally, the diameter of the vein, which is expanded by arterial blood pressure, is usually much greater than the diameter of the distal coronary artery at the graft anastomosis, a discrepancy that promotes blood stasis.

In the immediate postoperative period, these factors enhance the probability of thrombosis and probably play a role in the development of intimal hyperplasia during the months to years after surgery. Intimal hyperplasia is characterized by a concentric proliferation of smooth muscle cells and fibroblasts and the deposition of collagen in the intima of the vein. After several years, lipid deposition and atherosclerotic plaque formation can occur in the thickened intima of vein grafts, a process that is accelerated in patients with hyperlipidemia. Atherosclerosis is the most frequent cause of vein graft failure in patients who have had good graft function for several years after surgery.

Prosthetic Valves

In most patients with severe valve dysfunction, the best prospect for long-term symptomatic improvement is valve replacement. Operative mortality is low, especially for patients with good preoperative myocardial function. It is estimated that about half of all patients with prosthetic valves are free of complications after 10 years.

Heart-valve prostheses can be divided into two categories: those with tissue components and those that are entirely mechanical.

Tissue valves: The most commonly used tissue-valve prostheses are fabricated by using a mechanical frame, to which glutaraldehyde-fixed porcine aortic valve cusps or pieces of bovine pericardium are attached. These valves have good hemodynamic characteristics, cause little obstruction, and resist thromboembolic complications. The most common cause of valve failure with tissue-valve prostheses is tissue degeneration, with severe calcification of the prosthetic valve cusps. This complication affects virtually all porcine aortic valves within 5 years after implantation and is responsible for valve failure in 20% to 30% of patients within 10 years. The tissue-valve cusps can also become torn.

Mechanical valves: Mechanical prostheses include caged-ball valves, single tilting disk valves, and bileaflet tilting disk valves. The risk of thromboembolism with mechanical prostheses is high enough to require long-term anticoagulant therapy, whereas this complication is less frequent with tissue-valve prostheses. Failure of mechanical valves can occur because of the breakdown of mechanical components, but this is not significantly more frequent than failure due to paravalvular leaks, endocarditis, thrombosis, or tissue overgrowth. In some cases, fragments of valve material can break off and embolize to other organs.

Heart Transplantation

With the development of effective immunosuppressive regimens, cardiac transplantation has become an effective treatment for end-stage heart failure. Immediate graft failure can reflect injury sustained by the donor heart before it was excised or damage occurring during the lengthy period of cardioplegic arrest required to transport the donor heart to the transplant center. Donor hearts are often obtained from motor vehicle accident victims with severe head trauma. In this situation, there is often extreme lability of blood pressure and fluctuating endogenous catecholamine release, as well as possible exogenous catecholamine administration, all of which can produce myocyte injury.

In addition to generalized immediate contractile failure of the transplanted heart, isolated right ventricular failure can occur because of increased pulmonary vascular resistance in patients with chronic severe left ventricular failure. Typically, the right ventricle in the transplanted heart dilates in response to increased pulmonary vascular resistance, and a degree of tricuspid regurgitation may occur. However, the transplanted heart usually adapts, and pulmonary vascular resistance returns toward normal. Several days may be required for cardiac function to recover after transplantation.

Allograft rejection is the major life-threatening complication of cardiac transplantation.

Hyperacute rejection occurs on rare occasions in the presence of blood-group incompatibility or major histocompatibility differences. In these situations, preformed antibodies initiate vascular injury in the donor heart, with diffuse hemorrhage, edema, intracapillary fibrin–platelet thrombi, vascular necrosis, and infiltration of neutrophils.

Acute humoral rejection is another unusual form of allograft rejection, characterized by vascular deposition of immunoglobulin and complement, endothelial cell swelling, and edema. This form of rejection has a worse prognosis than does acute cellular rejection.

Acute cellular rejection is very common within the first month after transplantation, although it is rare within the first week. Mild cellular rejection begins as perivascular T-cell infiltration, which is generally focal and is not associated with acute myocyte necrosis. This reaction often resolves spontaneously and, therefore, does not necessitate a change in the immunosuppressive regimen.

Moderate cellular rejection is characterized by the extension of the perivascular T-cell infiltrate into adjacent interstitial spaces, where lymphocytes surround individual myocytes and expand the interstitium (Fig. 11-49). In this instance, focal acute myocyte necrosis is associated with a mononuclear interstitial inflammatory cell infiltrate. Moderate cellular rejection usually does not produce detectable functional impairment and tends to resolve within a few days to a week after treatment, with no residual functional changes and only small areas of fibrosis. However, additional immunosuppressive therapy is instituted because moderate cellular rejection can progress to severe rejection. The latter features vascular damage, widespread myocyte necrosis, neutrophil infiltration, interstitial hemorrhage, and functional impairment, which is difficult to reverse.

Significant cellular allograft rejection can occur without any symptoms, and necrotic myocytes cannot regenerate. It is, therefore, essential that routine monitoring be performed, especially during the early weeks after transplantation, to identify rejection at an early reversible stage. At present, the most reliable screening procedure is endomyocardial biopsy of the right side of the interventricular septum, performed by cardiac catheterization. Because cellular rejection is often focal, and endomyocardial

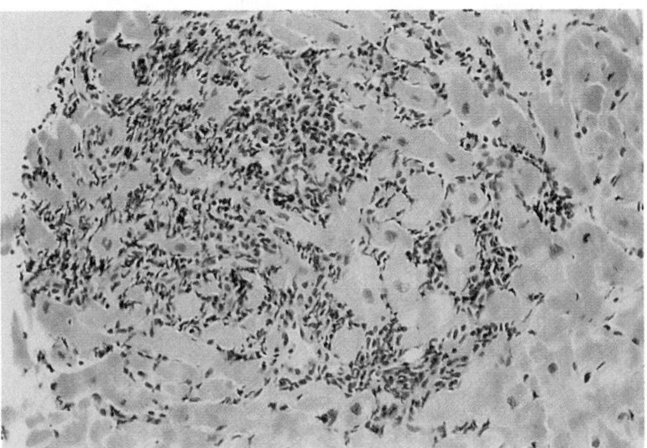

FIGURE *11-49*
Cardiac transplant rejection. An endomyocardial biopsy shows lymphocytes surrounding individual myocytes and expanding the interstitium.

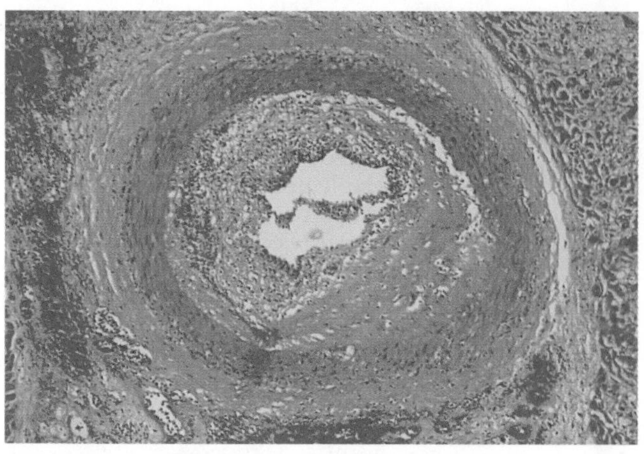

FIGURE *11-50*
Chronic cardiac transplant rejection. An intramyocardial branch of a coronary artery shows prominent intimal proliferation with narrowing of the lumen.

biopsy specimens are small, multiple biopsy samples are usually taken.

Accelerated coronary artery disease, which may represent a form of chronic humoral rejection, is the most common cause of death in heart transplant patients after the first year after transplantation. It affects the proximal and distal epicardial coronary arteries, the penetrating coronary artery branches, and even the arterioles. Microscopically, accelerated coronary artery disease is characterized by concentric intimal proliferation (Fig. 11-50). This process can lead to coronary occlusion and myocardial infarction, which is silent because the transplanted heart is denervated. Thus extensive myocardial damage can develop before the transplant patient is aware that ischemic injury has occurred.

SUGGESTED READING

BOOKS

Becker AE, Anderson RH: *Cardiac pathology.* New York: Raven Press, 1983.

Bloor CM: *Cardiac pathology.* Philadelphia: JB Lippincott, 1978.

Braunwald E (ed.): *Atlas of heart diseases. Heart failure: Cardiac function and dysfunction.* Vol 4. St. Louis: Mosby–Yearbook, 1995.

Braunwald E (ed.): *Heart disease,* 5th ed. Philadelphia: WB Saunders, 1997.

Fozzard HA, Haber E, Jennings RB, et al (eds.): *The heart and cardiovascular system: Scientificalave foundations.* New York: Raven Press, 1991.

Perloff JK: *The clinical recognition of congenital heart disease,* 4th ed. Philadelphia: WB Saunders, 1994.

Perloff JK, Child JS: *Congenital heart disease in adults.* Philadelphia: WB Saunders, 1991.

Schoen FJ: *Interventional and surgical cardiovascular pathology.* Philadelphia: WB Saunders, 1989.

Silver MD: *Cardiovascular pathology.* New York: Churchill Livingstone, 1983.

REVIEW ARTICLES

Aretz HT, Billingham ME, Edwards WD et al: Myocarditis. *Am J Cardiovasc Pathol* 1:3–14, 1987.

Dajani AS: Current status of non-suppurative complications of group A streptococci. *Pediatr Infect Dis J* 10:S25–S27, 1991.

Dare AJ, Veinot JP, Edwards WD, et al: New observations on the etiology of aortic valve disease. *Hum Pathol* 24:1330–1338, 1993.

Devereux RB: Recent developments in the diagnosis and management of mitral prolapse. *Curr Opin Cardiol* 10:107–116, 1995.

Dietz HC, Pyeritz RE: Molecular genetic approaches to the study of human cardiovascular disease. *Annu Rev Physiol* 56:763–796, 1994.

Hoffman JI: Congenital heart disease. *Pediatr Clin North Am* 37:25–43, 1990.

Jennings RB, Reimer KA, Steenbergen C: Myocardial ischemia revisited: The osmolar load, membrane damage, and reperfusion. *J Mol Cell Cardiol* 18:769–780, 1986.

Katz AM: The cardiomyopathy of overload: An unnatural growth response in the hypertrophied heart. *Ann Intern Med* 121:363–371, 1994.

Kelly DP, Strauss AW: Inherited cardiomyopathies. *N Engl J Med* 330:913–919, 1994.

Kushwaha SS, Fallon JT, Fuster V: Restrictive cardiomyopathy. *N Engl J Med* 336:267–276, 1997.

Roberts WC: Coronary thrombosis and fatal myocardial infarction. *Circulation* 49:1–3, 1974.

Stamler J: Epidemiology, established major risk factors, and the primary prevention of coronary heart disease. In: Chatterjee K, Cheitlin MP, Karlines J, et al, eds. *Cardiology: An illustrated text/reference.* Vol. 2. Philadelphia: JB Lippincott, 1991.

Watanakunakorn C, Burkert T: Infective endocarditis at a large community teaching hospital, 1980-1990: A review of 210 episodes. *Medicine (Baltimore)* 72:90–102, 1993.

CHAPTER 12

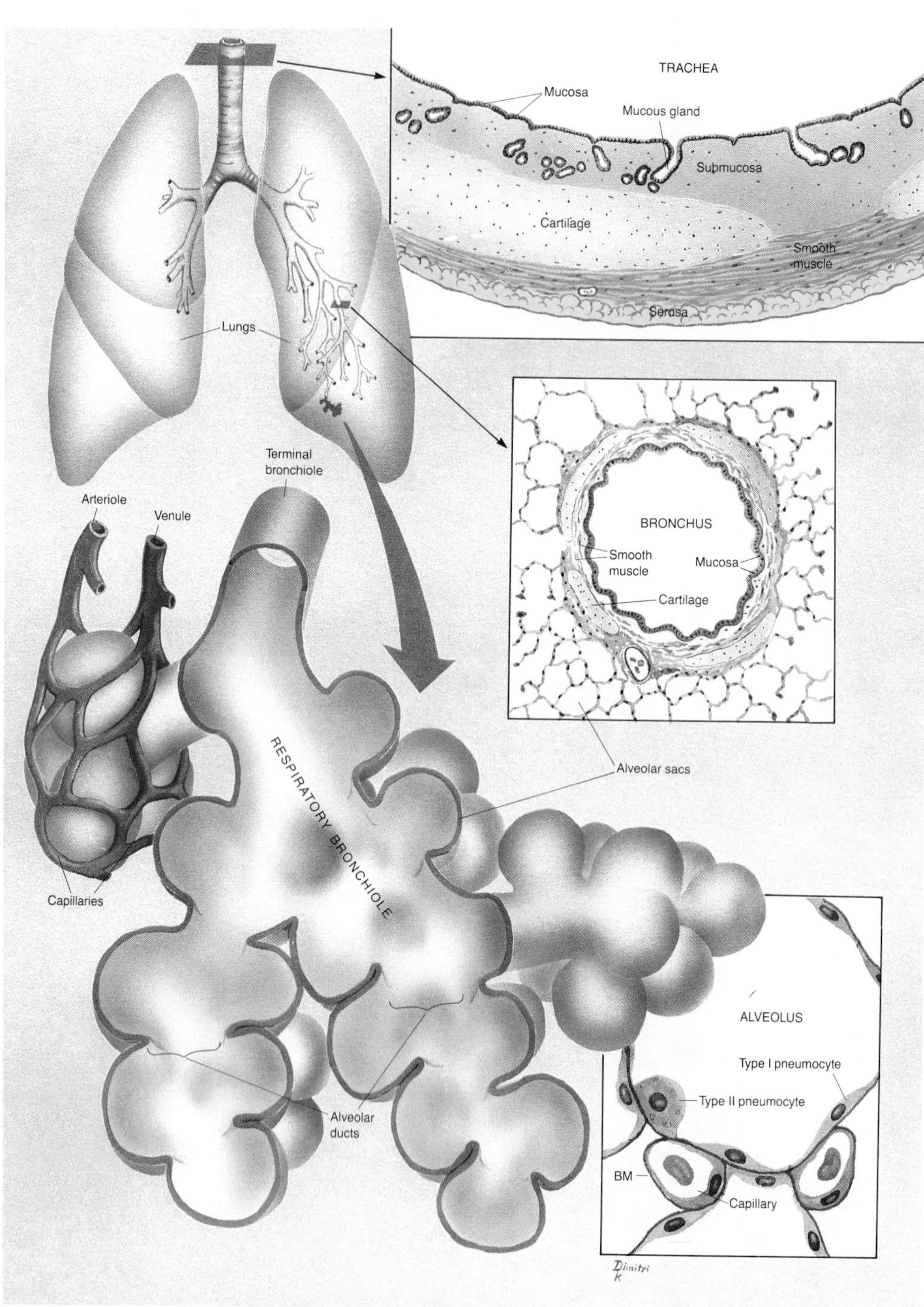

TRACHEA
Mucosa
Mucous gland
Submucosa
Cartilage
Smooth muscle
Serosa
Lungs
BRONCHUS
Smooth muscle
Mucosa
Cartilage
Terminal bronchiole
Arteriole
Venule
RESPIRATORY BRONCHIOLE
Alveolar sacs
Capillaries
ALVEOLUS
Type I pneumocyte
Type II pneumocyte
Alveolar ducts
BM
Capillary
Dimitri K

The Respiratory System

William D. Travis
John L. Farber
Emanuel Rubin

FIGURE *12-1 (see opposite page)*
Anatomy of the lung. The conducting structures of the lung include (1) the trachea, which has horseshoe-shaped cartilages; (2) the bronchi, which have plates of cartilage in their walls (both the trachea and bronchi have mucus-secreting glands in their walls); and (3) the bronchioles, which do not have cartilage in their walls and terminate in the terminal bronchioles. The gas-exchanging components compose the unit distal to the terminal bronchiole, namely, the acinus. Alveoli are lined by type I cells, which are large, flat cells that cover most of the alveolar wall, and by type II cells, which secrete surfactant and are the progenitor cells of the alveolar epithelium. Gas exchange occurs at the level of the alveolar wall.

EMBRYOLOGY

The respiratory system comprises the larynx, trachea, bronchi, bronchioles, and alveoli. During the fourth week of gestation, the laryngotracheal groove develops as a ventral outpouching of the foregut.

The embryonic period of lung development occurs between 4 and 6 weeks' gestation. During this period, the tracheobronchial bud divides to form the proximal airways complete to the segmental level.

The pseudoglandular period occupies weeks 6 to 16 of gestation, after which time the distal airways are formed up to the level of the terminal bronchioles.

The acinar or canalicular period encompasses weeks 17 to 28 of gestation. This is the time when (1) the framework of the gas-exchanging unit of the lung develops, (2) the acinus is formed, (3) the vascular system develops, (4) capillaries reach the epithelium, and (5) gas exchange becomes possible. It is at this point that extrauterine life becomes possible.

The saccular period extends from 28 to 34 weeks of gestation. The primary saccules become subdivided by secondary crests, a process that results in greater complexity of the gas-exchanging surface and thinning of air-space walls.

The alveolar period corresponds to 34 to 36 weeks of gestation and is the last step in lung development when alveoli begin developing. At birth, the number of alveoli is highly variable, ranging from 20 to 150 million. Most alveoli develop in the first 2 years of life.

ANATOMY

The Larynx

The larynx is attached to the most superior portion of the trachea and is specialized for the production of the voice. It is bounded above by the pharynx and oral cavity and below by the first tracheal ring. The supporting structures, or skeleton, of the larynx consist of four cartilaginous structures:

- **The epiglottic cartilage** is the most superior cartilage. In turn, the tip of the epiglottis is the most superior part of the larynx, projecting upward into the pharynx behind the base of the tongue.
- **The thyroid cartilage** is the largest laryngeal cartilage. It is located anteriorly and composed of bilateral plates, which are fused in the midline to form the laryngeal prominence ("Adam's apple").
- **The arytenoid cartilages** are paired triangular cartilages located posterolaterally at the level of the thyroid cartilage. The vocal cords are attached to the arytenoid cartilages, and their movement facilitates the vibration of the vocal cords.
- **The cricoid cartilage** is the most inferior laryngeal cartilage. Anteriorly, it is located between the inferior aspect of the thyroid cartilage and the first tracheal ring. Posteriorly, it is expanded upward to form a synovium-lined joint articulating with the arytenoid cartilages.
- **The epiglottis** forms the most superior aspect of the internal structure of the soft tissues of the larynx. Laterally and extending downward, the arytenoepiglottic folds separate the tubular larynx from the pyriform sinuses, which form part of the pharynx.

Midway between the epiglottis and the first tracheal ring are the ventricles, which are paired, groove-like outpouchings of the lumen of the larynx. The superior borders of the ventricles consist of the vestibular folds, or false cords, which have no important function in the production of voice. Immediately below the ventricles are the vocal folds, or true cords, which are responsible for speech. The **glottis** is composed of the false cords, ventricles, and true cords. The tissue above the false cords is termed the **supraglottis**, and the tissue below the true cords is called the **infraglottis**.

The superior aspect of the epiglottis, the arytenoepiglottic folds, and the true cords are lined by squamous mucosa. The remainder of the surface of the larynx is normally lined by ciliated respiratory mucosa. The submucosa throughout most of the larynx is composed of loose fibrous stroma and compound mucus-secreting glands, similar to those seen in the trachea and bronchi. The submucosa of the true cords is formed by skeletal muscle fibers from the thyroarytenoid muscle.

The Lung and Airways

TRACHEA AND BRONCHI: The trachea is a hollow tube measuring up to 25 cm in length and up to 2.5 cm in diameter. The right bronchus diverges at a lesser angle from the trachea than does the left, which is why foreign material is more frequently aspirated on the right side. On entering the lung, the bronchi divide into lobar bronchi and then into segmental bronchi, which supply the 19 segments of the lung. Because the segments are individual units with their own bronchovascular supply, they can be resected individually.

The tracheobronchial tree contains cartilage and submucosal mucous glands in the wall. The latter are compound tubular glands, which display both mucous cells (pale) and serous cells (granular, more basophilic). The tracheobronchial tree is lined by a pseudostratified epithelium, which appears as layers, although all cells reach the basement membrane. Most of the cells are ciliated, but mucus-secreting (goblet) cells also exist, as well as basal cells that do not reach the surface. The basal cells are thought to be precursor cells that differentiate to form the more specialized cells of the tracheobronchial epithelium. In addition, there are nonciliated columnar cells, or **Clara cells**, which accumulate and detoxify many inhaled toxic agents (e.g., nitrogen dioxide). Scattered in the tracheobronchial mucosa are **Kulchitsky cells**, which are neuroendocrine cells that contain a variety of hormonally active polypeptides and vasoactive amines.

BRONCHIOLES: Distal to the bronchi are bronchioles, which differ from the bronchi by the absence of cartilage and mucus-secreting glands. The epithelium of the bronchioles becomes thinner with progressive branchings, until only one cell layer is present. The last purely conducting structure free of alveoli is the terminal bronchiole, which has a circumferential layer of pseudostratified ciliated respiratory epithelium and a smooth muscle wall. Mucous cells gradually disappear from the lining of the bronchioles, until they are entirely replaced in the small bronchioles by the nonciliated, columnar Clara cells. The next branches of the airways are the **respiratory bronchioles**. The terminal bronchioles divide into the respiratory bronchioles, which merge into **alveolar ducts** and **alveoli**. The **acinus**, which is the unit of gas exchange in the lung, consists of respiratory bronchioles, alveolar ducts, and alveoli.

ALVEOLI: The alveoli are lined by two types of epithelium. **Type I cells cover 95% of the alveolar surface, although they compose only 40% of all the epithelial cells of the alveolus.** They are thin and have a large surface area, a combination that facilitates gas exchange. **Type II cells produce surfactant and account for 60% of the alveolar lining cells.** However, because they are more cuboidal, they contribute only 5% of the alveolar surface. Type I cells are particularly vulnerable to injury. When they are lost, type II pneumocytes multiply and differentiate to form new type I cells, thereby reconstituting the alveolar surface.

The alveolar epithelial and endothelial cells are arranged ideally for gas exchange. The cytoplasm of the epithelial and endothelial cells is spread very thinly on either side of a fused basement membrane, allowing efficient exchange of oxygen and carbon dioxide. An abundant capillary network covers 85% to 95% of the alveolar surface. Away from the site of gas exchange, there is more abundant interstitial connective tissue consisting of collagen, elastin, and proteoglycans. In addition, fibroblasts and myofibroblasts may be present. This expanded region forms the interstitial space of the alveolar wall, where significant fluid and molecular exchange occurs.

PULMONARY VASCULATURE: The lung has a dual blood supply, composed of the pulmonary circulation and the bronchial system. The pulmonary arteries accompany the airways in a sheath of connective tissue, termed the bronchovascular bundle. The more proximal arteries are elastic. They are succeeded by muscular arteries, the pulmonary arterioles, and eventually the pulmonary capillaries.

The smallest veins, which resemble the smallest arteries, join with other veins and drain into the lobular septa, connective tissue partitions that subdivide the lung into small respiratory units. The veins then continue in the lobular septa, joining other veins to form a network that is separate from the bronchovascular bundles.

The bronchial arteries arise from the thoracic aorta and nourish the bronchial tree as far as the respiratory bronchioles. These arteries are accompanied by their respective veins, which drain into the azygous or hemiazygous veins.

There are no lymphatics in most alveolar walls. The lymphatics commence in alveoli at the periphery of the acinus, which lies along a lobular septum, a bronchovascular bundle, or the pleura. The lymphatics of the lobular septa and bronchovascular bundle accompany these structures, and the pleural lymphatics drain toward the hilus through the bronchovascular lymphatics.

DEFENSE MECHANISMS

The respiratory system has effective defense mechanisms to cope with the numerous particulates and infectious agents inhaled on inspiration.

The nose and trachea warm and humidify the air entering the lung. The nose traps almost all particles more than 10 μm in diameter and about half of all particles with an aerodynamic diameter of 3 μm (Fig. 12-2). (Aerodynamic diameter refers to the way particles behave in air rather than to their actual size.)

The mucociliary blanket of the airway epithelium disposes of particles 2 to 10 μm in diameter. The ciliary beat drives the mucous blanket toward the trachea, and particles that land on it are thus removed from the lungs and swallowed or coughed up.

Alveolar macrophages protect the alveolar space. These cells are derived from the bone marrow, probably undergo a maturation division in the interstitium of the lung, and then enter the alveolar space. They are particularly effective in dealing with particles whose aerodynamic diameter is less than 2 μm. Very small particles are not phagocytosed and are exhaled.

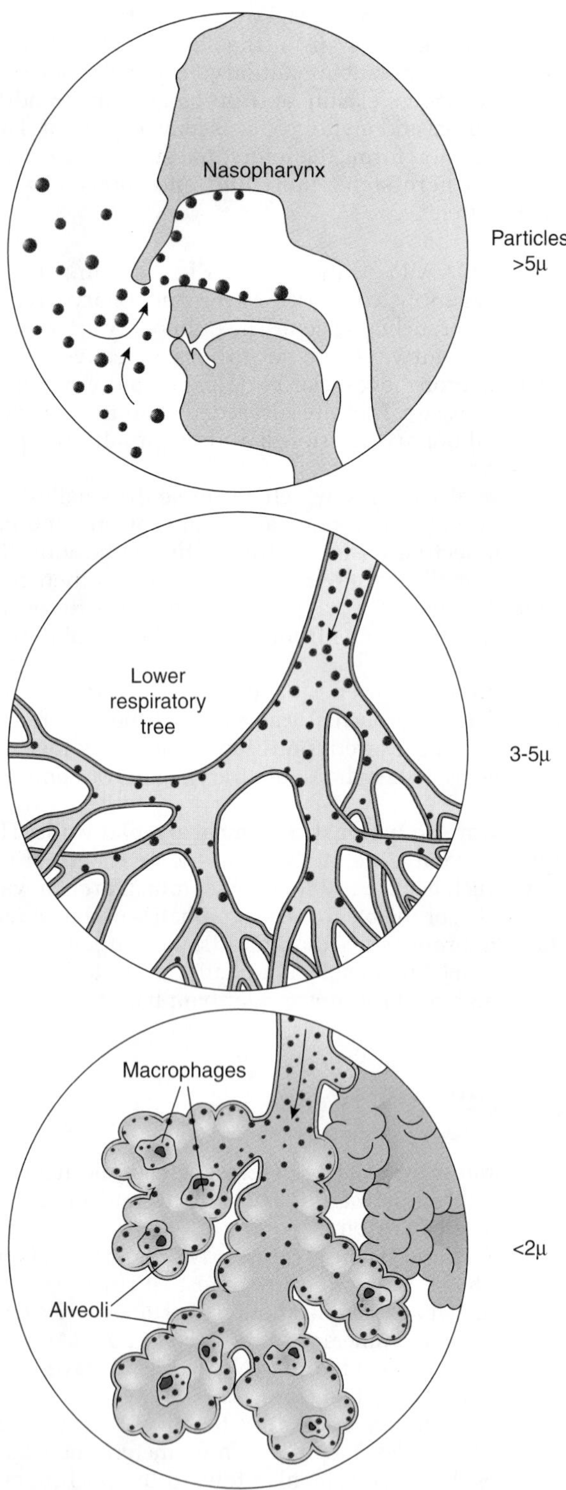

FIGURE 12-2
Deposition of particles in the respiratory tract. Large particles are trapped in the nose. Intermediate-sized particles deposit on the bronchi and bronchioles and are removed by the mucociliary blanket. Smaller particles terminate in the air spaces and are removed by macrophages. Very small particles behave as a gas and are breathed out.

Larynx

INFECTIONS

EPIGLOTTITIS: Inflammation of the epiglottis is a serious condition, most commonly caused by *Haemophilus influenzae,* type B. Occurring in infants and young children, it may be a life-threatening emergency. Swelling of the acutely inflamed epiglottis produces obstruction to airflow. Inspiratory stridor (a loud wheezing sound on inspiration) occurs, and the onset of cyanosis may indicate airway obstruction so severe as to require tracheostomy. Similar symptoms may be encountered in viral infections of the larynx and trachea, which are most commonly due to infection with parainfluenza viruses.

CROUP: This term refers to a syndrome in young children characterized by inspiratory stridor, cough, and hoarseness, resulting from varying degrees of laryngeal obstruction. Croup due to laryngotracheobronchitis is a complication of an upper respiratory tract infection and is marked by edema of the larynx.

LARYNGITIS AND TRACHEITIS: Inflammation of the larynx (laryngitis), which causes hoarseness, and inflammation of the trachea (tracheitis), which is associated with cough, are common at all ages. Both are caused by viral infections, varying from the common cold to influenza. The systemic effects of fever and malaise are usually more troublesome to the patient than the respiratory symptoms, and only supportive treatment is necessary.

NEOPLASMS

LARYNGEAL NODULE (SINGER'S NODULE): This frequently encountered benign lesion is actually reactive rather than neoplastic. It typically occurs on the anterior third of the true vocal cords and is usually single. A laryngeal nodule consists of a small polypoid structure covered by squamous mucosa. The histological appearance varies from a myxoid, edematous, fibroblastic stroma in the early stages to a hyalinized, densely fibrotic stroma in the later stages (Fig. 12-3). The lesion occurs most commonly in persons who use their voices more than most, particularly singers. Changes in the timbre of the voice and hoarseness are the main symptoms. Although a trivial biological lesion, laryngeal nodule may jeopardize a singer's career. Surgery is curative, but the quality of the voice may be impaired.

SQUAMOUS PAPILLOMA AND PAPILLOMATOSIS: Squamous papillomas of the larynx consist of papillary growths of mature squamous cells, which line the surface of fibrovascular cores (Fig. 12-4). These lesions may be solitary or multiple. Multiple papillomas (papillomatosis) are encountered in children or adolescents **(juvenile laryngeal papillomatosis)** and may extend into the trachea and bronchi. An etiological role for hu-

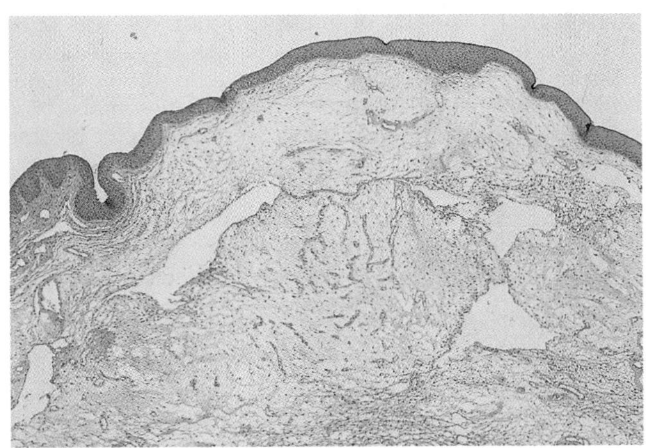

FIGURE 12-3
Laryngeal nodule. This vocal-cord lesion consists of a nodular expansion of the submucosa by an edematous fibroblastic stroma.

man papillomavirus (HPV) in juvenile laryngeal papillomatosis, especially types HPV-6 and HPV-11, is established. Similar to the HPV-related condylomatous lesions of the uterine cervix, the squamous cells may show koilocytosis, characterized by hyperchromatic nuclei and a halo of clear cytoplasm. Juvenile laryngeal papillomatosis may cause life-threatening respiratory obstruction and, rarely, may evolve into an overt squamous cell carcinoma, particularly in smokers and after radiation therapy. Surgical excision may not be curative, because there is often widespread viral infection of the mucosa, and the tumors tend to recur over many years. **Solitary laryngeal squamous papilloma** occurs in adults, predominantly in men, and there is a greater likelihood of curative removal than in juvenile laryngeal papilloma.

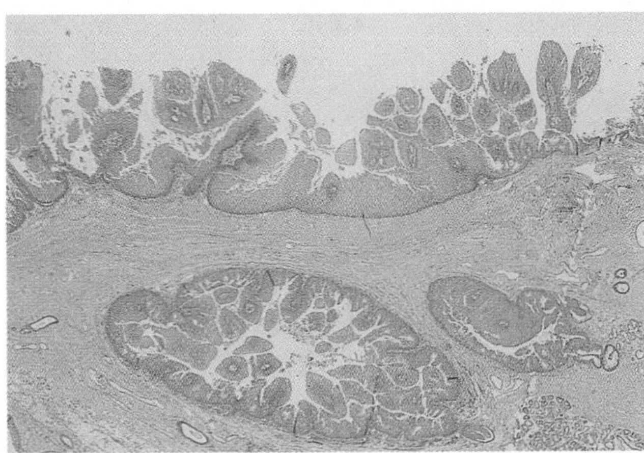

FIGURE 12-4
Laryngeal papillomatosis. The mucosal surface is covered by a carpet of papillary projections consisting of well-differentiated squamous epithelium with fibrovascular cores. The underlying submucosal glands are also involved.

SQUAMOUS CELL CARCINOMA: Almost all laryngeal cancers are squamous cell carcinomas; adenocarcinomas are very rare in this location. Precursor lesions of squamous dysplasia followed by squamous carcinoma *in situ* may be encountered. Virtually all of these patients are men, most of whom are cigarette smokers. Based on the location of the lesion, these cancers are divided into four groups, which have relevance to treatment and prognosis.

- **Glottic carcinoma** is a tumor limited to one or both true vocal cords and accounts for almost two thirds of laryngeal carcinomas. This cancer is slow to metastasize to lymph nodes and has a good prognosis. Early-stage carcinomas can often be effectively treated with radiation therapy or voice-saving surgery.
- **Supraglottic carcinoma** arises in the ventricle, false cords, or epiglottis and does not, by definition, involve the true cords. Up to one third of laryngeal carcinomas arise in this location. Nodal metastases are more common than in glottic tumors. Cancers in this location are treated by radiation or surgery.
- **Transglottic carcinoma**, by definition, involves the true and false cords (Fig. 12-5). This uncommon tumor is likely to metastasize to lymph nodes and often requires total laryngectomy.
- **Infraglottic carcinoma** is an infrequent tumor, which is located below the true cords or involves the true cords, with considerable infraglottic extension and frequent extension into the trachea. Nodal metastases are common, and total laryngectomy is generally required.

The rarity of tumors of the trachea remains unexplained. Because potent carcinogens in tobacco smoke reach the trachea in high concentrations, cancer should be common in this location. The reverse is actually true; cancer of the trachea is distinctly uncommon. Most tracheal

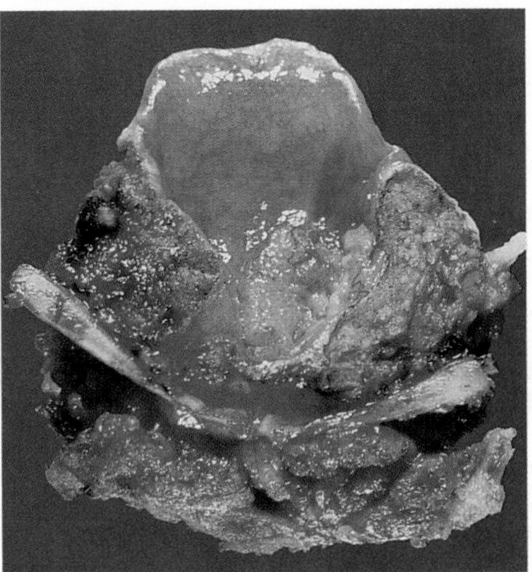

FIGURE 12-5
Carcinoma of the larynx. This transglottic carcinoma has an irregular, exophytic, indurated tan–white surface. It involves the right vocal cord and displays supraglottic extension.

• squamous cell
• cigarrette smoking

tumors are mucoepidermoid carcinomas and adenoid cystic carcinomas that arise from tracheal mucous glands, which are analogous to the salivary glands.

The Lungs

CONGENITAL ANOMALIES

BRONCHIAL ATRESIA: This abnormality most often involves the bronchus to the apical posterior segment of the left upper lobe. In infants, the lesion may result in an overexpanded part of the lung. In later life, the overexpanded lobe may also be emphysematous. Bronchial mucus, accumulating distal to the atretic region, may appear on radiological examination as a mass.

PULMONARY HYPOPLASIA: This condition reflects incomplete or defective development of the lung. The lung is smaller than normal in size, owing to fewer acini or a decrease in their size. Pulmonary hypoplasia is the most common congenital lesion of the lung, being found in 10% of neonatal autopsies. In the large majority of cases (90%), it occurs in association with other congenital anomalies, most of which impinge on the thorax. The lesion may be accompanied by hypoplasia of the bronchi and pulmonary vessels if the insult occurs early in gestation, as in congenital diaphragmatic hernia. Pulmonary hypoplasia also is seen in trisomies 13, 18, and 21.

Three major factors have been implicated as causes of pulmonary hypoplasia:

- **Compression of the lung** is usually caused by a congenital diaphragmatic hernia, typically on the left side, owing to failure of the pleuroperitoneal canal to close. Varying degrees of herniation of abdominal viscera are present in the affected hemithorax, and the degree of hypoplasia is variable. At one extreme, the lung on the affected side is reduced to a small nubbin of tissue, and the lung on the opposite side is severely hypoplastic. At the other extreme, the degree of hypoplasia is so slight that the infant has no symptoms, the abnormalities being noted incidentally on a routine chest radiograph. Other causes of hypoplasia in this category include diaphragmatic hernia, abnormalities of the chest wall, pleural effusions, and ascites, as in hydrops fetalis.
- **Oligohydramnios** (an inadequate volume of amniotic fluid) is usually due to genitourinary anomalies and is an important cause of pulmonary hypoplasia.
- **Decreased respiration** has been shown experimentally to produce hypoplastic lungs, which may be caused by a lack of repetitive stretching of the lung.

CONGENITAL CYSTIC ADENOMATOID MALFORMATION: *This common anomaly consists of abnormal bronchiolar structures of varying sizes or distribution.* The vast majority of cases are encountered in the first 2 years of life. The lesion usually affects one lobe of the lung and histologically consists of multiple cyst-like spaces lined by bronchiolar epithelium and separated by loose fibrous tissue (Fig. 12-6). By definition, acute or chronic inflammation and interstitial fibrosis should be absent, because a similar histological appearance can result in the healing phase of inflammatory or fibrotic pulmonary disorders. The most common presenting symptom is respiratory distress and cyanosis. Surgical resection is the treatment of choice. Some patients with congenital cystic adenomatoid malformation have other congenital anomalies.

BRONCHOGENIC CYST: *This lesion is a discrete, extrapulmonary, fluid-filled mass, which is lined by respiratory epithelium and delimited by walls that contain muscle and cartilage.* It is most commonly found in the middle mediastinum. In the newborn, a bronchogenic cyst may compress a major airway and cause respiratory distress. Secondary infection of the cyst in older patients may lead to hemorrhage and perforation. Many bronchogenic cysts are asymptomatic and are found on routine chest radiographs.

EXTRALOBAR SEQUESTRATION: *Extralobar sequestration is a mass of lung tissue that is not connected to the bronchial tree and is located outside the visceral pleura.* An abnormal artery, usually arising from the aorta, supplies the sequestered tissue (Fig. 12-7). This lesion is thought to originate from an outpouching of the foregut, which is separate from the pulmonary anlage but later becomes detached from the original foregut. The lesion occurs 3 to 4 times as often in male as in female infants, and in two thirds of the patients, it is associated with other anomalies.

On gross examination, extralobar sequestration appears as a pyramidal or round mass covered by pleura, ranging from 1 to 15 cm in greatest dimension. Microscopically, dilated bronchioles, alveolar ducts, and alveoli are noted. Infection or infarction may alter the histological appearance.

In half of the cases, extralobar sequestration is recognized in the first month of life, and by age 2 years, the di-

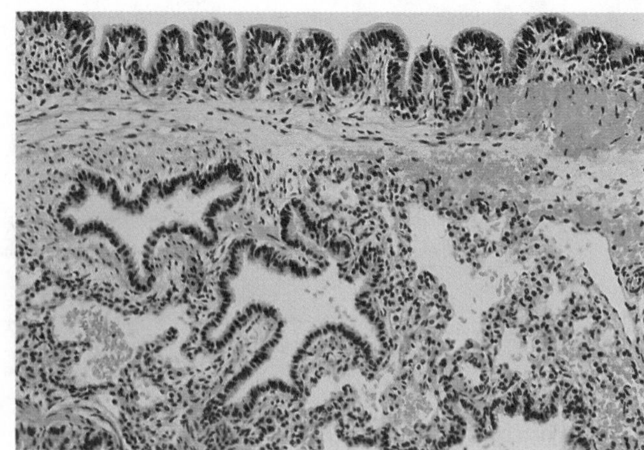

FIGURE 12-6
Congenital cystic adenomatoid malformation. Multiple gland-like spaces are lined by bronchiolar epithelium.

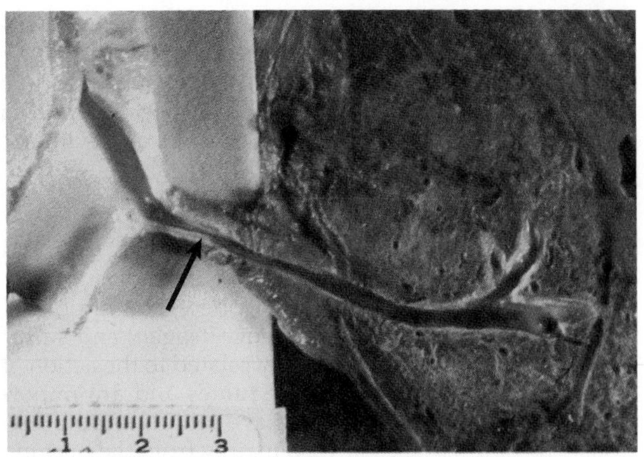

FIGURE 12-7
Extralobar sequestration. The sequestered pulmonary tissue is situated outside the lung parenchyma. It is supplied by an aberrant artery *(arrow)* from the aorta and is not connected to the bronchial tree.

agnosis has been made in 75% of the patients. In the neonatal period, often during the first day of life, the disorder may present as dyspnea and cyanosis. In older children, the lesion frequently comes to medical attention because of recurrent bronchopulmonary infections. Surgical excision is curative.

INTRALOBAR SEQUESTRATION: *Intralobar sequestration is a mass of lung tissue within the visceral pleura that is isolated from the tracheobronchial tree and is supplied by a systemic artery* (Fig. 12-8). For many years, this lesion was considered a congenital malformation, but it is now thought to be acquired. Intralobar sequestration is found in a lower lobe in almost all (98%) of the cases, and bilateral involvement is distinctly unusual. On gross examination, the sequestered pulmonary tissue shows the result of chronic recurrent pneumonias, with end-stage fibrosis and honeycomb cystic changes. The cysts range up to 5 cm in diameter and lie in a dense fibrous stroma. Microscopically, the cystic spaces are mostly lined by cuboidal or columnar epithelium, and the lumen contains foamy macrophages and eosinophilic material. Interstitial chronic inflammation and hyperplasia of lymphoid follicles is often prominent. Acute and organizing pneumonia may be seen.

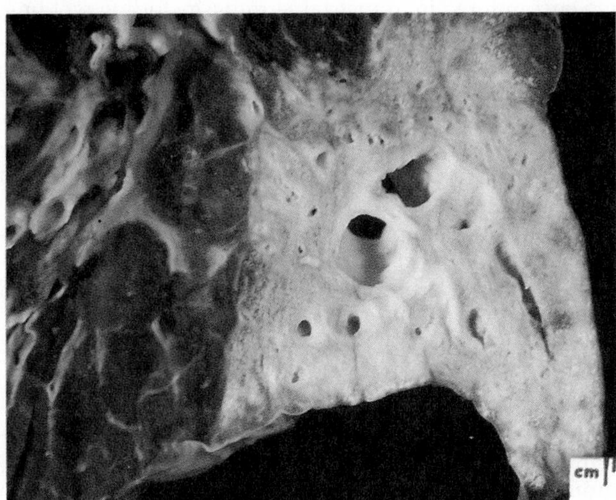

FIGURE 12-8
Intralobar sequestration. The sequestered tissue lies within the visceral pleura and exhibits cystic change and dense fibrosis. An aberrant arterial supply to this lesion was identified (not shown).

Symptoms of cough, sputum production, and recurrent pneumonia are noted in almost all patients. Most cases are discovered in adolescents or young adults. Only one fourth of patients are in the first decade of life, and the lesion is only rarely identified in infants. Surgical resection is often indicated.

DISEASES OF THE BRONCHI AND BRONCHIOLES

Most of the entities subsumed under bronchial and bronchiolar diseases deal with acute conditions and their sequelae. We reserve the discussion of chronic bronchitis for the section devoted to chronic obstructive pulmonary disease.

Infections

In this section, we distinguish between infections of the airways and parenchyma for reasons of classification and convenience, but this division should not be thought of as rigid. The agents causing these infections are discussed in detail in Chapter 9.

Many infectious agents that involve the intrapulmonary airways tend to affect the more peripheral airways **(bronchiolitis)**. The classic examples are adenovirus, measles, and respiratory syncytial virus. All appear to be more serious in malnourished children and populations not ordinarily exposed to these agents. Severe symptomatic illnesses are mostly confined to infants and children, and recovery is the rule. Symptoms include cough, a feeling of tightness in the chest, and, in extreme cases, shortness of breath and even cyanosis.

INFLUENZA: This is a characteristic example of tracheobronchitis, and in the occasional patient who dies with this infection, the appearance of the bronchi is dramatic. The surface of the airway is fiery red, reflecting acute inflammation and congestion of the mucosa.

ADENOVIRUS: Infection with this virus produces the most serious sequelae, including extensive inflammation of bronchioles (Fig. 12-9) and subsequent healing by fibrosis. Bronchioles may become obliterated or occluded by loose fibrous tissue (obliterative bronchiolitis).

RESPIRATORY SYNCYTIAL VIRUS: Infection with this agent tends to occur in epidemics in nurseries. It is usually a self-limited illness, but rare fatal cases occur. It

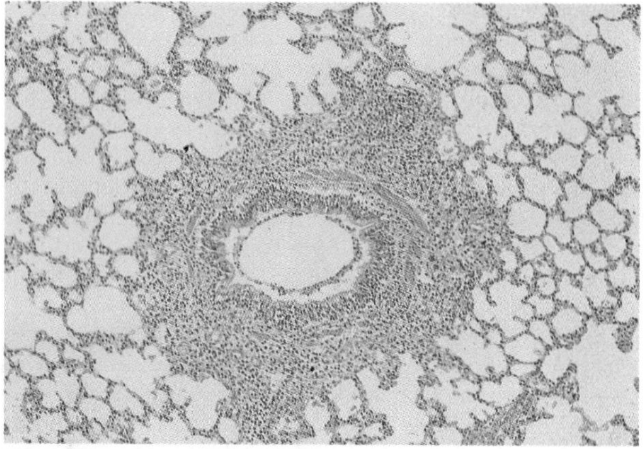

FIGURE 12-9
Bronchiolitis due to adenovirus. The wall of this bronchiole shows an intense chronic inflammatory infiltrate, with local extension into the surrounding peribronchial tissue.

can cause nosocomial infection in children and rarely in adults. Histologically, one encounters peribronchiolar inflammation and disorganization of the epithelium. Severe overdistention of the lung parenchyma may be found without obvious bronchiolar obstruction, possibly because of displacement of surfactant from the bronchiolar surface.

MEASLES: At one time a major cause of bronchiolitis, measles is no longer a problem in developed countries because of the advent of the measles vaccine. However, measles-induced bronchiolitis still remains a serious problem elsewhere, particularly in populations seldom exposed to the virus. Similar to adenovirus, it may result in bronchiolar obliteration and bronchiectasis.

BORDETELLA PERTUSSIS: This bacterium commonly infects the airways and is the cause of **whooping cough**. After the introduction of a pertussis vaccine, the disease became rare in the United States, but it has become increasingly common in England, where vaccination is no longer compulsory. Clinically, whooping cough is typified by fever and severe prolonged bouts of coughing, followed by a characteristic deep whooping inspiration. Severe bronchial and bronchiolar inflammation has been found in fatal cases. Whooping cough commonly preceded the development of bronchiectasis in the past, but this is no longer the case in areas where children are routinely immunized.

HAEMOPHILUS INFLUENZAE AND *STREPTOCOCCUS PNEUMONIAE:* These organisms have been implicated in exacerbations of chronic bronchitis. Such episodes contribute to the morbidity of chronic bronchitis and are treated with antibiotics.

CANDIDA ALBICANS: This fungus is a normal commensal organism in the oral cavity, gut, and vagina and is best known for its infection of those regions. *Candida* may also affect the lungs, usually as a noninvasive growth on the surface epithelium of the airways, where it may produce mucosal ulceration. Predisposing factors for invasive growth include trauma, burns, gastrointestinal surgery, and indwelling catheters, as well as neutropenia associated with a history of acute leukemia and cytotoxic chemotherapy.

Irritant Gases

Of the irritant gases in the atmosphere, the important ones are oxidants (ozone, oxides of nitrogen) and sulfur dioxide. Oxidants are particularly related to the action of sunlight on automobile exhaust fumes and are important in major urban areas that have temperature inversions. Sulfur dioxide is derived mainly from the burning of fossil fuels. Although the precise effects of these agents in low concentration is not certain, and although they clearly have a high nuisance value, it seems unlikely that they are a major cause of serious respiratory disease. However, they may compound the adverse effects of tobacco smoke. Indeed, persons living in urban and more polluted areas have worse pulmonary function, as expressed by reduced expiratory flow rates, than do those who reside in cleaner environments. Respiratory infections are also more common in young children in regions of high pollution. However, the decrement in function and increase in symptoms is small in the healthy population.

In persons with chronic pulmonary disease, the situation is different. Of particular relevance is the experimental observation that ozone makes the airways more reactive, an effect related to airway inflammation. Thus, air pollution may exacerbate the symptoms of asthmatic persons and of those with established respiratory disease. In high concentrations, irritant gases produce serious morphological and functional effects.

NITROGEN DIOXIDE (NO_2): Exposure to NO_2 is often encountered in industrial settings, including welding, electroplating, metal cleaning, and blasting. The gas is also produced by decaying grain stored in silos. Because NO_2 is heavier than air, it accumulates immediately above the surface of the grain. A worker entering the silo inhales high concentrations of the gas, with resulting injury to the lung, a condition known as **silo-filler disease**. The onset of respiratory symptoms is delayed for up to 30 hours, after which time the patient is seen with cough and dyspnea. Although most patients recover, some have developed progressive bronchiolitis obliterans and have died in respiratory failure.

SULFUR DIOXIDE (SO_2): This highly soluble gas, when inhaled over the long term by experimental animals, produces lesions in the more central airways that resemble chronic bronchitis and that may progress to squamous metaplasia. In humans, exposure to very high concentrations of SO_2 has been associated with severe inflammation and bronchiolitis.

CHLORINE AND AMMONIA: These gases are released in high concentrations in industrial accidents. On inhalation, they produce extensive bronchial and bronchiolar mucosal injury. Secondary inflammation may culminate in extensive bronchiectasis, in part from bronchiolar obliteration and in part from direct damage to the bronchi.

Bronchocentric Granulomatosis

Bronchocentric granulomatosis refers to nonspecific granulomatous inflammation centered on bronchi or bronchioles (Fig. 12-10). The histological pattern can be seen in a wide variety of clinical settings and is not a distinct clinical entity. Bronchocentric granulomatosis can be the predominant pulmonary pathological finding in two groups of patients, asthmatics and nonasthmatics.

Asthmatic patients, for the most part, have allergic bronchopulmonary aspergillosis (see later). In addition to the lesion of bronchocentric granulomatosis, such cases demonstrate bronchial mucous plugs, bronchiectasis and bronchiolectasis, and eosinophilic pneumonia. Irregular, fragmented *Aspergillus* hyphae may be seen in the mucous plugs. A nonspecific secondary vasculitis is centered on the airways rather than the vessels.

Nonasthmatic patients with bronchocentric granulomatosis are likely to have an infection, especially tuberculosis or fungal organisms such as *Histoplasma capsulatum.* Bronchocentric granulomatosis can also be a manifestation of rheumatoid arthritis, ankylosing spondylitis, and Wegener granulomatosis. In the absence of any of these potential causes, bronchocentric granulomatosis is regarded as *idiopathic*. Patients with *idiopathic* bronchocentric granulomatosis may respond well to corticosteroid therapy.

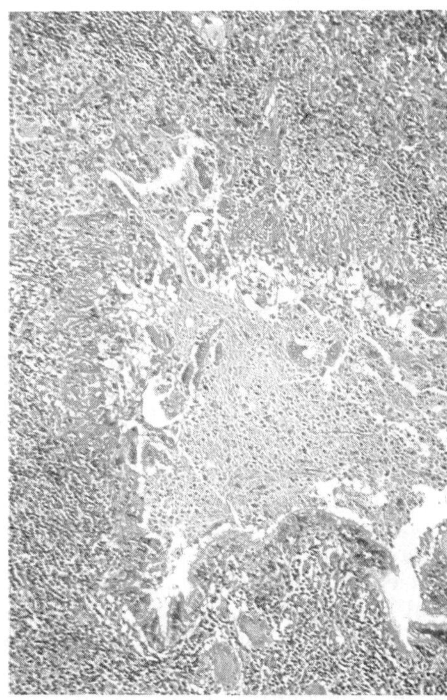

FIGURE *12-10*
Bronchocentric granulomatosis. The wall of a bronchiole is destroyed by necrotizing granulomatous inflammation. The lumen is filled with necrotic debris.

Obliterative Bronchiolitis

Obliterative bronchiolitis is an uncommon disorder in which an initial inflammatory bronchiolitis is followed by bronchiolar scarring and fibrosis, resulting in constrictive narrowing and eventually complete obliteration of the airway lumen (Fig. 12-11). Bronchioles show chronic mural inflammation and varying amounts of submucosal fibrosis. These lesions are often focal and may be difficult to identify. Elastic stains may assist in recognizing the scarred bronchioles. Bronchiolectasis and mucous plugs may be seen in adjacent airways. The surrounding lung is usually normal.

Patients may have dyspnea and wheezing owing to severe obstructive pulmonary function. The chest radiograph and computed tomography (CT) scan may be normal, or they may show overinflation, caused by air trapping distal to the obliterated bronchioles. This pattern of fibrosis is seen in a number of situations, including the following: (a) bone marrow transplant recipients (graft-versus-host disease), (b) heart–lung or single-lung transplant recipients (chronic rejection), (c) collagen vascular diseases (especially rheumatoid arthritis), (d) postinfectious disorders (mycoplasma and viral, especially adenovirus, respiratory syncytial virus, and influenza), (e) after inhalation of toxins (sulfur dioxide, ammonia, and phosgene), and (f) intake of certain drugs (penicillamine). It also may occur as an idiopathic entity. Most patients have a relentless progressive clinical course. Although many patients are treated with steroids, there is no known effective therapy for this disease.

Bronchial Obstruction and Atelectasis

Bronchial obstruction in adults is most often the consequence of the endobronchial extension of primary lung tumors, although mucous plugs from a variety of causes, aspirated gastric contents, or foreign bodies may be responsible. In children, foreign bodies are one of the most important causes of bronchial obstruction. In the case of

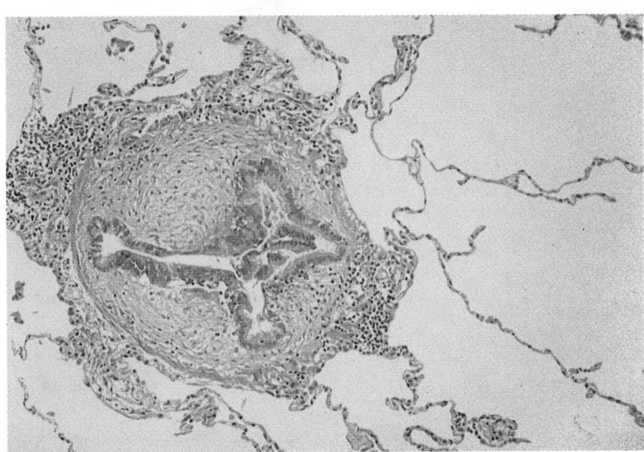

FIGURE *12-11*
Obliterative bronchiolitis. The lumen of a bronchiole is markedly narrowed, owing to marked submucosal fibrosis.

partial obstruction, the trapped air may lead to overdistention of the distal affected segment, whereas complete obstruction results in atelectasis. Areas distal to the obstruction are also susceptible to pneumonia, pulmonary abscess, and bronchiectasis (see later).

Atelectasis

Atelectasis refers to the collapse of expanded lung tissue (Fig 12-12). If the supply of air is obstructed, the loss of gas from the alveoli to the blood leads to collapse of the affected region. Atelectasis is an important postoperative complication of abdominal surgery, occurring because of (1) mucous obstruction of a bronchus and (2) diminished respiratory movement resulting from postoperative pain. It is often asymptomatic, but when severe, it results in hypoxemia.

Although atelectasis is usually caused by bronchial obstruction, it may also result from direct compression of the lung (e.g., hydrothorax or pneumothorax). Such compression, if severe enough, seriously compromises the function of the affected lung.

In long-standing atelectasis, the collapsed lung becomes fibrotic and the bronchi dilate, in part because of infection distal to the obstructed bronchus. Permanent bronchial dilatation (bronchiectasis) results.

Right middle lobe syndrome *refers to atelectasis secondary to obstruction of the bronchus to the right middle lobe.* The bronchial obstruction is usually due to external compression by hilar lymph nodes. The bronchus is particularly susceptible to external compression because it is long and slender and surrounded by lymph nodes. Histologically, the lung shows bronchiectasis, chronic bronchitis and bronchiolitis, lymphoid hyperplasia, abscess formation, and dense fibrosis. Acute and organizing pneumonia may be present. The lymph node enlargement can be due to tuberculous lymphadenitis or metastatic lung cancer. In a substantial proportion of cases, the cause of the bronchial obstruction remains undetermined.

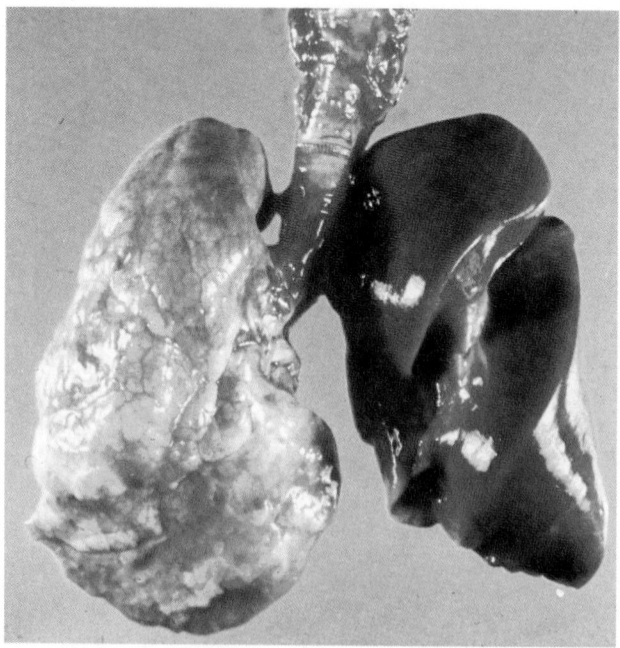

FIGURE *12-12*
Atelectasis. The right lung of an infant is pale and expanded by air, whereas the left lung is collapsed.

Bronchiectasis

Bronchiectasis is the irreversible dilatation of bronchi as a consequence of the destruction of the muscular and elastic elements of their walls.

☐ **Pathogenesis:** Bronchiectasis is either obstructive or nonobstructive.

Obstructive bronchiectasis is localized to a segment of the lung distal to a mechanical obstruction of a central bronchus by a variety of lesions, including tumors, inhaled foreign bodies, mucous plugs in asthma, and compressive lymphadenopathy. Nonobstructive bronchiectasis is usually a complication of respiratory infections or defects in the defense mechanisms that protect the airways from infection.

Nonobstructive bronchiectasis may be localized or generalized. Localized nonobstructive bronchiectasis was once a common disease, usually resulting from childhood bronchopulmonary infections, such as measles, pertussis, or other bacterial infections. Although vaccines and antibiotics have reduced the frequency of bronchiectasis, one half to two thirds of all cases still follow a bronchopulmonary infection. At present, adenovirus and respiratory syncytial virus infections are frequent causes of bronchiectasis in children. Childhood respiratory infections remain important causes of bronchiectasis in less developed parts of the world.

Generalized bronchiectasis is, for the most part, secondary to inherited impairments in host defense mechanisms or acquired conditions that permit the introduction of infectious organisms into the airways. The acquired disorders that predispose to bronchiectasis include (1) neurological diseases that impair consciousness, swallowing, respiratory excursions, and the cough reflex; (2) incompetence of the lower esophageal sphincter; (3) nasogastric intubation; and (4) chronic bronchitis.

The principal inherited conditions associated with generalized bronchiectasis are cystic fibrosis, the dyskinetic ciliary syndromes, hypogammaglobulinemias, and deficiencies of specific IgG subclasses.

Kartagener syndrome *is one of the immotile cilia (ciliary dyskinesia) syndromes and comprises the triad of dextrocardia (with or without situs inversus), bronchiectasis, and sinusitis.* This disorder is associated with a defect in the structure of cilia, characterized by an absence of inner or outer dynein arms. Other dyskinetic ciliary syndromes include radial spoke deficiency (Sturgess syndrome) and an absence of the central doublet of the cilium. Cilia are deficient throughout the body in immotile cilia syndromes. As a result, sterility in both men and women is usual, because of impaired ciliary mobility in the vas deferens and the fallopian tube. In the respiratory tract, ciliary defects lead to repeated upper and lower respiratory tract infections in the lung and, thus, to bronchiectasis.

Immunodeficiency diseases similarly predispose to repeated pulmonary infections and are associated with bronchiectasis. Hypogammaglobulinemia, owing to the absence of IgA or IgG antibodies that protect against viruses or bacteria, can result in recurrent pulmonary infections. Acquired and inherited disorders of neutrophils also lead to a greater risk of respiratory infections and bronchiectasis. Bronchiectasis is a potential complication of human immunodeficiency virus (HIV) infection in children.

☐ **Pathology:** On gross examination, bronchial dilatation is classified as saccular, varicose, or cylindrical.

- **Saccular bronchiectasis** affects the proximal third to fourth branches of the bronchi (Fig. 12-13). These bronchi are severely dilated and end blindly in dilated sacs, with collapse and fibrosis of the distal lung parenchyma.
- **Cylindrical bronchiectasis** involves the sixth to eighth bronchial branchings, which show uniform, moderate dilatation. It is a milder disease than saccular bronchiectasis and leads to fewer clinical symptoms.
- **Varicose bronchiectasis** results in bronchi that resemble varicose veins when visualized by radiological bronchography, with irregular dilatations and constrictions. Two to eight branchings of bronchi are recognized grossly, bronchiolar obliteration is not as severe, and parenchymal abnormalities are variable.

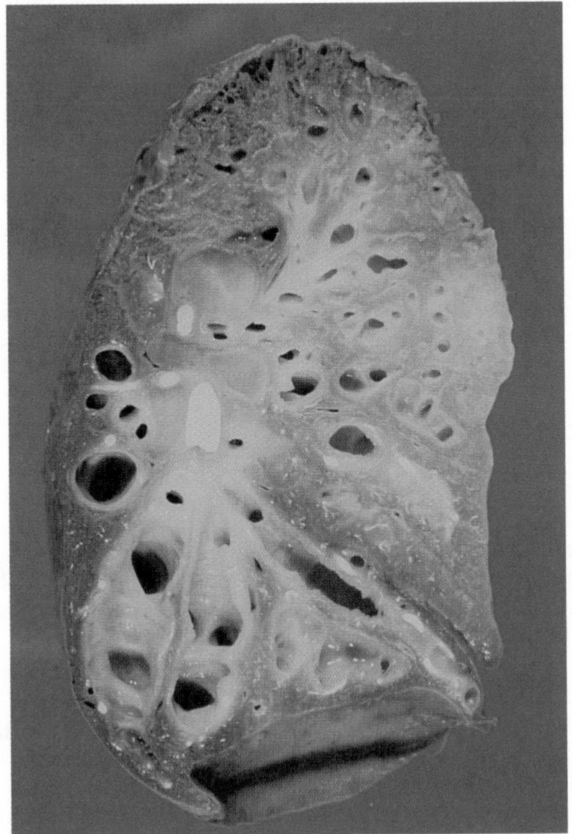

FIGURE *12-13*
Bronchiectasis. The resected upper lobe shows widely dilated bronchi, with thickening of the bronchial walls and collapse and fibrosis of the pulmonary parenchyma.

Generalized bronchiectasis is usually bilateral and most common in the lower lobes, the left more commonly involved than the right. Localized bronchiectasis may be situated wherever the obstruction or infection occurred. The bronchi are dilated and have white or yellow thickened walls. The bronchial lumen frequently contains thick, mucopurulent secretions. Microscopically, severe inflammation of bronchi and bronchioles results in destruction of all components of the bronchial wall. With the consequent collapse of distal lung parenchyma, the damaged bronchi dilate. Inflammation of the central airways leads to hypersecretion of mucus and abnormalities of the surface epithelium, including an increase in number of goblet cells and squamous metaplasia of the epithelium. Lymphoid follicles are often seen in the bronchial walls. The distal bronchi and bronchioles are scarred and often obliterated. The bronchial arteries increase in size and supply the inflamed bronchial wall and fibrous tissue. A vicious circle may be established, because a pool of mucus is liable to further infection, which leads to progressive destruction of the bronchial walls.

☐ **Clinical Features:** Patients with bronchiectasis are seen with chronic productive cough, often with several hundred milliliters of mucopurulent sputum a day. Hemoptysis is a common symptom, owing to erosion by the bronchial inflammation through the wall of the adjacent bronchial arteries. Dyspnea and wheezing are variable, depending on the extent of the disease. Pneumonia is a common complication, and long-standing cases are at risk of chronic hypoxia and pulmonary hypertension. Radiologically, the bronchi appear dilated with thickened walls. Today the definitive diagnosis is made by CT scans of the lung. Surgical treatment of localized bronchiectasis may be necessary, especially if complications such as severe hemoptysis or pneumonia arise. However, in the generalized disease, surgical resection is more palliative than curative.

It should be noted that acute, reversible dilatation of bronchi may occur as a consequence of bacterial or viral bronchopulmonary infection, and it may take months before the bronchi return to normal size. This is important to recognize because such patients do not require surgery.

INFECTIONS

Pulmonary infections are discussed in detail in Chapter 9. The major entities are described below, with particular emphasis on pathological features.

Bacterial Pneumonia

***Pneumonia** is a generic term that refers to inflammation and consolidation (solidification) of the pulmonary parenchyma.* Traditionally, bacterial pneumonias were classified as either lobar pneumonia or bronchopneumonia, but these terms have little clinical relevance today. In general, the term lobar pneumonia refers to consolidation of an entire lobe (Fig. 12-14); bronchopneumonia signifies scattered solid foci in the same or several lobes (Fig. 12-15).

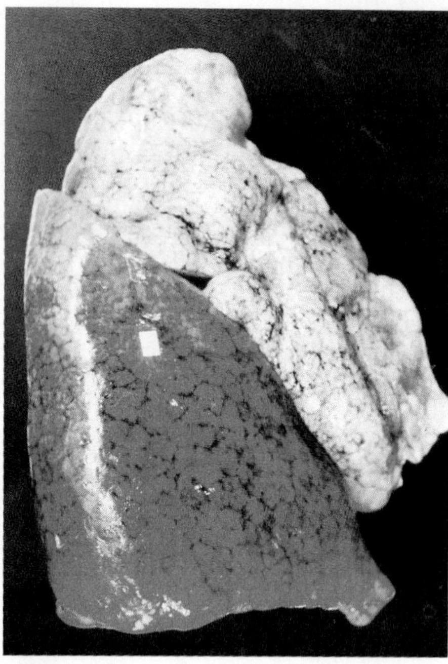

FIGURE 12-14
Lobar pneumonia. The entire left lower lobe is consolidated and in the stage of red hepatization. The upper lobe is normally expanded.

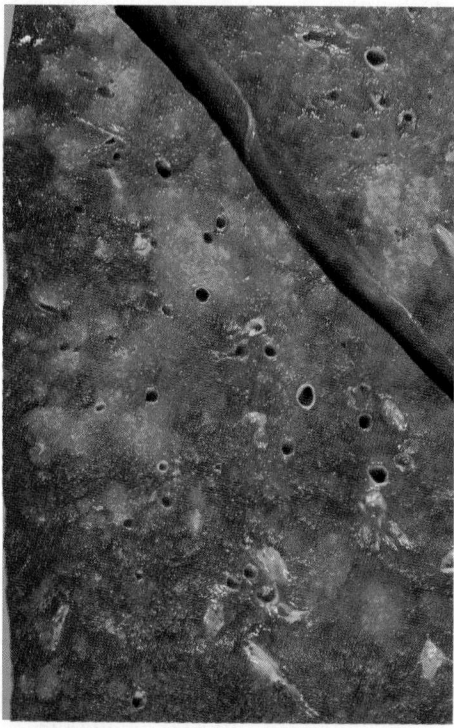

FIGURE 12-15
Bronchopneumonia. Scattered foci of consolidation are centered on bronchi and bronchioles.

Pneumococcal pneumonia was the classic example of lobar pneumonia, but today the involvement of a lobe tends to be incomplete, and more than one lobe is usually affected. By contrast, bronchopneumonia remains a common cause of death and is often found at autopsy. It typically develops in terminally ill patients, usually in the dependent and posterior portions of the lung. Scattered irregular foci of pneumonia are centered on terminal bronchioles and respiratory bronchioles. Bronchiolitis is present, with exudation of polymorphonuclear leukocytes into the adjacent alveoli. Large continuous areas of alveolar involvement do not occur in bronchopneumonia.

Bacterial pneumonias occur in three settings:

- **Community-acquired pneumonia** arises outside the hospital in persons with no primary disorder of the immune system.
- **Nosocomial pneumonia** represents an infection spread by organisms in the hospital environment to particularly susceptible patients.
- **Opportunistic pneumonia** afflicts persons whose immune status is compromised from whatever cause.

☐ **Pathogenesis:** Most bacteria that cause pneumonia are normal inhabitants of the oropharynx and nasopharynx and reach the alveoli by aspiration of secretions. Other routes of infection include inhalation of microorganisms from the environment, hematogenous dissemination from an infectious focus elsewhere, and rarely, spread of bacteria from an adjacent site. A change in the oropharyngeal flora from the normal commensals to a virulent organism often precedes the development of pneumonia. A number of conditions predispose to infection by depressing the host defenses, including cigarette smoking, chronic bronchitis, alcoholism, severe malnutrition, wasting diseases, and poorly controlled diabetes. Altered oropharyngeal flora commonly occurs in debilitated or immunosuppressed patients in the hospital, in whom nosocomial pneumonia can occur in as many as 25%.

It is important to classify bacterial pneumonias on the basis of the etiological agent, because the clinical and morphological features, and thus the therapeutic implications, often vary with the causative organism.

Pneumococcal Pneumonia

Despite the impact of antibiotic therapy, pneumonia caused by *Streptococcus pneumoniae* (pneumococcus) remains a significant problem. Pneumococcal pneumonia is principally a disease of young to middle-aged adults. It is rare in infants, less common in the elderly, and considerably more frequent in men than in women.

☐ **Pathogenesis:** Pneumococcal pneumonia is mostly a consequence of altered defense barriers in the respiratory tract. Frequently this pneumonia follows a viral infection of the upper respiratory tract (e.g., influenza). The bronchial secretions stimulated by a viral infection provide a hospitable environment for the proliferation of *S. pneumoniae* organisms, which are normal flora of the nasopharynx. The thin, watery secretions carry the organisms into the alveoli, thereby initiating an inflammatory

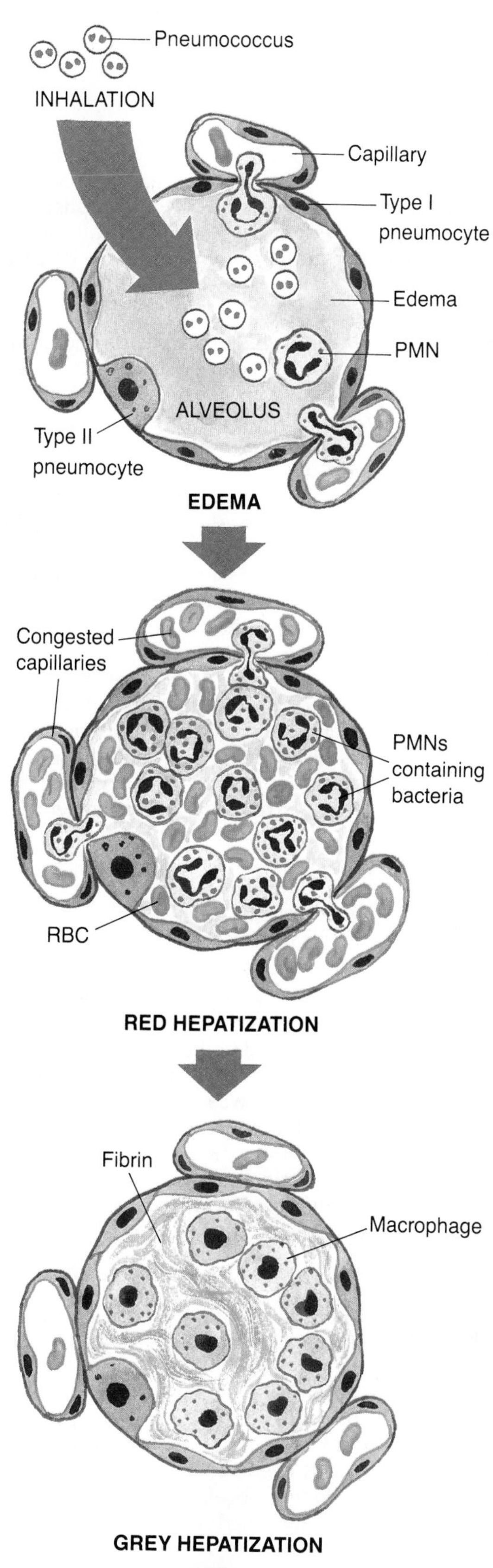

response. The remarkably severe acute inflammation with spreading edema has led to speculation that immunological mechanisms may be involved. The aspiration of pneumococci is also promoted by factors that impair the epiglottic reflex, including exposure to cold, anesthesia, and alcohol intoxication. Injury to the lung caused by factors such as congestive heart failure and irritant gases also renders the lung more susceptible to pneumococcal pneumonia.

The capsule of the pneumococcus provides a defense against phagocytosis by the alveolar macrophages, and the organisms must, therefore, be opsonized before they can be ingested and killed. In an immune-competent person, antipneumococcal antibodies function as opsonins, whereas a host that has not been exposed to the specific infecting strain of *S. pneumoniae* can achieve opsonization only through the alternative complement pathway.

□ **Pathology:** In the earliest stage of pneumococcal pneumonia, protein-rich edema fluid containing numerous organisms fills the alveoli (Fig. 12-16). Marked congestion of the capillaries is followed by a massive outpouring of polymorphonuclear leukocytes, accompanied by intra-alveolar hemorrhage (Fig. 12-17). Because the firm consistency of the affected lung is reminiscent of the liver, this stage has been aptly named "red hepatization."

The next phase, occurring after 2 or more days, depending on the success of treatment, involves the lysis of polymorphonuclear leukocytes and the appearance of macrophages. The latter phagocytose the fragmented polymorphonuclear leukocytes and other inflammatory debris. At this stage, the congestion has diminished, but the lung still remains firm ("gray hepatization"). The alveolar exudate is then removed, and the lung gradually returns to normal.

A number of complications may follow pneumococcal pneumonia:

- **Pleuritis**, often painful, is common, because the pneumonia readily extends to the pleura.
- **Pleural effusion** frequently occurs, but usually resolves.
- **Pyothorax** results from an infection of a pleural effusion and may heal with extensive fibrosis.
- **Empyema** (a loculated collection of pus with fibrous walls) results from the persistence of pyothorax.
- **Bacteremia** is present in more than 25% of patients in the early stages of pneumococcal pneumonia and may lead to endocarditis or meningitis. Patients whose spleens have been removed often die of this bacteremia.

FIGURE *12-16*
Pathogenesis of lobar pneumococcal pneumonia. Pneumococci, characteristically in pairs (diplococci), multiply rapidly in the alveolar spaces and produce extensive edema. They incite an acute inflammatory response, in which polymorphonuclear leukocytes and congestion are prominent (red hepatization). As the inflammatory process progresses, macrophages replace the polymorphonuclear leukocytes and ingest debris (gray hepatization). The process usually resolves, but complications may ensue.

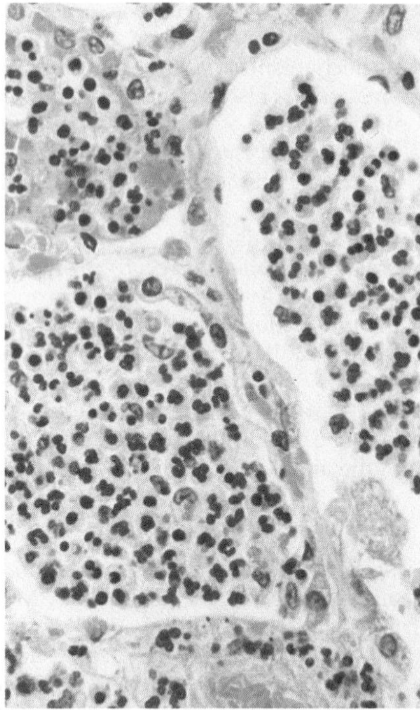

FIGURE 12-17
Pneumococcal pneumonia. The alveoli are packed with an exudate composed of polymorphonuclear leukocytes and occasional macrophages.

- **Pulmonary fibrosis** is a rare complication, in which the intra-alveolar exudate becomes organized as fibroblasts proliferate. Gradually, increasing alveolar fibrosis leads to a shrunken and firm lobe, a rare complication known as "carnification."
- **Lung abscess** is an unusual complication of pneumococcal pneumonia.

□ **Clinical Features:** The onset of pneumococcal pneumonia is acute, with fever and chills. Chest pain secondary to pleural involvement is common, as is hemoptysis, which is characteristically "rusty," because it is derived from altered blood in alveolar spaces. Radiological examination shows alveolar filling in large areas of lung, producing a solid appearance that extends to entire lobes or segments. Before antibiotic therapy, the clinical course was characterized by severe fever, dyspnea, debility, and even loss of consciousness. The dramatic event was the crisis, occurring 5 to 10 days after the onset of respiratory symptoms, when the moribund patient would suddenly become afebrile and return from death's door. The satisfactory resolution of the crisis was the result of the immune response to the infection. Unfortunately, all too often the outcome was not favorable, and in one third of the cases, the patient died. However, in the modern era, pneumococcal pneumonia is effectively treated with antibiotics. Although the symptoms of pneumonia respond rapidly to antibiotic therapy, radiologically, the lesion still takes several days to resolve.

Klebsiella Pneumonia

Other than *S. pneumoniae*, *Klebsiella pneumoniae* is the only other organism that causes lobar pneumonia with any frequency. However, it accounts for no more than 1% of all cases of community-acquired pneumonia. The disease is commonly associated with alcoholism and is seen most frequently in middle-aged men, although persons with diabetes and chronic pulmonary disease are also at risk.

□ **Pathology:** The stages in *Klebsiella* pneumonia are not so well described as those in pneumococcal pneumonia, but the congestion and hemorrhage in the acute phase are less pronounced. *Klebsiella pneumoniae* has a thick, gelatinous capsule, a feature that is responsible for the characteristic **mucoid appearance** of the cut surface of the lung. Another distinctive feature of *Klebsiella* pneumonia is an increase in the size of the affected lobe, so that the fissure "bulges" toward the unaffected region. There is a tendency toward necrosis of tissue and abscess formation. A serious complication is **bronchopleural fistula**, which is a communication between the bronchial airway and the pleural space.

The onset of *Klebsiella* pneumonia is less dramatic than that of pneumococcal pneumonia, but the disease may be more dangerous. Before the antibiotic era, mortality rates in *Klebsiella* pneumonia ranged from 50% to 80%. Even with prompt antibiotic treatment, the mortality is still considerable. The prognosis is dependent on the age of the patient and the severity of the underlying disease.

Staphylococcal Pneumonia

Staphylococcal pneumonia is an uncommon community-acquired disease, accounting for only 1% of these bacterial pneumonias. However, pulmonary infection with *Staphylococcus aureus* is common as a superinfection after influenza and other viral respiratory tract infections. In the 1918 influenza pandemic, it was a major cause of death. Repeated episodes of staphylococcal pneumonia are encountered in patients with cystic fibrosis, owing to colonization of the bronchiectatic airways. Nosocomial staphylococcal pneumonia typically occurs in weakened, chronically ill patients, who are prone to aspiration, and in intubated patients.

□ **Pathology:** Similar to staphylococcal infection elsewhere, staphylococcal pneumonia is characterized by the development of abscesses. In contrast to the classic solitary lung abscess, the multiple foci of staphylococcal pneumonia produce many small abscesses. In infants, and to a lesser extent in adults, these may lead to **pneumatoceles**, thin-walled cystic spaces lined primarily by respiratory tissue. Pneumatoceles may expand rapidly and compress the surrounding lung, or they may rupture into the pleural cavity and cause a tension pneumothorax. It is thought that a pneumatocele develops when an abscess breaks into an airway, thereby allowing the expansion of the former by the pressure of inspired air.

Cavitation and pleural effusions are common complications of staphylococcal pneumonia, but empyema is infrequent.

Staphylococcal pneumonia requires aggressive antibiotic treatment, particularly in view of the numerous antibiotic-resistant strains of *S. aureus*.

Streptococcal Pneumonia

Pulmonary infection with group A *Streptococcus pyogenes* was identified among soldiers as early as the 19th century, and its pathological features were described during World War I. Streptococcal pneumonia typically follows viral respiratory tract infections and is thought to have been the common superinfection in the 1918–1919 influenza pandemic. It is distinctly unusual in a community setting but may be encountered occasionally in debilitated persons.

On gross examination, the lungs of patients who die of streptococcal pneumonia are heavy and display bloody edema. Dry consolidation (hepatization) is not a feature of the disease. Microscopically, the alveoli are filled with fibrin-containing fluid, but neutrophils are few. After prolonged pneumonia, alveolar necrosis may be encountered. Empyema is a common complication.

Patients with streptococcal pneumonia have abrupt fever, dyspnea, cough, chest pain, hemoptysis, and often cyanosis. Radiologically, the pattern is that of bronchopneumonia, and lobar consolidation is not seen. Intensive antibiotic therapy is indicated.

Streptococcal pneumonia in the newborn is usually caused by group B streptococci (*S. agalactiae*), a normal resident of the female genital tract. The symptoms are similar to those of the infantile respiratory distress syndrome. However, the infants are often full term, have severe toxemia, and may die within a few hours.

Legionella Pneumonia

In 1976, a mysterious respiratory ailment, which carried a high mortality, broke out at an American Legion convention in Philadelphia. Speculation about the cause of this epidemic centered on toxic environmental agents and even poisoning with paraquat. However, the responsible organism, *Legionella pneumophila*, was soon identified as a fastidious bacterium, with special requirements to grow in culture. Serological and histological studies revealed that several previously unrecognized epidemics of the same disease had occurred.

Legionella organisms thrive in aquatic environments, and outbreaks of pneumonia have been traced to contaminated water in air-conditioning cooling towers, evaporative condensers, and construction sites. Person-to-person spread does not occur, and there is no animal or human reservoir.

☐ **Pathology:** In fatal cases of *Legionella* pneumonia, multiple lobes exhibit a bronchopneumonia, with large confluent areas. On microscopic examination, the alveoli contain fibrin and inflammatory cells, with either neutrophils or macrophages predominating. Necrosis of inflammatory cells (leukocytoclasis) may be extensive. If the patient survives for several weeks, the exudate may show fibrous organization. One third of the cases have been complicated by empyema. The *Legionella* organisms are usually abundant within and without the phagocytic cells. They are difficult to visualize with conventional stains and are gram negative with the Brown and Hopp's stain.

☐ **Clinical Features:** The onset of *Legionella* pneumonia tends to be abrupt, with malaise, fever, muscle aches and pains, and, curiously, abdominal pain. A productive cough is usual, and chest pain due to pleuritis occasionally occurs. The chest radiograph is variable, but the most common pattern is the presence of focal alveolar infiltrates, which may be bilateral. The symptoms are usually less severe than the chest radiographs suggest. Mortality has been high (10% to 20%), especially in immunocompromised patients. Erythromycin is the treatment of choice.

Pontiac fever, also caused by *Legionella* species, is mainly a febrile illness, with slight respiratory symptoms and radiological abnormalities and a good prognosis. It has occurred in epidemics in office buildings and affects apparently healthy persons.

Opportunistic Pneumonia Caused by Gram-Negative Bacteria

Pneumonias caused by gram-negative organisms have become more common with the advent of immunosuppressive and cytotoxic therapies, treatment with broad-spectrum antibiotics, and the epidemic of acquired immunodeficiency syndrome (AIDS). The most common bacteria are *Escherichia coli* and *Pseudomonas aeruginosa*.

ESCHERICHIA COLI: Pneumonia caused by *E. coli* is a recognized complication of bacteremia after gastrointestinal and urogenital surgery, even in patients who are not immunosuppressed. It also is encountered in cancer patients given chemotherapy and in persons with chronic lung or heart disease. It occurs as a bronchopneumonia and responds poorly to treatment.

PSEUDOMONAS AERUGINOSA: Pseudomonas pneumonia is most often seen in immunocompromised persons, in patients with burns, and in those with cystic fibrosis. A history of antibiotic treatment of another infection is common. Often an infectious vasculitis, in which large numbers of organisms can be seen in the wall of a blood vessel, results in pulmonary infarction. *Pseudomonas* infection is common in cystic fibrosis, probably because of the favorable environment provided by the abnormal bronchial secretions. Antibiotic treatment of *Pseudomonas* pneumonia is often unsatisfactory.

Pneumonia Caused by Anaerobic Organisms

Many anaerobic organisms are normal commensals of the oral cavity, especially in patients with poor dental hygiene. These include certain streptococci, fusobacteria, and *Bacteroides* species. Aspiration of these organisms commonly occurs with swallowing disorders, as seen in stuporous alcoholics, anesthetized patients, and persons subject to seizures. Pulmonary infection with anaerobic organisms leads to necrotizing pneumonias, which are frequently complicated by lung abscesses. The most dramatic complication is gangrene of the lung, a result of thrombosis of a branch of the pulmonary artery and consequent infarction. This is regarded as a medical emergency and requires resection of the affected lung.

Psittacosis

Psittacosis is a pulmonary infection that results from the inhalation of ***Chlamydia psittaci*** *in dust contaminated with excreta from birds, usually pets and often parrots.* It is characterized by severe systemic symptoms, with fever, malaise, and muscle aches, but surprisingly few respiratory symptoms other than cough. Chest radiographs may be negative, and when abnormal, they show irregular consolidation and an interstitial pattern. The morphological patterns in most cases are unknown, but the disease is likely to be an interstitial pneumonia. In fatal cases, varying degrees of diffuse alveolar damage are present, together with edema, intra-alveolar pneumonia, and necrosis.

Mycoplasma

Mycoplasma pneumoniae causes the syndrome of **atypical pneumonia**. Although *Mycoplasma* lacks a cell wall and is, therefore, not a true bacterium, it is discussed here for the sake of convenience. In contrast to lobar pneumonia, the onset of atypical pneumonia is insidious, leukocytosis is absent or slight, and the course is prolonged. Respiratory symptoms may be minimal or severe, and the chest radiograph shows a patchy intra-alveolar pneumonia or an interstitial infiltrate. Mycoplasma pneumonia is only rarely fatal. The infection characteristically causes a bronchiolitis with a neutrophilic intraluminal exudate and an intense lymphoplasmacytic infiltrate in the bronchiolar wall (Fig. 12-18). The diagnosis is often established clinically based on serology with acute and convalescent titers. Erythromycin is an effective antibiotic.

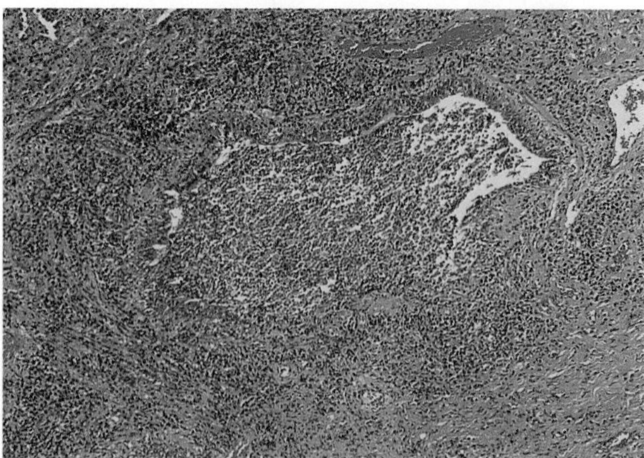

FIGURE *12-18*
Mycoplasma pneumonia. Chronic bronchiolitis with a neutrophilic luminal exudate.

Tuberculosis

No chest disease has had as dramatic a history as tuberculosis. Known since ancient Egypt, it became the scourge of 19th century Europe and North America. There has been an exponential decline in the prevalence of tuberculosis in the 20th century, and the advent of antituberculosis drugs has further diminished the impact of the disease. However, the recent resurgence of tuberculosis and the emergence of drug-resistant strains, particularly among patients with AIDS, has rekindled interest in this disease. The infection is discussed in detail in Chapter 9, and here we consider only the pulmonary pathology.

Tuberculosis represents infection with *Mycobacterium tuberculosis*, although atypical mycobacteria may mimic tuberculosis. The disease is divided into primary and secondary (or reactivation) tuberculosis.

PRIMARY TUBERCULOSIS: The disease is acquired from the initial exposure to *M. tuberculosis*, most commonly as a result of inhaling infected aerosols produced by coughing on the part of a person with cavitary tuberculosis. The inhaled organisms multiply in the alveoli, because the alveolar macrophages cannot readily kill the bacteria.

The Ghon complex is the first lesion of primary tuberculosis and consists of a peripheral parenchymal granuloma, often in the lower lobes, and a prominent, infected mediastinal lymph node (Fig. 12-19). On gross

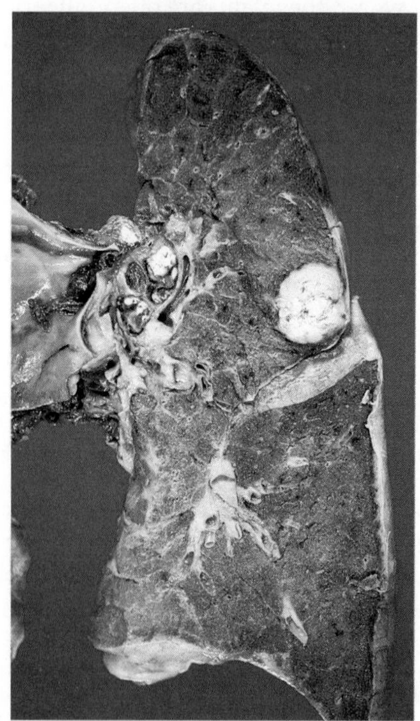

FIGURE *12-19*
Primary tuberculosis. A healed Ghon complex is represented by a subpleural nodule and involved hilar lymph nodes.

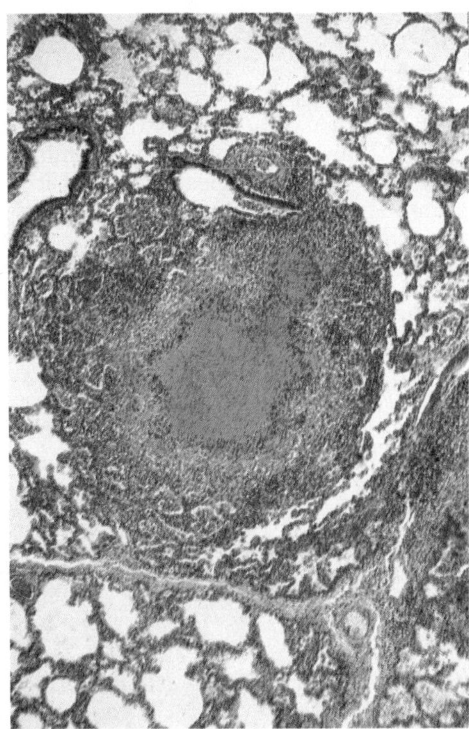

FIGURE 12-20
Necrotizing granuloma due to *M. tuberculosis*. A small tuberculous granuloma with conspicuous central caseation is present in the pulmonary parenchyma.

examination, the healed, subpleural Ghon nodule is 1 to 2 cm in diameter, well circumscribed, and centrally necrotic. In later stages, the lesion is fibrotic and calcified. Microscopically, a granuloma with central caseous necrosis (Fig. 12-20) shows varying degrees of fibrosis. The microscopic features of the draining hilar lymph nodes are similar to those of the peripheral parenchymal lesion.

The large majority (90% or more) of primary infections are asymptomatic, and the lesions remain localized and heal. In some instances, self-limited extension to the pleura, with secondary pleural effusion, occurs. However, less commonly primary tuberculosis does not remain limited but spreads to other parts of the lung **(progressive primary tuberculosis)**. This condition is usually seen in early childhood or in immunosuppressed adults. The initial lesion enlarges, producing necrotic areas up to 6 cm or more in greatest dimension. Central liquefaction results in cavities, which may expand to occupy most of the lower lobe. At the same time, the draining lymph nodes display similar histological changes. Erosion of a bronchus by the necrotizing process leads to further pulmonary dissemination of the disease.

SECONDARY TUBERCULOSIS: This stage represents either the reactivation of primary pulmonary tuberculosis or a new infection in a host previously sensitized by primary tuberculosis. The initial reaction to *M. tuberculosis* is different in secondary tuberculosis. A cellular immune response occurs after a latent interval and leads to the formation of many granulomas and extensive tissue necrosis. The apical and posterior segments of the upper lobes are most commonly involved, but the superior segment of the lower lobe is also often affected, and no part of the lung can be excluded. A diffuse, fibrotic, poorly defined lesion develops, which displays focal areas of caseous necrosis. Often these foci heal and calcify, but some erode into a bronchus, after which drainage of infectious material creates a tuberculous cavity.

Tuberculous cavities range in size from less than 1 cm in diameter to large, cystic areas that occupy almost the entire lung. Most cavities measure 3 to 10 cm in diameter and tend to be situated in the apices of the upper lobes (Fig. 12-21), although they may occur anywhere in the lung. The wall of the cavity is composed of an inner, thin, gray membrane encompassing soft necrotic nodules, a middle zone of granulation tissue, and an outer collagenous border. The lumen is filled with caseous material containing acid-fast bacilli. The tuberculous cavity often communicates freely with a bronchus, and release of the infectious material into the airways serves to disseminate the infection within the lung. The walls of healed tuberculous cavities eventually become fibrotic and calcified.

Secondary tuberculosis is associated with a number of complications:

- **Miliary tuberculosis** refers to the presence of multiple, small (size of millet seeds) tuberculous granulomas (Fig. 12-22) in many organs. It results from the hematogenous dissemination of the organisms, usually from secondary pulmonary tuberculosis, but occasionally from primary pulmonary tuberculosis or from other sites.
- **Hemoptysis** is caused by the erosion of small pulmonary arteries in the wall of a cavity. It may be severe enough to drown the patient in his own blood.
- **Bronchopleural fistula** occurs when a subpleural cavity ruptures into the pleural space. In turn, tuberculous empyema and pneumothorax result.

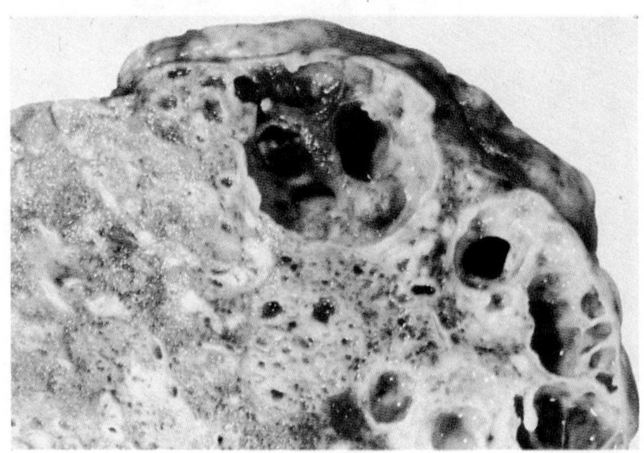

FIGURE 12-21
Cavitary tuberculosis. The apex of the left upper lobe shows tuberculous cavities surrounded by consolidated and fibrotic pulmonary parenchyma, which contains small tubercles.

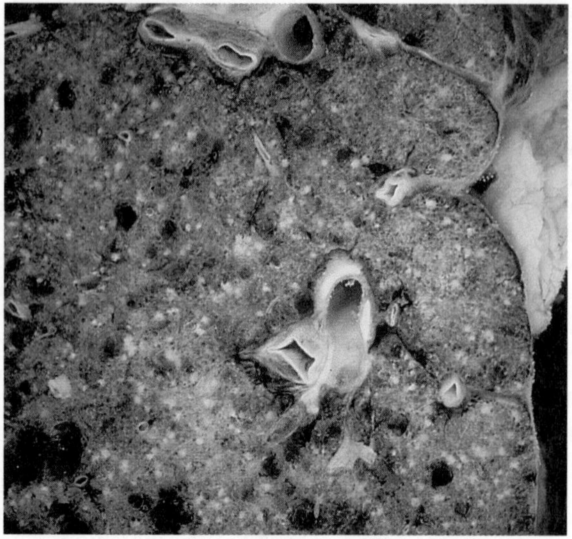

FIGURE 12-22
Miliary tuberculosis. Multiple millimeter-sized nodules are scattered throughout the lung parenchyma.

- **Tuberculous laryngitis** is a consequence of coughing up infectious material.
- **Intestinal tuberculosis** may follow the swallowing of the same tuberculous material.
- **Aspergilloma** is a fungal mass that follows superinfection of a persistent open cavity with *Aspergillus*; it may fill the entire cavity.

MYCOBACTERIUM AVIUM INTRACELLULARE (MAI) IN AIDS: In AIDS patients, the ability to form a granulomatous reaction may be impaired, and MAI pneumonia may be characterized by an extensive infiltrate of macrophages and innumerable acid-fast organisms (Fig. 12-23).

Actinomycosis

Actinomycosis is caused by infection with actinomycetes, and the usual pulmonary organism is *Actinomyces israelii*. Although actinomycetes resemble fungi in appearance, they are more closely related to bacteria. These gram-positive organisms, which normally inhabit the mouth and nose, infect the lung either by aspiration of oropharyngeal contents or by extension from an actinomycotic subdiaphragmatic abscess or liver abscess. The lung lesions consist of multiple interconnecting, small lung abscesses. The margin of an abscess is granulomatous, but the central necrotic area is purulent and contains colonies of organisms, which form "sulfur granules." The colonies consist of thin, branching, filamentous gram-positive bacteria. Clubbed basophilic filaments are noted at the margins of the colonies, which are visible to the naked eye as small yellow particles (sulfur granules). The abscesses invade the pleura and produce bronchopulmonary fistulas and empyema. They may also invade the chest wall.

Nocardia

Nocardia is a gram-positive bacillus that causes an acute progressive or chronic bacterial pneumonia. It is frequently encountered in immunocompromised persons, particularly patients with lymphomas, neutropenia, chronic granulomatous disease of childhood, and pulmonary alveolar proteinosis. *Nocardia asteroides* is the most common species to cause pneumonia. Histologically, the lungs show abscesses (Fig. 12-24A), which may have granulomatous features in chronic infections. The organisms are delicate, beaded, thin filaments, which branch mostly at right angles (see Fig. 12-24B). The highly branching pattern may resemble "Chinese characters." In

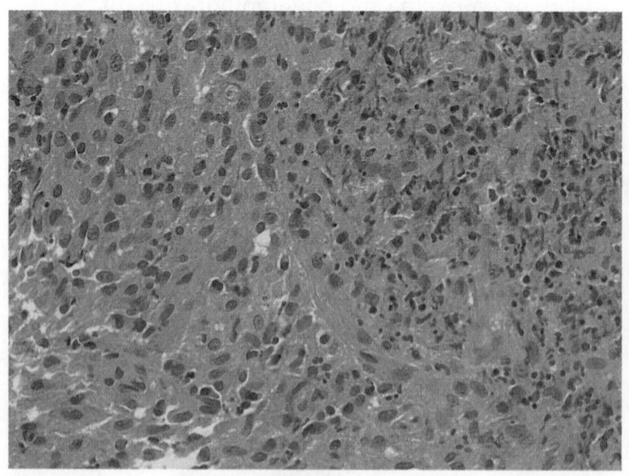

A

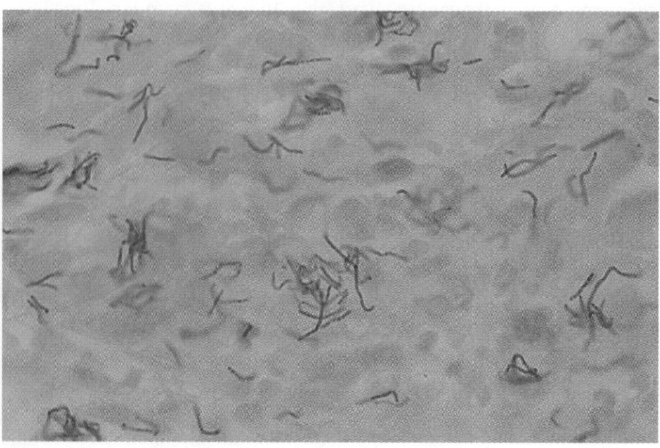

B

FIGURE 12-23
***Mycobacterium avium-intracellulare* pneumonia in AIDS. *(A)* The pneumonia is characterized by an extensive infiltrate of macrophages. *(B)* The Ziehl–Neelson stain shows numerous acid-fast organisms.**

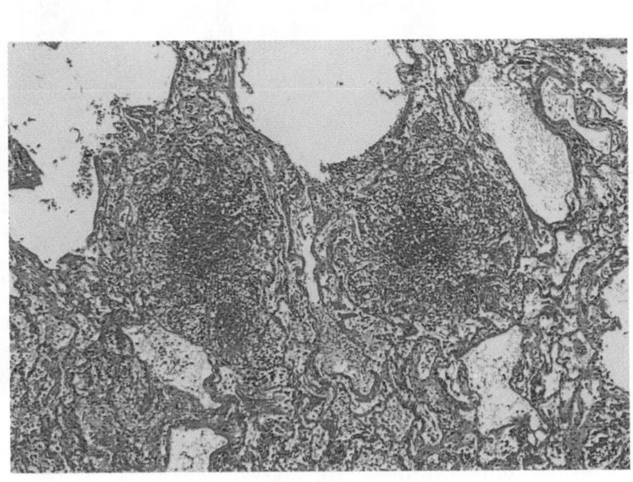

A

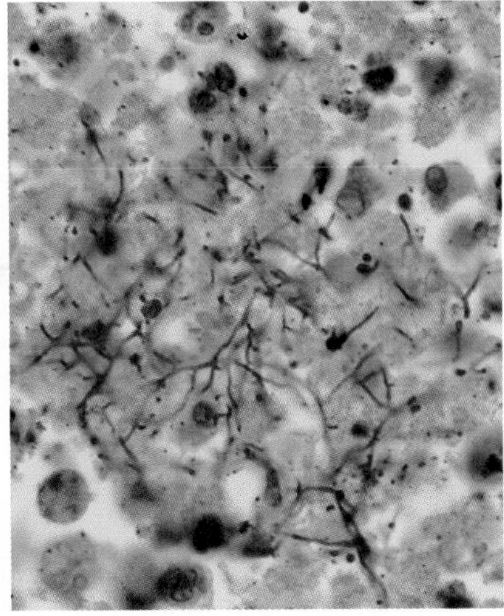

B

FIGURE *12-24*
Nocardiosis. *(A)* This lung shows abscesses consisting of focal collections of acute inflammation. *(B)* The organisms are thin, filamentous, branching bacteria (Gomori methenamine silver).

tissue sections, the organisms are best seen with the Gomori methenamine silver stain (see Fig. 12-24B) and a gram stain such as Brown and Brenn or Brown–Hopps. They are also weakly acid fast.

Fungal Infections

Histoplasmosis

Histoplasmosis is a disease of the midwestern and southeastern regions of the United States, particularly the Mississippi and Ohio valleys. The disease is caused by inhalation of *Histoplasma capsulatum* in infected dust, commonly from bird droppings.

☐ **Pathology:** Histoplasmosis has many clinical and pathological similarities to tuberculosis. The great majority of infections are asymptomatic and result in lesions comparable to the Ghon complex, including a parenchymal granuloma and similar lesions in the draining lymph nodes. The granulomas are particularly prone to calcify, often with a concentric laminar pattern. The acute phase, in which numerous organisms are seen within macrophages, is followed by granulomatous inflammation, with central areas of necrosis in the lesions. The granulomas heal by fibrosis and calcification, although the central necrotic areas may persist.

In a few cases, the pulmonary lesion progresses or reactivates, which leads to a progressive fibrotic and necrotic lesion that closely resembles reactivation tuberculosis. However, the lesion of histoplasmosis has a more fibrotic appearance than does that of tuberculosis, and cavitation is less common. The reason for progression is not known, although a large infective dose and a poor host response are usually considered to be responsible. Immunocompromised persons are at particular risk for dissemination of *Histoplasma* within the lungs and spread to other organs.

Coccidioidomycosis

Coccidioidomycosis, caused by the inhalation of spores of *Coccidioides immitis*, was originally known as San Joaquin Valley fever, after the location where the disease has been endemic for many years. However, the infection is widely spread throughout the southwestern part of the United States and shares many of the clinical and pathological features of histoplasmosis and tuberculosis. In most instances, the lesions are limited to a peripheral parenchymal granuloma, with or without lymph node granulomas. In a few instances, the lesion is progressive, although the rate of progression is slow. Immunocompromised persons may experience rapid progression of the disease, with release of endospores into the lung, in which case the tissue reaction may be purulent as well as granulomatous.

Cryptococcosis

Cryptococcosis results from the inhalation of spores of *Cryptococcus neoformans*, an organism frequently encountered in pigeon droppings. The pulmonary lesions range from small parenchymal granulomas to several large granulomatous nodules, pneumonic consolidation, and even cavitation. Most serious cases of pulmonary cryptococcosis occur in immunocompromised persons, in whom the organisms proliferate extensively within alveolar spaces, with little tissue reaction.

North American Blastomycosis

Blastomycosis is an uncommon condition caused by *Blastomyces dermatitidis*. It is concentrated in the basins of the Missouri, Mississippi, and Ohio rivers in the United States and in southern Manitoba and northwestern Ontario in Canada. The clinical and pathological features resemble those associated with the fungi mentioned earlier. The infection presents as a lesion resembling a Ghon complex or as a progressive pneumonitis. Unlike the tuberculous Ghon complex, the focal lesion of blastomycosis exhibits central necrosis with a purulent reaction, surrounded by granulomatous inflammation.

Aspergillosis

Infection of the lungs by *Aspergillus* species, usually *A. niger* or *A. fumigatus*, can occur under a number of circumstances.

- **Invasive aspergillosis:** This is the most serious manifestation of *Aspergillus* infection, occurring almost exclusively as an opportunistic infection in persons with compromised immunity, usually because of cytotoxic therapy or AIDS. The lungs exhibit patchy, multifocal areas of consolidation and occasionally cavities. Extensive blood vessel invasion (usually arterial [Fig. 12-25]) results in occlusion, thrombosis, and infarction of lung tissue. Invasive aspergillosis is a fulminant pulmonary infection that is not amenable to therapy.
- **Aspergilloma ("fungus ball" or mycetoma):** *Aspergillus* species may grow in preexisting cavities, such as those caused by tuberculosis or bronchiectasis. They proliferate to form a fungus ball within the cavities (Fig. 12-26). Radiological examination shows a large mass within a cavity that is separated from the wall by air. In most instances, the fungus ball is clinically unrecognized and represents merely an interesting radiological finding. However, sometimes it becomes clinically evident, the most important symptom being hemoptysis, owing either to the underlying condition, or less commonly, to fungal infection of the cavity wall.
- **Allergic bronchopulmonary aspergillosis (ABPA):** Certain asthmatic persons demonstrate an unusual immunological reaction to *Aspergillus* characterized by (1) transient pulmonary infiltrates on chest radiographs, (2) eosinophilia of blood and sputum, (3) skin sensitivity and serum precipitins to *A. fumigatus*, and (4) increased levels of serum IgE. Radiologically, thickened bronchial walls and mucous plugs in the bronchi are visualized. Morphologically, proximal (central) bronchiectasis, involving segmental bronchi and the next two to four orders of subsegmental bronchi, is almost invariable. Histologically, the lungs show bronchial and bronchiolar mucous plugs, with infiltrates of eosinophils (Fig. 12-27A,B). Bronchocentric granulomatosis and eosinophilic pneumonia may be present. The bronchial mucus may contain septate, branching fungal hyphae, with 45 degree–angle branching. Interestingly, the peripheral bronchial tree is spared. Clinically, patients with ABPA have wheezing, chest pain, and cough, commonly productive of thick mucous plugs. The administration of systemic corticosteroids usually controls the acute episode.

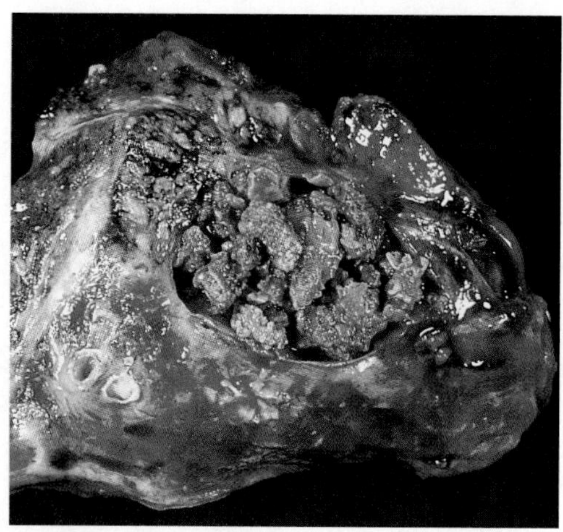

FIGURE *12-26*
Aspergillus fungus ball. The lung contains a cavity filled with a fungus ball.

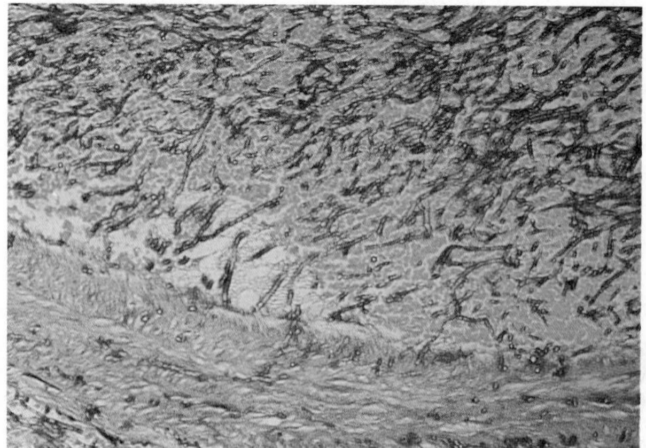

FIGURE *12-25*
Invasive pulmonary aspergillosis. A branch of the pulmonary artery shows fungal hyphae in the wall and within the lumen.

Pneumocystis carinii

First described as "plasma cell pneumonia," pulmonary infection with *Pneumocystis carinii* was identified in malnourished infants at the end of World War II. The disease came into prominence in North America with the advent of renal transplantation and immunosuppression. Since then, it has been recognized as a major pulmonary complication of chemotherapy for malignant disease. **It is also the most frequent cause of infectious pneumonia in patients with AIDS.**

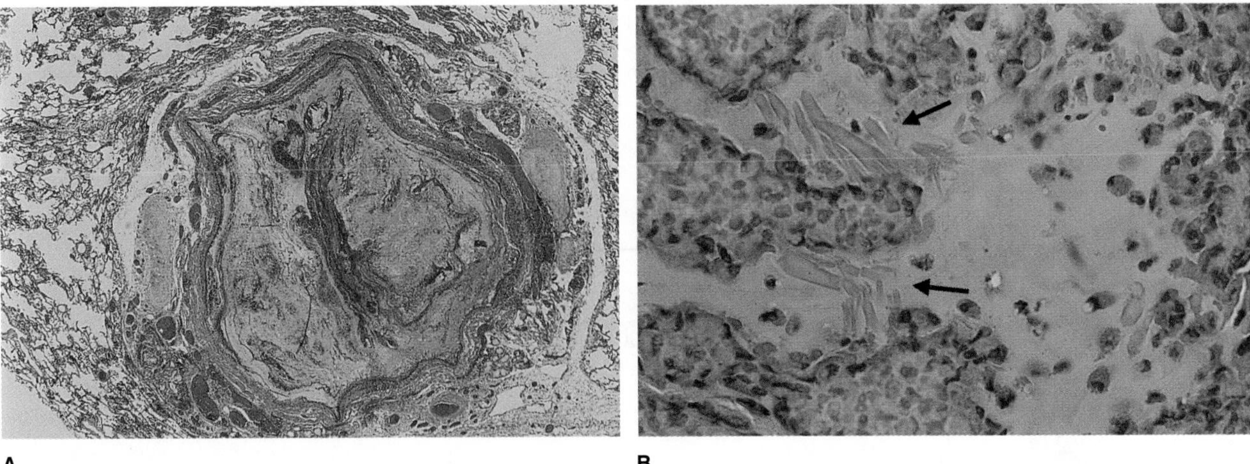

A B

FIGURE 12-27
Allergic bronchopulmonary aspergillosis. *(A)* A dilated bronchus is filled with a mucous plug, which has dense layers of eosinophilic infiltrates. *(B)* Higher magnification shows numerous eosinophils and Charcot–Leyden crystals *(arrows)*.

☐ **Pathology:** The classic lesion of *Pneumocystis* pneumonia comprises an interstitial infiltrate of plasma cells and lymphocytes, diffuse alveolar damage (see later), and hyperplasia of type II pneumocytes. The alveoli are filled with a characteristic foamy exudate, the organisms appearing as small bubbles in a background of proteinaceous exudate (Fig. 12-28A). With silver impregnation, the cysts appear as round or indented ("crescent moon") bodies, 5 μm in diameter (see Fig. 12-28B). A darkly stained focus represents focal thickening of the capsule. After sporozoites develop within the cyst, it ruptures and assumes an indented shape. The sporozoites develop into trophozoites, which may be recognized with stains such as Giemsa in cytological specimens; they are very difficult to see in routine histological sections. Granulomatous inflammation in *Pneumocystis* pneumonia is rare but may be seen in up to 5% of lung biopsies from HIV-infected patients.

☐ **Clinical Features:** Clinically and radiologically, the presentation of *Pneumocystis* pneumonia is variable. At one extreme, the symptoms are minimal, whereas at the other, there is rapidly progressive respiratory failure. In HIV-infected patients, thin-walled cysts may develop and predispose to pneumothorax. The diagnosis is made by identifying the organism with a variety of procedures including sputum examination, bronchoalveolar lavage, transbronchial biopsy, needle aspiration of the lung, and open-lung biopsy. Treatment is with trimethoprim–sulfamethoxazole or pentamidine.

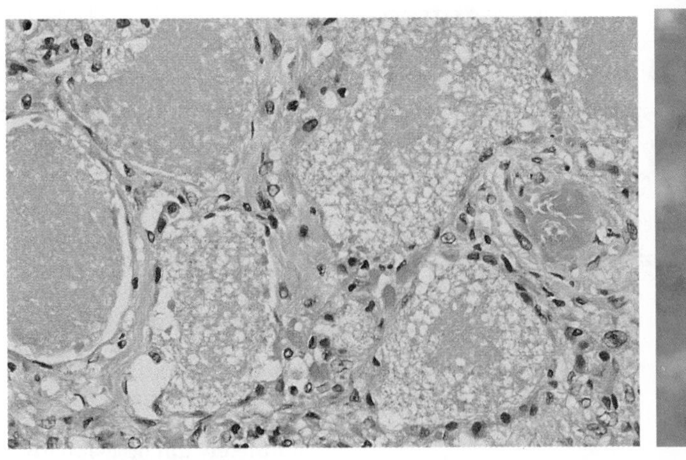

A

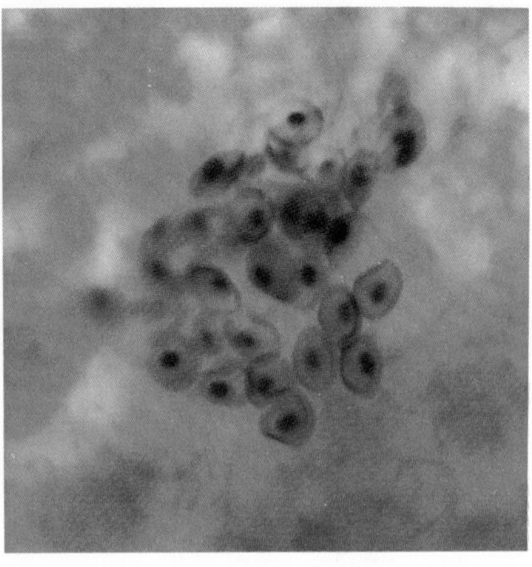

B

FIGURE 12-28
***Pneumocystis carinii* pneumonia. *(A)* The alveoli are filled with a foamy exudate, and the interstitium is thickened and contains a chronic inflammatory infiltrate. *(B)* A centrifuged bronchoalveolar lavage specimen impregnated with silver shows a cluster of *Pneumocystis* cysts.**

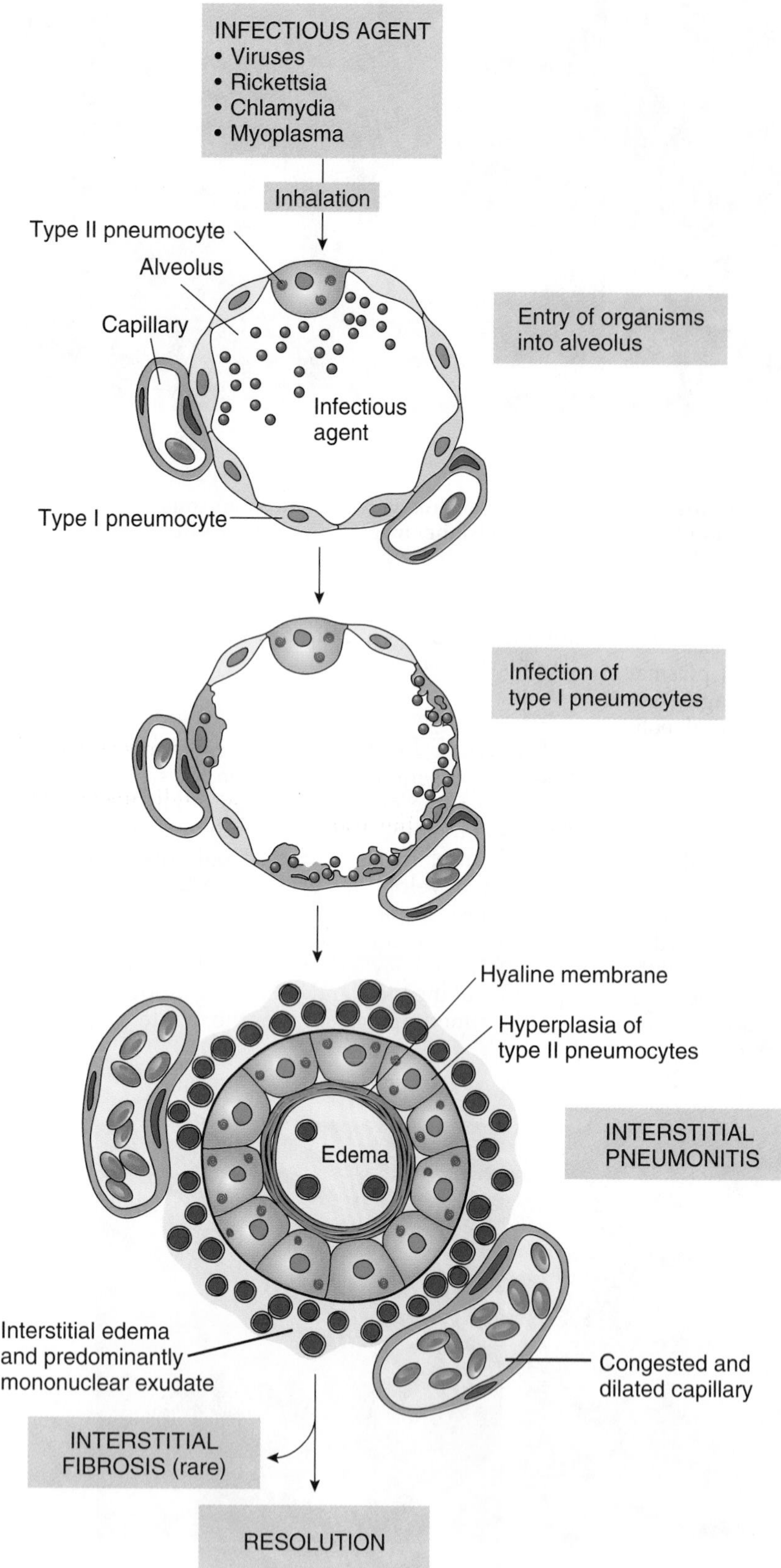

FIGURE *12-29*
Pathogenesis of interstitial fibrosis. Although interstitial pneumonia is most commonly caused by viruses, other organisms also may cause significant interstitial inflammation. Type I cells are the most sensitive to damage, and loss of their integrity leads to intra-alveolar edema. The proteinaceous exudate and cell debris form hyaline membranes, and type II cells multiply to line the alveoli. Interstitial inflammation is characterized mainly by mononuclear cells. The disease generally resolves completely but occasionally progresses to interstitial fibrosis.

Viral Pneumonia

Viral infections of the pulmonary parenchyma produce diffuse alveolar damage and interstitial (rather than alveolar) pneumonia. Viral bronchiolitis was discussed earlier. Initially, viral infections affect the alveolar epithelium and result in a mononuclear infiltrate in the interstitium of the lung (Fig. 12-29). Necrosis of type I epithelial cells and the formation of hyaline membranes result in an appearance that is indistinguishable from diffuse alveolar damage from other causes. In some instances, the alveolar damage may be indolent, in which case the disease is characterized by hyperplasia of type II pneumocytes and interstitial inflammation. This appearance contrasts with that of most bacterial infections, in which an intra-alveolar exudate predominates and in which the interstitium is only incidentally involved (Fig. 12-30).

Cytomegalovirus produces a characteristic interstitial pneumonia. Initially described in infants, it is now well recognized in immunocompromised persons. This viral pneumonia features an intense interstitial infiltrate of lymphocytes. The alveoli are lined by type II cells, which have regenerated to cover the epithelial defect left by necrosis of type I cells. The infected alveolar cells are very large (cytomegaly) and display a single, dark, basophilic nuclear inclusion with a peripheral halo and multiple indistinct cytoplasmic, basophilic inclusions (Fig. 12-31).

Measles infection, which involves both the airways and the parenchyma, is characterized by the presence of very large (100 μm across) multinucleated giant cells, which have nuclear inclusions and large eosinophilic cytoplasmic inclusions (Fig. 12-32). Although interstitial pneumonia is a well-characterized complication of measles, it is rarely fatal, except in immunocompromised, previously unexposed persons.

Varicella infection (both chickenpox and herpes zoster) produces disseminated, focally necrotic lesions

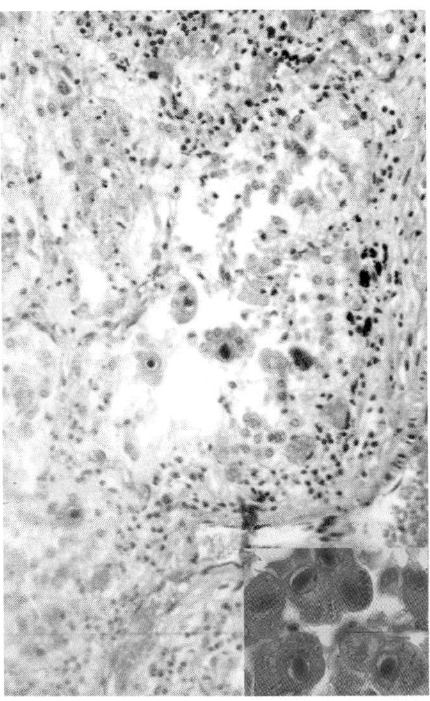

FIGURE 12-31
Cytomegalovirus pneumonitis. The infected alveolar cells are enlarged and display the typical dark-blue nuclear inclusions. *Inset:* A higher-power view shows infected alveolar cells, which display a single basophilic nuclear inclusion with a perinuclear halo and multiple, indistinct, basophilic, cytoplasmic inclusions.

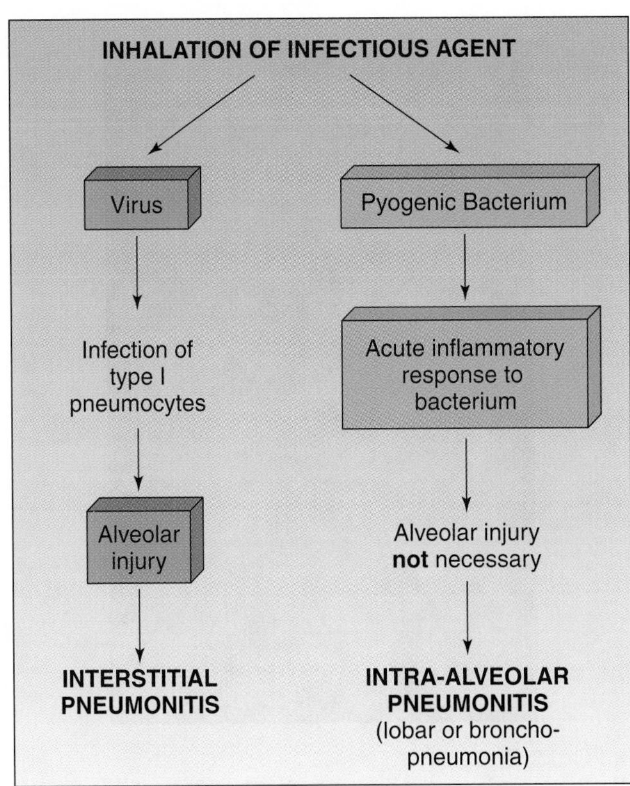

FIGURE 12-30
Pathogenesis of interstitial and intra-alveolar pneumonitis.

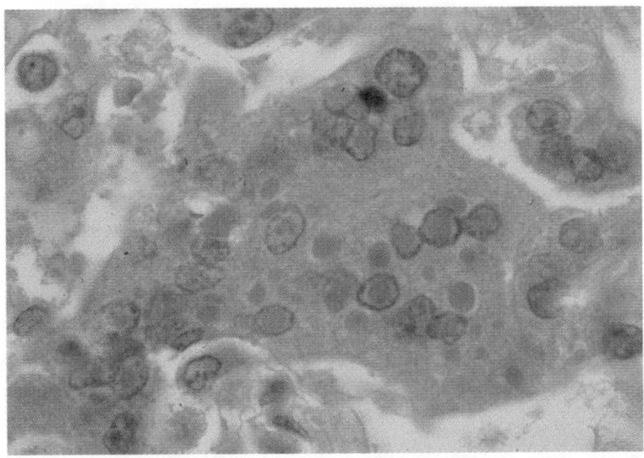

FIGURE 12-32
Measles pneumonitis. This multinucleated giant cell shows single, eosinophilic, refractile inclusions within each of the nuclei, as well as multiple, irregular, eosinophilic, cytoplasmic inclusions.

in the lung, as well as interstitial pneumonia. Pulmonary involvement is usually asymptomatic, except in immunocompromised hosts, in whom it may be fatal. The viral inclusions are nuclear, eosinophilic, and refractile, and are surrounded by a clear halo. Multinucleation can occur.

Herpes simplex can cause a necrotizing tracheobronchitis as well as diffuse alveolar damage. The viral inclusions are identical to those seen in varicella infection.

Adenovirus pneumonia results in a necrotizing bronchiolitis and bronchopneumonia. It can cause two types of inclusions: eosinophilic nuclear inclusions similar to those seen in herpes infections and smudge cells with indistinct, basophilic, nuclear inclusions (Fig. 12-33).

Lung Abscess

Lung abscess, recognized since the time of Hippocrates, is a localized accumulation of pus accompanied by the destruction of pulmonary parenchyma, including alveoli, airways, and blood vessels.

□ **Pathogenesis:** The most common cause of pulmonary abscess is aspiration, often in the setting of depressed consciousness. The large majority (>90%) of cases of lung abscess reflect the aspiration of anaerobic bacteria from the oropharynx. The infections are typically polymicrobial, with fusiform bacteria and *Bacteroides* species often isolated. Other organisms encountered in lung abscesses caused by aspiration include *S. aureus, K. pneumoniae, S. pneumoniae,* and *Nocardia.*

The deposition of sufficient bacteria to produce a lung abscess requires two conditions. A large number of anaerobic bacteria must be present in the oral flora, a situation encountered in persons with poor oral hygiene or periodontal disease. In addition, the cough reflex or tracheobronchial clearance must be impaired. Not surprisingly, alcoholism is the single most common condition predisposing to lung abscess. Persons with drug overdose, epileptics, and neurologically impaired patients are also at risk. Other causes of lung abscess include necrotizing pneumonias, bronchial obstruction, infected pulmonary emboli, penetrating trauma, and extension of infection from tissues adjacent to the lung.

□ **Pathology:** Lung abscesses mostly range from 2 to 6 cm in diameter, and 10% to 20% have multiple cavities, usually after a necrotizing pneumonia or a shower of septic pulmonary emboli. The right side of the lung is more prone than is the left to the development of a lung abscess, because the right main bronchus follows the direction of the trachea more closely at its bifurcation. Acute lung abscesses are not well separated from the surrounding pulmonary parenchyma. They exhibit abundant polymorphonuclear leukocytes and, depending on the age of the lesion, variable numbers of macrophages. Debris derived from necrotic tissue may be evident. The abscess is surrounded by hemorrhage, fibrin, and inflammatory cells. As the abscess ages, a fibrous wall forms around the margin. Lung abscesses differ from those elsewhere in their capacity for spontaneous drainage. The cavity thus formed contains air, necrotic debris, and inflammatory exudate (Fig. 12-34), creating a fluid level that is easily visualized radiographically. The lining of the cavity becomes covered with regenerating squamous epithelium. In an old abscess, ciliated respiratory epithelium may invade the wall, making the cavity difficult to distinguish from bronchiectasis.

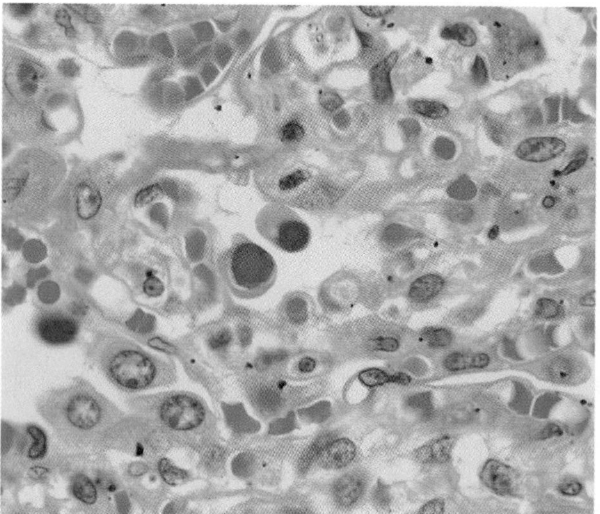

FIGURE *12-33*
Adenovirus pneumonia. The "smudge" cell in the center consists of a smudgy basophilic nuclear inclusion.

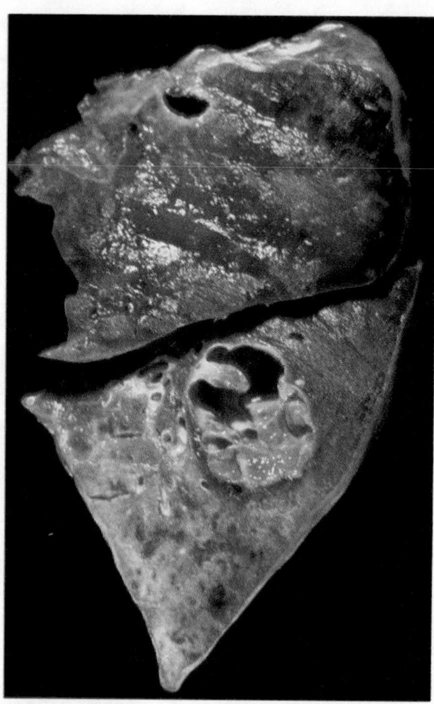

FIGURE *12-34*
Pulmonary abscess. A large, cystic abscess contains a purulent exudate and is contained by a fibrous wall. Pneumonia is present in the surrounding pulmonary parenchyma.

Clinical Features: Almost all patients with lung abscess are first seen with cough and fever. One of the most characteristic symptoms is the production of large amounts of foul-smelling sputum. Many patients complain of pleuritic chest pain, and 20% develop hemoptysis.

The differential diagnosis of lung abscess includes cancer of the lung and cavitary tuberculosis. Indeed, cancer is now a more common cause of cavitation than is lung abscess. About half of all cases of cavitation due to cancer reflect necrosis of the tumor; the others follow obstruction of the bronchi and subsequent infection. A tuberculous cavity only rarely displays the air–fluid level characteristic of a lung abscess.

Complications of lung abscess include rupture into the pleural space, with resulting empyema and severe hemoptysis. The abscess may drain into a bronchus, with subsequent dissemination of the infection to other parts of the lung. Despite vigorous antimicrobial therapy, principally directed against anaerobic bacteria, the mortality of lung abscess remains in the range of 5% to 10%.

DIFFUSE ALVEOLAR DAMAGE (ADULT RESPIRATORY DISTRESS SYNDROME)

Diffuse alveolar damage (DAD) refers to a nonspecific pattern of reaction to injury of alveolar epithelial and endothelial cells from a variety of acute insults (Table 12-1). The clinical counterpart of severe DAD is the adult respiratory distress syndrome (ARDS). In this disorder, a patient with apparently normal lungs sustains pulmonary damage and then develops rapidly progressive respiratory failure. The condition reflects decreased lung compliance (usually requiring mechanical ventilation), hypoxemia, and extensive radiological opacities in both lungs ("white-out"). The overall mortality of ARDS is more than 50%, and in patients older than 60 years, it is as high as 90%.

Pathogenesis: DAD is a final common pathway of pathological changes caused by a large variety of insults (see Table 12-1). These include respiratory tract infections, sepsis, shock, aspiration of gastric contents, inhalation of toxic gases, near-drowning, radiation pneumonitis, and a large assortment of drugs and other chemicals. Some patients have an idiopathic form of DAD in which no etiology can be found. Although these conditions are quite diverse, they are all capable of injuring the epithelial and endothelial cells of the alveoli, thereby producing DAD. **Importantly, the precise etiology of DAD cannot be determined from the morphological appearance of the lung alone, unless a specific infectious agent is identified.**

Injury to endothelial cells allows the leakage of protein-rich fluid from the alveolar capillaries into the interstitial space (Fig. 12-35). The destruction of type I pneumocytes permits the exudation of fluid into the alveolar spaces, where the deposition of plasma proteins results in the formation of fibrin-containing precipitates (hyaline membranes) on the injured alveolar walls (Fig. 12-36). Although it is denuded of type I pneumocytes, the alveolar basement membrane remains intact and functions as a scaffold for type II pneumocytes, whose proliferation replaces the normal epithelial lining of the alveoli. In response to the cell injury of DAD, inflammatory cells accumulate in the interstitial space.

If the patient survives the acute phase of ARDS, fibroblasts proliferate in the interstitial space and deposit collagen in the alveolar walls (Fig. 12-37). In those patients who recover completely, the lesions may heal, with resorption of the alveolar exudate and hyaline membranes and restitution of the normal alveolar epithelium. Fibroblastic proliferation ceases, and the extra collagen is metabolized. It is well documented that patients with ARDS who recover regain normal pulmonary function. In those patients who do not recover, DAD can progress to end-stage fibrosis; remodeling of the lung architecture produces multiple cyst-like spaces throughout the lung ("honeycomb lung"). These spaces are separated from each other by fibrous tissue and lined by type II pneumocytes, bronchiolar epithelium, or squamous cells.

The pathogenesis of DAD is not entirely clear. It is thought that activation of the complement system (e.g., by endotoxin in the case of gram-negative septicemia) results in the sequestration of neutrophils in the marginating pool. Only a small proportion, perhaps one third, of neutrophils actively circulate in the blood; most of the remainder are found in the lung. Normally, the neutrophils cause no damage, but after activation by complement, they release oxygen radicals and hydrolytic enzymes, which damage the capillary endothelium of the lung. The role of polymorphonuclear leukocytes in the pathogenesis of DAD is still debated, because ARDS has been reported in severely neutropenic patients.

In DAD produced by the inhalation of toxic gases or near-drowning, the damage occurs primarily at the alveolar epithelial surface. The alveolar epithelial junctions are usually very tight; damage to the epithelium disrupts these junctions, permitting exudation of fluid and proteins from the interstitium into the alveolar spaces. Endothelial damage may or may not occur in DAD caused by inhalation of toxic substances, but the sequence of events is similar to that resulting from endothelial damage after shock or septicemia.

TABLE *12-1* Important Causes of the Adult Respiratory Distress Syndrome

Nonthoracic trauma	**Drugs and therapeutic agents**
Shock due to any cause	Heroin
Fat embolism	Oxygen
	Radiation
Infection	Paraquat
Gram-negative septicemia	Cytotoxic
Other bacterial infections	
Viral infections	
Aspiration	
Near drowning	
Aspiration of gastric contents	

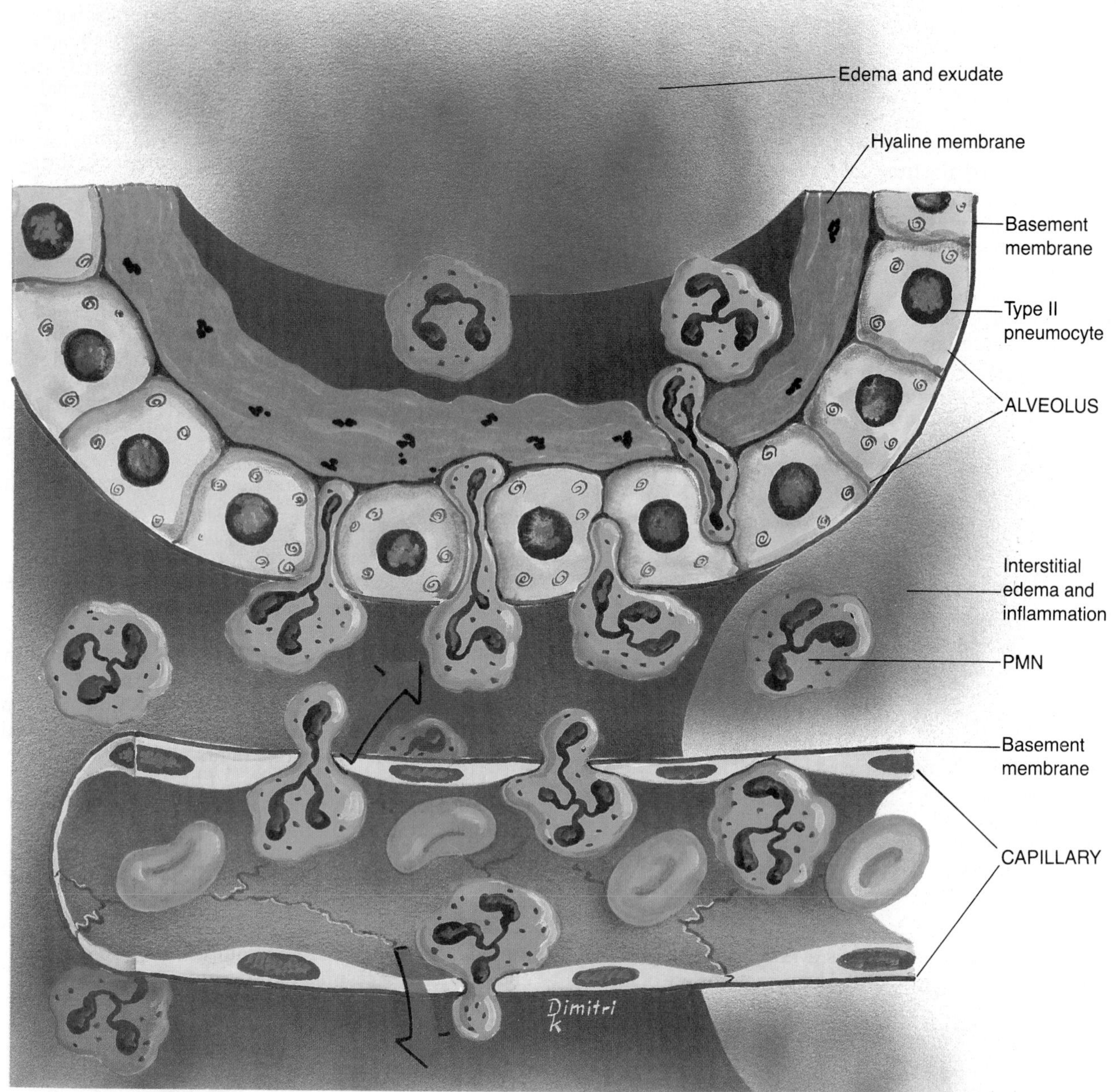

FIGURE 12-35
Diffuse alveolar damage (adult respiratory distress syndrome, ARDS). In ARDS, type I cells die as a result of diffuse alveolar damage. Intra-alveolar edema follows, after which there is formation of hyaline membranes composed of proteinaceous exudate and cell debris. In the acute phase, the lungs are markedly congested and heavy. Type II cells multiply to line the alveolar surface. Interstitial inflammation is characteristic. The lesion may heal completely or progress to interstitial fibrosis.

☐ **Pathology:** The evolution of DAD can be divided into two periods, the initial exudative phase, followed by an organizing phase.

The exudative phase of DAD develops during the first week after the pulmonary insult and features edema, the exudation of plasma proteins, the accumulation of inflammatory cells, and hyaline membranes (see Fig. 12-36). The earliest manifestation of alveolar injury is evidenced by electron microscopy, which reveals degenerative changes in both endothelial cells and type I pneumocytes. This is followed by the sloughing of type I cells and the appearance of denuded basement membranes. Interstitial and alveolar edema is prominent by the first day, but soon recedes. Hyaline membranes begin to appear by

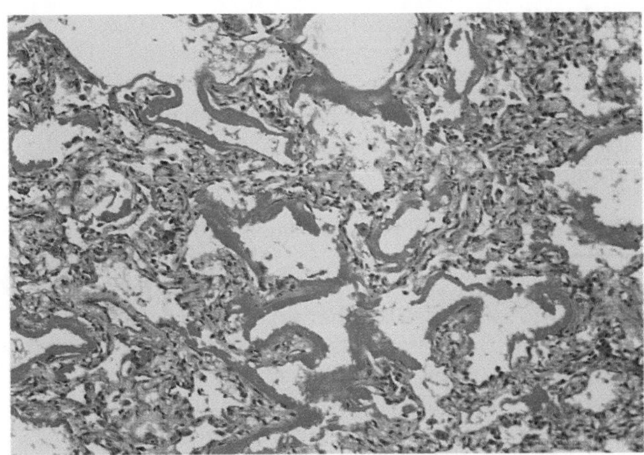

FIGURE 12-36
Diffuse alveolar damage, acute (exudative) phase. The alveolar septa are thickened by edema and a sparse inflammatory infiltrate. The alveoli are lined by eosinophilic hyaline membranes.

the second day and are the most conspicuous morphological feature of the exudative phase after 4 to 5 days. These eosinophilic, glassy "membranes" consist of precipitated plasma proteins and the cytoplasmic and nuclear debris from sloughed epithelial cells. Interstitial inflammation, consisting of lymphocytes, plasma cells, and macrophages, is apparent early and reaches its maximum in about a week. Toward the end of the first week, and persisting during the subsequent organizing stage, regularly spaced, cuboidal type II pneumocytes become arrayed along the denuded alveolar septa. The alveolar capillaries and pulmonary arterioles may exhibit fibrin thrombi. In fatal cases of DAD, the lungs are heavy, edematous, and virtually airless.

The organizing phase of DAD, beginning about a week after the initial injury, is marked by the proliferation of fibroblasts within the alveolar walls (see Fig. 12-37). During this phase, interstitial inflammation and proliferated type II pneumocytes persist, but hyaline membranes are no longer formed. Alveolar macrophages digest the remnants of hyaline membranes and other cellular debris. Loose fibrosis thickens the alveolar septa. Whereas this fibrosis resolves in mild cases, in severe ones it progresses to restructuring of the pulmonary parenchyma and cyst formation.

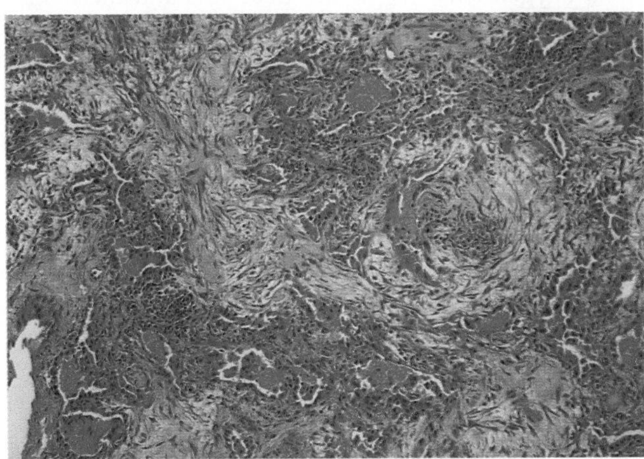

FIGURE 12-37
Diffuse alveolar damage, organizing phase. Fibroblasts and nascent connective tissue are present within the septa and alveoli.

☐ **Clinical Features:** Patients destined to develop ARDS have a symptom-free interval for a few hours after the initial insult, after which tachypnea and dyspnea mark the onset of the syndrome. At this time, arterial hypoxemia and decreased P_{CO_2} are evident on measurement of blood gases. As ARDS progresses, the dyspnea worsens, and the patient becomes cyanotic. Diffuse, bilateral interstitial and alveolar infiltrates are noted radiologically. The arterial hypoxemia at this stage cannot be reversed by simply increasing the oxygen tension of inspired air, and mechanical ventilation becomes necessary. In fatal cases, the combination of increasing tachypnea and decreasing tidal volume eventuates in alveolar hypoventilation, progressive hypoxemia, and increasing P_{CO_2}.

Patients who survive ARDS may recover normal pulmonary function, but in severe cases are left with scarred lungs, respiratory dysfunction, and, in some instances, pulmonary hypertension.

Specific Causes of Diffuse Alveolar Damage

Oxygen

During World War II, aviators were required to breathe increased concentrations of oxygen at high altitude. To study possible pulmonary damage, animal experiments were carried out and demonstrated harmful effects of oxygen on the lung. Later observations with patients who were administered high levels of oxygen for respiratory problems documented the development of DAD. Pulmonary lesions have developed in patients with long-term exposure to as little as 28% oxygen, but it is usually safe to breathe 40% to 60% oxygen for long periods. The mechanism of oxygen toxicity is thought to be related to increased production of activated oxygen species in the lung.

Shock

Adult respiratory distress syndrome often follows shock from any cause, including gram-negative sepsis, trauma, or blood loss, in which case, the pulmonary condition is colloquially referred to as "shock lung." Although the pathogenesis of DAD associated with shock is poorly understood, it is likely multifactorial. Tissue necrosis in organs damaged by trauma or by ischemia may lead to the release of vasoactive peptides into the circulation, which enhance vascular permeability in the lung. Disseminated intravascular coagulation may damage alveolar capillaries, and fat emboli from bone fractures may obstruct the distal capillary bed of the lung. The pathogenesis of endothelial cell injury in endotoxic shock is discussed in Chapter 7.

Aspiration

The aspiration of gastric contents introduces acid, with a pH less than 3.0, into the alveoli. As a result of the severe chemical injury to the alveolar lining cells, DAD develops. In near-drowning, the aspiration of water leads to pulmonary injury and the clinical picture of ARDS.

Drug-Induced Diffuse Alveolar Damage

The long list of drugs that cause DAD includes most chemotherapeutic agents. The best known is bleomycin, but other frequently used agents, such as 1,3-bis-(2-chloroethyl)-1-nitrosourea (BCNU), methotrexate, 5-fluorouracil, busulfan, and cyclophosphamide, are known causes. Thus, as a general rule, all cytotoxic agents should be suspected as a cause of DAD. With bleomycin, an imprecise dose-dependent relation has been demonstrated, but such an effect is not apparent with most other drugs.

Bizarre, atypical, hyperchromatic nuclei in type II cells are particularly common in cases of alveolar damage from chemotherapeutic agents (Fig. 12-38). The damage progresses despite discontinuation of the offending agent, although it may be modified by the administration of corticosteroids. Progressive interstitial fibrosis occurs, usually with retention of the lung structure. Methotrexate differs from the other chemotherapeutic agents in that it may sometimes cause a hypersensitivity reaction in the lung. Under these circumstances, DAD is reversible after the drug is discontinued. The lesions that reflect hypersensitivity are characterized by granulomatous inflammation and occasionally vasculitis.

Drugs other than chemotherapeutic agents also cause DAD. Examples are nitrofurantoin, amiodarone, and penicillamine.

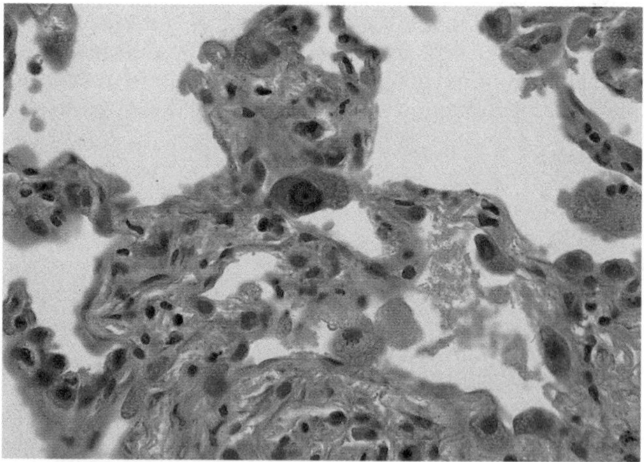

FIGURE *12-38*
Diffuse alveolar damage, associated with busulfan treatment. An atypical pneumocyte was encountered in a case of organizing diffuse alveolar damage (DAD) associated with busulfan therapy.

Radiation Pneumonitis

Radiation pneumonitis occurs in two forms, acute DAD and chronic pulmonary fibrosis. Alveolar injury is believed to be caused by the generation of oxygen radicals through the radiolysis of water.

Acute radiation pneumonitis occurs in as many as 10% of patients irradiated for cancer of the lung or breast or for mediastinal lymphoma. DAD caused by radiation is, for the most part, dose-related and appears 1 to 6 months after radiation therapy. Patients have fever, cough, and dyspnea. Microscopic examination of the lungs reveals atypical alveolar-lining cells, with enlarged hyperchromatic nuclei, and multinucleated cells. Most patients recover from acute radiation pneumonitis.

Chronic radiation pneumonitis is characterized by interstitial fibrosis and may follow acute DAD or may develop insidiously. Lung biopsy demonstrates interstitial fibrosis, radiation-induced vascular changes, and atypical type II pneumocytes. The disease remains asymptomatic unless a substantial volume of the lung is affected.

Paraquat

The inhalation of the widely used herbicide paraquat is associated with DAD. Pulmonary disease becomes apparent 4 to 7 days after ingestion, as ARDS develops. Patients rarely recover once pulmonary complications have evolved. A curious intra-alveolar exudate and organization occur, as well as the more usual interstitial fibrosis. The intra-alveolar exudate organizes in such a way that the alveolar framework persists and the airspaces are filled with loose granulation tissue.

Respiratory Distress Syndrome of the Newborn

The counterpart of ARDS in newborns is termed respiratory distress syndrome (RDS) of the newborn. The disease also is associated with DAD, which is known as **hyaline membrane disease** in this circumstance. Treatment of RDS with oxygen tensions greater than 80% and mechanical ventilation is associated with the development of **bronchopulmonary dysplasia**. This infantile disorder is caused initially by damage to the pulmonary acini and later by repair, which leads to atelectasis, fibrosis, and the destruction of clusters of acini. RDS of the newborn and bronchopulmonary dysplasia are discussed in further detail in Chapter 6.

RARE ALVEOLAR DISEASES

Alveolar Proteinosis

Alveolar proteinosis, also termed lipoproteinosis, is a rare condition in which the alveoli are filled with a granular eosinophilic material, which is periodic acid–Schiff (PAS)-positive, diastase-resistant, and rich in lipids. The disease was initially described as idiopathic, but recent studies have associated alveolar proteinosis with (1) compromised immunity; (2) a number of cancers, particularly leukemia and lymphoma; (3) respiratory infections; and (4) exposure to environmental inorganic dusts.

□ **Pathogenesis:** The origin of alveolar proteinosis is obscure, but it is suspected that impaired activity of alveolar macrophages, together with overproduction of lipid (surfactant) by type II pneumocytes, may be responsible. In particular, it has been suggested that alveolar lipoproteinosis is due to an excessive secretion of surfactant or to diminished removal of normal surfactant by macrophages. However, the large amount of protein in the material indicates an additional (although unknown) mechanism. A similar appearance was described in acute silicosis and in children treated for leukemia. In the great majority of cases, no etiological agent is identifiable, although patients with alveolar lipoproteinosis have a high frequency of occupational exposure to a variety of different substances. *Nocardia* and other mildly pathogenic organisms have been encountered in fatal cases, but they are thought to be superinfections rather than the causative agents.

□ **Pathology:** On gross examination, the lungs in alveolar proteinosis are very heavy and viscid, and yellow fluid leaks from the cut surface. Scattered, firm, yellow-white nodules vary in size from a few millimeters to 2 cm in diameter. On microscopic examination, the granular material is noted not only in the alveoli, but also in the respiratory bronchioles and alveolar ducts (Fig. 12-39). The intra-alveolar material often stains with an antibody to surfactant apoprotein, and electron microscopy reveals concentrically laminated myelin figures and lamellar bodies identical to the cytoplasmic inclusions of type II pneumocytes. Within the eosinophilic material may be found cellular debris, foamy macrophages, ghosts of degenerated cells, and detached type II pneumocytes. The presence of small, dense, globular clumps of eosinophilic material and cholesterol clefts assists in the histological distinction of alveolar proteinosis from pulmonary edema. Importantly, the interstitial architecture of the lung is intact, and little inflammation is present.

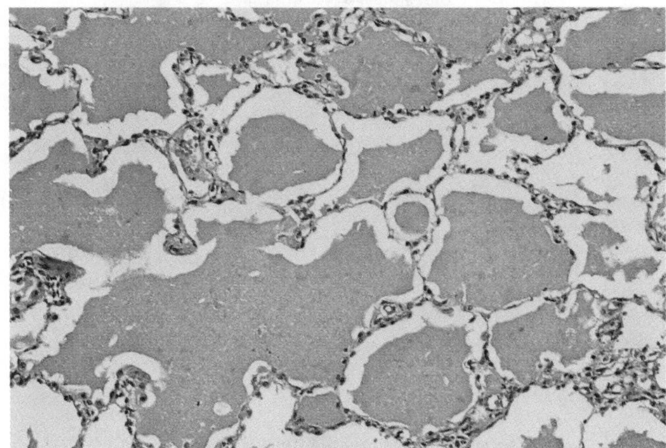

FIGURE *12-39*
Alveolar proteinosis. The alveoli and alveolar ducts contain a granular, eosinophilic material.

□ **Clinical Features:** Alveolar proteinosis is a disease of adults, although a few cases have been reported in infants and children. Patients have fever, a productive cough, and dyspnea. The most common finding on the lower chest radiograph is diffuse, bilateral, symmetric, alveolar infiltrates, which may radiate from the hilar regions. Repeated respiratory tract infections, often with fungi or *Nocardia,* are a common complication. Before treatment became available, alveolar proteinosis gradually progressed to respiratory failure in one third of the patients. Today, bronchoalveolar lavage is used to remove the alveolar material, and repeated lavage (sometimes for years) cures or halts the progress of the disease.

Diffuse Pulmonary Hemorrhage Syndromes

Diffuse alveolar hemorrhage can occur in a wide variety of clinical settings, including a group of disorders regarded as diffuse pulmonary hemorrhage syndromes (Table 12-2). Histologically, the diseases are characterized by diffuse acute (numerous intra-alveolar red blood cells) or chronic hemorrhage (hemosiderosis). Each of these syndromes is associated with acute or chronic intra-alveolar hemorrhage, manifested by the accumulation of red blood cells or hemosiderin-laden macrophages in the alveolar spaces. In virtually all of these disorders, a neutrophilic infiltrate of the alveolar wall **(neutrophilic capillaritis)** is present and is reminiscent of leukocytoclastic vasculitis seen in other organs such as the skin. This lesion tends to be most prominent in hemorrhagic syndromes associated with Wegener granulomatosis or systemic lupus erythematosus. Capillaritis may be seen in only a few cases of Goodpasture syndrome or idiopathic pulmonary hemorrhage.

Diffuse pulmonary hemorrhage syndromes can be classified according to the associated immunofluorescence patterns. A linear pattern of fluorescence is seen in anti–basement membrane antibody disease or Goodpasture syndrome. A granular pattern is present in immune complex–associated diseases, such as systemic lupus erythematosus. The immune complexes may also be demonstrated by electron microscopy as electron-dense deposits. Pauci-immmune disorders consist of anti–neutrophil cytoplasm antibody (ANCA)–associated diseases (e.g., Wegener granulomatosis or idiopathic pulmonary hemorrhage syndromes), in which no etiology or immunological mechanism can be determined (see Table 12-2).

Goodpasture Syndrome

Goodpasture syndrome refers to a triad of diffuse alveolar hemorrhage, glomerulonephritis, and a circulating cytotoxic autoantibody to a component of basement membranes. The cross-reactivity between the basement membrane of the

TABLE 12-2 **Classification of Pulmonary Hemorrhage**

Immunofluorescence Pattern	Immunological Mechanism	Common Terminology
Linear	Anti–basement membrane antibody	Goodpasture syndrome
Granular	Immune complexes	Systemic lupus erythematosus
		Mixed cryoglobulinemia
		Henoch-Schönlein purpura
		IgA disease
Negative or pauci-immune	Anti–neutrophil cytoplasmic antibody (ANCA)	Wegener granulomatosis
		Idiopathic glomerulonephritis
	No immunological marker	Idiopathic pulmonary hemorrhage

alveolus and the glomerulus accounts for the simultaneous attack on the lung and kidney. The pathogenesis of Goodpasture syndrome is discussed in greater detail in Chapter 16.

☐ **Pathology:** Patients with Goodpasture syndrome suffer extensive intra-alveolar hemorrhage (Fig. 12-40A). On gross examination, the lungs are dark red and heavy in the acute phase and rusty brown later, when the erythrocytes have been phagocytosed. Histologically, erythrocytes and hemosiderin-laden macrophages fill the airspaces. There is suggestive evidence of an "alveolitis" in the form of neutrophils in and around alveolar capillaries, although this reaction may be transient. The alveolar septa are mildly thickened by interstitial fibrosis and hyperplasia of type II pneumocytes. By immunofluorescence, linear deposition of IgG and complement is demonstrated in the basement membranes of the alveoli and glomeruli (see Fig. 12-40B).

☐ **Clinical Features:** Patients with Goodpasture syndrome are typically young men, although the disease may affect adults of either sex and of any age. The large majority (95%) of patients are seen initially with hemoptysis, often accompanied by dyspnea, weakness, and mild anemia. Evidence of glomerulonephritis follows the pulmonary manifestations in about 3 months (1 week to 1 year), although in some patients, renal disease does not

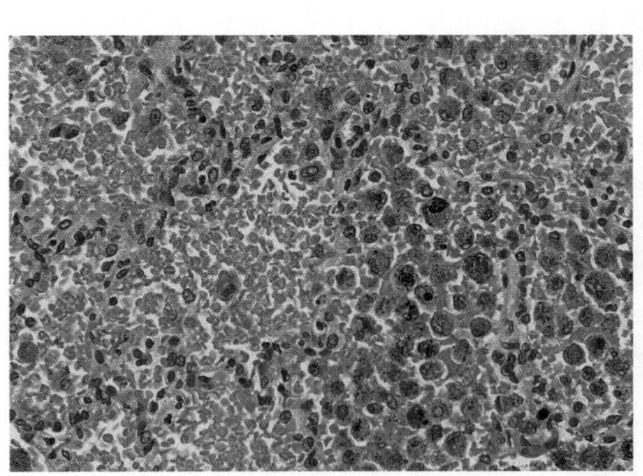

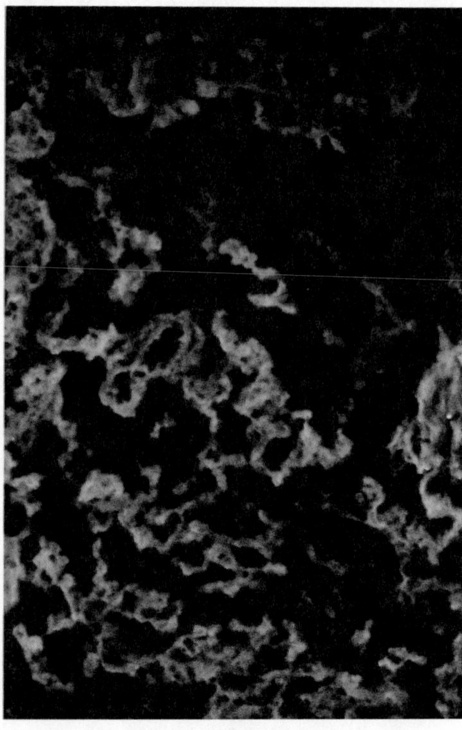

FIGURE 12-40
Goodpasture syndrome. *(A)* A section of lung shows extensive intra-alveolar hemorrhage. The alveolar septa are thickened, and the alveoli are lined by hyperplastic type II pneumocytes. *(B)* Linear deposition of IgG within the alveolar septa is demonstrated by immunofluorescence.

develop. Radiographic examination reveals diffuse, bilateral alveolar infiltrates, which may resolve rapidly in a matter of days as the erythrocytes lyse and are phagocytosed. The diagnosis is made on the basis of a renal or pulmonary biopsy. Hypoxemia and respiratory alkalosis are common, but respiratory function returns to normal as the hemorrhage resolves.

Goodpasture syndrome is treated by the administration of corticosteroids and cytotoxic drugs and by plasmapheresis. Before such aggressive treatment was instituted, the mortality of Goodpasture syndrome was 80%, but the prognosis is now considerably better. Even with current treatment, the 2-year survival is only 50%, and the outlook is worse when renal failure is present.

Idiopathic Pulmonary Hemorrhage

Idiopathic pulmonary hemorrhage (also known as idiopathic pulmonary hemosiderosis) is a rare disease characterized by diffuse alveolar bleeding similar to that of Goodpasture syndrome, but without renal involvement or the presence of anti–basement membrane antibodies. The malady primarily affects children, but 20% of patients are adults, usually younger than 30 years. There is a 2:1 male predominance in adults, but an equal sex distribution in children. The patients are first seen with cough (with or without hemoptysis), dyspnea, substernal chest pain, fatigue, and iron-deficiency anemia. Pulmonary hemorrhages are recurrent and intermittent, and the course is more protracted than that of Goodpasture syndrome.

Microscopically, idiopathic pulmonary hemorrhage is indistinguishable from the lung of Goodpasture syndrome. The response to corticosteroids is variable, and the mean survival is 3 to 5 years. One fourth of patients die rapidly of massive hemorrhage. Another fourth have persistent, active disease; repeated episodes of hemoptysis result in interstitial fibrosis and cor pulmonale. In another fourth of the patients, the disease remains inactive, but persistent dyspnea and anemia are troublesome. The remaining patients recover completely without recurrence.

Hypersensitivity to cow's milk in infants and children generally younger than 2 years can result in diffuse pulmonary hemorrhage similar to that seen in idiopathic pulmonary hemorrhage. Removal of milk from the diet ameliorates the condition.

Eosinophilic Pneumonia

Eosinophilic pneumonia refers to the accumulation of eosinophils in alveolar spaces. The disease is classified as idiopathic or secondary to an underlying illness (Table 12-3).

Idiopathic Eosinophilic Pneumonia

SIMPLE EOSINOPHILIC PNEUMONIA: Simple eosinophilic pneumonia (Löffler syndrome) is a mild condition characterized by fleeting pulmonary infiltrates, which usually resolve within a month. Patients typically have peripheral blood eosinophilia, but are often asymptomatic. Histologically, the lung shows eosinophilic pneumonia, but the diagnosis is usually established clinically, and lung biopsy is rarely performed.

TABLE 12-3 **Types of Eosinophilic Pneumonia**

Idiopathic

Chronic eosinophilic pneumonia
Acute eosinophilic pneumonia
Simple eosinophilic pneumonia (Löffler syndrome)

Secondary eosinophilic pneumonia

- Infection
  - Parasitic
    - Tropical eosinophilic pneumonia
      - *Ascaris lumbricoides, Toxocara canis,* filaria
    - Dirofilaria
  - Fungal
    - Aspergillus
- Drug-induced
  - Antibiotics
  - Cytotoxic drugs
  - Anti-inflammatory agents
  - Antihypertensive drugs
  - L-Tryptophan (eosinophilic fasciitis)
- Immunological or systemic diseases
  - Allergic bronchopulmonary aspergillosis
  - Churg–Strauss syndrome
  - Hypereosinophilic syndrome

ACUTE EOSINOPHILIC PNEUMONIA: In this disorder, patients are first seen with fewer than 7 days of symptoms, which include fever, hypoxemia, and diffuse interstitial and alveolar infiltrates on chest radiograph. The etiology of acute eosinophilic pneumonia is not known, but it is thought to be a type of hypersensitivity reaction. Although peripheral blood eosinophilia is frequently absent, bronchoalveolar lavage consistently demonstrates increased eosinophils. Leukocytosis is usually present. Histologically, the lung shows eosinophilic pneumonia accompanied by features of diffuse alveolar damage. Patients respond dramatically to corticosteroids, and (in contrast to chronic eosinophilic pneumonia) acute eosinophilic pneumonia does not recur.

CHRONIC EOSINOPHILIC PNEUMONIA: The etiology of chronic eosinophilic pneumonia is unknown, but an allergic diathesis is noted in some patients. The alveolar spaces are flooded with eosinophils, alveolar macrophages, and a proteinaceous exudate (Fig. 12-41). In some cases, there is also an eosinophilic interstitial pneumonia, and hyperplasia of type II pneumocytes may be prominent. Eosinophilic abscesses, formed by a central mass of necrotic eosinophils surrounded by palisaded macrophages, are sometimes encountered. A mild eosinophilic vasculitis may be seen. Bronchiolitis obliterans and organizing pneumonia are also occasionally described.

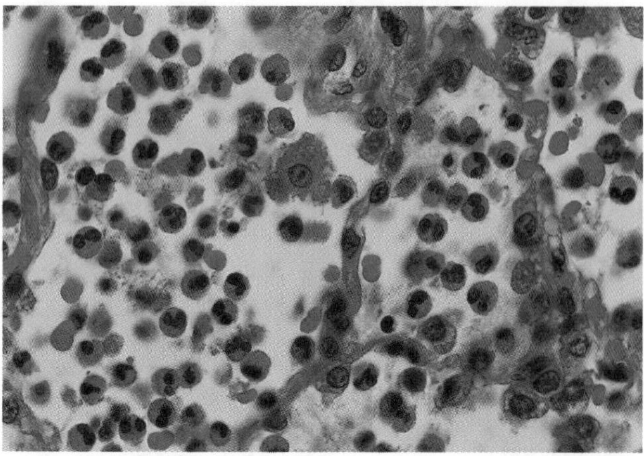

FIGURE 12-41
Eosinophilic pneumonia. The alveolar spaces are filled with an inflammatory exudate composed of eosinophils and macrophages. The alveolar septa are thickened by the presence of numerous eosinophils.

Patients have fever, night sweats, weight loss, cough productive of eosinophils, and dyspnea. Asthma is present in many of the patients, and circulating eosinophilia may be conspicuous. The chest radiograph is diagnostic and shows a photographic negative of pulmonary edema, characterized by peripheral alveolar infiltrates with sparing of the hilum. The response to corticosteroids is dramatic and helps to confirm the diagnosis.

Secondary Eosinophilic Pneumonia

Eosinophilic pneumonia can occur in a variety of known clinical settings, including parasitic or fungal infection, drug toxicity, and systemic disorders such as Churg–Strauss syndrome. In industrialized countries, the most frequent cause of eosinophilic pneumonia is drug hypersensitivity, including reactions to antibiotics, anti-inflammatory agents, cytotoxic drugs, and antihypertensive agents. The pulmonary disease resolves without long-term sequelae.

INFECTIOUS EOSINOPHILIC PNEUMONIA: The classic form of eosinophilic pneumonia associated with parasitic infection is *tropical eosinophilic pneumonia*. The migration of parasites through the lung is often accompanied by an acute, self-limited, respiratory illness, characterized clinically by (1) fever, (2) a cough productive of sputum containing eosinophils, and (3) transient pulmonary infiltrates.

In temperate zones, *Ascaris lumbricoides* is the usual inciting infection. Hypersensitivity to *Toxocara canis* is also occasionally encountered. However, the most distinctive infection associated with eosinophilic pneumonia is allergic bronchopulmonary aspergillosis (see earlier discussion on aspergillosis).

In tropical regions, eosinophilic pneumonia is most commonly a response to infestation with the filarial nematodes *Wuchereria bancrofti* and *Brugia malayi*, although other parasites may also produce this syndrome.

Endogenous Lipid Pneumonia (Obstructive Pneumonia)

Endogenous lipid pneumonia, also termed "golden pneumonia," is a localized condition distal to an obstructed airway, characterized by lipid-laden macrophages in the alveolar spaces. The size of the affected area corresponds to the caliber of the involved bronchus. Bronchial obstruction results in the retention of secretions and breakdown products of inflammatory and epithelial cells. Whereas the protein component is readily digested, lipids are phagocytosed by macrophages, which fill the alveoli distal to the obstruction.

On gross examination, endogenous lipid pneumonia has a characteristic golden-yellow color, which reflects the accumulation of fine lipid droplets within alveolar macrophages. Microscopically, alveoli are flooded by foamy macrophages, with needle-shaped clefts characteristic of cholesterol crystals. The alveolar walls typically remain intact. The pneumonia is accompanied by mild chronic inflammation and fibrosis. If the obstruction is relieved, the affected parenchyma can return to its normal state, unless bronchiectasis and chronic recurrent bronchopneumonia have led to irreversible parenchymal changes.

Exogenous Lipid Pneumonia (Aspiration of Mineral Oil)

Exogenous lipid pneumonia is the reaction of the pulmonary parenchyma to the aspiration of a variety of oils. Mineral oil is used as a laxative and as a carrier for medications in nose drops. Vegetable oils are used in cooking, and animal oils are ingested in the form of cod-liver oil and other vitamin preparations. Oil-based contrast media have also been used for radiological bronchography. Exogenous lipid pneumonia is most common in older persons who take

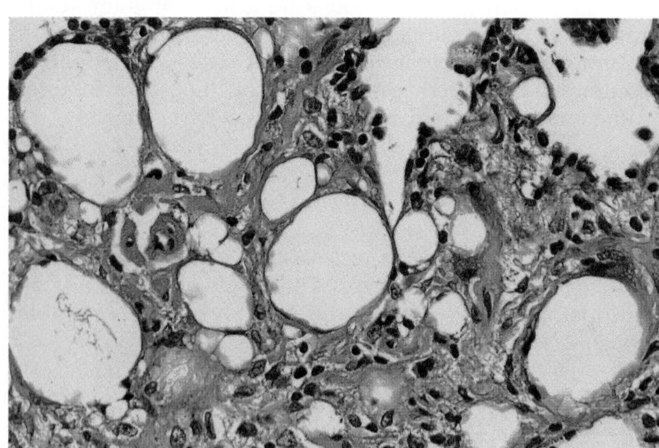

FIGURE 12-42
Exogenous lipoid pneumonia (mineral oil aspiration). The cystic spaces are empty, because the lipid was washed out during paraffin processing. A giant-cell reaction is also present.

nose drops or laxatives at bedtime and aspirate during sleep. Children have aspirated oily medications while vigorously resisting the dosing.

On gross examination, exogenous lipid pneumonia appears as a gray, poorly demarcated, greasy lesion. Microscopically, foamy macrophages are seen in the alveolar and interstitial spaces (Fig. 12-42). Large oil droplets in both locations are surrounded by a foreign-body granulomatous response. Because most of the oil washes out in paraffin processing, empty vacuolar spaces are noted in histological sections. In chronic cases, the affected areas may become densely fibrotic. Patients with exogenous lipid pneumonia are usually asymptomatic, and the condition is brought to medical attention when a mass simulating an infectious process or a tumor is noted on a chest radiograph.

OBSTRUCTIVE PULMONARY DISEASES

Several different diseases, including chronic bronchitis, emphysema, asthma, and in some classifications, bronchiectasis and cystic fibrosis, are grouped together because they have in common an obstruction to air flow in the lungs.

Chronic obstructive pulmonary disease (COPD) is a nonspecific term that describes patients with chronic bronchitis or emphysema who evidence a decrease in forced expiratory volume, measured by spirometric pulmonary-function tests.

Air flow has a hydraulic basis and can be reduced in two ways: by increasing the resistance to air flow or by reducing the outflow pressure. In the lung, narrowed airways produce increased resistance, whereas loss of elastic recoil results in diminished pressure. Airway narrowing occurs in chronic bronchitis or asthma, and emphysema causes loss of recoil.

Chronic Bronchitis

Chronic bronchitis is defined clinically as the presence of a chronic productive cough without a discernible cause for more than half the time over a period of 2 years. The pathological definition of the disease is less satisfactory, because the morphological alterations represent a continuum; in milder degrees of chronic bronchitis, they overlap with those seen in ostensibly normal persons.

☐ Pathogenesis: **Chronic bronchitis is primarily a disease of cigarette smoking (see Chapter 8), with 90% of all cases occurring in smokers**. The frequency of chronic bronchitis is less than 5% in nonsmokers, 10% to 15% in moderate smokers, and more than 25% in heavy smokers. Moreover, children and nonsmoking spouses of cigarette smokers are reported to have a slightly higher incidence of chronic respiratory symptoms, presumably owing to the passive inhalation of cigarette smoke. The frequency and severity of acute respiratory tract infections is increased in patients with chronic bronchitis, and recent epidemiological studies implicated such infections in the etiology and progression of the disease. Population studies also demonstrated a higher prevalence of chronic bronchitis among urban dwellers in areas of substantial air pollution and in workers exposed to toxic industrial inhalants. However, in both of these situations, the effects of cigarette smoking far outweigh other contributing factors.

The precise mechanisms by which cigarette smoke and other pollutants produce bronchial injury are poorly understood. Experimentally, rodents subjected to the inhalation of cigarette smoke or sulfur dioxide, or to the instillation of dilute acids, exhibit squamous metaplasia of the bronchial epithelium. A similar change is produced by the introduction of certain proteases into the bronchi, an effect that is prevented by pretreatment with antiproteases. Metaplasia of the bronchial epithelium can also be induced in rodents by adrenergic and cholinergic agonists, suggesting that autonomic stimulation may play a role in the pathogenesis of chronic bronchitis.

☐ Pathology: The principal morphological finding in chronic bronchitis is an increase in the size of the mucus-secreting apparatus (Fig. 12-43). Most mucus is produced by the subepithelial bronchial mucous glands, which consist of a series of branched tubules. The tubules, which resemble glands on cross-section, drain into a duct leading to the epithelial surface. Two types of cells line the acini: pale mucous cells, which are the most common, and serous cells, which are more basophilic and contain granules. **Chronic bronchitis is characterized by hyperplasia**

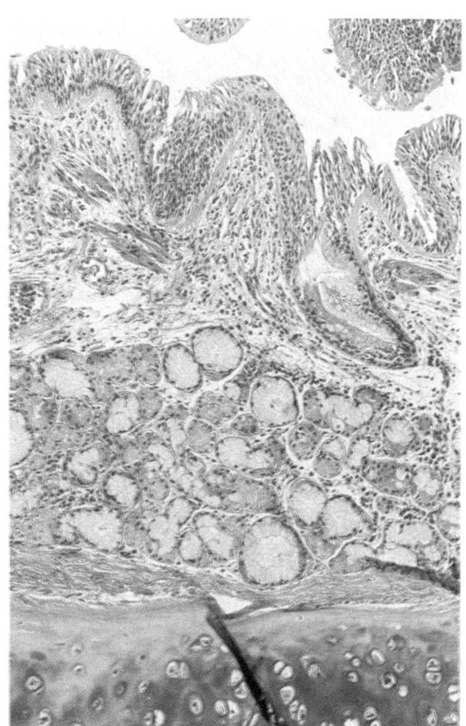

FIGURE *12-43*
Chronic bronchitis. The bronchial wall is thickened and shows hyperplasia of the mucus-secreting glands. The Reid index is greater than 0.5. The submucosa shows increased smooth muscle and mild chronic inflammation.

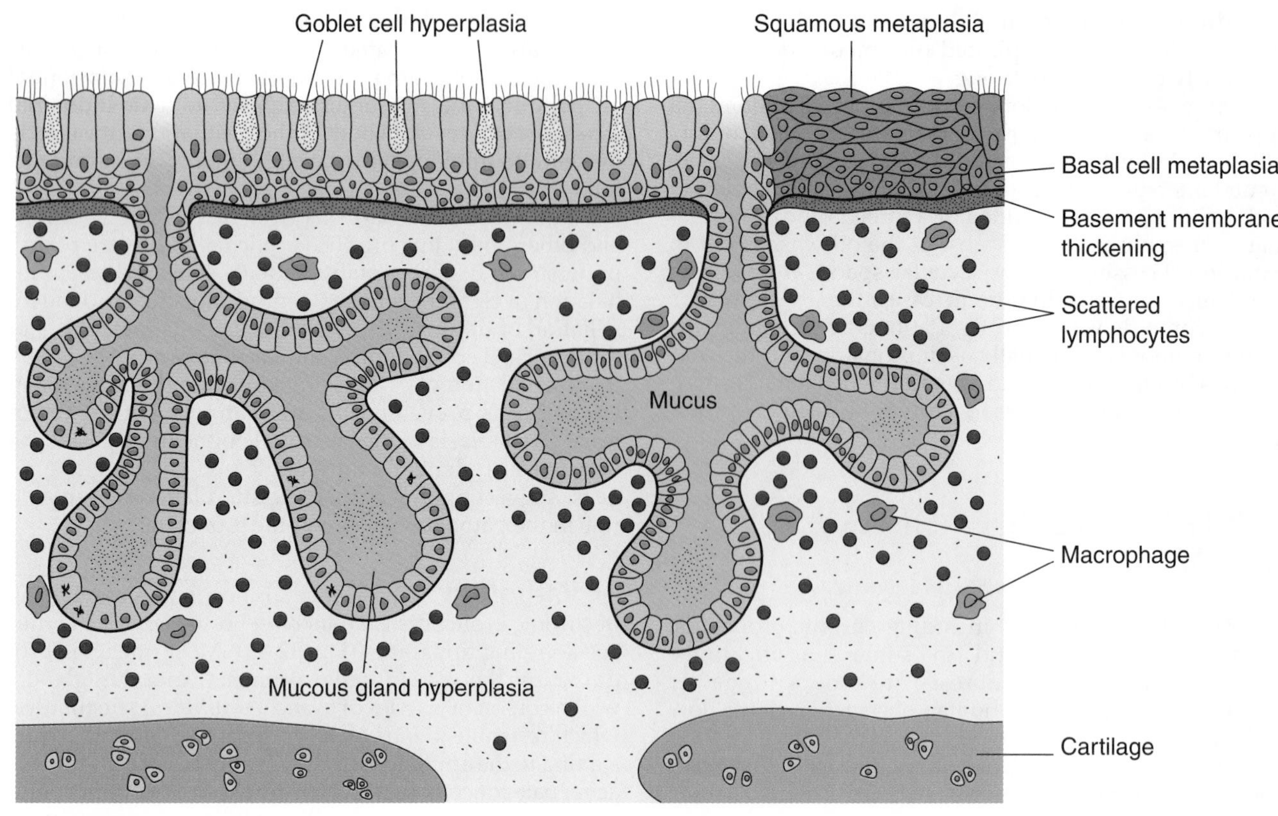

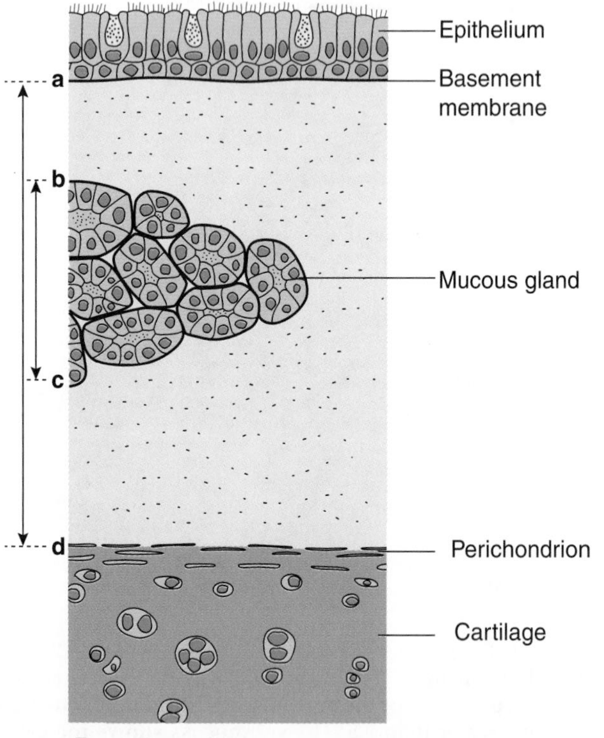

FIGURE 12-44
Chronic bronchitis. *(A)* Morphological changes in chronic bronchitis. *(B)* Reid index. The Reid index is the ratio of the thickness of the glands *(b–c)* to that of the bronchial wall (basement membrane to inner perichondrium; *a–d)*. It is increased in chronic bronchitis.

and hypertrophy of the mucous cells and an increased proportion of mucous to serous cells. As a result, both the individual acini and the glands become larger.

The Reid index is a measure of the increase in the size of the mucous glands (Fig. 12-44). The area occupied by the glands in the plane vertical to the cartilage and epithelium is expressed as a proportion of the thickness of the entire bronchial wall (basement membrane to inner perichondrium). The normal value of the Reid index is 0.4 or less, whereas it is more than 0.5 in chronic bronchitis.

Other morphological changes in chronic bronchitis are variable and include the following:

- Excess mucus in the central and peripheral airways
- "Pits" on the surface of the bronchial epithelium, which represent dilated bronchial gland ducts into which open several glands
- Thickening of the bronchial wall by mucous gland enlargement and edema, which leads to encroachment on the bronchial lumen
- An increase in the number of goblet cells
- Increased amounts of smooth muscle, which may indicate bronchial hyperreactivity
- Squamous metaplasia of the bronchial epithelium in chronic bronchitis reflects epithelial damage from tobacco smoke, an effect that is probably independent of the other morphological features of chronic bronchitis

☐ **Clinical Features:** Chronic bronchitis is often accompanied by emphysema (see later); it is often difficult to separate the relative contribution of each disease to the clinical presentation. In general, patients with predominantly chronic bronchitis have had a productive cough for many years. Cough and sputum production are initially more severe in the winter months, but as the malady becomes more chronic, it progresses from hibernal to perennial. Exertional dyspnea and cyanosis supervene, and cor pulmonale may ensue. The combination of cyanosis and edema secondary to cor pulmonale has led to the label "blue bloater" for such patients.

Acute respiratory failure in patients with advanced chronic bronchitis, with progressive hypoxemia and hypercapnia, may be precipitated by pulmonary infections, thromboembolism, and left ventricular failure, and by major episodes of air pollution. Because of retained mucous secretions, patients with chronic bronchitis are at an increased risk of bacterial infections of the lung, particularly with *H. influenzae* and *S. pneumoniae*.

Patients with chronic bronchitis must be admonished to stop smoking. Prompt antibiotic treatment of pulmonary infections, administration of bronchodilator drugs, and occasionally bronchopulmonary drainage are the mainstays of treatment.

Emphysema

Emphysema is a chronic lung disease characterized as enlargement of the airspaces distal to the terminal bronchioles, with destruction of their walls but without fibrosis. Emphysema is classified in anatomical terms, but the classification should not obscure the fact that the **severity of emphysema is more important than the type.** In practical terms, as emphysema becomes more severe, it becomes more difficult to classify, a situation similar to that of end-stage renal disease or cirrhosis of the liver. Moreover, several anatomical patterns may be present in the same lung.

☐ **Pathogenesis:** **The major cause of emphysema is cigarette smoking, and moderate to severe emphysema is rare in nonsmokers (see Chapter 8).** The dominant hypothesis concerning the pathogenesis of emphysema is the proteolysis–antiproteolysis theory (Fig. 12-45). It is thought that there is a balance between elastin synthesis and catabolism in the lung. In other words, emphysema results when elastolytic activity increases or antielastolytic activity is reduced.

Increased numbers of neutrophils, which contain serine elastase and other proteases, are found in the bronchoalveolar lavage fluid of smokers. Smoking also reduces α_1-antitrypsin activity, owing to the oxidation of methionine residues in the enzyme. In this way, unopposed and increased elastolytic activity leads to the destruction of elastic tissue in the walls of the distal airspaces, thereby impairing elastic recoil. At the same time, other cellular proteases may be involved in injury to the airspace walls. Although the proteolysis–antiproteolysis theory is attractive as an explanation for smokers' emphysema, it awaits further confirmation.

α_1-ANTITRYPSIN DEFICIENCY: A hereditary deficiency in α_1-antitrypsin (α_1-AT) accounts for about 1% of all patients with a clinical diagnosis of COPD and is considerably more common in young persons with severe emphysema. α_1-AT, a circulating glycoprotein produced in the liver, is a major inhibitor of a variety of proteases, including elastase, trypsin, chymotrypsin, thrombin, and bacterial proteases. In fact, it accounts for 90% of antiproteinase activity in the blood. In the lung, the most important action of α_1-AT is its inhibition of neutrophil elastase, an enzyme that digests elastin and other structural components of the alveolar septa.

The amount and type of α_1-AT is determined by a pair of co-dominant alleles, referred to as Pi (protease inhibitor). The most common genotype, PiM, and some 75 variants are now recognized. The most serious abnormality is associated with the PiZ allele, which occurs in some 5% of the population. It is more common in persons of Scandinavian origin, and is rare in Jews, blacks, and Japanese. PiZZ homozygotes have only 15% to 20% of the normal plasma concentration of α_1-AT, because the abnormal protein is poorly secreted by the liver. These persons are at risk for the development of both cirrhosis of the liver (see Chapter 14) and emphysema. **In fact, the majority of all patients with clinically diagnosed emphysema younger than age 40 years have α_1-AT deficiency (PiZ).** PiZZ homozygotes who do not smoke show a mean age at onset of emphysema between ages 45 and 50 years, whereas those who smoke develop emphysema at about age 35 years. It deserves emphasis that two thirds of nonsmoking, PiZZ homozygotes show no evidence of emphysema. The association of α_1-AT deficiency with emphysema supports the concept that cigarette smoking

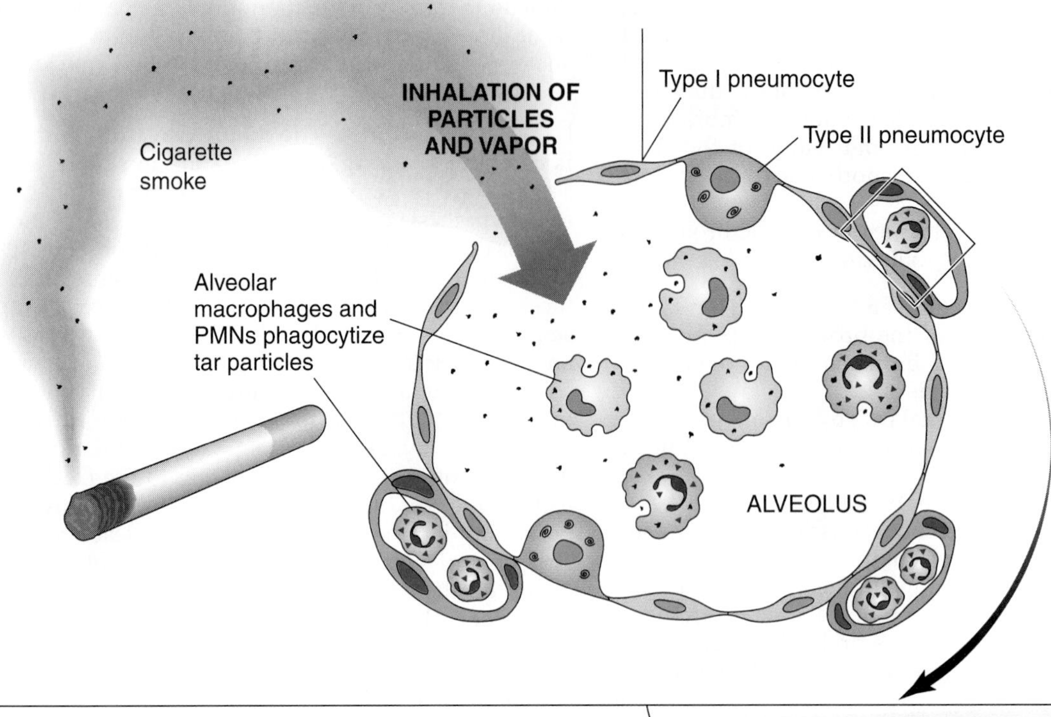

INHALATION OF PARTICLES AND VAPOR
Cigarette smoke
Type I pneumocyte
Type II pneumocyte
Alveolar macrophages and PMNs phagocytize tar particles
ALVEOLUS

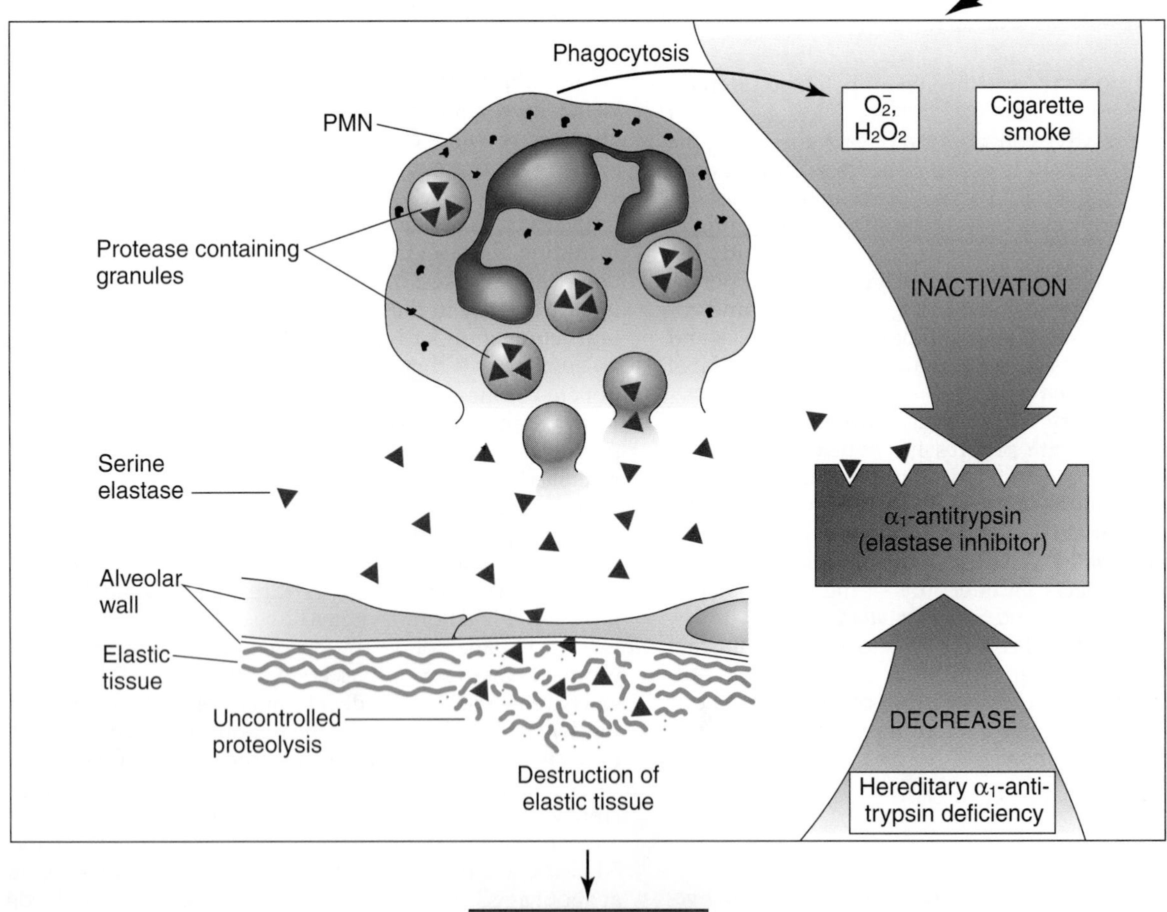

Phagocytosis
O_2^-, H_2O_2
Cigarette smoke
PMN
Protease containing granules
INACTIVATION
Serine elastase
α_1-antitrypsin (elastase inhibitor)
Alveolar wall
Elastic tissue
Uncontrolled proteolysis
Destruction of elastic tissue
DECREASE
Hereditary α_1-antitrypsin deficiency
EMPHYSEMA

FIGURE **12-45**

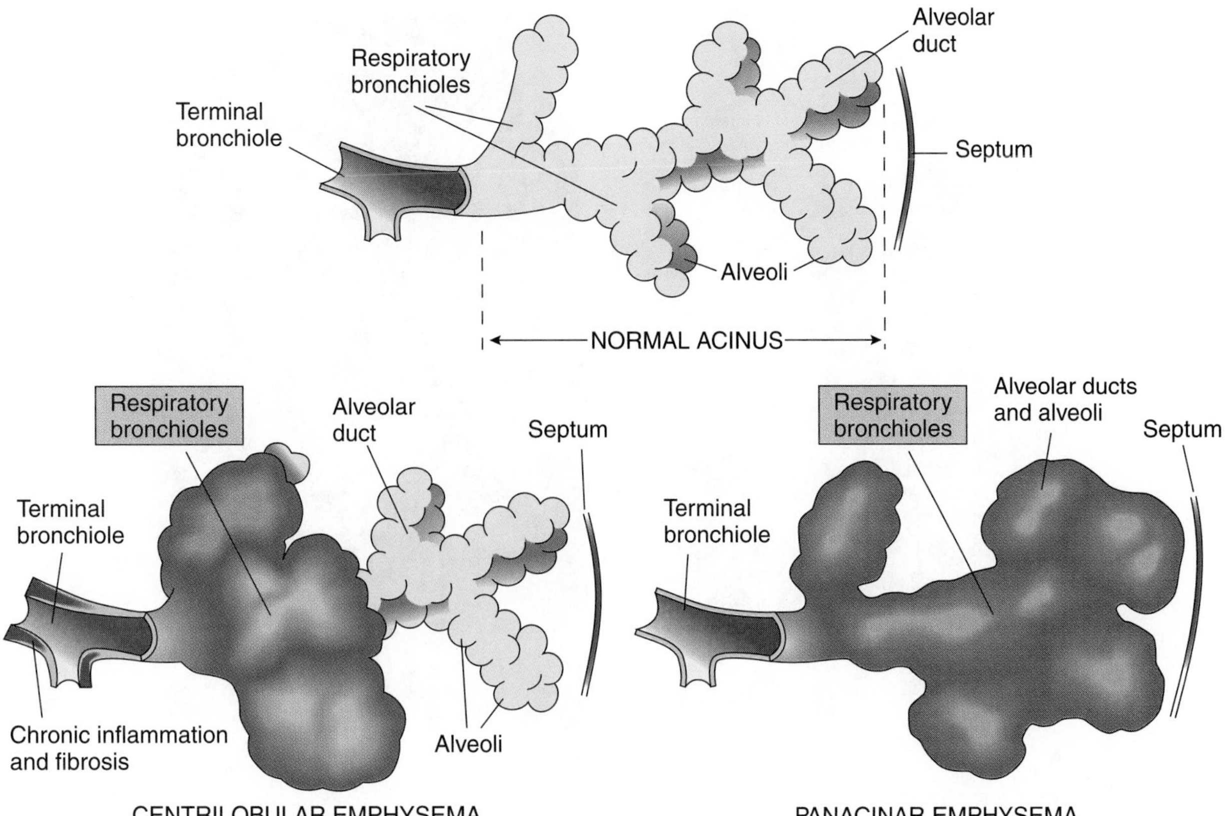

FIGURE *12-46*
Types of emphysema. The acinus is the unit gas-exchanging structure of the lung distal to the terminal bronchiole. It consists of, in order, respiratory bronchioles, alveolar ducts, alveolar sacs, and alveoli. In centrilobular (proximal acinar) emphysema, the respiratory bronchioles are predominantly involved. In paraseptal (distal acinar) emphysema, the alveolar ducts are particularly affected. In panacinar (panlobular) emphysema, the acinus is uniformly damaged.

by itself causes emphysema by altering the balance of the protease–antiprotease system in the lung.

☐ **Pathology:** Emphysema is morphologically classified according to the location of the lesions within the pulmonary acinus (Fig. 12-46). Only the proximal part of the acinus (respiratory bronchiole) is selectively involved in centrilobular emphysema, whereas the entire acinus is destroyed in panacinar emphysema.

CENTRILOBULAR EMPHYSEMA: This form of emphysema is the most frequently encountered variant and the one usually associated with cigarette smoking and with clinical symptoms. Centrilobular emphysema is characterized by destruction of the cluster of terminal bronchioles near the end of the bronchiolar tree in the central part of the pulmonary lobule (Fig. 12-47A). The lobule is the smallest portion of the lung bounded by septa and includes several acini. The enlarged respiratory bronchioles form enlarged airspaces that are separated from each other and from the lobular septa by normal alveolar ducts and alveoli. As centrilobular emphysema progresses, these distal structures also may be involved (see Fig. 12-47B). The bronchioles proximal to the emphysematous spaces are inflamed and narrowed. Centrilobular emphy-

FIGURE *12-45*
The proteolysis–antiproteolysis theory of the pathogenesis of emphysema. Cigarette (tobacco) smoking is closely related to the development of emphysema. Some product in tobacco smoke induces an inflammatory reaction. The serine elastase in polymorphonuclear leukocytes, which is a particularly potent elastolytic agent, injures the elastic tissue of the lung. Normally, this enzyme activity is inhibited by α_1-antitrypsin, but tobacco smoke, directly or through the generation of free radicals, inactivates α_1-antitrypsin (protease inhibitor).

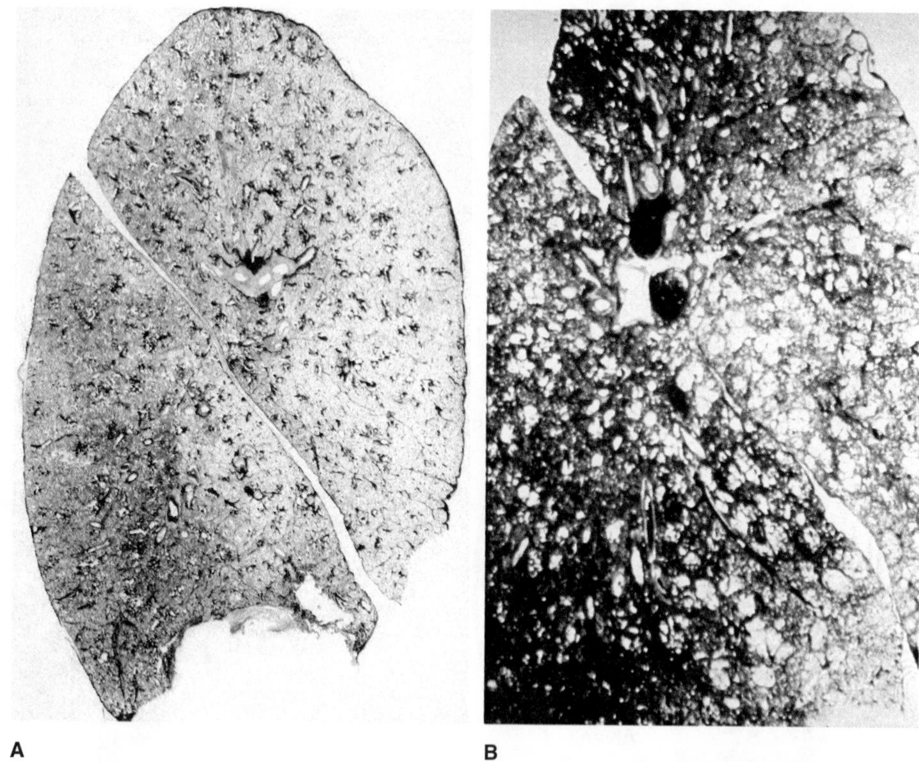

FIGURE 12-47
Centrilobular emphysema. ***(A)*** **A whole mount of the left lung of a smoker with mild emphysema shows enlarged air spaces scattered throughout both lobes, which represent destruction of the terminal bronchioles in the central part of the pulmonary lobule. These abnormal spaces are surrounded by intact pulmonary parenchyma.** ***(B)*** **In a more advanced case of centrilobular emphysema, the destruction of the lung has progressed to produce large, irregular air spaces.**

sema is most severe in the upper zones of the lung, the upper lobe, and the superior segment of the lower lobe.

Focal dust emphysema, a disease of coal miners, resembles centrilobular emphysema but differs in that the enlarged spaces are smaller and more regular, and inflammation of the bronchioles is not apparent. Importantly, the lesion is primarily distensive rather than destructive. Focal dust emphysema is discussed later in the section on coal worker's pneumoconiosis.

PANACINAR EMPHYSEMA: In this type of emphysema, the acinus is uniformly involved, with destruction of the alveolar septa from the center to the periphery of the acinus (Fig. 12-48A,B). The loss of alveolar septa is illustrated in the histological comparison of lung affected by α_1-AT deficiency with normal lung at the same magnification (Fig. 12-49). In the final stage, panacinar emphysema leaves behind a lacy network of supporting tissue ("cotton-candy lung"). This variant occurs in several different situations. Diffuse panacinar emphysema is the typical lesion associated with α_1-AT deficiency. It is also often found in cigarette smokers in association with centrilobular emphysema. In such cases, the panacinar pattern tends to occur in the lower zones of the lung, whereas centrilobular emphysema is seen in the upper zones.

LOCALIZED EMPHYSEMA: This condition, previously known as "paraseptal emphysema," is characterized by the destruction of alveoli and resulting emphysema in only one or at most a few locations. The remainder of the lungs is normal. The lesion is usually found at the apex of an upper lobe, although it may occur anywhere in the pulmonary parenchyma, such as in a subpleural location (Fig. 12-50). Although it is of no clinical significance itself, rupture of an area of localized emphysema produces spontaneous pneumothorax (see later). Progression of localized emphysema can result in a large area of destruction, termed a *bulla.* Bullae range in size from as small as 2 cm to large lesions that occupy an entire hemothorax.

☐ **Clinical Features:** Most patients with symptomatic emphysema are seen at age 60 years or older with a prolonged history of exertional dyspnea, but with minimal, nonproductive cough. They have lost weight and use the accessory muscles of respiration to breathe. Weight loss is probably due less to the lack of calories than to the increased work of breathing. Tachypnea and a prolonged expiratory phase are typical. The most prominent radiological abnormality is overinflation of the lung, as evidenced by enlarged lungs, depressed diaphragms, and an

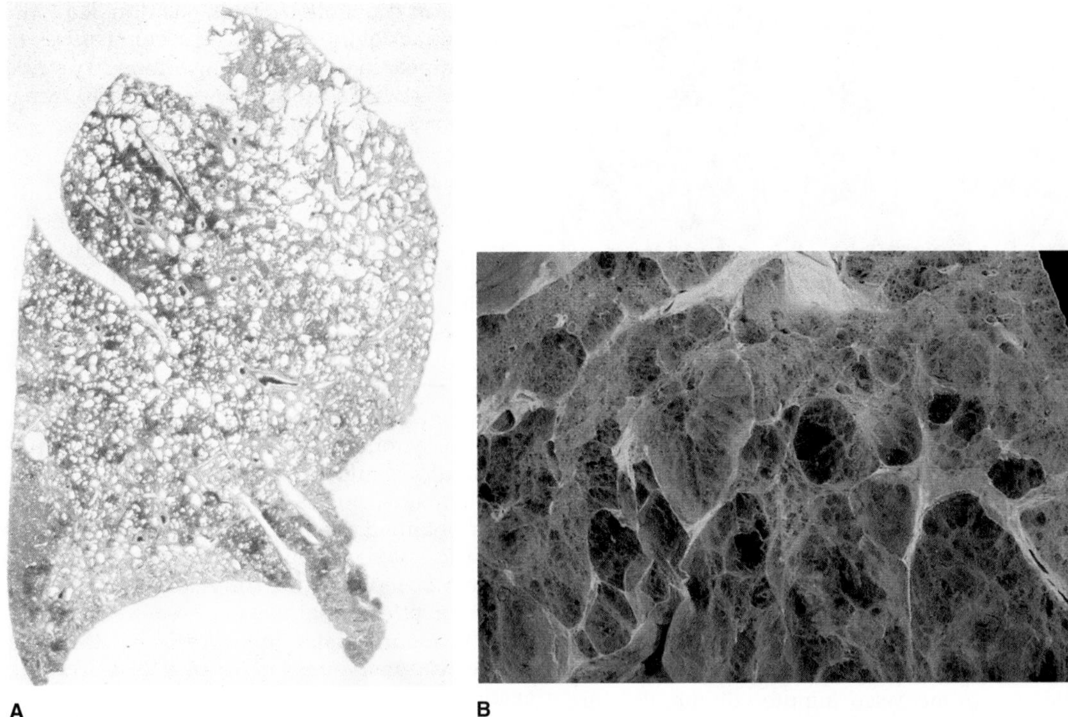

FIGURE 12-48
Panacinar emphysema. *(A)* A whole mount of the left lung from a patient with severe emphysema reveals widespread destruction of the pulmonary parenchyma, which in some areas leaves behind only a lacy network of supporting tissue. *(B)* The lung from this patient with α_1-antitrypsin deficiency shows a panacinar pattern of emphysema. The loss of alveolar walls has resulted in markedly enlarged air spaces.

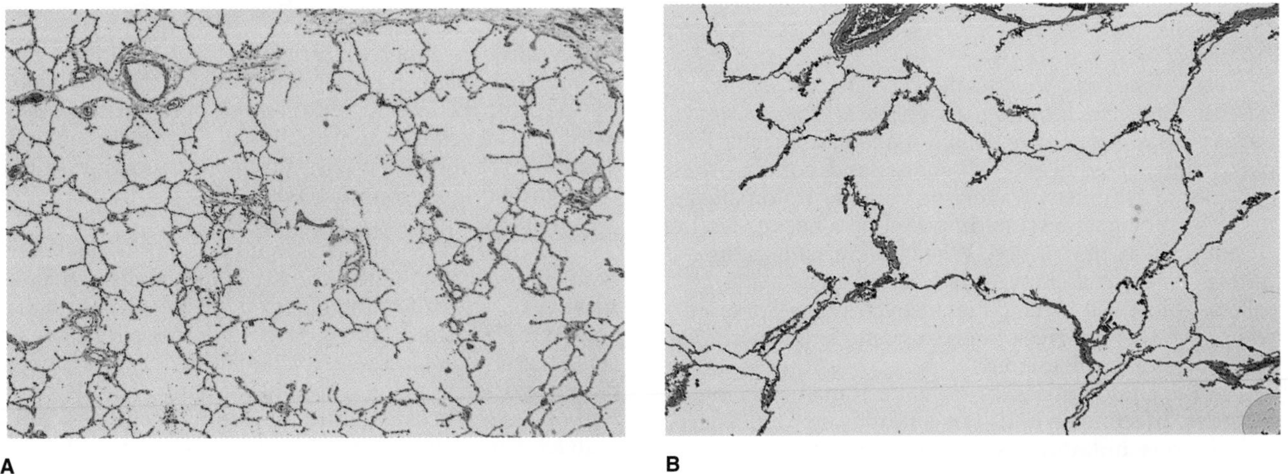

FIGURE 12-49
Panacinar emphysema. *(A)* This lung, from a patient with α_1-antitrypsin deficiency, shows large, irregular air spaces and a markedly reduced number of alveolar walls. *(B)* The extensive loss of alveolar walls in *A* is emphasized by comparison with this section of normal lung at the same magnification.

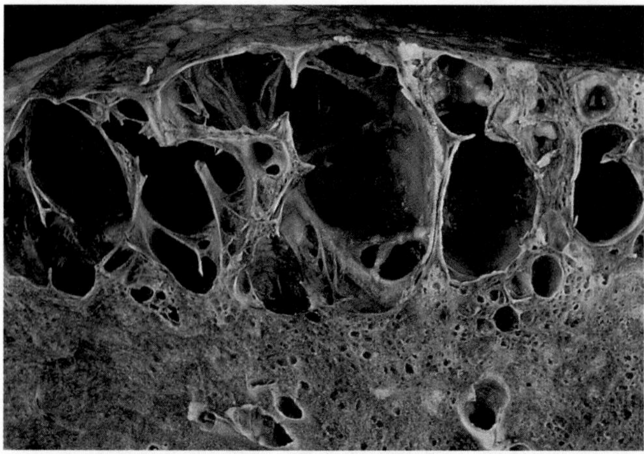

FIGURE *12-50*
Localized emphysema. The subpleural parenchyma shows markedly enlarged air spaces owing to the loss of alveolar tissue.

increased posteroanterior diameter ("barrel chest"). The bronchovascular markings do not extend to the peripheral lung fields. Because these patients have a higher respiratory rate and an increased minute volume, they are able to maintain arterial hemoglobin saturation at near-normal levels and are therefore referred to as "pink puffers." In contrast to patients with predominantly chronic bronchitis, those with emphysema are at lesser risk of recurrent pulmonary infections and are not so prone to the development of cor pulmonale. The clinical course of emphysema is marked by an inexorable decline in respiratory function and progressive dyspnea, for which no treatment is adequate.

Asthma

Asthma is a chronic lung disease characterized by periodic episodes of air-flow obstruction and increased responsiveness of the airways to a variety of stimuli. Patients typically have paroxysms of wheezing, dyspnea, and cough. Acute episodes of asthma may alternate with asymptomatic periods, or they may be superimposed on a background of chronic airway obstruction. When severe acute asthma is unresponsive to therapy, it is referred to as *status asthmaticus.* Most asthmatic patients, even when apparently well, have some degree of persistent air-flow obstruction and morphological lesions.

In the United States, bronchial asthma is a common disorder, affecting up to 10% of children and 5% of adults. For reasons unknown, since 1980, the prevalence of asthma in the United States has doubled. Although the initial attack of the disease can occur at any age, half of the cases appear in patients younger than 10 years, and the incidence is twice as high in boys as in girls. By age 30 years, both sexes are affected equally.

☐ **Pathogenesis:** Asthma was classically divided into two major categories depending on the inciting factors. Extrinsic (allergic) asthma referred to a condition in which bronchospasm is induced by inhaled antigens, usually in children with a personal or family history of allergic disease (e.g., eczema, urticaria, or hay fever). By contrast, intrinsic (idiosyncratic) asthma was a disease of adults in which bronchial hyperreactivity was produced in persons who had no apparent allergic diathesis by a variety of factors unrelated to immune mechanisms. These distinctions implied rigid differences in pathogenetic mechanisms, but as greater knowledge of asthma has been obtained, such distinctions have been blurred. At this time, it seems more appropriate simply to discuss asthma in terms of the different inciting factors and the common effector pathways.

The consensus hypothesis attributes bronchial hyperresponsiveness in asthma to an inflammatory reaction to diverse stimuli. As a result of exposure to an inciting factor (e.g., allergens, drugs, cold, exercise), inflammatory mediators are released by activated macrophages, mast cells, eosinophils, and basophils. These molecules induce bronchoconstriction, increased vascular permeability, and mucous secretions. Moreover, the resident inflammatory cells may be activated to release chemotactic factors, which in turn recruit more effector cells and amplify the response of the airways. Inflammation of the bronchial walls also may injure the epithelium, thereby stimulating nerve endings and initiating neural reflexes that further aggravate and propagate the bronchospasm.

A large number of inflammatory mediators and chemotactic factors has been implicated in the production of the bronchospasm and mucous hypersecretion of asthma. The relative contributions of the different substances probably vary with the inciting stimulus. The best-studied situation associated with the induction of asthma is the inhalation of allergens.

It is thought that in a sensitized person, an inhaled allergen interacts with IgE antibody bound to the surface of mast cells, which are interspersed among the epithelial cells of the bronchial mucosa (Fig. 12-51). As a result, mast cells degranulate and release mediators of type I (immediate) hypersensitivity, including histamine, bradykinin, leukotrienes, prostaglandins, thromboxane A_2, and platelet-activating factor (PAF). These substances lead to

FIGURE *12-51*
Pathogenesis of asthma. *(A)* Immunologically mediated asthma. Allergens interact with immunoglobulin E (IgE) on mast cells, either on the surface of the epithelium or, when there is abnormal permeability of the epithelium, in the submucosa. Mediators are released and may react locally or by reflexes mediated through the vagus. *(B)* The discharge of eosinophilic granules further impairs mucociliary function and damages epithelial cells. Epithelial cell injury stimulates nerve endings in the mucosa, thereby initiating an autonomic discharge that contributes to airway narrowing and mucous secretion.

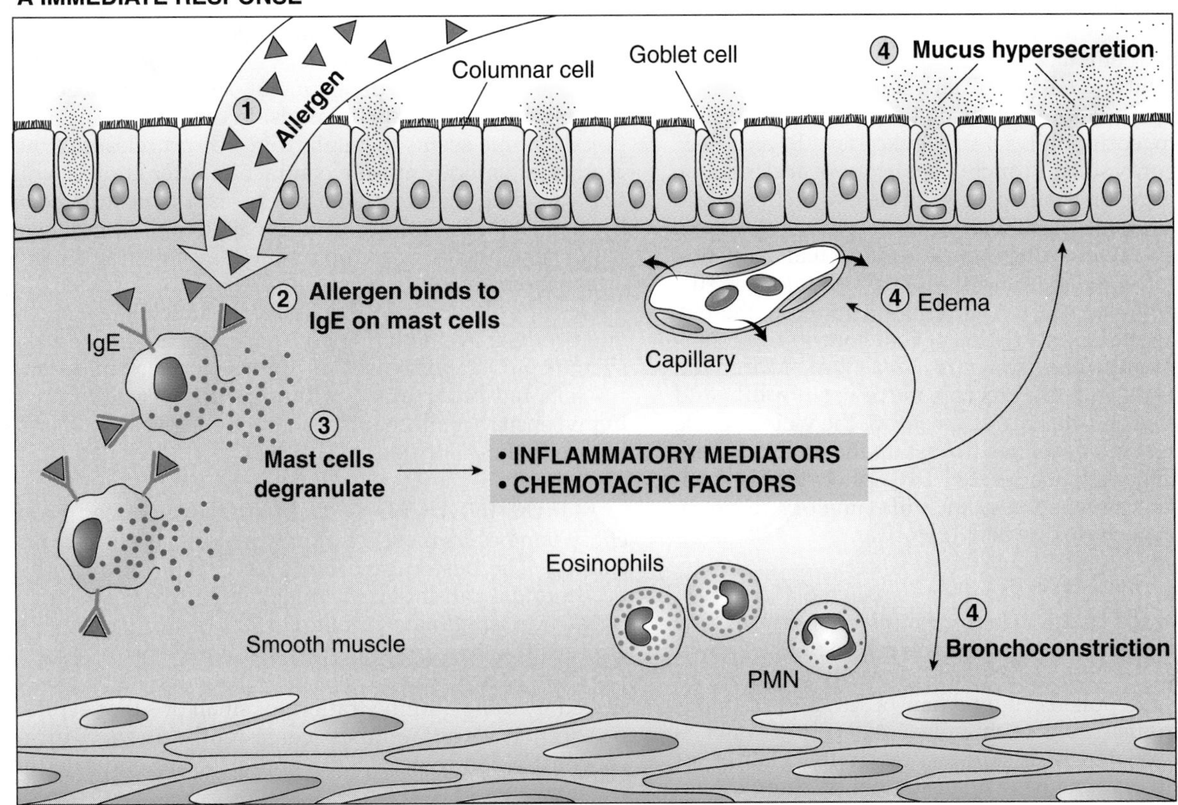
A IMMEDIATE RESPONSE
① Allergen
Columnar cell
Goblet cell
④ Mucus hypersecretion
② Allergen binds to IgE on mast cells
IgE
Capillary
④ Edema
③ Mast cells degranulate
• INFLAMMATORY MEDIATORS
• CHEMOTACTIC FACTORS
Eosinophils
Smooth muscle
PMN
④ Bronchoconstriction

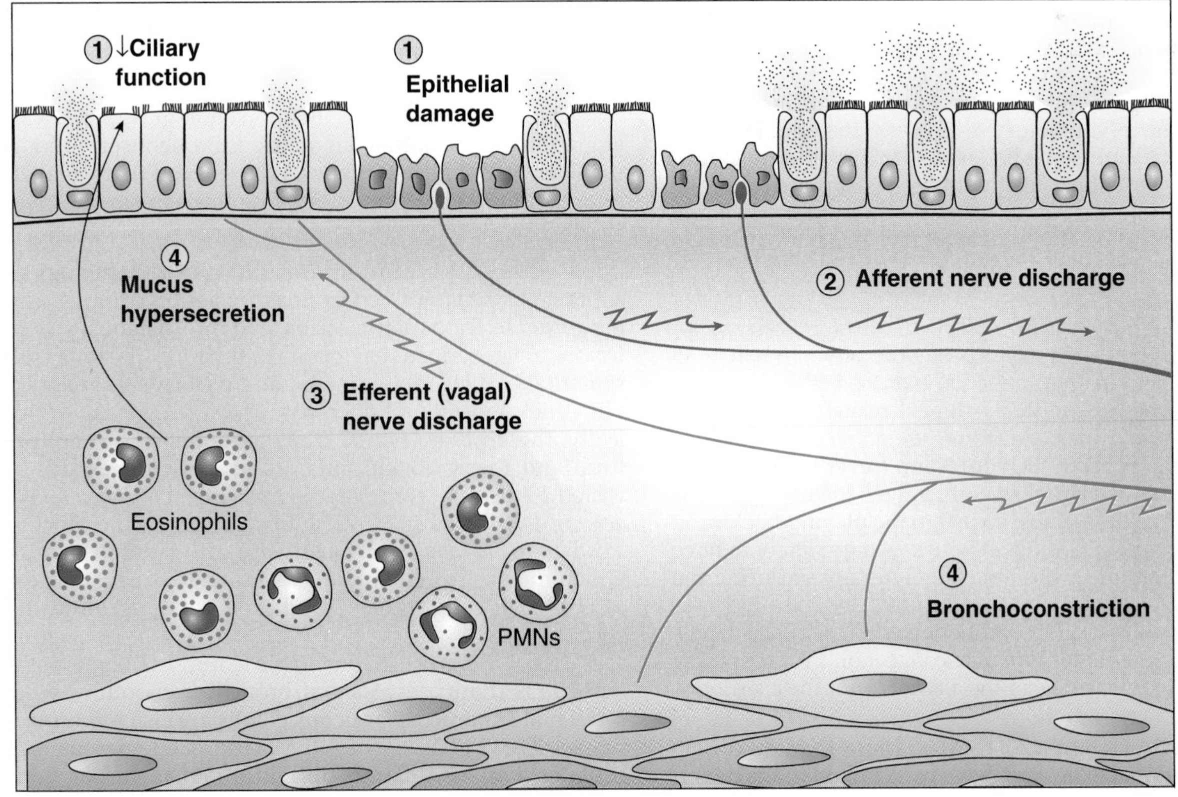
B DELAYED RESPONSE
① ↓Ciliary function
① Epithelial damage
④ Mucus hypersecretion
② Afferent nerve discharge
③ Efferent (vagal) nerve discharge
Eosinophils
PMNs
④ Bronchoconstriction

FIGURE *12-51*

(1) smooth muscle contraction, (2) mucous secretion, and (3) increased vascular permeability and edema. Each of these effects is a potent, albeit reversible, cause of airway obstruction. Chemotactic factors, including leukotriene B_4 and neutrophil and eosinophil chemotactic factors, attract neutrophils, eosinophils, and platelets to the bronchial wall. In turn, eosinophils release leukotriene B_4 and PAF, thereby aggravating bronchoconstriction and edema. The discharge of eosinophil granules, which contain eosinophil cationic protein and major basic protein into the bronchial lumen further impairs mucociliary function and damages epithelial cells. Epithelial cell injury is suspected to stimulate nerve endings in the mucosa, thereby initiating an autonomic discharge that contributes to airway narrowing and mucous secretion. Moreover, leukotriene B_4 and PAF recruit more eosinophils and other effector cells, thereby augmenting the vicious circle that prolongs and amplifies the asthmatic attack. Recent evidence suggests that activated T lymphocytes also contribute to the propagation of the inflammatory response through various cytokine networks.

ALLERGIC ASTHMA: This is the most common form of asthma and is usually found in children. One third to one half of all patients with asthma have known or suspected reactions to airborne allergens. Common allergens include pollens, animal hair or fur, and contamination of house dust with mites. Allergic asthma is strongly correlated with skin-test reactivity. Half of all children with asthma have a substantial or complete remission of symptoms by age 20 years, but a considerable number have a recurrence after age 30 years.

INFECTIOUS ASTHMA: A common precipitating factor in childhood asthma is a viral respiratory tract infection rather than an allergic stimulus. In children younger than age 2 years, respiratory syncytial virus is the usual agent, whereas in older children, rhinovirus, influenza, and parainfluenza are the common inciting organisms. The inflammatory response to the viral infection in a susceptible person is believed to trigger the episode of bronchoconstriction. This hypothesis is supported by the demonstration that nonasthmatic persons also show bronchial hyperreactivity, which may persist for as long as 2 months after a viral infection.

EXERCISE-INDUCED ASTHMA: Exercise can precipitate some degree of bronchospasm in more than half of all asthmatics, and in some patients, exercise is the only inciting factor. Exercise-induced asthma is related to the magnitude of heat or water loss from the epithelium of the airways. The more rapid the ventilation (severity of exercise) and the colder and drier the air breathed, the more likely is an attack of asthma. Thus, an asthmatic playing hockey on an outdoor rink in Canada in winter is more likely to have an attack than one swimming slowly in Texas during the summer. The mechanisms underlying exercise-induced asthma are unclear. The condition may be the consequence of mediator release or vascular congestion in the bronchi secondary to rewarming of the airways after the exertion.

OCCUPATIONAL ASTHMA: More than 80 different occupational exposures have been linked to the development of asthma. In some instances, these substances provoke allergic asthma by IgE-related hypersensitivity mechanisms. Examples of those affected by this malady include animal handlers, bakers, and workers exposed to wood and vegetable dusts, metal salts, pharmaceutical agents, and industrial chemicals. In other cases, occupational asthma seems to result from a direct release of mediators of smooth muscle contraction after contact with the offending agent. Such a mechanism is postulated in byssinosis ("brown lung"), an occupational lung disease in cotton workers. Some occupational exposures directly affect the autonomic nervous system. For instance, organic phosphorus insecticides act as anticholinesterases and produce overactivity of the parasympathetic nervous system. Substances such as toluene diisocyanate and western red cedar dust are thought to operate through hypersensitivity mechanisms, although specific IgE antibodies to these substances have not been identified.

DRUG-INDUCED ASTHMA: Drug-induced bronchospasm occurs most commonly in patients with known asthma. The best-known offender is aspirin, but other nonsteroidal anti-inflammatory agents also have been implicated. It is estimated that up to 10% of adult asthmatics are sensitive to aspirin. Immediate hypersensitivity does not seem to be involved, and these patients can be desensitized by daily administrations of small doses of aspirin. β-Adrenergic antagonists consistently induce bronchoconstriction in asthmatics and are contraindicated in such patients.

AIR POLLUTION: Massive air pollution, usually in episodes associated with temperature inversions, is associated with bronchospasm in patients with asthma and other preexisting lung diseases. Sulfur dioxide, oxides of nitrogen, and ozone are the commonly implicated environmental pollutants.

EMOTIONAL FACTORS: Psychological stress can aggravate or precipitate an attack of bronchospasm in as many as half of all asthmatics. It is believed that vagal efferent stimulation is the underlying mechanism.

☐ **Pathology:** Most information on the pathology of asthma has been derived from autopsies on patients who have died in status asthmaticus, and thus the most severe lesions are described. On gross examination, the lungs are remarkably distended with air, and the airways are filled with thick, tenacious, adherent mucous plugs. Microscopically, these plugs (Fig. 12-52A) contain strips of epithelium and many eosinophils, the extruded granules of which coalesce to form needle-like crystals *(Charcot–Leyden crystals)* (see Fig. 12-27B). In some cases, the mucoid exudate forms a cast of the airways *(Curschmann spirals),* which may be expelled with coughing. Compact clusters of epithelial cells ("Creola bodies") also are seen in the sputum.

One of the most characteristic features of status asthmaticus is the hyperplasia of bronchial smooth muscle. Bronchial submucosal mucous glands are also hyperplastic (see Fig. 12-52A). The submucosa is edematous and contains a mixed inflammatory infiltrate, including vari-

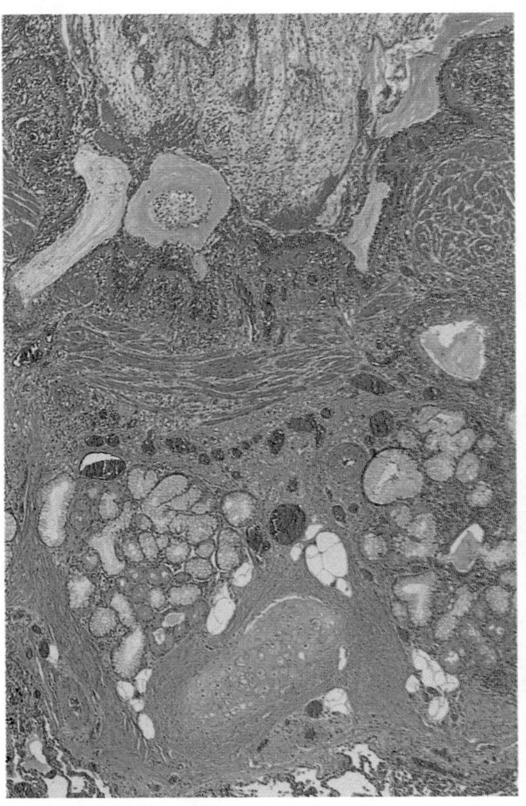

A

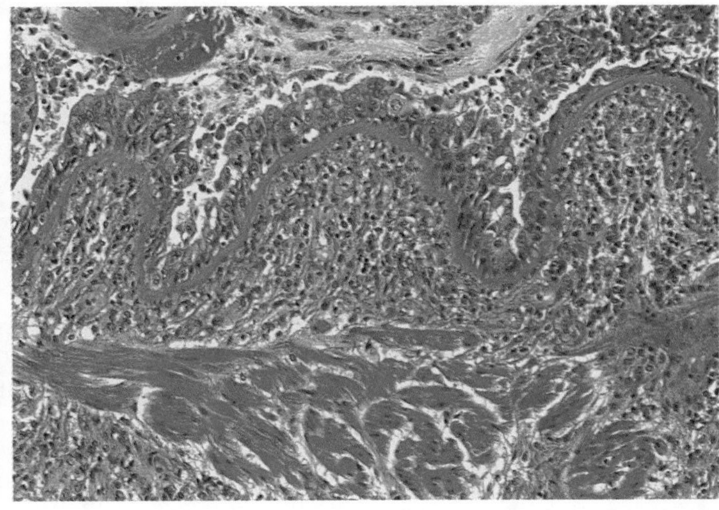

B

FIGURE *12-52*
Asthma. *(A)* A section of lung from a patient who died in status asthmaticus reveals a bronchus containing a luminal mucous plug, submucosal gland hyperplasia, and smooth muscle hyperplasia. *(B)* Higher magnification shows hyaline thickening of the subepithelial basement membrane and marked inflammation of the bronchiolar wall, with numerous eosinophils. The mucosa exhibits an inflamed and metaplastic epithelium.

able numbers of eosinophils. The epithelium does not display the normal pseudostratified appearance and may be denuded, with only the basal cells remaining (see Fig. 12-52B). The basal cells are hyperplastic, and squamous metaplasia is seen. An increase in goblet cells (goblet cell metaplasia) is also apparent. Characteristically, the epithelial basement membrane appears thickened, owing to an increase in collagen deep to the true basal lamina.

☐ **Clinical Features:** A typical attack of asthma begins with a feeling of tightness in the chest and a nonproductive cough. Both inspiratory and expiratory wheezes appear, the respiratory rate increases, and the patient becomes dyspneic. Characteristically, the expiratory phase is particularly prolonged. The end of the attack is often heralded by severe coughing and the expectoration of thick mucus-containing Curschmann spirals, eosinophils, and Charcot–Leyden crystals.

Status asthmaticus *refers to increasingly severe bronchoconstriction that does not respond to the drugs that usually abort the acute attack.* This situation is potentially serious and requires hospitalization. Patients in status asthmaticus have hypoxemia and often hypercapnia, and in particularly severe episodes, they may die. They require oxygen and other pharmacological interventions.

The cornerstone of treatment in asthma is pharmacological and includes the administration of β-adrenergic agonists, inhaled corticosteroids, cromolyn sodium, methylxanthines, and anticholinergic agents. Systemic corticosteroids are reserved for status asthmaticus or resistant chronic asthma. The inhalation of bronchodilators often provides dramatic relief.

PNEUMOCONIOSES

The pneumoconioses are pulmonary diseases caused by the inhalation of inorganic dusts. More than 40 inhaled minerals cause lung lesions and radiographic abnormalities. Most, such as tin, barium, and iron, are innocuous and simply accumulate in the lung. However, some lead to crippling pulmonary diseases. The specific types of pneumoconioses are named according to the substance inhaled (e.g., silicosis, asbestosis, talcosis). In certain instances, the offending agent is uncertain, and often the occupation is simply cited (e.g., "arc welder's lung"). Historically, occupations were recognized as predisposing to lung disease before an etiological agent was recognized. Thus, "knife grinder's lung" was used before this malady was recognized as silicosis.

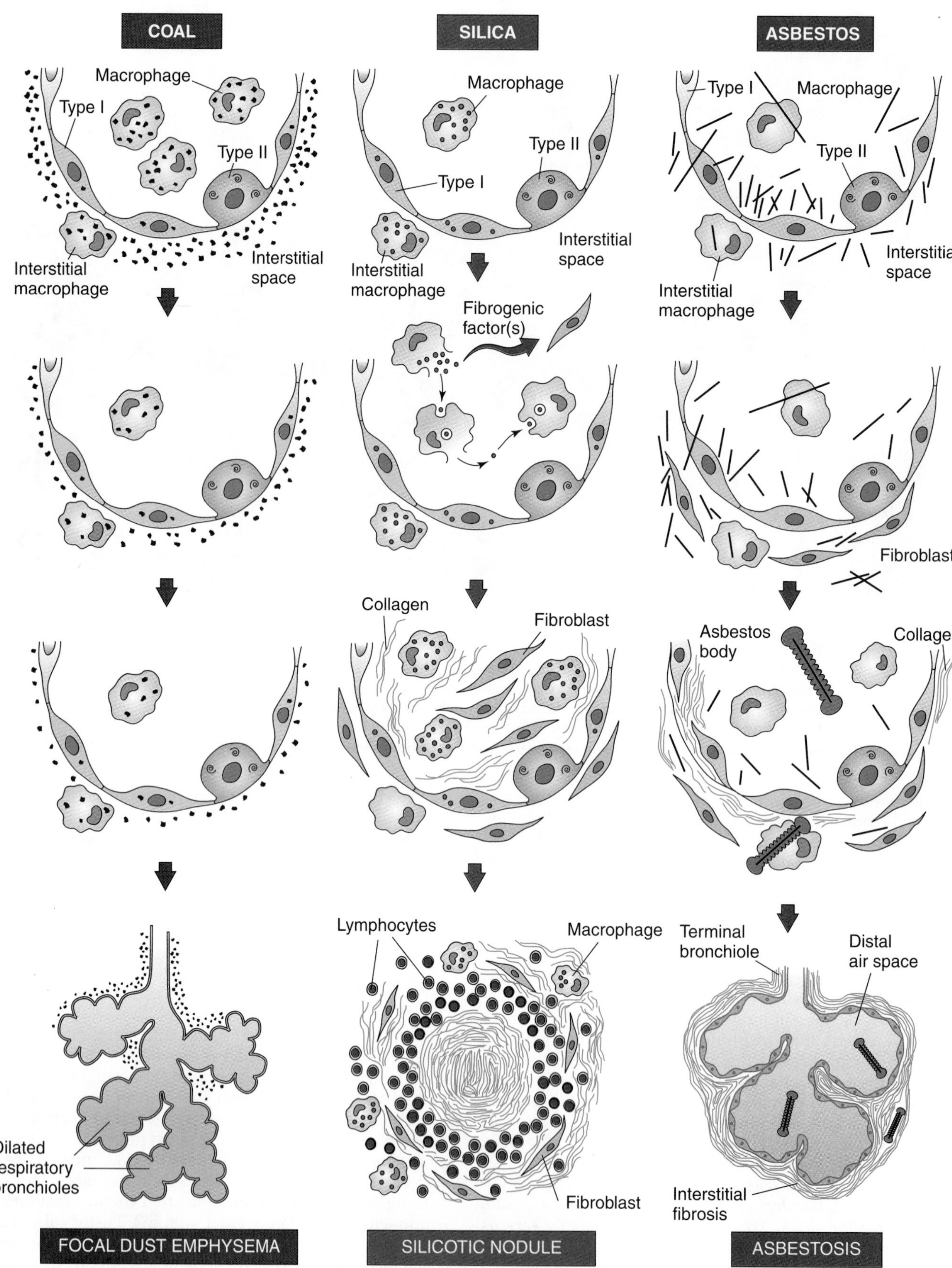
COAL
Macrophage
Type I
Type II
Interstitial macrophage
Interstitial space
FOCAL DUST EMPHYSEMA
Dilated respiratory bronchioles
SILICA
Macrophage
Type II
Type I
Interstitial space
Interstitial macrophage
Fibrogenic factor(s)
Collagen
Fibroblast
Lymphocytes
Macrophage
Fibroblast
SILICOTIC NODULE
ASBESTOS
Type I
Macrophage
Type II
Interstitial space
Interstitial macrophage
Fibroblasts
Asbestos body
Collagen
Terminal bronchiole
Distal air space
Interstitial fibrosis
ASBESTOSIS

FIGURE *12-53*

The most important factor in the production of symptomatic pneumoconioses is the capacity of inhaled dusts to stimulate fibrosis (Fig. 12-53). Thus, small amounts of silica or asbestos may produce extensive fibrosis, whereas coal and iron are weakly fibrogenic at best.

In general, lung lesions produced by inorganic dusts reflect the dose and size of the particles delivered to the lung. The dose is a function of the amount of dust in the ambient air and the time spent working in the environment. Because the inhaled particles are often irregular, it is important to express their size as aerodynamic particle diameter, a parameter that describes the motion of the particle in inspired air. The aerodynamic particle diameter determines where the inhaled dusts deposit in the lung (see Fig. 12-2). The most dangerous particles are those that reach the peripheral zones: the smallest bronchioles and the acini. The majority of large particles (>10 μm in diameter) deposit on the bronchi and bronchioles and are removed by the mucociliary escalator. The smaller particles terminate in the acinus, and the smallest ones behave as a gas and are exhaled.

The alveolar macrophages ingest the inhaled particles and constitute the primary defense mechanism of the alveolar space. Most of the phagocytosed particles ascend to the mucociliary carpet and are expectorated or swallowed. Others migrate into the interstitium of the lung and then into the lymphatics. A significant number of ingested particles accumulate in and about respiratory bronchioles and terminal bronchioles. Other particles are not phagocytosed but migrate through epithelial cells into the interstitium.

Silicosis

Silicosis is a pneumoconiosis caused by the inhalation of silicon dioxide (silica), usually in crystalline form as quartz. The earth's crust is composed largely of silicon and its oxides, and silicosis is one of the oldest recorded diseases, possibly having begun in the Paleolithic period when humans began to fashion flint instruments. Dyspnea in metal diggers was reported by Hippocrates, and early Dutch pathologists wrote that the lungs of stone cutters sectioned like a mass of sand. The 19th-century English literature provided numerous descriptions of silicosis, and the disease remained the major cause of death in workers exposed to silica dust for the first half of the 20th century.

Silicosis was described historically as a disease of sandblasters. Mining also involves exposure to silica, as do numerous other occupations, including stone cutting, polishing and sharpening of metals, ceramic manufacturing, foundry work, and the cleaning of boilers. The use of air-handling equipment and masks has substantially reduced the incidence of silicosis.

☐ Pathogenesis:

The biological effects of silica particles depend on a number of factors, some involving the particle itself and others related to the host response. Crystalline silica is more toxic than amorphous forms, and its biological activity is related to its surface properties. Particles of 0.2 to 2.0 μm are the most dangerous. Impurities, such as iron or aluminum, within the crystals decrease the potency of the particles. Silica particles also commonly exhibit a soluble surface layer that reduces their toxicity. Removal of this layer by acid washing or the creation of new surfaces by sandblasting enhances the biological activity of silica particles.

After their inhalation, silica particles are ingested by alveolar macrophages. Silicon hydroxide groups on the surface of the particles form hydrogen bonds with phospholipids and proteins, an interaction that is presumed to damage cellular membranes and thereby kill the macrophages. The dead cells release free silica particles and fibrogenic factors. The released silica is then reingested by macrophages, and the process is amplified.

☐ Pathology

SIMPLE NODULAR SILICOSIS: This is the most common form of silicosis and is almost inevitable in any worker with long-term exposure to silica. Twenty to 40 years after the initial exposure to silica (but sometimes after only 10 years), the lungs contain silicotic nodules. These characteristic lesions are less than 1 cm in diameter, and usually 2 to 4 mm. On histological examination, they have a characteristic whorled appearance, with concentrically arranged collagen that forms the largest part of the nodule (Fig. 12-54). At the periphery, there are aggregates of mononuclear cells, mostly lymphocytes and fibroblasts. Polarized light reveals doubly refractile needle-shaped silicates within the nodule.

The hilar nodes may become enlarged and calcified, often at the periphery of the node ("eggshell calcification"). Simple silicosis is not ordinarily associated with significant respiratory dysfunction.

PROGRESSIVE MASSIVE FIBROSIS: Progressive massive fibrosis is defined radiologically as nodular masses of more than 2 cm diameter in a background of simple silicosis. These larger lesions represent the coalescence of smaller nodules. Most of these lesions are 5 to 10 cm across and are usually located in the upper zones of

FIGURE *12-53*
Pathogenesis of pneumoconioses. The three most important pneumoconioses are illustrated. In simple coal workers' pneumoconiosis, massive amounts of dust are inhaled and engulfed by macrophages. The macrophages pass into the interstitium of the lung and aggregate around the respiratory bronchioles. Subsequently, the bronchioles dilate. In silicosis, the silica particles are toxic to macrophages, which die and release a fibrogenic factor. In turn the released silica is again phagocytosed by other macrophages. The result is a dense fibrotic nodule, the silicotic nodule. Asbestosis is characterized by little dust and much interstitial fibrosis. Asbestos bodies are the classic features.

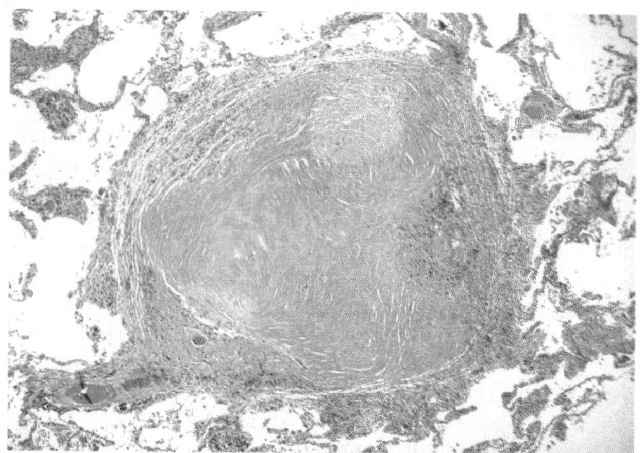

FIGURE 12-54
Silicosis. A silicotic nodule is composed of concentric whorls of dense, sparsely cellular collagen. At the edge of the nodule are dust deposits, which contain carbon pigment and silica particles.

the lungs bilaterally (Fig. 12-55). Morphologically, the lesions often exhibit central cavitation. Progressive massive fibrosis is related to the amount of silica in the lung. Disability is caused by the destruction of lung tissue that has been incorporated into the nodules.

ACUTE SILICOSIS: Now uncommon, acute silicosis results from heavy exposure to finely particulate silica during sandblasting or boiler scaling. It is associated with diffuse fibrosis of the lung, but silicotic nodules are not found. Dense eosinophilic material accumulates in alveolar spaces to produce an appearance that resembles alveolar lipoproteinosis. Indeed, experimental administration of finely particulate silica has been used as a model for that condition. The disease progresses rapidly over a few years, in contrast to other forms of silicosis, in which progression is measured in decades. On radiological examination, acute silicosis shows diffuse linear fibrosis and a reduction in lung volume. Clinically, there is a severe restrictive defect.

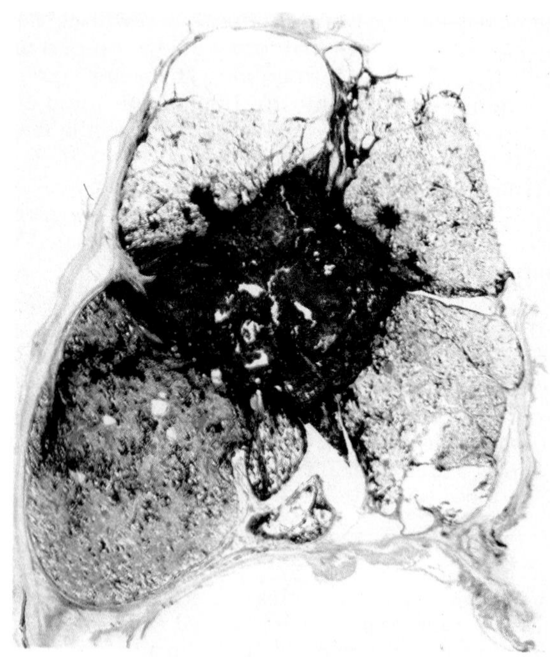

FIGURE 12-55
Progressive massive fibrosis. A whole mount of a silicotic lung from a coal miner shows a large area of dense fibrosis containing entrapped carbon particles.

☐ **Clinical Features:** Simple silicosis is usually a radiological diagnosis without significant symptoms. Dyspnea on exertion, and later at rest, suggests progressive massive fibrosis or other complications of silicosis. In acute silicosis, dyspnea may become rapidly disabling, after which respiratory failure ensues.

It is well recognized that tuberculosis is much more common in patients with silicosis than in the general population. The incidence of tuberculosis in patients with silicosis is higher in acute silicosis and among populations with a high prevalence of tuberculosis. Despite a decline in the incidence of tuberculosis in the general population, the association with silicosis has persisted. There is no increase in the incidence of lung cancer in patients with silicosis.

Coal Workers' Pneumoconiosis

Coal dust is composed of amorphous carbon and other constituents of the earth's surface, including variable amounts of silica. Anthracite (hard) coal contains significantly more quartz than does the bituminous variety (soft coal). Workers in certain occupations, such as those who work within mines, inhale more quartz particles than those working above ground or loading coal for transport. In this context, it is important to recognize that amorphous carbon by itself is not fibrogenic, owing to its inability to kill alveolar macrophages. It is simply a nuisance dust that causes an innocuous anthracosis. By contrast, silica is highly fibrogenic, and the inhalation of anthracotic particles may therefore lead to the lesions of anthracosilicosis.

☐ **Pathology:** The characteristic pulmonary lesions in coal workers are the coal-dust macules, which appear as scattered black areas, 1 to 4 mm across, throughout the lungs. The pigmented appearance of the lungs accounts for the term *black lung disease,* also termed *simple coal workers' pneumoconiosis.* Microscopically, the coal-dust macule exhibits numerous carbon-laden macrophages, which surround the distal respiratory bronchioles, extend to fill adjacent alveolar spaces, and infiltrate the peribronchiolar interstitial space. There is an accompanying mild dilatation of respiratory bronchioles *(focal dust emphysema),* which probably results from atrophy of smooth muscle.

Coal-dust macules appear on a chest radiograph as small nodular densities. Although simple coal workers' pneumoconiosis was once thought to cause severe disability, it is now clear that black lung causes at worst minor impairment of pulmonary function. When coal miners have severe air-flow obstruction, it is usually due to smoking.

The appearance of larger nodular lesions in lungs of coal workers suggests a change caused by silica in the inhaled dust, and the disease is now termed *anthracosilicosis* (Fig. 12-56). The silicotic component of this mixed disorder is no different from that encountered in silicosis itself and has the same evolution. In particular, cavitary lesions and progressive massive fibrosis may develop, and significant respiratory disability may ensue.

Caplan syndrome was originally described as the presence of rheumatoid nodules *(Caplan nodules)* in the lungs of coal miners with rheumatoid arthritis. However, the term Caplan syndrome is now also used for the association of pulmonary rheumatoid nodules with other pneumoconioses, such as silicosis or asbestosis. These nodular lesions are large (1 to 10 cm in diameter), multiple, bilateral, and usually peripheral. Microscopically, a Caplan nodule has the appearance of a rheumatoid nodule associated with inhaled dust deposits. Rheumatoid nodules consist of large, central, necrotic areas surrounded by a border of chronic inflammation and palisading macrophages. Caplan nodules are similar but not identical to rheumatoid nodules, and may represent a combination of silicotic and rheumatoid nodules.

Asbestos-Related Diseases

Asbestos is a generic term that embraces a group of fibrous silicate minerals that occur as long, thin fibers. This mineral has been used for a variety of purposes for more than 4000 years, since early Finns fashioned pottery from the material. The Roman vestal virgins used asbestos in the manufacture of oil-lamp wicks, and Marco Polo remarked on the asbestos-containing Chinese cloth that resisted fire. The mining of asbestos proceeded exponentially in the 20th century, until its deleterious effects elicited alarm in the medical community during the past few decades.

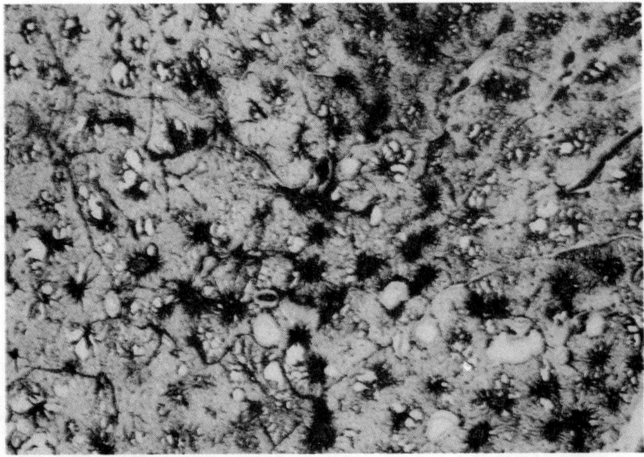

FIGURE 12-56
Anthracosilicosis. A whole mount of the lung of a coal miner demonstrates scattered, irregular, pigmented nodules throughout the parenchyma.

TABLE 12-4 **Asbestos-Related Lung Disease**

Pleural lesions	**Interstitial lung disease**
Benign pleural effusion	Asbestosis
Parietal pleural plaques	
Diffuse pleural fibrosis	**Malignant mesothelioma**
Rounded atelectasis	
	Carcinoma of the lung (in smokers)

Asbestos (Greek, *unquenchable*) occurs in three natural forms: crocidolite, which is found mainly in South Africa; chrysolite, the most common form of asbestos, most of which is mined in Quebec; and amosite. If coal is the classic example of much dust and little fibrosis, asbestos is the prototype of little dust and much fibrosis (see Fig. 12-53). Exposure to asbestos can result in a number of thoracic complications including asbestosis, benign pleural effusion, diffuse pleural fibrosis, pleural plaques, and rounded atelectasis (Table 12-4).

Asbestosis: *Asbestosis refers to the diffuse interstitial fibrosis that results from the inhalation of asbestos fibers.* The disease occurs as a result of the processing and handling of asbestos, rather than mining, which is a surface operation. Exposure starts with the baggers who package asbestos and continues with those who modify or use it, such as workers who make asbestos products (tiles, cement, insulation material) and those in the construction and shipbuilding industries.

☐ **Pathogenesis:** Asbestos fibers are long (up to 100 μm) but thin (0.5 to 1 μm), so that their aerodynamic particle diameter is small. They deposit in the distal airways and alveoli, particularly at the bifurcations of alveolar ducts. The smallest particles are engulfed by macrophages, but many of the larger fibers penetrate into the interstitial space. The first lesion is an alveolitis that is directly related to asbestos exposure. Release of inflammatory mediators by activated macrophages and the fibrogenic character of the free asbestos fibers in the interstitium promote interstitial pulmonary fibrosis.

☐ **Pathology:** Asbestosis is characterized by bilateral, diffuse interstitial fibrosis and asbestos bodies in the lung (Fig. 12-57). In the early stages, fibrosis occurs in and around alveolar ducts and respiratory bronchioles, as well as in the periphery of the acinus. Asbestos fibers that deposit in the bronchioles and respiratory bronchioles incite a fibrogenic response in these locations, which leads to mild chronic air-flow obstruction. Thus, asbestos may produce an obstructive as well as a restrictive defect. As the disease becomes more advanced, fibrosis spreads beyond the peribronchiolar location and eventually, results in an end-stage or ("honeycomb") lung. Asbestosis is usually more severe in the lower zones of the lung.

Asbestos bodies are found in the walls of the bronchioles or within alveolar spaces, often engulfed by alveolar macrophages. The particle has distinctive morpho-

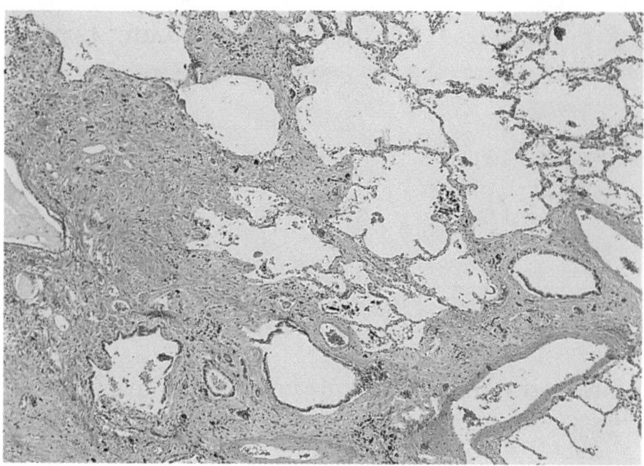

FIGURE 12-57
Asbestosis. The lung shows patchy, dense, interstitial fibrosis.

logical features, consisting of a clear, thin asbestos fiber (10 to 50 μm in length) surrounded by a beaded iron–protein coat. By light microscopy, it is golden brown (Fig. 12-58) and stains strongly with the Prussian blue stain for iron. The fibers are only partly engulfed by macrophages because they are too large for a single cell. The macrophages coat the asbestos fiber with protein, proteoglycans, and ferritin.

The incidental finding of asbestos bodies in autopsies does not warrant a diagnosis of asbestosis; the lungs must show diffuse interstitial fibrosis as well as asbestos bodies. Digests and concentrates of lung tissue show that asbestos bodies occur to varying degrees in the lungs of virtually all patients who come to autopsy.

BENIGN PLEURAL EFFUSION: Benign pleural effusion associated with the inhalation of asbestos is diagnosed by four criteria: (1) a history of asbestos exposure, (2) identification of a pleural effusion with radiographs or thoracentesis, (3) absence of other diseases that could cause effusion, and (4) no malignant tumor after 3 years of follow-up. Pleural effusions often occur within 10 years of initial exposure and have been observed in about 3% of workers exposed to asbestos.

PLEURAL PLAQUES: Pleural plaques typically occur on the parietal and diaphragmatic pleura, often 10 to 20 years after exposure to asbestos. Plaques may be found in up to 15% of the general population, and half of all patients with plaques at autopsy may not have a history of asbestos exposure. Plaques are found most often on the parietal pleura, in the posterolateral regions of the lower thorax, and on the domes of the diaphragm.

On gross examination, pleural plaques are pearly white and have a smooth or nodular surface (Fig. 12-59). They are usually bilateral, although not necessarily symmetric. Plaques may become quite large, measuring more than 10 cm in diameter, and may become calcified. Histologically, they consist of acellular, dense, hyalinized fibrous tissue, with numerous slit-like spaces in a parallel fashion (basket-weave pattern). Pleural plaques are not a predictor of asbestosis.

DIFFUSE PLEURAL FIBROSIS: Fibrosis limited to the pleura is usually detected at least 10 years after initial exposure to asbestos. It must be distinguished from asbestosis, in which fibrosis diffusely affects the interstitium of the underlying lung parenchyma. Plaques and pleural fibrosis can occur in association with all types of asbestos.

ROUNDED ATELECTASIS: Asbestosis exposure occasionally leads to a condition in which pleural fibrosis and adhesions are associated with atelectasis, which has a rounded appearance on chest radiograph. Radiographically, rounded atelectasis is characterized by a pleural-based, rounded or oval, 2.5- to 5.0-cm shadow, which usually lies along the posterior surface of a lower lobe. Pathologically, the lung shows pleural fibrosis or plaques, with curved pleural invaginations extending several centimeters into the underlying parenchyma. The condition is entirely benign.

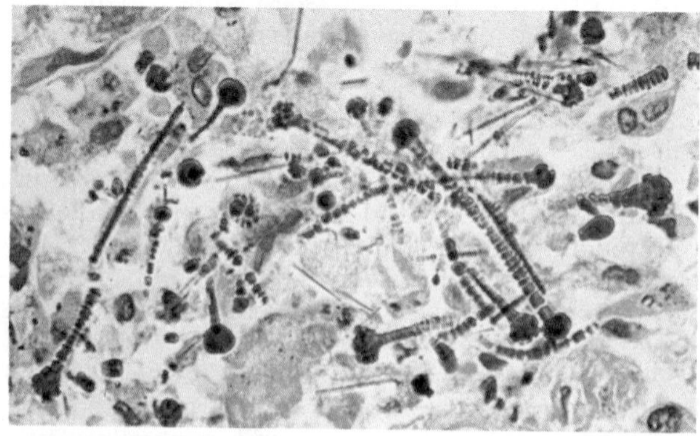

FIGURE 12-58
Asbestos bodies. These ferruginous bodies are golden brown and beaded, with a central, colorless, nonbirefringent core fiber. Asbestos bodies are encrusted with protein and iron.

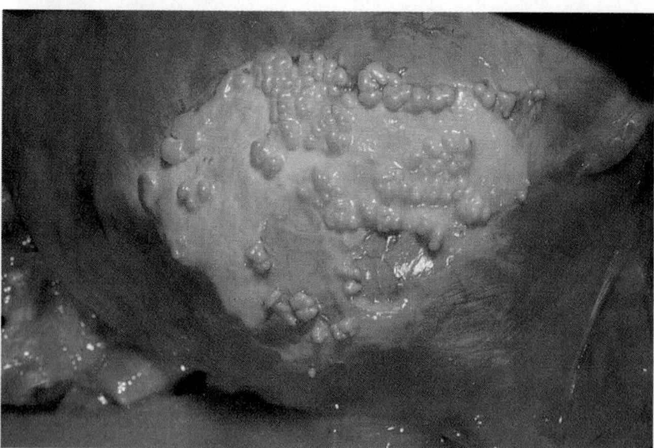

FIGURE 12-59
Pleural plaque. The dome of the diaphragm is covered by a smooth, pearly white, nodular plaque.

MESOTHELIOMA: **A clear-cut relation between asbestos exposure and malignant mesothelioma is firmly established.** Sometimes the exposure is slight, as in the wives of asbestos workers who wash their husbands' clothes. More often mesothelioma is found in workers heavily exposed to asbestos, predominantly of the crocidolite variety. The clinical and pathological features of this disease are discussed later with diseases of the pleura.

CARCINOMA OF THE LUNG: Lung cancer has been reported to be 3 to 5 times more common in nonsmoking asbestos workers than in similar workers not exposed to asbestos, although this figure is based on small numbers and remains to be firmly established. However, in asbestos workers who smoke, the incidence of carcinoma of the lung is vastly increased; the reported risk is increased up to 60 times that of the general population. The link between asbestos and lung cancer is most convincingly supported in the presence of asbestosis (diffuse interstitial fibrosis).

Berylliosis

Berylliosis refers to the pulmonary disease that follows the inhalation of beryllium. Today this metal is employed principally in structural materials used in aerospace industries, in the manufacture of industrial ceramics, and in atomic reactors. Exposure to beryllium also may occur during the mining and extraction of beryllium ores.

Berylliosis occurs as an acute, chemical pneumonitis or as a chronic pneumoconiosis. In the acute form, symptoms begin within hours or days after inhalation of metal particles and are reflected pathologically in diffuse alveolar damage. Of all persons with acute beryllium pneumonitis, 10% progress to chronic disease, although chronic berylliosis is often encountered in workers without any history of an acute illness.

Chronic berylliosis differs from other pneumoconioses in that the amount and duration of exposure may be small, and the lesion is suspected to be a hypersensitivity phenomenon. Pathologically, the pulmonary lesions are indistinguishable from those of sarcoidosis. Multiple noncaseating granulomas are distributed along the pleura, septa, and bronchovascular bundles (Fig. 12-60). Progression of the disease can result in end-stage fibrosis (honeycomb lung). Patients with chronic berylliosis have an insidious onset of dyspnea 15 or more years after the initial exposure. The disease appears to be associated with an increased risk of lung cancer.

Talcosis

Talcosis refers to a pneumoconiosis that is caused by prolonged and heavy exposure to talc dust. Talc consists of magnesium silicates that are used in a number of industries for their lubricant properties and in cosmetics and pharmaceuticals. Occupational exposure to talc occurs among workers engaged in the mining and milling of the mineral and in the leather, rubber, paper, and textile industries. Industrial talc is usually mixed with other minerals such as asbestos or silica. Cosmetic talc is more than 90% pure and rarely causes lung disease. On gross examination, the lesions of talcosis vary from minute nodules to severe fibrosis. Microscopically, foreign-body granulomas associated with birefringent plate-like talc particles are scattered throughout the parenchyma, which displays fibrotic nodules and interstitial fibrosis. The associated minerals, such as silica or asbestos, may contribute to the fibrotic changes.

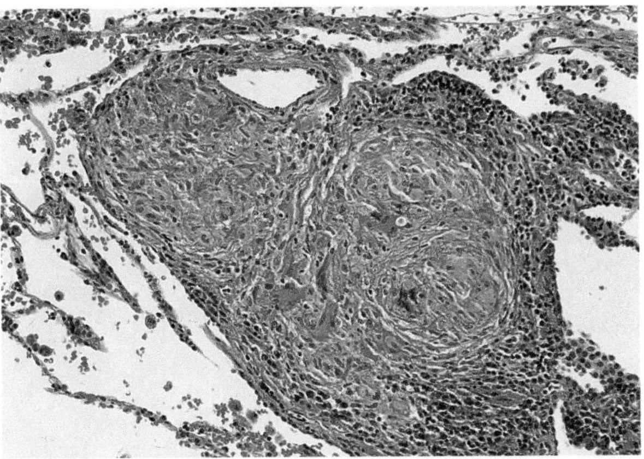

FIGURE *12-60*
Berylliosis. A noncaseating granuloma consists of a nodular collection of epithelioid macrophages and multinucleated giant cells.

Intravenous drug abusers who use talc as the carrier material for illicit drugs develop vascular and interstitial granulomas in the lung, together with variable degrees of fibrosis. Arterial changes of pulmonary hypertension are common, and persons with these changes may initially be seen with cor pulmonale.

INTERSTITIAL LUNG DISEASE

A large number of pulmonary disorders are grouped as interstitial, infiltrative, or restrictive diseases because they are characterized by inflammatory infiltrates in the interstitial space and have similar clinical and radiological presentations. These diverse maladies (a) are acute or chronic, (b) of known or unknown etiology, and (c) vary from minimally symptomatic conditions to severely incapacitating and lethal interstitial fibrosis.

Hypersensitivity Pneumonitis

Hypersensitivity pneumonitis, also termed extrinsic allergic alveolitis, is an immunological response in the lung to inhaled antigens.

☐ **Pathogenesis:** A wide variety of antigens is known to cause hypersensitivity pneumonitis. The inhalation of these antigens leads to acute or chronic interstitial inflammation in the lung. Most of the responsible antigens are encountered in occupational settings, and the diseases are often labeled according to the specific vocation. For example, *farmer's lung* occurs in farmers exposed to *Micropolyspora faeni* from moldy hay, *bagassosis* results from exposure to *Thermoactinomyces saccharii* in moldy sugar cane, *"maple bark–stripper's disease"* is seen in per-

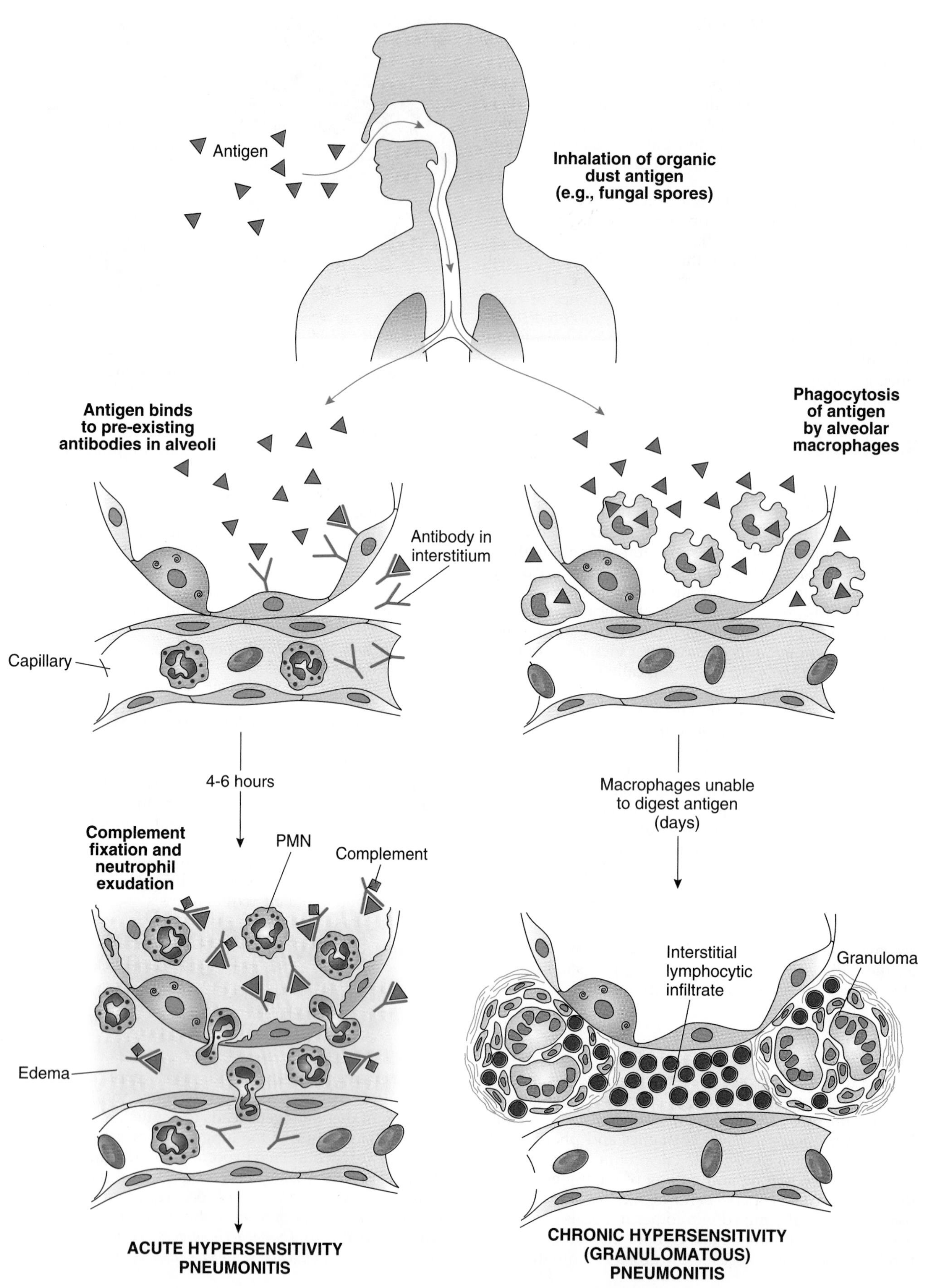
Antigen
Inhalation of organic dust antigen (e.g., fungal spores)
Antigen binds to pre-existing antibodies in alveoli
Phagocytosis of antigen by alveolar macrophages
Antibody in interstitium
Capillary
4-6 hours
Macrophages unable to digest antigen (days)
Complement fixation and neutrophil exudation
PMN
Complement
Edema
Interstitial lymphocytic infiltrate
Granuloma
ACUTE HYPERSENSITIVITY PNEUMONITIS
CHRONIC HYPERSENSITIVITY (GRANULOMATOUS) PNEUMONITIS

FIGURE 12-61

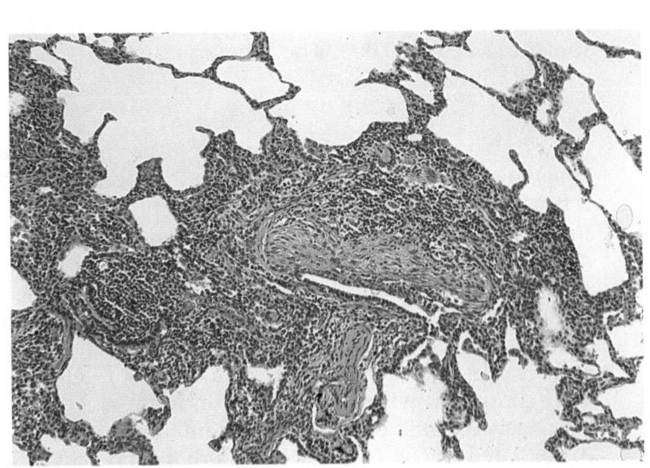

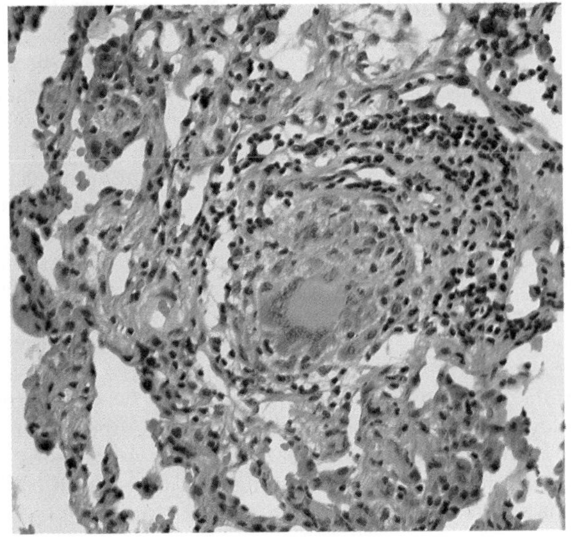

A B

FIGURE *12-62*
Hypersensitivity pneumonitis. ***(A)*** **A lung biopsy shows a mild peribronchiolar chronic inflammatory interstitial infiltrate, with a focus of intraluminal organizing fibrosis.** ***(B)*** **Focal poorly formed granulomas were scattered in the lung biopsy.**

sons exposed to the fungus *Cryptostroma corticale* from moldy maple bark, and *bird fancier's lung* affects bird keepers with long-term exposure to proteins from bird feathers, blood, and excrement. Other causes of hypersensitivity pneumonitis include the inhalation of pituitary snuff (*pituitary snuff taker's disease*), moldy cork (*suberosis*), and moldy compost (*mushroom worker's disease*). Hypersensitivity pneumonitis may also be caused by fungi growing in stagnant water in air conditioners, swimming pools, hot tubs, and central heating units. Skin tests and serum-precipitating antibodies are often used to confirm the diagnosis. In many cases, especially in the chronic form of hypersensitivity pneumonitis, the inciting antigen is never identified.

Acute hypersensitivity pneumonitis is characterized by a neutrophilic infiltrate in the alveoli and respiratory bronchioles, whereas chronic lesions display mononuclear cells and granulomas, typical of delayed hypersensitivity. In most cases, precipitating IgG antibodies against the offending agent are demonstrated in the serum. Hypersensitivity pneumonitis represents a combination of immune complex–mediated (type III) and cell-mediated (type IV) hypersensitivity reactions, although the precise contribution of each is still debated (Fig. 12-61). However, it is important to note that the large majority of persons with serum precipitins to inhaled antigens do not develop hypersensitivity pneumonitis on exposure, a fact that suggests a genetic component in host susceptibility.

☐ **Pathology:** In florid cases of hypersensitivity pneumonitis, the histological picture is strongly suggestive, whereas in subtle cases, the diagnosis may require careful clinical correlation; even then the diagnosis may remain tentative. The main microscopic features of chronic hypersensitivity pneumonitis include interstitial chronic inflammation, noncaseating granulomas, organization of the exudate within distal airways (intraluminal budding fibrosis), and interstitial fibrosis (Fig. 12-62A,B). The interstitial infiltrate, which tends to be peribronchiolar (bronchocentric) and varies from severe to subtle, consists of lymphocytes, plasma cells, and macrophages; eosinophils are distinctly uncommon. Poorly formed noncaseating granulomas are present in two thirds of cases (see Fig. 12-62B). Intraluminal budding fibrosis is found in two thirds of cases and may form the lesion of bronchiolitis obliterans (see Fig. 12-62A). In the end stage, the interstitial inflammation recedes, leaving nonspecific pulmonary fibrosis, resembling the final stage of usual interstitial pneumonia.

☐ **Clinical Features:** Hypersensitivity pneumonitis may be first seen as acute, subacute, or chronic pulmonary disease, depending on the frequency and intensity of exposure to the offending antigen. The prototype of hypersensitivity pneumonitis is "farmer's lung," caused by the inhalation of thermophilic actinomycetes,

FIGURE *12-61*
Hypersensitivity pneumonitis. An antigen–antibody reaction occurs in the acute phase and leads to acute hypersensitivity pneumonitis. If exposure is continued, this is followed by a cellular or subacute phase, with the formation of granulomas and chronic interstitial pneumonitis.

which grow in moldy hay. Typically, a farm worker enters a barn where hay has been stored for winter feeding. After a lag period of 4 to 6 hours, the worker rapidly develops dyspnea, cough, and mild fever. The symptoms remit within 24 to 48 hours, but return on reexposure; with time, they become chronic. Patients with the chronic form of hypersensitivity pneumonitis have a more nonspecific presentation, with the indolent onset of dyspnea and cor pulmonale.

Pulmonary-function studies show a restrictive pattern, characterized by decreased compliance, reduced diffusion capacity, and hypoxemia. In the chronic stage of hypersensitivity pneumonitis, airway obstruction may become troublesome. Bronchoalveolar lavage shows a T lymphocytosis, with a predominance of CD8+ suppressor/cytotoxic cells. Removal of the environmental antigen is the only adequate treatment for hypersensitivity pneumonitis. Steroid therapy may be effective in acute forms and for some chronically affected patients.

Sarcoidosis

Sarcoidosis is a multisystem disease of unknown etiology in which noncaseating granulomas occur in almost any organ of the body. The lung is the most frequently involved organ, but the lymph nodes, skin, and eye are also common targets (Fig. 12-63).

☐ **Epidemiology:** Sarcoidosis is a worldwide disease, affecting all races and both sexes. The differences in the prevalence of the disease among racial and ethnic groups are remarkable. In North America, sarcoidosis occurs much more frequently in blacks than in whites, the ratio being about 15:1. Whereas sarcoidosis is frequent among blacks in South Africa, it is reported to be uncommon in tropical Africa. The disease is often encountered in Scandinavian countries, where the prevalence is 64/100,000, compared with 10/100,000 in France, and 3/100,000 in Poland. It has been reported that the prevalence of sarcoidosis in Irish women in London is an astonishing 200/100,000. The illness is distinctly uncommon in China.

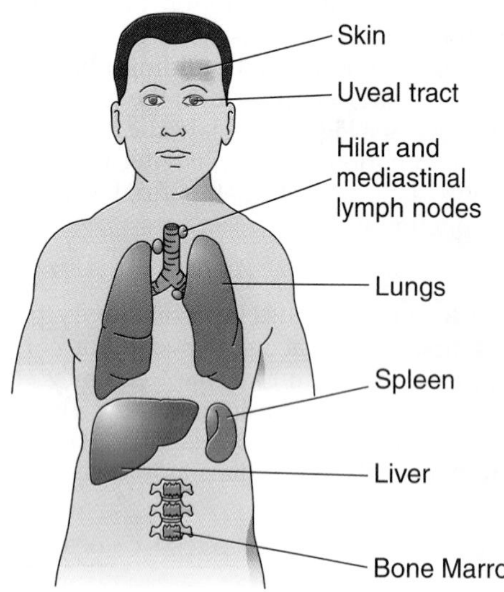

FIGURE *12-63*
Organs commonly affected by sarcoidosis. Sarcoidosis involves many organs, most commonly the lymph nodes and lung.

☐ **Pathogenesis:** Although the exact pathogenesis of sarcoidosis remains obscure, there is a consensus that it represents an exaggerated cellular immune response on the part of helper/inducer T lymphocytes to exogenous antigens or autoantigens. These cells accumulate in the affected organs, where they secrete lymphokines and recruit macrophages, which participate in the formation of noncaseating granulomas. The organs that contain sarcoid granulomas exhibit a CD4+ to CD8+ T-cell ratio of 10:1, compared with a ratio of 2:1 in uninvolved tissues. The basis for this abnormal accumulation of helper/inducer T lymphocytes is unclear. Perhaps a defect in suppressor-cell function permits unopposed helper-cell proliferation. In addition, inherited or acquired differences in immune-response genes may favor the response of one type of T cells as opposed to another. Nonspecific polyclonal activation of B cells by T-helper cells leads to hyperglobulinemia, a characteristic feature of active sarcoidosis.

☐ **Pathology:** Pulmonary sarcoidosis most commonly affects the lung and hilar lymph nodes, although either involvement may occur separately. Radiologically, a diffuse reticulonodular infiltrate is typical, but in occasional cases, larger nodules are present. Histologically, multiple sarcoid granulomas are scattered in the interstitium of the lung (Fig. 12-64). The distribution is distinctive: along the pleura and interlobular septa, and around the bronchovascular bundles (see Fig. 12-64A). Frequent bronchial or bronchiolar submucosal infiltration by sarcoid granulomas accounts for the high diagnostic yield (>90%) on bronchoscopic biopsy. Granulomas in the airways may occasionally be so prominent as to lead to airway obstruction (endobronchial sarcoid).

The cellular granulomatous phase of sarcoidosis can progress to a fibrotic phase. Fibrosis often begins at the periphery of the granuloma and may show an onion-skin pattern of lamellar fibrosis around the giant cells. Although necrosis is usually absent, small foci of necrosis are seen in one third of open lung biopsies. Interstitial chronic inflammation tends to be inconspicuous. Vasculitis can be demonstrated in two thirds of open lung biopsy specimens from patients with sarcoidosis. Asteroid bodies (star-shaped crystals) may be seen in the granulomas (see Fig. 12-64B). Schaumann bodies (small calcifications with a lamellar structure) may also be present.

In most cases of pulmonary sarcoidosis, interstitial fibrosis is not a prominent feature. However, in rare instances, progressive pulmonary fibrosis leads to a honeycomb lung and resulting respiratory insufficiency and cor pulmonale.

☐ **Clinical Features:** Sarcoidosis most commonly occurs in young adults of both sexes. **Acute sarcoidosis**

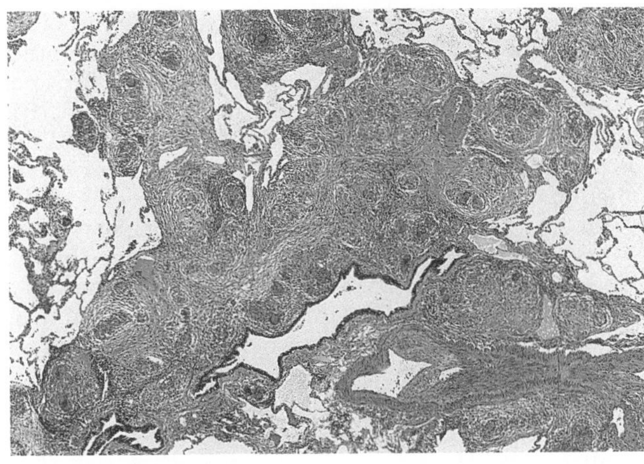
A

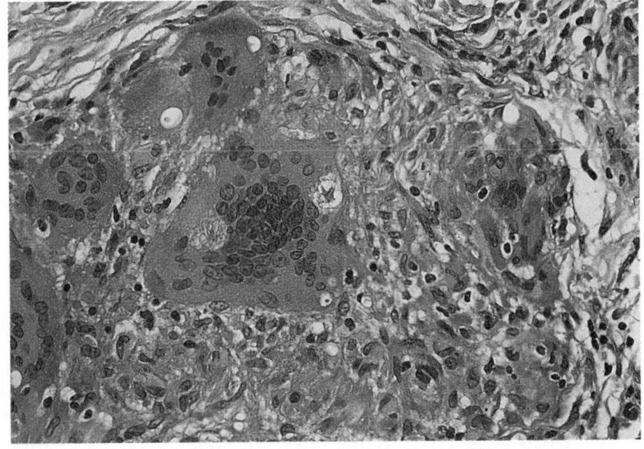
B

FIGURE *12-64*
Sarcoidosis. *(A)* Multiple noncaseating granulomas are present along the bronchovascular interstitium. *(B)* Noncaseating granulomas consist of tight clusters of epithelioid macrophages and multinucleated giant cells. Several asteroid bodies are present.

has an abrupt onset, usually followed by spontaneous remission within 2 years and an excellent response to steroids. **Chronic sarcoidosis** has an insidious onset, and patients are more likely to have persistent or progressive disease. Sarcoidosis causes several chest radiographic patterns, the most classic of which is bilateral hilar adenopathy, with or without interstitial pulmonary infiltrates. The malady may also affect the skin (erythema nodosum and lupus pernio), more commonly in women. Black patients tend to have more severe uveitis, skin disease, and lacrimal gland involvement. Cough and dyspnea are the major respiratory complaints. However, the disease can be mild, and the diagnosis may be discovered as an incidental finding on a chest radiograph in an asymptomatic patient.

No laboratory test is specific for the diagnosis of sarcoidosis. At one time, the skin reaction to the intradermal injection of Kveim antigen (an extract of spleen from a patient with sarcoidosis) was used. This test has been superseded by the more reliable transbronchial lung biopsy, a procedure in which granulomas are demonstrated in lung tissue obtained through a fiberoptic bronchoscope. Occasionally, the diagnosis is based on the finding of multiple noncaseating granulomas in the biopsy of a mediastinal lymph node by mediastinoscopy. Bronchoalveolar lavage often demonstrates an increase in the proportion of T lymphocytes that show a predominance of CD4+ cells. An increased uptake of gallium 67, a material phagocytosed by activated macrophages, can demonstrate granulomatous areas. The serum level of angiotensin-converting enzyme (ACE) is elevated in two thirds of the patients with active sarcoidosis, and the 24-hour urine calcium excretion is frequently increased. The laboratory data, together with the clinical and radiological findings, allow the diagnosis of sarcoidosis to be established with a high degree of probability.

The other organs commonly involved by sarcoidosis include the skin, eye, heart, central nervous system, extrathoracic lymph nodes, spleen, and liver. These are discussed separately in individual chapters.

The prognosis in pulmonary sarcoidosis is favorable, and most patients do not manifest clinically significant sequelae. Resolution occurs in 60% of patients with pulmonary sarcoidosis but is less likely in older patients and those with extrathoracic lesions, particularly the bone and skin. In up to 20% of the cases, the disorder does not remit or recurs at intervals, but it directly accounts for the death of the patient in only 10% of the cases. Corticosteroid therapy is effective for active sarcoidosis.

Usual Interstitial Pneumonia/ Idiopathic Pulmonary Fibrosis

Usual interstitial pneumonia (UIP) refers to a chronic interstitial disease of the lung of unknown etiology, characterized clinically by progressive respiratory insufficiency and pathologically by interstitial inflammation and fibrosis. UIP is one of the most common types of interstitial pneumonitis, with an annual incidence of 3 to 5 cases per 100,000 persons in the United States. A number of terms have been applied to this entity, including Hamman–Rich syndrome (which actually represents idiopathic DAD), cryptogenic fibrosing alveolitis, and idiopathic pulmonary fibrosis (IPF). IPF is actually a clinical term, which in the past embraced the pathological spectrum from desquamative interstitial pneumonia (DIP) to UIP. Currently, the term IPF is restricted to those cases that exhibit a morphological pattern characteristic of UIP. UIP has a slight male predominance and affects persons of all ages, with a mean age at onset of 50 to 60 years.

☐ **Pathogenesis:** The etiology of UIP is unknown, but viral, genetic, and immunological factors are thought to play a role. A viral etiology is favored by the history of a flu-like illness in some patients. A genetic role is suggested by cases of familial IPF and the association of UIP-like diseases in patients with inherited disorders such as neurofibromatosis and Hermansky–Pudlak syndrome.

An immunological component has been proposed because of the presence of an associated collagen vascular disease in about 20% of cases, including rheumatoid arthritis, systemic lupus erythematosus, and progressive systemic sclerosis. UIP also occurs in the context of other autoimmune disorders (e.g., Hashimoto thyroiditis, primary biliary cirrhosis, chronic hepatitis, idiopathic thrombocytopenic purpura, and myasthenia gravis). In addition, patients with UIP frequently exhibit circulating autoantibodies (e.g., antinuclear antibodies and rheumatoid factor). Immune complexes have been demonstrated in the circulation, the inflamed alveolar walls, and bronchoalveolar-lavage specimens, although the antigen has not been identified. It has been postulated that alveolar macrophages become activated on phagocytosis of immune complexes, after which they release cytokines that recruit neutrophils. In turn, polymorphonuclear leukocytes damage the alveolar walls, setting in motion a series of events that culminates in interstitial fibrosis.

□ **Pathology:** The lungs are small in UIP, and the fibrosis tends to be worse in the lower lobes, in the subpleural regions, and along the interlobular septa. Retraction of the scars, especially of lobular septa, gives the external surface of the lung a hobnail appearance, reminiscent of cirrhosis of the liver. Grossly, fibrosis is often patchy, with areas of dense scarring and honeycomb cystic change (Fig. 12-65A).

The histological hallmark of UIP is patchy chronic inflammation and interstitial fibrosis, with areas of normal lung adjacent to fibrotic areas (see Fig. 12-65B). This pattern of fibrosis is nonspecific, and the diagnosis of UIP is, therefore, one of exclusion. Because of alveolitis and subsequent fibrosis, the distal part of the acinus shrinks, and the proximal bronchioles dilate. The bronchiolar epithelium grows into the dilated air spaces, which may represent damaged proximal respiratory bronchioles but are no longer recognized as such. (Fig. 12-66). The areas of dense scarring fibrosis cause remodeling of the lung architecture, resulting in collapse of alveolar walls and formation of cystic spaces (see Fig. 12-65A). The cystic spaces are typically lined by bronchiolar or cuboidal epithelium and contain mucus, macrophages, or neutrophils. The edges of the dense scars may show small foci of loose fibroblastic connective tissue. Interstitial chronic inflammation is mild or moderate. Lymphoid aggregates, sometimes containing germinal centers, are occasionally noted, particularly in UIP associated with rheumatoid arthritis. Extensive vascular changes, particularly intimal fibrosis and thickening of the media, can be seen and may be associated with pulmonary hypertension.

□ **Clinical Features:** Usual interstitial pneumonitis begins insidiously, with the gradual onset of dyspnea on ex-

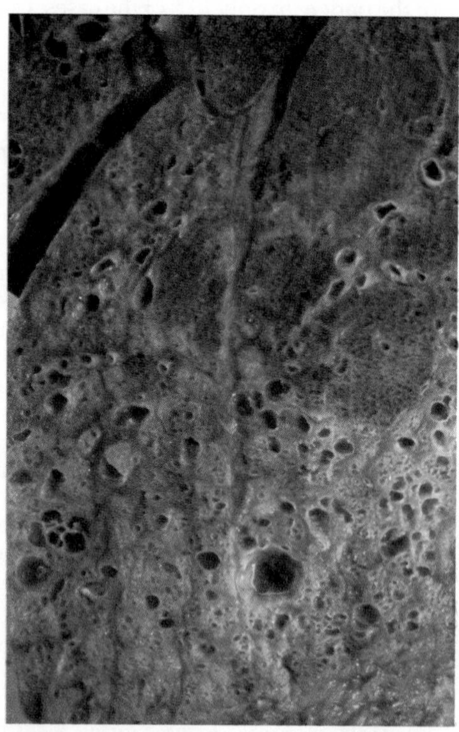

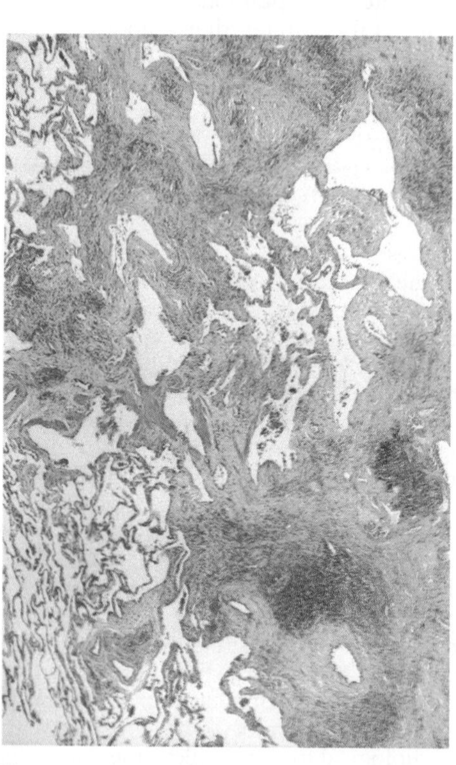

FIGURE *12-65*
Usual interstitial pneumonitis. *(A)* A gross specimen of the lung shows patchy dense scarring with extensive areas of honeycomb cystic change. *(B)* A microscopic view shows patchy interstitial dense fibrosis and interstitial chronic inflammation. The areas of dense fibrosis display remodeling, with loss of the normal lung architecture.

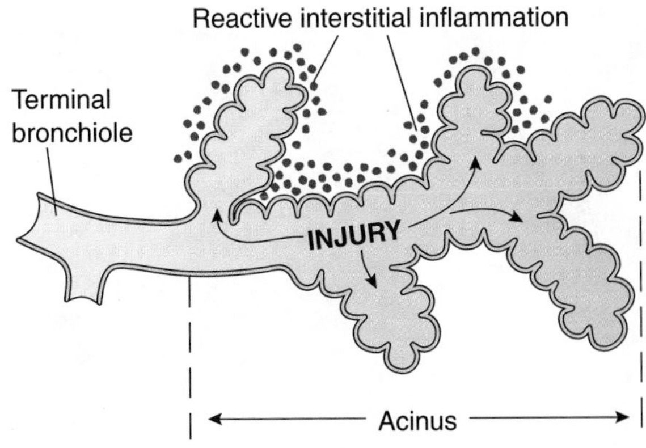

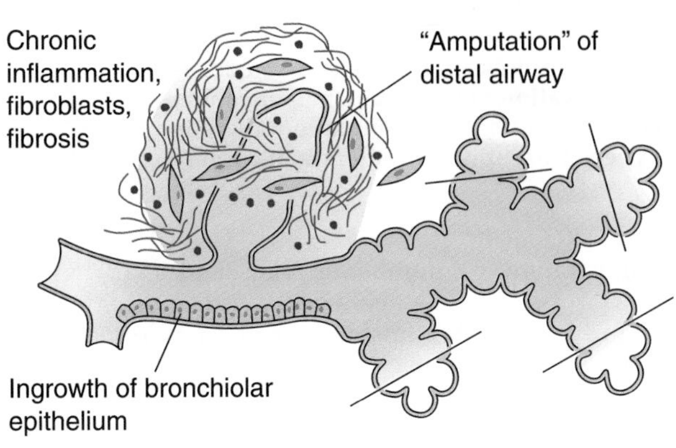

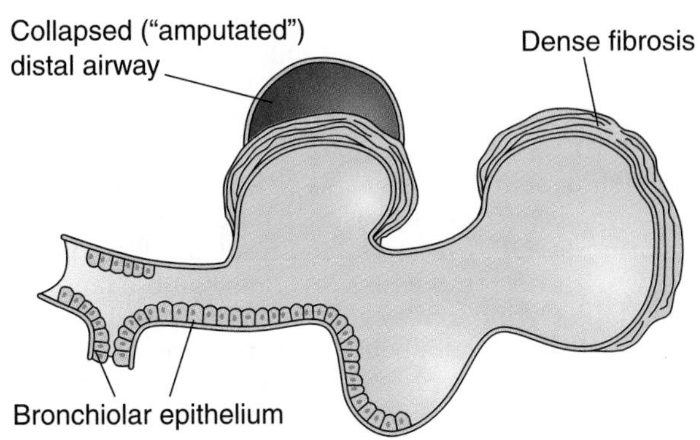

FIGURE *12-66*
Pathogenesis of honeycomb lung. Honeycomb lung is the result of a variety of injuries. Interstitial and alveolar inflammation destroys ("amputates") the distal part of the acinus. The proximal parts dilate and become lined by bronchiolar epithelium.

ertion and dry cough, usually over a period of 5 to 10 years. Clinically, patients have restrictive lung disease. Chest radiographs show diffuse bilateral infiltrates, predominantly in the lower lobes, and a reticular pattern. Clubbing of the fingers is common, especially late in the course of disease.

The classic auscultatory finding consists of late inspiratory crackles and fine ("Velcro") rales at the lung bases. Tachypnea at rest, cyanosis, and cor pulmonale eventually ensue. The prognosis is bleak, with a mean survival of 4 to 6 years. Patients are treated with corticosteroids and sometimes cyclophosphamide, but lung transplantation generally offers the only hope of a cure.

Desquamative Interstitial Pneumonia

Desquamative interstitial pneumonia (DIP) is a chronic, fibrosing, interstitial pneumonitis of unknown etiology that features marked intra-alveolar macrophage accumulation (Fig. 12-67A,B). Desquamative interstitial pneumonia is distinguished from UIP by the preservation of alveolar architecture in DIP and the lack of patchy scarring and remodeling of lung parenchyma characteristic of UIP. Alveolar walls in DIP may, however, show mild thickening by chronic inflammation and interstitial fibrosis (see Fig. 12-67B). Scattered lymphoid aggregates also may be present. Hyperplasia of type II pneumocytes is often prominent.

Opinion is equally divided on whether DIP is a separate entity or a stage of UIP. Patients with DIP tend to be younger (mean age, 42 years) than those with UIP, and the symptoms have been present for a shorter time (2 to 3 years) at the time of diagnosis. Most patients respond to corticosteroid therapy, and the mean survival in DIP is 12 years (i.e., twofold to threefold longer than in UIP). In addition, patients tend to have a milder restrictive defect on pulmonary-function tests than in UIP.

Respiratory Bronchiolitis–Interstitial Lung Disease

Respiratory bronchiolitis (RB) is a mild form of small airways disease, which occurs in cigarette smokers. Histologically, the process is patchy and consists of prominent accumulation of pigmented macrophages in the air spaces, centered on bronchioles (Fig. 12-68). The macrophages are present within the lumina of bronchioles and the adjacent alveolar spaces. The bronchiolar walls show mild chronic inflammation and fibrosis. However, interstitial fibrosis does not extend into the surrounding lung. The pigment within the macrophages is usually brown and finely granular.

Clinically, patients have mild respiratory dysfunction. Radiographically, bilateral interstitial infiltrates are seen. Patients with RB–interstitial lung disease have an excellent prognosis, and the symptoms may resolve after cessation of smoking.

Bronchiolitis Obliterans–Organizing Pneumonia

Bronchiolitis obliterans–organizing pneumonia (BOOP) is a clinicopathological entity of unknown etiology, which is associ-

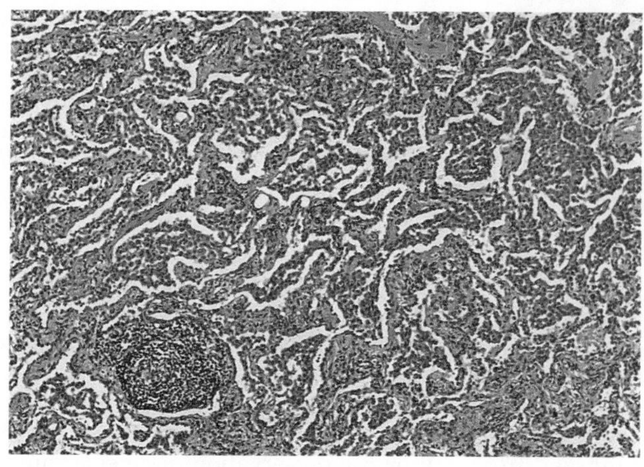

A

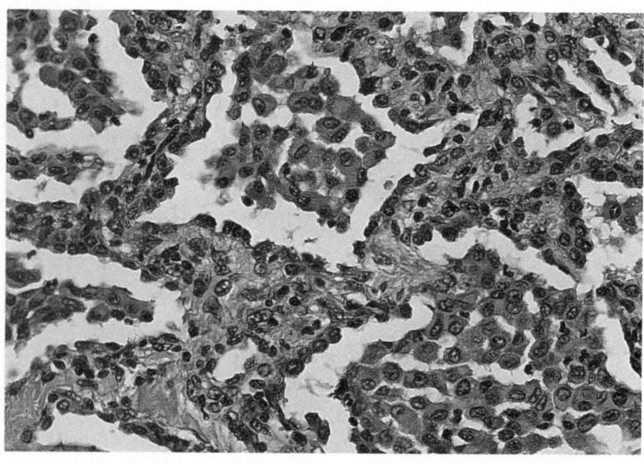

B

FIGURE *12-67*
Desquamative interstitial pneumonia (DIP). ***(A)*** **A diffuse process in the lungs is characterized by the accumulation of alveolar macrophages, preservation of the alveolar architecture, and a lymphoid aggregate.** ***(B)*** **In addition to alveolar macrophage accumulation, there is mild alveolar septal fibrosis, type II pneumocyte hyperplasia, and mild interstitial chronic inflammation.**

ated with a distinctive pattern of fibrosis that involves the distal airways and alveoli. Patients typically are first seen with cough or dyspnea and have bilateral nodular infiltrates on chest radiographs. Whereas *constrictive bronchiolitis obliterans* (see earlier) is characterized by severe obstructive pulmonary function and a progressive downhill clinical course, BOOP is regarded as *proliferative bronchiolitis obliterans* and features restrictive pulmonary function and an excellent response to corticosteroids.

The histological pattern seen in BOOP is nonspecific, and the etiology is not apparent from the morphological appearance. The BOOP pattern is observed in many settings, including respiratory tract infections (particularly viral bronchiolitis), the inhalation of toxic materials, the administration of a number of drugs, and several inflammatory processes (e.g., collagen vascular diseases). Importantly, a substantial number of cases remain idiopathic.

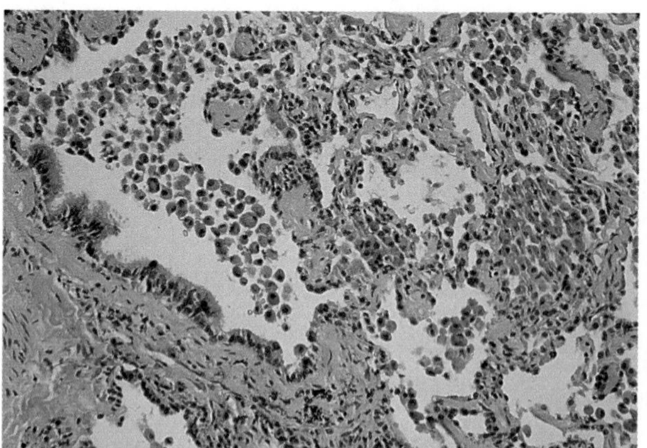

FIGURE *12-68*
Respiratory bronchiolitis–interstitial lung disease. There is marked accumulation of macrophages within the bronchioles and surrounding air spaces. Mild fibrotic thickening and chronic inflammation of the bronchiolar wall are present.

☐ **Pathology:** Histologically, BOOP features patchy areas of loose organizing fibrosis and chronic inflammatory cells in the distal airways adjacent to normal lung. The organizing fibrosis consists of plugs that occlude bronchioles (bronchiolitis obliterans), alveolar ducts, and surrounding alveoli (organizing pneumonia; Fig. 12-69A,B). The connective tissue plugs are primarily in the alveolar ducts and alveoli (see Fig. 12-69B), and there is relatively little connective tissue within bronchioles. Thus, BOOP is more an organizing pneumonia than a bronchiolitis obliterans. For this reason, the term *cryptogenic organizing pneumonia* has been used as a synonym for idiopathic BOOP. The architecture of the lung is preserved, with no remodeling or honeycomb changes as seen in UIP. Owing to the occlusion of the distal airways, an obstructive or endogenous lipid pneumonia may develop. The alveolar septa are only mildly thickened with chronic inflammatory cells, and there is only mild hyperplasia of type II pneumocytes. The BOOP histological pattern is nonspecific and may be seen as a reaction adjacent to many lesions in the lung, including infections, infarcts, neoplasms, abscesses, and hemorrhage.

☐ **Clinical Features:** BOOP is first seen with the acute onset of fever, cough, and dyspnea. Many patients have a history of a flu-like illness 4 to 6 weeks before the onset of symptoms. As noted earlier, some may have predisposing conditions. Chest radiographs reveal localized opacities or bilateral interstitial infiltrates, which may migrate over time. Corticosteroid therapy is effective, and some patients recover within weeks to months even without therapy.

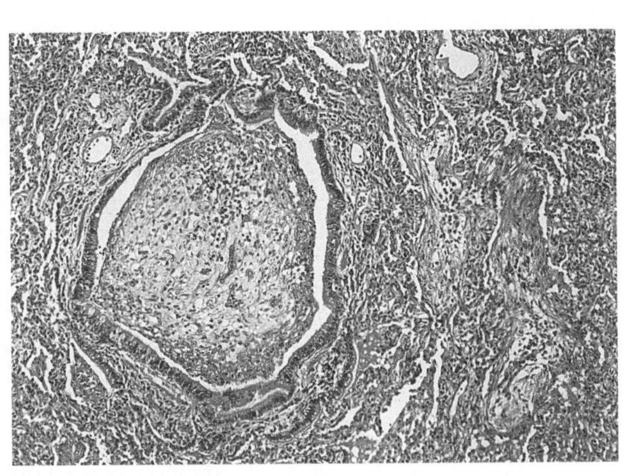

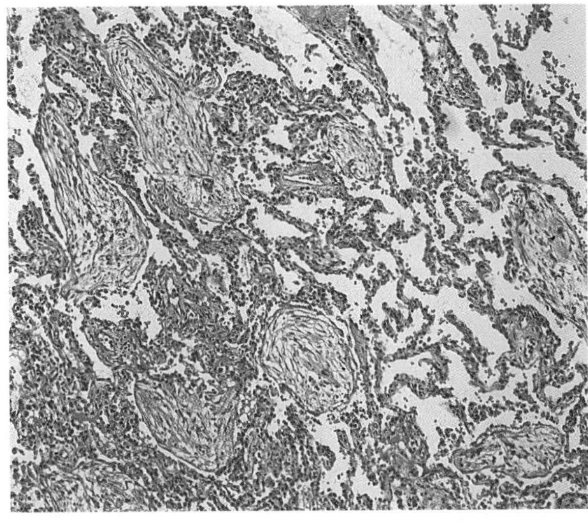

A B

FIGURE *12-69*
Bronchiolitis obliterans with organizing pneumonia (BOOP). *(A)* Polypoid plugs of loose fibrous tissue are present in a bronchiole and the adjacent alveolar ducts and alveoli. *(B)* The alveolar spaces contain similar plugs of loose organizing connective tissue.

Lymphoid Interstitial Pneumonia

Lymphoid interstitial pneumonia (LIP) is a rare pneumonitis in which lymphoid infiltrates are distributed diffusely in the interstitial spaces of the lung.

☐ **Pathology:** The hallmark of LIP is diffuse infiltration of alveolar septa and peribronchiolar spaces by chronic inflammatory cells (Fig. 12-70A,B). The infiltrate consists of lymphocytes, plasma cells, and macrophages. The alveolar architecture is preserved without dense scarring or remodeling of the lung architecture. Hyperplasia of type II pneumocytes may be conspicuous, and inconspicuous foci of organizing interstitial fibrosis are occasionally present. Sarcoid-like, noncaseating granulomas are often seen. The alveolar spaces tend to contain a proteinaceous exudate. In some cases, scattered lymphoid aggregates are present, some containing germinal centers. Hyperplasia of the peribronchiolar lymphoid tissue may be prominent.

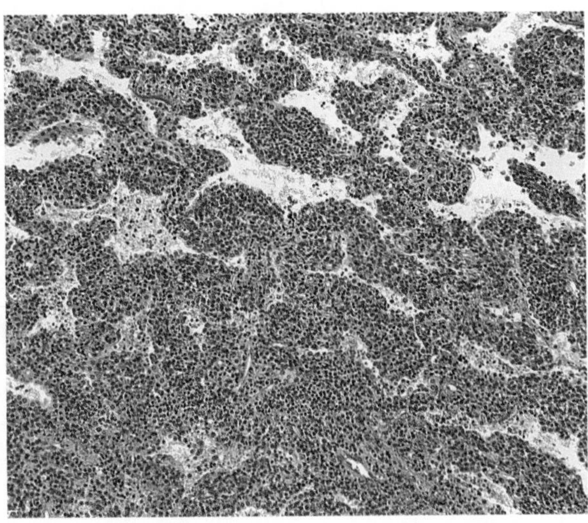

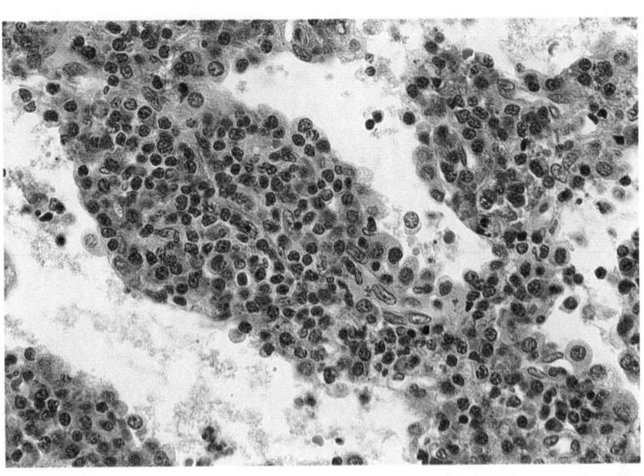

A B

FIGURE *12-70*
Lymphocytic interstitial pneumonia (LIP). *(A)* The walls of the alveolar septa are diffusely infiltrated by chronic inflammation. *(B)* The inflammatory infiltrate is composed of lymphocytes and plasma cells.

TABLE 12-5 **Conditions Associated with Lymphocytic Interstitial Pneumonia (LIP)**

Idiopathic	**Immunodeficiency**
Dysproteinemia	HIV infection
Polyclonal gammopathy	Severe combined immunodeficiency syndrome
Macroglobulinemia	
Hypogammaglobulinemia	**Infection**
Pernicious anemia	*Pneumocystis carinii* pneumonia
Collagen vascular disease	Epstein-Barr virus (lymphoproliferative disorder)
Sjögren syndrome	Chronic active hepatitis
Systemic lupus erythematosus	**Iatrogenic**
Rheumatoid arthritis	Bone marrow transplantation
	Phenytoin (Dilantin)

☐ **Clinical Features:** Lymphoid interstitial pneumonia may be idiopathic, but it often occurs in a variety of clinical settings (Table 12-5), particularly in patients with dysproteinemia, collagen vascular disease, and HIV infection. It is principally encountered in adults, although cases in children are recorded. In the latter, LIP is one of the defining criteria for the diagnosis of AIDS. Associated autoimmune manifestations include increased or reduced serum gamma globulins, a variety of dysproteinemias, and increased circulating autoantibodies, such as rheumatoid factor and antinuclear antibodies. Rarely lymphoma can develop in the setting of LIP, particularly in patients with Sjögren syndrome and AIDS.

Patients with LIP have cough and progressive dyspnea. The course of the disease varies from an indolent condition to one that progresses to end-stage lung and respiratory failure. Corticosteroids and cytotoxic agents have been of some benefit.

Langerhans Cell Histiocytosis (Histiocytosis X)

Langerhans cell histiocytosis (LCH) encompasses a spectrum of localized and systemic proliferations of Langerhans cells, which have been called eosinophilic granuloma, Hand–Schüller–Christian disease, and Letterer–Siwe disease. LCH can affect the lung as a distinctive form of interstitial lung disease. In adults, this occurs most often as an isolated form (also known as *pulmonary eosinophilic granuloma*), with extrapulmonary manifestations, such as bone lesions or diabetes insipidus, occurring in 10% to 15% of cases. **Virtually all of these patients are cigarette smokers.** In children, lung involvement may occur in association with Letterer–Siwe disease or Hand–Schüller–Christian disease.

☐ **Pathology:** Histologically, pulmonary eosinophilic granuloma appears as scattered nodular infiltrates, with a stellate border extending into the surrounding interstitium (Fig. 12-71A). These lesions are frequently centered on bronchioles or in a subpleural location. The cellular lesions consist of varying proportions of Langerhans cells admixed with lymphocytes, eosinophils, and macrophages. Langerhans cells are round to oval, with a moderate amount of eosinophilic cytoplasm and prominently grooved nuclei, which contain small inconspicuous nucleoli (see Fig. 12-71B). As the disease progresses, the lesions cavitate and become fibrotic. Eventually, honeycomb fibrosis can result. The lung parenchyma adjacent to the nodular lesions may show marked accumulation of intra-alveolar macrophages, owing to respiratory bronchiolitis, caused by smoking.

Langerhans cells have distinctive characteristics, including (1) cytoplasmic Birbeck granules (detected by electron microscopy), (2) C3, IgG-F_c receptors, CD1 (OKT6), CD1a (O10), and Ia antigens (HLA-DR), and (3) S-100 protein. Whether pulmonary histiocytosis X represents a neoplastic proliferation or an abnormal immuno-

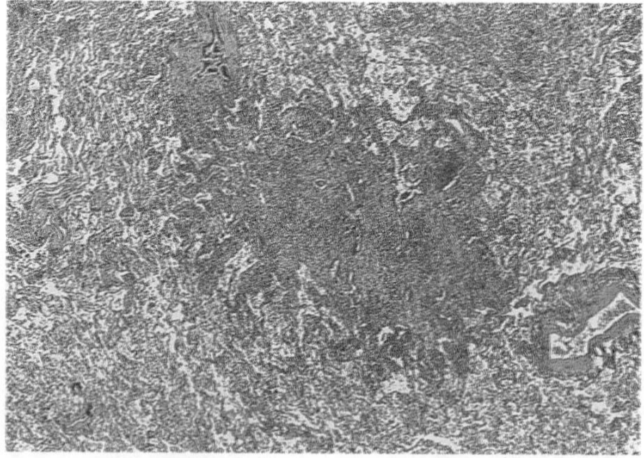
A

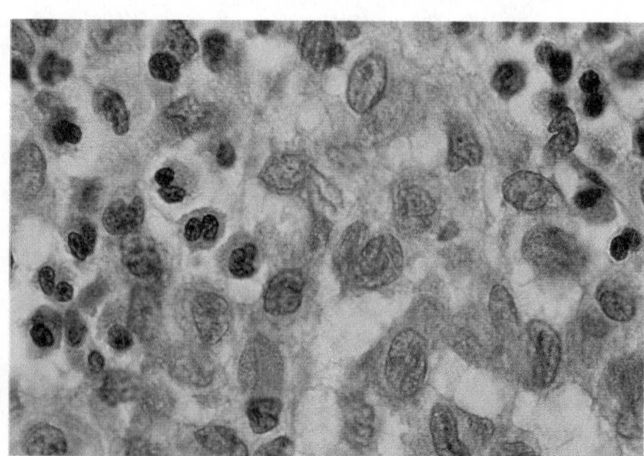
B

FIGURE 12-71
Langerhans cell histiocytosis. *(A)* The interstitial nodular infiltrate has a stellate shape, with extension of the cells into the adjacent alveolar septa. *(B)* The infiltrate has numerous Langerhans cells, which have a moderate amount of eosinophilic cytoplasm and prominently grooved nuclei. Several eosinophils are also present.

logical response to antigens within cigarette smoke remains to be determined.

☐ **Clinical Features:** Pulmonary eosinophilic granuloma usually affects patients in the third and fourth decades of life. The most common presenting manifestations are a nonproductive cough, dyspnea on exertion, and spontaneous pneumothorax. Some 25% of patients are asymptomatic at the time of diagnosis. Chest radiographs show diffuse bilateral reticulonodular lesions, usually in the upper lobes. The lesions frequently undergo cavitation. Although most patients have a good prognosis, some develop chronic pulmonary dysfunction. In a small subset of cases, progressive pulmonary fibrosis can lead to death. Cessation of smoking can be beneficial in the early stages of the disease.

Lymphangioleiomyomatosis

Lymphangioleiomyomatosis (LAM) is a rare interstitial lung disease, which occurs in women of childbearing age and is characterized by the widespread abnormal proliferation of smooth muscle in the lung, mediastinal and retroperitoneal lymph nodes, and the major lymphatic ducts. The etiology of LAM is unknown, but clinical responses to oophorectomy and progesterone therapy suggest that the smooth muscle proliferation is under hormonal control. The occurrence of LAM in patients with tuberous sclerosis and the association of LAM with renal angiomyolipomas have led to speculation that LAM may represent a *forme fruste* of tuberous sclerosis.

☐ **Pathology:** On gross examination, the lungs show bilateral, diffuse enlargement, with extensive cystic changes resembling those of emphysema (Fig. 12-72A). Histologically, numerous cystic spaces are lined by focal nodules or bundles of abnormal smooth muscle cells. These round or spindle-shaped cells (LAM cells) resemble immature smooth muscle cells and lack the parallel orientation of the normal smooth muscle surrounding airways and blood vessels (see Fig. 12-72B). The smooth muscle proliferation typically follows a lymphatic distribution in the lung, around blood vessels and bronchioles, and along the pleura and interlobular septa. Blood vessel walls, especially in small pulmonary veins, also may be infiltrated, resulting in microscopic hemorrhage and hemosiderin accumulation in alveolar macrophages. Immunohistochemical staining for HMB-45 (a melanoma antigen) specifically decorates the LAM cells but not other smooth muscle cells in the lung. Estrogen or progesterone receptors may occasionally be demonstrated in LAM cells.

☐ **Clinical Features:** Patients with LAM have shortness of breath, spontaneous pneumothorax, hemoptysis, cough, and chylous effusions. In early stages, the

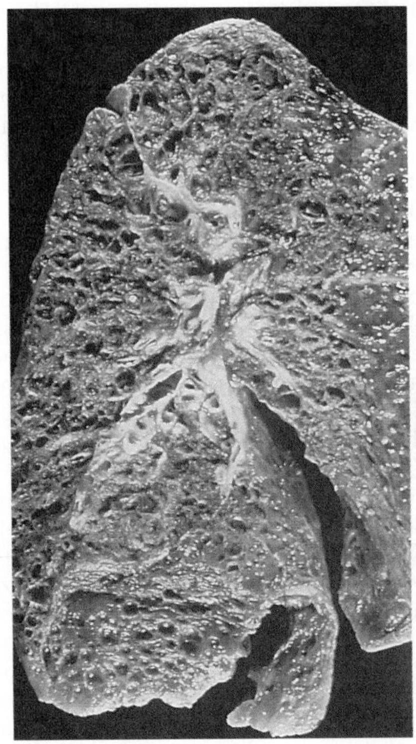

A

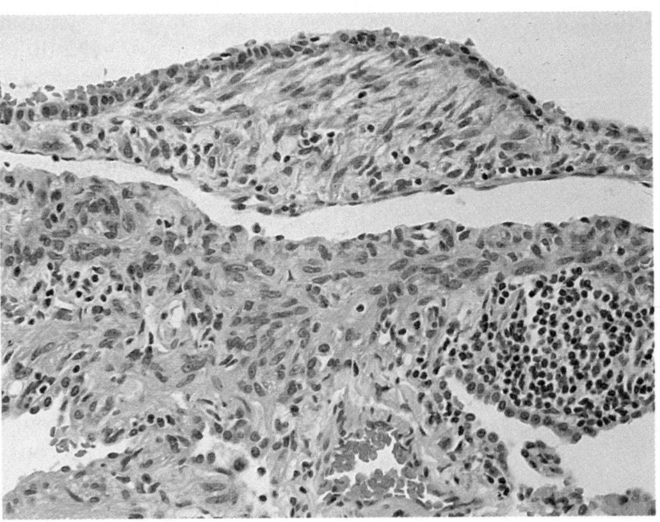

B

FIGURE *12-72*
Lymphangioleiomyomatosis. *(A)* The cut surface of the lung displays extensive cystic change, which resembles emphysema. *(B)* An abnormal cystic space is lined by smooth muscle bundles, in which the myocytes are haphazardly arranged.

chest radiograph may appear normal. However, as the disease progresses, a diffuse interstitial reticular or cystic pattern may appear on the radiograph, and pleural effusions, marked hyperinflation of the lungs, and pneumothorax may ensue. Pulmonary-function tests show markedly increased total lung capacity, decreased diffusing capacity, and obstructive or restrictive features. Although some patients have an indolent clinical course, many die of progressive respiratory failure. Hormonal manipulation through oophorectomy, as well as tamoxifen and progesterone therapy, have shown some promise.

LUNG TRANSPLANTATION

Patients who undergo lung transplantation develop pulmonary complications that have a specific set of pathological manifestations. The major problems encountered are acute and chronic rejection and infection. Histological clues to acute rejection include perivascular infiltrates of small round lymphocytes, plasmacytoid lymphocytes, macrophages, and eosinophils. In severe cases, the inflammation may spill over into adjacent alveoli, and hyaline membranes may be seen. In chronic rejection, the major pattern of injury is bronchiolitis obliterans, characterized by bronchiolar inflammation and varying degrees of fibrosis. The latter can take the form of polypoid plugs of intraluminal granulation tissue or concentric mural fibrosis, with the pattern of constrictive bronchiolitis (Fig. 12-73). Bronchiectasis is common in long-term survivors of lung transplants, an outcome that may be due to poor perfusion of the airways, denervation, and recurrent airway infection.

A spectrum of opportunistic infections, including bacteria, fungi, viral agents, and *P. carinii*, can be seen in transplant patients. The most common fungal pneumonias are due to *Candida* and *Aspergillus*. Cytomegalovirus is the most common cause of viral pneumonia. **Lymphoproliferative disorders** occur in 3% to 8% of lung-transplant patients who survive more than 30 days. These neoplasms are secondary to uncontrolled proliferation of B lymphocytes injected with the Epstein–Barr virus (EBV) as a result of immunosuppression by cyclosporine.

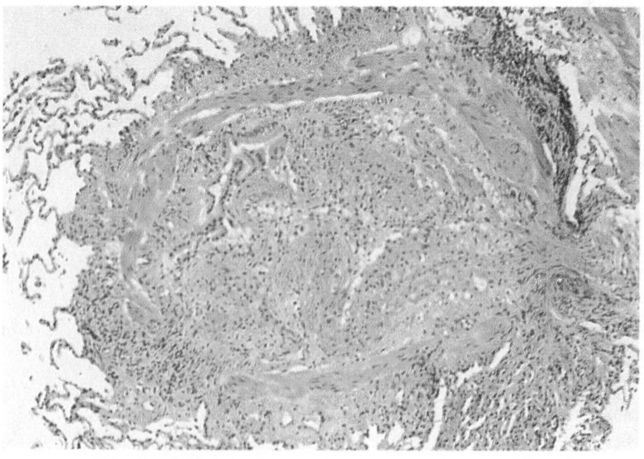

FIGURE *12-73*
Obliterative bronchiolitis, chronic rejection in lung transplantation. The lumen of this bronchiole is virtually entirely obliterated by concentric fibrosis.

VASCULITIS AND GRANULOMATOSIS

Many pulmonary conditions result in vasculitis, most of which are secondary to other inflammatory processes, such as necrotizing granulomatous infections. Only a few idiopathic vasculitis syndromes affect the lung, the most important of which are Wegener granulomatosis, Churg–Strauss granulomatosis, and necrotizing sarcoid granulomatosis.

Wegener Granulomatosis

Wegener granulomatosis (WG) is a disease of unknown cause, which is characterized by aseptic, necrotizing, granulomatous inflammation and vasculitis that affect the upper and lower respiratory tracts and the kidneys. The disease is described in Chapter 10. The glomerulonephritis associated with WG is discussed in Chapter 16, and the lesions of the upper respiratory tract are described in Chapter 25. In this section, we deal only with the pulmonary manifestations of WG.

☐ **Pathology:** The pulmonary pathology of WG features necrotizing granulomatous inflammation, parenchymal necrosis, and vasculitis. In most cases of pulmonary WG, multiple bilateral nodules, averaging 2 to 3 cm in diameter, are seen in the lungs. The nodules have an irregular edge, a tan–brown or hemorrhagic cut surface, and frequent central cavitation.

Although WG is generally regarded as a vasculitic syndrome, the most impressive findings are in the lung. Nodules of parenchymal consolidation consist of (1) tissue necrosis; (2) granulomatous inflammation with a mixed inflammatory infiltrate composed of lymphocytes, plasma cells, neutrophils, eosinophils, macrophages, and giant cells; and (3) fibrosis. Necrosis can take the form of neutrophilic microabscesses or large basophilic zones of "geographic" necrosis with irregular serpiginous borders (Fig. 12-74A). The granulomas may show several patterns, including palisading macrophages along the border of the large necrotic zones, loosely clustered multinucleated giant cells, and scattered giant cells. Vasculitis may affect arteries (see Fig. 12-74B), veins, or capillaries, and the vascular lesions may show acute, chronic, or granulomatous inflammation. The most common pattern of fibrosis consists of a nonspecific organizing pneumonia at the edges of the nodules of inflammatory consolidation. The lungs often show acute or chronic intra-alveolar hemorrhage. "Neutrophilic capillaritis," consisting of neutrophilic infiltration of alveolar walls, is often present.

☐ **Clinical Features:** Wegener granulomatosis most commonly affects the head and neck, followed by

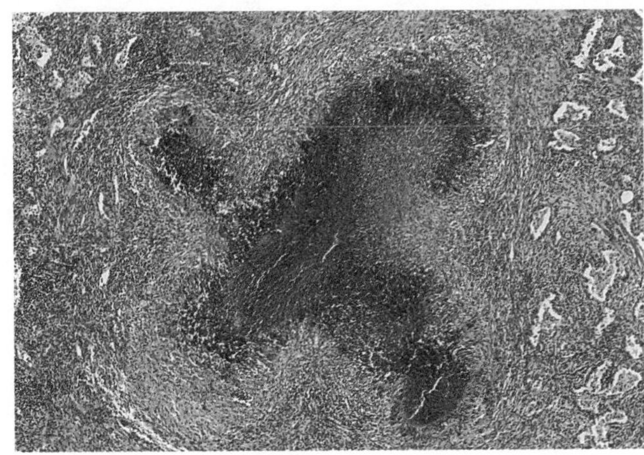

A

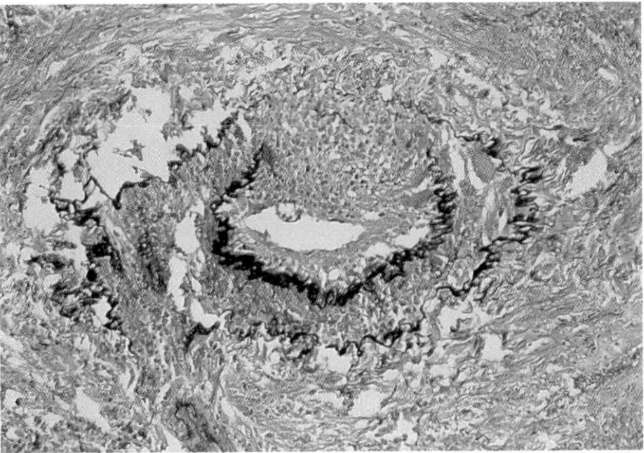

B

FIGURE *12-74*
(*A*) Wegener granulomatosis. This large area of necrosis has a "geographic" pattern with serpiginous borders and a basophilic center. (*B*) Vasculitis in this artery is characterized by a focal, eccentric, transmural chronic inflammatory infiltrate, which destroys the inner and outer elastic laminae (elastic stain).

the lung, kidney, and eye. Respiratory manifestations include cough, hemoptysis, and pleuritis. Chest radiographs commonly show multiple intrapulmonary nodules, although single nodules also may be encountered. Head and neck manifestations consist of sinusitis, nasal disease, otitis media, hearing loss, subglottic stenosis, ear pain, cough, and oral lesions. Other systemic manifestations include arthralgias, fever, skin lesions, weight loss, peripheral neuropathy, central nervous system abnormalities, and pericarditis.

Diffuse pulmonary hemorrhage is an important complication of WG, seen as a fulminant life-threatening crisis characterized by severe respiratory failure. It is usually accompanied by acute renal failure.

The serum anti–neutrophil cytoplasm antibody (ANCA) test is a useful marker for WG and other vasculitis syndromes. When these antibodies react with ethanol-fixed neutrophils, there are two major immunofluorescence patterns: cytoplasmic or classical (C-ANCA) and perinuclear (P-ANCA). C-ANCAs react with proteinase 3 and occur in more than 85% of patients with active generalized WG. Most P-ANCAs have a specificity for myeloperoxidase and are encountered in patients with idiopathic necrotizing and crescentic glomerulonephritis, as well as in patients with polyarteritis nodosa and Churg–Strauss syndrome.

The majority of patients with WG are effectively treated with corticosteroids and cyclophosphamide. Some patients are responsive to therapy with trimethoprim–sulfamethoxazole, suggesting the possibility of a bacterial infection.

Churg–Strauss Syndrome (Allergic Angiitis and Granulomatosis)

Churg–Strauss syndrome is a disorder of unknown etiology, which is defined by the triad of asthma, peripheral eosinophilia ($>1.5 \times 10^3/\mu L$), and systemic vasculitis.

☐ **Pathology:** The lungs of patients with Churg–Strauss syndrome show changes of asthmatic bronchitis or bronchiolitis (see earlier discussion of asthma). Histological features characteristic of Churg–Strauss syndrome include eosinophilic pneumonia, vasculitis (Fig. 12-75A), parenchymal necrosis (see Fig. 12-75B), and granulomatous inflammation. Infiltrates of eosinophils may be seen in any anatomic compartment of the lung. Involvement of blood vessel walls causes vasculitis and damage to airway walls and results in bronchitis or bronchiolitis. Alveolar damage leads to eosinophilic pneumonia. The vasculitis exhibits varying types of inflammatory cells, including eosinophils, lymphocytes, plasma cells, macrophages, giant cells, and neutrophils (see Fig. 12-75A). Fibrinoid vascular necrosis may be present. Necrotic foci have eosinophilic centers owing to the accumulation of dead eosinophils (see Fig. 12-75B).

☐ **Clinical Features:** Churg–Strauss syndrome passes through three clinical phases. During the **prodrome**, patients have one or more of the following: allergic rhinitis, asthma, peripheral eosinophilia, and eosinophilic infiltrative disease (eosinophilic pneumonia or eosinophilic enteritis). In the **systemic vasculitic phase**, extrapulmonary vasculitic manifestations are present, such as cutaneous leukocytoclastic vasculitis or peripheral neuropathy in the form of mononeuritis multiplex. In the **post-vasculitic phase**, patients may continue to have asthma and allergic rhinitis, and complications of neuropathy and hypertension may persist. Cardiovascular manifestations are common and often consist of pericarditis, hypertension, and cardiac failure. Renal disease and sinus involvement are usually less severe than those in WG.

Churg–Strauss patients usually are positive for P-ANCA during the vasculitic phase. Most patients respond to corticosteroid therapy, but cyclophosphamide may be needed in some who develop severe manifestations such as renal failure.

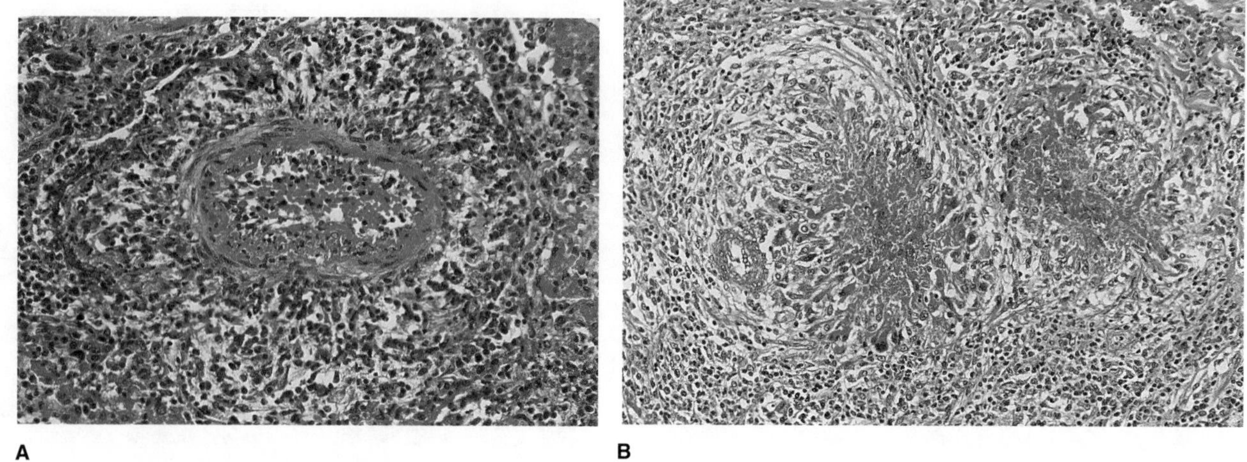

FIGURE 12-75
Churg–Strauss syndrome. ***(A)*** **An artery shows severe vasculitis, consisting of a dense infiltrate of chronic inflammatory cells and eosinophils.** ***(B)*** **A necrotic ("allergic") granuloma has a central eosinophilic area of necrosis surrounded by palisading macrophages and giant cells.**

Necrotizing Sarcoid Granulomatosis

Necrotizing sarcoid granulomatosis is a rare condition that features nodular confluent sarcoidal granulomas, large zones of necrosis (Fig. 12-76A), *and vasculitis* (see Fig. 12-82B). Three types of inflammation are seen in the vasculitis of necrotizing sarcoid granulomatosis: giant cells, necrotizing granulomas (see Fig. 12-82B), and chronic inflammation consisting of lymphocytes and plasma cells. Most patients are asymptomatic, and chest radiographs typically show multiple well-circumscribed pulmonary nodules. Extrapulmonary disease is uncommon, and localized lesions may be effectively treated by surgical removal. Corticosteroids are usually effective for patients with multiple lesions. The prognosis is excellent.

PULMONARY HYPERTENSION

In fetal life, the pulmonary arterial walls are thick, and pulmonary arterial pressure is correspondingly high. Blood is oxygenated through the placenta rather than through the lungs. Thus, the high fetal pulmonary arterial pressure serves to shunt the output of the right ventricle through the ductus arteriosus into the systemic circulation, effectively bypassing the lungs. After birth, the lungs

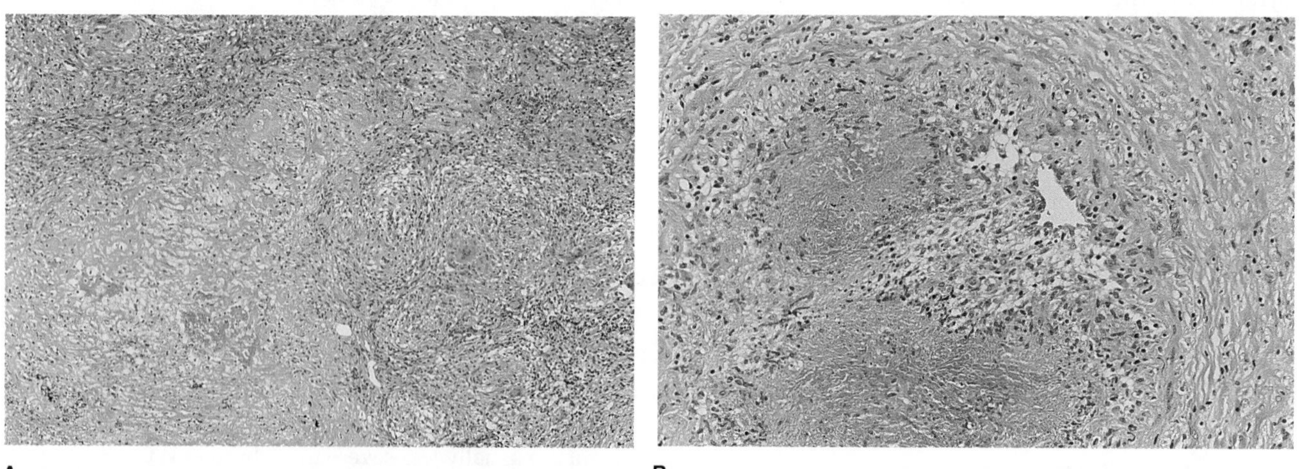

FIGURE 12-76
Necrotizing sarcoid granulomatosis. ***(A)*** **A large area of necrosis is surrounded by confluent sarcoidal granulomas.** ***(B)*** **The vasculitis consists of a necrotizing granuloma in the wall of an artery.**

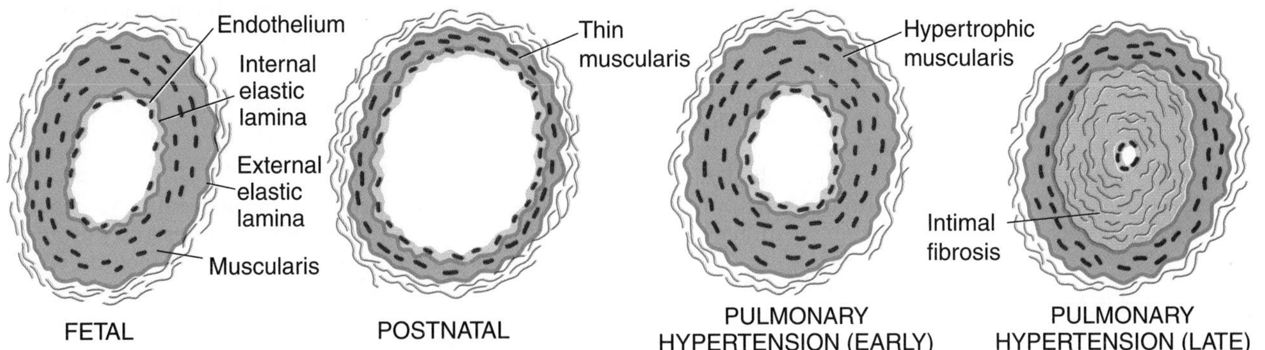

FIGURE *12-77*
Histopathology of pulmonary hypertension. In late gestation, the pulmonary arteries have thick walls. After birth, the vessels dilate and the walls become thin. Mild pulmonary hypertension is characterized by thickening of the media. As pulmonary hypertension becomes more severe, there is extensive intimal fibrosis and muscle thickening.

assume the obligation of oxygenating the venous blood, and the ductus arteriosus closes. Under these circumstances, the lungs must adapt to accept the entire cardiac output, a situation that demands the high-volume and low-pressure system of the mature lung. Accordingly, by the third day of life, the pulmonary arteries dilate, their walls become thin, and pulmonary arterial pressure correspondingly declines.

In the child or the adult, the pressure within the pulmonary arterial system may be increased either by augmented flow or by increased vascular resistance. Whatever the cause, characteristic morphological abnormalities result from increased pulmonary artery pressure (Fig. 12-77). In order of increasing severity, the grades of pulmonary hypertension, reflecting the changes in the pulmonary arteries, are as follows:

Grade 1. Medial hypertrophy of muscular pulmonary arteries and the appearance of smooth muscle in the pulmonary arterioles.
Grade 2. Intimal proliferation with increasing medial hypertrophy.
Grade 3. Intimal fibrosis of muscular pulmonary arteries and arterioles, which may be occlusive (Fig. 12-78A).
Grade 4. Formation of plexiform lesions together with dilatation and thinning of pulmonary arteries. These nodular lesions are composed of irregular interlacing blood channels and impose a further obstruction in the pulmonary circulation (see Fig. 12-78B).
Grade 5. Rupture of pulmonary arteries, with parenchymal hemorrhage and hemosiderosis.
Grade 6. Fibrinoid necrosis of the arteries and arterioles.

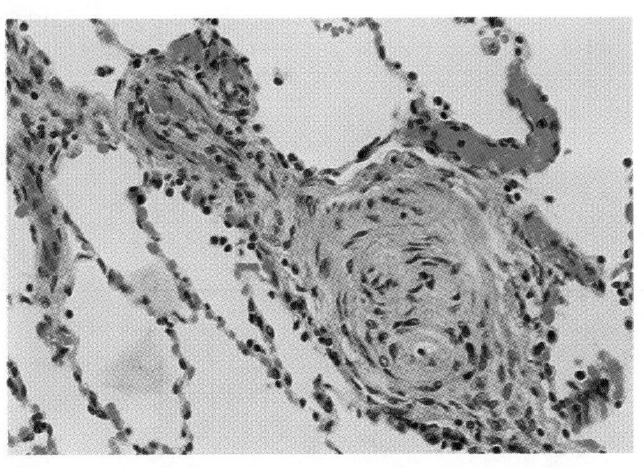
A

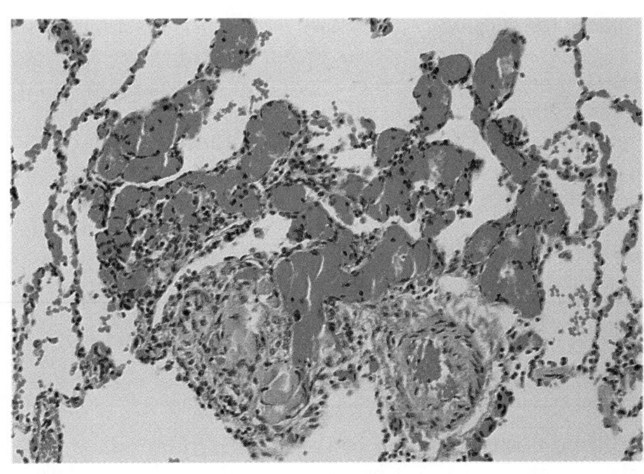
B

FIGURE *12-78*
Pulmonary arterial hypertension. *(A)* A small pulmonary artery is virtually occluded by concentric intimal fibrosis and thickening of the media. *(B)* A plexiform lesion is characterized by marked dilatation, congestion, and thinning of arterial walls, forming interconnected vascular channels adjacent to the small arteries. The latter show marked hypertensive changes of intimal fibrosis and medial thickening.

With all grades of pulmonary hypertension, atherosclerosis is seen in the largest pulmonary arteries. In this respect, even mild degrees of atherosclerosis are uncommon when pulmonary arterial pressure is normal.

Mild structural changes of the pulmonary vasculature are reversible (e.g., with corrective heart surgery). However, severe lesions (plexiform lesions, necrosis, and hemorrhage) indicate that pulmonary arterial hypertension has reached an irreversible stage. As a result of the increased pressure in the lesser circulation, hypertrophy of the right ventricle of the heart occurs (cor pulmonale).

Increased Flow

A shunt from the systemic circulation (including the heart) to the pulmonary circulation results in increased flow through the lungs. The great majority of cases represent congenital left-to-right shunts (see Chapter 11). Rarely an acquired condition, such as rupture of the interventricular septum, produces a left-to-right shunt. An additional lesion is present when hypertension exists from birth. At this time, the pulmonary artery and the aorta have about the same number of elastic lamellae in their media. In normal infants, there is a loss of elastic lamellae in the pulmonary artery after birth, but when pulmonary hypertension is present, the fetal pattern persists.

Precapillary Pulmonary Hypertension

Increased resistance to flow may be caused by obstruction proximal to the lung capillary bed (precapillary hypertension), destruction of the capillary bed, or obstruction distal to the capillary bed (postcapillary hypertension).

Primary Pulmonary Hypertension

Primary (or idiopathic) pulmonary hypertension is a rare condition caused by increased tone within the pulmonary arteries. It occurs at all ages, but is most common in young women in their 20s and 30s. The disorder is seen as an insidious onset of dyspnea. Physical signs and radiological abnormalities are initially slight, but with time they become more apparent. Severe morphological changes of pulmonary hypertension eventually ensue, and the patients die of cor pulmonale. Medical treatment is ineffective, and the disease is an indication for heart–lung transplantation.

Recurrent Pulmonary Emboli

Multiple thromboemboli in the smaller pulmonary vessels are often the result of asymptomatic, episodic showers of small emboli from the periphery. Gradually restricting the pulmonary circulation, they eventuate in pulmonary hypertension. Some patients have evidence of peripheral venous thrombosis, usually in the leg veins, or a history of circumstances predisposing to venous thrombosis. In addition to the vascular lesions of pulmonary hypertension, organized thromboemboli are evidenced by fibrous bands ("webs") that extend across the lumina of small pulmonary arteries. If the condition is diagnosed during life, placement of a filter in the inferior vena cava prevents further embolization.

Functional Resistance to Arterial Flow (Vasoconstriction)

Any disorder that produces hypoxemia can result in constriction of small pulmonary arteries and pulmonary hypertension. Predisposing conditions include chronic air-flow obstruction (chronic bronchitis), infiltrative lung disease, and living at high altitude. Severe kyphoscoliosis or extreme obesity *(Pickwickian syndrome)* may interfere with the mechanics of ventilation and can cause hypoxemia and pulmonary hypertension.

Cardiac Causes of Pulmonary Hypertension

Left ventricular failure from any cause increases pulmonary venous pressure and, to some extent, pulmonary arterial pressure. By contrast, mitral stenosis produces severe venous hypertension and significant pulmonary artery hypertension. In such cases, the lungs exhibit lesions of both pulmonary hypertension and chronic passive congestion (see Chapter 7).

Pulmonary Veno-Occlusive Disease

Pulmonary veno-occlusive disease is a rare condition of uncertain etiology characterized by extensive occlusion of small pulmonary veins and venules by loose, sparsely cellular, intimal fibrosis (Fig. 12-79). Some large veins may also be involved, and in half of the cases, similar but less severe lesions involve the pulmonary arteries. Canalization of the obstructive lesions suggests that they represent organized thrombi. The disease has been reported to follow viral infections, exposure to toxic agents, and chemotherapy.

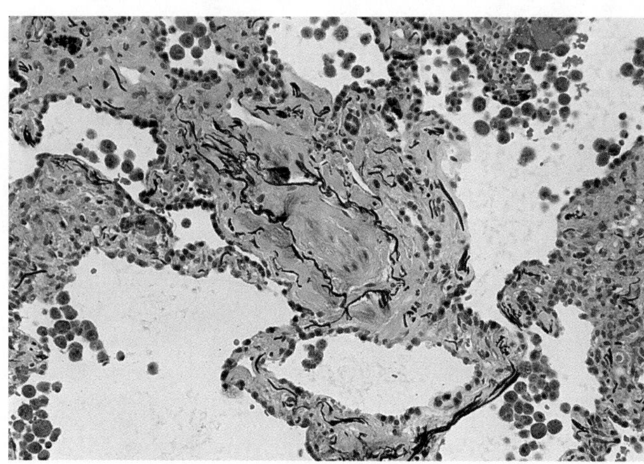

FIGURE *12-79*
Veno-occlusive disease of the lung. This pulmonary vein is occluded by intimal fibrosis (Movat stain).

More than half of the cases are encountered in the first 3 decades of life. In children, girls and boys are affected similarly, but after age 15 years, pulmonary veno-occlusive disease is more common in men.

Pulmonary veno-occlusive disease produces severe pulmonary hypertension. Gross examination reveals brown induration of the lung and atherosclerosis of large pulmonary arteries. Microscopic examination shows partial or total occlusion of small veins and venules and eccentric intimal thickening of larger veins. Moderate fibrosis of the alveolar walls is usually noted, and foci of hemosiderosis are common. The pulmonary arterial tree exhibits severe lesions of pulmonary hypertension, and recent thrombi are regularly observed.

The clinical presentation of progressive dyspnea is similar to that of primary pulmonary hypertension, but pulmonary veno-occlusive disease has a more fulminant course. Radiological examination reveals scattered infiltrates in the lung, representing hemorrhage and hemosiderosis, which increase with the progression of the disease. There is no effective therapy, and heart–lung transplantation should be contemplated.

TUMORS AND TUMOR-LIKE CONDITIONS

Pulmonary Hamartoma

Although the term hamartoma implies a malformation, **hamartomas are true tumors**, which typically occur in adults, with a peak in the sixth decade of life. They are the cause of some 10% of "coin" lesions discovered incidentally on chest radiographs. A characteristic ("popcorn") pattern of calcification is often seen in chest radiographs. Grossly, pulmonary hamartomas appear as solitary, circumscribed, lobulated masses, averaging 2 cm in diameter, with a white or gray, cartilaginous cut surface (Fig. 12-80A). The tumor consists of elements usually present in the lung, including cartilage, fibromyxoid connective tissue, fat, bone, and occasionally smooth muscle (see Fig. 12-80B). These components are interspersed with clefts lined by respiratory epithelium. The tumor is benign and well circumscribed, and shells out from the surrounding lung parenchyma. Most hamartomas occur in the peripheral parenchyma, but 10% occur in a central endobronchial location. The latter may be seen with symptoms due to bronchial obstruction.

Carcinoma of the Lung

Carcinoma of the lung is the most common cause of cancer death worldwide, including the United States. Regarded as a rare tumor as late as 1945, it now occurs in epidemic proportions. In the United States, it is the most common cause of cancer death in both men and women. Some 85% of lung cancers are a consequence of cigarette smoking (see Chapter 8). All histological types of lung cancer are associated with cigarette smoking, but the strongest association is with squamous cell carcinoma and small cell carcinoma. The nonsmoker who develops cancer of the lung usually has an adenocarcinoma. The peak age for lung cancer is between age 60 and 70 years, and most patients are between 50 and 80 years old. There is a male predominance, but the male-to-female ratio is decreasing, owing to the increase in smoking among women.

In the past, the term "bronchogenic" carcinoma was often used for primary lung cancer, but it is perhaps too specific, implying an origin from the bronchi. A substantial proportion, perhaps one fourth, of primary lung cancers do not have an obvious bronchial origin. The most important issue in the histological subclassification of lung cancer is the separation of small cell carcinoma from the other types (non–small cell carcinoma). Because small cell carcinoma is responsive to chemotherapy and other histological types of lung cancer are not, oncologists rely heavily on pathologists to make this distinction.

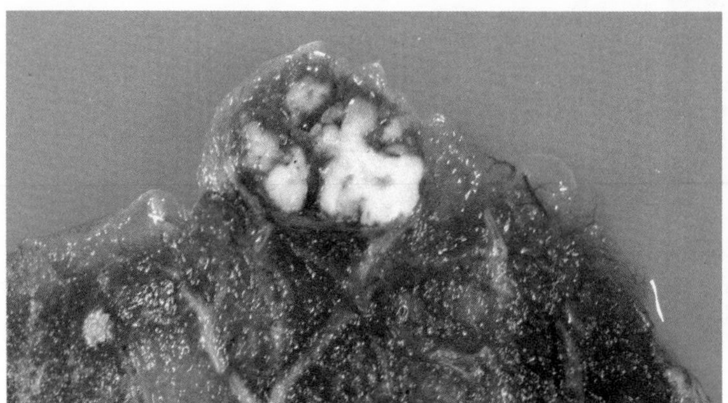

A

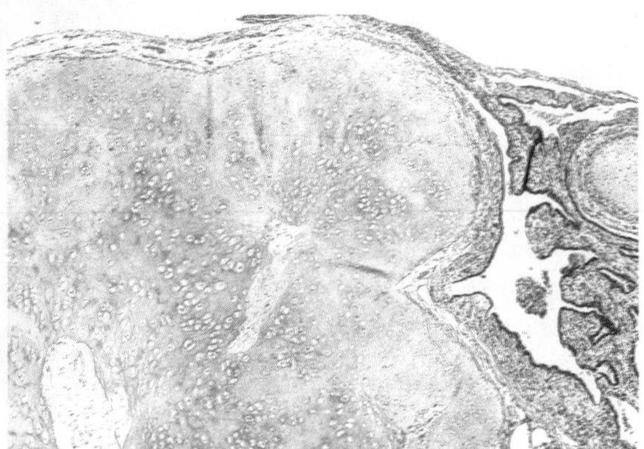

B

FIGURE *12-80*
Pulmonary hamartoma. ***(A)*** **The cut surface of a sharply circumscribed, peripheral pulmonary nodule shows a lobulated structure.** ***(B)*** **A photomicrograph reveals nodules of hyaline cartilage separated by connective tissue lined by respiratory epithelium.**

Histological subtyping of lung carcinoma is based on the best-differentiated component unless a component of small cell carcinoma is present. However, the differentiation of tumors is *graded* according to the worst differentiated component. For example, if a tumor consists mostly of poorly differentiated large cells but has foci of squamous cells or adenocarcinoma, it is classified as a poorly differentiated squamous cell or adenocarcinoma, respectively. Any tumor with a component of small cell carcinoma is regarded as a subtype of that tumor (see later).

Mutations in the K-*ras* oncogene occur in lung cancers, particularly in codons 12 and 13. They are found in 25% of adenocarcinomas, 20% of large cell carcinomas, 5% of squamous cell carcinomas, and only rarely in small cell lung carcinoma. Mutations in K-*ras* are correlated with cigarette smoking and have been reported to be associated with a poor prognosis in patients with adenocarcinoma. *Myc* oncogene overexpression occurs in 10% to 40% of small cell carcinomas but is rare in untreated non–small cell tumors. Two important tumor-suppressor genes in lung cancer are the p53 and retinoblastoma (Rb) genes. Mutations in the p53 gene are found in more than 80% of small cell carcinomas and 50% of non–small cell carcinomas. Rb mutations occur in more than 80% of small cell carcinomas and 25% of non–small cell cancers. Deletions in the short arm of chromosome 3 (3p) are frequently found in all types of lung cancers. The protooncogene bcl-2, which encodes a protein that inhibits programmed cell death (apoptosis), is expressed in 25% of squamous cell carcinomas and 10% of adenocarcinomas. Survival was reported to be improved in bcl-2–positive tumors compared with negative tumors.

The overall 5-year survival for all lung cancer patients has remained at 15% over the past 2 decades. The 5-year survival at all stages is 42% for bronchioloalveolar carcinoma, 17% for adenocarcinoma (not otherwise specified), 15% for squamous cell carcinoma, 11% for large cell carcinoma, and 5% for small cell carcinoma.

Squamous Cell Carcinoma

Squamous cell carcinoma accounts for 30% of all invasive lung cancers in the United States. After injury to the bronchial epithelium, such as occurs with cigarette smoking, regeneration from the pluripotent basal layer commonly occurs in the form of squamous metaplasia. The metaplastic mucosa follows the same sequence of dysplasia, carcinoma *in situ*, and invasive tumor as that observed in sites that are normally lined by squamous epithelium, such as the cervix, oral cavity, vocal cords, esophagus, and skin.

□ **Pathology:** Most squamous cell carcinomas arise in the central portion of the lung from the major or segmental bronchi, although 10% arise in the periphery. On gross examination, they tend to be firm, grey–white, 3- to 5-cm ulcerated lesions, which extend through the bronchial wall into the adjacent parenchyma (Fig. 12-81A). The appearance of the cut surface is variable, depending on the degree of necrosis and hemorrhage. Central cavitation is frequent. On occasion, a central squamous carcinoma is seen as an endobronchial tumor, which on bronchoscopy appears as a papillary, polypoid, or sessile mucosal mass.

The microscopic appearance of squamous cell carcinoma is highly variable. Well-differentiated squamous cell carcinomas have keratin "pearls," which appear as small round nests of brightly eosinophilic aggregates of keratin surrounded by concentric ("onion skin") layers of squamous cells (see Fig. 12-81B). Individual cell kera-

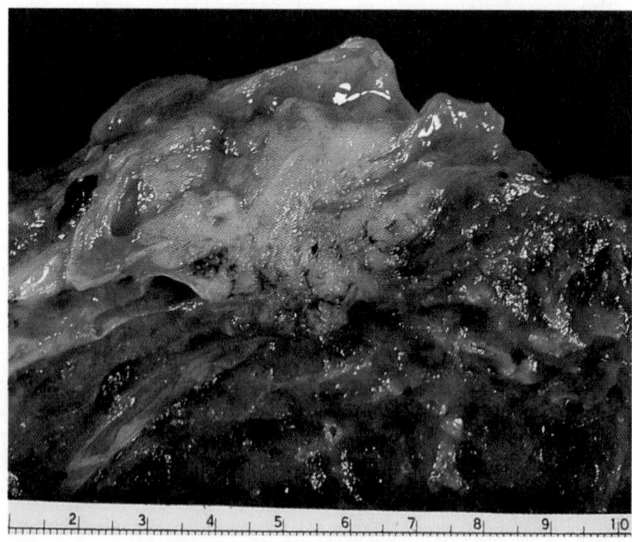

A

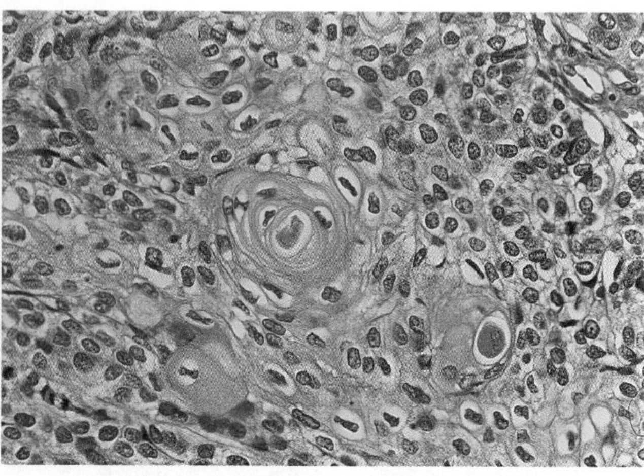

B

FIGURE *12-81*
Squamous cell carcinoma of the lung. *(A)* The tumor grows within the lumen of a bronchus and invades the adjacent intrapulmonary lymph node. *(B)* A photomicrograph shows well-differentiated squamous cell carcinoma, with a keratin pearl composed of cells with brightly eosinophilic cytoplasm.

tinization also occurs, in which the cytoplasm of the cell assumes a glassy, intensely eosinophilic appearance. Intercellular bridges are identified in some well-differentiated squamous cancers as slender gaps between adjacent cells, which are traversed by fine strands of cytoplasm. By contrast, some squamous tumors are so poorly differentiated that they do not exhibit even small foci of keratinization and are difficult to distinguish from large cell, small cell, or spindle cell carcinomas.

Tumor cells may be readily found in the sputum, and the diagnosis may be made by exfoliative cytology, even when the squamous cancer is not radiologically apparent. The resection specimens of these "occult" tumors reveal carcinoma *in situ* in one third of cases, whereas the rest show varying degrees of microscopic invasion.

The signs and symptoms of squamous carcinoma are representative of the other cell types and are due to (1) local or direct effects of the tumor, (2) mediastinal spread, (3) distant metastases, or (4) a variety of paraneoplastic syndromes.

LOCAL EFFECTS: Squamous cell carcinoma can produce cough, dyspnea, hemoptysis, chest pain, obstructive pneumonia, and pleural effusion. Growth of a lung cancer (usually squamous) in the apex of the lung *(Pancoast tumor)* may extend to involve the eighth cervical and first and second thoracic nerves, which results in shoulder pain radiating in an ulnar distribution down the arm *(Pancoast syndrome)*. A Pancoast tumor also may paralyze the cervical sympathetic nerves and cause *Horner syndrome*, characterized on the affected side by (1) depression of the eyeball (enophthalmos), (2) ptosis of the upper eyelid, (3) constriction of the pupil (miosis), and (4) absence of sweating (anhidrosis).

Most central endobronchial tumors produce symptoms related to bronchial obstruction: persistent cough, hemoptysis, and obstructive pneumonia or atelectasis. Effusions can result from extension of the tumor into the pleura or pericardium. Lymphangitic spread of the tumor within the lung may interfere with oxygenation. Tumors that arise in the periphery of the lung tend not to produce bronchial obstruction. They are more likely to be discovered either on routine chest radiographs in asymptomatic patients or after they have become advanced. The latter circumstance features invasion of the chest wall and resulting chest pain, the superior vena cava syndrome, and nerve-entrapment syndromes.

MEDIASTINAL SPREAD: Growth of the tumor within the mediastinum can cause the superior vena cava syndrome (owing to tumorous obstruction of this vein) and nerve-entrapment syndromes.

METASTASES: Carcinomas of the lung of all histological types metastasize most frequently to the regional lymph nodes, particularly the hilar and mediastinal nodes. The most frequent site of extranodal metastases is the adrenal gland, although adrenal insufficiency is distinctly uncommon. Lung cancer is sometimes initially detected as metastatic disease, with the brain, bone, and liver being common sites.

PARANEOPLASTIC SYNDROMES: Disorders associated with lung cancer include acanthosis nigricans, dermatomyositis/polymyositis, clubbing of the fingers, and myasthenic syndromes, such as Eaton–Lambert syndrome and progressive multifocal encephalopathy. Endocrine syndromes include Cushing syndrome (ectopic production of corticotropic hormone by a carcinoid tumor or small cell carcinoma), inappropriate release of antidiuretic hormone by small cell carcinoma, and hypercalcemia (secretion of a parathormone-like substance by squamous cell carcinoma).

Adenocarcinoma

Adenocarcinoma of the lung accounts for a third of all invasive lung cancers. It tends to arise in the periphery and is often associated with pleural fibrosis and subpleural scars, which can result in pleural puckering (Fig. 12-82). In the past, these cancers were thought to arise in scars secondary to old tuberculosis, healed infarcts, and so on. It is now recognized that most of these scars represent a desmoplastic response to the tumor.

☐ **Pathology:** At initial presentation, adenocarcinomas of the lung appear as irregular masses 2 to 5 cm in diameter, although they may be so large that they completely replace an entire lobe of the lung. On cut section, the tumor is greyish white and often glistening, depending on the amount of mucus production. Central adenocarcinomas may have predominantly endobronchial growth and invade bronchial cartilage.

There are four major subtypes of adenocarcinoma, as defined by the World Health Organization: acinar (Fig. 12-83A), papillary (see Fig. 12-83B), solid with mucus formation (see Fig. 12-83C), and bronchioloalveolar. Although some adenocarcinomas consist purely or predominantly of one of these patterns, it is common to encounter

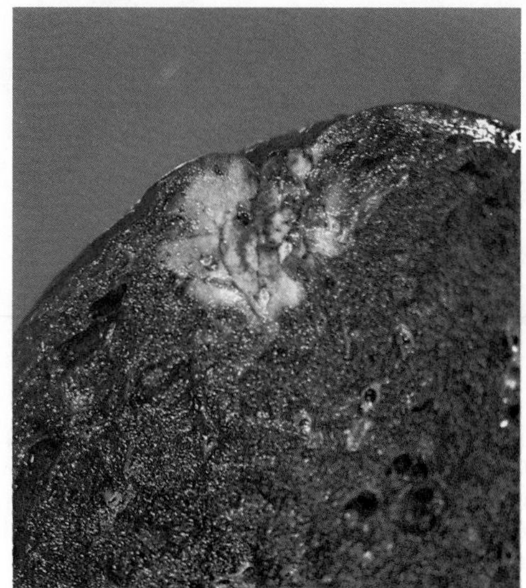

FIGURE *12-82*
Adenocarcinoma of the lung. A peripheral tumor of the right upper lobe has an irregular border and a tan or grey cut surface, and causes puckering of the overlying pleura.

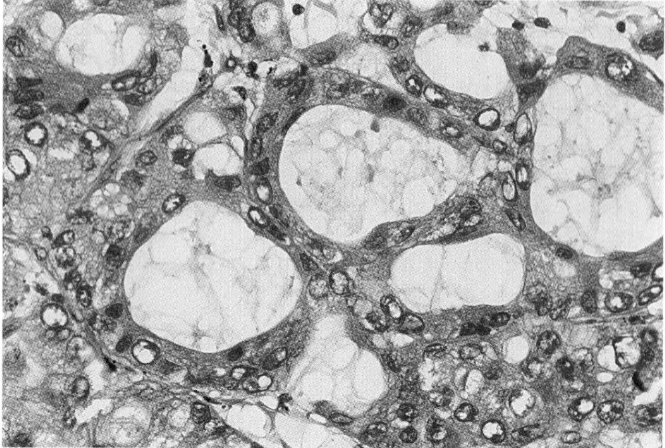

A

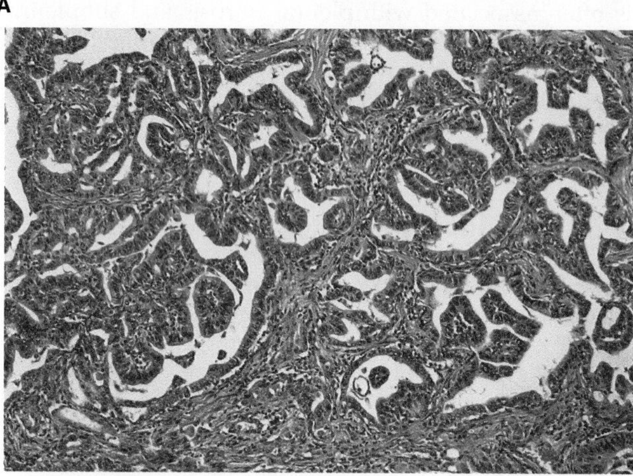

B

C

FIGURE *12-83*
Adenocarcinoma of the lung. ***(A)*** **The malignant epithelial cells of an acinar adenocarcinoma form glands.** ***(B)*** **A papillary adenocarcinoma consists of malignant epithelial cells growing along thin fibrovascular cores.** ***(C)*** **A tumor grows in the pattern of solid adenocarcinoma with mucin formation. Several intracytoplasmic mucin droplets stain positively with the mucicarmine stain.**

a mixture of these histological subtypes in a single tumor. Bronchioloalveolar carcinoma is sufficiently distinctive to merit special attention (see later).

Pulmonary adenocarcinoma can arise at different levels of the bronchial tree. Thus, an individual tumor may reflect the architecture and cell population of any part of the respiratory mucosa, from the large bronchi to the smallest bronchioles. The neoplastic cells may resemble ciliated or nonciliated columnar epithelial cells, goblet cells, cells of bronchial glands, or Clara cells.

The most common histological type of adenocarcinoma features the acinar pattern. Well-differentiated acinar carcinomas form regular glands, which are lined by cuboidal or columnar cells, with basal nuclei (see Fig. 12-83A). Papillary adenocarcinomas exhibit columnar to cuboidal cells and form a single cell layer on a core of fibrovascular connective tissue (see Fig. 12-83B). Solid adenocarcinomas with mucus formation are poorly differentiated tumors, which are distinguished from large cell carcinomas by the demonstration of mucin with the mucicarmine stain or PAS reaction (see Fig. 12-83C). Mucus production occurs in only half of adenocarcinomas, and the diagnosis may rest primarily on the histological pattern of the tumor.

Patients with stage I tumors (localized to the lung) who undergo complete surgical removal have a 5-year survival of 50% to 80%.

Bronchioloalveolar Carcinoma

Bronchioloalveolar carcinoma is a distinctive subtype of adenocarcinoma that grows along preexisting alveolar walls. Because this pattern is focally present in many lung tumors, a pure bronchioloalveolar pattern is required to make this diagnosis. Bronchioloalveolar cancers account for 1% to 5% of all invasive lung tumors. The presenting symptoms for patients with bronchioloalveolar carcinoma are similar to those in other lung cancer patients. Copious mucin in the sputum *(bronchorrhea)* is a distinctive sign of bronchioloalveolar carcinoma, but is seen in fewer than 10% of patients, usually in the setting of extensive lung involvement.

On gross examination, bronchioloalveolar carcinoma may appear as a single peripheral nodule or coin lesion (>50% of cases), multiple nodules, or a diffuse infiltrate indistinguishable from lobar pneumonia (Fig. 12-84). Histologically, the tumor has two major patterns: two thirds are nonmucinous, consisting of Clara cells and type II pneumocytes (Fig. 12-85A); the remaining third are mucinous tumors featuring goblet cells (see Fig. 12-85B). The nonmucinous tumors exhibit cuboidal cells growing along the alveolar walls. The mucinous tumors are composed of columnar cells with abundant apical cytoplasm filled with mucus. It is important to exclude the possibility of a metastasis, particularly for mucinous tumors.

Patients with stage I bronchioloalveolar carcinomas, detected as solitary coin lesions have a good prognosis, whereas those who have multiple nodules or diffuse lung involvement are more likely to have a poor outcome.

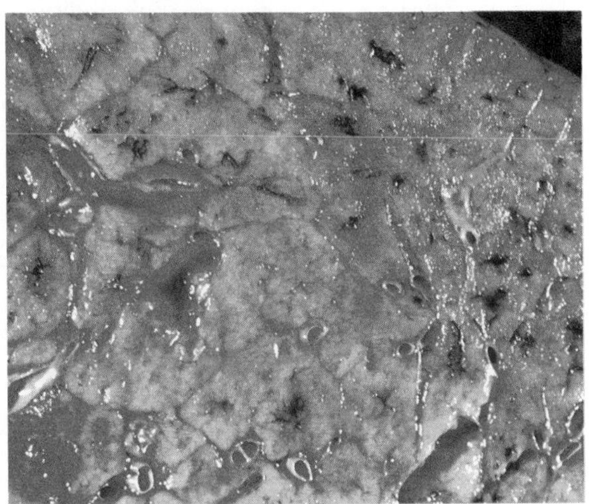

FIGURE 12-84
Bronchioloalveolar carcinoma. The cut surface of the lung is solid, glistening, and mucoid, an appearance that reflects a diffusely infiltrating tumor.

Small Cell Carcinoma

Small cell carcinoma (previously "oat cell" carcinoma) is a highly malignant epithelial tumor of the lung that exhibits neuroendocrine features. It accounts for 20% of all lung cancers and is strongly associated with cigarette smoking. In the past, the male-to-female ratio was 10:1, but it is now 2:1. The tumor grows and metastasizes rapidly, and 70% of patients are first seen in an advanced stage. A variety of paraneoplastic syndromes are distinctive for small cell carcinoma, including diabetes insipidus, ectopic ACTH (corticotropin) syndrome, and the Eaton–Lambert syndrome.

Small cell carcinoma usually appears as a perihilar mass, frequently with extensive lymph node metastases. On cut section, it is soft and white but often shows extensive hemorrhage and necrosis. The tumor typically spreads along the bronchi in a submucosal and circumferential fashion.

Histologically, small cell carcinoma consists of sheets of small round, oval or spindle-shaped cells. The tumor cells display scant cytoplasm and distinctive nuclear characteristics, which include finely granular nuclear chromatin and absent or inconspicuous nucleoli (Fig. 12-86). By electron microspy, many of the cells contain secretory neuroendocrine granules. A high mitotic rate is characteristic, with an average of 60 to 70 mitoses per 10 high-power fields. Necrosis is frequent and extensive. Basophilic nuclear staining of vascular walls by DNA from necrotic tumor cells (the Azzopardi effect) is common in necrotic areas. Although there is no absolute measure for the size of the tumor cells, a useful rule of thumb in small cell carcinoma is the diameter of three small lymphocytes.

The important difference between small cell carcinoma and other lung cancers is its more marked sensitivity to chemotherapy. From an oncologist's standpoint, therefore, all other lung cancers can be grouped together under the term "non–small cell carcinoma."

Large Cell Carcinoma

Large cell carcinoma is a diagnosis of exclusion in a poorly differentiated non–small cell carcinoma that does not show features of squamous or glandular differentiation (Fig. 12-87). This tumor type accounts for 10% of all invasive lung

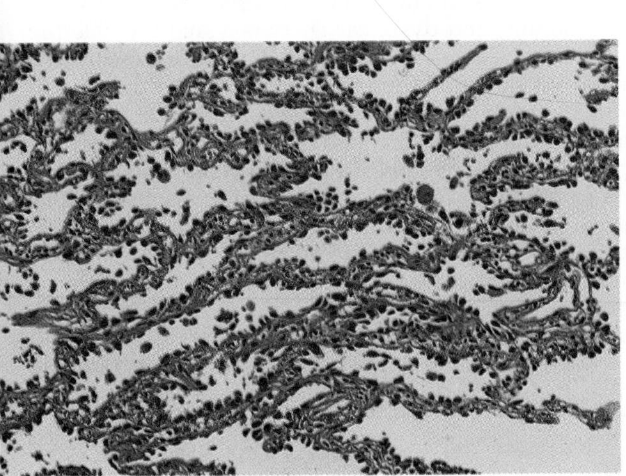

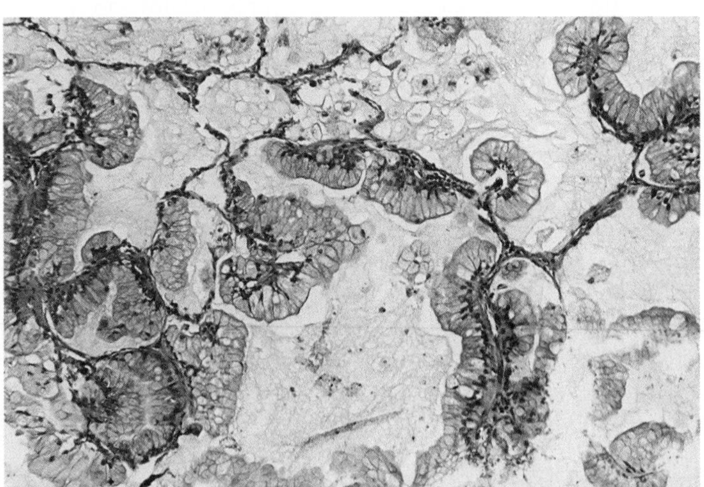

FIGURE 12-85
Bronchioloalveolar carcinoma. *(A)* Nonmucinous bronchioloalveolar carcinomas consist of atypical cuboidal to low columnar cells proliferating along the existing alveolar walls. *(B)* Mucinous bronchioloalveolar carcinoma consists of tall columnar cells filled with apical cytoplasmic mucin, which grow along the existing alveolar walls.

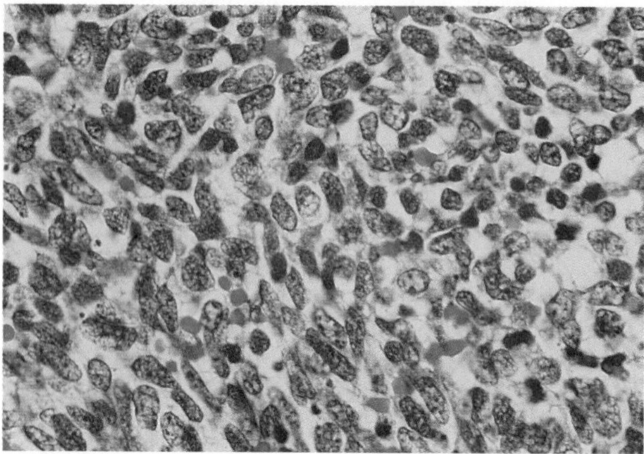

FIGURE 12-86
Small cell carcinoma of the lung. This tumor consists of small oval to spindle-shaped cells with scant cytoplasm, finely granular nuclear chromatin, and conspicuous mitoses.

tumors. The cells are large and exhibit ample cytoplasm. The nuclei frequently show prominent nucleoli and vesicular chromatin. Some large cell carcinomas have pleomorphic giant cells or spindle cells.

Carcinoid Tumors

Carcinoid tumors of the lung comprise a group of neuroendocrine neoplasms derived from the pluripotential basal layer of the respiratory epithelium. They exhibit a neuroendocrine differentiation similar to that of the resident Kulchitsky cells. In this respect, carcinoid tumors bear a resemblance to small cell carcinomas. These neoplasms account for 2% of all primary lung cancers, show no sex predilection, and are not related to cigarette smoking. Although neuropeptides are readily demonstrated in the tumor cells, the large majority are endocrinologically silent. A small subset of cases is associated with an endocrinopathy, such as Cushing syndrome with ectopic corticotropin production by tumor cells. The carcinoid syndrome occurs in 1% of cases, usually in the setting of hepatic metastases.

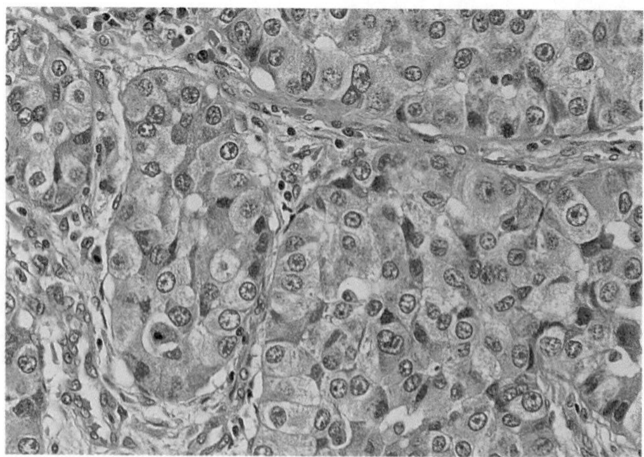

FIGURE 12-87
Large cell carcinoma of the lung. This poorly differentiated tumor is growing in sheets. The tumor cells are large and contain ample cytoplasm and prominent nucleoli.

☐ **Pathology:** One third of carcinoid tumors are central and one third are peripheral (subpleural); the remaining third are situated in the mid-portion of the lung. Central carcinoid tumors tend to have a large endobronchial component, with a fleshy, smooth, polypoid mass protruding into the bronchial lumen (Fig. 12-88A). The tumors average 3.0 cm in diameter, but range from 0.5 to 10 cm.

Carcinoid tumors are characterized histologically by an organoid growth pattern and uniform cytological features, consisting of an eosinophilic, finely granular cytoplasm and nuclei that display a finely granular chromatin pattern (see Fig. 12-88B). A variety of neuroendocrine patterns may be seen, including trabecular growth, peripheral palisading, and rosettes.

Atypical carcinoid tumors are distinguished from typical carcinoids by the following criteria: (1) increased mitotic activity, with 2 to 10 mitotic figures per 10 high-power fields, (2) tumor necrosis (Fig. 12-89), (3) areas of increased cellularity and disorganization of the architecture, and (4) nuclear pleomorphism, hyperchromatism, and an abnormal nuclear/cytoplasmic ratio.

☐ **Clinical Features:** The indolent nature of carcinoid tumors is reflected in the finding that half the patients are asymptomatic at presentation; the tumors are usually discovered because of a mass on radiograph. In symptomatic patients, the most common pulmonary manifestations include hemoptysis, postobstructive pneumonitis, and dyspnea. There is a slight female predominance. The mean age at the time of diagnosis is 55 years, but carcinoid tumors can occur at any age. In fact, bronchial carcinoids are the most common lung tumor in childhood. Atypical carcinoid tumors tend to be more malignant than typical ones. Regional lymph node metastases are found in 20% of patients with typical carcinoids and in 50% of those with atypical carcinoids. Patients with typical carcinoids have an excellent prognosis, with a 90% 5-year survival after surgery, compared with 60% for patients with atypical carcinoids.

Rare Pulmonary Tumors

INFLAMMATORY PSEUDOTUMOR: *Inflammatory pseudotumor of the lung is an uncommon lesion that consists of nodular masses of inflammatory cells and fibroblasts.* Most of these masses are contained within the lung, although the pleura may be involved. In 5% of cases, the tumor invades structures outside the lung such as the esophagus, mediastinum, chest wall, diaphragm, or pericardium.

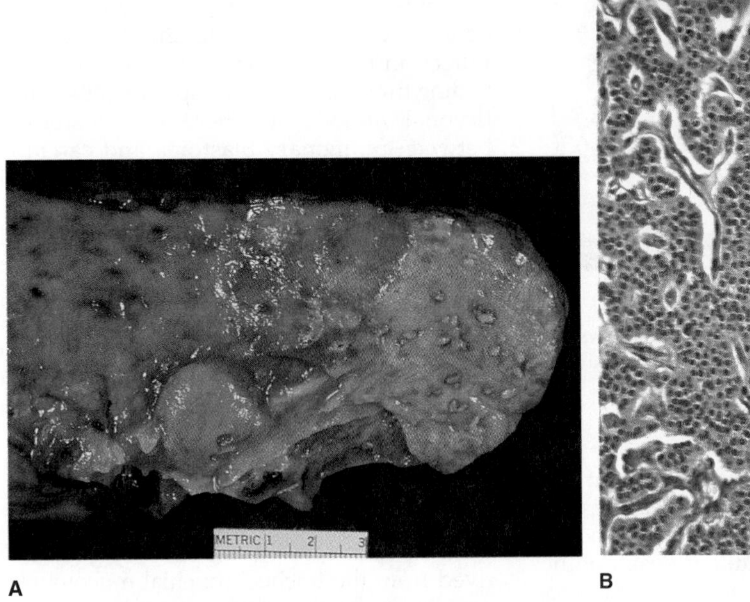

A

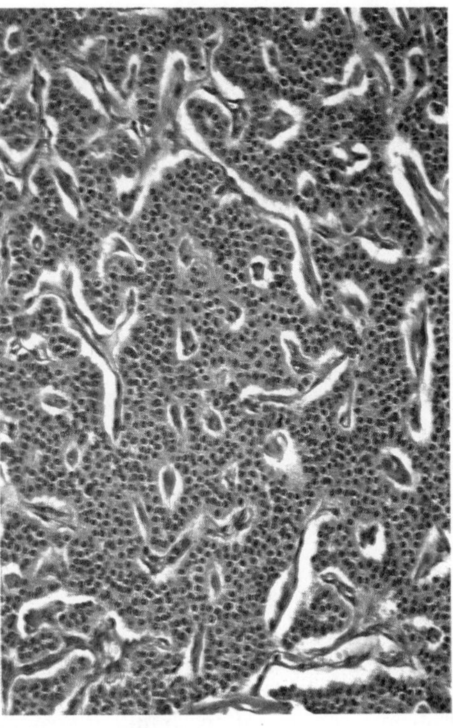

B

FIGURE *12-88*
Carcinoid tumor of the lung. *(A)* A central carcinoid tumor is circumscribed and protrudes into the lumen of the main bronchus. The compression of the bronchus by the tumor caused the postobstructive pneumonia seen in the distal lung parenchyma (right). *(B)* A microscopic view shows ribbons of tumor cells embedded in a vascular stroma.

Inflammatory pseudotumor is regarded as an inflammatory, non-neoplastic process, despite the occasional case that recurs and behaves in a locally aggressive fashion. A previous history of a pulmonary infection can be elicited in one third of patients. Some fibrohistiocytic variants exhibit clonality by cytogenetic studies, suggesting that some tumors may actually be neoplastic.

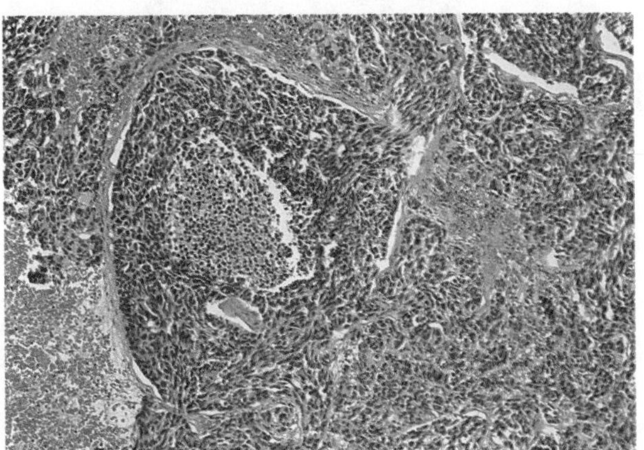

FIGURE *12-89*
Atypical carcinoid tumor of the lung. A cellular tumor shows central necrosis and a disorganized architecture.

The tumors are solitary and circumscribed, with a mean size of 4 cm. Virtually any inflammatory cells are present, including lymphocytes, plasma cells, macrophages, giant cells, mast cells, and eosinophils. Inflammatory pseudotumor causes consolidation of the lung parenchyma and loss of architecture. Two major histological patterns are fibrohistiocytic (Fig. 12-90) and plasma cell granuloma, depending on whether the predominant component consists of fibroblasts or plasma cells. In some cases, foamy macrophages impart a xanthomatous pattern.

Most patients are younger than 40 years, although inflammatory pseudotumor can occur at any age and is one of the most common lung tumors of childhood. Half of the patients are asymptomatic at presentation. The large majority of inflammatory pseudotumors are cured by surgical excision, but 5% recur within the chest.

PULMONARY EPITHELIOID HEMANGIOENDOTHELIOMA: *Pulmonary epithelioid hemangioendotheliomas are rare tumors that represent a low-grade vascular sarcoma.* Most patients are young adults, and 80% are women. The course tends to be indolent, and half of the patients are asymptomatic. The majority of patients are first seen with multiple pulmonary nodules. Histologically, the tumor consists of oval-shaped nodules, which have a central, sclerotic, hypocellular zone and a cellular peripheral zone. The tumor spreads within alveolar

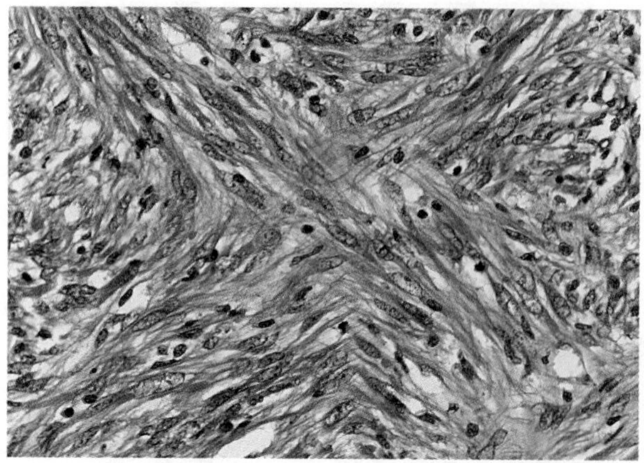

FIGURE *12-90*
Inflammatory pseudotumor. A photomicrograph shows intersecting spindle cells and scattered lymphocytes and macrophages.

spaces (Fig. 12-91). The tumor cells have abundant epithelioid cytoplasm, with frequent intracytoplasmic vascular lumina, which may contain red blood cells. The intercellular stroma consists of an abundant eosinophilic matrix. The tumors express vascular markers, such as factor VIII. Epithelioid hemangioendotheliomas with a histological pattern similar to that seen in the lung may occur in the liver, bone, and soft tissue. Pulmonary epithelioid hemangioendothelioma is a slow-growing tumor, with a mean survival of 5 years, ranging to 24 years.

CARCINOSARCOMA: Occasionally, cancers of the lung have the appearance of both a carcinoma and a sarcoma in different parts of the tumor, and the two are usually intimately mingled. In most cases, the epithelial component is a squamous carcinoma, and the sarcomatous one is composed of spindle cells. The sarcomatous portion may also exhibit heterologous elements, such as osteosarcoma, chondrosarcoma, and rhabdomyosarcoma. Metastases can contain both histological components of the primary tumor. The primary approach to therapy for carcinosarcoma is surgery, but the prognosis is poor, with a median survival of 9 to 12 months.

PULMONARY BLASTOMA: This malignant tumor resembles embryonal lung, with a glandular component consisting of poorly differentiated columnar cells arranged in tubules, without mucous secretion. The intervening tumor is formed by spindle cells that resemble embryonal mesoderm. There is a histological overlap between pulmonary blastoma and carcinosarcoma, including heterologous elements, and the clinical features are similar.

Despite the embryonal appearance of pulmonary blastoma, the tumor occurs primarily in adults (median age range, 35 to 43 years), and the large majority of patients are cigarette smokers. The prognosis for patients with biphasic tumors is poor and comparable to that for carcinoma of the lung. On the other hand, epithelial blastoma carries a much better prognosis, with an 80% 5-year survival.

MUCOEPIDERMOID CARCINOMA AND ADENOID CYSTIC CARCINOMA: These neoplasms resemble their namesakes in the salivary glands. They are derived from the tracheobronchial mucous glands and are seen in the trachea or proximal bronchus as a luminal mass, often associated with obstructive symptoms. Adenoid cystic carcinomas are difficult to resect locally and often metastasize.

PULMONARY ARTERY SARCOMA: Pulmonary artery sarcoma is a rare tumor of connective tissue (Fig. 12-92), which has a histological spectrum, including fibrosarcoma, leiomyosarcoma, osteosarcoma, rhabdomyosarcoma, angiosarcoma, or unclassifiable sarcoma. These tumors are rarely diagnosed during life and may be discovered because of pulmonary hypertension. The tumor often grows in an intraluminal fashion within proximal arteries and may extend in a worm-

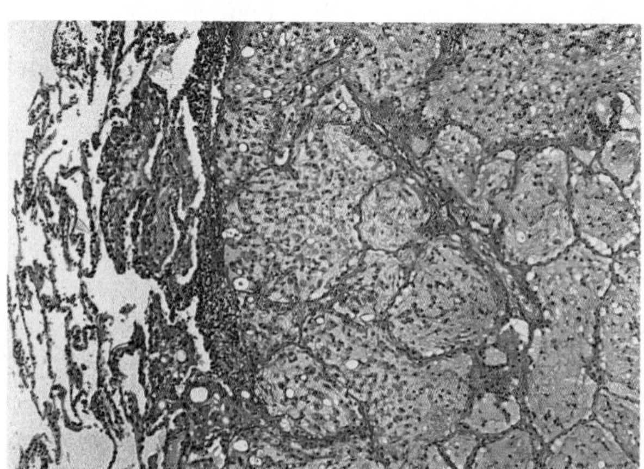

FIGURE *12-91*
Epithelioid hemangioendothelioma. A nodule of tumor has spread within alveolar spaces.

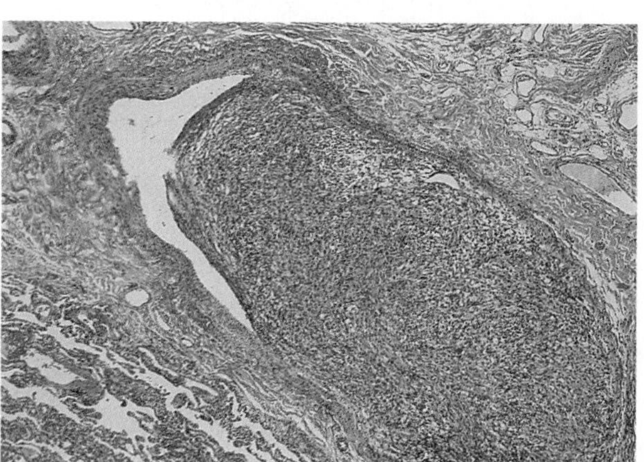

FIGURE *12-92*
Pulmonary artery sarcoma. A polypoid mass of malignant spindle cells is spreading within the lumen of this pulmonary artery.

like fashion to peripheral arteries, resulting in peripheral infarcts.

Lymphomatoid Granulomatosis

Lymphomatoid granulomatosis is a lymphoproliferative disorder characterized by pulmonary nodular lymphoid infiltrates, with frequent central necrosis and vascular permeation (Fig. 12-93). It is a disease of middle-aged persons. The lung is the major location, but the kidney, skin, and upper respiratory tract also may be involved. The lymphoid infiltrate is angiocentric and angioinvasive and consists of polymorphous, small to medium-sized lymphocytes. Scattered, large, atypical, immunoblast-like cells represent B cells infected with Epstein–Barr virus. The smaller cells are T lymphocytes.

Despite remissions induced by chemotherapy, half of all patients eventually develop large cell lymphoma. Even with aggressive treatment, the overall prognosis of lymphomatoid granulomatosis is poor.

Metastatic Tumor

The most common malignant neoplasm of the lung is a metastatic tumor. In fact, in one third of all fatal cancers, pulmonary metastases are evident at autopsy. Metastatic tumors in the lung are typically multiple and circumscribed. When large nodules are seen in the lungs radiologically, they are called "cannon ball" metastases (Fig. 12-94). The histological appearance of most metastases resembles that of the primary tumor. Uncommonly, metastatic tumors mimic widespread bronchioloalveolar carcinoma, the usual primary site being the pancreas or stomach.

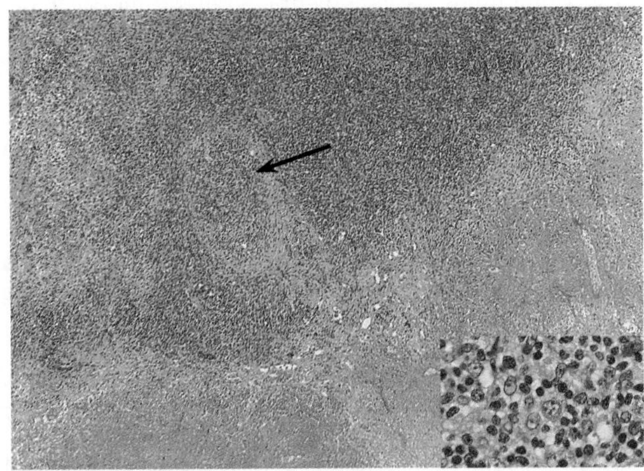

FIGURE *12-93*
Lymphomatoid granulomatosis. This extensively necrotic nodular mass consists of a cellular lymphoid infiltrate, which penetrates a blood vessel (*arrow*) at the edge of the lesion. *Inset:* The lymphoid infiltrate is composed of a polymorphous population of small, medium-sized, and large atypical lymphoid cells.

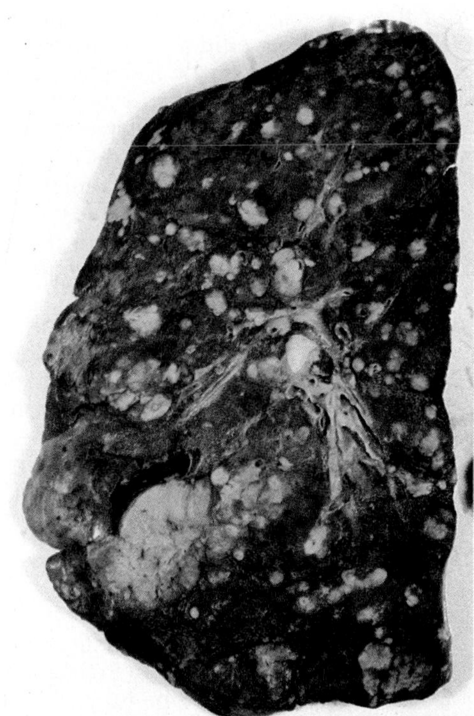

FIGURE *12-94*
Metastatic carcinoma of the lung. A section through the lung shows numerous nodules of metastatic carcinoma, corresponding to "cannon ball" metastases seen radiologically.

Lymphangitic carcinoma is a condition in which the metastatic tumor spreads widely through the pulmonary lymphatic channels to form a sheath of tumor around the bronchovascular tree and the veins. Clinically, patients suffer from cough and shortness of breath and display a diffuse reticulonodular pattern on the chest radiograph. The common primary sites are the breast, stomach, pancreas, and colon.

The Pleura

PNEUMOTHORAX

Pneumothorax is defined as the presence of air in the pleural cavity. It may be due to traumatic perforation of the pleura or may be "spontaneous." Traumatic causes include penetrating wounds of the chest wall (for example, a stab wound or a rib fracture). Traumatic pneumothorax is actually most commonly iatrogenic and is seen after aspiration of fluid from the pleura (thoracentesis), pleural or lung biopsies, transbronchial biopsies, and positive pressure–assisted ventilation.

Spontaneous pneumothorax is typically encountered in young adults. For example, while exercising vigorously, a tall young man develops acute chest pain and shortness of breath. A chest radiograph reveals collapse of the lung on the side of the pain and a large collection of air in the pleural space. The condition is due to the rupture of an emphysematous lesion, usually a subpleural emphysematous bleb. In most cases, spontaneous pneumothorax subsides by itself, but in some patients withdrawal of the air is required.

Tension pneumothorax refers to unilateral pneumothorax sufficiently extensive to shift the mediastinum to the opposite side, with compression of the opposite lung. The condition may be life-threatening and must be relieved by immediate drainage.

Bronchopleural fistula is a serious condition in which there is free communication between the airway and the pleura. It is usually iatrogenic, caused by the interruption of bronchial continuity by biopsy or surgery. It may also be due to extensive infection and necrosis of lung tissue, in which case the infection is more important than the air.

PLEURAL EFFUSION

Pleural effusion is the accumulation of excess fluid in the pleural cavity. Only a small amount of fluid in the pleural cavity lubricates the space between the lung and the chest wall. Fluid is secreted into the pleural space from the parietal pleura and absorbed by the visceral pleura. The severity of a pleural effusion varies from a few milliliters of fluid, which is detected only radiologically as obliteration of the costophrenic angle, to a massive accumulation that shifts the mediastinum and the trachea to the opposite side.

HYDROTHORAX: *This term refers to an effusion that resembles water and would be regarded as edema elsewhere.* It may be due to increased hydrostatic pressure within the capillaries, as occurs in patients with heart failure or in any condition that produces systemic or pulmonary edema. Hydrothorax also occurs in patients with low serum osmotic pressure, as in nephrotic syndrome, cirrhosis of the liver, or severe starvation. Other important causes of hydrothorax are the collagen vascular diseases (notably systemic lupus erythematosus and rheumatoid arthritis) and asbestos exposure.

PYOTHORAX: *A turbid effusion containing many polymorphonuclear leukocytes (pyothorax) results from infections of the pleura.* This may occasionally be caused by an external penetrating wound that brings pyogenic organisms into the pleural space. More commonly, it is a complication of bacterial pneumonia that extends to the pleural surface, the classic example of which is pneumococcal pneumonia. Pyothorax is a rare complication of medical procedures involving the pleural cavity.

EMPYEMA: *This is a variant of pyothorax in which thick pus accumulates within the pleural cavity, often with loculation and fibrosis.*

HEMOTHORAX: *This term refers to blood in the pleural cavity as a result of trauma or rupture of a vessel (for example, dissecting aneurysm of the aorta).* A pleural effusion may be blood-stained in tuberculosis, cancers involving the pleura, and pulmonary infarction.

CHYLOTHORAX: *This condition is the accumulation in the pleural cavity of a milky, lipid-rich fluid (chyle) as a result of lymphatic obstruction.* It has an ominous portent, because obstruction of the lymphatics suggests disease of the lymph nodes in the posterior mediastinum. Chylothorax is thus found as a rare complication of malignant tumors in the mediastinum, such as lymphoma. In tropical countries, chylothorax results from nematode infestations. Chylothorax can also be seen in pulmonary lymphangioleiomyomatosis.

PLEURITIS

Pleuritis, or inflammation of the pleura, may result from the extension of any pulmonary infection to the visceral pleura, bacterial infections within the pleural cavity, viral infections, collagen vascular disease, or pulmonary infarction that involves the surface of the lung. The most striking symptom is sharp, stabbing chest pain on inspiration. It is frequently associated with a pleural effusion.

TUMORS OF THE PLEURA

Localized (Solitary) Fibrous Tumor of the Pleura

Solitary fibrous tumor of the pleura is an uncommon localized neoplasm arising in association with the pleura. Most are benign, but one third are malignant. Eighty percent of the pleural tumors arise on the visceral pleura, with the remainder originating in the parietal pleura. Similar tumors can develop in any location associated with a mesothelial surface, including the mediastinum, peritoneum, pericardium, liver, and tunica vaginalis.

Of fibrous tumors of the pleura that are attached to the visceral pleura, more than half have a pedicle, often measuring 1 cm in length. The tumors range up to 40 cm, and more than 60% are greater than 10 cm in size. Weights up to 3800 g are recorded. The cut surface is grey–white, with a nodular, whorled, or lobulated appearance. Cysts are occasionally present, especially at the base near the pleural attachment.

The most common histological feature is the "patternless pattern," followed by hemangiopericytoma-like, storiform, herringbone, leiomyoma-like, or neurofibroma-like arrangements. The patternless pattern consists of fibroblast-like cells and connective tissue arranged in a random or disorderly pattern. The tumor cells are spindle- to oval-shaped, often with a fibroblast-like appearance. The collagen is compressed between the cells in a lace-like network, or it may form dense, wire-like bands. Histological features in favor of malignancy include increased cellularity, pleomorphism, necrosis, and more than four mitoses per 10 high-power fields.

The median age of patients diagnosed with localized fibrous tumor of the pleura is 55 years (range, 9 to 86 years) without any sex predominance. The most common presenting symptom is chest pain, followed by shortness of breath, cough, hypoglycemia, weight loss, hemoptysis, fever, and night sweats. Patients with benign fibrous tumors of pleura have an excellent prognosis. Half of histologically malignant tumors are cured if completely resected.

Malignant Mesothelioma

Malignant mesothelioma is a neoplasm of mesothelial cells, which is most common in the pleura but also occurs in the peritoneum and the tunica vaginalis of the testis. It affects some 2000 new persons a year in the United States. **In the United States, Great Britain, and South Africa, more than 80% of patients report exposure to asbestos.** The latency period between asbestos exposure and the appearance of malignant mesothelioma is 20 to 40 years, with a range of 15 to 60 years.

☐ **Pathology:** On gross examination, pleural mesothelioma characteristically encases and compresses the lung, extending into fissures and interlobar septa (Fig. 12-95A). Invasion of the pulmonary parenchyma is generally limited to the periphery adjacent to the tumor, and lymph nodes tend to be spared. Microscopically, classic mesothelioma exhibits a biphasic appearance, with epithelial and sarcomatous patterns (see Fig. 12-95B). Glands and tubules that resemble adenocarcinoma are admixed with sheets of spindle cells that are similar to a fibrosarcoma. In some instances, only the epithelial component is apparent, in which case, it is difficult to distinguish mesothelioma from adenocarcinoma. Less commonly, only the sarcomatous component is present. Useful criteria for the diagnosis of mesothelioma include the absence of mucin, the presence of hyaluronic acid (positive alcian blue staining), and the presence of long, slender microvilli by electron microscopy.

The application of immunohistochemistry provides more refined criteria for differentiating mesothelioma from adenocarcinoma. Adenocarcinomas are often, but not invariably, positive for carcinoembryonic antigen, Leu-M1, B72.3, and BER-EP4. Mesotheliomas are negative for these markers, but virtually all stain for cytokeratins. However, in some cases, histochemical analysis fails to distinguish between adenocarcinoma and mesothelioma.

☐ **Clinical Features:** The average age of patients with mesothelioma is 60 years. Patients are first seen with a pleural effusion or a pleural mass, chest pain, and nonspecific symptoms, such as weight loss and malaise. Pleural mesotheliomas tend to spread locally within the chest cavity, invading and compressing major structures. Metastases can occur to the lung parenchyma and media-

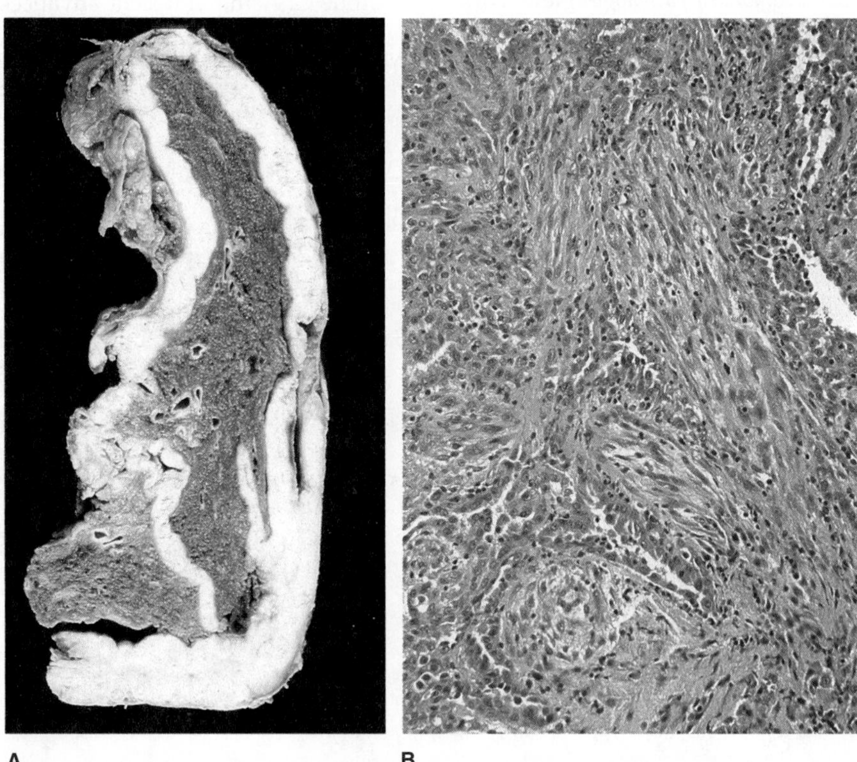

FIGURE 12-95
Pleural malignant mesothelioma. *(A)* The lung is encased by a dense pleural tumor, which extends along the interlobar fissures but does not involve the underlying lung parenchyma. *(B)* This mesothelioma is composed of a biphasic pattern of epithelial and sarcomatous elements.

stinal lymph nodes, as well as to extrathoracic sites such as the liver, bones, peritoneum, and adrenals. Treatment is ineffective, and the prognosis is hopeless.

Acknowledgment

The authors would like to gratefully acknowledge Mary Klassen for helpful comments in the review of this chapter.

SUGGESTED READING

BOOKS

Arnold W, Altermatt HJ: *Diseases of the head and neck.* Stuttgart: Thieme Medical Publishers, 1987.

Barnes L: *Surgical pathology of the head and neck.* New York: Marcel Dekker, 1985.

Barnes L, Peel RL: *Head and neck pathology.* New York: Igaku-Shoin Medical Publishers, 1990.

Churg A, Green FHY: *Pathology of occupational lung disease.* New York: Igaku-Shoin Medical Publishers, 1988.

Colby TV: *Atlas of pulmonary surgical pathology.* Philadelphia: WB Saunders, 1991.

Colby TV, Koss MN, Travis WD: *Tumors of the lower respiratory tract.* Armed Forces Institute of Pathology Fascicle, Third Series. Washington, DC: Armed Forces Institute of Pathology, 1995.

Dail DH, Hammar SP: *Pulmonary pathology.* New York: Springer-Verlag, 1994.

Fishman AP, Elias JA: *Pulmonary diseases and disorders.* New York: McGraw-Hill, Health Professions Division, 1997.

Katzenstein AL, Askin FB: *Surgical pathology of non-neoplastic lung disease.* Philadelphia: WB Saunders, 1990.

Murray JF, Nadel JA: *Textbook of respiratory medicine.* Philadelphia: WB Saunders, 1994.

Pass HI, Mitchell JB, Johnson DH, Turrisi AT, eds: *Lung cancer: Principles and practice.* Philadelphia: Lippincott–Raven Publishers, 1996.

Roggli VL, Greenberg SD, Pratt PC: *Pathology of asbestos-associated diseases.* Boston: Little, Brown, 1992.

Schwartz MI, King TE, eds: *Interstitial lung disease.* St. Louis: Mosby-Year Book, 1993.

Spencer H, Hasleton PS: *Spencer's pathology of the lung.* New York: McGraw-Hill, Health Professions Division, 1996.

Thurlbeck WM, Churg A: *Pathology of the lung.* New York: Thieme Medical Publishers, 1995.

Wenig BM: *Atlas of head and neck pathology.* Philadelphia: WB Saunders, 1993.

REVIEWS

Agostini C, Semenzato G: Immunology of idiopathic pulmonary fibrosis. *Curr Opin Pulm Med* 2:364–369, 1996.

Barnes P: The pathology of community-acquired pneumonia. *Semin Resp Infect* 9:130–139, 1994.

Bjoraker JA, Ryu JH, Edwin MK, et al: Prognostic signifigance of histopathologic subsets in idopathic pulmonary fibrosis. *J Resp Crit Care Med* 157:199–203, 1998.

Epler GR: Bronchiolitis obliterans organizing pneumonia. *Semin Resp Infect* 10:65–77, 1995.

Evans MD, Pryor WA: Cigarette smoking, emphysema, and damage to alpha 1-proteinase inhibitor. *Am J Physiol* 266:493–611, 1994.

Knight KR, Burdeon JG, Cook L, Brenton S, Ayad M, Janus ED: The proteinase-antiproteinase theory of emphysema: A speculative analysis of recent advances into the pathogenesis of emphysema. *Respirology* 2:91–95, 1997.

Leslie KO, Colby TV: Pathology of lung cancer. *Curr Opin Pulm Med* 3:252–256, 1997.

Luce JM: Acute lung injury and the acute respiratory distress syndrome. *Crit Care Med* 26:369–376, 1998.

Lynch JP 3rd, Kazerooni EA, Gay SE: Pulmonary sarcoidosis. *Clin Chest Med* 18:755–785, 1997.

Marone G: Asthma: Recent advances. *Immunol Today* 19: 5–9, 1998.

Murin S, Hilbert J, Reilly SJ: Cigarette smoke and the lung. *Clin Rev Allergy Immunol* 15:307–361, 1997.

Nicotra MB: Bronchiectasis. *Semin Resp Infect* 9:31–40, 1994.

Otto WR: Lung stem cells. *Int J Exp Pathol* 78:291–310, 1997.

Peak JK: The epidemiology of asthma: *Curr Opin Pulm Med* 2:7–15, 1996.

Salgia R, Skarin AT: Molecular abnormalities in lung cancer. *J Clin Oncol* 16:1207–1217, 1998.

Salvaggio JE: Extrinsic allergic alveolitis (hypersensativity pneumonitis): Past, present, and future. *Clin Exp Allergy* 27 (Suppl 1):18–25, 1997.

Schulger NW, Rom WN: The host immune response to tuberculosis. *Am J Resp Crit Care Med* 157: 679–691, 1998.

Schwartz DA, Peterson MW: Occupational lung disease. *Disease–A–Month* 44:41–84, 1998.

CHAPTER 13

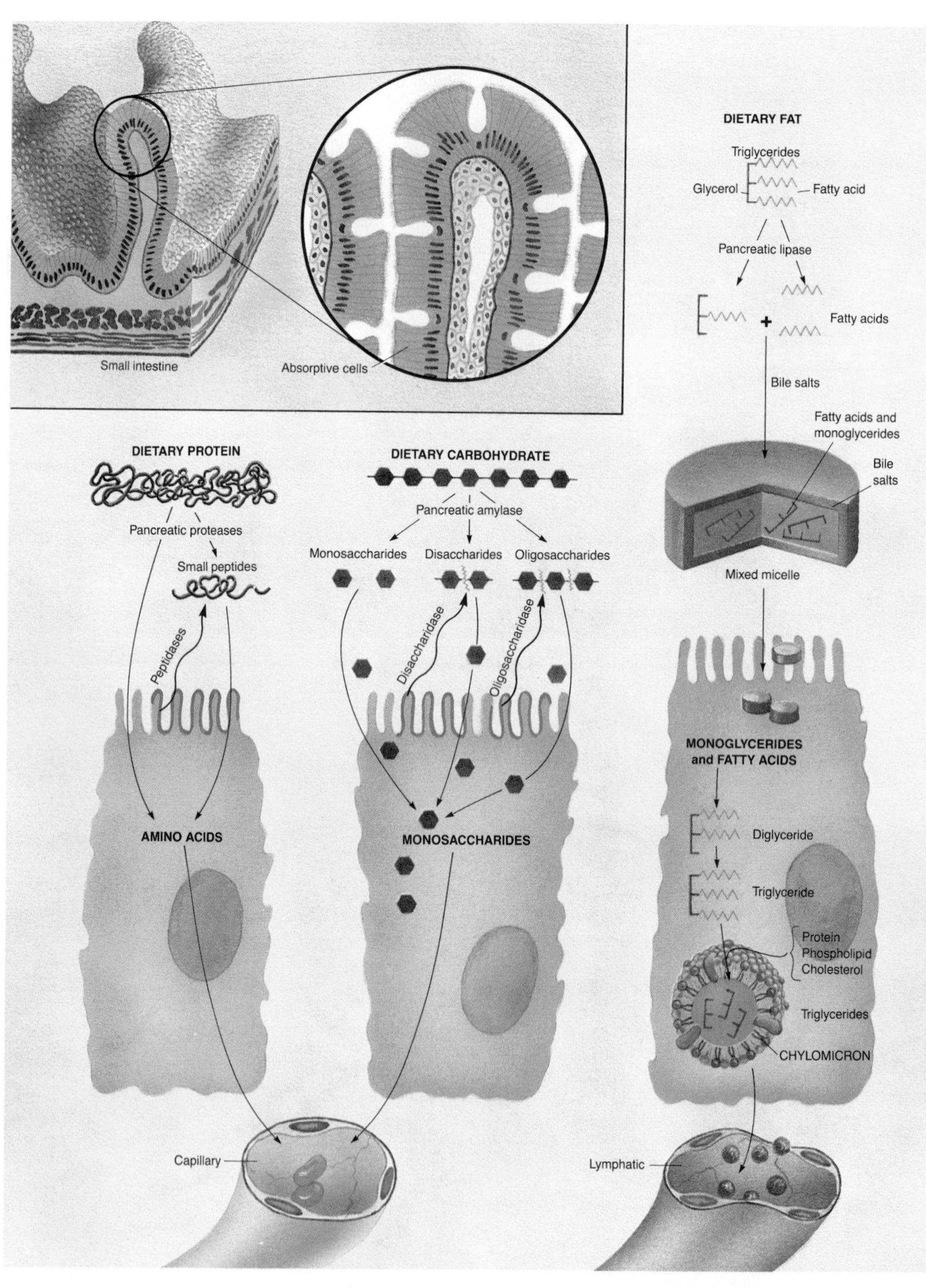

Small intestine
Absorptive cells
DIETARY FAT
Triglycerides
Glycerol
Fatty acid
Pancreatic lipase
Fatty acids
Bile salts
Fatty acids and monoglycerides
Bile salts
Mixed micelle
MONOGLYCERIDES and FATTY ACIDS
Diglyceride
Triglyceride
Protein
Phospholipid
Cholesterol
Triglycerides
CHYLOMICRON
Lymphatic
DIETARY PROTEIN
Pancreatic proteases
Small peptides
Peptidases
AMINO ACIDS
Capillary
DIETARY CARBOHYDRATE
Pancreatic amylase
Monosaccharides
Disaccharides
Oligosaccharides
Disaccharidase
Oligosaccharidase
MONOSACCHARIDES

The Gastrointestinal Tract

Stanley R. Hamilton
John L. Farber
Emanuel Rubin

FIGURE *13-1 (see opposite page)*
Mechanisms of nutrient absorption in the small intestine.

The Esophagus

ANATOMY

Embryologically, the gut and the respiratory tract arise from the same anlage and compose a single tube. This structure divides into two separate tubes, the esophagus being dorsal and the future respiratory tract ventral. Initially, a columnar epithelium lines the esophagus in its early embryonic development, but it is replaced by a stratified squamous epithelium.

The adult esophagus is a 25-cm tube that contains both striated and smooth muscle in its upper portion and smooth muscle alone in its lower portion. The organ is fixed superiorly at the cricopharyngeus muscle, which is considered the upper esophageal sphincter. It courses inferiorly through the posterior mediastinum behind the trachea and the heart and exits the thorax through the hiatus of the diaphragm. Tonic muscular contraction at the lower end of the esophagus creates an action similar to that of a one-way flutter valve. The so-called *lower esophageal sphincter* is not a true anatomical sphincter but rather a functional one.

The esophagus has a mucosa, submucosa, muscularis propria, and adventitia. The transition from the normal squamous mucosa of the esophagus to the gastric mucosa at the esophagogastric junction occurs abruptly at the level of the diaphragm. The esophageal submucosa contains mucous glands and a rich lymphatic plexus. The lymphatics of the upper third of the esophagus drain to the cervical lymph nodes, those of the middle third to the mediastinal nodes, and those of the lower third to the celiac and gastric lymph nodes. These anatomical features are significant in the spread of esophageal cancer.

The venous drainage of the esophagus is important in portal hypertension, in which esophageal varices occur. These varices are invariably found in the lower third of the esophagus, because the veins of the upper third drain into the superior vena cava, and those of the middle third drain into the azygous system. Only the veins of the lower third of the esophagus drain into the portal vein by way of the gastric veins.

The sole function of the esophagus is to serve as a conduit for the passage of food and liquid into the stomach. The act of swallowing, which is not entirely understood, is remarkably complex and requires precise coordination of a number of separate movements.

CONGENITAL DISORDERS

Tracheoesophageal Fistula

The most common esophageal anomaly is tracheoesophageal fistula (Fig. 13-2). It is frequently combined with some form of **esophageal atresia**, although isolated atresia is distinctly uncommon. The cause of esophageal atresia is unknown, but in some cases, it has been associated with a complex of anomalies identified by the acronym Vater syndrome (vertebral defects, anal atresia, tracheoesophageal fistula, and renal dysplasia). Maternal hydramnios has been recorded in some cases of esophageal atresia and, less commonly, in cases of tracheoesophageal fistula. Esophageal atresia and fistulas are often associated with congenital heart disease.

In the most common variety of tracheoesophageal fistula, accounting for about 90% of all such fistulas, the upper portion of the esophagus ends in a blind pouch, and the upper end of the lower segment communicates with the trachea. Because the walls of both the upper and the lower portions of the esophagus are more or less normal, surgical correction is feasible, albeit difficult. **In this type of atresia, the upper blind sac soon fills with mucus, which the infant then aspirates.**

Among the remaining 10% of cases, the most common fistula involves a communication between the proximal esophagus and the trachea; the lower esophageal pouch communicates with the stomach. **Infants with this condition develop aspiration immediately after birth.** In another variant, termed an H-type fistula, a communication exists between an intact esophagus and an intact trachea. In some cases, the lesion becomes symptomatic only in adulthood, when repeated pulmonary infections call attention to it.

When the proximal and distal portions of the esophagus are separated by a considerable distance, surgical correction is difficult because the ends of the esophageal pouches cannot be approximated. Repeated bougienage (mechanical dilation) of the proximal segment may be successful in elongating it enough to allow approximation

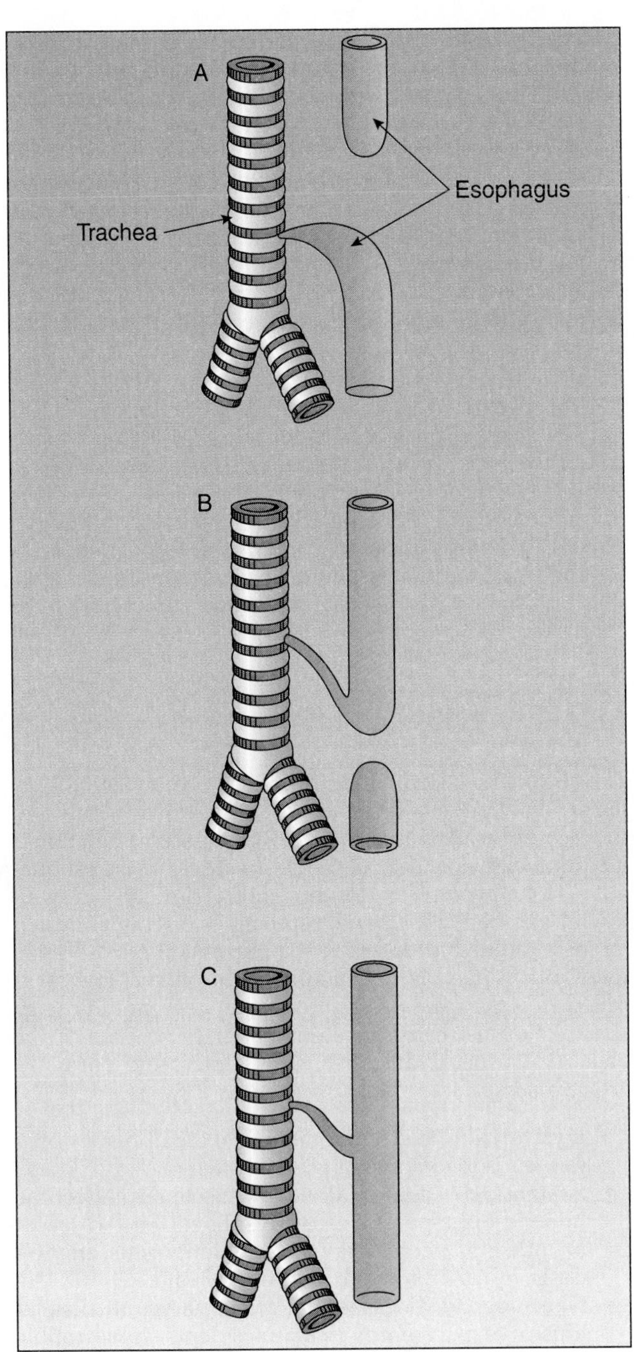

FIGURE 13-2
Congenital tracheoesophageal fistulas. *(A)* The most common type is a communication between the trachea and the lower portion of the esophagus. The upper segment of the esophagus ends in a blind sac. *(B)* In a few cases, the proximal esophagus communicates with the trachea. *(C)* The least common anomaly, the H type, is a fistula between a continuous esophagus and the trachea.

of the pouches. In some cases, steel dilators have been placed in both upper and lower pouches and subjected to strong magnetic fields. This has led to preoperative approximation of the segments and permitted successful surgical correction.

CONGENITAL ESOPHAGEAL STENOSIS: This rare condition is surprisingly resistant to mechanical dilation. In some instances, elements of pulmonary tissue are found in the stenotic region.

BRONCHOPULMONARY FOREGUT MALFORMATION: This uncommon tracheoesophageal developmental anomaly consists of a mass of abnormal pulmonary tissue within the lung. Such tissue is invested by its own separate pleural lining and communicates with the lower esophagus. Passage of esophageal contents into the lung leads to repeated pulmonary infections or an enlarging mediastinal mass.

Rings and Webs

ESOPHAGEAL WEBS: Occasionally, a thin mucosal membrane projects into the lumen of the esophagus. Usually single, the webs are sometimes multiple and can be found anywhere in the esophagus. Esophageal webs are generally successfully treated by dilation with large rubber bougies; occasionally, they can be excised with biopsy forceps during endoscopy.

PLUMMER–VINSON (PATERSON–KELLY) SYNDROME: *This disorder is characterized by (1) a cervical esophageal web, (2) mucosal lesions of the mouth and pharynx, and (3) iron-deficiency anemia.* Dysphagia, often associated with aspiration of swallowed food, is the most common clinical manifestation. Ninety percent of cases occur in women. The prevalence of this syndrome has significantly declined in recent years, possibly owing to improved nutrition and the addition of supplemental nutrients to food. **Carcinoma of the oropharynx and upper esophagus is a recognized complication of the Plummer–Vinson syndrome.**

SCHATZKI RING: *This lower esophageal narrowing is usually seen at the junction of the squamous and columnar epithelium* (Fig. 13-3). Because it occurs at the squamocolumnar junction, the upper surface of the mucosal ring exhibits stratified squamous epithelium, whereas the lower is lined by columnar epithelium. Mild chronic inflammation and fibrosis are common in the submucosa. Although it has been noted in as many as 14% of barium meal examinations, Schatzki ring is usually asymptomatic. Typically, patients with narrow Schatzki rings complain of intermittent dysphagia, and a food bolus may lodge in the lower esophagus and require endoscopic intervention. Esophageal bougienage is almost always effective in the treatment of a symptomatic Schatzki ring.

Esophageal Diverticula

A true esophageal diverticulum is an outpouching of the wall that contains all layers of the esophagus. When the sac lacks a muscular layer, it is known as a false diverticulum. Esophageal diverticula occur in the hypopharyngeal area above the upper esophageal sphincter, in the middle esophagus, and immediately proximal to the lower esophageal sphincter.

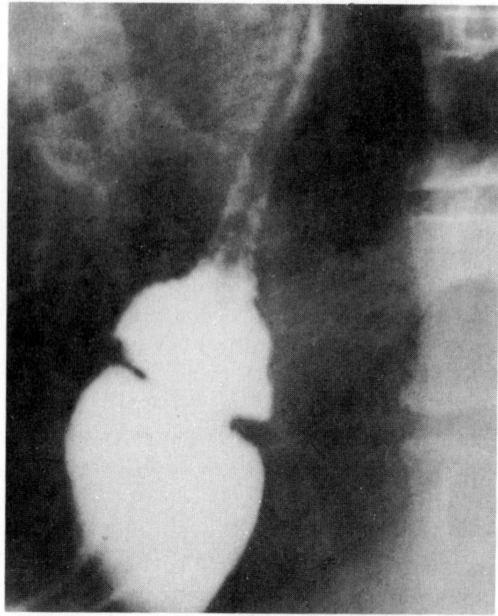

FIGURE 13-3
Schatzki mucosal ring. A contrast radiograph illustrates the lower esophageal narrowing.

ZENKER DIVERTICULUM: *Zenker diverticulum is an uncommon lesion that appears high in the esophagus and affects men more than women.* It was once believed to result from luminal pressure exerted in a structurally weak area and was therefore classed as a **pulsion diverticulum**. The cause is probably more complicated, but disordered function of the cricopharyngeal musculature is still generally thought to be involved in the pathogenesis of this false diverticulum. Most affected persons who come to medical attention are older than 60 years, an observation that supports the belief that this diverticulum is acquired.

Zenker diverticulum can enlarge conspicuously and accumulate a large amount of food. When drugs are trapped in the pouch, their bioavailability may be limited. The typical symptom is regurgitation of food eaten some time previously (occasionally days), in the absence of dysphagia. Recurrent aspiration pneumonia may be a serious complication. When symptoms are severe, surgical intervention is the rule.

TRACTION DIVERTICULA: *Traction diverticula are outpouchings that occur principally in the midportion of the esophagus.* They were so named because of their attachment to adjacent mediastinal lymph nodes, usually associated with tuberculous lymphadenitis. However, fibrous adhesions between midesophageal diverticula and diseased mediastinal nodes are today uncommon, and it is believed that these pouches often reflect a disturbance in the motor function of the esophagus. A diverticulum in the midesophagus ordinarily has a wide stoma, and the pouch is usually higher than its orifice. Thus, it does not retain food or secretions and remains asymptomatic, with only rare complications.

EPIPHRENIC DIVERTICULA: *These diverticula are located immediately above the diaphragm.* Motor disturbances of the esophagus (e.g., achalasia, diffuse esophageal spasm) are found in two thirds of patients with this true diverticulum. In addition, it has been speculated that reflux esophagitis plays a role in the pathogenesis of epiphrenic diverticula.

Unlike other diverticula, epiphrenic diverticula are encountered in young persons. Nocturnal regurgitation of large amounts of fluid stored in the diverticulum during the day is typical. When symptoms are severe, surgical intervention directed toward correcting the motor abnormality (e.g., myotomy to correct diffuse esophageal spasm) is appropriate.

INTRAMURAL PSEUDODIVERTICULOSIS: *This rare disorder is characterized by numerous small (1- to 3-mm) diverticula in the wall of the esophagus, commonly accompanied by a stricture of the upper esophagus.* The lesions are not true diverticula but rather dilated ducts of the submucosal glands. The condition is sometimes associated with esophageal candidiasis. The principal symptom is dysphagia; dilation of the stricture usually ameliorates the condition.

MOTOR DISORDERS

The automatic coordination of muscular movement during swallowing results in the free passage of food through the esophagus. Any failure of proper muscular function is included in the concept of motor disorders of the esophagus. The hallmark of motor disorders is difficulty in swallowing, termed *dysphagia*. Dysphagia is often manifested by an awareness of the lack of progression of a bolus of food and in itself is not painful. Pain on swallowing is called *odynophagia*. Disordered esophageal motility (e.g., spasm) may also cause substernal pain that radiates to the back, arms, neck, and jaw, thus simulating coronary artery disease.

- **Dysfunction of striated muscle** in the upper esophagus leads to dysphagia.
- **Systemic diseases of skeletal muscle** also affect the upper esophagus and cause dysphagia. Such diseases include myasthenia gravis, dermatomyositis, amyloidosis, hyperthyroidism, and myxedema.
- **Neurological diseases** that affect nerves to skeletal muscle (e.g., cerebrovascular accidents, amyotrophic lateral sclerosis) may impair swallowing.
- **Peripheral neuropathy** associated with diabetes or alcoholism may interfere with smooth muscle function and can lead to dysphagia.

Achalasia

Achalasia, at one time termed cardiospasm, is a disease characterized by failure of the lower esophageal sphincter to relax in response to swallowing and the absence of peristalsis in the body of the esophagus. As a result of these defects in both the outflow tract and the pumping mechanisms of the esophagus, food is retained within the esophagus, and the organ hypertrophies and dilates conspicuously (Fig. 13-4).

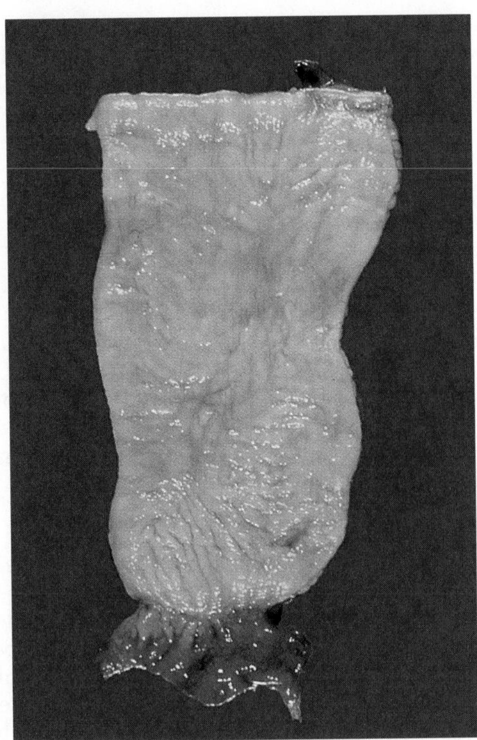

FIGURE *13-4*
Esophagus and upper stomach of a patient with advanced achalasia. The esophagus is markedly dilated above the esophagogastric junction, where the lower esophageal sphincter is located. The esophageal mucosa is redundant and has hyperplastic squamous epithelium.

Although the cause of achalasia is not precisely understood, there is a consensus that a loss or absence of ganglion cells in the myenteric plexus of the esophagus is involved. Degenerative changes in the dorsal motor nucleus of the vagus and the extraesophageal vagus nerves have also been described. Thus, it is not clear whether achalasia is a degenerative or infectious disease of the neurons in the medulla or in the myenteric plexus of the esophagus, or both.

It has also been suggested that the loss of neurons that release vasoactive intestinal peptide (VIP), which causes relaxation of the lower esophageal sphincter, may play a role. The loss of ganglion cells is occasionally accompanied by chronic inflammation. In Latin America, achalasia is a common complication of **Chagas disease**, the ganglion cells being destroyed by *Trypanosoma cruzi*.

Dysphagia, occasionally odynophagia, and regurgitation of material retained in the esophagus are common symptoms of achalasia. Aspiration of food may lead to pneumonia. Squamous carcinoma is also a complication. Treatment is by dilatation or surgical myotomy, which can lead to gastroesophageal reflux.

Scleroderma (Progressive Systemic Sclerosis)

Scleroderma causes fibrosis in many organs and produces a severe abnormality of esophageal muscle function. The disease affects principally the lower esophageal sphincter, which may become so impaired that the lower esophagus and upper stomach are no longer distinct functional entities and are visualized as a common cavity. In addition, there may be a lack of peristalsis in the entire esophagus.

Microscopically, fibrosis of the esophageal smooth muscle, especially the inner layer of the muscularis propria, and nonspecific inflammatory changes are seen. Intimal fibrosis of the small arteries and arterioles is common and may play a role in the pathogenesis of the fibrosis. Clinically, patients have dysphagia and heartburn caused by peptic esophagitis, owing to reflux of acid from the stomach.

HIATAL HERNIA

Hiatal hernia is a herniation of the stomach through an enlarged esophageal hiatus in the diaphragm. A common acquired condition, hiatal hernia is in most cases of unknown cause. Two basic types of hiatal hernia are the sliding, or axial, form, which accounts for most hiatal hernias, and the paraesophageal variety (Fig. 13-5).

SLIDING HERNIA: *An enlargement of the diaphragmatic hiatus and laxity of the circumferential connective tissue allows a cap of gastric cardia to move upward to a position above the diaphragm.* The condition is so common that, on appropriate manipulation by the radiologist, more than half of the population can be demonstrated to have a small sliding hernia. However, only 10% exhibit this abnormality on routine barium-swallow examination. Sliding hiatal hernia is asymptomatic in the large majority of patients, and only 5% of patients diagnosed radiologically complain of symptoms referable to gastroesophageal reflux.

PARAESOPHAGEAL HERNIA: *This form of hiatal hernia is characterized by herniation of a portion of the gastric fundus alongside the esophagus through a defect in the diaphragmatic connective tissue membrane that defines the esophageal hiatus* (see Fig. 13-5). The hernia progressively enlarges, and the hiatus grows increasingly wide. In extreme cases, most of the stomach herniates into the thorax, and it may even be accompanied by the colon or the small intestine. Interestingly, most large paraesophageal hernias do not cause significant symptoms.

☐ **Clinical Features:** Symptoms of hiatal hernia, particularly heartburn and regurgitation, are attributed to gastroesophageal reflux. However, evidence suggests that the reflux of gastric contents is primarily related to incompetence of the lower esophageal sphincter. Classically, the symptoms are exacerbated when the affected person is in the recumbent position, which facilitates acid reflux. Dysphagia, painful swallowing, and occasionally bleeding may also be troublesome. In cases of very large paraesophageal hernias, protrusion of the stomach into the thorax may embarrass respiration. In such large herniations, there is a risk of gastric volvulus or intrathoracic gastric dilatation.

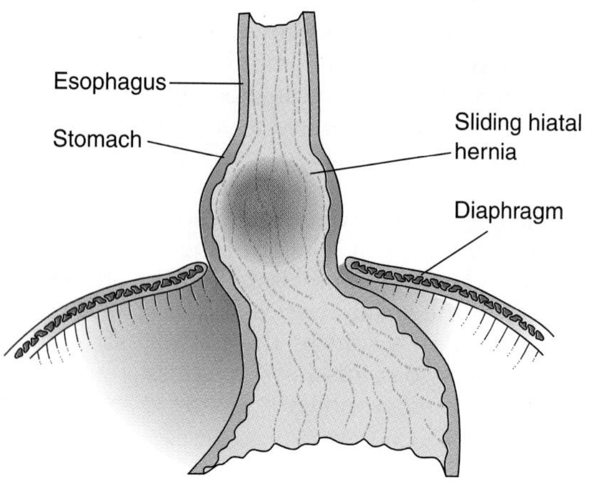

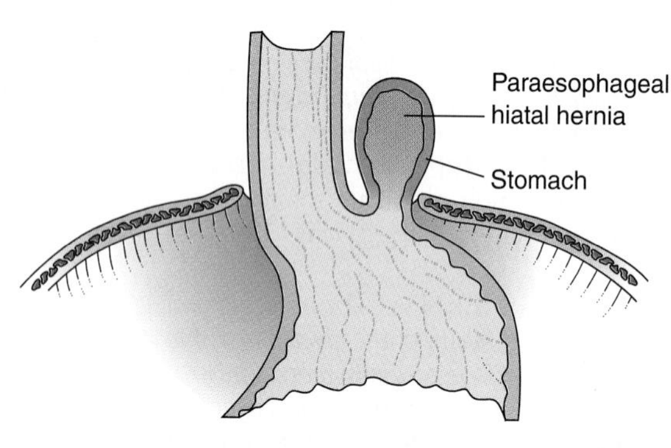

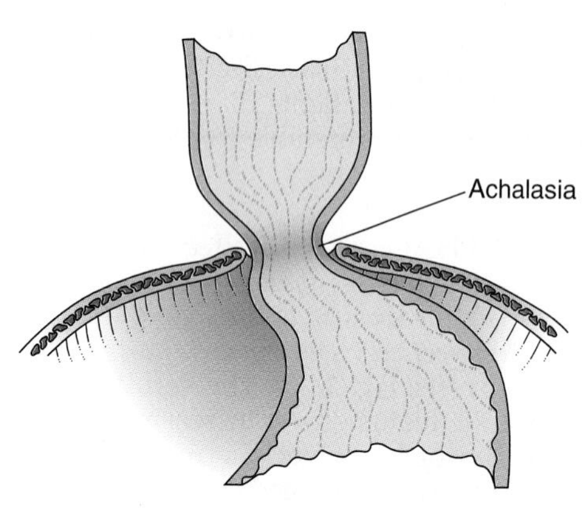

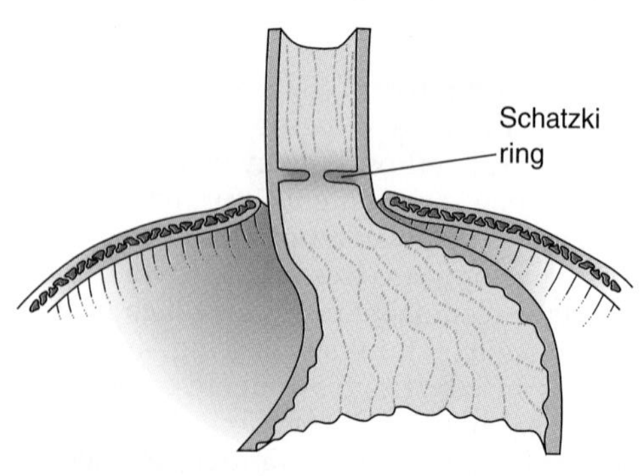

FIGURE *13-5*
Disorders of the esophageal outlet.

Sliding hiatal hernias generally do not require surgical repair; symptoms are often treated medically. By contrast, an enlarging paraesophageal hernia should be surgically treated, even in the absence of symptoms.

ESOPHAGITIS

Reflux Esophagitis

Reflux esophagitis refers to esophageal injury caused by the regurgitation of gastric contents into the lower esophagus. By far the most common type of esophagitis, it is often found in conjunction with a sliding hiatal hernia, although it may occur through an incompetent lower esophageal sphincter without any demonstrable anatomic lesion.

☐ **Pathogenesis:** The principal barrier to the reflux of gastric contents into the esophagus is the lower esophageal sphincter. Transient reflux is a normal event, particularly after a meal. When these episodes become more frequent and are prolonged, esophagitis results.

In addition to hiatal hernia, agents that cause a decrease in the pressure of the lower esophageal sphincter (e.g., alcohol, chocolate, fatty foods, cigarette smoking) are associated with reflux. Certain central nervous system depressants (e.g., morphine, diazepam [Valium], pregnancy, estrogen therapy, and the presence of a nasogastric tube) also lead to reflux esophagitis.

Although acid is damaging to the esophageal mucosa, the combination of acid and pepsin may be particularly injurious. Moreover, gastric fluid often contains refluxed bile from the duodenum, which is harmful to the esophageal mucosa. Alcohol, hot beverages, and spicy foods also may damage the mucosa directly.

☐ **Pathology:** The earliest grossly evident alteration produced by gastroesophageal reflux is hyperemia. When reflux is chronic, reactive thickening of the squamous epithelium, traditionally termed *leukoplakia*, is occasionally seen as irregular grayish white patches. Areas affected by reflux are susceptible to superficial mucosal erosions and ulcers, which often appear as vertical linear streaks. Microscopically, mild injury to the squamous epithelium is manifested by balloon cell (enlarged cells with clear cytoplasm due to intracellular edema and influx of plasma proteins). The basal-zone layer of the epithelium is thickened, and the papillae of the lamina propria are elongated and extend toward the surface because of reactive proliferation. Vascular papillae are often dilated. Eosinophils and neutrophils may be present within the squamous epithelium. A modest increase in lymphocytes is seen in the lamina propria and squamous epithelium.

Esophageal erosions and ulcers may result if reflux esophagitis is sufficiently severe. Such lesions usually heal, but on occasion, they may lead to life-threatening hematemesis or, rarely, perforation of the esophagus.

Esophageal stricture may eventuate in those cases in which the ulcer persists and damages the esophageal wall deep to the lamina propria. In this circumstance, fibrosis is stimulated and can narrow the esophageal lumen. Such a stricture is usually sharply localized and situated near the lower esophageal sphincter, although it may extend considerably higher. If an esophageal stricture seriously interferes with the passage of food, the esophagus becomes dilated above the narrowing. The most common clinical complaint is progressive dysphagia.

Barrett Esophagus

Barrett epithelium is defined as replacement of the squamous epithelium of the esophagus by columnar epithelium as a result of chronic gastroesophageal reflux. The incidence of Barrett esophagus has been increasing in recent years, particularly among white men. This disorder occurs in the lower third of the esophagus but may extend higher.

Barrett epithelium was originally considered to be a congenital lesion. **However, it is now established that it represents columnar replacement (metaplasia) of the squamous epithelium in response to the injury produced by chronic gastroesophageal reflux.** There is a slight male predominance and a greater than twofold increased risk for Barrett esophagus among smokers.

☐ **Pathology:** The metaplastic Barrett epithelium may partially involve the circumference of short segments or may line the entire lower esophagus (Fig. 13-6A). Histologically, the lesion is characterized by three types of metaplasia: (1) a distinctive intestine-like epithelium composed of goblet cells and surface cells similar to those of incompletely intestinalized gastric mucosa; (2) cardiac-like mucous glands, resembling those ordinarily seen at the gastroesophageal junction (no or very few parietal or chief cells are present); and (3) an epithelium similar to that of the fundus of the stomach, with short glands containing parietal and chief cells (see Fig. 13-6B). Complete intestinal metaplasia, with Paneth cells and absorptive cells, occurs occasionally in Barrett epithelium. Inflammatory changes are usually superimposed on the epithelial alterations, and in some cases, ulceration and even a stricture are found above the metaplastic epithelium. Reversion of Barrett epithelium to the normal squamous surface has been reported only rarely after correction of esophageal reflux.

As might be expected of a metaplastic epithelium, Barrett esophagus carries a serious risk of malignant transformation to adenocarcinoma (see later), and the risk correlates with the length of the involved esophagus.

Infective Esophagitis

Primary infections of the esophagus are rare, with the exceptions of candidiasis and herpes simplex.

CANDIDA ESOPHAGITIS: This fungal infection has become commonplace because of an increasing number of immunocompromised persons who (1) receive

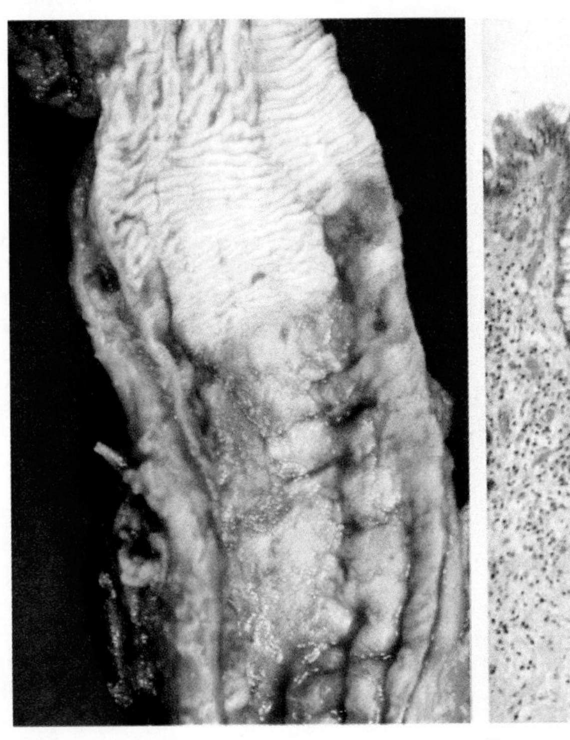

A

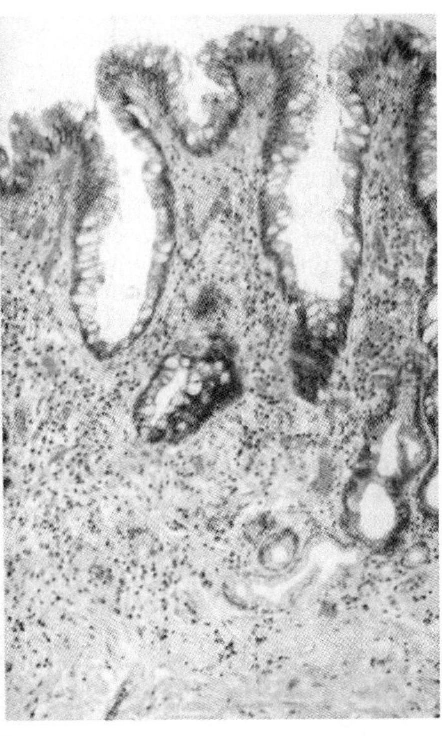

B

FIGURE *13-6*
Barrett esophagus. *(A)* The white squamous mucosa of the proximal esophagus (*top*) is contrasted with the columnar lining of the distal Barrett esophagus (*bottom*). *(B)* A microscopic section of the metaplastic epithelium in *A* shows a villiform surface with numerous goblet cells.

chemotherapy for malignant disease, (2) are treated with immunosuppressive drugs after organ transplantation, or (3) have contracted acquired immunodeficiency syndrome (AIDS). Esophageal candidiasis also occurs in patients with diabetes or those receiving antibiotic therapy, and in others with no known predisposing factors. Dysphagia and severe pain on swallowing are usual, and bleeding from the infected site, sometimes severe, can occur.

In mild cases of candidiasis, a few small, elevated white plaques, surrounded by a hyperemic zone, are present on the mucosa of the middle or lower third of the esophagus. In severe cases, confluent pseudomembranes lie on a hyperemic and edematous mucosa. If the pseudomembrane is removed, mucosal ulcerations and hemorrhages result. Microscopically, *Candida* sometimes involves only the superficial layers of the squamous epithelium. The candidal pseudomembrane contains fungal mycelia, necrotic debris, and fibrin. Involvement of the deeper layers of the esophageal wall can lead to disseminated candidiasis or fibrosis, sometimes severe enough to create a stricture.

HERPETIC ESOPHAGITIS: Esophageal infection with herpesvirus type I is most frequently associated with lymphomas and leukemias; indeed, the esophagus is the most common viscus involved with herpesvirus in those diseases. In such cases, the infection is often manifested by odynophagia. Herpetic infection of the esophagus also may occur in previously healthy persons, in whom it produces severe pain on swallowing.

The well-developed lesions of herpetic esophagitis are grossly similar to those of candidiasis. In early cases, vesicles, small erosions, or plaques are noted; as the infection progresses, these may coalesce to form larger lesions. Microscopically, the lesions are superficial, and the epithelial cells exhibit typical herpetic inclusions in their nuclei. Multinucleated epithelial cells are occasionally encountered, but stromal cells are spared. Necrosis of infected cells leads to ulceration, and candidal and bacterial superinfection results in the formation of pseudomembranes. The disease is self-limited in otherwise healthy persons but is protracted in immunocompromised patients.

CYTOMEGALOVIRUS ESOPHAGITIS: This condition was a curiosity until the AIDS epidemic, after which it has become common. Esophageal involvement with cytomegalovirus is usually a reflection of systemic viral disease in immunocompromised patients with AIDS. Ulceration of the mucosa, similar to that seen in herpetic esophagitis, is usual. Characteristic inclusion bodies of cytomegalovirus are present in the endothelial cells and fibroblasts of the granulation tissue but the epithelium is spared.

Chemical Esophagitis

Chemical injury to the esophagus is usually a result of accidental poisoning in children, attempted suicide in adults, or contact with medication. Ingestion of strong alkaline agents (e.g., lye) or strong acids (e.g., sulfuric or hydrochloric acid), both of which are used in various cleaning solutions, can produce chemical esophagitis. The alkaline solutions are particularly insidious, because they are generally odorless and tasteless and therefore easily swallowed before protective reflexes come into play. By contrast, acids are immediately painful and, at least in accidental cases, are usually rapidly expelled. Caustic alkaline solids adhere to mucous membranes and penetrate tissue much more rapidly than do acids.

☐ **Pathology:** Histologically, alkali-induced liquefactive necrosis is accompanied by conspicuous inflammation and saponification of the membrane lipids in the epithelium, submucosa, and muscularis propria of the esophagus and stomach. Thrombosis of small vessels adds ischemic necrosis to the injury. Severe injury is the rule with liquid alkali, but less than 25% of those who ingest granular preparations have severe complications.

Strong acids produce immediate coagulation necrosis, which results in a protective eschar that limits injury and penetration. Nevertheless, half of patients who ingest concentrated hydrochloric or sulfuric acid have severe esophageal injury. The severity of caustic injury to the esophagus is classified in a manner similar to that of a skin burn:

- **First-degree injury** is defined as erythema and edema of the mucosa and submucosa. The mucosa may slough, but no further complications ensue.
- **Second-degree injury** refers to penetration of the submucosa and muscularis. Sloughing of the tissue leads to ulceration, the formation of granulation tissue, and eventual fibrosis. Scar formation is usually complete within 2 months but can become severe during the next 6 months, often leading to stricture.
- **Third-degree injury** is characterized by necrosis of the full thickness of the esophageal wall.

Drug-related esophagitis is most often caused by direct chemical effects on the squamous-lined mucosa, especially with capsules; esophageal dysmotility and cardiac enlargement (which impinges on the esophagus) may be contributing factors. Allergic reactions to drugs may cause esophagitis. An impairment of the function of the lower esophageal sphincter caused by certain drugs may lead to reflux esophagitis.

Esophagitis in Systemic Illnesses

The squamous mucosa of the esophagus is similar to that of the skin and shares some reactions with that organ. Epidermolysis bullosa and pemphigoid produce bullous lesions in both the skin and esophageal mucosa.

The dystrophic form of epidermolysis bullosa involves all organs that are lined by or derived from squamous epithelium, including the skin, nails, teeth, and esophagus. The bullae, which occur episodically, evolve from fluid-filled vesicles to weeping ulcers. Dysphagia and painful swallowing are the rule. Severe cases result in stricture, usually in the upper esophagus. Corticosteroid therapy has been helpful but is not curative.

Pemphigoid produces subepithelial bullae in the skin and esophagus, but the disease does not lead to scarring. Other dermatological disorders associated with esophagitis include pemphigus, dermatitis herpetiformis, Behçet syndrome, and erythema multiforme.

Graft-versus-host disease in recipients of bone marrow transplants can occur as esophageal lesions causing dysphagia, painful swallowing, and symptoms of gastroesophageal reflux. Esophageal webs and strictures may develop. The upper and middle thirds of the esophageal mucosa are friable, and motor function of the esophagus is impaired.

Esophagitis Produced by Physical Agents

External irradiation for the treatment of thoracic cancers may include portions of the esophagus and lead to esophagitis and even stricture. **Nasogastric tubes** produce pressure ulcers of the esophageal mucosa in patients who have them in place for prolonged periods, although acid reflux also plays a role in these cases.

ESOPHAGEAL VARICES

Esophageal varices are dilated veins immediately beneath the mucosa (Fig. 13-7), *which are prone to rupture and hemorrhage.* They arise in the lower third of the esophagus, virtually always in the setting of portal hypertension resulting from cirrhosis of the liver. The lower esophageal veins are linked to the portal system through gastroesophageal anastomoses. If the portal pressure exceeds a critical level, these anastomoses become prominent in the upper stomach and lower esophagus. When the varices reach a size greater than 5 mm in diameter, they are likely to rupture, in which case, life-threatening hemorrhage ensues. Reflux injury or infective esophagitis can contribute to variceal bleeding. See Chapter 14 for a further discussion of esophageal varices.

LACERATIONS AND PERFORATIONS

Lacerations of the esophagus result from external trauma, such as automobile accidents and falls from great heights, and from medical instrumentation. However, the most common cause is severe vomiting, during which the intraesophageal pressure may rise as high as 300 mm Hg. The diaphragm descends rapidly, and a portion of the upper stomach is forced up through the hiatus. As a result, forceful retching may cause mucosal tears, beginning in the gastric epithelium and extending into the esophagus.

Mallory–Weiss syndrome *refers to severe retching, often associated with alcoholism, that leads to mucosal lacerations of the upper stomach and lower esophagus.* These

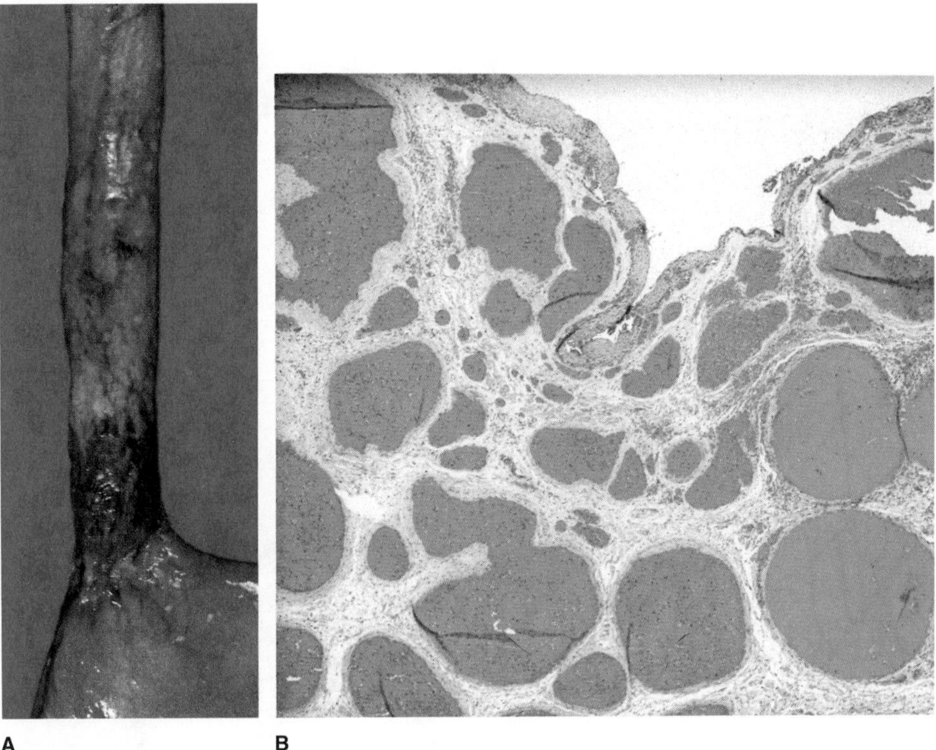

FIGURE *13-7*
Esophageal varices. *(A)* Numerous prominent blue venous channels are seen beneath the mucosa of the everted esophagus, particularly above the gastroesophageal junction. *(B)* Section of the esophagus reveals numerous dilated submucosal veins.

tears result in the vomiting of bright red blood, and bleeding may be so severe as to require the transfusion of many units of blood. The lacerations may also cause perforation into the mediastinum. Rupture of the esophagus as a result of vomiting is known as *Boerhaave syndrome*.

Perforation of the esophagus, whether from trauma or vomiting, can be catastrophic. It is a well-known occurrence in the newborn, in whom it is caused occasionally by suctioning or feeding with a nasogastric tube. However, it may also occur spontaneously.

The major non-neoplastic disorders of the esophagus are summarized in Figure 13-8.

NEOPLASMS

Benign Tumors

Benign tumors of the esophagus are uncommon and, with the exception of leiomyomas, are curiosities.

LEIOMYOMAS OF THE ESOPHAGUS: These tumors are only 10% as frequent as carcinomas and are usually discovered as an incidental finding during radiological or endoscopical examination of the upper gastro-

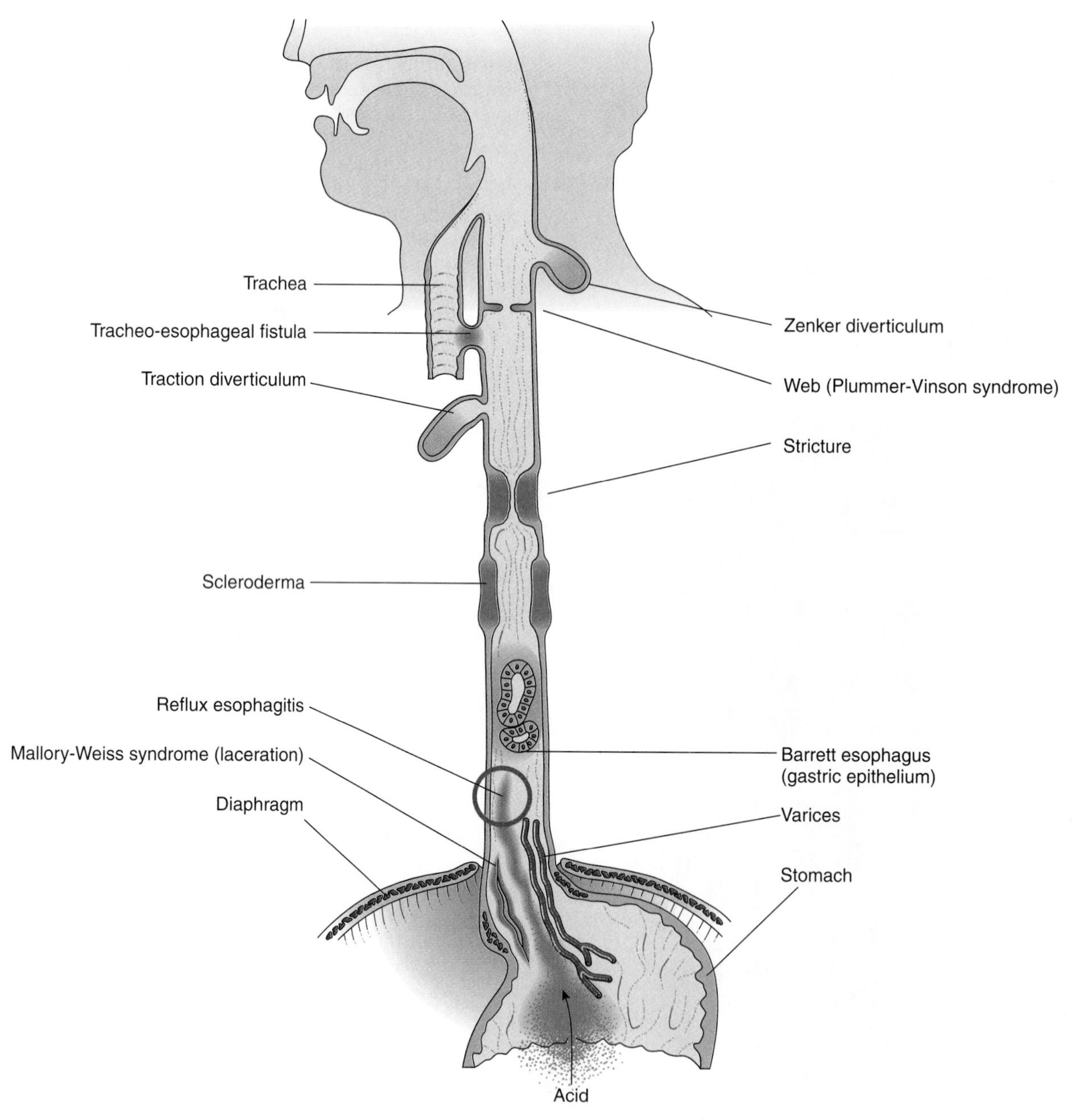

FIGURE *13-8*
Non-neoplastic disorders of the esophagus.

intestinal tract or at autopsy. The normal mucosa is elevated over an intramural mass, which on microscopic examination is similar to benign smooth muscle tumors in the stomach (see later). Most esophageal leiomyomas are properly left untreated, but if dysphagia or substernal pain is troublesome, simple surgical enucleation suffices.

Squamous cell papillomas of the esophagus are rare. They are asymptomatic and have no malignant potential. Some of these tumors have been related to infection with human papillomavirus, and when extensive are referred to as *papillomatosis*.

Carcinoma of the Esophagus

☐ **Epidemiology:** The majority of cancers of the esophagus worldwide are squamous cell carcinomas (Fig. 13-9). The incidence of this tumor in the United States is low, however, and esophageal cancer accounts for only about 2% of all cancer deaths. Adenocarcinoma is now more common in the United States (see later).

Worldwide geographic variations in the incidence of carcinoma of the esophagus are striking, and areas of high incidence are located adjacent to areas of low incidence. There is an esophageal cancer belt extending across Asia from the Caspian Sea region of northern Iran and the former Soviet Union through Central Asia and Mongolia to northern China. In parts of China, the mortality rate from esophageal cancer in men is reported to be some 70-fold greater than that in in the United States. By contrast, a Chinese province near one of these areas has a mortality rate comparable to that in the United States. Similarly, the Caspian region of Iran has an incidence of esophageal carcinoma about 30 times greater than that in the United States, whereas more southern zones of Iran have a low incidence. American blacks have a considerably greater incidence than do whites, and in the United States, urban dwellers are at greater risk than those in rural areas. Cancer of the esophagus is also common in certain regions of France, Finland, Switzerland, Chile, Japan, India, and Africa. By contrast, other Scandinavian countries, Holland, and Austria have low frequencies. In the United States, there is a male predominance of about 3:1.

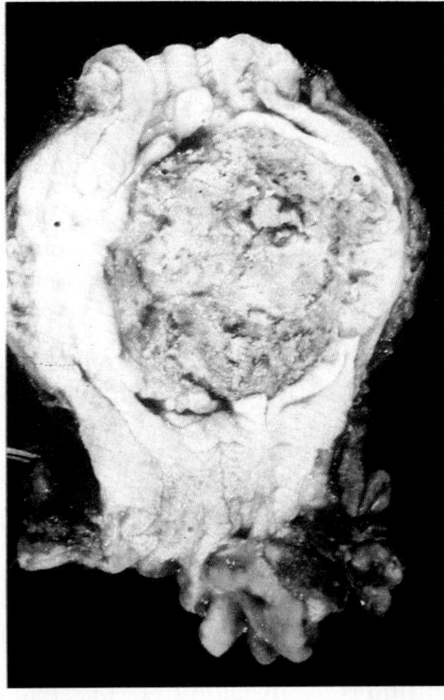

FIGURE 13-9
Carcinoma of the esophagus. A large, fungating, ulcerated squamous carcinoma of the esophagus is surrounded by apparently normal mucosa.

☐ **Pathogenesis:** The geographic variations in esophageal cancer, even in relatively homogeneous populations, suggest that environmental factors contribute strongly to the development of this disease. However, no single factor can be incriminated as the cause of esophageal cancer.

- **Excessive consumption of alcohol** is a major risk factor in the United States, even when cigarette smoking and degree of urbanization are taken into account.
- **Tobacco use, especially cigarette smoking,** is associated with an increased risk of esophageal cancer, and the number of cigarettes smoked correlates with the presence of dysplasia in the esophageal epithelium. However, the population in the Caspian littoral of Iran, which has one of the highest rates of esophageal carcinoma in the world, neither consumes alcohol nor smokes cigarettes excessively.
- **Nitrosamines** and aniline dyes produce esophageal cancer in animals. Although high levels of nitrosamines and other potentially carcinogenic compounds have been found in the diets of persons living in high-incidence areas, direct evidence for their contribution to esophageal cancer is lacking. Moreover, such chemical agents have not been detected in many high-risk areas, such as northern Iran.
- **Diets lacking in fresh fruits, vegetables, animal protein, and trace metals** have been described in areas with endemic esophageal cancer, and in some hyperendemic areas, deficiencies of various vitamins and minerals have been claimed. However, the close proximity of endemic and nonendemic areas renders a causative role for these dietary factors unlikely. Unproved environmental factors include spices, hot foods or liquids, betel nuts, asbestos, air pollution, and radiation.
- **Plummer–Vinson syndrome, celiac sprue, and achalasia** are associated with an increased incidence of esophageal cancer, but the cause for this risk has not been explained.
- **Chronic esophagitis** has been related to esophageal cancer in areas in which this tumor is endemic, but such an association has not been demonstrated in the ordinary reflux esophagitis seen in Western countries.
- **Chemical injury with esophageal stricture** is a risk factor. Five percent of persons who have an esophageal stricture after ingestion of lye develop cancer 20 to 40 years later.
- **Webs, rings, and diverticula** are sometimes associated with esophageal cancer.

Although the pathogenesis of esophageal cancer is not understood, it is tempting to speculate that irritation of the mucosa by gastric contents, food, alcohol, or other agents may stimulate cell proliferation and thereby act as a promoter for cells initiated by exposure to environmental carcinogens, such as those contained in tobacco smoke.

☐ **Pathology:** About half the cases of esophageal cancer involve the lower third of the esophagus; the middle and upper thirds account for the remainder. Grossly, the tumors are of three types: (1) polypoid, which projects into the lumen (see Fig. 13-9); (2) ulcerating, which is usually smaller than polypoid; and (3) infiltrating, in which the principal plane of growth is in the wall. Usually these features overlap. The bulky polypoid tumors tend to obstruct early, whereas the ulcerated ones are more likely to bleed. The infiltrating tumors gradually narrow the lumen by circumferential compression. Local extension of the tumor into adjoining mediastinal structures is commonly a major problem.

Microscopically, the neoplastic squamous cells range from well differentiated, with epithelial "pearls" (see Fig. 13-9), to poorly differentiated. The degree of differentiation does not correlate with the extent of the disease, the presence of metastases, or the prognosis. Occasional tumors have a spindle cell appearance (carcinosarcoma).

The rich lymphatic drainage of the esophagus provides a route for most metastases. The lymphatic vessels of the esophagus follow the blood supply. Accordingly, tumors of the upper third metastasize to the cervical, internal jugular, and supraclavicular nodes. Cancer of the middle third metastasizes to the paratracheal and hilar lymph nodes and to nodes in the aortic, cardiac, and paraesophageal regions. Because the lower third of the esophagus is fed by the left gastric artery, tumors in this portion of the esophagus spread to retroperitoneal, celiac, and left gastric nodes. "Skip" metastases may also involve distant lymph nodes. Visceral metastases to the liver and lung are common, and almost any organ may be involved.

☐ **Clinical Features:** The most common presenting complaint is dysphagia, which is usually not recognized until the diameter of the lumen of the esophagus is reduced by 30% to 50%. By this time, most tumors are unresectable. Patients with esophageal cancer are almost invariably cachectic, owing to anorexia, difficulty in swallowing, and the remote effects of a malignant tumor. Odynophagia occurs in half of the patients, and persistent pain suggests mediastinal extension of the tumor or involvement of spinal nerves. Compression of the recurrent laryngeal nerve produces hoarseness, and tracheoesophageal fistula is manifested clinically by a chronic cough.

Surgery and radiation therapy are useful for palliation, but the prognosis remains dismal. Only 40% of patients who undergo surgery have tumors that are potentially resectable, and of these, one third die as a result of the operation itself. Of the survivors, only 10% (4% of the total) live for 5 years. Newer combinations of surgery, radiation therapy, and chemotherapy have produced more promising results.

Adenocarcinoma of the Esophagus

Adenocarcinoma of the esophagus is now more common in the United States than squamous carcinoma because the incidence has increased in recent years. **Virtually all adenocarcinomas arise in Barrett epithelium**, although a few originate in mucous glands of the esophagus. Gastric cancers can extend upward into the esophagus. These may be difficult or impossible to distinguish from cancers arising in Barrett epithelium. The symptoms and clinical course of adenocarcinoma are similar to those of squamous cell carcinoma of the esophagus, but a 20% 5-year survival after radical surgery has been reported, and adjuvant therapy appears to improve the outcome.

Other Malignant Tumors

Rare primary malignant tumors of the esophagus include melanoma, endocrine tumors, and sarcoma. Metastases to the esophagus from distant tumors are rare, but direct extension from cancers of the lung and thyroid is occasionally encountered.

The Stomach

ANATOMY

The stomach, a J-shaped saccular organ with a volume of 1200 to 1500 mL, arises as a dilatation of the primitive foregut. It is continuous with the esophagus superiorly and the duodenum inferiorly. Situated in the upper abdomen, the stomach extends from the left hypochondrium across the epigastrium. The convexity of the stomach, extending leftward from the gastroesophageal junction, is termed the **greater curvature**. The concavity of the right side of the stomach, called the **lesser curvature**, is only about one fourth as long as the greater curvature. The entire stomach is invested in peritoneum, which descends from the greater curvature as the **greater omentum**.

The interior of the stomach has been divided into five regions, from superior to inferior (Fig. 13-10):

1. **The cardia** is a small, grossly indistinct zone that extends a short distance from the gastroesophageal junction.
2. **The fundus** is the dome-shaped part of the stomach, which is located to the left of the cardia and extends superiorly above a line drawn horizontally through the gastroesophageal junction.
3. **The body, or corpus,** constitutes two thirds of the entire stomach and descends from the fundus to the most inferior region, where the organ turns right to form the bottom of the J.
4. **The antrum** is the distal third of the stomach beginning at the incisura. It is positioned horizontally and extends from the body to the pyloric sphincter.
5. **The pyloric sphincter** is the most distal tubular segment of the stomach, which is entirely surrounded by the thick muscular layer that governs the passage of food into the duodenum.

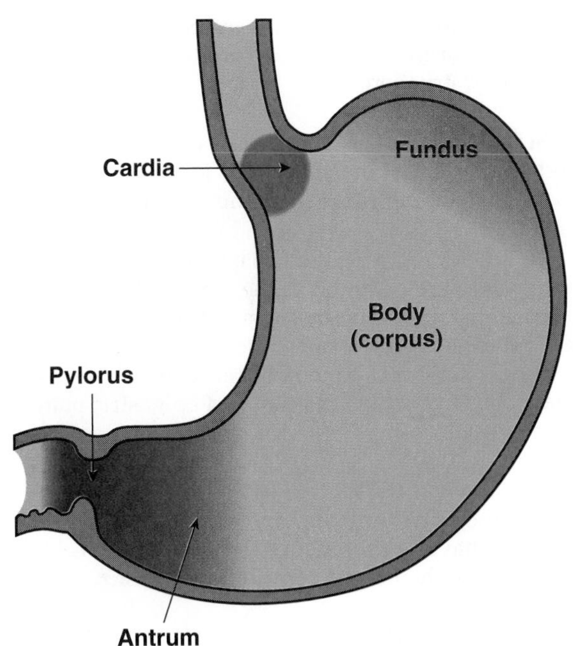

FIGURE 13-10
Anatomical regions of the stomach.

The wall of the stomach is composed of a mucosa, submucosa, muscularis, and serosa. The lining of the fundus and body of the stomach has prominent folds, the gastric rugae. When the stomach is distended, the rugae tend to be flattened and inconspicuous on radiological examination.

Branches of the celiac, hepatic, and splenic arteries supply blood to the stomach. The gastric veins drain either directly into the portal system or indirectly through the splenic and superior mesenteric veins. A rich plexus of lymphatic channels drains into the gastric and other regional lymph nodes. Both vagal nerves supply parasympathetic innervation to the stomach, and the celiac plexus supplies sympathetic innervation.

The histological appearance of the gastric mucosa varies according to the anatomical region. The surface has a mucus-secreting, columnar epithelium, which extends into numerous foveolae, or pits. These represent the orifices of millions of branched, tubular glands. There are three types of glands:

- **The cardiac glands** are located in the cardia.
- **The oxyntic (parietal) glands** are found in the body and fundus of the stomach.
- **The pyloric glands** are situated in the antrum and the pyloric canal.

The gastric glands, the principal secretory elements of the stomach, are densely arranged perpendicular to the mucosa and enter the base of the foveola through a narrowed segment called the neck of the gland. The gastric glands contain four cell types: zymogen (chief) cells, parietal (oxyntic) cells, mucous neck cells, and endocrine cells.

- **Zymogen, or chief, cells:** These cells reside primarily in the lower half of the gastric gland. They are pyramidal, basophilic cells filled with zymogen granules that contain pepsinogen. The basophilia reflects the rich content of ribosomes, a feature characteristic of cells that are actively engaged in protein synthesis.
- **Parietal, or oxyntic, cells:** These cells occupy the upper half of the gastric gland. They are oval or pyramidal eosinophilic cells that secrete hydrochloric acid. The eosinophilia is imparted by the presence of numerous mitochondria, which provide energy for the ion transport necessary for acid secretion. Ultrastructurally, parietal cells exhibit numerous invaginations of the surface membrane, termed **secretory canaliculi**, which vastly expand the surface area for acid secretion. In addition to being the source of acid, parietal cells in human beings are the source of intrinsic factor, which is necessary for the intestinal absorption of vitamin B_{12}.
- **Mucous neck cells:** These components are interspersed among the parietal cells in the neck of the gastric gland. These basophilic cells contain considerably more ribosomes and larger mucus granules than do the surface mucous cells, features that suggest more active secretion of mucus.
- **Endocrine cells:** These cells are scattered in the gastric glands, mostly between the zymogen cells and the basement membrane. They are small, round, or pyramidal cells filled with granules that are stained with silver salts. Those that reduce silver without prior treatment are termed **argentaffin cells**. These cells also reduce chromium salts and are therefore included in the designation **enterochromaffin cells**. In other endocrine cells, termed **argyrophil cells**, prior reaction with a reducing substance is necessary before the granules stain with silver. The reason for the differences in affinity for silver salts is not understood. Endocrine cells are scattered among the pyloric glands and contain biogenic amines such as serotonin and polypeptide hormones (e.g., gastrin and somatostatin). Vasoactive intestinal peptide (VIP) is found in neural elements of the mucosa, but not within endocrine cells.
- **Pyloric glands** are branched and conspicuously coiled structures, emptying into foveolae that are substantially deeper than those in other portions of the stomach. The glands are lined by pale cells similar in appearance to mucous neck cells and cells of Brunner glands in the duodenum. The endocrine cells include G cells, which secrete gastrin.
- **Cardiac glands** are lined by cells that are similar to mucous neck cells and those of the pyloric glands but lack G cells.

CONGENITAL DISORDERS

Congenital Pyloric Stenosis

Congenital pyloric stenosis is a concentric enlargement of the pyloric sphincter and narrowing of the pyloric canal that obstructs the outlet of the stomach. This disorder is the most common indication for abdominal surgery in the initial 6 months of life. It is four times more common in boys than in girls and affects first-born children more often than subsequent ones. Congenital pyloric stenosis occurs in 1 in 250 white infants but is rare in blacks and Asians.

☐ **Pathogenesis:** Congenital pyloric stenosis may have a genetic basis; there is a familial tendency, and the condition is more common in identical twins than in fraternal ones. Pyloric stenosis also has been recorded in the context of other developmental abnormalities, such as Turner syndrome, trisomy 18, and esophageal atresia. Embryopathies associated with rubella infection and maternal intake of thalidomide have been associated with congenital pyloric stenosis. In general, the disorder has been attributed to multifactorial inheritance. Evidence has been presented that, at least in some cases, congenital pyloric stenosis is associated with a deficiency of nitric oxide synthase in the nerves of pyloric smooth muscle (nitric oxide mediates relaxation of smooth muscle).

☐ **Pathology:** Gross examination of the stomach shows concentric enlargement of the pylorus and narrowing of the pyloric canal. The only consistent microscopic abnormality is extreme hypertrophy of the circular muscle coat. After pyloromyotomy, the tumor disappears, although occasionally a small mass remains.

☐ **Clinical Features:** The symptoms of pyloric stenosis usually become apparent within the first month of life, when the infant manifests projectile vomiting. Typically, after the stomach has emptied, the infant is ravenous and feeds avidly. The loss of hydrochloric acid via vomiting results in hypochloremic alkalosis in one third of the infants. Dehydration and wasting soon ensue. A palpable pyloric tumor and visible peristalsis are characteristic of the disorder. Surgical incision of the hypertrophied pyloric muscle is curative.

Hypertrophic pyloric stenosis is an uncommon disorder in adults. Some cases in adults may be due to prolonged pyloric spasm caused by peptic ulcer disease or gastritis; others represent mild cases of congenital pyloric stenosis. The symptoms and treatment are similar to those in the infant, although no abdominal mass is palpable.

Congenital Diaphragmatic Hernia

Congenital diaphragmatic hernias, of variable size and location, are associated with defective closure of embryological foramina or abnormalities of the esophageal hiatus. These hernias are often associated with congenital malrotations of the intestine. The stomach, together with other abdominal organs, may eventrate into the thoracic cavity. Herniation of the abdominal contents into the thorax may be asymptomatic or may lead to severe respiratory embarrassment, necessitating surgical intervention.

Rare Congenital Abnormalities

DUPLICATIONS, DIVERTICULA, AND CYSTS: These lesions are usually lined by normal gastric mucosa and are distinctly uncommon. Whereas all layers of the stomach wall tend to be present in congenital duplications, muscle coats are often deficient in diverticula and cysts. Patients with these disorders are generally asymptomatic. Acquired diverticula caused by inflammatory disorders near the pylorus may produce high (proximal) intestinal obstruction.

SITUS INVERSUS: This causes the stomach to be located to the right of the midline, as is the esophageal hiatus. Correspondingly, the duodenum is on the left.

ECTOPIC PANCREATIC TISSUE: Nodules of pancreatic tissue are common in the wall of the antrum and pylorus. Histologically, these islands of pancreatic rests are identical to normal pancreatic tissue, except that islets are rare. Heterotopic pancreatic tissue is usually asymptomatic, but pyloric obstruction and epigastric pain have been reported.

PARTIAL GASTRIC ATRESIAS: Lack of development of the body, antrum, and pylorus have been described, as have cases in which the stomach ends blindly. Intrauterine ischemia is a contributing factor.

CONGENITAL PYLORIC AND ANTRAL MEMBRANES: These lesions are presumably caused by failure of the stomach to canalize during embryogenesis. They may cause symptoms of obstruction in the neonatal period but more commonly become symptomatic in adults.

GASTRITIS

The terms *acute and chronic gastritis* are confusing, because to the pathologist, they refer only to the morphological appearance of gastric injury and do not connote a temporal difference. Yet acute gastritis is ordinarily a self-limited disorder, whereas chronic gastritis is typically present for many years. Gastritis is best classified on the basis of etiological factors and histopathology.

Acute Hemorrhagic (Erosive) Gastritis

Acute hemorrhagic gastritis is characterized by the presence of focal necrosis of the mucosa in an otherwise normal stomach. Erosion of the mucosa may extend into the deeper tissues to form an acute ulcer. The necrosis is accompanied by an acute inflammatory response and often by hemorrhage, which may be so severe as to result in exsanguination.

☐ **Pathogenesis:** Acute hemorrhagic gastritis is most commonly associated with the intake of aspirin, other nonsteroidal anti-inflammatory agents, excess alcohol, or ischemic injury. These agents are directly injurious to the gastric mucosa and exert their effects topically. The oral administration of corticosteroids is also occasionally complicated by acute hemorrhagic gastritis. Uncommonly, the accidental or suicidal ingestion of corrosive substances, such as those that produce erosive esophagitis, produces acute gastric injury. Any serious illness that is accompanied by profound physiological alterations, which require substantial medical or surgical intervention, renders the gastric mucosa more vulnerable to acute hemorrhagic gastritis because of mucosal ischemia. The factor common to all forms of acute hemorrhagic gastritis is thought to be the breakdown of the mucosal barrier, permitting acid-induced injury.

Stress ulcers and erosions, long known to occur in severely burned persons (*Curling ulcer*), commonly result in bleeding, which is occasionally severe. The ulceration may be so deep as to cause perforation of the stomach. Patients occasionally exhibit both gastric and duodenal ulcers.

Trauma to the central nervous system, either accidental or surgical (*Cushing ulcer*), is another cause of stress ulcers. These ulcers, which also may occur in the esophagus or duodenum, are characteristically deep and carry a substantial risk of perforation. Injury to the brain, particularly if it results in a decerebrate state, often leads to increased acid secretion in the stomach, presumably as a result of increased vagal tone. Enhanced production of gastrin may also contribute to enhanced acid secretion. **Severe trauma**, especially if accompanied by shock, **prolonged sepsis**, and **incapacitation** from many debilitating chronic diseases, also predispose to the development of acute hemorrhagic gastritis.

Stress ulcers have been produced experimentally in rats by restraint, forced exertion, and traumatic or hemorrhagic shock. In rats and other species, burns and neurological trauma also result in acute hemorrhagic gastritis. Certain types of prolonged psychological stresses have been reported to produce erosive lesions in the stomach and duodenum. Nonsteroidal anti-inflammatory compounds, corticosteroids, and concentrated ethanol consistently cause gastric erosions in rats.

Hypersecretion of gastric acid has been incriminated in the pathogenesis of acute hemorrhagic gastritis, but its role is not clear. Acid secretion is often increased in some circumstances, such as neurological trauma, but the development of stress ulcers is not generally accompanied by any such increase. Nevertheless, gastric acid plays a permissive role, because inhibition of gastric acid secretion (e.g., with histamine-receptor antagonists) protects against the development of stress ulcers.

Microcirculatory changes in the stomach induced by shock or sepsis suggest that ischemic injury may contribute to the development of acute hemorrhagic gastritis.

Because the contents of the stomach would be highly toxic to any tissue outside the gastrointestinal tract, the protective mechanisms of the gastric mucosa seem to be the important defense against mucosal injury. It follows that the pathogenesis of acute hemorrhagic gastritis likely involves, at least in part, impairment of these local defensive factors, which include gastric mucus, tissue prostaglandins, epithelial renewal, and intramural pH. Each of these defensive factors has been individually investigated as follows:

- **Decreased mucus production** and gastric ulcers have both been produced by the experimental administration of corticosteroids and aspirin.
- **Prostaglandin deficiency,** caused by nonsteroidal anti-inflammatory agents that inhibit prostaglandin synthesis, has been postulated to decrease the mucosal resistance to the contents of the stomach. By contrast, certain prostaglandins that stimulate mucus secretion also protect against gastric erosions.
- **Renewal of gastric epithelial cells** is clearly necessary for healing erosions of any etiology. In this respect, it is interesting that trophic agents, such as growth hormone, epidermal growth factor, and gastrin, not only stimulate DNA synthesis in the gastric mucosa but also protect against experimental erosions produced by restraint and by aspirin.
- **Reduction of the intramural pH of the gastric mucosa has been demonstrated** to protect against gastric erosions in hemorrhagic shock. It has also been shown experimentally that ethanol and aspirin injure the superficial gastric epithelial cells, thereby permitting back-diffusion of hydrogen ions. Acid-induced damage to the gastric mucosa thus is important in the pathogenesis of certain erosions.

☐ **Pathology:** The typical case of acute hemorrhagic gastritis is characterized grossly by widespread petechial hemorrhages in any portion of the stomach or regions of confluent mucosal or submucosal bleeding (Fig. 13-11). These lesions vary in size from 1 to 25 mm across and appear occasionally as sharply punched-out ulcers. Microscopically, patchy mucosal necrosis, which can extend to the submucosa, is visualized adjacent to normal mucosa. Fibrinous exudate, edema, and hemorrhage in the lamina propria are present in early lesions. The necrotic epithelium is eventually sloughed, but deeper erosions and hemorrhage may be present. In extreme cases, penetrating ulcers are associated with necrosis extending through to the serosa. However, in most cases, depending on the age of the process, there is only mild inflammation, initially neutrophilic and then mononuclear. Healing is usually complete within a few days.

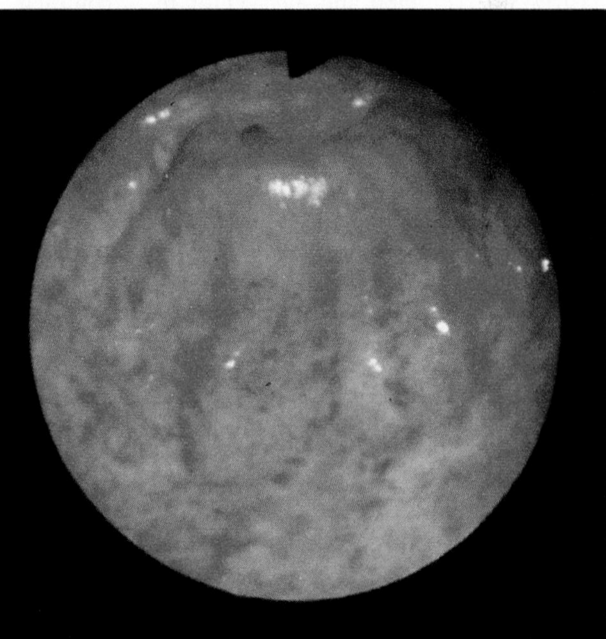

FIGURE *13-11*
Erosive gastritis. This endoscopic view of the stomach in a patient who was ingesting aspirin reveals acute hemorrhagic lesions.

☐ **Clinical Features:** The symptoms of acute hemorrhagic gastritis range from vague abdominal discomfort to massive, life-threatening hemorrhage or the clinical manifestations of gastric perforation. Patients with gastritis induced by aspirin and other nonsteroidal anti-inflammatory agents may be seen with hypochromic, microcytic anemia caused by undetected, chronic bleeding. However, in patients with a severe underlying illness, the first sign of stress ulcers may be exsanguinating hemorrhage. In critically ill patients, the overall mortality of acute hemorrhagic gastritis may reach 40% to 50%. Treatment with antacids and histamine-receptor antagonists has proved useful, particularly when these agents are given prophylactically.

Chronic Gastritis

Chronic gastritis refers to chronic inflammatory diseases of the stomach, which range from mild superficial involvement of the gastric mucosa to severe atrophy. The use of fiberoptic endoscopy has now clearly established that chronic gastritis actually comprises a heterogeneous group of disorders that have distinct anatomical distributions within the stomach, varying etiologies, and characteristic complications. At least four major entities, defined by their etiologies and histopathology, are subsumed under the rubric of chronic gastritis: (1) autoimmune atrophic gastritis (type A), (2) multifocal atrophic gastritis, (3) *Helicobacter pylori* gastritis (type B), and (4) chemical gastropathy, which includes duodenal reflux gastritis and the chronic effects of drugs such as nonsteroidal anti-inflammatory drugs.

☐ **Clinical Features of Chronic Gastritis:** The predominant symptom that has been ascribed to chronic gastritis has been dyspepsia. However, chronic gastritis is so common, and such symptomatic complaints so nonspecific, that any association with specific symptoms remains suspect. The diseases are also commonly discovered in asymptomatic persons undergoing routine endoscopic screening.

Autoimmune Atrophic Gastritis and Pernicious Anemia

Autoimmune atrophic gastritis refers to a chronic, diffuse inflammatory disease of the stomach that is restricted to the body and fundus and is associated with autoimmune phenomena. This disorder typically exhibits the following:

- Diffuse atrophic gastritis in the body and fundus of the stomach, with lack of or minimal involvement of the antrum.
- Antibodies to parietal cells and intrinsic factor.
- Significant reduction in or absence of gastric secretion, including acid.
- Increased serum gastrin due to G-cell hyperplasia of the antral mucosa.
- Enterochromaffin-like (ECL) cell hyperplasia in atrophic oxyntic mucosa due to gastrin stimulation.

***Pernicious anemia** is a megaloblastic anemia that is caused by malabsorption of vitamin B_{12}, occasioned by a deficiency of intrinsic factor.* **In the large majority of cases, pernicious anemia is a complication of autoimmune gastritis.** The latter disorder is also associated with extragastric autoimmune diseases, such as chronic thyroiditis, Graves disease, Addison disease, vitiligo, type I diabetes mellitus, and myasthenia gravis.

☐ **Pathogenesis:** Autoimmune gastritis is so named because of the presence of autoantibodies and the association with other diseases believed to have a similar pathogenesis. Chronic atrophic gastritis with metaplastic changes appears to result from autoimmune-mediated destruction of parietal cells.

CYTOTOXIC ANTIBODIES: Circulating antibodies to parietal cells, some of which are cytotoxic in the presence of complement, occur in up to 90% of patients with pernicious anemia. Parietal cell autoantibodies react with the alpha and beta subunits of the proton pump (H+/K+ ATPase). This enzyme, which is the major protein of the secretory canaliculi of parietal cells, mediates the secretion of H+ in exchange for K+. It is important to note that up to 20% of persons older than 60 years exhibit parietal cell antibodies, but few have pernicious anemia. However, such antibodies are distinctly uncommon in persons younger than 40 years in the absence of pernicious anemia.

INTRINSIC FACTOR ANTIBODIES: In addition to the postulated immunological destruction of parietal cells, the site of intrinsic factor synthesis in human beings, two types of autoantibodies to intrinsic factor are common in pernicious anemia. Some 70% of patients display an antibody to intrinsic factor that blocks its combination with vitamin B_{12}, thereby preventing the formation of the complex that is later absorbed in the ileum. About half of the patients with this blocking antibody also have an antibody that binds to the intrinsic factor–vitamin B_{12} complex and interferes with its absorption.

OTHER ANTIBODIES: Half of the patients with pernicious anemia have circulating antibodies to thyroid tissue. Conversely, about one third of patients with chronic thyroiditis possess gastric autoantibodies. Cell-mediated immunological abnormalities of various types also are present in many patients with pernicious anemia.

GENETIC FACTORS: Pernicious anemia shows a familial tendency. Concordance with respect to pernicious anemia has been observed in a dozen pairs of monozygotic twins. Ten percent to 15% of first-degree relatives of patients with pernicious anemia demonstrate severe atrophic gastritis, although they may not have megaloblastic anemia. Moreover, almost all of these relatives have achlorhydria, two thirds have circulating parietal cell antibodies, and one fifth manifest antibodies to intrinsic factor.

The histopathology of autoimmune gastritis is similar to that of multifocal atrophic gastritis (discussed later).

Multifocal Atrophic Gastritis (Environmental Metaplastic Atrophic Gastritis)

Multifocal atrophic gastritis is a disease of uncertain etiology that typically involves the antrum and adjacent areas of the body. This form of chronic gastritis has the following features:

- It is considerably more common than the autoimmune variety of atrophic gastritis, perhaps 4 times as frequent among whites as in other races.
- It is not associated with autoimmune phenomena.
- Similar to autoimmune gastritis, it is often associated with reduced acid secretion (hypochlorhydria).
- Complete absence of gastric secretion (achlorhydria) and pernicious anemia are uncommon.

☐ **Epidemiology and Pathogenesis:** The age and geographic distribution of environmental metaplastic atrophic gastritis are parallel to those of carcinoma of the stomach, and this type of gastritis is believed to be a precursor of this cancer. The disease exhibits a striking localization to certain populations, being particularly common in Asia, Scandinavia, and parts of Europe and Latin America. It also demonstrates an increasing incidence with age in all populations in which it is prevalent. In asymptomatic Japanese, environmental metaplastic atrophic gastritis was found in 90% of men and women older than 60 years. About half of the adult population of Finland, Italy, and Hungary has been reported to show evidence of chronic gastritis.

The offspring of emigrants from areas of high risk for stomach cancer to those of low risk lose their predisposition to this tumor. The environmental factors in its etiology include *Helicobacter pylori* infection (see later) and diet.

☐ **Pathology of Autoimmune and Multifocal Atrophic Gastritis:** The pathological features of autoimmune and multifocal atrophic gastritis are similar, except for the localization of the autoimmune type to the fundus and body and the multifocal variety mainly to the antrum. On gross examination, loss of the rugal folds in the body and fundus is often seen with the autoimmune type, but atrophy can be difficult to recognize; identification of the disorders is made on histopathological grounds.

SUPERFICIAL GASTRITIS: This is the mildest form of atrophic gastritis. Although superficial gastritis may occasionally revert to normal, it is estimated that it proceeds to atrophic gastritis in nearly half of the cases. Atrophic gastritis usually persists indefinitely, but in a few cases it terminates in **gastric atrophy**, a condition in which the inflammatory features of gastritis are often inconspicuous.

Superficial gastritis typically shows lymphocytes and plasma cells, and occasionally neutrophils, in the lamina propria of the mucosa of the antrum, or body of the stomach, or both. The inflammation is most intense around the gastric pits (foveolae), where small foci of neutrophils may also be seen, but the glands are spared. The normal columnar epithelium becomes more cuboidal and contains less mucin than normal. The process may be quiescent, in which case, the epithelial cells are little changed, and no neutrophils are present. Although superficial gastritis does not involve the gastric glands, histamine-stimulated secretion of acid and pepsin is impaired.

ATROPHIC GASTRITIS: This condition may evolve from superficial gastritis, but there is no sharp distinction between them. Like superficial gastritis, active atrophic gastritis is characterized by prominent chronic inflammation in the lamina propria. However, lymphocytes and plasma cells extend into the deepest reaches of the mucosa as far as the muscularis mucosae. Occasionally, lymphoid cells are arranged as follicles, an appearance that has led to an erroneous diagnosis of lymphoma, especially in patients with *Helicobacter pylori* infection (see later). Involvement of the gastric glands leads to degenerative changes in their epithelial cells and ultimately a conspicuous reduction in the number of glands (thus the name atrophic gastritis; Fig. 13-12). Eventually, the inflammatory process may abate, leaving only a thin atrophic mucosa, in which case, the term gastric atrophy is applied.

INTESTINAL METAPLASIA: This lesion is a common and important histopathological feature of both the autoimmune and multifocal types of atrophic gastritis. In this response of the injured gastric mucosa, the normal epithelium is replaced by one composed of cells of the intestinal type (Fig. 13-13). Numerous mucin-containing goblet cells and enterocytes line crypt-like glands, and many Paneth cells, which are not normal inhabitants of the gastric mucosa, are present. Intestinal-type villi may occasionally form. The various endocrine cells, normally situated on the basement membrane of the gastric glands, are clustered at the base of the crypts, similar to their location in the intestine. Mitoses are more numerous than in the normal gastric mucosa. In most cases of intestinal metaplasia, islands of metaplastic epithelium alternate with atrophic gastric glands, but in severe cases, large areas of the mucosa may resemble colon or small intestine, complete with villi and Paneth cells. Not only are the metaplastic cells morphologically similar to intestinal cells, but they also contain enzymes characteristic of the intestine but not of the stomach (e.g., alkaline phosphatase, aminopeptidase). Moreover, whereas gastric secretions contain principally neutral mucins, the goblet cells of the metaplastic epithelium produce the typical intestinal acid mucins.

In the fundus of the stomach with autoimmune atrophic gastritis, the normal parietal and zymogen cells

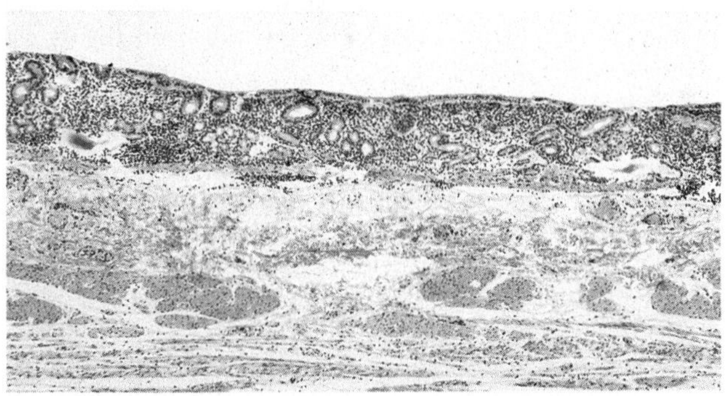

FIGURE *13-12*
Atrophic gastritis. The gastric mucosa is thinned and displays a conspicuous chronic inflammatory infiltrate that separates the atrophic glands.

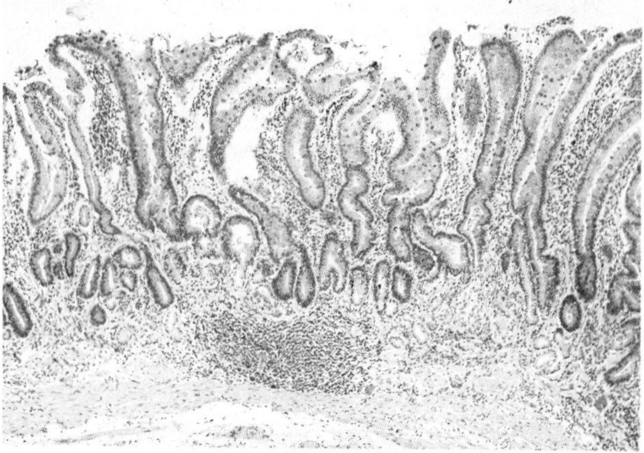

FIGURE 13-13
Chronic gastritis with intestinal metaplasia. The glands are of the intestinal type with an evident villous pattern. Chronic inflammation and atrophic gastric glands are seen immediately above the muscularis mucosae.

may be replaced by clear mucous glands similar to those of the cardia or antrum, a change termed *pseudopyloric metaplasia.* It is therefore important for the pathologist to know the precise location from which a biopsy specimen was taken, because fundal pseudopyloric metaplasia may be mistaken for gastritis of the antrum. Immunohistochemical analysis for gastrin-containing cells is helpful in determining the anatomical localization of the biopsy.

Atrophic Gastritis and Stomach Cancer

Persons with atrophic gastritis of the autoimmune or multifocal type have an increased incidence of carcinoma of the stomach. Reliable statistics about this relation are difficult to obtain, because atrophic gastritis is usually asymptomatic and therefore does not ordinarily come under medical scrutiny. However, patients with pernicious anemia, who invariably have atrophic gastritis, have a modestly increased risk (3 times) of developing gastric adenocarcinoma and a 13-fold increased risk for carcinoid tumors.

Cancer arises in the antrum several times more frequently than in the body of the stomach. Epidemiological studies, particularly from Japan, where gastric cancer is common, suggest that antral gastritis is related to the development of carcinoma of the stomach. However, direct evidence for a causal connection has not been firmly established.

Intestinal metaplasia of the stomach has been particularly identified as a preneoplastic lesion for several reasons: (1) stomachs that contain cancer have an increased incidence and severity of intestinal metaplasia; (2) gastric cancer has been shown to arise in areas of metaplastic epithelium; (3) half of all cancers of the stomach are of the intestinal cell type; and (4) many cases of carcinoma of the stomach show aminopeptidase activity similar to that seen in areas of intestinal metaplasia. Moreover, all grades of epithelial dysplasia, from mild cellular atypia to carcinoma *in situ,* have been observed in the metaplastic intestinal epithelium and are considered by many to be the precursor of invasive gastric cancer.

Helicobacter pylori Gastritis

Helicobacter pylori gastritis is a chronic inflammatory disease of the antrum and body of the stomach caused by H. pylori and occasionally by H. heilmannii. It is the most common type of chronic nonerosive gastritis in the United States, and the organism causes one of the most frequent chronic infections. In the United States, it is estimated that about one third of all asymptomatic adults have histological evidence of *H. pylori* gastritis. *H. pylori* infection is also strongly associated with peptic ulcer disease of the stomach and the duodenum (see later).

☐ **Pathogenesis:** *Helicobacter* species are small, curved, gram-negative rods (Proteobacteria) that bear polar flagella and display a corkscrew-like motion. *H. pylori* has been isolated from diverse populations throughout the world, and its genome has been sequenced. The prevalence of infection with this organism increases with age, and by age 60 years, it is estimated that up to half of the population has serological evidence of infection. Twin studies have shown genetic influences in susceptibility to infection with *H. pylori.* Intrafamilial clustering of *H. pylori* infection suggests that there may be person-to-person spread of these bacteria. Two thirds of those who have been infected with *H. pylori* manifest histopathological evidence of chronic gastritis.

The role of *H. pylori* in the pathogenesis of chronic gastritis is evidenced by the fulfillment of Koch postulates. Ingestion of the organism by healthy volunteers led to acute antral gastritis that progressed to chronic disease. Subsequently, the organism was recovered from the stomach. *H. pylori* also has been implicated in outbreaks of epidemic gastritis in volunteers who participated in studies requiring gastric intubation. Presumably contamination of the instruments introduced the organism into the stomach.

The reasons for accepting *H. pylori* as the pathogen responsible for chronic antral gastritis, rather than as a commensal that colonizes injured gastric mucosa, are as follows: (1) Gastritis develops in healthy persons after ingestion of the organism; (2) *H. pylori* is attached to the epithelium in areas of chronic gastritis, whereas it is absent from uninvolved areas of the gastric mucosa; (3) eradication of the infection with bismuth or antibiotics cures the gastritis; (4) antibodies against *H. pylori* are routinely found in persons with chronic gastritis; and (5) the prevalence of *H. pylori* infection with increasing age parallels that of chronic gastritis.

Helicobacter pylori has been found only in association with gastric-type epithelium and does not occur in other tissues. Although the bacterium is clearly associated with chronic gastritis, it is found only on the epithelial surface and does not invade the gastric mucosa.

The pathogenicity of *H. pylori* may relate to a pathogenicity island in the genome, also called the cag region, because it includes the cytotoxin-associated gene A (cag A). This virulence marker is putatively associated with duodenal ulcer and gastric cancer. A separate region of the genome contains the gene for vacuolating cytotoxin (vac A), which is also associated with duodenal ulcer disease.

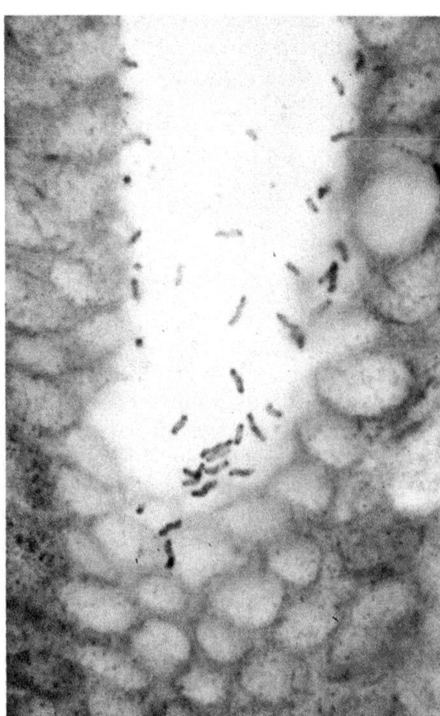

FIGURE 13-14
Infective gastritis. *Helicobacter pylori* appears on silver staining as small, curved rods on the surface of the gastric mucosa.

☐ **Pathology:** The curved rods of *H. pylori* are found in the surface mucus of the epithelial cells and in the gastric foveolae (Fig. 13-14). The uncommon bacterium, *H. heilmannii,* is long and has tight spirals, an appearance similar to that of spirochetes. Active gastritis features polymorphonuclear leukocytes in the neck glands and increased numbers of plasma cells and lymphocytes in the lamina propria. Lymphoid hyperplasia with germinal centers is frequent. Chronic infectious gastritis caused by *H. pylori* can lead to gastric atrophy and intestinal metaplasia. In addition, infection with *H. pylori* has been linked to the development of gastric adenocarcinoma and lymphoma (see later).

Chemical Gastropathy

Reflux gastropathy refers to chronic gastric injury (chemical gastropathy) that results from the reflux of alkaline duodenal contents, pancreatic secretions, and bile into the stomach. Whereas conspicuous reflux gastropathy is most common after gastroduodenostomy or gastrojejunostomy, a milder form is often identified in intact stomachs from patients with gastric ulcer, gallstone dyspepsia, postcholecystectomy syndrome, and various motor disturbances of the distal stomach.

The term "gastritis," as applied to chronic gastroduodenal reflux, is something of a misnomer, because it is not primarily a disorder characterized by inflammatory cell infiltration. The histopathological appearances are dominated by foveolar hyperplasia, edema, vasodilatation and congestion, fibromuscular proliferation in the lamina propria, and a paucity of inflammatory cells, which when present often include prominent eosinophils. Long-term exposure to nonsteroidal anti-inflammatory drugs also results in chronic chemical gastropathy.

Idiopathic Granulomatous Gastritis

Idiopathic granulomatous gastritis is defined as the presence of epithelioid granulomas in the gastric mucosa when specific granulomatous diseases have been excluded. Occasionally, the granulomas are found in association with mild superficial or atrophic gastritis, but usually little or no additional inflammation is present. The condition is benign and ordinarily asymptomatic. By definition, the cause is unknown, but granulomas are occasionally found in the vicinity of a peptic ulcer or carcinoma. Sometimes a foreign-body giant cell contains food debris. The condition is benign and ordinarily clinically silent. Granulomas can be seen occasionally with *H. pylori* gastritis.

Systemic granulomatous disorders (e.g., sarcoidosis, tuberculosis, Wegener granulomatosis, Crohn disease) on rare occasions affect the stomach.

Eosinophilic Gastritis

Eosinophilic gastritis, often in association with eosinophilic enteritis, is a rare disease in which eosinophilic inflammation involves all layers of the stomach wall or is selectively localized in a single layer. In classic cases, the disease affects principally the antrum and pylorus, where a diffuse thickening of the wall, presumably by muscular hypertrophy, may narrow the pylorus and cause symptoms of obstruction. These are occasionally severe enough to require surgical relief. In some cases, ulceration in the affected area leads to chronic blood loss and anemia. Peripheral eosinophilia and a history of food allergies are common, but many patients have neither. Treatment with corticosteroids is effective in some patients.

Allergic gastroenteropathy occurs in young children with a conspicuous allergic diathesis, who are seen with anemia, edema, and protein-losing enteropathy. Gastric biopsy in this disorder reveals an eosinophilic infiltrate limited to the mucosa. Eosinophilic inflammation is often seen with chemical gastritis.

Menetrier Disease (Hyperplastic Hypersecretory Gastropathy)

Menetrier disease is an uncommon disorder of the stomach characterized by enlarged rugae. It is often accompanied by a severe loss of plasma proteins (including albumin) from the altered gastric mucosa. The disease occurs in two forms, a childhood form due to cytomegalovirus infection and an adult form attributed to overexpression of transforming growth factor-alpha (TGF-α).

☐ **Pathology:** The stomach is increased in weight by as much as 900 to 1200 g. The folds of the greater curvature in the fundus and body of the stomach, and occasionally in the antrum, are increased in height and thickness, forming a convoluted surface-like brain (Fig. 13-15).

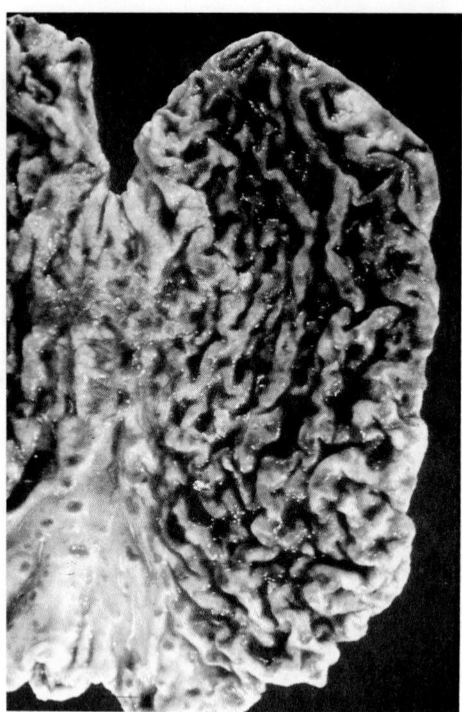

FIGURE 13-15
Menetrier disease. The folds of the stomach are increased in height and thickness, forming a convoluted surface similar to that of the brain.

Microscopically, Menetrier disease is restricted to the oxyntic mucosa. Hyperplasia of the gastric pits results in a conspicuous increase in their depth and a tortuous (corkscrew) structure. Mucus-secreting cells of the surface or neck type line the foveolae. The glands are elongated, and many appear cystic. These dilated glands, which are lined by superficial-type, mucus-secreting epithelial cells rather than parietal and chief cells, may penetrate the muscularis mucosae, in which case they resemble the sinuses of Rokitansky–Aschoff in the gallbladder. Pseudopyloric metaplasia is occasionally noted, but intestinal metaplasia does not occur. Lymphocytes, plasma cells, and occasional neutrophils are seen in the lamina propria.

□ **Clinical Features:** Menetrier disease is four times more common in men than in women and affects persons of all ages. The presenting symptom is usually postprandial pain, relieved by antacids. Weight loss, sometimes of rapid onset, occasionally occurs. Peripheral edema is common, and in some cases, ascites and cachexia simulate the presence of cancer.

These manifestations of the disease are related to a loss of plasma proteins from the gastric mucosa. The cause of the enormous protein loss into the lumen of the stomach is obscure. Amelioration of protein loss has been reported after treatment with anticholinergic agents or cimetidine. Although gastric acidity is usually low, severe peptic ulceration associated with hyperacidity has occasionally been observed. In such cases, the diagnosis of Zollinger–Ellison syndrome is suggested, but this condition can be ruled out by the absence of an increased serum gastrin level.

Menetrier disease does not usually resolve spontaneously in adults, and in intractable cases, partial gastrectomy is necessary. The disorder is considered to be a precancerous condition, and periodic endoscopic surveillance is recommended. Cytomegalovirus-associated Menetrier disease in children is often self-limited.

PEPTIC ULCER DISEASE

"Peptic ulcer disease" refers to breaks in the mucosa of the stomach and small intestine, principally the proximal duodenum, that are produced by the action of gastric secretions. Peptic ulcers of the stomach and duodenum are estimated to afflict 10% of the population of Western industrialized countries at some time during their lives. Although peptic ulceration can occur as high as Barrett esophagus and as low as Meckel diverticulum with gastric heterotopia, **for practical purposes, peptic ulcer disease affects the distal stomach and proximal duodenum**. Many clinical and epidemiological features distinguish gastric from duodenal ulcers; the common factor that unites them is the gastric secretion of hydrochloric acid. **With rare exceptions, a person who does not secrete acid will not develop a peptic ulcer anywhere.**

□ **Epidemiology:** Gastric and duodenal ulcers were distinctly uncommon in the 19th century, and those that occurred were usually gastric ulcers in young women. After World War I, the occurrence of duodenal ulcers changed from a rare event to an exceptionally common one, whereas gastric ulcers decreased in incidence and became a disorder of elderly men and women.

It has been widely perceived that both the incidence and the prevalence of duodenal ulcers declined substantially during the past 25 years. Certainly mortality from this disease, as well as the number of admissions to hospitals, has fallen. However, careful population studies in the United States and Europe have not supported the notion that the disease itself is less common today. The decreased hospitalization and mortality may reflect earlier diagnosis, more accurate discrimination of duodenal ulcer disease from other entities that cause ulcer-like symptoms, improved pharmacological management, and an increase in medical rather than surgical treatment. Only detailed prospective epidemiological studies can resolve this question. The incidence of gastric ulcers, at least as measured by hospital admissions and outpatient visits, seems to have remained essentially stationary over the past few decades.

The age profile of peptic ulcer disease has progressively increased in the past 50 years. The peak incidence of duodenal ulcer disease is now between the ages of 30 and 60 years, although the disorder may occur in persons of any age, and even in infants. Gastric ulcers afflict the middle-aged and elderly more than the young.

The sex distribution of duodenal ulcers has shown a striking change, from a marked female predominance in the 19th century to a predominantly male predominance today. By contrast, the incidence of gastric ulcers is similar in men and women.

Racial differences in the incidence of peptic ulcers have been observed, but the studies of different ethnic populations are confounded by variations in many other environmental factors. For example, in Africa, duodenal ulcers are rare among blacks, whereas in the United States, the incidence is the same in blacks and whites. In India, the disease is uncommon in the arid plains but more frequent in certain mountainous areas. The preponderance of evidence suggests that in an urban Western setting, all ethnic groups are susceptible.

The common stereotype of the patient with a peptic ulcer is that of a highly motivated executive operating in a stressful environment. However, careful epidemiological surveys in the United States and Great Britain have actually suggested an inverse relation between duodenal ulcers and socioeconomic status and education, although the trends are not marked.

☐ **Pathogenesis:** Numerous etiological factors have been implicated in the pathogenesis of peptic ulcers, but no single agent seems to be responsible.

Environmental Factors

Despite the folk wisdom that holds that spicy food and caffeine are ulcerogenic, the evidence to support the contention that the consumption of any food or beverage, including coffee, contributes to the development or persistence of peptic ulcers is surprisingly meager. This lack of evidence for a commonly held assumption extends to alcohol intake, which is also widely considered to be an important determinant in the pathogenesis of peptic ulcer disease. Although high concentrations of alcohol can result in hemorrhagic gastritis and may stimulate acid secretion, no data link the consumption of alcohol to either gastric or duodenal ulcers. However, cirrhosis from any cause is associated with an increased incidence of peptic ulcers.

The intake of certain drugs is widely held to lead to peptic ulcers, although close analysis of the epidemiological data has undermined the strength of some of these associations. Both prospective and cross-sectional studies indicate that **aspirin** is an important contributing factor in the genesis of duodenal and especially gastric ulcers. **Other nonsteroidal anti-inflammatory agents and analgesics** have been incriminated in the production of peptic ulcers. Prolonged treatment with high doses of corticosteroids has been claimed to increase slightly the risk of peptic ulceration.

Cigarette smoking is a definite risk factor for duodenal and gastric ulcers, particularly gastric ulcers. The mechanisms by which smoking predisposes to peptic ulcers are controversial.

Genetic Factors

Peptic ulcer disease illustrates the importance of genetic factors and their interaction with environmental mechanisms. First-degree relatives of patients with duodenal ulcers have a threefold increased risk of developing a duodenal ulcer but do not have a similar increase in the risk of developing a gastric ulcer. Patients with gastric ulcers similarly breed true. These data are confirmed by the finding of a considerably higher concordance for these ulcers in monozygotic than in dizygotic twins. The fact that identical twins show only a 50% concordance indicates that genetic factors alone are not sufficient to produce an ulcer; environmental factors must also be involved.

Blood-group antigens provide further evidence for the role of genetic factors. The risk of duodenal ulcer is about 30% higher in persons with type O blood than in those with types A, B, and AB. Interestingly, patients with gastric ulcers do not exhibit a greater frequency of blood group O. The fourth of the population who do not secrete blood-group antigens in the saliva and gastric juice are at a 50% increased risk of developing a duodenal ulcer. The risk of duodenal ulceration is increased (2.5:1) when nonsecretory status is combined with blood group O, a combination that occurs in 10% of the white population. Associations between certain histocompatibility antigens and peptic ulcers have been claimed but are still debated.

Pepsinogen I is secreted by the chief and mucous neck cells of the gastric mucosa and appears in the gastric juice, blood, and urine. Serum levels of this proenzyme correlate with the gastric capacity for acid secretion and are considered a measure of parietal cell mass. **A person with a high circulating level of pepsinogen I is at five times the normal risk of developing a duodenal ulcer.** Hyperpepsinogenemia I is present in half of the children of ulcer patients with hyperpepsinogenemia and has been attributed to autosomal dominant inheritance. Thus, not only is hyperpepsinogenemia considered a marker for an ulcer diathesis, but it is also thought to indicate a genetically predetermined increase in parietal cell mass.

Familial tendencies for other features are reported in ulcer patients. Many patients with peptic ulcer have normal pepsinogen I secretion, and familial aggregation has also been demonstrated among such persons. Familial clustering of duodenal ulcers and rapid gastric emptying have been demonstrated, and familial hyperfunction of gastrin-secreting cells (G cells) in the antrum is also reported. Patients with a childhood duodenal ulcer are considerably more likely to have a family history of an ulcer diathesis than are persons in whom the disease begins when they are adults.

Psychological Factors

Stress has been anecdotally related to peptic ulcers for at least a century, and repressed stress has been considered particularly ulcerogenic. Closer scrutiny of the epidemiological and experimental evidence supporting these concepts has cast serious doubt on their validity, and many today discount any relation between stress and ulcers. Whatever the final outcome of this debate may be, there is no need to incriminate stress in the pathogenesis of peptic ulcers.

Hydrochloric Acid

The formation and persistence of peptic ulcers in both the stomach and duodenum require the gastric secretion of acid. This is evidenced principally by the following: (1) all patients with duodenal ulcers and almost all with gastric ulcers are gastric acid secretors; (2) the experimental production of ulcers in animals requires the production of acid; (3) hypersecretion of acid is present in many, but not all, patients with duodenal ulcers (there is no evidence that overproduction of acid by itself is necessary or sufficient to explain duodenal ulceration); and (4) surgical or medical treatment that reduces acid production results in the healing of peptic ulcers. The gastric secretion of pepsin, which may also play a role in the production of peptic ulcers, parallels that of hydrochloric acid.

Physiological Factors in Duodenal Ulcers

The maximal capacity for acid production by the stomach is a reflection of total parietal cell mass. Both parietal cell mass and maximal acid secretion are increased up to twofold in patients with duodenal ulcers. However, there is a large overlap with normal values, and **only one third of these patients secrete excess acid**. The increase in parietal cells is paralleled by a comparable increase in chief cells, a situation that is consistent with the increased prevalence of hyperpepsinogenemia in patients with ulcers.

The gastric secretion of acid stimulated by food is increased in magnitude and duration in patients with duodenal ulcer, although here, too, there is significant overlap with normal values. In a few patients, this may involve, at least in part, an altered response of the G cells to meals. Such persons exhibit postprandial hypergastrinemia and an increase in the number of G cells in the antrum. The majority of patients with duodenal ulcers, however, show no evidence of G-cell hyperfunction.

Acid secretion in patients with duodenal ulcers may also be more sensitive than normal to gastric secretagogues such as gastrin, possibly as a result of increased vagal tone or a greater than normal affinity of the parietal cells for gastrin. It is further possible that the brisk secretion of acid after a meal is stimulated by increased vagal tone.

Accelerated gastric emptying, a condition that might lead to excessive acidification of the duodenum, has been noted in patients with duodenal ulcers. However, as with other factors, there is substantial overlap with normal rates. Normally, acidification of the duodenal bulb inhibits further gastric emptying. It has been reported that in the majority of patients with duodenal ulcer, this feedback inhibitory mechanism is absent, and duodenal acidification results in continued, rather than delayed, gastric emptying. Rapid gastric emptying may in some cases be an inherited abnormality.

The pH of the duodenal bulb reflects the balance between the delivery of gastric juice and its neutralization by biliary, pancreatic, and duodenal secretions. The production of duodenal ulcers requires an acidic pH in the bulb, that is, an excess of acid over neutralizing secretions. In ulcer patients, the duodenal pH after a meal decreases to a lower level and remains depressed for a longer time than that in normal persons. This duodenal hyperacidity certainly reflects the gastric factors discussed earlier. The role of neutralizing factors, particularly secretin-stimulated bicarbonate secretion by the pancreas and production of bicarbonate by the duodenal mucosa, is uncertain, and the subject remains controversial.

Impaired mucosal defenses have been invoked as contributing to peptic ulceration. The mucosal factors, including the function of prostaglandins, may or may not be similar to those protecting the gastric mucosa (considered earlier in the section entitled Acute Hemorrhagic Gastritis).

Physiological Factors in Gastric Ulcers

Gastric ulcers almost invariably arise in the setting of *H. pylori* gastritis or chemical gastritis that results in injury to the epithelium. The mechanisms by which chronic gastritis predisposes to the development of stomach ulcers remain obscure. **Most patients with gastric ulcers secrete less acid than do those with duodenal ulcers, and even less than normal persons.** The genesis of gastric hyposecretion, and its relation to chronic gastritis, is controversial. The factors implicated include (1) back-diffusion of acid into the mucosa, (2) decreased parietal cell mass, and (3) abnormalities of the parietal cells themselves. A minority of patients with gastric ulcers exhibit acid hypersecretion. In these persons, the ulcers are usually near the pylorus and are considered variants of duodenal ulcers. Interestingly, the intense gastric hypersecretion that occurs in the Zollinger–Ellison syndrome is associated with severe ulceration of the duodenum and even the jejunum, but rarely with gastric ulcers.

The occurrence of gastric ulcers in the presence of gastric hyposecretion implies the following possibilities: (1) the gastric mucosa is in some way particularly sensitive to low concentrations of acid; (2) some material other than acid damages the mucosa, especially nonsteroidal anti-inflammatory drugs; or (3) the gastric mucosa is exposed to potentially injurious agents for an unusually long period. As discussed in the section on acute hemorrhagic gastritis, the mucosal barrier to the action of acid, and perhaps to other contents of the stomach, may be impaired in some patients with gastric ulcers, although the evidence is far from conclusive. Reflux of bile (particularly deoxycholic acid and lysolecithin) and pancreatic secretions have been suggested as causes of gastric ulcers.

In some patients with pyloric obstruction (e.g., persons with adult hypertrophic pyloric stenosis or scarring resulting from a duodenal ulcer), peptic ulcers of the stomach appear to be related to the retention of gastric contents. However, the precise elements of the retained gastric contents that precipitate such ulcers have not been elucidated.

The Role of *Helicobacter pylori*

***Helicobacter pylori* has been isolated from the gastric antrum of virtually all patients with duodenal ulcers.** It is important to emphasize that the converse is not true; that is, only a small minority of persons infected with *H. pylori* have duodenal ulcer disease. Thus, *H. pylori* infection may be accepted as a necessary, but not sufficient, condition for the development of peptic ulcer disease of the duodenum.

The mechanisms by which *H. pylori* infection predisposes to duodenal ulcers are unknown. Cytokines produced by the inflammatory cells that respond to *H. pylori* infection stimulate gastrin release and suppress somatostatin secretion. These effects, together with the release of histamine metabolites from the organism itself, may stimulate basal gastric acid secretion. In addition, luminal cytokines from the stomach may enter and injure the duodenal epithelium. There is some evidence that *H. pylori* infection blocks inhibitory signals from the antrum to both the gastrin-producing cells and the parietal cell region, resulting in increased gastrin release and impaired inhibition of gastric acid secretion. Such an effect might lead to an increased load of acid in the duodenum, thereby contributing to the development of duodenal ulcers. Owing to acidification of the duodenal bulb, islands of metaplastic gastric mucosa occur in many patients with peptic ulcers. This gastric epithelium in the duodenum sometimes shows the same colonization with *H. pylori* as does the gastric mucosa. It has been postulated that infection of the metaplastic epithelium by *H. pylori* might render the mucosa more susceptible to peptic injury (Fig. 13-16).

Infection with *H. pylori* is probably also important in the pathogenesis of gastric ulcers, because this organism is responsible for most cases of the chronic gastritis that underlies this disease. It is estimated that about 75% of patients with gastric ulcers harbor *H. pylori.* The remaining 25% of the cases may represent an association with other types of chronic gastritis. Conversely, it is possible that *H. pylori* has disappeared from the stomach in some cases.

The various gastric and duodenal factors that have been implicated as possible mechanisms in the pathogenesis of duodenal ulceration are summarized in Figure 13-17.

Associated Diseases

CIRRHOSIS: Chronic liver disease is associated with an increased frequency of duodenal ulcers. The incidence of duodenal ulcers in patients with cirrhosis is 10-fold greater than that in normal persons. Moreover, the death rate from duodenal ulcer is increased fivefold in patients with cirrhosis. The mechanisms responsible for the association of duodenal ulcers with cirrhosis are unclear.

CHRONIC RENAL FAILURE: End-stage renal disease with hemodialysis has been reported to result in a greater than normal risk for the development of peptic ulcers, although the data are not conclusive. Patients subjected to **renal transplantation** also show a substantially increased incidence of peptic ulceration and its complications, such as bleeding and perforation. Prophylactic treatment with histamine-receptor antagonists has been reported to reduce this risk.

HEREDITARY ENDOCRINE SYNDROMES: There is an increased incidence of peptic ulcers in persons with **multiple endocrine neoplasia, type I**. The presence of a

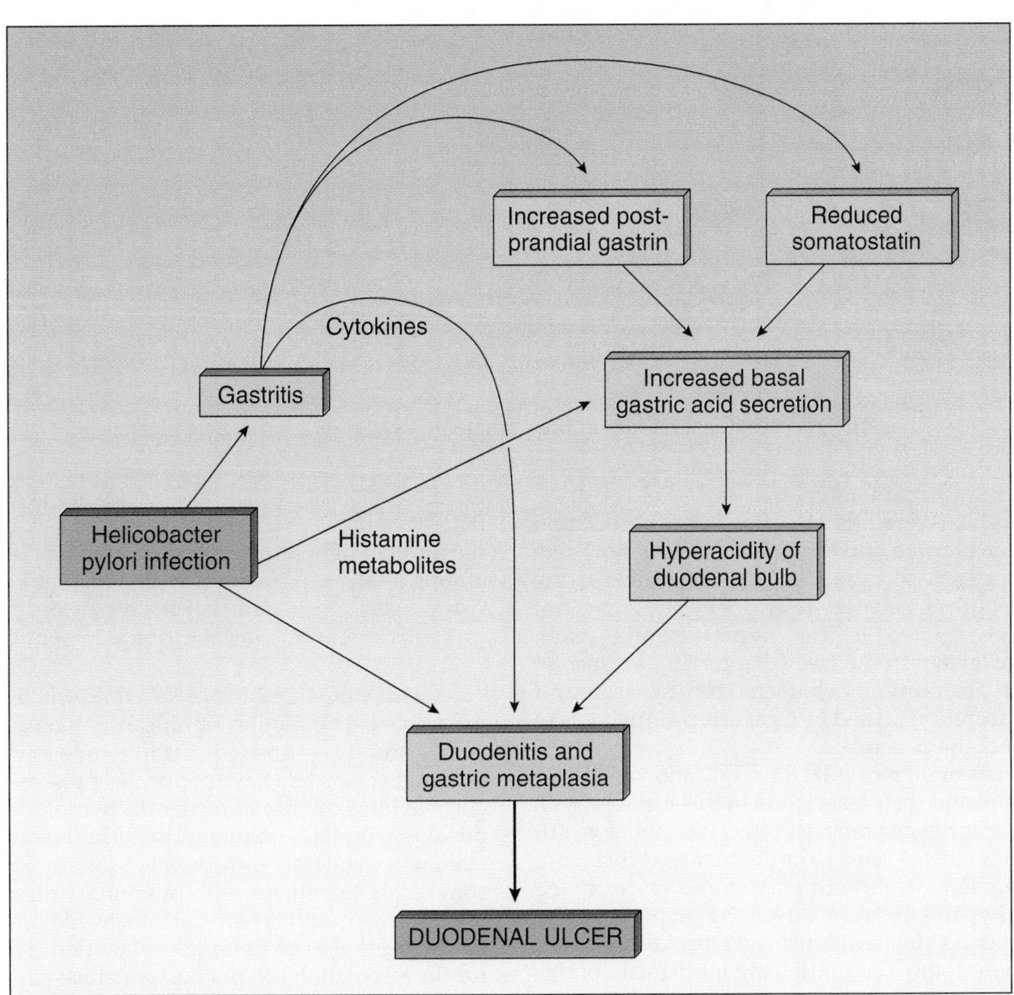

FIGURE 13-16
Possible mechanisms in the pathogenesis of duodenal ulcer disease associated with *Helicobacter pylori* infection.

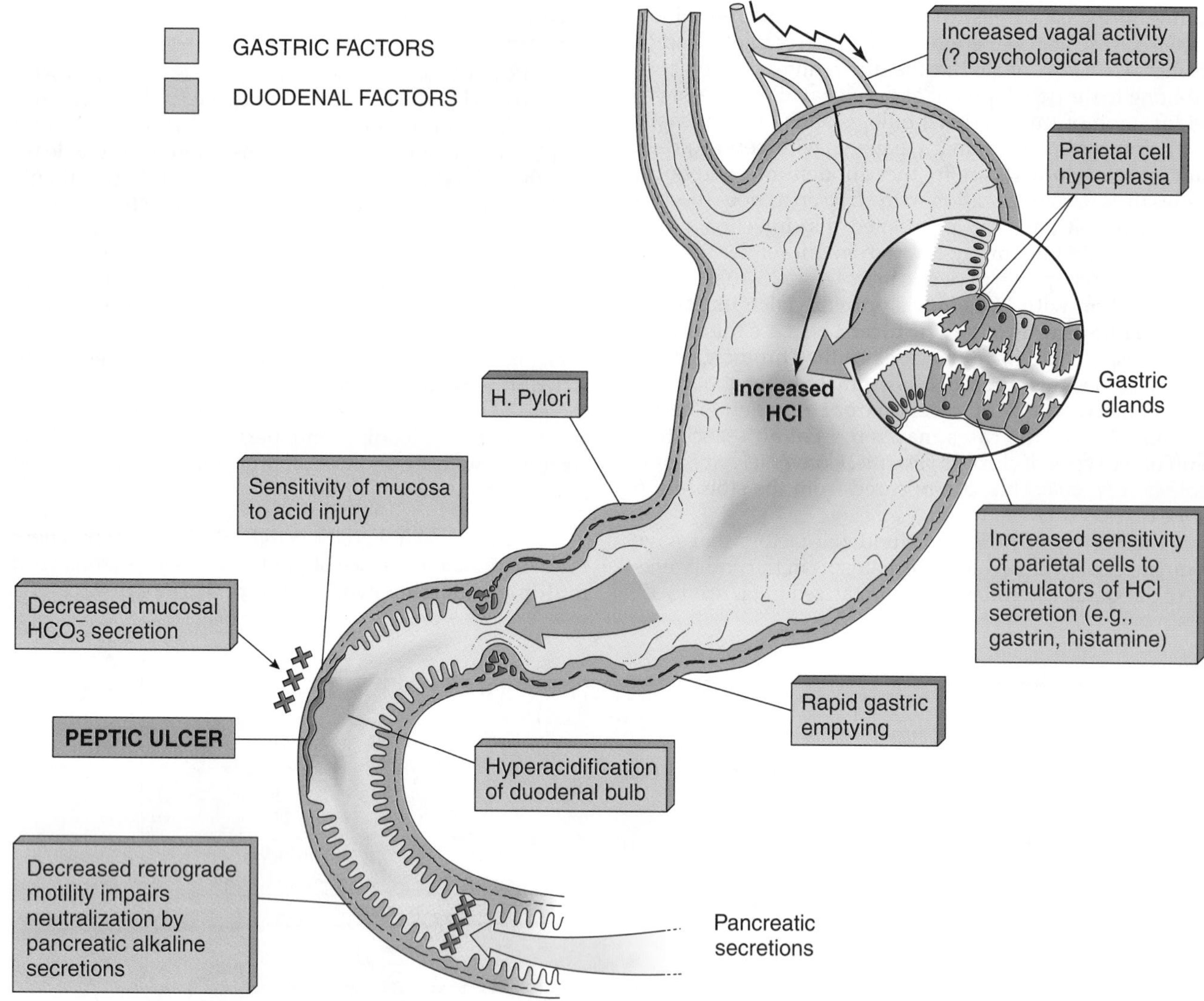

FIGURE *13-17*
Gastric and duodenal factors in the pathogenesis of duodenal peptic ulcers.

functioning parathyroid adenoma and the resulting hypercalcemia have been misinterpreted as an association between hypercalcemia and peptic ulcers. It is now recognized that this association is a consequence of the simultaneous presence of a gastrinoma and may not necessarily be related to the hypercalcemia itself. Zollinger–Ellison syndrome (see Chapter 15), a cause of severe peptic ulceration, is characterized by profound gastric hypersecretion caused by a gastrin-producing islet cell adenoma of the pancreas.

Renal stones are a recognized complication of hyperparathyroidism, and their association in this instance with peptic ulcer also probably reflects an accompanying gastrinoma. However, there seems to be an increased incidence of peptic ulcers in patients with renal stones unassociated with either hypercalcemia (caused by hyperparathyroidism) or an excess intake of milk and antacids for the relief of ulcer symptoms. The underlying mechanism of this association is obscure.

α_1-ANTITRYPSIN DEFICIENCY: This hereditary disorder is associated with peptic ulcers in almost one third of the patients, and this incidence is even higher in patients who have pulmonary disease as well. Moreover, the number of heterozygotes for α_1-antitrypsin deficiency among relatives of patients with peptic ulcer is increased. It has been speculated that in this disorder, unopposed proteolytic activity may contribute to peptic ulceration.

CHRONIC PULMONARY DISEASE: Long-standing pulmonary dysfunction significantly increases the risk of ulcers, and it is estimated that fully one fourth of patients with such disorders have peptic ulcer disease. Conversely, chronic lung disease is increased twofold to threefold in persons who have peptic ulcers. These correlations hold even when the data are corrected for smoking. Although some of these patients with pulmonary disease may have underlying α_1-antitrypsin deficiency, the correlation is too strong for this to be the sole explanation. The mechanism for the association has not been established.

☐ Pathology: **A peptic ulcer should be considered chronic when it does not heal readily and leads to scar-**

ring at the base of the ulcer, which precludes complete restoration of the normal submucosa and muscularis mucosae. Most peptic ulcers arise in the lesser curvature of the stomach, in the antral and prepyloric regions, and in the first part of the duodenum.

Gastric ulcers (Fig. 13-18) are usually single and less than 2 cm in diameter, although occasionally they reach a diameter of 10 cm or more, particularly if they are on the lesser curvature. Ulcers on the lesser curvature are usually associated with chronic gastritis, whereas those on the greater curvature are often related to nonsteroidal anti-inflammatory drugs. The edges tend to be sharply punched out, with overhanging margins. The flat base is gray and indurated and may exhibit clotted blood or an eroded vessel when the ulcer is active. Deeply penetrating ulcers produce a serosal exudate, which may cause adherence of the stomach to the surrounding structures. Scarring of ulcers in the prepyloric region may be severe enough to produce pyloric stenosis. **On gross examination, it may be exceedingly difficult to distinguish chronic peptic ulcer from an ulcerating gastric carcinoma.** Thus, when examining the stomach, the endoscopist is required to take multiple biopsy specimens from the edges and bed of any gastric ulcer.

Duodenal ulcers (Fig. 13-19) are ordinarily located on the anterior or posterior wall of the first part of the duodenum, within a short distance of the pylorus. The lesion is usually solitary, but it is not uncommon to find paired ulcers on both walls, so-called kissing ulcers.

Microscopically, gastric and duodenal ulcers have a similar appearance (Fig. 13-20). From the lumen outward, the following are noted: (1) a superficial zone of fibrinopurulent exudate; (2) necrotic tissue; (3) granulation tissue; and (4) fibrotic tissue at the base of the ulcer, which exhibits variable degrees of chronic inflammation. The ulceration sometimes penetrates the muscle layers, thereby causing them to be interrupted by scar tissue after healing. Blood vessels on the margins of the ulcer are often thrombosed. The mucosa at the margins of the ulcer is often hyperplastic, and with healing grows over the ulcerated area as a single layer of epithelium. This process requires proliferation of stroma and epithelium to re-form the mucosa. However, in a large ulcer, the ingrowth of the epithelium may be insufficient to cover the defect completely. down-growth of the regenerating epithelium at the margins of the ulcer is visualized in cross-section as islands of epithelial cells surrounded by inflamed and fibrotic tissue. This appearance may be confused with that

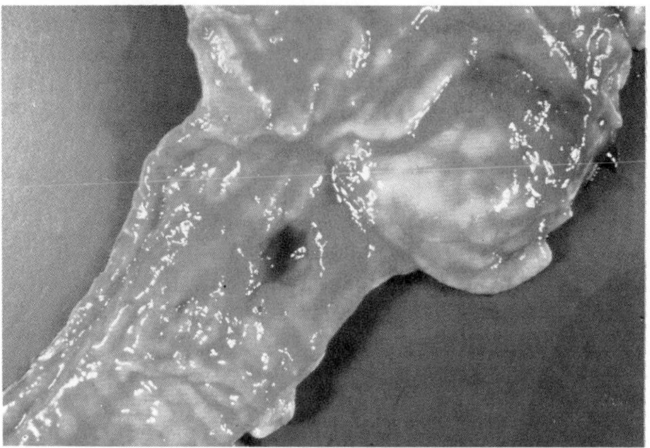

FIGURE *13-19*
Duodenal ulcer. A sharply punched-out peptic ulcer of the duodenum is situated immediately below the pylorus.

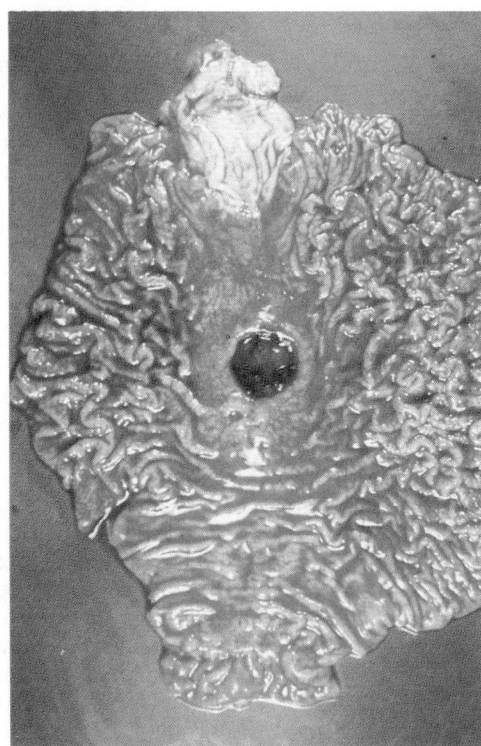

FIGURE *13-18*
Gastric ulcer. The stomach has been opened to reveal a sharply demarcated, deep peptic ulcer on the lesser curvature.

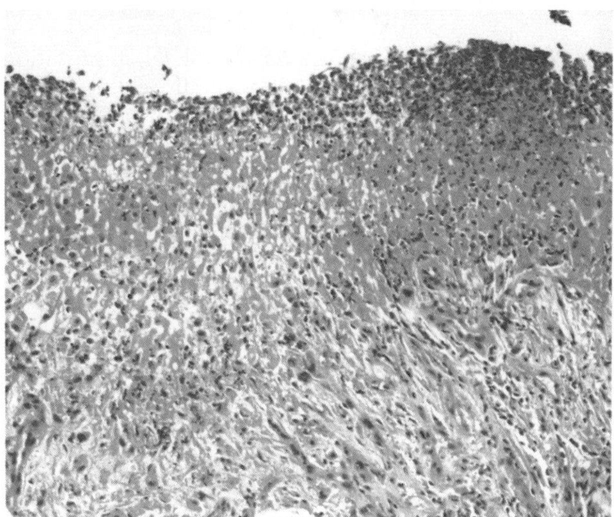

FIGURE *13-20*
Peptic ulcer of the stomach. A photomicrograph of the ulcer shows the mucosa to be denuded. The surface is covered with a fibrinous exudate containing neutrophils, below which is inflamed granulation tissue.

of an infiltrating carcinoma. Gastric ulcers are commonly accompanied by *H. pylori* gastritis or chemical gastritis. Duodenal ulcers are usually accompanied by peptic duodenitis, with Brunner gland hyperplasia and gastric mucin cell metaplasia.

□ **Clinical Features:** The symptoms of gastric and duodenal ulcers are sufficiently similar so that the two conditions are generally not distinguishable by history or physical examination. The classic case of duodenal ulcer is characterized by burning epigastric pain that is experienced 1 to 3 hours after a meal or that awakens the patient at night. Both alkali and food are said to relieve the symptoms. However, detailed studies have demonstrated that the majority of patients do not conform to the classic presentation. Half do not describe their pain as related to meals, and fewer than half report that the pain is relieved by food or alkali. Dyspeptic symptoms commonly associated with gallbladder disease, including fatty food intolerance, distention, and belching, occur in half of patients with peptic ulcers. The major complications of peptic ulcer disease are hemorrhage, perforation, penetration, and obstruction.

HEMORRHAGE: The most common complication of peptic ulcers is bleeding, occurring in up to 20% of the patients. In many cases, bleeding is occult and, in an otherwise asymptomatic ulcer, may be manifested as iron-deficiency anemia or as occult blood in the stools. **Massive life-threatening hemorrhage is a well-recognized danger in patients with active peptic ulcers.** Indeed, the first indication that a patient has an ulcer may come from a massive bleeding episode. Disorders of coagulation, whether from a primary clotting disorder or induced by anticoagulant drugs, increase the risk of bleeding from peptic ulcers. Despite improvements in surgical and endoscopic management, transfusion therapy, and the availability of drugs such as H_2-receptor antagonists and proton-pump inhibitors, the mortality from bleeding peptic ulcers has not changed over the past 30 years and remains at about 10%.

PERFORATION AND PENETRATION: Perforation is a serious complication of peptic ulcer disease, which occurs in 5% or less of patients; in one third of the cases, there are no antecedent symptoms referable to peptic ulcer. Perforations are seen more commonly with duodenal than with gastric ulcers, the large majority occurring on the anterior wall of the duodenum. Perforations result in the luminal contents freely escaping into the peritoneal cavity. Penetrations are sealed by surrounding structures or peritoneum. Because the anterior walls of the stomach and duodenum are undefended by contiguous tissue, ulcers in these locations are more likely to be complicated by free perforation, which leads to generalized peritonitis and the accumulation of air in the abdominal cavity, called *pneumoperitoneum*. Posterior gastric ulcers perforate into the lesser peritoneal sac, where the inflammatory reaction may be contained. When ulcers penetrate into the pancreas, liver, or greater omentum, they cause intractable symptoms. They may also penetrate the biliary tract and fill it with air.

Perforated ulcers continue to be associated with a high mortality. The overall mortality for perforated gastric ulcers is 10% to 40%, two to three times more than that for duodenal ulcers (5% to 13%). Perforations are occasionally complicated by hemorrhage, in which case, about half of the patients die. Although shock, abdominal distention, and pain are common symptoms, perforations are occasionally diagnosed for the first time at autopsy, particularly in institutionalized, elderly patients.

PYLORIC OBSTRUCTION (GASTRIC OUTLET OBSTRUCTION): Pyloric obstruction occurs in 5% to 10% of ulcer patients, and peptic ulcer disease is its most common cause in adults. Narrowing of the pyloric lumen by an adjacent peptic ulcer may be caused by muscular spasm, edema, muscular hypertrophy, or contraction of scar tissue; most commonly it is due to a combination of these. Retention of gastric contents results in epigastric distress, anorexia, and early satiety. Eventually obstruction may ensue. In many patients, a succussion splash is elicited in the fasting state because of retention of gastric contents. Most patients with symptomatic pyloric obstruction eventually require surgical relief.

DEVELOPMENT OF COMBINED ULCERS: The simultaneous occurrence of gastric and duodenal ulcers in the same patient is far greater than can be accounted for by chance alone. In prospective studies, patients with gastric ulcers have been found to have a substantially increased risk of developing a subsequent duodenal ulcer. Persons with duodenal ulcers are also at higher than normal risk of developing a subsequent gastric ulcer, although they are at lesser risk than those in the reverse situation. Nonsteroidal anti-inflammatory drugs are important causes of combined ulcers.

MALIGNANT TRANSFORMATION OF A BENIGN GASTRIC ULCER: It is extremely difficult to distinguish a cancer arising in a preexisting gastric ulcer from an ulcerated primary carcinoma. This difficulty does not complicate the study of duodenal ulcers, because **malignant transformation of a duodenal ulcer is virtually unknown.** However, although cancers originating in well-recognized benign peptic ulcers probably account for considerably fewer than 1% of all malignant tumors in the stomach, such cancers have been well documented.

BENIGN NEOPLASMS

Leiomyoma

Leiomyoma, a benign tumor of smooth muscle cells, is the most common tumor of the stomach (Fig. 13-21). Careful study of autopsy specimens reveals its presence in 25% to 50% of the population older than 50 years. The tumors range in size from barely detectable nubbins to large masses more than 20 cm in diameter. Leiomyomas smaller than 2 cm in diameter are usually asymptomatic. Larger tumors may ulcerate and bleed or may cause pain, in which case, the disorder is clinically indistinguishable from a peptic ulcer.

Leiomyomas are submucosal and covered by intact mucosa or, when they project externally, by peritoneum. The cut surface has a whorled appearance and often shows cystic spaces. Microscopically, gastric leiomyomas

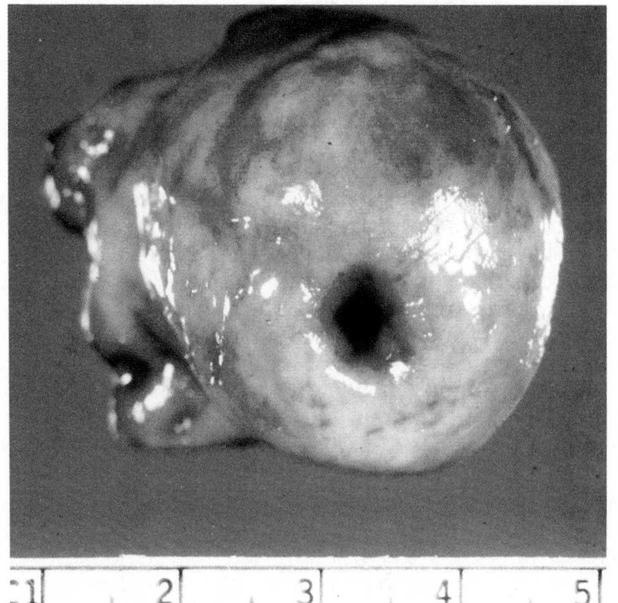

FIGURE 13-21
Leiomyoma of the stomach. The resected tumor is submucosal and covered by a focally ulcerated mucosa.

show variable cellularity and are composed of spindle-shaped smooth muscle cells embedded in a collagenous stroma, similar to their appearance elsewhere. The cells are disposed in whorls and interlacing bundles. The nuclei are often arranged in parallel rows, which resemble the palisading of neurilemomas. The presence of bizarre and giant nuclei is not necessarily a sign of malignancy. Local excision is curative.

Leiomyoblastoma

Leiomyoblastoma, a variant of leiomyoma, appears macroscopically similar to the usual smooth muscle cell tumor. However, the cells are polygonal rather than spindle shaped and have a substantial eosinophilic cytoplasm, a perinuclear clear zone, and no myofibrils. Thus, they are not easily recognized as smooth muscle cells, and the term *epithelioid leiomyoma* also has been suggested for these tumors. For the most part, leiomyoblastomas are benign, but metastases have been recorded. The histological criteria for malignancy, particularly the number of mitoses, are the same as for other smooth muscle sarcomas (see later). Even when metastases are present, the growth of the tumors is often indolent, and long-term survival after resection is common.

Epithelial Polyps

Epithelial polyps of the stomach, classed as either hyperplastic/inflammatory or adenomatous, account for almost half of all benign gastric tumors. The large majority of gastric polyps are found in patients with achlorhydria, and both types occur in association with atrophic gastritis and pernicious anemia, as well as in stomachs that harbor carcinoma.

HYPERPLASTIC/INFLAMMATORY POLYPS: These tumors represent the large majority of gastric polyps. They may be single or multiple and are seen as pedunculated or sessile lesions of variable sizes. Hyperplastic/inflammatory polyps are not true neoplasms but result from chronic inflammation and regenerative hyperplasia of the mucosa. They are common in the atrophic oxyntic mucosa of the body and fundus of patients with autoimmune metaplastic atrophic gastritis, but they occur in the antrum of patients with *H. pylori* gastritis. Microscopically, the polyps consist of elongated, branched crypts lined by normal foveolar epithelium, beneath which pyloric or gastric glands mingle with collagen and smooth muscle fibers. Cystic dilatation of the glands, granulation tissue in the lamina propria, and chronic inflammation may be conspicuous. **Hyperplastic polyps have no malignant potential.**

ADENOMATOUS POLYPS: These are true neoplasms, which occur most commonly in the antrum. The polyps range from less than 1 cm in diameter to a considerable size, the average being about 4 cm. Most adenomatous polyps are sessile and more often single than multiple. Microscopically, adenomas are composed of villous structures or a combination of tubular and villous glands. The glands are usually lined by dysplastic epithelium, which is sometimes intestinalized. Occasionally, an adenomatous polyp is composed solely of tubular glands, similar to those that arise in the colon.

Adenomatous polyps manifest a malignant potential, variably reported at 5% to 75%. This danger increases with the size of the polyp and is greatest for lesions larger than 2 cm in diameter. As in the colon, villous adenomas seem to undergo malignant transformation more frequently than do tubular adenomas. Adenomas sometimes accompany separate gastric adenocarcinomas. Dysplasia can also occur in flat gastric mucosa.

FUNDIC GLAND POLYPS: Fundic gland polyps are characterized by dilated oxyntic glands, with flattening of the parietal cells and chief cells and with mucous cell metaplasia. They are common in patients with familial adenomatous polyposis and patients treated with proton-pump inhibitors, but their pathogenesis is obscure.

Miscellaneous Benign Tumors

Benign lipomas, vascular tumors, fibromas, and heterotopic pancreatic tissue are occasionally encountered in the stomach.

MALIGNANT NEOPLASMS

Carcinoma of the Stomach

☐ **Epidemiology:** As recently as the mid-20th century, carcinoma of the stomach was the most common cause of death from cancer among men in the United States. For reasons that have not been explained, the incidence of gastric carcinoma has steadily decreased. It accounts for about 3% of cancer deaths in the United States. The incidence of stomach cancer remains exceedingly high in such countries as Japan and Chile, where the rates are seven to eight times that in the United States. Although the cause of gastric cancer is unknown, as discussed in Chapter 5, emigrants from high-risk to low-risk areas show a decline in the incidence of cancer of the stomach, an observation that strongly implicates environmental factors in its pathogenesis.

☐ **Pathogenesis:** Although correlations have been demonstrated with a number of factors, the cause of gastric cancer remains elusive.

DIETARY FACTORS: Ingredients in the diet have been invoked to account for geographic variations in the incidence of gastric cancer. Studies of dietary habits are complicated by the fact that they require retrospective analyses over a very long time, and it is often difficult to isolate nutritional factors from other environmental influences. Nevertheless, carcinoma of the stomach is more common among persons who eat large amounts of starch, smoked fish and meat, and pickled vegetables. Benzpyrene, a potent carcinogen, has been detected in smoked foods.

NITROSAMINES: Attention has been focused on the possible role of nitrosamines, which are powerful animal carcinogens, in the pathogenesis of cancer of the stomach. Secondary amines are converted nonenzymatically to nitrosamines in the presence of nitrates or nitrites. High nitrate concentrations have been found in the soil and water in certain areas where the incidence of gastric cancer is high, and processed meats and vegetables are high in nitrates and nitrites. In addition, certain persons at increased risk of gastric cancer, such as patients with atrophic gastritis and intestinal metaplasia, have a high intragastric pH and high stomach concentrations of bacteria that can convert nitrates to nitrites, favoring the production of nitrosamines.

The decreased incidence of gastric cancer in the United States has been paralleled by an increased use of refrigeration, a practice that inhibits the conversion of nitrates to nitrites and also obviates the need to add such compounds for food preservation. The consumption of whole milk and fresh vegetables rich in vitamin C is inversely related to the occurrence of stomach cancer. Vitamin C has been shown to inhibit the nitrosation of secondary amines *in vivo*.

GENETIC FACTORS: Hereditary traits have not been identified in most cases of carcinoma of the stomach. A few familial clusters of gastric cancer and several cases in twins have been reported. Gastric cancer occurs in hereditary nonpolyposis colorectal cancer syndrome, a disorder caused by germline mutations of genes responsible for DNA nucleotide mismatch repair. Blood type A is found in 38% of the general population, whereas half of the patients with gastric cancer display this blood type.

AGE AND SEX: Gastric cancer is uncommon in persons younger than 30 years and shows a sharp peak in incidence in persons older than 50 years. However, the age at onset seems to be somewhat lower in Japan, where the disease is endemic. In the United States, there is only a slight male predominance, but in countries with a high incidence of this tumor, the male-to-female ratio is about 2:1.

HELICOBACTER PYLORI: **Serological studies have demonstrated a high prevalence of gastric infection with *H. pylori* many years before the appearance of stomach cancer.** Persons seropositive for *H. pylori* were three times more likely than seronegative persons to develop gastric adenocarcinoma in the ensuing 1 to 24 years of follow-up. In view of the observation that the risk of stomach cancer is determined largely by environmental factors in the first decades of life, it is noteworthy that populations at high risk for this tumor exhibit a high prevalence of infection with *H. pylori* in children, whereas those at low risk do not. Because gastric adenocarcinoma develops in only a small proportion of persons infected with *H. pylori*, and because some stomach cancers are found in noninfected persons, this infection alone is neither sufficient nor necessary for gastric carcinogenesis. It is probable that the other environmental factors discussed earlier play an important role.

LOW-SOCIOECONOMIC SETTINGS: These situations pose an increased risk of gastric cancer, an observation that has been used to explain the high frequency of the tumor among American blacks and the fact that the incidence of the disease in that population has not declined as rapidly as it has among whites.

Atrophic gastritis, pernicious anemia, subtotal gastrectomy, and gastric adenomatous polyps were discussed earlier as factors associated with a high risk of stomach cancer.

☐ **Pathology:** Adenocarcinoma of the stomach accounts for more than 95% of all malignant gastric tumors. It occurs in two major but overlapping types: diffuse and intestinal types. Cancers are most common in the distal stomach, on the lesser curvature of the antrum, and in the prepyloric region. Adenocarcinoma is rare in the fundus but may occur in any location. In occasional cases, these tumors may arise at several sites simultaneously.

ADVANCED GASTRIC CANCER: By the time most gastric cancers in the Western world are detected, they are advanced; that is, they have penetrated beyond the submucosa into the muscularis propria and may extend through the serosa. The macroscopic appearance of these advanced cancers is of great importance not only to the pathologist but also to the radiologist and the endoscopist, who may be called on to distinguish carcinomas from benign lesions and to assess the degree of spread.

Advanced gastric cancers are divided into three major macroscopic types:

- **Polypoid (fungating) adenocarcinoma** accounts for one third of advanced cancers. It is a solid mass, often several centimeters in diameter, that projects into the lumen of the stomach. The surface may be partly ulcerated, and the deeper tissues may or may not be infiltrated.
- **Ulcerating adenocarcinoma** constitutes another third of all gastric cancers. It is visualized as a shallow ulcer of variable size (Fig. 13-22). The surround-

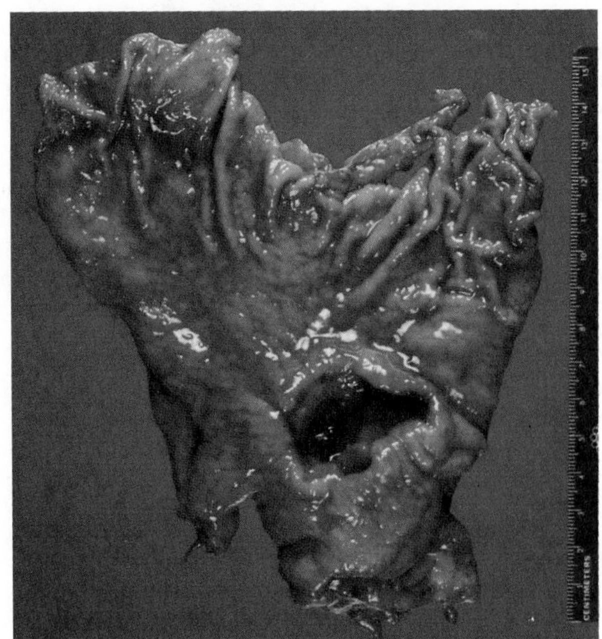

FIGURE 13-22
Ulcerating carcinoma of the stomach. The stomach has been opened along the greater curvature to reveal a large, centrally ulcerated adenocarcinoma in the antrum, characterized by raised, indurated margins.

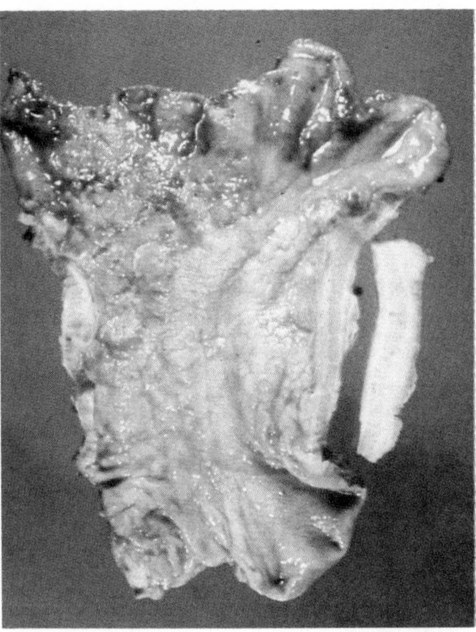

FIGURE 13-23
Infiltrating gastric carcinoma (linitis plastica). The wall of the stomach is thickened and indurated by diffusely infiltrating cancer.

ing tissue is firm, raised, and nodular. Characteristically, the lateral margins of the ulcer are irregular, and the base is ragged. This appearance stands in contrast to that of the usual benign peptic ulcer, which exhibits punched-out margins and a smooth base. Despite these differences, the radiological differentiation of ulcerating cancer from peptic ulcer is occasionally difficult. Endoscopic biopsy specimens from the margins and bed of the ulcer usually provide a correct diagnosis, but the absence of malignant cells does not guarantee a benign lesion, because necrotic or reactive tissue may predominate in the areas in which the biopsy is performed.

- **Diffuse or infiltrating adenocarcinoma** composes one tenth of all stomach cancers. No true tumor mass is seen macroscopically; instead, the wall of the stomach is conspicuously thickened and firm (Fig. 13-23). When the entire stomach is involved, the term *linitis plastica* (leather-bottle stomach; see Fig. 13-19) is applied. In the diffuse type of gastric carcinoma, the invading tumor cells induce extensive fibrosis in the submucosa and muscularis. As a result, the wall is stiff and may be more than 2 cm thick. Whereas the normal stomach has a volume greater than 1 L, the leather-bottle stomach contains as little as 150 mL. Interestingly, because tumor cells are often scarce in well-developed linitis plastica, this condition was historically not recognized as a tumor; instead it was believed to represent an infectious or inflammatory disease.

Microscopically, the histological pattern of advanced gastric cancer varies from a well-differentiated adenocarcinoma with gland formation (intestinal type) to a totally anaplastic tumor. The polypoid variant typically contains well-differentiated glands, whereas linitis plastica is characteristically poorly differentiated. Particularly in the ulcerated type of cancer, the tumor cells may be arranged in cords or small foci. Tumor cells may contain clear mucin that displaces the nucleus to the periphery of the cell, resulting in the so-called *signet ring cell* (Fig. 13-24). Extracellular mucinous material may be so prominent that the malignant cells seem to float in a gelatinous matrix, in which case it is called a *mucinous (colloid) carcinoma*. Cancers that display papillary infoldings are termed *papillary*

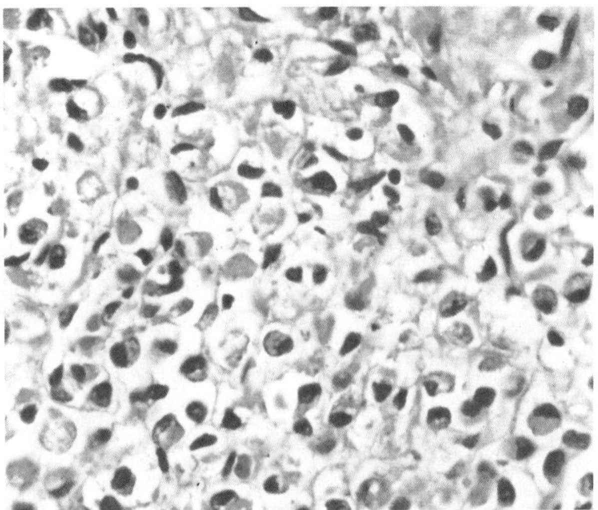

FIGURE 13-24
Signet ring cells of gastric adenocarcinoma. Intracellular mucin (red) displaces the nuclei to the periphery of the tumor cells (mucicarmine stain).

adenocarcinomas, and those that form solid tumor masses are referred to as *medullary carcinomas.* Gastric cancers commonly contain intestinal-type mucin on histochemical staining.

EARLY GASTRIC CANCER: In the early 1960s, Japanese gastroenterologists, alarmed by the high incidence of stomach cancer in their country, began to screen the adult population endoscopically for early evidence of that disease. They defined early gastric cancer as a tumor that is confined to the mucosa or submucosa (Fig. 13-25). An earlier term, *superficial spreading carcinoma,* is synonymous with early gastric cancer. In Japan, early gastric cancer accounts for fully one third of all stomach cancers, whereas in the United States and Europe, it constitutes only about 5% of diagnosed cancers.

Early gastric cancer is strictly a pathological diagnosis based on depth of invasion; the term does not refer to the duration of the malignant tumor, its size, the presence of symptoms, the absence of metastases, or the curability. In fact, 5% to 20% of early gastric cancers are already metastatic to lymph nodes at the time of detection.

Similar to advanced cancer, most early gastric cancers are found in the distal stomach and have been classified by Japanese investigators according to their macroscopic appearance. Three major types are recognized:

- **Type I** protrudes into the lumen as a polypoid or nodular mass.
- **Type II** is a superficial, flat lesion that may be slightly elevated or depressed.
- **Type III** is an excavated malignant ulcer that does not ordinarily occur alone but rather represents ulceration of type I or type II tumors.

The polypoid and the superficial elevated varieties of early gastric cancer are typically well-differentiated intestinal-type adenocarcinomas. In the flattened or depressed superficial early cancers, the pattern ranges from well differentiated to anaplastic. The excavated lesions have the highest proportion of undifferentiated tumors.

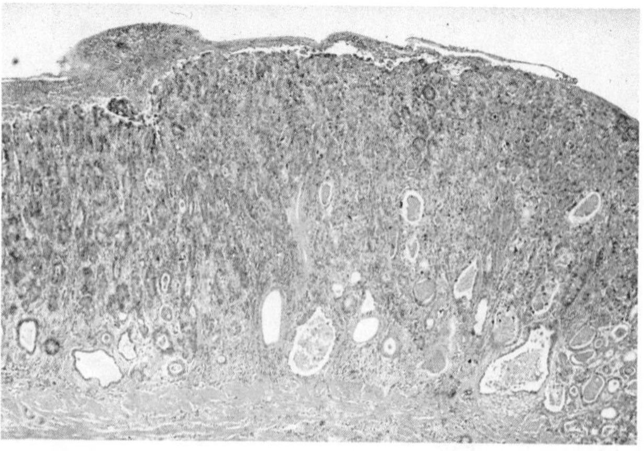

FIGURE *13-25*
Early gastric cancer. Irregular neoplastic glands are seen in the mucosa superficial to the muscularis mucosae.

It is generally accepted that most gastric cancers of the intestinal type originate from epithelium that has undergone intestinal metaplasia. The endoscopic studies of early gastric cancer established the validity of this concept and demonstrated that well-differentiated adenocarcinomas usually arise in the context of intestinal metaplasia, commonly associated with atrophic gastritis. By contrast, less differentiated and anaplastic tumors of the diffuse type are more likely to originate from the the necks of gastric glands without intestinal metaplasia. However, considerable overlap occurs, and no firm rules can be applied.

Intuitively, one would suppose that early gastric cancer would be the precursor of advanced gastric cancer. However, this is not always the case, and early gastric cancer may sometimes be a different disease from advanced cancer. It may exhibit a more benign course and greater curability because of an inherently lower biological potential for invasion, possibly related to the differences between the intestinal and gastric cell types. For example, even in the presence of lymph node metastases, early gastric cancer has a considerably better prognosis than advanced cancer. The 10-year survival rate for surgically treated advanced gastric cancer is about 20%, compared with 95% for early gastric cancer. Moreover, the mean age at onset of early gastric cancer is uniformly younger than that of advanced cancer, and the early variety shows a striking geographic distribution. Nevertheless, it is true that some cases of well-documented early gastric cancer have indeed progressed to advanced cancer.

Gastric cancer metastasizes principally by the lymphatic route to regional lymph nodes of the lesser and greater curvature, the porta hepatis, and the subpyloric region. Distant lymphatic metastases also occur, the most common being an enlarged supraclavicular node, called *Virchow node* or *sentinel node.* Hematogenous spread may seed any organ, including the liver, lung, or brain. Direct extension to nearby organs is often encountered. Carcinoma of the stomach can also spread to the ovary, where it commonly elicits a desmoplastic response, in which case it is termed a *Krukenberg tumor.* Figure 13-26 schematically depicts the major types of gastric cancer.

☐ Clinical Features:

In the United States and Europe, most patients with gastric cancer have metastases by the time they are seen for examination. Thus, the symptoms and course are usually those of advanced cancer. The most frequent initial symptom is weight loss, usually associated with anorexia and nausea. The majority of patients complain of epigastric or back pain, a symptom that mimics benign gastric ulcer and is often relieved by antacids or H_2-receptor antagonists. However, as the disease advances, symptomatic amelioration with medical therapy disappears.

Obstruction of the gastric outlet may occur with large tumors of the antrum or prepyloric region. Massive bleeding is uncommon, but chronic bleeding is often reflected in the finding of occult blood in the stools and anemia. Tumors that involve the esophagogastric junction result in dysphagia and occasionally mimic achalasia and esophageal adenocarcinoma.

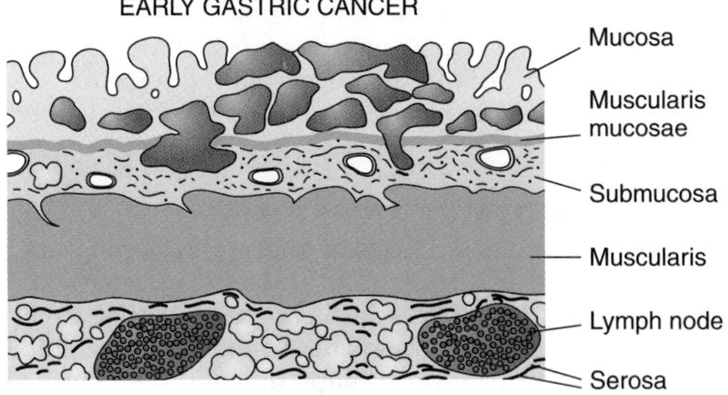

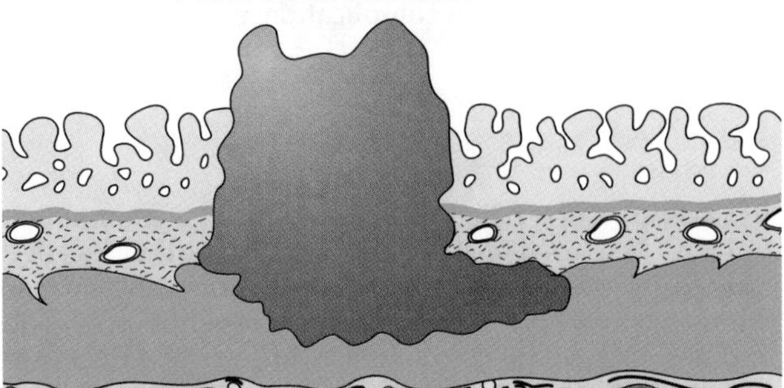

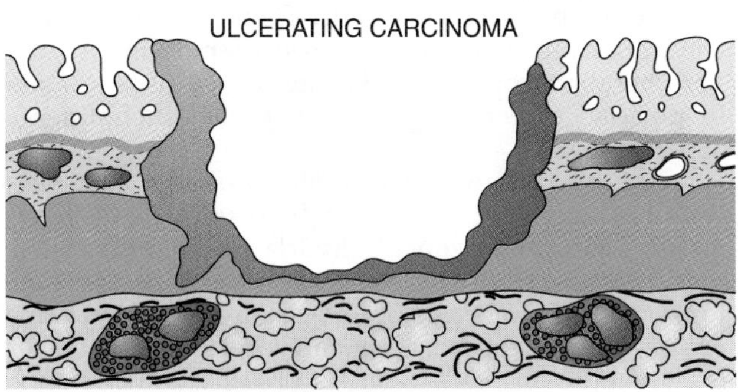

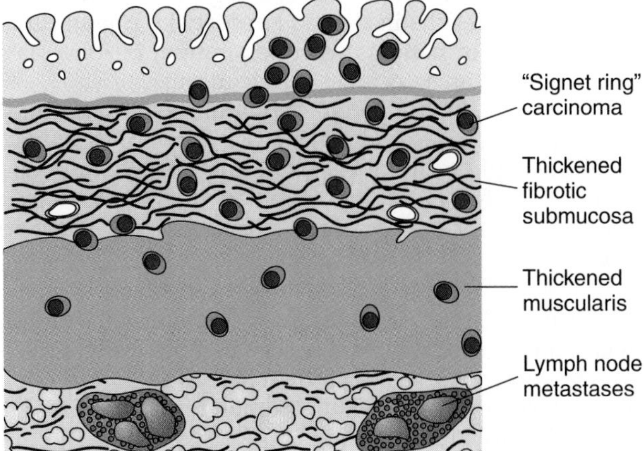

FIGURE *13-26*
The major types of gastric cancer.

Patients with early gastric cancer may be asymptomatic but usually complain of dyspepsia or epigastric pain. Weight loss, melena, and anemia are present in a minority of patients. Two thirds of patients with stomach cancer have fasting achlorhydria, compared with fewer than 25% of normal persons of the same age.

Carcinoembryonic antigen is increased in the blood of one fourth of patients with advanced gastric cancer. This test has little value in the diagnosis of stomach cancer, but it may be helpful in monitoring the course of metastatic disease or of postoperative recurrence.

Carcinoid Tumors

Various endocrine cells in the normal gastric mucosa may give rise to neoplasms, collectively termed *carcinoid tumors*. Most pathologists consider all carcinoid tumors of the gastrointestinal tract to be of low-grade malignancy. The probability of metastases depends more on the size than on the histopathological characteristics. Most of these tumors do not display hormonal function, although an occasional one secretes serotonin, and their metastases can cause the carcinoid syndrome. Many gastric carcinoids occur in the setting of autoimmune metaplastic atrophic gastritis and pernicious anemia. The features of carcinoid tumors are discussed later in this chapter.

Gastric Lymphoma

Primary lymphoma of the stomach accounts for about 5% of all malignant stomach tumors, but it is the most common of all extranodal lymphomas, constituting 20% of such neoplasms. **Clinically and radiologically, gastric lymphoma mimics gastric adenocarcinoma.** The presenting symptoms of gastric lymphoma of weight loss, dyspepsia, and abdominal pain are similar to those of gastric adenocarcinoma. The age at diagnosis is usually 40 to 65 years, and there is no sex predominance. Radiologically, the tumors often cannot be differentiated from carcinoma, because they may be polypoid, ulcerating, or diffuse. Most gastric lymphomas are low-grade B-cell neoplasms of the MALToma type (**m**ucosa-**a**ssociated **l**ymphoid **t**issue) and arise in the setting of chronic *H. pylori* gastritis with lymphoid hyperplasia. Some of these lymphomas regress after eradication of the infection with *H. pylori*. Other histopathological varieties are similar to those in primary nodal lymphomas, as described in Chapter 20.

The prognosis for gastric lymphoma is considerably better than that for adenocarcinoma. The overall 5-year survival is about 50%, depending on the extent of disease at the time of diagnosis. The treatment of favorable cases is primarily surgical; the value of postoperative radiation therapy is uncertain. More widespread lesions are treated with chemotherapy.

Malignant Stromal Tumor (Leiomyosarcoma)

Malignant stromal tumors, which constitute about 1% of gastric malignant tumors, are seen as palpable masses in up to half of the patients with this cancer. It is often difficult to predict the biological behavior of a stromal tumor from its morphological appearance in the absence of infiltration or metastases. Although there is no precise correlation between the size of a gastric stromal tumor and prognosis, tumors larger than 8 cm in diameter are more likely to have spread by the time of diagnosis. Macroscopically, a malignant stromal tumor is similar to a benign leiomyoma, except that it is often larger and softer. Microscopically, the malignant stromal tumors often have smooth muscle differentiation. Cellular pleomorphism and hyperchromasia may be present in both benign and malignant tumors, but the number of mitoses is usually greater in malignant stromal tumors than in leiomyomas. In some cases, the true nature of the tumor becomes apparent only after long-term follow-up.

Metastases are usually to the liver and the peritoneal surfaces, and direct spread to adjacent tissues may occur. Lymph node metastasis is rare. Treatment is surgical, and the 5-year survival rate is 25%.

Metastatic Tumors

Metastases to the stomach from tumors elsewhere are uncommon. The stomach is occasionally secondarily involved in lymphomas and leukemias. The most common metastases from solid tumors are from malignant melanoma, although examples of many other tumors have occasionally also been recorded. A metastasis may ulcerate and mimic a primary tumor of the stomach.

MECHANICAL DISORDERS

RUPTURE OF THE STOMACH: This catastrophe is rare and most commonly associated with blunt abdominal trauma from automobile accidents.

Spontaneous gastric perforation typically occurs in middle-aged women and follows gastric overdistention, severe vomiting, labor and delivery, or the production of excess carbon dioxide after ingestion of sodium bicarbonate or after consumption of unusually large quantities of carbonated beverages. Distention of the stomach during cardiopulmonary resuscitation has resulted in rupture of the stomach. Spontaneous perforation of the stomach in the newborn has also been described. The consequences of rupture and spontaneous perforation are disastrous, and early surgical repair is crucial for survival. Pneumoperitoneum after endoscopy has been recorded but does not necessarily indicate a clinically significant perforation.

VOLVULUS OF THE STOMACH: This rare condition refers to torsion of the stomach upon itself. Volvulus may be asymptomatic if the vascular supply of the stomach is not compromised. However, severe abdominal pain, upper gastrointestinal obstruction, and shock accompany interruption of blood flow and blockage of the lumen. A gastric tumor or pressure from an extragastric mass may warp the anatomy of the stomach and allow it to twist. Gastric volvulus has also occurred in association with a large hiatal hernia. Nasogastric decompression and surgical repair are the usual treatment.

DIVERTICULA OF THE STOMACH: These outpouchings of the gastric wall are rare, developing after prolonged stress from tumors, ulcers, gastritis, and surgery. Diverticula in the cardia are not associated with such conditions; they presumably result from congenital weakness of the wall or perhaps unusual intraluminal pressure at this site. Patients are either asymptomatic or complain of nonspecific symptoms. Hemorrhage and perforation are uncommon complications.

BEZOARS

Bezoars are foreign bodies in the stomach of animals and humans that are composed of food or hair that has been altered by the digestive process. Historically, bezoars were esteemed for their alleged therapeutic properties and aesthetic value, and one was included in the crown jewels of Queen Elizabeth I.

PHYTOBEZOAR: These vegetable concretions are unusual in the normal stomach, except in persons who eat many persimmons or swallow unchewed bubble gum. Phytobezoars are usually found in persons with conditions that cause delayed gastric emptying, such as peripheral neuropathy of diabetes or gastric cancer, and in persons undergoing therapy with anticholinergic agents.

In the past few decades, phytobezoars have been found principally in patients who display delayed gastric emptying and hypochlorhydria after partial gastrectomy, particularly when the surgery has included vagotomy. Wandering bezoars may cause small intestinal obstruction. Plant bezoars contain vegetable or fruit fibers (e.g., potato skins, corn, celery) and seeds. Unripe pulp or ripe skin of persimmons contains tannin monomers that polymerize at low pH to form tannin–cellulose–protein complexes. These complexes act as a glue that binds other material and results in a dark, hard, sticky phytobezoar. The majority of patients with persimmon bezoars have bleeding from an associated gastric ulcer.

The preferred treatment of phytobezoars is chemical attack with cellulase; in some cases, manual disruption by endoscopic techniques, including jets of water, has been successful. However, enzymatic therapy is usually not effective for persimmon bezoars, and surgery is required.

TRICHOBEZOAR: This mass is a hairball within a gelatinous matrix; it is usually seen in long-haired girls or young women who eat their own hair as a nervous habit. Such a bezoar may grow by accretion to form a complete cast of the stomach, reaching a size of up to 3 kg (Fig. 13-27). Strands of hair may extend into the bowel as far as the transverse colon, the so-called *Rapunzel syndrome*. Most trichobezoars require surgical removal.

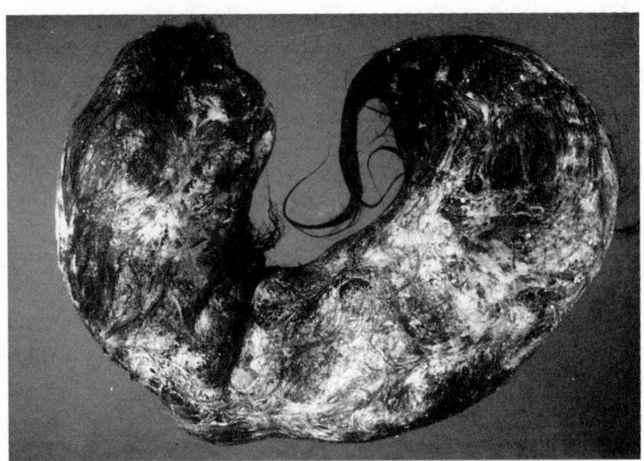

FIGURE 13-27
Trichobezoar (hairball). A mass of hair in a gelatinous matrix forms a cast of the stomach.

The Small Intestine

ANATOMY

Early in development, the intestinal tract begins as a tube that joins the stomach to the cloaca. This tube progressively elongates, and its cephalic portion becomes the segment that extends from the distal duodenum to the proximal ileum. The more caudal portion develops into the distal ileum and the proximal two thirds of the transverse colon. The vitelline duct, which connects the primitive duct with the yolk sac, may persist as a Meckel diverticulum. To achieve the final position of the intestine, the fetal gut undergoes a complex series of rotations.

The small intestine extends from the pylorus to the ileocecal valve and, depending on the tone of its muscle, measures from 3.5 to 6.5 m in length. It is divided into three regions:

1. **The duodenum** extends to the ligament of Treitz.
2. **The jejunum** is the proximal 40% of the remainder of the small intestine.
3. **The ileum** is the distal 60%.

The entire length of the small intestine, which is disposed in redundant loops, is movable, except for the duodenum, which is almost entirely retroperitoneal and therefore fixed.

The C-shaped duodenum surrounds the head of the pancreas and receives the biliary drainage of the liver and the pancreatic secretions through the common bile duct at the ampulla of Vater. The distal duodenum becomes invested by mesentery and merges with the jejunum at the ligament of Treitz. The proximity of the duodenum to its neighbors means that it may be affected by disorders such as cancer of the pancreas and cholecystoduodenal fistulas. Conversely, duodenal ulcers may penetrate into the pancreas or liver. There is no demarcation between the jejunum and ileum, which merge gradually. The wall of the jejunum is thicker and its lumen wider than that of the ileum.

The plicae circularis, the spiral folds that consist of mucosa and submucosa, are most prominent in the distal duodenum and proximal jejunum, usually disappearing in the terminal ileum. **Peyer patches** are lymphoid aggregates in the submucosa measuring up to 3 cm in diameter. They are located in the antimesenteric aspect of the distal half of the ileum. The ileocecal valve is not a true valve but rather a muscular sphincter that regulates the flow of intestinal contents into the cecum.

The duodenum is served by the pancreaticoduodenal branch of the hepatic artery, which arises from the celiac artery. The jejunum and ileum are supplied by the superior mesenteric artery (a branch of the aorta), which is arranged in arcades in the mesentery, thereby providing abundant collateral circulation in its distal reaches. The veins draining the small intestine empty into the portal venous system. The lymphatic channels of the duodenum drain to the portal and pyloric lymph nodes, whereas those of the jejunum and ileum communicate with the mesenteric lymph nodes. The lymphatics of the terminal ileum empty into the ileocolic nodes. The small intestine is innervated by sympathetic fibers from the celiac plexus and ganglia and by parasympathetic fibers from the vagus nerve.

Histology

An understanding of the microscopic anatomy of the small intestine is crucial for an appreciation of its function in health and disease. Similar to that of the stomach and the colon, the wall of the small intestine is composed of four layers: the mucosa, the submucosa, the muscularis, and the serosa. In the retroperitoneal duodenum, however, only the anterior wall is covered by a serosa.

SEROSA AND MUSCULARIS PROPRIA: The serosa consists of loose connecting tissue bounded by a single layer of mesothelial cells. The muscularis propria has an outer longitudinal layer and an inner circular layer, both of which function in a coordinated manner to propel the intestinal contents by peristalsis.

SUBMUCOSA: This region consists of vascularized connective tissue and a few scattered lymphocytes, plasma cells, and macrophages, with an occasional mast cell and eosinophil. In the duodenum, the submucosa is occupied by the Brunner glands, branched structures that contain mucous and serous cells. These secrete mucus and bicarbonate, which protect the duodenal mucosa from peptic ulceration. The lymphatic and venous capillaries of the mucosa drain into a highly developed system of lymphatic and venous plexuses in the submucosa.

The myenteric nerve plexus of Auerbach, which lies between the two layers of the muscularis, and Meissner plexus in the submucosa are interconnected.

MUCOSA: The distinctive feature of the intestinal mucosa is its arrangement in villi, finger-like projections 0.5 to 1 mm in length, which expand the absorptive area enormously. The macroscopic structure of the villi varies in different regions of the small intestine. In the proximal duodenum, the villi tend to be broad and blunted, whereas in the distal duodenum and proximal jejunum, they exhibit a more slender, leaf-shaped appearance. Shorter, finger-shaped villi are the rule in the distal jejunum and ileum. There are also geographic variations in the normal appearance of villi. For example, the populations of Southeast Asia and the Caribbean tend to exhibit shorter villi, deeper crypts, and increased cellularity of the lamina propria than do those of the United States and Europe, probably reflecting differences in diet, bacterial flora, or frequency of infection.

The villi are composed of a columnar epithelium resting on a basement membrane, a lamina propria, and a muscularis mucosae, which separates the mucosa from the submucosa. The connective tissue of the lamina propria forms the core of the villus and surrounds the crypts of Lieberkuhn at the base of the villi. The normal lamina propria is home to a variety of mesenchymal cells, including lymphocytes, plasma cells, and macrophages. Plasma cells in this location principally secrete immunoglobulin A (IgA) into the intestinal lumen or the lamina propria itself. Occasional eosinophils and mast cells are scattered throughout. A few smooth muscle cells and fibroblasts are also present. The cellular composition of the lamina propria reflects its role in protecting against invasion by bacteria that may penetrate the mucosa and segregating foreign material that breaches the mucosa.

Some IgA is produced by plasma cells in the lamina propria as a dimer that diffuses through the basement membrane of the crypt. IgA then reaches the basal or lateral surface of the epithelial cell, where it combines with the secretory component produced by that cell. The resulting *secretory IgA* molecule is taken up by the epithelial cell and secreted into the lumen. Secretory IgA, which is more resistant to proteolysis than is serum IgA, binds food antigens and prevents bacterial adherence to the intestinal epithelial cells. Moreover, IgA can neutralize bacterial toxins and inhibit the replication and mucosal penetration of viruses.

Lymphoid nodules (MALT) are scattered throughout the mucosa and aggregate into visible Peyer patches. The columnar epithelial cells of the villi are principally absorptive, whereas those lining the crypts are the source of cell renewal and secretion.

Absorptive cells, or enterocytes (see Fig. 13-1), are the principal lining cells of the intestinal villi. The villi also exhibit a few goblet and endocrine cells. Enterocytes are tall and display basally situated nuclei. Numerous microvilli extend from the surface of these cells into the lumen, thereby hugely increasing the absorptive surface. The plasma membrane of the microvilli is covered by a glycocalyx (fuzzy coat) produced by the absorptive cell. Disaccharidases and peptidases reside in this glycocalyx. Certain receptors, such as that for the intrinsic factor–vitamin B_{12} complex in the ileum, are also present in the membrane–glycocalyx complex. The cytoplasm immediately beneath the microvilli contains a network of actin microfilaments, termed the **terminal web**. These filaments, which are also associated with myosin and other contractile proteins, insert into the core of the microvilli and presumably serve as a contractile apparatus. The lateral borders of adjacent plasma membranes form tight junctions, which are impermeable to macromolecules but permit passive transport of small molecules by the paracellular route. Absorbed material is transported from the epithelial cell into the intercellular space between absorptive cells through the lateral or basal plasma membranes. It then penetrates the basement membrane, traverses the lamina propria, and enters a capillary or a lymphatic channel.

Four cell types are recognized in the crypts: Paneth, goblet, endocrine, and undifferentiated cells.

- **Paneth cells** at the base of the crypts are similar to the zymogen cells of the pancreas and salivary glands that are actively engaged in exocrine secretion. Within Paneth cells, eosinophilic secretory granules fill a basophilic cytoplasm. These cells play a role in mucosal defense, as evidenced by the presence of lysozyme, antimicrobial products, including peptides called crypt defensins (cryptdins), and CD95 ligand, which is a member of the tumor necrosis factor (TNF) family of cytokines.
- **Goblet cells** of the lateral walls of the crypts are flask-shaped and filled with mucus granules. They are similar in structure and function to goblet cells elsewhere and contain neutral and acid mucins.
- **Endocrine cells**, both argentaffin and argyrophilic, appear inverted, with an apical nucleus and basal granules. The basal location of the granules implies that they are secreted into the lamina propria rather than the lumen. These cells produce numerous gastrointestinal hormones and peptides, including gastrin, secretin, cholecystokinin, glucagon, VIP, and serotonin. The secretion of such hormones in response to appropriate stimuli is presumed to regulate many gastrointestinal functions. As in other tissues, primary tumors derived from these cells are often characterized by striking hormone secretion.
- **Undifferentiated cells** are located in the lateral walls of the crypts and are interspersed between the Paneth cells at their bases. They are the most numerous cells of the crypts. Small glycoprotein secretory granules are grouped in the apical cytoplasm of some of the undifferentiated cells. These cells function as the reserve cells from which all the other mucosal cells are renewed, and thus mitoses are numerous among them.

Cell renewal in the small intestine is limited to the crypts, where undifferentiated cells divide. The newly formed cells migrate up the villus, where they terminally differentiate into absorptive cells and goblet cells and eventually undergo apoptosis or slough into the lumen at the tip of the villus. Their absorptive capacity is maximal when the cells reach the upper third of the villus. The mucosal epithelium of the small intestine is replaced within a period of 4 to 7 days. This rapid cell proliferation explains why the intestinal epithelium is particularly sensitive to radiation and chemotherapeutic agents.

CONGENITAL DISORDERS

Atresia and Stenosis

Intestinal atresia and stenosis, although rare, are the most frequent causes of neonatal intestinal obstruction.

ATRESIA: Atresia is defined as a complete occlusion of the intestinal lumen, which may be manifested as (1) a thin intraluminal diaphragm, (2) blind proximal and distal sacs joined by a cord, or (3) disconnected blind ends. Multiple intestinal occlusions may give the appearance of a string of sausages. Although the majority of cases of congenital atresia are believed to reflect intrauterine ischemia during fetal development, one fourth of the cases are associated with meconium ileus, and cystic fibrosis is discovered in one tenth of the cases of atresia.

STENOSIS: This abnormality is an incomplete stricture of the small intestine, which narrows but does not occlude, the lumen. Stenosis may also be caused by an incomplete diaphragm. Although the condition is usually symptomatic in infancy, cases in middle-aged adults have been recorded.

One fourth of mothers of fetuses with high intestinal atresia develop polyhydramnios during the last trimester, presumably because the fetus does not swallow amniotic fluid. Intestinal atresia or stenosis is diagnosed on the basis of persistent vomiting of bile-containing fluid within the first day of life. Meconium is not passed. The obstructed fetal intestine is dilated and filled with fluid, a condition detectable with imaging techniques. Surgical correction is usually successful, but coexistent anomalies often complicate the course.

Duplications

Gastrointestinal duplications (enteric cysts), which may occur from the esophagus to the anus, are spherical or tubular structures attached to the alimentary tract. They may be seen as cystic structures or may communicate with the lumen of the gastrointestinal tract. Intestinal duplications are most common in the ileum and less so in the jejunum. The duplications have a smooth muscle wall and an epithelium of the gastrointestinal type. Communicating duplications are often lined by gastric mucosa, a situation that may lead to peptic ulceration, bleeding, or perforation. The cystic duplications may cause intestinal obstruction by extrinsic pressure or may be associated with intussusception. Many duplications are silent, but those that become symptomatic are treated with surgical removal.

Meckel Diverticulum

Meckel diverticulum, caused by persistence of the vitelline duct, is an outpouching of the gut on the antimesenteric border of the ileum, 60 to 100 cm from the ileocecal valve in adults. It is the most common and the most clinically significant congenital anomaly of the small intestine (Fig. 13-28). Two thirds of the patients are younger than 2 years.

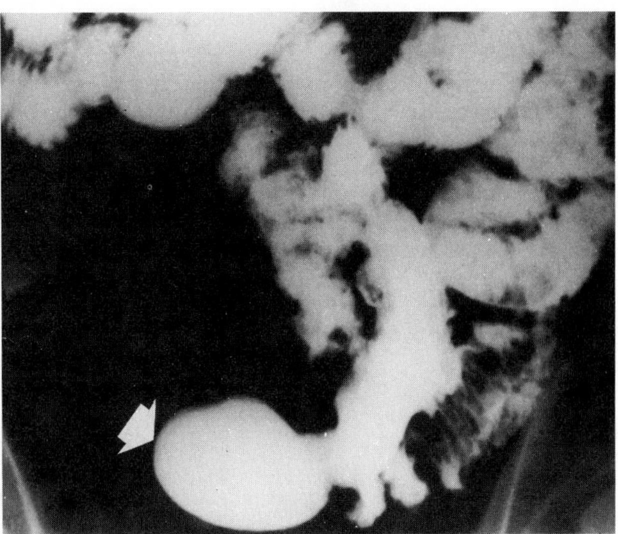

FIGURE *13-28*
Meckel diverticulum. A contrast radiograph of the small intestine shows a barium-filled diverticulum of the ileum *(arrow)*.

☐ **Pathology:** Meckel diverticulum is about 5 cm in length, with a diameter slightly less than that of the ileum, but considerably larger than that of the appendix. A fibrous cord may hang freely from the apex of the diverticulum or may be attached to the umbilicus, and fistulas between Meckel diverticulum and the umbilicus have been described.

Meckel diverticulum is a true diverticulum in that it possesses all the coats of the normal intestine, and the mucosa is similar to that of the adjoining ileum. Most Meckel diverticula are asymptomatic and discovered only as incidental findings at laparotomy for other causes or at autopsy. Of the minority that become symptomatic, about half contain ectopic gastric, duodenal, pancreatic, biliary, or colonic tissue. Of these, more than three fourths exhibit gastric ectopic tissue.

☐ **Clinical Features:** Meckel diverticulum may lead to a number of complications.

- **Hemorrhage:** The most common complication is bleeding, which is responsible for half of all lower gastrointestinal hemorrhage in children. Bleeding results from **peptic ulceration** of the ileum adjacent to the ectopic gastric mucosa.
- **Intestinal obstruction:** The diverticulum may act as a lead point for **intussusception** and thereby cause intestinal obstruction. Obstruction can also be caused by **volvulus** around the fibrotic remnant of the vitelline duct.
- **Diverticulitis:** Inflammation of a Meckel diverticulum, that is, diverticulitis leads to symptoms indistinguishable from those of appendicitis. Thus, the surgeon who operates for acute appendicitis, but encounters a normal appendix, is well advised to search for a Meckel diverticulum.

- **Perforation:** Peptic ulceration, either in the diverticulum or in the ileum, may cause perforation, complicated by a rapidly spreading peritonitis.
- **Fistula:** A fecal discharge from the umbilicus may be observed.

Traditionally, surgery was recommended even for an asymptomatic Meckel diverticulum; this advice has now been questioned, because the incidence of surgical complications may be greater than the risk of an untreated diverticulum.

Malrotation

Defective intestinal rotation in fetal life leads to abnormal positions of the small intestine and colon, anomalous attachments, and bands. The clinical importance of such rotational anomalies in children and adults lies in their propensity to cause catastrophic volvulus of the small and large intestine and incarceration of the bowel in an internal hernia.

Meconium Ileus

Cystic fibrosis often has as its earliest manifestation neonatal intestinal obstruction, caused by the accumulation of tenacious meconium in the small intestine. The abnormal consistency of the meconium reflects a deficiency in pancreatic enzymes and a high viscosity of the intestinal mucus. Usually the distal ileum is contracted beyond the obstruction, whereas the midileum proximal to the inspissated meconium is dilated. In half of affected infants, meconium ileus is complicated by (1) volvulus, (2) perforation with meconium peritonitis, or (3) intestinal atresia. Meconium ileus must be differentiated from the distal intestinal obstruction syndrome associated with cystic fibrosis, in which a small plug of meconium in the distal colon may eventually be passed, thereby relieving the obstruction.

Successful treatment of meconium ileus without complications may be accomplished by means of a hypertonic enema containing a detergent. Complicated meconium ileus always requires surgical intervention and is associated with a significant mortality.

INFECTIONS

Bacterial Diarrhea

Bacterial diarrhea has plagued humans since the dawn of recorded history and continues to be an important clinical problem. Despite advances in the identification of organisms, antibiotic therapy, and fluid and electrolyte replacement, infectious diarrhea still causes many deaths worldwide. This is particularly true in underdeveloped countries and in infants. The normal small bowel has few microorganisms (usually $<10^4$/mL), mostly aerobic bacilli such as lactobacilli. These organisms travel in the food stream and ordinarily do not colonize the small intestine. Infectious diarrheal states are caused by colonization with bacteria such as toxigenic strains of *Escherichia coli* and *Vibrio cholerae.*

The most significant factor in infectious diarrhea is increased intestinal secretion, stimulated by bacterial toxins and enteric hormones. Decreased absorption and increased peristaltic activity contribute less to the diarrhea.

The colon harbors an abundant bacterial flora, with a concentration seven orders of magnitude greater than that of the small intestine. In the colon, anaerobic bacteria (e.g., *Bacteroides* and *Clostridium* species) outnumber aerobic organisms by a factor of 1000. With the more rapid transit of intestinal contents during a diarrheal episode, the flora are shifted to a more aerobic population, including *E. coli, Klebsiella,* and *Proteus.* Moreover, the offending organisms themselves become conspicuous, and pathogens of the small intestine such as *V. cholerae* may be the major isolate in the stools.

The paucity of bacteria in the stomach and small intestine is accounted for by a number of protective mechanisms: (1) gastric acid production is inimical to bacterial growth, an effect that explains the overgrowth of bacteria in the stomach in the presence of achlorhydria; (2) bile has antimicrobial activity; (3) the peristaltic propulsion of intestinal contents limits the time available for bacterial accumulation; (4) the normal flora secrete their own antimicrobial substances to maintain an ecological balance (indeed, treatment with broad-spectrum antibiotics alters the natural flora and allows overgrowth of ordinarily harmless organisms); and (5) the plasma cells of the lamina propria secrete IgA into the intestinal lumen.

The individual agents responsible for infectious diarrhea are discussed in Chapter 9. Here we only briefly review the major entities. The agents of infectious diarrhea are conveniently classified into toxigenic organisms, which produce diarrhea by elaborating toxins, adherent bacteria, and invasive bacteria.

Toxigenic Diarrhea

The prototypic organisms that produce diarrhea by secreting toxins are *V. cholerae* and toxigenic strains of *E. coli.* Toxigenic diarrhea is characterized by the following:

- Damage to the intestinal mucosa is minimal or absent.
- The organism remains on the mucosal surface, where it secretes its toxin.
- Fluid secreted into the small intestine causes watery diarrhea, which can lead to dehydration, particularly in the case of cholera.

Although many organisms have been isolated in so-called *travelers' diarrhea,* the most common pathogen in almost all studies is toxigenic *E. coli.* Enteroadherent *E. coli* has been implicated as a diarrheal pathogen.

Diarrhea Caused by Invasive Bacteria

Invasive bacteria, as their name implies, cause diarrhea by directly injuring the intestinal mucosa. Among these organisms, *Shigella, Salmonella,* and certain strains of *E. coli, Yersinia,* and *Campylobacter* are the most widely recognized. Invasive organisms tend to infect the distal ileum and colon, whereas toxigenic bacteria mainly involve the upper intestinal tract. Curiously, despite the obvious morphological lesions associated with these invasive organisms, the mechanism by which they produce diarrhea has not been clarified. Enterotoxins have been identified, but their role in causing diarrhea has not been established. Invasion of the mucosa by bacteria increases the synthesis of prostaglandins in the affected tissue, and inhibitors of prostaglandin synthesis seem to block fluid secretion. It is also possible that the damaged mucosa is unable to resorb fluid from the lumen.

SHIGELLOSIS: Shigellosis principally affects the colon, although the terminal ileum is occasionally involved. Microscopically, a granular and hemorrhagic mucosa exhibits numerous shallow serpiginous ulcers. The inflammation, which is especially severe in the sigmoid colon and rectum, is usually superficial. In the early stage, the accumulation of neutrophils in damaged crypts (crypt abscesses) is similar to that in ulcerative colitis, and the lymphoid follicles of the mucosa break down to form ulcers. As the infection recedes, the ulcers heal and the mucosa returns to normal.

TYPHOID FEVER: Typhoid fever (*Salmonella* enteritis) is today uncommon in the industrialized world but still presents a problem in underdeveloped countries. Necrosis of lymphoid tissue, principally in the terminal ileum, leads to scattered ulcers. Infection of Peyer patches results in oval ulcers, in which the longer dimension is in the long axis of the intestine. Occasionally, lymphoid follicles in the large bowel or the appendix are ulcerated. The base of the ulcer is composed of black necrotic tissue mixed with fibrin.

Microscopically, the early lesions of typhoid fever contain large basophilic macrophages filled with typhoid bacilli, erythrocytes, and necrotic debris. Necrosis of lymphoid follicles becomes confluent, and mucosal ulceration follows. Similar lymphoid hyperplasia and necrosis are seen in the regional lymph nodes. Healing of the ulcers is complete within a week of the acute symptoms and leaves little fibrosis or other sequelae. **Intestinal hemorrhage and perforation**, principally in the ileum, are the most feared complications of typhoid fever and tend to occur in the third week and during convalescence.

NONTYPHOIDAL SALMONELLOSIS: Formerly known as *paratyphoid fever,* this enteritis is caused by *Salmonella* strains other than *S. typhi* and is generally a far less serious illness than typhoid fever. In addition to causing diarrhea, bacteremia, and fever, nontyphoidal salmonellosis also involves localized infections at other sites. The principal target is the ileum, although minor involvement of the colon may also take place. The organisms invade the mucosa, which shows mild ulceration, edema, and infiltration with neutrophils. Hematogenous dissemination from the intestine may carry the infection to bones, joints, and meninges. Interestingly, there seems to be a relation between sickle cell anemia and *Salmonella* osteomyelitis, presumably because phagocytosis of the products of hemolysis prevents further ingestion of the *Salmonella* organisms and allows their dissemination through the bloodstream.

ENTEROINVASIVE AND ENTEROHEMORRHAGIC STRAINS OF *E. COLI*: These organisms are uncommon causes of a bloody diarrhea that resemble shigellosis. Certain strains of *E. coli*, particularly serotype 0157:H7, produce *Shigella*-like toxins, but the role of these proteins in the pathogenesis of the enterocolitis is not understood. Serotype 0157:H7 has also been implicated in the pathogenesis of the hemolytic–uremic syndrome in children.

YERSINIA ENTEROCOLITIS: *Yersinia enterocolitica* and *Y. pseudotuberculosis* are transmitted by pets or contaminated food, and infection is most common in young children. *Yersinia* infection causes diarrhea, cramps, and fever and lasts 1 to 3 weeks. The disease is characterized by hyperplasia of Peyer patches, with acute ulceration of the overlying mucosa. The fibrinopurulent exudate that covers the ulcers often contains many organisms.

In addition to causing enterocolitis, *Yersinia* causes acute mesenteric adenitis and pain in the right lower quadrant. Infected children have undergone laparotomy because of a mistaken diagnosis of appendicitis. In such cases, the ileocecal nodes are enlarged and matted together. On section, small yellow microabscesses are seen. These correspond microscopically to epithelioid granulomas with central necrotic zones in the case of infection with *Y. pseudotuberculosis.* Langhans or foreign body–type giant cells are sometimes present. In addition to submucosal edema and an inflammatory infiltrate, the ileum and appendix may contain similar granulomas, causing an appearance that has been mistaken for Crohn disease.

Adults, who are less susceptible to infection with *Yersinia* than are children, have an acute diarrhea, often followed within a few weeks by erythema nodosum, erythema multiforme, or polyarthritis. Patients with chronic debilitating diseases may develop a fatal *Yersinia* bacteremia, which is resistant to antibiotic treatment. Interestingly, persons with thalassemia have a propensity for *Y. enterocolitica* infection.

CAMPYLOBACTER JEJUNI: Infection with *C. jejuni* is now recognized as one of the most important causes of bacterial diarrhea. Some investigators have reported a higher incidence of *Campylobacter* than of nontyphoidal *Salmonella* and *Shigella* infections in the United States, and in one survey from Great Britain, half of all bacterial diarrhea was caused by *Campylobacter.* Humans are involved mainly by contact with infected domestic animals or through ingestion of poorly cooked or contaminated food. Adults usually recover from the diarrheal illness in less than 1 week.

Food Poisoning

Infectious agents can produce gastroenteritis not only by infecting the bowel directly but also by elaborating enterotoxins in contaminated food, which is then ingested.

STAPHYLOCOCCUS AUREUS: This widespread bacterium is a common cause of food poisoning. Symptoms result from the ingestion of food contaminated with strains of *Staphylococcus* that produce an exotoxin that damages the epithelium of the gastrointestinal tract. Within 6 hours of the ingestion of tainted food, severe vomiting and abdominal cramps occur, often followed by diarrhea. Most victims recover in 1 to 2 days.

CLOSTRIDIUM PERFRINGENS: This bacterium elaborates an enterotoxin that causes vomiting and diarrhea. Although the organism is anaerobic, it can tolerate exposure to air for as long as 3 days. Maximal activity of the clostridial enterotoxin is in the ileum. In most cases, watery diarrhea and severe abdominal pain, which begin 8 to 24 hours after ingestion of the contaminated food, last only about 1 day. However, outbreaks of a necrotizing enteritis with high mortality are associated with contamination of undercooked pork in New Guinea, where the disease is known as **pigbel**.

Viral Gastroenteritis

ROTAVIRUS: Infection with this virus is a common cause of infantile diarrhea and accounts for about half of the cases of acute diarrhea in hospitalized children younger than 2 years. Rotavirus has been demonstrated in duodenal biopsy specimens and is associated with injury to the surface epithelium and impaired intestinal absorption for periods of up to 2 months.

NORWALK VIRUSES: These agents account for one third of the epidemics of viral gastroenteritis in the United States. Norwalk viruses have not been propagated in culture but have been demonstrated in the stools by electron microscopy. The virus targets the upper small intestine, where it causes patchy mucosal lesions and malabsorption. Vomiting and diarrhea are usual, but the symptoms resolve within 2 days. The morphological and absorptive alterations require 1 or 2 weeks for reversal.

Other viruses that have been implicated as etiological agents of infective diarrhea include echovirus, coxsackievirus, cytomegalovirus, adenovirus, and coronavirus.

Tuberculosis

Historically an important disease, gastrointestinal tuberculosis is now uncommon in industrialized countries, although it is still a problem in underdeveloped areas. At one time, a large proportion of intestinal tuberculosis involved infection with *Mycobacterium bovis,* which was principally transmitted by contaminated milk. However, the control of tuberculosis in dairy herds and the pasteurization of milk have made infection with this organism a curiosity. Today virtually all cases of intestinal tuberculosis in western countries are caused by *M. tuberculosis.*

Most cases of intestinal tuberculosis are caused either by the ingestion of bacteria in food or by the swallowing of infectious sputum. After it is ingested, the tubercle bacillus, protected from digestion by its waxy capsule, passes into the small bowel. The bacterium then establishes a locus of infection, usually (90% of patients) in the ileocecal region, where lymphoid tissue is abundant. Infection also occurs in the colon, jejunum, appendix, rectum, and duodenum, in that order of frequency. Esophageal and gastric tuberculosis are rare. Although there is a strong correlation between the frequency of intestinal tuberculosis and the severity of pulmonary disease, as many as half the patients with intestinal tuberculosis do not have radiological evidence of pulmonary involvement.

□ **Pathology:** The macroscopic presentation of intestinal tuberculosis is divided into three categories: ulcerative, hypertrophic, and ulcerohypertrophic.

- **Ulcerative intestinal tuberculosis:** This type is seen in more than half of the patients and is characterized by one or more circular or oval ulcers of varying size in the transverse plane of the bowel. As the ulcers heal, reactive fibrosis may cause a circumferential ("napkin ring") stricture of the bowel lumen. The involved bowel is indurated and the serosa studded with grayish white nodules. Mesenteric lymph nodes are typically enlarged and, on cut section, display caseous necrosis. Before antibiotic treatment, ulcerative tuberculosis was associated with a particularly high mortality.
- **Hypertrophic intestinal tuberculosis:** In pure form, this variety is uncommon (10% of patients). It affects the ileocecal region or the colon, which exhibits an exuberant inflammatory and fibroblastic reaction throughout the thickness of the wall. Adhesions between the bowel, mesentery, and lymph nodes may form a palpable mass, and the mass or a secondary stricture may cause intestinal obstruction. Protrusion of the hypertrophic lesion into the bowel lumen may mimic carcinoma.
- **Ulcerohypertrophic intestinal tuberculosis:** This variant is seen in about one third of the patients and combines the features of the ulcerative and hypertrophic forms. Microscopically, typical tuberculous granulomas are found in all layers of the bowel wall, particularly in Peyer patches and lymphoid follicles, and in the mesenteric lymph nodes. Occasionally, tuberculous granulomas are visualized only in the lymph nodes, and the bowel wall displays only nonspecific inflammatory lesions. In old lesions, the granulomas become hyalinized and then disappear, leaving only a dense scar containing small foci of lymphocytes. Seen at autopsy or in surgical specimens, old tuberculous strictures are difficult to distinguish from other causes of stricture, such as ischemic enterocolitis or Crohn disease.

Crohn disease exhibits virtually all the changes produced by intestinal tuberculosis, and indeed these entities have often been confused by pathologists. Unfortunately, the bacilli and caseating granulomas in tuberculous enteritis are often not demonstrable, thus adding to the occasional difficulty in making a correct diagnosis.

□ **Clinical Features:** Almost all patients with intestinal tuberculosis complain of chronic abdominal pain, and about two thirds have a palpable abdominal mass, usually in the right lower quadrant. Weight loss, fever, and weakness are common. Tuberculosis of the appendix has been mistakenly diagnosed as acute appendicitis. Diarrhea occurs in a minority of patients, and about the same number have constipation. Complications of intestinal tuberculosis include obstruction, fistulas, perforation, and abscess. Anorexia and malabsorption may lead to severe malnutrition. The disease is treated with antituberculosis drugs.

Fungi

The gastrointestinal tract is not normally a hospitable environment for fungi. The number of commensal organisms is miniscule, and such agents are restricted to yeasts and anaerobic actinomycetes. **Therefore, fungal infection of the gastrointestinal tract occurs almost exclusively in immunocompromised persons.** Suppression of the normal bacterial flora by antibiotics also favors fungal growth. Under these circumstances, the most common mycosis is caused by *Candida*. Other fungi, including *Histoplasma* and *Mucor*, are occasionally described.

Candidiasis and mucormycosis typically cause mucosal erosions; these may progress to larger ulcers, which are surrounded by hemorrhage and necrosis. The inflammation is characteristically neutrophilic, and there may be remarkably little reaction to the fungi due to immunosuppression. Mucormycosis often exhibits invasion of blood vessels with thrombosis and infarction, but hematogenous dissemination from the intestine is rare. Disseminated histoplasmosis may involve the bowel, where it causes elevated plaques that ulcerate and may even perforate.

Parasites of the Small Intestine

Parasitic diseases of the small bowel are discussed in detail in Chapter 9 and summarized in Figure 13-29. These parasites include (1) **protozoa**, such as *Giardia lamblia*, *Coccidia* species, and cryptosporidia; (2) **nematodes (roundworms)** such as *Ascaris*, *Strongyloides*, and hookworms; and (3) **flatworms**. The flatworms are divided into tapeworms (cestodes), which include *Diphyllobothrium latum*, *Taenia solium*, *Taenia saginata*, and *Hymenolepis nana*. Flukes (trematodes) include various schistosomes and the giant intestinal fluke *Fasciolopsis buski*. In addition, trichinosis has an intestinal phase, during which vomiting, diarrhea, and colic mimic acute food poisoning or bacterial enteritis.

VASCULAR DISEASES

Decreased blood flow to the intestines from any cause can lead to ischemic bowel disease. Analogous to coronary heart disease, there is a spectrum of manifestations. The most common type of ischemic bowel disease is acute intestinal ischemia, which is associated with injury ranging from mucosal necrosis to transmural infarction of the bowel. Chronic intestinal ischemic syndromes are considerably less common and generally require the severe compromise of two or more major arteries, usually by atherosclerosis.

Acute Intestinal Ischemia

☐ Pathogenesis

ARTERIAL OCCLUSION: The sudden occlusion of a large artery by thrombosis or embolization leads to infarction of the small bowel before collateral circulation comes into play. Depending on the size of the artery, infarction may be segmental or may lead to gangrene of virtually the entire small bowel (Fig. 13-30). Occlusive intestinal infarction is most often caused by embolic or thrombotic occlusion of the superior mesenteric artery. A lesser number are the result of arteritis, which often involves small arteries. Transmural infarction of the colon as a result of embolization to the inferior mesenteric artery is uncommon because of the (1) oblique takeoff of this vessel from the aorta, (2) its relatively smaller caliber, and (3) its richer collateral circulation. In addition to intrinsic vascular lesions, volvulus, intussusception, and incarceration of the intestine in a hernial sac may all lead to arterial as well as venous occlusion.

NONOCCLUSIVE INTESTINAL ISCHEMIA: Intestinal ischemic necrosis in which no acute vascular occlusion is evident is today more common than the occlusive type. Nonocclusive intestinal infarction may be extensive and is seen in hypoxic patients with reduced cardiac output from shock of a variety of causes including hemorrhage, sepsis, or acute myocardial infarction, and in uremia. Reduced renal blood flow activates the renin–angiotensin system. Angiotensin reduces blood flow via vasoconstriction, resulting in redistribution of blood flow to the brain and other vital organs. In addition, patients in shock often receive α-adrenergic agents, which may further shunt blood away from the intestine. The drastically lowered perfusion pressure in the arterioles leads to their collapse, thereby aggravating the ischemia.

THROMBOSIS OF THE MESENTERIC VEINS: This cause of intestinal ischemia occurs under a variety of conditions, including hypercoagulable states, stasis, and inflammation (pylephlebitis) Almost all thromboses affect the superior mesenteric vein, and only 5% of the cases involve the inferior mesenteric vein. The collateral flow in the distribution of the superior mesenteric vein is usually sufficient to preclude infarction of the intestine. However, the thrombosis of smaller veins can also lead to transmural infarction.

KAYEXYLATE: Hyperkalemia may be treated with the oral administration of sodium polystyrene sulfonate (Kayexylate). The osmotic effect of the sorbital carrier for the drug can produce catastrophic ischemic necrosis of the gastrointestinal tract.

☐ **Pathology:** The findings depend on the cause, time course, and severity of the ischemia. Infarcted bowel is edematous and diffusely purple. The demarcation between infarcted bowel and normal tissue is usually sharp, although venous occlusion may lead to a more diffuse ap-

CATEGORY	ORGANISMS	TRANSMISSION
PROTOZOON	Giardia 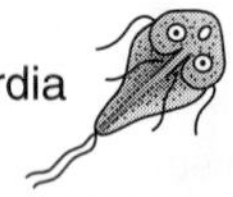	Fecal-oral
ROUND WORMS (NEMATODES)	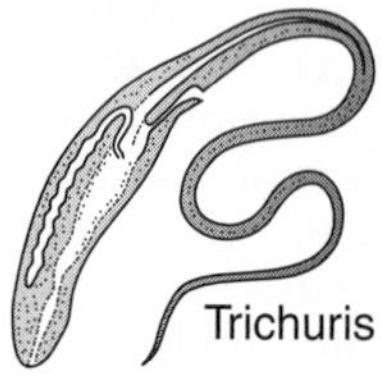 Trichuris; 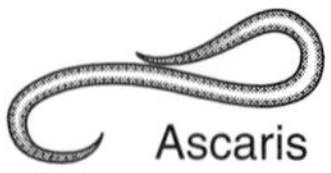 Ascaris	Fecal-oral
	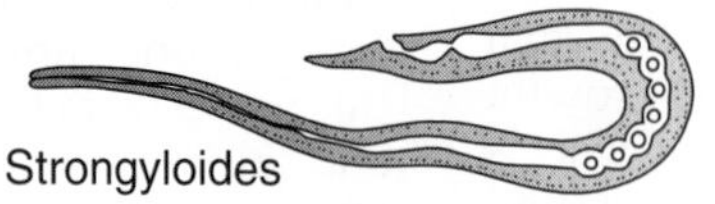 Strongyloides; 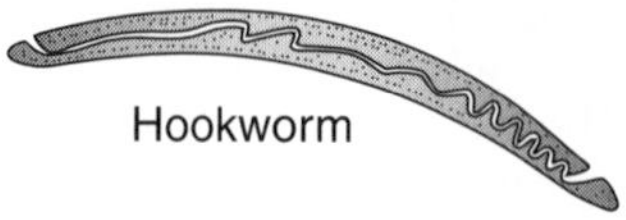 Hookworm	Free living larvae in soil penetrate skin
TAPEWORMS (CESTODES)	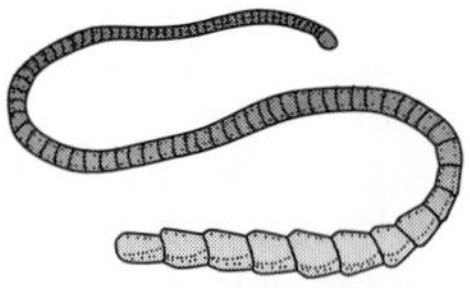 Pork tapeworm *Taenia solium* (2-4 meters); 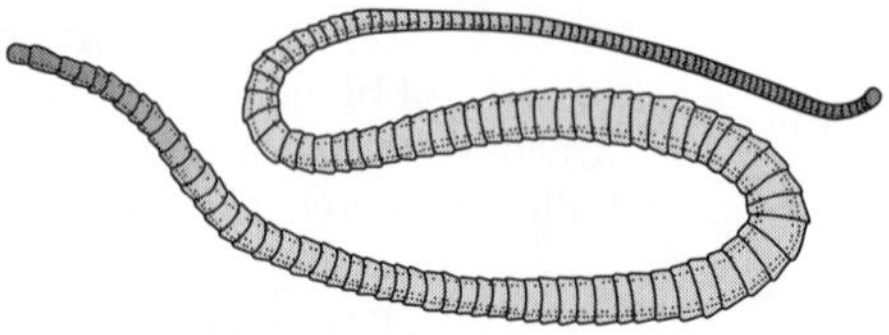 Fish tapeworm *Diphyllobothrium latum* (3-10 meters); 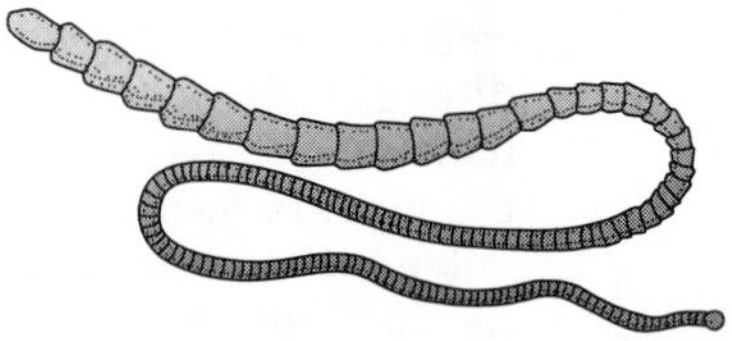 Beef tapeworm *Taenia saginata* (4-8 meters)	Undercooked or raw flesh containing cysts
	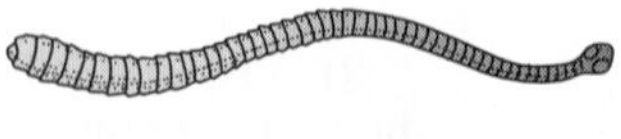 Human tapeworm *Hymenolepis nana* (0.5-5 meters)	Fecal-oral
FLUKE (TREMATODE)	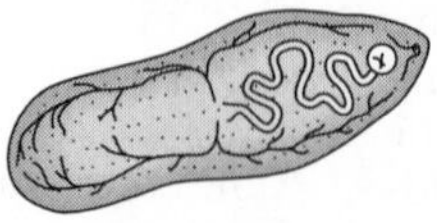 *Fasciolopsis buski*	Fecal-oral (with intermediate host)

FIGURE 13-29
Parasites of the small bowel.

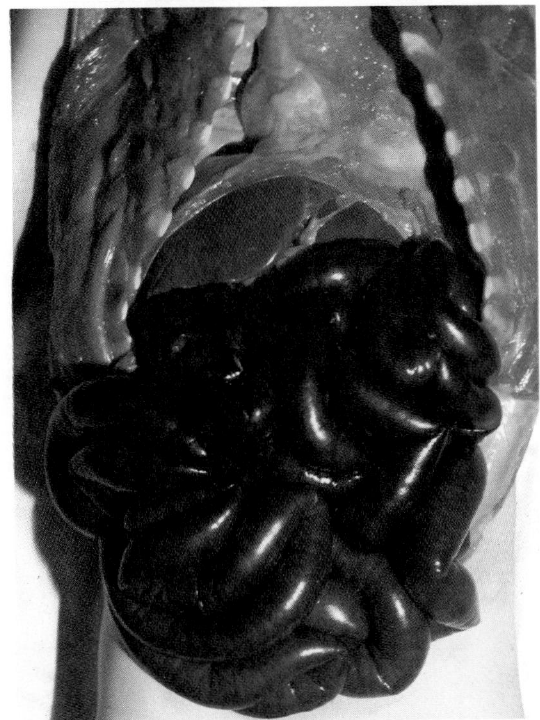

FIGURE 13-30
Infarct of the small bowel. This young boy died after an episode of intense abdominal pain and shock. Autopsy demonstrated volvulus of the small bowel, which had occluded the superior mesenteric artery. The entire small bowel is dilated, gangrenous, and hemorrhagic.

pearance. Extensive hemorrhage is seen in the mucosa and submucosa, the former becoming necrotic. Hemorrhage is prominent in the case of predominantly venous occlusion (e.g., mesenteric vein thrombosis). Although the deep muscle layers are initially preserved, they eventually also become necrotic. The mucosal surface shows irregular white sloughs, the wall becomes thin and distended, and bubbles of gas (pneumatosis) may be present in the bowel wall and mesenteric veins. The serosal surface is cloudy and covered by an inflammatory exudate.

The dysfunction of smooth muscle interferes with peristalsis and leads to **adynamic ileus**, a condition in which the bowel proximal to the lesion is dilated and filled with fluid. Intestinal organisms may pass through the damaged wall and cause **peritonitis** or **septicemia**.

In nonocclusive intestinal ischemia, the principal lesion is restricted initially to the mucosa. Mucosal changes range from foci of dilated capillaries with a few extravasated erythrocytes to severe hemorrhagic necrosis and bleeding into the lumen. Ulcers of varying size may result. In some cases, greenish yellow soft plaques slough into the bowel lumen or are easily scraped off the underlying viable tissue. If the patient survives the episode of hypoperfusion, the bowel may be completely repaired, or it may heal with granulation tissue and fibrosis, with eventual **stricture formation**.

☐ **Clinical Features:** In mesenteric artery occlusion, the abrupt onset of abdominal pain is virtually invariable. Bloody diarrhea, hematemesis, and shock are common, and in untreated cases, perforation is frequent. **As the infarction progresses, systemic manifestations become more severe (multiple organ failure syndrome), and death is inevitable without surgical intervention.** In extensive infarction, as a result of occlusion in the proximal portion of the superior mesenteric artery, almost the entire small bowel must be resected, a situation that is also not compatible with ultimate survival.

Chronic Intestinal Ischemia

Atherosclerotic narrowing of the major splanchnic arteries leads to chronic intestinal ischemia. As in the heart, the result is intermittent abdominal pain, termed *intestinal (abdominal) angina*. Characteristically, the pain begins within a half hour of eating and lasts for a few hours. Presumably this reflects the need for greater blood flow during periods of active digestion. Many cases of frank infarction of the intestine are preceded by abdominal angina. Recurrent abdominal pain has also been ascribed to pressure on the celiac axis from surrounding structures and has been labeled the *celiac compression syndrome*.

Chronic ischemia of the small bowel may lead to fibrosis and the formation of a stricture. Ischemic strictures of the small bowel, which may be single or multiple, produce intestinal obstruction or, occasionally, malabsorption resulting from stasis and bacterial overgrowth. These strictures are concentric, and the mucosa of this region is atrophic and often exhibits one or more small ulcers. The submucosa is thickened and fibrotic and displays granulation tissue, which may extend into the muscular layers.

CROHN DISEASE

Historically, Crohn disease, a chronic inflammatory disorder of the bowel wall, was considered to be restricted to the small intestine. However, it is now clear that the disease may involve all other parts of the gastrointestinal tract, particularly the colon and anorectal region. Therefore, the subject is treated with ulcerative colitis under the rubric of **idiopathic inflammatory bowel disease**.

MALABSORPTION

Malabsorption is a general term used to describe a number of clinical conditions in which important nutrients are inadequately absorbed by the gastrointestinal tract. Although some nutrient absorption occurs in the stomach and colon, only absorption from the small intestine, mainly in the proximal portion, is clinically important. The two substances that are preferentially absorbed by the distal small intestine are bile salts and vitamin B_{12}.

Normal intestinal absorption is characterized by a luminal phase and an intestinal phase (Fig. 13-31). The **luminal phase**, consisting of those processes that occur within the lumen of the small intestine, alters the physicochemical state of the various nutrients such that they can be taken up by the absorptive cells in the small bowel epithelium. **The intestinal phase** includes those processes that occur in the cells and transport channels of the in-

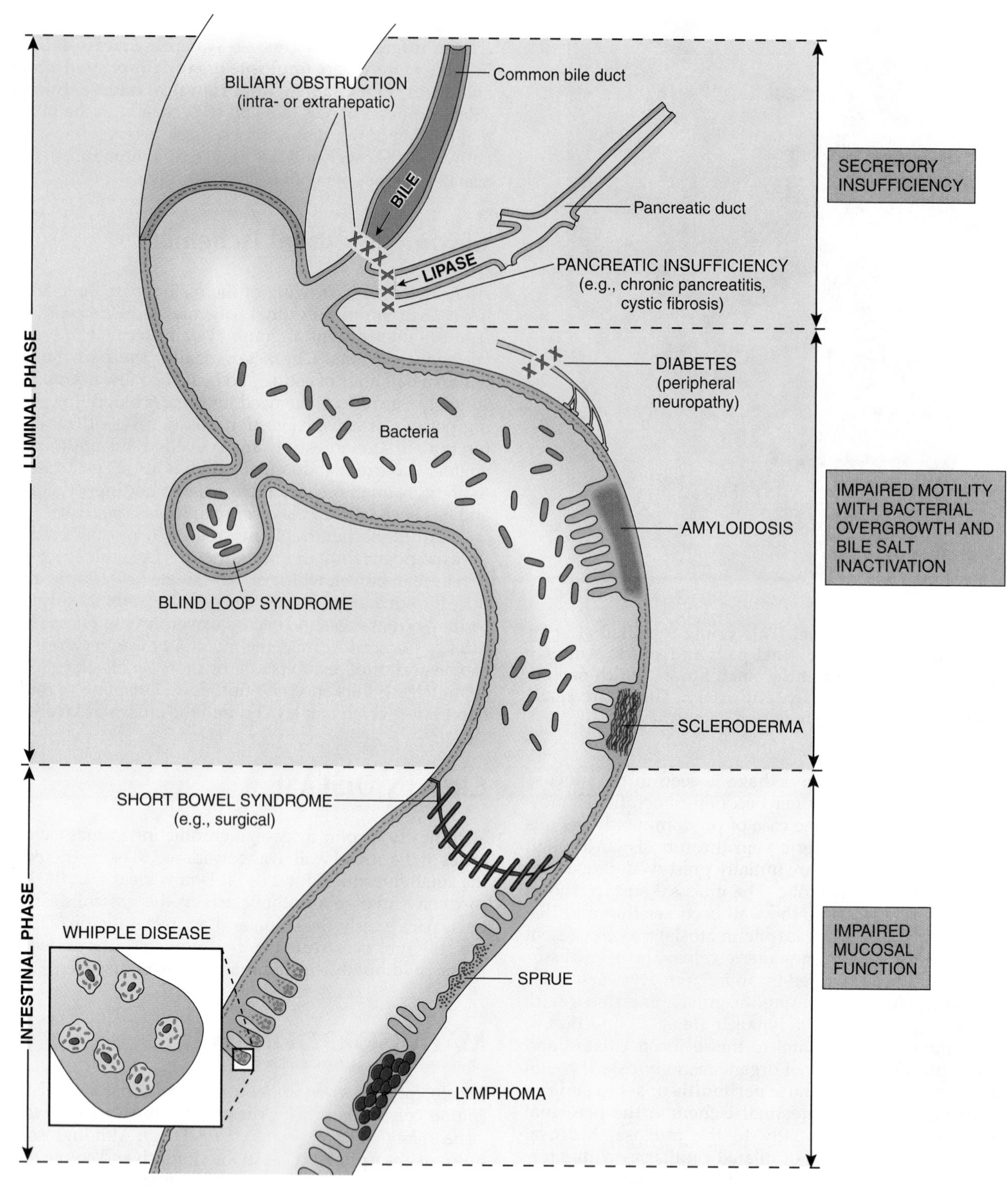

FIGURE 13-31
Causes of malabsorption.

testinal wall. Each of the two phases includes several critical components, and derangement of one or more leads to impaired absorption.

In the luminal phase of intestinal absorption, it is critical that **pancreatic enzymes** and **bile acids** be secreted into the duodenal lumen in adequate amounts and in a normal physicochemical condition. Two additional factors are important for optimal activity of both pancreatic enzymes and bile salts: a normal and regulated flow of gastric contents into the duodenum and an appropriately high pH of the duodenal contents. Normal pancreatic enzyme excretion into the duodenum requires adequate pancreatic exocrine function and an unobstructed flow of pancreatic juice.

The supply of a normal quantity and quality of bile to the duodenum requires (1) adequate hepatocellular function, (2) unobstructed flow of bile, and (3) an intact enterohepatic circulation of bile salts. The enterohepatic circulation of bile begins with absorption of most of the intestinal bile salts from the distal ileum and ends with their excretion into the duodenum through the bile ducts. Normally, 95% of intestinal bile salts are recycled through the enterohepatic circulation, with the remaining 5% being excreted in the stools. The essential conditions for the normal functioning of the enterohepatic circulation are (1) normal intestinal microflora, (2) normal ileal absorptive function, and (3) an unobstructed biliary system.

Causes of Luminal-Phase Malabsorption

Interruption of the normal continuity of the distal stomach and duodenum occurs after gastroduodenal surgery (gastrectomy, antrectomy, pyloroplasty).

Pancreatic dysfunction can occur as a result of chronic pancreatitis, pancreatic carcinoma, or cystic fibrosis.

Deficient or ineffective bile salts may result from three possible causes:

- **Impaired excretion of bile** resulting from liver disease.
- **Bacterial overgrowth** from a disturbance in the motility of the gut. This condition is seen in such conditions as blind-loop syndrome, multiple diverticula of the small bowel, and muscular or neurogenic defects of the intestinal wall (e.g., amyloidosis, scleroderma, diabetic enteropathy). When gastrointestinal motility is defective, bile salts are deconjugated by the excess bacterial flora. The deconjugated bile salts are absorbed and cycled normally through the enterohepatic circulation. However, they are ineffective in the process of micelle formation, which is essential for the normal absorption of monoglycerides and free fatty acids.
- **Deficient bile salts** as a consequence of the absence or bypass of the distal ileum caused by surgical excision, surgical anastomoses, fistulas, or ileal disease (e.g., Crohn disease, lymphoma).

Causes of Intestinal-Phase Malabsorption

Although abnormalities in any one of the four components of the intestinal phase may cause malabsorption, some diseases affect more than one of these components. Figure 13-31 summarizes the major causes of malabsorption.

MICROVILLI: The intestinal disaccharidases and oligopeptidases are integrally bound to the microvillous membranes. Disaccharidases are essential for sugar absorption, because only monosaccharides can be absorbed by the intestinal epithelial cells. Oligopeptides and dipeptides may be absorbed by alternate mechanisms that do not require peptidases. Abnormal function of the microvilli may be primary, as in the primary disaccharidase deficiencies, or secondary, when there is damage to the villi, as in celiac disease (sprue). The various enzyme deficiencies (e.g., of lactase) are characterized by intolerance for the corresponding disaccharides.

ABSORPTIVE AREA: The considerable length of the small bowel and the amplification of its surface wall by the intestinal folds (valves of Kerkring) provide a large absorptive surface. Moreover, the presence of villi and microvilli creates an additional absorptive area that is equivalent to the area of a basketball court. If sufficiently severe, a diminution in this area results in malabsorption. The surface area may be diminished by (1) small bowel resection (short bowel syndrome), (2) gastrocolic fistula (bypassing the small intestine), or (3) mucosal damage due to a number of small intestinal diseases (celiac disease, tropical sprue, Whipple disease).

METABOLIC FUNCTION OF THE ABSORPTIVE CELLS: Nutrients within the absorptive cells are dependent for their subsequent transport to the circulation on their metabolism within these cells. There, monoglycerides and free fatty acids are reassembled into triglycerides and coated with proteins (apoproteins) to form chylomicrons and lipoprotein particles. Specific metabolic dysfunction is seen in abetalipoproteinemia (associated with erythrocyte acanthocytosis), a disorder in which the absorptive cells are unable to synthesize the apoprotein required for the assembly of lipoproteins and chylomicrons. Nonspecific damage to small intestinal epithelial cells occurs in celiac disease, tropical sprue, Whipple disease, and hyperacidity due to gastrinoma.

TRANSPORT: Nutrients are transported from the intestinal epithelium through the intestinal wall by way of blood capillaries and lymphatic vessels. Impaired transport of nutrients through these conduits is probably an important factor in the malabsorption associated with Whipple disease, intestinal lymphoma, and congenital lymphangiectasia.

☐ **Clinical Features:** Malabsorption may be either specific or generalized.

- ***Specific or isolated malabsorption*** *refers to an identifiable molecular defect that causes malabsorption of a single nutrient.* Examples of this group are the disaccharidase deficiencies (notably lactase deficiency) and deficiency of gastric intrinsic factor, which causes malabsorption of vitamin B_{12} and consequently pernicious anemia. Specific deficiency states may be manifested by anemia resulting from a deficiency of iron, folic acid, or vitamin B_{12} or from a combination of these three. Patients may have a bleeding diathesis due to vitamin K deficiency, or malabsorption of vitamin D and calcium may lead to tetany, osteomalacia (in adults), or rickets (in children). In some persons, a deficiency of water-soluble vitamins of the B group is responsible for glossitis, cheilosis, dermatitis, and peripheral neuropathy.

- ***Generalized malabsorption*** *(sometimes referred to as panmalabsorption) describes a condition in which the absorption of several or all major nutrient classes is impaired.* This condition leads to generalized malnutrition. In adults, this is manifested by weight loss and sometimes cachexia; in children, it is expressed as "failure to thrive" with poor growth and weight gain.

Secondary effects of nonabsorbed or partially absorbed substances may lead to diarrhea. In disaccharidase deficiency, the unhydrolyzed sugars in the gut are metabolized by colonic bacteria to lactic acid, carbon dioxide, and water, a process that results in explosive fermentative diarrhea. In patients with ileal dysfunction, bile salts that are not absorbed pass into the colon and cause choleretic diarrhea, a reflection of the stimulation of colonic secretion.

Laboratory Evaluation

Laboratory tests are available to detect specific forms of malabsorption. For example, disaccharidase deficiency is diagnosed by measurement of blood sugar after the oral administration of a standard amount of disaccharide, as in the **lactose-tolerance test**, or by measurement of the activity of disaccharidase in a small bowel biopsy specimen. Vitamin B_{12} absorption is assessed by the **Schilling test**, in which isotopically labeled vitamin B_{12} is administered orally and its blood level then determined. This test also helps to distinguish between malabsorption resulting from intrinsic-factor deficiency and other causes of vitamin B_{12} malabsorption.

In generalized malabsorption, there is almost always impaired absorption of dietary fat. Quantitative fecal fat analysis is the most reliable and sensitive test of overall digestive and absorptive function and serves as a standard for all other tests for malabsorption. Steatorrhea (fat in the stools) is the hallmark of generalized malabsorption, and the two terms are often used interchangeably.

A few of the tests currently in use for the evaluation of various causes of malabsorption merit mention.

- ***d*-Xylose Absorption:** Xylose is a 5-carbon sugar, the absorption of which does not require any of the components of the luminal phase. Blood levels and urinary excretion of this compound after ingestion of a defined amount thus serve as useful tests for the intestinal phase of absorption.
- **$^{14}CO_2$-cholyl-glycine breath test:** Measurement of $^{14}CO_2$ in exhaled air after oral administration of $^{14}CO_2$-cholyl-glycine is a test of bile salt absorption by the ileum. It is used in the diagnosis of the blind- or stagnant-loop syndrome (caused by bacterial overgrowth) and of ileal absorptive function. A newer test to detect bacterial overgrowth is the ^{14}C-xylose breath test.
- **Schilling test**: Originally devised for the diagnosis of pernicious anemia, the Schilling test has been modified for additional use as a test of ileal absorptive function, bacterial overgrowth, and pancreatic function.

Lactase Deficiency

The intestinal brush border contains disaccharidases that are important for the absorption of carbohydrates. As a prominent constituent of milk and many other dairy products, lactose is one of the most common disaccharides in the diet. Acquired lactase deficiency is a widespread disorder of carbohydrate absorption. In fact, two thirds of Asian and African adults manifest evidence of this deficiency.

Typically, symptoms of the disease begin in adolescence. Patients complain of abdominal distention, flatulence, and diarrhea after the ingestion of dairy products. These symptoms are relieved by eliminating milk and its products from the diet.

Diseases that injure the intestinal mucosa (e.g., celiac disease or radiation enteritis) may also lead to acquired lactase deficiency. Congenital lactase deficiency is rare but may be lethal if not recognized.

Celiac Disease (Celiac Sprue)

Celiac disease (gluten-sensitive enteropathy, nontropical sprue), is a syndrome characterized by (1) generalized malabsorption; (2) a typical, but nonspecific, small intestinal mucosal lesion; and (3) a prompt clinical, and slower histopathological, response to the withdrawal of gluten-containing foods from the diet.

☐ **Epidemiology:** The prevalence of celiac sprue is highly variable, ranging from 1 in 300 in western Ireland to 1 in 3000 in other countries. The true incidence of the disease is not known because of the high frequency of latent disease. The disorder is worldwide and affects all ethnic groups. There is a slight female predominance, the sex ratio being 1.3:1. The malady may be seen at any time after the introduction of cereals into the diet. Most cases are diagnosed during childhood, although the disease may become clinically apparent for the first time as late as the seventh decade of life. The frequency of clinically overt disease among first-degree relatives has been estimated at 8%, but biopsy studies have indicated that the true familial frequency may be over 20%.

☐ **Pathogenesis:** Genetic predisposition and gliadin exposure are crucial factors in the development of celiac disease.

ROLE OF CEREAL PROTEINS: Experiments on successfully treated, asymptomatic patients with celiac disease have shown that the ingestion or instillation of wheat, barley, or rye flour into the histopathologically restored small intestine is followed by the clinical features and histopathological changes typical of celiac sprue. Other grains, such as rice and corn flour, do not have such an effect. Both the water-insoluble portion of wheat flour, **gluten**, and an alcoholic extract called **gliadin** have the same effect.

GENETIC FACTORS: Studies during the past 2 decades suggest that the pathogenesis of celiac sprue may involve the interplay of complex genetic factors and an abnormal immunological response to ingested cereal antigens. Although overt celiac sprue and latent disease are frequent among family members, a definite genetic pattern of inheritance has not been established, and both concordance and discordance for celiac sprue have been documented in identical twins. About 90% of patients with celiac disease carry the class I histocompatibility antigen, human leukocyte antigen–B8 (HLA-B8); a comparable frequency has been reported for the class II HLA antigens DR3 and DQw2. These are among the strongest associations of any illness with specific HLA molecules. These antigens occur in fewer than 20% of the adult population and are frequent in other diseases associated with an altered immune response.

IMMUNOLOGICAL FACTORS: The intestinal lesion in celiac disease is characterized by damage to the epithelial cells and a marked increase in the number of T lymphocytes within the epithelium and of plasma cells in the lamina propria. *In vivo* gliadin challenge of persons with treated celiac sprue stimulates local immunoglobulin synthesis. Moreover, gliadin applied to an organ culture of jejunal mucosa *in vitro* induces the proliferation of T cells.

A region of amino acid sequence homology has been found between α-gliadin and a protein of an adenovirus (serotype 12) that infects the human gastrointestinal tract. The large majority (90%) of untreated patients with celiac disease have serological evidence of prior infection with this virus, and in such patients, an antigenic determinant in the region of gliadin shares amino acid sequence homology with the viral protein. An attractive, but otherwise unsupported, hypothesis holds that infection with adenovirus 12 sensitizes T cells to an antigenic determinant that is shared with gliadin. Subsequent exposure to gluten-containing cereals in a genetically susceptible person might then stimulate an immunological reaction to gliadin bound to the surface of intestinal epithelial cells.

Antigliadin and anti-endomysial antibodies in the serum are present in almost all patients with celiac disease. However, it is likely that these antibodies result from the increased permeability of the injured mucosa, and their role in the pathogenesis of the disease remains to be established.

ASSOCIATION WITH DERMATITIS HERPETIFORMIS: Celiac disease is occasionally associated with dermatitis herpetiformis, a vesicular skin disease that typically affects the extensor surfaces and the exposed parts of the body. In this disorder, subepidermal neutrophilic infiltration leads to local edema and blister formation. Deposits of IgA are detected in the region of the basement membranes. Almost all patients with dermatitis herpetiformis have a small bowel mucosal lesion similar to that of celiac disease, although only 10% have overt malabsorption. However, only a few patients who have celiac disease develop dermatitis herpetiformis. Treatment with a strict gluten-free diet is followed by improvement in both the gastrointestinal symptoms and the skin lesions. The histocompatibility antigen HLA-B8 is much more frequent in patients with dermatitis herpetiformis than in normal persons.

Malabsorption in celiac disease probably results from multiple factors, including a reduction in the surface area of the intestinal mucosa (due to the blunting of villi and microvilli) and impairment of intracellular metabolism within the damaged epithelial cells. A probable aggravating factor is secondary disaccharidase deficiency, related to damage to the microvilli. A hypothetical mechanism for the pathogenesis of celiac disease is presented in Figure 13-32.

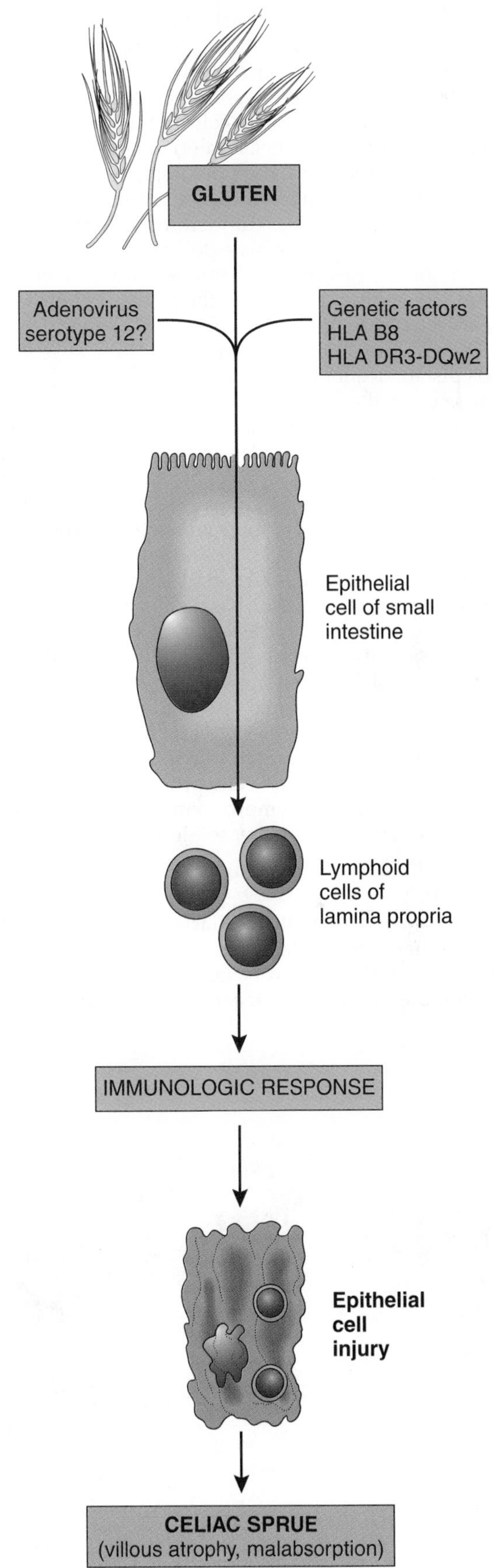

FIGURE *13-32*
Hypothetical mechanisms in the pathogenesis of celiac disease.

☐ **Pathology:** The hallmark of celiac disease is a flat small intestinal mucosa, with (1) blunting or total disappearance of villi, (2) damaged epithelial cells on the mucosal surface with numerous intraepithelial lymphocytes (T cells), (3) increased plasma cells in the lamina propria but not in the deeper layers, and (4) marked reactive epithelial proliferation in the crypts (Fig. 13-33). The most severe histological abnormalities in untreated celiac disease usually occur in the duodenum and proximal jejunum. There is a progressive decrease in severity distally; in some cases, the ileal mucosa appears virtually normal. The clinical severity of the disease is believed to be related to the length of the affected intestine.

The villi are short and blunt or entirely absent, and the crypts are deeper than normal (see Fig. 13-33). The total thickness of the mucosa may not be decreased, because lengthening of the crypts compensates for shortening of the villi. Thus, the term *villous atrophy*, which has been used to describe this appearance, is considered by many to be inappropriate, particularly because the rates of epithelial cell renewal and migration in celiac disease are increased sixfold.

The absorptive cells are flattened and more basophilic than normal, and the basal polarity of their nuclei is lost. Electron-microscopic examination reveals shortening and fusion of the microvilli. The epithelial cells lining the crypts of Lieberkuhn appear to be normal, but the crypts are longer than usual and contain numerous mitotic figures. The numbers of lymphocytes and plasma cells in the lamina propria is markedly increased (see Fig. 13-33). Most of the plasma cells produce IgA (as in the normal small bowel). Polymorphonuclear leukocytes and eosinophils may also be increased in the epithelium and lamina propria.

☐ **Clinical Features:** **Celiac disease is characterized by generalized malabsorption.** Children sometimes come to medical attention because they cease to thrive soon after the introduction of cereals into the diet. Not infrequently, overt signs of malabsorption are lacking, and the disease is suspected only because of growth retardation. Often the symptoms and signs of generalized malabsorption are initially manifested in older children, adolescents, and adults.

The systemic manifestations of celiac disease are related to the various deficiency states that result from generalized malabsorption. Late complications in some cases include ulcerative jejunitis and T-cell lymphoma of the small bowel. Adenocarcinoma of the small bowel and squamous carcinoma of the esophagus also occur. Treatment with a strict gluten-free diet is usually followed by a complete and prolonged clinical and histopathological remission. Some patients have refractory sprue and respond only to corticosteroids.

Collagenous sprue *refers to a rare disorder characterized by the deposition of collagen in the lamina propria of the samll bowel.* The disorder initially mimics celiac disease but is unresponsive to the removal of gluten from the diet. Unlike celiac disease, the prognosis in collagenous sprue is grave, and all reported patients have died of the disease.

Whipple Disease

Whipple disease is a rare, infectious disorder of the small intestine in which malabsorption is the most prominent feature. It most commonly affects white men in their 30s and 40s. The disease is systemic, and other clinical findings include fever, increased skin pigmentation, anemia, lymphadenopathy, arthritis, pericarditis, pleurisy, endocarditis, and central nervous system involvement.

☐ **Pathogenesis:** **Whipple disease typically shows infiltration of the small bowel mucosa by large macrophages that are packed with small, rod-shaped bacilli.** Dramatic clinical remissions occur with antibiotic therapy. The causative organism has been identified as a previously uncharacterized Actinomycetes and has been

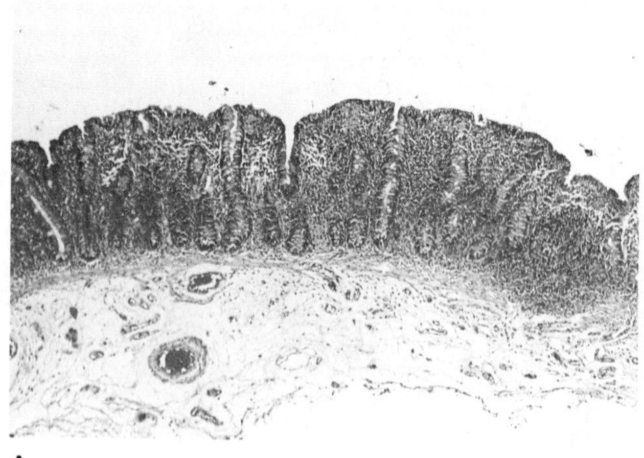

A

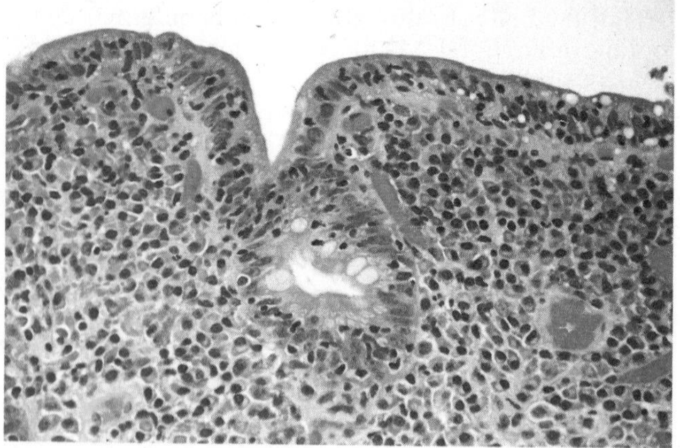

B

FIGURE *13-33*
(*A*) Villous atrophy with a flat surface, elongation of the crypts, and chronic inflammation of the lamina propria are characteristic of long-standing disease. (*B*) A higher-power view shows damaged, cuboidal surface epithelium with numerous intraepithelial lymphocytes. The lamina propria is heavily infiltrated by plasma cells.

named *Tropheryma whippelii*. Interestingly, *T. whippelii* is distantly related to mycobacteria such as *M. avium-intracellulare* and *M. paratuberculosis*, both of which have been associated with illnesses resembling Whipple disease. The sporadic nature of the disease and the lack of evidence for direct transmission have not permitted the establishment of an epidemiological pattern. The results of several studies suggest that host susceptibility factors, possibly defective T-lymphocyte function, may be important in predisposing toward the disease. Macrophages from patients with Whipple disease exhibit a decreased ability to degrade intracellular microorganisms. Patients have reduced numbers of circulating cells expressing CD11b, a cell-adhesion and complement-receptor molecule on macrophages, which is involved in the activation of intracellular killing of pathogens.

☐ **Pathology:** The bowel wall is thickened and edematous, and the mesenteric lymph nodes are usually enlarged. Histological examination of the small intestine reveals flat, thickened villi and extensive infiltration of the lamina propria with large foamy macrophages (Fig. 13-34A). **The cytoplasm of these macrophages is filled with large glycoprotein granules that stain strongly**

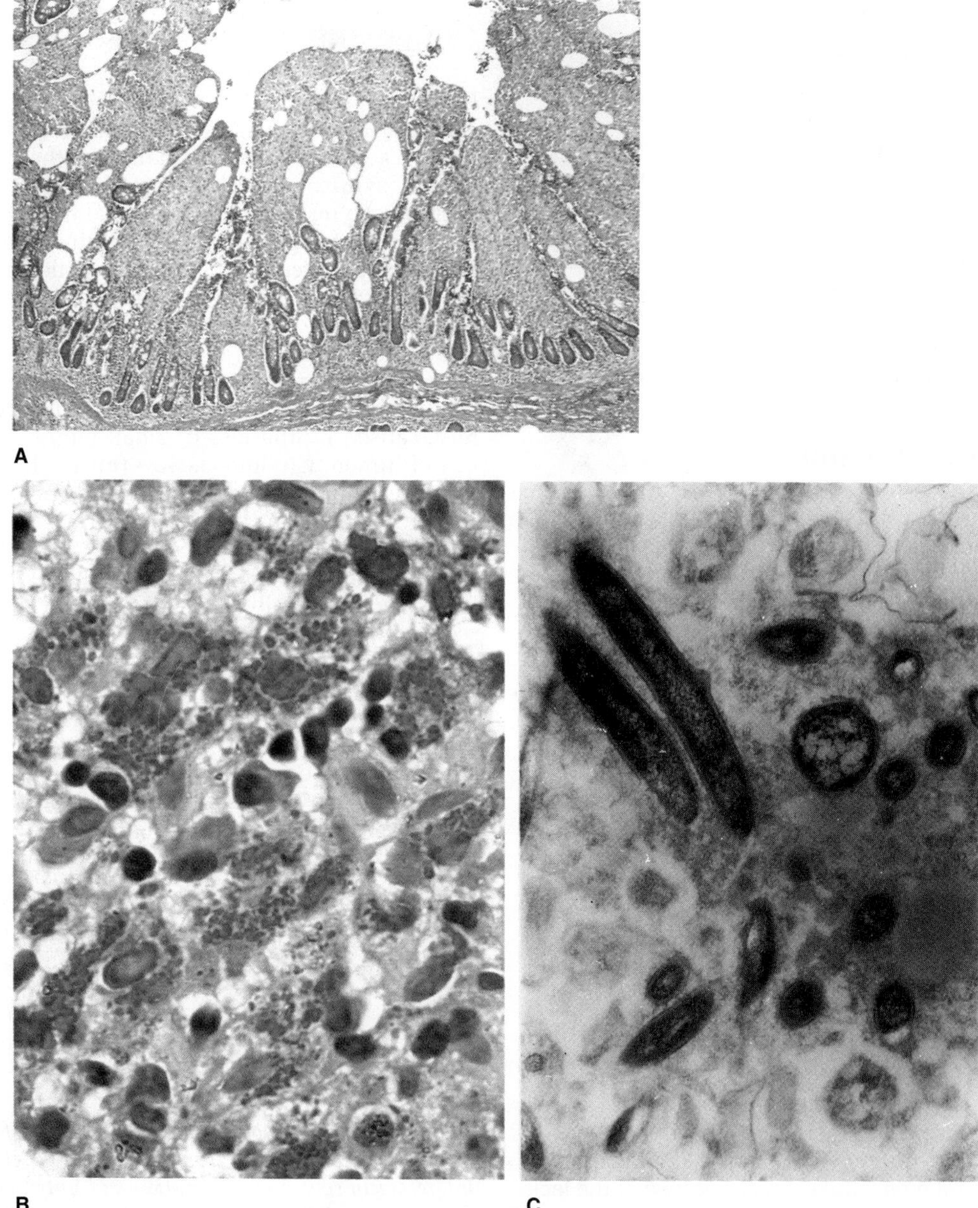

FIGURE 13-34
Whipple disease. *(A)* A photomicrograph of a section of jejunal mucosa shows distortion of the villi. The lamina propria is packed with large, pale-staining macrophages. Dilated mucosal lymphatics are prominent. *(B)* A periodic acid–Schiff (PAS) reaction shows abundant large macrophages filled with granular cytoplasmic material. *(C)* An electron micrograph shows small bacilli in a macrophage.

with periodic acid–Schiff (PAS) stain. Importantly, the other normal cellular components of the lamina propria (i.e., plasma cells and lymphocytes) are depleted. The lymphatic vessels in the mucosa and submucosa are dilated, and large lipid droplets abound within lymphatics and in extracellular spaces, a finding that suggests obstruction of the lymphatics. In contrast to the striking distortion of the villous architecture, the epithelial cells show only patchy abnormalities, including attenuation of the microvilli and an accumulation of lipid droplets within the cytoplasm.

Electron-microscopic examination reveals numerous small bacilli within macrophages and free in the lamina propria (see Fig. 13-34B). The PAS-positive granules seen by light microscopy correspond to lysosomes engorged with bacilli in various stages of degeneration. Many bacilli cluster immediately beneath the epithelial basement membrane.

The mesenteric lymph nodes draining the affected segments of small bowel reveal similar microscopic changes. A characteristic infiltration by macrophages containing bacilli also may be found in other organs, notably the lung, heart, spleen, liver, endocrine glands, brain, bone, and synovial membranes. Heart lesions may include vegetations on the heart valves, which contain bacilli-laden macrophages, sometimes with superimposed streptococcal endocarditis. Treatment of Whipple disease is with antibiotics that cross the blood–brain barrier.

Abetalipoproteinemia

Abetalipoproteinemia is an autosomal recessive inherited disease characterized by a failure to synthesize apoprotein B, a constituent of the membrane coat of low-density lipoproteins. It is an example of malabsorption resulting solely from a metabolic defect within the absorptive cells. Small intestinal absorptive cells that lack apoprotein B fail to assemble chylomicrons, an essential component of lipid transport out of the cell. The other manifestations of the disease result from defects in cell-membrane structure. These are manifested in erythrocytes as acanthocytosis and in the central nervous system as selective demyelinization, particularly of the posterior columns. Typical neurological manifestations are loss of deep tendon reflexes, sensory ataxia, and a mild form of retinitis pigmentosa. The serum shows a total absence of chylomicrons, very-low-density lipoproteins, and low-density lipoproteins. In addition, serum levels of cholesterol and triglycerides are low, and the bulk of serum lipids is carried within high-density lipoprotein particles.

Histologically, the villi, lamina propria, and submucosa appear normal. The epithelial cells contain lipid vacuoles, but no lipid is seen in the intestinal lymphatics. This lipid probably represents triglyceride, which has been assembled within the cell but which cannot be transported into the basolateral intercellular space because of the lack of apoprotein B.

Malabsorption in abetalipoproteinemia is partially reversed by ingestion of medium-chain (rather than the usual long-chain) triglycerides; these lipids are transported through the absorptive cells without an apoprotein coat.

Hypogammaglobulinemia

Malabsorption occurs frequently in patients with acquired hypogammaglobulinemia. The histopathological appearance of the small intestine includes paucity or lack of plasma cells in the lamina propria and often nodular lymphoid hyperplasia. Occasionally, there is a flat mucosa, similar to the lesion of celiac sprue; in this case, the disorder is termed *hypogammaglobulinemic sprue.*

Most hypogammaglobulinemic patients with malabsorption are found to be infected in the small intestine with *Giardia lamblia*. Appropriate treatment with metronidazole is followed by improved intestinal absorption.

Congenital Lymphangiectasia

Congenital lymphangiectasia is a poorly understood disease that usually begins in childhood and probably reflects a generalized malformation of the lymphatic system. A syndrome of intestinal lymphangiectasia and peripheral lymphedema is known as *Milroy disease*. In addition to steatorrhea caused by impaired transport of chylomicrons by intestinal lymphatics, patients with congenital lymphangiectasia have **protein-losing enteropathy**, a condition characterized by excessive loss of plasma proteins into the gut.

Other important features of congenital lymphangiectasia are lymphopenia and impaired cell-mediated immunity, caused by the loss of small lymphocytes into the bowel lumen. Chylous ascites (milky, lipid-containing peritoneal fluid) occurs in some cases as a result of leakage of lymph from the mesenteric or serosal lymphatic vessels into the peritoneal cavity.

The lesions of congenital lymphangiectasia are recognized macroscopically as opalescent white spots and microscopically as **dilated lymphatics (lacteals)** in the lamina propria. The submucosal lymphatics also tend to be dilated. The epithelium is normal, but the villi may be blunted or even absent in areas overlying severe lymphatic dilatation.

Acquired intestinal lymphangiectasia, with all or some of the associated clinical features described earlier, also occurs as a secondary manifestation of small intestinal or retroperitoneal lymphoma, other retroperitoneal tumors, tuberculosis, sarcoidosis, chronic pancreatitis, and retroperitoneal fibrosis.

Protein-losing enteropathy also may occur in association with certain gastrointestinal tumors, Whipple disease, Crohn disease, bacterial overgrowth, parasitic infestations of the bowel, and Menetrier disease.

Tropical Sprue

Tropical sprue is a poorly understood disease of obscure cause that is endemic in certain tropical areas and is characterized by progressively severe malabsorption and nutritional deficiency. Cure, or at least amelioration of the symptoms, usually follows treatment with oral tetracycline and folic acid. The disease is endemic to Puerto Rico, Cuba, the Dominican Republic, and Haiti but is uncommon in other parts of the Caribbean. It also occurs in the northern parts of South America and many Far Eastern countries.

The cause of tropical sprue is not known. Some studies suggest that **long-standing contamination of the bowel with bacteria**, perhaps toxigenic strains of *E. coli*, may be important, and that the resultant **folate deficiency** may play a role in perpetuating the intestinal lesion.

The histological findings are variable, ranging from mild widening and blunting of villi to a completely flat mucosa similar to that seen in celiac sprue. The morphological injury in the epithelium and the inflammation of the lamina propria usually parallel the severity of the alterations in the villi.

Typically, steatorrhea, anemia, and weight loss are followed by progressively severe manifestations of folic acid and vitamin B_{12} deficiencies and hypoalbuminemia. Laboratory findings include increased fecal fat, impaired *d*-xylose absorption, megaloblastic anemia, and decreased disaccharidase activity in the intestinal mucosa.

Radiation Enteritis

Abdominal irradiation may cause transient damage to the small intestinal mucosa. Anorexia, abdominal cramps, and changes in bowel habits occur frequently during the course of abdominal radiation therapy, and laboratory studies in such patients indicate malabsorption of bile salts and disaccharides. Transient histological changes in the small bowel include shortening of the villi, increased cellularity in the lamina propria, and submucosal edema. These changes usually revert to normal within 12 days of cessation of radiation therapy.

Chronic radiation damage is less common in the small intestine than in other parts of the gastrointestinal tract, probably because the mobility of the loops of small intestine reduces their continued exposure to the radiation beam. Occasionally, subacute or chronic radiation damage does occur, especially when (1) the radiation dose is very high, (2) segments of small bowel become fixed as a result of postoperative or inflammatory adhesions, (3) the blood supply to the bowel is impaired, or (4) the radiation is combined with chemotherapeutic agents that may augment radiation damage. Malabsorption in such situations may result from a combination of mucosal damage and impaired motility, resulting in bacterial overgrowth.

The major histological features of subacute and chronic radiation damage to the small intestine are similar to those seen elsewhere in the gastrointestinal tract; they include (1) mucosal ulceration, (2) swelling and detachment of endothelial cells of the small arterioles in the submucosa, (3) obliteration by fibrin plugs of the lumina of the arterioles, and (4) the presence of large foam cells beneath the intima. Thickening and fibrosis of the submucosa ensue, together with signs of progressive ischemia, to produce stricture.

MECHANICAL OBSTRUCTION

Mechanical obstruction to the passage of intestinal contents can be caused by (1) a luminal mass, (2) an intrinsic lesion of the bowel wall, or (3) extrinsic compression.

INTUSSUSCEPTION: *This is a form of intraluminal small bowel obstruction in which a segment of bowel (intussusceptum) protrudes distally into a surrounding outer portion (intussuscipiens), much in the way that one segment of a telescope inserts into the adjacent one.* This condition is usually a disorder of infants or young children, in whom it occurs without a known cause. In adults, the leading point of an intussusception is usually a lesion in the bowel wall, such as Meckel diverticulum or a polypoid tumor. Once the leading point is entrapped in the intussucepiens, peristalsis drives the intussusceptum forward. In addition to acute intestinal obstruction, intussusception compresses the blood supply to the intussusceptum, which may become infarcted. If the obstruction is not relieved spontaneously, treatment requires surgery.

VOLVULUS: *This is a cause of an acute abdomen and is an example of intestinal obstruction in which a segment of gut twists on its mesentery, thereby kinking the bowel and usually interrupting the blood supply.* Volvulus is virtually always a consequence of an underlying congenital abnormality. Malrotation of the bowel permits undue mobility of the bowel loops and predisposes to **midgut volvulus**. When the cecum or right colon is invested with a mesentery rather than being retroperitoneal, the result may be **cecal volvulus**. An unusually long sigmoid colon, which occurs sometimes in patients with idiopathic chronic constipation, permits the development of **sigmoid volvulus**.

ADHESIONS: Fibrous scars caused by previous surgery or peritonitis are a common cause of obstruction by kinking or angulating the bowel or by directly compressing the lumen.

HERNIAS: Loops of small bowel may be incarcerated in an inguinal or femoral hernia, in which case, the lumen may become obstructed and the vascular supply compromised. Similarly, portions of the bowel may be trapped internally by hernias that represent congenital or surgically acquired defects in the mesentery.

NEOPLASMS

The small intestine is curiously resistant to neoplasia, despite the fact that it is the longest portion of the alimentary tract. Tumors of the small intestine constitute less than 5% of all gastrointestinal tumors. Although many factors have been proposed as the cause, none have been proved and all are speculative. The following are the most credible of the theories, which are not mutually exclusive.

- **The rapid transit time** in the small bowel limits the length of exposure of the mucosa to carcinogens in the food.
- **The concentration of carcinogens** may be lower in the large liquid volume of the small intestine than in the more solid contents of the colon.
- **Detoxifying enzymes** in the small intestine may be more active than those in the stomach or colon.

- **The bacterial flora** of the colon are far more voluminous than those of the small intestine. Moreover, the colonic bacteria are principally anaerobes, which have been shown to convert bile acids into mutagens.
- **Humoral and cellular immune systems** are more active in the small intestine than at other sites in the gastrointestinal tract. IgA has been theorized to protect in some unknown way against the development of neoplasms. The lymphoid nodules of the small bowel contain abundant T lymphocytes, which may participate in immune surveillance.
- **The kinetics of cell renewal** are different in the small intestine than at other sites in the alimentary tract. It has been suggested that fewer cells in the small intestine retain a proliferative potential as they migrate up the villus than do cells of the crypts of the stomach or colon.

Benign Tumors

The most common benign tumors of the small intestine are adenomas, leiomyomas, and lipomas. As in other portions of the gastrointestinal tract, neurogenic tumors, fibromas, angiomas, and hamartomas may be encountered. Benign tumors of the small intestine rarely become malignant.

Adenomas

Adenomas of the small intestine resemble those of the colon (see later). As in the colon, adenomatous polyps in the small intestine may be tubular or villous or a mixture of these types. The villous adenoma is rare in the small intestine, usually occurring in the duodenum, especially the periampullary region. Although most adenomas remain benign, some, especially the villous type, undergo malignant transformation. Benign adenomas are ordinarily asymptomatic, but bleeding and intussusception are occasional complications.

Peutz–Jeghers Syndrome

Peutz–Jeghers syndrome is an autosomal dominant hereditary disorder characterized by intestinal hamartomatous polyps and mucocutaneous melanin pigmentation, which is particularly evident on the face, buccal mucosa, hands, feet, and perianal and genital areas. Except for the buccal pigmentation, the freckle-like macular lesions usually fade at puberty. The polyps occur most commonly in the proximal regions of the small intestine but are sometimes seen in the stomach and the colon. Patients usually have symptoms of obstruction or intussusception; in as many as one fourth of the cases, however, the diagnosis is suggested by pigmentation alone in an otherwise asymptomatic person. Acute upper gastrointestinal tract hemorrhage and occult bleeding with anemia may complicate the course.

Peutz–Jeghers syndrome apparently results from inactivating mutations of a gene (LKB1) on chromosome 19p, which encodes a protein kinase. Carriers of the defective gene are also at an increased risk for cancers of the breast, pancreas, testis, and ovary.

The polyps in Peutz–Jeghers syndrome are not true neoplasms but rather hamartomas. Histologically, a branching network of smooth muscle fibers continuous with the muscularis mucosae supports the glandular epithelium of the polyp (Fig. 13-35). Peutz–Jeghers polyps are generally considered benign; however, 2% to 3% of patients develop adenocarcinoma, although not necessarily in the hamartomatous polyps.

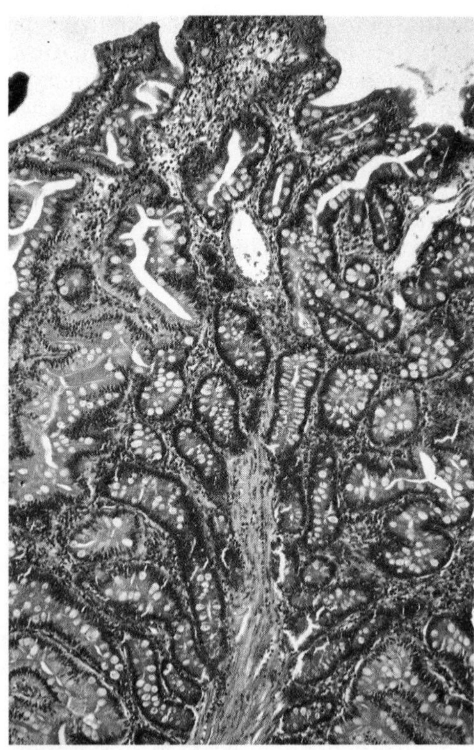

FIGURE *13-35*
Peutz–Jeghers polyp. In this hamartomatous polyp, the glandular epithelium, composed of both goblet cells and absorptive cells, is supported by a network of smooth muscle.

Leiomyomas

Leiomyomas are smooth muscle tumors that occur at all levels but are most common in the jejunum. This lesion ordinarily is seen as an intramural mass covered by intact mucosa. However, it may protrude into the lumen, where necrosis of tumor tissue and ulceration of the overlying mucosa give rise to bleeding. Intestinal obstruction is uncommon, but volvulus may be a complication. Histologically, leiomyomas of the small intestine are similar to those occurring elsewhere in the body. Surgical removal of large tumors is advisable because of bleeding and the fact that the risk of malignancy increases with size.

Lipomas

Lipomas are fatty tumors that occur throughout the length of the small intestine but are most common in the distal ileum. Although for the most part asymptomatic, these submucosal tumors may become large and produce intestinal obstruction, usually as a result of intussusception. The overlying mucosa may become ulcerated and bleed.

Malignant Tumors

Adenocarcinoma

☐ **Epidemiology:** Although adenocarcinoma of the small intestine accounts for only a minute proportion of all gastrointestinal tumors, it constitutes half of all malignant small bowel tumors. The large majority of adenocarcinomas are located in the duodenum and jejunum. Most occur in middle-aged persons, and there is a moderate male predominance. Interestingly, the geographic variation in the incidence of small bowel adenocarcinoma correlates with that of colon cancer but not with that of stomach cancer. For instance, Japanese who migrate to Hawaii have a lower than normal incidence of stomach cancer but a higher than normal incidence of both colon cancer and small bowel adenocarcinoma.

A risk factor for adenocarcinoma is inflammatory disease of the small bowel. Patients with Crohn disease are known to be at a significantly increased risk, perhaps as high as 100-fold. Moreover, the mean age for the appearance of an adenocarcinoma of the small intestine is 10 years younger than average in patients with Crohn disease, and the cancer tends to occur in the same area as the inflammatory lesions, the ileum. Adenocarcinomas occur in patients with familial adenomatous polyposis and hereditary nonpolyposis colorectal cancer syndrome (Warthin–Lynch syndrome) and is a rare complication of celiac disease.

☐ **Pathology and Clinical Features:** Adenocarcinoma of the small intestine may be polypoid or ulcerative or simply annular and stenosing. In addition to causing intestinal obstruction directly, a polypoid tumor may be the lead point of an intussusception. Microscopically, adenocarcinomas, which originate from the epithelium of the crypts rather than the villi, resemble colorectal cancers.

The symptoms of adenocarcinoma of the small bowel are commonly those of progressive intestinal obstruction. Occult bleeding is common and often leads to iron-deficiency anemia. Acute bleeding and perforation are infrequent. Adenocarcinoma of the duodenum may involve the papilla of Vater, in which case it is termed *ampullary carcinoma.* This tumor causes obstructive jaundice or pancreatitis. By the time the patient becomes symptomatic, most adenocarcinomas have metastasized to local lymph nodes, and overall 5-year survival is less than 20%. This neoplasm is the second most common cause of death in patients with familial adenomatous polyposis.

Primary Lymphoma

Primary lymphoma originates in nodules of lymphoid tissue normally present in the mucosa and superficial submucosa (MALT). Lymphoma represents the second most common malignant tumor of the small intestine in industrialized countries, where it accounts for about 15% of small bowel cancers. By contrast, another type of primary lymphoma comprises more than two thirds of all cancers of the small intestine in underdeveloped countries. The latter variety of intestinal lymphoma was originally described in Mediterranean populations, but it is now clear that it is distributed throughout the poorer parts of the world. Because these two types of lymphoma have distinct epidemiological, clinical, and pathological features, they are labeled, respectively, the western type and the Mediterranean variety. The small intestine may be secondarily involved in disseminated lymphomas, but symptoms are uncommon. The classification of primary intestinal lymphoma is identical with that of nodal lymphoma, which is discussed in Chapter 20.

The cause of primary lymphoma of the small bowel is unknown, but an association with celiac disease is well documented, occurring in as many as one tenth of patients with primary lymphoma. It is assumed that the persistent activation of lymphocytes in the bowel is related to the subsequent development of T-cell lymphoma. However, although a gluten-free diet usually improves the inflammatory component of the enteropathy, T-cell lymphoma can occur.

The risk of intestinal lymphoma is also increased in conditions that favor the development of nodal lymphoma, particularly immunodeficiency following treatment with immunosuppressive drugs.

MEDITERRANEAN LYMPHOMA: Mediterranean lymphoma typically occurs in poor countries in young men of low socioeconomic status; it is therefore thought by some to have an environmental cause. **This neoplasm has been associated with a proliferative disorder of intestinal B lymphocytes that secrete the heavy chain of immunoglobulin A without light chains, termed α-heavy chain disease.** Mediterranean lymphoma and α-chain disease are believed by some to be the same disorder, termed *immunoproliferative small intestinal disease.*

Mediterranean intestinal lymphoma, which typically affects men younger than 30 years, predominantly involves the duodenum and proximal jejunum. A long segment of small intestine, or even the entire small bowel, is characteristically affected. The lymphoma typically is seen as a diffuse infiltration of the mucosa and submucosa by plasmacytoid lymphocytes or plasma cells (Fig. 13-36). Lymphomatous infiltration of the mucosa leads to mucosal atrophy and severe malabsorption.

WESTERN-TYPE INTESTINAL LYMPHOMA: The western type of intestinal lymphoma usually affects adults older than 40 years and children younger than 10 years. It is most common in the ileum, where it is seen as (1) a fungating mass that projects into the lumen, (2) an elevated ulcerated lesion, (3) a diffuse segmental thickening of the bowel wall, or (4) plaque-like mucosal nodules. As a result, intestinal obstruction, intussusception, and perforation are important complications. Occult bleeding is common, although massive acute hemorrhage may also occur. Microscopically, all varieties of malignant lymphoma are encountered. When the disease is localized and confined to the small intestine, it does not recur after surgical removal in more than half the patients. When extraintestinal spread is present, the 5-year survival rate is less than 10%.

Chronic abdominal pain, diarrhea, and clubbing of the fingers are the most frequent clinical signs of intestinal lymphoma. Diarrhea and weight loss reflect the underlying malabsorption. Chemotherapy and occasionally radi-

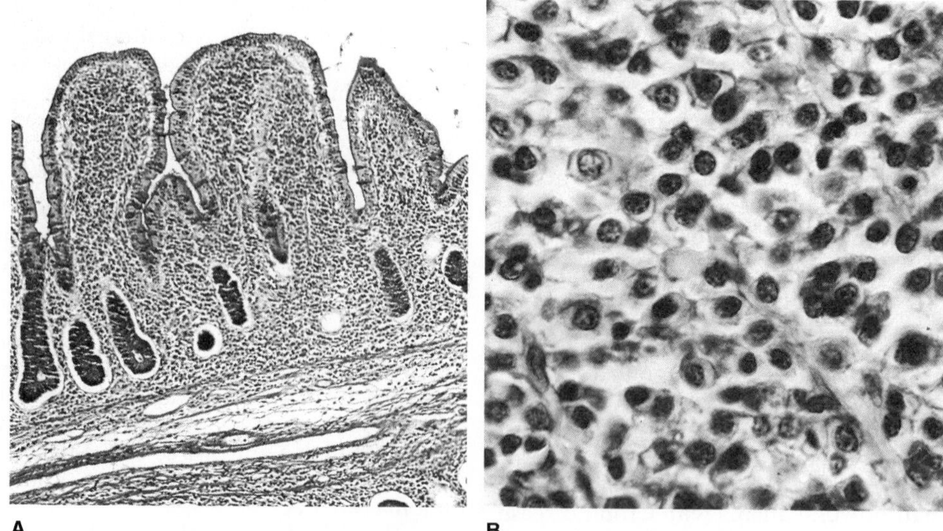

FIGURE *13-36*
Mediterranean intestinal lymphoma. *(A)* The villi are short and blunted, and the lamina propria is filled with lymphoid cells. The goblet cells are red with this periodic acid–Schiff stain. *(B)* A high-power view of *A* shows neoplastic plasmacytoid lymphocytes.

ation therapy are used as treatment, because the disease is usually too diffuse to permit surgery. Patients with Mediterranean lymphoma tend to survive longer than those with the western type of lymphoma.

Carcinoid Tumor

Carcinoid tumors of the gastrointestinal tract have differentiation characteristics of the neuroendocrine system of the gut. They are capable of secreting all the peptides and amines produced by their normal counterparts. The most commonly secreted hormone is serotonin.

Carcinoid tumors account for about 20% of all malignant tumors of the small intestine. Because neuroendocrine cells are most numerous in the appendix and terminal ileum, it is not surprising that carcinoid tumors are most frequent at these sites. **In fact, the majority of all carcinoid tumors are found incidentally in the appendix, and most of the remainder occur in the ileum.** Interestingly, 2% of carcinoid tumors of the small bowel arise in a Meckel diverticulum.

All carcinoid tumors are potentially malignant. **However, for practical purposes, carcinoid tumors of the appendix smaller than 2 cm in diameter do not metastasize.** In general, the malignant potential of intestinal carcinoid tumors appears to be related to their size. Those smaller than 1 cm in diameter are rarely malignant, 50% of those between 1 and 2 cm in diameter metastasize, and 80% of those larger than 2 cm in diameter metastasize.

Carcinoid tumors of the gastrointestinal tract, especially those of the small intestine, are often multicentric; that is, multiple primary tumors arise, either simultaneously or at different times. They are also seen in association with the multiple endocrine neoplasia (MEN) syndromes, most commonly with type I. Because neuroendocrine cells are widespread, carcinoid tumors are found in a variety of other locations, including the pancreas, bronchus, gallbladder, ovary, and testis. Carcinoid tumors of the gastrointestinal tract are also associated with a significantly increased frequency of nonendocrine malignant tumors, both in the alimentary tract and elsewhere.

□ **Pathology:** Macroscopically, small carcinoid tumors present as submucosal nodules covered by intact mucosa. Large tumors may grow in a polypoid, intramural, or annular pattern (Fig. 13-37A) and often undergo secondary ulceration. The cut surface is firm and white to yellow. As they enlarge, carcinoid tumors invade the muscular coat and penetrate the serosa, often causing a conspicuous desmoplastic reaction. This fibrosis is responsible for peritoneal adhesions and kinking of the bowel, which may lead to intestinal obstruction.

Microscopically, the neoplasms appear as nests, cords, and rosettes of uniform small, round cells (see Fig. 13-37B). Occasional glandlike structures are also encountered. The nuclei exhibit a remarkable regularity, and mitoses are rare. In the solid nests, the cells on the periphery tend to have smaller and more hyperchromatic nuclei than those in the center. An abundant eosinophilic cytoplasm contains cytoplasmic granules, which by electron microscopy are typically of the neurosecretory type. Goblet cell carcinoids or adenocarcinoid tumors have glandular differentiation. These tumors have a higher rate of aggressive behavior than do typical carcinoids.

Carcinoid tumors metastasize first to regional lymph nodes. Subsequently, hematogenous spread produces metastases at distant sites, particularly the liver. Surgical resection, the only therapy for the primary tumor, accomplishes a 5-year cure in about half of the cases of small bowel carcinoid tumors.

□ **Clinical Features:** **Carcinoid syndrome** is a unique clinical condition that marks carcinoid tumors. The disorder is caused by the release of a variety of active tumor products. Although most carcinoids are to some

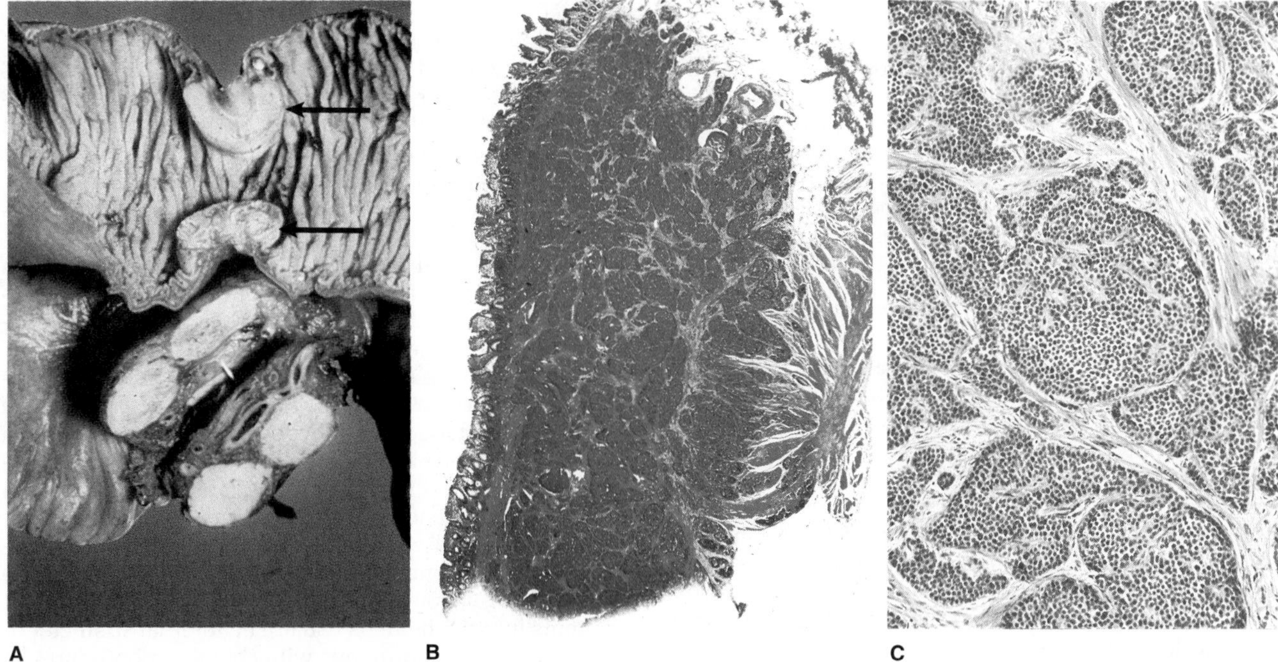

FIGURE 13-37
Carcinoid tumor of the small intestine. ***(A)*** **A bisected annular carcinoid tumor** ***(arrows)*** **constricts the lumen of the small intestine. Lymph node metastases are evident.** ***(B)*** **A photomicrograph of the lesion in** ***A*** **shows an intact mucosa** ***(left)*** **and the predominant submucosal location of the malignant tumor.** ***(C)*** **A higher-power photomicrograph demonstrates nests and cords of uniform small, round cells.**

extent functional, this syndrome ordinarily occurs only in cases with extensive hepatic metastases. **The classic symptoms of the carcinoid syndrome include diarrhea (often the most distressing symptom), episodic flushing, bronchospasm, cyanosis, telangiectasia, and skin lesions.** Half of the patients also have right-sided cardiac valvular disease. Diarrhea is thought to be caused by serotonin, but the tumor secretory products involved in the other symptoms have not been clearly identified.

After its release into the blood, serotonin is metabolized to 5-hydroxyindoleacetic acid (5-HIAA) by monoamine oxidase either in the tumor or in other tissues. The presence of 5-HIAA in the urine is a diagnostic test for the carcinoid syndrome. Whereas the liver, lung, and brain all have high levels of activity of monoamine oxidase and (presumably) of enzymes that inactivate other tumor secretions, the right side of the heart is exposed to the full effects of tumor products that have been released into the vena cava from hepatic metastases. As a result, endocardial fibrosis occurs, probably as a reaction to endothelial damage. Fibrous plaques form on the tricuspid and pulmonic valves, the endocardium of the right-sided cardiac chambers, the vena cava, the coronary sinus, and the pulmonary artery. **Distortion of the valves leads to pulmonic stenosis and tricuspid regurgitation.**

Malignant Gastrointestinal Stromal Tumors (Leiomyosarcomas)

Leiomyosarcomas in the small intestine, similar clinically and pathologically to those in the stomach, are rare. This cancer has a slower course than small bowel adenocarcinoma, and the 5-year survival rate has been reported to be better than 50%. Rare instances of other cancers of mesenchymal origin have been reported in the small intestine.

Metastatic Tumors

The most common malignant tumors that involve the small intestine are metastatic. Cancer of adjacent organs (e.g., stomach, pancreas, or colon) may spread to the small intestine by direct extension. Cancers of the lung and female genital organs and melanomas are the most frequent primary sites of small-intestinal metastases. Secondary involvement of the small intestine with systemic lymphoma may simulate metastatic carcinoma. Solitary, submucosal metastatic tumors may easily be mistaken for a primary cancer, and the symptoms may be indistinguishable.

PNEUMATOSIS CYSTOIDES INTESTINALIS (GAS CYSTS)

Pneumatosis cystoides intestinalis is an uncommon disorder in which numerous pockets of gas are found in the wall of the gut anywhere in the gastrointestinal tract. Most cases are associated with an underlying gastrointestinal disease, including intestinal obstruction, peptic ulcer, Crohn disease, mesenteric ischemia, volvulus, and neonatal necrotizing enterocolitis. Some are associated with chronic obstructive pulmonary disease or mechanical ventilation. Pneumatosis in adults is ordinarily benign, depending on the underlying disease. However, intestinal pneumatosis associated with neonatal necrotizing enteritis has a high mortality.

The cause of intestinal pneumatosis depends on the associated conditions. A mechanical break in the continuity of the mucosa allows the entry of air from the lumen to the submucosa. Alternatively, the gas can be a product of bacterial action, particularly in neonatal necrotizing enterocolitis. Dissection of air bubbles along the mesentery is common in patients with obstructive pulmonary disease or ventilation.

□ **Pathology:** Macroscopically, the cysts appear as bubbles under the serosa of the intestine, and the bowel wall feels spongy. In some cases, the air cysts are located principally in the submucosa, in which case, the cut surface of the bowel wall appears to be honeycombed. The cysts vary from a few millimeters to several centimeters in diameter. In addition to appearing in the small and large intestines, cysts may occur in the stomach and the mesentery. Microscopic examination reveals cystic spaces in the submucosa or beneath the serosa, and these spaces are often lined by large macrophages and multinucleated giant cells. Little or no other inflammation is elicited by the cysts. The mucosa overlying submucosal cysts is attenuated and may contain small hemorrhages. Microscopic pneumatosis is sometimes seen in the absence of grossly evident cysts.

□ **Clinical Features:** Many cases are found during investigation of symptoms unrelated to the pneumatosis. Some patients have episodic diarrhea. Constipation and diminished caliber of the stools may be related to intestinal obstruction by the cysts. There is often blood in the stools, and rectal bleeding may be brisk. When intestinal pneumatosis is a complication of neonatal necrotizing enterocolitis, bowel perforation and peritonitis are frequent; these complications are rare in adults.

Gas cysts may disappear spontaneously or may persist for years. Relief of symptoms may be obtained by oxygen inhalation or treatment with the antimicrobial agent metronidazole.

The Large Intestine

ANATOMY

The large intestine, defined as the portion of the gastrointestinal tract from the ileocecal valve to the anus, is 90 to 125 cm in length in adults and comprises the colon and rectum. The proximal part shares a common embryological origin with the small intestine, both being derived from the embryonic midgut and supplied by the superior mesenteric artery. The distal half of the large intestine is embryologically distinct. It is derived from the embryonic hindgut, is supplied by the inferior mesenteric artery, and serves principally as a storage organ.

MACROSCOPIC FEATURES: The large intestine is traditionally divided into six regions in a sequence that proceeds from the ileocecal valve distally: (1) cecum, (2) ascending colon, (3) transverse colon, (4) descending colon, (5) sigmoid colon, and (6) rectum. The bend between the ascending and transverse colon in the right upper quadrant is called the *hepatic flexure* and that between the transverse and descending segments in the left upper quadrant is termed the *splenic flexure*. The caliber of the lumen progressively diminishes from the cecum to the sigmoid colon.

Like the small intestine, the colon is endowed with outer longitudinal and inner circular muscle coats. However, in the colon, the longitudinal muscle has three separate bundles, termed the *taeniae coli*. Evaginations of the colonic wall between the taeniae, called the haustra, appear as external saculations. The *appendices epiploicae* are small serosal masses of fat, invested by peritoneum. The *vermiform appendix* arises at the apex of the cecum and terminates as a blind tube; it averages about 8 cm in length but occasionally measures up to 20 cm.

The ileocecal valve functions as a sphincter to regulate the flow of intestinal contents into the cecum. However, it is an incompetent sphincter, and reflux of cecal contents into the ileum is usual. The internal sphincter of the anal canal is continuous with colonic smooth muscle. The external anal sphincter, the major mechanism by which continence of the bowel is maintained, surrounds the anal canal with a layer of skeletal muscle. The mucosal surface of the large bowel has prominent folds, which are less pronounced in the rectum.

MICROSCOPIC FEATURES: Histologically, the surface of the colonic mucosa is flat and punctuated by numerous pits, termed crypts of Lieberkuhn. The mucosa of the surface and crypts is lined by a tall columnar epithelium. The surface epithelium consists primarily of simple columnar cells and occasional goblet cells. The crypts are lined mostly by goblet cells, except at their bases, where a few undifferentiated cells and a variety of neuroendocrine cells are located. The basal undifferentiated cells constitute the reserve cell population of the colonic mucosa and exhibit numerous mitoses. Mucosal cells migrate from the bases of the crypts toward the luminal surface. Programmed cell death (apoptosis) and sloughing of the mucosal cells balance proliferation in maintaining the crypt epithelial cell population. The ultrastructural appearance of the mucosal cells is similar to that in the small intestine, except that the microvilli of the absorptive cells are much shorter and narrower in the colon.

The lamina propria of the colonic mucosa contains lymphocytes, plasma cells, macrophages, and fibroblasts. Eosinophils and an occasional neutrophil also may be encountered. Lymphoid aggregates and nodules with follicles, grossly visualized as small nodules, interrupt the continuity of the muscularis mucosae and extend into the submucosa. Mucosal lymphatics are inconspicuous. The submucosa is similar to that in the small intestine, but lymphatic channels are far less prominent. The lymphatics drain into paracolic nodes in the serosal fat, intermediate nodes located along the course of the colic blood vessels, and central nodes clustered near the aorta. Parasympathetic and sympathetic innervations terminate in Meissner submucosal and Auerbach myenteric plexuses.

CONGENITAL DISORDERS

Congenital Megacolon (Hirschsprung Disease)

Hirschsprung disease is an uncommon, but not rare, disorder in which colonic dilatation (Fig. 13-38) *results from a defect in the innervation of the rectum.* **The lesion is a congenital absence of ganglion cells in the wall of the rectum** (Fig. 13-39). In one fourth of the cases, ganglion cells are deficient in more proximal portions of the colon, and in unusual instances, the lesion may extend as far as the small intestine. The incidence of the disorder is estimated to be 1 in 5000 live births, and 80% of the patients are male.

☐ **Pathogenesis:** The pathogenesis of Hirschsprung disease can be traced to an interruption of the developmental sequence that leads to innervation of the colon. The normal caudal migration of cells from the neural crest that eventually gives rise to the intramural ganglion cells is interrupted. Because the internal anal sphincter marks the terminus of this migration, the aganglionic segment always includes the rectum and may extend for variable distances proximally, depending on the point at which the primitive neuroblasts are halted. Given that the aganglionic rectum and occasionally the adjacent colon are permanently contracted because of the absence of relaxation stimuli, the fecal contents do not readily enter this stenotic area. The proximal bowel becomes dilated because of functional distal obstruction.

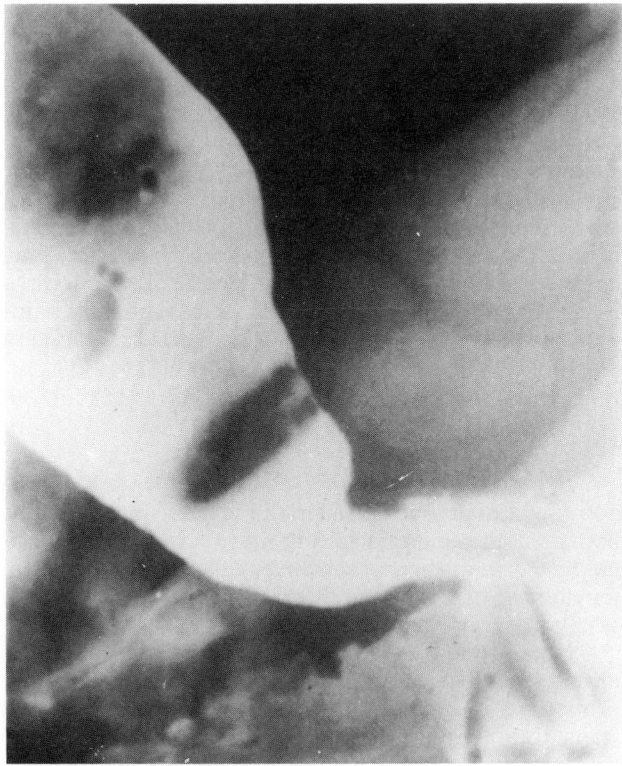

FIGURE 13-38
Hirschsprung disease. A contrast radiograph shows marked dilatation of the rectosigmoid colon proximal to the narrowed rectum.

Most cases of Hirschsprung disease are sporadic, but 10% of cases are familial. Half of the familial cases and 15% of sporadic ones are assoicated with inactivating gene mutations of the RET receptor tyrosine kinase on chromosome 10q11.2 (see MEN2 syndrome, Chapter 21). Some cases involve mutations of the gene for the endothelin-B receptor on chromosome 13q22. Finally, a few instances of the disease are due to mutations in the genes that code for the ligands of the RET receptor and the endothelin-B receptor.

The incidence of congenital megacolon is 10 times higher than normal in infants with **Down syndrome**, and 2% of patients with Down syndrome are born with Hirschsprung disease. Eighty percent of patients are male. Although most cases of aganglionosis of the colon are uncomplicated by other lesions, the disorder also has been reported in conjunction with a number of other congenital abnormalities, including anomalies of the kidneys and lower urinary tract, imperforate anus, and ventricular septal defect.

☐ **Pathology:** The colon and rectum in Hirschsprung disease reveal a constricted and spastic segment that corresponds to the aganglionic zone. Proximal to this area, the bowel is conspicuously dilated.

The definitive diagnosis of Hirschsprung disease is made on the basis of absence of ganglion cells in a rectal biopsy specimen. Additionally, there is a striking increase in nonmyelinated cholinergic nerve fibers in the submucosa and between the muscle coats (neural hyperplasia). The absence of ganglion cells leads to an accumulation of the enzyme acetylcholinesterase and acetylcholine. The histochemical demonstration of this enzyme, which is not visualized in the normal rectal mucosa, enhances the reliability of the diagnosis based on rectal biopsy. **Neuronal dysplasia** has features of Hirschsprung disease, but ganglion cells, often histopathologically abnormal, are present. Interestingly, similar to achalasia, which is caused by the destruction of esophageal ganglion cells, Chagas disease may cause aganglionic megacolon.

☐ **Clinical Features:** Hirschsprung disease is the most common cause of congenital intestinal obstruction. The clinical signs of congenital megacolon are delayed passage of meconium by the newborn and the development of vomiting in the first few days of life. In some cases, complete intestinal obstruction requires immediate surgical relief. In others, repeated enemas ameliorate the obstruction; however, fulminant enterocolitis has occasionally followed treatment with multiple enemas. In children who have short rectal segments lacking ganglion cells and who have only partial obstruction, constipation, abdominal distention, and recurrent fecal impactions characterize the clinical course.

The most serious complication of congenital megacolon is an enterocolitis, in which necrosis and ulceration affect the dilated proximal segment of the colon and may extend into the small intestine. The treatment for Hirschsprung disease is surgical removal of the aganglionic segment and reconstruction.

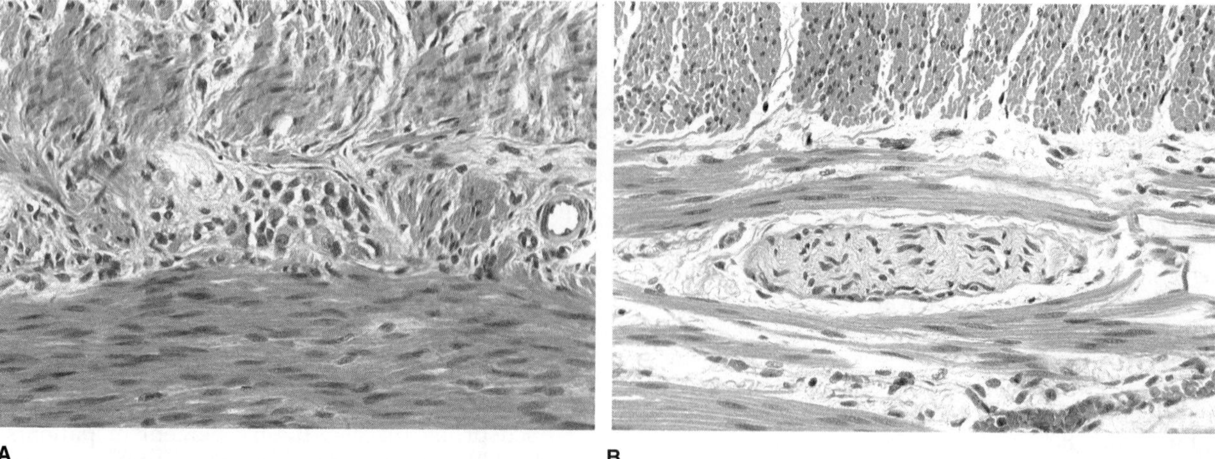

FIGURE *13-39*
Hirschsprung disease. *(A)* A photomicrograph of ganglion cells in the wall of the rectum. *(B)* A rectal biopsy in a case of Hirschsprung disease shows a nonmyelinated nerve in the mesenteric plexus and an absence of ganglion cells.

Acquired Megacolon

This disorder sometimes occurs in children and often has a psychogenic background. Acquired megacolon is also frequently associated with chronic constipation and the prolonged use of laxatives ("cathartic colon"). However, some cases, in which ganglion cells are demonstrated by rectal biopsy, begin in infancy and are associated with fecal incontinence. The cause of this apparently organic disturbance is not well understood, but the disorder is believed to represent a functional abnormality of colonic motility. Acquired megacolon in adults can result from disorders that interfere with the innervation of the bowel or smooth muscle function. Examples include diabetic neuropathy, parkinsonism, myotonic dystrophy, scleroderma, amyloidosis, and hypothyroidism.

Anorectal Malformations

Anorectal malformations are among the most common developmental defects and vary from minor narrowing to serious and complex anomalies. These lesions result from arrested development of the caudal region of the gut in the first 6 months of fetal life. The classification of these defects is based on the relation of the terminal bowel to the levator ani muscle. The classes are (1) high or supralevator deformities, in which the bowel ends above the pelvic floor; (2) intermediate deformities; and (3) low or translevator deformities, in which the bowel ends below the pelvic floor.

- **Anorectal agenesis and rectal atresia** are supralevator deformities.
- **Anal agenesis and anorectal stenosis** are classified as intermediate deformities.
- **Imperforate anus** is a low or translevator deformity in which the opening is covered by a cutaneous membrane behind which meconium is visible. **Anal stenosis** is a variant of imperforate anus.
- **Fistulas** between the malformation and the bladder, urethra, vagina, or skin may or may not occur in all types of anorectal anomalies.

***Pilonidal cyst* is an acquired lesion in the gluteal cleft superior to the anus consisting of cysts or sinus tracts containing hair**. The lesion is thought to be initiated by the penetration of hair beneath the skin. In a young adult, this lesion must occasionally be distinguished from an anorectal fistula. However, its location and the absence of a tract leading to the anus clearly mark it as an entity distinct from anorectal fistula.

Abnormal Positions of the Colon

Abnormal positions of the colon are principally the result of malrotation of the small intestine. The cecum may come to lie in the left lower quadrant or may be located in the middle of the abdomen, in which case, it remains attached to its mesentery. Volvulus is a catastrophic complication.

INFECTIONS

Many of the principal bacterial and parasitic infections that affect the colon, including tuberculosis and amebiasis, have been discussed either in Chapter 9 or earlier in the context of infectious diarrhea in the section on the small intestine.

Most of the remaining infectious diseases are transmitted sexually, principally affect male homosexuals, and primarily involve the anorectal region. These diseases are transmitted by anal intercourse and oral–anal or oral–genital contact. They include gonorrhea, syphilis, lymphogranuloma venereum, anorectal herpes, and venereal warts (condylomata acuminata). There is also a high incidence of colonic infections, such as amebiasis and shigellosis, among male homosexuals.

Pseudomembranous Colitis

Pseudomembranous colitis is a generic term for an inflammatory disease of the colon characterized by exudative plaques superimposed on a congested and edematous mucosa. The term is often used synonymously with *Clostridium difficile* toxin–induced colitis.

☐ **Pathogenesis:** Before the antibiotic era, pseudomembranous colitis was considered primarily a complication of intestinal surgery. After the introduction of antibiotics in the early 1950s, the administration of these drugs, principally tetracycline and chloramphenicol, was recognized to predispose to pseudomembranous colitis. At that time, it was thought that the eradication of certain bacteria in the gut allowed the overgrowth of *S. aureus,* and the term *staphylococcal enterocolitis* was used synonymously with *pseudomembranous enterocolitis.* However, in studies dating to the early 1970s, it became clear that *S. aureus* contributes little to the pathogenesis of antibiotic-associated colitis. It is now recognized that *C. difficile,* which has also been implicated in neonatal necrotizing enterocolitis, is the offending organism. *Clostridium difficile* is not invasive, but it produces toxins that damage the colonic mucosa. Interestingly, although almost all antibiotics have been inplicated in colitis associated with *C. difficile,* particularly ampicillin, clindamycin, and the cephalosporins, the bacteria usually remain sensitive to these antibiotics.

Most cases of pseudomembranous colitis are today associated with antibiotic therapy, but other conditions also may cause this disorder. Gastrointestinal surgery remains an important risk factor. Other predisposing conditions include various diseases of the colon (e.g., adenocarcinoma, obstruction, ischemic colitis, Crohn disease, Hirschsprung disease, shigellosis), shock, spinal fractures, burns, uremia, heavy metal poisoning, and therapy with antineoplastic agents.

The mechanism by which *C. difficile* becomes pathogenic is not entirely clear. Alteration of fecal flora by antibiotics contributes. Only 2% to 3% of healthy adults harbor the organism, whereas 10% to 20% of persons who have recently been treated with antibiotics are infected. By contrast, the microbe can be isolated from the stools of 95% of patients with antibiotic-associated pseudomembranous colitis. Half of healthy newborns are colonized by *C. difficile,* but the isolation rate decreases to adult levels by 1 year of age. The low prevalence of colonization by *C. difficile* in normal adults suggests that the pathogen is transferable. Indeed, outbreaks of pseudomembranous colitis associated with this organism in hospitalized patients have been traced to contaminated sigmoidoscopes, toilets, bed pans, and floors, and treatment of hospitalized carriers with vancomycin has helped to control the disease.

☐ **Pathology:** Macroscopically, the colon, particularly the rectosigmoid region, exhibits raised yellowish plaques up to 2 cm in diameter that adhere to the underlying mucosa (Fig. 13-40). The intervening mucosa appears congested and edematous but is not ulcerated. In severe cases, the plaques coalesce to form extensive pseudomembranes. Microscopic examination of the lesions discloses necrosis of the superficial epithelium, which is believed to be the initial pathological event, especially due to *C. difficile* toxins. Subsequently, the crypts become disrupted and are expanded by mucin and neutrophils. The pseudomembrane consists of the debris of necrotic epithelial cells, mucus, fibrin, and neutrophils.

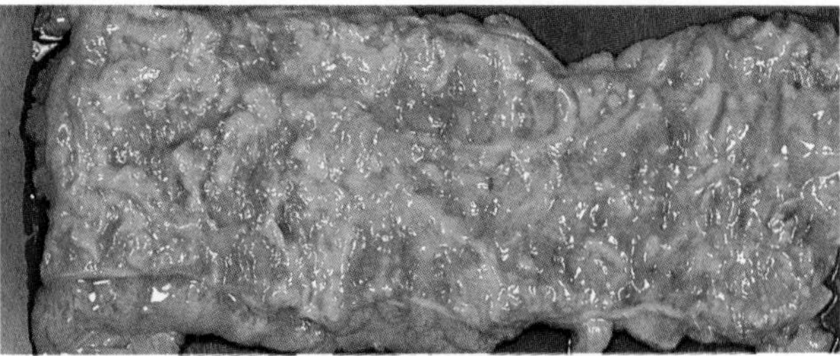

FIGURE *13-40*
Pseudomembranous colitis. The mucosal surface of the colon is covered by raised, irregular plaques composed of necrotic debris and an acute inflammatory exudate.

The lesions are occasionally restricted to the small intestine, in which case the term *pseudomembranous enteritis* is applied. When both the small and the large bowel are involved, the condition is referred to as *pseudomembranous enterocolitis.* Pseudomembranes are occasionally encountered in other enteric infections, such as those involving *S. aureus, Candida,* invasive bacteria, and verotoxin-producing *E. coli;* ischemic bowel disease also produces pseudomembranes.

☐ **Clinical Features:** Antibiotic-associated infections with *C. difficile* are virtually always accompanied by diarrhea, but in most cases, the disorder does not progress to colitis. In patients who develop pseudomembranous colitis, fever, leukocytosis, and abdominal cramps are superimposed on the diarrhea. In the preantibiotic era, this form of colitis was a catastrophic event, and many patients died within hours or days from ileus and irreversible shock. Today pseudomembranous colitis, although still a serious disease, is usually controlled with oral vancomycin therapy (also metronidazole and bacitracin) and supportive fluid and electrolyte therapy.

Neonatal Necrotizing Enterocolitis

Necrotizing enterocolitis is one of the most common acquired surgical emergencies in newborns. It is particularly common in premature infants after oral feeding and is believed to be related principally to an ischemic event involving the intestinal mucosa, which is followed by bacterial colonization, usually with *C. difficile.* The lesions vary from those of typical pseudomembranous enterocolitis to gangrene and perforation of the bowel.

DIVERTICULAR DISEASE

Diverticular disease refers to two entities: a bland, asymptomatic condition termed *diverticulosis,* and an inflammatory complication called *diverticulitis.*

Diverticulosis

Diverticulosis is an acquired herniation (diverticulum) of the mucosa and submucosa through the muscular layers of the colon.

☐ **Epidemiology:** **Diverticulosis shows a striking geographic variation**, being common in Western societies and infrequent in Asia, Africa, and underdeveloped countries. Within the same geographic area, high socioeconomic groups exhibit a considerably higher prevalence than do their poorer neighbors, and emigrants from a low-incidence area to a high-incidence one acquire the increased predilection for the disorder. Diverticulosis is unusual in persons younger than 40 years and increases in frequency with age. Some 10% of persons in western countries are afflicted. Interestingly, this disorder was distinctly uncommon in the last century but now has been demonstrated in one third to one half of persons older than 60 years.

☐ **Pathogenesis:** **The striking variation in the prevalence of diverticulosis implies that environmental factors are primarily responsible for the disease.** Western populations consume a diet in which refined carbohydrates and meat have replaced crude cereal grains, and it is widely assumed that the lack of indigestible fibers in some way predisposes to the formation of diverticula in susceptible persons. In this respect, the larger fecal mass in those who ingest a high-fiber diet diminishes spontaneous motility and intraluminal pressure in the colon. This concept has been supported by the observation that in a carefully matched British population, vegetarians had a threefold lesser prevalence of diverticulosis than did their meat-eating counterparts.

INCREASED INTRALUMINAL PRESSURE: Humans are the only species to develop diverticulosis coli. Although the colons of some other mammals, such as rabbits, horses, and subhuman primates, also have discontinuous bundles of longitudinal muscle (i.e., the taeniae coli), these animals are all herbivorous and clearly ingest large amounts of indigestible fiber. According to the fiber hypothesis, a lack of dietary residue in the Western diet leads to sustained bowel contractions and a consequent increase in intraluminal pressure. Such prolonged increased pressure is believed to lead to a herniation of the superficial coats of the colon through the muscular layers into the serosa.

DEFECTS IN THE WALL OF THE COLON: It is probable that, in addition to pressure, defects in the wall of the colon are required for the formation of a diverticulum. The circular muscle of the colon is interrupted by connective tissue clefts at the sites of penetration by the nutrient vessels that supply the submucosa and mucosa. In persons of advancing age, this connective tissue loses its resilience and, therefore, its resistance to the effects of increased intraluminal pressure. This concept is supported by the observation that persons with heritable disorders of connective tissue (e.g., Marfan syndrome or Ehlers–Danlos syndrome) acquire precocious diverticulosis, primarily of the small bowel. Wide-mouthed diverticula occur in scleroderma.

☐ **Pathology:** The abnormal structures that characterize diverticulosis are not true diverticula, which contain all layers of the intestinal wall, but rather **pseudodiverticula**, in which only the mucosa and submucosa are herniated through the muscle layers. **The sigmoid colon is affected in 95% of the cases**, but diverticulosis can affect any segment of the colon, including the cecum. When more proximal segments of the colon are involved, it is almost always in association with diverticula of the sigmoid.

Diverticula vary in number from a few to several hundred (Fig. 13-41). Most appear in parallel rows between the mesenteric and lateral taeniae. The diverticula, which measure up to 1 cm in greatest dimension, are connected to the intestinal lumen by necks of varying length and caliber. Hardened fecal material (fecalith) is frequently present in the diverticula but does not signify diverticulitis. The muscular wall of the affected colon is consistently thickened, but whether this thickening precedes the diverticulosis or results from it is unknown.

Microscopically, a diverticulum characteristically is seen as a flasklike structure that extends from the lumen through the muscle layers. The wall of the diverticulum is in continuity with the surface mucosa and therefore displays an epithelium and a submucosa. The base of the diverticulum is formed by serosal connective tissue.

☐ **Clinical Features:** **Diverticulosis is generally asymptomatic, and 80% of affected persons remain symptom free.** However, a significant number of those with diverticulosis complain of episodic colicky abdominal pain. Both constipation and diarrhea, sometimes alternating, may occur, and flatulence is common. **Sudden, painless, and severe bleeding from colonic diverticula** is a cause of serious lower gastrointestinal hemorrhage in

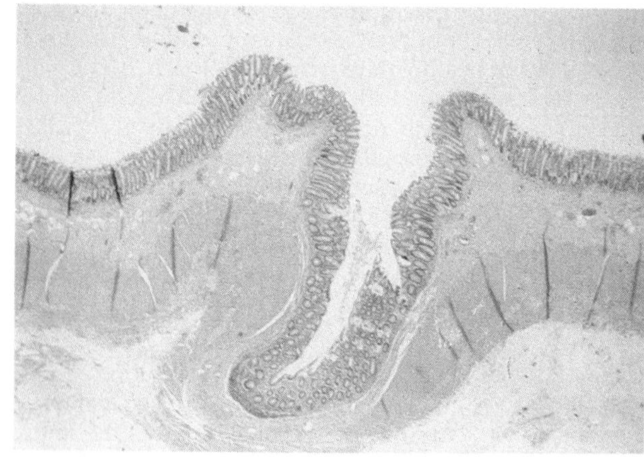

FIGURE *13-41*
Diverticulosis of the colon. A low-power photomicrograph shows a diverticulum, which extends through the muscle layers.

the elderly, occurring in as many as 5% of persons with diverticulosis. Chronic blood loss may lead to anemia.

Diverticulitis

Diverticulitis refers to inflammation at the base of a diverticulum, presumably in response to the irritation caused by retained fecal material. Although the large majority of persons with diverticulosis remain asymptomatic, in 10% to 20%, diverticulitis supervenes at some time in their lives.

☐ **Pathology:** Diverticulitis produces necrosis of the wall of the diverticulum, an event that results in perforation and the release of fecal contents containing bacteria into the peridiverticular tissues. The resulting abscess is usually contained by the appendices epiploicae, the pericolonic fat, the mesentery, or adjacent organs, but infrequently, free perforation leads to **generalized peritonitis**. Fibrosis in response to repeated episodes of diverticulitis may constrict the lumen of the bowel, thereby causing colonic obstruction. **Fistulas** may form between the colon and adjacent organs, including the bladder, vagina, small intestine, and skin of the abdomen. Additional complications include pylephlebitis and liver abscesses.

☐ **Clinical Features:** The most common symptoms of diverticulitis, usually following microscopic or gross perforation of the diverticulum, are persistent lower abdominal pain and fever. Changes in bowel habits, ranging from diarrhea to constipation, are frequent, and dysuria indicates irritation of the bladder. Most patients exhibit tenderness in the left lower quadrant, and a mass in that area is not infrequently palpated. Leukocytosis is the rule. Antibiotic treatment and supportive measures are usually successful in alleviating acute diverticulitis, but about 20% of patients eventually require surgical intervention.

IDIOPATHIC INFLAMMATORY BOWEL DISEASE

Idiopathic inflammatory bowel disease is a term that describes two diseases: Crohn disease and ulcerative colitis. Although these two disorders usually differ sufficiently to be clearly distinguishable, they have many common features, and it is still debated whether they are two distinct entities or merely ends of a continuum. Until more definitive information becomes available, it is convenient to consider both diseases within a single conceptual framework because of the following common features: (1) inflammation of the bowel, (2) lack of a proven causal agent, (3) pattern of familial occurrence, and (4) systemic manifestations. **Similarities apart, Crohn disease and ulcerative colitis have different clinical courses and natural histories.**

Crohn Disease

Crohn disease is a transmural, granulomatous, inflammatory disease that may affect any part of the digestive tract but occurs principally in the small intestine and occasionally the colon. The malady has acquired a multitude of names, owing to the confusion that has resulted from its varied anatomical and clinical features. It has variously been referred to as terminal ileitis and regional ileitis when it involves mainly the ileum, and granulomatous colitis and transmural colitis when it principally affects the colon. **Today, the eponym Crohn disease is most commonly used because the disorder may involve any part of the gastrointestinal tract and even tissues in other organs.**

☐ **Epidemiology:** Crohn disease occurs throughout the world, with an annual incidence of 0.5 to 5 per 100,000. Reports from various countries indicate that the incidence has increased dramatically over the past 30 years. The disease usually appears in adolescents or young adults and is most common among persons of European origin, with a considerably higher frequency among Jews. There is a slight female predominance (up to 1.6:1).

☐ **Pathogenesis:** Epidemiological studies, particularly concordance rates in twin pairs and siblings, strongly implicate genetic susceptibility in the pathogenesis of Crohn disease. In fact, the relative contribution of genetic factors to the pathogenesis of this disorder may be greater than that in schizophrenia, asthma, or hypertension, and at least equivalent to that in insulin-dependent diabetes. A family history of inflammatory bowel disease (Crohn disease or ulcerative colitis) has been found in as many as 40% of cases, with the greatest frequency among close relatives. A putative susceptibility locus for Crohn disease has been assigned to the centromeric region of chromosome 16, at least in non-Jewish patients. Other susceptibility loci may reside on chromosomes 3, 7, and 12. Crohn disease has only rarely been described in both a husband and a wife, a fact that indicates that environmental factors alone are not a sufficient cause of the disease. Interestingly, most patients with Crohn disease are smokers. Intensive research since the disease was first described in 1932 has failed to elucidate the etiology of Crohn disease. Several infectious agents have been suggested as possible causative agents. Bacteria that have been cultured from tissue involved with Crohn disease include a variant of *Pseudomonas* and atypical mycobacteria. The possibility of a viral cause also has been raised. None of these studies has given consistently reproducible results, and the excitement that has accompanied each new discovery of a possible causal pathogen has waned with failure to confirm the initial results.

If an infectious agent is not responsible for the disease, perhaps altered host susceptibility plays a role. Several studies have shown impairment of cell-mediated immunity in patients with Crohn disease. Some investigators have suggested increased suppressor T-cell activity, and others have claimed impaired phagocytic function. None of these findings has been confirmed. Inconsistent results have also been reported from studies of histocompatibility antigens in this disease.

The possibility that Crohn disease might be caused by immune-mediated damage to the intestine has been suggested by the chronic and recurrent nature of the inflammation and by the occurrence of systemic manifestations that are frequently associated with autoimmune diseases. However, no consistent evidence has been produced in favor of abnormal humoral immune responses or of circulating immune complexes as a cause of the disease. In recent years, most immunological studies have been concerned with the possible role of cell-mediated cytotoxicity. Some studies support the hypothesis that cytotoxic T cells sensitized to bacterial or other antigens damage the intestinal wall. In this respect, cyclosporine, a potent inhibitor of cell-mediated immunity that is widely used to prevent rejection of transplanted organs, has been reported to ameliorate the symptoms of Crohn disease.

The production of TNF-α is increased *in vitro* in mucosal cells derived from patients with Crohn disease. Moreover, in these patients, a shift in the mucosal balance of cytokine production by T cells toward TNF-α was observed. Importantly, the administration of anti–TNF-α antibodies to patients with Crohn disease provided effective short-term symptom remission.

The possibility that dietary factors or emotional stress may play a role in the pathogenesis of Crohn disease has led to a number of studies that, again, have produced inconsistent results. The fecal stream appears to be of prime importance, as evidenced by (1) the beneficial effects of surgical bypass, (2) the pattern of preanastomotic recurrence in patients with side-to-end anastomotic sites, and (3) the frequency of early inflammatory lesions (apthoid erosions) in association with phagocytic follicle-associated epithelium of mucosal lymphoid tissue.

☐ **Pathology:** Two major features characterize the pathology of Crohn disease and serve to differentiate it from other inflammatory diseases of the gastrointestinal tract. First, the inflammation usually involves all layers of the bowel wall and is, therefore, referred to as **transmural** inflammatory disease. Second, the inflammation of the intestine is discontinuous; that is, segments of inflamed tissue are separated by apparently normal intestine. The inflamed areas are frequently (and paradoxically) referred to as "skip" areas by surgeons and endoscopists.

It is convenient to classify Crohn disease into four broad macroscopic patterns, although many patients do not fit precisely into any one of them: the disease involves (1) mainly the ileum and cecum in about 50% of cases, (2) only the small intestine in 15%, (3) only the colon in 20%, and (4) principally the anorectal region in 15%. Disease of the ileum and cecum is more frequent when the onset of Crohn disease occurs in young persons, whereas colitis is common in older patients. Crohn disease is occasionally observed in the duodenum and stomach as a focal chronic inflammatory process, and more rarely in the esophagus and oral cavity, almost always in association with small intestinal Crohn disease. In women with anorectal Crohn disease, the inflammation may spread to involve the external genitalia.

The macroscopic and microscopic pathology of Crohn disease is variable and may comprise almost any combination of features considered characteristic of the disease. The following description relates to the typical morphological alterations encountered. On gross examination, the bowel affected by Crohn disease appears thickened and edematous, as does the adjacent mesentery. Mesenteric fat often wraps around the bowel ("creeping fat"). Mesenteric lymph nodes are frequently enlarged, firm, and matted together. The lumen is narrowed by edema in early cases and by a combination of edema and fibrosis in long-standing disease. Nodular swelling, fibrosis, and ulceration of the mucosa lead to a "cobblestone" appearance (Fig. 13-42). Ulcers vary in depth. In early cases, the ulcers have either an apthous or a serpiginous appearance; later they become deeper and appear as linear clefts or fissures.

The cut surface of the bowel wall shows the transmural nature of the disease, with thickening, edema, and fibrosis of all layers. Involved loops of bowel often become adherent, and fistulas between such segments are frequent. These fistulas, presumably a late result of the deep mural ulcers, may also penetrate from the bowel into other organs, including the bladder, uterus, vagina, and skin. Most fistulas end blindly, forming abscess cavities within the peritoneal cavity, in the mesentery, or in retroperitoneal structures. Lesions in the distal rectum and anus may create perianal fistulas, a well-known presenting feature of Crohn disease.

Microscopically, Crohn disease appears as a chronic inflammatory process that typically extends through all layers of the bowel wall (Fig. 13-43). During early phases of the disease, the inflammation may be confined to the mucosa and submucosa. Small, superficial mucosal ulcerations (aphthous ulcers) are seen, together with mucosal and submucosal edema and an increase in the number of lymphocytes, plasma cells, and histiocytes. Destruction of the mucosal architecture, with regenerative changes in the crypts and villous distortion, are frequent. Pyloric metaplasia and Paneth cell hyperplasia are common in the small intestine, and Paneth hyperplasia or metaplasia in the colorectum. Endothelial swelling in small blood vessels and lymphatics is usually prominent. Later, long, deep, fissure-like ulcers are seen, and vascular hyalinization and fibrosis become apparent.

The microscopic hallmark of Crohn disease is transmural nodular lymphoid aggregates, accompanied by proliferative changes of the muscularis mucosae and nerves of the submucosal and myenteric plexuses. **Discrete, noncaseating granulomas, mostly in the submucosa, are often present.** Indistinguishable from those of sarcoidosis, these granulomas consist of focal aggregates

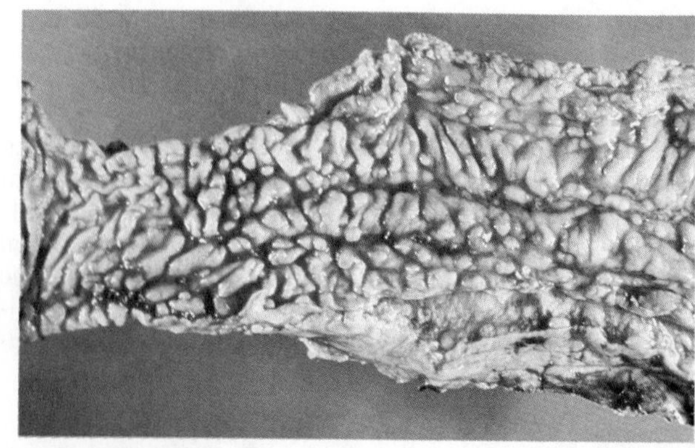

FIGURE *13-42*
Crohn disease. The mucosal surface of the colon displays a "cobblestone" appearance owing to the presence of linear ulcerations and edema and inflammation of the intervening tissue.

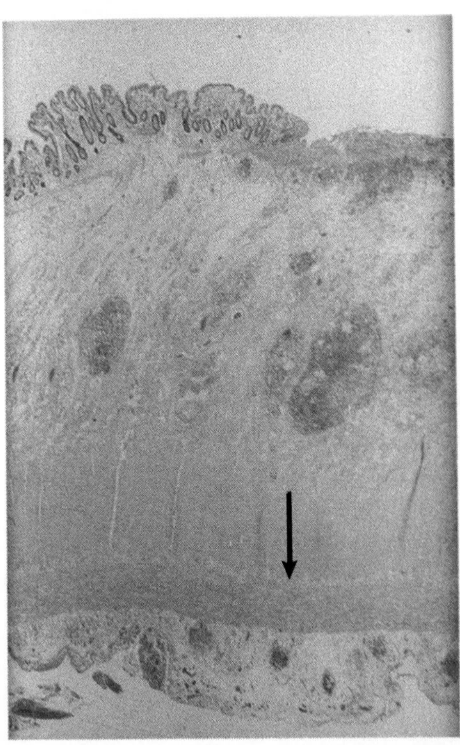

FIGURE 13-43
Crohn disease. A section of the colon shows mucosal ulceration *(right)*, a submucosa thickened by edema and nodular aggregates of chronic inflammatory cells, prominence of the myenteric plexus *(arrow)*, and an expanded and congested serosa.

of epithelioid cells, vaguely limited by a rim of lymphocytes. Multinucleated giant cells may be present, and the center of the granulomas usually displays hyaline material, but no caseation, and only very rarely necrosis.

Although the presence of discrete granulomas is strong evidence in favor of Crohn disease, the absence of granulomas by no means excludes the diagnosis. Indeed only half the cases show the typical granulomas, whereas the others show either a diffuse granulomatous reaction or nonspecific transmural inflammation. Thus, the diagnosis of Crohn disease is made principally on the basis of the **transmural** nature of the inflammation rather than on the basis of granulomas.

The pathological features of Crohn disease are summarized in Figure 13-44.

□ **Clinical Features:** The clinical manifestations and the natural history of Crohn disease are highly variable and are related to the anatomical localization of the disease. The most frequent symptoms are **abdominal pain and diarrhea**, which occur in more than 75% of patients, and recurrent **fever**, evident in 50%. The onset of the malady is usually insidious, although symptoms may occur acutely. When the disease involves mainly the ileum and cecum, the sudden onset may mimic appendicitis, and the diagnosis of Crohn disease is occasionally made first at the time of abdominal surgery. If the disease involves the ileum predominantly, the major clinical features are right lower quadrant pain, intermittent diarrhea and fever, and frequently a tender mass in the right lower quadrant of the abdomen. In cases of diffuse small intestinal involvement, **malabsorption** and malnutrition may be the major features. Lipid malabsorption may also result from interruption of the enterohepatic cycle of bile salts because of ileal disease. Crohn disease of the colon leads to **diarrhea** and sometimes **colonic bleeding**. In a few patients, the major site of involvement is the anorectal region, and recurrent anorectal fistulas are the presenting sign.

When Crohn disease begins in childhood, its major manifestation may be retardation of growth and physical development. The most frequent extraintestinal inflammatory features are in the eye (episcleritis or uveitis), the medium-sized joints (arthritis), and the skin (erythema nodosum).

Intestinal obstruction and fistulas are the most common intestinal complications of Crohn disease. Occasionally, free perforation of the bowel occurs. **The risk of intestinal cancer is increased at least threefold in patients with Crohn disease, and the disease also predisposes to colorectal cancer.** Systemic complications (in addition to the eye, joint, and skin lesions mentioned earlier) include liver disease (pericholangitis, sclerosing cholangitis), cholelithiasis, oxalate stones in the kidneys, and amyloidosis.

In the differential diagnosis of Crohn disease, one must consider bacterial infections, especially *Campylobacter* or *Y. enterocolitica* infection and tuberculosis; amebic colitis; schistosomiasis; and, less commonly, inflammation due to *Chlamydia*. Other conditions that may mimic Crohn disease (especially Crohn colitis) are pseudomembranous colitis, radiation injury, lymphoma, and ulcerative colitis.

No curative treatment is available for Crohn disease. Several medications are effective in suppressing the inflammatory reaction, including corticosteroids, sulfasalazine, metronidazole, 6-mercaptopurine, and cyclosporine. Surgical resection of obstructed areas or of severely involved portions of intestine and drainage of abscesses caused by fistulas are required in some cases. Preanastamotic or prestomal recurrence of the disease after resection is a hallmark of Crohn disease, a feature that makes clinical management difficult. The need for repeated resections can lead to short-bowel syndrome in some patients.

Ulcerative Colitis

Ulcerative colitis is an inflammatory disease of the large intestine characterized by chronic diarrhea and rectal bleeding, with a pattern of exacerbations and remissions, and with the possibility of serious local and systemic complications. The disorder is common in the Western world, occurring principally, but not exclusively, in young adults. The terms **nonspecific** and **idiopathic** have also been applied to this condition.

□ **Epidemiology:** In Europe and North America, ulcerative colitis has an annual incidence of 4 to 7 per 100,000 population and a prevalence of 40 to 80 per 100,000. There appears to be no sex predominance. The disease usually begins in early adult life, with a peak incidence in the third decade of life. However, it also occurs

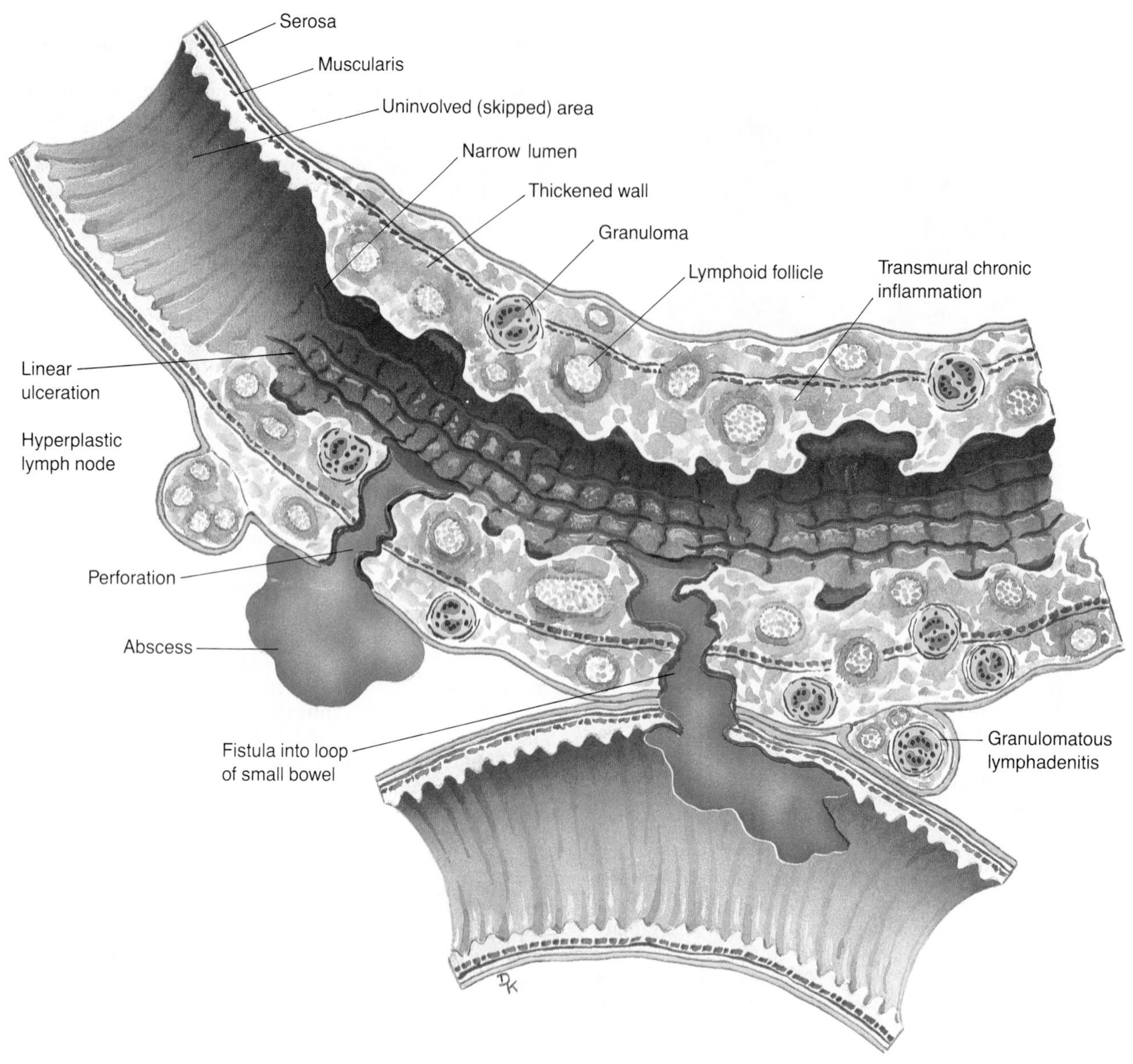

FIGURE *13-44*
Crohn disease. A schematic representation of the major features of Crohn disease in the small intestine.

in childhood and in old age. In the United States, whites are affected more commonly than blacks. It has been reported that the disease is especially common among Jews in the United States, although a study in Israel has shown a lower incidence and prevalence of the disease in Tel Aviv than in Baltimore, Copenhagen, or Oxford.

☐ **Pathogenesis:** **The cause of ulcerative colitis is not known.** Attempts to implicate a viral or bacterial agent have given only inconsistent results. The higher than normal incidence of ulcerative colitis in first-degree relatives of patients with the disease (up to 40% familial incidence) points to a genetic predisposition. Indeed, in some families, as many as six patients with this disease have been described, and concordance has been reported in monozygotic twins. However, available family studies do not suggest any distinct mode of genetic transmission, and studies of HLA distribution in patients with ulcerative colitis have not demonstrated a consistent pattern.

A possible role for so-called psychosomatic factors in the pathogenesis of ulcerative colitis was entertained for many years, but several well-planned studies during the past 20 years have failed to incriminate specific psychological traits, other than those to be expected in any long-term chronic disease.

The possibility that an abnormal immune response may play a role in the pathogenesis of ulcerative colitis has been extensively studied. The presence of abundant lymphoid tissue throughout the colon has made such a possibility attractive, as has the documented association of this disorder with immunorelated features, such as uveitis, erythema nodosum, and vasculitis. Several studies have demonstrated an increased frequency of circulating antibodies against antigens in colonic epithelial cells and against cross-reacting antigens in enterobacteria. Furthermore, *in vitro* studies of cell-mediated immune function have shown that mononuclear cells from the colonic mucosa and from the blood of patients with ulcerative colitis are toxic for autologous colonic epithelial cells. Perinuclear antineutrophil cytoplasmic antibodies (P-ANCA) have also been demonstrated in patients with ulcerative colitis. However, these abnormalities are not found exclusively in patients with ulcerative colitis, nor are any of these changes a prerequisite for the development of ulcerative colitis. It is, therefore, possible that all of these immune features are merely epiphenomena (that is, the result, rather than the cause, of the mucosal damage).

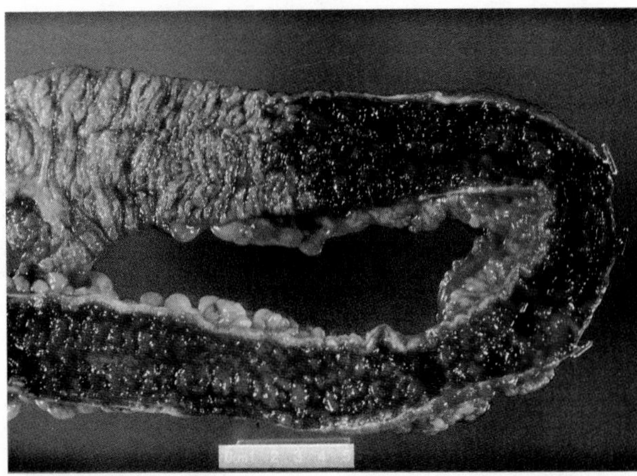

FIGURE *13-45*
Ulcerative colitis. Prominent erythema and ulceration of the colon begin in the ascending colon and are most severe in the rectosigmoid area.

☐ **Pathology:** Three major pathological features characterize ulcerative colitis and help to differentiate it from other inflammatory conditions:

- **Ulcerative colitis is a diffuse disease.** It usually extends from the most distal part of the rectum for a variable distance proximally. When the disease involves the rectum alone, it is referred to as *ulcerative proctitis.* When the inflammatory process extends toward the splenic flexure, the terms *proctosigmoiditis and left-sided colitis* are applied. *Universal colitis* or *pancolitis* describes disease involving the entire colon, from the anorectal junction to the ileocecal valve. Sparing of the rectum or involvement of the right side of the colon alone is rare and suggests the possibility of another disorder, such as Crohn disease.
- **The inflammatory process of ulcerative colitis is limited to the colon.** It does not involve the small intestine, stomach, or esophagus. When the cecum is affected, the disease ends at the ileocecal valve, although minor inflammation of the adjacent ileum is sometimes noted (backwash ileitis).
- **Ulcerative colitis is essentially a disease of the mucosa.** Involvement of deeper layers is uncommon, occurring only in fulminant cases, usually in association with toxic megacolon.

The macroscopic appearance of the mucosa throughout the colon has been extensively documented through the increasingly widespread use of fiberoptic colonoscopy. The following morphological sequence may develop rapidly or over a course of years.

EARLY COLITIS: Early in the evolution of the disease, the mucosal surface appears raw, red, and granular. It is frequently covered with a yellowish exudate and bleeds easily when touched by an instrument or a cotton swab. Later small, superficial erosions or ulcers may appear. These occasionally coalesce to form irregular, shallow, ulcerated areas that appear to surround islands of intact mucosa (Fig. 13-45). Raised areas of mucosa, corresponding to inflammatory polyps ("pseudopolyps") can be seen. In cases of toxic megacolon, the lumen is widely dilated, and the wall is thin and friable. Single or multiple perforations are common in **toxic megacolon**, and the serosal surface is often covered by a fibrinopurulent exudate.

The microscopic features of early ulcerative colitis correlate well with the colonoscopic appearances. Although they are not specifically diagnostic, they represent a highly characteristic pattern of injury. The early histopathological features are (1) mucosal congestion, edema, and microscopic hemorrhages; (2) a diffuse chronic inflammatory infiltrate in the lamina propria; and (3) damage and distortion of the colorectal crypts, which are often surrounded and infiltrated by neutrophils (Fig. 13-46). Suppurative necrosis of the crypt epithelium gives rise to the characteristic **crypt abscess**, which appears as a dilated, degenerated crypt filled with neutrophils.

PROGRESSIVE COLITIS: As the disease progresses, mucosal folds are lost (atrophy). Lateral extension and coalescence of crypt abscesses can undermine the mucosa, leaving areas of ulceration adjacent to hanging fragments of mucosa. Such mucosal excrescences surrounded by ulceration are seen by endoscopy or roentgenographic examination as *inflammatory polyps.* Tissue destruction is accompanied by manifestations of tissue repair. Highly vascular granulation tissue develops in denuded areas (Fig. 13-47). Collagen deposition is sparse and patchy, and fibrosis is not a prominent feature. Importantly, the strictures characteristic of Crohn disease are absent. Microscopically, the colorectal crypts may appear tortuous, branched, and shortened in the late stages, and the mucosa may be diffusely atrophic.

ADVANCED COLITIS: In long-standing cases, the large bowel is often shortened, especially in the left side. The mucosal folds are indistinct and are replaced by a granular or smooth mucosal pattern. Microscopically, advanced ulcerative colitis is characterized by mucosal atrophy and a chronic inflammatory infiltrate in the mucosa

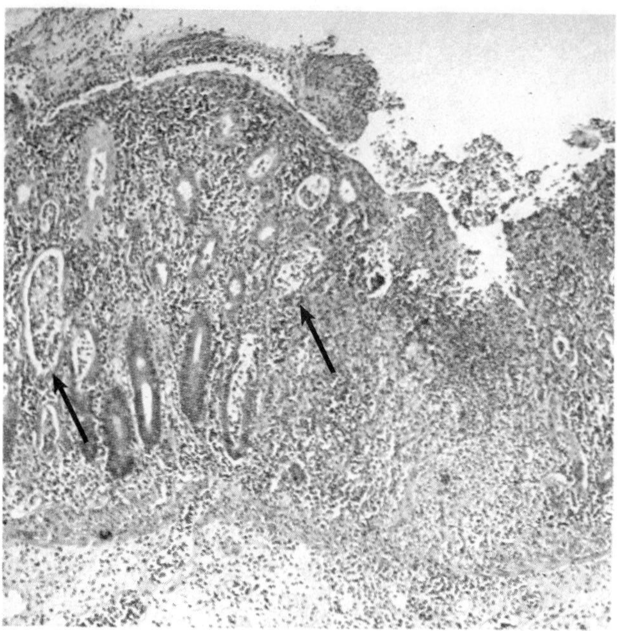

FIGURE 13-46
Ulcerative colitis. A section of the colonic mucosa from a patient with active ulcerative colitis shows purulent exudate on the surface, ulceration *(center)*, diffuse inflammation superficial to the muscularis mucosae, and numerous crypt abscesses *(arrows)*.

and superficial submucosa (see Fig. 13-42). Paneth cell hyperplasia and metaplasia are common.

☐ **Clinical Features:** The clinical course and manifestations of ulcerative colitis are highly variable. Most patients (70%) have intermittent attacks, with partial or complete remission between attacks. A small number (<10%) have a very long remission (several years) after their first attack. The remaining 20% have continuous symptoms without remission.

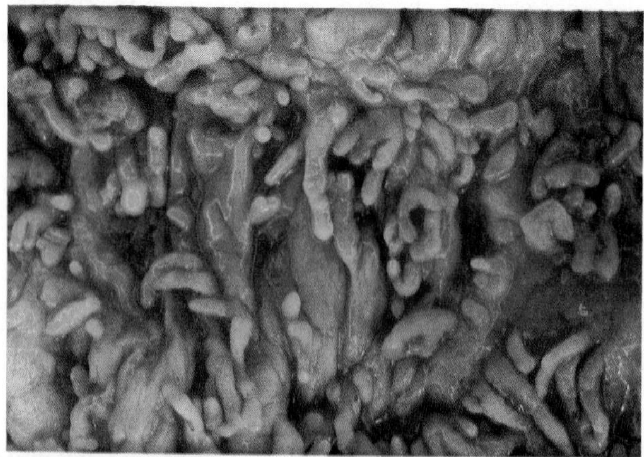

FIGURE 13-47
Inflammatory polyps of the colon in ulcerative colitis. Islands of regenerative mucosa surrounded by denuded areas provide a polypoid appearance.

It is convenient to classify the disease into three arbitrary clinical categories: mild, moderate, and severe (fulminant).

MILD COLITIS: Half of the patients with ulcerative colitis have mild disease. Their major symptom is rectal bleeding, sometimes accompanied by tenesmus (rectal pressure and discomfort). The disease in these patients is usually limited to the rectum but may extend to the distal sigmoid colon. Extraintestinal complications are uncommon, and in most patients in this category, the disease remains mild throughout their lives.

MODERATE COLITIS: About 40% of patients are categorized as having moderate ulcerative colitis. They usually have recurrent episodes of loose bloody stools, crampy abdominal pain, and frequently low-grade fever, lasting days or weeks. Moderate anemia is a common result of chronic fecal blood loss.

SEVERE COLITIS: A small minority (10%) of patients have severe or fulminant ulcerative colitis, sometimes from its onset but often during a flare of activity. They have more than 6, and sometimes more than 20, bloody bowel movements daily, frequently accompanied by fever and other systemic manifestations. The loss of blood and fluids rapidly leads to anemia, dehydration, and electrolyte depletion. Massive hemorrhage is occasionally life threatening. A particularly dangerous complication of fulminant colitis is toxic megacolon, which is characterized by extreme dilatation of the colon. Patients with this condition are at high risk for perforation of the colon. Fulminant ulcerative colitis is a medical emergency requiring immediate, intensive medical therapy and, in some cases, prompt colectomy. About 15% of patients with fulminant ulcerative colitis die of the disease.

Extraintestinal Manifestations

Arthritis is seen in 25% of patients with ulcerative colitis. Eye inflammation (mostly **uveitis**) develops in about 10%, and skin lesions occur in about the same number. The most common cutaneous lesions are **erythema nodosum** and **pyoderma gangrenosum**, the latter being a serious, noninfective disorder characterized by deep, purulent, necrotic ulcers in the skin.

Liver disease occurs in 3% of patients, the most common pathological findings being pericholangitis and fatty liver. Chronic active hepatitis is occasionally encountered in conjunction with ulcerative colitis, and sclerosing cholangitis and carcinoma of the bile ducts are both associated with the colorectal disease. Thromboembolic phenomena, mostly deep vein thromboses of the lower extremities, occur in 6% of ulcerative colitis patients.

The various complications of ulcerative colitis are shown in Figure 13-48.

Differential Diagnosis

The most important conditions to be distinguished from ulcerative colitis are other forms of chronic colitis due to specifically treatable causes and Crohn disease of the

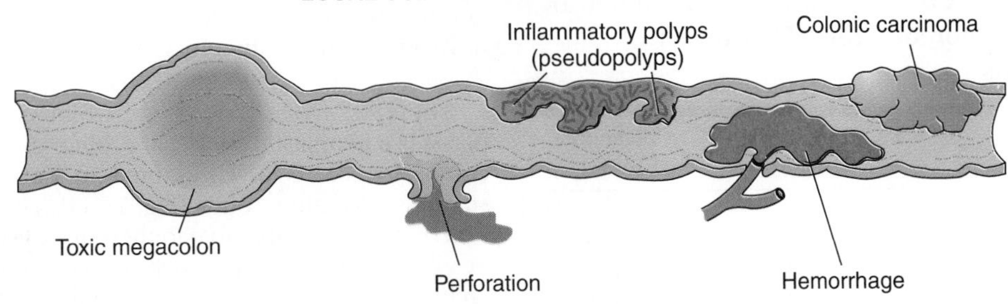

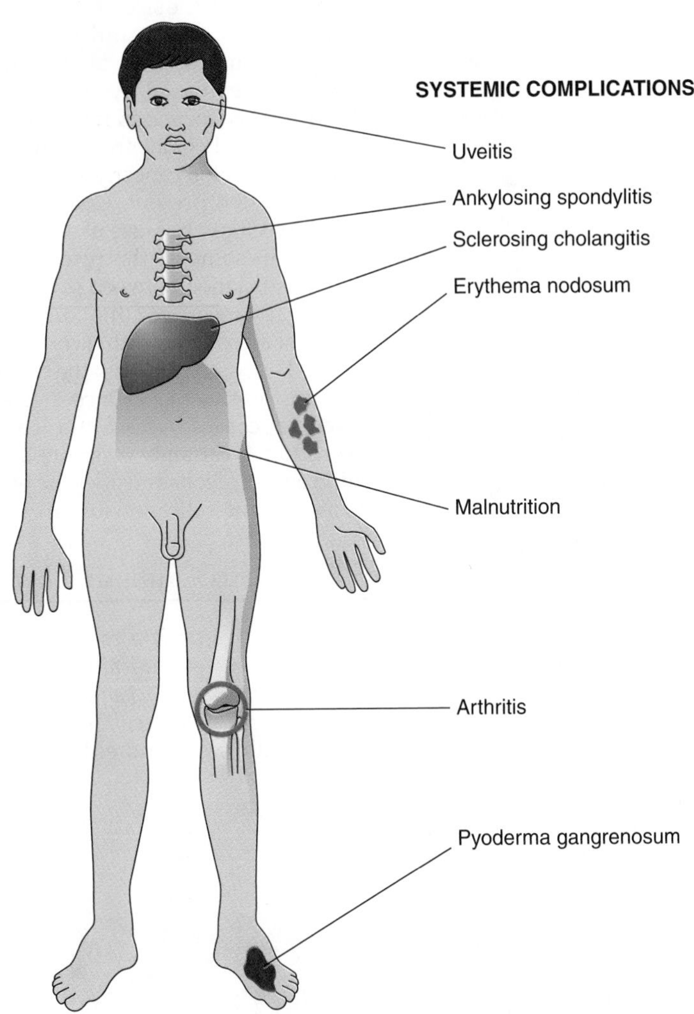

FIGURE *13-48*
Complications of ulcerative colitis.

colon (Crohn colitis, granulomatous colitis). Other conditions that should be considered in the differential diagnosis of ulcerative colitis are bacterial infections (e.g., with *Shigella, Salmonella, Campylobacter*) and amebic colitis, especially in areas in which it is endemic. When the inflammation is limited to the rectum, other infectious agents, including viruses, *Chlamydia*, fungi, and other parasites should be considered. Proctitis due to these agents is common in male homosexuals, and a variety of opportunistic infections of the bowel are encountered in patients with AIDS. Other conditions that may mimic ulcerative colitis are ischemic colitis, antibiotic-associated colitis, radiation injury, and the solitary rectal ulcer syndrome.

The distinction between ulcerative colitis and Crohn colitis is based on the difference in anatomical localization and histopathological appearance (Table 13-1). Ulcerative colitis is a diffuse process, usually more severe distally. By contrast, Crohn colitis is a patchy or segmental disease,

TABLE *13-1* **Comparison of the Pathological Features in the Colon of Crohn Disease and Ulcerative Colitis**

Lesion	Crohn Disease	Ulcerative Colitis
Macroscopic		
Thickened bowel wall	Typical	Uncommon
Luminal narrowing	Typical	Uncommon
"Skip" lesions	Common	Absent
Right colon predominance	Typical	Absent
Fissures and fistulas	Common	Absent
Circumscribed ulcers	Common	Absent
Confluent linear ulcers	Common	Absent
Pseudopolyps	Absent	Common
Microscopic		
Transmural inflammation	Typical	Uncommon
Submucosal fibrosis	Typical	Absent
Fissures	Typical	Rare
Granulomas	Common	Absent
Crypt abscesses	Uncommon	Typical

with frequent sparing of the rectum. The inflammation in ulcerative colitis is superficial (i.e., usually limited to the mucosa) and is characterized by an acute inflammatory infiltrate, with neutrophils and crypt abscesses. By contrast, Crohn colitis is transmural and involves all layers, with granulomas in many, although not all, specimens.

Demarcation of the disease at the ileocecal valve, or in the colon distal to it, favors ulcerative colitis. Involvement of the terminal ileum (a cobblestone-like gross appearance, discrete ulcers, and fistulas) suggest Crohn colitis.

In 10% of cases, a precise diagnosis of ulcerative colitis versus Crohn colitis cannot be made, and the idiopathic inflammatory bowel disease is termed indeterminant colitis. The distinction between ulcerative colitis and Crohn colitis is important because of (1) different surgical therapy (Crohn disease often has recurrences, so that continent ileostomy and ileoanal pouch procedures may be contraindicated), (2) a higher risk of cancer in ulcerative colitis, and (3) different medical therapy. Rare patients with both diseases have been reported.

Ulcerative Colitis and Colorectal Cancer

Persons with long-standing, extensive ulcerative colitis have a higher risk of colorectal cancer than do those of the general population. The risk is related to the extent of colorectal involvement and the duration of the inflammatory disease. Thus, persons with involvement of the entire colon are at the greatest risk of developing colorectal cancer. In patients with inflammatory disease limited to the rectum, colorectal cancer is no more common than in the general population. An incidence of colorectal cancer in the range of 5% to 10% for each decade of pancolitis is seen in the United States. Young age at the onset of colitis does not seem to be an independent risk factor, but because patients in whom ulcerative colitis develops at a young age have a longer duration of disease, they also have a high cumulative incidence of cancer.

EPITHELIAL DYSPLASIA: Colorectal epithelial dysplasia is a neoplastic epithelial proliferation and is the precursor to colorectal carcinoma in patients with long-standing ulcerative colitis (Fig. 13-49). The histopathological criteria are comparable to those for dysplasia in tubular or villous adenomas and include (1) alteration of mucosal architecture, (2) epithelial abnormalities (hypercellularity and stratification of nuclei), and (3) cytological abnormalities (variation in the size, shape, and staining qualities of nuclei). Dysplasia can be difficult to distinguish from reactive changes resulting from activity of the ulcerative colitis. High-grade epithelial dysplasia reflects a high probability of cancer or an increased risk of development of such a cancer. In resected colons from patients with ulcerative colitis that contain colon cancer, severe dysplasia distant from the tumor is often present. Conversely, in patients who undergo colectomy because of severe dysplasia, cancer is discovered in some of the resected colons. Because of the strong association between severe epithelial dysplasia and colorectal cancer, routine surveillance by colonoscopic biopsy of all patients with ulcerative colitis has been recommended by some, although the cost–benefit ratio of this procedure is controversial. Once severe dysplasia has been detected, a careful search for cancer elsewhere in the colorectum is certainly warranted, and many gastroenterologists and surgeons consider the presence of severe dysplasia a sufficient indication for proctocolectomy.

Collagenous Colitis and Lymphocytic Colitis

Collagenous colitis is a rare, inflammatory disorder of the colon characterized clinically by chronic watery diarrhea and pathologically by a thickening of the collagen table immediately below the surface epithelium. The disorder mainly afflicts middle-aged and elderly women.

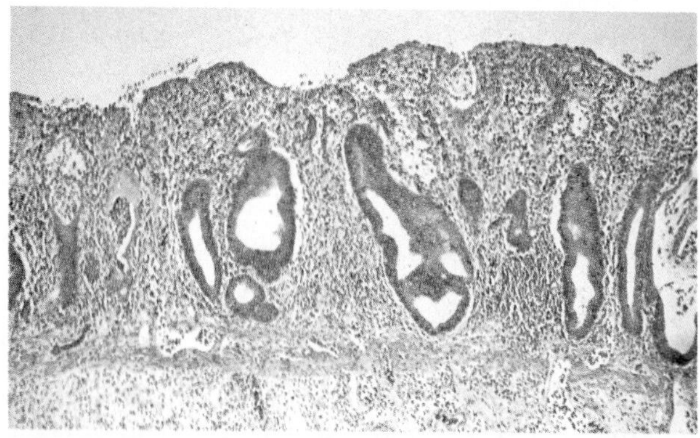

FIGURE *13-49*
Epithelial dysplasia in ulcerative colitis. The colonic mucosa exhibits severe inflammation and irregular crypts lined by dysplastic epithelial cells. The epithelial cells exhibit hyperchromatic nuclei and basophilic cytoplasm and are focally stratified.

The histopathological diagnosis of collagenous colitis is made by the demonstration of inflammatory disease with a band of acellular collagen immediately beneath the surface epithelium (Fig. 13-50). The surface epithelium displays flattened or cuboidal cells and even separation of the epithelial cells from the underlying structures. Intraepithelial lymphocytes and eosinophils are frequent. The lamina propria contains increased numbers of chronic inflammatory cells, but polymorphonuclear leukocytes are also found in some patients. ***Lymphocytic colitis*** also has the prominent infiltration of the damaged colonic epithelium by lymphocytes but lacks the collagen table and has an equal sex distribution.

The etiology of collagenous colitis and lymphocytic colitis is unknown. It has been postulated that the fibrosis of collagenous colitis may be the result of persistent inflammation. Although the diseases have not been consistently linked to other systemic disorders, an autoimmune etiology also has been suggested, based on a putative association with inflammatory polyarthritis and thyroiditis. Compared with patients with collagenous colitis, those with with lymphocytic colitis have an increased frequency of HLA-A1 and a decreased frequency of A3. Many patients with these diseases have taken nonsteroidal anti-inflammatory drugs.

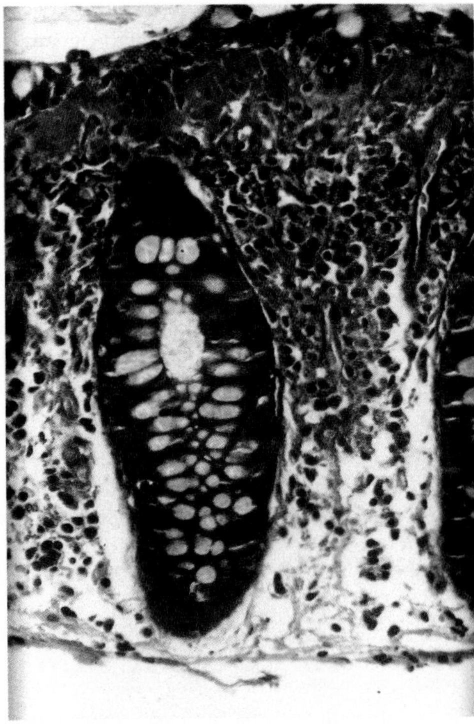

FIGURE *13-50*
Collagenous colitis. A band of acellular collagen is evident beneath the surface epithelium with the trichrome stain for connective tissue.

VASCULAR DISEASES

Ischemic Colitis

The colon is subject to the same types of ischemic injury as is the small intestine. Unlike the small bowel, extensive infarction of the colon is uncommon; chronic segmental disease is the rule. The most vulnerable areas are those between adjacent arterial distributions, so-called watershed areas. For example, the splenic flexure lies between the regions supplied by the superior and inferior mesenteric arteries, and the rectosigmoid area shares the blood from the inferior mesenteric and internal iliac arteries. However, the rectum itself is usually spared in ischemic colitis.

Because most cases of ischemic colitis are caused by atherosclerosis, the intestinal disease usually occurs in persons older than 50 years. Colonic ischemia also occurs in about 2% of patients undergoing aortoiliac reconstruction and has been reported in association with hypercoagulable states, vasculitis, and colorectal cancer.

☐ **Pathology:** Some patients are seen with the symptoms and complications of bowel infarction and require immediate surgical intervention. However, in the majority of patients, the acute signs stabilize, and radiographic examination shows only the pattern associated with intramural hemorrhage and edema. On sigmoidoscopy, multiple ulcers, hemorrhagic nodular lesions, or a pseudomembrane is seen. Biopsy reveals the characteristic changes of ischemic necrosis of the bowel: mucosal ulcerations, crypt abscesses, collapse of the lamina propria, edema, and hemorrhage. Acute and chronic inflammation and fibrosis develop as the disease proceeds. Such patients may recover completely or may develop a colonic stricture, in which case, surgical removal of the obstructing segment becomes necessary. Segments of ischemic stricture show variable mucosal ulceration and inflammation, as well as widening of the submucosa by granulation tissue and fibrosis. Hemosiderin-laden macrophages may be noted, and patchy fibrosis of the muscular coats also may be present. Submucosal arterioles are characteristically thick walled and tortuous.

☐ **Clinical Features:** Ischemic disease of the rectosigmoid area is typically manifested as abdominal pain, rectal bleeding, and a change in bowel habits. On clinical grounds alone, ischemic colitis often cannot be distinguished from certain forms of infective colitis (verotoxin-producing *E. coli, Clostridium difficile* toxin–induced inflammatory disease), ulcerative colitis, and Crohn disease of the colon.

Angiodysplasia (Vascular Ectasia)

Angiodysplasia refers to localized arteriovenous malformations, predominantly in the cecum and ascending colon, which produce lower intestinal bleeding. The mean age at presentation is 60 years. Younger persons preferentially exhibit lesions at other sites, including the rectum, stomach, and small bowel. Interestingly, angiodysplasia is associated with aortic valve disease in some patients. It has been suggested that the disorder may be the result of chronic circulatory insufficiency of the intestine, intestinal muscle hypertrophy, and resulting venous obstruction. Patients typically complain of multiple bleeding episodes, although the lesions also may cause chronic occult bleeding. Radiological studies and examination at laparotomy are usually negative. Thus, the diagnosis is difficult and often requires selective mesenteric arteriography or colonoscopy. Surgical removal of the affected segment is curative.

☐ **Pathology:** The resected specimen displays small, often multiple hemangiomatous lesions, usually less than 0.5 cm in diameter. Microscopically, the veins and capillaries of the submucosa are tortuous, thin walled, and dilated. The attenuated walls of these vessels are presumably responsible for their propensity to bleed. On resection of the colon, the ectatic vessels tend to collapse; their demonstration is facilitated by vascular injection of the specimen with silicone rubber or radiographic contrast material.

Hemorrhoids

Hemorrhoids are dilated venous channels of the hemorrhoidal plexuses that result from the downward displacement of the anal cushions. These cushions are composed of submucosal connective tissue and are believed to aid in anal continence. *Internal hemorrhoids* arise from the superior hemorrhoidal plexus above the pectinate line, whereas *external hemorrhoids* originate from the inferior hemorrhoidal plexus below that line. The fact that bleeding from hemorrhoids is bright red (i.e., arterial) suggests that these vessels are not truly varicose veins but rather a form of arteriovenous shunt similar to those of the corpus cavernosum of the genitalia.

Hemorrhoids are common in Western countries, to some degree afflicting at least half the population older than 50 years. By contrast, they are infrequent in populations who consume high-fiber diets. Hemorrhoids are common in pregnancy, presumably because of the increased abdominal pressure. Contrary to historical assumptions, hemorrhoids are now reported not to be more frequent than usual in patients with portal hypertension, although such patients may have rectal varices.

☐ **Pathology:** Microscopic examination of hemorrhoidectomy specimens discloses dilated vascular spaces with excess smooth muscle in their walls. Hemorrhage and thrombosis of varying severity are common. Squamous metaplasia of the overlying transitional zone may be noted. The result of thrombosis and the organization of an internal hemorrhoid is a **fibrous polyp of the anal canal**; a similar process in an external hemorrhoid results in an anal tag.

☐ **Clinical Features:** The salient clinical feature of hemorrhoids is **bleeding**, and chronic blood loss may lead to **iron-deficiency anemia. Rectal prolapse** often develops in patients with hemorrhoids. Prolapsed hemorrhoids may become irreducible, a situation that leads to painful strangulated hemorrhoids. **Thrombosis** of external hemorrhoids is exquisitely painful and requires evacuation of the intravascular clot.

RADIATION ENTEROCOLITIS

Radiation therapy for malignant disease of the pelvis or abdomen is not uncommonly complicated by injury to the small intestine and colon.

☐ **Pathology:** Clinically significant radiation colitis is most common in the rectum. The lesions produced by radiation therapy range from a reversible injury of the intestinal mucosa to chronic inflammation, ulceration, and fibrosis of the intestine.

In the short term, radiation results in epithelial and endothelial damage including decreased mitoses and, in the small bowel, shortening of the villi. Mucosal inflammation is conspicuous, and in the colorectal crypt, abscesses may be seen. Failure of epithelial renewal may lead to ulceration. Subacute changes, occurring 2 to 12 months after radiation therapy, are noted after the mucosa has healed. Damage to submucosal vessels leads to thrombosis. The submucosa becomes fibrotic and often contains bizarre fibroblasts. As a result of radiation vascular injury, progressive ischemia further damages the bowel. Telangiectases are commonly present.

Complications of radiation enterocolitis include perforation and the subsequent development of internal fistulas, hemorrhage, and stricture, occasionally severe enough to lead to intestinal obstruction. A slightly increased risk of colorectal cancer has been reported in persons who have undergone radiation therapy.

SOLITARY RECTAL ULCER SYNDROME

Internal mucosal prolapse of the rectum can produce mucosal changes that can be mistaken clinically and pathologically for chronic inflammatory disease or a neoplasm. The hallmark of solitary rectal ulcer syndrome is smooth muscle proliferation from the muscularis mucosae into the lamina propria. Despite the name, some patients have no ulcers, whereas others display multiple erosions or ulcers. Mucosal abnormalities often appear as a mass that can simulate a neoplasm. Glands can be entrapped in the rectal wall, a condition termed *colitis cystica profunda.*

POLYPS OF THE COLORECTUM

A gastrointestinal polyp is defined as a mass that protrudes into the lumen of the gut. Polyps are subdivided according to their attachment to the bowel wall (e.g., sessile or pedunculated), their histopathological appearance (e.g., hyperplastic or adenomatous), and their neoplastic potential (i.e., benign or malignant). By themselves, benign polyps are only infrequently symptomatic, and their clinical importance lies in their potential for malignant transformation.

Colorectal polyps are classified broadly as neoplastic and non-neoplastic. The neoplastic polyps are adenomas and carcinomas; the non-neoplastic ones include hyperplastic, juvenile, inflammatory, hamartomatous, and other polyps.

Adenomatous Polyps

Adenomatous polyps (adenomas) are benign neoplasms that arise from the mucosal epithelium. They are composed of neoplastic epithelial cells that have migrated to the surface and have accumulated beyond the needs for replacement of the cells sloughed into the lumen.

□ **Epidemiology:** The precise prevalence of adenomatous polyps of the colon is difficult to ascertain worldwide, but it is certainly highest in Western countries. As in diverticular disease, the diet is the only consistent environmental difference between high-risk and low-risk populations that has been identified. In the United States, it appears that at least one adenomatous polyp is present in half of the adult population, a figure that increases to more than two thirds among persons older than 65 years. There is a modest male predominance (1.4:1), and blacks have a higher proportion of right-sided adenomas and cancers. In about one fourth of those who have at least one adenoma, two or more are present.

□ **Pathology:** **Almost half of all adenomatous polyps of the colon in the United States are located in the rectosigmoid region and can therefore be detected by digital examination or by sigmoidoscopy.** The remaining half are evenly distributed throughout the rest of the colon. The macroscopic appearance of an adenoma varies from a barely visible nodule or small, pedunculated adenoma to a large, sessile adenoma. Adenomas are classified by their architecture into tubular, villous, and tubulovillous types.

TUBULAR ADENOMAS: These polyps constitute two thirds of benign large bowel adenomas. Tubular adenomas are typically smooth-surfaced spheres, usually less than 2 cm in diameter, which are often attached to the mucosa by a stalk (Fig. 13-51A). Some tubular adenomas, particularly the smaller ones, are sessile.

Microscopically, tubular adenoma exhibits closely packed epithelial tubules, which may be uniform or may be irregular and excessively branched (see Fig. 13-51B). The tubules are embedded in a fibrovascular stroma similar to the normal lamina propria. The tubules often show focal cystic dilatation. The stalk of the pedunculated tubular adenoma is lined by non-neoplastic colorectal mucosa, and its interior is composed of fibrovascular tissue continuous with the normal submucosa.

Although the majority of tubular adenomas display little epithelial dysplasia, one fifth, particularly the larger tumors, show a range of more pronounced dysplastic features, which vary from mild nuclear pleomorphism to frank invasive carcinoma (Fig. 13-52). Adenomatous

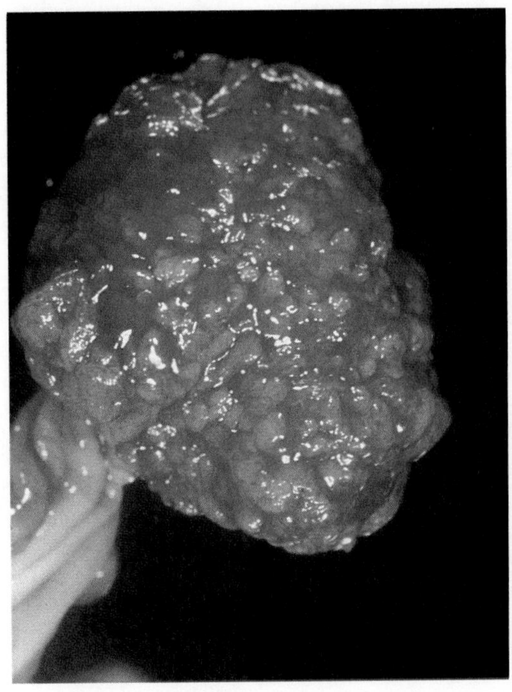
A

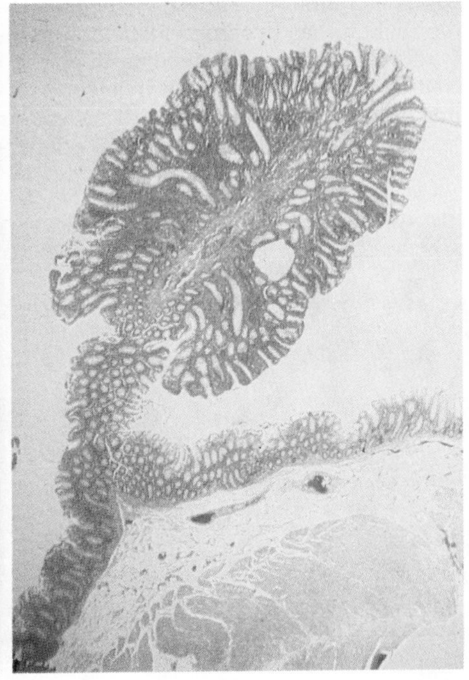
B

FIGURE *13-51*
Tubular adenoma of the colon. ***(A)*** **A pedunculated tubular adenoma.** ***(B)*** **A low-power photomicrograph of a tubular adenoma of the colon shows closely packed epithelial tubules. The fibrous stalk is vascular and covered by normal colonic epithelium.**

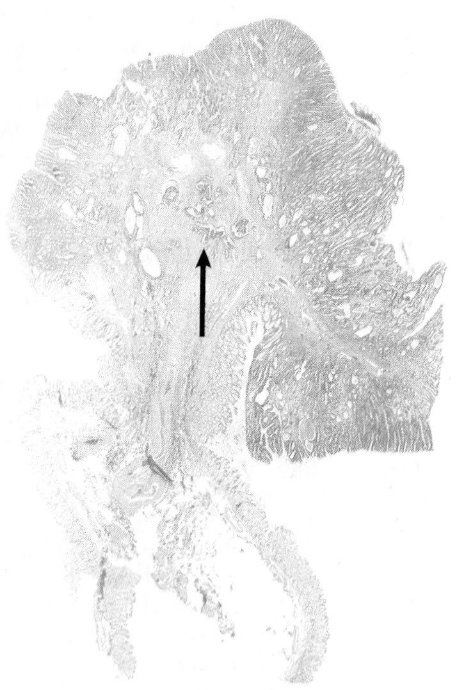

FIGURE 13-52
Adenocarcinoma arising in a pedunculated adenomatous polyp. A low-power photomicrograph shows irregular neoplastic glands *(arrow)* invading the stalk.

epithelium is characterized by hypercellularity, with elongated nuclei that are often stratified. Dysplasia is classified on the basis of alterations in mucosal epithelial cells. Adenomatous epithelium has hyperchromatic and pleomorphic nuclei, which sometimes lose their basal polarity and exhibit increased numbers of mitoses. In severe dysplasia, the glands become crowded and highly irregular in size and shape. Papillary or cribriform (sievelike or perforated) growth patterns are common. Nuclei are more rounded and irregular, often with prominent nucleoli.

The neoplastic glands must show no invasion through the muscularis mucosae for the adenoma to be considered benign. Penetration through this muscle layer is considered evidence of malignant transformation.

Intramucosal lesions that are severely dysplastic are classified by some pathologists as carcinoma *in situ*. They are found in about 10% of resected tubular adenomas. **As long as the dysplastic focus remains superficial to the muscularis mucosae, the lesion is invariably cured by resection of the polyp.**

The risk of invasive carcinoma correlates with the size of the tubular adenoma. Only 1% of tubular adenomas smaller than 1 cm across contain invasive carcinoma at the time of resection; among those between 1 and 2 cm, about 10% are found to have malignancy, and among those greater than 2 cm, 35% are cancerous. Given that only few tubular adenomas are more than 2 cm in diameter, the overall risk of invasive carcinoma in these growths is still small.

VILLOUS ADENOMAS: These polyps constitute one tenth of colonic adenomas and are found predominantly in the rectosigmoid region. They are typically large, broad-based, elevated lesions that grossly display a shaggy, cauliflower-like surface (Fig. 13-53A) but can be small and pedunculated. More than half are larger than 2 cm in diameter, and on occasion, they reach a size of 10 to 15 cm across. Microscopically, villous adenomas are composed of thin, tall, finger-like processes that superficially resemble the villi of the small intestine. They are lined externally by neoplastic epithelial cells and are supported by a core of fibrovascular connective tissue corresponding to the normal lamina propria (see Fig. 13-53B).

The histopathology of dysplasia in villous adenomas is comparable to that in tubular adenomas. **However, in contrast to tubular adenomas, villous adenomas commonly contain foci of carcinoma.** In polyps less than 1 cm

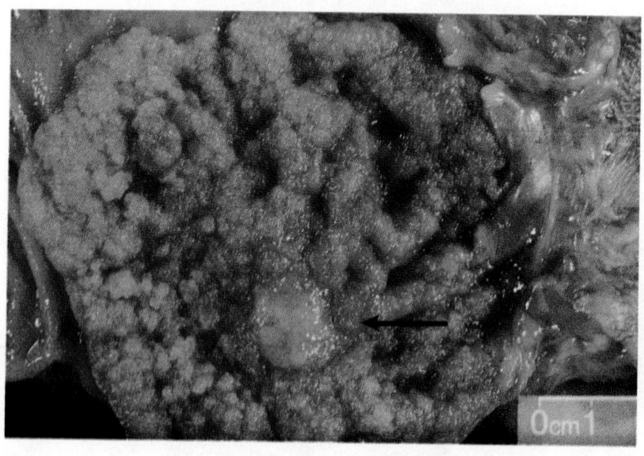

A

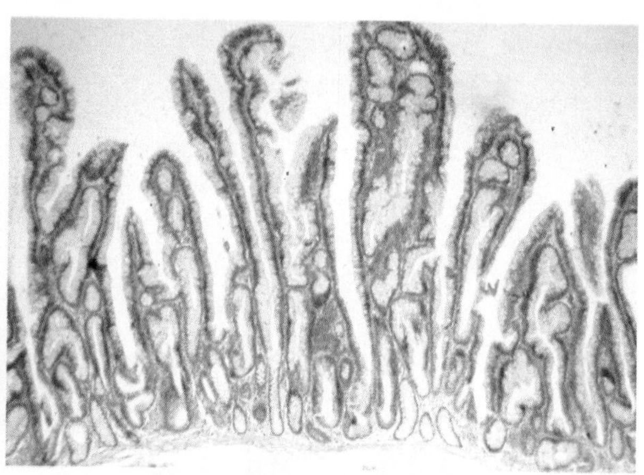

B

FIGURE 13-53
Villous adenoma of the colon. *(A)* The colon contains a large, broad-based, elevated lesion that has a cauliflower-like surface. A firm area near the center of the lesion (*arrow*) proved on histological examination to be an adenocarcinoma. *(B)* A photomicrograph shows finger-like processes that resemble the villi of the small intestine. The villi are supported by cores of fibrovascular connective tissue.

across, the risk is 10 times higher than that for comparably sized tubular adenomas. Of greater importance is the fact that villous adenomas greater than 2 cm in size have a 50% prevalence of invasive carcinoma at the time of resection. **Given that most villous adenomas measure more than 2 cm in greatest dimension, more than one third of all resected villous adenomas contain invasive cancer.**

TUBULOVILLOUS ADENOMAS: Many adenomatous polyps manifest both tubular and villous features. Polyps with more than 20% and less than 80% villous architecture are termed tubulovillous adenomas. These adenomas tend to be intermediate in distribution and size between the tubular and villous forms, one fourth to one third being larger than 2 cm across. Tubulovillous polyps are also intermediate between tubular and villous adenomas in the risk of invasive carcinoma.

□ **Pathogenesis:** The precursor to colorectal carcinoma is dysplasia, usually in the form of an adenoma. The pathogenesis of adenomas of the colon and rectum involves a neoplastic alteration of crypt epithelial homeostasis characterized by (1) diminished apotosis, (2) persistence of cell replication, and (3) failure of maturation and differentiation in the epithelial cells that migrate toward the surface of the crypts (Fig. 13-54). Normally, DNA synthesis ceases when the cells reach the upper third of the crypts, after which they mature, migrate to the surface, and become senescent. They then undergo apoptosis or are sloughed into the lumen. Adenomas arise from a focal disruption of this orderly sequence, such that the epithelial cells maintain their proliferative capacity throughout the entire depth of the crypt. Thus, mitotic figures are initially visualized, not only along the entire length of the crypt, but also on the mucosal surface. As the lesion evolves, cell proliferation exceeds the rate of apoptosis and sloughing, and the cells begin to accumulate in the upper crypts and on the surface. Eventually, the accumulated cells on the surface of the mucosa form tubules or villous structures, in concert with stromal elements.

The differences in histogenesis between tubular and villous adenomas have been theorized to result from differences in mesenchymal cell proliferation in the lamina propria. It has been postulated that, in the absence of mesenchymal cell proliferation beneath the altered mucosa, the proliferating epithelial cells fold in to form tubules. The resistance to outward expansion could also explain why tubular adenomas tend to remain small. By contrast, if growth of the lamina propria is stimulated parallel to that of the epithelium, the latter folds outward to produce villous structures. Without the constraint of an immobile lamina propria, the lesion can grow to a larger size.

ADENOMATOUS POLYPS AND COLORECTAL CANCER: Although it is now generally accepted that invasive carcinoma can arise in an adenomatous polyp, there has been controversy as to whether such benign tumors are necessary precursors of colorectal cancer. A better question is not whether adenomatous polyps are the **only** precursors of cancer (analogous to the relation between epithelial dysplasia in the uterine cervix and squamous cell carcinoma) but whether **most** colorectal cancers arise in preexisting polyps. The weight of evidence, which supports the latter hypothesis, can be summarized as follows:

- **The geographic coincidence** in the frequencies of adenomatous polyps and colorectal cancer suggests a causal relation. For example, the prevalence of both adenomatous polyps and colorectal cancer is extremely low in African blacks. By contrast, both polyps and cancer are more frequent in American blacks. Moreover, Japanese born in Hawaii display a higher frequency of both diseases than those born in

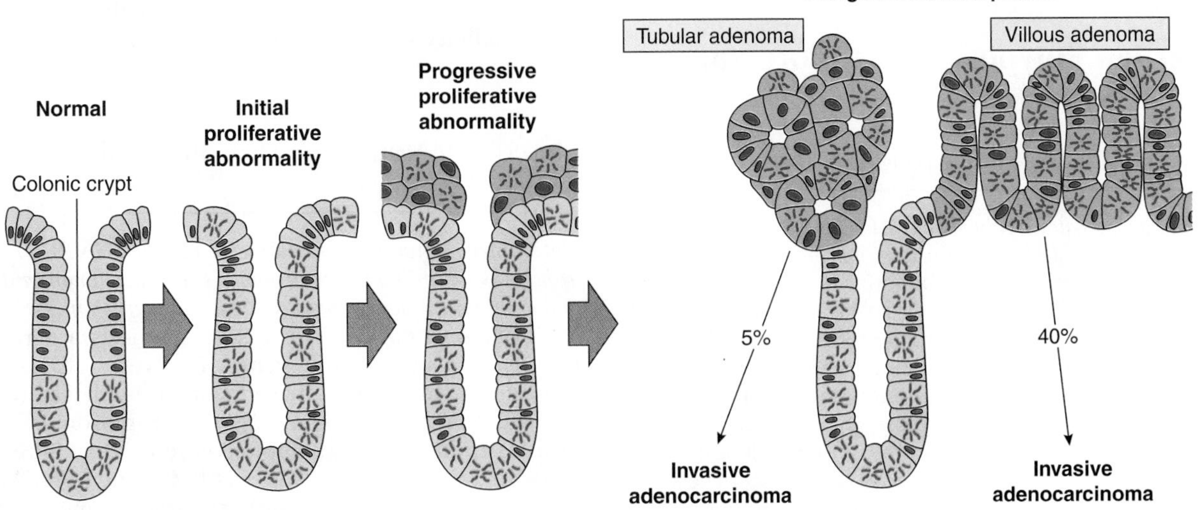

FIGURE *13-54*
The histogenesis of adenomatous polyps of the colon. The initial proliferative abnormality of the colonic mucosa, the extension of the mitotic zone in the crypts, leads to the accumulation of mucosal cells. The formation of adenomas may reflect epithelial–mesenchymal interactions.

Japan. In geographic regions in which there is a high risk of colorectal cancer, adenomatous polyps tend to be larger, are more often villous, and display more severe dysplasia than those in low-risk areas. The anatomical distribution of adenomas and carcinomas is similar, both being most frequent in the sigmoid colon in Western countries.

- **The average age at onset** of adenomatous polyps is earlier than that of colorectal cancer, suggesting that the latter follows the former. Adenomatous polyps tend to antedate colon cancer by 10 to 15 years.
- **Carcinomas are found in adenomas**, and some carcinomas have adenomatous remnants at their periphery.
- **An associated carcinoma** is commonly found in colons that harbor adenomas. Conversely, one third of colons resected for cancer contain an adenomatous polyp. Moreover, the presence of an adenomatous polyp in the same colon specimen resected for cancer doubles the risk that another carcinoma will develop in the remaining colon.
- **In familial polyposis coli** (see later), the innumerable adenomatous polyps are initially benign, but cancer of the colorectum invariably develops at a later age.

An argument can be made that the preceding points simply reflect the fact that the same stimulus that promotes the growth of adenomatous polyps independently leads to cancer in an otherwise normal mucosa. However, epithelial dysplasia and early invasive cancer are simply not found arising from normal mucosa. In this context, it should be emphasized that the uncommon finding of small invasive cancers that are not surrounded by adenomatous tissue and are bordered by normal mucosa may reflect destruction of a preexisting adenomatous polyps by the malignancy.

The most powerful support for the concept that most colorectal cancers arise in adenomatous polyps comes from studies in which prophylactic polypectomies have drastically reduced the risk of subsequent cancer development.

Inherited Polyposis and Colorectal Cancer Syndromes

Familial Adenomatous Polyposis

Familial adenomatous polyposis (FAP), also termed adenomatous polyposis coli (APC), a rare, autosomal dominant inherited trait, is characterized by the progressive development of innumerable adenomatous polyps of the colorectum, particularly in the rectosigmoid region. The disorder reflects a germline mutation of the APC gene on the long arm of chromosome 5 (5q21). Although young patients with FAP have no polyps, in a matter of a few years, the colorectal mucosa becomes carpeted, sometimes throughout its length, with hundreds to thousands of adenomas (Fig. 13-55). These are mostly of the tubular variety, although tubulovillous and villous adenomas also are present. Microscopic adenomas, sometimes involving a single crypt, are numerous. **Carcinoma of the colon and rectum is inevitable, often by age 40 years, unless a total colectomy is performed.**

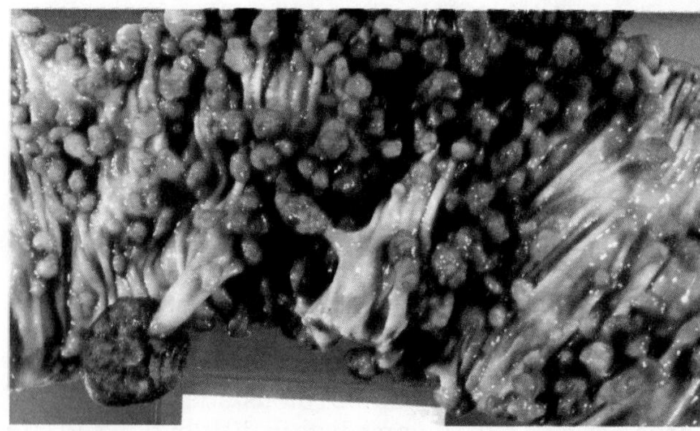

FIGURE *13-55*
Familial polyposis. The mucosal surface of the colon is carpeted by innumerable adenomatous polyps.

Although a few polyps are usually present by age 10 years, the mean age for the occurrence of symptoms is 36 years, by which time cancer is already present in many patients. In addition to having colonic polyps, some persons with familial polyposis have polyps in the small intestine and stomach, although malignant transformation at these sites is rare.

Gardner Syndrome

Gardner syndrome is familial adenomatous polyposis with extracolonic lesions: osteomas of the skull, mandible, and long bones, and soft tissue tumors of the skin. APC gene mutations do not predict this phenotype.

Turcot syndrome refers to the rare combination of adenomatous polyposis of the colorectum with malignant tumors of the central nervous system. Many cases, especially those with medulloblastoma, are due to germline mutation of the APC gene. Some cases, especially those with glioblastoma multiforme, are part of the spectrum of the hereditary nonpolyposis colorectal cancer syndrome (see later).

Hereditary Nonpolyposis Colorectal Cancer Syndrome

Hereditary nonpolyposis colorectal cancer (HNPCC) syndrome (Warthin–Lynch syndrome) is an uncommon, autosomal dominant inherited disease, which accounts for 3% to 5% of all colorectal cancers. This disorder reflects a germline mutation in one of four genes involved in DNA nucleotide mismatch repair. In most cases, these are the hMSH2 (human MutS homolog) on chromosome 2P and hMLH1 (human MutL homolog) chromosome 3P. Some cases are caused by mutations in hPMS1 and hPMS2 (human postmeiotic segregation) on chromosomes 2q and 7q, respectively. The syndrome is characterized by (1) the onset of colorectal cancer at a young age; (2) few adenomas (hence "nonpolyposis"); (3) a high frequency of carcinomas proximal to the splenic flexure (70%); (4) the common occurrence of poorly differentiated and mucinous colorectal carcinomas; (5) multiple synchronous or metachronous colorectal cancers; and (6) the presence of extracolonic cancers including adenocarcinomas of the stomach, small intestine, and hepatobiliary tract; gliomas (Turcot syndrome); transitional cell carcinomas of the renal pelvis and ureter; and endometrial and ovarian cancers.

In patients with HNPCC, the tumors have numerous DNA replication errors (RER), including microsatellite instability and ubiquitous somatic mutation, owing to the inability of the tumor cells to repair nucleotide mismatches and an increase in the mutation rate. The adenoma–carcinoma sequence occurs more rapidly than usual in these patients, but survival from the tumors is better than that in the usual cancers of the same stage.

Non-Neoplastic Polyps

Whereas all adenomatous polyps, and possibly colorectal cancer, may be considered to occupy places on the same developmental spectrum, the non-neoplastic polyps are entirely different entities from one another and are grouped together solely because of their gross appearance as raised lesions of the colonic mucosa.

Hyperplastic Polyps (Metaplastic Polyps)

Hyperplastic polyps are small, sessile mucosal excrescences that display an exaggerated crypt architecture. They are the most common polypoid lesions of the colon and are particularly frequent in the rectum. Because the polyps are benign, and because the term *hyperplastic* carries a connotation of neoplastic growth, the term *metaplastic polyp* also has been used to emphasize the fact that this type of polyp is not a forerunner of cancer.

Hyperplastic polyps are remarkably common, being present in 40% of rectal specimens in persons younger than 40 years and in 75% of older persons. The association of hyperplastic polyps with rectal cancer is striking; 90% of rectal specimens removed for cancer contain such polyps. Moreover, hyperplastic polyps seen in association with rectal cancer are often grouped around the tumor. In addition, hyperplastic polyps are more common than usual in colons that contain adenomatous polyps and in populations with higher rates of colorectal cancer. Thus, these asymptomatic lesions reflect an increased risk of colorectal cancer. Ras mutations and overexpression of Bcl-2 (which protects cells from apoptosis) have been found in a substantial minority of hyperplastic polyps.

☐ **Pathogenesis:** The pathogenesis of the hyperplastic polyp is believed to involve a defect in the proliferation and maturation of the normal mucosal epithelium. In a hyperplastic polyp, proliferation occurs at the base of the crypt, and the upward migration of the cells is slowed. Thus, the epithelial cells differentiate and acquire absorptive characteristics lower in the crypts. Moreover, the cells persist on the surface mucosa longer than do normal cells.

☐ **Pathology:** Hyperplastic polyps are seen macroscopically as small, sessile, raised mucosal nodules, which are up to 0.5 cm in diameter but occasionally larger. They are almost always multiple and have even been mistaken for familial polyposis coli. Histologically, the crypts of the hyperplastic polyp are elongated and may exhibit cystic dilatation (Fig. 13-56). The overall appearance is superficially similar to that of a villous adenoma, but focal infolding of the crowded epithelium imparts a saw-toothed, serrated appearance to the mucosal lining. The epithelium is composed of well-differentiated goblet cells and absorptive cells, without any atypical features. The lamina propria is also unremarkable.

Juvenile Polyps (Retention Polyps)

Juvenile polyps are classified as hamartomatous proliferations of the colonic mucosa, which are most common in children younger than 10 years, although one third occur in adults. They are not observed during the first year of life and are, therefore, believed to be acquired.

☐ **Pathology:** Juvenile polyps may be single or rarely multiple and occur most commonly in the rectum, although they may be seen anywhere in the small or large bowel. Grossly, most polyps are pedunculated lesions up to 2 cm in diameter. They have a smooth, rounded surface, in contrast to the fissured surface of an adenomatous polyp. Histologically, dilated and cystic epithelial tubules filled with mucus (hence the name "retention polyp") are embedded in a fibrovascular lamina propria (Fig. 13-57). Surface epithelial erosion is common, and reactive epithelial proliferation is evident, but the epithelium usually lacks dysplasia.

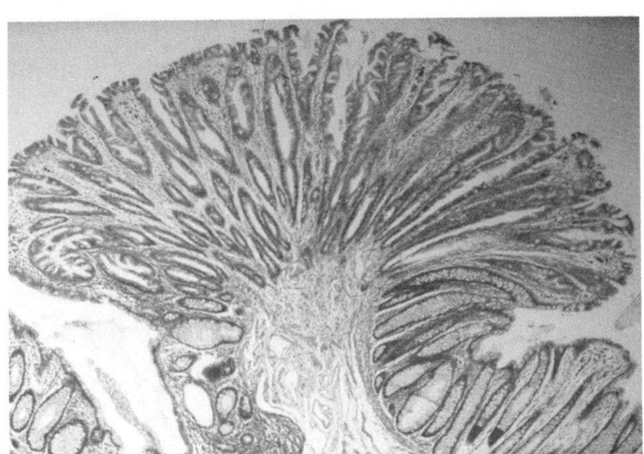

FIGURE *13-56*
Hyperplastic polyp of the colon. A low-power photomicrograph shows elongated crypts, which create an appearance somewhat similar to that of a villous adenoma.

Pedunculated juvenile polyps in the rectum may prolapse during defecation, and their ready autoamputation may deposit them on the toilet paper. Because of their tendency to bleed, they are usually surgically removed. Importantly, sporadic juvenile polyps do not progress to cancer.

Inflammatory Polyps

Inflammatory polyps are not neoplasms but rather elevated masses of chronically inflamed and regenerating epithelium over ulcerations caused by an inflammatory disease of the colon. Such polyps are commonly found in association with ulcerative colitis and Crohn disease; they are also encountered in cases of amebic colitis and bacterial dysentery. Microscopically, inflammatory polyps are composed of a variable component of distorted and inflamed mucosal glands, which may be intermixed with granulation tissue. Regenerating large, basophilic epithelial cells are frequent. When the surface of the polyp is ulcerated, granulation tissue may be prominent.

As healing proceeds, epithelial regeneration restores the mucosal architecture. Although these lesions are themselves not precancerous, they occur in chronic inflammatory diseases that are associated with a high incidence of cancer (e.g., ulcerative colitis) and must therefore be distinguished from adenomatous and malignant polyps.

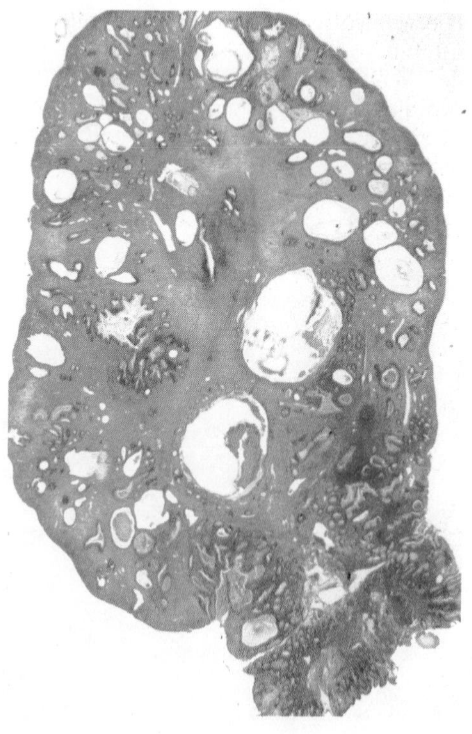

FIGURE 13-57
Juvenile polyp of the colon. A low-power photomicrograph shows cystic epithelial tubules embedded in a fibrovascular stroma.

Lymphoid Polyps

Lymphoid polyps refer to submucosal accumulations of lymphoid tissue, almost invariably in the rectum, which are seen as single, sessile nodules measuring from a pinpoint size to as large as 5 cm in diameter. On occasion, multiple lesions impart a cobblestone appearance to the mucosa. Microscopically, these polyps are covered by intact mucosa and are composed of prominent lymphoid follicles with germinal centers. In this context, lymphoid tissue, in the form of follicles or as scattered lymphocytes or plasma cells in the lamina propria, is normally present in the colorectal mucosa.

Lymphoid polyps are more common in female than in male subjects and are seen in persons of any age, including children. The lesions are usually asymptomatic and are unrelated to malignant lymphomas, although in rectal biopsies, they may superficially resemble malignant lymphoid tissue.

***Nodular lymphoid hyperplasia**, a condition seen primarily in children or with common variable immunodeficiency syndrome, features an excessive accumulation of the normal follicular lymphoid tissue of the colon.* Macroscopically, the mucosa exhibits numerous small sessile or polypoid nodules up to 0.5 cm in diameter. The microscopic appearance is similar to that of lymphoid polyps. The condition is only rarely related to malignant lymphoma, but the radiological appearance can be mistaken for familial adenomatous polyposis.

MALIGNANT TUMORS

Adenocarcinoma of the Colon and Rectum

In Western industrialized societies, colorectal cancer is the most common cause of cancer deaths that are not directly attributable to tobacco use. Some 5% of Americans develop this cancer during their lifetime. Although the widely used term *colorectal* implies a common biology, the differences between cancers of the colon and rectum seem to be more fundamental than simple location. For instance, whereas colonic cancer is much more common in the United States than in Japan, the incidence of rectal carcinoma in the two populations is nearly the same. In general, rectosigmoid carcinoma accounts for a considerably higher proportion of all large bowel cancers in populations at high risk for cancer of the large bowel, including the United States, than in low-risk populations. Moreover, cancer of the colon shows a slight female preponderance, whereas cancer of the rectum is somewhat more common in men. The proportion of cancer in the distal colorectum has been declining in recent decades, a shift that has implications for screening by sigmoidoscopy.

☐ **Pathogenesis:** Most cancers of the colon and rectum arise in adenomatous polyps, and therefore factors associated with the development of such polyps are probably relevant to the genesis of colorectal cancer. The importance of environmental factors in the pathogenesis of colorectal cancer is emphasized by the high incidence of the disease in industrialized countries and among emigrants from low-risk to high-risk regions.

DIETARY FIBER: The major environmental risk factor for colorectal cancer has been suggested to be the diet, specifically **a diet low in indigestible fiber and high in animal fat**. As previously discussed, such a diet also has been implicated in the etiology of other colonic diseases, including diverticulosis, appendicitis, and ulcerative colitis.

Compared with a high-fiber diet, a low-fiber one is associated with a slower transit of fecal contents through the colon, thereby permitting longer exposure of the mucosa to substances in the stools. It has been suggested that fiber may bind potential mutagens and, by increasing the bulk of the stools, dilute their concentration. In addition, dietary fiber may affect the production of bile acids and other potential cancer-related compounds in the stool.

Newer analyses of the epidemiological data have, however, weakened the case for an association between the fiber content of the diet and the incidence of colorectal cancer. Moreover, clinical trials have found that dietary fiber exerts little protective effect against colorectal adenomas.

DIETARY FAT: An increase in the consumption of animal fats (for example, that associated with the recent change in dietary habits in Japan) is paralleled by an increased incidence of colorectal cancer. Moreover, a lower content of animal fat in the diet of certain ethnic groups in the United States has been accompanied by a decreased incidence of colorectal cancer. The ingestion of fat elicits the secretion of bile into the intestine, and some bile acids have been claimed experimentally to enhance the tumorigenicity of experimental intestinal carcinogens. In this context, cholecystectomy, a procedure that increases the colonic content of secondary bile acids, has been claimed in some studies (although not in others) to be associated with an increased risk of right-sided colon cancer. High-temperature cooking has been implicated in generating mutagens such as heterocyclic aromatic amines.

ANAEROBIC BACTERIA: It has also been demonstrated that the feces of persons in high-risk populations have a higher content of anaerobic bacteria than those of persons in low-risk populations. Such microorganisms, particularly *Bacteroides* species, can convert bile salts into compounds that are potentially mutagenic. Repopulation of the colon with *Lactobacillus* protects experimental animals against chemically induced colon cancer.

OTHER DIETARY FACTORS: A low prevalence of colorectal cancer has been correlated with **high levels of selenium** in the soil and plants of certain geographic areas. The endogenous antioxidant glutathione peroxidase is a selenium-containing enzyme. **Exogenous antioxidants** (e.g., butylated hydroxytoluene and vitamin E) and a reducing agent such as ascorbic acid have protected animals against the experimental production of colonic cancer. **Diets rich in cruciferous vegetables** (for instance, cauliflower, brussels sprouts, and cabbage, and those that provide vitamin A) are said to be associated with a lower incidence of colorectal cancer.

MOLECULAR BIOLOGY OF COLORECTAL CANCER: Adenocarcinoma of the colorectum is a particularly favorable neoplastic system in which to study the progression of molecular events that underlie malignant transformation. This tumor (1) develops slowly, (2) is easily accessible, (3) shows a reproducible progression from benign precursor lesions, and (4) has clearly defined hereditary and sporadic variants. These features have allowed understanding of the progressive genetic changes that eventuate in invasive and metastatic colorectal cancer.

It is now believed that accumulated alterations of protooncogenes and suppressor genes are required for the development of colorectal cancers. Two major pathways are evident. One occurs in 85% of cancers, whereas the other, involving defects in DNA mismatch repair, is present in 15%.

- **APC gene**: Germline mutations in the APC gene, a putative tumor-suppressor gene, are responsible for familial adenomatous polyposis. Moreover, the majority of sporadic colorectal cancers contain a mutation in the same gene. Some of the tumors that lack an APC defect display mutations in the β-catenin gene, whose product binds with APC protein. It was recently reported that a specific APC mutation (T $\rightarrow$ A, 1307) is found in 6% of Ashkenazi Jews and renders surrounding gene regions susceptible to frame-shift mutations that inactivate the APC gene. These data suggest an important role for the APC gene in the early development of most colorectal neoplasms.
- **Ras oncogene:** Many colorectal cancers and adenomas demonstrate point mutations that activate the *ras* protooncogene.
- **p53 tumor-suppressor gene:** The p53 gene is mutated or deleted in many cases of colorectal cancer.
- **DCC gene:** A putative tumor-suppressor gene, labeled "deleted in colon cancer" (DCC) and located on chromosome 18, is often missing in colorectal cancers. However, its contribution to the development of colorectal cancer is controversial.

Numerous other genes have increased or decreased levels of expression in colorectal carcinomas, indicating the complexity of the process.

- **Mismatch repair genes:** Mutations in a group of genes involved in the early steps of DNA nucleotide mismatch repair lead to DNA replication errors (RER), including microsatellite instability and ubiquitous somatic mutations. Colorectal tumors accumulate large numbers of subtle mutations in repetitive nucleotide sequences and have a mutator phenotype that further enhances mutational events. APC mutations occur as early events, but the role of the alterations shown in Figure 13-58 is less important than mutations in nucleotide repeats in coding regions (TGF-β receptor, E2F4 transcription factor, Bax gene, etc.) and regulatory sequences that alter gene expression. RER-positive cancers exhibit a high frequency of poor differentiation, mucinous and signet ring cell histology, and prominent lymphoid inflammatory response.

It has been estimated that a minimum of 8 to 10 mutational events must accumulate during multistep carcinogenesis to produce an invasive colorectal cancer. A model of the genetic events that accompany the evolution of colorectal cancer is presented in Figure 13-58.

Risk Factors

AGE: Increasing age is probably the single most important risk factor for colorectal cancer in the general population. The risk is low before age 40 years and increases steadily to age 50 years, after which it doubles with each decade.

PRIOR COLORECTAL CANCER: Patients who have previously had colorectal cancer have an increased risk of a subsequent tumor. In fact, 5% to 10% of patients treated for colorectal cancer subsequently develop a second malignant lesion of the colorectum. Moreover, 2% to 5% of patients in whom a colorectal cancer is discovered harbor a second primary (synchronous) malignant tumor of the colorectum. As previously mentioned, patients who have had an adenomatous polyp removed, or who demonstrate the presence of such a polyp, are at increased risk for the subsequent development of colorectal cancer.

ULCERATIVE COLITIS AND CROHN DISEASE: These chronic inflammatory diseases increase the risk of colorectal cancer in proportion to their duration and extent within the large bowel.

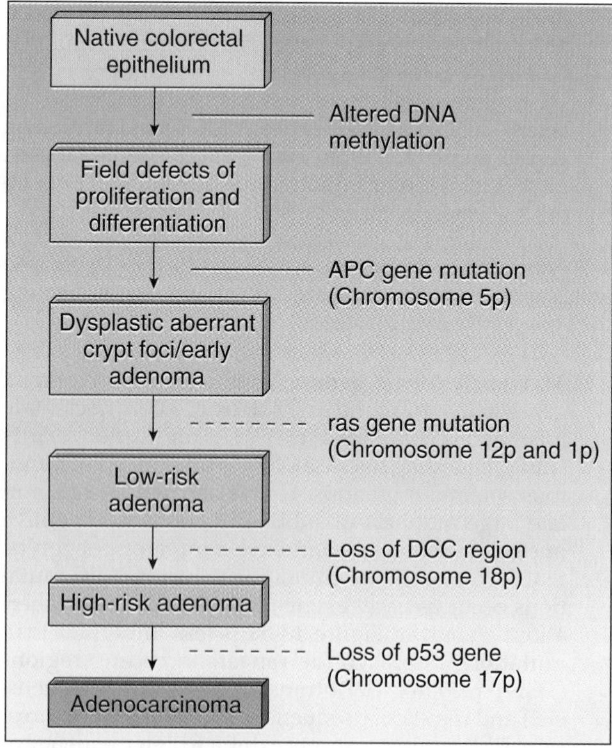

FIGURE *13-58*
Model of some of the genetic alterations involved in sporadic colorectal carcinogenesis.

HEREDITARY POLYPOSIS AND COLORECTAL CANCER SYNDROMES: See Prior Colorectal Cancer (previous column).

GENETIC FACTORS: Colorectal cancer is increased in frequency among relatives of patients with the disease, a finding that suggests some genetic contribution to the development of the cancer. A history of cancer at other sites, particularly breast or genital cancer in women, is associated with a higher than normal frequency of colorectal cancer.

DIET: As previously noted, prospective studies involving large populations in various countries have reported that the daily consumption of red meat and animal fat leads to an increased risk of colorectal cancer, compared with that in persons who eat little or no meat.

☐ **Pathology:** The gross appearance of colorectal cancers is similar to that of adenocarcinomas elsewhere in the gastrointestinal tract. They tend to be **polypoid, ulcerating, or infiltrative, and may be annular and constrictive** (Fig. 13-59A). Polypoid cancers are more common on the right side of the colon, particularly in the cecum, where the large caliber of the colon allows unimpeded intraluminal growth. Annular constricting tumors occur more often in the distal portions of the colon. Ulceration of tumors, irrespective of the growth pattern, is usual.

The vast majority of colorectal cancers are adenocarcinomas (see Fig. 13-59B), which are microscopically similar to their counterparts in other portions of the gastrointestinal tract. Most are well differentiated and secrete small amounts of mucin. Ten percent to 15% secrete considerable quantities of mucin, in which case, they are classed as mucinous adenocarcinomas. The degree of differentiation influences the prognosis; the better differentiated tumors are associated with a more favorable outlook. Occasionally, the predominant mucus-producing cell is of the signet ring variety, in which case, the cancer is associated with a particularly poor prognosis.

Colorectal cancer spreads by direct extension or invasion of vessels, an event that can be initiated by surgical manipulation. **Direct spread of colorectal cancer** is commonly observed in resected specimens. In its penetration of the muscular layers, colorectal cancer can exploit the gaps that house the penetrating arteries, as does the process that results in diverticulosis. The connective tissues of the serosa offer little resistance to the spread of the tumor, and cancer cells are often found in the fat and serosa at some distance from the primary tumor. The peritoneum is occasionally involved, in which case, there may be multiple deposits throughout the abdomen.

Colorectal cancer invades lymphatic channels and initially involves the lymph nodes immediately underlying the tumor. Lymphatic metastases tend to spread to adjacent nodes, and only rarely are so-called "skip metastases" encountered. Venous invasion leads to bloodborne metastases, which involve the liver in most patients with metastatic disease. The lungs are also a common metastatic site.

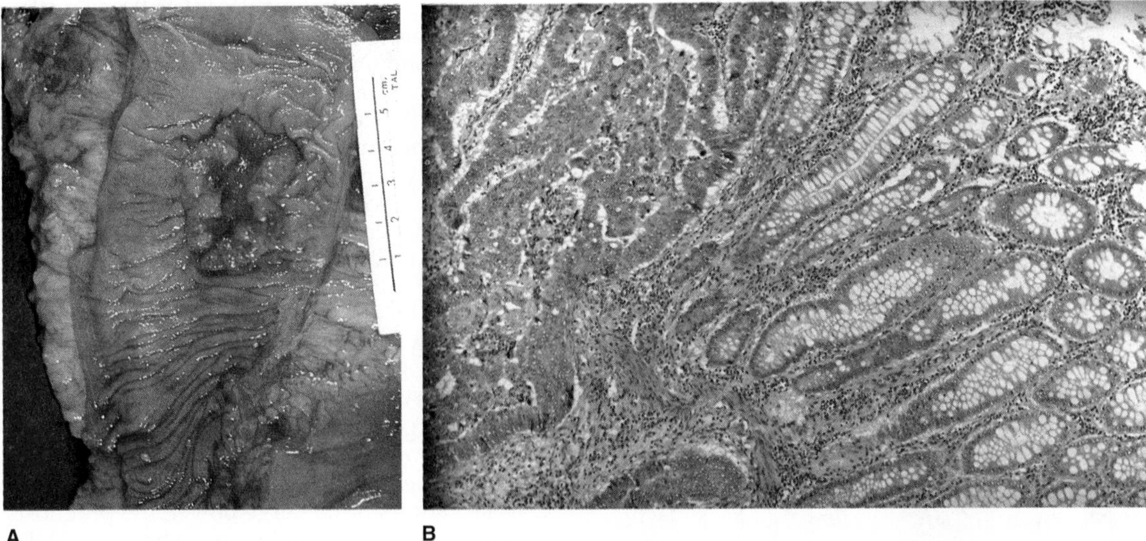

FIGURE *13-59*
Adenocarcinoma of the colon. *(A)* The opened colon contains an elevated, centrally ulcerated, infiltrating mass. *(B)* A section taken at the margin of the tumor shows infiltrating adenocarcinoma *(left)* adjacent to non-neoplastic colonic mucosa.

The prognosis of colorectal cancer is more closely related to the extension of the tumor through the wall of the large bowel than to its size or histopathological characteristics. Colorectal cancers are usually staged according to the Dukes classification or its variants (Fig. 13-60).

- **Dukes A** cancer (15% of symptomatic cases) is confined to the bowel wall in the original classification and does not penetrate through the muscularis propria.
- **Dukes B** classification (40%) refers to a tumor that has penetrated the muscle wall and possibly invaded the pericolic fat but has not metastasized to lymph nodes.
- **Dukes C** tumor (25%) shows lymph node metastases.
- **Dukes D** stage (20%) signifies distant metastases.

Since the original classification by Cuthbert Dukes in 1932, this scheme has undergone numerous modifications, although the basic concept has remained unchanged. The modification proposed by Astler and Coller is today the most popular and uses the following criteria:

- **Stage A:** Tumor confined to the mucosa.
- **Stage B_1:** Tumor invading the muscularis propria, but not penetrating to the serosa.
- **Stage B_2:** Tumor invading to the serosa without lymph node metastases.
- **Stage C_1:** B_1 tumors with metastases to regional lymph nodes.
- **Stage C_2:** B_2 tumors with metastases to regional lymph nodes.
- **Stage D:** Distant metastases.

In the tumor, nodes, metastasis (TNM) classification, stage I is equivalent to Dukes A, stage II to Dukes B, stage III to Dukes C, and stage IV to Dukes D.

Screening and surveillance lead to earlier stages at the time of diagnosis, thereby improving survival. Patients with Dukes A colon cancer are usually cured by surgical resection. The 5-year survival of patients with Dukes B tumors is 70%, whereas that of patients with stage C disease is 50%. In striking contrast, patients with disseminated disease have 5-year survival rates of only about 5%. In general, cancers of the distal colon and rectum tend to be more infiltrative than those on the right side and, therefore, are usually seen at a more advanced Dukes stage, with a correspondingly poorer prognosis.

☐ Clinical Features:

In its initial stages, colorectal cancer is clinically silent. As the tumor grows, the most common sign is **occult blood in the feces** when the tumor is in the proximal portions of the colon. Both occult blood or **bright red blood** may occur in the feces when the lesion is in the distal colorectum. In the right side of the colon, particularly in the cecum, where the diameter of the lumen is large and the fecal contents liquid, tumors can grow to large size without causing symptoms of obstruction. In this situation, chronic asymptomatic bleeding typically causes **iron-deficiency anemia**, which is often the first indication of colorectal cancer. By contrast, cancers on the left side of the colon, where the caliber of the lumen is small and the fecal contents more solid, often constrict the lumen, producing **obstructive symptoms**. These are manifested as changes in bowel habits, gaseousness, and abdominal pain. Rectal cancer is often signaled by tenesmus (straining at stool) and a reduction in the caliber of the stools. Occasionally, colorectal cancer **perforates** early and produces symptoms indistinguishable from those of diverticulitis. When the tumor has extended beyond the confines of the colorectum, it may produce en-

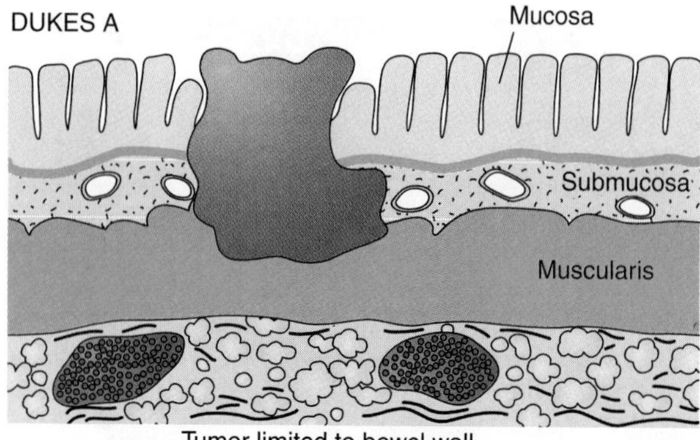

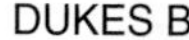

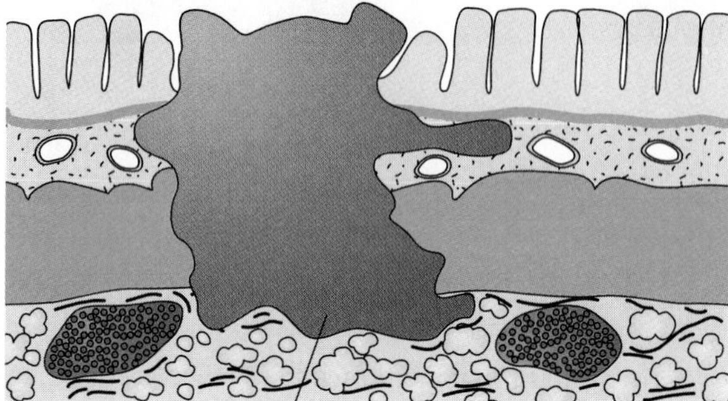

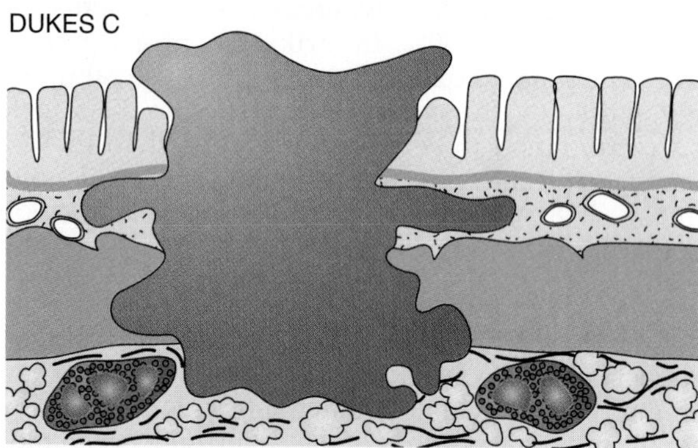

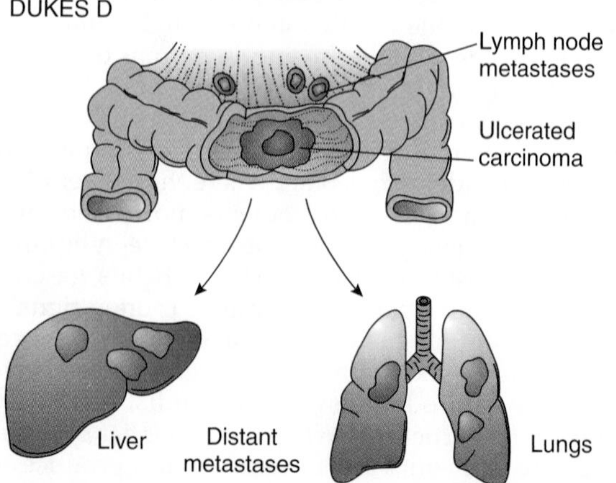

FIGURE 13-60
Dukes classification of the stages of carcinoma of the colon.

terocutaneous and rectovaginal **fistulas**, tumor masses in the abdominal wall, bladder symptoms, and sciatic nerve pain. Intra-abdominal spread may cause **small intestinal obstruction** and **ascites**.

A positive test for occult blood in the feces with reagent-impregnated paper predicts the presence of a cancer or an adenoma in 40% to 50% of the cases. For persons who are inclined to comply with an effective screening program, periodic fiberoptic sigmoidoscopy and testing for occult blood in the feces is believed to improve the prognosis of colorectal cancer, because these methods can often detect the disease at an early stage.

The only curative treatment for colorectal cancer is surgery. Small polyps are easily removed endoscopically; large lesions require segmental resection. Tumors close to the anal verge often necessitate abdominal–perineal resection and colostomy, although newer surgical techniques frequently allow sphincter preservation. In Dukes C rectal cancers of the large bowel, the prognosis is bettered by adjuvant chemotherapy, whereas in Dukes B and C rectal cancers, the combination of chemotherapy and radiation therapy improves the outlook.

Carcinoid Tumors

Carcinoid tumors of the colorectum constitute a small proportion of these tumors in the entire gastrointestinal tract. They behave in a manner similar to that of carcinoid tumors of the small intestine, in which malignancy correlates with size. About half of the carcinoid tumors of the colorectum have metastasized by the time they are discovered. The pathological and clinical features were discussed earlier in the context of small bowel tumors.

Large Bowel Lymphoma

Primary lymphoma of the colorectum is distinctly uncommon, constituting only about one tenth of all primary gastrointestinal lymphomas. The neoplasm may be seen as (1) segmental involvement of the mucosa, (2) diffuse polypoid lesions, or (3) a mass extending beyond the confines of the colorectum. The presenting symptoms in the case of large tumors are similar to those of other primary intestinal cancers, but the diffuse polypoid form may endoscopically and radiologically resemble the inflammatory polyps of ulcerative colitis or the adenomatous polyps of familial adenomatous polyposis.

Cancers of the Anal Canal

Carcinomas of the anal canal, which constitute 2% of cancers of the large bowel, may arise at or above the dentate line. These tumors occur in both sexes, but are more common in women, usually older than 50 years, and in blacks. Because the tumors tend to grow upward, they may be misdiagnosed clinically as rectal carcinomas.

☐ **Pathology:** Although anal cancers have various histological patterns, such as squamous, basaloid (cloacogenic), or mucoepidermoid, there are few clinical differences in behavior among the different tumor types, and they can be conveniently classed as *epidermoid carcinoma.* Bowen disease of the anus represents carcinoma *in situ,* whereas extramammary Paget disease at this site reflects intraepithelial invasion by adenocarcinoma.

Carcinoma of the anus penetrates directly into the surrounding tissues, including the internal and external sphincters, perianal soft tissues, prostate, and vagina. Lymphatic spread carries the tumor to the pelvic and inguinal nodes, and hematogenous dissemination may lead to distant metastases.

☐ **Clinical Features:** Infection with human papilloma virus (HPV) and chronic inflammatory disease of the anus (e.g., venereal disease), fissures, and trauma produced by anal intercourse predispose to anal cancer. In fact, receptive anal intercourse among male homosexuals is associated with a marked increase in the risk of anal cancer. It has been observed that factors associated with genital carcinoma (cancer of the penis, scrotum, cervix, or vulva), poor hygiene, indiscriminate sexual practices, and genital warts, also contribute to the development of anal cancer. In addition, cigarette smoking is associated with an increased risk.

The usual symptoms of anal cancers include bleeding, pain, and an anal or rectal mass. Often the tumor is not clinically recognized as a malignant lesion and may be discovered only in a hemorrhoidectomy specimen. Combined chemotherapy and radiation therapy is the customary treatment, although abdominal–perineal resection is sometimes carried out. More than half of the patients survive for at least 5 years.

Miscellaneous Cancers

Malignant melanoma of the anus is rare but well recognized. Because of its location and early metastasis, it is infrequently diagnosed before it has spread distantly.

Malignant counterparts of the various benign mesenchymal tumors (e.g., leiomyosarcoma and neurogenic sarcoma) have been occasionally reported but are far less common in the colorectum than in other parts of the alimentary tract.

MISCELLANEOUS DISORDERS

Endometriosis

Endometriosis involves the colon and rectum in 15% to 20% of the cases but is ordinarily asymptomatic and is discovered only incidentally during laparotomy for other reasons. When symptoms do occur (abdominal pain, constipation, and even intestinal obstruction), they may be mistaken for those of colorectal cancer. The pathology of endometriosis is described in detail in Chapter 18.

In brief, endometriomas generally are seen as indurated tumors of up to 5 cm in diameter in the serosa and muscularis propria of the bowel, although they may penetrate the submucosa. As a result of repeated hemorrhage, the lesions are surrounded by reactive fibrosis. Symptomatic endometriomas of the colon and rectum usually project into the lumen as polypoid masses covered by intact mucosa.

Melanosis Coli

Melanosis coli is a medical curiosity that refers to the occurrence of dark brown pigment in the colonic mucosa. Despite the name, the pigment is not melanin, but rather lipofuscin. Persons with prominent melanosis coli are chronic users of anthracene-type cathartics, including cascara sagrada, rhubarb, senna, and aloe, and the finding can be an indication of surreptitious laxative abuse. Although melanosis coli has been reported in association with partially obstructing colon cancers, many patients with such cancers use laxatives.

The gross appearance of the pigmented mucosa in melanosis coli has been likened to tiger or crocodile skin or, as in chronic passive congestion of the liver, a section of natural nutmeg. Microscopically, macrophages in the lamina propria contain brown pigment granules. The pigment is lysosomal and is derived from breakdown of cellular membranes.

Cathartic Colon

Women who have used the laxatives listed in the section on melanosis coli and other irritant cathartics (e.g., castor oil and phenolphthalein) for many years may develop intractable constipation and lower abdominal pain, without diarrhea. Grossly, the transverse colon is pendulous, and the sigmoid is dilated. In some cases, there is only mild thickening of the terminal ileum or no abnormalities at all. Melanosis coli is often present. Interestingly, there is sometimes a loss of myenteric neurons in cathartic colon, which is believed to reflect a neurotoxic effect of the irritant laxative.

Stercoral Ulcers

Incomplete evacuation of the feces, usually in association with debilitating disease or old age, may lead to the formation of a large mass of stool that cannot be passed, termed fecal impaction. Stercoral ulcers result from pressure necrosis of the mucosa caused by the fecal impaction. Although such ulcers are most common in the rectosigmoid region, they have also been reported as proximal as the transverse colon. The most feared complications are severe rectal bleeding, even exsanguination, and perforation leading to peritonitis. Chronic blood loss may lead to iron-deficiency anemia.

Gastrointestinal Diseases in AIDS

The epidemic of AIDS due to infection with the human immunodeficiency virus (HIV) has resulted in numerous

TABLE 13-2 **Gastrointestinal Pathogens Associated with AIDS**

Bacteria	Protozoa
Mycobacterium avium-intracellulare	*Cryptosporidia*
Shigella	*Toxoplasma*
Salmonella	*Giardia*
Clostridium difficile	*Entameba histolytica*
	Microsporidia
Viruses	*Isospora belli*
Cytomegalovirus	
Herpes simplex	**Helminths**
	Strongyloides
Fungi	*Enterobius*
Candida	
Aspergillus	

gastrointestinal infections previously considered rare. The majority of patients with AIDS (50% to 90%) have chronic diarrhea. Virtually all forms of infectious agents, including bacteria, fungi, protozoa, and viruses, afflict patients with AIDS (Table 13-2).

Two neoplasms, Kaposi sarcoma and lymphoma, occur in the gastrointestinal tract of patients with AIDS. Kaposi sarcoma in the gastrointestinal tract is found almost exclusively in patients with AIDS. One third to one half of AIDS patients with cutaneous Kaposi sarcoma exhibit involvement of the gastrointestinal tract. In most patients, intestinal Kaposi sarcoma does not lead to symptoms, although gastrointestinal bleeding, obstruction, and malabsorption have been reported.

A common presentation of lymphoma complicating AIDS is involvement of the gastrointestinal tract. Any portion may be affected. The histological appearance and prognosis of these tumors are similar to those elsewhere in AIDS patients.

The Appendix

ANATOMY

The vermiform appendix, which is usually 8 to 10 cm in length, typically has a retrocecal attachment to the cecum, but its tip is generally not fixed and can therefore move freely. The appendix is invested with a mesentery called the mesoappendix. The wall of the appendix is composed of the same layers as the rest of the intestine: mucosa, submucosa, muscularis, and serosa. The most prominent microscopic feature is the predominance of submucosal lymphoid tissue, which develops in early infancy, reaches its largest size during adolescence, and then progressively atrophies. Because of its presumed homology with the avian bursa of Fabricius, the appendix is considered by some to have an immune function, although such a role remains to be established. Thus, although the appendix has historically been considered a vestigial structure, its status is a matter of debate.

APPENDICITIS

Acute appendicitis is an inflammatory disease of the wall of the vermiform appendix that often results in transmural necrosis and perforation, with subsequent localized or generalized peritonitis. This condition, by far the most common disease of the appendix, is the most frequent cause of an abdominal emergency. Although the incidence peaks in the second and third decades, acute appendicitis may occur in persons of any age. For reasons unknown, the incidence of the disease seems to be declining.

☐ Pathogenesis: **Acute appendicitis is believed to relate to obstruction of its orifice, with secondary distention of the lumen and bacterial invasion of the wall.** Mechanical obstruction by fecaliths or solid fecal material in the cecum is demonstrated in one third of the cases. Occasionally tumors, parasites such as *Enterobius vermicularis*, or foreign bodies are incriminated. Lymphoid hyperplasia as a result of bacterial or viral infection (e.g., by *Salmonella* or measles) may obstruct the lumen and lead to appendicitis. **However, no obstruction is demonstrated in up to half of patients with appendicitis,** and the factor that precipitates the disease in these cases is unknown. The higher incidence of appendicitis in industrialized countries has been attributed to the fact that fecaliths and viscid fecal material are more common in persons who consume a low-fiber diet than in those who eat a high-fiber diet.

As secretions distend the obstructed appendix, the intraluminal pressure increases and eventually exceeds the venous pressure, thereby causing venous stasis and ischemia. As a result, the mucosa ulcerates and permits invasion by intestinal bacteria. The accumulation of neutrophils produces microabscesses, and arterial thromboses aggravate the ischemia. The infected necrotic wall can become gangrenous and may perforate, often in 24 to 48 hours.

☐ Pathology: Macroscopically, the resected appendix is congested, tense, and covered by a fibrinous exudate. The lumen often contains purulent material, and a fecalith may be evident (Fig. 13-61). Microscopically, early cases show mucosal microabscesses and a purulent exudate in the lumen. As the infection progresses, the entire wall becomes infiltrated with neutrophils, which eventually reach the serosa. Necrosis of the wall leads to perforation and release of the luminal contents into the peritoneal cavity. In patients who do not undergo surgery and survive, chronic abscess can occur or the inflammatory process may subside, leaving a scarred appendix.

The complications of appendicitis are principally related to perforation, which is reported to occur in about one third of children and young adults. Almost all children younger than 2 years have a perforated appendix at the time of operation, as do up to three fourths of patients older than 60 years.

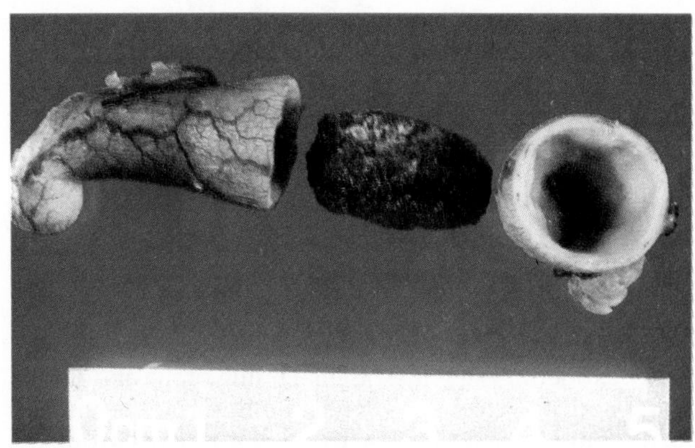

FIGURE 13-61
Acute appendicitis. The lumen of this acutely inflamed appendix is dilated and contains a large fecalith.

- **Periappendiceal abscesses** are common, although abscesses may develop anywhere in the abdominal cavity.
- **Fistulous tracts** may appear between the perforated appendix and adjacent structures, including the small and large bowel, bladder, vagina, or abdominal wall.
- **Pylephlebitis** (thrombophlebitis of the intrahepatic portal vein radicals) and **secondary hepatic abscesses** may occur, because venous blood from the appendix drains into the superior mesenteric vein.
- **Diffuse peritonitis and septicemia** are dangerous sequelae.
- **Wound infection** is the most common complication of acute appendicitis after surgery; it occurs in up to one fourth of patients with perforation and in one third of those who develop a periappendiceal abscess.

☐ **Clinical Features:** Acute appendicitis is typically manifested as epigastric or periumbilical cramping pain, but the pain may be diffuse or initially restricted to the right lower quadrant. Shortly thereafter, nausea and vomiting occur, and the patient develops a low-grade fever and a moderate leukocytosis. The pain shifts to the right lower quadrant, where point tenderness is the rule. A diseased retrocecal appendix is shielded from the anterior abdominal wall by the cecum and ileum; atypical symptoms are therefore easily misinterpreted because of their poor localization. In the elderly, appendicitis may produce only vague symptoms, and the diagnosis is often not made until perforation occurs. A number of conditions that do not require surgery are not infrequently misdiagnosed as appendicitis; these include mesenteric adenitis in children, Meckel diverticulitis, mittelschmerz (ovulatory rupture of an ovarian follicle), and acute salpingitis.

The treatment of acute appendicitis is surgical in the vast majority of cases. Because perforation carries a much higher risk of death than does laparotomy, early surgical intervention is warranted, even when the diagnosis of acute appendicitis is not entirely secure. In fact, at least 10% of all resected appendices should be normal. In remote locations where surgical facilities are not available, or when accompanying illnesses prohibit laparotomy, antibiotic treatment has occasionally been attempted.

Chronic appendicitis as a cause of symptoms is rare. However, recurrent appendicitis, although uncommon, is documented.

Other Causes of Appendicitis

***Yersinia* infection** of the ileum may also involve the appendix.

Tuberculous appendicitis is usually found in association with tuberculous enteritis, and rare cases of **actinomycotic infections** are recorded.

Crohn disease of the terminal ileum involves the appendix in one fourth of the cases and may affect it even when the inflammatory lesions are localized to distant sites in the small intestine or colon. Ulcerative colitis may also affect the mucosa of the appendix.

MUCOCELE

Mucocele refers to a dilated mucus-filled appendix. The pathogenesis may be neoplastic or non-neoplastic. In the non-neoplastic variety, the mucosa of the appendix is often ulcerated. Chronic obstruction leads to the retention of mucus in the appendiceal lumen.

In the presence of a cystadenoma (Fig. 13-62) or a cystadenocarcinoma, the dilated appendix is lined by a villous adenomatous mucosa or, in the case of cystadenocarcinoma, may exhibit infiltrating neoplastic glands.

The mucus-filled appendiceal mass may be large enough to be palpable and require exploratory laparotomy. A mucocele may become secondarily infected and rupture, thus discharging mucin and debris into the peritoneal cavity. This material may be mistaken at laparotomy for tumor implants on the peritoneum, but it will invariably be reabsorbed without incident. However, when the mucocele results from mucus secretion by a cystadenoma or cystadenocarcinoma of the appendix, perforation may lead to seeding of the peritoneum by mucus-secreting

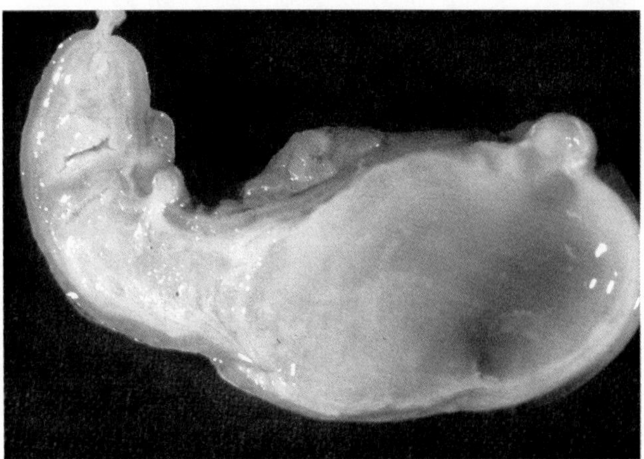

FIGURE 13-62
Mucocele of the appendix. The appendix is conspicuously dilated by mucinous material secreted by a cystadenoma.

tumor cells, a condition known as **pseudomyxoma peritonei**. In fewer than one third of the cases, pseudomyxoma peritonei is caused by disease of the appendix; in half, it originates from ovarian mucinous cystadenocarcinoma.

NEOPLASMS

The most common neoplasm of the appendix is carcinoid tumor, which in this location rarely metastasizes. Benign epithelial tumors (e.g., cystadenomas, adenomatous polyps; see Mucocele section earlier) are rare. The appendix infrequently gives rise to adenocarcinoma, mucinous cystadenoma, lymphoma, metastasizing malignant carcinoid tumors, and sarcomas. As in the other parts of the gastrointestinal tract, leiomyomas, fibromas, lipomas, and benign neurogenic tumors are encountered.

Figures 13-63 through 13-66 summarize the causes of gastrointestinal bleeding and obstruction and the major benign and malignant tumors of the gastrointestinal tract.

The Peritoneum

The peritoneum is the mesothelial lining of the abdominal cavity and its viscera. As the name implies, the visceral peritoneum invests the gastrointestinal tract from the stomach to the rectum and encircles the liver. The parietal

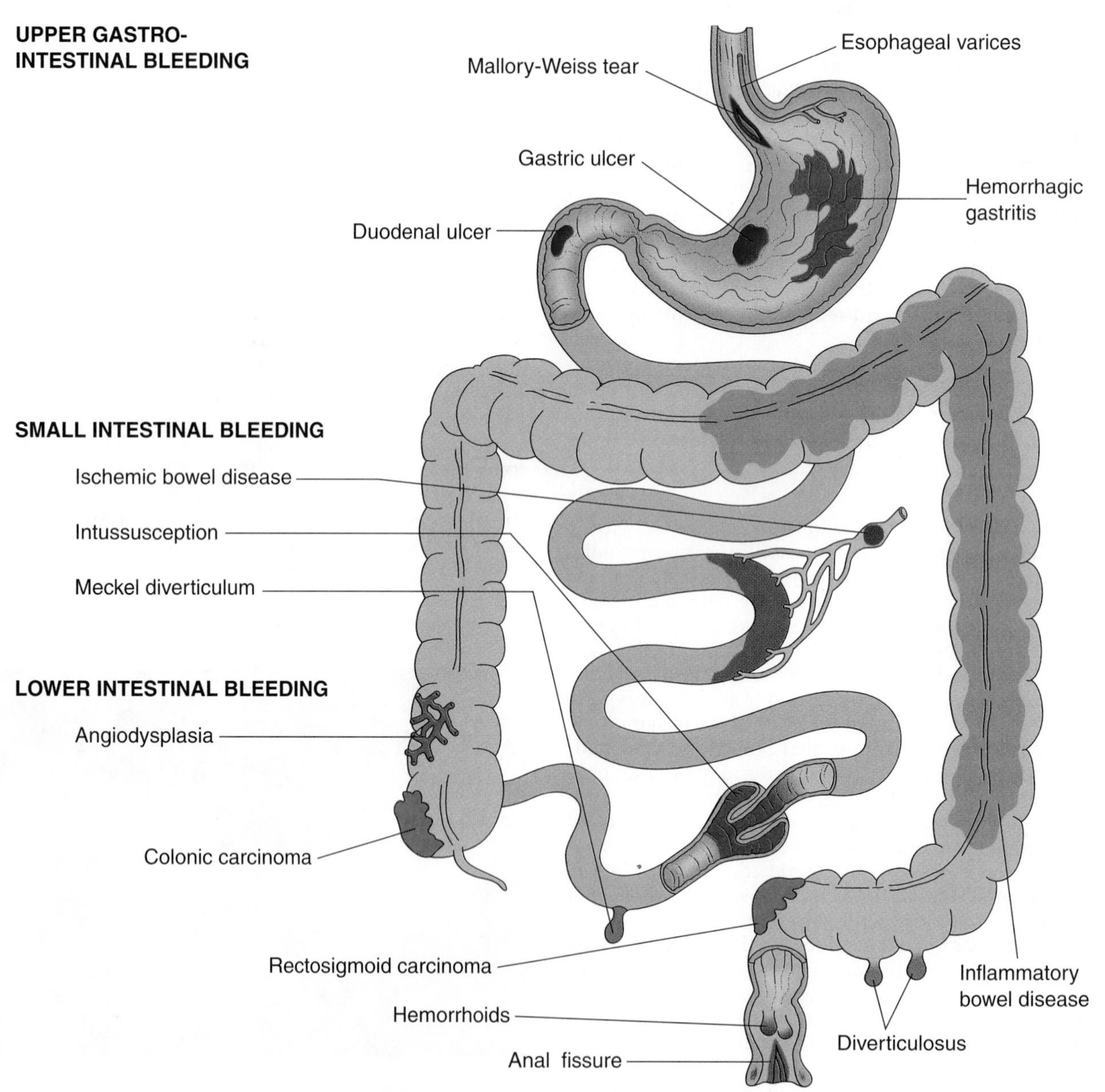

FIGURE *13-63*
Causes of gastrointestinal bleeding.

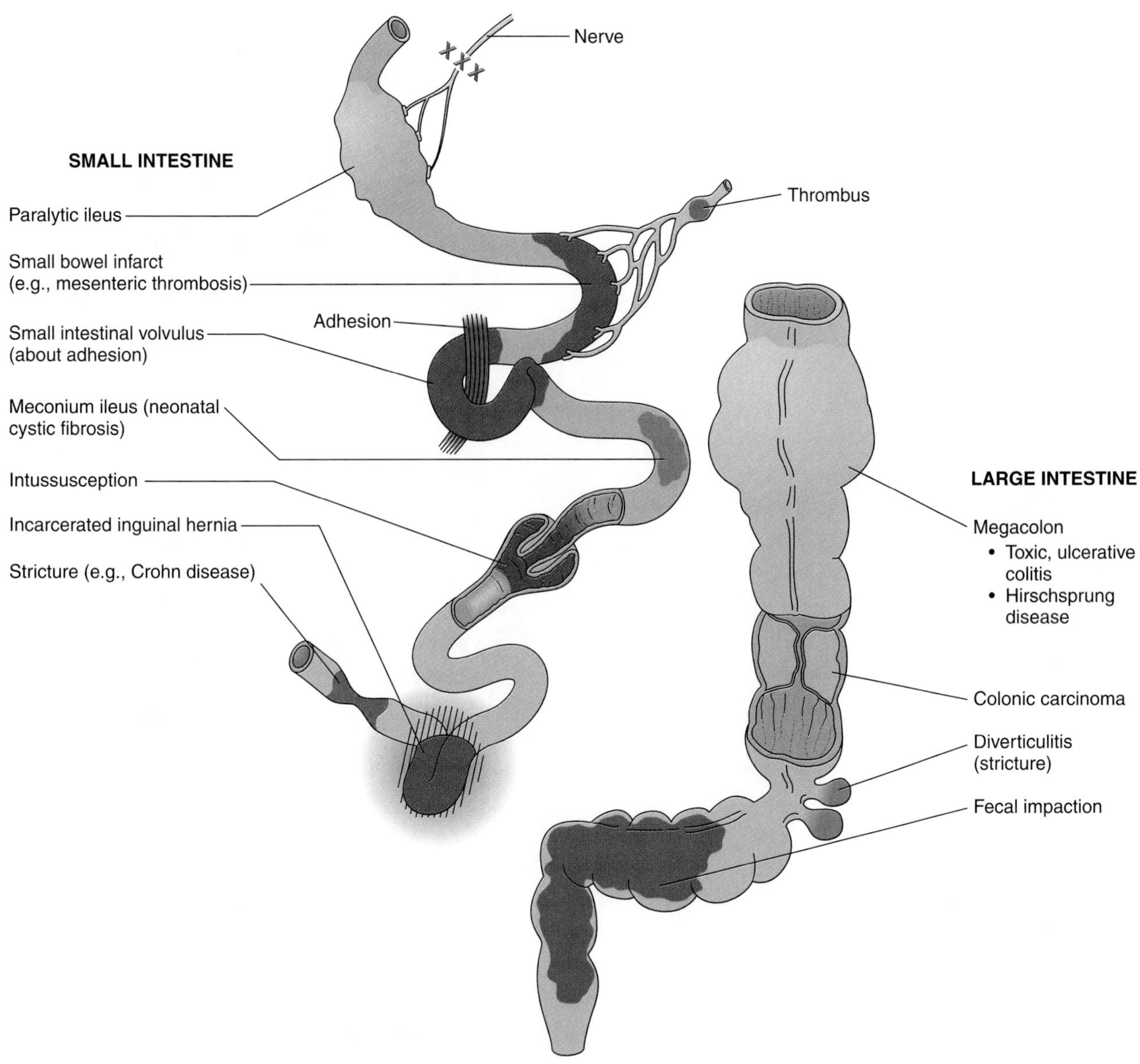

FIGURE *13-64*
Causes of gastrointestinal obstruction.

peritoneum lines the abdominal wall and the retroperitoneal space. The omentum, which has a double layer of peritoneum, encloses blood vessels and a variable amount of fat.

PERITONITIS

Bacterial Peritonitis

□ Pathogenesis

PERFORATION: A number of situations are associated with the introduction of microorganisms into the peritoneal cavity. **The most common cause of bacterial peritonitis is perforation of an abdominal viscus,** as in an inflamed appendix, peptic ulcer, or colonic diverticulum. Peritonitis results in an acute abdomen, in which severe abdominal pain and tenderness predominate. Nausea, vomiting, and a high fever are usual, and in severe cases, generalized peritonitis, paralytic ileus, and septic shock ensue. Often the perforation becomes "walled off," in which case, a peritoneal abscess results.

The bacteria released into the peritoneal cavity from the gastrointestinal tract vary according to the site of perforation and the duration of the peritonitis. Commonly, several aerobic and anaerobic species are cultured, including *E. coli, Bacteroides* species, various *Streptococcus* species, and *Clostridium.* Despite treatment with antibiotics, surgical drainage and debridement, and supportive measures, generalized peritonitis is still associated with substantial mortality and is especially dangerous in the elderly.

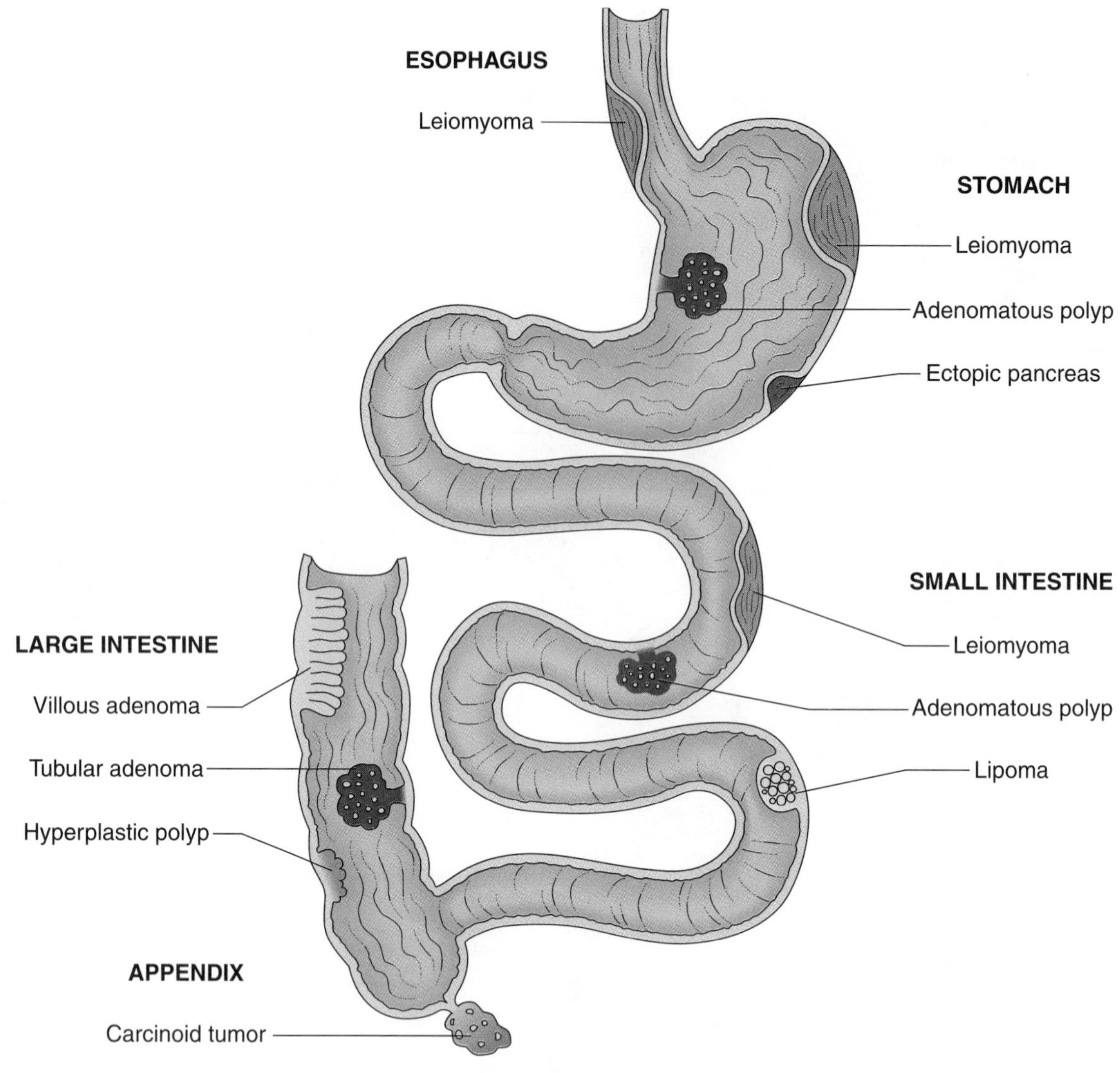

FIGURE *13-65*
Major benign tumors of the gastrointestinal tract.

PERITONEAL DIALYSIS: Chronic peritoneal dialysis is today a frequent cause of bacterial peritonitis, owing to contamination of instruments or dialysate. The clinical course is usually more mild than that noted with a perforated viscus, and the offending organisms are mostly *Staphylococcus* and *Streptococcus* species. Candidal peritonitis occurs occasionally. One fourth of the cases of peritonitis associated with chronic dialysis are aseptic; they are presumably caused by some chemical in the dialysate to which the peritoneum is sensitive.

SPONTANEOUS BACTERIAL PERITONITIS: This term refers to a peritoneal infection in the absence of a clear precipitating circumstance, such as a perforated viscus. **The most common cause of spontaneous bacterial peritonitis in adults is cirrhosis complicated by portal hypertension and ascites.** The pathogenesis appears to involve translocation of enteric organisms, mainly gram-negative bacilli, from the gut to mesenteric lymph nodes. Seeding of ascitic fluid then ensues, with depressed phagocytic activity and low antibacterial activity in ascitic fluid.

Spontaneous bacterial peritonitis in children can be a complication of the **nephrotic syndrome**, in part because ascites is more common in nephrotic children than in adults. Since the advent of the antibiotic era, most cases of spontaneous peritonitis in children are caused by gram-negative organisms, usually derived from urinary tract infections. The disease causes symptoms of an acute abdomen and ordinarily leads to surgical intervention, unless the child is known to have the nephrotic syndrome. Even with antibiotic treatment, the mortality remains at 5% to 10%.

TUBERCULOUS PERITONITIS: This infection is an unusual form of bacterial peritonitis. It is rarely seen in industrialized countries today, but occasionally complicates tuberculosis in developing countries. Many patients with

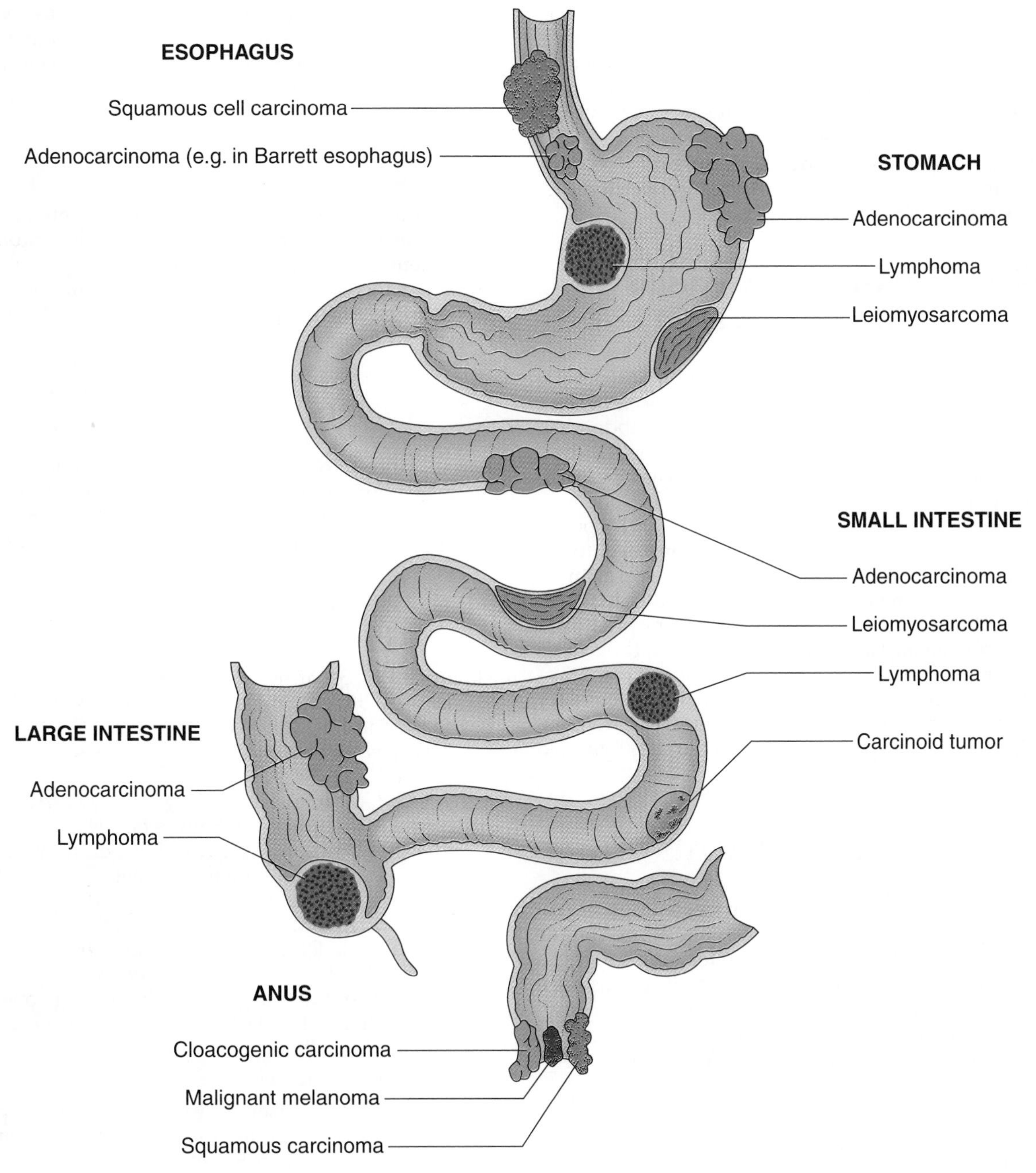

FIGURE *13-66*
Major malignant tumors of the gastrointestinal tract.

tuberculous peritonitis do not have apparent pulmonary or miliary tuberculosis, an observation that suggests the activation of latent tuberculous foci in the peritoneum derived from previous hematogenous dissemination.

□ **Pathology:** The macroscopic appearance of bacterial peritonitis is similar to that of purulent infection elsewhere. A fibrinopurulent exudate covers the surface of the intestines, and on organization, fibrinous and fibrous adhesions form between loops of bowel, which become joined to each other. Such adhesions may eventually be lysed, or they may lead to **volvulus** and **intestinal obstruction**. Bacterial salpingitis, usually gonococcal, may lead to pelvic peritonitis and adhesions, which define **pelvic inflammatory disease**.

Chemical Peritonitis

Bile peritonitis results from the escape of bile into the peritoneum, usually from a perforated gallbladder but sometimes from a needle biopsy of the liver. This abrupt insult may lead to shock.

Hydrochloric acid or hemorrhage from a perforated

peptic ulcer of the stomach or duodenum may elicit an inflammatory reaction in the peritoneum.

Acute pancreatitis causes the release and activation of potent lipolytic and proteolytic enzymes, which produce a severe peritonitis and fat necrosis. Shock is common and may be lethal unless adequately treated.

Foreign materials, introduced by surgery (e.g., talc) or by trauma are unusual causes of chemical peritonitis.

Leakage of urine can produce ascites.

Familial Paroxysmal Polyserositis (Familial Mediterranean Fever)

Familial Mediterranean fever (FMF) is an inherited autosomal recessive disorder, which features recurrent episodes of aseptic peritonitis, with fever and abdominal pain. The disease reflects mutations in a gene on the short arm of chromosome 16. FMF initially is seen as a peritonitis in about half of the cases and as arthritis in about one fourth. Pleuritis is the first complaint in only 5% of patients. However, almost all affected persons eventually manifest peritonitis, and more than half develop arthritis and pleuritis at some time. The disease predominates in Sephardic Jews and other Mediterranean populations, such as Armenians, Turks, and Arabs. The pathogenesis of FMF remains obscure, but in the absence of complications, the prognosis is good. Unfortunately, **secondary amyloidosis**, which results in renal failure, is a frequent complication. Therapy with colchicine has yielded promising results.

RETROPERITONEAL FIBROSIS

Idiopathic retroperitoneal fibrosis, an uncommon fibrosing condition of the abdomen, becomes symptomatic when it causes obstruction of the ureters. Although no cause is discernible in most cases, the disorder has been linked to treatment of migraine headaches with methysergide. A similar idiopathic fibrosis also has been described in the mediastinum and may affect the mesentery.

NEOPLASMS

Mesenteric and Omental Cysts

Mesenteric and omental cysts are generally of lymphatic origin but may derive from other embryonic tissues. Usually a slowly enlarging, painless mass is discovered in a child older than 10 years. The cyst may come to medical attention because of rupture, bleeding, torsion, or intestinal obstruction. Surgical excision is curative.

Mesothelioma

One fourth of all mesotheliomas arise in the peritoneum, and mesotheliomas are the most common primary tumor of that tissue. **Like pleural mesotheliomas, most of these malignant tumors are associated with exposure to asbestos.** The pathological characteristics of peritoneal mesotheliomas are identical to those of their pleural counterparts (see Chapter 12).

Metastatic Carcinoma

Metastatic carcinoma is by far the most common malignant disorder of the peritoneum, although peritoneal involvement is also common in intestinal lymphoma. Ovarian and pancreatic carcinomas are particularly likely to seed the peritoneum, but any intra-abdominal carcinoma can spread to the peritoneum.

Rare Tumors

Rarely, large retroperitoneal soft tissue tumors, such as lipomas, fibromas, myxomas, and mixtures of these mesenchymal elements, are encountered. They may attain a very large size and are not uncommonly sarcomatous.

SUGGESTED READING

BOOKS

Haubrich WS, Schaffner F, Berk JE (eds.): *Bockus gastroenterology,* 5th ed. Philadelphia: WB Saunders, 1991.

Lewin K, Riddell RH, Weinstein WM: *Gastrointestinal pathology and its clinical implications.* New York: Igaku-Shoin, 1992.

Ming S-C, Goldman H: *Pathology of the gastrointestinal tract.* Philadelphia: WB Saunders, 1992.

Morson BC, Dawson IMP, Day DW, et al: *Morson and Dawson's gastrointestinal pathology,* 3rd ed. Oxford: Blackwell Scientific, 1990.

Sleisenger MH, Fordtran JS (eds.): *Gastrointestinal disease,* 5th ed. Philadelphia: WB Saunders, 1993.

Whitehead R (ed.): *Gastrointestinal and oesophageal pathology,* 2nd ed. Edinburgh: Churchill Livingstone, 1995.

Yamada T (ed.): *Textbook of gastroenterology,* 2nd ed. Philadelphia: JB Lippincott, 1995.

REVIEW ARTICLES

Brandtzaeg P, Haraldsen G, Rugtveit J: Immunopathology of human inflammatory bowel disease. *Semin Immunopathol* 18:555–589, 1997.

Calam J: *Helicobacter pylori* and hormones. *Yale J Biol Med* 69:39–49, 1996.

Carter PS: Anal cancer: Current perspectives. *Dig Dis* 11:239–251, 1993.

Cave DR: Transmission and epidemiology of *Helicobacter pylori. Am J Med* 100:12S–17S, 1996.

Coffey RJ, Romano M, Goldenring J: Roles for transforming growth factor-alpha in the stomach. *J Clin Gastroenterol* 21(suppl 1):S36–S39, 1995.

Czinn SJ, Nedrud JG: Immunopathology of *Helicobacter pylori* infection and disease. *Semin Immunopathol* 18:495–514, 1997.

Dixon MF, Genta RM, Yardley JH, Correa P: Classification and grading of gastritis: The updated Sydney System. International Workshop on the Histopathology of Gastritis, Houston 1994. *Am J Surg Pathol* 20:1161–1181, 1996.

Foulkes WD: A tale of four syndromes: Familial adenomatous polyposis, Gardner syndrome, attenuated APC and Turcot syndrome. *Q J Med* 88:853–863, 1995.

Giardiello FM, Lazenby AJ, Bayless TM: The new colitides, collagenous, lymphocytic and diversion colitis. *Gastroenterol Clin North Am* 24:717–729, 1995.

Guarner C, Runyon BA: Spontaneous bacterial peritonitis: Pathogenesis, diagnosis, and management. *Gastroenterologist* 3:311–328, 1995.

Halter F, Zetterman RK: Long-term effects of *Helicobacter pylori* infection on acid and pepsin secretion. *J Biol Med* 69:99–104, 1996.

Ho SB: Premalignant lesions of the stomach. *Semin Gastrointest Dis* 7:61–73, 1996.

Howden CW: Clinical expressions of *Helicobacter pylori* infection. *Am J Med* 100:27S–32S, 1996.

Kinzler KW, Vogelstein B: Lessons from hereditary colorectal cancer. *Cell* 87:159–170, 1996.

Kozol RA, Dekhne N: *Helicobacter pylori* and the pathogenesis of duodenal ulcer. *J Lab Clin Med* 124:623–626, 1994.

Labigne A, deReuse H: Determinants of *Helicobacter pylori* pathogenicity. *Infect Agents Dis* 5:191–202, 1996.

Livneh A, Langevitz P, Zemer D, et al: The changing face of familial Mediterranean fever. *Semin Arthritis Rheum* 26:612–627, 1996.

Mittal RK, Balaban DH: The esophagogastric junction. *N Engl J Med* 336:924–932, 1997.

Quellette AJ, Selsted ME: Paneth cell defensins: Endogenous peptide components of intestinal host defense. *FASEB J* 10:1280–1289, 1996.

Savarino SJ: Diarrhoeal disease: Current concepts and future challenges: Enteroadherent *Escherichia coli:* a heterogeneous group of E. coli implicated as diarrhoeal pathogens. *Trans R Soc Trop Med Hyg* 87(suppl 3):49–53, 1993.

Schneider T, Ullrich R, Zeitz M: Immunopathology of human immunodeficiency virus infection in the gastrointestinal tract. *Semin Immunopathol* 18:515–534, 1997.

Scott H, Nilsen E, Sollid LM, et al: Immunopathology of gluten-sensitive enteropathy. *Semin Immunopathol* 18:535–554, 1997.

Sipponen P, Kekki M, Seppala K, Siurala M: The relationships between chronic gastritis and gastric acid secretion. *Aliment Pharmacol Ther* 10(suppl 1):103–118, 1996.

Spigelman AD, Arese P, Phillips RK: Polyposis: The Peutz-Jeghers syndrome. *Br J Surg* 82:1311–1314, 1995.

Thomas RM, Sobin LH: Gastrointestinal cancer. *Cancer* 75:154–170, 1995.

Veenendaal RA, Gotz JM, Lamers CB: Mucosal inflammation and disease in *Helicobacter pylori* infection. *Scand J Gastroenterol Suppl* 218:86–91, 1996.

Winawer SJ, Fletcher RH, Miller L, et al: Colorectal cancer screening: Clinical guidelines and rationale. *Gastroenterology* 112:594–642, 1997.

CHAPTER 14

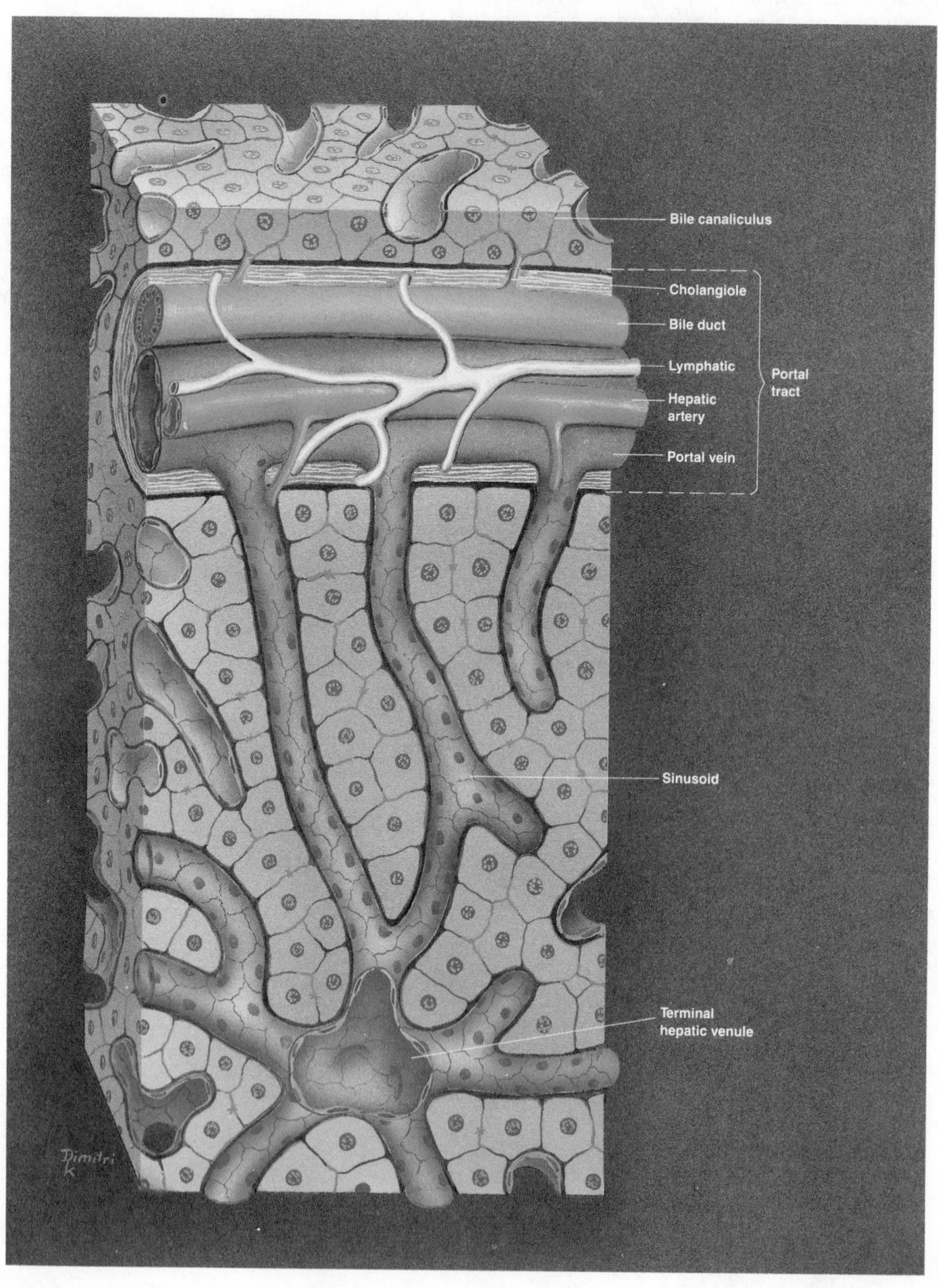

Bile canaliculus
Cholangiole
Bile duct
Lymphatic
Hepatic artery
Portal vein
Portal tract
Sinusoid
Terminal hepatic venule
Dimitri K

The Liver and Biliary System

Emanuel Rubin
John L. Farber

FIGURE *14-1 (see opposite page)*
Microanatomy of the liver.

The Liver

ANATOMY

The liver arises from the embryonic foregut as an entodermal bud, which differentiates into the hepatic diverticulum. Strands of entodermal cells mingle with proliferating mesenchymal cells to form all the structures of the adult liver, the gallbladder, and the extrahepatic biliary ducts.

The liver is the largest visceral organ in the body; in the average adult man it weighs about 1500 g. Situated in the right upper quadrant of the abdomen immediately below the diaphragm, it consists of two lobes, a larger **right lobe** and a smaller **left lobe,** which meet at the level of the gallbladder bed. Inferiorly, the right lobe exhibits lesser segments, the **caudate** and **quadrate lobes**. The **gallbladder** is located inferiorly in a fossa of the right hepatic lobe and normally extends slightly beyond the inferior margin of the liver.

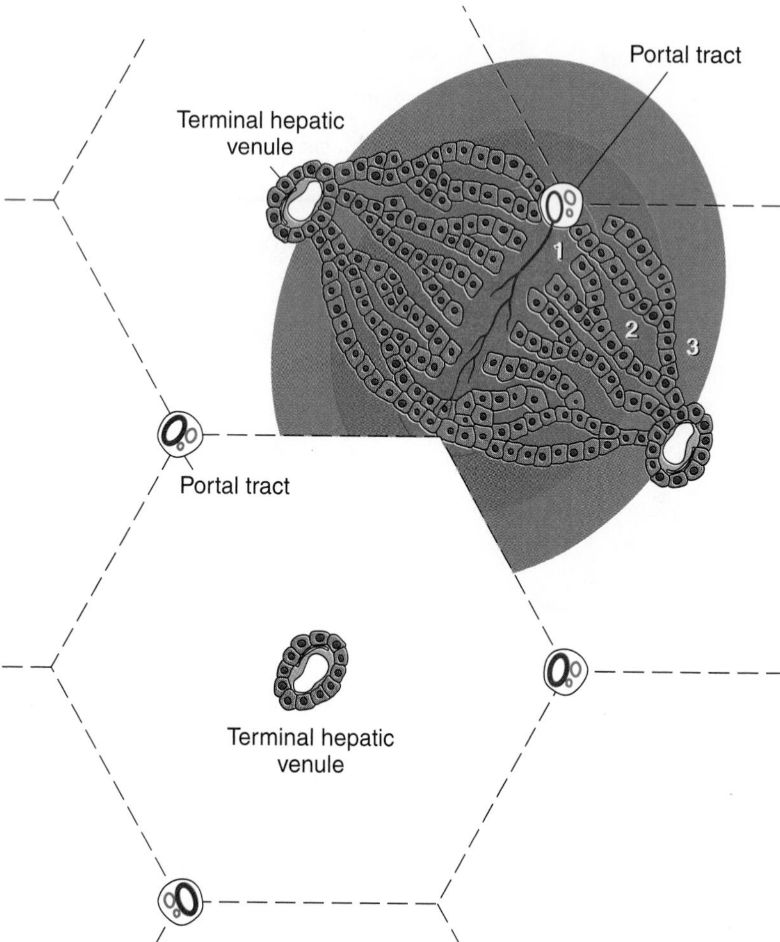

FIGURE *14-2*
Morphological and functional concepts of the liver lobule. In the classic, morphological liver lobule, the periphery of the hexagonal lobule is anchored in the portal tracts, and the terminal hepatic venule is in the center. The functional liver lobule is an acinus derived from the gradients of oxygen and nutrients in the sinusoidal blood. In this scheme, the portal tract, with the richest content of oxygen and nutrients, is in the center (*zone 1*). The region most distant from the portal tract (*zone 3*) is poor in oxygen and nutrients and surrounds the terminal hepatic venule.

The liver has a dual blood supply consisting of (1) the hepatic artery, a branch of the celiac axis, and (2) the portal vein, formed by the convergence of the splenic and superior mesenteric veins. The hepatic veins drain into the inferior vena cava, which is in intimate contact with and partly surrounded by the posterior surface of the liver. The hepatic lymphatics drain principally into lymph nodes of the porta hepatis and the celiac axis. The hepatic nerve plexus is innervated from the vagus and phrenic nerves and the lower thoracic sympathetic ganglia.

The common hepatic duct, formed by the union of the right and left hepatic ducts, receives the cystic duct from the gallbladder to form the common bile duct. Just before entering the duodenum, the common bile duct joins with the pancreatic duct. It terminates in the ampulla of Vater, where its lumen is guarded by the sphincter of Oddi.

The Liver Lobule

The basic unit of the liver is the polyhedral lobule (Figs. 14-1 through 14-3), classically depicted as a hexagon. **Portal triads** (or portal tracts) are found peripherally at the angles of the polygon. These portal triads—so named because they contain intrahepatic branches of the **bile ducts, hepatic artery, and portal vein**—are collagenous zones surrounded by an adjacent circumferential layer of hepatocytes called *the limiting plate*. As its name implies, the **central vein** (also known as the terminal hepatic venule) resides in the center of the lobule. Radiating from it are **one-cell-thick plates of hepatocytes**, which extend to the perimeter of the lobule, where they are continuous with the plates of other lobules. Between the plates of hepatocytes are the hepatic sinusoids, which are lined by endothelial cells and Kupffer cells.

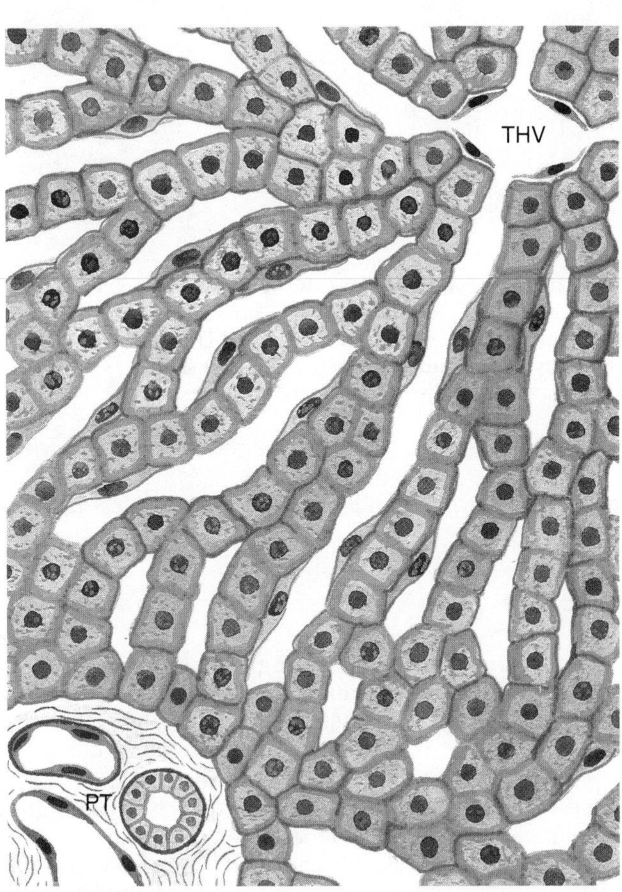

FIGURE 14-3
Schematic representation of the normal liver lobule. The portal tract (PT) contains branches of the hepatic artery, portal vein, and interlobular bile duct. The liver cell plates converge to the terminal hepatic venule (THV).

The large blood vessels that enter the liver at the porta hepatis eventually divide into the small interlobular branches of the hepatic artery and portal vein in the portal triads. From the portal triads, the interlobular vessels distribute blood to the hepatic sinusoids, where it flows centripetally into the central vein. The central veins coalesce to form sublobular veins, which eventually merge into the hepatic veins.

Bile flows in a direction opposite to that of the blood. Bile is secreted by hepatocytes into the bile canaliculi, formed by the apposed lateral surfaces of contiguous hepatocytes. Contraction of the bile canaliculus, mediated by the pericanalicular cytoskeleton of the hepatocytes, propels the bile toward the portal tract.

From the canaliculi, the bile flows into the bile ductules (canals of Hering or cholangioles) at the border of the portal tract and then enters a branch of the intrahepatic bile duct. Within each lobe of the liver, smaller bile ducts progressively merge, eventually forming the right and left hepatic ducts.

The Liver Acinus

The classic lobule described above is depicted as arranged around the central vein simply because of the histological appearance of the liver. **However, from a functional point of view, the lobule can also be thought of as an acinus with its center in the portal tract** (see Fig. 14-2). Such a concept takes into account the functional gradients that exist within the lobule. Concentrations of oxygen, nutrients, and hormones in the blood are highest at the portal tracts and progressively decline as the blood courses through the sinusoids to the central vein. This functional heterogeneity of the liver lobule can be expressed in terms of concentric functional zones around portal tracts. **Zone 1**, the most highly oxygenated zone, encircles the portal tracts, whereas **zone 3**, which surrounds the central veins, is oxygen poor. The intermediate or midlobular area is referred to as **zone 2**. For convenience, pathological changes in the liver are usually designated in relation to the classic histological lobule. For example, centrilobular necrosis refers to a lesion around the central veins, whereas periportal fibrosis is seen at the periphery of the classic lobule.

The Hepatocyte

About 60% of the total cell population of the liver consists of hepatocytes, although these cells account for 90% of the volume of the liver. The hepatocyte, roughly 30 μm across, has three specialized surfaces, sinusoidal, lateral,

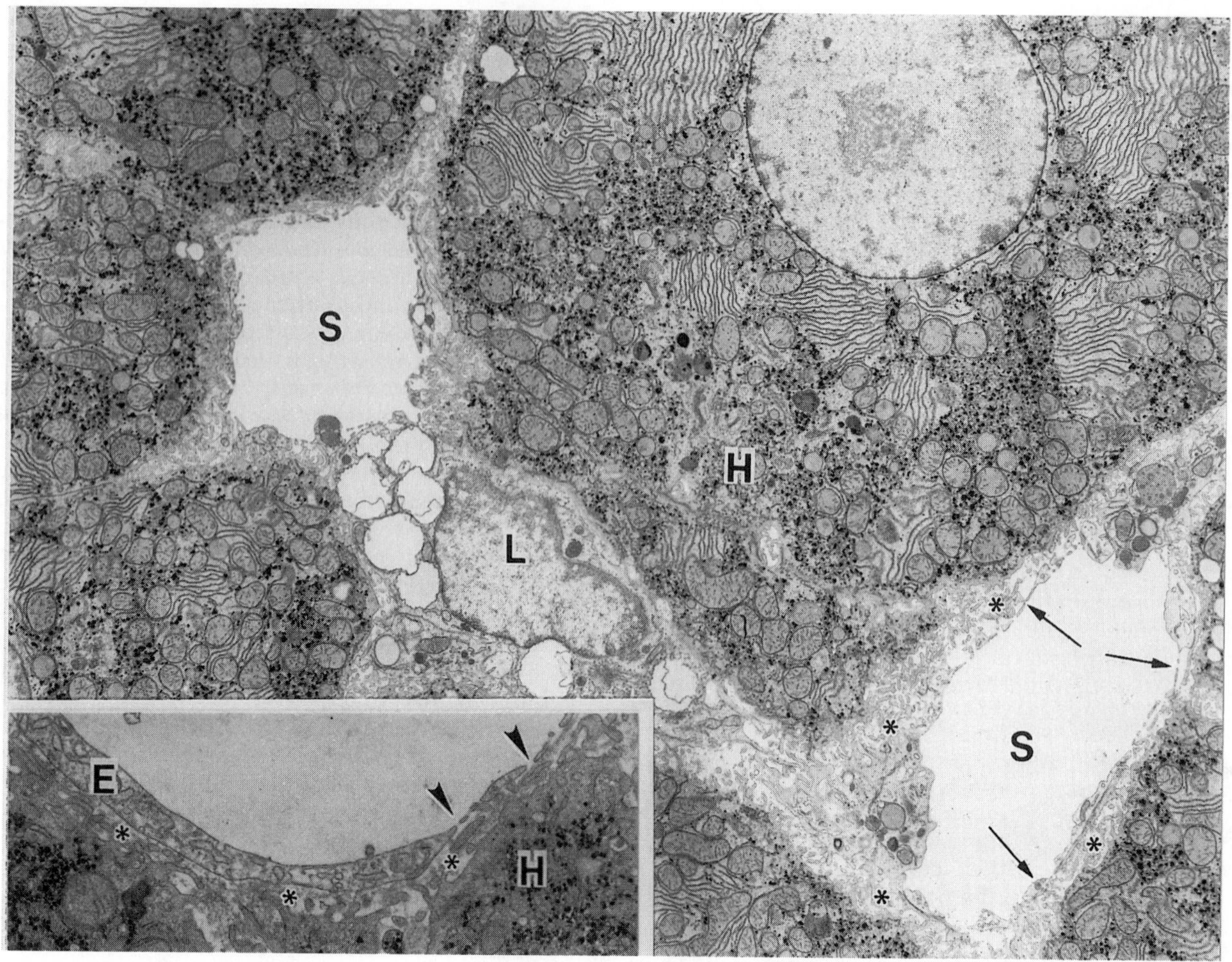

FIGURE 14-4
Hepatic sinusoids and space of Disse. An electron micrograph illustrates the relationship between hepatocytes, sinusoids, the space of Disse, and lipocytes (stellate cells, fat-storing cells). H, hepatocyte; S, sinusoid; L, lipocyte; *arrow*, endothelial cell; *asterisk*, space of Disse. The *inset* illustrates the relationship between hepatocytes (H) and endothelial cells (E). The *arrowheads* indicate fenestrae in the endothelial cells, whereas the *asterisks* are in the space of Disse.

and canalicular. Each cell has two sinusoidal surfaces, which exhibit numerous slender microvilli. The sinusoidal surface is separated from the endothelial cells that line the sinusoids by the space of Disse (Fig. 14-4). The canalicular surfaces of adjacent hepatocytes form the **bile canaliculus**, a collecting structure that is actually an intercellular space without a separate and distinct wall. The canalicular surface displays microvilli extending into the lumen. Leakage of bile from the canaliculus is prevented by a tight junctional complex between adjacent hepatocytes. The lateral, or intercellular, surfaces of adjacent hepatocytes are in close contact and contain gap junctions.

The centrally placed, spherical nucleus of the hepatocyte exhibits one or more nucleoli. The nuclei vary in size in ratios of 2 (diploid), 4 (tetraploid), and 8 (octaploid), with the majority being diploid. The cytoplasm is rich in organelles and shows prominent rough and smooth endoplasmic reticulum, Golgi complexes, mitochondria, lysosomes, and peroxisomes. In addition, in the fed state, abundant glycogen and occasional fat droplets are evident.

The Sinusoid

The hepatic sinusoids, through which blood flows through the liver, contain three cell types, namely endothelial, Kupffer, and stellate cells.

ENDOTHELIAL CELLS: The hepatic sinusoid is lined by a sheet of endothelial cells, which is penetrated by numerous holes called fenestrae. Unlike their counterparts in other tissues, adjacent endothelial cells do not form junctions, and there are many gaps between them. The result is a sievelike structure that affords free communication between the sinusoidal lumen and the space of Disse. Free access of sinusoidal plasma to the hepatocyte is further facilitated by the absence of a basement membrane between the endothelial cells and liver cells.

KUPFFER CELLS: The phagocytic Kupffer cells, which lack fenestrae, are located either in the gaps between adjacent endothelial cells or on their surfaces. Kupffer cells belong to the monocyte/macrophage system derived from the bone marrow. For that reason, after liver transplantation, the Kupffer cell population eventually originates from the recipient rather than the donor. Similar to other macrophages, activated Kupffer cells release a variety of cytokines, including tumor necrosis factor (TNF), interleukins, interferons, and transforming growth factor (TGF) alpha and beta.

STELLATE CELLS: Beneath the endothelial cells in the space of Disse are found occasional stellate cells (also known as Ito cells), which have specialized storage capacities. These cells contain fat, vitamin A, and other lipid-soluble vitamins. The stellate cell also secretes extracellular matrix components, including various collagens, laminin, and proteoglycans. In addition, under certain conditions, some growth factors are secreted by stellate cells. In a number of pathological states, these matrix constituents are formed in great excess, leading to the hepatic fibrosis characteristic of cirrhosis.

The most abundant extracellular matrix component in the space of Disse is normally fibronectin. Occasional bundles of type I collagen fibers provide the scaffold of the liver lobule. There is no continuous basement membrane barrier between the plasma and the surface of the hepatocyte, although by light microscopy reticulin stains impart the false impression of a continuous membrane.

FUNCTIONS

Although the hepatocyte is clearly a highly differentiated cell, it subserves a wide variety of functions. These can be broadly categorized as metabolic, synthetic, storage, catabolic, and excretory functions, with the understanding that there is substantial overlap between these divisions. The following are representative functions in each category.

METABOLIC FUNCTIONS: The liver is the central organ of **glucose homeostasis** and responds rapidly to fluctuations in the concentration of blood glucose. In the fed state, excess blood glucose is shunted to the liver to be stored as glycogen; in the fasting state, the liver maintains blood glucose levels by glycogenolysis and gluconeogenesis. For **gluconeogenesis**, the liver uses amino acids, lactate, and glycerol. The nitrogenous portion of amino acids is converted to urea. In the fasting state, during which energy is derived from the oxidation of fat, free fatty acids are taken up by the liver, converted to triglycerides, and secreted in the form of **lipoproteins** to be used elsewhere.

SYNTHETIC FUNCTIONS: Most serum proteins, with the major exception of the immunoglobulins, are synthesized in the liver. **Albumin** is the principal source of plasma oncotic pressure, and its decrease in chronic liver disease contributes to the development of edema and ascites. Blood coagulation depends on the continuous production of **clotting factors**, most of which, including prothrombin and fibrinogen, are synthesized by hepatocytes. Liver failure is thus characterized by a severe and often life-threatening bleeding diathesis. It is also interesting that endothelial cells of the liver manufacture **factor VIII**, and hemophilia has been reported to be ameliorated by liver transplantation. **Complement** and other acute-phase reactants are also secreted by the liver, as are numerous specific binding proteins—for example, the **binding proteins** for iron, copper, and vitamin A. Again, Wilson disease, a disorder of copper metabolism that is (among other abnormalities) associated with deficient ceruloplasmin production by the liver, is cured by liver transplantation.

STORAGE FUNCTIONS: The liver is an important storage site for glycogen, triglycerides, iron, copper, and lipid-soluble vitamins. Severe liver disease can result from excessive storage—for instance, abnormal glycogen in type IV glycogenosis and excess iron in hemochromatosis.

CATABOLIC FUNCTIONS: Endogenous substances, including hormones and serum proteins, are catabolized by the liver to maintain a balance between their production and their elimination. Thus, in chronic liver disease, impaired catabolism of estrogens contributes to feminization in men. The liver is also the principal site for the **detoxification of foreign compounds** (xenobiotics), such as drugs, industrial chemicals, environmental contaminants, and perhaps products of bacterial metabolism in the intestine.

EXCRETORY FUNCTIONS: The principal excretory product of the liver is **bile**, an aqueous mixture of conjugated bilirubin, bile salts, phospholipids, cholesterol, and electrolytes. Bile not only provides a repository for the products of heme catabolism but is also vital for fat absorption in the small intestine. Bile also contains IgA, which is involved in an enterohepatic circulation.

BILIRUBIN METABOLISM AND THE MECHANISMS OF JAUNDICE

Normal Bilirubin Metabolism

Bilirubin, the major end product of heme catabolism, has no known physiological function, although a role as an antioxidant has been suggested. **Up to 85% of bilirubin is derived from senescent erythrocytes,** which are removed from the circulation by mononuclear phagocytes of the spleen, bone marrow, and liver. The remaining bilirubin arises from the degradation of heme produced from other sources, the most important of which is the premature breakdown of hemoglobin in developing erythroid cells in the bone marrow. The amount of bilirubin produced from the turnover of nonhemoglobin hemoproteins—for instance, the mitochondrial and microsomal cytochromes—is small and does not ordinarily contribute to the development of jaundice.

Bilirubin is released from phagocytes and other cells

into the circulation, where it is bound to albumin for transport to the liver. Albumin in the circulation and the extracellular space constitutes a large binding reservoir for bilirubin and ensures a low extracellular concentration of free (unbound) bilirubin. Free bilirubin, unlike that bound to albumin or conjugated with glucuronic acid, is toxic to the brain in newborns and in high concentrations causes irreversible brain injury (kernicterus). In this respect, it is important to note that certain drugs that compete with bilirubin for binding sites on albumin (e.g., sulfonamides and salicylates) tend to shift bilirubin from the plasma into tissues and thereby increase its cytotoxicity.

The transfer of bilirubin from the blood to the bile involves a number of steps:

1. **Uptake:** On reaching the sinusoidal plasma membrane of the hepatocyte, the albumin–bilirubin complex is dissociated, and bilirubin is transported across the plasma membrane. This transport system seems to be carrier mediated and likely involves specific recognition of bilirubin by a plasma membrane receptor.
2. **Binding:** Within the hepatocyte, bilirubin is bound to cytosolic proteins, in this case a group of proteins known collectively as glutathione-S-transferases (also termed ligandin). These anion-binding proteins function within the cell in a manner similar to that of albumin in the blood. Ligandin binds bilirubin and prevents its reflux into the circulation and its nonspecific diffusion into inappropriate compartments of the hepatocyte.
3. **Conjugation:** Bilirubin is transferred to the endoplasmic reticulum, which contains the uridine diphosphate-glucuronyl transferase (UGT) system responsible for the conjugation of bilirubin with glucuronic acid. This reaction principally forms water-soluble bilirubin diglucuronide and a small amount (<10%) of the monoglucuronide.
4. **Excretion:** Conjugated bilirubin diffuses through the cytosol to the bile canaliculus, where it is excreted into the bile by a carrier-mediated process, which is the rate-limiting step for overall transhepatic transport of bilirubin.

After its excretion into the small intestine in bile, conjugated bilirubin is not absorbed and remains intact until it reaches the distal small bowel and colon, where it is hydrolyzed by the bacterial flora to free bilirubin. In turn, free bilirubin (now unconjugated) is reduced to a mixture of pyrroles, known collectively as *urobilinogen*. Whereas most of the urobilinogen is excreted in the feces, a small proportion is absorbed in the terminal ileum and colon, returned to the liver, and reexcreted into the bile; this entire process is termed the *enterohepatic circulation of bile*. Some urobilinogen escapes reabsorption by the liver and reaches the systemic circulation, after which it is excreted in the urine.

- **Hyperbilirubinemia** refers to an increased concentration of bilirubin in the blood (>1.0 mg/dL).
- **Jaundice** or **icterus** describes yellow skin and sclerae (Fig. 14-5), the color of which becomes apparent when the circulating bilirubin concentration attains levels greater than 2.0 to 2.5 mg/dL.
- **Cholestasis** is the presence of plugs of inspissated bile in dilated bile canaliculi and visible bile pigment in hepatocytes.
- **Cholestatic jaundice** is characterized by histological cholestasis and hyperbilirubinemia.

As shown in Figure 14-6, many conditions are associated with hyperbilirubinemia. Overproduction of bilirubin, interference with hepatic uptake or intracellular metabolism of bilirubin, and impairment of bile excretion are all causes of jaundice.

Overproduction of Bilirubin

An increased production of bilirubin results from increased destruction of erythrocytes (i.e., hemolytic anemia) or ineffective erythropoiesis (dyserythropoiesis). In unusual circumstances, the breakdown of the erythrocytes in a large hematoma (e.g., after trauma) may also provide excess bilirubin.

In the adult, even severe hemolytic anemia does not produce a sustained rise in serum bilirubin concentration beyond 4.0 mg/dL, provided that hepatic bilirubin clearance remains normal. However, the combination of prolonged hemolysis, as in sickle cell anemia, and intrinsic liver disease, such as viral hepatitis, leads to extraordinarily high levels of circulating bilirubin (up to 100 mg/dL) and pronounced jaundice.

The hyperbilirubinemia of uncomplicated hemolytic disease principally involves unconjugated bilirubin, whereas in parenchymal liver disease both conjugated and unconjugated bilirubin participate. Although the unconjugated hyperbilirubinemia of hemolytic disease is of little clinical significance in the adult, in the newborn it may be catastrophic. As discussed in Chapter 6, hemolytic disease of the newborn may result in concentrations of unconjugated bilirubin high enough to cause damage to the brain (*kernicterus*). Kernicterus has generally been associated with bilirubin concentrations over 20 mg/dL, but subtle degrees of psychomotor retardation may follow considerably lower bilirubin concentrations.

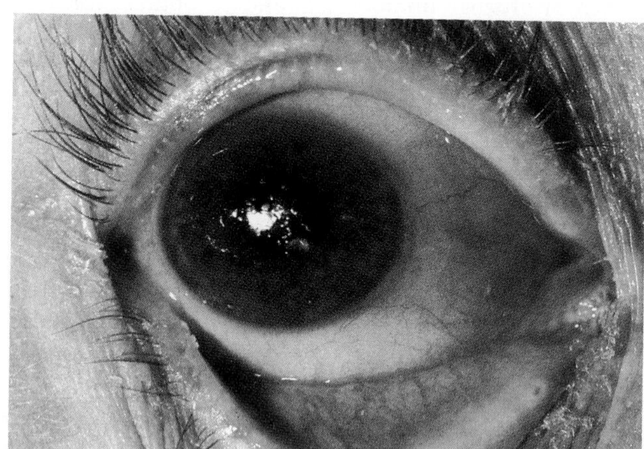

FIGURE *14-5*
Jaundice. A patient in hepatic failure displays a yellow sclera.

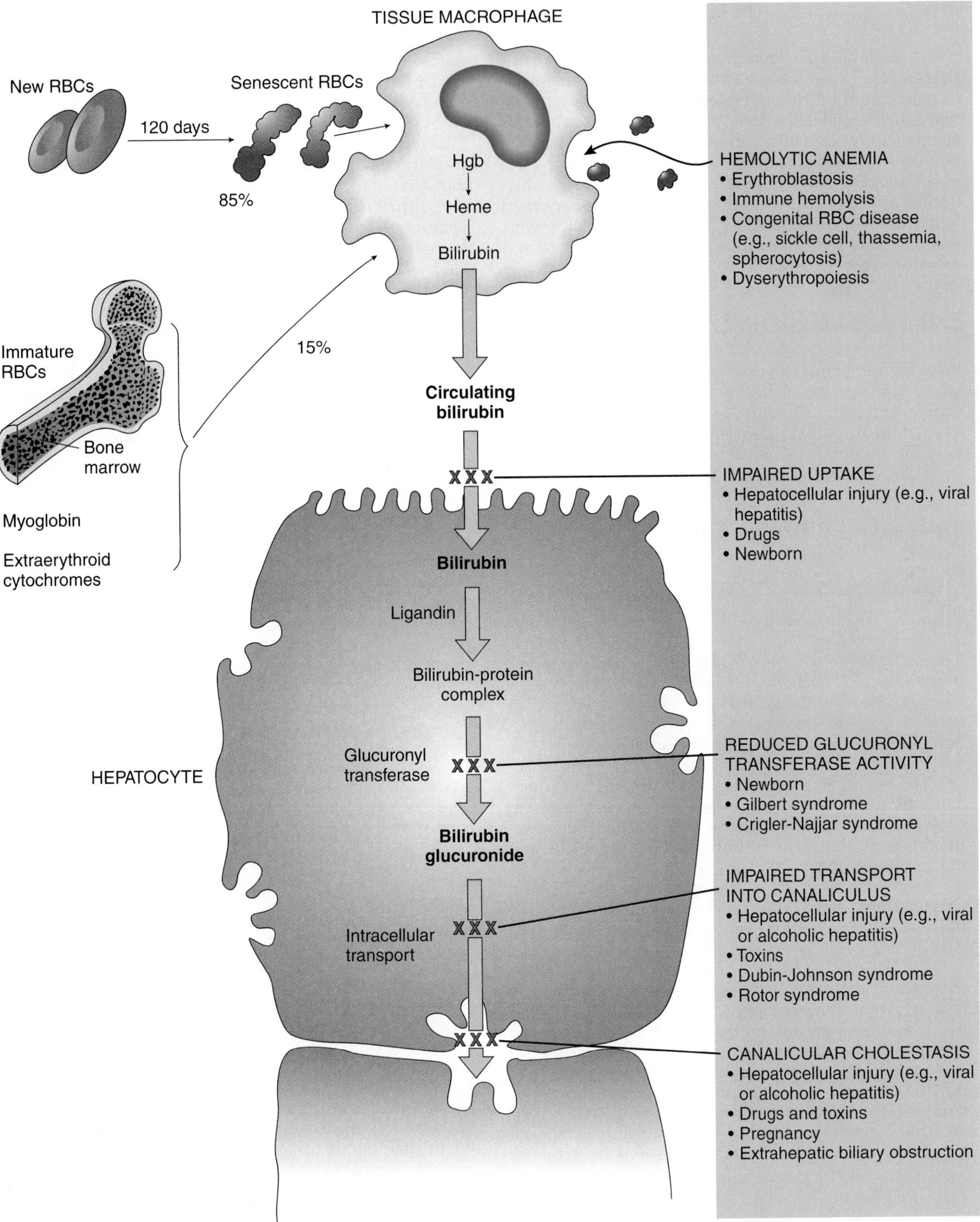

FIGURE *14-6*
Mechanisms of jaundice at the level of the hepatocyte. Bilirubin is derived principally from the senescence of circulating red blood cells, with a smaller contribution from the degradation of erythropoietic elements in the bone marrow, myoglobin, and extraerythroid cytochromes. Jaundice results from overproduction of bilirubin (hemolytic anemia) or defects in its hepatic metabolism. The locations of specific blocks in the metabolic pathway of bilirubin in the hepatocyte are illustrated.

In disorders characterized by ineffective erythropoiesis (e.g., megaloblastic and sideroblastic anemias), the fraction of bilirubin derived from the bone marrow may be increased to the point that hyperbilirubinemia develops. A rare hereditary disease of unknown etiology, *primary shunt hyperbilirubinemia*, or *idiopathic dyserythropoietic jaundice*, is characterized by massive overproduction of bilirubin in the bone marrow and is associated with chronic unconjugated hyperbilirubinemia. The bone marrow shows conspicuous erythroid hyperplasia and erythrophagocytosis, and iron turnover is augmented.

Decreased Hepatic Uptake of Bilirubin

Hyperbilirubinemia can result from impaired hepatic uptake of unconjugated bilirubin. Such a situation occurs in generalized liver cell injury, exemplified by viral hepatitis. Certain drugs (e.g., rifampin and probenecid) interfere with the net uptake of bilirubin by the liver cell and may produce a mild unconjugated hyperbilirubinemia.

Decreased Bilirubin Conjugation

Crigler-Najjar Syndrome

Crigler-Najjar syndrome type I is a recessively inherited malady characterized by chronic, severe unconjugated hyperbilirubinemia, owing to the complete absence of hepatic glucuronyl transferase (*UGT*) *activity.* A variety of mutations in the UGT gene lead to the synthesis of a completely inactive enzyme. As a result, treatment with phenobarbital, an inducer of microsomal enzymes (including UGT), is without effect.

The bile in this condition, which contains no conjugated bilirubin and no more than trace amounts of unconjugated bilirubin, is colorless. **The morphological appearance of the liver is normal, both by light and electron microscopy.**

In the era before liver transplantation, infants with Crigler-Najjar syndrome type I invariably developed bilirubin encephalopathy and usually died in the first year of life.

Crigler-Najjar syndrome type II is similar to but less severe than type I and manifests only a partial decrease in the activity of UGT. Autosomal recessive mutations in the UGT gene result in only a partial inactivation of the enzyme, and treatment with phenobarbital induces a decrease in unconjugated hyperbilirubinemia. This feature is the most reliable criterion for distinguishing type II from type I Crigler-Najjar syndrome. Almost all patients with type II syndrome develop normally, but in some, neurological changes resembling kernicterus are observed.

Gilbert Syndrome

Gilbert syndrome is an inherited, mild, chronic unconjugated hyperbilirubinemia (<6 mg/dL) that is caused by impaired clearance of bilirubin, in the absence of any detectable functional or structural liver disease. The syndrome runs in families, although only one member may have jaundice. Both autosomal dominant and recessive patterns of inheritance have been suggested, although the latter is favored today. The coding region of the UDP-glucuronyl transferase (UGT) gene is normal, but mutations in the promotor region lead to reduced transcription of the gene and, consequently, inadequate synthesis of the enzyme. Interestingly, the variant promotor is necessary, but by itself is not sufficient for the phenotypic expression of Gilbert syndrome. It has long been known that factors that increase serum bilirubin concentrations in normal persons, such as fasting or an intercurrent illness, produce an exaggerated increase in serum bilirubin levels in persons with Gilbert syndrome. This effect probably reflects the initially higher bilirubin level rather than any intrinsic difference in the physiological response to stress. Mild hemolysis, which also tends to increase bilirubin levels, is believed to occur in more than half of persons with Gilbert syndrome, but the mechanism is unclear.

Gilbert syndrome is exceptionally common, occurring in 5% to 10% of the population. It is seen more often in men than in women and is usually recognized after puberty. The sex differences and the age at onset suggest that hormones influence the modulation of bilirubin metabolism in the liver.

Gilbert syndrome is harmless, and for the most part without symptoms. Vague complaints of lassitude and weakness are common. However, these symptoms are possibly related to the anxiety engendered by the discovery of a chronically elevated bilirubin level rather than to the disease itself.

Decreased Intracellular Transport of Conjugated Bilirubin

Dubin-Johnson Syndrome

Dubin-Johnson syndrome is a benign autosomal recessive disease characterized by chronic conjugated hyperbilirubinemia and conspicuous melanin-like pigment deposition in the liver. This disorder is caused by a defect in the hepatocellular secretion of bilirubin glucuronides and other organic anions into the canalicular lumen. Specifically, it is thought that an impairment in an ATP-dependent mechanism for the transport of bilirubin glucuronides into the bile canaliculus is responsible for the jaundice. As a result of the widely diminished organic anion excretion, the transhepatic transport of a number of anionic dyes (sulfobromophthalein [BSP], rose bengal, indocyanine green) is also affected. In addition, there is an accompanying defect in the hepatic excretion of coproporphyrins and a consequent alteration in urinary coproporphyrin excretion.

The syndrome is rare among most populations, but certain groups that tend to have high rates of intermarriage, such as Iranian Jews and Japanese in remote areas, have a considerably higher incidence.

Dubin-Johnson syndrome can be distinguished from other conditions associated with conjugated hyperbilirubinemia by studies of **urinary coproporphyrin excretion**. There are two forms of human coproporphyrins, termed **isomer I** and **isomer III**. Normally, isomer I comprises

25% of urinary coproporphyrins. In Dubin-Johnson syndrome, although total urinary coproporphyrin excretion is normal, this isomer accounts for fully 80%. By contrast, in most hepatic disorders associated with jaundice, total urinary coproporphyrin excretion is increased, but coproporphyrin I comprises less than 65%. Thus, a finding of normal excretion of total urinary coproporphyrins combined with more than 80% as isomer I is diagnostic of Dubin-Johnson syndrome.

☐ **Pathology:** The microscopic appearance of the liver is entirely normal in Dubin-Johnson syndrome, except for the accumulation of coarse, iron-free, **dark-brown granules** in hepatocytes and Kupffer cells, primarily in the centrilobular zone (Fig. 14-7). By electron microscopy, the pigment is seen in enlarged lysosomes. Since hepatocytes do not synthesize melanin, it has been suggested that the pigment reflects the autooxidation of anionic metabolites (e.g., tyrosine, phenylalanine, tryptophan) and possibly of epinephrine. The accumulation of this intracellular pigment is reflected in a grossly pigmented, or "black," liver.

☐ **Clinical Features:** Except for mild intermittent jaundice, most patients with Dubin-Johnson syndrome do not complain of any symptoms. As in Gilbert syndrome, vague nonspecific complaints are common. Half of those affected have dark urine. In women, the disease may be discovered when jaundice appears during pregnancy or as a result of the use of oral contraceptives. The serum bilirubin value varies from 2 to 5 mg/dL, although it may be much higher transiently. About 60% of the increased bilirubin in the serum is conjugated.

Rotor Syndrome

Rotor syndrome is a *familial conjugated hyperbilirubinemia, which is clinically similar to Dubin-Johnson syndrome but without the associated pigmentation of the liver*. The disease is inherited as an autosomal recessive trait. Although the disorder clinically resembles Dubin-Johnson syndrome, it is a distinct entity. A defect in hepatic uptake or intracellular binding of organic ions has been postulated as the basis of Rotor syndrome. In addition, the pattern of urinary coproporphyrin excretion is similar to that of most hepatobiliary disorders accompanied by conjugated hyperbilirubinemia (i.e., increased total urinary coproporphyrins with 65% of isomer I). As in the Dubin-Johnson syndrome, patients with Rotor syndrome have few symptoms and lead normal lives.

Benign Recurrent Intrahepatic Cholestasis

Benign recurrent intrahepatic cholestasis is characterized by self-limited, periodic episodes of intrahepatic cholestasis preceded by malaise and itching. The cause of this disorder is unknown. Symptoms may last from several weeks to several months, although symptoms lasting for several years have been reported. The mean number of attacks in a lifetime is 3 to 5, but a significant proportion of affected persons have as many as 10 attacks. Recurrences have been noted at intervals of weeks to years. Serum bilirubin levels during the acute episodes are in the range of 10 to 20 mg/dL, and most of the bilirubin is conjugated. Serum alkaline phosphatase activity is significantly increased, whereas levels of aminotransferases are only slightly elevated.

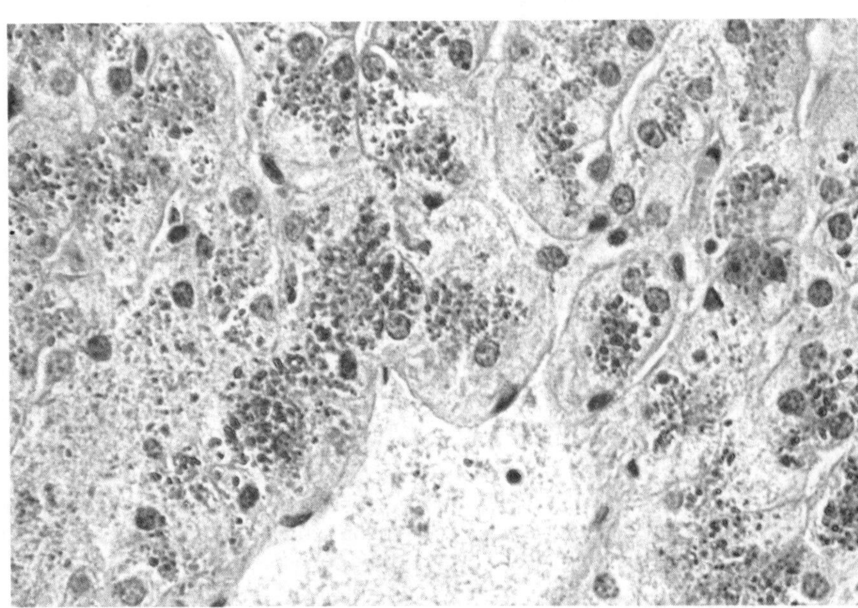

FIGURE *14-7*
Dubin-Johnson syndrome. The hepatocytes contain coarse, iron-free, dark-brown granules.

The liver shows centrilobular cholestasis (bile plugs in bile canaliculi) and a few mononuclear inflammatory cells in the portal tracts. All the structural and functional alterations disappear during remissions, and no permanent sequelae have been reported.

Intrahepatic Cholestasis of Pregnancy

Intrahepatic cholestasis of pregnancy is a familial disorder characterized by pruritus and cholestatic jaundice, which usually occurs in the last trimester of each pregnancy and promptly disappears after delivery. A variant of this condition without jaundice is referred to as *pruritus gravidorum*. Half of the patients with intrahepatic cholestasis of pregnancy have other family members who have experienced jaundice during pregnancy or after the use of oral contraceptives. It is likely that the increase in gonadal and placental hormones during pregnancy is responsible for the cholestasis in susceptible women. Maternal health is unaffected by this disease, but the effects on the fetus are often grave and include fetal distress, stillbirth, prematurity, and an increased risk of intracranial hemorrhage during delivery. The liver of the mother exhibits no specific changes other than centrilobular cholestasis.

Familial Intrahepatic Cholestasis (Byler Syndrome)

Byler syndrome is an uncommon, inherited, autosomal recessive disorder of infancy or early childhood in which intrahepatic cholestasis relentlessly progresses to cirrhosis. The pathogenesis of the disease is not understood. Although Byler syndrome was originally described in several Amish families, all of whom were named Byler, it is not limited to that ethnic group. There is an associated high incidence of retinitis pigmentosa, and the children are often mentally retarded. Most affected children die within the first 2 years of life.

Jaundice Associated with Sepsis

Severe conjugated hyperbilirubinemia may be associated with septicemia involving both gram-positive and gram-negative bacteria, although the latter infection is more common. In these situations, the serum alkaline phosphatase activity and cholesterol levels are usually low, suggesting the possibility of an isolated defect in the excretion of conjugated bilirubin. In jaundice associated with sepsis, the histological changes in the liver are nonspecific and include mild canalicular cholestasis and slight fat accumulation. The portal tracts may contain excess inflammatory cells, and varying degrees of proliferation of bile ductules may be seen. Occasionally, dilated ductules are filled with inspissated bile.

Neonatal (Physiological) Jaundice

Almost 70% of full-term, normal newborns exhibit hyperbilirubinemia in the absence of any specific disorder, and are said to suffer from physiological jaundice.

☐ **Pathogenesis:** In the fetus, the transhepatic clearance of bilirubin is negligible; hepatic uptake, conjugation, and biliary excretion are all much lower than in children and adults. Hepatic UGT activity is less than 1% of that in adults, and ligandin levels are low. Nevertheless, fetal bilirubin levels remain low because bilirubin traverses the placenta, after which it is conjugated and excreted by the maternal liver.

The liver of the newborn assumes the responsibility for bilirubin clearance before its conjugating and excretory capacities are fully developed. Moreover, the demands on the liver in the newborn are actually increased because of an augmented destruction of circulating erythrocytes during this period. **As a consequence, the normal newborn exhibits a transient, physiological, unconjugated hyperbilirubinemia.** This physiological jaundice is more pronounced in premature infants, both because the hepatic clearance of bilirubin is less developed and because the turnover of erythrocytes is more pronounced than in the term infant. The hepatic bilirubin conjugating capacity reaches adult levels about 2 weeks after birth; the ligandin level takes somewhat longer to reach adult values. As a result of this hepatic maturation, serum bilirubin levels rapidly decline to adult values shortly after birth.

In cases of maternal–fetal blood group incompatibilities that lead to erythroblastosis fetalis (see Chapter 6), a striking overproduction of bilirubin in the fetus results from immune-mediated hemolysis. However, although newborns with erythroblastosis fetalis display increased bilirubin levels in cord blood, jaundice becomes severe only after birth, because maternal metabolism of bilirubin no longer compensates for the immaturity of the neonatal liver.

Impairment of Canalicular Bile Flow (Cholestasis)

Cholestasis is defined morphologically as the demonstration of visible biliary pigment, caused either by extrahepatic or intrahepatic obstruction to the flow of bile (Fig. 14-8). Functionally, cholestasis represents a decrease in bile flow through the canaliculus and a reduction in the secretion of water, bilirubin, and bile acids by the hepatocyte. The clinical diagnosis is based on the accumulation in the blood of materials normally transferred to the bile, including bilirubin, cholesterol, and bile acids, and the presence in the blood of elevated activities of certain enzymes, typically alkaline phosphatase. Cholestasis may be produced by intrinsic liver disease, in which case the term *intrahepatic cholestasis* is used, or by obstruction of the large bile ducts, a condition known as *extrahepatic cholestasis*. In any event, cholestasis is caused by a defect in the transport of bile across the canalicular membrane.

The secretion of bile into the canaliculus and its passage into the biliary collecting system is an active process that depends on a number of factors, including (1) the functional and structural characteristics of the canalicular microvilli, (2) the permeability of the canalicular plasma membrane, (3) the intracellular contractile system surrounding the canaliculus (microfilaments, microtubules), and (4) the interaction of bile acids with the secretory apparatus.

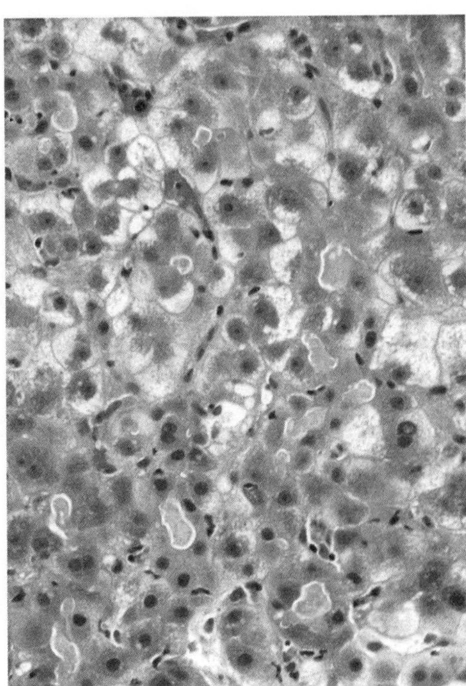

FIGURE *14-8*
Bile stasis. A photomicrograph of the liver shows prominent bile plugs in dilated bile canaliculi.

Cellular Mechanisms of Cholestasis

The biochemical basis of cholestasis is not entirely clear, but a number of abnormalities in the formation and movement of bile have been described. In the case of extrahepatic biliary obstruction, the effects clearly begin with increased pressure in the bile ducts. However, in the early stages the biochemical and morphological events at the canalicular level are similar to those that occur with intrahepatic cholestasis, including **a centrilobular predilection for the appearance of canalicular bile plugs**.

The invariable presence of bile constituents in the blood of persons with cholestasis implies regurgitation from the hepatocyte into the bloodstream. The hepatic clearance of unconjugated bilirubin in cholestasis is normal, and the increase in the levels of bile pigments in the plasma is due to a reflux of monoconjugates and diconjugates of bilirubin into the blood. Even in the presence of complete bile duct obstruction, the serum bilirubin level rises only as high as 30 to 35 mg/dL. Renal excretion of bilirubin prevents further accumulation.

Alterations at the canalicular level include the following:

LOBULAR DISTRIBUTION OF CHOLESTASIS: Both intrahepatic and extrahepatic cholestasis are characterized by an initially preferential **localization of visible bile pigment in the centrilobular zone**. Although the basis for this distribution remains enigmatic, it may relate to (1) the gradient from portal tract to central zone in the formation of bile acids, and (2) the particularly high levels of microsomal mixed-function oxidases in pericentral hepatocytes. Fluid secretion into the canalicular bile is divided into two components: one dependent on the secretion of bile acids and the other independent of bile acid secretion. Since the periportal hepatocytes secrete most of the bile acids, the fluid content in the periportal zone of the canaliculus is greater than that in the central zone, a condition that tends to keep bilirubin in solution. Moreover, the bile acids themselves, which act as detergents in the intestine, also solubilize aggregates of bilirubin. These properties may serve to limit the extent of peripheral, as opposed to central, bile deposition in cholestatic conditions. To the above factors is added the higher activity of microsomal mixed-function oxidases in the central zone, which predisposes central hepatocytes to injury by activated oxygen species formed during the biotransformation of drugs and other toxins. Such an effect may favor the deposition of bile in the centrilobular areas in cholestatic disorders.

DAMAGE TO THE CANALICULAR PLASMA MEMBRANE: The canalicular plasma membrane is the site of sodium (and therefore fluid) secretion into the bile. In addition, this membrane participates in the secretion of bile acids and bilirubin. The secretion of fluid is under the control of the Na^+-K^+ ATPase of the canalicular membrane. Alterations in the canalicular membrane by agents capable of perturbing its lipid structure (e.g., chlorpromazine) inhibit Na^+-K^+ ATPase and decrease bile flow. Similarly, ethinyl estradiol increases the cholesterol content of the canalicular membrane, inhibits ATPase, and interferes with bile flow. Clinically, both chlorpromazine and ethinyl estradiol cause cholestasis in some persons. Morphological alterations in the canalicular membrane (e.g., those associated with the infusion of certain monohydroxy bile acids, such as taurolithocholate) are also accompanied by a decreased bile flow. Although correlations between the physical structure and chemical composition of the canalicular membranes and bile flow are imperfect, the evidence suggests a causal relationship.

ALTERATION IN THE CONTRACTILE PROPERTIES OF THE CANALICULUS: It has been shown by cinematography that bile is propelled along the canaliculus by a **peristalsis-like contractile activity of the hepatocytes**. Agents that interact with the pericanalicular actin microfilaments (e.g., cytochalasin, phalloidin, and possibly chlorpromazine) inhibit this peristalsis and may cause cholestasis.

ALTERATIONS IN THE PERMEABILITY OF THE CANALICULAR MEMBRANE: It has been suggested that certain agents that produce cholestasis, including estrogens and taurolithocholate, permit back-diffusion of bile components by making the canalicular membrane more permeable, or "leaky."

Morphological Features of Cholestasis

The morphological hallmark of cholestasis is the presence of brownish bile pigment within dilated canaliculi and in hepatocytes. By electron microscopy the canaliculus is enlarged, and the microvilli are blunted and decreased in number, or even absent (Fig. 14-9). Although back-diffusion of bile may occur, the canalicular tight junctions are almost invariably preserved. By light microscopy, the biliary concretions appear homogeneous, but at the ultrastructural level they may have a variable appearance, including lamellar, crystalline, and granular forms. The pericanalicular zone of the hepatocyte is widened by an apparent increase in the number of microfilaments. Bile stasis in the hepatocyte is reflected in the presence of large, inhomogeneous, bile-laden lysosomes.

When cholestasis persists, secondary morphological abnormalities develop. Scattered necrotic hepatocytes probably reflect a toxic effect of excess intracellular bile. Within the sinusoids, macrophages and lymphoid cells appear. The macrophages and resident Kupffer cells contain bile pigment and cellular debris. In general, these changes parallel the severity and duration of the cholestasis. **Whereas early cholestasis is restricted almost exclusively to the central zone, chronic cholestasis is also marked by the appearance of bile plugs in the periphery of the lobule.** Cholestasis in the periphery of the lobule may reflect mechanical obstruction of the canaliculi by secondary proliferation of and damage to the bile ductules, which link the canaliculi with the smallest branches of the portal bile ducts. Periportal fibrosis further aggravates obstruction to bile flow into the biliary ducts. Although the exact mechanism responsible for this fibrosis in chronic cholestasis is not clear, injury to the ductular cells, ductular proliferation, and the escape of bile may contribute.

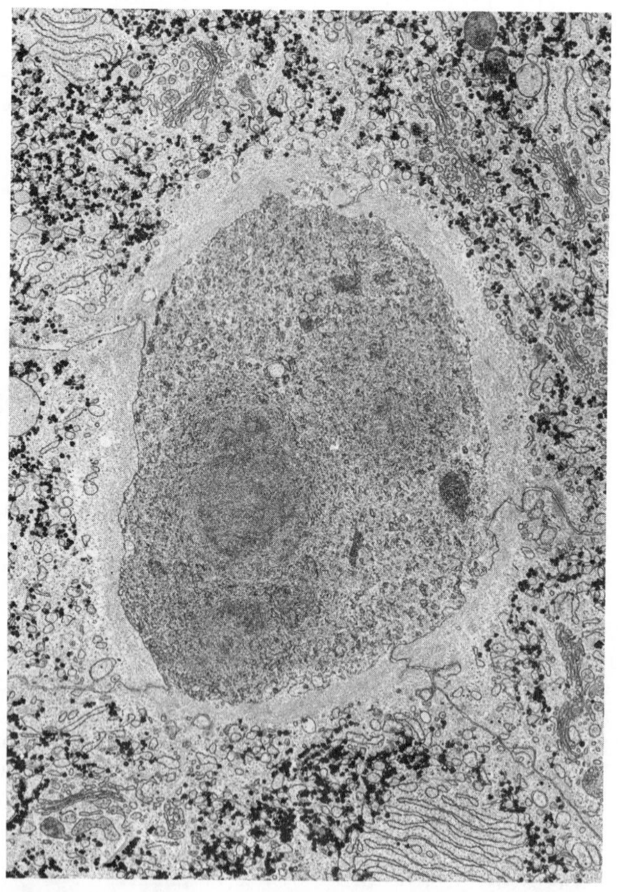

FIGURE *14-9*
Cholestasis. An electron micrograph reveals a distended bile canaliculus that has a thickened, filamentous ectoplasmic zone and encloses a granular bile plug.

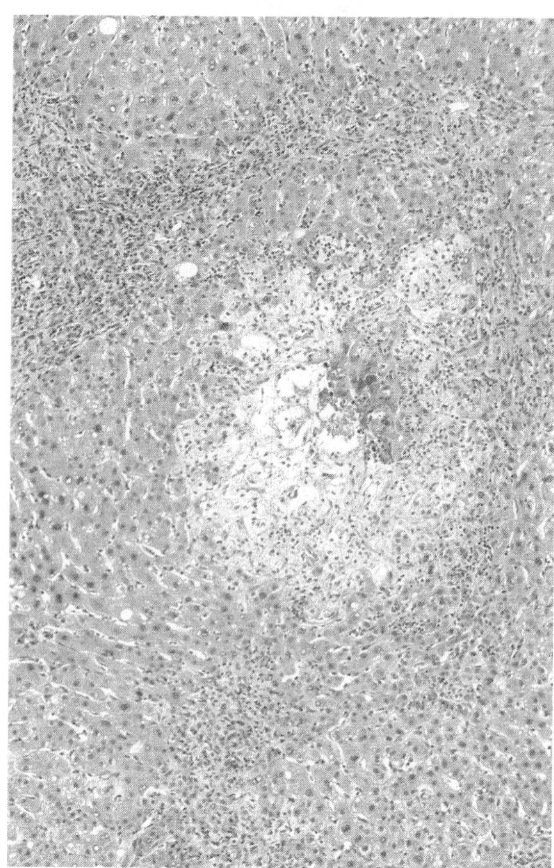

FIGURE *14-10*
Bile infarct (bile lake). A photomicrograph of the liver in a patient with extrahepatic biliary obstruction shows an area of necrosis and the accumulation of extravasated bile.

In long-standing cholestasis (usually the result of extrahepatic biliary obstruction), groups of hepatocytes manifest (1) hydropic swelling, (2) a diffuse impregnation with bile pigment, and (3) a reticulated appearance, a triad termed *feathery degeneration*. The necrosis of such cells, together with the accumulation of extravasated bile in the area, results in a golden-yellow focus of extracellular pigment and debris known as a *bile infarct or bile lake* (Fig. 14-10).

The sites of obstruction to the flow of bile in the liver are depicted in Figure 14-11.

HEPATIC FAILURE

Hepatic failure is the clinical syndrome that occurs when the mass of liver cells or their function is inadequate to sustain the vital metabolic, detoxifying, and synthetic activities dependent on the liver. Liver failure may develop acutely, most com-

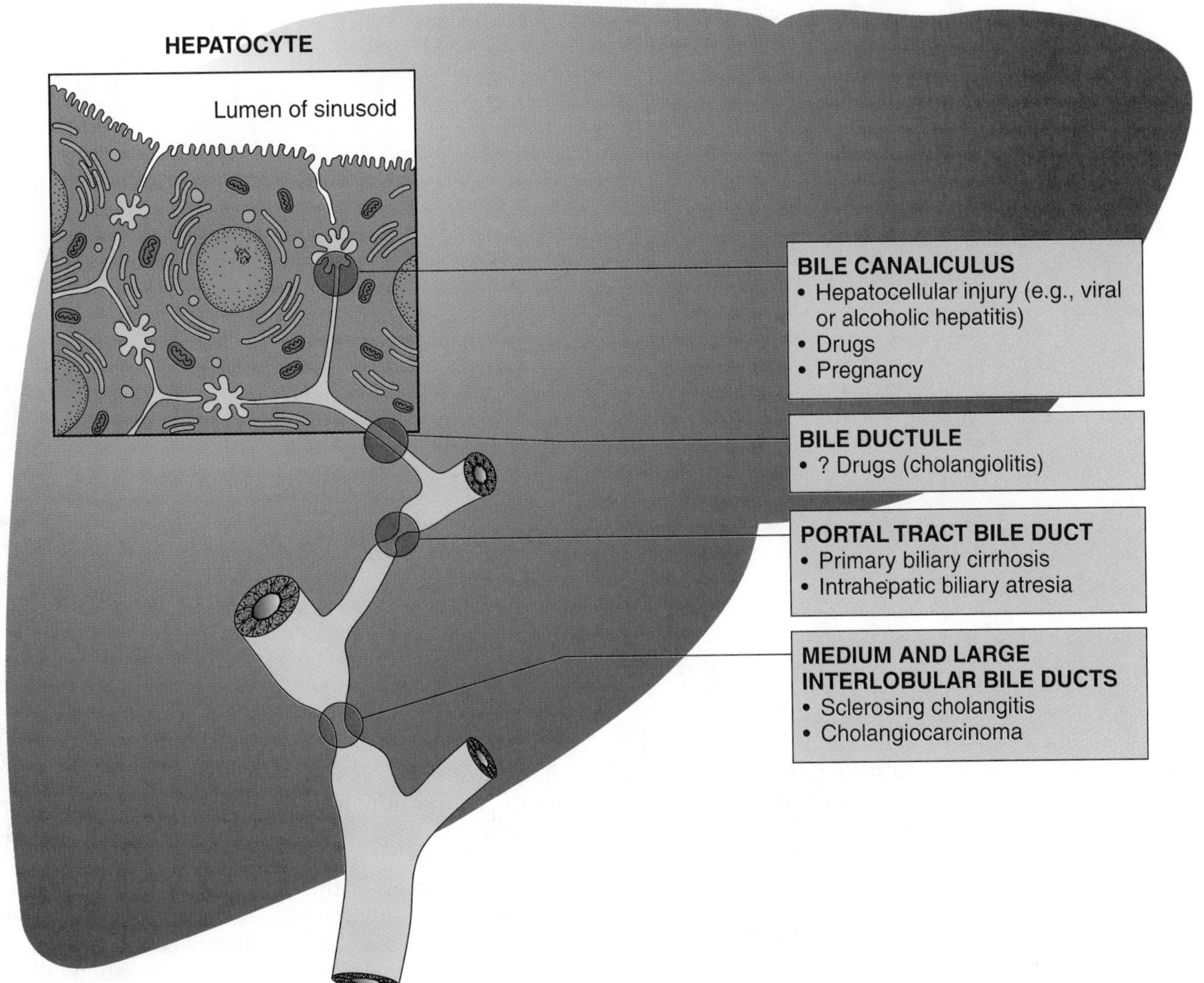

FIGURE *14-11*
Sites of intrahepatic cholestasis.

monly as a result of viral hepatitis or toxic liver injury. By contrast, chronic liver diseases, such as chronic viral hepatitis or cirrhosis, may lead to the insidious onset of hepatic failure. The consequences of acute and chronic failure are depicted in Figure 14-12, which deals with the complications of cirrhosis, the most common cause of hepatic failure. Although survival in acute hepatic failure has been improved by advances in supportive care, the mortality rate for this condition remains above 50%.

Jaundice

Hepatic failure is always associated with jaundice as a result of an inadequate clearance of bilirubin by the diseased liver. The hyperbilirubinemia is for the most part conjugated, but on occasion, increased erythrocyte turnover may lead to unconjugated hyperbilirubinemia, thereby aggravating the jaundice.

Hepatic Encephalopathy

Hepatic encephalopathy refers to a variety of neurological signs and symptoms in patients who suffer chronic liver failure or in whom the portal circulation is diverted. With unrelenting liver failure, hepatic encephalopathy may progress according to the following stages: stage I: sleep disturbance, irritability, and personality changes; stage II: lethargy and disorientation; stage III: deep somnolence; stage IV: coma. This sequence may occur over a period of many months or evolve rapidly in days or weeks in cases of fulminant hepatic failure. Associated neurological symptoms include (1) a flapping tremor of the hands, called asterixis, and hyperactive reflexes in the earlier stages, (2) extensor toe responses later, and (3) a decerebrate posture in the terminal stages. Whereas intensive supportive measures may be adequate therapy in the early stages of hepatic encephalopathy, patients with stages III and IV encephalopathy are usually salvaged only by liver transplantation.

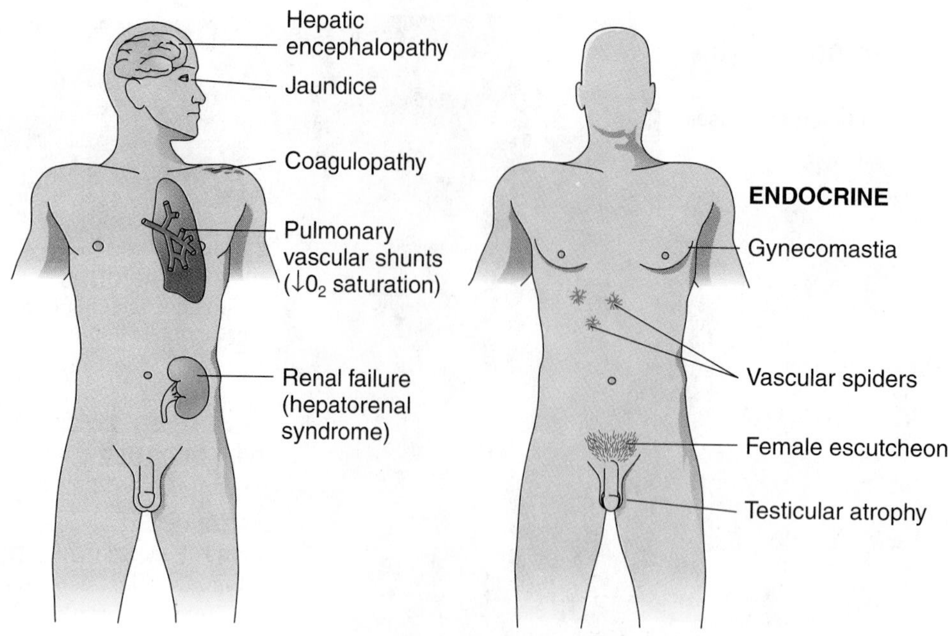

FIGURE *14-12*
Complications of hepatic failure.

☐ **Pathogenesis:** The pathogenesis of hepatic encephalopathy remains elusive, and no single factor has been proved to account for the clinical syndrome. It is probable that the encephalopathy is caused in part by toxic compounds absorbed from the intestine that have escaped hepatic detoxification because of hepatocyte dysfunction or the existence of structural or functional vascular shunts. The latter mechanism is particularly evident after the surgical construction of a portal-systemic anastomosis (portal vein to inferior vena cava or its equivalent) for the relief of portal hypertension, which accounts for the synonym *portasystemic encephalopathy*.

AMMONIA: Levels of ammonia are usually increased in the blood and brain of patients with hepatic encephalopathy. Most of the body's ammonia is of dietary origin, coming from ingestion of ammonia in foods, digestion of proteins in the small intestine, and bacterial catabolism of dietary protein and urea secreted into the intestine. The hypothesis that ammonia has an important role in the pathogenesis of hepatic encephalopathy is supported by the finding that patients with cirrhosis or a portacaval shunt display the symptoms and signs of hepatic encephalopathy after ingesting ammonium salts, urea, or protein. However, the correlation between the increased concentration of blood ammonia and the severity of hepatic encephalopathy is inexact.

In the brain, glutamine is formed by the reaction of ammonia with the excitatory neurotransmitter glutamate, thereby leading to a reduction in brain glutamate. Impaired glutamate-dependent neurotransmission in hepatic encephalopathy has been demonstrated. Interestingly, the glutamine concentration in cerebrospinal fluid correlates better with the degree of hepatic encephalopathy than does the blood level of ammonia.

GABA: There is now substantial evidence that increased neural inhibition, mediated by the γ-aminobutyric acid (GABA)–benzodiazepine receptor complex, plays an important role in hepatic encephalopathy. Neurons from animals with hepatic encephalopathy exhibit an increased sensitivity to benzodiazepine and GABA-receptor agonists. In addition, benzodiazepine-receptor antagonists excite these neurons at concentrations that do not affect control neurons, and the symptoms of hepatic encephalopathy are ameliorated by such antagonists. There is now substantial evidence that endogenous benzodiazepine-like substances contribute to the encephalopathy of liver failure by stimulating GABAergic neurotransmission.

OTHER SUBSTANCES: A number of other molecules have been suggested as contributing to the pathogenesis of hepatic encephalopathy. Among these are **mercaptans**, which result from the breakdown of sulfur-containing amino acids in the colon. The characteristic breath odor of patients with hepatic failure, termed *fetor hepaticus*, reflects the presence of mercaptans in saliva. Patients with cirrhosis who are fed methionine develop hepatic encephalopathy and the odor of mercaptans, both of which regress after methionine withdrawal. Another hypothesis for the pathogenesis of hepatic encephalopathy holds that increased blood levels of aromatic amino acids, typical of hepatic failure, lead to decreased synthesis of normal neurotransmitters, such as norepinephrine, and augmented production of **false neurotransmitters**, such as octopamine. A toxic effect of **phenols** and **short-chain fatty acids** on the brain has also been postulated. Finally, there is experimental evidence for a disturbance in the blood–brain barrier in hepatic failure.

☐ **Pathology:** Morphological changes in the brains of patients with acute or chronic hepatic encephalopathy are not large enough to account for the functional disturbances. **In patients who have died with chronic liver disease and hepatic coma, the most striking changes are found in the astrocytes.** These cells are increased in number and size and show the swelling, nuclear enlargement, and nuclear inclusions characteristic of *Alzheimer type II astrocytes*. Interestingly, such changes can be produced in animals by portacaval shunts and chronic administration of ammonia. The deep layers of the cerebral cortex and subcortical white matter, the basal ganglia, and the cerebellum exhibit laminar necrosis and a spongiform appearance.

In patients with acute hepatic failure, **cerebral edema** is the major cause of death, occurring in more than half the cases, often in conjunction with uncal and cerebellar herniation. This edema is not regarded as simply a terminal event but is rather considered a specific lesion associated with hepatic coma, although the precise mechanism is obscure.

Hepatorenal Syndrome

Hepatorenal syndrome refers to renal failure secondary to acute hepatic failure and is characterized by the features of renal hypoperfusion, namely oliguria, azotemia, and increased plasma creatinine levels. Although the severity of kidney dysfunction does not necessarily parallel the extent of hepatic failure, renal failure usually indicates a poor prognosis. Curiously, the kidneys clearly maintain the ability to function normally. Kidneys from patients who have died of the hepatorenal syndrome function well when transplanted into recipients with chronic renal failure. Conversely, in patients with the hepatorenal syndrome, liver transplantation can restore renal function.

☐ **Pathogenesis: The major determinant of the hepatorenal syndrome seems to be a decrease in renal blood flow and a consequent reduction in glomerular filtration rate.** It is thought that a reduction in the effective circulating blood volume leads to compensatory renal vasoconstriction. The resulting decrease in renal perfusion and the shunting of blood from the cortex to the medulla cause reduced glomerular filtration. It is also suspected that vasoactive substances produced by the failing liver, or inadequately cleared by it, contribute to the renal hemodynamic changes.

Elevated levels of renin, a potent vasoconstrictor, have been found in patients with acute hepatic failure and may contribute to the pathogenesis of hepatorenal syndrome. Whereas the urinary excretion of prostaglandins is considerably increased in patients with cirrhosis, it is markedly reduced in those with hepatorenal syndrome. Accordingly, it has been theorized that reduced renal production of vasodilating prostaglandins may contribute to the impaired hemodynamics in hepatorenal syndrome. Additional mediators that may be involved in hepatorenal syndrome include endotoxin, vasoactive intestinal peptide, and other poorly characterized vasoactive substances.

☐ **Pathology:** In hepatorenal syndrome, no intrinsic renal disease can be demonstrated morphologically. At autopsy, jaundiced patients with the hepatorenal syndrome show bile staining of renal tubular cells and bile casts in the lumina, so-called *biliary nephrosis*. However, these morphological alterations are not believed to contribute to the renal dysfunction.

Defects of Coagulation

Bleeding often accompanies hepatic failure, in part because of defects in hemostasis that parallel the severity of the liver disease. **Reduced hepatic synthesis of coagulation factors and thrombocytopenia** are the principal causes for the impairment of hemostasis. Decreased production of clotting factors (fibrinogen, prothrombin, and factors V, VII, IX, and X) reflects the generalized impairment of protein synthesis by the liver. The prolonged prothrombin time is most closely related to the decrease in the plasma concentration of factor VII.

Disseminated intravascular coagulation (DIC) may also occur in liver failure, and at least mild DIC may be universal in severe end-stage liver failure. Intravascular coagulation may reflect necrosis of liver cells, activation of factor XII (Hageman factor) by endotoxin, or inadequate hepatic clearance of activated clotting factors from the circulation.

A low platelet count ($<80{,}000/\mu L$) occurs commonly in hepatic failure and is accompanied by qualitative abnormalities in platelet function. The thrombocytopenia may result from (1) hypersplenism, (2) bone marrow depression, or (3) the consumption of circulating platelets by intravascular coagulation.

Hypoalbuminemia

Decreased levels of circulating albumin almost invariably complicate hepatic failure. Hypoalbuminemia, secondary to impaired synthesis of albumin, is an important factor in the pathogenesis of the edema often noted in chronic liver disease. Occasionally, albumin synthesis is normal, but in such cases, the rate of albumin production does not correlate well with the concentration of albumin in the blood. Alcohol appears to inhibit albumin synthesis directly.

Pulmonary Complications

Decreased arterial oxygen saturation occurs in about half of the patients with chronic liver disease. Occasionally, this is severe enough to result in cyanosis. Several explanations for the decrease in arterial oxygen saturation have been advanced: (1) microscopic arteriovenous fistulas with a right-to-left shunt; (2) a shift in the hemoglobin dissociation curve to the right (reduced affinity for oxygen); (3) alveolar hypoventilation; (4) a reduction in pulmonary diffusion capacity; and (5) alterations in ventilation–perfusion ratios. Of these proposed explanations, arteriovenous shunts and a shift in the hemoglobin dissociation curve have been shown to exist, although the reduction in oxygen affinity is not large enough to explain the arterial desaturation by itself. Arterial desaturation is responsible for the clubbing of the fingers occasionally encountered in chronic liver disease.

Endocrine Complications

Endocrine changes are associated with chronic hepatic failure rather than acute failure. In this context, it is important to distinguish between the direct effects of alcohol abuse, a common cause of liver disease, and changes that are better attributed to hepatic dysfunction. Chronic liver failure almost always leads to feminization, characterized by gynecomastia, a female body habitus, and a female distribution of pubic hair (female escutcheon). In addition, vascular manifestations of hyperestrogenism are common and include **spider angiomas** in the territory drained by the superior vena cava (upper trunk and face) and **palmar erythema. Feminization is attributed to a reduction in the hepatic catabolism of estrogens and weak androgens, such as androstenedione and dehydroepiandrosterone.** The weak androgens are converted to estrogenic compounds in peripheral tissues, thereby adding to the burden of circulating estrogens. Moreover, the extrahepatic portal–systemic shunts spontaneously develop as a result of portal hypertension in cirrhosis. These shunts permit the estrogens and weak androgens excreted in the bile to bypass the liver when they are reabsorbed from the intestine. It is also possible that an increase in the sensitivity of estrogen-responsive tissues may contribute to the feminization of men with chronic liver disease.

Men who suffer from alcoholic liver disease are more likely to be feminized than those with liver disease from other causes, and the severity of feminization is usually greater. The reason for this increased tendency to feminization in alcohol-induced liver disease is not clear. However, there is evidence to suggest that alcohol, either directly or as a consequence of alcohol-induced hypogonadism, reduces the hepatic content of an estrogen-binding protein that may protect the cell from excess estrogenic stimulation.

In addition to feminization, the large majority of men with chronic alcoholism also suffer hypogonadism, manifested by testicular atrophy, impotence, and loss of libido. Alcoholic women also exhibit gonadal failure, presenting as oligomenorrhea, amenorrhea, infertility, ovarian atrophy, and loss of secondary sex characteristics. These effects on gonadal function in both sexes reflect a direct toxic action of alcohol independent of chronic liver disease.

VIRAL HEPATITIS

Viral hepatitis is an infection of hepatocytes that produces necrosis and inflammation of the liver. The disease has been recognized as "epidemic jaundice" for millennia. Many viruses and other infectious agents are capable of producing hepatitis and jaundice (Table 14-1), but in the industrialized world, more than 95% of the cases of viral hepatitis involve a limited number of hepatotropic viruses, named from A to G. Hepatitis F virus seems to be a variant of hepatitis B. There remain patients who apparently suffer from viral hepatitis, both clinically and by liver biopsy, but who do not display any of the markers for the aforementioned viruses. Thus, it appears that there may be hepatotropic viruses that remain to be identified.

TABLE *14-1* **Infectious Agents that Cause Hepatitis**

Hepatitis A virus
Hepatitis B virus
Hepatitis C virus
Hepatitis E virus
Yellow fever virus
Epstein-Barr virus (infectious mononucleosis)
Lassa, Marburg, and Ebola viruses
Rubellavirus
Herpes simplex virus
Cytomegalovirus
Enteroviruses other than hepatitis A virus
Leptospires (leptospirosis)
Entamoeba histolytica (amebic hepatitis)

The following discussion will emphasize the illnesses commonly termed *viral hepatitis*, and the reader is referred to Chapter 9 for consideration of the other agents. The pathological changes encountered in all types of viral hepatitis are discussed together.

Historical Considerations

The outbreaks of jaundice that were recorded in association with military campaigns from ancient times to the modern era were almost certainly caused by hepatitis A virus. Historical evidence for transmission of hepatitis by inoculation with human serum dates to the mid 19th century. At that time, shipyard workers in Germany experienced jaundice after being vaccinated against smallpox with a vaccine that contained human lymph. During and after World War II, two distinct modes of transmission of human hepatitis were conclusively established. One type spread in epidemic form and the other was transmitted parenterally, especially by blood transfusion or inoculation by contaminated needles. In the 1960s, an antigen in an Australian aborigine (Australia antigen) was found and was later shown to be a component of the virus associated with parenteral inoculation of hepatitis. This discovery led directly to the identification of hepatitis B virus. Subsequently, hepatitis A virus was identified in human feces by immunological techniques combined with electron microscopy.

It soon became apparent that the elimination of blood containing hepatitis B virus from donor blood did not ensure against posttransfusion hepatitis. Subsequently, a virus was identified in the large majority of patients with transfusion-associated hepatitis and was named hepatitis C virus. Today, screening of blood for hepatitis B and hepatitis C eliminates most of the risk of transfusion-associated hepatitis. Another viral disease, hepatitis E, is transmitted enterically and is responsible for epidemics in underdeveloped countries. Hepatitis G virus is a relative of hepatitis C virus.

Hepatitis A

Hepatitis A virus (HAV) is a small **RNA-containing enterovirus** of the picornavirus group (which includes the polio virus). It can be demonstrated in the feces of patients with hepatitis A by its immune precipitation with convalescent serum or immune serum globulin (Fig. 14-13). The hepatocyte is the sole site of viral replication, and presumably shedding of progeny virus into the bile accounts for its appearance in the feces. On the basis of indirect evidence, it has been assumed that, like many other picornaviruses, HAV is directly cytopathic, although this remains to be established with certainty.

☐ **Epidemiology:** For hepatitis A, as for other viral diseases that do not lead to a chronic carrier state, the only reservoir for the disease seems to be the acutely infected person. **Transmission depends primarily on serial transmission from person to person by the fecal–oral route.** Epidemics of hepatitis A occur under crowded and unsanitary conditions, such as exist in warfare, or by fecal contamination of water and food. Edible shellfish concentrate the virus in contaminated waters and may also lead infection if eaten after being inadequately cooked. Although hepatitis A is not ordinarily a sexually transmitted disease, the infection rate is particularly high among male homosexuals, as a result of oral–anal contact.

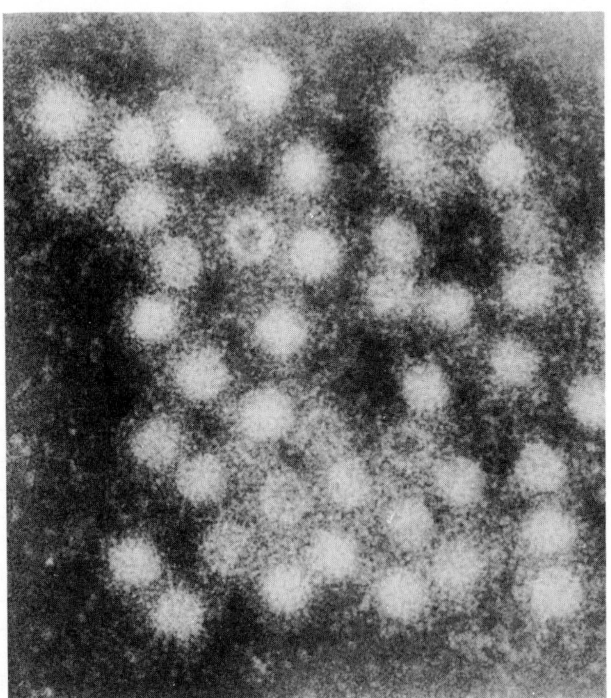

FIGURE *14-13*
Electron micrograph of hepatitis A virus (HAV). A fecal extract was treated with convalescent serum containing anti-HAV.

The patterns of HAV transmission are considerably different in various parts of the world. In the United States and other industrialized countries, which have relatively low rates of infection, most cases of hepatitis A are seen in older children and adults. By contrast, in less developed regions, where the disease is endemic, most of the population is infected before the age of 10 years.

In the United States, about 10% of the population younger than 20 years of age have serological evidence of previous HAV infection. **This circumstance indicates that the large majority of infections with HAV are anicteric.** Most symptomatic cases of HAV in Western countries are the consequence of community-wide epidemics, rather than secondary to point-source outbreaks. In the United States, such epidemics occur predominantly among persons of low socioeconomic status, the highest rates of infection being observed among American Indians and Alaskan natives. Childhood hepatitis A is also common in institutions for the mentally retarded and in day-care centers in the United States.

Every year, some 35 million persons from industrialized countries visit less developed regions where hepatitis A is endemic. These travelers make up a substantial proportion of symptomatic hepatitis A infections in the Western world; 60% of all hepatitis in travelers returning from endemic areas is caused by HAV. In fact, hepatitis A in travelers is 100 times more common than typhoid fever and 1000 times more frequent than cholera. The prevalence of hepatitis A is likely to be substantially reduced as the newly developed vaccines for this infection become more widely available.

☐ **Clinical Features:** Following an incubation period of 3 to 6 weeks, with a mean of about 4 weeks, patients infected with HAV develop nonspecific symptoms, including fever, malaise, and anorexia. Concomitantly, liver injury is evidenced by a rise in the serum aminotransferase activity (Fig. 14-14). As the activities of aminotransferases begin to decline, usually 5 to 10 days later, jaundice may appear. It remains evident for an average of 10 days but may persist for more than a month. In most cases, the elevated levels of aminotransferases return to normal by the time jaundice has disappeared. **Hepatitis A never pursues a chronic course. There is no carrier state, and infection provides lifelong immunity.** Moreover, virtually all patients recover without hepatic encephalopathy, and fatal fulminant hepatitis occurs only rarely.

Hepatitis A virus can be detected in the liver about 2 weeks after infection, it reaches a maximum in another 2 weeks, and it disappears shortly thereafter (see Fig. 14-14). Fecal shedding of HAV follows its appearance in the liver by about a week and lasts for only a brief time. The period of viremia is also short, occurring early in the course of the disease.

The first detectable antibody response to HAV infection is the appearance of IgM anti-HAV in the blood during the acute illness (see Fig. 14-14). The antibody titer begins to fall within a few weeks and generally disappears by 3 to 5 months. IgG anti-HAV is detected as the patient recovers and the IgM anti-HAV titer has begun to fall; it maintains peak levels after the IgM antibody has disappeared and persists for life. The finding of IgM anti-HAV

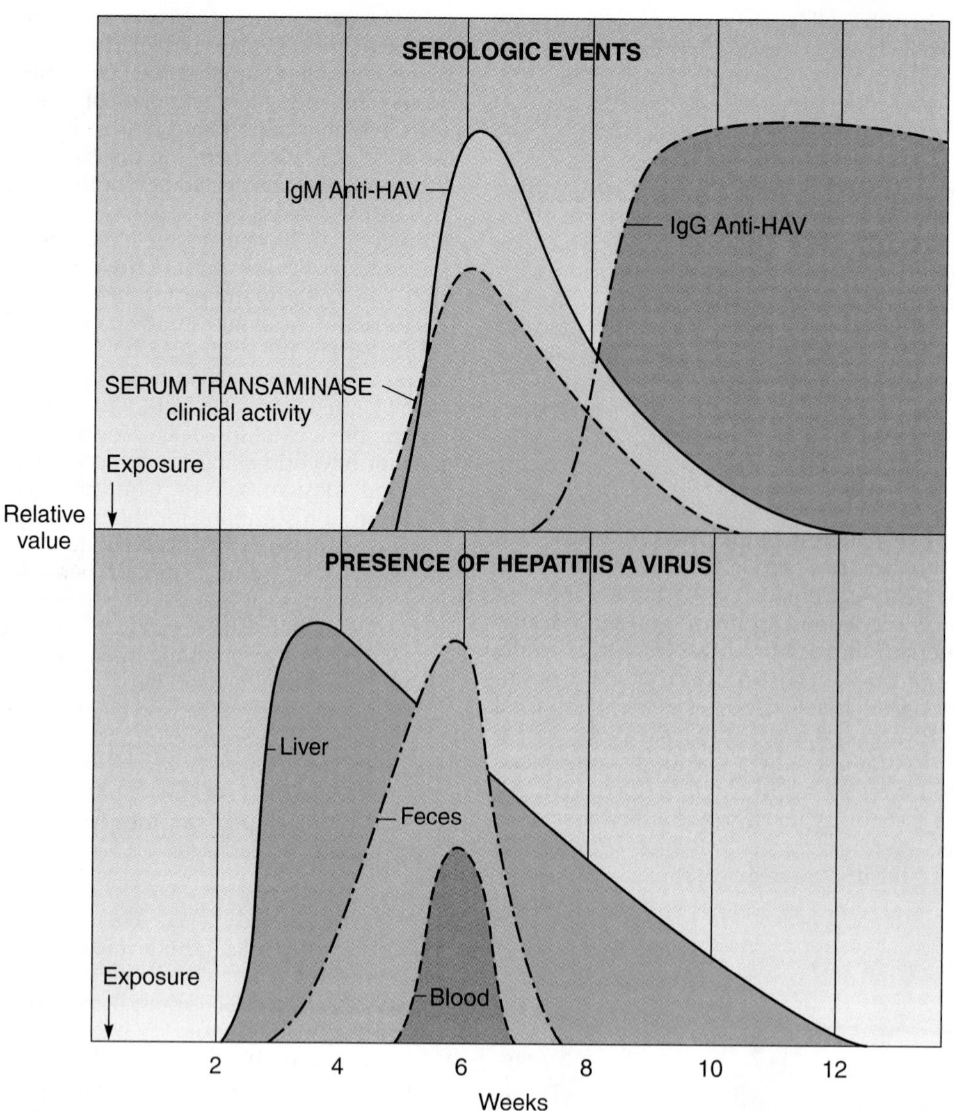

FIGURE *14-14*
Typical serological events associated with hepatitis A.

in the serum of a patient with acute hepatitis confirms HAV as the cause.

Hepatitis B

Hepatitis B virus (HBV) is a hepatotropic DNA virus that was the first of the so-called *hepadnaviruses*. Other members of this family include hepatotropic viruses that affect woodchucks, ground squirrels, and Pekin ducks. The genomes of the hepadnaviruses are among the smallest of all known viruses. The DNA of HBV consists of one long circular strand of about 3200 nucleotides, containing the entire genome, and a shorter complementary strand, which varies from 50% to 85% of the length of the longer strand. Thus, the DNA is predominantly double-stranded, with a variable single-stranded segment (Fig. 14-15). The HBV genome contains four open reading frames (genes):

- **Core (C) gene:** The core of the virus contains the **core antigen (HBcAg)** and the **e antigen (HBeAg)**. Both HBcAg and HBeAg are products of the C gene. The C gene includes two consecutive open reading frames, the pre-core and core regions, with separate start codons. Transcription of the core frame yields HBcAg, whereas HBeAg is derived from the proteolysis of the translation product of the entire C gene open reading frame, including the pre-core region.
- **Surface gene:** The core of HBV is enclosed in a coat that contains lipid, protein, and carbohydrate and expresses an antigen termed **hepatitis B surface antigen (HBsAg)**. The surface coat is synthesized by the infected hepatocyte independently from the viral core and is secreted into the blood in vast amounts. This material is visualized by electron microscopy in centrifuged serum as two distinct particles (see Fig. 14-15), one a 22-nm sphere and the other a tubular structure 22 nm in diameter and 40 to 400 nm in

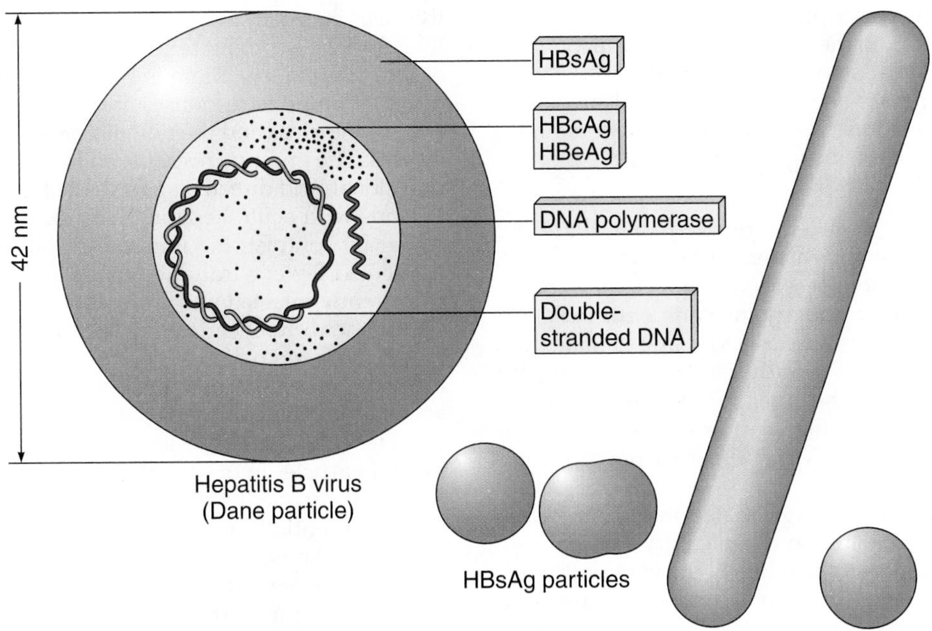

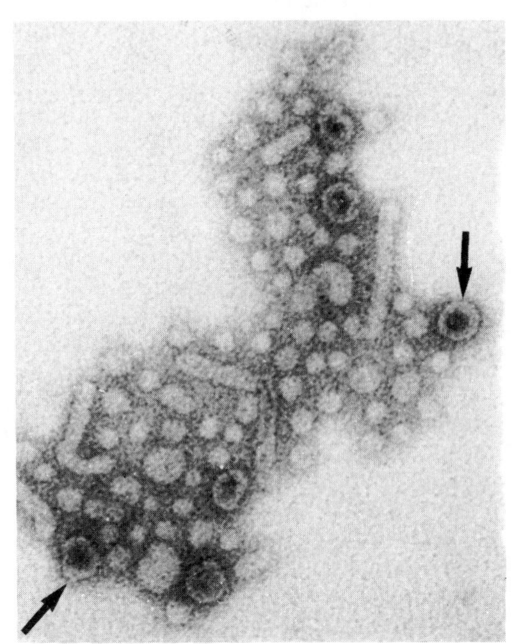

FIGURE 14-15
(*A*) Schematic representation of the hepatitis B virus (HBV) and serum particles associated with HBV infection. (*B*) Electron micrograph of particles from centrifuged serum in a case of hepatitis B. Rodlike and spherical particles containing HBsAg are evident. The complete virion, composed of the viral core and its surrounding envelope, is represented by Dane particles (*arrows*).

length. **HBsAg particles are immunogenic but not infectious. The intact and infectious virus** is also found in the same preparations as a 42-nm sphere (*Dane particle*), consisting of a 27-nm inner core and an outer shell 7 nm in thickness.

- **Polymerase gene:** The P gene encodes the virion-associated DNA polymerase.
- **X gene:** The small X protein is thought to activate viral transcription and possibly to play a role in the pathogenesis of hepatocellular carcinoma associated with chronic HBV infection. Interestingly, infection with rare strains of HBV containing mutations in the X gene have been reported to result in hepatitis that is serologically negative for HBV antigens ("silent hepatitis").

The life cycle of HBV is unique among known animal DNA viruses in its utilization of a reverse transcriptase mechanism. After infection of the hepatocyte, the viral genome enters the nucleus, where it serves as an episomal (not integrated into host DNA) template for the formation of viral mRNA. This RNA encodes a unique viral polymerase, which serves three different functions in the cytosol, namely reverse transcriptase, DNA polymerase, and RNase activities. Upon translocation to the cytoplasm, the RNA transcript is used to generate a DNA strand by reverse transcription. The mRNA is degraded by the RNase activity of the same enzyme. The incomplete complementary DNA strand is then synthesized by the viral DNA polymerase activity. This unusual process of replication shares many features with the reverse transcriptase mechanism of oncogenic retroviruses.

☐ **Epidemiology:** It is estimated that there are about 200 million chronic carriers of HBV in the world, constituting an enormous reservoir of infection. Depending on the incidence of primary infection with HBV, the carrier rates vary from as little as 0.3% (United States and western Europe) to 20% (Southeast Asia, sub-Saharan Africa, and Oceania). In the latter populations, an important avenue by which the high carrier rate is sustained is vertical transmission of the virus from a carrier mother to her newborn.

In the United States, it is estimated that there are between 500,000 and 1.5 million chronic HBV carriers, and 200,000 to 300,000 persons are newly infected with HBV annually. Of these new cases, only one fourth are clinically recognized because of jaundice. Fulminant hepatitis B results in 250 to 300 deaths a year.

Before the advent of routine screening of blood for HBsAg, chronic HBV carriers posed a public health hazard as a source of post-transfusion hepatitis. The threat of HBV-positive post-transfusion hepatitis has been largely eliminated by routine screening for HBsAg.

Whereas no more than 10% of adults infected with HBV become carriers, neonatal hepatitis B is, as a rule, followed by persistent infection. Males exhibit an increased tendency to become carriers. It has been suggested that immunosuppressed persons are more susceptible to persistent HBV infection, and the carrier state is more common in renal dialysis patients and in persons afflicted with Down syndrome, leprosy, and chronic lymphocytic leukemia. In the United States, chronic HBV carriers are particularly common among male homosexuals, drug addicts, certain health care workers, and institutionalized mentally retarded children. Of particular public health concern is the fact that paid blood donors are far more likely to harbor HBV than is the general population.

Humans are the only significant reservoir of HBV. Unlike hepatitis A, hepatitis B is not transmitted by the fecal–oral route, nor does it contaminate food and water supplies. **Although HBsAg is found in most secretions, infectious virus has been demonstrated only in blood, saliva, and semen.** Historically, transmission of hepatitis B was believed to be limited to direct transfer of blood products, either by transfusion or by the use of contaminated needles. However, it is now clear that the large majority of cases of hepatitis B result from transmission associated with intimate contact. The routes by which contact-transmission occurs are not entirely defined, but it seems probable that a direct transfer of the virus through breaks in the skin or mucous membranes is most common. In this respect, sexual contact—occasionally heterosexual but particularly homosexual—is an important mode of transmission.

☐ **Pathogenesis:** HBV is not directly cytopathic, as reflected in the fact that asymptomatic chronic carriers of the virus maintain a large burden of infectious virus in the liver for years without functional or biochemical evidence of liver cell injury. There is substantial evidence to indicate that immune responses are responsible for the clearance of the virus and the destruction of the infected hepatocytes. The immune response to HBV infection is potent, polyclonal, and directed against all of the viral proteins in persons with acute hepatitis who clear the virus and recover. By contrast, the immune response is weaker and limited to fewer viral antigens in persons who remain persistently infected and suffer chronic hepatitis. The basis for the difference in the strength of the immune response between patients who clear the virus and recover from the infection and those who fail to eradicate the agent and suffer chronic hepatitis is not well understood.

The antibody to the surface antigen (anti-HBs) binds to viral particles in the circulation, thereby preventing the infection of susceptible hepatocytes. This antibody is present in essentially all patients who recover from acute hepatitis, whereas it generally cannot be found in patients with chronic hepatitis B. Antibodies directed against the core proteins (anti-HBc and anti-HBe) are not thought to be important in viral clearance or the destruction of infected liver cells.

Cytotoxic (CD8+) lymphocytes directed against multiple HBV epitopes are generally regarded as the major mediators of the destruction of hepatocytes and consequent clinical liver disease. In conjunction with HLA class I molecules, the target viral antigens are expressed on the surface of infected hepatoyctes. In that location, they are recognized by CD8+ cytotoxic T lymphocytes (CTL), which in turn kill the infected hepatocytes. Patients who successfully clear HBV demonstrate a vigorous CTL response to all of the viral antigens in the circulation. By contrast, chronic persistence of HBV is associated with a feeble or undetectable CTL response. The weakness of the cellular immune response to HBV antigens in patients with chronic hepatitis is held to be the cause of the indolent necrosis and inflammation characteristic of this disorder.

In acute viral hepatitis, the immune response is directed against viral antigens that are synthesized in the course of episomal viral replication. The situation is more complicated in the case of chronic hepatitis B. In the early stages of chronic disease, the CTL response remains primarily directed against antigens synthesized during viral replication. However, as the disease continues, in most cases there is a progressive decline in viral replication as a result of the immune-mediated destruction of infected hepatocytes. During this time, fragments of the viral genome may be randomly integrated into host DNA, where they can serve as a template for the production of viral antigens. Importantly, the entire viral genome is never integrated into host DNA. Thus, patients who have lost episomal replicating DNA no longer produce infectious viral particles, despite the fact that they may synthesize prodigious amounts of HBsAg. With increasing duration of chronic hepatitis B, the extent of liver injury and thus the severity of the disease is probably determined by the expression pattern of integrated fragments of the viral genome. The precise viral targets of the variable immunological response during long-standing chronic hepatitis remain obscure.

☐ **Clinical Features:** There are three well-recognized clinical courses associated with HBV infection (Fig. 14-16):

- Acute hepatitis
- Fulminant hepatitis
- Chronic hepatitis

ACUTE HEPATITIS B: The large majority of patients have acute, self-limited hepatitis similar to that produced by HAV, in which complete recovery and lifelong immunity are the rule. The acute onset and symptoms of hepatitis B are for the most part similar to those of hepatitis A, although acute hepatitis B tends to be somewhat more severe. In addition, the incubation period is considerably longer. Typically, symptoms do not appear until 2 to 3 months after exposure, but incubation periods of less than 6 weeks and as long as 6 months are occasionally encountered. As in hepatitis A, serological studies have shown that many cases, including virtually all infections in infants and children, are anicteric and therefore not clinically apparent.

HBsAg is the first marker to appear in the serum of patients with acute hepatitis B, being detected 1 week to 2 months after exposure and 2 weeks to 2 months before the onset of symptoms (see Fig. 14-16). HBsAg disappears from the blood during the convalescent phase in patients who recover rapidly from the acute hepatitis. It should be noted that an occasional patient with unquestionable hepa-titis B is consistently negative for HBsAg in the blood. Nevertheless, such patients display considerable HBsAg in the liver. In this situation, the clinical course tends to be mild and brief.

Simultaneously with or shortly after the disappearance of HBsAg, antibody to HBsAg (anti-HBs) is found in the blood. Its appearance heralds complete recovery, and its presence provides lifelong immunity. Antibody to HBcAg (anti-HBc) appears shortly after HBsAg, roughly at the time that serum aminotransferase activities begin to rise. HBcAg itself does not circulate freely in the serum of such infected persons. Anti-HBc also remains elevated for life and is a useful marker of previous HBV infection. Unlike anti-HBs, anti-HBc does not seem to play a role either in clearing the virus or in protecting against reinfection.

HBeAg, the second circulating antigen to appear in hepatitis B, is seen before the onset of clinical disease and after the appearance of HBsAg. HBeAg generally disappears within about 2 weeks, while HBsAg is still present. Anti-HBe appears shortly after the disappearance of the antigen and is detectable for up to 2 years or more after resolution of the hepatitis. **The presence of HBeAg in the serum correlates with a period of intense viral replication and, hence, maximal infectivity of the patient.**

Circulating HBsAg–anti-HBs immune complexes cause a variety of extrahepatic ailments, including a serum sickness–like syndrome (fever, rash, urticaria, acute arthritis), polyarteritis, glomerulonephritis, and cryoglobulinemia. In fact, one third to one half of patients with biopsy-proven polyarteritis nodosa are carriers of HBV. On rare occasions, hepatitis B and hepatitis C have been followed by aplastic anemia.

FULMINANT HEPATITIS B: More often than hepatitis A, but still only rarely, acute hepatitis B pursues a fulminant course, characterized by massive liver cell necrosis, hepatic failure, and a high mortality. It was reported that strains bearing mutations in the pre-core region of the HBV genome may be associated with fulminant hepatitis B. However, pre-core mutants have not been found in other series, and the subject remains controversial.

CHRONIC HEPATITIS B: *Chronic hepatitis refers to the presence of necrosis and inflammation in the liver for more than 6 months.* In 5% to 10% of patients with hepatitis B, HBs antigenemia does not resolve. Accordingly, the infection persists, the patients do not recover, and the disease progresses to chronic hepatitis B. If high-risk groups (e.g., male homosexuals, intravenous drug addicts) are excluded from consideration, the risk of chronic hepatitis is closer to 5%. For reasons unknown, 90% of patients with chronic hepatitis B are male.

Most patients with chronic hepatitis B do not have detectable anti-HBs in the blood. Some chronic HBV carriers manifest HBsAg-anti-HBs complexes in their serum, indicating that although they produce antibody, the level is inadequate to clear the virus from the circulation. A few chronic carriers, who were initially negative for anti-HBs, eventually develop measurable antibody (often after many years), clear the virus, and are restored to full health. Others (no more than 3% of patients with hepatitis B) never develop anti-HBs and suffer from a relentless and progressive chronic hepatitis that leads to cirrhosis. **All patients with persistent HBV infection develop anti-HBc, and chronic hepatitis B is characterized by the presence of anti-HBc and HBsAg.** Hepatitis associated with persistent HBsAg antigenemia is often accompanied by the continued presence of HBeAg.

Some of the patients who do not produce anti-HBs have at first only an inapparent or mild, transient episode of acute hepatitis, after which they remain asymptomatic despite the presence of high levels of HBsAg in the blood. The hepatocytes of these chronic asymptomatic carriers remain infected with HBV, and both the liver and blood contain infective virus. Such persons seem to be immunologically tolerant to HBV antigens. As will be discussed in detail under the heading of hepatocellular carcinoma, chronic hepatitis B is associated with a significant risk of liver cancer.

The possible outcomes of infection with hepatitis B virus are summarized in Figure 14-17.

Hepatitis B Vaccine

The immunogenicity of HBsAg and the fact that anti-HBs protects against HBV infection have allowed the development of effective vaccines against hepatitis B. The original vaccine was prepared by purifying HBsAg particles from the blood of HBV carriers. Synthetic vaccines, composed of HBsAg or its immunogenic epitopes, have been produced using recombinant DNA. It is likely that worldwide use of these vaccines will eventually reduce the prevalence of HBV infection and relegate hepatitis B to the status of a minor disease. It will also serve to prevent the major cause of hepatocellular carcinoma in the world.

Hepatitis D

A distinct hepatotropic virus, hepatitis D virus (HDV, delta agent) is associated exclusively with HBV infection. It was first described in 1977, but studies of immune

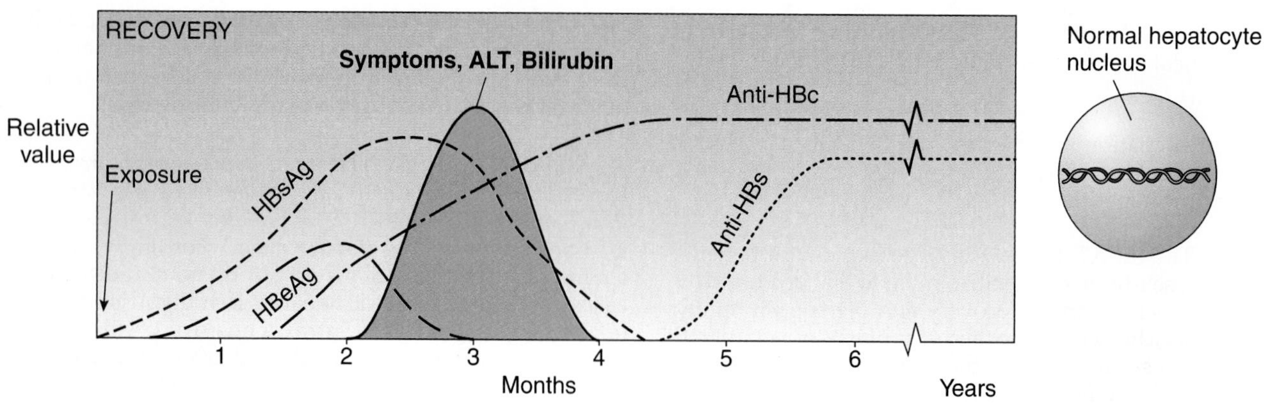

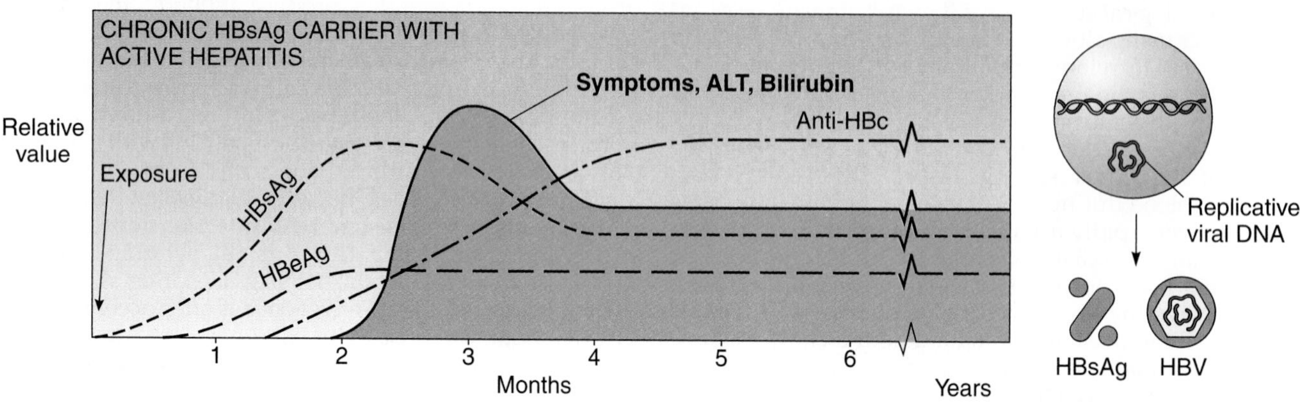

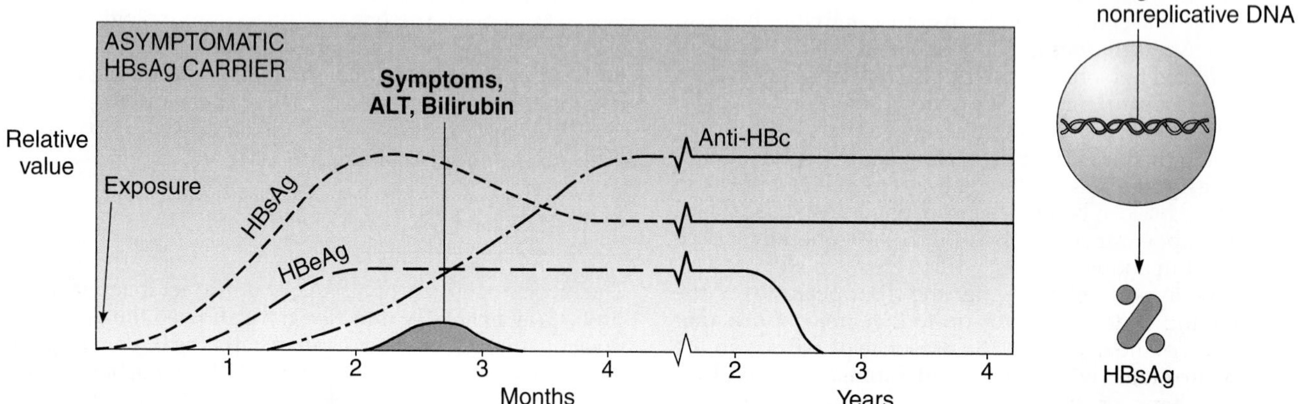

FIGURE *14-16*
Typical serological events in three distinct outcomes of hepatitis B.
(*Top panel*) In most cases, the appearance of anti-HBs ensures complete recovery. Viral DNA disappears from the nucleus of the hepatocyte.
(*Middle panel*) In about 10% of cases of hepatitis B, HBs antigenemia is sustained for longer than 6 months, owing to the absence of anti-HBs. Patients in whom viral replication remains active, as evidenced by sustained high levels of HBeAg in the blood, develop active hepatitis. In such cases, the viral genome persists in the nucleus but is not integrated into host DNA.
(*Lower panel*) Patients in whom active viral replication ceases or is attenuated, as reflected in the disappearance of HBeAg from the blood, become asymptomatic carriers. In these individuals, fragments of the HBV genome are integrated into the host DNA, but episomal DNA is absent.

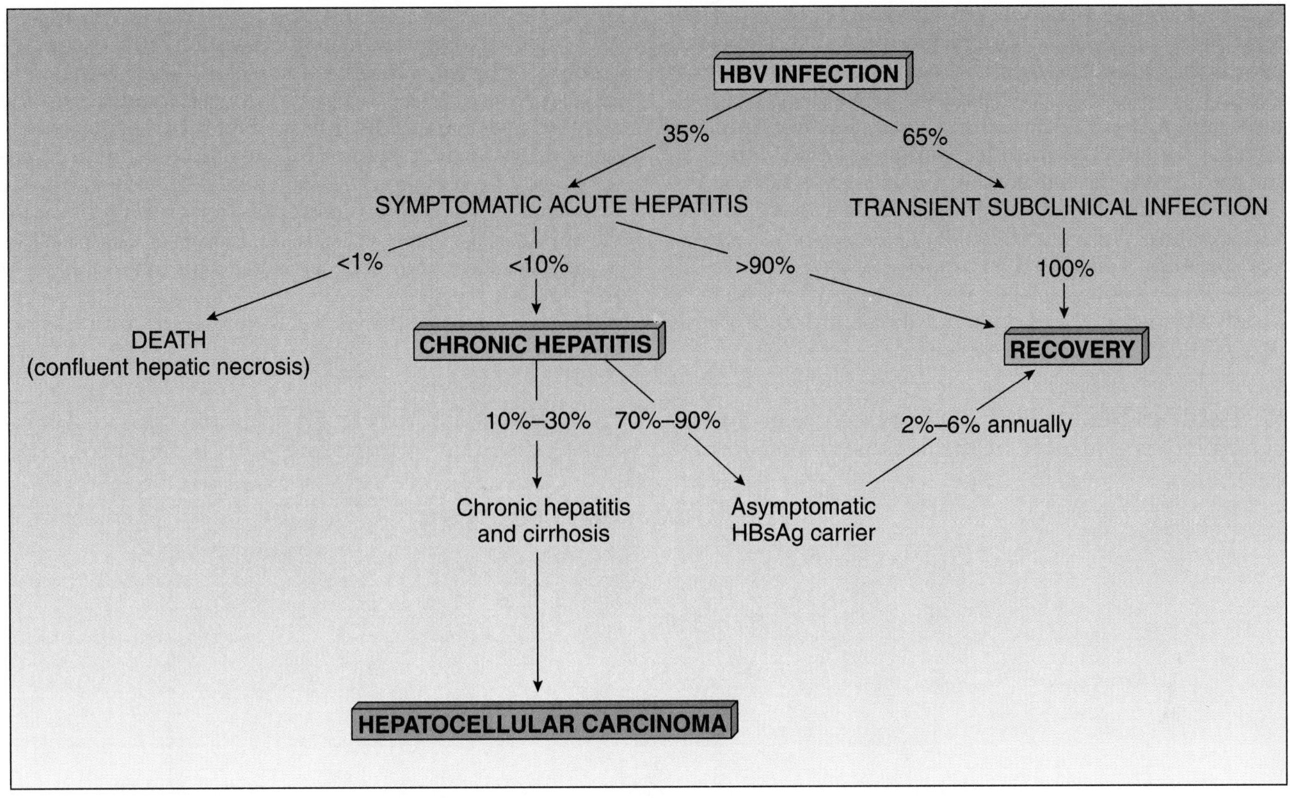

FIGURE *14-17*
Possible outcomes of infection with the hepatitis B virus.

globulin obtained in the United States in 1944 have shown that the virus has been present at least since that date and presumably earlier. HDV is a single-stranded RNA virus, visualized in hepatocytes as a 0.25-nm particle that is present predominantly in the nucleus. In the blood, HDV is coated with HBsAg and appears as a 37-nm particle.

Hepatitis D virus is a defective virus for which HBV is the helper. Assembly of HDV in the liver requires the synthesis of HBsAg, and, therefore, infection with this agent is limited to persons (and subhuman primates) infected with HBV.

Infection with HDV may occur either simultaneously with HBV infection (co-infection) or following HBV infection (superinfection). In cases of co-infection, the replication of HDV is limited to the period of HBsAg synthesis. HDV and HBsAg are cleared together, and the clinical course is generally no different from that of the usual acute hepatitis B. However, it has been reported that in some cases of co-infection with HBV, the presence of HDV leads to severe, fulminant, and often fatal hepatitis, particularly in intravenous drug abusers. **Superinfection of an HBV carrier with HDV typically increases the severity of an existing chronic hepatitis.** In fact, 70% to 80% of cases of HDV superinfection of HBsAg carriers develop chronic hepatitis.

Hepatitis C

Hepatitis C is today the most common cause of chronic hepatitis, cirrhosis, and hepatocellular carcinoma in the world. The advent of routine screening of blood for HBsAg led to an expectation that post-transfusion hepatitis would virtually disappear. This prediction proved inaccurate, since the incidence of post-transfusion hepatitis was only modestly reduced. It was discovered that there is a form of hepatitis that is not associated with HAV or HBV or any of the serological markers for these viruses. This form of the disease was termed *non-A, non-B hepatitis*.

Recombinant DNA technology led to the cloning and sequencing of hepatitis C virus (HCV), the agent responsible for most cases of non-A, non-B hepatitis. The virus is classified as a new genus of the flavivirus family and contains a single strand of RNA, 9.4 kB in length, which codes for about 3000 amino acids. There are only three structural genes (one core and two envelope genes) and four nonstructural genes. At least six different HCV genotypes are recognized, type 1 being the most common (72%). There is no relationship between the HCV genotype and the course or severity of hepatitis C.

☐ **Epidemiology:** HCV is present worldwide, and the prevalence of infection with this agent is remarkably similar in different geographic areas. The prevalence of anti-HCV antibodies ranges from a low of 0.3% in Canada, to 1.5% in Japan and European countries bordering on the Mediterranean, to as high as 6% in selected populations of Africa and the Middle East. In the United States, the incidence of hepatitis C has declined by 80% since 1989, but there remain about 3.5 million persons chronically infected with HCV. Furthermore, HCV still accounts for more than 90% of non-A, non-B hepatitis secondary to blood transfusions, although only 5% of patients with hepatitis C give a history of exposure to blood products. Other important risk factors include intravenous drug abuse, hemodialysis, and sexual (particularly homosexual) or household contact with persons infected with HCV. Vertical transmission of HCV from an infected mother to her newborn baby seems to be infrequent, although it is more common in the case of HIV-infected women. Importantly, half of all cases of hepatitis C are community acquired, sporadic, and occur in the absence of any known risk factors. These patients tend to be of low socioeconomic status, but the significance of this observation remains to be explained.

☐ **Pathogenesis:** HCV does not seem to be directly cytopathic, as evidenced by the fact that chronic carriers of the virus often have no evidence of liver cell injury. Moreover, cytopathic effects are absent in HCV tissue culture. By contrast, HCV-specific CD4+ T-cell clones and HLA-restricted CD8+ T cells have been identified in the peripheral blood and liver tissue of patients with chronic hepatitis C. Further support for the role of immune mechanisms in the pathogenesis of hepatitis C comes from the observation that immunosuppression in patients with chronic disease is often beneficial. However, understanding the viral and immunological basis for liver injury and the persistence of HCV infection, despite a number of polyclonal humoral- and cell-mediated immune responses, remains a challenge.

☐ **Clinical Features:** The incubation period of hepatitis C is similar to that of hepatitis B. Elevated serum

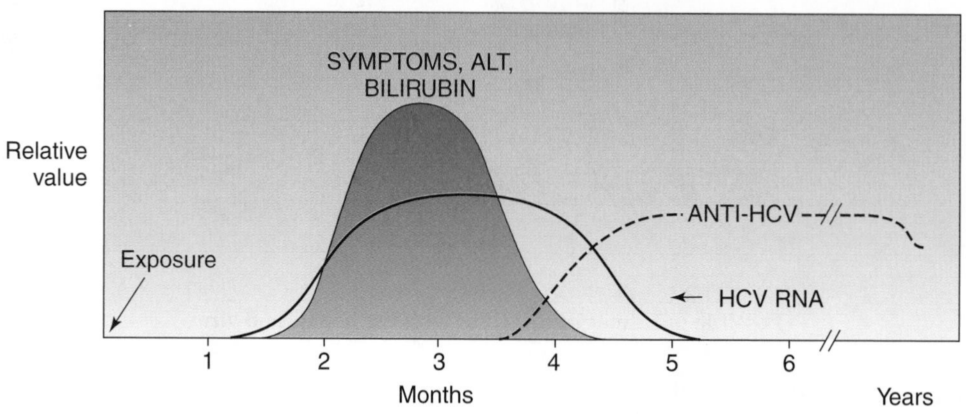

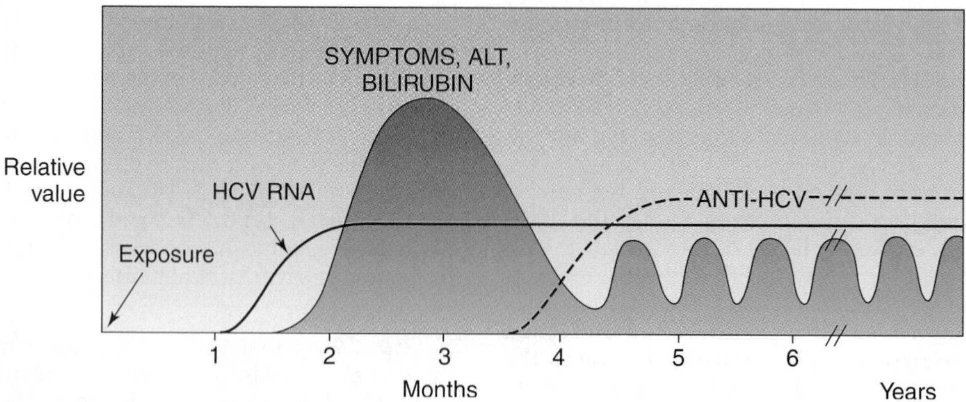

FIGURE *14-18*
Clinical course of hepatitis C. Typical serological events in two distinct outcomes.
(*Top panel*) About half of the patients with acute hepatitis C have a self-limited infection, which resolves in a few months. Anti-HCV appears at the end of the clinical course and persists.
(*Bottom panel*) The other half of the patients with hepatitis C develop chronic illness, with exacerbations and remissions of clinical symptoms. The development of anti-HCV does not affect the clinical outcome. Chronic active hepatitis often eventuates in cirrhosis.

aminotransferase activities (Fig. 14-18) are usually detected within 1 to 3 months of exposure to the virus (range, 2 to 26 weeks), and in most patients, anti-HCV becomes measurable a few weeks later. The clinical course of acute hepatitis C is surprisingly mild and is only very rarely complicated by fulminant hepatitis. In fact, only 10% of patients become jaundiced.

The major consequences of infection with HCV relate to chronic disease (Fig. 14-19). Despite complete recovery from clinical and biochemical acute liver disease, the probability of persistent HCV infection is at least 80% and may be higher. Moreover, chronic hepatitis ensues in 50% to 70% of infected persons. In such patients, histological evidence of hepatic inflammation and necrosis are unlikely to abate. Nevertheless, clinical morbidity in many patients remains mild for at least 10 years, and in many cases for 20 or more years. In fact, only about one third of chronically infected persons have clinically overt liver disease, and after 20 years only 20% to 35% manifest cirrhosis.

Liver disease in patients with chronic HCV infection tends to be more severe in the face of concurrent hepatitis B, alcoholic liver disease, hemochromatosis, and α_1-antitrypsin deficiency. Interestingly, up to 70% of patients with advanced alcoholic liver disease have antibodies to HCV. Although the relationship is unexplained, the possibility that HCV actually accounts for a proportion of cases otherwise classified as alcoholic cirrhosis is intriguing. In any event, alcohol consumption has been shown to worsen the course of chronic hepatitis C. Chronic HCV infection is also an important risk factor for the development of hepatocellular carcinoma, a topic discussed below.

Extrahepatic manifestations of hepatitis C are well recognized. Chronic HCV infection has been associated with essential mixed cryoglobulinemia, membranoproliferative glomerulonephritis, porphyria cutanea tarda, and possibly autoimmune thyroiditis.

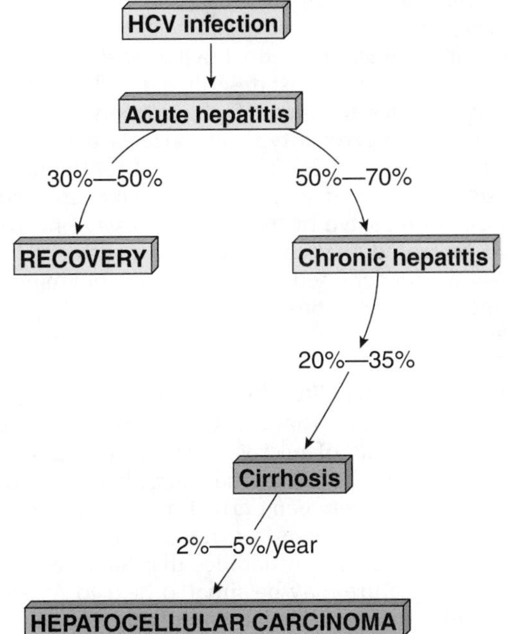

FIGURE *14-19*
Possible outcomes of infection with the hepatitis C virus.

Treatment with α-interferon has been beneficial in many cases of chronic hepatitis C, although relapses are common upon discontinuation of this therapy.

Hepatitis E

Major epidemics of hepatitis in underdeveloped countries are caused by infection with hepatitis E virus (HEV), which is an enteric virus transmitted by the fecal–oral route. HEV is now recognized to account for more than half of the cases of acute viral hepatitis in young to middle-aged persons in poor regions of the world. Large outbreaks have been reported in India, Nepal, Burma, Pakistan, the former Soviet Union, Africa, and Mexico. Most of these epidemics have followed heavy rains in areas with inadequate sewage disposal. Similar to hepatitis A, clinical illness from hepatitis E is far more common in adults than in children, suggesting that infection in the latter is often subclinical. The disease is especially dangerous in pregnant women, with mortality rates as high as 20% to 40% reported. No chronic disease or carrier state has been identified.

Hepatitis E virus is a 32-nm-diameter, nonenveloped, single-stranded RNA virus, which is similar to but not identical with caliciviruses. Hepatitis E is a self-limited acute, icteric disease similar to hepatitis A. The average incubation period is 35 to 40 days. Jaundice, hepatomegaly, fever and arthralgias are common. The symptoms and biochemical evidence of abnormal liver function usually resolve within 6 weeks. Although the mortality rate was as high as 12% in one study, it is reported to be less than 1% in others.

Hepatitis G

The persistence of transfusion-associated and community-acquired hepatitis that was negative for all antigens of hepatitides A through E suggested the existence of other hepatropic viruses. Recently, an agent was cloned from patients with hepatitis whose blood transmitted a disease similar to one in primates. Hepatitis G virus (HGV) has been placed in the Flaviviridae family and has some sequence homology (<25%) with HCV.

Hepatitis G virus is parenterally transmitted and has a high prevalence in intravenous drug users, hemophiliacs, and patients on dialysis. The agent has been detected in 1% to 2% of voluntary blood donors in the United States, a value higher than that for HCV. Although the use of the term hepatitis G implies an inflammatory condition, the large majority of patients with prospectively observed HGV infections have no evidence of liver disease. At this time, it is unclear whether HGV is, in fact, a cause of acute or chronic human hepatitis.

PATHOLOGY OF VIRAL HEPATITIS

Acute Viral Hepatitis

The morphological appearance of the liver in acute infection is similar in all forms of viral hepatitis (A–E). The hallmark of viral hepatitis is liver cell injury and necrosis (Fig. 14-20). Within the hepatic lobule, scattered necrosis of single cells or of small clusters of hepatocytes is seen. A few necrotic liver cells appear as small, deeply eosinophilic bodies (*Councilman or acidophilic bodies*), sometimes containing pyknotic nuclear material, that have been extruded from the liver cell plate into the sinusoid. They are now recognized to be apoptotic bodies. Although acidophilic bodies are characteristic of viral hepatitis, they are also occasionally encountered in other diseases associated with liver cell necrosis. In acute viral hepatitis, many liver cells appear normal, but others show varying degrees of hydropic swelling (balloon cells) and differences in size, shape, and staining qualities. Concomitantly, regenerative liver cells, which display a larger nucleus and an expanded basophilic cytoplasm, are also seen. The resulting irregularity of the liver cell plates is termed **lobular disarray**.

Chronic inflammatory cells, principally lymphoid, infiltrate the lobule diffusely, surround individual necrotic liver cells, and accumulate in areas of focal necrosis. In addition to the lymphoid cells, macrophages may be prominent, and eosinophils and polymorphonuclear leukocytes are not uncommon. These changes tend to be somewhat more pronounced in the centrilobular zones, although they are present throughout the lobule. Characteristically, lymphoid cells infiltrate between the wall of the central vein and the liver cell plates, an appearance termed *central phlebitis*. Swelling and proliferation of the endothelial cells of the central vein (*endophlebitis*) often develop. The Kupffer cells are enlarged, project into the lumen of the sinusoid, and contain lipofuscin pigment and phagocytosed debris (seen particularly well with the periodic acid–Schiff [PAS] reaction), including fragments of acidophilic bodies. Cholestasis is sometimes seen, in which case the term *cholestatic hepatitis* is applied. In this variant of acute viral hepatitis, and occasionally in the more classic case, many liver cells are arranged around a lumen, thereby presenting an acinar or glandular appearance. The lumen of such an "acinus" may contain a large bile plug.

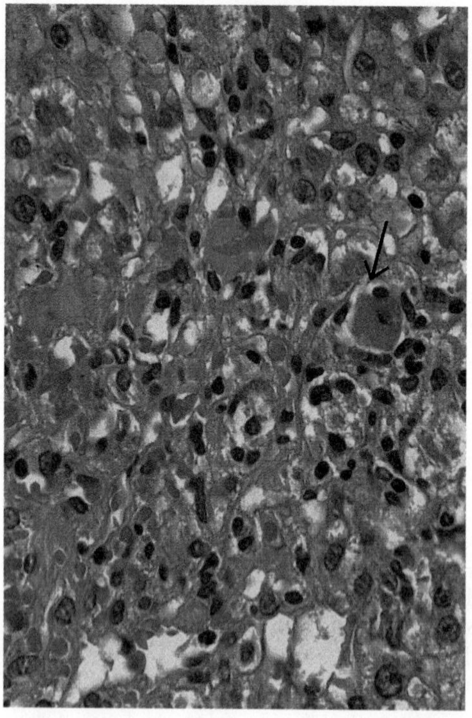

FIGURE *14-20*
Acute viral hepatitis. A photomicrograph shows disarray of liver cell plates, swollen (ballooned) hepatocytes, and an infiltrate of lymphocytes and scattered mononuclear inflammatory cells. The remnants of necrotic hepatocytes have been extruded into the sinusoids, where they appear as acidophilic, or Councilman, bodies (*arrow*).

The portal tracts are almost always enlarged and edematous. As a rule, chronic inflammatory cells accumulate within the portal tracts, but the severity of this inflammatory reaction varies from mild to pronounced. The inflammatory cells in the portal tracts mirror the distribution of those in the lobule. Occasionally, aggregates of lymphoid cells within the portal tracts assume a follicular form, particularly in hepatitis C. The limiting plate of hepatocytes around the portal tracts is usually intact and presents a sharp border with the portal tract. In some instances of acute viral hepatitis that resolve without complications, the inflammatory infiltrate extends from the portal tracts into the lobular parenchyma, thereby disrupting the limiting plate and simulating the appearance of chronic hepatitis. The portal tracts commonly exhibit only a few proliferated bile ductules, although occasionally this phenomenon may be more conspicuous. During recovery, hepatic regeneration is reflected in the presence of mitotic figures in the liver cell plates. All of the pathological changes are gradually reversed and the normal hepatic architecture is completely restored.

Confluent Hepatic Necrosis

The term confluent hepatic necrosis refers to particularly severe variants of acute viral hepatitis, which are characterized by the death of numerous hepatocytes in a geographic distribution and, in extreme cases, by the death of almost all the liver cells (massive hepatic necrosis). In contrast to the most common form of acute viral hepatitis just described, in which the necrosis of hepatocytes appears to be random and patchy, **confluent hepatic necrosis typically affects whole regions of the lobule** (Fig. 14-21). The lesions of confluent hepatic necrosis, in order of increasing severity, are bridging necrosis, submassive necrosis, and massive necrosis. It should be noted that the lesions of confluent hepatic necrosis are not confined to viral hepatitis but may also be encountered after exposure to a variety of hepatotoxic agents (see later).

BRIDGING NECROSIS: At the milder end of the spectrum of lesions that constitute confluent hepatic necrosis are bands of necrosis (bridging necrosis) that stretch between adjacent portal tracts, between adjacent central veins, and between portal tracts and central veins. These bands of necrosis are not necessarily uniform throughout the liver, and lobules that have retained the normal architecture may be situated next to severely affected ones. Curiously, the lobular inflammatory infiltrate is often scanty, although the portal tracts are generally inflamed and often contain an appreciable number of poly-

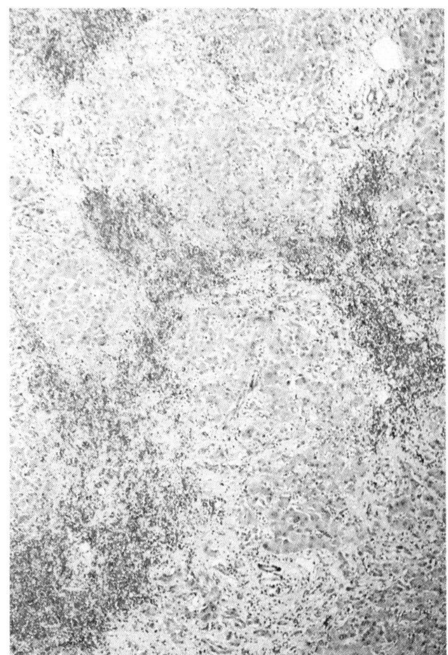

FIGURE *14-21*
Confluent hepatic necrosis. Hemorrhagic zones of necrosis bridge adjacent portal tracts (bridging necrosis).

morphonuclear leukocytes. The death of adjacent plates of hepatocytes results in the collapse of the collagenous stroma to form bands of connective tissue, best visualized with a reticulin stain. Increased collagen synthesis may also contribute to the formation of these connective tissue bands. When such bands encircle an area of liver cells, a nodular pattern, similar to that seen in cirrhosis, may be apparent. The presence of bridging necrosis in younger persons (younger than 30 years of age) has no adverse prognostic significance. However, when this lesion occurs in patients older than 40, as many as half eventually die in hepatic failure. This type of confluent hepatic necrosis was formerly termed *subacute hepatitis*, but the term is inappropriate, since it has a temporal, rather than a purely morphological, connotation.

SUBMASSIVE CONFLUENT NECROSIS: This form of acute hepatitis defines an even more severe injury involving necrosis of entire lobules or groups of adjacent lobules. Clinically, these patients manifest severe hepatitis, which may rapidly proceed to hepatic failure, in which case the disease is classed as *fulminant hepatitis*. In about one fifth of the cases that eventually prove fatal, the course is protracted, with death from hepatic failure occurring in 2 to 5 months.

MASSIVE HEPATIC NECROSIS (ACUTE YELLOW ATROPHY): Although uncommon, massive hepatic necrosis is the most feared variant of acute viral hepatitis, because it is a form of fulminant hepatitis that is almost invariably fatal. Grossly, the liver is shrunken to as little as 500 g (one third of the normal weight). The capsule is wrinkled, and the mottled, red-tan parenchyma is soft and flabby. Microscopic examination reveals that virtually all the hepatocytes are dead (Fig. 14-22), and the hepatic lobule is represented only by the reticulin framework, which in many areas has collapsed. Often the only viable hepatocytes are disposed as a thin rim surrounding the portal tracts. Macrophages, erythrocytes, and necrotic debris fill the sinusoids and impinge on the necrotic remnants of the liver cell plates. For unknown reasons, the massive necrosis does not elicit a vigorous inflammatory response in either the parenchyma or the portal tracts. A few proliferated bile ductules are common, and occasionally small ductular structures lined by altered hepatocytes are present in the remnants of the lobules.

Young patients who survive submassive or massive confluent hepatic necrosis generally do not develop cirrhosis and, in the case of hepatitis B, do not become HBs-Ag carriers. By contrast, older persons who recover from fulminant hepatitis are more likely to progress to chronic hepatitis and cirrhosis.

Chronic Hepatitis

Before the etiological agents of chronic viral hepatitis were identified, attempts were made to assign prognostic value to classifications of morphological features. However, later studies revealed a significant discordance between the morphological subtypes of chronic hepatitis and the prognosis of the infection. Today it is recognized that the lesions are not necessarily static but simply reflect varying degrees of severity. Thus, mild lesions can progress to severe ones, and vice versa.

Morphologically, the spectrum of chronic viral hepatitis (B and C) ranges from mild, portal inflammation with little or no evidence of liver cell necrosis (Fig. 14-23) to a widespread inflammatory, necrotizing, and fibrosing condition (Figs. 14-24 and 14-25). The pathological features of chronic hepatitis are common to both HBV and HCV infections and include piecemeal necrosis, portal inflammation, periportal fibrosis, and lobular inflammation, necrosis, and regeneration.

PIECEMEAL NECROSIS: This lesion is essentially periportal and refers to focal destruction of the limiting plate of hepatocytes. A periportal chronic inflammatory infiltrate, which creates an irregular border between the portal tracts and the lobular parenchyma (see Fig. 14-24).

PORTAL TRACT LESIONS: Chronic hepatitis is characterized by variable infiltration of the portal tracts by lymphocytes, plasma cells, and macrophages. The expanded portal tracts often display mild to severe proliferation of bile ductules, which represents a nonspecific response to chronic liver injury. In the case of chronic hepatitis C, lymphoid aggregates or follicles with reactive centers are often present (Fig. 14-26). Another feature that distinguishes the portal tracts in hepatitis C is the presence of bile duct damage, characterized by necrosis of epithelial cells and intraepithelial inflammation. Such injured bile ducts are often located within lymphoid aggregates, similar to the appearance of primary biliary cirrhosis (see later).

FIGURE 14-22
Massive hepatic necrosis. (*A*) The liver is soft and reduced in size and shows mottled, irregularly hemorrhagic, cut surfaces. (*B*) A photomicrograph shows the loss of most of the hepatocytes. Necrotic lobules are hemorrhagic, and the reticulin framework has collapsed. A sparse chronic inflammatory infiltrate is present within the lobules and portal tracts. The portal tracts are expanded and contain numerous proliferated bile ducts and ductules (*arrows*).

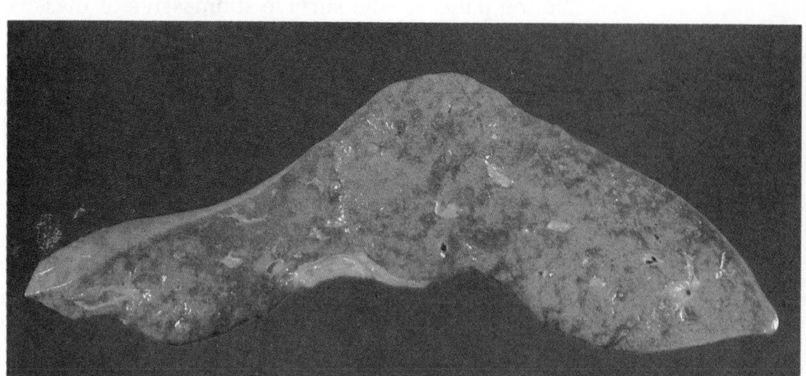
A

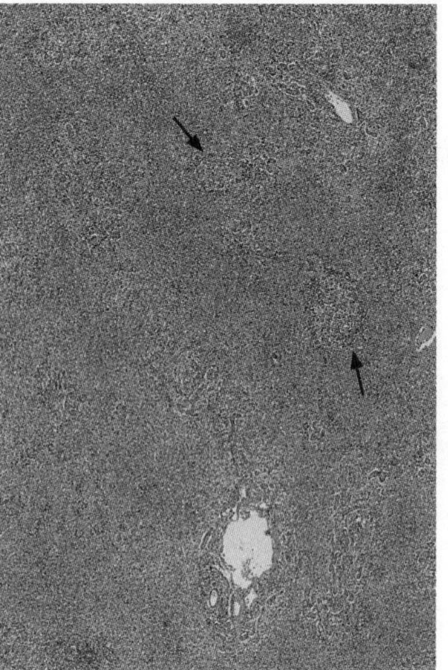
B

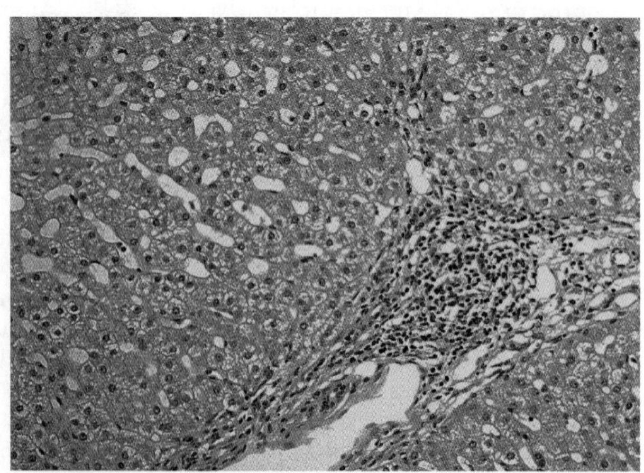

FIGURE 14-23
Mild chronic hepatitis. A photomicrograph shows a portal tract infiltrated by mononuclear inflammatory cells. The lobular parenchyma is intact.

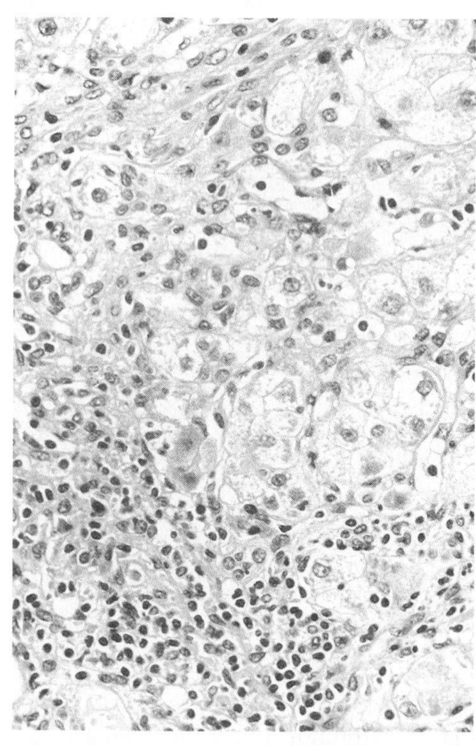

FIGURE 14-24
Severe chronic hepatitis. A photomicrograph discloses a mononuclear inflammatory infiltrate in an expanded portal tract. The inflammation penetrates the limiting plate and surrounds groups of hepatocytes on the border of the portal tract.

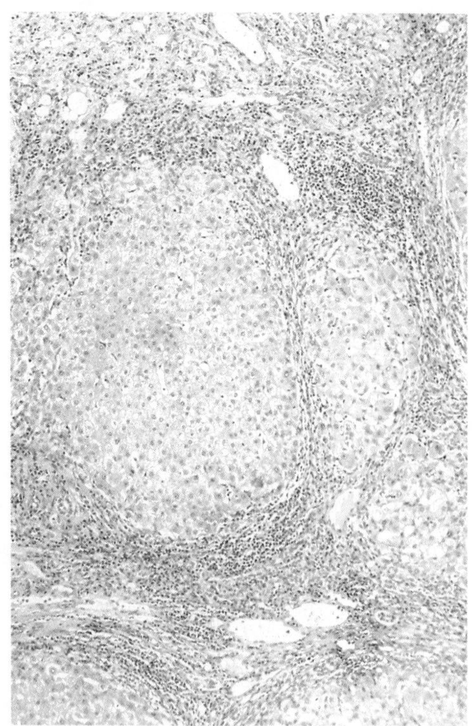

FIGURE 14-25
Chronic hepatitis with cirrhosis. A photomicrograph of the liver from a patient with long-standing chronic active hepatitis B shows hepatocellular nodules and chronically inflamed fibrous septa.

INTRALOBULAR LESIONS: Focal necrosis and inflammation within the parenchyma are typical of chronic hepatitis. Scattered acidophilic bodies are common, and enlarged Kupffer cells are seen within the sinusoids. When seen in the context of chronic hepatitis, confluent hepatic necrosis in the form of bridging necrosis is an ominous predictor of rapid progression to cirrhosis.

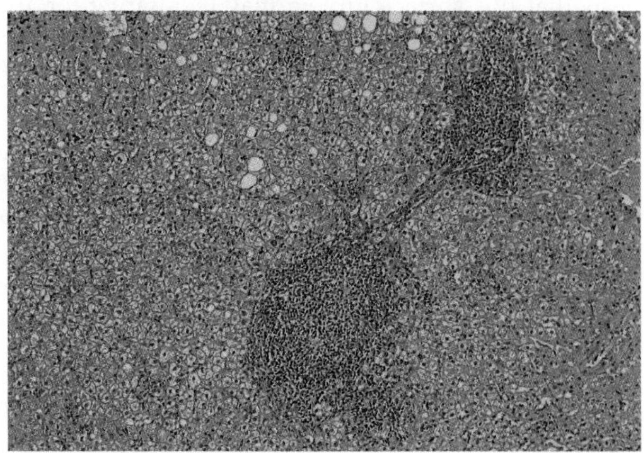

FIGURE 14-26
Chronic hepatitis C. A photomicrograph of the liver from a patient with long-standing hepatitis C exhibits two portal tracts connected by a fibrous bridge containing nodular aggregates of lymphoid cells.

The liver in chronic hepatitis B often exhibits scattered hepatocytes with a large granular cytoplasm containing abundant HBsAg (*ground-glass hepatocytes*) (Fig. 14-27). In the case of chronic hepatitis C, moderate fat accumulation within hepatocytes (steatosis) is frequently observed. Characteristically, the persistent hepatocellular necrosis stimulates regenerative changes, which are evidenced by increased numbers of binucleated hepatocytes and two-cell-thick liver cell plates.

PERIPORTAL FIBROSIS: The progressive erosion of the periportal hepatocytes by piecemeal necrosis leads to the deposition of collagen, which gives the portal tract a stellate (star-shaped) appearance. Threads of connective tissue also envelop single hepatocytes and groups of cells, particularly adjacent to the portal tracts. With time, the fibrosis may extend to adjacent portal tracts or into the lobule itself towards the central vein. The end-stage of chronic hepatitis is characterized by dense collagenous septa, which destroy the lobular architecture and divide the liver into hepatocellular nodules, an appearance termed *cirrhosis* (see later). In the cirrhotic stage, the activity of chronic hepatitis is evidenced by continued inflammation and liver cell necrosis.

The mildest form of chronic hepatitis is characterized by lymphocytic infiltration limited to the portal tracts (see Fig. 14-23). Many but not all patients with mild chronic hepatitis do not progress to more severe disease. A substantial number of cases manifest only minimal or sporadic increases in serum aminotransferase levels and are often referred to as "asymptomatic" HBV or HCV carriers.

In evaluating patients with chronic active hepatitis, it is important to realize that the clinical activity of this disease does not necessarily correlate with the morphological appearance of the liver. On liver biopsy, persons with only mild symptoms and modest elevations of serum aminotransferase activities may display severe chronic active hepatitis with progression to cirrhosis. **Although imperfect and subject to sampling errors, the liver biopsy remains the most important predictor of the course of chronic hepatitis.** Table 14-2 compares the major features of the common forms of viral hepatitis.

AUTOIMMUNE HEPATITIS

Autoimmune hepatitis is a severe type of chronic hepatitis of unknown cause, which is associated with circulating autoantibodies and high levels of serum immunoglobulins. The disease is distinct from any of the known types of viral hepatitis, although some 5% of patients with autoimmune hepatitis are falsely positive for HCV antibodies. Conversely, 10% of patients with chronic viral hepatitis exhibit circulating autoantibodies. In Western countries, autoimmune hepatitis accounts for 20% of all cases of chronic hepatitis. Autoimmune hepatitis occurs predominantly among young women, but up to one third of the patients are men, and the disease may appear at any age.

☐ **Pathogenesis:** Autoimmune hepatitis may represent a response to an environmental insult in a genetically

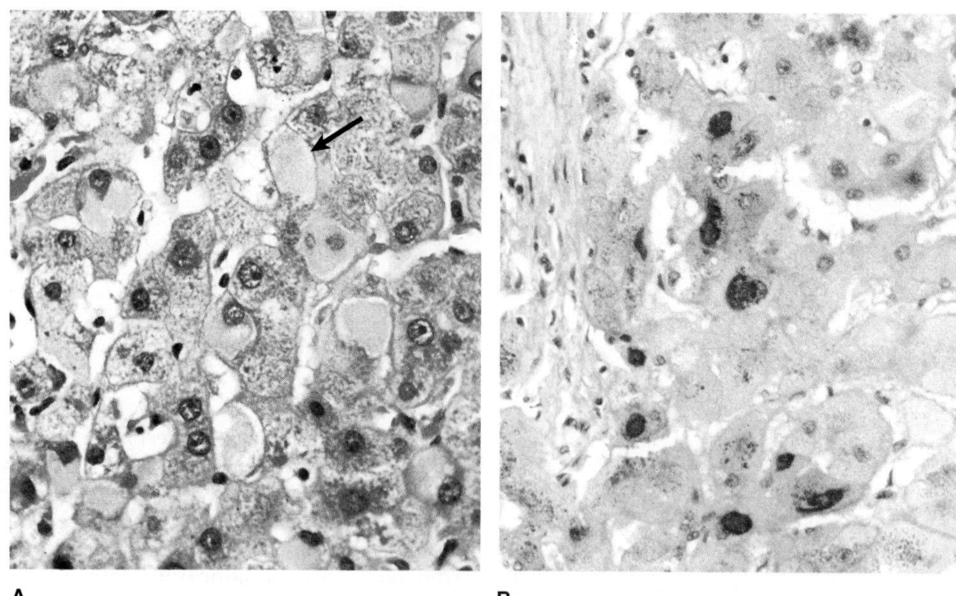

FIGURE 14-27
"Ground-glass" hepatocytes. (*A*) A photomicrograph of a case of chronic persistent hepatitis B shows scattered hepatocytes (*arrow*) with an abundant granular cytoplasm containing HBsAg. (*B*) The same case has been stained for HBsAg by the immunoperoxidase method. The abundant cytoplasmic HBsAg appears brown.

TABLE 14-2 **Comparative Features of the Common Forms of Viral Hepatitis**

	Hepatitis A	Hepatitis B	Hepatitis C
Genome	RNA	DNA	RNA
Incubation period	3–6 weeks	6 weeks to 6 months	7–8 weeks
Transmission	Oral	Parenteral	Parenteral
Blood	No	Yes	Yes
Feces	Yes	No	No
Vertical	No	Yes	?
Fulminant hepatic necrosis	Very rare	Yes	Rare
Chronic hepatitis	No	10%	50%
Carrier state	No	Yes	Yes
Liver cancer	No	Yes	Yes

predisposed person. According to this scenario, an environmental agent triggers an autoimmune attack against liver antigens, thereby producing progressive necrosis and inflammation in the liver. Like patients with autoimmune diseases in general, most patients with autoimmune hepatitis are positive for HLA-B8, DR3, or DR4. In addition, the genetic predisposition may include loci that encode complement products, immunoglobulins, and T-cell receptors. Relatives of patients with autoimmune hepatitis demonstrate an increased prevalence of circulating autoantibodies. The putative environmental agent has not been identified, but previous infections with the measles virus, Epstein-Barr virus, and hepatitis viruses have been proposed.

Autoimmune hepatitis is subclassified according to the predominant autoantibodies present in the patients serum. The most common or classic form **(type I)** exhibits circulating antinuclear, anti–smooth muscle, antiactin, and anti–asialoglycoprotein receptor antibodies. Except for the last, these antibodies are not organ specific and are not thought to injure the liver directly, although they serve as markers of the disease. In addition to these antibodies, a number of other autoantibodies directed against certain liver and pancreatic proteins, mitochondria, cytoskeletal elements, and the cytoplasm of neutrophils are occasionally present. The presence of antibodies against the liver-specific asialoglycoprotein receptor suggests that this surface protein may be a target for antibody-dependent cell-mediated cytotoxicity. It has also been postulated that defective suppressor-T-cell function plays a role in the pathogenesis of autoimmune hepatitis. **Type II autoimmune hepatitis** occurs most often in girls and young women and demonstrates circulating antibodies against liver–kidney microsomes (anti-LKM) and anti-liver cytosolic proteins.

☐ **Pathology:** In general, the histological appearance of autoimmune hepatitis resembles that of chronic viral hepatitis. In some patients, numerous plasma cells infiltrate the portal tracts. There may be a disparity between the severity of the clinical and histological manifestations of the disease, but the latter seems to be more important for prognosis.

☐ **Clinical Features:** Autoimmune hepatitis presents a variable clinical picture, ranging from an asymptomatic condition discovered by the finding of abnormal liver function tests during routine screening, to a severe, acute, and even fulminant liver disease. In most cases, the disease begins insidiously with nonspecific symptoms and progressive jaundice. As the disorder progresses, serum aminotransferase levels become conspicuously elevated and liver failure may ensue. In many patients, autoimmune hepatitis progresses to cirrhosis, which is similar to that produced by other causes. Thus, autoimmune hepatitis resembles the clinical course of chronic viral hepatitis and must be distinguished from that disease by appropriate serological studies. Pronounced hyperglobulinemia is characteristic of autoimmune hepatitis.

In contrast to viral hepatitis, autoimmune hepatitis is responsive to therapy with corticosteroids, particularly when combined with immune suppression with azathioprine. The initial remission rate is 80%. About half of these patients remain in remission after withdrawal of therapy, but the majority of patients require long-term maintenance on drugs. Liver transplantation is an option for those patients whose disease progresses to end-stage cirrhosis.

ALCOHOLIC LIVER DISEASE

The deleterious effects of excess alcohol (ethanol, ethyl alcohol) consumption have been recognized since the early days of recorded history. The prophet Isaiah warned, "Woe to him that is mighty to drink wine." The specific association of alcohol abuse and cirrhosis was noted by the English physician Thomas Heberden in 1699, when he linked "scirrhous livers" with the consumption of "spirituous liquors." Until the middle of the 20th century, the high incidence of liver disease in alcoholics was generally attributed to a toxic effect of ethanol. Subsequently, however, the similarity between (1) the experimental nutritional liver disease in rats induced by dietary choline deficiency and human alcoholic liver disease, and (2) the fact that some alcoholics are malnourished, led to the assumption that alcohol per se is not hepatotoxic. Rather, it was thought that the nutritional deficiencies associated with alcohol abuse are responsible for the liver disease commonly seen in alcoholics. This notion was subsequently questioned on clinical grounds, when it became clear that only a very small proportion of all alcoholics are socially deteriorated (*"skid row" alcoholics*) and that the majority are apparently adequately nourished or even obese. Experiments in which alcohol was given together with nutritionally adequate diets to rats, subhuman primates, and human volunteers demonstrated that alcohol is indeed toxic to the liver, as evidenced by the production of fatty liver and ultrastructural changes in the hepatocytes. Moreover, cirrhosis was produced in baboons fed alcohol with a diet containing all essential nutrients. Thus, today alcohol is again recognized as a direct hepatotoxic agent.

☐ **Epidemiology:** As in the relationship between smoking and cancer, the evidence linking alcoholism to cirrhosis of the liver in humans is derived from epidemiological data. The prevalence of cirrhosis is highest in those countries with the highest per capita consumption of alcohol. This relationship between alcohol consumption and chronic liver disease is valid regardless of the specific nature of the preferred beverage (e.g., wine in France, beer in Australia, and spirits in Scandinavia). A quantitative correlation between total alcohol consumption in the population and death from cirrhosis of the liver has also been established in the various states of the United States. When the consumption of alcoholic beverages was restricted, as occurred during the prohibition era in the United States and during World War II in France, deaths from cirrhosis of the liver declined. Although only a minority of chronic alcoholics develop cirrhosis, a dose–response relationship between the lifetime dose of alcohol (duration of exposure in years and the daily amount of alcohol consumed) and the appearance of cirrhosis has been established (Fig. 14-28).

It is estimated that in the United States about 7% of the total population is alcoholic. However, when one considers only the population at risk, eliminating children, the aged, institutionalized persons, and ethnic or religious groups that abjure the use of alcohol, the prevalence of alcoholism is considerably higher. **About 15% of alcoholics can be expected to develop cirrhosis, and many of these persons die in hepatic failure or from the extrahepatic complications of cirrhosis.** In fact, in many urban areas of the United States with high alcoholism rates, cirrhosis of the liver, about 70% of which is associated with alcoholism, is now the third or fourth leading cause of death in men younger than 45 years of age.

The amount of alcohol required to produce chronic liver disease varies widely depending on body size, age,

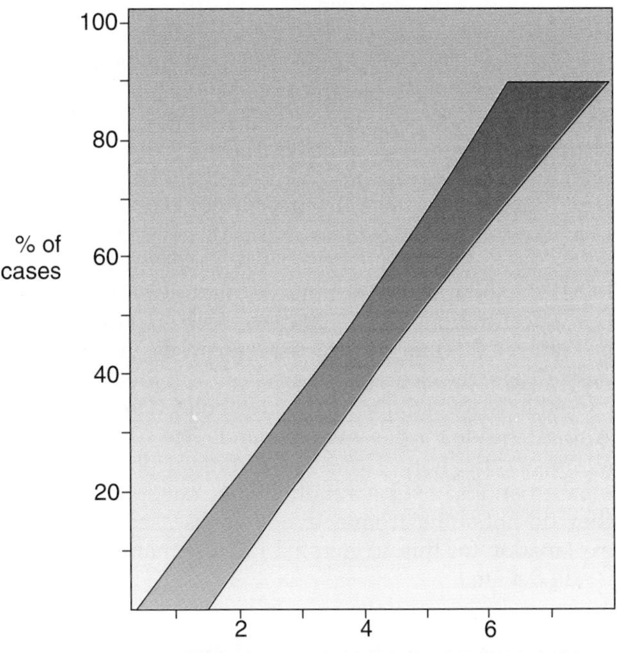

FIGURE *14-28*
Dose–response relationship between the amount of alcohol consumed in a lifetime and the incidence of cirrhosis. Only a minority of all alcoholics develop cirrhosis, but those who drink very large amounts are at high risk of developing the disease.

sex, and race, but the lower range seems to be about 80 g/day (235 mL of 86-proof alcoholic beverage) for men and is probably lower for women. In fact, there is some evidence that women are constitutionally more susceptible to the ravages of alcoholism than men, and the threshold dose for the development of cirrhosis in women has been claimed to be as low as 20 g/day, although this value seems unrealistically low. The daily amount of alcohol in established cirrhotic patients is usually in the range of 160 to 220 g. In general, more than 10 years of alcoholism is required to produce cirrhosis, although a few cirrhotic patients give shorter histories of heavy alcohol use. It has been suggested that, for practical purposes, a pint of whiskey a day (or its equivalent in other beverages) for 15 years is a threshold for the development of cirrhosis.

The epidemiology of alcoholic liver disease has recently been complicated by the discovery of its association with hepatotropic viruses. The prevalence of serum HBV markers is two- to fourfold higher in alcoholics than in corresponding control populations. The prevalence of anti-HCV is up to 10% among alcoholics, compared to about 1% in the general population. The significance of these data with respect to the pathogenesis of alcoholic cirrhosis remains unknown.

Metabolism of Ethanol

Ethanol is rapidly absorbed from the stomach and is eventually distributed in body water space. Almost all of the ethanol consumed is metabolized by the liver to acetaldehyde and acetate. Between 5% and 10% is excreted unchanged, principally in the urine and in the expired breath. The principal route of ethanol oxidation in the liver (Fig. 14-29) is through cytosolic alcohol dehydrogenase (ADH), a nicotinamide adenine dinucleotide (NAD)-dependent enzyme. A minor but nevertheless important metabolic pathway is a microsomal ethanol oxidizing system (MEOS) in the smooth endoplasmic reticulum, which is a mixed-function oxidase that utilizes NADP as a cofactor. Since the K_m of ADH is only about 1 mM and that of MEOS about 7 mM, at clinically significant blood alcohol concentrations (20 to 100 mM), both enzyme systems are saturated. Thus, for practical purposes, in contrast to most drugs, the clearance of alcohol from the body is linear—that is, a fixed quantity is metabolized per unit time. A rough guide for the average man is 7 to 10 g of alcohol eliminated per hour. However, chronic alcoholics metabolize ethanol at a substantially higher rate, provided that they do not suffer from active liver disease. The precise explanation for this accelerated rate of ethanol oxidation is still debated.

Liver Diseases Produced by Alcohol Consumption

The spectrum of alcoholic liver disease spans three major morphological and clinical entities: **fatty liver, alcoholic hepatitis, and cirrhosis**. Although these lesions usually occur sequentially, they may coexist in any combination and may actually be independent entities.

Fatty Liver and Associated Lesions

☐ **Pathogenesis:** Virtually all chronic alcoholics accumulate fat in hepatocytes (steatosis). The pathogenesis of fatty liver is not precisely understood, and the relative contributions of different pathways may vary, depending on the amount of alcohol consumed, dietary lipid content, body stores of fat, hormonal status, and other variables. Nevertheless, the accumulation of fat clearly depends on the intake of ethanol, since it is fully and rapidly reversible on discontinuation of alcohol ingestion. To understand the factors that may be involved in the accumulation of lipid, it is helpful to review briefly lipid metabolism in the liver.

Dietary fat, in the form of chylomicrons and free fatty acids, is transported to the liver, where it is taken up by the hepatocyte. Triglycerides are then hydrolyzed to free fatty acids. These, in turn, undergo β-oxidation in the mitochondria or are converted to triglycerides in the endoplasmic reticulum. The newly synthesized triglycerides are secreted in the form of lipoproteins or retained for storage.

Most of the fat deposited in the liver after chronic alcohol consumption is derived from the diet. However, in the fasting state, much of the fat in the liver has been accumulated from endogenous fat depots. Ethanol increases lipolysis and thus the delivery of free fatty acids to the liver. This effect may be accomplished through hormonal mechanisms, for example through epinephrine, corticotropin, or prostaglandins. Within the hepatocyte, ethanol (1) increases fatty acid synthesis, (2) decreases mitochondrial oxidation of fatty acids, (3) increases the production of triglycerides, and (4) impairs the release of lipoproteins (Fig. 14-30). Collectively, these metabolic consequences produce a fatty liver, but the quantitative role for each is not established and may be variable.

☐ **Pathology:** In the alcoholic, the liver becomes yellow and enlarged, sometimes massively, to as much as three times the normal weight. The increased weight does not reflect fat accumulation alone, since protein and water content are also increased. Microscopically, the extent of visible fat accumulation varies from minute droplets scattered in the cytoplasm of a few hepatocytes to distention of the entire cytoplasm of most cells by coalesced droplets (Fig. 14-31). In the latter situation, the liver cell is scarcely recognizable as such and bears a resemblance to an adipocyte, the cytoplasm being represented by a distended clear area and the nucleus flattened and displaced to the periphery of the cell. When steatosis is mild, centrilobular hepatocytes are preferentially affected, but as the lesion progresses the entire lobule is involved. A few thin strands of connective tissue may extend from the portal tracts or the central veins, but usually there is no increase in connective tissue. Occasionally, cholestasis is observed in the fatty liver, although the pathogenesis is unclear.

The ultrastructural appearance of the hepatocyte in alcohol-induced fatty liver reflects the cytotoxicity of ethanol, rather than an effect of the fat per se. The mitochondria are enlarged, with occasional bizarre giant forms. The smooth endoplasmic reticulum exhibits

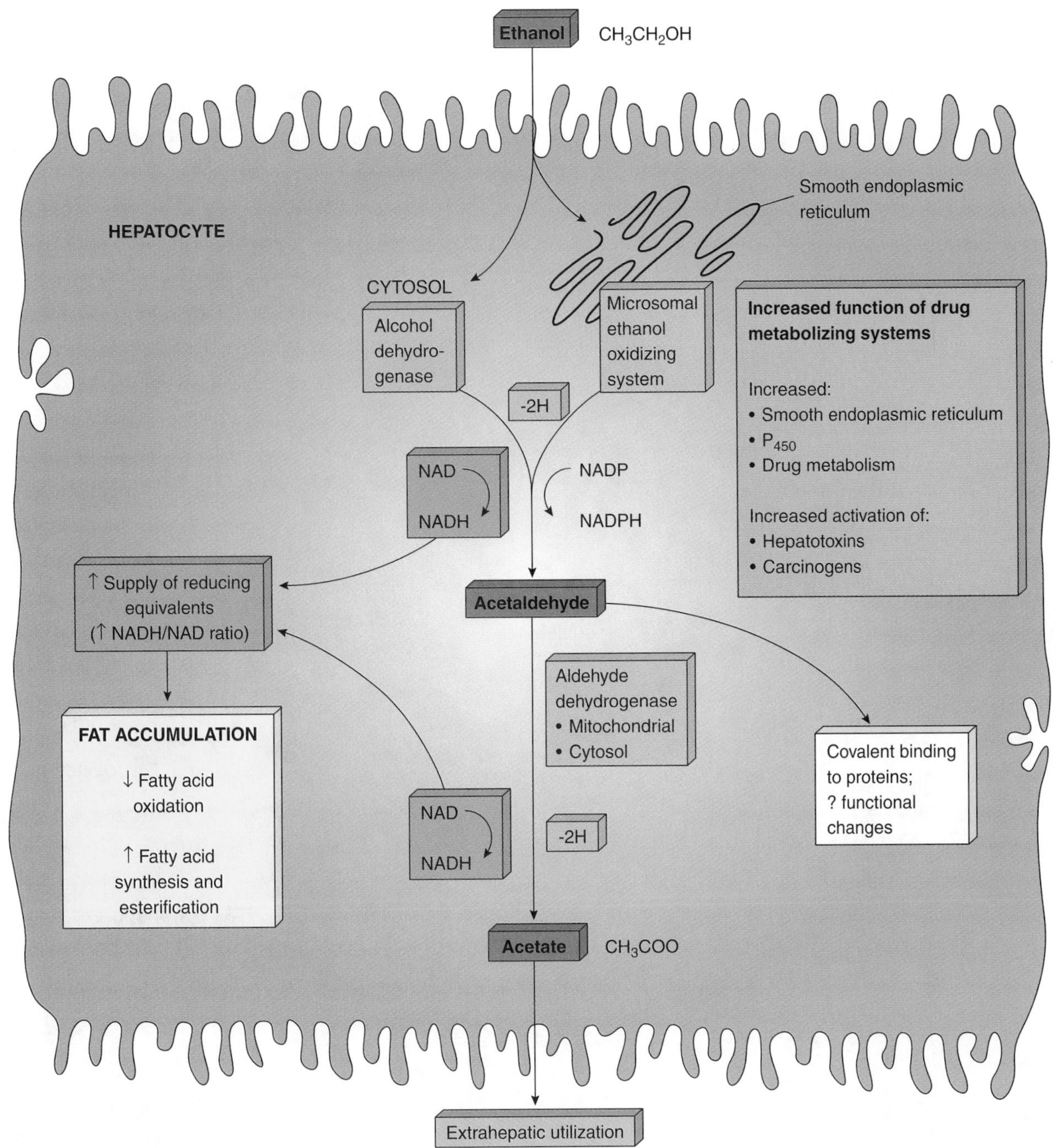

FIGURE *14-29*
The metabolism of ethanol and its hepatocellular effects.

hyperplasia resembling that produced by other inducers of microsomal drug-metabolizing enzymes. Initially, the fat accumulates as globules, which eventually merge to form large, cytoplasmic bodies of variable electron density.

The ultrastructural changes in mitochondria and endoplasmic reticulum produced by chronic ethanol ingestion are paralleled by functional alterations. Hepatic mitochondria show decreased rates of substrate oxidation (e.g., of fatty acids) and impaired formation of ATP. Hyperplasia of the smooth endoplasmic reticulum is accompanied by an increase in the activity of the cytochrome P_{450}-dependent mixed-function oxidases. Not only is the microsomal ethanol-oxidizing system induced, but the metabolism of a wide variety of drugs is also enhanced. The increased microsomal function also augments the metabolism of potential hepatic toxins. This results in an exaggeration of the toxicity of agents such as carbon tetrachloride and acetaminophen. In contrast to chronic alcohol consumption, which promotes microsomal functions, the presence of ethanol in the blood and

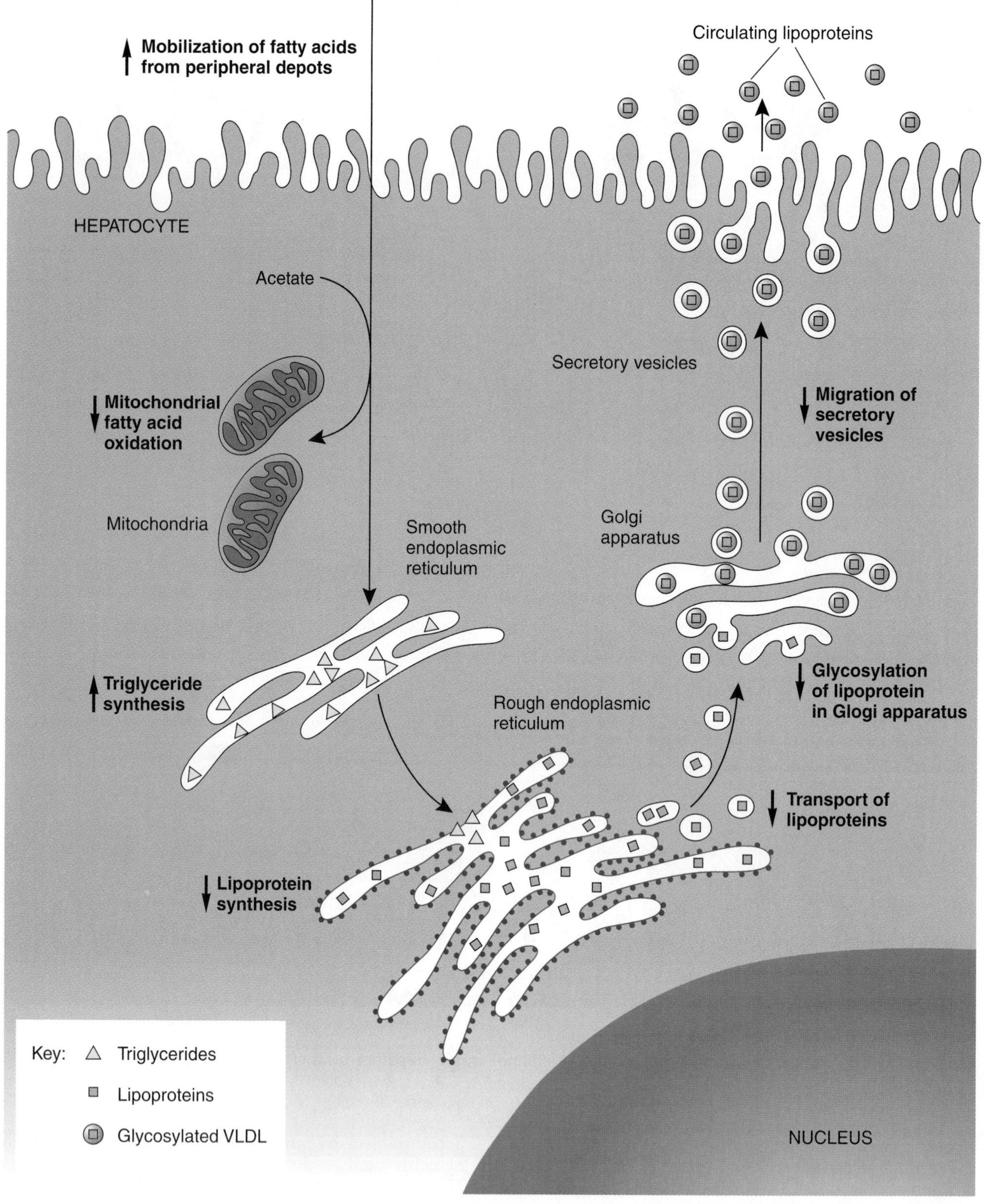

FIGURE *14-30*
Pathogenesis of alcoholic fatty liver.

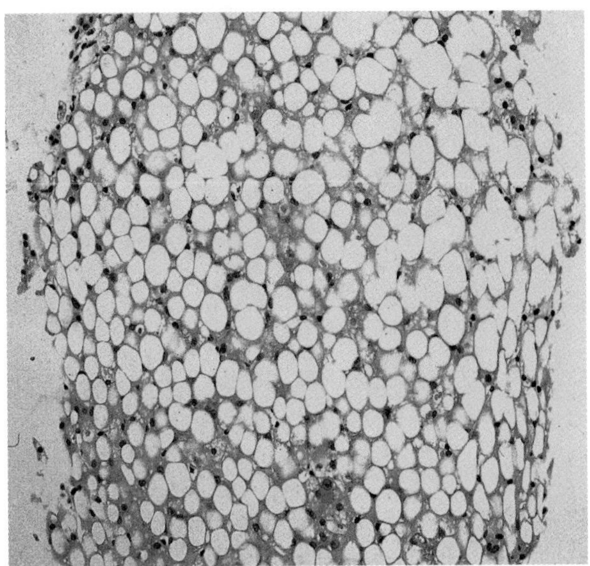

FIGURE *14-31*
Alcoholic fatty liver. A photomicrograph shows the cytoplasm of almost all the hepatocytes to be distended by fat, which displaces the nucleus to the periphery. Note the absence of inflammation and fibrosis.

hepatocytes after acute alcohol ingestion inhibits the activity of mixed-function oxidases and acutely reduces the rate of clearance of drugs from the body.

☐ **Clinical Features:** Patients with uncomplicated alcoholic fatty liver have surprisingly few symptoms of liver disease. Except for the unusual combination of fatty liver and cholestasis, the bilirubin level is normal, and the serum aminotransferase levels are only minimally elevated—up to twice normal at most. It is important to recall that, despite the striking morphological change in the liver, alcoholic fatty liver is a fully reversible lesion and does not by itself progress to more severe disease, notably cirrhosis.

A fatty liver, although characteristic of alcoholism, is not restricted to that condition but is also noted in obesity, uncontrolled diabetes, and kwashiorkor and following prolonged administration of corticosteroids.

Alcoholic Hepatitis

Alcoholic hepatitis is an acute necrotizing lesion characterized by (1) necrosis of hepatocytes, predominantly in the central zone, (2) cytoplasmic hyaline inclusions within hepatocytes, (3) a neutrophilic inflammatory response, and (4) perivenular fibrosis (Fig. 14-32). The pathogenesis of alcoholic hepatitis is mysterious. Alcoholics may have mild fatty liver for many years and, without any change in drinking habits, suddenly develop acute alcoholic hepatitis. The basis for the conversion of the benign fatty liver into the necrotizing lesion of alcoholic hepatitis may be the key to the eventual solution of the riddle of alcoholic liver injury.

☐ **Pathology:** In the typical case of acute alcoholic hepatitis, the hepatic architecture is basically intact, with a normal relation of portal tracts to central venules. The hepatocytes show variable hydropic swelling, which gives them a heterogeneous appearance. Isolated necrotic liver cells, or clusters of them, exhibit pyknotic nuclei and karyorrhexis. Scattered hepatocytes contain Mallory bodies (i.e., so-called alcoholic hyalin) (see Fig. 14-32). These cytoplasmic inclusions, which are more common in visibly damaged, swollen hepatocytes, are visualized as irregular skeins of eosinophilic material or as solid eosinophilic masses, often in a perinuclear location. Ultrastructurally, they are composed of aggregates of intermediate (cytokeratin) filaments (Fig. 14-33). The damaged, ballooned hepatocytes, particularly those containing Mallory bodies, are surrounded by neutrophils, although a more diffuse, intralobular inflammatory infiltrate is also present. Cholestasis, varying from mild to severe, is present in as many as one third of the cases. Importantly, alcoholic hepatitis is usually superimposed on an existing fatty liver, although there is no evidence that fat accumulation predisposes or contributes to the development of alcoholic hepatitis.

Collagen deposition is a constant feature of alcoholic hepatitis, especially around the central vein (terminal hepatic venule). In severe cases, the venule and perivenular sinusoids are obliterated and surrounded by dense fibrous tissue, in which case the lesion has been termed *central hyaline sclerosis* (Fig. 14-34). This fibrotic lesion may persist after recovery from an episode of alcoholic hepatitis and is, therefore, occasionally seen in a liver that does not display the other morphological stigmata of alcoholic hepatitis. This finding may also explain the presence of portal hypertension in some alcoholics who do not have cirrhosis. Small strands of collagen are commonly noted in the sinusoidal walls and in the periphery of the portal tracts. Characteristically, threads of connective tissue surround individual or groups of damaged hepatocytes.

The appearance of the portal tracts in alcoholic hepatitis is highly variable. In some instances, they are virtually normal, whereas in others they are enlarged and contain a mononuclear infiltrate and proliferated bile ductules. The altered portal tracts often display spurs of fibrous tissue that penetrate the lobules. The inflammation may be so severe that it spills over into the lobule and obscures the limiting plate, an appearance similar to that of so-called piecemeal necrosis in chronic active hepatitis.

The histological appearance of the liver in alcoholic hepatitis, when combined with an appropriate history, presents no diagnostic problem. However, a similar pattern of liver injury, termed *nonalcoholic steatohepatitis,* is occasionally seen in other conditions, including Wilson disease, diabetes, Indian childhood cirrhosis, and post-jejunoileal bypass for morbid obesity. Sometimes it occurs in persons with no other apparent disease. In addition, Mallory bodies are also occasionally encountered in primary biliary cirrhosis, extrahepatic biliary obstruction, drug-induced hepatic injury, and primary hepatocellular carcinoma.

☐ **Clinical Features:** The classic clinical features associated with alcoholic hepatitis are malaise and anorexia, fever, right upper quadrant abdominal pain, and jaundice. A mild leukocytosis is common. The serum aminotransferase activities, particularly that of aspartate aminotransferase, are moderately elevated, but not to the levels often noted in viral hepatitis. Serum alkaline phos-

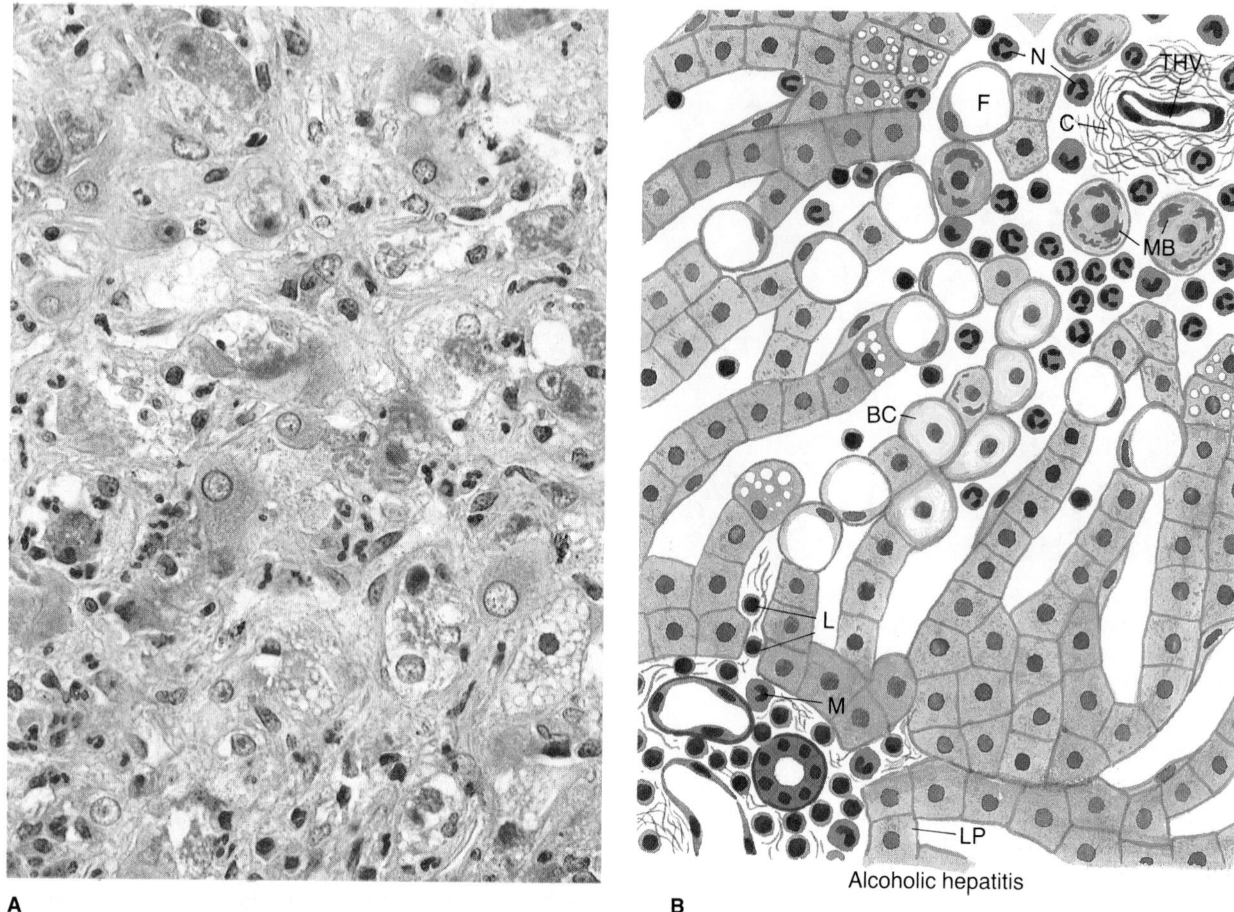

FIGURE 14-32
Alcoholic hepatitis. (*A*) A photomicrograph shows necrosis and degeneration of hepatocytes; Mallory bodies (eosinophilic inclusions) in the cytoplasm of injured hepatocytes; and infiltration by neutrophils. (*B*) Schematic representation of the major pathological features of alcoholic hepatitis. The lesions are predominantly centrilobular and include necrosis and loss of hepatocytes, ballooned cells (BC), and Mallory bodies (MB) in the cytoplasm of damaged hepatocytes. The inflammatory infiltrate consists predominantly of neutrophils (N), although a few lymphocytes (L) and macrophages (M) are also present. The central vein, or terminal hepatic venule (THV), is encased in connective tissue (C) (central sclerosis). Fat-laden hepatocytes (F) are evident in the lobule. The portal tract displays moderate chronic inflammation, and the limiting plate (LP) is focally breached.

phatase activity is usually increased. The sudden onset of jaundice, leukocytosis, and an elevated serum alkaline phosphatase level has on occasion led to the erroneous diagnosis of obstructive jaundice. In severe cases, the prothrombin time may be prolonged to such an extent that liver biopsy is not feasible, a situation associated with an ominous prognosis.

The prognosis in patients with alcoholic hepatitis correlates with the severity of the liver cell injury. In some patients, the disease rapidly progresses to hepatic failure and death. The mortality in the acute stage of alcoholic hepatitis ranges from 10% to 30%. If the patient survives and continues to drink, the acute stage may be followed by persistent alcoholic hepatitis, and more than one third of such patients progress to cirrhosis in only 1 or 2 years. Among those who abstain from alcohol after recovery from acute alcoholic hepatitis, only about one fourth have no morphological residuals by 6 months, and about one in five progresses to cirrhosis. Recovery in the remaining abstainers is slow, and most show histological lesions more than a year after the initial episode. As a group, patients with alcoholic hepatitis are at severe risk of permanent liver disease; up to 70% may ultimately develop cirrhosis. No specific treatment for acute alcoholic hepatitis is available, although in selected patients corticosteroids and dietary supplementation may improve short-term survival.

Alcoholic Cirrhosis

In about 15% of alcoholics, hepatocellular necrosis, fibrosis, and regeneration eventually lead to the formation of fibrous septa surrounding hepatocellular nodules, the two features that define cirrhosis (Fig. 14-35). The other

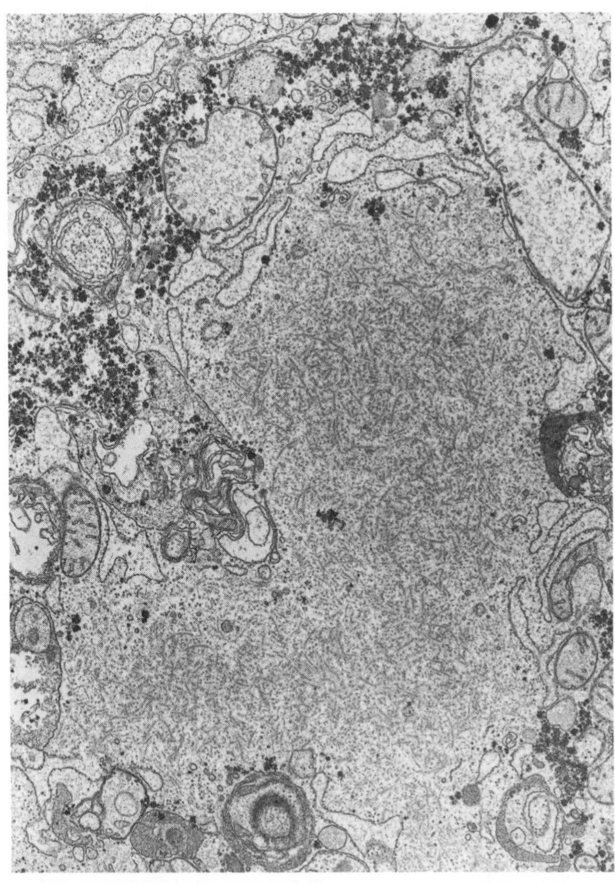

FIGURE 14-33
Mallory body. An electron micrograph shows an aggregate of filamentous material in the cytoplasm of a hepatocyte. The mass displaces the cytoplasmic organelles peripherally.

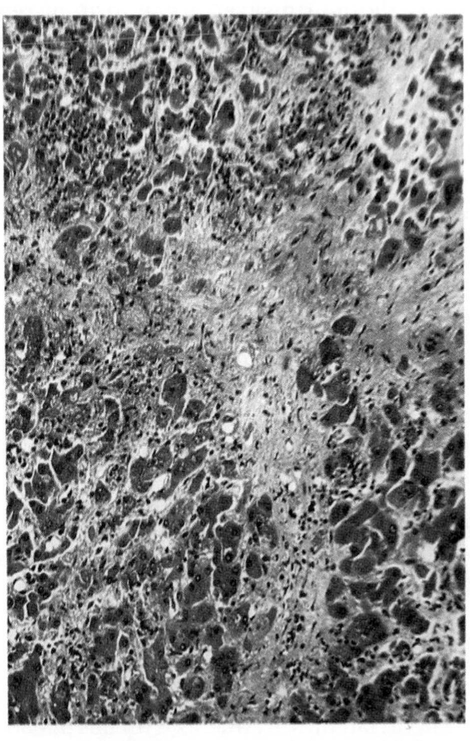

FIGURE 14-34
Central hyaline sclerosis. This photomicrograph from the liver of a patient with alcoholic liver disease shows the central terminal venule to be obliterated by fibrous tissue.

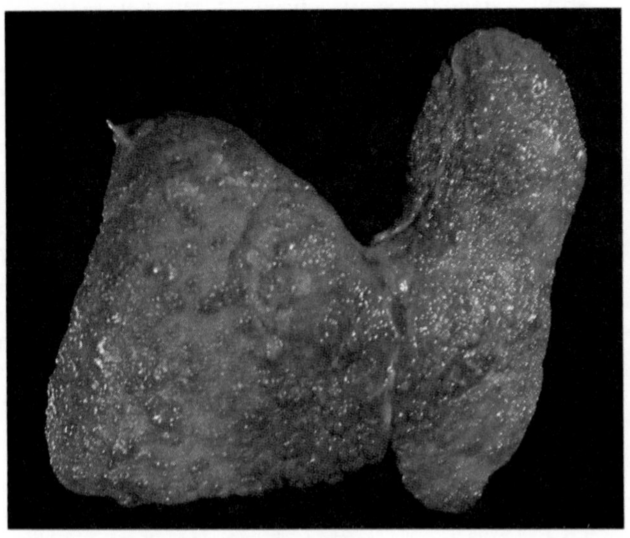

A

B

FIGURE 14-35
Alcoholic cirrhosis. (*A*) The surface of the liver displays innumerable small, regular nodules. (*B*) A photomicrograph shows small regular nodules surrounded by uniform fibrous septa.

lesions of alcoholic liver disease—namely, fatty liver and acute or persistent alcoholic hepatitis—are often seen in conjunction with cirrhosis. It is an open question whether typical alcoholic hepatitis—that is, an acute, inflammatory and necrotizing hepatic injury—is a necessary precursor of cirrhosis. **However, some form of persistent necrosis clearly precedes the development of cirrhosis.** The prognosis in cases of established alcoholic cirrhosis is for the most part considerably better in those who abstain from alcohol abuse. Nevertheless, many patients progress to end-stage liver disease, and alcoholic liver disease is the single most common cause for liver transplantation among adults in the United States.

PRIMARY BILIARY CIRRHOSIS

Primary biliary cirrhosis (PBC) is a chronic progressive cholestatic liver disease characterized by destruction of the intrahepatic bile ducts (nonsuppurative destructive cholangitis). PBC occurs principally in middle-aged women (10:1 female predominance). The use of the term *cirrhosis* in the designation of this malady is somewhat misleading, in that cirrhosis is actually a late complication of the disease.

Primary biliary cirrhosis accounts for up to 2% of deaths from cirrhosis. It shows no apparent ethnic predilection, but several familial clusters of the disease have been reported. A hereditary predisposition is also suggested by the finding of characteristic immunological abnormalities in some unaffected relatives. The prevalence of PBC in families of patients with this malady is 4%, a value considerably higher than that in the general population.

☐ **Pathogenesis:** **PBC is associated with many immunological abnormalities and is, therefore, widely held to be an autoimmune disease.** Although this may be probable, it should be stated at the outset that direct proof for this conjecture is lacking. The large majority (85%) of patients with primary biliary cirrhosis have at least one other disease usually classed as autoimmune, and almost half (40%) have two or more such ailments. Among these disorders are chronic thyroiditis, rheumatoid arthritis, scleroderma, Sjögren syndrome, and systemic lupus erythematosus.

Both humoral and cellular immunity appear to be altered. Serum immunoglobulin levels are increased, especially the level of IgM. **More than 95% of the patients have circulating antimitochondrial antibodies, a finding commonly used in the diagnosis of PBC.** These autoantibodies recognize epitopes associated with the mitochondrial pyruvate dehydrogenase complex.

Despite the specificity of the antimitochondrial antibodies, they have no inhibitory effect on mitochondrial function and play no known role in the pathogenesis or progression of the disease. Other circulating autoantibodies are antinuclear, antithyroid, antiplatelet, antiacetylcholine receptor, and antiribonucleoprotein antibodies. The complement system is chronically activated, the increased complement turnover reflecting activation of the classical pathway.

The most attractive explanation for the initial destruction of bile ducts in PBC is an attack on the biliary epithelial cells by cytotoxic T lymphocytes. The infiltrating lymphocytes in the portal tracts are mostly T cells, both helper and suppressor. Interestingly, the cells surrounding and infiltrating the sites of bile duct damage are predominantly suppressor/cytotoxic (CD8+) lymphocytes, suggesting that they may mediate the destruction of the ductal epithelium.

☐ **Pathology:** Three major pathological stages in the evolution of PBC are recognized. These are characterized, respectively, by ductal lesions, scarring, and cirrhosis.

STAGE I: THE DUCT LESION: Early stage I PBC is characterized by a unique lesion, namely a *chronic destructive cholangitis* affecting the intrahepatic small- and medium-sized bile ducts (Fig. 14-36). The injury to the bile ducts is segmental and therefore appears focal in histological sections. The bile ducts are surrounded principally by lymphocytes, but plasma cells and macrophages are also seen. In some patients, eosinophils are conspicuous in the portal tracts, although neutrophils are rare. Characteristically, the bile duct epithelium is irregular and hyperplastic, with stratification of epithelial cells and occasional papillary ingrowths. Foci of necrotic epithelial cells and ulceration of the epithelium are not uncommon. **In some portal tracts, lymphoid follicles, occasionally containing germinal centers, are conspicuous.** Discrete epithelioid granulomas often occur in the portal tracts and may impinge on the bile ducts. In stage I PBC, the lobular parenchyma tends to be normal, but in a minority of cases mild central cholestasis is present.

STAGE II: SCARRING: As a result of the destructive inflammatory process characteristic of stage I PBC, **the small bile ducts virtually disappear, and scarring of medium-sized bile ducts is common.** Such scarring constitutes stage II disease. Chronic inflammation persists in the portal tracts but is not as severe as in stage I. The chronic inflammatory infiltrate, both in stage I and stage II, may spill over into the periportal parenchyma, disrupt the limiting plate, and create a ragged border between portal tracts and the hepatic parenchyma—an appearance that may be mistaken for chronic active hepatitis. The presence of large amounts of copper and occasional Mallory bodies in the peripheral zone of the lobule assists in the differentiation from chronic active hepatitis. **Proliferation of bile ductules within the portal tracts is usual and may be florid.** Relatively acellular collagenous septa extend from the portal tracts into the lobular parenchyma and begin to encircle some lobules. Cholestasis, when present, may be severe and is now located at the periphery of the portal tracts.

STAGE III: CIRRHOSIS: The disease terminates as **end-stage liver disease**—namely, cirrhosis—characterized by fibrous septa that encompass regenerative nodules. Grossly, the bile-stained liver is dark green and exhibits a fine nodularity. Microscopically, small bile ducts are scarce and medium-sized ducts are conspicuously reduced in number. There is little inflammation within either the fibrous septa or the parenchymal nodules.

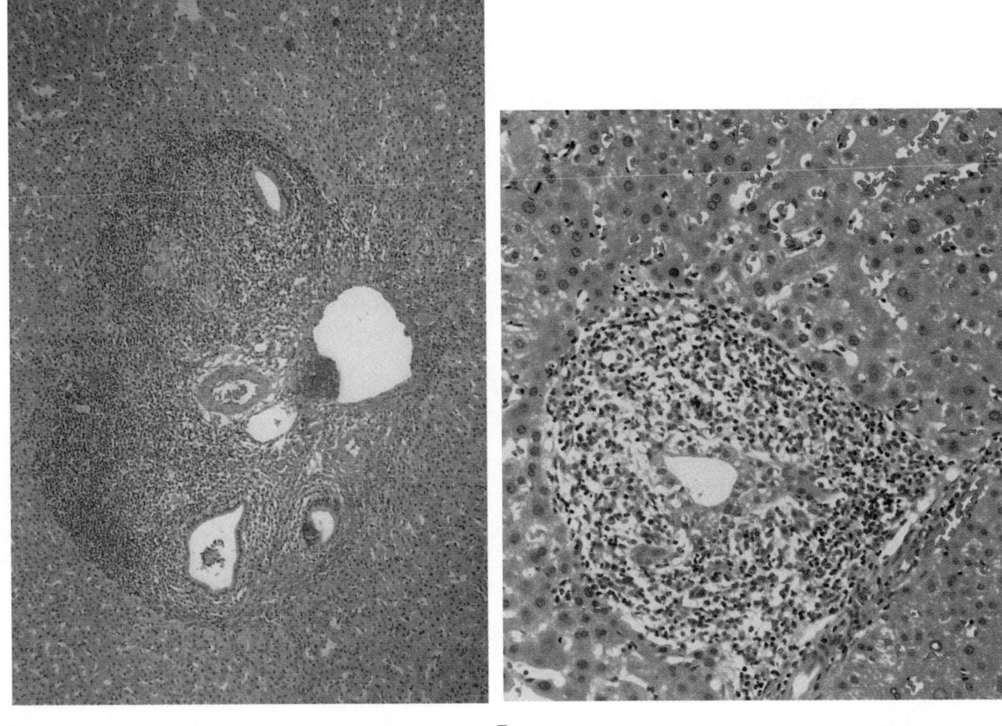

FIGURE *14-36*
Primary biliary cirrhosis (PBC), stage 1. (*A*) A photomicrograph shows that a large portal tract containing three bile ducts is expanded by a lymphocytic infiltrate. (*B*) A higher-power view of a liver biopsy from a patient with PBC displays a small bile duct with epithelial damage surrounded by a lymphoid infiltrate.

☐ Clinical Features: **Women, usually between 30 and 65 years of age, comprise some 90% to 95% of those afflicted with PBC.** In many patients, the initial symptoms are fatigue and pruritus without jaundice, although about one fifth of patients have jaundice when first seen. The cause of the severe pruritus is unknown, but it is relieved by oral treatment with resins (e.g., cholestyramine) that bind bile acids and other anions in the gut. On the other hand, a substantial proportion of patients with PBC have no symptoms during the early stages of the disease; some of these patients remain asymptomatic and appear to have an excellent prognosis, whereas others ultimately present with advanced cirrhosis and its complications.

In a typical case, a high serum alkaline phosphatase activity is accompanied by a normal or only slightly elevated serum bilirubin level. As the disease advances, most patients have a progressive increase in serum bilirubin level. Serum aminotransferase activities are only moderately elevated. The serum cholesterol level is strikingly increased, and an abnormal lipoprotein (lipoprotein-X) which is found in many forms of chronic cholestasis, appears. In the precirrhotic stages, most of the excess cholesterol is in the high-density lipoprotein fraction, a fact that may account for the rarity of atherosclerosis in these patients. Nevertheless, cholesterol-laden macrophages accumulate in the subcutaneous tissues, where they appear as localized lesions termed *xanthomas*. The impairment in the excretion of bile into the intestine often leads to severe **steatorrhea**, owing to fat malabsorption. Because of associated malabsorption of vitamin D and calcium, **osteomalacia** and **osteoporosis** are important complications of PBC. About one third of patients develop gallstones. Those patients who eventually develop cirrhosis die in hepatic failure or of the complications of **portal hypertension.**

Primary biliary cirrhosis generally pursues an indolent course. Patients who develop cirrhosis usually survive 10 to 15 years, whereas in those without symptoms, life expectancy may not be curtailed. Medical treatment of PBC with corticosteroids, immunosuppressive agents, and a variety of anti-inflammatory compounds has not convincingly shown a risk-to-benefit ratio that justifies the use of these drugs. By contrast, liver transplantation is highly effective in end-stage disease, with a 75% 1-year survival and a projected 5-year survival of over 65%.

PRIMARY SCLEROSING CHOLANGITIS

Primary sclerosing cholangitis (PSC) is a chronic cholestatic liver disease of unknown cause, in which an inflammatory and fibrosing process narrows and eventually obstructs the intrahepatic and extrahepatic bile ducts. The majority of patients are men younger than the age of 40 years. **Progressive biliary obstruction typically leads to persistent obstructive jaundice and eventually to secondary biliary cirrhosis.**

Although the cause of PSC is unknown, about two thirds of the patients also have ulcerative colitis. A few cases have been described in patients with Crohn disease of the colon. PSC has also been reported in association with retroperitoneal fibrosis, lymphoma, and the fibrosing variant of chronic thyroiditis (Riedel struma). In one fourth of the cases, no underlying disease is discerned.

Recent data suggest a possible role for genetic and immunological factors in the pathogenesis of PSC. The disease occasionally occurs in families and shows an association with certain HLA haplotypes, including HLA B8 and DR3. Hypergammaglobulinemia is common, as are circulating antineutrophil cytoplasmic antibodies (ANCA), immune complexes in the serum, and activation of the complement system by the classic pathway. The total number of circulating T cells is reduced, whereas the portal tracts exhibit an increased number of T cells. The ratio of CD4/CD8 lymphocytes in the blood is increased.

□ **Pathology:** The liver disease associated with PSC can be divided into four histological stages.

- **Stage I:** The initial lesion is periductal inflammation and fibrosis in the portal tracts (Fig. 14-37). The mucosa of the bile ducts remains normal, in contrast to early lesions of PBC.
- **Stage II:** Connective tissue extends into the periportal parenchyma, and chronic periductal inflammation is still present.
- **Stage III:** Many bile ducts become obliterated and fibrous septa extend into the parenchyma.
- **Stage IV:** Secondary biliary cirrhosis eventually develops.

Similar inflammatory and fibrotic changes may be seen in the large intrahepatic bile ducts and the extrahepatic biliary tree, where they lead to obstruction of the lumen and true extrahepatic biliary obstruction. Since the disease tends to be segmental, a characteristic beaded appearance of the intrahepatic biliary tree is noted by contrast radiography. The wall of the gallbladder is often thickened, presumably because it is affected by the same inflammatory process.

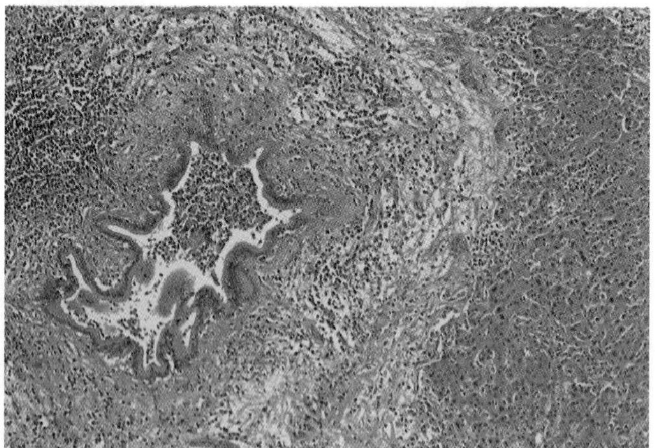

FIGURE *14-37*
Primary sclerosing cholangitis. A photomicrograph of a liver removed for hepatic transplantation shows an edematous, fibrotic, and chronically inflamed portal tract. Inflammatory debris is present within the lumen of the bile duct.

□ **Clinical Features:** Primary sclerosing cholangitis has a poor prognosis: the mean survival after the appearance of symptoms is 6 years. Cholangiocarcinoma has been reported to develop in as many as 10% of patients with primary sclerosing cholangitis. Surgical dilatation of the common bile duct, insertion of a stent, and biliary bypass operations have been successful in only a few cases. However, liver transplantation is curative.

CIRRHOSIS

The end stage of chronic liver disease is cirrhosis, defined as the destruction of the normal hepatic architecture by fibrous septa that encompass regenerative nodules of hepatocytes. This morphological pattern invariably results from persistent liver cell necrosis. Advanced cases of cirrhosis all tend to have a similar appearance, and often the cause can no longer be ascertained by morphological examination alone. During earlier stages, on the other hand, the characteristic features of the inciting pathogenic insult may be evident, as, for example, the fat and Mallory bodies typical of alcoholic liver injury or the chronic inflammation and periportal necrosis characteristic of chronic active hepatitis. Histological examination of the liver may also allow the diagnosis of PBC, extrahepatic biliary obstruction, α_1-antitrypsin deficiency, glycogen storage disease type IV, hemochromatosis, and chronic hepatic venous obstruction.

Morphological Classification

The number of terms applied to the different forms of cirrhosis rivals the number of causative agents incriminated in chronic liver disease. Out of this apparent complexity, we can extract a simple spectrum of nodular patterns. At one end of this spectrum, usually in the early evolution of cirrhosis, is the *micronodular* type, characterized by small, uniform nodules separated by thin fibrous septa (see Fig. 14-35). At the other end of the spectrum, ordinarily late in the course of the disease, is *macronodular cirrhosis,* in which grossly visible, coarse, irregular nodules are mirrored histologically by large nodules of varying size and shape that are encircled by bands of connective tissue (Fig. 14-38). These collagenous septa also vary conspicuously in width. Between these two extremes are many cases that show features of both types and for which the term *mixed cirrhosis* is appropriate.

MICRONODULAR CIRRHOSIS: This form of cirrhosis was previously termed *Laennec, portal, septal, or nutritional cirrhosis.* With the exception of the term *Laennec cirrhosis,* which honors the French physician who provided the first accurate description of this disease, these terms have little to recommend them, and the last is actually misleading.

Micronodular cirrhosis exhibits nodules scarcely larger than a lobule, measuring less than 3 mm in diameter. The micronodules show no landmarks of lobular ar-

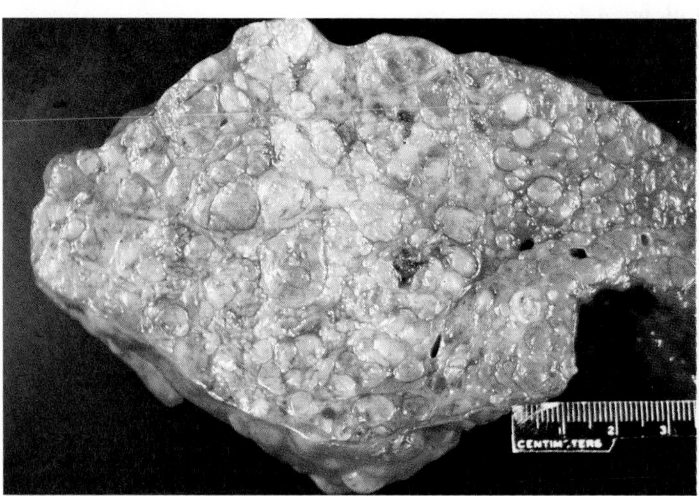

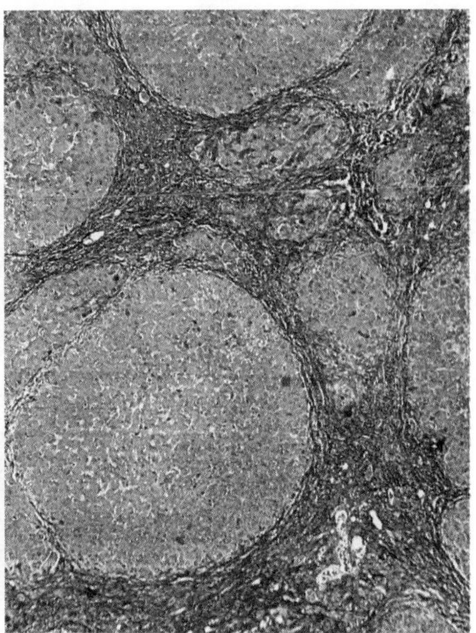

A B

FIGURE 14-38
Macronodular cirrhosis. (*A*) The liver is misshapen, and the cut surface reveals irregular nodules and connective tissue septa of varying width. (*B*) A photomicrograph shows nodules of varying size and irregular fibrous septa.

chitecture in the form of portal tracts or central venules. The connective tissue septa separating the nodules are usually thin, but irregular focal collapse of parenchyma may lead to the presence of wider septa. In active stages of the cirrhotic process, numerous mononuclear inflammatory cells and proliferated bile ductules inhabit the septa. The close approximation within the septa of capillaries and venules, fibroblasts, mononuclear inflammatory cells, and young connective tissue is similar to the appearance of granulation tissue in other organs. It is reasonable to assume that the same mechanisms that control the healing of wounds by granulation tissue in extrahepatic sites are also operative in the cirrhotic liver. The prototype of micronodular cirrhosis is alcoholic cirrhosis, but this pattern may also be observed in primary and secondary biliary cirrhosis, hemochromatosis, Wilson disease, chronic obstruction to the venous outflow of the liver (Budd-Chiari syndrome), and certain inherited metabolic disorders.

MACRONODULAR CIRRHOSIS: This morphological variety of cirrhosis was formerly labeled *postnecrotic, posthepatitic*, or *multilobular cirrhosis.* The large, irregular nodules often contain portal tracts and efferent venous channels, evidence that the original process was characterized by multilobular necrosis that healed with the formation of large scars surrounding more than a single lobule. **However, it is now recognized that the micronodular pattern can be converted into a macronodular one by continued regeneration and expansion of existing nodules.** This is particularly the case in alcoholics who abstain from drinking after the diagnosis of cirrhosis has been made. Given sufficient time, almost all (90%) cases of micronodular cirrhosis, even in those who continue to drink, will be converted to the macronodular pattern, usually within 2 to 3 years. The connective tissue septa in macronodular cirrhosis are characteristically broad and contain elements of preexisting portal tracts, mononuclear inflammatory cells, and proliferated bile ductules. In a variant, formerly termed *posthepatitic cirrhosis*, the macronodules are separated by slender strands of connective tissue that join widely separated portal tracts. Macronodular cirrhosis is classically associated with chronic active hepatitis. It is also occasionally a result of submassive hepatic necrosis, in which case the liver may be grossly misshapen.

TABLE *14-3* **Causes of Cirrhosis**

Alcoholic liver disease
Chronic active hepatitis
Primary biliary cirrhosis
Extrahepatic biliary obstruction
Hemochromatosis
Wilson disease
Cystic fibrosis
α_1-Antitrypsin deficiency
Glycogen storage disease, types III and IV
Galactosemia
Hereditary fructose intolerance
Tyrosinemia
Hereditary storage diseases: Gaucher, Niemann-Pick, Wolman, mucopolysaccharidoses
Zellweger syndrome
Indian childhood cirrhosis

☐ **Pathogenesis:** The diseases associated with cirrhosis are listed in Table 14-3. It is clear that they have little in common, except for the fact that they are all accompanied by persistent liver cell necrosis. Most cases of cirrhosis are attributable to alcoholism and chronic viral hepatitis, although a significant contribution from unexplained chronic active hepatitis is a factor. The following discussion will focus on less common causes of cirrhosis.

EXTRAHEPATIC BILIARY OBSTRUCTION

The extrahepatic biliary system may be obstructed by a number of lesions. These include gallstones passing through the cystic duct to lodge in the common bile duct, cancer of the bile duct or surrounding tissues (pancreas or ampulla of Vater), external compression by enlarged neoplastic lymph nodes in the porta hepatis (as in Hodgkin disease), benign strictures (postoperative scarring or primary sclerosing cholangitis), and congenital biliary atresia (Fig. 14-39).

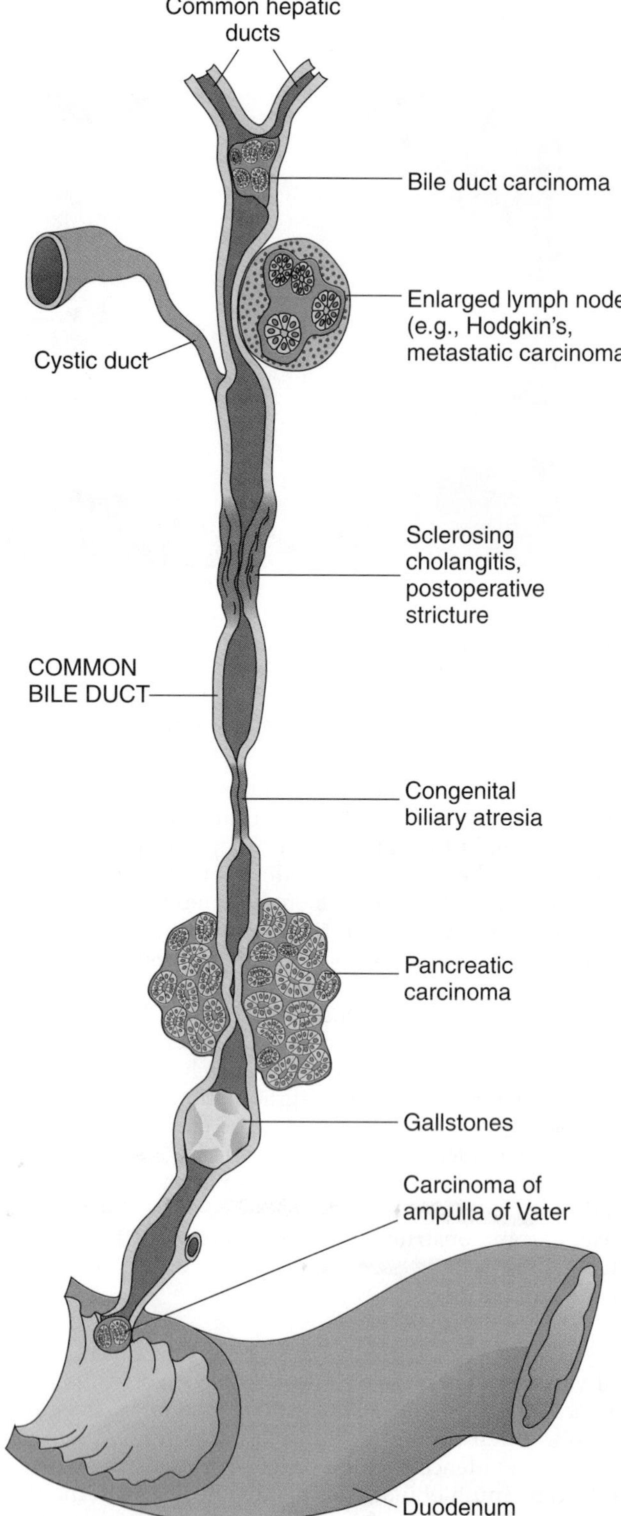

FIGURE *14-39*
Major causes of extrahepatic biliary obstruction.

☐ **Pathology:** Early in the precirrhotic stage of extrahepatic biliary obstruction, the liver is swollen and bile stained. In prolonged obstruction, the bile becomes almost colorless ("white bile"), because of the suppression of the secretion of bilirubin, although the liver remains green. Initially, centrilobular cholestasis is accompanied by edema of the portal tracts, and in biopsy specimens early extrahepatic obstruction is difficult to differentiate from the various forms of intrahepatic cholestasis. As obstruction proceeds, mononuclear inflammatory cells infiltrate the portal tracts. Tortuous and distended bile ductules, characterized by a high cuboidal epithelium, proliferate (Fig. 14-40). These stand in contrast to the bile ductules seen in other chronic liver diseases, in which the cells are flattened. The cholestasis eventually extends to the periphery of the lobule. Dilated bile ducts may rupture, leading to the formation of *bile lakes* (see Fig. 14-10), a feature diagnostic of extrahepatic biliary obstruction. Bile lakes appear as focal, golden-yellow deposits that are surrounded by degenerating hepatocytes. Leakage of bile into the portal tracts also causes the appearance of foamy, lipid-laden macrophages, often aggregated as *granulomas*. Damaged hepatocytes containing large amounts of bile show a characteristic reticulated cytoplasm, termed *feathery degeneration*. Single-cell necrosis within the lobules is common, and periportal necrosis, associated with the portal inflammatory reaction, may be prominent. Infection of the obstructed biliary passages often leads to a superimposed suppurative cholangitis, intraluminal pus, and even intrahepatic abscesses. Within bile ducts and proliferated ductules, biliary concretions may be conspicuous, again a diagnostic feature of extrahepatic biliary obstruction.

With time, the portal tracts become enlarged and fibrotic. Typically, the *periductal fibrosis* is concentric, giving rise to the term *onion-skin fibrosis*. As in other forms of cirrhosis characterized by periportal necrosis, in 10% of cases of prolonged extrahepatic biliary obstruction, septa eventually extend between the portal tracts of contiguous lobules and form a **micronodular cirrhosis**. In the early stage of this cirrhotic phase, the portal-to-portal linkage distinguishes this disease from the portal-to-central pattern typical of alcoholic cirrhosis or from that of macron-

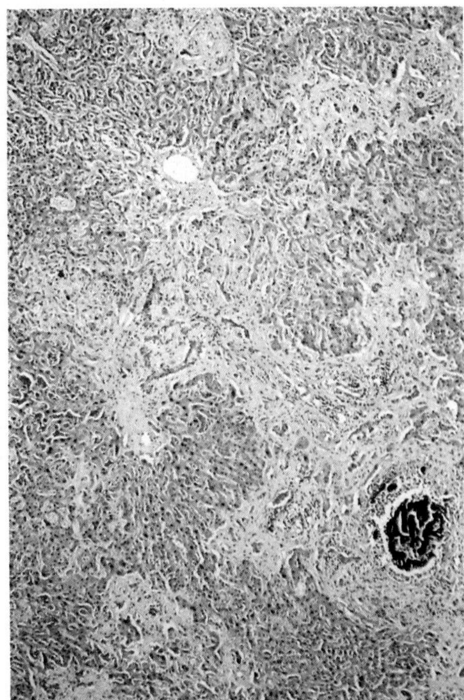

FIGURE 14-40
Secondary biliary cirrhosis. A photomicrograph of the liver from a patient with a carcinoma of the pancreas that obstructed the common bile duct. Irregular fibrous septa extend from an enlarged portal tract (*lower right*), containing a dilated interlobular bile duct, which encloses a dense biliary concretion. Numerous proliferated bile ductules are seen within the septa.

odular cirrhosis. However, in the late stage of extrahepatic biliary obstruction, further alterations make the distinction difficult.

IRON OVERLOAD SYNDROMES

A number of conditions are characterized by the excessive accumulation of iron in the body (siderosis). There is no major physiological mechanism for the excretion of iron. Therefore, iron overload results either from inordinate intestinal absorption of iron or from its parenteral administration. Iron overload is divided into two major categories based on the etiology of the increased body iron. **Hereditary hemochromatosis** is caused by a common genetic alteration in the control of the intestinal absorption of iron. **Secondary iron overload** is a condition that (1) complicates certain hematological disorders; (2) is associated with parenteral iron overload, in which the iron is obtained from multiple blood transfusions or the parenteral administration of iron itself; or (3) is caused by an enormous dietary intake of iron.

Iron Metabolism

The body of a normal man contains 3 to 4 g of iron, two thirds of which is present in hemoglobin, myoglobin, and iron-containing enzymes. The remainder is represented by storage iron, which exists in two forms, namely, soluble ferritin and insoluble hemosiderin. **Ferritin**, the primary iron storage protein, is present in the cytoplasm of all cells and, in small amounts, in the circulation. **Hemosiderin** is a product of the degradation of ferritin but, unlike the latter, is visualized by light microscopy as golden-yellow granules that stain with the Prussian blue reaction. The liver is an important organ for the storage of iron, although a comparable amount of storage iron exists in the bone marrow.

The absorption of iron from the gastrointestinal tract is controlled by the need to maintain appropriate iron stores. Thus, in the face of iron deficiency, small-intestinal absorption of iron increases, whereas when body stores of iron are adequate, iron absorption is relatively constant. The obligatory daily iron loss through the urine and desquamated cells of the gut and skin is about 1 mg in men. Women suffer extra losses during menstruation and pregnancy. The possible range of daily iron absorption is from less than 0.5 mg in the person with a normal iron balance to an upper limit of 4 mg in those with iron deficiency. Dietary ascorbate is important in iron absorption, because ferric iron in the diet is reduced by ascorbic acid to ferrous iron, the form in which it can be absorbed by the small intestine. The absence of dietary vitamin C significantly decreases the amount of iron that can be absorbed.

It is thought that iron absorption by the enterocyte is facilitated by a membrane iron-binding protein distinct from the transferrin receptor. In the blood, most of the iron is bound to transferrin, but a lesser amount circulates bound to another protein(s). Iron is then transferred to all cells of the body through the transferrin receptor and, to a lesser extent, by the uptake of non–transferrin bound iron.

Hereditary Hemochromatosis

Hereditary hemochromatosis (HHC) is a common autosomal recessive disorder of iron metabolism characterized by excessive iron absorption and the toxic accumulation of iron in parenchymal cells, particularly of the liver, heart, and pancreas. In this disease, 20 to 40 g of iron (i.e., up to 10 times the normal content) accumulates in the body. The excess iron in HHC is located exclusively within the storage compartment, and thus iron stores are increased up to 50 times normal. **The clinical hallmarks of advanced HHC are cirrhosis, diabetes, skin pigmentation, and cardiac failure** (Fig. 14-41). The disease is most often manifested clinically in patients between 40 and 60 years of age, and men are afflicted 10 times as often as women. This striking male predilection may be attributed to the increased loss of iron in women during the reproductive years. However, given sufficient time to absorb additional iron, postmenopausal women also seem to be at risk for the development of hemochromatosis. Since maximum daily iron absorption is about 4 mg, it is clear that hemochromatosis takes years to develop.

☐ **Pathogenesis:** HHC is inherited as an **autosomal recessive** disorder. Although only a few families have been reported in which more than one member has hemochromatosis, lesser degrees of iron overload are often found in relatives of those with the disease.

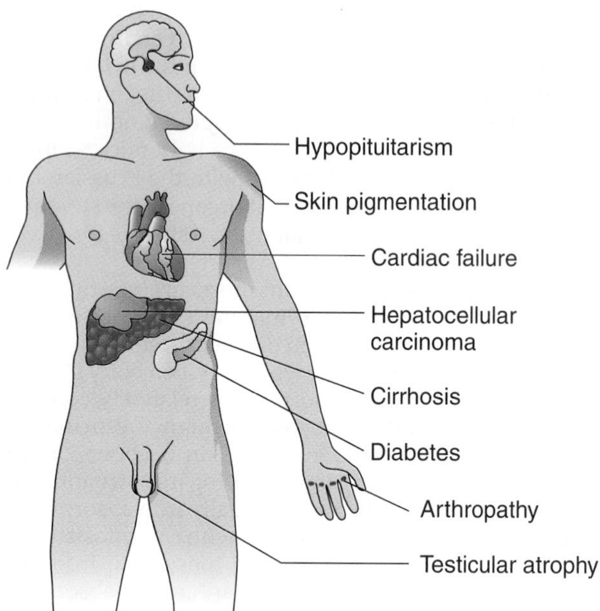

FIGURE *14-41*
Complications of hemochromatosis.

The HHC gene is located on the short arm of chromosome 6. There is a linkage between this gene and the HLA locus of the human major histocompatibility complex (MHC). The HLA-A3 antigen is present in 70% of persons with HHC but in only 25% of the normal population. Recently, a 250-kb region telomeric to the MHC locus on chromosome 6 has been sequenced and a novel MHC class I–like gene, termed HLA-H, was found to be mutated in 83% of all patients with HHC. The mechanism by which the product of the HLA-H gene regulates iron metabolism is not as yet understood.

It is now apparent that the HHC gene is far more common than previously suspected. It has been estimated that in white populations the heterozygous frequency is about 11% and that 1 person in every 220 is homozygous. Not all patients who exhibit this genetically determined increase in iron absorption develop hemochromatosis. Thus, only 1 in 400 persons develops clinically apparent hemochromatosis.

An increased uptake of iron by the duodenal mucosa has been documented as the most likely mechanism underlying the increased deposition of iron in parenchymal organs in HHC. The pathway by which increased iron absorption is accomplished has not been fully elucidated. An attractive hypothesis holds that there is increased expression of the iron-binding protein in the enterocyte. As a result, the transfer of iron across the mucosal cell is accelerated, leading to an increased concentration of non–transferrin bound iron in the blood. At the same time, the amount of the same iron binding protein is increased in the organs that accumulate iron in hemochromatosis, such as the liver, heart, and pancreas. The result is increased uptake of non–transferrin bound iron by these organs.

The pathogenesis of the cell injury that results from the excessive intracellular iron is not fully understood. However, as noted in Chapter 1, iron is an essential factor in the cell injury mediated by activated oxygen species. It is reasonable to speculate that the presence of excess iron in cells renders them more susceptible to injury by partially reduced oxygen species generated during the normal metabolism of oxygen.

□ Pathology: **HHC is characterized pathologically by the accumulation of very large amounts of iron in the parenchymal cells of a variety of organs and tissues.**

THE LIVER: The liver is always affected in HHC. It contains more than 0.5 g iron per 100 g wet weight and is usually cirrhotic. The liver is enlarged and reddish brown and exhibits a uniform micronodular cirrhosis. In most respects, the pattern is similar to that of alcoholic cirrhosis, which may explain the occasional confusion in the differentiation of these entities when alcoholic cirrhosis is accompanied by superimposed iron accumulation. The hepatocytes and bile duct epithelium are filled with iron granules, and lipofuscin pigment is increased (Fig. 14-42A,B). The excess cellular iron is stored predominantly in lysosomes in the ferric form. Late in the disease, many Kupffer cells contain large deposits of iron derived from the phagocytosis of necrotic hepatocytes. Within the fibrous septa, iron is conspicuous in proliferated bile ductules and macrophages. Eventually, as in micronodular cirrhosis of other causes, the pattern is transformed to that of a macronodular cirrhosis.

SKIN: The skin in patients with HHC is typically pigmented, but only half of the patients exhibit increased iron deposition in the skin. Most patients display increased melanin in the basal melanocytes. The accumulation of hemosiderin pigment is particularly severe in the sweat glands.

PANCREAS: Diabetes, a common complication of hemochromatosis, results from the deposition of iron in the pancreas (see Fig. 14-42C). Grossly, the organ appears rust colored and is firm, reflecting underlying fibrosis. Both the exocrine and endocrine cells are affected, particularly the former. Frequently, there is degeneration of acinar cells and a reduction in the number of islets of Langerhans. The combination of pigmented skin and glucose intolerance in patients with HHC is often referred to as *bronze diabetes*.

FIGURE *14-42*
Hemochromatosis. (*A*) A Prussian blue stain demonstrates considerable iron in a nodule of a cirrhotic liver. (*B*) A higher-power view of the liver in (*A*) shows iron in the bile duct epithelial cells. (*C*) Iron accumulation in a pancreatic islet of Langerhans and (*D*) in the myocardium.

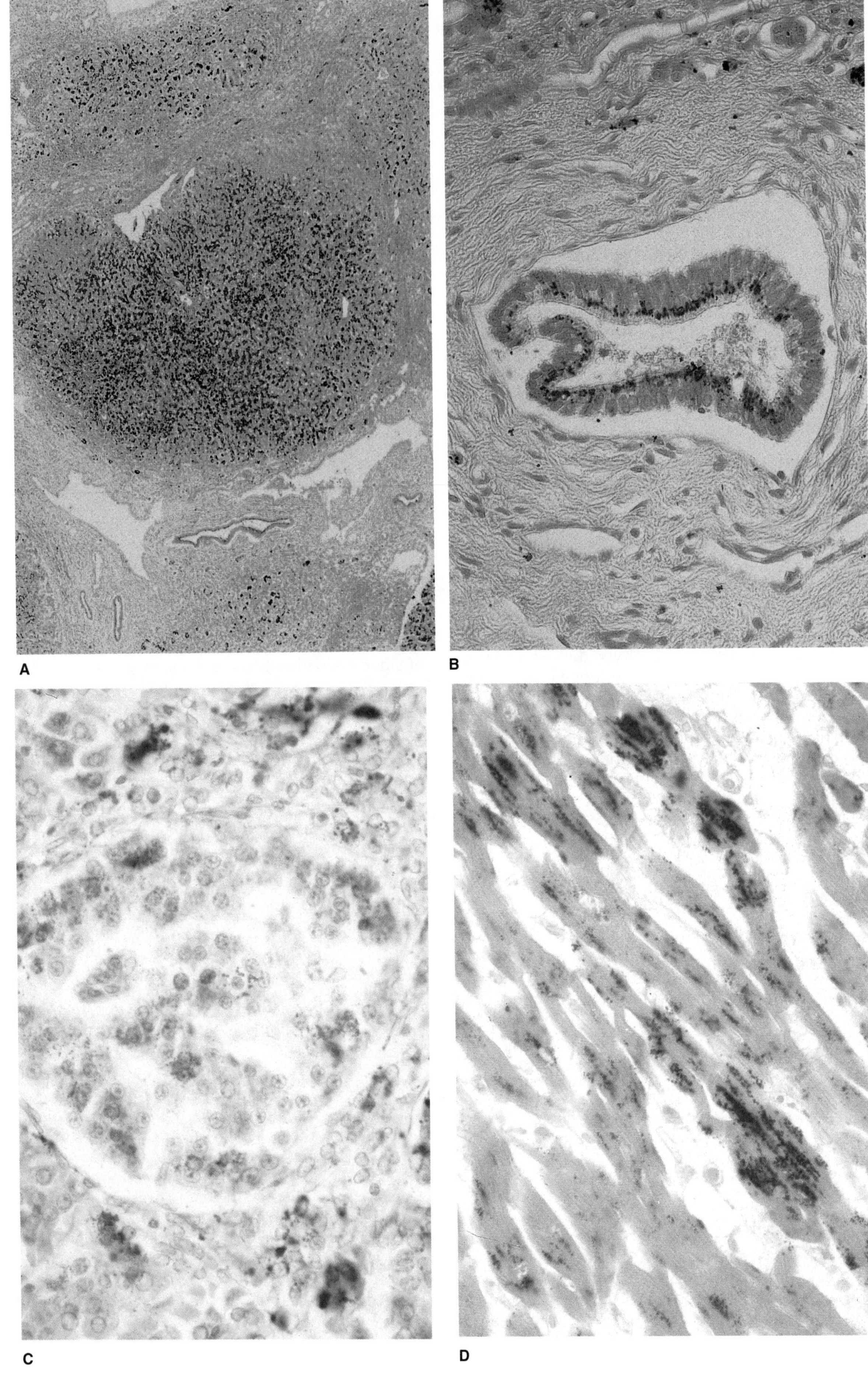

FIGURE **14-42**

HEART: Congestive heart failure is a common cause of death in patients with hemochromatosis. The heart is often enlarged, sometimes weighing more than twice normal. Microscopically, the myocardial fibers contain iron pigment (see Fig. 14-42D), which is more extensive in the ventricles than in the atria. Necrosis of cardiac myocytes and accompanying interstitial fibrosis are common.

ENDOCRINE SYSTEM: Numerous endocrine glands are typically involved in hemochromatosis. Iron is deposited in the pituitary, adrenal, thyroid, and parathyroid glands. However, tissue damage is not a usual feature in these organs, except for the pituitary, in which the release of gonadotropins is impaired. As a result, testicular atrophy is seen in a fourth of the male patients, even without iron deposition in the testes. The disturbance in the pituitary–gonadal axis is characterized by loss of libido and amenorrhea in women and impotence and sparse body hair in men. These effects are often manifested well before the onset of symptoms of liver disease.

JOINTS: Arthropathy, most severe in the fingers and hands, occurs in 25% to 75% of patients with HHC and is sometimes the initial symptom. When arthritis affects the larger joints, such as the knee, it may be severe enough to be disabling. Although deposits of hemosiderin may be seen in the synovium and articular cartilage, the pathogenesis of the arthritis is unclear.

□ **Clinical Features:** The liver disease in HHC generally pursues an indolent and prolonged course, but a fourth of patients eventually die in hepatic coma or from gastrointestinal hemorrhage. **Hepatocellular carcinoma is a significant late complication of hemochromatosis-induced cirrhosis.** In fact, among patients with cirrhosis, the 10-year cumulative probability of developing liver cancer is as high as 30%. By contrast, noncirrhotic patients with HHC treated by phlebotomy are not at increased risk of hepatocellular carcinoma.

Laboratory Diagnosis

The normal value for plasma iron is 80 to 100 g/dL, and transferrin is normally about one third saturated. In patients with HHC, the serum iron concentration is more than doubled, and transferrin is entirely saturated. The concentration of circulating transferrin, like that of other proteins whose synthesis is impaired in chronic liver disease, is reduced. The concentration of ferritin in the blood, which parallels the amount of storage iron, is greatly increased in hemochromatosis. Urinary excretion of iron after the administration of an iron chelator (deferoxamine) is a useful diagnostic test.

Treatment

The treatment of HHC is based on the removal of iron from the body, most effectively by repeated phlebotomy. Weekly phlebotomies for 2 to 3 years can remove 20 to 40 g of iron, after which phlebotomies every 2 to 3 months maintain iron balance. The beneficial effect of repeated phlebotomies is impressive. In homozygotes who have neither cirrhosis nor diabetes, iron depletion results in a life expectancy identical to that of the general population. By contrast, the 10-year survival of untreated patients with HHC is a mere 6%.

Secondary Iron Overload Syndromes

Many of the features of HHC may also occur in persons who do not carry the gene for that disease.

□ **Pathogenesis:** Within certain limits, the amount of iron absorbed bears a relation to the amount of iron ingested. For example, a low iron content in the diet renders the development of hemochromatosis unlikely. Whether excess dietary iron can produce iron overload in a normal person is still debated. Many patients with secondary iron overload (up to 40%) have a long history of **alcohol abuse**, and it is thought that alcohol may enhance both the accumulation of iron and its associated cell injury. The possible mechanisms are not clear, but the high iron content of many alcoholic beverages, the increased iron absorption in some patients with cirrhosis, and a putative synergism between two hepatotoxins (i.e., alcohol and iron) have been suggested.

An interesting example of secondary hemochromatosis is presented by the well-recognized iron accumulation in blacks of sub-Saharan Africa, commonly misnamed *Bantu siderosis*. These populations show a high incidence of siderosis without tissue damage, presumably because of the consumption of large amounts of iron-containing alcoholic beverages. A small proportion of these populations show both severe siderosis and tissue injury, an appearance similar to that of hereditary hemochromatosis. With the recent replacement of "home-brewed" beverages (of low alcoholic but high iron content) by Western spirits (of higher alcohol but lower iron content), the incidence of siderosis has fallen while that of alcoholic cirrhosis has increased. Thus, under some conditions, excess dietary iron appears to play a role in the development of secondary iron overload, although the contributions of other exogenous and genetic factors have not been fully elucidated.

Massive iron overload occurs in patients with certain anemias, such as thalassemia major, sideroblastic anemias, and other anemias associated with ineffective erythropoiesis. As a result, secondary iron overload may develop even in children and adolescents. The source of the excess iron is the patient's diet or transfused blood. Increased iron absorption occurs despite the saturation of transferrin; the release of iron by intravascular hemolysis adds a further burden of iron. It is important to note that patients with thalassemia often develop secondary iron overload whether or not they have received blood transfusions. On the other hand, multiple blood transfusions alone are generally insufficient to produce secondary iron overload, even in patients with hypoplastic anemia given many transfusions (250 mg iron/500 mL unit of blood). In these patients, iron is concentrated principally in mononuclear phagocytes, and cirrhosis is rare.

The causes of iron overload are summarized in Table 14-4.

TABLE *14-4* **Causes of Iron Overload**

Increased Iron Absorption
Hereditary hemochromatosis
Chronic liver disease
Iron-loading anemias
Porphyria cutanea tarda
Congenital diseases (e.g., atransferrinemia)
Dietary iron overload (Bantu siderosis)
Excess medicinal iron
Parenteral Iron Overload
Multiple blood transfusions
Injectable medicinal iron
Focal Iron Overload
Idiopathic pulmonary hemosiderosis
Renal hemosiderosis

☐ **Pathology:** Cirrhosis with secondary iron overload shows varying degrees of iron accumulation, but iron deposition in the liver is generally less extensive than that in HHC and is often restricted to the periphery of the nodules. The absence of iron deposition in the septa suggests that the cirrhosis preceded the iron accumulation. Transfusional and other types of siderosis are characterized by the uniform, initial deposition of iron in Kupffer cells, with eventual spillover into the hepatocytes.

HERITABLE DISORDERS ASSOCIATED WITH CIRRHOSIS

Wilson Disease (Hepatolenticular Degeneration)

Wilson disease (WD) is an autosomal recessive disorder of copper metabolism in which injury to the liver and brain is associated with deposition of excess copper. The carrier rate is in the vicinity of 1 in 100, and the incidence of clinical disease is about 30 per million, with a slight predilection for males. The gene appears to have a worldwide distribution.

☐ **Pathogenesis:** The WD gene on chromosome 13 encodes a copper-transporting ATPase. It is 70% homologous with the gene responsible for Menke disease, an X-linked neurological and connective tissue disorder characterized by congenital copper deficiency. A variety of distinct mutations in the WD gene have been identified in patients with WD.

In the fetus, most of the body copper is contained in the liver, principally in lysosomes and bound to metallothionien. After birth, the hepatic copper concentration falls, and by age 3 months the liver copper reaches adult concentrations (about 8% of total body copper). The daily copper requirement for the normal adult is between 1 and 2 mg. Since the intake of copper in the diet is ordinarily considerably greater, copper balance is easily maintained.

Unlike iron absorption, body copper homeostasis is not regulated at the level of the intestine. Copper absorbed from the intestine is bound to albumin and amino acids and transported to the liver. Within the hepatocyte, copper is (1) utilized for the synthesis of copper-containing enzymes (e.g., cytochrome oxidase and superoxide dismutase); (2) bound to metallothionien for storage in lysosomes; (3) complexed with the copper-binding protein ceruloplasmin for return to the blood; and (4) excreted into the bile. Biliary excretion of copper is the primary mechanism by which body copper balance is maintained, since negligible amounts of copper are reabsorbed by the intestine. **As a result, copper accumulates in the liver during prolonged cholestasis from any cause, such as, for example, primary biliary cirrhosis or extrahepatic biliary obstruction.** Between 90% and 95% of circulating copper is bound to ceruloplasmin, from which it is made available to peripheral tissue as well as returned to the liver.

Wilson disease is characterized by a striking reduction in the serum levels of ceruloplasmin. However, this deficiency is thought to be secondary to hepatic copper overload and does not explain the pathogenesis of WD.

It is now clear that intestinal absorption of copper is unaltered in WD. On the other hand, biliary, and therefore fecal, excretion of copper is reduced to about one fourth of the normal rate. It has been argued that the WD protein is responsible for excretion of copper from the hepatocyte into the bile canaliculus.

The similarity between copper metabolism in WD and that in the fetus is interesting, in that both are characterized by low concentrations of copper and ceruloplasmin in the blood and high levels in the liver. In the early stages of WD, the copper content of the liver is 30 to 50 times normal. It has been suggested that the transition from fetal to adult copper metabolism is regulated by the WD gene, which controls copper excretion from the liver cell. In any event, the primacy of the liver as the seat of WD is attested to by its cure with liver transplantation.

Although the total serum copper concentration is low in WD, the fraction not bound to ceruloplasmin (albumin-bound or free copper) is greater than normal, both relatively and absolutely. It is possible that this increased concentration of free copper plays a role in the excess deposition of copper in extrahepatic tissues.

The mechanism by which excess copper injures cells remains elusive. Like iron, copper may catalyze the formation of potent oxidizing species from superoxide anions and hydrogen peroxide produced by normal oxygen metabolism. In this regard, copper can replace iron in the Fenton reaction, in which ferrous iron and hydrogen peroxide generate hydroxyl radicals (see Chapter 1).

☐ **Pathology:** The initial alterations in the liver of children are nonspecific and include mild to moderate fat accumulation, lipofuscin deposition, and glycogen in the nuclei of hepatocytes. Subsequently, the disease progresses from mild to severe **chronic hepatitis**, with all of the typical histological features of that disease. The periportal hepatocytes often contain Mallory bodies, and cholestasis, with bile casts in proliferated bile ductules, is not infrequent. Occasional acidophilic bodies may be present. Kupffer cells are enlarged and contain hemosiderin, derived from phagocytosis during episodes of intravascular hemolysis. **Cirrhosis may develop rapidly, even in childhood.** An initial micronodular cirrhosis eventually assumes a macronodular pattern. **In young adults, the presence of fat, Mallory bodies, hepatocellular necrosis, and cholestasis may lead to an erroneous diagnosis of alcoholic liver disease.** By electron microscopy, the hepatocytes exhibit large, distorted mitochondria and numerous vacuolated and enlarged lysosomes.

The staining of the liver with rubeanic acid or rhodanine demonstrates copper granules in hepatocytes in some patients; most cases do not stain positively, however, even when hepatic copper concentrations are high. Copper stains are also positive in cholestatic states and neonatal livers, in which hepatic copper levels are also high. Chemical measurement of liver copper in unfixed tissue from livers of patients with WD demonstrates more than 250 μg of copper per gram of dry weight.

In the brain, the corpus striatum and occasionally the subthalamic nuclei display a reddish-brown discoloration. The central white matter of the cerebral or cerebellar hemispheres may manifest spongy softening or cavitation, in which case the overlying cortex is atrophic. The astrocytes proliferate in the putamen, and the number of neurons is decreased.

□ **Clinical Features:** Half of the patients with WD display some symptoms by adolescence, and the remainder become ill in their early adult years. A few instances have been recorded in which the disease did not become apparent until middle age. The presenting symptoms are referable to chronic liver disease in about half the patients, whereas one third initially present with neurological complaints and about one tenth are seen because of psychiatric manifestations. One fourth of the patients show symptoms related both to the liver and to the central nervous system.

LIVER: The liver disease begins insidiously with nonspecific symptoms and progresses to chronic liver disease indistinguishable from that of other forms of chronic hepatitis. WD should, therefore, be included in the differential diagnosis of chronic hepatitis. Eventually, chronic hepatitis and cirrhosis result in jaundice, portal hypertension, and hepatic failure. Unlike hemochromatosis, WD is not associated with an increased risk of primary hepatocellular carcinoma.

BRAIN: The neurological disease begins with mild incoordination and tremors. In untreated cases, dysarthria and dysphagia appear, and in late stages, disabling dystonia and spasticity occur. Progressive behavioral abnormalities and dementia may lead to the institutionalization of patients before the diagnosis of WD becomes evident.

EYE: Ophthalmic manifestations invariably accompany the neurological disease. *Kayser-Fleischer ring* is a golden-brown, bilateral discoloration of the cornea that encircles the periphery of the iris and obscures its muscular pattern (Fig. 14-43). It represents a deposition of copper in Descemet membrane. This ophthalmic sign is not

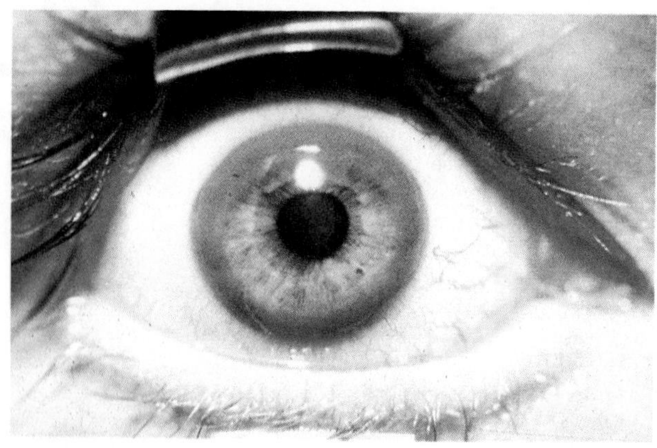

FIGURE *14-43*
Kayser-Fleischer ring. The deposition of copper in Descemet membrane is reflected in a peripheral brown color, which obstructs the view of the underlying iris.

diagnostic of WD unless it is accompanied by neurological disease. Kayser-Fleischer rings may be absent in patients with WD who suffer only from hepatic disease and in presymptomatic children. Corneal rings may also be present in other cholestatic liver diseases characterized by copper accumulation, including primary biliary cirrhosis, biliary atresia, and chronic active hepatitis with cirrhosis. In some patients, Kayser-Fleischer rings are accompanied by *sunflower cataracts*, which are green disks of copper deposition in the anterior capsule of the lens.

BONES: Skeletal lesions are commonly found on radiographic examination. They include osteomalacia, osteoporosis, spontaneous fractures, and various arthropathies. Clinical symptoms of bone disease are less common but are occasionally the presenting complaint.

KIDNEY: Renal glomerular and tubular dysfunction, manifested by proteinuria, lowered glomerular filtration, aminoaciduria, and phosphaturia, is common in WD. Although it was proposed that the aminoaciduria represents a primary gene defect in WD, it is now thought to be secondary to copper deposition in the renal tubules. This concept is supported by the observation that the renal disease disappears with removal of excess copper by chelating agents.

BLOOD: Transient acute hemolytic episodes, presumably related to a sudden release of free copper from the liver, occur in as many as 15% of patients with WD. This hematological complication commonly precedes the development of overt liver disease, and, therefore, WD should be included in the differential diagnosis of nonimmune hemolytic anemia in young persons. With the development of severe liver disease, hypersplenism and coagulation defects often supervene.

Treatment of WD not only prevents the accumulation of tissue copper but also extracts copper that has already been deposited. d-Penicillamine, a copper-chelating agent, augments the excretion of copper in the urine. Both central nervous system dysfunction and the symptoms of liver disease are often reversed by treatment. When d-penicillamine treatment is initiated during the early, asymptomatic phase, the clinical disease is entirely prevented. Patients who do not tolerate d-penicillamine can be treated with another copper chelator, triethylene tetramine. Liver transplantation has been effective in a number of cases of fulminant liver disease associated with WD.

Cystic Fibrosis

Historically, cystic fibrosis was almost invariably fatal in childhood, as a result of repeated pulmonary infections and respiratory insufficiency. However, the advent of antibiotic therapy and techniques for respiratory toilet have allowed many patients to survive into adult life. Concomitantly, hepatic complications of cystic fibrosis have become far more common. Cystic fibrosis is discussed in detail in Chapter 6.

Newborns with cystic fibrosis may present with obstructive jaundice within the first few weeks of life. Biliary obstruction results from the accumulation of tenacious mucous plugs in the intrahepatic biliary tree, and in that sense it is analogous to the meconium ileus found in half of these patients. Recovery typically occurs in 1 to 6 months, but some infants die in hepatic failure.

In children who survive to adolescence, clinically symptomatic liver disease develops in as many as 15%, and cirrhosis is found in 10% of patients who survive beyond the age of 25 years. The pattern of cirrhosis closely resembles that seen with extrahepatic biliary obstruction, but the lesions characteristically are focally accentuated in different parts of the liver. Cirrhosis is assumed to result from the obstruction of fine biliary passages by inspissated mucus. The interlobular bile ducts are focally dilated and contain eosinophilic, PAS-positive material. Portal hypertension and splenomegaly may accompany the cirrhosis and may indeed be the basis of the presenting complaints.

α_1-Antitrypsin Deficiency

The liver disease associated with α_1-antitrypsin (α_1-AT) deficiency is characterized by the accumulation of the mutant α_1-AT in hepatocytes and the development of chronic hepatitis and cirrhosis in early childhood. α_1-AT deficiency is inherited as an autosomal recessive trait and was initially described as a cause of emphysema (see Chapter 12). Thereafter, cases of liver disease without pulmonary involvement were described, and disease of both organs has also been recognized.

In infants and children, α_1-AT deficiency is the most common genetic cause of liver disease and is the most frequent genetic disease for which liver transplantation is indicated. Although the disorder is found in 1 out of 2000 live births, only 10% to 15% of those affected develop liver injury.

☐ **Pathogenesis:** α_1-AT is synthesized in the liver, and both the pulmonary and hepatic disorders result from a defect in the secretion of the mutant protein from the liver. The α_1-AT gene locus is termed *Pi*, and over 75 variants have been identified. The two most frequent variants associated with a deficiency of the circulating levels of this inhibitory protein are designated *PiS* and *PiZ*. In the PiS variant, the major defect most likely results from an aberrant splice site (introduced by the responsible point mutation) that results in the incorrect processing of mRNA transcripts. By contrast, the substitution of a lysine for a glutamate in the PiZ variant causes the mutant protein to fold abnormally and accumulate as an insoluble aggregate within the lumen of the endoplasmic reticulum of the hepatocyte. Although the precise mechanism of liver cell injury remains controversial, the accumulation of abnormal α_1-AT is the most likely culprit.

☐ **Pathology:** **The characteristic feature in the liver of patients with α_1-AT deficiency is the presence of faintly eosinophilic, PAS-positive cytoplasmic droplets** (Fig. 14-44). These tend to be small in infancy, but they may reach the size of the nucleus in older patients. By electron microscopy, these inclusions are visualized as amorphous material within dilated cisternae of the endoplasmic reticulum. Since cytoplasmic globules resembling those in α_1-AT deficiency are occasionally encountered in other disorders, a definitive diagnosis is made by demonstrating their reactivity with antibody to α_1-AT.

α_1-Antitrypsin deficiency is a cause of neonatal hepatitis and cannot be distinguished morphologically from other forms of neonatal hepatitis or from chronic active hepatitis. As in neonatal hepatitis from other causes, hepatocellular giant cells are prominent in some cases and often disappear within 6 to 12 months. Canalicular cholestasis is frequently striking. In infancy, conspicuous proliferation of bile ductules and fibrosis may lead to an erroneous diagnosis of extrahepatic biliary atresia. The increasing portal fibrosis is accompanied by a decrease in the number of bile ducts, again confusing the diagnosis with intrahepatic biliary atresia. **Micronodular cirrhosis**

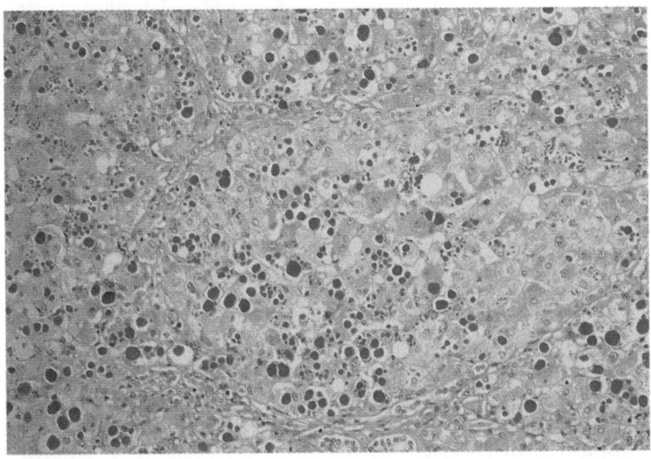

FIGURE *14-44*
α_1-Antitrypsin deficiency. A photomicrograph of a section of liver stained by the periodic acid–Schiff (PAS) reaction shows the presence of numerous cytoplasmic globules in the hepatocytes.

develops by the age of 2 to 3 years in these children and may ultimately become macronodular.

☐ **Clinical Features:** The clinical expression of liver disease in α_1-AT deficiency is highly variable, ranging from a rapidly fatal neonatal hepatitis to an absence of any hepatic dysfunction. **Of those infants with the ZZ genotype—that is, those who are susceptible to the development of clinical disease—about 10% develop neonatal cholestatic jaundice (conjugated hyperbilirubinemia).** This condition is far more common than previously recognized and accounts for 15% to 30% of all cases of neonatal conjugated hyperbilirubinemia. Most infants recover within 6 months, but a few progress to cirrhosis within 1 or 2 years. Moreover, about half of the patients with the ZZ phenotype have other intermittent abnormalities of liver function, and 10% to 20% develop permanent liver disease. Children with cirrhosis usually die before the age of 10 years from hepatic failure or other complications of α_1-AT deficiency. However, liver transplantation is curative.

Some children manifest hepatic dysfunction but develop cirrhosis only slowly. These patients may be asymptomatic until early adulthood, when they may present with symptoms of cirrhosis as the initial complaint. Another group of other children recover entirely from the acute illness in infancy and have no further evidence of liver disease. **The cirrhosis of α_1-AT deficiency is complicated by a very high incidence of hepatocellular carcinoma.**

Inborn Errors of Carbohydrate Metabolism

Glycogen Storage Diseases

The biochemical basis of the glycogen storage diseases has been discussed in Chapter 6. These disorders are inherited as autosomal recessive traits. **Only glycogenosis type IV (brancher deficiency, Andersen disease) is always complicated by cirrhosis.** A slowly developing cirrhosis may occur in glycogenosis type III (debrancher deficiency, Cori disease) but is not inevitable. Glycogenosis type I (glucose-6-phosphatase deficiency, von Gierke disease) is associated with striking hepatomegaly, and type II (acid-glucosidase deficiency, Pompe disease) features mild hepatomegaly. Neither type I nor type II is complicated by cirrhosis.

GLYCOGENOSIS TYPE I: The hepatocytes are distended by large amounts of glycogen, which appears pale in sections stained with hematoxylin and eosin. The enlarged liver cells compress the sinusoids and may obscure the normal arrangement of the hepatic cell plates. The PAS stain is heavily positive, and electron microscopy demonstrates masses of glycogen particles in the cytoplasm. Glycogen is present within the nuclei as well. Fat accumulation varies from mild to severe, but fibrosis is usually absent. A high incidence of hepatic adenomas, usually developing in adolescence, has been noted. Interestingly, these adenomas regress on dietary therapy.

GLYCOGENOSIS TYPE II: Only mild distention of hepatocytes, without fat or fibrosis, is noted. The cytoplasm of the hepatocytes contains small clear areas, which correspond to lysosomes distended with glycogen.

GLYCOGENOSIS TYPE III: Infants with this malady show severe hepatomegaly, and the liver morphologically resembles that seen in type I. Fat is less conspicuous, but fibrosis is present and may progress to cirrhosis.

GLYCOGENOSIS TYPE IV: Infants present with severe hepatomegaly and usually die of cirrhosis by the age of 4 years. Sharply circumscribed, PAS-positive inclusions are present in enlarged hepatocytes. By electron microscopy these inclusions consist of fibrillar material. The brancher enzyme deficiency responsible for glycogenosis type IV leads to the synthesis of an abnormal glycogen molecule that has fewer branch points than normal. This glycogen is less soluble than the normal one and therefore has an unusual ultrastructural appearance. Unlike normal glycogen, it is only partially digested by diastase. Deposits of abnormal glycogen are also found in the heart, skeletal muscle, and brain. **Extensive fibrosis eventually progresses to cirrhosis,** which is initially micronodular but may develop macronodular features. Liver transplantation is curative for glycogenosis type IV.

Galactosemia

Galactosemia, inherited as an autosomal recessive trait, is caused by a deficiency of galactose-1-phosphate uridyl transferase, the enzyme that catalyzes the second step in the conversion of galactose to glucose. As a result of this metabolic defect, galactose and its metabolites accumulate in the liver and other organs. Infants with this disorder who are fed milk rapidly develop **heptosplenomegaly, jaundice, and hypoglycemia**. Cataracts and mental retardation are common.

Microscopically, within 2 weeks of birth the liver shows **extensive and uniform fat accumulation and striking proliferation of bile ductules in and around the portal tracts.** Cholestasis is often present in canaliculi and bile ductules. Within several weeks the hepatic cell plates become arranged around a lumen, thus assuming a glandular or acinar appearance. Bile plugs fill many of these pseudoacini. At about 6 weeks of age, fibrosis begins to extend from the portal tracts into the lobule and **within 6 months progresses to cirrhosis**. The institution of a galactose-free diet has been reported to ameliorate the disease and reverse many of the morphological alterations. The basis of the liver cell injury and necrosis in this disorder is mysterious.

Hereditary Fructose Intolerance

Hereditary fructose intolerance is an autosomal recessive disease caused by a deficiency of fructose-1-phosphate aldolase; rare instances of fructose 1,6-diphosphate phosphatase deficiency have also been recorded. When fructose is fed early in infancy, hepatomegaly, jaundice, and ascites develop. However, the feeding of fructose after the age of 6 months results in far less severe disease, and the only clinical impairment is spontaneous hypoglycemia. Infants who suffer from liver disease show many of the changes of neonatal hepatitis: hepatocellular necrosis, giant hepatocytes, inflammation, ductular proliferation, and cholestasis. Fat accumulation may be marked, in which case the appearance resembles that of galactosemia. Progressive fibrosis culminates in cirrhosis.

Tyrosinemia

Tyrosinemia is an autosomal recessive trait that interferes with the catabolism of tyrosine to fumarate and acetoacetate. The biochemical defect is believed to be a deficiency of fumarylacetoacetate hydrolase. It is assumed that damage to the liver and kidney is caused by the accumulation of succinyl acetone and succinyl acetoacetate, both of which are potent electrophiles that can react with the sulfhydryl groups of glutathione and proteins. Tyrosinemia occurs in acute and chronic forms.

Acute tyrosinemia, which begins within a few weeks or months of birth, is characterized by hepatosplenomegaly and is associated with liver failure and death, usually before the age of 12 months. The appearance of the liver is remarkably similar to that of galactosemia, including progression to cirrhosis.

Chronic tyrosinemia begins in the first year of life and is characterized by growth retardation, renal disease, and hepatic failure. Death usually supervenes before the age of 10 years. The incidence of hepatocellular carcinoma associated with chronic tyrosinemia is extraordinarily high. In one series of patients who survived beyond 2 years of age, 37% manifested neoplastic transformation in the liver. Tyrosinemia is treated by liver transplantation.

Miscellaneous Inherited Causes of Cirrhosis

A wide variety of inborn errors of metabolism have been associated with cirrhosis, including storage diseases, such as Gaucher disease, Niemann-Pick disease, mucopolysaccharidoses, neonatal adrenoleukodystrophy, and Wolman disease. Zellweger syndrome, in which peroxisomes are lacking, has also been linked to cirrhosis.

INDIAN CHILDHOOD CIRRHOSIS

Indian childhood cirrhosis (ICC) is a fatal disorder largely restricted to preschool children on the Indian subcontinent. The disorder affects predominantly boys between the ages of 1 and 4 years from middle-class Hindu families. The liver in this **micronodular cirrhosis** displays hydropic swelling of hepatocytes, focal necrosis, and fibrosis connecting portal tracts and central venules. Diffuse fibrosis around injured hepatocytes and groups of cells is usual. Characteristically, Mallory bodies are abundant, but little fat is present. **This constellation of morphological features is almost identical to that seen in alcoholic liver disease.**

The etiology and pathogenesis of ICC are not well understood. Familial cases have been reported, but no hereditary pattern has been established. A search for viruses, toxins, and nutritional deficits has been fruitless.

Interestingly, children with this disease display a marked excess of copper and copper-binding protein in the liver. Indeed, the highest levels of hepatic copper have been reported in ICC. Asymptomatic siblings of patients with ICC cirrhosis also exhibit moderate increases in the liver content of copper and copper-binding protein. It has been proposed that excessive dietary copper in genetically susceptible children may be responsible for ICC.

PORTAL HYPERTENSION

Portal hypertension is defined as a sustained increase in portal venous pressure and is almost always a result of obstruction to blood flow somewhere in the portal circuit. The portal vein, arising at the junction of the superior mesenteric vein with the splenic vein, carries the major venous drainage from the gastrointestinal tract, the pancreas, and the spleen into the liver. The portal vein delivers two thirds of the hepatic blood flow but accounts for less than half of the total oxygen supply, the remainder being supplied by the hepatic artery. Normally, the pressure in the portal vein is only 7 to 14 cm H_2O (5 to 10 mm Hg). A pressure greater than 30 cm H_2O is considered evidence of portal hypertension.

Complications of portal hypertension arise from the increased pressure and dilatation of the venous bed behind the obstruction. **The major complications of this increased pressure and the opening of collateral channels are bleeding from gastroesophageal varices, ascites, and splenomegaly.**

For the sake of convenience, obstruction to the flow of portal blood can be pictured as (1) prehepatic, occurring before the blood enters the hepatic sinusoids; (2) intrahepatic, occurring during transit through the portal tracts and lobules; and (3) posthepatic, occurring after exit of the blood from the lobules (Fig. 14-45). In this scheme, the term **hepatic** refers to the lobule rather than to the entire liver.

Intrahepatic Portal Hypertension

By far the most common cause of portal hypertension is cirrhosis. Regenerative nodules impinge on and deform the hepatic veins, thereby obstructing blood flow distal to the lobules. The small portal veins and venules are trapped, narrowed, and often obliterated by scarring of the portal tracts. Moreover, blood flow through the hepatic artery is increased and small arteriovenous communications become functional. In this way, portal hypertension due to obstruction of blood flow distal to the sinusoid is augmented by an increase in arterial blood flow. In addition, an increase in splanchnic arterial blood flow, the cause of which is unclear, is an important factor in the maintenance of portal hypertension. Central vein sclerosis and sinusoidal fibrosis also contribute to the development of portal hypertension in alcoholic liver disease. In fact, portal hypertension can result from alcoholic central sclerosis even in cases that do not progress to cirrhosis.

Worldwide, hepatic schistosomiasis (*Schistosoma mansoni and S. japonicum*) is a major cause of portal

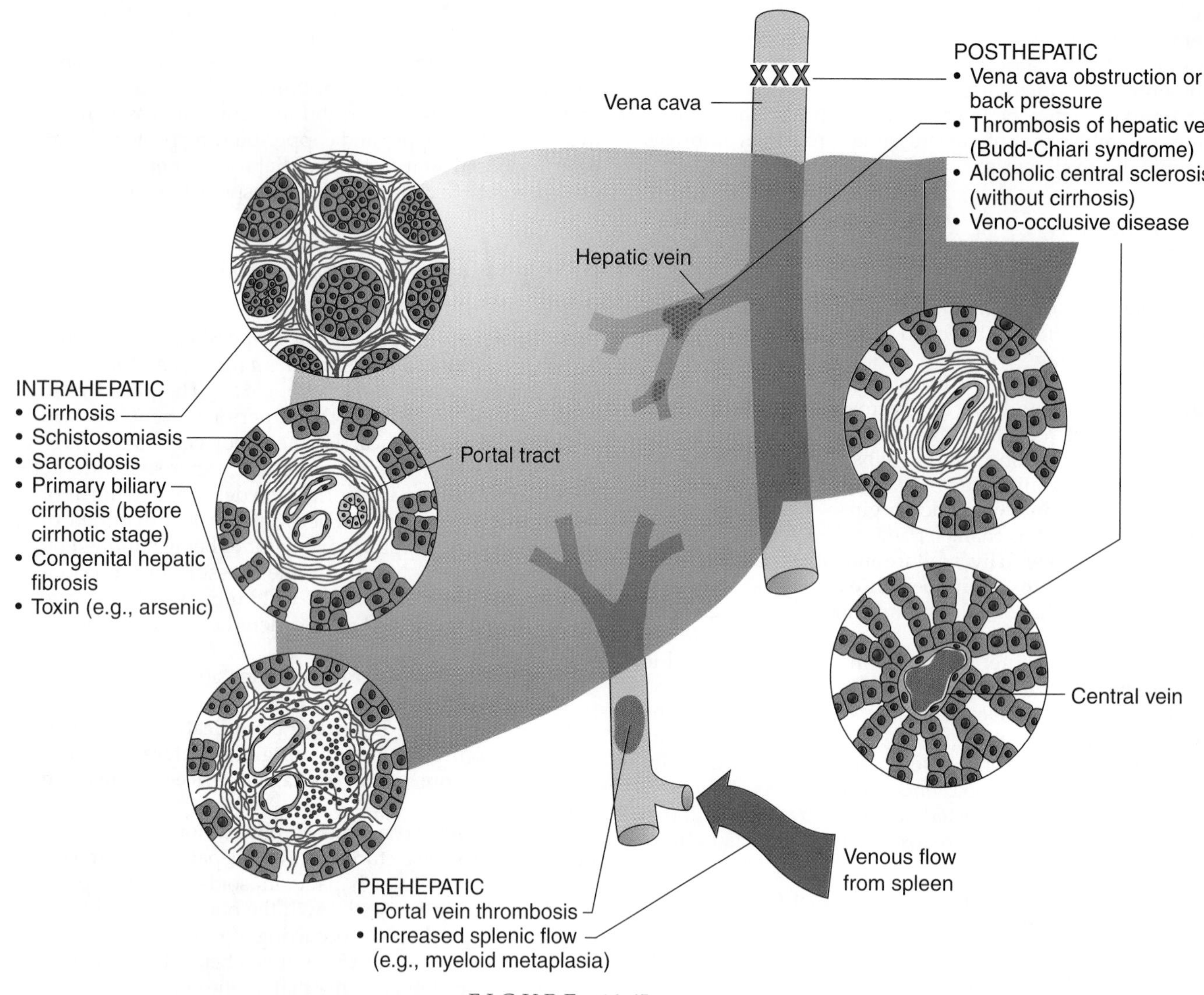

FIGURE *14-45*
Causes of portal hypertension.

hypertension. The ova released from the intestinal veins traverse the portal system and lodge in the intrahepatic portal venules, where they elicit a granulomatous reaction that heals by scarring. Because the obstruction within the liver occurs predominantly before the portal blood enters the hepatic sinusoids, **hepatic schistosomiasis is functionally similar to prehepatic portal hypertension**. Thus, hepatic function is well maintained, but the intrahepatic presinusoidal vascular obstruction leads to severe portal hypertension.

Idiopathic portal hypertension refers to occasional cases of intrahepatic portal hypertension with splenomegaly that occur in the absence of any demonstrable intrahepatic or extrahepatic disease. Historically, increased portal blood flow from the enlarged spleen was incriminated, but this now seems unlikely. In some cases, portal fibrosis and compression of portal veins, together with the deposition of collagen in the space of Disse, have been described. In prolonged idiopathic portal hypertension, portal fibrosis may be conspicuous. However, as the name indicates, the etiology is still being sought. In some countries (England, Japan), idiopathic portal hypertension accounts for 15% to 35% of all cases that require surgery to decompress the portal circulation.

Intrahepatic portal hypertension can be caused by other conditions that interfere with the flow of blood through the liver, including (1) cystic disease of the liver (see Chapter 16, which includes a discussion of cystic disease of the kidney), (2) partial nodular transformation of the liver in the region of the porta hepatis, (3) nodular regenerative hyperplasia (small regenerative nodules without fibrosis that compress the intervening hepatic parenchyma), and (4) metastatic or primary carcinoma of the liver. In rare instances, sarcoidosis involving the liver has been associated with portal hypertension, either because the granulomas directly obstruct blood flow by compressing the portal venules or sinusoids or because portal and periportal scarring distort the portal vein radicals.

Prehepatic Portal Hypertension

PORTAL VEIN THROMBOSIS: **The classic example of prehepatic portal hypertension is portal vein thrombosis,** commonly in association with cirrhosis. Other causes of portal vein thrombosis include tumors, infections, hypercoagulability states associated with oral contraceptive use and pregnancy, pancreatitis, and surgical trauma. Some cases are of unknown etiology. Primary hepatocellular carcinoma characteristically invades branches of the portal vein and occasionally reaches and occludes the main portal vein. When the portal vein is obstructed by a septic thrombus, bacteria may seed the intrahepatic branches of the portal vein (*suppurative pylephlebitis*) and cause multiple hepatic abscesses.

Occlusion of the portal vein may be manifested in the neonatal period or in early childhood. In some cases, umbilical sepsis is an important cause, but other local and systemic infections may also play a role. Sometimes the thrombosed portal or splenic vein is replaced by a fibrous cord or interlacing vascular channels, a process termed *cavernous transformation.*

INCREASED PORTAL BLOOD FLOW: The liver normally offers little resistance to the outflow of blood through the sinusoids and can, therefore, accommodate substantial increases in blood flow without a secondary increase in pressure. However, under some uncommon circumstances, increased portal venous blood flow can be associated with, or increase the severity of, portal hypertension. An arteriovenous fistula (i.e., an abnormal communication between an artery and the portal vein) may lead to prehepatic portal hypertension. It generally arises from trauma or rupture of an aneurysm of the splenic or hepatic artery. Such a fistula may also be found in association with hereditary hemorrhagic telangiectasia (Osler-Weber-Rendu syndrome). Portal hypertension also occasionally occurs in patients with splenomegaly from a variety of causes, including polycythemia vera, myeloid metaplasia, and chronic myelogenous leukemia. Although increased blood flow is the etiological factor in this form of portal hypertension, the liver also responds with increased resistance to blood flow, particularly with sclerosis of the smaller portal vein radicals. In cirrhosis, the accompanying splenomegaly may further aggravate portal hypertension.

Posthepatic Portal Hypertension

Posthepatic portal hypertension is defined as any obstruction to blood flow through the hepatic veins beyond the liver lobules, either within or distal to the liver.

Budd-Chiari Syndrome

Budd-Chiari syndrome refers to a congestive disease of the liver caused by occlusion of the hepatic veins and their tributaries. The disease was originally described in the large hepatic veins but is now known to occur in venous tributaries of any size, including central hepatic venules.

☐ **Pathogenesis:** The principal cause of the Budd-Chiari syndrome is thrombosis of the hepatic veins, in association with such diverse conditions as polycythemia vera and other myeloproliferative disorders, hypercoagulable states associated with malignant tumors, the use of oral contraceptives, pregnancy, bacterial infections, paroxysmal nocturnal hemoglobinuria, metastatic and primary tumors in the liver, and trauma. In 20% of the cases, no specific cause is evident. Thrombosis is most common in the large hepatic veins close to their exit from the liver and in the intrahepatic portion of the inferior vena cava. In parts of Africa and the Orient, membranous webs of unknown cause, presumably congenital, compromise the vena cava above the orifices of the hepatic veins and commonly cause the Budd-Chiari syndrome. Increased back-pressure in the venous system caused by severe congestive heart failure, tricuspid stenosis or regurgitation, or constrictive pericarditis may mimic the Budd-Chiari syndrome, although such complications of heart disease have been rendered uncommon by contemporary medical and surgical treatment.

Hepatic veno-occlusive disease is a variant of the Budd-Chiari syndrome and is caused by occlusion of the central venules and small branches of the hepatic veins. Most commonly this disorder is traced to the ingestion of toxic pyrrolizidine alkaloids present in plants of the *Crotalaria* and *Senecio* families, which are used in the formulation of "bush teas" in primitive societies. It is also seen in patients treated with certain antineoplastic chemotherapeutic agents, after hepatic irradiation, and in association with bone marrow transplantation, possibly as a manifestation of graft-versus-host disease.

☐ **Pathology:** In the early acute stage of **hepatic vein thrombosis**, the liver is swollen and tense and the cut surface exhibits a mottled appearance and oozes blood (Fig. 14-46A). In the chronic stage, the cut surface is paler, and the liver is firm, owing to an increase in connective tissue. Microscopically, the hepatic veins display thrombi in varying stages of evolution, from recent clots to well-organized thrombi that have been recanalized (see Fig. 14-46B). In veno-occlusive disease, similar thrombotic occlusions are present within the terminal hepatic venules, although some investigators have claimed that the proliferation of endothelial cells, rather than thrombosis, represents the initial lesion.

In the acute stage of both the Budd-Chiari syndrome and veno-occlusive disease, the sinusoids of the central zone are dilated and packed with erythrocytes. The liver cell plates are compressed, and necrosis of centrilobular hepatocytes is accompanied by the deposition of fibrin (see Fig. 14-46C). In long-standing venous congestion, fibrosis of the central zone radiating into the more peripheral portions of the lobules is conspicuous. The sinusoids are dilated, and the central to midzonal hepatocytes show pressure atrophy. Erythrocytes may be dislocated into the space of Disse and may be grouped in areas of hepatocyte necrosis. Eventually, connective tissue septa link adjacent central zones to form nodules with a single portal tract in the center, a process known as reverse lobulation. The fibrosis is usually not severe enough to justify a label of cirrhosis, although on rare occasions nodular transforma-

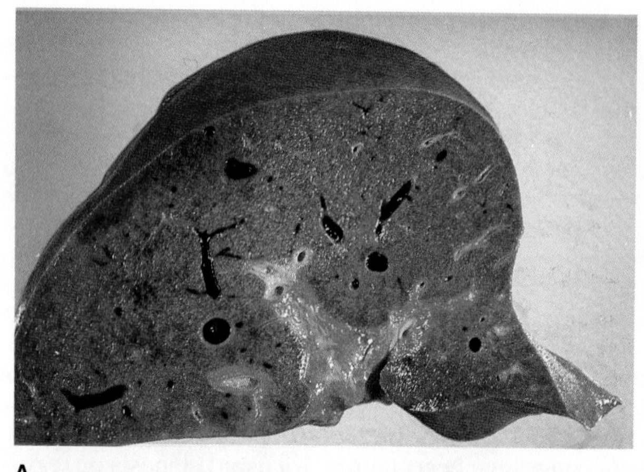
A

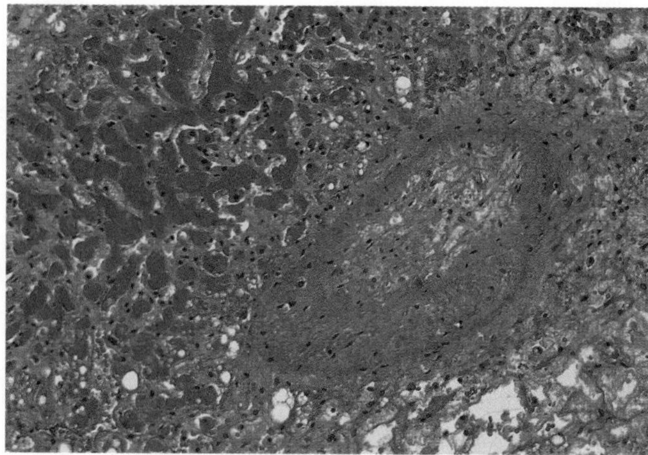
B

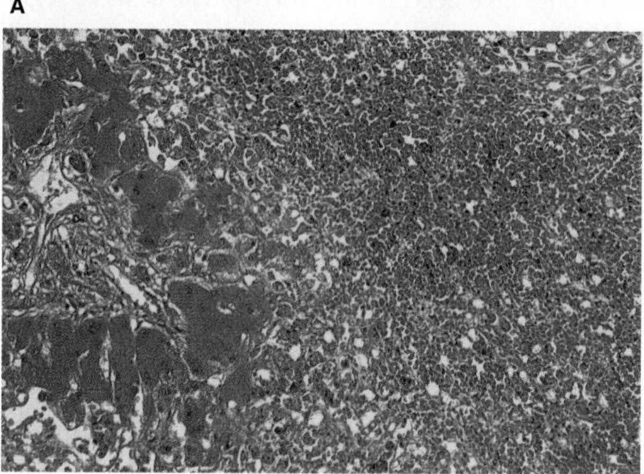
C

FIGURE 14-46
Budd-Chiari syndrome. (*A*) The cut surface of the liver from a patient who died from Budd-Chiari syndrome shows thrombosis of the hepatic veins and diffuse congestion of the parenchyma. (*B*) A photomicrograph from the same patient shows a hepatic vein occluded by an organized thrombus. (*C*) A photomicrograph of the liver from a patient with acute Budd-Chiari syndrome reveals centrilobular necrosis and hemorrhage.

tion of the architecture is significant enough to warrant this appellation.

☐ Clinical Features: **Complete thrombosis of the hepatic veins presents as an acute illness characterized by abdominal pain, enlargement of the liver, ascites, and mild jaundice.** Acute hepatic failure and death often occur rapidly. The more usual course, in which the obstruction of the hepatic venous circulation is incomplete, is marked by similar symptoms but may pursue a protracted course over periods ranging from a month to a few years. More than 90% of these patients develop ascites, usually severe, and splenomegaly is seen in over 30%. The liver is usually enlarged. Typically, the serum bilirubin and aminotransferase activities are only modestly increased. Most patients eventually die in hepatic failure or from the complications of portal hypertension. Liver transplantation has been successful in curing the disease.

Complications of Portal Hypertension

Portal hypertension leads to several systemic complications (Fig. 14-47). The classic complications are esophageal varices, splenomegaly, and ascites.

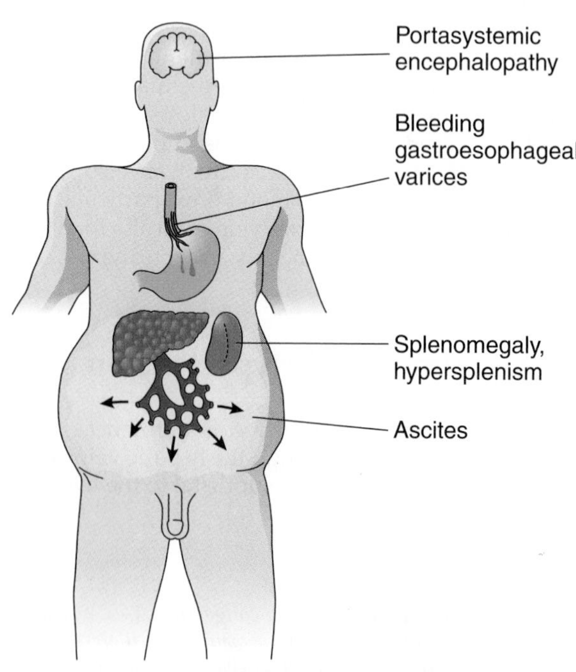

FIGURE 14-47
Complications of portal hypertension.

Esophageal Varices

Esophageal varices represent the most important complication of portal hypertension and arise from the opening of portal–systemic collaterals as an adaptation to decompress the portal venous system. One of the most common causes of death in patients with cirrhosis and other disorders associated with portal hypertension is exsanguinating upper gastrointestinal tract hemorrhage from **bleeding esophageal varices**.

☐ **Pathogenesis:** The collaterals of most clinical significance, located in the submucosa of the lower esophagus and upper stomach, are a result of communications between the portal vein and the gastric coronary vein. Because of the increased blood flow and higher pressure that follow the opening of these collaterals, the submucosal veins in the vicinity of the esophagogastric junction become dilated and protrude into the lumen. In cases of bleeding esophageal varices, the precise cause of hemorrhage is uncertain, since there is no simple correlation between portal venous pressure and the risk of variceal bleeding. However, the risk of bleeding does rise with increasing size of the varices.

☐ **Clinical Features:** The prognosis in cases of bleeding esophageal varices is poor, and the acute mortality may be as high as 40%. In patients with cirrhosis who survive an initial episode of variceal bleeding, long-term survival is unlikely because of a high risk of rebleeding or a worsening of liver failure. By contrast, patients in whom the portal hypertension is caused by a presinusoidal block, such as hepatic schistosomiasis, have a much better prognosis than those with cirrhosis because of the absence of underlying liver dysfunction. Importantly, death associated with bleeding esophageal varices is frequently not attributable directly to exsanguination and shock. Rather it is the result of hepatic failure precipitated by stress, ischemic necrosis of the liver, and the encephalopathy caused by the acute nitrogenous load imposed by blood in the intestinal tract.

Acute variceal hemorrhage may be treated by direct tamponade with an inflatable balloon, injection of varices with sclerosing agents through an endoscope, endoscopic variceal ligation, or intravenous administration of vasopressin to reduce splanchnic blood flow and portal venous pressure. For patients with repeated episodes of variceal bleeding in whom sclerotherapy has failed, permanent decompression of the portal circulation can be achieved by surgically constructed portasystemic shunts. These procedures divert blood from the high-pressure portal circulation to the lower-pressure systemic venous circulation. Portasystemic shunt surgery is generally reserved as a last resort for patients who continue to bleed from varices, in part because of the high operative mortality and in part because of the risk of portasystemic encephalopathy following diversion of the portal blood from the liver. The surgical diversion of portal blood from the liver may also increase the risk of subsequent hepatic failure. Intrahepatic portasystemic shunts can also be constructed by invasive angiography, in which a catheter in a hepatic vein is thrust through hepatic parenchyma into a dilated branch of the portal vein (transjugular intrahepatic portasystemic shunt [TIPS]) The communication is maintained by means of a stent. **Liver transplantation is now increasingly being considered as an alternative to shunt surgery.**

The back-pressure in the portal vein is also transmitted to its tributaries, including the inferior hemorrhoidal veins, which become dilated and tortuous (*anorectal varices*). Although the umbilical vein in the falciform ligament does not carry blood in the adult circulation, it remains probe patent. In portal hypertension, blood flows from the portal vein through this channel to the epigastric veins of the anterior abdominal wall. Clinically, visible collateral veins radiate from the umbilicus to produce the pattern known as *caput medusae*. On occasion, the left renal vein also becomes enlarged through anastomoses from the splenic vein or other channels.

Splenomegaly

The spleen in portal hypertension enlarges progressively, and splenomegaly is considered by some as the single most important diagnostic sign of portal hypertension. The enlarged spleen often gives rise to the syndrome of *hypersplenism*—that is, a decrease in the life span of all of the formed elements of the blood and, therefore, a reduction in their circulating numbers. Hypersplenism is attributed to an increased rate of removal of erythrocytes, leukocytes, and platelets because of the prolonged transit time through the hyperplastic spleen.

On gross examination, the spleen is firm and enlarged, up to 1000 g, and its cut surface is uniformly deep red, with an inapparent white pulp. Microscopically, the sinusoids are dilated and their walls are thickened by fibrous tissue and lined by hyperplastic endothelial cells and macrophage. Focal hemorrhages lead to the formation of fibrotic, iron-laden siderotic nodules, known as *Gamna-Gandy bodies*.

Ascites

Ascites refers to the accumulation of fluid in the peritoneal cavity. It often accompanies portal hypertension, most commonly in patients with decompensated cirrhosis. The amount of fluid may be so great, frequently many liters, that it not only distends the abdomen but also interferes with breathing. The onset of ascites in cirrhosis is associated with a poor prognosis.

☐ **Pathogenesis:** There is a consensus that, in addition to portal hypertension itself, sodium and water retention in cirrhosis is clearly important in the pathogenesis of ascites. The mechanisms for altered sodium and water homeostasis in cirrhosis remain controversial, but three major hypotheses can be considered:

- **Hypovolemia:** It was initially held that the increased pressure in the portal system caused sodium and water transudation into the abdominal cavity. The resulting hypovolemia was postulated to stimulate increased renal sodium and water retention (Fig. 14-48).
- **Overflow:** Subsequently, it was shown that the total

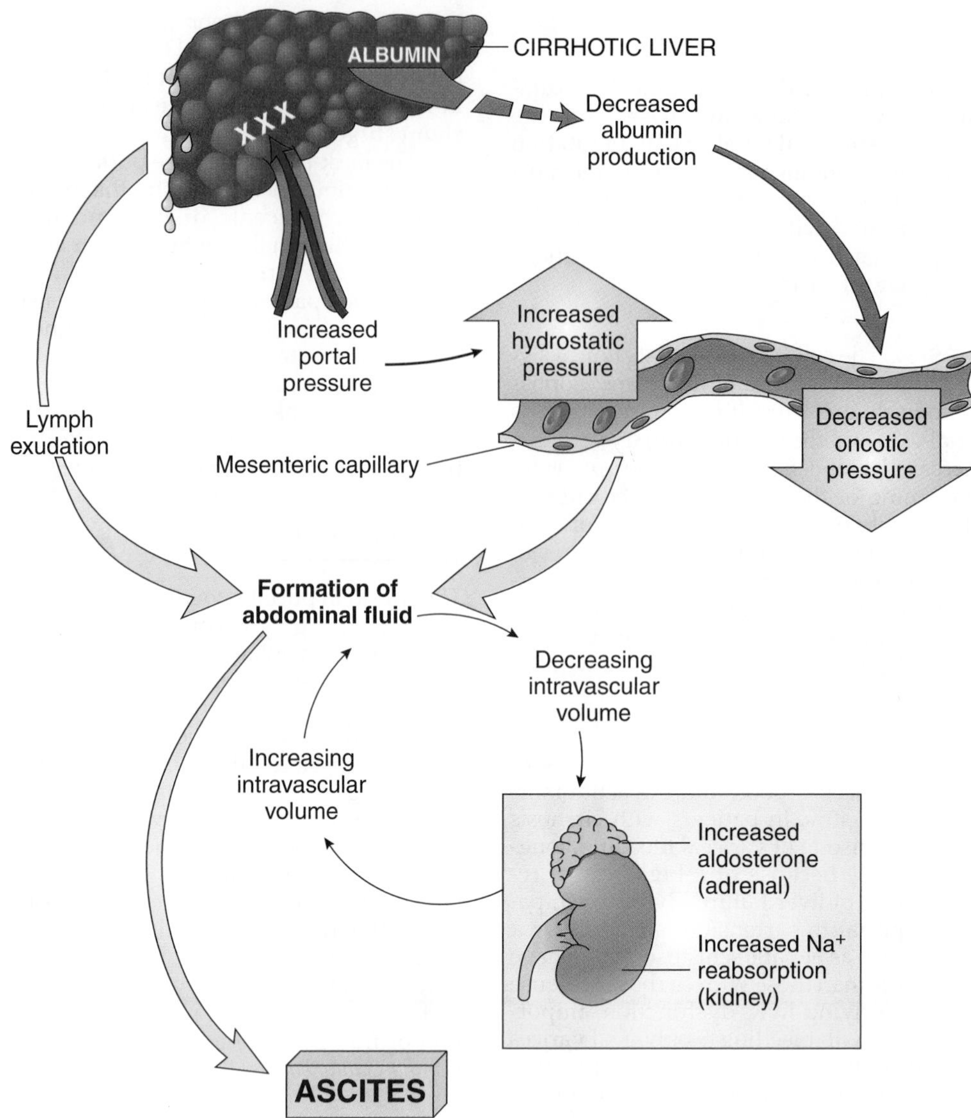

FIGURE *14-48*

Traditional concept (hypovolemic hypothesis) of the pathogenesis of ascites. In addition to the other factors depicted, the traditional concept holds that renal retention of sodium is a response to a decreased "effective" blood volume. It should be noted that an alternative view (overflow hypothesis) considers the increased renal reabsorption of sodium to be a primary effect of cirrhosis that precedes the formation of ascites. Peripheral vasodilatation is an additional factor to be considered.

blood volume in cirrhotic patients with ascites is actually increased rather than decreased. In fact, experimental studies have demonstrated that blood volume expansion and sodium and water retention by the kidney precede the formation of ascites. These findings suggested that the renal sodium and water retention in decompensated cirrhosis results from some as-yet-undefined alteration in volume regulation that is not secondary to a decrease in intravascular volume.

- **Vasodilatation:** It has recently been proposed that peripheral arterial vasodilatation is an initiating event in the renal retention of sodium and water in cirrhosis. This vasodilatation, while accommodating an increased total intravascular volume, also results in a decreased effective arterial blood volume, owing to the diversion of blood to the periphery. A decreased arterial blood volume is a potent stimulus for the renal retention of sodium and water.

Other factors also contribute to the formation of ascites in cirrhosis. Portal hypertension increases the hydrostatic pressure in the mesenteric capillaries. At the same time, the low serum albumin, characteristic of cirrhosis, is associated with decreased plasma oncotic pressure. As in the formation of peripheral edema (see Chapter 7), the resulting imbalance in Starling forces leads to transudation of fluid into the peritoneal cavity. Finally, the rate of formation of hepatic lymph exceeds the capacity of the lymphatics to remove it, and the liver "weeps" lymph into the abdomen.

Spontaneous Bacterial Peritonitis

Spontaneous bacterial peritonitis is an important complication in patients with both cirrhosis and ascites. The infection is extremely dangerous and carries a very high mortality, even when treated with antibiotics. Presumably, the ascitic fluid is seeded with bacteria from the blood or lymph or by the passage of bacteria through the bowel wall. No underlying infectious source is found, and the pathogenesis remains obscure. Typically, the leukocyte count in the ascitic fluid of spontaneous bacterial peritonitis is greater than 500/μL, and more than half are neutrophils. The diagnosis depends on the presence of bacteria, principally *Escherichia coli* and group D streptococci, in the ascitic fluid or on culture.

TOXIC LIVER INJURY

The spectrum of acute, chemically induced hepatic injury is so broad that it spans the entire spectrum of liver disease, from clinically trivial, transient cholestasis, to fatal fulminant hepatitis. Chronic toxic injury to the liver is equally diverse, being expressed, at one extreme, as a mild chronic hepatitis and, at the other, as an active cirrhosis. Although hepatic injury caused by drugs accounts for less than 5% of all cases of jaundice, it comprises up to 25% of cases of fulminant hepatic necrosis.

The multiplicity of drugs that cause liver injury, the differences in their chemical structure and metabolism, and the diverse patterns of injury all preclude a simple classification of toxic injury. In general, certain hepatotoxic chemicals invariably produce liver cell necrosis—that is, their action is entirely predictable. Among such agents are substances as diverse as yellow phosphorus, the organic solvent carbon tetrachloride, the mushroom poison phalloidin, and the analgesic acetaminophen. The defining characteristics of the liver injury produced by "predictable" hepatotoxins are as follows:

- The agent, in sufficiently high doses, always produces liver cell necrosis.
- The extent of hepatic injury is dose-dependent.
- These compounds produce the same lesions in different species.
- The liver necrosis is characteristically zonal—often, but not exclusively, centrilobular.
- The period between administration of the toxin and the development of liver cell necrosis is brief.

Historically, predictable hepatic necrosis was encountered principally in an industrial or occupational context, but today a greater awareness of the potential danger of liver damage and better occupational safety regulations have rendered such accidents uncommon.

Chapter 1 includes a discussion of the possible mechanisms by which these toxins produce liver necrosis. Briefly, toxic liver necrosis is, in most cases, a consequence of the metabolism of the compound by the mixed-function oxidase system of the liver, by which activated oxygen species and reactive metabolites are produced. The rate of drug metabolism is influenced by many factors, including age, sex, nutritional status, interactions with other drugs, and prior induction of hepatic drug-metabolizing activity.

In contrast to the aforementioned classic poisons, **most reactions to drugs are unpredictable** and seem to represent idiosyncratic events or manifestations of unusual sensitivity to a dose-related side effect. Sensitive persons may be predisposed to idiosyncratic reactions either because they possess metabolic pathways different from those of the general population or because they are unusually sensitive to a uniform pharmacological effect of the drug other than the desired therapeutic response.

It is now evident that genetic variations in systems of biotransformation and in the production or detoxification of reactive metabolites may determine the toxicity of some drugs. An immunological reaction to drugs, their metabolites, or modified liver cells has not been ruled out, although direct evidence is weak. Drugs that are principally cholestatic do not necessarily depend on metabolism for their action.

With these considerations in mind, we shall discuss toxic liver injury in terms of the morphological patterns of the resulting reaction.

Zonal Hepatocellular Necrosis

Drugs and chemicals that are predictable hepatotoxins and act through their metabolites typically cause centrilobular necrosis. This localization presumably reflects the greater activity of drug-metabolizing enzymes in the central zones. Examples of such agents are carbon tetrachloride, acetaminophen (Fig. 14-49), and the toxins of the mushroom *Amanita phalloides*. A minority of predictable hepatotoxins cause periportal necrosis, including yellow phosphorus, allyl alcohol, and ferrous sulfate.

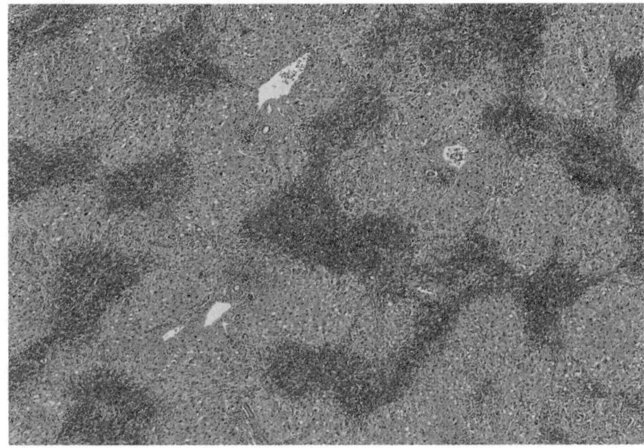

FIGURE *14-49*
Toxic centrilobular necrosis. The autopsy specimen in a case of acetaminophen discloses prominent hemorrhagic necrosis of the centrilobular zones of all liver lobules.

In the affected zones, hepatocytes show coagulative necrosis, hydropic swelling, and variable amounts of fat. Occasional acidophilic bodies, the remnants of necrotic hepatocytes, are free in the sinusoids. Inflammation is often sparse, although if the patient survives, a secondary inflammatory response becomes more conspicuous. If the dose of the hepatotoxin is sufficiently large, necrosis may extend to involve the entire lobule, leaving only a thin rim of viable hepatocytes surrounding the portal tracts. Patients either die in acute hepatic failure or recover without sequelae.

The chronic administration of hepatotoxins that cause zonal necrosis, exemplified by carbon tetrachloride, produces cirrhosis in experimental animals. However, this is generally not a problem in humans: once the acute toxic injury has been recognized, measures are usually taken to preclude reexposure to the offending agent.

Fatty Liver

The accumulation of triglycerides within the hepatocytes (i.e., hepatic steatosis or fatty liver) occurs in response to a variety of hepatotoxins, generally in a predictable fashion. Although substantial overlap may exist, two morphological patterns occur: *macrovesicular and microvesicular steatosis.*

Macrovesicular Steatosis

In macrovesicular steatosis, light microscopy shows the cytoplasm of the liver cell to be occupied by fat, seen as a large clear area that distends the cell and displaces the nucleus to the periphery.

In addition to its association with chronic ethanol ingestion, macrovesicular fat results from the experimental administration of, or accidental exposure to, such direct hepatotoxins as carbon tetrachloride and the poisonous constituents of certain mushrooms. Moreover, corticosteroids and some antimetabolites, such as methotrexate, may cause macrovesicular steatosis. There is no reason to believe that the presence of fat per se is injurious to the hepatocyte. Rather, its accumulation reflects the underlying liver cell damage. In many instances of toxic steatosis, the basis for fat accumulation is impaired secretion of lipoproteins as a consequence of an interference with protein synthesis.

STEATOHEPATITIS: A puzzling variant of toxic macrovesicular steatosis, termed steatohepatitis, resembles alcoholic hepatitis, not only in the distribution of fat but also in the presence of Mallory bodies and an acute inflammatory response. This unusual combination has been associated with the administration of the antiarrhythmic agent amiodarone, the coronary vasodilator perhexilene maleate, and synthetic estrogens used in the treatment of prostatic carcinoma. Experimentally, Mallory bodies have also been produced in mice with the antifungal agent griseofulvin. More commonly, steatohepatitis occurs spontaneously, especially in middle-aged, obese women, often in association with diabetes.

Microvesicular Steatosis

In contrast to macrovesicular steatosis, which by itself tends to be clinically inconsequential, microvesicular fatty liver is commonly associated with severe, and sometimes fatal, liver disease, although milder forms are recognized. In microvesicular steatosis, small fat vacuoles are dispersed throughout the cytoplasm and the nucleus retains its central position. Again, it is not the presence of fat but the underlying metabolic defects that produce the liver dysfunction.

REYE SYNDROME: *The most common and widely feared example of liver disease associated with microvesicular steatosis is Reye syndrome, an acute disease of children characterized by hepatic failure and encephalopathy.* The symptoms usually begin after a febrile illness, commonly influenza or varicella infection, and have been claimed to correlate with the administration of **aspirin**. Clearly, Reye syndrome is more complex than simple aspirin toxicity, because it almost always occurs after a febrile illness and the doses of aspirin consumed are far too small to produce liver injury in otherwise normal children. These observations suggest a possible synergism between aspirin and viral infection in the causation of Reye syndrome, but the precise mechanisms remain to be elucidated. In any event, with the decline in the use of aspirin in children, and possibly a reduced incidence of influenza, Reye syndrome is now distinctly uncommon.

Under the light microscope, the liver in a patient with Reye syndrome displays a typical microvesicular steatosis without accompanying hepatocellular necrosis or inflammation (Fig. 14-50). **Electron microscopy demonstrates characteristic alterations in mitochondria of the**

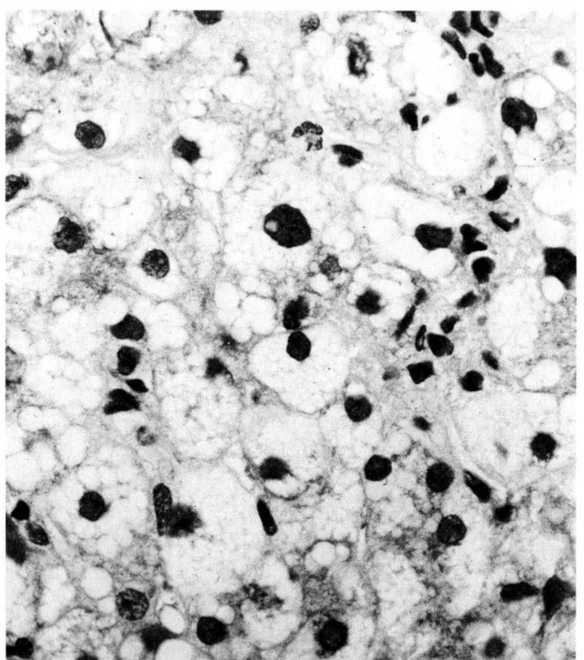

FIGURE *14-50*
Microvesicular fatty liver. A liver biopsy specimen in a case of Reye syndrome shows small droplet fat in hepatocytes and centrally located nuclei.

liver and brain, including large budding and branching forms. Mitochondrial dysfunction, characterized principally by a decrease in intramitochondrial enzymes, leads to impaired oxidation of fatty acids and hyperammonemia. Cerebral edema and fat accumulation are reported in the brain.

Reye syndrome has been compared with **Jamaican vomiting illness**, caused by the ingestion of **hypoglycin**, a poison in the unripened fruit of the ackee tree. The toxic principal binds to coenzyme A, thereby inhibiting fatty acid oxidation. A toxic microvesicular steatosis that is similar morphologically and functionally to Reye syndrome has been associated in Thailand with the intake of **aflatoxin**, a fungal product *(Aspergillus)* that contaminates the diet. Intravenous administration of **tetracycline** in high doses, particularly in pregnant women, has also resulted in microvesicular steatosis and hepatic failure.

FATTY LIVER OF PREGNANCY: Microsteatosis, not infrequently associated with hepatic failure, is a feature of the so-called fatty liver of pregnancy, the pathogenesis of which is unknown. In this condition, the morphological appearance of the liver is similar to that in Reye syndrome, but the characteristic mitochondrial abnormalities of the latter are not present. Many of the patients exhibit preeclampsia, and some cases have occurred in association with accompanying disorders (e.g., pancreatitis and disseminated intravascular coagulation). The condition ordinarily improves on delivery, although in some cases progressive hepatic failure could not be averted. Women who have suffered fatty liver of pregnancy may complete subsequent pregnancies without untoward effects.

PHOSPHOLIPIDOSIS: Triglycerides are not the only lipids that can accumulate in the liver in response to toxic injury. Phospholipidosis, which resembles certain heritable disorders of lipid metabolism (e.g., Niemann-Pick and Tay-Sachs disease), occurs after the administration of drugs such as perhexilene maleate and amiodarone. By light microscopy, both hepatocytes and Kupffer cells are enlarged and show a foamy cytoplasm. By electron microscopy, crystalloid or lamellated inclusions are found within distended lysosomes. Drugs that cause phospholipidosis are amphiphilic and bind to phospholipids, thereby inhibiting their catabolism. Changes similar to those in the liver occur in extrahepatic sites, including the lung, bone marrow, and lymphoid tissues.

Intrahepatic Cholestasis

Acute intrahepatic cholestasis is one of the most frequent manifestations of idiosyncratic types of drug-induced liver disease.

Bland centrilobular cholestasis, with virtually no hepatocellular necrosis or inflammation, is caused by a few drugs, principally sex steroids of the contraceptive or anabolic type. Except for mild jaundice, pruritus, and an elevated serum alkaline phosphatase level, the patients feel well.

Centrilobular cholestasis with slight to moderate inflammation and mild hepatocellular injury is associated with many other drugs, of which chlorpromazine is the prototype. Eosinophils are often conspicuous in the portal tracts, a feature that suggests a hypersensitivity reaction to chlorpromazine or its metabolites. In addition, as previously noted, chlorpromazine has been shown to inhibit bile flow directly in animals.

Proliferation of bile ductules in the portal tracts and the appearance of inspissated bile within the lumina compose an unusual pattern of cholestatic liver injury.

In some cases, continued administration of a drug that has produced acute cholestasis may lead to a chronic cholestatic syndrome resembling primary biliary cirrhosis, although the long-term prognosis is clearly more favorable than that of PBC if the drug is discontinued.

Mild Intralobular Hepatitis

A wide variety of drugs (e.g., aspirin and synthetic penicillins) may produce a mild liver injury, frequently dose dependent, that is rapidly reversible on discontinuation of the drug. Small foci of liver cell necrosis are scattered throughout the lobule and are associated with a few mononuclear inflammatory cells. A sparse infiltrate in the portal tracts is common. The morphological characteristics of viral hepatitis (lobular disarray, acidophilic bodies, hydropic swelling, cholestasis, and significant inflammation) are lacking, and the disease does not become chronic. A similar pattern is not uncommon in systemic diseases that do not primarily affect the liver, such as sepsis and ulcerative colitis.

Lesions Resembling Viral Hepatitis

All the typical clinical and morphological features of acute viral hepatitis can be seen after the administration of some drugs that cause idiosyncratic (unpredictable) liver injury. The most widely appreciated examples are the inhalation anesthetic halothane, the antituberculosis agent isoniazid, and the antihypertensive drug methyldopa. Although the incidence of these viral hepatitis–like reactions is low, they are far more dangerous than viral hepatitis itself, causing more severe disease and a much higher mortality rate. The entire range of acute liver injury, from mild anicteric hepatitis to rapidly fatal fulminant hepatic necrosis, is encountered. It deserves repetition that, for practical purposes, the pattern of liver injury is morphologically indistinguishable from that of documented acute viral hepatitis. As in viral hepatitis, when the offending agent is removed (i.e., when the virus is cleared or the drug is withdrawn), complete recovery is the rule.

The fact that hepatitis caused by halothane is typically more severe after a second or third exposure suggests that an allergic or immunological mechanism mediates the injury. The frequent occurrence of peripheral eosinophilia and eosinophils in the liver in cases of halothane hepatitis supports this concept. However, it has not been definitively established that an immunological mechanism produces halothane hepatitis. Alternatively, exposure to halothane may alter the response of the liver to subsequent exposures.

Chronic Hepatitis

Persistent intake of hepatotoxic drugs can lead to a syndrome indistinguishable from chronic hepatitis. Like chronic hepatitis caused by persistent viral infection, drug-induced chronic hepatitis may progress to cirrhosis. On discontinuation of drug administration, the lesion usually resolves, although this may require many months. In cases that have progressed to cirrhosis, the scarring remains, but the inflammatory and necrotizing activity is halted. Among the drugs incriminated in the production of chronic hepatitis are the laxative oxyphenisatin, the antihypertensive agent methyldopa, the antituberculosis drug isoniazid, and certain sulfonamides.

Granulomatous Hepatitis

A number of drugs occasionally associated with hepatotoxicity may also induce noncaseating, "sarcoid-like" granulomas in the portal tracts and the lobular parenchyma. In some instances, other organs also display granulomas. Focal necrosis and minimal intrahepatic cholestasis may complicate the granulomatous hepatitis. The liver damage is transient and does not lead to chronic lesions. Among the many drugs that have been associated with granulomatous hepatitis are the anti-inflammatory agent phenylbutazone, the antiarrhythmic drug quinidine, and allopurinol, used in the treatment of gout.

Vascular Lesions

As noted in the discussion of portal hypertension, occlusion of the hepatic veins (*Budd-Chiari syndrome*) has been reported to follow the use of oral contraceptive agents, presumably a reflection of the general hypercoagulable state associated with the use of these steroids. Obstruction at the level of the terminal venules (central veins), termed *veno-occlusive disease*, may result from the ingestion of certain alkaloids in "bush teas" or from the administration of some agents used in the chemotherapy of cancer.

Peliosis hepatis *is a peculiar hepatic lesion, characterized by cystic, blood-filled cavities that are not lined by endothelial cells* (Fig. 14-51). Anabolic sex steroids, and occasionally contraceptive steroids, sometimes produce this lesion. In some cases, peliosis caused by anabolic steroids, such as methyltestosterone and norethandrolone, is associated with mild intrahepatic cholestasis. Other agents that have been associated with peliosis are the antiestrogen tamoxifen and excess vitamin A.

Hyperplastic and Neoplastic Lesions

The spectrum of hepatic lesions caused by chemicals extends to benign and malignant tumors. Although preneoplastic hepatic nodules and hepatocellular carcinoma are regularly produced by chemicals in experimental animals, examples in humans are few.

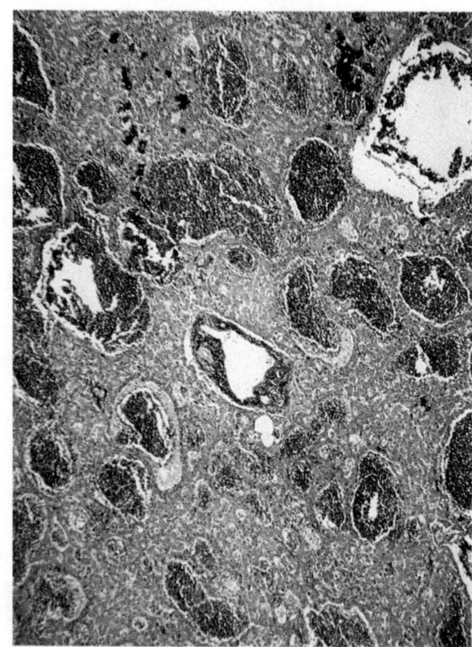

FIGURE *14-51*
Peliosis hepatis. The liver contains numerous large, irregular, blood-filled spaces.

Hepatic adenomas are recognized as a complication of the use of oral contraceptives and uncommonly of anabolic steroids. These tumors of hepatocytes are benign, and their greatest danger lies in their propensity to rupture and then bleed profusely. A few cases of primary hepatocellular carcinoma have been reported in persons taking oral contraceptives or anabolic steroids, but an etiological association is controversial.

Hemangiosarcomas of the liver appeared many years after the intravenous administration of thorium dioxide (Thorotrast), a radioactive compound used in the past to visualize the liver. This particulate isotope is engulfed by Kupffer cells, where it remains inert indefinitely, emits local radiant energy, and thereby produces neoplastic transformation. Chronic exposure to inorganic arsenic, usually in the form of insecticides, and the inhalation of vinyl chloride in an industrial setting have also been linked to the development of hemangiosarcoma of the liver.

THE PORPHYRIAS

The porphyrias comprise both acquired and inherited conditions that are caused by deficiencies in the pathway of heme biosynthesis and are characterized by the accumulation of porphyrin intermediates. The porphyrias are divided into two types, namely hepatic and erythropoietic porphyrias, based on the locations of defective heme metabolism.

Porphyrins are intermediate products in heme biosynthesis that are composed of four pyrrole rings surrounding a center that avidly binds iron (also cobalt and magnesium). A block at any point in the pathway, which requires eight enzymes to synthesize heme, leads to the accumulation of porphyrin intermediates; the consequent metabolic abnormalities are referred to as the porphyrias.

Hepatic Porphyrias

The hepatic porphyrias include three acute illnesses (acute intermittent porphyria, hereditary coproporphyria, variegate porphyria) and one chronic disease (porphyria cutanea tarda). All of the hepatic porphyrias are inherited as autosomal dominant traits and are often precipitated by the administration of drugs, sex hormones, starvation, and alcohol consumption. Acute hepatic porphyrias feature abdominal pain and neuropsychiatric symptoms, and two (variegate porphyria, coproporphyria) are also complicated by photosensitivity.

ACUTE INTERMITTENT PORPHYRIA: This malady is the most common genetic porphyria and reflects a deficiency of porphobilinogen deaminase activity in the liver. However, only 10% of gene carriers suffer clinical symptoms, which generally affect young adults. Colicky abdominal pain and neuropsychiatric symptoms predominate. Attacks of the disease can be prevented by proper nutrition and the avoidance of offending drugs and alcohol.

PORPHYRIA CUTANEA TARDA: This chronic hepa-tic porphyria is the most frequent porphyria and is either acquired or inherited as an autosomal dominant trait. All types of the disorder reflect deficient uroporphyrinogen decarboxylase activity in the liver, although one genetic variant also exhibits the enzyme deficiency in extrahepatic sites. The typical patient is middle-aged or elderly, displays cutaneous photosensitivity, and suffers from liver disease with hepatic iron overload. Alcohol consumption and estrogen administration may aggravate the condition. Porphyria cutanea tarda is best treated by phlebotomy, a procedure that mobilizes iron from the liver.

Erythropoietic Porphyrias

ERYTHROPOIETIC PROTOPORPHYRIA: This disease is inherited as an autosomal dominant trait and is associated with a deficiency in ferrochelatase, the enzyme that inserts iron into protoporphyrin. The bone marrow and immature red blood cells (reticulocytes) are the principal sources for the increased protoporphyrin in erythrocytes, plasma, bile, and feces. Cutaneous photosensitivity is the hallmark of the condition, and chronic liver disease with cirrhosis occurs in up to 10% of patients. No effective treatment is available, but the avoidance of, or protection from, sunlight is recommended.

CONGENITAL ERYTHROPOIETIC PORPHYRIA: This rare malady is inherited as an autosomal recessive trait. The expression of the defective gene, which encodes uroporphyrinogen cosynthase, is primarily in the erythropoietic cells of the bone marrow. Cutaneous photosensitivity begins in infancy and results in blisters on sun-exposed skin. Eventually, the necrotic lesions become scarred, resulting in mutilating distortions of the affected areas. Chronic hemolysis, variably accompanied by anemia, is typical of the disease. The treatment for erythropoietic porphyria is unsatisfactory, but avoidance of sunlight offers some palliation.

VASCULAR DISORDERS

Congestive Heart Failure

In the Western world, in which ischemic heart disease is endemic, congestive heart failure is the major cause of liver congestion.

Acute Passive Congestion

At autopsy, it is common for the liver to be acutely congested, presumably because of a failing heart in the agonal period. On cut section, the liver is diffusely speckled with small red foci. Microscopically, these foci are centrilobular zones with dilated and congested sinusoids and terminal venules. These changes are not clinically significant.

Chronic Passive Congestion

In the face of persistent congestive heart failure, the pressure in the peripheral venous circulation increases, impeding venous outflow from liver and producing chronic passive congestion of that organ. Unlike the acutely congested liver, which is somewhat enlarged, the chronically congested liver is often reduced in size. On gross examination, the cut surface of the liver exhibits an accentuated lobular pattern, with a mottled appearance of alternating light and dark areas (Fig. 14-52). Because this pattern is reminiscent of a cut nutmeg, it has been termed *nutmeg liver*. In severe cases, the centrilobular terminal venules and adjacent sinusoids are markedly dilated and filled with erythrocytes. The liver cell plates in this zone are thinned by pressure atrophy and may even be absent, leaving a collapsed reticulin framework. In extreme cases, frank hemorrhagic necrosis of the hepatocytes in the centrilobular zones is conspicuous. These changes are far less prominent in the periphery of the lobule, but periportal hepatocytes often contain increased amounts of fat.

Chronic passive congestion of the liver is of more pathological than clinical interest, since the condition has little effect on hepatic function. However, moderate increases in serum aminotransferase activities are common. Serum bilirubin levels may be mildly elevated, but jaundice is only partly of hepatic origin. Jaundice in such cases may also be caused in part by pulmonary infarcts, which are often found in jaundiced patients suffering from cardiac failure. Features of portal hypertension, including splenomegaly and ascites, sometimes accompany chronic passive congestion of the liver, but bleeding from esophageal varices is distinctly uncommon.

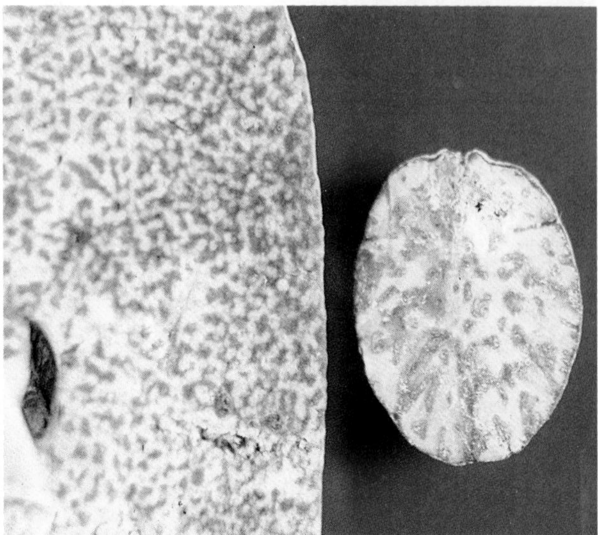

FIGURE 14-52
Chronic passive congestion of the liver. The surface of this fixed liver exhibits an accentuated lobular pattern, an appearance resembling that of a nutmeg (*right*).

Cardiac Fibrosis of the Liver

In cases of particularly severe and long-standing **right-sided heart failure** (e.g., tricuspid valvular disease or constrictive pericarditis), chronic passive congestion progresses to varying degrees of hepatic fibrosis. Delicate fibrous strands envelop terminal venules, and septa radiate from the centrilobular zones. The walls of the terminal venules and occasionally the sublobular veins may be thickened (phlebosclerosis). In prolonged cases of heart failure, the septa may link adjacent central veins, thereby producing a "reverse lobulation." Pressure atrophy of the centrilobular hepatocytes remains prominent. The older term *cardiac cirrhosis* is inappropriate, since the complete septa and regenerative nodules of true cirrhosis are rarely encountered.

Shock

Shock from any cause results in decreased perfusion of the liver and often leads to ischemic necrosis of the centrilobular hepatocytes. The centrilobular zone, referred to as zone 3 in the functional concept of the hepatic acinus (see Fig. 14-2), is most distal to the blood supply from the portal tracts and normally has a low oxygen tension. As a consequence, centrilobular hepatocytes are most vulnerable to the ischemia of hypoperfusion. Microscopically, coagulative necrosis of centrilobular hepatocytes is accompanied by frank hemorrhage. If shock is prolonged, or the patient survives, acute inflammatory cells accumulate in the necrotic zones. The lesion superficially resembles chronic passive congestion but is distinguished from it by a lack of dilatation and congestion of the veins and an absence of pressure atrophy.

Infarction

Infarcts of the liver are uncommon because of its dual blood supply and the anastomotic structure of the hepatic sinusoids. Acute occlusion of the hepatic artery or its branches is unusual but can occur as a result of embolism, polyarteritis nodosa, or accidental ligation during surgery. Under such circumstances, irregular pale areas, often surrounded by a hyperemic zone, reflect the underlying ischemic necrosis.

Thrombosis of the extrahepatic portal vein and the hepatic veins has been discussed in the context of portal hypertension. The acute occlusion of intrahepatic branches of the portal vein, generally in the presence of elevated hepatic venous pressure, classically produces the *Zahn infarct*, a dark-red, triangular area with its base on the surface of the liver. There is a surprising discrepancy between this distinctive gross appearance and the paucity of microscopic changes. In particular, hepatocellular necrosis is absent and the only abnormality is dilatation and congestion of the sinusoids. Thus, the traditional term "infarct" is actually a misnomer. The interruption of portal blood flow through the sinusoids allows a backflow of venous blood into the sinusoids and perhaps stimulates a compensatory increase in arterial flow, thereby creating stasis in and distention of the sinusoids.

BACTERIAL INFECTIONS

Bacterial infections are uncommon causes of liver disease in the industrialized countries and are for the most part complications of infections elsewhere. **The characteristic reactions in the liver are granulomas, abscesses, and diffuse inflammation.** Infections associated with granulomatous inflammation elsewhere (e.g., tuberculosis, tularemia, and brucellosis) also cause granulomatous hepatitis.

Pyogenic liver abscesses are produced by staphylococci, streptococci, and gram-negative enterobacteria. The morphological appearance of a pyogenic abscess in the liver is similar to that in other sites. It is increasingly recognized that anaerobic inhabitants of the gastrointestinal tract, particularly *Bacteroides* species and microaerophilic streptococci, are common causes of liver abscesses. Organisms reach the liver in arterial or portal blood or through the biliary tract. In cases of septicemia, seeding of the liver with organisms from distant sites is through the arterial blood.

Pylephlebitic abscesses (Fig. 14-53) result from intra-abdominal suppuration, as in peritonitis or diverticulitis, with the organisms being transmitted to the liver in portal blood. At one time, pylephlebitis was the most common cause of hepatic abscesses, but the control of abdominal sepsis with antibiotics has rendered this route of infection uncommon.

Cholangitic abscesses in the liver are today the most common form of hepatic abscess in Western countries. Biliary obstruction from any cause is often complicated by bacterial infection of the biliary tree, termed *ascending cholangitis*. The retrograde biliary dissemination of organ-

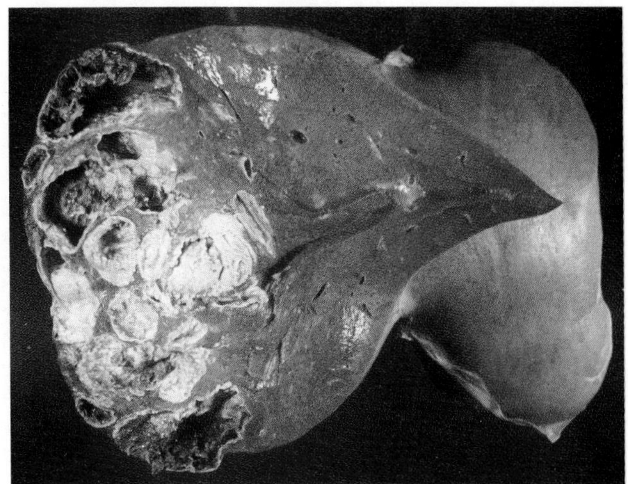

FIGURE *14-53*
Pylephlebitic abscesses of the liver. The cut surface of the liver shows large, confluent, irregular abscess cavities.

isms (usually *E. coli*) then leads to the formation of cholangitic abscesses. Nevertheless, in about half of all cases of hepatic abscess, the source of infection cannot be demonstrated.

Hepatic abscesses are more commonly located in the right lobe of the liver, presumably because of its larger mass. Diffuse inflammation of the liver from bacterial infection is distinctly uncommon today and may be encountered in various septicemic states, particularly in immunocompromised patients.

☐ **Clinical Features:** A patient with a hepatic abscess typically presents with high fever, rapid weight loss, right upper quadrant abdominal pain, and hepatomegaly. Jaundice occurs in a fourth of the cases, but the serum alkaline phosphatase level is almost always elevated. Solitary abscesses are treated with surgical drainage and antibiotics, but multiple abscesses present a difficult therapeutic problem. The complications of hepatic abscess relate principally to rupture and direct spread of the infection. Pleuropulmonary fistulas, from the rupture of an abscess through the diaphragm, and peritonitis, from leakage into the abdominal cavity, occur. The dissemination of organisms in the blood may lead to septicemia and metastatic abscesses in other parts of the body. The mortality from hepatic abscess, even in treated cases, remains high, ranging from 40% to 80%. However, early diagnosis and aggressive treatment can significantly reduce the mortality.

PARASITIC INFESTATIONS

Parasitic infestations of the liver are a serious public health problem worldwide, although they are uncommon in industrialized countries. These diseases are discussed in Chapter 9. Here we summarize the major parasitic diseases that involve the liver.

Protozoal Diseases

AMEBIASIS: In the United States, the carrier rate for *Entamoeba histolytica* is probably less than 5%, but a prevalence up to 35% has been reported in homosexual men. Amebiasis of the liver, the most common extraintestinal complication, leads to amebic abscesses, which are multiple in about half of the cases (Fig. 14-54).

On gross examination, an amebic abscess typically ranges from 8 to 12 cm in diameter, appears well circumscribed and contains thick, dark material, which has been likened to anchovy paste or chocolate. Microscopically, the border between the necrotic abscess and the surrounding liver parenchyma is not as sharp as implied by the gross appearance. The trophozoites are not apparent in the necrotic debris but may be visualized in the periphery.

The symptoms associated with amebic abscesses are similar to those that characterize pyogenic abscesses, but the former are ordinarily less severe. Secondary infection of an amebic abscess with pyogenic organisms is common. With appropriate treatment (tissue amebicides), the abscess may heal and leave only residual scar tissue. Alternatively, if the abscess continues to grow, it may rupture into the peritoneal cavity, where it produces peri-

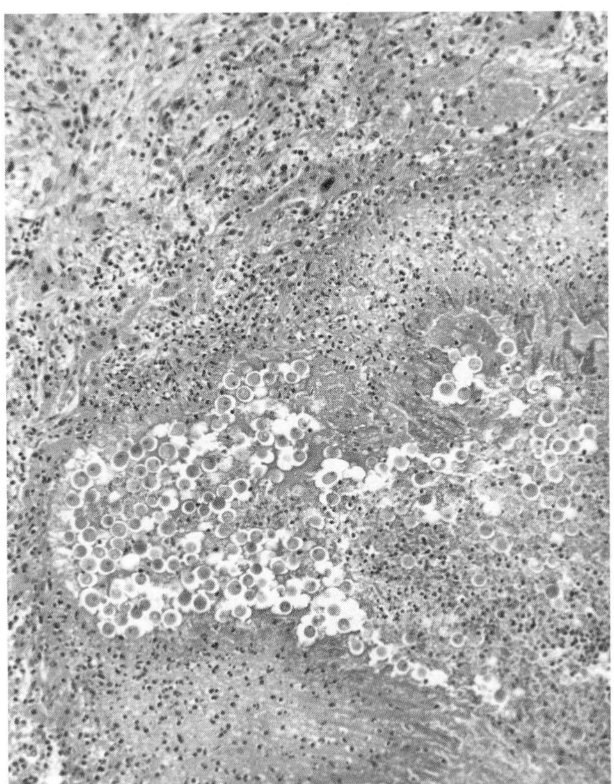

FIGURE *14-54*
Amebic abscess of the liver. A photomicrograph of the margin of an amebic abscess shows fibroblastic proliferation surrounding the cavity and amebic trophozoites in the lumen.

tonitis, a complication associated with a mortality as high as 40%. The amebae may also invade the blood, in which case abscesses of the brain and lung may ensue.

MALARIA: Hepatic involvement in malaria is a frequent cause of hepatomegaly in endemic areas. It reflects Kupffer cell hypertrophy and hyperplasia secondary to the phagocytosis of the debris resulting from the rupture of parasitized erythrocytes. The Kupffer cells are heavily pigmented and protrude into the sinusoidal lumen, which is often congested with parasitized erythrocytes. This hepatic involvement does not give rise to significant hepatic dysfunction.

VISCERAL LEISHMANIASIS (KALA-AZAR): As in malaria, the hepatomegaly of chronic visceral leishmaniasis results from hyperplasia of mononuclear phagocytes in the liver. In contrast to malaria, however, the Kupffer cells ingest the parasitic organisms themselves, which appear as *Donovan bodies*. These organisms are demonstrated in almost three fourths of liver biopsy specimens from patients with leishmaniasis. Macrophages containing Donovan bodies are often present in the portal tracts, where lymphocytes and eosinophils also accumulate. Clinically, there is little evidence of hepatic dysfunction.

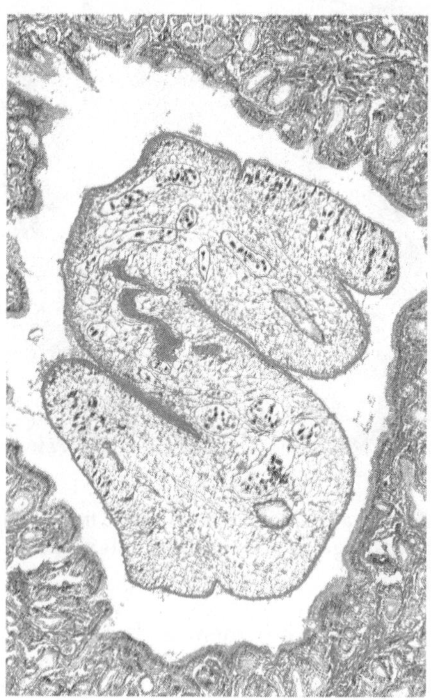

FIGURE *14-55*
Infection of the liver by *Clonorchis sinensis*. The lumen of a bile duct contains an adult liver fluke, and the mucosa is hyperplastic.

Helminthic Diseases

The major helminthic infestations of the liver are ascariasis, liver flukes, echinococcosis, and schistosomiasis. *Hepatic schistosomiasis* has already been discussed in the context of portal hypertension.

ASCARIASIS: From the duodenum, the worms of *Ascaris lumbricoides* gain access to the biliary tree, where they may produce an acute biliary colic. When the parasites retreat or are endoscopically removed from the common bile duct, the symptoms subside. However, when the worms lodge in the intrahepatic biliary passages, their disintegration results in the liberation of innumerable eggs, which precipitate a severe, suppurative cholangitis. As in the usual pyogenic abscess, the resulting cholangitic abscesses may rupture into the peritoneal cavity or into the pleural space. Spread of the infection into the hepatic or portal veins causes pylephlebitis, a highly dangerous complication. Ascaridic cholangitis, in general, carries a grave prognosis.

At autopsy, the liver is enlarged and numerous irregular cavities contain foul-smelling material, in which the remnants of degenerated parasites are found. The periphery of the abscess often displays a granulomatous response and sometimes an eosinophilic infiltrate.

LIVER FLUKES: The major parasitic flukes that involve the human liver are *Clonorchis sinensis* and *Fasciola hepatica*. Humans are the definitive host for *C. sinensis*, whereas sheep and cattle are the principal reservoir of *F. hepatica*. Both parasites lodge in the intrahepatic biliary tree, where they provoke hyperplasia of the biliary epithelium, particularly severe in clonorchiasis (Fig. 14-55). Although periductal fibrosis is common, most patients remain asymptomatic. However, in severe infestation with *C. sinensis*, the accumulation of material from degenerated worms, parasite eggs, and viscid mucus secreted by metaplastic goblet cells in the biliary epithelium obstructs intrahepatic bile flow and leads to intrahepatic pigment gallstones. Secondary infection of the bile with *E. coli* causes cholangitis and cholangitic abscesses, common causes of surgical emergencies in some Asian countries. Migration of *C. sinensis* into the pancreatic duct produces pancreatitis. **Biliary infestation with *C. sinensis* is an etiological factor in the development of cholangiocarcinoma.**

ECHINOCOCCOSIS (CYSTIC HYDATID DISEASE): Infection with the tapeworms of the genus *Echinococcus*, principally *E. granulosus*, is an important zoonosis that involves the human liver. Larvae, termed *onchospheres*, pass from the intestine into the portal circulation and lodge in the liver, where they encyst. In a few days, a germinal membrane develops, from which brood capsules containing innumerable scolices (the future head of the adult worm) arise. The cyst expands slowly and produces symptoms only after many years. Within the liver, the cyst behaves as a space-occupying lesion; systemic manifestations reflect toxic or allergic reactions to the absorption of constituents of the organisms. Mechanical obstruction of intrahepatic bile ducts may be complicated by secondary infection, namely cholangitis. Rupture of the cysts into the bile ducts commonly leads to pain and jaundice.

Leptospirosis (Weil Disease)

Infection of humans with organisms of the genus *Leptospira* is accidental, the reservoir being a wide variety of domestic animals. However, fewer than one fifth of patients who contract leptospirosis give a history of direct contact with animals. **Weil syndrome** refers to leptospirosis complicated by prolonged fever and jaundice and often azotemia, hemorrhages, and altered consciousness. Weil syndrome occurs in only 1% to 6% of all cases of leptospirosis. The morphological alterations of the liver in fatal cases are nonspecific and include focal necrosis, enlarged Kupffer cells, and centrilobular cholestasis. The organisms are generally not demonstrable in the liver.

Syphilis

Hepatic lesions from syphilis were at one time common, but with effective antibiotic treatment of the initial infection they are now rarely encountered.

Congenital syphilis causes neonatal hepatitis, which results in diffuse fibrosis in the portal tracts and around individual liver cells or groups of hepatocytes. Up to 10% of patients with secondary syphilis develop a hepatitis that is clinically similar to viral hepatitis. Focal necrosis of hepatocytes, Kupffer cell hyperplasia, and mild portal and parenchymal inflammation are present. The organisms are demonstrated in the liver in about half of these cases.

Tertiary syphilis is characterized by single or multiple hepatic gummas (i.e., focal lesions resembling granulomas), which heal with dense scars. Retraction of the scars in severe cases with multiple gummas produces deep clefts and a gross pseudolobation of the liver, termed *hepar lobatum*, a condition that should not be confused with cirrhosis.

CHOLESTATIC SYNDROMES OF INFANCY

Diseases characterized by prolonged cholestasis and jaundice in infants represent either diseases primarily affecting the hepatocytes or obstruction of the biliary system.

NEONATAL HEPATITIS

Neonatal hepatitis is a poorly defined clinical and pathological entity of multiple etiologies, which features prolonged cholestasis, morphological evidence of liver cell injury, and inflammation.

☐ **Pathogenesis:** In about half of all cases of neonatal hepatitis, the cause is discernible (Table 14-5), and about 30% of cases are assigned to α_1-antitrypsin deficiency alone. Most of the other cases with known causes can be attributed to viral hepatitis B and infectious agents such as those of the TORCH group (*to*xoplasmosis, *r*ubella, *c*ytomegalovirus, and *h*erpes simplex). A few cases represent hepatic injury associated with metabolic defects, for instance, galactosemia or fructose intolerance. Occasional cases of neonatal hepatitis are seen in association with Down syndrome and other chromosomal disorders. The remaining 50% of all cases of neonatal hepatitis are of unexplained etiology, but it is likely that as-yet-unidentified viruses and metabolic defects will be recognized. Rare familial cases of neonatal hepatitis have been reported.

TABLE *14-5* **Causes of Neonatal Hepatitis**

Idiopathic

- Idiopathic neonatal hepatitis
- Prolonged intrahepatic cholestasis
  1. Arteriohepatic dysplasia (Alagille syndrome)
  2. Paucity of intrahepatic bile ducts not associated with specific syndromes
  3. Zellweger syndrome (cerebrohepatorenal syndrome)
  4. Byler disease

Mechanical Obstruction of the Intrahepatic Bile Ductal

- Congenital hepatic fibrosis
- Caroli disease (cystic dilatation of intrahepatic ducts)

Metabolic Disorders

- Defects of carbohydrate metabolism
  1. Galactosemia
  2. Hereditary fructose intolerance
  3. Glycogenosis type IV
- Defects of lipid metabolism
  1. Gaucher disease
  2. Niemann-Pick disease
  3. Wolman disease
- Tyrosinemia (defect of amino acid metabolism)
- α_1-Antitrypsin deficiency
- Cystic fibrosis
- Parenteral nutrition

Hepatitis

- Hepatitis B
- TORCH agents
- Varicella
- Syphilis
- ECHO viruses
- Neonatal sepsis

Chromosomal Abnormalities

- Down syndrome
- Trisomy 18

Extrahepatic Biliary Atresia

☐ **Pathology:** The characteristic hepatic lesion of neonatal hepatitis is giant cell transformation of hepatocytes, hence the former term *giant cell hepatitis* (Fig. 14-56). The giant cells contain as many as 40 nuclei and may appear detached from other cells in the liver plate. The pale, distended cytoplasm contains large amounts of glycogen and, for unexplained reasons, iron. The number

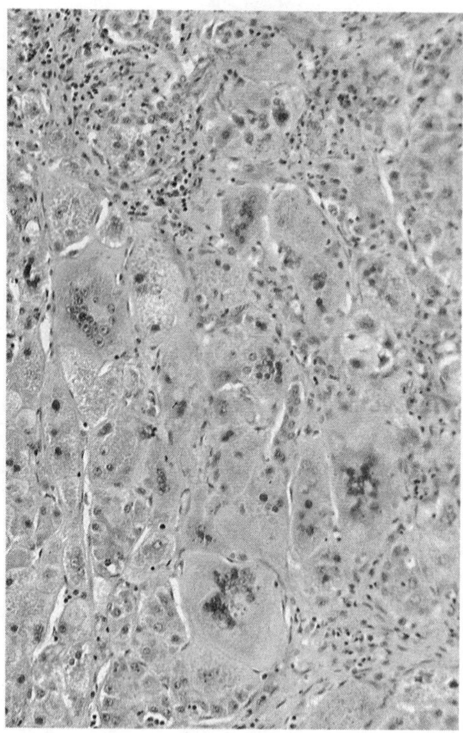

FIGURE *14-56*
Neonatal hepatitis. A photomicrograph shows multinucleated giant hepatocytes, liver cell injury, and a mild chronic inflammatory infiltrate.

of giant cells decreases with time, and they are rare in children older than 1 year of age. Bile pigment is often prominent within canaliculi and hepatocytes. Ballooned hepatocytes, acinar transformation, and acidophilic bodies are also typical of neonatal hepatitis. Extramedullary hemopoiesis is often conspicuous. Chronic inflammatory infiltrates are seen in the portal tracts as well as in the lobular parenchyma. Pericellular fibrosis around degenerating hepatocytes, singly or in groups, is common, and fibrous tissue septa extend from the portal tracts.

Biliary Atresia

Biliary atresia refers to the lack of a lumen in some part of the intrahepatic or extrahepatic biliary tree. Both extrahepatic and intrahepatic biliary atresias are often associated with the morphological features of neonatal hepatitis.

Extrahepatic Biliary Atresia

Extrahepatic biliary atresia is a cholestatic disease characterized by obliteration of the lumen of all or part of the extrahepatic biliary tree. Extrahepatic biliary atresia accounts for almost half of all infants who demonstrate persistent cholestasis in the neonatal period. Of these cases, about 20% exhibit associated congenital anomalies, including abnormalities of the heart, intestinal defects, and splenic malformations. Other cases of extrahepatic biliary obstruction are associated with known causes of neonatal hepatitis, such as chromosomal abnormalities (trisomies) and a number of viral infections.

☐ **Pathology:** Extrahepatic biliary atresia may involve all the extrahepatic bile ducts or may be restricted to segments of the proximal or distal biliary tree. Histologically, the activity of the inflammatory and necrotizing process in the bile ducts is variable. At one extreme, acute and chronic periluminal inflammation is prominent. Epithelial necrosis is evident and cellular debris is found in the obstructed or narrow lumen. At the other extreme, the original lumen is completely replaced by mature connective tissue, and little or no inflammation is present. Histologically, within the liver, cholestasis and periportal bile ductular proliferation are prominent. A minority of cases display multinucleated giant hepatocytes, identical to those seen in neonatal hepatitis. Although the intrahepatic bile ducts may initially appear normal, they are gradually obliterated with the persistence of cholestasis. Eventually, secondary biliary cirrhosis supervenes.

Intrahepatic Biliary Atresia

Intrahepatic biliary atresia refers to a paucity of intrahepatic bile ducts in the absence of extrahepatic biliary obstruction. The disorder occurs under three different circumstances:

- In association with known causes of neonatal hepatitis, for example, α_1-antitrypsin deficiency, various chromosomal anomalies, and metabolic derangements
- **Alagille syndrome** (arteriohepatic dysplasia), an autosomal dominant disease characterized by congenital facial abnormalities, cardiac anomalies, vertebral defects, and a variety of other anomalies
- Unassociated with other conditions (idiopathic)

☐ **Pathology:** The major histological feature of intrahepatic biliary atresia is paucity of the intrahepatic bile ducts. Whereas the normal ratio of intralobular bile ducts to portal tracts is 0.9 to 1.8, in affected infants this ratio is between 0 and 0.4. As the disease progresses, there is a progressive loss of intrahepatic bile ducts. Cholestasis, giant cell transformation, and bile ductular proliferation are usual. In contrast to extrahepatic biliary atresia, cirrhosis is uncommon, although it is occasionally encountered.

It has been suggested that biliary atresia in the newborn, whether intrahepatic or extrahepatic, is secondary to neonatal hepatitis, at least in those instances in which there are no other congenital anomalies. Alternatively, the etiological agent of neonatal hepatitis may independently cause biliary atresia. At one end of the spectrum are cases in which a striking paucity of intrahepatic bile ducts is seen in a liver that exhibits little cell injury and inflammation. At the other extreme, a comparable scarcity of bile ducts is accompanied by severe neonatal hepatitis. Moreover, the cordlike remnant of the common bile duct in cases of extrahepatic biliary atresia often displays chronic inflammation. Instances have been recorded in which a chronically inflamed but patent bile duct has closed and scarred. Last, extrahepatic biliary atresia, like pure intrahepatic biliary atresia, is often associated with full-blown neonatal hepatitis. Embryologically, the bile ducts differentiate from hepatocytes, and it is, therefore, possible that primary liver cell damage in the fetus retards or prevents the development of intrahepatic biliary passages. **These observations support the concept that neonatal hepatitis, intrahepatic biliary atresia, extrahepatic biliary atresia, and possibly choledochal cyst all result from a common inflammatory process (*infantile obstructive cholangiopathy*).**

☐ **Clinical Features:** Most patients who have uncomplicated neonatal hepatitis recover without sequelae. Intrahepatic biliary atresia associated with neonatal hepatitis carries a grave prognosis, since many of these children progress to biliary cirrhosis. By contrast, Alagille syndrome caries a good prognosis. Uncorrected extrahepatic biliary atresia invariably results in progressive secondary biliary cirrhosis and is incompatible with survival. Although surgical correction has been successful in some anatomically favorable cases, the majority of cases of extrahepatic, as well as intrahepatic, biliary atresia can be cured only by liver transplantation.

BENIGN TUMORS AND TUMOR-LIKE LESIONS

Hepatic Adenoma

Hepatic adenomas are benign tumors of hepatocytes that occur principally in women in the reproductive years. These tumors were exceedingly rare before the availability of oral contraceptives, but since their introduction, many such neoplasms have been reported. Today, hepatic adenomas are a well-recognized, although uncommon, complication of the use of oral contraceptives. It appears that the incidence of this tumor has been reduced by the use of low-dose formulations, but sporadic cases are still occasionally encountered.

☐ **Pathology:** Hepatic adenomas usually occur as solitary, sharply demarcated masses, up to 40 cm in diameter and 3 kg in weight (Fig. 14-57). In a fourth of the cases, multiple smaller adenomas are present. On gross examination, the tumor is encapsulated and paler than the surrounding parenchyma. Occasionally, hemorrhage and necrosis are present in the center of the tumor.

Microscopically, the neoplastic hepatocytes resemble their normal counterparts, except that they are not arranged in a lobular architecture (see Fig. 14-57). Portal tracts and central venules are not present. The cells composing the adenoma may be very large and eosinophilic or filled with glycogen, which makes the cytoplasm appear clear. By electron microscopy, the neoplastic hepatocytes have a "simplified" appearance. The tumor is circumscribed by a fibrous capsule of variable thickness, and the adjacent hepatocytes appear compressed. Large, thick-walled arteries are often seen in the vicinity of the capsule, and arteries and veins traverse the tumor.

☐ **Clinical Features:** In about one third of patients with hepatic adenomas (particularly in pregnant women

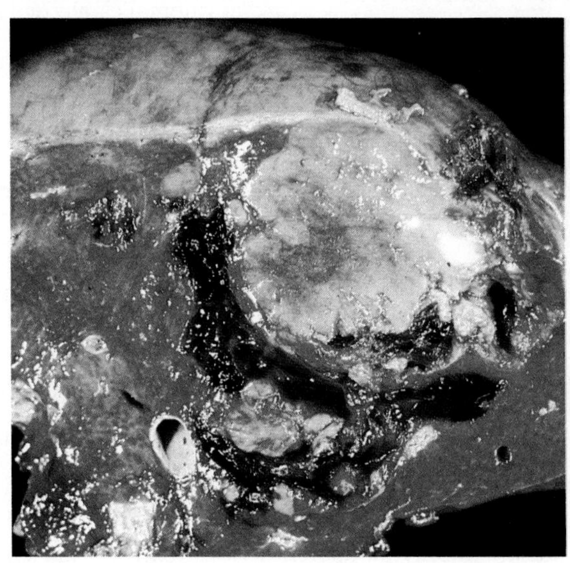
A

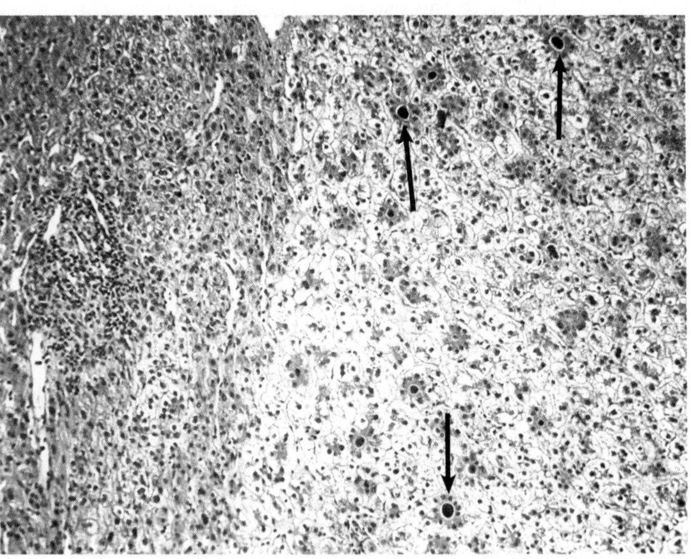
B

FIGURE 14-57
Hepatic adenoma. (*A*) A surgically resected portion of liver shows a tan, lobulated mass beneath the liver capsule. Hemorrhage into the tumor has broken through the capsule and also into the surrounding liver parenchyma. The patient was a woman who had taken birth control pills for a number of years and presented with sudden intraperitoneal hemorrhage. (*B*) There is a clear border between normal liver (*left*) and the adenoma. The adenomatous hepatocytes are arranged without discernible lobular architecture and show a clear cytoplasm filled with glycogen. Occasional cells are arranged in acini, which contain inspissated bile (*arrows*).

who have used oral contraceptives), **the tumors bleed into the peritoneal cavity and require treatment as a surgical emergency**. Some women report episodes of sudden abdominal pain, presumably a reflection of hemorrhage into the tumor. Even large adenomas have been reported to disappear after discontinuation of oral contraceptive use. A few adenomas are encountered in men, and they have occasionally been reported in association with the use of anabolic steroids. Despite isolated reports of progression to hepatocellular carcinoma, hepatic adenoma is not generally believed to be a premalignant lesion.

Focal Nodular Hyperplasia

Focal nodular hyperplasia is a nodular lesion in an otherwise normal liver, which is histologically characterized by a cirrhotic appearance. The hepatic mass varies in size from 5 to 15 cm in diameter and weighs as much as 700 g. On occasion, it protrudes from the surface of the liver, and it may even be pedunculated. The cut surface exhibits a characteristic central scar from which fibrous septa radiate. The division of the mass by multiple fibrous septa accounts for the older term **focal cirrhosis**. Microscopically, hepatocytic nodules are circumscribed by fibrous septa (Fig. 14-58), which contain numerous tortuous bile ducts and mononuclear inflammatory cells. Within the nodules, lobular architecture is absent. The lesion exhibits large arteries and veins in the septa, but hemorrhage is uncommon. The mass is not truly encapsulated, although the border is distinct on gross examination.

Focal nodular hyperplasia occurs in both sexes and at all ages, but most often in young women. It is not thought to be associated with the use of oral contraceptives. The lesion does not progress to cancer.

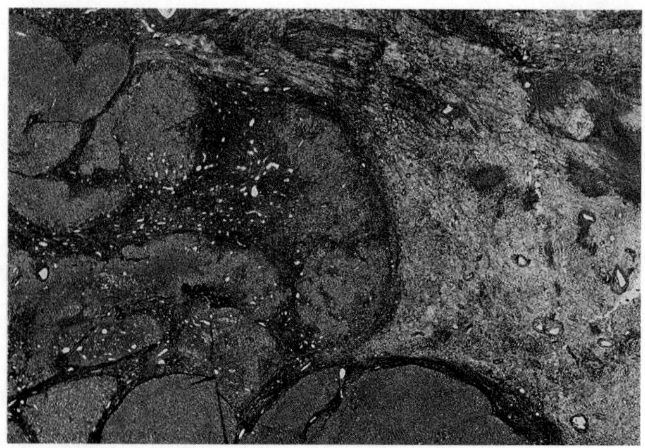

FIGURE *14-58*
Focal nodular hyperplasia. A photomicrograph of a surgically resected mass from the liver demonstrates a vascular central scar and irregular fibrous septa dissecting hepatic parenchyma, accounting for the resemblance to cirrhosis.

Nodular Regenerative Hyperplasia (Nodular Transformation of the Liver, Partial Nodular Transformation)

Nodular regenerative hyperplasia occurs in noncirrhotic livers and is characterized by small, hyperplastic nodules without fibrosis. The lesion may be partial and located predominantly in the perihilar region or may be diffuse throughout the liver. The nodules, composed of liver cells arranged in plates that are two and three cells thick, compress the surrounding parenchyma. Liver cell dysplasia (i.e., enlargement of the cells, nuclear pleomorphism, and the presence of multinucleated hepatocytes) is occasionally noted within the nodules.

The clinical importance of nodular regenerative hyperplasia relates to portal hypertension, which accounts for the older term *noncirrhotic portal hypertension*. The etiology of nodular regenerative hyperplasia is unknown, but it has been reported in association with the use of oral contraceptives or anabolic steroids, extrahepatic infections, neoplasms, chronic inflammatory disorders, and autoimmune diseases. The lesion is not considered to be preneoplastic.

Hemangioma

Hemangiomas, occurring at all ages and in both sexes, are the most common benign tumors of the liver, being found in up to 7% of autopsy specimens. They are ordinarily small and asymptomatic, although larger tumors have been reported to cause abdominal symptoms and even hemorrhage into the peritoneal cavity. Grossly, the tumor is usually solitary and less than 5 cm in diameter, but multiple hemangiomas and giant forms have been described. Microscopically, the tumor is similar to cavernous hemangiomas found elsewhere.

Infantile hemangioendothelioma, a rare cellular tumor that appears during the first 2 years of life, and sometimes at birth, contains arteriovenous shunts that may be large enough to cause congestive heart failure. Malignant transformation has been reported in a few cases.

Cystic Disease of the Liver

BILE DUCT MICROHAMARTOMAS (VON MEYENBURG COMPLEXES): These lesions consist of anomalous, small cystic bile ducts embedded in a fibrous stroma. They are usually multiple and vary from barely visible grayish-white foci to nodules 1 cm in diameter. Microscopically, the cysts are lined by bile duct epithelium and sometimes contain inspissated bile. It is thought that these clinically inapparent lesions represent one end of the spectrum of cystic disease of the liver.

SOLITARY AND MULTIPLE SIMPLE CYSTS: Simple cysts of the liver are lined by cuboidal to columnar epithelium and are often associated with adult polycystic disease of the kidney, an autosomal dominant trait. They are not infrequently seen in livers that contain von Meyenburg complexes.

CONGENITAL HEPATIC FIBROSIS: *This recessively inherited disorder is marked by enlarged portal tracts, which exhibit extensive fibrosis and numerous bile ductules that communicate with the biliary tree.* It is seen predominantly in children and adolescents. The bile ductules may be so dilated that they resemble microcysts, but even in these cases they retain their communication with the biliary system. The area involved by congenital hepatic fibrosis is sharply demarcated from the normal liver parenchyma. Regenerative nodules are absent, an appearance that distinguishes this condition from cirrhosis. The origin of the lesion is unknown, but it has been postulated that it may arise as a result of abnormal differentiation of primitive duct structures. The principal complication of congenital hepatic fibrosis is severe portal hypertension, with recurrent bleeding from esophageal varices. **Infantile polycystic disease** of the liver resembles congenital hepatic fibrosis and is also inherited as an autosomal recessive trait.

MALIGNANT TUMORS OF THE LIVER

Hepatocellular Carcinoma

Hepatocellular carcinoma (HCC) refers to malignant tumors that derive from hepatocytes or their precursors.

☐ **Epidemiology and Pathogenesis:** HCC is probably the most common malignant tumor of humans. It occurs in all parts of the world, but its incidence shows a striking geographic variability. In Western industrialized countries, the tumor is uncommon; in sub-Saharan Africa, Southeast Asia, and Japan, the rates are up to 50 times greater. For example, in Mozambique, which seems to have the highest incidence in the world, two thirds of all cancers in men and one third in women are HCC.

HEPATITIS B: **An association between HCC and infection with the hepatitis B virus (HBV) is clearly established.** The geographic incidence of this tumor correlates strongly with the prevalence of the carrier state for HBV. Moreover, in areas of high incidence, HBV infection was previously documented in some 80% of patients with HCC. Most patients had chronic HBV infection for many years, the disease often being transmitted from an infected mother to her newborn child perinatally. The carrier state is indeed dangerous, since such persons are estimated to have as much as a 200-fold increased risk of developing HCC. One fourth of those with chronic hepatitis B acquired at or near birth ultimately develop HCC.

Although most cases of HCC associated with HBV infection occur in patients with cirrhosis, numerous cases in noncirrhotic livers have also been reported. However, in most instances of HCC in HBsAg-positive persons who do not have cirrhosis, the liver shows some degree of chronic hepatitis. This suggests that persistent cell injury is crucial in the pathogenesis of HCC.

Further evidence that HBV has an important role in the development of hepatocellular carcinoma comes from the demonstration that **the genome of HBV is integrated into the host DNA of both the non-neoplastic liver cells and the tumor cells.** The prospective worldwide use of a vaccine for hepatitis B may significantly decrease the prevalence of HCC in the future. The role of HBV itself in the pathogenesis of liver cancer is discussed in Chapter 5.

HEPATITIS C: It has recently been demonstrated that two thirds to three fourths of patients with primary HCC in areas not endemic for HBV demonstrate antibodies to HCV. Interestingly, in some countries, notably Japan, in which HBV infection is endemic and has been the major cause of HCC, there has been a remarkable shift in the pattern of viral infection. Whereas in Japan, HBsAg-positive cases accounted for about half of all HCC in the early 1970s, fewer than one fifth of the cases today exhibit evidence of HBV infection. At the same time, about three quarters of Japanese patients with HCC now have evidence of infection with HCV. By contrast, in less-developed countries, HBV is still the predominant etiological factor in the pathogenesis of HCC. **Thus, in industrialized countries with low rates of HBV prevalence, the major cause of HCC is hepatitis C.**

The risk of liver cancer in persons who have anti-HCV and anti-HBc together is three times higher than in those with either antibody alone. It is possible that HBV and HCV can act synergistically to predispose to hepatocellular carcinoma.

Alcoholic cirrhosis has been considered by some to be an important predisposing condition for hepatocellular carcinoma. However, the high prevalence of infection with HBV and HCV in patients with alcoholic cirrhosis suggests that neither alcohol per se nor alcoholic cirrhosis alone is the culprit.

Other forms of cirrhosis are also associated with a high incidence of HCC. Liver diseases occurring in conjunction with hemochromatosis and α_1-antitrypsin deficiency carry a substantial risk of HCC: about 10% of patients with hemochromatosis may be expected to develop the tumor. On the other hand, HCC is rare in patients with "autoimmune" chronic hepatitis and cirrhosis, Wilson disease, and primary biliary cirrhosis. Hepatitis A has not been incriminated as a predisposing factor for hepatocellular carcinoma.

Aflatoxin B_1, a contaminant of many foods, particularly in less-developed countries, produces HCC in a number of mammalian species. The incidence of liver cancer in humans has been roughly correlated with the content of aflatoxin in the diet, although significant exceptions have been found. Since areas in which the diet is heavily contaminated with aflatoxin are also areas in which hepatitis B is endemic, the contribution of this toxin to the development of HCC in humans remains enigmatic.

Analyses of DNA from HCC in Africa and China, two areas with a high incidence of this cancer, revealed that as many as half of the samples had mutations in the p53 gene. Interestingly, most of these mutations were G-to-T substitutions in one particular codon (249), a change known to be produced experimentally by aflatoxin B_1.

☐ **Pathology:** HCCs appear grossly as soft and hemorrhagic tan masses in the liver (Fig. 14-59). Occasionally,

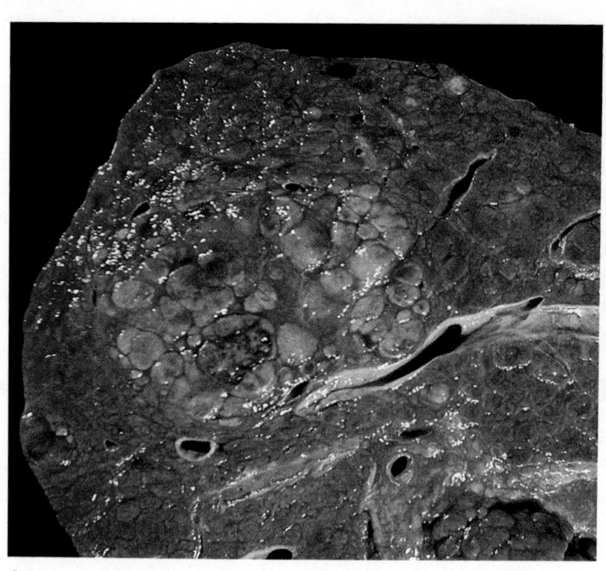

A

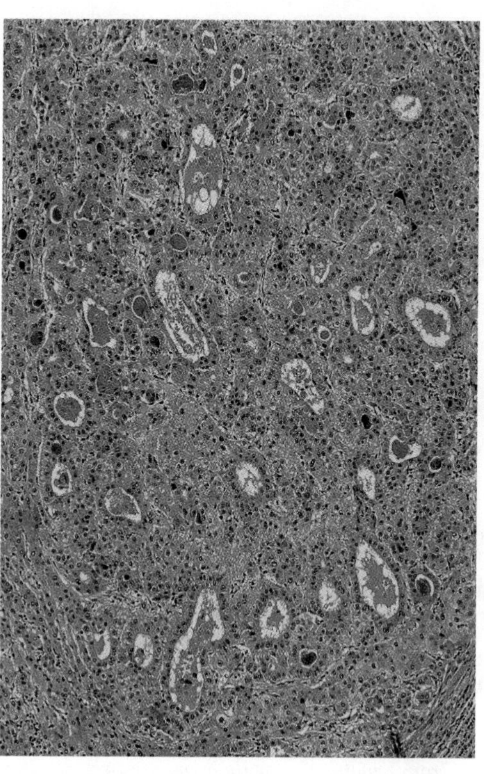

B

FIGURE *14-59*
Hepatocellular carcinoma. (*A*) Cross-section of a cirrhotic liver shows a poorly circumscribed, nodular area of yellow, partially hemorrhagic hepatocellular carcinoma. (*B*) A photomicrograph of the tumor shows a trabecular pattern of malignant hepatocytes. Many are arranged in an acinar pattern and surround concretions of inspissated bile.

a green color is present, indicating bile staining. In some cases, a large solitary tumor occupies a portion of the liver, whereas in other cases many smaller tumors are found. Multiple lesions are believed to indicate a multicentric origin of the tumor, although intrahepatic metastases from a single HCC cannot be excluded. The tumor has a tendency to grow into portal veins and may extend to the vena cava, and even the right atrium, through the hepatic veins.

A number of histological patterns are recognized, but no prognostic significance can be attributed to any of them. Most HCCs exhibit a *trabecular pattern,* that is, the tumor cells are arranged in trabeculae or plates that resemble the normal liver (see Fig. 14-59). The plates are separated by endothelium-lined sinusoids, but Kupffer cells are absent. Occasionally, tumor growth in the trabecular variant compresses the sinusoids to such an extent that the lesion appears solid. A second histological variant is termed the *pseudoglandular* (*adenoid, acinar*) *pattern.* In this variety, malignant hepatocytes are arranged around a lumen and thus resemble glands. The lumen may contain bile, and biliary canaliculi are often seen between the tumor cells. Endothelium-lined sinusoids are interspersed between the pseudoglandular structures. It is important to bear in mind that the acini formed by the tumor cells are not true glands, and the lesion should not be confused with adenocarcinoma. Some HCCs contain a considerable fibrous stroma, which separates tumor cell plates, accounting for the term *scirrhous carcinoma.*

***Fibrolamellar hepatocellular carcinoma** has a distinctive histological appearance and arises in an apparently normal liver, principally in adolescents and young adults.* The tumor is composed of large, eosinophilic, neoplastic hepatocytes arranged in clusters and surrounded by delicate collagen fibers (Fig. 14-60). As with oncocytes in other tumors, the eosinophilic character of the cytoplasm reflects an accumulation of mitochondria. The prognosis is said to be better than for other varieties of HCC.

Cytologically, some hepatocellular tumors are highly pleomorphic and exhibit conspicuous variation in the size and staining properties of the tumor cell nuclei, multinucleated cells, and giant cells. These changes may lead to disarray of the tumor cell plates, so that the trabecular pattern is obscured. Other HCCs may be partly or entirely composed of clear cells, which usually contain glycogen but may contain fat. Such clear cell tumors have been on occasion mistakenly identified as metastatic renal cell or adrenal carcinomas. Mallory bodies are seen in a minority of HCCs, although in some cases they are particularly conspicuous. Occasional carcinomas exhibit eosinophilic globules in the cytoplasm of tumor cells, some of which contain α-fetoprotein or α_1-antitrypsin.

Hepatocellular carcinoma may reach a large size be-

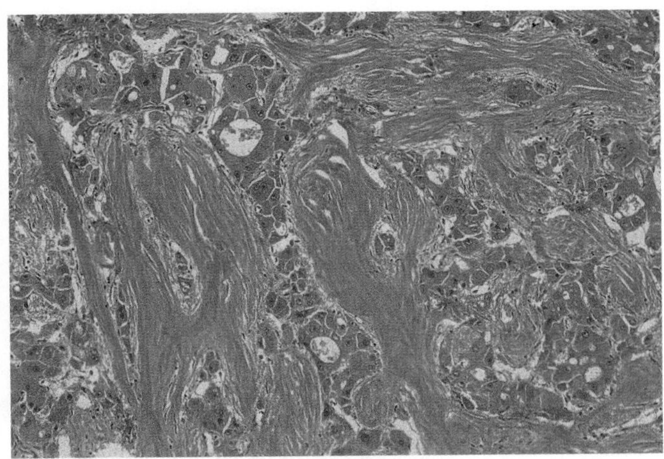

FIGURE 14-60
Fibrolamellar hepatocellular carcinoma. Eosinophilic tumor cells show a lamellar pattern and are surrounded by collagen fibers.

fore metastasizing. Metastases occur widely, but the most common sites are the lungs and portal lymph nodes.

□ **Clinical Features:** HCC usually presents as a painful and enlarging mass in the liver. Ascites, portal vein thrombosis, occlusion of hepatic veins, and hemorrhage from esophageal varices are common. The prognosis is dismal, and patients die of malignant cachexia, rupture of the tumor with catastrophic bleeding into the peritoneal cavity, bleeding esophageal varices, or hepatic failure.

Hepatocellular carcinoma may be associated with a variety of paraneoplastic manifestations (e.g., polycythemia, hypoglycemia, hypercalcemia) as a result of hormone production by the tumor. α-Fetoprotein, a circulating marker produced by hepatocellular carcinomas, is particularly important because of its diagnostic value. Normally, this fetal protein falls to very low levels (<10 ng/mL) by 1 year of age. In patients with HCC, levels above 4000 ng/mL are reported, and in most cases, the value is over 400 ng/mL. Since elevated levels of α-fetoprotein are also encountered in other neoplastic and non-neoplastic liver diseases and in some extrahepatic disorders, the finding of high concentrations of this oncofetoprotein is not absolutely diagnostic of HCC. Nevertheless, it remains an excellent screening measure for detection of this tumor and is used to monitor treated patients for recurrence.

In the cases of small tumors confined to one hepatic lobe, segmental resections of the liver have been successful in curing HCC in as many as half of the patients. In larger tumors, hepatic transplantation has been employed, but with generally disappointing results.

Cholangiocarcinoma (Bile Duct Carcinoma)

Cholangiocarcinoma is a malignant hepatic tumor of biliary epithelium, which arises anywhere from the large intrahepatic bile ducts at the porta hepatis to the smallest bile ductules at the periphery of the hepatic lobule. Cholangiocarcinoma occurs predominantly in older persons of both sexes, with an average age at presentation of 60 years. This cancer is particularly frequent in those parts of Asia in which the liver fluke *(C. sinensis)* is endemic, although cholangiocarcinoma is encountered in all parts of the world.

Peripheral cholangiocarcinomas are tumors that arise at the lobular level and frequently occur in association with cirrhosis. Cancers of the larger intrahepatic ducts are rare.

Hilar cholangiocarcinomas are extrahepatic lesions arising at the convergence of the right and left hepatic ducts. They produce symptoms of extrahepatic biliary obstruction.

□ **Pathology:** Peripheral cholangiocarcinomas are composed of small cuboidal cells arranged in a ductular or glandular configuration (Fig. 14-61). Characteristically, they show substantial fibrosis, and on liver biopsy they may be confused with metastatic scirrhous carcinoma of the breast or pancreas. A combined form of hepatocellular carcinoma and peripheral cholangiocarcinoma has been labeled *cholangiohepatocellular carcinoma.*

Hilar cholangiocarcinomas present three histological patterns: (1) a small sclerosing tumor that obliterates the duct, (2) a tumor that spreads within the wall of the duct, and (3) a rare intraductal papillary variant.

Cholangiocarcinomas show a lesser tendency to invade the portal and hepatic veins than do hepatocellular carcinomas. They metastasize to a wide variety of extra-

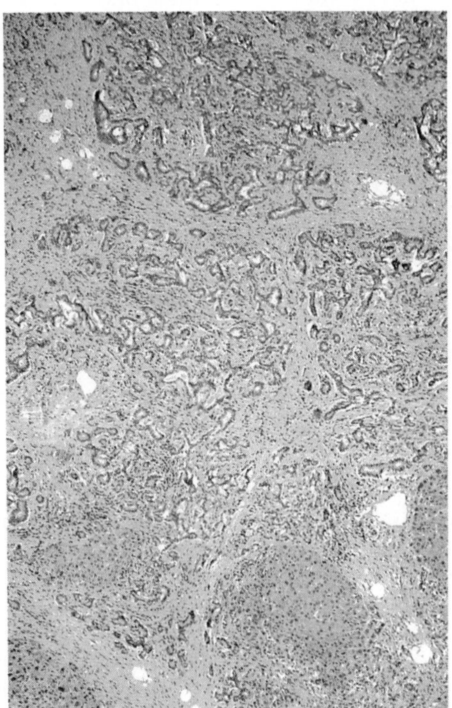

FIGURE 14-61
Cholangiocarcinoma. Well-differentiated neoplastic glands are embedded in a dense fibrous stroma. A few islands of hepatocytes are present.

hepatic sites and show a greater predilection for the portal lymph nodes than do hepatocellular carcinomas. Liver transplantation has been attempted in cases of cholangiocarcinoma but is rarely successful in eradicating the tumor.

Hepatoblastoma

Hepatoblastoma is a rare malignant tumor of the liver in children, found from birth to the age of 3 years.

☐ **Pathology:** The tumor presents as a partially necrotic and hemorrhagic circumscribed mass up to 25 cm in diameter. Microscopically, cells of epithelial and mesenchymal appearance are seen, but occasionally the latter are missing. The epithelial component of hepatoblastoma includes cells resembling embryonal and fetal cells. The "embryonal" cells are small and fusiform and are arranged in ribbons or rosettes. The "fetal" cells more closely resemble hepatocytes, contain glycogen and fat, and are arranged in trabeculae with intervening sinusoids. Extramedullary hemopoiesis is usually seen in the area populated by "fetal" cells. Foci of squamous epithelium are occasionally encountered. The mesenchymal elements include those often present in teratomas, including connective tissue, cartilage, and osteoid.

☐ **Clinical Features:** Attention is called to the presence of a hepatoblastoma by enlargement of the abdomen, vomiting, and failure to thrive. The serum α-fetoprotein level is almost invariably elevated, and occasionally secretion of ectopic gonadotropin leads to sexual precocity. Some of these children also exhibit congenital anomalies, including cardiac and renal malformations, hemihypertrophy, and macroglossia. Untreated hepatoblastomas are invariably fatal, but surgical resection by partial hepatectomy has been curative in many instances.

Hemangiosarcoma

Hemangiosarcoma is historically the only significant sarcoma of the liver. As noted earlier, it may result from exposure to thorium dioxide, vinyl chloride, or inorganic arsenic. With the increased awareness of the hazard posed by these agents, hemangiosarcoma of the liver has become distinctly uncommon.

☐ **Pathology:** On gross examination, hemangiosarcoma is characteristically multicentric, presenting as multiple hemorrhagic nodules, which may coalesce. Microscopic examination reveals spindle-shaped, neoplastic, endothelial cells that line the sinusoids and compress the liver cell plates. The tumor may form cavernous blood spaces and solid masses of neoplastic cells. Extramedullary hemopoiesis is almost invariable. Hemorrhage, thrombosis, and infarction often complicate the morphological pattern of this tumor. The tumor metastasizes widely.

☐ **Clinical Features:** Patients with hemangiosarcoma of the liver present with hepatomegaly, jaundice, and ascites. Hematological abnormalities, including pancytopenia and hemolytic anemia, are often prominent and in many cases reflect splenomegaly from noncirrhotic portal hypertension. The tumor may rupture and bleed vigorously into the abdominal cavity. The prognosis is poor.

Other rare malignant mesenchymal tumors of the liver include embryonal rhabdomyosarcoma, leiomyosarcoma, fibrosarcoma, and malignant mesenchymoma.

Metastatic Cancer

Metastatic cancers are by far the most common malignant neoplasms of the liver. The liver is involved in a third of all metastatic cancers, including half of those of the gastrointestinal tract, breast, and lung. Other tumors that characteristically metastasize to the liver are pancreatic carcinoma and malignant melanoma.

☐ **Pathology:** The liver may show only a single nodule of tumor or may be virtually replaced by metastases (Fig. 14-62), and liver weights of 5 kg or more are not uncommon. **In fact, liver metastases are the most common cause of massive hepatomegaly.** Metastatic carcinomas are often seen on the surface of the liver as umbilicated masses, a reflection of central necrosis and hemorrhage. The metastatic deposits tend to be histologically similar to the primary tumor, but on occasion are so undifferentiated that the primary site cannot be determined.

☐ **Clinical Features:** Weight loss is a common early finding in cases of metastatic cancer in the liver. Portal hypertension with splenomegaly, ascites, and gastrointestinal bleeding may occur. Obstruction of the major bile ducts or replacement of most of the liver parenchyma leads to jaundice. If the patient lives long enough, hepatic failure may ensue. Often the first indication of a

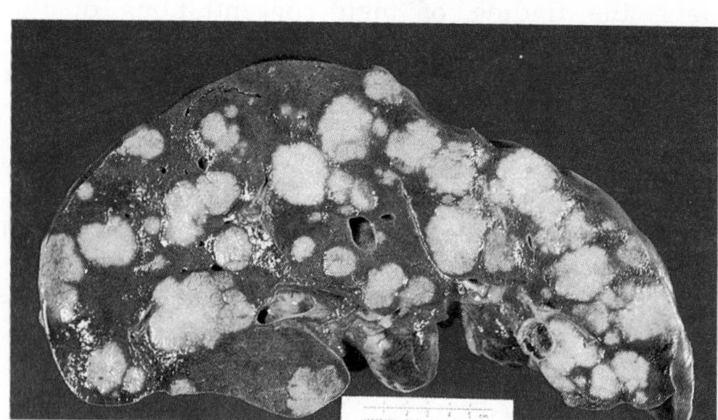

FIGURE *14-62*
Metastatic carcinoma in the liver. The cut surface of the liver shows many firm, pale masses of metastatic colon cancer.

metastatic tumor is an unexplained increase in the serum alkaline phosphatase level. The majority of patients die within a year of the diagnosis of liver metastases.

LIVER TRANSPLANTATION

The increasing availability of hepatic transplantation and the accompanying problems related to allograft rejection have focused attention on the morphological criteria by which the outcome can be assessed and therapy recommended. In this respect, it is clear that serial liver biopsies are the best means of clinical assessment after liver transplantation. Despite immunosuppressive therapy, about three fourths of patients subjected to hepatic transplantation may be expected to develop some morphological evidence of graft rejection in as little as 2 days or as long as 6 months.

☐ **Pathology:** Early rejection is characterized by chronic inflammation and enlargement of the portal tracts (Fig. 14-63). Large and small lymphocytes, plasma cells, and macrophages are present, and a few neutrophils and eosinophils are common. Occasionally, the inflammatory infiltrate extends beyond the borders of the portal tracts and is associated with necrosis of periportal hepatocytes, an appearance similar to that of so-called piecemeal necrosis of chronic hepatitis.

Early rejection results in distortion of the bile ducts by the portal inflammatory infiltrate, atypism of bile duct epithelial cells, and often inflammation of the ductal epithelium itself. Hyperplasia and chronic inflammation of bile ductules within the portal tracts may be conspicuous. Most cases exhibit moderate cholestasis, principally in the centrilobular zones.

In almost all cases of early rejection, lymphocytes are adherent to the endothelium of terminal venules and small branches of the portal veins, with or without subendothelial inflammation. This appearance has been termed *endothelialitis*. Varying degrees of centrilobular necrosis are accompanied by collapse of the reticulin framework; in severe cases, collapsed zones may link adjacent central venules.

This combination of mixed portal inflammation, mononuclear infiltration of venous endothelium, and injury to intrahepatic bile ducts has been compared with graft-versus-host disease. Intensive treatment with immunosuppressive agents generally causes most of these changes to subside.

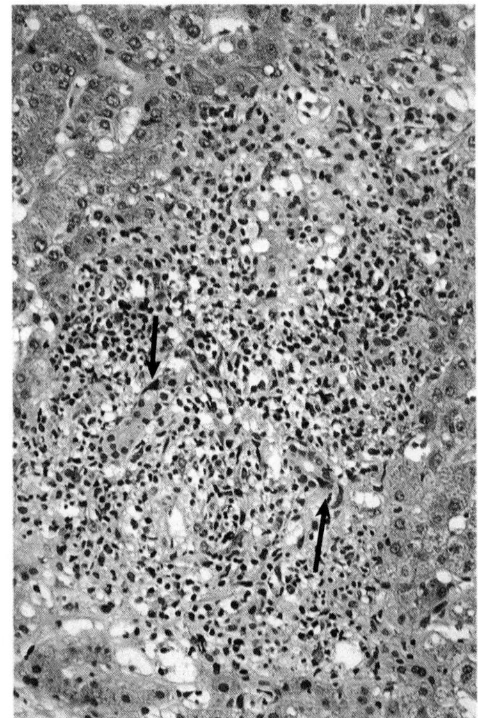

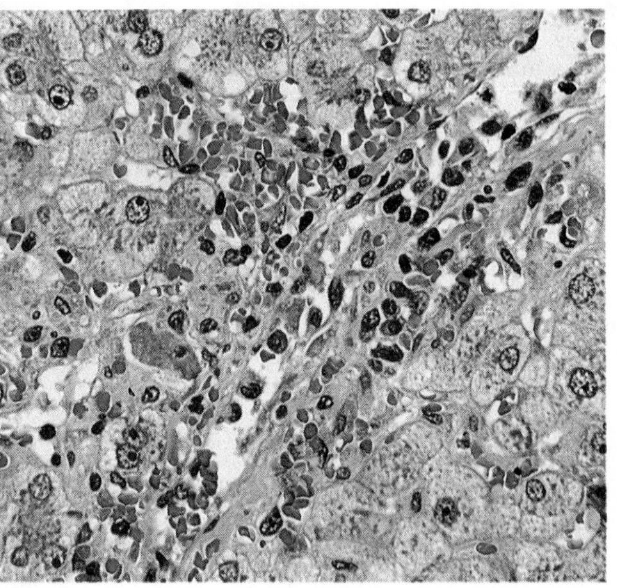

FIGURE *14-63*
Acute rejection of a liver transplant. (*A*) A portal tract is expanded by a polymorphous inflammatory infiltrate consisting of large and small lymphocytes, plasma cells, macrophages, and neutrophils. The bile ducts (*arrows*) are damaged and inflamed. (*B*) A central vein from the same biopsy exhibits endothelialitis, characterized by swollen endothelial cells and infiltrating lymphocytes.

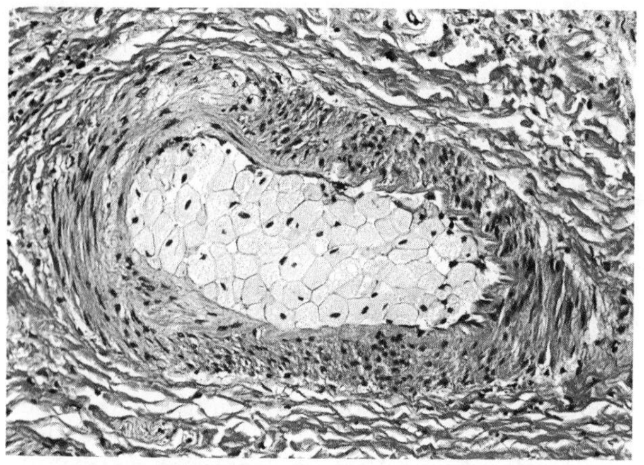

FIGURE *14-64*
Arterial lesions in chronic rejection of a liver transplant. Subintimal foam cells, intimal sclerosis, and myointimal hyperplasia virtually obliterate the lumen of a hepatic artery.

Allograft rejection persisting for more than 2 months generally exhibits a less intense inflammatory reaction, although in some cases it may remain severe. Periportal hepatocellular necrosis, however, is usually more conspicuous. **Damage to interlobular bile ducts** is now more prominent. As the lesion progresses, these small bile ducts are destroyed, and persistent cholestasis, similar to that seen in primary biliary cirrhosis, ensues. The end stage of this process is referred to as the *vanishing bile duct syndrome*.

On occasion, usually in late rejection but even in early rejection, medium-sized arteries in the porta hepatis display a **vasculitis**, with fibrinoid necrosis, disruption of the elastic lamina, and an infiltrate of lymphocytes and macrophages. Within several months, subintimal foam cells, intimal sclerosis, and myointimal hyperplasia may narrow or occlude these arteries (Fig. 14-64).

A serious complication of liver transplantation is the occasional occurrence of infection with cytomegalovirus or herpes simplex virus type 1 in the transplanted liver. When the transplant recipient has been a carrier of HBV or HCV, infection of the new liver is usual.

The Gallbladder and Extrahepatic Bile Ducts

ANATOMY

The gallbladder originates from the same foregut diverticulum that gives rise to the liver. In about one week, the gallbladder and cystic duct are discernible. The lumen of the gallbladder is formed in the 12th week of gestation.

The adult gallbladder, a thin elongated sac about 8 cm in length and about 50 mL in volume, occupies a fossa on the inferior surface of the liver between the right and the quadrate lobes. The primary function of the gallbladder is the storage, concentration, and release of bile. The cystic duct, which empties the gallbladder into the hepatic duct, is about 3 cm long. Its mucosa is arranged in a series of folds, termed the *valves of Heister*. Dilute bile from the hepatic duct passes into the gallbladder through the cystic duct, where it is concentrated and subsequently discharged into the common bile duct. The gallbladder is usually supplied by a branch of the right hepatic artery. Anatomical variations in the vascular anatomy may bring the parent artery into the surgical field of a cholecystectomy, in which case the surgeon must take great care not to ligate it. A similar caution must be exercised to avoid ligation of the common bile duct. A rich plexus of lymphatics drains the gallbladder and serves as a convenient route for metastases from gallbladder carcinoma.

The wall of the gallbladder is composed of a mucous membrane, a muscularis, and an adventitia and is covered by a reflection of the visceral peritoneum. The mucosa is thrown into folds and consists of a columnar epithelium and a lamina propria of loose connective tissue. Dipping into the wall of the gallbladder are mucosal diverticula, termed *Rokitansky-Aschoff sinuses*. Branched mucous glands are found near the neck of the gallbladder. *The ducts of Luschka*, presumably remnants of aberrant embryonic bile ducts, are located in the connective tissue between the liver and the gallbladder and connect with the cystic duct.

CONGENITAL ANOMALIES

Developmental anomalies of the gallbladder are rare and of little clinical significance except for the surgeon. **Agenesis** and **atresia** occur, and **duplication** is occasionally noted. **Heterotopic tissue**, including gastric, adrenal, pancreatic, and thyroid elements, has been recorded in the gallbladder, usually in conjunction with cholelithiasis and cholecystitis. Although the gallbladder is usually partially embedded in the liver, it floats free in about 4% of the normal population. Ectopic locations of the gallbladder, including the left lobe of the liver and the falciform ligament, are seen uncommonly.

The cystic duct may be absent or duplicated. On occasion, it is abnormally long and enters the bile duct close to its termination, or it may join the right hepatic duct. Again, these are important considerations for the surgeon.

Anomalies of the bile duct include **duplication** and **accessory bile ducts**. **Extrahepatic biliary atresia** was discussed earlier. Congenital dilatations of the bile duct are termed *choledochal cyst* (85% of all cases), *choledochal diverticulum*, and *choledochocele* (Fig. 14-65). Multiple cysts may occur as segmental dilatations in the entire extrahepatic biliary tree. Similar multiple dilatations in the intrahepatic portion of the biliary tree, termed *Caroli disease*, predispose to bacterial cholangitis. It has been suggested that choledochal cysts form part of the same complex as neonatal hepatitis and biliary atresia.

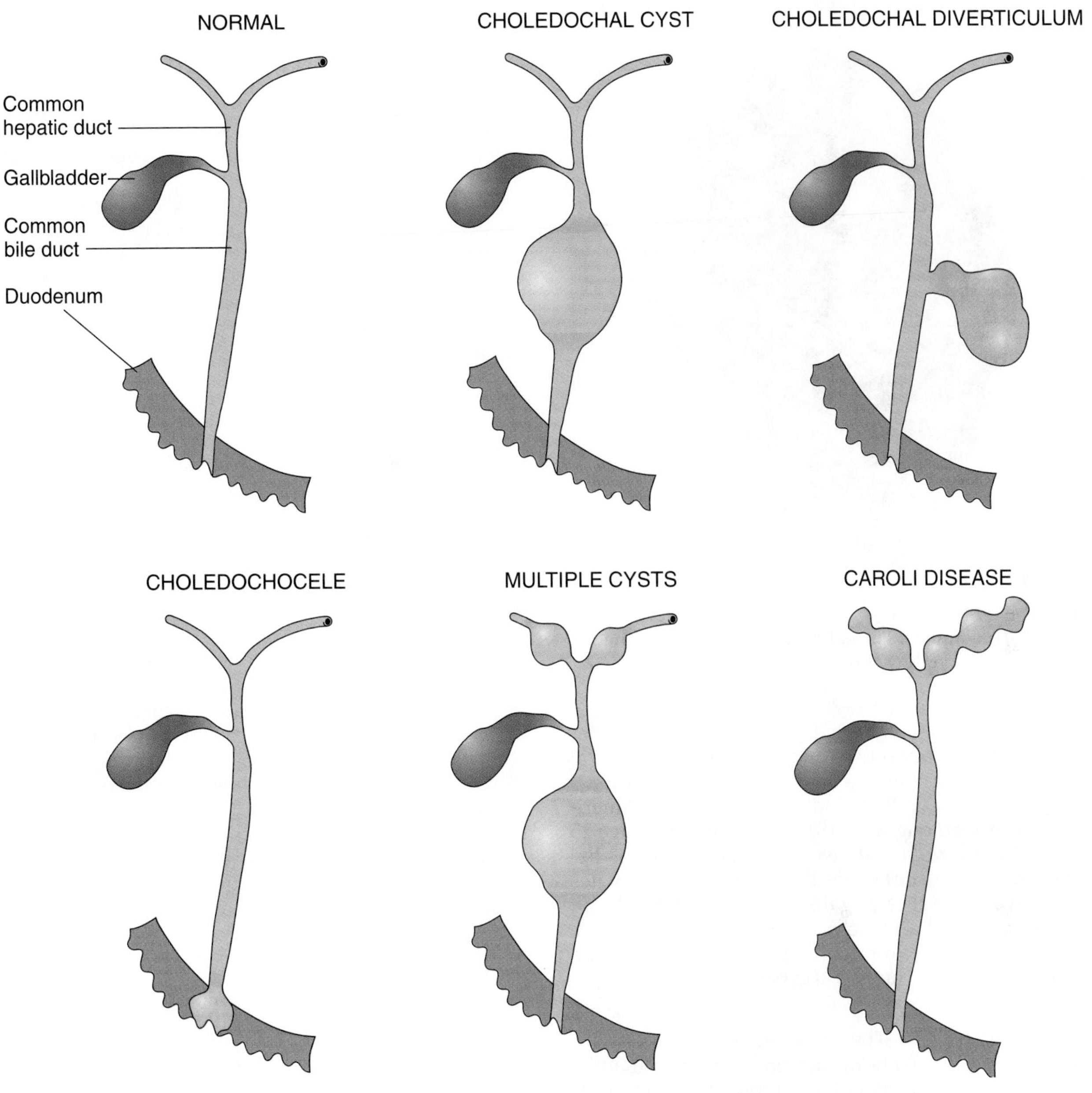

FIGURE *14-65*
Congenital dilatations of the bile ducts.

CHOLELITHIASIS

Cholelithiasis is defined as the presence of stones within the lumen of the gallbladder or in the extrahepatic biliary tree. Three fourths of gallstones in the industrialized countries consist primarily of cholesterol, and the remainder are composed of calcium bilirubinate and other calcium salts (pigment gallstones). However, pigment stones predominate in the tropics and the Orient. Most gallstones are not radiopaque, but they are readily visualized by ultrasound examination. Although gallstones are frequently asymptomatic, they often cause mild to severe pain (*biliary colic*) as a result of impaction in the cystic duct, or less frequently in the common bile duct.

Cholesterol Stones

Cholesterol stones are round or faceted, yellow to tan, and single or multiple and vary from 1 to 4 cm in greatest dimension (Fig. 14-66). Well over 50% of the stone is composed of cholesterol; the rest consists of calcium salts and mucin.

☐ **Epidemiology:** Cholesterol gallstones are common in the United States: 20% of American men and 35% of women older than the age of 75 years have gallstones at autopsy. **However, during their reproductive period, women are three times more likely to develop choles-**

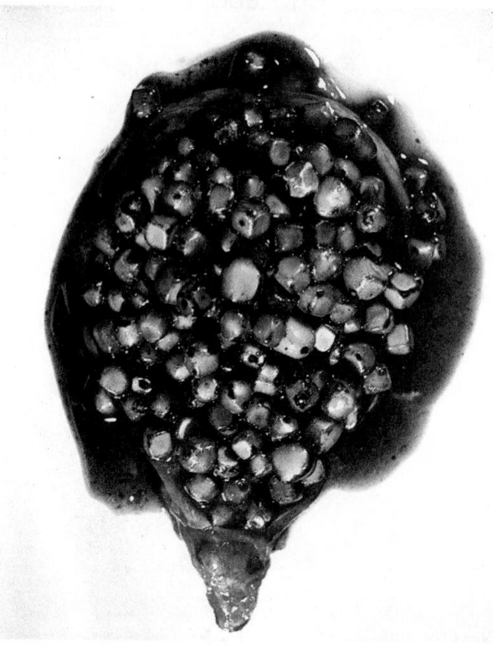

FIGURE *14-66*
Cholesterol gallstones. The gallbladder has been opened to reveal numerous yellow cholesterol gallstones.

terol gallstones than are men, the incidence being higher in users of oral contraceptives and in women with several pregnancies. Interestingly, cholesterol gallstones are exceedingly common in Pima Indian women of the American Southwest, among whom 75% are affected by age 25 and 90% by the age of 60 years. This occurrence is believed to reflect genetic factors. Blacks in the United States have a lower incidence of gallstones than whites, but a higher incidence than blacks in Africa. This difference probably reflects environmental influences, although a role for genetic admixtures is also possible.

☐ **Pathogenesis:** The pathogenesis of cholesterol stones relates principally to the composition of the bile (Fig. 14-67). Normally, cholesterol, a compound highly insoluble in water, is secreted by the hepatocytes into the bile, where it is held in solution by the combined action of bile acids and lecithin and carried in the form of mixed lipid micelles. If the bile contains excess cholesterol or is deficient in bile acids, the bile becomes supersaturated, and under some circumstances the cholesterol precipitates as solid crystals. **The bile of persons afflicted with cholesterol gallstones has more cholesterol as it leaves the liver than that of normal persons, pointing to the liver, rather than the gallbladder, as the culprit in the genesis of cholesterol stones.** The hepatocytes of patients with cholesterol gallstones are deficient in 7-hydroxylase, the enzyme involved in the rate-limiting step by which bile salts are formed from cholesterol. **As a result, the total size of the bile salt pool is reduced.** The resulting decrease in bile salt secretion contributes to the stone-forming (lithogenic) properties of the bile. **Furthermore, in obese persons, cholesterol secretion by the liver is augmented,** further adding to the supersaturation of the bile with cholesterol.

Although cholesterol supersaturation of the bile is apparently needed for gallstone formation, additional factors are also required. Cholesterol does not precipitate from saturated bile obtained from patients without gallstones, even after prolonged incubation. On the other hand, bile from persons without gallstones, but with properties similar to those in the bile of patients with gallstones, crystallizes without difficulty. It has been demonstrated that the precipitation of cholesterol crystals in a mucous gel to form *sludge* precedes the formation of stones. Moreover, all cholesterol stones contain a central nidus of calcium bilirubinate.

Risk Factors

The higher prevalence of gallstones in premenopausal women has been attributed to the fact that estrogens stimulate the formation of lithogenic bile by the liver. Estrogens increase the hepatic secretion of cholesterol and may decrease the secretion of bile acids. These effects are augmented during pregnancy because the gallbladder empties more slowly in the last trimester, thereby causing stasis and increasing the opportunity for precipitation of cholesterol crystals. Indeed, progesterone has been shown to inhibit the discharge of bile from the gallbladder. These mechanisms are also invoked to explain the increased incidence of gallstones in users of oral contraceptives.

Other major risk factors for the development of cholesterol gallstones can be divided into those that relate to increased biliary cholesterol secretion, those that contribute to decreased secretion of bile salts and lecithin, and those that reflect a combination of the two.

Risk factors associated with **increased biliary cholesterol secretion** include the following:

- Increasing age
- Obesity
- Membership in certain ethnic groups (e.g., Chilean women, some northern European groups)
- Familial predisposition
- Diet high in calories and cholesterol
- Certain metabolic abnormalities associated with high blood cholesterol levels (e.g., diabetes, some genetic hyperlipoproteinemias, and primary biliary cirrhosis)

There is a linear correlation between the magnitude of obesity and the risk of symptomatic gallstones, reaching a value as high as five times the risk in nonobese persons. Hepatic cholesterol synthesis is stimulated by insulin, and the increased biliary excretion of cholesterol associated with obesity may relate to the hyperinsulinism that accompanies increased body fat.

Decreased secretion of bile salts and lecithin occurs in nonobese whites who develop gallstones. Gastrointestinal absorptive disorders that interfere with the enterohepatic circulation of bile acids, for instance, pancreatic insufficiency secondary to cystic fibrosis and Crohn disease, also decrease secretion of bile acids and favor gallstone formation.

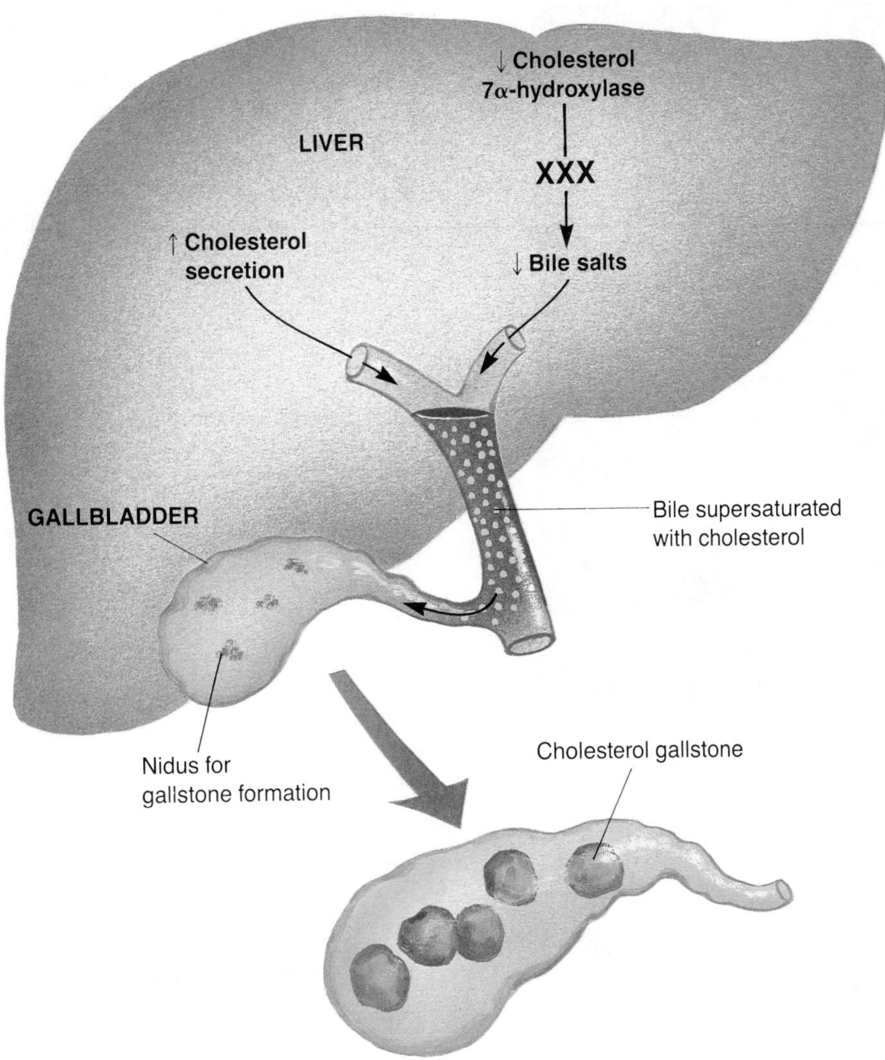

FIGURE *14-67*
Pathogenesis of cholesterol gallstones.

In American Pima Indians and in those who take certain drugs (e.g., clofibrate), **cholesterol synthesis is increased, whereas that of bile salts and lecithin is reduced**.

The risk of gallstones is decreased by moderate alcohol consumption both clinically and experimentally. The mechanism for this protective effect of alcohol is not understood, but it has been related to a reduced biliary cholesterol concentration.

Pigment Stones

Pigment stones are classed as black or brown stones, which have different characteristics.

Black Pigment Stones

Black pigment stones are irregular and measure less than 1 cm across. On cross-section, the surface appears glassy (Fig. 14-68). Black stones contain calcium bilirubinate, bilirubin polymers, calcium salts, and mucin.

☐ **Pathogenesis:** The incidence of black stones is increased in old and undernourished persons, but no correlations with gender, ethnicity, or obesity have been made. Chronic hemolysis, such as occurs with sickle cell anemia and thalassemia, predisposes to the development of black pigment stones. Cirrhosis, either because it leads to increased hemolysis or because of damage to liver cells, is also associated with a high incidence of black stones. However, in most instances, no predisposing cause for the formation of black pigment stones is evident.

The pathogenesis of black pigment stones is related to an increased concentration of unconjugated bilirubin in the bile. Unconjugated bilirubin is insoluble in bile and is usually present in only trace amounts. When increased amounts are secreted by the hepatocyte, the unconjugated bilirubin precipitates as calcium bilirubinate, probably around a nidus of mucinous glycoproteins. For unex-

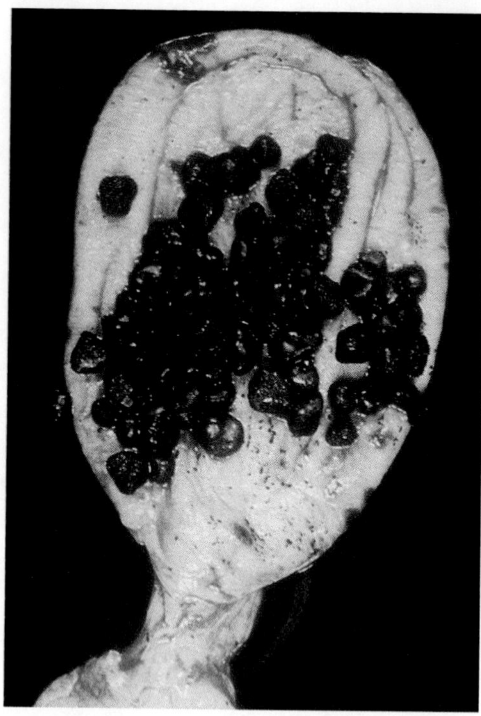

FIGURE *14-68*
Pigment gallstones. The gallbladder has been opened to reveal numerous small, dark stones composed of calcium bilirubinate.

plained reasons, patients without known predisposing factors who develop black pigment stones have increased concentrations of unconjugated bilirubin in the bile.

Brown Pigment Stones

Brown pigment stones are spongy and laminated and contain principally calcium bilirubinate mixed with cholesterol and calcium soaps of fatty acids. In contrast to the other types of gallstones, brown pigment stones are found more frequently in the intrahepatic and extrahepatic bile ducts than in the gallbladder.

☐ **Pathogenesis:** Brown stones are almost always associated with bacterial cholangitis, in which *E. coli* is the predominant organism. Rare or uncommon in Western countries, brown stones are not infrequent in Asia, where they are almost entirely restricted to persons infested with *Ascaris lumbricoides* or *Clonorchis sinensis*, helminths that may invade the biliary tract. In the rare cases in Western countries, brown stones are found only in patients with chronic mechanical obstruction to the flow of bile, as in sclerosing cholangitis, or as a result of a catheter in the common bile duct after common bile duct surgery.

The pathogenesis of brown pigment stones also relates to an increased concentration of unconjugated bilirubin in the bile. It has been proposed that conjugated bilirubin is hydrolyzed to unconjugated bilirubin by the action of bacterial β-glucuronidase or other hydrolytic enzymes.

Clinical Features of Gallstones

Gallstones may remain "silent" in the gallbladder for many years, and few patients ever die of cholelithiasis itself. One study that followed patients with initially asymptomatic gallstones for up to 11 years found that half remained asymptomatic, one third developed significant symptomatology, and fewer than 20% developed serious complications. The incidence of severe complications rose with increasing age. However, more recent studies indicate that the 15-year cumulative probability that asymptomatic stones will lead to biliary pain or other complications is less than 20%. These statistics bear on the question of whether to perform cholecystectomy for asymptomatic gallstones. In some otherwise healthy persons, the small risk associated with cholecystectomy may justify elective surgery. However, in the presence of diseases that increase the operative risk, such as cardiac or pulmonary disorders, there is little reason not to manage "silent" gallstones conservatively.

More cautious physicians recommend that *all* asymptomatic patients be treated medically unless symptoms supervene. Diabetics present a special case, because acute cholecystitis in these patients carries a high risk of serious complications, and cholecystectomy during the acute disease is far more dangerous than elective surgery. Medical treatment of gallstones is often effective with oral administration of the bile acids ursodeoxycholate and chenodeoxycholic acid. Retrograde instillation of cholesterol solvents into the gallbladder has been successful in dissolving gallstones. Extracorporeal lithotripsy (ultrasonic disruption of gallstones) has also been effective in some

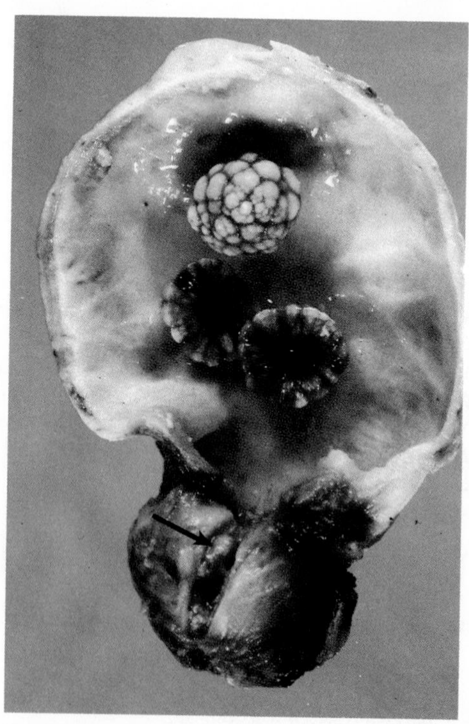

FIGURE *14-69*
Hydrops of the gallbladder. The lumen of the dilated gallbladder is filled with clear mucus and contains cholesterol stones. Note the stone (*arrow*) obstructing the cystic duct.

patients. Finally, the development of laparoscopic cholecystectomy, which is far less traumatic than a laparotomy, has changed the approach to cholecystectomy and in many instances has become the treatment of choice.

Most of the complications of cholelithiasis relate to the obstruction of the cystic duct or common bile duct by gallstones. Passage of a stone into the cystic duct often, but not invariably, causes severe biliary colic and may lead to acute cholecystitis. Repeated episodes of acute cholecystitis then produce chronic cholecystitis. The latter condition can also result from the presence of stones alone. Gallstones may pass into the common duct (*choledocholithiasis*), where they may lead to obstructive jaundice, cholangitis, and pancreatitis. In fact, in populations in whom alcoholism is not a factor, gallstones are the most common cause of acute pancreatitis. Passage of a large gallstone into the small intestine may cause intestinal obstruction, a condition called *gallstone ileus*. In obstruction of the cystic duct, with or without acute cholecystitis, the bile in the gallbladder is reabsorbed, to be replaced by a clear mucinous fluid secreted by the gallbladder epithelium. The term *hydrops of the gallbladder* (*mucocele*) (Fig. 14-69) is applied to the distended and palpable gallbladder, which may become secondarily infected.

ACUTE CHOLECYSTITIS

Acute cholecystitis is a diffuse inflammation of the gallbladder, usually secondary to obstruction of the gallbladder outlet.

☐ **Pathogenesis:** The pathogenesis of acute cholecystitis is related to the presence of concentrated bile and gallstones within the gallbladder. In fact, 90% to 95% of cases are associated with the presence of gallstones. The remaining cases (*acalculous cholecystitis*) occur in conjunction with sepsis, severe trauma, infection of the gallbladder with *Salmonella typhosa*, and polyarteritis nodosa. Bacterial infection is usually secondary to biliary obstruction, rather than a primary event.

It has been theorized that obstruction of the cystic duct by a gallstone leads to the release of phospholipase from the epithelium of the gallbladder. In turn, this enzyme may hydrolyze lecithin and release lysolecithin, a membrane-active cellular toxin. At the same time, disruption of the mucous coat of the epithelium renders the mucosal cells vulnerable to damage by the detergent action of concentrated bile salts. It has also been suggested that bile supersaturated with cholesterol is toxic to the epithelium.

☐ **Pathology:** The external surface of the gallbladder in acute cholecystitis is congested and layered with a fibrinous exudate. The wall is remarkably thickened by edema, and opening the viscus reveals a fiery-red or purple mucosa. Gallstones are usually found within the lumen, and a stone is often seen obstructing the cystic duct. On rare occasions, when obstruction of the cystic duct is complete and bacteria have invaded the gallbladder, the cavity may be distended by cloudy, purulent fluid, a condition termed *empyema of the gallbladder*. However, in some cases, fluid that grossly appears purulent actually consists simply of an emulsion of cholesterol crystals.

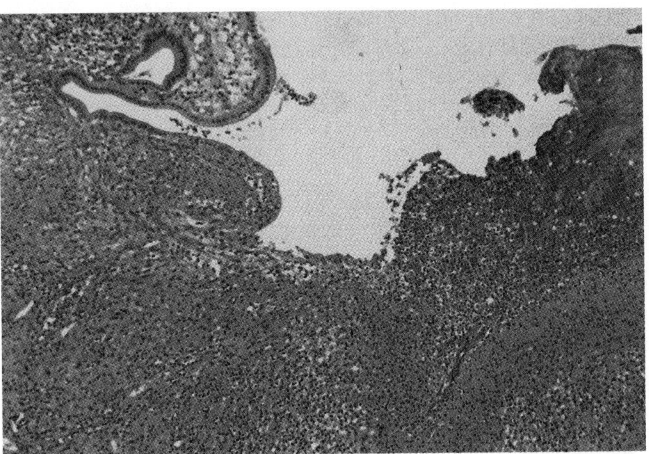

FIGURE *14-70*
Acute cholecystitis. A photomicrograph of a gallbladder removed from a patient with acute cholecystitis demonstrates ulceration of the mucosa, edema, and acute and chronic inflammation.

Microscopically, edema and hemorrhage in the wall are striking, with accompanying acute and chronic inflammation (Fig. 14-70). Secondary bacterial infection may lead to true suppuration in the gallbladder wall. The mucosa shows focal ulcerations or, in severe cases, widespread necrosis, in which case the term *gangrenous cholecystitis* is applied.

Perforation is a feared complication in severe cases and may occur after secondary bacterial infection, most commonly of the fundus. Discharge of bile into the abdominal cavity results in *bile peritonitis*. More commonly, the contents of the perforated gallbladder are localized by inflammatory adhesions, a lesion known as a *pericholecystic abscess*. The gallbladder contents may also erode into the small or large intestine, creating a *cholecystenteric fistula*. The prognosis for acute acalculous cholecystitis is not as favorable as that associated with stones, because perforation and other complications are more frequent.

☐ **Clinical Features:** The initial symptom of acute cholecystitis is abdominal pain in the right upper quadrant, and most patients have already experienced episodes of biliary colic. In a third of the cases, the gallbladder is palpable. Mild jaundice, caused by stones in or edema of the common bile duct, is evident in 20% of patients. In most cases, the acute illness subsides within a week, but persistent pain, fever, leukocytosis, and shaking chills indicate progression of the acute cholecystitis and the need for cholecystectomy. As the inflammatory process resolves, the gallbladder wall becomes fibrotic and the mucosa heals. However, the function of the gallbladder usually remains impaired.

CHRONIC CHOLECYSTITIS

Chronic cholecystitis, that is, a persistent inflammation of the gallbladder wall, is almost invariably associated with gallstones. It is the most common disease of the gallbladder.

Chronic cholecystitis may result from repeated attacks of acute cholecystitis, or, more often, from long-standing gallstones. In the latter case, the pathogenesis probably relates to chronic irritation and chemical injury to the gallbladder epithelium.

□ **Pathology:** Grossly, the wall of the chronically inflamed gallbladder is thickened and firm (Fig. 14-71A), and the serosal surface may show fibrous adhesions to surrounding structures as a result of previous episodes of acute cholecystitis. Gallstones are usually found within the lumen, and the bile often contains *gravel* (i.e., fine precipitates of calculous material). The bile is infected with coliform organisms in about half of the cases. The mucosa may be focally ulcerated and atrophic or may appear intact. Microscopically, the wall is fibrotic and often penetrated by sinuses of Rokitansky-Aschoff (see Fig. 14-71B). Chronic inflammation of variable degree may be seen in all layers. In long-standing chronic cholecystitis, the wall of the gallbladder may become calcified, in which case the term *porcelain gallbladder* is used.

□ **Clinical Features:** Many patients with chronic cholecystitis complain of nonspecific abdominal symptoms, although it is not at all clear that these are necessarily related to the gallbladder disease. On the other hand, pain in the right hypochondrium is typical and often episodic. The diagnosis is best made by ultrasound examination, which demonstrates gallstones in a thick, contracted gallbladder. Cholecystectomy is the definitive treatment.

CHOLESTEROLOSIS

Cholesterolosis of the gallbladder is defined as the accumulation of cholesterol-laden macrophages within the submucosa. It is a common incidental finding at autopsy but is not ordinarily associated with symptoms. Because cholesterolosis is often reported in conjunction with cholesterol gallstones, it is believed to reflect the presence of bile supersaturated with cholesterol. Grossly, the appearance of scattered, yellow mucosal flecks accounts for the term *strawberry gallbladder*. Microscopically, the mucosal folds are swollen with large, foamy macrophages, in which a small nucleus is displaced to the periphery.

TUMORS

Benign Tumors

Benign tumors of the gallbladder and extrahepatic biliary ducts are rare. In the gallbladder, **papillomas** are the most common benign tumors and may be single or multiple. In

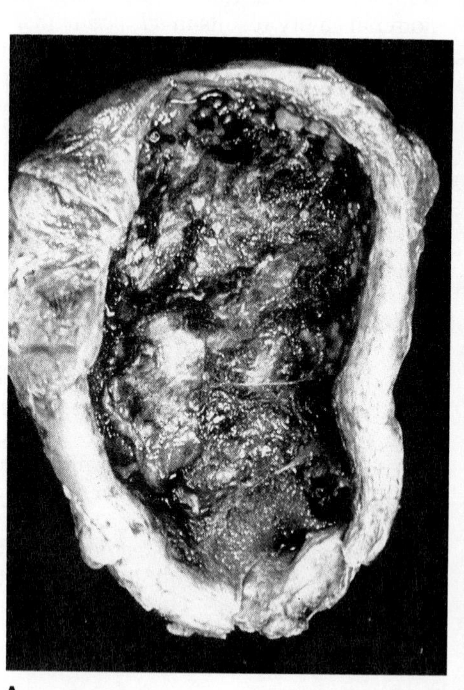

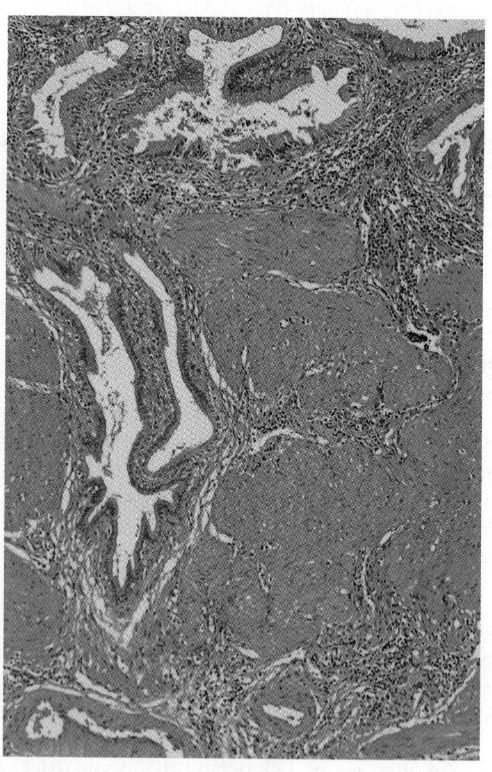

A B

FIGURE *14-71*
Chronic cholecystitis. (*A*) Gallbladder is thickened and fibrotic, and the lumen contains several gallstones. (*B*) A photomicrograph of (*A*) shows chronic inflammation of the gallbladder and a sinus of Rokitansky-Aschoff extending into the muscularis.

three fourths of the cases, they are associated with gallstones. **Mucous gland adenomas** in the infundibulum are reported and are also often associated with gallstones. The combination of smooth muscle proliferation and an adenoma has been termed *adenomyoma*. Fibromas, lipomas, leiomyomas, and myxomas have also been recorded.

The bile ducts are affected by the same benign tumors that occur in the gallbladder. Such tumors are clinically more important, since they may obstruct biliary flow and cause jaundice.

Carcinoma of the Gallbladder

The most common tumor of the gallbladder is adenocarcinoma (Fig. 14-72). Although it is not one of the more frequent cancers, it is not rare, being incidentally found in 2% of patients who undergo gallbladder surgery. **Because this cancer is usually associated with cholelithiasis and chronic cholecystitis, it is considerably more common in women than in men.** In addition, populations that have a high incidence of cholelithiasis, such as Native Americans, have a higher risk of carcinoma of the gallbladder. The calcified gallbladder (porcelain gallbladder), which represents an extreme variant of chronic cholecystitis, is particularly prone to the development of gallbladder cancer.

☐ **Pathology:** Gallbladder carcinoma may occur anywhere in the gallbladder but most frequently appears in the fundus. **The tumor is characteristically an infiltrative, well-differentiated adenocarcinoma** (see Fig. 14-72). It is usually desmoplastic, and thus the wall of the gallbladder becomes thickened and leathery. Squamous metaplasia may be so conspicuous that the tumor is believed to be a squamous carcinoma. Occasionally, the tumor grows into the lumen of the gallbladder and assumes a papillary configuration. Anaplastic, giant cell, and spindle cell forms of gallbladder carcinoma are reported. The rich lymphatic plexus of the gallbladder provides the most common route of metastasis, although vascular dissemination and direct spread into the liver and contiguous structures occurs.

☐ **Clinical Features:** The symptoms produced by carcinoma of the gallbladder are similar to those encountered with gallstone disease. However, by the time the tumor becomes symptomatic, it is almost invariably incurable, the 5-year survival rate being less than 3%. For practical purposes, surgical cure is obtained only in patients who undergo cholecystectomy for gallbladder disease and in whom the cancer is an incidental finding.

Carcinoma of the Bile Duct and the Ampulla of Vater

Cancer of the extrahepatic bile ducts, almost always adenocarcinoma, typically presents as obstructive jaundice. **It may occur anywhere along the length of the bile duct, including the location where the right and left hepatic ducts join to form the common hepatic duct.**

The tumor is less common than gallbladder cancer, and the female predominance of gallbladder cancer is not evident. The cause of bile duct cancer is unknown, but

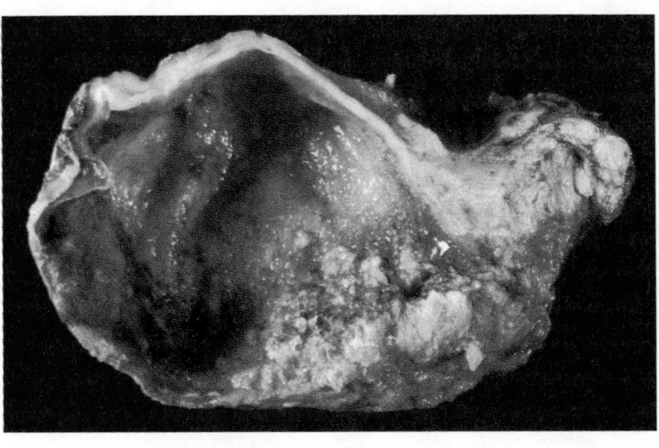

A

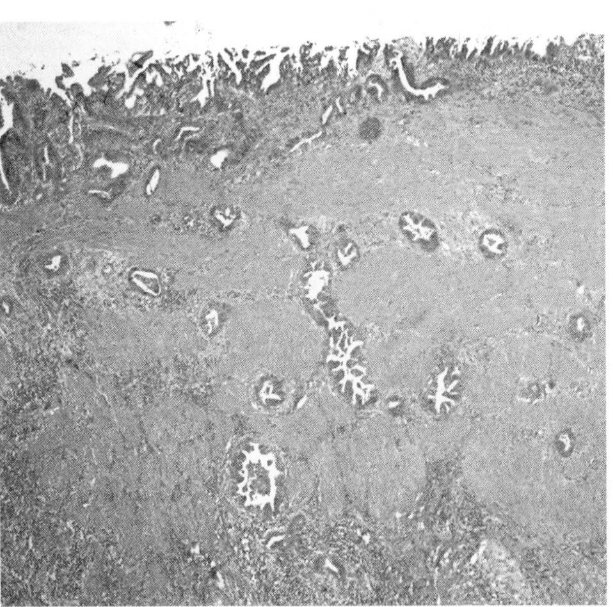

B

FIGURE *14-72*
Carcinoma of the gallbladder. (*A*) A surgically resected gallbladder has been opened to reveal a thickened wall infiltrated by adenocarcinoma, which also demonstrates exophytic growth into the lumen. (*B*) The gallbladder wall is thickened and infiltrated by a well-differentiated adenocarcinoma, which has stimulated a desmoplastic response.

gallstones are frequently found in those affected, and there is an association with idiopathic inflammatory disease involving the colon. The tumor has also been reported to arise in choledochal cysts and in Caroli disease. In the Orient, bile duct carcinoma is associated with biliary infestation by the fluke *C. sinensis*. As in carcinoma of the gallbladder, growth may be endophytic (into the lumen) or diffusely infiltrative. The prognosis is poor, but because symptoms arise early in the course of the disease, the outcome is somewhat better than that of gallbladder carcinoma.

The bile duct may also be obstructed by **adenocarcinoma of the ampulla of Vater**. The initial symptom is again obstructive jaundice, although a few patients present with pancreatitis. In contrast to bile duct carcinoma, surgical treatment of cancer of the ampulla of Vater leads to a 35% 5-year survival rate.

SUGGESTED READING

BOOKS

MacSween RNM, Anthony PP, Scheuer PJ: *Pathology of the liver,* 3rd ed. Edinburgh: Churchill Livingstone, 1994.

Schiff L, Schiff ER (eds): *Diseases of the liver,* 7th ed. Philadelphia: JB Lippincott, 1993.

Sherlock S: *Diseases of the liver and biliary system,* 10th ed. Oxford: Blackwell Scientific, 1997.

Zakim D, Boyer TD (eds): *Hepatology: A textbook of liver disease,* 3rd ed. Philadelphia: WB Saunders, 1996.

Zimmerman HJ: *Hepatotoxicity: The adverse effects of drugs and other chemicals on the liver.* New York: Appleton-Century-Crofts, 1978.

REVIEW ARTICLES

The familial conjugated hyperbilirubinemias. *Semin Liv Dis* 14:386–394, 1994.

Chisari FV, Ferrari C: Hepatitis B virus immunopathogenesis. *Annu Rev Immunol* 13:29–60, 1995.

Feitelson MA, Zern MA: Hepatitis and chronic liver disease. *Clin Lab Med* 16, 1996.

Ishak KG: Chronic hepatitis: Morphology and nomenclature. *Mod Pathol* 7:690–713, 1994.

Krawitt EL: Autoimmune hepatitis. *N Engl J Med* 334: 897–903, 1996.

Lee WM: Drug-induced hepatotoxicity. *N Engl J Med* 333:1118–1127, 1995.

Lee Y-M, Kaplan MM: Primary sclerosing cholangitis., *N Engl J Med* 332:924–933, 1995.

Okuda K: New trends in hepatocellular carcinoma. *Int J Clin Lab Res* 23:173–178, 1993.

Polish LB, Gallagher M, Fields HA, Hadler SC: Delta hepatitis: Molecular biology and clinical and epidemiological features. *Clin Microbiol Rev* 6:211–229, 1993.

van der Poel CL, Cuypers HT, Reesink HW: Hepatitis C virus: Six years. *Lancet* 344:1475–1479, 1994.

van Doorn L-J: Molecular biology of the hepatitis C virus. *J Med Virol* 43:345–356, 1994.

Vierling JM: Immune disorders of the liver and bile duct. *Gastroenterol Clin North Am* 21:427–449, 1992.

CHAPTER 15

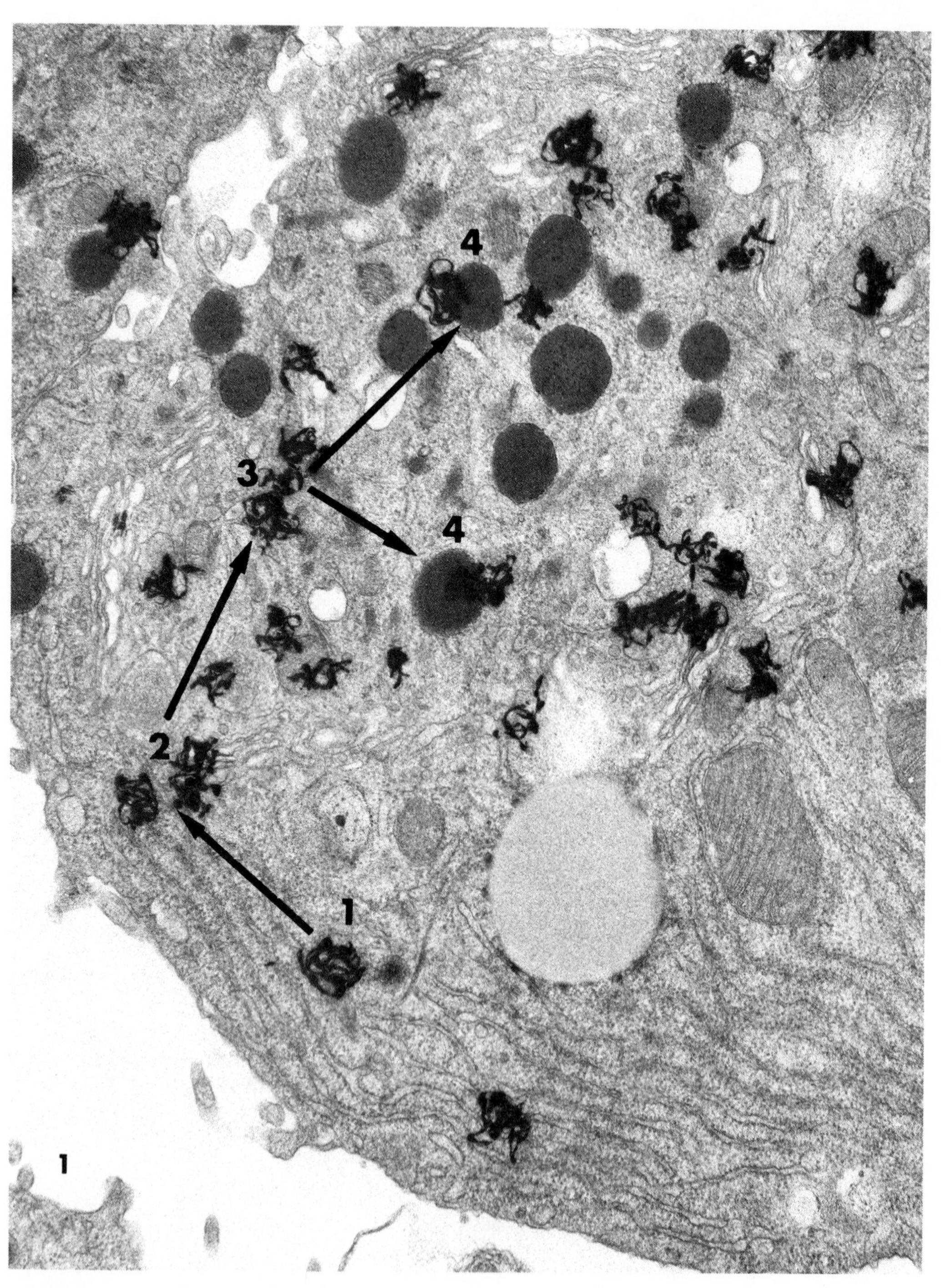

The Pancreas

Dante G. Scarpelli

FIGURE 15-1 *(see opposite page)*
Protein synthesis in the pancreatic acinar cell. An electron microscopic autoradiograph of a rat pancreatic acinar cell 30 minutes after a pulse label of [^{3}H]leucine shows serpentine silver grains that delineate the localization of (*1*) synthesis, (*2*) intracellular transport, (*3*) concentration, and (*4*) storage of digestive proenzymes. The *arrows* show the vectorial movement of the secretory product.

EMBRYOLOGY

The pancreas begins as two endodermal outpouchings that arise on the dorsal and ventral sides of the embryonic duodenal tube. The dorsal pancreas grows more rapidly than the ventral pancreas, and at the sixth week of embryonic development it becomes an elongated structure. The ventral pancreas fuses with the dorsal anlage during the seventh week to become a single organ. Most of the adult pancreas is derived from the dorsal pancreas, except for the head, which arises largely from the ventral rudiment. The duct systems of the two embryonic pancreases also fuse, giving rise to a single duct, the precursor of the major pancreatic duct (*the duct of Wirsung*). The unfused segment of the duct of the ventral pancreas remains to become the smaller accessory *duct of Santorini*, which enters the duodenum through a separate orifice. When fusion is complete, Santorini's duct is absent.

Cytological differentiation of the pancreas begins with the appearance of ducts, originating from nests of endodermal cells surrounded by mesenchyme. The ducts branch into elongate ductules, which arborize to form a complex duct system. At the third month of development, acinar cells arise from the ductules and acquire their complement of distinctive zymogen granules.

Islet cells are also derived from larger ducts. This derivation occurs about a month before the development of acinar cells. Islets arise as elongated and serpentine lateral extensions and consist of solid masses of cells that rapidly acquire small, dense, secretory granules characteristic of the endocrine pancreas. The sequence of acinar and islet cell development and differentiation, once accomplished, has generally been considered to be fixed. However, studies suggest that this may not be so and that pancreatic acini may, under the proper stimuli, convert to structures indistinguishable from preexisting ductules. Such plasticity of differentiation of pancreatic cells in the adult has interesting implications when one considers the pathogenesis of some pancreatic diseases, especially cancer of the pancreas.

ANATOMY AND PHYSIOLOGY

The pancreas is a mixed exocrine–endocrine gland that extends transversely in the upper abdomen and is cradled between the loop of the duodenum and the hilum of the spleen. It is retroperitoneal, lying behind the lesser omental sac and the stomach, a location that renders it largely inaccessible to physical examination and other modalities of direct clinical assessment. The adult pancreas is 10 to 15 cm long and weighs 60 to 150 g. It is divided into three anatomical subdivisions: (1) *the head*, which lies in the concavity of the duodenum and extends to the superior mesenteric vessels immediately behind the organ; (2) *the body*, which includes most of the gland; and (3) *a tapered tail*, which ends at the hilum of the spleen.

The secretions of the exocrine pancreas drain by way of the duct of Wirsung, which begins by the convergence of several small ducts in the tail and extends into the head, collecting secretions from ductal tributaries along the way. It then turns downward and backward, where it empties into the duodenum at the ampulla of Vater. Occasionally, in addition to the major duct, an accessory duct of Santorini is present. The major pancreatic duct usually drains into the common bile duct immediately proximal to the ampulla of Vater, but in a minority of persons it enters the duodenum directly. The common channel that carries bile and pancreatic secretions is invested with a circular complex of smooth muscle fibers, which condense into the sphincter of Oddi as they pass through the duodenal wall.

Exocrine tissue, comprising 80% to 85% of the pancreas, consists of secretory cells organized as acini that connect with ductules. These in turn merge into small ducts that empty into medium and large ducts and finally form the main pancreatic duct. Pancreatic acini consist of a single layer of pyramidal cells, whose basophilic cytoplasm is filled with acidophilic zymogen granules. By electron microscopy, the acinar cells exhibit conspicuous rough endoplasmic reticulum and numerous electron-dense zymogen granules in the apical portion of the cell (Fig. 15-1). **Acinar cells synthesize some 20 different digestive enzymes, which are secreted into the intestine following both neural and hormonal stimulation.** These include trypsin, chymotrypsin, amylase, carboxypeptidase, lipase, phospholipase, and elastase.

Stimulation of the vagus nerves increases the flow of pancreatic juice. Amino acids and a duodenal–jejunal pH of less than 3.0 trigger the release of the polypeptide hormone cholecystokinin, and antral distention stimulates the release of secretin. Cholecystokinin binds to specific surface receptors of acinar cells and stimulates their secretion of digestive enzymes. Secretin, on the other hand, binds to receptors on the surface of duct cells and triggers the release of bicarbonate ions and water into the pancreatic ducts. Bicarbonate ions serve to neutralize the highly acidic gastric chyle in the intestine and to achieve an optimum pH for the function of pancreatic digestive enzymes. The daily secretion of 1.5 to 3 liters of pancreatic juice attests to the remarkable synthetic and secretory capacity of acinar cells and the transport of ions and water by ductal cells.

The endocrine pancreas consists of cells organized into islets that are distributed throughout the organ but make up only 2% of the total mass of the pancreas. Islets contain several cell types, each of which synthesizes one or more hormones, including, among others, insulin and glucagon. Following an appropriate stimulus, the hormones are secreted directly into the blood. The major endocrine disorder of the pancreas is diabetes mellitus, a disease of such importance that it is accorded a separate chapter (see Chapter 22).

CONGENITAL ANOMALIES

Developmental defects of the pancreas include the following:

- **Aberrant or accessory pancreas,** in which pancreatic tissue is present outside its normal location
- **Annular pancreas,** characterized by encirclement of the duodenum by pancreatic tissue and less frequently by the bile duct or portal vein
- **Pancreas divisum,** in which failure of fusion of the two pancreatic anlagen, including the ducts, results in separation of the gland into two parts
- **Absence of the parts of adult gland** derived from the dorsal pancreas, namely, the body and tail
- **Congenital cysts**

ABERRANT (ECTOPIC) PANCREAS: This anomaly is an incidental finding in 2% of autopsies and is most commonly localized in the wall of the duodenum, stomach, and jejunum. More rarely, aberrant pancreas has been found in Meckel diverticulum of the ileum, the common bile duct, gallbladder, liver, spleen, and various other foci in the abdominal cavity. In the wall of the gastrointestinal tract, pancreatic nodules localize immediately below the mucosa, in the muscularis, beneath the serosa, or in small diverticula. The tissue contains all the components of normal pancreas, namely, acini, ducts, and islets.

The most plausible theories of the origin of aberrant pancreas are (1) incomplete atrophy of the left ventral anlage; (2) regression to a more primitive pattern of differentiation, reminiscent of that seen in lower vertebrates; (3) inappropriate expression of the pluripotent developmental capacity of the embryonic gut; and (4) buds of embryonic pancreatic tissue that have penetrated the intestinal wall. In that location, they become isolated from the main mass and thus misplaced by rapid longitudinal growth of the intestine. Of these theories, the last two seem most probable.

ANNULAR PANCREAS: This is an uncommon condition in which the head of the gland surrounds the second portion of the duodenum; encirclement may be complete or incomplete. Annular pancreas may be associated with duodenal atresia, an anomaly that requires surgery immediately after birth. Such infants frequently have other congenital anomalies, including trisomy 21 (Down syndrome). Many patients with annular pancreas do not require surgery in early life but develop symptoms at 60 or 70 years of age. More commonly, the diagnosis is made incidental to radiological studies for a duodenal ulcer. Annular pancreas is probably due to a failure of the ventral anlage to migrate behind the duodenum.

PANCREAS DIVISUM: Failure of fusion of the rudiments of the pancreas results in pancreas divisum. This defect leads to two separate glands, each with its separate duct draining into the duodenum.

CYSTS: True cysts of the pancreas are believed to arise from faulty development of pancreatic ducts. Although their origin is not understood, it is postulated that congenital cysts are caused by the failure of embryonic ducts to regress as they are replaced by more permanent ones. Remnants of persistent ducts presumably become obstructed and form cysts that fill with fluid. Congenital cysts can be single or multiple and range in size from a few millimeters to large cysts that fill the upper abdomen. Such cysts are lined by cuboidal to flat epithelium and contain fluid with both amylase and proteolytic enzyme activity.

ACUTE PANCREATITIS

Pancreatitis is defined as an inflammatory condition of the exocrine pancreas that results from injury to acinar cells. In 1925, the devastation of acute pancreatitis was justly described as the "most terrible of all calamities that occur in connection with the abdominal viscera. The suddenness of its onset, the illimitable agony which accompanies it, and the mortality attendant upon it render it the most formidable of catastrophes." Sadly, for reasons unknown, the incidence of the disease has increased by an order of magnitude in the past few decades.

Depending on its severity and duration, pancreatitis presents in a variety of clinical forms. At one end of the clinical spectrum is a mild, self-limited disease, consisting of acute inflammation and edema of the stroma, with little or no acinar cell necrosis. At the other extreme is a severe and sometimes fatal acute hemorrhagic pancreatitis with massive necrosis. In some cases, repeated episodes of acute pancreatitis lead to chronic pancreatitis, which is characterized by recurrent attacks of severe abdominal pain and progressive fibrosis, ultimately leading to pancreatic insufficiency. However, in about half the cases of chronic pancreatitis, no acute episodes are recognized clinically.

Interstitial or edematous pancreatitis is the mild and presumably reversible form of acute pancreatitis. It has not been extensively studied because of its brief and benign clinical course. An infiltrate of polymorphonuclear leukocytes and edema of the connective tissue between lobules of acinar cells constitute the initial lesion. There is no necrosis of acinar cells, fat necrosis, or hemorrhage.

Acute hemorrhagic pancreatitis is a condition of middle age, with a peak incidence at 60 years. It is often associated with alcoholism (more commonly in men) or chronic biliary disease (more commonly in women). Acute pancreatitis erupts abruptly, usually following a heavy meal or excessive alcohol intake.

☐ **Pathogenesis:** Acinar cell injury and duct obstruction are the major processes involved in the initiation of acute pancreatitis. These processes allow the inappropriate extracellular leakage of activated digestive enzymes and the consequent autodigestion of pancreatic and extrapancreatic tissues. Normally, host acinar cells are shielded from the potentially destructive action of their digestive enzymes (proteases, nucleases, amylase, lipase, and phospholipase A) through an intricate, intracellular, cavitary system of endoplasmic reticulum, Golgi complex, and zymogen granule membranes that physically isolate the various enzymes from other cytoplasmic components. Further protection is afforded by the fact that some of the digestive enzymes are synthesized as inactive forms (e.g., chymotrypsinogen, proelastase, prophospholipase, and trypsinogen) and the presence of specific enzyme inhibitors, such as that for trypsin. The mechanisms that initiate pancreatitis are not completely understood, although a number of factors have been implicated.

SECRETION AGAINST OBSTRUCTION: Most of the fluid secreted by acinar cells, which is rich in digestive enzymes, is discharged into the duct system and enters the duodenum. A small amount diffuses back into the periductular extracellular fluid and eventually into the plasma. Any condition that narrows the lumen of the pancreatic ducts, or that impairs the easy outflow of exocrine secretions, can raise the intraductal pressure and exacerbate back-diffusion across the ducts. This effect has been postulated to result in an inappropriate activation of digestive proenzymes.

Gallstones can cause pancreatic duct obstruction, and autopsy studies almost a century ago established the association of cholelithiasis with acute hemorrhagic pancreatitis. In some cases, gallstones were found lodged near the orifice of the common duct beyond the point where it is joined by the pancreatic duct. In recent years, however, it has become increasingly apparent that although pancreatitis may be accompanied by conditions that obstruct the flow of pancreatic juice into the duodenum, fewer than 5% of patients with acute pancreatitis have an impacted stone at the ampulla of Vater. Moreover, neither ligation of the pancreatic duct nor its occlusion by tumor results in acute pancreatitis.

BILE REFLUX: The association with cholelithiasis also led to the suggestion that reflux of bile into the pancreatic duct is a factor in the pathogenesis of acute pancreatitis. It has been postulated that intraductal phospholipase hydrolyzes the lecithin contained in the bile to form lysolecithin, a potent toxin. This mechanism is possible only if a common channel exists for the discharge of both bile and pancreatic secretions into the duodenum. Such a configuration of the common bile duct occurs in fewer than 20% of persons, and there is no predilection for this anatomical variant in patients with acute pancreatitis. In addition, the experimental instillation of bile into the pancreatic duct at physiological pressures does not provoke acute pancreatitis. Thus, it seems more likely that the association between cholelithiasis and acute pancreatitis reflects transient pancreatic duct obstruction rather than bile reflux.

REFLUX OF DUODENAL CONTENTS: The retrograde injection of a mixture of bile and activated pancreatic enzymes into the pancreatic duct has been shown experimentally to produce acute pancreatitis. Furthermore, under some experimental conditions, the instillation of such a mixture in a forward direction from the tail of the pancreas results in acute pancreatitis. Despite a number of problems with the hypothesis of duodenal reflux, it remains a possibility in at least some patients with acute pancreatitis.

INTRACELLULAR ACTIVATION OF PROTEASES: Heavy alcohol intake and certain types of experimental toxic pancreatic injury (ethionine, cerulein) produce acute pancreatitis. In these instances, a block in the secretion of zymogen granules by acinar cells seems to be an early event. The retained zymogen granules are removed by autophagy. However, in the case of the pancreas, the secretory products include nascent proteases, such as trypsinogen, which can be activated by lysosomal hydrolases. Thus, the intracellular activation of potent digestive enzymes may lyse the cell or result in the secretion of prematurely activated enzymes.

ACTIVATED PANCREATIC ENZYMES: Although the precise sequence of events by which activated pancreatic enzymes exert their harmful effects is not fully established, it is thought that the activation of trypsin is central to this process. Although activated trypsin by itself does not produce cell necrosis and pancreatitis, it does activate other pancreatic proenzymes, including prophospholipase A_2 and proelastase. Under the appropriate circumstances, phospholipase A_2 attacks membrane phospholipids to cause necrosis, and elastase digests the walls of blood vessels, thereby leading to hemorrhage. Moreover, the liberation of pancreatic lipase into the interstitium contributes to fat necrosis. Whatever the role for any of these postulated mechanisms, it is clear that the inappropriate activation of pancreatic proenzymes is the common feature in the pathogenesis of all variants of pancreatitis.

PROTEASE INHIBITORS: The various inhibitors of proteolytic enzymes present in many body fluids and tissues constitute a defense against the inappropriate activation of the digestive proenzymes of the pancreas. On activation of trypsin, the balance between activated proteases and protease inhibitors determines the extent of pancreatic injury. Four potent protease inhibitors have been identified in human plasma: α_1-antitrypsin, α_2-macroglobulin, C_1 esterase inhibitor, and pancreatic secretory trypsin inhibitor. Although collectively these proteins inhibit trypsin, chymotrypsin, and elastase, they are without effect on two other potent proteases, namely, carboxypeptidases A and B. α_2-Macroglobulin reduces the capacity of trypsin to digest protein but does not completely prevent it from cleaving small synthetic peptides. Thus, tryptic activity is demonstrable in plasma even when trypsin is bound by the inhibitor. Furthermore, a trypsin inhibitor in pancreatic juice is only partially effective, even when it is present in excess. Apparently, the inhibitor is digested by the trypsin to which it is bound. Despite the variety of trypsin inhibitors in different body compartments, it is clear that the protection they render is less than complete. Since activated trypsin is also able to activate other pancreatic proenzymes, such as chymotrypsinogen, proelastase, prophospholipase, and procarboxypeptidase, its incomplete inhibition in pancreatic juice and plasma poses a hazard.

ETHANOL: Chronic alcohol abuse of many years' duration accounts for one third of the cases of acute pancreatitis, although only 5% of chronic alcoholics develop this complication. Ethanol is well recognized as a chemical toxin, but a significant injurious effect on pancreatic

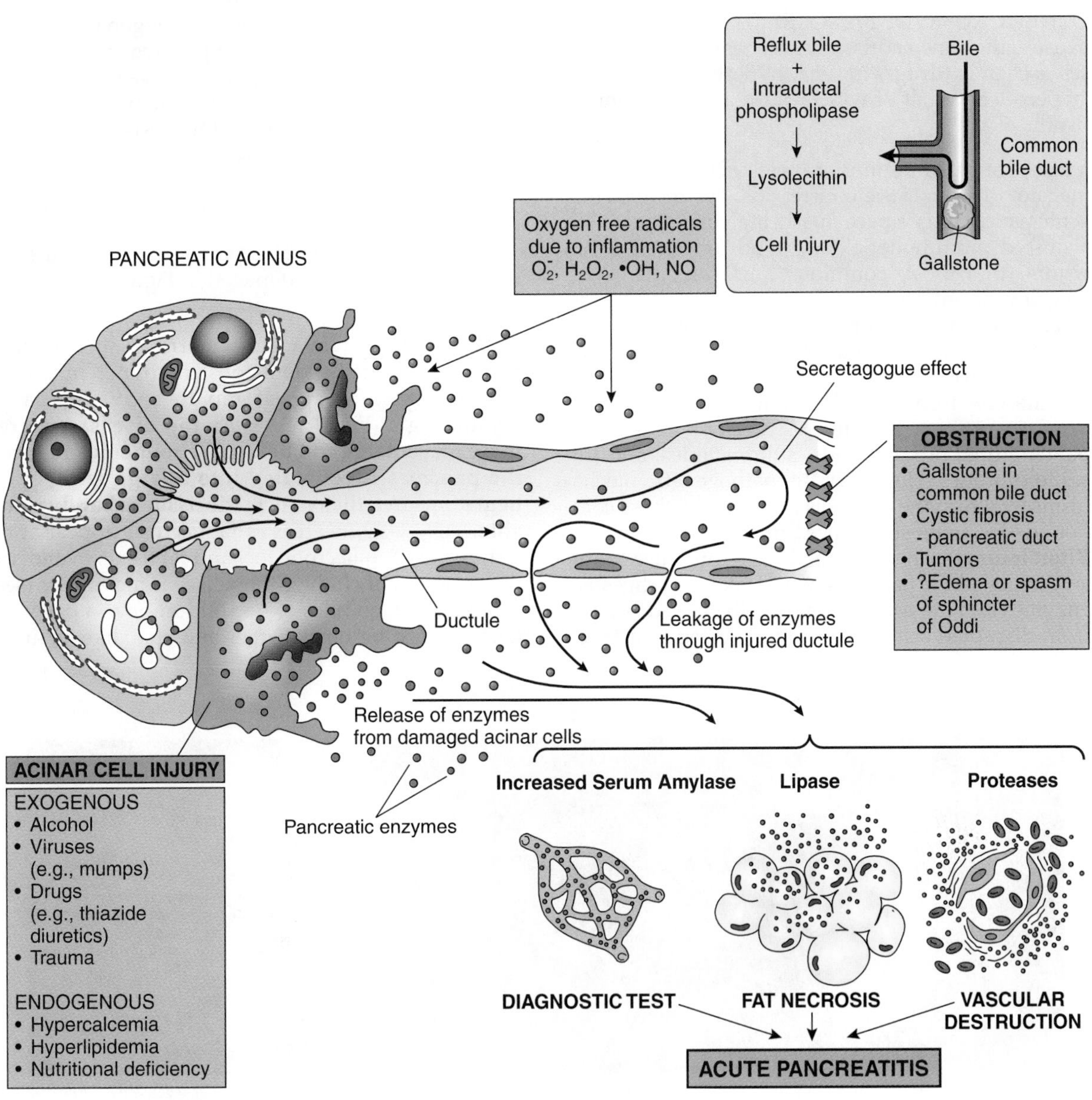

FIGURE *15-2*
The pathogenesis of acute pancreatitis. Injury to the ductules or the acinar cells leads to the release of pancreatic enzymes. Lipase and proteases destroy tissue, thereby causing acute pancreatitis. The release of amylase is the basis of a test for acute pancreatitis.

acinar or duct cells has yet to be demonstrated. Ethanol can adversely affect the pancreas by causing spasm or acute edema of the sphincter of Oddi, especially following an alcoholic binge. Ethanol also stimulates secretion from the small intestine, which in turn triggers the exocrine pancreas to release pancreatic juice. When these effects occur together (enhanced secretion into an obstructed duct), the results may be disastrous.

GALLSTONES: Some 45% of all patients with acute pancreatitis have cholelithiasis, and the risk of developing acute pancreatitis in patients with gallstones is 25 times higher than that in the general population. Furthermore, unless the gallstones are eliminated after the first attack, recurrent pancreatitis can be expected in 50% of the cases.

OTHER CAUSES OF PANCREATITIS: Other factors that cause acute pancreatitis, albeit uncommonly, include viruses, ischemia, drugs, trauma, hypertriglyceridemia, and hypercalcemia, all of which cause acinar cell injury and death.

- **Viruses** such as mumps, coxsackievirus, and cytomegalovirus can cause pancreatitis. The incidence of acute pancreatitis is particularly high in patients with acquired immunodeficiency syndrome (AIDS), in whom the most common cause is the cytomegalovirus infection.
- **Therapeutic drugs:** More than 85 drugs have been reported to cause acute pancreatitis, the highest incidence occurring with azathioprine and mercaptourine (3% to 5%), and didanosine (23%). Other drugs incriminated include estrogens, furosemides, pentamidine, procainamide, sulfonamides, and thiazide diuretics. However, the pathogenetic mechanisms by which the pancreas is injured by these compounds are, in most instances, unclear.
- **Blunt trauma** to the upper abdomen can cause contusive injury to the pancreas, with leakage of digestive enzymes into the pancreas and peripancreatic tissues from disrupted acinar cells and pancreatic ducts. Of patients undergoing endoscopic retrograde cholangiopancreatography (ERCP), 1% to 10% develop acute pancreatitis.
- **Hyperlipidemia** on occasion can precipitate the onset of acute pancreatitis. The mechanism is thought to involve the hydrolysis of triglycerides in the extracellular space by lipase inappropriately leaked by pancreatic cells, which releases cytotoxic free fatty acids. The same pathogenesis is postulated for pancreatitis associated with other disturbances of lipid metabolism that result in elevated levels of serum triglycerides. These include familial hyperlipoproteinemia (especially type V), chronic renal failure, and estrogen therapy.
- **Hypercalcemia** regardless of cause may be associated with acute pancreatitis. In this context, Ca^{2+} is necessary for the activation of trypsinogen by trypsin.
- **Obesity** is a risk factor for pancreatitis, especially for severe disease. Obese persons have increased deposition of peripancreatic fat, which may predispose them to more extensive fat necrosis after the local release of pancreatic lipase.
- **Idiopathic pancreatitis** is still the third most common form of the disease, accounting for 10% of all cases.

Factors involved in the pathogenesis of acute hemorrhagic pancreatitis are depicted in Figure 15-2.

☐ **Pathology:** In acute hemorrhagic pancreatitis, the pancreas is initially edematous and hyperemic. Within a day, pale, gray foci appear, rapidly becoming friable and hemorrhagic (Fig. 15-3A). **As the disease progresses, these foci enlarge and become so numerous that most of the pancreas is converted into a large retroperitoneal hematoma in which pancreatic tissue is barely recognizable.** Yellow-white areas of fat necrosis appear at the interface between necrotic foci and fat tissue in and around the pancreas, including the adjacent mesentery (see Fig. 15-3B). These nodules of necrotic fat have a pasty consistency, which becomes firmer and chalklike as more cal-

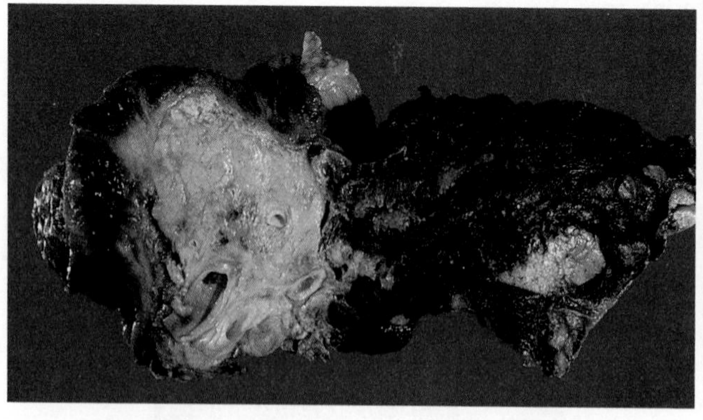

A

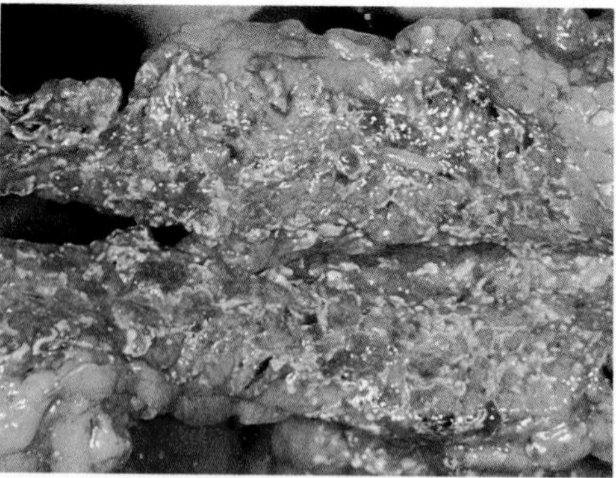

B

FIGURE *15-3*
Acute hemorrhagic pancreatitis. (*A*) Large areas of the pancreas are intensely hemorrhagic. (*B*) The cut surface of the pancreas in a less severe case of acute pancreatitis, and at a somewhat later stage than in (*A*), shows numerous yellow-white foci of fat necrosis.

cium and magnesium soaps are produced. Saponification reflects the interaction of cations with free fatty acids released by the action of activated lipase on triglycerides in fat cells. As a result, the level of blood calcium may be depressed, sometimes to the point of causing neuromuscular irritability, expressed as facial tics. Distant extrapancreatic fat necrosis, arising as a consequence of the release of lipase from the injured pancreas into the blood, has been reported in subcutaneous fat, skeletal muscle, and bone marrow.

The most prominent tissue alterations in acute pancreatitis are acinar cell necrosis, an intense acute inflammatory reaction, and foci of necrotic fat cells (Fig. 15-4). Irregular fibrosis of the pancreas and occasionally calcification are the residuals of healed acute pancreatitis.

PANCREATIC PSEUDOCYST: Patients who survive acute pancreatitis are at risk for the development of pancreatic abscesses and pseudocysts (Fig. 15-5), the latter with an incidence as high as 50%. Pancreatic pseudocysts exhibit large spaces limited by connective tissue, which contain degraded blood, debris of necrotic pancreatic tissue, and fluid rich in pancreatic enzymes. Pseudocysts may enlarge to compress and even obstruct the duodenum. They may become secondarily infected and form an abscess. Rupture of a pseudocyst is a rare complication that leads to a chemical or septic peritonitis, or both.

□ **Clinical Features:** The patient with acute pancreatitis presents with severe epigastric pain that is referred to the upper back and is accompanied by nausea and vomiting. Within a matter of hours, catastrophic peripheral vascular collapse and shock ensue. When shock is sustained and profound, pancreatitis may be complicated within the first week of onset by the adult respiratory distress syndrome and acute renal failure. Early in the disease, pancreatic digestive enzymes are released from injured acinar cells into the blood and the abdominal cavity. Elevation of serum amylase and lipase levels as early as 24 to 72 hours after onset is diagnostic for acute pancreatitis, as are high enzyme levels in the abdominal ascitic fluid. The necrotic pancreas becomes infected with gram-negative bacteria from the intestinal tract in half of the cases of acute pancreatitis. This complication increases the mortality associated with abdominal surgery.

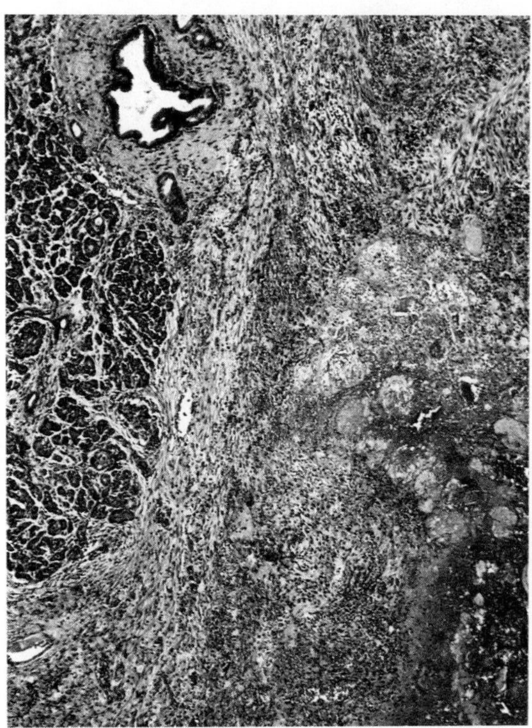

FIGURE *15-4*
Acute hemorrhagic pancreatitis. A photomicrograph of the pancreas shows areas of acinar cell necrosis and hemorrhage. An intact lobule is seen on the left.

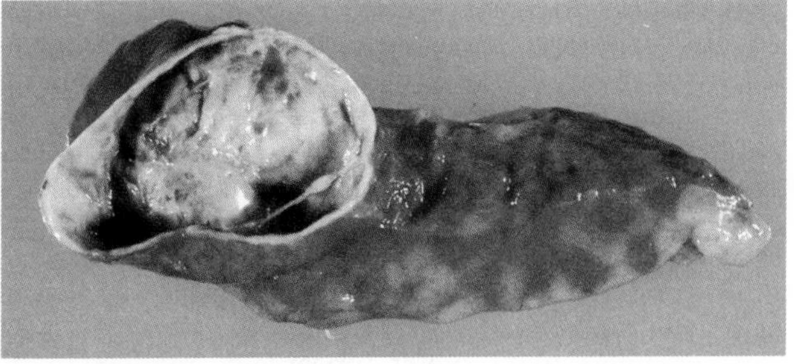

FIGURE *15-5*
Pancreatic pseudocyst. A cystic cavity arises from the head of the pancreas.

CHRONIC PANCREATITIS

Chronic pancreatitis is characterized by the progressive destruction of the pancreas with accompanying irregular fibrosis and chronic inflammation. Since the original description of the disease and its associated stones some two centuries ago, chronic pancreatitis "remains an enigmatic process of uncertain pathogenesis, unpredictable clinical course, and unclear treatment." Clinically, the disorder presents as recurrent or persisting abdominal pain or as evidence of pancreatic exocrine or endocrine insufficiency in the absence of pain.

□ **Pathogenesis:** **Long-standing alcohol abuse** is today the major cause of chronic pancreatitis, being responsible for two thirds of adult cases. In almost half of alcoholics who had no symptoms of chronic pancreatitis during life, autopsy reveals evidence of this disease. This is consistent with the finding that during life a comparable proportion of asymptomatic alcoholics manifest abnormal results of tests for pancreatic exocrine function. Although the etiological role of alcohol is undisputed, the mechanism by which it causes chronic pancreatitis is still debated. **In most cases of chronic pancreatitis that occur in the absence of alcohol abuse, the cause remains obscure.**

The earliest morphological abnormality in alcoholic chronic pancreatitis is generally the precipitation of protein plugs in the ducts, which serve as the nidus for subsequent calculi. It is speculated that these stones chronically obstruct the ductal system. Since alcohol is a secretagogue for the pancreas, early chronic pancreatitis features hypersecretion of protein by acinar cells, without concomitantly increased fluid release. As a result, protein plugs are precipitated in the small branches of the pancreatic ducts. These plugs, which are initially composed of degenerating cells within a reticular framework, enlarge to form laminar aggregates through the accretion of amorphous material. Intraductal stones form when calcium carbonate is precipitated in the plugs.

Two interesting proteins appear to be involved in the formation of the ductal plugs and stones. *Lithostathine*, formerly termed pancreatic-stone protein, is secreted by acinar cells and is detected in large amounts in ductal plugs and stones. *GP2* is a homologue of the protein involved in the formation of renal tubular casts. This protein is also secreted by acinar cells and is found in ductal plugs. The precipitation of both lithostathine and GP2 is facilitated by low pH and appropriate salt concentrations. Since lithostathine prevents the precipitation of calcium carbonate from pancreatic juice, its sequestration in ductal proteinaceous plugs reduces its concentration in pancreatic juice and may, thereby, favor stone formation. In any event, secretion against obstruction is thought to mediate the early lesions of chronic pancreatitis.

Cholelithiasis does not seem to be an etiological factor in chronic pancreatitis, and cholecystectomy does not alter the course of the disease. The distribution of idiopathic chronic pancreatitis is bimodal. A juvenile form of the disease occurs in young persons, with a mean age of 25 years. In the older group of patients with chronic pancreatitis, the disease peaks at age 60 years. Although genetic susceptibility has been suggested as an etiological factor for the juvenile form and vascular disease has been proposed as a cause for the senile form of chronic pancreatitis, neither theory has been proved.

Functional obstruction of the pancreatic duct caused by pancreas divisum or mechanical obstruction by cancer or by the inspissated mucus of cystic fibrosis leads to chronic pancreatitis. Chronic injury to the acinar cells (e.g., in hemochromatosis) is also associated with fibrosis and atrophy of the pancreas. Hypercalcemia and hyperlipidemia have been nominated as causes of chronic pancreatitis, but such a relationship is not firmly established.

The fact that chronic pancreatitis is often characterized by intermittent "acute" attacks followed by periods of quiescence suggests that in many patients the pathogenesis involves repeated bouts of acute pancreatitis, followed by scarring. However, in patients without a history of acute episodes, the pathogenesis of chronic pancreatitis may relate to persistent necrosis and insidious scarring, similar to the progression of cirrhosis of the liver.

□ **Pathology:** By the time chronic pancreatitis becomes clinically evident, it is usually well advanced. ***Chronic calcifying pancreatitis*** is the most common type of chronic pancreatitis and is associated with chronic alcoholism in more than 90% of cases. On gross examination, the pancreas is firm, and the cut surface lacks the

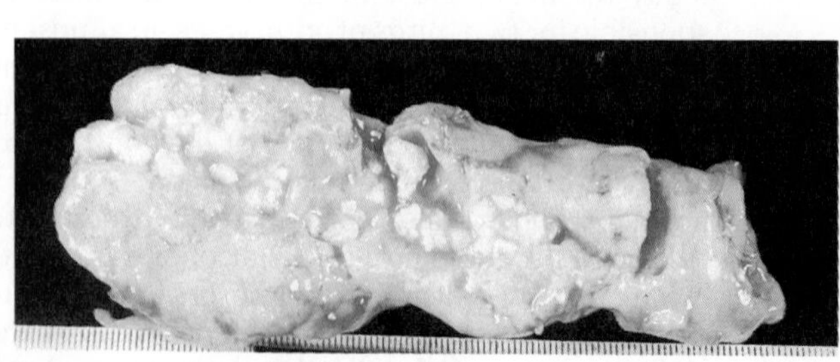

A

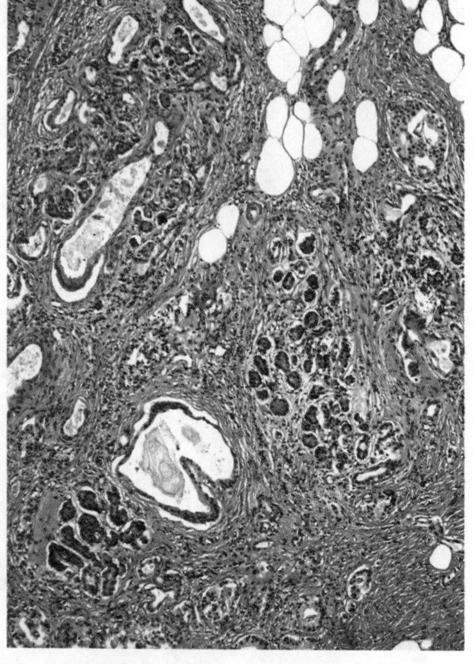

B

FIGURE *15-6*
Chronic calcifying pancreatitis. (*A*) The pancreas is shrunken and fibrotic, and the dilated duct contains numerous stones. (*B*) Atrophic lobules of acinar cells are surrounded by dense fibrous tissue infiltrated by lymphocytes. The pancreatic ducts are dilated and contain inspissated proteinaceous material.

usual lobular appearance (Fig. 15-6A). Often the pancreatic duct and its tributaries are dilated, owing to obstruction by thick proteinaceous plugs, intraductal stones, or strictures. True cysts and poorly defined pseudocysts are common and have presumably formed distal to ductal obstructions.

Microscopically, large regions of the pancreas display irregular areas of fibrosis, and the exocrine and endocrine elements are reduced in number and size (see Fig. 15-6B). Fibrotic areas exhibit activated fibroblasts, adjacent to which are zones of dense chronic inflammation, with infiltrates of lymphocytes, plasma cells, and macrophages, particularly around surviving pancreatic lobules. Pancreatic ducts of all sizes contain variably calcified proteinaceous material. ***Chronic obstructive pancreatitis*** is morphologically similar to alcoholic pancreatitis, but ductal stones are rare.

□ **Clinical Features:** Half of the patients with chronic pancreatitis suffer repeated episodes of acute pancreatitis. One third of the cases are characterized by the gradual onset of continuous or intermittent pain, without any acute attacks (Fig. 15-7). In a few patients, chronic pancreatitis is initially painless but is heralded by the appearance of diabetes or malabsorption. By the time that pancreatic calcifications are visible radiologically, the majority of patients have developed diabetes, malabsorption, or both. Conspicuous weight loss is common, and unrelenting epigastric pain, radiating to the back, may cripple the patient. The mortality rate in chronic pancreatitis is 3% to 4% per year, and it approaches 50% within 20 to 25 years. One fifth of the patients die of complications associated with attacks of pancreatitis. The remainder of the deaths are secondary to other causes, since the large majority of the patients are alcoholics.

Familial Hereditary Pancreatitis

Hereditary pancreatitis is a rare autosomal dominant disease characterized by recurring episodes of severe abdominal pain, often presenting in childhood. In some instances, hereditary pancreatitis is accompanied by aminoaciduria, although the two conditions are not necessarily linked etiologically. Some cases exhibit hypercalcemia, secondary to hyperplasia or adenomas of the parathyroid glands. It is noteworthy that about 15% of patients with hereditary pancreatitis subsequently develop ductal adenocarcinoma of the pancreas. The clinical and pathological features of hereditary pancreatitis are indistinguishable from other forms of chronic pancreatitis, including ductal stones and all the late complications.

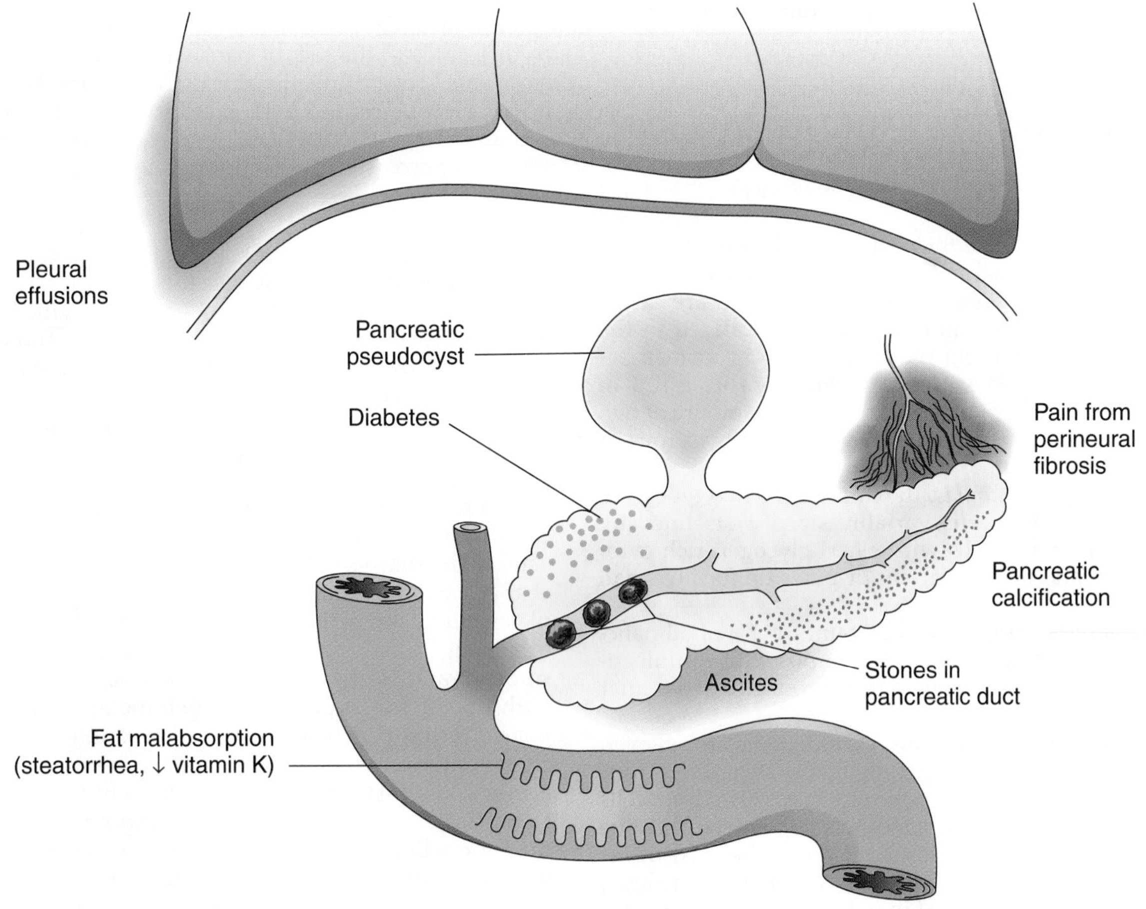

FIGURE *15-7*
Complications of chronic pancreatitis.

Hereditary pancreatitis is associated with an arginine-to-histidine substitution at residue 117 of the trypsinogen molecule. Interestingly, the normal arginine 117 residue is a trypsin-sensitive site. Cleavage at this location is probably part of a fail-safe mechanism by which trypsin may be inactivated. Failure to inactivate trypsin allows its activation within the pancreas, resulting in autodigestion and pancreatitis.

Cystic Fibrosis

Cystic fibrosis is briefly reviewed here because it manifests as a form of chronic pancreatitis. A full discussion of this disorder is presented in Chapter 6. Cystic fibrosis is an inherited, autosomal recessive disease of children, affecting all mucus-secreting tissues and exocrine sweat glands. The functional derangement is defective transport of chloride ions across the plasma membranes of epithelial cells. In the case of mucus-producing cells, such as those that line the ducts of the pancreas, the lack of chloride secretion is linked to impaired secretion of sodium and water. As a result, the intraductal secretions are abnormally viscid, accounting for the older name, *mucoviscidosis*. Plugs of inspissated mucus obstruct the pancreatic ducts, thereby leading to chronic pancreatitis and its complications. In children, malabsorption is an important feature of cystic fibrosis. Such children have bulky and fatty stools (steatorrhea), and they fail to thrive. Death usually results from the pulmonary complications of the disease.

PANCREATIC CYSTADENOMA

Benign tumors of the exocrine pancreas are rare. The most common ones, which present as large cystic tumors, deserve mention because they must be differentiated from the various congenital and acquired cysts that are not true neoplasms. **Cystadenomas of the pancreas are large, multiloculated, cystic tumors, usually localized in the body or tail.** They occur most frequently in women between the ages of 50 and 70 years and constitute 10% of cystic lesions of the pancreas. These neoplasms are of two types, depending on whether they are lined by serous or mucinous epithelium.

Serous cystadenomas, the rarer of the two types, are composed of numerous variably sized cysts lined by cuboidal epithelial cells with clear, glycogen-rich cytoplasm. The microcystic variant displays uniformly small cysts.

Mucinous cystadenomas account for 1% of all pancreatic exocrine tumors and are composed of multiloculated cysts lined by a high mucin-producing, columnar epithelium.

Both variants of pancreatic cystadenoma are believed to originate from the pancreatic duct system, the serous type from ductular cells and the mucinous form from cells lining the larger ducts. Mucinous cystadenomas must be strictly separated from the serous variety because of the malignant potential of the former. Mucinous cystadenocarcinomas have developed in patients several years after the surgical removal of apparently benign mucinous cystadenomas.

PANCREATIC CARCINOMA

Carcinoma of the pancreas is the fourth most common cause of cancer deaths in men and the fifth in women. Unfortunately, it remains virtually incurable. The incidence of pancreatic cancer seems to be increasing in all countries studied, and in the United States, it has tripled in the past 50 years. Ductal adenocarcinoma accounts for 90% of all pancreatic cancers.

☐ **Epidemiology:** The distribution of pancreatic adenocarcinoma is worldwide, with the highest incidence (twice that in the United States) among male Maoris, Polynesian aborigines of New Zealand, and female natives of Hawaii. Cancer of the pancreas shows a significant male predominance (up to 3:1) in younger age groups but an almost equal distribution in old age. In the United States, the disease is more common in native Americans and blacks than in whites. Pancreatic carcinoma is a disease of late life, with the greatest incidence in persons older than 60 years of age, although its appearance as early as the third decade is not rare.

☐ **Pathogenesis:** The factors involved in the causation of pancreatic cancer are obscure. Epidemiological studies have implicated both host and environmental factors as being of possible etiological significance.

SMOKING: There is a significant increase (twofold to threefold) in the risk of pancreatic cancer in cigarette smokers. A causal relationship is further implied by an apparent dose–response relationship associated with the number of cigarettes smoked per day and the demonstration of hyperplastic pancreatic ducts in autopsy studies of smokers.

CHEMICAL CARCINOGENS: Experimental studies in animals lend support to a role for chemical carcinogenesis in pancreatic cancer. 7,12-Dimethylbenz[a]anthracene (DMBA), a polycyclic hydrocarbon, and a number of β-oxidized dipropylnitrosamines are pancreatic carcinogens in rodents. The nitrosamines are of particular interest because in hamsters they induce adenocarcinoma of the pancreatic ducts, the predominant human type of pancreatic cancer.

Chronic exposure of experimental animals to chemicals that induce pancreatic cancer also cause metaplasia of acini to ductlike structures. In the hamster, preneoplastic changes and frank malignant tumors develop in the metaplastic ducts and in the larger pancreatic ducts. Comparable changes may be seen in the pancreas of cigarette smokers and in the noncancerous pancreas of patients with ductal adenocarcinoma. Such metaplastic acini in noncancerous pancreatic tissue fail to stain with a monoclonal antibody to a surface antigen present on normal acinar cells. Instead they stain intensely with a monoclonal antibody to a surface antigen expressed on normal duct epithelium. Although this evidence is circumstantial, it suggests that both preexisting ducts and ductules, and those arising from metaplastic acinar cells, may be involved in the pathogenesis of pancreatic ductal adenocarcinoma.

DIETARY FACTORS: Epidemiological studies suggest that dietary factors may be involved in the development of pancreatic cancer. A high intake of meat and fat, especially the latter, may be of particular significance. Dose–effect relationships between the level of fat consumption and experimental pancreatic ductal carcinogenesis support an etiological role for dietary factors.

DIABETES MELLITUS: Diabetics, especially women, may be at increased risk for the development of carcinoma of the pancreas, although the relationship is not firmly established. Proliferative lesions of the pancreatic ducts, such as papillary hyperplasia and metaplasia, have been reported in diabetics. However, whereas almost 15% of diabetics contract pancreatic cancer, more than half of these patients have had diabetes for no more than 3 months. Thus, in some patients, diabetes may be caused by pancreatic cancer, rather than the reverse.

CHRONIC PANCREATITIS: Recent studies have established that chronic pancreatitis is a risk factor for the development of pancreatic adenocarcinoma. When this association is considered in the light of an estimated annual incidence of only four cases of chronic pancreatitis per 100,000 population, it appears that the latter disease accounts for only few cases of pancreatic cancer. However, some cases of chronic pancreatitis are mild and present as vague attacks of indigestion or are clinically silent. In this regard, the prevalence of chronic pancreatitis at autopsy is a thousand times greater than that expected from the clinical incidence of disease. Thus, the risk of developing pancreatic cancer as a consequence of antecedent chronic pancreatitis may not be as modest as once thought.

MOLECULAR GENETICS: Pancreatic duct cancers exhibit a number of genetic alterations with considerable frequency. Mutational activation of K-*ras* (G to A transition in the second position of codon 12) and overexpression of *erb* B2 are common. The detection of this characteristic K-*ras* mutation in pancreatic cells obtained endoscopically has been used for the early diagnosis of pancreatic cancer. In addition, mutational inactivation or deletion may be noted in tumor suppressor genes, namely p53, p16 (MST1), and DPC-4 (deleted in pancreatic cancer, locus 4). Interestingly, deletions in chromosome 18 are present in 90% of pancreatic cancers. Although DPC-4 is located on chromosome 18, only half of all pancreatic cancers show loss or inactivation of this gene, suggesting that another nearby tumor suppressor gene contributes to the development of the remaining 40%. Overactivity or inappropriate expression of several growth factors and their receptors are described, including epidermal growth factor (EGF) and its receptor, transforming growth factor-alpha (TGF-α), and fibroblast growth factor (FGF) and its receptor.

☐ **Pathology:** Adenocarcinoma arises anywhere in the pancreas, the most frequent focus being in the head (60%), followed by the body (10%) and the tail (5%). In the remaining 25%, the pancreas is diffusely involved, a finding that suggests either late diagnosis or a multicentric origin. Carcinomas of the head of the pancreas tend to be smaller than those of the body and tail and show a more limited spread to regional lymph nodes and more distant sites. In large part, these differences reflect earlier diagnosis of cancer of the head of the pancreas, which causes early biliary obstruction and jaundice by compressing the ampulla of Vater and the common bile duct.

On gross examination, pancreatic carcinoma is a firm, gray, poorly demarcated multinodular mass (Fig. 15-8), often embedded in a dense connective tissue stroma. Tumors of the head of the pancreas may invade the common duct and the duodenal wall. When they penetrate the duodenum, they often compress or invade the ampulla of Vater. Carcinoma localized in the head of the pancreas

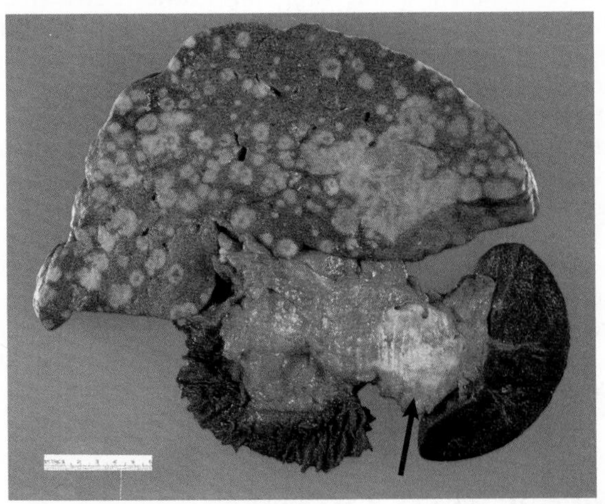
A

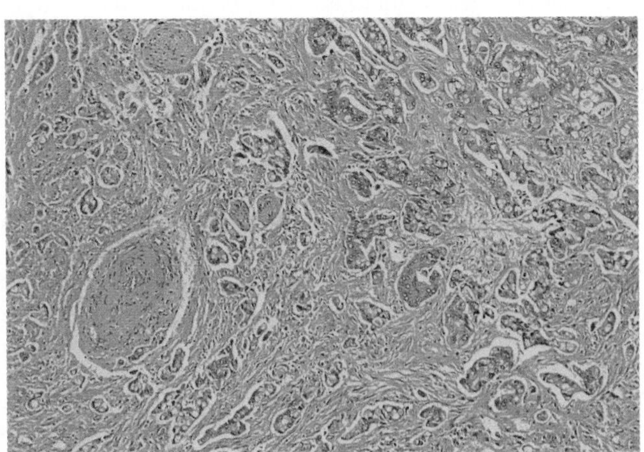
B

FIGURE *15-8*
Carcinoma of the pancreas. (*A*) An autopsy specimen shows a large tumor in the tail of the pancreas (*arrow*) and extensive metastases in the liver. (*B*) A section of the tumor reveals malignant glands embedded in a dense fibrous stroma. A nerve (*left*) shows perineural invasion.

may obstruct the duct of Wirsung and cause atrophy of the body and tail. Cancers of the pancreas often permeate the retroperitoneal space and appear as small, grayish, firm nodules in the mesentery and on the surface of intraperitoneal organs. The tumor may invade the splenic vein, showering the liver with metastases.

Microscopically, more than 75% of ductal adenocarcinomas of the pancreas are well differentiated, secrete mucin, and stimulate a florid deposition of collagen, a process referred to as a desmoplastic reaction. These tumors resemble mucinous adenocarcinomas of most other organs, such as the gallbladder, colon, and ovary. The remaining 25% of cancers that originate from pancreatic ducts and ductules are giant cell carcinoma, adenosquamous carcinoma, and small cell carcinoma.

Pancreatic cancer metastasizes most commonly to the regional lymph nodes and the liver. Other frequent metastatic locations include the peritoneum, lungs, adrenals, and bones. Direct extension into neighboring organs, such as the stomach and duodenum, occasionally occurs. Perineural infiltration by tumor is characteristic of pancreatic cancer and accounts for the early and persistent pain of this disease.

□ **Clinical Features:** Early diagnosis of cancer of the pancreas is unusual because the tumor does not ordinarily give rise to characteristic signs and symptoms until it is well advanced. Most pancreatic cancers have already metastasized by the time they have been diagnosed, and curative surgery is an option for only a trivial number of patients. Half of the patients die within 6 weeks of the diagnosis of pancreatic cancer, and the overall 5-year survival rate is less than 1%.

Patients with carcinoma of the pancreas present with anorexia, conspicuous weight loss, and a gnawing pain in the epigastrium, which often radiates to the back. Jaundice is present in about half of all patients with cancer localized to the head of the pancreas and in less than 10% of those in whom the body or tail is the site of the tumor. Progressive deterioration almost invariably ensues, with intractable pain, cachexia, and death.

Courvoisier sign refers to an acute painless dilatation of the gallbladder accompanied by jaundice, owing to obstruction of the common bile duct by tumor. It may be the first indication of pancreatic cancer in about one third of patients.

Migratory thrombophlebitis (deep venous thrombosis) develops in 10% of patients with pancreatic cancer, especially when the tumor involves the body and tail of the pancreas. It is not uncommon for migratory thrombophlebitis, also known as *Trousseau syndrome*, to be the first evidence of an underlying pancreatic malignancy, although it may be seen with other cancers as well. In fact, unexplained thrombophlebitis in an otherwise healthy person mandates a careful search for an occult malignancy. Thrombi develop in multiple veins, including the deep veins of the legs, the subclavian vein, the inferior and superior mesenteric veins, and even the vena cava. Portal vein thrombosis may also occur, occasionally as the presenting event. Although the mechanisms responsible for the hypercoagulable state that leads to migratory thrombophlebitis are not completely understood, the following facts are known: (1) a serine protease synthesized and released by malignant tumor cells directly activates plasma factor X; (2) tumor cells spontaneously shed plasma membrane vesicles, which exhibit procoagulant activity; and (3) intracellular tissue thromboplastin is released from necrotic tumor.

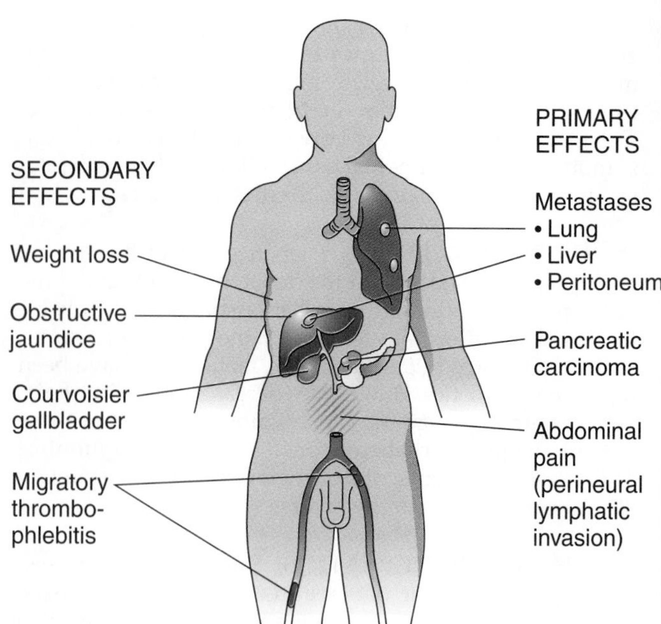

FIGURE 15-9
Complications of pancreatic carcinoma.

The complications of pancreatic ductal carcinoma are summarized in Figure 15-9.

Acinar Cell Carcinoma

Acinar cell carcinoma is principally a disease of mature adults in their fifth to eighth decades of life. The tumors are usually large and show foci of necrosis. They tend to metastasize locally to regional lymph nodes and liver and more distantly to the lungs and other body sites. Although most acinar cell carcinomas consist of well-differentiated tumor cells containing zymogen granules, some less-differentiated tumors are devoid of granules. The acinar cell origin of the latter tumors can be established either by demonstrating elevated serum levels of pancreatic digestive enzymes, such as α-amylase or lipase, or their immunocytochemical localization in the tumor cells.

Some patients with acinar cell carcinoma develop a curious syndrome consisting of fat necrosis in subcutaneous tissues and bone marrow and polyarthralgia. The resemblance of this complication to the extrapancreatic lesions encountered in acute pancreatitis suggests that it is attributable to the unregulated release of pancreatic enzymes into the serum.

NEOPLASMS OF THE ENDOCRINE PANCREAS

Islet cell tumors are rare, comprising less than 10% of all pancreatic neoplasms. Of these, many are nonfunctional and are only discovered as incidental findings at autopsy.

Functional islet cell tumors may occur alone or as part of the multiple endocrine neoplasia syndrome type I (MEN I). The secretion of hormones by functional endocrine tumors of the pancreas results in distinctive clinical syndromes. Before considering islet cell tumors, a brief discussion of the development and function of normal islets is appropriate.

Normal Pancreatic Islets

The islets of Langerhans, which form the endocrine portion of the pancreas, are scattered throughout the organ and consist of richly vascularized globular masses of cells. Six distinct cell types have been identified and correlated with hormone synthesis and storage:

- **Alpha cells:** These cells synthesize glucagon and are located in the outer rim of the islets. They constitute 15% to 20% of the total islet cell population (Fig. 15-10A). Glucagon induces glycogenolysis and gluconeogenesis in the liver, thereby raising the blood glucose level. Its secretion is stimulated by hypoglycemia and by the ingestion of a low-carbohydrate, high-protein meal. By virtue of these responses, glucagon, together with insulin, serves to maintain fuel homeostasis.
- **Beta cells:** These cells synthesize insulin and comprise 60% to 70% of all islet cells. Beta cells are distributed throughout the islet and can be visualized by their affinity for certain stains, such as aldehyde fuchsin or pseudoisocyanin, or by the use of specific antibody to insulin (see Fig. 15-10B). By electron microscopy, the insulin is resolved into characteristic polygonal and rhomboidal crystals enclosed in secretory vesicles. The major obligatory stimulus for insulin secretion is the binding of glucose to receptors on the surface of the beta cell.
- **Delta cells:** The delta cells are subdivided into D and D_1 types, secreting somatostatin and vasoactive intestinal polypeptide, respectively. Delta cells are fewer in number and slightly larger than alpha cells and, like them, tend to be localized at the periphery of the islets (see Fig. 15-10C). Delta cells are situated between the alpha and the beta cells, so that the three cell types are often contiguous. Pancreatic somato-

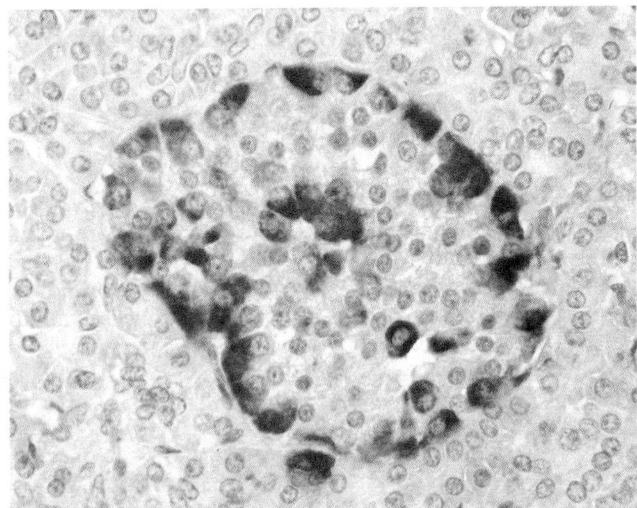

A

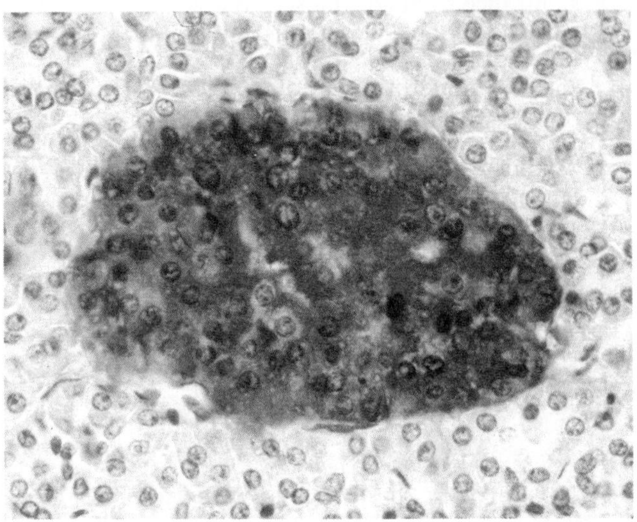

B

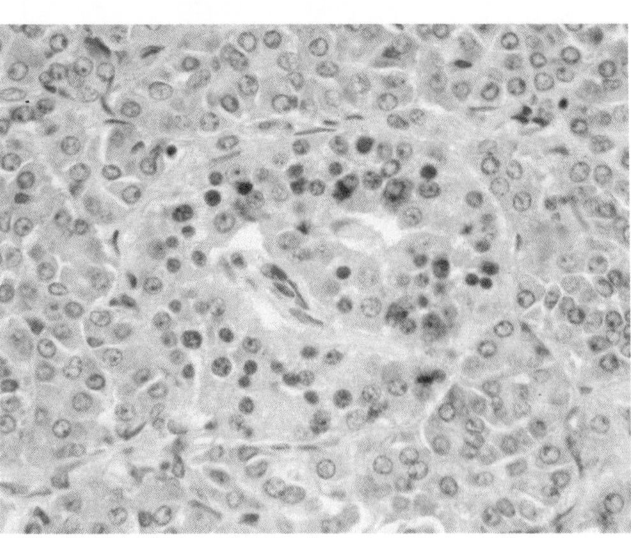

C

FIGURE *15-10*
Localization of hormones of the pancreatic islet by specific antibodies. The immunoperoxidase technique reveals (*A*) glucagon in alpha cells at the periphery of the islet, (*B*) insulin in beta cells distributed throughout the islet, and (*C*) somatostatin in sparsely distributed delta cells.

statin, a peptide identical to the one in the hypothalamus, inhibits the pituitary release of growth hormone. Somatostatin also inhibits secretion by alpha and beta cells, D_1 cells, acinar cells of the exocrine pancreas, and certain hormone-secreting cells in the gastrointestinal tract. Coupled with the topographical cell–cell relations noted earlier, these hormonal interactions suggest that somatostatin plays a regulatory role in alpha and beta cell secretion, which is reflected in the stability of glucose homeostasis.

- **D_1 cells:** D_1 cells are smaller than the other islet cell types and are rare in the islets of the normal human pancreas. Vasoactive intestinal polypeptide (VIP) has also been localized in ganglion cells and nerve fibers of the pancreas, gut, and brain. In a manner similar to that of glucagon, it induces glycogenolysis and hyperglycemia, and in addition it regulates the tone, motility, and ion and water secretion by epithelial cells of the gastrointestinal tract.
- **Pancreatic polypeptide-secreting cells:** These cells are located primarily in the islets of the head of the pancreas and synthesize a polypeptide that appears to have variable and opposed functions. These include stimulation of the secretion of enzymes from the gastric mucosa and inhibition of a variety of functions, such as smooth muscle contraction in the intestine and gallbladder, production of gastric acid, and secretion by the exocrine pancreas and biliary system.
- **Enterochromaffin cells:** These cells are rare components of the islet cell population in the head of the pancreas. They synthesize serotonin and the peptide motilin, a hormone that stimulates motility of gastric smooth muscle and increases the tone of the sphincter at the gastroesophageal junction.

The various types of islet cells, the products they secrete, and their physiological actions are summarized in Table 15-1.

Beta Cell Tumors (Insulinomas)

Beta cell tumors, the most common of the islet cell neoplasms (75%), may release sufficient insulin to induce severe hypoglycemia. Neoplastic beta cells, unlike their normal counterparts, are not regulated by the blood glucose level and continue to secrete insulin autonomously, even when the blood level of glucose is very low. Beta cell tumors and other islet cell neoplasms occur both sporadically and in the context of the MEN I syndrome (see Chapter 21).

☐ Pathology: **Most beta cell tumors are benign lesions in the body or tail of the pancreas** (Fig. 15-11). They are generally less than 3 cm in diameter and occasionally as small as 1 mm. The large majority (90%) are solitary and can be surgically excised. Only a minority (5% to 15%) demonstrate malignant behavior. Histologically, insulinoma cells resemble normal beta cells but are dispersed in trabecular or solid patterns (Fig. 15-12). The tumor often elicits a desmoplastic reaction, and amyloid (derived from a peptide hormone secreted with insulin and termed *amylin*) may be found in the stroma. Electron microscopy shows pleomorphic, paracrystalline granules surrounded by a clear halo, an appearance typical of insulin stored in normal beta cells. A reliable distinction between benign and malignant insulinomas is usually not possible on histological grounds and in most cases awaits the appearance of metastases.

Although overexpression of some genes (*ras*, *rig*) has been described in islet cell neoplasms, no mutational activation of such oncogenes has been detected. Inactivation of tumor suppressor genes (MEN I, Rb, p53, APC) has been found in some islet cell tumors.

☐ Clinical Features: Low blood sugar produces a syndrome of sweating, nervousness, and hunger, which may progress to confusion, lethargy, and coma. Since these symptoms are relieved by eating, it is common for patients with insulinomas to be overweight. Frequently, the diagnosis is delayed by abnormal behavior that causes some patients to seek psychiatric care. Most cases are characterized by only a mild hypoglycemia, and in some the tumor is not functional at all. The diagnosis is established by the demonstration of high levels of insulin in the blood and in the tumor cells (see Fig. 15-12B).

TABLE *15-1* **Secretory Products of Islet Cells and their Physiological Actions**

Cell	Secretory Product	Mol. Wt. (Daltons)	Physiological Actions
Alpha	Glucagon	3500	Catabolic, stimulates glycogenolysis and gluconeogenesis, raises blood glucose
Beta	Insulin	6000	Anabolic, stimulates glycogenesis, lipogenesis, and protein synthesis, lowers blood glucose
Delta	Somatostatin	1600	Inhibits secretion of alpha, beta, D_1, and acinar cells
D_1	Vasoactive intestinal polypeptide (VIP)	3800	Same as glucagon; also regulates tone and motility of GI tract and activates cAMP of intestinal epithelium
PP	Human pancreatic polypeptide (hPP)	4300	Stimulates gastric enzyme secretion, inhibits intestinal motility and bile secretion
EC	Serotonin, substance P (motilin)	176	Induces vasodilatation, increases vascular permeability, stimulates motility of gastric muscle and tone of lower esophageal sphincter

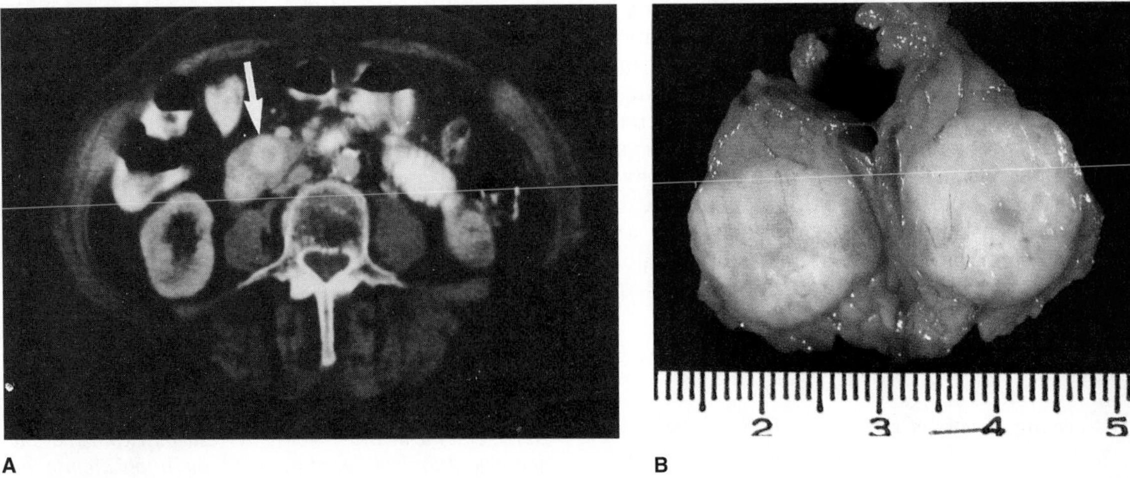

FIGURE 15-11
Insulinoma. (*A*) A computed tomography (CT) scan of the abdomen shows a solitary insulinoma (*arrow*). (*B*) An insulinoma is embedded in tan, lobular pancreatic tissue.

Pancreatic Gastrinoma (Zollinger-Ellison Syndrome)

Pancreatic gastrinoma is an islet cell tumor consisting of so-called G cells, which secrete gastrin, a potent hormonal stimulus for the secretion of acid by the stomach. The location of this tumor in the pancreas is curious, because gastrin-containing cells have not been demonstrated in normal islets. By electron microscopy, G cells bear a strong resemblance to the gastrin-secreting cells that normally reside in the duodenal mucosa. The pancreatic tumor is believed to arise from multipotent primitive endocrine cells that have undergone inappropriate differentiation to form G cells in the islets. Pancreatic gastrinoma is the cause of Zollinger-Ellison syndrome, a disorder characterized by (1) intractable gastric hypersecretion, (2) severe peptic ulceration of the duodenum and jejunum, and (3) high levels of gastrin in the blood.

Among islet cell tumors, pancreatic gastrinomas are

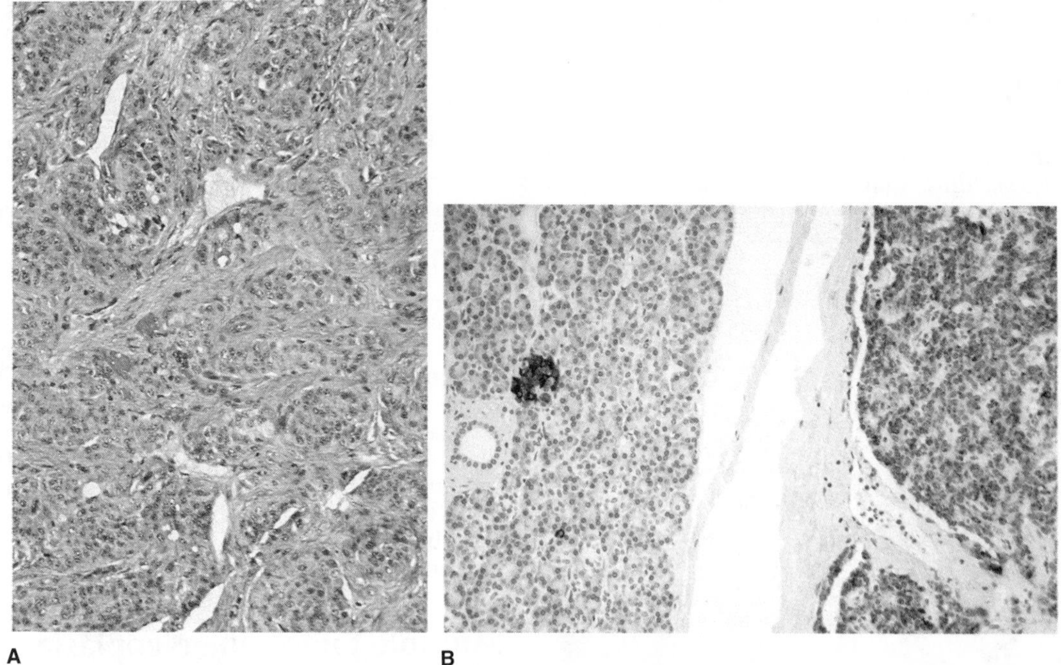

FIGURE 15-12
A functional insulinoma. (*A*) Nests of tumor cells are surrounded by numerous capillaries. (*B*) Immunochemical localization of insulin in an insulinoma (*right*) and in an islet in the adjacent normal pancreas.

second in frequency only to insulinomas, accounting for one fourth of islet cell tumors. They are most common between the ages of 30 and 50 years, with a slight male predominance. Fifteen percent of cases of the Zollinger-Ellison syndrome are due to gastrinomas outside the pancreas, particularly in the duodenum. The majority of gastrinomas are malignant (70% to 90%). The tumor may be solitary or multiple, the latter usually in the context of MEN I. Histologically, gastrinomas are remarkably similar to intestinal carcinoid tumors. Metastases to regional lymph nodes and the liver are often functional.

Alpha Cell Tumors (Glucagonomas)

Glucagon-secreting tumors of the alpha cells (glucagonomas) are associated with a syndrome consisting of (1) mild diabetes; (2) a necrotizing, migratory, erythematous rash; (3) anemia; (4) venous thromboses; and (5) severe infections. These tumors are rare (1% of functional islet cell tumors) and occur between the ages of 40 and 70 years, with a slight female predominance. Two thirds of symptomatic glucagonomas are malignant.

Functional glucagonomas are usually large tumors that invade surrounding structures. Microscopically, they resemble the trabecular and solid patterns of insulinomas. The presence of glucagon within the tumor is demonstrated immunocytochemically and by the demonstration of characteristic alpha cell granules by electron microscopy (Fig. 15-13). In addition to glucagon, some alpha cell tumors contain other hormones, such as insulin, somatostatin, and pancreatic polypeptide.

In patients with alpha cell tumors, plasma glucagon levels are elevated up to 30 times above normal. In addition to the characteristic hyperglycemia, fasting plasma amino-acid levels are decreased to as low as 20% of normal.

Delta Cell Tumors (Somatostatinomas)

Delta cell tumors are rare and produce a syndrome consisting of mild diabetes mellitus, gallstones, steatorrhea, and hypochlorhydria. These effects result from the inhibitory actions of somatostatin on other cells of the pancreatic islets and on neuroendocrine cells of the gastrointestinal tract, which secrete insulin, cholecystokinin, glucagon, and gastrin. Thus, the levels of insulin and glucagon in blood are decreased. In addition to producing somatostatin, some delta cell tumors also secrete calcitonin or adrenocorticotropic hormone (ACTH). The tumor is usually solitary, and the majority have been malignant, with metastases already present at the time of diagnosis.

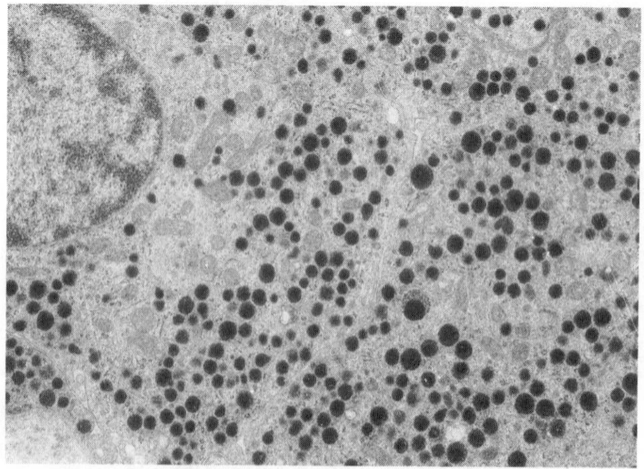

FIGURE 15-13
Alpha cells in a functional glucagonoma. The granules are indistinguishable from those of normal alpha cells.

D_1 Tumors (VIPomas, Verner-Morrison Syndrome)

D_1 tumors secrete VIP and give rise to the Verner-Morrison syndrome, a disorder characterized by explosive and profuse watery diarrhea, accompanied by hypokalemia and hypochlorhydria. The syndrome has also been referred to as pancreatic cholera. VIPomas are rare tumors (less than 5% of all islet tumors), are usually large and solitary, and in most cases are malignant.

High levels of circulating VIP and severe diarrhea have also been encountered in patients with a variety of nonpancreatic neoplasms containing different types of neuroendocrine cells (e.g., ganglioneuroma, pheochromocytoma of the adrenal medulla, medullary thyroid carcinoma, and bronchogenic carcinoma). In some patients, the Verner-Morrison syndrome is caused by MEN I.

Pancreatic Polypeptide-Secreting Tumors

Pancreatic polypeptide-producing tumors are rare and are not associated with a clinical syndrome, despite the fact that they are functional and secrete high levels of pancreatic polypeptide in the blood. The tumors are usually single and benign, although a few have metastasized to the liver. In addition to their own specific hormones, other islet cell tumors may secrete pancreatic polypeptide.

Enterochromaffin Cell (Carcinoid) Tumors

Carcinoid tumors of the pancreas are rare malignant neoplasms. They resemble intestinal carcinoids, contain enterochromaffin cells, and secrete serotonin. When confined to the pancreas, they may induce the so-called atypical carcinoid syndrome, consisting of a severe facial flush, hypotension, periorbital edema, and lacrimation. Carcinoid tumors that have metastasized to the liver cause the classic carcinoid syndrome (see Chapter 13).

The syndromes and complications of the major types of islet cell tumors are summarized in Figure 15-14.

Multiple Endocrine Neoplasia Syndrome Type I

Multiple endocrine neoplasia syndrome type I is an infrequent familial disorder characterized by multiple adenomas of the pituitary, parathyroids, and endocrine pancreas. It is frequently

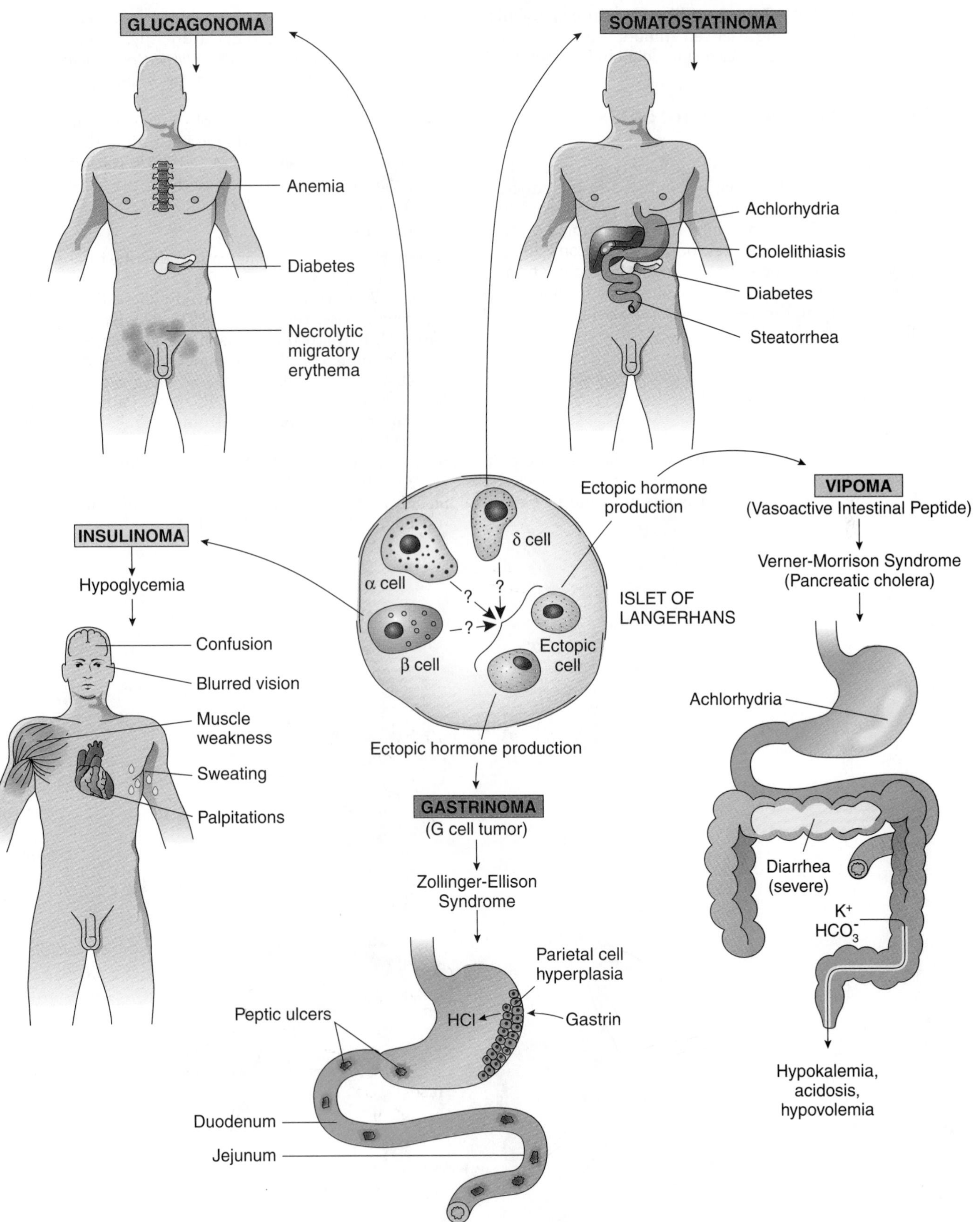

FIGURE 15-14
Syndromes associated with islet cell tumors of the pancreas.

associated with the Zollinger-Ellison syndrome, in which case gastrin-secreting islet cell tumors are present. The MEN syndromes are described in detail in Chapter 21.

Ectopic Hormone Syndromes

Islet cell tumors may secrete a variety of normal hormones that are not ordinarily produced in the pancreas (ectopic hormones), including ACTH, parathyroid hormone, calcitonin, and vasopressin. The ectopic hormone may be produced either alone or in combination with normally occurring pancreatic hormones. Endocrine tumors of the pancreas account for 10% of paraneoplastic Cushing syndrome, in this respect being second only to small cell carcinoma of the lung.

SUGGESTED READING

BOOKS

Cubilla AL, Fitzgerald PJ: Tumors of the exocrine pancreas. In: *Atlas of tumor pathology,* series 2, fascicle 19. Washington, DC: Armed Forces Institute of Pathology, 1984.

Klöppel G: Pathology of nonendocrine pancreatic tumors. In: Go VL, DiMagno E, Gardner JD, Lebenthal E, Reber HA, Scheele GA (eds), *The pancreas. Biology, pathobiology and disease,* 2nd ed, pp 871–897, New York: Raven Press, 1993.

Steer ML: Etiology and pathophysiology of acute pancreatitis. In: Go VL, DeMagno E, Gardner JD, Lebenthal E, Reber HA, Scheele GA (eds), *The pancreas. Biology, pathobiology and disease,* 2nd ed, pp 581–591, New York: Raven Press, 1993.

REVIEW ARTICLES

Klöppel G, Heitz PU: Pancreatic endocrine tumors. *Pathol Res Pract* 183:155–175, 1988.

Mallory A, Kern F: Drug-induced pancreatitis: A critical review. *Gastroenterology* 78:813–820, 1980.

Sarles H, Barnard JP, Chonson C: Pathogenesis and epidemiology of chronic pancreatitis. *Annu Rev Med* 40:453–468, 1989.

Solcia E, Capella C, Buffa R, et al: Pathology of the Zollinger-Ellison syndrome. *Prog Surg Pathol* 1:119–133, 1980.

Steinberg W, Tenner S. Acute pancreatitis. *N Engl J Med* 330:1198–1210, 1994.

Steer ML, Waxman I, Freedman S. Chronic pancreatitis. *N Engl J Med* 332:1482–1490, 1995.

CHAPTER 16

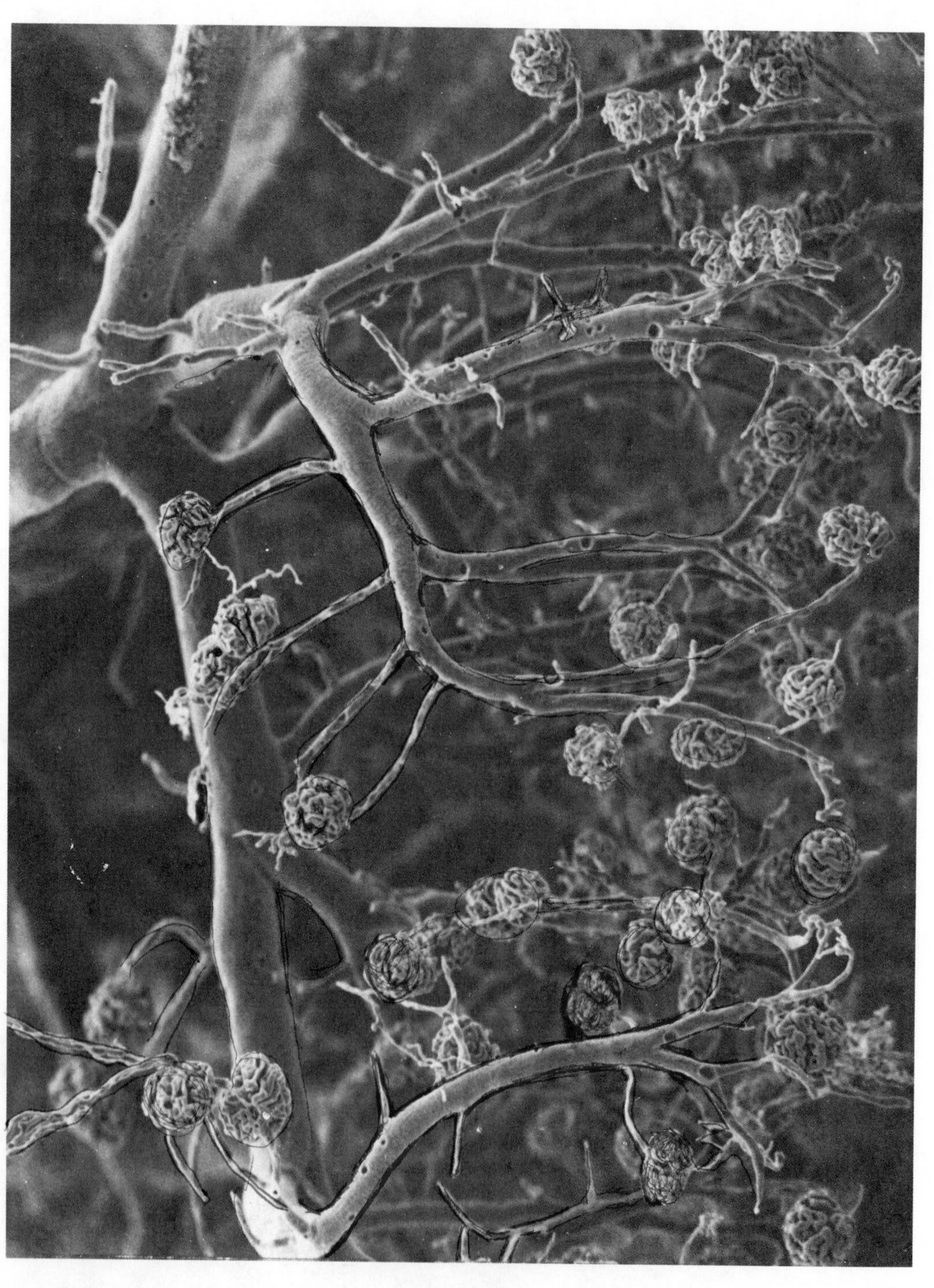

The Kidney

J. Charles Jennette
Benjamin H. Spargo

(continued)

FIGURE *16-1* *(see opposite page)*
The renal cortical vascular system. A scanning electron micrograph of a corrosion cast of the renal vasculature shows terminal arborizations of the blood vessels, including the capillaries of the glomerular tufts.

ANATOMY

The kidneys are paired, bean-shaped organs located on both sides of the vertebral column in the retroperitoneal space. The adult kidney weighs an average of 150 g and is approximately 11 cm long, 6 cm wide, and 3 cm thick. Each kidney consists of an outer cortex and an inner medulla. When the kidney is bisected, it is apparent that the medulla is composed of approximately 12 pyramids, the bases of which are at the corticomedullary junction. Each pyramid has an inner and an outer zone. The inner zone, called the papilla, empties into a calyx. The outer zone is divided into the outer stripe and the inner stripe. The medullary rays are faint vertical striations in the pyramids that consist of collecting ducts and ascending thick limbs of the loops of Henle.

Blood Vessels

In most kidneys, the blood supply is derived from a single renal artery, which arises from the aorta. About one quarter have one or more accessory renal arteries. Before entering the renal parenchyma, the renal artery divides into anterior and posterior branches, which in turn give rise to the interlobar arteries. The latter branch into the arcuate arteries, which course parallel to the renal surface between the medulla and the cortex. The interlobular arteries arise from the arcuate arteries and extend toward the renal surface. The interlobular arteries give off the afferent arterioles, each of which supplies a single glomerulus (Fig. 16-1). After emerging from the glomerulus, the efferent arteriole branches into capillaries.

The inner and outer zones of the cortex have their own characteristic capillary plexuses. The outer cortex receives branches from the efferent arterioles of the superficial glomeruli, whereas the deeper zones are fed by the efferent arterioles of the juxtamedullary glomeruli. The blood supply to the medulla is from thin-walled vessels, termed the *vasa recta*, which are looping vessels with few anastomoses that supply the papillae.

The Glomerulus

The nephron is the architectural unit of the kidney and includes the glomerulus and its tubule, the latter terminating at the common collecting system. The glomerulus is a specialized network of capillaries, with an arteriole at either end (Figs. 16-2 through 16-4). The glomerulus has a central connective tissue mesangium, which is inhabited by specialized mesangial cells. The glomerular capillaries are lined by fenestrated endothelial cells lying on a basement membrane, the outer surface of which is covered by specialized epithelial cells.

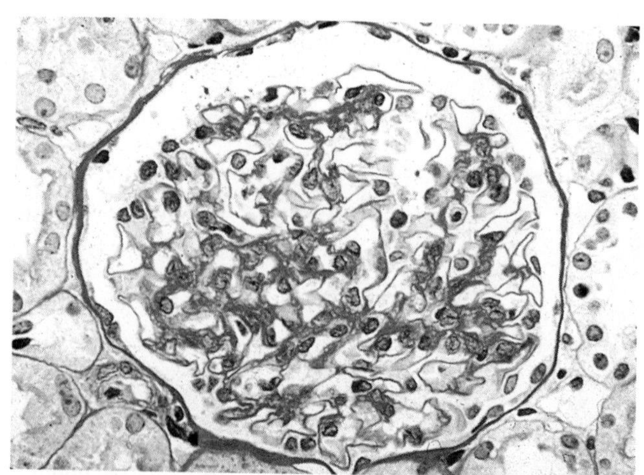

FIGURE *16-2*
Normal glomerulus, light microscopy. The periodic acid–Schiff (PAS) stain highlights the delicate basement membranes and the mesangial matrix.

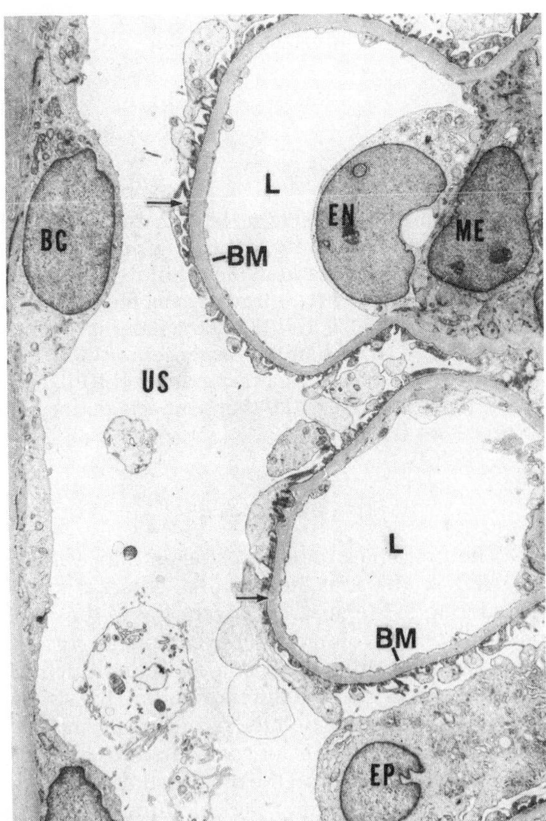

FIGURE 16-3
Normal glomerulus. In this electron micrograph, the normal glomerular capillary is covered by epithelial cells (EP), with foot processes (*arrows*) in contact with the basement membrane (BM). The endothelial cell (EN) has large pores and surrounds the capillary lumen (L). The mesangial cell (ME) is bordered by the endothelial cell on the luminal surface and the stalk basement membrane on the lateral areas. (US, urinary space; BC, Bowman capsule).

Glomerular Basement Membrane

The glomerular basement membrane (GBM) (Fig. 16-5) is a continuation of the arteriolar basement membrane, which merges at the hilus of the glomerulus with the membrane of Bowman capsule. In turn, Bowman capsule is continuous with the basement membrane of the proximal tubule. The GBM does not completely surround each capillary, the latter being separated from the mesangial cells only by endothelial cell cytoplasm. Thus, a potential pathway exists for mediators and molecular debris in the blood to enter the mesangium without crossing the GBM.

Although morphologically similar to many other basement membranes, the GBM is functionally and chemically distinct. Ultrastructurally, it is approximately 300 nm thick and has three definable layers (see Fig. 16-5):

- **Lamina densa:** a central electron-dense zone
- **Lamina rara interna:** a thin inner electron-lucent zone
- **Lamina rara externa:** a thin outer electron-lucent zone

The GBM has a strong negative charge, owing to the presence of polyanionic glycosaminoglycans, which are rich in heparan sulfate. This property allows charge-selective filtration of electrically neutral and cationic molecules and relative exclusion of negatively charged molecules, such as albumin. The GBM also discriminates between molecules on the basis of size.

The Endothelial Cells

Glomerular capillaries have a fenestrated endothelial layer, approximately 40 nm thick, with numerous 60 to 100 nm openings, some of which are closed by a thin membrane (see Fig. 16-5). These openings are not a major filtration barrier to constituents of the plasma. Endothelial surface membrane proteins, such as adhesion molecules, and their secretory products (e.g., prostaglandins) have

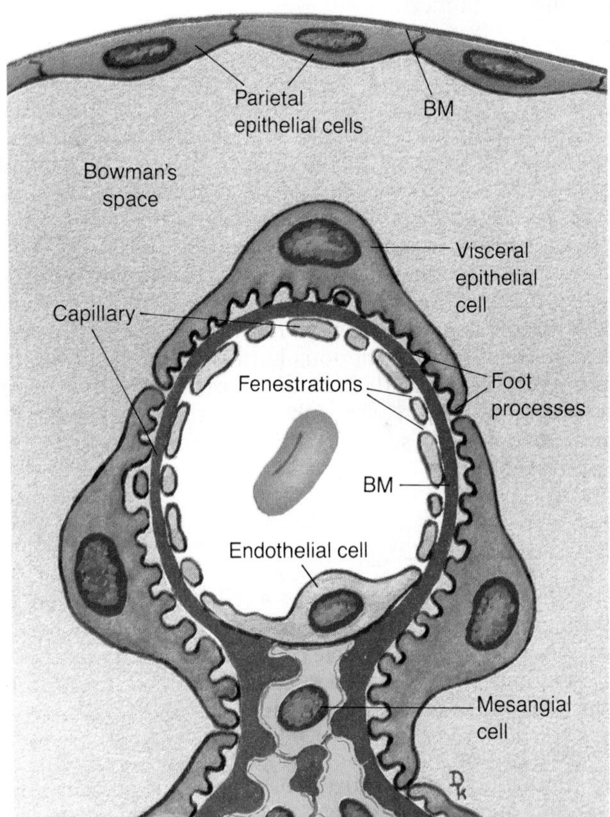

FIGURE 16-4
Normal glomerulus. The relationship of the different glomerular cell types to the significant stroma is illustrated using a single glomerular loop. The entire outer aspect of the glomerular basement membrane (BM) (peripheral loop and stalk) is covered by the epithelial cell foot processes. The outer portions of the endothelial cell, which surround the capillary lumen, are in contact with the inner surface of the basement membrane, whereas the central part is in contact with the mesangial cell of the stalk. The relationship of the mesangial cell to its stroma is unique to the glomerulus and has not been entirely clarified.

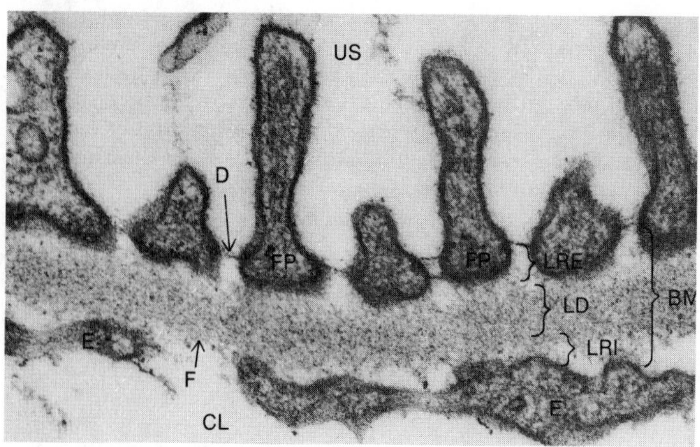

FIGURE 16-5
The glomerular filter. An electron micrograph illustrates the structures of the glomerular filter. Molecules that pass from the capillary lumen (CL) to the urinary space (US) traverse the fenestrations (F) of the endothelial cell (E), the trilaminar basement membrane (BM) (lamina rara interna [LRI], lamina densa [LD], and lamina rara externa [LRE]), and the slit pore diaphragm (D) that connects podocyte foot processes (FP).

important roles in the pathogenesis of inflammatory and thrombotic glomerular diseases.

The Epithelial Cells

Glomerular epithelial cells line Bowman space. Visceral epithelial cells rest on the GBM and the parietal epithelial cells on Bowman capsule. The visceral epithelial cell, or *podocyte*, sends cytoplasmic projections, termed *foot processes*, onto the lamina rara externa of the GBM (see Fig. 16-5). Between adjacent foot processes is a thin membrane called the filtration slit diaphragm. The visceral epithelial cells are the major glomerular filtration barrier. The parietal epithelium is continuous both with the visceral epithelium and the epithelium of the proximal convoluted tubule. At the origin of the tubule, the flat parietal epithelium abruptly gives way to the tall columnar cells of the proximal tubule.

The Mesangium

The glomerulus is supported by a cellular and matrix network, collectively termed the mesangium. Mesangial cells are modified smooth muscle cells situated in the center of the glomerular tuft between capillary loops. Important functions of the mesangium include the following:

- Mechanical support for the glomerulus
- Endocytosis and processing of plasma proteins, including immune complexes
- Maintenance of basement membrane and matrix elements
- Modulation of glomerular filtration by the contractility of mesangial cells
- Generation of molecular mediators (e.g., prostaglandins and cytokines)

The Tubules

The initial segment of the renal tubule that drains the urinary space of the glomerulus is the proximal convoluted tubule. The proximal tubule becomes a thin-walled segment as it descends into the medulla, where it forms the U-shaped loop of Henle. After ascending to the cortex, it forms the distal convoluted tubule. Within the cortex, several distal tubules unite to form a collecting duct, which ultimately empties into the ducts of Bellini, the structures that discharge urine through the papillae into the calyces.

The proximal tubule is longer and more conspicuous in histological sections than the distal tubule. The luminal membrane of the proximal tubular epithelial cells has a characteristic brush border composed of microvilli that provide a large surface area for salt and water reabsorption.

The Juxtaglomerular Apparatus

The juxtaglomerular apparatus, located at the hilus of the glomerulus, is a complex that consists of the following:

- **Afferent arteriole**
- **Macula densa,** a region of the thick ascending limb of the loop of Henle
- **Lacis cells,** located between the macula densa and the hilar arterioles

The wall of the afferent arteriole contains characteristic granular cells involved in the synthesis and secretion of renin and angiotensin. The secretion of renin appears to be influenced by changes in the stretch of the arteriole and the sodium or chloride load at the macula densa.

Interstitium

The renal interstitium is composed of interstitial cells and surrounding matrix. The interstitium occupies 10% of the cortical volume but comprises 20% to 30% of medullary volume. The interstitium offers structural support, whereas the interstitial cells have homeostatic secretory functions. For example, some cortical interstitial cells secrete erythropoietin and some medullary cells elaborate prostaglandins.

CONGENITAL ANOMALIES

Renal Agenesis

Renal agenesis is the complete absence of renal tissue. The absence of both kidneys is clearly not compatible with life. Most infants born with bilateral renal agenesis are stillborn, and the mother usually suffers from oligohydramnios (insufficient amniotic fluid). Bilateral agenesis is often associated with other congenital anomalies, including low-set ears, receding chin, beaklike nose, and pulmonary hypoplasia. Congenital anomalies of the genitalia are also common, as are lower limb anomalies. The pattern of malformations associated with oligohydramnios is known as *Potter syndrome* (see Chapter 6). If there are no associated anomalies, unilateral renal agenesis is not a serious matter, because the single kidney undergoes sufficient hypertrophy to maintain normal renal function.

Renal Hypoplasia

Renal hypoplasia refers to a reduction in renal mass without any histological malformation, with six or fewer renal lobes (medullary pyramids with overlying cortex). Renal hypoplasia must be differentiated from small kidneys secondary to atrophy or scarring.

Ectopic Kidney

Renal ectopia defines an abnormal location of the kidney, usually in the pelvis. Most commonly, this condition results from failure of the fetal kidney to migrate from the pelvis to the flank. Renal ectopia may involve only one kidney, or it may be bilateral. In *simple ectopia,* the ureters drain into the appropriate side of the bladder. In *crossed ectopia,* the ectopic kidney is on the same side as its normal mate, and the ectopic ureter crosses the midline and drains into the contralateral side of the bladder.

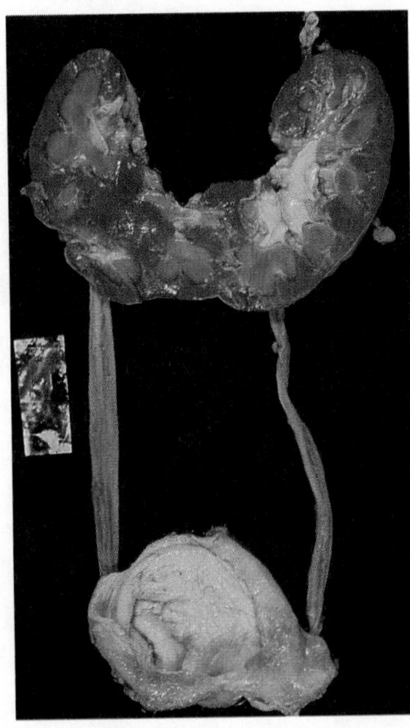

FIGURE 16-6
Horseshoe kidney. The kidneys are fused at the lower pole.

Horseshoe Kidney

Horseshoe kidney is a single, large, midline organ, which results from failure of the renal anlage to divide. The infant is born with fusion of the two kidneys, usually at the lower poles. (Fig. 16-6). This anomaly usually has no clinical consequences.

RENAL DYSPLASIA

Renal dysplasia is a developmental disorder of the kidney, characterized by the persistence of immature and abnormal structures, such as cartilage and undifferentiated mesenchyme.

☐ **Pathogenesis:** Renal dysplasia results from an abnormality in metanephric differentiation and is almost always (90%) accompanied by other urinary tract abnormalities. This association suggests that an obstruction to the flow of urine *in utero* causes dysplasia. The associated anomalies include the following:

- Ureteral agenesis
- Ureteral atresia
- Ureteropelvic junction obstruction
- Ureterovesical stenosis or posterior urethral valves

☐ **Pathology:** Histologically, the hallmark of renal dysplasia is undifferentiated tubules and ducts lined by cuboidal or columnar epithelium. These structures are surrounded by mantles of undifferentiated mesenchyme, which sometimes contain smooth muscle and islands of cartilage (Fig. 16-7). Rudimentary glomeruli may be present, and the tubules and ducts may be cystically dilated. Renal dysplasia can be unilateral or bilateral, and the involved kidney can be abnormally large or very small.

- **Aplastic renal dysplasia** results in tiny rudimentary dysplastic kidneys.
- **Multicystic renal dysplasia,** which is usually unilateral, is characterized by renal enlargement by multiple cysts, ranging from microscopic to several centimeters in diameter. The kidney does not show the usual beanlike (reniform) shape but rather resembles an irregular mass of cysts (Fig. 16-8).
- **Diffuse cystic renal dysplasia** is characterized by more-uniformly sized cysts and preservation of a reniform shape.

☐ **Clinical Features:** In most patients with multicystic renal dysplasia, a palpable flank mass is discovered

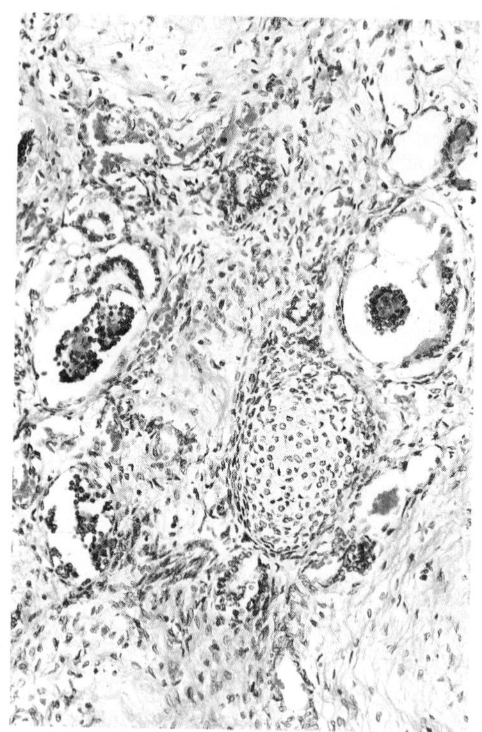

FIGURE 16-7
Renal dysplasia. Immature glomeruli, tubules, and cartilage are surrounded by loose, undifferentiated mesenchymal tissue.

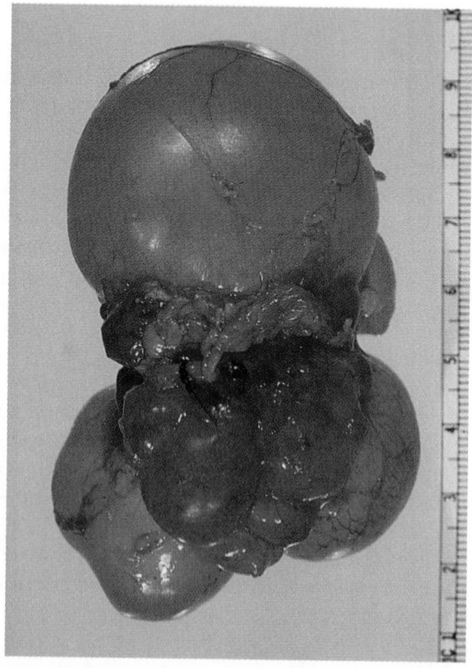

FIGURE 16-8
Multicystic renal dysplasia. An irregular mass of variably sized cysts does not have a reniform shape.

shortly after birth, although small multicystic kidneys may not become apparent until many years later. **Unilateral renal multicystic dysplasia is the most common cause of an abdominal mass in newborns.** Unilateral dysplasia is adequately treated by removal of the affected kidney. Bilateral aplastic dysplasia causes oligohydramnios and the resultant Potter syndrome and is incompatible with life. Aplastic renal dysplasia and diffuse cystic dysplasia are more often hereditary, especially if they are associated with multiple anomalies in other organs, as in Meckel syndrome.

POLYCYSTIC KIDNEY DISEASES

The polycystic kidney diseases are a heterogeneous group of congenital and acquired disorders characterized by distortion of the renal parenchyma by numerous cysts (Fig. 16-9). These in-

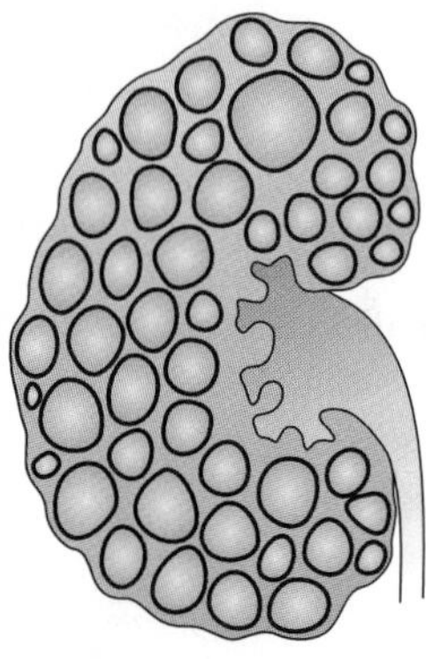

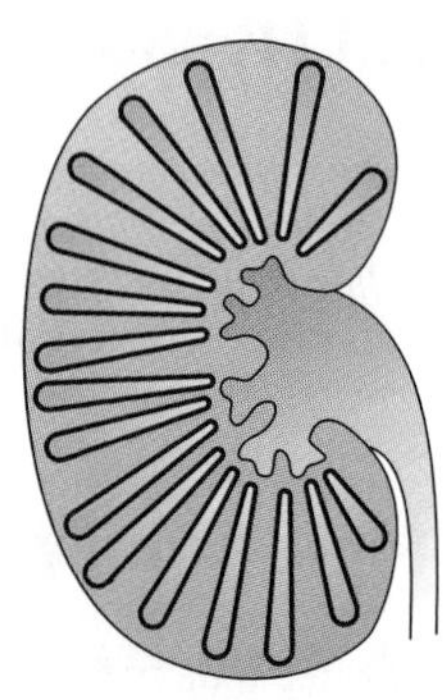

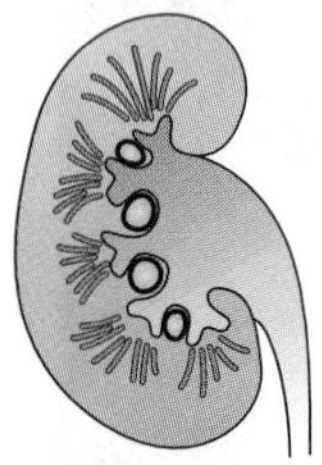

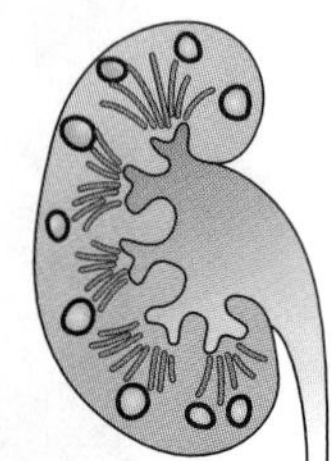

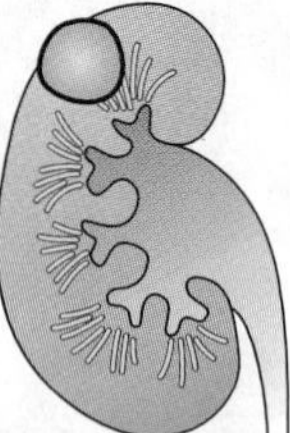

FIGURE 16-9
Cystic diseases of the kidney.

clude the following:

- Autosomal dominant polycystic kidney disease
- Autosomal recessive polycystic kidney disease
- Nephronophthisis-medullary cystic disease complex
- Medullary sponge kidney
- Acquired cystic renal disease

Autosomal Dominant (Adult) Polycystic Kidney Disease

Autosomal dominant polycystic kidney disease (ADPKD) is the most common monogenic renal disorder that is potentially fatal. ADPKD affects 1:400 to 1:1000 persons in the United States. Half of all patients with this disease eventually develop end-stage renal failure. It is estimated that ADPKD is responsible for 10% of all cases of renal disease that require dialysis or transplantation.

☐ **Pathogenesis:** This form of polycystic kidney disease is usually familial, although there is a significant incidence of spontaneous mutation. Mutations in the ADPKD-1 gene on the short arm of chromosome 16 account for 85% of the cases. The gene is very large (at least 54 kb), thereby creating a substantial target for a variety of mutations. The function of the gene product, termed *polycystin*, has not been elucidated. However, there is evidence to suggest that it is an integral membrane protein involved in cell–cell and cell–matrix interactions.

Although the precise pathogenesis of ADPKD remains unclear, it is held that cysts arise in segments of renal tubules from a few cells that proliferate abnormally. The wall of the tubule becomes covered by an undifferentiated epithelium composed of cells with a higher nucleus-to-cytoplasm ratio and only few microvilli. Concomitantly, a defective basement membrane immediately underlying the abnormal epithelium allows dilatation of the affected portion of the tubule. Initially, the fluid in the cysts is derived from the glomerular filtrate, but eventually most of the cysts become disconnected from the tubules, in which case the fluid accumulates by transepithelial secretion. Historically, end-stage renal disease in ADPKD has been attributed to the pressure exerted by the dilating cysts on the surrounding normal parenchyma. However, it is now appreciated that cysts originate in less than 2% of nephrons, and that factors other than crowding of normal tissue by the expanding cysts likely contribute to the loss of functioning renal tissue. Apoptotic loss of renal tubules and the accumulation of inflammatory mediators have been incriminated in the destruction of normal renal mass.

Two other genes associated with ADPKD have been identified, namely ADPKD-2 on chromosome 4 and ADPKD-3, whose location is still to be determined.

☐ **Pathology:** The kidneys in ADPKD are markedly enlarged bilaterally, each weighing as much as 4500 g (Fig. 16-10). The external contours of the kidneys are distorted by the presence of numerous cysts, filled with a straw-colored fluid, which are as large as 5 cm in diameter. Microscopically, the cysts are lined by a cuboidal and columnar epithelium. The cysts arise from virtually any

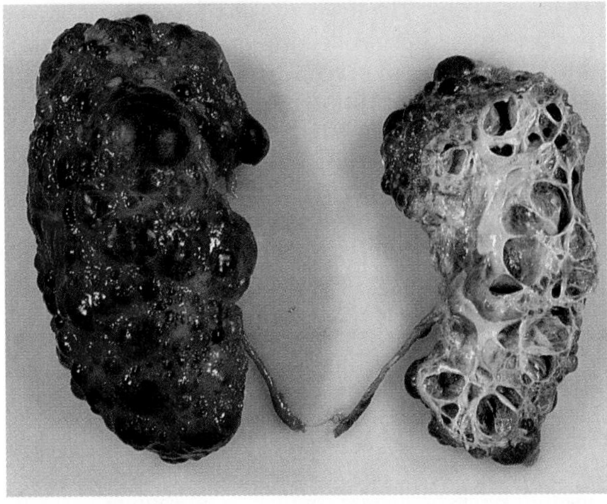

FIGURE *16-10*
Adult polycystic disease. The kidney is enlarged, and the parenchyma is almost entirely replaced by cysts of varying size.

point along the nephron, and some contain glomeruli. Areas of normal renal parenchyma are found between the cysts.

One third of patients with ADPKD also have **hepatic cysts**, the lining of which resembles bile duct epithelium. Cysts occur in the spleen in 10% of patients and in the pancreas in 5%. One fifth of the patients have an associated cerebral aneurysm, and intracranial hemorrhage is a frequent cause of death. Interestingly, the large majority of patients with ADPKD also develop colonic diverticula.

☐ **Clinical Features:** By the fourth decade, patients with ADPKD typically present with symptoms, such as a sense of heaviness in the loins, bilateral flank and abdominal masses, and the passage of blood clots in the urine. Azotemia (elevated blood urea nitrogen) is common and in half the patients it progresses to uremia (clinical renal failure) over a period of several years.

Autosomal Recessive (Infantile) Polycystic Kidney Disease

Autosomal recessive polycystic kidney disease (ARPKD) is a disease of infants that is rare compared with the adult variety, occurring in about 1 in 10,000 to 50,000 live births. Of these infants, 75% die in the perinatal period, often because the large kidneys compromise expansion of the lungs. Although ARPKD occurs primarily in infants, exceptional cases present in older children and adults. Cystic transformation in this hereditary condition targets the collecting ducts. A candidate gene has been proposed to reside on the short arm of chromosome 6.

☐ **Pathology:** In contrast to adult polycystic kidney disease, the external surface of the kidney in the infantile disorder is smooth. The involvement is invariably bilateral. The kidneys are often so large that the delivery of the infant is impeded. The cysts are fusiform dilatations of cortical and medullary collecting ducts and have a striking radial arrangement perpendicular to the renal capsule (Fig. 16-11). Interstitial fibrosis and tubular atrophy are common, particularly in children who present with the disorder at an older age. As in adult polycystic disease, the calyceal system is normal. There are usually associated liver changes, termed *congenital hepatic fibrosis*, which are characterized by enlargement of portal areas, with an increase in connective tissue and proliferation of bile ducts (see Chapter 14).

Nephronophthisis—Medullary Cystic Disease Complex

The medullary cystic disease complex is a group of autosomal recessive diseases characterized by renal medullary cysts, sclerotic kidneys, and progressive renal failure. There is evidence that the pathogenesis may involve a developmental defect in tubular basement membranes.

☐ **Pathology:** The kidneys are small and when sectioned display multiple, variably sized cysts (up to 1 cm in diameter) at the corticomedullary junction (see Fig. 16-9). The cysts arise from the distal portions of the nephron. Atrophic tubules with markedly thickened basement membranes and loss of tubules out of proportion to the glomerular loss are early histological features of the disease. At this stage, the kidneys may not yet be cystic; in fact, variants of this disorder that remain noncystic have been described. Eventually, corticomedullary cysts develop, and the remainder of the parenchyma becomes increasingly atrophic. Secondary glomerular sclerosis, interstitial fibrosis, and a nonspecific inflammatory infiltrate dominate the histological picture.

☐ **Clinical Features:** Medullary cystic disease complex accounts for 10% to 20% of renal failure in childhood. Most of the patients are in the first or second decade of life at the time of diagnosis. Patients present initially with deteriorating tubular function, such as impaired concentrating ability and sodium wasting, manifested as polyuria, polydipsia, and enuresis (bed wetting). Progressive azotemia and renal failure follow, usually within 5 years of the onset of symptoms.

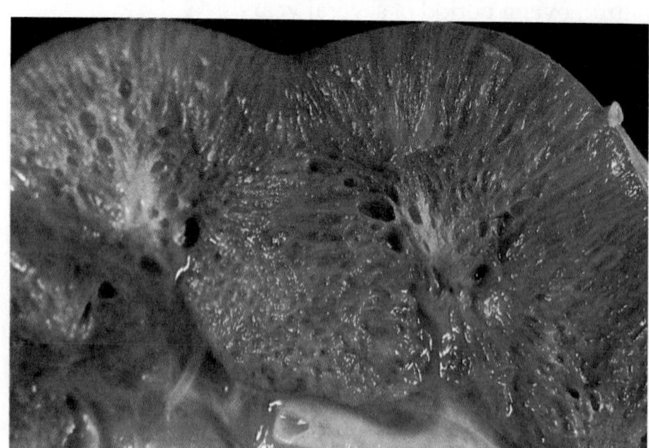

FIGURE *16-11*
Infantile polycystic disease. The dilated cortical and medullary collecting ducts are arranged radially, and the external surface is smooth.

Medullary Sponge Kidney

Medullary sponge kidney is a disorder characterized by small (<5 mm in diameter) cysts in one or more of the renal papillae (see Fig. 16-9). The cysts are lined by cuboidal or columnar epithelium and communicate with the collecting ducts in the renal papillae. In 75% of patients, the disease is bilateral. A few familial cases have been described.

Medullary sponge kidney is asymptomatic in young adults. Symptomatic cases are usually discovered between the ages of 30 and 60, when the affected person complains of flank pain, dysuria, hematuria, or "gravel" in the urine caused by stone formation in the cysts. Although the disease itself does not pose a threat to health, the cysts may predispose to secondary pyelonephritis.

Simple Renal Cysts

Simple renal cysts are very common acquired lesions, found in about half of persons over 50 years of age. They are usually incidental findings at autopsy and rarely produce clinical symptoms unless they are very large. These cysts, which are fluid-filled and may be solitary or multiple, are usually found in the outer cortex, bulging the capsule, or less commonly in the medulla. Microscopically, they are lined by a flat epithelium.

Acquired Cystic Kidney Disease

Multiple cortical and medullary cysts may form in the kidneys of patients with end-stage renal disease who undergo long-term dialysis. **In fact, after 5 years of dialysis, over 75% of patients acquire bilateral cystic kidneys.** The cysts are initially lined by flat to cuboidal epithelium, but hyperplastic and neoplastic epithelial proliferation may develop.

GLOMERULAR DISEASES

The functional complexity of the glomerulus and the varied pathogenic mechanisms that can injure the glomerulus cause a wide variety of clinical signs and symptoms that result from glomerular diseases. A glomerular disease may be the only major site of disease (primary glomerular disease; e.g., IgA nephropathy) or may be a component of a disease that affects multiple organs (secondary glomerular disease; e.g., lupus glomerulonephritis). The signs and symptoms of glomerular disease fall

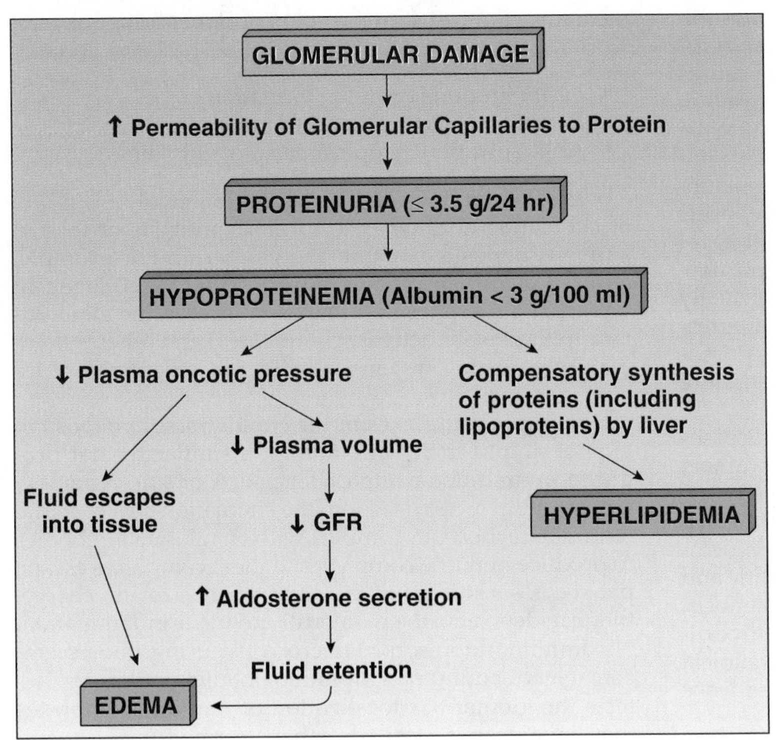

FIGURE 16-12
Pathophysiology of the nephrotic syndrome. (GFR, glomerular filtration rate).

into one of the following categories:

- Asymptomatic proteinuria
- Nephrotic syndrome
- Asymptomatic hematuria
- Acute nephritic syndrome
- Rapidly progressive nephritic syndrome
- Chronic nephritic syndrome

Nephrotic Syndrome

Nephrotic syndrome is characterized by heavy proteinuria (>3.5 g protein/24 hours), hypoalbuminemia, edema, hyperlipidemia, and lipiduria. The major pathogenetic abnormality is a permeability defect in the glomerular capillaries that allows protein to be lost from the plasma into the urine (proteinuria). Many different glomerular diseases cause proteinuria by a variety of pathogenetic mechanisms, most associated with reduced polyanionic charge of the capillary basement membrane.

Severe proteinuria causes the nephrotic syndrome (Fig. 16-12), but lower levels of proteinuria may be asymptomatic. Table 16-1 lists the major causes of the nephrotic syndrome in adults and children. There are important differences in the frequencies of specific glomerular diseases that produce the nephrotic syndrome in adults versus children. For example, minimal change glomerulopathy is responsible for the great majority (70%) of the nephrotic syndrome in children, but for only 20% of cases in adults. Systemic diseases that involve the kidney, such as diabetes, amyloidosis, and systemic lupus erythematosus, are responsible for a considerable proportion (20% to 30%) of cases of nephrotic syndrome in adults, whereas in children this condition is rarely caused by a systemic disease.

Nephritic (Glomerulonephritic) Syndrome

Nephritic syndrome is characterized by hematuria (either microscopic or visible grossly), variable degrees of proteinuria, and decreased glomerular filtration rate, with elevations in the levels of blood urea nitrogen and serum creatinine, oliguria, salt and water retention, edema, and hypertension. Glomerular diseases that cause the nephritic syndrome are character-

TABLE 16-1 **Frequency of Causes for the Nephrotic Syndrome Induced by Primary Glomerular Diseases in Children and Adults**

Cause	Children (%)	Adults (%)
Minimal change glomerulopathy	75	20
Membranous glomerulopathy	5	40
Focal segmental glomerulosclerosis	10	15
Type I membranoproliferative glomerulonephritis	5	5
Other glomerular diseases[a]	5	20

[a] Includes many forms of mesangioproliferative and proliferative glomerulonephritis, such as IgA nephropathy, that often also cause nephritic features.

ized by inflammatory changes in glomeruli, such as infiltration by leukocytes, hyperplasia of glomerular cells, and, in severe lesions, necrosis. This inflammation causes sufficient injury to the glomerular capillaries to result in the spillage of protein and blood cells (hematuria) into the urine. The glomerular inflammatory injury may also impair glomerular flow and filtration, resulting in renal insufficiency, fluid retention, and hypertension. Nephritic manifestations may (1) develop rapidly and result in reversible renal insufficiency (acute glomerulonephritis), (2) progress rapidly, with severe renal failure that usually resolves only with aggressive treatment (rapidly progressive glomerulonephritis), or (3) persist continuously or intermittently for years and progress slowly to renal failure (chronic glomerulonephritis).

As shown in Table 16-2, some glomerular diseases tend to cause the nephrotic syndrome, whereas others lead to the nephritic syndrome. However, with the possible exception of minimal change glomerulopathy (which almost always causes the nephrotic syndrome), on occasion all glomerular diseases produce mixed nephritic and nephrotic manifestations that confound clinical diagnosis. Renal biopsy evaluation is the only means of definitive diagnosis for most glomerular diseases, although clinical and laboratory data may provide presumptive evidence for a specific disease.

Pathogenesis of Glomerulonephritis

Glomerular inflammation (glomerulonephritis) is frequently caused by immunological mechanisms. Both antibody-mediated and cell-mediated types of immunity have roles in the production of glomerular inflammation; however, three mechanisms of antibody-induced inflammation have been incriminated as the major pathogenic mediators in most forms of glomerulonephritis (Fig. 16-13):

- *In situ* immune complex formation
- Deposition of circulating immune complexes
- Antineutrophil cytoplasmic autoantibodies

***In situ* immune complex formation** involves binding of circulating antibodies to intrinsic antigens or foreign antigens deposited within the glomeruli. For example, anti-GBM autoantibodies bind to type IV collagen in GBMs. The resultant immune complexes in the glomerular capillary walls activate complement and other inflammatory mediator systems, resulting in inflammatory injury.

Immune complexes in the circulation can deposit in glomeruli and incite inflammation similar to that produced by immune complex formation *in situ*. As an example, antigens released into the circulation by a bacterial or viral infection can complex with circulating antibodies to produce immune complexes. If these complexes escape phagocytosis and are of the appropriate size and charge, they can deposit in the glomeruli and incite inflammation.

Immunofluorescence microscopy, using fluorescein-conjugated, antihuman, immunoglobulin antibodies, detects the glomerular localization of immune complexes that have been deposited or have formed *in situ*. Anti-GBM antibodies produce linear staining of GBMs, whereas other immune complexes produce granular staining in capillary walls, mesangium, or both.

Antineutrophil cytoplasmic autoantibodies (*ANCA*) cause a frequent form of severe glomerulonephritis, which exhibits no glomerular immunofluorescent staining for immunoglobulins. These patients have a high frequency of circulating autoantibodies specific for antigens in the cytoplasm of neutrophils, which can mediate glomerular inflammation by activating neutrophils. The formation of glomerular immune complexes *in situ*, the deposition of immune complexes, and ANCA-induced inflammation all share a final common pathway of glomerular injury,

TABLE *16-2* **Tendencies of Glomerular Diseases to Manifest Nephrotic and Nephritic Features**

Disease	Nephrotic	Nephritic
Minimal change glomerulopathy	+ + + +	−
Membranous glomerulopathy	+ + + +	+
Focal segmental glomerulosclerosis	+ + +	+ +
Mesangioproliferative glomerulonephritis[a]	+ +	+ +
Membranoproliferative glomerulonephritis	+ +	+ + +
Proliferative glomerulonephritis[a]	+	+ + +
Crescentic glomerulonephritis[a]	+	+ + + +

[a] These histological phenotypes can be caused by many categories of glomerular disease, including IgA nephropathy, postinfectious glomerulonephritis, lupus glomerulonephritis, antineutrophil cytoplasmic autoantibody glomerulonephritis, and antiglomerular basement membrane glomerulonephritis.

Pathology of Glomerular Diseases

There are many specific glomerular diseases that have distinctive pathological features, as well as different natural histories and appropriate treatments. **Accurate pathological diagnosis of glomerular diseases requires evaluation of renal tissue by light microscopy, immunofluorescence microscopy, and electron microscopy.** Table 16-3 shows features that are useful for diagnosing glomerular diseases.

In general, the pathological features that indicate acute inflammation, such as endocapillary and extracapillary hypercellularity, leukocyte infiltration, and necrosis, are more common in the glomerular diseases that have predominantly nephritic clinical features than in those with predominantly nephrotic features. In patients with glomerulonephritis, the presence of **glomerular crescent formation** (extracapillary proliferation) correlates with a more rapidly progressive course. Crescent formation is

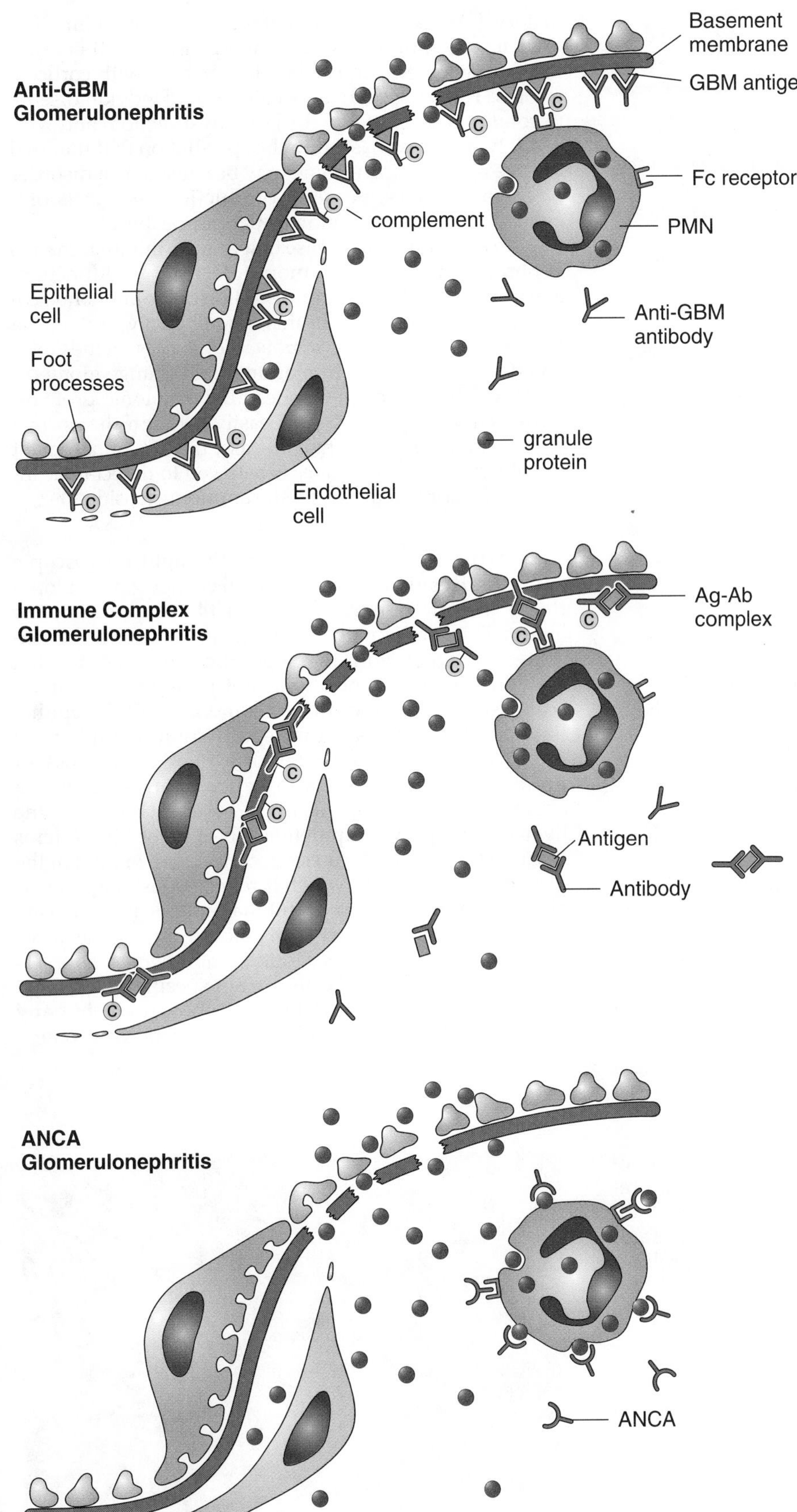

FIGURE 16-13
Antibody-mediated glomerulonephritis. ***Top panel:*** **Anti-glomerular basement membrane (GBM) antibodies cause glomerulonephritis by binding** ***in situ*** **to basement membrane antigens. This activates complement and recruits inflammatory cells.** ***Middle panel:*** **Immune complexes that deposit from the circulation also activate complement and recruit inflammatory cells.** ***Bottom panel:*** **Antineutrophil cytoplasmic antibodies (ANCA) are thought to cause inflammation by activating leukocytes, by direct binding of the antibodies to the leukocytes, or by Fc receptor engagement, or by both.**

TABLE 16-3 **Diagnostic Features of Glomerular Diseases**

I. Light Microscopic Features

A. Increased cellularity
  - Infiltration by leukocytes (e.g., neutrophils, monocytes, macrophages)
  - Proliferation of "endocapillary" cells (i.e., endothelial and mesangial cells)
  - Proliferation of "extracapillary" cells (i.e., epithelial cells) (crescent formation)

B. Increased extracellular material
  - Localization of immune complexes
  - Thickening or replication of glomerular basement membrane (GBM)
  - Increases in collagenous matrix (sclerosis)
  - Insudation of plasma proteins (hyalinosis)
  - Fibrinoid necrosis
  - Deposition of amyloid

II. Immunofluorescence Features

A. Linear staining of GBM
  - Anti-GBM antibodies
  - Multiple plasma proteins (e.g., in diabetic glomerulosclerosis)
  - Monoclonal light chains

B. Granular immune complex staining
  - Mesangium (e.g., IgA nephropathy)
  - Capillary wall (e.g., membranous glomerulopathy)
  - Mesangium and capillary wall (e.g., lupus glomerulonephritis)

C. Irregular (fluffy) staining
  - Monoclonal light chains (AL amyloidosis)
  - AA protein (AA amyloidosis)

III. Electron Microscopic Features

A. Electron-dense immune complex deposits
  - Mesangial (e.g., IgA nephropathy)
  - Subendothelial (e.g., lupus glomerulonephritis)
  - Subepithelial (e.g., membranous glomerulopathy)

B. GBM thickening (e.g., diabetic glomerulosclerosis)

C. GBM replication (e.g., membranoproliferative glomerulonephritis)

D. Collagenous matrix expansion (e.g., focal segmental glomerulosclerosis)

E. Fibrillary deposits (e.g., amyloidosis)

not specific for a particular cause of glomerular inflammation. It is rather a marker for severe injury that has resulted in extensive rupture of capillary walls, which allows inflammatory mediators to enter Bowman space and stimulate macrophage infiltration and epithelial proliferation.

Minimal Change Glomerulopathy

Minimal change glomerulopathy is characterized clinically by the nephrotic syndrome and pathologically by the fusion of visceral epithelial foot processes.

☐ **Pathogenesis:** The pathogenesis of minimal change glomerulopathy is unknown. Involvement of the immune system has been postulated (1) because this disease occurs occasionally in association with an allergic history, (2) because the onset of the disease sometimes follows infection or exposure to allergens, and (3) because the disease enters remission when treated with corticosteroids. The occasional association with Hodgkin disease (a condition associated with T-cell dysfunction) and with T-cell lymphomas has led to the speculation that minimal change nephrotic syndrome may be caused by a disorder of T lymphocytes, possibly production by T cells of a cytokine that increases glomerular permeability.

An experimental disease that mimics minimal change nephrotic syndrome both morphologically and functionally is produced by the administration of the aminonucleoside puromycin to rats. In this model, heavy proteinuria has been related to a loss of polyanionic sites on the GBM, an effect also noted in human minimal change glomerulopathy. The loss of these sites allows anionic proteins, particularly albumin, to pass easily through the normal barrier. In the experimental disease, the loss of basement membrane polyanionic sites is believed to reflect toxic injury to the epithelial cells by the aminonucleoside.

☐ **Pathology:** By definition, the light microscopic appearance of glomeruli in minimal change glomerulopathy is essentially normal (Fig. 16-14). The presence of "normal" or "minimally changed" glomeruli in the majority of children with the nephrotic syndrome puzzled early investigators, and it was not until electron microscopic studies showed diffuse obliteration of the epithelial cell foot processes that speculation about a nonglomerular origin of proteinuria ended. The loss of protein in the urine leads to hypoalbuminemia, and a compensatory increase in lipoprotein secretion by the liver results in hyperlipidemia. The loss of lipoproteins through the glomeruli causes accumulation of lipid in the proximal tubular cells, which is reflected histologically as glassy (hyaline) droplets in tubular epithelial cytoplasm. This appearance, together with lipid droplets in the urine, is responsible for the older term *lipoid nephrosis*. Droplets in the tubular epithelial cells are not specific for minimal change glomerulopathy but are produced by any glomerular disease that causes the nephrotic syndrome.

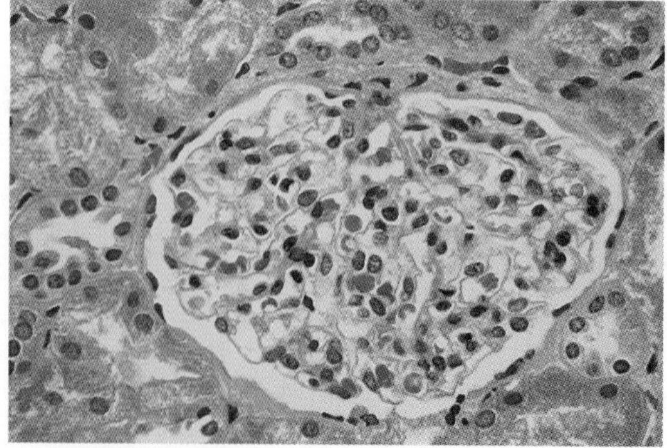

FIGURE *16-14*
Minimal change glomerulopathy. A light micrograph shows no abnormality.

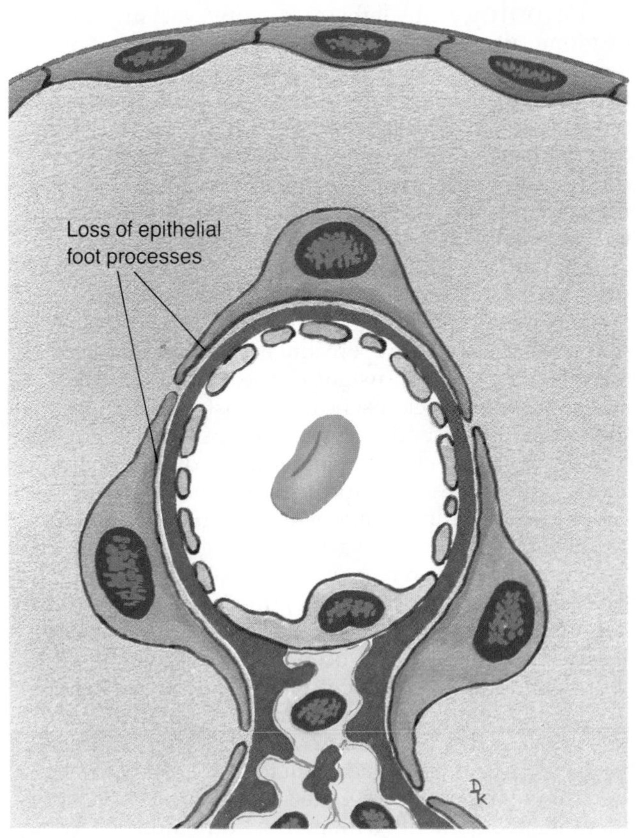

FIGURE *16-15*
Minimal change glomerulopathy. This condition is characterized predominantly by epithelial cell changes, particularly the effacement of the foot processes. All other glomerular structures appear intact.

Electron microscopic examination of the glomeruli reveals total **effacement of visceral epithelial cell foot processes,** an effect caused by their retraction into the parent epithelial cell bodies (Figs. 16-15 and 16-16). This retraction is presumably the result of extensive cell swelling and occurs in virtually all cases of proteinuria in the nephrotic range. It is, therefore, not specific for minimal change glomerulopathy. Numerous microvilli protrude from the surface of the epithelial cells. Immunofluorescence microscopy for immunoglobulins and complement are most often negative, but there is occasional weak mesangial staining for IgM and the complement component C3.

☐ Clinical Features: **Minimal change glomerulopathy causes 90% of the nephrotic syndrome in young children, 50% in older children, and 20% in adults**. Proteinuria is generally more selective (albumin > globulins) than in the nephrotic syndrome caused by other diseases, but there is too much overlap for this selectivity to be used as a diagnostic criterion. Over 90% of children and slightly fewer adults with minimal change glomerulopathy have complete remission of proteinuria within 8 weeks of the initiation of corticosteroid therapy. However, after withdrawal of corticosteroids, many patients suffer intermittent relapses for up to 10 years. A subgroup of a few patients show only partial remission with corticosteroid therapy and continue to lose protein in the urine, with the degree of proteinuria depending on the dose of corticosteroids. In an even smaller group that is totally resistant to corticosteroid therapy, the diagnosis of minimal change glomerulopathy may not be accurate, and focal segmental glomerulosclerosis may be present.

Death from infection was frequent before antibiotics and corticosteroids became readily available, but fatal outcome is now exceptional. The development of azotemia in a patient diagnosed as having minimal change nephrotic syndrome should always suggest an in-

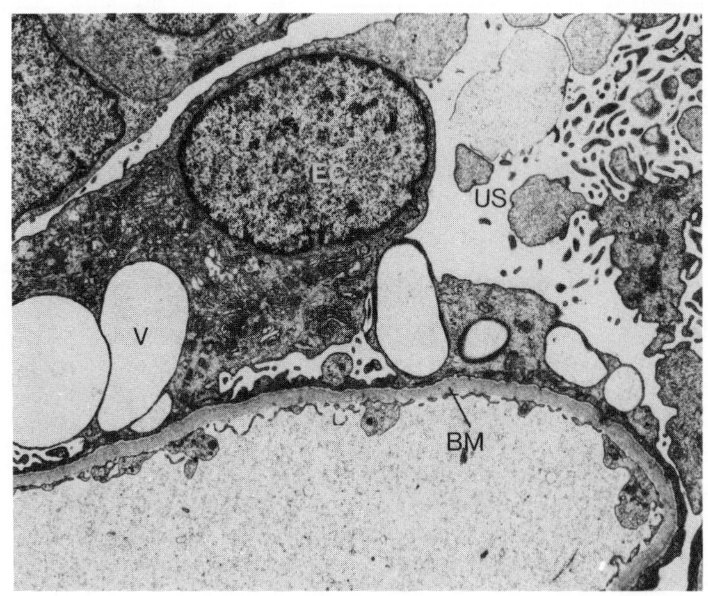

FIGURE *16-16*
Minimal change glomerulopathy. In this electron micrograph, the epithelial cells (EC) display effacement of foot processes, microvilli, and numerous vacuoles (V). (BM, basement membrane; US, urinary space).

correct diagnosis, usually focal segmental glomerulosclerosis or perhaps a complication such as interstitial nephritis. In the absence of complications, the long-term outlook for patients with minimal change glomerulopathy is no different from that of the general population.

Focal Segmental Glomerulosclerosis

Focal segmented glomerulosclerosis is characterized by glomerular scarring (sclerosis) that affects some (focal), but not all, glomeruli and initially involves only part of an affected glomerular tuft (segmental).

☐ **Pathogenesis:** The term focal segmental glomerulosclerosis has been applied to a heterogeneous group of glomerular diseases that most likely have several different causes, as suggested by varied histological patterns and different associated conditions. The disease occurs as an idiopathic (primary) process or secondary to a number of conditions (Table 16-4).

Congenital and acquired reductions in renal mass, which place adaptive stress on the reduced number of nephrons, appear to cause focal segmental glomerulosclerosis as a consequence of increased glomerular capillary pressure and filtration. A normal amount of renal tissue can also be stressed by too much body mass (obesity), resulting in focal segmental glomerulosclerosis. Reduced oxygen in the blood, for example as caused by sickle cell disease or cyanotic congenital heart disease, also causes a similar pattern of glomerular injury. In all of these settings, glomerular enlargement suggests a response to overwork.

Infection with human immunodeficiency virus (HIV), especially in blacks, is associated with a variant of focal segmental glomerulosclerosis that is characterized by a collapsing pattern of sclerosis. The causal relationship between the HIV infection and the glomerular disease is unclear. A similar pattern of glomerular injury also occurs in intravenous drug abusers.

In most patients with focal segmental glomerulosclerosis, however, none of these recognized causes are identified. Recently, a serum permeability factor has been detected in patients with focal segmental glomerulosclerosis, which suggests a systemic cause for the glomerular injury. This is further supported by the recurrence of focal segmental glomerulosclerosis in renal transplants.

TABLE *16-4* Causes of Focal Segmental Glomerulosclerosis

Primary (idiopathic)
Secondary
Obesity
Acquired renal mass reduction
Congenital unilateral renal agenesis or aplasia
Sickle cell disease
Cyanotic congenital heart disease
Human immunodeficiency virus infection
Intravenous drug abuse

☐ **Pathology:** By light microscopy, varying numbers of glomeruli show segmental obliteration of capillary loops by increased collagen and the accumulation of lipid and proteinaceous material (Fig. 16-17). The proteinaceous material, which is probably derived from insudation of plasma proteins, has a glassy appearance, and the condition is, therefore, called *hyalinosis*. In some patients, the sclerosis has a predilection for perihilar segments within glomeruli, and for glomeruli in the deep cortex (juxtamedullary glomeruli). Adhesions to Bowman capsule occur adjacent to the sclerotic lesions. Uninvolved glomeruli may appear entirely normal, although on occasion mild mesangial hypercellularity is present. Because uninvolved glomeruli usually appear normal, focal segmental glomerulosclerosis can be mistaken for minimal change glomerulopathy in small biopsy specimens that contain only nonsclerotic glomeruli. A differential diagnostic consideration is focal glomerular scarring secondary to a prior inflammatory glomerular disease.

Several histological variants of segmental glomerulosclerosis have been recognized. A collapsing pattern of sclerosis with hypertrophied epithelial cells adjacent to sclerotic segments is typical for HIV-associated nephropathy, and it also occurs with intravenous drug abuse and as an idiopathic process. This collapsing variant has a poor prognosis, with half of the patients reaching end-stage disease within 2 years. Sclerosis confined to the glomerular segment adjacent to the origin of the proximal tubule has been designated *tip lesion* and is most frequent in older patients with marked proteinuria.

By electron microscopy, focal segmental glomerulosclerosis exhibits diffuse effacement of epithelial cell foot processes, with occasional focal detachment of epithelial cells from the GBM. Increased matrix material, folding and thickening of the basement membranes, and capillary collapse are present in the sclerotic segments. Accumulation of electron-dense material within the sclerotic segments represents insudative trapping of plasma

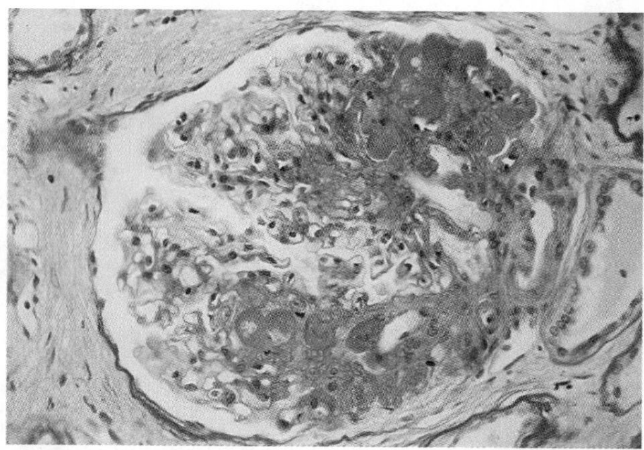

FIGURE *16-17*
Focal segmental glomerulosclerosis. A PAS stain shows perihilar areas of segmental sclerosis and adjacent adhesions to Bowman capsule.

proteins, which corresponds to the hyalinosis seen by light microscopy. Immune complexes are not visualized.

Immunofluorescence microscopy demonstrates trapping of IgM and C3 in the segmental areas of sclerosis and hyalinosis. IgG, C4, and C1q are less frequently found in sclerotic segments. Nonsclerotic segments have no staining or only trace mesangial staining, usually for IgM and C3.

□ **Clinical Features:** Focal segmental glomerulosclerosis is the cause of the nephrotic syndrome in 15% of children and adults. The disease is more common in blacks than in whites. The typical clinical presentation is an insidious onset of asymptomatic proteinuria, which frequently progresses to the nephrotic syndrome. Many patients are hypertensive, and microscopic hematuria is frequent. In a minority of patients, focal segmental glomerulosclerosis is diagnosed after prolonged proteinuria that has been variably sensitive to the administration of corticosteroids.

Most patients have persistent proteinuria and a progressive decline in renal function, leading to end-stage renal disease after 5 to 20 years. Corticosteroid therapy remains controversial. Renal transplantation is the preferred treatment for end-stage renal disease, but focal segmental glomerulosclerosis recurs in half of the transplanted kidneys.

HIV-Associated Nephropathy

Nephropathy associated with aquired immunodeficiency syndrome (AIDS) is a severe and rapidly progressive form of focal glomerular sclerosis.

□ **Pathogenesis:** The occurrence of nephropathy in patients with HIV infection has raised the possibility that it is caused by the virus within the renal parenchyma, although this concept remains to be proved. A different hypothesis proposes that the nephropathy is caused by another virus that has infected the kidney of an immunocompromised person.

□ **Pathology:** By light microscopy, HIV-associated nephropathy is characterized by focal sclerosis, which may be segmental or global (Fig. 16-18). Sclerotic segments display collapse of capillaries, frequently with adjacent swollen visceral epithelial cells, which contain numerous protein droplets. In addition to the glomerular injury, interstitial fibrosis and infiltration by mononuclear leukocytes are noted. Tubular epithelial atrophy and degeneration are conspicuous, and cystically dilated tubules contain proteinaceous casts. By electron microscopy, numerous tubuloreticular inclusions are seen in endothelial cells, similar to those in lupus nephritis.

□ **Clinical Features:** Some 10% of HIV patients develop nephropathy, of whom over 90% are black. The disease presents with marked proteinuria (over 10 g/day) and renal insufficiency. Patients typically progress to end-stage renal disease in less than a year.

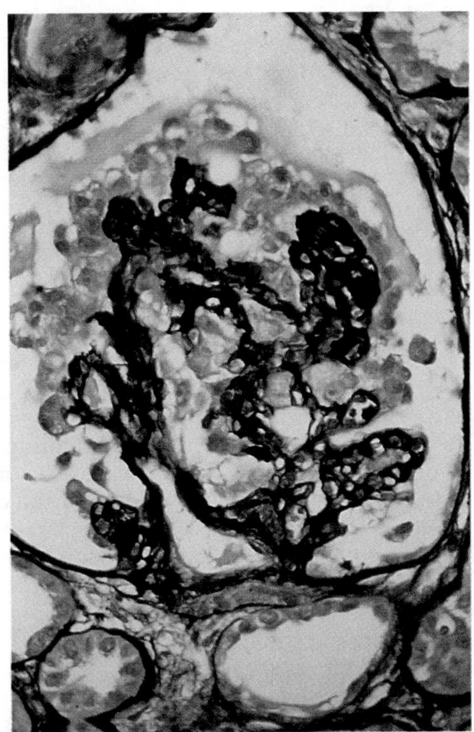

FIGURE *16-18*
HIV-associated nephropathy. A silver stain shows advanced collapse of glomerular capillaries, with an increase in matrix material (sclerosis) and hypertrophy of visceral epithelial cells.

Membranous Glomerulopathy

Membranous glomerulopathy is a frequent cause of the nephrotic syndrome in adults and is caused by the accumulation of immune complexes in the subepithelial zone of glomerular capillaries.

□ **Pathogenesis:** Membranous glomerulopathy displays localization of immune complexes in the **sub-epithelial zone** (between the visceral epithelial cell and the GBM) as a result of immune complex formation *in situ* or the deposition of circulating immune complexes. Formation *in situ* is the favored hypothesis because of the resemblance between membranous glomerulopathy and the experimental animal disease called *Heymann nephritis.* In the latter, mice are immunized with a renal epithelial antigen and develop autoantibodies. The antibodies cross GBMs and bind to antigens on visceral epithelial cells. The resultant immune complexes are shed into the adjacent subepithelial zone and produce membranous glomerulopathy. An analogous pathogenesis has been postulated for human idiopathic membranous glomerulopathy, even though no comparable autoantibody has been identified in patients.

Membranous glomerulopathy is also induced in animals by chronic injection of foreign proteins. This procedure results in the formation of circulating immune complexes, and, in some circumstances, free antigens and antibodies that can form immune complex *in situ*. The result is a chronic serum sickness model which may be analogous to certain forms of secondary membranous glomerulopathy. The following are general causes of membranous glomerulopathy, and specific examples:

- Idiopathic (primary) membranous glomerulopathy
- Secondary membranous glomerulopathy
  - Autoimmune disease (systemic lupus erythematosus)
  - Infectious disease (hepatitis B)
  - Therapeutic agents (penicillamine)
  - Neoplasms (lung cancer)

□ **Pathology:** By light microscopy, the glomeruli are slightly enlarged, yet normocellular. Depending on the duration of the disease, the capillary walls are normal or thickened (Fig. 16-19). In the early stages of the disease, silver stains (which demonstrate basement membrane material) reveal multiple projections or "spikes" of argyrophilic material on the epithelial surface of the basement membrane (Fig. 16-20). Such spikes represent projections of basement membrane material that is deposited around the subepithelial immune complexes, which do not stain with silver. As the disease progresses, the capillary lumens are encroached on and glomerular obsolescence eventually ensues. In advanced states of glomerular sclerosis, the lesions of membranous glomerulopathy cannot be distinguished from other forms of chronic glomerular disease. Atrophy of tubules and interstitial fibrosis parallel the degree of glomerular sclerosis.

By electron microscopy, immune complexes in the capillary walls appear as electron-dense deposits (Figs. 16-21 and 16-22). The progressive ultrastructural alterations that are induced by the subepithelial immune complexes are divided into stages:

- **Stage I:** Subepithelial dense deposits without adjacent projections of GBM material
- **Stage II:** Projections of GBM material around the subepithelial dense deposits (see Fig. 16-22)

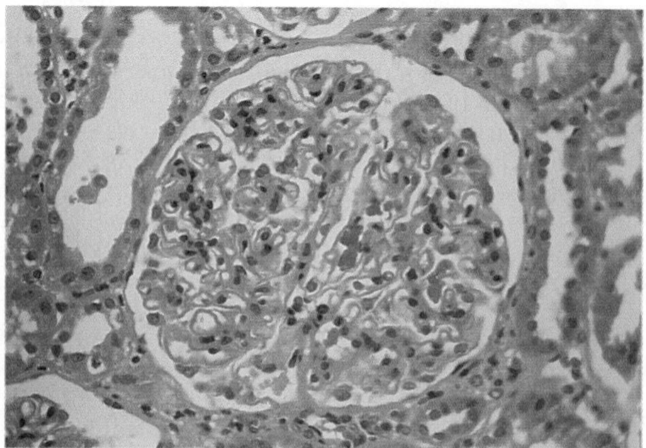

FIGURE *16-19*
Membranous glomerulopathy. The glomerulus is slightly enlarged and shows diffuse thickening of the capillary walls. There is no hypercellularity.

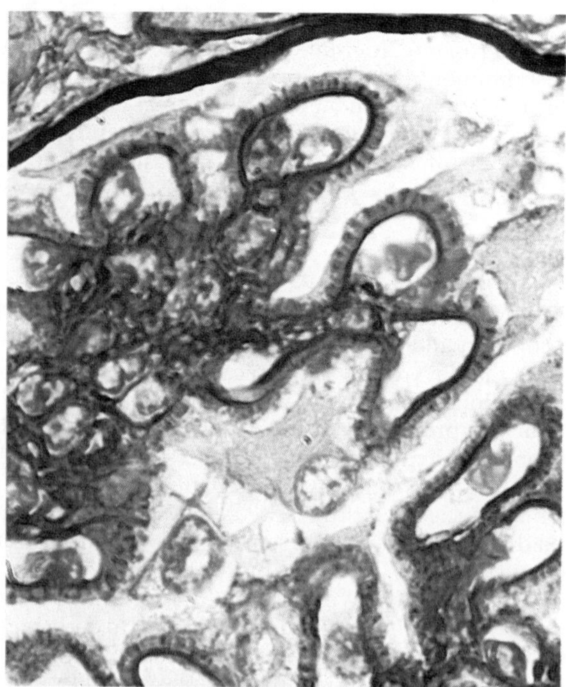

FIGURE *16-20*
Membranous glomerulopathy. A silver stain reveals multiple "spikes" diffusely distributed in the glomerular capillary basement membranes. This pattern corresponds to the stage II lesion illustrated in Figure 16-22. The appearance is produced by the deposition of silver-positive basement membrane material around silver-negative immune complex deposits.

- **Stage III:** Enclosure of the dense deposits within GBM material
- **Stage IV:** Rarefaction of the deposits within a thickened GBM

Mesangial electron-dense deposits are rare in idiopathic membranous glomerulopathy but are frequent in secondary membranous glomerulopathy (e.g., as seen in lupus erythematosus). This may reflect the fact that idiopathic disease is caused by antigens present only in the subepithelial zone (as in Heymann nephritis), whereas the secondary type is produced by circulating antigens.

Immunofluorescence microscopy reveals diffuse granular staining of capillary walls for IgG and C3 (Fig. 16-23). There is intense staining for terminal complement components, including the membrane attack complex, which are important in the induction of glomerular injury.

□ **Clinical Features:** Membranous glomerulopathy is the most frequent cause (40%) of the nephrotic syndrome in adults. The course of membranous glomerulopathy is highly variable, with a range of possible outcomes. When followed for 20 years, 25% of patients have spontaneous remission, 50% have persistent proteinuria and stable or only partial loss of renal function, and 25% develop end-stage renal failure. The treatment of idiopathic membranous glomerulopathy is controversial.

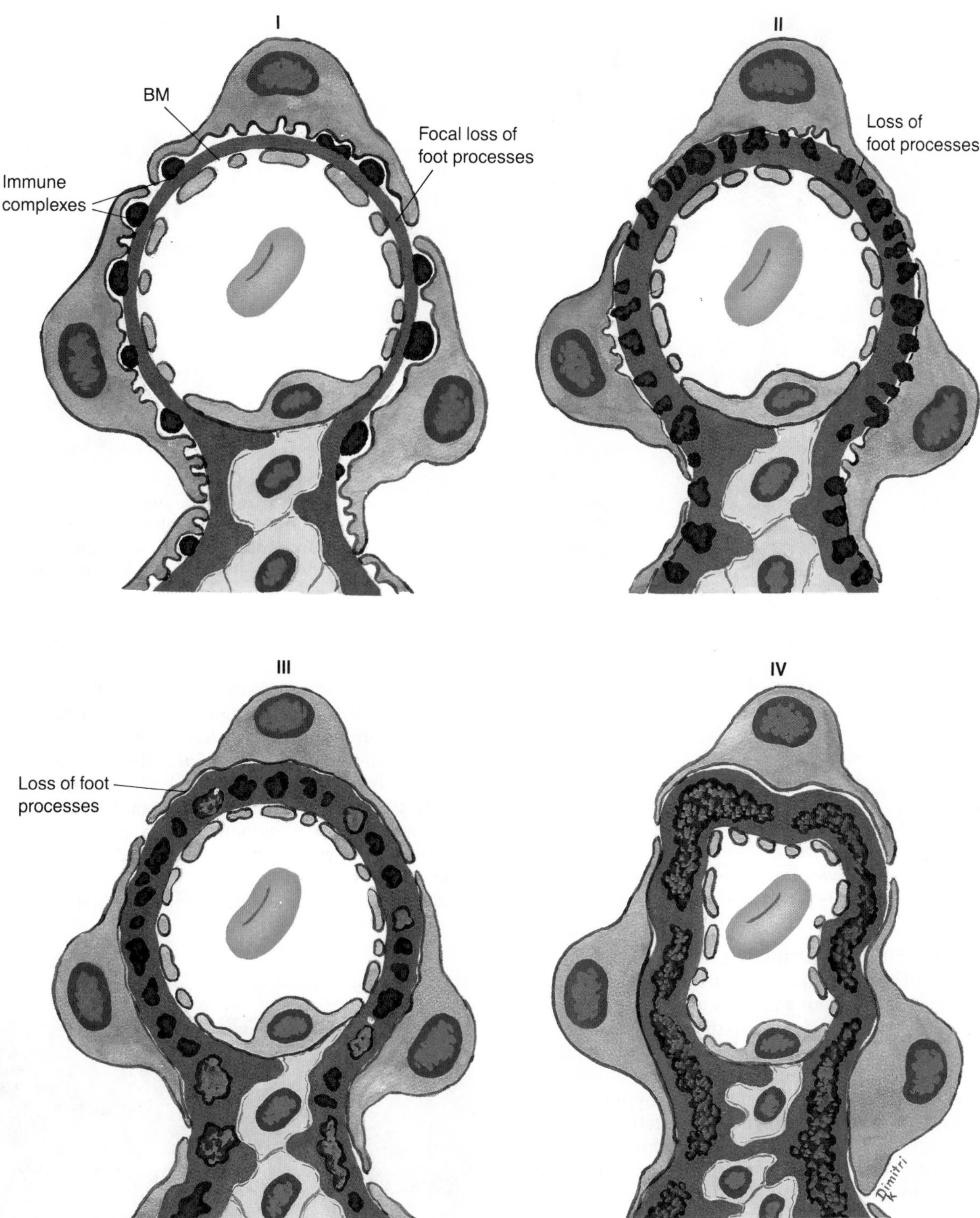

FIGURE *16-21*
Membranous glomerulopathy. This disease is caused by the subepithelial accumulation of immune complexes and the accompanying changes in the basement membrane. Stage I exhibits scattered subepithelial deposits. The outer contour of the basement membrane remains smooth. Stage II disease has projections (spikes) of basement membrane material adjacent to the deposits. In stage III disease, newly formed basement membrane has surrounded the deposits. With stage IV disease, the immune complex deposits lose their electron density, resulting in an irregularly thickened basement membrane with irregular electron-lucent areas.

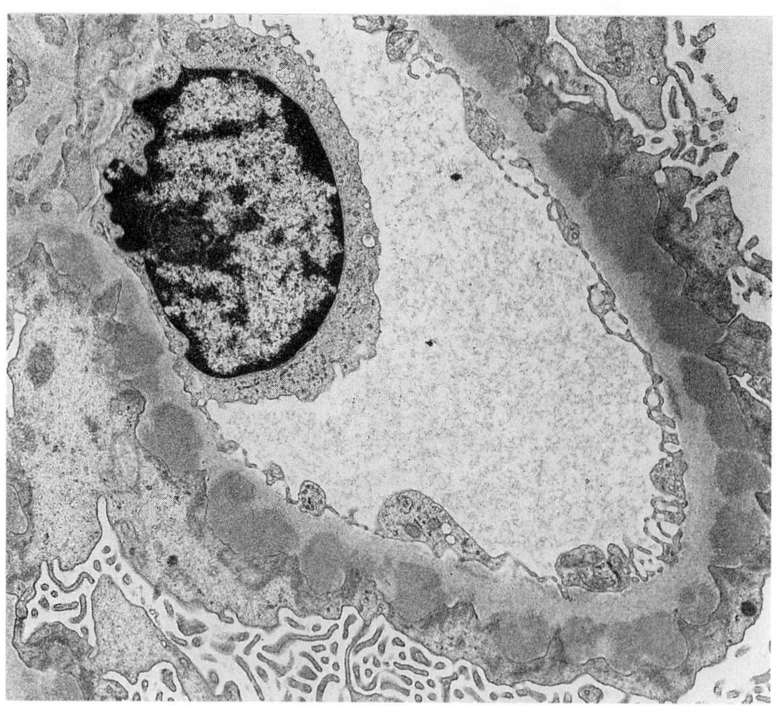

FIGURE 16-22
Stage II membranous glomerulopathy. An electron micrograph shows deposits of electron-dense material, with intervening delicate projections of basement membrane material.

Patients who develop progressive renal failure are treated with corticosteroids or other immunosuppressive drugs. The prognosis is better in children because of a higher rate of permanent remission.

Diabetic Glomerulosclerosis

Glomerular sclerosis caused by diabetes mellitus results in proteinuria and progressive renal failure.

☐ **Pathogenesis:** Diabetic glomerulosclerosis is a component of the vascular sclerosis that involves many small vessels throughout the body in patients with diabetes mellitus (see Chapter 22). In diabetes, there is a generalized increase in the synthesis of basement membrane material by the microvasculature, which in some way reflects the abnormal metabolic state. One hypothesis proposes that abnormal **nonenzymatic glycation** of matrix proteins, including those of the GBM and mesangial matrix, induces binding of plasma proteins, such as immunoglobulins, and thereby stimulates excessive matrix production. Less than 50% of patients with diabetes develop glomerulosclerosis, suggesting the possibility that, in addition to the diabetic state, synergistic factors are present in some but not all patients.

☐ **Pathology:** The earliest lesions of diabetic glomerulosclerosis are GBM thickening and expansion of the mesangial matrix (Fig. 16-24). Mild mesangial hypercellularity may also be present. In patients who develop symptomatic disease, GBM thickening and especially the expansion of the mesangial matrix result in changes that can be seen by light microscopy. Overt diabetic glomerulosclerosis is characterized by diffuse global thickening of GBMs and diffuse mesangial matrix expansion, with focal, segmental, nodular, sclerotic lesions called *Kimmelstiel-Wilson nodules* (Fig. 16-25). These nodules have an acellular core, with mesangial cells and capillaries pushed to the periphery. Insudation of proteins forms rounded nodules between Bowman capsule and the parietal epithelium ("capsular drops") or subendothelial accumulations along the capillary loops ("fibrin caps"). Sclerosing and insudative changes also occur in both the afferent and

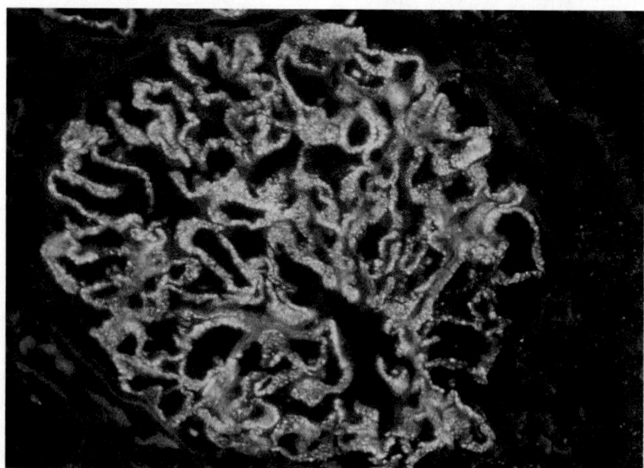

FIGURE 16-23
Membranous glomerulopathy. Immunofluorescence microscopy shows granular deposits of IgG outlining the glomerular capillary loops.

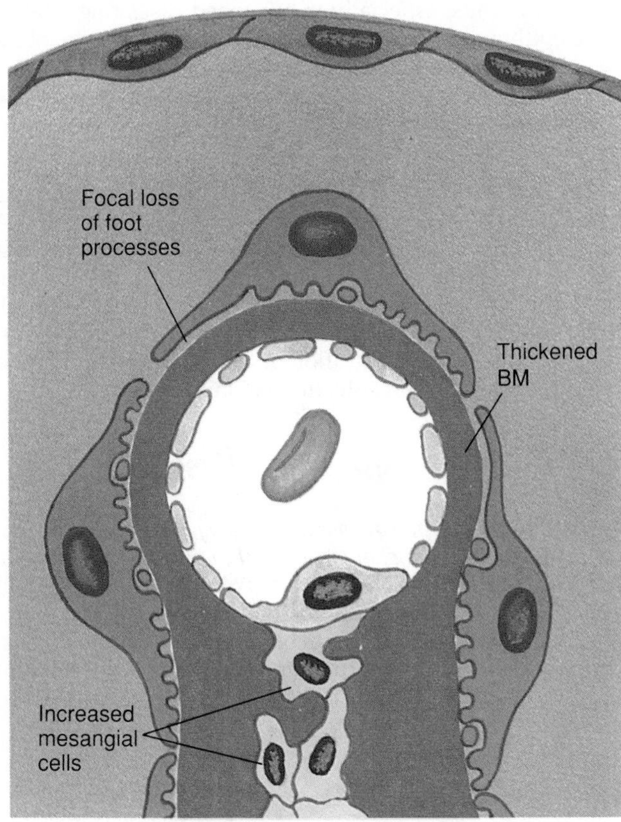

FIGURE *16-24*
Diabetic glomerulosclerosis. The lamina densa of the glomerular basement membrane is thickened, and there is an increase in mesangial matrix material.

efferent arterioles, resulting in hyaline arteriolosclerosis. Tubular basement membranes are also thickened.

Electron microscopy reveals widening of the basement membrane lamina densa, which may be thickened 5- to 10-fold, as well as an increase in mesangial matrix, particularly in the nodular lesions (Fig. 16-26). The insudative lesions appear as electron-dense masses, which contain lipid debris.

Immunofluorescence microscopy demonstrates diffuse linear trapping of IgG, albumin, fibrinogen, and other plasma proteins in the GBM. This is thought to result from the nonimmunological adsorption of these proteins to the thickened GBM, possibly as a result of nonenzymatic glycation of GBM proteins.

☐ Clinical Features: **Diabetic glomerulosclerosis is the leading cause of end-stage renal disease in the United States, accounting for a third of all patients with chronic renal failure.** It occurs in both type I and type II diabetes mellitus. The earliest manifestation is microalbuminuria (slightly increased proteinuria below the usual detection range). Overt proteinuria occurs between 10 and 15 years after the onset of diabetes and often becomes severe enough to cause the nephrotic syndrome. In time, diabetic glomerulosclerosis always progresses to renal failure. Strict glucose control reduces the likelihood of developing diabetic glomerulosclerosis but does not prevent progression once it develops. Control of hypertension and dietary protein restriction retard progression of the disease.

Renal Amyloidosis

Renal disease is a frequent complication of the amyloidosis associated with a variety of disorders.

☐ Pathogenesis: Amyloid may be formed from a number of different polypeptides (see Chapter 23). In each case, however, the amyloid has the same characteristic histological and ultrastructural appearance, and immunohistochemical tests are required to differentiate between the different forms. The two varieties of amyloid that affect the kidneys are termed *AL* and *AA*. **AA amyloid** is derived from a serum protein termed *SAA*, which increases markedly during inflammatory processes. The deposition of AA amyloid is often associated with chronic inflammatory disorders (e.g., rheumatoid arthritis and chronic tuberculosis). AA amyloid deposition also occurs in familial Mediterranean fever. **AL amyloid** is derived from lambda or, less often, kappa immunoglobulin light chains. It is frequently associated with, or is the harbinger of, multiple myeloma or other plasma cell dyscrasias. Renal diseases caused by the deposition of

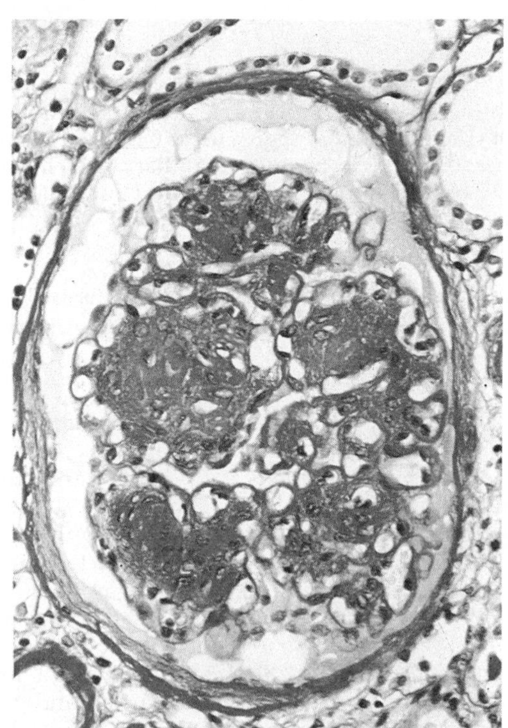

FIGURE *16-25*
Diabetic glomerulosclerosis. The PAS stain reveals a prominent increase in the mesangial matrix, forming several nodular lesions. Dilatation of glomerular capillaries is evident, and some capillary basement membranes are thickened.

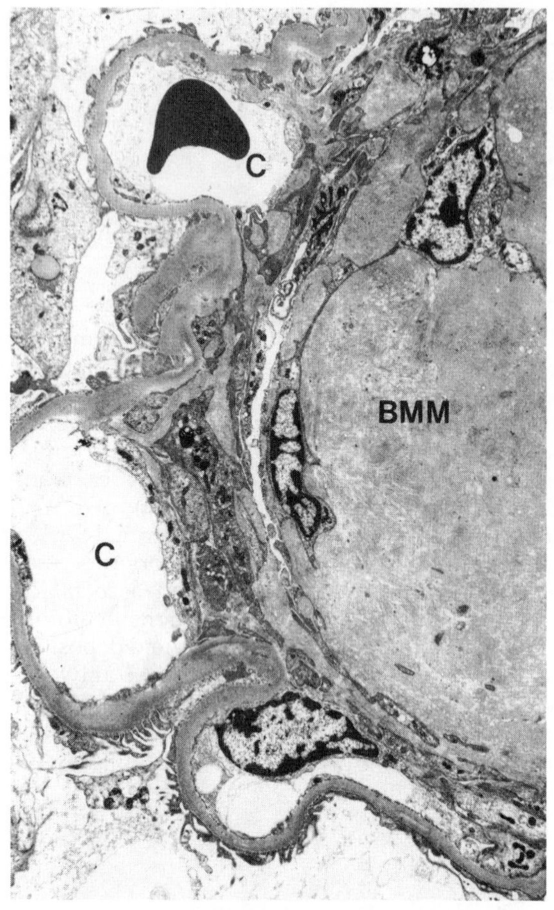

FIGURE *16-26*
Advanced diabetic glomerulosclerosis. An electron micrograph shows a nodular aggregate of basement membrane material (BMM). The peripheral capillary (C) demonstrates diffuse basement membrane widening but a normal texture.

monoclonal immunoglobulin light chains include AL amyloidosis, light-chain deposition disease, and light-chain cast nephropathy.

□ **Pathology:** Histologically, amyloid is an eosinophilic, amorphous material that has a characteristic apple-green color in sections stained with Congo red and examined by polarized light microscopy. Ultrastructurally, it is composed of nonbranching fibrils, approximately 10 nm in diameter. X-ray diffraction analysis shows primarily a β-pleated sheet configuration.

Renal amyloid deposition initially tends to be mesangial, but it progressively spreads to obliterate capillary lumens (Figs. 16-27 and 16-28). With increasing amyloid deposition, the glomeruli become enlarged and contain nodular deposits of eosinophilic material, which stain with Congo red (Fig. 16-29). In advanced amyloidosis, the glomerular structure is completely obliterated, and the glomeruli appear as large eosinophilic spheres.

By electron microscopy, amyloid fibrils are most prominent in the mesangium, but they often extend into capillary walls, especially in advanced cases (Fig. 16-30). The epithelial foot processes overlying the GBM are obliterated, and the epithelial cells may be tented by the amyloid fibrils, which are often oriented perpendicularly to the basement membrane.

□ **Clinical Features:** Renal involvement is a prominent feature in most cases of systemic AL and AA amyloidoses. Proteinuria is commonly the initial manifestation. The proteinuria is nonselective (i.e., both albumin and globulins appear in the urine), and it is severe enough to produce the nephrotic syndrome in 60% of patients. Eventually, severe infiltration of the glomeruli and blood vessels by amyloid results in renal failure.

Light-Chain Deposition Disease

Light-chain deposition disease is caused by the deposition of immunoglobulin light chains, usually kappa light chains, in GBMs, glomerular mesangial matrix, and tubular basement membranes. The deposition of this protein stimulates increased matrix production in basement membranes, causing thickening of glomerular and tubular basement mem-

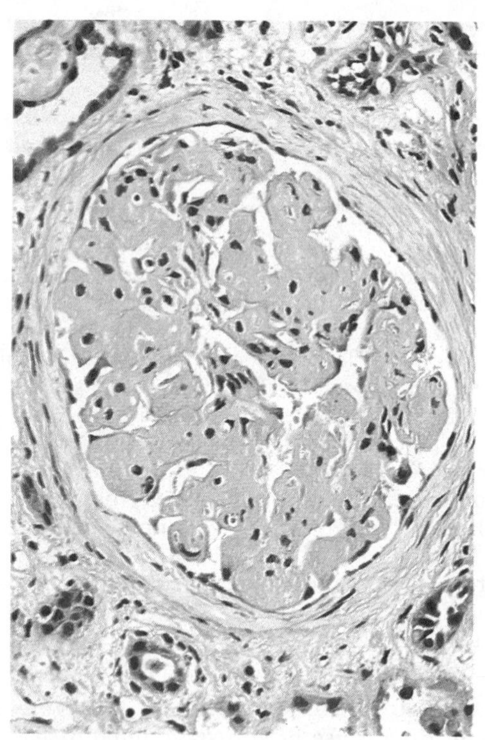

FIGURE *16-27*
Amyloid nephropathy. The mesangial areas are expanded and the glomerular capillaries are obstructed by amorphous acellular material. The deposits of amyloid may take on a nodular appearance, somewhat resembling those of diabetic glomerulosclerosis (see Fig. 16-25). However, amyloid deposits are not PAS-positive and are identifiable by Congo red staining.

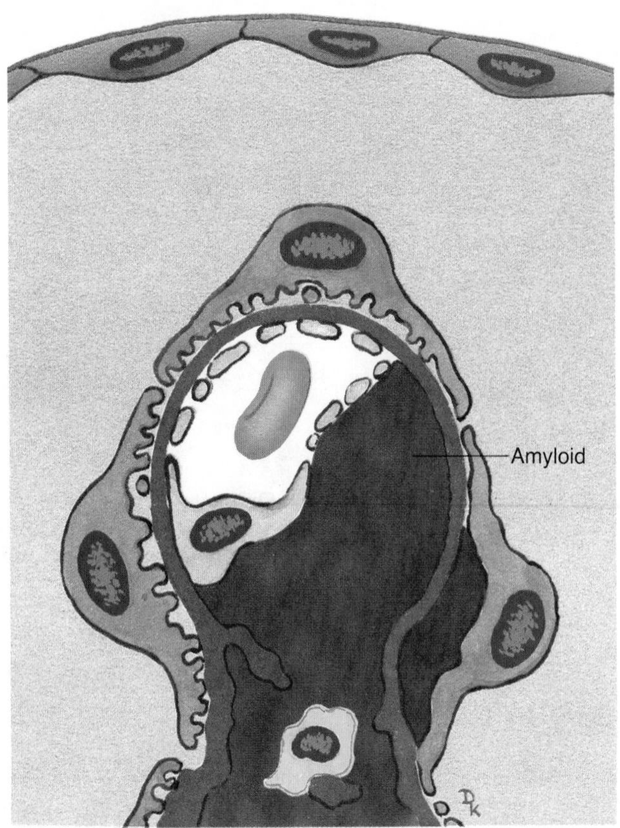

FIGURE 16-28
Amyloid nephropathy. This disorder is initially associated with the accumulation of characteristic fibrillar deposits in the mesangium. These inert masses, which are fibrillar by electron microscopy, extend along the inner surface of the basement membrane, frequently obstructing the capillary lumen. Focal extension of amyloid through the basement membrane may elevate the epithelial cell, in which case irregular spikes along the outer surface of the basement membrane are seen.

branes. Nodular expansion of mesangial regions resembles diabetic glomerulosclerosis. Importantly, the increased extracellular material does not stain with Congo red. Electron microscopy reveals a uniform, finely granular, electron-dense material along the glomerular and tubular basement membranes and within the mesangial matrix. Amyloid fibrils are not present. Immunofluorescence microscopy demonstrates linear staining for monoclonal light chains along the involved basement membranes. Light-chain deposition disease manifests clinically as nephrotic syndrome and renal failure.

Hereditary Nephritis (Alport Syndrome)

Alport syndrome is a proliferative and sclerosing glomerular disease, often accompanied by defects of the ears or occasionally the eyes, which is caused by a genetic abnormality in type IV collagen.

□ **Pathogenesis:** A variety of genetic abnormalities can lead to molecular defects in the GBM that produce the renal lesions of hereditary nephritis. The most common defect is X-linked and is caused by a mutation (e.g., point mutation, deletion, splicing error) in the COL4A5 gene, which codes for type IV collagen. A deletion at the 5′ end of COL4A5 that extends into the COL4A6 gene, which codes for the $\alpha6$ chain of collagen, also causes Alport syndrome and leiomyomas.

Because of disturbed basement membrane structure, many hereditary nephritis patients have defective expression of the target antigen in anti-GBM antibody disease (e.g., Goodpasture syndrome). Thus, serum from patients with anti-GBM disease fails to react with GBMs from patients with Alport syndrome. Conversely, patients with Alport syndrome who are subjected to renal transplantation are at risk for developing antibodies that react with kidney allograft GBMs.

□ **Pathology:** Early glomerular lesions of Alport syndrome show mild mesangial hypercellularity and matrix expansion. Progression of renal disease is associated with increasing focal and eventually diffuse glomerular sclerosis. Advanced glomerular lesions are accompanied by tubular atrophy, interstitial fibrosis, and the presence of foam cells in the tubules and interstitium. The most diagnostic morphological lesion is apparent only by electron microscopy: an irregularly thickened GBM exhibits splitting of the lamina densa into interlacing lamellae that surround electron-lucent areas (Fig. 16-31).

□ **Clinical Features:** Hereditary nephritis affects both sexes but is typically more severe in males. Hematuria is present early in life, even at birth. Proteinuria, progressive renal failure, and hypertension develop later in

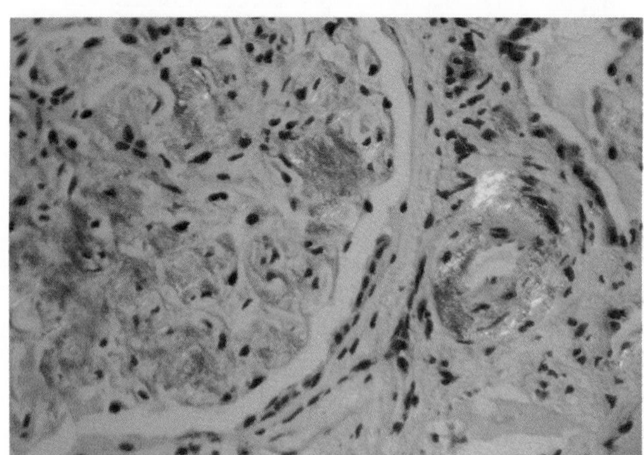

FIGURE 16-29
Amyloid nephropathy. In a section stained with Congo red and examined under polarized light, the amyloid deposits in the glomerulus and the adjacent arteriole show a characteristic apple-green birefringence.

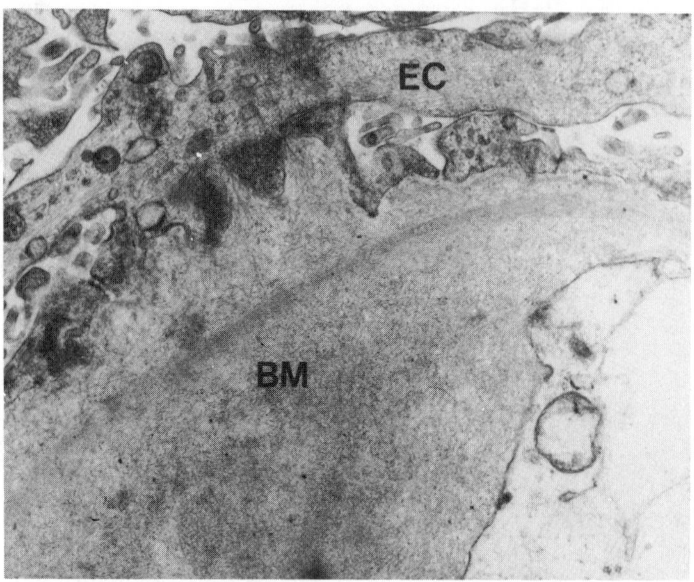

FIGURE 16-30
Amyloid nephropathy. Deposits of fibrils (10 nm diameter) accumulate in the mesangium and capillary walls of glomeruli. (BM, basement membrane; EC, epithelial cells).

the course of the disease. Virtually all men and about one fifth of women will develop end-stage renal disease by ages 40 to 50. Up to one half of the patients exhibit a progressive hearing impairment, initially manifested as high-frequency deafness. A smaller proportion of patients suffer ocular defects, most often involving the lens.

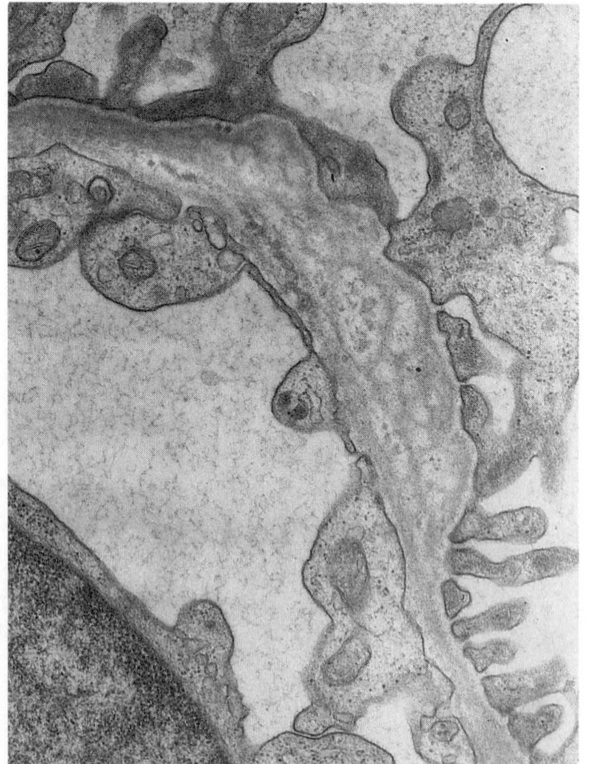

FIGURE 16-31
Hereditary nephritis (Berger disease). The lamina densa of the GBM is laminated rather than forming a single dense band (compare this electron micrograph with Fig. 16-5).

Thin Glomerular Basement Membrane Nephropathy

Thin basement membrane nephropathy, also termed benign familial hematuria, is a common, autosomal dominant, hereditary disorder of GBMs, which typically presents as asymptomatic microscopic hematuria and occasionally with intermittent gross hematuria. In fact, this disease and IgA nephropathy are the two major diagnostic considerations in patients with asymptomatic glomerular hematuria. Patients with thin basement membrane nephropathy do not develop renal failure and do not suffer substantial proteinuria. By light microscopy, the glomeruli are unremarkable. Electron microscopy reveals a reduced thickness of the GBM (200 to 300 nm, compared to the normal 350 to 450 nm).

Acute Postinfectious Glomerulonephritis

Acute postinfectious glomerulonephritis usually occurs after an infection with group A (β-hemolytic) streptococci and reflects the deposition of immune complexes in the GBM.

☐ **Pathogenesis:** Acute postinfectious glomerulonephritis is most often caused by certain ***nephritogenic*** **strains of group A (β-hemolytic) streptococci**. Occasional cases are related to staphylococcal infection (e.g., acute staphylococcal endocarditis), and rare cases result from viral (e.g., hepatitis B) or parasitic (e.g., malaria) infections. The exact mechanism by which infection causes the characteristic inflammatory changes in the glomeruli is not completely understood, although similarities to the experimental model of acute serum sickness suggest that the disease is caused by glomerular localization of immune complexes generated by an antibody response to circulating antigens. Both poststreptococcal glomerulonephritis in patients and acute serum sickness caused by injecting foreign proteins into animals have a latent period of 9 to 14 days between the time of exposure to a new antigen and the occurrence of glomerulonephritis. The granular immunofluorescence pattern of immune complex staining and the ultrastructural appearance of dense deposits are similar in the human and experimental diseases. However, streptococcal antigen has been difficult to demonstrate in the glomeruli of patients with this disease, possibly because the antigen is quickly removed from the inflamed glomeruli or is "masked" by immunoglobulin and complement. However, circulating immune complexes are demonstrable in half of the patients with acute poststreptococcal glomerulonephritis. There is also evidence for glomerular immune complex formation *in situ* between bacterial antigens trapped in the glomeruli and circulating antibodies.

Immune complexes within glomeruli initiate inflammation by activating complement, as well as other humoral and cellular inflammatory mediator systems. Complement activation is so extensive that over 90% of patients develop hypocomplementemia because of consumption within the glomeruli. The inflammatory mediators attract and activate neutrophils and monocytes, and they stimulate the proliferation of mesangial and endothelial cells. These effects result in marked glomerular hypercellularity, which defines acute diffuse proliferative glomerulonephritis. Importantly, the hypercellularity in proliferative glomerulonephritis is caused not only by proliferation of glomerular cells, but also by the influx of leukocytes. Rarely, the inflammatory injury is so severe that it disrupts capillaries and stimulates epithelial cell proliferation (crescent formation).

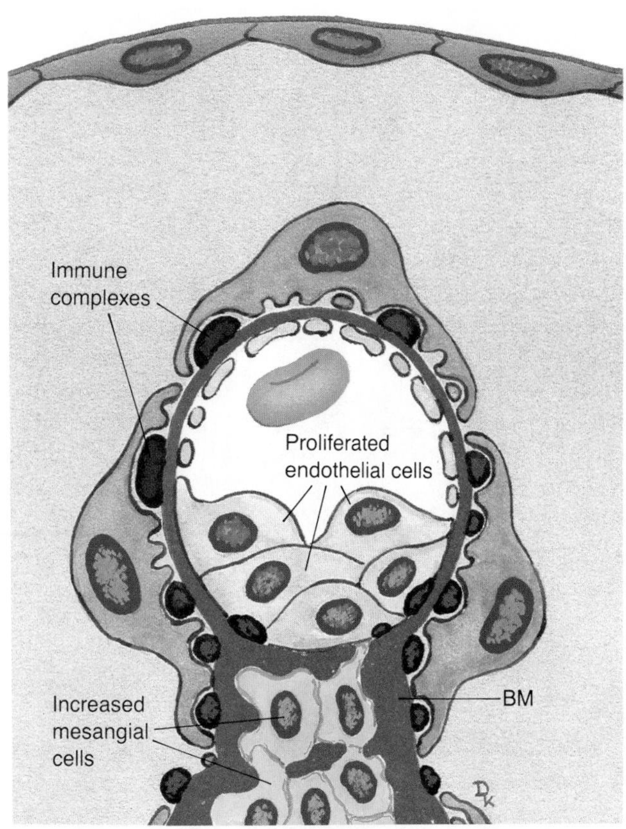

FIGURE *16-33*
Postinfectious glomerulonephritis. Trapping of immune complexes in a subepithelial pattern ("lumpy-bumpy") is seen, together with focal effacement of foot processes. Less prominent subendothelial immune complexes are associated with endothelial cell proliferation and are related to increased capillary permeability and narrowing of the lumen. Frequently, proliferation of mesangial cells and a thickened mesangial basement membrane (BM) result in widening of the stalk and conspicuous trapping of immune complexes.

☐ **Pathology:** The acute phase of postinfectious glomerulonephritis is characterized by diffuse enlargement and hypercellularity of the glomeruli (Fig. 16-32). Hypercellularity reflects the proliferation of both endothelial and mesangial cells (Fig. 16-33) and the infiltration of neutrophils and monocytes. Crescents are uncommon. Interstitial edema and mild infiltration of mononuclear leukocytes occur in parallel with the glomerular changes.

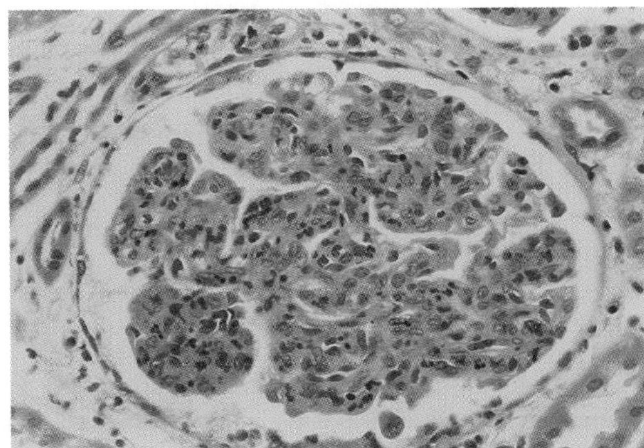

FIGURE *16-32*
Acute poststreptococcal glomerulonephritis. The glomerulus of a patient who developed glomerulonephritis after a streptococcal infection is hypercellular because of the proliferation of endothelial and mesangial cells and infiltration by neutrophils.

The acute phase begins 1 or 2 weeks after the onset of the nephritogenic infection and resolves in over 90% of patients after several weeks. Neutrophils and endothelial hypercellularity disappear first, leaving only mesangial hypercellularity and matrix expansion. After several months, most patients experience resolution of all histological abnormalities.

The most distinctive ultrastructural features of acute postinfectious glomerulonephritis are **subepithelial dense deposits that are shaped like "humps"** (Figs. 16-33 and 16-34). These deposits are invariably accompanied by mesangial and subendothelial deposits, which may be more difficult to find but are probably more important in pathogenesis because of their proximity to the inflammatory mediator systems in the blood. The variably sized, dome-shaped humps are situated on the epithelial side of the basement membrane. They are not as diffusely distributed as are the deposits of membranous glomerulopathy (compare Figs. 16-21 and 16-33).

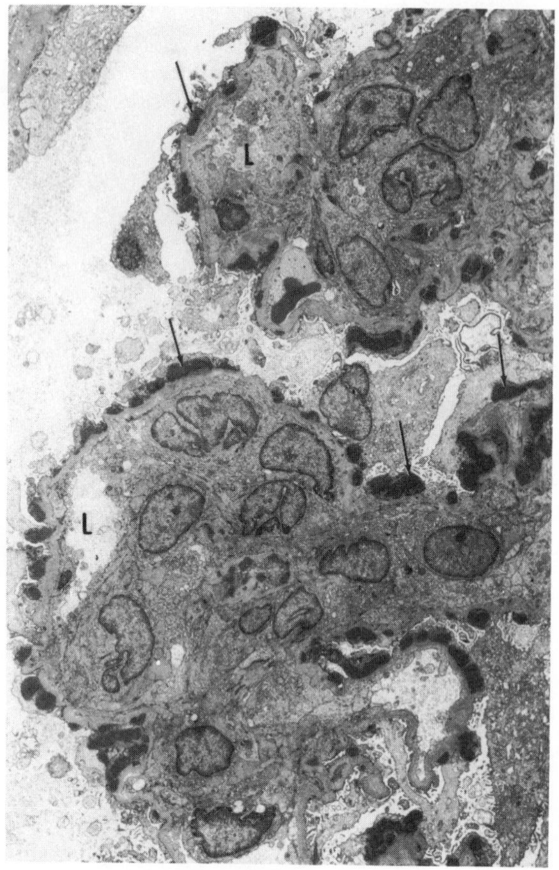

FIGURE 16-34
Acute postinfectious glomerulonephritis. An electron micrograph demonstrates numerous subepithelial humps (*arrows*). The capillary lumina (L) are markedly narrowed.

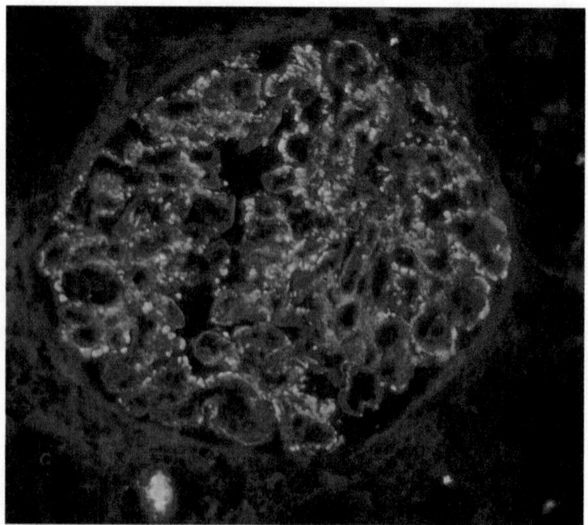

FIGURE 16-35
Acute postinfectious glomerulonephritis. An immunofluorescence micrograph demonstrates granular staining for C3 in capillary walls and the mesangium.

In the first few weeks of disease, immunofluorescence microscopy typically reveals granular deposits corresponding to IgG and C3 along the basement membrane, in locations corresponding to the humps. Later in the disease, C3 is present without IgG, because immune complexes containing IgG no longer accumulate in the glomeruli after the infection clears (Fig. 16-35).

☐ **Clinical Features:** Acute poststreptococcal glomerulonephritis most commonly affects children. In developed countries, it is not seen as frequently as in the past, but it remains one of the most common renal diseases in childhood. The primary infection involves the pharynx or, in hot and humid environments, the skin. Because the organisms may not be recoverable at the time of the nephritis, the diagnosis depends on the serological evidence of a rise in antibody titers to streptococcal products. The nephritic syndrome typically begins abruptly with oliguria, hematuria, facial edema, and hypertension. Depression of serum C3 during the acute syndrome, returning to normal within 1 to 2 weeks, is typical. Overt nephritis resolves after several weeks, although hematuria and especially proteinuria may persist for several months. A few patients have abnormal urinary sediment for years after the acute episode, and rare patients (particularly adults) develop progressive renal failure.

Type I Membranoproliferative Glomerulonephritis

Type I membranoproliferative glomerulonephritis is characterized by hypercellularity and capillary wall thickening; deposition of mesangial and subendothelial immune complexes causes mesangial proliferation and extension into the subendothelial zone.

☐ **Pathogenesis:** Type I membranoproliferative glomerulonephritis, also called *mesangiocapillary glomerulonephritis*, is caused by the localization of immune complexes to the mesangium and capillary walls. Half of the patients have detectable circulating immune complexes, and there is evidence for the activation of complement (which would mediate inflammatory changes) within glomeruli. In most patients, the origin of the nephritogenic antigen is unknown, but some have associated conditions that are the apparent source of the antigen (Table 16-5).

Elimination of the associated condition leads to reso-

TABLE 16-5 **Classification of Type I Membranoproliferative Glomerulonephritis**

Primary (idiopathic)
Secondary
Subacute bacterial endocarditis
Infected ventriculoatrial shunt
Osteomyelitis
Hepatitis C virus infection
Mixed cryoglobulinemia
Neoplasia

lution of glomerulonephritis, which supports a causal relationship between the two. Unlike the infections that cause acute postinfectious glomerulonephritis, those that are responsible for type I membranoproliferative glomerulonephritis are persistent, indolent infections, which are associated with chronic antigenemia.

☐ **Pathology:** The glomeruli in type I membranoproliferative disease are diffusely enlarged and display marked mesangial cell proliferation. The resulting lobular distortion ("hypersegmentation") of the glomeruli (Fig. 16-36) has in the past been termed *lobular glomerulonephritis*. Among these patients, 20% will have crescents, usually involving only a minority of glomeruli. Capillary walls are thickened, and silver stains show a doubling or complex replication of GBMs.

Electron microscopy demonstrates that the capillary wall thickening and replication of GBMs are a consequence of the marked expansion of the mesangial area, with extension of mesangial cytoplasm into the subendothelial zone and deposition of new basement membrane material between the mesangial cytoplasm and endothelial cell (Figs. 16-37 and 16-38). Subendothelial and mesangial electron-dense deposits, corresponding to immune complexes, are the likely cause for the mesangial response. Variable numbers of subepithelial dense deposits may also be seen. Immunofluorescence microscopy demonstrates granular deposition of immunoglobulins and complement in glomerular capillary loops and mesangium (Fig. 16-39).

☐ **Clinical Features:** Type I membranoproliferative glomerulonephritis is most frequent in older children and young adults, although it can occur at any age. The clinical presentation may be either the nephrotic or the nephritic syndrome or a combination of both. Type I disease accounts for 5% of the nephrotic syndrome in children and adults. Patients often have low levels of C3. Acute postinfectious glomerulonephritis and lupus glomerulonephritis, both of which can cause nephritis with hypocomplementemia, are in the differential diagnosis. Type I membranoproliferative glomerulonephritis is usually a persistent but slowly progressive disease. Half of the patients reach end-stage renal disease after 10 years.

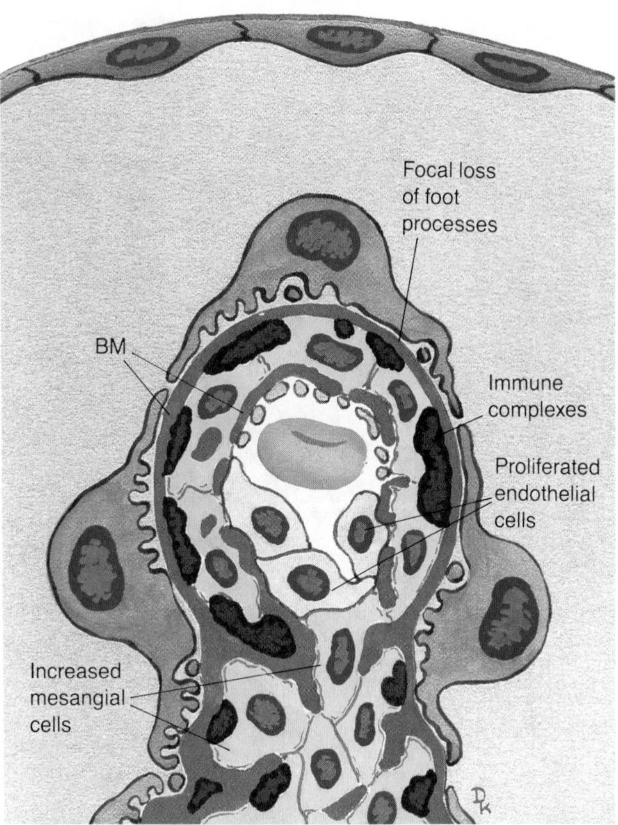

FIGURE 16-37
Membranoproliferative glomerulonephritis, type I. In this disease, the glomeruli are enlarged. Hypercellular tufts and narrowing or obstruction of the capillary lumen are seen. Large subendothelial deposits of immune complexes extend along the inner border of the basement membrane. The mesangial cells proliferate and migrate peripherally into the capillary. Basement membrane (BM) material accumulates in a linear fashion parallel to the basement membrane in a subendothelial position. The interposition of mesangial cells and basement membrane between the endothelial cells and the original basement membrane creates a double-contour effect. The accumulation of mesangial cells and stroma in the tufts narrows the capillary lumen. The stalk is also widened by the proliferation of mesangial cells and the accumulation of basement membrane stroma. The entire process leads progressively to lobulation of the glomerulus. Note the proliferation of endothelial cells and focal effacement of foot processes.

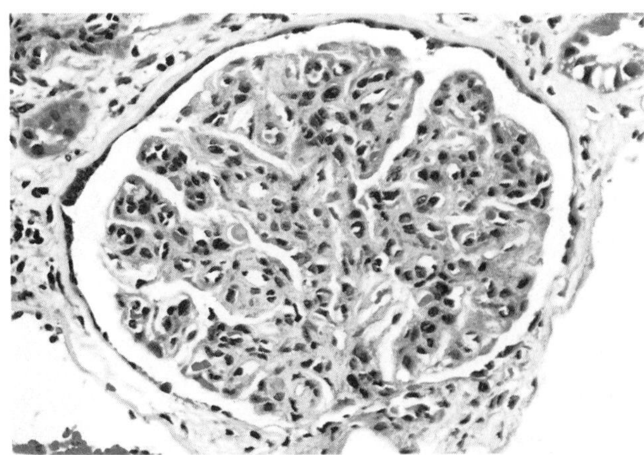

FIGURE 16-36
Type I membranoproliferative glomerulonephritis. The glomerular lobulation is accentuated. Increased cells and matrix in the mesangium and thickening of capillary walls are noted.

Type II Membranoproliferative Glomerulonephritis (Dense Deposit Disease)

Type II membranoproliferative glomerulonephritis is characterized by a pathognomonic electron-dense transformation of GBMs and extensive complement deposition.

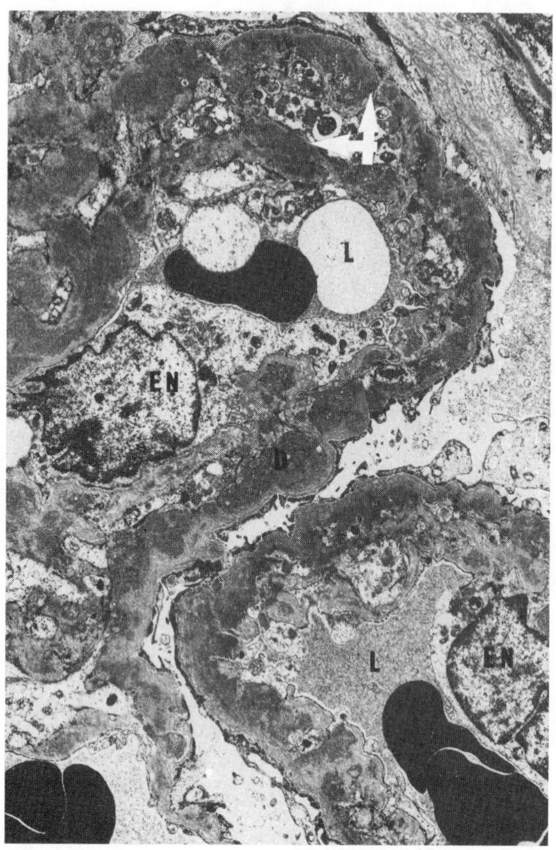

FIGURE *16-38*
Type I membranoproliferative glomerulonephritis. An electron micrograph demonstrates a double-contour basement membrane (*arrows*), with mesangial interposition and prominent subendothelial deposits. EN, endothelial cell; L, capillary lumen.

□ **Pathogenesis:** Although the cause of the extensive localization of complement in the GBMs and mesangial matrix in this disease suggests that complement activation is a major mediator of the structural and functional abnormalities, the basis for the complement deposition is unknown. The virtual absence of immunoglobulin in the glomeruli probably excludes mediation by immune complexes. Most patients have a circulating IgG autoantibody, termed *C3 nephritic factor*, that stabilizes the activated C3 convertase enzyme (C3bBb) of the alternative complement activation pathway. The result is a prolongation of C3 cleaving activity. A similar C3 nephritic factor is also present in a minority of patients with type I membranoproliferative glomerulonephritis and lupus nephritis. The role of this factor, if any, in the pathogenesis of type II membranoproliferative glomerulonephritis remains obscure. The common recurrence of type II membranoproliferative glomerulonephritis in renal transplants suggests that glomerular injury is mediated through some unknown humoral factor.

□ **Pathology:** The histological appearance of type II membranoproliferative disease may be similar to that of type I, with capillary wall thickening and hypercellularity (Fig. 16-40). However, many patients have less pronounced or absent hypercellularity, which makes the term "proliferative" problematic. The distinctive ribbonlike zone of increased density in the center of a thickened GBM and in the mesangial matrix (Fig. 16-41), justifies the alternative name *dense deposit disease*. Areas of density may also be found in the membranes of peritubular capillaries and in the elastic laminae of arterioles. Immunofluorescence microscopy shows linear or bandlike staining of capillary walls for C3, with little or no staining for immunoglobulins (Fig. 16-42).

□ **Clinical Features:** Type II membranoproliferative glomerulonephritis is rare and the clinical presentation and course are similar to type I disease. The frequency of hypocomplementemia is, however, higher, and

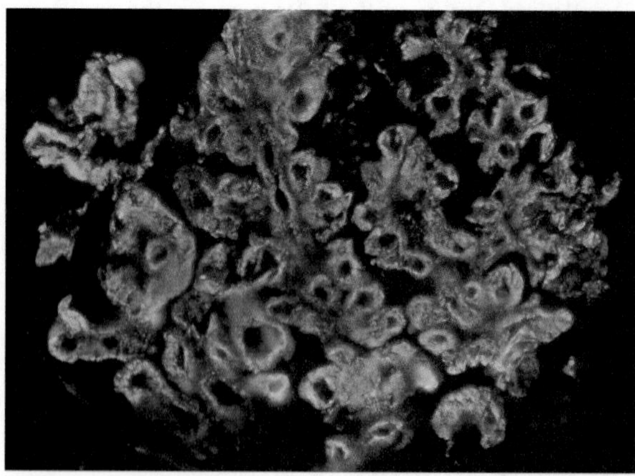

FIGURE *16-39*
Type I membranoproliferative glomerulonephritis. An immunofluorescence micrograph demonstrates granular to bandlike staining for C3 in the capillary walls and mesangium.

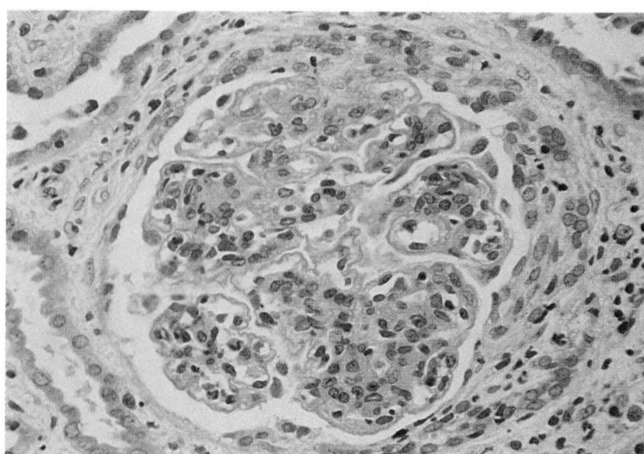

FIGURE *16-40*
Type II membranoproliferative glomerulonephritis (dense deposit disease). Capillary wall thickening, hypercellularity, and a small crescent are evident.

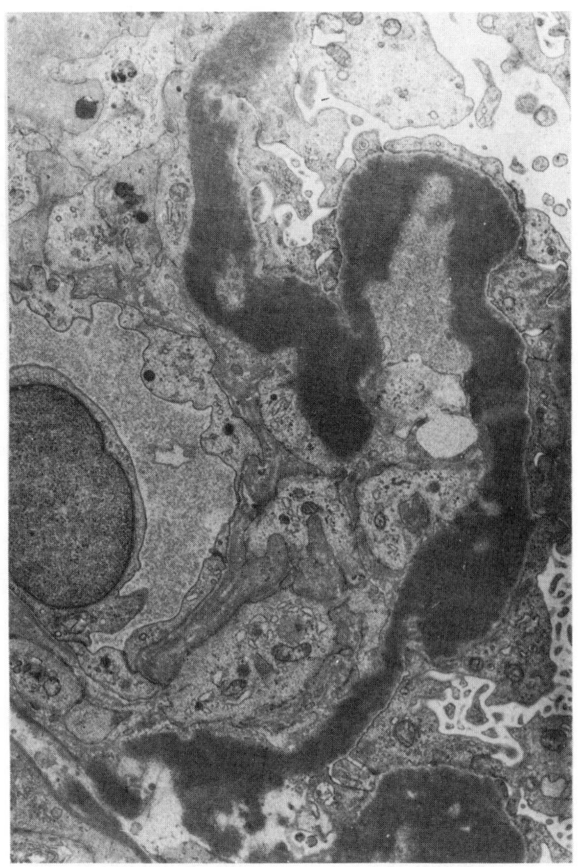

FIGURE *16-41*
Type II membranoproliferative glomerulonephritis (dense deposit disease). An electron micrograph demonstrates thickening of the basement membrane and intramembranous dense deposits.

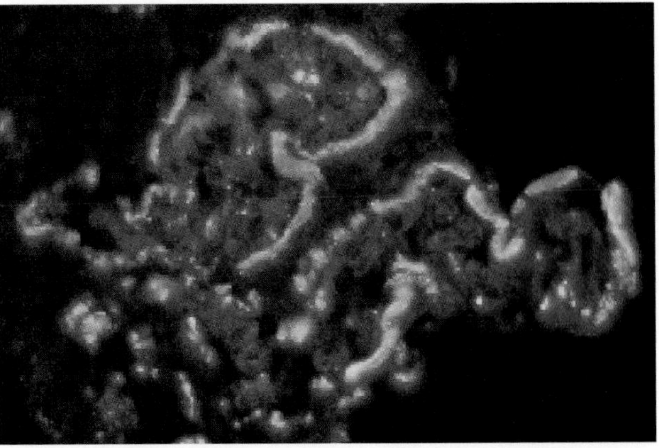

FIGURE *16-42*
Type II membranoproliferative glomerulonephritis (dense deposit disease). An immunofluorescence micrograph demonstrates bands of capillary wall staining and coarsely granular mesangial staining for C3.

the prognosis is slightly worse. No effective treatment has been identified.

Lupus Glomerulonephritis

Systemic lupus erythematosis (SLE) is an autoimmune disease characterized by a generalized dysregulation and hyperactivity of B cells, with production of autoantibodies to a variety of nuclear and nonnuclear antigens, including DNA, RNA, nucleoproteins, and phospholipids. Nephritis is one of the most common complications of SLE. There is a wide range of patterns of immune complex deposition in the glomeruli of lupus nephritis. Immune complexes confined to the mesangium cause less inflammation than subendothelial immune complexes. The latter are more exposed to the cellular and humoral inflammatory mediator systems in the blood and are, therefore, more likely to initiate inflammation. Subepithelial localization of immune complexes causes proteinuria but does not stimulate overt glomerular inflammation.

☐ **Pathogenesis:** Immune complexes may localize in glomeruli by deposition from the circulation, formation *in situ*, or both. There is experimental evidence that circulating immune complexes formed by high avidity antibodies deposit in the subendothelial and mesangial zones, and that low affinity antibodies form immune complexes *in situ* in the subepithelial zone. Formation of immune complexes *in situ* may involve antigens, such as DNA, that have become planted on GBMs or mesangial matrix by charge interactions. Glomerular immune complexes activate complement and initiate inflammatory injury. Complement activation in the kidneys and elsewhere often results in hypocomplementemia. Immune complexes also localize in the renal interstitium, the walls of interstitial vessels, and along tubular basement membranes. These complexes may be involved in the production of tubulointerstitial inflammation in patients with lupus nephritis.

☐ **Pathology:** The pathological and clinical manifestations of lupus nephritis are highly variable because of variable patterns of immune complex accumulation in

TABLE *16-6* **Pathological and Clinical Features of Lupus Nephritis**

Class	Location of Immune Complexes	Clinical Manifestations
I: No lesion	None	No glomerular dysfunction
II: Mesangial	Mesangial	Mild hematuria and proteinuria
III: Focal proliferative	Mesangial and subendothelial	Moderate nephritis
IV: Diffuse proliferative	Mesangial and subendothelial	Severe nephritis
IV: Membranous	Subepithelial	Nephrotic syndrome
VI: Chronic	Variable	Chronic renal failure

different patients (Table 16-6) and in the same patient over time. Immune complexes confined to the mesangium cause no changes by light microscopy, or varying degrees of mesangial hypercellularity and matrix expansion (**class II lupus nephritis**). Immune complex accumulation in the subendothelial zone, which is always accompanied by mesangial immune complexes, stimulates inflammation with proliferation of mesangial and endothelial cells and the influx of neutrophils and monocytes. In more severe disease, necrosis and crescent formation develop. This overt glomerular inflammation is called *focal proliferative lupus glomerulonephritis* **(class III lupus nephritis)** if less than 50% of glomeruli are involved, and *diffuse proliferative lupus glomerulonephritis* **(class IV lupus nephritis)** if 50% or more are involved (Fig. 16-43). When immune complexes are predominantly in the subepithelial zone, the pathological phenotype is a membranous glomerulopathy **(class V lupus nephritis)**. Some patients have a background of class V injury and a concurrent class II, III, or IV injury because of the presence of numerous subepithelial immune complexes, as well as mesangial and subendothelial immune complexes. Even pure class V lupus nephritis has mesangial immune complexes that can be detected by electron microscopy.

Electron microscopy demonstrates the varied locations of immune complex dense deposits in mesangial, subendothelial, and subepithelial locations. Class II lesions have only mesangial deposits. Classes III and IV have mesangial and subendothelial deposits, and usually scattered subepithelial deposits (Fig. 16-44). Class V lesions have numerous subepithelial dense deposits. The dense deposits of lupus glomerulonephritis occasionally have a patterned appearance that resembles a fingerprint. Some 80% of specimens have *tubuloreticular inclusions* in endothelial cells. Lupus nephritis and HIV-associated nephropathy are the only renal diseases with a high frequency of these structures.

Immunofluorescence microscopy also demonstrates the varied locations of immune complexes. The subepithelial complexes are granular, and the subendothelial deposits appear granular or bandlike (Fig. 16-45). The immune complexes often stain most intensely for IgG, but IgA and IgM are also almost always present. In addition, intense staining for C3, C1q, and other complement components is noted. Granular staining along tubular basement membranes and interstitial vessels is present in over 50% of patients.

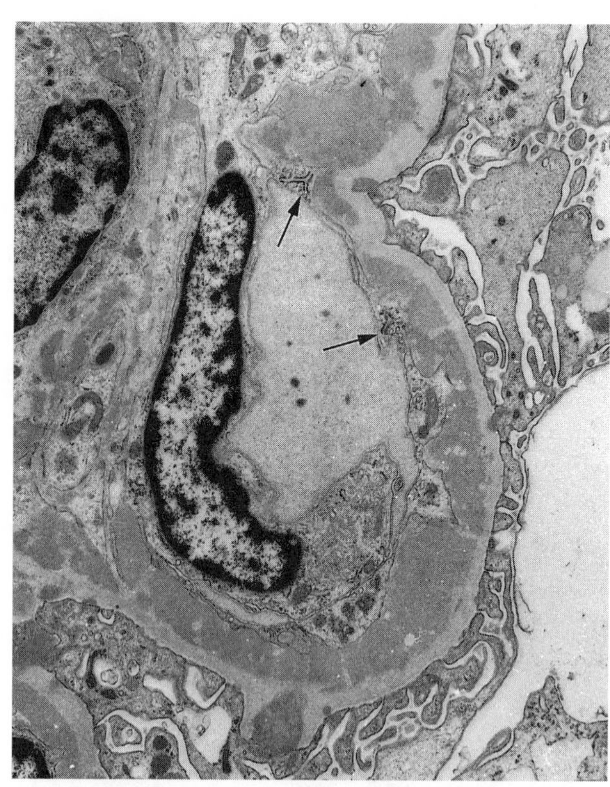

FIGURE *16-44*
Diffuse proliferative lupus glomerulonephritis. An electron micrograph reveals large subendothelial and mesangial dense deposits, and a few subepithelial deposits. Endothelial tubuloreticular inclusions (*arrows*) are present.

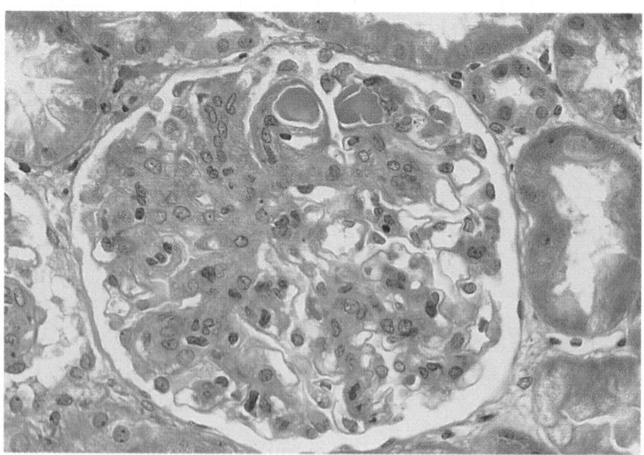

FIGURE *16-43*
Proliferative lupus glomerulonephritis. Segmental endocapillary hypercellularity and thickening of capillary walls are present.

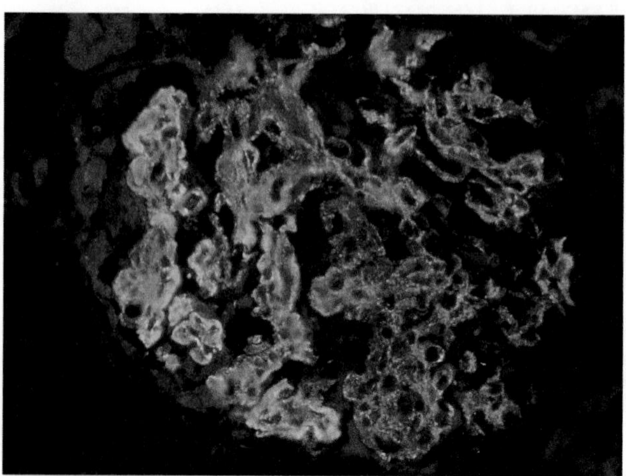

FIGURE *16-45*
Diffuse proliferative lupus glomerulonephritis. An immunofluorescence micrograph demonstrates segmental staining for IgG in the capillary walls and mesangium.

☐ **Clinical Features:** Of all patients with SLE, 70% develop renal disease, which is the major cause for morbidity and mortality in many patients. The disease is most common in black women. As noted in Table 16-6, the clinical manifestations and prognosis of renal dysfunction are varied and depend on the pathological nature of the underlying renal disease. **Renal biopsy specimens from lupus patients are usually evaluated to assess disease category, activity, and chronicity, rather than merely to make a diagnosis of lupus glomerulonephritis.** Class III and class IV lupus nephritis have the poorest prognosis (class IV being worse) and are the categories that are treated most aggressively, usually with high doses of corticosteroids and other immunosuppressive drugs. Over time, sometimes prompted by treatment, there can be transitions from one type of lupus nephritis to another, with the expected changes in clinical manifestations. Prior to the use of current immunosuppressive regimens, more than 75% of patients with class IV disease reached end-stage renal failure within 5 years, compared to less than 25% with current treatment.

IgA Nephropathy

IgA nephropathy (Berger disease) is glomerulonephritis caused by the accumulation of immune complexes composed predominantly of IgA.

☐ **Pathogenesis:** Glomerular IgA-dominant immune complexes are the apparent cause of IgA nephropathy, but the constituent antigens and the mechanism of accumulation (deposition versus *in situ* formation) have not been determined. Patients with IgA nephropathy often have elevated blood levels of IgA, and circulating IgA-containing immune complexes have been detected. **Exacerbations of IgA nephropathy are often initiated by infections of the respiratory or gastrointestinal tracts.** A leading hypothesis proposes that mucosal exposure to viral, bacterial, or dietary antigens stimulates a nephritogenic IgA-dominant immune response, which results in the glomerular accumulation of immune complexes. Possible involvement of dietary antigens is supported by the association between IgA nephropathy and gluten-sensitive enteropathy, and by the improvement in both diseases produced by eliminating dietary gluten. There is evidence for major histocompatibility complex (MHC)–linked susceptibility to IgA nephropathy, possibly mediated through dysregulation of IgA immune responses. Abnormal IgA glycosylation may also predispose to IgA nephropathy.

IgA-containing immune complexes within the mesangium most likely activate complement through the alternative pathway. This concept is supported by the finding by immunofluorescence microscopy of C3 and properdin in the IgA deposits, in the absence of C1q and C4.

☐ **Pathology:** Immunofluorescence microscopy is essential for the diagnosis of IgA nephropathy. The diagnostic finding is mesangial staining that is most intense for IgA (Fig. 16-46). This is usually accompanied by staining for C3, and sometimes by lower-intensity staining for IgG, IgM, or both. IgA deposition in the glomerular capillary wall (in addition to the mesangium) may be present in more severe cases and suggests a less favorable prognosis.

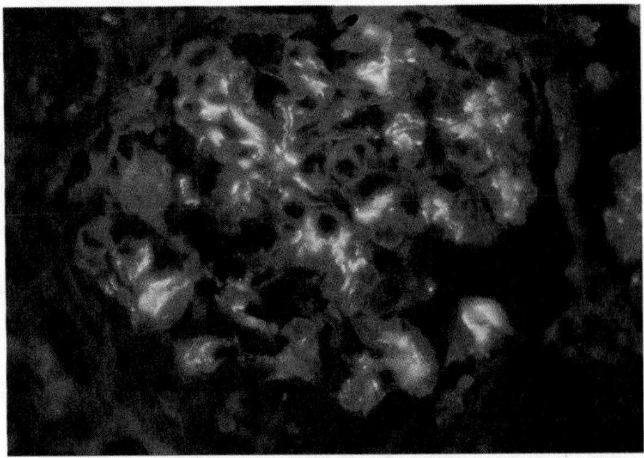

FIGURE *16-46*
IgA nephropathy. An immunofluorescence micrograph shows deposits of IgA in the mesangial areas.

Depending on the severity and duration of glomerular inflammation, IgA nephropathy manifests a continuum of histological appearances, ranging from (1) no discernible light microscopic changes, to (2) focal or diffuse mesangial hypercellularity, to (3) focal or diffuse proliferative glomerulonephritis with or without crescents (Fig. 16-47), to (4) chronic sclerosing glomerulonephritis. At the time of initial diagnosis, focal proliferative glomeru-

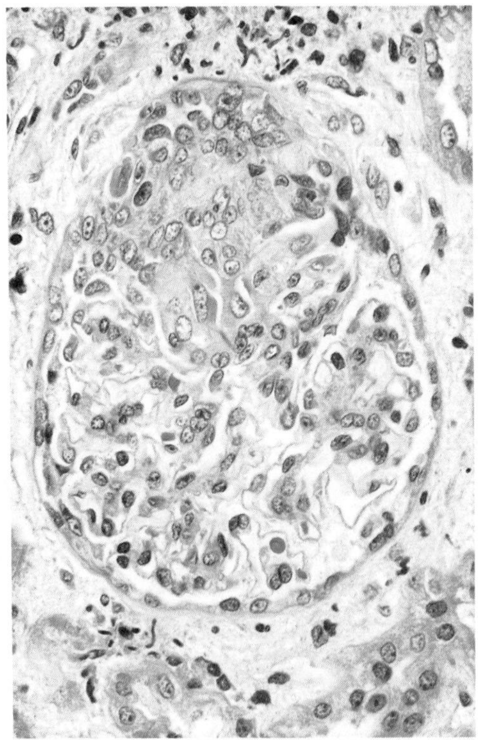

FIGURE *16-47*
IgA nephropathy. Segmental endocapillary hypercellularity and slight adjacent epithelial proliferation (crescent formation) are noted.

lonephritis is the most frequent manifestation. Crescent formation is uncommon, except in unusually severe cases.

Ultrastructural examination reveals electron-dense deposits (Figs. 16-48 and 16-49) typically located immediately beneath the mesangial basement membrane. A minority of patients, usually those with severe disease, have dense deposits in the capillary walls.

☐ **Clinical Features:** **IgA nephropathy (Berger disease) is the most common form of glomerulonephritis in the world.** Among patients who are found to have glomerulonephritis by renal biopsy, it accounts for 10% in the United States, 20% in Europe, and 40% in Asia. IgA nephropathy has a high frequency in Native Americans and is rare in blacks. It is most common in young men, with a peak age of 15 to 30 years at diagnosis. The clinical presentations are varied, which reflects the varied pathological severity: 40% of patients have asymptomatic microscopic hematuria, 40% have intermittent gross hematuria, 10% have nephrotic syndrome, and 10% have renal failure. The disease rarely completely resolves but may follow an episodic course with exacerbations often occurring at the time of an upper respiratory tract infection. IgA nephropathy has a slowly progressive course, with 20% of patients reaching end-stage renal failure after 10 years. When these patients are treated by renal transplantation, IgA deposits frequently recur in the allograft, although graft function is usually not impaired.

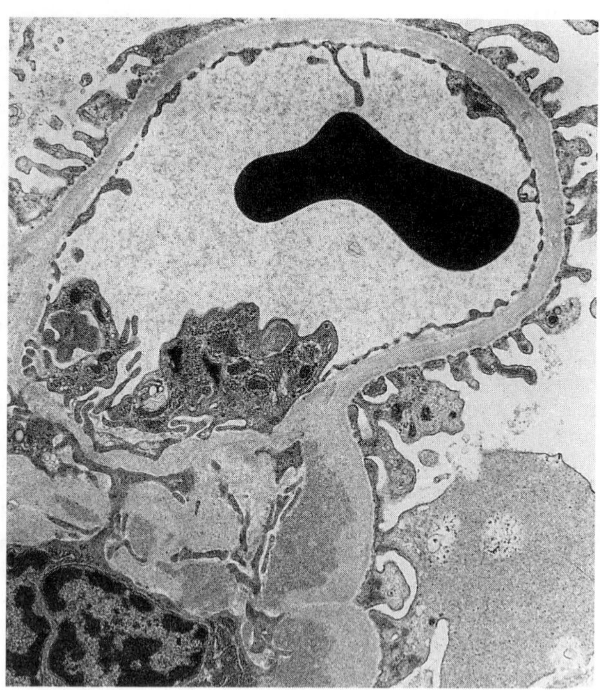

FIGURE *16-49*
IgA nephropathy. An electron micrograph demonstrates prominent dense deposits in the mesangial matrix.

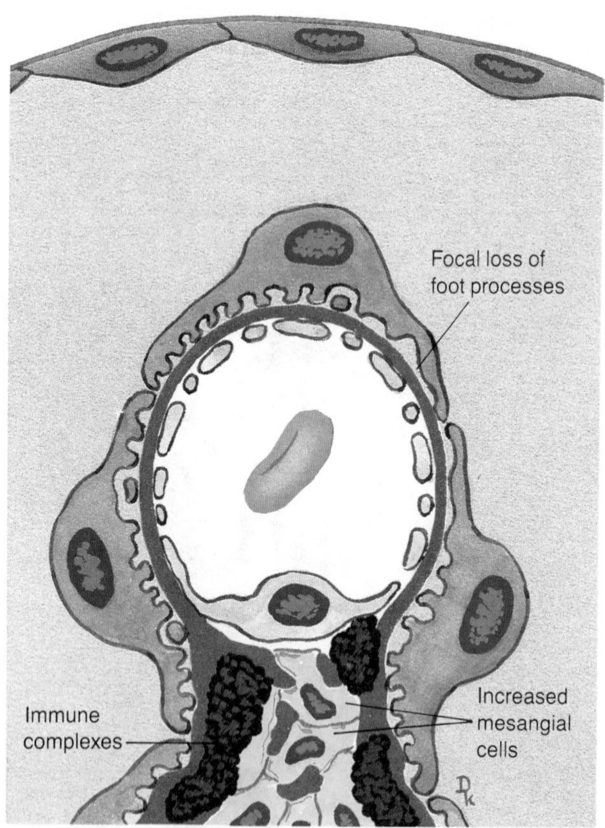

FIGURE *16-48*
IgA nephropathy. Significant accumulation of IgA is seen in the stalk and, most commonly, between the mesangial cells and the basement membrane. The disease is associated with a variable inflammatory reaction.

Antiglomerular Basement Membrane Antibody Glomerulonephritis

Anti-GBM antibody glomerulonephritis is an uncommon but aggressive form of glomerulonephritis caused by the binding of these autoantibodies.

☐ **Pathogenesis:** Anti-GBM is mediated by an autoantibody directed against a component of the GBM that is located within the **globular noncollagenous domain of type IV collagen**. The autoantibodies bind to the autoantigens *in situ*, and the resultant immune complexes initiate acute inflammation by activating mediator systems, such as complement. Because of cross reactivity of the autoantibodies with the pulmonary alveolar capillary basement membranes, many patients simultaneously suffer from pulmonary hemorrhages and recurrent hemoptysis, sometimes severe enough to be life-threatening. When both the lungs and kidneys are involved, the eponym *Goodpasture syndrome* is used. Genetic susceptibility to anti-GBM disease is associated with HLA-DR2 genes. The onset of disease often follows viral upper respiratory tract infections, and the development of the pulmonary component of Goodpasture syndrome is associated with cigarette smoking.

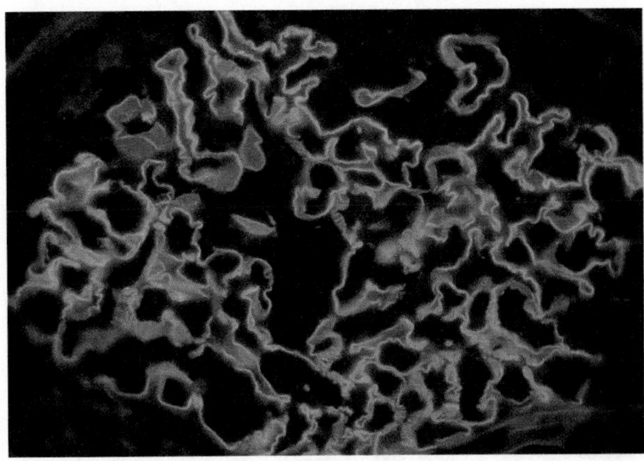

FIGURE *16-50*
Anti-GBM glomerulonephritis. Linear immunofluorescence for IgG is seen along the glomerular basement membrane. Contrast this linear pattern of staining with the granular pattern of immunofluorescence typical for most types of immune complex deposition within capillary walls (see Fig. 16-35).

□ **Pathology:** The pathological *sine qua non* of anti-GBM glomerulonephritis is the presence of diffuse linear staining of GBMs for IgG, which is indicative of autoantibodies bound to the basement membrane (Fig. 16-50). Linear staining for IgG, however, is not entirely specific. For example, nonimmunological binding of IgG to basement membranes is frequent in diabetic glomerulosclerosis. The diagnosis should, therefore, be confirmed by serological detection of circulating anti-GBM antibodies. By light microscopy, over 90% of patients with anti-GBM glomerulonephritis have glomerular crescents (*crescentic glomerulonephritis*) (Figs. 16-51 and 16-52), usually involving over 50% of glomeruli. Focal glomerular fibrinoid necrosis is common. Involved lungs exhibit marked intra-alveolar hemorrhage. Electron microscopy demonstrates focal breaks in GBMs, but no immune complex–type deposits.

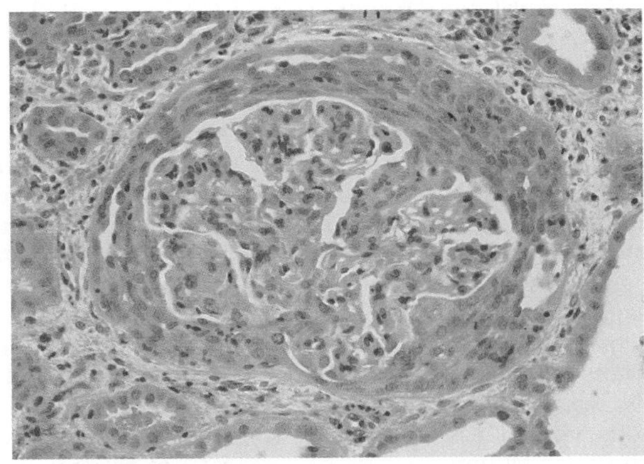

FIGURE *16-51*
Crescentic anti-GBM glomerulonephritis. A crescent that surrounds the periphery of the glomerulus is composed of cells contiguous with the lining of Bowman capsule.

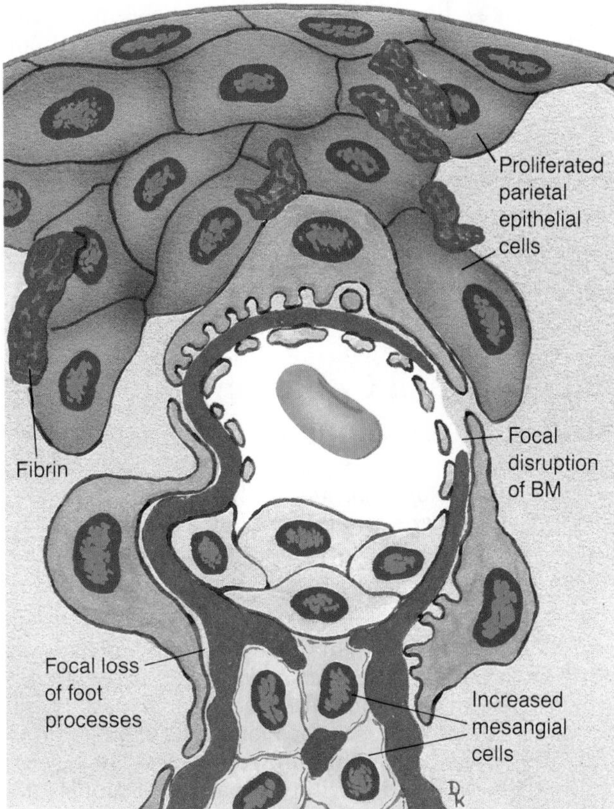

FIGURE *16-52*
Crescentic (rapidly progressive) glomerulonephritis. This severe variety of glomerulonephritis shows not only changes in the glomerular tuft but also conspicuous proliferation of capsular epithelial cells, which, together with visceral epithelial cells and macrophages that have entered the glomerulus, form cellular "crescents." Fibrin is also a significant component of many active cellular crescents. Focal disruption of the peripheral capillary basement membrane may result in red blood cells entering Bowman space and is manifest clinically as hematuria. Crescentic glomerulonephritis is not a specific diagnostic entity but describes the morphological counterpart of a highly active disease, which may have one of a number of causes, as listed in Table 16-7.

TABLE *16-7* **Frequency (%) of Immunopathological Categories of Crescentic Glomerulonephritis[a] in Different Age Groups**

	Age (years)		
Category	**<20**	**20–64**	**>65**
Antiglomerular basement membrane	10	10	10
Immune complex	55	40	10
Antineutrophil cytoplasmic autoantibody (ANCA)	30	45	75
No evidence for the three categories above	5	5	5

[a] Glomerulonephritis with crescents in >50% of glomeruli.

☐ **Clinical Features:** Anti-GBM glomerulonephritis typically presents with rapidly progressive renal failure and nephritic signs and symptoms. It accounts for 10% to 20% of rapidly progressive (crescentic) glomerulonephritis (see Table 16-7). Treatment is with immunosuppressive therapy and plasma exchange, which are most effective when the disease is in an early stage before severe renal failure has occurred. If end-stage renal failure develops, renal transplantation is frequently successful, with little risk of loss of the allograft to recurrent glomerulonephritis.

Antineutrophil Cytoplasmic Autoantibody Glomerulonephritis

Antineutrophil cytoplasmic autoantibody (ANCA) glomerulonephritis is an aggressive, neutrophil-mediated disease that is characterized by glomerular necrosis and crescents but no immunoglobulin deposits.

☐ **Pathogenesis:** This category of glomerulonephritis was once called *idiopathic crescentic glomerulonephritis* because immunofluorescence microscopy did not demonstrate evidence for glomerular deposition of anti-GBM antibodies or immune complexes. The discovery that 90% of patients with this pattern of glomerular injury have circulating ANCAs has prompted the hypothesis that these autoantibodies cause the disease. **ANCAs are specific for proteins in the cytoplasm of neutrophils and monocytes, usually myeloperoxidase or proteinase 3.** *In vitro,* these autoantibodies activate neutrophils and cause them to adhere to endothelial cells, release toxic oxygen metabolites, degranulate, and kill the endothelial cells. If these events take place *in vivo,* necrotizing vascular inflammation would result. As yet, however, there is no proof that ANCAs are actually pathogenic.

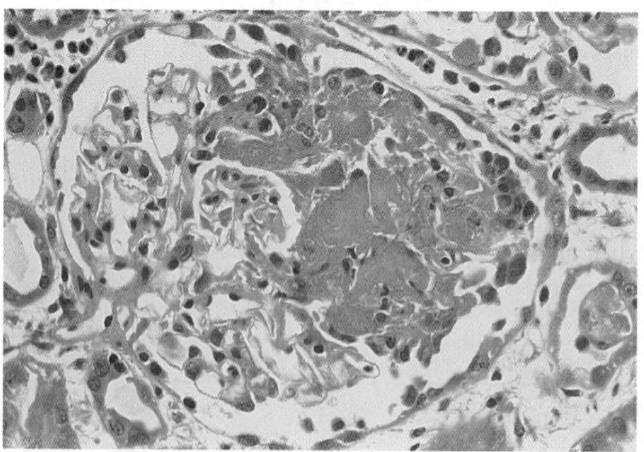

FIGURE 16-53
ANCA glomerulonephritis. Segmental fibrinoid necrosis is illustrated. In time, this lesion would stimulate crescent formation.

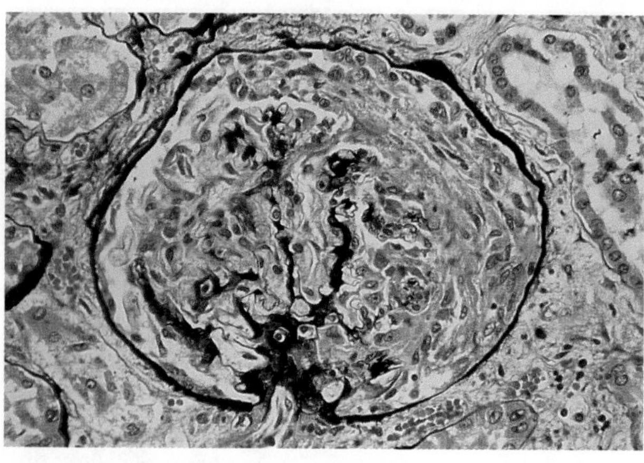

FIGURE 16-54
ANCA glomerulonephritis. A silver stain shows focal disruption of glomerular basement membranes, and crescent formation.

☐ **Pathology:** Over 90% of patients with ANCA glomerulonephritis have focal glomerular necrosis (Fig. 16-53) and crescent formation (Fig. 16-54), with many patients having over 50% of glomeruli involved with crescents. Non-necrotic segments may appear normal or have slight neutrophil infiltration or mild endocapillary hypercellularity. Immunofluorescence microscopy demonstrates an absence or paucity of staining for immunoglobulins and complement, which distinguishes ANCA glomerulonephritis from anti-GBM glomerulonephritis and immune complex glomerulonephritis. However, a minority of patients with crescentic glomerulonephritis have serological and pathological evidence for overlapping expression of ANCA glomerulonephritis with anti-GBM glomerulonephritis or immune complex glomerulonephritis. Electron microscopy demonstrates no immune complex–type dense deposits in ANCA glomerulonephritis.

☐ **Clinical Features:** The most common clinical presentation for ANCA glomerulonephritis is rapidly progressive renal failure, with nephritic signs and symptoms. The disease accounts for approximately 75% of rapidly progressive (crescentic) glomerulonephritis in patients over 60 years old, 45% in middle-aged adults, and 30% in young adults and children (see Table 16-7). **Three quarters of patients with ANCA glomerulonephritis have systemic small vessel vasculitis** (see later), which has many manifestations, including pulmonary hemorrhage. Therefore, ANCA glomerulonephritis with pulmonary vasculitis can cause a *pulmonary-renal vasculitic syndrome* identical to Goodpasture syndrome. In fact, ANCA vasculitis is a much more frequent cause for pulmonary-renal vasculitic syndrome than Goodpasture syndrome. Without treatment, over 80% of patients develop end-stage renal disease within 5 years. Immunosuppressive therapy decreases the development of end-stage disease at 5 years to less than 25%.

TABLE 16-8 Types of Vasculitis that Involve the Kidneys

Type of Vasculitis	Major Target Vessels in Kidney	Major Renal Manifestations
Small Vessel Vasculitis		
Immune complex vasculitis		
Henoch-Schönlein purpura	Glomeruli	Nephritis
Cryoglobulinemic vasculitis	Glomeruli	Nephritis
Anti-GBM vasculitis		
Goodpasture syndrome	Glomeruli	Nephritis
ANCA-vasculitis		
Wegener granulomatosis	Glomeruli, arterioles, interlobular arteries	Nephritis
Microscopic polyangiitis	Glomeruli, arterioles, interlobular arteries	Nephritis
Churg-Strauss syndrome	Glomeruli, arterioles, interlobular arteries	Nephritis
Medium-Sized Vessel Vasculitis		
Polyarteritis nodosa	Interlobar, arcuate and interlobular arteries	Infarcts and hemorrhage
Kawasaki disease	Interlobar, arcuate and interlobular arteries	Infarcts and hemorrhage
Large Vessel Vasculitis		
Giant cell arteritis	Renal arteries	Renovascular hypertension
Takayasu arteritis	Renal arteries	Renovascular hypertension

ANCA, antineutrophil cytoplasmic antibody; GBM, glomerular basement membrane.

VASCULAR DISEASES

Renal Vasculitis

The kidney is involved in many types of systemic vasculitis (Table 16-8). **In a sense, glomerulonephritis is a local form of vasculitis that affects glomerular capillaries.** The glomeruli may be the only site of vascular inflammation, or the renal disease may be a component of a systemic vasculitis.

Small Vessel Vasculitis

Small vessel vasculitis affects small arteries, arterioles, capillaries, and venules. Glomerulonephritis is a very frequent component of small vessel vasculitides. Other common manifestations include purpura, arthralgias, myalgias, peripheral neuropathy, and pulmonary hemorrhage. Small vessel vasculitides can be caused by immune complexes, antibasement membrane antibodies, or ANCAs (see Table 16-8).

Henoch-Schönlein purpura *is the most common type of childhood vasculitis and is caused by vascular localization of immune complexes containing predominantly IgA.* The glomerular lesion is identical with that of IgA nephropathy.

Cryoglobulinemic vasculitis affects the kidney in the form of a proliferative glomerulonephritis, usually with a type I membranoproliferative glomerulonephritis phenotype. By light microscopy, aggregates of cryoglobulins ("hyaline thrombi") can often be seen within capillary lumina (Fig. 16-55).

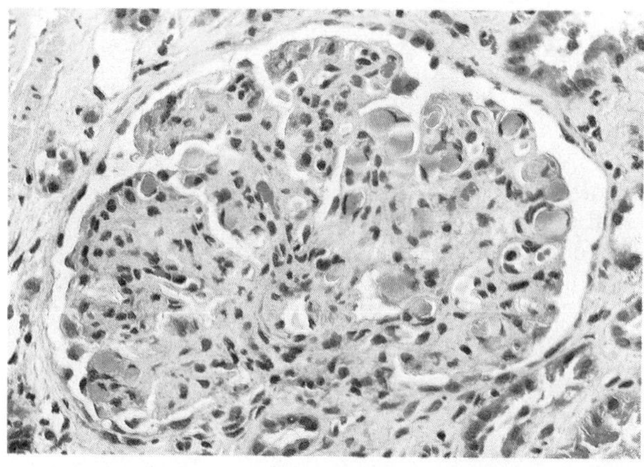

FIGURE 16-55
Cryoglobulinemic glomerulonephritis. The pattern of glomerular inflammation is similar to that of type I membranoproliferative glomerulonephritis, with hyaline thrombi within capillary lumina. These are not true thrombi but are rather aggregates of cryoglobulins.

In 25% of patients with ANCA-glomerulonephritis, the renal lesion is the only manifestation of vascular inflammation. However, in 75% of patients, ANCA glomerulonephritis is a component of a systemic small vessel vasculitis, as follows:

- **Wegener granulomatosis,** if there is necrotizing granulomatous inflammation, usually in the respiratory tract
- **Churg-Strauss syndrome,** if there is eosinophilia and asthma
- **Microscopic polyangiitis,** if there is no asthma or granulomatous inflammation

In addition to causing necrotizing and crescentic glomerulonephritis, the ANCA vasculitides are often

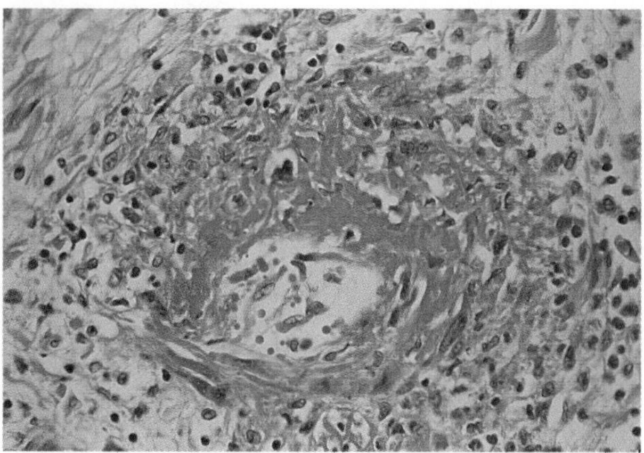

FIGURE *16-56*
ANCA necrotizing arteritis. Fibrinoid necrosis and inflammation involve a small artery in the renal cortex.

responsible for necrotizing inflammation in other renal vessels, such as arteries (Fig. 16-56), arterioles, and peritubular capillaries.

Medium-Sized Vessel Vasculitis

Medium-sized vessel vasculitides affect arteries, but not arterioles, capillaries, or venules. **Polyarteritis nodosa** (see Fig. 10-29), which occurs mainly in adults, and **Kawasaki disease**, which occurs principally in children, are rare causes of renal dysfunction. These diseases are characterized by necrotizing arteritis, which can involve renal arteries and result in pseudoaneurysm formation and renal thrombosis, infarction, and hemorrhage.

Large Vessel Vasculitis

Large vessel vasculitides, such as **giant cell arteritis** and **Takayasu arteritis**, affect the aorta and its major branches. These disorders may cause renovascular hypertension by involving the renal arteries or the aorta at the origin of the renal arteries. Narrowing or obstruction of these vessels results in renal ischemia, which stimulates increased renin production and consequent hypertension (Table 16-8).

Benign Nephrosclerosis (Hypertensive Nephrosclerosis)

Benign nephrosclerosis refers to renal vascular and glomerular sclerosis caused by mild to moderate hypertension.

☐ **Pathogenesis:** No precise definition is completely accepted for hypertension, but a sustained systolic pressure of greater than 140 mm Hg and a diastolic of greater than 90 mm are generally considered to be abnormal. Mild to moderate degrees of hypertension are called benign hypertension, which is the cause of typical hypertensive nephrosclerosis. The pathogenesis of hypertension is discussed in Chapter 10.

☐ **Pathology:** The kidneys are smaller than normal (atrophic) and usually affected bilaterally. The cortical surfaces have a fine granularity (Fig. 16-57), but coarser scars are occasionally present. On cut section, the cortex is thinned. Microscopically, many glomeruli appear normal, whereas others show varying degrees of ischemic

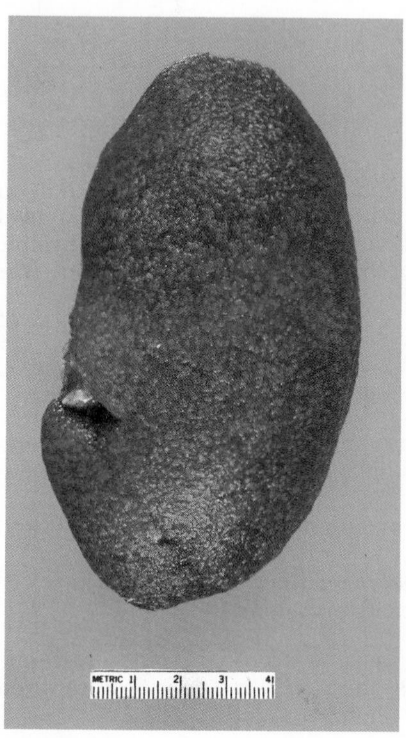

A

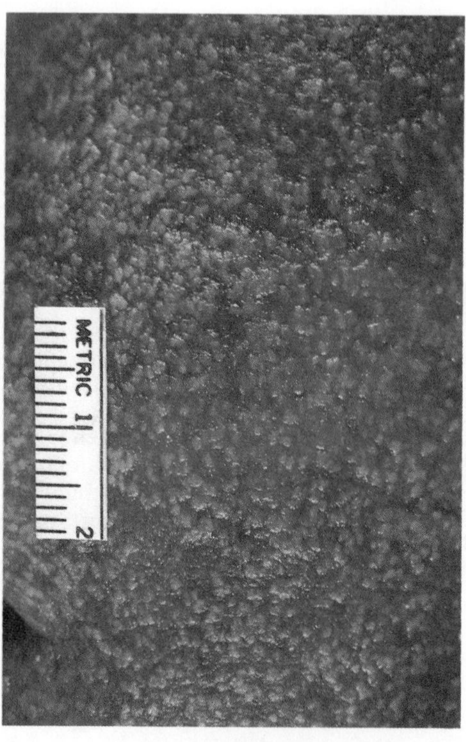

B

FIGURE *16-57*
Hypertensive nephrosclerosis. (*A*) The kidney is reduced in size, and the cortical surface exhibits fine granularity. (*B*) High magnification of the renal surface.

change. Initially, the glomerular capillaries are thickened because of thickening, wrinkling, and collapse of GBMs. Cells of the glomerular tuft are progressively lost, and collagen and matrix material are deposited within Bowman space. Eventually, the glomerular tuft is obliterated by a dense, eosinophilic globular mass enclosed in a scar, all within Bowman capsule. Tubular atrophy, a consequence of the obsolescence of the glomerulus, is associated with interstitial fibrosis and infiltration by chronic inflammatory cells. Globally sclerotic glomeruli and surrounding atrophic tubules are often clustered in focal subcapsular zones, with adjacent zones of preserved glomeruli and tubules (Fig. 16-58), an effect that is the basis for the granular surfaces of nephrosclerotic kidneys.

The pattern of change in the blood vessels of the kidney depends on the size of vessel involved. Large arteries down to the size of the arcuate arteries display fibrotic thickening of the intima, with replication of the elastica, and partial replacement of the muscularis with fibrous tissue. In addition to these changes, interlobular arteries exhibit medial hyperplasia. Arterioles feature concentric hyaline thickening of the wall, often with the loss of smooth muscle cells or their displacement to the periphery. This arteriolar change is termed *hyaline arteriolosclerosis*.

☐ **Clinical Features:** Although benign nephrosclerosis is ordinarily not associated with significant abnormalities of renal function, a few of the many persons with "benign" hypertension develop progressive renal failure, which may terminate in end-stage renal disease. Because "benign" hypertension is so prevalent, even the small proportion of these patients who develop renal insufficiency amounts to one third of all patients with end-stage renal disease. Benign nephrosclerosis is most prevalent and aggressive among blacks. **In fact, among blacks in the United States, hypertension without any evidence of a malignant phase is the single leading cause of end-stage renal disease.**

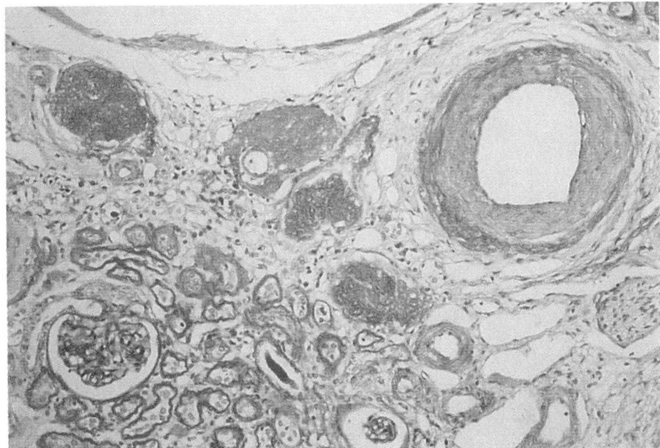

FIGURE *16-58*
Hypertensive nephrosclerosis. Several subcapsular globally sclerotic glomeruli are illustrated, together with adjacent tubular atrophy, interstitial fibrosis, and chronic inflammation.

Malignant Nephrosclerosis

Malignant nephrosclerosis refers to renal injury caused by malignant hypertension.

☐ **Pathogenesis:** There is no specific blood pressure that defines malignant hypertension, but a diastolic pressure greater than 125 mm Hg, retinal vascular changes, papilledema, and renal functional impairment are usual criteria. About half the patients with malignant hypertension have an antecedent history of benign hypertension, and many others have a background of chronic renal injury caused by many different diseases. Occasionally, malignant hypertension arises *de novo* in apparently healthy persons, particularly young black men. The pathogenesis of the vascular injury in patients with malignant hypertension is not completely elucidated. One hypothesis proposes that the extremely high blood pressures, combined with microvascular vasoconstriction, causes injury to endothelium as the blood slams into the narrowed small vessels. At sites of vascular injury, plasma constituents leak into the injured walls of arterioles (resulting in fibrinoid necrosis), into the intima of arteries (causing edematous intimal thickening), and into the subendothelial zone of glomerular capillaries (leading to glomerular consolidation). At these sites of vascular injury, thrombosis can result in focal cortical necrosis (infarcts).

☐ **Pathology:** The size of the kidneys in malignant hypertension varies from small to enlarged, depending on the duration of preexisting benign hypertension. The cut surface is mottled red and yellow and occasionally exhibits small cortical infarcts. Microscopically, malignant nephrosclerosis often exhibits a background of benign nephrosclerosis, with superimposed edematous (myxoid, mucoid) intimal expansion in arteries, fibrinoid necrosis of arterioles, and variable glomerular changes, ranging from capillary congestion, to consolidation, to necrosis (Fig. 16-59). Severe cases show thrombosis and focal ischemic cortical necrosis (infarction). Electron microscopy demonstrates electron-lucent expansion of the subendothelial zone in glomeruli. Immunofluorescence microscopy documents focal insudation of plasma proteins into injured vessel walls. These pathological changes are identical to those observed in other forms of thrombotic microangiography (see below).

☐ **Clinical Features:** Malignant hypertension occurs more frequently in men than in women, typically around the age of 40 years. Patients suffer headache, dizziness, and visual disturbances and may develop overt encephalopathy. Hematuria and proteinuria are frequent. Progressive deterioration of renal function develops if the malignant hypertension persists. The outlook for patients with malignant hypertension was previously dismal, but aggressive antihypertensive therapy now often controls the disease.

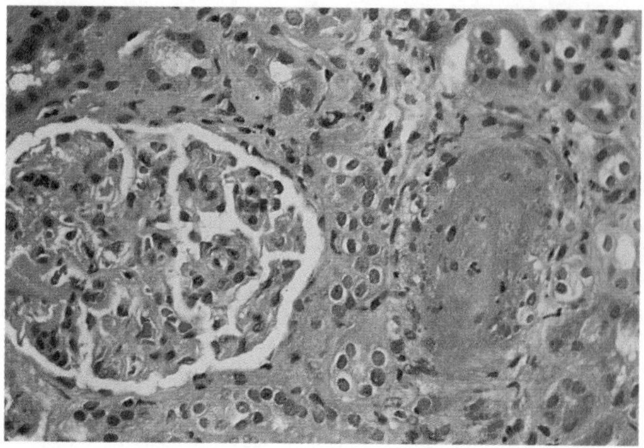

FIGURE *16-59*
Malignant nephrosclerosis. Arteriolar fibrinoid necrosis and glomerular consolidation are present.

Renovascular Hypertension

Renovascular hypertension refers to elevated systemic blood pressure secondary to renal ischemia caused by narrowing of a renal artery.

☐ **Pathogenesis:** Stenosis or total occlusion of a main renal artery produces a type of hypertension that is potentially curable by reconstitution of the arterial lumen. The initial experiments that led to the understanding of this syndrome were carried out in rats more than a half century ago by Goldblatt, and since that time the kidney deprived of vascular supply has been known as the *Goldblatt kidney.* Patients with renal artery stenosis have hypertension caused by increases in the production of renin, angiotensin II, and aldosterone. Renal vein renin from the ischemic kidney is elevated, whereas it is normal in the contralateral kidney. The majority (95%) of cases are caused by atherosclerosis, which explains why this disorder is twice as common in men as in women and is seen primarily in older age groups (average age, 55 years). Fibromuscular dysplasia and vasculitis are less common causes.

☐ **Pathology:** When vascular stenosis is caused by atherosclerosis, atherosclerotic plaques impinge on the aortic ostium or narrow the renal artery lumen, more frequently on the left than on the right. Occasionally, an atherosclerotic aneurysm of the abdominal aorta compromises the origin of the renal arteries.

Fibromuscular dysplasia*, the other major lesion that produces renovascular hypertension, is characterized by fibrous and muscular stenosis of the renal artery.* There are several patterns of renal artery involvement that are lumped under the heading of fibromuscular dysplasia. The most common is characterized by bilateral fibrosis of the media of the distal two thirds of the renal artery and its main branches. In some cases, the fibrosis is principally in the proximal one third to two thirds of the media, and the irregular pattern results in a beaded appearance on an angiogram. In these cases, which may be bilateral or unilateral, the intima is typically spared. In 20% of cases, hyperplasia of smooth muscle in short lengths of the media results in marked stenosis, whereas the other layers of the artery are not affected. Although the condition frequently does not worsen in those persons who display principally medial fibrosis, the subgroup with medial hyperplasia often exhibits clinical progression. Rarely, the major lesion is intimal fibroplasia, which consists of an accumulation of loose, cellular fibrous tissue.

No matter what the cause of renal artery stenosis, the kidney parenchymal changes are the same. The size of the involved kidney is reduced. The glomeruli appear normal, but because the intervening tubules show marked ischemic atrophy without extensive interstitial fibrosis, the glomeruli are closer than normal to each other. The juxtaglomerular apparatus is prominent and reveals hyperplasia and increased granularity.

☐ **Clinical Features:** Renovascular hypertension is characterized by mild to moderate elevations in blood pressure. A bruit over the renal artery may be heard. The diagnosis requires some type of imaging, such as angiography. In over half of the patients, hypertension is cured by surgical revascularization, angioplasty, or nephrectomy. However, when there is long-standing renovascular hypertension, the uninvolved kidney may become damaged by hypertensive nephrosclerosis.

Renal Atheroembolism

In patients with severe aortic atherosclerosis, embolization of atheromatous debris into the renal arteries and vascular tree as far as the glomerular capillaries may cause renal failure. Atheroembolization may be spontaneous or initiated by trauma, such as angiographic procedures. **Cholesterol clefts** are observed within vessel lumina (Fig. 16-60), and early lesions are surrounded by atheromatous material or thrombus. Later, they may elicit a foreign body reaction and may stimulate fibrosis in the adjacent vessel wall.

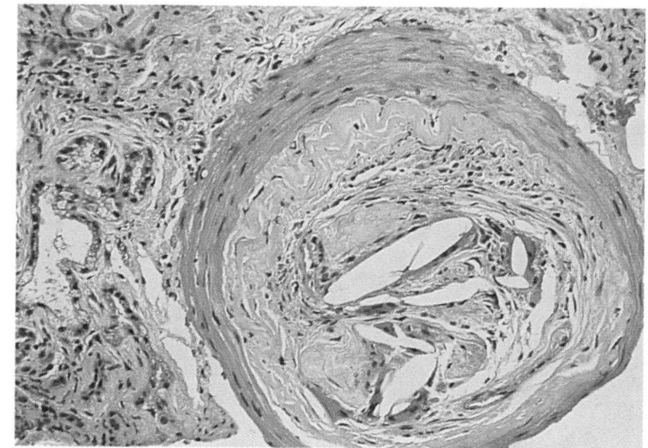

FIGURE *16-60*
Atheroembolus. An atheroembolus obstructs an arcuate artery. Note the cholesterol clefts.

Thrombotic Microangiopathy

Thrombotic microangiopathy refers to a group of diseases that share similar renal microvascular lesions, including thrombosis, arterial intimal expansion, arteriolar fibrinoid necrosis, and glomerular consolidation.

☐ **Pathogenesis:** Thrombotic microangiopathy reflects injury from a variety of factors, all of which cause endothelial damage that initiates a final common pathway of vascular changes. A leading theory holds that endothelial damage allows plasma constituents to enter the intima of arteries, the walls of arterioles, and the subendothelial zone of glomerular capillaries, resulting in narrowing of vessel lumina and ischemia. The injured endothelial surfaces also promote thrombosis, which worsens ischemia and may cause focal ischemic necrosis. The passage of blood through the injured vessels leads to a nonimmune (Coombs negative) hemolytic anemia, characterized by misshapen and disrupted erythrocytes (schistocytes) and thrombocytopenia. This pattern is termed *microangiopathic hemolytic anemia*. The kidneys are ubiquitous targets of thrombotic microangiopathies, but other organs may be injured as well.

☐ **Pathology:** The pathological changes in the kidney are comparable to those in malignant nephrosclerosis, which itself is a form of thrombotic microangiopathy. The basic renal lesions are the following:

- Arteriolar fibrinoid necrosis
- Arterial edematous intimal expansion
- Glomerular consolidation, necrosis, or congestion
- Vascular thrombosis

Electron microscopy of glomeruli demonstrates electron-lucent expansion of the subendothelial zone (Figs. 16-61 and 16-62), which results from the insudation of plasma proteins under injured endothelial cells. Immunofluorescence microscopy demonstrates the accumulation of fibrin and insudation of plasma proteins in injured vessel walls.

☐ **Clinical Features:** Various clinical presentations, associated conditions, and distributions of involved vessels allow the recognition of different categories of thrombotic microangiopathy. The various clinical disorders share microangiopathic hemolytic anemia, thrombocytopenia, hypertension, and renal failure, although these features are expressed to different degrees.

***Hemolytic-uremic syndrome* (*HUS*)** shows no evidence for significant vascular disease outside the kidneys. HUS is a common cause of acute renal failure in children. Major causes for HUS are certain *Shiga* toxin–producing strains of *Escherichia coli*, which are ingested in contaminated food, such as poorly cooked hamburger. The toxin injures endothelial cells, thereby setting in motion the sequence of events that produces thrombotic microangiopathy. These patients present with hemorrhagic diarrhea and rapidly progressive renal failure.

***Thrombotic thrombocytopenic purpura* (*TTP*)** is characterized by systemic microvascular injury, accompanied by purpura, fever, and changes in mental status.

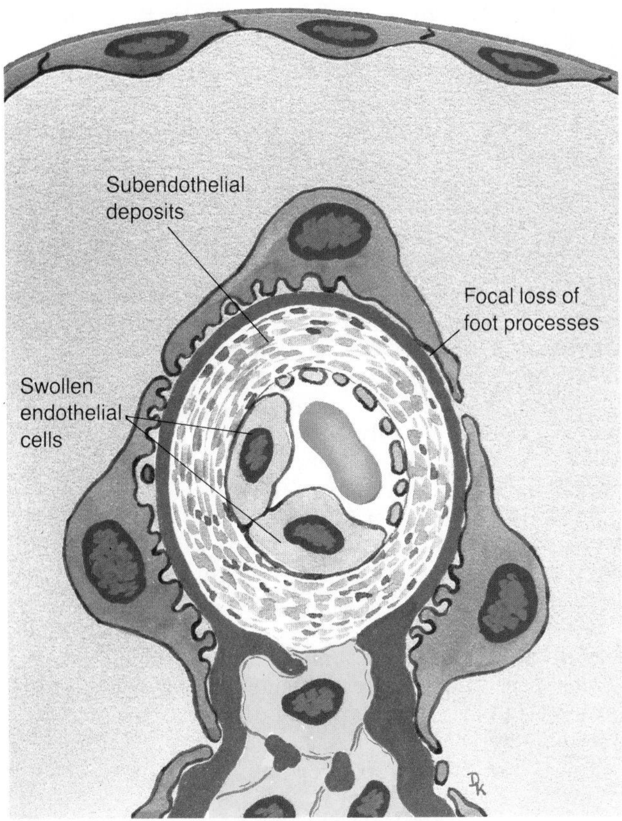

FIGURE *16-61*
Hemolytic-uremic syndrome. A wide band of subendothelial electron-lucent material narrows the capillary lumen. Moderate endothelial cell proliferation and focal irregular areas of endothelial cell swelling contribute to narrowing of the lumen. Focal effacement of epithelial foot processes is noted.

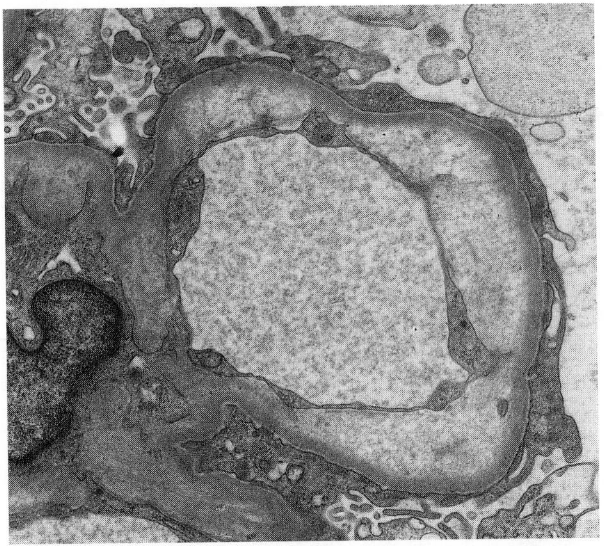

FIGURE *16-62*
Thrombotic microangiopathy. An electron micrograph shows lucent expansion of the subendothelial zone.

Systemic sclerosis renal crisis occurs in the context of scleroderma systemic sclerosis.

Malignant nephrosclerosis is usually preceded by a history of benign hypertension.

Causes of thrombotic microangiopathy are listed in Table 16-9.

Preeclampsia

Preeclampsia is a complication of the third trimester of pregnancy that is characterized by the triad of hypertension, proteinuria, and edema. When these features are complicated by convulsions, the term ***eclampsia*** *is applied* (see Chapter 18). The kidney is by definition involved in preeclampsia. The glomeruli are uniformly enlarged, and the endothelial cells are swollen, an appearance that results in an apparently bloodless glomerular tuft (Fig. 16-63 and 16-64). An increase in the number and size of mesangial cells is usual. By electron microscopy the swollen endothelial and mesangial cells contain large, irregular vacuoles. Vacuoles are also present in the foot processes and the trabeculae of the epithelial cells. Mild and moderate disease can be controlled with bed rest and antihypertensive agents. Severe cases may require induction of delivery. Hypertension and proteinuria typically disappear 1 to 2 weeks after delivery.

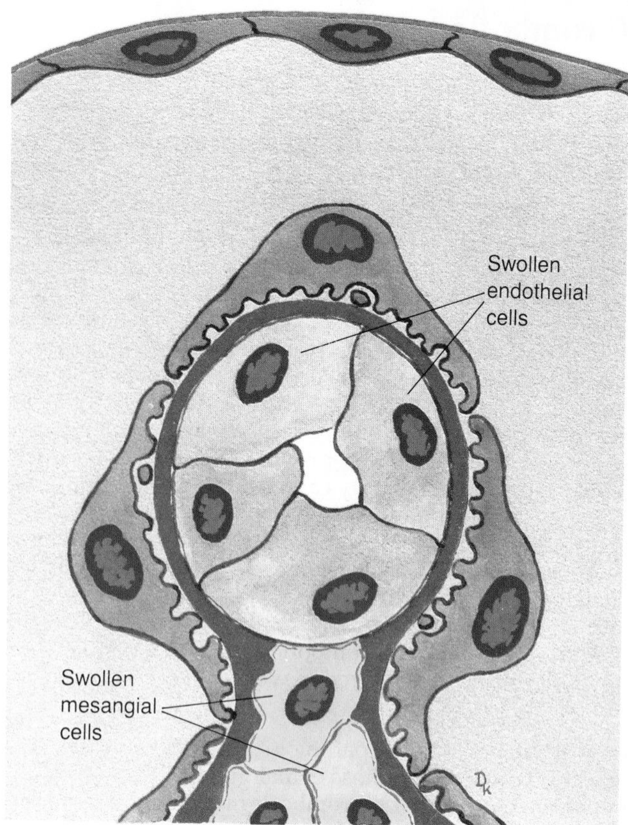

FIGURE 16-63
Preeclamptic nephropathy. Preeclamptic nephropathy, or pregnancy-induced nephropathy, exhibits marked swelling of endothelial cells with narrowing of the lumina. Both endothelial and mesangial cells are enlarged and have multiple vacuoles and vesicular structures.

Sickle Cell Nephropathy

Apart from the hematological abnormalities, the most common manifestations of sickle cell disease and sickle cell trait are in the kidney. The interstitial tissue in which the vasa recta course is hypertonic and has a low oxygen tension. As a result, the erythrocytes in the vasa recta tend to sickle and occlude the lumen. Infarcts in the medulla and papilla ensue, sometimes severe enough to cause papillary necrosis. Ischemic scarring of the medulla leads to focal tubular loss and atrophy. The glomeruli are conspicuously congested with sickle cells. Focal segmental glomerulosclerosis or, less commonly, membranoproliferative glomerulonephritis occurs in a minority of patients and may cause the nephrotic syndrome.

TABLE 16-9 **Causes of Thrombotic Microangiopathy**

Infections
Escherichia coli
Shigella
Pseudomonas
Drugs
Mitomycin
Cisplatin
Cyclosporin
FK506
Autoimmune diseases
Systemic sclerosis (scleroderma)
Systemic lupus erythematosus
Antiphospholipid antibody syndrome
Malignant hypertension
Pregnancy and postpartum factors

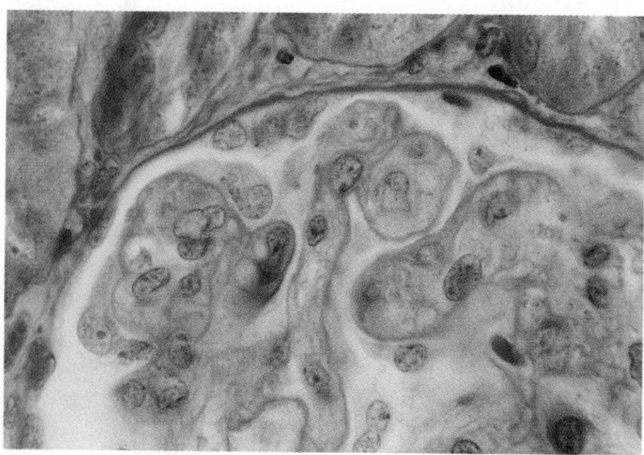

FIGURE 16-64
Preeclampsia. Capillary lumina are obliterated by swollen endothelial cells (Masson trichrome stain).

Renal Infarcts

Renal infarcts are, for the most part, caused by arterial obstruction, and the majority represent embolization to the branches of the main renal artery. The size of the infarct varies with the size of the occluded vessel. Common sources of emboli include the following:

- **Mural thrombi** overlying myocardial infarcts or caused by atrial fibrillation
- **Infected valves** in bacterial endocarditis
- **Complicated atherosclerotic plaques** in the aorta

Occasionally, a branch of the renal artery is occluded by thrombosis superimposed on underlying atherosclerosis or arteritis. The lumina of the small branches of the renal artery may be so severely compromised in malignant hypertension, scleroderma, or HUS that the blood supply is insufficient to maintain the viability of the tissue. Occlusion of small vessels by sickled erythrocytes in sickle cell anemia commonly causes renal infarcts, especially in the papillae. Hemorrhagic renal infarction caused by renal vein thrombosis may complicate severe dehydration, particularly in small infants, but it is also seen in adults with septic thrombophlebitis and conditions associated with hypercoagulability. Typically, an acute infarct is manifested clinically as sharp flank or abdominal pain and hematuria.

Infarction of an entire kidney by occlusion of the main renal artery is uncommon. When the main renal artery is occluded, it is more common for the kidney to remain viable because of collateral circulation. Clearly, in such a circumstance renal function ceases.

☐ **Pathology:** Variably sized, wedge-shaped areas of pale ischemic necrosis, with the base on the capsular surface, are typical (Fig. 16-65). All structures within the affected zone show coagulative necrosis. Acute infarcts are bordered by a hemorrhagic zone. As in other tissues, the histological response to the infarct progresses through phases of acute inflammation, granulation tissue, and fibrosis. Healed infarcts appear as sharply circumscribed and depressed cortical scars, containing ghosts of obliterated glomeruli, atrophic tubules, interstitial fibrosis, and a mild chronic inflammatory infiltrate. Dystrophic calcification is occasionally encountered in old infarcts. At the margins of a healed infarct, the viable tissue resembles that seen in chronic ischemia, with tubular atrophy, interstitial fibrosis, and infiltration by chronic inflammatory cells.

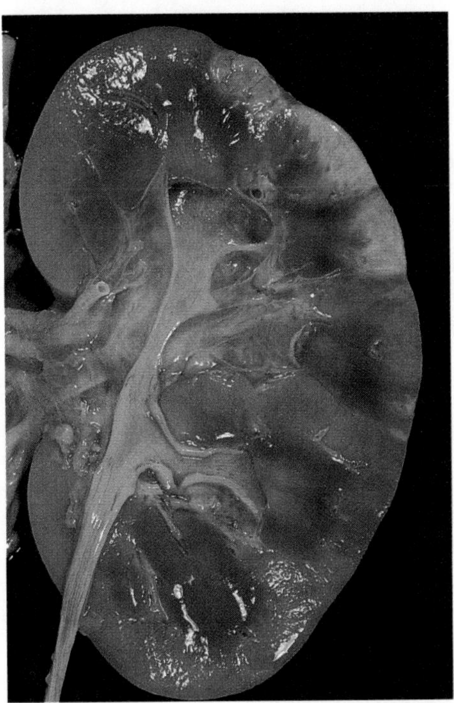

FIGURE *16-65*
Renal infarct. A cross-section of the kidney shows multiple areas of infarction characterized by marked pallor, which extends to the subcapsular surface.

Bilateral Cortical Necrosis

Cortical necrosis refers to ischemic necrosis of part or all of the renal cortex, with sparing of the medulla. The term infarct is used when there is one area (or a few areas) of necrosis caused by occlusion of arteries, whereas cortical necrosis implies more widespread ischemic necrosis.

☐ **Pathogenesis:** Historically, the most common clinical circumstance associated with renal cortical necrosis was premature separation of the placenta (abruptio placentae), a complication of the third trimester of pregnancy. Renal cortical necrosis can also complicate any clinical condition associated with hypovolemic or endotoxic shock. Since all forms of shock are associated with acute tubular necrosis, it is not surprising that there is an overlap between that condition and cortical necrosis, both clinically and pathologically.

The vasa recta that supply arterial blood to the medulla arise from the juxtamedullary efferent arterioles, proximal to the vessels supplying the outer cortex. Thus, occlusion of the outer cortical vessels, for example by vasospasm, fibrin thrombi, or a thrombotic microangiopathy, leads to cortical necrosis and sparing of the medulla. Experimentally, vasoconstrictors, such as vasopressin and serotonin, produce cortical necrosis. The experimental Schwartzman phenomenon, which is characterized by disseminated intravascular coagulation with widespread fibrin thrombi, also results in cortical necrosis.

☐ **Pathology:** The extent of the necrosis varies from patchy to confluent (Fig. 16-66). The mildest variety is characterized by scattered areas of cortical necrosis less than 1 mm in diameter. In the most severely involved areas, all parenchymal elements have coagulative necrosis. The proximal convoluted tubules are invariably necrotic, as are most of the distal tubules. In the viable portions of the cortex, the glomeruli and distal convoluted tubules are unaffected, but many of the proximal convoluted tubules are necrotic.

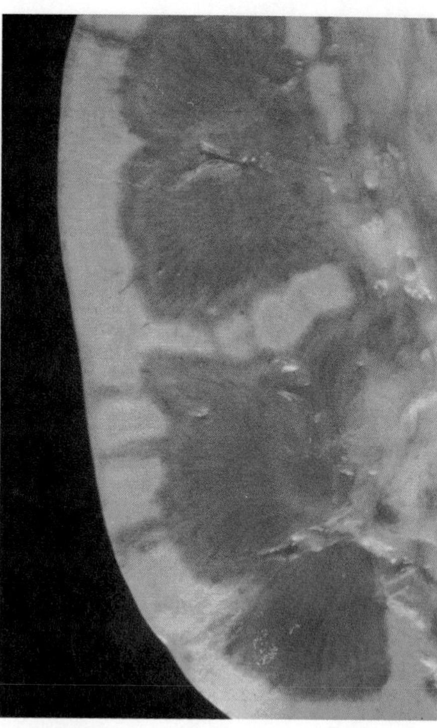

FIGURE *16-66*
Renal cortical necrosis. The cortex of the kidney is pale yellow and soft, owing to diffuse cortical necrosis.

TABLE *16-10* **Causes of Acute Tubular Necrosis**

Causes
Ischemia
Massive hemorrhage
Septic shock
Severe burns
Dehydration
Prolonged diarrhea
Congestive heart failure
Volume redistribution (e.g., pancreatitis, peritonitis)
Nephrotoxins
Antibiotics (e.g., aminoglycosides, amphotericin B)
Radiographic contrast agents
Heavy metals (e.g., mercury, lead, cisplatin)
Organic solvents (e.g., ethylene glycol, carbon tetrachloride)
Poisons (e.g., paraquat)
Heme proteins
Myoglobin (from rhabdomyolysis, e.g., with crush injury)
Hemoglobin (from hemolysis, e.g., with transfusion reaction)

With more extensive necrosis, the cortex shows a marked pallor. The cortex is diffusely necrotic, except for thin rims of viable tissue immediately beneath the capsule and at the corticomedullary junction, which are supplied by capsular and medullary collateral blood vessels respectively. Patients who survive may develop striking dystrophic calcification of the necrotic areas.

□ **Clinical Features:** Severe cortical necrosis manifests as acute renal failure, which may be indistinguishable from that produced by acute tubular necrosis. A renal arteriogram or biopsy may be required for diagnosis. Recovery is determined by the extent of the disease, but there is a significant incidence of hypertension among survivors.

DISEASES OF TUBULES AND INTERSTITIUM

Acute Tubular Necrosis

Acute tubular necrosis (ATN) is a severe but potentially reversible impairment of tubular epithelial function caused by ischemia or toxic injury, which results in acute renal failure.

□ **Pathogenesis:** The causes of ATN are listed in Table 16-10.

Ischemic ATN results from reduced renal perfusion, usually associated with hypotension. Tubular epithelial cells, with their high rate of energy-consuming metabolic activity and numerous organelles, are particularly sensitive to hypoxia and anoxia, which cause rapid depletion of intracellular ATP in the tubular epithelium.

Nephrotoxic ATN is caused by chemically induced injury to epithelial cells. Tubular epithelial cells are preferred targets for certain toxins because they absorb and concentrate the toxins. The high rate of energy consumption by epithelial cells also makes them susceptible to injury by toxins that perturb oxidative or other metabolic pathways. Hemoglobin and myoglobin can be considered endogenous toxins that can induce ATN (*pigment nephropathy*) when they are present in the urine in high concentrations.

The pathophysiology of ATN appears to involve some or all of the following perturbations (Fig. 16-67), various combinations of which result in a reduced glomerular filtration rate and tubular epithelial dysfunction:

- Intrarenal vasoconstriction
- Alteration of arteriolar tone by tubuloglomerular feedback
- Decreased glomerular hydrostatic pressure
- Decreased glomerular capillary permeability (K_f)
- Tubular obstruction by cellular debris with increased hydrostatic pressure
- Backleak of glomerular filtrate into the interstitium through damaged tubular epithelium

□ **Pathology:** **Ischemic ATN** is characterized by swollen kidneys, which have a pale cortex and a congested medulla. No pathological changes are seen in the glomeruli or blood vessels. Tubular injury is focal and is most pronounced in the proximal tubules and ascending limb of the loop of Henle. The tubules have focal flattening of the epithelium, with dilatation of the lumina and loss of the brush border (epithelial simplification). This re-

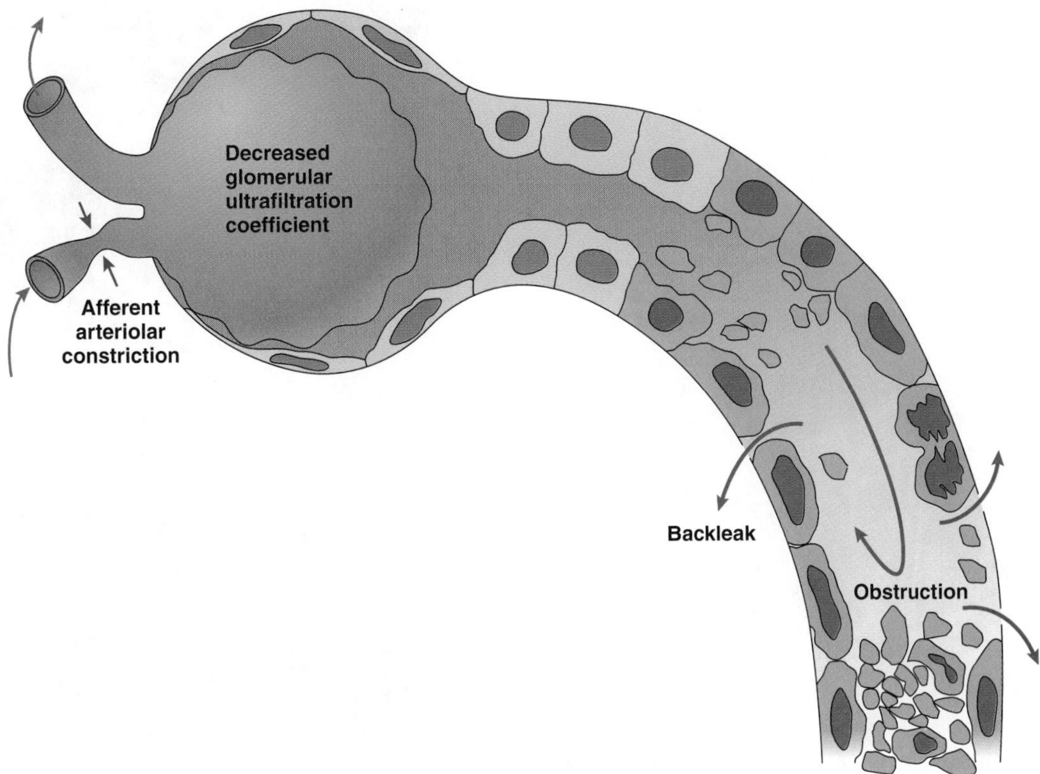

FIGURE *16-67*
Pathogenesis of acute tubular necrosis. Sloughing and necrosis of epithelial cells result in cast formation. The presence of casts leads to obstruction and increased intraluminal pressure, which reduce glomerular filtration. Afferent arteriolar vasoconstriction, caused in part by tubuloglomerular feedback, results in decreased glomerular capillary filtration pressure. Tubular injury and increased intraluminal pressure cause fluid backleak from the lumen into the interstitium.

sults in part from sloughing of the apical cytoplasm, which appears in the distal tubular lumina and urine as brown granular casts. The color reflects cytochrome pigments. Electron microscopy confirms the loss of the proximal tubular brush border and also demonstrates decreased infoldings at the basolateral membrane of proximal tubular epithelial cells. A characteristic feature of ischemic ATN is the absence of widespread necrosis of tubular epithelial cells (although simplification may be prominent). Instead, "necrosis" is more subtle and is reflected in individual necrotic cells within some proximal or distal tubules. These single necrotic cells are shed into the tubular lumen, with resulting focal denudation of the tubular basement membrane (Fig 16-68). Interstitial edema is common. The vasa recta of the outer medulla are congested and frequently contain nucleated cells, which are actually mononuclear leukocytes.

Toxic ATN differs morphologically from ischemic ATN in that the former is characterized by more extensive necrosis of the tubular epithelium (compare Figs. 16-68 and 16-69). In most cases, however, the necrosis is limited to certain tubular segments (most often all or specific portions of the proximal tubule) that are most sensitive to the toxin. ATN caused by hemoglobin or myoglobin has the added feature of numerous red-brown tubular casts, colored by heme pigments.

During the recovery phase of ATN, the tubular epithelium regenerates, leading to the appearance of mitoses, increased size of cells and nuclei, and cell crowding. Survivors eventually display complete restoration of normal renal architecture.

☐ Clinical Features: **ATN is the leading cause of acute renal failure.** It manifests as rapidly rising serum creatinine, which is usually associated with decreased urine output (oliguria). Less commonly, ATN induces nonoliguric acute renal failure. Urinalysis demonstrates degenerating epithelial cells and **dirty brown granular casts** (acute renal failure casts), which contain cellular debris that is rich in cytochrome pigments. Urinalysis is useful in differentiating among the three major intrinsic renal diseases that cause acute renal failure (Table 16-11).

In patients with ATN, the duration of renal failure depends on many factors, especially the nature and reversibility of the cause. Many patients, at least transiently develop uremia, with azotemia, fluid retention, metabolic acidosis, and hyperkalemia, and may require dialysis. If the cause is immediately removed after the initiation of the injury, recovery of renal function often occurs within 1 to 2 weeks, although it may be delayed for months. The recovery phase is heralded by an increase in urine output and a fall in serum creatinine.

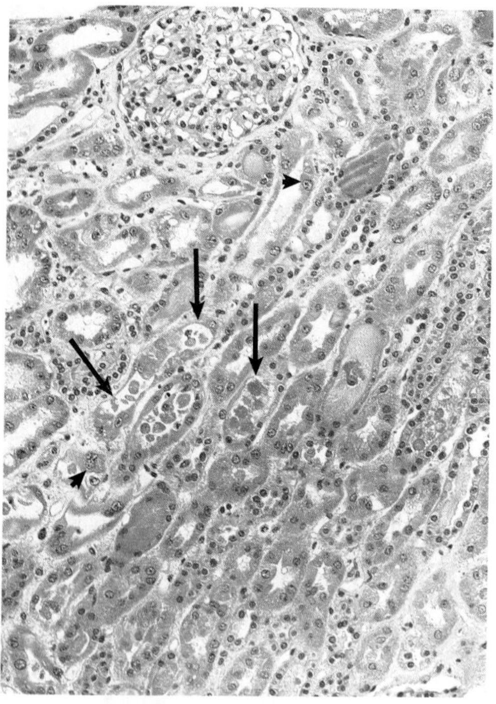

FIGURE 16-68
Ischemic acute tubular necrosis. Necrosis of individual tubular epithelial cells is evident both from focal denudation of the tubular basement membrane (*arrows*) and from the individual necrotic epithelial cells present in some tubular lumina. Some enlarged, regenerative-appearing epithelial cells are also present (*arrowheads*). Note the lack of significant interstitial inflammation.

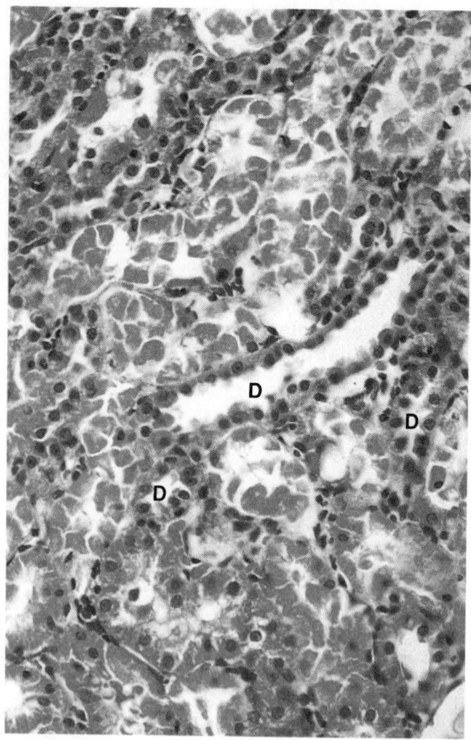

FIGURE 16-69
Toxic acute tubular necrosis due to mercury poisoning. There is widespread necrosis of proximal tubular epithelial cells, with sparing of distal and collecting tubules (D). Interstitial inflammation is minimal.

Pyelonephritis

Pyelonephritis refers to inflammation of the renal parenchyma, calyces, and pelvis caused by bacterial infection.

Acute Pyelonephritis

☐ **Pathogenesis: Gram-negative bacteria from the feces, most commonly *E. coli*, cause 80% of acute pyelonephritis.** The infection reaches the kidney by ascending through the urinary tract, a process that depends on several factors:

- Bacterial infection of the urine
- Reflux of the infected urine up the ureters into the renal pelvis and calyces
- Entry of the bacteria through the papillae into the renal parenchyma

Infection of the bladder precedes acute pyelonephritis. Bladder infection is more common in females because of a short urethra, lack of antibacterial prostatic secretions, and facilitation of bacterial migration by sexual intercourse. In some women who are unusually vulnerable to recurrent attacks of urinary tract infection, the normal commensal flora of the urethra is replaced by fecal organisms. This change in bacterial flora may reflect poor hygiene, hormonal effects, and genetic predisposition (e.g., increased numbers of receptors for *E. coli* on urothelial cells).

Asymptomatic bacteriuria occurs in 10% of pregnant women, one fourth of whom develop acute pyelonephritis. This increased incidence of acute pyelonephritis in pregnancy can also be attributed to an increased residual urine volume. Under the influence of high levels of progesterone, the bladder musculature becomes flaccid and does not expel the urine with its customary efficiency.

During micturition, the bladder normally empties all but 2 to 3 mL of residual urine. The subsequent addition of sterile urine from the kidneys dilutes any bacteria that may have found their way into the bladder. Under some circumstances, the residual urine volume is increased, for

TABLE 16-11 **Urinalysis in Acute Renal Failure**

Causes of Acute Renal Failure	Urinalysis Findings
Acute tubular necrosis	Dirty brown casts and epithelial cells
Acute glomerulonephritis	Red blood cell casts and proteinuria
Acute tubulointerstitial nephritis	White blood cell casts and pyuria

example, in prostatic obstruction or in an atonic bladder caused by neurogenic disorders, such as paraplegia or diabetic neuropathy. As a result, the bladder contents are not sufficiently diluted with sterile urine from the kidneys to prevent the accumulation of bacteria. The glycosuria of diabetes also predisposes to infection by providing a rich medium for bacterial growth.

Bacteria in the bladder urine usually do not gain access to the kidneys. The ureter commonly inserts into the bladder wall at a steep angle (Fig. 16-70) and in its most distal portion courses parallel to the bladder wall between the mucosa and muscularis. The intravesicular pressure produced by micturition occludes the distal lumen of the ureter, thereby preventing reflux of urine. In many persons who are particularly susceptible to pyelonephritis, an abnormally short passage of the ureter within the bladder wall is associated with an angle of insertion that is more perpendicular to the mucosal surface of the bladder. Thus, on micturition, rather than occluding the lumen, intravesicular pressure forces urine into the patent ureter. This reflux is sufficiently powerful to force the urine into the renal pelvis and calyces.

Even when present in the calyces, bacteria are not necessarily carried into the renal parenchyma by the reflux pressure. The simple papillae of the central calyces are convex and do not readily admit reflux urine (see Fig. 16-70). By contrast, the concave shape of the peripheral compound papillae allows easier access to the collecting

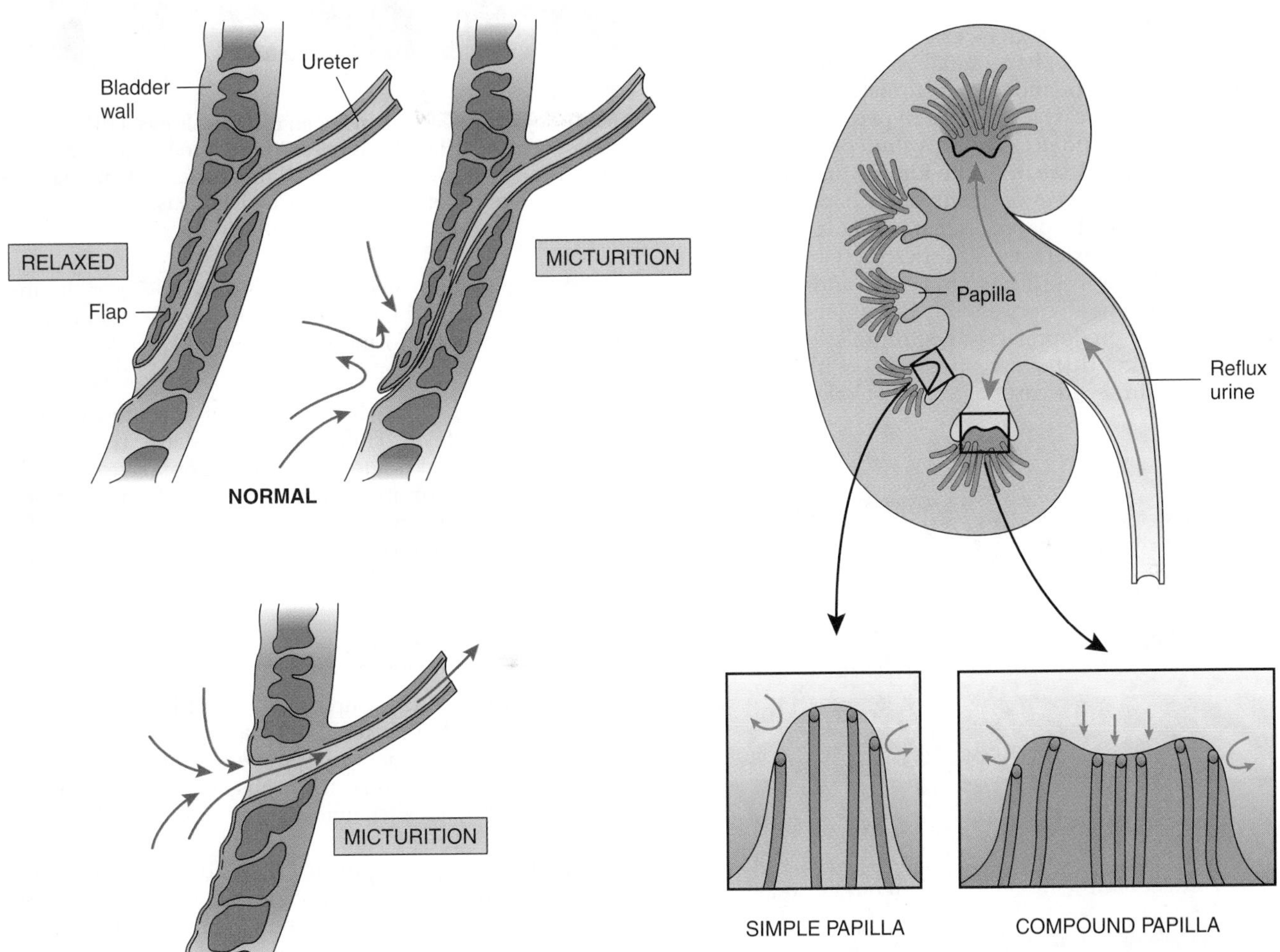

FIGURE *16-70*
Anatomical features of the bladder and kidney in pyelonephritis caused by ureterovesical reflux. In the normal bladder, the distal portion of the intravesical ureter courses between the mucosa and the muscularis, forming a mucosal flap. On micturition, the elevated intravesicular pressure compresses the flap against the bladder wall, thereby occluding the lumen. Persons with a congenitally short intravesical ureter have no mucosal flap, because the angle of entry of the ureter into the bladder approaches a right angle. Thus, micturition forces urine into the ureter. In the renal pelvis, simple papillae of the central calyces are convex and do not readily allow reflux of urine. By contrast, the peripheral compound papillae are concave and permit entry of refluxed urine.

system. However, if the pressure is prolonged, as in obstructive uropathy, even the simple papillae are eventually rendered vulnerable to the retrograde entry of urine. From the collecting tubules, the bacteria gain access to the interstitial tissue and other tubules of the kidney.

In addition to ascending through the urine, bacteria and other pathogens can gain access to the renal parenchyma through the blood. For example, gram-positive organisms, such as staphylococci, can disseminate from an infected valve in bacterial endocarditis and establish a focus of infection in the kidney. The kidney is commonly involved in miliary tuberculosis. Fungi, such as *Aspergillus*, can seed the kidney in an immunocompromised host. Hematogenous infections of the kidney preferentially affect the cortex.

☐ **Pathology:** On gross examination, the kidneys of acute pyelonephritis have small white abscesses on the subcapsular surface and on cut surfaces. The urothelium of the pelvis and calyces may be hyperemic and covered by a purulent exudate. **Acute pyelonephritis often is a focal disease, and much of the kidney may appear normal.** Most infections involve only a few papillary systems. Microscopically, the parenchyma, particularly the cortex, typically shows extensive focal destruction by the acute inflammatory process, although vessels and glomeruli often are preferentially preserved. The inflammatory infiltrates contain predominantly neutrophils. Tubules, especially collecting ducts, are often filled with neutrophils (Fig. 16-71). In severe cases of acute pyelonephritis, necrosis of the papillary tips may occur (Fig. 16-72) or the infection may extend beyond the renal capsule, resulting in perinephric abscess formation.

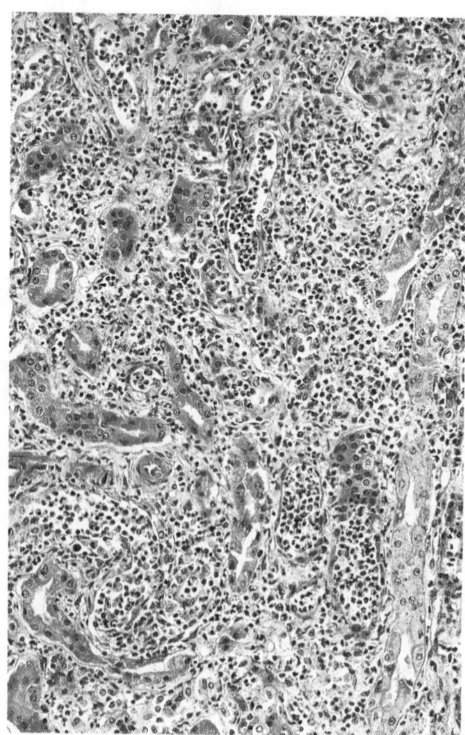

FIGURE *16-71*
Acute pyelonephritis. An extensive infiltrate of neutrophils is present in the collecting tubules and interstitial tissue.

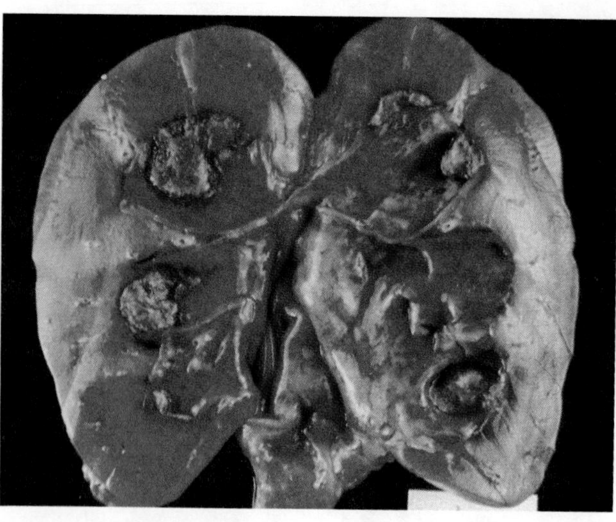

FIGURE *16-72*
Papillary necrosis. The bisected kidney shows a dilated renal pelvis and dilated calyces secondary to urinary tract obstruction. The papillae are all necrotic and appear as sharply demarcated, ragged, yellowish areas.

☐ **Clinical Features:** Symptoms of acute pyelonephritis include fever, chills, sweats, malaise, flank pain, and costovertebral angle tenderness. Leukocytosis with neutrophilia is common. The differentiation of upper from lower urinary tract infection is often clinically difficult, but the finding of **leukocyte casts** in the urine supports a diagnosis of pyelonephritis.

Chronic Pyelonephritis

☐ **Pathogenesis:** Chronic pyelonephritis is caused by recurrent and persistent bacterial infection secondary to urinary tract obstruction, urine reflux, or both (Fig. 16-73). Whether urine reflux in the absence of infection can produce pathological changes identical to chronic pyelonephritis is controversial.

In chronic pyelonephritis caused by either reflux or obstruction, the medullary tissue and overlying cortex are preferentially injured by recurrent acute and chronic inflammation. Progressive atrophy and scarring ensue, with resultant contraction of the involved papillary tip (or sloughing if there is papillary necrosis) and thinning of the overlying cortex. **This process results in the distinctive gross appearance of a broad depressed area of cortical fibrosis and atrophy overlying a dilated calyx (*caliectasis*)** (Fig. 16-74).

☐ **Pathology:** The histology of chronic pyelonephritis is nonspecific. Many diseases that cause chronic injury to the tubulointerstitial compartment induce chronic interstitial inflammation, interstitial fibrosis, and tubular atrophy. Thus, chronic pyelonephritis is only one of many causes of the pattern of injury termed *chronic tubulointer-*

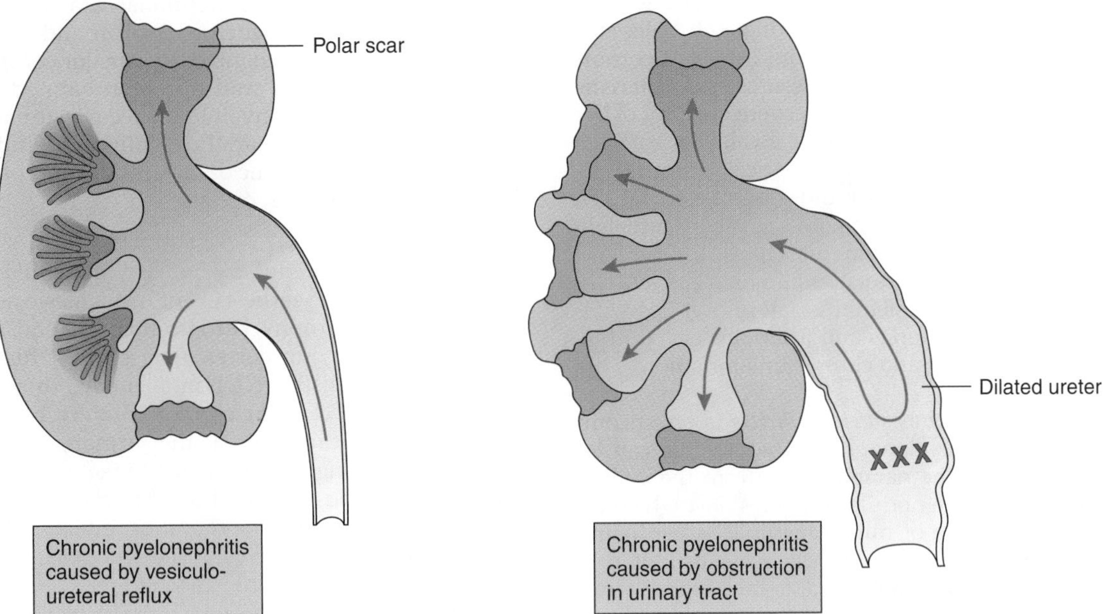

FIGURE 16-73
The two major types of chronic pyelonephritis. (*Left*) Vesicoureteral reflux causes infection of the peripheral compound papillae and, therefore, scars in the poles of the kidney. (*Right*) Obstruction of the urinary tract leads to high-pressure backflow of urine, which causes infection of all papillae, diffuse scarring of the kidney, and thinning of the cortex.

stitial nephritis. The gross appearance of chronic pyelonephritis is more distinctive. Only chronic pyelonephritis and analgesic nephropathy produce a combination of calyceal deformity and dilatation (*caliectasis*) with overlying corticomedullary scarring. In obstructive uropathy, all of the calyces and the renal pelvis are dilated, and the parenchyma is uniformly thinned (see Fig. 16-74). In cases associated with vesicoureteral reflux, the calyces at the poles of the kidney are preferentially expanded and are associated with overlying discrete, coarse

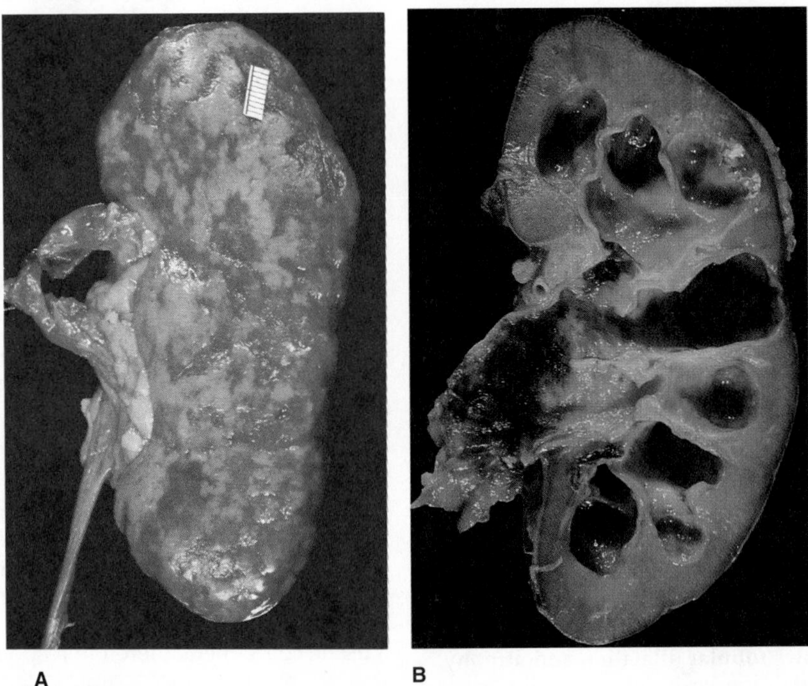

FIGURE 16-74
Chronic pyelonephritis. (*A*) The cortical surface contains many irregular, depressed scars (*reddish areas*). (*B*) There is marked dilatation of calyces (caliectasis) caused by inflammatory destruction of papillae, with atrophy and scarring of the overlying cortex.

scars, which cause an indentation of the renal surface. Microscopically, the scars have atrophic dilated tubules surrounded by interstitial fibrosis and infiltrates of chronic inflammatory cells (Fig. 16-75). The most characteristic (but not specific) tubular change is severe atrophy of the epithelium, with diffuse, eosinophilic, hyaline casts. Such tubules, which are "pinched-off" spherical segments, resemble colloid-containing thyroid follicles, a pattern called "thyroidization." The glomeruli may be completely uninvolved, may have periglomerular fibrosis, or may be sclerotic. The loss of most functioning nephrons may induce secondary focal segmental glomerulosclerosis. Fibrosis of the walls of arteries and arterioles is common. There is marked scarring and chronic inflammation of the calyceal mucosa.

Xanthogranulomatous pyelonephritis is an uncommon form of chronic pyelonephritis that is often caused by *Proteus* infection. The name derives from the yellow gross appearance of the nodular renal lesions, which results from the presence of numerous lipid-laden foamy macrophages *(xanthoma cells)*. The disease is usually unilateral. The clinical and pathological features can be confused with renal cell carcinoma.

☐ **Clinical Features:** Most patients with chronic pyelonephritis have recurrent manifestations of urinary tract infection or acute pyelonephritis, such as recurrent fever and flank pain. Occasional patients have a silent course until end-stage renal disease develops. Urinalysis demonstrates leukocytes, and imaging studies reveal caliectasis and cortical scarring.

Analgesic Nephropathy

Analgesic nephropathy is defined as chronic inflammation and scarring of the renal parenchyma caused by the use of analgesic drugs. **Patients typically have consumed more than 2 kg of analgesic compounds.** Incriminated analgesics often occur in combinations, such as aspirin and phenacetin. Phenacetin has been recognized as a major contributor to analgesic nephropathy and has been banned in many countries. The pathophysiological basis for analgesic nephropathy is not clear. Possibilities include direct nephrotoxicity or ischemic damage as a result of drug-induced vascular changes, or both.

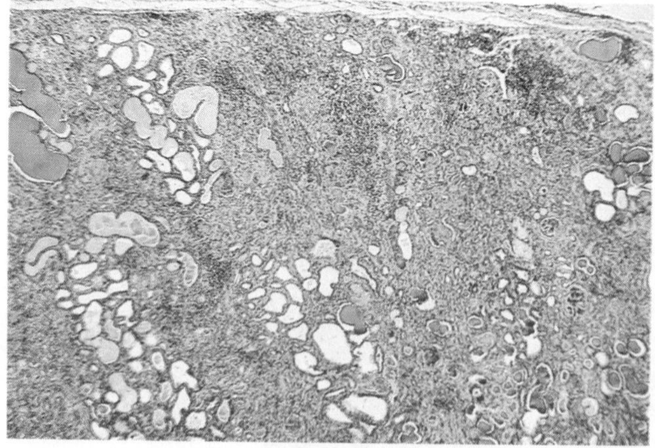

FIGURE *16-75*
A light micrograph shows tubular dilatation and atrophy, with many tubules containing eosinophilic hyaline casts resembling the colloid of thyroid follicles (so-called thyroidization). The interstitium is scarred and contains a chronic inflammatory cell infiltrate.

☐ **Pathology:** Medullary injury with papillary necrosis appears to be the earliest event in analgesic nephropathy, followed by atrophy, chronic inflammation, and scarring of the overlying cortex. The earliest histological abnormality is a distinctive **homogeneous thickening of the walls of the capillaries immediately beneath the transitional epithelium** of the urinary tract. Early parenchymal changes are confined to the papillae and the inner medulla and consist of focal thickening of tubular and capillary basement membranes, interstitial fibrosis, and focal coagulative necrosis. These necrotic areas eventually become confluent and extend to the corticomedullary junction, after which the collecting ducts become involved. Few inflammatory cells are found around the necrotic foci. Eventually, the entire papilla becomes necrotic (*papillary necrosis*), often remaining in place as a structureless mass. In such circumstances, dystrophic calcification of the necrotic papilla is common. Papillae may have incomplete detachment at the demarcation zone, or they may be completely sloughed. There is secondary tubular atrophy, interstitial fibrosis, and chronic inflammation in the overlying cortex.

☐ **Clinical Features:** Signs and symptoms occur only in the late stages of analgesic nephropathy and include an inability to concentrate the urine, distal tubular acidosis, hematuria, hypertension, and anemia. Sloughing of necrotic papillary tips into the renal pelvis may result in colic as they pass through the ureters. Progressive renal failure often develops and may lead to end-stage renal disease.

Drug-Induced (Hypersensitivity) Acute Tubulointerstitial Nephritis

Drug-induced acute nephritis refers to an acute inflammation of tubules and interstitium characterized by infiltrating lymphocytes and eosinophils.

☐ **Pathogenesis:** Acute drug-induced tubulointerstitial nephritis is characterized histologically by infiltrates of activated T lymphocytes and admixed eosinophils, a pattern that indicates a type IV cell-mediated immune response. The immunogen could be the drug itself, the drug bound to certain tissue components, a drug metabolite, or a tissue component altered in response to the drug. Drugs that are most commonly implicated include nonsteroidal anti-inflammatory drugs, diuretics, and certain antibiotics, especially β-lactam antibiotics, such as synthetic penicillins and cephalosporins.

☐ **Pathology:** Microscopically, there is patchy infiltration of the cortex, and to a much lesser extent the medulla, by lymphocytes and a small number of eosinophils (5% to 10% of the total leukocytes in the tissue) (Fig. 16-76). The eosinophils tend to be concentrated in small foci and may be seen within tubular lumina and in the urine. Neutrophils are rare, and their presence should raise suspicion of the possibility of pyelonephritis or hematogenous bacterial infection. Foci of granulomatous inflammation may be present, especially in the later phase of the disease. Proximal and distal tubules are focally invaded by white blood cells ("tubulitis"). Glomeruli and vessels are not inflamed, although some instances of drug-induced tubulointerstitial nephritis, usually caused by nonsteroidal anti-inflammatory drugs, are accompanied by minimal change glomerulopathy.

☐ **Clinical Features:** Acute tubulointerstitial nephritis usually presents as acute renal failure, typically about 2 weeks after drug administration is started. The urine contains erythrocytes, leukocytes (including eosinophils), and sometimes leukocyte casts. Tubular defects are common, including sodium wasting, glucosuria, aminoaciduria, and renal tubular acidosis. Systemic allergic symptoms such as fever and rash may also be present. Most patients recover fully within several weeks or months if the drug is discontinued.

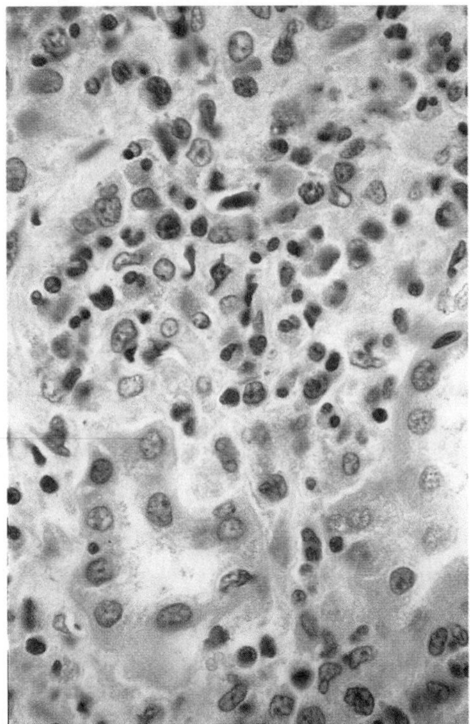

FIGURE *16-76*
Hypersensitivity tubulointerstitial nephritis. There is interstitial edema and infiltration by mononuclear leukocytes, with admixed eosinophils.

Multiple Myeloma Cast Nephropathy

Multiple myeloma cast nephropathy refers to renal injury caused by monoclonal immunoglobulin light chains in the urine that produce tubular epithelial injury and numerous tubular casts.

☐ **Pathogenesis:** As discussed earlier, multiple myeloma may produce AL amyloidosis, light-chain deposition disease, and light-chain cast nephropathy. The last is the most common form of renal disease associated with multiple myeloma and is caused by glomerular filtering of circulating light chains. At the acidic pH typical of urine, and possibly through interaction with other proteins in the urine (e.g., Tamm-Horsfall protein), light chains precipitate and cause obstruction. Renal dysfunction also results from the toxic effects of free light chains on tubular epithelial cells.

☐ **Pathology:** The characteristic tubular lesion exhibits numerous dense, hyaline casts in the distal tubules and collecting ducts (Fig. 16-77). These casts are brightly eosinophilic and glassy (hyaline) and often have fractures and angular borders. Occasionally, the casts have a crystalline appearance. The casts may induce a foreign body reaction, characterized by macrophages and multinucleated giant cells. Interstitial infiltrates of chronic inflammatory cells, as well as interstitial edema, typically accompany the tubular lesions. More chronic lesions show interstitial fibrosis and tubular atrophy. Focal calcium deposits (nephrocalcinosis) are also frequently noted in the fibrotic interstitium of the tubules. Immunohistochemical

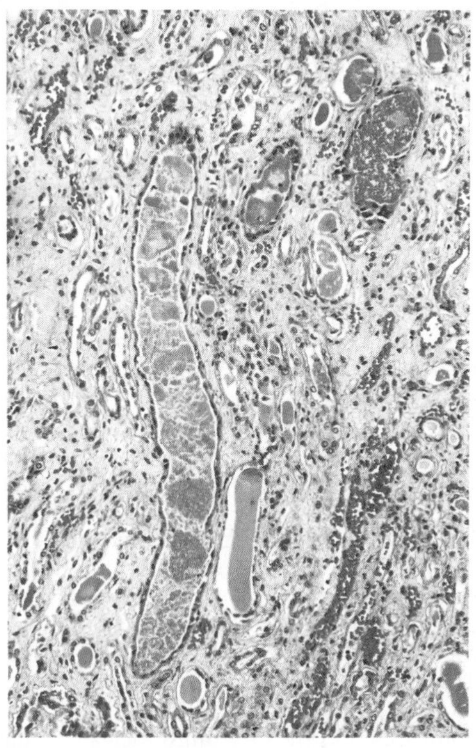

FIGURE *16-77*
Light-chain cast nephropathy. A light micrograph shows numerous casts within tubular lumina.

staining shows that the casts contain light-chain material, usually κ light chains.

☐ **Clinical Features:** Light-chain cast nephropathy may present as either acute or chronic renal failure. Proteinuria is usually present, although not in the nephrotic range, and most often consists predominantly of immunoglobulin light chains. If nephrotic range proteinuria is present in a patient with multiple myeloma, either AL amyloidosis or light-chain deposition disease is more likely than light-chain cast nephropathy.

Urate Nephropathy

Urate nephropathy is a renal disease caused by the deposition of urate crystals in the tubules and interstitium. Any condition associated with elevated levels of uric acid in the blood may cause urate nephropathy. The classic chronic disease in this category is primary gout, in which the biochemical basis of the hyperuricemia has not been fully established (see Chapter 26).

☐ **Pathogenesis:** **Chronic urate nephropathy** caused by gout is characterized by tubular and interstitial deposition of crystalline monosodium urate. **Acute urate nephropathy** can be caused by increased cell turnover (e.g., leukemia or polycythemia). For example, chemotherapy for malignant neoplasms results in a sudden increase in blood uric acid because of the massive necrosis of cancer cells (tumor lysis syndrome). Hepatic catabolism of large amounts of purines released from the DNA of necrotic cells leads to hyperuricemia. Acute renal failure reflects the obstruction of the collecting ducts by precipitated crystals of uric acid. This precipitation is promoted by the acidic pH of the urine in the presence of increased concentrations of uric acid. Conditions that interfere with the excretion of uric acid can also result in hyperuricemia, for example, the chronic intake of certain diuretics. Chronic lead intoxication also interferes with the proximal tubular secretion of uric acid and leads to *saturnine gout*.

☐ **Pathology:** In acute urate nephropathy, the precipitated uric acid in the collecting ducts is seen grossly as yellow streaks in the papillae. Histologically, the tubular deposits appear amorphous, but in frozen sections, birefringent crystals are apparent (Fig. 16-78). The tubules proximal to the obstruction are dilated. Penetration of collecting ducts by uric acid crystals may provoke a foreign-body giant cell reaction.

The basic disease process of chronic urate nephropathy is similar to that of the acute form, but the prolonged course results in a more substantial deposition of urate crystals in the interstitium, interstitial fibrosis, and cortical atrophy. The most diagnostic feature is the *gouty tophus*. Tophi are focal accumulations of urate crystals surrounded by inflammatory cells, which may appear granulomatous and include multinucleated giant cells. Uric acid stones, which account for one tenth of all cases of urolithiasis, occur in 20% of patients with chronic gout and in 40% of those with acute hyperuricemia.

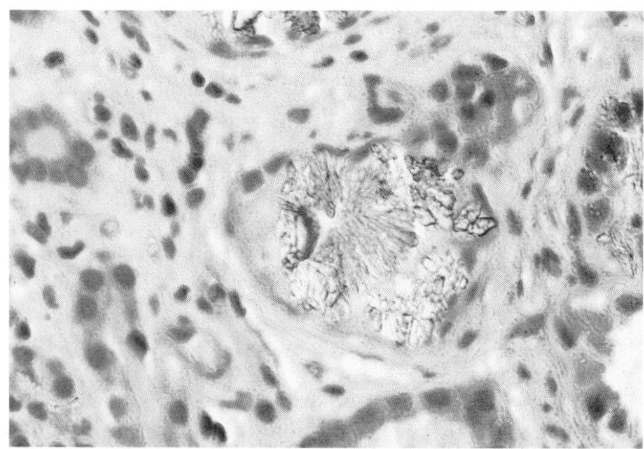

FIGURE *16-78*
Urate nephropathy. A frozen section demonstrates tubular deposits of uric acid crystals.

☐ **Clinical Features:** Acute urate nephropathy presents as acute renal failure, whereas chronic urate nephropathy causes chronic renal tubular defects. Although histological renal lesions are found in most persons with chronic gout, a significant compromise of renal function is seen in fewer than half.

Nephrocalcinosis

Nephrocalcinosis is defined as the deposition of calcium in the renal parenchyma.

☐ **Pathogenesis:** **Hypercalciuria** may result in nephrocalcinosis (Table 16-12) or the formation of calcium-containing stones (nephrolithiasis), or both. Nephrocalcinosis may cause abnormal renal function, especially tubular defects, such as impaired concentrating ability, salt wasting, and renal tubular acidosis.

Nephrocalcinosis caused by hypercalcemia is categorized as *metastatic calcification,* in contrast to calcification at sites of renal parenchymal injury (e.g., infarcts or cortical necrosis), which represents *dystrophic calcification*.

TABLE *16-12* **Causes of Hypercalcemia that Lead to Nephrocalcinosis**

Increased resorption of calcium from bone
Renal osteodystrophy
Primary hyperparathyroidism
Neoplasms producing parathormone or parathormone-like protein
Osteolytic neoplasms and metastases
Increased intestinal absorption of calcium
Idiopathic hypercalcemia
Vitamin D excess
Milk-alkali syndrome
Sarcoidosis

☐ **Pathology:** One fifth of kidneys at autopsy have small calcium deposits, which have no functional significance or recognized association with hypercalcemia. In patients with nephrocalcinosis caused by hypercalcemia, the extent of calcification varies from microscopic deposits to marked calcium accumulation visible grossly and radiologically. In the presence of severe hypercalcemia, typified by primary hyperparathyroidism, gross examination characteristically reveals wedge-shaped scars interspersed in relatively normal renal tissue. These scars reflect tubular atrophy and dilatation, with interstitial fibrosis secondary to obstruction of the larger collecting tubules by calcium concretions. There is also striking calcification of the basement membranes of the renal tubules, particularly those of the proximal convoluted tubules. The interstitial tissue also contains calcium deposits. Calcium deposits accumulate in the cytoplasm of tubular epithelial cells, which eventually degenerate and are sloughed into the lumina to aggregate as calcified casts. Scattered glomeruli show calcification of Bowman capsule, and the walls of intrarenal arteries may also be calcified. With hematoxylin, renal calcium deposits are deeply basophilic; with the more specific von Kossa stain, they are black. By electron microscopy, the mitochondria of renal tubular epithelial cells contain abundant calcium deposits.

RENAL STONES (NEPHROLITHIASIS AND UROLITHIASIS)

Nephrolithiasis and urolithiasis refer to stones within the collecting system of the kidney (nephrolithiasis) or elsewhere in the collecting system of the urinary tract (urolithiasis). The pelvis and calyces of the kidney are common sites for the formation and accumulation of calculi. Stones vary in composition, depending on individual factors, geography, metabolic alterations, and the presence of infection. For unknown reasons, renal stones are more common in men than in women. They vary in size from gravel (< 1 mm in diameter) to large stones that dilate the entire renal pelvis. Kidney stones may be well tolerated, but in some cases, they lead to severe hydronephrosis and pyelonephritis. Moreover, they can erode the mucosa and cause hematuria. The passage of a stone into the ureter causes excruciating flank pain, termed *renal colic*. Until recently, most kidney stones required surgical methods for their removal, but ultrasonic disintegration (lithotripsy) and endoscopic removal are now effective alternatives.

In most cases, the presence of a urinary stone is associated with an increased blood level and urinary excretion of its principal component. This is clearly the case with uric acid and cystine stones. However, in many patients with calcium stones, hypercalciuria is found in the absence of hypercalcemia. Mixed uric acid and calcium stones are common in the presence of increased uric acid excretion, because urate crystals act as a nidus around which calcium salts precipitate.

- **Calcium stones**: Some 75% of kidney stones contain calcium complexed with oxalate or phosphate, or a mixture of these anions. In the United States, calcium oxalate is more common, whereas in England, calcium phosphate predominates. A calcium oxalate stone is hard and occasionally dark, because it is covered by hemorrhage from the mucosa of the renal pelvis injured by the sharp calcium oxalate crystals. The calcium phosphate stone tends to be softer and paler.
- **Infection stones:** In the presence of infection with urea-splitting bacteria, usually *Proteus* or *Providencia* species, the resulting alkaline urine favors the precipitation of magnesium ammonium phosphate (struvite) and calcium phosphate (apatite). These stones vary in consistency from hard to soft and friable. Infection stones occasionally fill the pelvis and calyces to form a cast of these spaces, referred to as a *staghorn calculus* (Fig. 16-79). Infection stones are the most troublesome category of stones because they cause frequent complications, such as intractable urinary tract infection, pain, bleeding, perinephric abscess, and urosepsis.
- **Uric acid stones:** These stones occur in 25% of patients with hyperuricemia and gout, but most patients with uric acid stones do not have either condition (idiopathic urate lithiasis). The stones are smooth, hard, and yellow and are usually less than 2 cm in diameter. Importantly, in contrast to calcium-containing stones, pure uric acid stones are radiolucent.

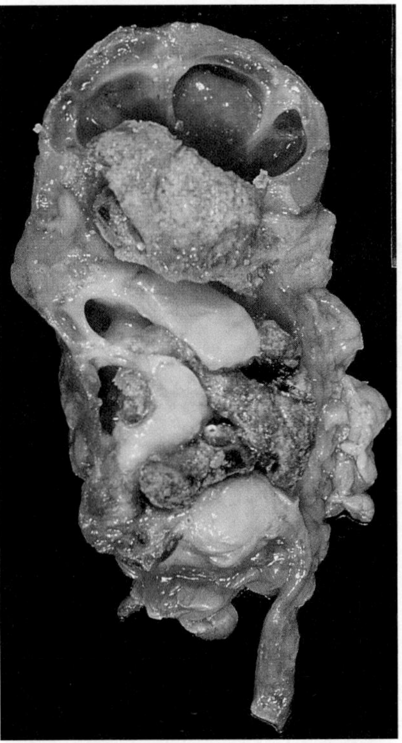

FIGURE *16-79*
Staghorn calculi. The kidney shows hydronephrosis and stones that are casts of the dilated calyces.

- **Cystine stones:** These stones are uncommon but represent a significant proportion of childhood calculi and occur exclusively with hereditary cystinuria. Although the stones are composed entirely of cystine, they may be enveloped by a layer of calcium phosphate.

OBSTRUCTIVE UROPATHY AND HYDRONEPHROSIS

Obstructive uropathy is caused by structural or functional abnormalities in the urinary tract that impede urine flow, which may cause renal dysfunction (obstructive nephropathy) and dilatation of the collecting system (hydronephrosis). The causes of urinary tract obstruction are discussed in detail in Chapter 17.

☐ **Pathology:** In early hydronephrosis, the most prominent microscopic finding is dilatation of the collecting ducts, followed by dilatation of the proximal and distal convoluted tubules. Eventually, the proximal tubules become widely dilated and loss of tubules is common. The glomeruli are usually spared. Grossly, progressive dilatation of the renal pelvis and calyces occurs, and atrophy of the renal parenchyma ensues (Fig. 16-80). In the presence of hydronephrosis, the kidney is more susceptible to pyelonephritis, which causes additional injury.

☐ **Clinical Features:** Bilateral acute urinary tract obstruction causes acute renal failure (*postrenal acute renal failure*). Unilateral obstruction is frequently asymptomatic and missed clinically. Because many causes of acute obstruction are reversible, prompt recognition is important. Left untreated, an obstructed kidney undergoes atrophy, and in the case of bilateral obstruction, chronic renal failure ensues.

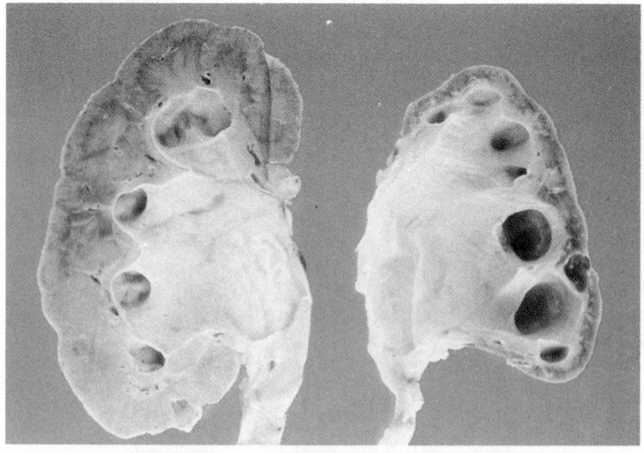

FIGURE *16-80*
Hydronephrosis. Bilateral urinary tract obstruction has led to conspicuous dilatation of the ureters, pelves, and calyces. The kidney on the right shows severe parenchymal atrophy.

RENAL TRANSPLANTATION

Renal transplantation is the treatment of choice for most patients with end-stage renal disease. The major obstacle is immunological rejection, but recurrence of the disease that destroyed the native kidneys and nephrotoxicity from immunosuppressive drugs also injure the renal allograft. Table 16-13 lists distinct, but often coexisting, patterns of humoral and cellular renal allograft rejection.

ABO blood group antigens and **human leukocyte antigens (HLAs)** are the two major groups of tissue antigens that are the principal targets of immune attack directed against the transplanted kidney. Incompatible ABO blood group antigens, expressed on endothelial cells as well as erythrocytes, are absolute barriers to a successful transplant. ABO-incompatible grafts encounter preformed, circulating antibodies, which bind to endothelial cells and cause immediate (hyperacute) rejection. The more commonly encountered (and more gradual) patterns of acute rejection and chronic rejection are caused primarily by donor–recipient differences in HLAs (major histocompatibility complex antigens, MHC), which are expressed on most cell membranes and are controlled by several closely related loci on chromosomes 6. Sensitization of kidney allograft recipients to HLAs produces both cell-mediated and antibody-mediated reactions. The pathogenesis of allograft rejection is discussed in detail in Chapter 4.

HYPERACUTE REJECTION: Hyperacute rejection is rare because of current compatibility testing, occurring in less than 0.5% of allografts. When recipient blood containing antibodies to major alloantigens (usually ABO or class I HLAs) begins flowing through allograft vessels, immediate binding of the antibodies to endothelial cells causes prompt and irreversible injury in minutes, which may become apparent intraoperatively by mottling, cyanosis, and poor tissue turgor of the graft. The complexing of antibodies with endothelial alloantigens induces complement activation, which attracts neutrophils. The cytotoxic effects of complement and neutrophil activation cause endothelial cell swelling, vacuolization, and lysis. The accumulation of neutrophils in glomerular capillaries is regarded as a sign of impending rejection. Endothelial cell changes are followed by platelet thrombi and later by fibrin thrombi. Interstitial

TABLE *16-13* **Patterns of Renal Allograft Rejection**

Category	Most Characteristic Lesions
Hyperacute rejection	Neutrophils, hemorrhage, and necrosis
Acute rejection	Tubulointerstitial or vascular inflammation
Mild (grade I)	Interstitial lymphocytes and tubulitis
Moderate (grade II)	Intimal arteritis
Severe (grade III)	Necrotizing arteritis with fibrinoid necrosis
Chronic rejection	Arterial intimal fibrosis, cortical atrophy

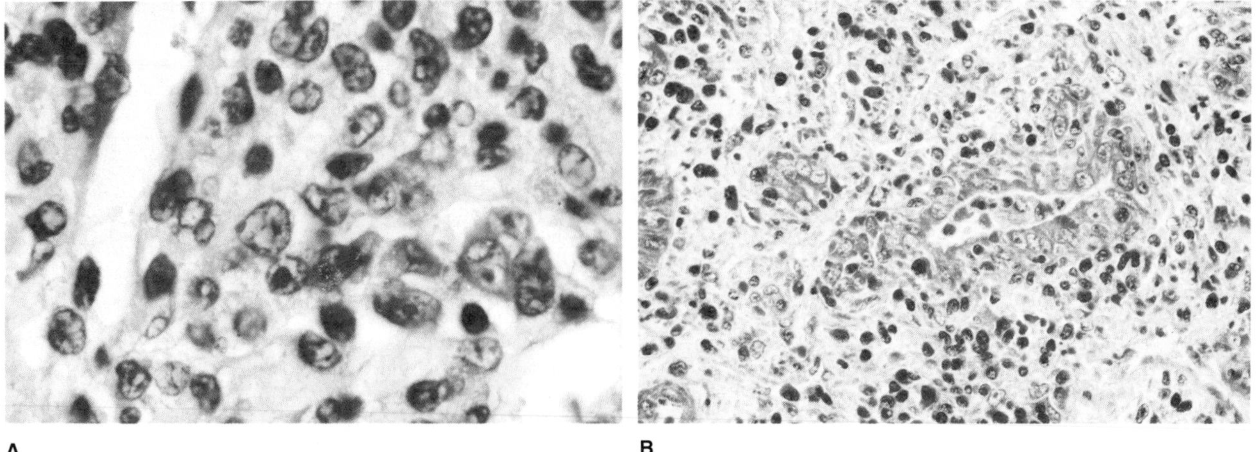

FIGURE 16-81
Acute cellular allograft rejection. (*A*) Large, activated lymphoid cells, including immunoblasts, are prominent in the interstitial infiltrate. (*B*) Lymphoid cells infiltrate through the wall of a tubule ("tubulitis"). The interstitium is edematous.

edema, hemorrhage, and cortical necrosis develop over the following 12 to 24 hours.

ACUTE REJECTION: The most severe but least common pattern of acute rejection is characterized by **necrotizing arteritis**, with fibrinoid necrosis involving the media. It occurs in less than 1% of allografts in patients whose immunosuppression includes cyclosporine A, although it occurred in 5% of renal allografts prior to the introduction of cyclosporine A therapy. Acute necrotizing rejection is mediated predominantly by antibodies, such as those to class I HLA antigens, although in some instances T cells play a major role. Once necrotizing arteritis develops, the chances of graft survival for 1 year are less than 25% even with aggressive immunosuppressive treatment.

Acute cellular rejection is the most common form of acute rejection and is characterized by infiltration of the interstitium, tubules, arteries, arterioles, or glomeruli by T lymphocytes and macrophages. The nuclei of the infiltrating lymphocytes are of variable sizes and shapes because the cells are at various stages of activation (Fig. 16-81A). Occasional cells are completely transformed into immunoblasts. Interstitial infiltrates are typically patchy rather than diffuse. Involvement of tubules (*tubulitis*) is manifested by lymphocytes crossing tubular basement membranes and lying between tubular epithelial cells (see Fig. 16-81B). Arterial involvement by cellular rejection results in the penetration of T lymphocytes and monocytes across the endothelium, resulting in an expanded intima filled with mononuclear leukocytes (*intimal arteritis*) (Fig. 16-82). Arterioles are occasionally involved by similar infiltration. Glomerular infiltration by mononuclear leukocytes with obliteration of capillary lumens (*acute transplant glomerulopathy*), is an uncommon manifestation of acute cellular rejection, and it indicates a worse prognosis than tubulitis or intimal arteritis. Renal transplants found to have tubulitis or intimal arteritis have a 65% to 75% chance for 1-year survival, compared to less than 40% with acute transplant glomerulopathy.

CHRONIC REJECTION: The pathological changes attributed to chronic rejection are listed in Table 16-14.

The arterial changes of chronic rejection affect a wide spectrum of vessels, ranging from small arteries to the main renal artery. There is prominent initial widening, caused by stromal cell proliferation and matrix deposition (Fig. 16-83). Mononuclear leukocytes within the vessel wall are much less prominent than with active intimal arteritis. Foam cells may be conspicuous, and there may be interruption of the internal elastic lamina. Peritubular capillaries have thickening and replication of basement membranes. Tubular atrophy and interstitial fibrosis may

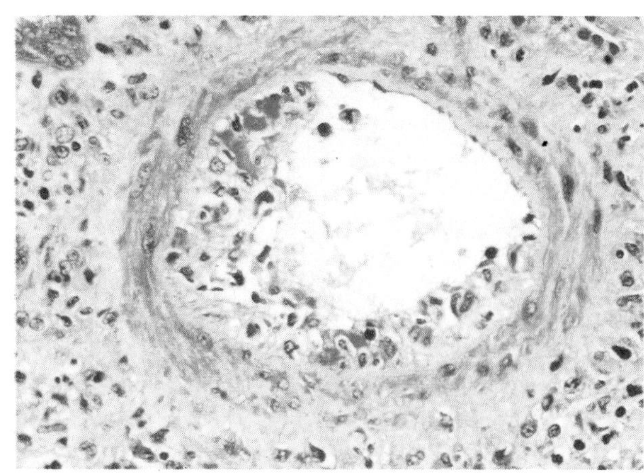

FIGURE 16-82
Acute allograft rejection with intimal arteritis. The intima is edematous and contains leukocytes and fibrin.

TABLE *16-14* **Histological Features of Chronic Renal Allograft Rejection**

Fibrotic intimal thickening of arteries
Tubular atrophy
Interstitial fibrosis
Interstitial mononuclear leukocytes
Glomerular capillary wall thickening and mesangial expansion
Glomerular sclerosis

be caused at least in part by ischemia secondary to the narrowing of arteries and peritubular capillaries. Tubulointerstitial injury may also result from indolent tubulitis. Glomerular involvement (*chronic transplant glomerulopathy*) manifests as thickening of capillary walls and mesangial widening. Electron microscopy demonstrates electron-lucent expansion of the subendothelial zone and occasional mesangial interposition and replication of basement membranes. The arterial, peritubular capillary, and glomerular injury all may result from persistent, low-level, immune injury to the vascular endothelium.

RECURRENCE OF KIDNEY DISEASE: The same disease that caused end-stage disease in the native kidneys can recur in a renal transplant. The frequency and significance of recurrence varies among different types of glomerular disease (Table 16-15).

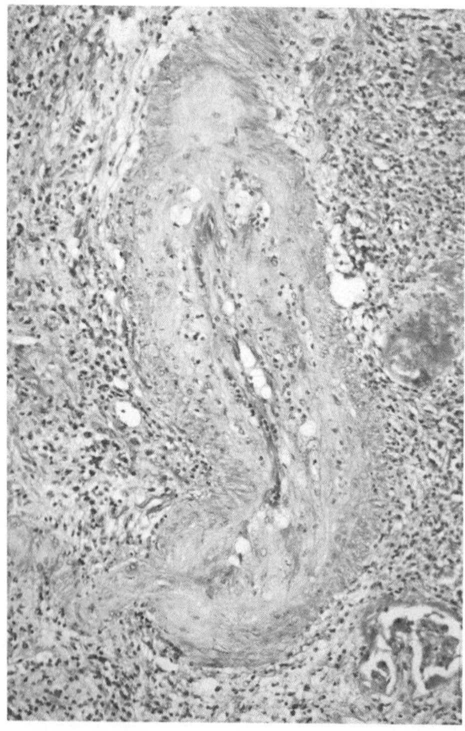

FIGURE *16-83*
Chronic allograft rejection. The lumen of this medium-sized artery is occluded by a thickened and fibrotic intima, which contains a few inflammatory cells.

TABLE *16-15* **Recurrence of Disease in Renal Allografts**

Disease	Recurrence Rate (%)	Rate of Graft Loss (%)
Type II membranoproliferative glomerulonephritis	>90	15
Diabetic glomerulosclerosis	>90	<5
IgA nephropathy	40	<10
Focal segmental glomerulosclerosis	35	30
Type I membranoproliferative glomerulonephritis	30	<10
Membranous glomerulopathy	20	<5
ANCA glomerulonephritis	10	<5
Anti-GBM glomerulonephritis	5	<5
Lupus glomerulonephritis	5	<5

ANCA, antineutrophil cytoplasmic autoantibody; GBM, glomerular basement membrane.

NEPHROTOXICITY OF CYCLOSPORINE A AND TACROLIMUS (FK506): Cyclosporine A and FK506 are effective immunosuppressive drugs that have dramatically improved not only the survival of kidney allografts, but also that of other allografts (e.g., liver, heart, and lungs). Unfortunately, both drugs injure kidney allografts, as well as the native kidneys of patients who are receiving immunosuppressive treatment for other reasons. The toxicity can cause acute or chronic renal failure.

The most characteristic renal lesion is an *arteriolopathy* that begins with smooth muscle cell degeneration and necrosis. The destroyed arteriolar muscle cells are replaced by acidophilic hyaline material (Fig. 16-84). In fulminant cases, the vascular lesions take on the appearance of a full-blown thrombotic microangiopathy, with circumferential fibrinoid necrosis of arterioles. Chronic toxicity has zones of interstitial fibrosis and tubular atrophy ("striped fibrosis").

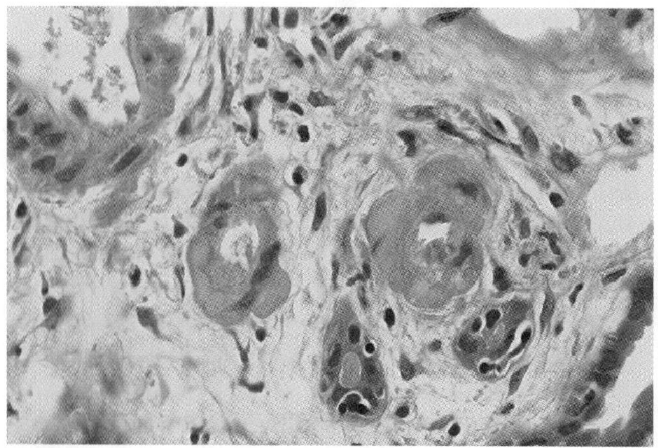

FIGURE *16-84*
Cyclosporine nephrotoxicity and arteriolopathy. Marked destructive hyalinosis of arterioles is present.

BENIGN TUMORS OF THE KIDNEY

RENAL ADENOMA: Whether any renal epithelial cell neoplasm should be designated an adenoma, a term that signifies no malignant potential, is controversial. Tumor size has been used as a criterion to separate adenomas from carcinomas, but this is problematic because all carcinomas begin as small lesions. Renal epithelial neoplasms less than 3 cm in diameter rarely metastasize, but "rarely" is not "never." Such small tumors are termed adenomas when they have well-demarcated margins and are composed of small cuboidal cells with round, regular nuclei. The cells may be arranged in closely packed tubules or papillary configurations. Neoplasms with clear cells that resemble renal cell carcinomas (clear cells) or oncocytomas (oncocytes) should not be designated adenomas even if they are small. When these criteria are used, most renal adenomas are in the outer cortex and are less than 1 cm in diameter.

RENAL ONCOCYTOMA: This tumor is composed of plump cells with abundant, finely granular, acidophilic cytoplasm, and with round nuclei without atypia. Electron microscopy demonstrates numerous mitochondria as the basis for the distinctive appearance of the cytoplasm. Grossly, oncocytomas have a characteristic mahogany-brown color, caused by the lipochrome pigments in the mitochondria.

MEDULLARY FIBROMA: Medullary fibromas (renomedullary interstitial cell tumors) are typically small (<0.5 cm in diameter), pale gray, well-circumscribed tumors, which are usually located in the midportion of the medullary pyramid. Histologically, the neoplasms are composed of small stellate to polygonal cells lying in a loose stroma. Renal medullary fibromas can be identified in half of all adult autopsies.

ANGIOMYOLIPOMA: Angiomyolipomas exhibit a haphazard admixture of well-differentiated adipose tissue, smooth muscle, and thick-walled vessels. Grossly, the tumors are yellow and bosselated and may resemble renal cell carcinoma. However, they are always well encapsulated and lack areas of necrosis. **Angiomyolipomas have a strong association with tuberous sclerosis.** Fully 80% of patients with tuberous sclerosis have angiomyolipomas, although less than 50% of patients with angiomyolipomas have tuberous sclerosis.

MESOBLASTIC NEPHROMA: Mesoblastic nephromas are congenital benign neoplasms, which are usually recognized during the first 3 months of life and must be differentiated from Wilms tumor. The tumors range from less than 1 cm in diameter to over 15 cm. Histologically, they are composed of spindle cells of fibroblastic or myofibroblastic lineage. Characteristically, the tumor margins are irregular, with bands of cells interdigitating with adjacent parenchyma. If some of these tongues of tumor tissue are left behind after surgical resection, local recurrence is possible.

MALIGNANT TUMORS OF THE KIDNEY

Wilms Tumor (Nephroblastoma)

Wilms tumor is a malignant neoplasm of embryonal nephrogenic elements composed of mixtures of blastemal, stromal, and epithelial tissue. It is the most frequent abdominal solid tumor in children, with a prevalence of 1 in 10,000.

☐ **Pathogenesis:** In the large majority (90%) of cases of Wilms tumor, the neoplasm is sporadic and unilateral. In 5% of the cases, however, Wilms tumor arises in the context of three different congenital syndromes, all of which include an increased risk for the development of this cancer at an early age and often bilaterally:

- **WAGR syndrome** (for **W**ilms tumor, **a**niridia, **g**enitourinary anomalies, mental **r**etardation)
- **Denys-Drash syndrome (DDS)** (Wilms tumor, intersexual disorders, glomerulopathy)
- **Beckwith-Wiedemann syndrome (BWS)** (Wilms tumor, overgrowth ranging from gigantism to hemihypertrophy, visceromegaly, and macroglossia)

Some 6% of cases of Wilms tumor are familial, have an early onset, and are bilateral but are not associated with any other syndrome.

Two decades ago, karyotypic analysis of children with WAGR syndrome revealed a deletion in the short arm of one copy of chromosome 11 (11p13). We now understand that the WAGR deletion affects contiguous genes, including PAX6, the aniridia gene, and **WT1, the Wilms tumor gene**. The loss or mutation of one WT1 allele leads to genitourinary anomalies, whereas a defect in the PAX6 gene is responsible for aniridia. One third of children with WAGR syndrome eventually develop Wilms tumor. The presence of a germline mutation in one WT1 allele and loss of heterozygosity at this locus in the tumors of WAGR syndrome imply that a second mutation in the normal WT1 allele is responsible for the appearance of Wilms tumor (similar to the pathogenesis of hereditary retinoblastoma) (see Chapter 5). In contrast to the deletions in WAGR syndrome, specific mutations of the WT1 gene characterize DDS. The fact that the phenotypic expression of the abnormalities in DDS is far more severe than that in WAGR syndrome suggests that mutated WT1 is actually a dysfunctional gene (dominant negative mutation).

WT1 is a tumor suppressor gene that functions as a regulator of the transcription of a number of other genes, including insulin-like growth factor-2 (IGF-2) and platelet-derived growth factor (PDGF). The WT1 gene protein also forms a complex with the p53 protein. **Whereas Wilms tumors arising in the context of WAGR syndrome all display defects of WT1, less than 10% of sporadic tumors exhibit abnormalities of WT1**. Thus, it is believed that other genes play a more critical role than does WT1 in the genesis of sporadic Wilms tumors.

A second gene for susceptibility to Wilms tumor (**WT2**) was discovered in sporadic tumors that showed loss of heterozygosity (LOH) on chromosome 11 (11p15), a site distinct from, but close to, the WT1 gene. WT2 is also linked to BWS. Interestingly, in LOH of the WT2 locus in sporadic Wilms tumors, the allele lost is invariably the maternal one. Importantly, some patients with BWS show a germline duplication of the paternal WT2 allele, and others have inherited both apparently normal copies of this gene from the father and none from the mother (*paternal uniparental isodisomy*). One possibility is that WT2 is normally expressed only by the paternal allele (*genomic imprinting*), and, therefore, overexpression of WT2 may be responsible for the overgrowth characteristic of BWS. Since the IGF-2 gene has also been mapped to chromosome 11p15 and is also paternally imprinted, it is possible that an increased dosage of IGF-2 might contribute both to BWS and to tumorigenesis. Another possibility is that WT2 is expressed only by the maternal allele acting as a tumor suppressor. Thus, loss of the maternal allele would contribute to tumorigenesis.

Nephrogenic rests (i.e., small foci of persistent primitive blastemal cells) are found in the kidneys of all children with syndromic Wilms tumors and in one third of sporadic cases. Since such rests in the nontumorous kidney have been demonstrated to contain the same somatic mutations in WT1 as are present in the tumors, it is thought that these rests represent clonal precursor lesions that are at least one step along the pathway to tumor formation.

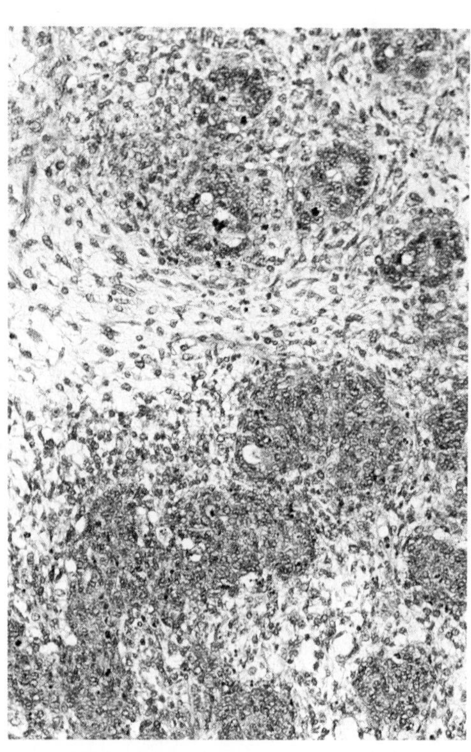

FIGURE *16-86*
Wilms tumor (nephroblastoma). This photomicrograph of the tumor shows highly cellular areas composed of undifferentiated blastema, loose stroma containing undifferentiated mesenchymal cells, and immature tubules.

☐ **Pathology:** Wilms tumor tends to be large when detected, with a bulging, pale-tan, cut surface enclosed within a thin rim of renal cortex and capsule (Fig. 16-85). Histologically, the tumor is composed of elements that resemble normal fetal tissue (Fig. 16-86), including (1) metanephric blastema, (2) immature stroma (mesenchymal tissue), and (3) immature epithelial elements.

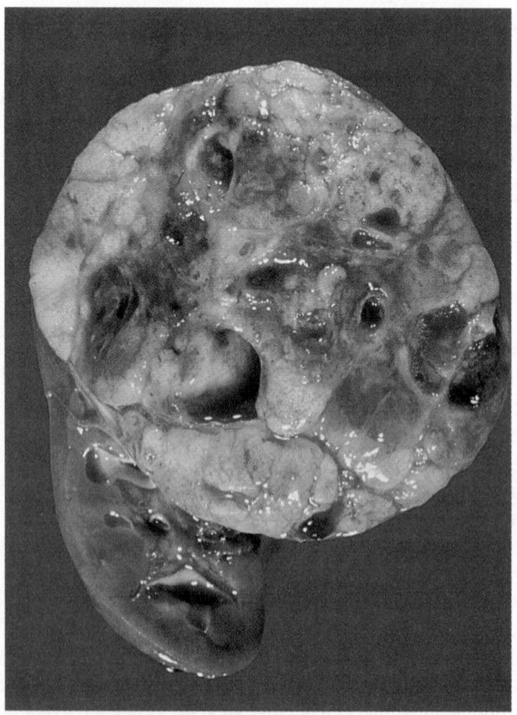

FIGURE *16-85*
Wilms tumor. A cross-section of a pale tan neoplasm is attached to a residual portion of the kidney.

Although most Wilms tumors contain all three elements in varying proportions, occasional ones contain only two elements or even only one. The component corresponding to blastema is composed of small ovoid cells with scanty cytoplasm, growing in nests and trabeculae. The epithelial component appears as small tubular structures. In some cases, structures resembling immature glomeruli are found. The stroma between the other elements is composed of spindle cells, which are mostly undifferentiated but occasionally display smooth muscle or fibroblast differentiation. Skeletal muscle is the most common heterotopic stromal element, although bone, cartilage, fat, or neural tissue may rarely be encountered.

☐ **Clinical Features:** Wilms tumor usually presents between 1 and 3 years of age, and 98% occur before 10 years of age. The large majority (99%) of all cases are sporadic. The few familial cases usually exhibit autosomal dominant inheritance. Only 5% of sporadic cases are bilateral, contrasted with 20% of familial cases. Most often, the diagnosis is made after the recognition of an abdominal mass. Additional manifestations include abdominal pain, intestinal obstruction, hypertension, hematuria, and symptoms of traumatic rupture of the tumor.

A number of histological and clinical parameters have been used with varying success to predict the behavior of Wilms tumor. Patients younger than 2 years of age tend to have a better prognosis. Invasion of the tumor beyond the renal capsule, noted at the time of surgery, is a negative prognostic indicator. Anaplasia (nuclear enlargement, hyperchromasia, and atypical mitotic figures) also indicates a poorer prognosis. Anaplasia is more common in older patients, a feature that contributes to the overall worse prognosis in these cases. Chemotherapy and radiation therapy, combined with surgical resection, have dramatically improved the outlook of patients with this tumor, and many centers now report an overall long-term survival rate of 90%.

Renal Cell Carcinoma

Renal cell carcinoma (RCC) is a malignant neoplasm of renal tubular or ductal epithelial cells. RCC is the most common cancer of the kidney (90%), accounting for more than 11,000 cases a year in the United States. The incidence of this tumor worldwide has recently been increasing 2% annually.

□ **Pathogenesis:** The large majority of cases of RCC are sporadic, but about 5% are inherited. Hereditary RCC occurs in the context of three distinct syndromes:

- **Autosomal dominant RCC**, in which a clear cell tumor is the primary manifestation and occurs in half of the persons at risk.
- **von Hippel-Lindau (VHL) disease**, an autosomal dominant cancer syndrome, characterized by the development of hemangioblastomas in the brain, retinal angiomas, clear cell RCC (40% of all cases of VHL disease), pheochromocytoma, and cysts in various organs.
- **Hereditary papillary RCC.**

All forms of hereditary RCC tend to be multifocal and bilateral, and they appear at a younger age than sporadic RCC.

In genetic studies of autosomal dominant RCC, a variety of translocations involving a breakpoint on chromosome 3 were recognized. Subsequently, studies of patients with sporadic RCC demonstrated consistent deletions and LOH in the short arm of chromosome 3 (3p) in the tumor tissue. Finally, the position of the VHL gene was similarly localized to 3p. The VHL gene is small, and its product exhibits no homology with other known proteins. Although its function remains to be determined, it is known to inhibit transcription elongation and to serve as a tumor suppressor gene. **Loss of one allele of the VHL gene occurs in virtually all (98%) of sporadic clear cell RCC, and mutations in the gene are found in more than half of these tumors**. Thus, the evidence strongly suggests that loss of the tumor suppressive function of the VHL is an important event in the genesis of clear cell RCC.

Unlike clear cell RCC, hereditary papillary RCC shows no association with the VHL gene. Trisomies of chromosomes 7, 16, and 17, and translocations involving chromosome 1 have been demonstrated in some cases.

Tobacco, whether smoked or chewed, is associated with an increased risk of RCC, and one third of these tumors are linked to tobacco use. Both inherited and acquired cystic diseases of the kidney may be complicated by the development of renal cell carcinoma. The cancer has also been tied to analgesic nephropathy. It is estimated that some 4% of cases of RCC are hereditary, and a family history of RCC places a person at a four- to fivefold increased risk for this malignancy.

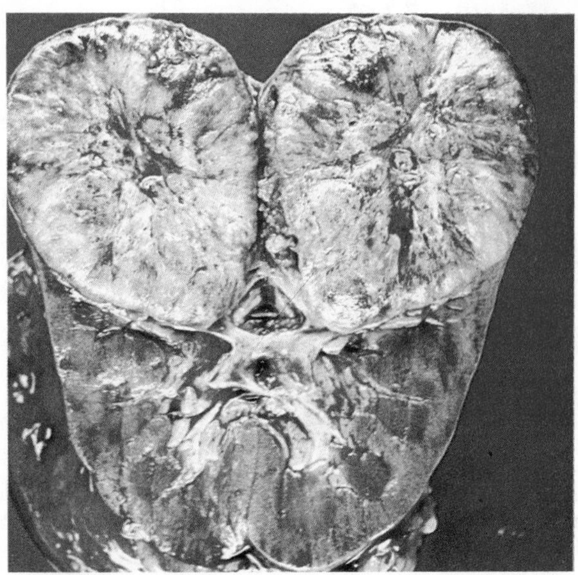

FIGURE *16-87*
Renal cell carcinoma. The kidney contains a large irregular neoplasm with a variegated cut surface, including yellow areas that correspond to lipid-containing cells.

□ **Pathology:** RCC is typically yellow-orange and often shows conspicuous focal hemorrhage and necrosis (Fig. 16-87). The tumors are solid or focally cystic. The various histological patterns are shown in Table 16-16.

Clear cell RCC is the most common type. The clear cytoplasm of the neoplastic cells (Fig. 16-88) reflects the removal of abundant cytoplasmic lipids and glycogen by the water and solvents used in the preparation of the tissue. The cells often are arranged in round or elongated collections demarcated by a network of delicate vessels, and little cellular or nuclear pleomorphism is present. By electron microscopy, the neoplastic cells often resemble proximal tubular epithelial cells, with microvilli, membrane-associated vesicles involved in pinocytosis, and infolding of the plasma membrane.

TABLE *16-16* **Patterns of Renal Cell Carcinoma**

Category	Frequency (%)
Clear cell type	70
Papillary type	15
Granular cell type	8
Chromophobe type	5
Sarcomatoid type	1.5
Collecting duct type	0.5

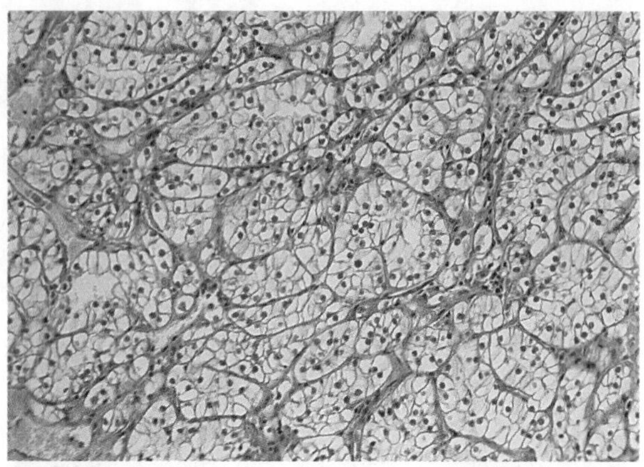

FIGURE 16-88
Renal cell carcinoma. Photomicrograph showing rounded collections of neoplastic cells with abundant clear cytoplasm.

The papillary type of RCC is characterized by neoplastic cells arranged on fibrovascular stalks. The tumor cells are typically cuboidal, with small round nuclei. These cancers are generally greater than 3 cm in greatest dimension and have a mean diameter of almost 10 cm.

The granular cell type of RCC features abundant acidophilic cytoplasm, frequently with marked nuclear pleomorphism, hyperchromasia, and atypia. Grossly, these tumors are brown because of the phospholipids in the numerous cytoplasmic organelles.

Chromophobe RCC shows a mixture of acidophilic granular cells and pale transparent cells with prominent cell borders, which impart a plant cell–like appearance. The cytoplasm contains numerous vesicles filled with a distinctive type of mucopolysaccharide that can be stained with the Hale colloidal iron technique. In the pale cells, these vesicles displace other organelles to the periphery, causing a central cytoplasmic pallor.

The sarcomatoid type of RCC is the most anaplastic and poorly differentiated form. These tumors are often widely disseminated at the time of diagnosis. Histologically, interlacing and whorled bundles of atypical spindle cells are present.

The collecting duct type is a rare form of RCC that usually arises in the medulla but may extend into the cortex. Histologically, it is composed of tubular and papillary structures lined by a single layer of cuboidal cells.

The recommended histological grading system for renal cell carcinomas is the Fuhrman system:

- **Grade I:** Nuclei round, uniform, 10 μm; nucleoli inconspicuous or absent
- **Grade II:** Nuclei irregular, 15 μm; nucleoli evident
- **Grade III:** Nuclei very irregular, 20 μm; nucleoli large and prominent
- **Grade IV:** Nuclei bizarre and multilobated, 20 μm or greater; nucleoli prominent

☐ Clinical Features: The incidence of RCC peaks in the sixth decade and is twice as frequent in men as in women. **The classic clinical triad of hematuria, flank pain, and a palpable abdominal mass** occurs in less than 10% of patients. Hematuria is the single most common presenting sign. Known in clinical medicine as one of the great mimics, RCC is a potential source of ectopic hormone production and is frequently associated with paraneoplastic syndromes. For example, secretion of a parathormone-like substance leads to hyperparathyroidism, production of erythropoietin causes erythrocytosis, and the release of renin results in hypertension. Often a patient with RCC initially presents with symptoms due to a metastasis. For instance, a sudden convulsion or development of a cough in a previously healthy person leads to the discovery of an unsuspected tumor in the brain or lung, which proves on further examination to be RCC.

The overall survival in cases of RCC is 40% at 5 years. The prognosis is influenced by many factors, including tumor size, extent of invasion and metastasis, histological type, and nuclear grade. Few patients with the sarcomatoid type survive for more than 1 year. By contrast, survival after nephrectomy for clear cell RCC is 50%. The papillary and chromophobe types have a better prognosis than the clear cell type, and the granular cell type a worse prognosis. Tumor stage (a measure of invasion and metastasis) is the most important prognostic factor. Distant metastases are found most frequently in the lung and the bones.

Transitional Cell Carcinoma

Between 5% and 10% of primary neoplasms of the kidney are transitional cell carcinomas of the renal pelvis or calyces. These are morphologically identical to the more common transitional cell carcinomas of the urinary bladder and are associated with them in half of the cases. Less than 5% of transitional cell carcinomas occur in the collecting system proximal to the bladder. Transitional cell carcinomas are discussed in detail in Chapter 17.

SUGGESTED READING

BOOKS

Churg J, Bernstein J, Glassock RJ: *Renal disease: Classification and atlas of glomerular disease,* 2nd ed. New York: Igaku-Shoin, 1995.

Jennette JC, Olson JL, Schwartz MM, Silva FG: *Heptinstall's pathology of the kidney,* 5th ed. Boston: Little, Brown, 1997.

Murphy WM, Beckwith JB, Farrow GM: *Tumors of the kidney, bladder and related urinary structures.* Washington, DC: Armed Forces Institute of Pathology, 1994.

Silva FG, D Agati VD, Nadasdy T: *Renal biopsy interpretation.* New York: Churchill Livingstone, 1996.

Tisher CC, Brenner BM: *Renal pathology,* 2nd ed. Philadelphia: JB Lippincott, 1994.

REVIEW ARTICLES

Austin HA, Boumpas DT, Vaughan EM, Balow JE: Predicting renal outcome in severe lupus nephritis: Contributions of clinical and histologic data. *Kidney Int* 45:544–550, 1994.

Brady HR: Leukocyte adhesion molecules and kidney diseases. *Kidney Int* 45:1285–1300, 1994.

Colvin RB: The renal allograft biopsy. *Kidney Int* 50:1069–1082, 1996.

Couser WG: Pathogenesis of glomerulonephritis. *Kidney Int* 44(suppl 42):S19–S26, 1993.

D'Agati VD: Morphologic features of cyclosporin nephrotoxicity. *Contrib Nephrol* 114:84–110, 1995.

Freedman BI, Iskandar SS, Appel RG: The link between hypertension and nephrosclerosis. *Am J Kidney Dis* 25:207–221, 1995.

Glassock RJ, Cohen AH: The primary glomerulopathies. Disease-A-Month 42:329–383, 1996.

Harris PC, Ward CJ, Peral B, Hughes J: Polycystic kidney disease 1: Identification and analysis of the primary defect. *J Am Soc Nephrol* 6:1125–1133, 1995.

Jennette JC, Falk RJ: The pathology of vasculitis involving the kidney. *Am J Kidney Dis* 24:130–141, 1994.

Linehan WM, Lerman MI, Zbar B: Identification of the von Hipple-Lindau (VHL) gene. Its role in renal cancer. *JAMA* 273:564–570, 1995.

Reddy JC, Licht JD: The WT1 Wilms tumor suppressor gene. How much do we really know? *Biochim Biophys Acta* 1287:1–28, 1996.

Ruggenenti P, Remuzzi G: Malignant vascular disease of the kideny: Nature of the lesion, mediators of disease progression, and the case for bilateral nephrectomy. *Am J Kidney Dis* 27:459–475, 1996.

Silva FG, Hogg RJ: Glomerular lesions associated with the acute nephritic syndrome and hematuria. *Semin Diagn Pathol* 5:4–38, 1988.

Weber M: Rapidly progressive glomerulonephritis: Recent advances in pathogenesis, diagnosis and therapy. *Clin Invest* 71:825–829, 1993.

Weiss LM, Gelb AB, Medeiros LJ: Adult renal epithelial neoplasms. *Am J Clin Pathol* 103:624–635, 1995.

CHAPTER 17

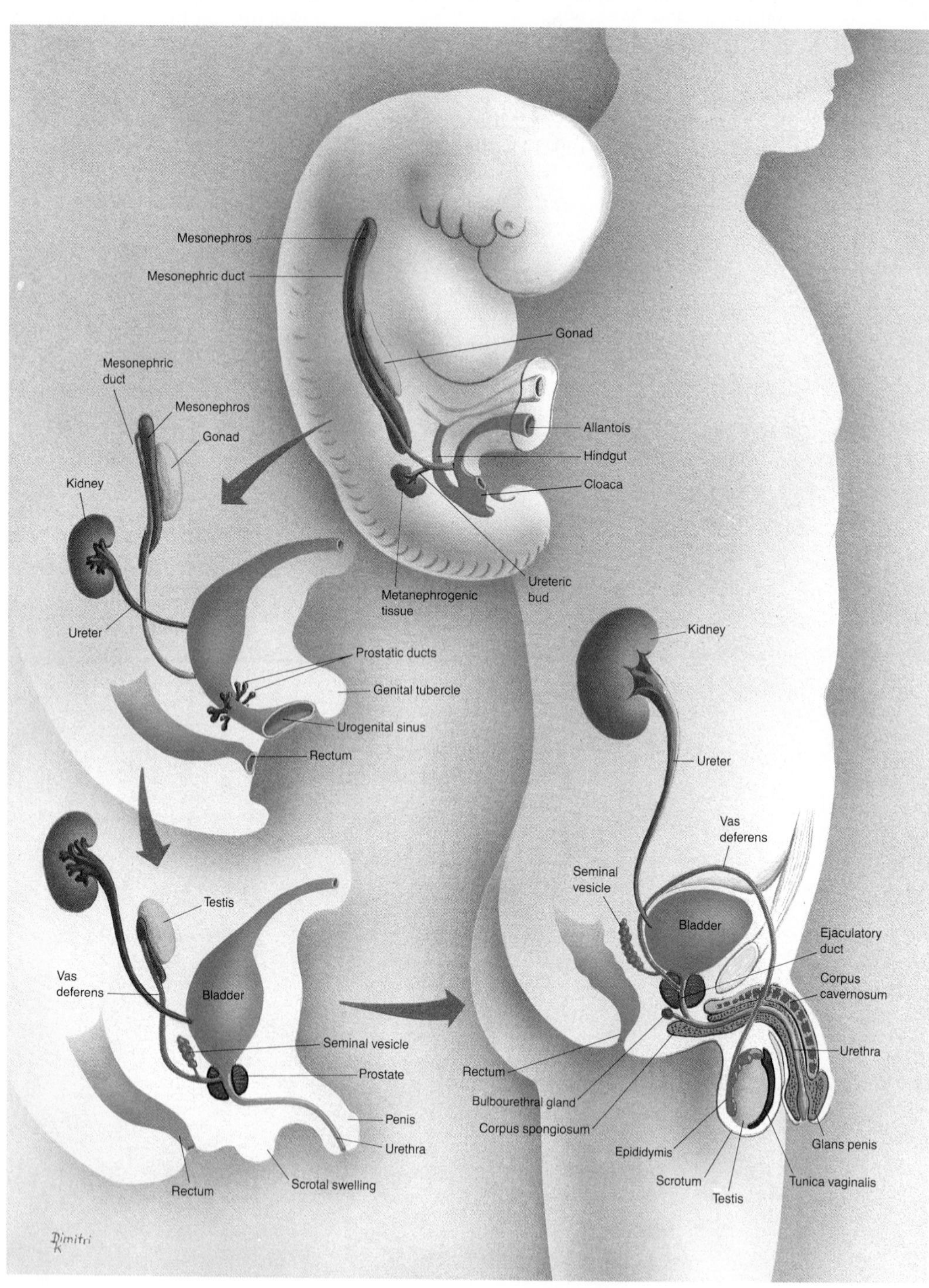

Mesonephros
Mesonephric duct
Gonad
Mesonephric duct
Mesonephros
Gonad
Kidney
Allantois
Hindgut
Cloaca
Ureter
Metanephrogenic tissue
Ureteric bud
Prostatic ducts
Genital tubercle
Urogenital sinus
Rectum
Kidney
Ureter
Testis
Vas deferens
Bladder
Seminal vesicle
Prostate
Penis
Urethra
Rectum
Scrotal swelling
Vas deferens
Seminal vesicle
Bladder
Ejaculatory duct
Corpus cavernosum
Urethra
Rectum
Bulbourethral gland
Corpus spongiosum
Epididymis
Scrotum
Testis
Tunica vaginalis
Glans penis
Dimitri K

The Urinary Tract and Male Reproductive System

Robert O. Petersen

FIGURE 17-1 *(see opposite page)*
Embryological development of the urinary tract and male reproductive system.

Renal Pelvis and Ureter

ANATOMY AND EMBRYOLOGY

The metanephric duct, the structure that ultimately develops into the ureter and renal pelvis, begins as the metanephric diverticulum and grows cephalad after a mass of metanephrogenic mesenchyme envelops its blind end. It emerges from the distal mesonephric duct near its entrance into the cloaca (Fig. 17-1) and then induces the development of nephrons in the metanephric mesenchyme. The metanephric duct and the differentiating metanephric mesenchyme migrate cephalad as a unit. The metanephric mesenchyme induces the blind end of the metanephric duct to subdivide, thereby progressively forming the major and minor calyces. The minor calyces give rise to the collecting tubules, which ultimately connect with the tubular system of the nephron. After the metanephric duct has developed, the distal mesonephric duct from which it arose is partially absorbed into the lateral wall of the urogenital sinus. This process separates the ostia of the metanephric duct (which becomes the ureter) from the mesonephric duct (which becomes the male ejaculatory duct system).

The mucosa of the calyceal system and renal pelvis rests on a basement membrane and is composed of a transitional epithelium of two or three cell layers. This increases to three to five cell layers in the ureter. The lamina propria is evident only in the ureters, where it is composed of loose collagenous fibers and thin-walled vessels. In the renal pelvis, the smooth muscle immediately under the basement membrane is arranged in interlacing spirals, which are continuous with the musculature of the ureter. In the distal ureter, an additional longitudinal muscle layer is observed between the circular muscle bundles and the adventitia. Contraction of the muscle layers of the ureter produces the characteristic mucosal infoldings when viewed in cross section. External to the muscularis of both the renal pelvis and the ureter is a well-vascularized, loose fibroadipose tissue, which comprises the adventitia.

Branches of the renal, gonadal, and common iliac arteries, which have numerous anastomoses, form the vascular supply to the renal pelvis and ureter. The lymphatics of the renal pelvis and proximal ureter drain to the regional periaortic lymph nodes (lateral lumbar nodes), whereas those of the distal ureter lead to the internal iliac lymph nodes.

CONGENITAL DISORDERS

AGENESIS OF THE URETER: This anomaly results from the failure of the metanephric diverticulum to develop from the mesonephric duct and is invariably associated with agenesis of the kidney on the same side.

URETERAL DUPLICATION: A more common condition than agenesis, ureteral duplication is caused either by the formation of multiple metanephric buds (complete duplication) or by a premature bifurcation of a single bud (incomplete duplication). The result is a duplicated renal pelvis and two incomplete or complete ureters, which course to the urinary bladder adjacent to each other. Most duplications are unilateral and are rarely of clinical significance.

ECTOPIC URETER: This congenital anomaly describes a ureter that has a distal terminus located somewhere other than the normal posterolateral wall of the urinary bladder. The condition reflects anomalous development of the distal mesonephric duct. This portion of the duct ultimately forms part of the proximal urethra, ejaculatory duct, seminal vesicle, and vas deferens. Thus, any abnormal juxtaposition of the mesonephric duct and the ostium of the metanephric duct (which forms the ureter) may lead to the abnormal insertion of the ureter into any of these mesonephric structures.

URETEROPELVIC JUNCTION OBSTRUCTION: The most common cause of hydronephrosis in infants and children is ureteropelvic junction obstruction. The etiology is not well understood, but a documented congenital stricture only rarely explains the obstruction. Abnormal smooth muscle function with deficient motility of the ureteral wall has been proposed as a cause of this disorder. Alternatively, mechanical factors (e.g., unusual insertion of the ureter into the renal pelvis or aberrant renal vessels) have been documented in some cases.

Ureteropelvic junction obstruction is principally

found in boys, although in the few cases in adults, women are more commonly affected. Interestingly, in young children, the left ureter is more commonly involved than the right, and only 30% of cases in the first year of life are bilateral. The contralateral kidney is absent or anomalous in one fifth of the cases. Treatment is surgical correction.

DIVERTICULUM OF A RENAL CALYX: Usually at the upper pole of the kidney, this abnormality is characterized by a cystic dilatation of a single calyx of the kidney, which retains continuity with the rest of the calyceal system through a narrow channel. A congenital defect in the embryological formation of the calyx is the probable underlying cause. Most diverticula of the calyces are identified as incidental findings during retrograde pyelography. Only rarely do they enlarge sufficiently to create a flank mass. Diverticula are uncommon in the renal pelvis or the ureter.

CONGENITAL URETERAL VALVES: These structures are rare and must be differentiated from acquired valves, which are secondary to distal ureteral obstruction. True congenital ureteral valves show transverse folds of ureteral mucosa containing smooth muscle, with obstructive changes above the valve and a normal ureter below it.

CONGENITAL MEGAURETER: This term is applied to many distinct entities that have only recently been classified on the basis of etiology and pathogenesis. Regardless of the underlying cause, the markedly enlarged ureter is associated with hydronephrosis and ultimate functional impairment of the kidney if the structural defect is left uncorrected.

URETERAL OBSTRUCTION

Obstruction to the flow of urine in the ureter results in hydroureter, hydronephrosis, and functional impairment of the kidney. Unilateral ureteral obstruction ultimately leads to a marked reduction in renal parenchyma and a nonfunctional (end-stage) kidney. Acute, bilateral ureteral obstruction is a medical emergency, which requires therapeutic, most frequently surgical, intervention.

The causes of ureteral obstruction are either intrinsic or extrinsic to the ureter (Fig. 17-2).

Intrinsic causes of ureteral obstruction include calculi, intraluminal blood clots, fibroepithelial polyps, inflammatory strictures of the ureteral wall, amyloidosis, and tumors originating in the wall of the ureter.

Extrinsic causes of ureteral obstruction include aberrant renal vessels to the lower pole of the kidney that cross the ureter, endometriosis, and tumors in adjacent lymph nodes. In addition, the pregnant uterus is capable of compressing the ureters.

Ureteral obstruction may also result from diseases that involve the urinary bladder, prostate, and urethra. Such disorders include cancer of the bladder in the vicinity of the ureteral orifice or bladder neck, neurogenic bladder, and prostatic hyperplasia.

Proximal causes of ureteral obstruction tend to be unilateral, whereas more distal causes of obstruction,

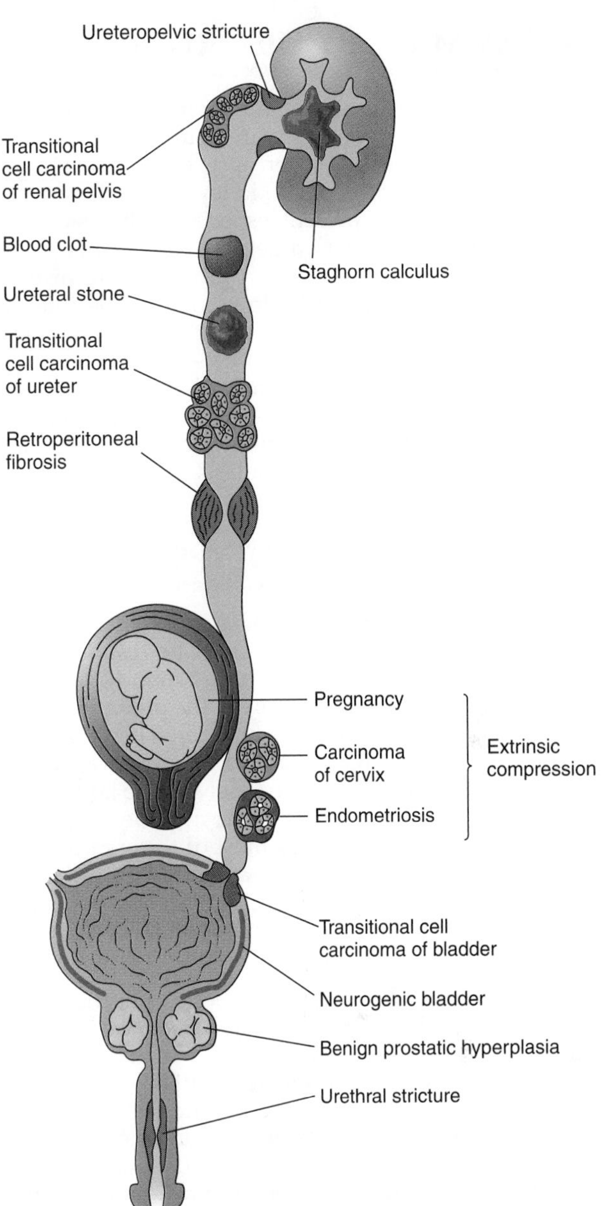

FIGURE 17-2
Causes of ureteral obstruction.

such as prostatic hyperplasia, cause bilateral hydronephrosis, with the possibility of renal failure in untreated cases.

Idiopathic retroperitoneal fibrosis, *a distinctly uncommon cause of ureteral obstruction, is characterized by dense fibrosis of the retroperitoneal soft tissues and a modest, nonspecific, chronic inflammatory reaction.* As the name implies, the etiology is unknown, although the use of certain drugs (methysergide, β-adrenergic blockers) and autoimmunity have been proposed as causes. On occasion, idiopathic retroperitoneal fibrosis is accompanied by inflammatory fibrosis in other areas, including Riedel's struma (thyroid), sclerosing cholangitis (liver), and mediastinal fibrosis. The disease is responsive to treatment with corticosteroids and immunosuppressive agents.

INFLAMMATORY DISORDERS

Pyelitis and ureteritis are inflammatory disorders of the renal pelvis and ureter. They are commonly associated with ascending infection, often as a complication of partial ureteral obstruction or of kidney stones. Frequently, pyelonephritis is also present, especially when stones occupy the renal pelvis. Gram-negative organisms are implicated in most instances of pyelitis and urethritis. A chronic inflammatory cell infiltrate of variable intensity occurs in the lamina propria of the affected urinary tract segment. On occasion, mucosal ulceration is observed. Chronic inflammation of the renal pelvis and ureter is associated with changes of the urothelium, including Brunn's buds and nests, pyelitis cystica and glandularis, and urethritis cystica and glandularis.

FIBROEPITHELIAL POLYPS

Fibroepithelial polyps are uncommon exophytic lesions of the urothelial mucosa, which may be responsible for urinary obstruction. These lesions are found throughout the urinary tract, most commonly in the ureter but also in the urethra, renal pelvis, and bladder. There is a male predilection for the ureter, bladder, and urethra, but a female preponderance in the renal pelvis. The large majority of urethral polyps (80%) occur in patients younger than 10 years of age, whereas most of those in the renal pelvis and ureter arise in young and middle-aged adults. Curiously, there is a predilection for fibroepithelial polyps to occur in the left ureter and left renal pelvis.

☐ **Pathogenesis:** The histogenesis of fibroepithelial polyps is still debated. They have been variously regarded as congenital, inflammatory, hamartomatous, or neoplastic. Thus, synonyms include inflammatory polyp, fibroma, and hamartoma. The absence of clinical and histological evidence of inflammation in many cases suggests that the polyps do not have an inflammatory origin. The presence of smooth muscle in some lesions points to a hamartomatous proliferation rather than a true tumor. It is possible that some of these lesions evolve in a manner analogous to that of polypoid cystitis with stromal fibrosis (see the discussion of proliferative and metaplastic variants in the section on the urinary bladder).

☐ **Pathology:** Fibroepithelial polyps are either smooth nodules or filiform projections, varying in size from a few millimeters to several centimeters. Histologically, the urothelium covering the centrally edematous stromal stalk is either normal or hyperplastic. The stroma contains collagen fibers, variable numbers of small blood vessels, and, on occasion, smooth muscle fibers. Acute and chronic inflammatory cells, focal hyalinization of the stroma, and calcification are all inconstant features.

☐ **Clinical Features:** The exophytic growth of fibroepithelial polyps produces ureteral obstruction of variable severity, corresponding to the size of the lesion. Patients present with flank pain, with or without hematuria. The combination of clinical and radiological findings has often led to the erroneous preoperative diagnosis of cancer of the renal pelvis or ureter, in which case unnecessarily radical surgery has been performed. Segmental resection of the ureter for fibroepithelial polyps is curative.

TUMORS

Tumors arising in the upper urinary tract (renal pelvis and ureter) are uncommon and are most frequently (90%) **transitional cell carcinoma** (Fig. 17-3). Mesenchymal tumors are distinctly rare. The etiological factors associated with epithelial tumors of the renal pelvis and ureter are similar to those observed in bladder cancer, suggesting that the entire urothelial mucosa represents a continuous "target organ."

Patients, most frequently in their sixth and seventh decades, present with flank pain and hematuria. The intrinsic obstruction produced by the tumor can be visualized by intravenous pyelography. Transitional cell carcinoma of the ureter or renal pelvis requires radical nephroureterectomy. Excision of the entire ureter is necessary because of the high frequency of concurrent and subsequent transitional cell carcinomas. **The ultimate prognosis is most closely related to the tumor stage at the time of diagnosis.**

In contrast to the high frequency of noninvasive or superficially invasive transitional cell carcinoma in the renal pelvis and ureter, the rare squamous cell carcinomas

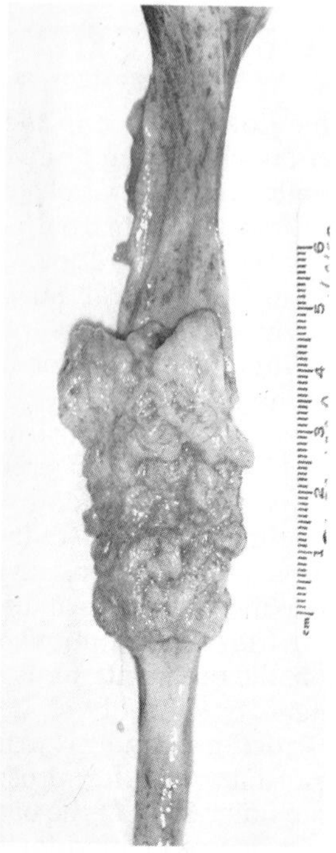

FIGURE *17-3*
Transitional cell carcinoma of the ureter. The neoplasm is an irregular exophytic mass, which obstructs the ureteral lumen and results in proximal dilatation (*top*).

and adenocarcinomas are invariably deeply invasive (higher stage) and associated with a correspondingly lower survival rate. Metastatic cancers and malignant lymphomas that involve the para-aortic lymph nodes may produce extrinsic compression of the ureter.

Urinary Bladder

ANATOMY AND EMBRYOLOGY

The urinary bladder is located in the retroperitoneum of the lower anterior abdominal wall. In females, it is anterior to the lower uterine corpus and anterior vaginal fornix. In males, the bladder is superior to the prostate and leads into the prostatic urethra. The paired seminal vesicles are adjacent to the inferior posterior wall of the bladder.

The urinary bladder develops in two stages from the cloaca and the urogenital sinus. The urogenital sinus arises from the partitioning of the cloaca into the dorsal rectum and the more ventral urogenital sinus (see Fig. 17-1). The urogenital sinus serves as the origin of the urachus, urinary bladder, and proximal urethra. Progressive attenuation of the urachus forms the umbilical ligament in the adult, which retains an attachment to the bladder dome.

The caudal urogenital sinus makes contact with an ectodermal invagination at the urogenital membrane, thereby forming the complete urethral lumen. **Thus, the bladder and the urethral urothelium are of endodermal origin, with the exception of the most distal segment, which is ectodermal. Each ureter, originating from the mesonephric duct in the form of a metanephric diverticulum, is of mesodermal origin.** The incorporation of the mesonephric duct into the bladder wall in the region of the trigone results in a transient mesonephric contribution to the bladder mucosa. This mesonephric urothelium is replaced by urothelium of endodermal derivation from the urogenital sinus. With the growth and enlargement of the bladder, the mesonephric duct is absorbed into the wall of the urogenital sinus at a location that ultimately becomes the proximal urethra. The muscular investments of the ureters, bladder, and urethra are of mesodermal origin.

The mucosal lining of the urinary bladder from the basal cells to the surface is composed of five to seven layers of urothelium. The bladder urothelium is continuous with that of the ureters and the urethra, which tend to have fewer layers. A basal lamina beneath the urothelium separates it from the richly vascularized subjacent lamina propria. The most superficial cells, the so-called "umbrella cells," are large and flat. Each covers several smaller cells of the intermediate layer.

The lamina propria, composed principally of loose collagen, overlies the interweaving bundles of the smooth muscle and comprises the muscularis propria layer. The muscularis mucosae is incomplete and poorly developed. The anatomical areas of the bladder are the following: (1) dome, (2) anterior and posterior walls, (3) lateral walls, (4) trigone region, and (5) bladder neck. Urachal remnants, usually in the form of small tubular structures, are commonly observed in the dome of bladder wall, and less frequently in the anterior wall.

CONGENITAL MALFORMATIONS

Exstrophy

Exstrophy of the bladder is a developmental abnormality characterized by the absence of a portion of the lower abdominal wall and the anterior wall of the bladder. This anomaly allows eversion of the posterior wall of the bladder through the defect. The estimated frequency of this congenital anomaly is 1 per 50,000 births.

☐ **Pathogenesis:** The development of exstrophy of the bladder centers around the fate of the embryonic cloacal membrane. This structure represents the anterior plate of the embryonic cloaca and provides the substrate for the formation of the lower abdominal musculature following the ingrowth of mesodermal tissue. In this process, the cloacal membrane is normally obliterated. In some embryos, however, the invasion of the cloacal membrane by mesodermal elements does not occur properly, and the cloacal membrane persists. With further development of the urogenital organs, this thin membrane ultimately ruptures, thereby exposing the posterior bladder mucosa to the exterior through the defect in the anterior abdominal wall. The failure of closure of the anterior abdominal wall may also extend to the external genitalia. In such cases, associated anomalies include failure of fusion of the labia in girls and epispadias in boys.

☐ **Pathology:** Abrasion by clothing and the continuous escape of urine results in chronic infection of the bladder mucosa. The externalized mucosa exhibits acute and chronic inflammation and metaplastic changes, most frequently squamous and glandular metaplasia (Fig. 17-4). Although the congenital defect may be surgically repaired, the inflammation and the established metaplastic changes in the bladder mucosa tend to persist.

☐ **Clinical Features:** The condition of the patient with an uncorrected exstrophic bladder is lamentable. There is continuous leakage of urine, persistent or recurrent local infection, and an increased risk of ascending urinary tract infection. Moreover, there is a substantial incidence of neoplastic transformation of the metaplastic urothelium, with resultant adenocarcinoma, squamous cell carcinoma, and, least frequently, transitional cell carcinoma. The median age of patients who develop cancer of the bladder as a complication of exstrophy is the fifth decade, with 75% of patients aged 30 to 60 years.

Bladder Diverticulum

Bladder diverticula are saclike evaginations of the bladder wall, which are most frequently small and of no clinical significance.

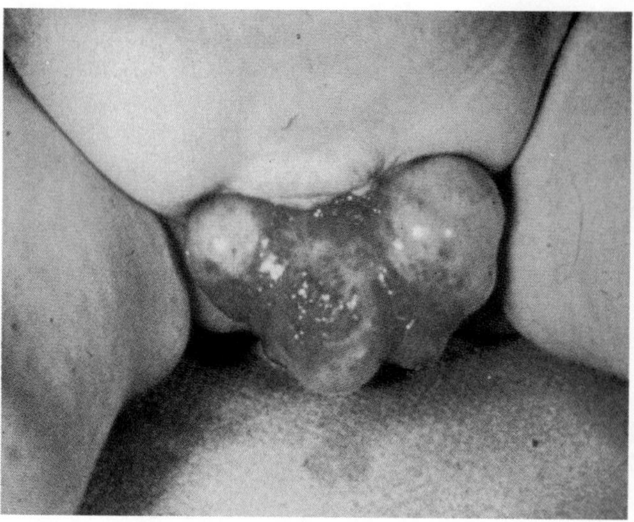
A

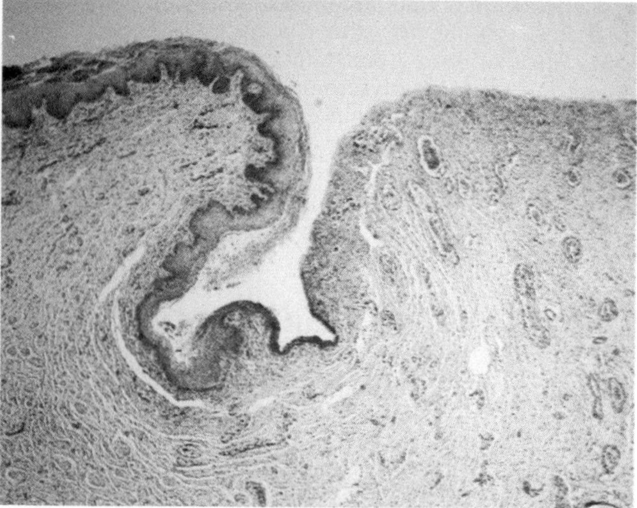
B

FIGURE *17-4*
Exstrophy of the urinary bladder. (*A*) The bladder mucosa is everted through the defect in the anterior abdominal wall. (*B*) A histological section shows that the exstrophic urinary bladder (*right*) is continuous with the epidermis of the skin (*left*). Inflammation and fibrosis are present in the lamina propria of the bladder.

On occasion, the complications of larger diverticula bring these lesions to clinical attention. The majority of bladder diverticula are observed in men older than age 50 years and are commonly associated with obstruction secondary to prostatism. Congenital bladder diverticula are also occasionally encountered in infants and children who have no evidence of obstruction.

☐ **Pathology:** A typical bladder diverticulum extends from the mucosal surface through a narrow orifice that opens into a larger cavity and distorts the external contour of the urinary bladder. The narrow intramural neck extends between bundles of the inner layer of the bladder muscle. The distended wall of the diverticulum contains attenuated muscle fibers, which are most commonly observed in young patients. This difference in the frequency with which smooth muscle is seen has led to the impression that congenital diverticula may be identified by the presence of smooth muscle and that acquired diverticula have no muscle within the diverticular wall. In practice, all diverticula with long-standing chronic inflammation, independent of the patient's age, show fibrosis of the wall that may have replaced the original muscle. Superimposed chronic inflammation, with or without squamous metaplasia, is observed in the majority of excised specimens.

☐ **Clinical Features:** The most common location of a bladder diverticulum is the vicinity of the ureteral orifices, frequently immediately superior to them. In this location, enlargement of a bladder diverticulum results in secondary ureteral obstruction or vesical reflux. Small saccules and diverticula are without symptoms or clinical significance, whereas progressive enlargement leads to stagnation of urine, infection, and the formation of bladder stones, conditions that require surgical intervention. The most serious complication of a bladder diverticulum, fortunately rare, is the development of cancer within it. Transitional cell and squamous cell carcinomas are the most frequently encountered types. The prognosis is poor, because of the occult location of the growth and the ease of invasion into the attenuated wall of the diverticulum.

Persistent Urachus

The urachus is a tubular embryonic structure that connects the urogenital sinus (later to become the bladder) with the allantois. Following birth, the urachus normally atrophies as it descends with the urinary bladder, to which it remains attached at the dome. The regression of the urachus converts it into a solid fibrous cord that extends from the dome of the bladder to the umbilicus.

In rare instances, the urachus fails to regress, either partially or completely. The clinical disorders associated with persistent urachus relate to the extent and location of the part that remains patent. Persistence of the entire urachus results in drainage of urine from the umbilicus, and supervening infection is common. Alternatively, incomplete persistence of the urachus forms a blind pouch, open only at one end, either to the skin at the umbilicus or to the urinary bladder. Segmental persistence of the lumen with closure at both ends leads to a urachal cyst.

The least common but most serious complication of persistent urachal segments is cancer, 90% of which is adenocarcinoma. The other tumors are transitional cell and squamous cell carcinomas.

Diagnostic criteria that favor cancer of urachal origin rather than the more common type that arises from the bladder mucosa include the following:

- The tumor is located within the dome or anterior wall of the bladder.
- The bulk of the tumor is located within the muscularis, without involvement of the bladder mucosa.
- Most of the infiltrating tumor is external to the bladder wall and involves the anterior abdominal wall.
- The presence of a urachal remnant associated with the tumor supports a urachal origin.

The practical application of these criteria to distinguish tumors of urachal origin from those of bladder origin is often difficult, especially with large tumors that show extensive ulceration of the bladder mucosa and conspicuous intramural infiltration. Patients with urachal carcinomas have a poorer prognosis than those with the corresponding histological type of bladder cancer.

CYSTITIS

Acute and Chronic Cystitis

Cystitis refers to inflammation of the urinary bladder. It is the most common disorder of this organ encountered in clinical practice.

☐ **Pathogenesis:** In most cases, cystitis is secondary to infection of the bladder. Factors related to bladder infection and the development of cystitis include the age and sex of the patient, presence of bladder calculi, bladder outlet obstruction, diabetes mellitus, immunodeficiency, prior instrumentation or catheterization, and radiation therapy or chemotherapy. The risk of cystitis in females is increased because of a short urethra, especially during pregnancy. Bladder outlet obstruction associated with prostatic hyperplasia predisposes men to cystitis. Introduction of pathogens into the bladder may also occur during instrumentation (cystoscopy) and is particularly common in patients in whom indwelling catheters remain for prolonged periods.

In the large majority of cases, coliform bacteria are the cause of cystitis, most frequently *Escherichia coli, Proteus, Pseudomonas,* and *Enterobacter*. Tuberculosis of the bladder is almost always secondary to renal tuberculosis. Fungal cystitis may be seen in immunosuppressed patients. Gas-forming bacilli, usually in persons with diabetes, may produce characteristic interstitial bubbles in the lamina propria of the urinary bladder (*emphysematous cystitis*). Schistosomiasis as a cause of cystitis is virtually unknown in the western world but is common in areas where *Schistosoma haematobium* is endemic, namely, Africa and the Middle East.

☐ **Pathology:** The cystoscopic and histological features of acute and chronic cystitis reflect the inflammatory process and are usually nonspecific. Stromal edema and a neutrophilic infiltrate of variable intensity are typical of acute cystitis. Lack of resolution of the inflammatory reaction is associated with the hallmarks of chronic inflammation, including a predominance of lymphocytes (Fig 17-5) and fibrosis of the lamina propria.

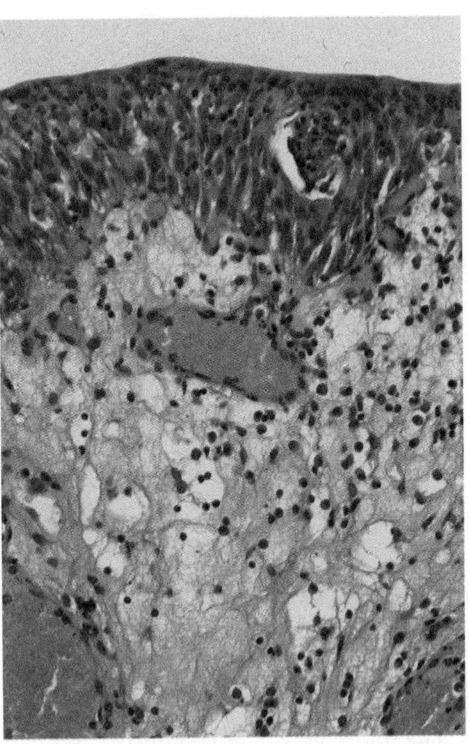

FIGURE *17-5*
Chronic cystitis. A nonspecific chronic inflammatory infiltrate of lymphocytes and plasma cells is present in the edematous stroma of the lamina propria.

☐ **Clinical Features:** Virtually all patients with acute or chronic cystitis complain of excessive frequency of urination, pain on urination (dysuria), and lower abdominal or pelvic discomfort. Examination of the urine usually reveals inflammatory cells, and culture identifies the causative agent. Most cases of cystitis are treated with antimicrobial agents.

Polypoid Cystitis

Polypoid cystitis is an inflammatory lesion characterized by papillary projections of the bladder mucosa (Fig. 17-6). When these mucosal elevations are broad based, they are described as *bullous* cystitis. These polypoid lesions reflect severe submucosal edema, which in most cases is associated with indwelling catheters. Some lesions persist long after removal of the catheter but are ultimately reversible. On cystoscopic examination, polypoid cystitis may be mistaken for papillary transitional cell carcinoma of the bladder.

Eosinophilic Cystitis

Eosinophilic cystitis is a rare bladder inflammation of middle-aged adults characterized histologically by eosinophilic infiltrates. The disease has been observed in all age groups. In many patients, this disorder is a manifestation of an allergic diathesis, which includes involvement of the lungs or gastrointestinal tract and peripheral eosinophilia.

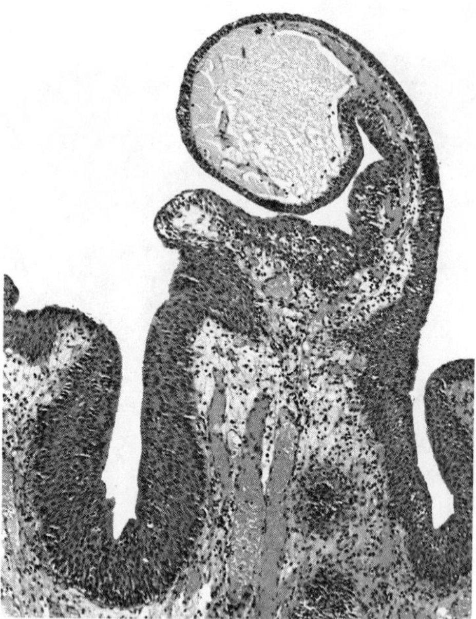

FIGURE 17-6
Polypoid cystitis. The polypoid structure is lined by a focally hyperplastic urothelial surface devoid of dysplastic changes. The underlying lamina propria has a chronic inflammatory cell infiltrate against a background of marked stromal edema.

Eosinophilic cystitis in older men is often associated with bladder injury (e.g., treatment for bladder cancer or transurethral resection of the prostate).

On histological examination, variable degrees of eosinophilic infiltration of the bladder wall, fibrosis, chronic inflammation, and muscle necrosis are present. The clinical presentation, with dysuria, frequency, and occasional hematuria, is similar to that in other forms of cystitis.

Chronic Interstitial Cystitis (Hunner Ulcer)

Chronic interstitial cystitis is a disorder of unknown cause, typically affecting middle-aged women, which features transmural inflammation of the bladder wall and is occasionally associated with mucosal ulceration (Hunner ulcer). The disease is typically persistent and refractory to all forms of therapy. Chronic inflammation and fibrosis are commonly observed within the muscularis. When present, a Hunner ulcer displays an intense acute inflammatory reaction.

The most common symptoms of chronic interstitial cystitis are long-standing suprapubic pain, frequency, and urgency, with or without hematuria. At cystoscopy, mucosal edema, focal petechiae, and irregular hemorrhagic areas, most often in the dome and posterior wall, are characteristic. Urine cultures are usually negative.

Malakoplakia

Malakoplakia (Gk. malakos, soft; plax, plaque) is an uncommon inflammatory disorder of unknown etiology that is identified by the accumulation of characteristic macrophages. The disorder was originally described in the bladder, but it has since been observed in numerous other sites, both within and outside the urinary tract. Malakoplakia is found in all age groups, the peak frequency occurring in the fifth to seventh decades. There is a marked preponderance of cases in women, regardless of the site of occurrence.

Malakoplakia is often associated with an infection of the urinary tract by *E. coli*, although a direct causal relationship is dubious. A clinical background of immunosuppression, chronic infections, or cancer is common.

☐ **Pathology:** Malakoplakia is characterized by soft, yellow plaques on the mucosal surface of the bladder, measuring up to 4 cm in diameter. On histological examination, the most striking feature of malakoplakia is a chronic inflammatory cell infiltrate composed predominantly of large macrophages with abundant, eosinophilic cytoplasm containing periodic acid–Schiff (PAS)-positive granules (*von Hansemann cells*). Some of these macrophages exhibit laminated, basophilic calcospherites termed *Michaelis-Gutmann bodies* (Fig. 17-7). Ultrastructurally, the granules of the von Hansemann cells are engorged lysosomes that contain fragments of bacteria, suggesting that malakoplakia may reflect an acquired defect in lysosomal degradation. The Michaelis-Gutmann bodies result from the deposition of calcium salts in these enlarged lysosomes.

The urinary bladder is the most common site of malakoplakia, with half the cases occurring in this organ. This enigmatic disorder has also been reported in other regions of the genitourinary system, including the kidney, renal pelvis, ureter, testis, epididymis, and prostate. The colon, bones, and lungs have also been sites of occurrence of malakoplakia.

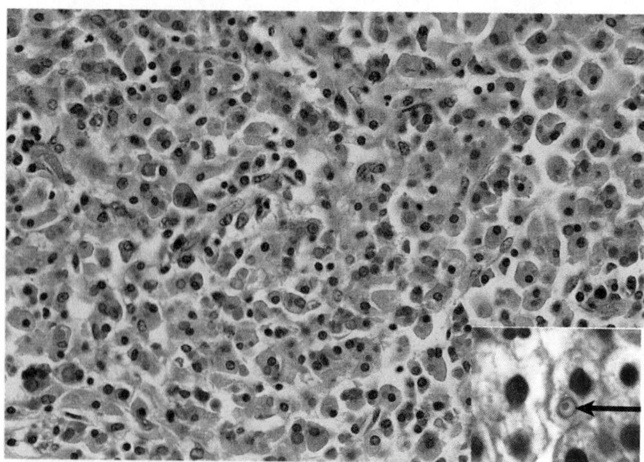

FIGURE 17-7
Malakoplakia. Numerous Michaelis-Gutmann bodies are seen as well-defined spherical structures in the cytoplasm. The background inflammatory cells are composed principally of macrophages, with fewer lymphocytes. (*Inset*) A Michaelis-Gutmann body (*arrow*) is seen at high magnification.

The clinical symptomatology of malakoplakia is nonspecific and suggests cystitis.

Iatrogenic Cystitis

Radiation-induced cystitis may complicate the treatment of pelvic malignancies. It is characterized by the vascular lesions typical of radiation-induced injury (endothelial proliferation, subendothelial accumulation of macrophages) and by atypical fibroblasts within the stroma of the bladder.

Cyclophosphamide-induced cystitis is a hemorrhagic lesion that may be accompanied by severe bleeding into the bladder lumen. It may be associated with cytological atypia of the urothelial cells, and there is a substantial increase in the incidence of bladder cancer in patients treated with cyclophosphamide.

Multiple endoscopic biopsy specimens of the bladder have resulted in foreign body granulomas and lesions resembling rheumatoid nodules.

ENDOMETRIOSIS

The urinary bladder is the most common site of endometriosis (see Chapter 18) of the urinary tract. Endometriosis of the urinary tract usually appears during the second to fifth decades of life, with a peak frequency in the fourth decade.

The diagnosis of vesical endometriosis requires the identification of endometrial glandular epithelium in association with endometrial stromal cells (Fig. 17-8). Past hemorrhage is indicated by the deposition of hemosiderin in the stroma.

Women with emdometriosis of the bladder present with pelvic pain, frequency, and urgency. Hematuria is reported in only one fourth of the patients. Conservative surgical excision of the lesions is appropriate therapy.

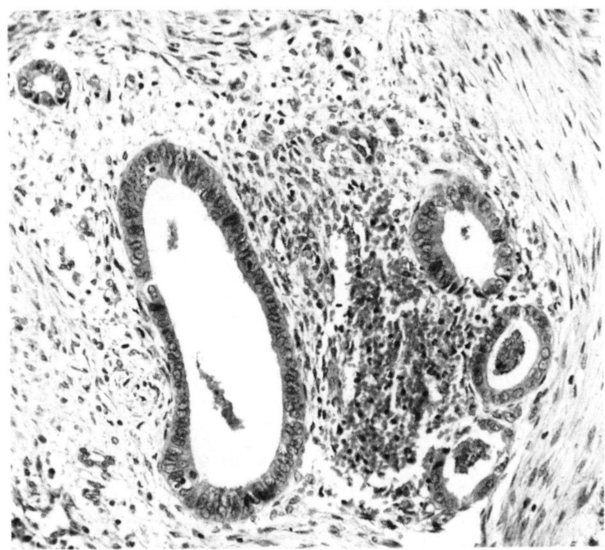

FIGURE *17-8*
Endometriosis of the bladder. A section of the bladder wall shows endometrial glands and stroma, with a focus of hemorrhage.

BLADDER OBSTRUCTION

Obstruction to the flow of urine from the bladder, most commonly as a result of prostatic hyperplasia in men and cystocele in women, is a far more common cause of hydronephrosis than obstruction of the upper urinary tract. Regardless of the cause of the obstruction, the bladder reacts in a similar manner, with dilatation, muscular hypertrophy, diverticula, and trabeculation of the mucosal surface.

BENIGN PROLIFERATIVE AND METAPLASTIC LESIONS

A spectrum of hyperplastic and metaplastic changes of the urothelium occurs throughout the urinary tract, from the renal pelvis to the urethra. These non-neoplastic lesions of the urothelium are characterized either by hyperplasia or by combined hyperplasia and metaplasia (Fig. 17-9). Mucosal lesions that are only hyperplastic include simple hyperplasia, Brunn's invaginations and nests, and cystic alterations. Cystic lesions are further identified by their site of occurrence (e.g., pyelitis cystica, ureteritis cystica [Fig. 17-10], or cystitis cystica). The urothelial changes that combine hyperplasia and concurrent metaplasia include (1) glandular lesions (pyelitis glandularis, ureteritis glandularis, cystitis glandularis, urethritis glandularis), (2) mucinous (or colonic) metaplasia, (3) nephrogenic metaplasia, and (4) squamous metaplasia.

These proliferative and metaplastic lesions are found in association with chronic inflammation, caused by urinary tract infections, calculi, neurogenic bladder, and exstrophy. However, they are occasionally observed in the absence of any documented preexisting inflammatory condition.

Proliferative Lesions

Simple hyperplasia refers to an increase in the number of cell layers of the mucosal transitional epithelium. This lesion has a flat configuration, with neither papillary features nor invaginations into the lamina propria.

Brunn's buds are bulbous invaginations of the surface urothelium into the lamina propria.

Brunn's nests are similar to Brunn's buds, but the urothelial cells have detached from the surface and are seen within the lamina propria.

Cystic lesions of the urinary tract (e.g., pyelitis cystica, ureteritis cystica, cystitis cystica) are characterized by small slits or round spaces in otherwise solid Brunn nests. Cystitis cystica is actually very common, being found in 60% of otherwise normal adult bladders. The size of the central lumen varies, as does the number of surrounding cell layers. Eosinophilic, proteinaceous material is present within the lumina of the cysts. Pyelitis cystica and urethritis cystica may achieve sufficient size to be apparent on cystoscopy.

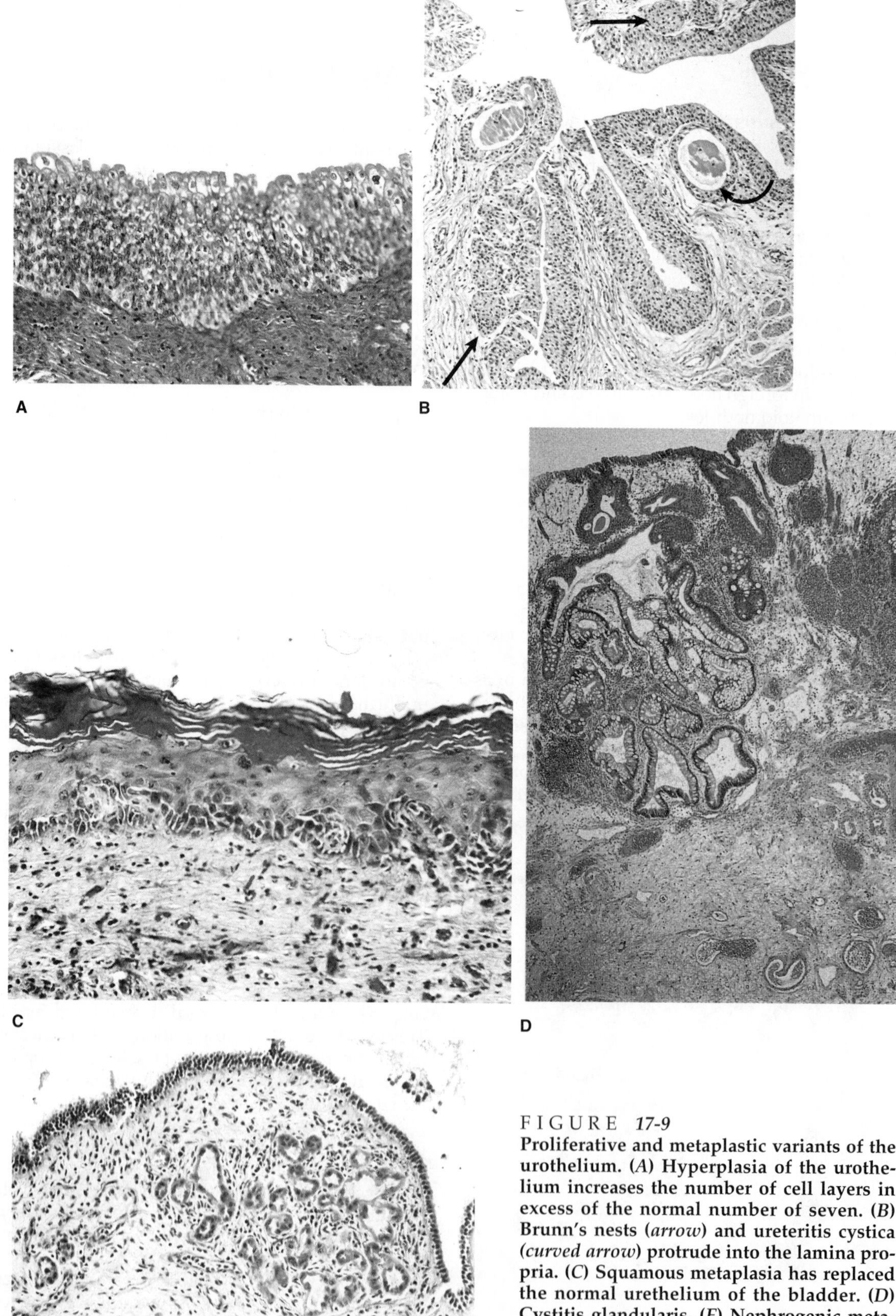

FIGURE 17-9
Proliferative and metaplastic variants of the urothelium. (*A*) Hyperplasia of the urothelium increases the number of cell layers in excess of the normal number of seven. (*B*) Brunn's nests (*arrow*) and ureteritis cystica (*curved arrow*) protrude into the lamina propria. (*C*) Squamous metaplasia has replaced the normal urethelium of the bladder. (*D*) Cystitis glandularis. (*E*) Nephrogenic metaplasia is characterized by clustered simple tubular structures lined by epithelium similar to that of the tubular epithelium.

Metaplastic Lesions

CYSTITIS GLANDULARIS: This lesion of the bladder mucosa is characterized by glandular structures lined by mucin-secreting columnar epithelial cells. The glands are haphazardly arranged or are clustered within the lamina propria, frequently in proximity to Brunn's nests and cystitis cystica. Cystitis glandularis differs from cystitis cystica only in the nature of the lining cells. In fact, structures with the columnar cells of cystitis glandularis and the transitional cells of cystitis cystica are not uncommon. In cystitis glandularis, the overlying surface epithelium usually remains one of transitional cells. Yet, metaplastic, mucus-secreting columnar cells similar to those in the underlying glandular structures may also be observed in the surface epithelium.

MUCINOUS (COLONIC) METAPLASIA: Particularly conspicuous glandular metaplasia of the urinary tract is referred to as mucinous metaplasia, and it occurs most frequently in the bladder. In this condition, the glands are lined by an epithelium resembling that of the colon, composed of goblet cells and occasionally Paneth cells.

SQUAMOUS METAPLASIA: The urinary tract may react to chronic injury and inflammation with squamous metaplasia, particularly when it is associated with calculi. It is now apparent that squamous metaplasia of the urinary tract, presumably associated with infections, is considerably more common than previously appreciated and is present in as many as 50% of normal adult women and 10% of men.

NEPHROGENIC METAPLASIA: The most recently described metaplastic change of urothelium, nephrogenic metaplasia, occurs most frequently in the urinary bladder but it has been reported uncommonly in the urethra and in the ureter. Numerous small tubules clustered in the lamina propria produce a papillary exophytic nodule (see Fig. 17-9E). These lesions are usually in the trigone region, but they have been observed in all locations within the bladder. The histogenesis of nephrogenic metaplasia is unsettled. Ultrastructural studies confirm the epithelial nature of the tubular lining cells, which show microvilli, complex intracellular interdigitations, and tight junctions. These features have been interpreted as recapitulations of different segments of the renal tubules, including the proximal convoluted tubules, the thin limb of the loop of Henle, and the collecting tubules.

Nephrogenic metaplasia is often associated with chronic cystitis. It has no age predilection and is reported from infancy to the eighth decade. There is a pronounced male predominance (3:1). Transurethral resection is the most common form of therapy, but recurrences are not uncommon.

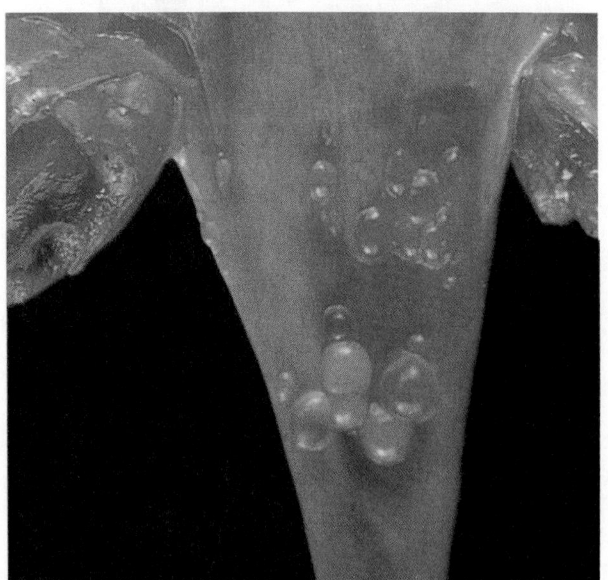

FIGURE *17-10*
Ureteritis cystica. The mucosa of the proximal ureter exhibits small cystic structures.

The Relation of Proliferative and Metaplastic Lesions to Cancer of the Urinary Tract

The clinical significance of proliferative and metaplastic lesions of the urothelium is limited to their possible neoplastic potential. Patients with these changes have a significantly increased risk for the development of transitional cell carcinoma of the bladder and, in the case of cystitis glandularis, of adenocarcinoma as well. However, there is no evidence to suggest that these lesions themselves are preneoplastic. Rather, the persistence of the injury related to the development of proliferative and metaplastic urothelial lesions is more likely the important factor in the pathogenesis of bladder cancer.

NEOPLASTIC DISORDERS

Epithelial tumors, the large majority of which are transitional cell carcinomas, comprise more than 98% of all primary tumors of the bladder. Neoplastic transitional cell epithelial lesions arising from the bladder mucosa constitute a spectrum that begins with benign papillomatous lesions and extends through carcinoma *in situ* to invasive and metastatic transitional cell carcinomas. The occurrence of any epithelial tumor in the bladder indicates a general propensity for further neoplastic transformation in other areas of the bladder mucosa. **In other words, bladder tumors seem to arise in a background of an unstable urothelium.** The epithelium of the urinary tract may be particularly sensitive in this regard, because it is constantly exposed to potentially carcinogenic chemicals in the urine. Early diagnosis of bladder tumors is facilitated by easily visible hematuria and the convenience of cystoscopic examination.

Transitional Cell Papilloma

Transitional cell papilloma of the urinary bladder is an uncommon benign lesion that is often encountered incidentally or after painless hematuria. Papillomas comprise 2% to 3% of bladder epithelial tumors and occur most frequently in men older than the age of 50 years.

The papillary fronds of this tumor are lined by a transitional epithelium that is virtually indistinguishable from normal urothelium (Fig. 17-11A). Papillary tumors that meet this criterion are uncommon, and they have been only recently accepted as papillomas rather than as low-grade transitional cell carcinomas. On cystoscopy, the majority of cases show single lesions, 2 to 5 cm in diameter, although multiple lesions are not unusual. Recurrent papillomas are common (70%), and invasive carcinoma develops in 7% of patients.

Transitional cell papillomas are not malignant, but they arise in a urothelial mucosa that is not at rest, and evolving tumors can be detected only by repeated examinations for many years. In most instances, "recurrences" represent new tumors that develop elsewhere in the urinary bladder.

Inverted papillomas are rare, benign tumors of the urothelial mucosa, which typically present as nodular mucosal lesions. They are most commonly found in the urinary bladder, usually in the trigone region. They have also been observed in the renal pelvis, ureter, and urethra. Inverted papillomas are covered by normal urothelium, from which cords of transitional epithelium descend into the lamina propria (see Fig. 17-11B). These lesions are more frequent in men, with a peak incidence in the sixth and seventh decades. Hematuria of recent onset is the usual clinical presentation.

Transitional Cell Carcinoma *in Situ*

The term carcinoma in situ is reserved for full-thickness, malignant changes confined to a flat (nonpapillary) urothelium. The term is not applied to a noninvasive papillary transitional cell carcinoma, in spite of the fact that the latter tumor is, by definition, confined to the mucosal surface. Carcinoma *in situ* is characterized by a urothelium of variable thickness that exhibits cellular atypia of the entire mucosa, from the basal layer to the surface (Fig. 17-12). This atypia is manifested as nuclear changes, including enlargement, hyperchromatism, irregular shape, prominent nucleoli, and coarse chromatin. Occasional multinucleated cells are present. A disorganized appearance, reflecting variation in nuclear polarity, is a constant feature.

Carcinoma *in situ* of the bladder, occurring in the absence of papillary carcinoma, is associated with the subsequent development of invasive carcinoma in one third of the cases. Confined to the mucosal surface, this lesion is most frequently observed endoscopically as multiple, red, velvety, flat patches topographically close to ex-

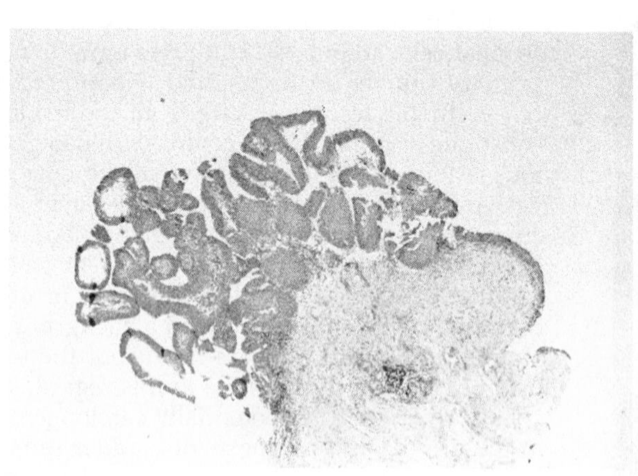
A

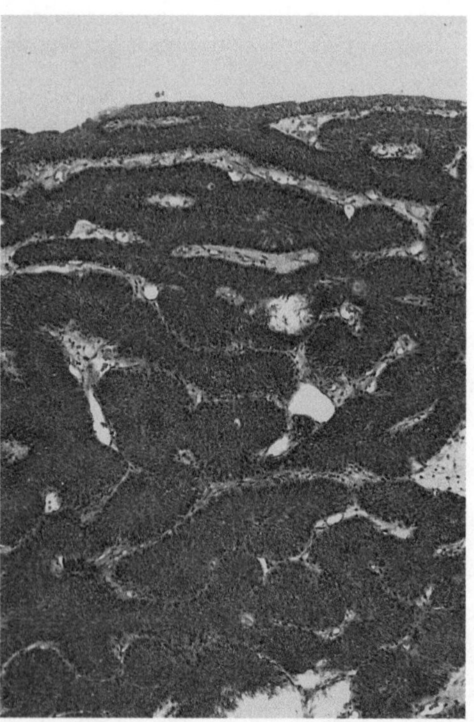
B

FIGURE *17-11*
Transitional cell papilloma of the bladder. (*A*) In this exophytic papilloma, branching papillary fronds project from the mucosal surface. (*B*) An inverted transitional cell papilloma shows an endophytic growth pattern and is composed of anastomosing cords of urothelial cells entirely within the lamina propria.

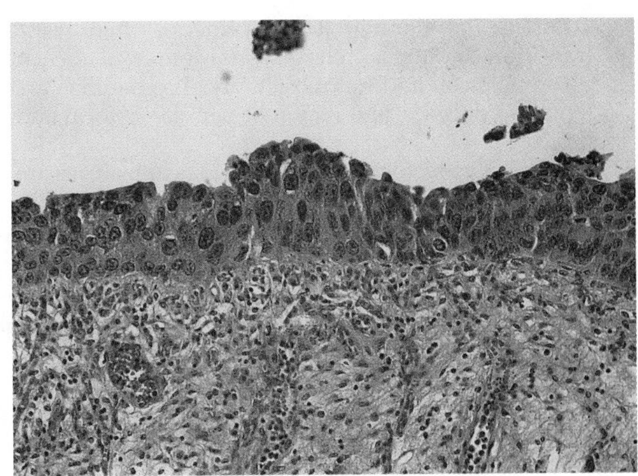

FIGURE 17-12
Transitional cell carcinoma *in situ*. The urothelial mucosa shows nuclear pleomorphism and lack of polarity from the basal layer to the surface, without evidence of maturation.

ophytic papillary transitional cell carcinoma. Concurrent involvement of the *in situ* lesion elsewhere in the bladder, or in the ureters, urethra, and prostatic ducts, is common. When confined to the urinary bladder, transitional cell carcinoma *in situ* is currently treated with intravesical chemotherapy agents or BCG. Patients are followed very closely, and only when repeat biopsy evidence indicates progression (bladder wall invasion or prostate involvement) is radical surgery, such as cystoprostatectomy, performed. The majority of invasive transitional cell carcinomas arise from flat lesions of carcinoma *in situ,* rather than from noninvasive papillary transitional cell carcinomas. Carcinoma *in situ* is often multifocal when it is discovered, or similar lesions may develop shortly thereafter. The growing respect for the aggressive nature of carcinoma *in situ* of the urinary bladder has prompted advocacy of radical cystectomy for such lesions.

Papillary Transitional Cell Carcinoma

☐ **Epidemiology:** The incidence of bladder carcinoma shows significant geographic and sex differences throughout the world. The highest frequencies are recorded among urban whites in the United States and western Europe, whereas a low prevalence prevails in Japan and among American blacks. Men are affected three to four times as often as women. Bladder cancer may be encountered at any age, but most patients (80%) are 50 to 80 years old. The association of transitional cell carcinoma of the bladder with similar tumors of the upper urinary tract is well known.

☐ **Pathogenesis:** The association of bladder cancer with occupational exposure to certain organic chemicals among workers in the German aniline dye industry was described in 1895 and was subsequently confirmed in similar workers in the United States. Later, an increased risk of bladder cancer was identified in the leather, rubber, paint, and organic chemical industries. Tobacco smokers have a fourfold increased risk compared to nonsmokers. Iatrogenic causes include analgesics (phenacetin), chemotherapeutic agents (cyclophosphamide), and radiation therapy (most frequently for cervical or prostate cancer). The role of *Schistosoma haematobium* in the development of squamous cell carcinoma will be discussed later.

Possible hereditary contributions and cytogenetic abnormalities in bladder carcinoma are the most recent developments in our understanding of this malignancy. There is evidence that multiple bladder tumors that arise either simultaneously or at different times are all derived from the same clone of neoplastic cells and thus represent seeding of additional sites within the vesical mucosa from a single original tumor. Previously, the presence of multiple tumors was regarded as a "field effect" on a urothelial mucosa pervasively "not at rest."

The influence of heredity on the risk of bladder cancer is limited to the identification of rare clusters of families who demonstrate autosomal dominant inheritance for this tumor. Such cases are rare, and the vast majority of patients with bladder cancer show no hereditary influence.

Specific cytogenetic abnormalities have been observed in a large proportion of bladder cancers. Chromosomal deletions in the long arm of chromosome 9 (9q−) are commonly observed in noninvasive tumors, and the Y chromosome may also be lost. Deletions have been observed in a variety of other chromosomes, including chromosome 17, the site of the p53 tumor suppressor gene. Overexpression of the *ras* oncogene and epidermal growth factor receptor has been reported in transitional cell carcinoma of the bladder.

A role for chemicals in the origin of bladder cancer has been strengthened by the demonstration that the administration of β-naphthylamine, a compound to which the dye industry workers were exposed, produces bladder cancer in dogs. The metabolic pathway of naphthylamines explains the organ specificity of their carcinogenic action. The arylamines are oxidized and then conjugated with glucuronic acid in the liver, after which the conjugates are excreted in the urine. In the bladder, β-glucuronidase hydrolyzes the glucuronic acid conjugate at the acidic pH of urine, thereby producing reactive arylnitrenium ions. These species are presumably carcinogenic by virtue of their ability to bind to the guanine moiety of DNA of the mucosal cells.

☐ **Pathology:** Bladder cancer arises most frequently from the lateral walls and less often from the posterior wall. At cystoscopy, the tumors vary from small, delicate, low-grade papillary lesions that are limited to the mucosal surface to larger, higher-grade, solid, invasive masses, which are often ulcerated (Fig. 17-13). The papillary and exophytic cancers tend to be more differentiated, whereas the infiltrating tumors are usually more anaplastic. Histologically, transitional cell carcinomas of the bladder are classified according to the World Health Organization grading system (Fig. 17-14):

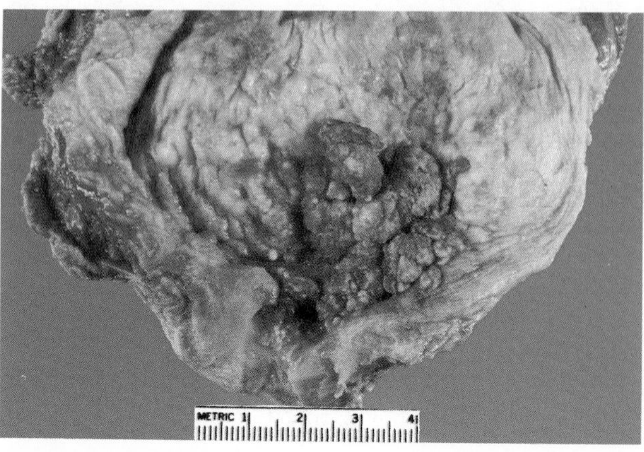

FIGURE 17-13
Transitional cell carcinoma of the urinary bladder. A large exophytic tumor is situated above the bladder neck.

- **Grade 1:** Papillary projections lined by neoplastic transitional epithelial cells that show minimal nuclear pleomorphism and mitotic activity. The papillae are long and delicate, and fusion of papillae is focal and limited.
- **Grade 2:** The histological and cytological features are intermediate between those of grade 1 (the best differentiated) and grade 3 (the most poorly differentiated).
- **Grade 3:** Significant nuclear pleomorphism, frequent mitoses, and fusion of papillae are typical. Occasional bizarre cells may be present, and focal sites of squamous differentiation are often seen. Although invasion of the underlying bladder wall may occur with any grade of transitional cell carcinoma, it is most frequent in grade 3 tumors.

☐ Clinical Features: **Transitional cell carcinoma of the bladder typically presents as sudden hematuria**

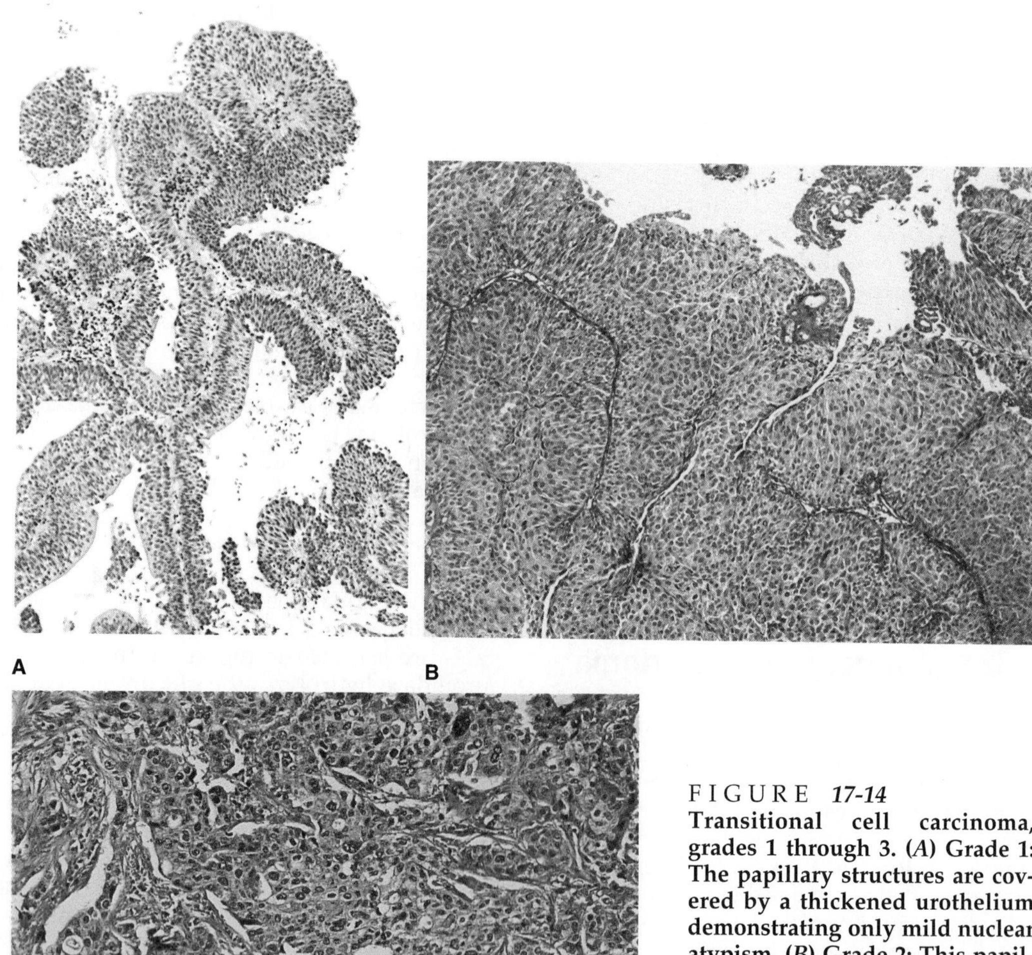

FIGURE 17-14
Transitional cell carcinoma, grades 1 through 3. (*A*) Grade 1: The papillary structures are covered by a thickened urothelium demonstrating only mild nuclear atypism. (*B*) Grade 2: This papillary neoplasm is characterized by nuclear pleomorphism and uncommon mitoses. (*C*) Grade 3: Marked nuclear pleomorphism and frequent mitoses, associated with blunting and fusing of the papillae, are present.

TABLE 17-1 **Clinical Staging of Transitional Cell Carcinoma of the Bladder**

Stage O: Tumor limited to the mucosa. The overall 3-year survival of patients with stage 0 disease is 97% for grade 1 lesions and 90% for grade 2 lesions.
Stage A: Invasion of the lamina propria. The 3-year prognosis of patients with stage A cancers varies with the grade of the tumor, from 92% for grade 1 lesions to 57% for grade 3 lesions.
Stage B: Invasion of muscle. The 5-year survival for patients with stage B disease is 35% to 40%.
B1: Superficial muscle invasion
B2: Deep muscle invasion
Stage C: Perivesical invasion. The 5-year survival of patients with stage C cancer is only 16%.
Stage D: Metastases
D1: Regional metastases
D2: Distant metastases

and less frequently as dysuria. Cystoscopy reveals single or multiple tumors. The extent of transitional cell carcinoma is described according to a staging classification (Table 17-1 and Fig. 17-15).

At the time of initial presentation, 85% of patients have tumor confined to the urinary bladder (stages O, A, B, and C) and 15% have regional or distant metastases. Therapeutic decisions referable to bladder cancer are related to the tumor stage. Papillary lesions limited to the mucosa (stage O) or lamina propria (stage A) are commonly treated conservatively by transurethral resection. Close follow-up is obligatory to detect "recurrences," that is, the development of new tumors. Radical cystectomy is performed on patients who demonstrate muscle invasion (stages B1 and B2) and occasionally on those with stage C tumors.

The probability of tumor extension and subsequent recurrence is associated with a number of factors:

- Large size
- High stage
- High grade
- The presence of multiple tumors
- Vascular or lymphatic invasion
- Urothelial dysplasia, including carcinoma *in situ*, at other sites in the bladder

Noninvasive or superficially invasive transitional cell tumors are treated conservatively, despite the fact that as many as 30% of such patients eventually exhibit extension of the tumor. It is now apparent that up to 90% of all patients with muscle wall invasion already had such invasion at the time of initial presentation. Patients with invasion of muscle or perivesical adipose tissue at the time of initial diagnosis often have regional lymph node metastases, with a median survival of 1 year. However, recent advances in chemotherapy have significantly improved the prognosis. In order of decreasing frequency, metastases of bladder cancer occur in regional and periaortic lymph nodes, liver, lung, and bone. The most common causes of death are uremia from ureteral obstruction and carcinomatosis.

Squamous Cell Carcinoma

Squamous cell carcinoma of the urinary bladder is distinctly uncommon in the Western world, whereas it is frequent in Egypt and other areas of the Middle East where schistosomiasis is endemic (Fig. 17-16A). Squamous metaplasia of the nontumorous vesical urothelium is common in cases of squamous cell carcinoma. The clinical presentation of patients with this type of bladder cancer is

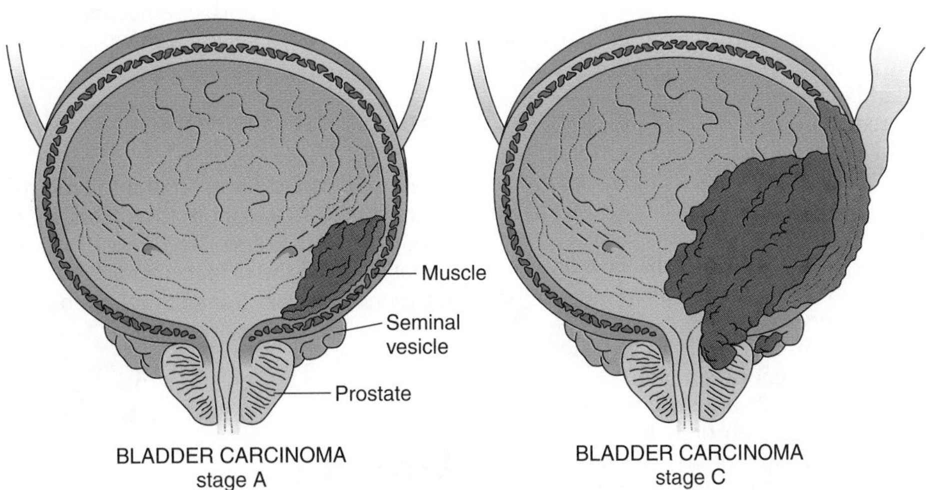

FIGURE 17-15
Clinical staging of bladder carcinoma. Carcinoma of the bladder, stage A, is restricted to the mucosa and lamina propria. Advanced carcinoma, stage C, exhibits a larger intravesical mass and invasion of the bladder wall, where it may obstruct the ureter and produce hydroureter. In this stage, the tumor extends beyond the bladder to the prostate and seminal vesicles.

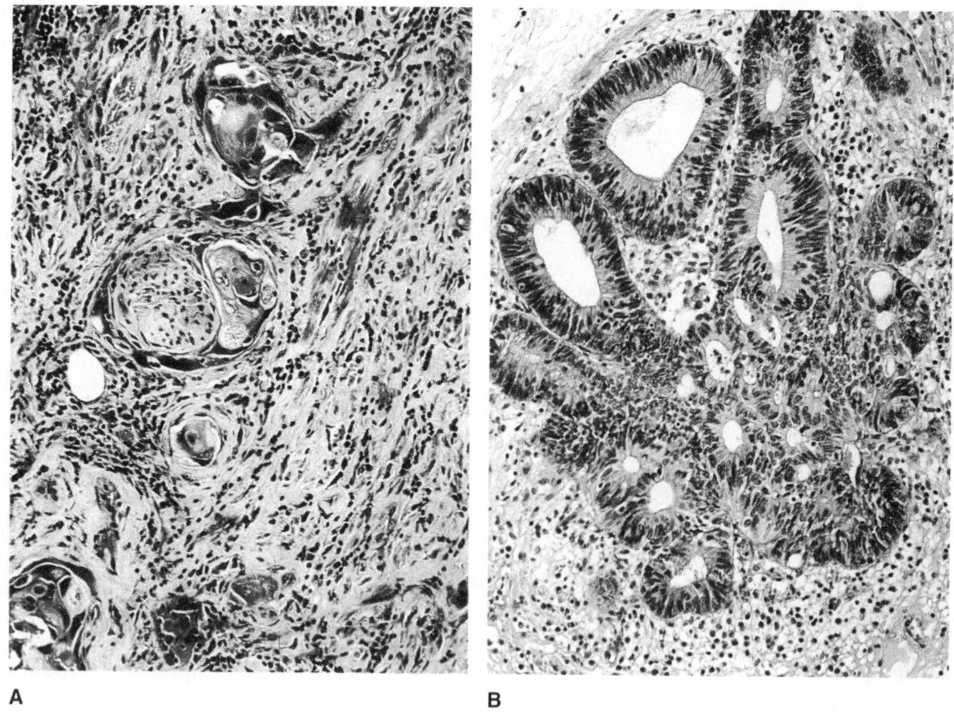

FIGURE 17-16
Unusual histological types of bladder carcinoma. (*A*) Squamous cell carcinoma. (*B*) Adenocarcinoma.

similar to that seen in the more common transitional cell carcinomas. **However, virtually all patients with squamous cell carcinoma demonstrate invasion of the bladder wall at the time of initial presentation and thus have a worse prognosis than the majority of patients with transitional cell carcinoma.**

Adenocarcinoma

Adenocarcinoma of the bladder is uncommon and most cases have been reported in the past two decades. As with the other forms of bladder cancer, adenocarcinoma shows a pronounced male predilection. Bladder adenocarcinoma must be distinguished from urachal adenocarcinoma and from prostatic cancer. The histological patterns encountered in primary adenocarcinoma of the bladder include papillary, glandular, mucinous, adenoid cystic, signet-ring cell, and clear cell types (see Fig. 17-16B). Foci of transitional cell carcinoma, with or without areas of squamous cell carcinoma, may be observed. An association with cystitis cystica and cystitis glandularis has been reported in a minority of cases of bladder adenocarcinoma.

The presenting symptoms are not specific, and most patients experience hematuria, with or without dysuria. The majority of bladder adenocarcinomas are deeply invasive at the time of initial presentation and are not curable.

Mesenchymal Tumors

Leiomyomas, hemangiomas, granular cell tumors, and neurofibromas have occasionally been reported to arise within the urinary bladder. The rare malignant mesenchymal tumors are usually rhabdomyosarcomas and leiomyosarcomas.

Rhabdomyosarcomas, typically of the embryonal type, occur most commonly in children, and 90% are seen in patients younger than the age of 40 years. Bladder rhabdomyosarcoma of childhood is an edematous mucosal polypoid mass, which has been likened to a cluster of grapes. Recent advances in combined treatment with radiation therapy and chemotherapy have resulted in greatly increased survival rates.

Metastatic Tumors

The urinary bladder is often involved by direct extension of cancers of adjacent organs, including the uterine cervix, prostate, and colon. The most common tumors that metastasize to the urinary bladder, in order of decreasing frequency, are malignant melanoma and carcinomas of the stomach, breast, and lung.

Urethra

ANATOMY

The male urethra is divided into proximal (posterior) and distal (anterior) segments. The posterior urethra begins at the internal urethral orifice of the prostatic urethra and continues to the membranous urethra. Prostatic duct ostia are present on the posterior and lateral walls throughout the length of the prostatic urethra. The distal urethra is divided into the proximal portion, called the bulbous urethra, and the more distal penile urethra. The latter terminates in the fossa navicularis, immediately proximal to the external orifice, or meatus.

The transitional cell epithelium lining the proximal urethra is continuous with the bladder urothelium, gradually changing to stratified columnar epithelium in the membranous and bulbous potions. In the male, the more distal portion of the urethra, the fossa navicularis, is lined by stratified squamous epithelium continuous with the meatus. Mucous glands (Cowper's glands) are situated in the bulbous portion of the anterior urethra. The female urethra is shorter than that in the male and displays a similar change from transitional to squamous epithelium.

CONGENITAL DISORDERS

Congenital disorders of the urethra predominantly involve the location of the external urethral orifice.

- **Hypospadias** is a condition in which the urethra opens on the underside of the penis.
- **Epispadias** refers to a urethra that opens on the upper side of the penis.
- **Urethral valves,** with associated bladder outlet obstruction, are only rarely encountered.

BENIGN CONDITIONS

Urethritis

The classic cause of urethritis is infection with *Neisseria gonorrhoeae*. However, the disease results more commonly from infection with *Chlamydia, E. coli,* or *Mycoplasma*. In males, urethritis typically complicates prostatitis, whereas in females it follows cystitis. In many cases, no organisms can be identified. A complex of unknown etiology, characterized by urethritis, arthritis, and conjunctivitis, is known as *Reiter syndrome.* Urinary frequency, dysuria, and urethral discharge characterize urethral inflammation regardless of etiology.

Diverticulum

Diverticula of the urethra, usually in the dorsolateral wall of the mid urethra, are virtually limited to women, in whom they are most frequently diagnosed in the third to sixth decades. The majority are probably acquired secondary to trauma or obstruction of a periurethral duct. Patients present with postmicturition dribbling and urinary frequency and urgency. Physical examination reveals a compressible bulge in the anterior vaginal wall.

Urethral Caruncle

Urethral caruncles are inflammatory lesions near the female urethral meatus that produce pain and bleeding. They occur exclusively in women, most frequently after menopause. The etiology and pathogenesis are unclear; prolapse of the urethral mucosa and associated chronic inflammation have been suggested as the cause.

A urethral caruncle typically presents as an exophytic, often ulcerated, polypoid mass, 1 to 2 cm in diameter, at or near the urethral meatus. Histologically, caruncles exhibit acutely and chronically inflamed granulation tissue and ulceration and hyperplasia of transitional cell or squamous epithelium (Fig. 17-17). Although complex patterns of papillomatosis and occasional dysplastic epithelium may give this inflammatory lesion a superficial resemblance to carcinoma, it does not lead to urethral cancer. Treatment is surgical excision.

Adenomatous Polyps with Prostatic Epithelium

Adenomatous polyps are exophytic, villous, and glandular proliferations of prostatic tissue in the prostatic urethra (Fig. 17-18). Patients present with hematuria, hemospermia (blood in the semen), or both. The peak age frequency is the second to fourth decades. Microscopically, these polyps are lined by typical prostatic acinar epithelium. The lesions are not premalignant, and treatment is by conservative transurethral resections.

Benign Tumors

Benign epithelial tumors of the urethra are uncommon and include squamous cell papillomas, transitional cell papillomas, and inverted papillomas. The histological features of these tumors are identical to their counterparts in the urinary bladder.

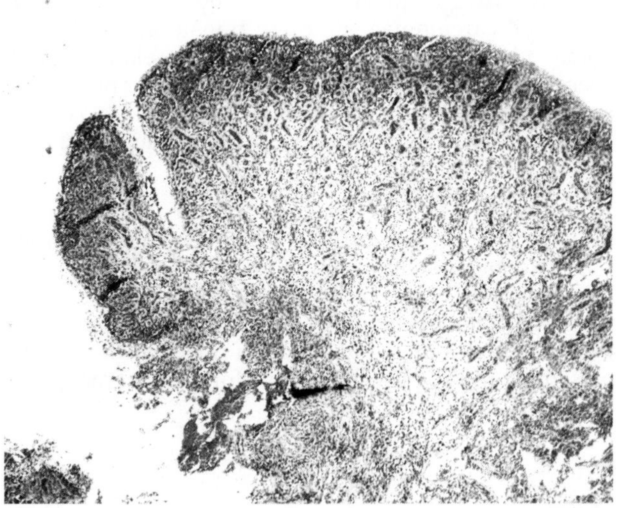

FIGURE *17-17*
Urethral caruncle. The submucosa of the distal urethral segment contains many thin-walled blood vessels. Numerous acute and chronic inflammatory cells are present in the stroma. Hyperplasia of the overlying mucosa can be seen at the top.

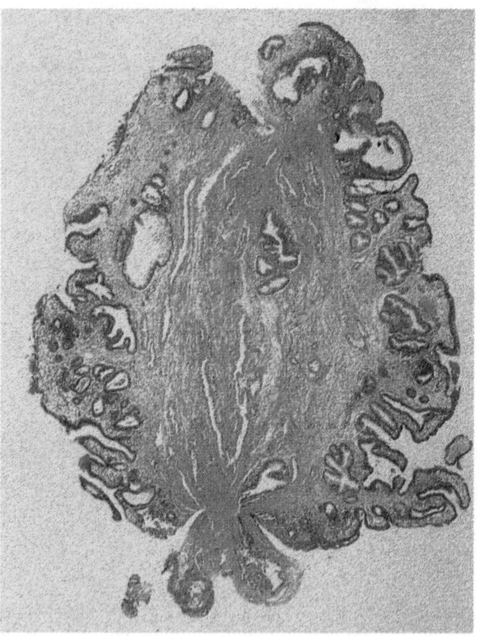

FIGURE 17-18
Adenomatous polyp of the urethra. The polypoid structure consists of glandular epithelium identical to that lining the prostatic acini.

CARCINOMA OF THE URETHRA

Carcinoma of the urethra is unusual, with a female predominance of 2:1. Disorders frequently associated with urethral carcinoma include urethral stricture, prior instrumentation, venereal disease, and, most importantly, prior or concomitant bladder cancer.

□ **Pathology:** Most cancers of the urethra are squamous cell carcinomas, although transitional cell carcinoma, adenocarcinoma, and malignant melanoma have been reported. Transitional cell carcinomas tend to arise in the proximal urethra, squamous cell carcinomas in the distal urethra, and adenocarcinoma in the mid urethra.

□ **Clinical Features:** Urethral carcinoma is most frequently observed in the sixth and seventh decades. Most patients present with urethral bleeding and dysuria. In spite of the accessible location and associated symptoms, the majority of urethral carcinomas have spread to adjacent tissues or regional lymph nodes at the time of presentation. The primary therapy for urethral malignancies is radical surgery.

Penis

PHIMOSIS

Phimosis refers to the congenital or acquired inability to retract the prepuce. Some cases are congenital, but most are the residual of previous infections and scarring of the prepuce. Regardless of cause, phimosis increases the risk of further inflammation of the glans and prepuce (*balanoposthitis*). Circumcision is effective therapy for phimosis.

SEXUALLY TRANSMITTED LESIONS

Infections of the penis acquired by sexual congress include syphilis, chancroid, granuloma inguinale, lymphogranuloma venereum, genital herpes, and the wart-like lesions associated with human papillomavirus (HPV) infection. These diseases are discussed in Chapter 9.

PEYRONIE DISEASE

Peyronie disease is a malady of unknown etiology characterized by focal, asymmetric, fibrous induration of the shaft of the penis. The resulting penile curvature is accompanied by pain during erection. Rare examples appear to be inherited as an autosomal dominant trait. The typical case appears as an ill-defined induration of the penile shaft in a young or middle-aged man, without any change in the overlying skin. On microscopic examination, dense dermal fibrosis is associated with a nonspecific chronic inflammatory cell infiltrate. Collagen focally replaces muscle in the septum of the corpus cavernosum. No reliable therapy has emerged.

CONDYLOMA ACUMINATUM (VENEREAL WART)

Condylomata acuminata of the penis are circumscribed, exophytic, cauliflower-like lesions that occur on the glans and are also occasionally are found on the shaft (Fig. 17-19A). They tend to spread to involve other sites of the anogenital region. Venereal warts are caused by sexually transmitted infection with HPV, most commonly types 6 and 11. The sexual partners of men with condylomata acuminata of the penis often have similar genital lesions that accord with the same strain of HPV.

Histologically, the lesions are papillomatous and exhibit conspicuous acanthosis and parakeratosis (see Fig. 17-19B). In the superficial zone of the epithelium, prominent clearing of the cytoplasm (koilocytosis) is interpreted as evidence of HPV infection. Importantly, cell atypism is absent, and the lesion is not a precursor of squamous carcinoma.

SQUAMOUS CELL CARCINOMA *IN SITU*

Historically, squamous cell carcinoma *in situ* of the skin of the penis was described in two forms: Bowen disease and erythroplasia of Queyrat. Almost a century ago, Bowen described precancerous dermatoses in extragenital sites. Contemporaneously, Queyrat reported similar lesions on the glans and prepuce. Although these diseases were traditionally accorded independent status, they are now viewed as variants of the same disease. Dysplastic epidermal lesions on the shaft of the penis are referred to as

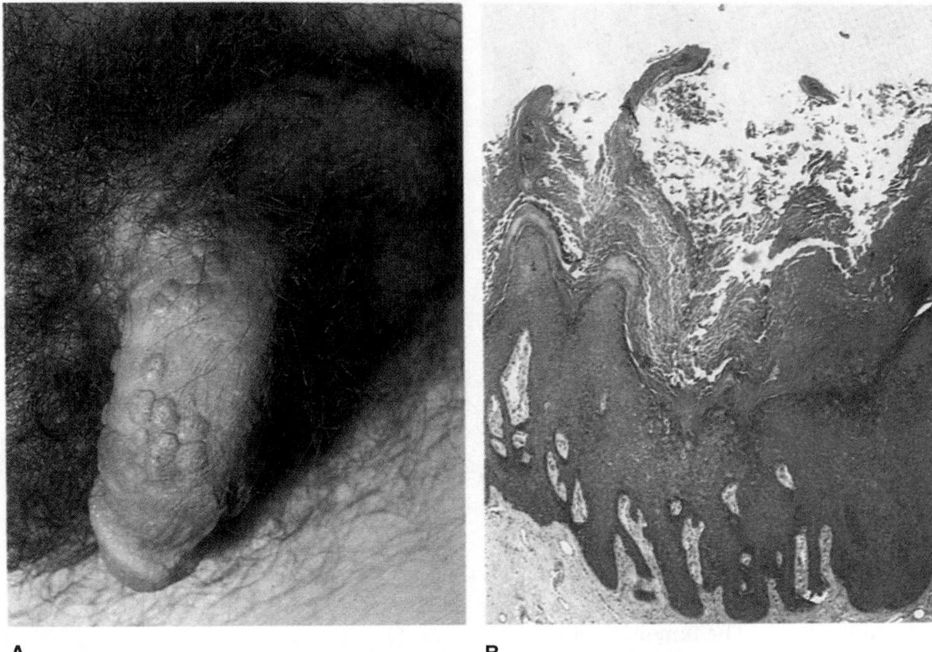

FIGURE 17-19
Condyloma acuminatum of the penis. (*A*) Raised, circumscribed, cauliflower-like lesions are seen on the shaft of the penis. (*B*) Section of a lesion shows epidermal hyperkeratosis, parakeratosis, acanthosis, and papillomatosis.

Bowen disease, whereas those on the glans and prepuce are termed erythroplasia of Queyrat.

Bowen disease appears as a sharply demarcated, erythematous plaque, usually occurring in middle-aged or elderly men.

Erythroplasia of Queyrat occurs in uncircumcised men who are younger than those with Bowen disease; it presents as shiny, soft, erythematous plaques on the glans and foreskin.

Both of these conditions are characterized histologically by squamous cell carcinoma *in situ*, similar to that in other sites. The lesions show cytological atypia of the keratinocytes of all layers of the epidermis, with parakeratosis and hyperkeratosis, papillomatosis with broad epidermal papillae, and thinning of the granular layer. By definition, the atypical keratinocytes do not invade the underlying dermis. A chronic inflammatory cell infiltrate within the subjacent dermis is characteristic of squamous carcinoma *in situ*. The frequency with which Bowen disease and erythroplasia of Queyrat progress to invasive squamous cell carcinoma remains unsettled but is estimated to be less than 10% of cases.

Bowenoid papulosis is another disease of the penile skin that is associated with squamous carcinoma *in situ*. It occurs in men in the third and fourth decades of life, that is, two decades earlier than the appearance of Bowen disease or erythroplasia of Queyrat. Bowenoid papulosis presents clinically as multiple violaceous papules on the shaft of the penis. Microscopically, the disorder resembles the other variants of carcinoma *in situ* but typically exhibits lesser cytological atypia. Bowenoid papulosis is likely a venereal disease. HPV type 16 antigens (but not type 18) have been demonstrated in the majority of lesions. The sexual partners of the patients tend to suffer from condylomata acuminata and cervical dysplasia, disorders also associated with HPV type 16. Virtually all lesions of bowenoid papulosis regress spontaneously or after topical therapy. The potential invasiveness of bowenoid papulosis is not established.

The distinctions between Bowen disease, erythroplasia of Queyrat, and bowenoid papulosis may simply reflect a sterile academic debate, and there is an increasing tendency to refer to any noninvasive, neoplastic lesion of the penile skin as *penile intraepithelial neoplasia*.

VERRUCOUS CARCINOMA (GIANT CONDYLOMA OF BUSCHKE-LÖWENSTEIN)

Verrucous carcinoma of the penis is a cytologically benign, but clinically malignant, exophytic squamous cell cancer. In 1925, Buschke and Löwenstein described a penile lesion that was grossly and cytologically similar to condyloma acuminatum, but unlike the latter, it showed deep local invasion. The lesion is today recognized as a low-grade squamous cell carcinoma. It does not, as a general rule, metastasize, although a few such cases have been reported.

Verrucous carcinoma of the penis invariably occurs in uncircumcised men (Fig. 17-20). The tumor may enlarge to form a substantial warty mass, which destroys the end of the penis. The histological features are similar to those of condyloma acuminatum, but at the base of the tumor the rete ridges are conspicuously enlarged. Although the basement membrane is not breached, the rete ridges extend into the underlying connective tissue. It is only late in the evolution of the tumor that true invasion through

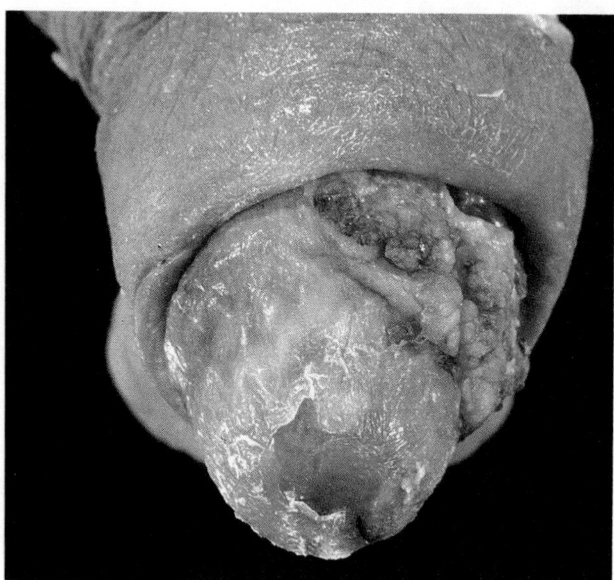

FIGURE *17-20*
Verrucous carcinoma of the penis. The tumor arises on the glans and presents as an exophytic mass.

the basement membrane occurs. Surgical removal of a verrucous carcinoma is curative.

SQUAMOUS CELL CARCINOMA OF THE PENIS

□ **Epidemiology:** In the United States, invasive squamous cell carcinoma of the penis is an uncommon tumor, accounting for less than 0.5% of all cancers in men. The average age of patients with invasive squamous cell carcinoma is 60 years. Penile cancer is much more common in less-developed countries, and in some parts of Africa and Asia it comprises 10% of male cancers. Since this tumor is virtually unknown in men circumcised at birth, these geographic variations have been attributed to differences in the frequency of circumcision. Interestingly, a few Muslims who delayed circumcision until prepubertal years have developed penile cancer.

No single causal agent has been identified, but current interest centers on the possible influence of the accumulated keratin debris and the inflammatory exudate (smegma) that accumulates beneath the prepuce. More than half of the patients with cancer of the penis have had phimosis since an early age, suggesting that a prolonged contact between smegma and the penile epithelium may play a role. HPV types 16 and 18 have also been suggested as factors in the pathogenesis of penile cancer.

□ **Pathology:** Squamous cell carcinoma of the penis presents as an ulcerated and hemorrhagic mass on the glans or the prepuce. It may be an exophytic fungating tumor or principally infiltrating. Extensive destruction of penile tissue, including the urethral meatus, is occasionally observed. Microscopically, the typical example is a well-differentiated, focally keratinizing, squamous cell carcinoma. Only rarely are these cancers poorly differentiated. Invasive tumors are associated with a dense, chronic inflammatory cell infiltrate in the dermis. The adjacent epithelium of the epidermis often shows dysplastic changes. The tumor may invade deeply along the penile shaft and may spread to inguinal lymph nodes, then to the iliac nodes, and ultimately to distant organs.

□ **Clinical Features:** Most squamous cell cancers are confined to the penis at the time of initial presentation, but occult metastases to inguinal lymph nodes are not uncommon. Conversely, half of the patients with clinically enlarged regional lymph nodes have no nodal metastases but rather reactive changes secondary to the inflammation associated with the primary tumor.

The survival of patients with penile cancer is related to the clinical stage and, to a lesser degree, to the histological grade of the tumor. Most patients with stage I cancer (superficial lesion of the glans or prepuce) can be cured, but the prognosis is progressively worse with more extensive cancers. Amputation of the penis is usually necessary.

SCROTUM

Sclerosing Lipogranuloma

This inflammatory process is directed toward exogenous lipids and waxes that gain access to the dermis. It has been reported most commonly among young men, in the penis and scrotum. The exogenous lipids prompt a foreign body giant cell reaction, which is associated with variable fibrosis. In most instances, there is a previous history of trauma to the genital region.

Squamous Cell Carcinoma of the Scrotum

The identification in 1775 of scrotal cancer as an occupational disease of chimney sweeps by Sir Percival Pott introduced the concept of chemical carcinogenesis (see Chapter 5). Pott implicated constant exposure to soot as the causative agent, but later investigators incriminated a large variety of industrial chemicals in the pathogenesis of this tumor. Owing to refinements in industrial hygiene, scrotal cancer is today uncommon.

Squamous cell carcinoma of the scrotum is most frequent in the sixth and seventh decades. It is typically a well-differentiated tumor. At the time of initial presentation, many patients demonstrate invasion of the scrotal contents and metastases to regional nodes. Therapy for scrotal cancer is surgical excision.

Testis

EMBRYOLOGY

The testis develops from the undifferentiated tissue of the gonadal ridge. During the third gestational week, the germ cells migrate from the yolk sac endoderm to assume residence in the gonadal ridge. Differentiation of the undifferentiated ridge to a testis requires aggregation of germ cells in the sex cords, which later become the seminiferous tubules.

The origin of the sex cords containing the Leydig cells and the Sertoli cells is debated. One view regards Sertoli cells of the seminiferous tubules and the Leydig cells of the gonadal interstitium as derivatives of a common gonadal stromal cell precursor. Others hold that the sex cords result from the downgrowth of the surface epithelium into the gonad. The unsettled state of this embryological question is reflected in the World Health Organization classification, in which tumors of Leydig and Sertoli cells are termed *sex cord/stromal neoplasms.*

During gestation, there is a progressive transition of the sex cords to recognizable seminiferous tubules, which ultimately connect to the testicular excretory ductal system, derived from the mesonephric (wolffian) duct. Within the testis, the seminiferous tubules converge and become continuous with the rete testis tubules, which connect to the efferent ductules of the proximal epididymis. The epididymis, in turn, continues as the vas deferens and its distal diverticular outpouching, the seminal vesicles.

The normal descent of the testes from their intra-abdominal point of origin progresses in late gestation. The size and structure of the adult testes are achieved only after a period of dramatic growth and maturation at puberty under the influence of pituitary gonadotropins. The hormonally induced changes initiate (1) spermatogenesis, (2) the reemergence of interstitial Leydig cells, and (3) their synthesis of testosterone, with a conspicuous increase in the level of circulating testosterone.

ANATOMY

The adult testis is 4 cm long and 3 cm wide. The attached epididymis is longitudinally oriented along the lateral–posterior aspect of the testis. The testis is invested with the tunica vaginalis, a layer of mesothelial cells that covers the outer fibrous capsule of the testis, the tunica albuginea. This capsule has internal septal ramifications that divide the testis into about 250 lobules. Within each of the lobules, the coiled seminiferous tubules and interstitium are intermingled.

The arterial supply to the testis is through the testicular arteries, which originate from the abdominal aorta. The venous drainage is a dual system: the right internal spermatic vein empties into the vena cava, and the left drains into the ipsilateral renal vein. This anatomical difference has several clinical implications, which are discussed later.

Following puberty, active spermatogenesis is apparent throughout the seminiferous tubules. Within the tubules, Sertoli cells and germ cells are seen in varying stages of maturation to sperm. The Sertoli cells are elongated and oriented with their base at the tubular basement membrane. Irregularly shaped nuclei with a prominent nucleolus distinguish Sertoli cells from the adjacent spermatogonia.

The precise role of Sertoli cells in the maturation of the germ cells remains unknown. Spermatogonia undergo mitosis to become primary spermatocytes, which in turn give rise to the transient secondary spermatocytes by meiotic division. Secondary spermatocytes mature to spermatids, and the latter to spermatozoa. Germ cells far outnumber Sertoli cells, and primary spermatocytes are the most numerous germ cells present.

The polygonal Leydig cells (interstitial cells), located within the intertubular interstitium, are frequently found in clusters. They have round nuclei and an abundant eosinophilic cytoplasm. Characteristic rectangle-shaped crystalloids, termed *Reinke crystals,* are observed in a few Leydig cells. Their significance is unknown. Leydig cells are stimulated by pituitary luteinizing hormone (LH) to synthesize testosterone. Old age is associated with advanced regressive changes, characterized by decreased spermatogenesis, increased Leydig cells, and tubular and interstitial fibrosis.

CRYPTORCHIDISM

Cryptorchidism refers to the failure of a testis to descend completely into its normal position within the scrotum. The descent of the testis may be arrested at any point from the abdomen to the upper scrotum (Fig. 17-21). At term, 4% of male newborns are cryptorchid. In the large majority of these infants, the testis descends within the first year of life, and the prevalence of cryptorchidism among adults is less than 0.4%.

Cryptorchidism is most commonly unilateral, but it is bilateral in one fourth of the cases. It is usually an isolated anomaly, although in rare instances it is associated with other congenital anomalies. The cause of testicular maldescent is largely unknown.

☐ **Pathology:** The histological changes in the cryptorchid testis are related to age. From birth to 5 years of age, the earliest changes are reduced diameters of the seminiferous tubules and decreased numbers of germ cells. Indeed, complete absence of germ cells has been observed in patients as young as 3 years old. If surgical repositioning of the testis (orchiopexy) is delayed beyond puberty, a decreased number of germ cells, hyaline thickening of the tubular basement membrane, and stromal fibrosis are observed (Fig. 17-22). Eventually, the tubules are reduced to hyalinized cords of connective tissue. Interestingly, the scrotal testis of 25% of adult men with untreated unilateral cryptorchidism demonstrates similar changes.

☐ **Clinical Features:** The clinical significance of cryptorchidism relates not to the abnormal position *per se* (patients are asymptomatic) but to the associated risk of infertility and germ cell tumors (see Fig. 17-21). **The risk of developing germ cell tumors in untreated cryptorchidism, most commonly seminomas and embryonal carcinomas, is increased 35-fold.** Germ cell tumors have not been reported in patients in whom orchiopexy was performed before age 5 years, and it is, therefore, crucial to treat this disorder early. Virtually all patients who have developed germ cell tumors after orchiopexy had the operation postponed to age 10 years or later. Nevertheless, there are troubling reports of germ cell tumors arising in testes that have been surgically positioned in the scrotum

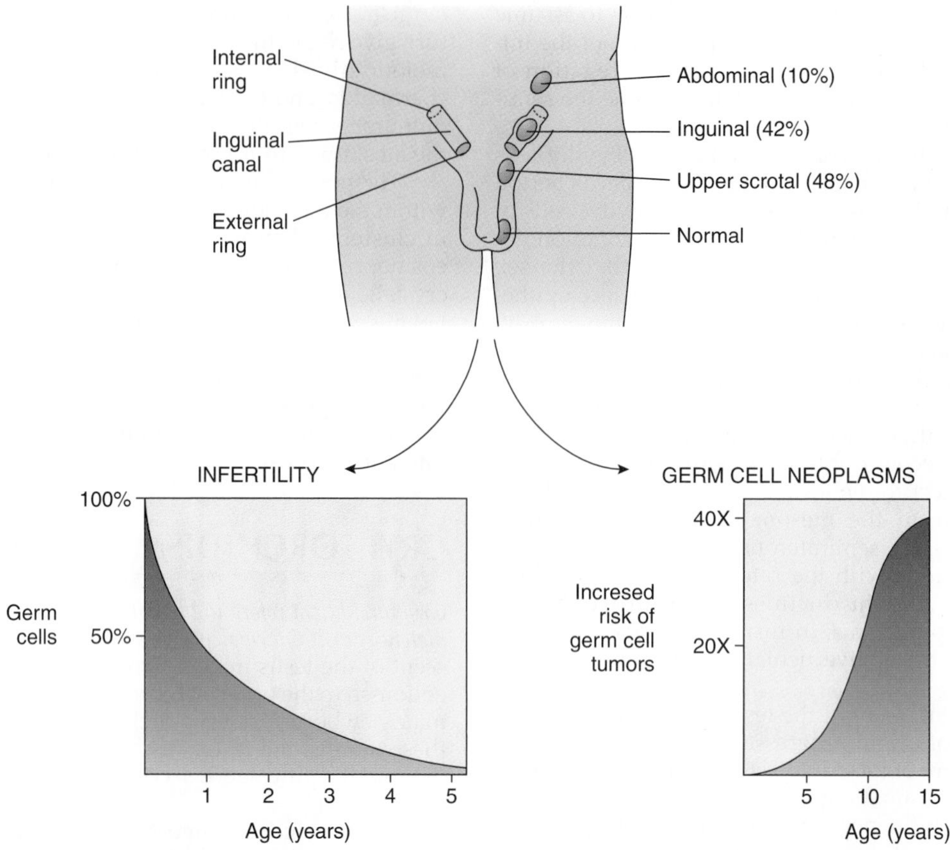

FIGURE *17-21*
Cryptorchidism and associated complications. There is a 50% reduction in germ cell number after the first year of life and a virtually complete loss by 4 to 5 years of age. After age 5, the risk of germ cell tumors increases steeply.

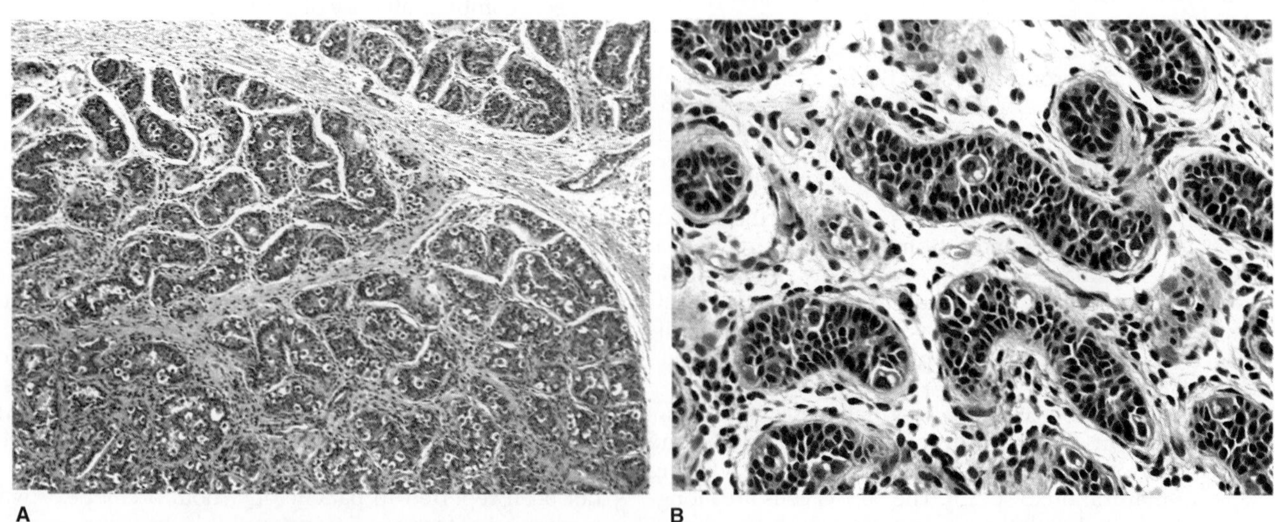

FIGURE *17-22*
Cryptorchidism. (*A*) The diameter of the seminiferous tubules is smaller than normal in this testis from a 2-year-old infant. (*B*) A high-power view shows that the germ cells are reduced in number.

at an early age, and even in the contralateral, normally descended testis.

Adult men with untreated bilateral cryptorchidism are infertile. Orchiopexy before the age of 2 years generally prevents this complication, but if surgery is postponed, only one fourth will be fertile (see Fig. 17-21). Infertility is also a risk in patients with a single undescended testis because of the previously noted changes in the scrotal testis. The combination of involutional changes and the occasional occurrence of germ cell tumors in the normally descended testis suggest the possibility that at least in some cases of cryptorchidism an inherent developmental defect is involved.

DISORDERS OF GENETIC SEX

Disorders of genetic sex refer to phenotypic abnormalities caused by chromosomal aberrations (see Chapter 6).

Turner syndrome (45,X karyotype) is distinguished by a female phenotype and bilateral streak gonads, which are composed of fibrous stroma and are devoid of germ cells.

Mixed gonadal dysgenesis refers to a condition in which a well-defined testis, varying from rudimentary to normal, is associated with a contralateral streak gonad. The latter is identical to that in Turner syndrome. Mixed gonadal dysgenesis is the second most common cause of ambiguous genitalia in the newborn, ranking only after congenital adrenal hyperplasia.

True hermaphrodites have bilateral gonads that consist of varying combinations of ovarian and testicular tissue. Such "ovotesticular" structures show testicular seminiferous tubules in proximity to ovarian primordial follicles.

DISORDERS OF PHENOTYPIC SEX

Disorders of phenotypic sex refer to patients with ambiguous external genitalia but normal male or female gonads.

Male pseudohermaphroditism (XY karyotype) may result from autosomal recessive disorders of testosterone biosynthesis. Five distinct metabolic disorders of testosterone synthesis are included under the rubric of the male

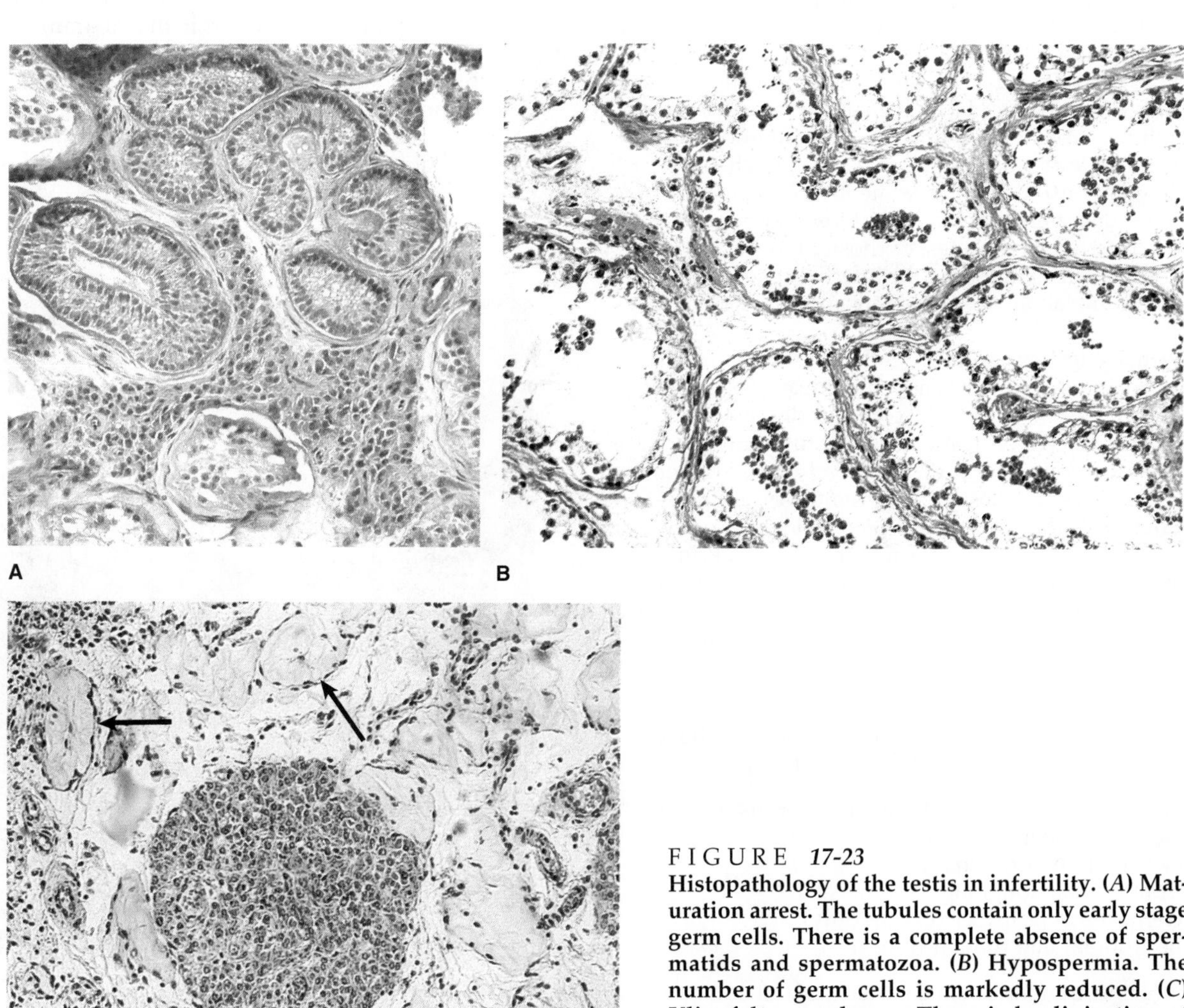

FIGURE 17-23
Histopathology of the testis in infertility. (*A*) Maturation arrest. The tubules contain only early stage germ cells. There is a complete absence of spermatids and spermatozoa. (*B*) Hypospermia. The number of germ cells is markedly reduced. (*C*) Klinefelter syndrome. There is hyalinization of the tubules (*arrows*) with absence of spermatogenesis and rare Sertoli cells. A large cluster of interstitial cells is present.

adrenogenital syndrome. These patients exhibit varying degrees of genital abnormalities, encompassing minimal to severe ambiguity of the genitalia, hypospadias, and adrenal cortical insufficiency. Alternatively, male pseudohermaphroditism may result from androgen insensitivity of peripheral organs, the classic example being **testicular feminization**. Such patients, although genetically male, are marked by a female phenotype, with the development of breast tissue, a clitoris, and a poorly developed vagina. Most patients with testicular feminization are initially discovered in the course of an evaluation for primary amenorrhea.

Female pseudohermaphroditism is caused by an autosomal recessive trait that leads to adrenal hypersecretion of androgens (adrenogenital syndrome) and the virilization of a genetic female (XX). An enlarged clitoris, resembling a penis, and fusion of the labia, similar to a scrotum, create ambiguity of the external genitalia.

INFERTILITY

The causes of male infertility can be broadly categorized into testicular damage, primary testicular failure, and post-testicular infertility.

Testicular damage is the most common cause of male infertility. It is produced by diverse mechanisms, including orchitis, varicocele, cryptorchidism, radiation, alcohol abuse, and a variety of drugs, in particular, chemotherapeutic agents used in the treatment of cancer. Systemic metabolic disorders that may interfere with male fertility encompass uremia, diabetes, cirrhosis, and malnutrition. The mechanisms underlying the infertile states associated with these metabolic disorders are incompletely understood.

Primary testicular failure reflects varied genetic disorders, including Turner syndrome, mixed gonadal dysgenesis, and Klinefelter syndrome. As discussed earlier, deleterious effects on testicular structure and function may result from a group of recessively inherited enzymatic disorders of testosterone biosynthesis.

Post-testicular infertility refers to blockage of the excretory ducts that convey sperm to the urethra. Prior vasectomy or infections of the epididymis or the vas deferens are often responsible. Less frequently the excretory duct obstruction is due to previous trauma or congenital atresia.

☐ **Pathology:** Morphological alterations of the testis in infertile males include the following (Fig. 17-23):

- Structural immaturity of the seminiferous tubules
- Decreased spermatogenesis
- Germ cell maturation arrest
- Intratubular sloughing of germ cells
- Germ cell aplasia (Sertoli cells only)
- Peritubular and tubular fibrosis

Not uncommonly, mixed patterns of testicular abnormalities are observed. Alternatively, morphological changes in the testis may be absent despite demonstrable infertility, in which case testicular biopsy provides no information relating to the underlying cause.

ORCHITIS

Orchitis refers to acute or chronic inflammation of the testis, frequently in association with inflammation of the epididymis.

Gram-negative bacterial orchitis is the most common form of the disease and is often secondary to urinary tract infections.

Syphilitic orchitis, in which the testis is infected with spirochetes and displays gummas, is a well-known complication of syphilis.

Mumps orchitis is the most frequent form of acute testicular inflammation caused by a virus, occurring in 20% of adult males with mumps. The disorder is characterized by testicular pain and gonadal swelling, most commonly unilateral.

Granulomatous orchitis of unknown cause is an infrequent disorder of middle-aged men that presents as painful enlargement of the testis or insidiously with testicular induration. The disease is characterized microscopically by noncaseating granulomas, which fail to reveal any organisms or the presence of sperm remnants that may act as possible inciting agents. This is in contrast to sperm granulomas of the epididymis, which characteristically show sperm phagocytosis in the inflammatory focus. Variable numbers of seminiferous tubules are destroyed by the granulomatous inflammatory process.

Malakoplakia of the testis is another form of granulomatous orchitis. It has the same histological features and presumably the same histogenesis as malakoplakia elsewhere.

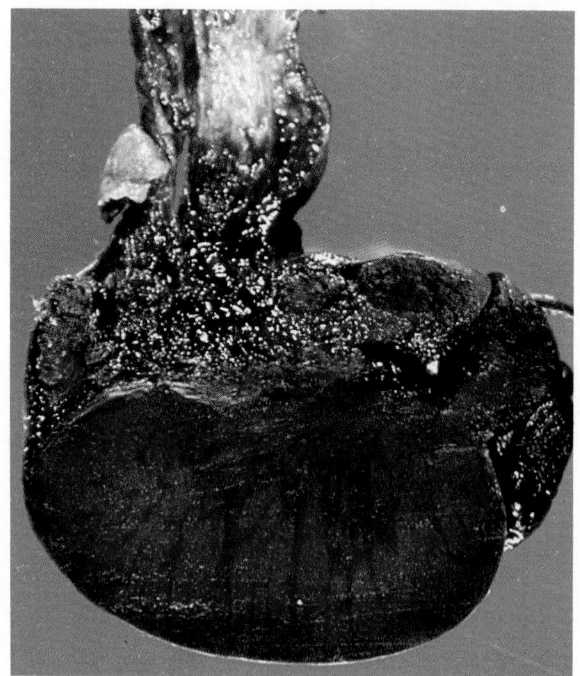

FIGURE *17-24*
Testicular torsion. A cut section of the testicle from a man who experienced sudden excruciating scrotal pain shows diffuse hemorrhage and necrosis of the testis and adnexal structures.

Chronic orchitis is currently uncommon, although chronic inflammation of the testis in tuberculosis and in infections with a variety of fungal agents has been well documented.

TORSION OF THE TESTIS

Torsion of the spermatic cord, if complete, produces severe pain and infarction of the testicular germ cells within a few hours. Most commonly, torsion presents shortly after vigorous physical exercise, although such a history is not always obtained. Torsion of the spermatic cord is often associated with congenital abnormalities that contribute to increased mobility of the testis and epididymis, for example, a high attachment of the tunica vaginalis on the spermatic cord, incomplete descent of the testis, or absence of the scrotal ligaments.

An abrupt onset of scrotal pain followed by swelling heralds testicular torsion. The swollen, firm testis shows the gross and microscopic features of hemorrhagic infarction (Fig. 17-24). Recurrent incomplete torsion of the spermatic cord results in a small fibrotic testis.

TESTICULAR TUMORS

Tumors of the testes are divided into two major histogenetic categories: germ cell tumors and gonadal stromal/sex cord tumors (Fig. 17-25). Tumors of germ cell origin constitute more than 90% of testicular tumors, and most of the remaining ones are of stromal/sex cord origin.

Germ Cell Tumors

Germ cell tumors originate from the neoplastic transformation of germ cells and reflect their capacity to differentiate along many histogenetic lines. Thus, germ cell tumors are characterized by either somatic or extraembryonic differentia-

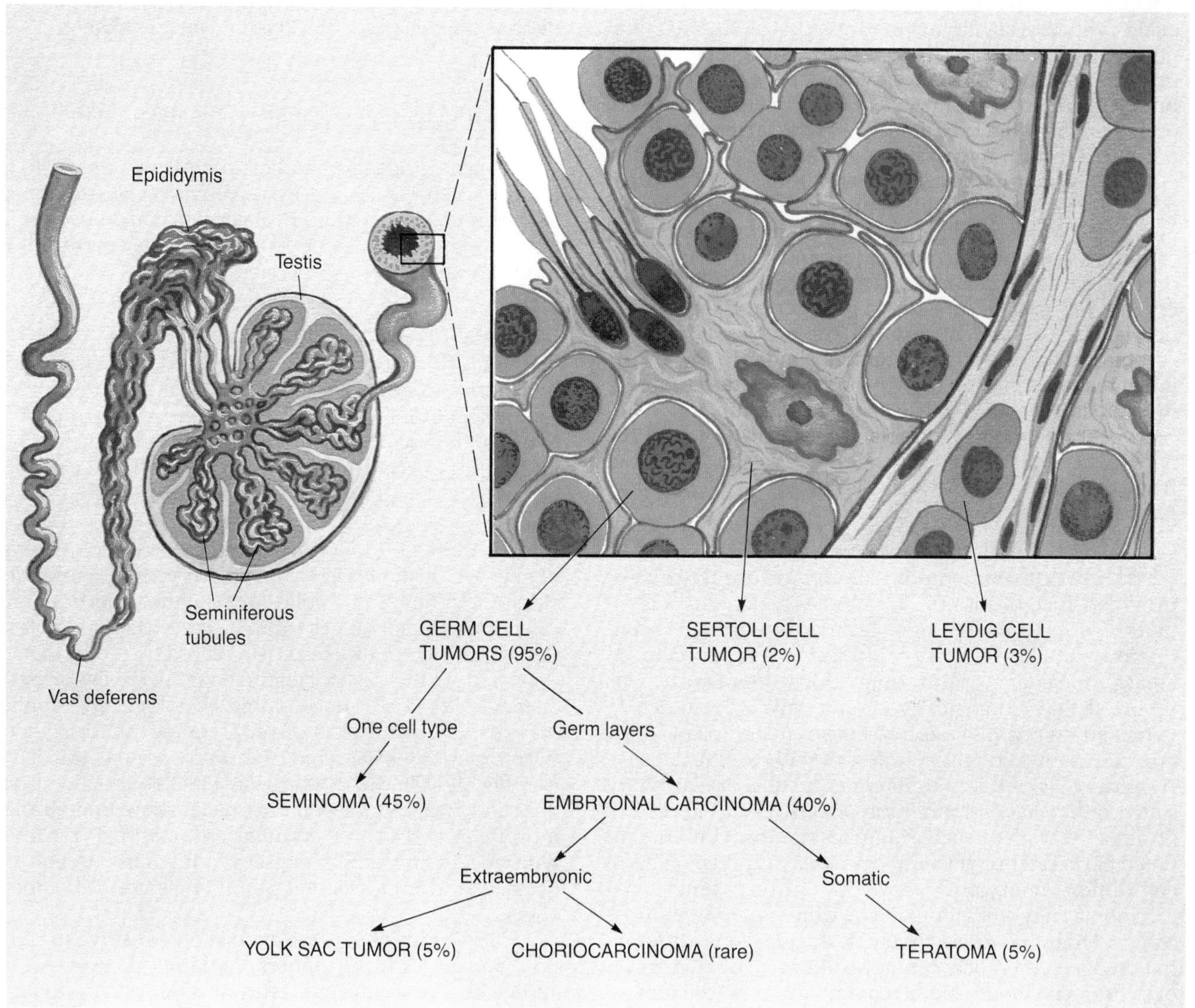

FIGURE 17-25
Histogenesis of testicular neoplasms.

tion, or by both. Alternatively, some germ cell tumors show no identifiable differentiation.

☐ **Epidemiology:** The worldwide incidence of germ cell testicular cancers has more than doubled in the last 40 years. There are intriguing geographic and racial differences in the frequency of testicular germ cell tumors. High rates are observed in the United States, in contrast to a low incidence in Japan. The frequency is consistently reported to be higher in whites than in blacks in all geographic locations, and in the United States Army the ratio is 40 to 1. The incidence of germ cell tumors peaks in infants and children (teratomas, yolk sac tumors) and in adults in the third and fourth decades (principally seminomas). The frequency of these tumors declines after the age of 40 years, although there is a modest increase after the age of 50.

☐ **Pathogenesis:** The cause of germ cell tumors is unknown. A role for previous trauma and infection cannot be entirely excluded, although such a history is rarely elicited. Studies suggesting increased risk associated with numerous different occupations, specific socioeconomic groups, and environmental exposures have been reported but none are proven. However, three circumstances have been demonstrated to be associated with an increased risk of testicular germ tumors: (1) prior diagnosis of testicular germ cell tumor in the contralateral testis; (2) prior diagnosis of testicular germ cell tumor in a first-degree family member; (3) abnormal germ cells in gonadal dysgenesis, especially testicular feminization and Klinefelter syndrome, and cryptorchidism. In the last case, the higher the cryptorchid testis is arrested in its descent, the greater is the risk of a subsequent germ cell tumor.

Interestingly, germ cell tumors similar to those arising in the testis may occur in extragonadal sites, primarily in midaxial locations such as the mediastinum and sacrococcygeal region. Such tumors are thought to reflect the neoplastic transformation of germ cells that migrated from their endodermal yolk sac origin to these extragonadal sites.

☐ **Histogenesis:** Studies of cryptorchid testes have provided insight into the histogenesis of germ cell tumors. Cytological atypism of germ cells within the seminiferous tubules of cryptorchid testes was noted to increase in severity with time. Subsequently, it was reported that cytologically similar cells were noted to demonstrate microinvasion of the stroma adjacent to the affected seminiferous tubules in cryptorchid testes. Atypical cells within seminiferous tubules are currently called *intratubular germ cell neoplasia (IGCN)* (Fig. 17-26). Stromal invasion by such cells gives rise to an undifferentiated germ cell tumor (seminoma) or a totipotential germ cell tumor (embryonal carcinoma). In turn, embryonal carcinoma may undergo somatic differentiation and become a teratoma. Alternatively, extraembryonic differentiation of an embryonal tumor results in a yolk sac tumor or a choriocarcinoma. Not uncommonly, germ cell tumors exhibit more than one type of differentiation, both within the primary testicular tumor and the metastatic sites. In addition, metastases of germ cell tumors may show a form of differentiation not present in the primary testicular tumor.

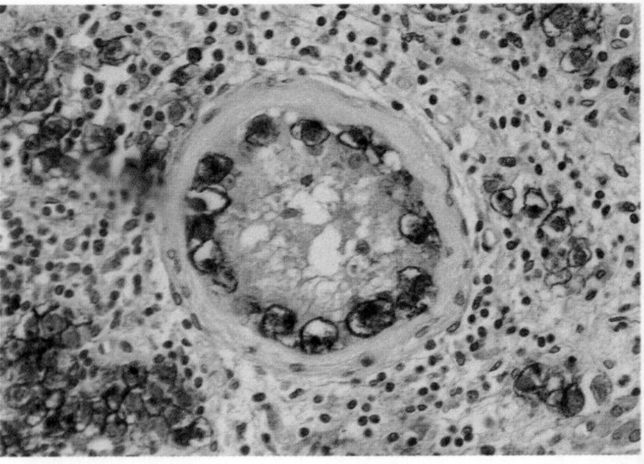

FIGURE *17-26*
Intratubular germ cell neoplasia (IGCN). The cytologically atypical germ cells are characteristically dispersed as a garland adjacent to the basement membrane of the seminiferous tubule. The IGCN cells stain intensely with placental alkaline phosphatase (PLAP) as demonstrated here.

Recent cytogenetic studies lend further weight to the link between IGCN and invasive germ cell tumors. An isochromosome of the short arm of chromosome 12, i(12p), is present in some 90% of testicular germ cell tumors and in IGCN.

Seminoma

Seminoma accounts for half of all germ cell tumors. The tumor is not found before puberty, and most patients are between the ages of 25 and 55 years. The peak incidence is in the fourth decade. Most are of the so-called classic type, but two less common variants are encountered.

CLASSIC SEMINOMA: Ninety percent of all seminomas are of the classic variety. On gross examination, classic seminoma is a solid, gray-white, poorly demarcated growth that bulges from the cut surface of the testis (Fig. 17-27). The entire testis is replaced by tumor in more than half of the cases. Hemorrhage, necrosis, or cystic change is distinctly uncommon. Histologically, seminomas display solid nests of proliferating tumor cells between randomly scattered, thin fibrovascular trabeculae (see Fig. 17-27). The tumor cells have well-defined borders and clear cytoplasm. The nuclei show limited pleomorphism and coarse granular chromatin. Typically, a lymphocytic infiltrate is present in the fibrovascular trabeculae, and noncaseating granulomas are occasionally seen.

Classic seminomas are exquisitely sensitive to radiation, and in localized tumors, radiation therapy has resulted in 5-year survival rates of 85% to 95%. Even in more advanced cases, chemotherapy is curative in 90%.

Up to 15% of seminomas contain rare, scattered syncytiotrophoblastic giant cells, which are capable of elevat-

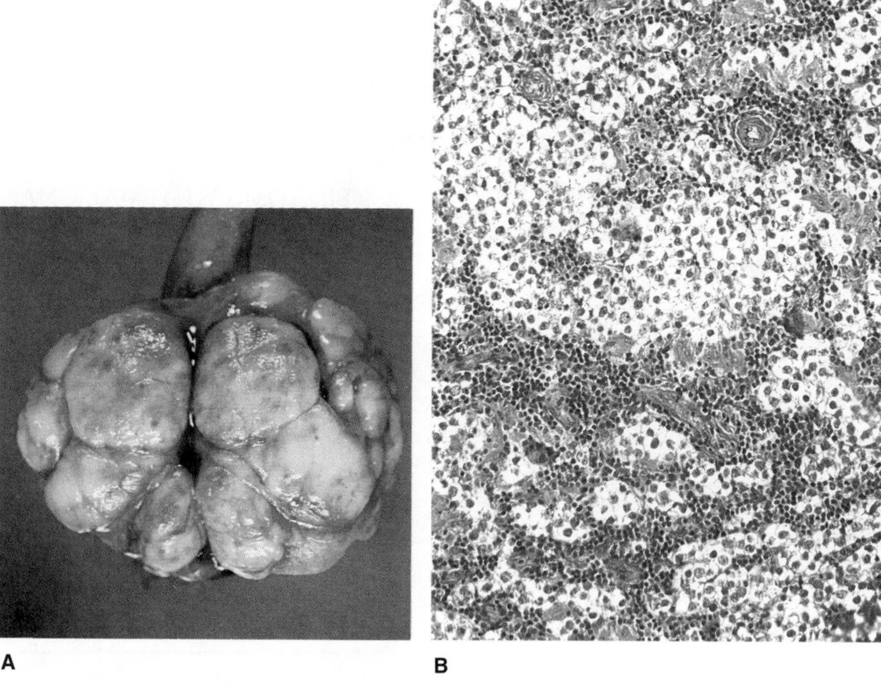

FIGURE 17-27
Classic seminoma. (*A*) The cut surface of the nodular tumor is tan and shows punctate hemorrhages in an otherwise solid mass. (*B*) Nests of tumor cells are confined by fibrous septa containing numerous lymphocytes.

ing serum levels of human chorionic gonadotropin (hCG). The presence of such giant cells does not justify the diagnosis of a mixed germ cell tumor.

ANAPLASTIC SEMINOMA: This tumor accounts for only 5% of all seminomas. The gross features of anaplastic seminoma are comparable to those of the classic variety. The tumor is composed of cells that exhibit marked nuclear pleomorphism and increased mitoses. Three or more mitotic figures per high-power field are required for the diagnosis of anaplastic seminoma. As a group, these tumors tend to be of higher stage at the time of diagnosis than classic seminomas. Stage for stage, the prognosis for anaplastic seminoma is the same as that for classic seminoma.

SPERMATOCYTIC SEMINOMA: This tumor comprises 5% of all seminomas and exhibits distinct morphological and clinical differences from classic seminoma. Spermatocytic seminomas arise in an older patient population than classic seminoma; most patients are older than 50 years of age. On gross examination, the size of spermatocytic seminoma is variable, and some examples have reached a diameter of 15 cm. The tumor tends to be poorly demarcated, soft, yellow-gray, and gelatinous. Small cystic areas are common, but hemorrhage and necrosis are unusual.

Spermatocytic seminomas are composed of three populations of neoplastic cells: (1) small cells, (2) intermediate cells (the most numerous and most similar to the tumor cells of classic seminoma), and (3) scattered large cells with clumped, coarse chromatin. All the cells of a spermatocytic seminoma show poor cohesiveness and lack the lymphocytic infiltrate characteristic of classic seminomas. Spermatocytic seminomas can be confused with lymphoma of the testis, which has a much graver prognosis than the germ cell tumor. Spermatocytic seminoma is rarely if ever malignant and is probably an entity distinct from classic seminoma.

Embryonal Carcinoma

Embryonal carcinoma is the second most common testicular germ cell tumor and accounts for 15% to 35% of these neoplasms, depending on the diagnostic criteria. As a rule, they do not occur before puberty, and most are found between the ages of 20 and 35 years. The cut surface of the tumor discloses a gray-white, bulging, poorly demarcated mass, with variable degrees of necrosis and hemorrhage. The tunica albuginea and the epididymis are extensively invaded in 20% of the cases.

Embryonal carcinomas show variable histological patterns. In many cases, they form sheets of cells, with clefts, acini, and papillary structures (Fig. 17-28). The cell borders are ill defined, and the nuclei have prominent nucleoli and coarse chromatin. Cellular pleomorphism and mitoses are more prominent than in classic seminomas. Occasional cells may stain positively for hCG and α-fetoprotein, in which case choriocarcinoma and yolk sac tumor elements are minor components of an otherwise typical embryonal carcinoma.

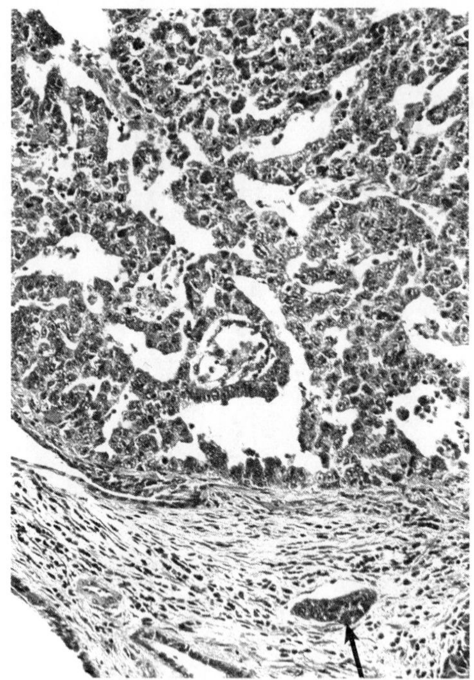

FIGURE 17-28
Embryonal carcinoma. A cystic space contains neoplastic cells that lack distinct cell membranes. A cluster of tumor cells is seen in a lymphatic (*arrow*).

Chemotherapy results in cure rates of 95% to 98% for localized tumors. Although many patients with embryonal carcinoma of the testis already have metastases at the time of initial diagnosis, half of the patients with advanced disease can expect a permanent cure.

Teratoma

Testicular teratomas are germ cell tumors characterized by tissues from all three germ layers: ectoderm, endoderm, and mesoderm (Fig. 17-29). They comprise almost half of the germ cell tumors in infants and children but less than 5% of all germ cell tumors in adults. Based on morphological features, teratomas are classified by the World Health Organization into mature teratomas, immature teratomas, and teratomas with malignant transformation.

MATURE TERATOMA: This tumor is characteristically a solid and multicystic lesion that enlarges the testis. The cut surface displays mucinous cysts, and the solid components often exhibit cartilaginous foci or, less frequently, bone formation. Although not typical, hemorrhage and necrosis are occasionally noted. The component tissues of mature teratomas are sufficiently differentiated to be virtually indistinguishable from their normal counterparts. Mature teratomas are characterized by the haphazard juxtaposition of a bewildering variety of cells and organoid structures, including neural elements, skeletal muscle, thyroid follicles, respiratory epithelium, cartilage, nests of squamous cells, and other tissues. The teratomatous elements are dispersed in a fibrous or myxoid stroma.

IMMATURE TERATOMA: This tumor is much more common in adults than in children. It demonstrates the same incongruous arrangement as mature teratomas, but the component tissues are less differentiated and more primitive. Pure immature teratomas are rare, and the immature components are frequently admixed with more mature tissue elements.

TERATOMA WITH MALIGNANT TRANSFORMATION: The presence of squamous cell carcinoma or a sarcomatous mesenchymal component identifies the malignant transformation of a teratoma.

The most important predictor of the biological behavior of a testicular teratoma is the age of the patient. In adult men, morphologically well-differentiated, mature teratomas, which would ordinarily be interpreted as benign, are commonly malignant and metastasize. In fact, all such tumors in the adult should be considered potentially malignant. By contrast, teratomas in infants and children, even those with foci of immature cells, are invariably benign.

Yolk Sac Tumor (Endodermal Sinus Tumor)

Yolk sac tumor, also termed endodermal sinus tumor, is the most common germ cell tumor of infants, and its name reflects the histological similarity to structures of the rat placenta. These tumors enlarge the testis and present as poorly defined, lobulated masses. On cut section, the lesions tend to be yellow-gray, focally cystic, solid masses of variable

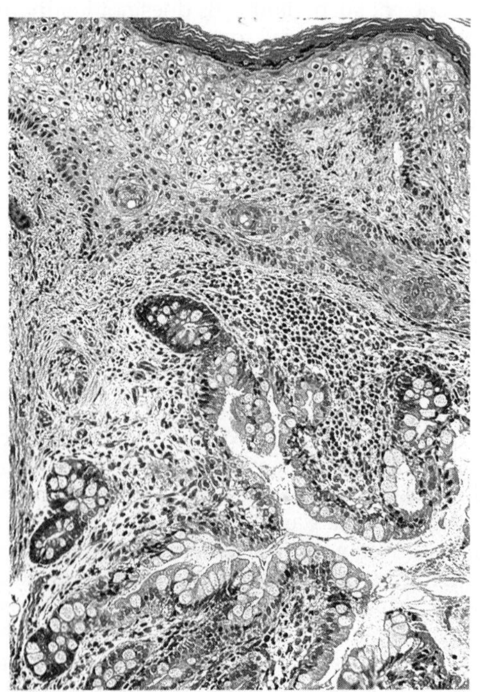

FIGURE 17-29
Teratoma. A cyst lined by well-differentiated squamous epithelium (*top*) is in proximity to a focus of endodermal glands that resembles colonic mucosa.

consistency. Focal areas of hemorrhage are common. Yolk sac tumors display a reticulated pattern of tumor cells, with multiple microcysts and papillary clusters, all in the background of a myxoid stroma. The tumor cells surround a characteristic structure, the *Schiller-Duval body*, which consists of a microcyst containing a glomerulus-like structure with a central fibrovascular core (Fig. 17-30). The tumor cells contain α-fetoprotein and α_1-antitrypsin. Yolk sac tumors typically exhibit extracellular eosinophilic globules, which also contain these marker proteins.

Testicular Choriocarcinoma

Choriocarcinoma is a highly malignant testicular tumor, which represents germ cell extraembryonic differentiation to the components of the placenta, namely, syncytiotrophoblast and cytotrophoblast (Fig. 17-31). The tumor is comparable to those that arise from placental tissue in pregnant women (see Chapter 18). Testicular choriocarcinoma typically presents as a small, painless nodule in the testis, although on occasion large bulky tumors are encountered. The cut surface is typically necrotic and hemorrhagic.

Microscopically, the neoplastic syncytiotrophoblasts and cytotrophoblasts are found in the areas of hemorrhage. Syncytiotrophoblasts are large multinucleated giant cells of irregular configuration, with abundant vacuolated cytoplasm, which contains hCG. Cytotrophoblasts are polygonal cells, with round hyperchromatic nuclei and sparse cytoplasm, which are clustered with the syncytiotrophoblasts. Pure testicular choriocarcinoma is rare, and the tumor is most frequently observed as a component of a mixed germ cell tumor. On occasion, hemorrhagic necrosis may be so extensive that viable tumor cells are found only with great difficulty or not at all. In fact, testicular choriocarcinoma may be reduced to a fibrous scar. In such a circumstance, the identification of the primary site of widely disseminated choriocarcinoma may be problematic.

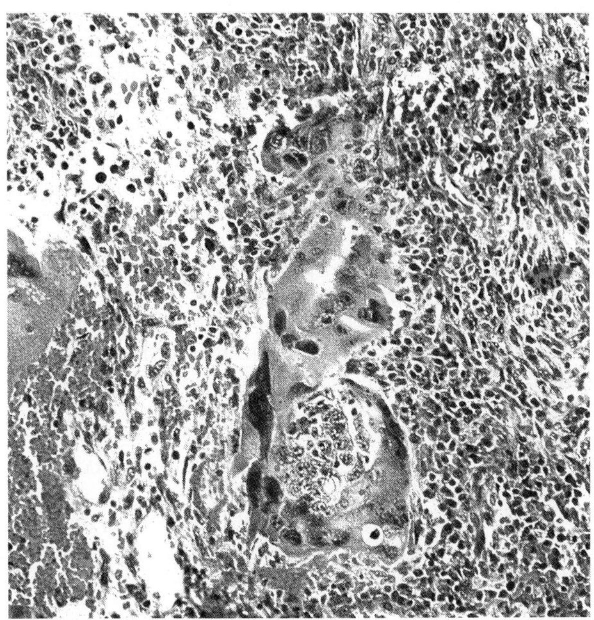

FIGURE *17-31*
Choriocarcinoma. The syncytiotrophoblast cell surrounds a cluster of cytotrophoblast cells. Hemorrhage is evident in the adjacent tissue.

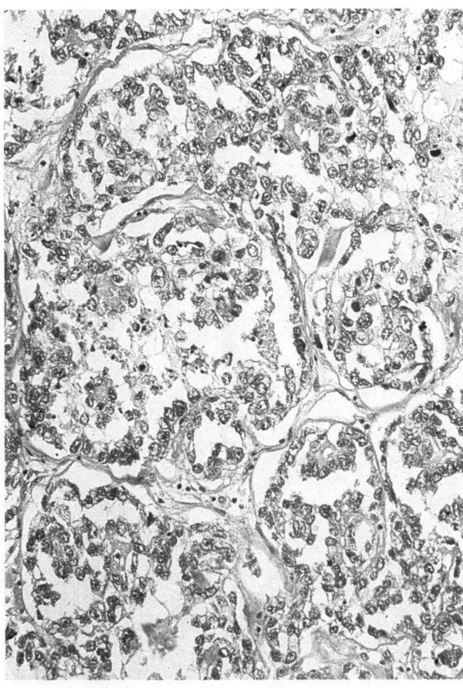

FIGURE *17-30*
Yolk sac (endodermal sinus tumor). The tumor is composed of dilated tubular spaces lined by flattened cells with an edematous stroma.

Mixed Germ Cell Tumor

Half of testicular germ cell tumors exhibit more than one type of neoplastic germ cell and are, therefore, referred to as mixed germ cell tumors. There are more than a dozen possible combinations, but the most frequent patterns are (1) teratoma with embryonal carcinoma (teratocarcinoma); (2) teratoma, embryonal carcinoma, and seminoma; and (3) embryonal carcinoma and seminoma. A surprisingly high frequency of yolk sac tumor components has been noted in mixed germ cell tumors. Twenty percent of patients with a teratocarcinoma initially present with metastases, most frequently in the form of embryonal carcinoma. Metastases from teratomatous elements or from foci of choriocarcinoma are less frequent.

Clinical Features of Germ Cell Tumors

Germ cell tumors present clinically as testicular swelling or pain, although on occasion the first symptoms derive from metastases.

TUMOR MARKERS: The presence of characteristic products of certain germ cell tumors in the blood assists in the diagnosis and follow-up of patients with germ cell neoplasms. These include hCG and α-fetoprotein. Elevations of serum hCG are typically found in patients with choriocarcinoma, whereas those with increased α-fetoprotein generally have yolk sac tumors or embryonal carcinomas (with yolk sac components). Following orchiectomy, a fall in the serum levels of these tumor markers is observed, and tumor recurrences are frequently associated with a return to elevated levels.

METASTATIC PATTERN: Germ cell tumors spread by invading the epididymis and by metastasizing, primarily to the regional lymph nodes and to the lungs (Table 17-2). **In contrast to other germ cell tumors, choriocarcinoma disseminates to the lung by hematogenous routes.** In order of decreasing frequency, metastases involve retroperitoneal lymph nodes, lungs, liver, and mediastinal lymph nodes. Distant metastases are most often observed in the first 2 years following the initial diagnosis and surgical therapy.

The fact that the histological features of the metastatic tumor may diverge from those of the primary testicular tumor has therapeutic implications. Metastases that do not resemble the original tumor are particularly common in cases of nonseminomatous germ cell tumors treated with orchiectomy and adjuvant chemotherapy. Two reasons may explain this observation: chemotherapy allows the patient to survive long enough to allow metastases to become clinically apparent, and the germ cell component least susceptible to the chemotherapeutic regimen may emerge as the "surviving" clone. In such cases, the germ cell component in the metastases is represented by teratomatous components.

Gonadal Stromal/Sex Cord Tumor

Primary tumors of Sertoli, Leydig, and granulosa cells constitute 5% of testicular tumors (see Fig. 17-25). These tumors may appear in "pure" form or as mixtures of neoplastic Sertoli and Leydig cells.

Leydig Cell Tumor (Interstitial Cell Tumor)

Leydig cell tumors are rare neoplasms that arise from interstitial (Leydig) cells of the testis. They are particularly interesting because they are functionally active, secreting androgens, estrogens, or both. These tumors occur in two age groups: boys older than 4 years of age and men in their third to sixth decades.

TABLE *17-2* **Clinical Staging of Testicular Cancer**

Stage	
Stage I: Local spread	
A	Confined to testis
B	Involves testicular adnexae
C	Involves scrotal wall
Stage II: Confined to retroperitoneal lymphatics	
A	Microscopic
B	Gross involvement without capsular invasion
C	Gross involvement with capsular invasion
D	Massive involvement of retroperitoneum
Stage III	
A	Solitary metastases
B	Multiple metastases

☐ **Pathology:** Leydig cell tumors are well circumscribed, and some appear encapsulated. They vary in size from 1 to 10 cm in diameter. The cut surface is yellow to brown, and the larger tumors have fibrous trabeculae, which imparts a lobular appearance. Microscopically, the tumor reveals sheets of polygonal cells with variably abundant eosinophilic or vacuolated cytoplasm, which may contain lipofuscin pigment. Central round nuclei are typical (Fig. 17-32). *The Reinke crystal,* which is observed in half of these tumors, is a characteristic rectangular, eosinophilic, cytoplasmic inclusion. Although the large majority (90%) of Leydig cell tumors are benign, it is difficult to predict their biological behavior on histological grounds. Of the few reported cases of Leydig cell tumors that proved to be clinically malignant, 25% showed neither capsular penetration nor vascular invasion in the surgical specimen.

☐ **Clinical Features:** The endocrine effects of testicular Leydig cell tumors in prepubertal boys lead to precocious physical and sexual development. By contrast, feminization and gynecomastia are observed in some adults with this tumor. Either estrogen or testosterone levels may be elevated, but there is no characteristic pattern. All Leydig cell tumors in children and almost all in adults are cured by orchiectomy.

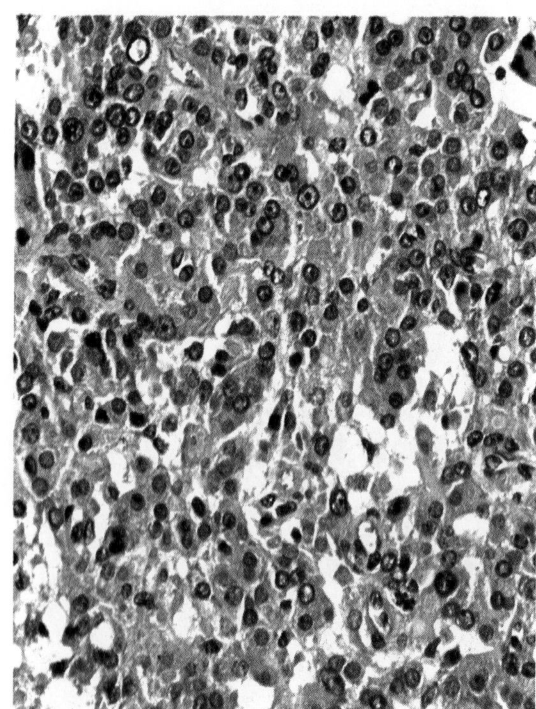

FIGURE *17-32*
Leydig cell (interstitial cell) tumor. The tumor cells, arranged in sheets, are moderately pleomorphic and have abundant eosinophilic cytoplasm. No mitoses are present.

Sertoli Cell Tumor

Sertoli cell tumors are even more infrequent than those of Leydig cells, and 20% are malignant. These neoplasms usually develop in the first four decades of life, with only a few cases reported in older patients.

□ **Pathology:** Sertoli cell tumors tend to be small (1 to 3 cm), but rare examples of larger bulky tumors are recorded. They are solid, well circumscribed, and yellow-gray. Microscopically, they demonstrate a tubular arrangement, with solid cords of cells and a fibrous trabecular framework (Fig. 17-33). The neoplastic Sertoli cells are columnar with a clear cytoplasm and relatively uniform nuclei. Nuclear chromatin tends to be most prominent near the nuclear membrane. One third of Sertoli cell neoplasms have admixed Leydig cells and are regarded as examples of mixed gonadal stromal tumors. Similar to Leydig cell tumors, malignant Sertoli cell tumors present a diagnostic challenge. The rare malignant variant exhibits greater cellular pleomorphism, areas of necrosis, and a reduced tendency to form cords and tubules.

□ **Clinical Features:** Most patients with Sertoli cell tumors come to medical attention because of a mass in the scrotum or endocrine effects (gynecomastia). Orchiectomy is curative.

Gonadoblastoma

Gonadoblastomas are rare tumors that are composed of an admixture of germ cell and immature sex cord and gonadal stromal elements, including Sertoli cells and, less frequently, Leydig cells. Virtually all gonadoblastomas arise in dysgenetic testes. Half of the reported cases are associated with an overgrowth of the germ cell component, and 10% of these have demonstrated metastatic spread.

Histologically, the diagnostic feature of gonadoblastoma is an intimate admixture of gonadal stromal cells and germ cells. When germ cell overgrowth occurs, the tumor presents the pattern of a seminoma.

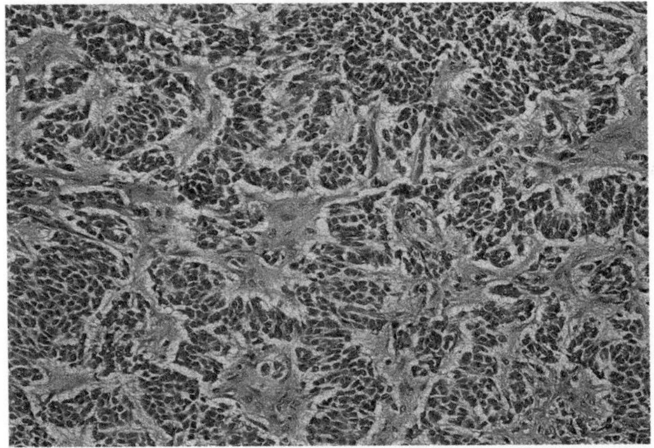

FIGURE *17-33*
Sertoli cell tumor. The neoplastic cells are arranged in cords of variable size in a fibrous stroma.

Lymphoma of the Testis

Malignant lymphoma is the most frequently encountered neoplasm in the testes of men older than 60 years. It usually occurs in the context of systemic disease, but a few cases of apparently primary lymphoma of the testis have been reported. The majority of patients with lymphomatous involvement of the testis have a poor prognosis, although some patients with primary testicular lymphoma have survived for many years.

TESTICULAR ADNEXAE

The testicular adnexae comprise the epididymis, the vas deferens, and the seminal vesicles. All are of mesonephric origin and, in continuity with the rete testes, serve as the excretory ducts of the testes. Similar to the tunica albuginea of the testis, the epididymis and proximal vas deferens are covered by a mesothelial cell lining, the tunica vaginalis. The seminal vesicles are located posterior to the prostate gland, and their excretory ducts join the distal vas deferens, immediately proximal to its entrance into the prostatic urethra.

Disorders of the Testicular Tunicae

HYDROCELE: *Defined as a collection of serous fluid in the scrotal sac, hydrocele is the most common cause of scrotal swelling* (Fig. 17-34). Hydroceles are either congenital and associated with a patent processus vaginalis or acquired secondary to an inflammatory disorder of the epididymis or testis. Uncomplicated hydroceles present as unilateral scrotal swelling, and ultrasound examination discloses fluid accumulation between the layers of the tunica vaginalis.

HEMATOCELE: This term refers to hemorrhage into a hydrocele.

SPERMATOCELE: *A cystic enlargement of the efferent ducts or ducts of the rete testis is termed a spermatocele and is clinically indistinguishable from a hydrocele.* The presence of sperm in the fluid of a spermatocele differentiates this cystic enlargement from a hydrocele.

VARICOCELE: *This term refers to dilatation of testicular veins, which is usually asymptomatic.* Most varicoceles are detected during the physical examination of infertile men. They may be accompanied by testicular atrophy and result in infertility. Varicoceles are treated by surgical ligation of the internal spermatic vein. Subsequent fertility is inversely related to the duration and severity of injury to the testicular germ cells prior to treatment.

FIBROUS PSEUDOTUMOR: Fibrous plaques or nodules, frequently with dystrophic calcification, may occur in the tunica albuginea. Such lesions are regarded as a late result of an inflammatory process. Half of the cases of fibrous pseudotumor are associated with a hydrocele, and many have a history of trauma or orchitis. These lesions

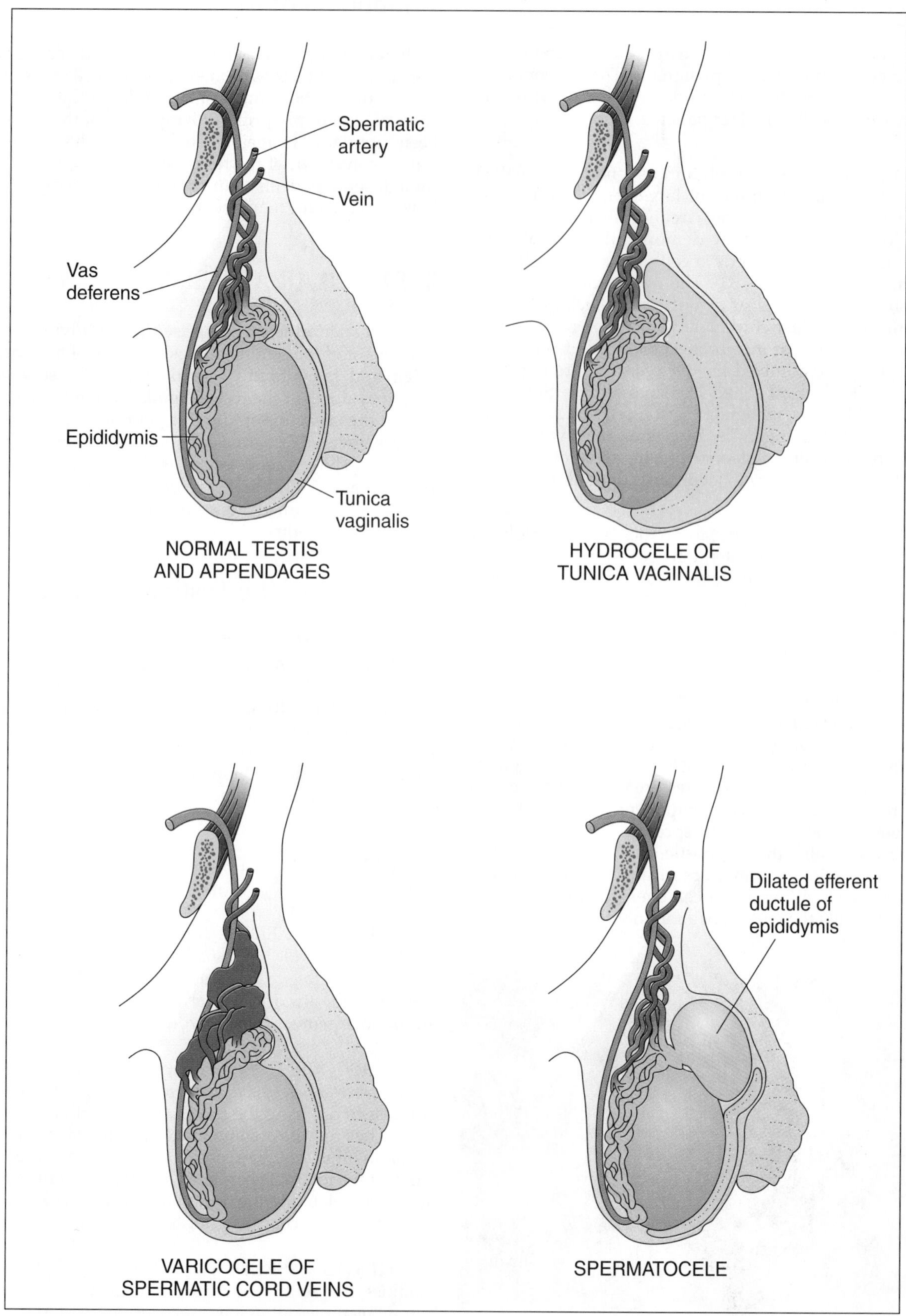

FIGURE *17-34*
Hydrocele, varicocele, and spermatocele.

are not neoplastic, but their gross features and clinical presentation simulate a testicular neoplasm.

MESOTHELIAL CELL PROLIFERATION: Local or diffuse benign mesothelial cell proliferation as a result of intrascrotal inflammation is not uncommon. It is mostly encountered as an incidental finding in surgical specimens, usually in hydrocele sacs.

Disorders of the Epididymis

The epididymis is affected by inflammatory disorders and rare neoplasms. An increased frequency of epididymal cysts has been reported in men exposed *in utero* to diethylstilbestrol. These lesions are commonly associated with testicular abnormalities, including hypoplasia and cryptorchidism. Acquired cysts (spermatoceles) are more common and reflect cystic dilatation of the efferent ducts or the more proximal rete testes.

Epididymitis

Most cases of acute epididymitis, that is, inflammation of the epididymis, in young men are due to gonorrhea and infection with *Chlamydia*. In older men, *E. coli* from associated urinary tract infections is the most common causative agent. Patients present with intrascrotal pain and tenderness, with or without associated fever. Epididymitis of recent origin shows the usual hallmarks of acute inflammation. Persistent epididymitis is associated with the accumulation of plasma cells, macrophages, and lymphocytes and, ultimately, with fibrotic obstruction of the infected ducts. **In fact, epididymal inflammation caused by gonorrhea is a common cause of male infertility.**

Tuberculous epididymitis is now infrequent and is usually associated with previously established pulmonary and renal infections. Concurrent prostatic and testicular involvement in these cases is common. Tuberculous epididymitis is manifested clinically by a palpable beading of the vas deferens and microscopically by typical tuberculous granulomas.

Spermatic granulomas result from an intense inflammatory response to sperm that have gained entrance to the interstitium of the epididymis. The underlying cause of this sperm extravasation is obscure, but trauma to or infection of the epididymal ducts may play a role. Patients present with scrotal pain and swelling, frequently lasting weeks or months. Histologically, a mixed inflammatory cell infiltrate is associated with numerous extravasated sperm fragments and phagocytosis of sperm by macrophages. Ultimately, the inflammatory process results in interstitial fibrosis, ductal obstruction, and infertility.

Adenomatoid Tumor

A nonpapillary form of benign mesothelioma, termed adenomatoid tumor, has a controversial histogenesis, but it is now believed to arise from mesothelial cells. These neoplasms are usually located in the upper pole of the epididymis, with fewer cases involving the tunica vaginalis of the testis or the spermatic cord. The lesions are well-demarcated tan nodules, which vary in size from a few millimeters to 2 cm, although rare examples have been reported up to 6 cm. The microscopic patterns of adenomatoid tumor have been classified into three patterns: plexiform, tubular, and mixed. The lesion resembles a vascular tumor, with innumerable small, irregular cysts or tubules and interstitial dense fibrous tissue. The lining cells in all forms vary from flat to cuboidal.

Disorders of the Spermatic Cord

The spermatic cord is composed of the vas deferens and the accompanying arteries, veins, lymphatics, and nerves within loose fibromuscular and adipose tissue. The most frequent clinical disorders are dilatation of the venous plexus (varicocele), inflammatory lesions, and a variety of benign and malignant mesenchymal tumors.

VASITIS NODOSA: *This term refers to the presence of sperm-containing ductules within the muscularis and the periadventitial fibroadipose tissue of the vas deferens, which communicate with the lumen* (Fig. 17-35). Most examples are encountered as incidental findings at the time of reconstruction of a vas deferens previously ligated for contraceptive purposes. Nodular or fusiform enlargements of the ends of the previously severed vas deferens are typical gross features. The intramural location of the proliferating ductules superficially resembles invasive adenocarcinoma, but the presence of sperm within the tubules, in association with chronic inflammation (including spermatic granulomas), suggests the diagnosis of vasitis nodosa.

LIPOMAS: These lesions of the spermatic cord are common, and most are discovered during the repair of an inguinal hernia. The absence of an identifiable capsule raises the possibility that some of these "lipomas" are not neoplasms but rather abundant retroperitoneal adipose tissue associated with the hernial sac.

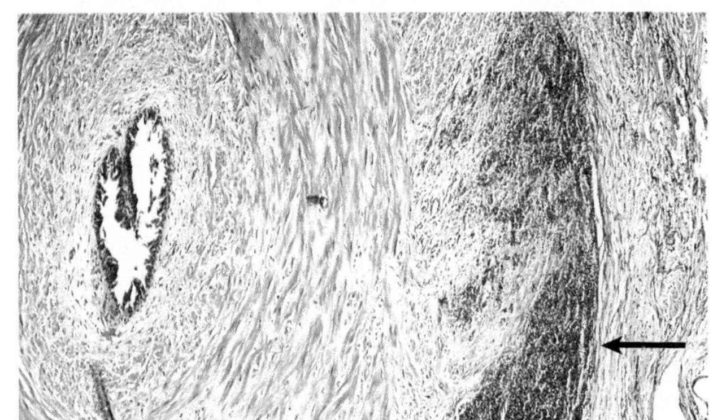

FIGURE *17-35*
Vasitis nodosa. Extravasated sperm (*arrow*) are present in the outer muscle layers of the vas deferens.

SARCOMAS: Malignant tumors of the spermatic cord have been observed. The most frequent include rhabdomyosarcoma, leiomyosarcoma, and fibrosarcoma. These neoplasms tend to disseminate by the hematogenous route. A notable exception is rhabdomyosarcoma of the spermatic cord, which demonstrates regional lymph node metastases.

Prostate

ANATOMY

The prostate develops from epithelial evaginations that appear along the distal urethra during the third gestational month (see Fig. 17-1). They give origin to five independent groups of tubules, which ultimately form the prostate gland. Between birth and puberty, there is little prostatic development. Under the influence of testosterone, the prostate at puberty enlarges to achieve a weight of about 20 g. After the age of 50 years, the prostate undergoes either progressive atrophy or enlargement in the form of nodular hyperplasia. Both atrophy and hyperplasia are present in the prostates of many elderly men. By the age of 80 years, half of the prostatic acini are obliterated.

The traditional concept of separate prostatic lobes has now been replaced by the identification of five histologically distinct regions.

- The anterior zone corresponds to the originally described anterior lobe. It is composed principally of fibromuscular stroma and a few prostatic glands.
- The peripheral zone is roughly equivalent to the lateral and posterior lobes and constitutes 75% of the glandular component of the prostate. It consists of simple glands and loose stroma, and the majority of prostatic adenocarcinomas originate in this zone.
- The central zone lies between the ejaculatory ducts, approximating the previously named middle lobe. It is separated from the peripheral zone by fibrous trabeculae.
- The periurethral glands are confined to a sleeve of the proximal urethra and comprise a separate zone.
- The transitional zone contains glands that terminate in the proximal urethra and grow laterally around the distal end of the internal urethral sphincter. This zone lies anterior to the central zone and gives rise to most of the hyperplastic nodules of the prostate.

Microscopically, the prostate of the newborn exhibits simple tubules radiating from the urethra, with abundant intervening primitive fibromuscular stroma. During the postnatal growth period, the microscopic features of the mature adult prostate are achieved. Tubuloalveolar glands are clustered in a fibromuscular stroma, which is continuous with the enveloping fibrous capsule. The acini are lined by a pseudostratified columnar epithelium, with the basal cell layer resting on a basement membrane. Similar epithelium lines the excretory ducts through most of their length to the urethra, where there is a change to transitional cell epithelium. The fibromuscular stroma contains smooth muscle, collagen, and elastic fibers in circumferential orientation around the acini and ducts. Occasional skeletal muscle fibers are incorporated into the prostate gland, most often in the anterolateral areas of the prostate.

Progressive acinar obliteration occurs in old age during the period of senescent atrophy of the prostate gland. The remaining acini are smaller and are lined by cuboidal or flattened epithelium, which has diminished secretory activity. Focal areas of epithelial hyperplasia occur in glands that are otherwise lined by atrophic epithelial cells.

HORMONAL INFLUENCES ON GROWTH OF THE PROSTATE

The normal growth and differentiation of the prostate is principally under the control of testicular androgens. Testosterone secreted by the Leydig cells of the testis is converted to 5-dihydrotestosterone (DHT) by 5α-reductase, an enzyme located primarily in the nuclei of prostatic epithelial cells. DHT is the most potent androgen with respect to the control of both normal prostatic growth and to the proliferative disorders of prostate, namely, nodular hyperplasia and adenocarcinoma.

Prior to puberty, little growth of the prostate occurs. With puberty the prostate enlarges in response to the increased synthesis of testosterone by the testis. Prostatic growth does not occur following prepubertal castration or in the rare patients with an inherited form of pseudohermaphroditism (5α-reductase deficiency), in which testosterone is not converted to DHT. Similarly, patients with these conditions do not develop nodular hyperplasia or prostatic adenocarcinoma in later life.

PROSTATITIS

Bacterial Prostatitis

Infections of the prostate usually follow lower urinary tract infections and result from the reflux of infected urine into the prostate.

Acute bacterial prostatitis is most commonly caused by gram-negative bacteria, especially *E. coli*, although gram-positive cocci are not infrequent. The morphological features of acute prostatitis are nonspecific, consisting of an acute inflammatory infiltrate in the prostatic acini and stroma (Fig. 17-36). The disorder presents as intense discomfort on urination and is associated with fever, chills, and perineal pain. The specific causative agent is identified by culture of urine and prostatic secretions. Acute prostatitis is treated with antibiotics.

Chronic bacterial prostatitis may be preceded by an episode of acute prostatitis, but many patients do not recall a previous infection of the prostate. Most patients with chronic prostatitis complain of suprapubic, perineal, and low back discomfort and experience dysuria and nocturia. Their urine usually contains bacteria. In addition to reflux

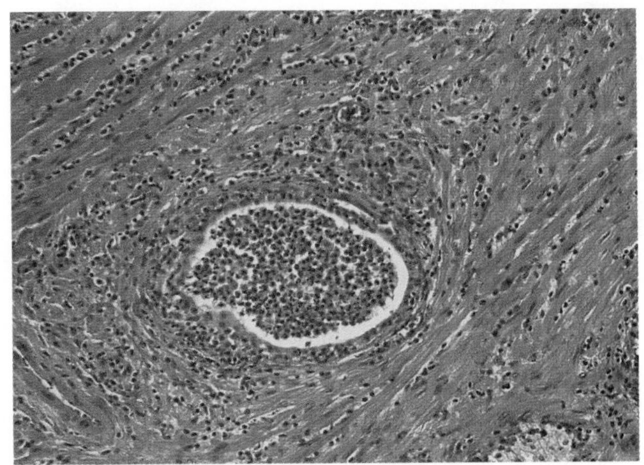

FIGURE 17-36
Acute prostatitis. A section of the prostate shows neutrophils in the lumen of an acinum and in the stroma.

of urine, additional factors such as prostatic calculi and local prostatic duct obstruction may contribute to the development of chronic bacterial prostatitis. In contrast to acute prostatitis, lymphocytes, plasma cells, and macrophages are the rule, and the inflammation tends to be more focal and less intense (Fig. 17-37). Prolonged antibiotic therapy is often, but not necessarily, curative, since the drugs have poor access to the organisms.

Nonbacterial Prostatitis

In the majority of cases of chronic prostatitis, no causative agent is identified. Nonbacterial prostatitis is most common in men older than age 50 years, but it has been reported in virtually all age groups. Some cases may be due to *Chlamydia trachomatis, Mycoplasma, Ureaplasma urealyticum*, and *Trichomonas vaginalis*. The most common histological pattern consists of dilated glands filled with neutrophils and foamy macrophages and surrounded by chronic inflammatory cells. The symptoms are similar to those in chronic bacterial prostatitis. No specific therapy is available.

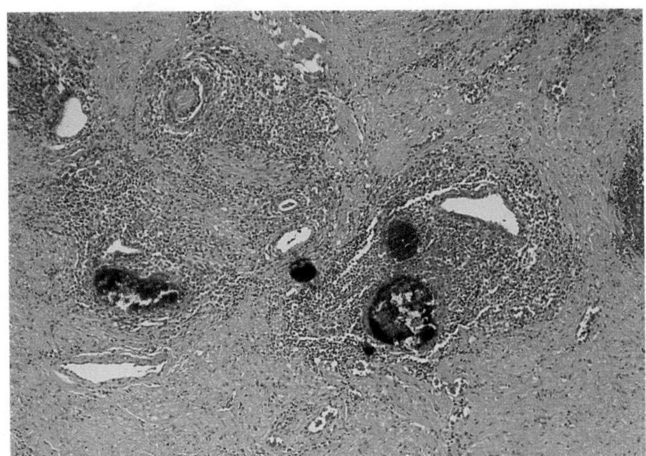

FIGURE 17-37
Chronic prostatitis. A section of prostate shows a diffuse infiltrate of lymphocytes and plasma cells in the stroma and invading several acini. Foci of dystrophic calcification are present in the inflammatory sites.

Granulomatous Prostatitis of Unknown Cause

The symptoms of chronic granulomatous prostatitis are vague, and the diagnosis is made histologically. The pathogenesis is not understood but may involve an inflammatory reaction to inspissated secretions or bacterial products in localized prostatic duct obstruction. Histologically, noncaseating granulomas are associated with localized destruction of prostatic ducts and acini and in later stages with fibrosis.

Granulomatous Prostatitis of Specific Cause

On rare occasions, granulomatous prostatitis is caused by specific causative agents, including tuberculosis and a wide variety of fungal infections. A granulomatous lesion resembling rheumatoid nodules has been recognized and related to previous transurethral resection of a portion of the prostate gland.

NODULAR HYPERPLASIA

Nodular hyperplasia of the prostate is a common disorder characterized clinically by enlargement of the gland, with obstruction to the flow of urine through the bladder outlet, and pathologically by the proliferation of glands and stroma.

☐ **Epidemiology: Three epidemiological factors, geography, race, and age, are related to the incidence of prostatic hyperplasia.** The disorder is least frequent in the Orient and most frequent in western Europe and the United States. The prevalence of prostatic hyperplasia in the United States is higher among blacks than among whites. Clinical prostatism, that is, nodular prostatic hyperplasia of sufficient degree to interfere with urination, peaks in the seventh decade. However, the prevalence of prostatic hyperplasia in all age groups is far greater at autopsy than is suggested by clinically apparent prostatism (Fig. 17-38). In fact, 75% of men 80 years of age or older have some degree of prostatic hyperplasia. The disorder is rarely observed in men younger than 40 years of age.

☐ **Pathogenesis:** Prior to the recognition of its hyperplastic nature, prostatic enlargement in elderly men was variously interpreted as a neoplastic, hypertrophic, inflammatory, or vascular disorder. The earliest histogenetic events in the evolution of nodular hyperplasia of the prostate are still not understood. It has been postulated that stromal–epithelial interactions ultimately give rise to the hyperplastic nodules, although it is not clear

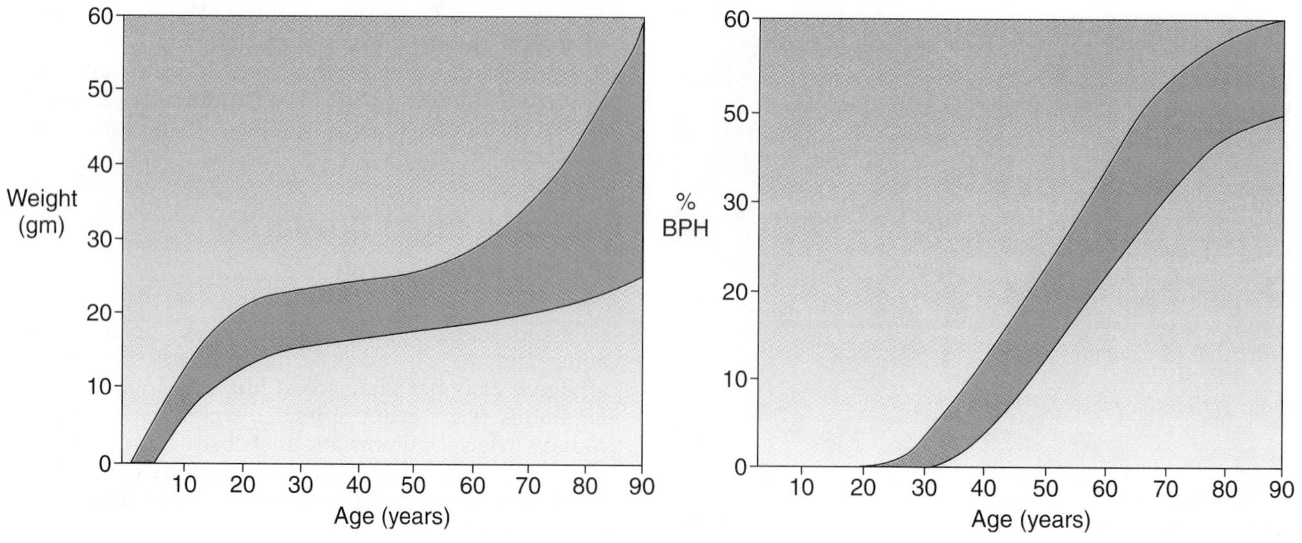

FIGURE 17-38
Growth of the prostate (*left*) and frequency of nodular hyperplasia (*right*). By 80 years of age, most men have benign prostatic hyperplasia.

whether the stroma induces epithelial proliferation or vice versa. However, stromal hyperplasia in a nodular configuration and virtually pure epithelial nodules are both observed, and a relationship between the two remains speculative.

As noted previously, prepubertal castration prevents the subsequent development of nodular hyperplasia of the prostrate. Yet, exogenous testosterone has no observable effect either on the histological appearance of the hyperplastic nodules or on the areas of the prostate that

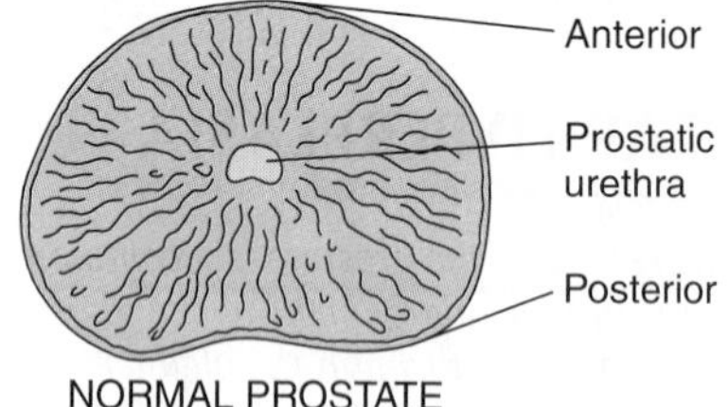

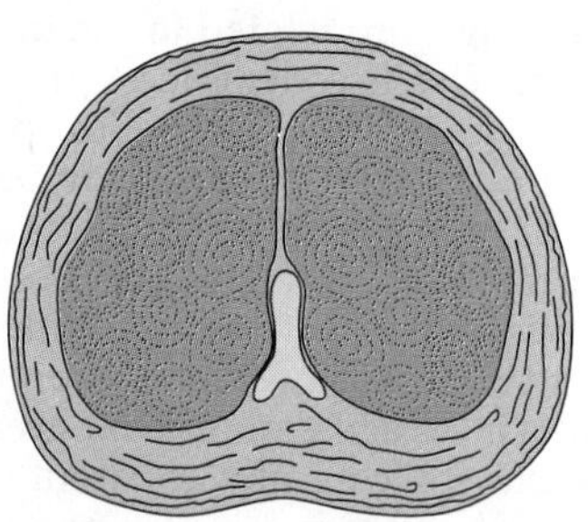

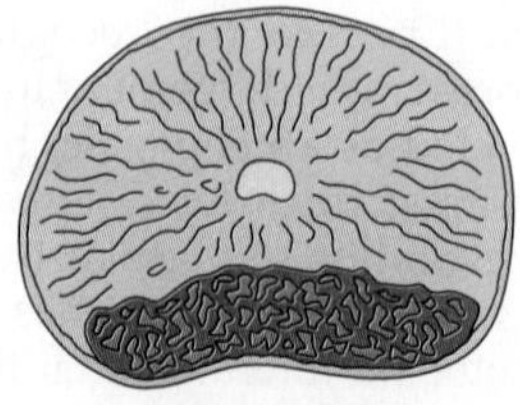

FIGURE 17-39
Normal prostate, nodular hyperplasia, and adenocarcinoma. In prostatic hyperplasia, the nodules distort and compress the urethra and exert pressure on the surrounding normal prostatic tissue. Prostatic carcinoma usually arises from peripheral glands, in which case it does not compress the urethra.

provide evidence of senile atrophy. Advancing age is associated with a comparable reduction in circulating testosterone both in normal men and in those with prostatic hyperplasia. Moreover, no change in the serum dihydrotestosterone (DHT) level is observed in men with prostatic hyperplasia, although the ratio of circulating testosterone to DHT may be abnormally low. Interestingly, changes resembling this lesion have been produced in dogs by the administration of dihydrotestosterone.

There is now evidence that the control of DHT synthesis from testosterone by 5α-reductase in the prostate may have therapeutic value. Indeed, the administration of a drug that blocks 5α-reductase has reduced the size of the prostate in men with clinical prostatism.

□ Pathology: **Early nodular hyperplasia of the prostate begins in the submucosa of the proximal urethra (the transitional zone).** The developing prostatic nodules compress the centrally located urethral lumen and the more peripherally located normal prostate (Figs. 17-39 and 17-40A). In well-developed nodular hyperplasia, the normal prostate is actually limited to an attenuated rim of tissue beneath the prostatic capsule. On cut section, an individual nodule is clearly demarcated by an enveloping fibrous pseudocapsule (Fig. 17-40A). Focal hemorrhage and infarction may be present, especially in the larger nodules. On occasion, small stones are present within the dilated hyperplastic acini. The secondary changes result from nodular prostatic hyperplasia related to bladder outlet obstruction (Fig. 17-41).

Histologically, nodular hyperplasia reflects the proliferation of epithelial cells of the acini and ductules, smooth muscle cells, and stromal fibroblasts, all in variable proportions. Accordingly, five types of nodules have been described: (1) stromal (fibrous), (2) fibromuscular, (3) muscular, (4) fibroadenomatous, and (5) fibromyoadenomatous, the most common type. A rare variant, frequently associated with the development of macroscopic prostatic cysts, resembles cystosarcoma phyllodes of the breast, hence the name *phyllodes type of hyperplasia.*

In the typical fibromyoadenomatous nodule, variably sized hyperplastic prostatic acini are randomly scattered throughout the stroma of the nodule. The epithelial (adenomatous) component is composed of a double layer of cells, with tall columnar cells overlying the basal layer (see Fig. 17-40B). Papillary hyperplasia of the glandular epithelium is characteristic. Hyperplastic nodules often contain chronic inflammatory cells, and corpora amylacea (eosinophilic, laminated concretions) are frequently seen within the acini. The glands of the uninvolved peripheral region of the prostate are frequently atrophic and compressed by the expanding nodules. The stroma of each type of nodule differs in composition, but elastic fibers are always absent. Immunoperoxidase staining of the hyperplastic epithelium is consistently positive for prostate-specific antigen (PSA) and prostatic acid phosphatase.

A nonspecific prostatitis is frequently encountered in specimens that exhibit nodular hyperplasia. There is a dense intraglandular and periglandular infiltrate of lymphocytes, plasma cells, and macrophages, frequently accompanied by acute inflammatory cells and focal gland

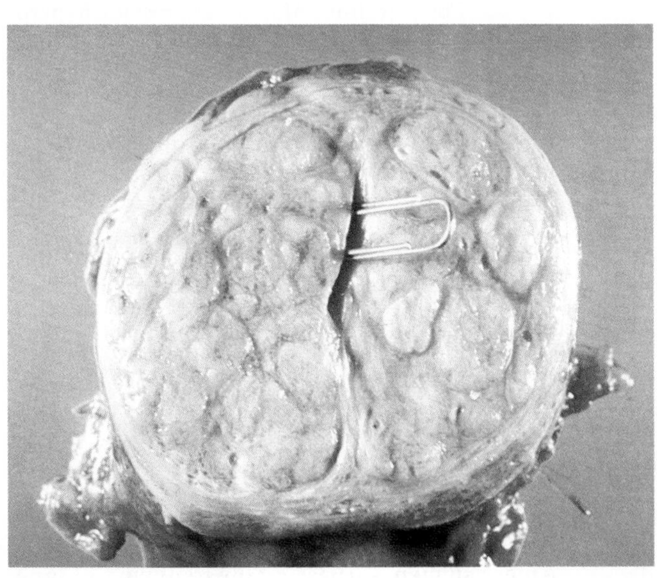
A

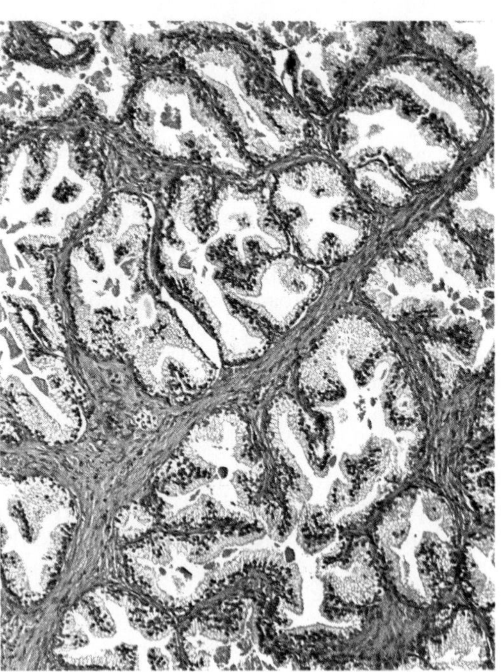
B

FIGURE *17-40*
Nodular hyperplasia of the prostate. (*A*) The cut surface of a prostate enlarged by nodular hyperplasia shows numerous, well-circumscribed nodules of prostatic tissue. The prostatic urethra (*paper clip*) has been compressed to a narrow slit. (*B*) The columnar epithelium lining the acini is composed of two cell layers. Numerous papillary projections are present in the enlarged acini.

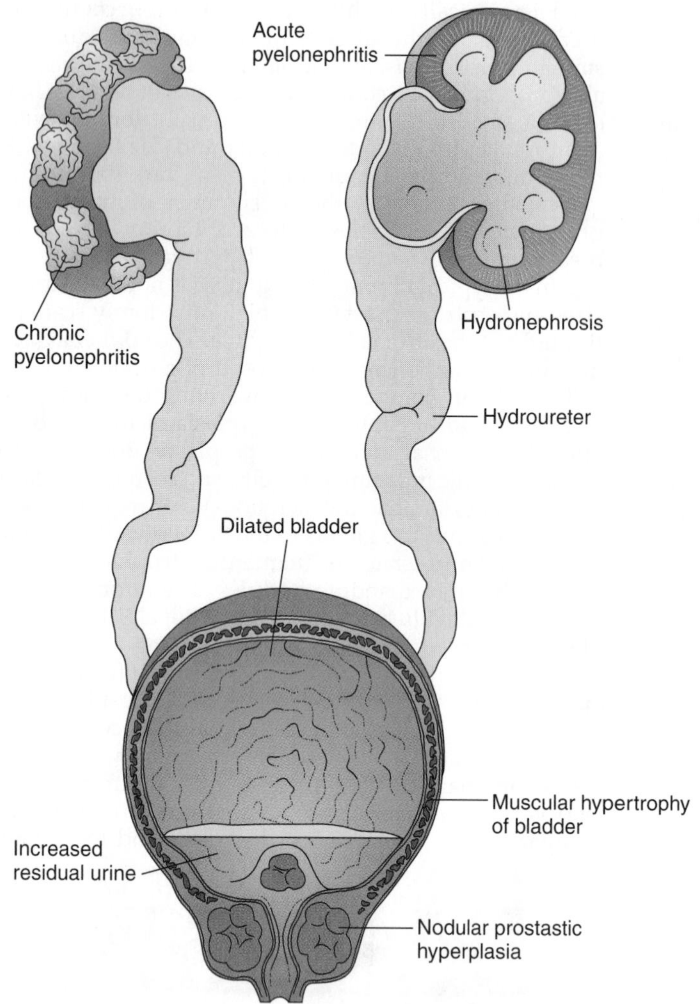

FIGURE *17-41*
Complications of nodular prostatic hyperplasia.

destruction. Focal infarcts of varying age are observed in 20% of cases. Squamous metaplasia of the epithelium of ducts at the periphery of infarcts is typical.

Incidental foci of prostatic adenocarcinoma are found in 10% of surgical specimens submitted with the preoperative diagnosis of prostatic hyperplasia. Such clinically occult adenocarcinomas are regarded as stage A prostate cancer.

☐ **Clinical Features:** The clinical symptoms of nodular hyperplasia result from compression of the prostatic urethra and the consequent obstruction to the bladder outlet. A history of decreased vigor of the urinary stream and increasing urinary frequency is typical. Rectal examination reveals a firm, enlarged, and nodular prostate. If the duration of severe obstruction is prolonged, back-pressure results in hydroureter, hydronephrosis, and, ultimately, renal failure and death.

The classic treatment of prostatic hyperplasia was surgical. Transurethral resection of the prostate, or less commonly suprapubic enucleation of the hyperplastic tissue, alleviated the symptoms of prostatism. Both procedures result in the surgical excision of the central hyperplastic nodules, leaving behind the more peripheral (subcapsular) prostatic glandular tissue. Currently, the surgical treatment of nodular hyperplasia has largely been replaced by administration of drugs that inhibit 5α-reductase, with resultant diminution of prostate size. α-Adrenergic blockers decrease muscular tone in the prostate and ameliorate symptoms of urinary obstruction.

ADENOCARCINOMA OF THE PROSTATE

☐ **Epidemiology: In 1990, prostatic adenocarcinoma became the cancer most frequently diagnosed in American men, surpassing the frequency of lung cancer for the first time.** An estimated 30,000 American men die annually of this malignancy, a figure that is still far lower than that for death from lung cancer. Prostatic cancer is a disease of elderly men, and of all patients with this diagnosis, 75% are 60 to 80 years of age. Patients younger than 50 years of age constitute less than 1% of cases in the United States. At the age of 50 years, the estimated lifetime probability of developing clinically apparent prostatic carcinoma is about 10% for American men.

Autopsy studies have shown that the true frequency of prostatic carcinoma is actually considerably higher than is indicated by its clinical incidence. Most cases (70% to 90%) are incidental microscopic findings at autopsy or are discovered in a specimen resected for prostatic hyperplasia. **The prevalence of prostatic carcinoma at autopsy progressively increases with age, rising from less than 10% among men 40 to 50 years of age to between one third and one half of those older than 80 years of age.**

There is considerable geographic variation in the age-related death rates for adenocarcinoma of the prostate throughout the world. The highest frequencies are reported in the United States and the Scandinavian countries, whereas the lowest are described in Mexico, Greece, and Japan. Most western European countries have intermediate rates. The highest incidence in the world is recorded in American blacks, who exhibit a rate twice as high as that of white Americans. Migrant studies have shown that in the United States, the descendants of Polish and Japanese immigrants demonstrate a higher incidence of prostatic carcinoma than do men in their original countries. Similarly, the mortality rate from prostatic carcinoma among black American men exceeds that among blacks in Africa.

In addition to geographic, racial, and age differences, heredity and diet influence the risk of prostate cancer. One tenth of the cases are familial, with a significantly increased risk in persons whose first-degree relatives are afflicted with prostate cancer. The large majority of cases of prostate cancer are random and the patients have no family history of this neoplasm. There is some evidence that dietary fat content may increase the risk of developing prostate cancer, but further studies are required to confirm this relationship. Multiple other factors, including sexually transmitted diseases, occupation, smoking, and viral causes, are not associated with any increased risk for the development of prostate cancer.

☐ **Pathogenesis:** The cause of prostatic adenocarcinoma is unknown, but the principal focus of research interest is directed toward endocrine influences. The androgenic control of normal prostatic growth and the responsiveness of prostatic cancer to castration and exogenous estrogens support a role for male hormones. However, higher levels of serum androgens have not been demonstrated consistently in patients with prostatic cancer. Elevated urinary estrone-to-testosterone ratios have been reported. Prostatic adenocarcinoma has been produced experimentally by a chemical carcinogen [3,2′-dimethyl-4-aminobiphenyl (DMAB)]. In addition, rats have developed the tumor following the prolonged administration of testosterone.

The histogenesis of prostatic adenocarcinoma is somewhat clearer than its cause. There is no evidence that this tumor originates from hyperplastic nodules. Current attention addresses intraductal dysplastic foci termed *prostatic intraepithelial neoplasia (PIN). PIN refers to resident prostatic ducts lined by cytologically atypical luminal cells and a concomitant diminution in the number of the basal cells.* **Substantial evidence now supports the contention that PIN lesions are premalignant changes that progress to prostatic adenocarcinoma.** PIN lesions precede the appearance of invasive cancer by two decades, and their severity increases with increasing age.

Morphological evidence linking PIN to invasive prostate cancer includes (1) the preponderance of the peripheral location of both lesions, (2) the cytological similarity of high-grade PIN to invasive cancer, and (3) the close topographic proximity of high-grade PIN to invasive cancer. Finally, PIN lesions are observed more frequently in prostates harboring cancer than in those without tumors. Certain markers are similar in high-grade PIN and invasive cancer (e.g., aneuploidy, TGF-α, type IV collagenase, and expression of the *bcl*-2 and c-*erb*-2 oncogenes).

High-grade PIN functions as an important marker for carcinoma when identified in needle biopsies of the prostate. Many patients who show only high-grade PIN on initial biopsy are demonstrated to harbor invasive carcinoma in subsequent follow-up biopsies performed within weeks to months.

☐ **Pathology:** Prostatic adenocarcinomas, which account for 98% of all primary prostatic tumors, are commonly multicentric and located in the peripheral zones. The cut surface of the prostate shows irregular, yellow-white, indurated, subcapsular nodules.

PROSTATIC INTRAEPITHELIAL NEOPLASIA: **Low-grade PIN** lesions are characterized by crowding and overlapping of luminal cells which exhibit a prominent variation in nuclear size. Nucleoli are frequently present but are not enlarged. The basal cell layer is present. By contrast, **high-grade PIN** foci are characterized by more pronounced cell crowding, greater prevalence of nuclear enlargement, and prominent enlarged nucleoli (Fig. 17-42). Fewer basal cells are demonstrated by immunohistochemical stains for high-molecular-weight cytokeratin (MA-903). The atypical cells within PIN-affected ducts may show a flat, papillary, or cribriform pattern.

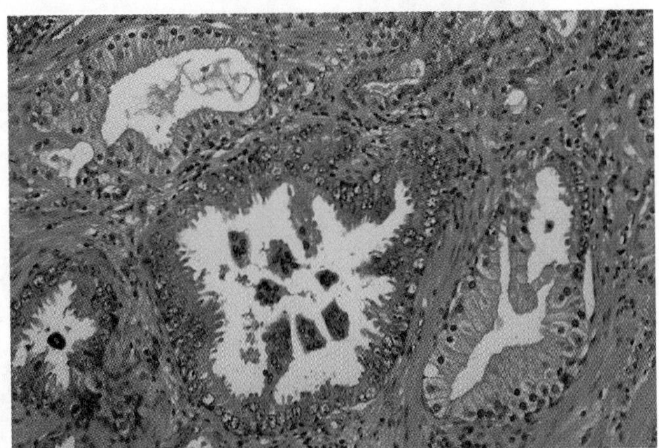

FIGURE **17-42**
High-grade prostatic intraepithelial neoplasia (PIN). The large duct in the center is lined by atypical cells with enlarged nuclei and prominent nucleoli. Two normal ducts are located adjacent to the neoplastic one.

HISTOLOGICAL FEATURES OF INVASIVE CARCINOMA: The majority of prostatic adenocarcinomas are of acinar origin and are characterized by small to medium-sized glands, which lack organization and infiltrate the stroma. Well-differentiated tumors show uniform medium-sized or small glands (Fig. 17-43), which are lined by a single layer of uniform neoplastic epithelial cells. **In fact, a single layer of cuboidal cells lining neoplastic acini is the most frequently employed criterion to establish the diagnosis of prostatic adenocarcinoma.** Progressive loss of differentiation of prostatic adenocarcinomas is characterized by (1) increasing variability of gland size and configuration, (2) papillary and cribriform patterns, and (3) rudimentary (or no) gland formation, with only solid cords of infiltrating tumor cells. Uncommonly, a prostatic cancer is composed of small undifferentiated cells, growing individually or in sheets, without evidence of any structural organization.

CYTOLOGICAL FEATURES: The prominence of pleomorphic and hyperchromatic nuclei is highly variable. One or two conspicuous nucleoli in the background of chromatin clumped near the nuclear membrane is the most frequent nuclear feature. The cytoplasm stains slightly eosinophilic, or it may be so vacuolated as to simulate the clear cells of renal cell carcinoma. Cell borders are distinct in the better-differentiated tumors but are indistinct in the more poorly differentiated ones.

GRADING: Prostatic adenocarcinoma is most commonly classified according to the **Gleason grading system** (see Fig. 17-43), which is based on five histological patterns of tumor gland formation and infiltration. Recognizing the high frequency of mixed tumor patterns, the Gleason score is the sum of the grade (1 to 5) attributed to the most prominent pattern and that of the minority pattern. The best-differentiated tumors have a Gleason score

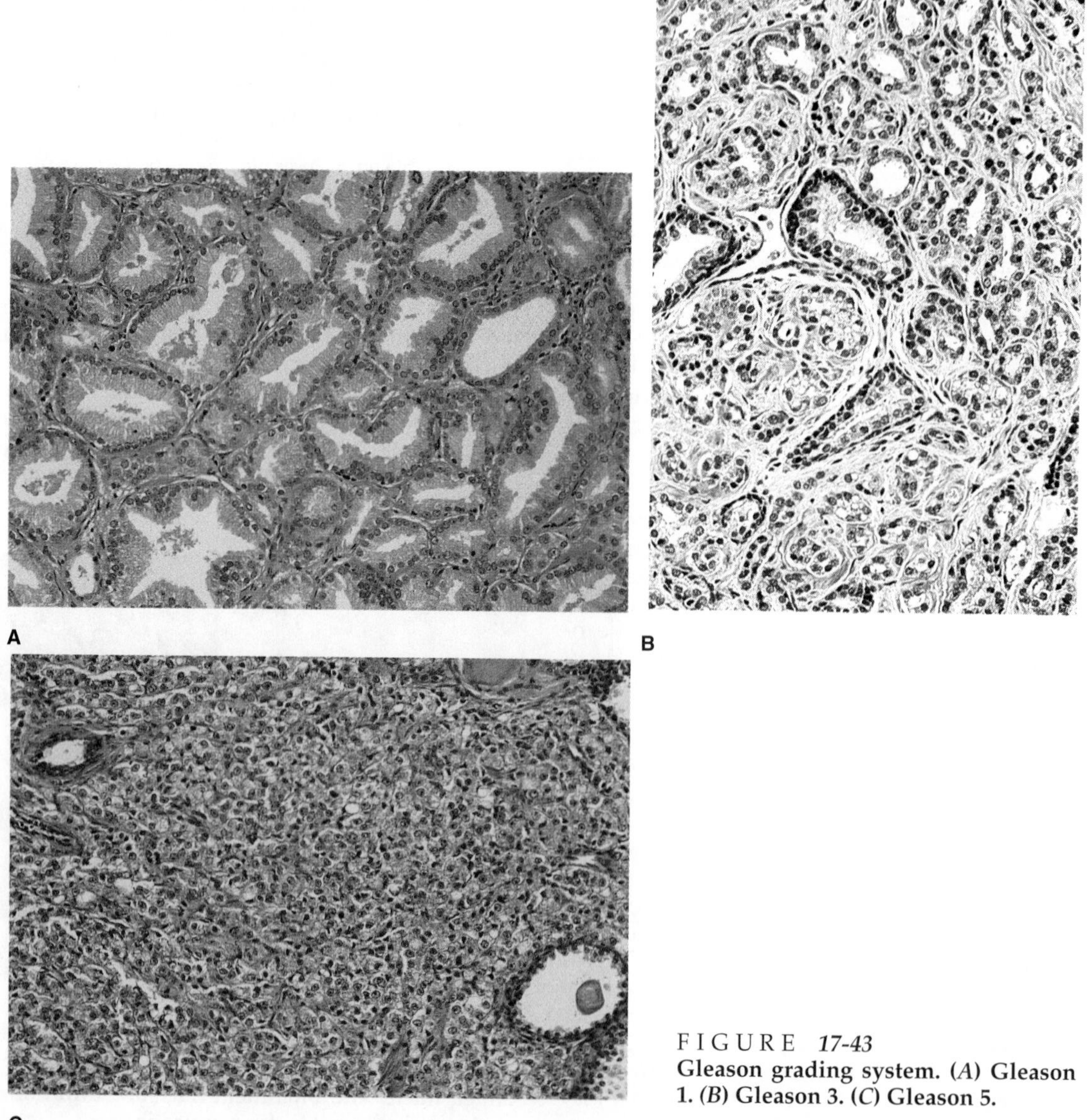

FIGURE *17-43*
Gleason grading system. (*A*) Gleason 1. (*B*) Gleason 3. (*C*) Gleason 5.

of 2 (1 + 1), whereas the most poorly differentiated cancers yield a Gleason score of 10 (5 + 5). The majority of prostate cancers have Gleason scores of 4 to 7 (2 + 2, to 3 + 4 or 4 + 3). When combined with the tumor stage, the Gleason grading system has prognostic value: the lower the score, the better the outlook.

INVASION AND METASTASIS: The high frequency of invasion of the prostatic capsule by adenocarcinoma relates to the subcapsular location of the tumor (Fig. 17-44). Perineural tumor invasion within the prostate and adjacent tissues is usual. Since peripheral nerves are devoid of perineural lymphatic channels, this mode of invasion represents contiguous spread of the tumor along a tissue space that offers the plane of least resistance.

The seminal vesicles are almost always involved by direct extension of prostatic cancer. Invasion of the urinary bladder is less frequent until late in the clinical course. The earliest metastases occur in the obturator lymph node, with subsequent dissemination to the iliac and periaortic lymph nodes. Metastases to the lung reflect further lymphatic spread through the thoracic duct and through dissemination from the prostatic venous plexus to the inferior vena cava. Bony metastases, particularly to the vertebral column (Fig. 17-45), ribs, and pelvic bones, are painful and present a thorny clinical problem.

Uncommon histological variants of acinar adenocarcinoma of the prostate include mucinous adenocarcinoma, carcinoid tumor, small cell undifferentiated carcinoma, ductal adenocarcinoma, transitional cell carcinoma, and squamous cell carcinoma. Rare mesenchymal tumors of the prostate have been reported.

☐ **Clinical Features:** The clinical presentation of prostatic cancer is variable. One tenth of the cases are initially discovered in the fragments of tissue obtained at the time of transurethral resection for prostatic hyperplasia. The current widespread screening programs for prostate cancer, which employ digital rectal examination in combination with serum PSA, serves to detect this malignancy in the majority of cases. Patients who demonstrate elevations of serum PSA with or without the detection of a nodule on rectal examination are further evaluated by needle biopsies of the prostate. Uncommonly, patients present with bladder outlet obstruction or symptoms referable to metastatic tumor.

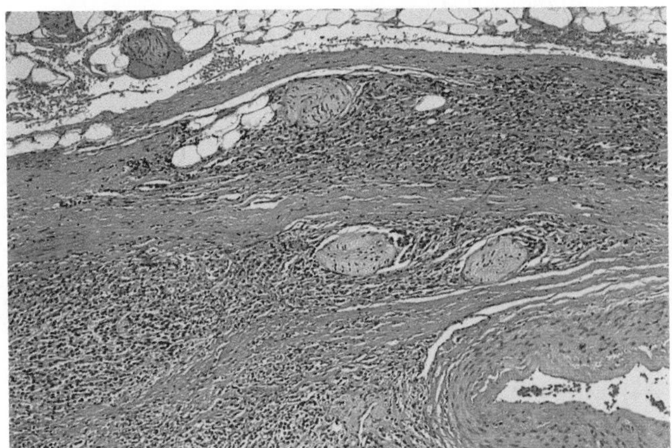

FIGURE *17-44*
Penetration of prostate capsule. Tumor cells show perineural invasion and penetration of the capsule, with invasion of periprostatic adipose tissue.

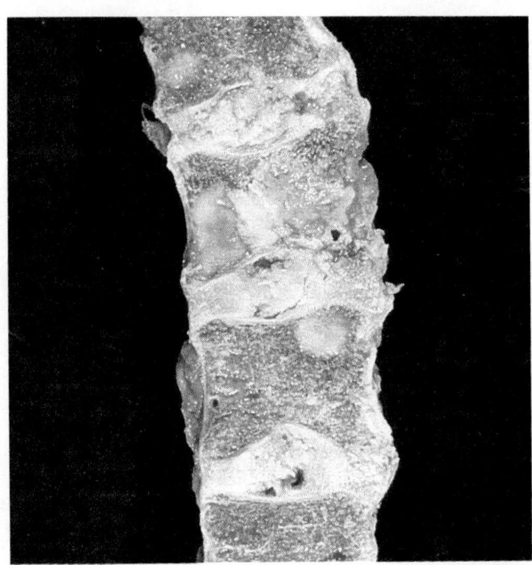

FIGURE *17-45*
Metastatic prostatic carcinoma. A section of the spine from a patient with prostatic adenocarcinoma shows pale, osteoblastic metastases in several vertebral bodies.

Staging

The clinical staging of prostate cancer is shown in Figure 17-46 and Table 17-3.

At the time of initial presentation, 10% of prostatic cancers are stage A. Of those patients with tumors clinically judged to be localized to the prostate, 60% show evidence of capsular penetration or seminal vesicle invasion (stage C). Metastases of prostate cancer, in order of decreasing frequency, are observed in lymph nodes, bones, lung, and liver. Widespread dissemination of the tumor (carcinomatosis), frequently with terminal pneumonia or sepsis, is the most common cause of death.

The demonstration of PSA and prostatic acid phosphatase (PAP) by immunoperoxidase staining of biopsy specimens of metastatic sites has proved valuable in identifying the prostate as the primary site of the tumor. These tumor markers are also detectable in the serum of patients with prostatic cancer. Serum PSA serves as a useful screening test for the presence of the disease and an indicator of the response to treatment. Serum PAP levels are elevated only in cases of metastatic prostate cancer, especially in patients with osteoblastic bony metastases.

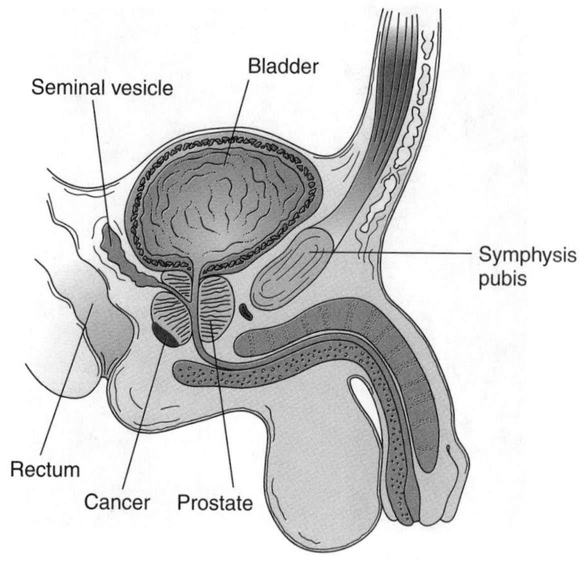

Lymph node metastases

EXTENSIVE CARCINOMA
stage C or D

FIGURE *17-46*
Clinical staging of prostatic carcinoma. In stages A and B, the tumor is confined to the prostate. In stage C, the cancer has extended beyond the prostatic capsule to involve adjacent structures. Metastases to lymph nodes or distant sites are present in stage D.

Treatment

Therapy for prostate cancer is stage-dependent. Patients with stage A and B cancers are treated by radical prostatectomy or radiation therapy. In stage C tumors, radiation therapy is the treatment of choice, acknowledging that half of these patients have occult pelvic lymph node metastases (and possibly further systemic dissemination), which cannot be cured by surgical means.

For those patients whose tumors progress clinically, and for all patients judged to have regional or distant metastases at initial presentation, the principal form of therapy is hormonal. This treatment involves orchiectomy or the administration of antagonists of pituitary luteinizing hormone (LH) releasing hormone (LHRH). LHRH suppression reduces the release of LH, thereby decreasing testosterone production by the testis and resulting in pharmacological castration. In either case, the goal is androgen deprivation.

TABLE *17-3* **Clinical Staging of Prostate Cancer**

Stage A: Incidental microscopic foci in otherwise benign specimens of prostatic tissue
- **A1:** Focal tumor
- **A2:** Cancer in a high proportion of prostatic chips

Stage B: Clinically palpable nodules confined to the prostate
- **B1:** Focal lesions
- **B2:** Involvement of more than one lobe of the prostate

Stage C: Local invasion beyond the capsule

Stage D: Metastases
- **D1:** Metastases to regional pelvic lymph nodes
- **D2:** Distant metastases

SUGGESTED READING

BOOKS

Petersen RO: *Urologic pathology,* 2nd ed. Philadelphia: JB Lippincott, 1992.

Scully RE: Tumors of the ovary and maldeveloped gonads. In: *Atlas of tumor pathology,* 2nd series, fascicle 16. Washington, DC: Armed Forces Institute of Pathology, 1979.

REVIEW ARTICLES

Damjanov I, Katz SM: Malacoplakia. *Pathol Annu* 16:103, 1981.

Mostofi FK: Pathology of germ cell tumors of testis: A progress report. *Cancer* 45:1735, 1980.

Wilson JD: The pathogenesis of benign prostatic hyperplasia. *Am J Med* 68:745, 1980.

REVIEW ARTICLES

Amin MB, Young RH: Primary carcinomas of the urethra. *Sem Diag Pathol* 14:147, 1997.

Bostwick DG, Brawer MK: Prostatic intra-epithelial neoplasia and early invasion in prostate cancer. *Cancer* 59:788, 1987.

Brawn PN: The origin of invasive carcinoma of the bladder. *Cancer* 50:515, 1982.

Geurts van Kessel A, Suijkerbuijk RF, Sinke RJ, et al: Molecular cytogenetics of human germ cell tumors: i(12p) and related chromosome anomalies. *Eur Urol* 23:23, 1993.

Gleason DF: Atypical hyperplasia, benign hyperplasia, and well-differentiated adenocarcinoma of the prostate. *Am J Surg Pathol* 9:53, 1985.

Helpap BGT, Bostwick DG, Montironi R: The significance of atypical adenomatous hyperplasia and prostatic intraepithelial neoplasia for the development of prostate cancer: an update. *Virchows Arch* 426:425, 1995.

Ilson DH, Bosl GJ, Motzer R, et al: Genetic analysis of germ cell tumors: Current progress and future prospects. *Hematol Oncol Clin North Am* 5:1271, 1991.

Koss LG: Mapping of the urinary bladder: Its impact on the concepts of bladder cancer. *Hum Pathol* 5:533, 1979.

Kovi J, Mostofi FK: Atypical hyperplasia of prostate. *Urology* 34(suppl):23, 1989.

Kunze E, Schauer A, Schmitt M: Histology and histogenesis of two different types of inverted urothelial papillomas. *Cancer* 51:348, 1983.

Martin DC: Germinal cell tumors of the testis after orchiopexy. *J Urol* 121:422, 1979.

McNeal JE: Normal histology of the prostate. *Am J Surg Pathol* 12:619, 1988.

Melamed MR, Vousta NG, Grabstald H: Natural history and clinical behavior of *in situ* carcinoma of the human urinary bladder. *Cancer* 17:1533, 1964.

Mostofi RK: Potentialities of bladder epithelium. *J Urol* 71:705, 1954.

Rueter VE: Sarcomatoid lesions of the urogenital tract. *Sem Diag Pathol* 10:188, 1993.

Ritchey ML, Novicki DE, Schultenover SJ: Nephrogenic adenoma of bladder: A report of cases. *J Urol* 131:537, 1984.

Sandberg AA, Berger CS: Review of chromosome studies in urological tumors. II. Cytogenetics and molecular genetics of bladder cancer. *J Urol* 151:545, 1994.

Utz DC, Hanash KA, Farrow GM: The plight of the patient with carcinoma *in situ* of the bladder. *J Urol* 103:160, 1970.

Werth DD, Weigel JW, Mebust WK: Primary neoplasms of the ureter. *J Urol* 125:632, 1981.

Wong T-W, Strauss FH II, Warner NE: Testicular biopsy in the study of male infertility: I. Testicular causes of infertility. *Arch Pathol* 95:151, 1973.

Woolf SH: Screening for prostate cancer with prostate specific antigen: an examination of the evidence. *N Eng J Med* 33:1401, 1995.

Young RH, Eble JN: Unusual forms of carcinoma of the urinary bladder. *Hum Pathol* 22:948, 1991.

CHAPTER 18

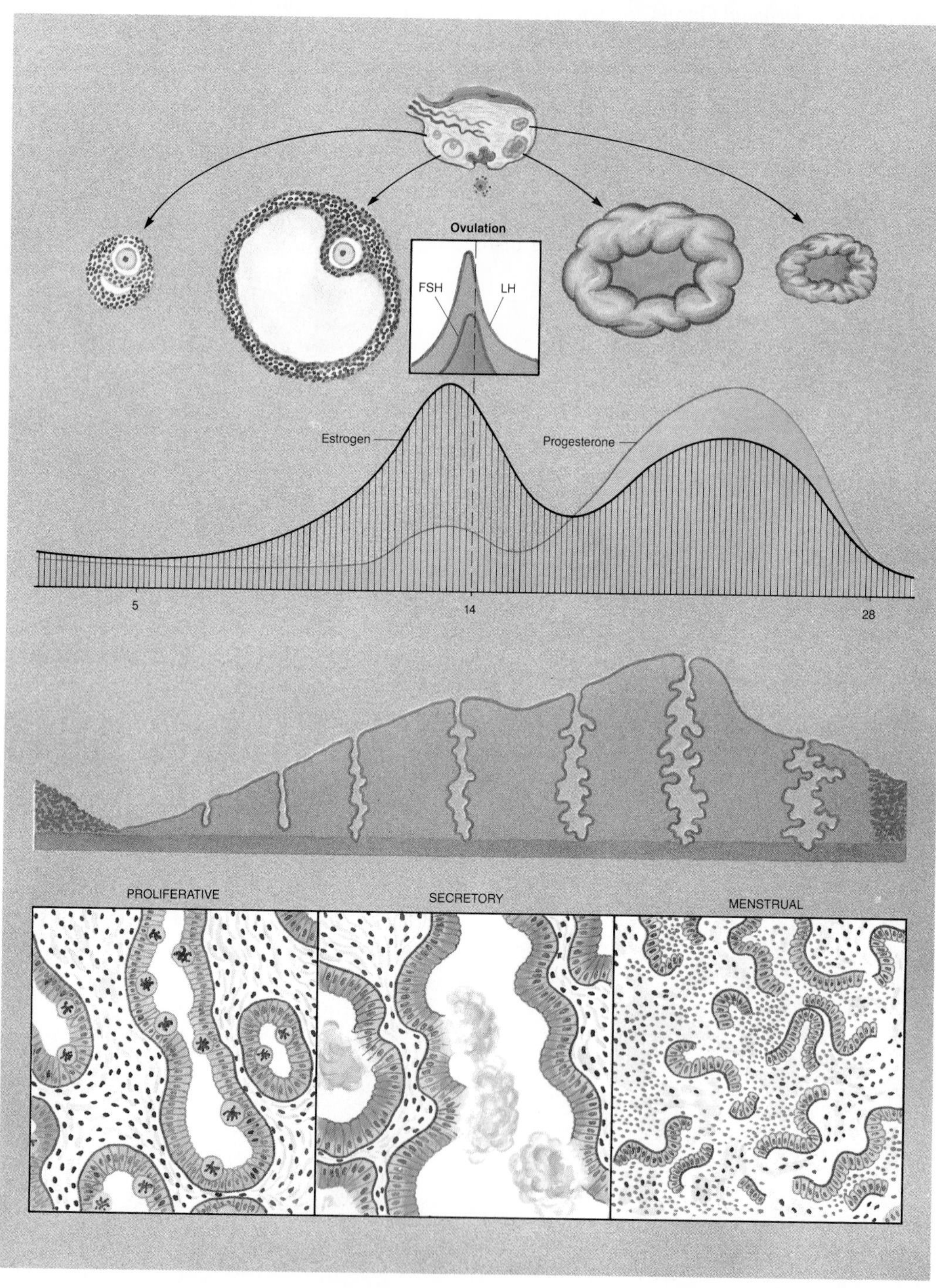

Ovulation
FSH
LH
Estrogen
Progesterone
5
14
28
PROLIFERATIVE
SECRETORY
MENSTRUAL

The Female Reproductive System

Stanley J. Robboy
Maire A. Duggan
Robert J. Kurman

(continued)

FIGURE *18-1* *(see opposite page)*
Menstrual cycle with correlation of hormonal, ovarian, and endometrial changes.

EMBRYOLOGY

The anlage of the human gonad, which forms as a swelling of the embryonic urogenital ridge, is initially in an indifferent state. Both sex chromosomes and autosomal chromosomes in the stromal cells of the gonad determine whether it will differentiate into a testis or an ovary. If the gonadal stroma is male, a gene on the Y chromosome (testis-determining gene) interacts with somatic components in the primitive gonad and initiates the development of seminiferous tubules. If the gonadal stroma is female, an ovary develops. The ovary is derived from mesoderm, except for the germ cells, which are endodermal. By about the 40th day, the ovaries and testes are histologically distinct.

The wolffian (mesonephric) ducts begin their development at about day 25, regardless of the sex of the embryo. If stimulated by testosterone (secreted by Leydig cells starting at about day 70), the ducts differentiate into vas deferens, epididymis, and seminal vesicle. If not stimulated by day 84, the ducts regress and remain as vestigial rests in the female. They may form cysts in the cervix (mesonephric cyst) or vagina (Gartner duct cyst).

The müllerian ducts (or paramesonephric ducts) comprise the anlage of the fallopian tubes, uterus, and vaginal wall. They appear at about day 37 as funnel-shaped openings of celomic epithelium. These develop into paired, undifferentiated tubes, using the wolffian ducts as guide wires to reach the region of the future hymen. If the wolffian duct is absent, as in renal agenesis, the vagina and cervix are almost always abnormal or absent. At day 54, the müllerian ducts fuse to become a straight uterovaginal canal.

A central tenet of genital tract development in both sexes is that the müllerian tubes will develop along female lines, unless specifically impeded by embryonic testicular factors. In males, Sertoli cells in the developing testis produce müllerian-inhibiting substance, a protein that causes the müllerian ducts to regress. This protein is first secreted in effective amounts 2 weeks after the testis has become anatomically distinct. In the absence of müllerian-inhibiting substance, the müllerian ducts develop "passively" into their adult form.

The development of the external genitalia into a masculine form depends on the local conversion of testosterone to dihydrotestosterone. A lack of dihydrotestosterone results in the persistence of female external genitalia. The genital tubercle develops into the clitoris, the genital folds into the labia minora, and the genital swellings into the labia majora. Even in the absence of hormones secreted by the fetal ovary, the female internal organs and external genitalia develop partially. Female development also occurs even when the gonads are not present at all. The basic architecture of the female genital tract is completed by day 120.

Genital Infections

SEXUALLY TRANSMITTED GENITAL INFECTIONS

Infectious diseases of the female genital tract are common and are caused by a wide variety of pathogenic organisms (Table 18-1). These diseases are also discussed in Chapter 9. **Most of the important infectious diseases of the female genital tract are sexually transmitted.**

Bacterial Infections

Gonorrhea

Gonorrhea is caused by *Neisseria gonorrhoeae*, a fastidious, gram-negative diplococcus. A million cases of gonorrhea occur yearly in the United States. It is a frequent cause of acute salpingitis and pelvic inflammatory disease (Fig. 18-2).

The squamous epithelium of the mature vulva and vagina is resistant to infection by *N. gonorrhoeae*. Juvenile vulvovaginal epithelium is thinner and is bathed by an alkaline vaginal secretion, rendering it more susceptible to infection. The organisms adhere to the mucous membranes of the lower genital tract and reach the tubal lumen by ascending through the cervix and the endometrial cavity. An acute endometritis results during this passage. The organisms attach to nonciliated cells in the fallopian tube and are engulfed within 3 hours by the microvilli. They then elicit a pronounced, acute, fibrinous, inflammatory reaction, which is confined to the mucosal surface (acute salpingitis). From the tubal lumen, the infection

TABLE *18-1* **Infectious Diseases of the Female Genital Tract**

Organism	Disease	Diagnostic Feature
Sexually Transmitted Diseases		
Gram-negative rods and cocci		
Calymmatobacterium granulomatis	Granuloma inguinale	Donovan body
Gardnerella vaginalis	*Gardnerella* infection	Clue cell
Haemophilus ducreyi	Chancroid (soft chancre)	
Neisseria gonorrhoeae	Gonorrhea	Gram-negative diplococcus
Spirochetes		
Treponema pallidum	Syphilis	Spirochete
Mycoplasmas		
Mycoplasma hominis	Nonspecific vaginitis	
Ureaplasma urealyticum	Nonspecific vaginitis	
Rickettsiae		
Chlamydia trachomatis type D–K	Various forms of PID	
Chlamydia trachomatis type L_{1-3}	Lymphogranuloma venereum	
Viruses		
Human papillomavirus (HPV)	Condyloma acuminatum/planum	Koilocyte
	Neoplastic potential	
Types 6, 11, 40, 42, 43, 44, 57	Low risk	
Types 16, 18, 31, 33, 35, 39, 45, 51, 52, 56, 58, 66	High risk	
Herpes simplex, type 2	Herpes genitalis	Multinucleated giant cell with intranuclear homogenization and inclusion bodies
Cytomegalovirus (CMV)	Cytomegalic inclusion disease	Bulbous intranuclear inclusion body
Molluscum contagiosum	Molluscum infection	Molluscum body
Protozoa		
Trichomonas vaginalis	Trichomoniasis	Trichomonad
Selected Nonsexually Transmitted Diseases		
The actinomyces and related organisms		
Actinomyces israelii	PID (one of many organisms)	Sulfur granules
Mycobacterium tuberculosis	Tuberculosis	Necrotizing granulomas
Fungi		
Candida albicans	Candidiasis	*Candida* species

PID, pelvic inflammatory disease.

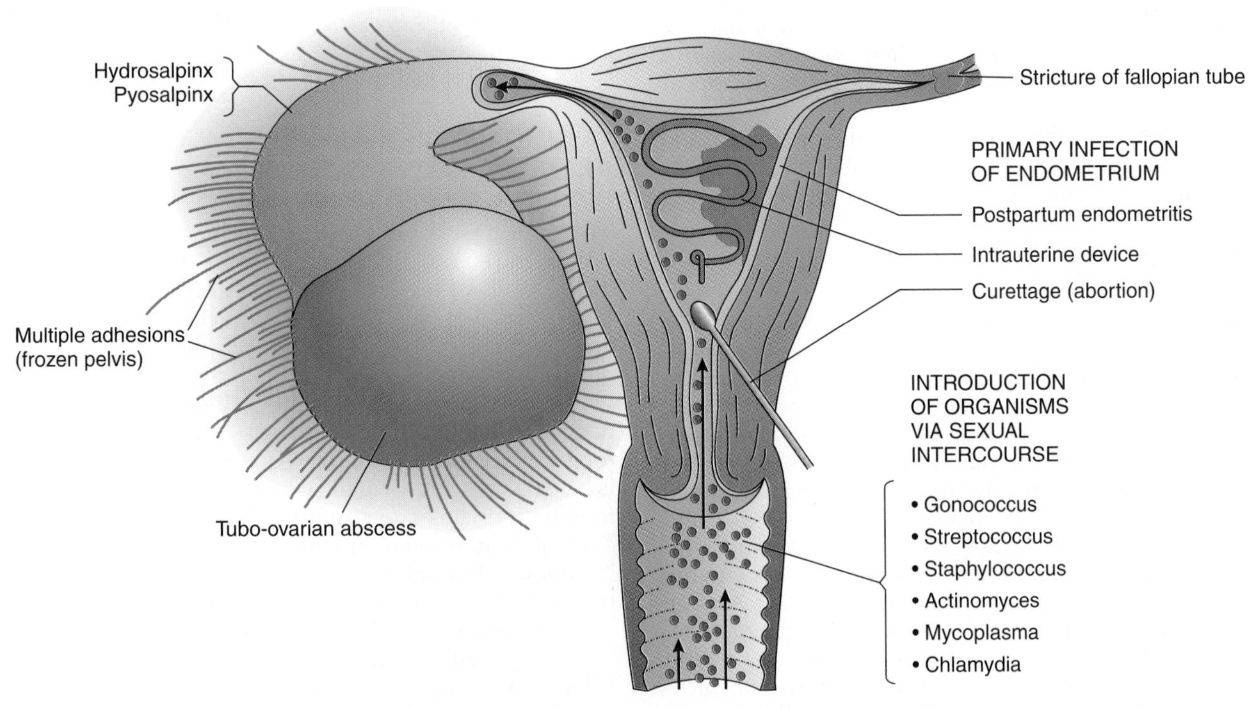

FIGURE *18-2*
Pelvic inflammatory disease.

spreads to involve the ovary, thereby creating a tubo-ovarian abscess. It may also spread more widely to involve the pelvic and abdominal cavities, with the formation of subdiaphragmatic and pelvic abscesses.

Systemic complications of gonorrhea include septicemia and septic arthritis. The organisms induce a purulent inflammatory reaction at all sites of infection. Resolution is rarely complete, and dense fibrous adhesions remain. The healing process distorts and destroys the plicae of the fallopian tube and often leads to sterility.

Syphilis

Syphilis is a venereal disease caused by *Treponema pallidum*, a thin, motile, spiral-shaped bacterium, commonly known as a spirochete. The disease is acquired through sexual contact with an infected person or as a result of transplacental spread (congenital syphilis). *T. pallidum* penetrates small abrasions in the skin or normal mucosal membranes. Because of a complex immunological reaction to the bacterium, which results in a chronic host–parasite relationship, untreated syphilis may wax and wane, progressing through primary, secondary, and tertiary stages.

- **The primary stage** is characterized by the *chancre*, which usually appears at the portal of entry after an incubation period of about 3 weeks. The chancre presents as a painless, indurated papule, 1 cm to several centimeters in diameter. It is surrounded by an inflammatory cuff, which breaks down to form an ulcer. The chancre may persist for 2 to 6 weeks and then heals spontaneously.
- **The secondary stage** of syphilis appears after a latent period of several weeks to months. It is characterized by low-grade fever, headache, malaise, lymphadenopathy, and the reappearance of highly contagious syphilitic lesions called *condylomata lata* (syphilitic warts). The secondary infectious lesions heal after 2 to 6 weeks, and the symptoms disappear spontaneously.
- **The tertiary stage** develops any time thereafter and may be complicated by involvement of the cardiovascular and nervous systems.

Granuloma Inguinale

Granuloma inguinale is caused by *Calymmatobacterium granulomatis*, a sexually transmitted, gram-negative, nonmotile, encapsulated rod related to the Enterobacteriaceae. The disease occurs with equal frequency in men and women. The primary lesion begins as a painless, ulcerated nodule involving the genital, inguinal, or perianal skin. The organisms invade through skin abrasions and spread locally by direct extension, destroying the skin and its underlying tissues. Extensive local spread and lymphatic permeation occur later. Vacuolated histiocytes are packed with characteristic intracellular bacteria (*Donovan bodies*). The organism, best seen with the Wright stain, resembles a closed safety pin. The squamous epithelium overlying the involved area may demonstrate conspicuous hyperplasia, sometimes exuberant enough to be misinterpreted as a squamous cell carcinoma. Relapses are common following antibiotic therapy and reflect an inadequate duration of therapy.

Chancroid

Chancroid, also called *soft chancre*, is caused by *Haemophilus ducreyi*, a gram-negative, nonmotile bacillus. This disease is rare in the United States but common in underdeveloped countries, such as those in Africa. Sexual congress with an infected man is followed in 3 to 5 days by the appearance of single or sometimes multiple small, vesiculopustular lesions on the cervix, vagina, vulva, or perianal region. Histological examination reveals a granulomatous inflammatory reaction. The lesion often ruptures to form a purulent ulcer, which is painful and bleeds easily. There may be associated inguinal lymphadenopathy, fever, chills, and malaise. A major complication is scar formation during the healing phase, an outcome that sometimes causes urethral stenosis. The diagnosis is confirmed by culture of the organism.

Gardnerella

A substantial proportion of cases of **nonspecific vaginitis** are caused by sexual transmission of *Gardnerella vaginalis*, a gram-negative coccobacillus. A biopsy specimen is usually normal, because the organism neither penetrates the mucosa nor elicits an inflammatory reaction. The squamous cells are covered with coccobacilli (*clue cells*), which are best seen in a wet mount specimen of the vaginal discharge or in a Papanicolaou-stained smear. The diagnosis of *Gardnerella* infection can be established either by identifying the organisms in the vaginal discharge or by cytological examination. Other aids to the diagnosis are a thin, homogeneous (milk-like) vaginal discharge, a vaginal pH greater than 4.5, and the presence of a fishy odor from the discharge after alkalinizing it with 10% potassium hydroxide.

Mycoplasma

Mycoplasmas are minute pleomorphic organisms that resemble the so-called L bacterial forms. They are common commensals of the oropharyngeal and urogenital tracts. Colonization of the lower genital tract by *Mycoplasma* occurs through sexual contact. Ureaplasma urealyticum can be isolated from the lower genital tract in 40% of healthy women and may cause infertility, adverse effects on pregnancy, and perinatal infections. *Mycoplasma hominis*, found in the lower genital tract of 5% of healthy women, is responsible for a small proportion of cases of symptomatic cervicitis and vaginitis. *M. hominis* is frequently cultivated in association with *G. vaginalis* or *Trichomonas* infection. Although the role of mycoplasmas in genital tract infection is not completely understood, the organisms are encountered in pelvic inflammatory disease, acute salpingitis, spontaneous abortion, and puerperal fever. The histological appearance of the affected tissue is usually unremarkable.

Chlamydia Infections

Chlamydia trachomatis is a common, venereally transmitted organism. It is an obligate, gram-negative, intracellular rickettsia, which was previously considered to be a virus because of its small size and its intracellular replication. Fifteen serotypes are known. Infection with *C. trachomatis* results in a wide variety of disorders in women, men, and infants. This organism has been found in the genital tract of about 8% of asymptomatic women and in 20% of women presenting with symptoms of a lower genital tract infection. In the more common genital infections, which involve serotypes D through K, the cervical mucosa is severely inflamed and the endocervical and metaplastic squamous cells reveal small inclusion bodies. Complications include ascending infection of the endometrium, fallopian tube, and ovary. Tubal occlusion and infertility may result. *Chlamydia* also gives rise to infections of Bartholin gland and acute urethritis. Infections of infants delivered vaginally may lead to conjunctivitis, otitis media, and pneumonia.

Lymphogranuloma Venereum

Lymphogranuloma venereum is a sexually transmitted infection in both men and women, which is endemic in tropical countries. The disease is caused by the L form of *C. trachomatis*, serotypes L1 through L3. After a few days to a month, a small painless vesicle forms at the site of inoculation. It heals rapidly, and in many instances the vesicle is not even noticed. The second stage presents with bilaterally enlarged inguinal lymph nodes, which may rupture and form suppurative fistulas. The inguinal nodes in men and perirectal nodes in women become matted and painful. In some untreated patients, a third stage appears after a latency of several years. This chronic phase is characterized by scarring, which causes lymphatic obstruction and resulting genital elephantiasis and rectal strictures. In the second and third stages, infected tissues contain necrotizing granulomas, neutrophilic infiltrates, and, occasionally, inclusion bodies within macrophages.

Viral Infections

Human Papillomavirus

Human papillomavirus (HPV) is a DNA virus that infects a wide variety of skin and mucosal surfaces to produce wartlike lesions, referred to as verrucae and condylomata. Over 70 types of this virus have been identified, one third of which cause lesions of the genital tract. In the United States, more than 10% of all men and women between the ages of 15 and 50 years have genital HPV infections, usually as a result of sexual contact with an infected person. HPV types 6 and 11 are detected in over 80% of the macroscopically visible condylomata.

Of particular concern is the possible etiological role of several strains of HPV in the development of cancer of the female lower genital tract. Types 16 and 18, and to a lesser degree types 31, 33, and 35, have been linked to intraepithelial neoplasia and to invasive cancer (see later section on the cervix).

Condyloma Acuminatum

Condyloma acuminatum is a benign, exophytic, papillomatous lesion on the skin or mucous membranes of the lower female genital tract caused by HPV. It is occasionally visible with the naked eye but usually requires visualization with the colposcope. This endoscopic instrument allows magnified observation of the vagina and cervix *in vivo*. Condylomata acuminata occur on the vulva, perianal region, perineum, vagina, and cervix. They may also involve the urethra, bladder, and rectum. Condylomata grow as papules, plaques, or nodules and eventually as spiked or cauliflower-like excrescences. Microscopic examination usually exhibits a striking papillomatous proliferation of squamous epithelium (Fig. 18-3). A characteristic finding is the koilocyte (Greek *koilos*, hollow), an epithelial cell with a perinuclear halo and a wrinkled nucleus that contains HPV particles. Parakeratosis, dyskeratosis, and sometimes hyperkeratosis may also occur.

Herpesvirus

Herpes simplex, type 2 is a double-stranded DNA virus, which is a common cause of sexually transmitted, genital infections. Although herpes simplex, type 1 is usually associated with lesions of the skin and mouth, it occasionally infects the female genital tract. After an incubation period of 1 to 3 weeks, small vesicles develop on the vulva and erode into painful ulcers. Similar lesions occur in the vagina and cervix. On biopsy of a lesion, epithelial cells adjacent to intraepithelial vesicles show ballooning degeneration, and many contain large nuclei with eosinophilic inclusions. The inclusions are not pathognomonic of herpes simplex, type 2, since similar inclusions are found in varicella-zoster infections.

Genital herpes tends to become latent, with the virus remaining in the sacral ganglia. Reactivation of the virus during pregnancy can result in its transmission to the newborn during passage through the birth canal, a complication that is often fatal.

Cytomegalovirus

Cytomegalovirus is a double-stranded DNA virus of the herpesvirus family. The virus is ubiquitous, and more than 80% of persons older than the age of 35 years have antibodies to cytomegalovirus. Several lines of evidence suggest that many cases are sexually transmitted: (1) the seroprevalence of cytomegalovirus has risen in young adults, (2) the virus is recovered more frequently from cervical secretions and semen than from any other body sites, and (3) viral titers in semen are 100,000 times greater than those in urine. However, cytomegalovirus is only rarely identified as causing genital infections in women. Infection in the endometrium may result in spontaneous abortion or infection of the newborn. Infected cells exhibit characteristic large, eosinophilic, intranuclear inclusions and, occasionally, cytoplasmic inclusions.

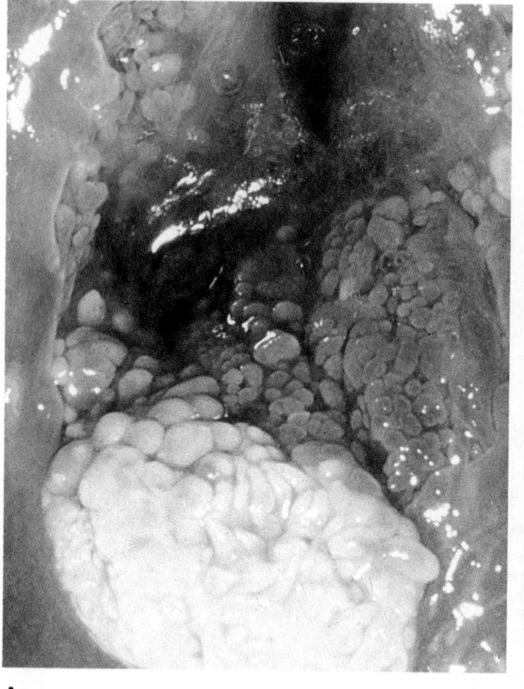
A

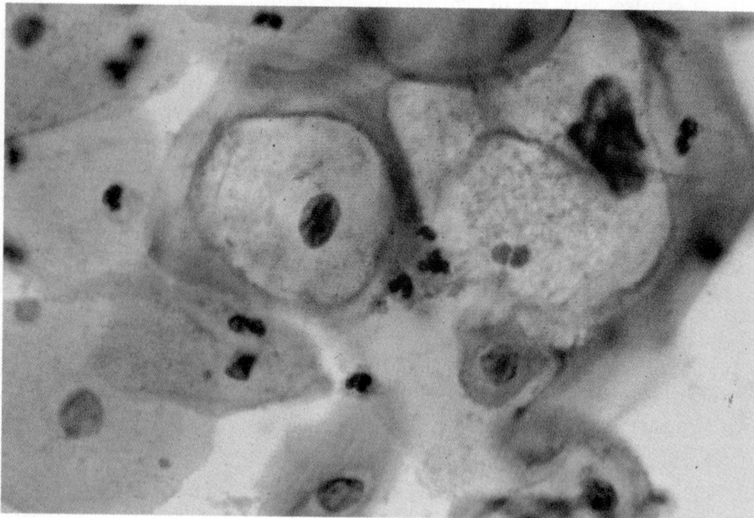
B

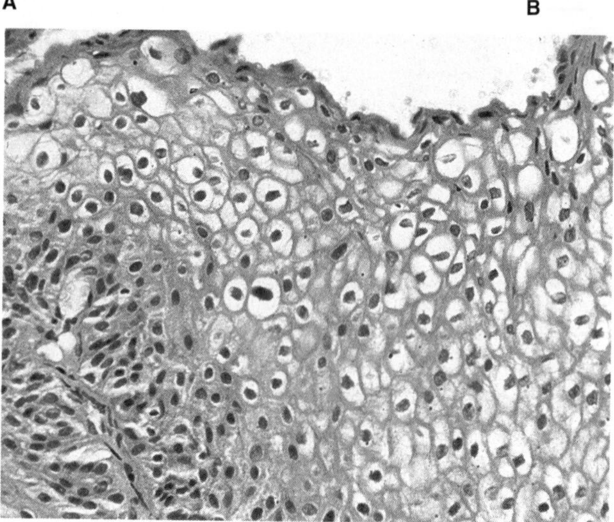
C

FIGURE 18-3
Human papillomavirus–induced condylomatous infections. (*A*) Condyloma acuminatum on the cervix, visible with the naked eye as cauliflower-like excrescences. (*B*) A cervical smear contains characteristic koilocytes, with a perinuclear halo and a wrinkled nucleus that contains viral particles. (*C*) Biopsy of the condyloma shows koilocytes with perinuclear halos but lacking nuclear atypia.

Molluscum Contagiosum

Molluscum contagiosum is a double-stranded DNA virus of the highly contagious poxvirus group. Infection with this virus leads to the appearance of multiple smooth, gray-white nodules that are centrally umbilicated and exude a cheesy material. The lesions occur predominantly in the genital region but may be found elsewhere on the body. Characteristic large, cytoplasmic viral inclusions ("molluscum bodies") are found in the infected epithelial cells. Most lesions regress spontaneously, but untreated ones may persist for years.

Trichomoniasis

Trichomonas vaginalis is a large, pear-shaped, flagellated protozoan, which commonly causes vaginitis. The disease is sexually transmitted, and 25% of infected women are asymptomatic carriers. The infection presents as a heavy, yellow-gray, thick, foamy discharge, which is accompanied by severe itching, dyspareunia (painful intercourse), and dysuria (painful urination). The diagnosis is confirmed by a wet mount preparation in which the motile trichomonads are seen. The organisms are also demonstrated in Papanicolaou-stained cervical smears.

Pelvic Inflammatory Disease

Pelvic inflammatory disease (PID) describes an infection of the pelvic organs that follows the extension of any of a variety of microorganisms beyond the uterine corpus (see Fig. 18-2). Ascent of the infection results in bilateral acute salpingitis, pyosalpinx, and tubo-ovarian abscesses. *N. gonorrhoeae* is the principal single organism causing PID, but most infections are polymicrobial. Although it has been claimed that users of intrauterine devices are at an increased risk of developing PID, in actuality this hazard is usually related to sexually transmitted infections. The incidence of PID is far greater in sexually promiscuous women than in those who are monogamous. Occasionally, PID is a sequel to postpartum endometritis or an infection after endometrial curettage.

Patients with PID usually present with lower abdominal pain. Physical examination reveals bilateral adnexal tenderness and marked discomfort when the cervix is manipulated (*chandelier sign*). Complications of PID include (1) rupture of a tubo-ovarian abscess, which may result in a life-threatening peritonitis; (2) infertility from scarring of the healed tubal plicae; (3) increased rates of ectopic pregnancy; and (4) intestinal obstruction, owing to fibrous bands and adhesions.

GENITAL INFECTIONS NOT TRANSMITTED SEXUALLY

Tuberculosis

Mycobacterium tuberculosis may infect any segment of the female genital tract. Genital tuberculosis is found in 1% of infertile women in the United States and in more than 10% of such women in less-developed countries.

TUBERCULOUS SALPINGITIS: Inflammation of the fallopian tube is the initial lesion in most cases of tuberculous genital infection. The mycobacteria usually reach the tube by hematogenous dissemination from the lung. Tuberculous salpingitis results in fibrinous adhesions and scarring of the fallopian tube; in turn, these complications lead to multiple functional abnormalities (e.g., infertility, ectopic gestation, and pelvic pain). The tubes may become nodular and mimic salpingitis isthmica nodosa. Pyosalpinx (fallopian tube distended with pus) and hydrosalpinx (fluid-filled tube) are late sequelae, and the adjacent ovary may become infected.

TUBERCULOUS ENDOMETRITIS: This condition complicates half of the cases of tubercular infection of the tube. Noncaseating, poorly formed granulomas with rare giant cells are typical. In other areas of the body afflicted with this infection, granulomas have time to develop caseous necrosis and characteristic Langhans giant cells. By contrast, tuberculous granulomas that develop in the endometrium are no more than one cycle old, owing to menstrual shedding, and thus are at an early stage of development.

Candidiasis

Ten percent of women are asymptomatic carriers of fungi in the vulva and vagina, with *Candida albicans* being the most common offender. However, only 2% of women present with clinically apparent candidal vulvovaginitis. Pregnant women are considerably more susceptible to candidal vulvovaginitis, and 10% of such women are symptomatic. Diabetes mellitus and the use of oral contraceptives also promote vaginal candidiasis. The infection presents as vulvar itching and a whitish discharge. Clinical examination reveals firmly adherent, small white plaques on the mucous membranes. Biopsy discloses submucosal edema and a chronic inflammatory infiltrate. The fungi do not penetrate the epithelium, and the white patches correspond to foci of desquamated, necrotic epithelial cells, cellular debris, bacterial flora, and the candidal spores and pseudohyphae. If untreated, the infection waxes and wanes, and it frequently disappears following delivery. The diagnosis is made by finding characteristic spores and pseudohyphae in a wet mount preparation or with a Papanicolaou stain.

Actinomycosis

Genital tract actinomycosis is uncommon but has been increasingly reported in association with the use of intrauterine devices. *Actinomyces israelii*, the causative organism, is a gram-positive rod found in about 4% of normal genital tracts. The bacterium is believed to enter the uterine cavity by way of the tail of the intrauterine device. It ascends to infect the fallopian tube, ovary, and broad ligaments and forms a tubo-ovarian abscess. Suppurating lesions display drainage tracts that contain dense microcolonies of organisms ("sulfur granules"). Actinomycosis results in extensive fibrosis and scarring of the female genital tract.

Toxic Shock Syndrome

Toxic shock syndrome is an acute, sometimes fatal disorder characterized by fever, shock, and a desquamative erythematous rash. In addition, vomiting, diarrhea, myalgias, neurological signs, and thrombocytopenia are common. It was initially believed to be related to the use of tampons during menstruation, but it is now recognized to occur with staphylococcal infection. Certain strains of *Staphylococcus aureus* release an exotoxin called toxic shock syndrome toxin-1. This toxin exerts its own effects and also alters the function of mononuclear phagocytes, thereby impairing the clearance of other potentially toxic substances, such as endotoxin. In addition to the pathological alterations characteristic of shock, the lesions of disseminated intravascular coagulation (microthrombi in many organs) are usually prominent. The occurrence of toxic shock syndrome has decreased markedly since the recognition of the role of tampons in promoting colonization of the vagina by *S. aureus*.

Vulva

ANATOMY

The vulva is composed of the mons pubis, labia majora and minora, clitoris, and vestibule. With the onset of puberty, the mons pubis and the lateral borders of the labia

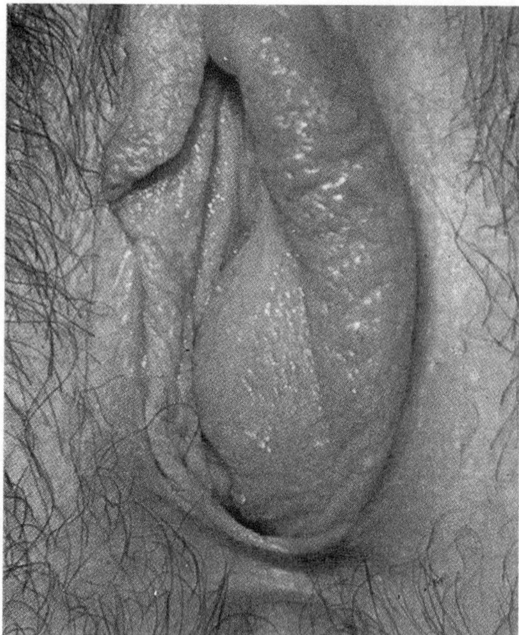

FIGURE 18-4
Bartholin gland cyst. The 4-cm lesion is located to the right of and posterior to the vaginal introitus.

majora acquire increased subcutaneous fat and develop coarse hair. The sebaceous and apocrine glands in these regions develop concomitantly. The paired external openings of the paraurethral glands (Skene glands) lie on either side of the urethral meatus. Bartholin glands, located immediately posterolateral to the introitus, are branching, mucus-secreting, tubuloalveolar glands, drained by a short duct. In addition, microscopic mucous glands are scattered throughout the area bounded by the labia minora. The inguinal and femoral lymph nodes provide the primary lymph drainage routes, except for the clitoris (the homologue of the penis), which shares the lymphatic drainage of the urethra.

DEVELOPMENTAL ANOMALIES AND CYSTS

ECTOPIC BREAST TISSUE: Small, isolated nodules of ectopic breast tissue may extend in the "milk line" to the vulva and enlarge during pregnancy.

BARTHOLIN GLAND CYST: The paired Bartholin glands produce a clear mucoid secretion, which continuously lubricates the vestibular surface. The ducts are prone to obstruction and consequent cyst formation (Fig. 18-4). In turn, infection of the cyst leads to abscess formation. Bartholin gland abscess was formerly associated commonly with gonorrhea, but it is now more frequently caused by staphylococci, chlamydia, and anaerobes. Treatment consists of incision, drainage, marsupialization, and appropriate antibiotics.

KERATINOUS CYSTS: Also termed *epithelial inclusion cysts* or *sebaceous cysts*, keratinous cysts are frequently seen on the vulva, especially the labia majora. They contain a white cheesy material and typically are lined by stratified squamous epithelium. Some cysts originate from occluded sebaceous glands that have undergone squamous metaplasia.

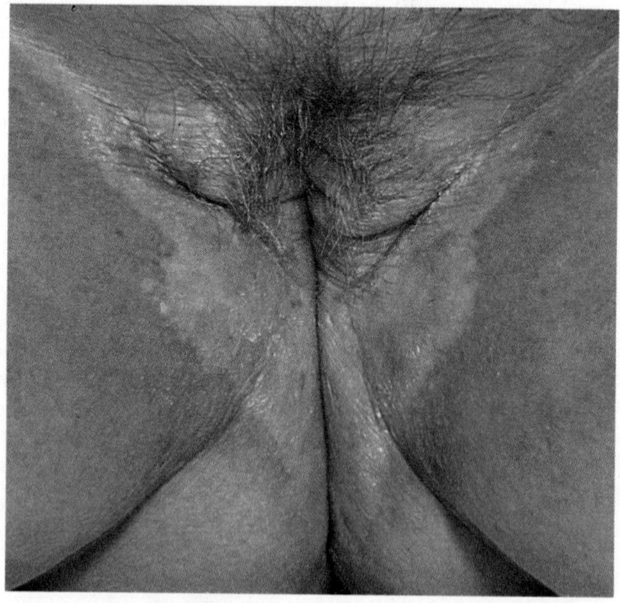

A

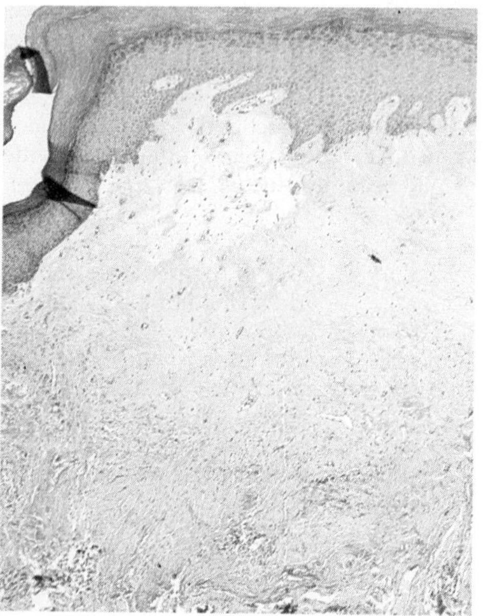

B

FIGURE 18-5
Lichen sclerosus of vulva. (*A*) The sharply demarcated white lesion affects the vulva and perineum. (*B*) The epidermis is thin and exhibits hyperkeratosis and a lack of the normal rete pattern. The dermis displays an acellular, homogeneous zone overlying a mild chronic inflammatory infiltrate.

MUCINOUS CYSTS: Mucinous glands of the vulva occasionally become obstructed and subsequently cystic. Mucinous columnar cells line the cyst and produce mucinous secretions, which may become infected.

DERMATOLOGICAL DISEASES

The term *non-neoplastic epithelial disorders of skin and mucosa* replaces the older usage *vulvar dystrophy*. The conditions usually present as white lesions of the vulva, usually in middle-aged or older women.

LICHEN SCLEROSUS: *This abnormal growth of the vulvar skin is characterized by white plaques, atrophy of the skin, and a parchment-like or crinkled appearance, and occasionally by marked contracture of the vulvar tissues (kraurosis).* Histologically, there is hyperkeratosis, blunting or loss of rete ridges, and a homogeneous, acellular zone in the upper dermis (Fig. 18-5). The acellular zone results from swelling and splitting of the collagen bundles into individual fibers and fibrils, which are enveloped by a gel-like matrix. A band of chronic inflammatory cells typically lies beneath this layer. Itching is the most common symptom, and dyspareunia is frequent. **Although slowly developing, insidious, and progressive, lichen sclerosus is not premalignant.**

SQUAMOUS HYPERPLASIA: The squamous epithelium of the vulva may become hyperplastic (acanthosis), in which case the epidermal rete ridges may become enlarged and confluent. Squamous hyperplasia is often a nonspecific reaction to vulvar irritants. The thickened epithelium displays a marked increase in superficial keratin (*hyperkeratosis*), which imparts a white appearance to the vulva. Since squamous carcinomas may also appear as white plaques, the previously used term *leukoplakia* has caused considerable confusion and is best avoided. Biopsy is required to distinguish benign squamous hyperplasia from intraepithelial neoplasia and carcinoma.

BENIGN TUMORS

HIDRADENOMA: This benign tumor of apocrine sweat gland origin appears chiefly in the labia majora as a sharply circumscribed nodule, rarely larger than 1 cm. Microscopically, the lesion is composed of papillary tubules and acini lined by two layers of cells: an inner layer of apocrine columnar cells and an outer one of myoepithelial cells.

SYRINGOMA: An adenoma of eccrine glands, syringoma presents as a flesh-colored papule within the dermis of the labia majora. This asymptomatic tumor is composed of two layers of cells: an inner layer of serous cells and an outer one of myoepithelial cells.

CONNECTIVE TISSUE TUMORS: ***Senile hemangiomas*** (cherry hemangiomas) are small, purple skin papules, which on surface trauma may bleed. ***Pyogenic granuloma***, previously thought to be a reaction to superficial wound infection, is a variant of hemangioma. Secondary infection occurs because the surface of the lesion is easily traumatized. Soft tissue tumors found elsewhere in the body also occur in the vulva, including granular cell tumor, leiomyoma, fibroma, lipoma, and histiocytoma.

MALIGNANT TUMORS AND PREMALIGNANT CONDITIONS

Vulvar Intraepithelial Neoplasia

Intraepithelial neoplasia of the vulva reflects a spectrum of neoplastic changes that range from minimal cellular atypia to the most marked cellular changes short of invasive cancer. Since 1980, there has been a 5- to 10-fold increase in the frequency of vulvar intraepithelial neoplasia (VIN) and a 10-fold increase in the number of women with the disease who are younger than 40 years of age. In addition, younger women have increasingly developed an undifferentiated form of VIN, sometimes called warty or basaloid dysplasia, commonly associated with HPV infection. A second form of VIN, which is found more frequently in older women, is more differentiated. If left untreated, many of these women develop invasive squamous cell carcinoma after 6 to 7 years. Thus, similar to comparable lesions in the cervix (CIN), **VIN is a precursor lesion of squamous cell carcinoma.**

☐ **Pathology:** VIN has a variable gross appearance. The lesions may be single or multiple, and macular, papular, or plaquelike. Microscopically, the grades are labeled VIN I, II, and III, corresponding to mild, moderate, and severe dysplasia. Grade III also includes carcinoma *in situ*. The criteria used in establishing the grade of VIN include (1) nuclear size and atypia, (2) the number and degree of atypical mitoses, and (3) loss of cytoplasmic differentiation toward the epithelial surface. In the undifferentiated form seen in younger women, the entire epithelium consists of cells with highly atypical nuclei and negligible cytoplasm. Mitoses, including many atypical forms, are frequent. The more differentiated form seen in older women shows atypia confined more to the basal or parabasal wells with keratin pearls often seen in the rete pegs. This latter form is more frequently associated with invasive carcinoma but less commonly with HPV infection. *Bowen disease*, a term that still appears in the dermatological literature, is a synonym for VIN III but is better replaced by the latter term.

Vulvar intraepithelial neoplasia, even if locally excised, often recurs (25%), in which case it may progress to invasive squamous cell carcinoma (6%). Women with VIN may have squamous neoplasms elsewhere in the lower genital tract.

Squamous Cell Carcinoma

Squamous cell carcinoma of the vulva (Fig. 18-6) is the end result of a multistep process that has its origin in VIN. This tumor accounts for 3% of all genital cancers in women and is the most common cancer of the vulva

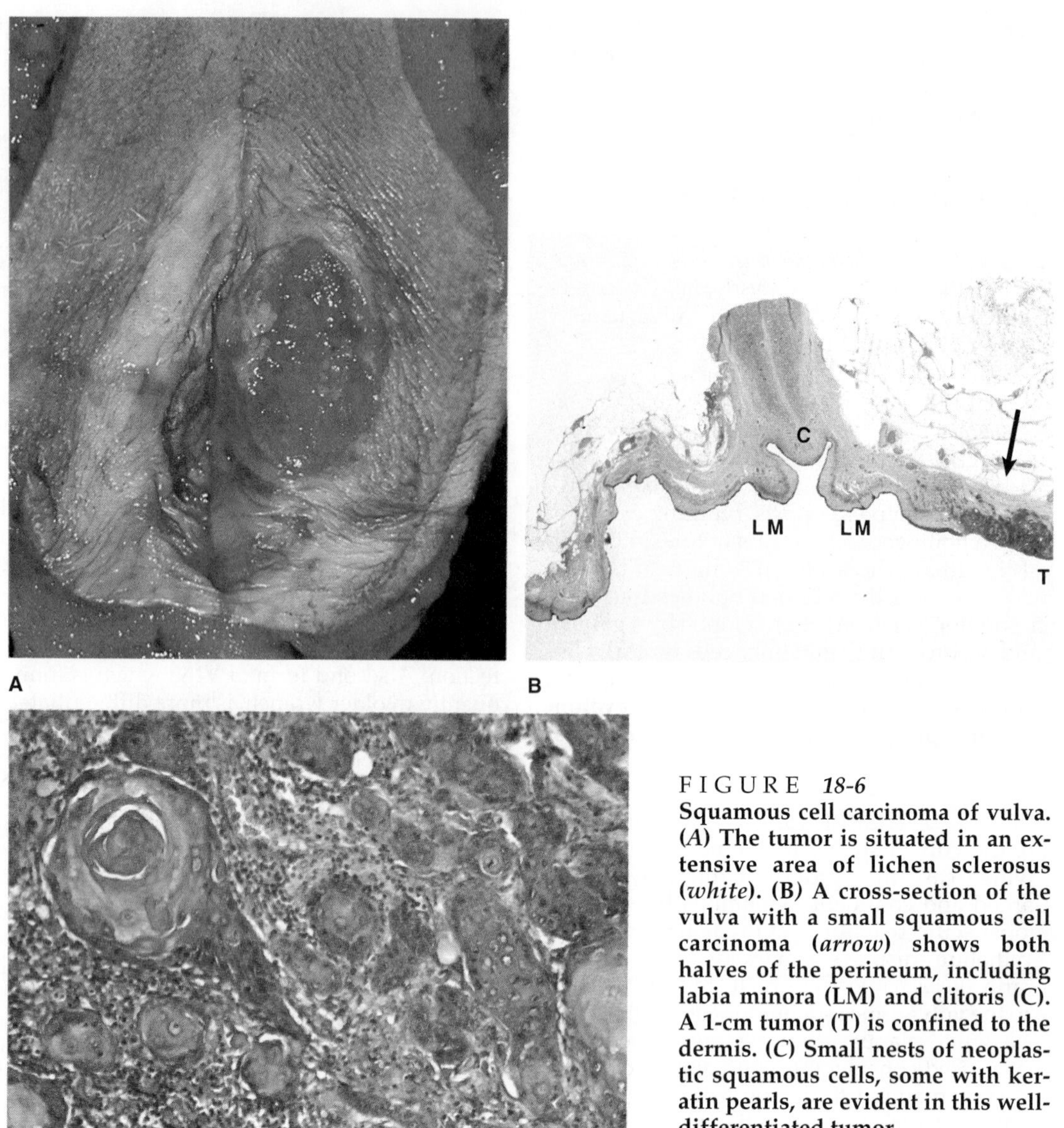

FIGURE *18-6*
Squamous cell carcinoma of vulva. (*A*) The tumor is situated in an extensive area of lichen sclerosus (*white*). (B) A cross-section of the vulva with a small squamous cell carcinoma (*arrow*) shows both halves of the perineum, including labia minora (LM) and clitoris (C). A 1-cm tumor (T) is confined to the dermis. (*C*) Small nests of neoplastic squamous cells, some with keratin pearls, are evident in this well-differentiated tumor.

(86%). In the past, it mainly affected older women, but like VIN it now occurs with increasing frequency in younger women. Two thirds of larger tumors are exophytic; the others are ulcerative and endophytic. Pruritus of long duration is commonly the first symptom. Ulceration, bleeding, and secondary infection may develop. The tumors grow slowly; extend to the contiguous skin, vagina, and rectum; and metastasize to the superficial inguinal and then the deep inguinal, femoral, and pelvic lymph nodes.

A staging system for vulvar cancer employs 2 cm in greatest dimension as the critical size that differentiates stage I and stage II lesions (Table 18-2). In addition to increased size (in one series, each centimeter of tumor size increased the risk of death by nearly 50%), factors affecting patient survival include tumor grade and the presence of lymph node metastases (relative risk of 8). More-differentiated tumors have a higher mean survival, and the survival rate approaches 90% when nodes are uninvolved. Two thirds of women with inguinal node metastases survive for at least 5 years, whereas only a fourth of those with pelvic node metastases live that long.

Verrucous Carcinoma

Verrucous carcinoma of the vulva is a distinct variety of squamous cell carcinoma that presents as a large fungating mass resembling a giant condyloma acuminatum. HPV, usually type 6, is commonly identified. The tumor is very well differentiated, being composed of large nests of squamous cells with abundant cytoplasm and small, bland nuclei. Squamous pearls are common, and mitoses are rare. The tumor invades with broad tongues, and the stromal interface frequently exhibits a heavy infiltrate of lymphocytes and plasma cells. Verrucous carcinoma invades locally but typically does not metastasize. Wide local surgical excision is the treatment of choice, and recurrence usually results from inadequate prior excision.

TABLE *18-2* **Clinical Staging of Carcinoma of Vulva (1994 Revised)**

Stage	Description
0	Carcinoma *in situ*
I	Tumor ≤2 cm, confined to vulva
Ia	Stromal invasion ≤1 mm
Ib	Stromal invasion >1 mm
II	Tumor >2 cm confined to vulva
III	Tumor of any size extending to the lower urethra, vagina, or anus; or ulilateral regional lymph node metastasis
IV	Tumor extension
IVa	Mucosa of bladder or rectum; bone or upper urethra; or bilateral regional lymph nodes
IVb	Distant metastases, including pelvic lymph nodes

Malignant Melanoma

Although uncommon, malignant melanoma is the second most frequent cancer of the vulva (5%). It occurs in the sixth and seventh decades but occasionally is found in younger women. The tumor has biological and microscopic characteristics of melanoma occurring elsewhere in the body. It is highly aggressive, and the prognosis is poor.

Extramammary Paget Disease

Paget disease of the vulva is a rare neoplasm characterized by the presence of intraepithelial, large, clear cells. It is named after similar-appearing tumors in the nipple and extramammary sites, such as the axilla and perianal region. The disorder usually occurs on the labia majora in older women. Women with Paget disease of the vulva complain of pruritus or a burning sensation for many years.

The lesion of Paget disease is large, red, moist, and sharply demarcated. The exact origin of the diagnostic cells (Paget cells) remains controversial; they are thought to arise in the epidermis or in epidermally derived adnexal structures. Paget cells are usually confined to the epidermis and appear as large single cells or, less commonly, as clusters of cells, which lack intercellular bridges. The typical Paget cell has a pale, vacuolated cytoplasm (Fig. 18-7), which contains glycosaminoglycans, and it stains with periodic acid–Schiff (PAS) and mucicarmine. These neoplastic cells also express carcinoembryonic antigen (CEA).

Intraepidermal Paget disease may have been present for many years and is often far more extensive throughout the epidermis than is apparent on preoperative biopsy. In contrast to Paget disease of the breast, which is almost always associated with an underlying duct carcinoma, extramammary Paget disease is only rarely associated with an adenocarcinoma of the skin adnexae. Since metastases rarely occur, treatment requires only wide local excision or simple vulvectomy.

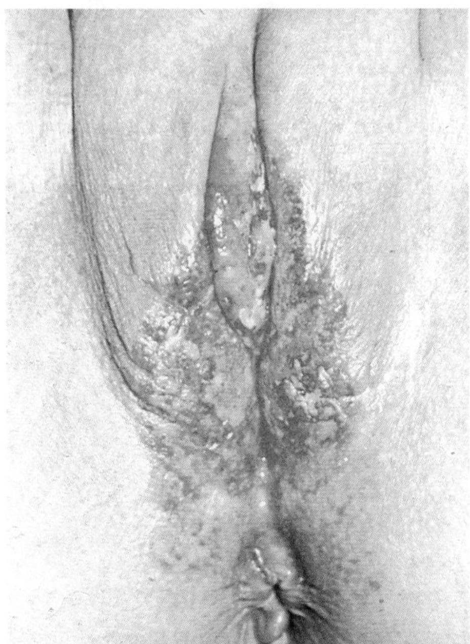

A

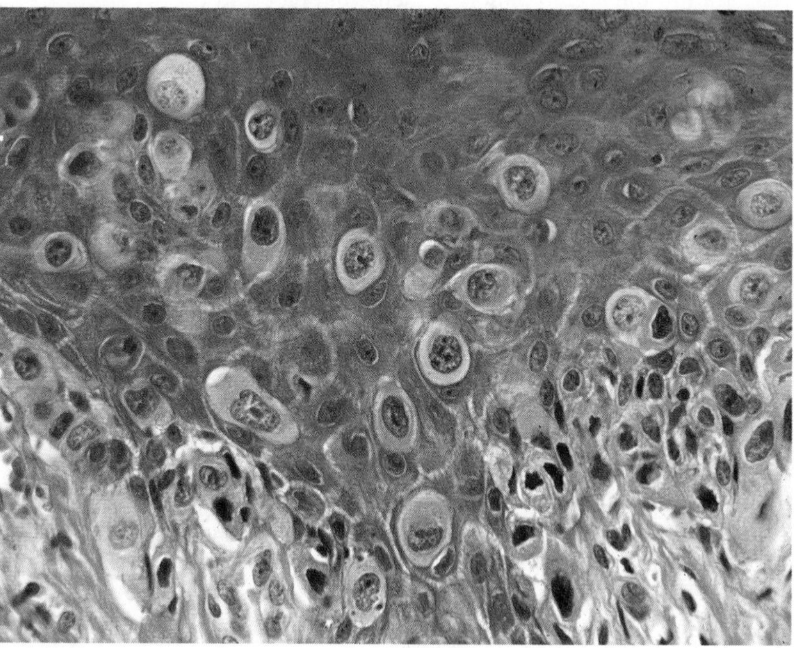

B

FIGURE *18-7*
Paget disease of the vulva. (*A*) The lesion is red, moist, and sharply demarcated. (*B*) Individual Paget cells, characterized by an abundant pale cytoplasm, infiltrate the epithelium and are interspersed among normal keratinocytes.

Vagina

ANATOMY

The vagina extends from the uterus to the vestibule of the vulva and is lined by a hormone-responsive squamous epithelium. Estrogens stimulate the proliferation and maturation of vaginal epithelial cells. Maturation is marked by the accumulation of glycogen, which imparts a clear appearance to the cytoplasm of the epithelial cells. By contrast, the maturation of vaginal epithelium is inhibited by progesterone. As a result, during the secretory phase of the menstrual cycle or during pregnancy, when progesterone levels are high, the intermediate cells, rather than the superficial ones, predominate in vaginal smears.

Lymph drains through the lateral perivaginal plexus. The lymphatics from the vaginal vault and upper vagina communicate with branches from the cervix to drain into the pelvic and then the para-aortic nodes. The lower vagina drains in addition to the inguinal/femoral nodes.

NON-NEOPLASTIC CONDITIONS AND BENIGN TUMORS

Congenital Anomalies

Congenital anomalies of the vagina are rare.

Congenital absence of the vagina is generally associated with anomalies of the uterus and urinary tract. In the presence of a functional uterus, the absence of a vagina may lead to the accumulation of menstrual blood in the uterus.

Septate vagina results from the failure of the embryonic müllerian ducts to fuse.

Vaginal atresia and imperforate hymen prevent the transformation of the lining of the embryonic vagina from a müllerian to a squamous epithelium, an effect that is a cause of vaginal adenosis.

Atrophic Vaginitis

Atrophic vaginitis is a thinning and atrophy of the vaginal epithelium that results from diminished estrogenic stimulation and superimposed infection. The thinned epithelium in the estrogen-deficient woman is a poor barrier to infections or abrasions. Atrophic vaginitis occurs most commonly in postmenopausal women in whom estrogen levels are low. Dyspareunia and vaginal spotting are common symptoms. The latter must be distinguished from signs of uterine cancer, which also occurs in older women.

Vaginal Adenosis

Vaginal adenosis refers to failure of the normal glandular epithelium that lines the embryonic vagina to be replaced during fetal life by squamous epithelium. Prior to the use of diethylstilbestrol (DES), which began in the 1940s, for the treatment of high-risk pregnancies, vaginal adenosis was a curiosity. However, in the 1970s there was a substantial increase in the incidence of this disorder in young daughters of women who had received DES during pregnancy. Up to 2 million women were exposed *in utero* to DES between 1940 and 1971. It is now accepted that exposure to DES during early prenatal life is associated with the development of multiple changes in the genital tract. These lesions include (1) vaginal adenosis and cervical ectropion (presence of glandular tissue in the vagina or exocervix, respectively), (2) gross structural changes in the vagina and cervix, and (3) structural and functional abnormalities of the upper genital tract. Rare cases of clear cell adenocarcinoma of the vagina have also occurred in the daughters of women treated with DES.

☐ **Pathogenesis:** At the 10th week of gestation, the upgrowth of a squamous epithelium derived from the urogenital sinus replaces the glandular (müllerian) epithelium lining the vagina and exocervix. DES exposure at any time during this critical window, which lasts until about the 18th week, arrests the transformation process. Hence, some glandular tissue (i.e., adenosis) remains. The frequency of DES-related vaginal adenosis in the offspring correlates directly with the time in pregnancy that the mother was first given the drug (the earlier the use, the greater the risk) and with the total dose of the drug. One third of women exposed to DES *in utero* have foci of adenosis or secondary metaplastic squamous cells, both of which are usually asymptomatic.

☐ **Pathology:** Adenosis presents as red, granular patches on the vaginal mucosa. Microscopically, it comprises two types of cells: mucinous columnar cells, resembling those lining the endocervix, and ciliated cells with eosinophilic cytoplasm, similar to those lining the endometrium and fallopian tubes (Fig. 18-8). The glandular cells ultimately undergo squamous metaplasia.

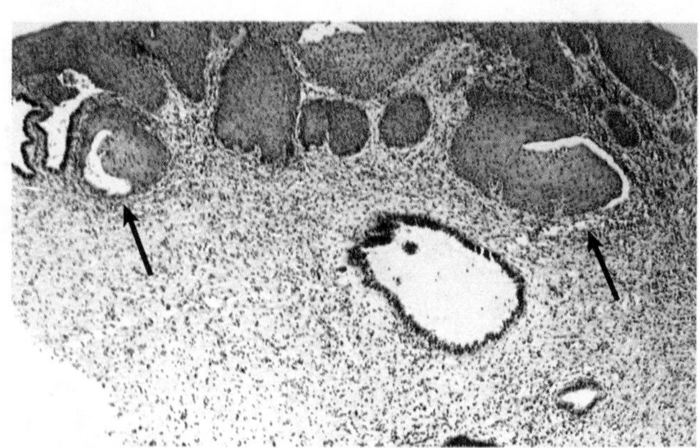

FIGURE *18-8*
Vaginal adenosis. A section of the vagina shows glands in the chronically inflamed lamina propria, lined by ciliated, darkly staining cells similar to tubal or endometrial epithelium. Some glands merge with metaplastic squamous pegs (*arrows*). The surface epithelium consists of metaplastic glycogen-free squamous cells, accounting for the abnormal iodine staining.

Fibroepithelial Polyp

Vaginal polyps are uncommon benign growths composed of a connective tissue core and an outer lining of vaginal squamous epithelium. They are usually single, gray-white, and less than 1 cm in diameter. Simple excision is usually curative.

Benign Mesenchymal Tumors

Most benign tumors in the vagina resemble those in other parts of the female genital tract and include leiomyomas, rhabdomyomas, and neurofibromas. These are solid submucosal tumors usually less than 2 cm in diameter. The granular cell tumor is an unusual tumor of Schwann cell origin. Granular cell tumors that impinge on the overlying squamous epithelium can elicit pseudoepitheliomatous hyperplasia, which may be confused with squamous cell carcinoma.

MALIGNANT TUMORS

Primary malignant tumors of the vagina are uncommon, constituting about 2% of all genital tract tumors. Because the vagina is in close anatomical relation to the cervix and vulva, the large majority (80%) of all vaginal malignancies represent secondary spread. The most common symptoms are a vaginal discharge, which often is foul smelling, and bleeding during coitus. Depending on the extent of tumor spread, symptoms may include pelvic or abdominal pain and swelling of the legs. Tumors that are confined to the vagina are usually treated by radical hysterectomy and vaginectomy.

Squamous Cell Carcinoma

Squamous cell carcinoma of the vagina accounts for over 90% of all primary malignant tumors of the vagina. It is generally a disease of older women, with a peak incidence between the ages of 60 and 70 years. Squamous cell carcinoma appears most commonly in the posterior wall of the upper third of the vagina, where it usually presents as an exophytic mass. *Vaginal intraepithelial neoplasia* (VAIN), a term replacing both *vaginal dysplasia* and *carcinoma in situ*, frequently occurs in conjunction with squamous cell carcinoma and may precede the development of invasive carcinoma. Not infrequently, squamous cell carcinoma of the vagina develops some years after cervical or vulvar carcinoma, a sequence that supports the concept of a field effect of carcinogenesis in the lower genital tract related to HPV infection.

Since most preinvasive and early invasive cancers are clinically silent, the routine use of Papanicolaou smears remains the most effective method to detect squamous cell carcinoma of the vagina. The prognosis is to a large extent related to the spread of the tumor at the time of its discovery (Table 18-3). The 5-year survival rate for tumors confined to the vagina (stage I) is 80%, whereas it is only 20% for those with extensive spread (stages III/IV).

TABLE *18-3* **Clinical Staging of Carcinoma of Vagina**

Stage	Description
0	Carcinoma *in situ*
I	Limited to vaginal wall
II	Involves subvaginal tissue, but does not extend to pelvic wall
III	Extends to pelvic wall
IV	Extends beyond true pelvis or involves mucosa of bladder or rectum
IVa	Spread to adjacent organs
IVb	Spread to distant organs

Clear Cell Adenocarcinoma

Clear cell adenocarcinoma of the vagina is a rare tumor encountered almost exclusively in women exposed in utero to DES. It develops most frequently on the anterior wall of the upper third of the vagina. The tumor is unusual before age 13 and is most common between ages 17 and 22. Although almost all clear cell adenocarcinomas are associated with vaginal adenosis, very few women with adenosis develop this cancer. Atypical adenosis of the tuboendometrial type is suspected of being the precursor lesion. The abundant clear cytoplasm, reflecting the presence of glycogen, accounts for the name clear cell adenocarcinoma (Fig. 18-9). Its other pattern shows cells with bulbous nuclei that line the glandular lumina (hobnail cells). Clear cell adenocarcinomas are almost invariably curable when they are small and asymptomatic, but in more advanced stages they may spread by hematogenous or lymphatic routes.

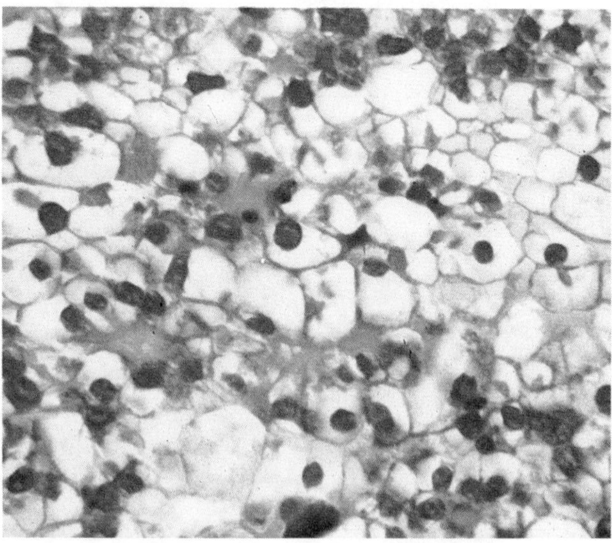

FIGURE *18-9*
Clear cell adenocarcinoma of the vagina in the daughter of a woman treated with diethylstilbestrol.

Embryonal Rhabdomyosarcoma (Sarcoma Botryoides)

Embryonal rhabdomyosarcoma is a rare vaginal tumor that appears as confluent polypoid masses resembling a bunch of grapes, hence the name sarcoma botryoides (Greek botrys, *grapes)* (Fig. 18-10). It occurs almost exclusively in children younger than the age of 4 years. The tumor is of mesenchymal (stromal) origin and arises in the lamina propria of the vagina. It is composed of primitive spindle rhabdomyoblasts, some of which display cross striations. Myofibrils composed of myosin and actin are often demonstrable. A dense zone of round rhabdomyoblasts, referred to as the cambium layer, is present beneath the vaginal epithelium. Deep to this layer the stroma is myxomatous and shows fewer rhabdomyoblasts.

The tumor is usually detected because of spotting found on the child's diaper. Tumors less than 3 cm in greatest dimension tend to be localized and may be cured by wide excision and chemotherapy. Larger tumors are likely to have invaded adjacent structures, metastasized to regional lymph nodes, and spread hematogenously to distant sites. Even in advanced cases, half the patients survive following radical surgery and chemotherapy.

Yolk Sac Tumor

Yolk sac tumor (previously termed endodermal sinus tumor) is a rare, highly malignant germ cell neoplasm, which occurs almost exclusively in girls younger than 4 years of age. It presents as a mass filling the vagina and protruding through the introitus; consequently, it may be confused with em-

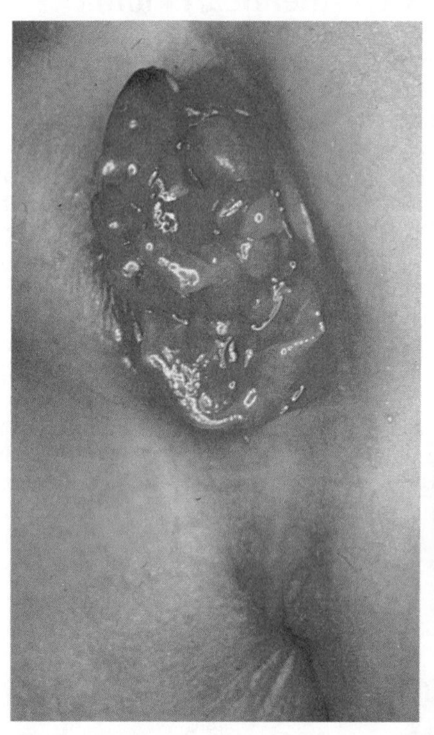

A

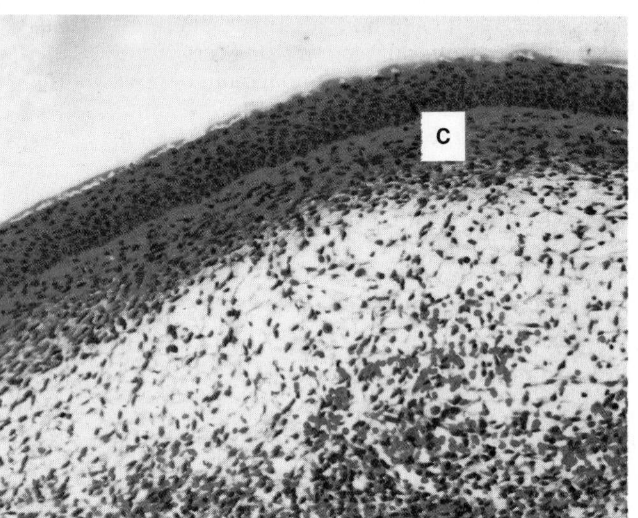

B

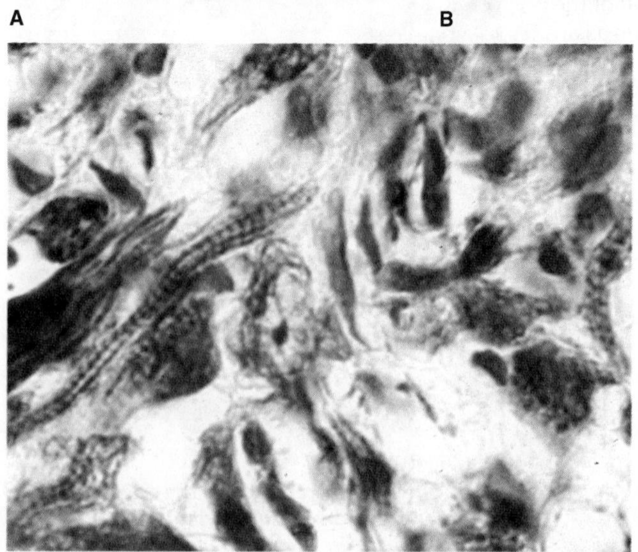

C

FIGURE *18-10*
Embryonal rhabdomyosarcoma (sarcoma botryoides) of vagina. (*A*) The grape-like tumor protrudes through the introitus. (*B*) A section of the tumor shows a dense layer of neoplastic stroma termed the cambium layer (c) beneath the surface epithelium of the vagina. A loose neoplastic stroma is present beneath the cambium layer. (*C*) The tumor contains rhabdomyoblasts characterized by cross striations (PTAH stain).

bryonal rhabdomyosarcoma. Histologically, it resembles its counterpart in the ovary or testis and synthesizes alpha-fetoprotein. This tumor marker can be measured in the serum and serves as an aid in diagnosis and monitoring for recurrence. The prognosis of yolk sac tumor is poor.

Cervix

ANATOMY

The cervix (Latin *collare*, neck) is the inferior portion of the uterus that connects the corpus to the vagina (Fig. 18-11). Its exposed portion, called interchangeably the exocervix, ectocervix, or portio vaginalis, protrudes into the upper vagina and is covered by glycogen-rich squamous epithelium. The endocervix, the canal leading to the endometrial cavity, is lined by longitudinal mucosal ridges, which are composed of fibrovascular cores lined by a single layer of mucinous columnar cells. The external os is the macroscopically visible junction between the exocervix and endocervix. The squamocolumnar junction is the anatomical junction of the squamous and mucinous epithelia. The area between the endocervix and endometrial cavity is called the isthmus or lower uterine segment.

The Transformation Zone

The exocervix remodels continuously during life. During embryonic development, the upward migration of squamous cells meets the columnar epithelium of the endocervix to form the initial squamocolumnar junction (Fig. 18-12). In some young women, this "original" squamocolumnar junction is located at the internal os. In most young women, however, the columnar epithelium extends onto the exocervix, in which case the squamocolumnar junction is also located on the exocervix. In the latter situation, the areas of the exocervix lined by columnar epithelium are referred to as endocervical ectropion and appear by colposcopic examination as reddish discolorations. The term *erosion* for such areas is a misnomer, since they are lined by normal columnar epithelium. An endocervical ectropion is particularly prominent in young women after the birth of the first child. With age, the columnar epithelium of the ectropion undergoes squamous metaplasia (see Fig. 18-12), a process by which the columnar epithelium is replaced or transformed into a stratified squamous epithelium. As a result, the new squamocolumnar junction is located at the internal os. **The area between the original squamocolumnar junction on the exocervix and the new squamocolumnar junction at the internal os is termed the *transformation zone*.**

The progression of the squamous transformation of the endocervical ectropion is primarily dependent on the environment of the vagina, the initial stimulus being the conversion to an acidic pH following puberty. Trauma and cervicitis are also factors that influence conversion of the ectropion to a squamous epithelium. Occasionally, the outlet of the endocervical glands becomes blocked. As a result, mucin is retained and produces macroscopically visible cystic dilations of these glands, termed *nabothian cysts*.

The immature squamous epithelium of the transformation zone displays progressive nuclear maturation and

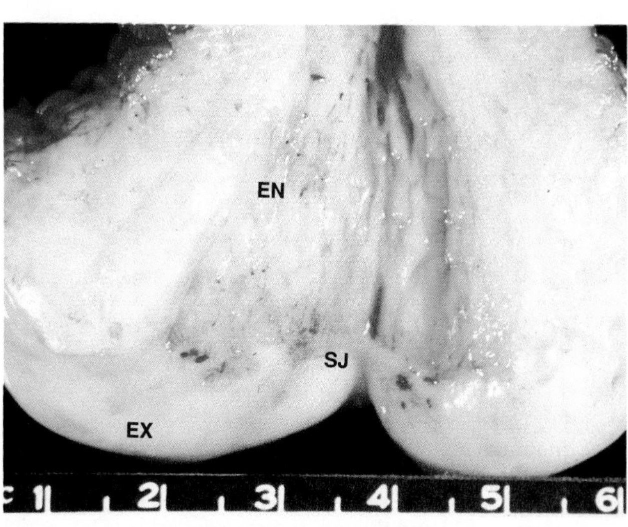

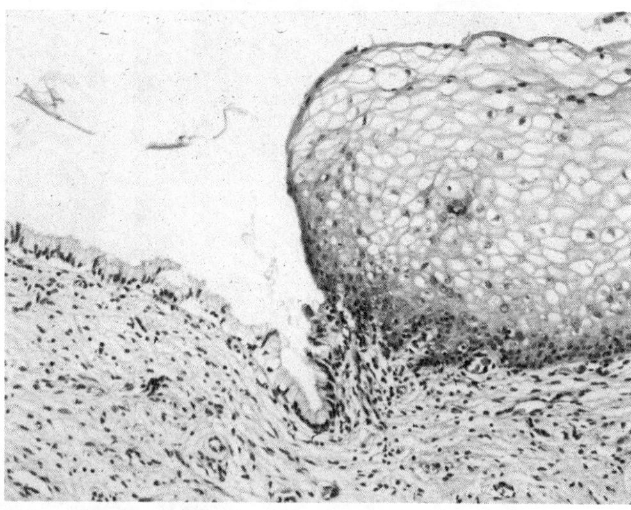

FIGURE *18-11*
Anatomy of the cervix. (*A*) The cervix has been opened to show the endocervix (EN), squamocolumnar junction (SJ), and exocervix (EX). The thick layer of squamous cells covering the exocervix accounts for its white color. (*B*) A microscopic view of the squamocolumnar junction. The endocervix is lined by a single layer of columnar mucus-producing cells, which abruptly meets the exocervix lined by mature squamous cells. *Note:* In specimens where the squamocolumnar junction is on the ectocervix or in the endocervical canal, the region between it and the external os is called the *transformation zone* (see Fig. 18-12).

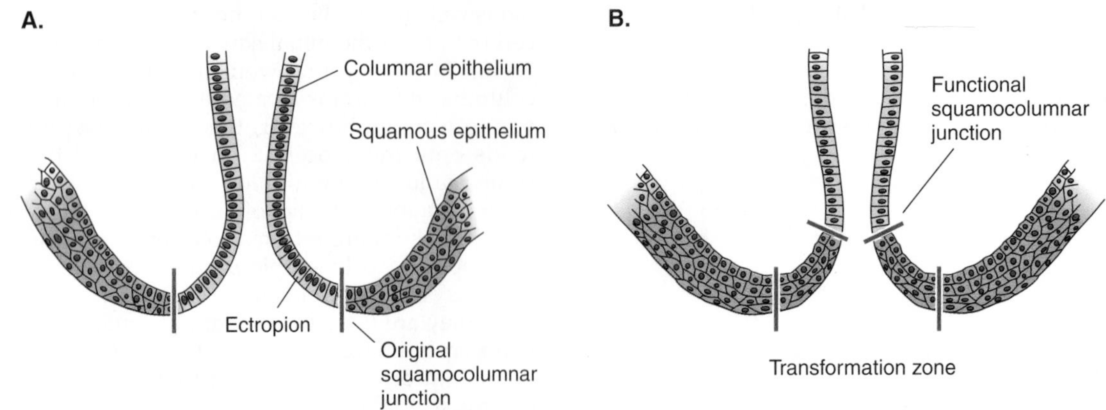

FIGURE 18-12
The transformation zone of the cervix.

increasing amounts of glycogen-free cytoplasm toward the surface. Colposcopy reveals the development of a thin white membrane, which eventually becomes thicker and whiter as the squamous epithelium matures (Fig. 18-13). Subsequently, the cells accumulate glycogen and are indistinguishable from the normal squamous epithelium lining the exocervix.

Examination of the transformation zone by iodine staining forms the basis of the Schiller iodine test. If the squamous cells lining the exocervix are mature (glycogen rich), which is normal, they stain with iodine and the exocervix appears mahogany brown. If the cells lining the exocervix are immature (glycogen poor), no iodine staining occurs and the exocervix is pale.

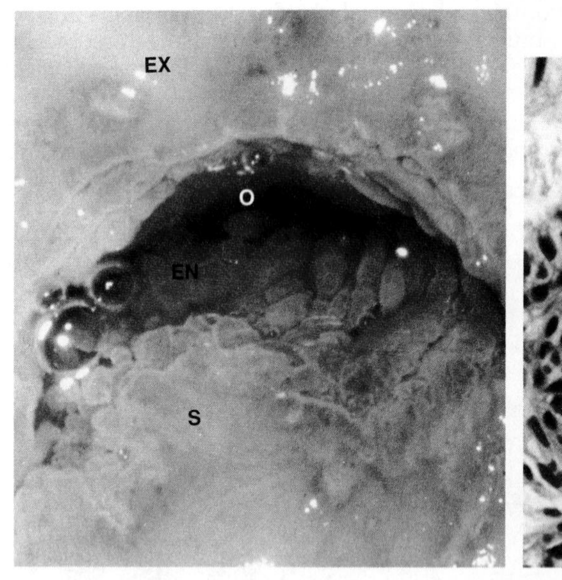

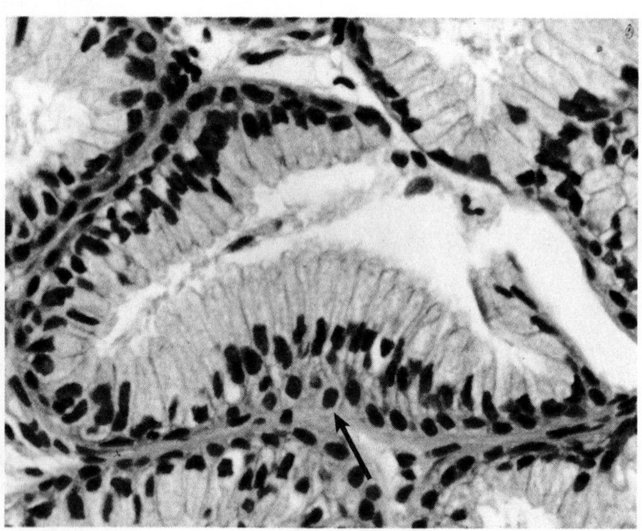

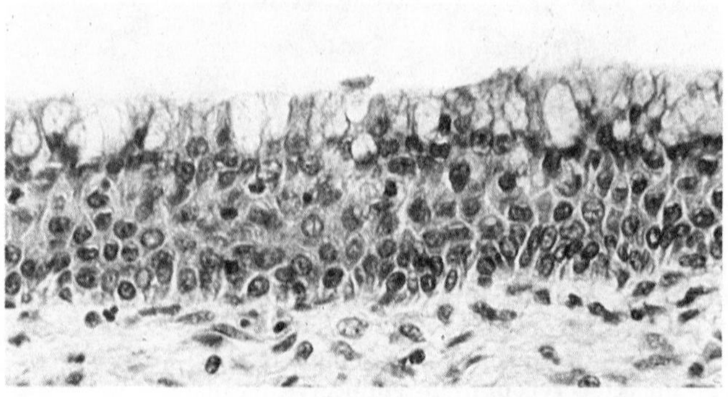

FIGURE 18-13
Squamous metaplasia in the transformation zone. (*A*) In this colposcopic view of the cervix, a white area of metaplastic squamous epithelium (S) is situated between the exocervix (EX) and the mucinous endocervix (EN), which terminates at the internal os (O). (*B*) In the early stages of squamous metaplasia of the transformation zone, the reserve cells, which normally constitute a single layer, begin to proliferate (*arrow*). (*C*) At a later stage, the proliferating reserve cells displace the glandular epithelium. As a final step, the metaplastic cells mature into glycogen-rich squamous cells, resembling those in Figure 18-11B.

Exfoliative Cytology

Exfoliative cytopathology is the study of normal and disease-altered desquamated cells from various body sites. This field of study has grown largely from the effectiveness of the Papanicolaou cytological test, the "Pap smear." The most superficial epithelial cells are exfoliated either spontaneously (e.g., vaginal smear) or artificially (i.e., when the epithelium is scraped with a spatula, brush, or swab, such as with the cervicovaginal smear). Traditionally, the smears are stained by the Papanicolaou method. Cervicovaginal cytology is an effective screening procedure for the early detection of premalignant and malignant cervical lesions. With the use of a spatula, brush, or swab, the transformation zone is circumferentially sampled. Recommendations for the frequency of cervicovaginal screening vary, but in general the first smear should be at age 18 years or whenever sexual activity commences, and thereafter on an annual basis. Exfoliative cytology is treated in greater detail in Chapter 30.

CERVICITIS

Inflammation of the cervix is exceedingly common and is related to its constant exposure to the bacterial flora in the vagina. Acute and chronic cervicitis result from infection with many microorganisms, particularly the endogenous vaginal aerobes and anaerobes, *Streptococcus, Staphylococcus,* and *Enterococcus*. Other specific organisms include *Chlamydia trachomatis, Neisseria gonorrhoeae,* and *Herpes simplex, type 2.* Some agents are sexually transmitted, whereas others may be introduced by foreign bodies, such as residual fragments of tampons and pessaries. Excluding *N. gonorrhoeae*, the organisms that most commonly cause cervicitis are *Streptococcus* and *Staphylococcus*, which are usually encountered after parturition.

In acute cervicitis, the cervix is grossly red, swollen, and edematous, with copious pus "dripping" from the external os. Microscopically, the tissues exhibit an extensive infiltrate of polymorphonuclear leukocytes and stromal edema.

In chronic cervicitis, which is more common, the cervical mucosa is hyperemic (Fig. 18-14), and there may be true epithelial erosions. Microscopically, the stroma is infiltrated by mononuclear cells, principally lymphocytes and plasma cells. The metaplastic squamous epithelium of the transformation zone may extend into the endocervical glands, forming clusters of squamous epithelium with slightly enlarged nuclei, which must be differentiated from carcinoma.

BENIGN TUMORS AND TUMOR-LIKE CONDITIONS

Endocervical Polyp

Endocervical polyp, the most common cervical growth (Fig. 18-15), appears as a single, smooth, or lobulated mass, typically less than 3 cm in greatest dimension. It occurs in less than 5% of adult women, often presenting as vaginal bleeding or discharge. The lining epithelium is mucinous, with varying degrees of squamous metaplasia in asymptomatic women, but often discloses areas of true

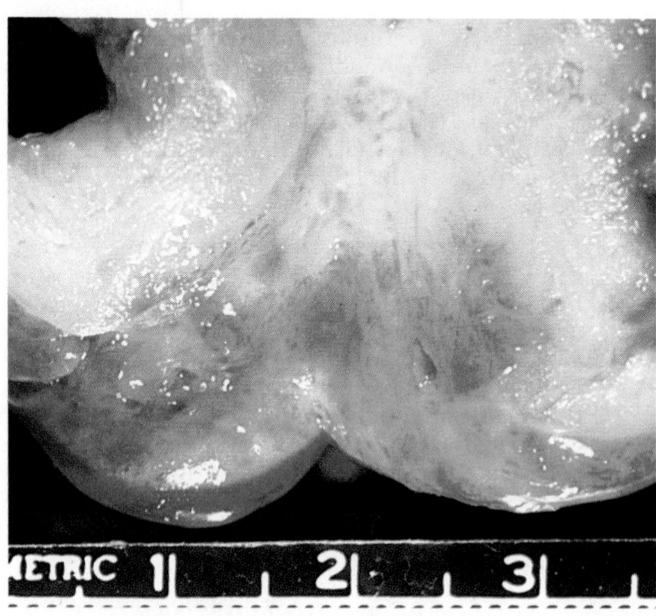

A

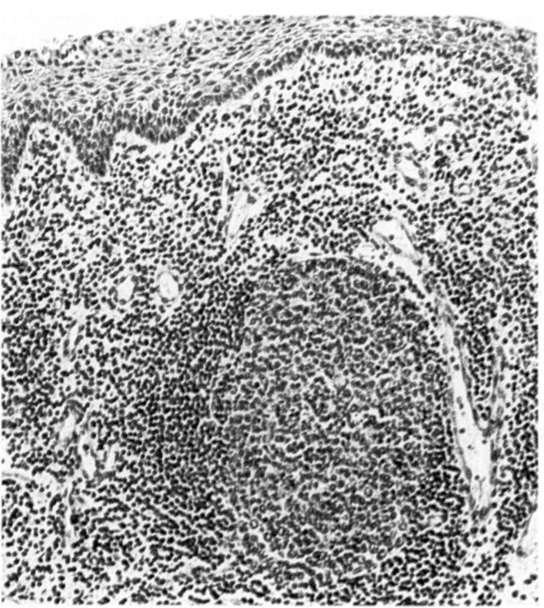

B

FIGURE *18-14*
Chronic cervicitis. (*A*) The cervix has been opened to reveal the reddened exocervix. (*B*) Microscopic examination discloses chronic inflammation and the formation of a lymphoid follicle.

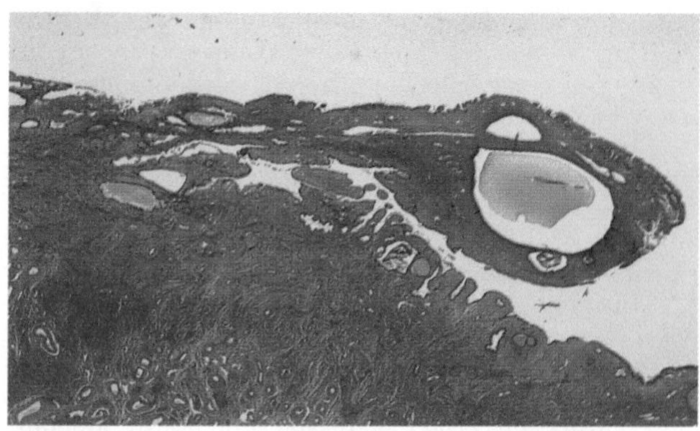

FIGURE 18-15
Endocervical polyp. A low-power photomicrograph shows cystic endocervical glands in a chronically inflamed stroma.

erosion with granulation tissue in women with symptoms. The stroma is edematous and contains thick-walled blood vessels. Simple excision or curettage is curative. Cancer rarely arises in an endocervical polyp (0.2% of cases).

Microglandular Hyperplasia

Microglandular hyperplasia of the cervix is a benign condition characterized by closely packed glands that lack an intervening stroma and display a neutrophilic infiltrate. It is important that it not be confused with well-differentiated adenocarcinoma. Microglandular hyperplasia is usually asymptomatic and typically caused by progestin stimulation. It usually occurs during pregnancy and the postpartum period and in women taking oral contraceptives. There have been no recorded cases of malignant transformation. It is less commonly encountered now than in the past because the progestin content of oral contraceptives has been reduced.

Leiomyoma

Leiomyoma of the cervix accounts for one tenth of all uterine leiomyomas. It can become symptomatic by bleeding or by prolapsing into the endocervical canal, an event that leads to uterine contractions and pain resembling the early phases of labor. The gross and microscopic appearance of cervical leiomyomas is similar to that of uterine leiomyomas (described later in this chapter).

SQUAMOUS CELL NEOPLASIA

Fifty years ago, cervical cancer was the leading cause of cancer death in American women. With the introduction and widespread application of cytological screening, the incidence of cervical cancer has decreased by 50% to 85% in Western countries, and the mortality rate in the United States has fallen by 70%. Nevertheless, worldwide, cervical cancer remains the second most common cancer in women, although in the United States it is sixth among female cancers. With improved surveillance, there has been a marked increase in the incidence of its precursor lesions, cervical intraepithelial neoplasia (CIN), also known as cervical dysplasia and carcinoma *in situ*. The Papanicolaou smear detects premalignant disease long before invasion has occurred. Even one smear during a woman's lifetime, a number which is clearly inadequate, reduces the risk of invasive cancer 10-fold.

Cervical Intraepithelial Neoplasia

Cervical intraepithelial neoplasia is defined as a spectrum of intraepithelial changes that begins with minimal atypia and progresses through stages of more marked intraepithelial abnormalities to invasive squamous cell carcinoma. CIN, dysplasia, carcinoma *in situ*, and squamous intraepithelial lesion (SIL) are today synonymous terms. **Dysplasia in the cervical epithelium implies an alteration that carries with it the potential for malignant transformation.** Carcinoma *in situ* refers to a malignant lesion that involves the entire thickness of the squamous epithelium but is confined to the epithelium. Importantly, the term *in situ* signifies that it has not invaded the underlying stroma. The term *cervical intraepithelial neoplasia* emphasizes that dysplasia and carcinoma *in situ* are points on a disease spectrum rather than separate entities. The grades of CIN are related to the previous terminology as follows:

- CIN-1: mild dysplasia
- CIN-2: moderate dysplasia
- CIN-3: severe dysplasia and carcinoma *in situ*

The recently promulgated "Bethesda System for Reporting Cervical/Vaginal Cytologic Diagnoses" further groups these lesions into two groups, called low- and high-grade squamous intraepithelial lesions. Low-grade SIL reflects conditions that should rarely progress in severity and commonly disappear (CIN-1). High-grade SIL corresponds to higher-grade histological lesions (CIN-2 and CIN-3), which tend to progress and require treatment. Chapter 30 illustrates the cytological characteristics that correspond to different grades of CIN.

□ **Epidemiology and Pathogenesis:** The epidemiological features of CIN and invasive cancer are similar. Whereas cervical cancer usually presents between the ages of 40 and 60 years, with a mean age of 54 years, CIN generally occurs in women under the age of 40 years. **Multiple sexual partners and early age at first coitus are the most important factors.** As a consequence, CIN is considered to be a sexually transmitted disease. The incidence of cancer of the cervix is also higher in women who smoke. An important role for HPV in the pathogenesis of cervical cancer has now emerged, although other factors are certainly contributory.

HUMAN PAPILLOMAVIRUS INFECTION: A substantial body of clinical and laboratory evidence strongly supports the view that HPV infection is involved in the pathogenesis of CIN and cervical cancer (Fig. 18-16). Infection with HPV is widespread, being present in one third of American female college students and in 8% of men between 15 and 50 years of age. Of CIN-1 lesions,

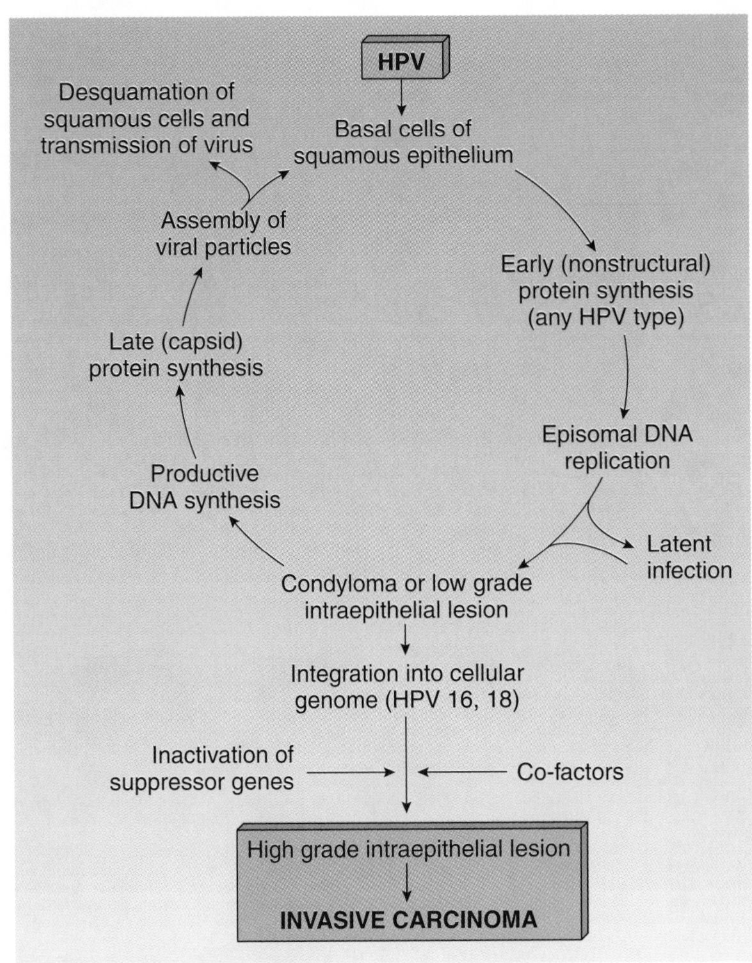

FIGURE *18-16*
Role of human papillomavirus (HPV) in the pathogenesis of cervical neoplasia.

80% demonstrate cytological features of HPV infection. Low-grade CIN is an example of a permissive infection, wherein HPV is episomal and freely replicates, thereby causing cell death. The virus in these lesions can be seen by electron microscopy, and the capsid protein can be detected by immunocytochemical techniques. By contrast, in higher-grade CIN, viral regulation is disrupted; in cervical cancer, the virus is integrated into the cell genome. The E6 and E7 genes of HPV 16 have transforming functions *in vitro*, which may be related to the inactivation of suppressor gene products (p53 and Rb respectively) by the E6 and E7 proteins (see Chapter 5). Interestingly, in the minority of cervical cancers that do not contain HPV, p53 is inactivated by mutation.

Genital warts (condylomata acuminata) on the cervix usually contain HPV 6 or 11; these are regarded as low-risk HPV types, since they are found in over 90% of condylomas but only rarely in invasive cancers. By contrast, cells in high-grade CIN usually contain HPV types 16, 18, 31, 33, or 35. **HPV types 16 and 18 are found in 70% of invasive cancers, and types 31, 33, and 35 in 20%, and are therefore considered to be high-risk types.**

☐ **Pathology:** CIN is a disease of the metaplastic squamous epithelium of the transformation zone and areas of squamous metaplasia in the endocervix. **Thus, the extent of the transformation zone determines the distribution of CIN, and hence cervical cancer, on the exposed portion of the cervix.**

The normal process of maturation of the squamous epithelium of the cervix is disturbed in CIN, as evidenced morphologically by changes in cellularity, differentiation, polarity, nuclear features, and mitotic activity. In CIN-1 (mild dysplasia), the most pronounced changes are seen in the basal third of the epithelium. Those cells with abnormal nuclei migrate toward the surface, are sloughed, and as a result can be detected in Papanicolaou smears. In CIN-1, substantial cytoplasmic differentiation occurs in cells in the upper two thirds of the epithelium. In CIN-2 (moderate dysplasia), most of the cellular abnormalities are in the lower and middle thirds of the epithelium. Cytodifferentiation occurs in cells in the upper third, but it is less than in CIN-1.

As noted earlier, CIN-3 is synonymous with severe dysplasia and carcinoma *in situ*. Severe dysplasia is characterized by abnormal cells that diffusely involve more than two thirds of the epithelium, whereas carcinoma *in situ* involves all layers of the epithelium. Cytodifferentiation is negligible in CIN-3. The sequence of histological changes from CIN-1 to CIN-3 is illustrated in Figure 18-17.

Dysplasia and carcinoma *in situ* can often be detected on colposcopic examination by signs associated with their altered vasculature and epithelial changes. Punctation (vascular dots differentiated from the surrounding tissue

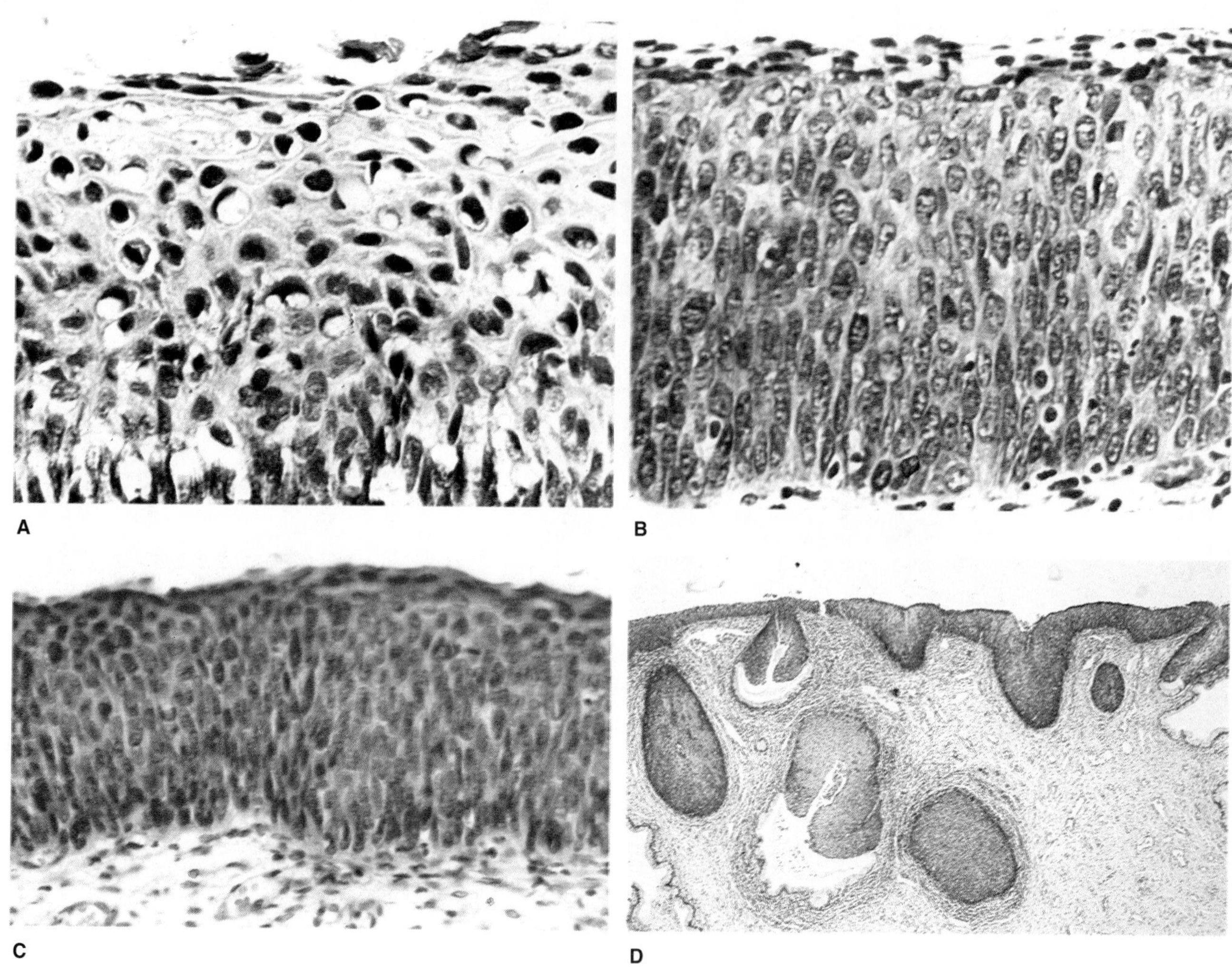

FIGURE *18-17*
Cervical intraepithelial neoplasia (CIN). (*A*) CIN-1: The cervical epithelium shows pronounced cellular atypia in the basal third. Some cells in the upper two thirds of the epithelium have abnormal nuclei, but all show cytoplasmic differentiation. (*B*) CIN-2 to CIN-3: The lower two thirds of the epithelium displays pronounced cell atypia. Although cytodifferentiation occurs in the upper third of the epithelium, it is less pronounced than in CIN-1. (*C*) CIN-3 (carcinoma *in situ,* CIS): Neoplastic cells are present throughout the entire epithelium. (*D*) CIN-3: CIS partially or completely replaces the columnar epithelium of the endocervical glands.

surface by color and texture) and mosaicism (irregular surface resembling inlaid woodwork) (Fig. 18-18) are the two patterns most often found in high-grade CIN. The neoplastic process occurs more commonly on the anterior than on the posterior lip of the cervix and often extends to involve the endocervical glands, an area that cannot be evaluated by colposcopy.

The mean age at which women develop CIN is 24 to 27 years for CIN-1 and CIN-2, and 35 to 42 for CIN-3. Based on morphological criteria, half of the cases of CIN-1 regress, 10% progress to CIN-3, and less than 2% eventuate in invasive cancer. The frequency of progression is much greater for initially higher grades of CIN. Similarly, the required time for progression to a higher grade of CIN depends on the initial grade. Higher grades of dysplasia require shorter times to progress to carcinoma *in situ.* The average time for all grades of dysplasia to progress to carcinoma *in situ* is about 10 years. **At least 20% of cases of CIN-3 progress to invasive carcinoma within 10 years.**

☐ **Clinical Features:** When CIN is discovered, colposcopic examination, in combination with a Schiller test, is important to delineate the extent of the lesion and to indicate the areas to be biopsied. Diagnostic endocervical curettage is also useful for determining the extent of endocervical involvement. Women with CIN-1 are often followed conservatively (i.e., repeated Pap smears plus close

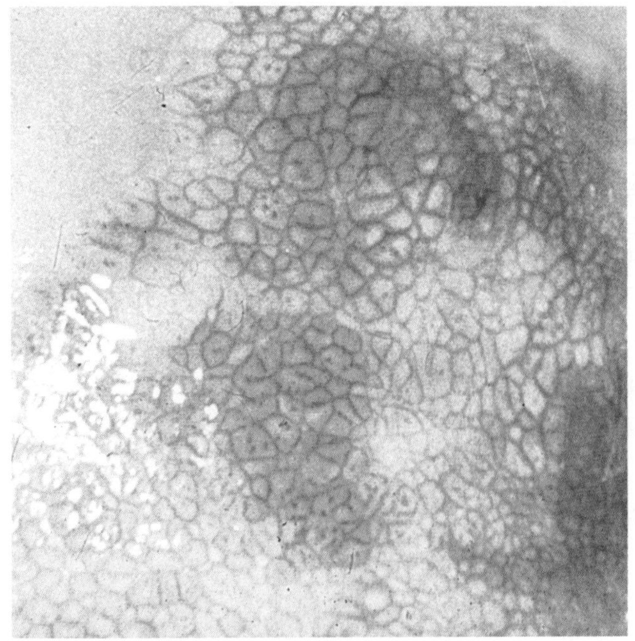

FIGURE 18-18
Dysplasia of the cervix. Examination with the colposcope discloses a mosaic pattern resembling inlaid woodwork.

follow-up), although some gynecologists now advocate local ablative treatment. High-grade lesions are treated according to the extent of disease. Laser therapy, which can be performed on an outpatient basis, is commonly used. In certain situations cervical conization (removal of a cone of tissue around the external os), cryosurgery, and (rarely) hysterectomy are performed. Follow-up smears and clinical examinations should continue for life, since vaginal or vulvar squamous cancer may develop later.

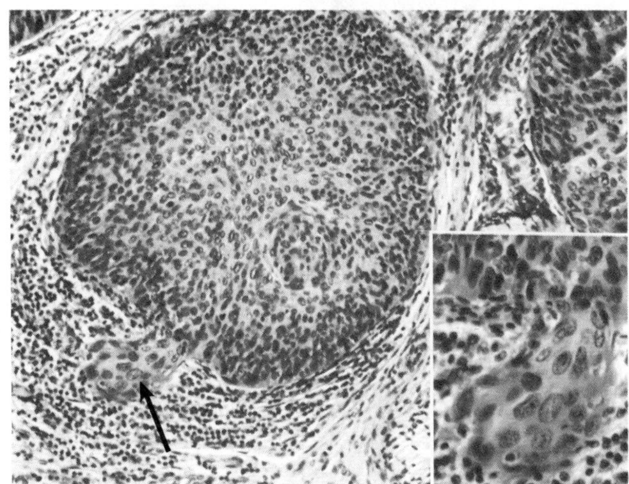

FIGURE 18-19
Microinvasive squamous cell carcinoma. Section of the cervix shows that carcinoma *in situ* in an endocervical gland has broken through the basement membrane (*arrow*) to invade the stroma. *Inset:* A higher-power view of the microinvasive focus.

Microinvasive Squamous Cell Carcinoma

Microinvasive carcinoma is an early stage in the spectrum of cervical cancer (stage Ia) and is characterized by minimal invasion of the stroma by neoplastic cells (Fig. 18-19). About 7% of specimens removed for carcinoma *in situ* demonstrate foci of microinvasive cancer. Through continual refinement of definition, most recently revised by the Federation of International Gynecologists and Obstetricians (FIGO) in 1994 (see Table 18-5), small clusters of cells or solid lesions in the stroma have the following characteristics :

- Invasion to a depth of less than 5 mm below the basement membrane (3 mm in the system used by most American gynecologic oncologists)
- Lack of vascular invasion
- No lymph node metastases

Conization or simple hysterectomy is generally sufficient for the cure of microinvasive cancers less than 3 mm deep. Radical hysterectomy is often recommended for larger cancers.

Invasive Squamous Cell Carcinoma

□ **Epidemiology:** Squamous cell carcinoma is by far the most common type of cervical cancer. Despite its declining frequency in the United States (Table 18-4), it still accounts for some 13,000 new cases annually (15 new cases annually per 100,000 women), which is less than the incidence of either endometrial or ovarian cancer. By contrast, in Central and South America, parts of Asia, and Africa, squamous cell cancer of the cervix remains a major cause of cancer death. In some high-risk areas, its incidence is 100 new cases annually per 100,000 women.

TABLE *18-4* **Incidence of Gynecologic Cancer in the United States**

	New Cases		Death	
	Cases	**%**	**Cases**	**%**
Endometrium	34,000	6	6000	2
Ovary	27,000	4	15,000	6
Cervix, invasive	16,000	3	5000	2
Vulva, invasive	3000	<1		
Vagina, invasive	1000	<1		
Other	2000	<1		

Carcinoma *in situ* of cervix >50,000 new case/yr.
%, percent of all cases of cancer in females.

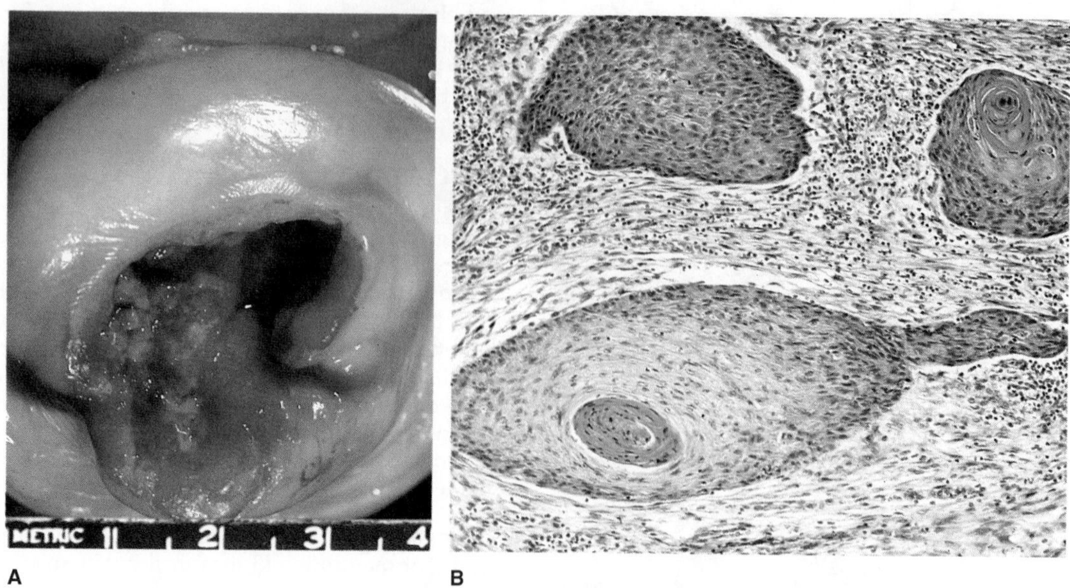

FIGURE 18-20
Squamous cell cancer. (*A*) The cervix is distorted by the presence of an exophytic, ulcerated squamous cell carcinoma. (*B*) The keratinizing pattern of the tumor is manifested as whorls of keratinized cells ("keratin pearls").

□ **Pathology:** Cervical cancer in its early stages often presents as a poorly defined, granular, and eroded lesion or as a nodular and exophytic mass (Fig. 18-20A). If it is predominantly within the endocervical canal, cervical cancer may appear as an endophytic mass, infiltrating the stroma and causing diffuse enlargement and hardening of the cervix (barrel-shaped cervix). On microscopic examination, the majority of tumors display a large cell nonkeratinizing pattern, which is characterized by solid nests of large malignant squamous cells with no more than individual cell keratinization. Most of the remaining cancers are keratinizing, exhibiting nests of keratinized cells that are organized in concentric whorls, so-called *keratin pearls* (see Fig. 18-20B).

The least common pattern of squamous cell cancer is small cell carcinoma. This is the most aggressive type of squamous cell cancer of the cervix and is associated with the poorest prognosis. It consists of infiltrating masses of small, cohesive, nonkeratinized, malignant cells.

Cervical cancer spreads by direct extension and through lymphatic vessels (Fig. 18-21) and only rarely by the hematogenous route. Local extension into surrounding tissues results in ureteral compression (stage IIIb, Table 18-5); the corresponding clinical complications are hydroureter, hydronephrosis, and renal failure, the last being the most common cause of death (50% of patients). Bladder and rectal involvement (stage IVa) may lead to fistula formation. Metastases to regional lymph nodes involve the paracervical, hypogastric, and external iliac nodes. Overall, the cancer's growth and spread are relatively slow, since the average age for stage 0 tumor (CIN-III) is 35 to 40 years, whereas the average age for stage IV is 17 years older.

□ **Clinical Features:** In the earliest stages of cervical cancer, patients complain most frequently of vaginal bleeding after intercourse or douching. With more advanced cancer, the symptoms are referable to the route and degree of spread. The Papanicolaou smear is the most

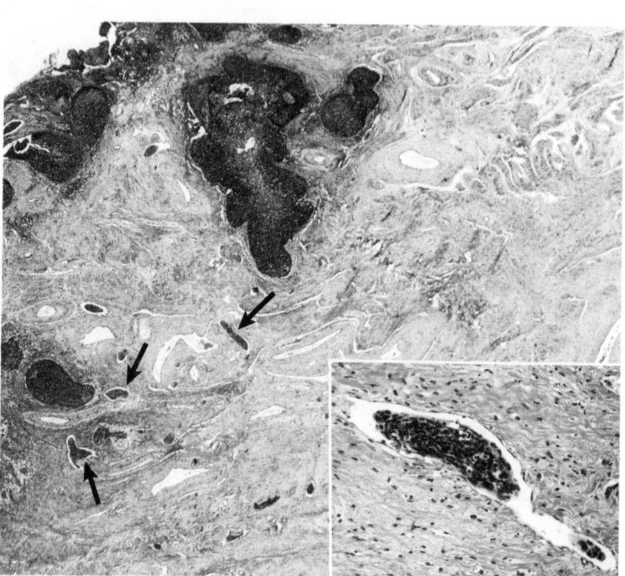

FIGURE 18-21
Squamous cell cancer of the cervix with lymphatic invasion. Low magnification shows a squamous cell carcinoma that has invaded the stroma and permeated the lymphatics (*arrows*). *Inset*: A high-power view of lymphatic invasion.

TABLE *18-5* **Clinical Staging of Cervical Cancer (FIGO, 1995)**

Stage	Description
0	Carcinoma *in situ* (cervical intraepithelial neoplasia III)
I	Carcinoma confined to cervix (extension to corpus disregarded)
Ia	Invasive cancer identified *only* microscopically. Maximum depth, 5.0 mm; maximum width, 7.0 mm.
1a1	Depth ≤3.0 mm
1a2	Depth >3.0 mm
Ib	Any cancer *grossly* visible
1b1	Clinical size ≤4.0 cm
1b2	Clinical size >4.0 cm
II	Carcinoma extending beyond cervix, but not to lateral pelvic wall; involvement of vagina limited to upper two thirds
IIa	Paracervical extension not suspected
IIb	Paracervical extension suspected
III	Invasive carcinoma extending to lateral pelvic wall or lower one third of vagina
IIIa	No extension to the pelvic wall
IIIb	Extension to pelvic wall, hydronephrosis, or nonfunctioning kidney
IV	Extended spread involving
IVa	Mucosa of urinary bladder or rectum
IVb	Tissues beyond true pelvis

reliable clinical screening test for the detection of the tumor. A newer test used in detection and follow-up is an assay for squamous cell carcinoma antigen (SCC-Ag), which is positive in one third of cases of stage I tumor and in over half of cases of higher stage and greater bulk.

The clinical stage of the tumor is the best prognostic index of survival (see Table 18-5). The overall 5-year survival rate is 60%, and for each stage it is as follows: I, 90%; II, 75%; III, 35%; and IV, 10%. About 15% of patients develop recurrences on the vaginal wall, bladder, pelvis, or rectum within 2 years of appropriate therapy. Treatment depends on cancer staging. Radical hysterectomy is favored for localized tumor, especially in younger women, whereas radiation therapy or combinations of the two are used for more advanced tumors.

Adenocarcinoma

Adenocarcinoma of the endocervix accounts for 10% of malignant cervical tumors. An increased incidence has been reported, but whether this is due to better recognition or a real increase is not clear. The mean age at presentation is 56 years. Most adenocarcinomas are of the endocervical cell (mucinous) type. While the epidemiological data are not entirely compelling, adenocarcinoma appears to share epidemiological factors with squamous cell carcinoma of the cervix and spreads in a fashion similar to it. The tumors are often associated with adenocarcinoma *in situ* and are frequently infected with HPV types 16 and 18.

□ Pathology

ADENOCARCINOMA *IN SITU*: This lesion generally arises in the region of the squamocolumnar junction and extends into the endocervical canal. It is composed of tall columnar cells with eosinophilic or mucinous cytoplasm, sometimes resembling goblet cells. Its pattern of spread and involvement of endocervical glands resemble those of CIN. Adenocarcinoma *in situ* typically is an intraepithelial proliferation, and the normal architecture of the endocervical glands is maintained. The cells show slight enlargement, atypical hyperchromatic nuclei with an increased nuclear-to-cytoplasmic ratio, and variable numbers of mitoses. Abrupt transitions help distinguish neoplastic from neighboring, normal endocervical cells. Associated high-grade squamous cell CIN occurs in 40% of cases of adenocarcinoma *in situ*.

INVASIVE ADENOCARCINOMA: This tumor typically presents as a fungating polypoid or papillary mass. In addition to the characteristic features of an adenocarcinoma, exophytic tumors often have a papillary pattern, whereas endophytic ones display tubular or glandular patterns. Poorly differentiated tumors are predominantly composed of solid sheets of cells.

As does squamous carcinoma, invasive adenocarcinoma of the endocervix spreads by local invasion and lymphatic metastases. However, the overall survival is somewhat less than that for squamous carcinoma. Adenocarcinoma is treated in a manner similar to that of squamous carcinoma.

Uterine Body

ANATOMY

The uterine corpus (body) is smaller than the cervix at birth and during childhood but increases rapidly in size after puberty. The endometrium, composed of glands and stroma, is thin at birth, consisting of a continuous surface of cuboidal epithelium that dips to line a few sparse tubular glands. After puberty, the endometrium thickens. The superficial two thirds, the zona functionalis, is responsive to hormones and is shed with each menstrual phase. The deepest third, the basal layer, is the germinative portion, and with each cycle it regenerates a new functional zone.

The endometrium is supplied by arcuate arteries, which traverse the outer myometrium and give off two sets of vessels, one to the myometrium and the other, the radial arteries, to the endometrium. In turn, the radial arteries branch into two types of vessels. The basal arteries supply the basal endometrium and the spiral arteries nourish the superficial two thirds.

NORMAL MENSTRUAL CYCLE

The normal endometrium undergoes a series of sequential changes that support the growth of the implanted fertilized ovum (zygote). In the absence of conception, the endometrium is shed and is then regenerated to support a fertilized ovum.

PROLIFERATIVE PHASE: During the first 14 days of the menstrual cycle, the endometrium is under estrogenic stimulation. The superficial or functional zone exhibits tubular to coiled glands, which are evenly distributed and supported by a cellular, monomorphic stroma (Figs. 18-1 and 18-22). Early during the proliferative phase, the glands are of narrow diameter, but as proliferation progresses, the glands coil more and increase slightly in caliber. The cells lining the tubules are columnar. They increase from one cell layer in thickness to a pseudostratified epithelium and are mitotically active. The glands produce a watery alkaline secretion, which facilitates passage of the sperm through the fallopian tubes and into the endometrial cavity. The stroma is mitotically active. The spiral arteries are narrow and usually inconspicuous.

SECRETORY PHASE: After ovulation, which occurs about 14 days after the last menstrual period, the graafian follicle that has discharged its ovum becomes a corpus luteum. The granulosa cells of the corpus luteum begin to secrete substantial amounts of progesterone, the hormone that transforms the endometrium from a proliferative to a secretory state.

- Days 17 to 19 (postovulatory days 3 to 5): The endometrial glands enlarge and become more coiled. The cells lining the glands develop abundant and prominent, glycogen-rich, subnuclear vacuoles (day 17). Over the next several days, the endometrial glandular cells produce copious secretions, which are intended to bathe the implanted zygote. The secretions support the zygote, while it develops early chorionic villi capable of invading the endometrium.
- Days 20 to 22 (postovulatory days 6 to 8): The endometrium displays prominent glandular secretions and stromal edema. The glands dilate, have serrated borders, and are more tortuous.
- Day 23 (postovulatory day 9): The stromal cells enlarge and exhibit large, round vesicular nuclei and abundant eosinophilic cytoplasm. These cells, which normally appear first about the spiral arterioles, are the precursors of the decidual cells of pregnancy and are sometimes referred to as "predecidua."
- Day 27 (postovulatory day 13): The full thickness of the stroma has become significantly predecidualized.

MENSTRUAL PHASE: In the absence of pregnancy, a series of regressive events occurs. Without a blastocyst to elaborate human chorionic gonadotropin (hCG), the granulosa and thecal cells of the corpus luteum degenerate. As the corpus luteum degenerates, progesterone levels fall, the endometrium becomes desiccated, the spiral arteries collapse, and the stroma disintegrates. Menses commence on day 28, last 3 to 7 days, and result in a flow of about 35 mL of blood. The denuded surface is reepithelialized by extension of the residual glandular epithelium.

ATROPHIC ENDOMETRIUM: After the menopause, the number of glands and the amount of stroma progressively decrease. The remaining glands often are oriented parallel to the surface, and the stroma contains

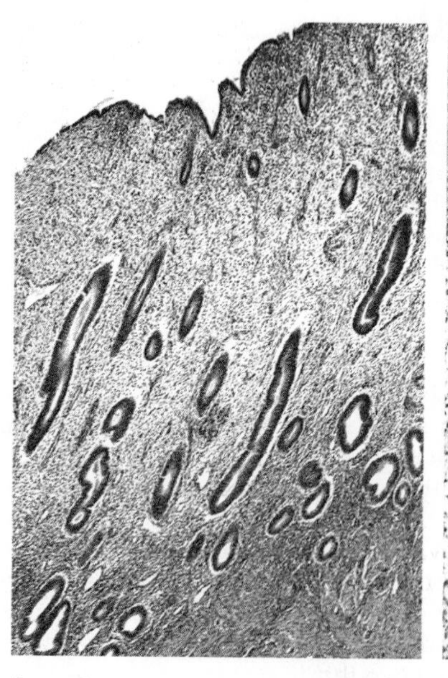
A

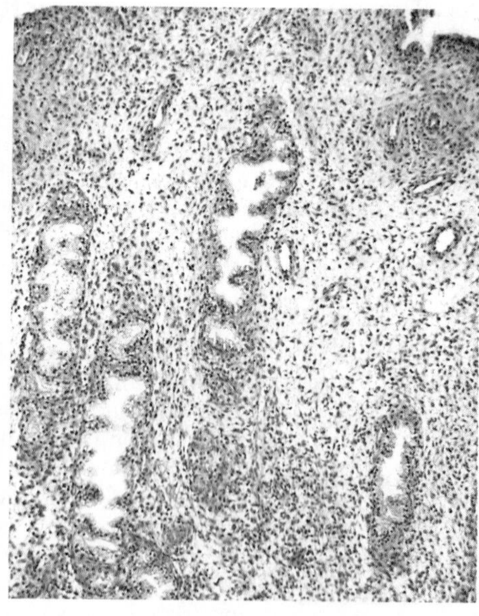
B

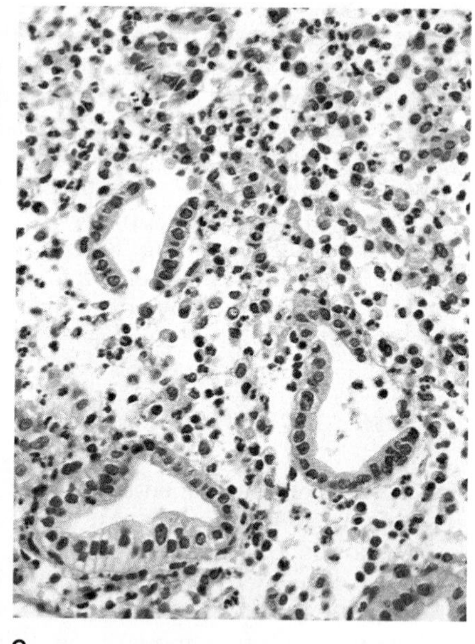
C

FIGURE *18-22*
Endometrial phases of the normal menstrual cycle. (*A*) Proliferative phase. Straight tubular glands are embedded in a cellular, monomorphic stroma. (*B*) Secretory phase, day 24. Dilated tortuous glands with serrated borders are situated in a predecidual stroma. (*C*) Menstrual endometrium. Fragmented glands, dissolution of the stroma, and numerous neutrophils are evident.

abundant collagen. For reasons unknown, the glands of the atrophic endometrium are often conspicuously dilated, an appearance termed *senile cystic atrophy of the endometrium.*

ENDOMETRIUM OF PREGNANCY

The development and maintenance of the corpus luteum of pregnancy depends on continuous stimulation by hCG secreted by the trophoblast of the developing embryo. In the usual pregnancy, the trophoblast begins to develop about day 23. At that time, under the influence of hCG, the corpus luteum increases its output of progesterone, thereby stimulating secretion by the endometrial glands. The hypersecretory endometrium of pregnancy is characterized by widely dilated glands lined by cells with abundant glycogen. These features can persist for up to 8 weeks after delivery.

The hypersecretory response may become exaggerated with intrauterine pregnancy, ectopic pregnancy, or trophoblastic disease. In this circumstance the nuclei of the glandular cells become enlarged, bulbous, and polyploid, because the DNA has replicated but the cells have not divided. The nuclei protrude beyond the apparent cytoplasmic limits of the cell into the gland lumen, an appearance referred to as the *Arias-Stella reaction* (Fig. 18-23). This change should not be confused with adenocarcinoma.

CONGENITAL ANOMALIES

Congenital anomalies of the uterus are rare, but some affect a woman's ability to carry a pregnancy to term. Most malformations reflect the aberrant development of one or more stages of uterine growth during fetal life.

Congenital absence of the uterus (agenesis) is caused by a failure of the müllerian ducts to develop. Since elongation of the müllerian ducts during embryonic life depends on the presence of the wolffian ducts as guide wires, uterine agenesis is almost always accompanied by anomalies of the genital tract, agenesis of the vagina, and poorly developed or aplastic fallopian tubes.

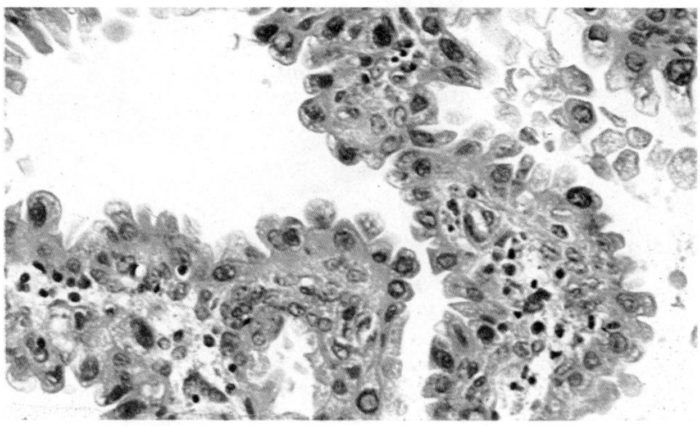

FIGURE *18-23*
Arias-Stella reaction of pregnancy associated with human chorionic gonadotropin (hCG) stimulation. A section of endometrium shows enlarged, bulbous nuclei, which protrude into the gland lumen.

Uterus didelphys refers to a completely double uterus (didelphoid, double), which results from a lack of fusion of the two müllerian ducts. This anomaly may be accompanied by a double vagina.

Uterus duplex bicornis is a uterus with a common fused wall between two distinct endometrial cavities. It reflects the failure of the common wall between the apposed müllerian ducts to break down and form a single uterine cavity.

Uterus septus is a single uterus with a partial remaining septum, owing to a partial failure of resorption of the fused müllerian ducts. Patients with a uterine septum are at increased risk for habitual abortion.

Bicornuate uterus refers to a uterus with two cornua (horns) and a common cervix. Didelphic and bicornuate uterine fusion defects lead to a small increase in the incidence of premature birth.

ENDOMETRITIS

Endometritis, or inflammation of the endometrium, is a histological diagnosis based on the finding of an abnormal inflammatory cell infiltrate in the endometrium. It must be distinguished from the normal presence of polymorphonuclear leukocytes during menstruation and a mild lymphocytic infiltrate at other times. The findings in most cases of endometritis are nonspecific, since they do not usually point to a specific etiological cause.

ACUTE ENDOMETRITIS: This condition is defined as the abnormal presence of polymorphonuclear leukocytes in the endometrium. Most cases of acute endometritis result from an ascending infection from the cervix, such as occurs after the usually impervious cervical barrier is compromised by abortion, delivery, or medical instrumentation. Curettage is diagnostic and often curative, because it removes the necrotic tissue that has served as the nidus of ongoing infection. Nowadays, the condition is of little significance, contrasted with the dangers that it presented before the antibiotic era.

CHRONIC ENDOMETRITIS: Plasma cells in the endometrium identify chronic endometritis (Fig. 18-24). Although lymphocytes and lymphoid follicles are occasionally found scattered in the normal endometrium, their presence alone is not considered diagnostic of chronic endometritis. Chronic endometritis is associated with intrauterine device (IUD) use, PID, and retained products of conception after an abortion or delivery. In the absence of cultures, the pathological findings alone are insufficient to distinguish between infective and noninfective causes. Patients usually complain of bleeding, pelvic pain, or both. The condition is generally self-limited.

PYOMETRA: Defined as pus in the endometrial cavity, pyometra is associated with any lesion that causes cervical stenosis, such as a tumor or scarring from surgical treatment (conization) of the cervix. Long-standing

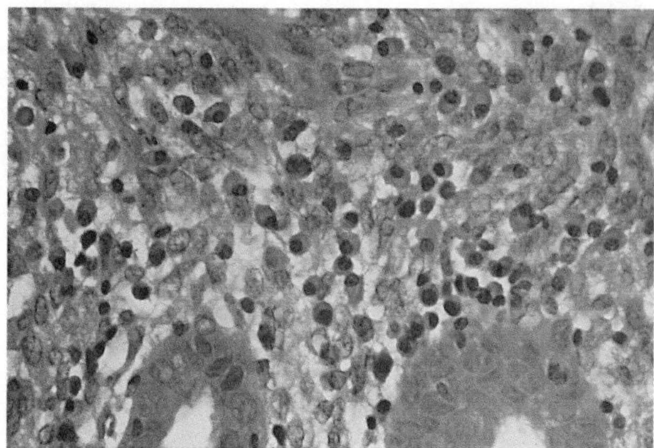

FIGURE *18-24*
Chronic endometritis. The inflammatory infiltrate is composed largely of lymphocytes and plasma cells.

pyometra may be associated with the rare development of squamous cell cancer of the endometrium.

TRAUMATIC LESIONS

INTRAUTERINE DEVICE (IUD): The presence of an IUD is associated with several risks, including (1) increased menstrual flow, (2) uterine perforation, (3) spontaneous abortion when conception occurs with an IUD in place, and (4) PID, particularly salpingitis.

INTRAUTERINE ADHESIONS (ASHERMAN SYNDROME): Intrauterine fibrous adhesions sometimes develop after curettage of the uterus, particularly for postpartum complications or therapeutic abortion. These bands traverse, but do not necessarily obliterate, the endometrial cavity. Additional complications include amenorrhea or, in the event of a subsequent pregnancy, increased abortion rates, preterm labor, and placenta accreta.

ADENOMYOSIS

Adenomyosis refers to the presence of endometrial glands and stroma within the myometrium (Fig. 18-25). While commonly defined as a presence more than 3 mm beneath the endometrial–myometrial junction, recent studies have shown that more than two thirds of women will be symptomatic with pain, dysmenorrhea, or menorrhagia if the glands are as little as 1 mm deep to the basalis. The most clinically significant correlation occurs if the glands are located 2 mm or greater into the myometrium. One fifth of all uteri removed at surgery show some degree of adenomyosis, the etiology of which is unknown.

☐ **Pathology:** On gross examination, the myometrium contains small, soft, red areas, some of which are cystic. Microscopic examination of these lesions reveals glands lined by mildly proliferative to inactive endometrium and surrounded by endometrial stroma. Secretory changes are rare, except during pregnancy and in patients treated with progestins. Sometimes the uterus is enlarged by smooth muscle hypertrophy around the foci of adenomyosis. Over time, the uterus may also become enlarged from cyclic bleeding into these foci. Varying degrees of glandular hyperplasia may be seen, and occasionally hyperplastic surface endometrium extends into the foci of adenomyosis.

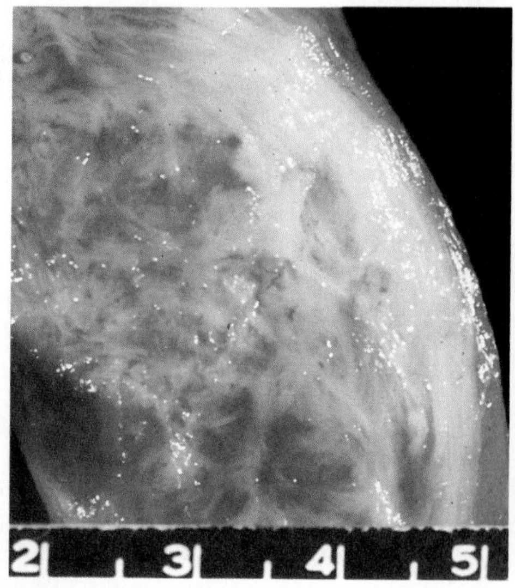

FIGURE *18-25*
Adenomyosis. (*A*) The cut surface of the uterus reveals small, red areas corresponding to endometrial glands in the myometrium. (*B*) A microscopic view shows an endometrial gland and stroma in the myometrium.

☐ **Clinical Features:** Although many patients with adenomyosis are asymptomatic, it is not uncommon for patients to present with varying degrees of pelvic pain, dysfunctional uterine bleeding, dysmenorrhea, and dyspareunia. These symptoms appear in parous women of reproductive age and regress after the menopause.

ENDOMETRIOSIS

Endometriosis is defined as the presence of benign endometrial glands and stroma outside the uterus. It afflicts 3% of women of reproductive age and regresses following natural or artificial menopause. The mean age at diagnosis is 25 to 29 years of age, although it may appear at any time after menarche. The sites most frequently involved are the ovaries (80%) and the other uterine adnexae, including the uterine ligaments, the rectovaginal septum, the pouch of Douglas, and the pelvic peritoneum covering the uterus, fallopian tubes, rectosigmoid colon, and bladder (Fig. 18-26). Endometriosis, however, can be more widespread and occasionally involves the cervix, vagina, perineum, bladder, and umbilicus. Even the pelvic lymph nodes may contain foci of endometriosis. On rare occasions, distant areas such as lungs, pleura, small bowel, kidneys, and bones may be affected.

☐ **Pathogenesis:** The pathogenesis of endometriosis has long been controversial. Several theories have been proposed, and they are not mutually exclusive.

MENSTRUAL IMPLANTATION: The most widely accepted theory holds that foci of menstrual endometrium reflux through the fallopian tubes and implant on the various pelvic organs. Retrograde menstruation through the fallopian tubes has been demonstrated to occur in 90% of women. Since the fimbrial openings are in the posterior area of the pelvis, most deposits from the menstrual "spill" implant on structures located in the posterior pelvis.

INTRAOPERATIVE IMPLANTATION: Endometriosis has been documented in hysterotomy and episiotomy scars, in which case it has been attributed to the implantation of endometrial fragments during surgery.

LYMPHATIC AND HEMATOGENOUS DISSEMINATION: The occurrence of endometriosis at distant sites such as the lungs and kidneys has been attributed to hematogenous spread from the endometrium. This concept is supported by the observation that pulmonary endometriosis occurs almost exclusively in women who have been subjected to uterine surgery. The presence of endometriosis in lymph nodes is consistent with similar lymphatic dissemination.

CELOMIC METAPLASIA: Endometriosis has been proposed to arise by celomic metaplasia of the epithelium (the lining of peritoneal cavity), in view of the müllerian potential of this tissue. This theory has gained support by the occurrence of endometriosis in persons with Turner syndrome (gonadal dysgenesis), who have primary

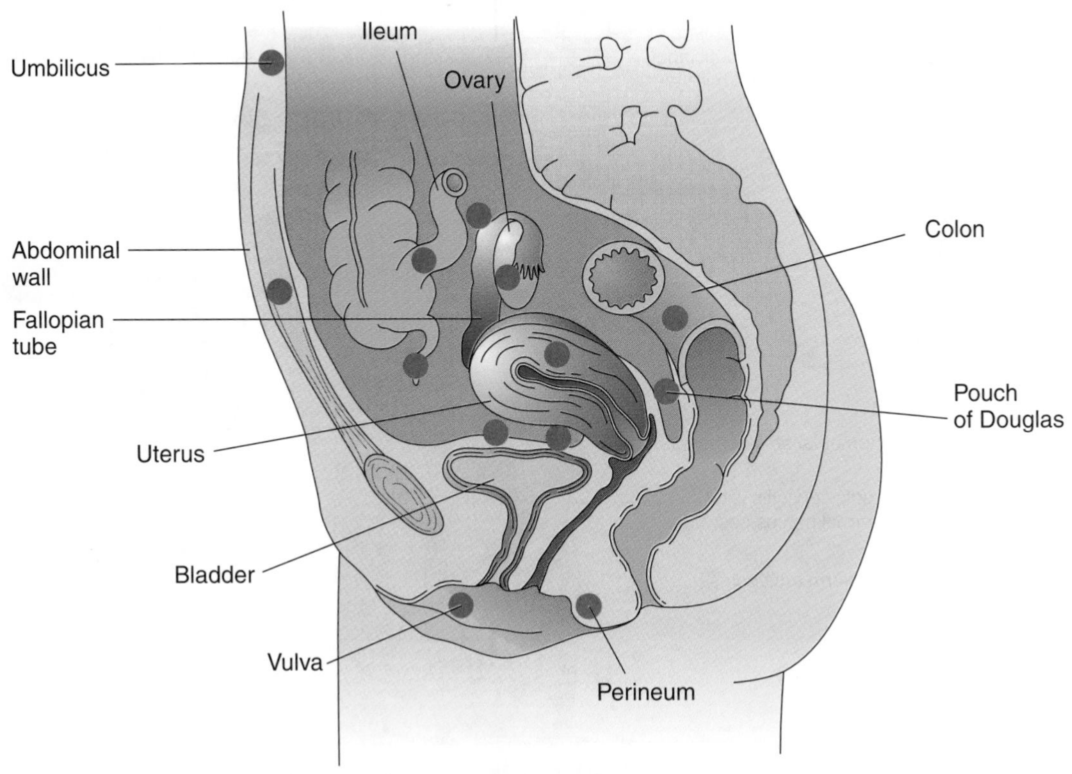

FIGURE *18-26*
Sites of endometriosis.

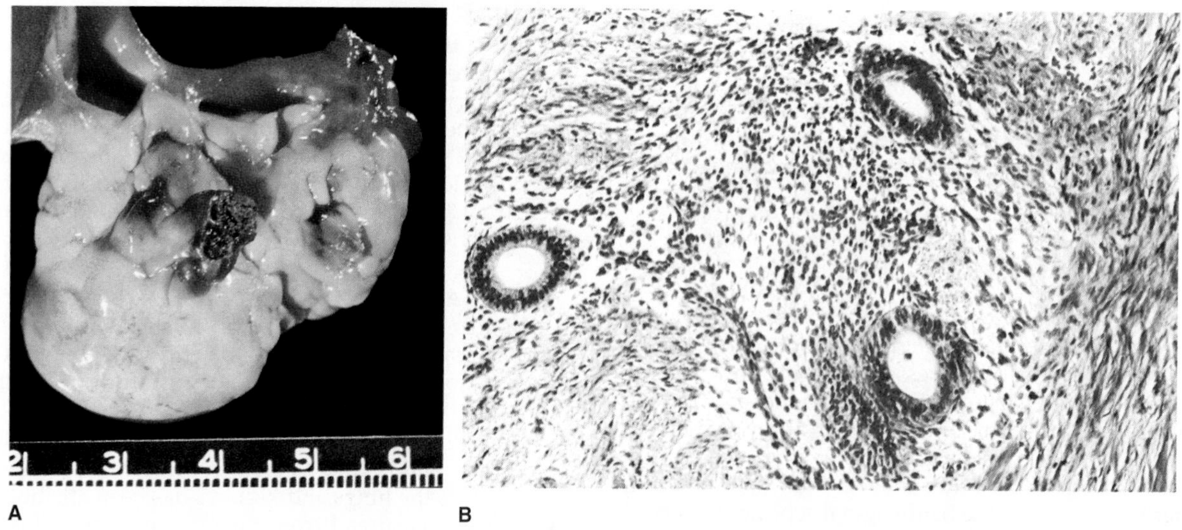

FIGURE *18-27*
Endometriosis. (*A*) Implants of endometriosis on the ovary appear as red-blue nodules. (*B*) A microscopic section from the broad ligament shows endometrial glands and stroma in the ovary.

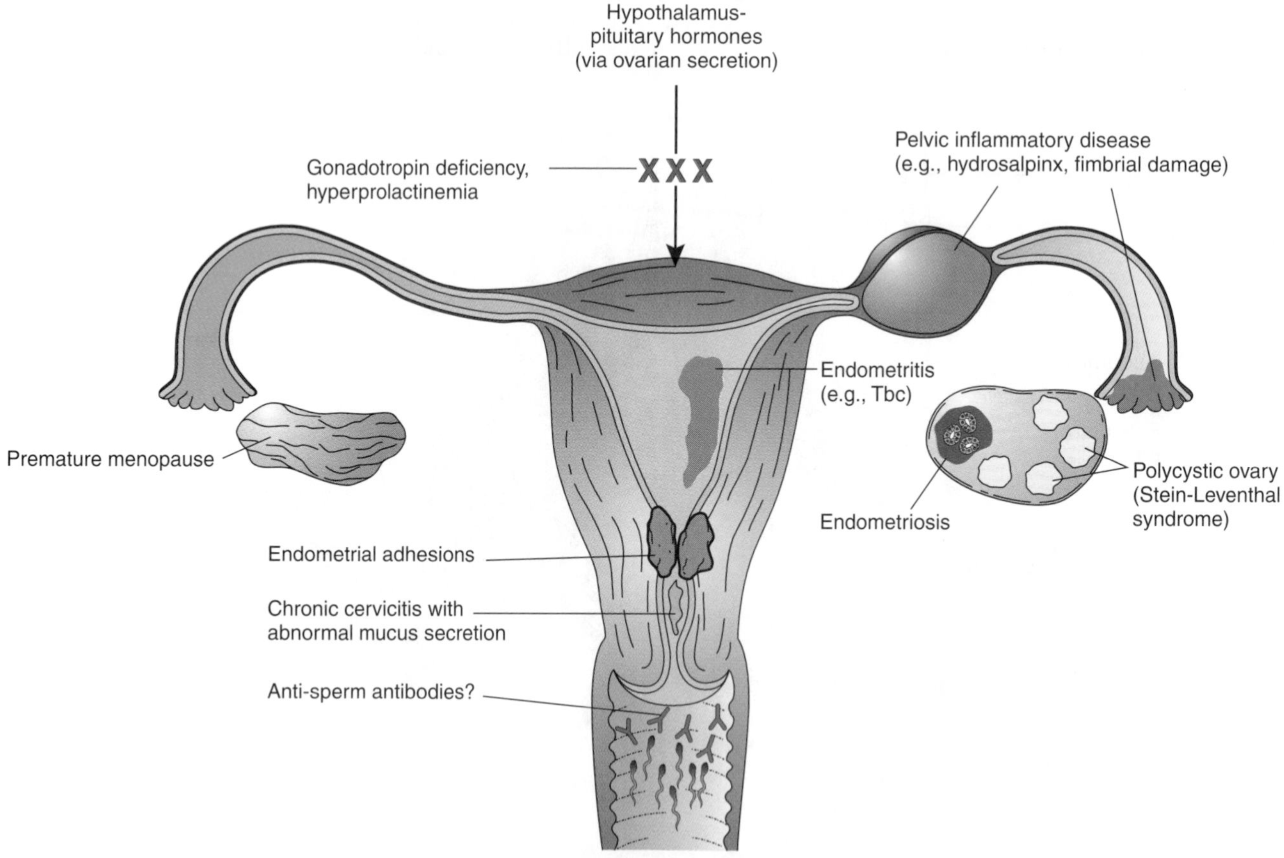

Hypothalamus-pituitary hormones (via ovarian secretion)

Gonadotropin deficiency, hyperprolactinemia

XXX

Pelvic inflammatory disease (e.g., hydrosalpinx, fimbrial damage)

Endometritis (e.g., Tbc)

Premature menopause

Polycystic ovary (Stein-Leventhal syndrome)

Endometriosis

Endometrial adhesions

Chronic cervicitis with abnormal mucus secretion

Anti-sperm antibodies?

FIGURE *18-28*
Causes of acquired infertility.

amenorrhea and hypoplastic uteri. Moreover, endometriosis has also been reported in men, involving the bladder, prostate, and scrotum.

☐ **Pathology:** Early foci of endometriosis on the ovary or peritoneal surfaces are red or bluish ("mulberry") nodules, which vary from 1 to 5 mm (Fig. 18-27A). Since the ectopic endometrial glands often participate in the menstrual cycle, repeated bleeding leads to the deposition of hemosiderin and a grossly brown discoloration ("powder burns"). Fibrous adhesions often surround endometriotic foci and may cause adjacent structures, such as loops of bowel, to adhere.

In the ovaries, repeated hemorrhage may cause enlargement of the endometriotic foci to form cysts up to 15 cm in diameter. The cyst often contains inspissated, chocolate-colored material (*chocolate cysts*).

Microscopically, endometriosis is diagnosed by the presence of ectopic endometrial glands and stroma (see Fig. 18-27B). On occasion, healed foci of endometriosis consist only of fibrous tissue and hemosiderin-laden macrophages.

☐ **Clinical Features:** The signs and symptoms of endometriosis depend on the location of the implants. The most common complaint is dysmenorrhea, related to implants on the uterosacral ligaments. These implants swell immediately prior to or during menstruation, producing pelvic pain. **Half of all women with dysmenorrhea have endometriosis.** Infertility is the primary complaint in a third of women with endometriosis (Fig. 18-28). With conservative surgery to restore the pelvic anatomy, many of these women eventually become pregnant. Dyspareunia and cyclical abdominal pain may be troublesome.

HORMONAL EFFECTS

Contraceptive Steroids

Oral contraceptive agents induce a wide variety of endometrial changes that reflect the types, potencies, and dosages of estrogens and progestins used in these formulations. Combined preparations generally contain potent progestins and weak estrogens. The decidual change, therefore, appears early and overshadows the weak glandular growth. Over time (i.e., after a number of cycles), the endometrial glands atrophy. More recently developed contraceptive combinations contain lower doses of hormones and correspondingly elicit less change. **Women who use contraceptive steroids have significantly reduced rates of both endometrial and ovarian cancer, effects that reflect the growth-inhibiting properties of progesterone.**

Dysfunctional Uterine Bleeding

Dysfunctional uterine bleeding is defined as abnormal bleeding during or between menstrual periods, in which the cause lies outside the uterus. It is one of the most common gynecological disorders of women of reproductive age, but one that is still poorly understood. After excluding the uterus as the cause, most cases appear to be related to an endocrine disturbance that involves any aspect of the hypothalamic–pituitary–ovarian axis (Table 18-6). Ovarian dysfunction is usual, especially when on the basis of anovulation.

Some causes of menstrual irregularity that are not considered dysfunctional are intrinsic to the uterus itself, such as (1) growths (e.g., carcinoma, hyperplasia, and polyps), (2) inflammation (e.g., endometritis), (3) pregnancy (e.g., complications of intrauterine or ectopic pregnancy), and (4) the effect of IUDs (see Table 18-6).

Anovulatory Bleeding

Anovulatory bleeding is a complex syndrome of many causes that presents as the absence of ovulation during the reproductive years. It is the most common form of dysfunctional uterine bleeding and is most often noted at either end of reproductive life (i.e., menarche and menopause). In an anovulatory cycle, the failure of ovulation leads to excessive and prolonged estrogen stimulation, without the postovulatory rise in progesterone levels. The end result is an endometrium that is in a proliferative state but with a disordered, fragmented appearance. In the absence of adequate progesterone, the spiral arteries of the endo-

TABLE *18-6* Causes of Abnormal Uterine Bleeding (Including Uterine and Extrauterine Causes)

Newborn	Maternal estrogen
Childhood	Iatrogenic (trauma, foreign body, infection of vagina)
	Vaginal neoplasms (sarcoma botryoides)
	Ovarian tumors (functional)
Adolescence	Hypothalamic immaturity
	Psychogenic and nutritional problems
	Inadequate luteal function
Reproductive age	Anovulatory
	Central: psychogenic, stress
	Systemic: nutritional and endocrine disease
	Gonadal: functional tumors
	End-organ: endometrial hyperplasia
	Pregnancy: ectopic, retained placenta, abortion, mole
	Ovulatory
	Organic: neoplasia, infections (PID), leiomyomas
	Polymenorrhea: short follicular or luteal phases
	Iatrogenic: anticoagulants, IUD
	Irregular shedding
Menopause	Organic: carcinoma, hyperplasias, polyps
Postmenopause	Organic: carcinoma, hyperplasias, polyps
	Endometrial atrophy

IUD, intrauterine device; PID, pelvic inflammatory disease.

metrium do not develop normally. When the level of estrogen falls, "breakthrough bleeding" occurs. Since estrogen maintains the stromal fluid turgescence that supports the endometrial blood vessels, a fall in the estrogen level results in stromal fluid loss and hence a loss of vascular support. The subsequent compression of the poorly developed spiral arteries leads in turn to stasis, thrombosis, infarction, and hemorrhage. Bleeding can also occur if the endometrium continues to proliferate in the presence of an unchanged estrogen level. In this case, the proliferative endometrium is not adequately nourished and withdrawal bleeding also ensues. On microscopic examination, the glands in anovulatory bleeding are frequently disordered and appear crowded because of severe stromal necrosis and collapse of the proliferative endometrium.

Luteal Phase Defect

Luteal phase defect refers to inadequate progesterone secretion by the corpus luteum. This dysfunction results in an abnormally short menstrual cycle in which menses occur 6 to 9 days after the surge of luteinizing hormone associated with ovulation. A luteal phase defect occurs when the corpus luteum does not develop properly or regresses prematurely. The disorder is primarily of interest in the investigation of infertility and occasionally of abnormal uterine bleeding. In fact, luteal phase defects are responsible for 3% of cases of infertility. The diagnosis of a luteal phase defect is confirmed by endometrial biopsies in which the microscopic findings are more than 2 days out of synchrony with the chronological day of the menstrual cycle.

TUMORS

Endometrial Polyp

Endometrial polyps are benign localized overgrowths that project from the endometrial surface into the endometrial cavity. They occur most commonly in the perimenopausal period and are virtually unknown before menarche. Endometrial polyps are thought to arise from endometrial foci that are hypersensitive to estrogenic stimulation or unresponsive to progesterone. In either case, such foci would not slough during menstruation and would continue to grow.

☐ **Pathology:** Most endometrial polyps arise in the fundus (Fig. 18-29A), although they may originate in any location within the endometrial cavity. The majority are solitary, but 20% are multiple. They vary in size from several millimeters in length to a growth that fills the entire endometrial cavity.

Microscopically, the core of a polyp is composed of (1) endometrial glands, which often are cystically dilated and hyperplastic; (2) a fibromatous endometrial stroma; and (3) thick-walled, coiled, dilated blood vessels, thought to be derived from one of the straight arteries that normally supply the basal zone of the endometrium (see Fig. 18-29B). A mantle of endometrial epithelium covers the polyp. The glandular epithelium is usually not at the same stage of the cycle as that of the adjacent, normal endometrium.

☐ **Clinical Features:** Endometrial polyps typically present with intermenstrual bleeding, owing to surface

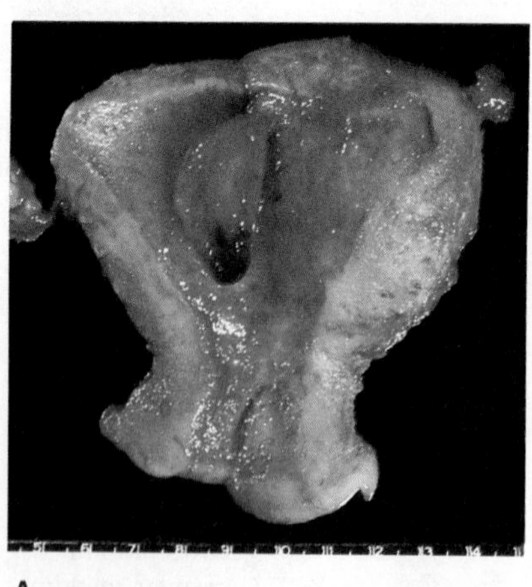

A

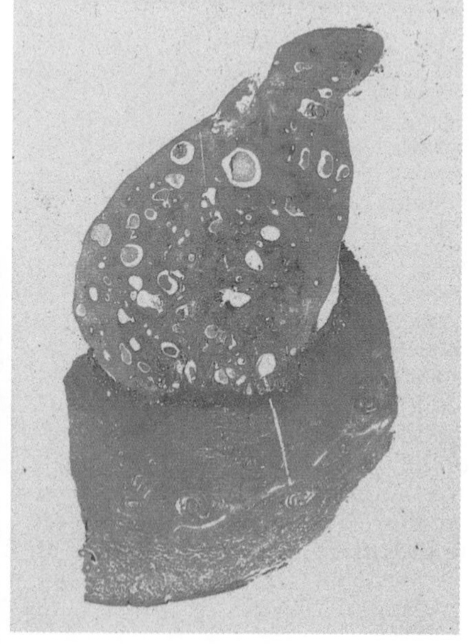

B

FIGURE *18-29*
Endometrial polyp. (*A*) A single polyp extends into the endometrial cavity. The necrotic tip is responsible for clinical bleeding. (*B*) On microscopic section, a polyp (from a different case) exhibits slightly dilated endometrial glands embedded in a markedly fibrous stroma.

ulceration or hemorrhagic infarction. Since bleeding in an older woman is not uncommonly due to cancer, the presence of this sign must be thoroughly evaluated. Endometrial polyps are not believed to be preneoplastic, but up to 0.5% harbor adenocarcinoma.

Endometrial Hyperplasia and Adenocarcinoma

Endometrial hyperplasia and adenocarcinoma represent a broad spectrum of proliferative disease that constitutes a morphological and biological continuum, similar to multistep carcinogenesis in other tissues. Thus, the lesions progress from the mildest degrees of hyperplasia of endometrial glands to invasive cancer. Proliferative lesions of the endometrium often result from endogenous estrogens produced by hormonally functioning tumors, such as granulosa cell tumor of the ovary, or in polycystic ovary syndrome. Hyperestrinism also results from the administration of exogenous estrogens to control the symptoms of the menopause.

Endometrial Hyperplasia

Endometrial hyperplasia refers to a morphological continuum that ranges from simple glandular crowding to a conspicuous proliferation of atypical glands, which are difficult to distinguish from early carcinoma. It is generally agreed that the risk of developing carcinoma increases with progressively higher degrees of endometrial hyperplasia.

☐ **Pathology:** The most recent classification of endometrial hyperplasia is based on the presence of cytological atypia and abnormal glandular architecture. **The most important prognostic feature is the presence of cytological atypia.**

- **Simple hyperplasia:** This term encompasses the older terms *cystic* and *mild.* It is a proliferative lesion that shows minimal glandular complexity and crowding and no cytological atypia. The epithelial lining is usually one cell layer thick, and the stroma between the glands is abundant. **One percent of cases of simple endometrial hyperplasia progress to adenocarcinoma.**
- **Complex hyperplasia:** Formerly termed *moderate hyperplasia,* this variant exhibits severe glandular complexity and crowding but no cytological atypia (Fig. 18-30). The glands are increased in number but may vary in size. The stroma between the glands is scanty. **Three percent of such lesions progress to adenocarcinoma.**
- **Atypical hyperplasia:** This lesion, which was previously called "severe," displays cytological atypia and marked glandular crowding, frequently as back-to-back glands. The glands may have a complex architecture, with an intraluminal papillary arrangement or the appearance of budding glands in the stroma. The epithelial cells are enlarged and hyperchromatic and have prominent nucleoli and an increased nuclear-to-cytoplasmic ratio. **One third of the cases of atypical endometrial hyperplasia progress to adenocarcinoma.** If papillary or budding glands are not present, the lesion is classified as simple atypical hyperplasia, and only 8% progress to carcinoma.

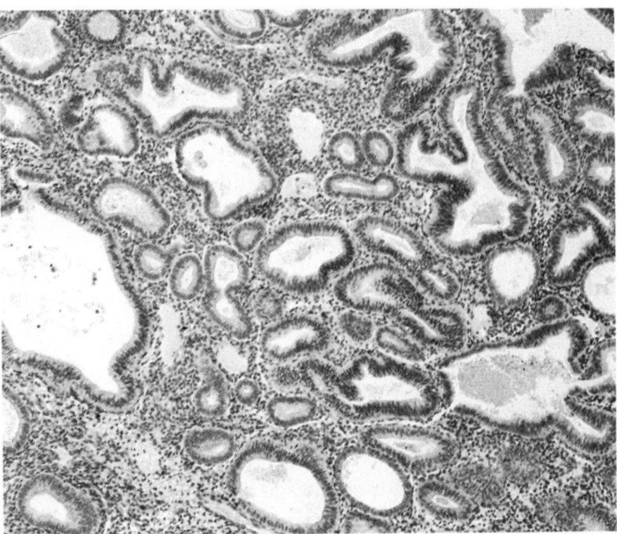

FIGURE *18-30*
Complex endometrial hyperplasia. The endometrial glands, which are in the proliferative phase, are closely packed and display moderate architectural disarray (budding and branching). No cytological atypia is present.

The progression from hyperplasia free of atypia to invasive cancer requires about 10 years. The corresponding time for hyperplasia with cytological atypia is roughly 4 years.

☐ **Clinical Features:** The treatment of endometrial hyperplasia depends on the severity of the lesion, the patient's age, her desire to retain fertility, and the ability to control the risk factors associated with the development of endometrial carcinoma. It is important to recognize that about one sixth of uteri harbor small foci of adenocarcinoma when endometrial curettage discloses only advanced degrees of hyperplasia. In these cases, the tumor is always well differentiated and, at worst, is superficially invasive. Endometrial hyperplasia may result from anovulatory cycles, polycystic ovary syndrome, an estrogen-producing tumor, or obesity. In such cases, therapy aimed at the primary disease may alleviate the estrogenic stimulation. Treatment with large doses of progestins can produce objective remissions, although more than 60% of cases recur when the initial degree of hyperplasia is severe. Hysterectomy is usually considered the therapy of choice in a woman who has completed child bearing and in whom curettage reveals a significant degree of hyperplasia.

Endometrial Adenocarcinoma

Endometrial carcinoma is the fourth most frequent cancer in American women and the single most common gynecological cancer. An estimated 34,000 cases and 6000 deaths occurred in the United States in 1996 (7% of all cancers in women). The incidence of this cancer was stable between 1950 and 1970 (23 per 100,000) but then increased 40% by 1975 (33 per 100,000). The rise was attributed to the common practice of prescribing estrogens for menopause. By 1985, the rates had returned nearly to 1950 levels, a trend that reflected the administration of lower doses of estrogen, the incorporation of progestins (estrogen antagonists) into estrogen replacement regimens, and increased surveillance of women treated with estrogens. With recognition that hyperplasia is the precursor of cancer, timely treatment has led to the prevention of many cancers.

The occurrence of endometrial cancer varies with age. Whereas the incidence is 12 cases per 100,000 women at 40 years of age, it is sevenfold higher at age 60. Three quarters of women with endometrial cancer are postmenopausal, and the median age at diagnosis is 63 years.

☐ **Pathogenesis:** **Endometrial cancer is linked to prolonged estrogenic stimulation of the endometrium.** With the exception of treatment of menopausal symptoms with exogenous estrogens, the most common risk factors for endometrial cancer are obesity, diabetes, nulliparity, early menarchy, and late menopause. Each risk factor points to relative hyperestrinism. Women with ovarian agenesis do not develop endometrial cancer unless treated with exogenous estrogens. A high frequency of endometrial cancer is also found in women with estrogen-secreting granulosa cell tumors. In the case of obesity, the degree of risk correlates with body weight, the risk being increased 10-fold for women who are more than 23 kg (50 lb) overweight. This effect of obesity is related to the enhanced aromatization of androstenedione to estrone in adipocytes. Interestingly, cigarette smoking, which interferes with the hepatic conversion of estrone to its active metabolite estriol (see Chapter 8), is associated with a reduced risk of endometrial cancer. Treatment of breast cancer with tamoxifen, a synthetic anti-estrogen that also has agonist activity, increases somewhat the risk of endometrial cancer.

Endometrial cancer occurs in association with a higher incidence of both breast and ovarian cancer in closely related women, suggesting a genetic predisposition. Moreover, endometrial cancer is the most common extracolonic cancer in women with the hereditary nonpolyposis syndrome (*Lynch syndrome II*), which is also associated with breast and ovarian cancers.

☐ **Pathology:** Endometrial cancer may grow in a diffuse or polypoid pattern (Fig. 18-31). Regardless of its site of origin, the tumor often involves multiple areas, since the anterior and posterior walls of the endometrium are in contact. Large tumors are often hemorrhagic and necrotic.

PURE, OR ENDOMETRIOID, ADENOCARCINOMA OF THE ENDOMETRIUM: This type of endometrial cancer is composed entirely of glandular cells and is the most common histological variant (60%). The FIGO system divides this tumor into three grades based on the ratio of the glandular to the solid elements in the tumor, the latter being a sign of decreasing differentiation (Table 18-7; Fig. 18-32).

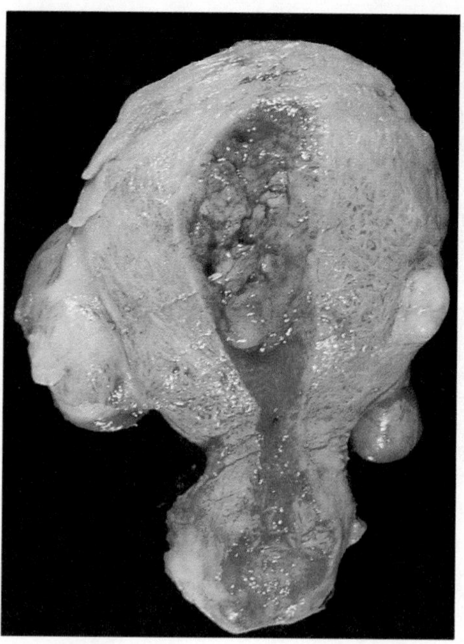

FIGURE *18-31*
Adenocarcinoma of the endometrium. The uterus has been opened to reveal a partially necrotic, polypoid endometrial cancer.

- **Grade 1:** highly differentiated; composed almost exclusively of neoplastic glands, with only minimal (<5%) solid areas.
- **Grade 2:** moderately differentiated; formed partly by glandular elements and partly (<50%) by solid tumor.
- **Grade 3:** poorly differentiated; shows large (>50%) areas of solid tumor.

TABLE *18-7* **Surgical Staging and Histopathological Grading of Endometrial Cancer**

Stage	Description
O	Atypical hyperplasia or carcinoma *in situ*
I	Confined to corpus
Ia	Confined to endometrium
Ib	Invades <½ myometrium
Ic	Invades >½ myometrium
II	Involves cervix
IIa	Endocervical glandular involvement only (i.e., *in situ* in glands)
IIb	Cervical stromal invasion
III	Extends beyond uterus but not outside true pelvis
IIIa	Involves serosa or adnexa, or has positive peritoneal cytology
IV	Extends beyond true pelvis or involves the mucosa of bladder or rectum
IVa	Spread to adjacent organs
IVb	Spread to distant organs

Grading (FIGO) of glandular tissue: G1, <5% solid (highly differentiated); G2, 5%–50% solid (differentiated with partly solid areas); G3, >50% solid (predominantly solid or entirely undifferentiated).

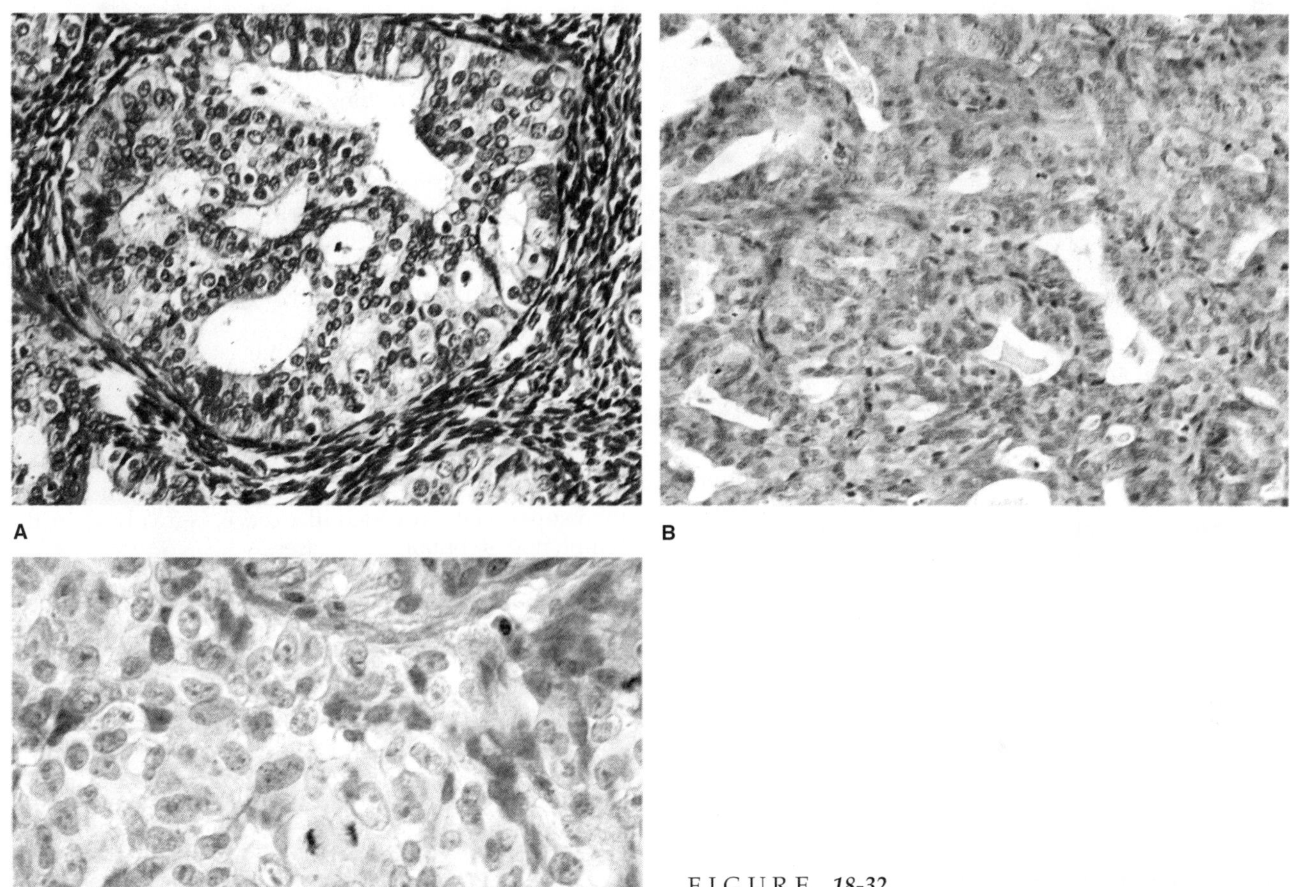

A B C

FIGURE 18-32
Adenocarcinoma of the endometrium (FIGO grades 1 to 3). (*A*) Grade 1: The tumor is well differentiated and composed entirely of glands. (*B*) Grade 2: The cancer is moderately differentiated and shows both glands and solid sheets of cells. (*C*) Grade 3: The tumor is poorly differentiated and is composed entirely of sheets of cells. Numerous mitoses are present.

The nuclei of endometrial adenocarcinoma are vesicular and may be markedly pleomorphic and show prominent nucleoli. Mitotic figures are abundant and frequently abnormal. Tumor cells growing in solid sheets generally are poorly differentiated.

ENDOMETRIOID ADENOCARCINOMA WITH SQUAMOUS DIFFERENTIATION: One third of all endometrial carcinomas contain squamous cells in addition to the glandular element. If the squamous element is well differentiated and exhibits minimal atypia, the tumor is called *well-differentiated adenocarcinoma with squamous differentiation* (formerly adenoacanthoma) (Fig. 18-33). If the squamous element appears malignant, the tumor is labeled *poorly differentiated adenocarcinoma with squamous differentiation* (formerly adenosquamous carcinoma). These two variants represent 22% and 7% of all endometrial cancers, respectively.

OTHER TYPES OF ENDOMETRIAL CARCINOMA: Other types of endometrial carcinoma are less common and include the following:

- **Serous carcinoma of the endometrium** histologically resembles papillary serous adenocarcinoma of the ovary (Fig. 18-34A). It also behaves more like an ovarian carcinoma than an endometrial tumor, and it generally behaves as a poorly differentiated carcinoma.
- **Clear cell adenocarcinoma,** a tumor typically of elderly women, is composed of large cells with copious cytoplasmic glycogen (*clear cells*) or of cells with bulbous nuclei that line glandular lumina (*hobnail cells*) (see Fig. 18-34B). The serous and clear cell carcinomas and the poorly differentiated adenocarcinoma with squamous differentiation are associated with adverse outcomes.
- **Secretory carcinoma** is characterized by cells with subnuclear vacuolization. It usually occurs in pre-

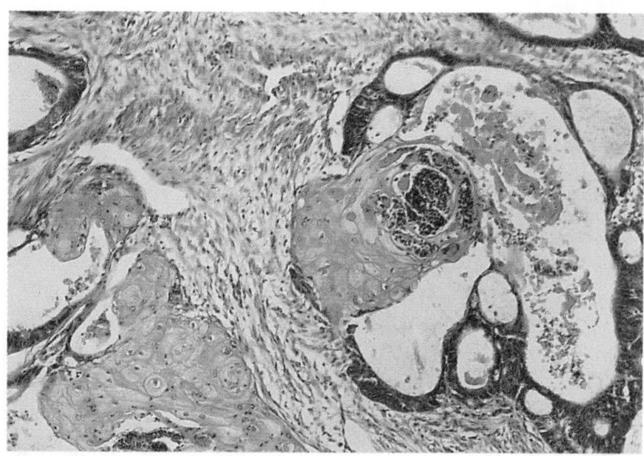

FIGURE *18-33*
Squamous differentiation in endometroid adenocarcinoma of the endometrium. The well-differentiated squamous cells show minimal atypia, a pattern that has also been called adenoacanthoma.

menopausal women. Secretory carcinoma is an extremely well differentiated, but otherwise typical, adenocarcinoma. The tumor cells manifest their responsiveness to progesterone by forming large subnuclear vacuoles of glycogen. Secretory carcinoma has the most favorable outcome of any adenocarcinoma, presumably since the cells are so well differentiated.

□ **Clinical Features:** Endometrial carcinoma typically occurs in perimenopausal or postmenopausal women. The chief complaint is usually abnormal uterine bleeding, especially when the tumor is in its early stages of growth (i.e., confined to the endometrium). Unfortunately, cervicovaginal cytological screening is unsuitable for the early detection of endometrial carcinoma. Fractional curettage is necessary to assess spread to the cervix, whereas peritoneal washing detects tubal reflux and abdominal contamination. Transvaginal ultrasonography has become a valuable diagnostic modality because of its usefulness in measuring the thickness of the endometrium; a thickness greater than 5 mm is highly predictive of endometrial hyperplasia or cancer. Unlike cervical cancer, endometrial cancer may spread directly to para-aortic lymph nodes, thereby skipping the pelvic nodes. Patients with advanced cancers may also develop pulmonary metastases (40% of cases with metastases), indicative of hematogenous dissemination.

Patients with well-differentiated tumors confined to the endometrium are usually treated by simple hysterectomy. Postoperative radiation is administered if the tumor is poorly differentiated, the myometrium is more than superficially invaded, the cervix is involved, or the lymph nodes contain metastases.

Survival in endometrial carcinoma is related to multiple factors, including (1) the stage and grade of the tumor, (2) the age of the patient, and (3) other measurable risk factors, such as progesterone receptor activity, depth of myometrial invasion, and results of peritoneal cytological washings. High levels of estrogen and progesterone receptors correlate with a significantly better prognosis. The actuarial survival rate of all patients with endometrial cancer following treatment (regardless of history of estrogen usage) is 80% after the second year, decreasing to 65% after 10 years. Tumors that penetrate into the myometrium, especially its deeper layers, or invade lymphatics, are more likely candidates for extrauterine dissemination. Endometrial cancers involving the cervix have a poorer prognosis, and those extending outside the uterus have the worst prognosis (Table 18-8).

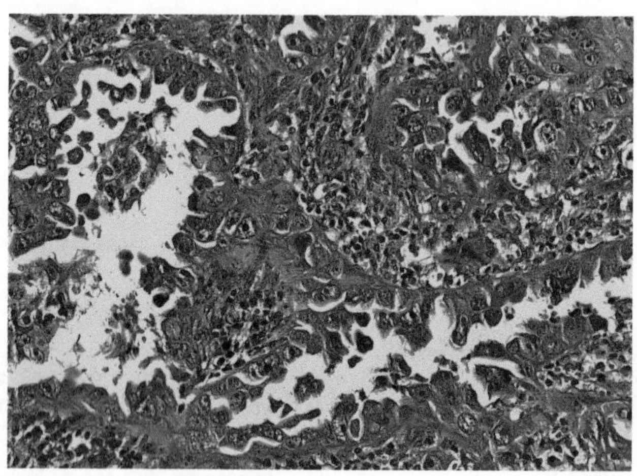

A

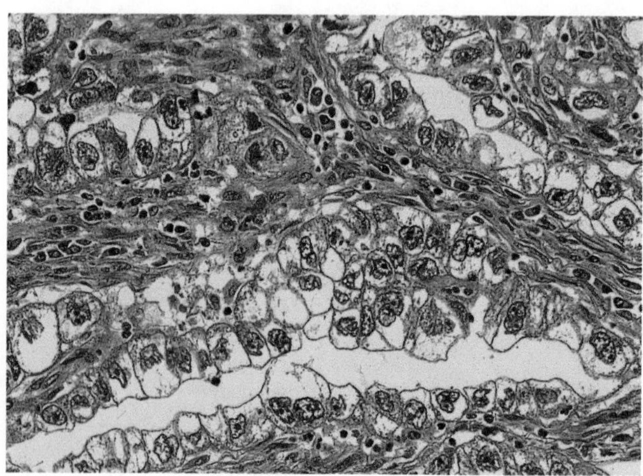

B

FIGURE *18-34*
Variants of endometrial adenocarcinoma. (*A*) Serous adenocarcinoma shows large cells with bulbous, pleomorphic nuclei growing in a papillary configuration. (*B*) Clear cell adenocarcinoma. The clear appearance of the cytoplasm is due to the dissolution of glycogen when the specimen is processed for microscopic examination. Hobnail cells with bulbous nuclei line glandular lumina.

TABLE *18-8* **Stage, Grade, and Survival for Endometrial Cancer**

Stage	5-Year Survival (%) G-1	G-2	G-3
I	90	69	52
II	80	42	12
III, IV	25	33	17

G, FIGO grade.

Endometrial Stromal Tumors

Endometrial stromal tumors account for less than 2% of all uterine malignancies. Some are pure stromal sarcomas, whereas others exhibit intimate admixtures of sarcomatous (stromal) and carcinomatous (epithelial) elements. In the latter case, the prognosis depends on the relative maturity or malignancy of each component. The nomenclature of these tumor types, the spectrum of their histological components, and the correlation of each tumor type with its potential for malignant behavior are presented in Table 18-9.

Endometrial Stromal Sarcoma

Pure stromal tumors are divided into two major categories, based on whether the tumor margin is expansile or infiltrating. Expansile lesions that do not invade are *benign stromal nodules*, which are of little clinical significance. Tumors with infiltrating margins are termed *stromal sarcomas*.

☐ **Pathology:** Endometrial stromal sarcoma may be polypoid and fill the endometrial cavity, or it may diffusely invade the uterus. Large masses of spindle cells with scant cytoplasm dissect the myometrium and invade vascular channels. The neoplastic cells resemble endometrial stromal cells in the proliferative phase. A characteristic feature of all endometrial stromal tumors is a rich vascular supporting framework, with the neoplastic cells concentrically arranged around blood vessels (Fig. 18-35). Nuclear atypism may be minimal to severe. Mitotic activity may be restrained (low-grade stromal sarcoma) or exuberant (high-grade stromal sarcoma). As the tumor becomes progressively less differentiated, it may lose its resemblance to endometrial stroma and may be classified as an undifferentiated sarcoma.

☐ **Clinical Features:** Endometrial stromal sarcoma may recur even if confined to the uterus at initial surgery. Recurrences usually involve the pelvis initially and are followed later by pulmonary metastases. In small tumors or low-grade sarcomas (also called *endolymphatic stromal myosis* and *endometrial stromatosis*), many years may elapse before recurrent disease becomes clinically evident. In these cases, prolonged survival and even cure are feasible, despite metastases. By contrast, high-grade sarcomas recur early, generally with widespread metastases, even if there has been little myometrial invasion.

UTERINE ADENOSARCOMA: Uterine (müllerian) adenosarcoma is a distinctive low-grade tumor characterized by a combination of benign (but neoplastic) glandular epithelium and malignant stroma. It should be distinguished from carcinosarcoma, which has malignant epithelial and stromal elements and is highly aggressive.

TABLE *18-9* **Nomenclature of Uterine Tumors**

Tumor	Epithelium	Stroma	Clinical Behavior
Epithelium and Stroma			
Endometrial hyperplasia	Hyperplastic	—	Benign
Endometrial adenocarcinoma	Malignant	—	Malignant
Endometrial stromal nodule	—	Benign	Benign
Endometrial stromal sarcoma			
Low grade	—	Malignant	Low-grade malignant
High grade	—	Malignant	Malignant
Adenosarcoma	Benign	Malignant	Low-grade malignant
Carcinosarcoma			
Homologous type	Malignant	Malignant	Malignant
Heterologous type[a]	Malignant	Malignant	Malignant
Smooth Muscle			
Leiomyoma	—	Benign	Benign
Cellular leiomyoma	—	Benign	Benign
Intravenous leiomyomatosis	—	Benign	Benign
Leiomyosarcoma	—	Malignant	Malignant

[a] Formerly called rhabdomyosarcoma if composed predominantly of embryonal rhabdomyoblasts, or malignant mixed mesodermal tumor if other heterologous components (e.g., cartilage, bone) were present.

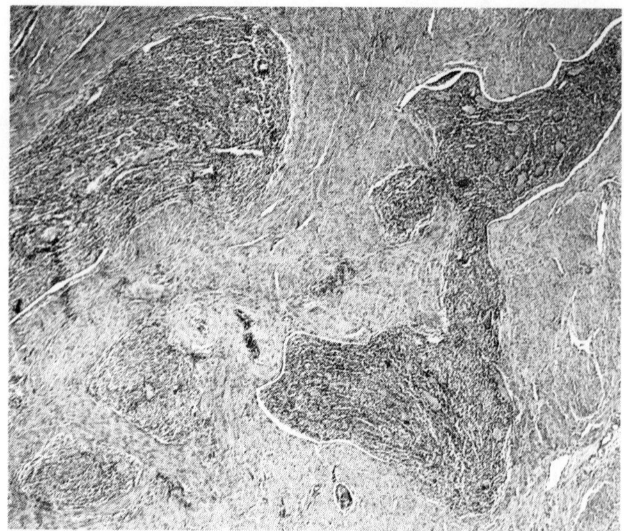

FIGURE *18-35*
Endometrial stromal sarcoma. The myometrium is irregularly invaded by the tumor, which displays a rich vascular network.

Adenosarcoma typically presents as a polypoid mass within the endometrial cavity. The glandular epithelium resembles endometrial glands in the proliferative phase, but occasionally squamous epithelium and mucinous-type epithelium may be encountered. The stroma is cellular, may exhibit mitotic activity, and hugs the glandular epithelium. The stromal cells are malignant and resemble endometrial stromal cells in the proliferative phase of the cycle. One fourth of the patients with adenosarcoma eventually succumb to local recurrence or metastatic spread.

CARCINOSARCOMA (MALIGNANT MIXED MESODERMAL TUMOR): In this mixed tumor, the epithelial and stromal components are both highly malignant. These neoplasms are derived from multipotential stromal cells. If they contain mesenchymal components foreign to the uterus, such as striated muscle, bone, osteoid, cartilage, and fat, they are termed *heterologous*. If the stromal component is present without an admixture of other elements, and thus homologous to the uterus, the tumor is classified as *homologous*. Whether heterologous or homologous, these tumors have many similarities with poorly differentiated adenocarcinoma of the endometrium, and the presence or absence of heterologous elements has no prognostic significance. The overall 5-year survival is 25%.

Leiomyoma

Leiomyoma, defined as a benign tumor of smooth muscle origin, is the most common tumor of the female genital tract. Colloquially, it is also known as a myoma or a fibroid. If minute tumors are included, leiomyomas occur in 75% of women older than 30 years of age. They are rare before age 20, and most regress after the menopause. Although often multiple, each leiomyoma is clonal in origin, a conclusion based on the patterns of glucose-6-phosphate dehydrogenase isoenzymes (see Chapter 5). A genetic predisposition may also exist. Estrogens enhance the growth of leiomyomas, although they do not initiate them.

☐ **Pathology:** Grossly, leiomyomas of the uterus are firm, pale gray, whorled, and without encapsulation (Figs. 18-36 and 18-37A). They range in size from 1 mm to more than 30 cm in diameter. Typically, the cut surface bulges, and the borders are smooth and distinct from the neighboring myometrium. Most leiomyomas are intramural, but some are submucosal, subserosal, or pedunculated. Leiomyomas with low mitotic activity (four or fewer mitoses per 10 high-power fields) and lacking nuclear atypia and coagulative necrosis have little or no malignant potential.

Leiomyomas are composed of interlacing fascicles of uniform spindle cells, in which the nuclei are elongated and have blunt ends (see Fig. 18-37B). The cytoplasm is abundant, eosinophilic, and fibrillar. The myocytes of leiomyomas and adjacent myometrium are cytologically identical, but leiomyomas are easily distinguished by their circumscription, nodularity, and denser cellularity.

☐ **Clinical Features:** Submucosal leiomyomas may cause bleeding, an effect due to ulceration of the thinned, overlying endometrium. Some submucosal leiomyomas pedunculate and protrude through the cervical os, eliciting cramping pains. Many intramural leiomyomas are symptomatic, owing to sheer bulk, and large ones may interfere with bowel or bladder function or cause dystocia in labor. Pedunculated leiomyomas on the serosal surface of the uterus may also interfere with the function of neighboring viscera. If they undergo torsion, they may become infarcted and painful.

Leiomyomas usually grow slowly, but occasionally they increase rapidly in size during pregnancy. Large symptomatic leiomyomas are removed by myomectomy or hysterectomy.

Intravenous Leiomyomatosis

Intravenous leiomyomatosis is a rare condition characterized by the growth of benign smooth muscle within the uterine and pelvic veins. The condition originates either from vascular invasion by a preexisting uterine leiomyoma or as a result of the growth of venous smooth muscle. The condition may be evident at surgery as wormlike extensions near the external uterine surface or as projections into uterine veins in the broad ligament. Despite extensive intravascular growth, these neoplasms do not metastasize. Rare fatalities have resulted from the direct extension of leiomyomatous tissues within pelvic veins into the inferior vena cava and right atrium. Treatment consists of total abdominal hysterectomy.

Leiomyosarcoma

Leiomyosarcoma is a malignancy of smooth muscle origin. This cancer accounts for nearly 2% of uterine malig-

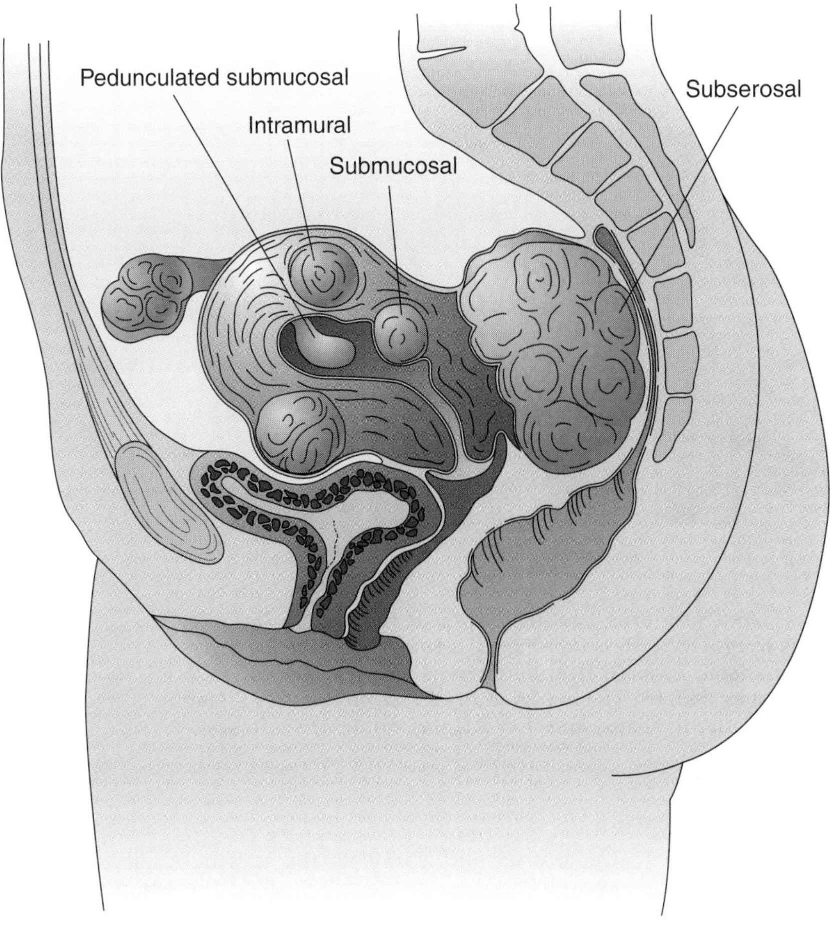

FIGURE 18-36
Leiomyomas of the uterus. The leiomyomas are intramural; submucosal, with a pedunculated one appearing in the form of an endometrial polyp; and subserosal, with one compressing the bladder and the other the rectum.

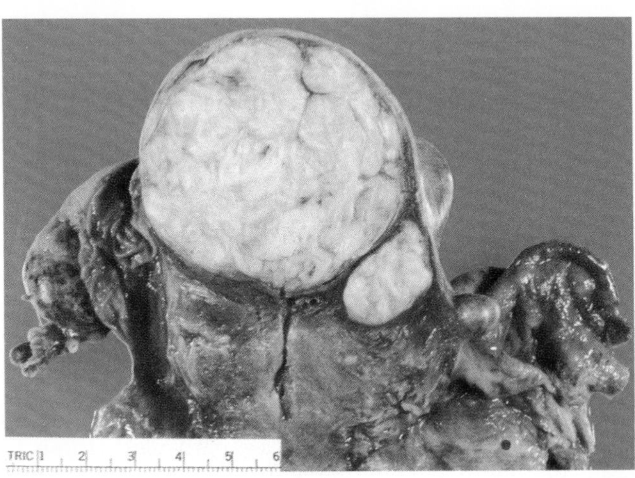

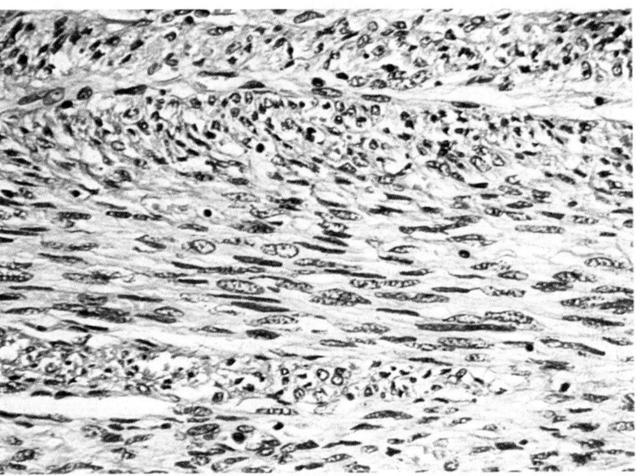

FIGURE 18-37
Leiomyoma of the uterus. (*A*) A bisected uterus displays a prominent, sharply circumscribed, fleshy tumor. (*B*) Microscopically, smooth muscle cells intertwine in bundles, some of which are cut longitudinally (elongated nuclei) and others transversely.

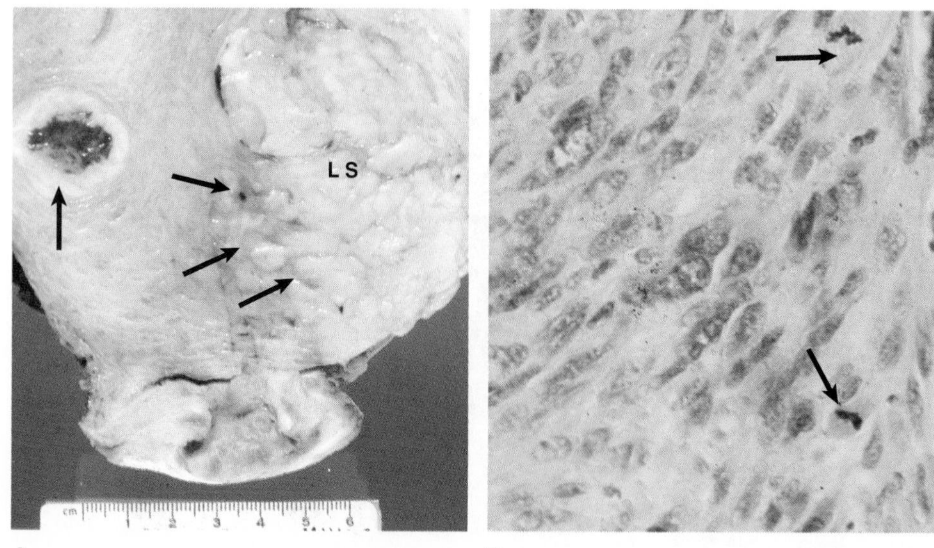

FIGURE 18-38
Leiomyosarcoma of the uterus. (*A*) The uterus has been opened to reveal a large, soft leiomyosarcoma (LS), which has irregular borders (*horizontal arrows*) and invades the surrounding myometrium. By comparison, a small, firm leiomyoma (*vertical arrow*), with a hemorrhagic center, is sharply demarcated. (*B*) The malignant cells are moderately disorganized in arrangement, they are irregular in shape, and they display numerous mitoses (*arrows*).

nancies and is rare in comparison to its benign counterpart (1 : 1000 compared with leiomyoma). The pathogenesis of leiomyosarcoma is uncertain, but some appear to arise from within leiomyomas. Women with leiomyosarcomas are on average more than a decade older (age above 50) than women with leiomyomas, and the malignant tumors are larger (10 to 15 cm versus 3 to 5 cm).

Leiomyosarcoma should be suspected if a "leiomyoma" is soft, shows areas of necrosis on gross examination, has irregular borders (invasion into neighboring myometrium), or does not bulge above the surface when cut (Fig. 18-38). Mitotic activity and cellular atypia are the best diagnostic criteria. Smooth muscle tumors with no mitotic activity are leiomyomas. The following features are considered evidence for the diagnosis of leiomyosarcoma: (1) 10 or more mitoses per 10 high-power fields; (2) 5 or more mitoses per 10 high-power fields and nuclear atypia; and (3) myxoid and epithelioid smooth muscle tumors with 5 or more mitoses per 10 high-power fields. Since most leiomyosarcomas are large and at an advanced stage when detected, they are usually fatal despite combinations of surgery, radiation therapy, and chemotherapy.

Fallopian Tube

ANATOMY

The fallopian tubes extend from the uterine fundus to the ovaries. An interstitial portion lies within the cornua of the uterus and connects the uterine cavity with the straight portion of the tube, called the isthmus. As the tube extends to the ovary, it increases in diameter to form the ampulla, which merges with the infundibulum. The fimbriated end, which opens like the bell of a trumpet, has numerous finger-like extensions. These envelop the ovary and facilitate passage of the ovum from the ruptured graafian follicle. The majority of cells lining the fallopian tube are ciliated and play an important role in transport of the ovum.

SALPINGITIS

Salpingitis refers to inflammation of the fallopian tubes, typically the result of ascending infections of the lower genital tract. The most common causative organisms are *Neisseria gonorrhoeae, Escherichia coli, Chlamydia,* and *Mycoplasma. Clostridium perfringens* and various other anaerobes are less commonly encountered. The infection is typically polymicrobial. The acute episodes, particularly those associated with chlamydial infection, may be asymptomatic. A fallopian tube damaged by prior infection is particularly susceptible to reinfection. In most cases, chronic salpingitis develops only after repeated episodes of acute salpingitis. Uncommonly, salpingitis is a primary infection within the fallopian tube or represents a secondary spread of infection from a nearby perforated viscus, such as the appendix.

☐ **Pathology and Clinical Features:** In acute salpingitis, microscopic examination reveals a marked inflammatory infiltrate of polymorphonuclear leukocytes, in association with pronounced edema and congestion of the mucosal folds (plicae). The inflammatory infiltrate in chronic salpingitis is composed of lymphocytes and plasma cells, and edema and congestion tend to be minimal. In late stages, the fallopian tube may seal and become distended with pus (*pyosalpinx*) or an acellular transudate (*hydrosalpinx*).

The fallopian tube allows ascending microorganisms from the lower genital tract to reach the peritoneal cavity, a journey that leads to peritonitis and PID. Fibrinous adhesions between the serosa of the fallopian tube and surrounding peritoneal surfaces may organize into thin, fibrous adhesions ("violin string" adhesions). The adjacent ovary may also be involved in the process, sometimes giving rise to a *tubo-ovarian abscess*.

Complications also ensue from damage to the fallopian tube itself. Destruction of the epithelium or deposition of fibrin on the mucosal plicae of the fallopian tube results in the formation of fibrin bridges, which cause adherence of the plicae to one another. In severe chronic salpingitis, the adhesions are dense and form a blunted, clubbed end of the tube. The consequence of the blocked lumen may be hydrosalpinx or pyosalpinx. **The damage wrought by chronic salpingitis often poses a mechanical obstruction to the passage of sperm, in which case infertility results. Chronic salpingitis is a common cause of ectopic pregnancy,** since adherent mucosal plicae create pockets in which ova can become entrapped.

ECTOPIC PREGNANCY

Ectopic pregnancy refers to any implantation that develops outside the endometrium. The frequency of this disorder in the United States has increased threefold to 1.5% of live births during the past decade, although mortality has sharply declined. **Over 95% of ectopic pregnancies occur in the fallopian tube, mostly in the distal and middle thirds** (Fig. 18-39). An ectopic pregnancy results when the passage of the conceptus along the fallopian tube is impeded, for example, by mucosal adhesions or abnormal tubal motility secondary to inflammatory disease or endometriosis. The trophoblast readily penetrates the mucosa and wall of the tube. Thus, ectopic pregnancy resembles placenta increta and placenta percreta of the uterus (see later). Blood from the implantation site in the tube enters the peritoneal cavity, causing abdominal pain. In addition, ectopic pregnancy is often associated with anomalous uterine bleeding following a period of amenorrhea. The thin tubal wall usually ruptures by the 12th week of gestation. **Tubal rupture is life-threatening, because it can result in rapidly exsanguinating hemorrhage.**

Rupture of the interstitial portion of the fallopian tube carrying an ectopic pregnancy generally produces greater intra-abdominal hemorrhage than in other locations because the vasculature is richer in that region and the rupture occurs later in gestation. In the isthmus, the tube ruptures early (within the first 6 weeks), because its thick, rigid muscular wall does not allow for much distention. Tubal pregnancies in the ampulla tend to be of longer duration, since the distensible tubal wall can accommodate a growing pregnancy for a longer time.

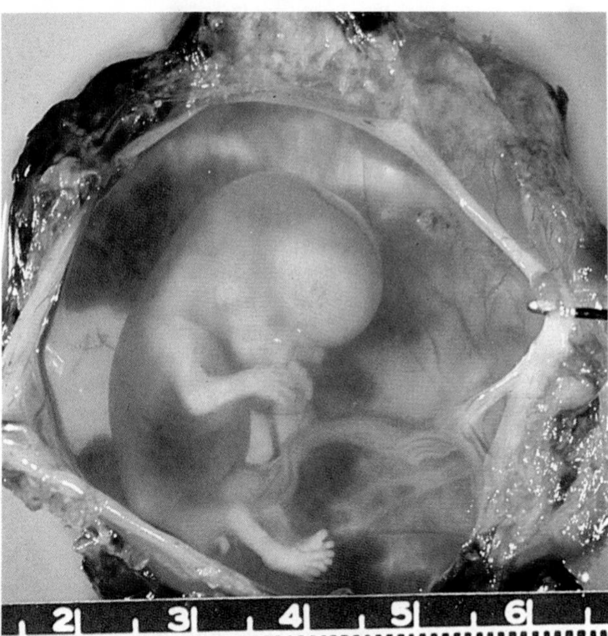

FIGURE *18-39*
Ectopic pregnancy. An enlarged fallopian tube has been opened to disclose a minute fetus.

Ectopic pregnancy should be treated promptly with surgical or chemotherapeutic intervention. The administration of methotrexate terminates ectopic pregnancy and is used when the conceptus is smaller than 4 cm and the tube has not ruptured.

TUMORS

Tumors of the fallopian tube are rare. The most common is the small, circumscribed *adenomatoid tumor*, which is of mesothelial origin. It arises in the mesosalpinx and is composed of benign mesothelial cells that line slitlike spaces.

Tubal involvement by metastases or implants from adjacent ovarian and uterine neoplasms far exceeds the frequency of the rare primary cancer of the fallopian tube. Most primary malignancies are adenocarcinomas, and the peak incidence is in the 50- to 60-year age group. The tumor is bilateral in 25% of cases. The prognosis is poor, because the disease is almost always detected at a late stage.

Ovary

ANATOMY AND EMBRYOLOGY

The ovaries are paired organs that lie on either side of the uterus. They are attached to the posterior surface of the broad ligament in a shallow peritoneal fossa between the external iliac vessels and the ureter. Each ovary is composed of (1) an epithelial surface, (2) a mesenchymal stroma containing steroid-producing cells, and (3) germ cells. It is divided into an outer cortex and an inner medulla.

The ovaries appear early in fetal life as swellings of the genital ridges. At the 19th day of gestation, germ cells migrate from the primitive yolk sac to the gonads and multiply by mitotic division. By the 40th day, the ovaries and testes are histologically distinct. Toward the third trimester of fetal life, the germ cells stop multiplying and instead continue to develop by meiosis. Of the 1 million primordial follicles present at birth, only 70% remain by puberty, and fewer than 15% remain by age 25 years. Only some 450 ova are actually shed during a reproductive lifetime of 35 years.

The mesenchyme of the ovarian cortex consists of spindle-shaped, fibroblast-like cells. These give rise to the granulosa and theca cells, which form the functional unit about each ovum (theca interna and theca externa). The complex of the germ cell and supporting granulosa cells is known first as a primordial follicle. During the reproductive period, a dominant follicle develops every month into a *graafian follicle*, which then ruptures during ovulation. Ovulation itself is often associated with mild cramping pain and, if severe, is called *mittelschmerz* (i.e., mid [cycle] pain). It is not infrequently confused with appendicitis. Following ovulation the granulosa cells of the follicle luteinize, a change characterized by hypertrophy and lipid accumulation, and secrete progesterone in addition to estrogens. The collapsed follicle turns bright yellow and becomes the *corpus luteum* (yellow body).

The cells of ovarian stromal origin include hilus cells and those resembling luteinized cells of the theca interna, both of which respond to pituitary hormones. These specialized cells synthesize and secrete both androgenic and estrogenic hormones, which stimulate proliferation in end-organs, such as the uterus. They inhibit hypothalamic function by negative feedback loops.

CYSTIC LESIONS

Cysts are the most common cause of enlarged ovaries. Excluding cysts that arise from the invaginated surface epithelium of the ovary (serous cysts), almost all arise from ovarian follicles.

Follicle Cyst

Follicle cysts are thin-walled, fluid-filled structures that are lined internally by granulosa cells and externally by a layer of theca interna cells. They occur at any age up to the menopause. Follicular cysts are unilocular and may be single or multiple, unilateral or bilateral. They arise from ovarian follicles and are probably related to abnormalities in the release of pituitary gonadotropins.

Follicle cysts rarely exceed 5 cm in diameter. In an unstimulated state, the granulosa cells have uniform, round nuclei and little cytoplasm. The thecal cells are small and spindle-shaped. Occasionally, the layers may be luteinized, in which case the lumen contains fluid with a high estrogen or progesterone content. If the cyst persists, the hormonal output can lead to precocious puberty in a

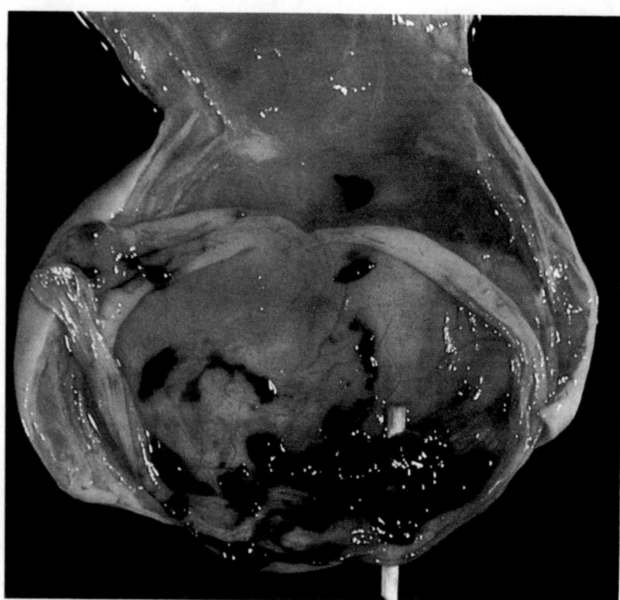

FIGURE *18-40*
Follicle cyst of the ovary. The rupture of this thin-walled follicular cyst (dowel stick) led to intra-abdominal hemorrhage.

child and menstrual irregularities in the adult. The only significant complication is mild intraperitoneal bleeding (Fig. 18-40).

Corpus Luteum Cyst

A corpus luteum cyst results from the delayed resolution of the central cavity of a corpus luteum. Continued progesterone synthesis leads to menstrual irregularities. Rupture of a corpus luteum cyst can cause mild hemorrhage into the abdominal cavity. A corpus luteum cyst is typically unilocular and 3 to 5 cm in diameter, with a yellow wall. The contents of the cyst vary from serosanguineous fluid to clotted blood. Microscopic examination shows numerous, large, luteinized granulosa cells. The condition is usually self-limited.

Theca Lutein Cyst

Theca lutein cysts, also known as hyperreactio luteinalis, are multiple, bilateral, luteinized follicular cysts. They are commonly associated with conditions characterized by high levels of circulating gonadotropin (e.g., pregnancy, hydatidiform mole, choriocarcinoma, and exogenous gonadotropin therapy). The excessive gonadotropin levels lead to exaggerated stimulation of the theca interna and extensive cyst formation. Both ovaries are replaced by multiple thin-walled cysts filled with clear fluid. Microscopically, the cysts show marked luteinization of the theca interna layer. The parenchyma of the ovaries shows edema and foci of luteinized stromal cells. Intra-abdominal hemorrhage secondary to torsion or rupture of the cyst may require surgical intervention.

POLYCYSTIC OVARY SYNDROME

Polycystic ovary syndrome, originally known as Stein-Leventhal syndrome, describes (1) clinical manifestations related to the secretion of excess androgenic hormones, (2) persistent anovulation, and (3) ovaries containing many small subcapsular cysts. It was described initially as a syndrome complex of *secondary amenorrhea, hirsutism, and obesity*. However, it is now recognized that the clinical presentation is far more variable and includes amenorrheic women who appear otherwise normal and, even rarely, have ovaries lacking polycystic features. Up to 7% of women experience the polycystic ovary syndrome, making this condition one of the most common causes of infertility.

☐ **Pathogenesis:** The pathophysiology of the polycystic ovary syndrome is complex and remains to be completely defined. However, it is known that the syndrome represents a state of functional ovarian hyperandrogenism associated with increased levels of luteinizing hormone (LH), although the increase in LH is probably a result rather than a cause of the ovarian dysfunction (Fig. 18-41).

1. The central abnormality is thought to be an increased ovarian production of androgens, although adrenal hypersecretion of androgens may contribute to the clinical manifestations of the disorder. The precise defect responsible for ovarian dysfunction remains elusive, but there is ample evidence for abnormal regulation of the rate-limiting enzyme in the biosynthesis of androgens, namely cytochrome P-$_{450c17\alpha}$ (17α-hydroxylase). This enzyme is expressed in both the ovary and the adrenal gland, and an intrinsic abnormality in its activity could explain androgen hypersecretion in both organs.
2. Excess ovarian androgens act locally to cause premature follicular atresia, multiple follicular cysts, and a persistent anovulatory state. The impairment in follicular maturation results in a lowered secretion of progesterone. Peripherally, hyperandrogenism results in hirsutism, acne, and a male-pattern (androgen-dependent) alopecia.
3. Excess androgens are converted to estrogens in peripheral adipose tissue, an effect that is exaggerated by obesity. Acyclical estrogen production and progesterone deficiency increase the pituitary secretion of LH.
4. Patients with polycystic ovary syndrome exhibit marked peripheral insulin resistance, which is out of proportion to the degree of obesity. The mechanism appears to involve a post–insulin receptor defect, possibly related to decreased expression of a glucose

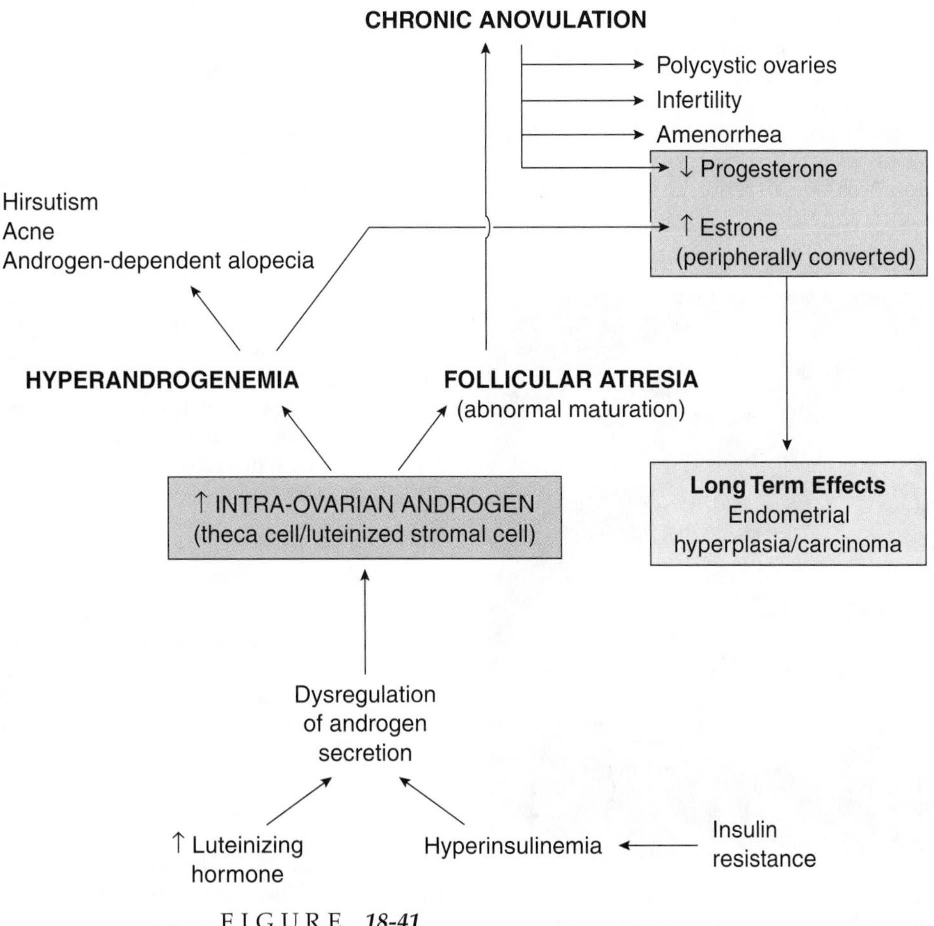

FIGURE *18-41*
Pathogenesis of the polycystic ovary syndrome.

transporter. In any event, the resulting hyperinsulinemia is thought to contribute both to an increase in ovarian hypersecretion of androgens and to a direct stimulation of pituitary LH production.

Pathology: On gross examination, both ovaries are enlarged. The surface is smooth, an appearance reflecting the absence of ovulation. On cut section, the cortex is thickened and discloses numerous cysts, typically 2 to 8 mm in diameter arranged peripherally around a dense core of stroma, or scattered throughout an increased amount of stroma (Fig. 18-42). Microscopically, the following features are present: (1) numerous follicles in early stages of development, (2) follicular atresia, (3) increased stroma, occasionally with luteinized cells (hyperthecosis), and (4) morphological signs of an absence of ovulation (thick, smooth capsule and absence of corpora lutea and corpora albicantiae). Many of the subcapsular cysts are lined by thick zones of theca interna, some cells of which may be luteinized.

□ **Clinical Features:** Infertility afflicts 15% of married couples in the United States. Of those with anovulatory infertility, nearly three quarters have polycystic ovary syndrome. Patients with this disorder are typically in their twenties and give a history of early obesity, menstrual problems, and hirsutism. Half of the women with polycystic ovary syndrome are amenorrheic, whereas most of the others have irregular menstrual periods. Only 75% of affected women are actually infertile, indicating that some of these women do occasionally ovulate. Unopposed acyclic estrogen secretion results in an increased incidence of endometrial hyperplasia and adenocarcinoma.

The treatment of polycystic ovary syndrome encompasses two common problems in reproductive endocrinology—hirsutism and anovulation. Today's therapy is mostly hormonal and is directed toward interruption of the steady state of excess androgen production. Wedge resection of the ovary has also provided temporary remission of the syndrome but is rarely employed today.

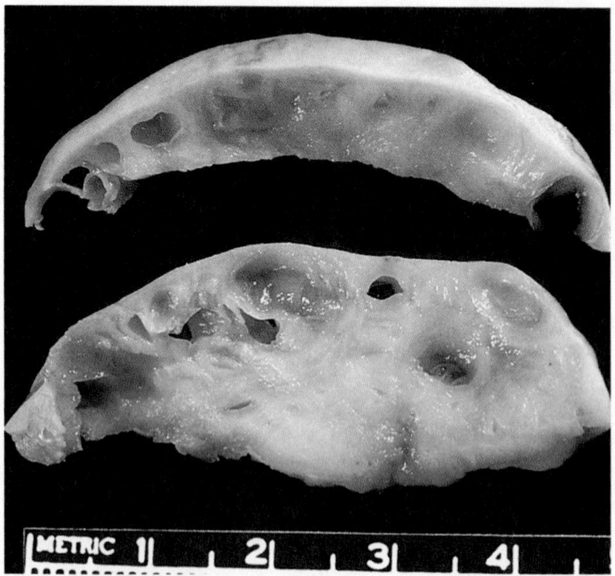

FIGURE 18-42
Polycystic disease of the ovary. Cut sections of an ovary show numerous cysts embedded in a sclerotic stroma.

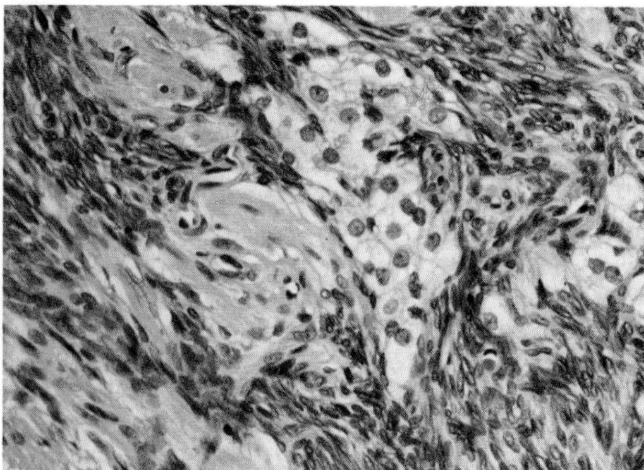

FIGURE 18-43
Hyperthecosis of the ovary. Nests of luteinized (lipid-rich) stromal cells are present.

STROMAL HYPERTHECOSIS

Stromal hyperthecosis refers to focal luteinization of ovarian stromal cells. It is an important condition, since the luteinized stromal cells are often functional and cause virilization. The condition occurs most commonly in postmenopausal women, and, in a microscopic form, it is found in one third of postmenopausal ovaries that are carefully examined.

In women in whom the condition is detected clinically, usually on the basis of masculinizing signs, both ovaries may be enlarged, sometimes up to 8 cm in greatest dimension. The capsule is smooth, and the cut surface is homogeneous, firm, and brown to yellow. Microscopically, single nests or nodules of luteinized stromal cells are present in the cortex or medulla of the ovary (Fig. 18-43). The cytoplasm of these cells is deeply eosinophilic and often vacuolated. The luteinized cells have a central, large nucleus, with a prominent nucleolus.

TUMORS

Cancer of the ovary is the second most frequent gynecological malignancy after endometrial cancer, but in the United States it carries a higher mortality rate than all other genital cancers combined (see Table 18-4). It is difficult to detect this cancer early in its evolution, when it is still curable. More than three fourths of patients already have extragonadal spread of tumor to the pelvis or abdomen at the time of diagnosis.

There are more than 25 major types of ovarian neoplasms. With variants and rare entities, they number nearly 100. The most common malignant tumor, the serous adenocarcinoma (also called serous cystadenocarcinoma), occurs in about 1% of women.

The broad range of histological features displayed by ovarian tumors reflects the diverse anatomical structure of the ovary itself. The classification of ovarian tumors identifies them by the tissue of origin (Fig. 18-44). The most frequently encountered tumors arise from the surface epithelium and are termed *common epithelial tumors*. Other important groups include germ cell tumors, sex cord/stromal tumors, steroid cell tumors, and tumors metastatic to the ovary. About one sixth of ovarian tumors are of a mixed type.

Epithelial Tumors

Tumors of common epithelial origin can be broadly classified as benign, of borderline malignancy (also called atypical proliferating or of low malignant potential), and malignant. They account for over 90% of ovarian cancers and nearly 60% of all ovarian tumors.

☐ **Pathogenesis:** It is generally accepted that most common epithelial tumors arise from the surface epithelium, or serosa, of the ovary. During embryonic life, the celomic cavity is lined by a mesothelium, parts of which become specialized to form the serosal epithelium covering the gonadal ridge. The same mesothelial lining gives rise to the müllerian ducts, from which arise the fallopian tubes, uterus, and vagina.

As the ovary develops, the surface epithelium may extend into the ovarian stroma to form glands and cysts. In some cases, these inclusions become neoplastic and exhibit a variety of müllerian-type differentiations. In order of decreasing frequency, the common epithelial tumors are as follows:

- **Serous tumors,** which resemble the epithelium of the fallopian tube
- **Mucinous tumors,** which mimic the mucosa of the endocervix
- **Endometrioid tumors,** which are similar to the glands of the endometrium
- **Clear cell tumors,** glycogen-rich cells that resemble endometrial glands in pregnancy
- **Transitional cell tumors**

Epidemiological studies suggest that common epithelial neoplasms are associated with the repeated dis-

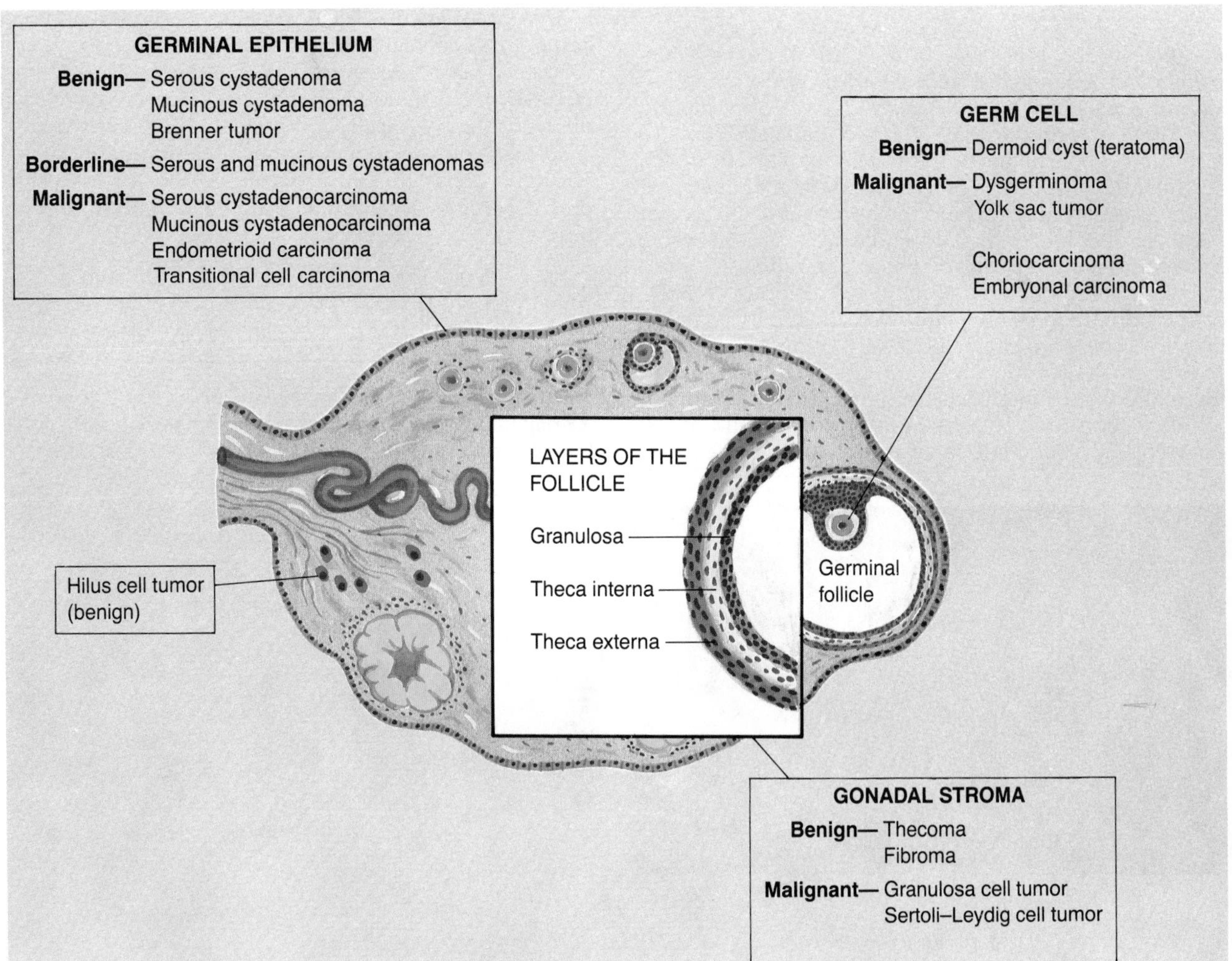

FIGURE *18-44*
Classification of ovarian neoplasms based on cell of origin.

ruption of the epithelial surface that results from cyclic ovulation. Thus, the tumors most commonly afflict women who are nulliparous and, conversely, occur least often in women in whom ovulation has been suppressed (e.g., by pregnancy or oral contraceptives). Irritants such as powder, which is used for feminine hygiene and easily transported up the reproductive tract to come into contact with the ovaries, have also been implicated.

A family history of ovarian carcinoma is occasionally elicited. Women with a first-degree relative with ovarian cancer have a 3.5-fold increased risk of developing the same disease. Women who have a history of ovarian carcinoma are also at greater risk for breast cancer, and vice versa. The same gene implicated in hereditary breast cancers, namely *BRCA-1* (17q12-q23), has been incriminated in the pathogenesis of familial ovarian cancers. As noted for endometrial carcinoma, women who suffer from hereditary nonpolyposis colon cancer are also at greater risk for ovarian cancer. Women who bear the *BRCA-1* gene or the one for hereditary nonpolyposis colon cancer tend to develop ovarian cancer considerably earlier than women who have sporadic ovarian cancer, but their prognosis appears to be considerably better.

Benign Epithelial Tumors

Benign common epithelial tumors are almost always serous or mucinous and generally arise in women between the ages of 20 and 60 years. They are frequently large, often growing to 15 to 30 cm in diameter. Some of these tumors, particularly the mucinous variety, reach truly massive proportion, exceeding 50 cm in diameter, in which case they may mimic the appearance of a term pregnancy. Benign epithelial tumors are typically cystic, hence the term *cystadenoma*. Serous cystadenomas are more commonly bilateral (15%) than mucinous cystadenomas and tend to be unilocular (Fig. 18-45). By contrast, *mucinous tumors* are characteristically composed of hundreds of small cysts (locules) (Fig. 18-46). As opposed to their malignant counterparts, benign epithelial tumors of the ovary tend to have thin walls and lack solid areas. Microscopically, a single layer of tall columnar epithelium lines the cysts. Papillae, when present, consist of a fibrovascular core covered by a single layer of tall columnar epithelium identical to that of the cyst lining.

PSEUDOMYXOMA PERITONEI: *Pseudomyxoma peritonei is a condition characterized by implants of mucus-producing cells on the peritoneal surfaces.* These result in the massive accumulation of gelatinous material in the abdominal cavity. During the past few years, it has been documented that many, if not most, of these tumors actually arise from the appendix, rather than from the ovary, as was originally thought. This subject, however, remains controversial. The peritoneal implants are composed of well-differentiated, mucous, columnar cells, without atypism or mitoses, thus resembling borderline tumors of the ovary (see later). Implants that histologically resemble adenocarcinoma most often arise from appendiceal cancers. Treatment of pseudomyxoma peritonei is primarily surgical and usually requires repetitive operations. Intraperitoneal alkylating agents have also been used successfully. The 5-year survival rate is less than 50%.

Transitional Cell Tumor (Brenner Tumor)

Brenner tumor, unlike other common epithelial tumors, has two components. The typical Brenner tumor is benign and occurs at all ages, with half of the cases presenting in women over 50 years of age. The size varies from a microscopic focus to masses as large as 8 cm or more in diameter. Histologically, Brenner tumor is composed of solid nests of transitional-like (urothelium-like) cells encased in a dense, fibrous stroma (Fig. 18-47). The most superficial epithelial cells may exhibit mucinous differentiation.

Borderline Tumors (Tumors of Low Malignant Potential)

The designation of borderline malignancy refers to a group of ovarian tumors that share an excellent prognosis, despite certain histological features that suggest cancer. A surgical cure is al-

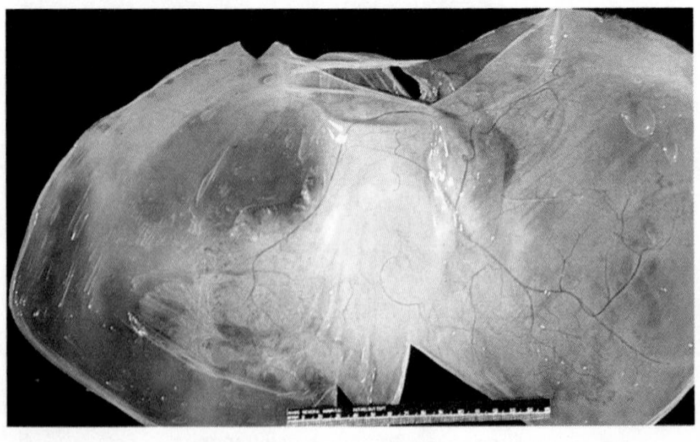

A

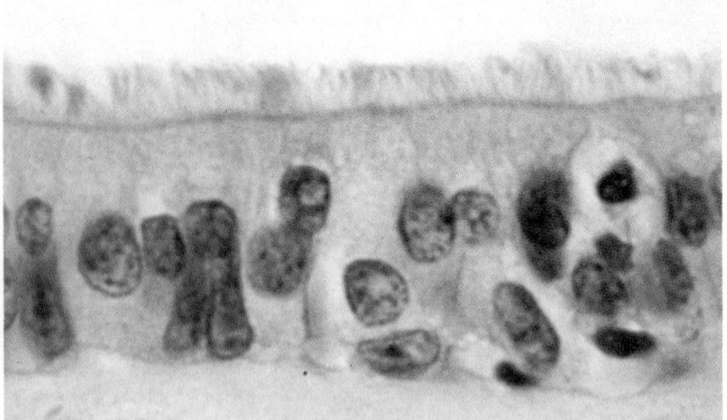

B

FIGURE *18-45*
Serous cystadenoma of the ovary. (*A*) The fluid has been removed from this huge, unilocular serous cystadenoma. The wall is thin and translucent. (*B*) On microscopic examination, the cyst is lined by a single layer of ciliated tubal-type epithelium.

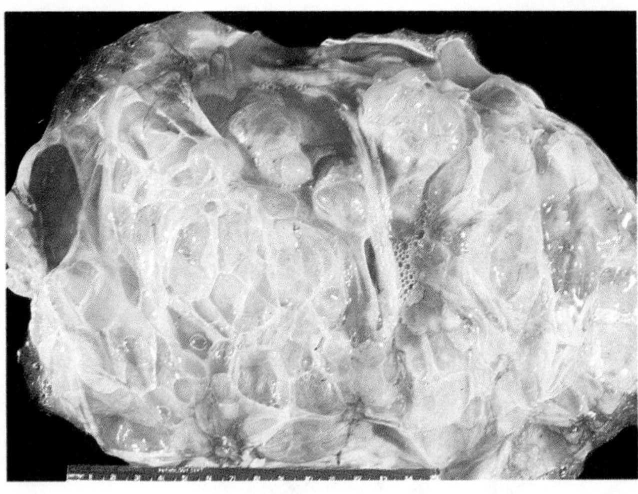

A

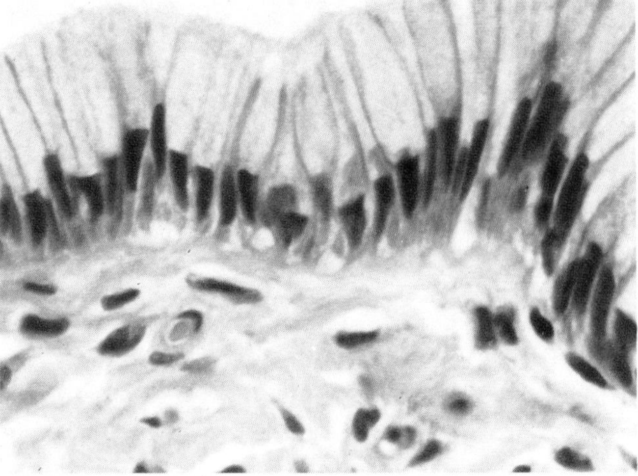

B

FIGURE *18-46*
Mucinous cystadenoma of the ovary. (*A*) The tumor is characterized by numerous cysts filled with thick, viscous fluid. (*B*) A single layer of mucinous epithelial cells lines the cyst.

most always possible if the tumor is confined to the ovaries. Even when it has spread to the pelvis or abdomen, 80% of patients are alive after 5 years, although there is a significant rate of late recurrence. Borderline tumors generally occur in women between the ages of 20 and 40 years but may also be encountered in older women.

Serous tumors of borderline malignancy are more commonly bilateral (34%) than mucinous ones (6%) or other types. The tumors are of variable size. Mucinous tumors sometimes achieve gigantic size (100+ kg). In serous tumors of borderline malignancy, it is common to find papillary projections, ranging from fine and exuberant to clusters of grapelike structures arising from one or several sites on the cyst wall (Fig. 18-48). Microscopically, these structures resemble the papillary fronds in benign cystadenomas, but they are distinguished from them by (1) epithelial stratification, (2) nuclear atypism, and (3) mitotic activity. The same criteria apply to borderline mucinous tumors, although papillary projections are less conspicuous. **By definition, the presence of more than focal microinvasion by the primary tumor removes it from the category of borderline malignancy and identifies it as frankly malignant.**

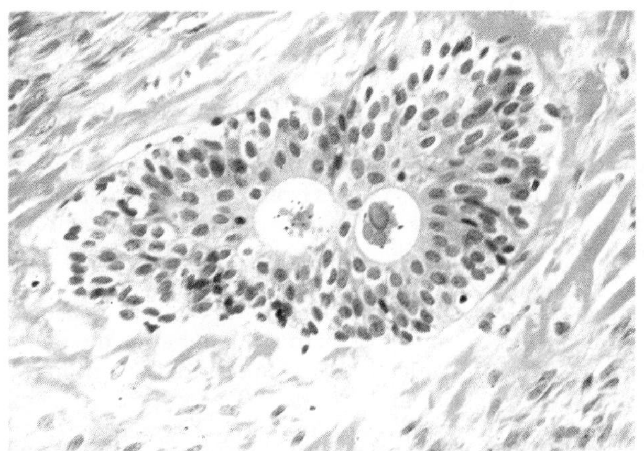

FIGURE *18-47*
Brenner tumor. A nest of transitional-like cells is embedded in a dense, fibrous stroma.

PERITONEAL LESIONS OF SEROUS EPITHELIUM: Primary peritoneal tumors that resemble ovarian serous cystadenoma of borderline malignancy (also called peritoneal serous micropapillomatosis of low malignant potential) are well described, although controversy as to their histogenesis persists. There is evidence that borderline tumors can arise *de novo* from the peritoneal surface, but only in a small proportion of cases (possibly as low as 3%). In most patients, peritoneal serous tumors appear to be implants from an ovarian epithelial tumor.

Malignant Epithelial Tumors

Malignant epithelial tumors of the ovary are most common between the ages of 40 and 60 years and are rare under the age of 35. By the time a carcinoma reaches a size of 10 to 15 cm, it often has already spread beyond the ovary and seeded the peritoneum.

SEROUS CYSTADENOCARCINOMA: Serous cystadenocarcinoma is the most common malignant ovarian tumor, accounting for a third of all cancers of the ovary. Since tumors of advanced stage are bilateral more than twice as often as tumors of low stage, it is thought that in many cases the cancer spreads to the other ovary by implantation. Two thirds of serous cancers that have spread beyond the confines of the ovary are bilateral. On gross examination, serous cystadenocarcinomas usually present as multiloculated tumors, with soft, delicate papillae lining the entire surface. Solid areas, often with areas of necrosis and hemorrhage, are commonly present (Fig. 18-49).

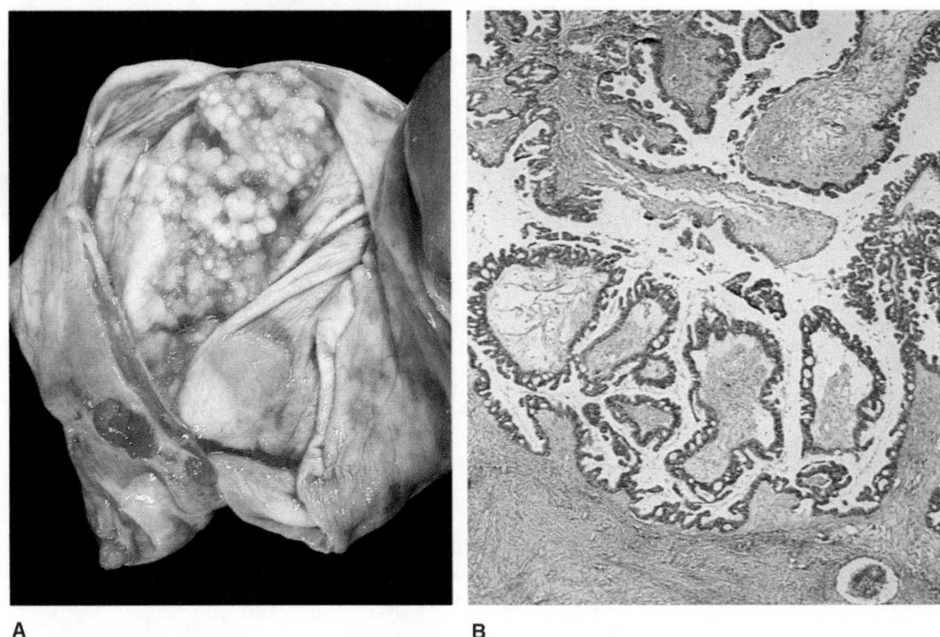

FIGURE *18-48*
Serous ovarian tumor of borderline malignancy. (*A*) Papillary excrescences project from the cyst wall. (*B*) A microscopic view demonstrates the papillary structure of the tumor.

Microscopically, serous cystadenocarcinomas vary from well-differentiated to poorly differentiated tumors. In the latter, the papillary pattern may be inconspicuous, with most areas being composed of solid sheets of malignant cells. Stromal and capsular invasion by the tumor cells is evident. Laminated calcified concretions, referred to as *psammoma bodies*, are present in one third of the cases (see Fig. 18-49c).

MUCINOUS CYSTADENOCARCINOMA: Mucinous cystadenocarcinomas constitute up to 10% of all ovarian cancers. In one sixth of cases in which the tumor is confined to the ovary, the tumor is bilateral. Mucinous cancers are typically cystic and multilocular, with many solid areas and papillary projections. Microscopically, as in serous cancers, the appearance ranges from well differentiated to poorly differentiated. The well-differentiated tumors are characterized by neoplastic glands lined by tall columnar, mucin-producing, malignant cells (Fig. 18-50). Poorly differentiated mucinous adenocarcinomas show irregular nests and cords of tumor cells and numerous mitoses. Stromal invasion is the rule, and infiltration of the capsule is common.

ENDOMETRIOID ADENOCARCINOMA: Endometrioid adenocarcinoma is a tumor of the ovary that histologically is identical to carcinoma of the endometrium. It is second only to serous cystadenocarcinoma in frequency, accounting for 20% of all ovarian cancers. The tumor occurs most commonly after the menopause. In contrast to serous and mucinous neoplasms, most endometrioid tumors are malignant. One third to one half of endometrioid carcinomas are bilateral.

On gross examination, endometrioid carcinomas vary in size from 2 cm to more than 30 cm in diameter. They tend to be cystic, although some are completely solid, and exhibit necrotic areas. Microscopically, the tumors are graded according to the same scheme used for endometrial adenocarcinoma. Interestingly, a concomitant endometrial cancer is frequently encountered, the rates in various series ranging from 15% to 50%. The favorable outcome in many cases of such synchronous tumors and the focal nature of many of the uterine neoplasms strongly suggest that both the ovarian and endometrial cancers arise independently, rather than as metastases from one or the other. As with all other forms of epithelial tumors, the prognosis depends on the stage at which the tumor presents.

CLEAR CELL ADENOCARCINOMA: Clear cell adenocarcinoma, which is thought to be closely related to endometrioid adenocarcinoma, is often found in association with endometriosis. It constitutes 5% to 10% of all ovarian cancers, usually occurring after the menopause. The size of the tumors ranges from 2 to 30 cm in diameter, and 40% are bilateral. The majority are partially cystic and exhibit necrosis and hemorrhage in the solid areas.

Microscopically, clear cell adenocarcinoma is composed of sheets of malignant cells with clear cytoplasm, or tubules lined by cancer cells. In the latter case, the malignant cells often display bulbous nuclei that protrude into the lumen of the tubule (*hobnail cell*), an appearance similar to the Arias-Stella reaction in the gestational endometrium. The microscopic appearance of clear cell adenocarcinoma of the ovary resembles that of its counterpart in the vagina. The clinical course parallels that of endometrioid carcinoma.

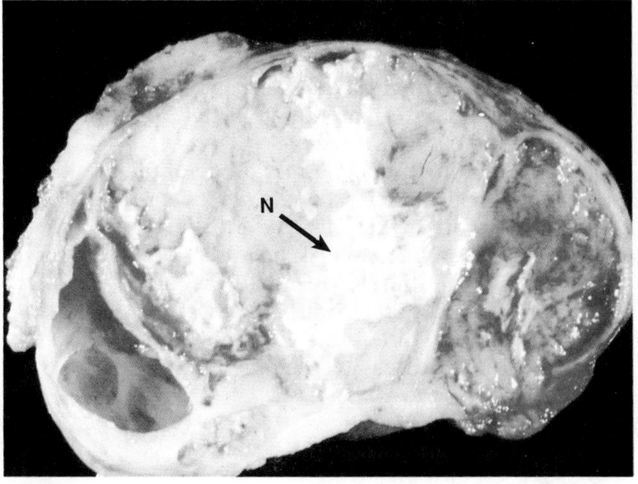

A

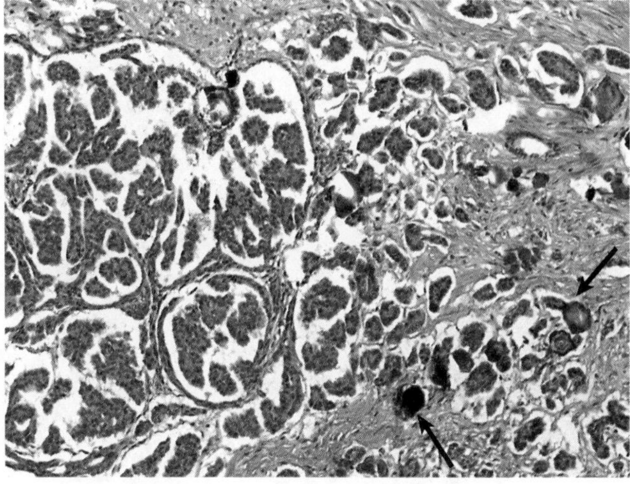

B

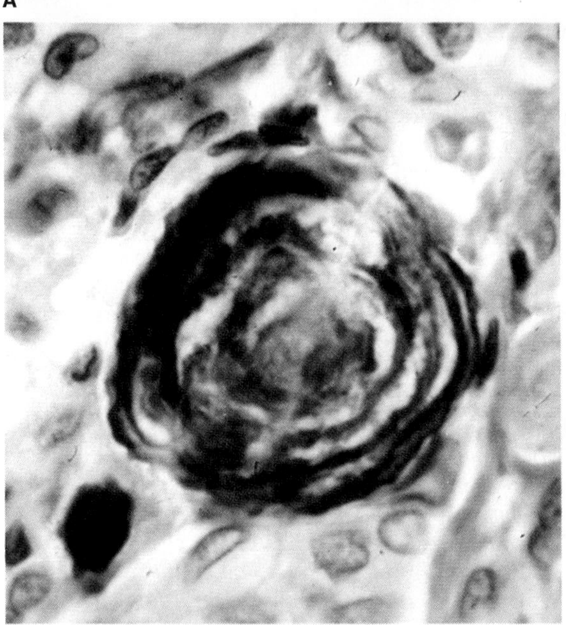

C

FIGURE *18-49*
Serous cystadenocarcinoma. (*A*) The ovary is enlarged by a solid tumor, which exhibits extensive necrosis (*N*). (*B*) Microscopic examination shows a papillary cancer invading the ovarian stroma. Several psammoma bodies are present (*arrows*). (*C*) A higher-power view shows the laminated structure of a psammoma body.

☐ **Clinical Features:** The vast majority of ovarian tumors are nonfunctional, that is, they do not secrete hormones. However, an antibody (OC-125) to a cancer antigen (CA-125) in the serum detects about half of the epithelial tumors that are still confined to the ovary and about 90% that have already spread. The specificity of this test is near 90%, whereas the sensitivity is about 75%. Ovarian masses rarely cause symptoms until they are large. When they distend the abdomen, they cause pain, pelvic pressure, or compression of regional organs. By the time the tumors are diagnosed, many have metastasized (implanted) to the surfaces of the pelvis, abdominal organs, or bladder. In addition to specific symptoms, metastatic cancers are associated with ascites, weakness, weight loss, and cachexia.

Evaluation of a patient with an ovarian cancer of epithelial origin requires an intimate knowledge of staging, grading, and routes of spread of the tumor. For example, ovarian tumors have a tendency to implant in the peritoneal cavity on the diaphragm, paracolic gutters, and omentum. Lymphatic dissemination carries malignant cells preferentially to the para-aortic lymph nodes near the origin of the renal arteries and to a lesser extent to the external iliac (pelvic) or inguinal lymph nodes.

In general, survival for patients with malignant ovarian tumors is poor. The single most important prognostic index is the surgical stage of the tumor at the time it is first detected (Table 18-10). Overall, the 5-year survival is only 35%, because more than half the tumors have spread to the abdominal cavity (stage 3), or elsewhere, by the time they are discovered. Important prognostic indices for epithelial tumors also include grade and histological type and the size of the residual neoplasm. Cell kinetics, DNA profiles, and possibly morphometric analysis are becoming of prognostic significance.

The cornerstone to the management of ovarian cancer is surgery. It not only removes the primary tumor but also is important in establishing the diagnosis and assessing

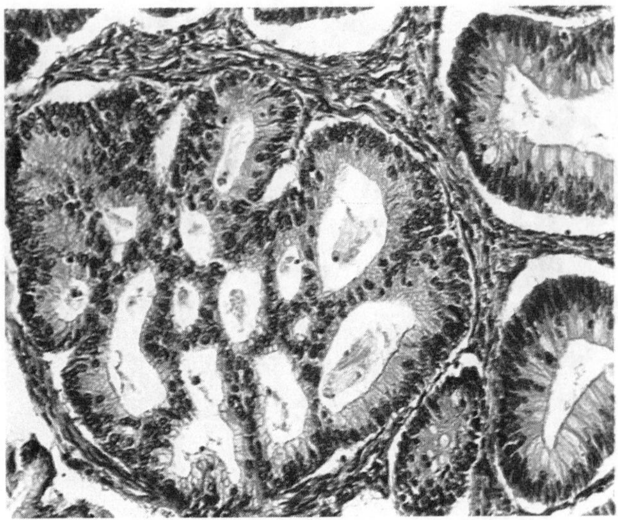

FIGURE *18-50*
Mucinous cystadenocarcinoma. The malignant glands are arranged in a cribriform pattern and are composed of mucin-producing columnar cells.

TABLE *18-10* **Clinical Staging of Ovarian Cancer**

Stage	Description
I	Limited to ovaries; capsule intact; no tumor on the external surface
Ia	Limited to one ovary; ascitic fluid, if present, lacks malignant cells
Ib	Limited to both ovaries; capsule intact; no tumor on the external surface; ascitic fluid, if present, lacks malignant cells
Ic	Any of above, but with ascites or positive peritoneal washings
II	With pelvic extension
IIa	Extension or metastases to uterus or tubes
IIb	Extension to other pelvic tissues
IIc	Any of above, but with ascites or positive peritoneal washings
III	With intraperitoneal metastases outside the pelvis, or positive retroperitoneal nodes, or both. Tumor limited to true pelvis with histologically proven malignant extension to small bowel or omentum.
IIIa	Microscopic seeding on abdominal peritoneal surface
IIIb	Implants $\leq$2 cm on abdominal peritoneal surface
IIIc	Implants >2 cm on abdominal peritoneal surface
IV	With distant metastases. If pleural effusion present, positive cytology required. Liver metastases must be parenchymal.

the extent of spread. At laparotomy, the surgeon is required to examine the peritoneal surfaces, omentum, liver, subdiaphragmatic recesses, and all abdominal regions so as to remove as much of the metastatic tumor as possible. Adjuvant chemotherapy is used to treat distant occult sites of tumor spread.

At some time after the initial operation, another exploratory laparotomy (second-look laparotomy) is used in some institutions to assess the effectiveness of therapy. However, even when no residual disease is apparent, one third of older patients eventually develop later recurrences. Risk factors for recurrence include (1) high-stage tumor, (2) poorly differentiated tumor, and (3) more than 2 cm of residual disease remaining after the primary operation.

Germ Cell Tumors

Tumors derived from the germ cells of the ovary constitute a fourth of all ovarian tumors. In adult women, germ cell tumors are virtually all benign (mature cystic teratoma, dermoid cyst), whereas in children and young adults, they are largely malignant. In children, germ cell tumors are the most common form of ovarian cancer (60%); they are rare after the menopause.

The neoplastic germ cell may follow one of several lines of differentiation, giving rise to tumors analogous to those found in the male testis (Fig. 18-51). *Dysgerminoma* is a tumor composed of neoplastic germ cells, resembling the oogonia of the fetal ovary. Tumors that differentiate toward somatic (embryonic) tissues are *teratomas*. When extraembryonic differentiation of a tumor provides a resemblance to the placental mesenchyme or its precursors, a *yolk sac tumor* results. When differentiation leads to cells similar to those covering the placental villi, the tumor is termed *choriocarcinoma*.

The age of the patient provides a clue to the tumor type. Tumors in infants tend to be solid and immature (e.g., yolk sac tumor and immature teratoma). Tumors in young adults show greater differentiation, as in the mature cystic teratoma. Malignant germ cell tumors in women older than 40 years of age usually result from the transformation of one of the components of a benign cystic teratoma.

Malignant germ cell tumors are usually highly aggressive. At one time, solid germ cell tumors of the ovary were uniformly fatal, but with the advent of chemotherapy, survival rates for many exceed 80%.

Dysgerminoma

Dysgerminoma is the ovarian counterpart of testicular seminoma and is composed of primordial germ cells. Although it accounts for less than 2% of all ovarian cancers, dysgerminoma is responsible for 10% of these cancers in women younger than 20 years of age. Most patients are between 10 and 30 years of age. The tumors are bilateral in about 15% of cases.

On gross examination, dysgerminomas are often large and firm and have a bosselated external surface. The

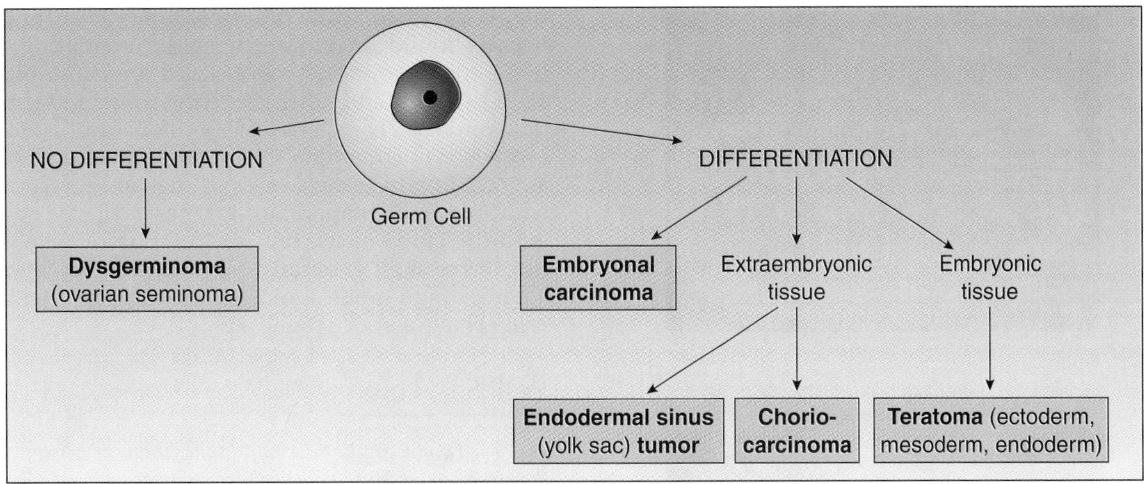

FIGURE 18-51
Classification of germ cell tumors of the ovary.

cut surface is soft and fleshy. Microscopic examination reveals large nests of monotonous tumor cells, which have a clear glycogen-filled cytoplasm and irregularly flattened central nuclei (Fig. 18-52). Fibrous septa containing lymphocytes traverse the tumor.

Dysgerminoma is treated surgically. The 5-year survival rate for patients with stage I tumors approaches 100%. Because the tumor is highly radiosensitive, 5-year survival rates for higher-stage tumors exceed 80%.

Teratoma

Teratoma is a tumor of germ cell origin that shows differentiation toward somatic structures. Most teratomas contain tissues representing at least two, and usually all three, embryonic layers.

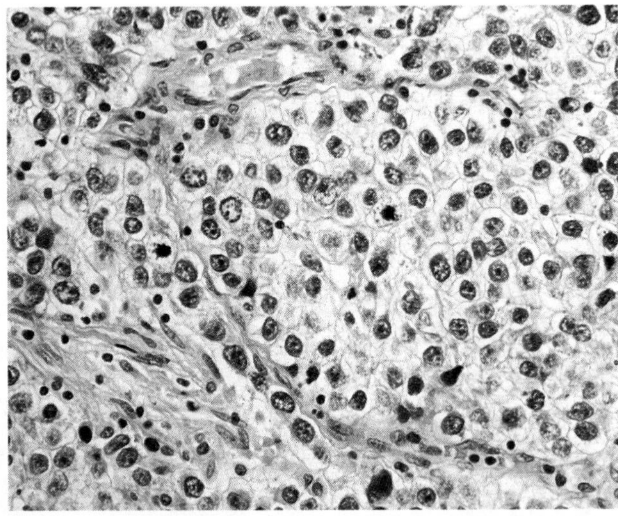

FIGURE 18-52
Dysgerminoma. The neoplastic germ cells have clear, glycogen-filled cytoplasm and central nuclei. Fibrous septa containing lymphocytes traverse the tumor.

MATURE TERATOMA (MATURE CYSTIC TERATOMA, DERMOID CYST): The most common germ cell tumor, the mature cystic teratoma (dermoid cyst) is a benign neoplasm, which accounts for one fourth of all ovarian tumors. The peak incidence occurs in the third decade. Mature teratomas develop by parthenogenesis: haploid (postmeiotic) germ cells autofertilize to give rise to diploid tumor cells that are genetically female (46,XX).

The tumor is cystic, and more than 90% contain skin, sebaceous glands, and hair follicles (Fig. 18-53). Half of the tumors exhibit smooth muscle, sweat glands, cartilage, bone, teeth, and respiratory tract epithelium. Tissues such as gut, thyroid, and brain are encountered less frequently. Nodular foci in the cyst wall (mammary tubercles or Rokitansky nodules), when present, contain the tissue elements of the three germ cell layers. These are (1) ectoderm (e.g., skin and glia), (2) mesoderm (e.g., smooth muscle or cartilage), and (3) endoderm (e.g., respiratory epithelium).

Struma ovarii refers to a cystic lesion composed predominantly of thyroid tissue (5% to 20% of mature cystic teratomas). It is not clear in some of these tumors whether thyroid tissue has overgrown all other elements or whether only thyroid tissue initially developed. Rare cases of hyperthyroidism have been associated with struma ovarii.

A small minority (1%) of dermoid cysts undergo malignant transformation. These cancers usually occur in older women and correspond to the tumors that arise in other differentiated tissues of the body. Three fourths of all cancers that arise in dermoid cysts are squamous cell carcinomas. The remainder include carcinoid tumor, basal cell carcinoma, thyroid cancer, adenocarcinoma, and others. In rare cases, derivatives of the gut may be functional, producing the carcinoid syndrome. The overall prognosis of patients with malignant transformation of a mature cystic teratoma is variable and related largely to

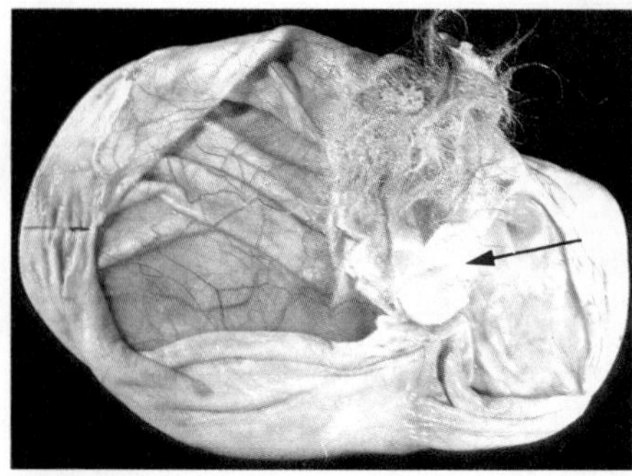

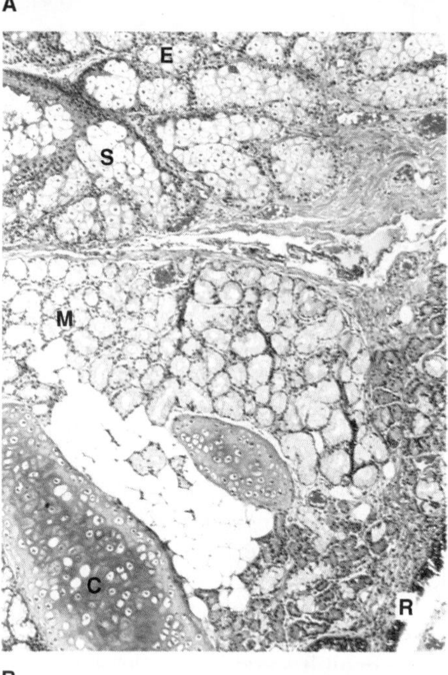

FIGURE 18-53
Mature cystic teratoma of the ovary. (*A*) A mature cystic teratoma has been opened to reveal a solid knob (*arrow*) from which hair projects. (*B*) A photomicrograph of the solid knob shows epidermal and respiratory components. Tissue resembling the skin shows an epidermis (E) with underlying sebaceous glands (S). The respiratory tissue consists of mucous glands (M), cartilage (C), and respiratory epithelium (R).

whether the cancer is confined to the ovary at the time of initial diagnosis.

IMMATURE TERATOMA: Immature teratoma of the ovary is composed of elements derived from the three germ layers. However, unlike mature cystic teratoma, immature teratoma contains immature or embryonal tissues. The pathogenesis of these tumors is unknown. Immature teratoma accounts for 20% of malignant tumors at all sites in women younger than the age of 20 years and becomes progressively less common in older women.

Immature teratoma is predominantly solid and lobulated and contains numerous small cysts. The solid areas may contain grossly recognizable immature bone and cartilage. Microscopically, multiple tumor components are usually found, including those differentiating toward nerve (neuroepithelial rosettes and immature glia) (Fig. 18-54), glands, and other structures found in mature cystic teratomas. The metastases in immature teratoma are composed of embryonal tissues, unlike mature cystic teratomas, in which metastases, if they arise, resemble the adult-type malignancy. Survival has been well correlated with the grade of the tumor. Well-differentiated immature teratomas generally have a favorable outcome, whereas high-grade tumors (predominantly embryonal tissue) have a poor prognosis.

Yolk Sac Tumor

Yolk sac tumor is a highly malignant tumor of women younger than the age of 30 years that histologically resembles the mesenchyme of the primitive yolk sac. Typically, the yolk sac tumor is large and displays extensive necrosis and hemorrhage. Microscopic examination reveals multiple patterns. The most common appearance is a reticular, honeycombed pattern of communicating spaces lined by primitive cells. *Schiller-Duval bodies* (Fig. 18-55), which resemble the endodermal sinuses of the rodent placenta, are found sparingly in over half of tumors and are characteristic of the tumor. These structures consist of papillae that protrude into a space lined by tumor cells. The papillae are covered by a mantle of embryonal cells and contain a fibrovascular core and a central blood vessel.

Yolk sac tumor should not be confused with embryonal cell carcinoma, which is common in the testis. The former secretes α-fetoprotein, which can be demonstrated histochemically within eosinophilic droplets. Detection of α-fetoprotein in the blood is useful both for diagnosis and for monitoring the effectiveness of therapy. Prior to the era of chemotherapy, the yolk sac tumor was nearly al-

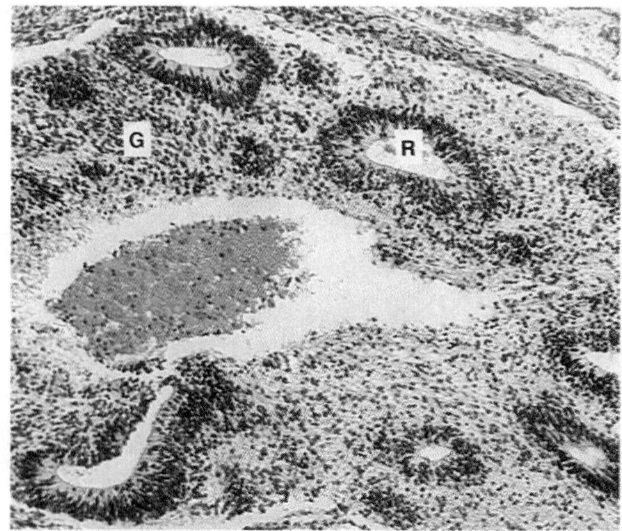

FIGURE 18-54
Immature teratoma of the ovary. Immature neural tissue exhibits rosettes (R) with multilayered nuclei. Embryonal glia (G) display densely packed, atypical nuclei.

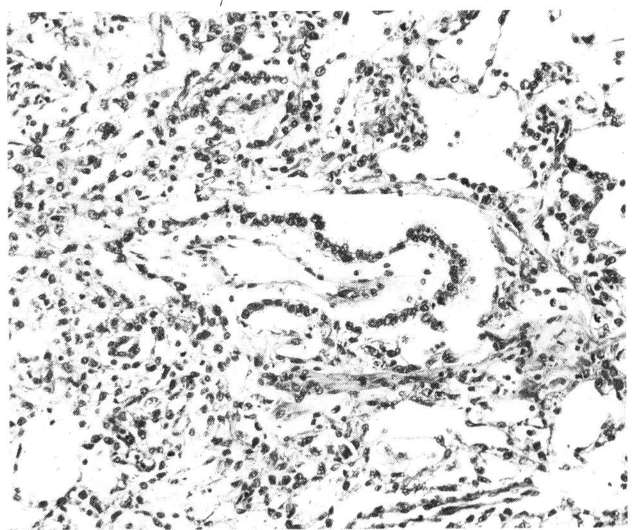

FIGURE 18-55
Endodermal sinus tumor (yolk sac carcinoma) of the ovary. The tumor cells are arrayed in a reticular pattern, and a Schiller-Duval body is present in the center. The latter resembles the endodermal sinuses of the rodent placenta and consists of a papilla protruding into a space lined by tumor cells.

ways fatal. Now 5-year survival rates exceed 80% for stage I tumors.

Choriocarcinoma

Choriocarcinoma of the ovary is a rare tumor that mimics the epithelial covering of placental villi, namely, cytotrophoblast and syncytiotrophoblast. A derivation from ovarian germ cells is assumed if the tumor arises before puberty or in combination with another germ cell tumor. On the other hand, in women of reproductive age, choriocarcinoma of the ovary may also represent a metastasis from an intrauterine gestational tumor. Choriocarcinoma of germ cell origin generally presents in young girls as precocious sexual development, menstrual irregularities, or rapid breast enlargement.

Choriocarcinoma of the ovary is unilateral, solid, and extensively hemorrhagic. Microscopically, it is composed of an admixture of malignant cytotrophoblasts and syncytiotrophoblasts (see Fig. 18-56). The syncytial cells secrete hCG, which accounts for the frequent finding of a positive pregnancy test. Bilateral theca lutein cysts, which result from the hCG stimulation, may also be found. Serial determinations of serum hCG levels are useful both for diagnosis and follow-up. The tumor is highly aggressive but is responsive to chemotherapy.

Gonadoblastoma

Gonadoblastoma is a rare ovarian tumor, which is distinctive because of its association with various types of gonadal dysgenesis, especially in women who bear a Y chromosome. It is seen in phenotypic women younger than 30 years of age, although 20% occur in phenotypic men with cryptorchidism, hypospadias, and female internal sex organs. The majority of affected women are virilized and suffer from primary amenorrhea and developmental abnormalities of the genitalia. The tumor is solid and often exhibits extensive calcification. Microscopically, the cellular nests are composed of a mixture of germ cells and sex cord derivatives which resemble immature Sertoli and granulosa cells, for which reason some considered the tumor to be an *in situ* form of germinoma. In half the cases, the gonadoblastoma is overgrown by dysgerminoma. The gonadoblastoma itself does not metastasize; its overgrowths do.

Sex Cord/Stromal Tumors

Tumors of the sex cord and stroma are derived from either the primitive sex cords or the mesenchymal stroma of the developing gonad. They account for 10% of all ovarian tumors. The tumors range from benign to low-grade malignant and frequently differentiate toward female (granulosa and theca cells) or male (Sertoli and Leydig cells) structures. **Sex cord/stromal tumors account for most of the clinically functional ovarian tumors.**

Fibroma

Fibromas are the most common ovarian stromal tumors (76% of all stromal tumors and 7% of all ovarian tumors). They occur at all ages, with a peak in the perimenopausal period, and are virtually always benign. The tumors are solid, firm, and white (Fig. 18-56). Microscopically, the cells resemble the stroma of the normal ovarian cortex, being composed of well-differentiated fibroblasts and variable amounts of collagen. Half of the larger tumors are associated with ascites and, rarely, with ascites and pleural effusions (*Meigs syndrome*).

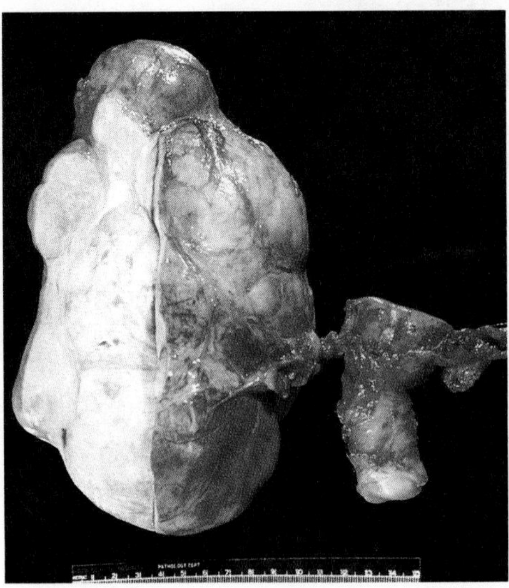

FIGURE 18-56
Fibroma of the ovary. The ovary is conspicuously enlarged by a firm, white, bosselated tumor.

Thecoma

Thecomas are functional ovarian tumors that arise in postmenopausal women. In the majority of cases, they produce signs of estrogen production. Thecomas are solid tumors, mostly 5 to 10 cm in diameter. The cut section is yellow, owing to the presence of many lipid-laden theca cells. Microscopically, the cells are large and oblong to round, with a vacuolated cytoplasm that contains lipid. Bands of hyalinized collagen separate nests of theca cells. Thecomas are virtually always benign. Because of estrogen output by the tumor, thecomas commonly cause irregularity in menstrual cycles and breast enlargement. Endometrial hyperplasia or cancer may be complications of the tumor.

Granulosa Cell Tumor

Granulosa cell tumor is the prototypical functional neoplasm of the ovary associated with estrogen secretion. This tumor should be considered malignant because of its potential for local spread and the rare occurrence of distant metastases. Most granulosa cell tumors occur after the menopause, and they are unusual before puberty. In contrast to common epithelial tumors, in which repeated ovulation is a contributing factor, there is experimental evidence that the development of granulosa cell tumors is linked to the loss of oocytes. Oocytes appear to regulate granulosa cells, and tumorigenesis occurs when the follicles are disorganized or atretic.

☐ **Pathology:** Granulosa cell tumors, like most ovarian tumors, are large and focally cystic to solid. Characteristically, the tumor has yellow areas, representing lipid-laden luteinized granulosa cells, white zones of stroma, and focal hemorrhages (Fig. 18-57A). Microscopically, granulosa cell tumors display an array of growth patterns: (1) diffuse (sarcomatoid), (2) insular (islands of cells), or (3) trabecular (anastomotic bands of granulosa cells). Haphazard orientation of the nuclei about a central degenerative space (*Call-Exner bodies*) results in a characteristic follicular pattern (see Fig. 18-57B). The tumor cells are typically spindle shaped and commonly have a cleaved, elongated nucleus (coffee bean appearance).

☐ **Clinical Features: Three fourths of granulosa cell tumors are functional, that is, they secrete estrogens.** Consequently, endometrial hyperplasia is a common presenting sign. Hyperplasia may progress to endometrial adenocarcinoma, if the functioning granulosa cell tumor remains undetected. When detected clinically, 90% of granulosa cell tumors are confined to the ovary (stage I). These patients have a greater than 90% 10-year survival. Tumors that have extended into the pelvis and lower abdomen have a poorer prognosis. Late recurrence after surgical removal is not uncommon after 5 to 10 years and is usually fatal

Sertoli-Leydig Cell Tumors

The Sertoli-Leydig cell tumor (arrhenoblastoma or androblastoma) is a rare mesenchymal neoplasm of the ovary of low malignant potential that resembles the embryonic testis. The Sertoli-Leydig cell tumor is the prototypical functional tumor associated with androgen secretion. It typically secretes weak androgens (dehydroepiandrosterone), which ac-

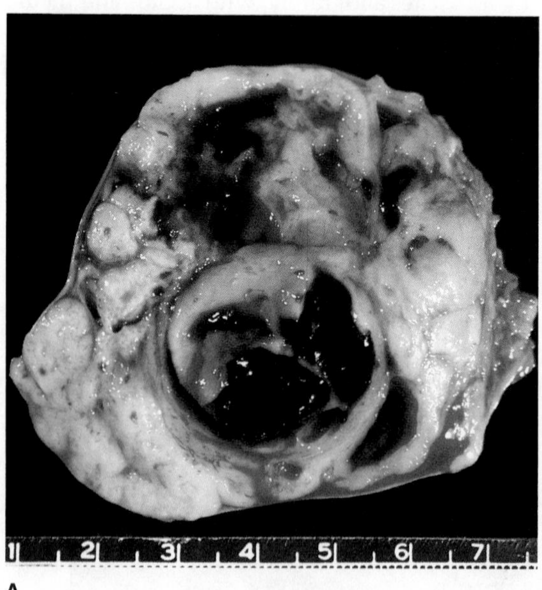

A

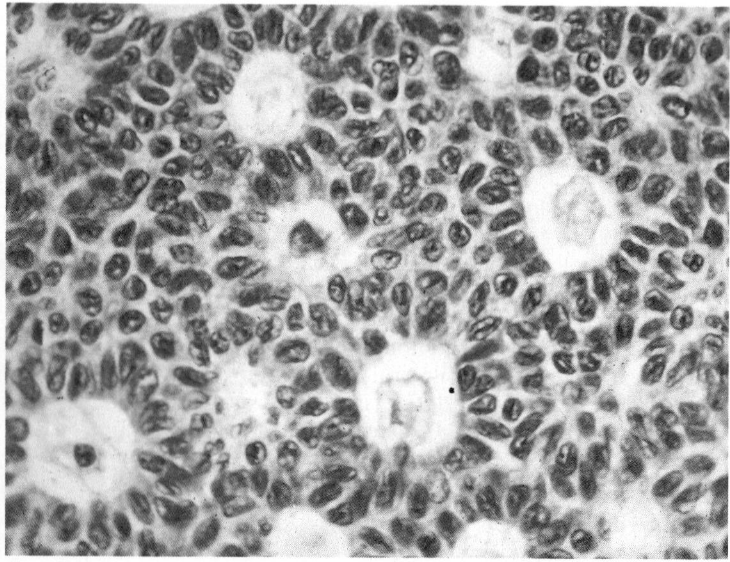
B

FIGURE *18-57*
Granulosa cell tumor of the ovary. (*A*) Cross-section of the enlarged ovary shows a variegated, solid tumor with focal hemorrhages. The yellow areas represent collections of lipid-laden luteinized granulosa cells. (*B*) The orientation of tumor cells about central spaces results in the characteristic follicular pattern (Call-Exner bodies).

counts for the large size required to achieve masculinizing signs. It occurs at all ages but is most common in young women of child-bearing age.

☐ **Pathology:** Sertoli-Leydig cell tumors are unilateral and vary in size, most measuring between 5 and 15 cm in diameter. They tend to be lobulated, solid, and brown to yellow or tan. Microscopically, the tumors vary from well differentiated to poorly differentiated, and some exhibit heterologous elements (e.g., mucinous glands and rarely even cartilage). The most characteristic features are large Leydig cells, which have abundant eosinophilic cytoplasm and a central round to oval nucleus with a prominent nucleolus, in a somewhat banal, sarcomatoid stroma (Fig. 18-58). The stroma in some areas often differentiates as fine trabeculae, which are sex cords composed of immature solid tubules of embryonic Sertoli cells.

☐ **Clinical Features:** Nearly half of all patients with Sertoli-Leydig cell tumors exhibit endocrine effects, that is, signs of virilization, evidenced by hirsutism, male escutcheon, enlarged clitoris, and deepened voice. The initial signs of the tumor are often defeminization, manifested as breast atrophy, amenorrhea, and loss of hip fat. Both virilization and defeminization result from the secretion of androgenic hormones by the Sertoli-Leydig cell tumor. Once the tumor is removed, the hormonally induced signs disappear or are at least ameliorated. Well-differentiated tumors are virtually always cured by surgical resection, but poorly differentiated ones may recur and metastasize.

Steroid Cell Tumor

Steroid cell tumors of the ovary, also known as *lipid cell* and *lipoid cell tumors*, are composed of steroid-type cells resembling lutein cells, Leydig cells, and adrenal cortical cells. Most steroid cell tumors are hormonally active, usually with androgenic manifestations. Some secrete testosterone, whereas others synthesize weaker androgens.

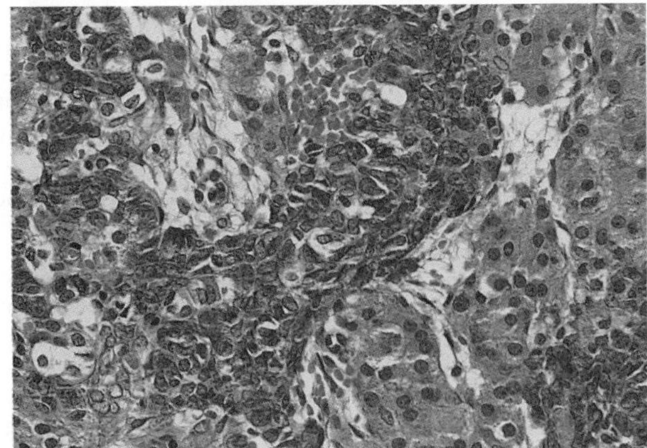

FIGURE *18-58*
Sertoli-Leydig cell tumor. Immature solid tubules of embryonic Sertoli cells are adjacent to clusters of Leydig cells, which exhibit abundant eosinophilic cytoplasm.

Hilus Cell Tumor

The hilus cell tumor, a specialized form of steroid cell tumor, is typically a benign neoplasm composed of Leydig cells, which arises in the hilus of the ovary, usually after the menopause. Testosterone, which is the most potent of the common androgens, accounts for the high frequency with which masculinizing signs are found in association with the tumor (75%) despite it being typically small. The majority of these tumors contain *crystalloids of Reinke* (rod-like structures with round or square ends).

Tumors Metastatic to the Ovary

About 3% of ovarian cancers (1% of all ovarian tumors) arise outside the ovary, the most common primary sites being, in descending order, breast, large intestine, endometrium, and stomach. The tumors vary in size from microscopic lesions to large masses. Metastases from the breast are in most cases microscopic and not clinically detectable. Such metastases are found in nearly 10% of ovaries removed prophylactically in cases of advanced breast cancer.

Of those metastatic tumors large enough to present clinically, the colon is the most frequent site of origin. In fact, metastases from colon cancer to the ovary nearly always mimic a primary ovarian mass. Commonly, the tumor cells stimulate the ovarian stroma to differentiate into hormonally active cells (luteinized stromal cells), thereby inducing androgenic and sometimes estrogenic symptoms.

***Krukenberg tumors** are ovarian metastases in which the tumor appears as nests of mucin-filled "signet-ring" cells within a cellular stroma derived from the ovary* (Fig. 18-59).

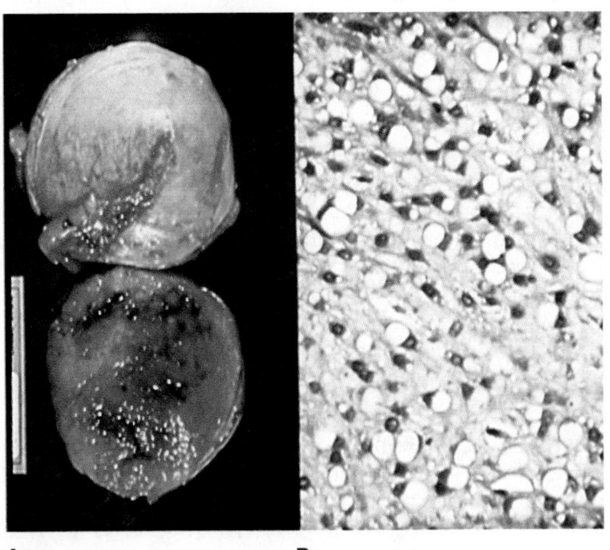

FIGURE *18-59*
Krukenberg tumor. (*A*) The ovary is enlarged and partially hemorrhagic. (*B*) A microscopic section of *A* reveals mucinous (signet-ring) cells infiltrating the ovary.

The stomach is the primary site in 75% of the cases, and most of the other Krukenberg tumors are from the colon.

Bilateral ovarian involvement and multinodularity are important clues to the diagnosis of metastatic carcinoma. Both ovaries are grossly involved in up to 75% of cases. In metastatic disease that is clinically unilateral, the seemingly normal ovary may also contain implants on the surface or tiny microscopic foci of tumor. Thus, when metastasis to one ovary is documented, it is important for the surgeon to remove the contralateral ovary.

Placenta and Gestational Disease

DEVELOPMENT

The fertilized ovum implants in the endometrium about 5 days after ovulation. The blastocyst gives rise to three layers of trophoblast: cytotrophoblast, intermediate trophoblast, and syncytiotrophoblast.

- **The cytotrophoblast** constitutes the germinative layer of the placenta and is devoid of hormones. This layer is composed of small, mononuclear cytotrophoblastic cells.
- **The syncytiotrophoblast** is the most differentiated form of trophoblast and is composed of large multinuclear cells. These cells contain numerous hormones, among them hCG and human placental lactogen (hPL).
- **The intermediate trophoblastic cells** are a transitional form between cytotrophoblasts and syncytiotrophoblasts. They are mononuclear cells but have an eosinophilic cytoplasm more closely resembling syncytiotrophoblast. Intermediate cells contain mainly hPL and small quantities of hCG.

The functions of the trophoblast are (1) fostering implantation of the blastocyst, (2) developing the uteroplacental circulation, and (3) synthesizing hormones.

Chorionic villi develop on day 21 from the primary villous stems that extend into the intervillous space. By the fourth month of gestation, the definitive placenta is developed and no further anatomic alterations occur, although growth continues until parturition.

ANATOMY

The placenta contains about 200 subunits called *lobules*. The primary stem villi originate from the chorionic plate and branch into secondary and then tertiary stem villi. The lobules are formed by the tertiary stem villi, which course through the intervillous space toward the basal plate. There they insert and reenter the intervillous space, dividing into a complex terminal villous network. Fetal blood enters the placenta through two umbilical arteries that spiral around the umbilical vein. Each artery supplies one half of the placenta.

The terminal villus is the functional unit of the placenta and is composed of an inner layer of cytotrophoblast (*Langhans cells*), a middle layer of intermediate trophoblast, and an outer layer of syncytiotrophoblast. The villous stroma consists of loose mesenchyme, which contains macrophages (*Hofbauer cells*). During the second trimester, the villi become smaller and more numerous, the cytotrophoblastic cells and intermediate trophoblast become less prominent, and the syncytiotrophoblast attenuates. The villous capillaries grow larger and more numerous and remain mainly within the center of the villi. This process continues until term.

In the third trimester, syncytiotrophoblastic nuclei aggregate to form multinuclear protrusions, referred to as syncytial knots. In other areas along the villous surface, the syncytium between the knots markedly thins and attenuates. At these points, the trophoblastic cytoplasm comes into direct contact with the endothelium of the fetal capillaries to form the vasculosyncytial membrane. These specialized zones facilitate gas and nutrient transfer across the placenta. Nonmembranous areas play a role in hormone synthesis.

INFECTIONS

Chorioamnionitis

Chorioamnionitis refers to inflammation of the placental amnion and chorion and the extraplacental membranes. It is usually the result of an ascending infection from the maternal birth canal, commonly owing to premature rupture of the membranes. In this type of infection, the inflammatory process affects primarily the membranes (chorioamnionitis) rather than the chorionic villi.

☐ **Pathology:** The amniotic fluid is usually cloudy. The membrane walls are slightly opaque, yellow, malodorous, edematous, and friable, and they microscopically disclose a neutrophilic infiltrate, often with fibrin deposition. With more extensive spread, the umbilical cord may become infected (*funisitis*) and exhibit vasculitis of one or more umbilical vessels or inflammation of the cord mesenchyme (*Wharton jelly*). Generally, the chorionic villi remain free of the inflammatory infiltrate. Microorganisms cultured from placentas with chorioamnionitis are group B streptococci, *E. coli, Gardnerella vaginalis,* and anaerobic organisms of the *Bacteroides* group.

☐ **Clinical Features:** Acute chorioamnionitis is important because of its occurrence in 20% of placentas and its clear association with preterm labor, fetal and neonatal infections, and intrauterine hypoxia. The risks of chorioamnionitis to the fetus include (1) pneumonia after inhalation of infected amniotic fluid, (2) skin or eye infections from direct contact with organisms in the fluid, and (3) neonatal gastritis, enteritis, or peritonitis from ingestion of infected fluid. Major risks to the mother are intrapartum fever, postpartum endometritis, and pelvic sepsis with venous thrombosis.

Villitis

Infection of chorionic villi results from endometritis or transplacental passage of organisms delivered by way of the maternal circulation. The process is frequently focal. While the infection cannot be demonstrated in most cases, the microorganisms causing this type of infection include (1) bacteria (*Treponema pallidum, Mycobacterium tuberculosis, Mycoplasma,* and *Chlamydia*), (2) viruses (rubella, cytomegalovirus, and herpes), (3) parasites and protozoa (*Toxoplasma*), and (4) fungi (*Candida*). The most important consequence of hematogenous placental infection is the establishment of an inflammatory focus, which can then secondarily infect the fetus. Approximately 30% of the villi must be destroyed before perinatal mortality is significantly increased.

PREECLAMPSIA AND ECLAMPSIA (TOXEMIA OF PREGNANCY)

The hypertensive disorders of pregnancy, known as preeclampsia and eclampsia, define a symptom-complex of hypertension, proteinuria, and pathological edema, and, in its most advanced stage, convulsions. It occurs in 6% of pregnant women as **preeclampsia** during the last trimester, especially with the first child. If convulsive seizures appear, the disorder is termed **eclampsia**.

☐ **Pathogenesis:** The pathogenesis of preeclampsia and eclampsia has not been fully elucidated (Fig. 18-60), but it is clear that the term *toxemia* is a misnomer, since no toxin has been identified. Immunological and genetic factors have been invoked, as well as altered vascular reactivity, endothelial injury, and coagulation abnormalities. Regardless of the precise cause, certain features are characteristic and must be incorporated into any theory proposed.

- Preeclampsia occurs with hydatidiform mole (discussed later), which suggests that the trophoblast is the most likely responsible tissue and that preeclampsia is a trophoblastic disease. Even though the hemodynamic, renal, or endothelial systems are essential for the development of this disorder, preeclampsia is not a primary disease of any of these systems.
- There is a marked reduction in maternal blood flow to the placenta, because the normal changes in the maternal spiral arteries of the placental bed do not take place.
- Renal involvement in preeclampsia contributes to hypertension and proteinuria.
- Disseminated intravascular coagulation is a prominent feature of preeclampsia, manifested as fibrin thrombi in the liver, brain, and kidneys. Treatment with antiplatelet agents, particularly aspirin in low doses, ameliorates or prevents the disease.
- The first pregnancy presents a risk for the syndrome that is many-fold higher than that associated with subsequent pregnancies. The incidence is also increased in women whose current pregnancy was conceived with a different partner than the first pregnancy, and in women with a history of using barrier contraception, suggesting that previous antigen exposure protects against the disease.

The pathological changes in the placenta reflect a reduced maternal blood flow to the uteroplacental unit. **The key factor resides in the spiral arteries of the uteroplacental bed, which never fully dilate in preeclampsia.** The arteries are smaller than normal and retain their musculoelastic wall, which is ordinarily attenuated by infiltrative trophoblasts. Normally, extravillous trophoblast invades these arteries and destroys their vascular tone. As a result, these vessels become dilated passive conduits of blood from the mother to the fetoplacental unit. However, in preeclampsia, up to half of the spiral arteries escape invasion by endovascular trophoblastic tissue and thus never dilate. The lack of trophoblastic invasion and the resulting lack of vascular dilatation appear to be critical. More likely than not, there is an inappropriate immune response between the trophoblastic tissue and the musculoelastic tissue of the spiral artery that prevents appropriate invasion by trophoblast, hence, less dilatation of these vessels. There is also some evidence that cytotrophoblastic cells do not differentiate properly and do not express the appropriate adhesion molecules that allow for vascular invasion.

In women with preeclampsia, the spiral arteries commonly exhibit *acute atherosis*, a lesion of the vessel wall consisting of fibrinoid necrosis with the accumulation of lipid-laden macrophages. Thrombosis of these vessels is frequent and results in focal placental infarctions. The combination of vasoconstriction and structural changes in the spiral arteries contributes to inadequate blood flow and placental ischemia.

☐ **Pathology:** The placenta and maternal organs of women with preeclampsia show conspicuous changes. Extensive infarction of the placenta (more than 10% of the parenchyma) occurs in nearly one third of patients with severe preeclampsia, although it is often negligible in mild preeclampsia. Retroplacental hemorrhage occurs in up to 15% of patients. Microscopically, the chorionic villi show signs of underperfusion: the cytotrophoblastic cells lining them are hyperplastic, and the basement membrane is thickened.

The kidneys always demonstrate glomerular changes. The glomeruli are enlarged, and the endothelial cells are swollen. Fibrin is present between the endothelial cells and the basement membrane of the glomerular capillaries. Mesangial cell hyperplasia is the rule. By electron microscopy, both the affected endothelial and mesangial cells exhibit large irregular vacuoles. The changes in the maternal kidneys are reversible on therapy or after delivery.

In fatal cases, cerebral hemorrhages ranging from petechiae to large hematomas are common.

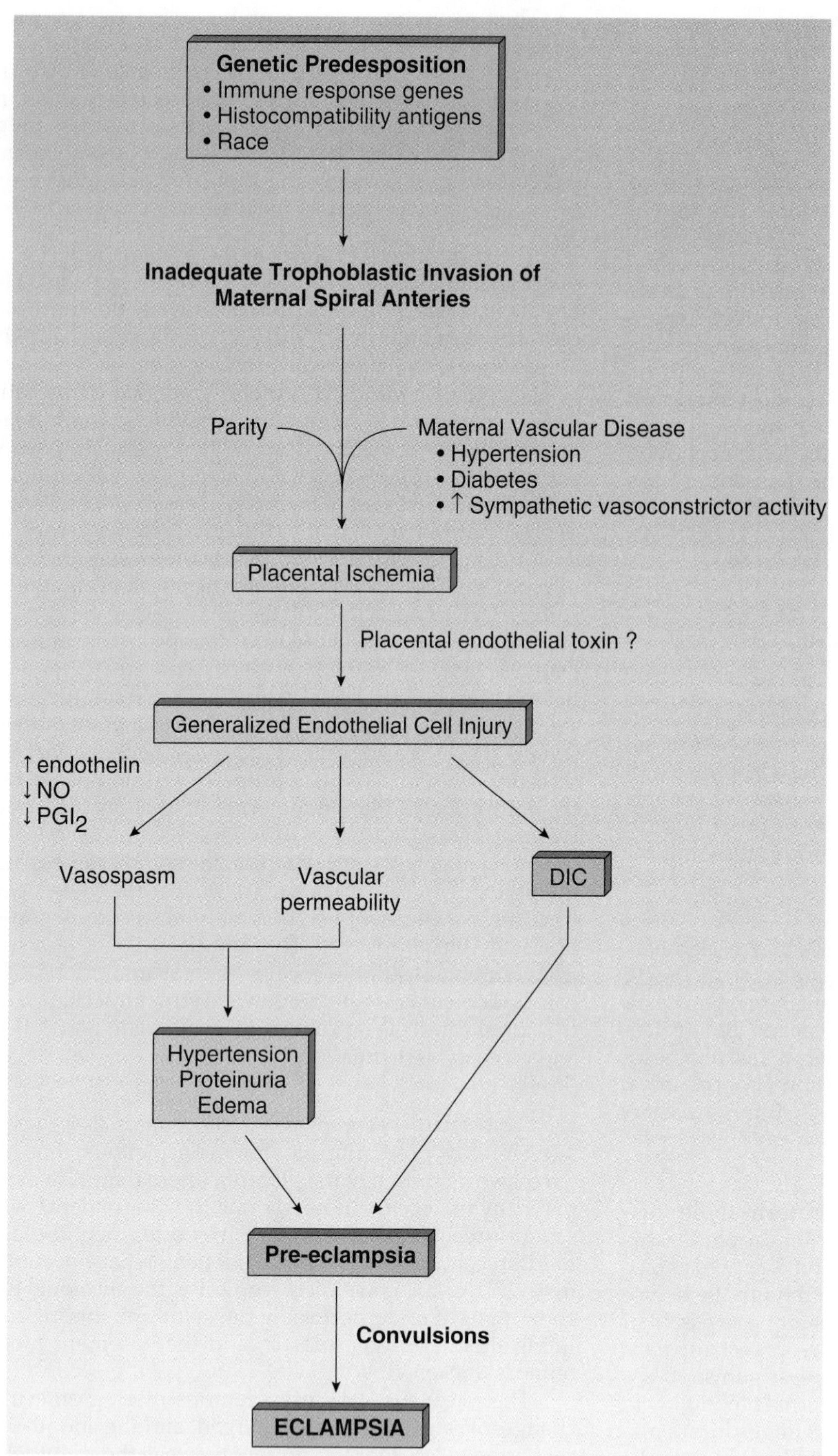

FIGURE *18-60*
Pathogenesis of preeclampsia and eclampsia.

☐ **Clinical Features:** Preeclampsia usually begins insidiously after the 20th week of pregnancy with excessive weight gain, occasioned by fluid retention, an increase in the maternal blood pressure, and the appearance of proteinuria. As the disease progresses from mild to severe preeclampsia, the diastolic pressure persistently exceeds 110 mm Hg, the protein excretion in the urine exceeds 3 g/day, renal function declines, changes of disseminated intravascular coagulation are present, and pulmonary edema and cerebral disturbances appear. Finally, convulsions and coma supervene (eclampsia). Preeclampsia is treated with antihypertensive agents and antiplatelet drugs, but the definitive therapy is the removal of the placenta, hopefully by normal delivery.

RETROPLACENTAL HEMATOMA

Retroplacental hematoma consists of blood between the basal plate of the placenta and the uterine wall. The source of the hemorrhage may be the rupture of a maternal artery, or premature separation of the placenta. In one third of cases, a retroplacental hematoma may occur in the absence of a clinical abruption (i.e., *abruptio placentae*, premature separation of the placenta) and the reverse is also true. Although the cause is uncertain, nearly half of cases are associated with maternal smoking, advanced maternal age, acute chorioamnionitis, and more recently with cocaine abuse. Retroplacental hematomas may be small, or they may occupy the entire maternal surface of the placenta. Recent hematomas are soft, red, and easily detached from the maternal surface. Older hematomas are firm, brown, and more adherent to the placental surface. Adverse perinatal outcome associated with retroplacental hematoma is related to the size of the lesion and the severity of accompanying disorders, particularly preeclampsia, systemic lupus erythematosus, and infarction. Retroplacental hematoma is one of the most common causes of perinatal mortality, accounting for 8% of perinatal deaths.

PLACENTA ACCRETA

Placenta accreta is defined as the *abnormal* adherence of part or all of the placenta to the underlying uterine wall (Fig. 18-61). A deficiency of decidua at the implantation site may result from implantation of the placenta close to or over the cervix (*placenta previa*). A similar situation may arise when implantation occurs on scars from a previous cesarean section. Owing to the absence of the decidua, the placenta does not separate normally from the underlying uterine wall following parturition, an event that can result in life-threatening bleeding.

Placenta accreta is subclassified according to the depth that the villi invade into the myometrium:

- **Placenta accreta** refers to the attachment of villi to the myometrium without further invasion.
- **Placenta increta** defines villi invading the underlying myometrium.
- **Placenta percreta** is a condition in which the villi penetrate the full thickness of the uterine wall.

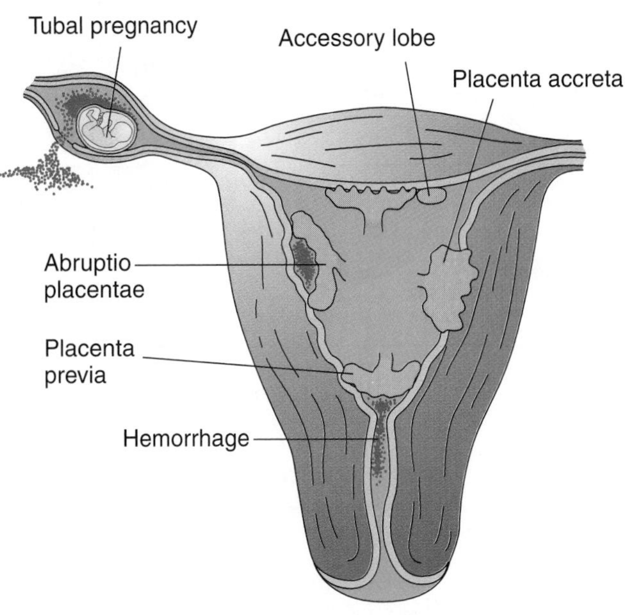

FIGURE *18-61*
Utero-placental abnormalities.

The placental villi in all these placental disorders are normal and show no evidence of trophoblastic proliferation.

Most patients with placenta accreta have a normal pregnancy and delivery. However, complications may occur during pregnancy, delivery, or especially in the immediate postpartum state. Bleeding in the third trimester is the most common presenting sign before delivery. Uterine rupture, before, during, or after labor, occurs in 15% of patients with placenta accreta. Substantial fragments of placenta may remain adherent following delivery and are a source of postpartum hemorrhage. The bleeding can be difficult to control and not uncommonly requires emergency hysterectomy. An attempt to remove the attached placental fragments can itself cause hemorrhage and even uterine inversion. Placenta accreta is a serious complication and is associated with a maternal death rate of 2%.

MULTIPLE GESTATION

Twinning occurs in slightly under 1% of pregnancies and may be dizygotic or monozygotic (Fig. 18-62).

DIZYGOTIC TWINS: The fertilization of two separate ova results in twins that are genetically different and that may be of the same or different sex. Dizygotic twinning has a strong hereditary component, which is confined to the maternal side. The frequency of dizygotic twinning and multiple gestations is increased in women who have undergone artificial induction of ovulation with hormones.

Separate placentas develop when two fertilized ova implant apart from one another. If the ova implant near one another, the two placentas show varying degrees of

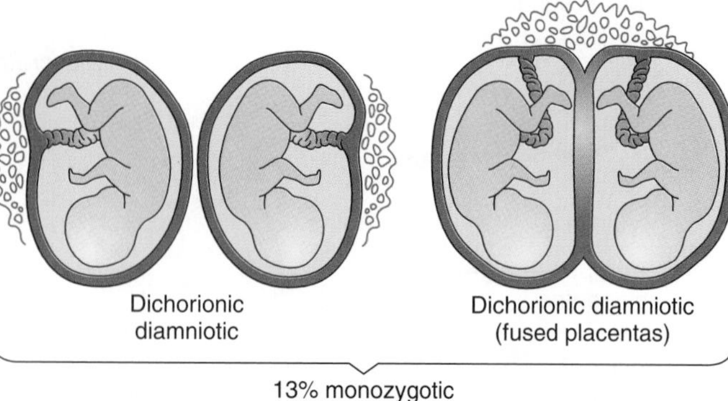

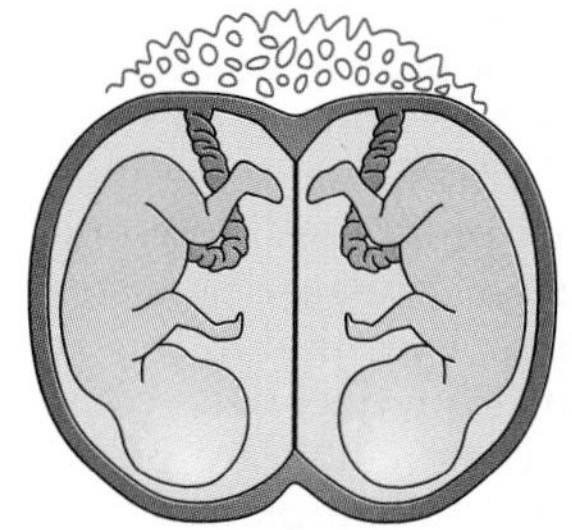

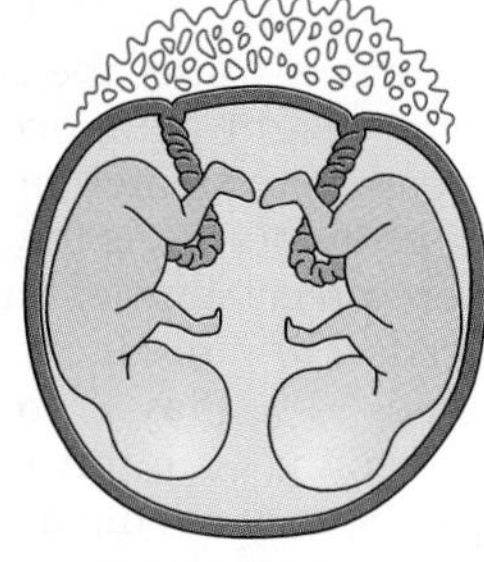

FIGURE *18-62*
Placental structure in twin pregnancies. The percentages in the figure refer to the proportion of total twin pregnancies (100%) accounted for by each variant.

fusion and may appear as one. When the ova implant apart, there are discrete conceptuses, each placenta having its own amniotic sac. In the case of placental fusion, microscopic examination of the intervening membranes between the two fetuses discloses two amnions and two chorions, that is, a diamnionic, dichorionic gestation.

MONOZYGOTIC TWINS: The early division of a single fertilized ovum results in twins that are genetically identical and therefore of the same sex. If a single fertilized ovum divides within 2 days of fertilization, before the trophoblast has differentiated, two separate embryos develop, each with its own placenta and amniotic sac (dichorionic, diamniotic twinning). Hence, scrutiny of the placenta cannot always distinguish between monozygotic and dizygotic twinning. If division occurs between the 3rd and 8th days after conception, the trophoblast, but not the amniotic cavity, has already differentiated, and a single placenta with two amniotic sacs develops (monochorionic, diamniotic twinning). A monochorionic, monoamniotic placenta is formed if division occurs between the 8th and 30th day after conception, because the amniotic cavity has already developed. Division at later periods results in conjoint (Siamese) twins.

SPONTANEOUS ABORTION

The term spontaneous abortion applies to a pregnancy that terminates before the fetus is capable of extrauterine life, which currently is about the 22nd week of gestation. Approximately 15% of recognized pregnancies spontaneously abort, and an additional 30% of women abort without being aware that pregnancy has occurred. **Thus, the overall spontaneous abortion rate is estimated to be 45%.** The principal factors responsible for abortion are maternal and fetal and include the following:

- Infection early in pregnancy
- Mechanical factors (e.g., submucous uterine leiomyoma or cervical incompetence)
- Endocrine factors (e.g., inadequate progesterone production)
- Immunological factors
- Fetal congenital abnormalities (e.g., neural tube defects)
- Chromosomal abnormalities

Pathological examination of the abortus and placenta in cases of spontaneous abortion is often difficult, because the aborted tissue is usually fragmented and/or macerated by the time it is received by the pathologist. Fetal products, if identified, should be examined for changes suggestive of chromosomal anomalies. An empty gestational sac with hydropic swelling of the chorionic villi (blighted ovum) is evidence of the early demise of the conceptus. Microscopically, the chorionic villi in spontaneous abortion may appear normal for gestational age or show intravillous fibrosis or hydropic change.

GESTATIONAL TROPHOBLASTIC DISEASE

The term *gestational trophoblastic disease* embraces the spectrum of trophoblastic disorders characterized by abnormal proliferation and maturation of trophoblast, as well as neoplasms derived from the trophoblast (Fig. 18-63).

Complete Hydatidiform Mole

Complete hydatidiform mole is a placenta that has grossly swollen chorionic villi, resembling bunches of grapes, in which there are varying degrees of trophoblastic proliferation. The villi are enlarged and generally exceed 1 mm in diameter (Fig. 18-64). Commonly the villi are between 5 mm and 10 mm in diameter. There is no embryo.

☐ **Pathogenesis:** Complete mole results from the fertilization of an empty ovum that lacks functional DNA. The haploid (23,X) set of paternal chromosomes duplicates to 46,XX. Hence, most complete moles are homozygous 46,XX but all the chromosomes are of paternal origin. Since the embryo dies at a very early stage, before

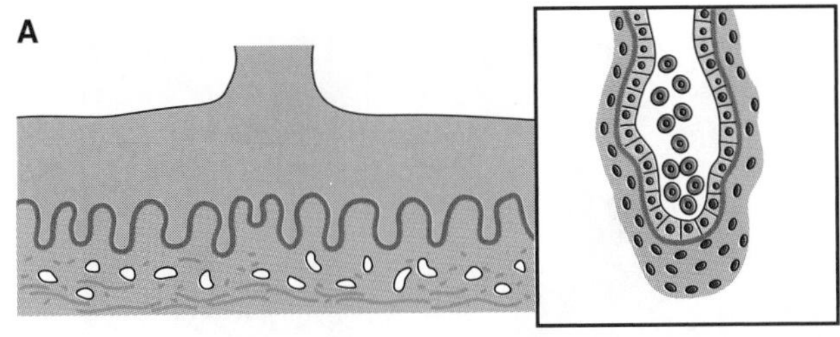

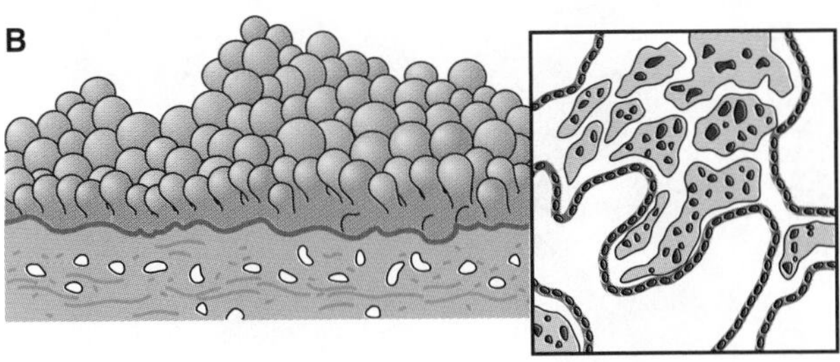

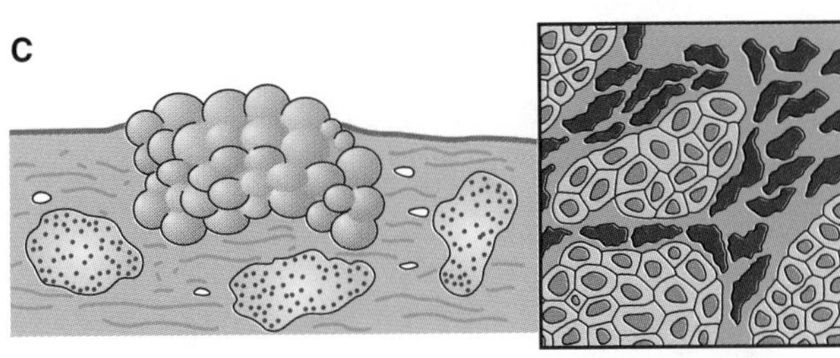

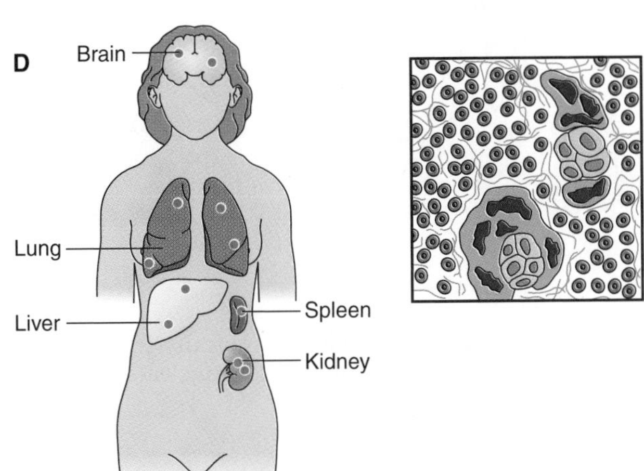

FIGURE *18-63*
Proliferative disorders of the trophoblast. *(A)* Normal chorionic villus of 8-week fetus, with blood vessel containing nucleated red blood cells. *(B)* Complete hydatidiform mole with hydropic villi. The villi are enlarged by an edematous stroma devoid of blood vessels. The trophoblastic epithelium is hyperplastic and exhibits variable atypia. *(C)* Choriocarcinoma, which has arisen in a molar pregnancy, invades the myometrium and consists of admixed syncytiotrophoblastic and cytotrophoblastic elements. *(D)* Common sites of metastasis from choriocarcinoma.

placental circulation has developed, few chorionic villi develop blood vessels, and fetal parts are always absent.

RISK FACTORS: The risk for the development of hydatidiform mole is related to maternal age and has two peaks. Girls younger than 15 years of age have a 20-fold higher risk than women of ages 20 to 35 years. The risk increases progressively for women older than 40 years of age. In fact, women older than 50 years of age have a risk 200 times greater than women between 20 and 40 years of age. Ethnic background and obstetric history also influence the risk of hydatidiform mole. The incidence of hydatidiform mole is manifold higher in Asian women than among white women, reaching an incidence in Taiwan that is 25 times greater than in the United States. Women who have had a previous hydatidiform mole are at more than 20-fold greater risk than the general population to develop a subsequent molar pregnancy.

☐ **Pathology:** Molar tissue is voluminous and consists of macroscopically visible villi that are obviously swollen. Microscopically, many of the individual villi have cisternae, which are central, acellular, fluid-filled spaces devoid of mesenchymal cells. The trophoblast is hyperplastic and is composed of syncytiotrophoblast, cytotrophoblast, and intermediate trophoblast. Considerable cellular atypia is present.

☐ **Clinical Features:** Patients with complete moles commonly present between the 11th and 25th weeks of pregnancy complaining of excessive uterine enlargement and often of abnormal uterine bleeding, sometimes accompanied by the passage of tissue fragments, which appear as small grapelike masses. The serum hCG concentration is markedly elevated, and serial determinations disclose rapidly increasing levels.

Complications of complete hydatidiform mole include uterine hemorrhage, disseminated intravascular coagulation, uterine perforation, trophoblastic embolism, and infection. **The most important complication of hydatidiform mole is the development of choriocarcinoma, which occurs in about 2% of patients after a complete mole has been evacuated.**

Treatment of hydatidiform mole consists of suction curettage of the uterus and subsequent monitoring of serum hCG levels. As many as 20% of the patients require adjuvant chemotherapy for persistent disease, as judged by stable or rising hCG levels. The presence of aneuploidy in the molar tissue may help to identify patients who require adjuvant treatment. With such management, the rate of survival approaches 100%.

Partial Hydatidiform Mole

Partial hydatidiform mole is now recognized to be a distinct form of mole. It is important to distinguish this lesion from complete hydatidiform mole, since it does not evolve into choriocarcinoma (see Table 18-11).

The karyotype of a partial hydatidiform mole has 69 chromosomes (triploidy). This abnormal chromosomal complement results from the fertilization of a normal

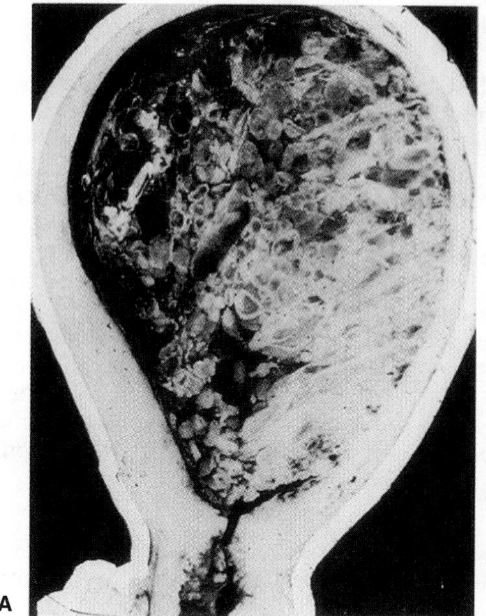

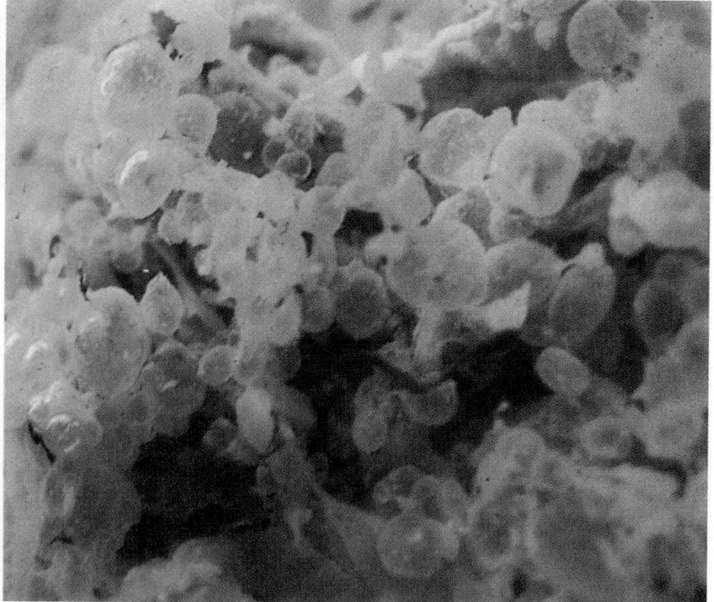

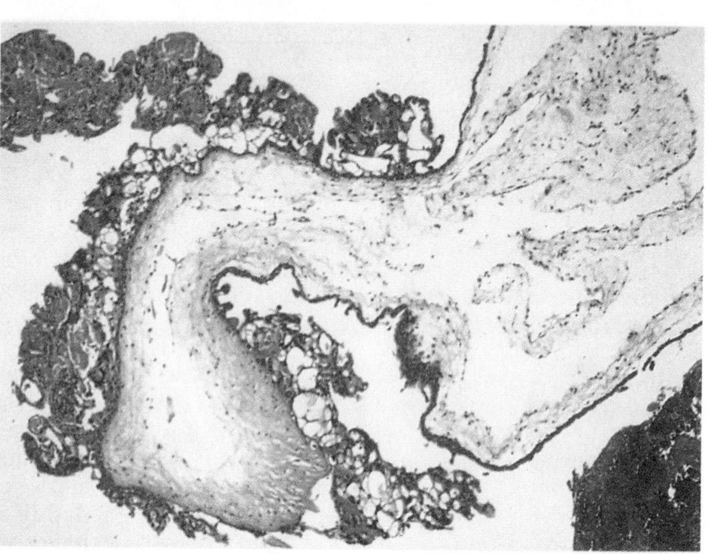

FIGURE *18-64*
Complete hydatidiform mole. (*A*) Complete mole in which the entire uterine cavity is filled with swollen villi. (*B*) The villi are each 1 to 3 mm in diameter and appear grapelike. (*C*) Individual molar villi, many of which have cavitated central cisterns, exhibit considerable trophoblastic hyperplasia and atypia. The blood vessels of the villi have atrophied and disappeared.

ovum (23,X) by two normal spermatozoa, each carrying 23 chromosomes, or a single spermatozoon that has not undergone meiotic reduction and bears 46 chromosomes. The fetus associated with a partial mole usually dies at about 10 weeks' gestation, and the mole is aborted shortly thereafter. In contrast to a complete mole, fetal parts are commonly present.

☐ **Pathology:** Partial moles have two populations of chorionic villi. Some villi are normal, whereas others are enlarged by hydropic swelling and may show central cavitation which result from tangential histological sections of invaginated surface epithelium ("fjord-like") (Fig. 18-65). Trophoblastic proliferation is focal and much less pronounced than in the complete mole. In partial hydatidiform mole, unlike complete mole, the embryo is sometimes present. Blood vessels are typically found within the chorionic villi and contain fetal (nucleated) erythrocytes.

Invasive Hydatidiform Mole

Invasive mole is a hydatidiform mole in which the villous trophoblast has invaded the underlying myometrium.

☐ **Pathology:** Invasive villi may extend only superficially into the myometrium or may penetrate the uterus and even involve the broad ligament. An invasive mole often penetrates dilated venous channels in the myometrium, and 25% to 40% of cases spread to distant sites, most frequently the lungs. Unlike choriocarcinoma (see

TABLE *18-11* **Comparative Features of Complete and Partial Hydatidiform Mole**

Features	Complete Mole	Partial Mole
Karyotype	46,XX	47,XXY or 47,XXX
Preoperative diagnosis	Mole	Missed abortion
Marked vaginal bleeding	3+	1+
Uterus	Large	Small
Serum hCG	High	Less elevated
Hydropic villi	All	Some
Trophoblast proliferation	Diffuse	Focal
Atypia	Diffuse	Minimal
hCG in tissue	3+	1+
Embryo present	No	Some
Blood vessels	No	Common
Nucleated erythrocytes	No	Sometimes
Persists after initial therapy	20%	7%
Choriocarcinoma develops	2% after mole	No choriocarcinoma

hCG, human chorionic gonadotropin.

later), distant deposits of an invasive mole do not penetrate beyond the confines of the blood vessels in which they are lodged, and death from such spread is unusual. However, it should be noted that the clinical distinction between invasive mole and choriocarcinoma is often difficult.

Histologically, invasive moles show less hydropic change than complete moles. Trophoblastic proliferation is usually prominent. Uterine perforation is the major complication, but this occurs in only a minority of cases. Theca lutein cysts may occur with any form of trophoblastic disease and, as they result from hCG stimulation, may be prominent with invasive moles.

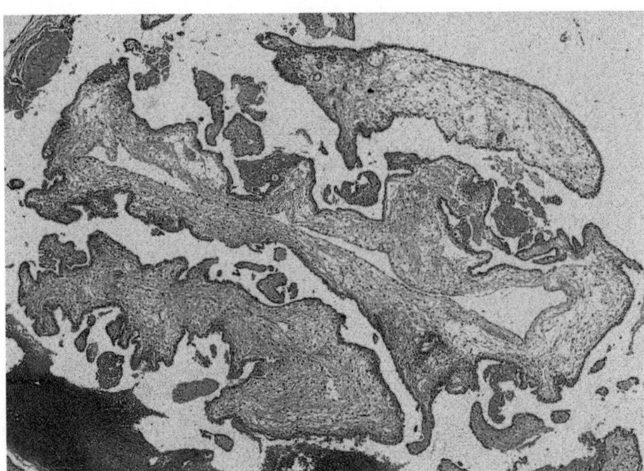

FIGURE *18-65*
Partial hydatidiform mole. Two populations of chorionic villi are evident; some are normal, whereas others are conspicuously swollen. Trophoblastic proliferation is focal and less conspicuous than in a complete mole.

Choriocarcinoma

Gestational choriocarcinoma is a malignant tumor derived from the trophoblast. It is actually a tumor allograft in the host mother and thus unique among human cancers.

☐ **Epidemiology:** Choriocarcinoma occurs with a frequency of about 1 in 30,000 pregnancies in the United States, whereas in areas with a high incidence of hydatidiform mole, such as the Orient, the frequency is far greater. The incidence of choriocarcinoma seems to be related to the degree of abnormality of the pregnancy. Thus, there is an incidence of 1 in 160,000 normal gestations, 1 in 15,000 spontaneous abortions, 1 in 5000 ectopic pregnancies, and 1 in 40 molar pregnancies. In whites, 25% of choriocarcinomas arise from term deliveries, 25% from spontaneous abortions, and 50% from hydatidiform moles. Although the risk that a hydatidiform mole will transform into a choriocarcinoma is only 2%, it is still several orders of magnitude higher than if the pregnancy were normal.

☐ **Pathology:** The uterine lesions of choriocarcinoma range from microscopic foci to huge necrotic and hemorrhagic tumors. Viable tumor is usually confined to the rim of the neoplasm because, unlike most other cancers, choriocarcinoma lacks an intrinsic tumor vasculature. Histologically, choriocarcinoma consists of a dimorphic population of cytotrophoblast and syncytiotrophoblast, with varying degrees of intermediate trophoblast (Fig. 18-66). The tu-

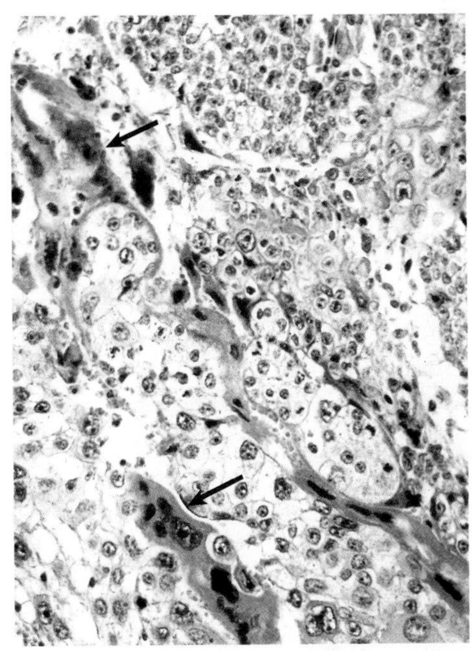

FIGURE *18-66*
Choriocarcinoma. Malignant cytotrophoblast and syncytiotrophoblast (*arrows*) are present.

mor resembles the trophoblast in the early implanting blastocyst. Rims of syncytiotrophoblast surround central cores of cytotrophoblast, in addition to being arranged around maternal blood spaces, which resemble the intervillous space of normal placentation. hCG is localized to the syncytiotrophoblastic element. By definition, tumors containing any villous structures, even if metastatic and predominantly composed of cytotrophoblast and syncytiotrophoblast, are considered hydatidiform mole and not choriocarcinoma.

Choriocarcinoma invades primarily through venous sinuses in the myometrium. It metastasizes widely by the hematogenous route, especially to lung (over 90%), brain, gastrointestinal tract, liver, and vagina (Table 18-12).

□ **Clinical Features:** The most frequent initial indication of the presence of choriocarcinoma is abnormal uterine bleeding. Occasionally, the first sign is occasioned by metastases to the lungs or brain. In some cases, a choriocarcinoma only becomes evident 10 or more years after the last pregnancy.

Prior to the era of chemotherapy, the cure rate for choriocarcinoma limited to the uterus was only 20%, and metastatic choriocarcinoma was virtually always fatal. Today, with both recognition of adverse risk factors (high hCG levels and prolonged interval since antecedent pregnancy) and early treatment, the large majority of patients are cured. Survival rates above 70% are now being achieved for tumors that have metastasized, and virtually 100% remission rates are to be expected if the tumor is localized. Serial serum hCG levels are used to monitor the effectiveness of treatment.

Placental Site Trophoblastic Tumor

Placental site trophoblastic tumor, the least common of the various forms of trophoblastic disease, is composed predominantly of intermediate trophoblastic cells.

□ **Pathology:** The gross appearance of the placental site trophoblastic tumor is more variable than that of the choriocarcinoma. Often, the myometrium shows an ill-defined tumor mass, which is yellow to tan and without striking hemorrhage. The degree of myometrial invasion is variable. Microscopically, the pattern of infiltration resembles that of normal trophoblast in the placental bed. In as much as the function of intermediate trophoblast in the normal developing pregnancy is to anchor the pregnancy into the superficial myometrium, the microscopic appearance is typically that of an exaggerated placental site. Mononuclear and multinuclear trophoblast may be present as single cells or as cords, islands, and sheets of cells interspersed among myometrial cells. Necrosis is not present, nor are chorionic villi. Placental site trophoblastic tumor is also distinguished from choriocarcinoma by its monomorphic (intermediate) trophoblastic proliferation, contrasted with the dimorphic pattern of trophoblast in choriocarcinoma. Most trophoblastic cells are positive for hPL, and only a small proportion are positive for hCG.

TABLE *18-12* **Clinical Staging of Gestational Trophoblastic Tumors**

I	Confined to the uterus
	Ia 0 risk factors
	Ib 1 risk factor
	Ic 2 risk factors
II	Extends outside of the uterus but limited to genital structures
III	Extends to lungs
IV	All other metastatic sites

Risk factors affecting stage include (1) hCG > 100,000 mIU/mL, and (2) duration of disease >6 months from termination of antecedent pregnancy.

hCG, human chorionic gonadotropin.

□ **Clinical Features:** The age and parity of patients with placental site trophoblastic tumor resemble those of patients with choriocarcinoma. Half of the patients with placental site trophoblastic tumor report amenorrhea, whereas vaginal bleeding usually occurs with choriocarcinoma. Compared with patients with choriocarcinoma, many fewer patients with placental site trophoblastic tumor have had a preceding molar pregnancy (5% versus 50%).

Placental site trophoblastic tumor generally behaves in a benign fashion, but on occasion it may metastasize and prove fatal. Because of the short half-life of hPL, serum levels of hCG are more useful in monitoring the response to treatment. Generally, conservative management suffices. If hCG persists, even at low levels, aggressive treatment with hysterectomy or chemotherapy is necessary.

SUGGESTED READING

BOOKS

Anderson MC, Robboy SJ: *Female reproductive system,* 4th ed. London: Churchill Livingstone, 1998.

Burghardt E, Webb MJ, Monaghan JM, Kindermann G: *Surgical gynecologic oncology.* New York: Thieme Medical, 1993.

Fox H: *Haines and Taylor gynecopathologic and obstetrical pathology,* 3nd ed. London: Churchill Livingstone, 1996.

Gompel C, Silverberg SG: *Pathology in gynecology and obstetrics,* 4th ed. Philadelphia: JB Lippincott, 1994.

Hoskins WJ, Perez CA, Young RC: *Principles and practice of gynecologic oncology,* 2nd ed. Philadelphia: JB Lippincott, 1997.

Kurman RJ: *Blaustein's pathology of the female genital tract,* 4th ed. New York: Springer-Verlag, 1994.

Pettersson F: *Annual report on the results of treatment in gynecologic cancer.* Federation Internationale of Gynecologists and Obstetricians (FIGO). Stockholm, Sweden: Radiumhemmet, vol 22, 1994.

Robboy SJ: *Kodachrome atlas of gynecologic pathology.* Durham, NC: Gyn-Path Assoc Publ, 1996.

Sternberg SS: *Diagnostic surgical pathology.* Female reproductive system and peritoneum. New York: Raven Press, vol 3 (sect 10):1487–1775, 1996.

REVIEW ARTICLES

Kosary C: FIGO stage, histology, histologic grade, age and race as prognostic factors in determining survival for cancers of the female gynecological system: An analysis of 1973-87 SEER cases of cancers of the endometrium, cervix, ovary, vulva, and vagina. *Semin Surg Oncol* 10:31–46, 1994.

Platz C, Benda J: Female genital tract cancer. *Cancer* 75:270–294, 1995.

Robboy S, Bentley R, Krigman H, et al: Synoptic reports in gynecologic pathology. *Int J Gynecol Pathol* 13:161–174, 1994.

VULVA

Baehrendtz H, Einhorn N, Pettersson F, Silfversward C: Paget's disease of the vulva: The Radiumhemmet series 1975–1990. *Int J Gynecol Cancer* 4:1–6, 1994.

Kaufman R. Intraepithelial neoplasia of the vulva. *Gynecol Oncol* 56:8–21, 1995.

Lawrence W: Non-neoplastic epithelial disorders of the vulva (vulvar dystrophies): Historical and current perspectives. *Pathol Annu* 28:23–51, 1993.

Lininger RA, Tavassoli FA: The pathology of vulvar neoplasia. *Curr Opin Obstet Gynecol* 8:63–68, 1996.

Lynch PJ, Edwards L: *Genital dermatology.* New York: Churchill Livingstone, 1994.

van der Putte S. Mammary-like glands of the vulva and their disorders. *Int J Gynecol Pathol* 13:150–160, 1994.

CERVIX

Anderson MC, Jordan JA, Morse A, Sharp F: A text and atlas of integrated colposcopy, 2nd ed. London: Chapman & Hall Medical, 1996.

Crowther M: Is the nature of cervical carcinoma changing in young women? *Obstet Gynecol Surv* 50:71–82, 1994.

Davey D, ML N, Frable W, Rosenstock W, Lowell D, Kraemer B: Improving accuracy in gynecologic cytology. *Arch Pathol Lab Med* 17:1193–1198, 1993.

Inman G, Cook I, Lau R: Human papillomaviruses, tumor suppressor genes and cervical cancer. *Int J STD AIDS* 4:128–134, 1993.

Oster A: Natural history of cervical intraepithelial neoplasia: A critical review. *Int J Gynecol Pathol* 12:186–192, 1993.

Oster A: Studies on 200 cases of early squamous cell carcinoma of the cervix. *Int J Gynecol Pathol* 12:193–207, 1993.

Oster A, Rome RM: Microinvasive squamous cell carcinoma of the cervix: A clinicopathologic study of 200 cases with long-term follow-up. *Int J Gynecol Cancer* 4:257–264, 1994.

Palefsky J, Holly E: Molecular virology and epidemiology of human papillomavirus and cervical cancer. *Cancer Epidemiol Biomarkers Prev* 4:415–428, 1995.

Park T, Fujiwara H, Wright T: Molecular biology of cervical cancer and its precursors. *Cancer* 76:1902–1913, 1995.

Robboy SJ, Norris HJ: *Cervical pathology. An interactive videodisc and expert system.* Santa Monica, CA: Intellipath, 1995.

Stock R, Zaino R, Bundy B, et al: Evaluation and comparison of histopathologic grading systems of epithelial carcinoma of the uterine cervix: Gynecologic Oncology Group studies. *Int J Gynecol Pathol* 13:99–108, 1994.

UTERINE BODY

Bell S, Kempson R, Hendrickson M: Problematic uterine smooth muscle neoplasms. *Am J Surg Pathol* 18:535–558, 1994.

Buckley C: The pathology of intra-uterine contraceptive devices. *Curr Top Pathol* 86:307–330, 1994.

Gusberg S. Estrogen and endometrial cancer: An epilogue a la Recherche du Temps Perdu. *Gynecol Oncol* 52:3–9, 1994.

Jones M, Norris H: Clinicopathologic study of 28 uterine leiomyosarcomas with metastasis. *Int J Gynecol Pathol* 14:243–249, 1995.

Longacre T, Chung M, Jensen D, Hendrickson M: Proposed criteria for the diagnosis of well-differentiated endometrial carcinoma. *Am J Surg Pathol* 19:371–406, 1995.

Major F, Blessing J, Silverberg S, et al: Prognostic factors in early-stage uterine sarcoma. *Cancer* 71:1702–1709, 1993.

Mazur MT, Kurman RJ: Diagnosis of endometrial biopsies and curettings: A practical approach. New York: Springer-Verlag, 1995.

Quade B: Pathology, cytogenetics and molecular biology of uterine leiomyomas and other smooth muscle lesions. *Curr Opin Obstet Gynecol* 7:35–42, 1995.

Rose PG: Endometrial carcinoma. *N Engl J Med* 335:640–649, 1996.

Sreenan J, Hart W: Carcinosarcomas of the female genital tract. *Am J Surg Pathol* 19:666–674, 1995.

Zaino R: Interpretation of endometrial biopsies and curettings. Philadelphia: Lippincott-Raven, 1996.

Zaino R, Kurman R, Diana K, Morrow C: The utility of the revised International Federation of Gynecology and Obstetrics histologic grading of endometrial adenocarcinoma using a defined nuclear grading system. *Cancer* 75:81–86, 1995.

Zaino R, Kurman R, Diana K, Morrow C. Pathologic models to predict outcome for women with endometrial adenocarcinoma. The importance of the distinction between surgical stage and clinical stage. A Gynecologic Oncology Group study. *Cancer* 77:115–1121, 1996.

FALLOPIAN TUBE

Nordin A: Primary carcinoma of the fallopian tube: a 20-year literature review. *Obstet Gynecol Surv* 49:349–361, 1994.

OVARY

Berchuck A, Elbendary A, Havrilesky L, Rodriguez G, Bast R: Pathogenesis of ovarian cancers. *J Soc Gynecol Invest* 1:181–190, 1994.

Brinkhuis M, Meijer G, Baak J: An evaluation of prognostic factors in advanced ovarian cancer. *Eur J Obstet Gynecol Reprod Biol* 63:115–124, 1995.

Ehrmann DA, Barnes RB, Rosenfield RL: Polycystic ovary syndrome as a form of functional ovarian hyperandrogenism due to dysregulation of androgen secretion. *Endocr Rev* 16:322–353, 1995.

Gordon M, Ireland K: New developments in sex cord-stromal and germ cell tumors of the ovary. *Clin Lab Med* 15:595–610, 1995.

Hempling RE: Tumor markers in epithelial ovarian cancer: Clinical applications. *Obstet Gynecol Clin North Am* 21:41–61, 1994.

O'Connor D, Norris J: The influence of grade on the outcome of stage 1 ovarian immature (malignant) teratomas and the reproducibility of grading. *Int J Gynecol Pathol* 13:283–289, 1994.

Russell P, Bannatyne P: *Surgical pathology of the ovaries,* 2nd ed. New York: Churchill Livingstone, 1997.

Silva EG, Kurman RJ, Russell P, Scully RE: Symposium: Ovarian tumors of borderline malignancy. *Int J Gynecol Pathol* 15:281–302, 1996.

Young R: New and unusual aspects of ovarian germ cell tumors. *Am J Surg Pathol* 17:1210–1224, 1993.

PLACENTA AND GESTATIONAL DISEASES

Baldwin VJ: *Pathology of multiple pregnancy.* New York: Springer-Verlag, 1993.

Berkowitz R, Goldstein D: Gestational trophoblastic disease. *Cancer* 76:2079–2085, 1995.

Brown MA: The physiology of pre-eclampsia. *Clin Exp Pharmacol Physiol* 22:781–791, 1995.

de Groot CJM, Taylor RN: New insights into the etiology of pre-eclampsia. *Ann Med* 25:243–249, 1993.

Lage JM, Wolf NG: Gestational trophoblastic disease. New approaches to diagnosis. *Clin Lab Med* 15:631–664, 1995.

Kaplan C: Placental pathology for the nineties. *Pathol Annu* 28:15–72, 1993.

Sander CM: What's new in placental pathology. *Pathol Annu* 30:59–93, 1995.

CHAPTER 19

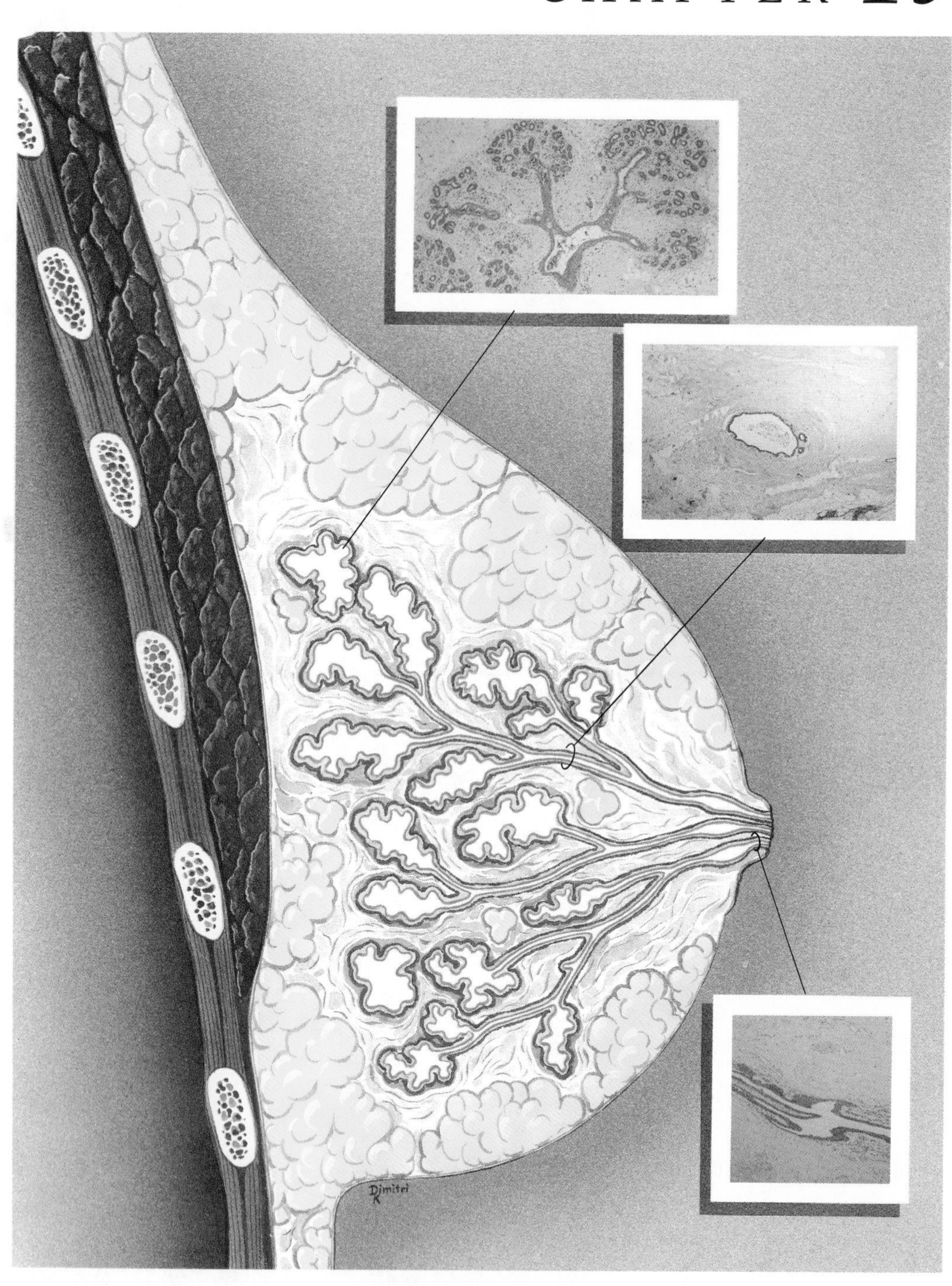

The Breast

Sue A. Bartow

FIGURE **19-1** **(*see opposite page*)**
Anatomy of the breast. The terminal duct lobular units (*top*) are the functional units of the breast. The conduits for the secretory products are the intermediate ducts (*center*) and the lactiferous sinuses (*bottom*). The lobular, ductal, and fibrous stroma components of the parenchyma are dispersed within the fatty tissue of the organ.

The breast has become biologically superfluous in advanced societies, and it is now a matter of choice whether to make use of its sole function of nursing the young. Nevertheless, cancer of the breast is common and remains one of the leading causes of death in women. It is, therefore, important to understand the biology of malignant tumors and of benign changes that are associated with an increased risk of cancer. In recent years, specific histological subsets of breast cancer have been correlated with varying prognoses, and the types of benign disease that predispose to the development of cancer have been delineated.

ANATOMY AND DEVELOPMENT

The human breast is first recognizable at about 6 weeks of embryonic development as an ectodermal, ridgelike thickening extending from the anterior limb bud to the posterior limb bud along either side of the ventral surface of the fetus. Most of this ridge undergoes regression. By the ninth week of gestation, the only persistent thickening is in the definitive breast areas of the anterior thorax. From these thickenings, solid epithelial cords begin to extend from the epidermis into the underlying mesenchyme. The cellular cords gradually form branching primary mammary ducts, which then canalize.

Breast development is still rudimentary at birth, and the ducts continue to elongate and branch throughout childhood. In the female breast, this development accelerates at puberty. Under the influence of increasing estrogen production, the large and intermediate-sized ducts and connective tissue stroma proliferate in the perimenarchal breast. This process establishes the overall architecture of the breast. The branching duct system consists of approximately 20 lobes that are radially distributed around the nipple. These lobes are further divided into terminal duct lobular units, which do not fully develop until after menarche. The glandular units consist of (1) the terminal ductules, the epithelium of which differentiates into the secretory "acini" of the pregnant or lactating breast; (2) the intralobular collecting duct; and (3) the specialized intralobular stroma. Each of the lobes drains into its own lactiferous duct, which opens onto the surface of the nipple.

The parenchyma of the female breast consists of the ducts and lobules (Fig. 19-1), together with their surrounding interlobular fibrous tissue. The parenchyma is diffusely distributed within the adipose tissue of the breast. The amount of adipose tissue varies considerably, depending on the age and general habitus of the woman. It is the variability in adipose tissue that is primarily responsible for differences in overall breast size.

Whereas adolescent women typically have dense, fibrous breasts, postmenopausal women generally have predominantly fatty breasts. Women of reproductive age, between the ages of 20 and 50, have much more variable patterns. In roughly half of the women in this age group, dense parenchyma constitutes more than 25% of the breast.

These differences in the ratio of parenchymal to fatty tissue have implications for the radiographical examination of suspected breast disease. Breasts containing abundant fibrous tissue are more difficult to evaluate radiologically than fatty breasts, because tumors of the breast also contain fibrous tissue and may appear similar to normal fibrous parenchyma in a "mammogram."

Response to Hormones

With the onset of menarche and the attendant hormonal changes, the terminal ducts, or acini, of the lobule develop (Fig. 19-2). Once formed, the large and intermediate duct systems of the breast are stable and are unaffected by the fluctuating hormone levels of the menstrual cycle, pregnancy, or lactation. By contrast, the terminal ducts of the lobule are dynamic structures that undergo marked alterations, not only at the time of pregnancy but, to a lesser degree, also during the regular menstrual cycles. These cyclical changes involve not only the epithelial cells of the lobule but also the intralobular stromal components. Thus, the terminal ducts and the adjacent specialized stroma of the terminal duct lobular units are the functional components of the adult female breast.

The female breast and endometrium are governed by many of the same hormones. However, unlike the endometrium, which shows mitotic activity during the first half of the menstrual cycle, the breast epithelium undergoes its greatest proliferation during the second half of the menstrual cycle.

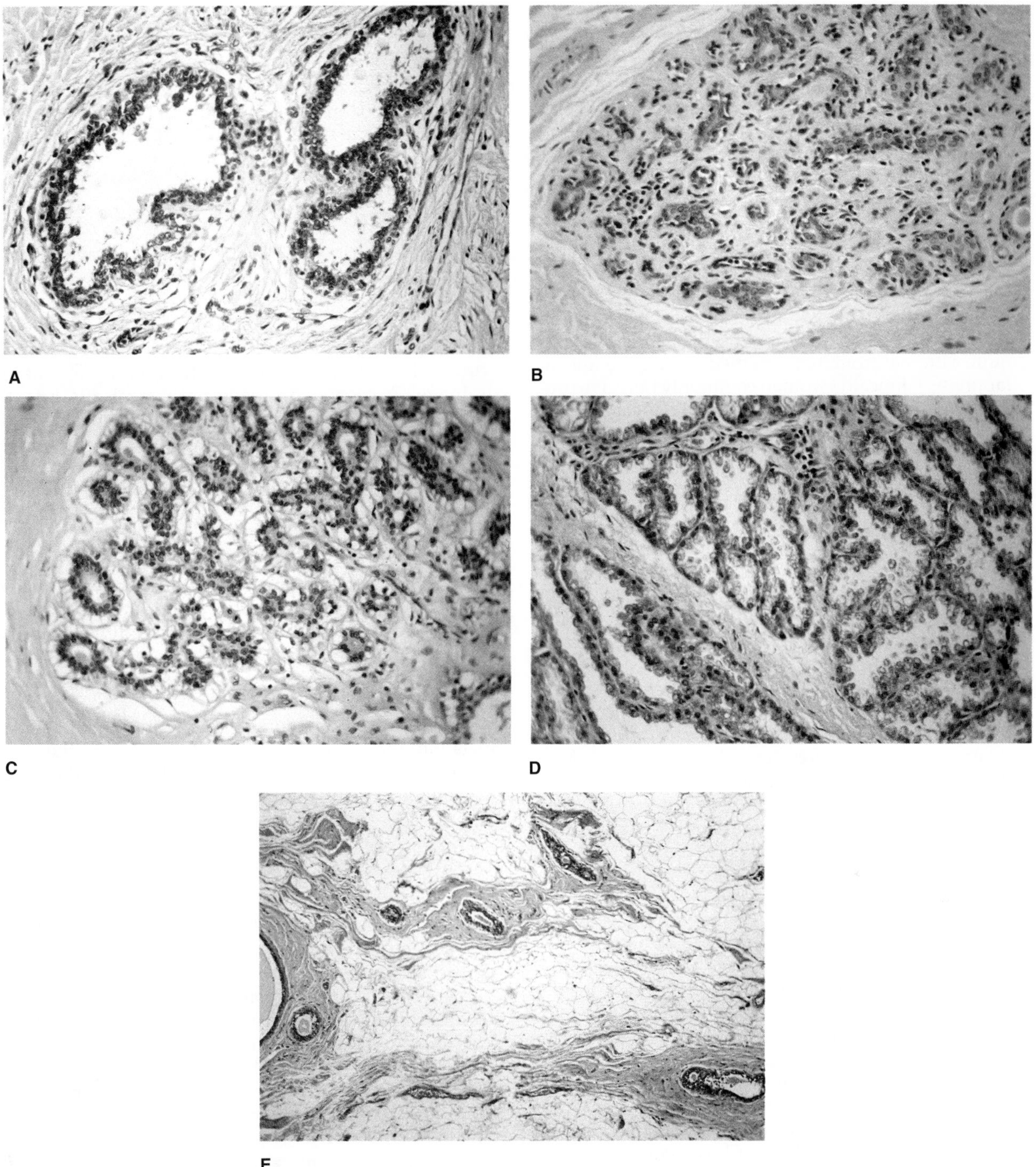

FIGURE 19-2
Normal breast architecture at various ages. (*A*) Adolescent breast: Large and intermediate size ducts are seen within a dense fibrous stroma. No lobular units are present. (*B*) Postpubertal breast, first half of the menstrual cycle: The terminal duct lobular unit consists of small ductules arrayed around intralobular duct. The two cell–layered epithelium shows no secretory or mitotic activity. The intralobular stroma is dense and confluent with the interlobular stroma. (*C*) Postpubertal breast, second half of the menstrual cycle: The terminal duct lobular units are enlarged, with increased numbers of terminal ducts. The basal epithelial cells are vacuolated, and mitoses are present. The intralobular stroma is edematous and distinct from the interlobular stroma. (*D*) Lactating breast: The terminal duct lobular units are conspicuously enlarged, with inapparent interlobular and intralobular stroma. The individual terminal ducts (now termed acini) show prominent epithelial secretory activity (cytoplasmic vacuolization). The acinar lumina contain secretory material. (*E*) Postmenopausal breast: The terminal duct lobular units are absent. The remaining intermediate ducts and larger ducts are commonly dilated. There is little interlobular fibrous connective tissue, and most of the breast is composed of fat.

- **Follicular phase:** During the first half, or follicular phase of the cycle, the terminal ducts are few and lined by a simple, two-cell layer of epithelium surrounded by a layer of myoepithelial cells.
- **Luteal phase:** After ovulation, enhanced mitotic activity in the terminal duct epithelium results in a conspicuous increase in the number of terminal ducts within a lobule. Simultaneously, the basal layer of epithelial cells becomes vacuolated. The intralobular stroma becomes edematous and distinct from the dense fibrous tissue that surrounds each lobule. As a result of these changes, the appearance of the lobules in the second half of the cycle (i.e., the luteal phase) is quite different from that observed during the follicular phase. Clinically, women commonly perceive progressive fullness and tenderness of the breast during the luteal phase of the menstrual cycle.
- **Menses:** With the onset of menstruation, as the levels of estrogen and progesterone fall, the lobules again undergo a change. There is an increase in apoptotic cell death in the terminal duct epithelium. Progressive lymphocytic infiltration occurs in the intralobular stroma. The functional unit of the breast ultimately regresses to the morphological state described in the follicular phase of the menstrual cycle.
- **Pregnancy:** In pregnancy, there is a pronounced hormonally induced increase in the number of terminal ducts. The lobular epithelium is increased to such a point that it is the major component of the breast tissue, while both the intralobular and interlobular stroma becomes almost inapparent. In contrast to the usual white, fibrous appearance of breast parenchyma, the parenchyma of the pregnant or lactating breast takes on an overall tan-brown color and a fleshy consistency.
- **Lactation:** During lactation, the breast epithelial cells become vacuolated and the lumina are distended with secretions. When lactation ceases, the lobular units involute and revert to their former state.
- **Postmenopause:** After menopause, the terminal duct lobular units atrophy. As a consequence, it is unusual to see more than small residual foci of the terminal ducts in women older than 60 years of age. The large and intermediate duct systems, formed in the prepubertal developmental stage, remain. Minor degrees of cystic dilatation of these residual ducts is common. Lobular atrophy is accompanied by a concomitant loss of the dense, interlobular, fibrous connective tissue. Thus, the amount of adipose tissue is relatively increased. By 80 years of age, 80% of women have predominantly fatty breasts. In some older women, cuffs of dense fibrous tissue persist around the remaining ducts.

Nipple

The nipple consists predominantly of dense fibrous tissue mixed with fascicles of smooth muscle. The latter component gives the nipple its "erectile" capability and contributes to the expression of the milk. The skin immediately surrounding the nipple is the areola, which becomes pigmented during pregnancy. The epidermal surfaces of the nipple and areola typically have a thick corneal layer, which protects against the traumatic and drying effects of nursing. The skin in this area has pilosebaceous units and is one of the few areas of the body that contains apocrine as well as eccrine sweat glands.

Lymphatic Drainage

The lymphatic drainage of the breast is derived from a plexus originating in the interlobular stroma and areas around the large ducts. This plexus communicates with a subareolar plexus. The efferent lymphatics extend around the anterior edge of the axilla into the lower pectoralis group of axillary nodes, which receive 75% of the drainage. A second drainage pathway leads into the parasternal nodes (internal mammary nodes) and receives the remaining 25% of the lymphatic flow from the breast.

Male Breast

The male breast develops in a manner similar to that of the female breast until puberty, at which time further development is arrested. Thus, the normal adult male breast resembles the immature female breast and consists of large- to intermediate-sized ducts embedded in a small amount of fibrous stroma.

The further development of the intermediate-sized ducts into the terminal duct lobular units and the abundant proliferation of stromal collagen typical of the female breast do not occur in the normal man.

CONGENITAL ANOMALIES

It is common for a tail of breast tissue to extend to the lower edge of the axilla. Uncommonly, breast or nipple tissue may be present elsewhere along the original embryonic breast ridge (*milk line*). Thus, breast tissue may be found along the anterior trunk, superior or inferior to the main breast, all the way to the inguinal area, and even occasionally into the vulva. These *supernumerary breasts and nipples*, or *accessory breast tissue*, may present as masses or, rarely, may be subject to the same diseases that affect the main breast.

The most frequent variant of the normal breast is *inversion of the nipple*. It is of clinical significance because of the difficulty it may cause in nursing and because secondary nipple inversion may be caused by traction from an underlying carcinoma.

JUVENILE HYPERTROPHY

Abnormal hypertrophy of the breast occasionally presents in the neonatal and peripubertal periods.

NEONATAL HYPERTROPHY: Hypertrophy of the breast in the neonatal period is induced by maternal hormones and resolves as levels of these hormones fall after birth.

JUVENILE (PUBERTAL) HYPERTROPHY: Hypertrophy of the breast at the time of puberty may occur in both girls and boys and may be bilateral or unilateral. Morphologically, the fibrous stroma expands and the ducts increase in number. The duct epithelium becomes hyperplastic, and the branching structures become more exaggerated. Since lobules are not yet formed, they do not participate in the hyperplastic process. Juvenile hypertrophy usually presents no major problem, except to the psyche of the adolescent girl or boy, and most often regresses spontaneously. Rarely, the process becomes severe and fails to resolve, in which case surgical correction is appropriate.

SECONDARY HYPERTROPHY: Hypertrophy of the breast may be secondary to abnormally high hormone levels, such as those induced by functioning ovarian, adrenocortical, or pituitary tumors. If the hormone levels are lowered, the hypertrophy resolves.

GYNECOMASTIA

Gynecomastia refers to an enlargement of the adult male breast and is morphologically similar to juvenile hypertrophy of the female breast (Fig. 19-3). The two terms may be used interchangeably when the process occurs in a pubertal boy. In the adult man, gynecomastia is caused by an absolute increase in circulating estrogens or by a relative increase in the estrogen/androgen ratio. Gynecomastia associated with excess estrogens occurs with (1) the intake of exogenous estrogens or estrogen-like agents (e.g., digitalis, opiates); (2) the presence of hormone-secreting adrenal or testicular tumors; (3) the paraneoplastic production of gonadotropins by cancers of the liver, lung, and other organs; and (4) metabolic disorders, such as liver disease and hyperthyroidism, that are characterized by increased conversion of androstenedione into estrogens. Low levels of androgens may be due to inadequate testicular secretion of testosterone (Klinefelter syndrome, castration, orchitis) or to androgen insensitivity (testicular feminization). Gynecomastia is often idiopathic, in which case it is commonly unilateral. There is no evidence that gynecomastia is associated with an increased risk of cancer.

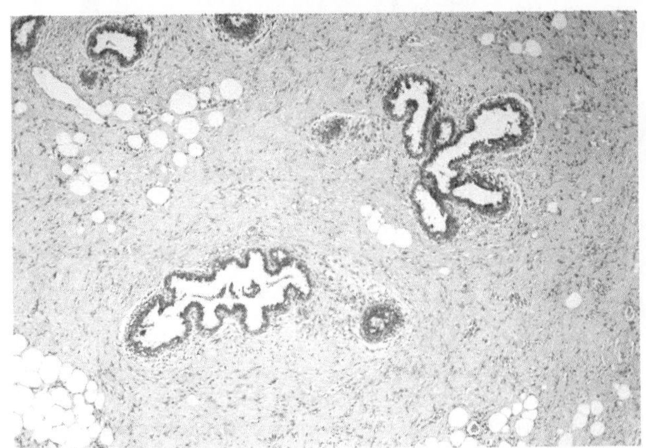

FIGURE *19-3*
Gynecomastia. There is a proliferation of branching, intermediate-sized ducts. The ductal epithelium is hyperplastic, and mitoses are present. A concomitant increase in the surrounding fibrous tissue causes a palpable mass. Note the resemblance to the normal adolescent breast (see Fig. 19-2A).

ACUTE MASTITIS AND ABSCESS

Acute mastitis is a bacterial infection of the breast. It may be seen at any age, but by far the most frequent setting is in the postpartum lactating or involuting breast. This disorder is usually secondary to obstruction of the duct system by inspissated secretion, with stasis of secretions. The most common organisms isolated are *Staphylococcus* and *Streptococcus*. As in other forms of acute inflammation, the infection may progress to abscess formation, a complication that necessitates surgical intervention. A firm, walled-off, nontender abscess may be mistaken for cancer. Acute bacterial mastitis may be treated successfully by aggressive mechanical suction, with frequent emptying of the breasts, and by the administration of antibiotics.

DUCT ECTASIA

Duct ectasia refers to the presence of dilated large and intermediate ducts of the breast containing pasty, inspissated material, with accompanying periductal inflammation and fibrosis. It is a common lesion in elderly women, in whom it affects the large collecting ducts immediately under the areola. The disease is rare in younger women, in whom it usually involves the peripheral intermediate-sized ducts. The peripheral form of duct ectasia is more often subjected to biopsy because it is clinically difficult to distinguish from cancer. The cause of duct ectasia is unknown.

Morphologically, the involved ducts are markedly dilated and contain acellular debris and foamy macrophages. These dilated ducts may rupture, and the escape of grumous material incites chronic inflammation, often with foreign body granulomas, in the surrounding stroma.

FAT NECROSIS

A history of trauma can usually be elicited in cases of fat necrosis occurring in the breast. Initially, the lesion consists of necrosis of adipocytes and hemorrhage. Subsequently, inflammatory cells phagocytize the lipid debris. As the process resolves, there may be marked fibroblastic proliferation. Healing leads to fingers of fibrous scar tissue that extend into the adjacent breast. **As a result, an irregular, fixed, hard mass may ensue and clinically resemble breast cancer. Dystrophic calcification, a common feature of breast cancer, may also be detected radiographically in areas of fat necrosis.** Thus, the lesions of fat necrosis often require biopsy to establish their benign character.

GRANULOMATOUS MASTITIS

Granulomatous inflammation is uncommon in the breast but is found in two settings. The first is in association with foreign material. Breast implants made of silicone, even when there is no evidence of rupture, slowly leak into the surrounding breast tissue. This results in formation of a fibrous capsule with associated macrophages and foreign body giant cells. The second diagnosis to be considered in granulomatous breast inflammation is infection, usually of the mycobacterial type. Fungal infection is much less common.

FIBROCYSTIC CHANGE

Fibrocystic change of the breast refers to a constellation of morphological features characterized by (1) cystic dilatation of terminal ducts, (2) relative increase in fibrous stroma, and (3) variable proliferation of terminal duct epithelial elements. The diagnosis of fibrocystic change should be made only by identifying specific morphological components in a biopsy specimen. Adherence to this guideline is very important because some, but not all, subsets of fibrocystic change may place a woman at increased risk for the development of breast cancer. The presence of diffuse radiographic densities in the breast (Fig. 19-4), *lumpy breasts* on physical examination, or premenstrual breast pain all correlate poorly with the presence and degree of fibrocystic change and should not be used to make the diagnosis.

The cause of fibrocystic change is unknown. It is most often diagnosed in women from their late 20s to the time of menopause. Autopsy studies have documented some

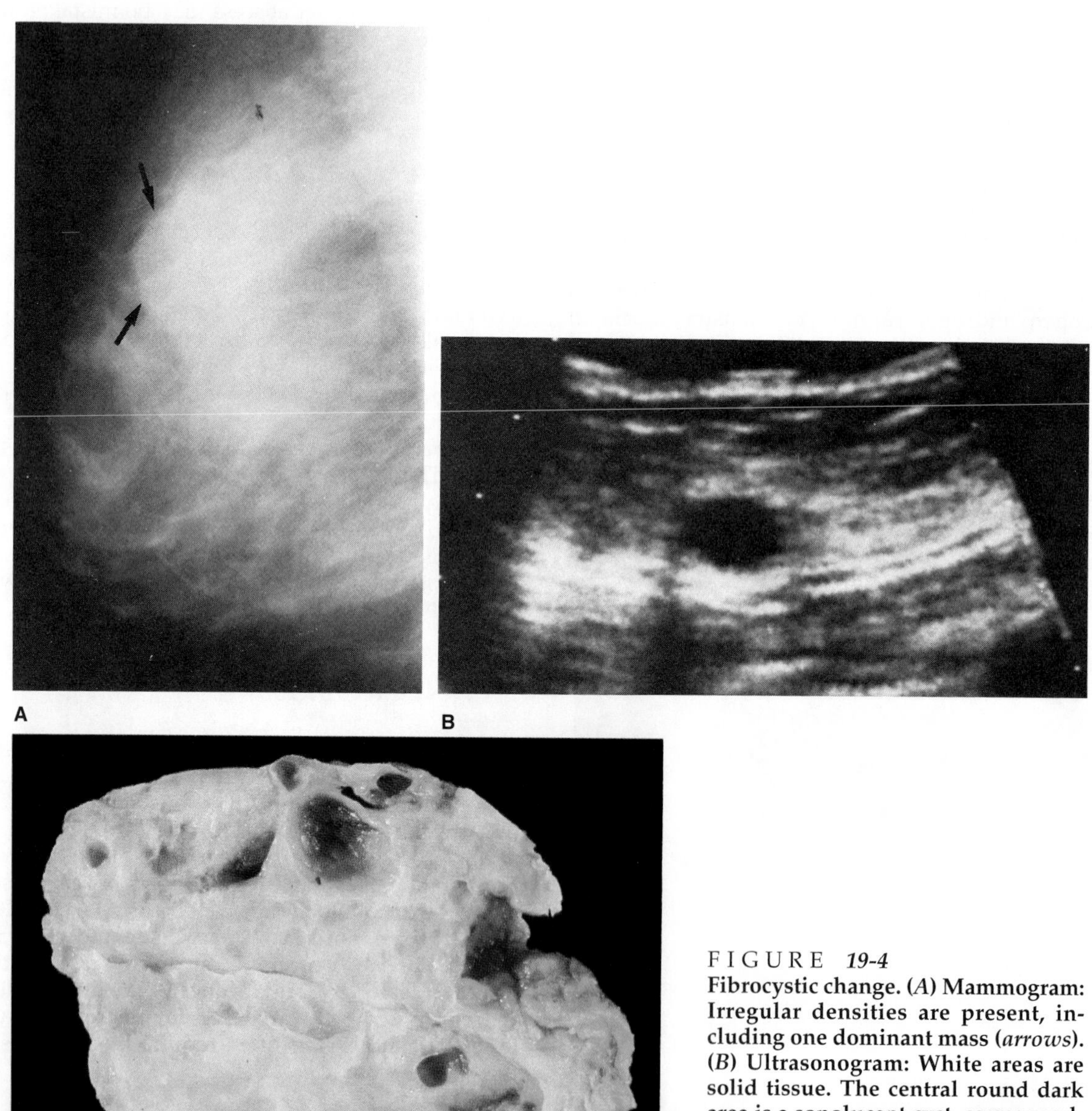

FIGURE *19-4*
Fibrocystic change. (*A*) Mammogram: Irregular densities are present, including one dominant mass (*arrows*). (*B*) Ultrasonogram: White areas are solid tissue. The central round dark area is a sonolucent cyst, corresponding to the dominant mass in the mammogram (*A*). (*C*) Surgical specimen: Cysts of various sizes are dispersed in dense, fibrous connective tissue.

degree of fibrocystic change in 60% to 80% of adult women in the United States. Mild fibrocystic change does not produce symptoms and should probably not be thought of as a "disease." Symptomatic fibrocystic change, in which large, clinically detectable cysts are formed, is much less common, occurring in 10% of adult women between the ages of 35 and 55 years. The frequency of both clinical and histological fibrocystic change decreases progressively after menopause.

Fibrocystic change with giant cysts and proliferative epithelial lesions is more common in populations that have an increased risk of breast cancer. Progression of fibrocystic change to carcinoma has not been documented. However, some of the florid manifestations appear to be indicators for women at increased risk for breast cancer. Such lesions are designated **proliferative** fibrocystic change. The forms of fibrocystic change that do not carry an increased risk for the development of cancer, termed *nonproliferative* fibrocystic change, are far more prevalent.

☐ **Pathology:** Fibrocystic change of both the nonproliferative and proliferative types involves the terminal ducts and surrounding stroma.

Nonproliferative Fibrocystic Change

The morphological hallmarks of nonproliferative fibrocystic change are an increase in dense, fibrous stroma and some degree of cystic dilatation of the terminal ducts (Fig. 19-5). Fibrocystic change is a generalized phenomenon. Although the degree may vary from one area of the breast to another, fibrocystic change always occurs in multiple areas of both breasts. Most often, cystic changes are minor and are not the cause of discrete masses. However, a dominant cyst, or aggregate of fibrous connective tissue containing smaller cysts, may present as a discrete "mass," prompting biopsy to exclude the possibility of cancer.

The large cysts, up to 5 cm in diameter, often contain dark, thin fluid, which imparts a blue color to the unopened cysts—the so-called *blue-domed cysts of Bloodgood.* Aspiration of a large cyst will usually cause it to collapse and the mass to disappear. In a small minority of women, the cyst recurs, a situation that raises the possibility of an associated cancer and requires a biopsy.

On microscopic examination, the epithelium lining the cysts varies from columnar to flattened or may be entirely absent. A frequent concomitant of nonproliferative fibrocystic change is an alteration of the epithelial lining, termed *apocrine metaplasia*. The metaplastic cells are larger and more eosinophilic than the cells that usually line the ducts and resemble apocrine sweat gland epithelium. These cells are usually arranged in a single layer, but on occasion they form papillary structures.

Proliferative Fibrocystic Change

Proliferative fibrocystic change refers to several forms of epithelial proliferation that occur in the context of nonproliferative fibrocystic change. It is, therefore, a microscopic finding, the presence of which cannot be predicted from clinical or radiographic studies. The most common proliferative change is an increase in the number of cells lining the dilated terminal ducts, described as *ductal epithelial hyperplasia*. The proliferation can at times become exuberant and form papillary structures within the lumen of the distended ductule (papillomatosis).

Hyperplasia of the duct epithelium involves the same cell type that gives rise to carcinoma of the breast. The morphological spectrum of ductal hyperplasia includes (1) minor degrees of hyperplasia; (2) florid, but cytologically benign, hyperplasia; (3) hyperplasia with cytological atypia not sufficient to warrant a diagnosis of malignancy (atypical hyperplasia); and (4) histological features that constitute carcinoma *in situ*.

SCLEROSING ADENOSIS: *This condition is a less common variant of proliferative fibrocystic change, which is characterized by a proliferation of small ducts and myoepithelial cells in the region of the terminal duct lobular unit (adenosis)* (Fig. 19-6). It is almost always associated with other forms of proliferative fibrocystic change. Because the lesion is commonly associated with fibrosis, the term *sclerosing* is added. Microscopically, the lobular units are deformed and enlarged by the proliferated epithelial cells, which appear as whorls and cords of tubules surrounded by fibrous stroma.

Sclerosing adenosis is of significance primarily to the surgical pathologist, who must distinguish it histologically from invasive carcinoma. **However, the condition is occasionally so florid that it gives rise to a distinct mass that can be mistaken clinically for cancer.**

Prognostic Significance

A number of conclusions can be drawn with respect to the relationship of fibrocystic change to breast cancer.

- The presence of nonproliferative fibrocystic change in a biopsy specimen does not indicate an increased risk of developing invasive breast cancer.
- The demonstration of proliferative fibrocystic change in a biopsy places a woman at a 1.5- to 2-fold increased risk for the development of invasive cancer.
- **"Atypical hyperplasia" increases the risk for the subsequent development of invasive carcinoma of the breast to four to five times that of the general population.** This risk is further increased if the woman has had a mother, sister, or daughter with breast cancer.
- The proliferative lesions may be multifocal and bilateral, and the risk of subsequent carcinoma is equal in both breasts, not just on the side of the biopsy.

BENIGN TUMORS

Fibroadenoma

Fibroadenoma is the most common benign neoplasm of the breast and is composed of epithelial and stromal elements that originate from the terminal duct lobular unit. Fibroadenomas usually are found in women between the ages of 20 and

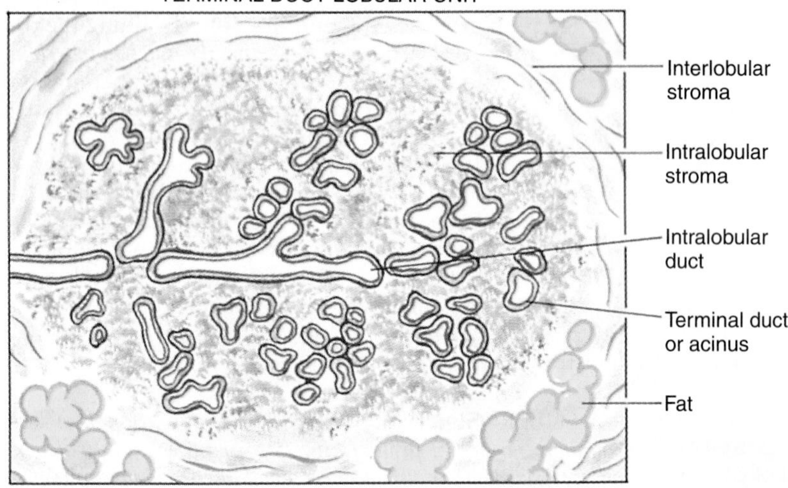

A

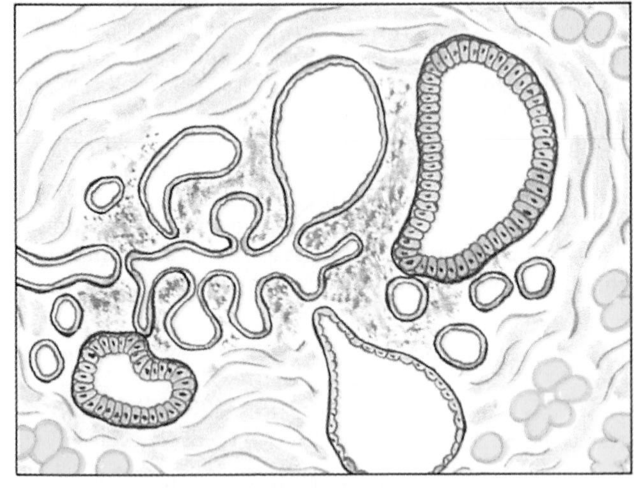

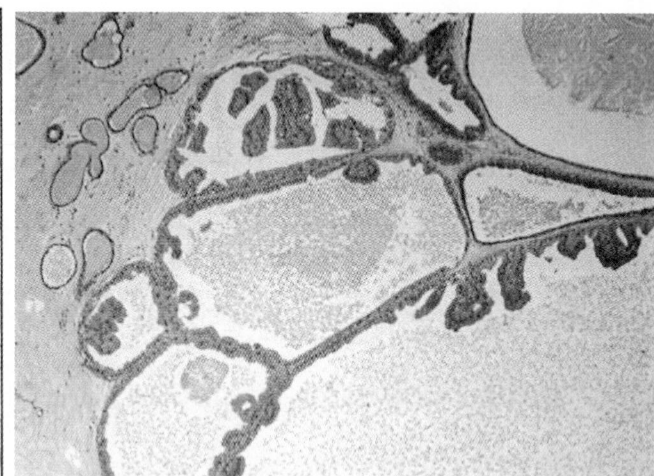

B

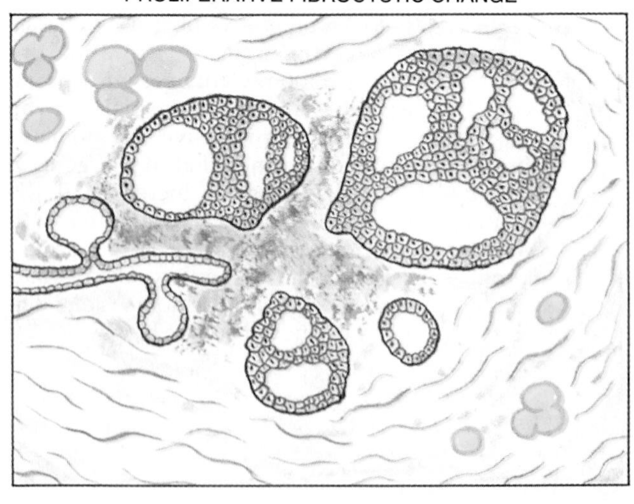

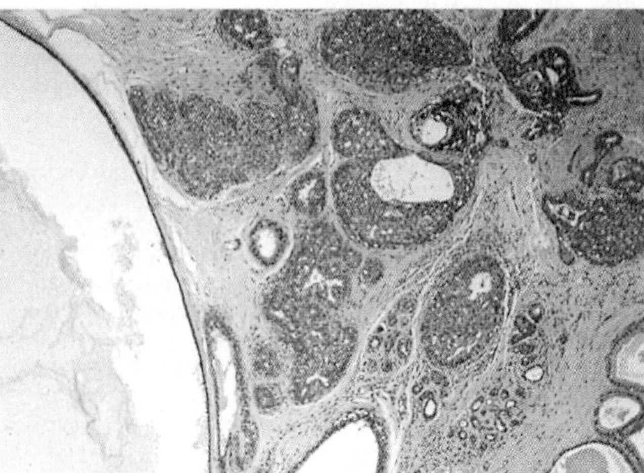

C

FIGURE *19-5* **(A–C)**

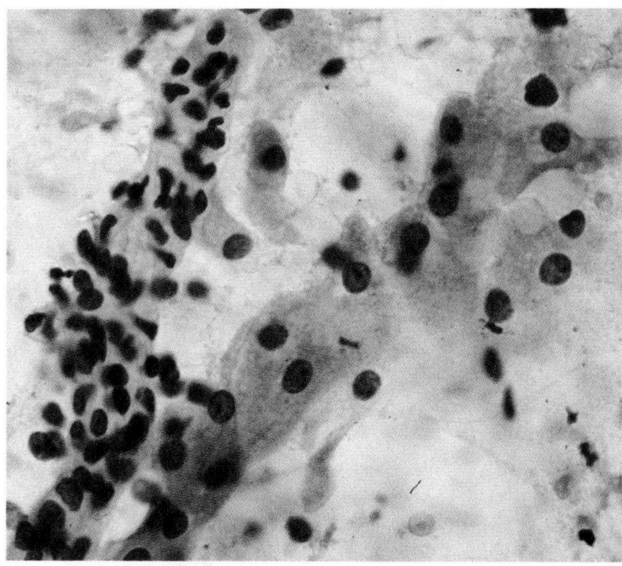

D

FIGURE 19-5
Histology of fibrocystic change. (*A*) The normal terminal lobular unit. (*B*) Nonproliferative fibrocystic change: This lesion combines cystic dilatation of the terminal ducts with varying degrees of apocrine metaplasia of the epithelium and increased fibrous stroma. (*C*) Proliferative fibrocystic change: Terminal duct dilatation and intraductal epithelial hyperplasia are present. (*D*) Fine-needle aspiration cytology: In this cytological preparation, the normal ductal epithelial cells display small, bland nuclei. Some epithelial cells have apocrine features, with eosinophilic cytoplasm and single nucleoli.

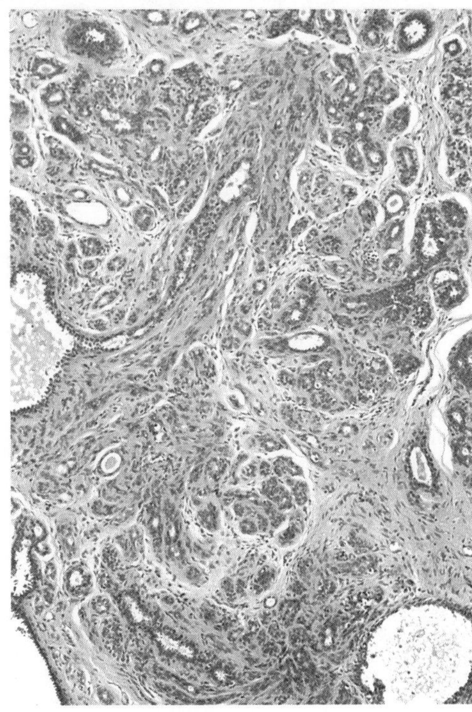

FIGURE 19-6
Sclerosing adenosis. A proliferation of small, abortive, duct-like structures and myoepithelial cells expands and distorts the lobule in which it arises.

35, although they also occur in adolescent girls. Some juvenile fibroadenomas attain great size, in which case they are termed giant fibroadenomas. They do not regress spontaneously and may not be detected until the woman is in her 40s or 50s.

Fibroadenomas commonly enlarge more rapidly during pregnancy and cease to grow after the menopause. Although they are hormonally responsive, a causal relationship between hormones and the development of fibroadenomas has not been established.

☐ **Pathology:** Fibroadenoma is a round, rubbery tumor, which is sharply demarcated from the surrounding breast and is thus freely movable. The cut surface appears glistening gray-white. Although it may vary in size from a microscopic lesion to a large tumor, it is usually 2 to 4 cm in diameter when first detected.

On microscopic examination, fibroadenomas are distinctive, being composed of a mixture of fibrous connective tissue and ducts (Fig. 19-7). The ducts may be either simple and round or elongate and branching, and are dispersed within a characteristic fibrous stroma. The fibrous stroma varies from loose and myxomatous to hyalinized collagen. This fibrous tissue, which forms most of the tumor, often compresses the proliferated ducts, reducing them to curvilinear slits. In other areas, the ducts remain patent because the stroma proliferates circumferentially around them. The appearance of the epithelium ranges from the double layer of epithelium of normal lobules to varying degrees of hyperplasia.

Although fibroadenomas are ordinarily solitary, occasionally they are multiple. Multifocal microscopic fibroadenomas are sometimes seen in a background of fibrocystic change. Rare cases of infiltrating carcinoma arising in a fibroadenoma have been documented. Interestingly, the risk of subsequent invasive cancer in a breast from which a fibroadenoma has been removed has been reported to be doubled. Proliferative fibrocystic disease in the parenchyma adjacent to a fibroadenoma further increases the risk of later breast cancer.

Intraductal Papilloma

Intraductal papilloma is a common tumor that occurs in the lactiferous ducts of middle-aged and older women. Because it is situated in the large, subareolar ducts, it may be associated with a serous or bloody nipple discharge. This lesion must be distinguished from papillomatosis, the form of epithelial hyperplasia that occurs in the peripheral ducts as a component of proliferative fibrocystic change. Solitary intraductal papilloma is not a premalignant lesion or a marker for increased risk of cancer in the breast.

☐ **Pathology:** Intraductal papilloma (Fig. 19-8) is a single tumor, usually a few millimeters in diameter. Histologically, it is attached to the wall of the duct by a fibrovascular stalk. The papillomatous portion consists of a double layer of epithelial cells, an outer one of cuboidal or columnar cells and an inner layer of more rounded myoepithelial cells. It is sometimes difficult to distinguish an atypical intraductal papilloma from a low-grade papillary carcinoma. The latter is an uncommon tumor.

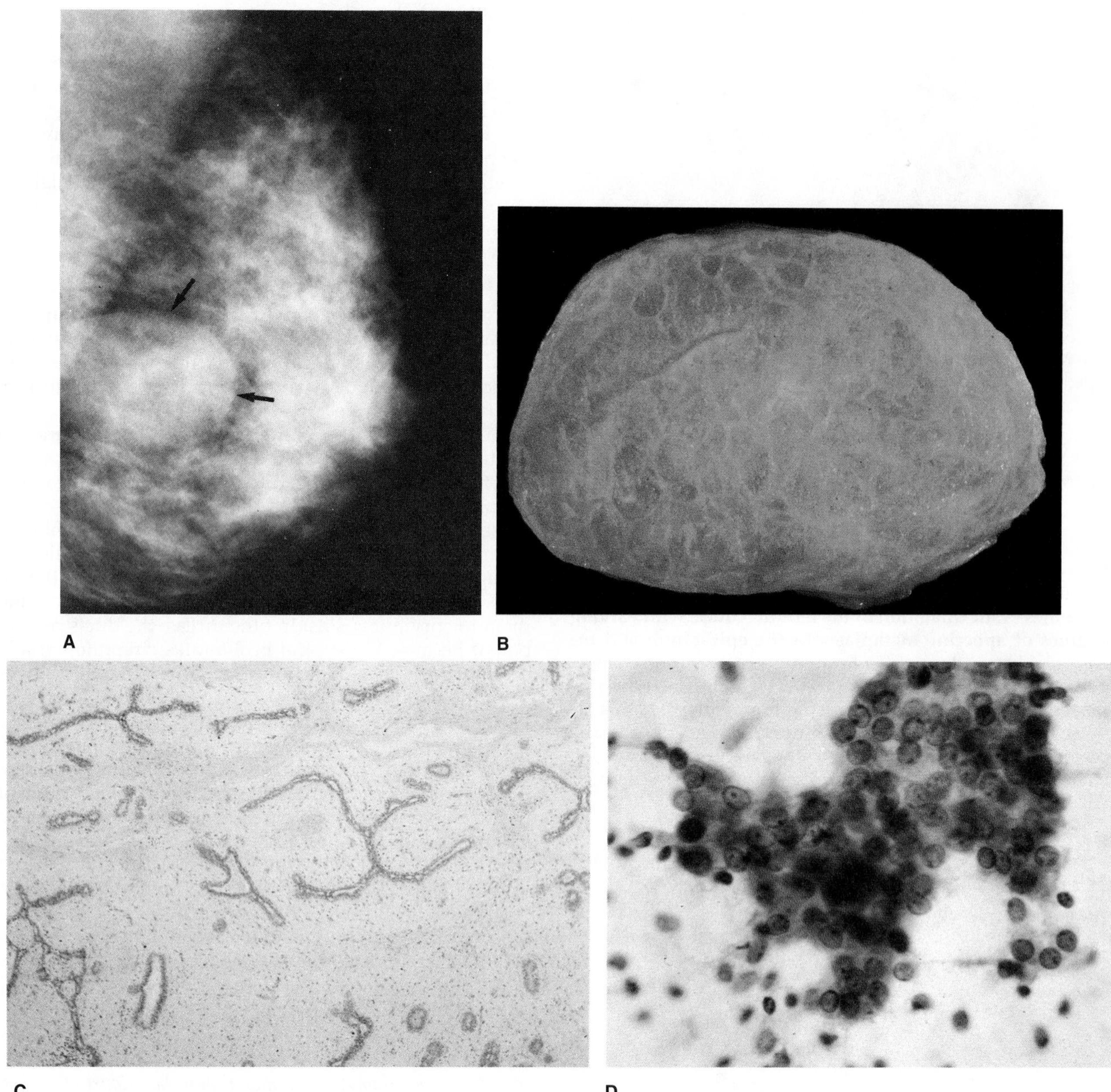

FIGURE 19-7
Fibroadenoma. (*A*) Mammogram. A dominant mass (*arrows*) with smooth borders is the same density as normal breast tissue in a young woman. (*B*) Surgical specimen. This well-circumscribed tumor was easily enucleated from the surrounding tissue. The cut surface is characteristically glistening tannish-white and has a septate appearance. (*C*) Microscopic section. Elongated epithelial duct structures are situated within a loose, myxoid stroma. (*D*) Fine-needle aspiration. This cytological preparation shows bland ductal cells arranged in cohesive clusters, which have an irregular "staghorn" shape.

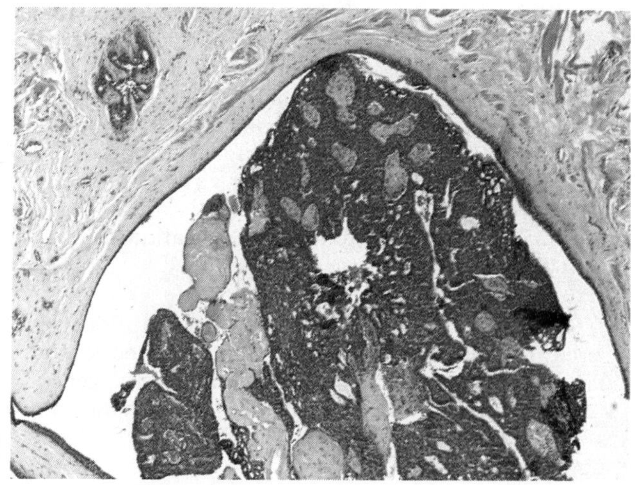

FIGURE *19-8*
Intraductal papilloma. A benign papillary growth occupies a subareolar duct.

Other Benign Tumors

Adenoma of the nipple *is a rare benign tumor of the breast that displays a complex proliferation of small ducts.* Its major significance is the risk of confusion with an infiltrating papillary carcinoma. Lipomas and, more rarely, fibromas, leiomyomas, and hemangiomas occur in the breast. Benign tumors that arise from the skin and adnexal structures also occasionally arise in the breast.

CARCINOMA OF THE BREAST

Breast cancer is the most common malignancy of women in the United States, and the mortality from this disease is second only to that of lung cancer as a cause of death from cancer among women.

☐ **Epidemiology:** The incidence of cancer of the breast has slowly increased over the past 50 years. Currently, one in nine American women may be expected to develop breast cancer, of whom one third will die of the disease. In Western industrialized countries with high rates of breast cancer, the incidence of this tumor continues to increase throughout life, albeit at a slower rate in elderly women. In populations at low risk for breast cancer, the incidence reaches a plateau prior to menopause and then does not increase further. Breast cancer is uncommon before the age of 35 years.

☐ **Pathogenesis:** The pathogenesis of breast cancer is poorly understood, but epidemiological, molecular and clinical genetic studies have implicated factors that are associated with an increased risk of breast cancer.

GENETIC FACTORS: **The strongest association with an increased risk for breast cancer is a family history, specifically breast cancer in first-degree relatives (mother, sister, daughter).** The risk is greater when the relative is afflicted at a young age or with bilateral breast cancer. A woman who has two sisters with breast cancer, one of whom had bilateral tumors, or a mother and sister who show the same pattern, has a greater than 25% chance of developing breast cancer by age 70.

The rare inheritance of breast cancer as an autosomal dominant trait has been documented in a few families. Mutations in several tumor suppressor genes have been identified in these families.

The p53 tumor suppressor gene is mutated in the Li-Fraumeni syndrome. This rare familial cancer syndrome features tumors of the brain and adrenals in children and breast cancer in young women. It is estimated that germline (inherited) mutations in p53 account for 1% of breast cancers among women in whom the tumor is detected before the age of 40 years. Somatic p53 mutations are commonly found in the breast cancers that arise in women who do not evidence a family history of this disease.

The BRCA1 gene (Breast Cancer 1), located on chromosome 17 (17q21), has been implicated in the pathogenesis of hereditary breast and ovarian cancers. Mutations in this gene are thought to be carried by 1 in 200 to 400 people in the United States. Germline point mutations and deletions in BRCA1 place a woman at a remarkable 85% lifetime risk of breast cancer. Moreover, breast cancer develops in more than half these women before the age of 50 years. Thus, although inherited BRCA1 mutations seem to be responsible for less than 2% of cases of breast cancer discovered after 70 years of age, some 30% of women in whom the tumor is detected before the age of 45 are carriers of these mutations. It is currently suspected that mutated BRCA1 is responsible for half of all cases of inherited breast cancer (up to 10% of all breast cancers). Somatic mutations in BRCA1 are uncommon in sporadic (nonfamilial) breast cancers, although the possibility of acquired alterations in other genes that may regulate BRCA1 is currently under study.

Women with BRCA1 mutations are also at greater lifetime risk of ovarian cancer, which has been estimated to range from 20% to 60%. There is some evidence that persons with mutations in this gene may also be at increased risk of prostate and colon cancers.

The BRCA2 gene, located on chromosome 13q, is incriminated in some 70% of cases of inherited breast cancer that are not secondary to mutations in BRCA1. Women with one copy of the a mutated BRCA2 gene have a 30% to 40% lifetime chance of developing breast cancer. Similar to the situation with BRCA1, these women also exhibit an increased risk of ovarian cancer, although the magnitude is not precisely known. Moreover, BRCA2 mutations place men at increased risk of breast cancer. Mutations in BRCA2 are particularly common among Ashkenazi Jewish women.

HORMONAL STATUS: A link between breast cancer and the hormonal status of women is strongly suggested by the conspicuous association between the incidence of this tumor and the age of menarche, menopause, and first pregnancy. **Early menarche, late menopause, and older age at first-term pregnancy all increase the risk of breast cancer.** Oophorectomy before age 35, but not after, dramatically lowers the risk of breast cancer.

Nulliparous women, or those who become pregnant for the first time after age 35, have a twofold to threefold increased risk of breast cancer compared with women whose first pregnancy occurred before age 25. The use of oral contraceptive agents has not been associated with an increased risk of breast cancer. The mechanisms underlying the observed associations between hormonal status and the risk of breast cancer remain controversial. It is likely, however, that they relate to the influence of female hormones on the proliferation or differentiation of the breast epithelium.

ENVIRONMENTAL INFLUENCES: The importance of environmental factors in the pathogenesis of breast cancer is indicated by the striking geographic distribution of this disease. There is a fourfold to fivefold greater incidence of breast cancer in Western industrialized countries than in less developed countries and in Native Americans in the United States. Furthermore, women who migrate to the United States from countries where the incidence of breast cancer is low (e.g., Japan), within one or two generations manifest a cancer risk as high as the white American population. It has been suggested that dietary factors, particularly the fat content, are responsible for the differences in the geographic distribution of breast cancer, but the concept remains controversial. Alternatively, by delaying menarche and accelerating the onset of menopause, poor nutrition in and strenuous physical activity by women in less-developed countries may contribute to the international differences in the incidence of breast cancer.

RADIATION: The female breast is susceptible to radiation-induced neoplasia, and the risk of breast cancer was increased in survivors of atomic bomb explosions, women irradiated for postpartum mastitis, and women subjected to multiple fluoroscopic examinations during treatment of tuberculosis. The increased risk of breast cancer is highest when exposure occurs in young children and pre and perimenarchal women; there is little hazard when women are exposed to radiation after the age of 40. Modern mammographic techniques use extremely low doses of radiation, and any possible increased risk of cancer is negligible.

FIBROCYSTIC CHANGE: Women with fibrocystic change have an increased risk of breast cancer only when specific proliferative lesions are identified in biopsy tissue. As discussed previously, the strongest association with increased risk appears to be in women with "atypical" hyperplasia (four to five times that of the general population). Women with both a first-degree family history of breast cancer and "atypical" hyperplasia have a 10-fold increased risk of developing cancer. Proliferative breast disease is more common in clinically normal women who have a first-degree relative with breast cancer, suggesting that genetic susceptibility may contribute to both proliferative breast disease and cancer.

PREVIOUS CANCER: Women who have previously had breast cancer have a 10-fold increased risk of developing a second primary breast cancer.

VIRUSES: The role of viruses in the etiology of breast cancer has been the subject of extensive research since the discovery of the *mouse mammary tumor virus*, or Bittner virus (see Chapter 5). This agent integrates into the host DNA and activates an array of mouse genes ("int" genes) that are implicated in growth and development. Although the mouse mammary tumor virus affords an interesting experimental model of viral carcinogenesis, there are no data to support viral causation of human breast cancer.

GENOMIC ALTERATIONS: Gene amplifications, overexpression, and allelic deletions are frequent and multiple in breast cancer. However, no specific genomic change has yet been conclusively implicated in the pathogenesis of sporadic breast cancer. The role of inherited mutations is discussed above.

☐ **Pathology:** Cancers of the breast are almost all adenocarcinomas, which are derived from the glandular epithelium of the terminal duct lobular unit. The various subtypes derive their names from a combination of their histological patterns and cytological characteristics, not their site of origin (Table 19-1).

Carcinoma *in situ*

The lesions called carcinoma *in situ* are controversial with regard to their biological behavior. The name implies that they are obligate precursors of invasive carcinoma, and, histologically, the various subtypes of carcinoma *in situ* do have invasive counterparts. However, only 20% to 30% of women who have demonstrated these lesions in a breast biopsy but who have received no further therapy subsequently developed invasive cancer. The likelihood of an invasive cancer arising after the diagnosis of "*in situ* carcinoma" varies with the histological subtype of this lesion.

Intraductal Carcinoma *in situ*

This lesion arises in the terminal duct lobular unit, greatly distending and distorting the ducts by its growth. The terminal ducts may become markedly enlarged, thereby resembling large ducts. Intraductal carcinoma *in situ* has

TABLE *19-1* Frequency of Histological Subtypes of Invasive Breast Cancer

Subtype	Frequency (%)
Invasive ductal carcinoma	
Pure	55
Mixed with other types (including lobular)	25
Invasive lobular carcinoma (pure)	10
Medullary carcinoma (pure)	<5
Mucinous carcinoma (pure)	2
Other pure types	2
Other mixed types	1

two main histological types namely comedo- and noncomedo carcinoma.

COMEDOCARCINOMA: This subtype is composed of very large, pleomorphic cells, which have abundant eosinophilic cytoplasm and irregular nuclei, commonly with prominent nucleoli. Comedocarcinoma *in situ* typically grows in a solid pattern and often becomes centrally necrotic. The necrotic debris may undergo dystrophic calcification (see Fig. 19-10A). On gross examination, the cut surface shows distended ducts containing pasty necrotic debris, resembling comedos, hence the term *comedocarcinoma.* Even though the malignant cells do not invade through the basement membrane of the ducts, this form of carcinoma *in situ* commonly incites a chronic inflammatory and fibroblastic response in the surrounding stroma.

The stromal inflammation and fibrosis in comedocarcinoma are sometimes sufficient to cause a clinically palpable or radiographically detectable mass. In addition, the microcalcifications that occur in the necrotic debris within the ducts have a distinctive, branching appearance by mammography. The extent of ductal involvement in comedocarcinoma is not always paralleled by that of surrounding fibrosis. Thus, the cancer may extend within the duct system beyond the clinically detectable tumor growth. For this reason, it is not uncommon for the surgical biopsy margins to contain cancer. The consequent difficulties in obtaining complete excision of the primary tumor frequently necessitates mastectomy rather than "lumpectomy."

NONCOMEDO INTRADUCTAL CARCINOMA: This tumor has multiple architectural patterns, which are often intermixed and exhibit a spectrum of cytological atypia. The patterns are classified as micropapillary, cribriform, and solid. The tumor cells and nuclei are smaller and more regular than those of the comedo type. Noncomedo intraductal carcinoma *in situ* is less likely than is comedocarcinoma to incite a desmoplastic response in the surrounding tissue. Necrosis is minimal or absent.

Intraductal carcinoma *in situ*, treated only by biopsy, carries a 30% chance of invasive carcinoma developing in the same breast over the ensuing 20 years. The risk of cancer in the contralateral breast is also increased, but not to the same degree. The chances of local recurrence, as either *in situ* or invasive cancer, is substantially greater in the case of the comedo than in noncomedo subtypes.

Lobular Carcinoma *in situ*

This tumor also arises in the terminal duct lobular unit. In lobular carcinoma *in situ* the cells tend to be smaller and more monotonous than those of the ductal type, with round, regular nuclei and minute nucleoli (see Fig. 19-12A). This neoplasm does not form papillary or cribriform structures. The malignant cells appear as solid clusters that pack and distend the terminal ducts, but not to the extent of ductal carcinoma *in situ*. Although lobular carcinoma *in situ* does not commonly undergo the central necrosis seen in intraductal carcinoma, it may also have microcalcifications in the ducts, which can be detected radiographically. Lobular carcinoma *in situ* does not usually incite the dense fibrosis and chronic inflammation so characteristic of intraductal carcinoma *in situ*. It is, therefore, less likely to cause a detectable mass. It is not uncommon for lobular carcinoma *in situ* to be an "incidental" finding in a biopsy that was prompted by benign changes.

As with intraductal carcinoma *in situ*, 20% to 30% of women with lobular carcinoma *in situ* receiving no further treatment after biopsy will develop invasive cancer within 20 years of diagnosis. In contrast to intraductal carcinoma *in situ*, however, about half of these invasive cancers will arise in the contralateral breast and may be either lobular or ductal cancers. Thus, lobular carcinoma *in situ*, more than ductal carcinoma *in situ*, serves as a marker for an enhanced risk of subsequent invasive cancer in both breasts.

Papillary Carcinoma *in situ*

This neoplasm is far less common than either intraductal carcinoma or lobular carcinoma *in situ*. Papillary carcinoma *in situ* is unusual in that it originates in the larger branches of the duct system. The tumor is very well differentiated and exhibits a papillary configuration. The cells are typically small and regular, making it in some instances difficult to distinguish this form of carcinoma from a benign intraductal papilloma. Provided that it is not accompanied by other forms of carcinoma, papillary carcinoma *in situ* does not carry an increased risk of subsequent invasive cancer after its complete local excision.

Invasive Carcinoma

Ductal Carcinoma

Invasive, or infiltrating, ductal carcinoma is the most common form of breast cancer (Fig. 19-9). In this cancer, stromal invasion by malignant cells usually incites a pronounced fibroblastic proliferation. This "desmoplasia" creates a palpable mass, which is the most common initial sign of ductal carcinoma. Invasive ductal carcinoma usually presents as a hard, fixed mass, which is often referred to as *scirrhous carcinoma.* On gross examination, the tumor is typically firm and shows irregular margins. The cut surface is pale gray and gritty and flecked with yellow, chalky streaks.

Microscopically, invasive ductal carcinoma grows as irregular nests and cords of epithelial cells, usually within a dense fibrous stroma (Fig. 19-10). The well-differentiated cancers may form abortive glands, whereas the less-differentiated forms consist of solid sheets of neoplastic cells. The cells show a variable degree of differentiation and mitotic activity and are cytologically indistinguishable from those of ductal carcinoma *in situ*. Necrosis of the tumor is not characteristic of well-differentiated cancers. However, poorly differentiated, more rapidly growing cancers may display extensive necrosis.

PAGET DISEASE OF THE NIPPLE: *Paget disease of the nipple refers to an uncommon variant of ductal carcinoma, either in situ or invasive, that extends to involve the epidermis of the nipple and areola* (Fig. 19-11). This condition usually

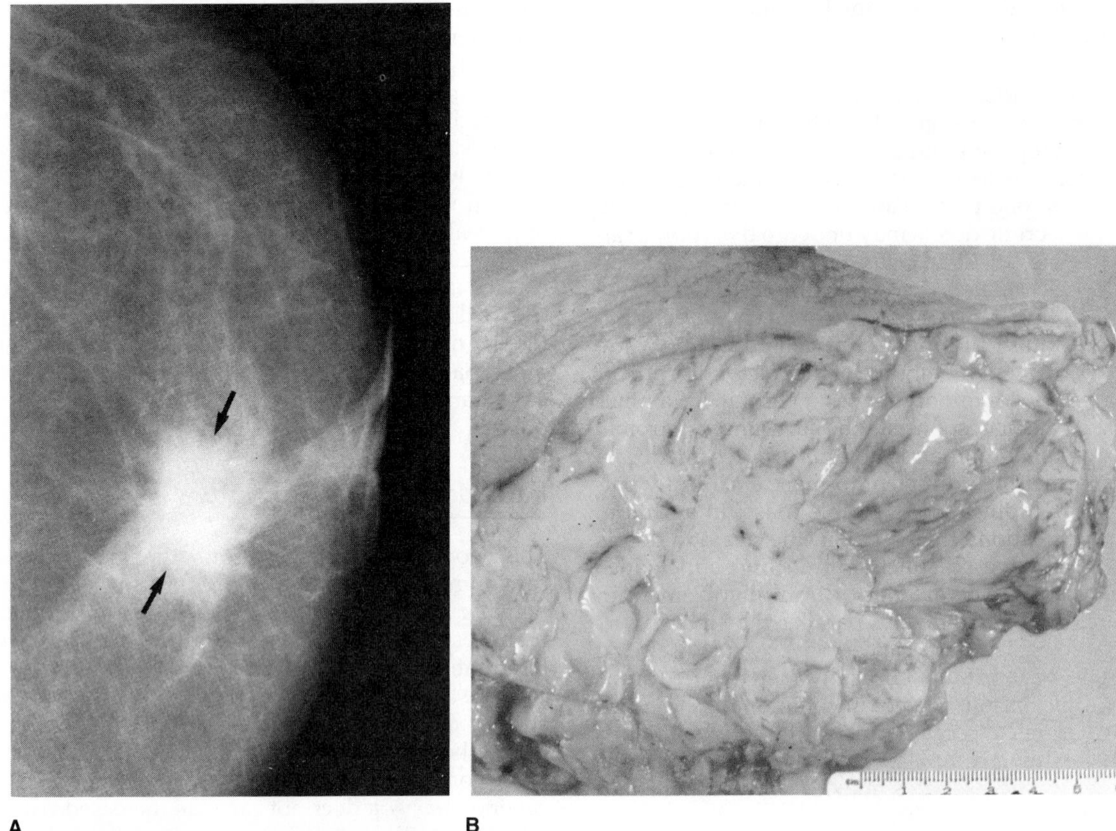

FIGURE 19-9
Carcinoma of the breast. (*A*) Mammogram. An irregularly shaped, dense mass (*arrows*) is seen in this otherwise fatty breast. (*B*) Mastectomy specimen. The irregular white, firm mass in the center is surrounded by fatty tissue.

comes to medical attention because of an eczematous change in the skin of the nipple and areola. Microscopically, large cells with clear cytoplasm (Paget cells) are found singly or in groups within the epidermis. The prognosis of Paget disease is related to that of the underlying ductal cancer.

Lobular Carcinoma

Invasive lobular carcinoma is the second most common form of invasive breast cancer (Fig. 19-12). It may occur alone or may be mixed with ductal carcinoma. Because the amount of fibrosis is variable, the clinical presentation of invasive lobular carcinoma varies from a discrete firm mass, similar to ductal carcinoma, to a more subtle, diffuse, indurated area. Microscopically, the classic invasive lobular carcinoma consists of single strands of malignant cells infiltrating between stromal fibers, a feature termed *Indian filing*. Occasionally, a more solid or trabecular growth pattern is observed. The small, bland cells are cytologically identical to those of the *in situ* form, and mitotic activity is rare. In spite of the innocuous cytological characteristics of this form of invasive carcinoma, it is biologically as aggressive as the invasive ductal type.

Variants of classical lobular carcinoma display an overall growth pattern that is identical to that of the ordinary invasive lobular carcinoma. However, the nuclear characteristics are different. In one form, the small, regular tumor cells possess intracellular mucin. The mucin commonly compresses the nucleus to one side, giving the cell a "signet ring" appearance, hence the term *signet ring carcinoma*. Another variant maintains the usual lobular growth pattern, but has more marked nuclear pleomorphism, and is referred to as *pleomorphic lobular carcinoma*. Ten percent of invasive carcinomas have mixed features of ductal and lobular carcinoma.

Uncommon Types of Invasive Breast Cancer

COLLOID (MUCINOUS) CARCINOMA: This invasive variant tends to occur in older women. On cut section, colloid carcinoma has a glistening surface and mucoid consistency. Histologically, it is composed of small clusters of epithelial cells, occasionally forming glands, floating in pools of extracellular mucin (Fig. 19-13). In its pure form, colloid carcinoma has a considerably better prognosis than infiltrating ductal or lobular carcinoma. However, colloid carcinoma is often admixed with infiltrating ductal carcinoma, in which circumstance the prognosis is determined by the ductal component.

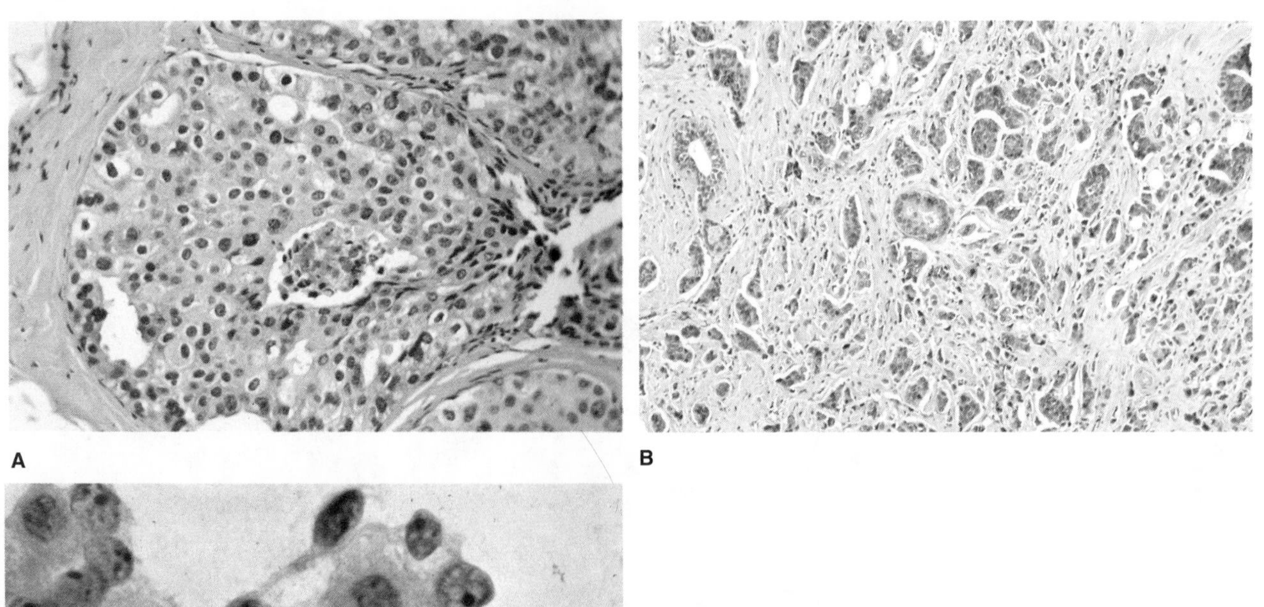

FIGURE 19-10
Ductal carcinoma. (*A*) Ductal carcinoma *in situ*. The terminal ducts are distended by carcinoma *in situ* (intraductal carcinoma). The tumor cells are large and have abundant cytoplasm. The center of the tumor mass is necrotic. (*B*) Invasive ductal carcinoma. Irregular cords and nests of tumor cells, derived from the same cells that compose the intraductal component (*A*), invade the stroma. Many of the cells form duct-like structures. (*C*) Fine-needle aspiration. This cytological preparation shows tumor cells, which exhibit nuclear pleomorphism and prominent nucleoli.

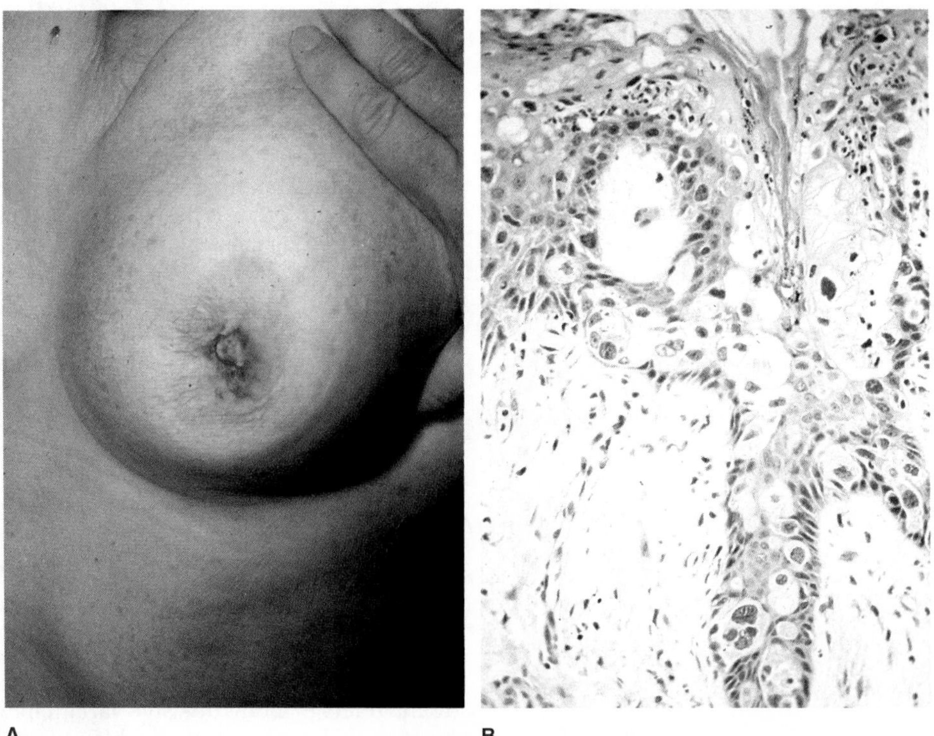

FIGURE 19-11
Paget disease of the nipple. (*A*) An erythematous, scaly, and weeping "eczema" involves the nipple. (*B*) The epidermis contains clusters of ductal type carcinoma cells, which are larger and have more abundant pale cytoplasm than the surrounding keratinocytes.

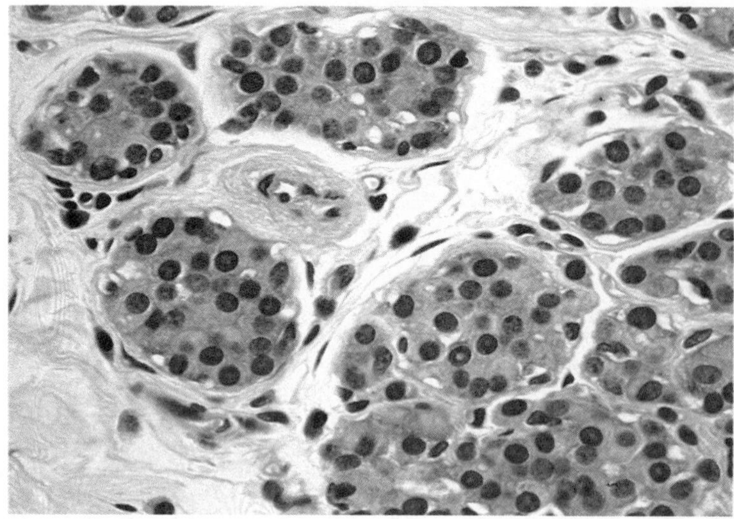

A

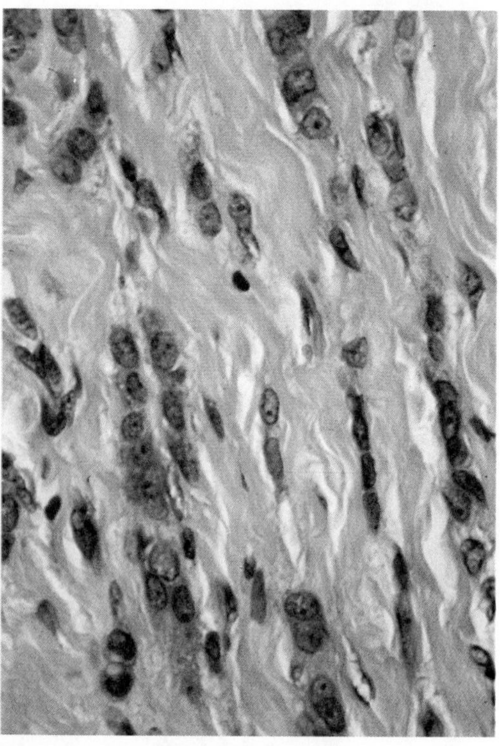

B

FIGURE 19-12
Lobular carcinoma. (*A*) Lobular carcinoma *in situ*. The lumina of the terminal duct lobular units are distended by tumor cells, which exhibit round nuclei and small nucleoli. The cancer cells in the lobular form of carcinoma *in situ* are smaller and have less cytoplasm than those in the ductal type. (*B*) Invasive lobular carcinoma. In contrast to invasive ductal carcinoma, the cells of lobular carcinoma tend to form single strands that invade between collagen fibers in a single pattern. The tumor cells are similar to those seen in lobular carcinoma *in situ*.

TUBULAR CARCINOMA: Also known as well-differentiated carcinoma, invasive tubular carcinoma is composed of randomly arranged, infiltrating, well-formed small ducts that consist of only one or two layers of small, regular cells. The prognosis of this cancer, when it is not admixed with other types, is excellent, and it is virtually always cured by mastectomy or wide excision.

FIGURE 19-13
Colloid (mucinous) carcinoma. Clusters of malignant cells float in large pools of extracellular mucin.

MEDULLARY CARCINOMA: Clinically and by mammography, this invasive tumor presents as a circumscribed mass, which lacks calcifications. Medullary carcinoma has a distinctive gross appearance, being a well-circumscribed, fleshy, pale gray mass. Microscopically, it is composed of sheets of cells, that are highly pleomorphic and have a high mitotic index (Fig. 19-14). The pathological definition of medullary carcinoma includes a lymphoid infiltrate encompassing the periphery of the tumor. In spite of the highly malignant histological appearance of this neoplasm, it has a distinctly better prognosis than that of the usual infiltrating ductal or lobular carcinoma.

METAPLASTIC CARCINOMA: Metaplastic carcinoma refers to a rare invasive variant in which the malignant epithelium has partially differentiated into either another type of epithelium or mesenchymal tissue. Such tumors may show areas of malignant squamous, fibrous, cartilaginous, or bony tissue, admixed with the malignant glandular component.

Metastatic Patterns of Breast Cancer

Invasive breast cancer spreads primarily through the lymphatics to regional lymph nodes, including the axillary, internal mammary, and supraclavicular nodes. In about half of all patients with breast cancer, the tumor has already metastasized to the axillary nodes at the time of diagnosis. The probability of spread to the axillary nodes is directly related to the size of the primary tumor. Involvement of the internal mammary and the supraclavicular lymph nodes is uncommon in the absence of metastases to the axillary nodes. Breast cancer also spreads to distant sites, most commonly the lung and pleura, liver, bone, adrenals, skin, and brain.

Prognostic Factors

Stage at Diagnosis

The most important prognostic factor in breast cancer is the stage (i.e., the extent of tumor spread) at the time of diagnosis. In general, small tumors localized to the breast have an excellent prognosis, whereas those that have spread to distant organs are incurable. Larger primary tumors and those that have metastasized to regional lymph nodes have an intermediate prognosis.

- **Stage I**: Tumors 2 cm or less in diameter without direct extension or nodal metastases
- **Stage II**: Tumors between 2 and 5 cm in diameter without nodal metastases, or any tumor less than 5 cm with ipsilateral axillary metastases in which the lymph nodes remain movable
- **Stage III**: A tumor greater than 5 cm in diameter with or without lymph node metastases; or any tumor with metastases in axillary lymph nodes and nodes fixed to one another or other structures; or any tumor with involvement of the underlying pectoral muscle or fascia (not including the chest wall)
- **Stage IV:** Any tumor with involvement of the chest wall (ribs and intercostal muscles) or skin of the breast (including, inflammatory carcinoma); any tumor with metastases to ipsilateral supraclavicular or infraclavicular nodes, or edema of the arm, or any distant metastases

The majority of breast cancers present as small tumors localized in the breast (stage I or II). There is a significant difference in survival between women who present with stage I disease, as opposed to those with axillary node metastases (stage II). Within stage II disease there is a decreasing survival with an increasing number of involved axillary nodes. Women with advanced local or regional disease (stage III) can be palliated, but not usually cured. The prognosis for women with distant metastases (stage IV) is poor in terms of survival, but palliative treatment may significantly prolong life.

With growing public awareness of breast cancer and the expanding use of screening mammography, more than half of the breast cancers currently diagnosed in the United States present as stage I disease. Some 70% of these women will be cured by surgery. The remaining 30%, if treated with surgery alone, will have recurrent disease.

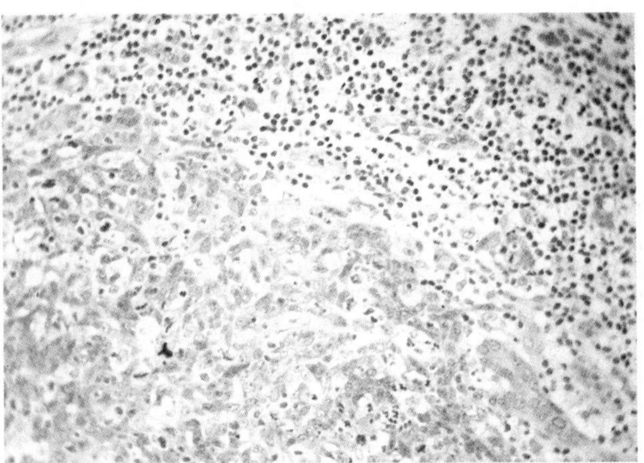

FIGURE *19-14*
Medullary carcinoma. The malignant cells are pleomorphic and grow in solid sheets, forming a blunt margin. There is no gland formation. Numerous mitoses are present. The tumor is surrounded by a dense lymphocytic infiltrate.

Clinical studies have shown that the benefit of routinely adding chemotherapy to surgery in the treatment of all stage I patients is marginal and not without morbidity. Thus, there is an impetus to identify specific subsets of women who might particularly benefit from chemotherapy in addition to surgery.

Histological Grade

In addition to the histological subtype and stage of the cancer, the histological grade of the primary tumor is also a useful prognostic indicator. The histological grade comprises: (1) the degree of glandular differentiation, (2) the degree of nuclear atypia and (3) the mitotic index. In the standard grading system, each of these parameters is given a score of one to three. The sum of the scores of these three parameters results in an overall grade as follows: 3 to 5, well-differentiated; 6 to 7, moderately differentiated; 8 to 9, poorly differentiated.

Estrogen and Progesterone Receptors

Over half of breast cancers exhibit nuclear estrogen receptor protein. A slightly smaller proportion also have progesterone receptors. The presence of these proteins has been used as a prognostic indicator and as a predictor of response to hormonal therapy. Women whose cancers possess hormone receptors have a longer disease-free survival and overall survival than those with early stage cancers who are negative for these receptors.

The beneficial effects of oophorectomy on survival in patients with breast cancer led to the use of estrogen antagonists in the treatment of breast cancer. In general, anti-estrogen therapy seems to prolong disease-free survival, particularly in postmenopausal and node-positive women. It also lowers the risk of cancer in the contralateral breast. The latter discovery has led to current studies of anti-estrogens as chemoprevention in women at "high risk" for developing breast cancer.

Proliferative Capacity and Ploidy

The measurement of proliferative capacity of breast cancers has prognostic value. In general, increased proliferative capacity is associated with a poorer prognosis. There are several methods used to evaluate the proliferative capacity of breast cancers, including (1) mitotic index, as judged by histological evaluation; (2) estimation of the proportion of cells in the S phase of the cell cycle by flow cytometry; and (3) immunohistochemical staining for nuclear proteins expressed in cells that are actively proliferating (Ki67 or mib1 antigens). When proliferative capacity is evaluated by flow cytometry, cell cycle analysis can also detect the presence of aneuploid cell populations. The presence of aneuploidy, which is found in two thirds of breast cancers, has also been associated with a worse prognosis.

Lymphatic and Vascular Invasion

The presence of lymphatic and vascular invasion within the breast is associated with a poorer prognosis. ***Inflammatory carcinoma of the breast*** describes dermal lymphatic invasion, a condition that carries a particularly poor prognosis. Such invasion causes obstruction of lymphatic drainage and, therefore, commonly correlates with clinical erythema and induration of the skin of the breast, so-called *peau d'orange* (because of the resemblance to the skin of an orange).

Oncogene Expression

Amplification of genes for growth factor receptors, related genes C-*erb* B2 (HER-2) and epidermal growth factor receptor (EGRF), as well as mutation and over-expression of the p53 tumor suppressor gene, correlates with recurrence of breast cancer and shortened survival.

Other Factors Related to Invasion and Metastasis

A number of enzymes, cell adhesion molecules, and angiogenic markers are related to breast cancer metastasis and recurrence. These include cathespin D, stromelysin, urokinase-plasminogen activator, laminin receptor and high vascular density.

Treatment

The cornerstone of effective treatment of breast cancer is early detection. Regular self-examination of the breasts, adherence to recommended guidelines for screening mammograms, and periodic examinations by a physician decrease mortality from breast cancer by 30%.

It is useful to evaluate a suspicious mass in as minimally invasive a way as possible, so that the greatest number of options for definitive therapy are maintained, not only for curing the cancer but also for preservation of the woman's breast. Fine-needle aspiration is now a widely accepted modality for evaluating a clinically palpable mass. This technique has a sensitivity of 80% to 90%, with virtually no false-positive results.

The treatment of breast cancer remains controversial. Historically, a significant advance in the treatment of this cancer was radical mastectomy (*en bloc* removal of the breast, all axillary lymph nodes, and underlying chest wall muscles). Although early detection has increased the proportion of tumors that are treated at more favorable stages, subsequent developments in the therapy for breast cancer have not greatly improved the prognosis of women with this disease. Today, the modified radical mastectomy, which differs from radical mastectomy in leaving the chest wall muscles intact and foregoing dissection of the superior axillary lymph nodes, is the treatment of choice for many breast cancers. In early-stage breast cancer, an acceptable alternative to mastectomy is the complete excision of the primary cancer ("lumpectomy" or segmental excision), leaving most of the breast intact. Separate surgical excision of the nearby axillary nodes is performed, followed by irradiation of the breast. This approach is as successful as a modified radical mastectomy, in terms of the 10-year survival for appropriately selected cases.

Cancer of the Male Breast

Cancer in the male breast accounts for less than 1% of all cases of breast cancer. As in women, by far the most common subtype is infiltrating ductal carcinoma. Rarely, lobular carcinoma is seen in men. Because there is less fat in the breast, invasion of chest wall muscles is more frequent at the time of diagnosis in men. For tumors of the same stage, however, the prognosis for male breast cancer is similar to that of the female. Predisposing factors for the development of breast cancer in men are largely unknown, although mutations in the BRCA2 gene (see earlier) increase the risk of this tumor.

PHYLLODES TUMOR

Phyllodes tumor of the breast is a proliferation of stromal elements accompanied by a benign growth of ductal structures (Fig. 19-15). These tumors usually occur in women between 30 and 70 years of age, with a peak in the fifth decade. The original term for this tumor, *cystosarcoma phyllodes*, implies malignant behavior, although only a minority of these tumors are capable of invasion and metastasis. Thus, current terminology refers to *phyllodes tumor*, with the additional designation of benign or malignant.

☐ **Pathology:** Phyllodes tumors resemble fibroadenomas in their overall architecture and the presence of glandular and stromal elements. Similar to fibroadenoma, benign phyllodes tumors are sharply circumscribed, and the cut surface is firm, glistening, and grayish white. Benign and malignant phyllodes tumors are similar in gross appearance. Whereas in the past they were described as very large tumors, the average size today is 5 cm in diameter, and many smaller tumors are encountered.

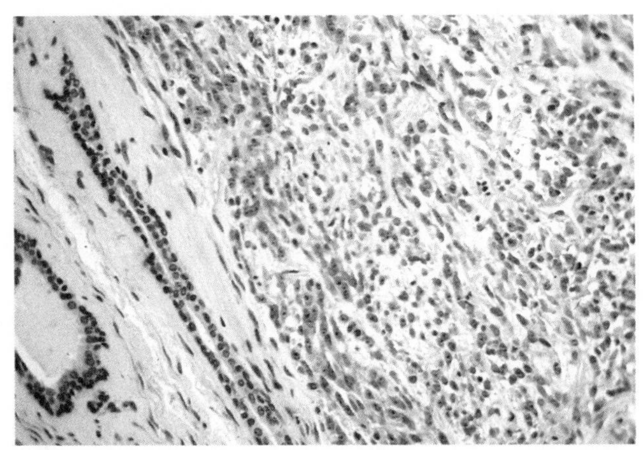

FIGURE 19-15
Malignant phyllodes tumor (cystosarcoma phyllodes). This tumor has stromal and epithelial components similar to fibroadenoma. The stroma is more cellular and in this case is clearly malignant. The residual ductal structures are benign.

Microscopically, the stroma of a benign phyllodes tumor is hypercellular and has mitotic activity. The distinction from fibroadenoma is made not on the size, but on the histological and cytological characteristics of the stromal component.

The diagnosis of a malignant phyllodes tumor is based on the appearance of the stromal component. Malignant phyllodes tumors have an obviously sarcomatous stroma with abundant mitotic activity, and the stromal component is increased out of proportion to the benign duct elements. They are usually poorly circumscribed, with invasion into the surrounding breast tissue. Malignant tumors may exhibit various sarcomatous tissue types, such as malignant fibrous histiocytoma, chondrosarcoma, and osteosarcoma.

□ **Clinical Features:** Benign phyllodes tumors are adequately treated by local excision. The initial treatment of a malignant phyllodes tumor is wide excision if the tumor is small, or a simple mastectomy if the tumor is large. An axillary lymph node dissection is not indicated. Malignant phyllodes tumors tend to recur locally, and 15% eventually metastasize to both distant sites and axillary lymph nodes.

MISCELLANEOUS TUMORS

Malignant tumors can originate from the mesenchymal elements of the breast. True sarcomas are rare and must be distinguished from malignant phyllodes tumor and metaplastic carcinoma. They include angiosarcoma, fibrosarcoma, and malignant fibrous histiocytoma. Malignant lymphoma may involve the breast, usually in addition to more common sites. Occasionally, lymphoma may be primary in the breast.

Metastases to the breast from primary tumors in other parts of the body are uncommon. When present, the site of origin is usually the opposite breast or melanoma.

SUGGESTED READING

BOOKS

Harris JR, Lippman ME, Morrow M, Hellman S: *Diseases of the breast.* Philadelphia: Lippincott–Raven, 1996.

Rogers K: Breast abscesses and problems with lactation. In Smallwood JA, Taylor I (ed): *Benign breast disease.* Baltimore: Urhan and Schwarztenberg, 1990.

Rosai J: Breast. In *Ackerman's surgical pathology*, 8th ed. St. Louis: Mosby, 1996.

Rosen PP: *Rosen's breast pathology.* Philadelphia: Lippincott–Raven, 1997.

Sharkey FE, Allred DC, Valente PT: Breast. In Damjanov I, Linder J (eds): *Anderson's pathology*, 10th ed. St. Louis: Mosby, 1996.

Tavassoli FA: *Pathology of the breast.* New York: Elsevier, 1992.

REVIEW ARTICLES

Association of Directors of Anatomic and Surgical Pathology: Recommendations in the reporting of breast carcinoma. *AJCP* 104:614–619, 1995.

Braunstein GD: Gynecomastia. *N Engl J Med* 328:490–495, 1993.

Fechner RE: One century of mammary carcinoma *in situ*. What have we learned. *AJCP* 100:654–661, 1993.

International conference series on nutrition and health promotion. Breast cancer research: Current issues-future directions. *Cancer* 74 (suppl):991–1192, 1994.

Kelsey JL, Horn-Ross PI: Breast cancer: Magnitude of the problem and descriptive epidemiology. *Epidemial Rev* 15:7–16, 1993.

Love SM, McGuigan KA, Chap L: The Revlon/UCLA breast center practice guidelines for the treatment of breast disease. *The Cancer Journal* 2:2–14, 1996.

Marshall E: Search for a killer. Focus shifts from fats to hormones. *Science* 259:618–621, 1993.

Mettler FA, Upton AC, Kelsey CA, et al: Benefits versus risks from mammography. A critical assessment. *Cancer* 77:903–909, 1996.

Rosen PP: Proliferative breast "disease." An unresolved diagnostic dilemma. *Cancer* 17:3798–3807, 1993.

Skolnick AA: New data suggest needle biopsies could replace surgical biopsy for diagnosing breast cancer. *JAMA* 271:1724–1728, 1994.

ORIGINAL ARTICLES

Bellamy COC, McDonald C, Salter DM, Chetty U, Anderson TJ: Non-invasive ductal carcinoma of the breast. The relevance of histologic categorization. *Hum Pathol* 24:16–23, 1993.

Ernster VL, Barclay J, Kurlikawshe K, Grady D, Henderson IC: Incidence of and treatment for ductal carcinoma *in situ* of the breast. *JAMA* 275:913–918, 1996.

Fisher B, Anderson S, Redmond CK, et al: Reanalysis and results after 12 years of follow-up in a randomized clinical trial comparing total mastectomy with lumpectomy with or without irradiation in the treatment of breast cancer. *N Engl J Med* 333:1456–1461, 1995.

Henson DE, Ries LA, Carriaga MT: Conditional survival of 56,268 patients with breast cancer. *Cancer* 76:237–242, 1995.

Page DL, Jensen RA: Ductal carcinoma *in situ* of the breast. Understanding the misunderstood stepchild (editorial). *JAMA* 275:948, 949, 1996.

Shattuck-Eidens D, McClure M, Simard J, et al: A collaborative survey of 80 mutations in the BRCA1 breast and ovarian cancer susceptibility gene. Implications for presymptomatic testing and screening. *JAMA* 273:535–541, 1995.

CHAPTER 20

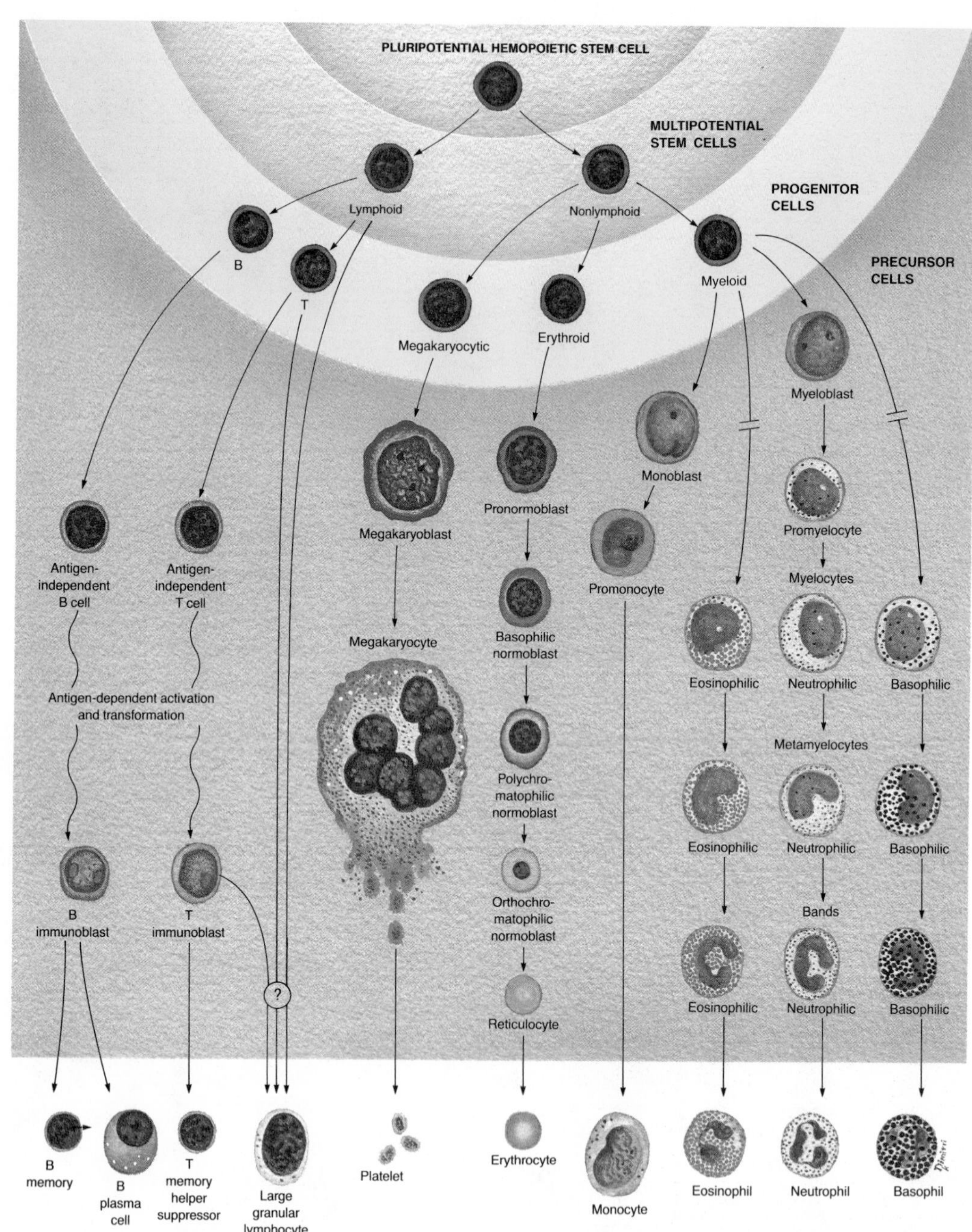

PLURIPOTENTIAL HEMOPOIETIC STEM CELL
MULTIPOTENTIAL STEM CELLS
PROGENITOR CELLS
PRECURSOR CELLS
Lymphoid
Nonlymphoid
B
T
Megakaryocytic
Erythroid
Myeloid
Myeloblast
Monoblast
Megakaryoblast
Pronormoblast
Promonocyte
Promyelocyte
Myelocytes
Antigen-independent B cell
Antigen-independent T cell
Megakaryocyte
Basophilic normoblast
Eosinophilic
Neutrophilic
Basophilic
Antigen-dependent activation and transformation
Metamyelocytes
Polychromatophilic normoblast
Eosinophilic
Neutrophilic
Basophilic
Orthochromatophilic normoblast
Bands
B immunoblast
T immunoblast
?
Reticulocyte
Eosinophilic
Neutrophilic
Basophilic
B memory
B plasma cell
T memory helper suppressor
Large granular lymphocyte
Platelet
Erythrocyte
Monocyte
Eosinophil
Neutrophil
Basophil

The Blood and the Lymphoid Organs

Hugh Bonner
Adam Bagg
Jeffrey Cossman

FIGURE *20-1* (*see opposite page*)
Cellular differentiation and maturation of the lymphoid (*left*) and myeloid (*right*) components of the hemopoietic system. Only the precursor cells (blasts and maturing cells) are visually identifiable in a light morphological evaluation of the bone marrow.

The cellular elements of the blood and the lymphoid organs are responsible for a number of vital functions, including transport of oxygen, defense against microorganisms and parasites, and preservation of vascular integrity. These cells are all derived from a single pool of pluripotential stem cells in the bone marrow (Fig. 20-1), which gives rise to two distinct types of multipotential stem cells, (1) **the nonlymphoid stem cells,** which differentiate in the bone marrow and (2) **the lymphoid stem cells,** which differentiate in the marrow (B cells) or thymus (T cells) and then migrate to the lymphoid organs.

The nonlymphoid stem cells differentiate into three committed progenitor cell lines: (1) erythroid, (2) granulocytic-monocytic, and (3) megakaryocytic. The lymphoid stem cells differentiate into two committed progenitor cell lines, giving rise to the B-cell and T-cell lineages. Stimulated and regulated by various growth factors, the progenitor cells proliferate and undergo further differentiation to morphologically distinctive precursor cells and, in turn, to mature circulating blood cells.

Structure and Function of the Blood and Lymphoid Organs

THE HEMOPOIETIC SYSTEM

Embryology

Hemopoiesis, or blood cell formation, first occurs in the fetal yolk sac (Fig. 20-2). "Blood islands," consisting of clusters of large nucleated erythrocytes, can be identified in the third week of embryogenesis. Shortly thereafter, erythrocyte formation shifts to the liver, where small, nonnucleated erythrocytes are produced. These cells contain fetal hemoglobins rather than the embryonic hemoglobins produced during the yolk sac phase. Hepatic erythrocyte production continues until the end of the third trimester, at which time bone marrow erythropoiesis has become fully established. During the second trimester, the spleen is also involved in the production of erythrocytes. At term, erythropoiesis in the liver and spleen has ceased. Nevertheless, these organs, especially the spleen, remain well suited for erythrocyte formation. Under conditions of increased demand for erythrocytes, as in the hemolytic disorders erythroblastosis fetalis or thalassemia, splenic and hepatic erythropoiesis continues into and beyond the neonatal period. The production of cellular elements other than erythrocytes also takes place in the liver and spleen, transferring to the newly formed bone cavities during the second trimester.

At birth and until 4 years of age, all bone cavities are densely packed with hemopoietic tissue. After that time, the size of the bone cavities outgrows the volume required for hemopoiesis and fat cells fill the available space. This imbalance between available and required bone marrow space continues to increase until early adulthood, when most cavities in the peripheral bone marrow have become fatty (yellow) and hemopoietically inactive. The cavities in the axial skeleton continue to be active and full of "red marrow" until old age, when resorption of cancellous bone further enlarges the marrow cavities and leads to replacement by fat.

Local expansion of red (cellular) marrow and reactivation of peripheral yellow marrow provide the hemopoietic system with a readily available capacity to meet acute and chronic demands for increased blood cell formation. Reactivation of hepatic and splenic hemopoiesis rarely occurs during adult life. **The finding of extramedullary hemopoiesis in soft tissue sites usually suggests a clonal (malignant) disorder, rather than a reactive one.**

Bone Marrow

The bone marrow consists of a complex network of solid cords separated by sinusoids (Fig. 20-3). It receives its blood supply from nutrient arteries and capillaries within the bone. In the marrow the vessels arborize into a network of sinusoids, which drain into a central vein. The cords consist of stromal cells and hemopoietic cells, knitted together by an adhesive and fertile extracellular matrix.

The semipermeable barrier between the sinusoids and the cords consists of a layer of endothelial cells, a thin basement membrane, and an outer interrupted layer of reticular adventitial cells. These reticular cells branch extensively throughout the cords and provide a scaffold for stromal and hemopoietic cells. They also have the capa-

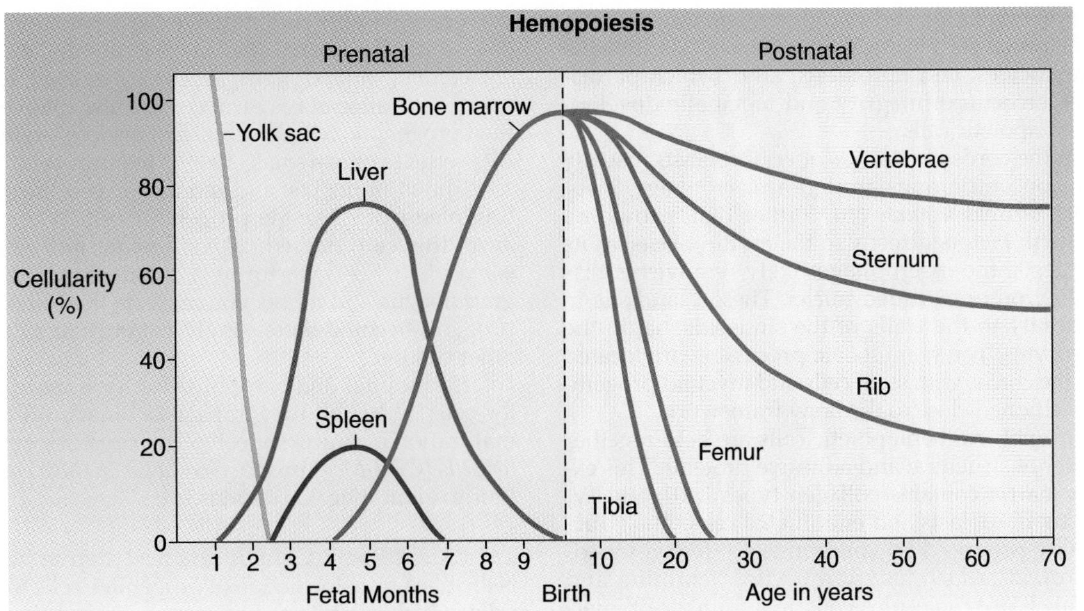

FIGURE 20-2
Hemopoiesis in various organs before and after birth.

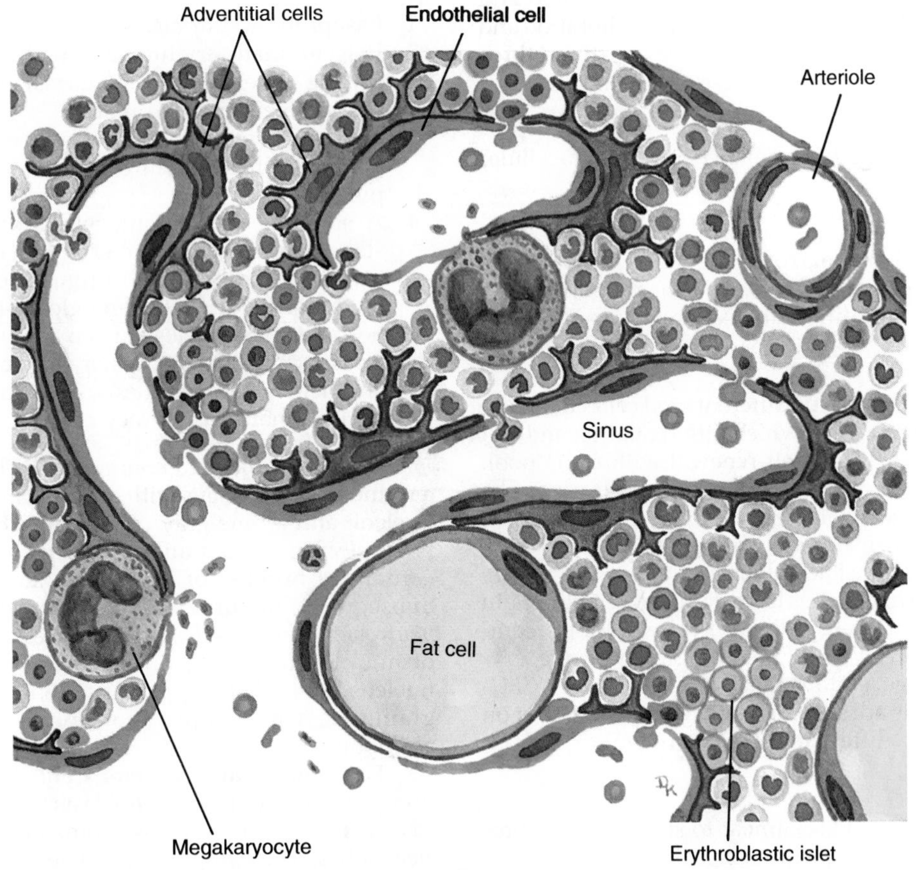

FIGURE 20-3
Structure of normal bone marrow.

city to synthesize lipids and to differentiate into fat cells. The other stromal cells include macrophages, endothelial cells, lymphocytes, and fibroblasts, all of which participate in the structural integrity and metabolic development of hemopoietic cells.

Within the cords are islands of erythroblasts, usually located in concentric rings around a macrophage, inappropriately termed a *nurse cell*. Rather than providing iron or growth factors directly to the erythroblasts, as its name suggests, the macrophage likely removes excess cytoplasmic iron or extruded nuclei. These islands lie in close proximity to the walls of the sinusoids, as do the megakaryocytes. The granulocyte precursors are located deeper in the cords, with stem cells and myeloid progenitor cells positioned close to the bony framework.

The stromal and hemopoietic cells are held together by a number of structural and adhesive proteins. This extracellular matrix contains collagen types I, III, and IV, produced by fibroblasts and endothelial cells. The structural stability produced by collagen is reinforced by adhesion proteins, such as fibronectin, laminin, and hemonectin. These molecules contain a number of interacting domains, including the common attachment peptide: arginine, glycine, aspartic acid, serine (RGDS). Receptors for these domains (the integrins) are present on most hemopoietic cells; fibronectin specifically binds erythroblasts and hemonectin binds myeloid precursor cells. The migration and release of mature cells reflect, at least in part, a gradual loss of these receptors. In addition, the adhesion proteins bind various proteoglycans and growth factors, which in turn control the proliferation and maturation of hemopoietic cells. There are, thus, three critical components of hematopoiesis:

- Stem cells (seed)
- Stroma, consisting of stromal cells and extracellular matrix (soil)
- Growth factors (fertilizer)

Hemopoietic bone marrow cells can be divided into pluripotential stem cells, bipotential or monopotential progenitor cells, and differentiated precursor cells (Fig. 20-4).

STEM CELLS: These undifferentiated cells constitute a self-perpetuating pool, in which differentiation and exit are carefully balanced by self-renewal within the pool. Stem cells are small mononuclear cells, which cannot be easily identified morphologically. However, they can be isolated by injecting marrow elements into radiated mice, in which they form visible colonies in the spleen (*colony forming unit, spleen*; *CFU-S*). In bone marrow cultures in semisolid medium, stem cells also form colonies composed of multiple cell types, including granulocyte, erythroid, macrophage, and megakaryocyte elements (*CFU-GEMM*). Stem cells are semidormant (noncycling), but on demand undergo differentiation to progenitor cells of specific cell lines.

PROGENITOR CELLS: Similar to stem cells, the progenitor cells are small to medium-sized mononuclear cells that cannot be morphologically distinguished from mature lymphocytes. When cultured *in vitro*, they give rise to colonies consisting of thousands of differentiated progeny. The progenitor cell committed to the production of erythrocytes forms luxuriant burst-shaped colonies and is named *burst forming unit, erythroid* (*BFU-E*) (Fig. 20-5). Each subsequent generation of BFU-E makes smaller colonies, until the final progenitor cell, *the colony forming unit, erythroid* (*CFU-E*), produces only a small clone of mature erythroblasts.

The granulocytic and monocytic cell lines appear to originate from a single progenitor cell. When grown *in vitro*, this cell, named *colony forming unit, granulocyte-monocyte* (*CFU-GM*), forms a colony consisting of both granulocytic and monocytic cells. As the cell matures, its progeny become increasingly committed to one or the other cell line.

Eosinophils and basophils also have specific progenitor cells, although they appear to branch off during the maturation of precursor cells. The *megakaryocytic progenitor cells* (*CFU-Meg*) produce colonies *in vitro* consisting of four to eight megakaryocytes.

PRECURSOR CELLS: The next step in hemopoiesis is the blast transformation of progenitor cells to precursor cells, which exhibit specific morphological characteristics (see Fig. 20-1). It is only at this stage and beyond that the cells are morphologically recognizable in terms of their lineage.

The Erythroid Precursor Cell: The proerythroblast is a large cell with intense blue cytoplasm and a round homogeneous nucleus, containing a few nucleoli. The proerythroblast matures sequentially as follows:

1. Basophilic erythroblasts without nucleoli
2. Polychromatic erythroblasts with grayish cytoplasm (owing to hemoglobin synthesis) and a nucleus with coarsely clumped chromatin
3. Smaller orthochromatic erythroblasts, with red hemoglobin-containing cytoplasm and a dense pyknotic nucleus
4. A nonnucleated reticulocyte, representing the last stage before the mature erythrocyte. The nucleus is extruded from the orthochromatic erythroblast, leaving mitochondria and hemoglobin-producing polyribosomes. After release from the bone marrow, the reticulocyte loses its capacity for aerobic metabolism and hemoglobin synthesis, and after 1 or 2 days becomes a mature erythrocyte.

The Granulocytic Precursor Cell: The *myeloblast* has a round to oval nucleus with delicate chromatin and a few nucleoli and a blue-gray cytoplasm. The next stage, the *promyelocyte*, has a similar nucleus, but the cytoplasm contains a number of primary (azurophilic) granules. Subsequent maturation from *myelocyte* to mature *neutrophil* involves (1) the progressive condensation of nuclear chromatin, (2) increasing lobulation of the nucleus, and (3) the appearance of secondary (specific) granules, which are neutrophilic, basophilic, or eosinophilic.

The Monocytic Precursor Cell: The parallel formation of monocytes from monoblasts involves a similar nuclear condensation but less prominent formation of nuclear lobes. The cytoplasm becomes grayish, containing only a few pink or purple granules. Subsequently, after the monocyte leaves the bloodstream and becomes a member of the mononuclear phagocyte system (formerly

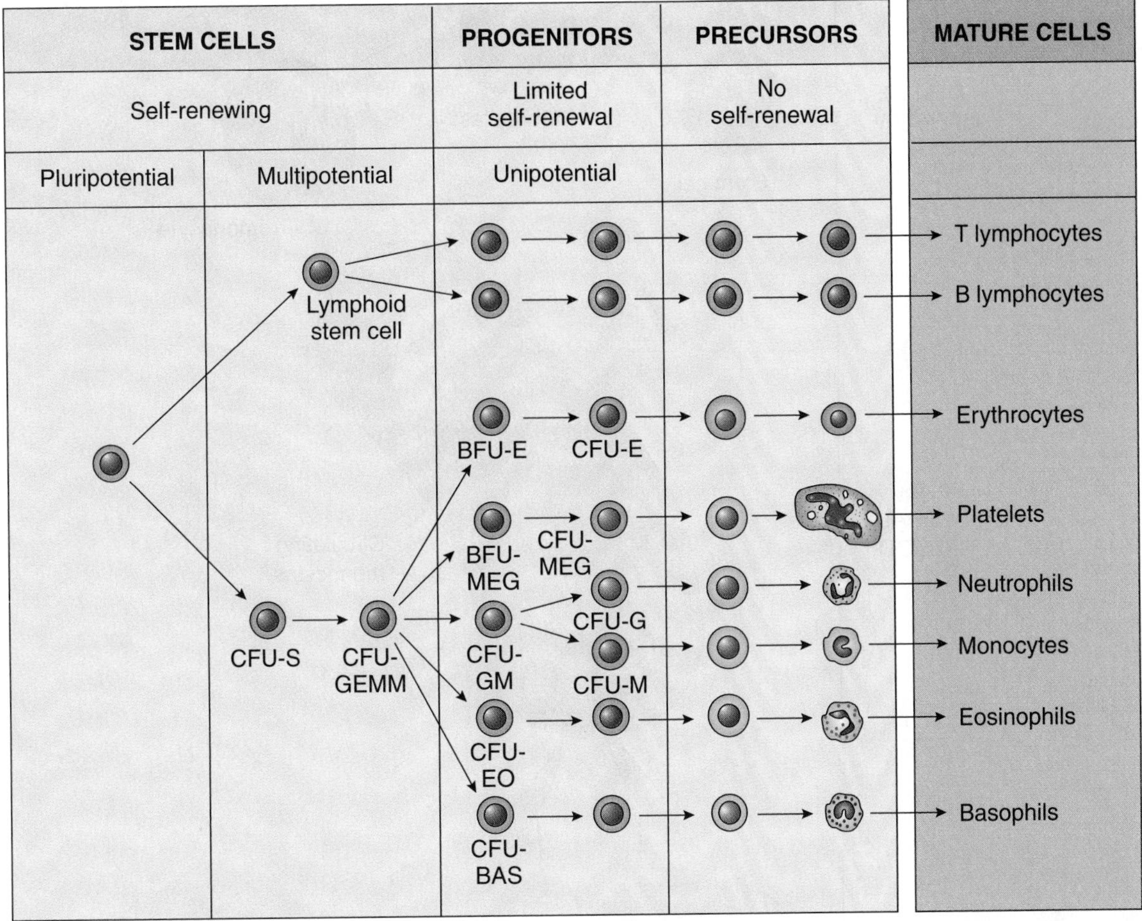

FIGURE 20-4
Differentiation of formed elements of the blood, with a simplified schema of some sites of action (→) of selected cytokines, interleukins, and colony stimulating factors. Note that the stem cells and progenitors are not readily identifiable in the routine examination of a bone marrow aspirate.

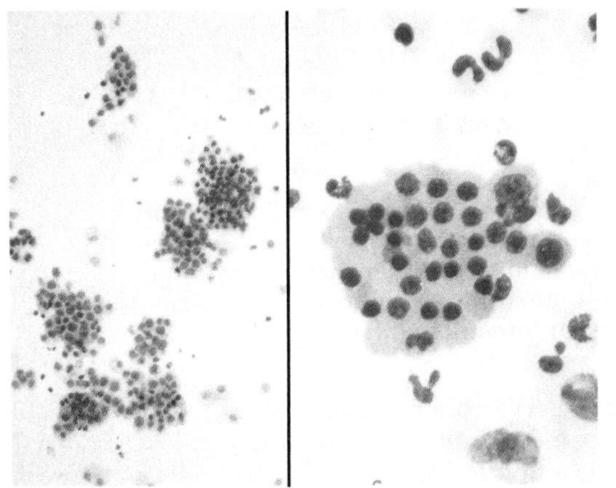

FIGURE 20-5
(*Left*) When grown *in vitro*, erythroid progenitor cells give rise to burst-shaped colonies consisting of differentiated progeny. (*Right*) A higher-power view. The progenitor cell committed to the production of erythrocytes forms luxuriant burst-shaped colonies and is named burst forming unit, erythroid (BFU-E).

called the reticuloendothelial system), it undergoes further morphological changes, depending on its tissue location and its function as either a phagocyte (fixed or wandering), or an immunoregulator (Fig. 20-6).

The Megakaryocytic Precursor: Megakaryocytes in the bone marrow mature into multilobed giant cells by a number of endomitotic divisions. After having reached a certain ploidy, the cytoplasm becomes stippled and azurophilic and is eventually released into the sinusoids in long platelet-containing ribbons. Some intact megakaryocytes are also released, and platelet production then occurs after the megakaryocytes have been trapped in the pulmonary microcirculation.

Examination of the Bone Marrow

The cellular elements of the bone marrow are commonly evaluated both by needle biopsy and aspiration of marrow from the posterior iliac crest. Marrow can also be obtained in infants from the anterior tibial bone and in adults from the sternum. The cellularity and histological architecture of the bone marrow is best evaluated on ex-

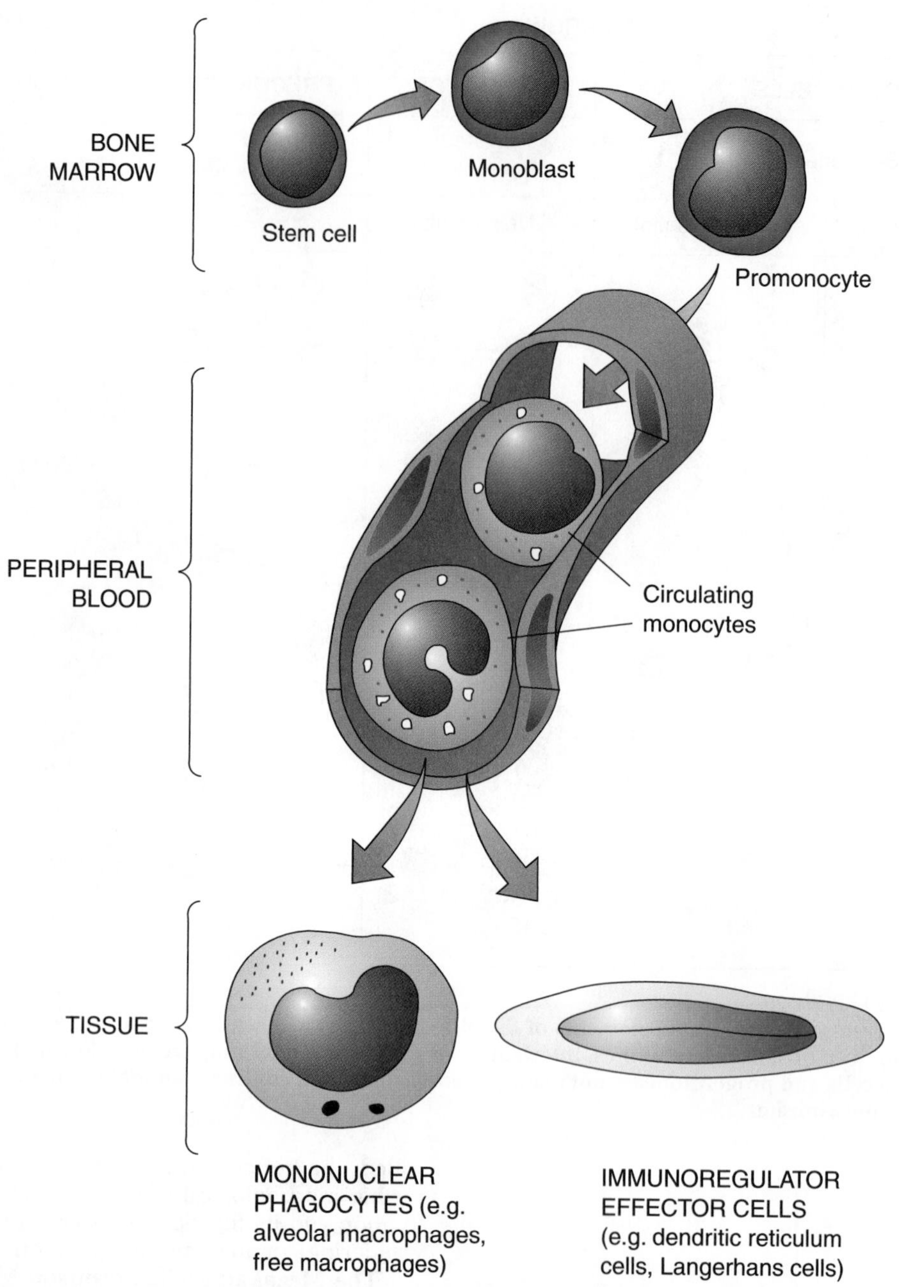

FIGURE *20-6*
The mononuclear phagocyte and immune regulator effector (M-PIRE) system. The cells of this system take origin in the bone marrow from hemopoietic stem cells, which give rise to monoblasts and then promonocytes. The last mature into monocytes, which circulate in the peripheral blood. These monocytes then exit the peripheral blood and enter the tissues, where they become the various specialized phagocytes or immunoregulator cells.

amination of biopsy sections (Fig. 20-7A), whereas identification of specific precursor cells is best made on a smear of the aspirate (see Fig. 20-7B). In a normal adult, half (range, one third to two thirds) of the biopsy surface area consists of fat cells and half of active hemopoietic tissue. The proportion of hemopoietic cells is referred to as the cellularity. Relative to a normal adult, the cellularity is increased in children and decreased in the elderly.

The normal ratio of granulocytic precursors (myeloid cells) to erythroblastic precursors (erythroid cells), or the myeloid:erythroid ratio, is between 2:1 and 7:1 (Table 20-1). Since the proliferation of both myeloid and erythroid cells is amplified at each step, blast cells are few and the most mature cells are plentiful. Changes in this distribution are designated as a "left shift" (toward immaturity) or a "right shift" (toward maturity). In normal bone marrow, two to five megakaryocytes can be identified per high-power field. The normal bone marrow contains fewer than 3% plasma cells, up to 20% lymphocytes, and only rare mast cells and macrophages. The reticulin silver

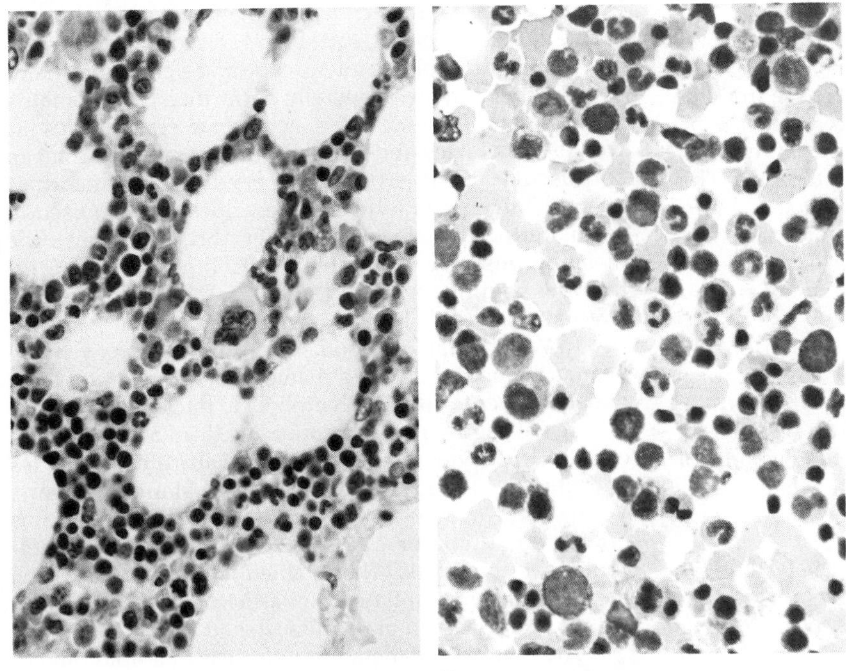

FIGURE 20-7
Normal bone marrow. (*A*) A photomicrograph of a tissue section shows the normal relationship (1:1) of cellular elements to fat, a normal myeloid:erythroid ratio, and a megakaryocyte in the center. (*B*) A smear of the bone marrow aspirate from the same patient demonstrates normal hemopoietic elements and varying stages of differentiation.

stain reveals scattered fibers in the hemopoietic stroma. With the trichrome stain for collagen, delicate perivascular fibrosis is usually observed.

Evaluation of bone marrow iron stores is most accurately made on an aspirate stained with Prussian blue. The normal bone marrow contains blue hemosiderin granules in macrophages and in the interstitium. Minute hemosiderin granules are found in the cytoplasm of 10% of the erythroid precursor cells (sideroblasts).

Functional Kinetics

The hemopoietic cells in the bone marrow maintain the size of the circulating blood cell mass. Under normal conditions, they produce daily 3 billion erythrocytes, 1 billion granulocytes, and 1.5 billion platelets per kilogram of body weight. This output is adjusted to compensate for senescence and destruction of blood cells and can be increased or decreased according to the needs of the body. Such regulation is mediated by a number of growth factors that affect the rate of cellular proliferation, primarily within the progenitor cell compartment.

TABLE *20-1* **Normal Adult Bone Marrow (Age 18–70 Years)**

Fat:cell ratio 50:50 ± 15%
Myeloid:erythroid ratio 2:1 to 7:1
Cell distribution (% surface area)
Fat cells 35–65%
Erythroid series 10–20%
Granulocytic (myeloid) series 40–65%
Megakaryocytes 2–5/high-power field
Plasma cells <3% of nucleated cells
Lymphocytes <20% of nucleated cells
No fibrosis

GROWTH FACTORS: Colony stimulating factors (CSF) and interleukins (IL) constitute a family of glycoproteins produced by macrophages, endothelial cells, fibroblasts, and T lymphocytes. They are members of a large group of hormone-like factors that mediate many immune and inflammatory responses.

IL-1, IL-3, IL-6, IL-11, and stem cell factor (SCF) primarily support the survival and proliferation of stem cells. The mechanisms underlying the differentiation of stem cells to lineage-committed progenitor cells are not well understood. However, the subsequent proliferation and maturation of the progenitor cells is affected by specific growth factors. Granulocyte-monocyte colony stimulating factor (GM-CSF) stimulates the growth of the granulocytic and monocytic cell lines, as well as the progenitors of megakaryocytes and erythrocytes. Granulocyte colony stimulating factor (G-CSF) promotes the growth of the granulocytic cell line, and monocyte colony stimulating factor (M-CSF) fosters that of the monocytic cell line. In addition to promoting expansion at the progenitor level, these growth factors influence the proliferation and maturation of precursor cells, as well as the function of mature cells.

Erythropoietin is released by the interstitial peritubular cells of the kidney in response to hypoxia and activates specific receptors on the cell membrane of erythroid progenitor cells. Erythropoietin promotes the growth of early erythroid progenitor cells (BFU-E), in conjunction with IL-3 and GM-CSF. However, erythropoietin alone determines the transformation of the late erythroid progenitor cells (CFU-E) to erythroblasts.

Whereas IL-3, IL-6, and IL-11, among others, affect the growth and differentiation of megakaryocytes, a more specific regulator of megakaryopoiesis has recently been identified. This factor, thrombopoietin, facilitates the production and maturation of megakaryocytes.

RELEASE FROM THE MARROW: There are also factors that regulate the release of mature cells into the circulating blood. The mature blood cell forms a very narrow migration channel through the endothelium. This pathway may participate in the extrusion of the nondeformable pyknotic nucleus of the orthochromatic erythroblast. The nuclei of other precursor cells can change their shape to accommodate even an extremely narrow opening.

In addition to facilitating a continuous exit of cells from the cords to the blood, the release mechanism can, in an emergency situation, provide the blood with a boost of mature cells stored in the bone marrow. Such release is of special importance for short-lived granulocytes but of much less significance for long-lived platelets and erythrocytes.

Circulating Blood

Erythrocytes

After entry into the circulation, erythrocytes survive for 120 days and platelets for 10 to 12 days. By contrast, granulocytes are short-lived and circulate for up to 12 hours (usually 4 to 6 hours), and may then take up residence in the tissues or participate in the response to infection. Monocytes circulate for 1 to 2 days before they take up residence in the tissues, where they remain for months.

The erythroid composition of the blood is evaluated by a blood cell count and an examination of a blood smear (Table 20-2). In the past, total blood cell counts were measured manually using a microscope and a counting chamber, but they are now generally performed by automated cell counters. These counters enumerate erythrocytes (as well as leukocytes and platelets) and measure the mean corpuscular volume (MCV) of erythrocytes and their hemoglobin concentration. These values are then used to calculate the hematocrit (MCV/erythrocyte count), the mean corpuscular hemoglobin (MCH; hemoglobin/erythrocyte count), and the mean corpuscular hemoglobin concentration (MCHC; hemoglobin/hematocrit).

In Wright-stained blood smears, the erythrocytes appear as round disks with a diameter of 7 μm, or approximately the same size as a lymphocyte nucleus (Fig. 20-8). An area of central pallor is about one third as wide as the cell. Reticulocytes are larger than mature erythrocytes and may not be visible on Wright-stained smears. Younger forms have a grayish blue hue, referred to as polychromophilia or diffuse basophilia, owing to their content of ribosomes. When stained with supravital dyes, the ribosomes precipitate into particles, thereby facilitating the identification of reticulocytes.

The erythrocyte membrane consists of a lipid bilayer studded with proteins (Fig. 20-9). Some proteins act as receptors, some have attached extracellular antigenic polysaccharides, some function as transmembrane channels for electrolytes, and others serve as anchors for a submembranous cytoskeletal scaffold. The supporting scaffold is composed of a hexagonal lattice of twisted spectrin dimers linked to each other and to other membrane proteins by actin and ankyrin. The cytoplasmic portion of the erythrocytes contains hemoglobin and en-

TABLE 20-2 The Complete Blood Count (CBC): Normal Adult Values

Erythrocytes		
Hemoglobin		Male, 14–18 g/dL Female, 12–16 g/dL
Hematocrit		Male, 40–54% Female, 35–47%
Red blood cell (RBC) count		Male, 4.5–6 × 10⁶/μL Female, 4–5.5 × 10⁶/μL
Reticulocytes		0.5–2.5%
Indices		
Mean corpuscular volume		82–100 μm³
Mean corpuscular hemoglobin		27–34 pg
Mean corpuscular hemoglobin concentration		32–36%
Leukocytes		
	Absolute Count/μL	Differential Count (%)
White blood cell (WBC) count	4000–11,000	
Neutrophil granulocytes	1800–7000	50–60
Neutrophil bands	0–700	2–4
Lymphocytes	1500–4000	30–40
Monocytes	0–800	1–9
Basophils	0–200	0–1
Eosinophils	0–450	0–3
Platelets		

Quantitative normal value: 150,000–400,000/μL
Qualitative estimation on smear: # platelets/oil immersion field × 10,000 = estimated platelet count
Normal ratio of RBC:platelets = 15:1 to 20:1

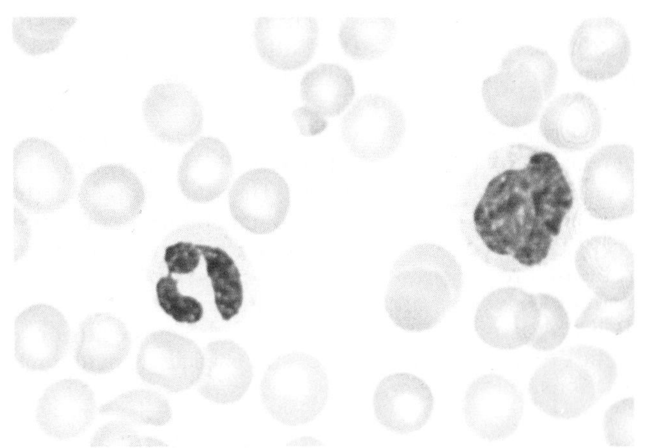

FIGURE 20-8
Normal peripheral blood smear. The mature erythrocytes are of normal size and show central pallor. A neutrophil and monocyte are also present.

zymes that maintain the integrity of the erythrocyte membrane and the functional competence of hemoglobin.

The erythrocytes are simple cells with one major function, namely, the transport of oxygen from the lungs to the tissues. The hemoglobin molecule contains four heme groups, which bind oxygen in the lungs and discharge it in the tissues. Hemoglobin A consists of two α chains and two β chains, each containing a heme pocket. The molecule undergoes allosteric changes, depending on the degree of oxygenation of the heme. Several factors affect the affinity of hemoglobin for oxygen:

- The oxygen affinity of deoxygenated hemoglobin is low, and a large increase in oxygen tension is required to oxygenate the first heme group. In turn, this oxygenation changes the conformation of the α-β chain contact and progressively facilitates the oxygenation of the remaining three heme pockets. This stepwise increase in oxygen affinity is reflected in the characteristically sigmoid oxygen dissociation curve (Fig. 20-10).
- The slope of the oxygen dissociation curve can be altered by the *p*H of the environment, with enhancement of oxygen delivery at the more acid *p*H of deoxygenated tissue.
- 2,3-Diphosphoglyceride (2,3-DPG), a sugar moiety released by hypoxic tissues, also affects the slope of the oxygen dissociation curve and enhances delivery of oxygen to the tissues.

The erythrocytes also facilitate the uptake and transport of carbon dioxide from the tissues to the lungs. This function, however, is less dependent on an adequate number of erythrocytes than is the transport of oxygen, and it is rarely disturbed, even in severe anemias.

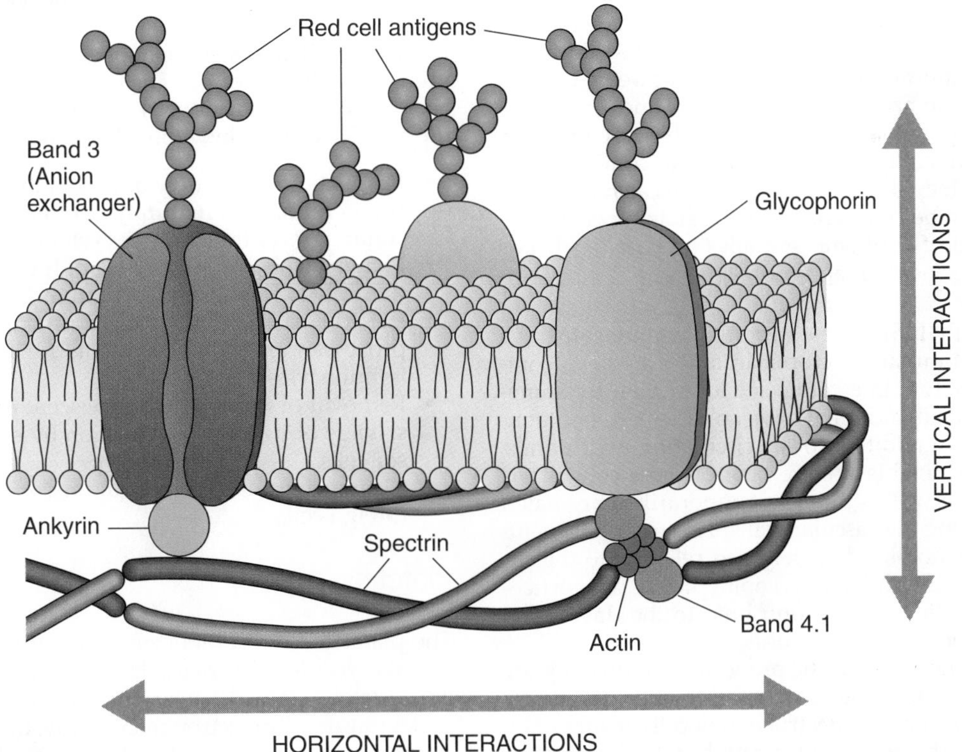

FIGURE 20-9
Structure of the erythrocyte plasma membrane. The membrane is stabilized by a number of interactions. The two vertical ones are spectrin-ankyrin-band 3 and spectrin-protein 4.1-glycophorin. The two horizontal interactions are spectrin heterodimer assembly and spectrin-actin-protein 4.1.

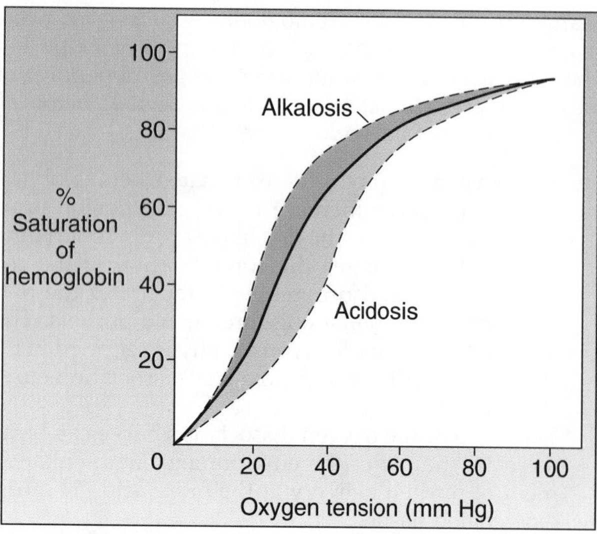

FIGURE *20-10*
Oxygen dissociation curve of hemoglobin. With decreasing *p*H (acidosis) the oxygen affinity declines (shifted to the right), whereas with increased *p*H (alkalosis) the affinity is increased (shifted to the left). Oxygen affinity is also increased by 2,3 DPG and lowered temperatures.

Granulocytes

Differential counts of leukocytes based on cell size, granularity, conductivity, cytochemical staining, and membrane properties are automated by electronic devices. However, the visual identification of cells on a smear treated with a Wright or a Giemsa polychrome stain and examined microscopically with an oil immersion objective provides more information. Because of their nuclear configuration, mature granulocytes are also termed *polymorphonuclear leukocytes*. Subtypes are defined by the staining characteristics of specific cytoplasmic granules and are labeled as neutrophils, eosinophils, and basophils.

NEUTROPHILS: The neutrophilic granulocyte has a pink, finely granulated cytoplasm and a nucleus composed of two to four interconnected lobes. Slightly immature neutrophils (band cells) have an indented, nonlobulated nucleus. In addition to the circulating neutrophils, there is a considerable storage pool of these cells in the bone marrow, as well as a pool of temporarily marginated neutrophils along the vascular walls. This reserve of neutrophils can be mobilized acutely and released to the circulating blood by endotoxins, epinephrine, or corticosteroids. Sporadic releases contribute to the day-to-day variations in the neutrophil counts.

Owing to their phagocytic properties, neutrophils are the first line of defense against invading microorganisms (see Chapter 2). The local destruction of cells at sites of infection causes the release of a number of chemotactic molecules. These substances bind to receptors on the surface of neutrophils and cause them to marginate, cross the endothelial barrier, and slowly move toward the infectious locus. Assisted by opsonins, they then engulf the bacteria, which are in turn killed and digested by lysosomal enzymes, in the presence of hydrogen peroxide, superoxide, and halides. The pathways by which neutrophils kill bacteria are discussed in Chapter 2.

EOSINOPHILS: The eosinophilic granulocytes contain large granules, which stain red with eosin because of their content of basic proteins. The nucleus is usually bilobed, with a thin connecting filament. Eosinophils are primarily tissue cells, with only a short intravascular stay. They are present primarily in the mucosa of the gastrointestinal, bronchial, and lower genitourinary tracts. Here their IgA receptors and toxic cationic proteins contribute to the defense against parasites and participate in allergic reactions.

BASOPHILS: Basophilic granulocytes contain prominent blue-black granules that often overlie and obscure the nucleus. The granules contain histamine and other substances, and their release is an important component of certain allergic disorders. Other inflammatory mediators, for example, leukotrienes (SRS-A), are produced upon appropriate stimulation.

MONOCYTES: These medium-sized to large cells exhibit a kidney-shaped or lobed nucleus and abundant gray cytoplasm with few granules. They are potentially phagocytic, but they do not become truly functional macrophages until they enter tissues and undergo a number of morphological and functional changes. The general transformation to a phagocytic macrophage is modulated by the final tissue location. Fully differentiated monocytes perform either phagocytic or immunoregulatory functions, accounting for the term M-PIRE system (*m*ononuclear-*p*hagocyte and *i*mmuno*r*egulatory *e*ffector). The IR arm includes Langerhans cells and other dendritic cells. The functions of these versatile M-PIRE cells include the following:

- Production of a variety of factors that control cellular proliferation and maturation, often referred to as the conductors of the immune system.
- Phagocytosis and processing of foreign antigens, and their class I and class II human leukocyte antigen (HLA) surface proteins facilitate the presentation of processed antigenic fragments for the activation of lymphocytes.
- Removal of abnormal or senescent erythrocytes and salvage of iron for reutilization by erythroid precursor cells.
- Clearance from the blood and tissues of neoplastic or foreign cells.

Platelets

The platelets, or thrombocytes, are derived from mature megakaryocytes. They circulate as 2- to 3-μ disks, which on a Wright-stained smear appear pale blue with faint pink granules. By electron microscopy, they contain mitochondria, glycogen particles, dense granules, and α granules. The dense granules contain various nucleotides, including the potent aggregating substance ADP, whereas the α granules contain many factors, including adhesive proteins, such as fibrinogen, von Willebrand factor, fibronectin, and thrombospondin.

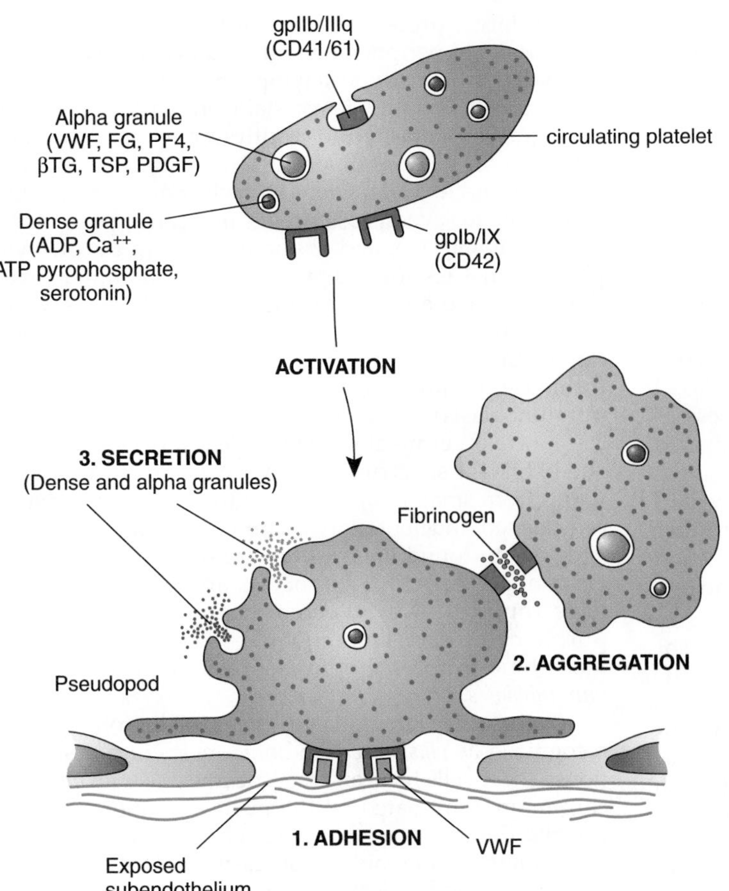

FIGURE *20-11*
Platelet activation involves three overlapping mechanism. (1) Adhesion to the exposed subendothelium is mediated by the binding of von Willebrand factor (VWF) to gpIb/IX (CD 42) and is the initiation signal for activation. (2) The exposure of gpIIb/IIIa (CD 41/61) to the fibrinogen (FG) receptor on the platelet surface allows for platelet aggregation. (3) At the same time, platelets secrete their granule contents, which facilitates further activation. Alpha-granules contain VWF, FG, platelet factor 4 (PF4), thromboglobulin (TG), thrombospondin (TSP), and platelet-derived growth factor (PDGF).

Platelets circulate freely for about 12 days. On exposure to subendothelial collagen and von Willebrand factor in areas of endothelial injury, platelets undergo morphological and functional changes and are said to be *activated* (Fig. 20-11). Platelet alterations that accompany activation include the following:

The platelets become angulated, display hairy processes, and *adhere* to the subendothelial tissues via their glycoprotein Ib/IX receptors for von Willebrand factor.

Concomitantly, a ring of microtubules contracts and expels the contents of dense granules and α granules.

The actions of the granule contents, the appearance on the platelet surface of the fibrinogen receptor *glycoproteins IIb/IIIa*, and the synthesis of thromboxane from membrane lipids cause new platelets to *aggregate* on the initially activated platelets.

All of these interrelated processes result in the formation of a hemostatic platelet plug, which then serves as an anchor and source of lipids for the prothrombinase complex and subsequent clot formation.

THE LYMPHOPOIETIC SYSTEM

The lymphopoietic system consists of circulating B and T lymphocytes and of lymphoid organs, including the lymph nodes, spleen, thymus, and mucosa-associated lymphoid tissue (MALT). The last comprises the oropharyngeal lymphoid tissue (Waldeyer's ring), the gut-associated lymphoid tissue (GALT), and the bronchus-associated lymphoid tissue (BALT).

Lymphocytes are all derived from bone marrow stem cells. Cells that undergo differentiation and maturation in the thymus are termed *T cells*, whereas those that develop in the bone marrow are called *B cells*. The differentiation and maturation of lymphocytes are associated with a sequential gain and loss of a number of cytoplasmic and surface antigens. The availability of antibodies to these antigens has been of special importance for the study of functional and neoplastic disorders of the lymphopoietic system. The pattern of expression of these antigens identifies the character of the cells or the stage at which the mutational event resulted in the emergence of a neoplastic clone.

T LYMPHOCYTES: The lymphocytic stem cells that migrate to the thymus are exposed to a number of thymic hormones. These hormones first induce the production of surface receptors (CD2) that bind sheep erythrocytes. At this point, recombination of the T-cell receptor genes leads to the production of a T-cell receptor that recognizes a single antigen. This receptor is present on the membrane in association with a CD3 molecule; the CD2 and CD3 markers define the cells as T cells. Other markers appear, such as CD5 and particularly either CD4 (helper) or CD8 (suppressor). The cells then migrate from the thymus to lymph nodes, spleen, and peripheral blood.

When exposed to antigens specific for their receptors, CD4 cells become activated. These antigens are peptide fragments derived from the partial digestion of proteins by macrophages or antigen presenting cells. When antigens are presented in association with a class 2 HLA molecule, CD4 cells become activated, release mitogenic growth factors (IL-1 and IL-2), and undergo transformation to a helper/inducer cell. These cells interact with B lymphocytes that express the same antigenic specificity, thereby promoting their proliferation and inducing their differentiation to immunoglobulin-producing plasma cells.

CD8 cells become activated when their receptors recognize peptides presented in association with a class I HLA antigen. The activated cells become suppressor-cytotoxic cells. CD8 cells limit the expansion of activated B cells and terminate their immune response.

A subpopulation of T lymphocytes activated by antigenic peptides become cytotoxic lymphocytes or killer cells (κ cells). These cells play a direct role in the elimination of foreign cells or viruses bearing the recognized antigen.

B LYMPHOCYTES: The B lymphocyte precursor cells acquire their repertoire of cytoplasmic and cell surface antigens in the bone marrow. Even the earliest pre-B progenitor cells display on their membrane certain antigens common to all subsequent B cells (CD19, CD20, and CD24). Similar to the surface membrane of all cells, the membrane of B cells expresses an HLA class I antigen. However, it also displays an HLA class II antigen, a feature shared only by antigen processing and presenting cells. At this early stage, the antigen CALLA (common acute leukemia/lymphoma antigen) is present for a short time, as is the nuclear antigen Tdt (terminal deoxynucleotidyl transferase).

As the B lymphocytes mature, the genes for the immunoglobulin heavy chains are rearranged in preparation for the synthesis of IgM molecules. In pre-B cells, these molecules are contained in the cytoplasm. In the early B cells, heavy chains are present on the membrane and light chains in the cytoplasm.

The mature B cells contain pan B-cell markers (CD19, CD20, CD24, HLA class II antigens), as well as heavy and light chains. When activated by an antigen and stimulated by an appropriate T-helper cell, B cells transform into plasma cells, which synthesize and export immunoglobulins. At this stage, they no longer display heavy or light immunoglobulin chains on the surface membrane.

NULL CELLS: A small proportion of lymphocytes do not express either B or T lymphocyte differentiation antigens and are, therefore, termed null cells. They may function as cytotoxic or natural killer cells (*NK cells*), which do not require antigenic recognition for their function. Morphologically, NK cells are recognized by their granular cytoplasm (large granular lymphocytes).

Lymphocytes exhibit a heterogeneous morphological appearance. Small to medium-sized lymphocytes may be primitive antigen-independent B and T cells or antigen-dependent, committed cells that have not been reexposed to the specific sensitizing antigen. When activated by an antigen, both B and T lymphocytes undergo transformation to large, protein-synthesizing cells, called *atypical lymphocytes* in peripheral blood smears and *immunoblasts* in tissue sections. Atypical lymphocytes in smears visualized with the Wright-Giemsa stain tend to have abundant blue-gray cytoplasm and multiple nucleoli. The same cells in tissue sections stained with hematoxylin and eosin have a round to oval nucleus with clear or vesicular chromatin, one to several eosinophilic nucleoli apposed to the nuclear membrane, and abundant clear to purple cytoplasm. In tissues affected by infections and immune reactions, the size and appearance of lymphocytes varies widely, owing to lymphocyte transformation and modulation. Small lymphocytes, partially activated (transformed) lymphocytes, and large activated lymphocytes (immunoblasts) are all observed.

Normal germinal centers (follicles) of lymphoid tissue exhibit a spectrum of B cells. The cell population varies from small lymphocytes with irregularly indented or "cleaved" nuclei to large lymphocytes with vesicular, irregular to round nuclei. In lymphoid tissue other than germinal centers, B lymphocytes are more regular and have round to oval hyperchromatic nuclei and blue-purple cytoplasm. Immunoblast-like cells with prominent blue-purple cytoplasm are termed *plasmacytoid immunoblasts.*

Terminally differentiated, effector B lymphocytes are recognized as *plasma cells* in both smears and tissue sections. These cells have an eccentric nucleus with clumped chromatin marginated on the nuclear membrane, traditionally described as "clockface chromatin." The abundant blue-purple cytoplasm of plasma cells often displays a clear paranuclear clear zone representing the Golgi complex.

T lymphocytes are usually indistinguishable from B cells in tissue sections. Infrequently, they show an irregularly contoured nuclear membrane and pale, clear cytoplasm.

In peripheral blood, 60% to 80% of circulating lymphocytes are of T-cell lineage and 10% to 15% are of B-cell lineage. The remainder are null cells lacking both B- and T-cell lineage differentiation markers.

Lymph Nodes

Lymph nodes consist of organized collections of lymphoid tissue located along the lymphatic vessels. Typically grayish white and ovoid or bean shaped, they vary from 2 mm to 2 cm in greatest dimension. A fibrous capsule and radiating trabeculae provide a supporting structure. A delicate reticulum network contributes internal support. Architecturally, lymph nodes exhibit an outer cortex and an inner medulla. The cortex contains defined B-cell and T-cell domains (Fig. 20-12).

THE B CELL–DEPENDENT CORTEX: This area consists of two types of follicles. Immunologically inactive follicles are termed *primary follicles,*whereas active ones are referred to as *secondary follicles or germinal centers.* Primary follicles consist of cohesive aggregates of small, normal-appearing lymphocytes. Germinal centers contain a spectrum of small, intermediate, and large activated lymphocytes. There are also scattered macrophages that

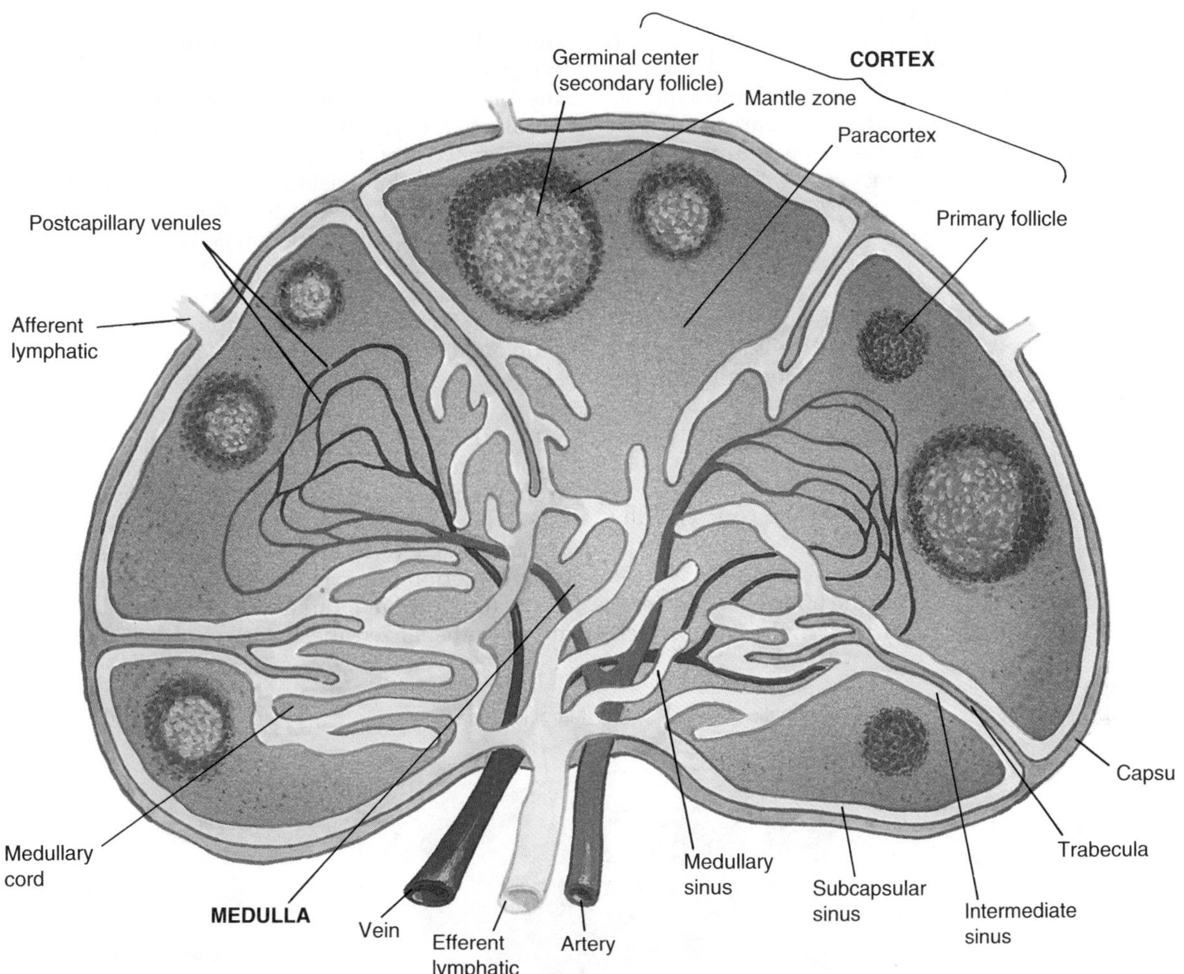

FIGURE *20-12*
Structure of a normal lymph node.

contain phagocytized nuclear and cytoplasmic debris ("tingible body" macrophages). The dendritic reticular cells are stellate cells with long cytoplasmic processes, which are located near the periphery of the germinal centers. Macrophages and, to a lesser extent, dendritic cells provide growth factors for activated B cells. Following activation and clonal expansion in the germinal centers, B lymphocytes migrate to the B cell–dependent medullary cords of the lymph nodes, and either become immunoglobulin-secreting plasma cells or exit the lymph nodes as memory B lymphocytes.

THE T CELL–DEPENDENT PARACORTEX: Also known as the deep cortex, this area is situated between the B-cell follicles and deep to them. In addition to T lymphocytes, scattered macrophages and interdigitating reticulum cells are found in the paracortex. The latter process and present antigen to T lymphocytes, which in turn proliferate and induce the transformation of both T cells and B cells.

Circulating B lymphocytes and T lymphocytes enter the lymph nodes by migrating through the tall endothelial cells of the postcapillary venules in the paracortex. T lymphocytes tend to remain in the paracortex, whereas B lymphocytes home to the germinal centers.

Lymph or interstitial fluid enters the lymph nodes through afferent lymphatics in the convexity of the cortex. Percolating first through the subcapsular sinuses and then the radial sinuses, lymph exits through efferent lymphatics. The sinuses are lined by cells that belong to the mononuclear phagocyte system. The arrangement of the sinuses maximizes the exposure of foreign antigen in lymph to macrophages and to immunoreactive B cells and T cells.

Lymphoid Tissue of the Intestine and Bronchus

Aggregates of lymphoid tissue are present along the course of the gastrointestinal tract, with prominent accentuation in the oropharynx and nasopharynx (*Waldeyer's ring*) and in Peyer's patches of the terminal ileum. Less prominent aggregates of lymphocytes are also distributed in the lamina propria of the bronchial tree (*BALT or bronchus associated lymphoid tissue*). In sites such as the tonsils and Peyer's patches, lymphocytes arrive by migration through tall endothelial cells of vessels comparable to the postcapillary venules of the lymph nodes. Mucosa-associated lymphoid tissue (*MALT*) plays an important role in immunological protection of the host in areas vulnerable to potential invaders. IgA secretion is a prominent component of this protective function.

Spleen

The spleen is a lymphoid organ that also serves as a versatile filter for abnormal or senescent cells. The normal weight of the spleen is 100 to 170 g; it is normally not palpable on clinical examination. The supporting structure of the organ consists of a fibrous capsule, radiating fibrous trabeculae, and a delicate stromal framework of reticulum fibers. The splenic artery enters at the hilum and branches into the trabecular arteries, following the course of the fibrous trabeculae.

THE WHITE PULP: Leaving the trabeculae, the central arteries become ensheathed by lymphocytes, which constitute the white pulp. The white pulp is further subdivided into a T-cell domain, located in the periarteriolar lymphoid sheath, and a B-cell domain, which comprises the follicles and perifollicular mantle zone (Fig. 20-13). Similar to the lymph nodes, the follicles are either inactive or activated, the latter being associated with germinal center formation. Arising from the central artery, follicular arteries enter the B-cell follicles and terminate in the marginal sinus at the junction between the white and red pulp. Circulating lymphocytes exit the vascular system from the marginal sinus and travel to their respective B-cell and T-cell domains. Lymphocytes leave the white pulp and enter the red pulp by way of the same marginal sinuses.

THE RED PULP: This region comprises a network of stromal cords and vascular sinuses. Most of the blood from the penicilliary arteries empties directly into the sinuses (closed circulation), with subsequent drainage to the trabecular veins and ultimately to the splenic vein. A small fraction, 5% to 10%, is diverted into the splenic cords (open circulation) and slowly percolates through a nonendothelialized meshwork studded with phagocytic

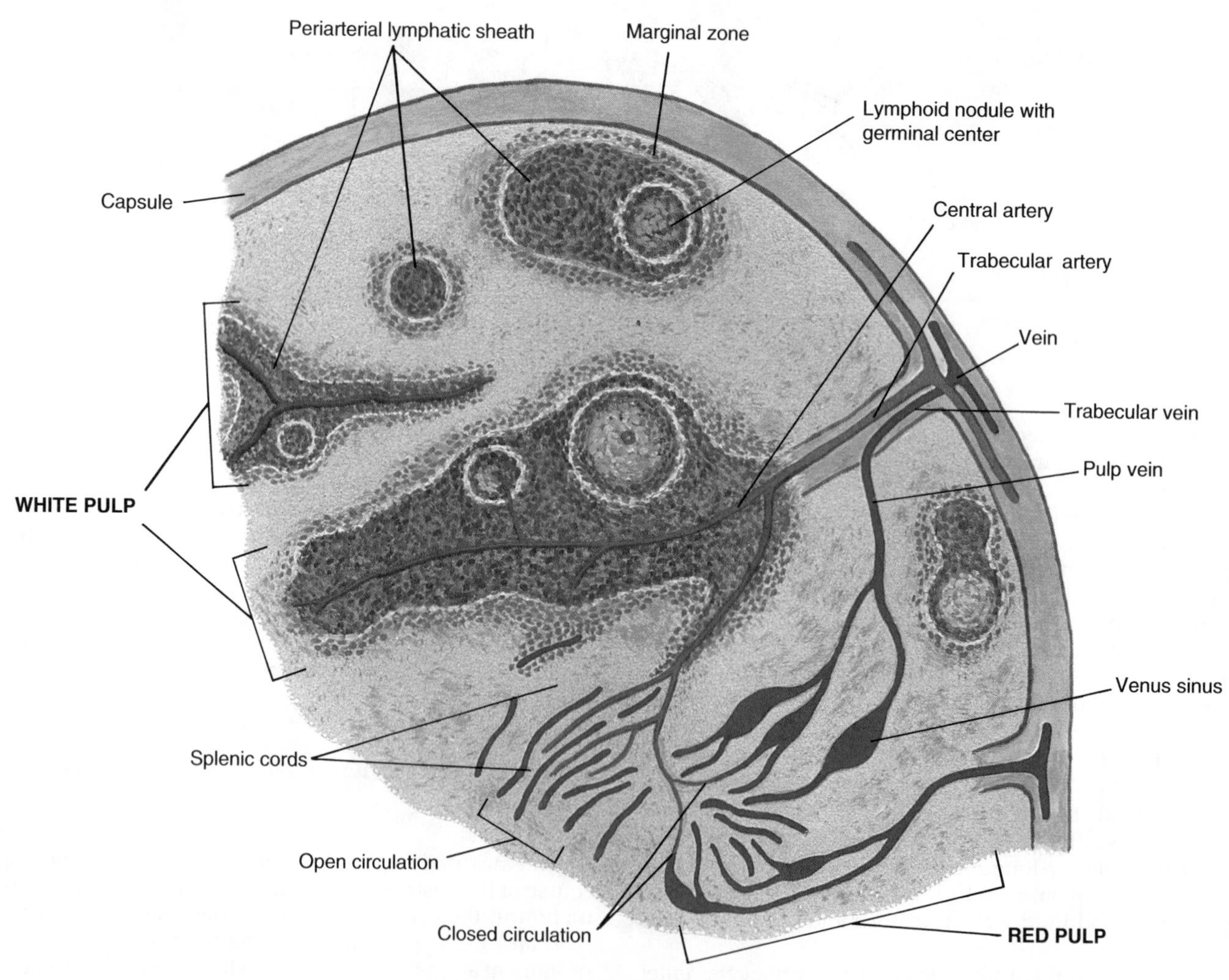

FIGURE *20-13*
Structure of the normal spleen.

macrophages. The blood then reenters the sinusoids through narrow slits composed of longitudinally oriented, slender endothelial cells and radially oriented ring fibers.

In the splenic cords, erythrocytes are subjected to the sustained scrutiny of mononuclear phagocytes and must exhibit deformability to traverse the narrow interstices between the lining endothelial cells. The erythrocytes must also be able to withstand the hypoxia, hypoglycemia, and acidosis that are characteristic of the stromal cord microenvironment. Most normal erythroid cells survive, as do granulocytes and platelets. They ultimately enter the trabecular veins and leave the hilum by way of the splenic vein.

The splenic white and red pulps have separate functions. As part of the peripheral lymphoid system, effector B and T lymphocytes of the white pulp perform an immunological function for the circulatory system comparable to the immunological function of the lymph nodes. The white pulp is (1) the source of protection from bloodborne infection, (2) a major site for the production of opsonizing IgM antibody, and (3) a site of production of lymphocytes and plasma cells.

The red pulp is primarily a filter designed to screen and eliminate defective or foreign cells. Senescent and damaged erythrocytes are recognized and phagocytosed by splenic macrophages. The spleen ordinarily accounts for the removal of about half of aged erythrocytes, the remainder being destroyed in the liver, bone marrow, and other components of the mononuclear phagocyte system. Following phagocytosis and breakdown of erythrocytes, the iron is first stored as hemosiderin in macrophages. It is then released, bound to transferrin, and transported to the bone marrow for reutilization in erythrocyte production. Abnormal erythrocyte inclusions, such as Howell-Jolly bodies (remnants of nuclear DNA), Heinz bodies (denatured hemoglobin), and siderotic granules (iron) are recognized and removed (pitted) by macrophages without destruction of the erythrocyte.

Some membrane lipids of the maturing erythrocyte are removed in the red pulp. In the absence of this function, such as after splenectomy, there may be excess erythrocyte membrane in relation to hemoglobin content, a situation that leads to central pooling of hemoglobin and a "target cell" appearance.

One third of the peripheral blood platelet pool and a small fraction of granulocytes are normally sequestered in the spleen without causing any damage to the cells. By contrast, there is no significant splenic sequestration of erythrocytes, and splenectomy is followed only by an increase in platelet and granulocyte counts.

HEMOSTASIS

Hemostasis refers to the arrest of bleeding. It depends on close interactions among three biological systems—the blood vessels, the platelets, and the plasma coagulation factors.

ENDOTHELIUM: The blood vessels provide the blood with a closed circuit covered internally by a smooth, nonthrombogenic monolayer of endothelial cells. Unstimulated platelets do not adhere to or penetrate the endothelial barrier. This nonthrombogenic property of the luminal surface is caused by the production or activation of antiplatelet agents and anticoagulants by the endothelium. The endothelial cells synthesize prostacyclin, which inhibits platelet function and is a potent vasodilator. Nitric oxide exerts similar effects. These actions maintain the blood in a fluid state until an accidental injury of the endothelium exposes subendothelial tissue.

SUBENDOTHELIAL MATRIX: The endothelial cells rest on a matrix that contains collagens, elastin, laminin, fibronectin, von Willebrand factor, and other structural and adhesive proteins. When exposed, the matrix of the intima is intensely thrombogenic. Its adhesive proteins bind the corresponding glycoprotein receptors on platelet membranes and cause their adherence to the exposed matrix.

PLATELETS: Once adherence has occurred, a series of changes in platelet metabolism and morphology takes place. The membrane phospholipase is activated, leading to the production of (1) thromboxane A_2, a platelet-aggregating factor, and (2) phospholipid metabolites, which are involved in calcium-dependent intracellular reactions. The contents of α granules, including fibrinogen and von Willebrand factor, and those of dense particles, including ADP, are released, thereby causing the adherence of additional platelets to those already aggregated. The platelet membrane spreads out, exposing the glycoprotein receptor IIb/IIIa. In turn, this receptor cross-links the adhesive proteins fibrinogen, von Willebrand factor, fibronectin, and other adhesive proteins. These processes all help to secure the formation of a firm, hemostatic platelet plug.

COAGULATION FACTORS: The hemostatic plug is unstable until reinforced by fibrin strands. The surface of the platelet plug is used as a scaffold for the assembly of a prothrombinase, composed of activated factors V and X and calcium (Fig. 20-14). This catalytic complex transforms prothrombin into thrombin, which in turn converts fibrinogen to fibrin. Unstable fibrin monomers become stabilized by factor XIII and transform a friable platelet plug into a firm thrombus.

In addition to supporting the production of prothrombinase, the lipid surface of activated platelets and the matrix of exposed subendothelium also promote the assembly of a second catalytic complex. This complex consists of activated factors IX and VIII and calcium; it activates factor X and causes the production of more prothrombinase. The crucial activation of factor IX was thought to be accomplished through the intrinsic pathway. This part of the coagulation cascade was believed to be primarily initiated when injured tissue activates factor XII, which in turn activates factor XI and factor IX. Recent observations, however, indicate that the intrinsic pathway plays a minor role in clotting and the activation of factor IX. It is more likely that factor VII, which is activated by exposure to a tissue factor, not only activates factor X, the usual extrinsic pathway, but also activates factor IX. Accordingly, the factor VII/tissue factor complex is primarily involved in the initiation of coagulation, whereas sustained coagulation requires the activities of the "intrinsic factors" VIII, IX, and XI.

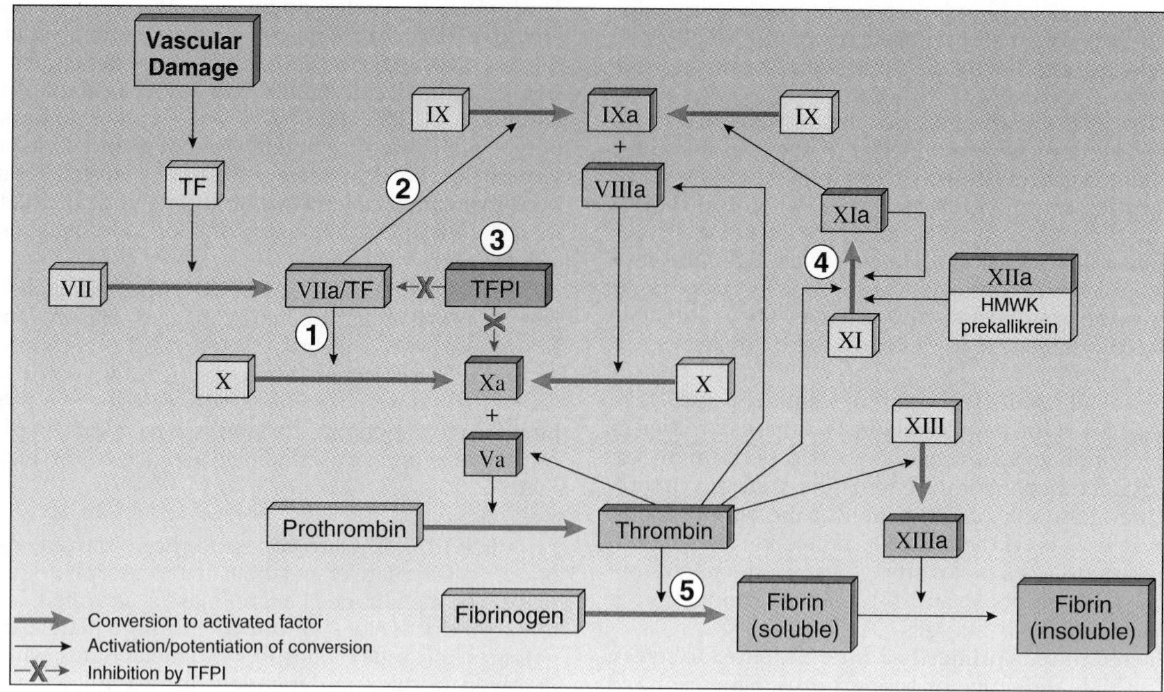

FIGURE 20-14

The coagulation cascade. Following injury to a vessel, coagulation is initiated when the factor VIIa/tissue factor (TF) complex (1) activates factor X to form Xa and (2) activates factor IX to form IXa. However, tissue factor pathway inhibitor (TFPI) (3) inhibits both (1) and (2), so that additional mechanisms are required for subsequent amplification of the cascade. Sustained amplification is achieved through the action of intrinsic factors VIII, IX, and XI. Activation of XI to form XIa (4) may occur via one of three pathways: thrombin, autoactivation, and perhaps classic contact activation (XII, high molecular weight kininogen (HMWK), and prekallikrein). Note the central and multiple roles of thrombin (5), which not only converts fibrinogen to fibrin, but also activates cofactors V and VIII, as well as XI and XIII.

NATURAL ANTICOAGULANTS AND THROMBOLYSIS: In addition to inhibitors of platelet aggregation (prostacyclin, NO), there are a number of other natural inhibitors of coagulation (Fig. 20-15). At least three mechanisms by which coagulation is held in check have been defined:

- Anti-thrombin III (ATIII)
- Protein C and protein S
- Tissue factor pathway inhibitor (TFPI)

In addition to its inhibition of thrombin, ATIII cleaves a number of activated factors, namely IXa, Xa, XIa, and XIIa. *In vivo,* this effect is accentuated by heparan sulfate proteoglycans and most dramatically by the therapeutic administration of heparin. Protein C is activated by thrombin, the function of which is, in turn, potentiated by thrombomodulin. Using protein S as a co-factor, protein C then inactivates factors Va and XIIIa. Finally, the inability of factor VII/tissue factor to sustain coagulation on its own is due to the presence of TFPI (see Fig. 20-14).

After the thrombus has become firmly established, further growth is curtailed by the removal of platelet activating factors and coagulation proteins. The endothelial cells in the vicinity of the thrombus produce plasminogen activators, which in turn activate circulating plasminogen to plasmin and initiate thrombolysis. The dissolution of the thrombus is accomplished by plasmin.

Functional Disorders of the Blood and Lymphoid Organs

ANEMIA

Anemia refers to a reduction in the total circulating erythrocyte mass. It is diagnosed by the demonstration of below normal values for the hemoglobin concentration, the hematocrit, or erythrocyte count. A decrease in erythrocyte mass leads to lesser transport of hemoglobin-bound oxygen from the lungs to the tissues and, in turn, to tissue hypoxia.

In mild anemias, with hemoglobin concentrations greater than 10 g/dL, compensatory mechanisms are highly effective and render the disorder virtually asymptomatic. In moderate anemias, with hemoglobin levels of 7 to 10 g/dL, the symptomatology is dominated by compensatory efforts, such as redistribution of blood from the skin to vital organs, tachycardia, and shortness of breath. In severe anemias, with hemoglobin levels less than 7

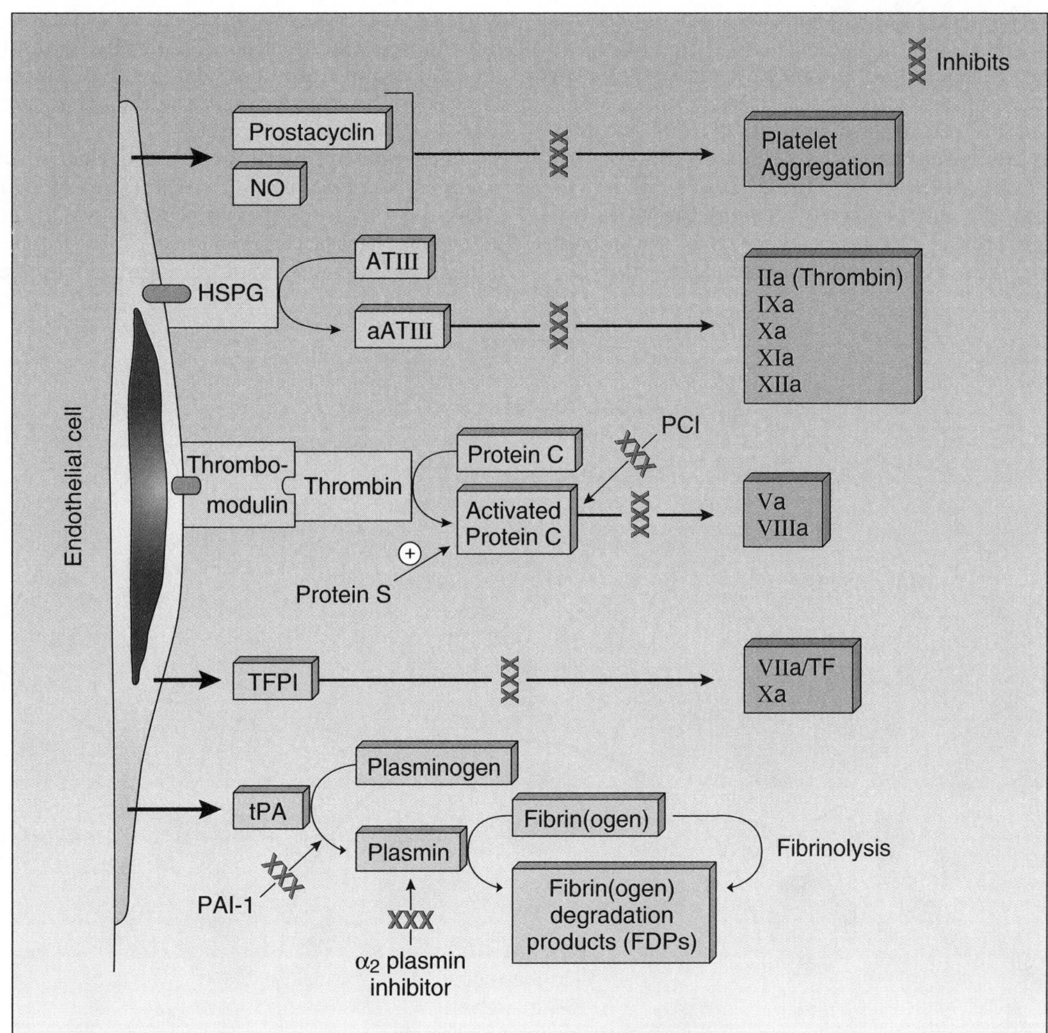

FIGURE *20-15*
The role of the endothelium in anticoagulation, platelet inhibition, and thrombolysis. The endothelial cell plays a central role in the inhibition of various of components of the clotting mechanism. Heparan sulfate proteoglycan (HSPG) potentiates the activation of ATIII 15-fold, whereas thrombomodulin stimulates the activation of protein C by thrombin 30-fold. NO, nitric oxide; HSPG, heparan sulfate proteoglycan; PCI, protein C inhibitor; TFPI, tissue factor pathway inhibitor; tPA, tissue plasminogen activator; PAI-I, plasminogen activator inhibitor-I. *Arrows* refer to products secreted by the endothelial cell, whereas *bars* indicate molecules bound to the surface of this cell. + indicates potentiation; − indicates inhibition.

g/dL, tissue hypoxia often remains uncompensated and may be manifested by angina, fainting spells, and extreme weakness.

The compensatory mechanisms are aimed at providing the capillaries with oxygen at a partial pressure high enough to allow it to diffuse into the surrounding tissues. This can be accomplished in several ways:

- **Decreased hemoglobin-oxygen affinity** (shift to the right in the oxygen dissociation curve of hemoglobin) caused by a more acid *p*H or by an increased erythrocyte concentration of 2,3-DPG occurs even in mild anemia (see Fig. 20-10).
- **Increased tissue perfusion of** vital organs, such as the heart and brain, is accomplished at the expense of blood supply to tissues with lower oxygen requirements.
- **Increased cardiac output** is particularly evident in severe anemia and is characterized by tachycardia and hemodynamic murmurs. Unfortunately, it is metabolically expensive and may eventually cause congestive heart failure.
- **Increased erythrocyte production** is a response to a reduction in the oxygen supply to the kidneys, which induces increased synthesis of erythropoietin. In turn, this hormone stimulates the production of erythrocytes in the bone narrow. This adaptive response may eventually restore the erythrocyte mass to normal, provided that bone marrow function is not compromised.

Classification of Anemias

Anemias can be classified either morphologically or pathophysiologically (Fig. 20-16).

The morphological classification divides anemias into three types based upon red cell size—macrocytic, microcytic, and normocytic (Table 20-3). Since the automated blood counters directly measure the MCV, it is convenient to relate the anemias to this parameter. Furthermore, this classification emphasizes the importance of the two most curable anemias, namely, the macrocytic anemias of vitamin B_{12} and folic acid deficiency and the microcytic anemia of iron deficiency. However, for most other anemias the morphological classification is less adequate.

The pathophysiological classification divides the anemias into two major groups: (1) those caused by decreased production of erythrocytes and (2) those that result from increased destruction (Table 20-4). These two general mechanism can be distinguished by measuring ef-

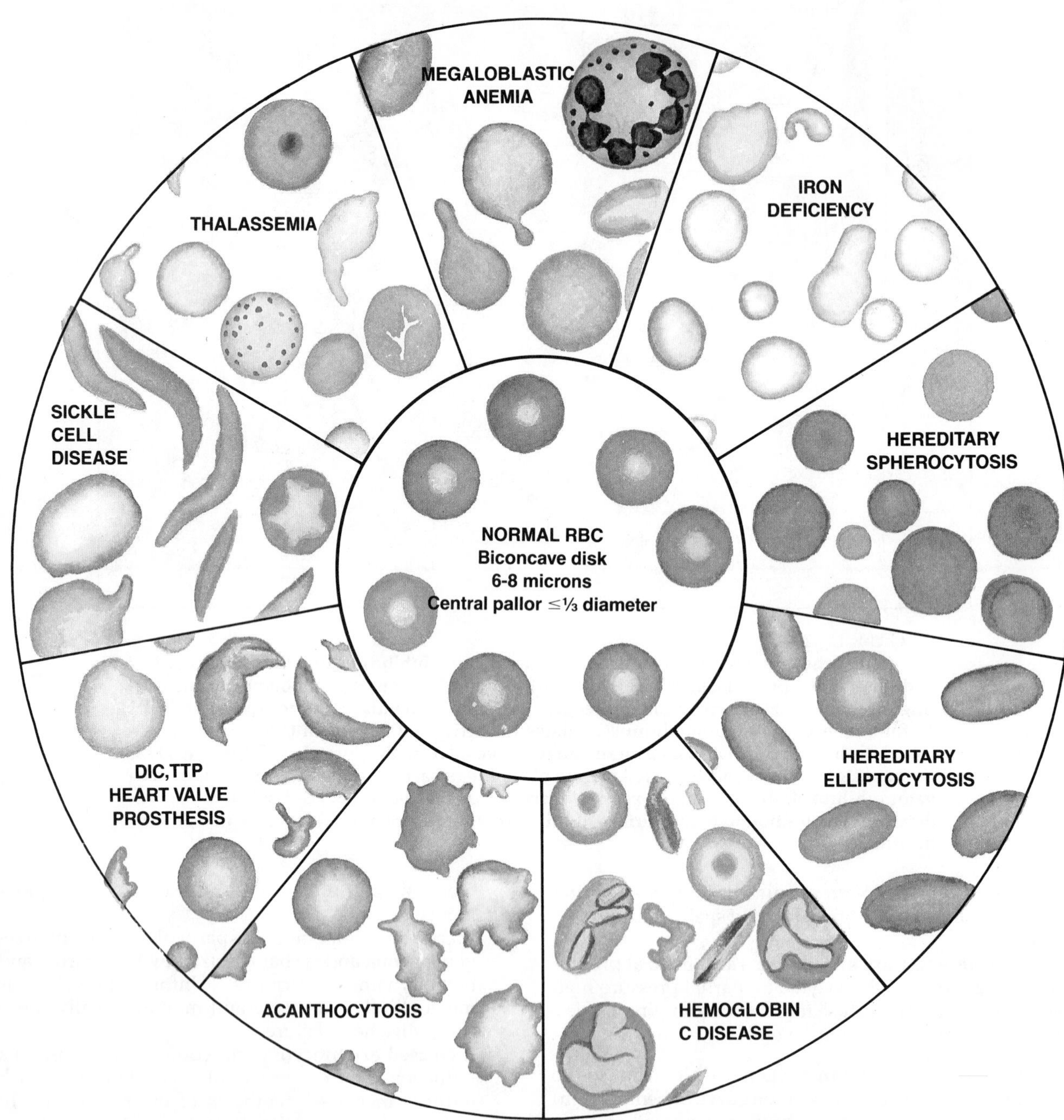

FIGURE 20-16
The anemias. The pathophysiology of characteristic morphological features of the various anemias are shown. The morphology of normal erythrocytes is contrasted in the central circle.

fective erythropoietic activity by the Reticulocyte Production Index (RPI). The RPI is typically low in those anemias caused by decreased production of erythrocytes and higher in those that result from increased destruction.

Decreased Production of Erythrocytes

Aplastic Anemia

Aplastic anemia is a chronic disorder of hemopoietic stem cells that results in the cellular depletion of the bone marrow and pancytopenia (a decrease in all circulating formed elements).

PATHOGENESIS: Although bone marrow aplasia can occur as an acute self-limited event following exposure to radiation or chemotherapeutic drugs, in aplastic anemia, marrow depletion continues indefinitely. In some patients, there is an initiating event, such as exposure to certain drugs, toxins, or viruses (Table 20-5). In most cases, however, no cause is found, the disorder arising in a previously healthy person with no known exposure to cytotoxic drugs or irradiation. In such a situation, the disease is termed *idiopathic* and is assumed to have been triggered by an unknown event in a genetically susceptible person.

Since bone marrow transplantation for aplastic

DISORDER	PATHOPHYSIOLOGY	MORPHOLOGY
Megaloblastic anemia	Disturbance in DNA synthesis	Oval macrocytes, teardrop poikilocytosis, hypersegmented polys
Iron deficiency	Disturbance in hemoglobin synthesis (lack of iron)	Hypochromic, microcytic
Hereditary spherocytosis	Membrane defect	Spherocytes
Hereditary elliptocytosis	Membrane defect	Elliptocytes
Hemoglobin C disease	Abnormal globin chain	Target cells, rhomboid crystals (HbC)
Acanthocytosis	Membrane lipid defect (abetalipoproteinemia)	Irregular spiculation (similar to spur cells of liver disease)
DIC, TTP, heart valve prosthesis sequela	Mechanical damage to erythrocytes	Schistocytes
Sickle cell disease	Abnormal globin chain	Sickle cells
Thalassemia	Disturbance in hemoglobin synthesis (defect of globin chain)	Hypochromic, microcytic,poikilocytosis, basophilic stippling
Myelophthisic anemia	Marrow replacement or infiltration	Teardrop poikilocytosis, immature WBC and RBC, large platelets
Anemia of chronic disease	Block in utilization of storage iron	Normochromic, normocytic to mild hypochromic, microcytic
Sideroblastic anemia	Defect in porphyrin and heme synthesis	Bimorphic population (normal and microcytic), Pappenheimer bodies
Anemia of renal disease	Multifactorial	Burr cells (uniform marginal scalloping)
Autoimmune hemolytic anemia	RBC destruction mediated by antibodies	Spherocytes
Acute blood loss anemia	Hemorrhage	Polychromasia (increased reticulocytes)

FIGURE *20-16 Continued.*

TABLE 20-3 **Morphological Classification of Anemia**

Macrocytic
Megaloblastic
Alcohol use
Liver disease
Hypothyroidism
Reticulocytosis
Primary bone marrow disease
Microcytic
Iron deficiency
Anemia of chronic disease/inflammation
Thalassemias
Sideroblastic anemias
Normocytic
Anemia of chronic disease/inflammation
Anemia of renal disease
Acute blood loss

anemia may be curative, the defect must be intrinsic to the hemopoietic cells. It is believed that the primary lesion involves an inability of stem cells to regenerate and repopulate the marrow. This defect is thought to involve the function of all stem cells, rather than specific clones. Nevertheless, many long-term survivors show chromosomal abnormalities. Moreover, monoclonal disorders may emerge, for example, paroxysmal nocturnal hemoglobinuria, myelodysplastic syndromes, and acute leukemia.

The successful therapeutic use of anti-T lymphocyte antibodies and other immunosuppressive agents for the treatment of aplastic anemia suggests that there is an immunological component either in the pathogenesis of the disease or in its subsequent progression. Since immunosuppression rarely cures the disease but only causes a variable remission, it seems likely that the immune system simply aggravates a preexisting defect in the stem cells.

TABLE 20-4 **Pathophysiological Classification of Anemia**

Decreased Production	Increased Destruction
Stem cell– and progenitor cell–based	Intracorpuscular
Aplastic anemia	Membrane defect
Pure red cell aplasia	Enzyme deficiency
Paroxysmal nocturnal hemoglobinuria	Hemoglobinopathies
Leukemia	Extracorpuscular
Myelodysplastic syndromes	Immunological
Marrow infiltration	Autoimmune
Anemia of chronic disease/inflammation	Alloimmune
Anemia of renal disease	Nonimmunological
Nutritional deficiency	Mechanical
Megaloblastic anemia (vitamin B_{12} and folic acid)	Hypersplenism
Iron deficiency	Infectious
	Chemical
	Acute blood loss

TABLE 20-5 **Etiology of Aplastic Anemia**

Idiopathic (2/3 of all cases)
Ionizing radiation
Drugs
Chemotherapeutic agents
Chloramphenicol
Anticonvulsants
Nonsteroidal anti-inflammatory agents
Gold
Chemicals
Benzene
Viruses
Hepatitis (HCV)
Epstein-Barr virus
HIV
Parvovirus B19
Hereditary
Fanconi anemia

☐ **Pathology:** The bone marrow in aplastic anemia is to a large extent replaced by fat (Fig. 20-17). Thin strands of cells contain scant granulocytic and erythroid elements, and stromal cells, such as lymphocytes, plasma cells, mast cells, and macrophages, predominate.

The peripheral blood invariably exhibits pancytopenia, although this may be of varying severity. The anemia tends to be macrocytic, with an increased erythrocyte content of fetal hemoglobin. Erythropoietin levels are usually elevated. Absolute granulocytopenia is often present, and the total lymphocyte count is frequently depressed. The platelet count is always reduced.

☐ **Clinical Features:** The diagnosis of aplastic anemia is suspected in a patient with pancytopenia and established after at least two bone marrow biopsies have demonstrated the characteristic morphological features of aplastic anemia. Nuclear magnetic resonance imaging of the bone marrow appears useful for estimating the extent of fatty replacement. Granulocytopenia and thrombocytopenia are the components of the pancytopenia that are most feared and least amenable to treatment.

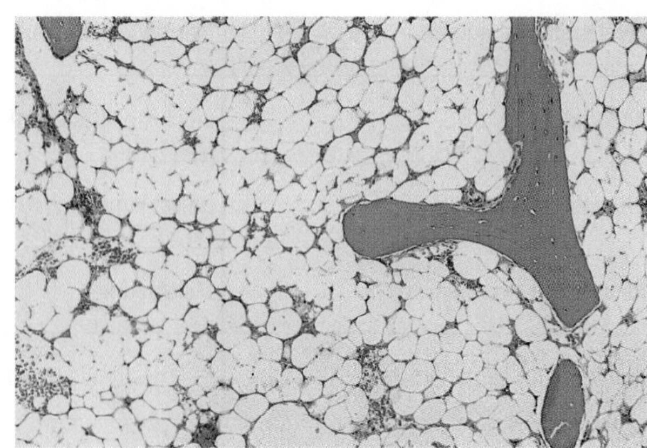

FIGURE 20-17
Aplastic anemia. The bone marrow consists largely of fat cells and lacks normal hemopoietic activity.

Untreated patients with severe aplastic anemia have a median survival of 3 to 6 months, and only 20% survive 1 year. The therapeutic use of blood components, immunosuppressive agents, and bone marrow transplantation has significantly improved the prognosis for patients with idiopathic aplastic anemia, although it remains a life-threatening disease.

Fanconi anemia is a constitutional form of aplastic anemia. It is an autosomal recessive disorder of the Fanconi Anemia Complementation (FAC) group C gene in some patients and presents clinically in the first decade of life. Fanconi anemia is associated with a variety of congenital malformations, including hypoplastic thumbs, absent radii, skin pigmentation, and renal anomalies. Chromosomal analysis reveals a number of nonspecific deletions and exchanges, which may reflect the observed instability of DNA when subjected to radiation or alkylating agents.

Paroxysmal Nocturnal Hemoglobinuria

Paroxysmal nocturnal hemoglobinuria (PNH) is a clonal stem cell disorder that affects all hemopoietic lineages and is characterized by the production of defective erythrocytes, as well as abnormal platelets and granulocytes. The defining characteristic of this acquired condition is an unusual predisposition of the faulty erythrocytes to complement-mediated lysis.

☐ **Pathogenesis:** Although PNH has previously been considered to be a hemolytic anemia caused by complement-induced erythrocyte destruction, it is actually an acquired clonal stem cell disorder in which all blood cell lineages are defective. Indeed it is unique among the intracorpuscular defects that cause anemia in that it is not heritable. Not infrequently, the abnormal clone of PNH emerges in the marrow of patients with aplastic anemia.

The erythrocyte defect in PNH relates to deficiencies of decay-accelerating factor (DAF or CD55) and membrane inhibitor of reactive lysis (MIRL or CD59) on the erythrocyte membrane. The absence of the latter appears to play a more critical role. These factors are membrane proteins that normally accelerate the degradation of surface-bound complement, thereby preventing complement-induced hemolysis. In PNH, the genes for these proteins are normal and functional. However, the anchorage of DAF, MIRL, and other proteins is faulty. The fundamental cause of these deficiences is defective synthesis of glycosyl phosphatidyl inositol (GPI), a lipid that anchors many proteins, including DAF and MIRL, to the plasma membrane. A mutant gene, termed PIG-A (phosphatidylinositol glycan class A), is a variant of 1 of 10 genes involved in the biosynthesis of GPI.

☐ **Clinical Features:** PNH is characterized by intermittent or sustained periods of hemolysis and hemoglobinuria, sometimes in a nocturnal pattern, in which patients excrete a red morning urine. However, in many patients hemolysis occurs at random intervals. Patients with PNH are usually anemic, sometimes with hemoglobin levels below 5 g/dL. Although the reticulocyte count is increased, the compensatory increase in erythrocyte production by the marrow is inadequate. The serum iron is decreased in PNH, owing to the loss of iron that accompanies hemoglobinuria. Since the membrane defect in PNH affects all hemopoietic cells, thrombocytopenia and granulocytopenia are usually present.

Thrombotic complications are frequent, especially in the deep abdominal veins. In fact, PNH should always be considered in the differential diagnosis of Budd-Chiari syndrome (hepatic venous thrombosis). The reason for this thrombotic diathesis is poorly understood, but it may reflect complement-mediated activation of platelets.

In PNH, the erythrocytes are excessively sensitive to a low ionic environment, such as occurs in plasma with added sucrose. If the sucrose hemolysis test for PNH is positive, it should be confirmed by the Ham acid hemolysis test, which identifies complement-sensitive cells.

The course of PNH is variable; some patients succumb within months of the diagnosis, whereas others live for decades. Many patients eventually die of the complications of pancytopenia and thrombosis, and a few develop a myelodysplastic syndrome or acute leukemia. Bone marrow transplantation has resulted in long-term remissions in some patients.

Myelodysplastic Syndromes

Myelodysplastic syndromes (MDS) encompass a heterogeneous group of disorders characterized by clonal proliferation of abnormal stem cells. Although it is quantitatively increased, hemopoiesis in the marrow is qualitatively ineffective, resulting in pancytopenia of varying severity. Accordingly, a diagnostic clue to the presence of MDS is the finding of peripheral cytopenia, in the face of hypercellularity of the bone marrow. Because of the clonal proliferation and frequent transformation to acute myelogenous leukemia, some authors preferred the term preleukemia for MDS. However, leukemia is not an invariable outcome, and a number of subgroups, which identify different prognoses, have been defined (Table 20-6).

The cause of MDS is obscure, but some of the patients have evidence of exposure to toxic chemicals. Benzene is the best defined of these agents, but it is suspected that gasoline and diesel fumes may also be etiological agents. The use of chemotherapeutic agents, usually alkylating agents, is associated with an increased risk of subsequent MDS.

☐ **Pathology:** In MDS, the cellularity of the bone marrow is normal or increased. The erythroblasts tend to be megaloblastoid, with numerous immature forms (shift to the left) and nuclear fragmentation. Ringed sideroblasts, characterized by iron-laden mitochondria encircling the nucleus, may be present (Fig. 20-18). The myeloid precursors may be morphologically normal, and the number of myeloblasts determines in part the classification (see Table 20-6). The megakaryocytes vary in number, and frequently have hyposegmented nuclei, although hypersegmented nuclei may also be encountered. Chromosomal abnormalities, especially 5q−, 7q−, and +8, are often found and are frequently used as diagnostic criteria.

The circulating erythrocytes vary in size and shape but display an increase in the mean volume. Basophilic stip-

TABLE *20-6* **The Myelodysplastic Syndromes: French-American-British (FAB) Classification**

	Refractory Anemia (RA)	**Refractory Anemia with Ringed Sideroblasts (RARS)**	**Refractory Anemia with Excess Blasts (RAEB)**	**Chronic Myelomonocytic Leukemia (CMML)**	**Refractory Anemia with Excess Blasts (RAEB) in Transformation**
Peripheral Blood					
% Myeloblasts	<1	<1	<5	<5	>5
Monocytes	—	—	—	Increased >1000/μL	—
Bone Marrow					
% Myeloblasts	<5	<5	5–20	≤20	20–30
Ringed sideroblasts	—	>15%	—	—	—

—, Not required for classification. The presence of Auer rods, no matter which other features are present, results in a designation of RAEB in transformation.

pling and nucleated erythrocytes are frequently observed. Hemoglobin abnormalities include an increased level of fetal hemoglobin and the presence of β4 complexes (acquired hemoglobin H disease). Granulocytes may show decreased nuclear lobation, mimicking the inherited Pelger-Huet anomaly. Cytoplasmic hypogranularity and an increase in mature and immature monocytes occur. Large and atypically granulated platelets may also be encountered.

☐ **Clinical Features:** MDS may smolder for years and only require occasional transfusions or antibiotics. However, MDS eventually transforms into acute myelogenous leukemia in 20% to 40% of patients. Attempts to modify this course with chemotherapeutic agents and growth factors have shown only limited success. The recent employment of growth factors, such as erythropoietin and myeloid and monocytic growth factors, has been encouraging but is of only temporary value. Bone marrow transplantation may offer the only hope for cure of this neoplastic disorder.

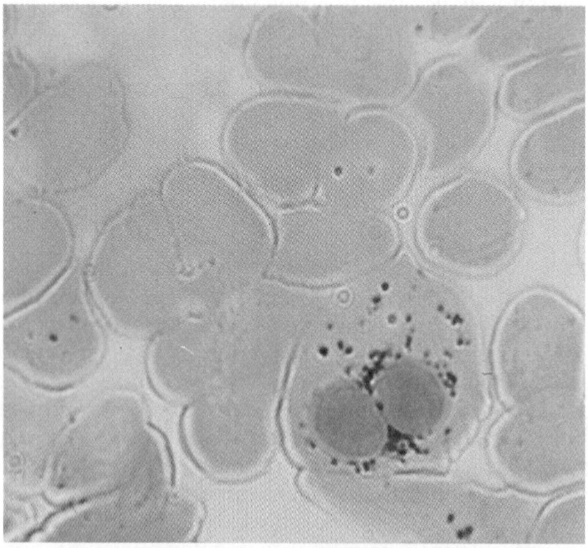

FIGURE *20-18*
Ringed sideroblast. Smear of a bone marrow aspirate stained with Prussian blue shows a binucleated erythroid precursor cell containing iron-laden mitochondria that encircle the nuclei.

Pure Red Cell Aplasia

Pure red cell aplasia (PRCA) is an autoimmune disease in which erythroid progenitor and precursor cells are suppressed, resulting in secondary anemia. Leukopenia and thrombocytopenia are absent. PRCA may present as an acute, self-limited disorder or as a chronic congenital or acquired disease.

ACUTE RED CELL APLASIA: The acute form of PRCA frequently follows a viral illness, especially infection with parvovirus B19, or exposure to one of a number of potentially toxic drugs. Parvovirus preferentially invades and destroys the erythroid progenitor cells.

Acute PRCA usually becomes clinically apparent only in patients with underlying disorders characterized by a shortened life span of circulating erythrocytes, for example, sickle cell anemia or hereditary spherocytosis. In such patients, a temporary decrease in the production of erythrocytes may cause a rapidly developing but brief anemia, the so-called aplastic crisis.

CHRONIC CONSTITUTIONAL PRCA (DIAMOND-BLACKFAN ANEMIA): This condition is usually detected in the first year of life and is caused by the inheritance of defective erythroid progenitor cells. In marrow cultures, the number of erythroid colonies (BFU-E and CFU-E) is decreased, and they are less responsive to erythropoietin.

The dramatic responsiveness to corticosteroids in the inherited type of PRCA suggests an immunological component, but no firm evidence for this concept has been obtained.

CHRONIC ACQUIRED PRCA: This disease usually presents in middle-aged adults, and has an intriguing but uncommon (5%) relationship to thymomas, suggestive of an immunological rejection of erythroid progenitor and precursor cells.

The marrow is usually depleted of erythroblasts, but

some cases of acquired PRCA are marked by a maturation arrest, with the presence of large abnormal proerythroblasts. The myeloid and megakaryocyte cell lines are unaffected; their involvement suggests the diagnosis of early aplastic anemia.

Thymic enlargement should be sought by computed tomography or magnetic resonance imaging, since the removal of an abnormal thymus may result in clinical remission. Even when enlarged and presumably responsible for the anemia, the thymus shows only an overgrowth of spindle cells.

Anemia Associated with Chronic Renal Failure

A normocytic, normochromic anemia occurs in almost all patients with chronic renal disease, with its severity roughly proportional to the degree of the uremia. The anemia is multifactorial and reflects both decreased production and increased destruction of erythrocytes, the former playing the major role. Decreased production results primarily from inadequate synthesis of erythropoietin by the damaged kidneys. Although a still unidentified uremic toxin may suppress the erythroid progenitor or precursor cells, the complete restoration of the erythrocyte mass by the administration of recombinant erythropoietin suggests that the latter effect is of minor importance.

The bone marrow usually appears normal in patients with chronic renal failure and does not show the compensatory erythroid hyperplasia expected with severe anemia. The circulating erythrocytes often show scalloped margins (burr cells) in cases of severe uremia and fragmentation in patients with severe renal hypertension. The widespread use of recombinant erythropoietin in the treatment of anemia of chronic renal disease has had a dramatic impact on this complication of uremia.

Anemia Associated with Chronic Disease

Mild to moderate normochromic or hypochromic anemia, with a hemoglobin of 9 to 11 g/dL, is common in (1) chronic inflammatory disorders (e.g., rheumatoid arthritis and systemic lupus erythematosus), (2) chronic infectious diseases (e.g., tuberculosis and acquired immunodeficiency syndrome [AIDS]), and (3) cancer. Anemia of chronic disease is one of the most common anemias worldwide, second only to iron deficiency anemia. Fortunately, it is not severe enough to cause major symptoms, but it may render the underlying disorders more difficult to endure.

Despite the heterogeneous etiologies, the anemias associated with chronic disease have certain common characteristics. The serum iron and iron-binding capacity are both decreased, despite a normal to high ferritin level. In other words, the abundant iron in macrophages is not released in amounts adequate to provide sufficient iron for circulating transferrin and, in turn, the bone marrow. The presence of impaired iron reutilization is also apparent from the finding of decreased sideroblast iron in developing erythroid cells, despite an increased iron content in bone marrow macrophages. Various cytokines (IL-1, TNF-α, and interferons) contribute to poor iron utilization.

Although a decreased iron supply to the developing erythroblast plays an important pathogenetic role, the anemia of chronic disease is also caused by a slightly shortened erythrocyte life span. Furthermore, there is an impaired bone marrow response to erythropoietin and an inadequate production of erythropoietin in response to anemia.

Megaloblastic Anemias

The megaloblastic anemias are caused by impaired DNA synthesis owing to a deficiency of either vitamin B_{12} or folic acid. In rare instances, these macrocytic anemias are due to a congenital or acquired disturbance in the synthesis of purines or pyrimidines.

Pernicious Anemia

Pernicious anemia is a megaloblastic anemia caused by chronic gastritis, which results in deficient secretion of intrinsic factor and consequent defective intestinal absorption of vitamin B_{12}. Vitamin B_{12} (cyanocobalamin) is synthesized by certain microorganisms and is present in the human diet in foods of animal origin, such as meat, fish, liver, milk, and eggs. After ingestion, it is bound to a gastric glycoprotein known as intrinsic factor (IF), which is secreted by the parietal cells in tandem with hydrochloric acid. IF protects vitamin B_{12} from degradation by intestinal enzymes until the B_{12}-IF complex reaches receptors in the terminal ileum. Here vitamin B_{12} is separated from IF and absorbed. In the circulation, it is again bound and protected by vitamin B_{12}-binding glycoproteins (transcobalamins), which carry the vitamin to the bone marrow (Fig. 20-19).

This transport chain can be broken in a number of places, in which case vitamin B_{12} deficiency ensues. Poor diet rarely causes vitamin B_{12} deficiency, since only about 1 μg is lost daily, and even a poor diet usually contains some food of animal origin.

Defective intestinal absorption of vitamin B_{12}, owing to a lack of production of IF, is the most common defect and causes pernicious anemia. This dramatic but treatable illness is believed to result from an autoimmune attack on the gastric mucosa, in particular on the gastric parietal cells (see Chapter 13). Pernicious anemia is consequently associated with a lack of secretion of gastric juice, gastric acid, and pepsin. In addition, blocking autoantibodies in the gastric juice can bind to the vitamin B_{12} binding site of IF and prevent the formation of the vitamin B_{12}-IF complex. Antibodies to parietal cells or IF are found in 50% of patients with pernicious anemia.

Vitamin B_{12} deficiency can also be caused by (1) gastrectomy, (2) overgrowth of vitamin B_{12}-consuming microorganisms in a surgically constructed intestinal blind loop, (3) a variety of inflammatory and neoplastic disorders involving the terminal ileum, (4) surgical removal of the site of absorption, the terminal ileum, and (5) intestinal infestation with the fish tapeworm (*Diphyllobothrium latum*) that consumes vitamin B_{12}.

After absorption, vitamin B_{12} is well utilized unless there is a rare congenital deficiency of the principal vitamin B_{12}-binding protein, transcobalamin II. Since only 1 μg of vitamin B_{12} per day is lost and the total body stores are 1000 to 5000 μg, it requires years of vitamin B_{12} deficiency for megaloblastic anemia to develop.

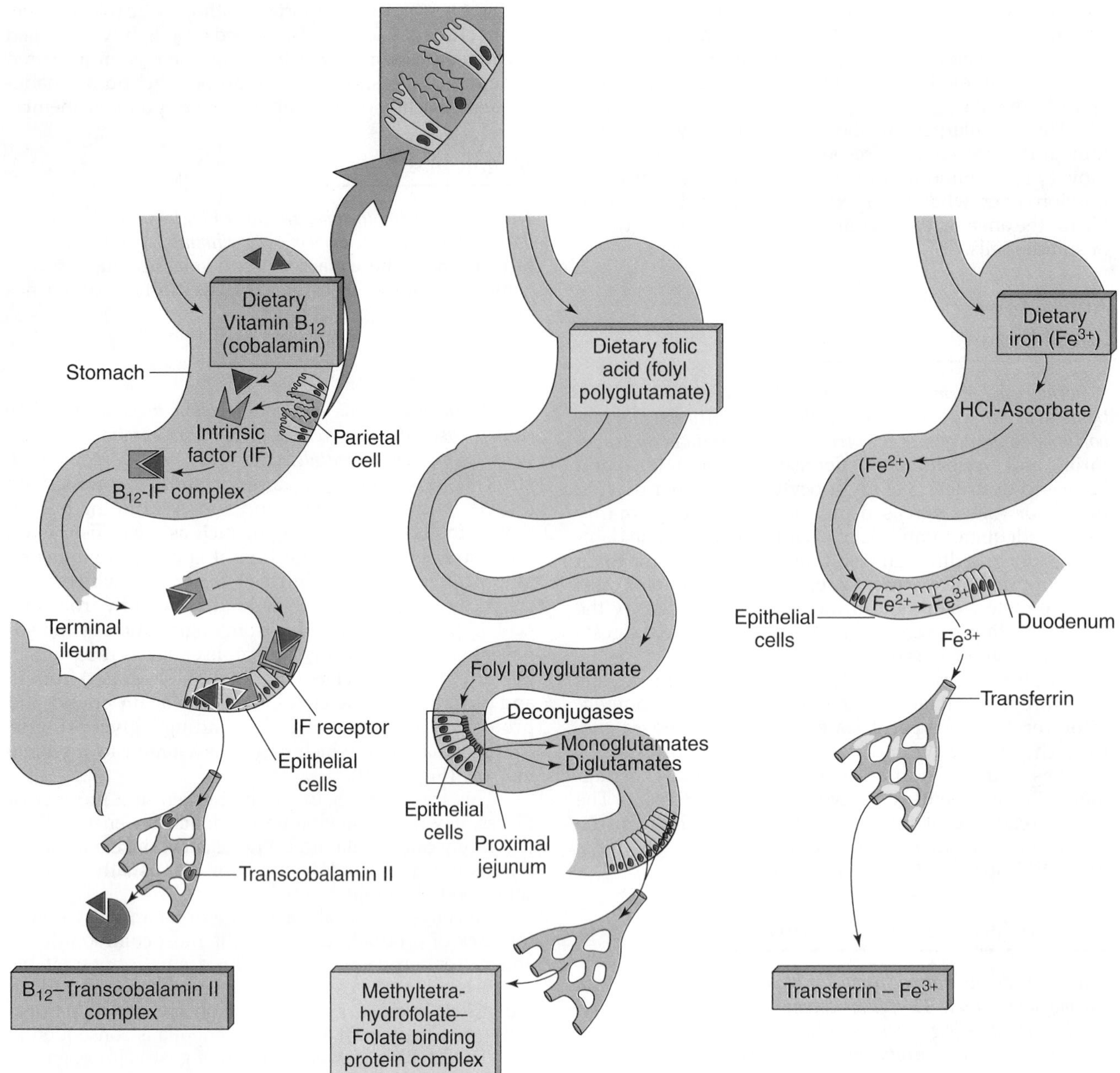

FIGURE *20-19*

Absorption of vitamin B_{12}, folic acid, and iron. Absorption of vitamin B_{12} requires initial complexing with intrinsic factor (IF), which is produced by the parietal cells of the gastric mucosa. Absorption then occurs in the terminal ileum, where there are receptors for the IF-B_{12} complex. Dietary folic acid is conjugated by conjugase enzymes to polyglutamate. Absorption occurs in the jejunum following deconjugation in the intestinal lumen. Reduction and methylation result in the generation of methyl tetrahydrofolate, which is then transported by folate binding protein. Dietary ferric iron is reduced to ferrous iron in the stomach and absorbed principally in the duodenum. Iron is transported by transferrin in the circulation.

Folic Acid Deficiency

Folic acid is a vital nutrient present in leafy vegetables and in meat and egg products. It is conjugated to a number of glutamic acid residues, which are split off in the intestinal lumen. Folic acid is absorbed in the jejunum as a monoglutamate and reduced and methylated in the blood to 5-methyl tetrahydrofolic acid (5-methyl FH4).

The most common cause of folic acid deficiency is an inadequate dietary intake. The daily requirement for folic acid is 50 μg, and the total body stores amount only to 2000 to 5000 μg. Accordingly, in contrast to vitamin B_{12} deficiency, it requires only months of folic acid deficiency for megaloblastic anemia to develop. Folic acid deficiency occurs most commonly in alcoholics and in recluses with poor nutrition. Impaired intestinal absorption of folic acid occurs in celiac disease and tropical sprue and may be responsible in part for the deficiency observed in some patients taking anticonvulsive drugs such as phenytoin. Deficiency develops more rapidly when there is an increased demand for folic acid, such as in pregnancy or in hemolytic anemias.

Impaired DNA Synthesis

Regardless of the cause, a deficiency of either vitamin B_{12} or folic acid results in impaired DNA synthesis, which in turn leads to a megaloblastic transformation of hemopoietic cells. In order to synthesize DNA, pyrimidine uridylate, a component of RNA, is converted to thymidylate, a component of DNA. Tetrahydrofolic acid is needed as a co-enzyme for this reaction. As shown in Figure 20-20, vitamin B_{12} is also required to generate and regenerate tetrahydrofolic acid from its transport form 5-methyl FH4. Consequently, impaired DNA synthesis occurs directly in folic acid deficiency and indirectly in vitamin B_{12} deficiency. Nevertheless, the hematological consequences are identical.

The defect in DNA synthesis associated with deficiencies of vitamin B_{12} or folic acid causes delayed nuclear maturation and abnormal mitotic activity. These consequences are mainly expressed in rapidly dividing cells, such as those in the bone marrow and in the gastrointestinal epithelium. Because of the delay in nuclear maturation, the nuclear chromatin is loose, and the maturations of the nucleus and the cytoplasm are asynchronous (nuclear-cytoplasmic dissociation).

☐ **Pathology:** In the erythroid precursor cells, the defect in DNA synthesis produces large megaloblasts, with loose immature nuclei, often with satellite pieces (Fig. 20-21A). The cytoplasm displays various degrees of maturation and hemoglobin synthesis. There is a considerable degree of cellular destruction and ineffective erythropoiesis in the bone marrow. The circulating erythrocytes are large, often with an oval shape, and are associated with prominent poikilocytosis and a teardrop configuration (see Fig. 20-21B).

The myeloid cells also show considerable changes. Large metamyelocytes with horseshoe-shaped nuclei are seen in the bone marrow, and neutrophils with six or

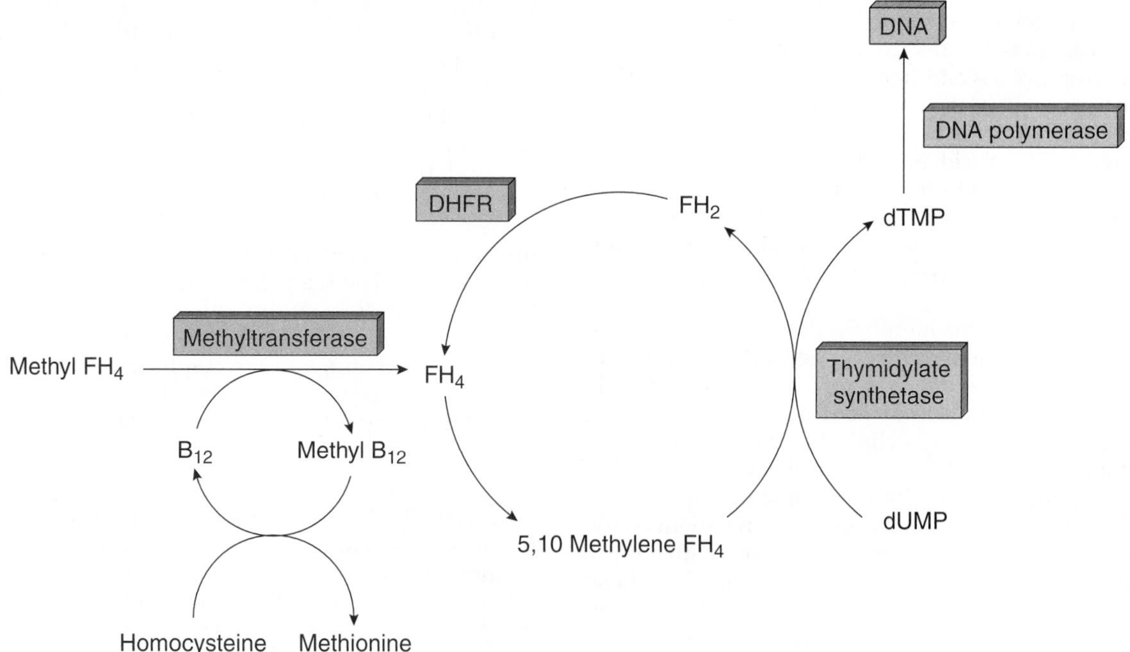

FIGURE *20-20*
Relationship of folic acid to vitamin B_{12}. A 1-carbon transfer mediated by folic acid methylates dUMP to dTMP, which is then used for the synthesis of DNA. To enter this cycle, folate (methyl FH4) is demethylated to FH4, vitamin B_{12} acting as the co-factor. Thus, both vitamin B_{12} and folic acid deficiency lead to impaired DNA synthesis and megaloblastic anemia. FH4, tetrahydrofolate; dUMP, deoxyuridine monophosphate; dTMP, deoxythymidine monophosphate; FH2, dihydrofolate; DHFR, dihydrofolate reductase.

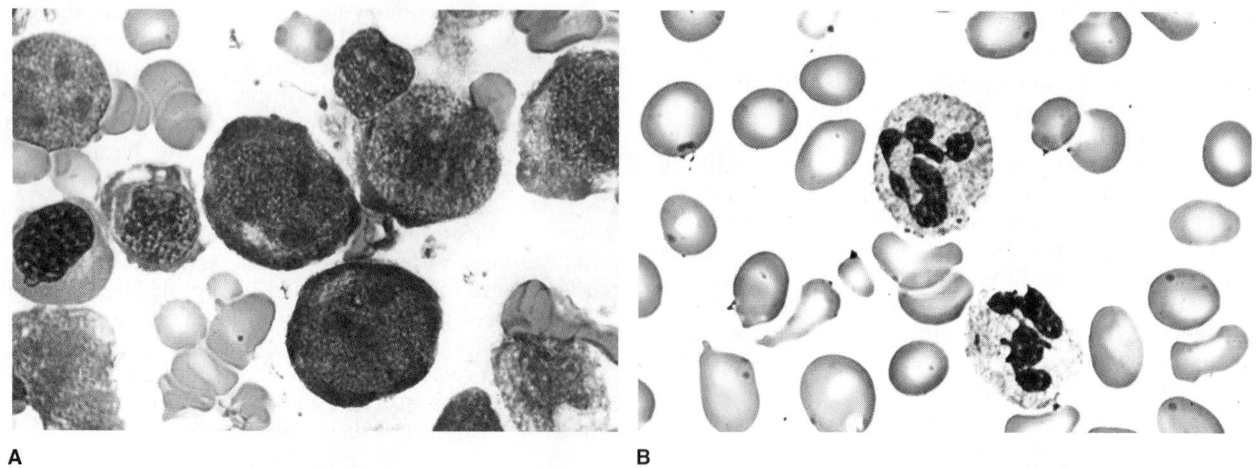

FIGURE 20-21
Megaloblastic anemia (*A*) A bone marrow aspirate from a patient with vitamin B_{12} deficiency (pernicious anemia) shows prominent megaloblastic erythroid precursors. (*B*) In this smear of peripheral blood from the same patient, the erythrocytes are large, often with an oval shape, and are associated with poikilocytosis and teardrop shapes. The neutrophils are hypersegmented.

more nuclear lobes (hypersegmentation or right shift) circulate in the blood. The megakaryocytes display nuclear abnormalities, including hypersegmentation and wide separation of the nuclear lobes.

☐ **Clinical Features:** Since all cellular proliferation is defective, patients with vitamin B_{12} or folic acid deficiencies can develop pancytopenia. Lactic dehydrogenase (LDH) isoenzymes 1 and 2 are elevated because of ineffective erythropoiesis and hemolysis. The differentiation between vitamin B_{12} deficiency and folic acid deficiency is made by specific immunoassays of the plasma for vitamin B_{12} and red cell folic acid. Newer diagnostic tests for vitamin B_{12} deficiency and serum homocysteine and methyl malonate may be very sensitive predictors of morbidity. Intestinal absorption of vitamin B_{12} is evaluated by means of the Schilling test, which measures absorption with and without added IF.

Some patients with vitamin B_{12} deficiency suffer **subacute combined degeneration of the posterior and lateral columns of the spinal cord**, which is associated with irreversible ataxia and other neurological defects (see Chapter 28). Thus, the two clinical features that distinguish vitamin B_{12} from folic acid deficiency are neurological abnormalities and the slower onset of the latter.

Megaloblastosis can also be observed in patients with adequate vitamin B_{12} and folic acid levels, but with inborn or acquired abnormalities of the bone marrow. The most common causes are drug therapy, such as phenytoin for seizures, antiretroviral agents for human immunodeficiency virus (HIV) infection, and chemotherapy of neoplastic disorders with methotrexate or hydroxyurea.

Iron Deficiency Anemia

Iron is utilized primarily in the production of hemoglobin, although it also functions as a co-factor for a variety of intracellular enzymes. An adequate diet provides about 20 mg of iron daily, of which 1 or 2 mg is absorbed, principally in the duodenum. The rate of absorption is finely tuned to admit enough iron to compensate for the normal loss of cells desquamated from the skin and intestinal mucosa. In anemias, regardless of cause, the duodenal absorption of iron is increased. This is a useful compensation in iron deficiency anemia but carries a potential for dangerous iron overload in patients with other types of anemias.

After absorption in the gut, iron binds to transferrin and is transported to specific transferrin receptors present on the surface of most cells. The greatest receptor density is found on the surface of erythroid precursor cells and reticulocytes, and 80% to 90% of circulating iron is used for hemoglobin synthesis. After their allotted life span, senescent erythrocytes are phagocytized by macrophages. The hemoglobin iron is then split off, released to transferrin, and reutilized for hemoglobin synthesis. Excess macrophage iron is packed densely inside shells of apoferritin, and the resulting ferritin molecules are deposited to provide a store of reserve iron. Ferritin molecules can be further packed into large lysosomal aggregates and become visible as hemosiderin particles.

☐ **Pathogenesis:** **Paradoxically, although iron is the most abundant metal in the world, iron deficiency is the most common cause of anemia.** The principal causes of iron deficiency are (1) impaired intake, owing to an iron-poor diet, or (2) excessive loss, caused by hemorrhage, pregnancy, lactation, or intravascular hemolysis. In Western countries, dietary intake of iron is frequently inadequate in infants and young children on iron-deficient milk diets. In adults, although the normal diet usually contains adequate iron, there is little reserve to compensate for increased iron loss.

Loss of iron by blood loss is by far the most common cause of iron deficiency anemia in adults, since 2

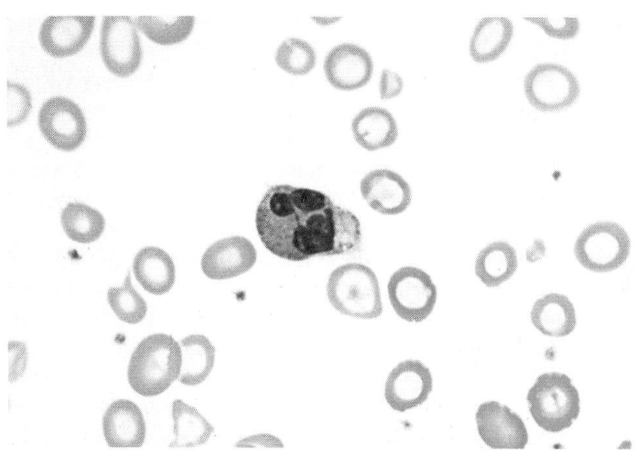

FIGURE 20-22
Iron deficiency anemia. A smear of peripheral blood shows hypochromic and microcytic erythrocytes. Poikilocytosis (irregular shape) and anisocytosis (irregular size) are also observed.

mL of whole blood contains 1 mg of iron. In women of reproductive age, iron loss is usually caused by menstruation or pregnancy, although the possibility of gastrointestinal or urinary blood loss should not be forgotten. The occurrence of iron deficiency anemia in an otherwise healthy man mandates a search for a gastrointestinal lesion, which may be leaking blood. Impaired iron absorption is rare and primarily limited to patients with extensive surgical resection of the upper gastrointestinal tract.

□ **Pathology:** On the peripheral blood smear, the erythrocytes are hypochromic and microcytic. In severe iron deficiency anemia, poikilocytosis (irregular shape) and anisocytosis (irregular size) can be observed (Fig. 20-22). The bone marrow smear reveals an increased number of small normoblasts with poorly hemoglobinized or ragged cytoplasm.

The laboratory findings include a low serum iron and increased total iron-binding capacity (TIBC). The most important finding is a decreased ferritin level (<20 ng/mL), which reflects a decrease in total tissue stores of iron. However, ferritin is an acute phase protein and is increased in febrile and toxic patients. Only ferritin levels above 100 ng/mL clearly rule out iron deficiency in such patients. A decrease in tissue iron can also be demonstrated by decreased or absent hemosiderin in macrophages, demonstrated in Prussian blue–stained smears of bone marrow.

□ **Clinical Features:** Chronic iron deficiency anemia is associated with nonspecific symptoms, such as weakness, malaise and shortness of breath. Abnormal cellular function caused by a decrease in iron-containing enzymes is uncommon but may cause atrophic glossitis, angular stomatitis, and spoon-shaped fingernails (koilonychia).

Thalassemia

The thalassemia syndromes are a heterogeneous group of heritable anemias that have in common quantitatively defective synthesis of either the α or the β chains of the normal hemoglobin A tetramer ($\alpha_2\beta_2$) (Fig. 20-23). The specific thalassemia syndromes are defined by the affected globin chain. In the β-thalassemias, synthesis of the β chain is impaired, whereas in the α-thalassemias, the defect involves the α chain.

All forms of thalassemia are characterized by a hypochromic, microcytic anemia, owing to reduced or

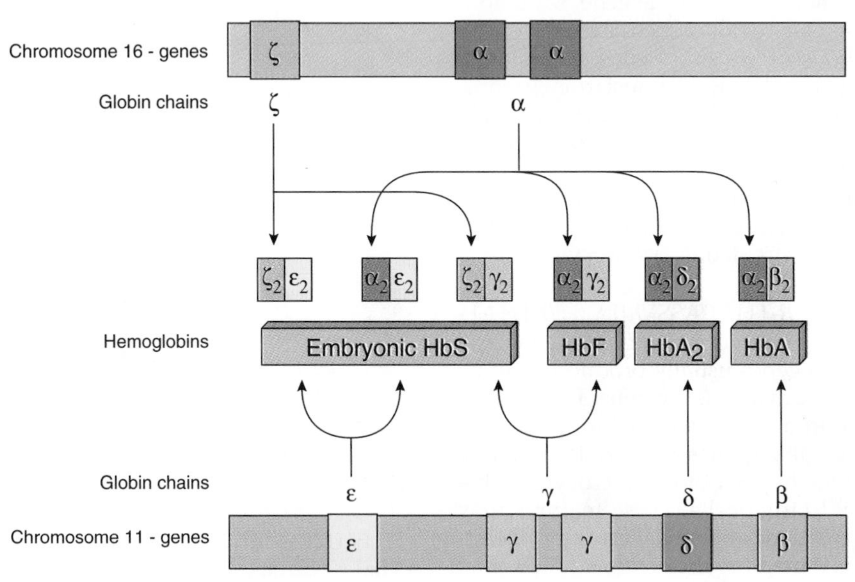

FIGURE 20-23
Assembly of subunit chains to form different hemoglobins.

absent synthesis of the complete hemoglobin molecule. In addition, the accumulation of unmatched globin chains leads to their precipitation. The consequent damage to the membrane of nucleated erythrocytes leads to ineffective erythropoiesis, and injury to mature erythrocytes results in hemolysis.

☐ **Epidemiology:** Thalassemia (Greek, *thalassa*, "sea") originally pertained to anemias observed in populations that inhabited the Italian and Greek coasts. However, it is now realized that in addition to the Mediterranean basin, thalassemias also occur in a belt that extends across the Middle East, through parts of Pakistan and India, to Southeast Asia. This belt also includes southern parts of the former Soviet Union, China, and the northern regions of the African continent. Importantly, sporadic mutations occasionally produce β-thalassemia among populations in whom the disease does not ordinarily occur.

Gene frequencies in endemic areas may be as high as 15%. Similar to sickle cell anemia and some other hemoglobinopathies, thalassemias are most frequent in regions where malaria was historically endemic. The high incidence of these anemias in such populations is attributed to heterozygote selection by malaria, owing to the fact that malaria-infected heterozygotes seem to have milder symptoms and, thus, greater reproductive fitness.

β-Thalassemia

At the molecular level, the β-thalassemias are extremely heterogeneous, and more than 100 distinct mutations have been associated with this phenotype. Specific molecular lesions are seen more commonly in specific ethnic groups.

☐ **Pathogenesis:** The β-thalassemias are caused by either a point mutation on chromosome number 11 or, less commonly, a deletion of part of the gene. Mutations in the upstream promoter region affect DNA transcription, whereas mutations in the splice sites, termination codons, or coding regions affect RNA translation. In some thalassemic persons, the deletion encompasses the neighboring delta gene ($\delta\beta$-thalassemia) and may even encroach on the upstream gamma genes.

Defective β-globin synthesis causes anemia, owing to impaired production of erythrocytes (ineffective erythropoiesis) and hemolysis of circulating erythrocytes.

HETEROZYGOUS *B*-THALASSEMIA (*B*-THALASSEMIA MINOR): The one normal β globin gene and the two normal δ globin genes usually produces β and δ chains to bind most of the available α chains. The result is a moderate reduction in normal hemoglobin ($A_2\beta_2$) and an increase in hemoglobin A_2 ($\alpha_2\delta_2$). There is usually a mild anemia, with some hypochromia, microcytosis, basophilic stippling, and target cells. These features may mimic those of iron deficiency anemia. However, the diagnosis of thalassemia is made by the demonstration of an increased amount of hemoglobin A_2 (>5%). Moreover, whereas erythrocyte counts are normal or even mildly elevated in β-thalassemia minor, they tend to be decreased in iron deficiency anemia (Fig. 20-24).

The situation is somewhat different in the case of patients with δ,β-thalassemia. In such persons, γ-chain synthesis is released from its normal neonatal suppression, and γ chains bind excess α chains. The result is the formation of an increased amount of fetal hemoglobin ($\alpha_2\gamma_2$).

HOMOZYGOUS *B*-THALASSEMIA (COOLEY ANEMIA): This severe disorder is caused by a pronounced reduction in (β^+) or absence (β^0) of β chain production. Hemoglobin electrophoresis reveals principally fetal hemoglobin. The hemoglobin A_2 concentration is normal or moderately elevated. Since the excess unpaired α chains readily precipitate within the erythroid cells, they destroy both erythroid precursor cells (ineffective erythropoiesis) and circulating erythrocytes (hemolysis). The peripheral blood erythrocytes are hypochromic and microcytic and show marked anisocytosis, poikilocytosis, and target cell configuration (see Fig. 20-24). Circulating nucleated erythrocytes are often observed, especially after splenectomy.

The increased oxygen affinity of HbF leads to increased production of erythropoietin and a consequent stimulation of erythropoiesis. The facial and cranial bones tend to be enlarged or distorted because of severe bone marrow hyperplasia. Extramedullary foci of blood formation may be present in the spleen, liver, and paraspinal regions. The spleen is increased in size because of both production and destruction of erythrocytes. The enlarged spleen may sequester and destroy leukocytes and platelets (hypersplenism). **Increased erythropoiesis enhances iron absorption and results in massive iron overload, the major cause of morbidity and mortality in these patients.**

Intensive transfusion therapy has diminished some of the effects of ineffective erythropoiesis and hemolysis in Cooley anemia, and the concomitant use of iron chelators (to prevent secondary iron overload) has resulted in

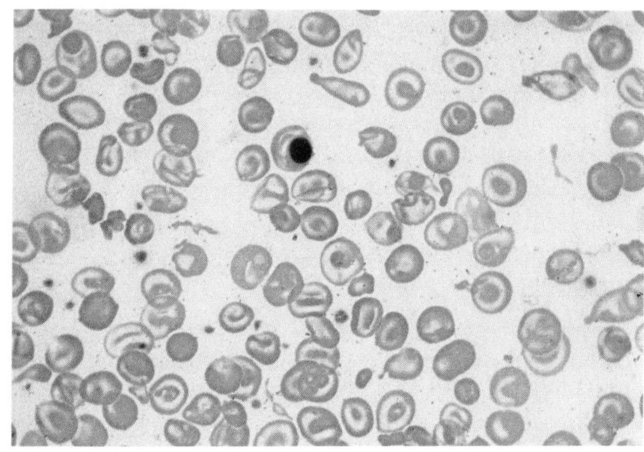

FIGURE *20-24*
Thalassemia. The peripheral blood erythrocytes are hypochromic and microcytic and show anisocytosis, poikilocytosis, and target cells.

a reasonably good prognosis for this formerly lethal disease.

α-Thalassemia

α-Thalassemia comprises four distinct syndromes, each of which reflects the failure of one or more of the four α gene loci on chromosome 16 to function. In contrast to β-thalassemia, 80% of cases of α-thalassemia reflect gene deletions, whereas the remainder are caused by point mutations. Over 30 different genetic lesions have been identified.

The content of the different hemoglobins in the diverse α-thalassemias differs. *In utero* and in the neonatal period, unbalanced synthesis of γ chains causes the precipitation of unmatched γ chains as hemoglobin Barts (γ_4), whereas in children and adults excess β chains are deposited as hemoglobin H (β_4). A minor component of hemoglobin γ_4 may be identified. The tetrameric hemoglobin Barts and hemoglobin H in α-thalassemia are more soluble and, therefore, less toxic than the unmatched α chains in the β-thalassemic syndromes. Consequently, ineffective erythrocyte production is less prominent and peripheral erythrocyte destruction is less severe in the α-thalassemias. However, these tetramers bind oxygen tightly, and, hence the erythrocytes function poorly in the delivery of oxygen.

The severity of the four α-thalassemias depends on the number of chains deleted.

- **The silent carrier state** is caused by the deletion of only one gene. The hematological parameters are normal, and in infants only 1% to 2% of the total hemoglobin is hemoglobin Barts.
- **α-Thalassemia trait** reflects the deletion of two genes. This results in only a mild hemolytic anemia, and in infants hemoglobin Barts accounts for no more than 5% of the total hemoglobin.
- **Hemoglobin H disease,** in which three genes are deleted, is characterized by a moderate hemolytic anemia, with hypochromia and microcytosis. In the first year of life, the erythrocytes may contain up to 25% hemoglobin Barts. In adults, hemoglobin A predominates, with a minor component of hemoglobin H.
- **Deletion of all four α-chain genes** causes death either *in utero* or at the time of delivery. The predominance of the high-affinity hemoglobin Barts produces a severe impairment of oxygen delivery *in utero*. Massive splenomegaly occurs as a result of a compensatory extramedullary hemopoiesis, and generalized edema (hydrops fetalis) is caused by severe heart failure.

Increased Destruction of Erythrocytes (Hemolytic Anemias) Associated with Hemoglobinopathies

Sickle Cell Disease

Sickle cell disease refers to a group of hereditary hemoglobinopathies in which deoxygenated erythrocytes undergo a transformation from the normal biconcave disk to a sickle-shaped structure. This shape change, caused by the polymerization of sickle hemoglobin (HbS), leads to hemolytic anemia and the occlusion of small blood vessels. The most important disorders associated with the presence of HbS include homozygous sickle cell anemia and the double heterozygote entities of sickle cell hemoglobin C disease and sickle cell β-thalassemia.

Sickled erythrocytes were first described in 1910, when James Herrick, a physician noted for his observations of hereditary disorders, reported the presence of these cells in the blood of an anemic black medical student. In 1949, Pauling and colleagues were the first to identify the molecular basis of an inherited trait when they reported a single amino acid substitution as the basis of sickle cell disease and christened the disorder as a molecular disease. In 1987, diagnosis by polymerase chain reaction (PCR) became available.

Sickle Cell Anemia

☐ **Epidemiology:** Persons with sickle cell anemia are homozygous for the HbS gene. The disease is particularly common among blacks, and in some regions of Africa as many as 40% of the population are heterozygotes. In the United States, about 10% of blacks are carriers of the trait, and 1 in 650 persons in this population (50,000 persons) has sickle cell anemia. The gene is also encountered in parts of the Mediterranean basin, the Middle East, and India.

It is noteworthy that the gene for HbS is prevalent in areas of the world in which falciparum malaria is endemic, suggesting that heterozygosity for the gene confers a selective advantage in persons who become infected with malaria. The benefit of HbS is apparently restricted to children, who are readily infected with *Plasmodium falciparum* but in whom parasite counts remain low. It is thought that parasitized erythrocytes preferentially sickle and are removed from the circulation by tissue macrophages in the spleen and liver, a process that also destroys the organism.

☐ **Pathogenesis:** HbS ($\alpha_2\beta S_2$) is the result of a point mutation in which valine is substituted for glutamic acid at the sixth position of the β-globin chain. The primary event in the molecular pathogenesis of sickle cell disease is the tendency of HbS to aggregate and polymerize at low oxygen tension to form a rigid filamentous gel (Fig. 20-25), which renders the erythrocyte rigid and less deformable. The membrane contracts around aggregated polymers of HbS, and the erythrocytes take on a characteristic appearance, resembling sickles or holly leaves (Fig. 20-26).

Since gel formation is reversible, most circulating erythrocytes do not sickle completely in the tissues before they are reoxygenated in the lungs. However, after many cycles of deoxygenation and reoxygenation, the erythrocytes become irreversibly sickled and tend to obstruct the microvasculature. Erythrocyte ghosts (devoid of hemoglobin) derived from irreversibly sickled cells retain the sickle shape, indicating that secondary alterations in the erythrocyte membrane have occurred. Indeed, a number of structural and functional membrane defects have been described, including phospholipid changes, altered

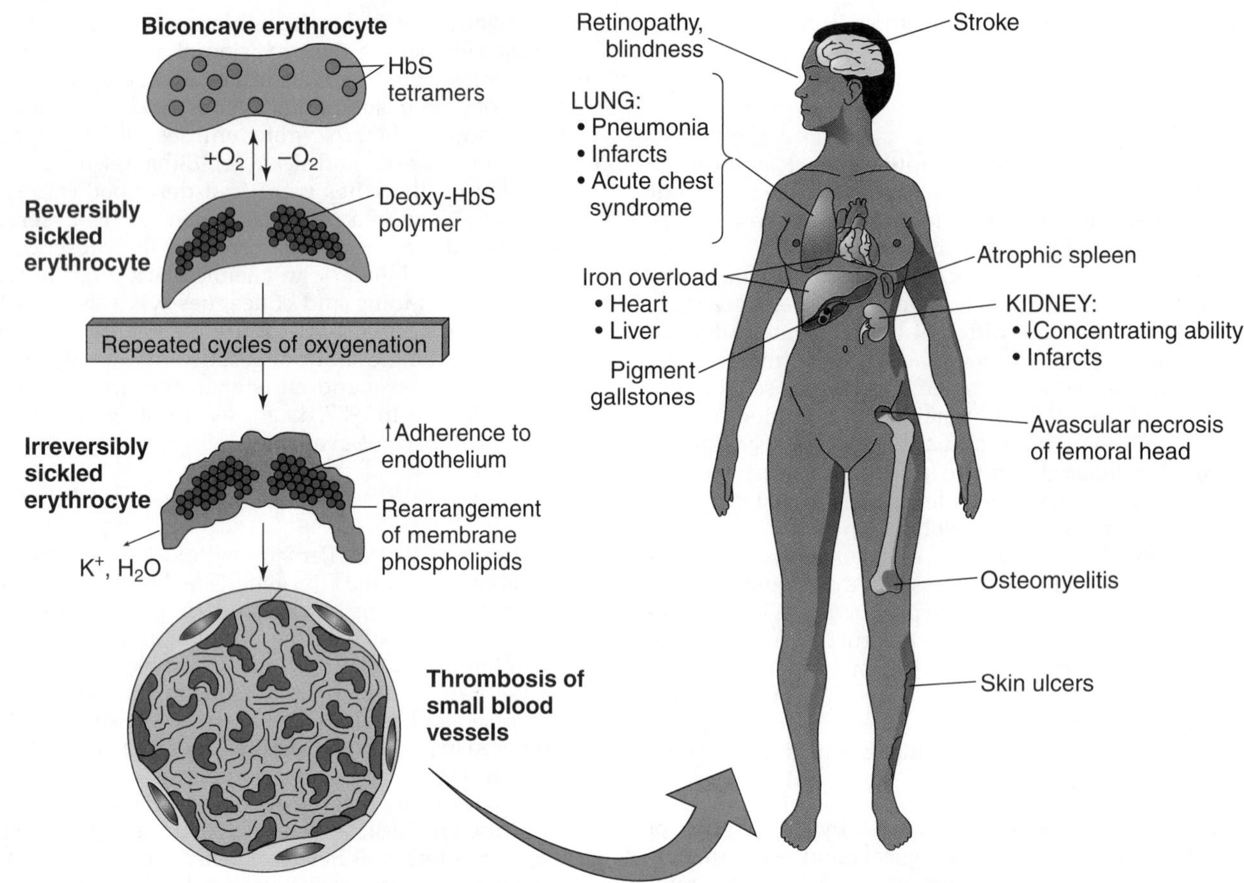

FIGURE *20-25*
Pathogenesis of the vascular complications of sickle cell anemia. Because of the substitution of valine for glutamic acid, there is an alteration in the charge on the surface of the hemoglobin molecule. Upon deoxygenation, sickle hemoglobin tetramers aggregate to form poorly soluble polymers. A change in the shape of the erythrocyte from a biconcave disk to a sickle form accompanies the polymerization of sickle hemoglobin (HbS). This process is initially reversible upon reoxygenation. However, with repeated cycles of deoxygenation and reoxygenation, the erythrocytes become irreversibly sickled. Irreversibly sickled cells display a rearrangement of phospholipids between the outer and inner monolayers of the cell membrane, in particular an increase in aminophospholipids in the outer leaflet. Potassium and water are lost from the cells. The erythrocytes are no longer deformable and are more adherent to endothelial cells, properties that predispose to thrombosis of small blood vessels. The resulting vascular occlusions lead to widespread ischemic complications.

ion transport, and enhanced adherence of sickled cells to vascular endothelium.

☐ **Pathology and Clinical Features:** Homozygous sickle cell anemia (hemoglobin SS) is a devastating illness. In this malady, hemoglobin S constitutes 80% to 95% of the total hemoglobin, with hemoglobins F and A_2 comprising the remainder. **The predominance of hemoglobin S leads to both severe chronic hemolytic anemia and to vaso-occlusive disease, the latter usually dominating the clinical course.**

The infant with sickle cell anemia is protected by the presence of fetal hemoglobin, which persists for 8 to 10 weeks, after which symptoms of the disease may become apparent. HbF is a potent inhibitor of the polymerization of HbS. Many afflicted persons are asymptomatic most of the time, only to suffer sudden episodes of sickle crises, which are sometimes fatal.

VASO-OCCLUSIVE CRISIS: This is the most frequent form of sickle crisis, occurring frequently or as uncommonly as once a year. **Sickled erythrocytes obstruct small blood vessels in many organs, producing severe pain, especially in the bones, abdomen, and chest.** SS red cells have a sticky surface and attach more readily than normal erythrocytes to endothelial cells. Repeated infarcts in the spleen cause progressive fibrosis, scarring and, eventually, splenic atrophy. By the time the affected

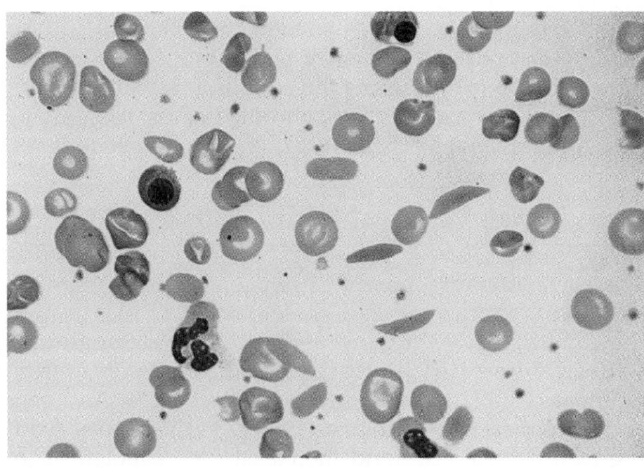

FIGURE *20-26*
Sickle cell anemia. A peripheral blood smear shows numerous sickled cells, as well as normoblasts and occasional target cells. The erythrocyte to the left of center contains a Howell-Jolly body, indicative of functional hyposplenism.

person has reached adulthood, the spleen is reduced to a small, functionless, fibrous nodule, weighing as little as 10 g. Ulceration of the skin in the region of the ankles is common and results from the obstruction of small dermal and subcutaneous vessels with consequent infarctions of the skin. Infarcts of the femoral head are especially common because of its limited vascularization.

APLASTIC CRISIS: Intercurrent infections, both viral and bacterial, tend to depress the normal rate of erythrocyte production. Infection by parvovirus B19 is most commonly incriminated. Since hemolysis continues unabated, the hemoglobin concentration falls rapidly, a condition termed aplastic crisis.

SEQUESTRATION CRISIS: This complication is typically seen in young children and infants, in whom sudden pooling of erythrocytes leads to a rapid fall in the hemoglobin level to less than 6 g/dL. The loss of circulating volume to sequestration may result in hypovolemic shock. This complication accounts for most of the deaths from sickle cell anemia in the early years of life.

Numerous organs demonstrate the ravages of sickle cell anemia.

- **Heart:** Chronic anemia leads to cardiac changes associated with the consequences of a persistently increased cardiac output. This may be complicated by myocardial ischemia as a result of occlusive disease of the coronary microvasculature. Secondary iron overload, caused by chronic hemolysis and multiple blood transfusions, may further compromise cardiac function. Thus, cardiomegaly and even congestive heart failure are not infrequent.
- **Lungs:** Pulmonary infarction and infections of the lungs are well-recognized complications of sickle cell anemia. In addition, a rapidly progressive decrease in pulmonary function associated with radiological infiltrates, a situation termed *acute chest syndrome,* occurs in almost one third of the patients and may be fatal.
- **Spleen**: Although splenomegaly is common in early childhood, it is rare in adults with sickle cell anemia, owing to recurrent infarction. Splenic atrophy results in functional asplenia, characterized by defective phagocytosis and abnormalities of the alternative complement pathway. Subsequent septicemic episodes secondary to infection with encapsulated bacteria, especially *S. pneumoniae,* can be life-threatening.
- **Brain:** As many as 25% of patients have some evidence of neurological disturbances, including strokes, often preceded by transient ischemic attacks, and cerebral hemorrhage.
- **Kidney:** Because the microenvironment of the renal medulla is hypoxic, acidotic, and hypertonic, sickling in the vasa recta is common. Many patients lose the ability to concentrate urine. Hematuria is frequent, and renal infarcts and papillary necrosis are encountered.
- **Hepatobiliary system:** Chronic hemolysis predisposes to **pigment gallstones**, which are present in over half of the adult patients and have been seen in children as young as 6 years of age. Massive hepatomegaly is occasionally observed, and secondary iron overload in the liver is common.
- **Bones:** A classic complication of sickle cell anemia is **osteomyelitis**, particularly with *Salmonella typhimurium.* The precise pathogenesis is not understood, but it is thought to relate to poor splenic function and microinfarcts of the bone marrow. In young children, marrow infarcts of the bones of the hands and feet also lead to self-limited swelling in those areas (*hand-foot syndrome*). In adults, avascular necrosis of the head of the femur leads to gait disturbances.
- **Eye:** Occlusion of the microvasculature of the retina is complicated by hemorrhage, proliferative retinopathy, retinal detachment, and eventually blindness.

Sickle Cell Trait

The heterozygous form of sickle cell disease (hemoglobin SA) is termed sickle cell trait. It is a benign disorder found in 10% of American blacks. HbS constitutes one third of the total hemoglobin of the erythrocyte, the remainder consisting of normal hemoglobin A. Because of the low content of HbS, the erythrocytes only sickle at a low unphysiological oxygen tension (unpressurized aircraft, deep-sea diving) and irreversibly sickled erythrocytes are rarely produced. The peripheral blood erythrocyte counts and the erythrocyte life spans are normal, and the patient does not experience painful ischemic attacks. Although there may be some effect on the kidneys, sickle cell trait rarely causes functional renal disease. The condition does not affect the life span of the patient, and no treatment is required.

Sickle Cell Disease and Other Hemoglobinopathies

The sickle gene is sometimes inherited with another abnormal globin gene or with a thalassemia gene. In such cases, the clinical presentation depends on the total amount of HbS present and on its interactions with the other abnormal hemoglobins.

Hemoglobin SC disease is characterized by a hemoglobin composed of 50% HbS and 50% hemoglobin C (see later). Hemoglobin C adds to the erythrocyte rigidity imparted by hemogloblin S. Hence, hemoglobin SC disease is associated with severe hemolytic anemia, painful crises, and bone marrow infarctions.

Sickle cell β-thalassemia presents variable clinical features, depending on the intracellular amount of hemoglobin F, which protects the erythrocyte from the deleterious effects of HbS. In both HbSC and this double heterozygote, splenomegaly commonly persists into adulthood.

Hemoglobin SD disease, in which there is 50% HbS and 50% hemoglobin D, is an extremely mild form of sickle cell disease. The molecular interactions between hemoglobin D and HbS actually prevent the sickling of erythrocytes.

Hemoglobin C Disease

Hemoglobin C (HbC) is the second most common abnormal hemoglobin, occurring in as many as one fourth of West Africans. Two to 3% of blacks in the United States are asymptomatic heterozygotes (hemoglobin AC). HbC results from the substitution of lysine for glutamic acid in the same sixth position of the hemoglobin β-globin chain involved in sickle cell anemia.

In homozygous hemoglobin C disease (hemoglobin CC), a chronic, mild hemolytic anemia is associated with dehydrated and rigid erythrocytes. These cells are removed primarily in the spleen, which is reflected in a shortening of the erythrocyte life span. They may even become fragmented in the circulation, leading to the formation of microerythrocytes.

The spleen is enlarged because of pooling and destruction of the abnormal erythrocytes. The anemia is mild and for the most part asymptomatic, possibly because a decreased oxygen affinity of hemoglobin C increases the delivery of oxygen to the tissues. The most prominent morphological feature in homozygous hemoglobin C disease is the presence of numerous target cells. Occasionally, rhomboid hemoglobin C crystals are observed in the erythrocytes, especially after splenectomy.

Unstable Hemoglobins

Well over one hundred amino acid substitutions or deletions in the globin chains that affect the stability of the hemoglobin molecule have been described. The various unstable hemoglobins are generally named after the location where they were first described (e.g., hemoglobins Köln, Caribbean, Belfast). These mutations result in a gene product in which the forces that maintain the structure of hemoglobin are weakened. As a result, hemoglobin becomes denatured and precipitates as insoluble globins, recognized as inclusions attached to the erythrocyte membrane, termed *Heinz bodies*. The "pitting" of Heinz bodies from the erythrocytes in the spleen damages the membrane and shortens the life span of the cell. Mild chronic hemolysis, with splenomegaly and jaundice, is common, although in most instances the condition is well compensated. In a minority of cases, chronic hemolysis is severe and is aggravated by oxidant drugs or viral infections.

Hemoglobins with Abnormal Oxygen Affinity

The reversible attachment of oxygen to heme causes a shift in the configuration of the globin molecules around the contacts between the α and β chains. **Hemoglobins with an abnormally high affinity for oxygen** result from aminoacid substitutions in these contact areas. As a consequence they release oxygen poorly to the tissues, leading to tissue hypoxia and increased erythropoietin production. The resulting erythrocytosis is usually benign, although the increased erythrocyte mass and the associated increased viscosity may cause symptoms.

Abnormal hemoglobins with low oxygen affinity release oxygen more readily than normal to the tissues, thereby leading to decreased erythropoietin production and a mild anemia. Because of the increased amount of deoxygenated heme, the patients may be cyanotic.

Hemolytic Anemias Associated with Membrane Defects

The erythrocyte membrane consists of a lipid bilayer and a supporting protein cytoskeleton (see Fig. 20-9). A defect in any component of this skeleton renders the membrane unstable, thereby leading to a shortened erythrocyte life span. An abnormality in the *vertical* plane of the cytoskeleton-membrane interaction leads to the membrane loss of *hereditary spherocytosis,* whereas a *horizontal* one results in the deformity associated with *hereditary elliptocytosis.*

Hereditary Spherocytosis

Hereditary spherocytosis (HS) refers to a heterogeneous group of inherited hemolytic anemias characterized by a genetic defect in the cytoskeleton of the erythrocyte that results in spherical red blood cells. The large majority of HS cases are autosomal dominant, but severe autosomal recessive forms are well documented.

☐ **Pathogenesis:** The heterogeneous molecular defects in HS involve one of four cytoskeletal proteins of the erythrocyte, allowing subdivision into four broad forms.

- **Combined Partial Deficiency of Spectrin and Ankyrin:** Ankyrin (band 2.1) anchors spectrin molecules to the major transmembrane protein (anion exchanger, band 3) of the erythrocyte membrane. In the common autosomal dominant variant of HS, mutations in the gene on chromosome 8 that codes for ankyrin result in abnormal cytoskeletal structure and function.
- **Isolated Partial Deficiency of Spectrin:** Spectrin is the major cytoskeletal protein of the erythrocyte. It is

a dimer of two protein chains, the α and β subunits, and, in addition to ankyrin, binds to both actin and glycophorin by way of protein 4.1. Ten percent of patients with autosomal dominant HS have a mutation in the β-spectrin gene on chromosome 14. In the rare autosomal recessive variant of severe HS, polymorphisms of the α-spectrin gene on chromosome 1 have been reported.

- **Protein 4.2 Deficiency:** This condition is common in Japan. Protein 4.2 binds to ankyrin and band 3, thereby stabilizing their association. A few patients with mild autosomal recessive HS have been shown to manifest a deficiency in this protein, although it seems that this may not be the primary defect.
- **Partial Deficiency of Band 3:** This abnormality is associated with a characteristic "pincered" red cell structure.

As a result of these abnormalities, the density of the cytoskeleton of the erythrocyte is decreased and the membrane bilayer is destabilized. The cell surface area is progressively reduced owing to the loss of bilayer phospholipids in the form of microvesicles. The decrease in the surface-volume ratio is reflected in the formation of spherical erythrocytes (spherocytes), which are poorly deformable and trapped in the spleen. In that organ, the spherocytes are further damaged ("splenic conditioning"), and after several such splenic passages, they are prematurely removed from the circulation. Although splenic conditioning has been attributed to impaired erythrocyte glycolysis and consequent ATP depletion, this theory no longer seems tenable, and the precise nature of the process remains obscure. Nevertheless, it remains clear that the spleen plays an important role in the pathogenesis of HS.

□ **Pathology and Clinical Features:** The anemia of hereditary spherocytosis is normocytic and also hyperchromic, reflecting cellular dehydration. The MCHC frequently exceeds 36%. The peripheral blood smear shows a mixture of erythrocytes with decreased diameter, intense staining, and no central pallor (spherocytes); large bluish erythrocytes (polychromasia, diffuse basophilia); and normal erythrocytes (Fig. 20-27). Hemolysis is reflected in a decrease in serum haptoglobin and an increase in lactic dehydrogenase. Bone marrow examination reveals marked erythroid hyperplasia.

The spleen is enlarged, owing to packing of the red pulp cords with macrophages and erythrocytes. The sinuses appear empty, although electron microscopic studies have revealed the presence of erythrocyte ghosts. Hemosiderin-laden macrophages are often prominent.

Clinically, HS is characterized by jaundice, anemia, and splenomegaly. The severity of these manifestations varies greatly but is consistent within each family. Because chronic hemolysis increases bilirubin production, pigment gallstones are present in half of the adult patients. Intercurrent infections may aggravate the anemia, either by reducing erythrocyte formation (aplastic crisis) or by increasing erythrocyte destruction (hemolytic crisis). The Coombs test, in which immunoglobulin coating of erythrocytes is evaluated, must be performed to distinguish hereditary spherocytosis (negative Coombs test) from acquired autoimmune hemolytic anemia (positive Coombs test). **Since the spleen is primarily responsible for the destruction of spherocytes, splenectomy is usually curative.**

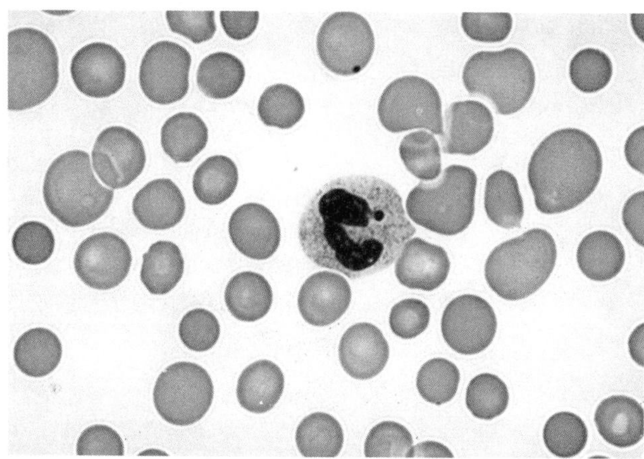

FIGURE *20-27*
Hereditary spherocytosis. The peripheral blood smear shows many erythrocytes with decreased diameter, intense staining, and no central pallor (spherocytes).

Hereditary Elliptocytosis

Hereditary elliptocytosis is the common name for a group of autosomal dominant disorders characterized by the presence of elliptical or oval-shaped erythrocytes in the circulation. Many different defects in the protein skeleton can cause elliptocytosis, and the clinical manifestations are equally varied. These abnormalities include (1) defective self association of spectrin subunits, (2) impaired binding of spectrin to ankyrin, (3) protein 4.1 defects, and (4) deficiency of glycophorin C. The common mechanism is a horizontal defect of the cytoskeleton. Interestingly, the red blood cells of camels and llamas are normally elliptical, although they do not suffer from hemolytic anemia.

In hereditary elliptocytosis, more than 75% of circulating erythrocytes appear elliptical (Fig. 20-28). In many cases, however, there are also teardrop-shaped erythrocytes, fragmented cells, and stomatocytes (a wide slit or mouthlike area replaces the normal central pallor). The hemolysis is usually moderate, but if it is severe, splenectomy is curative.

Acanthocytosis

Acanthocytosis refers to a group of anemias in which the erythrocyte membrane shows multiple irregular projections caused by defects in the lipid bilayer. A common cause of acanthocytosis is **liver disease**, in which free (nonesterified) cholesterol is deposited in the membrane. Acanthocytosis is also a feature of **abetalipoproteinemia**, an autosomal recessive lipid disorder. The acanthocytes, or spur cells, are morphologically impressive, but hemolysis is rarely pronounced (Fig. 20-29).

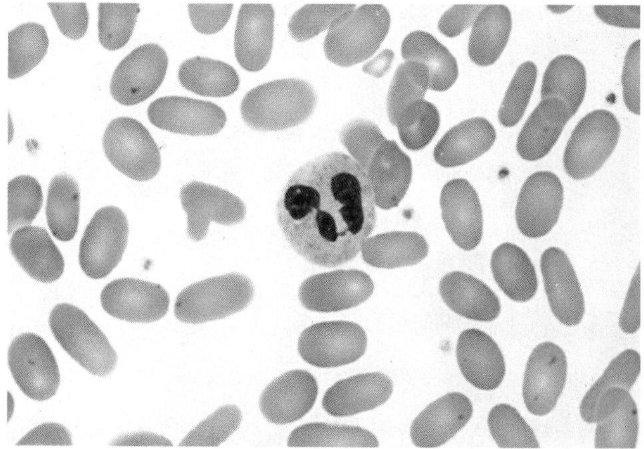

FIGURE 20-28
Hereditary elliptocytosis. A smear of peripheral blood reveals that virtually all of the erythrocytes have an elliptical shape.

Glucose-6-Phosphate Dehydrogenase Deficiency

Glucose-6-phosphate dehydrogenase (G6PD) deficiency refers to a group of X-linked, hereditary, hemolytic anemias in which an inadequate activity of erythrocyte G6PD predisposes to episodes of hemolysis precipitated by drugs or infections. Over 350 variants of G6PD have been described, many of which are associated with G6PD deficiency and hemolytic anemia. The persistence of G6PD deficiency in certain populations is believed to reflect the selective advantage afforded by resistance to malaria conferred by the lack of this enzyme.

The distribution of G6PD deficiency shows ethnic and geographic variations. For example, whereas northern Europeans have a prevalence of less than 1 in 1000, up to half of male Kurdish Jews are afflicted. The condition occurs in all populations but is particularly common among blacks of West African descent and among certain Mediterranean populations.

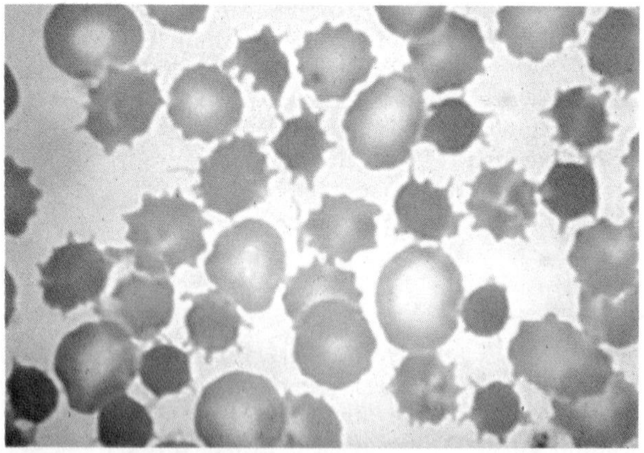

FIGURE 20-29
Acanthocytosis. In this smear of peripheral blood from a patient with abetalipoproteinemia, the erythrocytes display multiple irregular projections from the surface.

☐ **Pathogenesis:** G6PD is an enzyme of the hexose monophosphate shunt pathway that maintains glutathione in its reduced (active) form. Erythrocytes that are deficient in G6PD are less resistant to oxidation caused by infections or by exposure to oxidant drugs. Under such stress, hemoglobin is denatured and precipitates as Heinz bodies on the erythrocyte membrane. These abnormal erythrocytes are then phagocytized in the spleen. On occasion, Heinz bodies are removed from the erythrocytes, leaving a visible defect ("bite" cells).

The gene for G6PD is located on the X chromosome, and a deficiency is expressed only in males. Both the "normal" G6PD B enzyme and the G6PD A (A+) isozyme (found in 15% of American blacks) have the same biological activity. Another 10% to 15% of blacks, however, have a mutant enzyme designated as A−. In these persons, the erythrocytes contain only about 10% of the normal G6PD activity, owing to the instability of G6PD A−. As a result, hemolysis may occur when the patient is exposed to any one of a number of oxidizing drugs, such as the antimalarial agent primaquine.

In the Mediterranean population, a mutant gene encodes a severely deranged enzyme with barely detectable G6PD activity. Persons with this deficiency suffer sustained hemolytic anemia, which is aggravated by infections and drugs. Classically, they also develop a potentially lethal hemolysis after eating fava beans (*favism*).

Other hereditary enzyme deficiencies that impair the glycolytic pathways are rare, but when present they cause a mild hemolytic anemia. Most of these conditions are autosomal recessive, the most common being **pyruvate kinase deficiency**.

Autoimmune Hemolytic Anemias

Hemolytic anemia may be caused by autoantibodies with specificity for erythrocyte membrane proteins. They are either warm reacting, with maximal activity at 37°C, or less commonly cold reacting, in which case the activity increases at temperatures below 37°C.

Warm-Reacting Autoantibodies

Hemolytic anemia due to warm-reacting antibodies constitutes 80% of all autoimmune anemias. It occurs (1) as an idiopathic disorder, (2) in association with a variety of malignant or benign conditions, and (3) as a response to a number of drugs. Women are affected more than men, and the disease usually strikes in midlife.

☐ **Pathogenesis:** Warm-reacting antibodies are usually of the IgG class and are often directed at the core antigen of the Rh locus. If the density of antibodies is sufficiently high, they bind complement, although complement-induced intravascular hemolysis is rare. In hemolytic anemia mediated by warm-reacting antibodies, the erythrocytes are mostly destroyed in the splenic sinusoids by macrophages with receptors for the Fc portion of immunoglobulins or for the C3b component of complement. The macrophages phagocytize fragments of antibody-coated membrane, thereby reducing the size of the cell surface and causing spherocytosis. In turn, this promotes entrapment of erythrocytes in the spleen and eventually erythrocyte destruction.

Half of the cases of warm autoimmune hemolytic anemia (AIHA) are idiopathic, and the majority of the remainder are associated with the low-grade neoplasms small lymphocytic lymphoma and chronic lymphocytic leukemia. Autoimmune hemolytic anemia may also occur in association with collagen vascular diseases (particularly systemic lupus erythematosus), viral infections, some solid tumors (e.g., ovarian cancer) and certain inflammatory disorders (e.g., ulcerative colitis).

DRUG-INDUCED HEMOLYTIC ANEMIA: There are two pathogenetic variants of drug-induced autoimmune hemolytic anemia. In one type, the drug changes the antigen permanently, thereby eliciting the production of autoantibodies. These antibodies react with the altered antigen in the absence of the drug and produce complement-mediated hemolysis. The principal offender is the antihypertensive drug α-methyldopa, which alters an antigen of the Rh family.

In a second type of anemia associated with drug administration, the drug is only temporarily attached to an erythrocyte antigen and antibodies are formed against the drug-antigen complex. The antibodies bind to this complex and destroy the cell, but only as long as the drug is present in the form of a drug-antigen complex. The principal offender is the antiarrhythmic agent quinidine.

Drug-mediated immunological destruction of erythrocytes is usually a benign process, often incidentally recognized by a positive Coombs test. However, severe hemolysis may occur, especially in the immune complex–mediated injury of erythrocytes.

☐ **Pathology and Clinical Features:** Anemia and jaundice are prominent clinical features of warm-reacting autoimmune hemolysis. The blood smear shows a characteristic mixture of normal erythrocytes, large bluish polychromatic forms, and small, intensely stained spherocytes. The haptoglobin level is decreased, LDH is increased, and, most importantly, the Coombs test is positive. Immune suppressive agents and splenectomy are effective in the treatment of warm-reacting autoimmune hemolytic anemia, but the prognosis generally reflects the underlying disorder.

ERYTHROBLASTOSIS FETALIS: This immune disorder is another example of hemolytic anemia induced by warm-reacting antibodies (Fig. 20-30). Also termed *autoimmune hemolytic disease of the newborn,* erythroblastosis fetalis is usually caused by immunization of an Rh-negative mother by the erythrocytes of an Rh-positive fetus (see Chapter 6). In contrast to the autoantibodies of autoimmune hemolytic anemia, those seen in hemolytic disease of the newborn (and also hemolytic transfusion reactions) are alloantibodies.

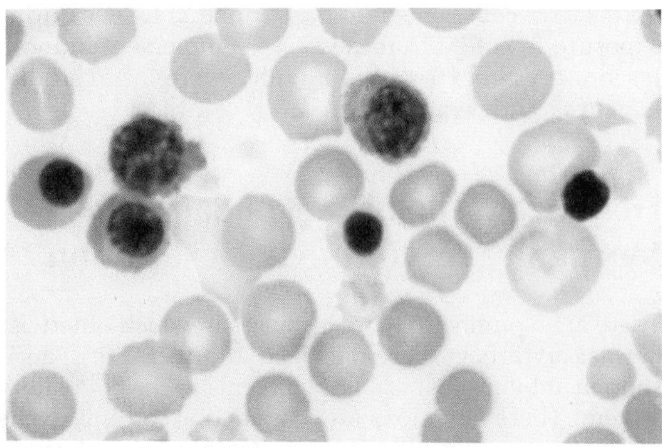

FIGURE *20-30*
Erythroblastosis fetalis. The peripheral blood contains numerous erythroid precursors normally confined to the bone marrow.

Cold-Reacting Autoantibodies

Cold-reacting autoantibodies account for 20% of cases of autoimmune hemolytic anemia. These antibodies are usually of the IgM type, with specificity for the I antigen present on most adult erythrocytes. When blood is cooled in the extremities, IgM autoantibodies fix complement C3 to the erythrocyte membrane. However, at warmer body temperatures, the antibodies dissociate from the erythrocyte membrane, leaving the erythrocyte coated only by complement. Since Kupffer cells have more receptors for complement than do splenic macrophages, the final erythrocyte destruction is hepatic rather than splenic.

Hemolytic anemia caused by cold-reacting autoantibodies occurs as an idiopathic chronic disorder in the elderly. Many of these patients eventually develop a malignant lymphoma. It also occurs in younger persons with mycoplasmal pneumonia or infectious mononucleosis.

The hemolytic anemia tends to be mild. The blood smear shows polychromasia and spherocytes, but not as pronounced as in the warm-reacting antibody type. Cold agglutinins and autoagglutination on the blood smear can be readily demonstrated. The disease can be prolonged and difficult to manage, since immunosuppressive agents or splenectomy are rarely effective.

PAROXYSMAL COLD HEMOGLOBINURIA: This form of hemolytic anemia is now rare. It is caused by the production of an IgG antibody (Donath-Landsteiner antibody) that has anti-P blood group specificity. Historically, the disorder was associated with syphilis, but today it usually follows a viral infection. The cold-reacting IgG antibody fixes complement in the peripheral tissues during exposure to cold. On rewarming, complement-induced lysis of erythrocytes occurs, with severe intravascular hemolysis and hemoglobinuria.

Hemolytic Anemia Secondary to Mechanical Erythrocyte Destruction

There are a number of circumstances in which otherwise normal erythrocytes are damaged and their life span is shortened by mechanical impediments in the circulatory system. These situations are classified according to the mechanism by which the erythrocytes are traumatized.

MACROANGIOPATHIC HEMOLYSIS: Circulating erythrocytes are vulnerable to shear forces exerted by intravascular prostheses in the heart and major arteries, particularly artificial heart valves. In such circumstances, erythrocyte fragmentation results in a macroangiopathic hemolytic anemia, characterized by the presence of many schistocytes (remnants of fragmented erythrocytes containing several spicules) on the blood smear.

MICROANGIOPATHIC HEMOLYSIS: Microangiopathic hemolytic anemia, which presents a similar morphological picture (Fig. 20-31), is caused by the fragmentation of erythrocytes by fibrin strands in partially obstructed small peripheral blood vessels. Disseminated intravascular coagulation (DIC; see later) is a frequent cause and is associated with a consumptive deficiency in platelets and coagulation factors. Thrombotic thrombocytopenic purpura (TTP) also leads to microangiopathic hemolysis, but this disorder is associated only with the consumption of platelets, whereas the concentration of coagulation factors remains normal.

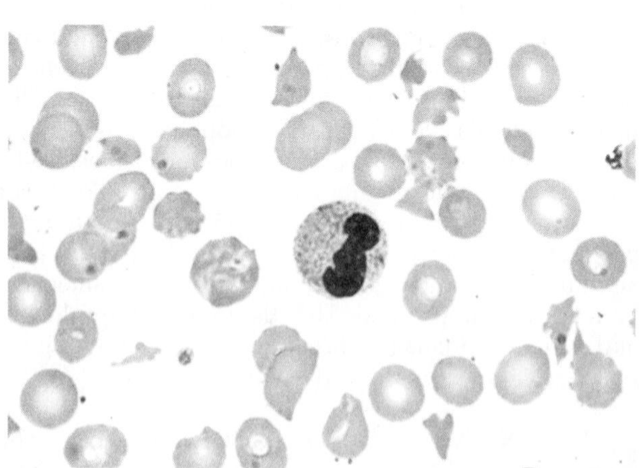

FIGURE *20-31*
Microangiopathic hemolytic anemia. Irregular, fragmented erythrocytes (schistocytes) are seen in the blood smear of a patient with disseminated intravascular coagulation.

MARCH HEMOGLOBINURIA: Erythrocytes are also vulnerable to mechanical impacts caused by external pressure. Vigorous exercise, particularly walking or running long distances in poorly fitting footwear, causes traumatic disruption of erythrocytes, with hemoglobinemia and hemoglobinuria. Athletes who engage in prolonged vigorous exercise but who are not exposed to external impacts, such as swimmers or bicycle competitors, may also develop hemoglobinuria.

HYPERSPLENISM: Hemolytic anemia associated with leukopenia and thrombocytopenia occurs in many patients with an enlarged spleen. This is especially true with congestive splenomegaly, as occurs in cirrhosis and (less prominently) when the spleen is infiltrated by leukemic cells. An enlarged spleen causes pooling and sequestration of all cellular elements. The erythrocytes, which depend critically on active intermediary metabolism to maintain their shape and viability, are especially vulnerable to stasis and are therefore lysed in the congested splenic cords. The resulting anemia stimulates compensatory erythroid hyperplasia in the bone marrow.

Blood Loss Anemia

The clinical manifestations of acute blood loss primarily reflect volume depletion and decreased perfusion pressure. During uncontrolled bleeding, the hemoglobin concentration actually remains normal for several hours, until a fluid shift from the interstitium to the intravascular compartment dilutes the remaining erythrocytes. This effect is gradual, and it may be 24 to 48 hours before the decrease in hemoglobin concentration accurately reflects the extent of the blood loss. If the bleeding is controlled, the erythrocyte mass and blood volume are restored to normal only slowly, since the rate of erythrocyte production cannot increase more than 6 to 10 times.

Chronic blood loss causes a loss of iron, but significant anemia occurs only after the body iron stores are depleted. Since inadequate intake or absorption of iron in otherwise healthy adults rarely causes anemia, a low ferritin level should always raise the suspicion of a blood loss anemia. In women of reproductive age, menstruation and frequent childbirth are the most likely causes of blood loss anemia. Nevertheless, in all patients with iron deficiency anemia, gastrointestinal and urogenital blood loss should be ruled out by testing the stool for blood and the urine for erythrocytes or hemosiderin.

ERYTHROCYTOSIS (POLYCYTHEMIA)

Erythrocytosis, usually but not accurately termed polycythemia, encompasses a number of conditions characterized by an increased hematocrit. In men, this value is higher than 54% and in women it is greater than 47%. The hematocrit reflects the total erythrocyte mass more accurately than other erythrocyte indices. At hematocrits above 50%, the viscosity of the blood increases exponentially, thereby interfering with cardiac output and peripheral blood flow. The concomitant increase in blood volume and oxygen-carrying capacity of the blood maintains the oxygen supply to most tissues until the hematocrit reaches 60%. Above this level, the blood flow decreases and the tissues become hypoxic. Erythrocytosis can be classified as relative or absolute.

RELATIVE ERYTHROCYTOSIS: This condition is characterized by a normal erythrocyte mass with a decreased plasma volume. **Dehydration is the most common cause of relative erythrocytosis.** In fact, in critical care units, the hematocrit is used as a convenient measure of fluid balance.

A decrease in plasma volume, designated as *spurious* or *stress* polycythemia, is sometimes observed in middle-aged, overweight, and often mildly hypertensive persons. However, the erythrocytosis is associated not so much with stress as with excessive smoking. Tobacco smoking can cause both a carbon monoxide–induced hypoxic stimulation of erythrocyte production and a nicotine-induced diuretic depletion of plasma volume.

ABSOLUTE ERYTHROCYTOSIS: A number of disorders feature an increase in the erythrocyte mass. Absolute erythrocytosis is classified as either primary or secondary. Primary absolute erythrocytosis **(polycythemia vera)** is a clonal stem cell disorder, in which all progenitor cells continuously proliferate in the absence of growth-stimulating factors (see myeloproliferative syndromes below).

In secondary absolute erythrocytosis, the proliferation of progenitor cells is due to increased erythropoietin. The production of erythropoietin can be elevated appropriately as a response to tissue hypoxia or inappropriately in the case of abnormal renal or extrarenal synthesis.

Appropriate secondary erythrocytosis is induced by arterial hypoxia under the following conditions:

- High altitude with low ambient PO_2
- Pulmonary disease with impaired gas exchange
- Cardiac anomalies with a right-to-left shunt
- Hemoglobinopathies with increased oxygen affinity of the abnormal hemoglobin

In all of the above situations, the resulting renal tissue hypoxia causes the release of erythropoietin and, in turn, an increased rate of erythrocyte production.

Inappropriate secondary erythrocytosis reflects the secretion of erythropoietin in the absence of generalized tissue hypoxia. Renal lesions such as cysts or hydronephrosis may produce localized renal hypoxia by a pressure effect, which in turn enhances erythropoietin production. Paraneoplastic erythrocytosis occurs in association with a variety of tumors that produce erythropoietin. Such neoplasms include renal cell carcinoma, cerebellar hemangioblastoma, primary hepatocellular carcinoma, and even uterine leiomyoma. In inappropriate secondary erythrocytosis, correction of the renal abnormality or excision of the primary tumor generally results in a prompt return of the erythrocyte mass to normal levels.

QUANTITATIVE DISORDERS OF NEUTROPHILS

Neutropenia

The term neutropenia or granulocytopenia refers to an absolute neutrophil count less than 1800/μL. However, even at this level, there is an adequate number of granulocytes to defend against microorganisms. When the absolute number of neutrophils declines to 1000/μL, the patient becomes vulnerable to microbial infections, but a serious risk is usually first experienced with absolute counts of less than 500/μL (severe granulocytopenia). The term *agranulocytosis* is reserved for severe granulocytopenias, in which both the marginated pool and the bone marrow reserve have been depleted.

Neutropenia is caused by decreased or ineffective production or by increased destruction of neutrophils (Table 20-7). Most cases of neutropenia are asymptomatic and unexplained, and the term *chronic benign neutropenia* is used. It appears that at least in some cases the total granulocyte pool is normal, but an excessive number of neutrophils are stored in the marrow or marginated in blood vessels.

DECREASED PRODUCTION OF NEUTROPHILS: Impaired formation of neutrophils is observed after exposure to radiation or to chemotherapeutic drugs and is part of an *expected* general suppression of cellular proliferation in the marrow. Certain drugs, such as phenothiazine, phenylbutazone, antithyroid drugs, and indomethacin, can cause an *idiosyncratic* suppression of the bone marrow. Viral infection and alcohol intake have also been associated with suppression of myelopoiesis. A decreased production of granulocytes is a feature of a number of hereditary disorders, including Kostmann

TABLE *20-7* **Principal Causes of Neutropenia**

Decreased production
Irradiation
Drug-induced (acute, chronic)
Viral infections
Congenital
Cyclic
Ineffective production
Megaloblastic anemia
Myelodysplastic syndromes
Increased destruction
Isoimmune neonatal
Autoimmune
Idiopathic
Drug-induced
Felty syndrome
Systemic lupus erythematosus
Dialysis (complement activation–induced)
Splenic sequestration
Increased margination

syndrome and infantile genetic agranulocytosis. Ineffective myelopoiesis appears to be involved in the neutropenia observed in megaloblastic anemias and myelodysplasias. In cyclic neutropenia, episodes regularly recur every 21 days.

INCREASED PERIPHERAL DESTRUCTION OF GRANULOCYTES: An acceleration of elimination of granulocytes is caused by the following:

- Increased consumption in overwhelming infections
- Increased sequestration in hypersplenism
- Increased destruction by antibodies

Neutropenia is a common feature in AIDS, and its etiology is multifactorial. Virus-induced depression of neutrophil production is aggravated by infectious consumption of neutrophils and often by drug-related mechanisms (e.g., by zidovudine).

A second type of drug-induced neutropenia is immunologically mediated. Many drugs may lead to this form of neutrophil destruction, especially sulfonamides, phenylbutazone, and indomethacin. The toxic effect seems to result from the attachment of circulating antigen–antibody complexes to the granulocyte surface, with subsequent complement-mediated injury.

Neutrophilia

Neutrophilia is defined as an increase in the absolute peripheral blood neutrophil count to more than 7000/μL. It has many causes (Table 20-8) and reflects (1) an increased mobilization of neutrophils from the bone marrow storage pool, (2) enhanced release from the peripheral blood marginal pool, or (3) stimulation of granulopoiesis in the bone marrow. Increased mobilization of neutrophils from the bone marrow storage pool or from the peripheral blood marginal pool occurs in acute traumatic or infectious disorders. A mild neutrophilia occurs in 20% of women during the third trimester of pregnancy, but the mechanism is poorly defined.

TABLE *20-8* Principal Causes of Neutrophilia

Infections
Primarily bacterial
Immunological inflammatory
Rheumatoid arthritis
Rheumatic fever
Vasculitis
Neoplasia
Hemorrhage
Drugs
Glucocorticoids
Colony stimulating factors (CSFs)
Lithium
Hereditary
CD18 deficiency
Metabolic
Acidosis
Uremia
Gout
Thyroid storm
Tissue necrosis
Infarction
Trauma
Burns

LEUKEMOID REACTION: In acute infections, neutrophilia may be so pronounced that it may be mistaken for leukemia, especially chronic myeloid leukemia, in which case it is termed a leukemoid reaction. Clues to the benign (or reactive) nature of a leukemoid reaction include the following: (1) the cells in the peripheral blood are usually more mature than myelocytes; (2) leukocyte alkaline phosphatase activity is high in a leukemoid reaction, but low in chronic myeloid leukemia; and (3) benign neutrophils often contain large blue cytoplasmic inclusions (Döhle bodies) or toxic granulation (Fig. 20-32).

QUALITATIVE DISORDERS OF NEUTROPHILS

If the functional competence of granulocytes is impaired, a decreased resistance to infection may occur despite a normal granulocyte count. A number of rare hereditary disorders of the chemotactic, migratory, phagocytic, and bactericidal functions of granulocytes have been described.

CHRONIC GRANULOMATOUS DISEASE: *Chronic granulomatous disease (CGD) refers to a group of rare, inherited, X-linked or autosomal recessive disorders characterized by a defect in bactericidal function of phagocytic cells, including neutrophils and macrophages.* All forms of CGD reflect the inability of these cells to undergo a respiratory burst and generate hydrogen peroxide on phagocytosis of microorganisms. The basic defect in the X-linked variant is a deficiency of the membrane-bound cytochrome b moiety of NADPH oxidase. In autosomal recessive CGD, a cytosolic factor necessary for the activation of NADPH oxidase is lacking.

In CGD, neutrophils and macrophages are capable of phagocytosis of microorganisms. However, they cannot kill catalase-positive microorganisms (e.g., *Staphylococcus aureus, Serratia marcescens, Salmonella* species), which are protected from their own endogenous hydrogen peroxide by catalase. The deficiency of NADPH oxidase activity impairs the generation of hydrogen peroxide by the inflammatory cell and the consequent hypochlorous acid-induced killing of the microorganisms mediated by myeloperoxidase. Catalase-negative microorganisms, such as *Lactobacillus*, are killed in a normal fashion. CGD becomes symptomatic at any age from infancy to adulthood, and recurrent infections lead to widespread microabscesses and granulomas. The neutrophils are morphologically normal in CGD. The diagnosis is made by measuring respiratory burst activity in the nitroblue tetrazolium (NBT) test.

MYELOPEROXIDASE DEFICIENCY: This is an inherited autosomal recessive disorder characterized by

NEUTROPHILS

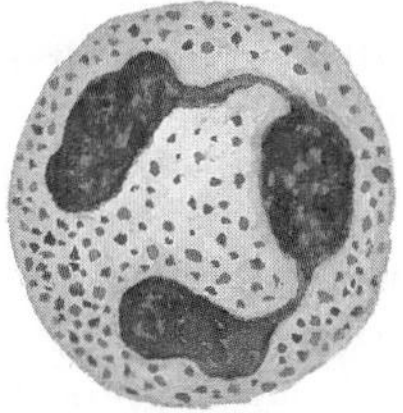

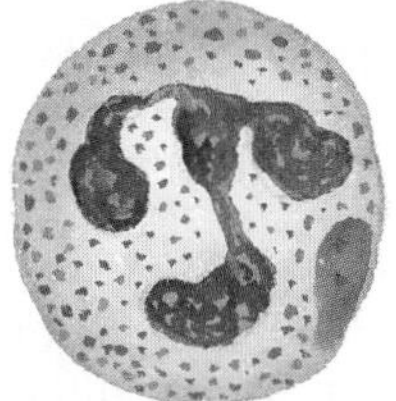

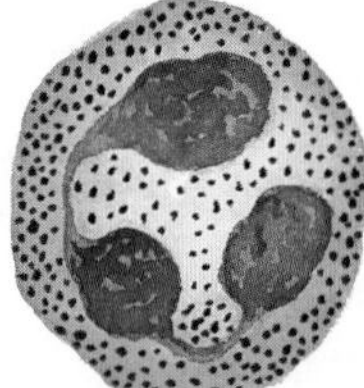

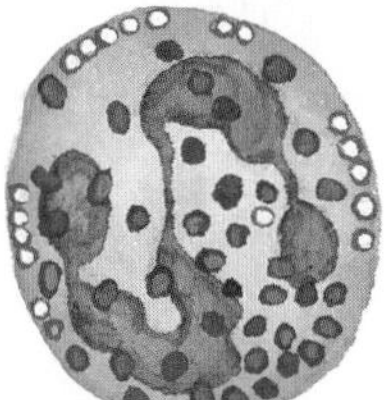

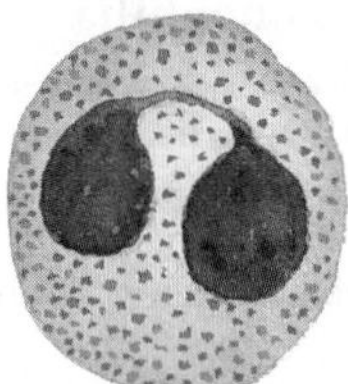

LYMPHOCYTES

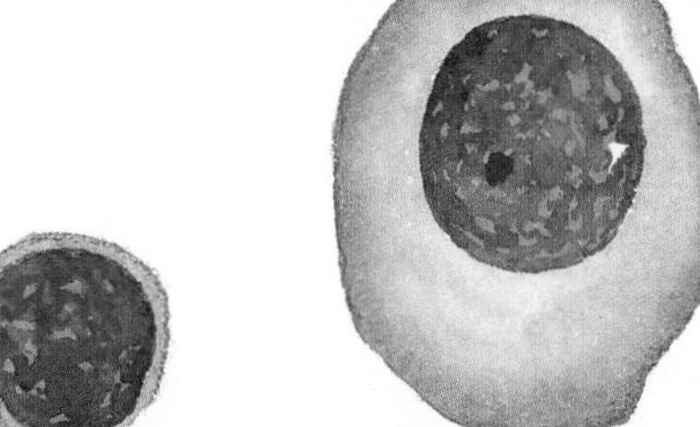

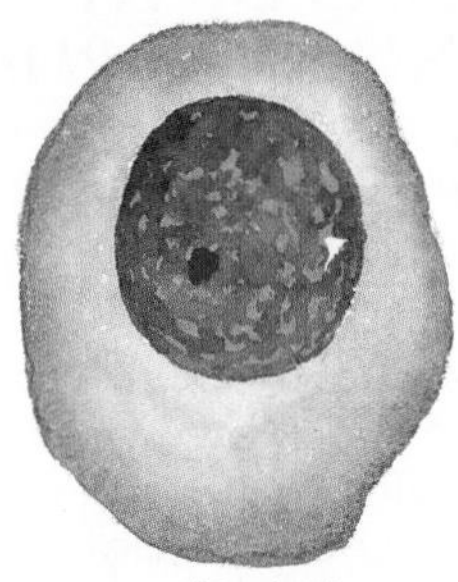

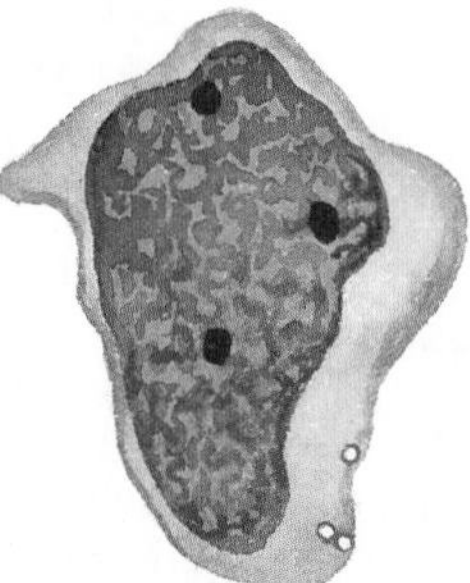

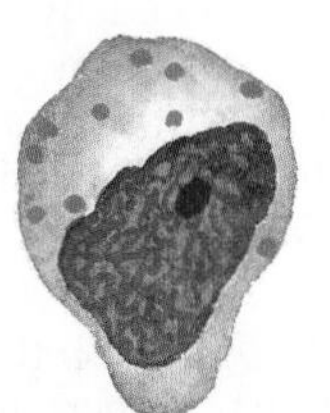

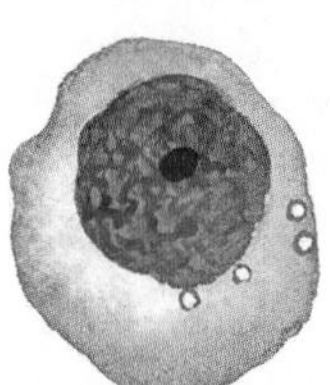

FIGURE *20-32*
Abnormal leukocyte morphology. Abnormal neutrophils and lymphocytes are contrasted with normal cells. Döhle bodies are blue cytoplasmic inclusions that represent ribosome-associated endoplasmic reticulum. In toxic granulation, there is prominent blue-black granulation in the cytoplasm. This represents persistence of prominent primary or azurophilic granules. Both Döhle bodies and toxic granulation are characteristic of benign or reactive processes. In the storage diseases or mucopolysaccharidoses, large, blocklike cytoplasmic inclusions are seen. The Pelger-Huet anomaly consists of nuclear hyposegmentation, frequently with bilobed nuclei, and dense chromatin. Atypical lymphocytes are large, with deep blue to pale gray cytoplasm; they are seen in benign reactive processes. Large granular lymphocytes are medium to large lymphoid cells with some pink cytoplasmic granules. They are suppressor T lymphocytes, some with natural killer function, and may be increased in benign or malignant disorders. Plasmacytoid lymphocytes have abundant blue cytoplasm and are seen in some reactive disorders.

lack of neutrophilic lysosomal myeloperoxidase. Bacterial infections are rarely observed, however, because there is a compensatory increase in intracellular hydrogen peroxide. Candidal infections are a significant problem in diabetic patients with this deficiency.

CHÉDIAK-HIGASHI SYNDROME: This disorder is a rare autosomal recessive condition characterized by abnormal, giant lysosomes in leukocytes and numerous cells in other tissues. In neutrophils, monocytes, and lymphocytes, the defect is manifested morphologically by the presence of huge cytoplasmic granules and functionally by neutropenia, decreased chemotaxis, impaired degranulation, and ineffective bactericidal activity. The disorder is attributed to a generalized increase in the fusion of cytoplasmic granules (lysosomes).

Clinically, patients with Chédiak-Higashi syndrome suffer recurrent **bacterial and fungal infections**, involving principally the skin, mucous membranes, and respiratory tract. Defective platelet aggregation is reflected in **prolonged bleeding times**. **Oculocutaneous albinism** (see Chapter 6) is related to the segregation of melanin in giant melanosomes. The disease may progress to a fatal *accelerated phase,* in which a lymphoproliferative syndrome leads to pancytopenia. This lymphoproliferative disease is likely a consequence of Ebstein-Barr virus infection. In a few patients, bone marrow transplantation has apparently cured Chédiak-Higashi syndrome.

EOSINOPHILIA

Eosinophils differentiate in the bone marrow under the influence of one or several eosinophil growth factors (e.g., IL-5). They circulate briefly in the peripheral blood and then migrate preferentially to the gastrointestinal and res-

TABLE 20-9 **Principal Causes of Eosinophilia**

Allergic disorders
Skin diseases
Parasitic (helminth) infestations
Malignant neoplasms
Hemopoietic
Solid tumors
Collagen vascular disorders
Miscellaneous
Hypereosinophilic syndromes
Eosinophilia-myalgia syndrome
IL-2 therapy

piratory tracts and to the skin. Eosinophils respond to chemotactic substances produced by mast cells or induced by the presence of persistent antigen–antibody complexes, such as occur in chronic parasitic, dermatological, and allergic conditions. The principal causes of eosinophilia are listed in Table 20-9.

IDIOPATHIC HYPEREOSINOPHILIC SYNDROME: *This term refers to heterogeneous disorders in which circulating eosinophils are increased above 1500/μL for more than 6 months and in which no underlying disease is evident.* The accumulation of eosinophils in tissue often leads to necrosis, particularly in the myocardium, where it leads to endomyocardial disease (see Chapter 11). Neurological dysfunction may also develop. The eosinophil-mediated cell injury is thought to be related to the cytotoxicity of the constituents of the eosinophil granules, particularly major basic protein and cationic protein (see Chapter 2). The prognosis of untreated idiopathic hypereosinophilic syndrome is serious, and only about 10% of patients survive for 3 years. Aggressive therapy with corticosteroids has markedly improved this situation; even in cases with cardiac involvement, 70% survive for more than 5 years.

TABLE 20-10 **Principal Causes of Basophilia**

Allergic (drug, food)
Inflammation
Juvenile rheumatoid arthritis
Ulcerative colitis
Infection
Viral (chickenpox, influenza)
Tuberculosis
Neoplasia
Myeloproliferative syndromes
Basophilic leukemia
Carcinoma
Endocrine
Diabetes mellitus
Myxedema
Estrogen administration

BASOPHILIA

The basophil is the least numerous of all leukocytes. It differentiates in the bone marrow, circulates briefly in the peripheral blood, and then passes to the tissues, where its fate is uncertain. Its relationship to mast cells is controversial. Basophil granules contain a number of preformed mediators of the inflammatory response, including histamine and chondroitin sulfate. Basophils also synthesize leukotriene and other mediators upon stimulation. The principal causes of basophilia are listed in Table 20-10. Basophilia is most commonly observed in immediate-type hypersensitivity reactions and in the chronic myeloproliferative syndromes.

DISORDERS OF THE MONONUCLEAR PHAGOCYTE SYSTEM

Monocytosis

Monocytosis is defined as a peripheral blood monocyte count greater than 800/μL. The principal causes of monocytosis include hematological disorders, immunological and inflammatory conditions, infectious diseases, and nonhemopoietic cancers. Hematological disorders account for at least half of the peripheral blood monocytoses. For example, monocytes may constitute a component of acute or chronic myelogenous leukemia. In such cases, they may be either morphologically normal or they may exhibit immature and dyspoietic cytological features. Monocytosis often occurs in neutropenic states, probably as a compensatory mechanism. Peripheral blood monocytosis may also accompany malignant lymphomas and Hodgkin's disease.

Sinus Histiocytosis

Sinus histiocytosis refers to an increase in tissue macrophages (histiocytes) of the subcapsular and trabecular sinuses of the lymph nodes (Fig. 20-33). The sinus histiocytes are derived from the sinus lining cells, which in turn originate from blood monocytes. Sinus histiocytes have eccentric, round to oval, indented nuclei, with delicate chromatin, punctate nucleoli, and abundant pink cytoplasm. Free macrophages as well as multinucleated giant cells may be observed in the expanded sinuses.

Sinus histiocytosis is a common finding in lymph nodes draining sites of cancer and, less commonly, inflammatory and infectious foci. The character of the phagocytic debris in the cytoplasm of the macrophages helps identify the origin of the sinus histiocytosis. For example, anthracotic pigment is frequently seen in the macrophages of mediastinal lymph nodes that exhibit sinus histocytosis. Macrophages containing erythrocytes and hemosiderin pigment occur with autoimmune hemolytic anemia. Radiopaque contrast material is observed in the macrophages of enlarged pelvic and abdominal lymph nodes after lymphangiographic staging of malignant lymphomas and Hodgkin's disease.

Sinus Histiocytosis with Massive Lymphadenopathy

Sinus histiocytosis with massive lymphadenopathy (SHML), also known as ***Rosai-Dorfman disease,*** *is a rare, self-limited disorder of unknown etiology characterized by striking bilateral, painless, cervical lymphadenopathy.* Other peripheral and central lymph node groups may also be involved, and in over a fourth of the cases extranodal soft tissue sites are affected. SHML occurs most commonly in blacks in the first two decades of life, although it may be encountered at any age. Males and females are equally susceptible.

☐ **Pathology:** On gross examination, the involved lymph nodes are enlarged and orange-brown. Characteristic histopathological features include (1) capsular and pericapsular fibrosis and chronic inflammation; (2) marked sinus histiocytosis, with dilatation of the subcapsular and trabecular sinuses and variable distortion of the lymph node architecture; and (3) prominent plasmacytosis of the intersinusoidal stroma. The sinus histiocytes have large, oval or indented, vesicular nuclei, with one to several small nucleoli. The abundant cytoplasm is pink and occasionally vacuolated. Numerous lymphocytes, and less commonly erythrocytes and plasma cells, are typically seen in the cytoplasm of the sinus histiocytes (see Fig. 20-33). This phenomenon may reflect phagocytosis but may also represent active penetration of the cytoplasm of sinus histiocytes by these cells (emperipolesis). The sinus histiocytes of SHML exhibit the usual immunological and cytochemical cell markers of mononuclear phagocytes. Additionally, they demonstrate strong immunohistochemical reactivity for S-100 protein.

Common accompanying clinical signs of inflammation include fever, an elevated erythrocyte sedimentation rate, neutrophilic leukocytosis, and polyclonal hypergammaglobulinemia. The clinical course is benign, with spontaneous resolution in months to years. There is no effective therapy.

Dermatopathic Lymphadenopathy

Dermatopathic lymphadenopathy refers to specific reactive changes in lymph nodes that are secondary to a variety of chronic dermatoses. This reaction is due to the drainage of lipid, melanin, and hemosiderin from the affected skin to the regional lymph nodes. Additionally, there is an immunological reaction in the lymph nodes to antigenic ma-

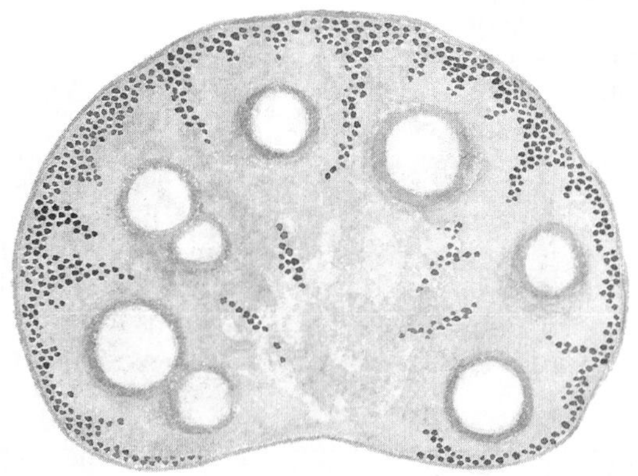

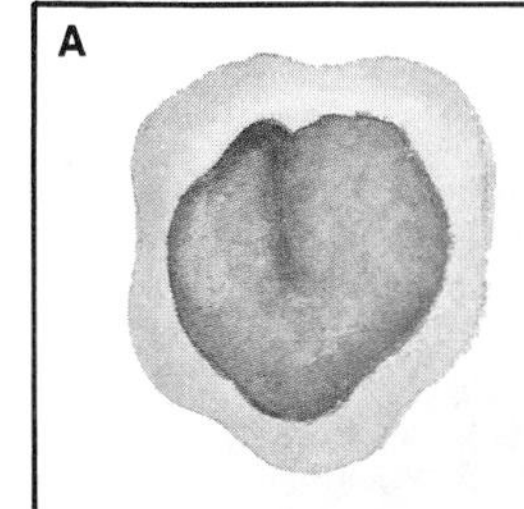

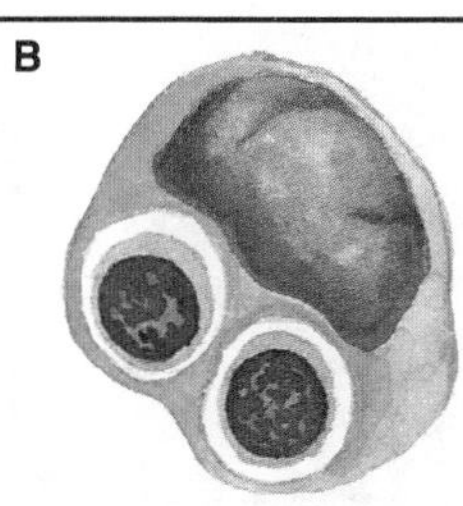

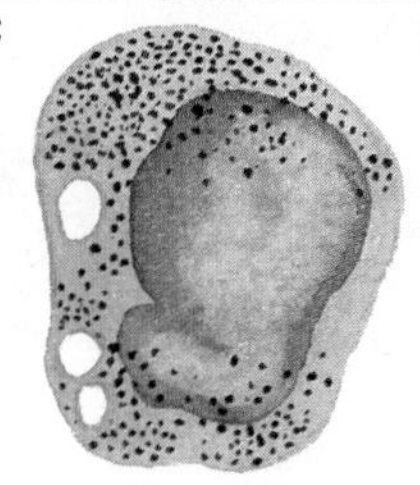

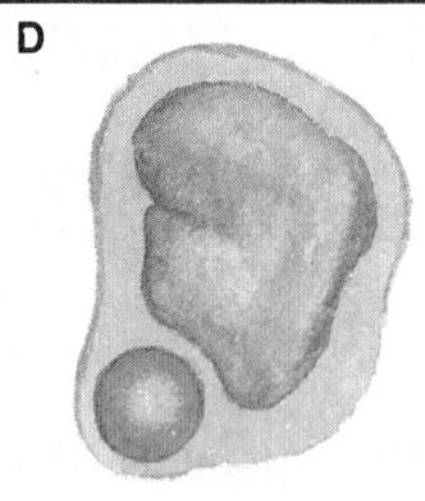

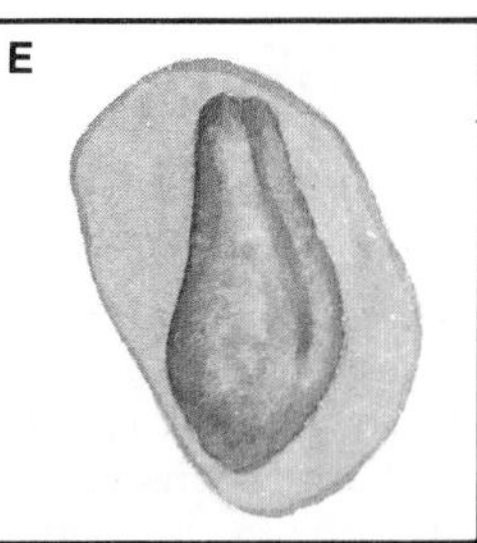

FIGURE *20-33*
Mononuclear phagocyte system: benign disorders. In the lymph nodes, benign proliferations of mononuclear phagocytes first involve the nodal sinuses (blue dots in lymph node cross-section) but may subsequently extend to involve the nodal stroma. (*A*) In benign sinus histiocytosis, the nodal sinuses are expanded by bland histiocytes or phagocytic macrophages. (*B*) In sinus histiocytosis with massive lymphadenopathy, the macrophages contain lymphocytes in cytoplasmic vacuoles. (*C*) In dermatopathic lymphadenopathy, the macrophages contain cytoplasmic lipid and melanin pigment. (*D*) In infection-induced hemophagocytic reticulosis, the macrophages contain phagocytosed red cells. (*E*) In the differentiated histiocytoses, the cells are bland, and a deep nuclear crease or fold is characteristic.

terial draining from the skin. The cutaneous drainage products in dermatopathic lymphadenopathy accumulate principally in macrophages of the paracortical region of the lymph nodes. The paracortex is expanded by a heterogeneous cell population, which consists principally of macrophages whose cytoplasm contains lipid or granular, brown, melanin pigment (see Fig. 20-33). There are increased Langerhans cells and interdigitating reticulum cells with delicate chromatin and folded nuclei. The paracortex also contains lymphocytes and some eosinophils, plasma cells, and immunoblasts. On low-power microscopy of the lymph node, the heterogeneous cell population imparts a characteristic mottled appearance to the paracortex.

Infection-Induced Hemophagocytic Syndrome

Infection-induced hemophagocytic syndrome is a rare disorder characterized by a generalized activation of tissue macrophages in immunosuppressed or immunodeficient persons. It occurs in a variety of viral, bacterial, fungal, and parasitic infections and rarely in some T-cell lymphomas. The common pathophysiological mechanism may be lymphokine-induced activation of benign tissue macrophages.

The principal histopathological feature of infection-induced hemophagocytic syndrome is a generalized hyperplasia of tissue macrophages in the splenic red pulp, hepatic sinusoids, lymph node sinuses, and the bone marrow. The macrophages exhibit active phagocytosis, principally of erythrocytes (see Fig. 20-33) but also of neutrophils and platelets.

Infection-induced hemophagocytic reticulosis is characterized by the acute onset of fever, hepatosplenomegaly, lymphadenopathy, rash, pulmonary infiltration, and pancytopenia. The disorder is generally self-limited but rarely may be fatal.

LANGERHANS CELL HISTIOCYTOSIS

Langerhans cell histiocytosis (LCH) refers to a spectrum of uncommon proliferative disorders of Langerhans cells. The disease ranges from an asymptomatic involvement of a single site, such as bone or lymph nodes, to an aggressive systemic disorder that involves multiple organs.

Langerhans cells are a component of the mononuclear phagocyte system derived from precursor cells in the bone marrow. They are found in the epidermis and in other sites such as the lymph nodes, spleen, thymus, and mucosal tissues. Langerhans cells ingest, process, and present antigens to T lymphocytes.

The etiology and pathogenesis of LCH are unknown. It has been thought that the disease may represent an atypical immunological reaction or an unusual manifestation of an autoimmune disorder. However, the recent demonstration of clonal proliferation of Langerhans cells in all forms of LCH suggests the possibility of a neoplastic disorder. In turn, the production of cytokines by neoplastic Langerhans cells may account for the polymorphous appearance of the lesions of LCH. Infants, children, and young adults are most commonly affected. The extent of the disease and the rate of progression correlate inversely with the age at presentation. Certain eponyms were traditionally attached to the various presentations of LCH.

- **Eosinophilic granuloma** is the term used for the localized, usually self-limited disorder of older children (5 to 10 years old) and young adults (younger than the age of 30 years). It accounts for up to 75% of all cases of LCH and afflicts males four times as frequently as females. The bones (Fig. 20-34) and the lungs are the principal organs affected.
- **Hand-Schüller-Christian disease** is a multifocal and typically indolent disorder, usually in children between 2 and 5 years of age, which represents about one fourth of all cases of LCH. Boys and girls are affected equally. Bony lesions tend to predominate, although involvement of endocrine glands may be prominent.
- **Letterer-Siwe disease** refers to the rare (less than 10% of cases) acute disseminated variant of LCH in infants and children younger than 2 years of age. There is no sex predominance. Skin lesions and involvement of visceral organs and the hemopoietic system are characteristic (Fig. 20-35).

☐ **Pathology:** Despite the clinical heterogeneity of the Langerhans cell histiocytoses, there are common histopathological findings. The Langerhans cells that accumulate in this disorder are large (15 to 25 μm in diameter), with round to indented nuclei, delicate vesicular chromatin, and small nucleoli. Marked nuclear folds and prominent grooves or creases (see Fig. 20-33) are cytological features lacking in other disorders of mononuclear phagocytes. The abundant cytoplasm is pink to red and in chronic disease may contain lipid vacuoles. Binucleated or multinucleated cells with similar nuclear and cytoplasmic features may be identified.

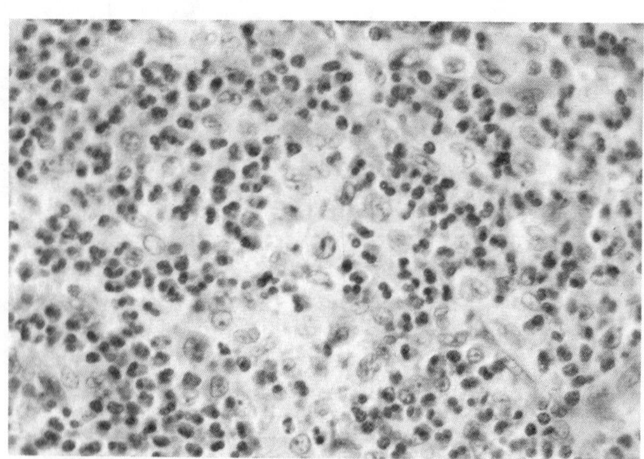

FIGURE *20-34*
Eosinophilic granuloma. A section of an affected rib shows proliferated Langerhans cells and numerous eosinophils.

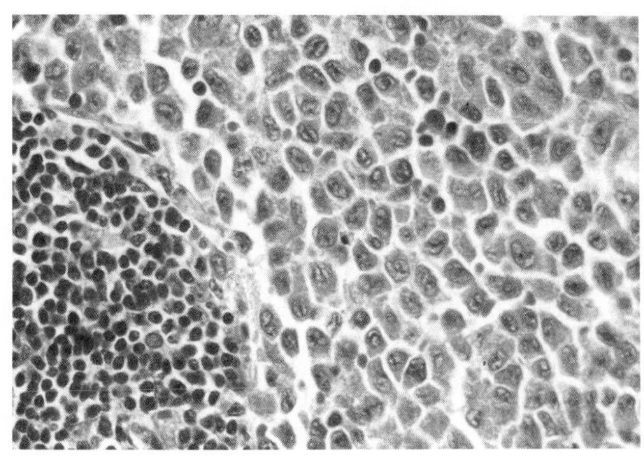

FIGURE 20-35
Letterer-Siwe disease. A section of the spleen illustrates sheets of proliferated Langerhans cells.

By electron microscopy, a distinctive cytoplasmic inclusion, the *Birbeck granule*, is commonly observed in the Langerhans cells. This inclusion is rod shaped or tubular, with a dense core and a double outer sheath. Frequently, one end is bulbous, in which case the granule resembles a tennis racket. Characteristic immunological cell markers identical to those of epidermal Langerhans cells include S-100 protein and CD1.

The infiltrating Langerhans cells are accompanied by variable numbers of inflammatory cells, principally eosinophils, and less commonly plasma cells and neutrophils. Foci of necrosis with surrounding eosinophils are called eosinophilic microabscesses. There are characteristic histopathological patterns of histiocytic infiltration in different organs.

- **The skin** initially shows involvement of the superficial papillary dermis. Invasion of the epidermis by Langerhans cells leads to secondary ulceration.
- **The lymph nodes** first exhibit involvement of the sinuses, although subsequent infiltration of the stroma is common.
- **The spleen** is infiltrated by Langerhans cells, predominantly in the red pulp.
- **The liver** displays Langerhans cells in the sinusoids.
- **The lungs** initially show infiltration in the alveolar septa and in peribronchial and perivascular areas.
- **The bone marrow** is infiltrated in the hemopoietic stroma.

☐ **Clinical Features:** The clinical manifestations of LCH reflect the sites of tissue involvement. Skin involvement, principally in the Letterer-Siwe variant, takes the form of seborrheic or eczematoid dermatitis, most prominently on the scalp, face, and trunk. Otitis media is a common finding. Painless localized or generalized lymphadenopathy and hepatosplenomegaly are frequent. Lytic lesions of bone cause pain or tenderness to palpation. Proptosis (protrusion of the eyeball) may be a complication of infiltration of the orbit. Diabetes insipidus occurs when the hypothalamic pituitary axis is affected. **The classic triad of diabetes insipidus, proptosis, and defects in membranous bones occurs in only 15% of cases of Hand-Schüller-Christian disease.**

The prognosis in LCH depends principally on the age at presentation, the extent of disease, and the rate of progression. In general, the disorder is self-limited and benign in older persons (eosinophilic granuloma), whereas children younger than the age of 2 years (Letterer-Siwe disease) tend to do poorly. Rarely, the clinical course is aggressive and indistinguishable from that of a malignant neoplasm.

PROLIFERATIVE DISORDERS OF MAST CELLS

Mast cells are thought to derive from precursor cells in the bone marrow and are found in the connective tissues, usually in close proximity to blood vessels. In sections stained with hematoxylin and eosin, mast cells are indistinguishable from fibroblasts or tissue macrophages. They are elongate or spindle shaped but may be polygonal or stellate. The nucleus is centrally situated, round to elongate, and frequently indented. The cytoplasm is pale pink and finely granular. With Giemsa or metachromatic stains, such as toluidine blue, mast cell granules are basophilic (blue-purple). The chloroacetate esterase (CAE) reaction stains the granules red.

Mast cell granules contain inflammatory mediators, such as histamine, heparin, eosinophil and neutrophil chemotactic factors, and certain proteases. The symptoms of mast cell proliferative diseases, including flushing, pruritus, hives, headaches, and vomiting, are due to the release of these substances. The secretion of heparin also causes bleeding from the nasopharynx or gastrointestinal tract. The spectrum of mast cell proliferative disorders comprises a variety of benign and malignant conditions.

MAST CELL HYPERPLASIA (REACTIVE MASTOCYTOSIS): This process occurs in immediate- and delayed-type hypersensitivity reactions and in lymph nodes that drain the sites of malignant tumors. It is also observed in Waldenström macroglobulinemia, in the bone marrow in women with postmenopausal osteoporosis, in myelodysplastic syndromes, and after chemotherapy for leukemia.

LOCALIZED MASTOCYTOSIS (MASTOCYTOMA): This lesion presents either as a single, tan-brown, cutaneous nodule in newborns or as several groups of skin nodules in young children. Microscopically, a diffuse dermal infiltrate of mast cells is noted. The disorder resolves spontaneously, and secondary extracutaneous involvement is rare.

URTICARIA PIGMENTOSA: This entity presents as multiple, symmetrically distributed, tan-brown, cutaneous macules or papules, most commonly in infants and young children. The skin of the trunk is predominantly affected, but any cutaneous site may be involved. Microscopically, a diffuse dermal infiltrate of mast cells is observed. Spontaneous resolution usually occurs at puberty, and systemic involvement is unusual.

SYSTEMIC MASTOCYTOSIS: This rare disorder is characterized by infiltration of many organs with mast cells, including the skin, lymph nodes, spleen, liver, bones and bone marrow, and gastrointestinal tract. Systemic mastocytosis occurs at any age, but adults in the sixth and seventh decades of life are most commonly affected. Systemic mastocytosis may accompany urticaria pigmentosa. It is not clear whether the disorder is a reactive process or represents a neoplastic proliferation of mast cells.

□ **Pathology:** In systemic mastocytosis, the lymph nodes initially show perifollicular and perivascular infiltration by mast cells. The spleen exhibits nodular aggregates of mast cells, with accompanying dense fibrosis in the red pulp, particularly in relation to the fibrous trabeculae and the capsule. In the liver, the portal triads are first involved. Involvement of the bone marrow may be paratrabecular, perivascular, or diffuse (Fig. 20-36), and there is often accompanying fibrosis.

On roentgenological examination, both osteolytic and osteoblastic lesions may be identified in systemic mastocytosis. The central axial skeleton, which includes the ribs, vertebrae, pelvis, skull, and proximal long bones, is most commonly affected.

□ **Clinical Features:** Patients with systemic mastocytosis suffer symptoms related to the overproduction of a number of mediators normally produced by mast cells and basophils, including histamine, prostaglandin D_2, and thromboxane B_2. The large majority experience gastrointestinal pain and diarrhea. Anaphylactic episodes, with pruritus, flushing, and asthmatic symptoms, are common. Extensive mast cell infiltration of the bone marrow leads to secondary anemia, leukopenia, and thrombocytopenia.

Systemic mastocytosis follows a chronic, indolent course, with about half of the patients surviving for 5 years. Symptomatic relief is obtained, at least partially, with H1- and H2-receptor antagonists. There is no effective therapy for the underlying disease process.

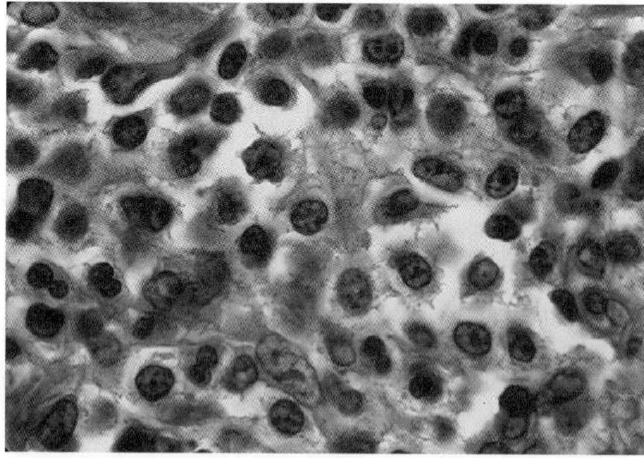

FIGURE *20-36*
Mastocytosis. A section of lymph node shows effacement of the normal architecture by sheets of mast cells. The centrally situated nuclei are round to elongated, and occasionally indented. The cytoplasm is pale pink and finely granular.

MAST CELL LEUKEMIA: This complication develops in 15% of cases of systemic mastocytosis. The circulating cells exhibit the typical cytological features of mast cells or of less differentiated variants. The leukocyte count may be markedly increased.

MAST CELL SARCOMA: This cancer is a rare malignant disorder of mast cells that is characterized by extensive infiltration of cutaneous and extracutaneous sites by anaplastic mast cell variants. The disease is rapidly progressive, and the prognosis is poor.

BENIGN DISORDERS OF LYMPHOID CELLS

Lymphocytosis

Peripheral blood lymphocytosis is defined as an increase in the absolute peripheral blood lymphocyte count above the normal range (>4000/μL in adults, 7000/μL in children, and 9000/μL in infants). The principal causes of absolute peripheral blood lymphocytosis are (1) acute infections (infectious mononucleosis, whooping cough, acute infectious lymphocytosis), (2) chronic bacterial infections (tuberculosis, brucellosis), and (3) lymphoproliferative diseases.

ATYPICAL LYMPHOCYTES: In addition to lymphocytosis, atypical lymphocytes are a hallmark of viral infections, particularly infectious mononucleosis, and some immunological disorders, such as drug reactions and serum sickness. Atypical lymphocytes are large cells with round to irregular nuclei, coarsely clumped chromatin, one to several distinct nucleoli, and abundant blue cytoplasm (Fig. 20-37). Occasionally, the cytoplasm is vacuolated. Frequently, the cytoplasmic membrane is in-

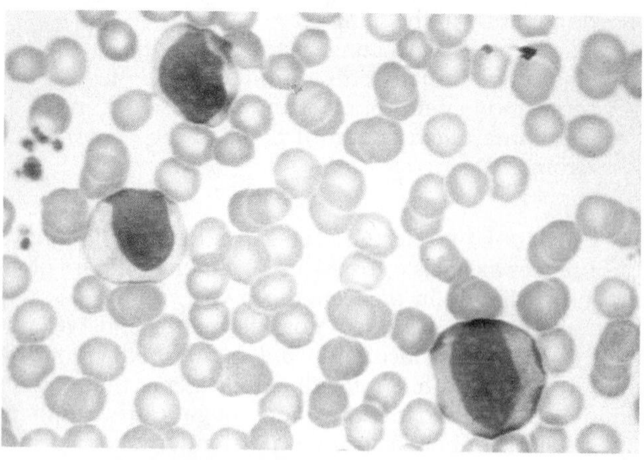

FIGURE *20-37*
Atypical lymphocytes in infectious mononucleosis.

dented by surrounding erythrocytes (ballerina-skirt phenomenon). The large majority of atypical lymphocytes are of the T-cell lineage (CD8+, cytotoxic/suppressor cells).

ACUTE INFECTIOUS LYMPHOCYTOSIS: This is a rare, self-limited, childhood disorder in which there is a marked peripheral blood lymphocytosis, principally T cells. Although lymphocytosis may persist for several weeks, affected children are usually asymptomatic. In a few cases of acute infectious lymphocytosis, mild fever, abdominal pain, and diarrhea occur. The etiology is unknown.

REACTIVE LYMPHOID HYPERPLASIA OF THE BONE MARROW: An increased number of lymphocytes in the marrow may accompany peripheral blood lymphocytosis, although either may occur alone. In normal bone marrow, lymphocytes are distributed interstitially in the hemopoietic stroma or in cohesive aggregates called lymphoid nodules. In biopsy sections of the marrow, lymphoid hyperplasia has been defined as four or more lymphoid aggregates in any low-power (4×) microscopic field or as the presence of a single aggregate that measures at least 0.6 cm in diameter. An adult with more than 20% lymphocytes in either bone marrow aspirates or biopsy sections is considered to have lymphocytosis.

Plasmacytosis

PERIPHERAL BLOOD PLASMACYTOSIS: An increase in plasma cells in the blood is uncommon. The most frequent cause is plasma cell neoplasia (multiple myeloma), usually in the terminal stages of the disease. Peripheral plasmacytosis may also be identified in some systemic immunological reactions and viral infections. On occasion, atypical lymphocytes resemble plasma cells, in which case they are called *Turk cells*.

REACTIVE BONE MARROW PLASMACYTOSIS: An increase in plasma cells in the marrow occurs in a variety of infectious, inflammatory, and neoplastic disorders. For example, it accompanies infections as diverse as bronchopneumonia and viral hepatitis. It also occurs in association with collagen vascular diseases and with epithelial cancers, such as carcinoma of the lung. Reactive bone marrow plasmacytosis is present when plasma cells comprise more than 3% of the total nucleated cell population in the bone marrow. In both reactive and neoplastic proliferation of plasma cells, immunoglobulin may accumulate in the cytoplasm to form a prominent eosinophilic globule called the *Russell body*. Uncommon, and usually in neoplastic disorders, the invagination of immunoglobulin-containing cytoplasm into the nucleus appears in cross section as an intranuclear eosinophilic globule called a *Dutcher body*.

Lymphocytopenia

Peripheral blood lymphocytopenia is defined as a decrease in the peripheral blood lymphocyte count to less than 1500/μL in adults or less than 3000/μL in children. Since the predominant lymphocyte in the peripheral blood is the T helper-inducer (CD4+) lymphocyte, lymphocytopenia generally indicates a decrease in these cells. There are several mechanisms by which lymphocytopenia occurs:

- **Decreased production of lymphocytes:** A variety of congenital and acquired immunodeficiency syndromes are characterized by a decreased production of lymphocytes. Decreased production of T lymphocytes occurs in Hodgkin's disease, particularly in advanced stages.
- **Increased destruction of lymphocytes:** Lymphocytes are destroyed by a number of medical treatments, including X-irradiation, chemotherapy for malignant tumors, and the administration of antilymphocyte globulin, corticotropin, or corticosteroids. Some viral infections, particularly AIDS, are characterized by the destruction of T cells.
- **Loss of lymphocytes:** Intestinal disorders that are associated with damage to lymphatics result in the loss of lymph and its lymphocytes into the intestinal lumen. Such maladies include the protein-losing enteropathies, Whipple disease, and disorders associated with increased central venous pressure (e.g., right-sided heart failure and chronic constrictive pericarditis). Immunological damage to lymphocytes may occur in the collagen vascular diseases such as systemic lupus erythematosus.

Reactive Hyperplasia of Lymph Nodes

The lymph nodes may exhibit hyperplasia of all cellular components or any combination of B lymphocytes, T lymphocytes, and mononuclear phagocytic cells in response to a variety of infectious, inflammatory, and neoplastic disorders (Fig. 20-38).

- **Hyperplasia of the secondary follicles,** or germinal centers, and plasmacytosis of the medullary cords are indicators of B lymphocyte immunoreactivity.
- **Hyperplasia of the deep cortex or paracortex** (interfollicular or diffuse hyperplasia) is characteristic of T lymphocyte immunoreactivity.

The histopathological features and degree of lymph node enlargement in immunoreactive hyperplasias reflect (1) the age of the patient (children tend to exhibit a more pronounced immunoreactivity than adults), (2) the immunological competence of the host, and (3) the type of infectious agent or inflammatory disorder.

Acute suppurative lymphadenitis occurs in the lymph nodes that drain a site of acute bacterial infection. Suppurative lymph nodes enlarge rapidly, because of edema and hyperemia, and are tender, owing to distention of the capsule. Microscopically, infiltration of the lymph node sinuses and stroma by polymorphonuclear leukocytes and prominent follicular hyperplasia are noted.

The anatomical site of the lymphadenopathy often provides a clue to the etiology. For example, the posterior auricular lymph nodes are commonly enlarged in rubella

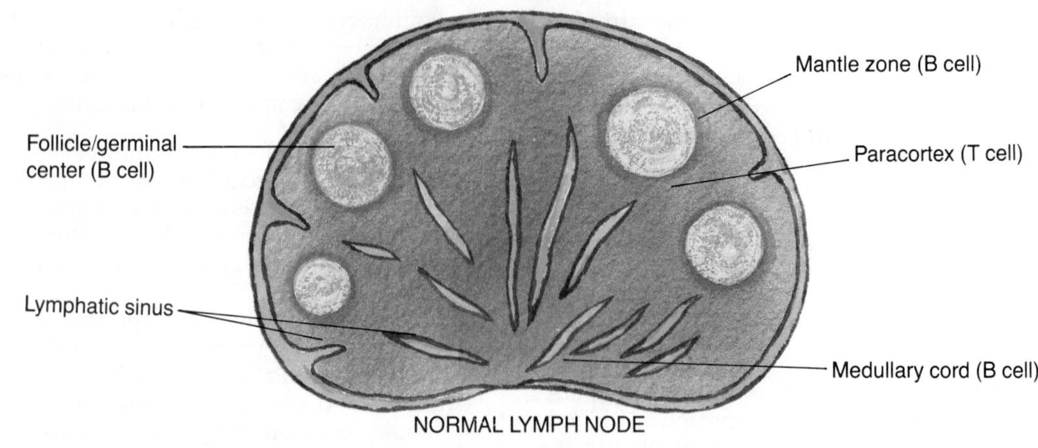
Mantle zone (B cell)
Follicle/germinal center (B cell)
Paracortex (T cell)
Lymphatic sinus
Medullary cord (B cell)
NORMAL LYMPH NODE

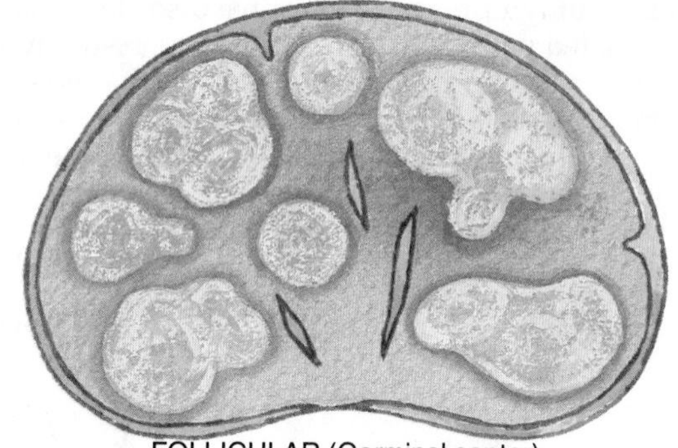
FOLLICULAR (Germinal center)

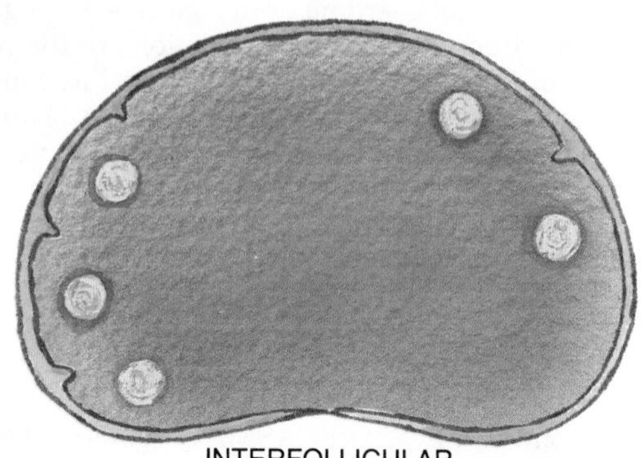
INTERFOLLICULAR

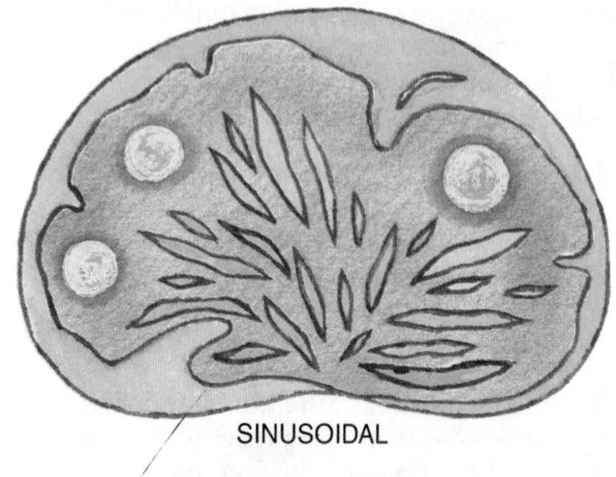
SINUSOIDAL

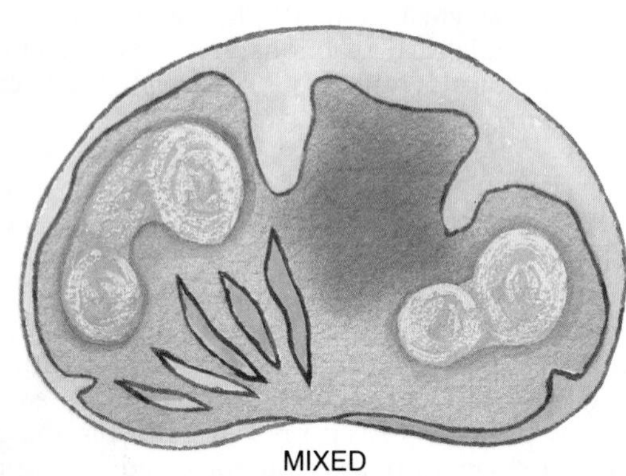
MIXED

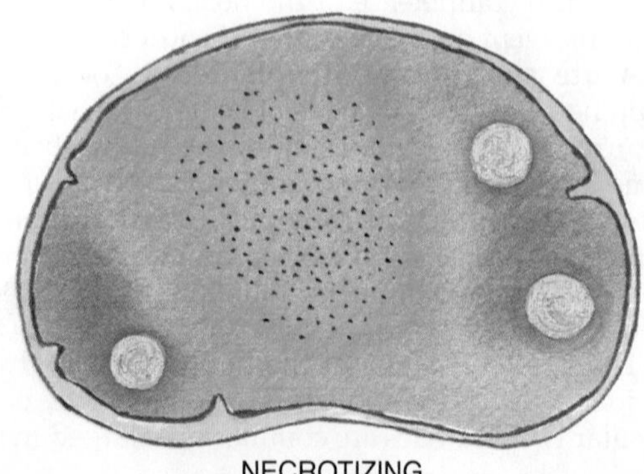
NECROTIZING

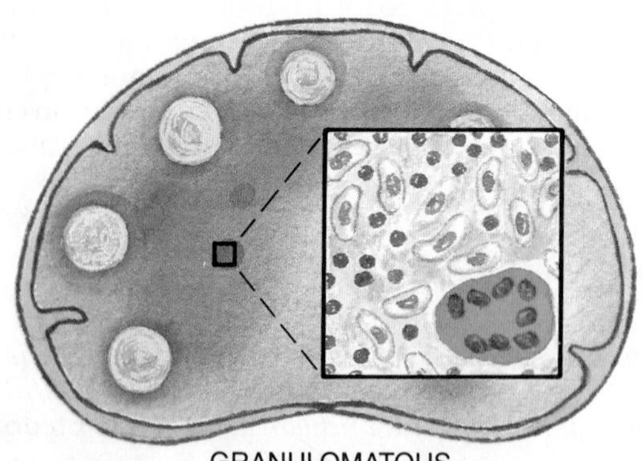
GRANULOMATOUS

FIGURE *20-38*

infection; the occipital lymph nodes in scalp infections; the posterior cervical lymph nodes in toxoplasmosis; the axillary lymph nodes in infections of the upper extremities or chest wall; and the inguinal lymph nodes in venereal infections and in infections of the lower extremities. Generalized lymphadenopathy may occur in systemic infections, hyperthyroidism, drug reactions, and the collagen vascular diseases.

Follicular Hyperplasia

NONSPECIFIC REACTIVE FOLLICULAR HYPERPLASIA: In this condition, prominent hyperplastic follicles occur principally in the cortex of the lymph node (Fig. 20-39). The follicles are round or irregular and may be confluent. The activated B lymphocytes in the follicles range from small cells with irregular, cleaved nuclei to large immunoblasts. Benign lymphoid follicles are characterized by "polarization," that is, the predominance of transformed lymphocytes or immunoblasts at one pole. Numerous mitotic figures reflect the rapid proliferation of activated B lymphocytes. Scattered benign macrophages, with abundant pale cytoplasm containing pyknotic nuclear and cytoplasmic debris, impart the characteristic "starry sky" pattern of benign follicles. Isolated dendritic reticulum cells, with round vesicular nuclei and abundant pink cytoplasm, may be identified near the margin of the follicle. A well-defined mantle of normal small B lymphocytes surrounds the follicles, sharply demarcating them from the interfollicular regions. A few partially transformed lymphocytes and immunoblasts and nonspecific inflammatory cells inhabit the interfollicular zone, and plasma cells may be increased in the medullary cords.

The etiology of nonspecific reactive follicular hyperplasia is frequently not known, although a viral or inflammatory etiology is often suspected. The clinical course is typically benign, with rapid and complete resolution of the lymphadenopathy.

LYMPHADENOPATHY OF RHEUMATOID ARTHRITIS: Lymphadenopathy, either localized or generalized, is a common finding in rheumatoid arthritis. Conspicuous follicular hyperplasia primarily involves the cortex, but occasionally may extend to the medulla. Prominent interfollicular plasmacytosis is also characteristic. Lymphadenopathy with histological features indistinguishable from those of rheumatoid arthritis may also occur in related disorders, such as Sjögren syndrome and Felty syndrome, and in unrelated diseases such as syphilis.

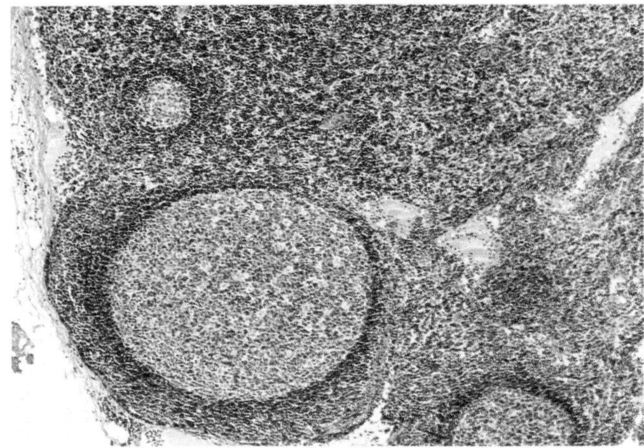

FIGURE *20-39*
Lymph node with reactive follicular hyperplasia. A section of a hyperplastic lymph node shows prominent follicles or germinal centers containing numerous macrophages with pale cytoplasm.

ANGIOFOLLICULAR LYMPH NODE HYPERPLASIA (CASTLEMAN DISEASE): This condition is a distinctive disorder of unknown etiology, which involves both lymph nodes and extranodal tissues. Two histopathological subtypes are recognized:

- **Hyaline-vascular angiofollicular lymph node hyperplasia:** This type comprises 90% of the cases. It usually presents as an asymptomatic mass, most commonly in the mediastinum, but also in other soft tissues. Young adult men are most commonly affected. The characteristic histopathological features include (1) numerous, small, follicle-like structures, frequently with radially penetrating, thick-walled, hyalinized vessels; (2) concentrically arranged small lymphocytes around the follicular structures, called "onion skinning"; and (3) extensive proliferation of capillaries in the interfollicular areas.
- **Plasma cell angiofollicular lymph node hyperplasia:** Accounting for 10% of the cases of Castleman disease, this type appears either as a localized mass or as a multicentric systemic disorder. The discrete mass may actually consist of multiple matted lymph nodes.

FIGURE *20-38*
Lymph nodes; patterns of benign reactive hyperplasia. The patterns of benign reactive hyperplasia in lymph nodes are contrasted with the structure of a normal lymph node. Follicular hyperplasia with prominent enlarged and irregular benign follicles is characteristic of B-cell immunoreactivity. Interfollicular hyperplasia is typical of T-cell immunoreactivity. The sinusoidal pattern with expansion of sinuses by benign macrophages is seen in reactive proliferations of the mononuclear-phagocyte system. Mixed patterns of follicular, interfollicular, and sinusoidal hyperplasia are common in a variety of complex mixed immune reactions. In necrotizing lymphadenitis, variable necrosis of the lymph node architecture with residual cell debris is present. In granulomatous inflammation, cohesive clusters of macrophages and occasional multinucleated giant cells are characteristic.

The histopathological features include (1) large hyperplastic follicles with less prominent penetrating vessels than in the hyaline-vascular type, (2) pronounced interfollicular plasmacytosis, and (3) prominent vascularity.

The multicentric form of the plasma cell variant of angiofollicular lymph node hyperplasia is more aggressive and occasionally exhibits a chronic course. Affected patients are at some risk for the development of Kaposi sarcoma or immunoblastic lymphoma. Clinical features of plasma cell angiofollicular hyperplasia include fever, polyclonal hypergammaglobulinemia, elevated sedimentation rate, and anemia.

AIDS LYMPHADENOPATHY: AIDS-associated lymphadenopathy is characterized by (1) marked follicular hyperplasia, with a distinctive loss of mantle zones; (2) infiltration of follicles by clusters of small lymphocytes; (3) foci of intrafollicular hemorrhage ("follicle lysis"); and (4) focal perisinusoidal monocytoid B-cell hyperplasia. Variable degrees of vascular proliferation, with subsequent depletion of lymphocytes in both follicles and interfollicular areas, may occur. Additionally, the lymph nodes in AIDS show a high incidence of superimposed malignant neoplasms, including diffuse B-cell lymphomas, Hodgkin's disease, and Kaposi sarcoma.

Interfollicular Hyperplasia

NONSPECIFIC INTERFOLLICULAR HYPERPLASIA: In this situation, the lymph nodal paracortex is expanded by a heterogeneous, reactive cell population. On low-power microscopy, the infiltrate imparts a typical mottled ("salt and pepper") appearance, reflecting an admixture of small lymphocytes, variably activated lymphocytes, immunoblasts, and scattered macrophages (Fig. 20-40). Isolated interdigitating reticulum cells, with grooved nuclei, can be identified. Prominent postcapillary venules exhibit conspicuous endothelial lining cells. Rarely, the immunoblastic component is so florid that reactive interfollicular hyperplasia must be distinguished from an evolving malignant lymphoma.

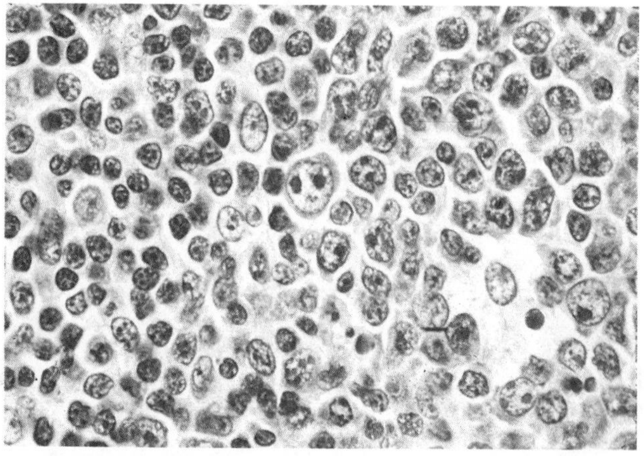

FIGURE *20-40*
Lymph node with reactive interfollicular hyperplasia. A high-power view of the T-dependent paracortex shows an admixture of small lymphocytes, variably activated lymphocytes, immunoblasts, and scattered macrophages.

Reactive nonspecific interfollicular hyperplasia is most commonly due to viral infections or to immunological reactions. Although the precise etiology is often not determined, the condition usually resolves promptly.

VIRAL LYMPHADENITIS: Interfollicular lymph node hyperplasia is a common finding in viral diseases, a few of which are characterized by specific histological features.

Infectious mononucleosis shows immunoblastic cells in lymph nodal sinuses. Rarely, extensive or even complete obliteration of the normal nodal architecture by proliferating immunoblasts occurs. Bizarre binucleated or multinucleated immunoblasts, which simulate the Reed-Sternberg cells of Hodgkin's disease, may be noted.

Varicella-herpes zoster infection features eosinophilic intranuclear inclusions surrounded by a clear zone or halo (Cowdry type A inclusions) in endothelial cells.

Measles in the prodromal phase is characterized by scattered multilobed or multinucleated lymphoid cells. These cells *(Warthin-Finkeldey cells)* display delicate chromatin, small punctate nucleoli, and scant pale cytoplasm.

Cytomegalovirus lymphadenitis is distinguished by the presence in endothelial cells of large, round, eosinophilic, intranuclear inclusions, which show a surrounding clear halo.

HISTIOCYTIC NECROTIZING LYMPHADENITIS (KIKUCHI DISEASE): This is an unusual lymphadenitis of young women, which most commonly involves the cervical lymph nodes. Focal infiltrates of immunoblasts and macrophages, both with distinctive angulated and twisted nuclei, are noted in the cortex and paracortex. Prominent karyorrhexis and cytoplasmic debris are characteristic, but granulocytes are absent. The lymphadenitis is usually self-limited and resolves in 3 to 4 months. A viral etiology is suspected.

PHENYTOIN-INDUCED LYMPHADENOPATHY: Phenytoin (Dilantin) is a drug commonly used in the treatment of epilepsy. Some patients chronically treated with this drug manifest lymphadenopathy characterized by interfollicular hyperplasia, with variable effacement of the lymph nodal architecture. A polymorphous cell population, consisting of small lymphocytes, immunoblasts, eosinophils, and plasma cells, is characteristic. Atypical binucleated immunoblasts, which are similar to the Reed-Sternberg cells of Hodgkin's disease, may be observed. Focal areas of necrosis are common. Systemic abnormalities include fever, rash, polyclonal hypergammaglobulinemia, and peripheral blood eosinophilia. Resolution usually occurs on withdrawal of the drug. There is a controversy whether there is an increased incidence of Hodgkin's disease or malignant lymphoma associated with phenytoin-induced lymphadenopathy.

SYSTEMIC LUPUS ERYTHEMATOSUS: Systemic lupus erythematosus is often associated with lymphadenopathy, characterized by interfollicular hyperplasia, with prominent immunoblasts and plasma cells, and focal to massive necrosis. Arteriolitis, with fibrinoid necrosis of vessel walls, is frequently observed. Hematoxylin bodies (see Chapter 4) are found in relation to foci of lymph nodal necrosis or in nodal sinuses.

Mixed Patterns of Reactive Hyperplasia of Lymph Nodes

Some infectious diseases are associated with mixed patterns of lymph node hyperplasia, in which several different features are prominent.

TOXOPLASMOSIS: This form of lymphadenitis is characterized by (1) prominent follicular hyperplasia; (2) small collections of epithelioid macrophages in the interfollicular regions of the lymph node (Fig. 20-41), which encroach on the follicles (Piringer-Kuchinka lesion); and (3) perisinusoidal monocytoid B-cell hyperplasia. Monocytoid B lymphocytes are medium-sized lymphoid cells, with round to indented nuclei, bland chromatin, and moderate pale cytoplasm.

CAT-SCRATCH DISEASE: This malady typically presents with lymphadenitis of the axillary and cervical lymph nodes, characterized by follicular hyperplasia and suppurative granulomatous foci. These areas consist of elongated or stellate abscesses, with central necrosis containing polymorphonuclear leukocytes and cell debris, and surrounded by palisaded macrophages and fibroblasts. Monocytoid B-cell hyperplasia and scattered immunoblasts may be observed in the interfollicular regions. The histological features of lymphadenitis caused by **lymphogranuloma venereum** and **tularemia** (see Chapter 9) are indistinguishable from those of cat-scratch disease.

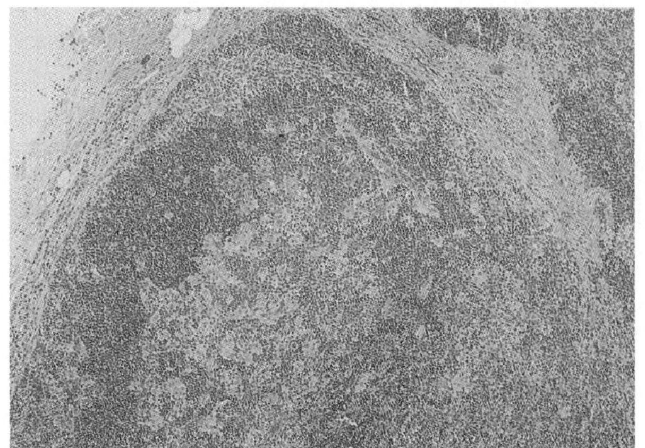

FIGURE *20-41*
Toxoplasmosis. A section of a lymph node shows clusters of pink epithelioid macrophages.

Angioimmunoblastic Lymphadenopathy

Angioimmunoblastic lymphadenopathy with dysproteinemia (AILD) is a disorder that features generalized lymphadenopathy, hepatosplenomegaly, anemia, and hypergammaglobulinemia. It was initially described as an unusual hyperimmune disorder of B lymphocytes, but it is now thought to represent a variant of postthymic (peripheral) T-cell lymphoma in most cases. In a few instances, the disease has followed the administration of certain drugs, and in other cases a viral pathogenesis has been suspected. In any event, it is believed that AILD probably represents a variable expression of an unstable lymphoproliferative state as a result of poor regulation by a defective immune system. According to this scenario, in a background of polyclonal lymphoid proliferation, malignant clones may eventually emerge and have a growth advantage over their benign counterparts.

☐ **Pathology:** The lymph nodes in AILD show (1) a diffuse effacement of the normal architecture; (2) a spectrum of transformed lymphocytes and immunoblasts; (3) arborizing thick-walled blood vessels; (4) a periodic acid–Schiff (PAS)-positive, eosinophilic proteinaceous material in the interstitium; and (5) admixed inflammatory cells, including eosinophils, plasma cells, and macrophages. AILD is a systemic disease that also involves extranodal sites, including the spleen, liver, skin, and bone marrow.

☐ **Clinical Features:** Patients with AILD tend to be middle-aged to elderly persons who present with generalized lymphadenopathy and hepatosplenomegaly, a maculopapular rash, fever, night sweats, and weight loss. Frequently, there is polyclonal hypergammaglobulinemia and peripheral blood eosinophilia. The clinical course is usually aggressive and characterized by progressive immune failure and a high mortality rate. Aggressive chemotherapy has resulted in complete remissions in more than half the patients.

Extranodal Lymphoid Hyperplasia (Pseudolymphoma)

Lymphocytes recirculate in the vascular and lymphatic systems and preferentially home to the lymphopoietic organs. However, they may be found in any organ or tissue site, where they are available to participate in local or systemic immune reactions. Rarely, hyperplasia of such lymphocytes occurs, with the formation of discrete mass lesions called extranodal lymphoid hyperplasia or pseudolymphoma. Extranodal lymphoid hyperplasias are of unknown etiology but may represent an exaggerated immune response to antigenic stimuli, possibly on the part of defective lymphocytes.

The diagnosis of pseudolymphoma originally rested on the lack of aggressive clinical behavior on the part of an extranodal lymphoid mass of polymorphous cellular composition. However, with more prolonged follow-up and the development of immunophenotyping and genotypng, it is now clear that many cases that would previously have been diagnosed as pseudolymphoma, particularly those arising in the lung, are actually low-grade, indolent lymphomas or MALTomas (tumors of *m*ucosa *a*ssociated *l*ymphoid *t*issue).

☐ **Pathology:** Common sites of extranodal lymphoid hyperplasias include the lungs, stomach, soft tissues of the orbit, and the skin. They are well demarcated from the surrounding soft tissues and measure 1 to 10 cm or larger in greatest dimension. On gross examination, pseudolymphomas are pale gray or yellow. Microscopically, scattered secondary lymphoid follicles, or germinal centers, are noted. The intervening polymorphous inflammatory cell infiltrate consists of small lymphocytes, transformed lymphocytes (including immunoblasts), plasma cells, macrophages, and eosinophils.

DISORDERS OF THE SPLEEN

Hypersplenism is a functional disorder, which, as previously noted (see hemolytic anemia), is characterized by anemia, leukopenia, thrombocytopenia, and compensatory bone marrow hyperplasia.

Hyposplenism refers to a situation in which normal splenic functions are reduced by disease or absent after splenectomy. Impaired filtering function causes an increased risk of severe bacteremia and a mild leukocytosis and thrombocytosis. Nuclear remnants and Howell-Jolly bodies are found in many of the circulating erythrocytes.

Congenital absence of the spleen (asplenia) is rare and is often associated with other congenital anomalies.

Acquired asplenia is seen most commonly in young adults with sickle cell anemia. Multiple infarctions eventually result in atrophy and hyposplenism. The infarctions are often painful, owing to the complication of fibrinous perisplenitis. As the result of the absence of splenic sequestration of erythrocytes, with consequent lack of removal of excess membrane and intracellular debris, many erythrocytes become targeted and contain nuclear remnants, Howell-Jolly bodies, or even intact nuclei.

Accessory spleens are common, occurring in 10% of normal persons. They may measure up to several centimeters in diameter and are most frequently found in the tail of the pancreas or in the gastrosplenic ligament. Following splenectomy, accessory spleens may increase considerably in size, but they rarely become large enough to restore the functions of the lost spleen.

Splenomegaly

The spleen is a prominent member of the lymphopoietic and mononuclear phagocyte systems, and splenomegaly is a common finding in a variety of unrelated pathological situations (Table 20-11).

Reactive Splenomegaly

Reactive hyperplasia of the spleen occurs in a number of acute and chronic inflammatory conditions. It is probably caused by phagocytosis of blood-borne bacteria, with the release of growth factors and other products of the inflammatory response. The spleen is moderately enlarged (up to 400 g), and macrophages and neutrophils abound in the red pulp. Mild hyperplasia of the lymphoid white pulp is common.

In acute and chronic parasitemias, the red pulp may be engorged with parasites and their breakdown products. The spleen may be massively enlarged in chronic malarial infections (up to 10 kg). It shows fibrous thickening of the capsule and trabeculae, with a slate gray to black coloration of the pulp, owing to the presence of phagocytosed malarial pigment (hematin).

In chronic immunological inflammatory disorders, splenomegaly is caused by hyperplasia of the white pulp. Germinal centers are prominent, as in rheumatoid arthritis, and there is an associated increase in mononuclear phagocytes, immunoblasts, plasma cells and eosinophils in the red pulp.

Systemic lupus erythematosus is characterized by fibrinoid necrosis of capsular and trabecular collagen and concentric, or "onion skin," thickening of the penicilliary arteries and central arterioles of the white pulp.

In infectious mononucleosis, transformed lymphocytes (immunoblasts) prominently infiltrate the red pulp, whereas the white pulp may no longer be evident. Infiltration of the capsular and trabecular systems and of blood vessels by lymphoid elements weakens the supporting structure of the spleen and accounts for **traumatic splenic rupture** in infectious mononucleosis.

TABLE *20-11* **Principal Causes of Splenomegaly**

Infections
Acute
Subacute
Chronic
Immunological inflammatory disorders
Felty syndrome
Lupus erythematosus
Sarcoidosis
Amyloidosis
Thyroiditis
Hemolytic anemias
Immune thrombocytopenia
Splenic vein hypertension
Cirrhosis
Splenic or portal vein thrombosis or stenosis
Right-sided cardiac failure
Primary or metastatic neoplasm
Leukemia
Lymphoma
Hodgkin's disease
Myeloproliferative syndromes
Sarcoma
Carcinoma
Storage diseases
Gaucher
Niemann-Pick
Mucopolysaccharidoses

Congestive Splenomegaly

Chronic passive congestion of the spleen causes splenomegaly and hypersplenism. This is most common in patients with portal hypertension due to cirrhosis, thrombosis of the portal or splenic veins, or right-sided heart failure.

☐ **Pathology:** The spleen is modestly enlarged (300 to 700 g) and has a thickened, fibrotic capsule. Focal accentuation of the capsular fibrosis leads to a "sugar-coated" appearance. The cut surface is firm, and the color varies from pink to deep red, depending on the extent of fibrosis. Microscopically, the red pulp initially shows dilated sinuses and an increased number of macrophages. Later, the parenchyma becomes fibrotic and the red pulp is hypocellular. Foci of old hemorrhages persist as *Gamna-Gandy bodies*, which are fibrotic nodules containing iron and calcium salts encrusted on collagenous and elastic fibers. The white pulp tends to be atrophic.

Infiltrative Splenomegaly

The spleen may be enlarged by an increase in the number of cellular elements or by the deposition of extracellular material, as in amyloidosis. Splenic macrophages accumulate in chronic infections, hemolytic anemias, and a variety of storage diseases, Gaucher disease being the prototype (see Chapter 6). A variety of neoplastic and reactive bone marrow disorders are accompanied by extramedullary hemopoiesis and a corresponding increase in the size of the spleen. Splenomegaly is also caused by the infiltration of malignant cells in hematological proliferative disorders, such as leukemias and lymphomas.

Splenomegaly Due to Cysts and Tumors

Splenic cysts are rare and the most common are actually pseudocysts. The latter are lined by a fibrous wall and are the residue of previous hemorrhage or infarction. Hydatid cysts are encountered in areas endemic for *Echinococcus granulosus* (see Chapter 9).

Primary splenic tumors are also distinctly uncommon. The most common primary benign tumors of the spleen are hemangiomas and lymphangiomas. Usually of the cavernous type, they contain large endothelial-lined spaces and vary from minute foci to lesions that occupy most of the spleen. The spaces in hemangiomas are occupied by erythrocytes, and in lymphangiomas by lymph.

Malignant tumors, such as lymphomas or Hodgkin's disease are usually not primary in the spleen but rather part of a generalized disease. Splenic hemangiosarcoma is a rare, highly malignant neoplasm of vascular endothelial cells, which frequently metastasizes to the liver by way of the portal drainage.

Despite its large blood supply and filtering function, the spleen is only rarely involved by metastatic tumors. The microenvironment, with its abundance of macrophages and lymphocytes, is apparently not favorable for tumor growth. Metastatic tumors are usually observed only late in the course of a widely metastasizing neoplasm. The primary tumors that most commonly metastasize to the spleen are carcinomas of the lung, breast, stomach, colon, and prostate, as well as malignant melanomas.

Disorders of Hemostasis

Normal hemostasis depends on three highly interactive systems—the blood vessels, the platelets, and the coagulation factors. Abnormal hemostasis may lead either to a hemorrhagic diathesis or to an increased tendency towards clotting (hypercoagulability). The clinical manifestations of hemorrhage associated with disorders of each component of the hemostatic system tend to be distinctive (Table 20-12).

Disorders of the blood vessels usually cause purpura, sometimes palpable. Platelet abnormalities result in both petechiae and purpuric hemorrhages in the skin (usually nonpalpable) and mucous membranes. Deficiencies of the coagulation factors are most commonly manifested as hemorrhage into muscles, viscera, and joint spaces.

TABLE *20-12* **Principal Causes of Bleeding**

Vascular disorders
- Senile purpura
- Purpura simplex
- Glucocorticoid excess
- Dysproteinemias
- Allergic (Henoch-Schönlein) purpura
- Hereditary hemorrhagic telangiectasia

Platelet abnormalities
- Thrombocytopenia (see Table 20-13)
- Qualitative disorders
  - Inherited
    - Glycoprotein IIb/IIIa deficiency (Glanzmann thrombasthenia)
    - Glycoprotein Ib/IX/V deficiency (Bernard-Soulier syndrome)
    - Storage pool diseases (alpha and delta)
    - Abnormal arachidonic acid metabolism
  - Acquired
    - Uremia
    - Drugs
    - Cardiopulmonary bypass
    - Myeloproliferative disorders
    - Liver disease

Coagulation factor deficiencies
- Inherited
  - von Willebrand disease
  - Hemophilia A
  - Hemophilia B
- Acquired
  - Vitamin K deficiency/antagonism
  - Liver disease
  - Disseminated intravascular coagulation

DISORDERS OF BLOOD VESSELS

Dysfunction of the extravascular or vascular tissues may cause hemorrhages, ranging from cosmetic blemishes to life-threatening blood loss.

Extravascular Dysfunction

The most common disorder in extravascular dysfunction is age-related atrophy of the supporting connective tissues. This condition is termed *senile purpura* and is associated with superficial, sharply demarcated and persistent purpuric spots on the forearms and other sun-exposed areas. A similar type of purpura *(purpura simplex)* occurs principally in women at the time of the menses. It is present in the deeper layers of the dermis and resolves quickly. Collagen synthesis is disturbed in *scurvy* (vitamin C deficiency) and purpura is a common manifestation. Perifollicular hemorrhages are particularly characteristic of vitamin C deficiency.

Vascular Dysfunction

The deposition of immunoglobulin fragments in vessel walls may occur in **amyloidosis, cryoglobulinemia, and other paraproteinemias** and can cause vessel wall weakness and purpura.

Hereditary Hemorrhagic Telangiectasia (Rendu-Osler-Weber Syndrome)

Hereditary hemorrhagic telangiectasia is an autosomal dominant disorder of blood vessel walls (venules and capillaries) that results in tortuous, dilated vessels (telangiectasias). The underlying defect is a thinning of the vessel walls, in which inadequate elastic tissue and smooth muscle permit dilatation of the vessels. Telangiectasias appear initially as punctate reddish spots on the lips and nose, measuring up to 0.5 cm in diameter. They can remain as telangiectasias or progress to arteriovenous malformations or aneurysmal dilatations found throughout the body.

Clinically, patients with hereditary hemorrhagic telangiectasia experience recurrent hemorrhage, which may be spontaneous or secondary to trivial trauma, and anemia. Although bleeding may occur at the site of any lesion, recurrent epistaxis ensues in over 80% of patients, beginning at an early age. Later in life, gastrointestinal hemorrhage may be the dominant symptom. Arteriovenous fistulas in the lung, brain, and retina may be troublesome and associated with hemorrhage or clinically significant shunting of blood. The patient's activities may be restricted by recurrent bleeding, but death from exsanguination is rare.

Allergic Purpura (Henoch-Schönlein Purpura)

Allergic purpura is a vascular disease that results from immunological damage to the blood vessel wall (see Chapter 16). In children, the disorder is of short duration and often follows a viral infection. In adults, it is associated with exposure to a variety of drugs and may be chronic, occasionally lasting for years.

Histologically, allergic purpura is characterized by leukocytoclastic vasculitis, with a perivascular infiltration of neutrophils and eosinophils. Fibrinoid necrosis of the vessel walls and plugging of the vascular lumina by platelets are observed. IgA and complement are often deposited in the vessel wall, and IgA complexes have been found in the circulating blood. The purpuric spots are often accompanied by raised urticarial lesions. Gastrointestinal involvement is indicated by intestinal cramps and bleeding, and renal involvement may lead to renal failure.

DISORDERS OF PLATELETS

Platelet abnormalities, whether qualitative or quantitative, result in a bleeding diathesis. Clinically, the most important are those conditions that lead to a decrease in the number of circulating platelets (thrombocytopenia).

Thrombocytopenia *is defined as a decrease in the platelet count to a level less than 150,000/μL.* A reduction in platelets to less than 50,000/μL increases the hazard of bleeding from trauma or surgical procedures. Spontaneous bleeding can be expected with a platelet count below 20,000/μL and is especially likely with a count below 10,000/μL. Thrombocytopenia can result from decreased production of platelets, increased destruction, splenic sequestration, or dilution (Table 20-13).

Decreased Production of Platelets

A decrease in the number of marrow megakaryocytes or ineffective thrombopoiesis leads to inadequate production of platelets. A reduced number of megakaryocytes occurs in aplastic anemia, infiltrative disorders of the marrow, or marrow hypoplasia produced by drugs, radiation, or viral infections. Chemotherapeutic agents are the most common drugs that cause a reduction in the number of megakaryocytes as a feature of general bone marrow

TABLE ***20-13*** **Principal Causes of Thrombocytopenia**

Decreased production
Aplastic anemia
Bone marrow infiltration (neoplastic, fibrosis)
Bone marrow suppression by drugs or radiation
Ineffective production
Megaloblastic anemia
Myelodysplasias
Increased destruction
Immunological (idiopathic, HIV, drugs, neonatal)
Nonimmunological (DIC, TTP, HUS, drugs)
Increased sequestration
Splenomegaly
Dilutional
Blood and plasma transfusions

hypoplasia. Thiazide diuretics, alcohol, and interferon have a more specific suppressive effect on megakaryocytes than on other marrow elements. Viral infections produced by live measles vaccine or human immunodeficiency virus also have a suppressive effect on megakaryocytes. HIV presumably enters megakaryocytes via the CD4 receptor on the surface of these cells.

Maturation arrest and premature destruction of megakaryocytes are observed most frequently in association with the megaloblastic anemias of vitamin B_{12} or folic acid deficiencies, presumably as a result of impaired DNA synthesis in megakaryocytes. Ineffective production of platelets is also seen in the myelodysplastic syndromes.

May-Hegglin anomaly is a hereditary defect in megakaryocyte maturation, in which thrombocytopenia is associated with circulating giant platelets and Dohle-like bodies in neutrophils (see Fig. 20-33).

Increased Destruction of Platelets

There are two major mechanisms that are responsible for an increased destruction of platelets. Many cases reflect immune-mediated damage and removal of circulating platelets, as in idiopathic thrombocytopenic purpura and drug-induced thrombocytopenia. Alternatively, intravascular platelet aggregation may produce thrombocytopenia, for example, in thrombotic thrombocytopenic purpura.

Idiopathic (Immune) Thrombocytopenic Purpura

Idiopathic thrombocytopenic purpura (ITP) is a quantitative disorder of platelets caused by antibodies directed against platelet or megakaryocytic antigens. It is, therefore, more appropriate to speak of immune thrombocytopenic purpura. ITP occurs in two forms, an acute, self-limited, hemorrhagic syndrome in children and a chronic bleeding disorder in adults.

☐ **Pathogenesis:** In a manner similar to autoimmune hemolytic anemia, the etiology of ITP is related to antibody-mediated immune destruction of platelets or their precursors. In the large majority of patients, the autoantibodies are of the IgG class, but IgM antiplatelet antibodies have also been reported in a few patients, although their clinical significance remains to be clarified.

Acute ITP typically appears in children (male:female = 1:1) after a viral illness and is likely caused by viral-induced changes in platelet antigens that elicit autoantibodies. Complement is then bound at the surface, after which the platelets are lysed in the blood or phagocytosed and destroyed by splenic and hepatic macrophages.

Chronic ITP occurs predominantly in adults (male:female = 1:2.6) and may be associated with a collagen vascular disease (e.g., systemic lupus erythematosus) or a malignant lymphoproliferative disease, especially chronic lymphocytic leukemia. It is also common in persons infected with HIV. The extent of thrombocytopenia in ITP is determined by the balance between three mechanisms: (1) the level of antiplatelet antibodies, (2) the degree of inhibition of platelet production in the bone marrow, since some antibodies may be directed against megakaryocytes, and (3) the expression of Fc and complement receptors on the surface of macrophages. This expression is up-regulated in infection and pregnancy, but is ameliorated by certain drugs, for example, corticosteroids, danazol, and intravenous gamma globulin, all of which are used to treat ITP.

☐ **Pathology:** In acute ITP, the platelet count is typically less than 20,000/μL. In chronic adult ITP, the platelet count varies from a few thousand to 100,000/μL. The peripheral blood smear in ITP exhibits numerous large platelets, which reflect an increased number of young platelets released by a bone marrow actively engaged in platelet production. Accordingly, examination of the bone marrow reveals a compensatory increase in megakaryocytes (Fig. 20-42). IgG is present on the platelets in more than 80% of patients with chronic ITP, and in half, increased levels of platelet-associated C3 can be demonstrated.

☐ **Clinical Features:** Children with acute ITP experience the sudden onset of petechiae and purpura but are otherwise asymptomatic. Spontaneous recovery can be expected in more than 80% of cases within 6 months. The major threat (1% of cases) is intracranial hemorrhage. In most cases, no treatment is necessary, but with serious disease corticosteroids and intravenous immunoglobulin may be needed. Glucocorticoids decrease the production of the antiplatelet antibodies and down-regulate Fc receptors on macrophages. γ-Globulin interferes with the clearance of IgG-coated platelets from the circulation.

Chronic ITP in adults presents as bleeding episodes, such as epistaxis, menorrhagia, or ecchymoses. Although life-threatening hemorrhages may occur, they are uncommon. Occasionally, asymptomatic persons are discovered to have thrombocytopenia on a routine blood cell count. Most adults with chronic ITP are improved by corticosteroid treatment and intravenous administration of

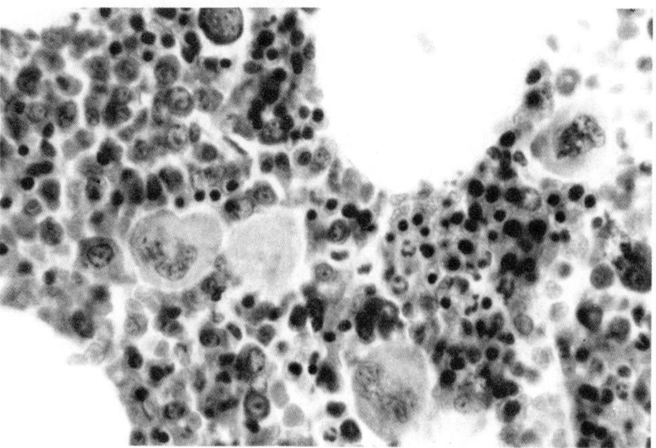

FIGURE *20-42*
Idiopathic thrombocytopenic purpura. A section of the bone marrow reveals increased megakaryocytes.

γ-globulin. Danazol (a synthetic anabolic steroid) acts in a manner similar to that of glucocorticoids. In patients who fail to respond adequately to drug therapy within 2 to 3 months, splenectomy produces a complete or partial remission in 60% to 80% of cases.

Drug-Induced Thrombocytopenia

A number of drugs, especially quinidine, sulfonamides, penicillin, cimetidine, and digoxin, combine with surface proteins on platelets to produce neoantigens. The latter elicit antibodies and, in turn, platelet destruction. This idiosyncratic reaction occurs weeks to months after the initial administration of the drug but may appear more rapidly if the patient has been previously exposed to the offending agent. Thrombocytopenia tends to be severe and symptomatic, with platelet counts less than 20,000/μL. The disorder usually resolves promptly on discontinuation of the drug.

Heparin is a common cause of drug-induced thrombocytopenia, affecting up to 5% of patients treated with this anticoagulant. There are two distinct thrombocytopenic syndromes associated with heparin therapy. A mild thrombocytopenia results from the direct interaction of heparin with surface proteins of platelets, which leads to activation and aggregation. Heparin administration may also cause a severe, idiosyncratic, immune-mediated thrombocytopenia, which is similar to other drug reactions. However, in contrast to other drug-induced thrombocytopenias, that associated with heparin is often accompanied by arterial and venous thromboses, leading to complications such as stroke, myocardial infarction, and iliofemoral arterial thrombosis. The pathogenesis of the thrombotic diathesis induced by heparin is poorly understood, but appears to be due to the stimulation of procoagulant activity by the heparin-antibody-platelet interaction.

Isoimmune Neonatal Purpura

Isoimmune neonatal purpura is characterized by an alloantibody-mediated thrombocytopenia that occurs in the fetus by a mechanism analogous to the destruction of erythrocytes in erythroblastosis fetalis. Unlike the situation in erythroblastosis fetalis, first-born children are often affected, owing to the ability of platelets to cross the placenta. Up to three fourths of cases in whites are associated with a platelet antigen termed *Pl^{A1}*. If the mother is Pl^{A1} negative and the fetus has inherited this antigen from the father, fetal Pl^{A1}-positive platelets cross the placenta and elicit the production of specific maternal IgG. In turn, these antibodies cross the placenta and destroy the fetal platelets. The major complication of isoimmune neonatal purpura is intracranial hemorrhage, which occurs in as many as 20% of affected infants, half of whom suffer this complication *in utero*. Spontaneous recovery of the platelet count usually occurs in a few weeks after delivery.

Post-Transfusion Purpura

As a consequence of a prior transfusion, Pl^{A1}-negative persons may develop alloantibodies to Pl^{A1}-positive platelets. Newly infused Pl^{A1}-positive platelets are destroyed by these antibodies. Curiously, the patient's own Pl^{A1}-negative platelets are also destroyed, perhaps related to the passive acquisition of the antigen by these platelets or the development of immune complexes. In any event, a self-limited thrombocytopenia occurs about a week after the transfusion.

Thrombotic Thrombocytopenic Purpura

Thrombotic thrombocytopenic purpura (TTP) is a rare syndrome featuring the pentad of thrombocytopenia, microangiopathic hemolytic anemia, neurological symptoms, fever, and azotemia. Platelet aggregation leads to the widespread deposition of platelets in the microvasculature as characteristic hyaline thrombi.

☐ **Pathogenesis:** The pathogenesis of TTP is obscure, but the most tenable hypothesis holds that it results from the introduction into the circulation of one or more platelet-aggregating substances. **The theory that has received the most attention is the inappropriate release of von Willebrand factor multimers from injured endothelial cells.** Von Willebrand factor monomers are normally assembled into multimeric molecules of varying size (up to millions of daltons) within endothelial cells and released locally in response to endothelial stimulation. In TTP, for unknown reasons unusually large multimers of von Willebrand factor are present in the plasma, where they presumably mediate intravascular platelet aggregation.

Although most cases of TTP arise in otherwise normal persons, the disease may also complicate autoimmune collagen vascular disorders (systemic lupus erythematosus, rheumatoid arthritis, Sjögren syndrome) and drug-induced hypersensitivity reactions. TTP has also apparently been triggered by infections, cancer chemotherapy, bone marrow transplantation, and pregnancy. In addition, the disease has been observed in siblings, suggesting the possibility of a hereditary predisposition. The diverse circumstances in which TTP arises argues for the view that it is a consequence of heterogeneous conditions that injure the microcirculation.

☐ **Pathology:** The morphological hallmark of TTP is the deposition throughout the body of PAS-positive hyaline microthrombi in arterioles and capillaries, principally in the heart, brain, and kidneys. The microthrombi contain platelet aggregates, fibrin, and a few erythrocytes and leukocytes. TTP is clearly distinguished from immune-mediated vasculitis by a lack of inflammation. On the peripheral blood smear, fragmented erythrocytes (schistocytes) are always evident and numerous reticulocytes are present.

☐ **Clinical Features:** TTP occurs at virtually any age, but is most common in women in the fourth and fifth decades of life. The disease may be chronic and recurrent over a period of years or more commonly occurs as an acute, fulminant disease, which is often fatal. Most patients present with neurological symptoms, including seizures, focal weakness, aphasia, and alterations in the state of consciousness. Widespread purpura is often present, and in women vaginal bleeding may occur. Anemia is a constant feature, often severe enough to reduce the hemoglobin below 6 g/dL. Jaundice secondary to hemolysis may be pronounced. Renal dysfunction is frequently prominent, half of the patients being azotemic.

Thrombocytopenia is invariable in TTP, and more than half of the patients have a platelet count less than 20,000/μL. Despite the presence of aggregated platelets, activation of the coagulation cascade does not occur. Consequently, the prothrombin time, partial thromboplastin time (PTT), and fibrinogen concentration remain normal, distinguishing this syndrome from disseminated intravascular coagulation (see later). Prior to modern therapy, acute TTP was ordinarily fatal. However, with the use of plasma infusion and plasmapheresis, the cure rate has increased to 80%.

Hemolytic Uremic Syndrome

Hemolytic uremic syndrome (HUS) is similar to TTP, and in its adult form it is thought by many to be a variant of the latter. Classic HUS occurs in children, usually after an acute enteric infection. It seems to be the consequence of glomerular endothelial cell injury produced by verotoxins elaborated by the offending microorganism (usually *E. coli* or *S. dysinteriae*) (see Chapter 16). In HUS, aggregated platelet thrombi are found primarily in the renal microvasculature, and renal failure, rather than neurological abnormalities, is the characteristic clinical feature. Adult HUS has not been linked to enteric infections, and, as with TTP, the pathogenesis of the underlying endothelial injury has not been elucidated.

Splenic Sequestration of Platelets

Many patients with splenomegaly, irrespective of the cause, manifest hypersplenism, a syndrome that includes sequestration of platelets in the spleen (see earlier). Whereas one third of platelets produced are normally sequestered temporarily in the spleen, in massive splenomegaly, up to 90% of the total platelet pool may be captured in that organ. Interestingly, the platelet life span is normal or only slightly reduced. Thrombocytopenia associated with hypersplenism is rarely severe and by itself does not produce a hemorrhagic diathesis.

Thrombocytosis

REACTIVE THROMBOCYTOSIS: An increase in platelets occurs frequently in association with the following conditions: (1) iron deficiency anemia, especially in children; (2) splenectomy; (3) cancer; and (4) chronic inflammatory disorders. Reactive thrombocytosis is rarely symptomatic, although it has been associated with thrombotic episodes, especially in bedridden patients after splenectomy.

CLONAL THROMBOCYTOSIS: Patients with chronic myeloproliferative syndromes, such as polycythemia vera and essential thrombocythemia, suffer a malignant proliferation of megakaryocytes. The resulting increase in circulating platelets may be associated with episodes of thrombosis or bleeding (see later).

Qualitative Disorders of Platelets

A number of hereditary disorders of platelet function have been described. Despite their clinical rarity, they are important because they provide insights into normal platelet function.

BERNARD-SOULIER SYNDROME (GIANT PLATELET SYNDROME): *This disorder is an autosomal recessive trait in which platelets have a quantitative or qualitative defect in the membrane glycoprotein complex (GPIb/IX [CD42] and sometimes GPV) that serves as a receptor for von Willebrand factor.* The complex plays a prominent role in the adhesion of normal platelets when exposed to injured subendothelial tissues. The platelets in Bernard-Soulier syndrome vary widely in size and shape, and the diagnosis is suggested by the presence of thrombocytopenia with giant platelets on the blood smear.

Bernard-Soulier syndrome manifests in infancy or childhood with a bleeding pattern characteristic of abnormal platelet function, namely ecchymoses, epistaxis, and gingival bleeding. At a later age, traumatic hemorrhage, gastrointestinal bleeding, and menorrhagia occur. Although many patients have only a mild bleeding disorder, others suffer more severe hemorrhage, which demands frequent platelet transfusions and may even be fatal.

GLANZMANN THROMBASTHENIA: *This autosomal recessive defect in platelet aggregation is caused by a quantitative or qualitative abnormality in the glycoprotein complex IIb/IIIa (CD41/61).* In normal platelets, this complex is activated during platelet adhesion and serves as a receptor for fibrinogen and von Willebrand factor, mediating platelet aggregation and the generation of a solid plug. In addition, the IIb/IIIa complex is linked to the platelet cytoskeleton and transmits the force of contraction to adherent fibrin, a mechanism that promotes clot retraction. In Glanzmann thrombasthenia, the lack of aggregation and clot retraction impairs hemostasis and causes bleeding, despite a normal platelet count. The disease becomes clinically apparent shortly after birth when the infant manifests mucocutaneous or gingival hemorrhage, epistaxis, or bleeding after circumcision. Later, patients may suffer unexpected hemorrhage after trauma or surgery. The severity of the disease is variable, and only a few patients experience life-threatening hemorrhage. Platelet transfusions temporarily correct the condition.

ALPHA STORAGE POOL DISEASE (GRAY PLATELET SYNDROME): *A rare inherited malady, this type of storage pool disease is characterized by the absence of morphologically recognizable α granules in the platelets.* The defect resides in abnormal granule membranes. Thrombocytopenia is common, and the platelets are large and pale. The bleeding diathesis tends to be mild.

DELTA STORAGE POOL DISEASE: *This heterogeneous malady affects the dense granules of platelets.* The disease is sometimes associated with other multisystem hereditary disorders, including Chediak-Higashi syndrome or Hermansky-Pudlack syndrome (a type of oculocutaneous albinism; see Chapter 6). Bleeding manifestations are mild to moderate.

ACQUIRED QUALITATIVE DISORDERS OF PLATELETS: A variety of acquired disorders may adversely affect platelet function (see Table 20-12). Many drugs compromise platelet function, including aspirin and other nonsteroidal anti-inflammatory agents. Aspirin irreversibly acetylates platelet cyclooxygenase, the enzyme required for the production of thromboxane A_2, an important aggregation factor. Although spontaneous purpura and bleeding are rare, there is an increased risk of bleeding after trauma and surgery. Considering the 10-day life span of platelets, aspirin ingestion should be avoided for at least a week prior to elective surgery.

Renal failure is often accompanied by a qualitative platelet defect, which results in a prolonged bleeding time and a hemorrhagic tendency. The platelet abnormality is heterogeneous and is aggravated by the uremic anemia per se. Restoration of a normal hematocrit by erythropoietin administration may return the bleeding time back to normal without affecting the degree of azotemia.

COAGULATION DISORDERS

Quantitative and qualitative disorders of all of the coagulation factors have been identified. These conditions may be hereditary or acquired. Of the hereditary deficiencies, only those of factor VIII (hemophilia A), factor IX (hemophilia B), and von Willebrand factor are common. Hemophilia A is discussed in Chapter 6.

Hemophilia B

Hemophilia B (Christmas disease) is an X-linked recessive bleeding disorder that results from a deficiency of factor IX activity. Hemophilia B accounts for at least 10% of all cases of hemophilia, occurring in 1:30,000 male births. The hemorrhagic diathesis is clinically indistinguishable from hemophilia A.

The gene for factor IX resides at band q26-qter of the X chromosome. A variety of mutations in the factor IX gene in patients with hemophilia B have been described, including complete or partial deletions, insertions, and missense and nonsense mutations. The same mutation is found in a given family, and the severity of the illness correlates closely with the level of factor IX activity. It is estimated that one third of cases of hemophilia B are not familial and represent new mutations.

Since the half-life of factor IX is 18 to 24 hours longer than that for factor VIII, it is easier to maintain therapeutic levels with exogenous factor IX. Highly purified factor IX concentrates have recently become available and provide a major advantage over the previously employed "prothrombin complex concentrates."

Von Willebrand Disease

von Willebrand disease (VWD) is the common name for a heterogeneous complex of hereditary bleeding disorders related to a deficiency or abnormality of von Willebrand factor (VWF). Over 20 distinct subtypes have been described. A simplified classification (see below) recognizes three major categories. Variable expression of VWF (especially type I) confounds estimates of prevalence, although some hold that VWD is the most common inherited coagulopathy. VWF, an adhesive molecule, is synthesized by endothelial cells and megakaryocytes as a 250-kd monomer that undergoes polymerization to multimers with molecular weights in the millions. VWF is stored in the cytoplasmic Weibel-Palade bodies of endothelial cells and is released into the subendothelial tissues and the plasma. After endothelial injury, subendothelial VWF binds to platelet glycoprotein receptors (Ib/IX or D42), thereby promoting the adherence of platelets and sealing off the endothelial injury. It can also bind to GPIIb/IIIa (CD41/61) to promote platelet aggregation.

In plasma, VWF binds to and protects factor VIII; its absence is always associated with a deficiency in the activity of factor VIII. Although the concentration of VWF can thus be estimated indirectly by the bleeding time and by the PTT, it is usually measured by its reactivity with an antibody (VWF:Ag) or by its capacity to induce platelet aggregation in the presence of the antibiotic ristocetin.

☐ **Pathogenesis:** Three types of VWD are recognized, each of which in turn represents a heterogeneous group of defects:

TYPE I VWD: These variants comprise 75% of all cases of VWD and are inherited as autosomal dominant traits with variable penetrance. Type I VWD is basically a partial quantitative deficiency of VWF, in which all the multimers found in the plasma are reduced, although their relative concentrations remain unchanged.

TYPE II VWD: Compared with type I VWD, qualitative defects in VWF characterize the type II variants, which account for 20% of all cases of VWD. In type II disease, the interactions of VWF and the blood vessel wall are defective. The plasma activities of both VWF and factor VIII are reduced. In type IIa, the higher molecular weight multimers are absent from the platelets and the plasma. Type IIb is caused by the synthesis of an abnormal VWF with an increased affinity for platelets and may be associated with thrombocytopenia.

TYPE III VWD: This severe form of VWD (also labeled type IS, for severe) is the least common variety and is inherited as an autosomal recessive trait or exhibits compound heterozygosity (different mutations in the two VWF alleles). VWF activity is absent, and the plasma levels of factor VIII are decreased to less than 10% of normal.

☐ **Clinical Features:** Most cases of VWD are associated with only a mild bleeding diathesis, with the exception of type III. Easy bruising, epistaxis, gastrointestinal bleeding, and, in women, menorrhagia are frequent. The presenting symptom is often excessive hemorrhage after trauma or surgery. Patients with type III VWD may experience life-threatening hemorrhage from the gastrointestinal tract, and hemarthroses comparable to those in hemophilia are not infrequent.

The bleeding tendency in all forms of VWD is successfully treated with Factor VIII, VWF concentrates, or cryoprecipitate. Vasopressin is the treatment of choice in type I and IIa VWD because it increases the release of preformed VWF from its endothelial storage pools.

Acquired Coagulation Disorders

Vitamin K Deficiency

Vitamin K is a necessary cofactor for the carboxylation and activation of prothrombin and factors VII, IX and X, as well as for the anticoagulant proteins C and S. In many cases, vitamin K deficiencies are caused by the elimination of vitamin K–producing bacteria in the gut after antibiotic treatment. Severe malnutrition and intestinal malabsorption are also causes of vitamin K deficiency. The deficiency was previously common in newborns because of a lack of intestinal bacteria, but all hospital-born infants in the United States are now given prophylactic vitamin K. In liver disease, a deficiency of vitamin K–dependent factors is due not to vitamin K deficiency but to inadequate hepatic synthesis of the factors themselves. Coumadin therapy exerts its anticoagulant effect by interfering with the enzymatic reduction of vitamin K. The bleeding manifestations associated with vitamin K deficiency can be mild or severe, with prolongation of both prothrombin time (PT) and activated PTT (aPTT).

Inhibitors of Coagulation Factors

Acquired inhibitors of coagulation factors, also termed *circulating anticoagulants*, are usually IgG autoantibodies. The large majority are directed against factor VIII and VWF, although rare cases of antibodies against most of the other coagulation factors are reported. In hereditary coagulation disorders, especially hemophilia, circulating anticoagulants arise in response to the chronic administration of concentrates of human plasma containing the deficient factor. Anticoagulants also develop in some patients with autoimmune disorders (e.g., systemic lupus erythematosus, rheumatoid arthritis), presumably as a result of abnormal immune regulation. Finally, many cases of acquired anticoagulants appear in apparently normal persons.

The consequences of acquired anticoagulants vary from an asymptomatic laboratory finding to life-threatening hemorrhage. These autoantibodies are difficult to eliminate, but one third of patients experience spontaneous remission. The condition is treated by the administration of plasma concentrates, corticosteroids, or immunosuppressive agents.

Lupus anticoagulants are antiphospholipid antibodies in patients with systemic lupus erythematosus and other autoimmune conditions, or in otherwise asymptomatic individuals. Bleeding is distinctly uncommon, but these patients have a **hypercoagulable (thrombotic) tendency** (see later).

Disseminated Intravascular Coagulation

Disseminated intravascular coagulation (DIC) refers to widespread ischemic changes secondary to microvascular fibrin thrombi, which are accompanied by the consumption of platelets and coagulation factors and a hemorrhagic diathesis. DIC is a serious and often fatal acquired disorder and typically occurs as a complication of massive trauma, septicemia from numerous organisms, and obstetric emergencies. It is also associated with metastatic cancer, hemopoietic malignancies, cardiovascular and liver disease, and numerous other conditions.

☐ Pathogenesis: **The central event in the initiation of DIC is the activation of the clotting cascades within the vascular compartment by tissue injury or damage to the endothelium, or both.** The subsequent generation of substantial amounts of thrombin (see Fig. 20-14), combined with the initial failure of the natural inhibitory mechanisms that neutralize thrombin, is responsible for the initiation of DIC. With the consequent uncontrolled intravascular coagulation, the delicate balance between coagulation and fibrinolysis is disrupted. This event leads to the consumption of clotting factors, platelets, and fibrinogen and a consequent hemorrhagic diathesis (Fig. 20-43).

Procoagulant tissue factor is released into the circulation following injury in a variety of circumstances, including direct trauma, brain injury, and obstetric accidents such as premature separation of the placenta (see Chapter 18). **Bacterial endotoxin** also stimulates macrophages to release tissue factor. **Certain neoplasms** are associated with DIC, owing to the release of tissue factor by the cancer cells. As a consequence of the activation of the clotting cascade, intravascular fibrin is deposited as microthrombi in the smallest blood vessels. The stimulation of the fibrinolytic system by fibrin generates fibrin split products that possess anticoagulant properties and contribute to the bleeding diathesis.

Endothelial injury plays an important role in the pathogenesis of many cases of DIC. The normal endothelium has anticoagulant properties (see Fig. 20-15) and shields platelets from activation by contact with the subendothelial connective tissue (see Chapters 2 and 10). The anticoagulant properties of the endothelium are impaired by widely varying injuries, including (1) tumor necrosis factor in gram-negative sepsis; (2) other inflammatory mediators, such as activated complement, IL-1, or neutrophil proteases; (3) viral or rickettsial infections; and (4) trauma (e.g., burns). As a result, platelet aggregates form in the microvasculature.

☐ Pathology and Clinical Features: Arterioles, capillaries, and venules in many parts of the body are occluded by **microthrombi** composed of fibrin and

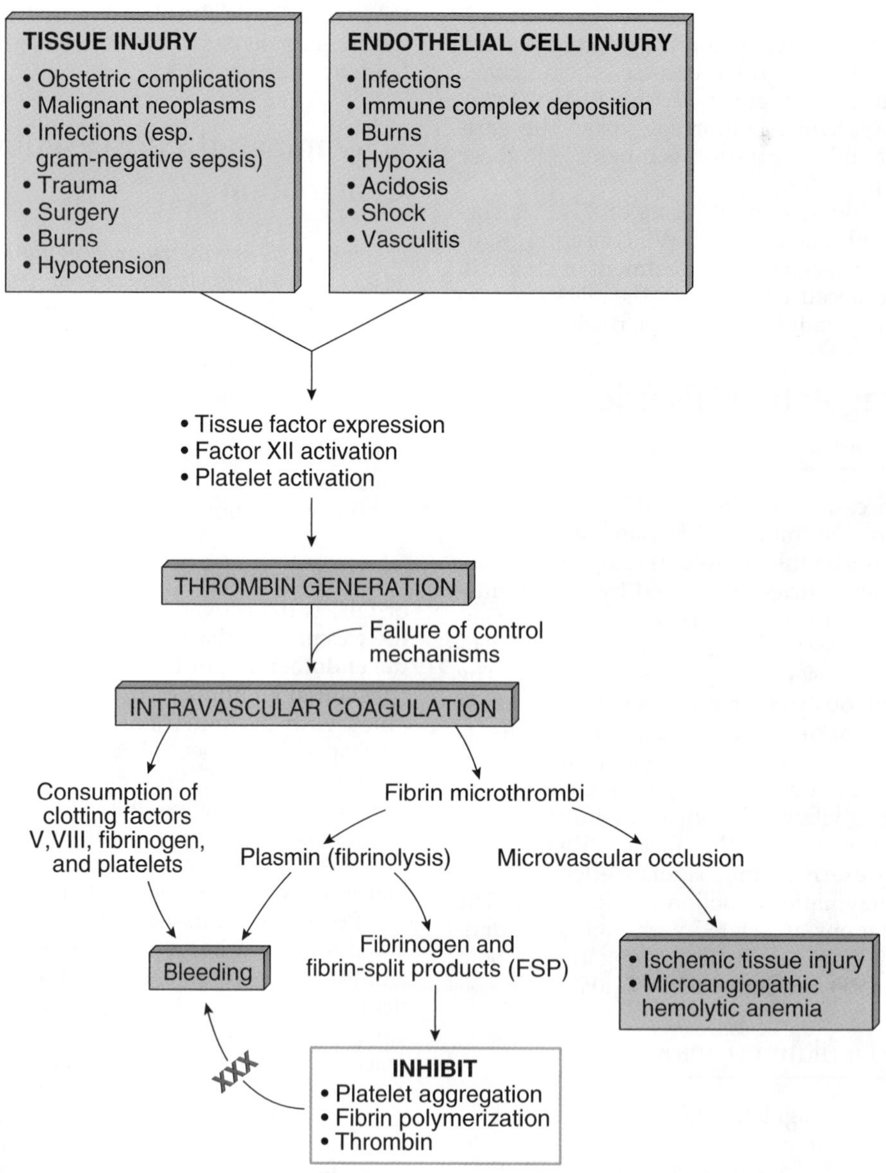

FIGURE *20-43*
The pathophysiology of disseminated-intravascular coagulation (DIC). The syndrome of DIC is precipitated by tissue injury, endothelial cell injury, or a combination of the two. These injuries trigger increased expression of tissue factor on cell surfaces, and activation of clotting factors (including XII and V) and platelets. With the failure of normal control mechanisms, the generation of thrombin leads to intravascular coagulation.

platelets (Fig. 20-44). However, owing to the enhancement of fibrinolysis, these thrombi may no longer be visualized at the time of autopsy. Microvascular obstruction is associated with **widespread ischemic changes**, particularly in the brain, kidneys, skin, lungs, and gastrointestinal tract. These organs are also the sites of bleeding, which in the case of the brain and gastrointestinal tract may be fatal.

Erythrocytes become fragmented (schistocytes) by passage through webs of intravascular fibrin strands, resulting in **microangiopathic hemolytic anemia**. The consumption of activated platelets leads to **thrombocytopenia**, whereas the **depletion of clotting factors** is reflected in a prolongation of the PT and PTT and a decrease in the plasma fibrinogen level. Plasma fibrin split products prolong the thrombin time. Laboratory tests that are useful in the diagnosis of DIC include the measurement of fibrinopeptide A and D-dimer, the levels of which are elevated (as markers of coagulation and fibrinolytic activation, respectively).

The symptoms of DIC reflect both microvascular thrombosis and the bleeding tendency. Ischemic changes in the brain lead to seizures and coma. Depending on the severity of DIC, renal symptoms range from mild azotemia to fulminant acute renal failure from bilateral cortical necrosis. The acute respiratory distress syndrome

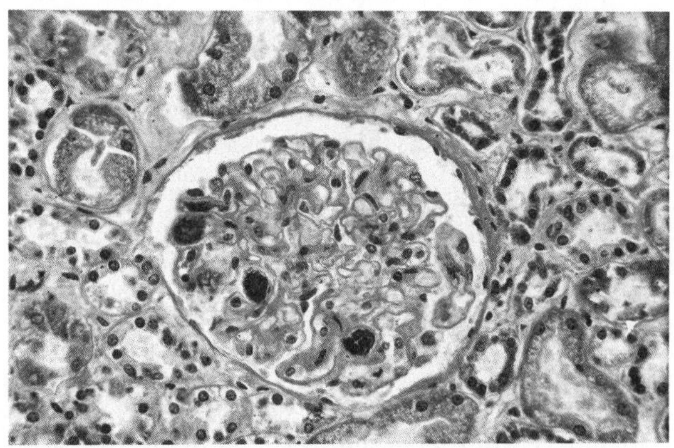

FIGURE 20-44
Disseminated intravascular coagulation. A section of a glomerulus stained with phosphotungstic acid hematoxylin (PTAH), which colors fibrin deep purple, demonstrates several microthrombi.

may supervene, and acute ulcers of the gastrointestinal tract may cause substantial hemorrhage. The bleeding diathesis is evidenced by cerebral hemorrhage, ecchymoses, and hematuria. Patients with DIC are treated with heparin anticoagulation, to interrupt the cycle of intravascular coagulation, and replacement of platelets and clotting factors, to control the bleeding.

Hypercoagulability

Hypercoagulability is defined as an increased risk of thrombosis in circumstances that would not cause thrombosis in a normal person. Laboratory evaluation of an underlying hypercoagulable state is warranted in persons who have unexplained thrombotic episodes, which show one or more of the following:

- Recurrence
- Development at a young age
- Family history of thrombotic episodes
- Thrombosis in unusual anatomic locations
- Difficulty in controlling with anticoagulants

Hypercoagulable states are divided into inherited and acquired forms (Table 20-14).

TABLE *20-14* **Principal Causes of Hypercoagulability**

Inherited
Activated protein C resistance
Anti-thrombin III deficiency
Protein C deficiency
Protein S deficiency
Dysfibrinogenemias
Acquired
Lupus inhibitor
Malignancy
Nephrotic syndrome
Therapy
Factor concentrates
Heparin
Oral contraceptives
Hyperlipidemia
Thrombotic thrombocytopenic purpura

Inherited Hypercoagulability

Inherited hypercoagulable states are due to genetic mutations that affect one of the natural anticoagulant mechanisms (see Fig. 20-15). The hereditary tendency to develop thrombosis, irrespective of its origin, is referred to as *thrombophilia.*

Antithrombin III (ATIII) deficiency: This autosomal dominant disorder, which has incomplete penetrance, occurs in 0.2% to 0.4% of the general population, and can result in either a quantitative or qualitative effect on ATIII. The risk of a thrombotic event (usually venous) is variable, ranging between 20% and 80% in different families.

Protein C and protein S deficiencies: Homozygous protein C deficiency causes life-threatening neonatal thrombosis with purpura fulminans. Up to 0.5% of the general population has heterozygous protein C deficiency, but many of these persons are symptom-free. The clinical presentations for deficiencies of protein C and protein S are similar to that for ATIII deficiency.

Activated protein C (APC) resistance: A point mutation in the gene encoding factor V renders it resistant to the inhibitory effect of APC. APC resistance is the commonest known genetic disorder associated with hypercoagulability, and its prevalence in patients with venous thrombosis has been reported to be as high as 10% to 65%. In the general population, its prevalence is 3% to 7%, making it 10 times more common than any other genetic defect that predisposes to thrombosis. Compared to normal persons, the risk for deep venous thrombosis is increased 7-fold in heterozygotes and 80-fold in homozygotes.

Acquired Hypercoagulability

Venous stasis contributes to the hypercoagulability associated with prolonged immobilization and congestive cardiac failure. Increased platelet activation probably accounts for the tendency to clot in patients with myeloproliferative disorders, heparin-associated thrombocytopenia and thrombotic thrombocytopenic purpura.

Antiphospholipid antibodies are antibodies directed against several negatively charged phospholipids, which may be associated with the development of *antiphospholipid antibody syndrome.* This disorder features (1) thromboembolic events, (2) spontaneous abortions, and (3) thrombocytopenia.

The lupus anticoagulant (which is not restricted to patients with systemic lupus erythematosus) is an antiphospholipid antibody that results in the paradoxical prolongation of aPTT *in vitro* (due to phospholipid inhibition), but hypercoagulability *in vivo* (probably through platelet activation). The latter accounts for the frequent occurrence of arterial thrombosis and is the most common of the acquired blood protein defects causing thrombosis.

Neoplastic Disorders of the Blood and Lymphoid Organs

Neoplastic disorders of the hemopoietic and lymphopoietic systems are a complex group of malignancies that reflect the heterogeneity of cell differentiation and maturation of these cell compartments. The hemopoietic malignancies include (1) the chronic myeloproliferative syndromes, which reflect the retention of capacity for differentiation and maturation, or (2) the acute myelogenous leukemias, which represent the inability to differentiate beyond the blast cell stage.

The varied presentations of the neoplastic diseases of the lymphopoietic system reflect the stages of differentiation and activation of the B- and T-cell compartments of the lymphoid system. They generally manifest mass lesions involving lymph nodes or other tissue sites. A leukemic distribution with involvement of bone marrow and peripheral blood may occur secondarily. However, certain neoplastic disorders of lymphocytes initially present as leukemias, including chronic lymphocytic leukemia and acute lymphoblastic leukemia.

CHRONIC MYELOPROLIFERATIVE SYNDROMES

The chronic myeloproliferative syndromes comprise a group of interrelated neoplastic disorders of multipotential marrow stem cells, commonly associated with increased production of hemopoietic cells and elevations of peripheral blood counts. As a result, all cell lineages—erythroid, granulocytic, monocytic, and megakaryocytic—are involved. Four subtypes are recognized, each of which features a predominant cell lineage:

- **Polycythemia vera:** Erythroid cells
- **Chronic myelogenous leukemia:** Granulocytes
- **Idiopathic thrombocythemia:** Megakaryocytes
- **Myelofibrosis with myeloid metaplasia:** All hemopoietic cell lines plus reactive marrow fibrosis (myelofibrosis)

Polycythemia Vera

Polycythemia vera is a neoplastic disorder of multipotential hemopoietic stem cells that features clonal proliferation, differentiation, and maturation of all hemopoietic cells, but predominantly those of the erythroid cell lineage. **As a result, the total body erythrocyte mass is markedly increased.** The corresponding increase in blood viscosity predisposes to vascular thrombosis and hemorrhage.

The annual incidence of polycythemia vera in Western countries is 1 per 100,000. The disorder most commonly occurs in middle-aged and elderly persons, although it may develop at any age. There is a slight male predominance. Hereditary factors may play a role, since there is a modest increase in the incidence of polycythemia vera in families of patients with the disease.

☐ **Pathogenesis:** Polycythemia vera is thought to derive from the malignant transformation of a single multipotential hemopoietic stem cell with primary commitment to the erythroid lineage. Proliferation of the neoplastic clone occurs predominantly in the bone marrow but may involve such extramedullary sites as the spleen, lymph nodes, and liver (myeloid metaplasia).

The neoplastic erythroid progenitor cells of polycythemia vera are sensitive to erythropoietin, similar to their normal counterparts. In semisolid culture media, they form luxuriant clusters of erythroid cells (BFU-E) when exposed to erythropoietin. However, at the more mature colony-forming stage (CFU-E), the neoplastic cells may form erythroid colonies in semisolid culture media even in the absence of exogenous erythropoietin stimulation. **These autonomous erythroid colonies are called endogenous CFU-E and are characteristic of polycythemia vera during the entire course of the disease.** By contrast, CFU-E formation in normal erythroid progenitor cells is erythropoietin-dependent (exogenous CFU-E). The autonomous proliferation of the more mature cells confers a proliferative advantage to the neoplastic clones since the increased erythrocyte mass suppresses normal erythropoietin secretion and the function of the remaining normal progenitors. As a result, serum erythropoietin levels are either normal or decreased in polycythemia vera. By contrast, in secondary (functional) erythrocytoses, serum erythropoietin levels are increased.

☐ **Pathology:** The bone marrow is homogeneously red-purple. The spleen is moderately enlarged, and its cut surface is uniformly red-purple, with expansion of the red pulp and obliteration of the white pulp. The liver tends to be enlarged. The lymph nodes are of normal size or slightly enlarged, owing to myeloid metaplasia.

The principal morphological features in polycythemia vera are outlined in Table 20-15. The bone marrow is hypercellular, with hyperplasia of all elements. However, erythroid precursor cells predominate, and the myeloid:erythroid ratio is less than 2:1. Erythroid maturation is normal (normoblastic), unless there is superimposed iron deficiency, in which case the erythrocytes are hypochromic and microcytic. There is normal maturation of the granulocytic cell lineage. Megakaryocytes are typically increased and tend to be clustered. The megakaryocytes are enlarged, and their nuclei are hyperchromatic. In 90% of cases, marrow stainable iron is decreased or absent. A mild to moderate increase in reticulin fibrosis is common, and 10% of the cases ultimately progress to severe collagenous fibrosis.

The spleen exhibits a prominent accumulation of erythrocytes in the red pulp cords and sinuses. There may be myeloid metaplasia, with erythroid precursor cells, immature granulocytes, and megakaryocytes. The lymphoid white pulp is atrophic or obliterated. Myeloid metaplasia is also common in the sinusoids of the liver and in the sinuses and paracortex of the lymph nodes.

On the peripheral blood smear, the erythrocytes tend to appear normal, although hypochromia and microcytosis are observed if iron deficiency is present. Iron deficiency anemia is a characteristic feature of polycythemia vera because of (1) diversion of storage iron to the increased developing erythron, (2) loss of iron in the gastrointestinal tract as a complication of gastric and duodenal ulcers, and (3) therapeutic phlebotomy. If the disease has progressed to myeloid metaplasia of the spleen, the

TABLE 20-15 **The Chronic Myeloproliferative Syndromes: Morphological Features**

	Polycythemia Vera	Chronic Myelogenous Leukemia	Myelofibrosis with Myeloid Metaplasia	Idiopathic Thrombocythemia
Bone Marrow				
Histopathology	Panhyperplasia (predominantly erythroid)	Panhyperplasia (predominantly granulocytic)	Panhyperplasia with fibrosis	Atypical megakaryocytes predominate
M:E ratio	≤2:1	10:1 to 50:1	2:1 to 5:1	2:1 to 5:1
Marrow iron	↓ or absent	Normal or ↑	Normal or ↑	Normal to absent
Marrow fibrosis	15–20%	<10%	90–100%	<5%
Liver, Spleen				
Extramedullary hemopoiesis (myeloid metaplasia)	Moderate (predominantly erythroid)	Moderate to marked (predominantly granulocytic)	Moderate to marked	Slight (predominantly megakaryocytic)

erythrocytes exhibit marked anisocytosis and poikilocytosis, with characteristic teardrop forms.

The common initial laboratory findings are outlined in Table 20-16. The hemoglobin concentration may be greater than 20 g/dL and the hematocrit higher than 60%. The erythrocyte count is 6 to 10 million/μL. Serum iron is usually decreased, and the total iron binding capacity is increased. The arterial oxygen saturation is typically normal, thereby excluding a cardiopulmonary cause for the polycythemia.

All formed elements of the blood are usually increased in polycythemia vera. A mild to moderate leukocytosis of 10,000 to 25,000/μL occurs initially in two thirds of the cases, but on rare occasions neutrophil counts of more than 100,000/μL may be observed. A mild shift to the left in the granulocytic cell series, with circulating immature granulocytes, is common. Circulating basophils and eosinophils are also usually increased. A mild to moderate thrombocytosis (400,000 to 800,000 platelets/μL) occurs initially in half of the cases. Rarely, there is a marked thrombocytosis (>1 million platelets/μL). The platelets often exhibit abnormal morphological features, including giant and hypogranulated forms. Abnormal aggregation of platelets on exposure to ADP, epinephrine, and collagen is observed in many cases. The leukocyte alkaline phosphatase (LAP) score is normal in 30% of cases and increased in 70%. The LAP score is useful in distinguishing the subtypes of the chronic myeloproliferative syndromes (see Table 20-16). Hyperuricemia may be present and is related to rapid cell turnover.

☐ **Clinical Features:** The criteria for the diagnosis of polycythemia vera serve to distinguish this neoplastic disorder from reactive erythrocytosis. These include the following:

- An elevated erythrocyte mass (elevated hemoglobin and hematocrit)
- Splenomegaly
- Marrow panhyperplasia and clusters of atypical enlarged megakaryocytes with hyperchromatic nuclei
- Depletion of marrow iron stores
- Decreased serum erythropoietin

TABLE 20-16 **The Chronic Myeloproliferative Syndromes: Laboratory Features**

	Polycythemia Vera	Chronic Myelogenous Leukemia	Myelofibrosis with Myeloid Metaplasia	Idiopathic Thrombocythemia
Hemoglobin	>20 g/dL	Mild anemia	Mild anemia	Mild anemia
RBC morphology	Slight aniso- and poikilocytosis	Slight aniso- and poikilocytosis	Immature erythrocytes and marked aniso- and poikilocytosis	Hypochromic microcytes
Granulocytes	Normal to mildly increased, may show a few immature forms	Moderate to markedly increased with spectrum of maturation Basophilia	Normal to moderately increased with some immature WBC	Normal to slightly increased
Platelets	Normal to moderately increased	Normal to moderately increased	Increased to decreased	Markedly increased with abnormal forms
Leukocyte alkaline phosphatase (LAP)	Normal to increased	Decreased to absent	Variable	Variable
Cytogenetics	Nonspecific	Philadelphia chromosome (Ph^1) (>95%)	Nonspecific	Nonspecific

RBC, red blood cells; WBC, white blood cells.

The onset of polycythemia vera tends to be insidious, and the symptoms are generally nonspecific, typically relating to the increased erythrocyte mass. Plethora and splenomegaly are early findings. Headache, dizziness, and visual disturbances result from vascular disturbances in the brain and retina. Angina pectoris, secondary to disturbances of coronary artery blood flow, and intermittent claudication, caused by sluggish peripheral blood flow in the lower extremities, may be observed. Gastric or duodenal ulcers may result from circulatory problems in the gastrointestinal tract, and possibly (in part) from histamine release by basophils. Major thrombotic complications occur in a third of the cases, including cerebrovascular accidents and myocardial infarction. The clinical features of polycythemia vera are outlined in Table 20-17.

The clinical course of polycythemia vera proceeds as a series of phases:

- **Proliferative phase:** Most patients experience a prolonged proliferative phase, which is dominated by erythroid proliferation and an increased erythrocyte mass. This phase often persists unchanged until the patient succumbs to complications or dies of extraneous causes. In one third of patients, the disease progresses to other stages.
- **Spent phase:** In 10% of cases, the excessive proliferation of erythroid cells ceases, resulting in a stable or decreased erythrocyte mass.
- **Postpolycythemic myelofibrosis with myeloid metaplasia:** An additional 10% of cases show progression to myelofibrosis, which is similar to that observed in other chronic myeloproliferative syndromes. Such patients display (1) progressively severe anemia; (2) increasing splenomegaly, owing to myeloid metaplasia; (3) a peripheral blood leukoerythroblastic reaction, with circulating immature erythroid and granulocytic cells and poikilocytosis and anisocytosis of erythrocytes; and (4) severe myelofibrosis, with depletion of hemopoietic cells. At this stage, the prognosis is poor, with a mean survival of only 2 years.
- **Acute myelogenous leukemia:** Acute myelogenous leukemia (AML) develops in 5% to 10% of cases of polycythemia vera. The risk of progression to AML appears to be increased if there has been prior treatment with ^{32}P or alkylating agents. However, it may also reflect the natural history of the disease, with treated patients surviving longer.

The median survival in polycythemia vera is 13 years, and the most common causes of death are those associated with old age. Specific causes of death related to the disease itself include thrombosis, hemorrhage, acute myelogenous leukemia, and the spent phase. Therapeutic reduction of the erythrocyte mass, either by repeated phlebotomy or by drug therapy, constitutes effective management in most cases.

Chronic Myelogenous Leukemia

Chronic myelogenous leukemia (CML) is a neoplastic disorder of multipotential hemopoietic stem cells that principally involves the granulocytic cell lineage. Accordingly, monoclonality has been demonstrated in other lineages, including lymphoid cells. Patients with CML display pronounced granulocytosis and immaturity of granulocytic elements, anemia, thrombocytosis, basophilia, and splenomegaly. CML constitutes 20% of all the leukemias in Western countries. The disorder is most common in middle-aged and elderly adults, with a median age at onset of 50 years, although it may occur at any age. There is a slight male predominance. No difference in ethnic susceptibility is observed.

☐ **Pathogenesis:** The etiology of CML is not known. Survivors of the atomic bomb explosions in Japan suffered an increased incidence of CML after a latent period of 3 years, the peak incidence occurring at 7 years. British patients who had been treated with spinal irradiation for ankylosing spondylitis also displayed an increased incidence of CML after a latent period of 13 years. Nevertheless, a history of exposure to radiation is elicited in less than 5% of cases of CML. Myelotoxic agents such as benzene are involved in a small minority of cases.

Chronic myelogenous leukemia is thought to derive from the malignant transformation of a single hemopoietic stem cell that has a principal commitment to the granulocytic cell lineage. In some cases, however, neoplastic transformation may occur in a pluripotential stem cell, since the Philadelphia (Ph^1) chromosome and restricted isoenzymes of G6PD have also been identified in the B lymphocytes of some patients with CML.

In more than 90% of cases of CML, the Ph^1 chromosome can be demonstrated in the karyotype (see Chapter

TABLE *20-17* **The Chronic Myeloproliferative Syndromes: Clinical Features**

	Polycythemia Vera	Chronic Myelogenous Leukemia	Myelofibrosis with Myeloid Metaplasia	Idiopathic Thrombocythemia
Male : female	1.2:1	3:2	1:1	1.2:1
Peak age range (years)	40–60	25–60	50–70	50–70
Clinical symptoms	Headache, dizziness, pruritus	Asymptomatic or LUQ discomfort, fatigability	Asymptomatic or LUQ discomfort, fatigability	Asymptomatic or LUQ discomfort
Splenomegaly	75%	90%	100%	30% (slight)
Hepatomegaly	40%	50%	80%	40% (slight)
Acute leukemic conversion	5–10%	80%	5–10%	2–5%
Median survival (years)	13	3–4	5	>10

LUQ, left upper quadrant.

5). This chromosome represents a balanced, reciprocal translocation of a portion of chromosome 9 to chromosome 22 [t(9:22)(q34:q11)]. As a result, the protooncogene c-*abl* on chromosome 9 is translocated to a site on chromosome 22 known as the breakpoint cluster region (*bcr*). A hybrid gene sequence (*bcr-abl*) is formed that encodes a unique, fusion protein (P210) with enhanced tyrosine kinase activity. P210 is thought to be important in the genesis of CML, perhaps conferring a growth advantage to the neoplastic clone. The importance of P210 in the pathogenesis of CML is supported by the production of a similar disease in mice transfected with a *bcr-abl* construct. Five percent of all cases of CML are characterized by variant Ph translocations, but the clinicopathological features in such patients are indistinguishable from those with the classic Ph^1 chromosome. **CML results in a 10- to 100-fold expansion of the total body granulocyte cell pool.**

☐ **Pathology:** The proliferation and expansion of neoplastic hemopoietic cells in CML occur primarily in the bone marrow and secondarily in the spleen. Extramedullary proliferation (myeloid metaplasia) may also be identified in sites such as the liver and the lymph nodes.

On gross examination, the bone marrow in CML is homogeneously red-purple. The spleen is enlarged, often to massive proportions. Splenic infarction is common, and the surface of the organ may display fibrinous perisplenitis. The cut surface of the spleen is uniformly red-purple, with marked expansion of the red pulp and obliteration of the white pulp. The liver is moderately enlarged. The lymph nodes usually appear normal, but they may be mildly enlarged, especially in blast crisis (see later).

Microscopically, the bone marrow is conspicuously hypercellular, owing to hyperplasia of all three lineages (Fig. 20-45). Granulocytic precursor cells predominate, and the myeloid:erythroid ratio is markedly increased. The absolute number of erythroid precursor cells is moderately increased. Megakaryocytes are typically numerous. However, the cohesive clustering and morphological atypia of the neoplastic megakaryocytes characteristic of the other chronic myeloproliferative syndromes may be inconspicuous in CML. A small minority of cases of CML display a mild reticulin fibrosis of the bone marrow, but progression to severe collagenous fibrosis is distinctly uncommon. Occasionally, macrophages with prominent pale cytoplasm, containing abundant sphingoglycolipid derived from the increased granulocytic cell turnover, simulate Gaucher cells. The principal morphological features of CML are outlined in Table 20-15.

In Wright-stained aspirates of bone marrow, the normal proportions of maturing granulocytic cells are observed. Myeloblasts and promyelocytes together constitute less than 10% of the total nucleated cell population. Basophils and eosinophils are typically increased, whereas erythroid precursor cells are relatively decreased. Megakaryocytes are numerous. The hemopoietic cells tend not to be dyspoietic.

The features on peripheral blood smears are similar to those of marrow aspirates, and the entire spectrum of maturing granulocytic cells is observed. **Indeed, the diagnosis of CML is made essentially on examination of a peripheral blood smear, in which granulocytes in all stages of maturation are predominant**. Mature granulocytes and myelocytes constitute the predominant cell types, and circulating basophils are increased. Less commonly eosinophils are also increased.

The spleen exhibits prominent myeloid metaplasia in the red pulp cords and less prominently in the sinusoids. Maturing hemopoietic precursor cells, principally of the granulocytic lineage, are observed. The lymphoid white pulp is generally obliterated.

In the liver, foci of myeloid metaplasia in the sinusoids are common. Myeloid metaplasia in the lymph nodes initially involves the sinuses and the paracortex and may progress to complete obliteration of the nodal architecture.

With the invariable progression to blast crisis, there is a loss of differentiation and maturation capacity of the

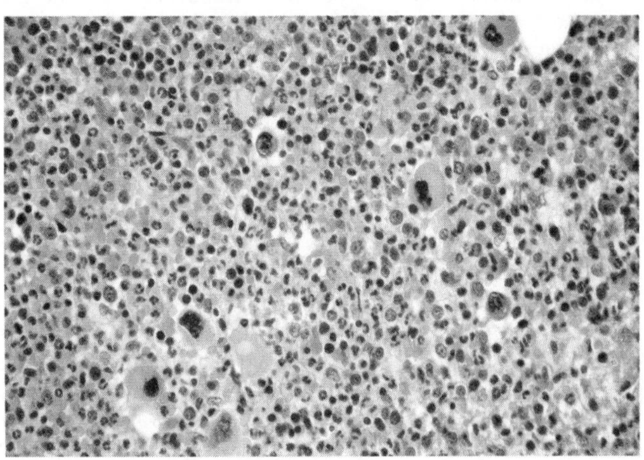

A

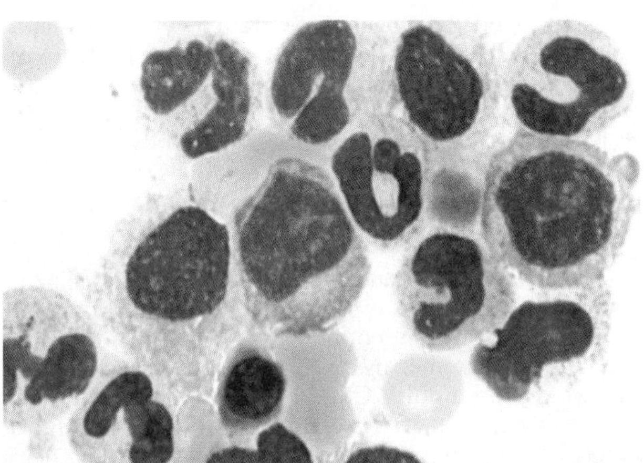

B

FIGURE *20-45*
Chronic myelogenous leukemia. (*A*) The bone marrow is conspicuously hypercellular, owing to an increase in granulocyte precursors, mature granulocytes, and megakaryocytes. (*B*) A smear of the bone marrow aspirate from the same patient reveals numerous granulocytes at various stages of development.

granulocytic precursor cells. If the initial neoplastic transformation has occurred in a pluripotential stem cell, the blast cell immunological phenotype may be either nonlymphopoietic (myeloid) or lymphopoietic. Medullary and extramedullary accumulation of primitive blast cells occurs. In a blast crisis, the initial focal infiltration of the marrow by primitive blast cells progresses to effacement of the marrow architecture. Given their pluripotential stem cell origin, the blast cells may have the morphological features of any of the subtypes of acute leukemia. Indeed, 70% are myeloblastic and 30% are lymphoblastic. Some are of mixed myeloid and lymphoid lineage. Additional cytogenetic abnormalities are common in blast crisis and include a second Ph^1 chromosome, isochromosome 17, and trisomies 8 and 19. Destructive tumor masses consisting of myeloblasts and promyelocytes *(granulocytic sarcomas or chloromas)* may occur in such sites as lymph nodes, bones, and meninges.

The common laboratory findings in early CML are outlined in Table 20-16. They include (1) a peripheral blood leukocytosis of 20,000 to 400,000/μL (mean, 200,000/μL), with the characteristic granulocytic lineage spectrum; (2) frequent basophilia; (3) mild normocytic and normochromic anemia; and (4) mild thrombocytosis of 400,000 to 800,000 platelets/μL in one third of the cases. Less commonly there is a marked thrombocytosis (>1 million platelets/μL). There may be abnormalities of platelet morphology (hypogranulation and large platelets), which are accompanied by abnormal platelet aggregation on exposure to ADP, epinephrine, or collagen. The LAP score is decreased to zero in most cases of CML, although it may increase with infection, remission, pregnancy, splenectomy, and blast crisis. The levels of uric acid in the serum and urine tend to be increased, owing to the turnover of leukemic cells and consequent increased production of purines. Elevated serum vitamin B_{12} levels and increased vitamin B_{12}–binding capacity are also due to increased granulocytic cell turnover.

☐ **Clinical Features:** The diagnosis of CML is established by the following findings:

- A sustained peripheral blood granulocytic leukocytosis (>20,000/μL) that involves the entire spectrum of maturing granulocytic cells (myeloblast to polymorphonuclear leukocyte)
- Trilineage hyperplasia of the bone marrow, with predominance of the granulocytic cell lineage
- A decreased LAP score
- The Ph^1 chromosome

The onset of CML tends to be insidious. In fact, the diagnosis in some cases is first suggested by abnormal findings in a blood cell count done for other reasons or by the detection of splenomegaly on a routine physical examination. More commonly, CML begins with nonspecific symptoms, including fatigue, malaise, and exercise intolerance. Fever, sweating, tremor, and weight loss reflect hypermetabolism. Symptoms due to splenomegaly include early satiety and left upper quadrant discomfort. Hemorrhagic manifestations may be caused by thrombocytopenia or qualitative platelet defects. Thrombosis may occur secondary to thrombocytosis. The clinical course of CML is characterized by an initially stable phase of 2 to 8 years or even longer (mean 3 to 4 years). During this period, the disorder is usually well tolerated. The salient clinical features of CML are outlined in Table 20-17.

In most cases of CML, the chronic stable phase is terminated by blast crisis, either abruptly or after an accelerated phase. The accelerated phase is characterized by increasing or decreasing leukocyte and platelet counts, progressive basophilia and eosinophilia, and increasing splenomegaly. Fever, weight loss, and other signs and symptoms of hypermetabolism are common. Blast crisis shows rapidly increasing blast cell counts in the marrow and peripheral blood, and progressive anemia and thrombocytopenia. The mean survival in blast crisis is measured in months. The treatment of choice for CML is bone marrow transplantation, chemotherapy, and the administration of interferon α to suppress the proliferation of hemopoietic progenitor cells.

Myelofibrosis with Myeloid Metaplasia

Myelofibrosis with myeloid metaplasia (MMM), originally termed agnogenic myeloid metaplasia, refers to neoplastic proliferation of multipotential hemopoietic stem cells in which the proliferation of all hemopoietic cell lineages stimulates a reactive fibrosis of the bone marrow. Myeloid metaplasia involves the sites of extramedullary hemopoiesis normally restricted to the fetus, principally the spleen, liver, and lymph nodes. Abnormally shaped erythrocytes abound in the peripheral blood, and circulating immature erythroid and granulocytic cells (leukoerythroblastic reaction) are typical.

Myelofibrosis with myeloid metaplasia is an uncommon disorder, with an annual incidence of 0.4 per 100,000 population. The disease usually afflicts middle-aged and elderly adults, the median age at onset being 60 years. There is no sex preference or differences in ethnic susceptibility.

☐ **Pathogenesis:** As the name indicates, the etiology of MMM is not known. In rare cases, prior bone marrow damage secondary to irradiation or to myelotoxic agents such as benzene has been documented. One third of cases of polycythemia vera, and a lesser proportion of chronic myelogenous leukemia, progress to a condition indistinguishable from MMM.

Myelofibrosis with myeloid metaplasia is a clonal disorder, which is thought to derive from the malignant transformation of a single multipotential hemopoietic stem cell that has no selective commitment to any particular hemopoietic cell lineage. The neoplastic cells proliferate primarily in the bone marrow. From that site, the progenitor cells gain access to the peripheral blood and hence to the tissues, where they proliferate and differentiate as foci of myeloid metaplasia. **Fibrosis of the bone marrow is thought to be reactive rather than neoplastic because the marrow fibroblasts are polyclonal and the proliferation of clonal hemopoietic cells may occur before the onset of myelofibrosis.** Myelofibrosis is attributed to the secretion of growth factors contained in the granules of megakaryocytes or platelets, including platelet-derived growth factor (PDGF) and transforming growth factor-beta (TGF-β), which stimulate fibroblasts to secrete collagen. The secretion of platelet factor 4, which inhibits collagenase, has also been suggested as a possible contributor to marrow fibrosis.

☐ **Pathology:** In the early hypercellular phase of MMM, the bone marrow is grossly a homogeneous red-brown color. With progression to myelofibrosis, the marrow becomes gray-white. At the time of presentation, the spleen is mildly or moderately enlarged in 75% of cases. Massive enlargement is noted in one fourth of the cases, with some splenic weights exceeding 4000 g. Splenomegaly reflects myeloid metaplasia, erythrocyte pooling, and fibrosis. Infarcts are common in the enlarged spleen and are covered by a fibrinous perisplenitis. On cut surface, the spleen shows marked expansion of the red pulp and obliteration of the white pulp. The liver is also moderately enlarged.

The bone marrow is difficult to aspirate because of myelofibrosis, and evaluation of the marrow is usually performed on sections of biopsies or clots, rather than on aspirates. The marrow is often hypercellular, with decreased or even absent fat cells. Less commonly, it is normocellular, and on occasion it is even hypocellular. Regardless of the degree of cellularity, the granulocytic and megakaryocytic cell lineages predominate, and the erythroid cell series is relatively, although not absolutely, decreased. As in all chronic myeloproliferative syndromes, basophils and eosinophils are frequently increased.

Although cells of the granulocytic series show normal maturation, mild dyspoietic features may be present, including nuclear lobe hyposegmentation or hypersegmentation, nuclear-cytoplasmic asynchrony, and cytoplasmic hypogranulation. Megakaryocytes are increased and tend to be distributed in characteristic cohesive clusters of more than five cells. Dyspoietic features of megakaryocytes include mononuclear or small forms (micromegakaryocytes) and large forms with bizarre hyperchromatic nuclei. Megaloblastoid change and hyperchromatic, irregular, or fragmented nuclei are dyspoietic features in erythroid precursor cells.

Myelofibrosis commonly involves the central flat bones and proximal long bones. Biopsy specimens demonstrate a moderate to marked increase in reticulin fibers, which progresses to collagenous fibrosis (Fig. 20-46). Because of the myelofibrosis, the marrow vascular sinusoids are distended with blood and hemopoietic cells. Thickening of bony trabeculae (osteosclerosis), owing to new bone formation, is a late complication.

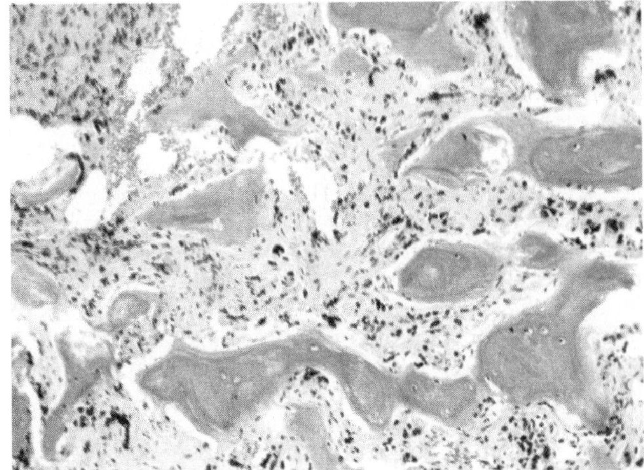

FIGURE *20-46*
Myelofibrosis with myeloid metaplasia. A section of bone marrow shows collagenous fibrosis, osteosclerosis, and numerous abnormal megakaryocytes.

The spleen exhibits prominent myeloid metaplasia of the red pulp sinusoids and less prominently of the cords, with infiltration by and proliferation of all hemopoietic cell lineages. The white pulp is atrophic. Myeloid metaplasia involving the sinusoids of the liver is frequently observed.

A smear of peripheral blood discloses a leukoerythroblastic reaction, with circulating immature erythroid and granulocytic cells and giant platelets. The erythrocytes exhibit pronounced anisocytosis and poikilocytosis. Teardrop-shaped erythrocytes (dacryocytes) are a characteristic finding in MMM and result from damage to or inadequate conditioning of erythrocyte membranes in the spleen. The principal morphological findings in MMM are outlined in Table 20-15.

The common initial laboratory findings in MMM are outlined in Table 20-16. The LAP score is low in 25% of cases, normal in 50%, and increased in 25%. The levels of serum uric acid, vitamin B_{12}, and vitamin B_{12}–binding protein may be elevated. Chromosomal aberrations are found in half of the cases but are nonspecific and are of no prognostic significance.

☐ **Clinical Features:** The diagnosis of MMM is established by the following:

- Trilineage hyperplasia in the bone marrow, with clustering of atypical megakaryocytes
- Myelofibrosis and/or osteosclerosis
- Conspicuous splenomegaly
- Pronounced morphological changes of erythrocytes (particularly teardrop forms)
- Leukoerythroblastic peripheral blood smear

Since the proliferative lesion in MMM involves particularly the granulocytic and megakaryocytic lineages, there is initially a mild peripheral blood granulocytosis and thrombocytosis. Anemia is common even early in the course of the disease. The anemia is multifactorial and due to ineffective erythropoiesis, erythrocyte pooling in the enlarged spleen, and a shortened erythrocyte survival (hemolysis).

The onset of MMM tends to be insidious. Nonspecific symptoms include fatigue, malaise, weight loss, and exercise intolerance. Left upper quadrant discomfort and early satiety with meals reflect splenomegaly. The clinical features of MMM are outlined in Table 20-17.

The clinical course in MMM is characterized by (1) progressively severe anemia, with gradually increasing transfusion requirements, (2) leukopenia with infections, and (3) thrombocytopenia with hemorrhages. The median survival in MMM is 5 years, the usual causes of death being infection and hemorrhage. Superimposed acute myelogenous leukemia occurs in 5% to 10% of cases, in which case the mean survival is only 2 to 3 months.

The treatment of MMM is variable and includes chemotherapy, splenic irradiation, or splenectomy. Although splenectomy may decrease transfusion requirements and prolong survival, it may also dramatically increase the platelet count, necessitating chemotherapeutic intervention. Alternatively, it may worsen the situation by removing an important source of hemopoiesis. Bone marrow transplantation is a promising therapy and in some patients has resulted in resolution of myelofibrosis and return of hemopoiesis to normal.

Primary Thrombocythemia

Primary thrombocythemia is an uncommon neoplastic disorder of multipotential hemopoietic stem cells, which is expressed as an uncontrolled proliferation of megakaryocytes. A marked increase in circulating platelets is accompanied by recurrent episodes of thrombosis and hemorrhage. The disease affects middle-aged persons. There is a slight male predominance.

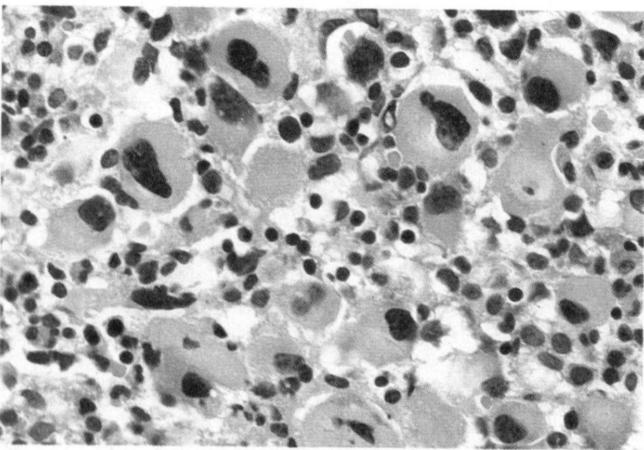

FIGURE *20-47*
Primary thrombocythemia. A section of bone marrow shows a conspicuous increase in the number of megakaryocytes, which exhibit atypical features and hypolobated forms.

☐ **Pathogenesis:** Thrombocythemia is a clonal disorder that is believed to derive from the malignant transformation of a single multipotential hemopoietic stem cell. The principal but not exclusive developmental commitment of this cell is to the megakaryocytic lineage.

Primary thrombocythemia features a marked proliferation of megakaryocytes, with up to a 15-fold or greater increase in platelet production. Megakaryocyte colony-forming units (CFU-Mega) are increased in number and have the capacity to proliferate autonomously without the addition of specific growth factors. In some cases, BFU-E are also increased, a finding that may explain some features that overlap polycythemia vera. However, unlike the latter disease, the erythrocyte mass in thrombocythemia is not increased.

Abnormalities of platelet function are common in primary thrombocythemia. Recurrent episodes of thrombosis are attributed to severe thrombocytosis and hemorrhage owing to defects in platelet function. Iron deficiency anemia reflects hemorrhages from the gastrointestinal and urogenital tracts.

Thrombosis may occur in any organ or tissue and may involve arteries or veins. Thromboses in the spleen, with consequent infarctions, may result in splenic atrophy. In turn, this effect reduces the size of the principal sequestration site for the increased blood platelet pool. The consequent enhancement of thrombocytosis worsens the prognosis. Similarly, splenectomy is generally contraindicated because it produces a marked increase in the platelet count.

☐ **Pathology:** The spleen is mildly enlarged in 50% of cases of primary thrombocythemia. The cut surface of the spleen is homogeneously red-purple, with expansion of the red pulp and atrophy of the white pulp.

The bone marrow is markedly hypercellular, with a decreased number of fat cells and increased megakaryocytes. Less commonly, hyperplasia of all three hemopoietic cell lineages occurs, but the megakaryocytic lineage predominates (Fig. 20-47). Megakaryocytes are distributed in cohesive clusters or sheets and exhibit atypical morphological features. These include forms with large, bizarre, hyperchromatic and hyperlobulated nuclei and abundant cytoplasm, as well as smaller micromegakaryocytic forms. Large clusters of free platelets are a characteristic finding. Reticulin fibers in the marrow are increased in one third of the cases, but overt fibrosis is rare. Iron stores are normal or decreased.

The spleen often displays myeloid metaplasia of the sinusoids of the red pulp and less prominently of the cords. Myeloid metaplasia of the hepatic sinusoids and of the lymph nodes is occasionally observed. The principal morphological findings in primary thrombocythemia are summarized in Table 20-15.

The common findings in the peripheral blood in primary thrombocythemia are outlined in Table 20-16 and include the following:

- A markedly increased platelet count (1 to 3 million/μL or more)
- Abnormal platelet morphology (microthrombocytes, macrothrombocytes, bizarre shapes, and megakaryocyte fragments)
- Mild hypochromic microcytic anemia
- Neutrophilic leukocytosis ($>$10,000/μL)

The LAP score is usually normal. The serum vitamin B_{12} or vitamin B_{12}–binding protein levels may be elevated. Nonspecific cytogenetic abnormalities, most commonly aneuploidy, are demonstrated in 20% of cases.

☐ **Clinical Features:** The clinical course of primary thrombocythemia is protracted, with a median survival of over 10 years. In untreated cases, thrombosis of large arteries and veins is a common complication, with the arteries of the lower extremities, heart, intestine, and kidneys being most frequently affected. Hemorrhage is usually mild and not life threatening. Acute myelogenous leukemia supervenes in 2% to 5% of the cases, the neoplastic blast cells being either of granulocytic or megakaryocytic lineage. The acute leukemia is aggressive, with a mean survival of only 2 months. In a small minority of patients, primary thrombocythemia becomes transformed into another chronic myeloproliferative syndrome. The clinical features of primary thrombocythemia are listed in Table 20-17. The disease is treated with plateletpheresis and myelosuppressive chemotherapy.

The myelodysplastic syndromes comprise a group of neoplastic disorders of hemopoietic stem cells, which are associated with ineffective hemopoiesis. The subject has been discussed in the section on anemias.

ACUTE MYELOGENOUS LEUKEMIAS

The acute myelogenous leukemias (AML) comprise a heterogeneous group of interrelated disorders in which neoplastic transformation occurs in a hemopoietic stem cell or in one of restricted lineage potential. Because these stem cells give rise to granulocytes, monocytes, erythrocytes, and megakaryocytes, any or all of these cell lineages may be affected in a specific case of AML. In general, the neoplastic clone fails to mature beyond the blast cell stage, leading to a progressive accumulation of myeloblasts in the bone marrow. By definition, in AML, more than 30% of the bone marrow aspirate nucleated cells consist of blasts.

☐ **Epidemiology:** AML constitutes 20% of all the leukemias in Western countries, the large majority occurring in adults. Whereas AML accounts for 20% of the acute leukemias in childhood, it is responsible for 85% of cases in adults. The incidence steadily increases after middle age. AML in the elderly appears to be increasing in frequency. The incidence is slightly greater in males than in females and is comparable in whites and blacks.

☐ **Pathogenesis:** The etiology of AML is not known. The risk factors include the following:

- **Myelotoxic agents:** The most important are benzene and the antineoplastic drugs (alkylating agents and epipodophyllotoxins).
- **Radiation:** In doses exceeding 100 rad (or cGy), there is a linear relationship between ionizing radiation dose and the development of AML.
- **Genetic abnormalities:** Trisomy 21 (Down syndrome) is characterized by an increased incidence of AML, although most cases of leukemia in this syndrome are acute lymphoblastic leukemia. In the chromosomal instability syndromes (Bloom syndrome, Fanconi anemia, ataxia telangiectasia), there is a small, but significant, increased risk for AML.
- **Hematological disorders:** Many "chronic" clonal hematological disorders, such as myeloproliferative syndromes, myelodysplastic syndromes, aplastic anemia, and paroxysmal nocturnal hemoglobinuria, carry an increased risk for AML.

Superimposed AML may constitute the terminal event in any of the chronic myeloproliferative syndromes. This is particularly important in chronic myelogenous leukemia, in which superimposed AML (blast crisis) occurs in 80% of cases. AML supervenes in 30% to 50% of cases of myelodysplastic syndromes, particularly when there are abnormalities of all three hemopoietic cell lineages and a peripheral blood pancytopenia. The risk of AML in myelodysplastic syndromes is dependent on the specific French-American-British (FAB) subtype of the latter (see above).

Cytogenetic abnormalities in the leukemic cells are demonstrated in most cases of AML. There are nonrandom chromosomal translocations in AML that are characteristic of specific FAB morphological subtypes and have prognostic relevance. For example, in M2 AML, t(8;21) is common and is associated with a favorable prognosis, as is the inv(16) of M4E0. In AML superimposed on a prior myelodysplastic syndrome, or following marrow damage produced by chemotherapy or radiation therapy, deletions of the long arm of chromosomes 5 and 7 and trisomy 8 are common.

In the M3 (acute promyelocytic) subtype, t(15;17) is invariably demonstrated, a translocation that results in the rearrangement of the gene for the retinoic acid receptor (RAR-α). The fusion gene (PML/RAR-α) encodes a truncated receptor, which does not bind retinoic acid efficiently, thereby interfering with cellular differentiation. Interestingly, the administration of large doses of a retinoic acid is clinically effective in the treatment of patients with promyelocytic leukemia.

The major problems associated with AML principally relate to the progressive accumulation in the marrow of immature myelogenous cells that lack the potential for further differentiation and maturation. Whereas leukemic myeloblasts replicate at a slower rate than do normal hemopoietic precursor cells, the frequency of spontaneous cell death is less than normal The expanded pool of abnormal leukemic blasts encroaches on the normal marrow and suppresses normal hemopoiesis. As a consequence, the major clinical problems in AML are granulocytopenia, thrombocytopenia, and anemia.

☐ **Pathology:** Nine variants of AML are recognized, reflecting the predominant lineage commitment of the neoplastic stem cells. The neoplastic blast cells of AML are identified with Wright's stain in peripheral blood and bone marrow aspirates and are classified according to cytological criteria proposed by the FAB group (Fig. 20-48). The most common subtypes are M2 and M4. The clinical presentations and natural histories of the AML subtypes are in general similar. However, there are clinicopathological features characteristic of specific FAB subtypes.

M0—MINIMALLY DIFFERENTIATED AML: The blasts, which may resemble lymphoblasts morphologically, are negative for the usual cytochemical stains that identify AML (myeloperoxidase and Sudan black B). Granules or Auer rods (see later) are absent. The diagnosis requires immunophenotypic analysis by flow cytometry to demonstrate the expression of myeloid antigens (e.g., CD13, CD33).

M1—AML WITHOUT MATURATION: The blast cells have round to oval nuclei and finely reticulated chromatin, usually two or more nucleoli, and scant to moderate, gray-blue, variably granular cytoplasm. Auer rods (azurophilic, rod-shaped, cytoplasmic inclusions) represent aberrant primary lysosomes and are observed in up

MORPHOLOGY	CLASSIFICATION	NUCLEUS	NUCLEOLUS	CHROMATIN	CYTOPLASM
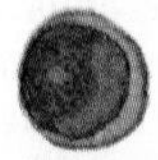	L1 ACUTE LYMPHOBLASTIC (principally pediatric)	Uniformly round, small	Single, indistinct	Slightly reticulated with perinucleolar clumping	Scant, blue
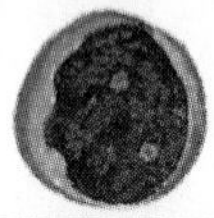	L2 LYMPHOBLASTIC (principally adult)	Irregular	Single to several, indistinct	Fine	Moderate, pale
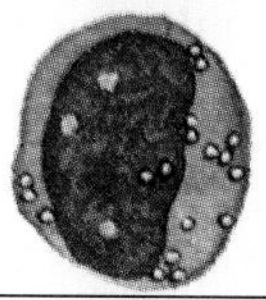	L3 BURKITT-TYPE	Round to oval	Two to five	Coarse with clear parachromatin	Moderate blue, prominently vacuolated
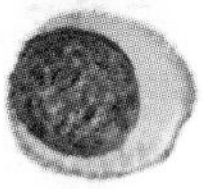	M0 MYELOBLASTIC (minimally differentiated)	Round to oval	Single to multiple, distinct	Fine to coarse	Scant, non-granulated
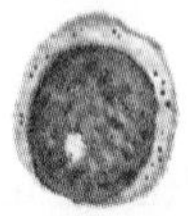	M1 MYELOBLASTIC (without maturation)	Round to oval	Single to multiple, distinct	Fine	Scant, variably granulated
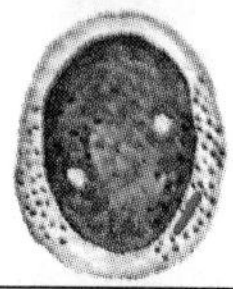	M2 MYELOBLASTIC (with maturation)	Round to oval	Single to multiple, distinct	Fine	Moderate azurophilic granules with or without Auer rods
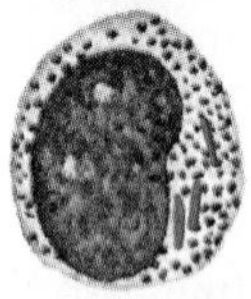	M3 MYELOCYTIC	Round to indented to lobed, "cottage-loaf"	Single to multiple, (granules may obscure)	Fine	Prominent azurophilic granules and/or multiple Auer rods
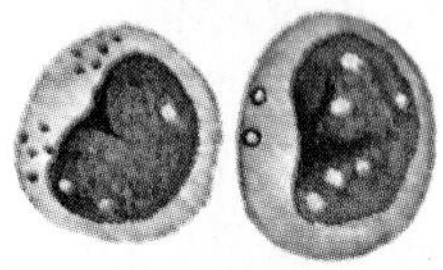	M4 MYELOMONOBLASTIC (biphasic M1 and M5)	Round to indented, folded	Single to multiple, distinct	Fine	Moderate, blue to gray, may be granulated
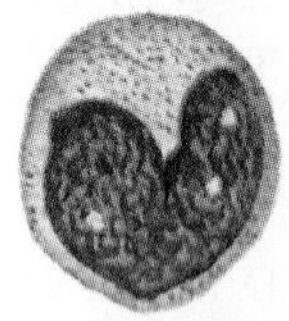	M5 MONOBLASTIC	Round to indented, folded	Single to multiple, distinct	Variable, lacy or ropy	Scant to moderate, gray-blue, dustlike lavender granules
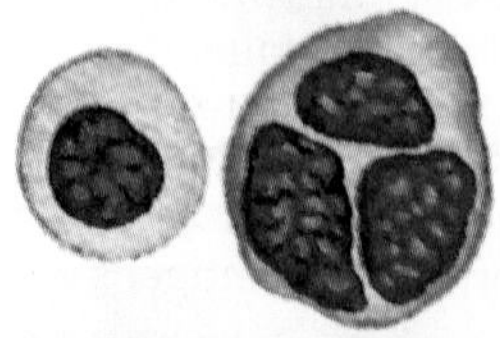	M6 ERYTHROBLASTIC	Single to bizarre multinucleated, multilobed	Single to multiple, distinct	Open "megaloblastoid"	Abundant, red to blue
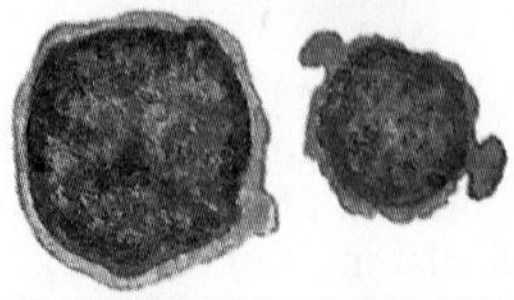	M7 MEGAKARYOBLASTIC	Round to oval	Single to multiple, distinct	Slightly to moderately reticulated	Scant to moderate, gray-blue, with blebbing

FIGURE 20-48
Acute leukemia: FAB classification.

to 10% of cases in any variant of AML except M6 (see Fig. 20-48).

M2—AML WITH MATURATION: A variable proportion of the blast cells have delicate, pink-purple (azurophilic) cytoplasmic granules, which represent primary lysosomes. More than 10% of the cells show evidence of myeloid maturation, from promyelocytes to mature neutrophils.

M3—PROMYELOCYTIC LEUKEMIA: Abundant cytoplasmic azurophilic granules, with or without numerous Auer rods, are characteristic of the M3 (acute promyelocytic) variant (Fig. 20-49). In M3 AML, a bleeding diathesis is secondary to the development of disseminated intravascular coagulation, possibly because of the release of cytoplasmic granules or Auer rods, which have tissue factor-like activity. The associated translocation, t(15;17), disrupts one of the retinoic acid receptor genes.

M4—MYELOMONOBLASTIC LEUKEMIA: Both myeloblasts (M1 and M2) and monoblasts are observed in M4 AML. Monocytic differentiation is suggested by indentation or lobation of the nucleus and a coarse or ropy chromatin. M4 is the most common variant of AML, accounting for one quarter of the cases. Of these, 25% are associated with abnormal eosinophils (M4E0).

M5—MONOBLASTIC LEUKEMIA: Acute monoblastic leukemia is characterized by prominent infiltration of soft tissue sites, such as the gingiva, skin, and central nervous system. Elevation of serum or urine lysozyme (muramidase) levels is a common finding in acute monocytic leukemia, since the lysosomes of leukemic monocytes contain abundant lysozyme. The FAB classification recognizes two variants of monocytic leukemia: primitive monoblastic (M5a) and more mature monocytic (M5b).

M6—ERYTHROBLASTIC LEUKEMIA: This variant is suggested by bizarre erythroblasts that display (1) single to multiple nuclei, (2) irregularly distributed and open (megaloblastoid) nuclear chromatin, and (3) variable cytoplasmic hemoglobinization, which imparts a pink color. In erythroleukemia, there are more than 50% marrow erythroblasts and 30% or more myeloblasts. Typically, the disease progresses to a state characterized by a predominance of myeloblasts. A rare, more chronic, form of this disease displays pure erythroblasts (M6b) and is referred to as *erythremic myelosis or diGuglielmo syndrome*.

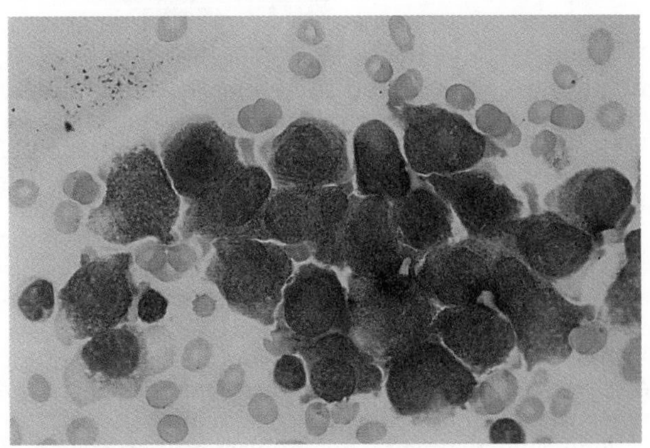

FIGURE *20-49*
Acute promyelocytic leukemia (M3). A bone marrow aspirate shows numerous hypergranular promyelocytes with irregular nuclei. The leukemic promyelocyte in the center of the top row of cells contains numerous Auer rods.

M7—ACUTE MEGAKARYOCYTIC LEUKEMIA: The blast cells range from small to large and show coarse chromatin, gray cytoplasm, and frequent budding of the cytoplasmic margins. Acute megakaryocytic leukemia presents as an aggressive, but otherwise typical, variant of AML. Immunophenotypic analysis is necessary for the diagnosis of M7 to show the expression of platelet-associated glycoproteins GPIIb/IIIa (CD41/61) or GPIb/IX (CD42). In addition, ultrastructural cytochemistry is advisable to demonstrate platelet peroxidase activity.

Acute myelofibrosis is an uncommon, rapidly fatal M7 variant, which is characterized by pancytopenia, hyperplasia of all marrow cell lines (panhyperplasia), conspicuous marrow fibrosis, absence of splenomegaly, and a rapid progression to acute megakaryocytic or myelogenous leukemia.

Although there may be morphological clues to the diagnosis of AML (Auer rods being the only definitive one), specific cytochemical stains (Fig. 20-50) are required to distinguish AML from ALL and to identify certain subtypes with monocytic differentiation, such as M4 and M5. Immunophenotypic (marker) studies are useful in the diagnosis of all FAB types, but they are essential for M0 and M7. Demonstration of the nuclear DNA-polymerizing enzyme, terminal deoxynucleotidyl transferase (Tdt), suggests a lymphoid origin (more than 90% Tdt positive) rather than a myelogenous one (5% to 10% Tdt positive).

Dyspoiesis (i.e., morphological abnormalities of residual maturing granulocytic, erythroid, and megakaryocytic precursor cells) is characteristic of AML and typically lacking in ALL. These morphological abnormalities in AML include (1) granulocytes with cytoplasmic hypogranulation and hyposegmentation of nuclear lobes (acquired Pelger-Huet anomaly); (2) erythroid cells with megaloblastoid nuclei, nuclear fragmentation, and basophilic stippling; and (3) small megakaryocytes with single-lobed nuclei and pink cytoplasm.

On gross examination, the bone marrow in AML is homogeneously red-tan or gray. The spleen and lymph nodes are moderately enlarged and firm. The cut surface of the spleen is uniformly red-purple, with prominence of the red pulp and partial to complete obliteration of the white pulp. The liver tends to be enlarged, and its cut surface is gray-tan.

The bone marrow in AML is typically hypercellular (Fig. 20-51) but may be normocellular or infrequently hypocellular (hypoplastic AML). Normal hemopoiesis is inconspicuous. Blast cells are increased (more than 30% of nucleated cells) and often efface the normal architecture. A moderate marrow reticulin fibrosis is commonly observed in most types of AML, but severe fibrosis is invariable in the acute megakaryocytic variant (M7).

The lymph nodes are initially infiltrated in the paracortex (Fig. 20-52), a condition that may progress to com-

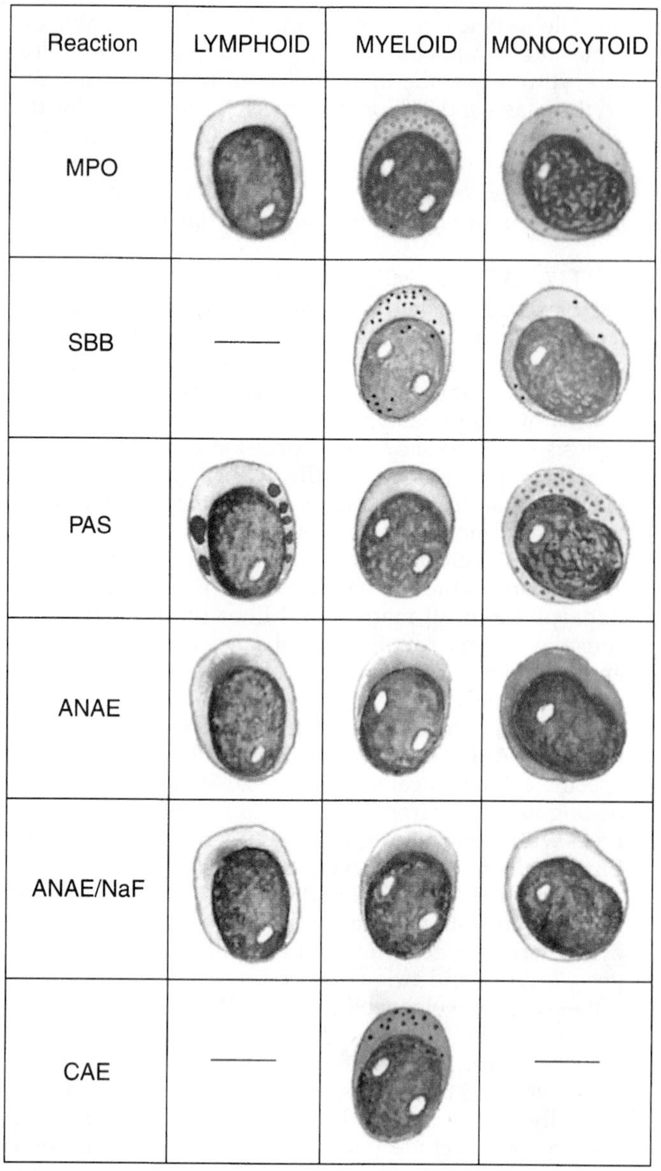

Reaction	LYMPHOID	MYELOID	MONOCYTOID
MPO			
SBB	—		
PAS			
ANAE			
ANAE/NaF			
CAE	—		—

FIGURE 20-50
Acute lymphoblastic, myeloblastic, and monocytic leukemias: cytochemical stains. *PAS*, periodic acid–Schiff; *CAE*, chloracetate esterase; *SBB*, Sudan black B; *APh*, acid phosphatase; *ANAE*, alphanapthol acetate esterase (with and without fluoride inhibition).

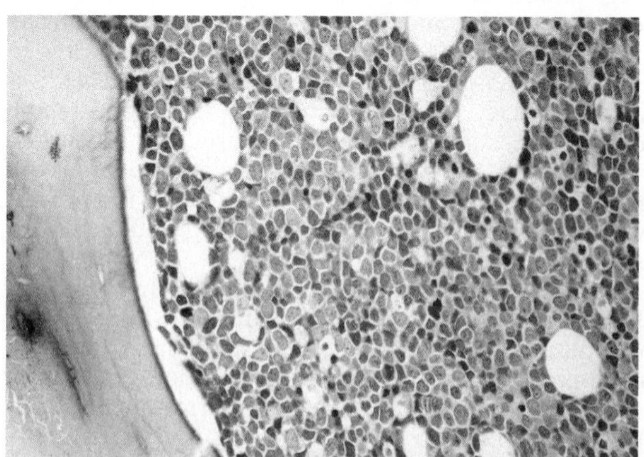

FIGURE 20-51
Acute myelogenous leukemia. A bone marrow section is hypercellular, owing to effacement of the normal architecture by myeloblasts.

plete obliteration of the nodal architecture. In the spleen, initially the red pulp and subsequently the lymphoid white pulp are eventually obliterated by leukemic cells. The liver contains blasts in the sinusoids. Infiltration of any visceral organ, the skin (leukemia cutis), and other sites, such as the central nervous system, may also occur.

In cases in which there is a marked elevation of the peripheral blood leukocyte count ($>$150,000/μL), myelogenous blasts may occlude the capillaries and small vessels of the central nervous system and the lungs (leukostasis). With subsequent infiltration and destruction of the vessel walls, there may be secondary hemorrhages in the brain and in the pulmonary parenchyma.

Leukemic meningitis due to blast cell infiltration of the leptomeninges may be mistaken for an infectious meningitis. Arthralgias and bone pain reflect leukemic infiltration of the synovia and periosteum and expansion of the medullary spaces. Hyperuricemia secondary to leukemic blast cell turnover predisposes to uric acid nephropathy and renal calculi.

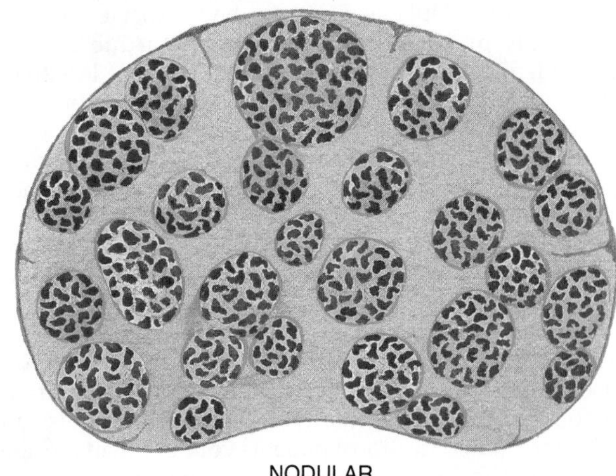

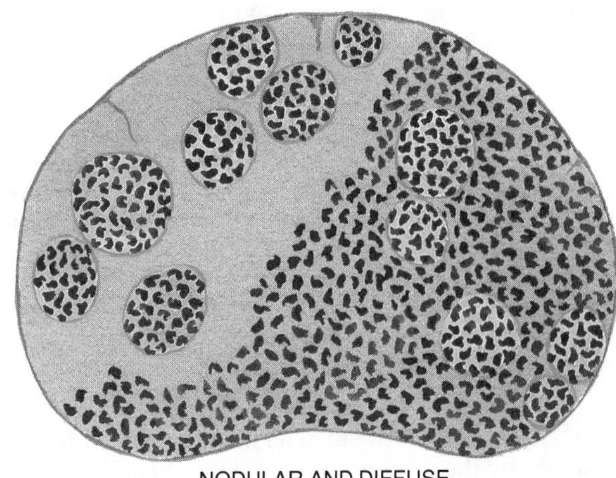

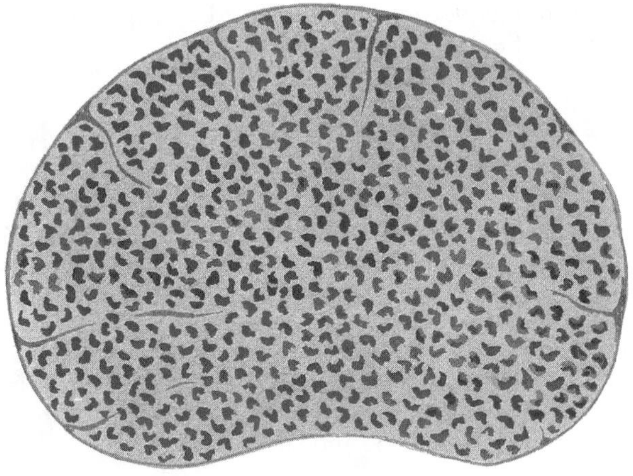

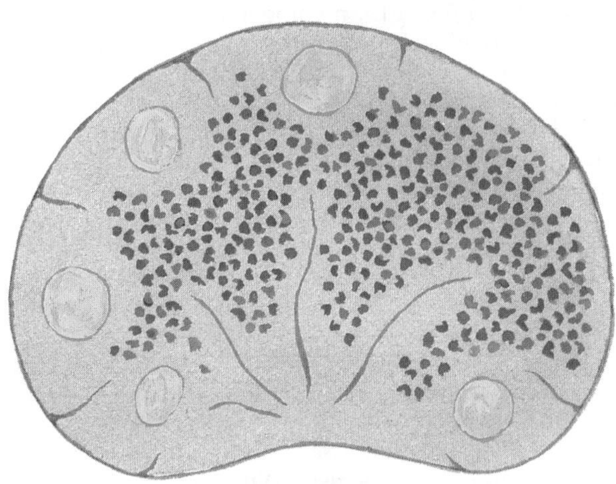

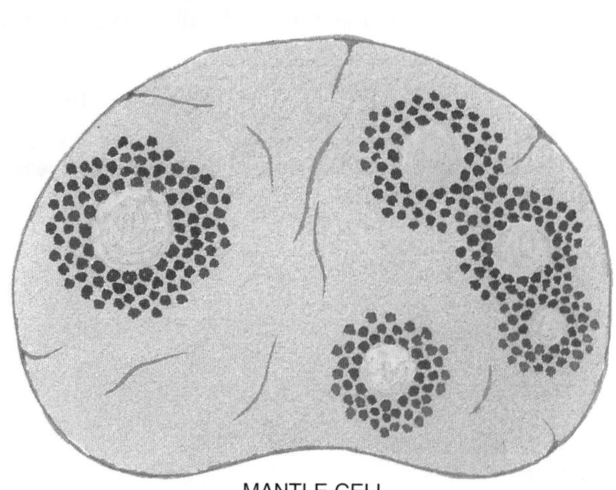

FIGURE *20-52*
The lymph node-patterns of involvement in leukemia and lymphoma. In the follicular lymphomas, there is replacement of the normal lymph node architecture by uniform nodular aggregates of neoplastic B lymphocytes. In the follicular and diffuse lymphomas, there is variable replacement of the node architecture by neoplastic B lymphocytes in both follicular and diffuse architectural patterns. In the diffuse lymphomas and in the leukemias, there is partial to (frequently) total obliteration of the normal nodal architecture by neoplastic B or T lymphocytes or leukemia cells. The architectural pattern is diffuse without proclivity to form follicles. With primary paracortical involvement, there is neoplastic cell infiltration of the T cell–dependent paracortex by neoplastic T lymphocytes or by leukemic cells. Involvement may progress to total effacement of the lymph node architecture. In mantle cell lymphomas, there is initial variable expansion of the B-cell cuff that surrounds normal germinal centers. Ultimately, there may be progression to total obliteration of the normal lymph node architecture.

GRANULOCYTIC SARCOMA: In a few cases of AML, discrete tumor masses composed of myeloblasts and promyelocytes occur in the bones, soft tissues adjacent to the orbit and facial bones, lymph nodes, and other soft tissue sites. These tumorous masses are called *granulocytic sarcoma or chloroma*, the latter because of the green color imparted by the cytoplasmic enzyme myeloperoxidase. The diagnosis of granulocytic sarcoma is suggested by the presence of primitive cells, with delicate round or lobated nuclei, and eosinophilic myelocytes (Fig. 20-53). The diagnosis of granulocytic sarcoma is confirmed by the demonstration in the leukemic cells of chloroacetate esterase or myelomonocytic lineage specific antigens.

□ **Clinical Features:** The diagnosis of AML is established by the demonstration of more than 30% myelogenous blasts in the bone marrow, with or without the presence of blasts in the peripheral blood. The total peripheral blood leukocyte count may be low, normal, or increased. If the peripheral blood leukocyte count is increased (>11,000/μL), myelogenous blasts are almost invariably demonstrated on the peripheral smear. At the time of presentation, there is usually some degree of thrombocytopenia, neutropenia, and anemia.

The clinical onset of AML is typically acute or subacute. However, in 20% of cases, there is a prodromal myelodysplastic syndrome, characterized by marrow dyspoiesis and variable peripheral blood cytopenias persisting for months to years. The most common initial symptoms and signs in AML are nonspecific and secondary to anemia. They include weakness, fatigue, decreased exercise tolerance, and pallor. On physical examination, splenomegaly and hepatomegaly are detected in one third of the cases of AML. Initial lymphadenopathy is uncommon, except in the monocytic variant (M5).

Bleeding secondary to thrombocytopenia occurs in one third or more of the cases. With platelet counts of less than 20,000/μL, and particularly less than 5,000/μL, there is a serious risk of hemorrhage in the gastrointestinal tract and central nervous system. Intracranial hemorrhage may also result from leukostasis when the leukocyte count is particularly high. There may be dyspnea due to pulmonary leukostasis. With neutrophil counts of less than 500/μL, secondary infectious episodes are common, and at levels below 200/μL, they are inevitable.

Adverse prognostic findings in AML include (1) advanced age at diagnosis (older than 60 years), (2) chromosomal abnormalities 5q− and 7q−, (3) a previous myelodysplastic syndrome, (4) prior chemotherapy or radiation therapy for cancer, and (5) severe leukocytosis (>100,000/μL).

Untreated AML is a rapidly fatal disease, the median survival being less than 2 months. The most common causes of death are infection or hemorrhage. With current chemotherapeutic regimens, a complete clinical remission can be anticipated in 70% of patients younger than the age of 60 years. The disease relapses in most patients, but with maintenance chemotherapy remissions longer than 8 years (and possibly complete cures) have been obtained in 15% of cases. Although the risk of allogeneic and autologous bone marrow transplantation is considerable, this procedure has become the preferred therapy in many younger patients with AML.

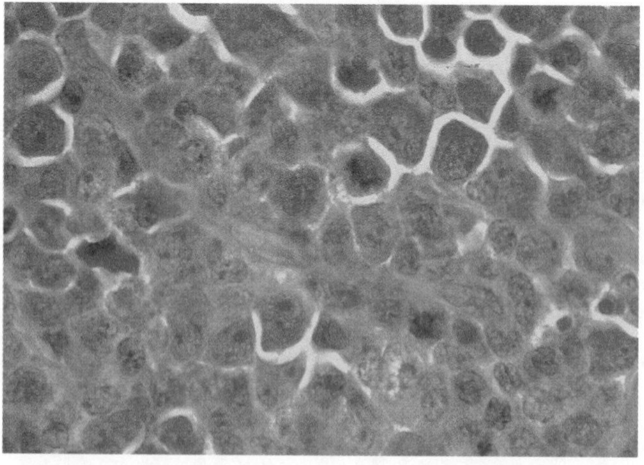

FIGURE *20-53*
Granulocytic sarcoma (chloroma). A diffuse soft tissue infiltrate of the orbit contains primitive blast cells with round to lobulated nuclei. The napthol-AS-D chloroacetate esterase stain is focally positive (*red*).

CHRONIC LYMPHOCYTIC LEUKEMIA

Chronic lymphocytic leukemia (CLL) is a neoplastic disorder characterized by clonal proliferation of small lymphocytes. B-cell lineage is demonstrated in more than 95% of cases. The spectrum of B-cell malignant lymphoproliferative disease is outlined in Table 20-18 and that of T-cell disorders is given in Table 20-19. The immunophenotypes of developmental stages in the maturation of B and T lymphocytes and their major neoplastic counterparts are illustrated in Figures 20-54 and 20-55, respectively.

B-Cell Chronic Lymphocytic Leukemia

In CLL of B-cell lineage (B-CLL), there is primary involvement of the bone marrow, with subsequent release

TABLE *20-18* **B-Cell Lymphoproliferative Diseases**

Precursor B-cell lymphoblastic leukemia/lymphoma
Mature (peripheral) B-cell neoplasms
B-cell chronic lymphocytic leukemia/lymphoma (95%)[a]
Prolymphocytic leukemia (80%)
Lymphoplasmacytoid lymphoma
Mantle cell lymphoma
Follicular center lymphoma
Marginal zone lymphoma
Extranodal (MALT-type)
Nodal (+/− monocytoid B cells)
Splenic with villous lymphocytes
Hairy cell leukemia
Diffuse large cell lymphoma (85%)
Anaplastic large cell lymphoma (<10%)
Burkitt and Burkitt-like lymphoma
Plasma cell neoplasia (plasmacytoma and multiple myeloma)

[a] %, percentage of B-cell lineage.

TABLE *20-19* **T-Cell and NK-Cell Lymphoproliferative Diseases**

Thymic-derived
Precursor T-cell lymphoblastic leukemia/lymphoma

Peripheral (mature) T-cell and NK-cell neoplasms
T-cell CLL/prolymphocytic leukemia
Large granular lymphocytic leukemia
  T-cell type
  NK-cell type
Mycosis fungoides/Sezary syndrome
Peripheral T-cell lymphomas, unspecified
Specific subtypes
  Angioimmunoblastic (AILD)
  Angiocentric
  Intestinal (+/− enteropathy)
  Adult T-cell leukemia/lymphoma (ATLL)
  Anaplastic large cell (Ki-1, CD30+)
  Hepatosplenic gamma delta
  Subcutaneous panniculitis-like

of neoplastic lymphocytes to the peripheral blood. As the disease progresses, a variable infiltration and enlargement of the lymph nodes, spleen, and, less prominently, the liver takes place. The hemopoietic and lymphopoietic tissues become compromised because of the gradual replacement of the bone marrow and extramedullary lymphoid tissues. B-CLL is typically an indolent neoplasm, and survival for years can be anticipated.

☐ **Epidemiology:** **B-CLL is the most common leukemia in Western countries, where it constitutes 30% of all leukemias.** The annual incidence in males (4 per 100,000 population) is roughly twice that in females. There is no difference in incidence between blacks and whites, but the disease is significantly less common in Japanese, Chinese, and other Asian populations. There is an increasing frequency of B-CLL with age, the median age at onset being in the seventh decade. The disorder strikes only occasionally in young adults and is exceptionally rare in children. Most cases of B-CLL occur sporadically, although rare examples of familial B-CLL have been reported.

☐ **Pathogenesis:** The etiology of B-CLL is not known. There is no demonstrated association with prior ionizing radiation or with myelotoxic drugs or chemicals. Neither retroviruses nor other oncogenic agents have been incriminated. The occurrence of occasional familial clustering of B-CLL and differences in ethnic susceptibility suggest that genetic influences may be important. The male predominance raises the possibility of hormonal influences.

Based on immunophenotypic analyses of surface antigens of B-CLL lymphocytes, it is believed that the neoplastic cell is the counterpart of a lymphocyte that is normally present in only small numbers in the adult but is more prominent in cord blood and fetal tissues. In addition to various pan B–cell antigens, this normal lymphocyte also expresses the pan T–cell marker CD5, an antigen

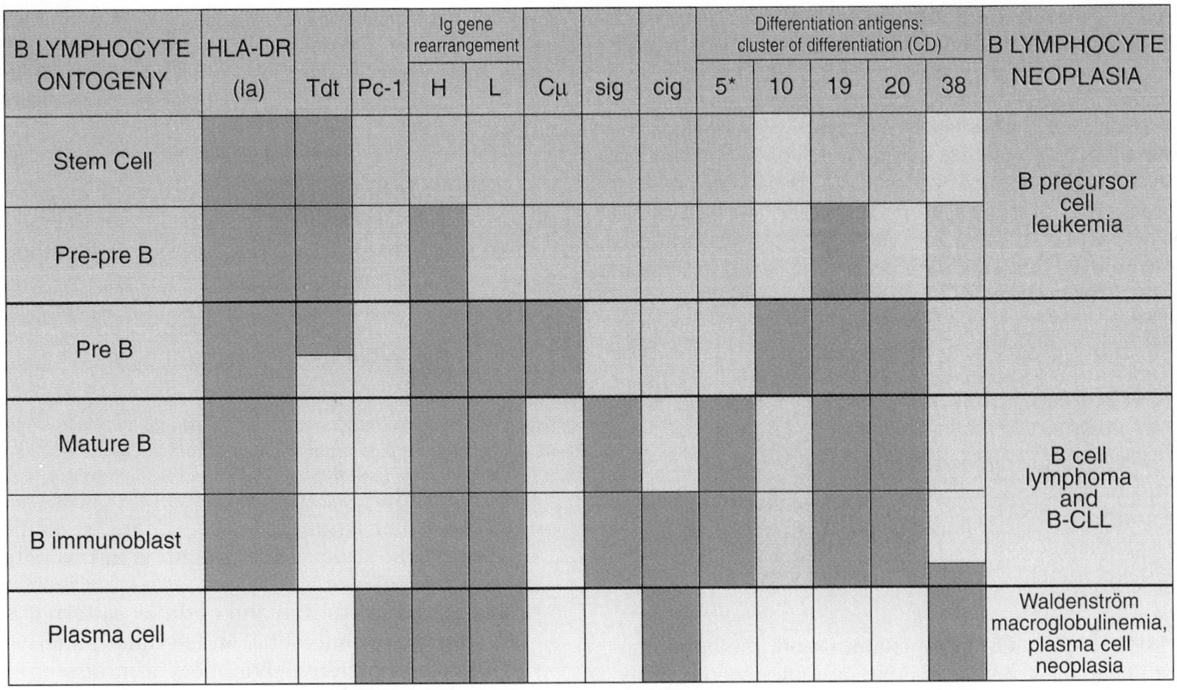

B LYMPHOCYTE ONTOGENY	HLA-DR (Ia)	Tdt	Pc-1	Ig gene rearrangement H	L	Cμ	sig	cig	Differentiation antigens: cluster of differentiation (CD) 5*	10	19	20	38	B LYMPHOCYTE NEOPLASIA
Stem Cell														B precursor cell leukemia
Pre-pre B														
Pre B														
Mature B														B cell lymphoma and B-CLL
B immunoblast														
Plasma cell														Waldenström macroglobulinemia, plasma cell neoplasia

*CLL/WDLL (SLL) only; H-Ig heavy chain gene; L-Ig light chain gene

FIGURE *20-54*
B-cell maturation: immunophenotypes and neoplastic counterparts. H, immunoglobulin heavy-chain gene; L, immunoglobulin light-chain gene.

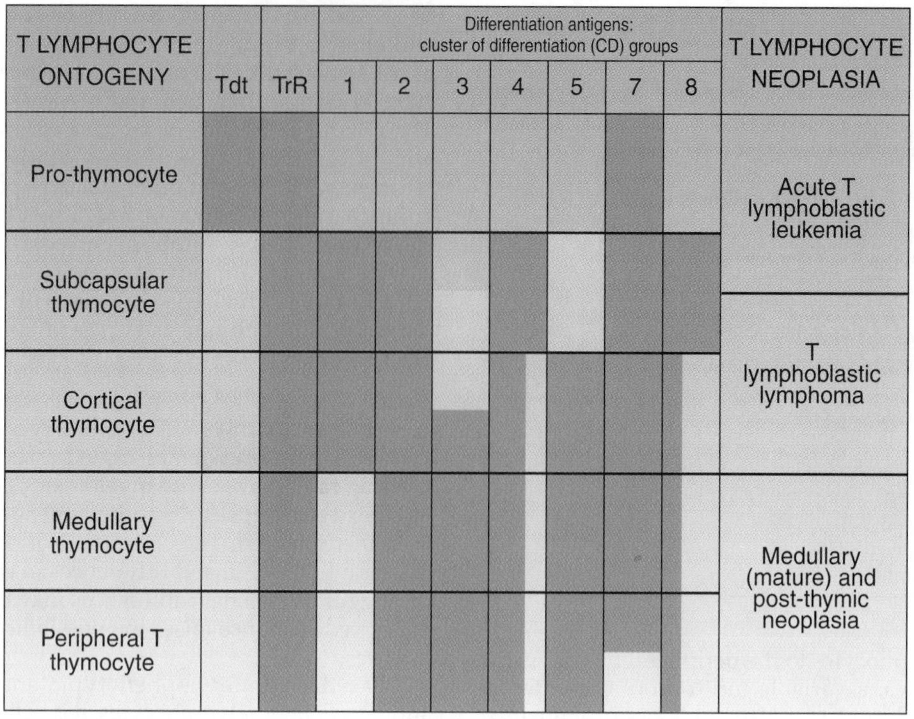

T LYMPHOCYTE ONTOGENY	Tdt	TrR	Differentiation antigens: cluster of differentiation (CD) groups 1	2	3	4	5	7	8	T LYMPHOCYTE NEOPLASIA
Pro-thymocyte										Acute T lymphoblastic leukemia
Subcapsular thymocyte										
Cortical thymocyte										T lymphoblastic lymphoma
Medullary thymocyte										Medullary (mature) and post-thymic neoplasia
Peripheral T thymocyte										

FIGURE *20-55*
T-cell maturation: immunophenotypes and their neoplastic counterparts.

that in this setting reflects activation of immature B cells. The presence of CD5 on B-CLL lymphocytes has been interpreted to signify the abnormal accumulation of a clone of neoplastic cells frozen at stage of normal B-cell differentiation. Interestingly, the expression of CD5 in B-CLL also helps explain the autoimmune phenomena that are often associated with this disease, since both normal and neoplastic CD5-positive B lymphocytes have been shown to produce IgM autoantibodies. CD23 is usually positive. Chromosomal abnormalities are present in half of the cases of B-CLL. These include trisomy 12, translocations, for example, t(11;14), and deletions (14q−) and inversions (14q) of chromosome 14.

The clinical signs and symptoms in B-CLL relate principally to the progressive infiltration of neoplastic lymphocytes in the bone marrow and extramedullary tissue sites and to secondary immunological deficiencies. In B-CLL, a relentless neoplastic replacement of the normal hemopoietic tissue by the neoplastic clone causes anemia, granulocytopenia, and thrombocytopenia. Autoimmune destruction of blood elements and, less commonly, hypersplenism secondary to splenomegaly also contribute to the development of peripheral blood cytopenias.

☐ **Pathology:** On gross examination, the bone marrow infiltrated by B-CLL exhibits a homogeneous, gray-tan color. Lymph nodes and other soft tissues involved by B-CLL typically display a homogeneous, soft, gray-white ("fish flesh") appearance. Peripheral lymphadenopathy is more often a cosmetic abnormality than a functional one. Occasionally, however, lymphadenopathy is massive and when it occurs in the central or axial nodes, it may cause organ dysfunction or obstruction of vital body conduits by direct pressure. The spleen is moderately enlarged, and the cut surface shows a generalized prominence of the white pulp. Occasionally, particularly in untreated cases, the spleen contains tumor nodules (Fig. 20-56).

Microscopically, characteristic changes in various organs are noted.

BONE MARROW: The proportion of marrow lymphocytes in B-CLL usually exceeds 40% of the nucleated cells (normal, up to 20%). There are four histopathological patterns of infiltration of the bone marrow:

- **The interstitial pattern of lymphocytic infiltration,** often the initial morphological finding, is characterized by an increased population of lymphocytes irregularly distributed among normally maturing hemopoietic cells. This pattern is associated with a favorable prognosis.
- **The nodular pattern** shows lymphocytes clustered into nodular aggregates and separated by normal hemopoietic stroma. The prognosis in this pattern is also good.
- **The mixed interstitial and nodular pattern** is a combination of the interstitial and nodular patterns.
- **The diffuse pattern** of lymphocytic infiltration, manifested as an obliteration of normal hemopoietic elements and fat cells, represents progression of the disease and is associated with a poor prognosis.

PERIPHERAL BLOOD: The peripheral blood smear demonstrates an increase in small to medium-sized lym-

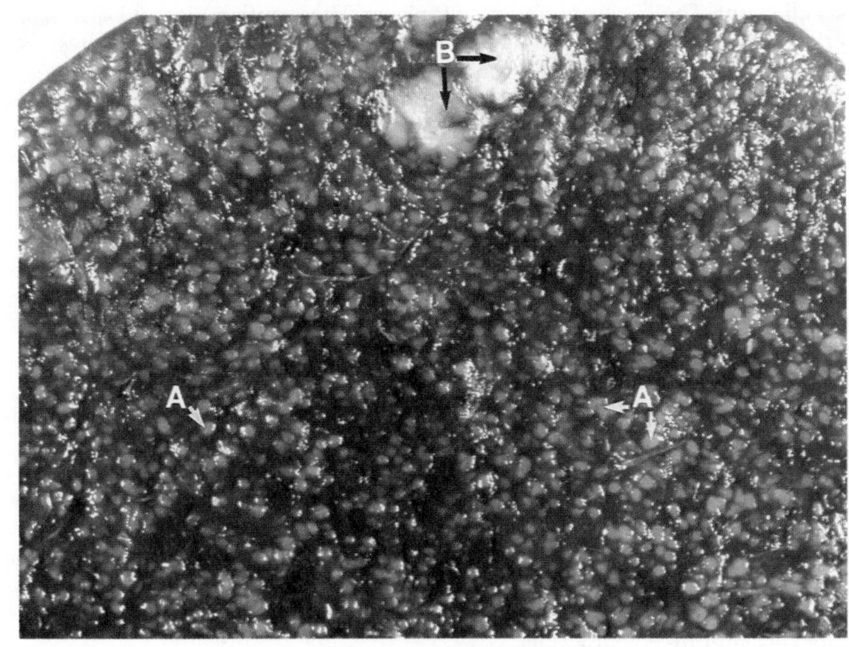

FIGURE 20-56
The spleen in chronic lymphocytic leukemia. There is diffuse enlargement of the white pulp (*A*), with focally prominent tumor nodules (*B*).

phocytes, which show round nuclei with compact chromatin, inconspicuous nucleoli, and scant blue cytoplasm (Fig. 20-57). Prolymphocytes, which constitute less than 15% of the total neoplastic cell population, have eccentric round to oval nuclei, coarsely reticulated chromatin, a distinctive single large nucleolus, and a moderate amount of gray-blue cytoplasm. Cells with prominent single to multiple nucleoli and delicate chromatin are occasionally observed.

The neoplastic lymphocytes in B-CLL are fragile and easily ruptured on preparation of the peripheral blood smear. The resultant amorphous, dark blue, nuclear remnant is called a "smudge cell" and is characteristic of B-CLL.

LYMPH NODES The histopathological features of lymph nodes and other soft tissue sites involved by B-CLL reflect a diffuse infiltration of small lymphocytes, with only rare mitotic figures (see Fig. 20-60). There are scattered pale foci of partially transformed lymphocytes, with more open chromatin and central nucleoli, representing foci of mitotically active prolymphocytes and paraimmunoblasts. These foci are called "proliferation centers" or "pseudoreaction centers."

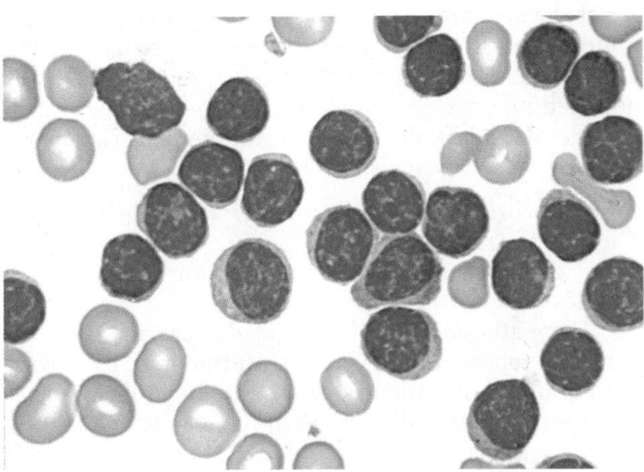

FIGURE 20-57
Chronic lymphocytic leukemia. A smear of peripheral blood shows numerous small-to-medium-sized lymphocytes. A smudge cell is seen at the upper left.

☐ **Clinical Features:** The diagnosis of B-CLL is established by the demonstration of a sustained peripheral blood lymphocytosis, generally greater than 15,000/μL, and a bone marrow lymphocytosis exceeding 40% of the nucleated cell elements. If the blood lymphocyte count is between 5,000 and 15,000/μL, the demonstration of monoclonality (light-chain restriction or clonal rearrangement of a light-chain gene) confirms the diagnosis of B-CLL.

The erythrocyte and platelet counts are initially normal, but with advanced disease, severe anemia, thrombocytopenia, and neutropenia develop. A positive Coombs test is observed at some time in up to 20% of cases.

Immunological deficiencies, principally of B cells but also of T cells, are common. Although the precise cause of B-cell dysfunction is not known, hypogammaglobulinemia occurs in 50% to 75% of cases at some time during the course of the disease. The degree of hypogammaglobulinemia generally correlates with the disease stage and is responsible for infectious complications.

Patients with B-CLL also manifest an increase in peripheral blood T cells (>3,000/μL). There is an increase in CD8+ T cells and a corresponding decrease in CD4+ cells, with a resulting decrease in the CD4+/CD8+ cell ratio. The T cells often show impaired delayed-type hypersensitivity *in vitro*, a defect that also contributes to the increased risk of infection. A small amount of monoclonal immunoglobulin, most commonly IgM κ, is found in the serum in a minority of patients with B-CLL.

Initially, most patients with B-CLL are asymptomatic, and the diagnosis is suggested by finding lymphadenopathy and splenomegaly on a routine physical examination or lymphocytosis on a blood cell count. The subsequent clinical course is highly variable. In some cases, the disease progresses rapidly and the patients die within 2 to 3 years. Other patients remain asymptomatic for 10 to 20 years. The most common complications are bacterial infections, and less frequently fungal and viral ones. Coombs-positive autoimmune hemolytic anemia and hemorrhagic episodes secondary to thrombocytopenia are often observed.

The overall mean survival in B-CLL is 6 years. The prognosis is related principally to (1) the extent of tumor burden at the time of initial diagnosis, (2) the pattern of bone marrow infiltration, and (3) the presence of cytogenetic abnormalities. Adverse prognostic findings include (1) advanced disease; (2) diffuse, as opposed to interstitial or nodular, patterns of marrow involvement; and (3) the presence of chromosomal abnormalities, particularly if multiple.

CONVERSION TO PROLYMPHOCYTIC LEUKEMIA: This complication occurs in 10% of cases of B-CLL and is characterized by a marked elevation in the blood lymphocyte count, 15% to 50% prolymphocytes, and increasing splenomegaly. Prolymphocytic conversion predicts a more aggressive clinical course, with a mean survival of less than 2 years. Rare instances of conversion to acute lymphoblastic leukemia have been described, with a rapidly fatal course. There is more than a twofold increase in the expected incidence of second cancers in B-CLL, including lung tumors, malignant melanoma, soft tissue sarcomas, and plasma cell neoplasms.

RICHTER SYNDROME: A large cell immunoblastic lymphoma (see later) is superimposed in 5% of cases of B-CLL. Patients with this complication, termed Richter syndrome, present with the rapid onset of fever, abdominal pain, and progressive lymphadenopathy and hepatosplenomegaly. Prominent enlargement of the retroperitoneal lymph nodes and neoplastic involvement of the gastrointestinal tract are common findings. Richter syndrome is aggressive and refractory to therapy, with a mean survival of 2 months.

Asymptomatic patients with B-CLL, who have stable lymphocyte counts, are ordinarily not treated. More advanced disease is treated with chemotherapeutic agents. Corticosteroids are used to control autoimmune hemolytic anemia and thrombocytopenia. Splenectomy or splenic irradiation may be necessary to manage refractory hypersplenism.

T-Cell Chronic Lymphocytic Leukemia

T-cell CLL (T-CLL) is a rare and poorly understood heterogeneous disorder, comprising less than 5% of all cases of CLL. It consists of two principal entities, T-CLL and T-large granulated lymphocytosis (T-LGL).

T-CLL has the immunological phenotype, CD2, 3, and (unusually) CD4. Natural killer (NK) cell markers are lacking. There is moderate peripheral blood lymphocytosis. The neoplastic lymphocytes are small to medium in size. They exhibit round to convoluted nuclei, and display an agranular cytoplasm. The lymph nodes and spleen are variably enlarged. The clinical course is aggressive and the prognosis is poor.

T-LGL has the immunological phenotype CD2, 3, 8, 16, and 57. The neoplastic cells are medium-sized to large lymphocytes, with abundant cytoplasm that contains coarse azurphilic granules. The clinical course is generally chronic and indolent, and there is an association with rheumatoid arthritis. Neutropenia with secondary repeated infections is characteristic. A minority of cases exhibit an aggressive clinical course (LGL leukemia). In some cases, only NK immunological markers are expressed.

Prolymphocytic Leukemia

Prolymphocytic leukemia is a distinctive variant of CLL. Some 80% are of B-cell and 20% of T-lymphocyte lineage. Neoplastic B prolymphocytes express more abundant surface membrane immunoglobulin than do B-CLL cells. They appear to be immunologically more mature than B-CLL cells.

Prolymphocytic leukemia is characterized clinically by massive splenomegaly and by a marked elevation of the leukocyte count (greater than 50% prolymphocytes). Lymphadenopathy is inconspicuous in B-cell prolymphocytic leukemia, whereas moderate lymphadenopathy is often observed in the T-cell variety. Prolymphocytic leukemia is most common in elderly men (4:1 male predominance). It is an aggressive disease, with a mean survival of 2 to 3 years.

Hairy Cell Leukemia

Hairy cell leukemia (HCL) is a distinctive variant of chronic lymphocytic leukemia that is named for the membranous filamentous projections or "hairs" on the surface of the neoplastic cells. A B-lymphocyte lineage is demonstrated by monoclonal surface Ig, immunoglobulin gene rearrangements, and B-cell markers.

Hairy cell leukemia is uncommon, comprising only 2% of all leukemias. The disease occurs most commonly in middle-aged to elderly men. The male-to-female ratio is 4:1 and the median age at diagnosis is 50 years. HCL has not been reported in children or teenagers. There are no well-defined ethnic or geographic differences in incidence.

☐ **Pathogenesis:** The etiology of HCL is unknown. There is no association with ionizing radiation, myelotoxic agents, oncogenic viruses, or chromosomal abnormalities.

The pathogenesis of clinical disease in hairy cell leukemia reflects principally (1) infiltration of the spleen, with consequent splenomegaly and functional hypersplenism, and (2) infiltration of the bone marrow, with resulting marrow failure.

☐ **Pathology:** Splenic enlargement occurs in almost all (85%) cases of HCL and is frequently massive. Splenic weights vary from 300 to 5000 g, with a mean of 1000 g. The cut surface is homogeneously firm and purple-red, reflecting primary involvement of the red pulp and obliteration of the white pulp . Moderate hepatomegaly occurs in half the cases. Mild lymphadenopathy, principally of the central or axial lymph node groups, is observed in 25% of cases.

Microscopically, in Wright- or Wright-Giemsa-stained blood smears, (Fig. 20-58), hairy cells are 10 to 20 nm in diameter and exhibit fine, irregular cytoplasmic projections. Ultrastructurally, the hairy projections are plasma membrane ruffles and microvilli. The round to oval nuclei are eccentrically situated. The nuclei may also be folded, bilobed, or, rarely, irregular and cerebriform. The nuclear chromatin is delicate or lacy. Nucleoli are usually not visualized. The cytoplasm is abundant and pale blue to gray-blue. Occasionally, cytoplasmic vacuoles are observed.

The tartrate-resistant acid phosphatase (TRAP) stain is positive in almost all (95%) cases of HCL. By contrast, in most lymphoproliferative disorders other than HCL, there is a marked diminution or total loss of acid phosphatase activity after tartaric acid pretreatment (TRAP negative). By electron microscopy, a characteristic cytoplasmic organelle, the ribosome-lamellar complex, is identified in half of the cases. This structure is a hollow cylinder with peripheral parallel lamellae and interlamellar ribosome-like granules. With Wright's stain, the complexes appear as purple cytoplasmic rods. Although the significance of these structures is not known, they are characteristic of, but not diagnostic for, HCL.

Bone marrow sections in HCL reveal a patchy or diffuse infiltration of medium-sized lymphoid cells, which have homogeneous round or indented nuclei. The most distinctive finding is a uniform, water-clear cytoplasm, which creates a perinuclear halo that appears to separate the nuclei of the neoplastic cells and produces a pattern described as "mosaic-like." Mitotic figures are rare. Plasma cells and mast cells are often scattered throughout the marrow. Islands of residual hemopoiesis commonly exhibit a decreased myeloid-erythroid ratio (<1:1) because of decreased granulocytopoiesis and normal to increased erythropoiesis. Silver stains demonstrate a characteristic diffuse pericellular reticulin fibrosis, but dense collagenous fibrosis is absent.

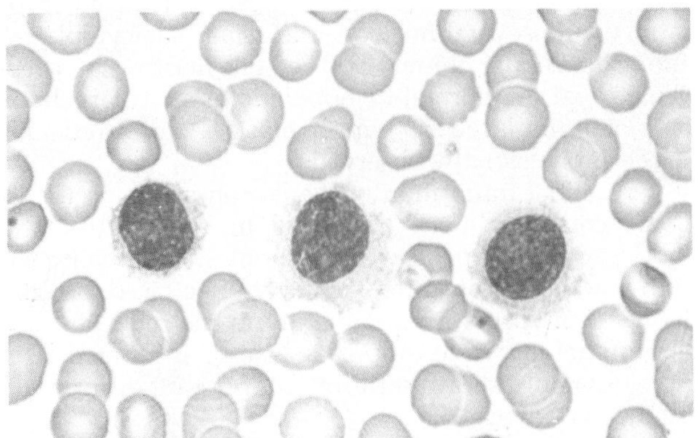

FIGURE *20-58*
Hairy cell leukemia. Hairy cells with fine, irregular cytoplasmic projections are seen in the peripheral blood.

The histological features of the spleen are also distinctive. The red pulp cords and sinuses are diffusely infiltrated by bland lymphoid cells similar to those in the marrow. The cytoplasm of hairy cells in the spleen is poorly visualized, and no cytoplasmic halo is noted. Scattered plasma cells are commonly observed. There is encroachment on or obliteration of the lymphoid white pulp. Blood-filled spaces lined by hairy cells, called venous lakes or pseudosinuses, are a characteristic finding in the spleen. The venous lakes are thought to be caused by destruction of endothelial cells and ring fibers of the sinus walls by hairy cells, with secondary dilatation of the sinuses and pooling of erythrocytes.

A variety of organs, with the notable exception of the central nervous system, may be involved in HCL. The liver often shows infiltration of the portal triads and hepatic sinusoids. In the lymph nodes, the sinuses, paracortex, and cortex are initially infiltrated. Ultimately, the normal nodal architecture may be completely effaced. Skin infiltration, initially around dermal blood vessels, occurs in 10% of cases. Destructive lesions of bone, most frequently of the head of the femur, are sometimes encountered.

☐ **Clinical Features:** The diagnosis of hairy cell leukemia is established by the demonstration of (1) the characteristic histopathological findings on bone marrow biopsy, (2) hairy cells on stained smears or imprints, (3) a positive TRAP stain, and (4) a CD5-negative, light-chain restricted B-lineage phenotype.

The laboratory findings in HCL include neutropenia (75% of cases), thrombocytopenia, monocytopenia, and anemia. Morphological and functional abnormalities of platelets are commonly observed. Circulating hairy cells can usually be identified on a peripheral blood smear, particularly in the 15% of cases that exhibit an increased leukocyte count.

The clinical onset of HCL is typically insidious. About 25% of patients are initially asymptomatic, and the diagnosis is suggested by the finding of isolated splenomegaly or by the results of a complete blood cell count. In the remaining patients, HCL presents as (1) abdominal fullness or discomfort, owing to splenomegaly; (2) bleeding, secondary to thrombocytopenia; (3) infection caused by granulocytopenia or monocytopenia; or (4) nonspecific signs and symptoms, including weight loss, fatigue, and weakness.

The course of HCL is characteristically chronic and indolent, but in 15% of cases it is aggressive, with severe peripheral blood cytopenias and progressive enlargement of visceral organs. The most frequent cause of death is infection. Infections due to atypical mycobacteria are particularly characteristic of HCL and are attributed to monocytopenia.

Prior to modern therapy, the mean survival in HCL was only 4 years, and the only treatment available was splenectomy. The introduction of interferon α and 2-CdA (2-chlorodeoxyadenosine), an inhibitor of DNA repair enzymes, has prolonged survival, and clinical cure can be anticipated in a substantial number of cases. In fact, with close follow-up and appropriate treatment the life span of patients with HCL approaches that of comparably aged persons.

ACUTE LYMPHOBLASTIC LEUKEMIA

The acute lymphoblastic leukemias (ALL) comprise a group of clonal disorders of lymphopoietic stem cells characterized by the accumulation of lymphoblasts. The progressive infiltration of malignant lymphoblasts in the bone marrow eventually suppresses the production of normal hemopoietic cells. B-cell subtypes (B-ALL) comprise 80% of all cases of ALL, whereas the remainder consist of T-cell (T-ALL) and rare null cell variants.

☐ **Epidemiology:** ALL comprises 10% of all leukemias in Western countries, with an annual incidence in the United States of 2 per 100,000 population. **Of these cases, 60% occur in children, and in Western countries, ALL is the most common malignancy of childhood.** The frequency of ALL is similar in males and females. ALL is less common in Africa and the Middle East than in Western and Asian countries. In the United States, it is twice as common in whites as in blacks. In Western countries, the peak age in whites is 3 to 7 years, after which the incidence remains stable. After the age of 50 years, there is a small but progressive increase in the frequency of ALL.

☐ **Pathogenesis:** The etiology of ALL is not known, and there is no demonstrated association with myelotoxic drugs, chemicals, or retroviruses. A modest increase in incidence has been reported to follow heavy exposure to ionizing radiation and is noted in some immunodeficiency states. Although Epstein-Barr virus is integrated in the genome of African Burkitt lymphoma, the viral genome has not been demonstrated in the Burkitt leukemia variant (L3) of ALL.

A genetic predisposition toward ALL is suggested in some cases. The incidence of acute leukemia, usually ALL and less commonly AML, is increased 15- to 20-fold in Down syndrome. If one identical twin develops ALL before the age of 8 years, the risk for the other twin is 20% within 1 year.

Cytogenetic studies reveal some abnormality of chromosome number or structure in the large majority (90%) of cases of ALL. In two thirds, the chromosome number is diploid (46 chromosomes), whereas one third are hyperdiploid (47 or more chromosomes). Certain consistent chromosomal translocations involving protooncogenes occur in ALL. **One of three chromosomal translocations is invariably identified in B-ALL (L3).** Most cases of B-ALL (L3) demonstrate a translocation of the c-*myc* protooncogene on chromosome 8 to the region of the immunoglobulin coding gene on chromosome 14 (t(8;14)(q24;q32)). The remainder of B-ALL (L3) cases manifest either t(2;8) or t(8;22). **Whatever the specific translocation, the c-*myc* locus is deregulated by an immunoglobulin promotor.**

In the pre-B cell variant of ALL (see later), a specific translocation, t(1;19), has been observed in one fourth of all cases. The resulting hybrid gene on chromosome 19 is thought to encode a fusion protein that perturbs transcriptional regulation. A number of other nonrandom translocations have been reported in ALL, especially involving chromosome 11 and T-cell receptor loci on chromosomes 14 and 7. Chromosomal deletions, principally involving chromosomes 6, 9, and 12, are present in 30% of patients with ALL, suggesting that some cases may involve the loss of tumor suppressor genes (see Chapter 5).

The Philadelphia chromosome, t(9;22), originally described in CML (see earlier), is detected in 20% of adult ALL but in less than 5% of children with the disease. The presence of this translocation is associated with a poorer prognosis. The fusion protein encoded by the hybrid oncogene in ALL is distinct from that in CML, suggesting that the ALL version of protein is particularly potent in lymphoid progenitors.

Clinical disease in ALL relates principally to the progressive accumulation in the bone marrow of lymphoblasts that lack the potential for differentiation and maturation. The population of leukemic lymphoblasts in any given patient derives from a single transformed lymphopoietic stem cell that has been arrested in a specific differentiation stage. Thus, the malignant cells closely approximate the phenotype of normal lymphoid progenitors. Leukemic lymphoblasts have a slower generation time (3 days) as compared with normal lymphoid precursors (1 day). However, because the lymphoblasts do not mature to more differentiated stages, they accumulate in the bone marrow. The relentless expansion of the clone of malignant lymphoblasts, possibly secreting inhibitory lymphokines, crowds out the normal marrow elements and, thereby, suppresses hemopoiesis. Thus, the clinical manifestations in ALL reflect anemia, granulocytopenia, and thrombocytopenia.

☐ **Pathology:** On gross examination, the involved bone marrow in ALL is homogeneously gray-tan. The lymph nodes are enlarged and firm, and the cut surface is uniformly gray-white. The spleen is moderately enlarged; the cut surface is pale gray-red, with blurring of the demarcation between the white and red pulp. The liver is moderately enlarged but is usually not macroscopically abnormal.

Microscopically, lymphoblasts vary from small to moderately large. They exhibit delicate reticulated chromatin, one to several nucleoli, and scant pale cytoplasm. Mitotic figures are numerous. The bone marrow is hypercellular, and the normal hemopoietic tissue is largely or completely replaced by lymphoblasts. A mild reticulin fibrosis is occasionally observed.

The initial infiltration of the lymph nodes occurs in the paracortex, following egress of lymphoblasts from the blood through the postcapillary venules. Eventually, the normal nodal architecture is completely effaced. Splenic involvement occurs predominantly in the red pulp, but the lymphoidal white pulp may also be infiltrated. The liver commonly shows infiltration of both the sinusoids and the portal areas.

CYTOLOGICAL SUBTYPES OF ALL: The lymphoblasts of ALL are morphologically, immunologically, and cytogenetically heterogeneous. With Wright's stain, the neoplastic lymphoblasts are classified according to criteria proposed by the FAB group. Three subtypes are recognized (see Fig. 20-48):

- **L1 lymphoblasts** are small and display round to oval nuclei, with finely reticulated chromatin, a single inconspicuous nucleolus, and scant blue cytoplasm.
- **L2 lymphoblasts** are moderate to large and contain irregular or indented nuclei, with finely reticulated chromatin, one to several prominent nucleoli, and scant to moderate gray-blue cytoplasm (Fig. 20-59).
- **L3 lymphoblasts** are uniformly large, with round to oval nuclei. They show coarsely reticulated chromatin, two to five small nucleoli, and scant, dark blue, and frequently vacuolated cytoplasm.

IMMUNOLOGICAL SUBTYPES OF ALL: Immunological markers define four major subtypes of ALL, three of B-cell origin and one that derives from T cells.

- **B-ALL:** Two subtypes of B-ALL are composed of B-cell precursors, namely, pre-pre-B cell ALL (morphologically L1) and pre-B cell ALL (L2). One subtype is composed of more mature B cells (L3). Rearrangements of immunoglobulin genes are seen in all cases of B-ALL, and rearrangements of T-cell receptor genes are present in some cases.
- **T-ALL:** Twenty percent of cases of ALL derive from T-cell precursors and are morphologically L2. Rearrangements of the β or γ chain genes of the T-cell receptor can usually be demonstrated. In 10% to 20% of cases of T-ALL, immunoglobulin heavy-chain gene rearrangements are observed.
- **Null cell ALL:** A small proportion of cases of ALL lack distinguishing B- or T-lymphocyte lineage markers and are called null or unclassified ALL.

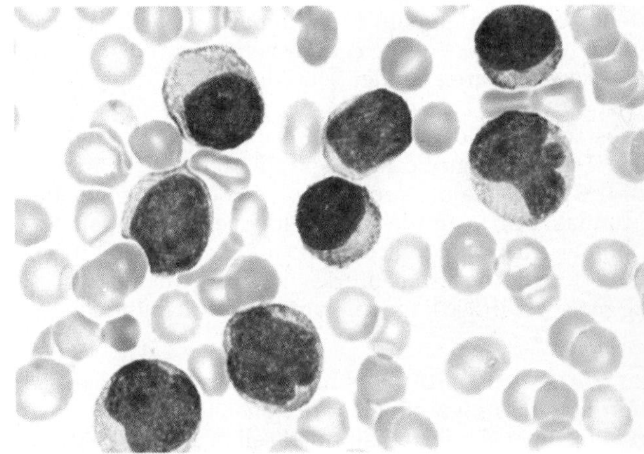

FIGURE *20-59*
Acute lymphoblastic leukemia (L2 ALL). The lymphoblasts in the peripheral blood contain irregular and indented nuclei with prominent nucleoli and a moderate amount of cytoplasm.

Terminal deoxynucleotidyl transferase (Tdt), a nuclear enzyme, is demonstrated in almost all (95%) cases of B-cell precursor (pre-pre-B and pre-B) ALL and T-ALL. This enzyme is uniformly lacking only in the mature B-cell or L3 variant. **The demonstration of Tdt activity suggests that a leukemic blast cell is of lymphoid rather than of myeloid lineage, since the enzyme is demonstrated in only 5% to 10% of cases of AML.** Because ALL has a more favorable prognosis than AML, and typically responds to a less intensive chemotherapeutic regimen, the demonstration of Tdt has therapeutic and prognostic implications.

□ **Clinical Features:** The diagnosis of ALL is established by the demonstration of lymphoblasts in the bone marrow, with or without circulating lymphoblasts in the peripheral blood smear. In half the cases, the initial leukocyte count is normal or decreased and lymphoblasts may or may not be identified on the peripheral smear. However, if the leukocyte count is increased above normal, lymphoblasts are almost invariably present. Normocytic, normochromic anemia, thrombocytopenia, and neutropenia are initially present in most cases.

Acute lymphoblastic leukemia usually presents with nonspecific signs and symptoms secondary to anemia, including weakness, pallor, malaise, and decreased exercise tolerance. Bleeding secondary to thrombocytopenia occurs in half the cases. Less commonly, bacterial infections secondary to neutropenia bring the patient to medical attention. Bone pain due to medullary or subperiosteal involvement, or joint pain secondary to infiltration of the synovium, occurs in one third of cases. **Generalized lymphadenopathy, particularly prominent in the cervical lymph nodes, is characteristic.** Hepatosplenomegaly is common. Involvement of the central nervous system, particularly the leptomeninges (leukemic meningitis), is frequent, even early in the course of the disease. This complication is now usually prevented by routine prophylactic irradiation of the craniospinal axis following the diagnosis of ALL.

PROGNOSTIC FEATURES: The two most important prognostic features of ALL are the age at onset and the initial blood leukocyte count (Table 20-20).

- **Infants younger than 1 year of age:** ALL is rarely observed in this age group, but when it does occur it carries a poor prognosis. In infants, adverse prognostic features include (1) a high initial leukocyte count; (2) extensive extramedullary disease, the so-called leukemia-lymphoma syndrome; (3) the chromosomal translocation t(4;11); and (4) L2 morphology, with the expression of both B-lymphocyte and myeloid differentiation antigens (lineage infidelity) in lymphoblasts.
- **Children 3 to 7 years of age:** The large majority (85%) of pediatric ALL occurs in this prognostically favorable group in which the disease responds to chemotherapy. L1 is the common morphological subtype, and B-cell precursor ALL is the most often associated immunological subtype.
- **Children 6 to 11 years of age:** L3 ALL, commonly

TABLE 20-20 Acute Lymphoblastic Leukemia: Clinicopathological Prognostic Features

Clinicopathological Features	Prognosis	
	Favorable	Unfavorable
FAB subtype	L1	L2, L3
Immunological subtype	B precursor ALL Pre-B Pre-pre-B	Mature B T
White blood cell count	<10,000/μL	>50,000/μL
Age (years)	3–7	<1 >10
Sex	Female	Male
Race	White	Black
Organ involvement	Minimal or absent	Prominent

known as **Burkitt leukemia**, is most commonly observed in these children. It is an infrequent disorder, constituting 3% of all cases of ALL. In some cases, L3 ALL arises in the setting of Burkitt lymphoma rather than as a primary leukemia. L3 ALL has a poor prognosis, and extramedullary involvement of many sites, including the central nervous system, is common.

- **Adolescents and young adults:** T-ALL most commonly occurs in males of this age group. It is an aggressive disorder, which typically presents with a high leukocyte count and a mediastinal mass, and carries a poor prognosis. T-ALL exhibits some overlapping clinicopathological features with lymphoblastic lymphoma, which in 90% of cases is of T-cell lineage. In fact, half of the cases diagnosed as T-ALL present as lymphoblastic lymphoma and a mediastinal mass, and they subsequently progress to a disorder indistinguishable from T-ALL.
- **Adults:** L2 ALL is the subtype in 65% of adults. The clinical presentation is similar to that in children, but the peripheral leukocyte count tends to be higher. Unlike young children, adults with ALL have a poor prognosis.

Prior to the introduction of chemotherapeutic agents for the treatment of malignant diseases, the median survival after the diagnosis of ALL was only 2 months. The natural history of ALL has been dramatically altered by modern aggressive chemotherapy. **A complete clinical remission can now be achieved in over 90% of children with favorable prognostic features (age 3 to 7 years, L1 morphology), and a permanent cure can be anticipated in the majority of such cases.** The prognosis in children with L2 ALL and especially L3 ALL is less favorable. Complete clinical remission can, however, be achieved in most L2 and L3 cases, and a cure is obtained in a substantial minority. In adults with ALL, a complete clinical remission can be achieved in over half of the cases but a cure occurs in only a minority.

THE MALIGNANT LYMPHOMAS

The malignant lymphomas are a heterogeneous group of neoplastic disorders of lymphoid cells. Their heterogeneity reflects the potential for malignant transformation at any stage of B or T lymphocyte differentiation. Malignant lymphomas are solid tumors that usually first involve the lymphoidal tissues. A secondary leukemic distribution, with lymphoma cells circulating in the peripheral blood, may occur. Malignant lymphomas have been divided into non-Hodgkin's lymphomas and Hodgkin's disease. The non-Hodgkin's lymphomas are characterized by the following:

- Homogeneous neoplastic lymphoid cell population
- Characteristic patterns of tumor cell growth, either as cohesive cell aggregates called follicles or nodules or in a diffuse pattern
- Unpredictable or random spread of the disease
- Frequent presentation as a widespread or systemic disorder
- Pronounced clinicopathological differences between children and adults

The histopathological subtypes of the lymphomas have been broadly divided into three major clinical subgroups; (1) low grade or clinically indolent, (2) intermediate grade, and (3) high grade or clinically aggressive. Low-grade lymphomas typically present as widespread or systemic chronic disorders in which cure usually cannot be achieved by conventional therapy. The intermediate- and high-grade lymphomas are more likely to present as localized disorders, and untreated cases usually progress rapidly to death. However, with appropriate treatment, a clinical cure can be achieved in a significant number of these patients.

☐ **Epidemiology:** The malignant lymphomas constitute 3% of all malignancies in Western countries. The annual incidence is 4.5 per 100,000 population with a steadily increasing incidence in the United States. The disease is slightly more common in males and in whites. There is a small peak in the incidence of malignant lymphoma in the preadolescent years, a decline during late adolescence, and a logarithmic increase with advancing age. The median age at onset is 50 years. The overall incidence of the malignant lymphomas, in particular, primary lymphomas of the central nervous system (even if cases of AIDS are excluded), has doubled or tripled in the past 30 years. The high risk of lymphoma in AIDS has substantially added to the increasing incidence.

There are significant geographic and racial variations in the incidence of specific subtypes of malignant lymphomas. For example, the incidence of indolent lymphomas, including follicular lymphomas, is lower in Asia than it is in Western countries, whereas the incidence of aggressive diffuse large cell lymphomas is higher in Asia.

☐ **Pathogenesis:** It is now well established that all non-Hodgkin's lymphomas are clonal, that is they are derived from a single, transformed cell of lymphoid origin. All of these tumors carry one or more genetic defects, and since some of them occurred prior to clonal expansion, they are presumably involved in the etiology of the neoplasm. Moreover, these clonal genetic abnormalities serve as unique markers of the lymphoma and are useful for monitoring minimal residual disease. The genetic defects are often seen as chromosomal translocations that juxtapose two genes. The new configuration may lead to overexpression of a gene, as in Burkitt lymphoma (see Fig. 20-66). In that disease, one of the immunoglobulin genes (active in the context of the B cell) is joined to the C-*myc* oncogene, which becomes constitutively overexpressed and drives the cell through continuous rounds of division. Successive mutations also impart biological changes to a lymphoma during the course of the disease. Some of these evoke an aggressive transformation of the neoplasm, a common event in patients with otherwise indolent lymphomas.

Two uncommon types of lymphoma are etiologically associated with specific viruses. First, there is evidence for Epstein-Barr virus (EBV) infection in 95% of cases of endemic Burkitt lymphoma in central equatorial Africa. By contrast, in sporadic Burkitt lymphoma in the United States and in other nonendemic areas, evidence for EBV infection is found in less than 10% of cases. Second, human T-cell leukemia/lymphoma virus (HTLV-1) is endemic in the southwestern islands of Japan and occurs sporadically in several other geographically restricted areas. Evidence for HTLV-1 infection is demonstrated in more than 90% of cases of adult T-cell leukemia/lymphoma in Japan.

The risk of malignant lymphoma is significantly increased in a variety of disorders, in particular the immunodeficiency and collagen vascular diseases (Table 20-21). **Congenital and acquired immunodeficiency disorders are particularly associated with an increased risk for the development of aggressive B-cell lymphomas.** This risk is further increased in situations in which there is both an immunodeficiency state and chronic antigenic stimulation. For example, renal and cardiac transplant recipients are clinically immunosuppressed to prevent allograft rejection and are simultaneously subjected to chronic antigenic stimulation by the allograft. Such transplant recipients are at significant risk for the development of B-cell immunoblastic lymphomas of the central nervous system. In AIDS, there is a markedly increased risk for the development of aggressive diffuse lymphomas, including undifferentiated, Burkitt and Burkitt-like, and large cell immunoblastic (B-cell type) lymphomas. The frequency of Hodgkin's disease is also increased.

TABLE *20-21* **Disorders with Increased Risk of Secondary Malignant Lymphoma**

Sjögren syndrome
Renal and cardiac transplant recipients
Acquired immunodeficiency syndrome (AIDS)
Congenital immune deficiency syndromes
Chediak-Higashi
Wiscott-Aldrich
Ataxia telangiectasia
IgA deficiency
Severe combined immune deficiency
Alpha heavy-chain disease
Celiac disease
Hodgkin's disease (post-treatment)

The risk of malignant lymphomas is variably increased in all of the collagen vascular disorders. The risk is greatest in Sjögren syndrome, in which malignant B-cell lymphomas, either low-grade or high-grade immunoblastic lymphoma, occurs in up to 10% of cases.

Treatment with alkylating agents and radiation in the therapy for cancer is associated with a risk for the development of malignant lymphomas. It has been reported that occupational exposure to a number of chemicals, including herbicides and benzene, is associated with an increased risk of lymphoma.

The malignant lymphomas are clonally derived from the malignant transformation of a single lymphocyte, which is arrested at a specific stage of B- or T-lymphoid cell differentiation. The neoplastic lymphocytes often express the functional and proliferative characteristics of their normal counterparts. For example, the cells of low-grade B-cell lymphomas may secrete monoclonal immunoglobulins. Low-grade B-cell lymphomas may also exhibit a follicular pattern, which recapitulates the structure of normal secondary follicles (germinal centers). The more mature T-helper cell lymphomas may display hypergammaglobulinemia, presumably because the neoplastic T cells exert a helper function on the non-neoplastic B lymphocytes. Additionally, the better differentiated lymphomas of both B- and T-cell types usually retain the migratory and homing characteristics of their normal counterparts. Low-grade B-cell lymphomas are, therefore, widespread at the time of diagnosis, and involvement is often initially restricted to the B cell–dependent regions of the lymph nodes and spleen. By the same token, T-cell lymphomas often preferentially involve the T cell–dependent regions of the lymph nodes and spleen.

The neoplastic cells in the intermediate- and high-grade lymphomas have a resemblance to normal activated lymphocytes. One third of diffuse large cell lymphomas are clinically localized disorders at the time of diagnosis, possibly reflecting a loss of normal lymphoid migratory characteristics.

☐ **Pathology:** Lymphomas principally involve the lymph nodes, spleen, liver, and bone marrow, although they may infiltrate any organ or tissue.

LYMPH NODES: The lymph nodes involved by malignant lymphoma are enlarged and soft, although they may be firm if there is associated fibrosis. On cut section, they are glistening gray-white, imparting a so-called fish-flesh appearance (Fig. 20-60A). Necrosis, particularly in the aggressive lymphomas, appears as areas of opaque yellow softening.

Microscopically, malignant lymphomas feature monotonous neoplastic lymphoid cells, which infiltrate and ultimately obliterate the normal lymph nodal architecture and that of other tissues. The lymphoma cells exhibit abnormal cytological features, except in the case of diffuse, small cell lymphocytic lymphoma, in which the cells resemble normal lymphocytes (see Fig. 20-60B).

In adult Americans, 40% of non-Hodgkin's lymphomas initially show uniform, cohesive aggregates of neoplastic cells, termed the *follicular or nodular pattern*

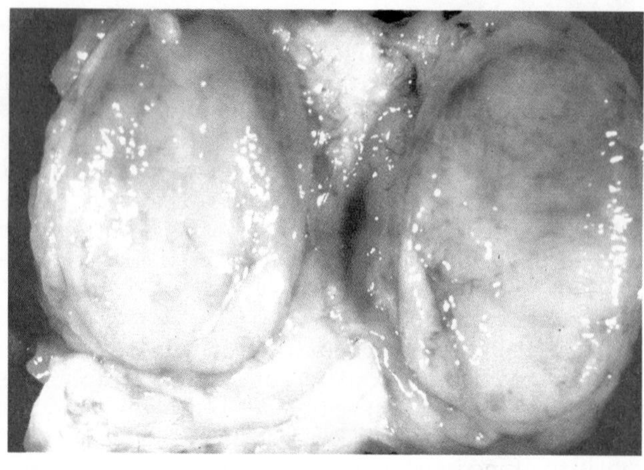

A

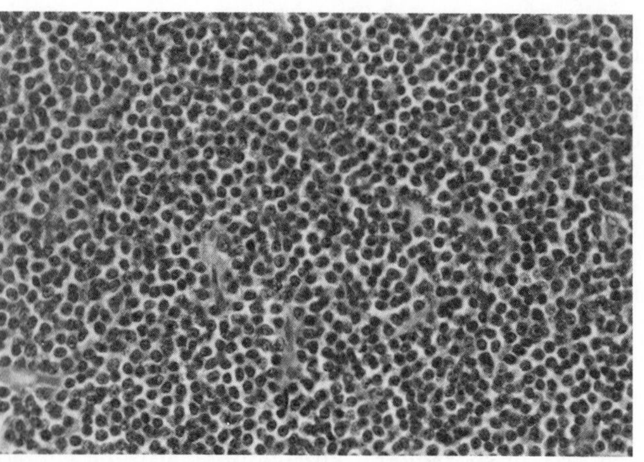

B

FIGURE *20-60*
Small lymphocytic lymphoma/leukemia. (*A*) The bisected, enlarged lymph node shows the characteristic uniform, glistening, gray color, which imparts a fish-flesh appearance. (*B*) On microscopic examination, the lymph nodal architecture is replaced by a diffuse infiltration of normal-appearing small lymphocytes.

(Fig. 20-61). Follicular lymphomas, which are all of B-lymphocyte lineage, must be distinguished from reactive follicular hyperplasia which they simulate. The neoplastic cells in follicular lymphoma progressively infiltrate the residual normal interfollicular areas, and may subsequently progress to a mixed follicular and diffuse pattern, and in many cases eventually to a uniformly diffuse pattern.

In 60% of adult lymphomas, the initial pattern of tumor cell growth is diffusely infiltrative, without the formation of follicles or nodules. In children, virtually all malignant lymphomas are high-grade aggressive neoplasms with a diffuse pattern. Patterns of neoplastic involvement of the lymph nodes are shown in Figure 20-52.

Varying degrees of fibrosis are observed in the involved lymph nodes and other soft tissue sites, particularly in the mediastinum, retroperitoneum, and inguinal area. Necrosis, usually involving single cells rather than broad zones, occurs particularly in the highly proliferative large cell lymphomas. Microscopically, the distinctive "starry sky" pattern observed in some aggressive diffuse lymphomas is due to phagocytosis of cellular debris from multifocal single cell necrosis by macrophages.

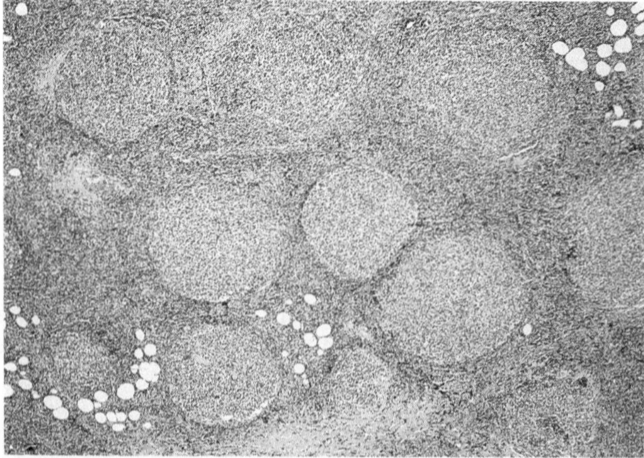

FIGURE *20-61*
Follicular lymphoma. The lymph nodal architecture is replaced by homogeneous nodular aggregates of neoplastic B lymphocytes.

SPLEEN: The involved spleen is mildly to moderately enlarged, and the cut surface shows a generalized expansion of the white pulp, particularly in low-grade lymphomas. Discrete, variably sized tumor masses are characteristic of the more aggressive intermediate- and high-grade lymphomas. Microscopically, B-cell lymphomas initially involve the B cell–dependent germinal centers and mantle zones of the spleen. By contrast, T-cell lymphomas first infiltrate the periarteriolar lymphoid sheaths and, less frequently, the marginal zones.

LIVER: The liver may be enlarged. One may observe a vague accentuation of the normal lobular pattern, owing to widespread involvement of the portal tracts, particularly in low-grade lymphomas. Alternatively, there may be discrete gray-tan tumor masses in the liver, especially in the intermediate and high-grade lymphomas. In the liver, both B- and T-cell lymphomas typically involve the portal tracts. In some T-cell lymphomas, however, neoplastic cells are located in the hepatic sinusoids (leukemic distribution).

BONE MARROW: The pattern of lymphomatous involvement in the bone marrow may be focal, multifocal, or diffuse. Focal paratrabecular involvement is a characteristic initial finding in the follicular lymphomas. Multifocal or diffuse involvement rather than selective paratrabecular involvement is seen in the aggressive diffuse large cell lymphomas.

Classification of Lymphomas

Because the malignant lymphomas are pathologically heterogeneous, a number of classification systems have been proposed and several of these have been widely accepted. In the 1960s and 70s, the prevailing classification systems were developed by hematopathologists and were called the Rappaport, Lukes-Collins and Kiel classifications. In 1982, the International Working Formulation grouped lymphomas by clinical categories into three grades according to overall survival:

- Low-grade or clinically indolent
- Intermediate grade
- High-grade or clinically aggressive

More recently a group of pathologists has proposed an updated classification called the "REAL" (revised European-American lymphoma) terminology. The REAL classification summarizes histopathological, immunological, cytogenetic, and molecular features of defined lymphoma entities.The REAL system does not divide the lymphomas into clinical grades and, as of this writing, has not been widely accepted by oncologists. The REAL classification does catalog several non-Hodgkin's lymphomas that have been recognized after the Working Formulation was initially established. Examples of these more recently described entities are mantle-cell lymphoma, marginal zone lymphoma including mucosal-associated lymphoid tissue lymphoma (MALToma). By recognizing and adding the more recently described entities, the Working Formulation remains in general use and is the basis for the classification of non-Hodgkin's lymphomas presented later. A summary of the Working Formulation is presented in Table 20-22.

TABLE *20-22* **Working Formulation of Non-Hodgkin's Lymphoma**

Working Formulation
Low Grade
A. Small lymphocytic
Consistent with CLL
Plasmacytoid
B. Follicular, predominately small cleaved cell
C. Follicular, mixed small cleaved and large cell
Intermediate Grade
D. Follicular, large cell
E. Diffuse, small cleaved cell
F. Diffuse, mixed small and large cell
G. Diffuse, large cell
High Grade
H. Large cell immunoblastic
I. Lymphoblastic
J. Small noncleaved cell
Burkitt
Non-Burkitt
Miscellaneous Categories
K. Cutaneous T cell
L. Adult T-cell leukemia/lymphoma

The Working Formulation facilitates comparison of the various classification systems but does not incorporate immunological concepts. Cytological features of the principal subtypes of malignant lymphomas following the schema of the Working Formulation are illustrated in Figure 20-62.

The Working Formulation attempts to predict the clinical behavior of lymphomas, particularly their response to chemotherapy. In general, low-grade lymphomas follow an indolent course but are difficult to eradicate, owing to a low proliferative index. By contrast, high-grade lymphomas are characterized by an aggressive natural history and yet are often cured by appropriate chemotherapy. In this case, a high proliferative rate renders the tumor more susceptible to cytotoxic agents.

Low-Grade Malignant Lymphoma

Low-grade malignant lymphomas include (1) small lymphocytic, (2) small lymphocytic plasmacytoid, (3) follicular small cleaved, and (4) follicular mixed small cleaved and large cell lymphomas.

Small Lymphocytic Lymphoma

Small lymphocytic lymphoma (SLL) is a diffuse lymphoma in which the neoplastic cells resemble normal small lymphocytes. B-lymphocyte lineage is found in nearly all cases, and a T-cell phenotype is very rare.

☐ **Pathogenesis:** The cells of SLL are closely related to those of CLL, both morphologically and immunophenotypically. The cells of both SLL and CLL express CD5, CD19, CD20, and CD23 and weakly display surface membrane immunoglobulin, usually IgM-κ. This immunophenotypic pattern indicates an intermediate stage of B-cell differentiation, similar to that of normal lymphocytes in the medullary cords of the lymph nodes. Thus, the distinction between SLL and CLL is made on the basis of the predominant distribution of the tumor cells, with SLL affecting principally lymph nodes and CLL, the bone marrow and the peripheral blood. Importantly, up to one third of patients who present with SLL eventually develop peripheral lymphocytosis and a clinical syndrome indistinguishable from CLL. In most cases, the tumor cells of SLL exhibit chromosomal aberrations, although none are unique. One third have trisomy 12.

☐ **Pathology:** Microscopically, the normal architecture of involved lymph nodes and other tissue sites is replaced by a monotonous population of small lymphocytes. There are randomly scattered pale foci of partially transformed lymphocytes, called "proliferation centers." Prolymphocytes in these centers have vesicular nuclei and distinctive single nucleoli. Also identified are paraimmunoblasts, which simulate immunoblasts but are smaller and have pale cytoplasm. Mitotic figures tend to be uncommon in SLL, and the presence of over 30 mitoses per 20 high-power fields predicts a more aggressive clinical course.

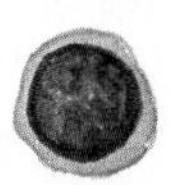

SMALL LYMPHOCYTIC
Nucleus: round
Chromatin: dense
Nucleolus: indistinct
Cytoplasm: scant, blue

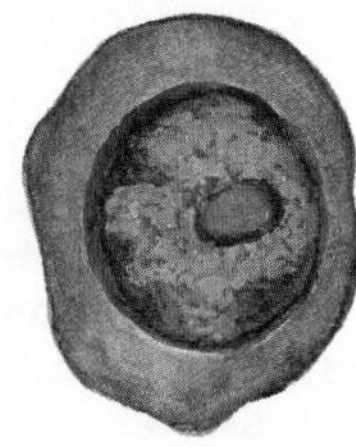

IMMUNOBLASTIC
Nucleus: round to oval
Chromatin: vesicular
Nucleolus: prominent
Cytoplasm: moderate, dense, blue

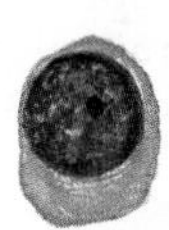

SMALL LYMPHOCYTIC, PLASMACYTOID
Nucleus: round, eccentric
Chromatin: dense
Nucleolus: variable
Cytoplasm: moderate, blue

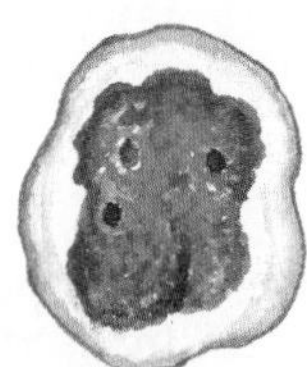

IMMUNOBLASTIC, T
Nucleus: round to irregular
Chromatin: variable
Nucleoli: variable
Cytoplasm: clear

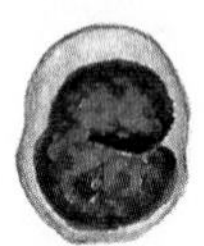

SMALL CLEAVED
Nucleus: indented
Chromatin: coarse
Nucleolus: small
Cytoplasm: scant

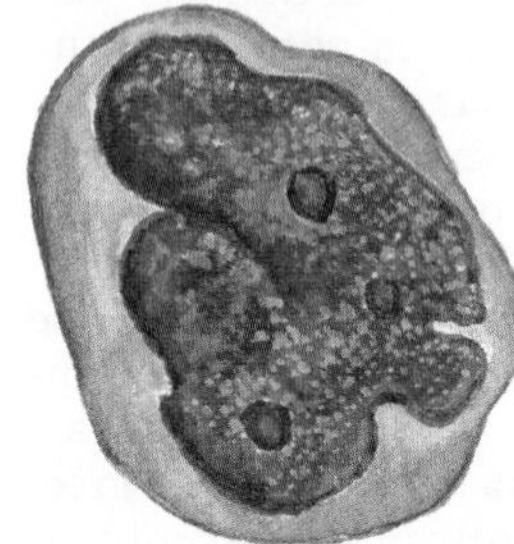

IMMUNOBLASTIC, POLYMORPHOUS
Nucleus: pleomorphic
Chromatin: variable
Nucleoli: variable
Cytoplasm: moderate

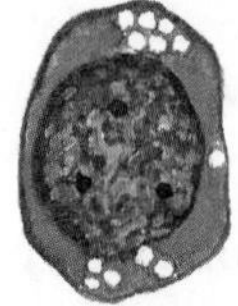

SMALL NONCLEAVED (BURKITT)
Nucleus: round to oval
Chromatin: coarsely reticulated
Nucleoli: small, 2-5
Cytoplasm: blue, vacuolated

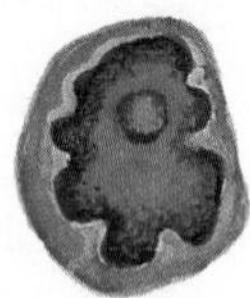

LYMPHOBLASTIC, CONVOLUTED
Nucleus: irregular
Chromatin: delicate
Nucleolus: variable
Cytoplasm: blue, scant

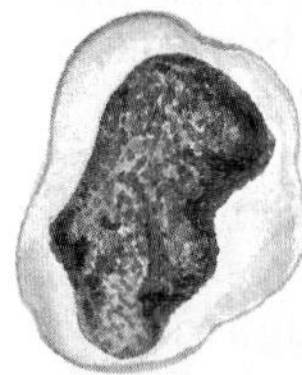

LARGE CLEAVED
Nucleus: irregular, indented
Chromatin: dense
Nucleoli: indistinct
Cytoplasm: scant, pale

LYMPHOBLASTIC, NONCONVOLUTED
Nucleus: round to oval
Chromatin: delicate
Nucleolus: variable
Cytoplasm: scant, blue

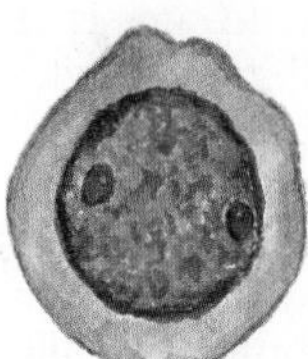

LARGE NONCLEAVED
Nucleus: round to oval
Chromatin: vesicular
Nucleoli: contiguous to membrane
Cytoplasm: moderate

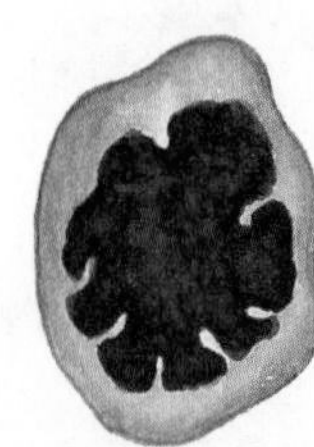

MYCOSIS FUNGOIDES
Nucleus: irregular, convoluted
Chromatin: dense
Nucleolus: indistinct
Cytoplasm: scant

FIGURE *20-62*
Malignant lymphomas: neoplastic cells.

When the spleen, liver, or bone marrow is involved, the microscopic appearance is indistinguishable from that of CLL.

☐ **Clinical Features:** Similar to the morphologic characteristics, the clinical features of SLL resemble those of CLL. The disorder is most common in middle-aged to elderly men and tends to be indolent and chronic. Generalized painless lymphadenopathy and moderate hepatosplenomegaly are typical.

Small Lymphocytic Lymphoma with Plasmacytoid Differentiation

WALDENSTRÖM MACROGLOBULINEMIA: This diffuse B-cell lymphoma exhibits plasmacytoid differentiation and secretes monoclonal IgM, usually with kappa light chains. The neoplastic cells are small to medium-sized lymphocytes, with eccentric nuclei and a moderate amount of purple cytoplasm.

Waldenström macroglobulinemia occurs most commonly in middle-aged to elderly adults. Generalized lymphadenopathy and hepatosplenomegaly are common presenting signs. A leukemic distribution of circulating plasmacytoid lymphocytes occurs in 10% to 20% of cases. Microscopic examination of the lymph nodes and bone marrow reveals focal to diffuse infiltration by normal-appearing small lymphocytes and plasmacytoid lymphocytes. Scattered transformed lymphocytes and mast cells are frequently observed. Evidence for immunoglobulin production includes refractile eosinophilic nuclear inclusions (*Dutcher bodies*) and cytoplasmic globules (*Russell bodies*).

Hyperviscosity syndrome in macroglobulinemia is secondary to the high-molecular-weight IgM paraprotein in the blood. Circulatory disturbances, principally in the central and peripheral nervous systems, are observed, including peripheral neuropathy, headache, dizziness, deafness, paresis, and coma. A bleeding tendency, with severe nosebleeds and ecchymoses, is caused by a reduced factor VIII level, owing to the combination of factor VIII with IgM paraprotein. The clinical course of Waldenström macroglobulinemia is indolent, with a mean survival of 3 to 4 years. The hyperviscosity syndrome is treated with plasmapheresis, and the lymphoma is treated with chemotherapy.

HEAVY-CHAIN DISEASES: These disorders are uncommon B-lymphocyte malignant lymphomas in which tumor cells secrete a portion of an immunoglobulin heavy-chain molecule. IgA, IgG, IgM, and IgD heavy-chain diseases have been described.

IgA heavy-chain disease (α chain disease) is the only common subtype, occurring endemically in some Middle Eastern countries. The disorder predominantly occurs in adults younger than 30 years of age. Males and females are equally affected. The pathogenesis appears to involve an acquired inability to assemble a complete secretory IgA molecule. The resulting impaired immune response to enteric microorganisms leads to a compensatory hyperplasia of defective plasma cells in the lamina propria of the duodenum and jejunum (immunoproliferative small intestinal disease). Frequently, there is an associated malabsorption syndrome, with diarrhea and steatorrhea. More significantly, the combined risk factors of immunodeficiency and chronic antigenic stimulation predispose to a high incidence of B-cell immunoblastic lymphoma, called *Mediterranean lymphoma* (see Chapter 13).

IgG heavy-chain disease is a clinically aggressive disorder characterized by generalized lymphadenopathy, hepatosplenomegaly, and prominent involvement of Waldeyer tonsillar ring. Secondary palatal edema is common. Variably transformed lymphocytes and plasmacytoid lymphocytes populate the involved organs.

Low-Grade Follicular Lymphoma

Low-grade follicular lymphomas are the most common type of lymphoma in the United States. They are classified into two types in the Working Formulation: follicular small cleaved and mixed small cleaved and large cell lymphoma.

FOLLICULAR SMALL CLEAVED CELL LYMPHOMA: This lymphoma, which is the most common subtype (60%) of the follicular lymphomas, is characterized by cohesive aggregates, or follicles, of neoplastic lymphocytes. The tumor cells are atypical, small to medium-sized (10 to 15 μ), lymphoid cells, with indented or cleaved nuclei, clumped chromatin, poorly defined nucleoli, and scant cytoplasm. Among the neoplastic cells, less than 20% are large and noncleaved. The mitotic rate is low. The immunological cell markers include prominent surface membrane monoclonal immunoglobulin, usually IgM-κ, and complement receptors (CD21). B-cell differentiation antigens, including CD19, CD20, CD22, and CD24, are usually expressed.

A translocation involving the long arms of chromosomes 14 and 18, t(14;18)(q32;q21), is identified in most cases of follicular lymphoma. The translocation involves the immunoglobulin heavy-chain locus on chromosome 14 and the protooncogene *bcl*-2 on chromosome 18. *Bcl*-2 acts to prevent the programmed cell death (apoptosis) of B lymphocytes. Interestingly, transgenic mice carrying the *bcl*-2 gene develop conspicuous lymphoid hyperplasia characterized by the abnormal persistence of a mature B-cell population and ultimately develop lymphoma. It has been suggested that the overexpression of *bcl*-2 confers a survival advantage on B cells by allowing them to remain in the G_0 nonproliferating state without undergoing apoptosis.

Follicular small cleaved cell lymphoma is typically an indolent disorder, with a median survival of 10 years. Middle-aged and elderly adults of either sex are affected. The disorder is usually disseminated at the time of diagnosis, with bone marrow involvement in most cases. Generalized lymphadenopathy and moderate hepatosplenomegaly are observed. A leukemic distribution of lymphocytes with notched and cleaved nuclei occurs in up to 20% of cases, usually late in the course of the disease. Follicular small cleaved cell lymphoma often progresses to a diffuse lymphoma.

FOLLICULAR MIXED SMALL CLEAVED AND LARGE CELL LYMPHOMA: This variant features a mixture of small cleaved and large noncleaved cells. The latter constitute 20% to 50% of the total neoplastic cell population. The mixed small cleaved and large cell type comprises 30% of follicular lymphomas, and its clinical course is similar to that of follicular lymphoma composed exclusively of small cleaved cells. Progression to more aggressive subtypes of malignant lymphoma may occur.

Intermediate-Grade Malignant Lymphoma

FOLLICULAR LARGE CELL LYMPHOMA: This is an uncommon disorder (less than 10% of follicular lymphomas), in which the malignant follicles are largely composed of either large cleaved or noncleaved transformed lymphoid cells. As the disease evolves, the follicular pattern is often progressively obliterated and the neoplasm becomes a diffuse large cell lymphoma. The median survival is about 4 years.

DIFFUSE SMALL CLEAVED CELL LYMPHOMA: This lymphoma features diffuse infiltrates of neoplastic cells with cleaved, or notched, nuclei and scant cytoplasm (Fig. 20-63). The neoplastic cells may be indistinguishable from those of follicular small cleaved cell lymphoma, and most cases are predictably of B-lymphocyte lineage. In some instances, diffuse small cleaved cell lymphoma reflects progression of a previous follicular lymphoma, whereas others are actually mantle cell lymphomas.

Diffuse small cleaved cell lymphoma accounts for fewer than 4% of malignant lymphomas in the United States. The disease is more common in men than in women, and the median age at diagnosis is 60 years. It is moderately aggressive, and patients tend to present with advanced disease, including generalized lymphadenopathy, hepatosplenomegaly, and anemia.

DIFFUSE, MIXED, SMALL AND LARGE CELL LYMPHOMAS: These lymphomas are a heterogenous mixture of small and large cells of either B- or T-lymphocyte lineage.

B-cell diffuse mixed cell lymphoma is composed of neoplastic cells analogous to those of the follicular mixed lymphomas. It is probable that in most cases the disease represents progression of a previous follicular tumor. The cells of diffuse, mixed small and large cell lymphoma are predominantly small cleaved lymphocytes, with large, noncleaved, lymphoid cells comprising 20% to 50% of the neoplastic population (Fig. 20-64). Diffuse, mixed, small and large cell lymphoma is usually widespread at the time of presentation.

T-cell diffuse lymphoma of mixed cell type is composed of mature (peripheral) post-thymic T cells. Unlike the B-cell diffuse, mixed lymphomas, the neoplastic T cells do not resemble the cells of follicular lymphomas but are a mixture of atypical small and large lymphocytes. The characteristic features of diffuse, mixed T-cell lymphomas include (1) diffuse infiltration by small-to-large lymphoid cells; (2) small clusters of neoplastic cells outlined by delicate reticulin fibers; (3) prominent postcapillary venules; and (4) admixed inflammatory cells, including eosinophils and plasma cells. Cells similar to Reed-Sternberg cells may be identified, thereby simulating Hodgkin's disease. In general, the clinical course of T-cell diffuse, mixed lymphoma is comparable to its B-cell counterpart, and the tumor is treated as an aggressive diffuse lymphoma.

DIFFUSE LARGE CLEAVED AND NONCLEAVED CELL LYMPHOMAS: Diffuse large cell lymphomas are the second most common lymphomas in the United States. They are composed of large transformed lymphoid cells of either B-lymphocyte (90%) or T-lymphocyte (10%) lineage. The nuclear contours are either irregular or indented (cleaved) or round to oval (noncleaved). The nuclei show vesicular to coarsely reticulated chromatin and one to several nucleoli apposed to the nuclear membrane. Scant to moderate pink cytoplasm is present. Numerous mitoses are typical.

Clinically, diffuse large cleaved and noncleaved cell lymphomas of both B- and T-cell types tend to behave aggressively. The disorder may occur at any age. Lymph nodes are commonly first involved. However, extranodal sites of origin such as the stomach, terminal ileum, thy-

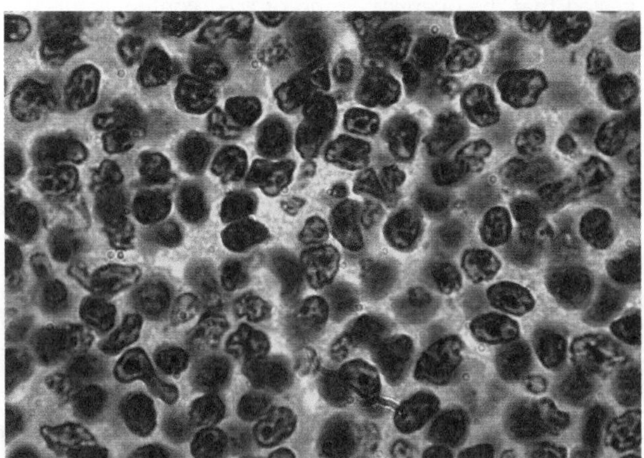

FIGURE *20-63*
Diffuse small cleaved cell lymphoma. The lymph node demonstrates a diffuse infiltrate of neoplastic B lymphocytes with cleaved or notched nuclei and scant cytoplasm.

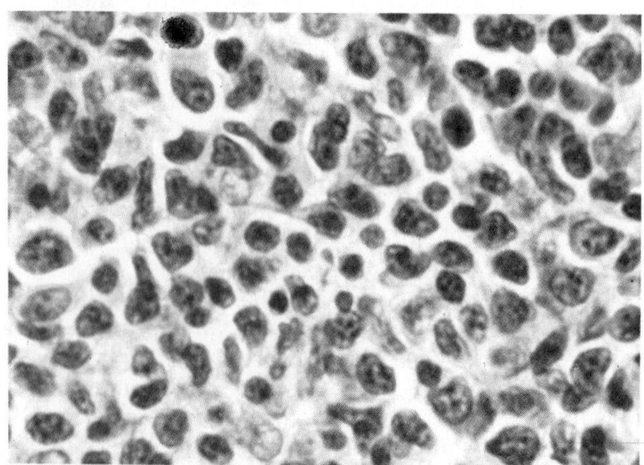

FIGURE *20-64*
Diffuse, mixed, small and large cell lymphoma. The lymph nodal architecture is replaced by a diffuse infiltrate of small cleaved and large noncleaved neoplastic B lymphocytes.

roid gland, bone marrow, and the skin are the primary sites of involvement in 30% of cases of diffuse, large cleaved and noncleaved cell lymphomas.

High-Grade Malignant Lymphoma

LARGE CELL IMMUNOBLASTIC LYMPHOMA: Immunoblast is a morphological term that refers to a transformed extrafollicular lymphoid cell that (1) is three to four times the size of a small lymphocyte, (2) displays a characteristic prominent nucleolus or nucleoli, and (3) exhibits abundant cytoplasm. Immunoblastic lymphomas are high-grade tumors whose cells resemble normal immunoblasts, although there is no conclusive evidence that they arise from the latter.

The REAL classification does not recognize distinct subtypes of large-cell lymphoma (immunoblastic vs. other), because pathologists find it difficult to distinguish among these subtypes morphologically. In addition, differences in clinical responses among the various subtypes are not compelling. Nevertheless, the following discussion incorporates the description provided through the Working Formulation.

Immunoblastic tumors are clinically aggressive, diffuse large cell lymphomas, arising in middle-aged or elderly persons of both sexes. They frequently occur in the setting of an immunodeficiency or disordered immune state, such as occurs in allograft recipients and patients with AIDS, chronic thyroiditis, and Sjögren syndrome. Most immunoblastic lymphomas are of B-cell lineage, and only a small minority derive from T cells. The Working Formulation recognizes four morphological variants of immunoblastic lymphomas:

- **Plasmacytoid:** This type is characterized by large, transformed cells with eccentric vesicular nuclei, a prominent eosinophilic nucleolus, and abundant blue-purple cytoplasm (Fig. 20-65).
- **Clear cell:** This form is identified by moderate to abundant clear cytoplasm.
- **Polymorphous:** This variety features the presence of tumor giant cells, with lobated or multilobed nuclei and prominent eosinophilic nucleoli, which may simulate the Reed-Sternberg cells of Hodgkin's disease.
- **Epithelioid cell component:** This disorder exhibits benign epithelioid macrophages, which in some cases are so numerous that they obscure the underlying neoplastic lymphoid cells.

Most plasmacytoid variants are of B-cell lineage, whereas the other immunoblastic lymphomas (clear cell, polymorphous, and epithelioid cell) usually originate from T cells. The morphological subtypes have no prognostic significance, and half of all patients with immunoblastic lymphoma die within 5 years.

Anaplastic large cell lymphoma (ALCL, Ki-1 lymphoma) is an uncommon variant of large cell lymphoma, which typically occurs in children or young adults and was not included in the original Working Formulation. The lymph node sinuses are often infiltrated by large transformed neoplastic cells with prominent nucleoli. The disorder is more commonly of T-lymphocyte than of B or null lymphocyte lineage, and the neoplastic cells are positive for the Ki-1 antigen (CD30). The neoplastic cells of T lineage often have a t(2;5) translocation involving a fusion of the genes *npm* and *alk*. In some cases, particularly in adults, ALCL lymphoma tends to be clinically aggressive, with frequent involvement of the skin, lungs, pleura, and central nervous system. This disorder is more clinically indolent in children.

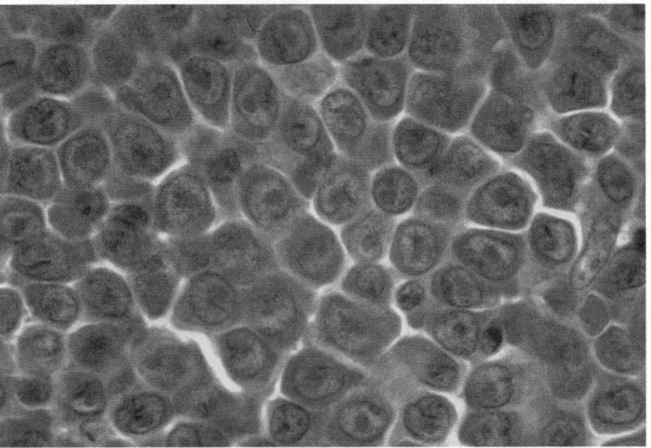

FIGURE *20-65*
Large cell immunoblastic lymphoma, plasmacytoid type. A lymph node displays uniform, large, transformed lymphocytes with vesicular nuclei, prominent nucleoli, and abundant basophilic cytoplasm.

LYMPHOBLASTIC LYMPHOMA: This variety of lymphoma is a clinically aggressive, diffuse, high-grade neoplasm of primitive lymphoblasts. The neoplastic cells are morphologically indistinguishable from those of ALL and are medium in size, measuring 10 to 15 μ in diameter. They have round or convoluted and cerebriform nuclei, with delicate chromatin, indistinct nucleoli, and scant cytoplasm. The mitotic rate is extremely high. The large majority of cases are of precursor T-lymphocyte lineage, whereas 10% are derived from B cells. The neoplastic T lymphocytes express the immunophenotype of a thymocyte. The cells express early T-cell markers (frequently common thymocyte marker CD-1) and the intranuclear enzyme terminal deoxynucleotidyl-transferase (Tdt), a phenotype indistinguishable from that of ALL.

Both T and B lineage lymphoblastic lymphomas exhibit overlapping clinicopathological features overlapping with their ALL counterparts. Nevertheless, the majority of lymphoblastic lymphomas differ in their clinical presentation and immunophenotype from ALL. The lymphoblastic lymphomas present initially as soft tissue masses and may subsequently progress to a leukemic distribution indistinguishable from ALL. However, the neoplastic cells of lymphoblastic lymphomas often have a more mature thymic immunophenotype than that of ALL.

T-lymphoblastic lymphomas occur most commonly in adolescent and young adult males, although the disease also occurs in young children and older adults. An anterior mediastinal mass occurs in at least half of the cases, apparently reflecting a thymic origin of the tumor.

Supradiaphragmatic lymphadenopathy is common. The clinical course is marked by rapid spread to the bone marrow, with secondary leukemic distribution and involvement of the central nervous system, in particular the lepto-meninges. The prognosis is poor.

Although precursor B-lymphoblastic lymphoma is morphologically indistinguishable from the T-cell variety, it exhibits somewhat different clinical features. These include (1) absence of a mediastinal mass, (2) lymph-adenopathy, (3) abdominal involvement, and (4) lytic bone lesions. The pronounced male predominance characteristic of T-lymphoblastic lymphoma is not observed.

DIFFUSE SMALL NONCLEAVED CELL LYMPHOMA (BURKITT LYMPHOMA): The diffuse, small noncleaved cell lymphomas include Burkitt lymphoma and Burkitt-like lymphoma. Both of these tumors are high-grade, clinically aggressive, neoplasms of B lymphocytes. They display extremely high mitotic rates and are among the most rapidly proliferative human tumors.

Diffuse small noncleaved cell lymphoma is composed of uniform, medium-sized lymphoid cells, with round nuclei, coarsely reticulated chromatin, 2 to 5 small nucleoli, and a rim of dense blue-purple cytoplasm. Scattered benign macrophages containing cellular debris impart a "starry sky" pattern (Fig. 20-66).

Morphologically, Burkitt lymphoma cells are indistinguishable from those of L3 ALL (Burkitt leukemia). The usual phenotype includes the B lymphocyte differentiation antigens CD19, CD20, CD22, and CD10 (CALLA). IgM heavy chains, with κ or λ light chains, are found on the cell surface. A characteristic chromosomal abnormality, t(8;14), is the translocation of the protooncogene c-*myc* on chromosome 8 to chromosome 14, which is noted in 80% of the tumors (see Chapter 5). In the remainder, the translocation involves chromosomes 8 and 2 or 8 and 22. **Whatever the translocation, the c-*myc* protooncogene is deregulated by its proximity to an immunoglobulin promotor sequence and by the loss of its own regulatory ele-ments.** Such an event seems to be necessary for the development of the malignant phenotype, and other genetic alterations are also probably involved.

Endemic Burkitt Lymphoma: This lymphoma is endemic in tropical equatorial Africa and in parts of New Guinea and occurs sporadically in other areas of the world. The Epstein-Barr viral genome is identified in the neoplastic cells in 95% of cases. The median age at onset in endemic areas is 7 years, and the common sites of involvement include the jaw bones (maxilla and mandible) and abdominal sites, such as the ileocecal region of the small bowel, kidneys, and ovaries.

Sporadic Burkitt Lymphoma: In nonendemic areas, fewer than 15% of cases of Burkitt lymphoma harbor the EBV genome. The median age at onset is 11 years, and abdominal sites are commonly first involved. Tumors of the jaw are rare. In both endemic and sporadic cases of Burkitt lymphoma, the lymph nodes tend to be spared. As the disease progresses, the bone marrow may be involved, with a leukemic distribution (L3ALL).

Burkitt lymphoma (endemic or sporadic) is a highly treatable lymphoma in patients with an intact immune system. Even in the case of advanced disease, 75% of the patients can be cured by chemotherapy.

Burkitt-Like Lymphoma: This is an uncommon diffuse lymphoma of B-cell lineage. The median age at onset is 34 years, compared with the childhood presentation of Burkitt lymphoma. The neoplastic lymphocytes of Burkitt-like lymphoma display a greater variability in cell size and nuclear membrane configuration than do those

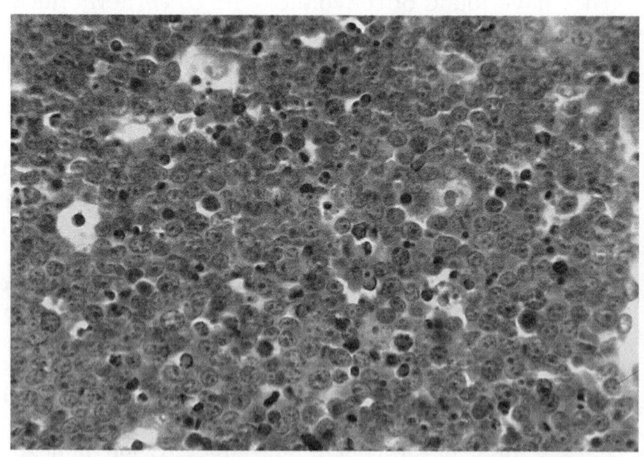

A

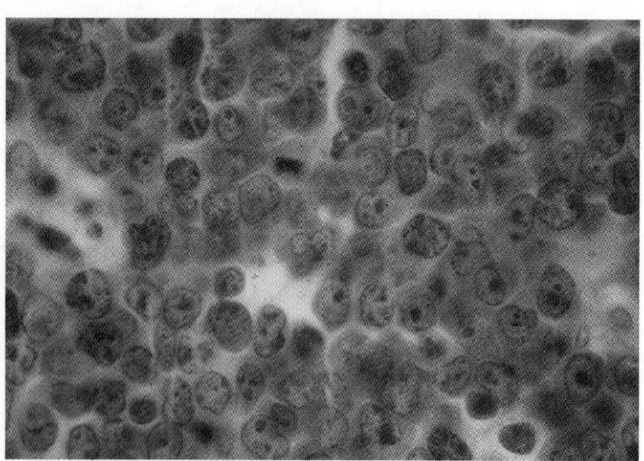

B

FIGURE *20-66*

Burkitt lymphoma. (*A*) Low-power view of a lymph node shows a uniform infiltrate of medium-sized lymphoid cells, with scattered, benign macrophages, which impart a starry-sky pattern. (*B*) High-power view illustrates the neoplastic lymphocytes, which contain round nuclei with coarsely reticulated chromatin and small nucleoli and abundant basophilic cytoplasm. Numerous mitoses are evident. Large macrophages with abundant clear cytoplasm containing cell debris are prominent.

in Burkitt lymphoma. The chromatin is delicate, a single eosinophilic nucleolus is often present, and the cytoplasm is pale. Lymph nodes are usually involved.

Burkitt and Burkitt-like lymphomas are the most common (40%) lymphomas in AIDS, the remainder equally divided between large cell lymphoma and Hodgkin's disease.

Miscellaneous Lymphomas

Several distinctive subtypes of malignant lymphoma are included in a miscellaneous category in the Working Formulation.

Cutaneous T-Cell Lymphoma (Mycosis Fungoides)

Cutaneous T-cell lymphoma (CTCL) is a primary lymphoma of the skin composed of mature post-thymic T-helper (CD4+) lymphocytes. CTCL is a chronic disorder, with a survival of years to decades. It is characterized by three well-defined clinicopathological stages.

- **The premycotic or eczematous stage** is of some years' duration and is not distinguishable from a variety of benign chronic dermatoses. The skin biopsy specimen is not diagnostic of lymphoma and shows a nonspecific perivascular and periadnexal lymphocytic infiltration, with accompanying eosinophils and plasma cells.
- **The plaque stage,** which follows the premycotic stage, is characterized by well-demarcated, raised cutaneous plaques. A definitive diagnosis of CTCL can usually be made in this stage. There is a dense subepidermal bandlike infiltrate of lymphoid cells, with irregular nuclear contours and a spectrum of cell size. Distinctive medium-to-large lymphoid cells with hyperchromatic nuclei and cerebriform nuclear contours, called *mycosis cells,* are typical. Often, clusters of mycosis cells in intraepidermal clear spaces, termed *Pautrier microabscesses,* are observed.
- *The tumor stage* features raised cutaneous tumors, most commonly on the face and in the body folds, which frequently ulcerate and become secondarily infected. The name *mycosis fungoides* initially derived from the raised, fungating, mushroom-like appearance of these cutaneous tumors. Extracutaneous involvement, particularly of the lymph nodes, spleen, liver, bone marrow, and lungs, commonly occurs.

Sézary syndrome is the leukemic variant of mycosis fungoides. The circulating neoplastic lymphoid cells (Sézary cells; Fig. 20-67) have cerebriform nuclei and a perinuclear ring of clear, PAS-positive vacuoles. Sézary cells are most commonly identified when there is generalized erythroderma and skin exfoliation, which occurs in 15% of cases of mycosis fungoides.

The predominant clinical manifestations in CTCL are extreme pruritus and recurrent cutaneous infections. The prognosis varies with the stage of the illness. Patients with early disease exhibit a 90% 5-year survival, whereas those with advanced CTCL (visceral and lymph node involvement) have a median survival of only 2 years. Infection and progressive lymphoma are the common causes of death. CTCL is treated with topical and systemic chemotherapy, photochemotherapy, and radiation.

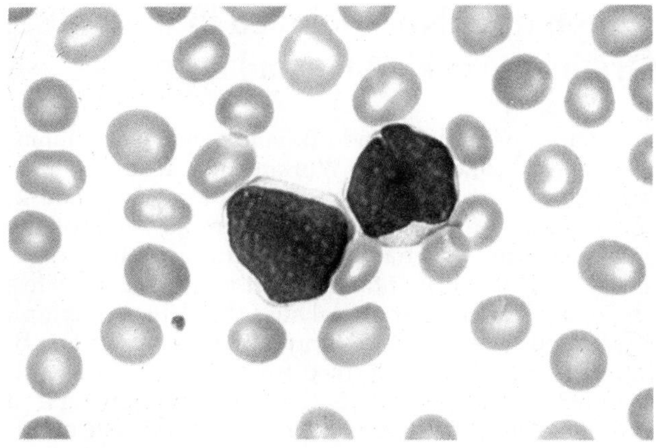

FIGURE *20-67*
Sézary cells. Two circulating neoplastic T- helper cells with irregular nuclei and a thin rim of cytoplasm are seen.

Adult T-Cell Leukemia/Lymphoma

Adult T-cell leukemia/lymphoma (ATLL) is an aggressive malignancy that is endemic in the southwestern islands of Japan and occurs with increased frequency in the Caribbean basin (including Florida) and West Africa. **ATLL is thought to be caused by a retrovirus, the human T-cell leukemia/lymphoma virus (HTLV-I)** (see Chapter 5). The virus is transmitted perinatally from infected mothers to their offspring or by sexual contact later in life. The risk of ATLL among carriers of HTLV-I is estimated to be no more than a few percent. The median age at onset of ATLL is 45 years, and in the Western hemisphere the disorder has occurred almost exclusively in blacks of West African ancestry. Carriers of HTLV-I are also at risk for the development of a distinctive myelopathy, characterized by progressive demyelination of the spinal cord.

ATLL is characterized by diffuse infiltration of many organs by (1) small lymphoid cells, (2) mixed small and large lymphoid cells, or (3) large lymphoid cells with irregular nuclear contours. The disease features involvement of the skin, lymph nodes, lungs, pleura, central nervous system, bone marrow, and blood.

ATLL carries a poor prognosis, although indolent variants have been described. The disease can begin acutely as a leukemia or with predominant involvement of the lymph nodes as in other lymphomas, followed by conversion to leukemia. Hypercalcemia is often prominent. Patients with aggressive acute leukemia have a 50% survival of less than 6 months, despite vigorous chemotherapy.

Lymphomas Not Included in the Original Working Formulation.

There are several low-grade B-lymphocytic lymphomas that are not included in the Working Formulation.

The marginal zone lymphomas are low-grade B-cell lymphomas derived from B lymphocytes of the marginal zone, which is located contiguous to and external to follicular mantle zones in various tissue sites. They may involve extranodal sites (MALToma), lymph nodes, and spleen. **MALT lymphoma** is a low-grade B-cell lymphoma that is derived from the ***m***ucosa-***a***ssociated ***l***ymphoid ***t***issue. It is the only common type of marginal zone lymphoma. The most common site of origin is the gastric mucosa. Characteristic histopathological features include (1) diffuse infiltration of small to medium-sized lymphocytes with slight nuclear irregularity and scant to moderate pale cytoplasm; (2) residual normal germinal centers; and (3) selective infiltration of the epithelium by clusters of tumor cells (lymphoepithelial lesion). Gastric MALT- oma is associated with *Helicobacter pylori* infection. The polyclonal T-cell immunological response to *H. pylori* secondarily drives B lymphocyte proliferation, with the resultant emergence of a B-cell neoplastic clone. In some cases, antibiotic treatment for *H. pylori* results in remission or cure of the B-cell proliferation.

In lymph nodes, marginal zone lymphomas tend to be disseminated indolent disorders with monocytoid B-cell differentiation of the neoplastic cells. Monocytoid B cells, which derive from the perisinusoidal zones of lymph nodes, are medium-sized cells with bland round to indented nuclei and moderate clear cytoplasm. The infiltration in this disorder is initially sinusoidal and perifollicular. Middle-aged and elderly men are most commonly affected.

Primary splenic marginal zone lymphoma is a rare indolent disorder. The neoplastic cells arise in the splenic marginal zone between the red pulp and the white pulp. They tend to be small to medium-sized, with moderate pale cytoplasm. A leukemic distribution with circulating lymphoid cells that display villous processes is common.

Mantle cell lymphoma is a B-cell neoplasm in which the neoplastic lymphocytes are morphologically and immunologically intermediate between small lymphocytes and small cleaved lymphocytes. The nuclei of the neoplastic cells are round to slightly irregular. The lymph nodes show either diffuse involvement with vaguely defined nodules or a broad expansion of the perifollicular mantle zones (see Fig. 20-52). The mantle cell lymphomas have a characteristic chromosomal translocation t(11;14), which joins the *bcl*-1 oncogene on chromosome 11 to the immunoglobulin heavy-chain gene locus on chromosome 14. The *bcl*-1 gene product is cyclin-D, a protein involved in the control of mitosis.

Middle-aged and elderly adults are affected by mantle cell lymphoma. Although originally considered to be an indolent lymphoma because of the cytological features, the disease is now known to be a clinically aggressive neoplasm with a poor prognosis. Several more aggressive subtypes, including a blastic variant, have recently been described.

HODGKIN'S DISEASE

Hodgkin's disease (HD) is a unique malignant neoplasm originating in lymphoid tissue that features the presence of characteristic Reed-Sternberg cells in association with an appropriate cellular background.

Hodgkin disease was first recognized by Thomas Hodgkin of Guy's Hospital, London, in 1832. The first descriptions of the distinctive malignant cell were by Sternberg in 1898 and by Reed in 1902. HD has traditionally been included with the malignant lymphomas and the terms *Hodgkin's lymphoma and non-Hodgkin's lymphoma* are commonly encountered. Historically, there has been uncertainty as to the histogenesis of HD. There is now accumulating evidence that most cases of HD are neoplasms of B lymphocytes. However, its unique clinicopathological features warrant its recognition as a distinctive neoplastic disorder.

☐ Epidemiology and Pathogenesis:

HD is the most common malignant neoplasm of Americans between the ages of 10 and 30 years. Some 8000 cases are reported annually in the United States, for an incidence of 3 per 100,000 population. The disorder is somewhat more common in men than in women (4.0:2.5) and in whites than in blacks (3.5:2.0). There is a distinctive **bimodal age distribution in developed countries**, with a peak in the late 20s, a decrease in frequency during the fourth and fifth decades, and a gradually increasing incidence after the age of 50 years.

Epidemiological patterns in HD suggest that early and increased exposure to an unidentified agent of low oncogenic potential may be important in its development. In underdeveloped countries and less advanced regions of developed countries, the overall incidence is low, but there is an increased frequency in children. There is also a different distribution of subtypes of HD in different areas. Compared with affluent societies, less-developed regions show an increase in the frequency of the more aggressive "mixed cellularity" and "lymphocyte depletion" subtypes. In developed countries, less aggressive variants (nodular sclerosis and lymphocyte predominant) are more common in young adults from small families and few neighborhood playmates during childhood.

These epidemiological patterns suggest the possibility that early exposure to an unidentified etiologic agent may predispose children to aggressive HD. According to this theory, delayed exposure results in a predisposition to indolent HD in young adults. This scheme does not explain whether the increasing incidence of HD after the age of 50 years reflects exposure to the same hypothetical etiological agent or has a different cause.

The geographic variation in the incidence of HD and some clinicopathological features that simulate an infectious process suggest a viral etiology, but proof is still lacking. The possibility of horizontal transmission (transmission by interpersonal contact) of an infectious agent has been suggested by several self-limited "mini-epidemics" of HD in children. However, such apparent case clustering is predictable on statistical grounds and has not been confirmed by broader epidemiological studies. A possible relationship between HD and infection with EBV has been suggested. Young adults who have experienced EBV infection (infectious mononucleosis) have a threefold increased risk of developing HD, and the EBV genome is frequently identified in the Reed-Sternberg cell.

Genetic factors may play a role. The frequency of certain HLA subtypes, particularly HLA-B18, is increased in patients with HD. Moreover, there is a 7-fold increased risk of HD in siblings of patients with this disorder, and a 100-fold increased risk when the sibling is a monozygotic twin.

Immune status seems to be a factor in at least some cases of HD. There is an increased incidence of HD in patients with compromised immunity and in persons with autoimmune diseases, such as rheumatoid arthritis. In fact, in patients with ataxia telangiectasia, who have a 100-fold increased incidence of cancer, 7% of the malignancies are HD.

Historically, the pathogenesis of HD has been difficult to study, in part because of the inability to define the lineage and clonality of the Reed-Sternberg cell. This failure is due in part to the rarity of this malignant cell in tumor tissue and to the problem of obtaining pure populations of neoplastic cells for study. Reed-Sternberg cells frequently constitute less than 1% of the total cell population. In fact, a salient feature of HD is the predominance in tumor tissue of reactive benign tissue components. Recent studies have indicated that EBV is present in Reed-Sternberg cells in the majority of cases of HD. Multiple independent lines of evidence have confirmed the clonality of the Reed-Sternberg cell, suggesting that it is, in fact, the neoplastic cell of HD. Many of the normal cell components of lymph nodes have been proposed as a candidate for the origin of the Reed-Sternberg cell. These include B and T lymphocytes and cells of the mononuclear phagocyte system, including macrophages, dendritic reticulum cells of the lymphoid follicles, and the interdigitating reticulum cells of the T cell–dependent paracortex. Cell markers characteristic of each of these cell lineages have been demonstrated in some, but not all, Reed-Sternberg cells, and the origin of the latter remains problematic. One subtype, namely, nodular lymphocyte predominance HD is clearly demonstrated to be a neoplasm of B-lymphoid origin, and the Reed-Sternberg cells of this variant express specific B-lymphocyte lineage markers. They lack the immunological cell markers CD15 (Leu-M1) and CD30 (Ki-1), which are usually but not always identified on the Reed-Sternberg cells of all other subtypes of HD. Nevertheless, recent evidence suggests that most cases of HD are neoplasms of aberrant B lymphocytes.

☐ **Pathology:** Most patients with HD present with lymphadenopathy. After an initial diagnosis of HD, a comprehensive evaluation is commonly performed to establish the extent, or stage, of the disease. In selected cases, an abdominal exploratory operation (staging laparotomy) is performed in which the spleen is removed and biopsies of lymph nodes, liver, and bone marrow are taken to search for abdominal involvement.

LYMPH NODES: On clinical examination, lymph nodes involved by HD are described as firm or rubbery, but on gross examination in the laboratory the consistency is variable. When fibrosis is not a prominent feature, and when there are broad areas of cell necrosis, the lymph nodes may even be soft. The cut surface is homogeneously gray-white, producing a "fish flesh" appearance. If tumor tissue extends beyond the confines of individual lymph nodes, groups of nodes may be matted together.

SPLEEN: The spleen is involved in one third of the cases of HD at the time of diagnosis, and in most patients at autopsy. On cut section, the splenic white pulp is enlarged by HD, and the red pulp is affected only secondarily by direct extension from the white pulp. The incidence of splenic involvement correlates directly with the size of the organ. A spleen that weighs more than 400 g is almost invariably involved by HD. By contrast, a smaller spleen may show HD or may exhibit only benign reactive hyperplasia.

In the spleen, HD occurs first in the T cell–dependent, periarteriolar lymphoid sheath of the white pulp or in the marginal zone between the white pulp and the red pulp. As the disease progresses, single or multiple discrete tumor nodules or confluent multinodular tumor masses in the spleen are common (Fig. 20-68). The prognosis in HD is adversely affected by the finding of multiple discrete tumor nodules in the spleen.

LIVER: At autopsy, the liver is involved with HD in two thirds of the patients with residual disease, although it is unusual at the time of presentation. The portal areas are first involved, without significant macroscopic findings. With time, multiple gray-white tumor nodules, often resembling metastatic carcinoma, may appear in the liver.

BONE MARROW: The bone marrow is only rarely involved initially. The initial changes in the bone marrow are characterized macroscopically by discrete foci of fibrotic tumor, without destruction of bony trabeculae. As the disease progresses, destruction of bone may produce an osteolytic appearance on radiological examination. Rarely, thickening of bony trabeculae (osteosclerosis) occurs. When present, osteosclerosis may be

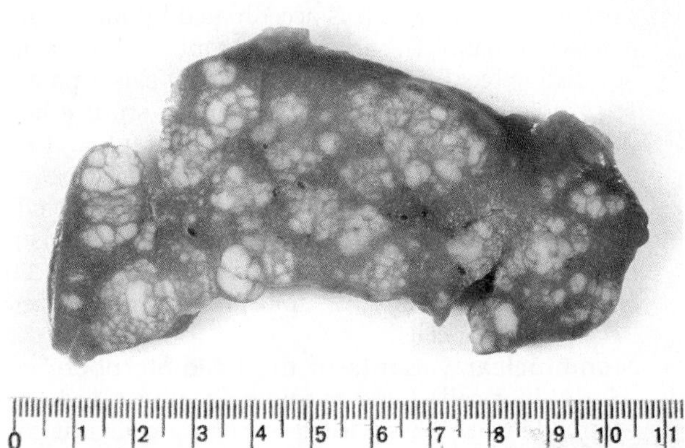

FIGURE *20-68*
Hodgkin's disease involving the spleen. Multinodular tumor masses replace the normal splenic parenchyma.

particularly prominent in the vertebrae, producing a densely sclerotic radiological appearance, described as "ivory vertebrae."

OTHER SYSTEMS: Pulmonary involvement is discovered at autopsy in more than half the patients with residual disease, and epidural spread of HD from paravertebral nodes through intervertebral foramina is a frequent neurological complication.

Classification of Hodgkin's Disease

The histopathological subtypes of HD are distinguished both by the morphological type of Reed-Sternberg cell and by the nature of the host immune response to the Reed-Sternberg cell. The Rye classification (Rye, New York, 1966) recognizes four types of HD.

- **Lymphocyte predominance**
- **Mixed cellularity**
- **Lymphocyte depletion**
- **Nodular sclerosis**

In Western countries, nodular sclerosis accounts for 60% to 70%, mixed cellularity for 20% to 30%, and lymphocyte predominance and lymphocyte depletion each for 5% to 10% of HD. The subtypes of HD have rather similar clinical behavior and response to therapy and, therefore, do no have strong implications for clinical stratification. However, precise histopathological criteria employed for each of the four subtypes is important to distinguish HD from benign reactive processes and non-Hodgkin's lymphomas with which it may be confused.

THE REED-STERNBERG CELL: Reed-Sternberg cell variants include (1) classic binucleated Reed-Sternberg cells, (2) mononuclear variants (Hodgkin's cells), and (3) variants that are each characteristic of, but not diagnostic for, specific subtypes of HD (Fig. 20-69).

- **The classic Reed-Sternberg cell** is a binucleated (or bilobed) cell with mirror image nuclei that contains clear chromatin and a large central eosinophilic nucleolus in each nuclear lobe (Fig. 20-70). Delicate strands of heterochromatin extend from each nucleolus to the nuclear membrane, which is accentuated by marginated heterochromatin. The abundant cytoplasm is pink and not distinctive. Electron microscopy reveals a paucity of cytoplasmic organelles. Cytogenetic studies have shown an aneuploid, frequently hypotetraploid, karyotype, but no consistent chromosomal abnormalities have been identified. The classic Reed-Sternberg cell is generally thought to be an end-stage cell, which is no longer capable of dividing. Thus, tumor tissue in HD often exhibits eosinophilic, amorphous, "mummified" Reed-Sternberg cells.
- **Mononuclear variants** of the Reed-Sternberg cell (Hodgkin's cell) have cytologic features indistinguishable from classic Reed-Sternberg cells but contain only a single nucleus (see Fig. 20-69). Hodgkin's cells may be identified in any subtype of HD but are not diagnostic of the disease. When a second biopsy is performed for pathological staging or for documentation of recurrence in a patient with known HD, the demonstration of Hodgkin's cells in an appropriate histopathological background is sufficient to confirm involvement by HD.

The three additional varieties of the Reed-Sternberg cell are each characteristic of, but not diagnostic for, a specific type HD (see Fig. 20-69).

- **The lymphocytic and histiocytic variant (L and H or "popcorn cell")** is typical of lymphocyte predominance HD. It has a single to multilobed nucleus, with delicate chromatin, inconspicuous nucleoli, and scant-to-moderate pale cytoplasm.
- **The lacunar variant** is prominent in nodular sclerosis HD. It has single to multiple nuclear lobes, occasionally in a horseshoe-shaped configuration, eosinophilic nucleoli, clear chromatin, and abundant pink cytoplasm. In formalin-fixed tissue, the abundant cytoplasm retracts toward the nucleus, which consequently appears to lie in a lake or lacuna (lacunar cell).
- **The pleomorphic variant** is often seen in the reticular variant of lymphocyte depleted HD. These cells exhibit bizarre multinucleated or multilobed nuclei, with prominent eosinophilic nucleoli.

The subtypes of HD are distinguished both by the nature of the Reed-Sternberg cell and by the accompanying cellular response (Fig. 20-71). The ratio of normal small lymphocytes to neoplastic cells determines the sequence of HD, namely, lymphocyte predominance to mixed cellularity to lymphocyte depletion. A decreasing number of normal lymphocytes might correlate with a diminished host immune response to Reed-Sternberg cells and constitute an adverse prognostic sign. A variable infiltration by reactive inflammatory cells, including eosinophils, neutrophils, plasma cells, and macrophages is seen in all types of HD. However, they are inconspicuous in LPHD, except for macrophages (histiocytes). There may be delicate or abundant loose fibrosis or, in the case of nodular sclerosis HD, dense bands of collagen.

LYMPHOCYTE PREDOMINANCE HD (LPHD): Small lymphocytes are the predominant cell type in LPHD. Benign macrophages, singly or in small clusters, may also be conspicuous. L and H (lymphocytic and histiocytic) variants of Reed-Sternberg cells are typical, whereas classic Reed-Sternberg cells and mononuclear variants are rare or lacking. Reactive inflammatory cells, fibrosis, and necrosis are lacking or inconspicuous.

LPHD has been traditionally subdivided into *nodular and diffuse subtypes.* In the nodular subtype, there is a vaguely nodular pattern on low-power microscopy, a feature that is not seen in the diffuse subtype of LPHD. In 25% of cases of nodular LPHD, a distinctive abnormality of B-cell germinal centers, called progressive transformation of germinal centers, occurs at any time in the course of the disease. In this process, germinal centers are unusually large, and there is a breakdown between the mantle zone and the germinal center. As a consequence, the germinal center consists of small lymphocytes and scattered islands of transformed or activated lymphocytes (immunoblasts).

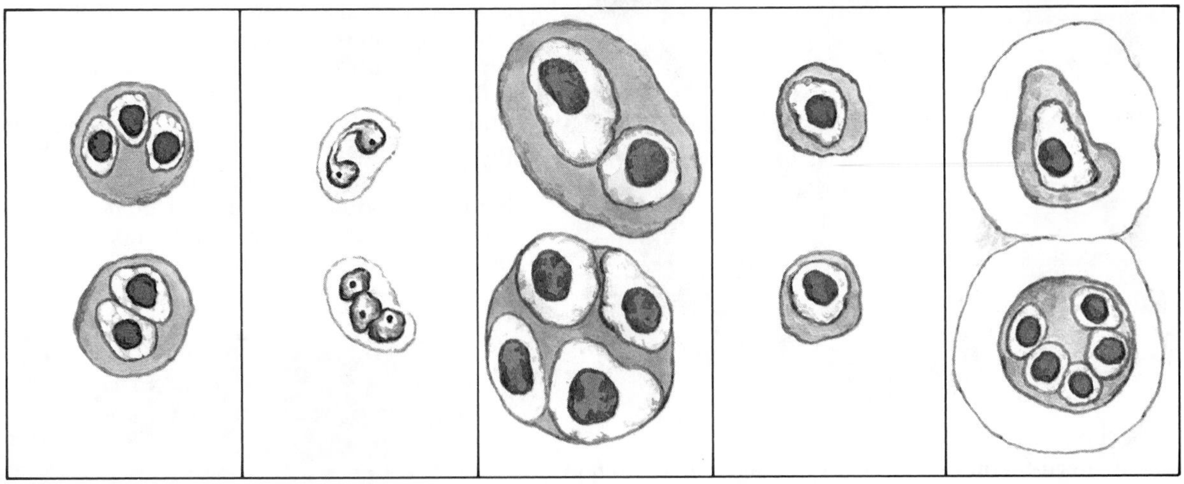

	CLASSIC	LP VARIANT	PLEOMORPHIC VARIANT	MONONUCLEAR	LACUNAR CELL
R-S cell morphology					
Nuclear Configuration	Binucleated to multinucleated to multilobulated	Single to multilobed	Single to multinucleated or multilobed	Single	Single to multilobed
Nucleoli	large (≥1/3 diameter of nucleus), eosinophilic	Small, punctate	Variable, prominent	large (≥1/3 diameter of nucleus), eosinophilic	Variable (generally <1/3 diameter of nucleus), eosinophilic
Chromatin	Clear parachromatin	Delicate	Variable, clear parachromatin to hyperchromatic	Abundant, clear parachromatin	delicate to clear parachromatin
Cytoplasm	Moderate to abundant, pale to pink	Scant, nodular	Moderate to abundant, eosinophilic	Moderate, pale to pink	Abundant, pale†
Associated histologic subtype	Diagnostic in mixed cellularity, may be seen (diagnostic) in lymphocyte depleted, nodular sclerosis	Lymphocyte predominance	Lymphocyte depleted‡	May be seen in any subtype	Nodular sclerosis§

Mononuclear R-S cell variants are not diagnostic of Hodgkin's disease. However, these cells, in the appropriate environment, indicate involvement either in the staging work-up or in relapse

† Formalin fixation artifact: the cytoplasm of these cells may retract and the cell appears to lie in a clear space (lacuna or lake).

‡ Pleomorphic large cell lymphoma of T-cell type must be ruled out

§ Similar cells may occasionally be seen in mixed cellularity

FIGURE *20-69*
Hodgkin's disease Reed-Sternberg cells. Morphology of the classic Reed-Sternberg cell of Hodgkin's disease and variants of the Reed-Sternberg cell that are characteristic of Hodgkin's disease subtypes. Criteria for the identification of each cell type are shown in the accompanying table.

The association of an abnormality of a B-cell germinal center with nodular LPHD is of interest, since it has been demonstrated that this type of HD appears to be a neoplasm of B-cell origin. In nodular LPHD, the L and H variants (1) express the B-cell marker CD20, (2) are positive for CD45 (leukocyte common antigen), (3) synthesize immunoglobulin J or joining chain, (4) express monoclonal surface membrane and cytoplasmic monotypic immunoglobulins, (5) have immunoglobulin gene rearrangements, and (6) are negative for the usual HD markers, CD15 (Leu-M1) and CD30 (Ki-1).

The diffuse variant of LPHD is an uncommon disorder. It has recently been redefined as lymphocyte-rich classic HD and is considered to be in the spectrum of lymphocyte predominance to mixed cellularity to lymphocyte-depleted HD. The rare Reed-Sternberg cells in this subtype of HD may express CD15 and CD30.

MIXED CELLULARITY HD (MCHD): This is the classic historic form of HD and exhibits (1) numerous, classic, binucleated Reed-Sternberg cells and mononuclear variants, (2) an intermediate number of lymphocytes, and (3) a prominent component of inflammatory cells, particularly eosinophils and neutrophils (Fig. 20-72). There may be focal necrosis and fibrosis, and a prominent granulomatous reaction is occasionally observed. Limited or focal involvement of the paracortical or interfollicular regions of lymph nodes is frequent in MCHD and has been termed **interfollicular HD**. Such cases have a better prognosis than other cases of MCHD.

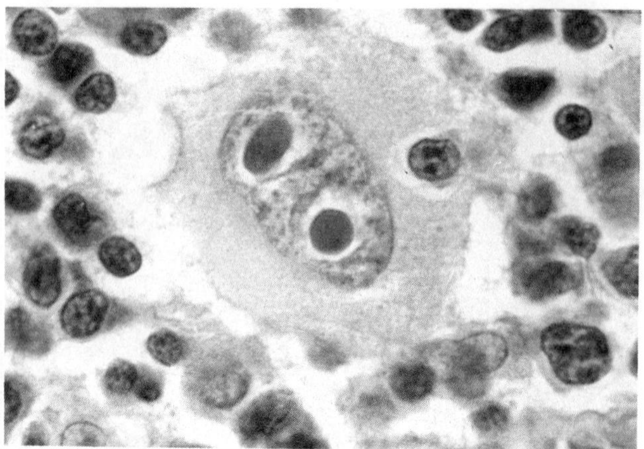

FIGURE *20-70*
Classic Reed-Sternberg cell. Mirror image nuclei contain large eosinophilic nucleoli.

LYMPHOCYTE DEPLETION HD (LDHD): This category is subdivided into *diffuse fibrosis* and *reticular subtypes*. Marked depletion of lymphocytes and inflammatory cells, is noted. The diffuse fibrosis subtype of LDHD is characterized by (1) an abundant loose and disorderly proteinaceous material, (2) rare classic Reed-Sternberg cells, and (3) scant lymphocytes and inflammatory cells. Foci of necrosis are common. The reticular subtype displays a predominance of either classic Reed-Sternberg cells or pleomorphic variants (Fig. 20-73). Commonly both subtypes of LDHD, namely, diffuse fibrosis and reticular, are seen in the same lymph node.

NODULAR SCLEROSIS HD (NSHD): This common form of HD is a distinctive subtype, which may be unrelated to any of the other subtypes. It is characterized by (1) broad bands of dense collagen, which extend from a thickened capsule into the substance of the lymph node and circumscribe residual nodules of lymphoid tissue, and (2) a predominance of the lacunar cell variant of the Reed-Sternberg cell (Fig. 20-74). In the lymphoid nodules of NSHD, the number of normal small lymphocytes varies from predominant to scant. The inflammatory cell component is also heterogeneous, and eosinophils are often conspicuous. Focal necrosis is a characteristic feature, typically with lacunar cell variants of Reed-Sternberg cells palisaded around the foci of necrosis. Three morphological subtypes of NSHD are recognized: cellular phase, syncytial variant, and obliterative fibrosis.

The cellular phase of NSHD shows vaguely defined lymphoid nodules containing lacunar cells, which are frequently clustered. However, the nodules in the cellular phase are not circumscribed by collagenous bands.

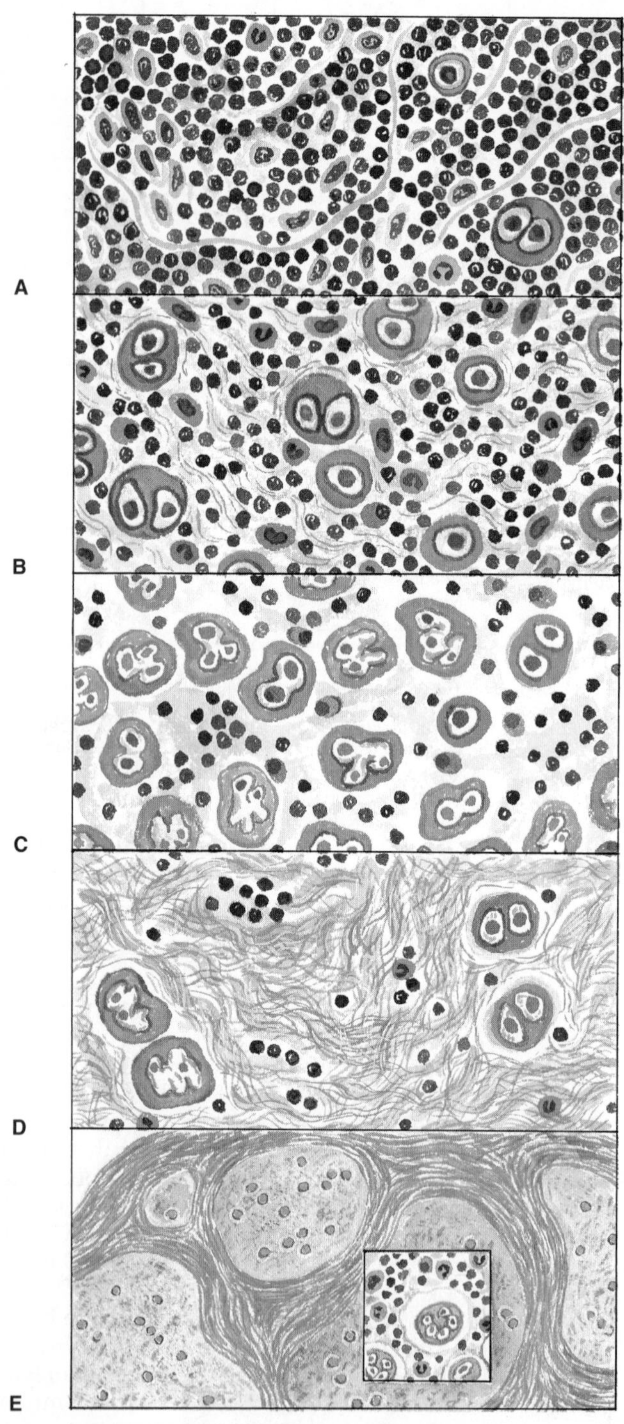

FIGURE *20-71*
Histopathological subtypes of Hodgkin's disease. (*A*) lymph-ocyte predominant; (B) mixed cellularity (*C*) lymphocyte depleted, reticular; (D) lymphocyte depleted, diffuse fibrosis; (*E*) nodular sclerosis. The characteristic histopathological appearance of each of the principal subtypes of Hodgkin's disease is shown. The sequence from lymphocyte-predominant Hodgkin's disease to lymphocyte-depleted Hodgkin's disease is characterized by progressively fewer normal lymphocytes and by increasing numbers of Reed-Sternberg cells. The subtype of lymphocyte-depleted diffuse fibrosis is characterized by few lymphocytes, few Reed-Sternberg cells, and abundant loose fibrosis. The subtype nodular sclerosing Hodgkin's disease is distinctive because of dense, bandlike, collagenous fibrosis, which envelops cellular aggregates that contain lymphoid and inflammatory cells and the specific lacunar cell variants of the Reed-Sternberg cell.

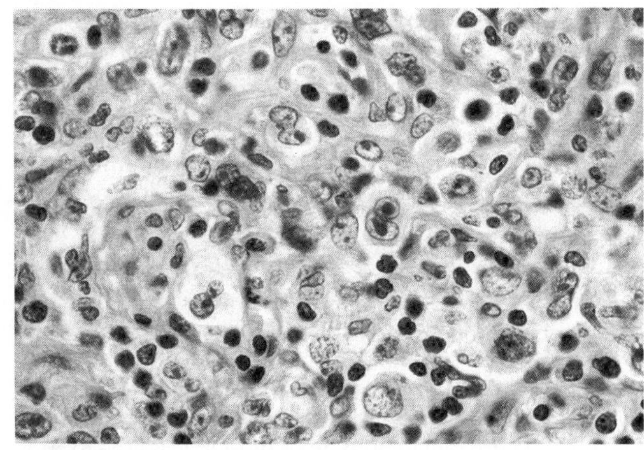

FIGURE 20-72
Hodgkin's disease, mixed cellularity. A photomicrograph of a lymph node shows classic, binucleated and mononuclear Reed-Sternberg cells, lymphocytes, and mild diffuse fibrosis.

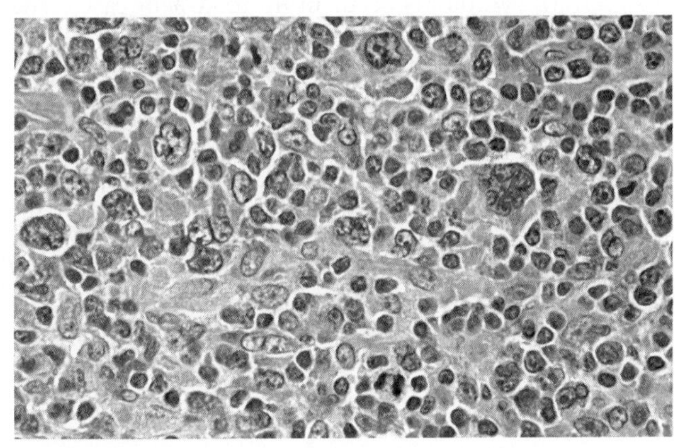

FIGURE *20-73*
Hodgkin's disease, lymphocyte depletion (reticular subtype). A photomicrograph of a lymph node shows numerous variants of Reed-Sternberg cells, whereas lymphocytes are sparse.

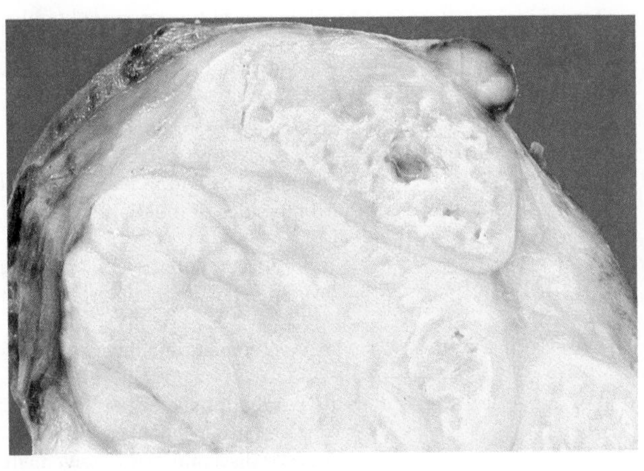

A B

FIGURE *20-74*
Hodgkin's disease, nodular sclerosis. (*A*) A cut section of matted lymph nodes shows broad bands of fibrosis that divide the parenchyma into distinct nodules. Several foci of necrosis are evident. (*B*) A low-power photomicrograph demonstrates broad bands of fibrosis.

The syncytial variant of NSHD exhibits sheets of lacunar cells and mononuclear variants, which may simulate a large cell lymphoma or other neoplasm. In such cases, immunohistochemical techniques may be required to establish the diagnosis of HD.

Obliterative fibrosis is the final phase, in which case only scant neoplastic and reactive cell components are present.

□ Clinical Features:

HD usually presents as nontender peripheral adenopathy, involving a single lymph node or groups of lymph nodes. The cervical and mediastinal nodes are involved in over half the cases, and the anterior mediastinum is frequently involved, especially in NSHD. Less commonly, the axillary, inguinal, and retroperitoneal lymph nodes are initially enlarged. Peripheral lymph node groups, such as the antecubital, popliteal, and mesenteric lymph nodes, tend to be spared.

Initially, HD spreads predictably between contiguous lymph node groups by way of the efferent lymphatics. As the disease progresses, spread is frequently unpredictable, owing to vascular invasion, with secondary hematogenous dissemination.

Constitutional ("B") symptoms are found in 40% of patients with HD. These include low-grade fever, which is occasionally cyclical (Pel-Ebstein fever), night sweats, and weight loss exceeding 10% of body weight in the 6 months prior to diagnosis. Pruritus may occur with disease progression. For unknown reasons, the ingestion of alcohol induces pain in involved sites in 10% of cases of HD.

The laboratory findings in HD are nonspecific. They include mild normocytic, normochromic anemia and moderate neutrophilia and eosinophilia. Elevation of the erythrocyte sedimentation rate correlates with disease activity.

A deficiency of T lymphocyte function is characteristic of HD. Subtle defects of delayed-type hypersensitivity, which can be detected in most patients even at the time of initial diagnosis, tend to become more pronounced as the disease progresses. Anergy to skin test antigens is often noted early in the course of HD. Such immune dysfunction is exacerbated by the immunosuppressive effects of therapy. An absolute lymphocytopenia (<1500 per μL) is observed in half of the cases, most commonly in advanced HD. Humoral immunity usually remains intact until late in the course of the disease.

Lymphocyte-predominance HD is the most indolent type. Adult men younger than 35 years of age are most commonly affected (male-to-female ratio of 4:1). At the time of initial diagnosis, the disease is usually localized (stage I), the high cervical, axillary, or inguinal lymph nodes being most commonly involved. B signs and symptoms are typically lacking, presenting in only 20% of cases. Visceral involvement is uncommon. The prognosis of LPHD is excellent, with a long-term, disease free-survival exceeding 90%.

Mixed cellularity HD is most common in the fourth and fifth decades of life, although any age group may be affected. The left cervical lymph nodes are the most common site of initial involvement. However, after staging the majority of patients are found to have stage II or III disease, and a minority have visceral involvement (stage IV). B signs and symptoms are present in half of the cases of MCHD. The prognosis is intermediate, with a cure rate of 75%.

Lymphocyte depletion HD is the most clinically aggressive type. Middle-aged to elderly men are most commonly affected. Advanced clinical stage (III–IV) and B signs and symptoms are characteristic, presenting in two thirds of the cases. Patients with the diffuse fibrosis subtype of LDHD commonly present with fever of undetermined origin, pancytopenia, and wasting. There is usually no peripheral or mediastinal adenopathy. However, retroperitoneal adenopathy is frequently prominent, and involvement of the spleen, liver, and bone marrow is common. Profound immunodeficiency develops, and death commonly results from inanition or secondary infections. The reticular subtype of LDHD is characterized by bulky peripheral adenopathy, which is most frequent above the diaphragm. Patients usually succumb because of tumor progression. The overall cure rate in both types of LDHD is 40% to 50%.

Nodular sclerosis HD is the most common form of HD and is often found in adolescent and young adult women, ages 15 to 34 years. It usually presents as lower cervical, supraclavicular, and mediastinal adenopathy (stage II). B symptoms occur in up to 40% of cases. The prognosis is good, with a cure rate of 80% to 85%.

If untreated, HD is a lethal disorder, with a 10-year survival rate of only 1%. With modern radiation therapy and chemotherapy, an overall 70% cure rate can be achieved. **The prognosis in HD is principally dependent on the age of the patient and the anatomical extent of the disease or the stage.** A better prognosis is associated with (1) younger age, (2) a lower clinical stage (localized disease), and (3) the absence of B signs and symptoms. In the assessment of stage, the comprehensive Ann Arbor staging system (Table 20-23), which is based on both clinical

TABLE *20-23* Ann Arbor Staging System

Stage I A or B[a]	I	Involvement of a single lymph node region
		or
	I_E	a single extralymphatic organ or site
Stage II A or B	II	Involvement of two or more lymph node regions on the same side of the diaphram
		or
	I_E	with localized contiguous involvement of an extralymphatic organ site
Stage III A or B	III	Involvement of lymph node regions on both sides of the diaphram
		or
	III_E	with localized contiguous involvement of an extralymphatic organ or site
		or
	III_S	with involvement of spleen
		or
	III_{ES}	both extralymphatic organ or site and spleen involvement
Stage IV A or B	IV	Diffuse or disseminated involvement of one or more extralymphatic organs with or without associated lymph node involvement

[a] A, asymptomatic; B, presence of constitutional symptoms (fever, night sweats, and weight loss exceeding 10% of baseline body weight in preceding 6 months).

evaluation and the pathological findings obtained from staging laparotomy, is employed.

Complications of HD include the compromise of vital organs by progressive tumor growth and secondary infections, owing both to the primary defect in delayed type hypersensitivity and to the immunosuppressive effects of therapy. The development of second malignancies as a consequence of therapy is of special concern, since more than 15% of treated patients may eventually suffer this complication. AML develops in up to 5% of cases, and aggressive large cell lymphomas occur in less than 5%.

PLASMA CELL NEOPLASIA

Plasma cell neoplasia comprises a group of related malignant disorders of terminally differentiated B lymphocytes (plasma cells).

Multiple myeloma (90% of cases) is characterized by a multifocal infiltration of malignant plasma cells in the bone marrow. In this condition, there are typically multiple destructive (lytic) lesions or diffuse demineralization of bone.

Solitary osseous myeloma (5% of cases) is a single destructive lesion of bone.

Extramedullary plasmacytoma (5% of cases) presents as an extramedullary soft tissue mass, most frequently in the upper respiratory tract.

In the large majority of cases of plasma cell neoplasia, the neoplastic cells secrete a homogeneous, complete or partial, immunoglobulin molecule, termed an *M-component* or *paraprotein.* Based on the type of M-component, multiple myeloma can be divided into the following types:

- **IgG, IgA, IgD, IgE, and IgM types**
- **Light-chain disease,** in which only κ or λ light chains are synthesized.
- **Biclonal multiple myeloma,** in which two distinct M-components are secreted (rare)
- **Nonsecretory myeloma,** in which no M-component is secreted (1%)

☐ **Epidemiology:** Plasma cell neoplasia constitutes 10% of all hematological malignancies. About 7500 cases are reported annually in the United States, yielding an overall incidence of 3 per 100,000 population. The disorder is more than twice as common in blacks (8 per 100,000 population) than in whites. The frequency of plasma cell neoplasia increases with age, the mean age at diagnosis of multiple myeloma being 65 years and that of solitary osseous myeloma and extramedullary plasmacytoma a decade earlier. Plasma cell neoplasia is distinctly uncommon before the age of 40 years. There is a slight male predominance in multiple myeloma, with an overall male-to-female ratio of 1.5:1. This male predominance is even more pronounced for solitary osseous myeloma and extramedullary plasmacytoma, each with a male-to-female ratio of 3:1.

☐ **Pathogenesis:** A number of risk factors for plasma cell neoplasia have been identified.

- **A genetic predisposition** is suggested by an increased incidence of multiple myeloma in first-degree relatives of patients with plasma cell neoplasia and the higher frequency of multiple myeloma in blacks.
- **Ionizing radiation** has been incriminated in the etiology of plasma cell neoplasia. Long-term survivors of the bombing of Hiroshima and Nagasaki suffered a fivefold increased incidence of multiple myeloma.
- **Chronic antigenic stimulation** may constitute a risk factor. For example, in Balb-C mice, intraperitoneal instillation of mineral oil or solid plastic material commonly induces the formation of a plasmacytoma. In humans, some cases of multiple myeloma have been associated with chronic infections, such as chronic osteomyelitis, and with chronic inflammatory disorders (e.g., rheumatoid arthritis). A two-hit hypothesis is proposed by which (1) antigenic stimulation leads to reactive, polyclonal proliferation of B lymphocytes and (2) a subsequent mutagenic event establishes a single malignant clone.
- **Chromosomal abnormalities** have been reported in some cases of multiple myeloma, including translocations, trisomy, and monosomy. The translocation t(11;14) (q13;q32), involving the protooncogene *bcl*-1 on chromosome 11 and the immunoglobulin heavy-chain gene on chromosome 14, has been observed in a variety of B-cell neoplasms, including multiple myeloma.

☐ **Pathology:** On gross examination, the osseous and extraosseous tumors of plasma cell neoplasia are variably red, tan, or gray and have a consistency that ranges from fleshy to gelatinous. The bony lesions are well demarcated from the surrounding normal tissue (Fig. 20-75). The cortical bone may be destroyed, with direct tumor extension into the surrounding soft tissues. In multiple myeloma, moderate enlargement of the lymph nodes, spleen, and liver is occasionally observed, although the gross appearance of these organs is not distinctive. The kidneys are often contracted in size.

BONE MARROW: Microscopically, the morphological hallmark of multiple myeloma in the bone marrow is the presence of diffuse sheets or nodular aggregates of plasma cells. A characteristic early feature is the encircling of fat cells by plasma cells. Ultimately, both normal hemopoietic tissues and fat cells are replaced by neoplastic plasma cells.

In smears of marrow aspirates, neoplastic plasma cells usually exceed 25% of the nucleated cell elements. The malignant cells may be morphologically normal, but more commonly they demonstrate cytological atypia (Fig. 20-76). The atypical cytological features include (1) prominent nucleoli, (2) irregular chromatin distribution, (3) binucleation and bizarre multinucleation, and (4) nuclear-cytoplasmic asynchrony, with immature nuclei and mature cytoplasm. Plasmablasts, characterized by large central nuclei, finely dispersed chromatin, prominent nucleoli, and scant blue cytoplasm, may be observed and in some cases constitute the predominant cell type. A distinctive reddish tint of the peripheral cytoplasm of the neoplastic plasma cells (flame cells) is commonly seen in IgA myeloma.

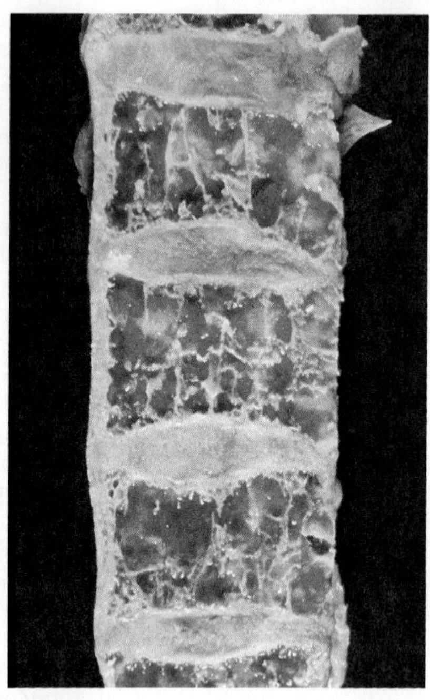

FIGURE 20-75
Multiple myeloma. Multiple lytic lesions of the vertebrae are present.

Cytoplasmic and nuclear inclusions, representing immunoglobulin accumulation, may be observed in neoplastic plasma cells. *Russell bodies* are globular, eosinophilic, refractile, cytoplasmic inclusions, and *Dutcher bodies* are similar intranuclear ones. Precipitates of crystalline immunoglobulin may also be observed in the cytoplasm of the neoplastic plasma cells.

BONES: Increased osteoclasts are commonly present in resorption lacunae along the scalloped margins of bony trabeculae. Mild myelofibrosis or thickening of the bony trabeculae (osteosclerosis) is occasionally encountered.

KIDNEYS: A constellation of renal abnormalities is seen in over half of the cases of plasma cell neoplasia (see Chapter 16).

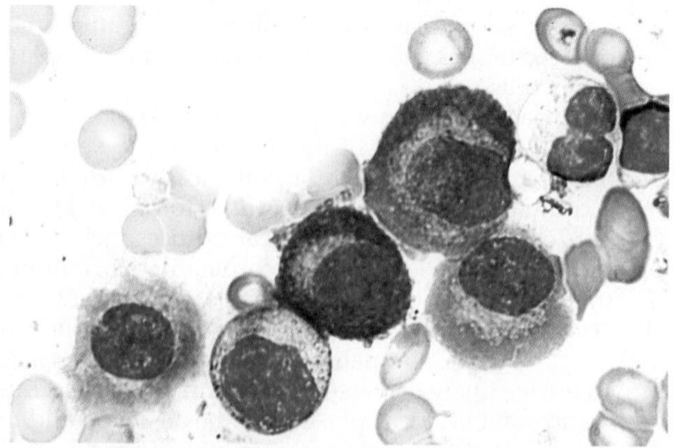

FIGURE 20-76
Multiple myeloma. A smear of a bone marrow aspirate illustrates a cluster of three neoplastic plasma cells.

Light-chain cast nephropathy is the most characteristic finding and is characterized by the precipitation of finely granular or lamellar protein casts, containing light chains and other proteins, in the distal convoluted and collecting tubules. Secondary injury to the tubules by the protein casts leads to tubular epithelial cell atrophy or hyperplasia, with the formation of epithelial cell syncytia. Destruction of tubular basement membranes induces tubulointerstitial inflammation and secondary interstitial fibrosis.

Glomerulopathy is the other important renal abnormality in plasma cell neoplasia. A diffuse deposition of M-component occurs in the renal glomeruli, tubular basement membranes, and in the vasculature. The glomerulopathy is characterized by proliferation of mesangial cells and an increase in the mesangial matrix. Additionally, there may be damage to both renal tubules and blood vessels.

Additional renal findings in multiple myeloma include the deposition of (1) amyloid in the glomeruli and blood vessels, (2) calcium (nephrocalcinosis), and (3) uric acid crystals (urate nephropathy). Acute and chronic pyelonephritis may be seen. Focal or (rarely) massive neoplastic plasma cell infiltration may occur in the interstitium.

LYMPH NODES: The lymph nodes may be infiltrated by neoplastic plasma cells, initially in the B cell–dependent medullary cords. This process may progress to a total obliteration of the normal nodal architecture.

SPLEEN AND LIVER: The spleen shows a variable infiltration of the red pulp cords and sinuses. In the liver, the portal triads may contain plasma cells, and in the case of a leukemic distribution, they are identified in the hepatic sinusoids.

☐ **Clinical Features:** The diagnosis of multiple myeloma requires the findings of (1) uniform diffuse sheets or nodular aggregates of plasma cells in the bone marrow, (2) the presence in the large majority of cases of a significant monoclonal serum M-component (>3 g/dL) or a urine M-component (>150 mg/dL), and (3) the radiological demonstration of lytic bone lesions or diffuse demineralization of bone. Lytic bone lesions of the skull and other flat bones, including the spine and ribs, are a characteristic (but not diagnostic) radiological finding in multiple myeloma (Fig. 20-77).

The most important disorder to consider in the differential diagnosis of multiple myeloma is the more common *monoclonal gammopathy of unknown significance (MGUS)* (Fig. 20-78). Also known as benign essential gammopathy, the term MGUS is preferred because the disorder is not necessarily benign. About 2% of patients with MGUS per year progress to a B-cell neoplasm (lymphoplasmacytic disorder or multiple myeloma). The strong link between MGUS and multiple myeloma supports the two-hit hypothesis for the origin of the latter. In this scenario, a first oncogenic event causes MGUS and a second event results in multiple myeloma.

Common initial laboratory findings in multiple myeloma include normocytic, normochromic anemia, hypercalcemia, and hyperuricemia. A sharp peak or spike representing the M-component is observed with serum or urine protein electrophoresis (see Fig. 20-78). The erythrocyte sedimentation rate is elevated, owing to the M-com-

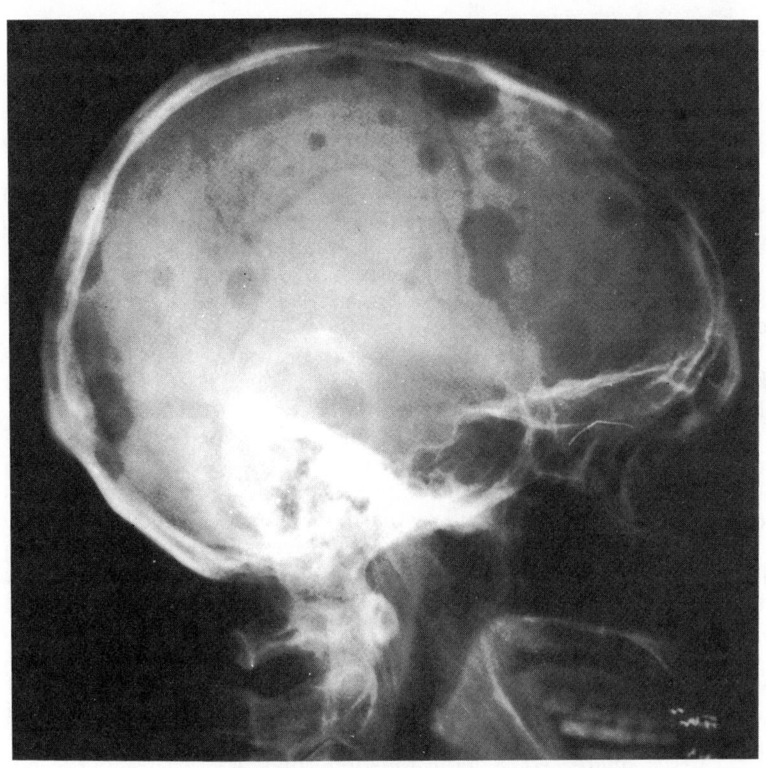

FIGURE *20-77*
Multiple myeloma. A radiograph of the skull shows numerous punched-out radiolucent areas.

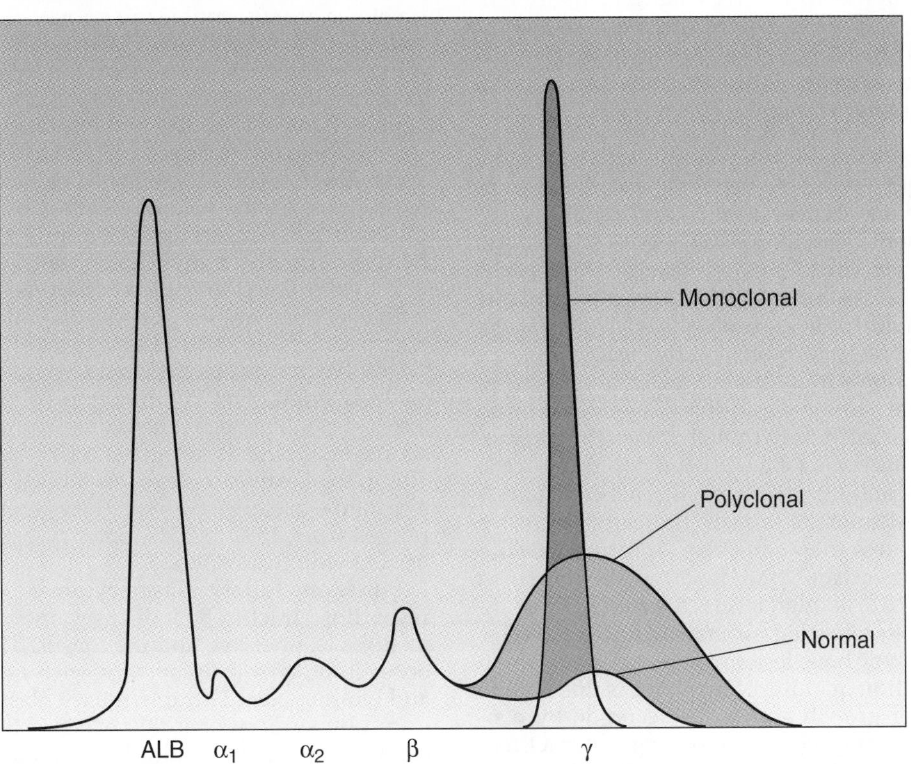

FIGURE *20-78*
Serum protein electrophoretic patterns. Abnormal serum protein electrophoretic patterns are contrasted with a normal pattern. In polyclonal hypergammaglobulinemia, which is characteristic of benign reactive processes, there is a broad-based increase in immunoglobulins due to immunoglobulin secretion by a myriad discrete reactive plasma cells. In monoclonal gammopathy, which is characteristic of monoclonal gammopathy of unknown significance or plasma cell neoplasia, there is a narrow peak, or spike, due to the homogeneity of the immunoglobulin molecules secreted by a single clone of aberrant plasma cells.

ponent. On the peripheral blood smear, the erythrocytes may appear stacked and clumped (rouleaux formation), also a reflection of the M-component.

The type of M-component is clinically relevant because of some commonly observed clinicopathological associations.

- **IgG myeloma** is "typical" myeloma, with a mean survival of 3 to 4 years. Infections are a common complication.
- **IgA myeloma** shows symptoms and signs due to serum hyperviscosity because of the tendency of the IgA molecule to form dimers.
- **IgD myeloma** is an aggressive clinical disorder, which tends to occur in middle-aged men. The mean survival is 1 year. Extramedullary involvement with soft tissue masses is common. Renal disease is also frequent, possibly because IgD heavy chains are almost invariably associated with an unbalanced synthesis of nephrotoxic λ light chains.
- **IgE myeloma** is an uncommon and aggressive clinical disorder, which also tends to occur in young adult men. A leukemic phase, with peripheral blood plasma cell counts exceeding 2000/μL, occurs in at least a fourth of the cases. Other than in IgE myeloma, plasma cell leukemia is an uncommon and usually preterminal manifestation of plasma cell neoplasia.
- **Light-chain disease** is an aggressive variant of multiple myeloma in which only κ or λ light chains are synthesized. The κ chain disease is twice as common as the λ chain disease. The serum protein pattern is normal until secondary renal disease prevents glomerular filtration of light chains.

Multiple myeloma typically presents with bone pain, most commonly involving the vertebrae and ribs. Symptoms due to anemia, hypercalcemia, and renal insufficiency are frequent. Amyloidosis of light-chain origin (principally λ) occurs in 15% of cases, and the hyperviscosity syndrome in less than 5%. There is a "primary" distribution of amyloid, with deposition in such sites as the tongue, the gastrointestinal tract, and the heart.

The clinical course in multiple myeloma tends to be biphasic. An initial chronic stable phase is followed by an aggressive or accelerated preterminal phase. The prognosis is dependent on (1) the total body tumor burden at the time of diagnosis and (2) the status of renal function. A high total body tumor burden is indicated by (1) a hemoglobin level less than 8.5 g/dL, (2) serum calcium concentration greater than 12 mg/dL, (3) an M-component higher than 5 gm/dL, (4) high levels of serum LDH or β_2-microglobulin, both reflecting turnover of nucleated cells, and (5) extensive lytic bone lesions.

Bone destruction in multiple myeloma is due both to progressive tumor growth and to the secretion by neoplastic plasma cells of osteoclast activating factor. Osteoclasts may also be activated by the IL-6 system, the activity of which is increased in patients with multiple myeloma. Common complications of bone destruction include vertebral collapse and pathological fractures of long bones. Additionally, calcium released from the injured bone may precipitate in the kidneys and cause renal damage (nephrocalcinosis).

The hyperviscosity syndrome (see macroglobulinemia) is particularly common in IgG and IgA myelomas, although it is far less frequent than in macroglobulinemia. An increase in serum viscosity to over 4 cp units (normal, 1.4 to 1.8) results in abnormalities of blood flow, with secondary complications in multiple organ systems. Neurological abnormalities and spontaneous bleeding episodes are observed.

Some M-components function as cryoglobulins, which are proteins and precipitate in the cold. As a consequence, blood flow to the distal extremities may be impaired, with resultant acrocyanosis and Raynaud phenomenon.

Coagulation abnormalities result from (1) complexes formed between the M-component and coagulation factors, (2) co-precipitation of M-component cryoglobulins with coagulation complexes, and (3) coating of platelets with the M-component.

Monoclonal light chains are present in the urine (Bence-Jones protein) in up to 75% of cases of multiple myeloma and in a minority of solitary osseous myelomas and extramedullary plasmacytomas. The neoplastic clone of plasma cells may secrete excess light chains, owing to an unbalanced synthesis of heavy and light chains. The light chains are rapidly filtered through the glomeruli and appear in the urine as Bence-Jones protein.

Humoral immune deficiency, with decreased levels of normal serum immunoglobulins, is characteristic of multiple myeloma. This defect is due to (1) suppression of normal B lymphocytes by the neoplastic clone and (2) an increased catabolic rate of normal IgG. Because of the low levels of normal antibodies, patients with multiple myeloma are susceptible to a variety of infectious complications, particularly pneumonia and pyelonephritis. The infections may be caused by either gram-negative or gram-positive bacteria and less commonly by such organisms as *Toxoplasma gondii* and *Pneumocystis carinii*.

Multiple myeloma is an incurable disease, with a mean survival of 6 months in untreated patients and 3 years with appropriate chemotherapy. Death is usually due either to infection or to renal failure. The disease may be complicated by a superimposed myelodysplastic syndrome or AML, usually attributed to the leukemogenic effect of treatment with alkylating agents. The risk of AML occurring 5 years after treatment is 14% and as high as 20% after 10 years.

Solitary osseous myeloma presents as a single lytic skeletal lesion, most commonly involving the ribs, vertebrae, or pelvic bones. The natural history of solitary osseous myeloma is progression to multiple myeloma (70%), local extension or recurrence (15%), or extension to a distant skeletal site (15%). The overall 10-year survival ranges from 15% to 25%. Solitary osseous myeloma is treated with irradiation.

Extramedullary plasmacytomas occur in the upper respiratory tract in 80% of cases, including the nasal sinuses, nasopharynx, and the tonsils. The remaining 20% occur in other soft tissue sites, such as the lungs, breast, and lymph nodes. Extramedullary plasmacytoma is eradicated by surgery or local radiation therapy. In 20% of cases progression to multiple myeloma occurs.

METASTATIC CANCER

Metastases to Bone

The incidence of metastatic cancer exceeds that of primary malignant tumors of the bone marrow and bone. The spread of malignant tumors to the bone marrow is typically hematogenous. Less commonly, tumors in contiguous soft tissues invade the bone. The axial skeleton (vertebrae, sacrum, cranium, and ribs) is involved in 70% of cases of bony metastases. In the appendicular skeleton, metastases are almost always proximal to the elbows and knees.

Cancers of the breast, lung, and prostate account for 80% of metastases to the bone marrow. In children, neuroblastoma, Ewing tumor, and embryonal rhabdomyosarcoma are the most common tumors that metastasize to the bone marrow. Sarcomas rarely metastasize to bone. Metastatic tumors in the bone marrow often induce conspicuous reactive fibrosis, particularly cancers of the breast and stomach.

A variety of secondary abnormalities due to metastatic cancer in the bone marrow may be observed. These include (1) increased bone destruction (osteolytic), (2) new bone formation (osteoblastic), (3) reactive fibrosis, and (4) abnormalities in hemopoiesis. Most metastatic tumors of the bone marrow are osteolytic, particularly those from the thyroid, kidney, and lung. Carcinomas of the prostate and breast and carcinoid tumors are particularly prone to produce osteoblastic metastases. Mixed osteolytic and osteoblastic foci may be encountered with any metastasis to the bone marrow.

Hemopoietic changes in the bone marrow adjacent to tumor deposits include hyperplasia or hypoplasia of any or all of the cell lineages. Hyperplasia of megakaryocytes and cells of the eosinophil lineage is particularly characteristic. Reactive bone marrow plasmacytosis is occasionally prominent and requires distinction from plasma cell neoplasia.

Reactive neutrophilia, eosinophilia, or thrombocytosis may be seen in the peripheral blood in cases of bony metastases. Alternatively, thrombocytopenia may be observed. A normocytic, normochromic anemia of chronic disease is common, and the presence of teardrop-shaped erythrocytes suggests bony metastases. A leukoerythroblastic reaction may occur, with immature circulating erythrocytes and leukocytes and large platelets.

An elevated serum level of alkaline phosphatase, secreted by osteoblasts actively laying down new bone, is usual in any osteoblastic bone marrow metastasis. The identification of specific bone and liver alkaline phosphatase isoenzymes is required to distinguish bony metastases from those in the liver. An elevated serum acid phosphatase level, due to enzyme secretion by the neoplastic cells, is typical of metastatic carcinoma of the prostate.

The principal clinical symptoms associated with metastases to the bone marrow are pain and tenderness, which are typically worse at night. Pathological fractures most commonly involve the weight-bearing bones such as the femur.

Metastases to Lymph Nodes

The regional lymph nodes that drain the sites of malignant tumors are frequently enlarged, owing either to immunological reactions to tumor antigenic products or to the presence of metastatic cancer. In lymphadenopathy secondary to immunological reactions to tumor, hyperplasia may be follicular or interfollicular. Other patterns of response to tumor products include sinus histiocytosis and a granulomatous response, in which well-defined, sarcoid-like granulomas occur within the node. In certain cancers (e.g., carcinomas of the breast and stomach), the findings of interfollicular hyperplasia and sinus histiocytosis in the regional lymph nodes have been associated with a more favorable prognosis and may indicate an effective immune response directed against the tumor.

Metastatic tumor cells enter the lymph nodes by invading tissue lymphatics at the primary site, and are carried by lymph flow into the subcapsular and then the trabecular sinuses. Thus, the location of palpable lymph nodes often suggests the primary site of malignancy. For example, the appearance of firm, enlarged nodes in the axilla of a woman suggests the presence of an occult breast cancer, whereas the enlargement of a supraclavicular node (sentinel node) is often associated with a primary cancer of the lung or stomach. The presence of cohesive nests and clusters of atypical cells that expand the sinuses of a lymph node, but spare the intervening normal lymphoidal stroma, is characteristic of metastatic cancer. As the lymph node stroma is invaded, the margin of advancing tumor is well demarcated from the surrounding normal nodal tissue (pushing margins). Ultimately, the entire normal nodal architecture is effaced.

Sarcomas usually disseminate by the hematogenous route and metastases to the lymph nodes are relatively less common. Yet some sarcomas (e.g., embryonal rhabdomyosarcoma, synovial sarcoma, and Kaposi sarcoma) often metastasize to lymph nodes.

SUGGESTED READING

BOOKS

Brunning RD, McKenna RW: *Atlas of tumor pathology: tumors of the bone marrow.* Armed Forces Institute of Pathology, Washington, 1994

Hoffman R, Benz EJ Jr, Shattik SJ, et al (eds): *Hematology: basic principles and practice.* New York: Churchill Livingstone, 1995.

Jaffe ES (ed): *Surgical pathology of the lymph nodes and related organs.* Philadelphia: WB Saunders, 1995.

Knowles DM (ed): *Neoplastic hematopathology.* Baltimore: Williams & Wilkins, 1992.

Stamatoyannopoulos G, Nienhuis AW, Leder P, Majerus PW (eds): *The molecular basis of blood diseases.* Philadelphia: WB Saunders, 1994.

Warnke RA, Weiss LM, Chan, JKC et al: *Atlas of tumor pathology: tumors of the lymph nodes and spleen.* Armed Forces Institute of Pathology, Washington, 1995.

Williams WJ, Beutler E, Erslev AJ, Lichtman MA (eds): *Hematology,* 5th ed. New York: McGraw-Hill, 1990.

REVIEW ARTICLES

Harris NL, Jaffe ES, Stein H, et al: A revised European-American classification of lymphoid neoplasms: a proposal from the International Lymphoma Study Group. *Blood* 84:1361–1392, 1994.

McGlave P., Verfaillie CM (eds): Biology and therapy of chronic myelogenous leukemia. *Hematology/oncology clinics of north america,* vol 12, Philadelphia: WB Saunders, February 1998.

Miller, T, Grogan T (eds): Lymphoma *Hematology/oncology clinics of north america,* vol 11, Philadelphia: WB Saunders, October 1997.

National Cancer Institute sponsored study of classification of non-Hodgkin's's lymphoma: Summary and description of a Working Formulation for Clinical Usage: the non-Hodgkin's's lymphoma pathologic classification project. *Cancer* 49:2112–2135, 1982.

Zon L (ed): Aplastic anemia and stem cell biology. *Hematolgy/oncology clinics of north america,* vol 11, Philadelphia: WB Saunders, December 1977.

CHAPTER 21

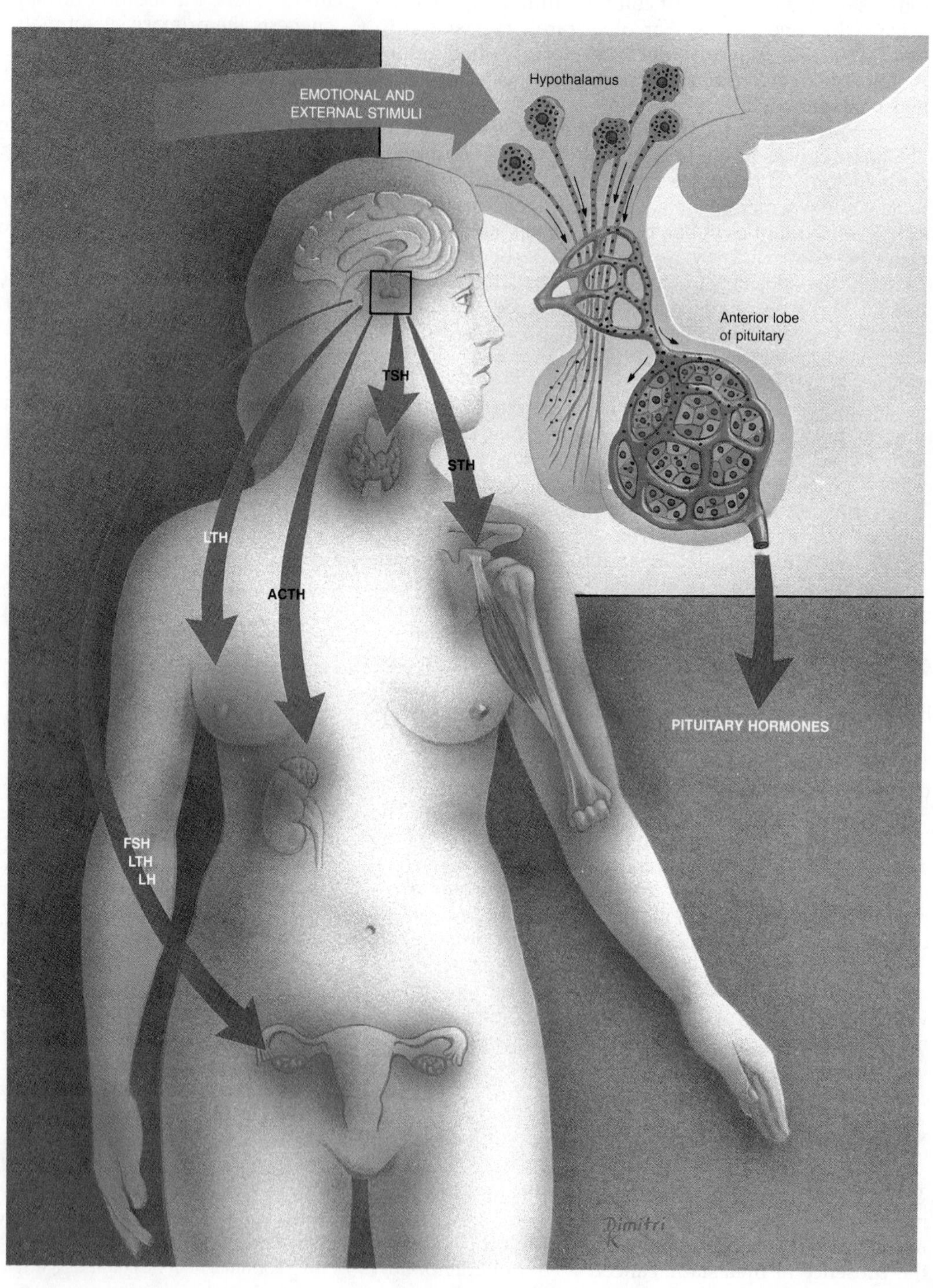

EMOTIONAL AND EXTERNAL STIMULI
Hypothalamus
Anterior lobe of pituitary
TSH
STH
LTH
ACTH
FSH
LTH
LH
PITUITARY HORMONES
Dimitri K

The Endocrine System

Ernest A. Lack
John L. Farber
Emanuel Rubin

FIGURE ***21-1*** ***(see opposite page)***
The pituitary releases a variety of hormones that stimulate hormone secretion by other endocrine glands or act directly. Pituitary activity is modulated by releasing factors from the hypothalamus, which in turn responds to emotional and external stimuli. ACTH, adrenocorticotropic hormone; FSH, follicle-stimulating hormone; LH, luteinizing hormone; LTH, luteotropic hormone (prolactin); STH, somatotropin (growth hormone); TSH, thyroid-stimulating hormone.

Multicellular organisms utilize two seemingly distinct systems for intercellular communication. It was recognized almost a century ago that one, the nervous system, is a structurally fixed network designed for rapid signaling. The other, the endocrine system, was described as acting more slowly and employing mobile chemical messengers that are effective at a distance from their site of production (Fig. 21-1). With the discovery of neurotransmitters and the recognition that signaling molecules can act locally on adjacent cells or even on the producing cell itself, it is today understood that a rigid distinction between the nervous and endocrine systems is inappropriate and that in many ways they act in an integrated manner as a *neuroendocrine system*.

The term *hormone* (Greek, "set in motion") originally referred to a chemical secreted in one location that produces effects, often at a distance, on another part of the body. The notion of "ductless" (i.e., endocrine) glands implied that the chemical messenger enters the circulation, which carries it to the target organ. Many hormones, such as thyroid hormone, corticosteroids, and pituitary hormones, conform to this classic definition. By contrast, some traditionally recognized hormones, such as catecholamines, are produced in a variety of sites and act either locally or through the circulation. Other mediators function only in restricted compartments. For example, hypothalamic hormones act only on the pituitary and reach this gland through portal tributaries without entering the systemic circulation. Finally, many hormones exert their effects in the same tissues in which they are formed, such as müllerian-inhibiting substance. These diverse forms of chemically mediated cell-to-cell communication are summarized in Figure 21-2.

To qualify as a hormone, a chemical messenger must bind to a receptor, either on the surface of the target or within it. Hormones act either on the final effector target or on other glands that in turn produce another hormone. For instance, thyroid hormone acts directly on many types of peripheral cells, whereas thyroid-stimulating hormone (TSH) is released by the pituitary and thereafter promotes the secretion of thyroid hormone by the thyroid gland. Diseases of the endocrine system result in overproduction or underproduction of hormones. In addition, insensitivity of target tissues leads to effects similar to those associated with underproduction of hormones.

Pituitary Gland

ANATOMY

The pituitary gland, also termed the *hypophysis*, resides within the sella turcica, located at the base of the skull within the sphenoid bone. The anterior lobe, which comprises 80% of the gland, is known as the *adenohypophysis*, and the posterior lobe is known as the *neurohypophysis*. The pituitary is in proximity to the optic chiasm and cranial nerves III, IV, V, and VI; thus, tumors of the gland may produce blindness or a number of cranial nerve palsies.

The two lobes of the pituitary are anatomically distinct and derived from different embryological anlage. The anterior lobe develops from ectoderm that grows upward from the oral cavity (Rathke duct). Along its tract, this craniopharyngeal duct leaves intrasphenoidal squamous epithelial rests, which may later serve as the origin of craniopharyngioma. The neurohypophysis (posterior lobe) originates as a downward projection of the brain and remains connected to the hypothalamus by the hypophyseal stalk. Between the anterior and posterior lobes is the vestigial intermediate lobe, composed of a few colloid-filled follicles.

The pituitary has a dual circulation, composed on the one hand of arteries and veins and on the other of a portal venous system between the hypothalamus and the anterior lobe. The latter supplies 80% to 90% of the blood to the pituitary. This portal system is the conduit for the transport of hypothalamic releasing hormones to the anterior pituitary. Short portal vessels also provide a vascular communication between the anterior and posterior lobes.

The posterior lobe is controlled by unmyelinated nerve fibers that originate in the hypothalamus and proceed along the pituitary stalk to the neurohypophysis. In addition to their conventional neural action, these nerves also secrete arginine vasopressin (antidiuretic hormone [ADH]) and oxytocin, which are synthesized in the hypothalamus, stored in the posterior lobe, and then released into the systemic circulation.

Microscopically, the glandular cells of the adenohypophysis are arranged in cords or nests within a highly vascular stroma. On the basis of staining with hema-

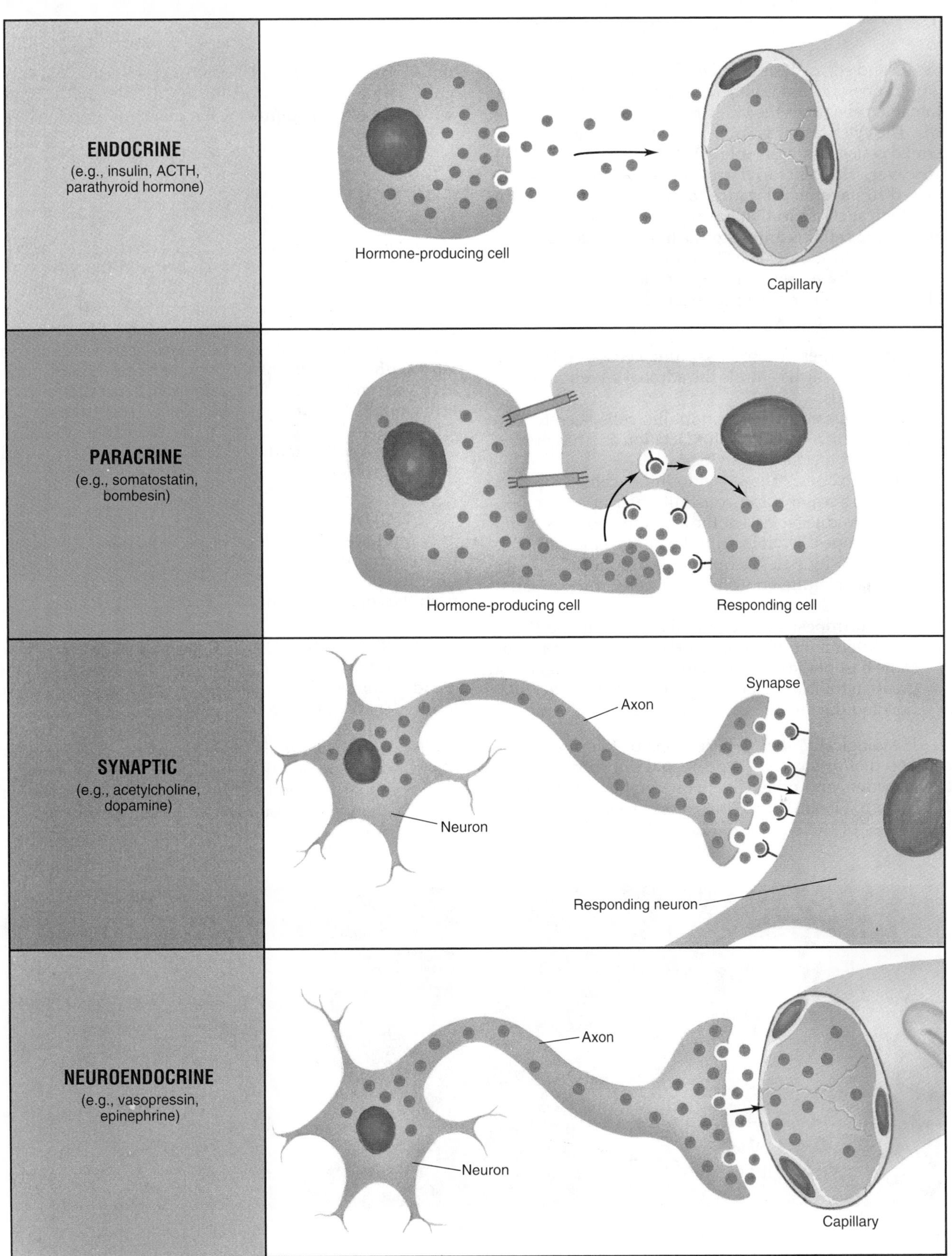

FIGURE 21-2
Mechanisms of chemically mediated cell-to-cell communication. Biological messages may be transmitted by mechanisms other than the classic endocrine pathway via the circulation. These include paracrine, synaptic, and neuroendocrine modes of communication.

toxylin and eosin, these cells were classically divided into two groups of equal number, namely, stainable and unstainable cells, with the latter referred to as *chromophobe cells*. The cytoplasmic granules of the stainable cells were termed *acidophilic* (eosinophilic) (40%) or *basophilic* (10%). **However, the tinctorial properties of the granules proved to have no relevance to their function, and the histological classification has been replaced by one that defines the cells according to the hormone secreted.** The cellular localization of specific pituitary hormones is accomplished by means of immunohistochemical staining (Fig. 21-3). The hormone-producing cells in the anterior pituitary are as follows:

- **Corticotropes:** These basophilic cells secrete corticotropin, which controls the adrenal secretion of corticosteroids.
- **Lactotropes:** Certain acidophilic cells secrete prolactin, which is essential for lactation and has numerous other metabolic activities.
- **Somatotropes:** These acidophilic cells elaborate growth hormone and constitute half of all the hormone-producing cells of the adenohypophysis.
- **Thyrotropes:** Thyroid-stimulating hormone (TSH) is produced by pale basophilic or amphophilic cells, which constitute only 5% of the cells of the anterior lobe.
- **Gonadotropes:** Follicle-stimulating hormone (FSH) and luteinizing hormone (LH) are secreted by the same basophilic cell. FSH stimulates the formation of graafian follicles in the ovary, and LH induces ovulation and the formation of corpora lutea in the ovary.

Histologically, the posterior lobe of the pituitary is composed of pituicytes, a type of glial cell without secretory function, and unmyelinated nerve fibers containing ADH and oxytocin. Both of these hormones are formed in the bodies of the nerve cells in the hypothalamus and transported axonally to the neurohypophysis. ADH promotes water resorption from the distal renal tubules, whereas oxytocin stimulates the pregnant uterus to contract at term.

HYPOPITUITARISM

Hypopituitarism refers to the deficient secretion of one or more of the hormones secreted by the pituitary. In the most common situation, only one or a few of the pituitary hormones are deficient. Occasionally, a total failure of pituitary function occurs, in which case the term *panhypopituitarism* is applied. The effects of hypopituitarism vary with the extent of the loss, the specific hormones involved, and the age of the patient. In general, the symptoms relate to deficient function of the thyroid and adrenal glands and that of the reproductive system. In children, growth retardation and delayed puberty are additional problems.

PITUITARY TUMORS: More than half of all cases of hypopituitarism in adults are caused by pituitary tumors, usually an adenoma. Even though the tumor itself may be functional, symptoms of hypopituitarism often result from the compression of adjacent tissue by the mass.

SHEEHAN SYNDROME: In this situation, panhypopituitarism is caused by ischemic necrosis of the gland, commonly, but not exclusively, after hypotension induced by postpartum hemorrhage. The pituitary is particularly susceptible at this time, because its enlargement during pregnancy renders it vulnerable to a reduction in blood flow. Amenorrhea, hypothyroidism, and inadequate adrenal function are frequent consequences (Fig. 21-4). With modern obstetric care, Sheehan syndrome has become rare.

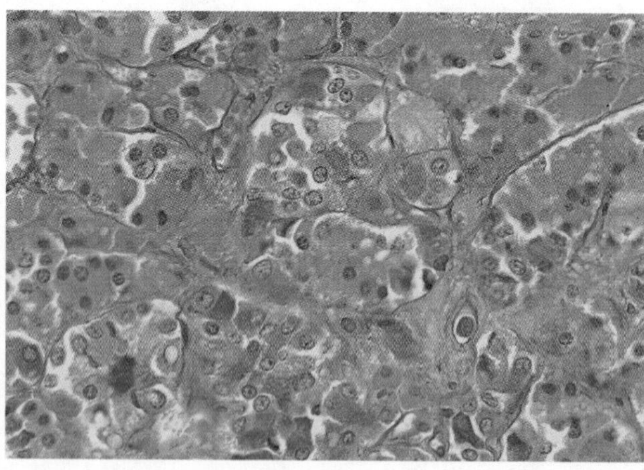

A

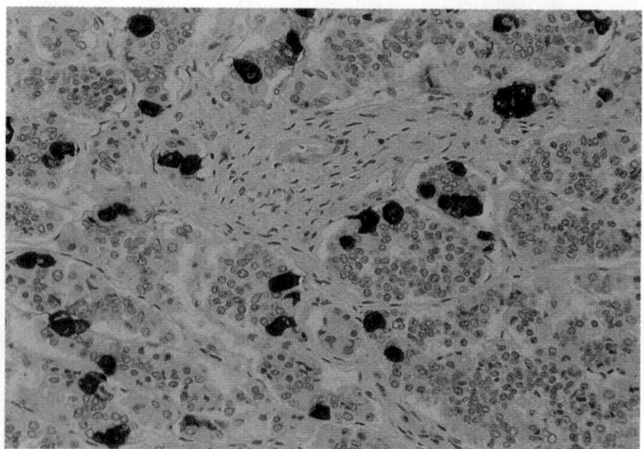

B

FIGURE 21-3
Normal anterior lobe of pituitary. (*A*) In a PAS-orange G stain, the cytoplasm of somatotropic and prolactin-secreting cells take up the orange G stain. Most of the cells with a lavender cytoplasm produce corticotropin (corticotropes). (*B*) An immunohistochemical stain demonstrates cells that synthesize growth hormone (somatotropes).

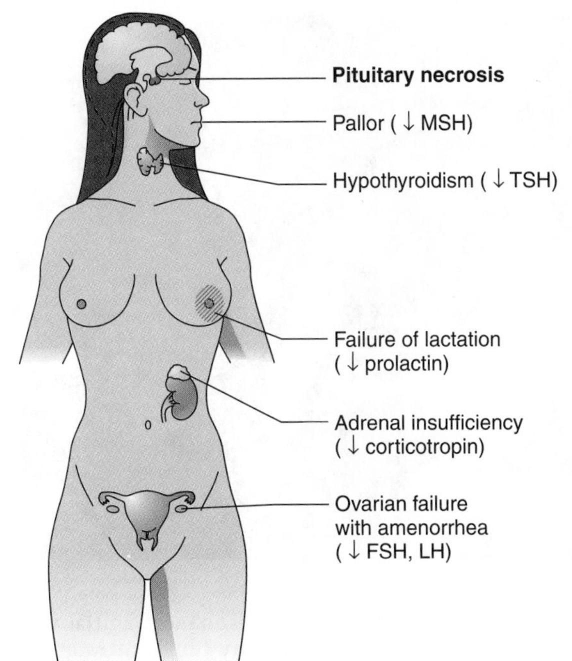

FIGURE 21-4
The major clinical manifestations of Sheehan syndrome.

PITUITARY APOPLEXY: Hemorrhagic infarction of a pituitary adenoma is usually without endocrine effects because sufficient functioning tissue remains. However, on occasion, pituitary apoplexy leads to hypopituitarism.

IATROGENIC HYPOPITUITARISM: Radiation therapy to the pituitary itself or to lesions of the adjacent head and neck regions can result in hypopituitarism. Similarly, neurosurgical procedures may involve the pituitary.

TRAUMA: Basal skull fractures and other trauma to the sella turcica may injure the pituitary.

INFILTRATIVE DISEASES: Bacterial and viral infections that lead to inflammation of the pituitary area can damage the gland. Hand-Schüller-Christian disease is associated with diabetes insipidus but may also cause hypopituitarism. Hemochromatosis leads to iron deposition in the pituitary and may result in panhypopituitarism.

ISOLATED GROWTH HORMONE DEFICIENCY (IGHD): Most dwarfs and midgets suffer from defects of nonpituitary origin, but a few are true pituitary dwarfs. IGHD may be associated with a number of familial disorders caused by defective growth hormone genes. In many cases, the condition reflects complete deletions of the growth hormone gene, whereas in others inactivating mutations are responsible. It may also be secondary to hypothalamic dysfunction of unknown etiology or caused by a variety of lesions. The availability of recombinant human growth hormone has permitted the safe and effective treatment of these children.

GROWTH HORMONE INSENSITIVITY (LARON SYNDROME): *Laron dwarfism is a rare, autosomal recessive, form of short stature due to extreme resistance to growth hormone (GH) secondary to abnormalities in the growth hormone receptor (GHR).* Clinically, these dwarfs tend to be obese and display high levels of serum GH and low concentrations of insulin-like growth factor-1 (IGF-1). The condition is seen predominantly in people of Mediterranean origin, especially Sephardic Jews. Interestingly, the same lesion is responsible for the dwarfism of *African pygmies*.

Laron syndrome is caused by diverse GHR mutations, including deletions, RNA processing defects, inappropriate stop codons, and missense mutations. All of the mutations involve the extracellular domain of the receptor, and most are unique to particular families or geographic areas. Since growth hormone exerts its effects by promoting the secretion of IGF-1, the latter hormone provides effective replacement therapy for Laron syndrome, mimicking most effects ascribed to GH itself.

ISOLATED GONADOTROPIN DEFICIENCY (KALLMANN SYNDROME): *Kallman syndrome is an X-linked disorder characterized by hypogonadotropic hypogonadism and anosmia (absent sense of smell).* Cleft palate and other anomalies may also be present. Kallman syndrome is usually diganosed at puberty because of a delay in the appearance of secondary sex characteristics. The syndrome is caused by a mutation in the KAL gene (Xp22.3), which codes for an extracellular matrix component with putative antiprotease activity and cell adhesion function. As a result of this mutation, neurons destined to secrete gonadotropin-releasing hormone (GnRH) fail to migrate from their origin in the olfactory anlage to their normal location in the hypothalamus.

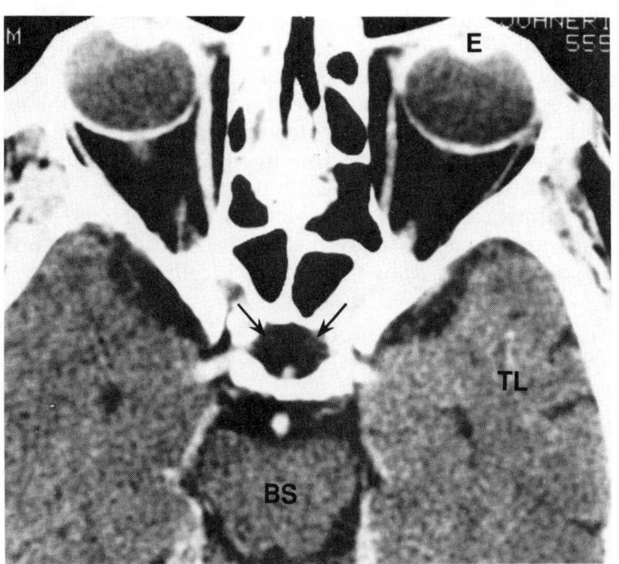

FIGURE 21-5
Empty sella syndrome. A CT scan of the cranium in an axial section demonstrates an empty sella turcica (*arrows*). E, eye; TL, temporal lobe; BS, brainstem.

EMPTY SELLA SYNDROME: This is a radiological term that describes an enlarged sella containing a thin, flattened pituitary at the base (Fig. 21-5). The empty sella syndrome is secondary to a congenitally defective or absent diaphragma sella, which permits the transmission of cerebrospinal fluid pressure into the sella. Hormonal abnormalities are usually minor, although some women develop mild hypopituitarism.

PITUITARY ADENOMAS

Pituitary adenomas are benign neoplasms of the anterior lobe of the pituitary and are often associated with the excess secretion of pituitary hormones and evidence of corresponding endocrine hyperfunction (Table 21-1). They occur in both sexes at almost any age but are more common in men between the ages of 20 and 50 years. Small, apparently nonfunctioning pituitary adenomas are found incidentally in as many as 25% of adult autopsies.

The etiology of pituitary adenomas is obscure. In rare instances, they occur in the context of multiple endocrine neoplasia (MEN) type 1, a hereditary disposition to the formation of adenomas of the pituitary, parathyroid hyperplasia or adenoma, and islet cell adenomas of the pancreas. Activating point mutations in the stimulatory subunit of the G protein (G_s) that activates adenylyl cyclase have been reported in 40% of pituitary adenomas that secrete growth hormone. The resultant elevation of intracellular cyclic adenosine monophosphate (cAMP) levels leads to hypersecretion of growth hormone and cellular proliferation. These mutations are presumably acquired, since they are present only in tumor cells and not in peripheral blood leukocytes from the same patients.

Pituitary adenomas have classically been subdivided histologically according to the tinctorial properties of their cells. Thus, they have been classified as acidophil, basophil, or chromophobe adenomas. In this scheme, acidophil adenomas were associated with the overproduction of growth hormone, basophil adenomas with the excess secretion of corticotropin, and chromophobe adenomas with no endocrine hyperfunction. In view of the lack of correlation between the staining properties of the tumor cells and the type of hormone secreted, pituitary adenomas are today classified according to the hormone(s) elaborated by the neoplastic cells.

TABLE *21-1* **Frequency of Adenomas of the Anterior Pituitary**

Cell Type	Hormone	Frequency (%)
Lactotrope	Prolactin	26
Null cell	None	17
Corticotrope	Corticotropin	15
Somatotrope	Growth hormone	14
Plurihormonal	Multiple	13
Gonadotrope	FSH, LH	8
Oncocytoma	None	6
Thyrotrope	TSH	1

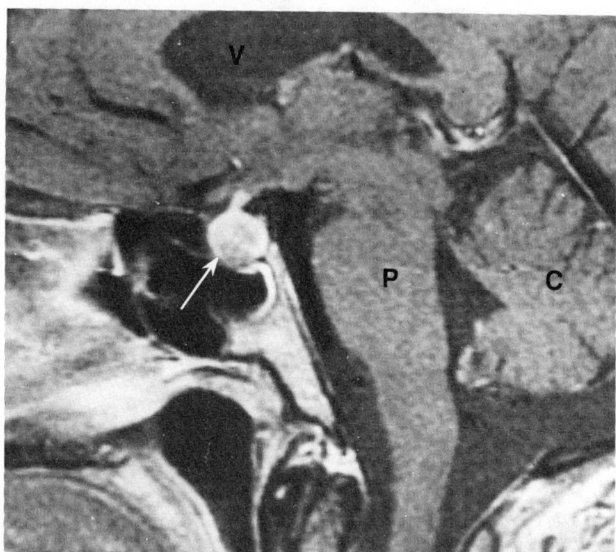

FIGURE *21-6*
Pituitary adenoma. A magnetic resonance sagittal view of the brain shows a distinct pituitary tumor (*arrow*). V, lateral ventricle; P, pons; C, cerebellum.

Pituitary adenomas range from small lesions that do not enlarge the gland to expansive tumors that erode the sella turcica and impinge on adjacent cranial structures (Fig. 21-6). In general, adenomas less than 10 mm in diameter are referred to as *microadenomas*, whereas larger ones are termed *macroadenomas*. Microadenomas do not produce symptoms unless they secrete hormones, but macroadenomas tend to cause both local symptoms, by virtue of their size, and systemic manifestations, as a result of the overproduction of hormones. The mass effects of pituitary macroadenomas include impingement on the optic chiasm, often with bitemporal hemianopsia and loss of central vision, oculomotor palsies when the tumor invades the cavernous sinuses, and severe headaches. Large adenomas may invade the hypothalamus and lead to loss of temperature regulation, hyperphagia, and hormonal syndromes caused by interference with the normal hypothalamic input to the pituitary.

Lactotrope Adenomas (Prolactinomas)

Hyperprolactinemia is the most common endocrinopathy associated with pituitary adenomas. Almost half of all pituitary microadenomas contain prolactin, but the number that secrete this hormone appears to be far lower. Prolactin-producing microadenomas are most often symptomatic in young women, whereas more than half of all macroadenomas that elaborate prolactin are found in men. This difference in sex distribution is related to the more frequent occurrence of endocrinological symptoms in women, and the true incidence in unselected autopsies is similar in both sexes. In general, the larger the adenoma the more prolactin is secreted.

☐ **Pathology:** Lactotrope adenomas tend to be chromophobic or slightly acidophilic. By immunohistochemistry, the Golgi region stains strongly for prolactin. The deposition of endocrine amyloid (see Chapter 23) and the presence of psammoma bodies (calcospherites) are characteristic of lactotrope adenoma but are not pathognomonic.

☐ **Clinical Features:** In women, functional lactotrope adenomas lead to amenorrhea, galactorrhea, and infertility. The consistently elevated blood prolactin levels inhibit the surge in the secretion of pituitary LH necessary for ovulation. Men tend to suffer from decreased libido and erectile dysfunction. Functional lactotrope microadenomas are successfully treated with dopamine agonists (bromocriptine) to inhibit prolactin secretion, whereas macroadenomas may require surgery or radiation therapy.

Somatotrope Adenomas

Pituitary adenomas that secrete growth hormone produce dramatic bodily changes. Should a somatotrope adenoma arise in a child or adolescent before the epiphyses close, the result is *gigantism*. By contrast, when a somatotrope adenoma occurs after the epiphyses of the long bones have fused and adult height has been achieved, the consequence is *acromegaly*.

☐ **Pathology:** In patients with acromegaly, 75% have a somatotrope macroadenoma at the time of diagnosis and most of the remainder have microadenomas. By light microscopy, somatotrope adenomas are either acidophilic or chromophobic. Electron microscopically, acidophilic tumors tend to contain abundant secretory granules, whereas the chromophobic ones are sparsely granular. Acidophilic somatotrope adenomas usually grow slowly and remain within the sella.

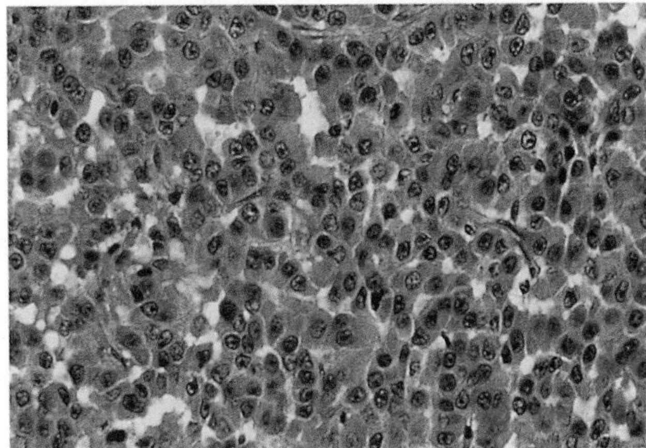

FIGURE *21-7*
Pituitary somatotropic adenoma from a man with acromegaly. The tumor cells are arranged in thin cords and ribbons.

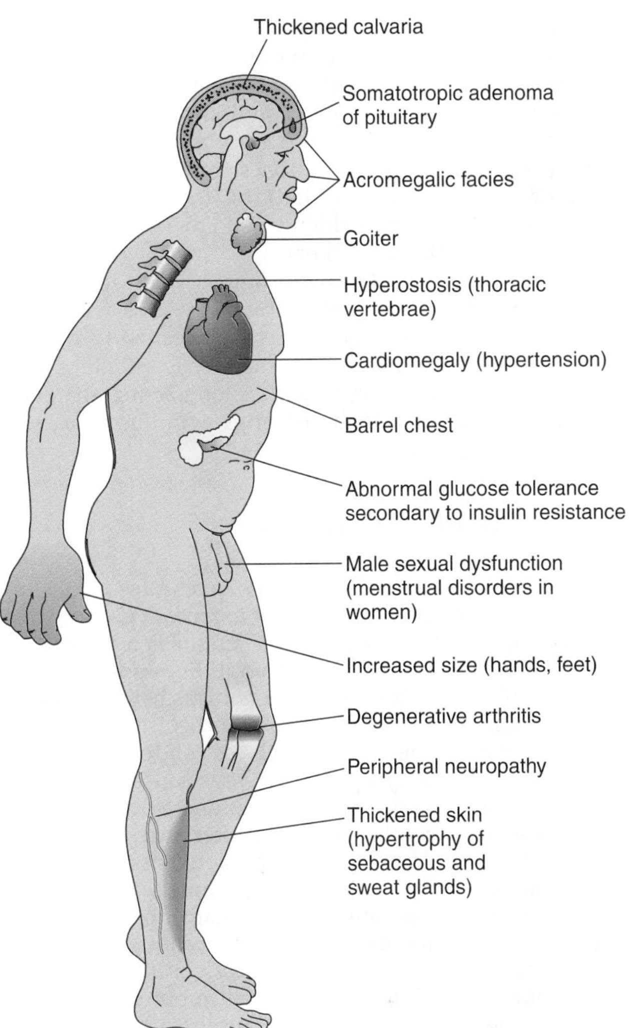

FIGURE *21-8*
The clinical manifestations of acromegaly.

Microscopically, sheets or trabeculae of regular eosinophilic cells are noted (Fig. 21-7). The chromophobic variant is typically faster growing and invasive and microscopically manifests cellular and nuclear pleomorphism.

☐ **Clinical Features:** Acromegaly is an uncommon disorder, with an annual incidence of only three cases per million. Over the course of many years, patients with acromegaly gradually develop coarse facial features (Fig. 21-8). They exhibit overgrowth of the mandible (prognathism) and maxilla, with spaces between the upper incisor teeth, and a thickened nose. The hands and feet become enlarged, and the hat size is increased.

Acromegaly has more implications for the health of the patient than simple cosmetic disfigurement, and the incidence of cardiovascular, cerebrovascular, and respiratory deaths is increased. Most acromegalics suffer from neurological and musculoskeletal symptoms, including headaches, paresthesias, arthralgias, and muscle weakness. One third have hypertension, and even half of nonhypertensive acromegalics have an increased left ventricular mass and may develop congestive heart failure in the absence of a defined cardiac condition. The viscera are also hypertrophied. Diabetes occurs in as many as 20%, and hypercalciuria and renal stones are present in another fifth of the patients. In half of the patients with acromegaly, hyperprolactinemia is sufficiently severe as to be symptomatic (see earlier).

The treatment of choice for somatotrope adenomas is transsphenoidal removal of the pituitary, after which circulating growth hormone levels may decline to normal levels within hours. Radiation therapy is an alternative when surgery is contraindicated. A long-acting analogue of somatostatin, an antagonist of growth hormone, is a useful adjunct to treatment.

Corticotrope Adenomas

Corticotrope adenomas secrete corticotropin, which in turn induces adrenal cortical hypersecretion to produce Cushing disease (see later). In most cases, the tumor is a microadenoma, which is intensely basophilic and periodic acid–Schiff (PAS) positive. Immunohistochemical analysis reveals not only the presence of corticotropin but also that of related peptides, such as endorphins and lipotropin, in the cytoplasm. A few functional corticotrope adenomas are chromophobic and tend to be more aggressive than their basophilic counterparts.

By electron microscopy, basophilic adenomas contain numerous secretory granules and perinuclear bundles of fine, keratin-positive, intermediate filaments (type I filaments). These filaments may be so abundant that they are visible by light microscopy as *Crooke hyalinization*, the morphological indicator of functional suppression of corticotropes by high levels of circulating cortisol. Crooke hyalinization was originally thought to occur only in the nontumorous corticotropes in patients with Cushing disease. However, their presence in some basophilic adenomas suggests that these tumors may not be entirely autonomous.

Nelson syndrome refers to a rapidly growing and often invasive corticotrope adenoma that appeared some years after the treatment of Cushing disease by bilateral adrenalectomy. The removal of the adrenals presumably eliminated a feedback suppression of neoplastic corticotropes by glucocorticoid hormones. The paucity of intermediate filaments in the corticotrope tumors of Nelson syndrome supports the hypothesis that excess glucocorticoids are essential for the appearance of Crooke hyalinization. Nelson syndrome is today uncommon, owing to the fact that corticotrope adenomas are now treated by surgical removal of the tumor.

Gonadotrope Adenomas

Gonadotrope adenomas secrete LH and FSH. Most of these tumors are macroadenomas and present in middle-aged men as headache, visual disturbance, and acquired hypogonadism. Since LH normally stimulates testosterone production in the testis, the hypogonadism in men with gonadotrope adenomas is seemingly paradoxic. This effect has been attributed to inadequate bioactivity of the secreted LH or abnormalities in the normal pulsatile pattern of LH release.

Gonadotrope adenomas are chromophobic or somewhat acidophilic. The tumor cells exhibit strong immunoreactivity for FSH, LH, or both. By electron microscopy, secretory granules are sparse, and there is no correlation between circulating levels of FSH or LH and immunoreactivity or ultrastructure. Surgical resection is the treatment of choice.

Thyrotrope Adenomas

Thyrotrope adenomas, the rarest of all pituitary adenomas, secrete TSH. The tumor comes to medical attention because of symptoms of hyperthyroidism, goiter, or a pituitary mass lesion. Typically, circulating levels of TSH and thyroid hormone are both increased, a situation unique to this tumor. Thyrotrope adenomas are chromophobic, with polyhedral or columnar cells that form pseudorosettes around blood vessels. They stain for the α- and β-subunits of TSH, and by electron microscopy the secretory granules are often arranged in a single row immediately beneath the plasma membrane.

In patients with long-standing hypothyroidism, hyperplasia of pituitary thyrotropes (thyroid deficiency cells) is a well-described entity and is presumably secondary to inadequate feedback inhibition by thyroid hormones. It is not known whether these hyperplastic thyrotropes are particularly susceptible to neoplastic transformation.

Nonfunctional Pituitary Adenomas

About one fourth of all pituitary tumors removed surgically do not secrete excess hormones and are not associated with endocrinopathies. The tumors are slowly growing macroadenomas that are diagnosed in older persons because of their mass effects. Two variants of nonfunctional pituitary adenomas are described, null cell adenomas (including oncocytomas) and silent adenomas.

Null cell adenomas are chromophobic, or only slightly acidophilic, and PAS negative. By immunohistochemistry, the tumors are either negative for all hormones of the anterior pituitary or display small clusters of cells that are immunoreactive for a number of hormones. By electron microscopy, they contain secretory granules. The lack of excess hormone secretion is attributed to deficiencies in hormone production and release.

Oncocytoma is a variant of nonfunctional null cell adenoma characterized by enlarged, eosinophilic, and often granular tumor cells. By electron microscopy, they are packed with mitochondria but are otherwise similar to other null cell adenomas.

Silent adenomas are distinguished from other nonfunctional pituitary adenomas by their well-differentiated appearance under the electron microscope and in many cases by immunoreactivity for corticotropin and other hormones. The reasons for the lack of hormone secretion are not understood. It has been speculated that at least some silent adenomas produce hormones that have not yet been characterized.

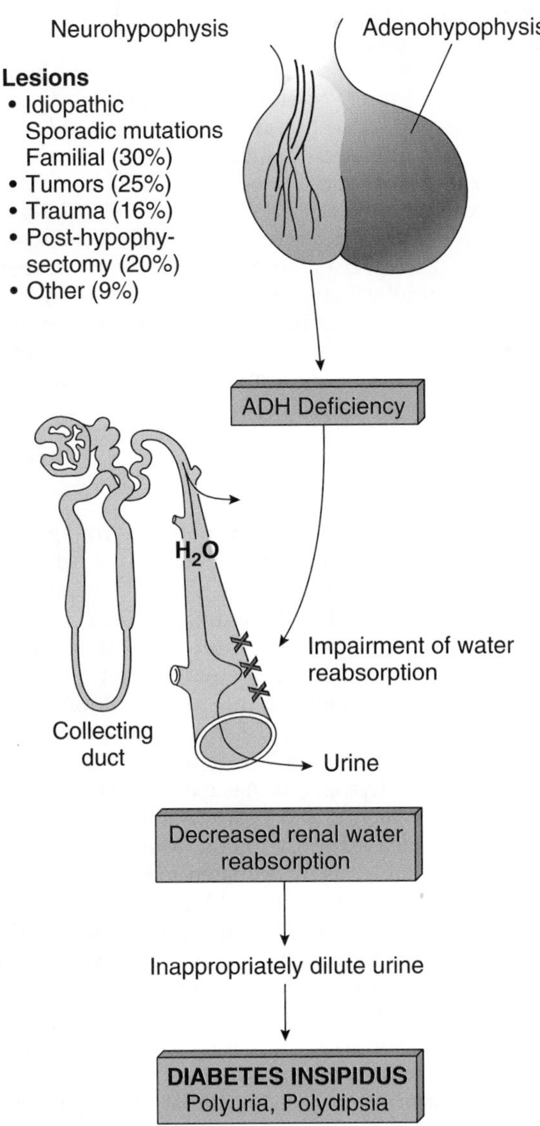

FIGURE *21-9*
The mechanism of diabetes insipidus.

POSTERIOR PITUITARY

Central diabetes insipidus (Fig. 21-9) is the only significant condition associated with disease of the posterior pituitary. This disorder is characterized by an inability to concentrate the urine and consequent chronic water diuresis (polyuria), thirst, and polydipsia. The biochemical basis of the disease is a deficiency of vasopressin (ADH), which is secreted by the posterior pituitary under the influence of the hypothalamus. About one third of the cases of central diabetes insipidus are still of unknown etiology or can be attributed to sporadic or familial mutations in the vasopressin-neurophysin II gene. Mutations in the vasopressin receptor and the vasopressin-sensitive water channel genes have also been described in the context of *nephrogenic diabetes insipidus*. One fourth of the cases of central diabetes insipidus are associated with brain tumors, particularly craniopharyngioma (Fig. 21-10). This

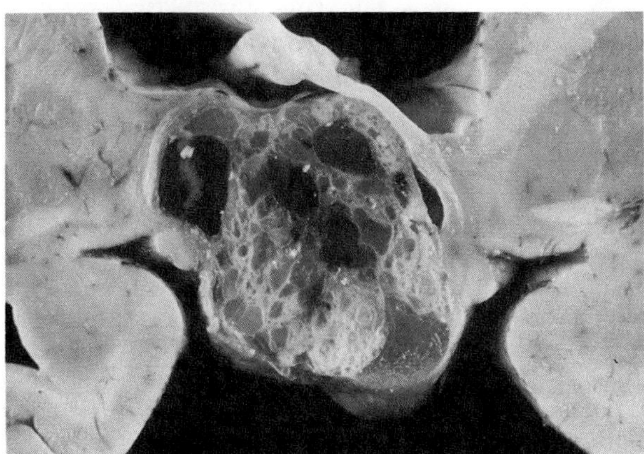

FIGURE *21-10*
Craniopharyngioma. A coronal section of the brain shows a large, cystic tumor mass replacing the midline structures in the region of the hypothalamus.

tumor arises above the sella turcica from remnants of Rathke pouch and invades and compresses adjacent tissues (see Chapter 28). Trauma and hypophysectomy for anterior pituitary tumors account for most of the remaining cases. Uncommonly, localized hemorrhage or infarction, Langerhans cell histiocytosis, or granulomatous infiltrates involve the posterior pituitary stalk or body. Polyuria may be controlled by powdered posterior pituitary or vasopressin administered as snuff.

HYPOTHALAMIC-PITUITARY AXIS

The hypothalamus, pituitary stalk, and pituitary gland constitute an integrated "neuroendocrine system," both anatomically and functionally. Neuron groups in the hypothalamus secrete a number of factors that stimulate

TABLE *21-2* **Hormones of the Hypothalamic-Pituitary-Target Gland Axis**

Hypothalamus	Pituitary	Target Gland	Peripheral Inhibitory Hormone
CRH	Corticotropin	Adrenal	Corticosteroids
AVP	Corticotropin	Adrenal	Corticosteroids
TRH	TSH	Thyroid	T_3, T_4
GHRH	Growth hormone	Varied	IGF 1
Somatostatin	Growth hormone	Varied	IGF 1
LHRH	LH	Gonads	Estradiol, testosterone
	FSH	Gonads	Inhibin, estradiol, testosterone
Dopamine	Prolactin	Breast	Unknown

AVP, arginine vasopressin; CRH, corticotropin-releasing hormone; GHRH, growth hormone–releasing hormone; IGF 1, insulin-like growth factor 1; LHRH, luteinizing hormone–releasing hormone; TRH, thyrotropin-releasing hormone.

the anterior pituitary lobe (Table 21-2). The secretion of these hypothalamic factors is, in turn, antagonized by the hormones secreted by the peripheral target organs, thereby completing a feedback loop. In addition, specific hypothalamic inhibitory hormones have been identified, for example, dopamine, which inhibits the pituitary secretion of prolactin. Secreted into the hypothalamic portal capillary network, the various releasing and inhibitory factors flow through the pituitary stalk to be redistributed in the second portal capillary network of the anterior pituitary lobe, where their specific function is exerted.

The relation of the hypothalamus to the posterior pituitary is different. The posterior pituitary hormones are synthesized in the supraocular and paraventricular regions of the hypothalamus. Neurons in these regions have axons that extend into the posterior pituitary lobe (see Fig. 21-1). The hormones are stored in the nerve terminals in the posterior pituitary and are released on appropriate stimulation.

The hypothalamus may be damaged by a variety of primary and metastatic tumors, viral infections and granulomatous inflammations, and several types of degenerative and hereditary disorders. In many instances, hypothalamic dysfunction occurs in the absence of an identifiable anatomic abnormality. Diverse conditions result from disturbances of hypothalamic function and include among others hypogonadism, precocious puberty, amenorrhea, and eating disorders (obesity or anorexia). Some pituitary disorders characterized by increased or decreased hormone secretion have their origin in hypothalamic dysfunction. A detailed description of the hypothalamic syndromes is beyond the scope of this chapter, and the reader is referred to the textbooks of endocrinology listed under Suggested Reading.

Thyroid Gland

EMBRYOLOGY AND ANATOMY

The thyroid gland develops from two separate anlagen. The medial portion originates from an invagination of the tongue, termed the *foramen cecum*. The primitive thyroid descends to its eventual location in the lower anterior neck by elongation of its tubular attachment to the tongue, known as the *thyroglossal duct*, which then atrophies. The lateral lobes derive from a portion of the fifth branchial pouch called the ultimobranchial body. The ultimobranchial bodies are joined to the medial anlage to form the adult thyroid.

The adult thyroid comprises two lobes connected by an isthmus and is situated below the thyroid cartilage anterior to the trachea. Each lobe is about 4 cm in greatest dimension, and the entire gland weighs some 20 g. The cut surface has a glistening, light brown, lobulated appearance. Microscopically, the parenchyma is arranged in acini or follicles averaging about 200 μm in diameter. They appear to vary considerably in size owing to the different planes of section of the spherical follicles. The follicles are lined by an epithelium whose appearance depends on the demand for thyroid hormone. The lining cells are columnar when the gland is actively secreting hormone and flatter when the thyroid is less active. The epithelial cells contain glycoprotein globules composed of thyroglobulin, which is well demonstrated with the PAS reaction. The lumen of the follicle contains a glassy, eosinophilic proteinaceous material termed *colloid*. This substance contains secreted thyroglobulin, from which active thyroid hormones are released.

In addition to the follicular epithelial cells, the thyroid also contains parafollicular or *C cells*, which produce calcitonin, a calcium-lowering hormone. These cells are derived from the ultimobranchial bodies and are found interspersed with follicular epithelial cells or in the interstitium. With routine stains, C cells are difficult to identify but are readily visualized with immunostaining for calcitonin.

FUNCTION

The principal metabolic products of the thyroid gland are triiodothyronine (T_3) and tetraiodothyronine (thyroxine, T_4). T_4 is principally a prohormone, and the major effector of thyroid function is T_3. These molecules are formed by the iodination of tyrosine residues of thyroglobulin within the follicular cells. Iodinated thyroglobulin is secreted into the lumen of the follicle. Alone among endocrine glands, the thyroid is thus equipped to store a large amount of preformed hormone.

On demand, thyroglobulin is reabsorbed by the follicular cells, after which T_4 and T_3 are liberated by proteolytic cleavage and released to the blood. Most of the secreted hormone is T_4, which is deiodinated in peripheral tissues to the more active form, T_3. In the blood, thyroid hormones circulate both free and bound to thyronine-binding globulin (TBG). The free thyroid hormone hypothesis holds that peripheral cells take up only free hormone, which is in equilibrium with the bound form. Within the target cells, thyroid hormone binds to nuclear receptors, initiating specific mRNA-directed protein synthesis.

Thyroid hormone affects almost all organs in the body. It stimulates the basal metabolic rate and the metabolism of carbohydrates, lipids, and proteins. Thyroid hormone augments thermogenesis and hepatic glucose production through enhanced gluconeogenesis and glycogenolysis. It promotes the synthesis of numerous structural proteins, enzymes, and other hormones. Glucose utilization, fatty acid synthesis in the liver, and adipose tissue lipolysis are all increased. In general, the overall metabolic activities of the body, both anabolic and catabolic, are upregulated by thyroid hormone.

Thyroid structure and function are governed principally by TSH secreted by the pituitary. In turn, thyroid hormone suppresses TSH secretion, to complete an autoregulatory feedback loop. For example, hypopituitarism leads to hypothyroidism, and thyroidectomy results in hyperplasia of pituitary thyrotropes and elevated blood levels of TSH. The maintenance of a normal rate of thyroid hormone production is also dependent on an adequate dietary supply of iodine. Within certain limits, the thyroid can compensate for either an acute increase or decrease in the availability of exogenous iodine. However, beyond this range, too little or too much iodine is associated with an inhibition of thyroid hormone secretion.

CONGENITAL ANOMALIES

LINGUAL THYROID: If the thyroid fails to descend during embryogenesis, it remains at its origin as a nodule at the base of the tongue. Its removal results in total hypothyroidism.

HETEROTOPIC THYROID TISSUE: *Nests of thyroid tissue may be found anywhere along the pathway of its descent into the lower neck.* Thyroid tissue is also occasionally encountered in the pericardium or mediastinum. Interestingly, conditions that lead to enlargement of the thyroid (e.g., thyroiditis or nodular goiter) also affect the heterotopic thyroid tissue.

LATERAL ABERRANT THYROID: *Ectopic thyroid tissue occasionally occurs in the lymph nodes and soft tissue adjacent to the normal gland.* The origin of lateral aberrant thyroid tissue is controversial. Some hold that all of these cases actually represent well-differentiated metastases from an occult thyroid cancer, whereas others accept the concept of embryonal rests lateral to the thyroid. In any event, the finding of thyroid follicles in enlarged lymph nodes must be treated as suggestive evidence for the presence of a primary thyroid cancer.

THYROGLOSSAL DUCT CYST: *Failure of the thyroglossal duct to involute completely can result in a cystic, fluid-filled remnant anywhere along the route of the duct.* The cysts, which are most common in children, are 1 to 3 cm in diameter and are lined by squamous or respiratory-type epithelium. The presence of thyroid follicles in the wall or adjacent soft tissue serves to distinguish thyroglossal duct cyst from branchial cleft cyst. Surgical excision is curative.

NONTOXIC GOITER

Nontoxic goiter (Latin, guttur, "throat"), also termed simple, colloid, or multinodular goiter, refers to an enlargement of the thyroid that is not associated with functional, inflammatory, or neoplastic alterations. Thus, patients with nontoxic goiter are neither hyperthyroid nor hypothyroid and do not suffer from any form of thyroiditis (see later). The disease is far more common in women than in men (8:1). The diffuse form is frequent in adolescence and during pregnancy, whereas the multinodular type usually presents in persons older than the age of 50 years.

☐ **Pathogenesis:** It is by no means evident that all cases of nontoxic goiter have the same etiology, although they are similar morphologically. It has been accepted that for unknown reasons the capacity of the thyroid to produce thyroid hormone is impaired. As a result, the increased secretion of TSH leads to enlargement of the gland, a situation that maintains the euthyroid state. However, this concept is challenged by the fact that circulating levels of TSH in patients with nontoxic goiter are usually normal, although in some instances the goiter regresses on administration of thyroid hormone. Experimentally, iodine depletion renders the thyroid hyperresponsive to TSH. This finding supports the theory that patients with nontoxic goiter have a subtle impairment of iodine utilization and respond in an exaggerated fashion to normal TSH levels. It is also possible that the cause of the goiter has disappeared and that normal TSH levels simply maintain the enlargement of the thyroid.

Although TSH stimulates both the growth and the function of the thyroid, these parameters are not necessarily coupled. It has been proposed that some patients with nontoxic goiter bear certain immunoglobulins (thyroid growth immunoglobulins) that promote thyroid growth without activating hormone production. According to this hypothesis, nontoxic goiter takes its place among autoimmune diseases, but such an explanation remains conjectural.

Simple nodular enlargement of the thyroid tends to be familial, suggesting a genetic contribution to the disorder. Indeed, mutations in the thyroglobulin gene have been detected in a number of families affected by simple goiter.

The cause of nodular transformation in nontoxic goiter (and in other goitrous conditions) is obscure. It may be related to cyclical variations in the need for thyroid hormone and alternating episodes of stimulation and involution. Alternatively, clonal heterogeneity among thyroid follicles may determine differential sensitivity to growth stimulation. In this regard, it has been demonstrated that the nodules in nontoxic goiter may be polyclonal or monoclonal, suggesting that monoclonal proliferation may emerge secondarily from a polyclonal population, owing to a growth advantage of a genetically altered follicular cell.

☐ **Pathology:** The size of nontoxic goiters ranges from a doubling in the size of the gland (40 g) to a massive enlargement in which the thyroid weighs a few hundred grams (Fig. 21-11).

Diffuse nontoxic goiter characterizes the early stages of the disease. The gland is diffusely enlarged and microscopically exhibits hypertrophy and hyperplasia of the follicular epithelial cells. On occasion, the epithelium has a papillary appearance. At this stage, the amount of colloid in the follicles is decreased.

Multinodular nontoxic goiter evolves as the disease becomes more chronic. The enlarged thyroid assumes an increasingly nodular configuration, and the cut surface is typically studded with numerous irregular nodules. When they contain large amounts of colloid, nodules tend to be soft, glistening, and reddish. Those composed of smaller follicles containing little colloid are typically grayish white and fleshy. Hemorrhagic, necrotic, and cystic areas are common, and fibrous bands often traverse the gland. Calcific foci, which impart a gritty surface, are frequent.

Microscopically, the nodules vary considerably in size and shape. Some are distended with colloid, whereas others are collapsed. Large colloid-containing follicles may fuse to form even larger "colloid cysts." The lining epithelial cells are flat to cuboidal and are occasionally arrayed as papillae that project into the follicular lumen. Hemosiderin deposition and cholesterol granulomas are

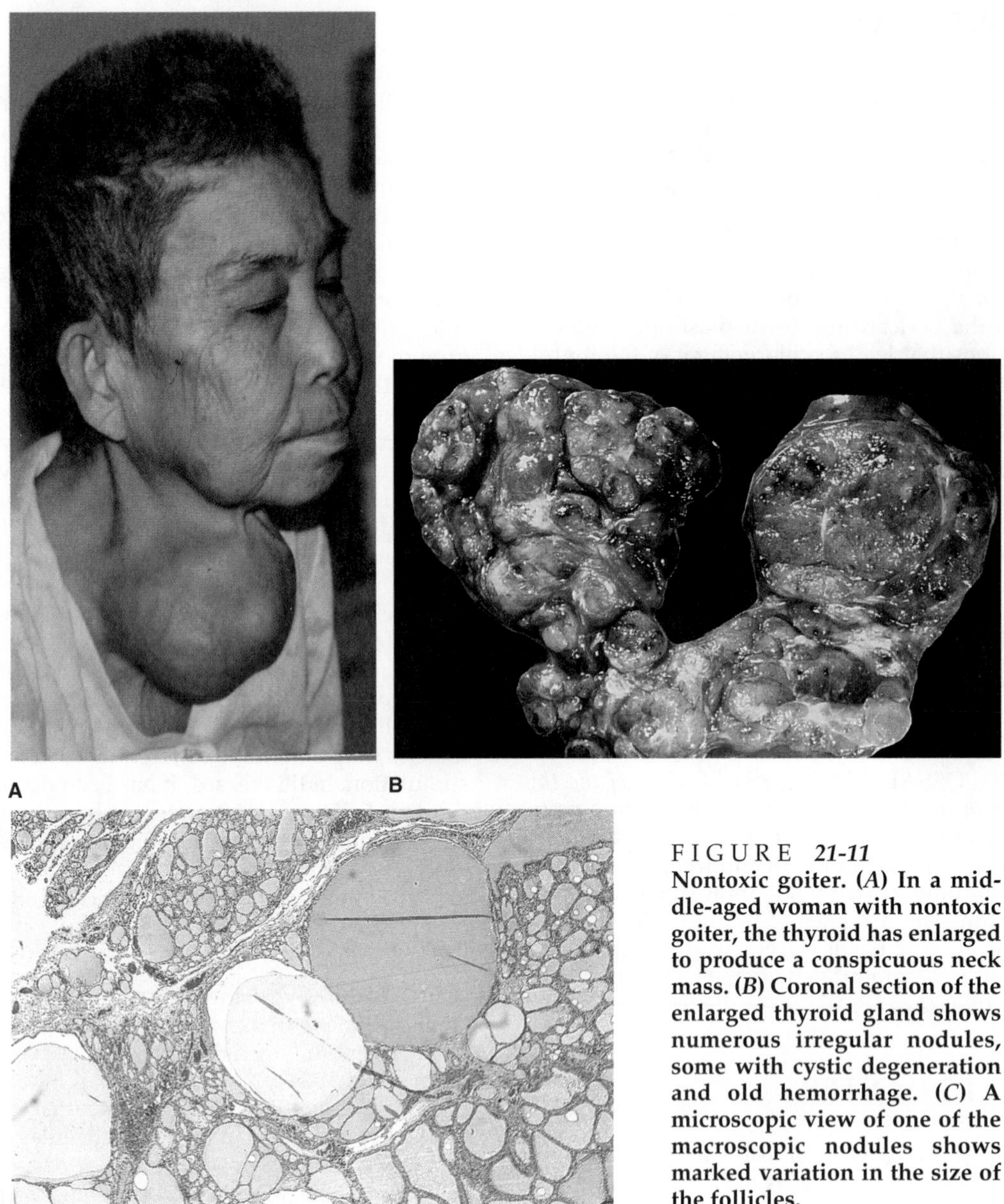

FIGURE 21-11
Nontoxic goiter. (*A*) In a middle-aged woman with nontoxic goiter, the thyroid has enlarged to produce a conspicuous neck mass. (*B*) Coronal section of the enlarged thyroid gland shows numerous irregular nodules, some with cystic degeneration and old hemorrhage. (*C*) A microscopic view of one of the macroscopic nodules shows marked variation in the size of the follicles.

evidence of old hemorrhage. The individual follicles or groups of follicles are separated by dense fibrosis, and dystrophic calcification of necrotic foci is noted.

□ **Clinical Features:** Patients with nontoxic goiter are typically asymptomatic and come to medical attention because of a mass in the neck. Large goiters may cause dysphagia or inspiratory stridor by compressing the esophagus or the trachea. Pressure by the goiter on the neck veins leads to venous congestion of the head and face. Hoarseness may result from compression of the recurrent laryngeal nerve. Occasionally, local pain is produced by hemorrhage into a nodule or cyst. Importantly, the concentrations of T_4 and T_3, and usually of TSH, in the blood are normal.

Nontoxic goiter is most commonly treated with the administration of thyroid hormone to reduce TSH levels and, thus, the stimulation to thyroid growth. In older patients with low TSH levels, further suppression by exogenous thyroid hormone may be ineffective and radioactive iodine therapy is indicated. Although surgery is ordinarily contraindicated, it may become necessary if local obstructive symptoms become troublesome. Many patients with nontoxic goiter eventually develop hyperthyroidism, in which case the term *toxic multinodular goiter* is applied (see later).

HYPOTHYROIDISM

Hypothyroidism refers to the clinical manifestations of thyroid hormone deficiency. It can be the consequence of three general processes:

- Defective synthesis of thyroid hormone, with compensatory goitrogenesis (goitrous hypothyroidism).
- Inadequate function of thyroid parenchyma, usually as a result of thyroiditis or surgical resection of the gland or the therapeutic administration of radioiodine.
- Inadequate secretion of TSH by the pituitary or of thyroid-releasing hormone (TRH) by the hypothalamus.

Hypothyroidism in Adults

The clinical symptomatology of hypothyroidism for the most part reflects only the level of circulating thyroid hormone rather than the cause of the hormone deficiency (Fig. 21-12). Symptoms of hypothyroidism develop insidiously, and often the first manifestations are tiredness, lethargy, sensitivity to cold, and an inability to concentrate. Many organ systems in the body are affected, but all are hypofunctional.

SKIN: Alterations in the skin are almost universal in patients with clinically apparent hypothyroidism. Proteoglycans accumulate in the extracellular matrix, binding water and resulting in a peculiar form of edema termed *myxedema*. Myxedematous patients have boggy facies, puffy eyelids, edema of the hands and feet, and an enlarged tongue. Thickening of the mucous membranes of the larynx causes the patient to be hoarse. A pale, cool skin reflects cutaneous vasoconstriction. The skin is also dry and coarse, because the secretions of the sebaceous and sweat glands are inadequate. Ecchymoses are common because of increased capillary fragility, and skin wounds heal slowly.

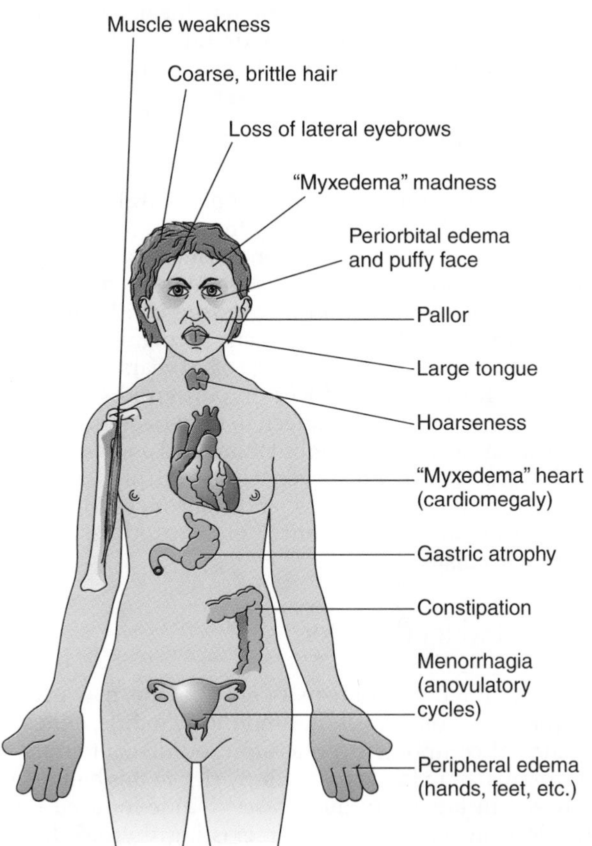

FIGURE *21-12*
The dominant clinical manifestations of hypothyroidism.

NERVOUS SYSTEM: Hypothyroidism in pregnant women has grave neurological consequences for the fetus, expressed after birth as cretinism (see later). The hypothyroid adult is lethargic and somnolent and suffers from memory loss and a general slowing of mental processes. Paranoid ideation or depression is frequent, and even severe agitation, termed *myxedema madness*, may develop. Sensory defects, including deafness and night blindness, occur. A cerebellar ataxia may appear, and tendon reflexes are dulled. Microscopic examination of the brain shows mucinous accumulations in nerve fibers and in the cerebellum.

HEART: In early hypothyroidism, the heart rate and stroke volume are both reduced, resulting in a decreased cardiac output. Since vascular resistance is also increased, the peripheral circulation is impaired, accounting for the cool, pale skin. In untreated hypothyroidism, so-called myxedema heart develops, which is characterized by a dilated heart and a pericardial effusion. Thyroid hormone deficiency decreases cardiac contractility, prolongs diastolic relaxation, and slows the heart rate. Hypothyroidism results in altered ratios of cardiac myosin isoforms and in decreases of transcription of the Ca^{2+}-adenosine triphosphatase (ATPase) that regulates relaxation. On pathological examination, the heart is flabby and microscopically shows interstitial edema and swelling of the myocytes. Coronary atherosclerosis is a common finding. Myxedema heart is entirely reversed by the administration of thyroid hormone.

GASTROINTESTINAL TRACT: Constipation, owing to decreased peristalsis, is a common complaint and may be so severe as to lead to fecal impaction (myxedema megacolon).

REPRODUCTIVE SYSTEM: Women with hypothyroidism suffer ovulatory failure, progesterone deficiency, and irregular and excessive menstrual bleeding. In men, erectile dysfunction and oligospermia are common.

Congenital Hypothyroidism

Congenital hypothyroidism, also termed *cretinism*, may be endemic, sporadic, or familial and is twice as frequent in girls as boys. In nonendemic regions, 90% of cases result from developmental defects of the thyroid (*thyroid dysgenesis*). The remainder have a variety of inherited metabolic defects, including a number of conditions that result in defective synthesis of thyroid hormone and unresponsiveness to thyroid hormone or TSH. A deficiency of TSH owing to pituitary or hypothalamic disease may also cause congenital hypothyroidism.

The clinical manifestations of congenital hypothyroidism are difficult to detect at birth, but symptoms appear in the early weeks of life. The infants are apathetic and sluggish. The abdomen is large and often exhibits an umbilical hernia. The body temperature is often below 35°C (95°F), and the skin is pale and cold. Refractory anemia and a dilated heart are frequent. By the age of 6 months, the clinical syndrome of congenital hypothyroidism is well developed. Mental retardation, stunted growth owing to defective osseous maturation, and characteristic facies are evident. The serum levels of T_4 and T_3 are low, and the serum TSH level is elevated (unless the problem relates to a lack of TSH secretion itself).

If thyroid hormone replacement therapy is not promptly provided, congenital hypothyroidism results in mentally retarded dwarfs. Although treatment may prevent dwarfism, the effects on mental development are more variable. Children in whom hypothyroidism is detected early in neonatal screening programs respond well to treatment with thyroid hormone and develop apparently normal mental capacity. By contrast, children treated at a later age may be left with irreversible brain damage.

Primary Hypothyroidism

In many cases of hypothyroidism, the cause of thyroid failure is uncertain. Primary hypothyroidism is most common in the fifth and sixth decades and, like most thyroid disorders, is more common in women than in men. Three fourths of the patients have circulating antibodies to thyroid antigens, suggesting that these cases represent the end stage of autoimmune thyroiditis (see later). Nongoitrous hypothyroidism may also result from antibodies that block TSH itself or the TSH receptor without activating the thyroid. Some cases of primary hypothyroidism are part of multiglandular autoimmune syndrome, including insulin-dependent diabetes, pernicious anemia, hypoparathyroidism, adrenal atrophy, and hypogonadism.

Goitrous Hypothyroidism

There are a number of conditions in which thyroid enlargement (goiter) is associated with hypothyroidism. The causes are diverse, but in all cases goiter is a compensatory response to the lack of adequate secretion of thyroid hormone. The etiology of goitrous hypothyroidism includes iodine deficiency, antithyroid agents (drugs or dietary goitrogens), chronic iodide intake, and a number of hereditary defects in the synthesis of thyroid hormone. The evolution of the pathological changes in goitrous hypothyroidism is similar to that described earlier for nontoxic goiter.

Endemic Goiter

Endemic goiter refers to the goitrous hypothyroidism of dietary iodine deficiency in locales with a high prevalence of the disease. In areas far from salt water and seafood, which are rich sources of iodides, goiters are (or were) common. The Great Lakes region of the United States, alpine Europe, central Africa, parts of China, and the Himalayas are such places. Iodized salt is an effective preventive dietary measure, and its wide availability has essentially eliminated endemic goiter in many areas. Nevertheless, it has been estimated that more than 200 million persons worldwide are still afflicted with the disease.

The pathological evolution of endemic goiter is comparable to that of nontoxic goiter discussed earlier. However, in contrast to the latter, endemic goiter rarely eventuates in hyperthyroidism, presumably because iodine protects against this complication. Although the administration of iodine may reverse the early, diffuse stage of endemic goiter, such therapy has little effect on a fully developed multinodular goiter. Replacement therapy with thyroid hormone is indicated, and surgical resection may be necessary if local symptoms are severe.

Endemic Cretinism

Endemic cretinism refers to congenital hypothyroidism in areas of endemic goiter. Both parents are usually goitrous. The disease encompasses two overlapping clinical presentations, a neurological syndrome and a predominantly hypothyroid one.

Neurological cretinism features mental retardation, ataxia, spasticity, and deaf-mutism. In the pure form of neurological cretinism, the children may be of normal stature and virtually euthyroid. Thus, it is postulated that iodine deficiency in the first trimester of pregnancy may damage the developing nervous system independently of its effect on thyroid hormone production.

Hypothyroid cretinism is thought to arise from iodine deficiency in late fetal life and in the neonatal period. The clinical course in these children is similar to that of other forms of congenital hypothyroidism (see earlier).

Goiter Induced by Antithyroid Agents

There are a number of drugs and naturally occurring chemicals in foods that are goitrogenic, owing to their suppression of thyroid hormone synthesis. Such goiters may or may not be associated with hypothyroidism. The most commonly used goitrogenic drug is **lithium**, which is employed in the management of manic-depressive states. Women older than the age of 40 years are at particular risk for lithium-induced hypothyroidism, with as many as one third being affected. Other common goitrogenic drugs include phenylbutazone and *p*-aminosalicylic acid. Certain cruciferous vegetables (turnips, rutabaga, cassava) contain goitrogens, and their ingestion can potentiate an iodine-deficient diet to produce goitrous hypothyroidism.

Iodide-Induced Goiter

Goiter and hypothyroidism, or either alone, may occur in persons who consume large amounts of iodide, either as a medicinal component (potassium iodide-containing expectorants) or in foods particularly rich in this halide (e.g., seaweed in Japan). In most cases, iodide-induced goiter develops in the context of preexisting thyroid disease, such as thyroiditis. Women given large doses of iodine during pregnancy may be delivered of goitrous infants.

Hereditary Defects in Thyroid Hormone

Goitrous hypothyroidism secondary to inherited defects in the synthesis of thyroid hormone is rare. These abnormalities include (1) defective iodide transport, (2) an inability of the thyroid to iodinate thyroglobulin, (3) impaired deiodination of iodotyrosines, and (4) abnormal secretion of iodoproteins. In addition, there exist several syndromes in which peripheral tissues are resistant to the action of thyroid hormone, secondary to mutations in the T_3-receptor gene.

Pendred syndrome refers to the combination of congenital goitrous hypothyroidism and nerve deafness. The disorder is inherited as an autosomal recessive trait and accounts for 10% of cases of hereditary deafness. The condition is the result of a defect in thyroid iodine organification, owing to a mutation on chromosome 7q31.

HYPERTHYROIDISM

Hyperthyroidism refers to the clinical consequences of an excessive amount of circulating thyroid hormone. In general, the signs and symptoms of hyperthyroidism reflect a hypermetabolic state of the target tissues. Prolonged hypersecretion of thyroid hormone can result from (1) an excess production of TSH (rare), (2) the presence of an abnormal thyroid stimulator (Graves disease), and (3) intrinsic disease of the thyroid gland (toxic multinodular goiter or functional adenoma). Rare instances of hyperthyroidism follow the release of preformed thyroid hormone during a bout of thyroiditis or the production of thyroid hormone by ectopic thyroid tissue.

Graves Disease

Graves disease, also known as Basedow disease in continental Europe, is an autoimmune disorder characterized by diffuse goiter, hyperthyroidism, and exophthalmos (Fig. 21-13). In the United States, Graves disease is the most frequent cause of hyperthyroidism in patients younger than age 40 years, affecting as many as 0.4% of the population. Taken together, autoimmune diseases of the thyroid (e.g., Graves disease, Hashimoto thyroiditis) are as common as diabetes mellitus.

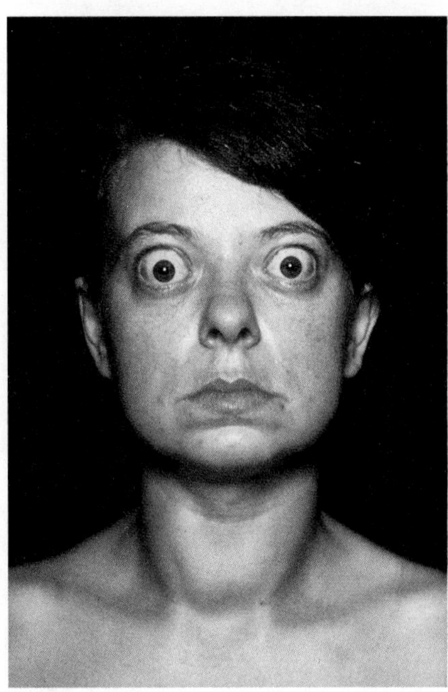

FIGURE *21-13*
Graves disease. A young woman with hyperthyroidism presented with a mass in the neck and exophthalmos.

☐ **Pathogenesis:** The etiology of Graves disease is not fully understood and seems to involve an interplay between immune mechanisms, heredity, sex, and possibly emotional factors. In addition, it is clear that the mechanisms underlying Graves ophthalmopathy are distinct from those that mediate hyperthyroidism.

IMMUNE MECHANISMS: Patients with Graves disease are hyperthyroid owing to the presence of IgG antibodies directed against components of the plasma membrane of thyroid follicular epithelium, presumably the TSH receptor (Fig. 21-14). These antibodies function as agonists, that is, they stimulate the TSH receptor, thereby activating adenylyl cyclase and increasing thyroid hormone secretion. Under this continued stimulation, the thyroid becomes diffusely hyperplastic and excessively vascular. The autoantibodies of Graves disease were originally termed *long-acting thyroid stimulator* (LATS), because the peak secretion of thyroid hormone occurs 16 hours after the exposure of thyroid tissue to antibody, compared with 2 hours for TSH.

Graves autoantibodies are actually heterogeneous, and those that stimulate thyroid hormone secretion represent only one component. Other antibodies seem to be cytotoxic and may account for the thyroid failure that often follows long-standing Graves disease. There is also a suggestion that sensitized T lymphocytes may stimulate B cells to elaborate thyroid-activating immunoglobulins.

The mechanism underlying the origin of the autoantibodies in Graves disease remains unclear, but there is evidence that sensitization to antigens of *Yersinia enterocolitica* plays a role. This gram-negative enteric pathogen displays a TSH binding site that also binds Graves autoantibodies, suggesting that antibodies to *Y. enterocolitica* may cross-react with thyroid tissue. There is reason to believe that an abnormality of T suppressor cell function permits the persistence of sensitized B-cell clones. Another theory holds that an antibody to anti-TSH antibody (anti-idiotypic antibody) mimics TSH and, thereby, stimulates the TSH receptor.

GENETIC FACTORS: Graves disease exhibits a higher concordance rate in monozygotic twins than in dizygotic ones. Moreover, patients with Graves disease and their relatives have a considerably higher incidence of other autoimmune diseases, including pernicious anemia and Hashimoto thyroiditis. Some asymptomatic, first-degree relatives of these patients also have an increased uptake of iodine-131. White patients with Graves disease display an increased frequency of HLA-B8 and HLA-DR3, whereas Chinese patients are more likely to manifest HLA-Bw46 and Japanese ones to exhibit HLA-Bw35.

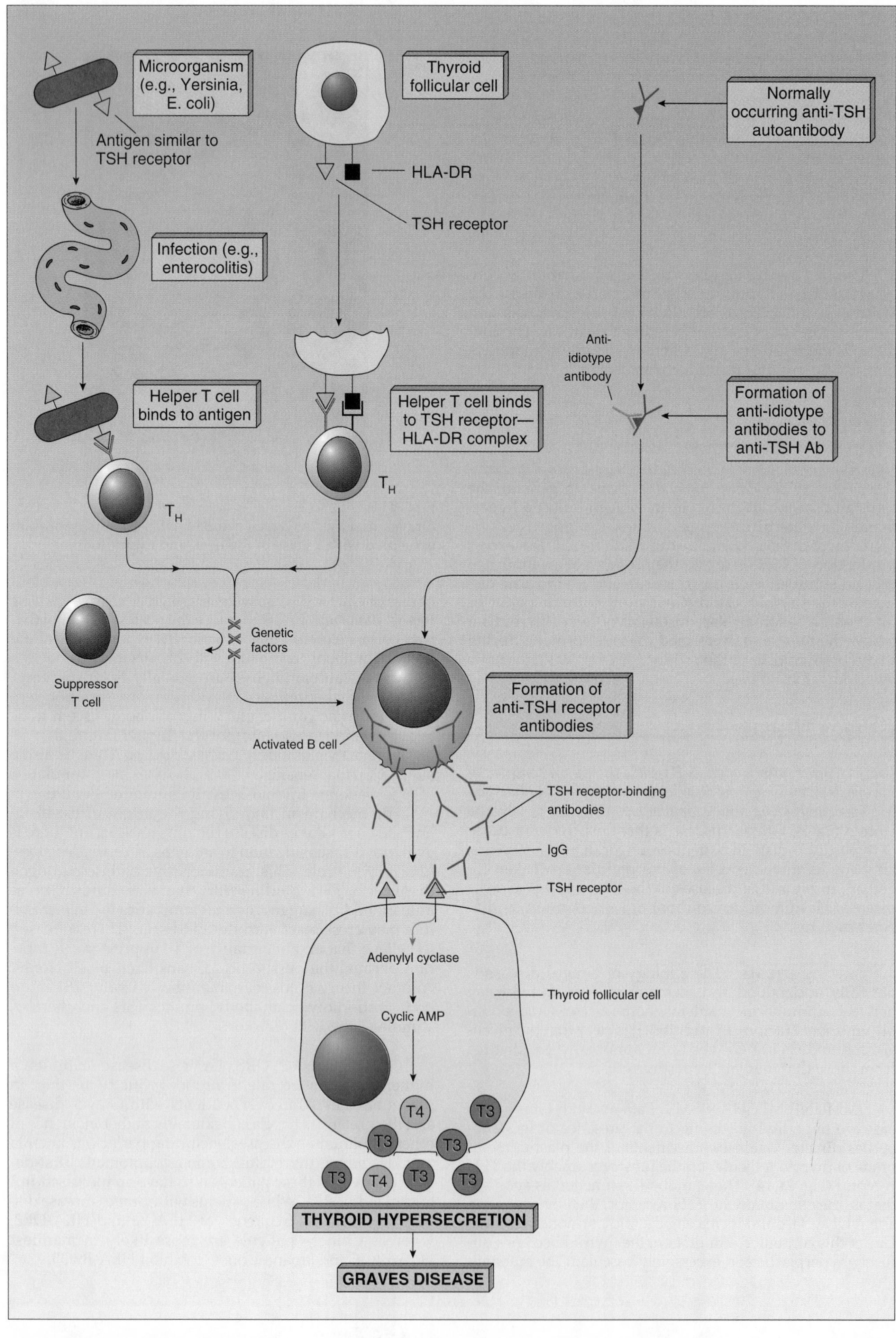

Microorganism (e.g., Yersinia, E. coli)
Antigen similar to TSH receptor
Thyroid follicular cell
HLA-DR
TSH receptor
Normally occurring anti-TSH autoantibody
Infection (e.g., enterocolitis)
Anti-idiotype antibody
Helper T cell binds to antigen
Helper T cell binds to TSH receptor—HLA-DR complex
Formation of anti-idiotype antibodies to anti-TSH Ab
T_H
T_H
Genetic factors
Suppressor T cell
Formation of anti-TSH receptor antibodies
Activated B cell
TSH receptor-binding antibodies
IgG
TSH receptor
Adenylyl cyclase
Thyroid follicular cell
Cyclic AMP
T4
T3
T3
T3
T3
T4
T3
T3
THYROID HYPERSECRETION
GRAVES DISEASE

SEX: Like other autoimmune diseases, Graves disease is far more common (7 to 10 times) in women than in men. Interestingly, the disorder tends to arise during periods of hormonal imbalance, including puberty, pregnancy, and menopause. Men with Graves disease are usually older, and although the degree of thyroid hyperfunction is often greater than in women, the symptoms tend to be less severe.

EMOTIONAL INFLUENCES: Quantitative data are lacking, but endocrinologists have long observed that the onset of Graves disease often follows a period of emotional stress, such as separation anxiety, death of a loved one, or near injury in an accident.

SMOKING: Smoking is associated with an increased risk of contracting Graves disease, and it increases the severity of the eye disease in cases that develop ophthalmopathy.

OPHTHALMOPATHY: Although exophthalmos (protrusion of the eyeballs) is a common complication of Graves disease, its occurrence and severity correlate poorly with the levels of thyroid hormone. It seems likely a combination of humoral and cell-mediated immune mechanisms are involved. T lymphocytes that are sensitized to antigens shared by thyroid follicular cells and orbital fibroblasts accumulate around the eye, where they secrete cytokines that activate fibroblasts. There is also evidence for the systemic or local production of antibodies that stimulate orbital fibroblasts to proliferate and produce collagen and glycosaminoglycans.

☐ **Pathology:** The thyroid in Graves disease is symmetrically enlarged, usually weighing 35 to 40 g. The cut surface is firm and dark red. The tan translucence of the normal cut surface of the thyroid, attributable to stored colloid, is notably absent. Microscopically, the thyroid is diffusely hyperplastic and highly vascular. The epithelial cells are tall and columnar and are often arranged as papillae that project into the lumen of the follicles. The colloid tends to be depleted and presents a scalloped or "moth-eaten" appearance where it abuts the epithelial cells (Fig. 21-15). Scattered lymphocytes and plasma cells infiltrate the interstitial tissue and may even aggregate to form germinal follicles.

Treatment of Graves disease with iodine, which is only rarely employed today, causes involutional changes in the thyroid. The vascularity is diminished, and dilated, colloid-containing follicles appear. These effects are often not uniform, and some hyperplastic areas persist. Therapy with antithyroid medication (e.g., methimazole or propylthiouracil) commonly results in increased thyroid hyperplasia and a complete absence of colloid.

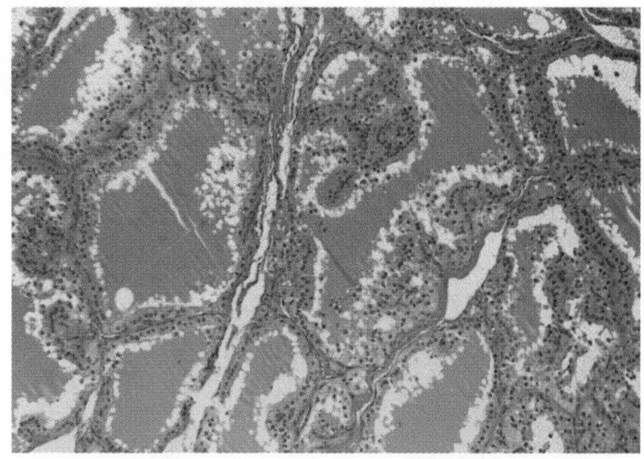

FIGURE *21-15*
Graves disease. The follicles are lined by hyperplastic, tall columnar cells. Colloid is pink and scalloped at the periphery adjacent to the follicular cells.

Exophthalmos is caused by enlargement of the extraocular muscles within the orbit. The muscles themselves are normal, but they are swollen by mucinous edema, the accumulation of fibroblasts, and infiltration by lymphocytes. The increased orbital contents cause forward displacement of the eye (*proptosis*).

☐ **Clinical Features:** Patients with Graves disease note the gradual onset of nonspecific symptoms, such as nervousness, emotional lability, tremor, weakness, and weight loss (Fig. 21-16). They are intolerant of heat, seek cooler environments, and tend to sweat profusely and may report palpitations . Excess thyroid hormone reduces systemic vascular resistance, enhances cardiac contractility, and increases the heart rate. In patients with preexisting heart disease, congestive heart failure may ensue. Women develop oligomenorrhea, which may progress to amenorrhea.

Physical examination reveals a symmetrically enlarged thyroid, often with an audible bruit and a palpable thrill. Protrusion of the eyeball and retraction of the eyelids expose the sclera above the superior margin of the limbus. The skin is warm and moist, and some patients exhibit Graves dermopathy, a peculiar pretibial edema caused by the accumulation of fluid and glycosaminoglycans. The diagnosis of Graves disease is documented by an increased uptake of radioactive iodine by the thyroid and elevated serum levels of T_4 and T_3.

The course of Graves disease is characterized by exacerbations and remissions. In untreated cases, hyperthy-

FIGURE *21-14*
Possible mechanisms of the autoimmune pathogenesis of Graves disease. The figure depicts three possible pathways by which B-cells are activated to produce anti-TSH receptor antibodies. These antibodies, in turn, stimulate thyroid follicular cells to secrete T_3 and T_4. The mechanisms of B-cell activation may be indirect (*left* and *middle*)—that is, they may involve activation of helper T cells in conjunction with genetic factors that inhibit suppressor T cells. The two pathways illustrated differ with respect to the mechanism of helper T-cell activation. In the pathway shown on the *right*, anti-idiotype antibodies formed against anti-TSH antibodies cross react with the TSH receptor.

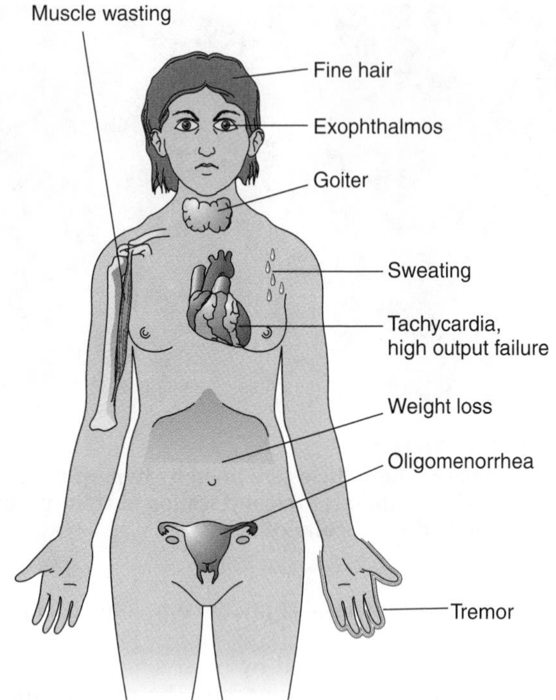

FIGURE *21-16*
The major clinical manifestations of Graves disease.

roidism may eventually be replaced by progressive thyroid failure and hypothyroidism, presumably as a result of chronic thyroiditis. Treatment of the disorder depends on many individual factors and includes the use of antithyroid medication, destruction of thyroid tissue with radioactive iodine, and adjunctive therapy with corticosteroids and adrenergic antagonists. Surgical ablation is not commonly performed today. Unfortunately, despite successful relief of hyperthyroidism, exophthalmos often persists and may even worsen.

Toxic Multinodular Goiter

Many patients with nontoxic multinodular goiter, usually older than the age of 50 years, eventually develop functional autonomy of the nodules and a toxic form of the disease. Like its precursor disease, toxic goiter is 10 times as frequent in women as in men.

☐ **Pathogenesis and Pathology:** The precise mechanisms by which a nontoxic multinodular goiter assumes functional autonomy are not clear, but two patterns are noted.

In some patients, the uptake of iodine is diffuse and not affected by the administration of thyroid hormone. Microscopic examination of the thyroid shows groups of small hyperplastic follicles mixed with other nodules of varying size that appear to be inactive.

The second pattern is characterized by focal accumulation of radiolabeled iodine in one or more nodules. Hyperfunction of these nodules suppresses the function of the remainder of the thyroid. As in the first type of toxic multinodular goiter, exogenous thyroid hormone produces no further suppression of iodine uptake, although the previously inactive areas will respond to TSH by sequestering iodine. On microscopic examination, the functional nodules are clearly demarcated from the inactive areas and consist of large hyperplastic follicles, thus resembling adenomas. Although there is little evidence to suggest that the functional nodules have neoplastic characteristics, the clinical presentation is similar to that of a normal thyroid with a single hyperfunctioning adenoma.

☐ **Clinical Features:** Patients with toxic multinodular goiter usually have less severe symptoms of hyperthyroidism than those with Graves disease and never develop exophthalmos. Since patients with a toxic goiter tend to be older, cardiac complications, including atrial fibrillation and congestive heart failure, may dominate the clinical presentation. Serum T_4 and T_3 levels are frequently only minimally elevated, and the uptake of radiolabeled iodine may be within the normal range or only slightly increased. Radiolabeled iodine administration after a course of antithyroid therapy is the most common therapy for toxic multinodular goiter.

Toxic Adenoma

Toxic adenoma is defined as a benign, solitary, hyperfunctioning, follicular neoplasm in an otherwise normal thyroid. It is an infrequent cause of hyperthyroidism. Such tumors display autonomous function, are not dependent on TSH, and are not suppressed by the administration of thyroid hormone. Hyperfunction of the toxic adenoma eventually suppresses the remainder of the thyroid, which then atrophies. Under these circumstances, a ^{131}I scintiscan shows a solitary focus of iodine uptake ("hot nodule") in a background of minimal uptake. Many, but not all, toxic adenomas exhibit a variety of activating somatic mutations of the TSH receptor gene, which result in constitutive upregulation of the cAMP cascade and less commonly the inositol phosphate-diacylglycerol system.

Toxic adenoma of the thyroid is most common in the fourth and fifth decades of life. Most patients do not suffer symptoms of hyperthyroidism until the adenoma has grown to a diameter of about 3 cm. On occasion, spontaneous necrosis and hemorrhage within the adenoma relieves the hyperthyroidism, after which the remainder of the gland resumes its normal function. In such cases, the adenoma appears as a "cold" nodule in a scintigram and may simulate thyroid cancer.

Since the normal thyroid tissue is suppressed, toxic adenoma is effectively treated with radiolabeled iodine. Alternatively, large nodules may be excised surgically, especially in young patients who are at risk for the development of thyroid cancer many years after radiolabeled iodine administration.

Hypersecretion of Thyroid-Stimulating Hormone

Pituitary adenomas that secrete TSH (thyrotrope adenomas) are rare causes of hyperthyroidism. Increased hypothalamic secretion of TSH has also been implicated in some cases of hyperthyroidism. Resistance on the part of thyrotropes in the pituitary to suppression by thyroid hormone has been documented on rare occasions. A thyroid stimulator distinct from TSH may also be produced by trophoblastic tumors, and hyperthyroidism may actually be the first manifestation of a molar pregnancy.

Iodine-Induced Hyperthyroidism

In areas of endemic iodine deficiency, treatment of a goiter with iodine infrequently leads to hypersecretion of thyroid hormone, a situation termed *jodbasedow*. It is now clear that jodbasedow occurs only in goiters that contain nodules capable of autonomous function independent of TSH stimulation. Even in areas in which iodine supplies are adequate, excessive iodine intake (e.g., iodide-containing expectorants in the treatment of pulmonary disease) may induce hyperthyroidism.

THYROIDITIS

Thyroiditis is a term that encompasses a heterogeneous group of inflammatory disorders of the thyroid gland, including those that are caused by autoimmune mechanisms and infectious agents.

Chronic Autoimmune Thyroiditis (Hashimoto Thyroiditis)

Hashimoto thyroiditis is an autoimmune disease characterized by the presence of circulating antibodies to thyroid antigens and features of cell-mediated immunity to thyroid tissue. The disease arises most commonly in the fourth and fifth decades, and women are six times more likely to be afflicted than men. Although autoimmune thyroiditis is rare in children, it accounts for half of the cases of adolescent goiter. In regions where supplies of iodine are adequate, Hashimoto thyroiditis is the most common cause of goitrous hypothyroidism.

□ **Pathogenesis:** It is generally agreed that immune mechanisms are responsible for the destruction of thyroid tissue in Hashimoto thyroiditis, although the details of the initiation of the autoimmune response and the progression of the disease remain to be fully elucidated. The autoimmune process is thought to arise from the activation of CD4 (helper) T lymphocytes that have been sensitized to thyroid antigens. Two hypotheses have been advanced to explain the origin of T-cell sensitization. One holds that cross reactivity with antigens of an infectious agent (molecular mimicry) accounts for the appearance of thyroid-specific CD4 cells, but the evidence for this theory is weak. Alternatively, it is thought that thyroid epithelial cells present their own antigens to helper T cells, thereby inducing the proliferation of specifically sensitized antithyroid T cells. This concept is supported by the observation that, in contrast to normal thyroid epithelial cells, those from patients with autoimmune thyroiditis express MHC class II antigens (HLA-DR, DP, DQ). These cell surface molecules are necessary for the presentation of antigens to CD4 cells.

Activated CD4 cells recruit both autoreactive B cells and cytotoxic (CD8) T cells. The principle mediator of the destruction of the thyroid gland is believed to be the CD8 cells. However, in some cases autoantibodies produced by B cells may also play a role. In Hashimoto thyroiditis, the major autoantibodies detected are directed against thyroid microsomal peroxidase (95%), thyroglobulin (60%), and the TSH receptor. Cytotoxic antibodies capable of fixing complement have been described in some patients, and antibody-dependent cell-mediated cytotoxicity (ADCC) may contribute to thyroid injury. In contrast to the agonist function of the anti-TSH receptor antibodies in Graves disease, the comparable antibodies in Hashimoto thyroiditis block the action of TSH. Such blocking antibodies have been described in 10% of patients with goitrous autoimmune thyroiditis and in 20% of those with end-stage atrophy of the gland.

A genetic predisposition to autoimmune thyroiditis is suggested by the familial nature of the disease. Half of all first-degree relatives of patients with this condition display thyroid antibodies, apparently transmitted as a dominant trait. Moreover, both Graves disease and chronic autoimmune thyroiditis have been described in these family members. A familial tendency for Hashimoto thyroiditis is further suggested by the higher prevalence of other autoimmune disorders in patients and their relatives, including multiple endocrine neoplasia syndrome type 2 (MEN 2), insulin-dependent diabetes, pernicious anemia, Addison disease, and myasthenia gravis. The high incidence of thyroid autoimmunity in persons with Down syndrome and familial Alzheimer disease has attracted attention to genes on chromosome 21. Interestingly, half of all patients with Turner syndrome, especially those with an X isochromosome, also suffer from Hashimoto thyroiditis.

Iodine intake is linked to the prevalence of Hashimoto thyroiditis, which is highest in regions with the greatest intake of iodine, for example, Japan and the United States. In iodine-deficient areas, iodine supplementation leads to significant increases in the prevalence of chronic inflammation of the thyroid and the presence of thyroid autoantibodies.

□ **Pathology:** On gross examination, the gland in cases of Hashimoto thyroiditis is diffusely enlarged, firm, and slightly lobular, weighing 60 to 200 g. The cut surface is pale tan and fleshy and exhibits a vaguely nodular pattern (Fig. 21-17). Microscopically, the thyroid displays (1) a conspicuous infiltrate of lymphocytes and plasma cells, (2) destruction and atrophy of the follicles, and (3) oxyphilic metaplasia of the follicular epithelial cells (*Hürthle* or *Askanazy cells*). The inflammatory infiltrates are focally arranged in lymphoid follicles, often with germinal centers. The Askanazy cells are filled with mitochondria and frequently display nuclear atypia, which may be mistaken for cancer. Interstitial fibrosis is present to a varying extent and in 10% of the cases is particularly conspicuous (fibrous variant). In some cases, the thyroid eventually undergoes atrophy, and the patient is left with a small, fibrotic gland infiltrated by lymphocytes.

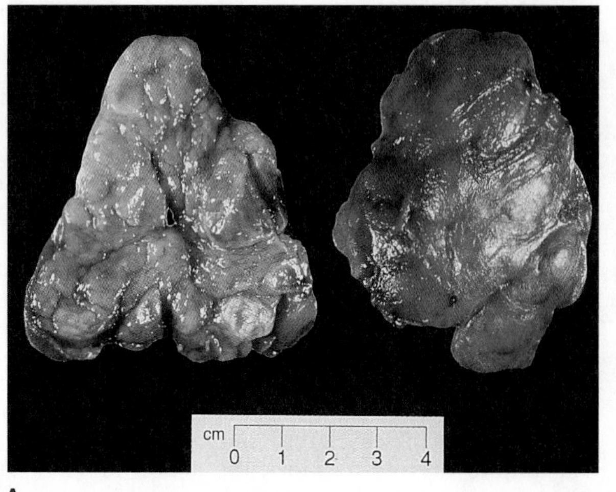

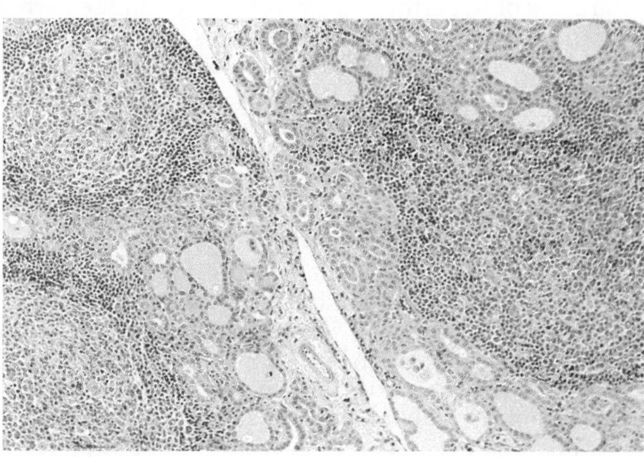

A B

FIGURE 21-17
Chronic autoimmune (Hashimoto) thyroiditis. The thyroid gland is symmetrically enlarged and coarsely nodular. (*A*) A coronal section of the right lobe shows irregular nodules and an intact capsule. (*B*) A microscopic section of the thyroid reveals a conspicuous chronic inflammatory infiltrate and many atrophic thyroid follicles. The inflammatory cells form prominent lymphoid follicles with germinal centers.

☐ **Clinical Features:** In most cases of Hashimoto thyroiditis, the patient notes the gradual onset of a goiter, although in a few cases the thyroid enlarges rapidly. The majority of these patients are initially euthyroid, but a few are hypothyroid when they present for medical attention. Eventually, one third to a half of all cases progress to an overt hypothyroid state, the risk being considerably greater among men then among women. On rare occasions, hyperthyroidism may develop (*hashitoxicosis*). The diagnosis of Hashimoto thyroiditis is now made by the detection of circulating antithyroid antibodies and an elevated TSH.

Many patients require no treatment for Hashimoto thyroiditis. Thyroid hormone is administered to alleviate hypothyroidism and to decrease the size of the gland. Surgery is reserved for cases that are unresponsive to suppressive hormone therapy or in which pressure symptoms are troublesome.

Subacute Thyroiditis (DeQuervain, Granulomatous, or Giant Cell Thyroiditis)

Subacute thyroiditis is an infrequent, self-limited viral infection of the thyroid characterized by granulomatous inflammation. The disease typically occurs after upper respiratory tract infections, including those caused by influenza virus, adenovirus, echovirus, and coxsackievirus. Mumps virus has also been incriminated in some cases. DeQuervain thyroiditis principally affects women between the ages of 30 and 50 years.

☐ **Pathology:** The thyroid gland is enlarged to 40 to 60 g, and the cut surface is firm and pale. Initially, microscopic examination reveals an acute inflammatory reaction, often with microabscesses. This is followed by the appearance of a patchy infiltrate of lymphocytes, plasma cells, and macrophages throughout the thyroid. Destruction of follicles allows the release of colloid, which elicits a conspicuous granulomatous reaction (Fig. 21-18). Numerous multinucleated giant cells of the foreign body type, often containing colloid, are present. Fibrosis of the thyroid may follow resolution of the inflammatory reaction, but the normal thyroid architecture is usually restored.

☐ **Clinical Features:** Patients with subacute thyroiditis typically notice pain in the anterior neck, sometimes accompanied by fever. The disorder is often mistaken for a pharyngitis, because of a preceding respiratory tract infection and the presence of hoarseness and dysphagia. On physical examination, the thyroid is moderately enlarged and exquisitely tender. Subacute thyroiditis generally resolves within a few months without any clinical sequelae.

The release of preformed thyroid hormone by destruction of the follicles often elevates serum T_4 and T_3 levels, occasionally to such an extent that transient clinical hyperthyroidism is produced. The consequent suppression of TSH leads to decreased uptake of radiolabeled iodine. This phase is followed by decreased serum T_4 and T_3 levels, but as subacute thyroiditis resolves a euthyroid state is restored.

Silent Thyroiditis

Silent thyroiditis, also termed *painless subacute thyroiditis* or *lymphocytic thyroiditis*, is a transient illness characterized by painless enlargement of the thyroid, self-limited

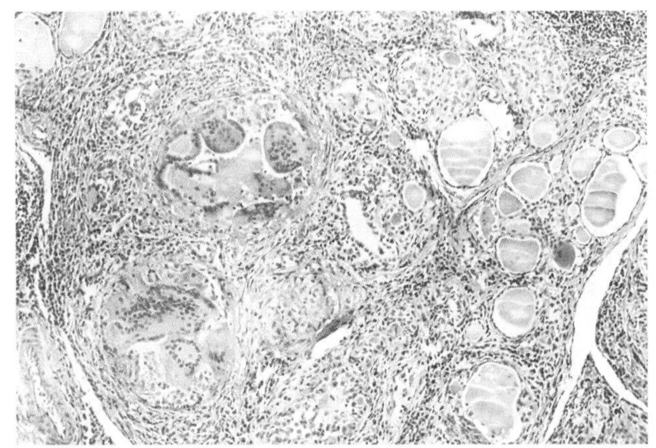

FIGURE *21-18*
Subacute thyroiditis. The release of colloid into the interstitial tissue has elicited a prominent granulomatous reaction, with numerous foreign body giant cells.

hyperthyroidism, and, on biopsy, destruction of thyroid parenchyma with a lymphocytic infiltrate. Thus, it clinically resembles subacute thyroiditis but pathologically is more similar to Hashimoto thyroiditis. Importantly, silent thyroiditis is distinguished from the latter by the lack of antithyroid antibodies or other evidence of autoimmune thyroiditis. However, an association with HLA-DR3 has been reported. As in subacute thyroiditis, the hyperthyroid state is a reflection of the release of preformed thyroid hormone from the injured gland.

Silent thyroiditis predominantly affects women, often in the postpartum period. Hyperthyroidism usually persists for 2 to 4 months. Treatment is symptomatic, and most patients become euthyroid.

Riedel Thyroiditis

Riedel thyroiditis is a rare disease characterized by dense fibrosis of the thyroid. The term thyroiditis is something of a misnomer since the disease also involves extrathyroidal soft tissues of the neck and is often associated with progressive fibrosis in other locations, including the retroperitoneum, mediastinum, and orbit. Riedel thyroiditis is primarily a disease of middle age, with a female-to-male ratio of 3:1. The etiology is unknown, but it does not appear to be related to other forms of thyroiditis.

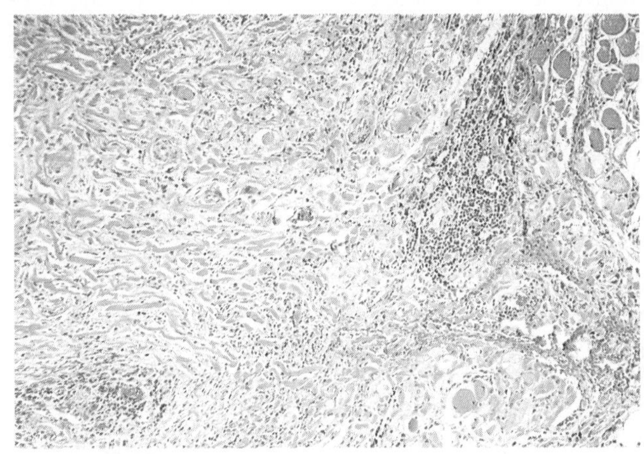

FIGURE *21-19*
Riedel thyroiditis. The thyroid parenchyma is largely replaced by dense, hyalinized fibrous tissue and a chronic inflammatory infiltrate.

☐ **Pathology:** On gross examination, part or all of the thyroid is stony hard and is described as "woody." In most instances, the process is asymmetric and often affects only one lobe. Characteristically, fibrosis extends beyond the borders of the gland, and the surgeon may have extreme difficulty in identifying a tissue plane. Microscopic examination reveals dense, hyalinized fibrous tissue and a chronic inflammatory infiltrate replacing the parenchyma in the involved portions of the thyroid (Fig. 21-19). The follicles are normal in the unaffected portions of the gland. Fibrous tissue also surrounds and infiltrates other tissues, including skeletal muscle, nerves, fat, and blood vessels. In some cases, the parathyroids are also embedded in the fibrosis.

☐ **Clinical Features:** Patients with Riedel thyroiditis notice the gradual onset of a painless goiter. Subsequently, they may suffer from the consequences of compression of the trachea (stridor), esophagus (dysphagia), and recurrent laryngeal nerves (hoarseness). In the unusual cases that involve the entire thyroid, hypothyroidism ensues. Treatment is primarily surgical to relieve the compression of the local organs.

FOLLICULAR ADENOMA OF THE THYROID

Follicular adenoma refers to a benign neoplasm that exhibits follicular differentiation. It is the most common tumor of the thyroid and typically presents in euthyroid persons as a solitary "cold" nodule, that is, a tumor that does not take up radiolabeled iodine. Follicular adenoma is an encapsulated neoplasm in which the cells are either arranged in follicles resembling normal thyroid tissue or mimic stages in the embryonic development of the gland. It deserves emphasis that up to 90% of palpable, solitary follicular lesions are actually the dominant nodule in a multinodular goiter and that follicular adenomas are correspondingly infrequent. Follicular adenoma is most common in the fourth and fifth decades, with a female-to-male ratio of 7:1. The clonal origin of follicular adenomas has been established.

☐ **Pathology:** On gross examination, follicular adenoma is a solitary, circumscribed nodule, 1 to 3 cm in diameter, which protrudes from the surface of the thyroid. The cut surface of the tumor is soft and paler than the surrounding parenchyma. Hemorrhage, fibrosis, and cystic change are common. Histologically, a number of distinctive patterns are observed (Fig. 21-20). Although these variants are of no particular clinical significance, their recognition may be important in separating them from thyroid cancers.

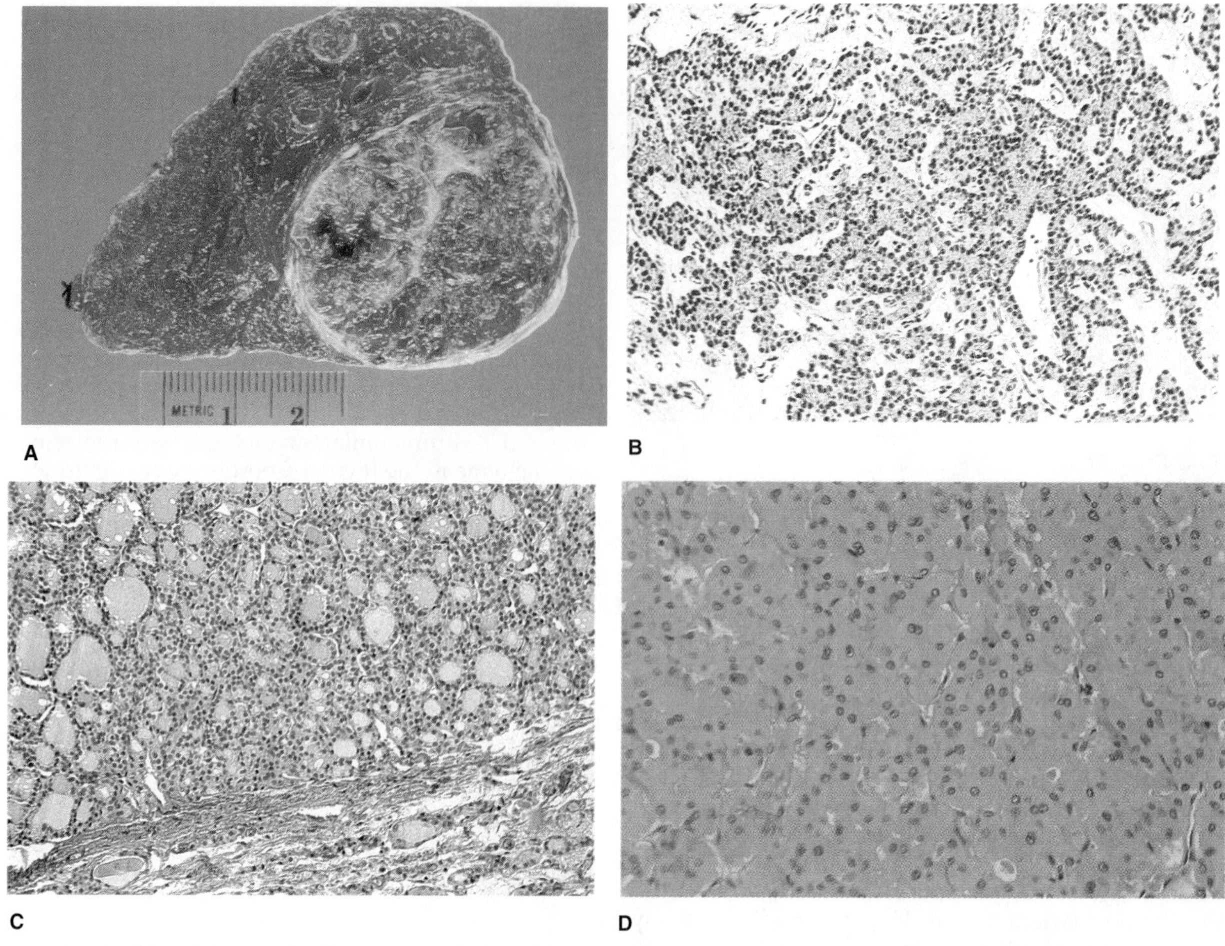

FIGURE 21-20
Follicular adenoma. (*A*) Colloid adenoma. The cut surface of an encapsulated mass reveals hemorrhage, fibrosis, and cystic change. (*B*) Embryonal adenoma. The tumor features a trabecular pattern with poorly formed follicles that contain little if any colloid. (*C*) Fetal adenoma. A regular pattern of small follicles is noted. (*D*) Hurthle cell adenoma. The tumor is composed of cells with small, regular nuclei and abundant eosinophilic cytoplasm.

- **Embryonal adenoma** is distinguished by a trabecular pattern in which poorly formed follicles contain little or no colloid.
- **Fetal adenoma** features cells that are similar to those of embryonal adenoma but tend to be arranged in microfollicles containing little colloid.
- **Simple adenoma** exhibits mature follicles with a normal amount of colloid.
- **Colloid adenoma** is similar to simple adenoma except that the follicles are larger and contain more abundant colloid.
- **Hürthle cell adenoma** is a solid tumor characterized by oxyphil cells, small follicles, and scanty colloid.
- **Atypical adenoma** is a follicular tumor that displays mitoses, excessive cellularity, nuclear atypism, or equivocal capsular invasion but in which a diagnosis of carcinoma cannot be established with certainty.

THYROID CANCER

The topic of thyroid neoplasia has aroused the interest of clinicians and pathologists out of proportion to the incidence of thyroid cancer. This attention can be attributed to the frequency of nontoxic thyroid nodules and the difficulty of distinguishing clinically between non-neoplastic lesions, benign tumors, and thyroid cancer. Whereas thyroid nodules are found in as many as 1% to 10% of the population, malignant tumors of the thyroid account for about 1% of all cancers and only 0.4% of cancer-related deaths. It is therefore clear that only a very small proportion of clinically evident thyroid nodules are malignant. Nevertheless, thyroid cancer is the most common malignant endocrine tumor.

The large majority of cases of carcinoma of the thyroid occur between the third and seventh decades. The prognosis is related to the morphological features of the tumor, ranging from a virtually benign clinical course to a rapidly fatal disease. The latter outcome is fortunately uncommon.

Before the advent of fine-needle aspiration, the definitive diagnosis of a thyroid nodule required open biopsy, often with the resection of a significant portion of the gland and consequent morbidity. Today, fine-needle biopsy of thyroid nodules is a safe and rapid procedure that provides a diagnosis in the majority of cases. As a result, the incidence of cancer in resected thyroid nodules has increased from 3% to over 70%.

Papillary Thyroid Carcinoma

Papillary carcinoma is the most common thyroid cancer, comprising more than three fourths of all cases in the United States. The tumor is most frequent between the ages of 20 and 50 years, with a female-to-male ratio of 3:1. However, papillary carcinoma may arise at any age, even in children. The reported incidence of this tumor has varied from 35% to 90% of all thyroid cancers because some pathologists consider the most mature variant to be a papillary adenoma and others classify papillary tumors with follicular elements as follicular carcinoma. **In this context, we consider all neoplasms with papillary elements to be papillary cancers.** Such a classification is of more than academic interest, since the biological behavior of papillary cancers is different from that of other malignant tumors of the thyroid.

☐ **Pathogenesis:** Although the etiology of papillary carcinoma of the thyroid remains to be established, a number of associations have been identified.

- **Iodine excess:** Papillary thyroid cancer has been produced in animals by administering excess iodine. In endemic goiter regions, the addition of iodine to the diet has increased the proportion of papillary carcinoma compared with follicular cancer.
- **Radiation:** External radiation to the neck of children and adults increases the incidence of later papillary carcinoma of the thyroid. Survivors of the atomic bomb explosions in Japan suffered more papillary cancers than would otherwise be expected. A substantially increased incidence of papillary thyroid carcinoma has been experienced by children living in contaminated areas surrounding Chernobyl, the site in Ukraine of a nuclear reactor catastrophe in 1986. On the other hand, treatment with radiolabeled iodine has not been shown to increase the risk of this tumor.
- **Genetic factors:** A concordance for papillary carcinoma of the thyroid has been described in monozygotic twins, and an association between this tumor and HLA-DR7 has been reported. Somatic rearrangements of the RET protooncogene on chromosome 10 (10q11.2) are common in papillary thyroid cancers, and 60% of such tumors in children exposed to radiation from the Chernobyl accident displayed this mutation. These rearrangements cause the fusion of the tyrosine kinase domain of RET to various other genes, creating the RET/PTC (papillary thyroid cancer) fusion oncogenes. Interestingly, transgenic mice that express the RET/PTC1 chimeric gene develop papillary carcinomas of the thyroid. Illegitimate recombination of the NTRK1 gene on chromosome 1, which encodes the high affinity nerve growth factor receptor (NGFR), with another gene on the same chromosome (TPM3) has also been described in papillary thyroid cancers. The fusion product is constitutively activated by phosphorylation of a tyrosine residue.

☐ **Pathology:** Papillary carcinomas of the thyroid vary from microscopic lesions to tumors larger than the normal gland. Serial sections of ostensibly normal thyroids obtained at autopsy have revealed a high proportion of papillary cancers that measure less than 1 mm across, but lymph node metastases in such cases are distinctly uncommon. On gross examination, most papillary carcinomas are pale and firm or hard and gritty lesions, with less than 10% being truly encapsulated (Fig. 21-21A). A few tumors display cystic changes.

Microscopic examination reveals branching papillae that are composed of a central fibrovascular core and a single or stratified lining of cuboidal to columnar cells (see Fig. 21-21B). In most instances, irregularly shaped or tubular neoplastic follicles are present within the tumor, but the proportions of the papillary and follicular elements are highly variable. Nuclear atypism is an important diagnostic feature and includes clear (*ground-glass* or *Orphan Annie*) nuclei, eosinophilic pseudoinclusions (which represent invaginations of the cytoplasm into the nucleus), and nuclear grooves. Many papillary cancers show dense fibrosis, and calcospherites (*psammoma bodies*) are present in half the cases. The latter feature is virtually diagnostic of papillary carcinoma, being rare in other conditions. The stroma may be infiltrated by lymphocytes and Langerhans cells. In over three fourths of the cases of papillary cancer, careful sectioning of the resected thyroid reveals multiple microscopic foci of tumor, but it is not clear whether this represents a multifocal origin of the tumor or lymphatic spread from a solitary primary. Vascular invasion is distinctly uncommon.

Papillary thyroid carcinoma typically invades lymphatics and spreads to the regional cervical lymph nodes. The lymph node metastases vary from microscopic foci in otherwise normal lymph nodes to large masses that dwarf the primary lesion. Direct extension of papillary carcinoma into the soft tissues of the neck occurs in one fourth of the cases. Although hematogenous metastases are less common than in other varieties of thyroid cancer, they occasionally occur, most commonly to the lungs.

☐ **Clinical Features:** Papillary carcinoma of the thyroid presents as (1) a painless, palpable nodule in an otherwise normal gland; (2) a nodule with enlarged cervical lymph nodes; or (3) cervical lymphadenopathy in the absence of a palpable thyroid nodule. Tumors larger than 0.5 cm can be detected as cold areas in a thyroid scintiscan.

In general, the prognosis of papillary carcinoma is excellent, and life expectancy for these patients differs little from that of the general population. The prognosis in individual cases is influenced by age, sex, and the size and differentiation of the tumor. The prognosis is more serious in patients older than 50 years of age, whereas in children, the outlook is good even when lung metastases are detected. Papillary cancer tends to be more aggressive in men than in women.

As a rule, the larger the size of the primary tumor, the more aggressive it is, and direct extension into the adjacent soft tissues points to a poorer prognosis. The proportion of papillary and follicular elements contributes little to the prognosis, but less-differentiated papillary carcino-

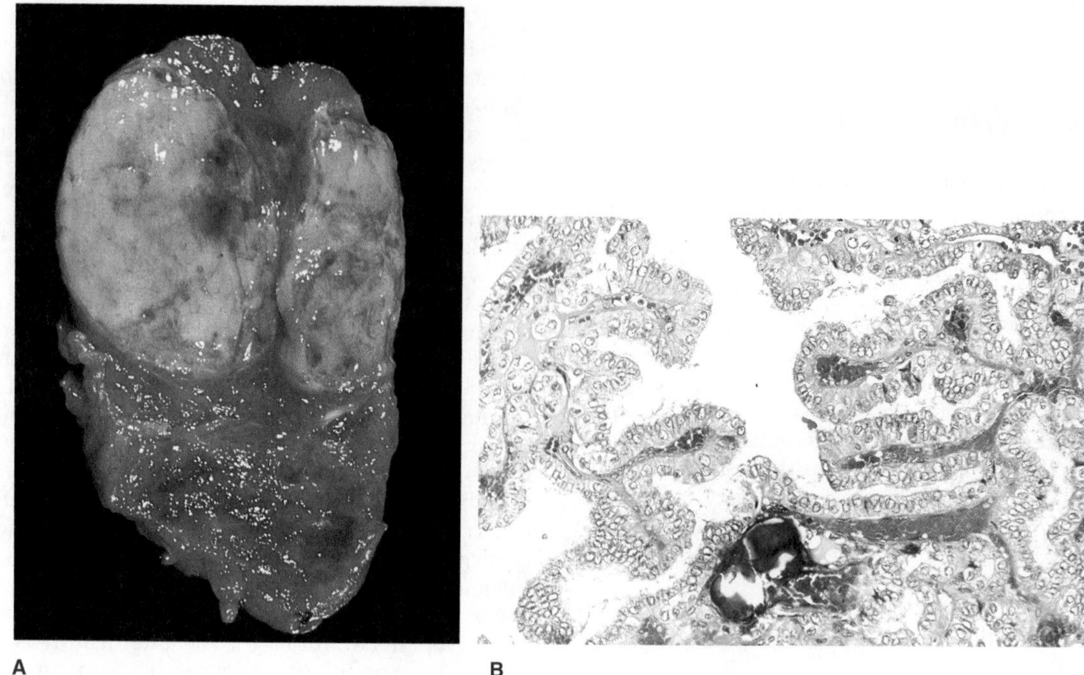

FIGURE 21-21
Papillary carcinoma of the thyroid. (*A*) The cut surface of a surgically resected thyroid displays a circumscribed pale tan mass with foci of cystic change. (*B*) Branching papillae are lined by neoplastic columnar epithelium containing clear nuclei. A calcospherite, or psammoma body, is evident.

mas tend to be more aggressive. The presence of metastases to cervical nodes at the time or surgery does not change the prognosis, and less than 10% of these patients succumb to the tumor. In fatal cases of papillary cancer, death is caused principally by metastases to the lungs or brain or by obstruction of the trachea or esophagus.

Follicular Thyroid Carcinoma

Follicular carcinoma of the thyroid is defined as a malignant neoplasm that is purely follicular and does not contain any papillary or other elements. This tumor represents about 15% of all thyroid cancers. Most patients are older than 40 years of age, and the female-to-male ratio is 3:1. The risk factors for follicular carcinoma are not as clear as those for papillary cancer, because many studies have classified tumors with both features as follicular. The incidence of follicular carcinoma seems to be increased in endemic goiter areas among persons who do not receive iodine supplements. The effect of radiation with respect to this tumor is controversial.

☐ **Pathology:** Follicular carcinomas are subdivided into minimally invasive and widely invasive variants.

Minimally invasive follicular carcinoma is seen grossly as a well-defined, encapsulated tumor, which on cut section is soft and pale tan to pink and bulges from the confines of its capsule. Microscopically, most lesions resemble follicular adenoma, although they tend more to a microfollicular or trabecular pattern. Occasionally, hemorrhagic necrosis is present in the center of the tumor. Mitoses are commonly encountered, a feature that distinguishes follicular cancer from a benign adenoma. The principal distinction from adenoma is in the interface of the capsule and the normal parenchyma. Minimally invasive cancer is diagnosed when the tumor extends into but not entirely through the capsule (Fig. 21-22).

Invasive follicular carcinoma usually presents few diagnostic problems, since it extends through the capsule or shows vascular invasion (see Fig. 21-22), often within or adjacent to the capsule. Interestingly, intravascular masses of follicular carcinoma are often covered by endothelium in a manner similar to that of an ordinary thrombus. The tumor may also extend into the surrounding soft tissues.

Follicular carcinoma differs from papillary cancer in being solitary and rarely occult. Metastases are blood borne rather than lymphatic and are directed principally to the bones of the shoulder and pelvic girdles, sternum, and skull. Whereas metastases in invasive follicular carcinoma are common, less than 5% of the minimally invasive tumors metastasize. The metastases may be so well differentiated that they are hardly recognizable as neoplastic tissue and at one time were referred to as *benign metastasizing struma.*

☐ **Clinical Features:** Most follicular cancers of the thyroid are detected clinically as a palpable nodule or as an enlarged thyroid, but in some cases the presenting sign is a pathological fracture through a bony metastasis or a

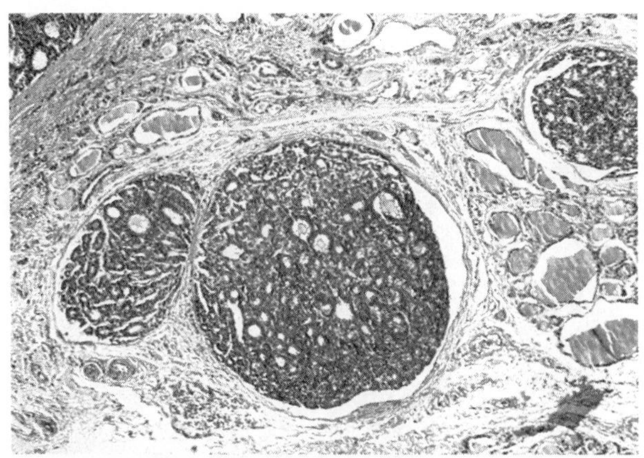

FIGURE *21-22*
Follicular carcinoma of the thyroid. A microfollicular tumor has invaded veins in the thyroid parenchyma.

pulmonary lesion. Both the primary tumor and the metastases have an affinity for radiolabeled iodine, although the thyroid scintiscan may indicate a cold nodule because the normal thyroid accumulates iodine more efficiently. However, the affinity for ^{131}I may be used therapeutically. Minimally invasive follicular tumors have a 10-year survival rate of 85%, compared with a rate of only 45% for the widely invasive form.

Medullary Thyroid Carcinoma

Medullary thyroid carcinoma (MTC) is a tumor derived from the parafollicular or C cells of the thyroid, which are distinguished by their secretion of the calcium-lowering hormone calcitonin. This tumor represents no more than 5% of all thyroid cancers, although the proportion in referral centers is higher. The disease occurs in sporadic and familial forms, the latter accounting for 20% of the cases. Patients with the familial form of medullary carcinoma are often afflicted with MEN type 2, which includes pheochromocytoma of the adrenal medulla and parathyroid hyperplasia or adenoma.

Somatic mutations in the RET protooncogene have been detected in more than half of the cases of sporadic MTC. Most of these occur at codon 918 (ATG to ACG) in the tyrosine kinase domain of the protein and indicate a poorer prognosis than in tumors without a RET mutation. The RET gene is discussed more fully in the section on MEN syndromes (see later).

The mean age of patients with medullary carcinoma is 50 years, but familial cases appear earlier (mean age, 20 years). There is a slight female predominance (1.5:1); in familial cases, the inheritance is autosomal dominant and the sex distribution is equal.

□ **Pathology:** On gross examination, MTC tends to arise in the superior portion of the thyroid, the regions that are richest in C cells. In the setting of MEN type 2, the tumors are often multicentric and bilateral. Although MTCs are not encapsulated, they are usually circumscribed. The cut surface is firm and grayish white. The histological appearance is highly variable. Characteristically, the tumor is solid and composed of polygonal, granular cells, which are separated by a distinctly vascular stroma (Fig. 21-23). **A conspicuous feature is the presence of stromal amyloid, representing the deposition of procalcitonin.** The nests of tumor cells are embedded in a hyalinized collagenous framework. Focal calcification is often present and may be sufficiently extensive to be detected radiologically.

The histological variability of MTC is evidenced by different architectural patterns, including trabecular, tubular, follicular, carcinoid-like, or pseudopapillary arrangements. The neoplastic cells may exhibit peripheral nuclei (plasmacytoid pattern) or may be spindle shaped, anaplastic, or oxyphilic. In addition, the stroma may feature hemorrhage or bone formation and amyloid may be absent.

By electron microscopy, the neoplastic C cells show dense-core secretory granules, which stain immunohistochemically for a variety of endocrine markers, including calcitonin, synaptophysin, chromogranin, and neuron-specific enolase. Almost all of these tumors are positive for carcinoembryonic antigen (CEA). Many cases are also positive for corticotropin, serotonin, substance P, glucagon, insulin, and human chorionic gonadotropin (hCG).

Medullary thyroid carcinoma extends by direct invasion into soft tissues and metastasizes to the regional lymph nodes and to lung, liver, and bone. In some instances, metastatic disease is responsible for the initial presentation. The metastatic deposits resemble the primary tumor and also tend to contain amyloid.

The precursor lesion of the familial variety of medullary carcinoma is C cell hyperplasia. Thus, patients with MEN types 2A and 2B (see section on adrenal medulla) who are at risk for the development of medullary carcinoma of the thyroid are monitored by periodic measurements of serum calcitonin, CEA, and sometimes chromogranin. When levels of these substances are elevated, the patient is subjected to total thyroidectomy.

□ **Clinical Features:** Patients with medullary carcinoma often suffer a number of symptoms related to endocrine secretion, including carcinoid syndrome (serotonin) and Cushing syndrome (corticotropin). Watery diarrhea in one third of the patients is caused by the secretion of vasoactive intestinal peptide, prostaglandins, and several kinins. In cases of familial medullary carcinoma, patients may exhibit hyperparathyroidism and episodic hypertension and other symptoms attributable to the secretion of catecholamines by pheochromocytoma.

The tumor usually presents as a firm thyroid nodule or as cervical lymphadenopathy. By scintiscan, a cold nodule is characteristic. The treatment is total thyroidectomy, but local recurrences follow in one third of the patients. The 5-year survival rate is 75%.

Anaplastic (Undifferentiated) Thyroid Carcinoma

Anaplastic carcinoma is a highly aggressive, undifferentiated thyroid cancer, which is usually rapidly fatal. This type of thyroid cancer principally afflicts women (female:male ratio

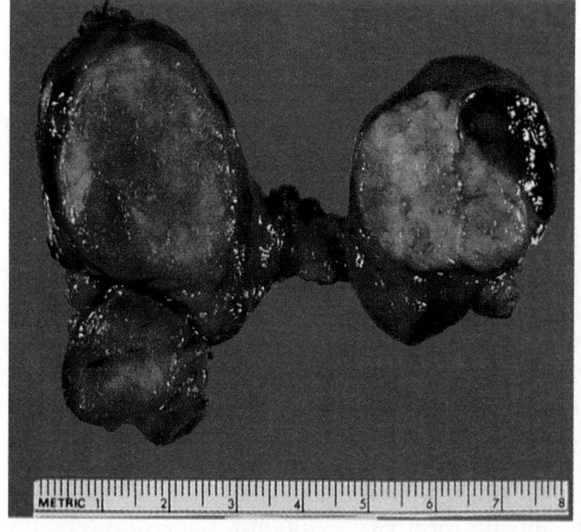

A

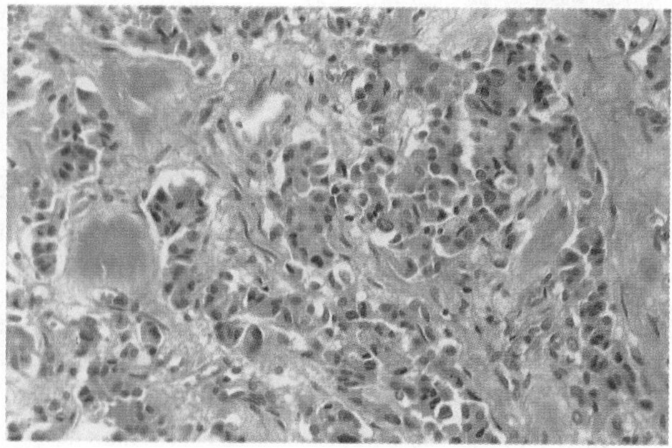

B

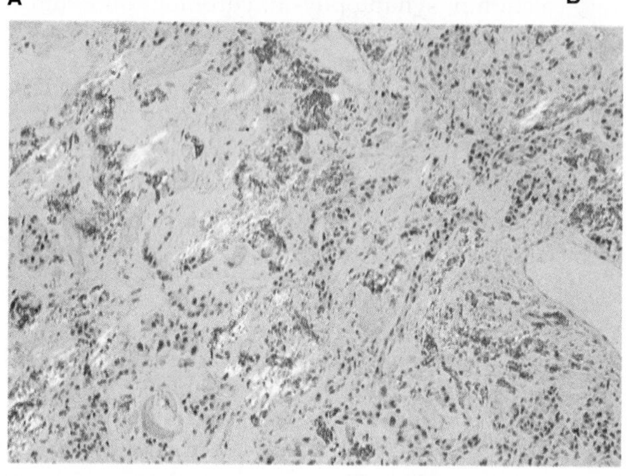

C

FIGURE 21-23
Medullary thyroid carcinoma. (*A*) Coronal section of a total thyroid resection shows bilateral involvement by a firm, pale tumor. (*B*) The tumor features nests of polygonal cells embedded in a collagenous framework. The connective tissue septa contain eosinophilic amyloid. (*C*) A section stained with Congo red and viewed under polarized light demonstrates the pale green birefringence of amyloid.

of 4:1) over the age of 60 years. The tumor comprises 10% of thyroid cancers and is more common in endemic goiter areas. In fact, overall at least half of the patients have a history of long-standing goiter. In addition, many cases of anaplastic carcinoma occur in patients with a history of a lower-grade thyroid cancer. Thus, it seems likely that anaplastic thyroid carcinoma often represents the transformation of a benign or low-grade thyroid neoplasm into a poorly differentiated and highly aggressive cancer. There is evidence that the risk of such an event is enhanced by external radiation.

☐ Pathology: Anaplastic carcinoma of the thyroid presents as large masses in the gland, which are poorly circumscribed and frequently extend into the soft tissues of the neck. The cut surface is hard and grayish white. The histological appearance is highly variable. The most common pattern is a sarcoma-like proliferation of bizarre spindle and giant cells, with polyploid nuclei, many mitoses, necrosis, and stromal fibrosis (Fig. 21-24). Other specimens reveal distinct epithelial differentiation. The tumor tends to invade veins and arteries, often occluding the vessels and producing foci of infarction within the tumor.

☐ Clinical Features: These highly malignant tumors compress and destroy local structures. Dysphagia and dyspnea are caused by tracheal compression or invasion. The prognosis is dismal and widespread metastases are frequent. Less than 10% of patients survive for 5 years.

Lymphoma of the Thyroid

Lymphoma originating in the thyroid is distinctly uncommon, accounting for 2% of all thyroid cancers. The large majority (95%) are B-cell tumors. Most if not all cases arise in the setting of chronic thyroiditis, and in regions where this disorder is frequent, up to 10% of malignant tumors of the thyroid are lymphomas. Similar to chronic thyroiditis, thyroid lymphoma is more common in women than in men (4:1), but the mean age at presentation (seventh decade) is older.

Thyroid lymphomas present as large, soft, tannish masses in the thyroid, usually extending beyond the confines of the gland. Microscopically, they present the spectrum of lymphomas seen at other sites, the most common subtype being the diffuse large cell pattern. A few tumors exhibit plasmacytoid differentiation, whereas others resemble immunoblastic lymphoma.

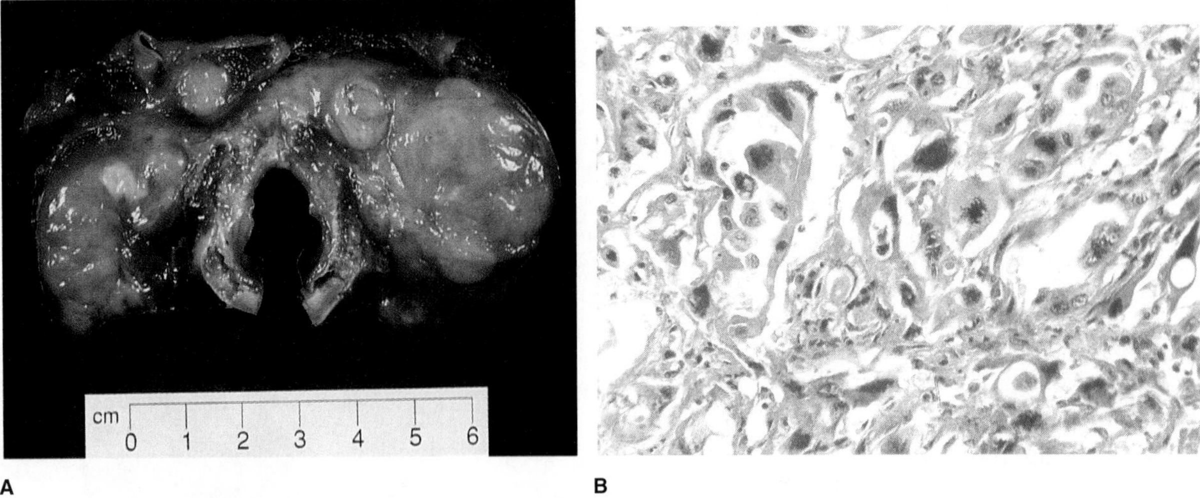

FIGURE *21-24*
Anaplastic carcinoma of the thyroid. (*A*) The tumor in transverse section partially surrounds the trachea and extends into the adjacent soft tissue. (*B*) The tumor is composed of bizarre spindle and giant cells with polyploid nuclei and numerous mitoses.

The prognosis of thyroid lymphoma depends on the stage at the time of diagnosis. If restricted to the thyroid gland, the prognosis is excellent, and three fourths of the patients now survive for 10 years. The outlook for patients with disseminated disease is poorer and is similar to that of other lymphomas.

Parathyroid Glands

ANATOMY AND PHYSIOLOGY

The parathyroid glands are derivatives of branchial clefts III and IV. Most persons have 4 glands, but the number varies from 1 to 12. Normally, they are found on the posterior thyroid surface, the lower two adjacent to the inferior thyroid arteries and the upper two adherent to the upper posterolateral third of each thyroid lobe. A parathyroid gland may be entirely intrathyroid or intrathymic. On occasion, a gland is located between the trachea and esophagus, or in other ectopic locations. Hence, surgical identification and removal of a functioning parathyroid tumor is at times difficult.

The parathyroid glands are the size and color of a grain of saffron-cooked rice. The combined weight of all the glands is about 130 mg. The weight of an individual gland varies considerably, but anything in excess of 50 mg probably represents enlargement. Microscopically, about three fourths of the parathyroids are composed of chief cells and oxyphil cells, with the remainder being adipose tissue scattered throughout the parenchyma. The parenchymal cells are variants of the same functional unit.

Chief cells are responsible for the secretion of parathyroid hormone (PTH). They are polyhedral cells that are characterized by a pale, eosinophilic to amphophilic cytoplasm, which contains glycogen and fat droplets. Electron microscopy reveals membrane-bound secretory granules in the cytoplasm.

Clear cells are chief cells whose cytoplasm is packed with glycogen.

Oxyphil cells, which appear after puberty, are larger than chief cells and display a deeply eosinophilic cytoplasm, owing to the presence of numerous mitochondria. They do not contain secretory granules and do not secrete PTH.

The parathyroids are responsive to the level of ionized calcium and magnesium in the blood. In turn, PTH controls the level of plasma calcium. Magnesium, a cation closely related to calcium, acts as a brake on PTH secretion.

HYPOPARATHYROIDISM

Hypoparathyroidism results from decreased secretion of PTH or end organ insensitivity to the hormone (pseudohypoparathyroidism).

Decreased Secretion of Parathyroid Hormone

The most common cause of hypoparathyroidism is surgical resection of the parathyroids as a complication of thyroidectomy. In patients undergoing surgery for primary hyperparathyroidism, 1% develop irreversible hypoparathyroidism. The symptoms of hypoparathyroidism relate to hypocalcemia. Increased neuromuscular excitability is reflected in symptoms that range from mild tingling in the hands and feet to severe muscle cramps, laryngeal stridor, and convulsions. Neuropsychiatric manifestations include depression, paranoia, and psychoses. An elevated cerebrospinal fluid pressure and papilledema may mimic a brain tumor. Patients with all forms of hypoparathyroidism are successfully treated with vitamin D and calcium supplementation. ***Idiopathic hypoparathyroidism*** is a heterogeneous group of rare disorders, sporadic and familial, that have in common a deficient secretion of PTH.

Familial isolated hypoparathyroidism is a rare disorder characterized by deficient secretion of PTH, which may be autosomal dominant, autosomal recessive, or X-linked. In the ***autosomal dominant*** form, activating mutations in the gene for the Ca^{2+}-sensing receptor (PCAR1) on chromosome 3q13 have been identified. The mutant receptor is hyperreactive to the level of extracellular Ca^{2+} and, therefore, interprets hypocalcemia as the normal state. In other words, the set point of the parathyroid glands for Ca^{2+} is decreased, and PTH secretion is correspondingly reduced. Interestingly, inactivating mutations of PCAR1 result in an insensitivity to extracellular Ca^{2+}, in which case the parathyroid fails to sense a normal Ca^{2+} level and severe hyperparathyroidism ensues. **The autosomal recessive** variant of familial isolated hypoparathyroid is the result of inactivating mutations in the PTH gene itself, which determine the deficiency in PTH activity.

Familial hypoparathyroidism may be part of a polyglandular syndrome that also includes adrenal insufficiency and mucocutaneous candidiasis. Antibodies specific for parathyroid antigens have been reported in a number of cases, and antiendothelial cell antibodies have also been recorded. These data suggest an autoimmune basis for the hypoparathyroidism associated with the polyglandular syndrome. This conclusion is bolstered by an association with other conditions presumed to have an autoimmune etiology, including insulin-dependent diabetes mellitus, pernicious anemia, primary hypothyroidism, and primary hypogonadism. The only pathological changes are lymphocytic infiltration, parathyroid atrophy, and replacement of parenchymal cells by fat.

Suppression of PTH secretion occurs in hypercalcemic states that do not involve the parathyroids. However, even in the face of continued hypercalcemia (e.g., renal disease), normal parathyroid function is restored within a week of return to normal calcium levels. Hypomagnesemia also impairs PTH release, as opposed to PTH synthesis.

Rare causes of inadequate PTH secretion include metastases to the parathyroids, iron storage disease, Wilson disease, and DiGeorge syndrome (parathyroid agenesis due to defective formation of branchial pouches).

Pseudohypoparathyroidism

Pseudohypoparathyroidism designates a group of hereditary conditions in which hypocalcemia is caused by target organ insensitivity to PTH. Most patients do not exhibit the normal increase in urinary excretion of cAMP on intravenous administration of PTH. The defect in these patients has been traced to mutations on the long arm of chromosome 20 that result in a decreased activity of G_s (the alpha subunit of the G protein that couples hormone receptors to the stimulation of adenylyl cyclase) in the renal tubular epithelium. Consequently, the production of cAMP in response to PTH is impaired, and inadequate resorption of calcium from the glomerular filtrate ensues. Patients with pseudohypoparathyroidism are also often resistant to the other hormones that are coupled to cAMP, including TSH, glucagon, and the gonadotropins FSH and LH. These patients demonstrate a characteristic phenotype (*Albright hereditary osteodystrophy*), including short stature, obesity, mental retardation, subcutaneous calcification, and a number of congenital anomalies of bone, particularly abnormally short metacarpals and metatarsals (Fig. 21-25).

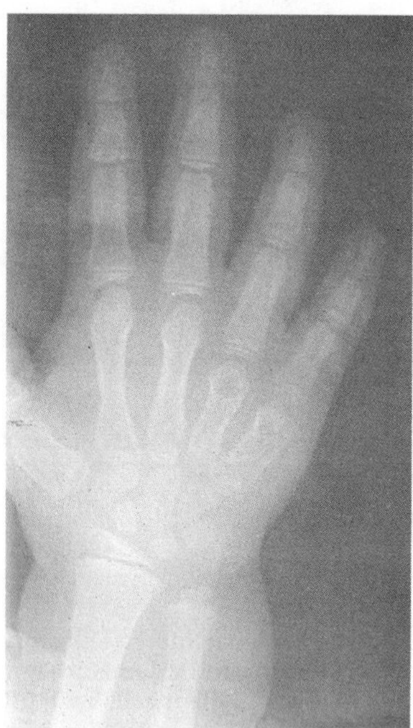

FIGURE *21-25*
Pseudohypoparathyroidism. A radiograph of the hand reveals the characteristic shortness of the fourth and fifth metacarpal bones.

Some patients with pseudohypoparathyroidism display normal G_s activity and have a normal phenotype. The basis for the resistance to PTH in these patients is undefined.

Pseudopseudohypoparathyroidism reads like a typographical error, but the term refers to rare cases in which the phenotype of Albright hereditary osteodystrophy is associated with a normal cAMP response to PTH. Yet these patients also have a reduction in G_s comparable to that reported in cases of pseudohypoparathyroidism. The basic defect underlying pseudopseudohypoparathyroidism has been suggested to involve a gene locus on chromosome 2q37.

PRIMARY HYPERPARATHYROIDISM

Primary hyperparathyroidism refers to the syndrome caused by excessive secretion of PTH by a parathyroid adenoma, primary hyperplasia of all the parathyroids, or in rare cases parathyroid carcinoma.

Parathyroid Adenoma

Parathyroid adenomas arise sporadically or in the context of multiple endocrine neoplasia syndrome type 1 (MEN-1, see later) and account for 80% of all cases of primary hyperparathyroidism. Genetic analysis of sporadic tumors has identified rearrangement and overexpression of the cyclin D1 (PRAD1) protooncogene on chromosome 11 in a subset of patients with such adenomas. A variety of other candidate tumor suppressor genes have been proposed to contribute to the development of parathyroid adenomas.

A parathyroid adenoma is a circumscribed, reddish-brown, solitary mass, measuring 1 to 3 cm in diameter. Hemorrhagic areas are common, and cystic changes are occasionally noted. On microscopic examination, parathyroid adenoma is composed of sheets of neoplastic chief cells embedded in a rich capillary network. A rim of normal parathyroid tissue is usually evident outside the capsule and serves to distinguish an adenoma from parathyroid hyperplasia (Fig. 21-26). For the most part, the cells resemble normal chief cells, but some clear cells and occasional oxyphilic foci may be present. In some instances, bizarre, multinucleated cells and other atypical nuclear and cytoplasmic features are noted. On occasion, the neoplastic cells are arranged in pseudorosettes around blood vessels or as follicles containing eosinophilic, colloid-like material. Rarely, the entire adenoma is composed of oxyphil cells. Regardless of the histological appearance, positive immunohistochemical stains for PTH attest to the secretory activity of the tumor. With a functioning parathyroid adenoma, the other three glands tend to be atrophic. Surgical resection of the tumor relieves the symptoms of hyperparathyroidism.

Primary Parathyroid Hyperplasia

Chief cell hyperplasia is responsible for some 15% of cases of primary hyperparathyroidism. Of these, about one third are associated with familial hyperparathyroidism or MEN syndromes (MEN types 1 and 2A). One third of the sporadic instances of primary parathyroid hyperplasia demonstrate monoclonality, suggesting a neoplastic basis for the proliferation of chief cells in these cases.

On gross examination, all four parathyroid glands are enlarged, the combined weights ranging from less than 1 g to as much as 10 g. In half the patients, one gland is noticeably larger than the others, in which case the distinction from adenoma may be difficult. Microscopically, the normal adipose tissue of the gland is replaced by hyperplastic chief cells arranged as sheets or in trabecular or follicular patterns (Fig. 21-27). Scattered oxyphil cells are common, and small foci of adipose tissue may remain. Rare cases of pure clear cell or oxyphil cell hyperplasia are also reported. An important feature that distinguishes hyperplasia from adenoma is the lack of cellular pleomorphism in the former.

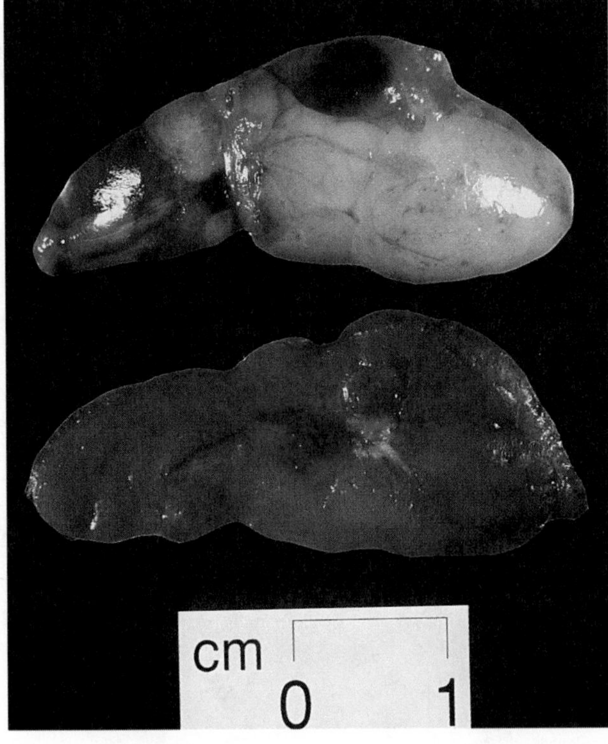

A

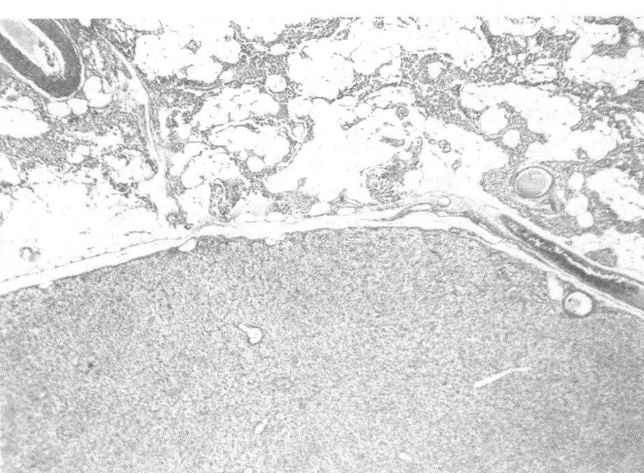

B

FIGURE *21-26*
Parathyroid adenoma. (*A*) The external (*top*) and cross-section (*bottom*) show a tan fleshy tumor. (*B*) The tumor consists of sheets of neoplastic chief cells and is separated from normal parenchyma by a thin capsule.

Parathyroid Carcinoma

Parathyroid carcinoma accounts for 1% of all cases of primary hyperparathyroidism, occurring principally between the ages of 30 and 60 years in both sexes. Parathyroid carcinoma is usually a functioning tumor, and most patients present with symptoms of hyperparathyroidism. Similar to functioning parathyroid adenomas, overexpression of cyclin D1 has also been described in some parathyroid carcinomas, suggesting that deregulation of this protooncogene is an important feature of parathyroid neoplasia in general. It has also been reported that most parathyroid carinomas have absent nuclear staining for Rb protein (another cell cycle regulator), whereas adenomas in this respect are normal.

Carcinomas tend to be somewhat larger than adenomas and appear as lobulated, firm, tannish, unencapsulated masses, often adherent to the surrounding soft tissues. Microscopically, most cases show a trabecular pattern, with significant mitotic activity and the presence of thick fibrous bands. Capsular or vascular invasion is occasionally noted. Importantly, the cell atypism often encountered in parathyroid adenoma is unusual in parathyroid carcinoma. Despite surgical removal of the tumor, local recurrence is common, and about a third of the patients develop metastases to regional lymph nodes, lungs, liver, and bone. In fatal cases, the cause of death is most often hyperparathyroidism rather than carcinomatosis.

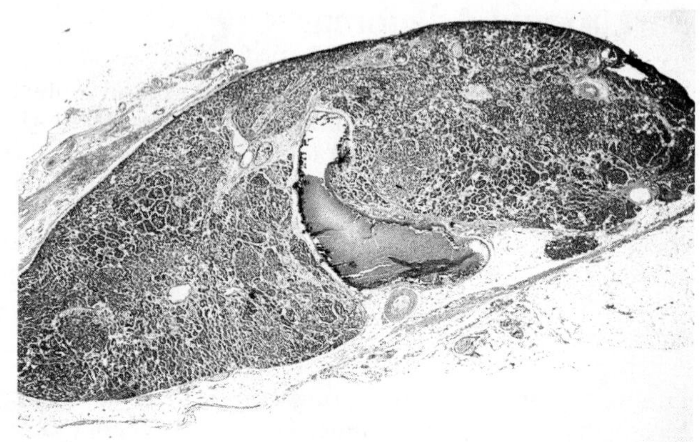

FIGURE *21-27*
Primary parathyroid hyperplasia. The normal adipose tissue of the gland has been replaced by sheets and trabeculae of hyperplastic chief cells.

Clinical Features of Hyperparathyroidism

The clinical manifestations of primary hyperparathyroidism are highly variable, ranging from asymptomatic hypercalcemia detected on routine blood analysis to florid systemic, renal, and skeletal disease (Fig. 21-28). Hypercalcemia and hypophosphatemia are the characteristic biochemical abnormalities. Excessive PTH leads to excessive loss of calcium from the bones and enhanced calcium resorption by the renal tubules. The production of the activated form of vitamin D (1,25[OH]$_2$D) by the renal tubules is also stimulated by PTH, an effect that results in increased intestinal absorption of calcium. The action of PTH on the kidney, together with hypercalcemia, leads to hypophosphatemia.

SKELETAL SYSTEM: The classic bone lesions of hyperparathyroidism, known as *osteitis fibrosa cystica* (see Chapter 26), are encountered in a minority of patients who follow an accelerated and serious form of the disease. Briefly, these patients present with bone pain, bone cysts, pathological fractures, and localized bone swellings (brown tumors and epulis of the jaw). Chondrocalcinosis may be a complication of hyperparathyroidism.

KIDNEY: Ten percent of patients with primary hyperparathyroidism present with renal colic as a result of kidney stones. Nephrocalcinosis, observed radiologically as diffuse renal calcification, may also occur (see Chapter 16). Polyuria is related to hypercalciuria, an effect that also leads to polydipsia.

NERVOUS SYSTEM: Hyperparathyroidism is often accompanied by mental changes, including depression, emotional lability, poor mentation, and memory defects. Hyperactive reflexes are common. Peripheral neuropathy results in type 2 fiber atrophy of skeletal muscles and consequent weakness.

GASTROINTESTINAL TRACT: The incidence of peptic ulcer disease is increased in patients with hyperparathyroidism, possibly because hypercalcemia increases serum gastrin, thereby stimulating gastric acid secretion. Peptic ulcers in the context of MEN type 1, which includes parathyroid hyperplasia or adenoma, may be secondary to Zollinger-Ellison syndrome (see Chapter 15). Chronic pancreatitis is also a recognized complication of prolonged hypercalcemia, but the pathogenesis is not understood. Hypercalcemia is also a cause of constipation.

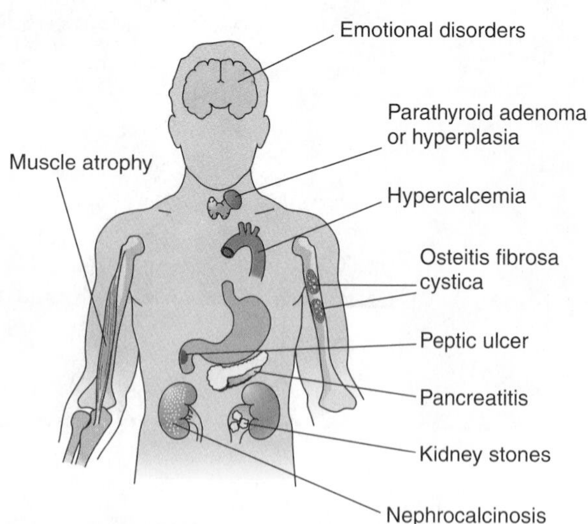

FIGURE *21-28*
The major clinical features of hyperparathyroidism.

OTHER SYSTEMS: Hypertension occurs in up to half of patients with hyperparathyroidism, although the underlying mechanism is not clear. Anemia of unknown cause is also frequent.

SECONDARY HYPERPARATHYROIDISM

Secondary parathyroid hyperplasia is encountered principally in patients with chronic renal failure, although the disorder also occurs in association with vitamin D deficiency, intestinal malabsorption, Fanconi syndrome, and renal tubular acidosis (Fig. 21-29). Chronic hypocalcemia owing to renal retention of phosphate, inadequate production of $1{,}25(OH)_2D$ by the diseased kidneys, and some degree of skeletal resistance to PTH all lead to compensatory hypersecretion of PTH. As a result, secondary hyperplasia of all four parathyroids occurs. In turn, the excess levels of PTH lead to osseous manifestations of hyperparathyroidism, termed *renal osteodystrophy* (see Chapter 26). The morphological appearance of the parathyroids in secondary hyperplasia is similar to that of primary hyperplasia.

Tertiary hyperparathyroidism refers to the development of autonomous parathyroid hyperplasia after long-standing hyperplasia secondary to renal failure. In such instances, parathyroid hyperplasia may not regress following renal transplantation, and surgical intervention to remove parathyroid tissue is required. In this context, it is interesting to note that monoclonality of hyperplastic parathyroid lesions in two thirds of patients with long-standing uremia has been described.

Adrenal Cortex

ANATOMY

Each adrenal gland consists of two independent endocrine organs, namely, the cortex and the medulla. Both components are distinct not only anatomically and functionally but also embryologically. The adrenal cortex arises from celomic mesenchymal cells near the urogenital ridge. The medulla is formed when the fetal adrenal is invaded by neuroectodermal cells. During the second trimester, the adrenal gland is larger than the kidney but the inner "fetal" zone degenerates shortly after birth and disappears by 1 year of age. The remaining outer zone becomes the adult adrenal cortex.

The adult adrenal glands are pyramidal organs situated at the upper pole of each kidney. Each gland is 4 to 6 cm in greatest dimension and weighs about 4 g. Microscopically, the cortex exhibits three layers or zones.

- **The zona glomerulosa** is the outermost layer and is the site of aldosterone secretion. It is stimulated by angiotensin and potassium and inhibited by atrial natriuretic peptide and somatostatin. The zona

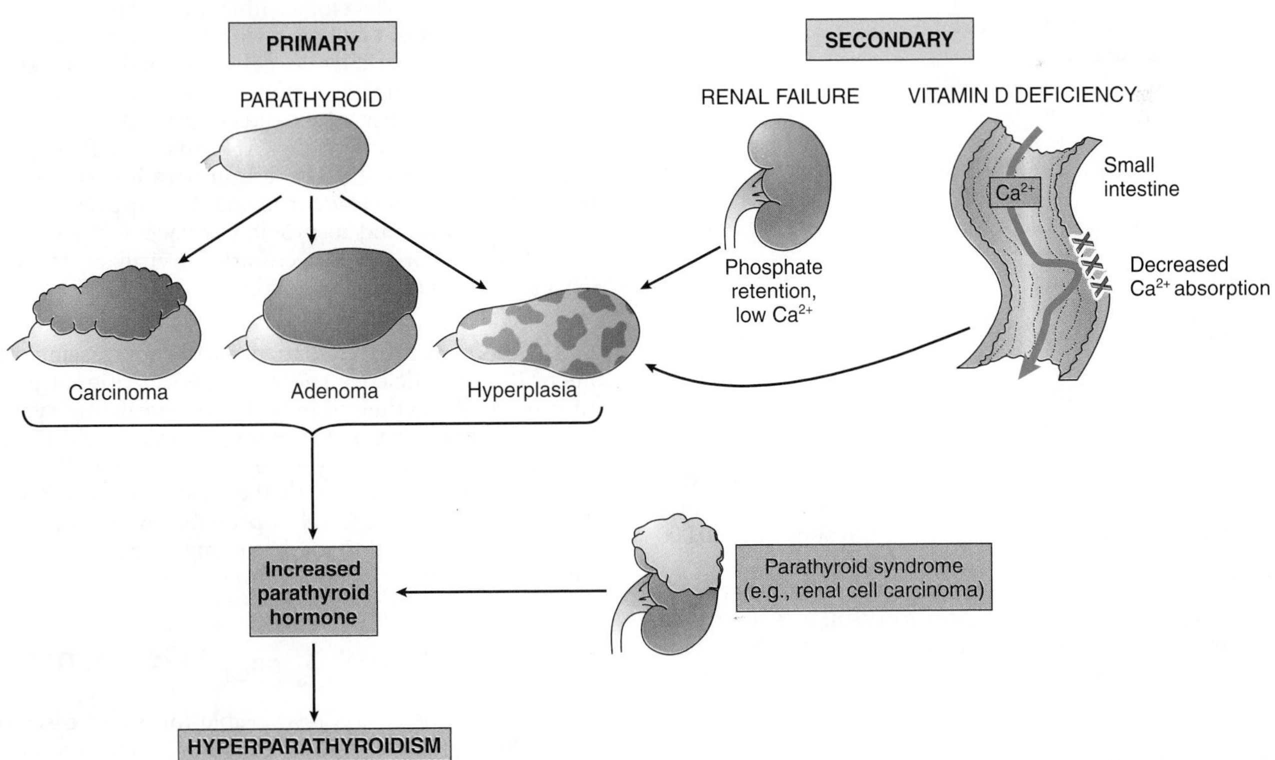

FIGURE 21-29
Major pathogenetic pathways leading to clinical primary and secondary hyperparathyroidism.

glomerulosa comprises 15% of the cortex and is composed of indistinct spherical nests of cells with dark-staining nuclei and a moderate number of fat droplets in the cytoplasm.
- **The zona fasciculata** accounts for 75% of the cortex and is not distinctly separated from the zona glomerulosa. Radial cords of cells, each containing a small nucleus and a large, foamy, clear cytoplasm, representing stored lipid, are readily appreciated.
- **The zona reticularis** is the innermost layer adjacent to the medulla. Irregular anastomosing cords are composed of compact cells with a lipid-poor, slightly granular cytoplasm and bland nuclei.

The cells of the zonae fasciculata and reticularis secrete glucocorticoids under the control of corticotropin. In addition, corticotropin stimulates adrenal growth. These zones also produce dehydroepiandrosterone, a weak adrenal androgen.

CONGENITAL ADRENAL HYPERPLASIA

Congenital adrenal hyperplasia (CAH) is a syndrome that results from a number of autosomal recessive, enzymatic defects in the biosynthesis of cortisol from cholesterol (Fig. 21-30). In general, a deficiency in the synthesis of corticosteroids results in the unopposed action of corticotropin and, hence, adrenal hyperplasia. CAH is the most common cause of ambiguous genitalia in newborn girls (Fig. 21-31A).

☐ **Pathology:** The adrenal glands are enlarged, weighing as much as 30 g (see Fig. 21-31B). The cut surface is soft, tan to brown, and either diffusely enlarged or nodular. Microscopically, the cortex is widened between the medulla and the zona glomerulosa (see Fig. 21-31C). The hyperplastic zone is filled by compact, granular, eosinophilic cells. In most cases, the zona glomerulosa is also hyperplastic, although not to the extent of the other zones.

21-Hydroxylase ($P_{450_{C21}}$) Deficiency

More than 90% of cases of CAH represent an inborn deficiency of 21-hydroxylase, more specifically termed $P_{450_{C21}}$. The gene for $P_{450_{C21}}$ is linked to the MHC locus on the short arm of chromosome 6 and is closely associated with HLA-B and the C4A and C4B complement genes. The incidence of this disease varies from about 1 in 10,000 among whites to 1 in 500 in Alaskan Eskimos.

$P_{450_{C21}}$ is a microsomal enzyme that converts 17-hydroxyprogesterone to 11-deoxycortisol. A deficiency in this enzyme activity impairs cortisol biosynthesis, and the accumulated precursors are instead converted to androgens.

☐ **Clinical Features:** Classic CAH caused by $P_{450_{C21}}$ deficiency presents as several genetically distinct syndromes. There are two variants that affect newborns. One is referred to as simple virilizing CAH and is associated with HLA-B5. The other is the salt-wasting form, which is linked to HLA-Bw47. There is also a late-onset (nonclassic) variant, which is less severe and associated with HLA-B14.

SIMPLE VIRILIZING CAH: Female infants are afflicted with pseudohermaphroditism, whereas males exhibit no abnormalities of the sexual organs. The conversion of cortisol precursors into adrenal androgens is amplified by the corticotropin-dependent increase in the size of the gland. Female newborns exposed to a large excess of adrenal androgens *in utero* are born with fused labia, an enlarged clitoris, and the presence of a urogenital sinus, which may be mistaken for a penile urethra. The sexual ambiguity may be so severe that the infant is mislabeled as male.

The female external genitalia are not necessarily abnormal at birth, but infant girls may develop a syndrome of androgen excess, characterized by enlargement of the clitoris and the presence of pubic hair. Infant boys exhibit sexual precocity. Eventually, the high levels of adrenal androgens lead to closure of the epiphyses and stunted growth. Adult women with CAH tend to be infertile, because the elevated levels of androgens and progestogens interfere with the hypothalamic-pituitary-gonadal axis and thereby inhibit ovulation and disturb the menstrual cycle. By contrast, men with CAH may be fertile, although some exhibit azoospermia.

SALT-WASTING CAH: Owing to $P_{450_{C21}}$ deficiency, aldosterone synthesis may be impaired. As a result, hypoaldosteronism develops within the first few weeks of life in two thirds of newborns with CAH, manifested as hyponatremia, hyperkalemia, dehydration, hypotension, and increased renin secretion. These effects may be rapidly fatal if the disease remains untreated.

Both infantile variants of CAH caused by $P_{450_{C21}}$ deficiency are treated by the administration of glucocorticoids and mineralocorticoids to suppress corticotropin secretion and to provide replacement steroids. Reconstructive surgery is necessary for virilized females with ambiguous external genitalia.

LATE-ONSET CAH: Patients with nonclassic variants of $P_{450_{C21}}$ deficiency show no abnormalities at birth but present at the time of puberty with virilizing symptoms. In young women, late-onset CAH may be difficult to distinguish from polycystic ovary syndrome. By contrast, most young men with the disorder are asymptomatic. This form of CAH is probably more common than classic CAH, particularly among Ashkenazi Jews, Italians, and persons from the former Yugoslavia.

11β-Hydroxylase ($P_{450_{C11}}$) Deficiency

A deficiency in $P_{450_{C11}}$ is responsible for 5% of cases of CAH. Although the disorder is distinctly uncommon in the general population, among Jews of Iranian or Moroccan ancestry in Israel, $P_{450_{C11}}$ deficiency is the most common cause of CAH. The gene for $P_{450_{C11}}$ is located on chro-

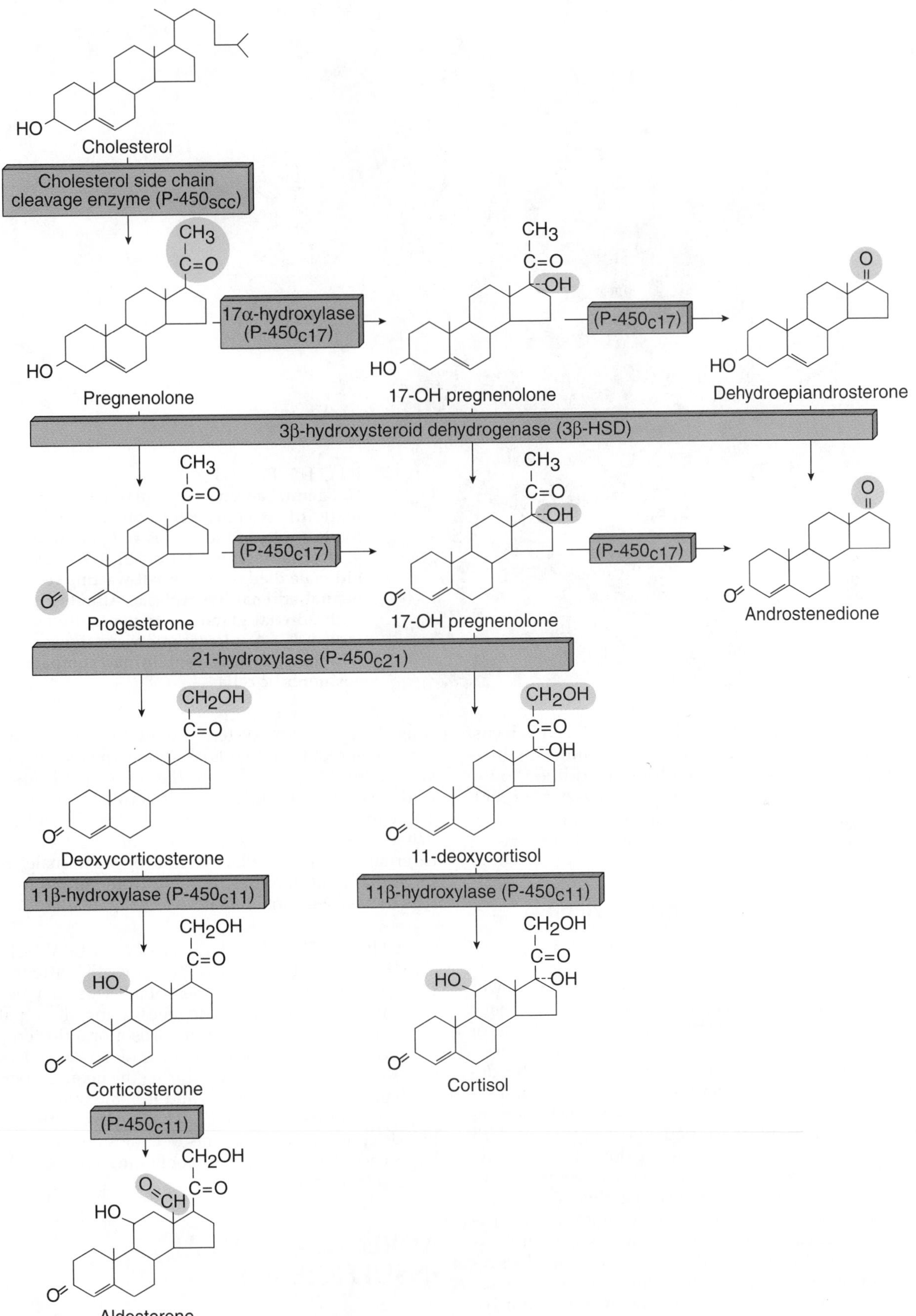

FIGURE *21-30*
Biosynthetic pathways in the synthesis of adrenal corticosteroids.

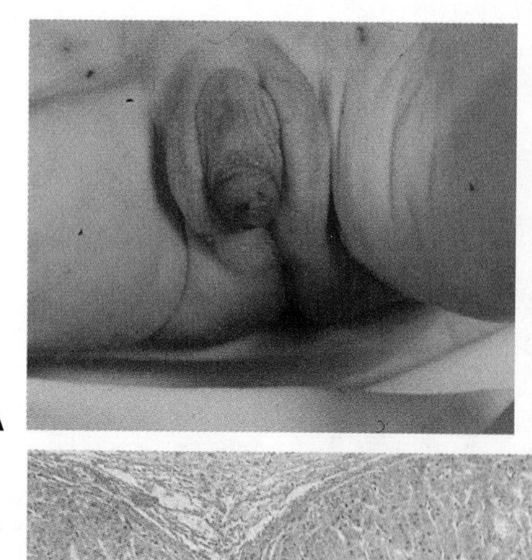
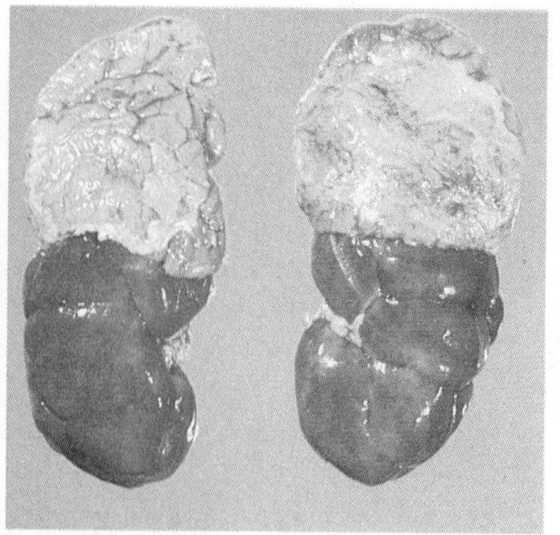
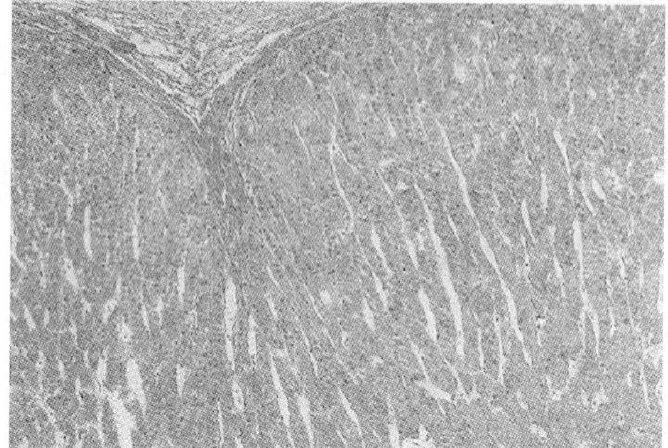

FIGURE 21-31
Congenital adrenal hyperplasia. (*A*) A female infant is markedly virilized with hypertrophy of the clitoris and partial fusion of labioscrotal folds. (*B*) A 7-week-old male died of severe salt-wasting congenital adrenal hyperplasia. At autopsy, both adrenal glands were markedly enlarged. (*C*) A microscopic view shows a widened cortex containing compact eosinophilic cells.

mosome 8 and, thus, there is no linkage to the HLA locus. $P_{450_{C11}}$ is the enzyme responsible for the terminal hydroxylation in the biosynthesis of cortisol. In addition to the androgenic complications of CAH, the presence of high levels of 11-deoxycortisol, a weak mineralocorticoid, causes sodium retention and accompanying hypertension in many cases.

Rarer Forms of Congenital Adrenal Hyperplasia

17α-HYDROXYLASE ($P_{450_{C17}}$) DEFICIENCY: Fewer than 50 patients with CAH caused by $P_{450_{C17}}$ deficiency have been reported. $P_{450_{C17}}$ is required for the synthesis of cortisol, androgens, and estrogens. The production of these steroid hormones is impaired in patients with a deficiency of this enzyme, whereas the levels of the mineralocorticoids, corticosterone and deoxycorticosterone are increased. As a result, these patients are afflicted with hypokalemic alkalosis and hypertension. Interestingly, $P_{450_{C17}}$ deficiency does not influence the development of female characteristics *in utero,* because this is a passive process that does not require female sex hormones. However, $P_{450_{C17}}$ deficiency does interfere with secondary sexual development in girls at puberty, an event that does require estrogens. By contrast, males are born with hypospadias, cryptorchidism, and other manifestations of pseudohermaphroditism.

3β-HYDROXYSTEROID DEHYDROGENASE DEFICIENCY: A few dozen patients with CAH in infancy caused by 3β-hydroxysteroid dehydrogenase deficiency have been reported. In this condition, the inability to convert δ5-hydroxysteroids into the respective ketosteroids leads to impaired synthesis of all steroid hormone classes. The clinical presentation features adrenal insufficiency. Whereas female infants show only mild virilization of the external genitalia, the lack of androgens in males results in genital abnormalities, ranging from simple hypospadias to nearly normal female external genitalia.

CHOLESTEROL SIDE-CHAIN CLEAVAGE ENZYME ($P_{450_{scc}}$) DEFICIENCY: Some 45 patients with $P_{450_{scc}}$ deficiency have been described. This enzyme is the rate-limiting step in steroidogenesis, and these patients have virtually no secretion of cortisol or aldosterone. In addition, the production of sex steroids is also deficient. Severe adrenal insufficiency during the neonatal period is the hallmark of the disease, and in male infants pseudohermaphroditism is noted. The hyperplastic adrenal glands contain large amounts of cholesterol, evident as a large vacuolated cytoplasm containing cholesterol clefts (*lipoid adrenal hyperplasia*).

ADRENAL CORTICAL INSUFFICIENCY

Deficient production of adrenal cortical hormones can result from (1) destruction of the adrenal gland, (2) pituitary or hypothalamic dysfunction, or (3) the intake of corticosteroids in the treatment of chronic inflammatory diseases.

Primary Chronic Adrenal Insufficiency (Addison Disease)

Addison disease is a fatal wasting disorder caused by the failure of the adrenal glands to produce glucocorticoids, mineralocorticoids, and androgens. If untreated, the disease is characterized by weakness, weight loss, gastrointestinal symptoms, hypotension, electrolyte disturbances, and hyperpigmentation.

☐ **Pathogenesis:** At the time that Addison initially described primary adrenal insufficiency in 1855, the most common cause of the syndrome that carries his name was tuberculosis of the adrenal glands. Worldwide, tuberculosis probably remains the most common cause of chronic adrenal insufficiency, but in advanced societies, autoimmune adrenalitis is responsible for 75% of the cases. Autoimmune adrenalitis occurs as an isolated disorder or as a part of two different polyglandular autoimmune syndromes. Other causes of adrenal destruction include metastatic carcinoma, amyloidosis, adrenal hemorrhage, sarcoidosis, and fungal infections. In idiopathic Addison disease, the biochemical defect of adrenoleukodystrophy (see Chapter 28) is often detected. Rarely, adrenal insufficiency is the result of congenital adrenal hypoplasia or familial glucocorticoid deficiency (defective corticotropin receptor).

The autoimmune pathogenesis of most cases of Addison disease is supported by the following:

- Lymphoid infiltrates in the adrenal gland.
- The presence of circulating antibodies to adrenal antigens.
- Abnormalities of cellular immunity.
- Associations with other autoimmune endocrinopathies.
- Genetic linkage with HLA loci.

HUMORAL IMMUNITY: Antiadrenal antibodies that react with tissue from all three zones of the adrenal cortex have been reported in two thirds of patients with chronic adrenal insufficiency that could not be attributed to a specific cause. Such antibodies often appear a few years prior to the onset of symptoms of adrenal insufficiency. The major autoantigens are members of the adrenal steroidogenic enzymes, particularly 21-hydroxylase, which is located in the class III segment of the major histocompatibility complex (MHC). Such autoantibodies are characteristic of adult-onset Addison disease and may contribute to adrenal failure by inhibiting the enzyme. Other specific target antigens have not been identified, but they presumably reside in the endoplasmic reticulum or plasma membrane. Immunoglobulins from patients with Addison disease inhibit corticotropin-induced stimulation of cortisol production and DNA synthesis *in vitro*.

CELLULAR IMMUNITY: Evidence for the participation of cell-mediated immune mechanisms in the pathogenesis of primary adrenal insufficiency includes increased numbers of Ia-positive T lymphocytes in the blood and decreased suppressor T-cell function. Inhibition of leukocyte migration is produced by adrenal homogenates from half of the patients with idiopathic Addison disease.

POLYGLANDULAR ENDOCRINOPATHIES: Half of the patients with autoimmune adrenal insufficiency suffer from other autoimmune endocrine diseases. These disorders are grouped into two polyglandular endocrine syndromes termed type I and type II.

Type I polyglandular autoimmune syndrome is a rare autosomal recessive condition, which exhibits a slight female predominance and is seen in older children and adolescents. In addition to adrenal insufficiency (60%), the large majority of patients are afflicted with hypoparathyroidism and chronic mucocutaneous candidiasis. Insulin-dependent diabetes (type I) is also frequent. Premature ovarian failure is common, and hypothyroidism, malabsorption syndromes, pernicious anemia, chronic active hepatitis, alopecia totalis, and vitiligo are also encountered with a higher frequency than in the general population.

Type I polyglandular disease is highly prevalent among the Finnish population and Iranian Jews. In these populations and in sporadic cases in other countries, a spectrum of mutations in a still unknown gene on chromosome 21q22.3 has been described. Interestingly, almost all cases in Finland and among Iranian Jews are attributable to two different founder mutations. Similar to the common form of autoimmune Addison disease, sera from patients with type I polyglandular disease recognizes steroidogenic autoantigens.

Type II polyglandular autoimmune syndrome (*Schmidt syndrome*) is more common than type I and always includes adrenal insufficiency. Women are affected twice as often as men, and the disorder usually presents between 20 and 40 years of age. Half of the cases are familial, but several modes of inheritance are known. Hashimoto thyroiditis and occasionally Graves disease occur in more than two thirds of the cases. Insulin-dependent diabetes mellitus and premature ovarian failure are common. Only rarely are other autoimmune diseases present, for example, pernicious anemia, Sjögren syndrome, rheumatoid arthritis, myasthenia gravis, and immune thrombocytopenic purpura.

GENETIC FACTORS: In half of the patients with autoimmune adrenal insufficiency as part of a polyglandular syndrome, there is a familial history of an autoimmune endocrinopathy. In those instances in which Addison disease occurs in the absence of other endocrinopathies, a third have an affected relative. There is a strong linkage between autoimmune adrenalitis and HLA-B8, HLA-DR3, and HLA-DR4, with the exception of cases occurring as part of polyglandular syndrome type I, which is not linked to any HLA alleles.

☐ **Pathology:** More than 90% of the adrenal gland must be destroyed before the symptoms of chronic adrenal insufficiency surface. Cases attributed to specific infectious, neoplastic, or metabolic disorders show corresponding evidence of the underlying disorder in the adrenals. Autoimmune adrenalitis leads to a pale, irregular, shrunken gland, weighing 2 to 3 g or less. Microscopically, an intact medulla is surrounded by fibrous tissue containing small islands of atrophic cortical cells (Fig. 21-32). Depending on the stage of the disease, lymphoid infiltrates of varying density are encountered.

☐ **Clinical Features:** The original description of the clinical features of chronic adrenal insufficiency by Addison remains valid for untreated cases today. The patients were reported as having "general languor and debility, remarkable feebleness of the heart's action, irritability of the stomach, and a peculiar change of the colour of the skin." In the typical case, the first symptom is the insidious onset of weakness, which may become so profound that the patient becomes bedridden. Anorexia and weight loss are invariable features of the disease. A diffuse, tan pigmentation usually, but not invariably, develops on the skin, and dark patches may appear on the mucous membranes. The hyperpigmentation is related to the stimulation of melanocytes in the skin by the melanocyte-stimulating activity of pituitary proopiomelanocortin (POMC), increased levels of which are characteristic of Addison disease. Hypotension, with blood pressures in the range of 80/50 mm Hg, is the rule. A variety of gastrointestinal symptoms, including vomiting, diarrhea, and abdominal pain, affects most patients and may be the presenting complaint. Patients with Addison disease often exhibit marked personality changes and even organic brain syndromes.

The lack of mineralocorticoid secretion, together with other metabolic derangements, leads to low serum levels of sodium and elevated potassium. The absence of glucocorticoids is reflected in lymphocytosis and mild eosinophilia. The diagnosis of chronic adrenal insufficiency is established by measuring corticosteroid blood levels after stimulation by corticotropin. Prior to the availability of corticosteroids, less than 20% of patients with a diagnosis of Addison disease survived for 2 years. Today, such patients live a normal life when treated with glucocorticoids and mineralocorticoids.

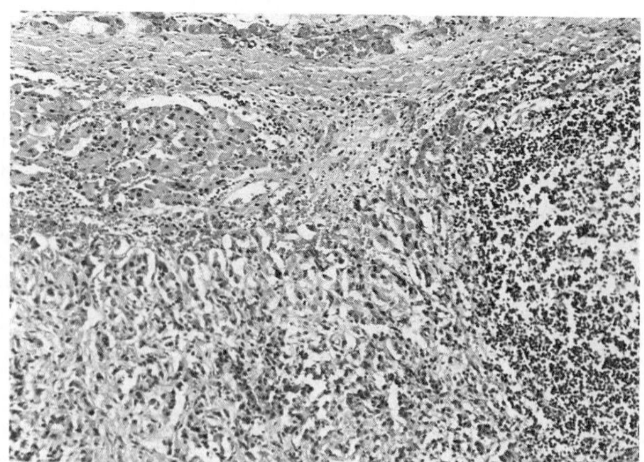

FIGURE *21-32*
Autoimmune adrenalitis. A section of the adrenal gland from a patient with Addison disease demonstrates chronic inflammation and fibrosis in the cortex, an island of residual atrophic cortical cells and an intact medulla.

Acute Adrenal Insufficiency

Acute adrenal insufficiency, or adrenal crisis, is a life-threatening medical emergency that reflects a sudden loss of adrenal cortical function. The symptoms are related more to mineralocorticoid deficiency than to inadequate glucocorticoids. Adrenal crisis occurs in three settings:

- Abrupt withdrawal of corticosteroid therapy in patients with adrenal atrophy secondary to chronic administration of these steroids is probably the most common cause of acute adrenal insufficiency.
- A sudden and devastating worsening of chronic adrenal insufficiency may be precipitated by the stress of infection or surgery.
- ***Waterhouse-Friderichsen syndrome*** *refers to acute, bilateral, hemorrhagic infarction of the adrenal cortex, most commonly secondary to meningococcal or pseudomonal septicemia* (see Fig. 7-24). Adrenal hemorrhage in these circumstances is thought to be a local manifestation of a generalized Shwartzman reaction with disseminated intravascular coagulation. Acute adrenal insufficiency secondary to adrenal hemorrhage is also seen in newborns who have been subjected to birth trauma and in patients undergoing anticoagulant therapy.

☐ **Clinical Features:** The initial manifestations of adrenal crisis are usually hypotension and shock. Nonspecific symptoms are also common, including weakness, vomiting, abdominal pain, and lethargy, which may progress to coma. In the typical case of Waterhouse-Friderichsen syndrome, a young person suddenly develops hypotension and shock, together with abdominal or back pain, fever, and purpura.

Adrenal crisis is almost invariably fatal unless the patient is promptly and aggressively treated with corticosteroids and supportive measures. In addition, antibiotics are needed to manage the infection of Waterhouse-Friderichsen syndrome.

Secondary Adrenal Insufficiency

Destruction of the pituitary and consequent panhypopituitarism lead to secondary adrenal insufficiency. Such lesions include pituitary tumors, craniopharyngioma, empty sella syndrome, and pituitary infarction. Trauma, surgery, and radiation therapy also may result in loss of pituitary function. Metastases to the pituitary rarely cause sufficient pituitary injury as to result in adrenal insufficiency.

Isolated corticotropin deficiency, which does not respond to corticotropin-releasing hormone (CRH), has also been described as a rare cause of secondary adrenal insufficiency. Isolated corticotropin deficiency is often associated with other autoimmune endocrinopathies, and antipituitary and anticorticotropin antibodies have been detected in this condition.

Any disorder that interferes with the secretion of CRH by the hypothalamus (e.g., tumors, sarcoidosis) can result in inadequate secretion of corticotropin and consequent adrenal insufficiency. Such a situation has been labeled by some as *tertiary adrenal insufficiency.*

Since the secretion of POMC (the precursor molecule of corticotropin that contains melanocyte-stimulating peptide sequences) is deficient in secondary adrenal insufficiency, the characteristic hyperpigmentation of primary insufficiency is absent. Aldosterone secretion is regulated by angiotensin and potassium rather than corticotropin, and therefore patients with secondary adrenal insufficiency do not require mineralocorticoid replacement therapy. Secretion of glucocorticoids in response to corticotropin serves to distinguish secondary from primary adrenal insufficiency.

ADRENAL HYPERFUNCTION

Excess secretion of corticosteroids occurs in the context of adrenal hyperplasia or neoplasia (Fig. 21-33). Such hyperfunction may take one of two forms, namely, hypercortisolism (Cushing syndrome) or hyperaldosteronism (Conn syndrome), disorders reflecting the two major classes of adrenal steroid hormones.

In the early part of the 20th century, the neurosurgeon Harvey Cushing associated "painful obesity, hypertrichosis, and amenorrhea" with the presence of a pituitary tumor. The combination of pituitary hyperfunction and the signs and symptoms produced by chronic glucocorticoid excess was termed *Cushing disease.* It is now recognized that the constellation of clinical features caused by high glucocorticoid levels can also result from an adrenal adenoma or carcinoma, ectopic production of corticotropin or CRH by a tumor, or the exogenous administration of corticosteroids. *Thus, the clinical features of hypercortisolism from any cause are now referred to as* ***Cushing syndrome****, and the term* ***Cushing disease*** *is reserved for excessive secretion of corticotropin by pituitary corticotrope tumors.*

The most common cause of Cushing syndrome in the United States is the chronic administration of corticosteroids in the treatment of immunological and inflammatory disorders. The second most common cause is a paraneoplastic effect associated with nonpituitary cancers that inappropriately produce corticotropin. Cushing disease is five times more frequent than the type of Cushing syndrome associated with adrenal tumors.

Corticotropin-Dependent Adrenal Hyperfunction

Bilateral hyperplasia of the adrenal cortex is found in 85% of patients with hyperadrenalism, with the exception of cases that result from the administration of exogenous corticosteroids. **With few exceptions, adrenal hyperplasia is secondary to chronic stimulation by corticotropin.** Women, usually between the ages of 25 and 45 years, are five times more likely than men to develop Cushing disease.

□ **Pathogenesis:** Corticotropin-dependent adrenal hyperfunction results from one of the following:

- Primary hypersecretion of corticotropin by the pituitary (Cushing disease).
- Ectopic corticotropin production by a nonpituitary tumor.
- Inappropriate secretion of CRH by tumors arising outside the hypothalamus, with secondary pituitary hypersecretion of corticotropin.

PRIMARY HYPERSECRETION OF CORTICOTROPIN: Cushing disease usually results from corticotrope microadenomas of the pituitary, although it is occasionally secondary to a macroadenoma or, in a few patients, diffuse corticotrope hyperplasia. Whereas adenomas are clearly monoclonal, arising from a single progenitor cell, corticotrope hyperplasia is caused by chronic CRH hypersecretion. Excessive secretion of corticotropin by pituitary adenomas leads to adrenal cortical hyperplasia; the subsequent increased levels of circulating corticosteroids suppresses both CRH secretion and the release of corticotropin from the non-neoplastic pituitary.

ECTOPIC PRODUCTION OF CORTICOTROPIN: Inappropriate secretion of corticotropin by a malignant tumor accounts for the majority of cases of corticotropin-dependent hyperadrenalism, although a lower incidence is usually given because few of these cases are recognized, and fewer still are reported. Cancer of the lung, particularly small cell carcinoma, is responsible for more than half of the cases of ectopic corticotropin syndrome. The remainder are attributable principally to carcinoids and neural crest tumors (pheochromocytoma, neuroblastoma, medullary carcinoma of the thyroid), thymoma, and islet cell adenoma of the pancreas. Hypersecretion of cortisol by the hyperplastic adrenals suppresses CRH secretion and pituitary release of corticotropin, whereas the corticotropin-producing tumor is not controlled by CRH and is, therefore, unresponsive to the excess glucocorticoids.

ECTOPIC PRODUCTION OF CRH: The ectopic CRH syndrome is similar to the ectopic corticotropin syndrome, except that a malignant tumor secretes CRH. In turn, CRH stimulates corticotropin secretion by the pituitary, thereby leading to adrenal hyperplasia. In some cases, the tumor produces both CRH and corticotropin, in which case adrenal hyperplasia is caused by the latter. Although rare, ectopic production of CRH has been reported most often with bronchial carcinoid tumors, as well as with medullary carcinoma of the thyroid, adenocarcinoma of the prostate, and intrasellar gangliocytoma.

□ **Pathology:** Cushing disease is characterized by bilateral, diffuse (75%) or nodular (25%) hyperplasia of the adrenal glands, each gland usually weighing 8 to 10 g but occasionally as much as 20 g.

Diffuse adrenal hyperplasia features a grossly visible, broadened cortex composed of an inner brown layer and a yellow, lipid-rich cap. Microscopically, the inner third of the cortex is composed of a compact cell layer, and the outer zone, corresponding to the zona fasciculata, displays large clear cells packed with lipid. The appearance of the zona glomerulosa is variable, sometimes being prominent and at other times difficult to identify.

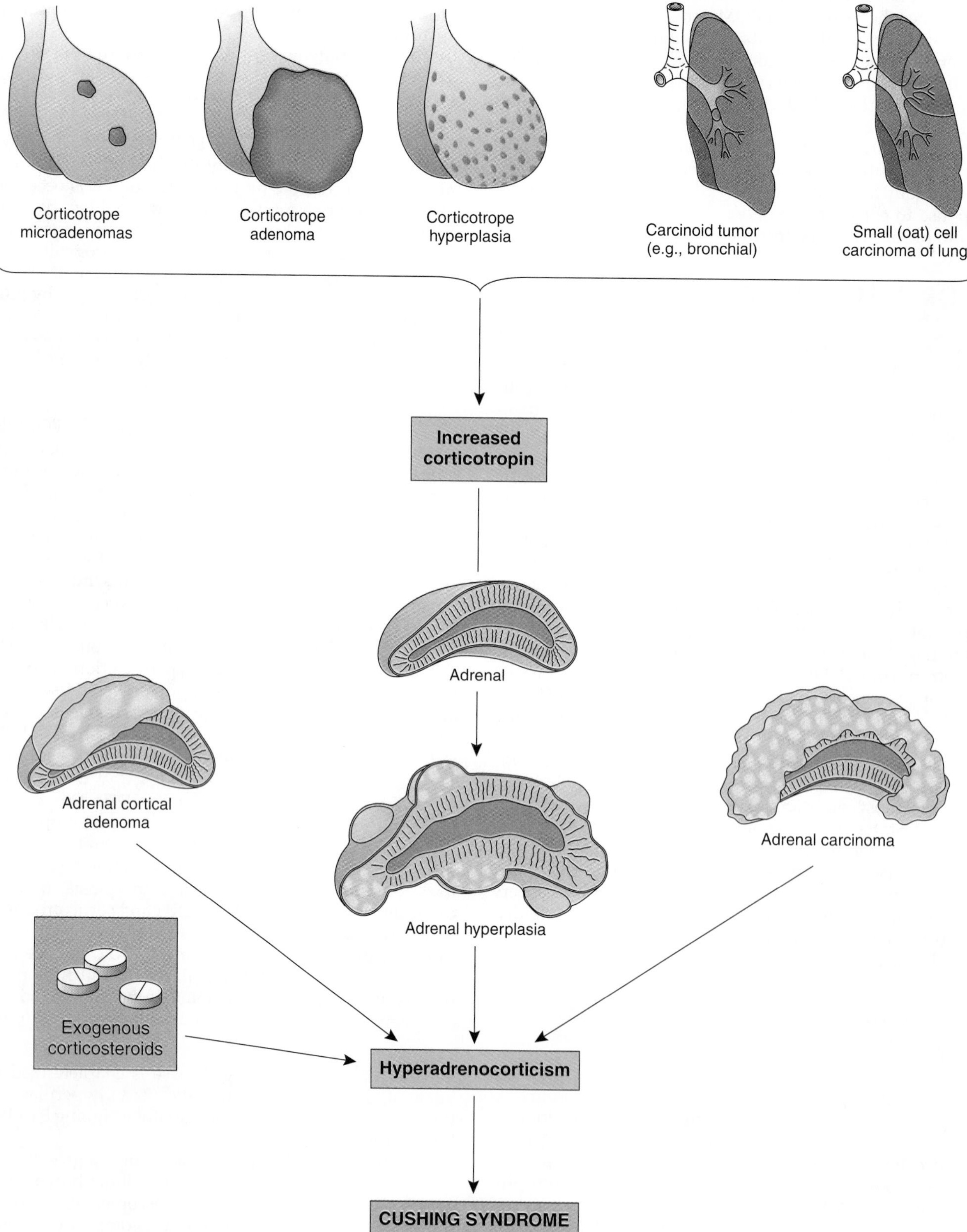

FIGURE *21-33*
The pathogenetic pathways of Cushing syndrome. The corticotropin-dependent pathway is referred to as Cushing disease.

Nodular adrenal hyperplasia is a term reserved for grossly visible nodules up to 2.5 cm in diameter, since microscopic nodules are common in diffuse hyperplasia. Bilateral, multiple nodules compress the overlying cortex, and the intervening parenchyma exhibits diffuse hyperplasia. However, nodular hyperplasia may be asymmetrical, and the two glands may differ significantly in weight. Microscopically, the nodules are composed of large, lipid-laden, clear cells.

Corticotropin-Independent Adrenal Hyperfunction

Benign or malignant adrenal cortical tumors are the most common cause of corticotropin-independent Cushing syndrome. In adults, the incidence of adrenal carcinoma peaks at 40 years of age and that of adenoma a decade later. In children, adrenal carcinoma accounts for fully one half of the cases of Cushing syndrome, whereas 15% are caused by adenoma. At all ages, the female-to-male ratio is 4:1. Despite anecdotal reports of adrenal neoplasms arising in a background of adrenal hyperplasia, there is no evidence that chronic stimulation by corticotropin plays a role in the pathogenesis of adrenal adenoma or carcinoma.

Adrenal Adenoma

Adenomas of the adrenal gland are uncommon, provided that minute nodules of the adrenal cortex are excluded. The typical adenoma is an encapsulated, firm, yellow, slightly lobulated, mass, measuring about 4 cm in diameter (Fig. 21-34). These tumors usually weigh between 10 and 50 g, although weights up to 100 g have been recorded. On cut section, the surface is mottled yellow and brown and occasionally black, owing to the deposition of lipofuscin pigment. A thin rim of compressed normal adrenal cortex surrounds the tumor. Necrosis and calcification may be present even in small tumors. Microscopically, adenomas exhibit clear, lipid-laden (fasciculata type) cells arranged in sheets or nests, often with interspersed clusters of compact, lipid-depleted, eosinophilic (reticularis type) cells. The nontumorous cortex of the involved and contralateral gland is generally atrophic.

Nonfunctional adrenal cortical adenoma is observed in as many as 5% of adult autopsies, but only less than 10% of surgically removed benign tumors of the adrenal are hormonally silent. Whether such tumors may be associated with hypertension as a "forme fruste" of Conn syndrome remains controversial. On morphological grounds alone, nonfunctional adenomas cannot be distinguished from their functional counterparts.

Adrenal Cortical Carcinoma

Eighty percent of adrenal cortical carcinomas are functional. They weigh more than 100 g, and weights up to 5 kg have been recorded. Adrenal carcinomas are soft, encapsulated, lobulated, and bulky tumors (Fig. 21-35). The cut surface has a variegated pink, brown, or yellow color, often with necrosis, hemorrhage, and cystic change. The tumor commonly invades locally, and remnants of normal adrenal tissue are difficult to identify. Microscopically, both clear and compact cells are present. Varying degrees of nuclear pleomorphism are seen. Mitotic figures and vascular invasion may or may not be apparent. In the case of functional carcinomas, the contralateral adrenal cortex is atrophic.

The large majority of adrenal cortical carcinomas cannot be resected completely, and even when the surgeon believes that the entire tumor has been removed, micrometastases in other organs are already present. Even with surgery, most patients survive for only 1 to 3 years.

Nonfunctional adrenal cortical carcinomas tend to be highly malignant tumors, with weights exceeding 1 kg. They are morphologically identical to functional cancers.

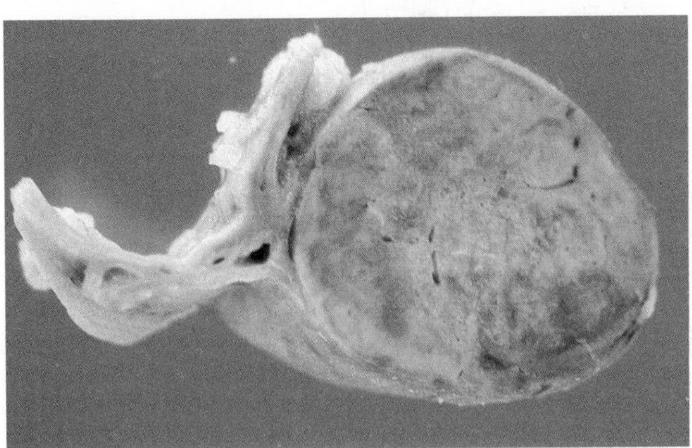

A

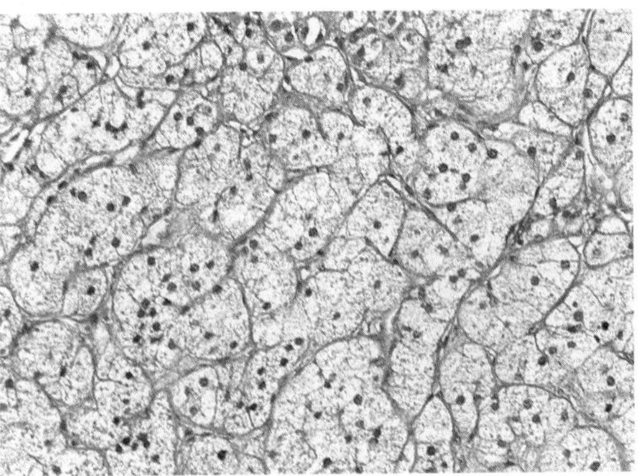

B

FIGURE *21-34*
Adrenal adenoma. (*A*) The cut surface of an adrenal tumor removed from a patient with Cushing syndrome is a mottled yellow with a rim of compressed normal adrenal tissue. (*B*) A microscopic view reveals nests of clear, lipid-laden cells.

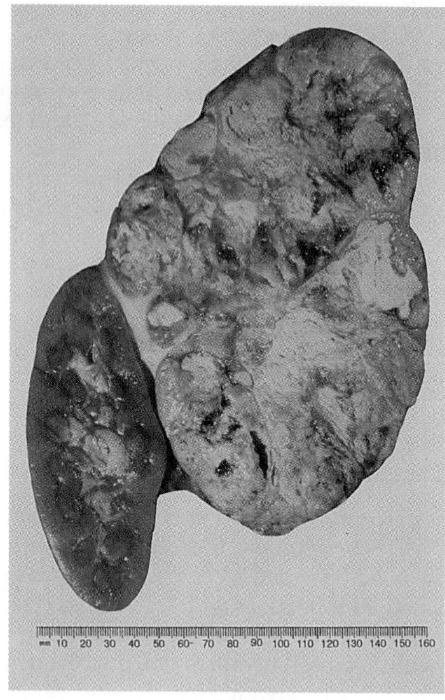

A

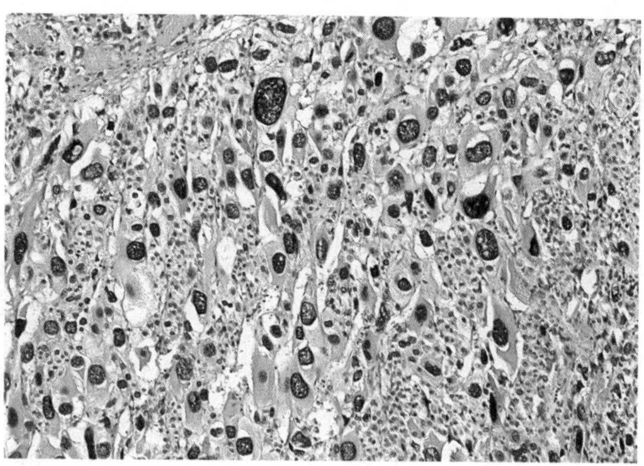

B

FIGURE 21-35
Adrenal cortical carcinoma. (*A*) The bulky tumor on section is yellow to tan with areas of necrosis and cystic degeneration. (*B*) A microscopic section demonstrates marked anisocytosis and nuclear pleomorphism.

Other Causes of Corticotropin-Independent Cushing Syndrome

Chronic administration of corticosteroids in the treatment of a variety of immunological and inflammatory diseases is today by far the most common cause of Cushing syndrome. The synthetic hormones ordinarily employed (e.g., dexamethasone, prednisone) have only glucocorticoid activity and little or no mineralocorticoid or androgen effects. As a result, hypertension and hirsutism, features commonly seen with Cushing syndrome secondary to adrenal hyperplasia or neoplasia, are usually absent in this iatrogenic disorder.

Bilateral micronodular hyperplasia of the adrenal cortex is a rare cause of corticotropin-independent Cushing syndrome. The patients are children or young adults. Half have an autosomal dominant disease characterized by pigmented skin lesions over much of the body, a variety of myxomas, testicular tumors, and somatotrope adenomas of the pituitary. The adrenal glands contain small, brown or black nodules, up to 0.5 cm in diameter, which consist of large eosinophilic cells laden with lipofuscin granules. Autoantibodies that promote adrenocortical growth and steroidogenesis are thought to underly the pathogenesis of this condition.

Clinical Features of Cushing Syndrome

The clinical manifestations of Cushing syndrome (Fig. 21-36) depend on the degree and duration of excessive corticosteroid levels, as well as on the levels of adrenal androgens.

OBESITY: Typically, the patient notes the gradual onset of obesity of the face (moon face), neck (buffalo hump), trunk, and abdomen (Fig. 21-37). The extremities are characteristically unaffected or even wasted.

SKIN: The skin is atrophic, and there is a loss of subcutaneous fat. Enlargement of the abdomen and other areas of fat deposition stretches the thin skin and produces purplish striae, which represent venous channels that are visible through the attenuated dermis. Hyperpigmentation of the skin, similar to but less severe than that in Addison disease, may occur, owing to pituitary hypersecretion of POMC. Acanthosis nigricans is seen with increased frequency in patients with Cushing syndrome.

MUSCULOSKELETAL SYSTEM: Increased bone resorption causes osteoporosis. Back pain is a common complaint, and up to a fifth of patients with Cushing syndrome have radiological evidence of compression fractures of the vertebrae. Fractures of the ribs and occasionally the long bones may occur. Proximal muscle wasting (*steroid myopathy*) causes weakness, which may be so severe that the patient is unable to rise from a sitting position or climb a flight of stairs.

CARDIOVASCULAR SYSTEM: Hypertension is a frequent feature of Cushing syndrome, often reflecting an

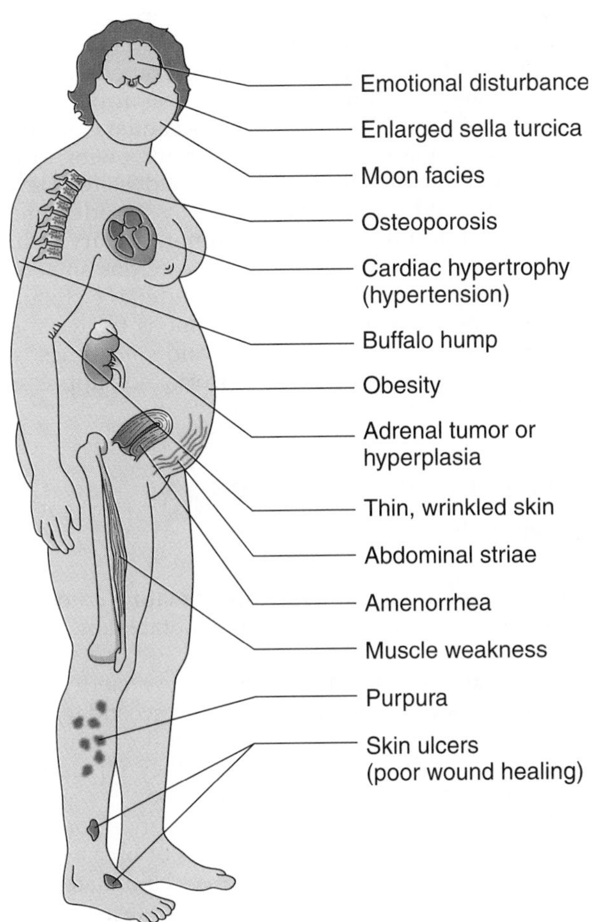

FIGURE 21-36
The major clinical manifestations of Cushing syndrome.

excessive mineralocorticoid activity. In older patients, congestive heart failure is a common sequel.

SECONDARY SEX CHARACTERISTICS: Females with Cushing syndrome tend to be virilized, showing increased facial hair, thinning of scalp hair, acne, and oligomenorrhea. Excess glucocorticoid levels in men cause erectile dysfunction and in both sexes decreased libido.

EYES: One fourth of the patients have an increased intraocular pressure, which may be a problem in the presence of preexisting glaucoma.

GLUCOSE INTOLERANCE: The stimulation of gluconeogenesis by glucocorticoids leads to glucose intolerance and hyperinsulinemia. Diabetes mellitus supervenes in 15% of the patients, but usually in those with a family history of diabetes.

PSYCHOLOGICAL CHANGES: The majority of patients with Cushing syndrome, both endogenous and iatrogenic, suffer distinct personality changes. These include irritability, emotional lability, depression, and paranoia. The disturbance in mentation may be so severe that the patient becomes suicidal.

LABORATORY FINDINGS: Half of the patients exhibit an absolute lymphopenia, and one third have abnormally low eosinophil counts. Hypercalciuria is common, although serum calcium levels remain unchanged. Serum cholesterol and triglyceride levels are frequently elevated.

All forms of Cushing syndrome are characterized by increased glucocorticoid levels. The dexamethasone suppression test is used to distinguish corticotropin-dependent from corticotropin-independent forms of Cushing syndrome. Dexamethasone suppresses pituitary corticotropin secretion, and hence hypercortisolism, whereas it is without effect on adrenal tumors.

Cushing syndrome is treated by (1) extirpation (surgery or irradiation) of pituitary, adrenal, or ectopic corticotropin-producing tumors, (2) discontinuation of corticosteroid therapy, or (3) the administration of adrenal enzyme inhibitors (e.g., aminoglutethimide, ketoconazole, metapyrone). At one time, the 5-year mortality for Cushing syndrome was 50%, but the prognosis is considerably better today. With the exception of ectopic corticotropin syndrome and adrenal carcinoma, in which patients die of the cancer rather than of hypercortisolism, Cushing syndrome is highly curable.

Primary Aldosteronism (Conn Syndrome)

The inappropriate secretion of aldosterone by an adrenal adenoma or hyperplastic adrenal glands produces Conn syndrome, characterized by hypertension and hypokalemia. Aldosterone-secreting adenomas are more common in women than in men (3:1) and usually occur between the ages of 30 and 50 years.

☐ **Pathogenesis:** Solitary adrenal adenoma has been previously reported to account for up to 90% of cases of hyperaldosteronism. However, bilateral hyperplasia of the adrenal zona glomerulosa now comprises as many as

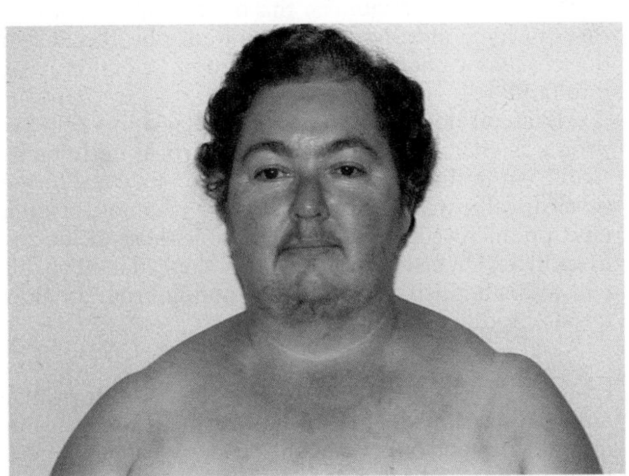

FIGURE 21-37
Cushing syndrome. A woman who suffered from a pituitary adenoma that produced ACTH exhibits a moon face, buffalo hump, increased facial hair, and thinning of the scalp hair.

half of the cases in some university hospitals, perhaps reflecting a more careful evaluation of hypertensive patients. Only a few cases of primary aldosteronism are caused by adrenal carcinoma.

Two types of familial hyperaldosteronism have recently been defined. Type I (glucocorticoid-suppressible) is an autosomal dominant disease in which the fusion of the corticotropin-responsive regulatory elements of the 11β-hydroxylase gene to the aldosterone synthase gene results in a hybrid gene. This gene is ectopically and constitutively activated in the zona fasciculata, with resulting bilateral hyperplasia of this zone. By suppressing the release of corticotropin, glucocorticoids ameliorate type I disease. In contrast to type I disease, type II familial hyperaldosteronism is associated with adrenal cortical adenomas and is, therefore, not suppressible by glucocorticoids.

The hypersecretion of aldosterone enhances sodium reabsorption by the renal tubules, thereby increasing body sodium. Hypertension is caused not only by the retention of sodium and consequent volume expansion but also by increased peripheral vascular resistance. Hypokalemia reflects aldosterone-induced loss of potassium in the distal renal tubule.

☐ **Pathology:** Most aldosterone-secreting adenomas measure less than 3 cm in diameter, weigh less than 6 g, and are yellow. However, the size is variable and tumors up to 50 g are reported. On microscopic examination, the dominant cell is clear, lipid-rich, and arranged in cords or alveoli. Little nuclear pleomorphism is noted. Some tumors contain "hybrid" cells, which are smaller than clear cells and are intermediate between cells of the normal zona glomerulosa and those of the zona fasciculata. Occasionally, hybrid cells predominate in the adenoma. A few nests of compact cells, similar to those observed in cortisol-producing adenomas, are encountered throughout the tumor. By electron microscopy, the mitochondria in some cases have platelike, stacked cristae, typical of the normal zona glomerulosa. Others have tubulovesicular mitochondrial plicae of the zona fasciculata type, since in humans this zone may also produce aldosterone. In contrast to cortisol-producing adenomas, the nontumorous cortex in cases of hyperaldosteronism is not atrophic, because aldosterone does not inhibit corticotropin secretion by the pituitary.

Bilateral nodular adrenal hyperplasia in Conn syndrome is characterized by yellow cortical nodules less than 2 cm in diameter. Microscopically, they are formed by clear cells, which show no nuclear pleomorphism. By electron microscopy, the cells resemble those of the zona fasciculata. On histological grounds alone, it may be difficult to distinguish a hyperplastic nodule from an aldosterone-producing adenoma.

☐ **Clinical Features:** Most patients with primary aldosteronism are diagnosed after the detection of asymptomatic diastolic hypertension. Muscle weakness and fatigue are produced by the effects of potassium depletion on skeletal muscle. Polyuria and polydipsia result from a disturbance in the concentrating ability of the kidney, probably secondary to hypokalemia. Metabolic alkalosis and elevation of serum bicarbonate levels reflect the loss of hydrogen ions into the urine and their migration into potassium-depleted cells. The excessive secretion of ammonium and bicarbonate ions, which compensate for the metabolic alkalosis, produces an alkaline urine. Primary aldosteronism is distinguished from secondary aldosteronism by a low plasma renin in the former, owing to suppression of renin secretion by elevated aldosterone levels.

Primary aldosteronism caused by an adenoma is cured by surgical removal of the tumor. Dietary sodium restriction and treatment with the aldosterone antagonist spironolactone are also frequently effective. Bilateral adrenal hyperplasia in Conn syndrome is treated medically with aldosterone antagonists and sometimes with dexamethasone in the case of glucocorticoid-suppressible hyperaldosteronism.

MISCELLANEOUS ADRENAL TUMORS

Adrenal myelolipoma is a mixture of mature adipose tissue and hemopoietic marrow and is notable for its occasional large size.

Adrenal cysts are rare, and the large majority are actually pseudocysts that have developed secondary to degenerative changes in benign adrenal tumors or the resolution of hemorrhage. In some cases, they represent the remnants of an underlying vascular lesion.

Metastatic cancer to the adrenal glands commonly originates from carcinomas of the lung or breast or from malignant melanoma. The glands may be unilaterally or bilaterally massively enlarged, up to 20 to 45 g each. They are largely replaced by carcinoma and often display necrosis and hemorrhage. Usually, enough adrenal cortical parenchyma remains to ensure that Addison disease does not develop, particularly in view of the limited survival of these patients.

Adrenal Medulla and Paraganglia

ANATOMY AND FUNCTION

The adrenal medulla is entirely contained within the adrenal cortex and comprises 10% of the weight of the gland. It consists of neuroendocrine cells, termed *chromaffin cells*, which are derived from primitive pheochromoblasts of the developing sympathetic nervous system (Fig. 21-38). Chromaffin cells are so named because the catecholamines contained in their cytoplasmic granules have an affinity for chromium salts and darken on oxidation by potassium dichromate. These cells are also present at extra-adrenal sites of the sympathetic nervous system, such as the preaortic sympathetic plexuses and the paravertebral sympathetic chain.

Chromaffin cells appear as nests of small polyhedral cells, which display pale amphophilic cytoplasm and vesicular nuclei. The cells of the adrenal medulla contain

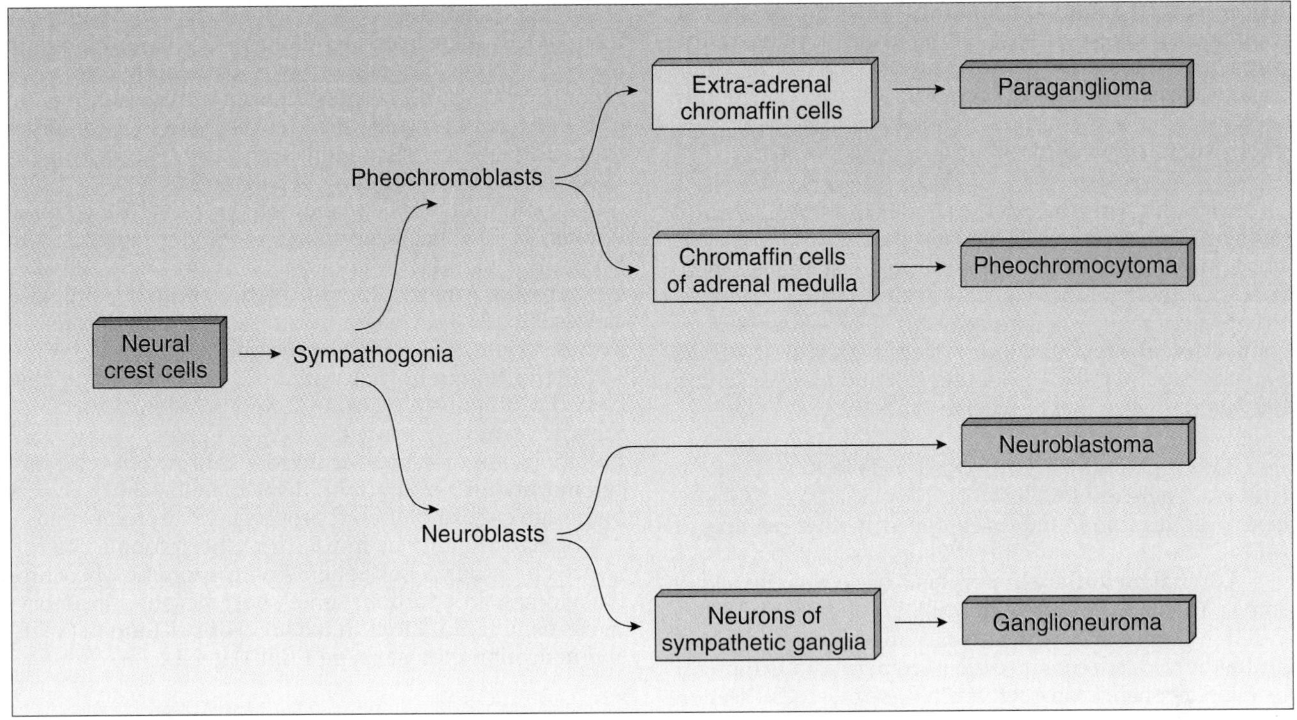

FIGURE *21-38*
Histogenesis of tumors of the adrenal medulla and extra-adrenal sympathetic nervous system.

numerous, electron-dense chromaffin (catecholamine-containing) granules, which are 100 to 300 nm in diameter and resemble those of the sympathetic nerve endings. Epinephrine constitutes 85% of the contents of the granules, with norepinephrine and a number of noncatecholamine hormones representing the remainder. Interspersed among the chromaffin cells are postganglionic neurons and small autonomic nerve fibers. Stored catecholamines are secreted on sympathetic stimulation as an arousal response to stress (exercise, cold, fasting, trauma) and to emotional excitation accompanying fear and anger.

The adrenal medulla is supplied by both arterial and portal venous circulations that originate in the zona reticularis of the cortex. Most of the blood to the hormonally active cells of the medulla is derived from the portal blood. The medulla is innervated from the splanchnic nerves by cholinergic preganglionic sympathetic neurons.

PHEOCHROMOCYTOMA

Pheochromocytoma refers to a rare tumor of chromaffin cells of the adrenal medulla that secretes catecholamines. Such tumors also originate in extra-adrenal sites, in which case they are termed *paraganglioma*. Other catecholamine-producing tumors (e.g., chemodectoma and ganglioneuroma) may also cause a syndrome similar to that seen with pheochromocytoma.

Pheochromocytomas are somewhat more frequent in women than in men and are observed at any age, including infancy, although they are uncommon after 60 years of age. **The presenting symptoms are related to sustained or episodic hypertension.** Despite the fact that pheochromocytoma accounts for less than 0.1% of cases of hypertension, it is important to consider this tumor in the evaluation of any hypertensive patient. When detected early, pheochromocytoma is amenable to surgical resection but when left untreated the patients can die of the complications of prolonged hypertension. This problem is emphasized by the observation that most pheochromocytomas are found unexpectedly at autopsy, indicating that some curable cases of hypertension escaped clinical detection.

☐ **Pathogenesis:** Most pheochromocytomas are sporadic, whereas a minority of cases are familial and arise alone or as part of several hereditary syndromes, including MEN types 2A and 2B, von Hippel-Lindau disease, neurofibromatosis type 1, and McCune-Albright syndrome.

The features of the autosomal dominant MEN syndromes are as follows:

- **MEN type 1 (Wermer syndrome)** includes (1) adenoma of the pituitary, (2) parathyroid hyperplasia or adenoma, and (3) islet cell tumor of the pancreas. Two thirds of the patients have adenomas of two or more endocrine systems, and one fifth develop tumors of three or more systems. Carcinoid, adrenal cortical, and lipoid tumors may also occur in MEN-1. The gene for MEN-1 has been mapped to chromosome 11q13, but has not yet been identified.
- **MEN type 2 syndromes** feature medullary thyroid carcinoma in virtually all patients and pheochromocytoma in more than half.

MEN-2A (SIPPLE SYNDROME): The large majority (95%) of MEN-2 patients are classified as 2A. In addition, to medullary thyroid carcinoma and pheochromocytoma, a quarter of these patients suffer from hyperparathyroidism as a result of parathyroid hyperplasia or adenoma. A variety of neural crest tumors are occasionally seen in patients with MEN type 2A, including gliomas, glioblastomas, and meningiomas.

MEN-2B: This disorder is similar to MEN-2A, but it develops some 10 years earlier and parathyroid disease is uncommon. The *mucosal neuroma syndrome* (ganglioneuromas of the conjunctiva, oral cavity, larynx, and gastrointestinal tract) is a feature of MEN-2B. Mucosal neuromas are always encountered, but only half of the patients express the full phenotype. Many patients have a habitus similar to that of Marfan syndrome.

FAMILIAL MEDULLARY THYROID CARCINOMA: There are families who have at least four members with this tumor and no evidence of other features of MEN-2.

Adrenal medullary hyperplasia has been reported in some patients with both both MEN-2A and 2B. Similar to C-cell hyperplasia as a precursor of medullary carcinoma of the thyroid, adrenal medullary hyperplasia is thought to antedate pheochromocytoma in these cases. Cut section of the enlarged adrenal shows an expanded medulla. Microscopically, the chromaffin cells are not unusual but are larger than normal and are arranged in distinct nests or cords.

The RET protooncogene on chromosome 10q11.2 is responsible for MEN-2 syndromes. This gene codes for a transmembrane receptor of the tyrosine kinase family, but the physiological ligand and the normal function of the receptor are unknown. A variety of germline, missense, activating mutations in the cysteine-rich extracellular domain of RET have been identified in 95% of families with MEN-2A and in 85% of those with familial thyroid carcinoma (Fig. 21-39). The most common mutation (codon 634) constitutively activates the receptor by promoting the dimerization of its monomer, thereby reproducing the effect caused by the binding of a ligand.

A point mutation at codon 918 of the tyrosine kinase domain of RET has been found in 95% of patients with MEN-2B. This mutation not only constitutively activates the tyrosine kinase function of the receptor, but also causes it to phosphorylate substrates ordinarily preferred by other kinases (e.g., c-src and c-abl).

Identification of RET mutations is now used to confirm the diagnosis of MEN-2 and to identify asymptomatic family members. Persons who carry RET mutations are screened for thyroid cancer, pheochromocytoma, and hyperparathyroidism from the age of 6 years to the age of 35 and offered prophylactic thyroidectomy.

Somatic mutations in RET have been found in a minority (10% to 20%) of patients with sporadic pheochromocytomas. In addition, some sporadic pheochromocytomas exhibit mutations in the von Hippel-Lindau (VHL) and neurofibromatosis, type 1 (NF1) genes.

☐ **Pathology:** In sporadic cases of pheochromocytoma, 80% of the tumors are unilateral, 10% are bilateral, and 10% are in extra-adrenal locations. By contrast, two thirds of those occurring in the context of MEN are bilateral. The tumors range in size from small lesions measuring 1 cm across to large masses of more than 2 kg. Most tumors are 5 to 6 cm in diameter and weigh 80 to 100 g.

Pheochromocytomas tend to be encapsulated, spongy, reddish masses, with prominent central scars,

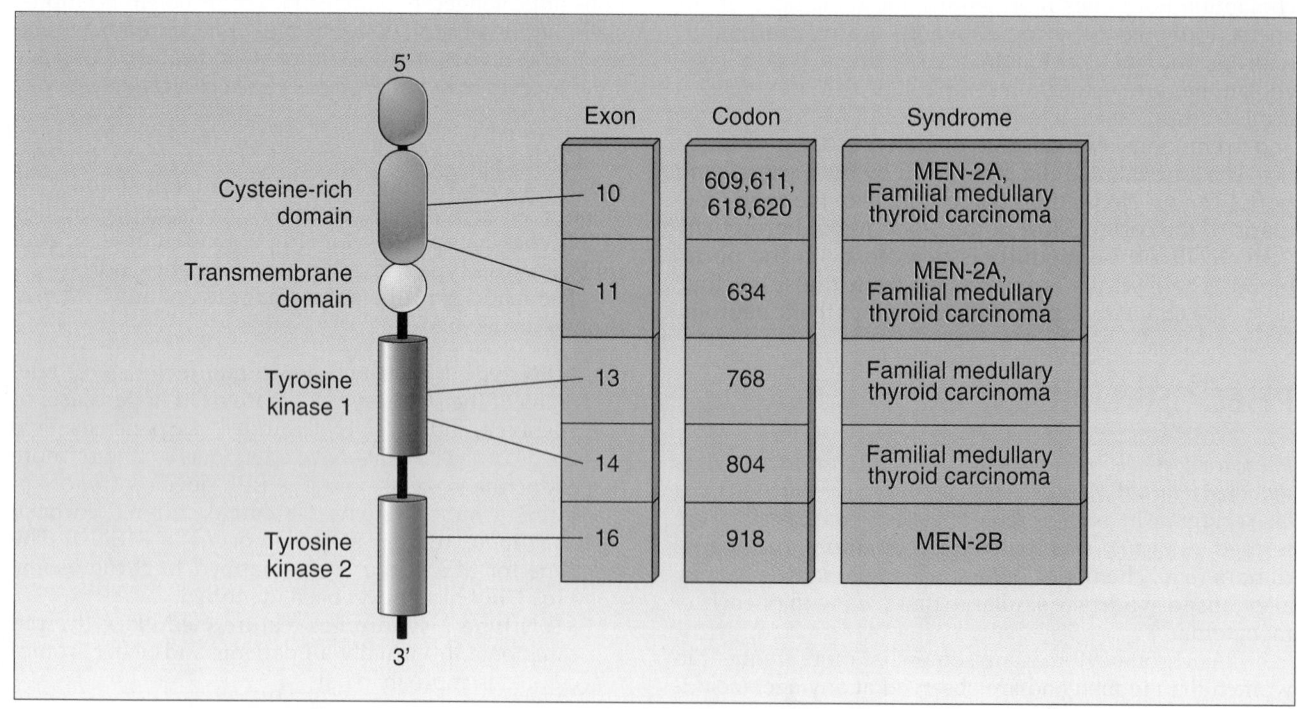

FIGURE *21-39*
RET protooncogene mutations in multiple endocrine neoplasia, type 2 (MEN-2).

hemorrhage, and foci of cystic degeneration (Fig. 21-40A). The histological appearance is highly variable. Typically, circumscribed nests ("zellballen") of neoplastic cells are present. The tumor cells range from polyhedral to fusiform and show a granular, amphophilic or basophilic cytoplasm and vesicular nuclei. Eosinophilic globules are usually seen in the cytoplasm. Cellular pleomorphism is often prominent and may include multinucleated tumor giant cells (see Fig. 21-40B). The tumor is traversed by numerous capillaries. Less commonly the architectural pattern features trabecular or solid formations, with only indistinct zellballen.

By electron microscopy, membrane-bound, dense core granules are seen, corresponding to stored catecholamines. Immunohistochemical stains attest to the neuroendocrine nature of the tumor and reveal the presence of neuron-specific enolase, chromogranin, and synaptophysin.

In 5% to 10% of the cases, pheochromocytoma proves to be malignant, although this figure may be higher for extra-adrenal tumors. There are no reliable histological criteria to distinguish malignant from benign pheochromocytoma, and malignancy is only determined by the biological behavior of the tumor, namely metastases. Both benign and malignant pheochromocytomas evidence mitoses, cellular pleomorphism, invasion of the capsule or blood vessels, and necrosis. Metastases are most common in the regional lymph nodes, bone, lung, and liver.

☐ **Clinical Features:** With few exceptions, the clinical features associated with pheochromocytoma are caused by the release of catecholamines by the tumor. Patients with pheochromocytoma come to medical attention because of (1) asymptomatic hypertension discovered on a routine physical examination, (2) symptomatic hypertension that is resistant to antihypertensive therapy, (3) malignant hypertension (e.g., encephalopathy, papilledema, proteinuria), (4) myocardial infarction or aortic dissection, or (5) paroxysms of convulsions, anxiety, or hyperventilation.

In the typical case, episodic catecholamine release leads to a paroxysm or crisis, lasting up to several hours, with severe throbbing headache, sweating, palpitations, tachycardia, abdominal pain, and vomiting. An elevated blood pressure, often to an extreme degree, is characteristic. A paroxysm is often precipitated by activities that place pressure on the abdominal contents (including the tumor), such as exercise, lifting, bending, or vigorous abdominal palpation. Although anxiety may be a prominent feature of a paroxysm, emotional stress is not an initiating factor.

More than 90% of patients with pheochromocytoma exhibit hypertension, which is sustained in two thirds of

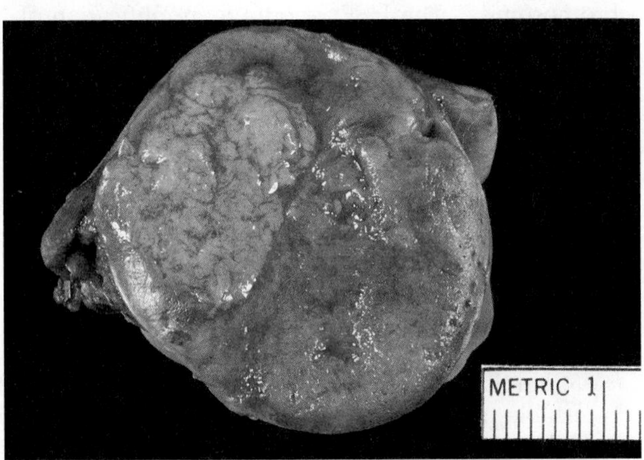

A

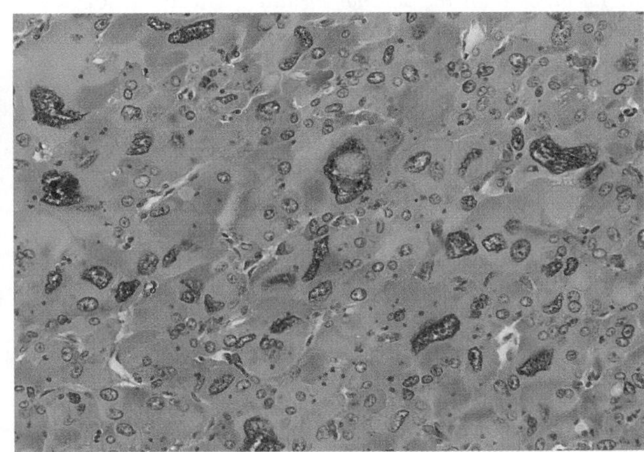

B

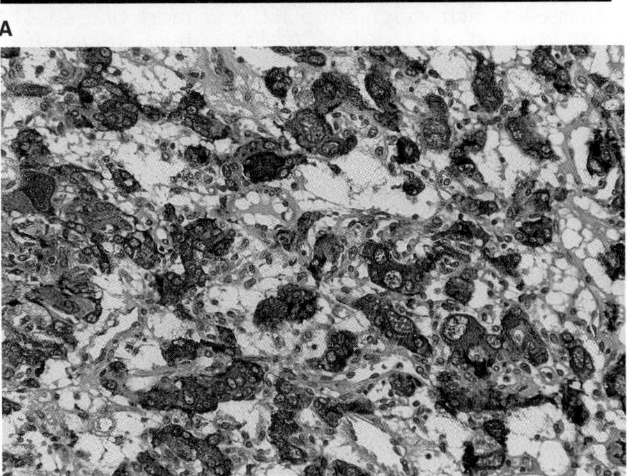

C

FIGURE *21-40*
Pheochromocytoma. (A) The cut surface of an adrenal tumor from a patient with episodic hypertension is reddish brown with a prominent area of fibrosis. Foci of hemorrhage and cystic degeneration are evident. (*B*) A photomicrograph of the tumor shows polyhedral tujor cells with ample finely granular cytoplasm. Note the enlarged hyperchromatic nuclei. (*C*) Many of the tumor cells show positive immunohistochemical staining for chromogranin A, a marker of neuroendocrine differentiation.

the patients and is similar to essential hypertension. In these patients, blood pressure rises to even higher levels during a paroxysm. In one third of the patients, hypertension is only episodic. Frequently, episodic hypertension becomes sustained, and in many untreated patients the condition evolves into malignant hypertension.

There are other consequences of excess catecholamine levels. Orthostatic hypotension results from a decrease in plasma volume and poor postural tone. An increased basal metabolic rate, sweating, heat intolerance, and weight loss may mimic hyperthyroidism. Angina and myocardial infarction occur in the absence of coronary artery disease. The cardiac complications are attributed to myocardial necrosis caused by elevated catecholamine levels (*catecholamine cardiomyopathy*).

Pheochromocytoma is diagnosed by finding increased urinary levels of catecholamine metabolites, particularly vanillylmandelic acid, metanephrine, and unconjugated catecholamines. The definitive treatment for pheochromocytoma is surgical extirpation of the tumor. α-Adrenergic blocking agents are used to control hypertensive crises, and β-adrenergic receptor antagonists are helpful adjuncts.

Paraganglioma

Paragangliomas are pheochromocytomas that develop in paraganglia other than the adrenal medulla. These tumors develop in virtually any location that harbors paraganglia, including the retroperitoneum, the posterior mediastinum, and the urinary bladder. Bladder paraganglioma may present as a peculiar syndrome of headaches and paroxysmal hypertension on urination. Paragangliomas may also arise in the base of the skull, in the neck, in vagal or aortic bodies, or in any organ that contains paraganglionic tissue, such as the larynx and small intestine. They arise in such paraganglia as the glomus jugulare, the carotid body, and other vasoreceptor bodies. Whereas the large majority (90%) of paragangliomas of the head and neck are benign, those in the retroperitoneum are more often malignant.

Carotid body tumor *is a prototypic paraganglioma, which arises at the carotid bifurcation, forming a palpable mass in the neck.* Interestingly, carotid body tumors are ten times more frequent in persons living at high altitude than those at sea level, suggesting that these tumors actually represent a hyperplastic response to prolonged sensing of hypoxia by the carotid body.

Autosomal dominant transmission of paragangliomas has been described in some families, and the genetic linkage is traced to chromosome 11q.23. Curiously, all affected persons, whether male or female, have inherited the disease from their father, indicating that genomic imprinting is involved.

NEUROBLASTOMA

Neuroblastoma is a malignant tumor of neural crest origin that is composed of neoplastic neuroblasts and originates in the adrenal medulla or sympathetic ganglia. The neuroblast is derived from primitive sympathogonia and represents an intermediate stage in the development of the sympathetic ganglion neurons (see Fig. 21-38). **Neuroblastoma is one of the most important malignant tumors of childhood, accounting for up to 10% of all childhood cancers and 15% of cancer deaths among children.** The peak incidence is in the first 3 years. The tumor is congenital in some cases and has even been found in premature stillborns. In fact, neuroblastoma accounts for half of all cancers diagnosed in the first month of life. Occasional cases are encountered in adolescents or adults. Although the occurrence of neuroblastoma is sporadic, a few instances of familial tumors are recorded.

☐ **Pathogenesis:** The adrenal glands of fetuses in the third trimester of pregnancy contain microscopic nodules of primitive neuroblasts. In infants who died before the age of 3 months of diverse causes, the prevalence of such neuroblastic islands, termed by some "neuroblastoma *in situ*," was up to 200 times their frequency in adults. Thus, it is clear that embryogenesis of the adrenal medulla, and presumably of other parts of the sympathetic nervous system, continues during the first year of life. Persistence and transformation of these embryonal structures may be related to the pathogenesis of neuroblastoma.

Neuroblastoma is characterized by frequent deletions on chromosome 1 (1p35-36), extrachromosomal double minutes, and homogeneously staining regions (HSRs) on chromosome 2. The HSRs represent amplification of N-*myc*, an abnormalitiy that plays a key role in determining the aggressiveness of neuroblastoma. It is thought that the locus on chromosome 1 encodes a gene that suppresses the amplification of N-*myc*.

☐ **Pathology:** Neuroblastoma can originate in any location where cells derived from the neural crest are present (i.e., from the posterior cranial fossa to the coccyx). One third of the tumors are in the adrenal gland, another third in other abdominal sites, and 20% in the posterior mediastinum.

Neuroblastomas range in size from minute, barely discernible nodules to tumors readily palpable through the abdominal wall. They are round, irregularly lobulated masses, which weigh 50 to 150 g or more (Fig. 21-41A). The cut surface is soft and friable, with a variegated maroon color. Areas of necrosis, hemorrhage, calcification, and cystic change are frequently present. In the case of small neuroblastomas, a yellow rim of compressed adrenal cortex may be noted.

Microscopically, the tumor is composed of dense sheets of small, round to fusiform cells with hyperchromatic nuclei and scanty cytoplasm, which are often compared with lymphocytes. Mitoses are frequent. Characteristic rosettes are defined by a rim of dark tumor cells in a circumferential arrangement around a central pale fibrillar core (see Fig. 21-41B). Pseudorosettes, featuring tumor cells clustered radially around small vessels, are also present. The electron microscopic appearance of neuroblastoma cells is distinctive. The malignant neuroblasts exhibit peripheral dendritic processes containing longitudinally oriented microtubules and neurosecretory granules and filaments in the cytoplasm.

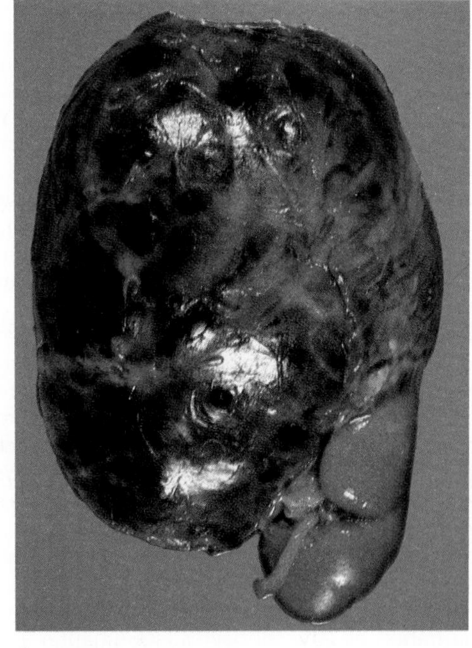

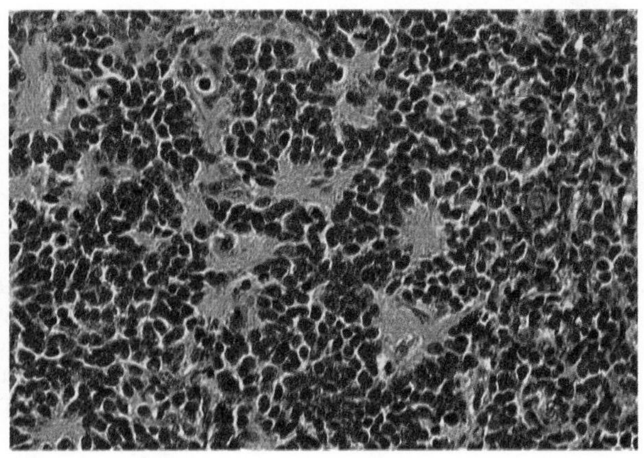

A B

FIGURE 21-41
Neuroblastoma. (*A*) A large, lobulated, hemorrhagic, and cystic tumor, adherent to the upper pole of the kidney, was removed from a child who presented with an abdominal mass. (*B*) A photomicrograph illustrates the characteristic rosettes, formed by small, regular, dark tumor cells arranged around a central, pale fibrillar core.

Neuroblastomas readily infiltrate the surrounding structures and metastasize to regional lymph nodes, the liver, lungs, bones, and other sites. Metastasis to the orbit may result in proptosis. Occasionally, metastases may be found earlier than the primary tumor.

☐ **Clinical Features:** The signs and symptoms of neuroblastoma are highly variable, owing to the numerous sites of the primary tumor and its metastases. The presenting sign is often an enlarging abdomen in a young child. Physical examination discloses a firm, irregular, and nontender mass. Hepatic metastases enlarge the liver and occasionally produce ascites. Marked irritability may reflect pain from bony metastases. Respiratory distress accompanies large masses in the thorax, and tumors in the pelvis obstruct the bowel or ureters. Spinal cord compression may lead to gait disturbance and sphincter dysfunction. Severe diarrhea may be caused by secretion of vasoactive intestinal peptide by the neuroblastoma.

The urinary excretion of catecholamines and their metabolites is almost invariably elevated in patients with neuroblastoma. The urine contains increased amounts of norepinephrine, vanillylmandelic acid (VMA), homovanillic acid (HVA), and dopamine. The catecholamine content of the tumor itself is not as great as that of pheochromocytoma, possibly because neuroblastoma cells metabolize these compounds.

A number of prognostic factors have been identified:

- **Age**: The best prognosis is seen in children under the age of 2 years.
- **Site**: Extra-adrenal tumors tend to be better differentiated and, accordingly, have a better prognosis.
- **Stage**: Survival is 90% in stage I (tumor confined to the organ of origin) and decreases to less than 3% in stage IV (widespread metastases). An exception is stage IVS (special), in which the characteristic chromosomal abnormalities of neuroblastoma are absent. Even with metastases to the liver and bone marrow, patients with stage IVS often undergo spontaneous remissions and have a 60% to 90% survival rate.
- **Grade**: Low-grade (better differentiated) tumors carry a better prognosis than do high-grade (undifferentiated) neuroblastomas.
- **VMA/HVA ratio**: A ratio of less than 1 indicates a deficiency of dopamine β-hydroxylase activity in aggressive tumors and suggests an unfavorable outcome.
- **Genomic alterations**: Amplification of N-*myc* occurs in 30% of the cases and, as noted earlier, is negatively correlated with survival. Some neuroblastomas express the nerve growth factor receptor that is encoded by the TRK gene. A high level of TRK expression is strongly predictive of prolonged survival.

Localized neuroblastomas are treated by surgical resection alone. Patients with disseminated tumor are subjected to chemotherapy and sometimes irradiation.

Ganglioneuroma

Ganglioneuroma, similar to neuroblastoma, is a tumor of neural crest origin and is the most mature variant of all the neuroblastic

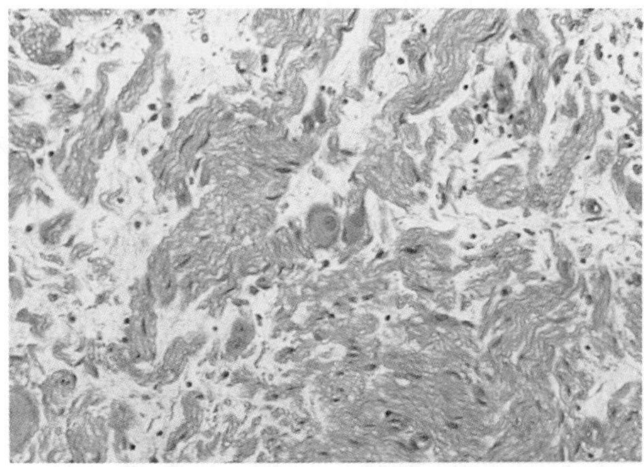

FIGURE *21-42*
Ganglioneuroma. A photomicrograph shows mature ganglion cells interspersed among wavy spindle cells embedded in a myxoid matrix.

tumors. It is found in older children and young adults. Ganglioneuroma is benign and arises in sympathetic ganglia, typically in the posterior mediastinum. Up to 30% of these tumors occur in the adrenal medulla. In keeping with its degree of differentiation, ganglioneuroma does not manifest the chromosomal abnormalities characteristic of neuroblastoma.

Ganglioneuromas are well encapsulated and display a myxoid, glistening, cut surface. Microscopically, they show well-differentiated, mature ganglion cells, associated with spindle cells in a loose and abundant fibrillar stroma (Fig. 21-42). The fibrils represent neurites extending from the tumor cell bodies. The cytoplasmic processes of the ganglion cells contain neurosecretory granules, and may even form synaptic junctions. Typical neuroendocrine substances, such as neuron-specific enolase and certain peptide hormones, are readily demonstrated. As previously mentioned, a neuroblastoma may differentiate into a ganglioneuroma.

Thymus

The theories underlying the historical categorization of the thymus as an endocrine organ have long been discredited. Nevertheless, we now know that the thymus elaborates a number of factors (thymic hormones) that play a key role in the maturation of the immune system and the development of immune tolerance. On this basis, the inclusion of the thymus in a chapter on endocrine pathology is appropriate.

ANATOMY AND FUNCTION

Embryologically, the thymus derives from the third pair of pharyngeal pouches, with an inconstant contribution from the fourth pair. The organ is irregularly pyramidal, with its base located inferiorly and its two lobes fused in the midline. Its fibrous capsule extends into the parenchyma, forming septa that delimit lobules. The thymus is largest in relation to total body size and weight at birth, at which time it averages about 25 g. It continues to grow until puberty, and then may weigh 45 g.

Microscopically, the lobules display an outer cortex and an inner medulla. The cortex consists of densely packed lymphocytes, which in this location are termed *thymocytes.* A few epithelial cells are interspersed among the thymocytes. The medulla contains many more epithelial cells and fewer thymocytes. By electron microscopy, the epithelial cells of the cortex display elongated cytoplasmic processes, whereas those of the medulla are more densely packed and have less prominent cytoplasmic projections. Desmosomes and dense tonofilaments are characteristic of the medullary epithelial cells, particularly in the *Hassall corpuscles.* These medullary structures are focally keratinized, concentric aggregates of epithelial cells characteristic of the thymus. The epithelial nature of these cells is documented by prominent staining for cytokeratins.

The thymus has now emerged as the key site for the differentiation of T lymphocytes (see Chapter 4). The surface antigens of uncommitted lymphocytes are rearranged or otherwise modified as a result of interaction with thymic epithelial cells. It appears that cell-to-cell contact and secretion of "thymic lymphopoietic factors" are required for T lymphocyte processing. Various thymic polypeptides include thymosin, thymopoietin, and thymin, which may be required for the development and maintenance of immunologically competent T lymphocytes.

The thymus has a small population of neuroendocrine cells, which may explain the occurrence of neuroendocrine tumors in this organ. The thymus also exhibits a complement of myoid cells, which have many structural and functional features of striated muscle cells but are nevertheless regarded as epithelial cells. Myoid cells may play a role in the autoimmune pathogenesis of myasthenia gravis.

Beginning at puberty, the thymus starts to involute and continues to diminish in size into adulthood. Initially, cortical thymocytes are decreased relative to the epithelial cells. Eventually, the thymus consists of islands of epithelial cells depleted of lymphocytes and contains aggregates of Hassall corpuscles separated by adipose tissue.

AGENESIS AND DYSPLASIA

Developmental abnormalities of the thymus are associated with congenital immune deficiency states. The alterations in the thymus vary from complete absence (*agenesis*) or severe *hypoplasia* to a situation in which the thymus is small but exhibits a normal architecture. Some small glands exhibit *thymic dysplasia,* characterized by an absence of thymocytes, few if any Hassall corpuscles, and the presence of only epithelial components. A number of developmental abnormalities of the thymus are associated with immune deficiencies (see Chapter 4) and hematological disorders.

Severe combined immunodeficiency features defects of both T and B lymphocytes and is associated with severe thymic dysplasia.

DiGeorge syndrome is caused by a failure in the development of the third and fourth branchial pouches, resulting in agenesis or hypoplasia of the thymus and parathyroid glands, congenital heart defects, dysmorphic facies, and a variety of other congenital anomalies. As a result, the patients suffer from hypocalcemia and a deficiency of cellular immunity, with a particular susceptibility to *Candida* infections.

Nezelof syndrome is similar to DiGeorge syndrome except for the absence of parathyroid and cardiac involvement.

Wiscott-Aldrich syndrome is a sex-linked recessive hereditary disease in which severe immunodeficiency is associated with a hypoplastic thymus, eczema, and thrombocytopenia.

Reticular dysgenesis refers to a severe form of immune deficiency characterized by a vestigial thymus and failure of the development of bone marrow stem cells, resulting in lymphopenia, granulocytopenia, and death *in utero* or in the neonatal period.

Swiss-type hypogammaglobulinemia is an autosomal recessive disorder featuring severe thymic hypoplasia or dysplasia. Infants with this condition have no lymphocytes or Hassall corpuscles in the thymus and die within a few years from a variety of infections. The anomaly represents a failure of the thymic anlage in the neck to descend into the mediastinum.

Ataxia telangiectasia is an autosomal recessive trait featuring diffuse telangiectasia and cerebellar ataxia and the frequent occurrence of lymphoma. The involuted thymus shows no epithelial differentiation or Hassall corpuscles.

HYPERPLASIA

Thymic hyperplasia refers to the presence of lymphoid follicles in the thymus irrespective of the size of the gland (Fig. 21-43). The total weight of the thymus is usually within the normal range, although it may be increased. The follicles contain germinal centers and are composed largely of B lymphocytes, which contain IgM and IgD. The follicles tend to occupy and distort the medullary zones.

The best known association of thymic hyperplasia is with **myasthenia gravis** (see Chapter 27), in which two thirds of the patients exhibit this thymic abnormality. Interestingly, thymic epithelial and myoid cells contain nicotinic acetylcholine receptor protein, suggesting a potential source for the development of antibodies directed against this receptor. Thymic follicular hyperplasia may also be found in other diseases in which autoimmunity is believed to play a role, including Graves disease, Addison disease, systemic lupus erythematosus, scleroderma, and rheumatoid arthritis.

THYMOMA

Thymoma is a neoplasm of thymic epithelial cells, without regard to the presence or number of lymphocytes. This tumor almost always occurs in adult life, and the large majority (up to 80%) are benign.

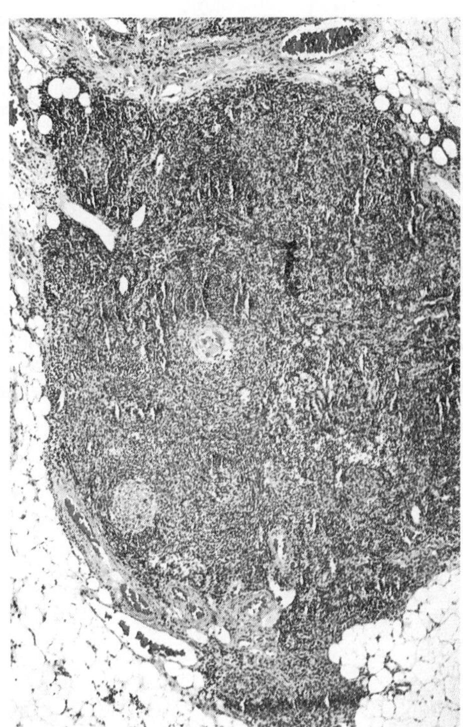

FIGURE *21-43*
Thymic hyperplasia. Lymphoid follicles with germinal centers are observed in this thymus removed from a patient with myasthenia gravis.

☐ **Pathology:** Most thymomas are located in the anterosuperior mediastinum, although a few have been described in other locations where thymic tissue is found, including the neck, middle and posterior mediastinum, and pulmonary hilus. Benign thymomas are irregularly shaped masses, which range from a few centimeters to 15 cm or more in greatest dimension. They are encapsulated, firm, and gray to yellow tumors, which are divided into lobules by fibrous septa (Fig. 21-44). Large tumors show foci of hemorrhage and necrosis and cystic degeneration. In some instances, the entire thymoma becomes cystic, and multiple sections are required to identify the true nature of the lesion.

On microscopic examination, thymomas consist of a mixture of neoplastic epithelial cells and nontumorous lymphocytes. The proportions of these elements vary in individual cases, and even among different lobules. The epithelial cells are plump or spindle shaped and show vesicular nuclei. In those cases in which epithelial cells predominate, they may exhibit an organoid differentiation, including perivascular spaces containing lymphocytes and macrophages, tumor cell rosettes, and whorls suggestive of abortive Hassal corpuscle formation. Many of the accompanying T lymphocytes are small, but others tend to be larger and have prominent vesicular nuclei, features suggestive of activation. Mitotic activity of the non-neoplastic lymphocytic component generally exceeds that of the neoplastic epithelial cells. Occasionally, the dominant lymphoid component of a thymoma may result in an erroneous diagnosis of lymphoma.

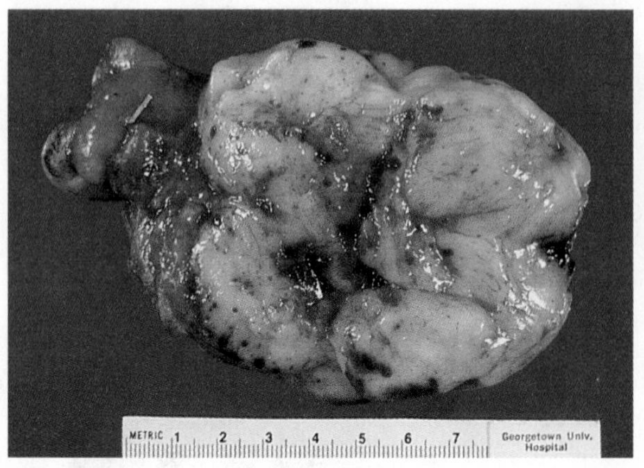

A

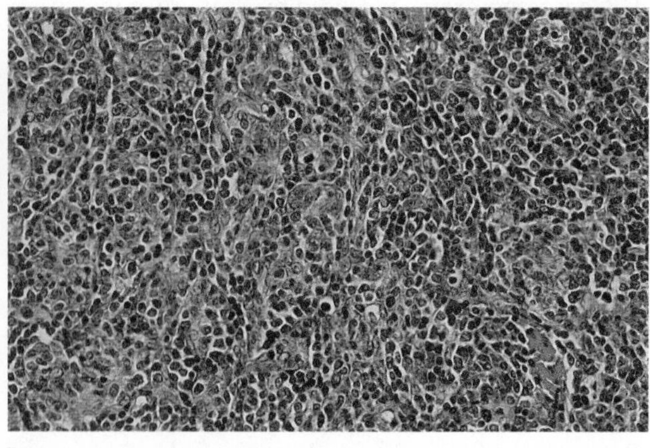

B

FIGURE *21-44*
Thymoma. (*A*) The tumor in cross-section is whitish and has a bulging surface with areas of hemorrhage. Note the attached portion of normal thymus. (*B*) Microscopically, the thymoma consists of a mixture of neoplastic epithelial cells and nontumorous lymphocytes.

MYASTHENIA GRAVIS: The most conspicuous clinical association of thymoma is with myasthenia gravis. Ten percent of patients with myasthenia gravis have thymoma. Conversely, one third to one half of patients with thymoma develop myasthenia gravis. The occurrence of thymoma in persons with myasthenia gravis is more common in men older than the age of 50 years.

In cases of thymoma associated with myasthenic symptoms, the epithelial cells are of the plump rather than the spindle cell variety. The antigens related to the nicotinic acetylcholine receptor have also been detected in thymomas. Thymic hyperplasia is almost always present in the nontumorous thymic tissue, and lymphoid follicles may even be present in the thymoma itself.

OTHER ASSOCIATED DISEASES: Thymoma is also associated with many other immune disorders. More than 10% of patients with thymoma are afflicted with hypogammaglobulinemia, and 5% suffer from erythroid hypoplasia. In contrast to the situation with myasthenia gravis, the epithelial component of the thymoma is spindle-shaped in these cases. Other associated diseases include myocarditis, dermatomyositis, rheumatoid arthritis, lupus erythematosus, scleroderma, and Sjögren syndrome. Certain malignant tumors have also been associated with thymoma, including T-cell leukemia-lymphoma and multiple myeloma.

Malignant Thymoma

Roughly one fourth of thymomas are not encapsulated and exhibit malignant features. Many of these invade locally within the thorax, and a few metastasize widely. Malignant thymomas have been divided into two general types.

Type I malignant thymoma is the most common cancer of the thymus and is virtually indistinguishable histologically from encapsulated, benign thymoma. However, it penetrates the capsule, implants on pleural or pericardial surfaces, and may metastasize to lymph nodes, lung, liver, and bone.

Type II malignant thymoma is a distinctly uncommon, invasive tumor, which is also termed *thymic carcinoma*. The morphological appearance of this tumor is highly variable and takes the form of squamous cell carcinoma, lymphoepithelioma-like carcinoma (identical to that found in the oropharynx; see Chapter 25), a sarcomatoid variant (carcinosarcoma), and a number of other rare patterns. The feature that these variants have in common is a distinct epithelial appearance, and a mediastinal tumor that lacks this feature is probably not a thymic carcinoma.

Malignant thymoma is treated by surgical excision and radiation therapy. Chemotherapy is added in cases with distant metastases. The prognosis for benign thymoma is excellent, and the presence or absence of myasthenic symptoms is of little prognostic value. In the case of type I malignant thymomas, the prognosis correlates with the extent of the disease. The majority of patients with type II thymomas die within 5 years of the diagnosis.

Other Tumors of the Thymus

CARCINOID TUMOR: The thymus gives rise to carcinoid tumor, which is similar in its morphological appearance and natural history to comparable tumors elsewhere. Thymic carcinoid tumors tend to invade locally and metastasize widely, although well-circumscribed tumors may be cured by local excision. Interestingly, one third of the patients manifest Cushing syndrome, whereas carcinoid syndrome does not occur. A thymic carcinoid tumor may also arise in the context of MEN-1 and 2A.

SMALL CELL CARCINOMA: The thymus may also be the site of another neuroendocrine tumor, namely, small cell carcinoma, which is indistinguishable from its counterpart in the lung. Of course, a primary pulmonary neoplasm must be ruled out before the diagnosis of thymic small cell carcinoma can be made.

GERM CELL TUMORS: Germ cell tumors in the thymus account for 20% of all mediastinal tumors. It is thought that the migration of germ cells during embryogenesis leaves misplaced germ cells in this location, which eventually give rise to germ cell neoplasms. The spectrum of germ cell tumors in the mediastinum parallels that in the gonads (see Chapters 17 and 18). Mature cystic teratoma is the most common of these thymic tumors. Seminoma, embryonal carcinoma, endodermal sinus tumor, teratocarcinoma, and choriocarcinoma all occur. With the exception of mature cystic teratoma, which afflicts both sexes equally, all the other tumors show a substantial male predilection, and thymic seminoma occurs only in men. In general, the prognosis is similar to that of comparable gonadal tumors.

Tumors consisting of admixtures of thymic and adipose tissues have been termed *thymolipomas*. Non-neoplastic tumors include thymic and mesothelial cysts and enteric-type cysts.

Pineal Gland

ANATOMY AND FUNCTION

The pineal gland is only 5 to 7 mm in maximal diameter and weighs barely 100 to 180 mg. Shaped like a minute pine cone, it is located below the posterior edge of the corpus callosum and between the superior colliculi. The gland develops as an outpouching of the posterior segment of the roof of the third ventricle, to which it remains linked by a stalk. The stalk is not a vestigial structure but rather is rich in nerve fibers and seemingly arises from the brain. The significance of these fibers is unclear, and their connection with pineal cells remains controversial.

Microscopically, the pineal gland is composed of cords and clusters of large epithelial-like cells, termed *pinealocytes*. As in paraganglia, interlacing cytoplasmic processes and neurosecretory granules are seen. A second cell type is similar to brain astrocytes. It is not clear whether these cells are simply glial or whether they represent an anatomically and functionally distinct cell class.

The pineal gland produces a number of neurotransmitter substances, among which the most abundant and readily demonstrable is melatonin. Although in lower animals melatonin has a significant depigmenting effect, such an action has not been shown in mammals. Melatonin is found in the blood, cerebrospinal fluid, and urine. Experimentally, in higher mammals and humans, it induces sleep and increases brain serotonin. Since melatonin levels are distinctly higher at night than during waking hours, it has been suggested that it may function as a sleep inducer.

Serotonin and several peptides are also produced by the pineal. Significant among the peptides is arginine vasotocin, a hormone that has been shown to have important antigonadotropic activity in animals. Melatonin may act as a releasing factor for arginine vasotocin.

About the time of puberty, calcifications in the pineal gland can be shown in autopsy specimens or by various radiological techniques. Focal cystic changes may also be seen, but these alterations do not seem to have clinical manifestations.

NEOPLASMS

Tumors of the pineal gland are curiosities, representing less than 1% of brain tumors.

- **Germ cell tumors:** These are the most frequent pineal neoplasms and are apparently derived from misplaced germ cells. Germinomas, or dysgerminomas, account for about 60% of pineal tumors and are indistinguishable from their gonadal counterparts. Other variants of germ cell tumors in the pineal gland are embryonal carcinoma, choriocarcinoma, endodermal sinus tumor, and teratoma.
- **Pineocytoma:** This benign tumor is a solid, well-circumscribed mass that replaces the pineal body. Microscopically, small tumor cells with round nuclei and eosinophilic cytoplasm appear as nests separated by thin strands of connective tissue. The overall appearance is similar to that of a paraganglioma, but neurosecretory granules are not present.
- **Pineoblastoma:** This highly malignant tumor is extremely rare and occurs in the young adults. Soft masses, often showing hemorrhagic and necrotic areas, invade and infiltrate the surrounding structures. Microscopically, pineoblastoma consists of small oval cells, with dark nuclei and scanty cytoplasm, resembling medulloblastoma or neuroblastoma. Mitoses are generally numerous.

Regardless of histological type, tumors of the pineal gland present with signs and symptoms related to their impact on the surrounding structures, including headaches and visual and behavioral disturbances. In children, these tumors are frequently associated with precocious puberty, predominantly in boys. The prognosis of pineal tumors is poor in the case of pineoblastoma but is also guarded in cases of pineocytoma. Even non-neoplastic pineal cysts pose a great threat to life because of the difficulties involved in their removal.

SUGGESTED READING

BOOKS

Bloodworth JMB Jr (ed): *Endocrine pathology: general and surgical*, 2nd ed. Baltimore: Williams & Wilkins, 1982.

DeGroot LJ (ed): *Endocrinology*. 3rd ed. Philadelphia: WB Saunders, 1994.

DeLellis RA: *Tumors of the parathyroid gland. Atlas to tumor pathology*, 3rd Series. Fascicle 16. Washington, DC: Armed Forces Institute of Pathology, 1993.

Felig P, Baxter JD, Frohman, LA (eds): *Endocrinology and metabolism*. New York: McGraw-Hill, 1995.

Lack EE (ed): *Pathology of the adrenal gland.* New York: Churchill Livingstone, 1990.

Lack EE: *Tumors of adrenal glands and extra-adrenal paraganglia. Atlas of tumor pathology*, 3rd Series. Fascicle. Washington, DC: Armed Forces Institute of Pathology, 1997.

LiVolsi VA: *Surgical pathology of the thyroid.* Philadelphia: WB Saunders, 1990.

Mendelsohn G: *Diagnosis and pathology of endocrine diseases.* Philadelphia: JB Lippincott, 1988.

Rosai J, Carcangina ML, DeLellis RA: *Tumors of the thyroid gland. Atlas of tumor pathology,* 3rd Series. Fascicle. Washington, DC: Armed Forces Institute of Pathology, 1992.

Wilson JD, Foster DW (eds): *Williams textbook of endocrinology,* 8th ed. Philadelphia: WB Saunders, 1992.

REVIEW ARTICLES

Broon EM, Pollak M, Seidman CE, et al: Calcium ion sensing cell-surface receptors. *N Engl J Med* 333:234–240, 1995.

Chen S, Sawicka J, Betterle C, et al: Autoantibodies to steroidogenic enzymes in autoimmune polyglandular syndrome, Addison's disease and premature ovarian failure. *J Clin Endocrin Met* 81:1871–1876, 1991.

Dayan, CM, Daniels GH: Chronic autoimmune thyroiditis. *N Eng J Med* 335:99–107, 1996.

Eng C: The RET proto-oncogene in multiple endocrine neoplasia type 2 and Hirschsprung's disease. *N Engl J Med* 335:943–951, 1996.

Farid NR, Zou M, and Shi Y: Genetics of follicular thyroid cancer. *Endocrinol Metab Clin North Am* 24:865–883, 1995.

Goodfellow PJ, Wells SA, Jr: RET gene and its implications for cancer. *J Natl Cancer Inst* 87:1515–1523, 1995.

Laron Z: Disorders of growth hormone resistance in childhood. *Curr Opin Pediatr* 5:474–480, 1993.

Orth DN: Cushing's syndrome. *N Engl J Med* 332:791–803, 1995.

Perez Jurado LA, Argente J: Molecular basis of familial growth hormone deficiency. *Horm Res* 42:189–197, 1994.

Schnabel P, Bohm M: Mutations of signal-transducing G proteins in human disease. *J Mol Med* 73:221–228, 1995.

CHAPTER 22

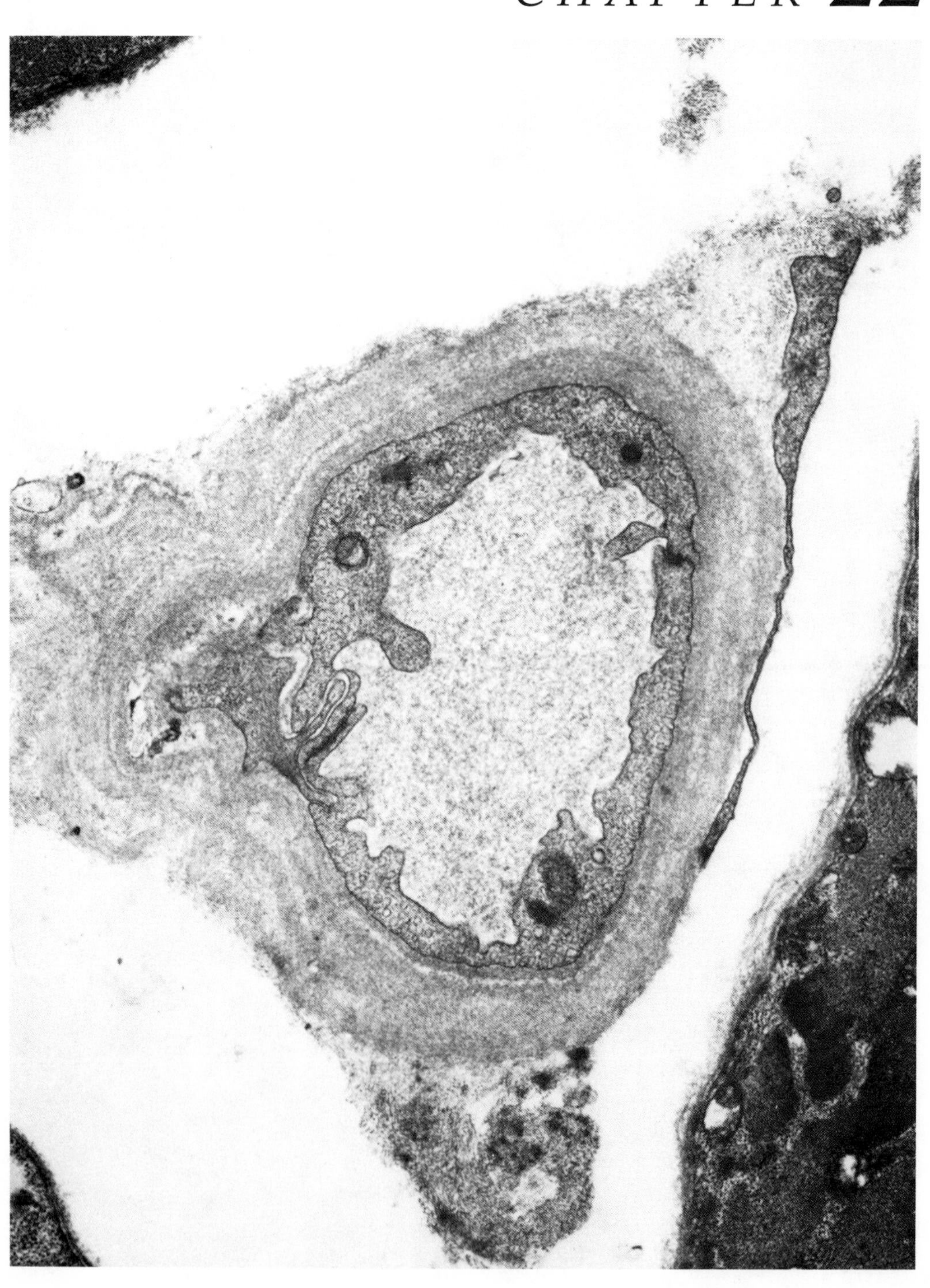

Diabetes

John E. Craighead

FIGURE *22-1 (see opposite page)*
Electron micrograph of a muscle capillary from a 56-year-old woman with type II diabetes mellitus. Note the thickened basement membrane, a characteristic late lesion in this disease.

Almost a century ago, the noted physician Sir William Osler defined diabetes mellitus as "a syndrome due to a disturbance in carbohydrate metabolism from various causes, in which sugar appears in the urine, associated with thirst, polyuria, wasting and imperfect oxidation of fats." Although he described the salient clinical features of the disease, Osler also emphasized the diverse etiologies of diabetes. Some years later, heritable predispositions to diabetes were described. In the 1970s, a Congressional commission concluded that diabetes is "a complex metabolic derangement, characterized by either relative or absolute insulin deficiency."

Various descriptors for diabetes were in vogue for periods of time and then discarded. Currently, two common forms of diabetes are recognized. Insulin-dependent diabetes mellitus (IDDM) is also referred to as type I or juvenile-onset diabetes. By contrast, noninsulin-dependent diabetes mellitus (NIDDM) is also known as type II or maturity-onset diabetes (Table 22-1).

Insulin-dependent diabetes mellitus customarily occurs in children and adolescents, but it occasionally develops in adults. By contrast, most cases of NIDDM appear during the later decades of life, although an uncommon heritable form of the disease (maturity onset diabetes of the young, MODY) is sometimes seen. IDDM is uncommon compared with NIDDM, which affects 5% of adult Americans (Fig. 22-2).

Diabetes occasionally develops during pregnancy but persists only infrequently after parturition. Glucocorticoid treatment can also cause a diabetes-like syndrome, which disappears after treatment is halted. A number of rare clinical syndromes are also associated with either frank hyperglycemia or abnormal glucose metabolism. Because these conditions are uncommon and have a genetic predisposition, they will not be considered in detail.

The current criteria for the diagnosis of diabetes pragmatically define a disease that exhibits enormous variability in its biochemical and clinical features. If a patient has typical symptoms and markedly elevated concentrations of blood glucose, the diagnosis is obvious. However, some patients have impaired glucose metabolism, but are not frankly diabetic. In such persons, a "challenge" consists of a large amount of glucose orally or intravenously (glucose tolerance test). If blood glucose concentrations increase excessively and remain persistently high, the findings are consistent with a disposition to diabetes mellitus. A few of these persons develop typical diabetes later in life. In the past, such patients often were considered to have "chemical," "latent," "borderline," "subclinical," or "asymptomatic" diabetes. These terms are rarely found in the medical literature today, and their use is discouraged because the impaired glucose metabolism in most of these patients does not progress to diabetes.

TABLE ***22-1*** **Comparison of Type I and Type II Diabetes**

	Type I	Type II
Age at onset	Usually before 20	Usually after 30
Type of onset	Abrupt; often severe	Gradual; usually subtle
Usual body weight	Normal	Overweight
Genetics (parents or siblings with diabetes)	<20%	>60%
Monozygotic twins	50% concordant	90% concordant
HLA associations	+	0
Islet cell antibodies	+	0
Islet lesions		
	Early—inflammation	
	Late—atrophy and fibrosis	Fibrosis, amyloid
Beta cells	Markedly reduced	Normal or slightly reduced
Blood insulin	Markedly reduced	Elevated or normal
Clinical management	Insulin and diet	Diet; occasionally drugs or insulin

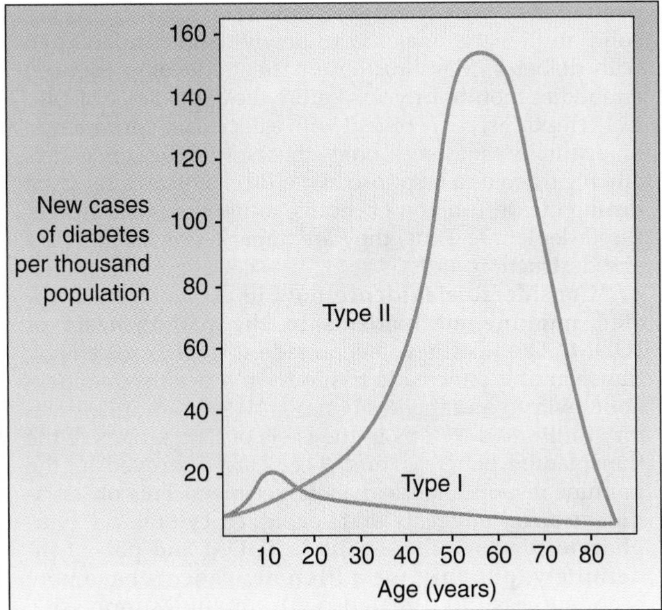

FIGURE 22-2
Age of onset of new cases of type I and type II diabetes. Type II diabetes is far more common than is type I.

INSULIN-DEPENDENT DIABETES MELLITUS

Insulin-dependent diabetes mellitus (IDDM) is a life-long disorder of glucose homeostasis that results from the autoimmune destruction of the β-cells in the islets of Langerhans. The disease is characterized by few if any functional β-cells in the islets of Langerhans and substantially reduced or nonexistent insulin secretion. As a result, body fat is metabolized as a source of energy. Oxidation of fat produces ketone bodies (acetoacetic acid and β-hydroxybutyric acid), which are released into the blood and lead to metabolic acidosis. Hyperglycemia and glucosuria produce fluid and electrolyte imbalances, which can ultimately lead to coma and death (Fig. 22-3). In fact, before insulin became commercially available, IDDM was usually fatal.

☐ **Epidemiology:** Insulin-dependent diabetes mellitus is most common among northern Europeans and their descendents, whereas it is not seen as frequently among Asians, blacks, and Native Americans. As an example, the incidence of IDDM in Finland is 20 to 40 times as great as that in Japan. Although the disorder can develop at any age, the peak age of onset coincides with puberty. An increased incidence in late fall and early winter has been documented in many geographic areas.

☐ **Pathogenesis:** A variety of factors have been incriminated in the pathogenesis of IDDM.

Genetic Factors

Many believe that susceptibility to IDDM is inherited as an autosomal recessive trait with variable penetrance, although this view is not universally accepted. Fewer than 20% of type I diabetics have a parent or sibling with the disease. In studies of identical (monozygotic) twins, in which one or both twins were diabetic, both members of the pair were affected in less than half of the cases. This lack of concordance suggests that environmental factors may contribute to the development of the disease, when superimposed on a heritable predisposition.

Additional genetic evidence has been provided by studies of the antigens of the major histocompatibility

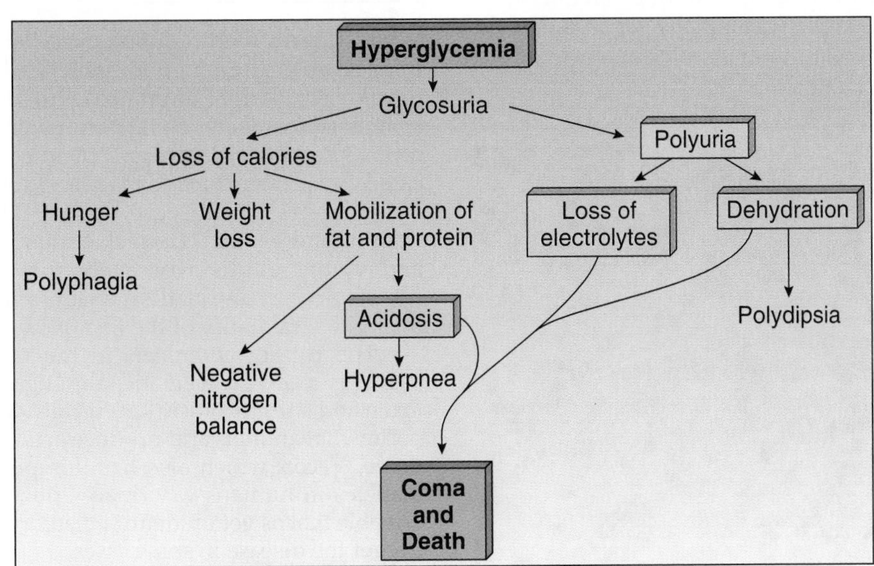

FIGURE 22-3
Symptoms and signs of uncontrolled hyperglycemia in diabetes mellitus.

complex (MHC). In fact, the only genes definitely associated with IDDM are those of the major histocompatibility complex. **In patients with IDDM, 95% express either HLA-DR3 or HLA-DR4, or both, compared with 20% of the general population.** The predisposition to IDDM is not caused by specific mutations in class II alleles, since the same nucleotide sequences in these patients are also found in normal persons.

There is evidence that susceptibility to IDDM is associated with the DQ locus and a single amino acid substitution at a specific site (codon 57) in the DQ β-chain domain. Fully 96% of patients with IDDM are homozygous for this polymorphism, compared with only 19% of healthy, unrelated persons. How this change in the composition of the class II antigen influences the development of diabetes is at present unknown. It could modulate an autoimmune T-cell response directed against the β-cell. However, there are clearly exceptions to the simple hypothesis that the disease solely reflects changes at codon 57. In fact, some 20 independent chromosomal regions have thus far been associated with susceptibility to IDDM. Interestingly, the children of fathers with IDDM are three times more likely to develop the disease than are those of diabetic mothers, an observation that indicates paternal imprinting.

Autoimmunity

The concept of an autoimmune pathogenesis for IDDM is supported by the observation that patients who die shortly after the onset of the disease often exhibit an infiltrate of mononuclear cells in and around the islets of Langerhans, termed *insulitis* (Fig. 22-4). Among the inflammatory cells, CD8+ T lymphocytes predominate, although some CD4+ cells are also present and are presumed to play a pathogenetic role. In addition, the infiltrating inflammatory cells elaborate cytokines, for example, IL-1, IL-6, interferon-α, and nitric oxide, that may further contribute to the pathogenesis of β-cell injury.

An autoimmune origin was initially suggested by the demonstration of circulating antibodies against components of the β-cells of the islets (and sometimes against insulin) in the large majority of newly diagnosed children with diabetes. Many of these patients develop islet cell antibodies months or years before the appearance of clinical symptoms, concomitant with a decreasing production of insulin by the islets. Today, these antibodies are generally regarded as a response to the β-cell antigens released during the destruction of β-cells, rather than the cause of β-cell depletion. Thus, they are a marker of β-cell injury and destruction.

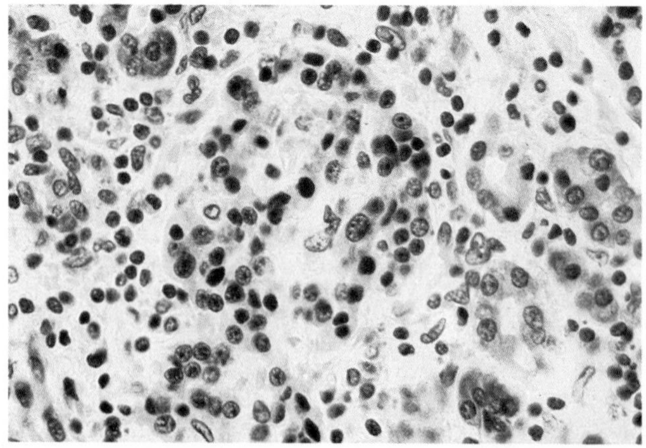

FIGURE 22-4
Insulitis in type I diabetes. A mononuclear inflammatory cell infiltrate is seen in and around the islet.

Considerable evidence now implicates cell-mediated immune mechanisms in the pathogenesis of IDDM. Attempts have been made to replace β-cells by transplanting pancreatic tissue from a healthy monozygotic twin to a diabetic sibling. However, an inflammatory infiltrate develops in the islets of Langerhans of the transplanted pancreas, and β-cells are destroyed by the immune response of the diabetic recipient. **This observation strongly suggests that sensitized cytotoxic T lymphocytes damage the β-cells in IDDM and persist indefinitely, possibly for a lifetime.** Patients have now been successfully treated with immunosuppressive drugs, particularly when such agents are administered early in the course of IDDM.

Ten percent of patients with IDDM manifest other organ-specific autoimmune diseases, for example, chronic thyroiditis, Graves disease, myasthenia gravis, Addison disease, and pernicious anemia. Interestingly, most patients with polyendocrine immune syndromes (see Chapter 22) possess HLA DR3 and DR4 histocompatibility antigens.

The lesions of IDDM develop slowly, and clinical disease becomes apparent after an average of 3 years, when insulin deprivation becomes severe. It has been estimated that a clinically significant metabolic abnormality appears only after at least 80% of the β-cells have been eliminated.

Environmental Factors

What triggers the immunological injury to the islets of Langerhans? Are diabetics genetically programmed to develop an aberrant immunological response, or do environmental insults to the islets initiate an autoimmune reaction? Recently, viruses and chemicals have been implicated as causative factors in at least some cases of IDDM. For example, the disease occasionally develops after mumps and group B coxsackievirus infections. Children and young adults who were infected *in utero* with rubellavirus occasionally develop diabetes, presumably owing to viral injury of the fetal pancreas.

The role of chemicals in the initiation of human IDDM is more problematic, although agents such as alloxan and streptozotocin specifically destroy β-cells in experimental animals and produce acute diabetes. A rodenticide, Vacor, which also has this property, has caused diabetes in humans who inadvertently ingested it. It is possible that as yet unidentified environmental chemicals trigger the disease in some cases.

Proteins in cow's milk may initiate IDDM. Breast-fed children have a lower incidence of IDDM than do those nurtured on cow's milk. Moreover, the elimination of cow's milk proteins from the diet of genetically diabetic rats reduces the incidence of the disease. It has been reported that a region of the bovine serum albumin molecule is homologous with subunits of MHC class II proteins. Bovine milk proteins may share antigenic epitopes with human cell surface proteins, thereby eliciting the production of autoreactive antibodies.

The geographic and seasonal differences in the incidence of IDDM discussed above further suggest that environmental factors are important in the pathogenesis of this disorder, although the mechanisms that mediate these effects remain obscure.

☐ **Pathology:** In children who suffer the acute onset of IDDM, the most characteristic lesion in the pancreas is an infiltrate of lymphocytes in the islets (insulitis), sometimes accompanied by a few macrophages and neutrophils (see Fig. 22-4). **As the disease becomes chronic, the β-cells of the islets are progressively depleted, and in many long-standing cases, insulin-producing cells are no longer discernible.** The loss of β-cells results in variably sized islets, many of which appear as ribbon-like cords, which are difficult to distinguish from the surrounding acinar tissue. Fibrosis of the islets may occur, but is uncommon. The amyloid deposition characteristic of NIDDM, which depends on β-cell secretion, is absent.

The exocrine pancreas in chronic IDDM often exhibits diffuse interlobular and interacinar fibrosis, accompanied by atrophy of the acinar cells.

☐ **Clinical Features:** In many patients, diabetes is discovered at the time of hospitalization because of the signs and symptoms of metabolic acidosis and ketosis, weight loss, dehydration, and electrolyte imbalance. These events sometimes occur unexpectedly and precipitously and may be life-threatening emergencies. Often the clinical onset of diabetes coincides with another acute illness, such as an infection. More frequently, patients with IDDM experience vague symptoms for weeks and months before the diagnosis is made. Prominent among these are an increase in urine output (polyuria) and thirst (polydipsia), owing to the diuresis resulting from glucosuria. In addition, many patients have an insatiable appetite (polyphagia). Nonetheless, they lose weight because of the inefficient energy utilization that results from defective carbohydrate metabolism.

NONINSULIN-DEPENDENT DIABETES MELLITUS

Noninsulin-dependent diabetes mellitus (NIDDM) is a heterogeneous disorder characterized by impaired insulin secretion and reduced tissue sensitivity to insulin. The disease usually develops in adults, its prevalence being increased in the obese and in the elderly. **Hyperglycemia in NIDDM is not caused by the destruction of β-cells but is rather a failure of the β-cells to meet an increased demand for insulin.** NIDDM affects 10 million Americans, about half of whom are undiagnosed. In fact, almost 10% of persons older than 65 years of age are affected, and 80% of patients with NIDDM are overweight (Fig. 22-5). The incidence of NIDDM is higher in women than in men, and in the United States it is greater among blacks and Hispanics than among whites.

☐ **Pathogenesis:** The common denominator in the pathogenesis of NIDDM is a reduction in glucose-stimulated insulin secretion compounded by peripheral resistance to the actions of insulin. The major controversy has focused on whether insulin resistance or insulin secretion is the primary defect in the pathogenesis of NIDDM. **The current consensus holds that NIDDM is a genetically programmed failure of the β-cell to compensate for peripheral insulin resistance** (Fig. 22-6).

Genetic Factors

Multifactorial inheritance is a key contributor to the development of NIDDM. Sixty percent of patients have either a parent or a sibling with the disease. In some popu-

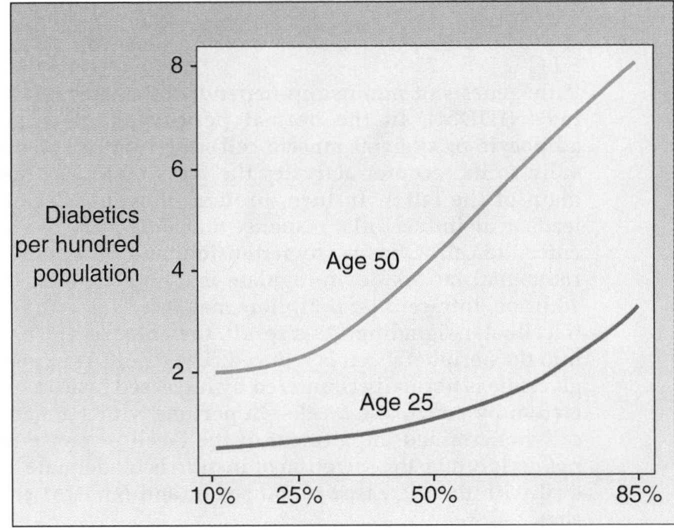

FIGURE 22-5
Occurrence of diabetes in relation to body weight in young and older adults. In persons over 50 years of age, the risk of diabetes increases linearly with body weight more than 25% above normal.

lations, notably the Pima Indians of Arizona and the natives of Nauru in the Gilbert Islands of the Pacific, one third to one half of all persons are afflicted with NIDDM. When one member of a monozygotic twinship has the disease, the second twin is almost invariably affected. However, an association with genes of the MHC, as seen in IDDM, is not found. Despite the high familial prevalence of the disease, the precise mode of inheritance remains to be defined. Constitutional factors such as obesity, which itself has strong determinants, hypertension, and the amount of exercise influence the expression of the disorder and thus complicate genetic analyses.

Glucose Metabolism

In a normal person, the extracellular concentration of glucose is exquisitely controlled, even though the amount of dietary carbohydrate fluctuates and the peripheral utilization of glucose also varies. This rigid control is medi-

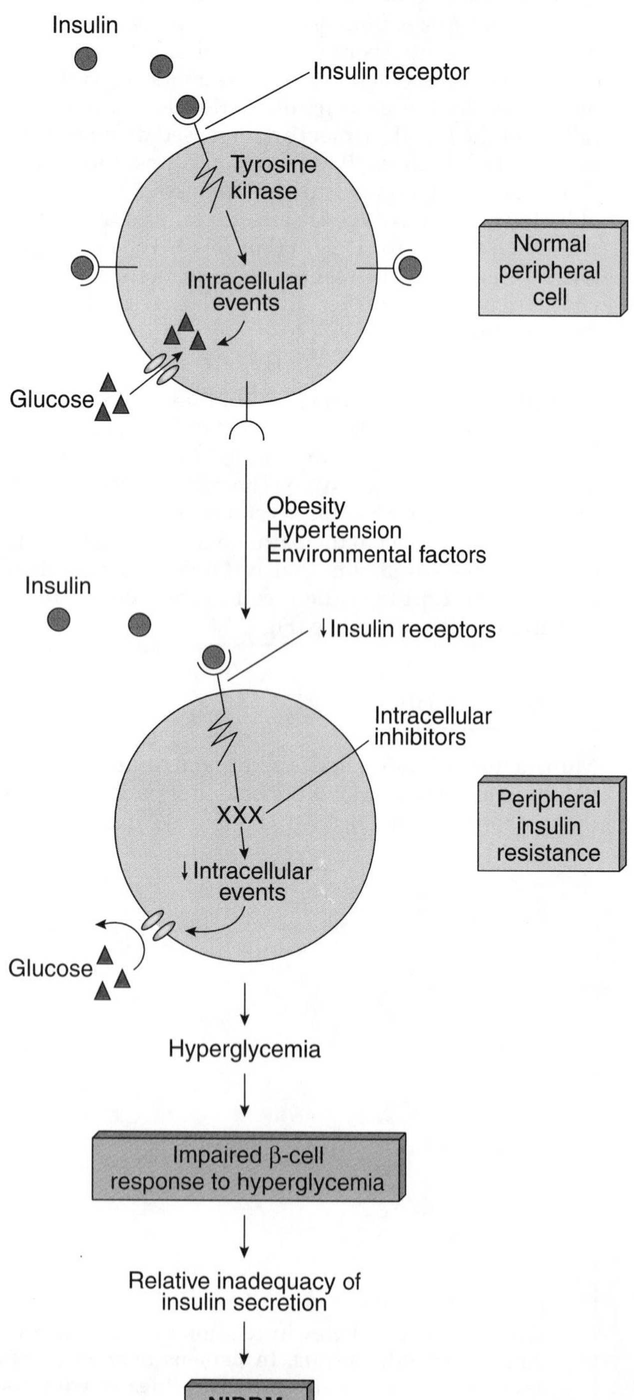

FIGURE 22-6
Pathogenesis of noninsulin-dependent diabetes mellitus (NIDDM). In the normal peripheral cell (e.g., adipocyte or skeletal muscle cell), the binding of insulin to its receptor activates the tyrosine kinase domain of the latter. In turn, protein phosphorylation leads to an intracellular response that allows glucose to enter the cell. Obesity, hypertension, and other environmental factors down-regulate insulin receptors. In addition, intracellular inhibitors may interfere with intracellualar signaling. As a result, the entry of glucose into the peripheral cell is reduced. The resulting hyperglycemia is normally countered by increased insulin secretion by pancreatic β-cells. In persons with a genetically determined impairment of the β-cell response to hyperglycemia, the secretion of insulin is inadequate to deal with the increased blood sugar, and NIDDM ensues.

ated by the opposing actions of insulin and glucagon. Following a carbohydrate-rich meal, the absorption of glucose from the gut leads to hyperglycemia, which is limited to 10 mM glucose; the fasting level of 5 mM glucose is restored within 2 hours. This response reflects the stimulation of insulin secretion by the pancreatic β-cells and the insulin-mediated increase in glucose uptake by the peripheral cells, principally adipose and muscle tissue. At the same time, insulin inhibits hepatic glucose production by antagonizing the release of glucagon from the islets and by blocking its effect on the liver.

β-Cell Function

Persons with NIDDM manifest impaired insulin release by the β-cell in response to glucose stimulation, a lesion that is most prominent in those with severe hyperglycemia. A similar lesion is also observed in a number of rodent strains that develop NIDDM. In these animal models, a deficiency in the glucose transporter (GLUT-2) in the plasma membrane of β-cells, and in its mRNA, was demonstrated, and it was initially proposed that this reduction in GLUT-2 was responsible for the impaired insulin response to hyperglycemia. However, current evidence suggests that the decrease in β-cell GLUT-2 expression is secondary to other more primary metabolic abnormalities and, thus, is not the cause of the impaired β-cell response to glucose, although it may aggravate it.

Studies of persons who develop autosomal dominant NIDDM at an early age (maturity-onset diabetes of the young, MODY) have documented mutations in the genes that code for glucokinase. It is, therefore, thought that glucokinase is an important glucose sensor of the β-cell, and impairment of its function causes the MODY phenotype. However, mutations in still other unidentified genes can also lead to the development of MODY. In any case, no link has been discovered between any of the genes involved in the pathogenesis of MODY and those associated with late-onset NIDDM. In this context, the genetic heterogeneity of MODY suggests that the more common late-onset forms of NIDDM will also prove to be similarly heterogeneous. In view of the dominant inheritance and strong penetrance of MODY, it is likely that the genes responsible for late-onset NIDDM are less important than the MODY genes and only result in overt diabetes in the presence of insulin resistance or environmental influences, such as sedentary behavior or a high-fat diet.

Insulin Resistance

Peripheral insulin resistance is a fundamental component in the pathogenesis of NIDDM. Importantly, insulin resistance is also associated with other conditions, most notably obesity (see Chapter 8). Despite the defect in insulin secretion by the β-cell, many patients with NIDDM exhibit an increased insulin concentration in the blood. This seemingly paradoxical situation is attributed to a reduction in the number of insulin receptors in the plasma membranes of adipocytes and skeletal muscle cells. Thus, patients with NIDDM are hyperglycemic, but their cells are relatively deficient in insulin and they metabolize glucose inefficiently.

The insulin receptor is composed of two linked glycoprotein subunits, a β-component that binds insulin and an α-subunit that serves as a transmembrane protein kinase (tyrosine kinase). In obese persons, for unknown reasons, the number of insulin receptors on the plasma membrane is reduced. This down-regulation of insulin receptors in obesity may account for the high circulating insulin levels. In turn, high insulin levels in the blood further down-regulate the expression of insulin receptors in fat and skeletal muscle. By contrast, receptor density is up-regulated by a low-calorie diet and exercise. Rarely, insulin resistance is caused by a mutation in the extracellular hormone-binding domain of the insulin receptor or in the cytoplasmic tyrosine kinase region. Finally, a number of intracellular inhibitors of insulin action have been postulated to play a role in the insulin resistance of NIDDM.

□ **Pathology:** A variety of microscopic lesions are found in the islets of Langerhans of many, but not all, patients with NIDDM. These changes are not diagnostic, since they are occasionally seen in nondiabetic persons. Unlike IDDM, there is no consistent reduction in the number of β-cells, and no morphological lesions of these cells have been identified by light or electron microscopy.

In some islets, fibrous tissue accumulates, sometimes to such a degree that the islets are obliterated. In other patients, amyloid is present (Fig. 22-7), particularly in those older than 60 years of age. This type of amyloid is composed of a polypeptide molecule known as *amylin*, which

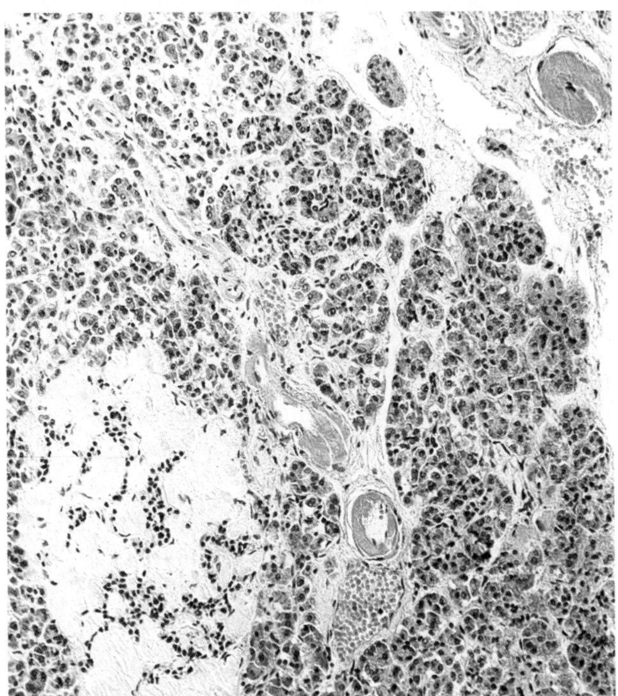

FIGURE 22-7
Amyloidosis (hyalinization) of an islet in the pancreas of a patient with type II diabetes. The blood vessel adjacent to the islet shows the advanced hyaline arteriolosclerosis characteristic of diabetes.

is secreted with insulin by the β-cell (see Chapter 23). Importantly, as many as 20% of aged nondiabetic persons also have amyloid deposits in their pancreas, a finding that has been attributed to the aging process itself.

Diabetes or impaired glucose tolerance is found in 80% of patients with pancreatic cancer. This condition is not due to a loss of β-cells as a result of the tumor, but appears to be caused by the release of amylin or an amylin-like protein by the malignant cells. This protein seems to produce insulin resistance in fat and muscle cells.

COMPLICATIONS OF DIABETES

The discovery of insulin in the early years of the 20th century promised to cure diabetes, but as diabetics lived longer it became apparent that they were subject to numerous complications (Fig. 22-8). For many years, a controversy raged as to whether these complications were effects independent of the disordered insulin and carbohydrate metabolism or whether they resulted from hyperglycemia itself. **It is today generally accepted that the development of secondary lesions in the diabetic patient relates largely to the severity and chronicity of hyperglycemia.** However, even with seemingly adequate management, many of the secondary effects of diabetes still evolve. **From a practical perspective, control of blood glucose remains the major means by which the development of diabetic complications can be minimized.**

The biochemical basis and the pathogenesis of the complicating lesions of diabetes differ from one tissue to another. Two distinct mechanisms have been proposed to account for the development of many of these changes.

PROTEIN GLYCOSYLATION: Glucose binds to a wide variety of proteins, roughly in proportion to the severity of hyperglycemia. Glycosylation is a process by which glucose attaches to a free amino group (typically a lysine or valine residue) on a protein without catalytic mediation by a specific enzyme. Numerous proteins in cells that are not insulin-dependent, as well as extracellular structural proteins and circulating molecules, may be modified in this manner. Such proteins include, but are not limited to, hemoglobin, components of the crystalline lens, collagen, myelin, fibrinogen, fibrin, cathepsin B, and antithrombin III. Assays for glycosylated hemoglobin (hemoglobin A_{1C}) are now used clinically to monitor the management of hyperglycemia. In a person with poorly regulated blood glucose, more than 10% of the hemoglobin is glycosylated.

The initial glycosylation products (Schiff bases) are labile and dissociate at the same rate at which they are formed. Thus, they accumulate only in proportion to the blood glucose concentration. With the passage of time, these labile products undergo complex chemical rearrangements to form stable *advanced glycosylation products.* These compounds are bound covalently to amino groups in proteins. As a result, the function of the protein is altered or inactivated. For example, albumin and IgG do not bind to normal collagen, whereas they attach to glycosylated collagen. The cross-linking of proteins is believed to contribute to the characteristic thickening of vascular basement membranes in diabetes. Moreover, the binding of glycosylated IgG may activate the membrane attack complex of complement, thereby producing cell injury.

Importantly, unlike the initial labile glycosylation products, advanced products can continue to cross-link proteins despite a return of blood glucose to a normal level. Thus, in a canine model of diabetic retinopathy (see later), this complication is prevented only if blood glucose is strictly controlled within two months of the initiation of hyperglycemia. The significance of advanced glycosylation products is underscored by the observation that patients with diabetic retinopathy have higher levels of these products than do diabetics without this complication. Moreover, aminoguanidine, a compound that inhibits the formation of advanced glycosylation products, has been found to provide some protection against diabetic complications in experimental animals, including damage to the kidneys, nerves, and retina.

THE POLYOL PATHWAY: Hyperglycemia also increases the uptake of glucose in tissues that are not dependent on insulin. The increased flux of glucose is handled by a number of metabolic routes, of which the polyol pathway is the best characterized:

$$\text{glucose} + \text{NADH} + \text{H}^+ \xrightarrow{\text{aldose reductase}} \text{sorbitol} + \text{NAD}^+$$

The polyol pathway leads to the accumulation of sorbitol, a sugar alcohol (polyol) that is suspected to be responsible for diabetic complications in a variety of tissues, including peripheral nerves, retina, lens, and kidney. Cells of these tissues contain aldose reductase, an enzyme that has a low affinity for glucose. Thus, in the normoglycemic state, the formation of sorbitol proceeds slowly. However, the presence of hyperglycemia drives the reaction forward, and sorbitol accumulates in the cells.

The mechanism by which an accumulation of sorbitol causes tissue injury is not fully understood. In the lens, the accumulation of this alcohol may simply create an osmotic gradient, which causes an influx of fluid and consequent swelling. Sorbitol may also be directly toxic to cells. Increased intracellular sorbitol has been linked to decreased myoinositol (a precursor of phosphoinositides), lowered activity of protein kinase C, and an inhibition of the plasma membrane sodium pump. In animals with experimentally induced diabetes, drugs that inhibit aldose reductase prevent the development of cataracts, retinal damage, peripheral neuropathy, and early functional derangements in the kidney. However, the results of experimental therapeutic studies in humans have been inconclusive.

Atherosclerosis

The extent and severity of atherosclerotic lesions in large and medium-sized arteries are increased in long-standing diabetes, and their development tends to be accelerated. **Cardiovascular disease, including atherosclerotic heart**

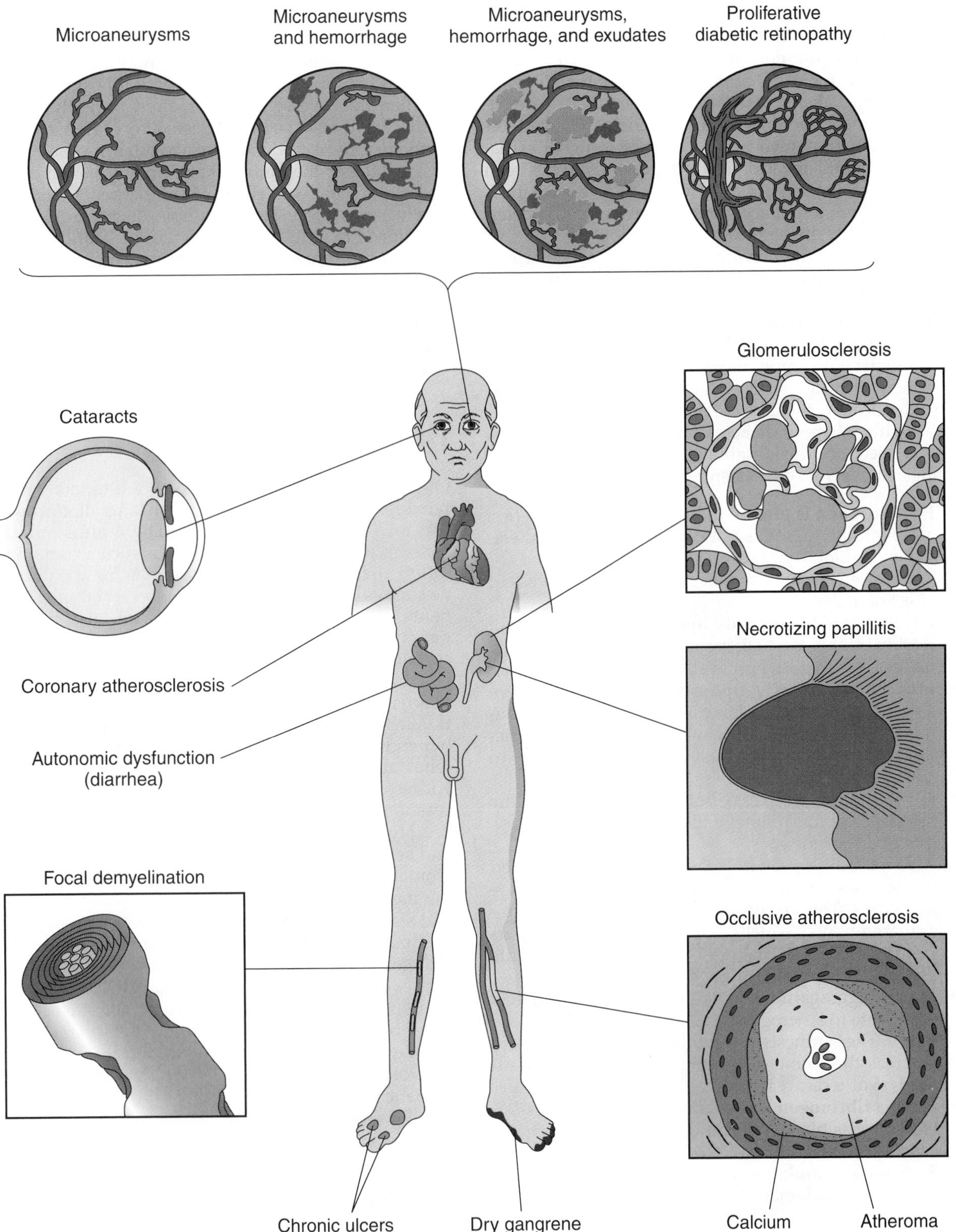

FIGURE *22-8*
Secondary complication of diabetes. The effects of diabetes on a number of vital organs result in complications that may be incapacitating (cerebral and peripheral vascular disease), painful (neuropathy), or life-threatening (coronary artery disease, pyelonephritis with necrotizing papillitis).

disease and ischemic stroke, is the major cause of death among adults with diabetes, accounting for half of all deaths in this population. With respect to coronary atherosclerosis, the usual protective effect of female sex is eliminated by diabetes, and coronary artery disease develops at a younger age than in nondiabetic patients. Moreover, mortality from myocardial infarction is higher in diabetic than in nondiabetic patients. Importantly, it has been shown that diabetes is a risk factor for these effects independent of conditions that commonly accompany diabetes, including obesity, hypertension, and dyslipidemias.

Occlusive peripheral vascular disease, particularly of the lower extremities, is a common complication of diabetes. Vascular insufficiency leads to ulcers and gangrene of the toes and feet, complications that ultimately necessitate amputation. Indeed, diabetes accounts for 40% of the nontraumatic limb amputations in the United States.

Atherosclerotic lesions in the diabetic are morphologically identical to those occurring in nondiabetics. The mechanisms whereby diabetes promotes atherosclerosis is the subject of considerable study, and a number of pathogenetic factors have been proposed:

- **Hypertension** is present in half of all adult diabetics, although the reason is not obvious. A sustained elevation in blood pressure is a known risk factor for atherosclerosis, and may aggravate the independent effect of diabetes.
- **Glycosylated low-density lipoproteins (LDL)** do not readily bind to the LDL receptor in the liver, thereby making LDL cholesterol available to the arterial wall.
- **Lower high-density lipoprotein (HDL) levels** in some diabetic subjects have been attributed to an enhanced turnover of glycosylated HDL. HDL is believed to exert a protective effect with respect to atherosclerosis.
- **Glycosylation and cross-linking of proteins in the arterial wall** may damage the vessel and predispose it to atherosclerosis.
- **A defect in lipoprotein lipase** has been documented in diabetics and leads to impaired lipolysis of chylomicrons. This results in the retention of chylomicron remnants, which is the basis for the hypertriglyceridemia of diabetes. Chylomicron remnants are considered to be atherogenic.
- **Platelet aggregation** is enhanced in diabetes and may contribute to atherogenesis at sites of endothelial cell injury. The synthesis of thromboxane A_2 is increased, whereas the counterbalancing effects of prostaglandin I_2 synthesis are reduced.
- **Plasma fibrinogen** levels tend to be increased in diabetics, possibly accelerating the development of atherosclerosis.
- **Sorbitol accumulation and advanced glycosylation** products may damage the cells of the vessel wall and may predispose to atherosclerosis.

Diabetic Microvascular Disease

Hyaline arteriolosclerosis (see Fig. 22-7) **and capillary basement membrane thickening** (see Fig. 22-1) **are characteristic vascular changes in diabetics.** Hypertension certainly contributes to the development of the arteriolar lesions. In addition, an increased deposition of basement membrane proteins, which also may become glycosylated, occurs in diabetes. Aggregation of platelets in the smaller blood vessels and impaired fibrinolytic mechanisms have also been suggested to play a role in the pathogenesis of diabetic microvascular disease.

Whatever the pathogenetic processes, the effects of disease in small vessels on tissue perfusion and wound healing are profound. For example, microvascular disease is believed to reduce blood flow to the heart, which is already compromised by coronary atherosclerosis. Healing of chronic ulcers that develop from trauma and infection of the feet in diabetic patients is commonly defective, in part because of microvascular disease. The major complications of diabetic microvascular disease involve the kidney and the retina.

Diabetic Nephropathy

Of patients with IDDM, 30% to 40% ultimately develop renal failure (Fig. 22-9). A somewhat smaller proportion (up to 20%) of patients with NIDDM are similarly affected. Conversely, since diabetes is such a common condition, diabetic nephropathy accounts for one third of all new cases of end-stage renal disease. Although some patients with IDDM die from uremia, the large majority of patients with this disorder who develop nephropathy succumb to cardiovascular disease, the risk of this complication being 40 times greater than in diabetics with normal renal function. The prevalence of diabetic nephropathy increases with the severity and duration of the hyperglycemia. Blacks who suffer from diabetes develop renal failure two to three times more often than do whites. **Kidney disease due to diabetes is now the most common reason for renal transplantation among adults.**

Hyperglycemia leads to glomerular hypertension and renal hyperperfusion. It is thought that increased glomerular pressure favors the deposition of protein in the mesangium, thereby resulting in glomerulosclerosis and eventually in renal failure. Advanced glycosylation products and lipoprotein abnormalities may contribute to changes in the chemical composition of basement membrane components of the glomerulus. Interestingly, cigarette smoking has been reported to increase the severity of both diabetic microvascular disease and glomerulopathy. Regardless of the underlying mechanism, strict control of blood glucose levels retards the development of diabetic nephropathy. Treatment with angiotensin-converting enzyme (ACE) inhibitors, which reduce blood pressure and renal perfusion, has resulted in a significant retardation of the progression of diabetic nephropathy.

The glomeruli in the kidney of the diabetic exhibit a unique lesion referred to as *Kimmelstiel-Wilson disease or diabetic glomerulosclerosis* (see Chapter 16). Two microscopic patterns are seen. In the more common one, spherical masses of basement membrane-like material accumulate in the lobules of the glomeruli (Fig. 22-10). The second form is characterized by a more diffuse, although somewhat irregular, deposition of this material throughout the glomerulus. The latter change must be differentiated from membranous nephropathy. The onset of

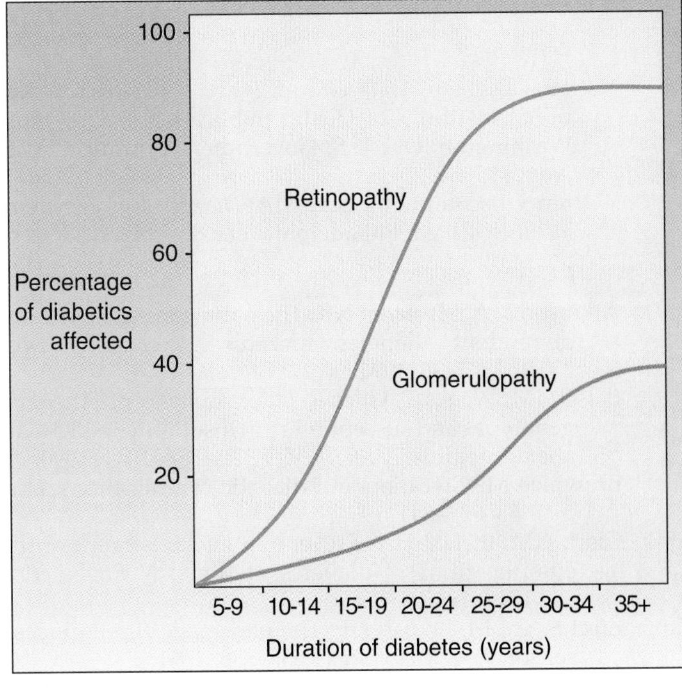

FIGURE 22-9
Frequency of retinopathy and glomerulopathy in type I diabetes.

glomerular disease is heralded clinically by the appearance of small amounts of protein in the urine. Proteinuria increases with the passage of time, after which a progressive decline in renal function ensues.

Diabetic Retinopathy

Diabetic retinopathy is the most important cause of blindness in the Unites States in persons under the age of 60 years, the risk being higher in IDDM than in NIDDM. In fact, 10% of patients with IDDM of 30 years' duration are legally blind. Nevertheless, since there are many more patients with NIDDM than IDDM, persons with the former condition comprise the majority of patients with diabetic retinopathy. Retinopathy is the most devastating ophthalmic complication of diabetes, although glaucoma, cataracts, and corneal disease occur with increased frequency (see Chapter 29). The prevalence of retinopathy relates to the duration and control of diabetes (see Fig. 22-9). Diabetic retinopathy is discussed in detail in Chapter 29.

Diabetic Neuropathy

Peripheral sensory impairment and autonomic nerve dysfunction are among the most common and distressing complications of diabetes. Changes in the nerves are complex, and abnormalities in axons, the myelin sheath, and Schwann cells have all been found. In addition, disease of the small blood vessels of the nerves contributes to the disorder. There is also evidence to suggest that hyperglycemia increases the perception of pain, independent of any structural lesions in the nerves.

Peripheral neuropathy is characterized by pain and abnormal sensations in the extremities. Fine touch, pain detection, and proprioception are ultimately lost. As a result, the diabetic tends to ignore irritation and minor trauma to the feet, joints, and lower extremities. Thus, peripheral neuropathy can be a major factor in the development of ulcers of the feet, which so commonly plague patients with severe diabetes. It also plays a role in the painless destructive joint disease that occasionally occurs.

Although autonomic nerve dysfunction is subtle, abnormalities in the neurogenic regulation of cardiovascular and gastrointestinal functions frequently result in pos-

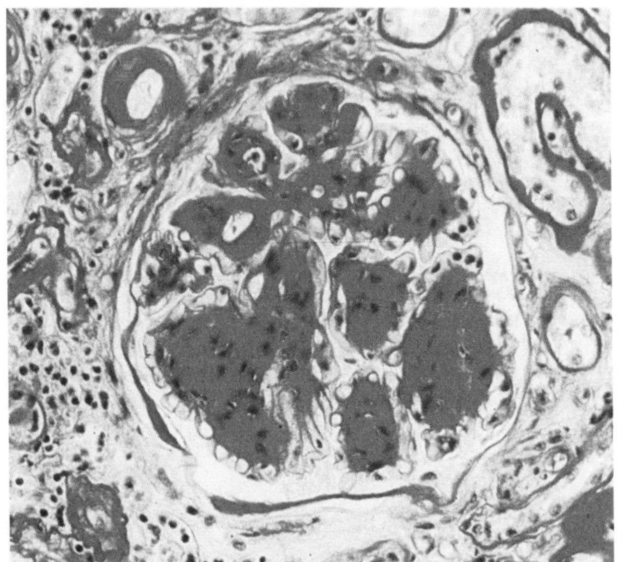

FIGURE 22-10
Diabetic glomerulosclerosis. A periodic acid–Schiff stain demonstrates nodular accumulations of basement membrane–like material in the glomerulus.

tural hypotension and problems of gut motility, such as diarrhea. Erectile dysfunction and retrograde ejaculation are common complications of autonomic dysfunction, although vascular disease is often a contributing factor. Occasionally, diabetics develop a hypotonic urinary bladder, which results in the retention of urine and predisposes to infection.

Infections

Bacterial and fungal infections complicate the life of the diabetic in whom hyperglycemia is poorly controlled. Multiple abnormalities in the host response to microbial invasion have been described in such patients. Leukocyte function is compromised, and the immune response is blunted. In the preinsulin era, tuberculosis and purulent infections were life-threatening. Fortunately, with good control, the diabetic patient today is much less susceptible to infections. However, urinary tract infections continue to pose a problem, in part because a dystonic bladder retains urine. Pyelonephritis is a constant threat for the patient with diabetes, and necrotizing papillitis may be a devastating complication of renal infection (see Chapter 17).

Pregnancy

Evidence of diabetes develops in 1% to 2% of seemingly healthy women during pregnancy, but it continues after parturition in only a small proportion of these patients. The metabolic basis for this syndrome, termed *gestational diabetes*, is uncertain.

Pregnancy is a metabolic challenge for a diabetic woman. In the preinsulin era, many diabetic women died during pregnancy, and fetal loss was substantial. Although this grim outlook has changed dramatically with modern treatment, the fetus continues to be at risk, and prenatal complications are common. **Diabetic mothers tend to give birth to large infants, making labor and delivery difficult.** These infants are often delivered by cesarean section, a procedure that increases the risk of respiratory distress syndrome of the newborn. In addition, infants of diabetic mothers frequently are hypoglycemic at birth. Their pancreatic islets are hyperplastic, because the insulin supply of the fetus was called upon by the mother during gestation.

Infants of diabetic mothers show a 5% to 10% incidence of major developmental abnormalities. These include anomalies of the heart and great vessels and neural tube defects, such as anencephaly and spina bifida. The frequency of these lesions relates to the control of maternal diabetes during early gestation.

SUGGESTED READING

BOOKS

National Diabetes Data Group: *Diabetes in America.* National Institutes of Health publication No. 85-1468. Washington, DC: U.S. Government Printing Office, August 1985.

Warren S, Lecompt PM, Legg MA: *The pathology of diabetes mellitus,* 4th ed. Philadelphia: Lea & Febiger, 1966.

REVIEW ARTICLES

Atkinson MA, Maclaren NK: The pathogenesis of insulin-dependent diabetes mellitus. *N Engl J Med* 331:1428–1436, 1994.

Baisch JM, Weeks T, Giles R, et al: Analysis of HLA-DQ genotypes and susceptibility in insulin-dependent diabetes mellitus. *N Engl J Med* 322:1836–1841, 1990.

Brownlee M: Glycation and diabetic complications. *Diabetes* 43: 836–841, 1994.

Clark CM, Jr, Lee DA: Prevention and treatment of the complications of diabetes mellitus. *N Engl J Med* 332:1210–1217, 1995.

Efrat S, Tal M, Lodish HF: The pancreatic β-cell glucose sensor. *Trends Biol Sci* 19:535–538, 1994.

Frank RN: The aldolase reductase controversy. *Diabetes* 43: 169–172, 1994.

Kahr R: Insulin action, diabetogenesis, and the cause of type II diabetes. *Diabetes* 43:1066–1079, 1994.

Kuhl C, Hornness PJ, Andersen O: Etiology and pathophysiology of gestational diabetes mellitus. *Diabetes* 34:66–70, 1985.

Merimee TJ: Diabetic retinopathy: A synthesis of perspectives. *N Engl J Med* 322:978–979, 1990.

Nathan DM: Long-term complications of diabetes mellitus. *N Engl J Med* 328:1676–1685, 1993.

Orchard TJ, Dorman JS, Maser RE, et al: Prevalence of complications in IDDM by sex and duration. Pittsburgh Epidemiology of Diabetes Complications Study II. *Diabetes* 39:1116–1124, 1990.

Partanen J, Niskanen L, Lehtinen J, et al: Natural history of peripheral neuropathy in patients with non-insulin-dependent diabetes mellitus. *N Engl J Med* 333:89–94, 1996.

Pimenta W, Korytkowski M, Mitrakou A, et al: Pancreatic beta-cell dysfunction as the primary genetic lesion in NIDDM. *JAMA* 273: 1855–1861, 1995.

Polonsky KS, Sturis J, Bell GI: Non-insulin-dependent diabetes mellitus—a genetically programmed failure of the beta cell to compensate for insulin resistance. *N Engl J Med* 334:777–783, 1996.

Seino S, Seino M, Bell GI: Human insulin-receptor gene. *Diabetes* 39:129–133, 1990.

CHAPTER 23

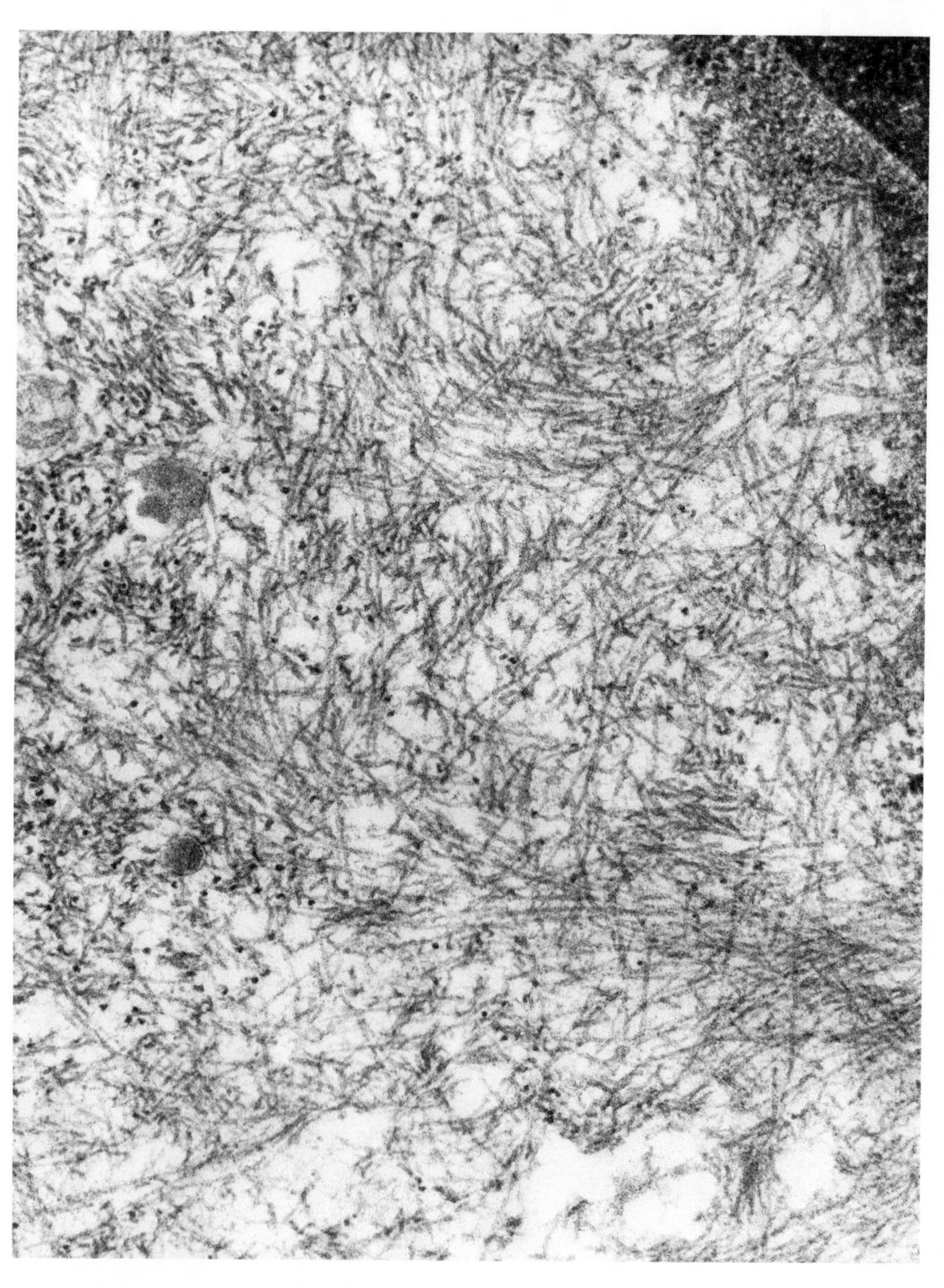

Amyloidosis

Robert Kisilevsky

FIGURE 23-1 *(see opposite page)*
Amyloid deposits in tissue. Parallel and interlacing arrays of fibrils are evident in this electron micrograph.

Amyloid, *refers to a group of diverse extracellular protein deposits, which have (1) common morphological properties, (2) affinities for specific dyes, and (3) a characteristic appearance under polarized light.* **Although they vary in amino acid sequence, all amyloid proteins are folded in such as way as to share common ultrastructural and physical properties.**

Disorders associated with amyloid deposition have been known for more than 300 years, but it was not until Virchow's time in the mid-19th century that attempts were made to define the nature of the tissue deposits by their staining properties. Amyloid stained blue with iodine, which was then in use for demonstrating cellulose or starch. This staining not only led to coining of the term *amyloid* (starch-like), but also incorrectly suggested its fundamental nature. Neither starch nor cellulose is a constituent of amyloid, and a different complex carbohydrate is responsible for its iodine-staining properties. Amyloid deposits are composed of two classes of constituents:

A DISEASE-SPECIFIC FIBRILLARY PROTEIN: The nature of this protein varies with the underlying disease. The tertiary structure of the protein and the manner in which it interacts with other molecules are responsible for the characteristics of amyloid. **The specific fibrillary protein in various types of amyloid is now the determining factor in the classification of amyloid.**

A SET OF COMMON COMPONENTS FOUND IN ALL AMYLOIDS:

- **The amyloid P component (AP)** is a pentagonal, doughnut-shaped protein, which is present in all types of amyloid. AP is identical with, and is derived from, a normal circulating serum protein, termed *serum amyloid P (SAP)*. SAP is also a structural component of normal basement membranes.
- **Other molecular building blocks of basement membranes** are present in amyloid and include laminin, collagen type-IV, and perlecan (a heparan sulfate proteoglycan). The glycosaminoglycan side-chain of perlecan is heparan sulfate. This carbohydrate side-chain is probably responsible for the iodine-staining properties of amyloid.
- **Apolipoprotein E (apoE)** is normally found as a constituent of high-density lipoproteins and plays a role in cholesterol transport.

It is important to emphasize that not all amyloids are the same and that the protein responsible for the fibrillary characteristics varies significantly. For example, in amyloid associated with multiple myeloma, the fibrillary component is a product of immunoglobulin light chains produced by myeloma cells. In amyloid associated with inflammatory diseases, the fibrillary component is derived from an acute phase protein, which is produced by the liver and is unrelated to immunoglobulins. In these two cases, amyloid is deposited systemically.

In other situations, amyloid is deposited only locally. Amyloid in medullary carcinoma of the thyroid is restricted to the tumor deposits, and its fibrillary component is derived from a polypeptide hormone related to calcitonin. In the pancreas, amyloid located either in an islet cell tumor or in the islets in type II diabetes is derived from a peptide hormone secreted with insulin (amylin or islet amyloid polypeptide [IAPP]). In Alzheimer disease, the amyloid is restricted to the brain and its blood vessels; yet it is derived from a plasma membrane protein, which is ubiquitously distributed in the body.

Despite the fact that the nature of amyloid deposits varies widely, and the conditions under which they occur are disparate, a century of usage has entrenched the term *amyloidosis* as connoting a single disease. This notion has today been replaced by the concept that the term should be used generically to designate a group of diseases. **Thus, amyloidosis is characterized by proteinaceous tissue deposits with common morphological, structural, and staining properties, but with variable protein composition.**

STAINING PROPERTIES OF AMYLOID DEPOSITS

The staining properties and general appearance of amyloid are governed primarily by the nature of its protein. Because of its compact structure, amyloid has few morphological features visible by light microscopy. When routine stains are used, amyloid is amorphous, glassy, and almost cartilage-like, properties that are responsible for its so-called hyaline appearance. On staining with hematoxylin and eosin, amyloid stains no differently from many other proteins. However, the specific nature and underlying organization of the amyloid proteins, as

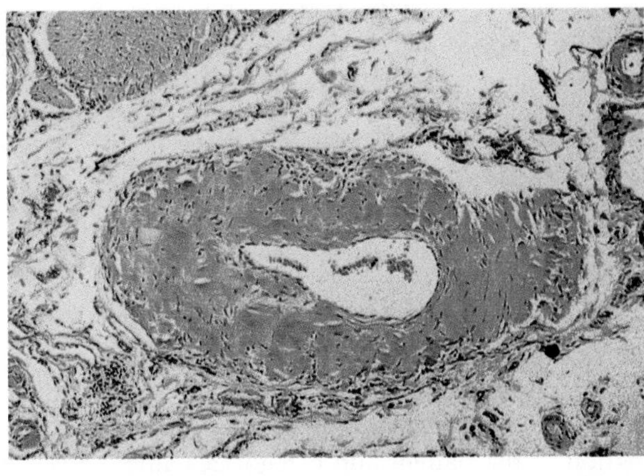

A

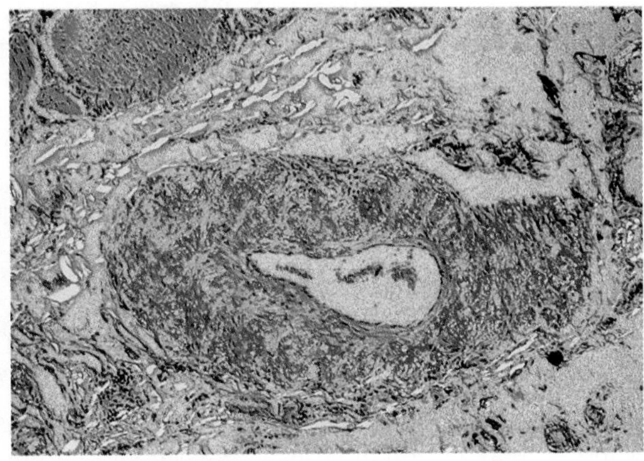

B

FIGURE 23-2
AL amyloid involving the wall of an artery, stained with Congo red. The appearance under ordinary light (*A*) and polarized light (*B*) is shown. Note the red-green birefringence of the amyloid. Collagen has a silvery appearance.

well as those of associated molecules (glycosaminoglycans and amyloid P component), allow amyloid to be stained in specific ways.

CONGO RED: All amyloids stain red with the Congo red dye (Fig. 23-2A). When the sections stained with Congo red are viewed under polarized light, the deposits exhibit a red-green birefringence (see Fig. 23-2B). The fibrillary deposits organized in one plane have one color, whereas those organized perpendicularly to that plane have the other color. **Congo red is the stain most commonly used for the diagnosis of amyloidosis.**

THIOFLAVIN T: Although not entirely specific for amyloid, staining with thioflavin T allows the amyloid to fluoresce when viewed in ultraviolet light.

ALCIAN BLUE: The presence of glycosaminoglycans in all amyloid deposits is demonstrated with a variety of alcian blue stains, which cause the glycosaminoglycans to appear blue.

SPECIFIC ANTIBODIES: The success in isolating various amyloid proteins has led to the preparation of both polyclonal and monoclonal antibodies directed against the different proteins. In turn, immunohistochemical techniques have been devised to demonstrate the presence of AP component, as well as the specific protein present in each type of amyloid.

STRUCTURE OF AMYLOID

All amyloids have a similar ultrastructural appearance, regardless of which protein is responsible for the fibrillary component. By electron microscopy, groups of fibers are arranged in parallel arrays, with each group having a different orientation (see Fig. 23-1). These parallel arrays orient the specific dyes, such as Congo red, and thus impart to amyloid the ability to rotate polarized light, a property that yields its classic birefringence. Although the individual fibrils vary considerably in length, all have a diameter of 7 to 13 nm. When isolated, individual fibrils usually consist of two intertwining strands, each 3.0 to 3.5 nm thick, which are twisted as a shallow helix. However, the structure of the fibril and the composition of amyloid *in situ* seem to be similar to those of basement membrane microfibrils, on the surface of which are the 1 to 2 nm protein-specific filaments.

The secondary and tertiary organization of the protein that constitutes the amyloid fibril has been explored by x-ray diffraction and infrared spectroscopy. The individual protein subunits appear to be organized primarily as a **β-pleated sheet**. However, in the case of the amyloid peptide found in inflammatory diseases, there is an abundant α-helical structure, as well as one segment that is organized into a β-pleated sheet. Similar findings have now been made with the amyloid peptides responsible for amyloid in Alzheimer disease and in the pancreatic islets in adult-onset (type II) diabetes. The individually folded polypeptide subunits are stacked into fibrils. The precise manner and mechanism by which this occurs may be different for each amyloid. The interactions between the polypeptide monomers are responsible for most of the crossed β-pleated sheet structure.

In all amyloids, highly charged glycosaminoglycans (as part of proteoglycans), SAP, and the other basement membrane components (laminin and collagen IV, and apoE) are present in close association with the amyloid deposits. In at least six types of amyloid, the basement membrane form of heparan sulfate proteoglycan (perlecan) has been identified as the charged component. The interaction of amyloid protein precursors with the common components probably influences the conformation of the disease-specific protein, shifting it in favor of amyloidogenic intermediates, which in turn interact as β-pleated sheets. Thus, the basic fibril seems not to be formed simply as a result of the primary structure of the precursor or the protein fragment. Fibril formation is most likely influenced by the manner in which the protein fragment interacts with additional components. The common secondary and tertiary organization of the proteins then results in uniform structural and staining properties.

Definition of Amyloid

The staining and structural properties of amyloid allow a general definition, based primarily on its morphological characteristics.

- All forms of amyloid stain positively with Congo red and show red-green birefringence when viewed under polarized light.
- Ultrastructurally, all forms of amyloid consist of interlacing bundles of parallel arrays of fibrils, which have a diameter of 7 to 13 nm.
- The protein in the amyloid fibrils contains a large proportion of crossed β-pleated sheet structure.

Types of Amyloid Deposits

The classification of amyloidosis has undergone a major change (Table 23-1), primarily because of the realization that the specific protein found in each type of amyloid overlaps previous groupings. For example, the amyloid protein of familial Mediterranean fever (an inherited disorder) and that deposited secondarily in a variety of inflammatory disease are one and the same. Similarly, the proteins found in "primary" amyloidosis and in amyloid associated with a variety of plasma cell dyscrasias are identical. The amyloid of isolated cardiac amyloidosis and that of senile systemic amyloidosis are also indistinguishable.

The older clinical classifications did not take protein structure into account. For example, familial Mediterranean fever and familial amyloidotic polyneuropathy were grouped together as "familial" forms of amyloid, a classification that implies a similar process in each disease. This concept is not supported by newer information. The older classification is still employed in clinical medicine, and the newer groupings, based on the protein type, are only now coming into general use. For this reason, both classifications need to be reviewed.

CLINICAL CLASSIFICATION OF AMYLOIDOSIS

The older classification is based on the clinical presentation of the patient and categorizes amyloidosis as primary, secondary, familial, or isolated. Primary, secondary, and familial amyloidoses are usually, but not always, systemic diseases, in which patients frequently present with renal dysfunction or heart failure. The liver, spleen, gastrointestinal tract, tongue, and subcutaneous tissues are also frequent sites of amyloid deposition. Isolated amyloidosis is, by definition, restricted to a single organ.

Primary Amyloidosis

Primary amyloidosis refers to the presentation of amyloid de novo, that is, without any preceding disease. In one third of these cases, primary amyloidosis is the harbinger of frank **plasma cell neoplasia**, such as multiple myeloma or other B-cell lymphomas. In this respect, primary amyloidosis forms part of the spectrum of amyloid disorders associated with B-cell dysfunction, but differs from other types in that the amyloid appears before, rather than after, the overt malignancy. Regardless of whether amyloidosis or multiple myeloma presents first, the type of amyloid protein is the same.

TABLE *23-1* **Classification of Amyloids**

Amyloid Protein	Protein Precursor	Clinical Setting
AA	apoSAA	Persistent acute inflammation
AL	κ or λ light chain	Multiple myeloma, plasma cell dyscrasias, and primary amyloid
AH	γ chain	Waldenström macroglobulinemia
ATTR	Transthyretin	Familial amyloidotic polyneuropathy (FAP), normal TTR in senile systemic amyloid
AApoAI	apoAI	FAP Iowa
AGel	Gelsolin	Familial amyloidosis, Finnish
ACys	Cystatin C	Hereditary cerebral hemorrhage with amyloid (HCHWA), Icelandic
ALys	Lysozyme	Hereditary systemic amyloidosis, Ostertag-type
AFib	Fibrinogen	Hereditary renal amyloidosis
Aβ	β-protein precursor	Alzheimer disease Down syndrome, HCHWA Dutch
APrP	Prion protein	CJD[a], scrapie, BSE[a], GSS[a], Kuru
ACal	(Pro)calcitonin	Medullary carcinoma of the thyroid
AANF	Atrial naturetic factor	Isolated atrial amyloid
AIAPP	Islet amyloid polypeptide	Type II diabetes, insulinomas
AIns	Insulin	Islet amyloid in the degu (a rodent)
AApoAII	ApoAII (murine)	Amyloid in senescence accelerated mice

[a] CJD, Creutzfelt Jacob disease; BSE, bovine spongiform encephalopathy; GSS, Gerstmann-Straussler-Sheinker syndrome.

Secondary Amyloidosis

Secondary amyloidosis is a complication of a previously existing chronic inflammatory disorder, which may or may not have an immunological basis. Patients with rheumatoid arthritis, ankylosing spondylitis, and occasionally systemic lupus erythematosus may develop secondary amyloidosis. Most other patients with secondary amyloidosis have conditions that are complicated by long-standing inflammation (e.g., lung abscess, tuberculosis, or osteomyelitis). These disorders were the most common causes of amyloidosis in the past, but the use of antibiotics and modern surgical techniques have drastically reduced the frequency of this complication.

Currently, secondary amyloidosis also occurs in persons who develop chronic skin abscesses as a result of subcutaneous self-administration of narcotics. Secondary amyloidosis is also seen in patients with specific cancers, such as Hodgkin disease and renal cell carcinoma. The amyloid protein deposited secondary to these malignancies is identical to that seen in rheumatoid arthritis, chronic infections, and familial Mediterranean fever.

Familial Amyloidosis

Several geographic populations display genetically inherited forms of amyloidosis.

FAMILIAL MEDITERRANEAN FEVER: This autosomal recessive disease is found predominantly in the Mediterranean basin among Sephardic Jews and Turks, although Armenians and Arabs may also be affected. More than 90% of the Jewish patients in Israel are of Sephardic origin. Familial Mediterranean fever is characterized by polymorphonuclear leukocyte dysfunction and recurrent episodes of serositis, including peritonitis. Since there is recurrent inflammation, the type of amyloid protein deposited is the same as that in amyloidosis secondary to acquired inflammatory disorders. The gene for Mediterranean fever (MEFV) has been mapped to the short arm of chromosome 16, encoding a protein termed "pyrin" or more poetically, "mare nostrin." It is expressed in neutrophils and is thought to be a transcription factor that regulates other genes involved in the suppression of inflammation.

FAMILIAL AMYLOIDOTIC POLYNEUROPATHY (FAP): This is usually an autosomal dominant genetic disorder, in which at least 60 mutations, scattered throughout the amyloidogenic protein, have been described. Each protein gives rise to a clinical variant of the disease. FAP exhibits a predilection for peripheral and autonomic nerves. The most common variant is due to a methionine for valine substitution at residue 30 in **transthyretin**, the protein which is responsible for this form of amyloidosis. This Met30 variant has been described in three nationalities, namely, Swedish, Portuguese, and Japanese. Interestingly, the demographic distribution of FAP in Japan occurs primarily in a region where the Portuguese had established a colony. In Portugal, the area where this disorder is most frequent was originally visited and settled by Viking seamen. Whether the mutation responsible for this form of familial amyloidosis originated in Scandinavia or whether identical mutations arose in different geographic populations remains to be determined.

HEREDITARY CONGOPHILIC ANGIOPATHY (ICELANDIC): Also termed hereditary cerebral hemorrhage with amyloid (HCHWA), this form of amyloidosis is the result of a mutation cystatin-C, a protease inhibitor.

HEREDITARY CONGOPHILIC ANGIOPATHY (DUTCH): HCHWA (Dutch) clinically and pathologically is similar to the Icelandic variety, but results from a mutation in the amyloid-forming segment of the β-protein of Alzheimer disease (see later). These patients do not, however, manifest dementia.

Isolated Amyloidosis

The isolated forms of amyloidosis tend to involve single organ systems. Isolated amyloidosis has been described in the lung, heart, and various joints, and in association with endocrine tumors that secrete polypeptide hormones. In endocrine tumors, the amyloid is usually part of a hormone or a prohormone. By far, the most common organ-specific amyloids are those found in Alzheimer disease and type II (insulin-independent) diabetes.

Alzheimer Disease

In the most common form of dementia, namely Alzheimer disease, the amyloid (called Aβ) is restricted to the brain and its vessels. The deposited protein, a 4kD peptide called the β-protein, is a fragment of a larger β-protein precursor (βPP), which is a normal cell membrane constituent. The longer part of βPP is extracellular, with the remainder traversing the cell membrane and ending in a cytoplasmic portion of approximately 100 amino acids. The β-protein itself is a segment of 42 to 43 amino acids that lies immediately outside and partially within the cell membrane. βPP is present not only in the cells of the central nervous system but also in most other tissues. There are at least five splicing products, several of which have been identified in the brain, but only one of which (βPP-695) is brain specific. It is generally accepted, but has never been demonstrated, that the β-protein giving rise to Aβ is derived from a cell in the central nervous system. Since βPP is produced by so many cell types, it is still possible that the source of Aβ for the vascular amyloid or the brain parenchymal amyloid in Alzheimer disease is extracerebral.

β-Protein is derived from βPP by a series of proteolytic steps, catalyzed by enzymes, termed secretases. The α-secretase cuts within the β-protein segment and, therefore, precludes its involvement in producing the β-protein fragment. The β- and γ-secretases respectively cut at the amino- and carboxy-terminal ends of β-protein, thereby generating the amyloidogeneic fragment. Mutations adjacent to these cleavage sites (but not within the β-protein) are associated with several familial forms of Alzheimer disease, suggesting that amyloid is important in the pathogenesis of Alzheimer disease.

The gene for βPP is located on chromosome 21, which likely explains the observation that patients with **Down syndrome** (associated with trisomy of part or all of chromosome 21) all develop the morphological lesions of Alzheimer disease by 35 years of age. Several other genes, in addition to βPP, have been implicated in both the pathogenesis of Alzheimer disease and the deposition of Aβ. These include a locus on chromosome 19, which codes for apoE, one of the common constituents of all amyloids. The E_4 isoform of apoE is linked to Alzheimer disease. Recently, loci on chromosomes 1 and 4, which code for two related proteins, called *presenilins*, have also been linked to Alzheimer disease. These proteins influence the production and processing of β-protein. In tissue culture, the β-protein in a random conformation is innocuous to neurons. However, folding of the protein into a β-sheet and its organization into Aβ *in vivo* confer neuronal toxicity. There is also evidence that the injury-response factor transforming growth factor-beta 1 (TGF-β1) may contribute to amyloid deposition in Alzheimer disease through its capacity to induce amyloid—binding proteins.

Diabetes

The amyloid deposited in the islets of Langerhans in type II diabetes is also derived from a larger precursor, a peptide related to a variant of calcitonin, termed *islet amyloid polypeptide (IAPP)*, or *amylin*. Similar to insulin, this novel hormone is produced by the β-cells of the islets and seems to have a profound effect on glucose uptake by the liver and striated muscle cells. In mice, transgenic for human amylin, which are fed a high-fat diet, overproduction of this protein leads to islet amyloid. These observations imply that islet amyloid is involved in the pathogenesis of type II diabetes, although the subject requires further study.

Senile Cardiac Amyloidosis

Isolated amyloid deposition may occur in the heart, particularly in men, after the age of 70 years. This disorder is usually asymptomatic, but occasionally extensive deposits in the myocardium may cause heart failure. The amyloid precursor responsible is normal **transthyretin**.

CLASSIFICATION OF AMYLOIDOSIS BY THE TYPE OF PROTEIN

The clinical classification of amyloidosis was useful until the early 1970s. However, isolation and characterization of many of the fibrillar proteins in the various forms of amyloid has prompted a reconsideration of the groupings into which each specific disorder should be placed. It is now apparent that (1) specific forms of secondary amyloidosis share a common protein with primary amyloidosis; (2) familial Mediterranean fever should be grouped with secondary forms occurring in association with inflammatory disorders and some cancers; and (3) there are isolated forms of amyloidosis that involve single organ systems, which have the same type of protein found in familial amyloidotic polyneuropathy. The presence of amyloid deposits with identical proteins in seemingly distinct clinical entities implies that common pathological processes occur. These various amyloid proteins are designated A (amyloid), followed by a letter or a word that refers to the specific origin of the protein.

The most common clinical associations of amyloid are (1) Aβ and Alzheimer disease, (2) AIAPP (islet amyloid polypeptide) and Type II diabetes, and (3) Aβ2M and chronic dialysis. The first two have been covered above. The last, and several important historical forms of amyloid, follow, since they put into perspective general mechanisms now thought to be operative in amyloidogenesis.

Aβ2M Amyloid

The deposition of amyloid formed from β-2-microglobulin (β2M) is a relatively new disease, characterized by a **destructive arthropathy, owing to amyloid deposition in the major joints of patients undergoing chronic renal dialysis.** Because dialysis has been in common use for only 20 to 25 years, and more than 8 to 10 years are required before the manifestations of Aβ2M, the disease did not appear as a clinical entity until the early 1980s. Today, the majority (50% to 75%) of patients undergoing dialysis for more than 10 years manifest this disorder. Aβ2M amyloid is deposited in the subchondral bone and periarticular tissues, as well as in the gastrointestinal tract. The circulating level of β2M, which serves as the precursor pool for amyloid deposition, is markedly increased in patients with renal failure. The intact normal protein is deposited, and neither proteolytic processing nor a mutation is involved in the pathogenesis of Aβ2M deposition.

AL Amyloid

The first amyloid protein to be isolated and sequenced was AL amyloid, which was derived from patients who had primary amyloidosis or multiple myeloma. **AL amyloid usually consists of the variable region of immunoglobulin light chains (L—light) and can be derived from either the κ or λ moieties.** Occasionally, the AL amyloid subunit is larger than the variable end of light chains, in which case it may represent the complete immunoglobulin light chain. Within an individual patient, the sequence of AL amyloid protein is constant, regardless of the organ from which the amyloid is isolated. The amino acid sequence of the variable region of urinary Bence Jones protein corresponds to the patient's AL protein. Since the light chains produced by the neoplastic cells in plasma cell dyscrasias are unique to each patient, **AL amyloid isolated from different persons differs in its amino acid sequence**.

AL protein is common to primary amyloidosis and amyloidosis associated with either multiple myeloma, B-cell lymphomas, or other plasma cell dyscrasias. AL protein in isolated nodules of lung amyloid is a product of focal aggregates of plasma cells. Since one third of the patients who first present with "primary" amyloidosis subsequently develop plasma cell abnormalities or frank myeloma, "primary" amyloidosis, multiple myeloma, and immunoblastic lymphomas apparently form a spectrum of a single disorder. In some cases, the malignant disease presents first as multiple myeloma or lymphoma, whereas in other cases it is announced by AL deposits in various tissues.

Only some patients with multiple myeloma develop AL amyloid, probably because some κ or λ chains are more fibrillogenic than others. The mechanism by which AL amyloid is deposited is summarized in Figure 23-3.

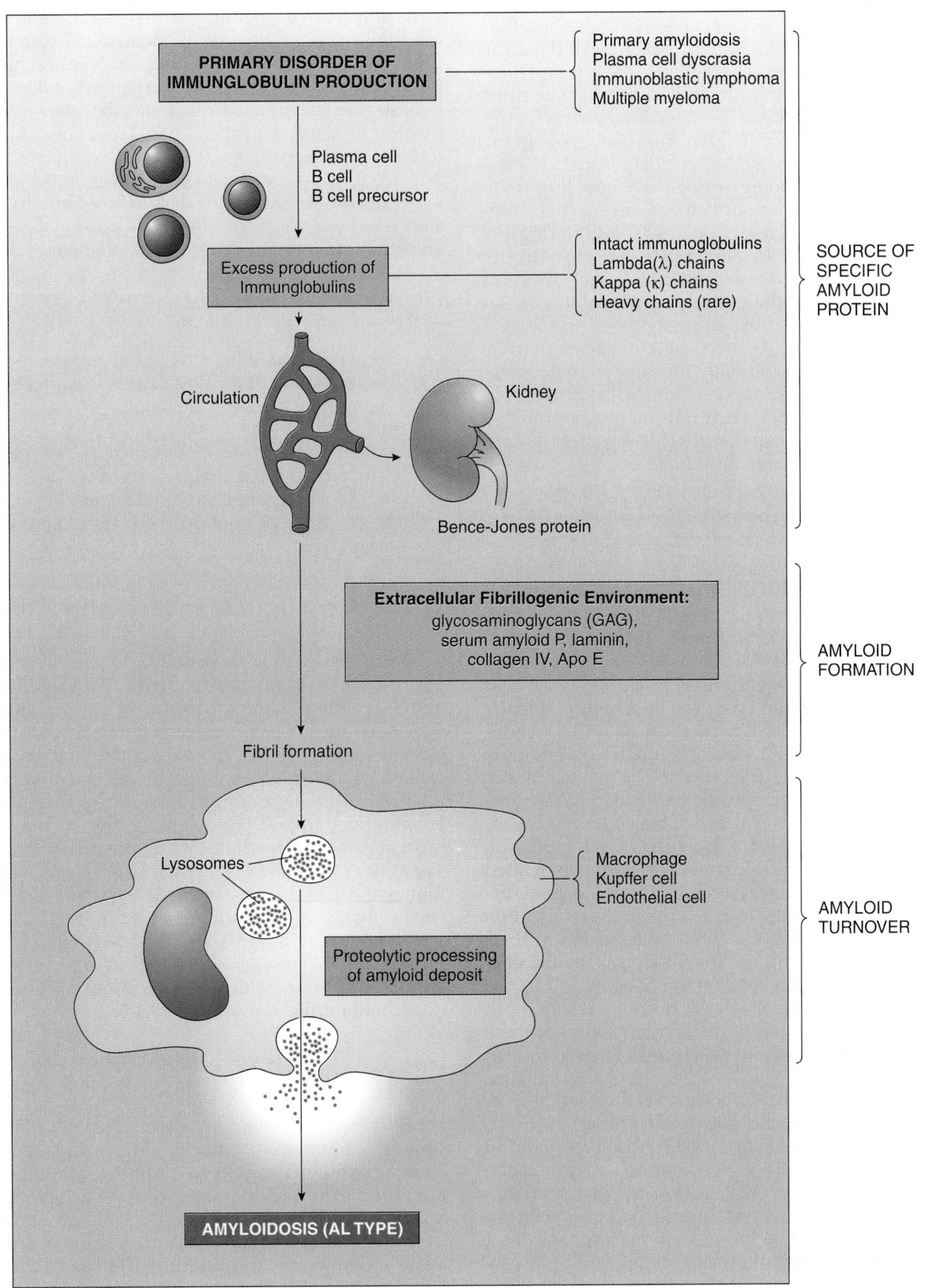

FIGURE 23-3
The mechanism of AL amyloid deposition.

AA Amyloid

AA amyloid is common to a host of seemingly unrelated, chronic inflammatory, neoplastic, and hereditary disorders that lead to so-called secondary amyloidosis. As with AL amyloid, there is a spectrum of AA peptides of differing size within AA deposits all of which have the same amino-terminal sequence. This includes the intact precursor of AA, namely serum amyloid A (SAA). The most prevalent size is a peptide of 76 amino acids, which corresponds to the amino terminal two thirds of SAA. In experimental animals, intact SAA is incorporated into AA fibrils, after which it undergoes postfibrillogenic proteolysis. SAA is an acute phase protein, the serum concentration of which rapidly increases up to 1000-fold during any inflammatory process. **In contrast to AL protein, the amino acid sequence of AA proteins is identical in all patients, regardless of the underlying disorder.** The AA protein has also been found in many other species, including ducks, guinea pigs, mice, and monkeys. In these animals AA protein is essentially the same as that seen in humans. The evolutionary preservation of the amino acid sequence reflects the important role that SAA probably plays during inflammation, which is apparently concerned with cholesterol metabolism.

Deposition of AA Amyloid and Inflammation

Circulating SAA is converted into AA. SAA has the characteristics of an apolipoprotein for a high-density lipoprotein (HDL); yet it is present in significant quantities only during inflammation. Denaturation of this lipoprotein, which releases a subunit termed apoSAA, renders it amyloidogenic. ApoSAA is synthesized primarily in the liver and binds to HDL on entering the circulation. Hepatic apoSAA mRNA synthesis is induced by IL-1, IL-6, and tumor necrosis factor (TNF), cytokines that are released by activated inflammatory cells at sites of inflammation. Thus, at least part of the pathway involved in AA deposition involves the normal reaction of the body to acute inflammatory stimuli. As in the case of AL amyloid, macrophages and endothelial cells are intimately related to AA amyloid deposition. Although the anatomical distribution of these cells seems to determine the localization of AA, amyloid deposition cannot be regarded as their normal activity. Why do inflammatory and endothelial cells fail to degrade SAA completely?

Whereas only a small proportion of patients with high levels of SAA actually develop amyloidosis, there are experimental models in which all animals deposit amyloid within a matter of days. Persistent acute inflammation induces not only the synthesis of the amyloid precursor SAA, but also the appearance of a substance termed *amyloid enhancing factor (AEF)*. In experimental models, amyloid deposition does not occur without the concomitant presence of AEF, which has characteristics analogous to those of a crystallization nidus. When injected intravenously AEF localizes to macrophages and endothelial cells, thereby altering their metabolic processing of SAA.

An additional element in the pathogenesis of murine AA amyloid is the co-deposition of apoE and the structural constituents of basement membranes (perlecan, laminin, collagen IV, and SAP). Despite the observation that these basement membrane components *in vitro* spontaneously organize to form basement membranes, no basement membranes are seen in amyloid deposits *in vivo*. At least two amyloid precursors, SAA and βPP, can bind to several of these components *in vitro* and prevent their normal interactions. Other evidence suggests that part of the process of amyloid formation is a derangement in basement membrane protein metabolism.

Recent work with apoE "knock-out" mice has shown that the presence of apoE does not determine whether or not AA amyloid is deposited. However, in the absence of apoE, the onset of amyloidosis is delayed and its progression is slowed considerably. These observations in mice are similar to those in patients with Alzheimer disease.

Thus, during inflammation, the following coincident processes are necessary for AA amyloid deposition (Fig. 23-4):

- The generation of the amyloid precursor apoSAA.
- The generation of AEF, which in turn affects the processing of apoSAA in macrophages and endothelial cells.
- A disturbance in the metabolism of basement membrane proteins, the components of which can bind to apoSAA and change its conformation.
- The presence of apoE in the progression of amyloidosis.

ATTR Amyloid (Transthyretin Amyloid)

Transthyretin (TTR) is secreted by the liver into the plasma, where it serves as a carrier of thyroid hormones and as a retinal binding protein. At least 60 mutants of TTR have been described, each being responsible for a clinical variant of FAP. The most common form of FAP is caused by a methionine for valine substitution in TTR at position 30. This mutation lowers the stability of the tetrameric native TTR, allowing the formation of a monomeric intermediate with altered conformation. There is a satisfying correlation between the mutations that give rise to the most unstable tetramers and the most severe forms of FAP. Interestingly, normal TTR is deposited in isolated cardiac amyloidosis and in a systemic form of amyloidosis associated with aging, indicating that an altered amino acid sequence is not an absolute requirement for the deposition of ATTR.

Other Amyloids

Other forms of amyloid are derived from a normal preprohormone or from a hormonal product secreted by endocrine tissue or endocrine tumors. Medullary carcinoma of the thyroid originates from the C-type cells of the thyroid, which normally secrete calcitonin. The amyloid in this tumor is a fragment of procalcitonin. In isolated atrial amyloid, the peptide is atrial natriuretic factor. Amyloid proteins have been characterized in the skin, where they are related to keratin. There are other examples of isolated forms of human amyloidosis for which

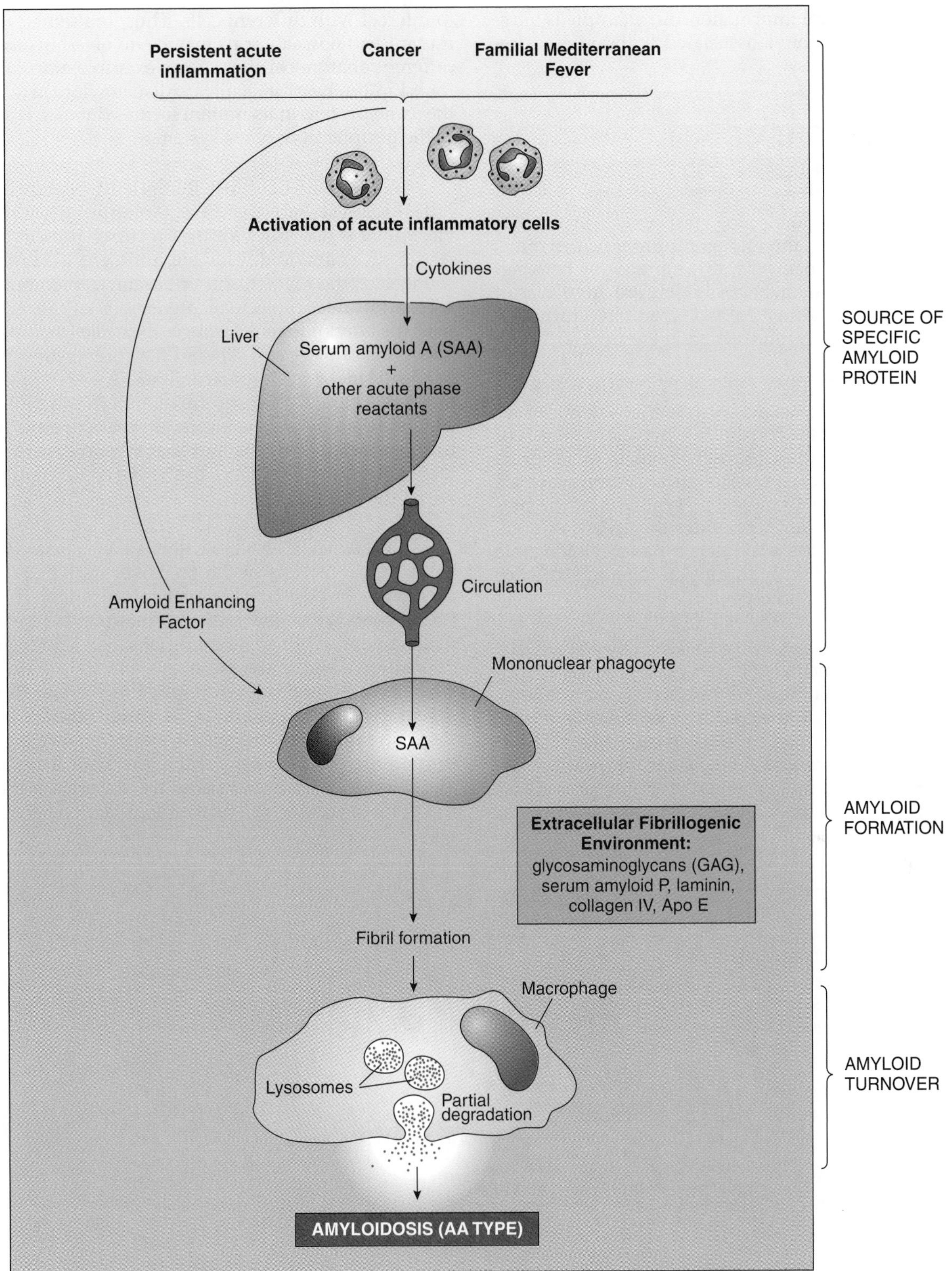

FIGURE *23-4*

The mechanism of AA amyloid deposition. A variety of diseases is associated with the activation of polymorphonuclear leukocytes and macrophages, which in turn leads to the synthesis and release of acute phase reactants by the liver, including SAA. SAA in the presence of amyloid enhancing factor (AEF) is likely released substantially intact by reticuloendothelial cells where in a fibrillogenic environment the released product complexes with glycosaminoglycans and SAP, as AA amyloid. This deposit is then processed by macrophages.

there is little structural information. An example is amyloid in osteoarthritic joints associated with aging, a frequent finding at autopsy.

A GENERAL SCHEME OF AMYLOIDOGENESIS

The requirements for amyloidogenesis *in vivo* include (1) an adequate pool of an amyloidogenic protein, (2) a nidus or nucleus for fibrillogenesis, (3) interactions between common components, most of which are involved in basement membrane structure, and (4) amyloid turnover. These are schematically interrelated in Figure 23-5.

AN ADEQUATE PRECURSOR POOL: In some settings, such as ATTR associated with senile systemic or senile cardiac amyloid, the constitutive hepatic synthesis of transthyretin provides the necessary pool. In other forms of amyloid, such as AA, a physiological response as part of inflammation leads to increased synthesis of the precursor, which inadvertantly provides the necessary pool. Alternatively, mutations may alter a nonamyloidogenic protein, providing it with an amyloidogenic sequence and generating the required pool.

ANATOMICAL LOCALIZATION OF AMYLOID: The physiological function of the amyloid precursor probably determines the location of the specific form of amyloid. For instance, SAA, the precursor of AA, may target HDLs to macrophages and endothelial cells. Mishandling of SAA by such cells would set the stage for local AA deposition. Similarly, a mutation may not only provide an amyloidogenic sequence, but may also cause the protein to interact with different cells. Thus, the same protein in mutant and normal forms may be involved in amyloid at different anatomical sites. As an example, normal TTR is found in the heart in senile cardiac amyloid. Yet in FAP, the same protein in its mutant form is deposited as ATTR in the peripheral nervous system.

AN ALTERED MICROENVIRONMENT AND FIBRILLIZATION NUCLEUS: An appropriate microenvironment is necessary for the precursor protein to manifest itself as amyloid. This environment likely involves changes in the metabolism of basement membrane proteins and direct molecular interactions of these proteins with the amyloidogenic protein. Examples include the interactions of SAA and Aβ and their interaction with the perlecan side-chain heparan sulfate. In both cases, this interaction changes the conformation of the amyloidogenic protein, thereby increasing its β-sheet content. A fibrillization nucleus may aid and abet this process by driving the equilibrium away from the native conformation in favor of the amyloid one.

PROTEOLYSIS AND TURNOVER: In some forms of amyloid, proteolysis of the precursor may be part of its processing or post-translational modification. These prefibrillogenic steps generate a normal peptide or protein, which under appropriate conditions may lead to amyloid deposition. The conversion of β protein into Aβ in Alzheimer disease is an example. Proteolysis of amyloid precursors, which generates the varied sizes of peptides found in individual deposits, is inferred to occur at a step beyond the incorporation of the precursor into the amyloid fibrils. Proteases in various tissues process the fibrils to a point beyond which further degradation becomes dif-

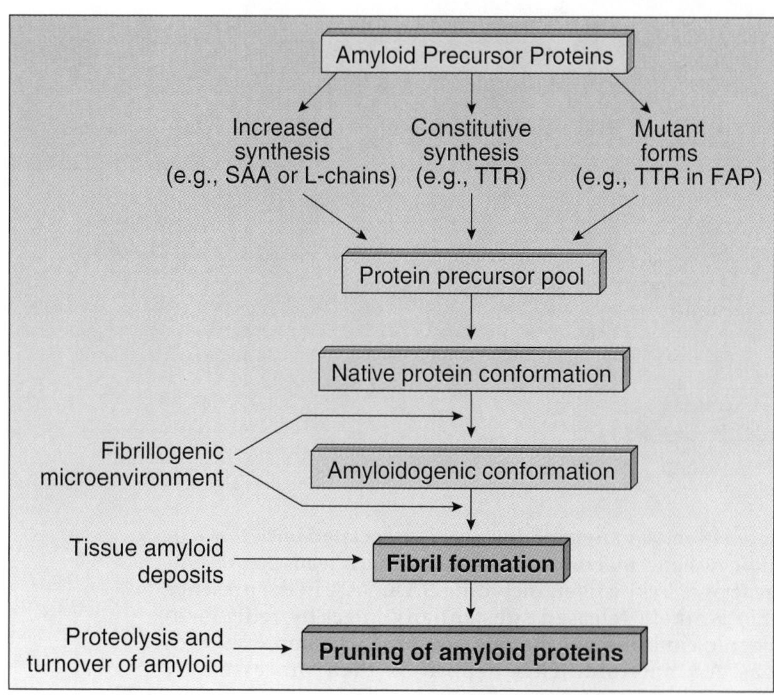

FIGURE 23-5
General scheme for amyloidogenesis.

ficult. Thus, the size of the residual amyloid peptides varies in any given deposit.

MORPHOLOGICAL FEATURES OF AMYLOIDOSIS

Amyloid fibrils, when first deposited, are usually in close association with subendothelial basement membranes (Fig. 23-6). **Because amyloid accumulates along stromal networks, the deposits take on the architectural framework of the organs involved.** The morphological differences in amyloid deposition from one organ to the next simply reflect the differing stromal organization of each tissue. For example, in the medulla of the kidney, amyloid is laid down in a longitudinal fashion, parallel to the tubules and vasa recta. By contrast, in the glomerulus (Figs. 23-7 and 23-8), amyloid appears in a pattern determined by the lobular architecture of that structure. Splenic amyloid may be associated either with the stroma of the red pulp or with that of the white pulp. On gross examination, amyloid in the red pulp imparts a diffusely pale and waxy appearance, the so-called *lardaceous spleen*. The cut surface of the spleen containing white pulp amyloid is different and shows multiple pale foci scattered throughout the organ, an appearance labeled *sago spleen*. Deposits in the liver follow the arteries of the portal triads or are laid down along central veins and radiate into the parenchyma along the liver cell plates.

Amyloid adds interstitial material to sites of deposition, thereby increasing the size of affected organs. This increase may be counterbalanced by the deposition of amyloid in blood vessels (Fig. 23-9), an effect that impairs circulation and may lead to organ atrophy. Affected organs may, therefore, increase or decrease in size. Since compact amyloid deposits are essentially avascular, the involved organs tend to be pale and firm.

Regardless of whether amyloid is laid down in a systemic or local fashion, the deposits tend to occur between

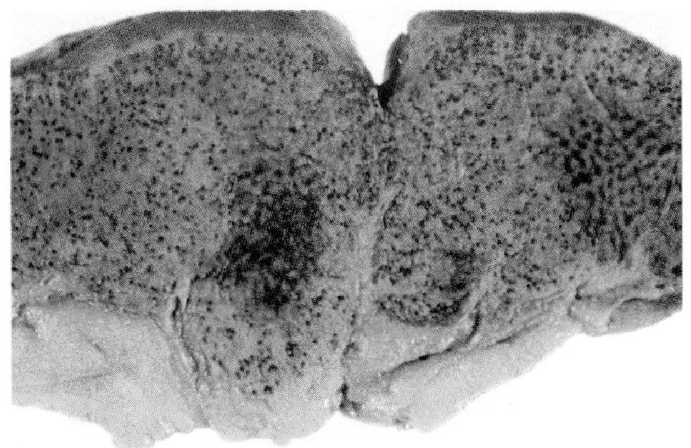

FIGURE 23-7
A kidney containing AA amyloid stained with the iodine reaction. Note the dot-like staining of the glomeruli in the cortex and the linear array in the medulla.

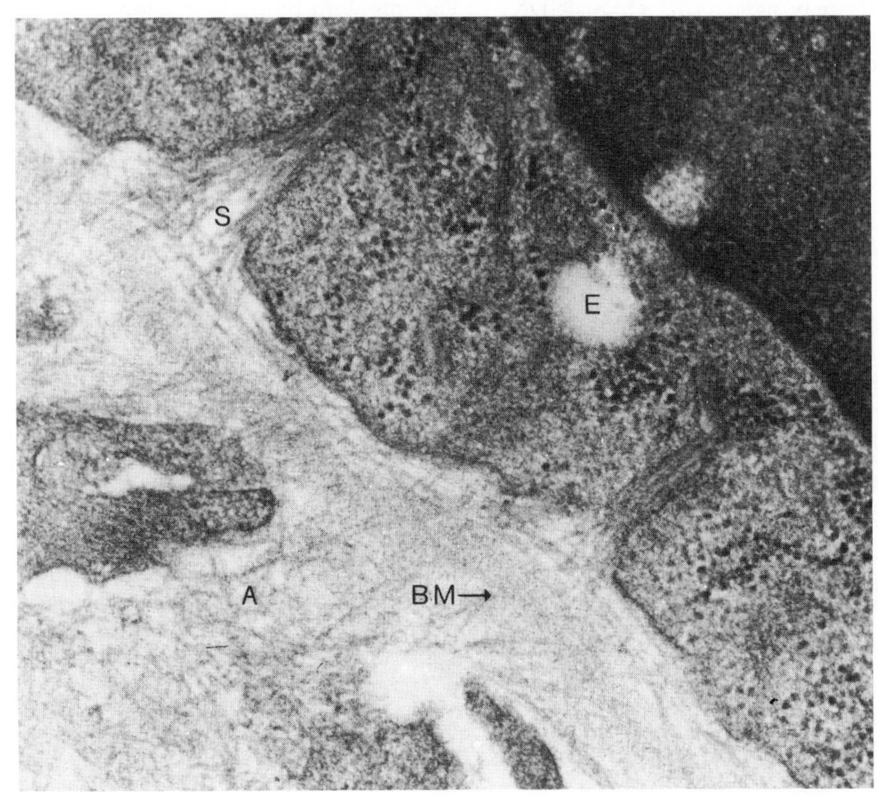

FIGURE *23-6*
Electron micrograph of glomerular amyloid (*A*) illustrating its location relative to the basement membrane (*BM*). Amyloid spicules (*S*) extend into the cytoplasm of the glomerular epithelial cells (*E*).

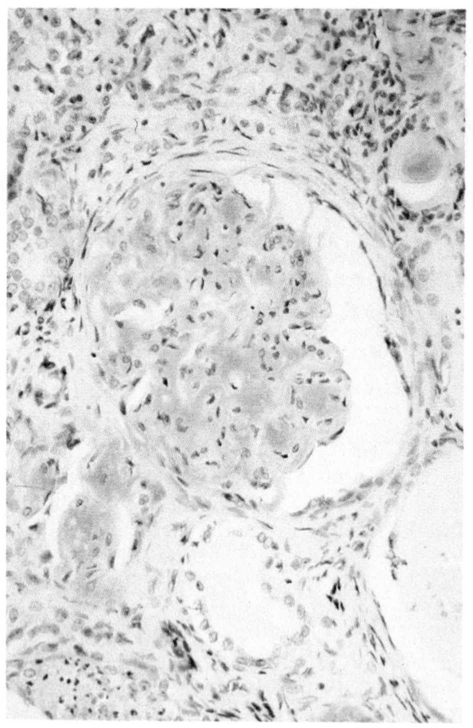

FIGURE 23-8
The microscopic appearance of AA amyloid from the glomeruli of the specimen in Figure 23-7. Note the lobular pattern of the amyloid deposit and the involvement of the afferent arteriole.

parenchymal cells and their blood supply. Amyloid may eventually entrap the parenchymal cells, may have a direct toxic effect on these cells, or may interfere with their nutrition. **In any event, amyloidosis leads to cell strangulation and atrophy** (Fig. 23-10).

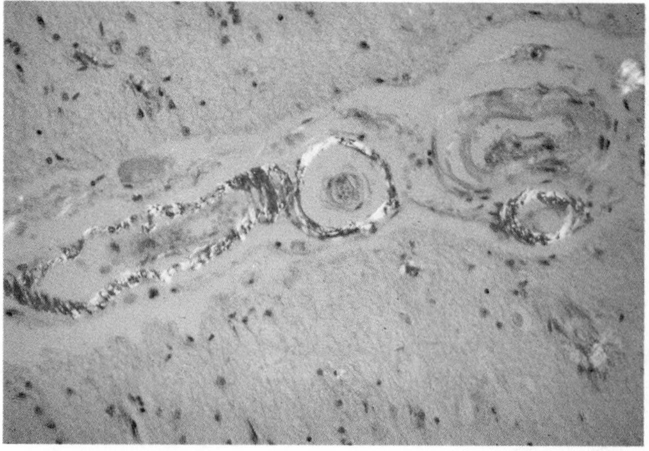

FIGURE 23-9
Cerebrovascular amyloid in a case of Alzheimer disease. The section was stained with Congo red and examined under polarized light.

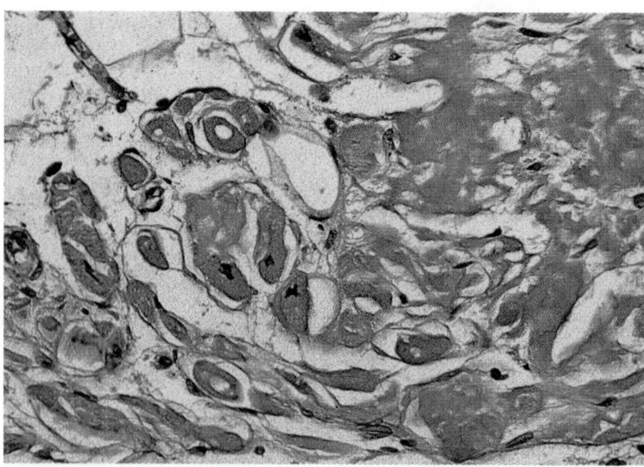

FIGURE 23-10
Myocardial amyloid (AL type), showing the encroachment upon and strangulation of individual myocardial fibers.

CLINICAL FEATURES OF AMYLOIDOSIS

No single set of symptoms points unequivocally to amyloidosis as a diagnosis. The symptomatology of amyloidosis is governed both by the underlying disease and the type of protein deposited. It is not uncommon for amyloidosis to be found as a completely unexpected disorder, with no clinical manifestations. In other cases, unexplained renal and cardiac complications are common, presenting conditions in several varieties of amyloidosis.

KIDNEY: Patients with multiple myeloma, chronic long-standing inflammatory disorders, or familial Mediterranean fever who develop the nephrotic syndrome should be suspected of having amyloidosis. Proteinuria, particularly in patients with plasma cell dyscrasias, may be overlooked if the patient is already excreting a Bence Jones protein. Progressive glomerular obliteration may ultimately lead to renal failure and uremia.

HEART: Amyloid involvement of the myocardium should be suspected in systemic forms of amyloidosis, in which congestive failure or cardiomegaly is associated with low voltage on the electrocardiogram. Entrapment of the conduction system leads to arrhythmias, which in turn can result in sudden death. Not only does congestive failure secondary to cardiac amyloidosis respond poorly to digitalis therapy, but amyloid fibrils also sequester and concentrate digoxin, thereby precipitating digitalis toxicity and fatal arrhythmias. Amyloid deposition within the myocardium may also impair ventricular distensibility and filling, an effect that appears clinically as a **restrictive form of cardiomyopathy**. In some instances, cardiac amyloidosis has masqueraded as constrictive pericarditis.

GASTROINTESTINAL TRACT: The ganglia, smooth muscle vasculature, and submucosa of the gastrointestinal tract may all be affected by amyloid. Deposits in these locations alter gastrointestinal motility and absorption. Patients complain of either constipation or diarrhea, occasionally in association with malabsorption. Enlargement of the tongue is classic, and interference with its motor function may be of sufficient degree to affect speech and swallowing.

PERIPHERAL NERVES: The familial polyneuropathic forms of amyloid usually present as paresthesias, with loss in temperature and pain sensation of the extremities.

In all systemic forms of amyloidosis, the patient's course is usually unremitting and ultimately fatal. Patients with multiple myeloma and AL amyloidosis generally die within 1 to 2 years, either from the malignancy itself or from cardiac or renal complications. Patients with AA amyloidosis secondary to long-standing inflammatory disease have a more protracted course, but death may be expected within 5 years of the diagnosis, usually from cardiac or renal failure. Persons who suffer deposition of ATTR of the familial type have an extended course of 15 to 25 years. Symptoms may begin at any age, but are usually postpubertal, with death most common in the fifth and sixth decades. Successful treatment of the underlying condition, such as multiple myeloma or an inflammatory disorder, may on occasion lead to the resorption and resolution of amyloid deposits. These clinical observations indicate that amyloid does turn over, albeit slowly.

Even when one suspects amyloidosis, the diagnosis ultimately rests on its histological demonstration in biopsy specimens. Amyloid is readily demonstrated in gingival and rectal biopsy specimens and in abdominal subcutaneous fat. It is commonly visualized in renal biopsies taken as part of a general investigation of impaired renal function. In the past, it was sufficient simply to make a diagnosis of amyloid on tissue biopsy. The availability of antisera specific for the various amyloid proteins now allows the determination of the specific forms of amyloid.

Persons who carry the genes for familial forms of amyloid can now be identified by demonstrating the amino acid or base substitution with appropriate molecular techniques. The detection of carriers is valuable in genetic counseling.

AMYLOID TREATMENT STRATEGIES

Strategies for antiamyloid therapy flow from the processes of amyloidogenesis outlined earlier.

REDUCTION IN THE AMYLOID PRECURSOR CONCENTRATION: Since an adequate amyloid precursor pool is necessary for fibrillogenesis, attempts have been made to limit the availability of such precursors. A clinical example involves mutant ATTR and familial amyloidotic polyneuropathy. Liver transplantation in patients with FAP replaces the abnormal TTR with its normal counterpart. In such patients, one can demonstrate a gradual reduction in amyloid load. It is, however, too early to conclude that such an approach leads to clinical improvement.

INHIBITION OF NIDUS (NUCLEUS) FORMATION: Colchicine is the drug of choice in preventing the development of amyloidosis in such patients. Experimentally, this drug acts by preventing the generation of AEF (the nidus), thereby preventing the appearance of amyloid.

INHIBITION OF MOLECULAR INTERACTIONS: The recent recognition that amyloid fibril formation may be the product of interactive processes between two or more molecular components suggested that interference with such interactions may inhibit amyloidogenesis. Experimentally, this approach has proved successful with several different forms of amyloid, but its effectiveness in human amyloidosis remains to be demonstrated.

ACCELERATION OF AMYLOID REMOVAL: Patients with AL amyloid who are treated with an iodinated analogue of doxorubicin resorb considerable amounts of their amyloid. The agent binds with high affinity to several amyloids, including AL. On theoretical grounds, displacement of some of the components from amyloid fibrils may make the remainder more susceptible to proteolytic digestion. Treatment of human amyloidosis has not been attempted.

SUGGESTED READING

Benson MD, Uemichi T: Transthyretin amyloidosis. *Amyloid* 3:44–56, 1996.

Breitner JCS: The role of anti-inflammatory drugs in the prevention and treatment of Alzheimer's disease. *Annu Rev Med* 47:401–411, 1996.

Castillo MJ, Scheen AJ, Lefebvre PJ: Amylin/islet amyloid polypeptide: Biochemistry, physiology, patho-physiology. *Diabete Metab* 21:3–25, 1995.

Glenner GG: Amyloid deposits and amyloidosis: The B-fibrilloses (Part I). *N Engl J Med* 302:1283–1292, 1980.

Glenner GG: Amyloid deposits and amyloidosis: The B-fibrilloses (Part II). *N Engl J Med* 302:1333–1341, 1980.

Haass C: The molecular significance of amyloid beta-peptide for Alzheimer's disease. *Eur Arch Psychiat Clin Neuros* 246:118–123, 1996.

Hardy J: Molecular genetics of Alzheimer's disease. *Acta Neurol Scand* 93:13–17, 1996.

Hendriks L, van Broeckhoven C: The βA4 amyloid precursor protein gene and Alzheimer's disease. *Eur J Biochem* 237:6–15, 1996.

Husby, G: Classification of amyloidosis. In Husby G (ed): Clinical rheumatology. Vol. 8, No. 3, *Reactive amyloidosis and the acute phase response.* London: Bailliere Tindall, pp. 503–511, 1994.

Kazatchkine MD, Husby G, Araki S, et al: *Nomenclature of amyloid and amyloidosis.* WHO-IUIS Nomenclature Sub-Committee. Bull WHO 71:105–108, 1993.

Kisilevsky R: Anti-amyloid drugs: Potential in the treatment of diseases associated with aging. *Drug Aging* 8:75–83, 1996.

Kisilevsky R, Gruys E, Shirahama T: Does amyloid enhancing factor (AEF) exist? Is AEF a single biological entity? *Amyloid* 2:128–133, 1995.

Kisilevsky, R, Young, ID: Pathogenesis of amyloidosis. In Husby G (ed): *Clinical rheumatology: reactive amyloidosis and the acute phase response.* London: Bailliere Tindall, pp. 613–626, 1994.

Kushner I, Rzewnicki DL: The acute phase response: General aspects. In Husby G (ed): Clinical rheumatology, Vol. 8, No. 3, *Reactive amyloidosis and the acute phase response.* London: Bailliere Tindall, pp. 513–530, 1994.

Kyle RA, Gertz MA: Primary systemic amyloidosis: Clinical and laboratory features in 474 cases. *Semin Hematol* 32:45–59, 1995.

Marhaug, G, Dowton, SB: Serum amyloid A: An acute phase apolipoprotein and the precursor of AA amyloid. In Husby G (ed): Clinical rheumatology, Vol. 8, No. 3, *Reactive amyloidosis and the acute phase response.* London: Bailliere Tindall, pp. 553–573, 1994.

Merlini G: Monoclonal gammapathies. *Cancer J* 8:173–180, 1995.

Roses AD: Apolipoprotein E alleles as risk factors in Alzheimer's disease. *Annu Rev Med* 47:387–400, 1996.

Sacks DB: Amylin: A glucoregulatory hormone involved in the pathogenesis of diabetes mellitus? *Clin Chem* 42:494–495, 1996.

Solomon A, Weiss DT: Protein and host factors implicated in the pathogenesis of light chain amyloidosis (AL amyloidosis). *Amyloid* 2:269–279, 1995.

Strittmatter WJ, Roses AD: Apolipoprotein E and Alzheimer's disease. *Annu Rev Neurosci* 19:53–77, 1996.

Young AA, Pittner R, Gedulin B, Vine W, Rink T: Amylin regulation of carbohydrate metabolism. *Biochem Soc Trans* 23:325–331, 1995.

CHAPTER 24

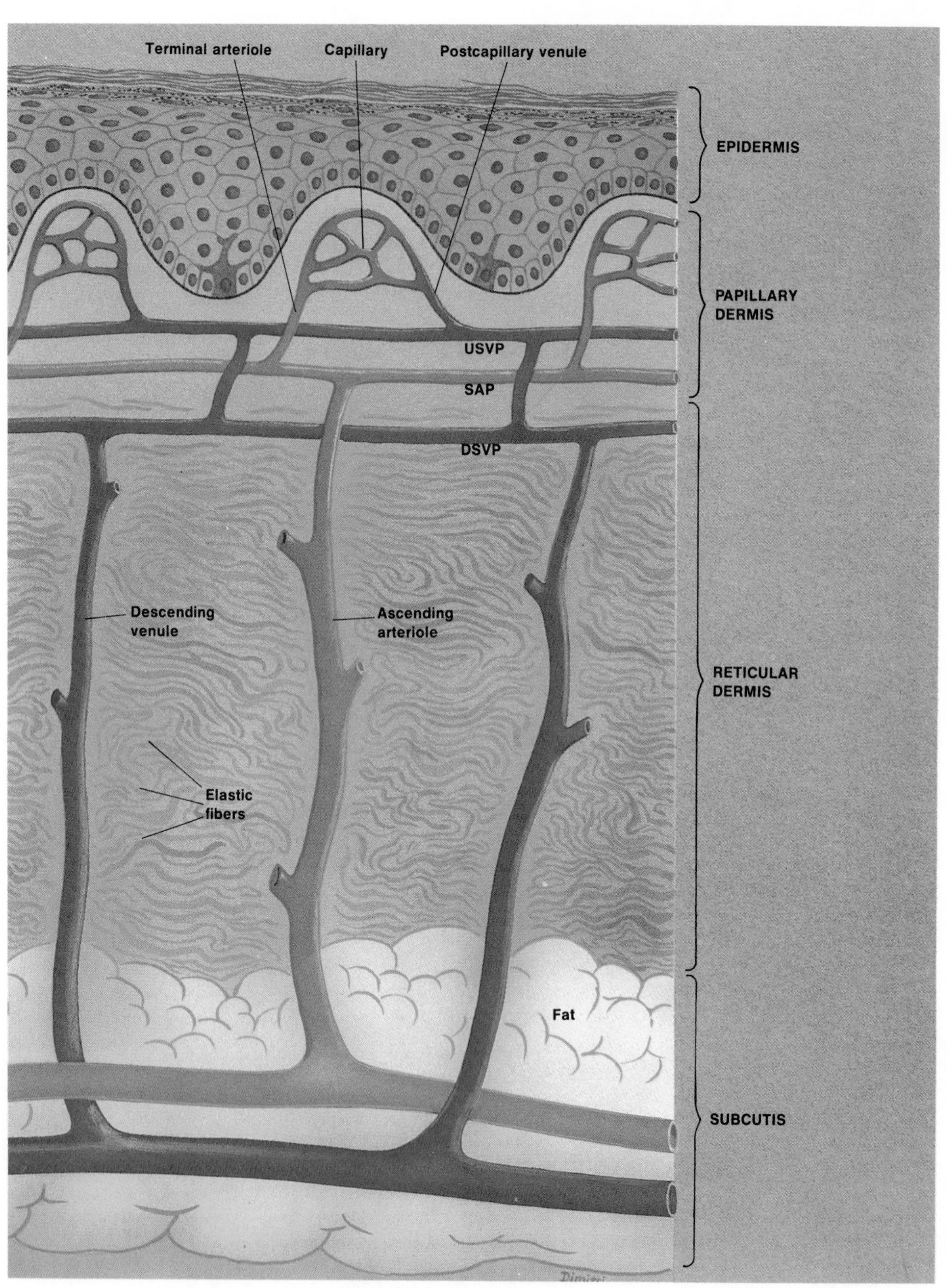

Terminal arteriole
Capillary
Postcapillary venule
EPIDERMIS
PAPILLARY DERMIS
USVP
SAP
DSVP
Descending venule
Ascending arteriole
RETICULAR DERMIS
Elastic fibers
Fat
SUBCUTIS

The Skin

Terence J. Harrist
Brian Schapiro
Timothy R. Quinn
Wallace H. Clark

FIGURE *24-1 (see opposite page)*
The dermis and its vasculature. The fact that the dermis is divided into two distinct anatomical regions is of importance in studying cutaneous pathology. The papillary dermis, with its vascular plexus, and the epidermis usually react together in most diseases that are primarily limited to the skin. The reticular dermis and subcutis are altered in association with systemic diseases that are manifested in the skin. DSVP, deep superficial venular plexus; SAP, superficial arterial plexus; USVP, upper superficial venular plexus.

The skin is a favorable organ for studying fundamental principles of pathology, because the lesions on its surface are readily appreciated and studied. Except for diseases of highly specialized tissues—for instance, those of the alveolus or the glomerulus, or the demyelinating diseases of the central nervous system—all classes of disease are seen in the skin. On the other hand, some diseases—the dyshesive, blistering ones quickly come to mind—are manifested only in the skin (except for some involvement of the mucous membranes).

Considering the imperatives of appearance in human relationships, it is not surprising that an alteration in the appearance of the skin may be the single most important feature of cutaneous disease. Many cutaneous diseases have minor symptomatology, whereas others have none at all. With notable exceptions, only few are life-threatening, and many are self-limited. However, even the self-limited, asymptomatic cutaneous diseases are of great concern to the patient. For example, the symptoms of acne are systemically minor, but the disease can totally change a life. Loss of some unneeded scalp hair has generated an industry of significant size. Vitiligo, a completely asymptomatic, progressive, depigmentary disorder, may convert a normal human being into a recluse or outcast.

ANATOMY AND PHYSIOLOGY OF THE SKIN

The skin serves a protective barrier function; microorganisms find it almost impossible to traverse the epidermis, and water loss is limited. The skin is also vital in regulating temperature and in protecting against ultraviolet light. A wide variety of sensory receptors communicate details related to the immediate environment. The skin plays a prominent role in immune regulation through the *skin-associated lymphoid tissues (SALT)* and the immune functions of keratinocytes and Langerhans cells. Epidermal keratinocytes produce a variety of cytokines, notably Il-1a and Il-1b, as well as eicosanoids. These diverse products of keratinocytes, which mediate immunity and inflammation, are necessary in an organ continuously exposed to the external environment. Langerhans cells, the dendritic antigen-presenting cells of the skin, are bone marrow-derived epidermal immigrant cells that are part of a widespread system involved in antigen presentation and processing. These play an important role in the development and regulation of contact hypersensitivity, allograft rejection, and graft-versus-host disease. Langerhans cells are also present in tissues other than the skin, for example, the genital mucosa, where they are thought to participate in the pathogenesis of human immunodeficiency virus (HIV) infections. All of these cells, together with other dermal cells, such as mast cells, lymphocytes, and macrophages, indicate that the skin is an important immunological organ.

The Epidermis and the Keratinocytic Cellular System

The human epidermis is a multilayered sheet of keratin-synthesizing cells. A progressive change in form proceeds from the lowermost basal layer to the outermost shedding cells of the stratum corneum (Fig. 24-2). The columnar basal cells are replicating stem cells. The nonviable, superficial, cornified cells are flattened plates, arrayed on the surface of the skin. The layering of keratinocytes is accomplished through an intrinsic stacking architecture related to (1) the rate of proliferation, (2) the order of desquamation, and (3) the regulation of water loss. Keratinocytes synthesize a sulfur-poor, filamentous protein, the *tonofibril*, which is related to the keratin molecule of the stratum corneum. Tonofibrils are formed of acidic and basic intermediate keratin filaments, comprising some 30 different keratins. The types of keratins and their organization are responsible for the structure of the stratum corneum, hair, and nails. In addition to various specialized attachment zones, the keratinocytes are distinguished by two structural products.

Keratohyaline granules, the defining hallmark of the stratum granulosum, are composed of a histidine-rich, electron-dense, basophilic protein, profillaggrin, which is associated with intermediate filaments. Keratohyaline granules form the electron-dense, amorphous matrix of the cornified cells and may be abnormal in some forms of harlequin ichthyosis, where fillaggrin is not expressed.

Odland bodies (keratinosomes, membrane-coating granules) are the only structurally distinctive, secretory product of the epidermis (Fig. 24-3). They form in the outer spinous and granular layers and discharge their uniquely lamellated contents into the intercellular spaces, there appearing as lamellar masses that parallel the sur-

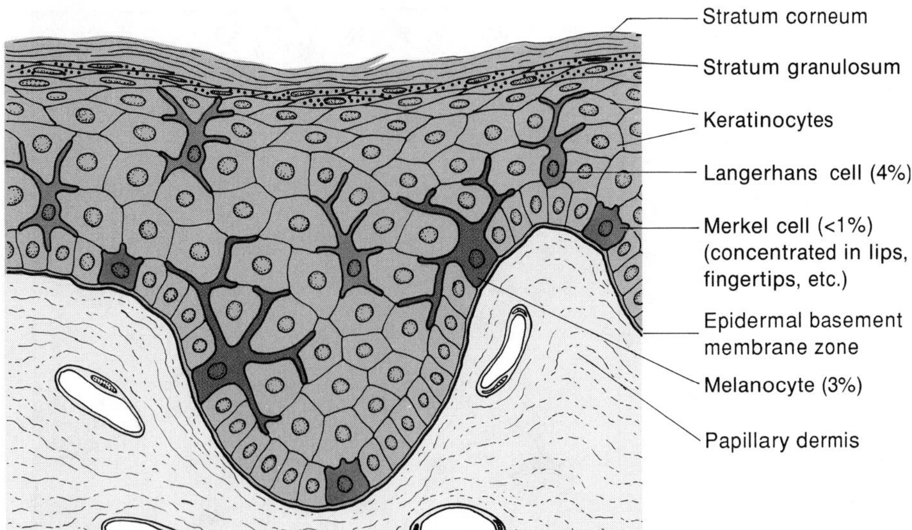

FIGURE 24-2
Normal epidermis and the epidermal immigrant cells. The keratinocytes form the multilayered epidermis, protecting against water loss and bacterial invasion. The melanocytes, forming some 3% of the cells of the epidermis, provide color, as well as protection against ultraviolet radiation. The Langerhans cells, which are slightly more numerous than melanocytes, are one of the cells responsible for the skin's function as an immunological organ. The Merkel cells may represent one of the markers of tactile function of the skin. They are confined to special sites, such as the lips.

face of the skin. Odland bodies and the discharged lamellated products, are most clearly manifested in the outer granular layer and are related to the epidermal barrier function. Although the primary barrier function is in the stratum corneum, Odland bodies may also be involved in cholesterol synthesis and storage, and may possibly induce the conversion of vitamin D_3 by ultraviolet light. An increase in Odland bodies and their intercellular products in some ichthyoses may play a role in the abnormal retention of the stratum corneum.

Epidermal Immigrant Cells

The epidermis harbors immigrant cells of neuroectodermal and mesenchymal origin. These cells do not synthesize keratin and have their own highly distinctive organelles. All appear in varying numbers and at varying levels of the epidermal strata as cells with a clear perikaryon. Two of these cells, melanocytes and Langerhans cells, are dendritic; the third, the Merkel cell, is associated with a terminal neuronal axon.

Melanocytes

Melanocytes, dendritic cells that are largely responsible for the color of human skin, originate in the neural crest. After traversing a mesenchymal migratory pathway, they take up residence in the epidermis from the eighth embryonic week forward and are the first immigrant cell to arrive in that location. By the fourth month of gestation, melanin synthesis begins, and the transfer of the synthesized pigment granules occurs by the sixth month. This is the beginning of the native color of a person. In postembryonic life, the melanocytes come to lie in the basal layer of the epidermis, where they tend to hang down as teardrops into the papillary dermis. However, they are separated from the dermis by the epidermal basement membrane zone. A given melanocyte supplies dendrites to some 36 keratinocytes, forming a complex known as the *epidermal-melanin unit* (Fig. 24-4).

The melanosome (see Fig. 24-4) is a membrane-bound complex in which melanin is synthesized. When melanin synthesis is active, the derigible-shaped melanosome contains filaments (melanofilaments), which have a distinctive 9 nm periodicity and are arranged in a parallel array along the long axis of the organelle. In some profiles, melanofilaments are cross-linked coincident with their periodic structure, a feature that results in a distinctive striated appearance. With melanization (a tyrosinase-dependent process), the orderly internal structure is progressively obliterated, and the melanosome then appears as an electron-opaque granule. This melanin granule provides protection from ultraviolet light and is responsible for the diverse coloration of humans and other animals. Interestingly, the black cloud that obscures the retreat of the squid is secreted by a gland that synthesizes massive quantities of melanin.

The color of the skin is largely based on the number, size, and packaging of melanosomes in keratinocytes and is not primarily dependent on variations in the chemical structure of melanin. There are only two basic melanins, namely, eumelanin (brown-black insoluble melanin) and pheomelanin (yellow-red melanin soluble in dilute alkali). Melanins move from the melanocytes to keratinocytes, where they form a supranuclear cap that absorbs light to shield the skin against ultraviolet radiation.

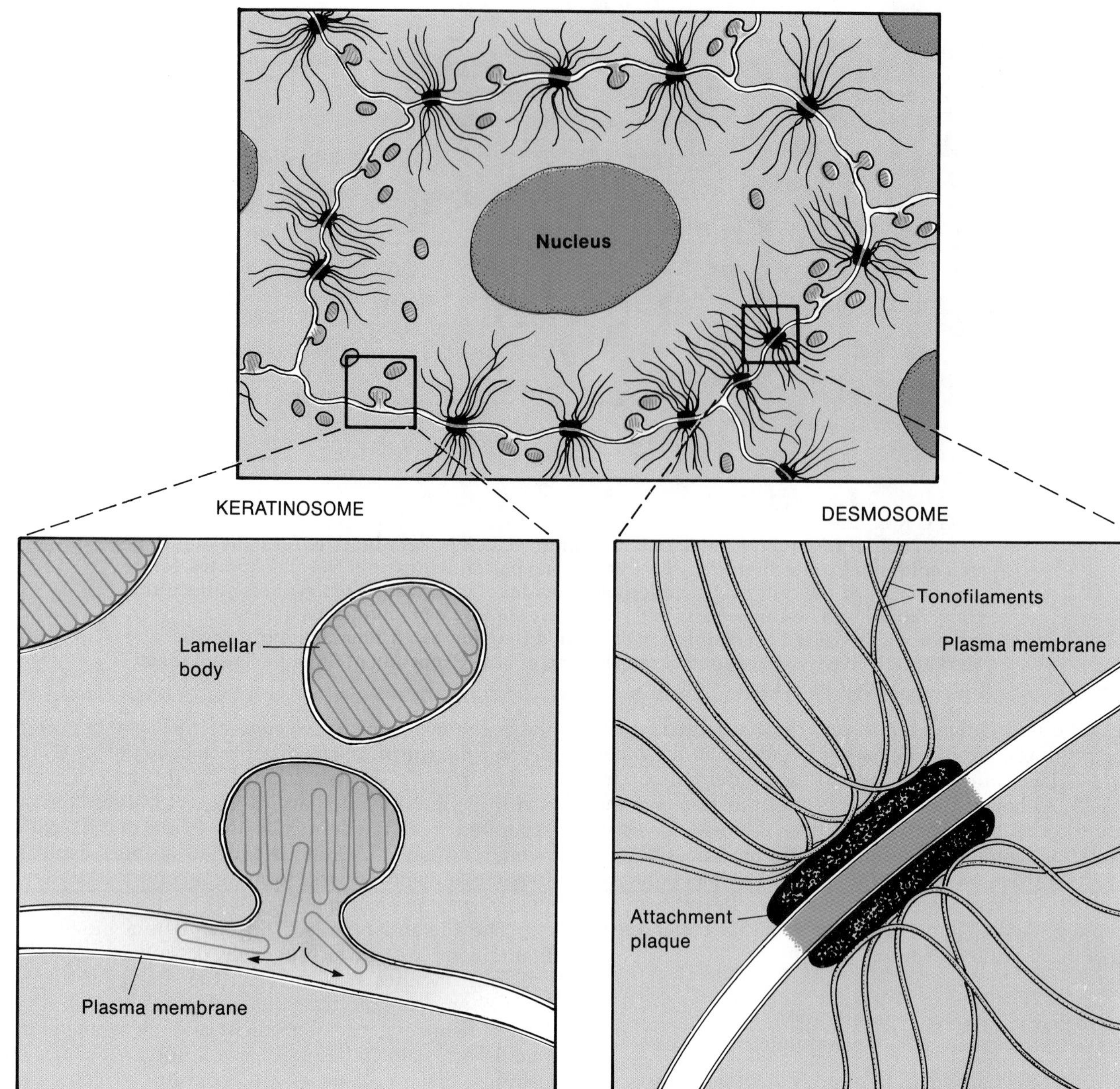

FIGURE 24-3
The keratinocyte, keratinosome, and desmosome. The keratinocyte cytoplasm is dominated by delicate keratin fibrils, the tonofilaments. These form a part of the cytoskeleton of the cell and loop within the attachment plaque of the desmosome. The lamellar body of the keratinocyte extrudes its contents into the intercellular space. The material probably has a role in cellular cohesion.

In hair and epidermal keratinocytes, melanins are packaged to variably absorb and reflect visible light, thereby forming the integumentary colors.

The Langerhans Cells

The next immigrants to the epidermis (and dermis) are the Langerhans cells. They arrive in embryonic skin in the last month of the first trimester, following the melanocytes by a month. With the arrival of these HLA-DR–positive cells, the skin acquires the ability to recognize and process antigens, at which time it becomes a part of the immune system. Uncommon in the dermis, these cells are distributed throughout the nucleated layers of the epidermis, where they constitute 4% of the cells. They are difficult to see in routine light microscopic preparations, because their cytoplasm is translucent and is formed of a perikaryon and dendrites. The Langerhans cells do not form specialized attachments to the apposed

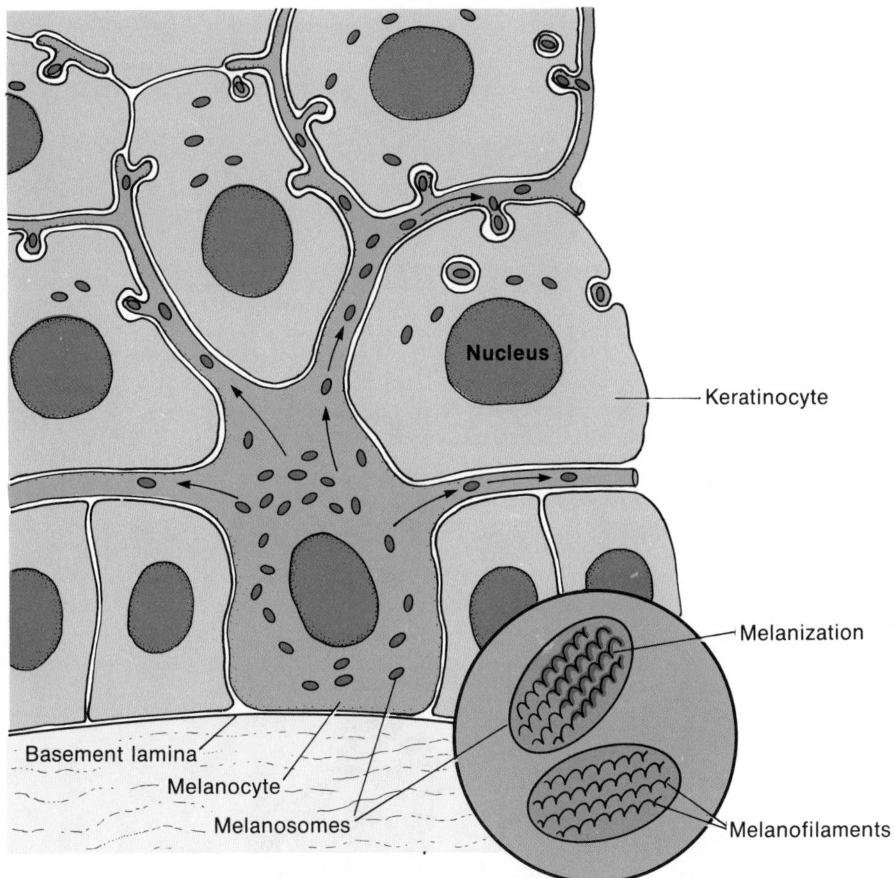

FIGURE *24-4*
The melanocyte supplies approximately 36 keratinocytes with melanin granules by way of complex dendritic cytoplasmic extensions. The melanin granules are transferred to keratinocytes and come to lie in a supranuclear cap, a site suggestive of the protective function of these pigment granules. Pigment is actually formed in the melanocytes within distinctive organelles—the melanosomes—which are the parents of the pigment granule. Pigment is synthesized on small filaments within this organelle (*inset*).

keratinocytes. In electron micrographs, the cytoplasm contains a moderate number of specialized organelles, the *Birbeck granules*. In two dimensions, these structures appear to be racquet-shaped, but three-dimensional reconstruction has shown them to be cup-shaped (Fig. 24-5). The function of these unique organelles, which are derived from the plasma membrane, is probably related to the role of Langerhans cells as antigen-presenting cells (antigenic material being internalized into Birbeck granules).

In the Langerhans cell histiocytoses (see Chapter 20), Birbeck granules are attached to the plasma membrane of the proliferating cells and are in direct communication with the extracellular space. Furthermore, they have a fuzzy coat of clathrin, a feature of "coated pits," suggesting a relationship to receptor-mediated antigen processing and recognition. Langerhans cells express MHC I, MHC II, and receptors for Fc IgG and Fc IgE. Langerhans cells are identified by the immunohistochemical demonstration of CD1 or less specifically by S-100.

Merkel Cells

Although still classed as "immigrant" cells, evidence is accumulating that Merkel cells may actually not be immigrants to the epidermis, but rather specialized basal keratinocytes. They form desmosomes with keratinocytes and express keratins 8, 18, and 20 in a fashion similar to that of keratinocytes. Merkel cells become evident in the basal layer at the beginning of the second trimester of pregnancy, indicating that specialization as neurosecretory keratinocytes begins at that gestational age. They do not appear in all areas of the epidermis, but are seen in special regions, such as the lips, oral cavity, external root sheath of the hair follicles, and the palmar skin of the digits. Merkel cells project short, blunt, cytoplasmic fingers into adjacent keratinocytes and are attached to them by desmosomes. Merkel cells have a distinctive organelle, a membrane bound, dense-core granule, 100 nm or larger in width Fig. 24-6). Immunohistochemical and ultrastructural studies suggest that the Merkel cell has a neurosecretory function. The basal aspect of the cell is apposed to

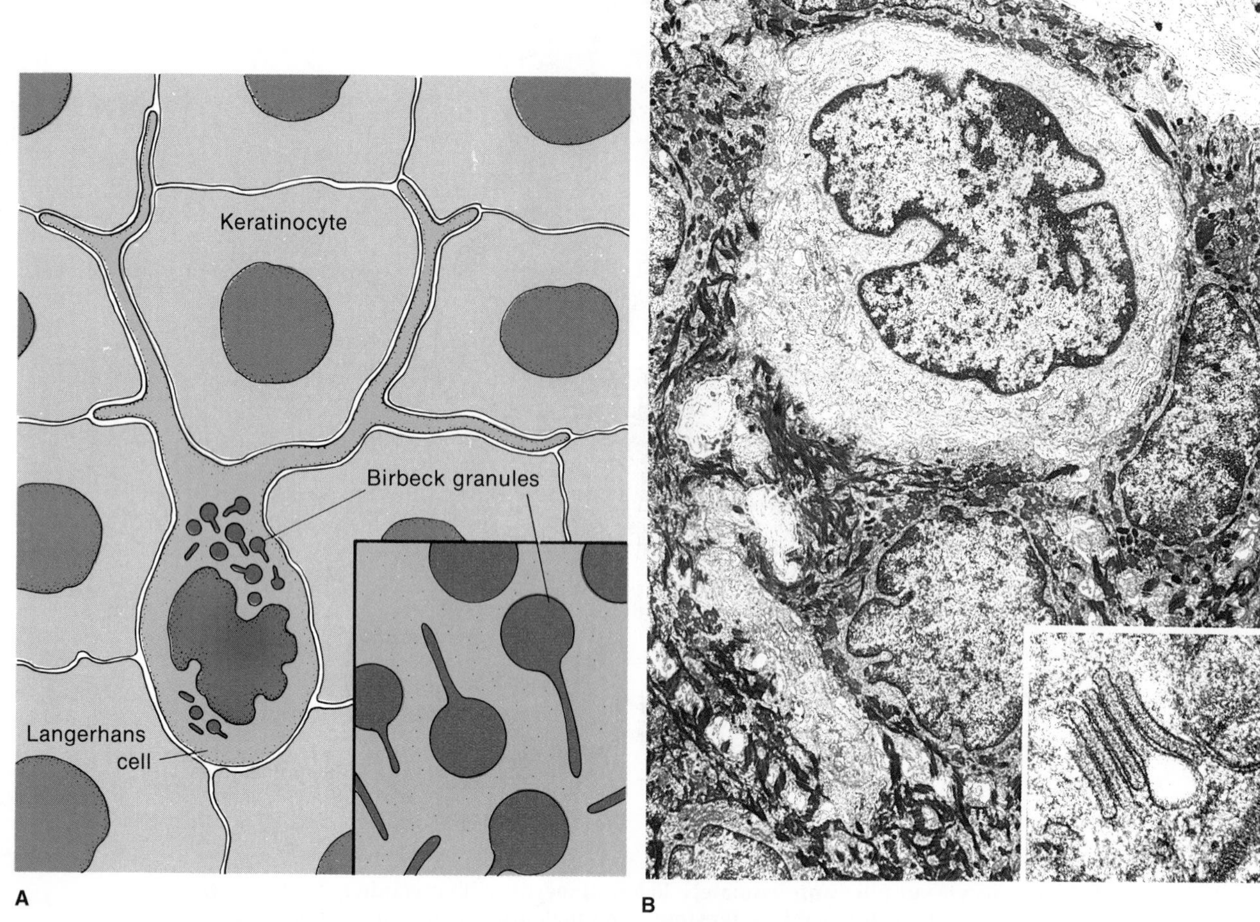

FIGURE 24-5
The dendritic Langerhans cell can recognize and process antigens. (*A*) The unique racket-shaped organelles, called Birbeck granules, may be important in antigen presentation. (*B*) An electron micrograph of a Langerhans cell is inset with a high-power view of the racket-shaped organelles. The Langerhans cell body, residing in the mid-lower portion, is pale when compared with the surrounding keratinocytes, whose cytoplasms contain electron-dense packets of tonofilaments. A dendrite is present in the upper right-corner.

a small nerve plate, which is connected to a myelinated axon by a short, nonmyelinated axon. This complex structure may function as a tactile mechanoreceptor.

Dermal-Epidermal Basement Membrane Zone and Basal Lamina

The basement membrane zone serves as an interface between the epidermis and dermis and is as diverse in function as it is complex in structure (Fig. 24-7). It is responsible for dermal-epidermal adherence and probably serves as a selective macromolecular filter. It is also a major site of immunoglobulin and complement deposition in cutaneous disease. The basal lamina organizes cells into tissues; is responsible for epithelial cell polarity; and directs some keratin gene expression. There is a "dynamic reciprocity" between the extracellular matrix, which includes the basal lamina, and the cytoskeleton and nuclear matrix of keratinocytes. The basement membrane zone includes the following:

- **The innermost part of the basal keratinocytes**, especially the tonofilaments that attach to the inner face of the hemidesmosome.
- **The hemidesmosome**, with its subdesmosomal dense plate.
- **The basal aspect of the plasma membrane** of keratinocytes that faces the dermis.
- **The anchoring filaments** that extend from the subdesmosomal dense plates across the lamina lucida and insert into the lamina densa.
- **The lamina lucida**, an electron lucent layer, where adherence proteins are located. (Recent studies indicate that the lamina lucida is an artifact of fixation for electron microscopy, but most texts still describe it as a definitive structure.)

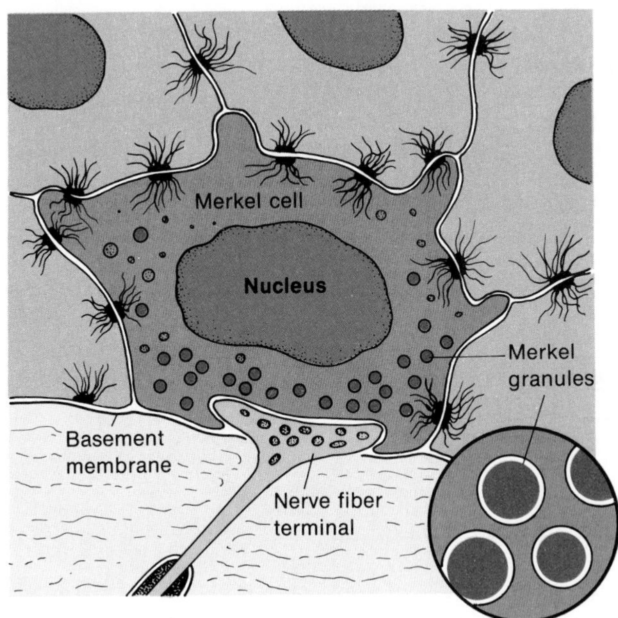

FIGURE 24-6
The Merkel cell, which differs from other immigrant cells, forms desmosomes with keratinocytes and is attached to a small nerve plate (nerve fiber terminal). The membrane-delimited, dense core granule is distinctive (*inset*).

- **The lamina densa**, composed principally of type IV collagen, as well as laminin, perlecan, and entactin.
- **Anchoring fibrils**, which are unstaggered arrays of type VII collagen, extending from the inner face of the lamina densa for a short distance into the papillary dermis.
- **Microfibrils**, which are delicate, long, elastic fibrils that blend with the underlying elastic fibrillary system of the skin.

All of the structures of the basement membrane zone are elaborated by the epidermis, except for the anchoring fibrils and microfibrils. Many antigenic components have been detected in the epidermal basement membrane zone, although the significance of some of these elements is unknown.

Lamina Lucida

LAMININ: This glycoprotein is present in the lamina densa and lamina lucida of all basement membrane zones and plays a role in the organization of the macromolecules of the basement membrane zone. It also promotes attachment of cells to the extracellular matrix. Laminin binds to type IV collagen, perlecan, and entactin.

BULLOUS PEMPHIGOID ANTIGENS: These antigens were identified with antibodies present in patients with bullous pemphigoid. The antigens BPAG1 and BPAG2 (type XVII collagen) are normal constituents of the dermal-epidermal junction, but are absent in basement membrane zones around skin appendages and cutaneous blood vessels. Bullous pemphigoid antigens are in the hemidesmosomes and the cytoplasm of the basal keratinocytes.

CICATRICIAL PEMPHIGOID ANTIGEN: Antibodies from patients affected by cicatricial pemphigoid identified this antigen, which is present within the lower part of the lamina lucida. In some cases of cicatricial pemphigoid, the antigen has been characterized as BPAG1, indicating that the disease is a variant of bullous pemphigoid.

Lamina Densa

TYPE IV COLLAGEN: This component is present in all basement membrane zones. It is the most superficial component of the complex collagen fiber network of the dermis and is important in dermal-epidermal attachment. Type IV collagen links to laminin, perlecan, and entactin.

Subbasal Lamina Densa Zone

TYPE VII COLLAGEN: This type of collagen is present on the deep aspect of the basal lamina in anchoring fibrils.

ANCHORING FIBRIL (AF-1 AND AF-2) ANTIGENS: These proteins appear to reside within anchoring fibrils and possibly within the lower lamina densa. The exact relationship to type VII collagen is unclear.

EPIDERMOLYSIS BULLOSA ACQUISITA ANTIGEN: This antigen is the globular carboxyl terminus of type VII procollagen. It is identical with the one that reacts with the antibody found in patients with bullous systemic lupus erythematosus.

The Dermis

The papillary dermis is a narrow zone immediately deep to the basement membrane zone of the epidermis. This region is pale-pink with the hematoxylin and eosin stain and has little organization when viewed with the light microscope (see Fig. 24-1). Its most prominent structures are delicate collagen fibrils, 0.4 to 0.6 mm wide. The delicate connective tissue of the papillary dermis extends as a narrow sheath about blood vessels, nerves, and skin appendages. The entire network of this collagen is termed the *adventitial dermis*.

The reticular dermis is deep to the papillary dermis and contains most of the dermal collagen, which is organized into coarse bundles (see Fig. 24-1). Each bundle is associated with elastic tissue fibers, which are demonstrated with special stains.

As a rule, the papillary dermis is altered in conjunction with epidermal disease and disorders that affect the superficial venular bed. The three structures—the epidermis, papillary dermis, and superficial capillary-venular bed—react jointly and influence each other in complex

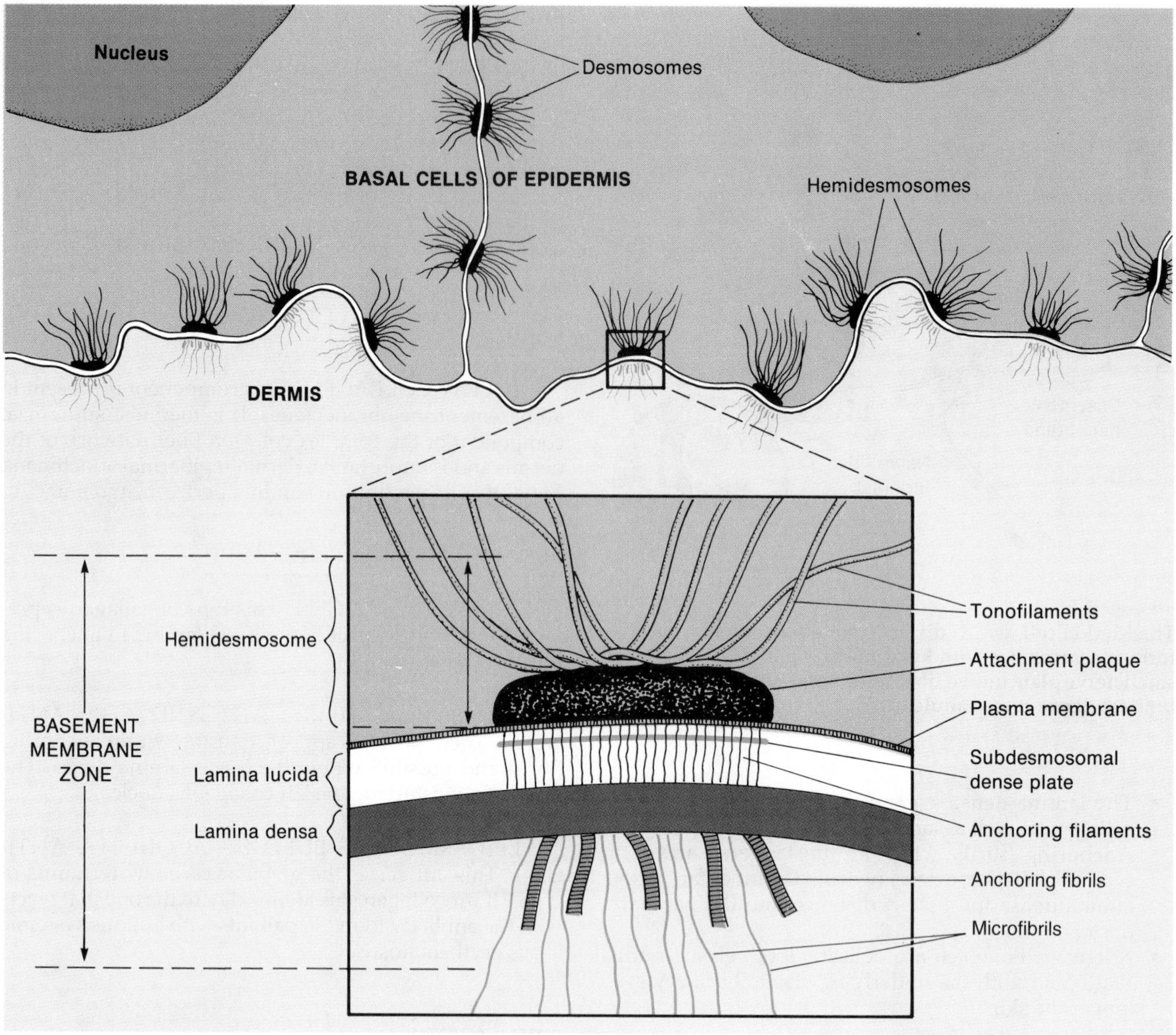

A

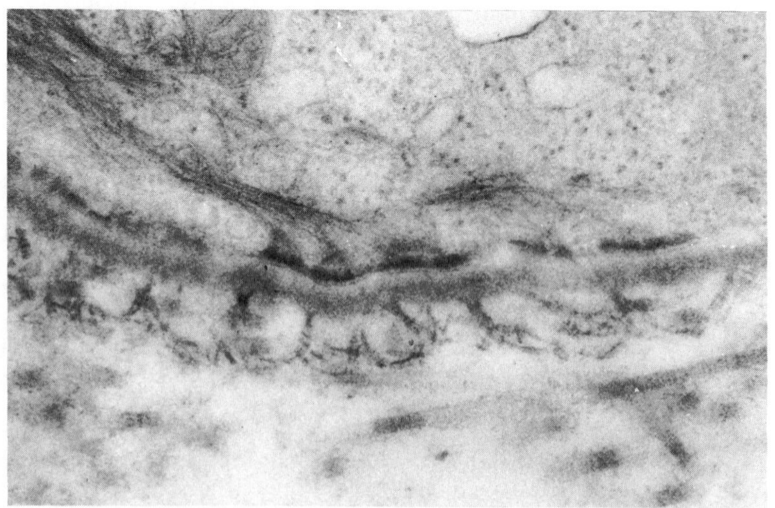

B

FIGURE *24-7*
The dermal-epidermal interface and the basement membrane zone. (*A*) This epithelial-mesenchymal interface is the site of the basement membrane zone, a complex structure that is mostly synthesized by the basal cells of the epidermis. Each of its complex structures, from tonofilaments and attachment plaques of basal cells to anchoring fibrils and microfibrils, attached to the inner face of the lamina densa, is a site of change in specific disease. (*B*) An electron micrograph shows the hemidesmosomal attachment plaques with their inserting tonofilaments (near the center). The subdemosomal dense plates, the lamina lucida, the lamina densa, and the subjacent anchoring fibrils are well demonstrated. The lamina lucida may be a fixation artifact. Compare this with *A*.

ways. Primary skin diseases with few or no systemic manifestations, for example, psoriasis and lichen planus, involve these superficial cutaneous structures. The reticular dermis and subcutis (also formally designated as a cutaneous structure) are less common sites of pathological change and, when diseased, are usually manifestations of systemic disease. Scleroderma (progressive systemic sclerosis) and erythema nodosum exemplify this principle of cutaneous pathology.

Cutaneous Vasculature

The skin receives 10 times the amount of blood needed for its nutrition, and its circulating blood has a number of other functions. For example, the skin is of great importance in temperature regulation. Many aspects of cutaneous inflammation involve the superficial cutaneous vascular unit.

An ascending arteriole arises from arteries in the subcutis and directly crosses much of the reticular dermis (see Fig. 24-1). In the outer part of the reticular dermis, in conjunction with other similar ascending arteries, a superficial arteriolar plexus is formed. From this plexus a terminal arteriole extends into each dermal papilla, where an arterial capillary is formed. The arterial capillary makes a U-turn and on its descent becomes a venous capillary and a postcapillary venule. The venules then join to form a complex venular plexus in the reticular dermis, immediately deep to the papillary dermis. The venular end of this vascular structure is important in the mediation of the cutaneous inflammatory response.

The lymphatic vessels of the skin form a random network, beginning as lymphatic capillaries near the epidermis. A superficial lymphatic plexus is then formed, from which lymphatic channels drain to regional lymph nodes. The lymphatic channels are involved in the metastasis of cutaneous cancers, especially malignant melanoma. Cutaneous lymphatics have no basal lamina, or an incomplete one.

Mast Cells

Mast cells are derived from the bone marrow and are normally present about the venules of the skin, where they provide for the immediate release of vasoactive and chemotactic substances. Mast cells mediate inflammation of all types (their function is discussed with urticaria and angioedema), and they proliferate in a spectrum of skin diseases termed *urticaria pigmentosa* (Fig. 24-8).

The Hair Follicles

Hair grows in a cyclical fashion. Growing hair of the scalp and beard have bulbs of epithelial and mesenchymal tissue firmly embedded within the subcutis. Cross-section of a bulb reveals a cap of actively dividing, keratin-synthesizing cells, which become arrayed in layers that join at the top of the bulb to form the cylindrical hair shaft. The differentiating hairs form the roof of the epithelial bulb and interact with an island of melanocytes, which contribute melanin to the passing keratinocytes. It is this process that results in hair color. The colored keratinocytes lose their nuclei as they form the final cylindrical hair shaft. Curly hair is formed from angulated bulbs, whereas straight hair develops from round bulbs.

THE HAIR CYCLE: Some 90% of hairs are normally in the *anagen phase*, the actively growing hair phase. The growing hairs have a mosaic distribution and are interspersed with hairs showing no evidence of growth, termed *telogen hairs*. Hairs in the process of ceasing growth, known as *catagen hairs*, still have a hair shaft. However they end in the lower reticular dermis as a slightly widened club-like structure, which is surrounded by a rim of nucleated keratinocytes. The hair bulb is no longer evident, and a strikingly thickened and widened lamina densa surrounds the catagen hair.

As the telogen phase (resting follicle) is reached, the

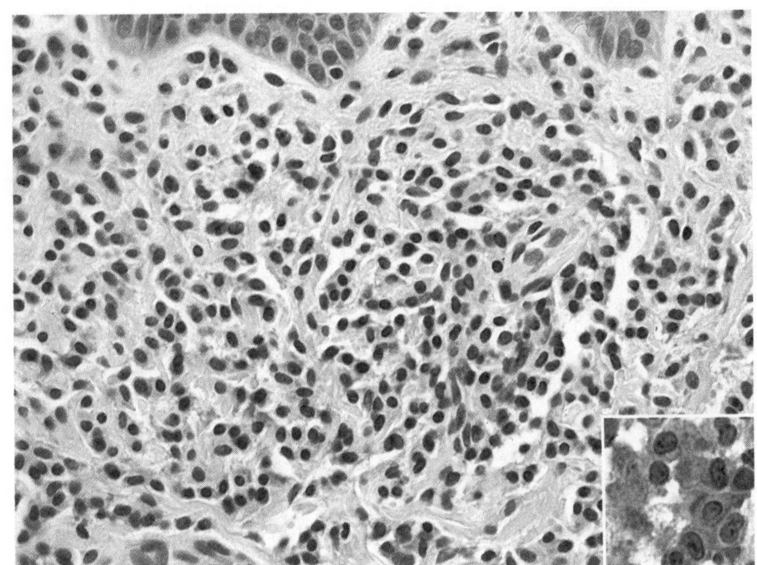

FIGURE *24-8*
Urticaria pigmentosa. Mast cells fill and expand the papillary dermis. The cytoplasms of mast cells contain chloracetate esterase-rich granules, giving them a red hue in this stain (*inset*), a useful distinguishing feature.

end of the hair retreats to the level of the arrectores pilorum. The hair shaft may be missing, since it is no longer tethered at the base, leaving but a rudiment of the original follicle. However, a delicate, vascularized mesenchymal tract, the *telogen tract*, extends from its attenuated tip. At the top of this tract, the early anagen hair forms again from the follicular stem cells. With growth, it follows the delicate pathway through the reticular dermis into the panniculus, there forming a mature anagen follicle and a new hair.

ALOPECIA: *Alopecia, usually known as baldness, refers to the loss of hair.* **Common alopecia** affects both men (male pattern baldness) and women (female pattern). It results from a complex and poorly understood interaction of heritable and hormonal factors. Men castrated before puberty do not lose scalp hair and fail to grow a beard. On the other hand, the administration of testosterone to such castrated men results in the growth of a beard and may lead to male pattern baldness. The loss of scalp hair results in the replacement of a large terminal hair follicle by a vellus hair follicle, the parent of the delicate fuzz on the cheeks of women and on the upper cheeks of men.

Growing hair is the site of active mitosis, and many systemic diseases cause cessation of mitosis in this location and thus alopecia. If the malady passes, mitotic activity is renewed and regrowth occurs. If a person is subjected to a potent antimitotic regimen, such as chemotherapy for advanced cancer, hair follicles stop growth, hair is lost, and a telogen follicle follows. With cessation of therapy, hair cycling resumes. Almost any kind of follicular inflammation can induce the telogen phase; if fibrosis distorts the telogen tract (the regrowth pathway), permanent loss of that follicle and alopecia result.

Alopecia areata is a circumscribed area of hair loss, usually on the scalp, although other body areas may be involved. Less commonly, there may be loss of all scalp hair (*alopecia totalis*), and rarely all hair (*alopecia universalis*). These diseases are characterized by a brisk lymphocytic infiltrate around the hair bulb, resulting in the formation of telogen hairs and hair loss. The combination of this histological pattern and the association of these forms of alopecia with the inheritance of HLA class II alleles (especially HLA-DQ3) has been interpreted as evidence for an autoimmune etiology. As a rule scarring does not occur, and hair may regrow normally after varying time periods. On occasion, especially when hair loss is extensive, alopecia is permanent. Alopecia areata does not result in scarring of the affected hair follicles and is, therefore, is a noncicatricial, reversible, alopecia.

VELLUS HAIRS: These fine hairs may play a role in touch perception in many mammals, but in humans they have no function. Microscopically, vellus hairs are diminutive anagen hairs, with a small active bulb high in the reticular dermis, together with small sebaceous glands.

SEBACEOUS FOLLICLES: These structures develop with puberty and are clinically important, because they are the site of acne. Sebaceous follicles have a minute vellus hair at the base. However, instead of the usual small sebaceous glands, they exhibit large sebaceous glands that dwarf the vellus hair and fill the follicular canal with sebum. They are present particularly on the central face.

DISEASES OF THE EPIDERMIS

Heritable Diseases Associated with Excessive Cornification

Icthyoses

The ichthyosiform dermatoses, many of which are heritable, are a heterogeneous group of cutaneous diseases characterized by striking thickening of the stratum corneum. The thickening of the stratum corneum is usually disproportionate to that of the nucleated epidermal layers. The term *ichthyosis* reflects the similarity of the diseased skin to coarse, fishlike scales. There are four major ichthyoses: (1) ichthyosis vulgaris, (2) X-linked ichthyosis, (3) lamellar ichthyosis, and (4) epidermolytic hyperkeratosis (localized and bullous forms). Several rare ichthyoses are associated with other abnormalities, such as abnormal lipid metabolism, neurological disorders, bone diseases, and cancer.

☐ **Pathogenesis and Pathology:** Three general defects seem to be involved in the excessive epidermal cornification of the ichthyoses:

- **Increased cohesiveness** of the cells of the stratum corneum (retention keratosis), possibly related to altered lipid metabolism. This defect is characteristic of ichthyosis vulgaris
- **Abnormal keratinization**, expressed as impaired tonofilament formation and keratohyaline synthesis and as excessive cornification.
- **Increased basal cell proliferation**, associated with a decrease in transit time of keratinocytes across the epidermis.

All ichthyoses (with the possible exception of lamellar ichthyosis) have a stratum corneum that is disproportionately thick in comparison with the nucleated epidermal layers. Virtually all diseases characterized by thickening of the nucleated epidermal layers also exhibit hyperkeratosis. For example, chronic scratching or rubbing of normal skin causes a thickened epidermis and dermal changes, a condition known as *lichen simplex chronicus*. In this ailment, both the nucleated epidermal layers and the compacted stratum corneum are likely to be three times the normal thickness. By contrast, in ichthyosis, although the stratum corneum may be four or five times thicker than normal, it commonly overlies a disproportionately thin nucleated epidermis.

Ichthyosis vulgaris *is an autosomal dominant disorder of keratinization characterized by mild hyperkeratosis and reduced or absent keratohyaline granules in the epidermis.* Scaly skin results from increased adhesiveness of the stratum corneum. The attenuated stratum granulosum consists of a single layer with small defective keratohyaline granules. Decreased or absent synthesis of profilaggrin, a keratin filament "glue," is responsible for the inadequate formation of keratohyaline granules and the increased adhesion.

Ichthyosis vulgaris is the prototype of disproportionate corneal thickening. The stratum corneum is loose and has a basket-weave appearance, which differs little from the normal, except in amount. The granular layer is greatly diminished and often seems absent (Fig. 24-9). Ultrastructurally, the keratohyaline granules are small and spongelike, an appearance indicative of defective synthesis. The basal and spinous layers seem entirely normal. Thus, the primary defect in ichthyosis vulgaris is in the granular and cornified layers, the epidermal zones responsible for the final stage of keratinization and cornification.

Ichthyosis vulgaris is the most common of the ichthyoses and begins in early childhood. A family history of a similar condition is often obtained. Small white scales occur on the extensor surfaces of the extremities and on the trunk and face. The disease is lifelong, but most patients can be maintained free of scales with topical treatment.

A clinical and histological state similar to ichthyosis vulgaris is occasionally associated with other diseases or may follow the use of drugs that affect cholesterol metabolism. Lymphomas and especially Hodgkin's disease may be associated with ichthyosis. However, other types of neoplasms, systemic granulomatous disorders, and connective tissue disease are also occasionally complicated by ichthyosis. It is possible that drugs produce ichthyosis by interfering with pathways of cholesterol metabolism similar to those involved in the rare ichthyoses. In these uncommon keratotic diseases, cutaneous changes are apparently due to abnormalities in lipid metabolism, for instance, phytanic acid storage disease (*Refsum disease*).

***X-linked ichthyosis** is a heritable epidermal disorder characterized by delayed dissolution of the desmosomal discs in the stratum corneum, owing to a deficiency of steroid sulfatase.* Steroid sulfatase normally degrades the Odland body product, cholesterol sulfate, which provides cellular adhesion in the lower stratum corneum. Failure of steroid sulfatase action on cholesterol sulfate leads to persistent cohesion of the stratum corneum.

***Lamellar ichthyosis** is an autosomal recessive congenital disorder of cornification characterized by severe and generalized ichthyosis.* It is typified by an increased cohesiveness of the stratum corneum, accompanied by numerous keratinosomes and an abnormally large amount of intercellular substance. The disease is genetically heterogeneous, and deficient transglutaminase acylation (TGM1 gene), with a defect in lamellar body secretion, underlies the disorder in many cases.

***Epidermolytic hyperkeratosis,** originally known as bullous congenital ichthyosiform erythroderma, is a congential, autosomal dominant disease that features generalized erythroderma, ichthyosiform skin, and blistering.* The disease results from mutations in the K1 and K10 keratin genes, the differentiation-specific keratins found in the suprabasal epidermis. Faulty assembly of keratin tonofilaments and their insertion into desmosomes result from mutations in the highly conserved carboxy-terminal rod domain of keratin 1 and the aminoterminal of the rod domain of keratin 10. These flaws prevent normal development of the cytoskeleton, resulting in dissolution and a tendency to vesiculation.

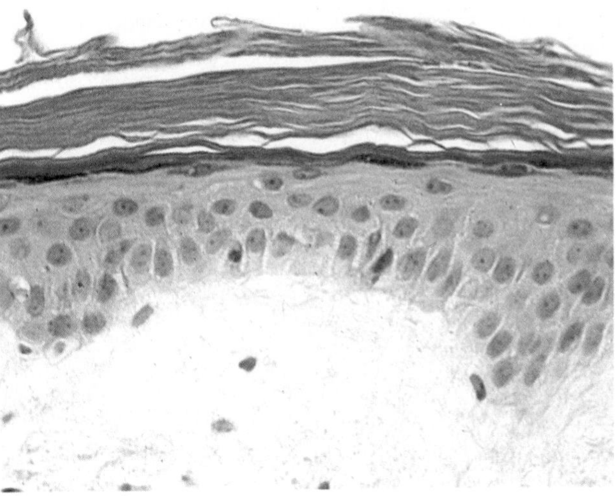

FIGURE 24-9
Ichthyosis vulgaris. There is disproportionate thickening of the stratum corneum in relationship to the normal thickness of the nucleated epidermal strata. The stratum granulosum is thin and focally absent.

In epidermolytic hyperkeratosis, the stratum spinosum has a faulty tonofilament structure, which readily explains the epidermal lysis and the tendency to vesiculation. The spinous keratinocytes contain thick, eosinophilic tonofilaments, which whorl around the nucleus in a concentric fashion (Fig. 24-10). The cytoplasm has a clear zone peripheral to the perinuclear tonofilaments, but at the periphery of the cell these filaments

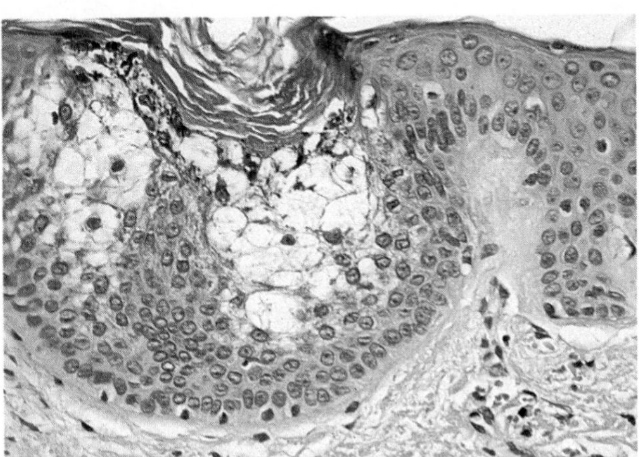

FIGURE 24-10
Epidermolytic hyperkeratosis. The keratinocytes of the stratum spinosum have clumped tonofilaments. As a result, their cytoplasms are relatively clear. In the outer stratum spinosum, the clumped fibrils are further compacted and whorl about the nuclei, resulting in dark cytoplasms condensed about the nuclei. These cells separate from each other to produce epidermolysis. A normal portion of epidermis is to the *right*.

again become condensed. Electron microscopy reveals a faulty insertion of tonofilaments into desmosomes. This flaw, together with other abnormalities in tonofilament structure, may be responsible for cell lysis and the formation of vesicles. The stratum corneum is again disproportionately thickened (Fig. 24-11).

Epidermolytic hyperkeratosis presents at or shortly after birth with blistering. The disease may be generalized or localized to only several areas of the body. The lesions tend to be dark and even verrucous. Other than the cosmetic disfigurement, the major problem is bacterial infection.

Ichthyosis vulgaris and epidermolytic hyperkeratosis are compared with the other ichthyotic disorders in Table 24-1.

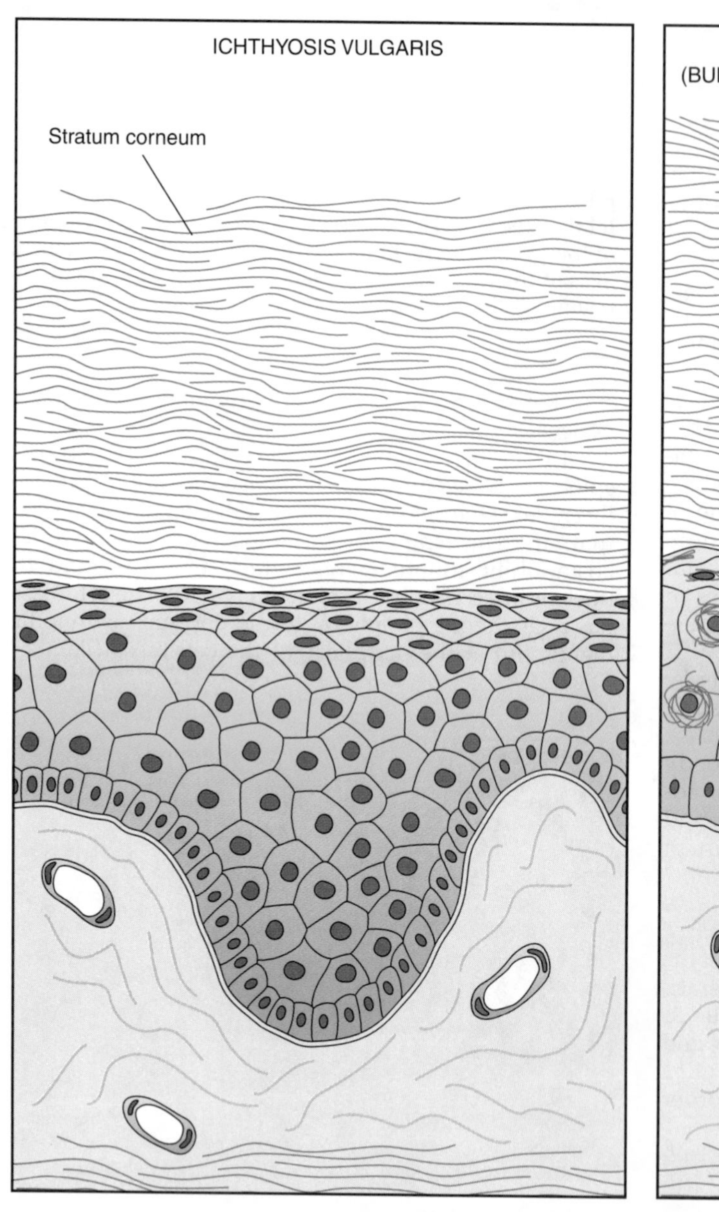

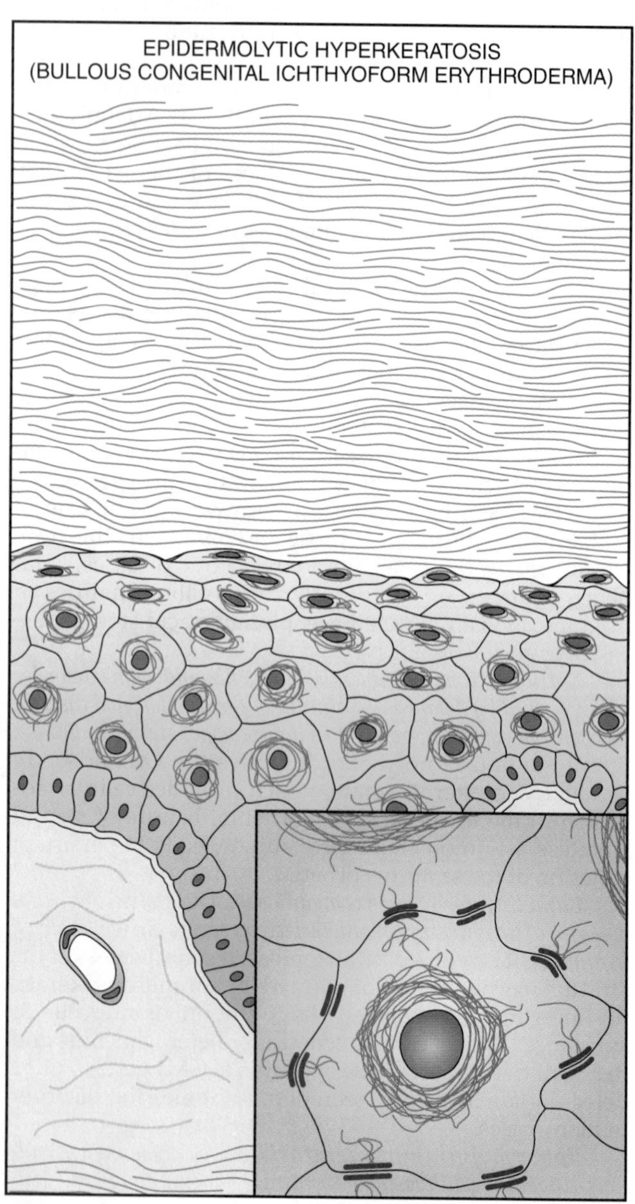

FIGURE *24-11*
(*A*) Ichthyosis vulgaris and (*B*) epidermolytic hyperkeratosis (bullous congenital ichthyosiform erythroderma). Both diseases are characterized by thickening of the stratum corneum relative to the nucleated layers. Epidermolytic hyperkeratosis is characterized by abnormal keratin synthesis, which is manifested by whorled keratin filaments about the nucleus (*inset*).

TABLE 24-1 A Comparison of the Major Ichthyoses

Type of Ichthyosis	Mode of Inheritance	Present at Birth	Pathogenetic Mechanism	Histology
Ichthyosis vulgaris	Autosomal dominant	No; onset in childhood	Normal epidermal turnover Retention keratosis due to defective dissolution of adhesive mechanisms in the stratum corneum.	Hyperkeratosis, loosely woven; disproportionately thick in relationship to a relatively thin stratum spinosum. Thin granular layer with abnormal keratohyaline granules.
Sex-linked ichthyosis	X-linked recessive	Yes; onset may be in infancy	Normal epidermal turnover Constitutional absence of steroid sulfatase and arylsulfatase-C. Retention keratosis due to a failure to break down cholesterol sulfate, an important substance in stratum corneum adhesion.	Compact, disproportionately thick stratum corneum. Normal granular layer. Stratum spinosum only slightly thick.
Epidermolytic hyperkeratosis (bullous congenital ichthyosiform erythroderma)	Autosomal recessive	Yes	Increased germinative cell replication and decreased cellular transit time through the epidermis. Defect in keratin genes K1 and K10, the differentiation specific keratins of the suprabasal epidermis.	Tonofilaments aggregate at the cell periphery and have a distorted association with desmosomes. This may lead to dyshesion (acantholysis) of epidermal keratinocytes and vesicle formation. Entire skin is rarely involved.
Lamellar ichthyosis (nonbullous congenital ichthyosiform erythroderma)	Autosomal recessive	Yes	Increased number of keratinosomes and increase in intercellular substance. Defects in transglutaminase acylation and in lamellar body secretion.	Moderate hyperkeratosis; normal or thickened granular layer. Moderate epidermal hyperplasia. May be psoriasiform with parakeratosis. Entire skin and nails are involved.

Darier Disease (Keratosis Follicularis)

Darier disease is an autosomal dominant disorder of keratinization characterized by numerous focal keratoses. Evidence points to a defect in the glycocalyceal intercellular matrix. Recently, the gene responsible has been localized to chromosome 12 (12q23-24.1).

☐ **Pathology:** Microscopically, the warty papule of Darier disease has a suprabasal cleft. Above and to the side of the cleft, dyskeratotic keratinocytes with eosinophilic cytoplasm contain keratin fibrils, which whorl about the nucleus (Fig. 24-12). The roof of the cleft is formed by a column of compact keratotic material. In the stratum spinosum, some of these cells, called *corps ronds*, have pyknotic nuclei. The eosinophilic seedlike remnants of dyskeratotic cells in the stratum corneum are termed *corps grains*.

☐ **Clinical Features:** Darier disease first appears late in childhood or in adolescence as skin-colored papules, which later become crusted. The affected area presents as numerous warty elevations, 2 to 4 mm in di-

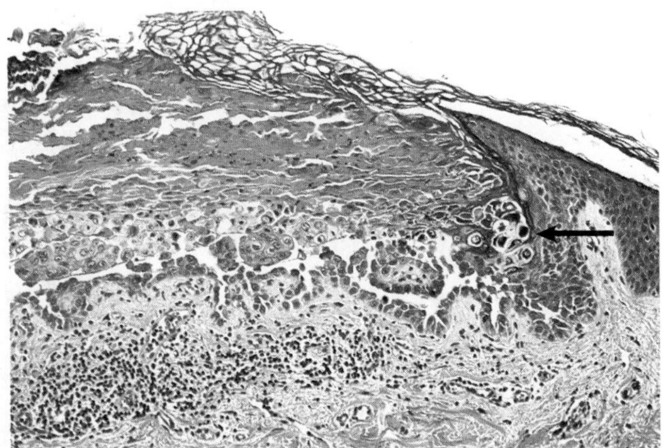

FIGURE 24-12
Darier disease. Virtually the entire epidermis exhibits focal acantholytic dyskeratosis. A small portion of normal epidermis is present (*right*). In the lesion, there is a suprabasal cleft with a few dyshesive (acantholytic) keratinocytes surmounted by hyperkeratosis and parakeratosis. The cleft is not a true vesicle, since most true vesicles contain inflammatory cells and tissue fluid. The dyskeratosis is characterized by an abnormal granular layer keratinocytes (*arrow*).

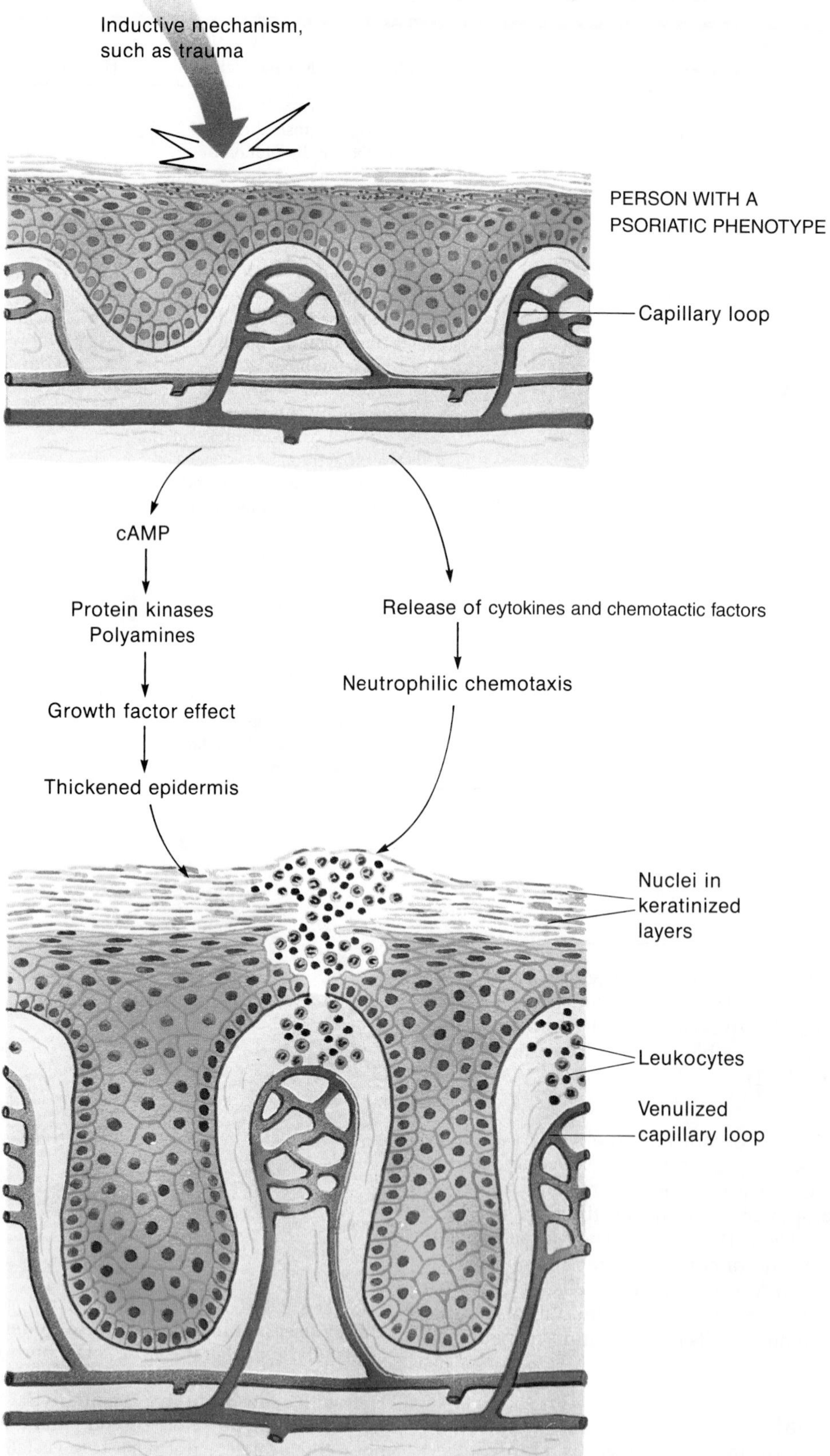
Inductive mechanism,
such as trauma
PERSON WITH A
PSORIATIC PHENOTYPE
Capillary loop
cAMP
Protein kinases
Polyamines
Growth factor effect
Thickened epidermis
Release of cytokines and chemotactic factors
Neutrophilic chemotaxis
Nuclei in
keratinized
layers
Leukocytes
Venulized
capillary loop

FIGURE 24-13

ameter. The chest, nasolabial folds, back, scalp, forehead, ears, and groin exhibit multiple lesions.

Psoriasis: Epidermal-Dermal Disease Characterized by Persistent Epidermal Hyperplasia

Psoriasis is a chronic, frequently familial disease characterized by large, erythematous, scaly plaques, commonly on the extensor dorsal cutaneous surfaces. Psoriasis is one of the oldest diseases of mankind. It is believed that the injunctions in the Old Testament directed against lepers inadvertently also pertained to persons suffering from psoriasis. The disease was known to Hippocrates, although its modern classification dates to the mid-19th century, when the several forms were recognized by the great Viennese dermatologist von Hebra.

Psoriasis is worldwide in distribution and affects 1% to 2% of the population. It may arise at any age and shows a peak in late adolescence. Interestingly, the disease is absent among Native Americans and shows a low incidence among Asians.

A psoriasiform appearance is one of the common patterns of cutaneous pathology. For example, seborrheic dermatitis, reaction to chronic trauma (lichen simplex chronicus), and cutaneous T-cell lymphoma (mycosis fungoides) all may exhibit a psoriasiform epidermal change.

☐ **Pathogenesis:** The pathogenesis of psoriasis remains poorly understood and is likely multifactorial.

GENETIC FACTORS: Psoriasis unquestionably has a genetic component, although only one third of patients with psoriasis have a positive family history of the disease. The more severe the illness, the greater is the likelihood of a familial background. The genetic basis for psoriasis rests on a number of observations: (1) an increased incidence of the disease among relatives and offspring of patients with psoriasis, (2) 65% concordance for psoriasis in monozygotic twins, and (3) the increased occurrence of certain HLA haplotypes in affected persons. The freqeuency of HLA-B13, HLA-B17. HLA-Bw16, and particularly HLA-Cw6, are all increased. In fact, persons with the HLA-Cw6 phenotype are 10 to 15 times more likely to develop psoriasis than the general population.

ENVIRONMENTAL FACTORS: **The entire epidermis of any person with the psoriatic phenotype has the capacity to express clinical lesions.** In this context, a variety of stimuli, such as physical injury, infection, certain drugs, and photosensitivity, may produce psoriatic lesions in apparently normal skin. The pathogenesis of the psoriatic plaques may be appreciated by contrasting the effect of chronic cutaneous trauma in persons with and without psoriasis. Chronic irritation of the skin of a normal person—for instance, that caused by repeated rubbing—produces a tough, scaly, cutaneous plaque, which is psoriasiform both clinically and histologically. However, with cessation of the trauma, the lesion disappears. In the psoriatic patient, even less trauma produces a psoriatic plaque that may persist for years after the initial injury.

ABNORMAL CELLULAR PROLIFERATION: There is evidence to suggest that deregulation of epidermal proliferation and an abnormality in the microcirculation of the dermis are responsible for the development of psoriatic lesions (Fig. 24-13). Abnormal proliferation of keratinocytes is possibly related to defective epidermal cell surface receptors. A decrease in the activity of adenylyl cyclase in the lower proliferative compartment of the epidermis has been attributed to faulty β-adrenergic receptors. The consequent decrease in cAMP alters cutaneous responses to trauma in complex ways that are not fully understood.

An increase in cAMP-regulated proteinases and augmented polyamines of low molecular weight are postulated to be associated with a growth factor–like effect and induction of neutrophilic inflammation. The induction of neutrophilic inflammation follows an increase in phospholipase A_2, which enhances the production of arachidonic acid. In turn, the lipooxygenase metabolites of arachidonic acid, notably leukotriene B_4, exert potent chemotactic effects (see Fig. 24-13).

MICROCIRCULATORY CHANGES: In psoriatic skin, the capillary loops of the dermal papillae become venular, showing multiple layers of basal lamina material, wide lumina, and "bridged" fenestrations between endothelial cells. The vascular change, which occurs in concert with a striking increase in neutrophilic chemotactic factors, leads to diapedesis of many neutrophils at the tips of dermal papillae and subsequent migration into the epidermis. This unusual pattern of neutrophilic inflammation is responsible for the dense collections of neutrophils in the stratum corneum (*Munro microabscesses*), as well as for the scattering of neutrophils throughout the epidermis (*spongiform pustules*).

FIGURE *24-13*
Pathogenetic mechanisms in psoriasis. The drawing depicts the deregulation of epidermal growth, venulization of the capillary loop, and a unique form of neutrophilic inflammation. The altered epidermal growth is thought to be caused by defective epidermal cell surface receptors. This results in a decrease in cAMP, together with the effects indicated. The decrease in cAMP is also likely to be related to the increased production of arachidonic acid which, in turn, leads to activation of LTB-4. This potent neutrophilic chemotactic agent acts on a venulized capillary loop. Neutrophils then emerge from the tips of the capillary loop at the apex of the dermal papilla, rather than from the postcapillary venule, as is the rule in most inflammatory skin diseases.

IMMUNOLOGICAL FACTORS: T lymphocytes have been proposed to contribute to pathogenesis of psoriatic lesions. The eruption of such lesions coincides with the infiltration of T cells into the epidermis. By contrast, resolution of psoriatic plaques, whether spontaneous or induced by treatment, is preceded by the disappearance of or reduction in the number of epidermal T cells. Recently, streptococcal superantigens have been reported to induce the expression of cutaneous lymphocyte antigens, which are believed to enable T cells to migrate to the skin. Finally, T lymphocytes from psoriatic patients are capable of producing lesional plaques in apparently normal skin from the same patients that has been transferred to nude mice.

In summary, the keratinocytes of persons afflicted with psoriasis possess a genetically determined phenotype that exhibits a capacity for hyperproliferation and altered differentiation. A number of environmental stimuli may trigger the release of cytokines and growth factors by the keratinocytes and other cell types in the epidermis. The ensuing immune and inflammatory responses contribute to the full development of psoriatic lesions. The complex pathogenetic mechanisms likely to be operative in psoriasis are depicted in Figure 24-13.

☐ **Pathology:** The most distinctive pathological changes are seen at the periphery of a psoriatic plaque. The epidermis is thickened and displays both hyperkeratosis and parakeratosis. Parakeratosis may present as circumscribed, ellipsoidal foci, or it may be diffuse, in which case the granular layer is diminished or absent. The nucleated layers of the epidermis are thickened several fold in the rete pegs and frequently are thinner over the dermal papillae (Fig. 24-14). In turn, the papillae are elongated and appear as sections of cones, with their apices toward the dermis. In chronic lesions, the papillae tend to appear as bulbous clubs with short handles (Fig. 24-15). The rete ridges of the epidermis have a profile reciprocal to that of the dermal papillae, resulting in interlocked mesenchymal and epithelial clubs with alternatively reversed polarity (see Fig. 24-15). The capillaries of the papillae are dilated and tortuous.

Ultrastructurally, the capillaries are venule-like; neutrophils may emerge at their tips and migrate into the epidermis above the apices of the papillae. Neutrophils may become localized in the epidermal spinous layer or in small Munro microabscesses in the stratum corneum and may be associated with circumscribed areas of parakeratosis (Fig. 24-16). The dermis below the papillae exhibits a varying number of mononuclear inflammatory cells, mostly lymphocytes, about the superficial vascular plexus. There is little extension of the inflammatory process into the subjacent reticular dermis.

☐ **Clinical Features:** The severity of psoriasis varies from annoying scaly lesions over the elbows to a serious debilitating disorder involving most of the skin and often associated with arthritis. A single lesion of psoriasis may be a small focus of scaly erythema or an enormous confluent plaque covering much of the trunk. A typical plaque is 4 to 5 cm in diameter, is sharply demarcated at

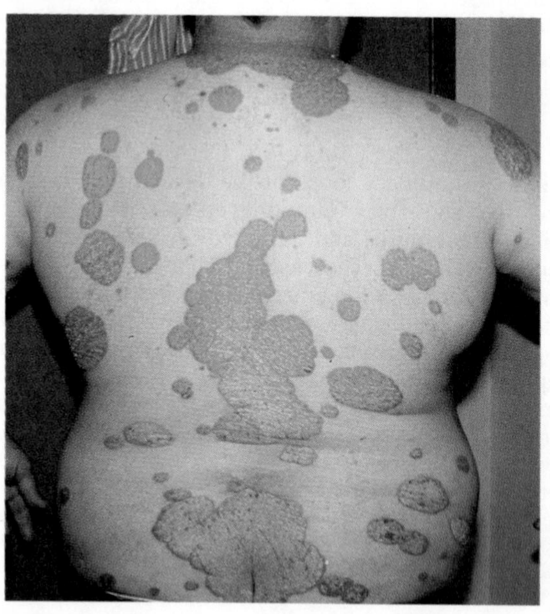
A

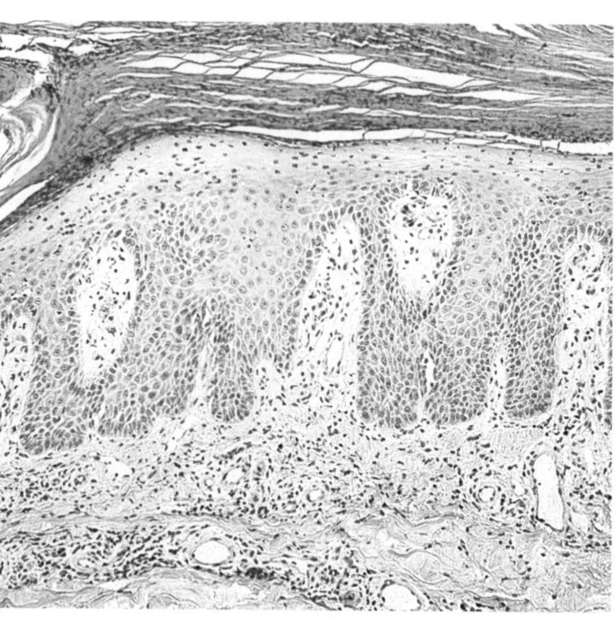
B

FIGURE *24-14*

Psoriasis. Psoriasis is the prototype of psoriasiform epidermal hyperplasia. (*A*) A patient with psoriasis shows large, confluent, sharply demarcated, erythematous plaques on the trunk. (*B*) Microscopic examination of a lesion demonstrates that the rete ridges are uniformly elongated, as are the dermal papillae, giving an interlocking pattern of alternately reversed "clubs." The dermal papillae are edematous and reside beneath a thinned epidermis (suprapapillary thinning) with striking parakeratosis. The parakeratosis is the scale observed clinically.

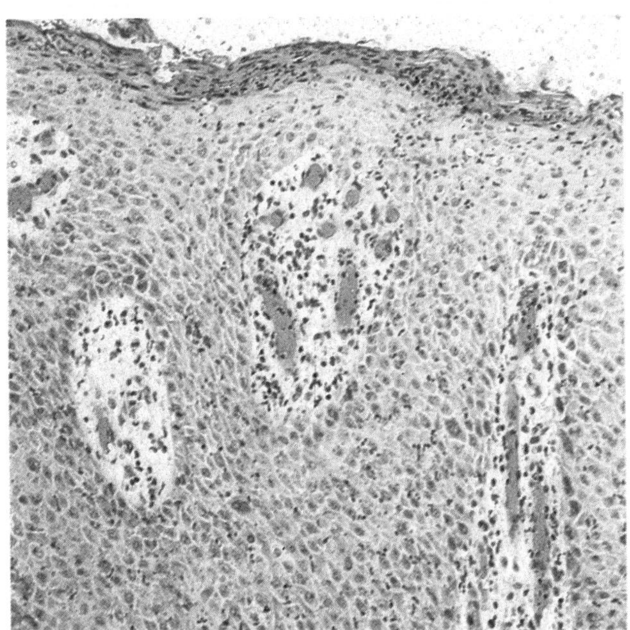

FIGURE 24-15
Psoriasis. The clubbed papillae contain tortuous dilated venules. The prominent venules are part of the venulization of capillaries, which may be of histogenetic importance in psoriasis. The papilla to the right has one cross-section of its superficial capillary venule loop, which is normal. The papilla in the center shows numerous cross-sections of its venule, indicating striking tortuosity.

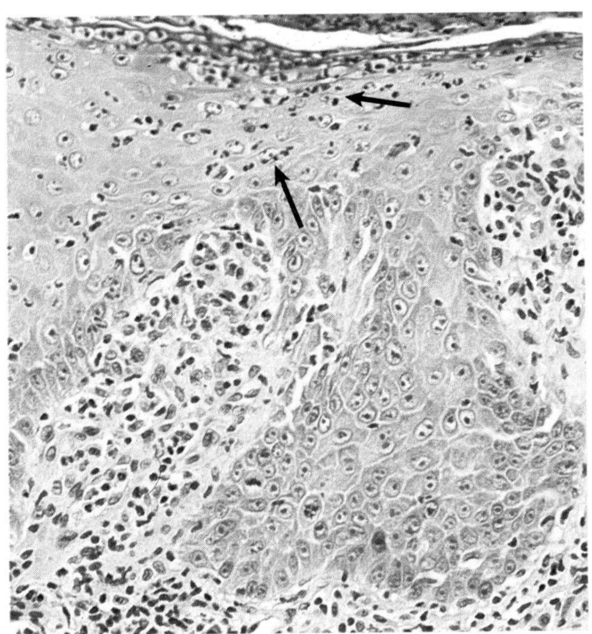

FIGURE 24-16
Psoriasis. Neutrophils migrate into the epidermis, emerging from the venulized capillaries at the tips of the dermal papillae. They migrate to the upper stratum spinosum and stratum corneum (*arrows*). In some forms of psoriasis, pustules are common clinical lesions.

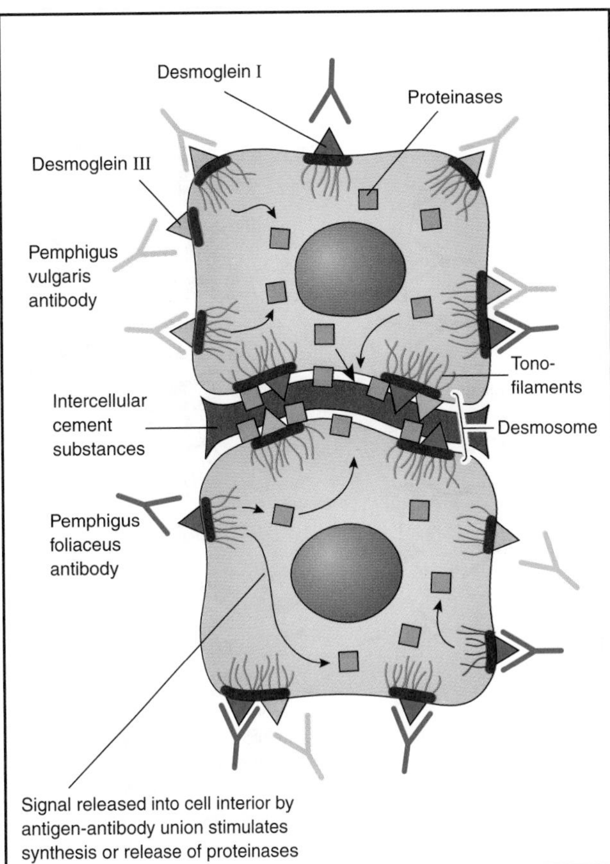

FIGURE 24-17
A pathogenetic mechanism of suprabasal dyshesion in pemphigus vulgaris. (*1*) A circulating autoantibody, whose stimulus for production is unknown, binds to an antigen on the outer leaflet of the plasma membranes (desmosomes) of keratinocytes, especially in the basal regions. *(figure continues)*

its margin, and is covered by a surface of silvery scales. When the scales are detached, pinpoint foci of bleeding dot the underlying glossy erythematous surface.

Of all patients with psoriasis, 7% develop **seronegative rheumatoid arthritis** (see Chapter 26). The tendency to arthropathy has a genetic component and is linked to several HLA haplotypes, particularly HLA-B27. Psoriatic arthritis closely resembles its rheumatoid counterpart, but it is usually milder and causes little disability.

Psoriasis is a disease of intermittent activity and variable presentation. Familial psoriasis is unusually severe. In some variations of the disease, neutrophilic pustules dominate the pathological process (*pustular psoriasis*). Severe intractable psoriasis has been observed in some patients with acquired immunodeficiency syndrome (AIDS), but the cause is not known.

Psoriasis has long been treated with coal tar or wood tar derivatives and anthralin, a strong reducing agent. Topical and systemic corticosteroids have also been employed. Severe, generalized psoriasis justifies systemic treatment with methotrexate, although hepatic toxicity remains a threat (see Chapter 14). Phototherapy after the

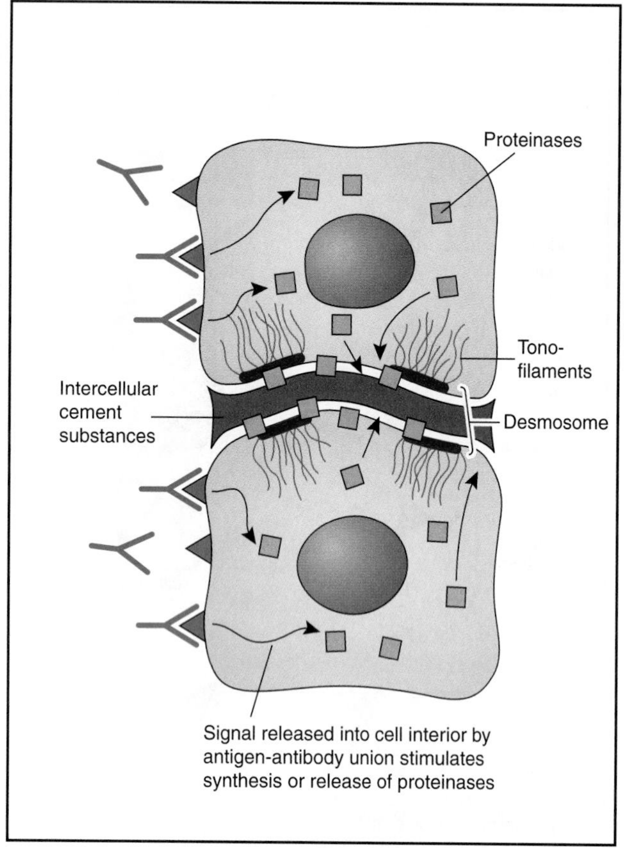

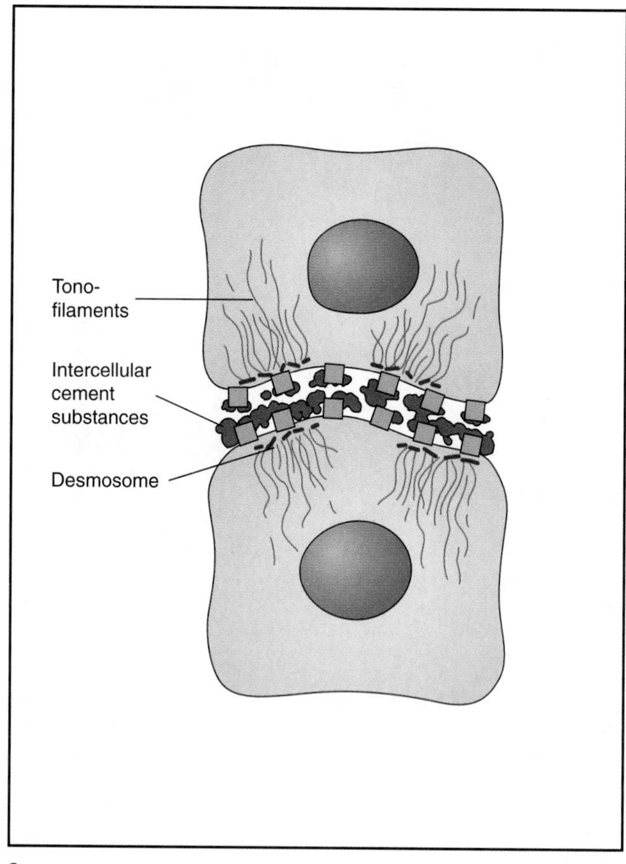

FIGURE *24-17 continued*
(2) Antigen-antibody union results in release of a proteinase (plasmin). (3) The proteinase interacts with intercellular cement, initiating dyhesion.

administration of psoralens (ultraviolet-absorbing compounds that bind to DNA) has proved effective in many severe cases. More recently, synthetic derivatives of vitamin A and vitamin D have been added to the list of effective pharmacological treatments of psoriasis.

Dyshesive Disorders

Dyshesive disorders are cutaneous maladies in which blister formation is secondary to diminished cohesiveness (dyshesion) of the epidermal keratinocytes.

Pemphigus Vulgaris

Pemphigus vulgaris (Greek, pemphix, "bubble"), the prototype of dyshesive diseases, is a chronic, blistering, skin disorder caused by the action of antibodies to surface antigens on stratified squamous cells. The malady occurs most commonly between 30 and 50 years of age, but it is reported in all age groups, including children. All races are susceptible to pemphigus vulgaris (PV), but persons of Jewish or Mediterranean extraction are at greater risk.

☐ **Pathogenesis:** **PV is an autoimmune disease caused by antibodies to a keratinocyte antigen.** Circulating IgG antibodies in patients with PV react with an epidermal surface antigen, which is also found in other mammals and birds. The antigen is a 130-kd protein (*desmoglein III*) associated with desmosomes and is intimately bound to a protein known as *plakoglobin*. The autoantibodies from patients with PV induce dyshesion in animal skin. Moreover, antibodies produced in rabbits in response to the administration of purified pemphigus antigen cause lesions similar to PV in the skin of the newborn mouse.

Antigen-antibody union results in dyshesion, which is augmented by the release of plasminogen activator and, hence, the activation of plasmin. This proteolytic enzyme acts on the intercellular substance and may be the dominant factor in dyshesion. Internalization of the pemphigus antigen-antibody complex, disappearance of attachment plaques, and retraction of perinuclear tonofilaments may all act in concert with proteinases to cause dyshesion and vesiculation (Fig. 24-17).

☐ **Pathology:** The blister in PV forms because of the separation of the stratum spinosum and outer epidermal layers from the basal layer. This suprabasal dyshesion results in a blister that has an intact basal layer as a floor and the remaining epidermis as a roof (Figs. 24-18 and 24-19). It appears that desmoglein III may be concentrated in the lower epidermis, explaining the location of the blister. The blister contains a moderate number of lymphocytes,

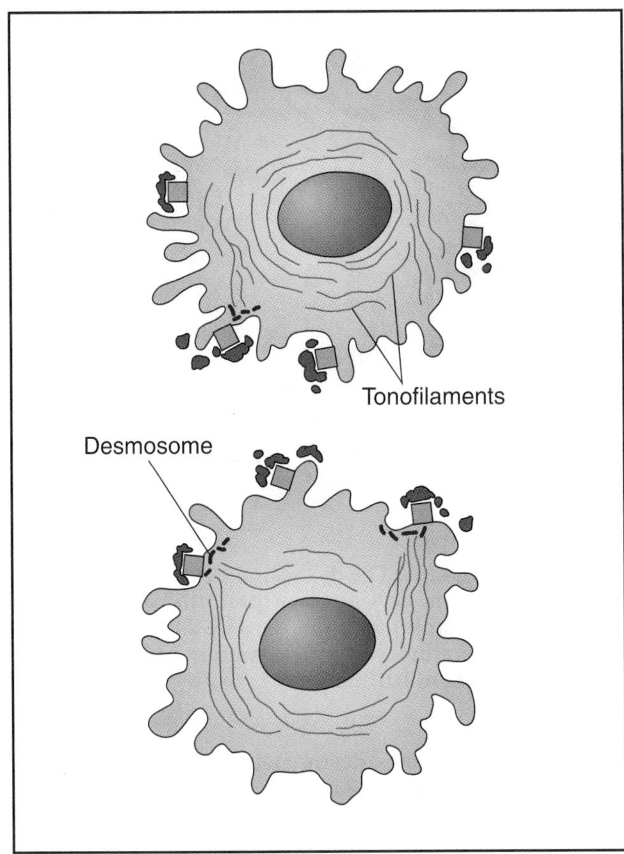

4

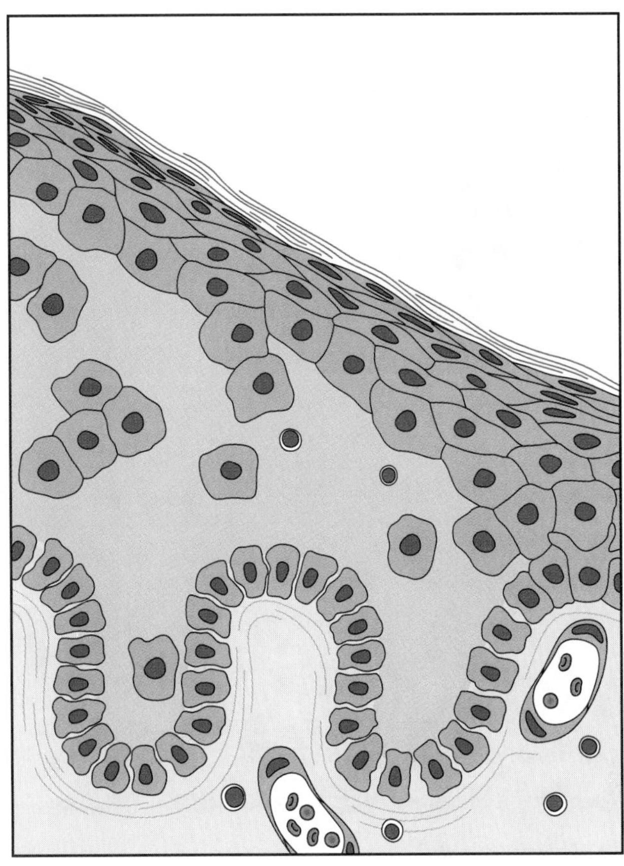

5

FIGURE 24-17 *continued*
(4) Desmosomes deteriorate, tonofilaments clump about the nucleus, the cells round up, and separation is complete. (5) A vesicle, which is usually suprabasal, forms. Alternatively, acantholysis may occur by direct interference with desmosomal and adherent junction attachments.

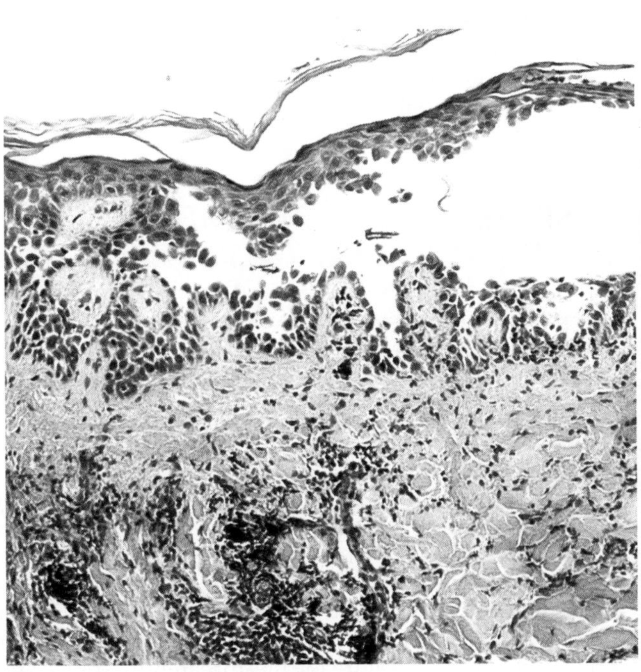

A

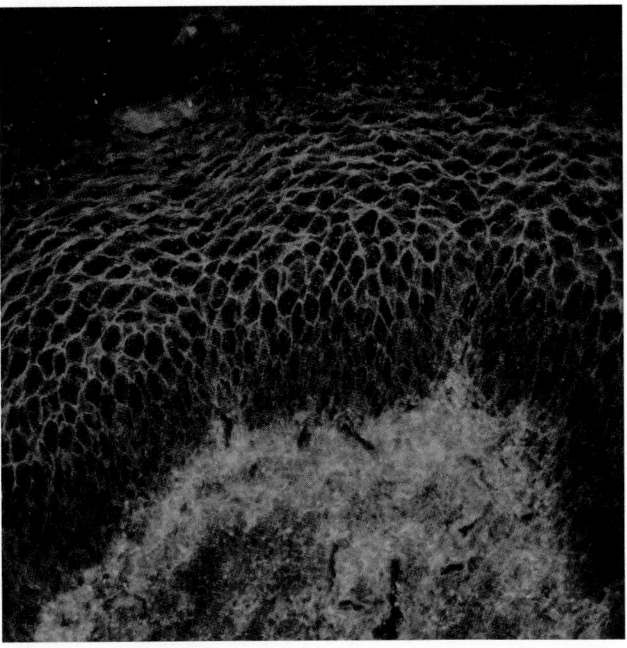

B

FIGURE 24-18
Pemphigus vulgaris. (*A*) Suprabasal dyshesion leads to an intraepidermal blister containing acantholytic keratinocytes. (*B*) Direct immunofluorescence examination of perilesional skin reveals antibodies, usually of IgG type, deposited in the intercellular substance of the epidermis, yielding a lace-like pattern outlining the keratinocytes.

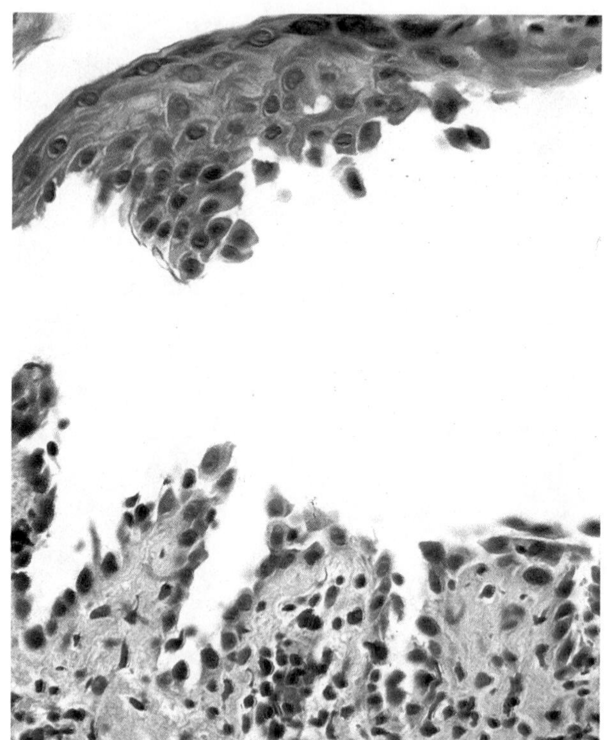

FIGURE 24-19
Pemphigus vulgaris. High-power magnification of the suprabasal dyshesion reveals crisply delineated basal keratinocytes slightly separated from each other and totally separated from the stratum spinosum. The basal keratinocytes are firmly attached to the epidermal basement membrane zone.

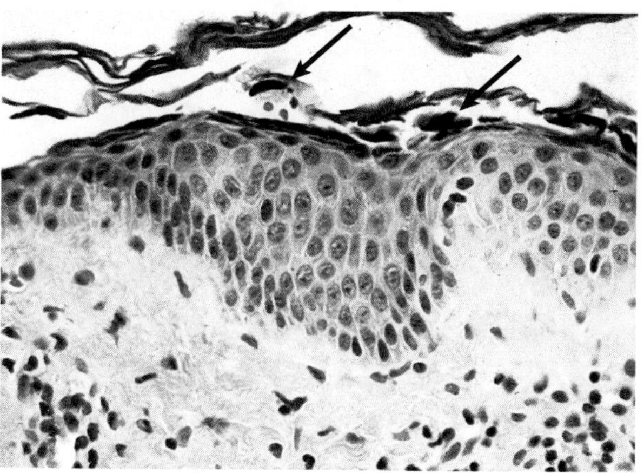

FIGURE 24-20
Pemphigus foliaceus. The dyshesion develops in the outer stratum spinosum and stratum granulosum. (Compare with that of pemphigus vulgaris; Fig. 24-19.) Dyshesive dyskeratotic keratinocytes of the stratum granulosum (*arrows*) are important hallmarks.

macrophages, eosinophils, and neutrophils. Distinctive, rounded keratinocytes, termed *acantholytic cells*, are shed into the vesicle during the process of dyshesion. The dyshesion may extend along the dermal adnexae and is not always strictly suprabasal. The subjacent dermis shows a moderate infiltrate of lymphocytes, macrophages, eosinophils, and neutrophils, predominantly about the capillary venular bed. Occasionally, eosinophils are particularly prominent.

☐ **Clinical Features:** The characteristic lesion of PV is a large, easily ruptured blister that leaves extensive denuded or crusted areas. The lesions are most common on the scalp and mucous membranes and in the periumbilical and intertriginous areas. Without corticosteroid treatment, the disease is progressive and usually fatal, and much of the cutaneous surface may become denuded. In addition to corticosteroid administration, immunosuppressive agents are useful for maintenance therapy. With appropriate therapy, the 10-year mortality rate for PV is less than 10%.

Disorders Related to Pemphigus Vulgaris

Other diseases caused by dyshesion that have a pathogenetic mechanism similar to that of PV include pemphigus vegetans, pemphigus foliaceus, Brazilian pemphigus foliaceus, pemphigus erythematosus, and drug-induced pemphigus (most commonly associated with penicillamine and captopril). The specific antigen of pemphigus foliaceus and Brazilian pemphigus is desmoglein I, a protein found in desmosomes. Autoantibodies to desmoglein I cause dyshesion in the outer spinous and granular epidermal layers (Fig. 24-20). The differences between the various forms of pemphigus are outlined in Table 24-2. Paraneoplastic pemphigus has recently been described in association with cancers, usually lymphoproliferative tumors.

Pemphigus may be associated with other autoimmune diseases, such as myasthenia gravis and lupus erythematosus, and may also be seen with benign thymomas. Other maladies may simulate the histological appearance of PV, notably familial benign chronic pemphigus and transient acantholytic dermatosis. However, in none of these disorders that simulate PV do IgG antibodies react with epidermal antigens.

DISEASES OF THE BASEMENT MEMBRANE ZONE (DERMAL-EPIDERMAL INTERFACE)

Blister Formation Due to Dermal-Epidermal Separation

Epidermolysis Bullosa

Epidermolysis bullosa (EB) embraces a heterogeneous group of at least 16 disorders, loosely held together by their hereditary nature and by a tendency to form blisters at the sites of minor trauma. EB may have been the cause of the biblical Job's skin disease, "my skin closeth up and breaketh out afresh." The clinical spectrum of EB ranges from a minor annoyance to a widespread, life-threatening, blistering disease. The blisters of almost all forms of EB are noted at birth or shortly thereafter. The classification of these disorders is based on the site of blister formation in the basement membrane zone (Table 24-3). The different mechanisms of blister formation that underlie each of the three major categories of EB are shown in Figure 24-21.

TABLE 24-2 **Diseases of the Pemphigus Group: Reactive Antibodies of the IgG Type to Antigen on the Plasma Membranes of Stratified Squamous Epithelia**

Type of Pemphigus	Clinical Features	Pathology
Pemphigus vulgaris	Flaccid, easily ruptured bullae commonly involving the scalp, periumbilical region, intertriginous areas, and mucous membranes. Commonly occurs during the fourth and fifth decades of life. Occurs predominantly in people of Jewish origin and other Mediterranean peoples.	Suprabasal dyshesive vesicle with a sparse infiltrate of lymphocytes, macrophages, and eosinophils. Antigen is desmoglein III in desmosomes.
Pemphigus vegetans	A variant of pemphigus vulgaris, but healing in intertriginous areas is characterized by complex papillary epidermal hyperplasia, resulting in verrucous or vegetating lesions.	The same as for pemphigus vulgaris with superimposed extensive epidermal hyperplasia. Eosinophils may be numerous.
Pemphigus foliaceus	Bullae occur early in the course of the disease but may not be present. The disease may be eczematoid, with shallow erosions, scales, and crusting. The scalp, face, throat, back, and abdomen are commonly involved, but mucous membrane involvement is uncommon. Not fatal if untreated. Question of slight predominance in Jews.	Dyshesion is in the spinous layer. Granular cells may peel apart; appearance is of shedding granular cells one by one. Variable number of inflammatory cells. Neutrophils may be numerous with formation of subcorneal pustules. Antigen is desmoglein I (in desmosomes).
Brazilian pemphigus foliaceus	Clinically and immunologically identical with pemphigus foliaceus. Occurs in two rural areas of south central Brazil as a common endemic disease. Two thirds of the patients are women. Common in children and young adults. Arthropod vector (? *Simulium* blackfly).	Same as for pemphigus foliaceus.
Pemphigus erythematosus	Similar to pemphigus foliaceus but dominated by lupus-like changes on the butterfly area of the face. Immunologically, patients have pemphigus antibodies, antinuclear antibodies, and immune complex deposits of lupus erythematosus.	Same as for pemphigus foliaceus.

Epidermolytic Epidermolysis Bullosa

Epidermolytic EB (also known as EB simplex) is a group of autosomal dominant skin diseases that feature blister formation as a result of disruption of basal keratinocytes. Epidermolytic EB has been attributed to mutations of genes encoding cytokeratin intermediate filaments, which are believed to provide mechanical stability to the epidermis. The blisters develop in response to minor trauma, such as merely rubbing the skin, but heal without scarring (the basis of the term *simplex*). Although epidermolytic EB is cosmetically disturbing and sometimes debilitating, it poses no threat to life.

TABLE 24-3 **Classification of Epidermolysis Bullosa (Selected Variants)**

Class	Site of Blister Formation	Name of Variant	Healing Residuum	Heredity	Molecular Defect	Chromosomal Defect
Epidermolytic	Within the basal keratinocytic layer	Localized epidermolysis bullosa simplex Generalized epidermolysis bullosa simplex	None None	Autosomal dominant Autosomal dominant	Keratins 5 and 14	12q11-13 and 17q21
Junctional	Lamina lucida	Epidermolysis bullosa letalis Generalized atrophic benign epidermolysis bullosa	None or atrophic scars Atrophic scars	Autosomal recessive Autosomal recessive	Laminin	1q25-31, 1q3, and 18q11.2 1q32 and 10q23.4
Dermolytic	Immediately deep to the lamina densa	Dystrophic epidermolysis bullosa Dystrophic epidermolysis bullosa	Scars, nails deformed Scars, teeth and nails deformed	Autosomal dominant Autosomal recessive	Collagen type VII	3q21

EPIDERMOLYTIC

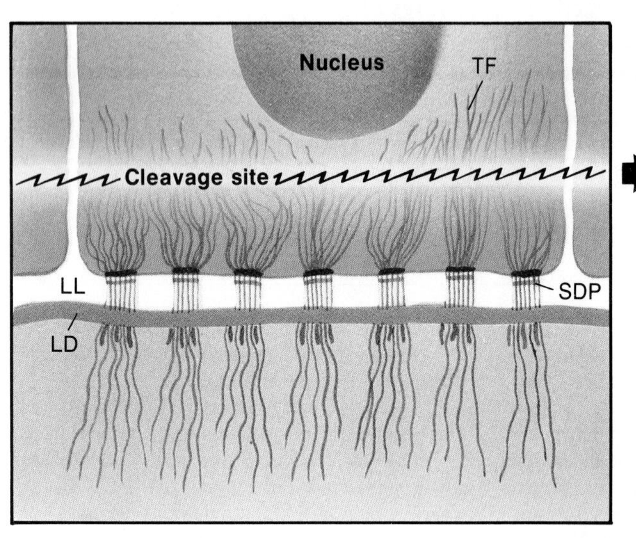

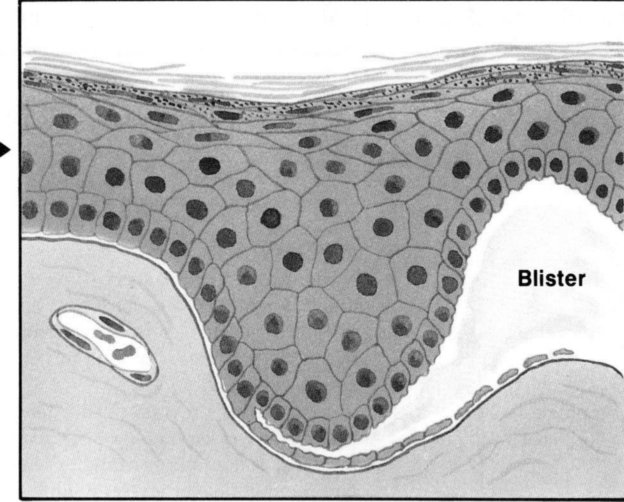

JUNCTIONAL

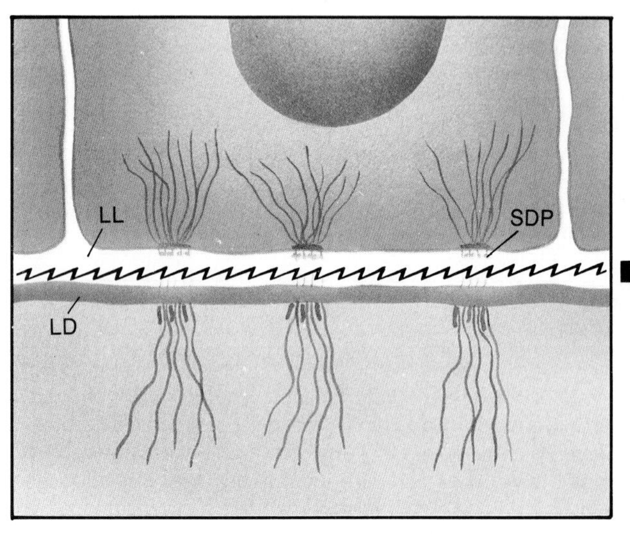

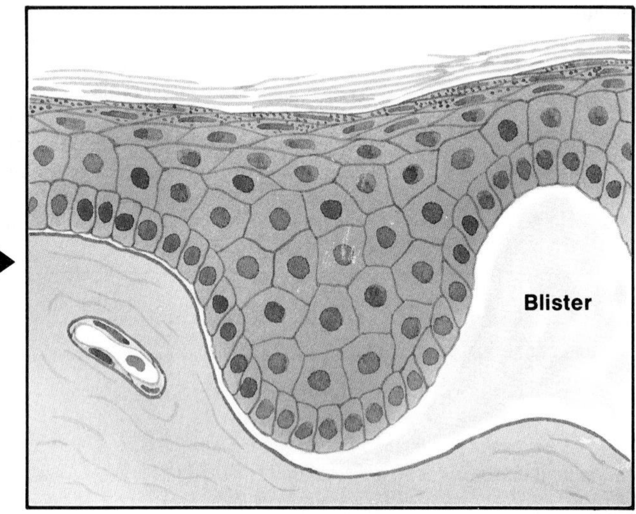

DERMOLYTIC

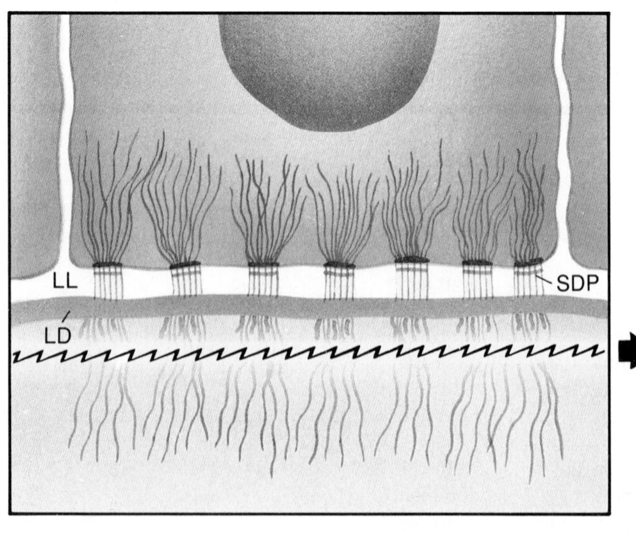

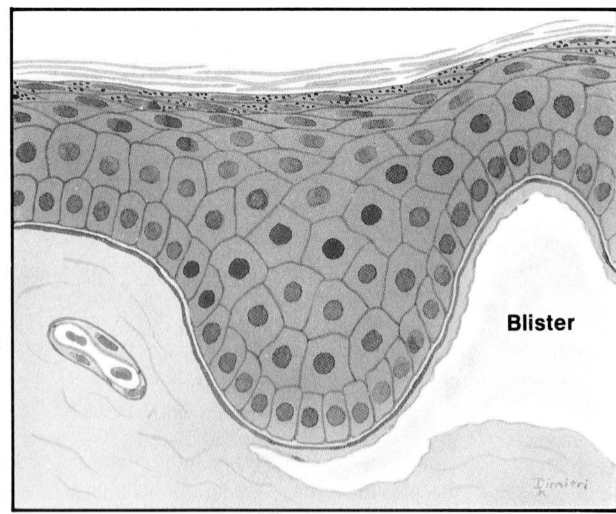

FIGURE *24-21*

☐ **Pathology:** Cytolysis of the basal keratinocytes is the basis of blister formation in the epidermolytic variety of EB. Initially, small, subnuclear, cytoplasmic vacuoles develop, increase in size, and coalesce. The formation of these vacuoles reflects the presence of abnormal keratins 4 and 5, which aggregate about the keratinocyte nuclei. The plasma membrane ruptures when the large vacuole reaches it, after which the cell is lysed. An intraepidermal vesicle results from the lysis of several basal keratinocytes. The roof of the vesicle is an almost intact epidermis with a fragmented basal layer. The floor of the vesicle shows bits of basal cell cytoplasm attached to the lamina densa, which is seen as a well-preserved pink line at the base of the vesicle. Inflammatory cells are sparse.

Junctional Epidermolysis Bullosa

Junctional EB is a heritable, autosomal recessive, skin disease in which blisters form within the lamina lucida. The clinical expression ranges from a benign disease that has no effect on life span to a severe condition that is fatal within the first 2 years of life. In the severe form of junctional EB, mutations in the genes for certain isoforms of laminin and the integrins have been reported. The blisters of the benign form of junctional EB heal without scarring but leave behind atrophic skin. There may be associated abnormalities of nails and teeth.

☐ **Pathology:** An intact epidermis forms the roof of the vesicle in junctional EB. The plasma membranes of the basal keratinocytes are unchanged. The floor of the vesicle is an intact lamina densa, as in epidermolytic EB, but the attached fragments of basal cell cytoplasm are lacking. The blister, therefore, occurs within the lamina lucida. Both lesional and uninvolved skin show fewer basal hemidesmosomes, which have poorly developed attachment plaques and subbasal dense plates. Recently, the absence of an isoform of laminin has been described.

Dermolytic Epidermolysis Bullosa

Dermolytic EB (also known as dystrophic EB) is a heritable skin condition in which blisters are located immediately deep to the lamina densa. Dermolytic disease may be either dominant or recessive, the latter being more severe. In both variants, healed blisters are characterized by atrophic ("dystrophic") scarring. There may be associated abnormalities of nails and teeth.

☐ **Pathogenesis:** The pathogenesis of dermolytic EB is attributed to a defect in anchoring fibrils. An abnormal architecture and a reduction in the number of these fibrils have been demonstrated in apparently normal skin of affected newborns. The basic defect is a mutation in the gene encoding collagen type VII on chromosome 3 (3p21). Anchoring fibrils comprise a net in the upper dermis, through which fibers of collagen types I and III course. This structure serves to anchor the epidermis to the underlying dermis, and its disruption results in subepidermal bullae, arising in the sublamina densa zone.

☐ **Pathology:** The roof of the vesicle is a normal epidermis with an attached, intact lamina lucida and lamina densa. The base of the vesicle is formed by the outer part of the papillary dermis. Ultrastructurally, there is a diminution in the number of anchoring fibrils in the dominant variant, and a virtual absence of fibrils in the recessive form. A corresponding decrease in the anchoring fibril proteins AF-1 and AF-2 occurs in the two variants.

Bullous Pemphigoid

Bullous pemphigoid (BP) is a common, autoimmune, blistering disease with clinical similarities to pemphigus vulgaris (hence the name "pemphigoid"), but in which acantholysis is absent. The disease has a predilection for the later decades of life, but it has no significant racial or sexual predilection.

☐ **Pathogenesis:** Similar to pemphigus vulgaris, BP is an autoimmune disease, but in this case IgG antibodies bind two glycoproteins (BPAG1 and BPAG2) in the lamina lucida. The antigen is a basal keratinocyte transmembrane molecule associated with the cytoplasmic plaques of the hemidesmosomes. A portion of the molecule traverses the plasma membrane and is found in the upper lamina lucida. BP antigen, together with laminin and anchoring filaments, contributes to dermal-epidermal adherence.

Virtually all cases of BP display linear deposits of IgG and C3 in the lamina lucida of the epidermal basement membrane zone. The BP antigen-antibody complex in the lamina lucida may injure the basal cell plasma membrane through the formation of the C5b-C9 membrane attack complex (see Chapter 4). In turn, this damage may interfere with the elaboration of adherence factors by

FIGURE *24-21*
Three distinct mechanisms of blister formation in epidermolysis bullosa. Electron microscopic images are on the *left;* light microscopic images are on the *right.* Epidermolytic epidermolysis bullosa is caused by disintegration of the lowermost regions of the epidermal basal cells. The bottom portions of the basal cells cleave, and the remainder of the epidermis lifts away. Small fragments of basal cells remain attached to the basement membrane zone. Junctional epidermolysis bullosa is characterized by cleavage in the lamina lucida. Dermolytic epidermolysis bullosa is associated with rudimentary and fragmented anchoring fibrils. The entire basement membrane zone and epidermis split away from the dermis in relationship to these flawed anchoring fibrils. LL, lamina lucida; LD, lamina densa; SDP, subdesomosomal dense plate.

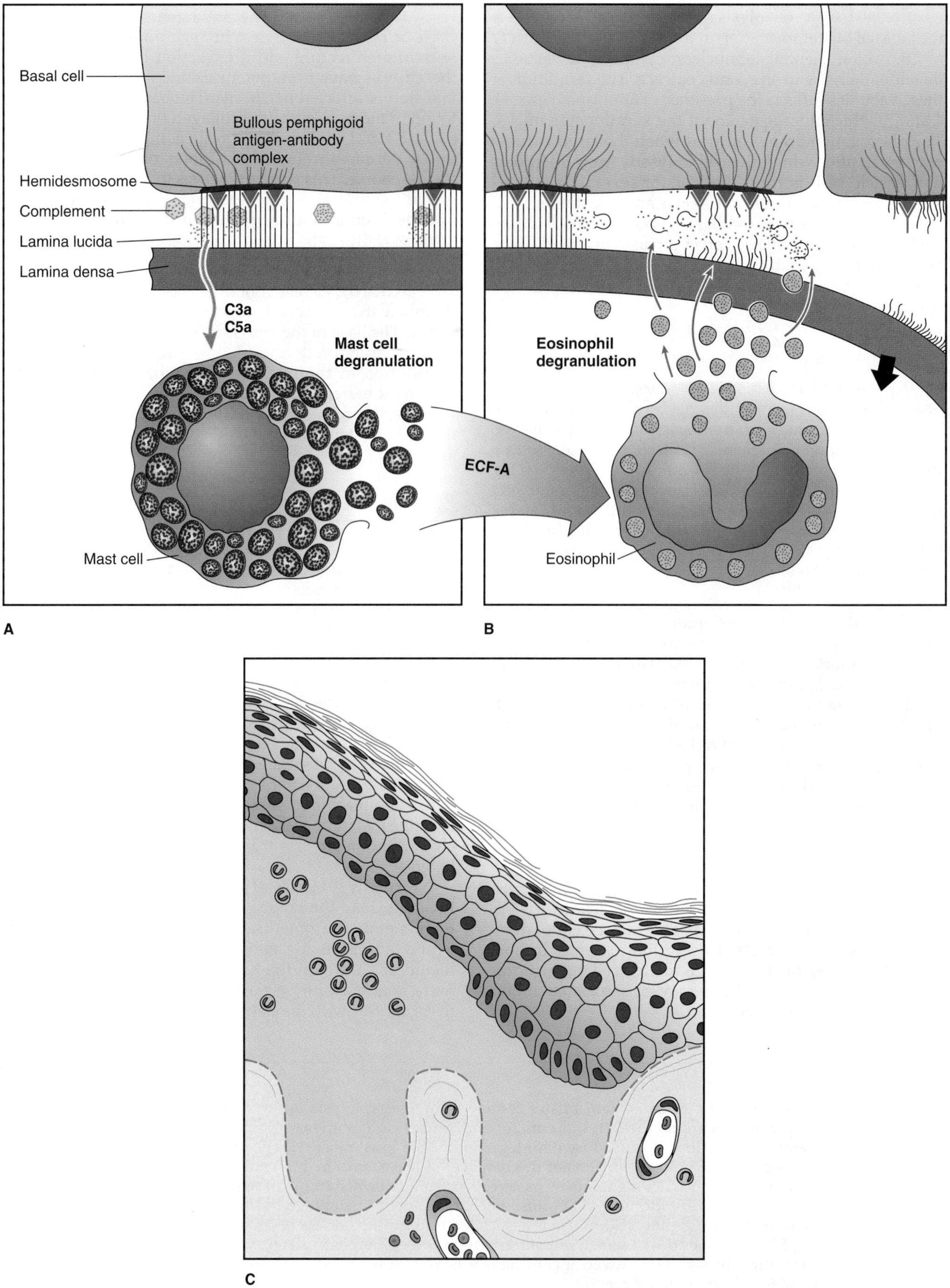

Basal cell
Bullous pemphigoid antigen-antibody complex
Hemidesmosome
Complement
Lamina lucida
Lamina densa
C3a
C5a
Mast cell degranulation
ECF-A
Mast cell

A

Eosinophil degranulation
Eosinophil

B

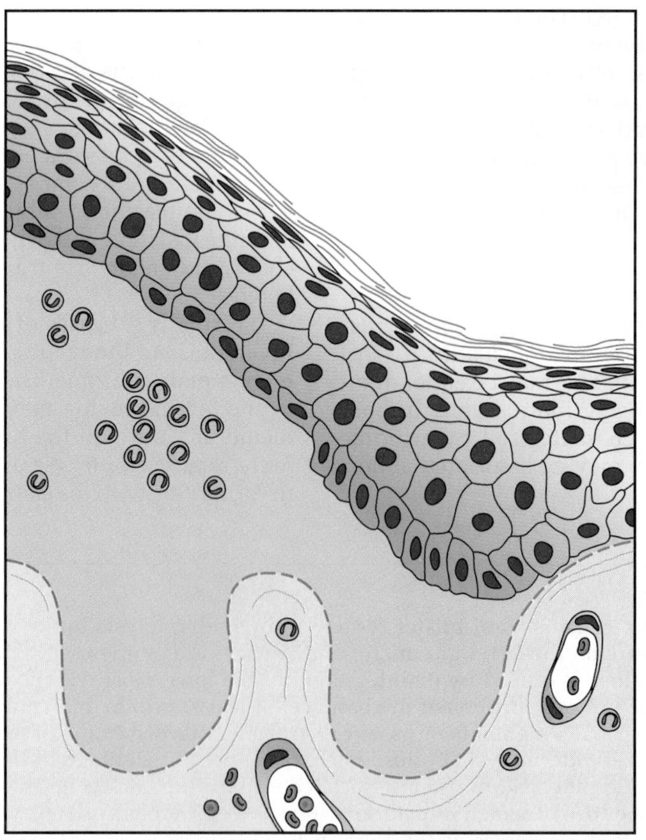

C

FIGURE *24-22*

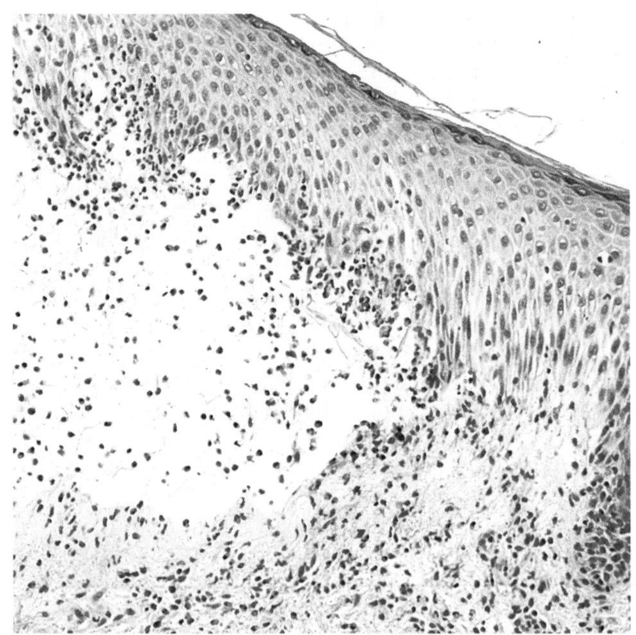

FIGURE *24-23*
Bullous pemphigoid. A subepidermal blister has an edematous papillary dermis as its base. The roof of the blister consists of the intact entire epidermis, including the stratum basalis. Inflammatory cells, fibrin, and tissue fluid fill the blister.

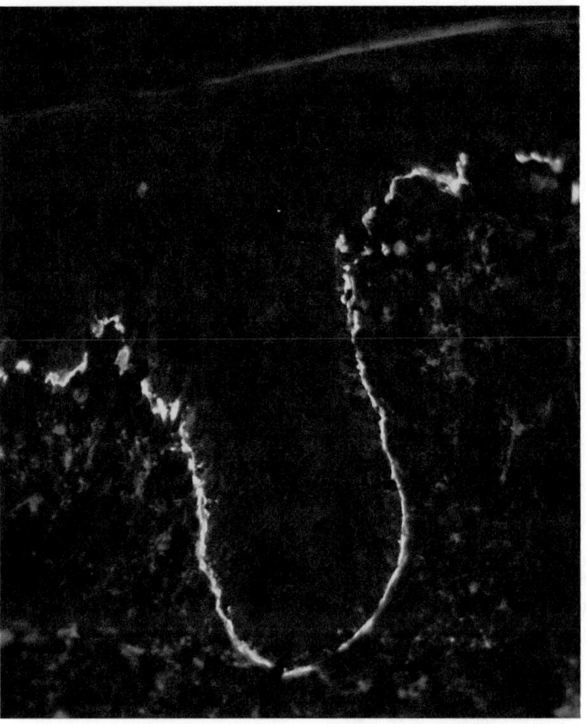

FIGURE *24-24*
Bullous pemphigoid. Direct immunofluorescence study discloses linearly deposited IgG (and C3) along the dermal-epidermal junction. Ultrastructurally, these antibodies and complement are present in the lamina lucida.

basal keratinocytes. Of greater importance is the production of the anaphylatoxins, C3a and C5a, following activation of the complement cascade. These anaphylatoxins cause degranulation of mast cells and the release of factors chemotactic for eosinophils, neutrophils, and lymphocytes. The eosinophil granules contain tissue-damaging substances, including eosinophil peroxidase and major basic protein. These molecules, together with proteases of neutrophilic and mast cell origin, cause dermal-epidermal separation within the lamina lucida (Fig. 24-22).

Protease inhibitors, such as α2-macroglobulin, block dermal-epidermal separation in normal skin cultured with fluid obtained from BP blisters. Although a dense inflammatory infiltrate doubtless causes extensive destruction of the entire basement membrane zone, the primary site of dermal-epidermal change in BP remains within the lamina lucida, the location of antigen-antibody union.

□ **Pathology:** The blisters of BP are subepidermal, with the roof of the blister formed by an intact epidermis and the base by the lamina densa of the basement membrane zone (Figs. 24-23 and 24-24). The blisters contain numerous eosinophils, together with fibrin, lymphocytes, and neutrophils.

Even before becoming erythematous, apparently normal skin shows migration of mast cells from the venule toward the epidermis. With the onset of erythema, eosinophils appear in the upper dermis and are occasionally arranged along the epidermal basement membrane zone. Ultrastructurally, the first site of dermal-epidermal separation is in the lamina lucida and is associated with the disruption of anchoring filaments. Immunofluorescent studies demonstrate linear deposition of C3 and IgG along the epidermal basement membrane zone and antibodies directed against BPAG1 and BPAG2 in the serum of patients with active disease.

□ **Clinical Features:** The blisters of BP are large and tense and may appear on normal-appearing skin or

FIGURE *24-22*
Pathogenetic mechanisms of blister formation in bullous pemphigoid. A circulating antibody to an apparently normal glycoprotein—BP antigen—in the lamina lucida precipitates the pathogenetic events in bullous pemphigoid. (*A*) Antigen-antibody union activates complement, and the anaphylatoxins C3a and C5a are produced. These degranulate mast cells, resulting in release of eosinophilic chemotactic factor. (*B* and *C*) The tissue-damaging substances of eosinophilic granules cause vesicle formation at the lamina lucida, with some breakdown of the lamina densa. ECF-A, eosinophil chemotactic factor-A.

on an erythematous base. The medial thighs and flexor aspect of the forearm are commonly affected, but the groin, axilla, and other cutaneous sites may also develop blisters. The disease is self-limited but chronic, and the patient's general health is usually unaffected. The course of the disease is greatly shortened by systemic administration of corticosteroids.

Dermatitis Herpetiformis

Dermatitis herpetiformis (DH) is an intensely pruritic cutaneous eruption related to gluten sensitivity, which is characterized by urticaria-like plaques and small vesicles over the extensor surfaces of the body.

□ **Pathogenesis:** DH is associated with gluten sensitivity in patients of the HLA-B8 and HLA-DRw3 haplotypes; most of these patients also have a subclinical gluten-sensitive enteropathy (see Chapter 14). The cutaneous lesions are related to granular deposits of IgA at the dermal-epidermal interface, mainly at the tips of dermal papillae. The HLA-B8/HLA-Dw3 locus is physically close to the immune response gene that determines gluten sensitivity. Gluten is a protein found in wheat, barley, rye, and oats, which may bind to a surface protein in the dermal papillae of the skin. IgA immune complexes at the tips of dermal papillae are more prominent in perilesional skin than in normal-appearing skin. Importantly, a gluten-free diet controls the disease, whereas reintroduction of gluten provokes new lesions.

It has been suggested that patients of the HLA-B8/HLA-DRw3 haplotype express two genes. One is responsible for gluten-sensitive enteropathy, and the other controls dimeric IgA antibody formation in response to partially digested forms of gluten and other dietary proteins. Such proteins might penetrate a defective mucosal epithelial barrier damaged by gluten sensitivity. The resultant IgA immune complexes form at gluten-binding sites in the skin, where they accumulate at locations that frequently sustain trauma (thereby increasing vascular permeability), such as the elbow.

IgA immune complexes are inefficient in complement activation (alternative pathway), and only a few neutrophils are attracted to the site. However, the neutrophils that do accumulate elaborate leukotrienes, which attract

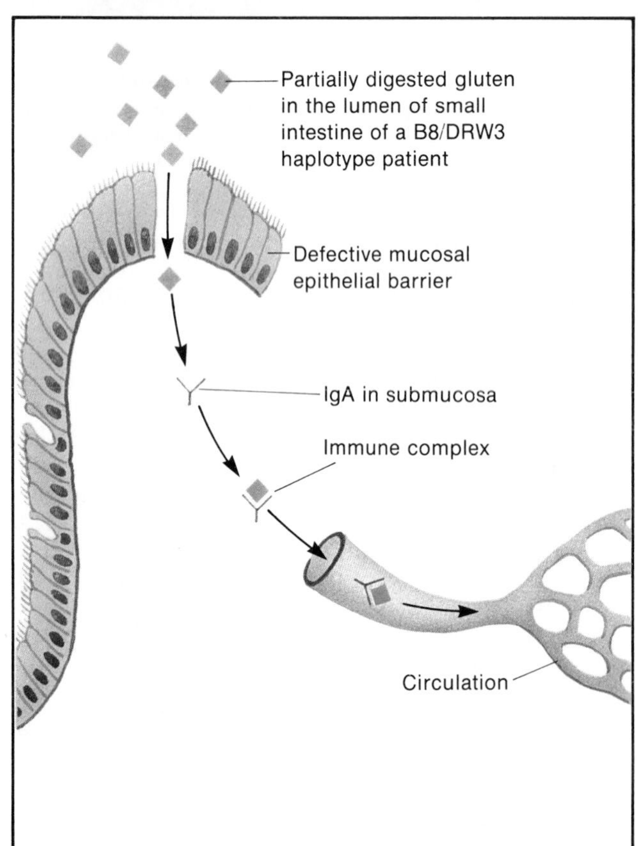

1. Formation of immune complexes in submucosa of small intestine. Passage of immune complexes into circulation.

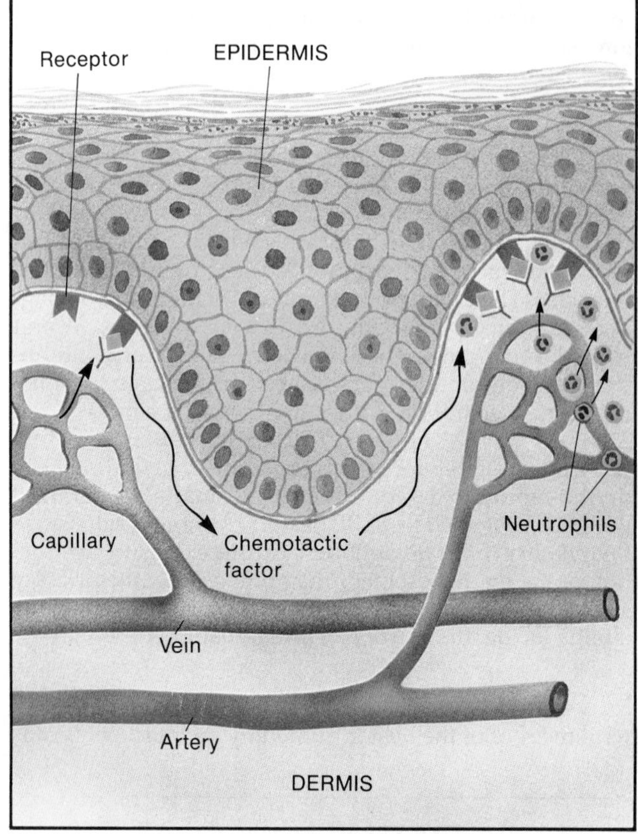

2. Receptor–immune complex union releases neutrophil chemotactic factor. Neutrophils migrate to the tips of the papillae.

FIGURE 24-25
Proposed pathogenesis for the cutaneous lesions in dermatitis herpetiformis. The disease is initiated in the small intestine and is likely expressed in the skin because of a gluten receptor immediately deep to the lamina densa.

more neutrophils. The release of lysosomal enzymes by the inflammatory cells cleaves the epidermis from the dermis. The immune complexes are deposited deep to the lamina densa in intimate relationship to the collagen rootlets (microfibrils), which, along with anchoring fibrils, are important in the attachment of the lamina densa to the subjacent papillary dermis (Fig. 24-25).

☐ Pathology: The pathological changes of DH are best appreciated by studying sequential biopsy specimens over a 72-hour period after cessation of dapsone therapy. Within 24 hours, erythematous, urticarial plaques develop about the elbows and knees. A delicate perivenular lymphocytic infiltrate appears, together with a row of neutrophils immediately deep to the lamina densa in the dermal papillae. During the next 12 hours, the neutrophils aggregate in clusters of 10 to 25 at the tips of the dermal papillae to create a diagnostic histological appearance.

There are two related mechanisms of dermal-epidermal separation. One is associated with the sheetlike spread of a layer or two of neutrophils at the dermal-epidermal interface. In this situation, the entire epidermis detaches from the papillary dermis (Fig. 24-26). The roof of such a vesicle contains the epidermis, whereas the floor is composed of the lamina densa and the papillary dermis, with a prominent neutrophilic infiltrate. In contrast to bullous pemphigoid, eosinophils are uncommon early in the course of DH.

In the second mechanism of vesicle formation, many neutrophils rapidly accumulate in the tips of the dermal papillae. The release of neutrophilic lysosomal enzymes in the outer portion of the dermal papillae results in (1) uncoupling of the epidermis from the dermis at the tips of dermal papillae, (2) disruption of the basement membrane zone in the lamina lucida and outer part of the papillae, and (3) tearing of the epidermis across the adjacent rete ridges. In the resulting vesicle, the roof has alternating tears across its epidermal covering, and the floor shows residual epidermal pegs alternating with the basal half of dermal papillae.

☐ Clinical Features: The lesions of DH are especially prominent over the elbows, knees, and buttocks. The intensely pruritic vesicles may become grouped in a fashion similar to that in herpes simplex infections (therefore, the term "herpetiformis") and are almost invariably rubbed until broken. Thus, patients may present with only crusted lesions and no intact vesicles. Although the disease is of varying severity and characterized by remis-

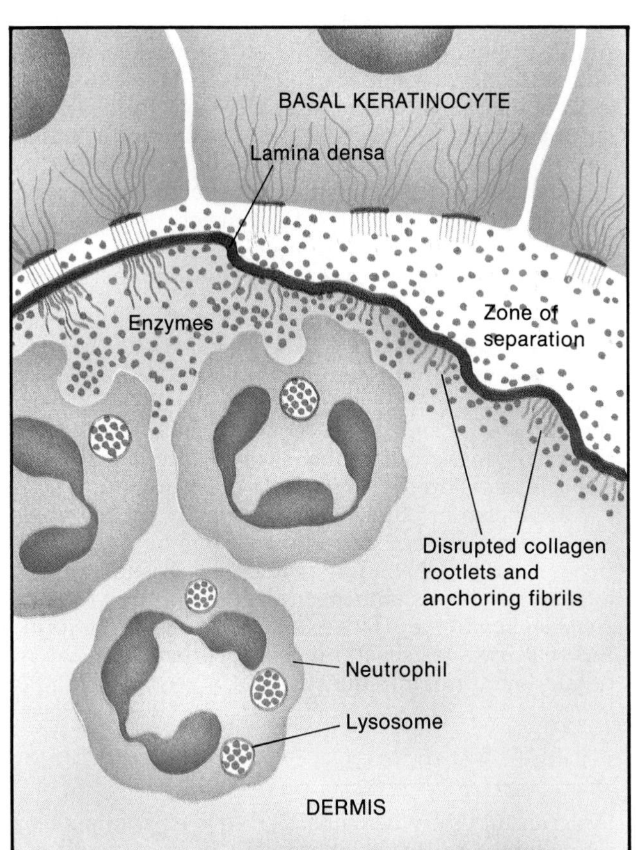

3. Dissolution of basal rootlets and anchoring fibrils by enzymes released by neutrophils. Early dermo-epidermal separation.

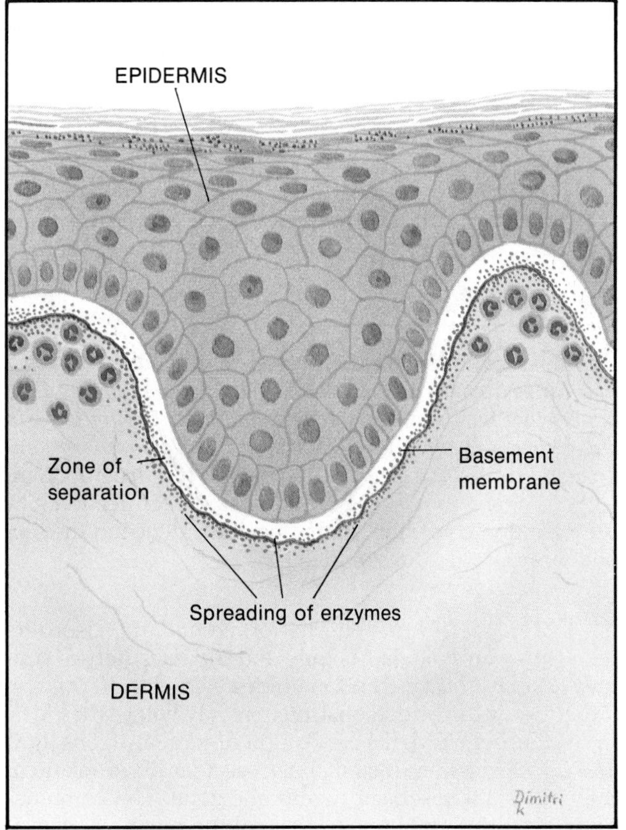

4. Concentration of neutrophils at the tips of the papillae. Spreading of enzymes along basement membrane. Lifting away of lamina densa.

FIGURE *24-25 continued*

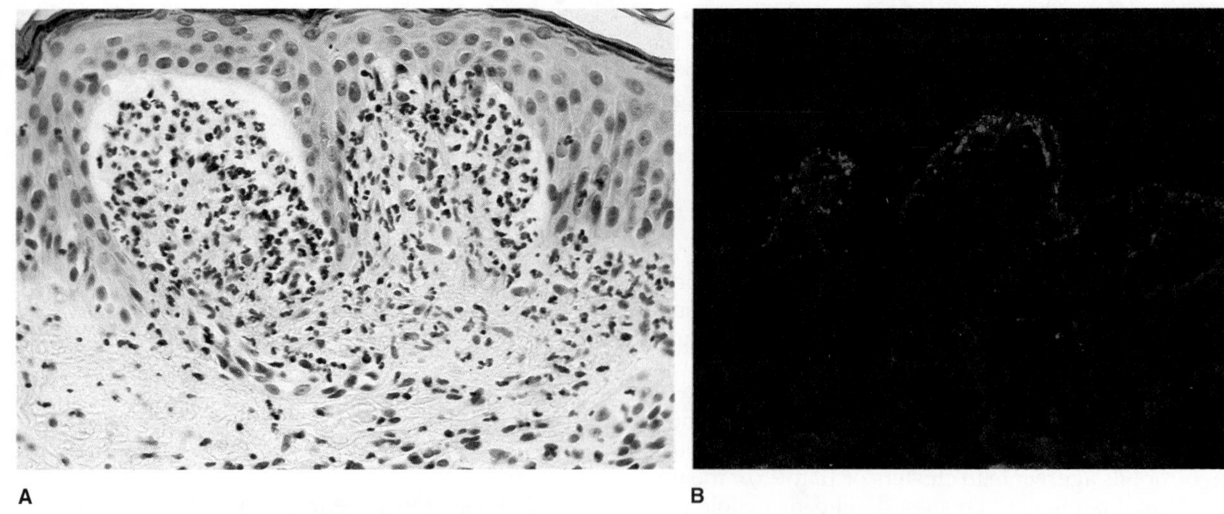

FIGURE 24-26
Dermatitis herpetiformis. (*A*) Dermal papillary abscesses of neutrophils with vesicle formation at the dermal-epidermal junction are characteristic. (*B*) Direct immunofluorescence study universally reveals IgA deposited in dermal papillae in association with (but not necessarily directly upon) anchoring fibrils and elastic tissue fibers. This is the exact site of neutrophil infiltration and subepidermal vesicle formation.

sions, it is disturbingly chronic. The healing lesions often leave scars. Treatment with dapsone or sulfapyridine completely controls the signs and symptoms of DH.

Basal Keratinocytic Injury, Excessive Synthesis of Lamina Densa, and Immune Reactants at the Basement Membrane Zone

Erythema Multiforme

Erythema multiforme (EM) is an acute, self-limited disorder that varies from a few erythematous macules and blisters (EM minor) to a life-threatening, widespread ulceration of the skin and mucous membranes (EM major; Stevens-Johnson syndrome). The disease is usually a reaction to a drug or an infectious agent, in particular, herpes simplex infection. EM is a common condition, with a peak incidence in the second and third decades of life.

☐ **Pathogenesis:** The list of agents and disorders thought to provoke EM is long and includes herpes simplex, *Mycoplasma*, and sulfonamides. However, a precipitating factor can be demonstrated in only half of the cases. In postherpetic EM, the deposition of viral antigens, IgM and C3, can be identified in a perivascular location and at the epidermal basement membrane zone. The combination of infiltrating lymphocytes and the presence of antigen-antibody complexes within the lesions suggest that both and humoral and delayed type hypersensitivity contribute to the pathogenesis of EM.

☐ **Pathology:** The dermis in EM shows a sparse infiltrate of lymphocytes about the superficial vascular bed and at the dermal-epidermal interface. The characteristic morphological feature in the epidermis is the presence of shrunken keratinocytes that have a pyknotic nucleus and an eosinophilic cytoplasm. Necrosis of keratinocytes may be extensive and associated with a subepidermal vesicle, the roof of which is an almost completely necrotic epidermis. Because of the acute onset of the disease, in most cases, there is little or no change in the stratum corneum.

☐ **Clinical Features:** The characteristic "target" or "iris" lesions of EM have a central, dark red zone, occasionally with a blister, surrounded by a paler area. In turn, the latter is encompassed by a peripheral red rim. Urticarial plaques are common. The presence of vesicles and bullae usually predicts a more severe course.

Erythema multiforme is occasionally encountered in association with other presumably immunological cutaneous disorders, including erythema nodosum, toxic epidermal necrolysis, and necrotizing vasculitis. ***Stevens-Johnson syndrome*** refers to an unusually severe form of EM that involves several mucosal surfaces and internal organs and is not infrequently fatal.

Lupus Erythematosus

Systemic lupus erythematosus (SLE), the paradigm of immune complex disease, is characterized by a variety of autoantibodies and other immune abnormalities indicative of B-cell hyperactivity (see Chapters 4 and 16). Although cutaneous involvement may be severe and cosmetically devastating, it is not life-threatening. However, the nature and pattern of immune reactants in the skin serve as an excellent guide to the likelihood of systemic disease.

☐ **Pathogenesis:** Although an impressive case can be made for the pathogenetic significance of immune complexes in renal diseases, they are not likely to be solely responsible for the production of the cutaneous lesions of SLE. In this respect, immune complexes are present in both lesional and normal-appearing skin in SLE. The deposition of immune reactants along the epidermal basement membrane zone (positive lupus band test) of "normal" skin is important in the diagnosis of SLE. The epidermal injury in the cutaneous lesions of SLE seems to be initiated by exogenous agents such as ultraviolet light and perpetuated by cell-mediated immune reactions similar to those in graft-versus-host disease. The manifestations of epidermal injury include (1) vacuolization of basal keratinocytes, with diminution in epidermal thickness and hyperkeratosis, (2) release of DNA and other nuclear and cytoplasmic antigens to the circulation, and (3) deposition of DNA and other antigenic determinants in the epidermal basement membrane zone (lamina densa and immediately subjacent dermis) (Fig. 24-27). Thus, epidermal injury, local immune complex formation, deposition of circulating immune complexes, and lymphocyte-induced cellular injury all seem to act in concert in the pathogenesis of skin disease in SLE.

☐ **Pathology and Clinical Features:** The various forms of cutaneous lupus erythematosus have been classified according to their chronicity. There is an in-

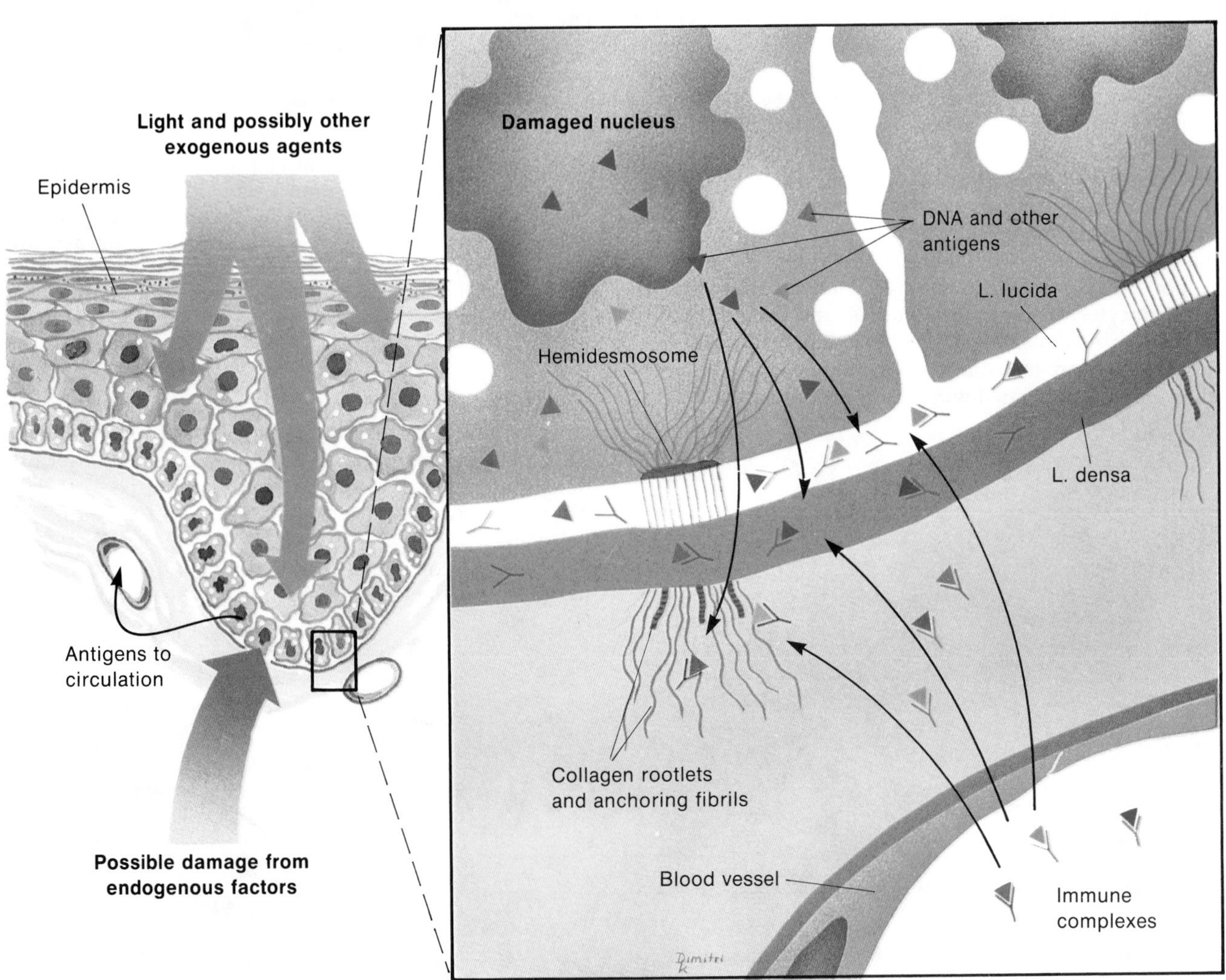

FIGURE 24-27
In lupus erythematosus, a cell-mediated immune reaction leads to epidermal cellular damage when initiated by light or other exogenous agents, as well as endogenous ones. Such injury releases a large number of antigens, some of which may return to the skin in the form of immune complexes. Immune complexes are also formed in the skin by a reaction of local DNA with antibody, which may also be deposited beneath the epidermal basement membrane zone.

verse relationship between the prominence of skin lesions and the extent of systemic pathology in lupus erythematosus.

CHRONIC CUTANEOUS (DISCOID) LUPUS ERYTHEMATOSUS: This form of lupus is usually a disease of the skin alone. The lesions of chronic cutaneous lupus erythematosus are generally above the neck and are found on the face (especially in the malar area), scalp, and ears. The lesions begin as slightly elevated violaceous papules, which have a rough scale of keratin. As they enlarge, they assume the shape of a disc, with a hyperkeratotic margin and a depigmented center. The cutaneous lesions may culminate in disfiguring scars.

Chronic cutaneous (discoid) lupus erythematosus presents distinctive histological changes. The nucleated epidermal layers are modestly thickened or somewhat thin. Hyperkeratosis and plugging of hair follicles are prominent. The rete-papillae pattern of the dermal-epidermal interface is partially effaced (Fig. 24-28). The basal keratinocytes are vacuolated, and karyolytic bodies (i.e., death of individual keratinocytes; see later section on lichen planus) are noted. The lamina densa is greatly thickened and reduplicated. On periodic acid–Schiff (PAS) staining, multiple layers of lamina densa extend into the subjacent dermis. The excessive quantity of lamina densa, a product of the basal keratinocytes, reflects a response of basal cells to damage. **The vacuolated basal keratinocytes, the apoptotic bodies, and the alterations of the lamina densa all suggest that injury to basal keratinocytes is an essential pathogenetic characteristic of skin disease associated with lupus erythematosus** (Figs. 24-29 and 24-30).

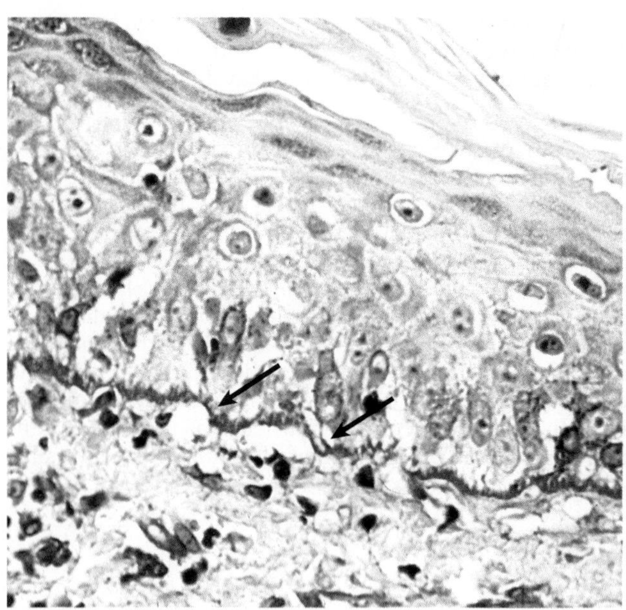

FIGURE *24-29*
Lupus erythematosus. Basal cell necrosis, with resultant basal keratinocytic migration and synthesis of new basement membrane zone, leads to thickening of the epidermal basement membrane zone, as defined in this periodic acid–Schiff (PAS) stain. Notice the vacuoles (*arrows*) on either side of the basement membrane zone, an indicator of cellular injury.

The basal keratinocytes and basement membrane zone contain a diffuse lymphocytic infiltrate, which focally penetrates the basal layer. Deeper in the dermis, dense patches of helper and cytotoxic/suppressor T lymphocytes are commonly disposed about skin appendages.

Immune complexes are predominantly located deep to the lamina densa, but they are also seen on the lamina

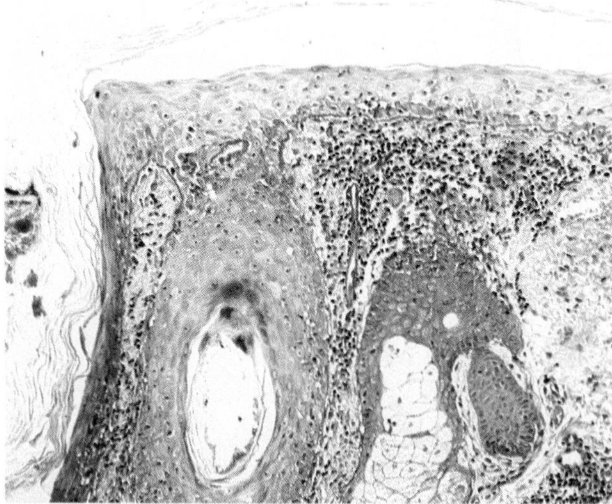

FIGURE *24-28*
Lupus erythematosus. A variably cell-rich to cell-poor, band-like lymphocytic infiltrate is present in the papillary and adventitial dermis. There is epidermal atrophy arising from damage to the epidermis, which is mediated by infiltrating lymphocytes.

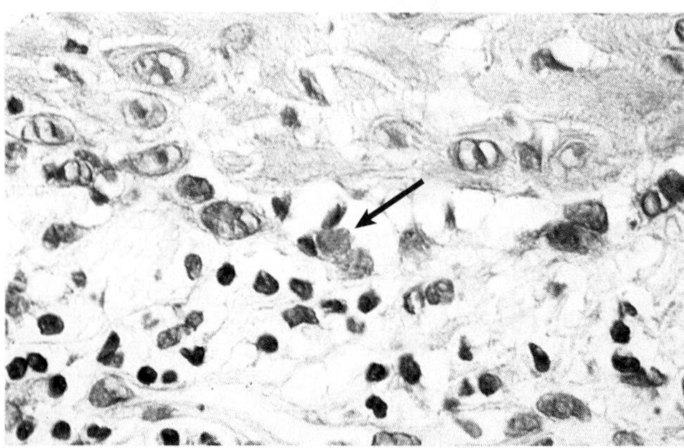

FIGURE *24-30*
Lupus erythematosus. In an active lesion, there is striking basal vacuolization, with keratinocyte necrosis (*arrow*) forming a dense eosinophilic body (apoptotic/fibrillary/colloid body) that is surrounded by lymphocytes (satellitosis).

densa and within the lamina lucida. This pattern contrasts with that of bullous pemphigoid, in which there are but two antigens, both precisely localized to the lamina lucida.

SUBACUTE CUTANEOUS LUPUS ERYTHEMATOSUS: This disorder primarily afflicts young and middle-aged white women. In contrast to chronic discoid lupus erythematosus, subacute cutaneous lupus may be accompanied by involvement of the musculoskeletal system and kidneys. Initially, scaly erythematous papules develop and then enlarge into psoriasiform or annular lesions, which in turn, may fuse. The lesions are seen in the "V" area of the upper chest, upper back, and extensor surfaces of the arms, a distribution indicating that light plays a role in the pathogenesis of subacute cutaneous lupus. Indeed, photosensitivity is common. Significant scarring does not occur. About 70% of patients have circulating anti-Ro (ss-A) antibody.

Histologically, subacute cutaneous lupus features edema of the papillary dermis, thickening of the lamina densa, and prominent vacuolar degeneration of the basal layer. There is some lymphocytic infiltration of the basement membrane zone, but deeper patches of lymphocytes are not observed. Occasional necrotic keratinocytes are noted.

ACUTE SYSTEMIC LUPUS ERYTHEMATOSUS: Over 80% of patients with SLE have cutaneous manifestations during the course of their illness, in association with disease of the kidneys and joints. The skin rash is often the first manifestation of the disease and may precede the onset of systemic symptoms by a few months. The typical butterfly rash of SLE is a delicate erythema of the malar area of the face, which may pass in a few hours or a few days. Many patients exhibit a maculopapular eruption of the chest and extremities, often developing after sun exposure. Both rashes heal without scarring. In 20% of patients with SLE, a lesion indistinguishable from that of discoid lupus occurs.

Histologically, the earliest malar blush of acute cutaneous lupus may show only edema of the papillary dermis. More commonly, the changes are similar to those in the subacute form of lupus. In SLE, blisters may occur subepidermally and beneath the lamina densa, where an autoantibody against type VII collagen, a component of anchoring fibrils, is deposited. This antibody is identical with that observed in an acquired adult form of epidermolysis bullosa (EB acquisita).

Basal Keratinocytic Injury with a Lymphocytic Infiltrate Obscuring the Dermal-Epidermal Interface: Lichen Planus

Lichenoid tissue reactions are so named because of a fancied resemblance to certain lichens that form a scaly growth on rocks or tree trunks. The prototypic disorder of this group is lichen planus. Other diseases in this category include lichen nitidus and lichenoid drug eruptions.

Lichen Planus

Lichen planus (LP) is a chronic papular eruption characterized by a dense band-like infiltrate of lymphocytes and macrophages at the dermal-epidermal interface. This infiltrate is so characteristic that the term *lichenoid* is used to describe other diseases that have a similar histological appearance.

☐ **Pathogenesis:** The etiology of LP is unknown. The disease is occasionally familial and is sometimes associated with glucose intolerance. It may also accompany a variety of disorders thought to be autoimmune, such as SLE and myasthenia gravis. LP is also more frequent in patients with ulcerative colitis. Drugs such as gold, chlorothiazide, and chloroquine may induce lichenoid reactions. External agents such as photographic color developer may also evoke a lichenoid response as a form of allergic contact dermatitis. Finally, LP-like lesions are commonly observed in the later stages of chronic graft-versus-host disease. These varied observations suggest that immunological mechanisms play a role in the pathogenesis of lichen planus (Fig. 24-31). The presence of apoptotic bodies and the demonstration of increased epidermal cell turnover provide evidence that the lesions of LP result from cell destruction followed by reactive epidermal proliferation.

☐ **Pathology:** The epidermis in LP features compact hyperkeratosis, with little or no parakeratosis. The stratum granulosum is thickened, frequently in a distinctive, focal, wedge-shaped pattern. The base of the wedge abuts the stratum corneum, and the stratum spinosum is variably thickened.

The distinctive pathological changes of LP are at the dermal-epidermal interface. The basal layer is no longer a distinctive row of cuboidal cells but is replaced by flattened or polygonal keratinocytes. **The undulating, interface between the dermal papillae and the rounded profiles of the rete ridges is obscured by a dense infiltrate of lymphocytes and macrophages, many of the latter containing melanin pigment (melanophages)** (Fig. 24-32). The lymphocytes are principally of the helper/inducer phenotype. Sharply pointed (saw-toothed) wedges of keratinocytes project into the inflammatory infiltrate.

Commonly admixed with the infiltrate (in the epidermis or dermis) are globular, fibrillary, eosinophilic bodies, 15 to 20 μm in diameter (Figs. 24-33 and 24-34), which represent apoptotic keratinocytes. These structures are variously termed *apoptotic, colloid, Civatte, Sabouraud,* or *fibrillary bodies*. The fibrils within the apoptotic bodies are keratin filaments. An increased number of epidermal Langerhans cells is seen in early LP.

☐ **Clinical Features:** LP is characterized by violaceous, flat-topped papules, usually on the flexor surfaces of the wrists. White patches or streaks may also be present on the oral mucous membranes. In most patients, the pruritic lesions resolve in less than a year, but may occasionally persist for longer periods.

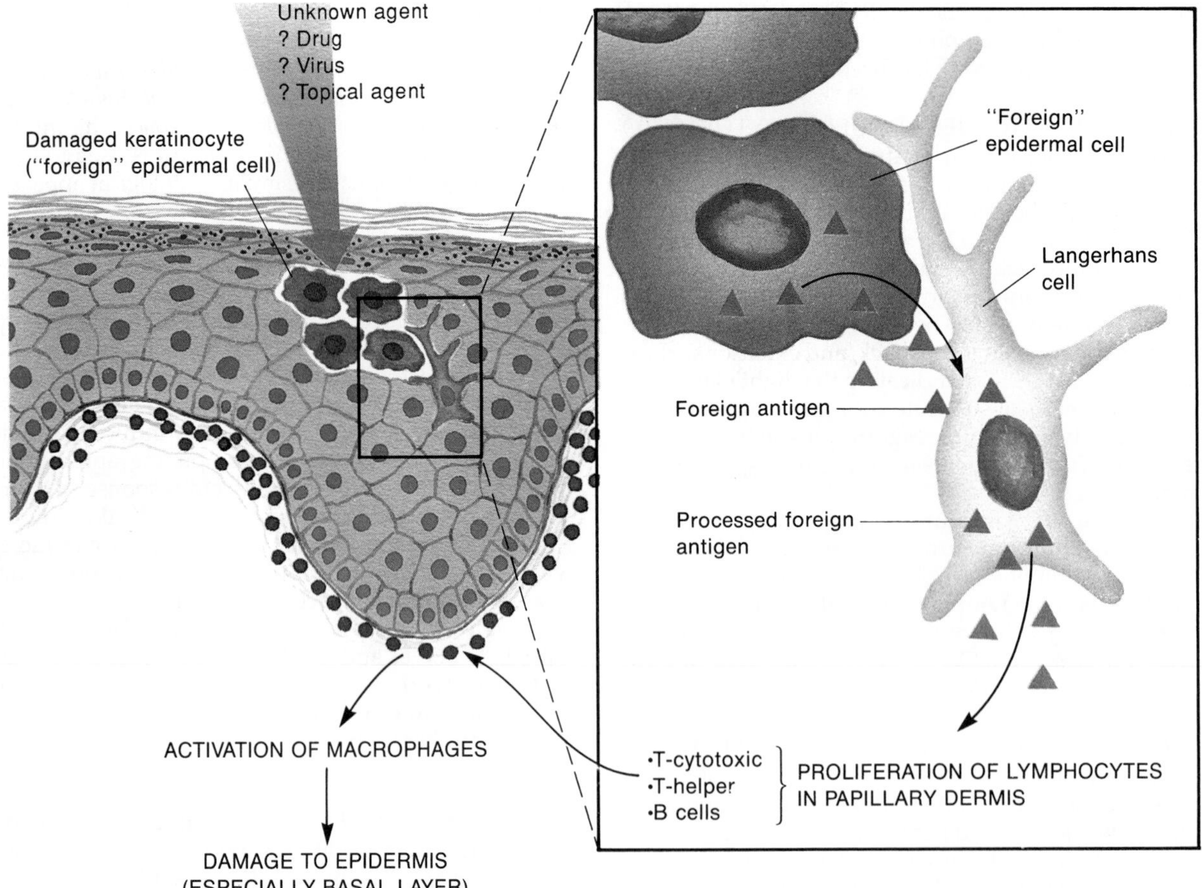

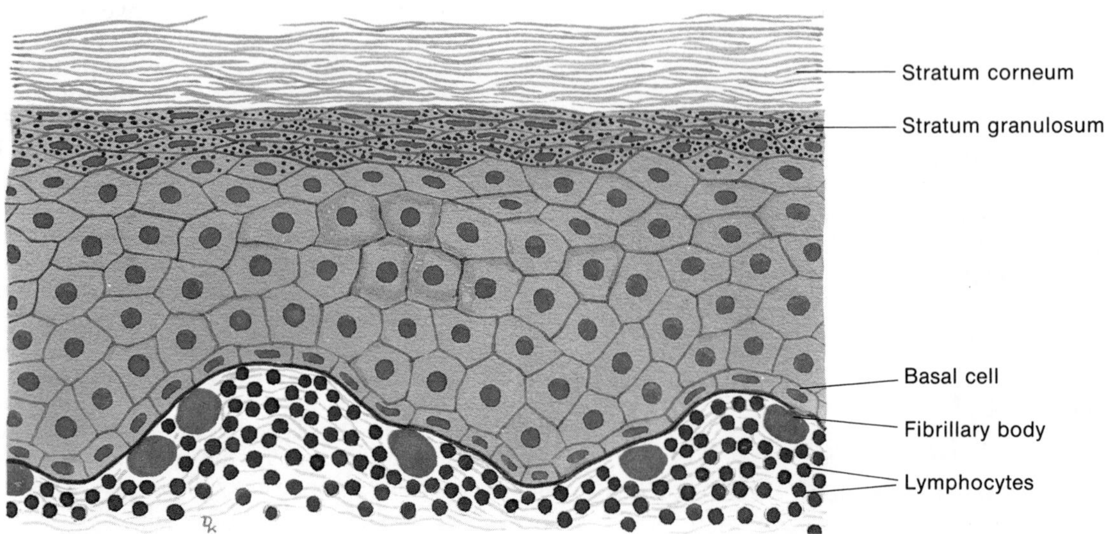

FIGURE *24-31*
Pathogenetic mechanisms in lichen planus. Lichen planus is apparently initiated by epidermal injury. This injury causes some epidermal cells to be treated as "foreign." The antigens of such cells are processed by Langerhans cells. The processed antigen induces lymphocytic proliferation and macrophage activation. Macrophages, along with T-lymphocytes, kill the epidermal basal cells, resulting in a reactive epidermal proliferation and the formation of fibrillary bodies.

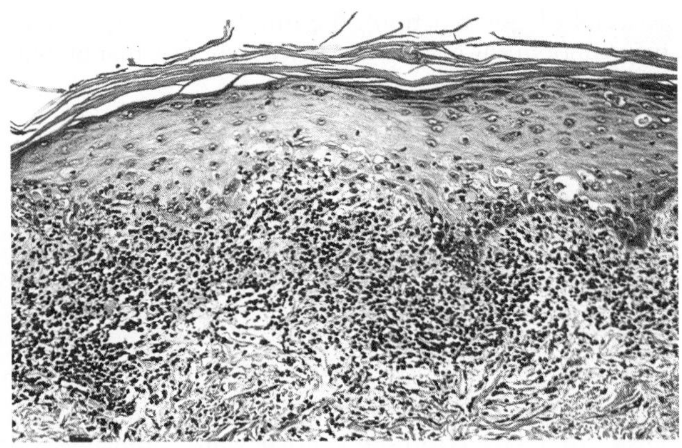

FIGURE 24-32
Lichen planus. A cell-rich, bandlike lymphocytic infiltrate disrupts the stratum basalis. Unlike lupus erythematosus, there is usually epidermal hyperplasia, with hyperkeratosis and wedge-like hypergranulosis.

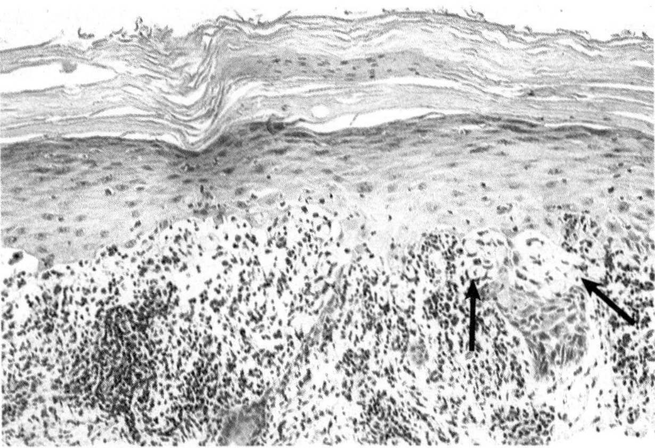

FIGURE 24-34
Lichenoid actinic keratosis. Apoptotic keratinocytes are evident (*arrows*).

INFLAMMATORY DISEASES OF THE SUPERFICIAL AND DEEP VASCULAR BED

Urticaria and Angioedema

Urticaria and angioedema are immediate-type immunological reactions (type I, anaphylactic, or IgE-dependent hypersensitivity) that reflect the degranulation of mast cells sensitized to a specific antigen.

Urticaria, or hives, *are raised, pale, well-delimited, pruritic papules and plaques that appear and disappear within a few hours.* The lesions represent edema of the superficial portions of the dermis.

Angioedema *refers to a condition in which the edema involves the deeper dermis or subcutaneous adipose tissue, resulting in an egglike swelling.*

Both urticaria and angioedema are of rapid onset and range in severity from simply annoying lesions to life-threatening allergic reactions. The mainstays of treatment are avoidance of the offending agent and prompt administration of antihistamines.

Dermatographism *is a linear hive with a rich pink flare produced by brisk stroking of the skin.* It is found in 4% of the population and represents an exaggerated IgE-dependent response. One may write on the skin of such persons and create a hive in the form of a legible word.

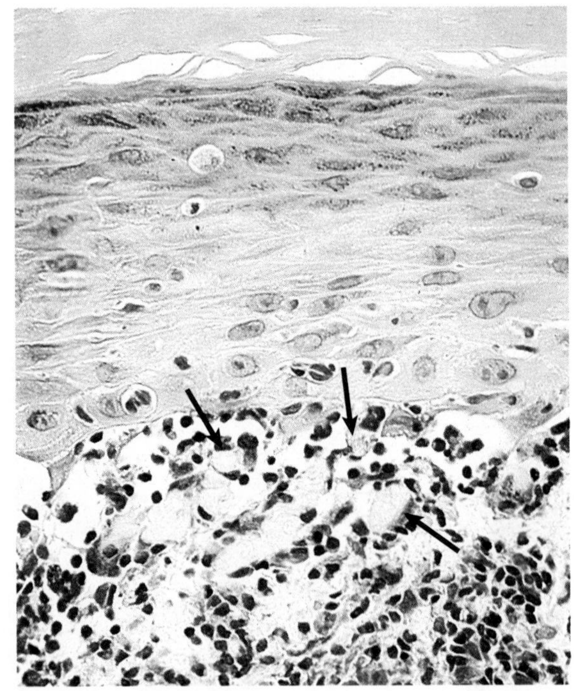

FIGURE 24-33
Lichen planus. Hypergranulosis and loss of rete ridges are noted. The site of pathological injury is at the dermal-epidermal junction, where there is a striking infiltrate of lymphocytes, many of which surround apoptotic keratinocytes (*arrows*).

☐ **Pathogenesis:** Most cases of urticaria are IgE dependent, and the final pathway is an exaggerated permeability of venules secondary to the degranulation of mast cells. The normal skin contains 7000 to 12,000 mast cells/mm^3, and an almost unending list of materials may react with IgE antibodies on the surface of the mast cell. Urticaria occur in both atopic and nonatopic persons. Atopic patients have intensely pruritic skin eruptions, a family history of similar eruptions, and a personal or family history of allergies, such as allergic rhinitis or asthma. They commonly exhibit an elevation of circulating IgE.

Initially, cutaneous venules react to the degranulation of mast cells and the release of their stored vasoactive mediators with increased permeability, thereby resulting in rapidly forming edema. If the reaction persists, inflammatory cells are attracted to the area and a persistent urticarial plaque (lasting for more that 24 hours) is the result. Such plaques occasionally show true venulitis.

☐ **Pathology:** In urticaria, the collagen fibers and fibrils are pushed apart and are separated by clear areas occupied by excess fluid. The lymphatic vessels are dilated, and the venules show margination of neutrophils and eosinophils, associated with a cuff of a few lymphocytes. Perivenular mast cell degranulation is an important feature. When the urticarial lesion persists for 24 hours (an urticarial plaque reaction), the number of lymphocytes and eosinophils is greatly increased, whereas that of neutrophils is diminished.

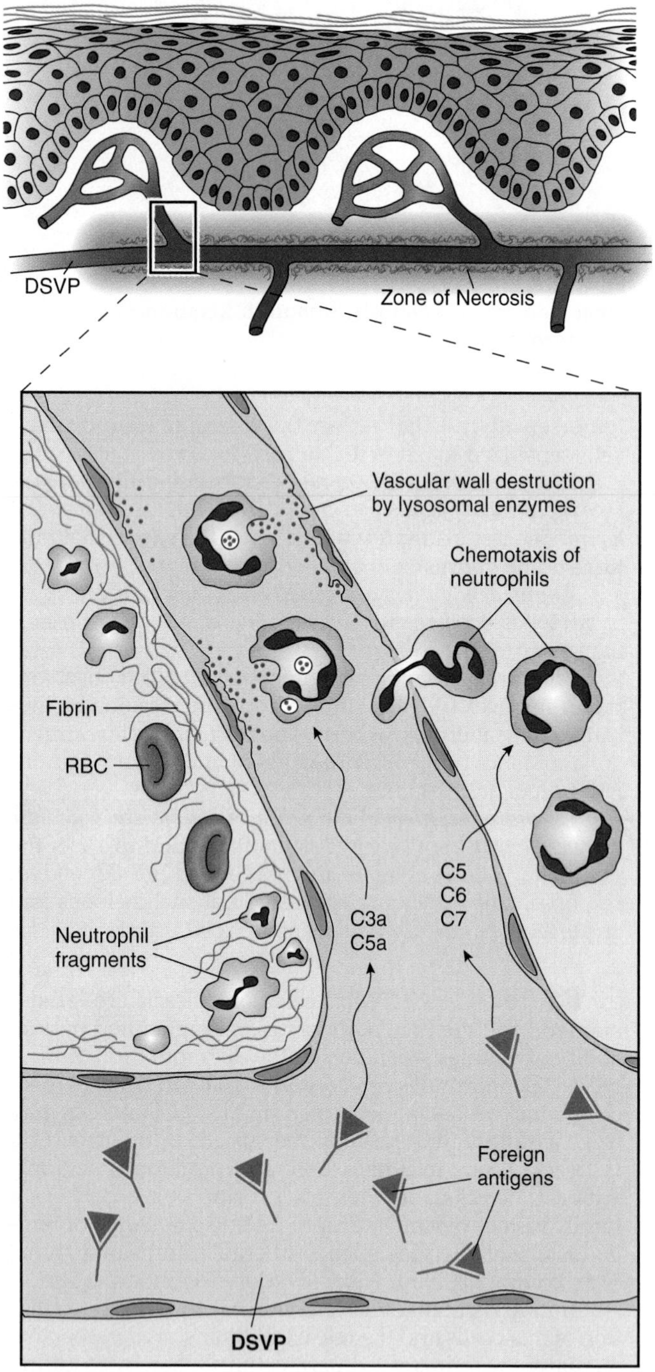

FIGURE 24-35
Pathogenesis of venular damage in cutaneous necrotizing venulitis. The site of the venular pathology is indicated in the upper diagram. Circulating immune complexes activate complement. There is neutrophilic chemotaxis (C3a and C5a) and neutrophilic destruction. Venular damage occurs with extravasation of erythrocytes, fibrin deposition, and luekocytoclasia. RBC, red blood cell; DSVP, deep superficial venular plexus.

Cutaneous Necrotizing Venulitis

Cutaneous necrotizing venulitis (CNV) is an immune complex vasculitis characterized by multiple, purpuric papules (palpable purpura). The disorder has also been termed *allergic cutaneous vasculitis, leukocytoclastic vasculitis, and hypersensitivity angiitis.*

☐ **Pathogenesis:** In CNV, circulating immune complexes are deposited in the venular walls, probably at a site of injury, at branch points where turbulence is increased, or where the venous circulation is slowed, as in the lower extremity. The elaborated C3a and C5a complement components attract neutrophils, which degranulate and release lysosomal enzymes, resulting in endothelial damage and fibrin deposition (Fig. 24-35).

Cutaneous necrotizing venulitis may be either primary (that is, without a known precipitating event) or associated with a specific infectious agent (such as hepatitis B or C virus) (see Chapter 10). It may also represent a secondary process in a wide variety of chronic illnesses, such as rheumatoid arthritis, SLE, and ulcerative colitis. Occasionally, CNV is associated with underlying malignancy, such as lymphoma.

☐ **Pathology:** The lesions of CNV show venular walls obliterated by a neutrophilic infiltrate (Fig. 24-36). The endothelial cells are difficult to visualize, and the damage to the vessel is manifested by fibrin deposition and the extravasation of erythrocytes (Fig. 24-37). Many of the neutrophils are also damaged, resulting in dustlike nuclear remnants, a process known as *leukocytoclasia* (Fig. 24-38). The collagen fibers between affected venules are separated by neutrophils, eosinophils, and leukocytoclastic cellular remnants.

☐ **Clinical Features:** CNV is distinguished by purpuric papules, which are red, palpable lesions, 2 to 4 mm

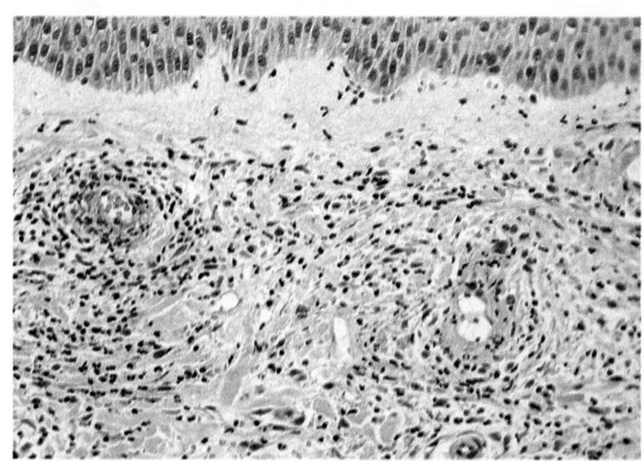

FIGURE 24-36
Cutaneous necrotizing venulitis (vasculitis). Two damaged venules are present within the papillary dermis. There is loss of endothelial lining in the venule to the *right*.

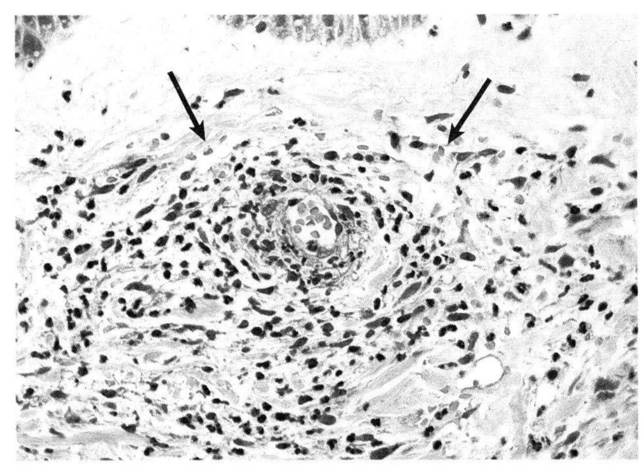

FIGURE 24-37
Cutaneous necrotizing venulitis (vasculitis). The venule is surrounded by pink fibrin and neutrophils, many of which have disintegrated (leukocytoclasis). Extravasated red blood cells (*arrows*) and inflammation give the classic clinical appearance of "palpable purpura."

in width, that do not blanch under pressure (palpable purpura). Multiple lesions characteristically appear in crops on the lower extremities or at sites of pressure. The lesions may be confined to the skin in an otherwise healthy person, or they may involve small blood vessels in the joints, gastrointestinal tract, or kidney. In half of the cases, the cause of vasculitis is unknown. In the other half, the vascular disorder is (1) secondary to an infectious disease, as in Henoch-Schönlein purpura, (2) an allergic reaction to a drug, or (3) associated with a chronic disease, such as SLE. Individual lesions persist for up to a month and then resolve, leaving hyperpigmentation or atrophic scars. Despite removal of the offending agent, episodes of CNV may recur.

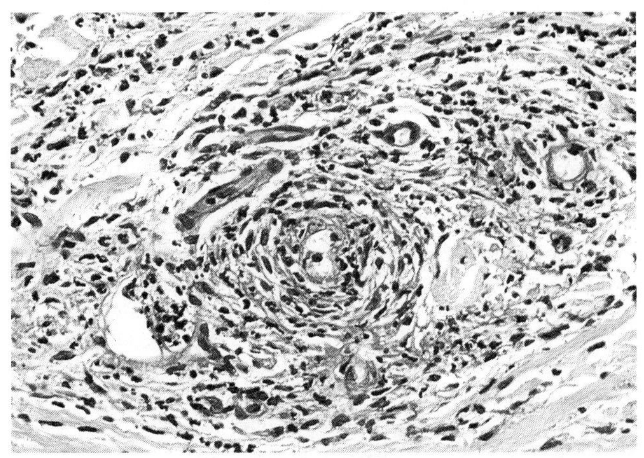

FIGURE 24-38
Cutaneous necrotizing venulitis. The pink fibrillary-to-amorphous material about the venules is called "fibrinoid." The principal component is fibrin, as corroborated by this periodic acid–Schiff (PAS) stain with diastase digestion. "Fibrinoid" also contains degenerated cellular components, complement, and other serum constituents.

Allergic Contact Dermatitis (Poison Ivy)

Allergic contact dermatitis refers to a cell mediated (type IV) hypersensitivity reaction in the skin that follows exposure to the sensitizing agent. One of the most common contact dermatitides is poison ivy, which is caused by exposure to members of the *Rhus* genus of plants. Some 90% of the population of the United States is sensitive to the common offenders, *R. radicans* (poison ivy), *R. diversiloba* (poison oak), and *R. vernix* (poison sumac). These plant dermatitides are so common that the resultant disease is synonymous with the offending plant. The patient states "I have poison ivy," and he comes to the physician for relief, not diagnosis.

☐ **Pathogenesis:** The offending plant contains low molecular weight compounds called haptens, in particular, oleoresins. These are not active in sensitization unless they combine with a carrier protein. This likely happens at the cell membrane of the Langerhans cell in the *sensitization phase*. Formation of the hapten-carrier complex requires about one hour, after which it is processed as an antigen by the Langerhans cells. These cells carry the antigen through the lymphatics to the regional lymph nodes and present the antigen to CD4+ T lymphocytes (Fig. 24-39). After 5 to 7 days, some clones of these T lymphocytes become sensitized to the antigen, become activated, multiply, and circulate as memory cells in the bloodstream. Some migrate to the skin, ready to react with the antigen if they encounter it. IL-1 produced by Langerhans cells supports proliferation of CD4+, Th1 lymphocytes. The ability to mount a delayed hypersensitivity response resides in this Th1 subset.

In the *elicitation phase*, the specifically sensitized T lymphocytes in the circulation enter the skin. At the site of challenge with the antigen, Langerhans cells, endothelial cells, perivascular dendritic cells and monocytes process the antigen and present it to the specifically sensitized T cells, which then migrate into the epidermis. Cytokine production leads to the accumulation of more T cells and macrophages. This inflammatory infiltrate is responsible for epidermal cell injury.

☐ **Pathology:** In the initial 24 hours following reexposure to the offending plant (elicitation phase), numerous lymphocytes and macrophages accumulate about the superficial venular bed and extend into the epidermis. The epidermal keratinocytes are partially separated, creating a spongelike appearance (spongiosis) (Fig. 24-40). The stratum corneum contains coagulated, eosinophilic fluid and plasma proteins. Later, numerous mononuclear inflammatory cells and eosinophils accumulate. Severe spongiosis of the epidermis, with vesicles containing lymphocytes and macrophages, is present. Large amounts of eosinophilic coagulated fluid accumulate in the stratum corneum.

☐ **Clinical Features:** When a person first comes into contact with poison ivy, no immediate reaction occurs. Five to 7 days after reexposure, the site of contact becomes intensely pruritic, after which erythema and small vesicles develop rapidly. Over the ensuing few days, the area enlarges, becomes fiery red, develops numerous

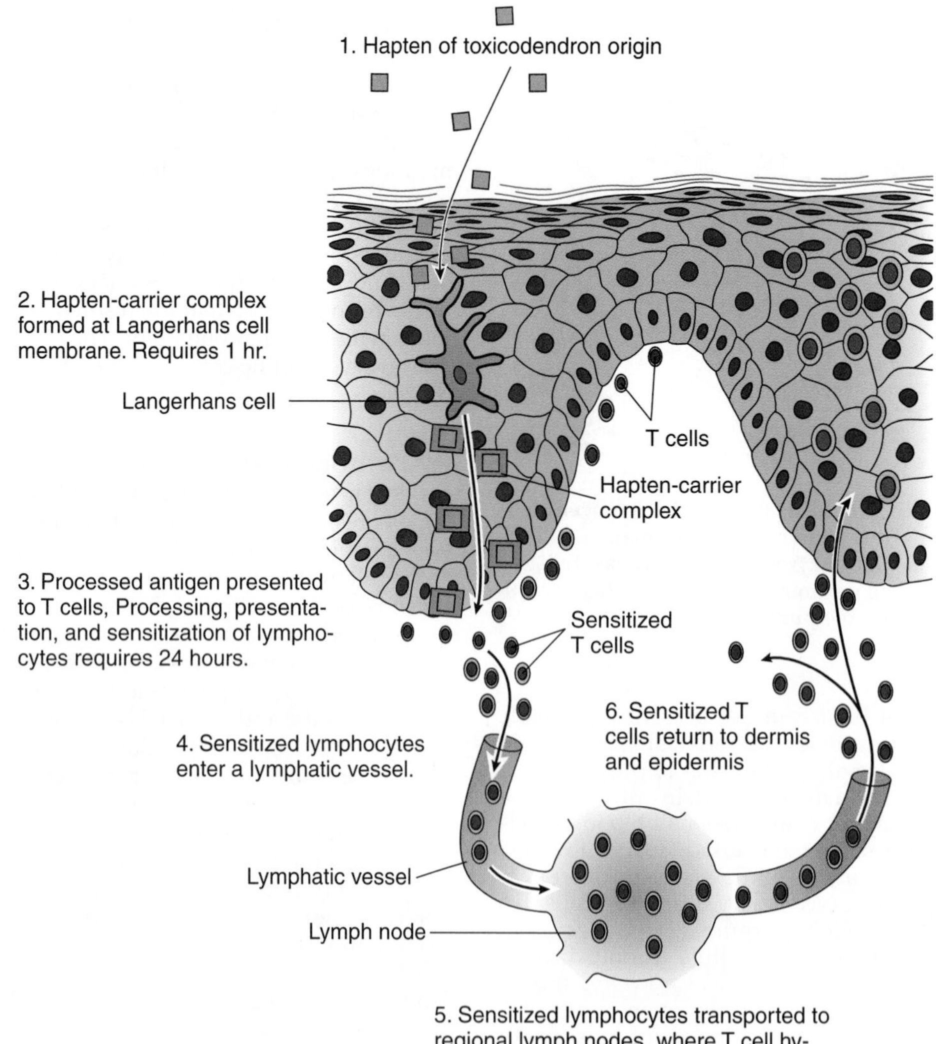

FIGURE *24-39*
Pathogenetic mechanisms in allergic contact dermatitis.

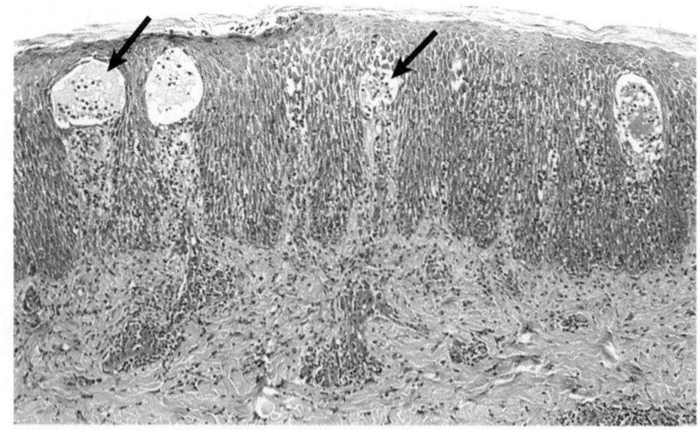

FIGURE *24-40*
Allergic contact dermatitis. Epidermal spongiosis and spongiotic vesicles (*arrows*) are present in this biopsy of "poison ivy." Infiltrating lymphocytes are apparent in the epidermis where they affect the cell-mediated delayed hypersensitivity reaction.

vesicles and exudes a large amount of clear proteinaceous fluid. During this evolution, pruritus is intense. The entire process lasts about 3 weeks. Exudation gradually subsides and the whole area is covered by an irregular crust, which eventually falls off. Pruritus diminishes, and healing occurs without scarring.

When a sensitized patient again comes into subsequent contacts with poison ivy, the entire process is greatly accelerated. Within 24 to 48 hours, the lesions appear, spread rapidly, and produce the same clinical appearance. However, the reaction is usually more intense. Again, the lesions clear in about 3 weeks. Allergic contact dermatitis is responsive to the topical or systemic administration of corticosteroids.

Granulomatous Dermatitis

Granulomatous dermatitis encompasses a variety of cutaneous inflammatory disorders characterized by dermal or subcutaneous granulomatous inflammation. Granulomas form as a response to insoluble or slowly released antigens that produce either a focal nonallergic response or an allergic response in sensitized persons. Implicated antigens include foreign substances accidently implanted into the skin, for example, silicone in breast implants or endogenous antigens such as keratin. However, in many cases of granulomatous dermatitis, the exact antigen is not well characterized.

Phagocytosis of the foreign particulate matter or processing of protein antigen is central to the activation of tissue macrophages to become the characteristic granulomatous epithelioid cells (see Chapter 2). Common causes of granulomatous dermatitis included mycobacterial and other infections (see Chapter 9), sarcoidosis, foreign bodies, and granuloma annulare.

Sarcoidosis

Sarcoidosis is a granulomatous disorder of unknown etiology that affects primarily the lungs, but also the skin, lymph nodes, spleen, eyes, and other organs (see Chapter 12). The granulomas of sarcoidosis are of the classic epithelioid cell type, but without caseation necrosis (Fig. 24-41). They involve both the dermis and the subcutaneous tissue. The cutaneous manifestations of sarcoidosis are characterized by asymptomatic papules, plaques and nodules of the dermis and subcutaneous tissue. Some dermal plaques may be annular, and those that involve the subcutaneous tissue present as irregular nodules. In severe cases, the cutaneous lesions are so prominent as to simulate a diffusely infiltrative neoplasm.

Granuloma Annulare

Granuloma annulare is a benign, self-limited, disorder of unknown etiology, characterized by palisading granulomas in the skin.

☐ **Pathogenesis:** It is postulated that granuloma annulare is an immunologically mediated reaction to an unknown antigen. The disease has been reported to follow various conditions such as insect bites, sun exposure, and viral infections. Antigenic stimuli are thought to include viral antigens, altered dermal collagen or elastic fibers, or proteins in the saliva of biting arthropods. The precise type of immune reaction is unclear, but both circulating immune complexes and cell mediated immunity may be involved. The activated macrophages may themselves contribute to the disease process by releasing lysosomal enzymes and cytokines, which, in turn, cause the focal collagen degeneration (so-called "necrobiosis") characteristic of granuloma annulare.

☐ **Pathology:** Well-developed lesions contain a central area of acellular degenerated collagen and mucin deposition in the superficial to mid-reticular dermis (Fig. 24-42). This central area is surrounded by palisaded macrophages, with the long axis of the nucleus radiating outwards. Occasional multinucleated cells are found, together with a superficial perivascular lymphocytic infiltrate.

☐ **Clinical Features:** The most common type of granuloma annulare occurs on the dorsum of the hands

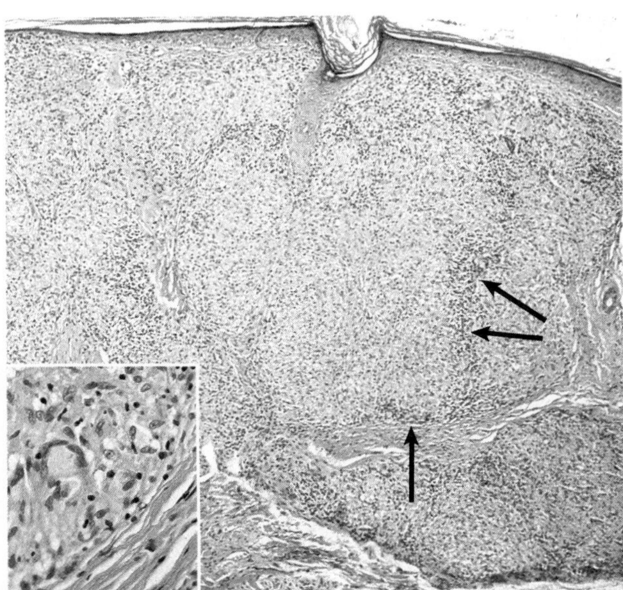

FIGURE 24-41
Sarcoidosis. Numerous large granulomas fill the reticular dermis. About some of the granulomas are small cuffs of lymphocytes (*arrows*). The granulomas are composed of epithelioid macrophages, some of which are multinucleated (*inset*).

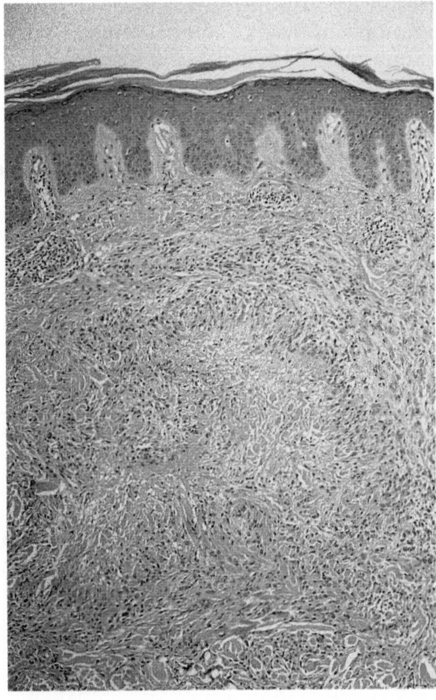

FIGURE 24-42
Granuloma annulare. A central area of acellular degenerated collagen is surrounded by palisaded macrophages, with the long axis of the nuclei radiating outwards.

and feet, primarily in children and young adults. The disease presents as asymptomatic, skin-colored or erythematous annular plaques. About 15% of patients have disseminated granuloma annulare, with 10 or more lesions involving the trunk and neck. Granuloma annulare rarely requires treatment and usually has no medical consequences. In cases with significant cosmetic disfigurement, lesional injection of steroids is usually effective.

DISORDERS OF THE DERMAL CONNECTIVE TISSUE

Scleroderma (Progressive Systemic Sclerosis)

Scleroderma (Greek, skleros, hard; and derma, skin) is defined by progressive sclerosis and tightening of the skin. The disorder also features varying structural and functional involvement of internal organs, including the kidneys, lungs, heart, esophagus, and small intestine. *Morphea* is similar to scleroderma, but it involves only patchy, circumscribed areas of the skin. The pathogenesis and systemic manifestations of scleroderma are discussed in Chapters 4 and 16.

□ **Pathology:** The initial cutaneous lesions of scleroderma are in the lower reticular dermis, but eventually the entire reticular dermis and even the papillary dermis are involved. There is a diminution of interbundle space in the reticular dermis and a tendency for the collagen bundles to be enlarged, hypocellular, and parallel to each other. A patchy lymphocytic infiltrate containing a few plasma cells is common and may also be present in the underlying subcutaneous tissue. Sweat ducts are entrapped in the thickened fibrous tissue, and there is loss of the normal fat around eccrine structures. Hair follicles are completely lost (Fig. 24-43). In late stages of the disease, large areas of subcutaneous fat are replaced by newly formed collagen.

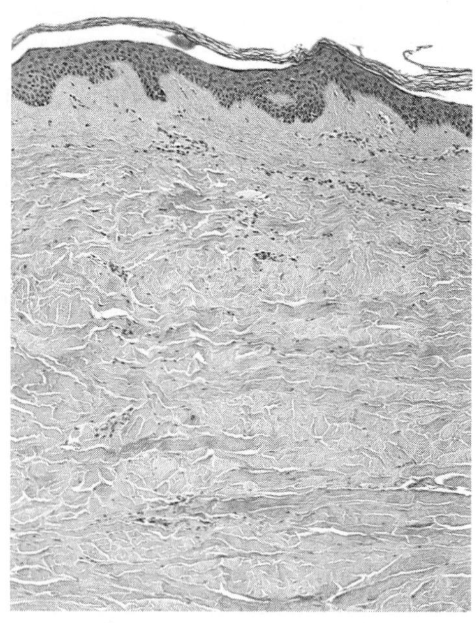

FIGURE *24-43*
Scleroderma. The dermis is characterized by large reticular dermal collagen bundles that are oriented parallel to the epidermis. The large size and loss of basket-weave pattern of these collagen bundles are abnormal. No appendages are apparent, as these are destroyed in the disease process.

□ **Clinical Features:** Scleroderma shows a peak incidence in persons between 30 and 50 years of age, and women are afflicted four times as often as men. All races are equally susceptible. Patients with early scleroderma usually present with Raynaud phenomenon (see Chapter 10) or nonpitting edema of the hands or fingers. As induration and stiffness of the skin involve the fingers, the affected areas become hardened and tense. The skin of the face becomes masklike and expressionless, and the skin around the mouth exhibits radial furrows. In late stages of the disease, the skin over large parts of the body is thickened, densely fibrotic, and fixed to the underlying tissue. The prognosis is related to the extent of disease in visceral organs, particularly the lung and kidney.

Eosinophilia-Myalgia Syndrome

The eosinophilia-myalgia syndrome (EMS) is an illness characterized by peripheral eosinophilia, myalgias, and a variety of neurological, cutaneous, and pulmonary features. Most of the persons afflicted with EMS have ingested dietary supplements of L-tryptophan containing trace amounts of contaminants, but the syndrome shares many similarities with ailments caused by the consumption of adulterated cooking oil and a diffuse fasciitis with eosinophilia of unknown etiology

Cutaneous lesions of EMS include erythematous macules, eosinophilic fasciitis, mucinous papules (owing to increased hyaluronic acid deposition in the dermis), and alopecia. There is dense fibrosis of the dermis and underlying fascia, associated with a perivascular infiltrate of lymphocytes. Numerous eosinophils may be present in the lesions, but are occasionally absent. However, peripheral blood eosinophilia is a constant.

Persons with EMS may also have complex neuromuscular involvement. The clinical spectrum extends from a primarily neuromuscular disorder with mild myalgia and weakness to quadriparesis. In addition, patients may develop Löffler syndrome (pulmonary infiltrates with eosinophilia).

Pseudoxanthoma Elasticum

Pseudoxanthoma elasticum is a hereditary disorder (autosomal recessive or dominant) of connective tissue characterized by cutaneous changes, angioid streaks in the retina, and involvement of blood vessels in visceral organs. The basic biochemical defect is not understood.

□ **Pathology:** Elastic fibers in the skin are fragmented and thickened. In routine preparations, the elastic fibers are deeply basophilic, owing to the deposition of calcium (Fig. 24-44). An inflammatory response dominated by foreign body giant cells is frequently observed about the altered elastic fibers.

☐ **Clinical Features:** The skin of patients with pseudoxanthoma elasticum is thickened, pebbled, and yellow-orange, in the axillary folds, about the neck, or in the inguinal area. The lesions have a fancied resemblance to xanthomas, hence, the term, "pseudoxanthoma." Elastic tissues in other organs of the body are also altered, including the fundus of the eye, where the disease appears as broad streaks ("angioid streaks") that radiate from the optic disc. Lesions in the walls of coronary arteries may lead to myocardial ischemia. Renal vessel involvement causes hypertension, and hemorrhage in the gastrointestinal tract is a common complication.

INFLAMMATORY DISORDERS OF THE PANNICULUS

Panniculitis *defines a heterogeneous group of diseases in which the principal focus of inflammation is in the subcutis (panniculus).* The various disorders subsumed under the rubric of panniculitis are classified according to their location. ***Septal panniculitis*** refers to inflammation in the connective tissue septa, whereas ***lobular panniculitis*** denotes major involvement of the fat lobules. These two entities may occur with or without an accompanying vasculitis. For example, polyarteritis nodosa (see Chapter 10) produces a septal panniculitis with vasculitis.

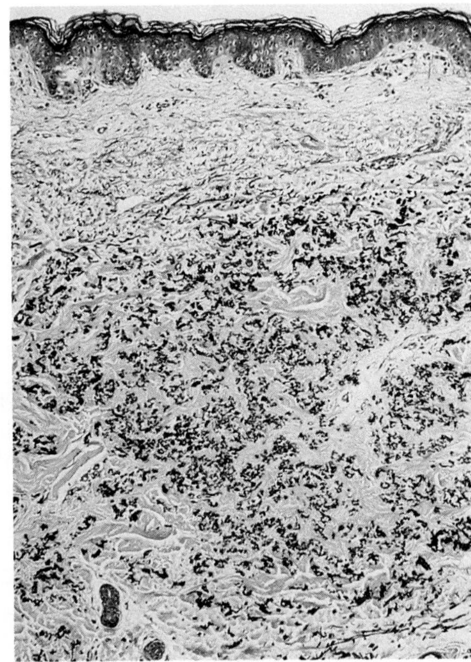

FIGURE **24-44**
Pseudoxanthoma elasticum. In this Verhoeff van Gieson preparation, there are numerous clumped and fragmented black elastic tissue fibers throughout the reticular dermis.

Erythema Nodosum: Septal Panniculitis Without Vasculitis

Erythema nodosum (EN) is a cutaneous disorder that presents as self-limited, nonsuppurative, tender nodules over the extensor surfaces of the lower extremities. The disease has a peak incidence in the third decade of life and is three times more common in women than in men.

☐ **Pathogenesis:** EN is triggered by exposure to a wide variety of agents, including drugs and microorganisms (bacteria, viruses, and fungi), and occurs in association with a number of benign and malignant systemic diseases. Common infections complicated by EN include streptococcal diseases (especially in children), tuberculosis, and *Yersinia* enterocolitis. In endemic areas, deep fungal infections (blastomycosis, histoplasmosis, coccidioidomycosis) are a common cause. EN is also frequent after acute respiratory tract infections of unknown etiology, which are likely viral. In drug-induced EN, the agents most commonly implicated are sulfonamides and oral contraceptives. Finally, Crohn disease and ulcerative colitis are occasionally complicated by EN.

It is thought that EN represents an immunological response to foreign antigens, although the evidence is indirect. For example, patients with tuberculosis or coccidioidomycosis do not develop EN until the skin test becomes positive, and testing with Frei antigen for lymphogranuloma venereum may itself induce EN. The early neutrophilic inflammation suggests that EN may be a response to the activation of complement, with resulting neutrophilic chemotaxis. The subsequent chronic inflammation is probably secondary to necrosis of adipose tissue at the interface of the septa and lobules, with a foreign body giant cell response to degraded fat and subsequent fibrosis.

☐ **Pathology:** Early in the course of the disease, the lesions of EN are in the fibrous septa of the subcutaneous tissue, where neutrophilic inflammation is associated with the extravasation of erythrocytes. In chronic lesions, the septa are widened, with focal collections of giant cell macrophages about small areas of altered collagen and an ill-defined lymphocytic infiltrate (Fig. 24-45). Giant cells and inflammation extend into the lobule at the interface between the septum and the surrounding fat lobule. Secondary vascular involvement is occasionally noted. No infectious organisms are identified in the lesions

☐ **Clinical Features:** EN typically presents acutely on the anterior aspects of the lower limbs as dome-shaped, exquisitely tender, erythematous nodules. The nodules eventually become firm and less tender and disappear in 3 to 6 weeks. As some nodules heal, others arise, but all lesions resolve without residual scarring within 6 weeks.

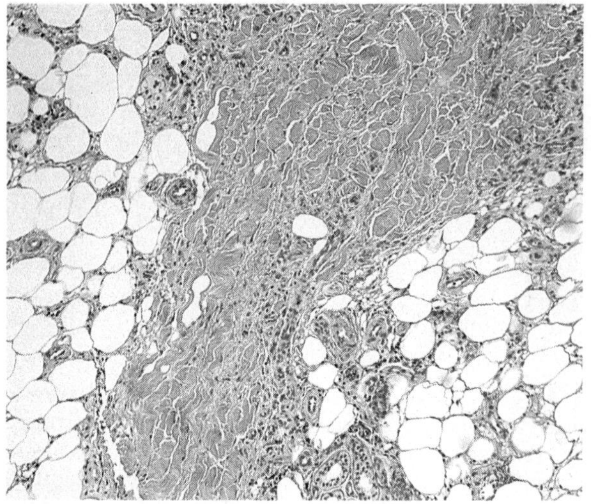

FIGURE 24-45
Erythema nodosum. The reticular dermis is present in the upper right. Within the panniculus (extending through the middle of the field) is a widened septum (see Fig. 24-1). Lymphocytes and macrophages are present at its border with the adipose tissue lobules. The vessels palisading along the border of the septum are infiltrated by lymphocytes.

Erythema Induratum (Nodular Vasculitis): Lobular Panniculitis with Vasculitis

Erythema induratum (EI) refers to chronic, recurrent subcutaneous nodules or plaques on the legs, predominantly in women. Historically, EI has been considered as a "tuberculid", a hypersensitivity reaction to mycobacteria or associated antigens at a distant site. Failure of lesional tissue to yield isolates of mycobacteria in culture or in laboratory animals had cast doubt on the validity of this concept. Recent investigations using the polymerase chain reaction have, however, detected a specific *M. tuberculosis* DNA sequence in over 75% of skin biopsy specimens with a histological diagnosis of EI.

☐ **Pathology:** In contrast to EN, EI presents initially as a lobular panniculitis. This lesion is secondary to a vasculitis, which produces ischemic necrosis of the fat lobule. The panniculus exhibits a dense chronic inflammatory infiltrate within the lobules, which can form prominent tuberculoid granulomas or result in areas of coagulative necrosis. The lobular septa within the panniculus are relatively spared. The vascular changes are usually extensive and include (1) prominent infiltration of small and medium-sized arteries and veins by a dense lymphoid or granulomatous infiltrate, (2) endothelial swelling, which may progress to thrombosis, and (3) fibrous thickening of the intima. Extensive ischemic necrosis leads to subsequent ulceration of the overlying epidermis. Eventually, the lesions heal by fibrosis.

☐ **Clinical Features:** Patients with erythema induratum present with recurrent, tender, erythematous, subcutaneous nodules on the legs, particularly in the area of the calf. The lesions tend to ulcerate and heal with an atrophic scar. The course may be prolonged for many years, and systemic steroids are usually necessary to control the disease.

ACNE VULGARIS: A DISORDER OF THE PILOSEBACEOUS UNIT

Acne vulgaris is a self-limited, inflammatory disorder of the sebaceous follicles that typically afflicts adolescents, results in the intermittent formation of discrete papular or pustular lesions, and may lead to scarring. In some cases, acne extends as long as the third decade. The condition is cosmetically disfiguring and often psychologically debilitating. Acne is so common that many regard it as a normal part of the maturing process.

☐ **Pathogenesis and Pathology:** The development of acne is related to (1) hormonally-induced, excessive production of sebum; (2) abnormal cornification of portions of the follicular epithelium; (3) a response to the anaerobic diphtheroid *Propionibacterium acnes*; and (4) rupture of the follicle and consequent inflammation. The sebaceous follicle contains a vellus hair and prominent sebaceous glands. The change in hormonal status at puberty leads to the production of sebum in the follicle and to altered cornification in the neck of the sebaceous follicule (infundibulum), effects that produce dilatation of the follicular canal. Another round of excessive sebum production is associated with the desquamation of squamous cells and the accretion of keratinous debris, a situation that provides a rich environment for the proliferation of *P. acnes*. These combined changes result in the formation of a distended, plugged follicle, termed a *comedone*. Neutrophils are attracted to the area by chemotactic factors released by *P. acnes*, where they release hydrolytic enzymes to form a follicular abscess (*pustule*). They also attack the wall of the follicle, thereby permitting the escape of sebum, keratin, and bacteria into the perifollicular tissue, where they stimulate further acute inflammation and a perifollicular abscess (Fig. 24-46). The development of allergy to *P. acnes* intensifies the inflammatory response. The fully evolved lesions show intense neutrophilic inflammation surrounding a ruptured sebaceous follicle. In addition, numerous macrophages, lymphocytes, and foreign body giant cells accumulate as a response to the rupture of the sebaceous follicle.

☐ **Clinical Features:** Acne vulgaris features a variety of skin lesions in different stages of development, including comedones, papules, pustules, nodules, cysts, and pitted scars. Comedones, which are the primary noninflammatory lesions of acne, are either open (blackheads) or closed (whiteheads). The more advanced inflammatory lesions vary from small, erythematous papules to large, tender, purulent nodules and cysts.

Acne vulgaris is treated with topical cleansing and keratolytic and antibacterial agents. Severe cases are managed with topical vitamin A, systemic antibiotics, and synthetic oral retinoids (isotretinoin).

ARTHROPOD INFESTATIONS

Human mites and lice, other insects, and spiders produce focal lesions that may be intensely pruritic.

- **Scabies:** *Sarcoptes scabiei*, a human mite, causes a severely pruritic, eczematous dermatitis. The female mite burrows beneath the stratum corneum on the fingers, wrists, trunk, and genital skin. An intense lymphoid and eosinophilic dermatitis is induced as a hypersensitivity reaction to the mite and to its eggs and feces.
- **Pediculosis:** Another pruritic dermatosis, namely pediculosis, may be caused by a variety of human lice. Eggs (nits) of the lice may be found attached to the hair shafts.
- **Arthropod bites:** The lesions produced by biting insects vary from small, pruritic papules to large, weeping nodules. The reaction depends on the arthropod species and the host immune response. For example, tick bites tend to be large, with a striking lymphocytic and eosinophilic infiltrate and on occasion the formation of lymphoid follicles. Flea bites are usually urticarial, with a scant neutrophilic infiltrate. The venoms injected by some arthropods (e.g., spiders) may lead to severe tissue necrosis at the site of the bites.

Lyme disease, a treponemal infection transmitted by the *Ixodes* tick, is discussed in Chapter 9.

PRIMARY NEOPLASMS OF THE SKIN

Neoplasia in the skin is an important paradigm for the understanding of cancer in general, particularly because it is known that the most important carcinogenic agent in most cutaneous cancers is ultraviolet light. The lesions of cutaneous neoplasia are on the body surface, where their development and evolution are readily observed. The pathology of most of the developmental stages of the specific skin neoplasms is known. The ready availability of tumor tissue from the sequential lesions has permitted *in vitro* studies of tumor cells to be correlated with the observed behavior of the clinical lesions.

Melanocytic Neoplasia

The incidence of malignant melanoma is increasing at a rate greater than that of any other form of human cancer. It is estimated that more than 1% of children born today will develop malignant melanoma. Although the tumor was once regarded as particularly malignant, this reputation is no longer deserved. The prognosis is excellent if the lesion is recognized before it enters into the vertical growth phase. However, when the tumor extends to a critical depth in the dermis, 75% of affected patients will die of metastatic disease. With proper awareness on the part of physicians and the general public, the mortality from malignant melanoma should be less than 5%.

The Initial Lesion: Common Acquired Melanocytic Nevi (Moles)

A mole is a pigmented skin lesion composed of a benign proliferation of melanocytes within the epidermis or dermis. Most people who are exposed to a significant amount of light in the first 15 years of life, regardless of their native skin color, develop some 10 to 50 moles on their skin. Black skin can develop moles, but they are uncommon and are not associated with progression to melanoma (except on the palms, soles, and genital skin). The moles do not ordinarily develop in areas protected from light by at least two layers of clothing, such as the breasts of women. A notable exception to the induction of melanocytic nevi by light occurs in red-haired, blue-eyed persons with milk-white skin. Such individuals are exquisitely sensitive to light and form freckles, but they do not exhibit a significant number of melanocytic nevi.

Although there is an unequivocal causal relationship between ultraviolet light and melanocytic nevi (and malignant melanoma), the relationship is clearly complex; some people with light sensitive skin form few nevi, whereas some with dark skin develop many moles. Recent epidemiological studies have shown the significance of precursor lesions (melanocytic nevi or moles) to the development of melanoma. A person with 100 or more moles that are 2 to 5 mm wide has a threefold greater risk of developing melanoma than one with fewer than 25 moles of similar size. Patients with clinically atypical nevi or histologically dysplastic nevi have an even greater risk of developing melanoma.

Melanocytic nevi begin to appear between the first and second years of life and continue to emerge for the first two decades of life. A mole is first recognized as a small tan dot, that does not exceed 0.1 to 0.2 cm in diameter. Over a period of 3 to 4 years, the dot enlarges as a uniform tan to brown area. During this enlargement, the outline of the melanocytic nevus is usually regular and either circular or oval. When the nevus is 4 to 5 mm in diameter, it is flat or slightly elevated and stops enlarging at the periphery. When peripheral enlargement ceases, the uniform, rich brown mole becomes sharply demarcated from the surrounding normal skin. Over the next 10 years, the lesion begins to elevate, and its color is slightly diminished. Gradually, the mole becomes a tan skin tag. For one to two decades, it gradually flattens, and the skin may return to a normal appearance. Most people show a gradual decrease in the number of their moles through the years, as reflected in the statement, "We come into this world without moles and we leave without moles." It is of note that melanoma patients retain significant numbers of moles, atypical ones at that, in the late decades of life.

☐ **Pathology:** At the inception of a melanocytic nevus, an increased number of melanocytes in the basal epidermis is associated with hyperpigmentation. Subsequently, the melanocytes form nests, frequently at the tips of rete ridges and migrate into the dermis, where they form small clusters. These small cells are oval and bear a superficial resemblance to a lymphocyte. In time, the lesion becomes clearly elevated. The dermal component

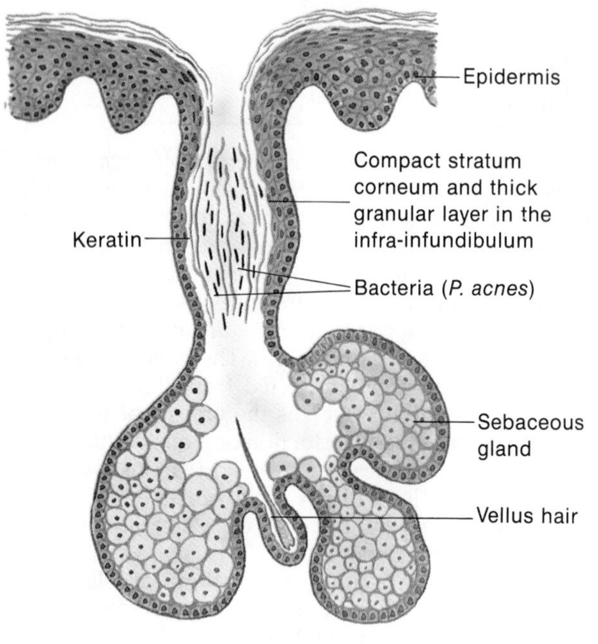

A. MICROCOMEDONE

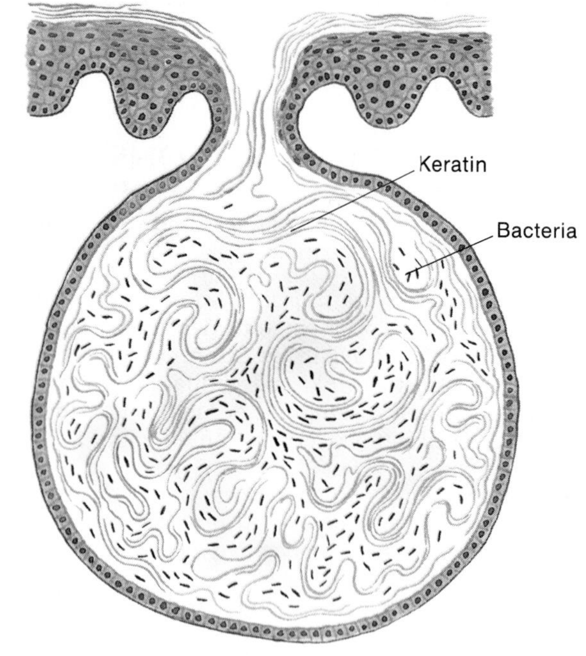

B. CLOSED COMEDONE

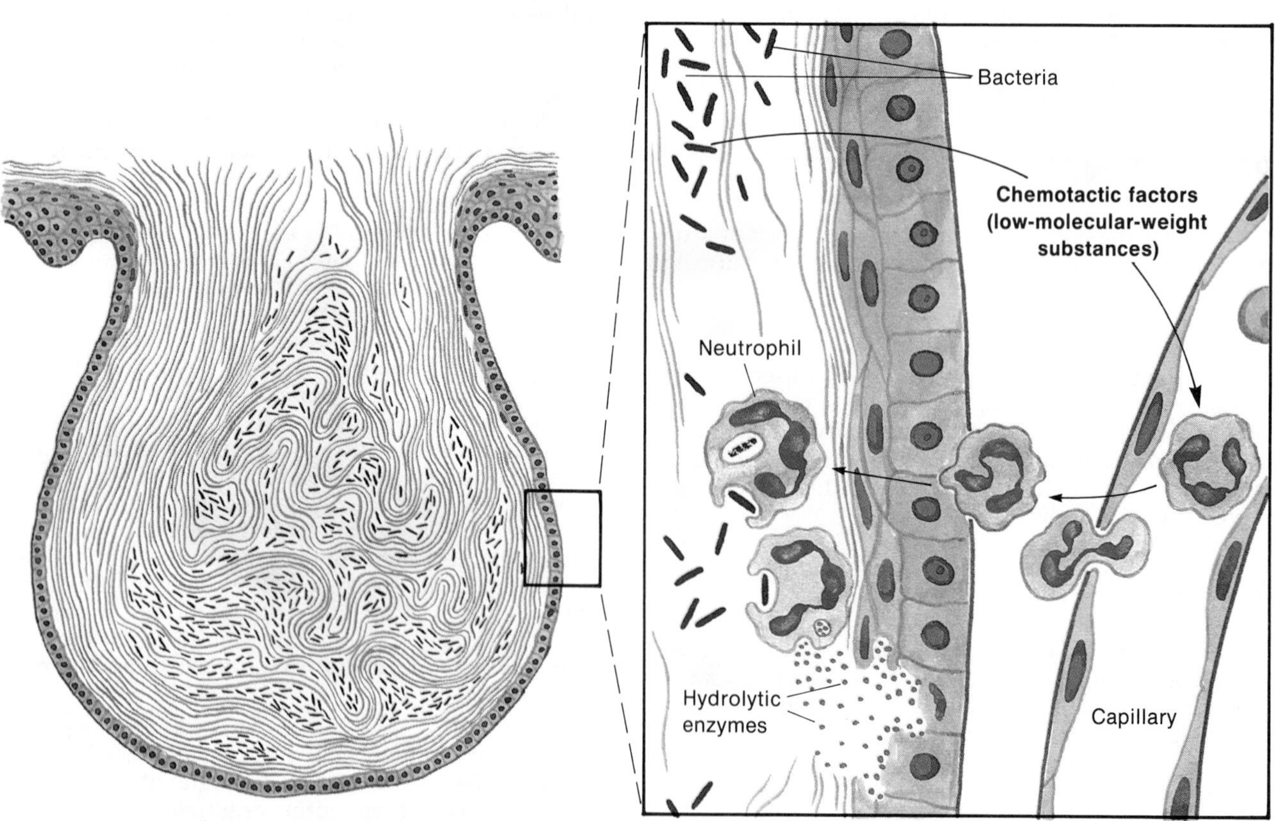

C. OPEN COMEDONE

D. INVASION OF FOLLICLE BY NEUTROPHILS

FIGURE *24-46*

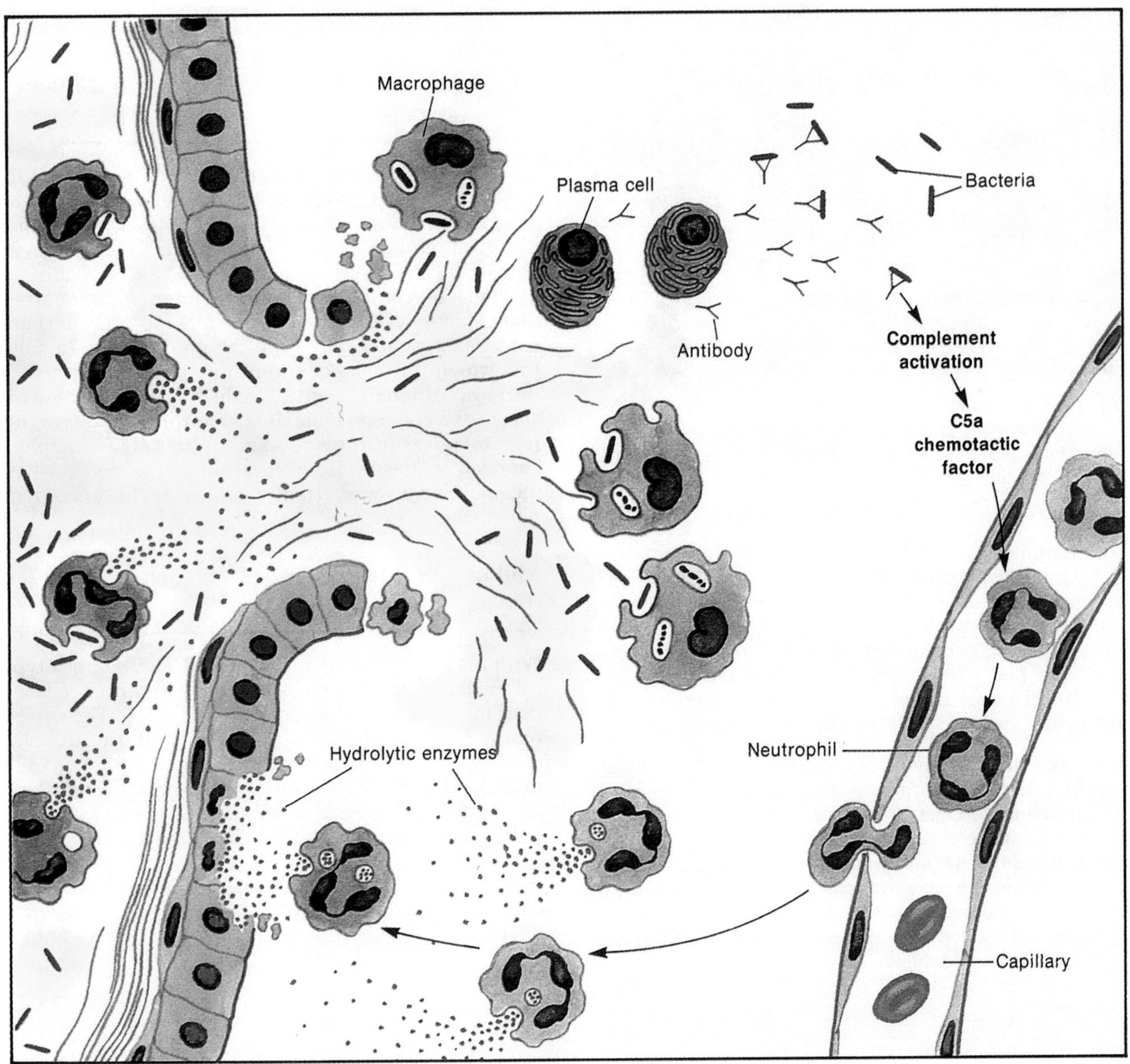

E. INFLAMMATION AND RUPTURE OF SEBACEOUS FOLLICLE

FIGURE *24-46*
Pathogenesis of follicular distention, rupture, and inflammation in acne vulgaris. Acne is a disease of the follicular canal of a sebaceous folicle. A compact stratum corneum and a thickened granular layer in the infrainfundibulum are the beginning of the formation of a comedone. Microcomedones (*A*) and closed (*B*) and open (*C*) comedones form. Excessive sebum secretion occurs, and the bacterium *P. acnes* proliferates. The organism produces chemotactic factors, leading to neutrophil migration into the intact comedone. Neutrophilic enzymes are released and the comedone ruptures, inducing a cycle of chemotaxis and intense neutrophilic inflammation (*D* and *E*).

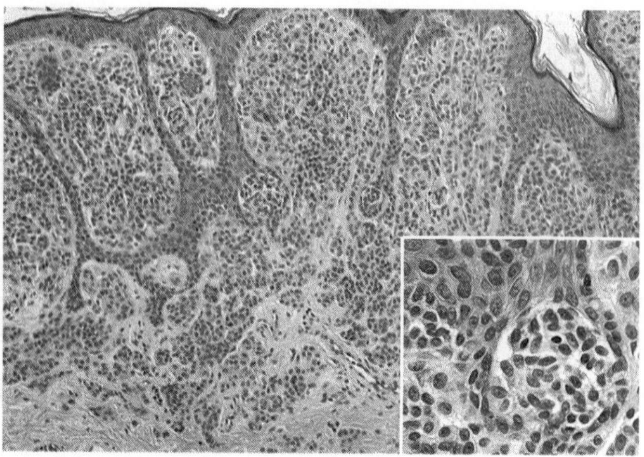

FIGURE 24-47
Compound melanocytic nevus. Melanocytes are present as nests within the epidermis and dermis. An intraepidermal nest of melanocytes is surrounded by keratinocytes (*inset*).

differentiates, and the cells evolve along the lines of Schwann cells, forming small structures similar to nerve endings. Gradually, this differentiation encompasses the entire dermal component of the lesion, and the core of a 20-year-old nevus may be composed of a delicate neuromesenchyme. Eventually, the nevus flattens and disappears.

The histological classification of melanocytic nevi distinguishes various stages of evolution of the lesion.

- **Lentigo**: The melanocytes are limited to the basal layer of the epidermis.
- **Junctional nevus**: The melanocytes form nests at the tips of the rete ridges in the epidermis.
- **Compound nevus**: Nests of melanocytes are seen in the epidermis and the cells have also migrated into the dermis (Fig. 24-47).
- **Dermal nevus**: Intraepidermal melanocytic growth has ceased (Fig. 24-48).
- **Skin tag**: The dermal component has differentiated into a delicate neuromesenchyme, and the lesion is indistinguishable from a small nonmelanocytic skin tag.

Atypical Nevus: Melanocytic Nevus with Aberrant Differentiation

Occasionally, common acquired nevi do not follow the normal pattern of growth, differentiation, and disappearance described above. Such lesions persist rather than disappear and are commonly greater than 5 mm across. One or several moles may show focal areas of aberrant melanocytic growth, and become larger and more irregular. The peripheral irregular area is flat (macular) and extends asymmetrically from the parent mole. Initially, the growth of melanocytes in the basal epidermis appears no different from that which occurs in the early stages of a common mole. **It is abnormal in pattern, not in cytological features.** A band of brightly eosinophilic connective tissue is seen around the rete, where melanocytes grow aberrantly and small clusters of lymphocytes are present.

Melanocytic Nevus with Dysplasia (Dysplastic Nevus)

With the passage of time, melanocytes with large atypical nuclei that have some similarities to cancer cells appear in the area of aberrant differentiation. The combination of an abnormal growth pattern and the cytological abnormality of melanocytes (melanocytic nuclear atypia) defines a dysplastic nevus (Figs. 24-49 and 24-50). These areas of dysplasia are also associated with a subjacent lymphocytic infiltrate and distinctive connective tissue changes. More than half of malignant melanomas 0.75 mm in thickness or larger have a precursor nevus, the majority of which show melanocytic dysplasia.

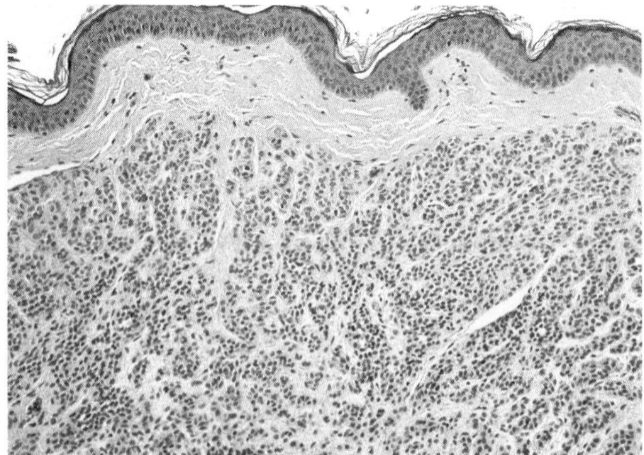

FIGURE 24-48
Dermal melanocytic nevus. The melanocytes are entirely confined to the dermis.

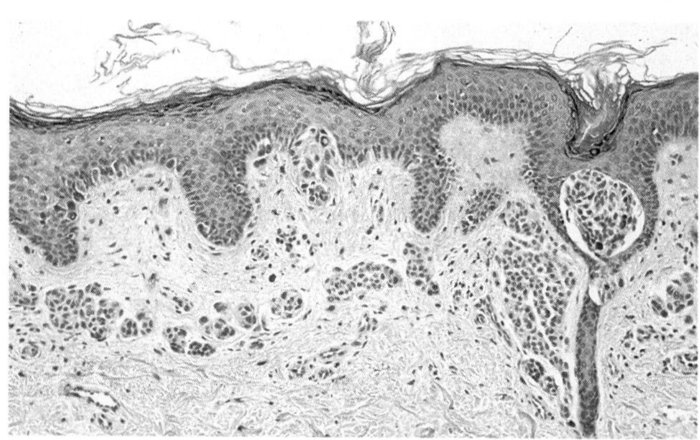

FIGURE 24-49
Compound nevus with melanocytic dysplasia. On the *right* a compound nevus is apparent with both intraepidermal and dermal components. To the *left* within the epidermis are single atypical melanocytes within the basal unit, as well as incipient lamellar fibroplasia. Dermal melanocytes are present below.

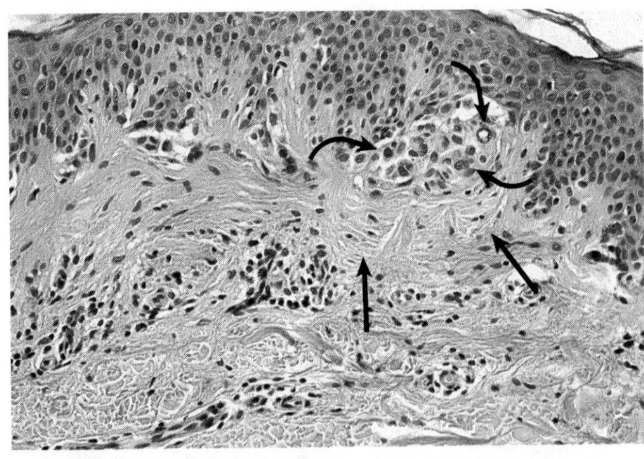

A

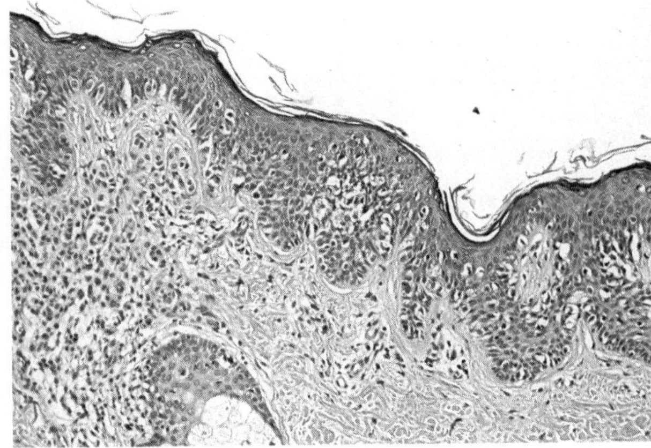

B

C

FIGURE 24-50
(*A*) Dysplastic nevus. There is bridging of rete by nests of melanocytes, melanocytes with cytological atypia (*curved arrows*), lamellar fibroplasia (*arrows*), and a scant perivascular lymphocytic infiltrate. (*B*) Dysplastic nevus. To the *left* is a zone containing typical dermal nevic cells of a compound melanocytic nevus. In the epidermis on the *right* is a lentiginous proliferation of atypical melanocytes with lamellar fibroplasia. This photomicrograph is taken from the junction of the papular and macular components of this dysplastic nevus. It is the macular portion, which takes up most of the field, in which dysplasia usually develops. (*C*) Dysplastic nevus. These ellipsoidal melanocytic nests resting above lamellar fibroplasia (*straight arrows*) exhibit large epithelioid melanocytes with atypia (*curved arrows*).

The Intermediate Lesions: Radial Growth Phase Melanoma (Superficial Spreading Melanoma)

The appearance of intermediate lesions heralds the very beginnings of malignancy (malignant melanoma). There are four common forms and several uncommon forms of malignant melanoma. Only the common forms are discussed here, with emphasis on the most frequently encountered variety—namely superficial spreading melanoma.

□ **Pathology:** Early melanomas in the radial growth phase have a slightly elevated and palpable border. The neoplasm is variably and haphazardly colored. Some parts are unusually black or dark brown, whereas lighter brown shades are mingled with pink and light blue tints. Occasionally, the entire lesion is purely dark brown (Fig. 24-51).

On microscopic examination, large epithelioid melanocytes are dispersed in nests and as individual cells throughout the entire thickness of the epidermis (Fig. 24-52). These melanocytes may be only in the epidermis (***in situ melanoma***), but focal extension into the papillary dermis is the rule. There is a characteristic disposition of the cells in

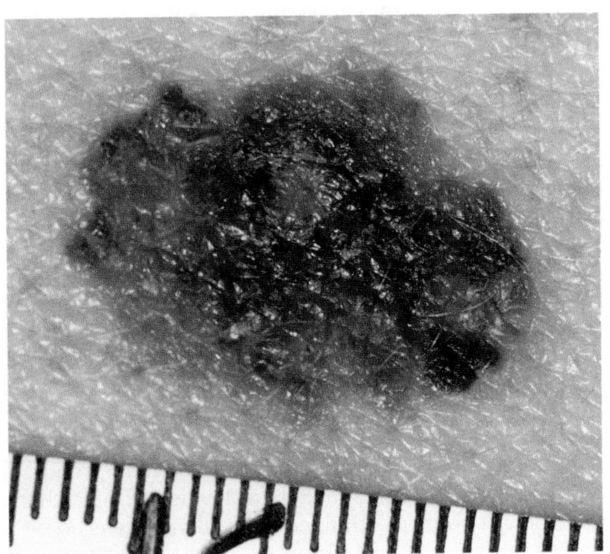

FIGURE 24-51
The clinical appearance of the radial growth phase in malignant melanoma of the superficial spreading type. The larger diameter is 1.8 cm.

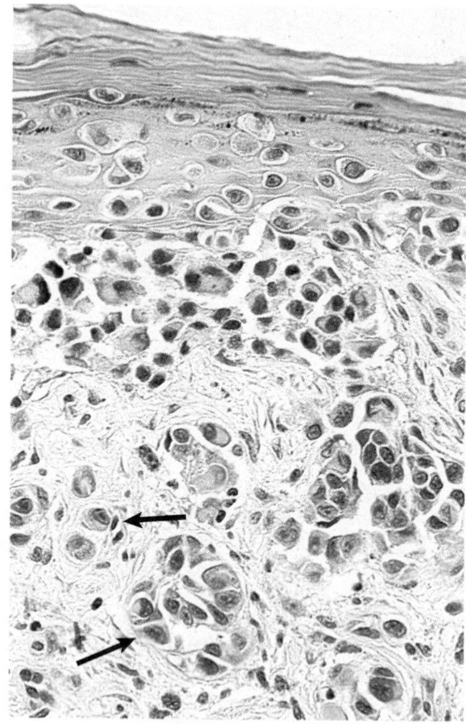

FIGURE 24-52
Malignant melanoma, superficial spreading type, radial growth phase. Melanocytes grow singly within the epidermis at all levels and as large, irregularly-sized nests at the dermal-epidermal junction. Tumor cells are present in the papillary dermis (*arrows*), but no nest shows preferential growth over the others.

the radial growth phase. The melanocytes are arranged in small nests or as individual cells, and no nest has growth preference (larger size) over the surrounding cells (see Fig. 24-52). The melanocytes of the radial growth phase are typically associated with a brisk lymphocytic response. Thus, melanocytes of the radial growth phase grow in all directions: upward in the epidermis, peripherally in the epidermis, and downward from the epidermis into the dermis. No dermal mitoses are noted. The enlargement of such circular lesions is at the periphery; hence the term radial growth phase. Importantly, melanomas in the radial growth phase have only rarely been observed to metastasize.

☐ **Clinical Features:** Except for the smallest lesions (<6 mm in diameter), superficial spreading melanoma can be diagnosed in the radial growth phase with considerable accuracy by clinical inspection, and it may be distinguished from a nevus, even an abnormal one. However, any clinical suspicion that a lesion may be melanoma warrants an excisional biopsy. With regard to lesions documented to be melanoma, patients frequently state that a change in a mole had developed. The change may be as subtle as itching, but usually there is some increase in size or darkening of the lesion.

Vertical Growth Phase Melanoma

After a variable time (usually 1 to 2 years), the character of growth of the radial growth phase changes focally.

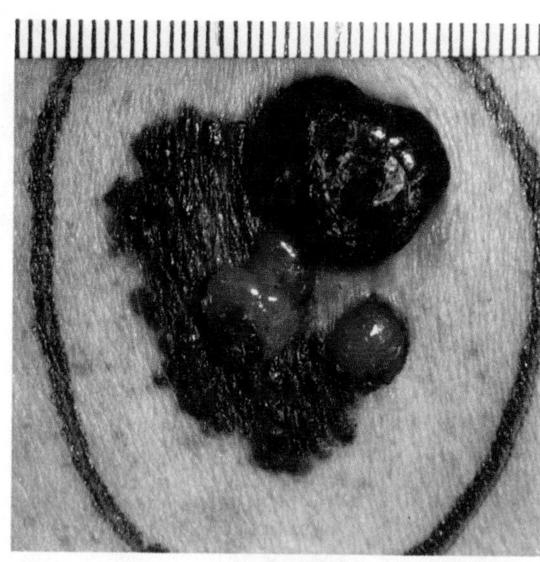

FIGURE 24-53
Clinically, the radial growth phase in malignant melanoma of the superficial spreading type is represented by the relatively flat, dark, brown-black portion of the tumor. There are three areas in this lesion that are characteristic of the vertical growth phase. All are nodular in configuration; two have a pink coloration, and the largest is a rich, ebony black.

Melanocytes exhibit focal mitotic activity and grow as spheroidal nodules, in a manner similar to the growth of metastatic lesions. The nodules expand more rapidly than the rest of the tumor in the surrounding papillary dermis (Fig. 24-53). The net direction of growth tends to be perpendicular to that of the radial growth phase, hence the term vertical growth phase (Figs. 24-54 through 24-56). The characteristics of the vertical growth phase are as follows:

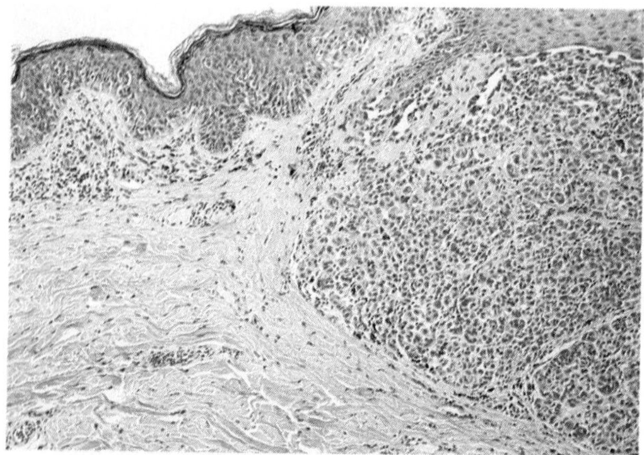

FIGURE 24-54
Malignant melanoma, superficial spreading type, vertical growth phase. Vertical growth is manifested by the distinct spherical tumor nodule to the *right*. A focus of melanocytes clearly has a growth advantage (larger-size) over other nests in the radial growth phase (*left*). The nodule distorts the papillary dermal-reticular dermal junction and therefore is level III.

- The cells tend to differ in appearance from those of the radial growth phase. For example, they may contain little or no pigment, whereas the cells of the radial growth phase are melanotic.
- The cellular aggregate that characterizes the vertical growth phase is larger than the clusters of cells that form the intraepidermal and invasive components of the radial growth phase. The dominant site of the tumor growth is shifted from the epidermis to the dermis.
- Tumors that extend into the lower half of the reticular dermis are, by definition, in the vertical growth phase.
- The cellular immune response of the host may be absent at the base of the vertical growth phase.

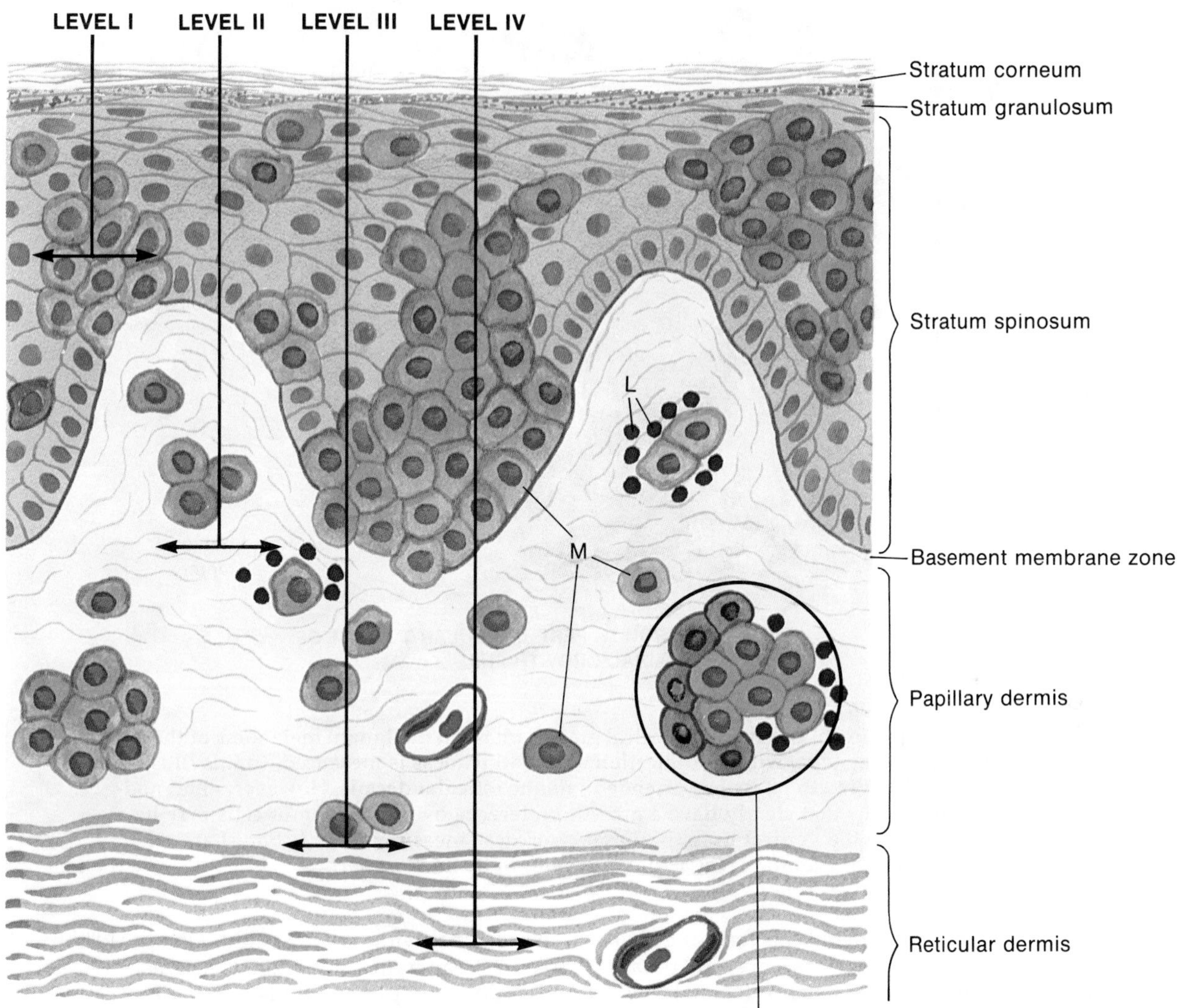

FIGURE *24-55*
Schematic depiction of the radial growth phase in malignant melanoma of the superficial spreading type. In the radial growth phase, cells grow in the epidermis and are present in the dermis. They grow in all directions: outward, peripherally, and downward. However, the net direction of growth is peripheral—along the radii of an imperfect circle. Growth, as manifested by mitotic activity, is largely in the epidermis. No cells in the dermis seem to have a growth preference over others. The nest depicted here will be shown as it evolves into the vertical growth phase in Figures 24-55 and 24-56. The anatomical landmarks of the levels of invasion are shown. Level III is not simply the occasional impingement of a tumor cell against the reticular dermis, but indicates a collection of cells that fills and widens the papillary dermis and broadly abuts the reticular dermis. Level III invasion is usually a manifestation of the vertical growth phase. Level IV invasion should be designated only when tumor cells clearly permeate between otherwise unaltered collagen bundles of the reticular dermis.

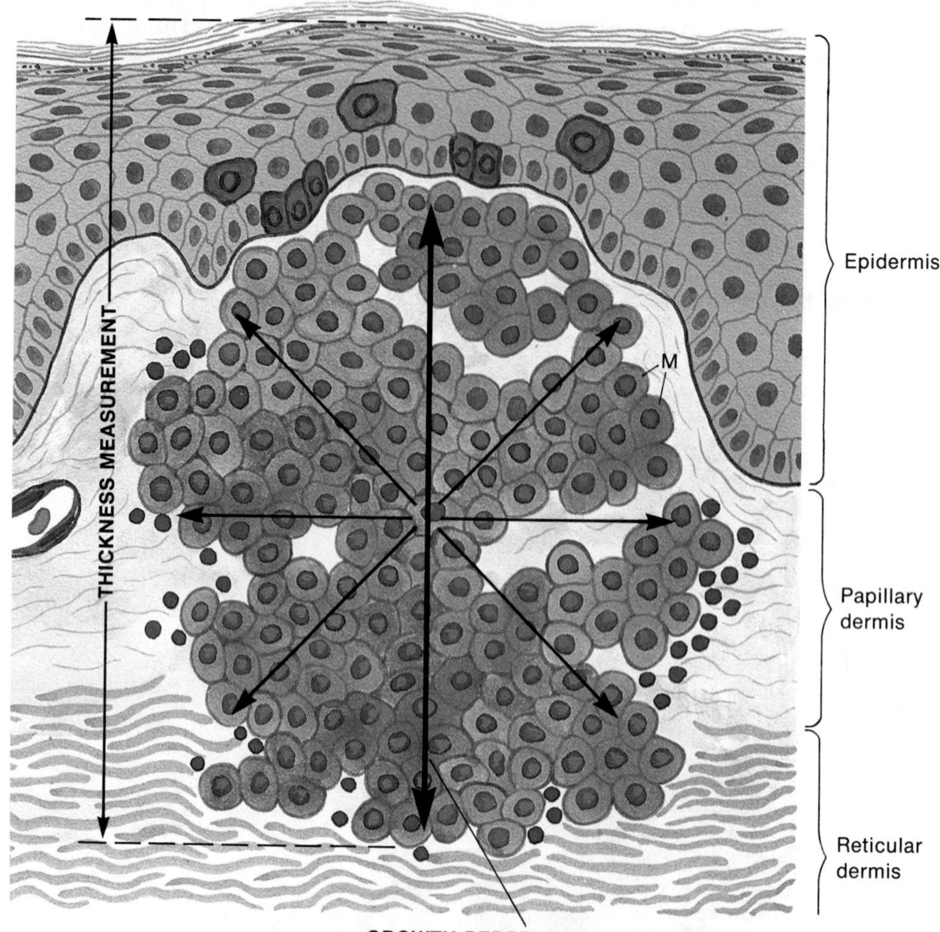

FIGURE *24-56*
Schematic depiction of the evolved vertical growth phase in malignant melanoma of the superficial spreading type, with an indication of how thickness is measured. In this illustration, the vertical growth phase has extended into the reticular dermis. However, small nodules of tumor cells that clearly have a growth preference over other tumor cells may be a manifestation of the vertical growth phase. Thickness measurements (*arrows*) are taken from the outermost granular layer across the tumor in its thickest part.

Even when tumors have entered the vertical growth phase, properties required for metastasis may still be lacking. Some tumors have little competence for metastasis, whereas others have a greater potential. For example, vertical growth phase melanomas that are more than 1.7 mm in thickness, have no evident mitoses, and exhibit a brisk infiltrate of lymphocytes rarely metastasize.

Vertical growth phase melanomas that are more than 3.6 mm thick, display more than 6 mitoses/mm^2, and do not contain tumor-infiltrating lymphocytes usually metastasize. The measurement of tumor thickness of the vertical growth phase tumors is made from the outermost layer of the stratum granulosum to the deepest part of the tumor (see Figs. 24-55 and 24-56).

Metastatic Melanoma

Metastatic melanoma arises from the melanocytes of the vertical growth phase. Initial metastases usually involve the regional lymph nodes, although spread through the blood stream is also common. When blood stream metastases do occur, they are unusually widespread in comparison with other neoplasms; virtually every organ system may be involved.

Nodular Melanoma

Even though a cancer generally acquires its properties in a stepwise fashion, occasional tumors arise with all of their malignant characteristics expressed in the initial lesion. Nodular malignant melanoma is such a tumor. This lesion, which is fortunately the rarest form of melanoma, appears as circumscribed, elevated nodule. It tends to be spheroidal initially, that is, it does not develop through a radial growth phase (Fig. 24-57). Histologically, nodular melanoma is composed of one or more nodules of cells that clearly grow in an expansile fashion in the dermis (Figs. 24-58 and 24-59). In other

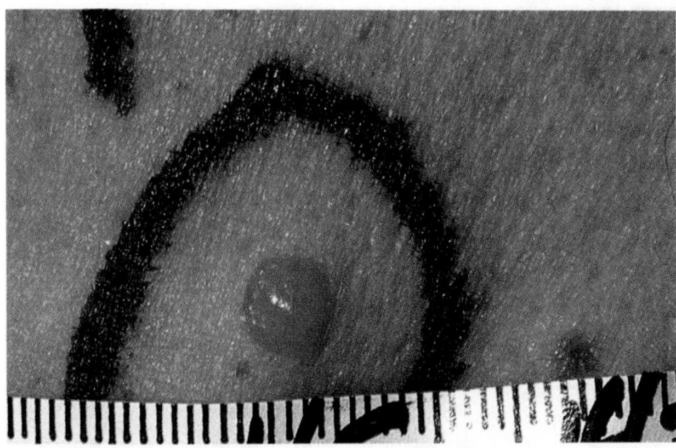

FIGURE 24-57
In malignant melanoma of the nodular type, the primary focus of growth of this 0.5-cm lesion is in the dermis.

words, the tumor is in the vertical growth phase when initially observed.

Lentigo Maligna Melanoma

Lentigo maligna melanoma, also known as ***Hutchinson's freckle,*** *is a large pigmented macule that occurs on sun damaged skin.* This lesion develops almost exclusively in fair, usually elderly, whites. It occurs on the exposed surfaces of the body and, similar to other forms of melanoma, is probably related to ultraviolet light exposure. In its radial growth phase, lentigo maligna is a flat, irregular, brown to black patch, which may cover a large part of the face or back of the hand (Fig. 24-60). The cells of the radial growth phase are predominantly in the basal layer, occasionally forming small nests that "hang-down" into the papillary dermis (Fig. 24-61). Invasion is not as prominent or as extensive in the radial growth phase of lentigo maligna melanoma as it is in superficial spreading melanoma. Cells of the radial growth phase, especially those disposed in nests, are of variable size. The subjacent dermis shows a modest lymphocytic infiltrate, and almost invariably, advanced solar degeneration of the connective tissue.

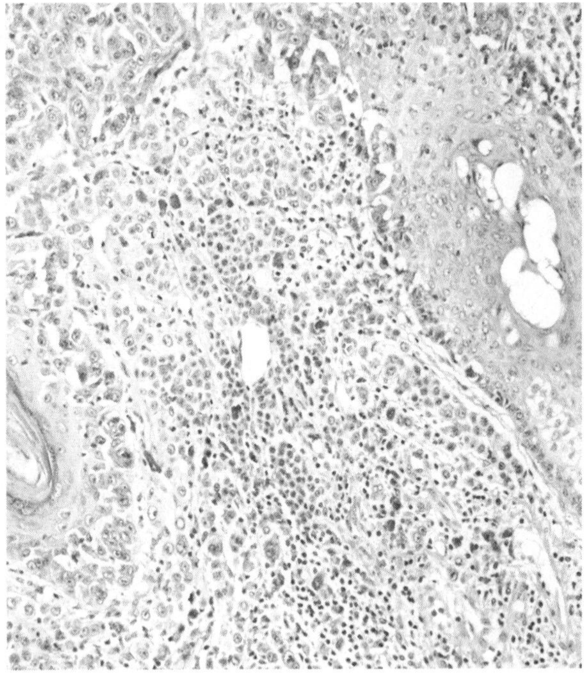

FIGURE 24-59
Malignant melanoma, vertical growth phase. The host response consists of lymphocytes infiltrating amidst the melanocytes (tumor-infiltrating lymphocytes).

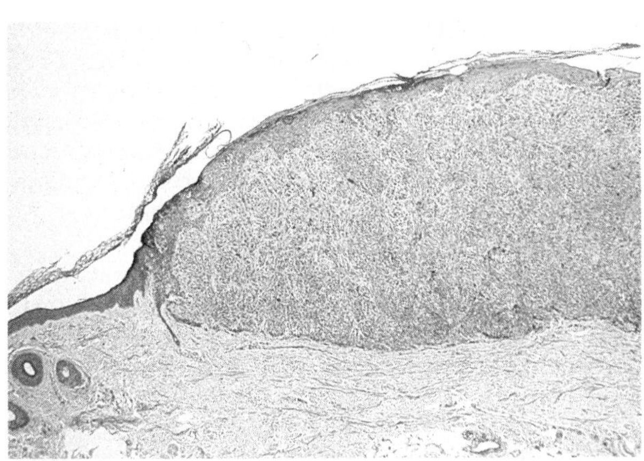

FIGURE 24-58
Malignant melanoma, nodular type. Intraepidermal growth is essentially absent. There is no radial growth lateral to the nodule. This tumor expands the papillary dermis and distorts the reticular dermal junction; it is therefore level III.

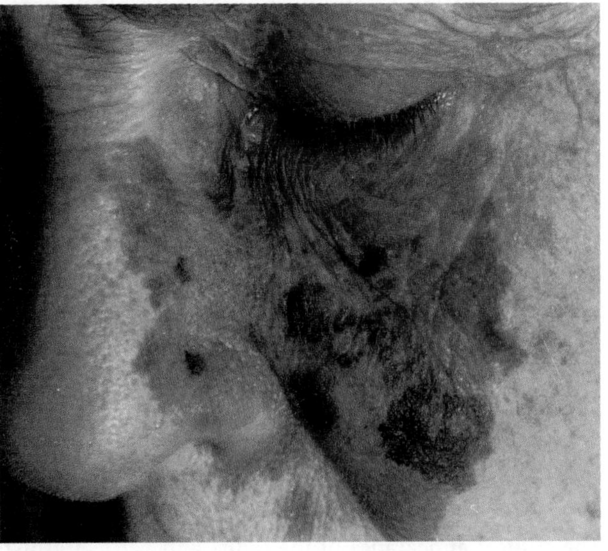

FIGURE 24-60
The radial growth phase in malignant melanoma of the lentigo maligna type.

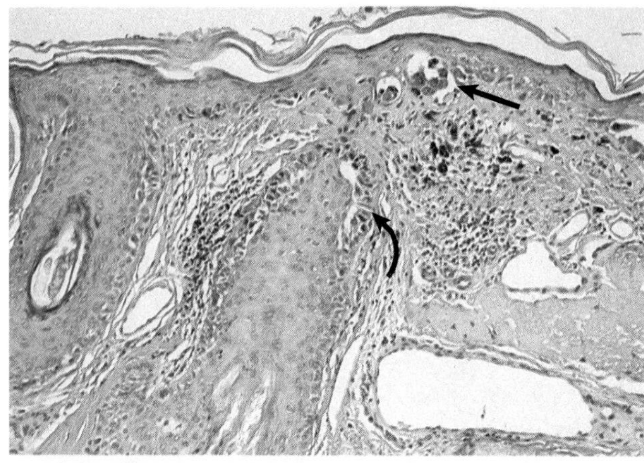

FIGURE *24-61*
Lentigo maligna. Atypical melanocytes grow largely at the dermal-epidermal interface (*straight arrow*), with extension down the external root sheath of follicles (*curved arrow*). Upward growth of melanocytes is much less prominent than in intraepidermal malignant melanoma of the superficial spreading type.

In the vertical growth phase (Fig. 24-62), the cells tend to be spindle-shaped. Occasionally, the cells of this phase provoke a connective tissue response to form a firm plaque (desmoplastic melanoma). Cells of the vertical growth phase may also grow along small nerves (neurotropic vertical growth phase).

Acral Lentiginous Melanoma

Acral lentiginous melanoma is the most common form of melanoma in dark-skinned people and is essentially limited to the palms, soles and subungual regions. Although rare, a similar tumor occurs, on the mucous membranes, and is termed *mucosal lentiginous melanoma.*

In the radial growth phase, acral lentiginous melanoma forms an irregular, brown to black patch, which covers a large part of the palm or sole, or arises under a nail, usually the large toe or thumb (Fig. 24-63). Microscopically, the cells are, for the most part, confined to the basal layer of the epidermis and maintain long dendrites (Figs. 24-64 and 24-65). Frequently, a brisk lichenoid lymphocytic response is present. As the vertical growth phase develops, cells may grow upward in the epidermis and be more epithelioid. The vertical growth phase (Fig. 24-66) is similar to that of lentigo maligna melanoma, commonly consisting of spindle cells (Fig. 24-67). Neurotropism is also occasionally seen.

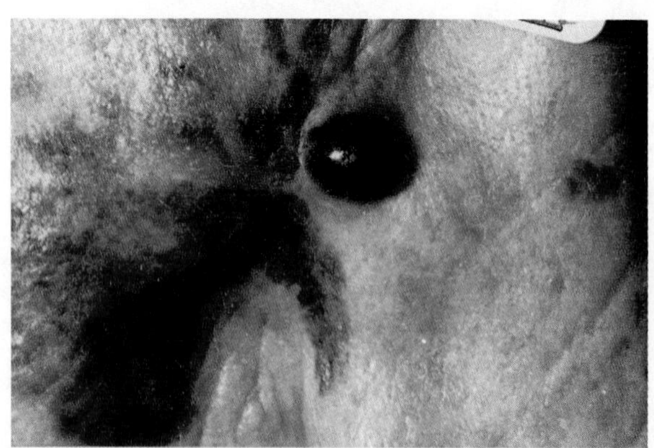

FIGURE *24-62*
The clinical appearance of the radial and vertical growth phase in malignant melanoma of the lentigo maligna type. The lesion is 1 cm in diameter.

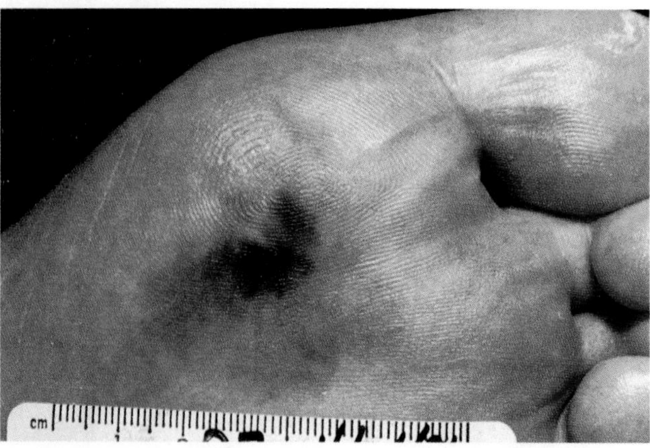

FIGURE *24-63*
Clinical appearance of the sole of the foot in a patient with malignant melanoma of the acral lentiginous type (radial growth phase).

Prognostic Features in Malignant Melanoma

Clinical changes in the appearance of new moles that warrant a biopsy to rule out melanoma are described by the ABCD rule: ***A***symmetry of shape, ***B***order irregularity, ***C***olor variation, and a ***D***iameter more than 6 mm. The prognosis of patients whose tumor has entered the vertical growth phase is based upon a number of different attributes.

MITOTIC RATE: The number of mitoses is an independent predictor of outcome for as long as 8 years after removal of the primary melanoma and, except for the growth phase of the primary tumor, is the most powerful prognostic feature. Patients whose tumors show no mitoses have a 12-fold greater chance of survival than those in whom the mitotic rate is greater than 6/mm^2.

LYMPHOCYTIC RESPONSE: The interaction of lymphocytes and tumor cells in the vertical growth phase is an important prognostic indicator. The cellular response is reported to be *infiltrative* when the lymphocytes actually infiltrate and disrupt the tumor, frequently forming rosettes about tumor cells (Fig. 24-68). If tumor-infiltrating lymphocytes are present throughout the vertical growth phase, or are seen across the entire base of the vertical growth phase, the infiltrate is said to be *brisk.* Patients whose tumors exhibit a brisk infiltrate have a survival probability 11 times greater than that of patients whose melanoma lacks tumor-infiltrating lymphocytes.

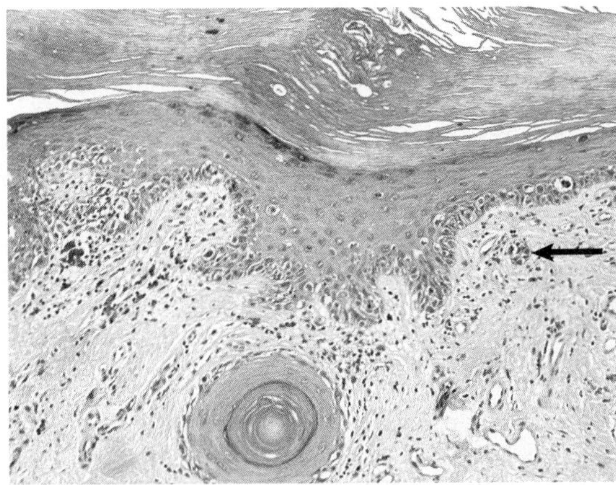

FIGURE 24-64
Malignant melanoma, acral lentiginous type, principally intraepidermal radial growth. Atypical melanocytes are present along the dermal-epidermal junction, with focal upward growth. A small dermal nest of atypical melanocytes is present (*arrow*).

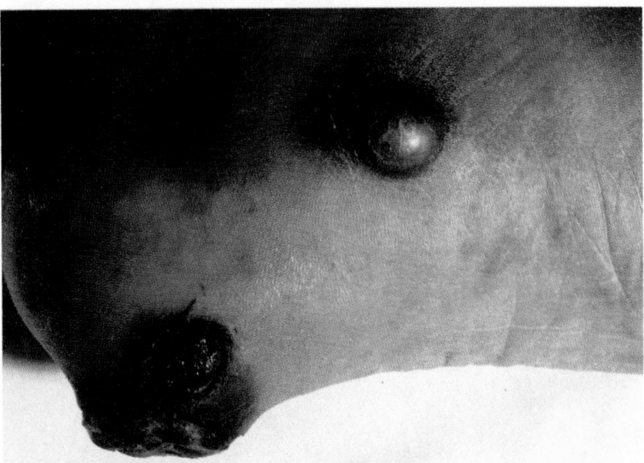

FIGURE 24-66
Clinical presentation of malignant melanoma of the acral lentiginous type (radial and vertical growth phases). The lesion on the heel is the primary tumor. The flat portion represents the radial growth phase, whereas the elevated portion is indicative of the vertical growth phase. The dark module on the instep is a metastasis.

TUMOR THICKNESS: The thickness of a melanoma is measured from the outermost layer of the stratum granulosum to the deepest penetration of the tumor in the dermis (see Fig. 24-55). In practice, the thickness is usually recorded, and it may be the only attribute used to determine outcome. In this circumstance, the outcome may be predicted with some accuracy by dividing the tumors into four thickness groups without regard to the growth phase of the tumor. The prognosis up to 8 years after removal of the primary lesion may then be estimated from Table 24-4.

LOCATION: Melanomas on the extremities have a better prognosis than those on the head, neck, or trunk (axial). However, melanomas on the sole of the foot or the subungual region have a prognosis similar to or worse than axial lesions.

SEX: For every site and thickness, women have a better prognosis than men. For example, women with axial melanomas that are 0.8 to 1.7 mm thick have a survival rate of almost 90% 10 years after excision of the lesion, whereas in men the comparable figure is only 60%.

REGRESSION: Many primary melanomas show some evidence of spontaneous regression, indicated clinically by a change to a blue-white or white color. Microscopically, such regression is characterized by a widened papillary dermis, with melanophages and a lymphocytic

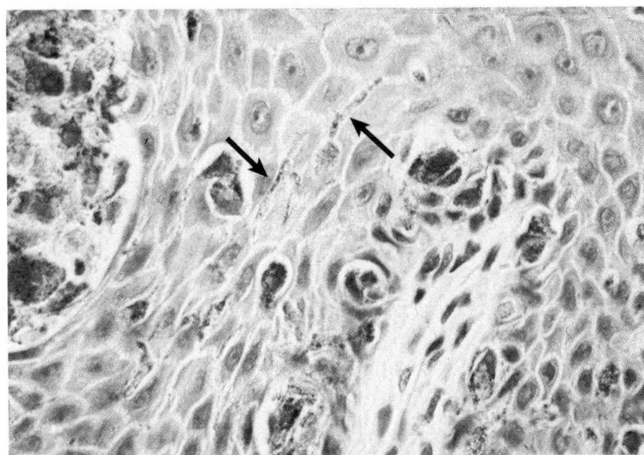

FIGURE 24-65
Malignant melanoma, acral lentiginous type. Large melanocytes with prominent dendrites (*arrows*) are present in the basilar region of the epidermis, with upward growth. The tumor cells contain numerous melanosomes, making the perinuclear and dendritic cytoplasms brown.

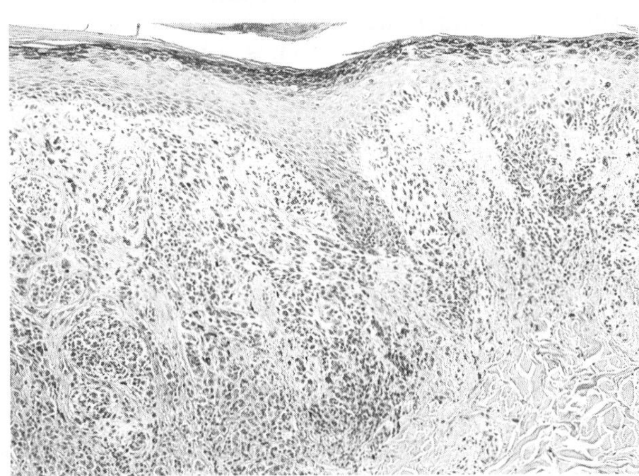

FIGURE 24-67
Malignant melanoma, acral lentiginous type, vertical growth phase. On the *left* is confluent growth of atypical dermal melanocytes filling and expanding the papillary dermis.

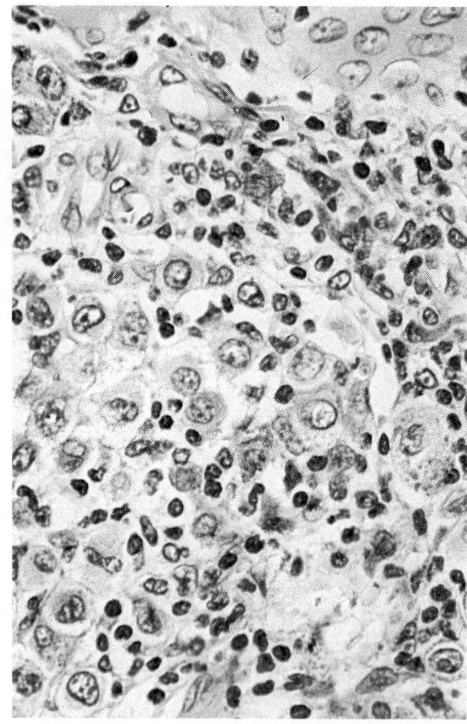

FIGURE *24-68*
A host response is apparent in the vertical growth phase of this malignant melanoma. Numerous tumor-infiltrating lymphocytes are arranged about individual tumor cells as satellites within the center of the field.

infiltrate. Patients whose tumors show such changes have a somewhat poorer prognosis than those in whom regression in absent.

LEVELS OF INVASION: The level of tumor invasion refers to the degree of tumor penetration within the anatomical layers of the skin. It is a predictor of the likelihood of metastasis, although it is not as accurate as tumor thickness. Although levels of invasion are not independent predictors of outcome, level IV invasion may predict lymph node metastases and may provide additional prognostic information for tumors greater than 1.7 mm.

TABLE *24-4* **Tumor Thickness as Sole Predictor of Outcome 8 Years After Definitive Therapy of Primary Melanoma**

Thickness (mm)	Survival (%)
<0.76	93
0.76–1.69	86
1.70–3.60	60
>3.60	33

- **Level I**: Tumor cells are situated entirely above the basement membrane (*in situ*).
- **Level II**: Invasive cells are present only in the papillary dermis (radial growth phase).
- **Level III**: The tumor has entered the vertical growth phase and impinges on the reticular dermis, forming small expansile nodules that widen the papillary dermis.
- **Level IV:** Tumor cells clearly invade between the collagen bundles of the reticular dermis.
- **Level V:** The tumor extends into the subcutaneous fat.

In excising a melanoma that is in the radial growth phase, it is common practice to include a margin of normal skin 8 to 10 mm around the lesion. Tumors in the vertical growth phase require excisions that have a radius of 2.5 cm around the lesion. Even though 8-year disease-free survival is commonly used as the baseline for prognosis in melanoma, recurrences up to 20 years are well known.

Other Benign Tumors of Melanocytic Origin

CONGENITAL MELANOCYTIC NEVI: About 1% of white children are born with some form of pigmented lesions on their skin, sometimes as inconspicuous as a small patch of pale tan hyperpigmentation. Rarely, the trunk or an extremity is covered by a large pigmented patch or plaque, which is cosmetically deforming. Such areas have a striking increase in intraepidermal and dermal melanocytes, which extends deeply into the subcutaneous tissue. Malignant melanoma may develop in these large congenital melanocytic nevi. Some physicians attempt to remove these large lesions, but in many instances their size makes surgical removal problematic.

SPITZ TUMOR (EPITHELIOID CELL NEVUS): Spitz tumors occur in children and, with somewhat less frequency, in adults. The Spitz tumor presents as an elevated, spheroid, pink, smooth nodule and grows rapidly, increasing to a diameter of 3 to 5 mm within 6 months. The lesion is composed of large epithelioid melanocytes that extend into the epidermis and into the dermis (Fig. 24-69). The cells are so atypical that a false diagnosis of melanoma may be made, although melanoma is exquisitely rare in childhood.

Benign Keratinocytic Neoplasms Related to Human Papillomavirus

Verrrucae or warts are benign cutaneous tumors induced by human papillomavirus (HPV). The lesions are circumscribed, symmetrical, epidermal neoplasms that are elevated above the skin and often appear papillary. Several clinicopathological entities exist under the general category of warts.

VERRUCA VULGARIS: Also known as common warts, these lesions are elevated papules with a verrucous (papillomatous) surface. They may be single or multiple and are most frequent on the dorsum of the hands or on the face. Histologically, verruca vulgaris is characterized by hyperkeratosis and papillary epidermal hyperplasia

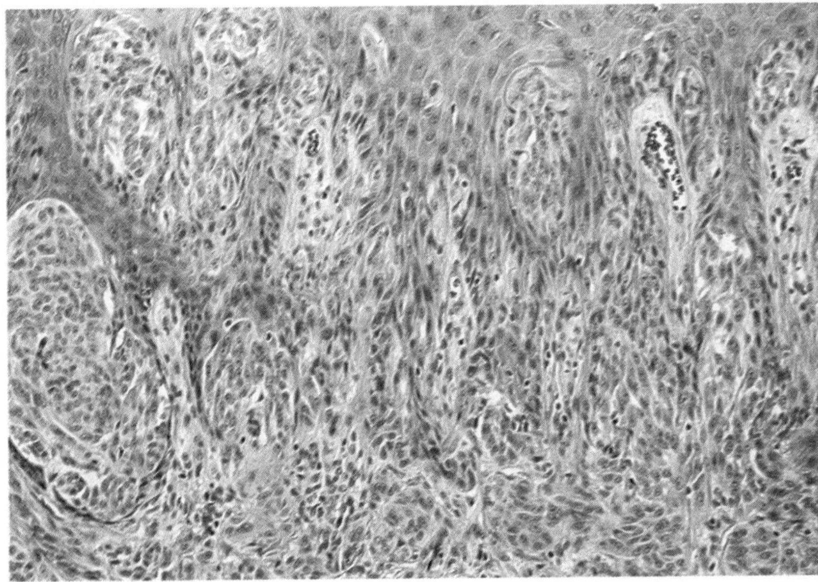

A

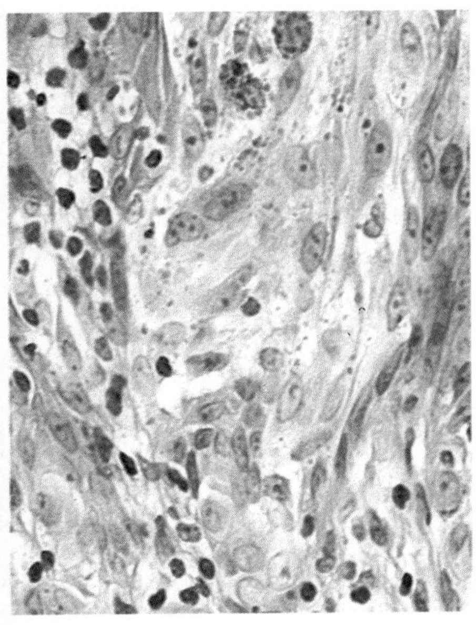

B

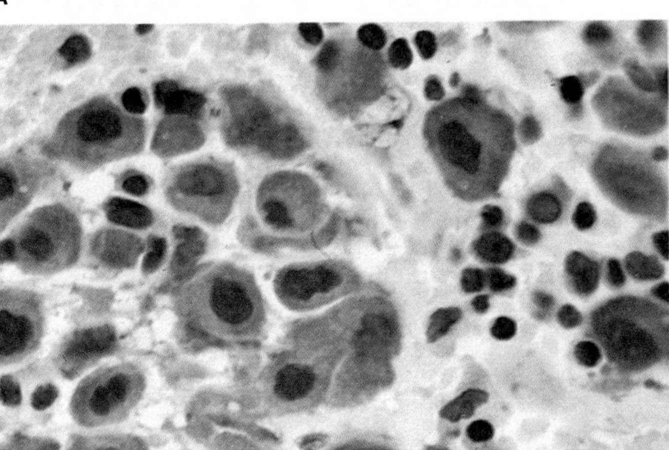

C

FIGURE *24-69*
Epithelioid cell nevus. (*A*) Spitz tumors are composed of large melanocytes with prominent nuclei. Within a hyperplastic epidermis, the melanocytes are disposed in large nests. Even though the cells are large and, at first glance, suggestive of melanoma, they are much more uniform than the cells of most malignant melanomas. (*B*) The melanocytes have amphophilic cytoplasms and prominent regular nucleoli. (*C*) Most melanocytic tumors, including Spitz tumors, are composed of cells that possess S100 antigen, as shown by the brown reaction product in them after immunohistochemical study. S100 antigen is found in high concentration in most tumors that are of neural crest origin.

(Fig. 24-70). Koilocytes (enlarged keratinocytes with a pyknotic nucleus surrounded by a halo), are observed within the upper epidermis, particularly on the sides of papillae. Viral inclusions are difficult to identify (Fig. 24-71). Several different HPV serotypes, including types 2 and 4, have been demonstrated in verrucae vulgaris.

PLANTAR WARTS: The lesions on the soles are hyperkeratotic nodules that are similar to a callus. They are frequently painful and difficult to eradicate. On occasion, similar lesions appear on the palms (*palmar wart*). Histologically, plantar warts are endophytic or exophytic, papillary, squamous, epithelial proliferations. The cells contain abundant cytoplasmic inclusions, which are similar to keratohyalin granules. The nuclei of keratinocytes near the base of these warts also contain bright pink nuclear inclusions. HPV serotype 1 is the etiological agent.

VERRUCA PLANA: These small flat papules appear on the face and are induced primarily by HPV-3. Microscopically, slight acanthosis, often with striking hypergranulosis and superficial koilocyte formation, are present.

CONDYLOMA ACCUMINATUM: These warts occur primarily about the genitalia and are associated with sexually transmitted infection by HPV type 6 and, less commonly, type 11. Histologically, they consist of a papillary squamous proliferation. Koilocytosis and an almost continuous cap of parakeratotic cells are usually present. Squamous carcinoma may develop in the lesions, in which case HPV-16 or HPV-18 is usually identified (also see Chapter 18).

BOWENOID PAPULOSIS: The disorder, also caused by HPV-16 and HPV-18, is characterized by multiple hyperpigmented papules on the genitalia. The lesions exhibit parakeratosis and irregular acanthosis, with scattered atypical keratinocytes. In some instances, the lesions are histologically identical with squamous carcinoma *in situ*. Characteristically, bowenoid papulosis regresses.

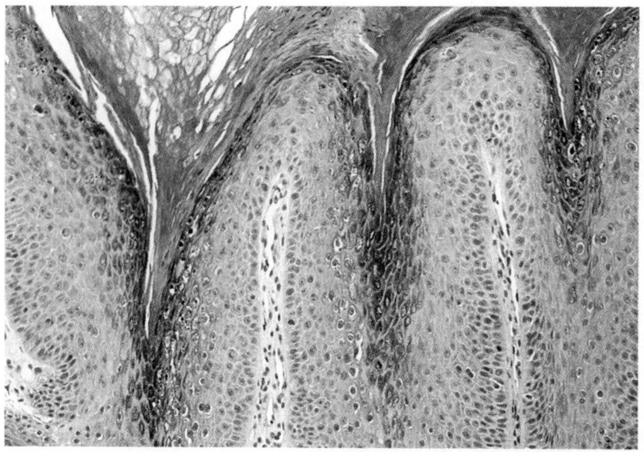

FIGURE 24-70
Verruca vulgaris. Verruca vulgaris is the prototype of papillary epidermal hyperplasia. Squamous epithelial-lined fronds have fibrovascular cores. The blood vessels within the cores extend close to the surface of verrucae, which makes them susceptible to traumatic hemorrhage and the resultant black "seeds" that patients observe.

EPIDERMODYSPLASIA VERRUCIFORMIS: This rare autosomal recessive disease is characterized by impaired cell-mediated immunity and enhanced susceptibility to HPV infection. Warts similar to those of verruca plana, with confluence into patches, are widespread. Epidermodysplasia verruciformis is first apparent in childhood, and in one third of the patients the warts progress to squamous carcinoma. HPV-5 in the most commonly encountered virus, but others, including types 3, 8, 9, and 10, have been observed. However, only HPV-5 and HPV-8 have been identified in the cancers.

Benign Keratoses

Keratosis refers to any horny growth or callosity composed of a benign, localized, proliferation of keratinocytes.

Seborrheic Keratosis

Seborrheic keratoses are scaly, frequently pigmented, elevated papules or plaques, the scales of which are easily rubbed off. Although they are among the most common keratoses, the etiology is unknown. The lesions generally present in the later years of life and tend to be familial. Microscopically, seborrheic keratoses appear tacked onto the skin and are composed of broad anastomosing cords of mature stratified squamous epithelium, associated with small cysts of keratin (horn cysts). Although the lesions are innocuous, they are a cosmetic nuisance.

Actinic Keratosis

Actinic keratosis ("from the sun's rays") is a keratinocytic neoplasm that develops in sun-damaged skin as a circumscribed keratotic patch or plaque, commonly on the backs of the hands or the face. Microscopically, the stratum corneum is no longer loose and basket-weaved, but is replaced by a dense parakeratotic scale. The underlying basal keratinocytes display significant atypia (Fig. 24-72). **With the passage of time, actinic keratosis may evolve into squamous cell carcinoma *in situ*, and finally into invasive squamous cell carcinoma.**

Keratoacanthoma

Keratoacanthomas are rapidly growing keratotic papules on sun-exposed skin that develop over a period of 3 to 6 weeks into centrally umbilicated, " volcano-like," nodules. They reach a

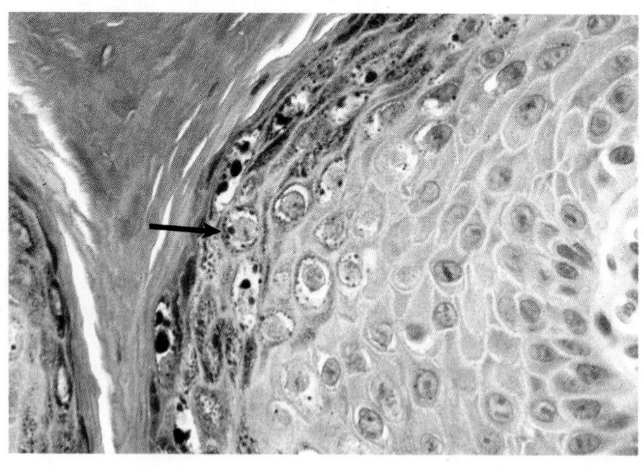

A

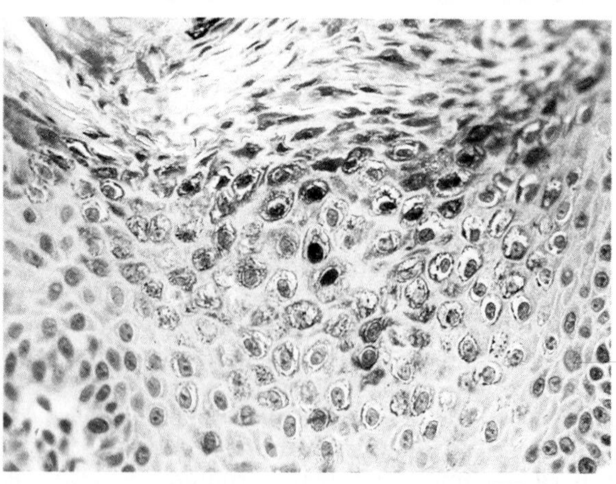

B

FIGURE 24-71
Verruca vulgaris. (*A*) Characteristic cytopathic changes occur in the outer portion of the stratum spinosum and stratum granulosum, in which there is perinuclear vacuolization and prominent keratohyaline granules, with homogeneous blue inclusions (*arrow*). (*B*) Papilloma virus surface antigen is demonstrated in an immunohistochemical preparation as brown intranuclear reaction product.

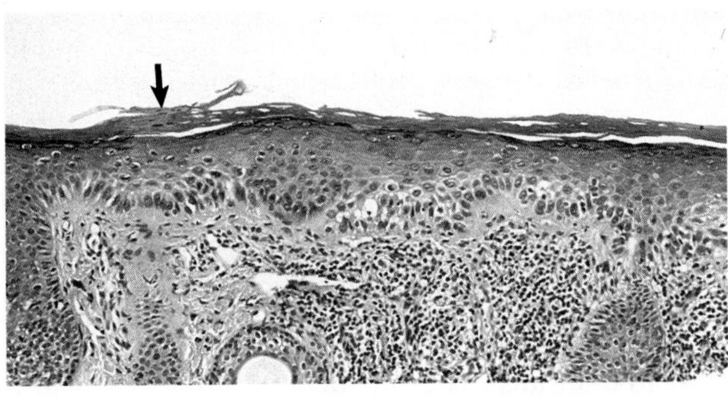

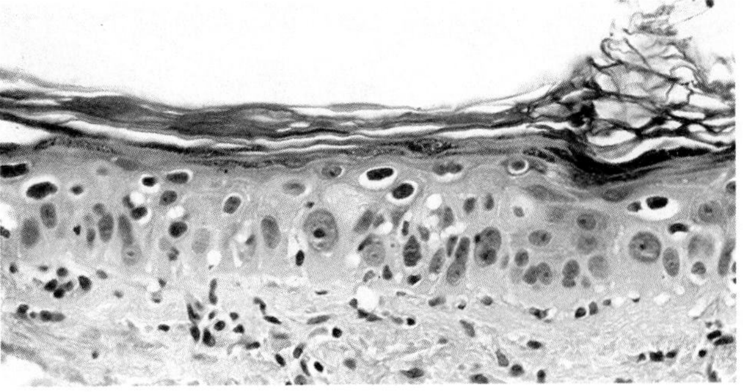

A B

FIGURE 24-72
Actinic keratosis. (*A*) A low-power view reveals cytological atypia within the stratum basalis and lower stratum spinosum, with loss of polarity. A lichenoid, bandlike, lymphocytic infiltrate is frequently present. Parakeratosis is present here only in a small focus (*arrow*). (*B*) High-power examination of an actinic keratosis reveals striking cytological atypia of the basal keratinocytes, the hallmark of actinic keratosis.

maximum diameter of 2 to 3 cm (some rare variants may measure up to 20 cm). Spontaneous regression usually ensues within 6 to 12 months, leaving an atrophic scar. At this time, keratocanthoma is best considered a variant of squamous cell carcinoma, which heals by itself or which heals spontaneously in the vast majority of patients.

☐ **Pathology:** Histologically, keratoacanthoma is an endophytic papillary proliferation of keratinocytes. The lesion is cup-shaped, with a central, keratin-filled umbilication and overhanging edges (Fig. 24-73). At the base of the keratin, the keratinocytes are large, with an abundance of homogeneous, eosinophilic ("glassy") cytoplasm. At the lower aspect of the lesion, irregular tongues of squamous epithelium infiltrate the collagen of the reticular dermis. Older lesions show active fibroplasia in the dermis around the epithelial tongues. There may be focal lichenoid inflammation, and the dermis may also be markedly infiltrated with neutrophils, lymphocytes, and eosinophils. Microabscesses of neutrophils and entrapped dermal elastic fibers may be apparent within the keratoacanthoma.

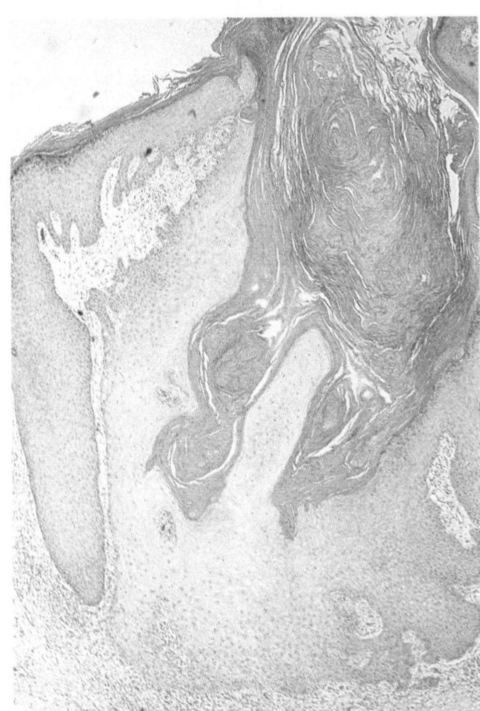

FIGURE 24-73
Keratoacanthoma. A keratin-filled crater (*right*) is lined by glassy proliferating keratinocytes that invade the dermis.

Basal Cell Carcinoma

Basal cell carcinoma (BCC) is a locally invasive epidermal neoplasm that derives its name from the histological similarity of the tumor cells to basal keratinocytes. **BCC is the most common malignant tumor in persons with pale skin**. Although the tumor may be locally aggressive, metastases are exquisitely rare.

☐ **Pathogenesis:** BCC usually develops on the sun-damaged skin of people with fair skin and freckles. However, unlike squamous cell carcinoma (see later), BCC also arises on areas not exposed to intense sunlight, but is unusual on the fingers and dorsum of the hands. BCC is also a component of a number of heritable syndromes in which the tumor originates on skin that has had little light exposure. It is thought that the tumor derives from pluripotential cells in the basal layer of the epidermis. Indeed, BCCs tend to differentiate along skin appendage lines.

☐ **Pathology:** BCCs feature prominent epithelial and mesenchymal components. Superficial BCCs are composed of multiple nests of deeply basophilic epithelial cells that are attached to the epidermis and protrude into the subjacent papillary dermis (Fig. 24-74). The central part of the nests is composed of closely-packed ker-

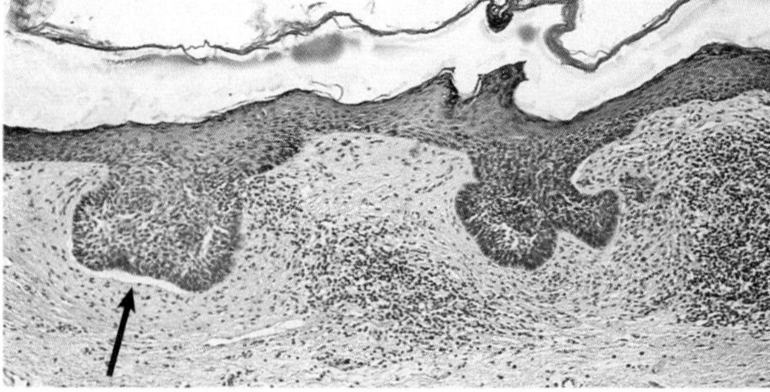

FIGURE 24-74
Basal cell carcinoma, superficial type. Buds of atypical basaloid keratinocytes extend from the overlying epidermis into the papillary dermis. The peripheral keratinocytes mimic the stratum basalis by palisading. The separation artifact (*arrow*) is present because of poorly formed basement membrane components and the hyaluronic acid-rich stroma that contains collagenase.

atinocytes, which are slightly smaller than the normal epidermal basal keratinocytes. The nuclei are deeply basophilic and are surrounded by a small rim of cytoplasm. The periphery of the nests is composed of an organized layer of polarized, columnar keratinocytes, with the long axis of each cell perpendicular to the surrounding basement membrane zone. A partially formed basement membrane zone separates the epithelial component from the mesenchymal one. The tumor parenchyma is surrounded by a whorled array of fibroblasts. Morphea-like BCCs have a dense, sclerotic stroma (Fig. 24-75).

☐ **Clinical Features:** BCC occurs in a number of common forms.

- **Pearly papule,** the prototypic lesion, resembles a 2- to 3-mm pearl. It is covered by tightly stretched epidermis and is laced with small, delicate, branching vessels (telangiectasia).
- **Rodent ulcer** is a small crater in the center of the pearl.
- **Superficial BCC** (see Fig. 24-74) appears as a scaly, red, sharply demarcated, plaque.
- **Morphea-like BCC** (see Fig. 24-75) is an ill-defined, pale, firm, scar-like tumor, which is particularly difficult to eradicate locally.
- **Pigmented BCC** grossly resembles malignant melanoma of the superficial spreading or nodular type.

Nevoid BCC syndrome *refers to the occurrence of multiple tumors in the context of a complex multisystem disease.* In addition to BCCs, the syndrome includes pits (dyskeratoses) on the palms and soles, mandibular cysts, hypertelorism, and a predisposition to other neoplasms, including medulloblastoma. The BCCs of the syndrome appear at a young age and may number over 100. The tumors involve both exposed and nonexposed cutaneous surfaces.

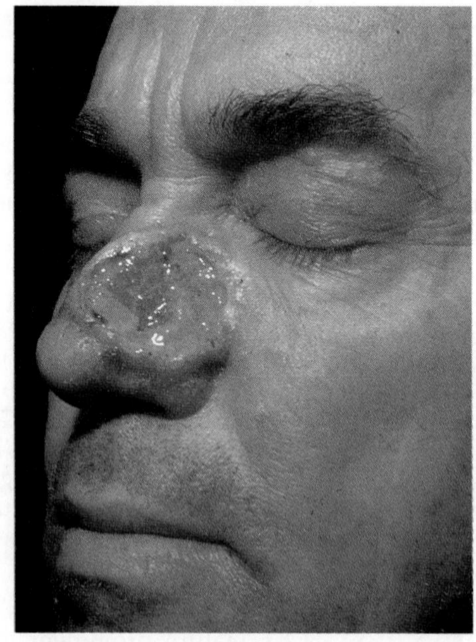

A

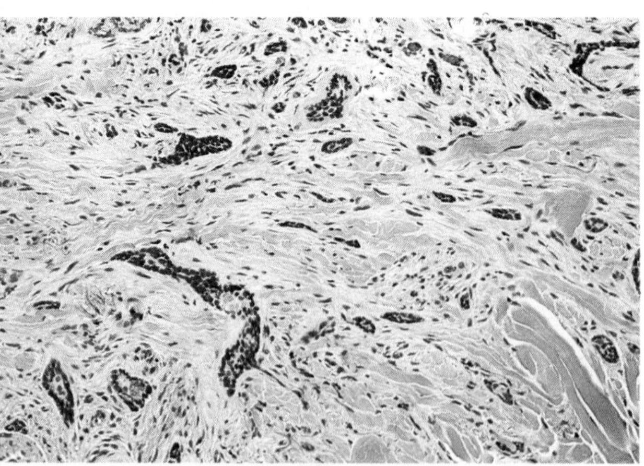

B

FIGURE 24-75
Basal cell carcinoma. (*A*) A neglected basal cell carcinoma of the skin overlying the nose has ulcerated and invaded the deeper tissues. (*B*) Microscopic examination shows a sclerosing and infiltrative lesion. Irregularly branching strands of tumor cells permeate the dermis, with induction of a cellular, fibroblastic, hyaluronic acid-rich stroma.

Squamous Cell Carinoma

Squamous cell carcinoma (SCC) is a cancer of the epidermis whose cells typically resemble differentiated keratinocytes. SCC is second only to basal cell carcinoma in incidence and may be caused by ultraviolet light, ionizing radiation, chemical carcinogens, and HPV. SCC is most common on the sun-damaged skin of fair persons with light hair and freckles and often originates in an actinic keratosis. The tumor is distinctly rare on normal black skin. SCC arising in sun-damaged skin has a low propensity to metastasize (less than 2%).

☐ **Pathogenesis:** Although SCC has multiple causes, by far the most common form is related to ultraviolet light. SCC may develop in association with chronic scarring processes, such as tracts of osteomyelitis and old burn scars. In this setting, the cancer has a greater propensity for metastases than does solar-related SCC.

☐ **Pathology:** SCC is composed of tumor cells that tend to mimic the epidermal stratum spinosum and extend into the subjacent dermis (Fig 24-76). The edge of most SCCs shows a precursor actinic keratosis, in which the epidermis is variably thickened and parakeratotic, with significant atypia of the basal keratinocytes.

☐ **Clinical Features:** SCC characteristically arises on the backs of the hands or the face, but they are also common on the lips and ears, the latter sites associated

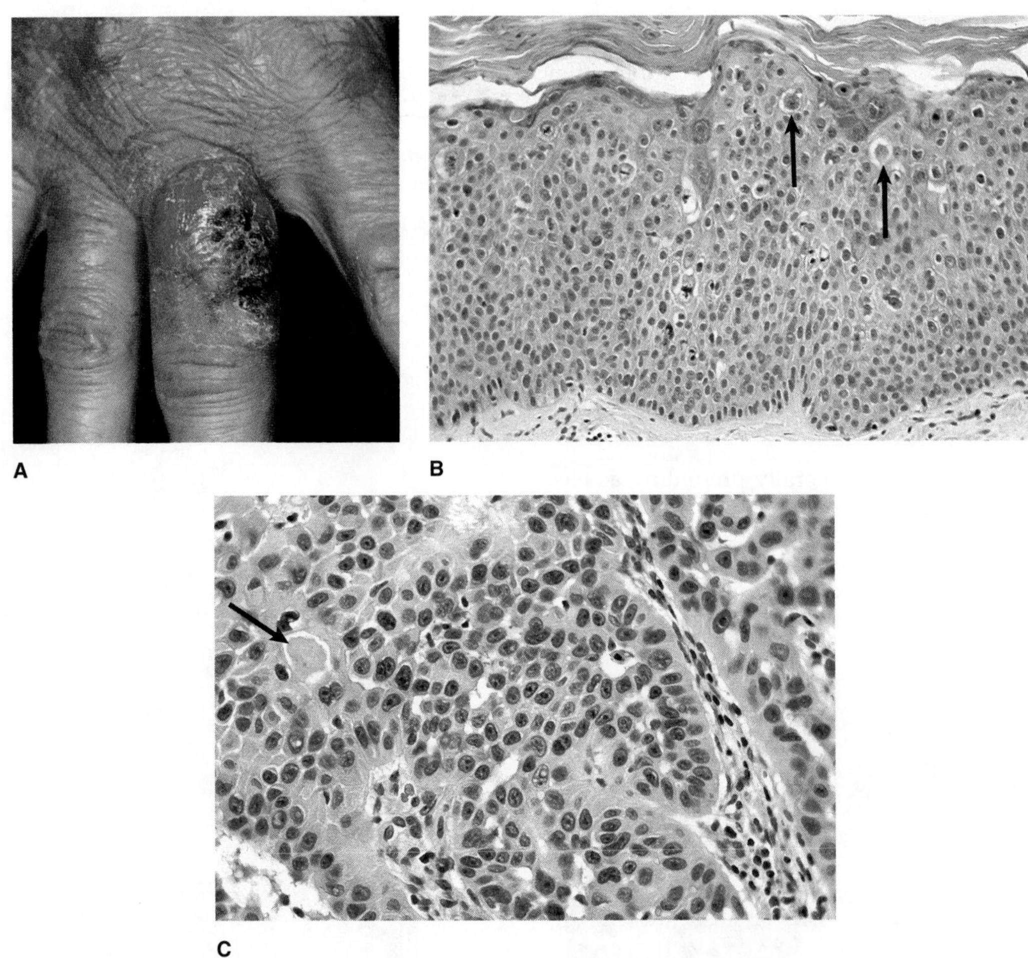

FIGURE *24-76*
Squamous cell carcinoma. (*A*) An ulcerated, encrusted, and infiltrating lesion is seen on the sun-exposed dorsal of a finger. (*B*) A microscopic view of the periphery of the lesion shows squamous cell carcinoma *in situ*. The entire epidermis is replaced by atypical keratinocytes. Mitoses and multinucleation of keratinocytes are apparent, as is apoptosis (*arrows*). (*C*) Squamous cell carcinoma, invasive component. High-power view reveals irregularly shaped lobules of strikingly atypical keratinocytes that have invaded to the level of the mid-reticular dermis. Apoptotic cells are present (*arrow*). The pink, plate-like cytoplasm, as well as intercellular bridges (desmosomes), are helpful diagnostic features in excluding other malignancies.

with more aggressive tumors. Early lesions are small, scaly or ulcerated, erythematous papules, which may by pruritic. Small SCCs may be treated by electrosurgery, chemosurgery, or excision, whereas larger lesions require excision or radiation therapy.

Merkel Cell Carcinoma

Merkel cell carcinoma (MCC) is an aggressive malignant tumor that arises from the neurosecretory cutaneous Merkel cell tumors and also display features of epithelial differentiation. The tumor typically is a solitary, dome-shaped, red to violaceous nodule or indurated plaque. MCC typically arises on the skin of the head and neck in elderly Caucasians. These tumors are dangerous, leading to death in one third of the patients.

☐ **Pathology:** Most MCCs consist of large solid nests of undifferentiated cells (Fig. 24-77), which resemble small cell carcinoma of the lung. At its periphery, the tumor may manifest a trabecular pattern. The nuclear chromatin pattern is dense and uniformly distributed, and the cytoplasm is scant. Frequent mitotic figures and nuclear fragmentation are observed. Immunohistochemical staining for cytokeratin 20 shows a characteristic "punctate globoid" cytoplasmic zone of immunoreactivity. MCC also stains for neuron-specific enolase and chromogranin.

Tumors of the Skin Appendages (Adenexal Tumors)

Several tumors of the skin, generally presenting as elevated, small nodules, differentiate toward the various skin appendages, including hair follicles and sebaceous, apocrine, or eccrine sweat glands. Many patients have a familial history of similar tumors. Frequently, the lesions appear at puberty. Although most of these tumors are benign, a few carcinomas arise is skin appendages (or differentiate in that direction).

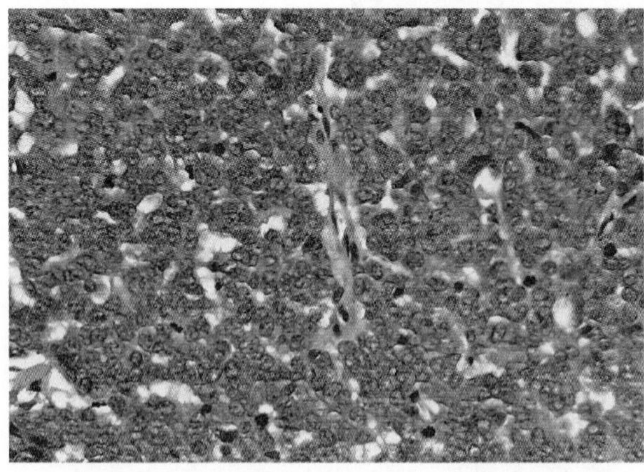

FIGURE *24-77*
Merkel cell carcinoma. The individual tumor cells are small with a dense basophilic nucleus and scant cytoplasm. Note the high mitotic index and numerous pyknotic nuclei.

Cylindroma

Cylindroma is a benign skin appendage tumor in which the cells differentiate into sweat gland structures. The tumor presents as a solitary lesion or as multiple elevated nodules about the scalp. An autosomal dominant, heritable variant features multiple tumors. Occasionally, cylindromas become large and cover the head as a cluster, in which case they are termed *turban tumors*. Microscopic examination reveals sharply circumscribed nests of deeply basophilic cells (Fig. 24-78). These cells are associated with hyalinized, thickened, basement membrane zones, which form a ring about the nests, accounting for the name of the tumor.

Syringoma

Syringoma is a benign sweat gland tumor that typically appears about the eyelid and upper cheek as an elevated small, flesh-colored papule. Microscopically, small ducts resembling the intraepidermal portion of the eccrine sweat ducts are observed (Fig. 24-79).

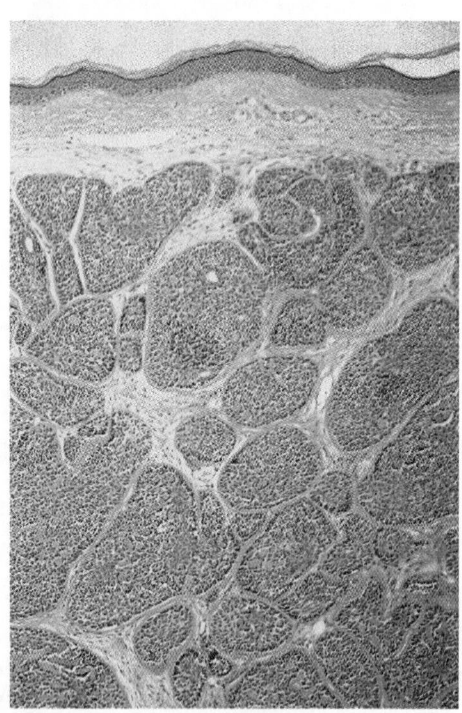

FIGURE *24-78*
Cylindroma. Sharply circumscribed islands of basophilic epithelial cells reside in a jigsaw-like array. Dense eosinophilic hyaline sheaths surround each island and form small circular cords within each one.

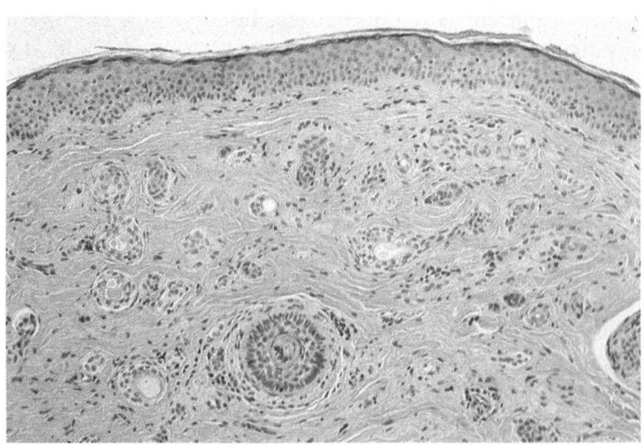
A

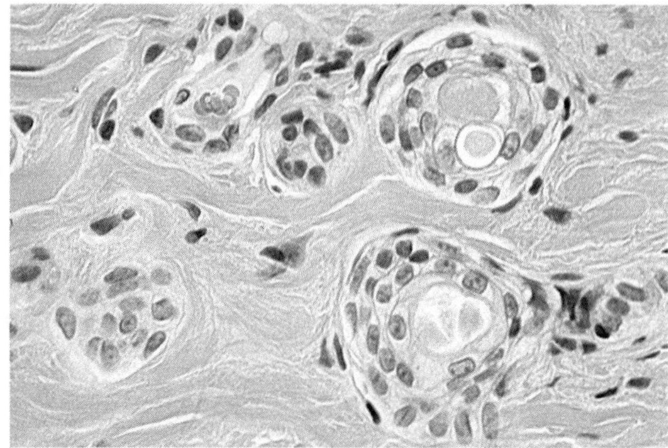
B

FIGURE *24-79*
Syringoma. (*A*) Within the upper dermis is a proliferation of epithelium-forming ducts, tubules, and solid islands amidst a dense fibrous stroma. (*B*) The ductal differentiation closely mimics that of the straight dermal eccrine duct, with a central lumen and cuticle formation. The enzyme complement of the cells and their immunophenotype support eccrine ductal differentiation or derivation.

Eccrine Poroma

Eccrine poroma is a common, benign, solitary tumor that histologically resembles seborrheic keratosis, but contains foci of eccrine gland differentiation. The tumor is a firm, raised lesion, usually less than 2 cm in diameter, that develops on the sole or sides of the foot, the hands, and the fingers. Microscopically, eccrine poroma extends from the lower portion of the epidermis into the dermis as broad anastomosing bands of uniform, cuboidal cells. Narrow ductal lumina and occasional cystic spaces indicate the eccrine differentiation of the tumor.

Tricoepithelioma

Trichoepithelioma is a benign skin appendage tumor that differentiates toward hair structures. It occurs as a solitary tumor or less commonly as multiple lesions, the latter transmitted as an autosomal dominant trait. Microscopically, trichoepithelioma resembles basal cell carcinoma, but contains numerous "horn cysts," which are composed of a keratinized center surrounded by basophilic epithelial cells. In the *multiple trichoepithelioma syndrome*, the lesions begin to appear at puberty, principally on the face, but sometimes on the scalp, neck, and upper trunk.

Fibrous Tumors

Dermatofibroma

Dermatofibroma is a common, benign dermal lesion composed of fibroblasts and macrophages, the former being the neoplastic cell. It occurs in the skin of the extremities as a dome-shaped, firm, rubbery nodule, with ill-defined borders and variable pigmentation, ranging from pink to dark brown. The lesions are usually no more than 3 to 5 mm in width, but an occasional large lesion is seen. Microscopically, the papillary and reticular dermis are replaced by fibrous tissue with a distinctive pattern. The fibroblasts tend to form ill-defined small cartwheels, with a small vascular space at the center. The tumors are not sharply circumscribed and blend with the surrounding dermis. The overlying epidermis is hyperplastic and frequently hyperpigmented, and from it small structures similar to basal cell carcinoma may develop.

Dermatofibrosarcoma Protruberans

This tumor occurs most frequently on the trunk of young adults as slowly growing nodule or indurated plaque. Local recurrence after incomplete excision is common, however metastasis is rare. The most common histological pattern is a poorly circumscribed, monotonous population of spindle cells arranged in a dense storiform array which extends into the subcutis along the fat septa and interstices creating a honey-comb like pattern. The tumor cells contain CD34, an antigen found in endothelium and some neural tumors, in contrast to the cells of dermatofibroma.

Atypical Fibroxanthoma (Superficial Malignant Fibrous Histiocytoma)

Atypical fibroxanthoma is a low-grade malignant skin tumor that presents as a dome-shaped nodule on the sun-damaged skin of elderly persons, the cells of which are characterized by bizarre cytological features. Historically, this tumor was known as *atypical fibroxanthoma*, but it is actually a superficial malignant fibrous histiocytoma (see Chapter 26). Microscopically, atypical spindle cells and epithelioid cells infiltrate and disrupt the dermis. Multinucleated cells, some with a finely vacuolated cytoplasm, may be prominent. Mitoses, including atypical forms, are numerous. The prognosis is dependent on the depth of invasion of the tumor.

Cutaneous Lymphoproliferative Disease

Cutaneous B-Cell Lymphoma

Cutaneous B-cell lymphoma may be a primary disease or may reflect secondary involvement of the skin from a primary nodal tumor (Chapter 20). Primary cutaneous B-cell lymphoma is most frequently derived from follicular center cells (follicular center cell lymphoma). In addition, new subtypes of cutaneous B-cell lymphomas have been recently described, including mantle zone lymphoma, marginal zone lymphoma, and cutaneous plasmacytoma.

Cutaneous B-cell lymphoma presents most commonly in middle-aged to elderly persons as erythematous or violaceous nodules and plaques on the scalp, trunk and back. Typically, a dense infiltrate of atypical lymphocytes is most concentrated in the deep dermis and extends into the panniculus. Germinal center formation is rare; when present, it should raise the possibility of a reactive lymphoid infiltrate (cutaneous lymphoid hyperplasia; pseudolymphoma). The prognosis of primary cutaneous B-cell lymphoma is excellent, and more than 90% of patients survive 5 years.

Secondary involvement of the skin occurs in up to 20% of patients with nodal lymphomas, most commonly lymphoblastic or diffuse centrocytic lymphoma. The histological features mimic the primary nodal disease. In contrast to primary cutaneous lymphoma, secondary skin involvement by systemic lymphoma has a poor prognosis.

Mycosis Fungoides (Primary Cutaneous T-Helper Cell Lymphoma

Mycosis fungoides is a T-cell lymphoma that originates in the skin (see Chapter 20).

Sézary syndrome *refers to systemic dissemination of mycosis fungoides, in which case it features circulating atypical lymphoid cells.*

In the early stages of mycosis fungoides, delicate, erythematous plaques, which are often psoriasiform, appear about the buttocks. The early cellular infiltrates in the dermis are polymorphic and may not be diagnostic of lymphoma. The tendency for lymphocyte involvement of the epidermis (*epidermotropism*) is the most important histological feature of this T-cell lymphoma. The cutaneous disease becomes progressively more prominent and more infiltrative. In late stages, it shows an unequivocal dense dermal infiltrate, forming tumor nodules. With progression, an increasing number of atypical lymphocytes is seen in the papillary dermis and there is extensive epidermotropism. Sharply circumscribed nests of atypical

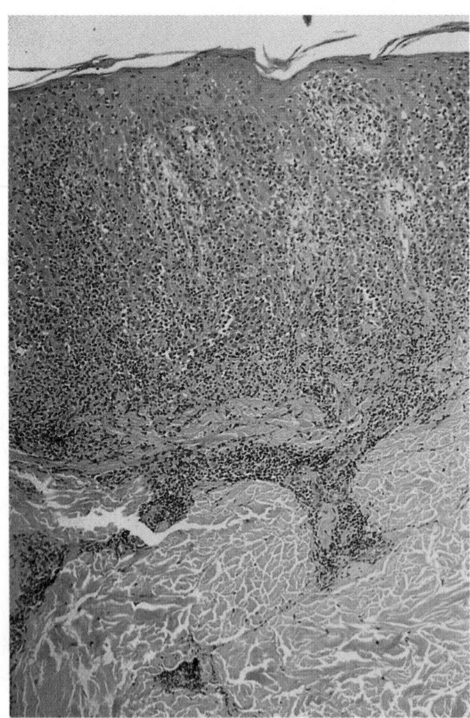

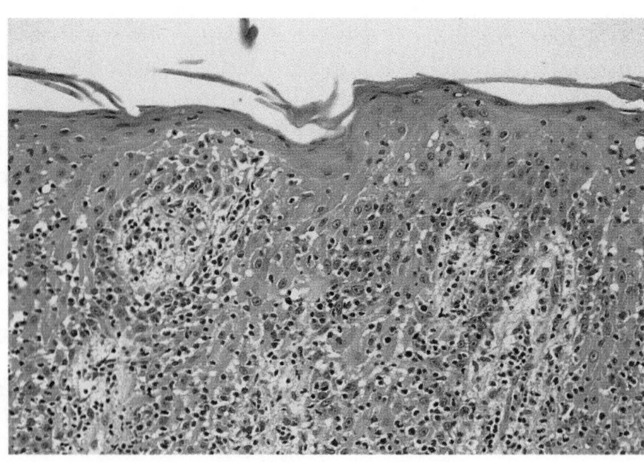

FIGURE *24-80*
Mycosis fungoides, plaque stage. (*A*) The papillary dermis is expanded by an infiltrate of atypical lymphocytes. Lymphocytes with hyperchromatic nuclei infiltrate the thickened epidermis. (*B*) The lymphocytes exhibit nuclear convolutions, some with cerebriform morphology and deep incisuras.

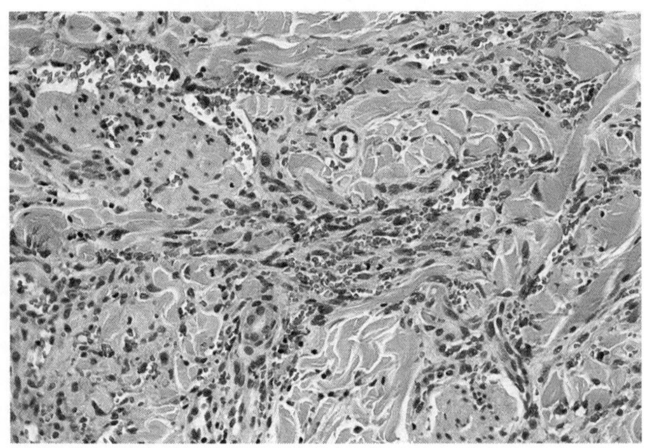

FIGURE *24-81*
Kaposi sarcoma, plaque. Extending along the vascular arcades and amidst reticular dermal collagen is a proliferation of endothelial cells. They form delicate vascular channels filled with red blood cells. Some endothelial cells are not canalized (have not formed lumens.)

CD4+ T cells in the epidermis, as well as a dense subjacent infiltrate, are characteristic of mycosis fungoides (Fig. 24-80).

CUTANEOUS MANIFESTATION OF HIV INFECTION

Kaposi Sarcoma

Kaposi sarcoma (KS) is a malignant tumor derived from endothelial cells. The neoplasm is the principal cutaneous sign observed in the AIDS pandemic and is discussed in Chapters 4 and 10.

All cases of Kaposi sarcoma, whether or not associated with HIV, evolve through three distinctive stages. (1) In the early patch stage, a subtle vascular proliferation of irregular vascular channels, lined by a single layer of mildly atypical endothelial cells, radiates from preexisting blood vessels and extends almost imperceptibly into the surrounding reticular dermis. Extravasated red blood cells, hemosiderin deposition, and a sparse inflammatory infiltrate composed of lymphocytes and plasma cells are commonly observed. Further histological clues include both the "promontory sign," in which normal blood vessels and adnexal structures protrude into newly formed vascular spaces, and intracellular or extracellular eosinophilic globules (fragmented red blood cells). (2) In the plaque stage (Fig. 24-81), there is involvement of the entire reticular dermis, with frequent extension into the subcutis and the formation of bundles of spindle cells. (3) In the nodule stage (Fig. 24-82), well-circumscribed, dermal nodules are composed of intersecting fascicles of spindle cells surrounding numerous slit-like spaces.

Bacillary Angiomatosis

Bacillary angiomatosis is a pseudoneoplastic proliferation of capillaries that arises in response to infection with Bartonella henselae, usually as a complication of AIDS. The lesions appear as red to brown papules, often in large numbers, and may be confused with Kaposi sarcoma. Morphologically, the tumors appear as cellular conjuries of capillaries. Plump, protuberant, endothelial cells are surrounded by an edematous stroma containing an inflammatory infiltrate of mononuclear cells and variable numbers of neutrophils and neutrophil debris. An additional characteristic feature is the extracellular deposition of pale, basophilic, granular material. Silver impregnation stains, such as Warthin-Starry stain, reveal dense masses of bacilli within the basophilic deposits. The lesions clear with antibiotic treatment.

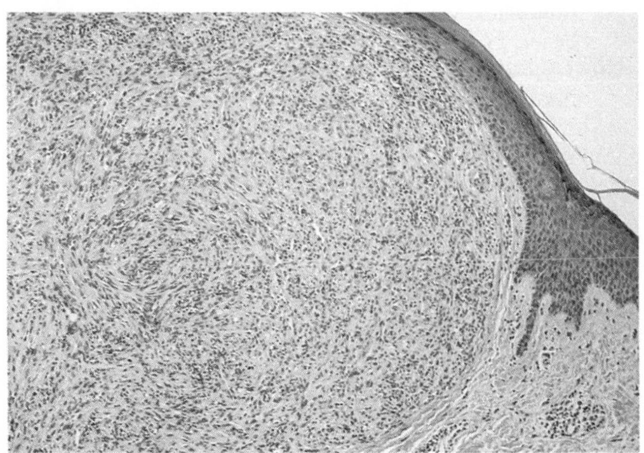

A

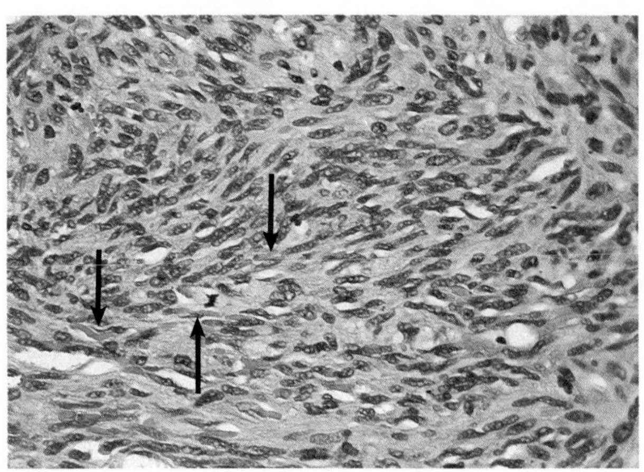

B

FIGURE *24-82*
Kaposi sarcoma, nodule. (*A*) A large nodule (low power) is composed of proliferated endothelial cells forming fascicles and vascular spaces. (*B*) A higher-power view of (*A*) shows mitoses and cytological atypia of the spindle cells. Red blood cells appear agglutinated (*arrows*). The endothelial cells, in which the agglutinated red blood cells are present, form so-called vascular slits.

Eosinophilic Pustular Folliculitis

Eosinophilic pustular folliculitis is a chronic pruritic eruption of papules centered on hair follicles that most commonly develop on the trunk and proximal extremities of AIDS patients. An infiltrate composed of lymphocytes, macrophages, and numerous eosinophils is present in the perifollicular adventitial dermis and around the dermal blood vessels. Eosinophilic pustular folliculitis commonly develops in patients with T-cell counts of less than 200/μL.

SUGGESTED READING

BOOKS

Balch CM, Milton GW, Soong S, et al (eds): *Cutaneous melanoma*, 2nd ed. Philadelphia: JB Lippincott, 1992.

Elder D, Elenitsas R, Jaworsky C, et al (eds): *Lever's histopathology of the skin*, 8th ed. Philadelphia: Lippincott-Raven, 1997.

Farmer ER, Hood AF (eds): *Pathology of the skin.* Norwalk, CT: Appleton and Lange, 1990.

Fitzpatrick TB, Eisen AZ, Wolff K, et al: *Dermatology in general medicine*, 4th ed. New York: McGraw-Hill, 1993.

Friedman RJ, Darrell SR, Koph AW, et al (eds): *Cancer of the skin.* Philadelphia: WB Saunders, 1991.

Murphy GF: *Dermatopathology.* Philadelphia: WB Saunders, 1995.

REVIEW ARTICLES

Burgeson RE: Type VII collagen, anchoring fibrils, and epidermolysis bullosa. *J Invest Derm* 101:252–255, 1993.

Chu T, Jaffe R: The normal Langerhans cell and the LCH cell. *Brit J Cancer* 23:S4–10, 1994.

Clark WH Jr, Elder DE, Van Horn M: The biologic forms of malignant melanoma. *Hum Pathol* 17:443–450, 1986.

Enzinger FM: Malignant fibrous histiocytoma 20 years after Stout. *Am J Sur Pathol* 10(suppl):43–53, 1986.

Favara BE, Jaffe R: The histopathology of the Langerhans cell histiocytosis. *Br J Cancer* 23:S17–23, 1994.

Fine JD: The skin basement membrane zone. *Adv Dermatol* 2:283–304, 1987.

Fletcher CDM: Pleomorphic malignant fibrous histiocytoma, fact or fiction? A critical reappraisal based on 159 tumors diagnosed as pleomorphic sarcoma. *Am J Surg Pathol* 16:213–228, 1992.

Fuchs E: The cytoskeleton and disease: Genetic disorders of intermediate filaments. *Ann Rev Genet* 30:197–231, 1996.

Galli SJ, Tsai M, Wershil Bk: The c-kit receptor, stem cell factor, and mast cells: What each is teaching us about the others. *Am J Pathol* 142:965–974, 1993.

Greene MH: Dysplastic nevus syndrome. *Hosp Pract* 19(January):91–108, 1984.

Inoue S: Ultrastructure of basement membranes. *Int Rev Cyt* 117:57–98, 1989.

Kerl H, Cerroni L: The morphological spectrum of cutaneous B-cell lymphomas. *Arch Dermat* 132:1376–1377, 1996.

Korge BP, Krieg T: The molecular basis for inherited bullous diseases. *J Mol Med* 74:59–70, 1996.

Kraemer KH, Lee MM, Scotto J: Xeroderma pigmentosum. *Arch Dermatol* 123:241–250, 1987.

Krigel RL, Friedman-Kien AE: Epidemic Kaposi's sarcoma. *Semin Oncol* 17:350–360, 1990.

LeBoit PE: Dermatopathologic findings in patients infected with HIV. *Dermat Clin* 10:59–1, 1992.

Pochi PE, Leyden JJ, Shalita AR, et al: Acne: Current concepts: A Scope publication of the Upjohn Company, 1987.

Rabinowitz LO, Zaim MT: A clinicopathologic approach to granulomatous dermatoses. *J Am Acad Dermatol* 35:588–600, 1996.

Rietschel RL: A simplified approach to the diagnosis of alopecia. *Dermat Clin* 14:691–695, 1996.

Smack DP, Korge BP, James WD: Keratin and keratinization. *J Am Acad Dermatol* 30:85–102, 1994.

Sprecher E, Becker Y: Role of Langerhans cells and other dendritic cells in disease states. *In Vivo* 7:217–228, 1993.

Syder AJ, Yu QC, Paller AS et al: Genetic mutations in the K1 and K10 genes of patients with epidermolytic hyperkeratosis: Correlations between location and disease severity. *J Clin Invest* 93:1533–1542, 1994.

Uitto J, Christiano AM: Molecular genetics of the cutaneous basement membrane zone: perspectives on epidermolysis bullosa and other blistering skin diseases. *J Clin Invest* 90:687–692, 1992.

Uitto J, Pulkkinen L: Molecular complexity of the cutaneous basement membrane zone. *Mol Biol Rep* 23:35–46, 1996.

Van den Hooff A: An essay on basement membranes and their involvement in cancer. *Perspectives in Biol and Med* 32:401–413, 1989.

Willemze R: New concepts in the classification of cutaneous lymphomas. *Arch Dermat* 131:1077–1080, 1995.

CHAPTER 25

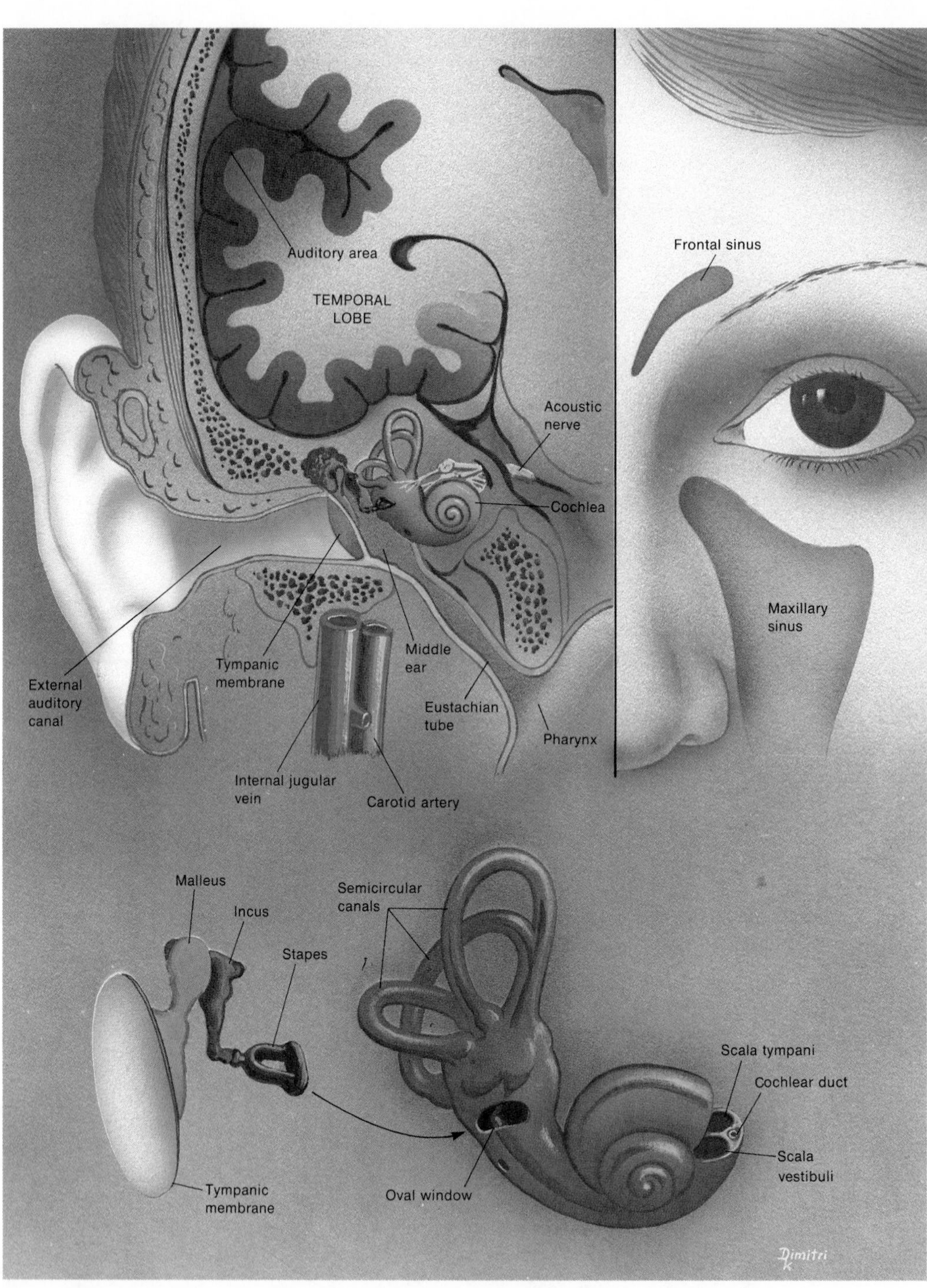

Auditory area
TEMPORAL LOBE
Acoustic nerve
Cochlea
Frontal sinus
Maxillary sinus
External auditory canal
Tympanic membrane
Middle ear
Eustachian tube
Pharynx
Internal jugular vein
Carotid artery
Malleus
Incus
Stapes
Semicircular canals
Scala tympani
Cochlear duct
Scala vestibuli
Oval window
Tympanic membrane
Dimitri

The Head and Neck

Károly Balogh

FIGURE 25-1 *(see opposite page)*
Anatomy of the ear. (*Top*) The relations of the external, middle, and inner ear. Note the tympanic membrane, the ossicles of the middle ear, the location of the eustachian tube, and the proximity of the meninges and the brain. (*Bottom*) Diagrammatic visualization of the tympanic membrane and the ossicles. The *arrow* indicates the normal position of the stapes in the oval window. A cross-section of the cochlea demonstrates the relation of the cochlear duct (carrying endolymph) to the scala tympani and scala vestibuli (filled with perilymph).

Head and neck pathology refers to commonly encountered congenital and acquired disorders in this region, rather than disease of a specific organ or system. In accord with the domain of a specific surgical specialty, we discuss the oral cavity (including dental diseases), salivary glands, nose and paranasal sinuses, nasopharynx, and ear.

Oral Cavity

The oral cavity is lined by nonkeratinized or only lightly keratinized squamous epithelium. The bacteria, spirochetes, viruses, fungi, and parasites normally found in the oral cavity are usually harmless. If the mucosa is injured or the defense mechanisms of the body are impaired, for instance by immunosuppression, the same organisms can cause disease, as in fusospirochetal gingivitis. Healthy persons may also carry pathogens such as *Corynebacterium diphtheriae* or meningococci in the oral cavity. Systemic diseases frequently affect the oral cavity, and although the oral mucosa is not necessarily a mirror to the body, it may reflect more than localized disease.

DEVELOPMENTAL ANOMALIES

The complex embryological development of the face, lips, and oral and nasal cavities gives rise to numerous anomalies, only the most important of which are discussed here.

FACIAL CLEFTS: Failure of fusion of facial structures in the seventh week of embryonic life leads to the formation of facial clefts, the most common of which is cleft upper lip (harelip). It may be unilateral or bilateral and frequently occurs in association with cleft palate (see Chapter 6).

LINGUAL THYROID NODULE: During its normal development, the thyroid gland descends from the base of the tongue to its final position in the neck. Heterotopic functioning thyroid tissue or a developmental cyst (thyroglossal duct cyst) may occur anywhere along the path of descent. The most common location is at the foramen cecum of the tongue.

BRANCHIAL CLEFT CYST: *Branchial cleft cysts originate from remnants of the branchial arches* (Fig. 25-2). They occur on the lateral anterior aspect of the neck or in the parotid gland, mostly in young adults. The cyst contains thin, watery fluid and mucoid or gelatinous material. It is usually lined by squamous epithelium, although foci of ciliated respiratory or pseudostratified columnar epithelium also are seen (Fig. 25-3).

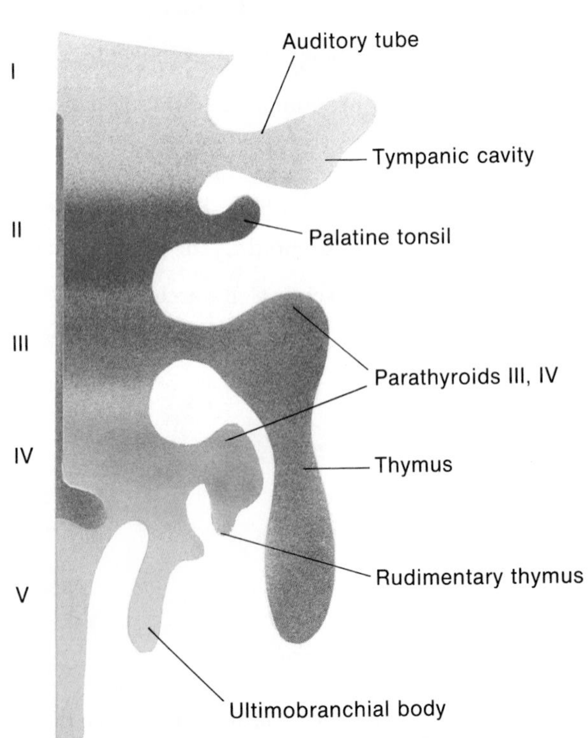

FIGURE 25-2
Branchial apparatus in humans. Schematic diagram of the pharyngeal pouches (*left half, ventral view*) in a human embryo of 6 weeks. Five pairs of pouches give rise to many important structures of the head, neck, and chest. A wide spectrum of congenital malformations results from abnormalities of the branchial apparatus.

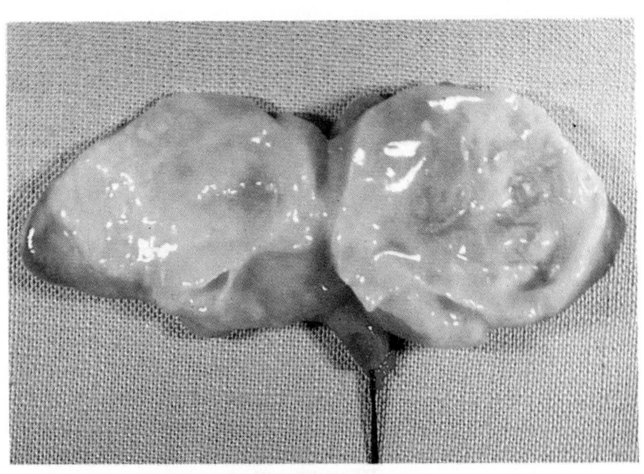

FIGURE 25-3
Branchial cyst. Most of these cysts arise from the second branchial cleft and occur laterally in the neck. The cysts have a thin wall, contain turbid fluid, and are lined by stratified squamous or respiratory-type epithelium.

INFECTIONS

The following terms are used to describe localized inflammation of the oral cavity:

- Cheilitis (lips)
- Gingivitis (gum)
- Glossitis (tongue)
- Stomatitis (oral mucosa)

Bacterial and Fungal Infections

The oral cavity can harbor many infections, some of which are briefly discussed here (see also Chapter 9).

SCARLET FEVER: Predominantly a disease of children, scarlet fever is caused by several strains of β-hemolytic streptococci (*Streptococcus pyogenes*). Damage to the vascular endothelium by the erythrogenic toxin results in a rash on the skin and in the oral mucosa. The tongue has a white coating, through which the hyperemic fungiform papillae project as small red knobs ("strawberry tongue").

APHTHOUS STOMATITIS (APHTHAE, CANKER SORES): *Aphthous stomatitis describes a common disease that is characterized by painful, recurrent, solitary or multiple, small ulcers of the oral mucosa.* The causative agent is unknown. Bacteria, mycoplasma, viruses, autoimmune reactions, and hypersensitivity have been implicated but are unproved. Microscopically, the lesion consists of a shallow ulcer covered by a fibrinopurulent exudate. The underlying inflammatory infiltrate is composed of mononuclear and polymorphonuclear leukocytes. The lesions heal without scar formation.

PYOGENIC GRANULOMA: *Pyogenic granuloma is a reactive vascular lesion that commonly occurs in the oral cavity.* Usually some minor trauma to the tissues permits invasion of nonspecific microorganisms. In the oral cavity, pyogenic granulomas, ranging from a few millimeters to a centimeter, are most frequent on the gingiva. The lesion is seen as an elevated, red or purple, soft mass, with a smooth, lobulated, ulcerated surface. Microscopically, the nodule consists of highly vascular granulation tissue that shows varying degrees of acute and chronic inflammation (Fig. 25-4). The lesion is occasionally difficult to distinguish from a malignant vascular neoplasm. With time, however, pyogenic granuloma becomes less vascular and comes to resemble a fibroma.

In pregnant women, particularly near the end of the first trimester, a gingival lesion may develop that grossly and microscopically is identical to pyogenic granuloma. Termed *pregnancy tumor*, it may or may not regress after delivery.

ACUTE NECROTIZING ULCERATIVE GINGIVITIS (VINCENT INFECTION OR VINCENT ANGINA): *Vincent angina represents an infection by two symbiotic organisms, one a fusiform bacillus and the other a spirochete (Borrelia vincentii).* The term fusospirochetosis is used to describe such an infection. The fact that these organisms are found in the mouths of many healthy persons suggests that predisposing factors are important in the development of acute, necrotizing, ulcerative gingivitis. The most important element appears to be decreased resistance to infection as a result of inadequate nutrition, immunodeficiency, or poor oral hygiene. Vincent infection is characterized by punched-out erosions of the interdental papillae. The ulceration tends to spread and eventually to involve all gingival margins, which become covered by a necrotic pseudomembrane.

***Noma** is a severe fusospirochetal infection in persons who are malnourished, debilitated from infections, or weakened by blood dyscrasias, and features a rapidly spreading gangrene of the oral and facial tissues.* Large masses of tissue slough and leave the bones exposed (see Fig. 9-39). This extreme complication of fusospirochetosis is more common in children.

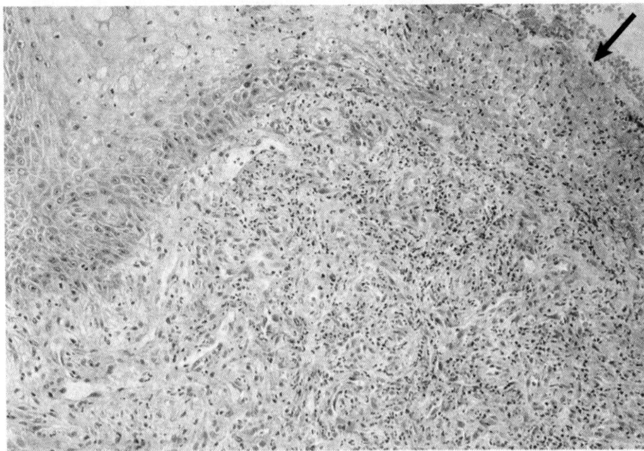

FIGURE 25-4
Pyogenic granuloma of the gingiva. The lesion displays vascular granulation tissue and inflammation. The epithelial surface is partly ulcerated (*arrow*).

LUDWIG ANGINA: *Ludwig angina is a rapidly spreading cellulitis, or phlegmon, which originates in the submaxillary or sublingual space but extends locally to involve both.* The bacteria responsible for this infection are believed to originate from the oral flora, but this potentially life-threatening inflammatory process is uncommon in developed countries. A variety of aerobic or anaerobic microorganisms have been implicated in Ludwig angina, and in many cases, mixed cultures are recovered. Systemic disease may play a role, because patients often have chronic illnesses associated with immunosuppression.

Ludwig angina is most often related to dental extraction or trauma to the floor of the mouth. After extraction of a tooth, hairline fractures may occur in the lingual cortex of the mandible, providing microorganisms ready access to the submaxillary space. By following the fascial planes, the infection may dissect into the parapharyngeal or pharyngomaxillary space and from there into the carotid sheath. An infected (mycotic) aneurysm of the internal carotid artery may result, and its erosion causes massive hemorrhage. The inflammation may also dissect into the superior mediastinum, involving the pleural space and pericardium.

DIPHTHERIA: Infection with *Corynebacterium diphtheriae* is characterized by the formation of a patchy pseudomembrane, which often begins on the tonsils and pharynx but may also involve the soft palate, gingiva, or buccal mucosa.

TUBERCULOSIS: Primary tuberculous lesions of the oral mucosa are rare, and most lesions are the result of pulmonary disease. The bacilli are carried in the sputum and enter the mucosa through a small break, where they produce irregular, painful ulcers, most commonly on the tongue. A biopsy reveals typical tuberculous granulomas (Fig. 25-5).

SYPHILIS: The chancre of primary syphilis may form on the lips, tongue, or oropharyngeal mucosa after oral–genital contact with an infected person. It is accompanied by a regional lymphadenitis and heals spontaneously in a few weeks. If syphilis is not treated adequately, a diffuse mucocutaneous eruption of the secondary stage develops. The lesions in the oral mucosa appear as multiple gray–white patches overlying the ulcerated surface. They may undergo spontaneous remission but may also recur. After years of syphilitic infection, gummas may appear on the palate and tongue. They are firm nodular masses that eventually ulcerate and may lead to perforation of the palate.

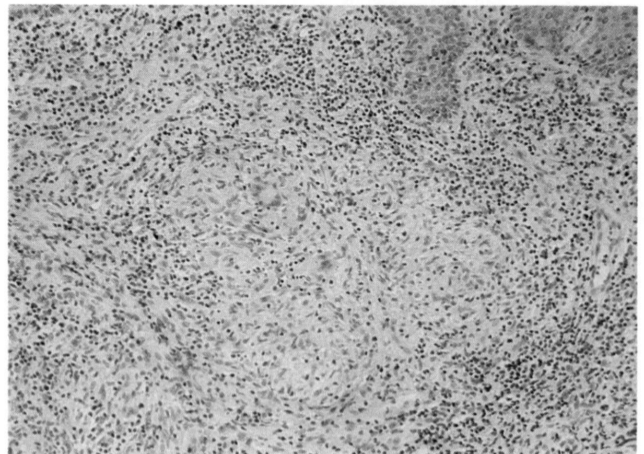

FIGURE 25-5
Tuberculosis of the tongue. The lesion was first seen as a persistent ulcer in a man with pulmonary tuberculosis. Chronic inflammation and a tubercle with Langhans giant cells are seen under the epithelium.

ACTINOMYCOSIS: Branched, filamentous bacteria of the Actinomyces group occasionally cause oral infections. The most common offender is *Actinomyces bovis*, but *A. israelii* is sometimes encountered. The organisms produce a chronic, granulomatous inflammation and abscesses, which drain by the formation of fistulas. Because actinomycetes are common inhabitants of the oral cavity of healthy persons, culture of the organism does not necessarily signify an infection. It is customary to distinguish cervicofacial (the most common form), pulmonary, and abdominal forms of actinomycosis, according to the site of the infection. In cervicofacial actinomycosis, the infection of the soft tissues may extend to adjacent bones, most commonly to the mandible.

CANDIDIASIS: Also termed thrush or moniliasis, candidiasis is caused by a yeast-like fungus, *Candida albicans*, which is a common surface inhabitant of the oral cavity, gastrointestinal tract, and vagina. To cause disease, the fungus must penetrate the tissues, albeit superficially. Oral candidiasis is most common in immunocompromised persons and diabetics, and the incidence in patients with acquired immunodeficiency syndrome (AIDS) is 40% to 90%. The oral lesions typically appear as white, slightly elevated, soft patches that consist mainly of fungal hyphae. Candidiasis may also be represented by pseudomembranous, hyperplastic, or erythematous lesions.

Viral Infections

HERPES SIMPLEX VIRUS TYPE 1: Herpes labialis (cold sores, fever blisters) and herpetic stomatitis are caused by herpes simplex virus type 1 and are among the most common viral infections of the lips and oral mucosa in both children and young adults. Transmission occurs by droplet infection, and the virus can be recovered from the saliva of infected persons. The disease starts with painful inflammation of the affected mucosa, followed shortly by the formation of vesicles. These vesicles rupture and form shallow, painful ulcers, ranging from a punctate size to a centimeter in diameter. Microscopically, the herpetic vesicle forms as a result of "ballooning degeneration" of the epithelial cells. Some epithelial cells show intranuclear inclusion bodies. The ulcers heal spontaneously without scar formation.

Once herpes simplex virus has been introduced into the body, it survives in a dormant state in the trigeminal ganglion. It can be reactivated to cause recurrent herpetic lesions in diverse ways, including trauma, allergy, menstruation, pregnancy, exposure to ultraviolet light, and other viral infections. In the oral cavity, the recurrent vesicles almost invariably develop on a mucosa that is tightly bound to the periosteum, for example, the hard palate.

OTHER VIRAL INFECTIONS: Coxsackievirus A causes herpangina, which is seen as an acute vesicular oropharyngitis. After a brief course, the infection confers immunity. Other viral infections that involve the oral mucosa are infectious mononucleosis (Epstein–Barr virus; EBV), measles, rubella, chickenpox, and herpes zoster.

BENIGN TUMORS

Benign tumors that are common in other regions of the body are seen also in the oral cavity. These include pigmented nevi, fibromas, hemangiomas, lymphangiomas, and squamous papillomas. Trauma may lead to ulceration of these lesions, in which case, they may bleed or become infected. Two entities distinctive to the oral cavity, peripheral giant cell granuloma and oral hairy leukoplakia, deserve mention.

PERIPHERAL GIANT CELL GRANULOMA: *Peripheral giant cell granuloma is not a neoplasm but rather an unusual proliferative reaction to local injury that is seen as a mass on the gingiva or the alveolar process.* This lesion has a variety of names, such as epulis, giant cell reparative granuloma, giant cell tumor of gum, and osteoclastoma. The adjective "peripheral" denotes the superficial, extraosseous location of the lesion, as opposed to the "central" giant cell granulomas that occur within the jawbones.

The prevailing view is that peripheral giant call granuloma is not a neoplasm but rather an unusual proliferative reaction to local injury. In a few cases, it is caused by hyperparathyroidism, in which case, it can be regarded as a brown tumor of soft tissues. The lesion always occurs on the gingiva or the alveolar process and seems to originate from the deeper soft tissues. The majority of patients are young or middle-aged adults, but the lesion occurs in children and has been reported in edentulous elderly patients.

☐ **Pathology:** Peripheral giant cell granuloma is seen as a mass covered by mucous membrane, which can be ulcerated. The tumor varies from brown to black, depending on the amount of hemorrhage. Histological examination reveals a nonencapsulated lesion, with numerous multinucleated giant cells embedded in a fibrous stroma, which also contains ovoid or spindle-shaped mesenchymal cells (Fig. 25-6). The lesion is vascular and shows foci of old hemorrhage, with hemosiderin-laden macrophages and chronic inflammation. The origin of the multinucleated giant cells remains unclear, although immunohistochemical evidence suggests they are derived from macrophages.

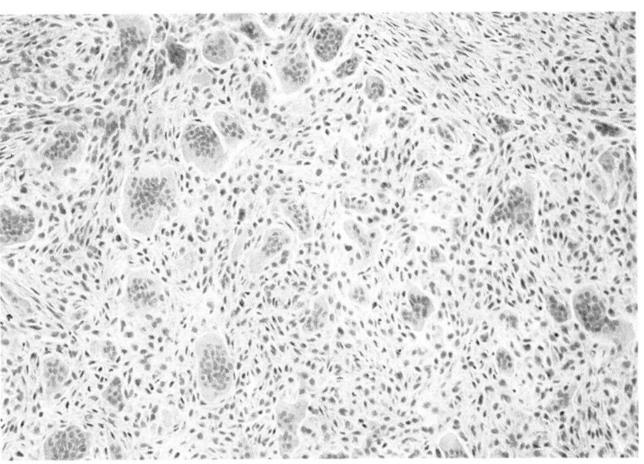

FIGURE 25-6
Peripheral giant cell granuloma. A protruding gingival mass contains multinucleated giant cells and spindle-shaped stromal cells.

ORAL HAIRY LEUKOPLAKIA: *Oral hairy leukoplakia refers to a raised white area of epithelial thickening of the oral and esophageal mucosa that occurs in persons infected with AIDS.* The lesion typically appears on the lateral border of the tongue. Microscopically, it reveals epithelial hyperplasia and marked hyperkeratosis; the prickle cell layer shows changes characteristic of viral infection. Oral hairy leukoplakia is thought to be caused by infection with EBV.

Leukoplakia

Leukoplakia (Greek, leukos, "white" and plax, "plaque") designates an asymptomatic white patch on the surface of a mucous membrane. Although not a tumor, oral leukoplakia is discussed here because some cases undergo transformation to squamous cell carcinoma. The disorder occurs with equal frequency in both sexes, mostly after the third decade of life. A variety of diseases appear clinically as leukoplakia, including various keratoses, hyperkeratosis, and squamous carcinoma *in situ*. Thus, leukoplakia is not a histological diagnosis but rather a descriptive clinical term. Other clinical entities may also feature a white plaque on the oral mucosa, for example, candidiasis, lichen planus, psoriasis, and syphilis.

The causes of leukoplakia are diverse, the most common factors being use of tobacco products, alcoholism, and local irritation. The same factors also appear important in the etiology of oral carcinoma. Leukoplakia occurs most often on the buccal mucosa, tongue, and floor of the mouth. The plaques may be solitary or multiple and vary in size from small lesions to large patches.

It deserves emphasis that there is no correlation between the clinical appearance of leukoplakia and the microscopic diagnosis, although most cases show some abnormality of the squamous epithelium (Fig. 25-7). Biopsies have revealed dysplasia or carcinoma *in situ* in 10% of the cases and invasive carcinoma in 8%. In cases of leukoplakia without epithelial dysplasia, 20% eventually become malignant. In view of these data, all cases of leukoplakia should clinically be considered precancerous.

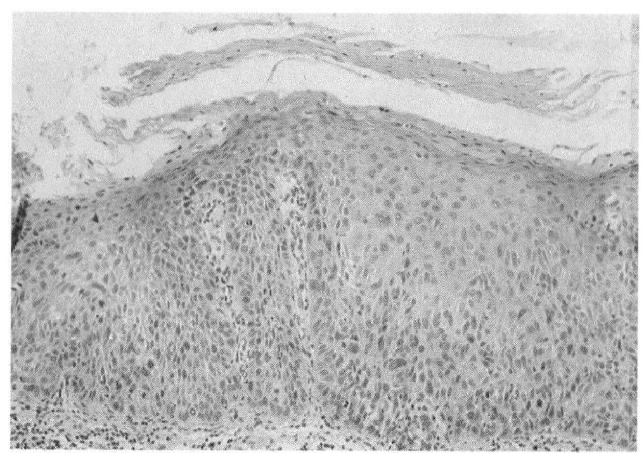

FIGURE *25-7*
Leukoplakia. The lesion was seen as a white patch on the buccal mucosa of a heavy smoker. Histologically, epithelial hyperplasia, marked atypia, and parakeratosis are evident.

SQUAMOUS CELL CARCINOMA

Squamous carcinoma is the most common malignant tumor of the oral mucosa and may occur at any site. It most frequently involves the tongue, followed in descending order by the floor of the mouth, alveolar mucosa, palate, and buccal mucosa. The male-to-female ratio is 2:1 for the gum but 10:1 for squamous carcinoma of the lip. There are substantial variations in the geographic distribution of oral cancer; for example, it is the single most common cancer of men in India.

□ **Pathogenesis:** Predisposing factors in the pathogenesis of oral cancer include the use of tobacco products, alcoholism, iron deficiency (Plummer–Vinson syndrome), physical and chemical irritants, chewing of betel nuts, ultraviolet light on the lips, and poor oral hygiene (craggy teeth and ill-fitting dentures). Not surprisingly, several of these factors also have been mentioned in connection with leukoplakia. Some squamous cell carcinomas of the head and neck have been associated with human papillomavirus infection. Multiple separate epidermoid carcinomas may be found at the same time (synchronous) or at intervals (metachronous) in the oral mucosa, a situation termed *field cancerization.*

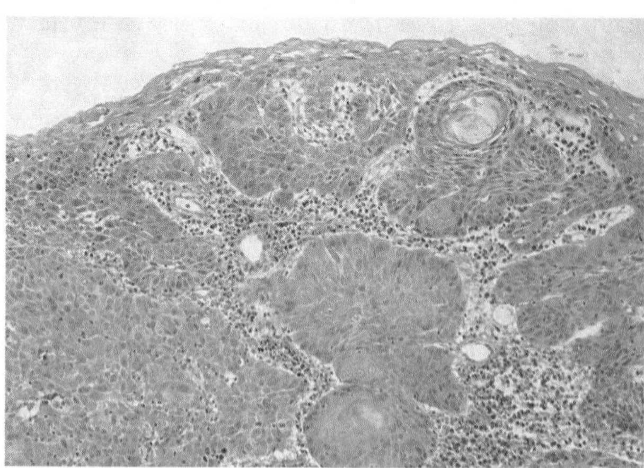

FIGURE *25-8*
Squamous cell carcinoma of the tongue. Nests and sheets of malignant epithelial cells have invaded the stroma. This well-differentiated tumor shows keratinization.

□ **Pathology:** Invasive squamous carcinoma of the oral cavity is similar to the same tumor in other sites and is generally preceded by carcinoma *in situ*. Variations in differentiation in squamous cell carcinoma have led to a system of grading tumors. Accordingly, grade I carcinoma is well differentiated and frequently keratinizing (Fig. 25-8). At the other end of the spectrum, grade IV carcinomas are so poorly differentiated that their origin is difficult to detect on morphological grounds.

Oral carcinoma metastasizes mainly to the submandibular, superficial, and deep cervical lymph nodes. More than half of patients who die of squamous cell carcinoma of the head and neck have distant, blood-borne metastases, most commonly in the lungs, liver, and bones.

Malignant melanoma, various sarcomas, lymphomas, and metastatic carcinomas uncommonly involve the oral cavity.

DISEASES OF THE LIPS

The lips are affected by a variety of degenerative, inflammatory, and proliferative processes. Some of these, particularly those expressed in the skin and mucous membranes, are systemic; others reflect localized disease (Figs. 25-9 and 25-10).

DISEASES OF THE TONGUE

MACROGLOSSIA: *All the components of the tongue may be involved by various localized or systemic diseases, some of which can lead to enlargement of the tongue, which is known as macroglossia.* If present at birth, macroglossia is usually due to diffuse lymphangioma or hemangioma, although rarely enlargement is caused by congenital neurofibromatosis or true muscle hypertrophy. An enlarged tongue that protrudes from the mouth occurs in congenital hypothyroidism, Hurler syndrome, glycogen-storage disease type II (Pompe disease), Beckwith–Wiedemann syndrome, and Down syndrome. Acquired macroglossia is due to amyloidosis, acromegaly, and infiltration or lymphatic obstruction by tumors.

GLOSSITIS: Inflammation of the tongue, termed glossitis, can be caused by various microorganisms, physical effects, chemical agents, or systemic diseases. Some forms of glossitis are associated with vitamin deficiencies, including pernicious anemia, riboflavin deficiency, pellagra, and pyridoxine deficiency.

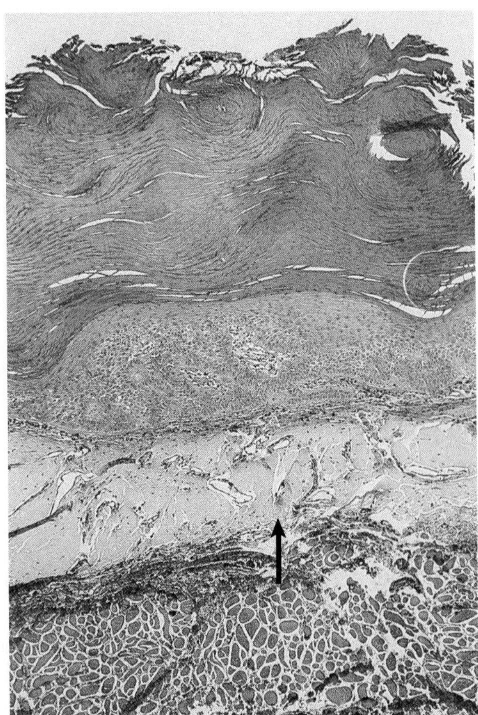

FIGURE 25-9
Solar cheilitis. A lesion analogous to a solar keratosis is present in the vermilion border of the lower lip. Hyperkeratosis and epithelial hyperplasia and dysplasia are evident. The light band under the epithelium (*arrow*) represents solar elastosis (damaged collagen) resulting from ultraviolet radiation.

DENTAL CARIES (TOOTH DECAY)

Caries is the most prevalent chronic disease of the calcified tissues of the teeth. It affects persons of both sexes and every age group throughout the world, and its incidence has markedly increased with modern civilization. Dental caries results from the interactions of several factors.

BACTERIA: Dental caries is a chronic infectious disease of the enamel, dentin, and cementum of teeth, the organisms being part of the indigenous oral flora. Tooth surfaces are normally colonized by numerous microorganisms, and unless the surface is cleaned thoroughly and frequently, colonies of bacteria coalesce into a soft mass known as dental plaque.

The essential characteristics of carious lesions result primarily from the dissolution of mineral in dental tissues by acids that are produced during the metabolism of food residues by microorganisms on tooth surfaces. Numerous streptococci, lactobacilli, and actinomyces in the oral flora have these characteristics. When all pertinent data are evaluated, indirect evidence points strongly to *Streptococcus mutans* as the primary etiological agent initiating caries. Deeper in the enamel and dentin, organisms other than *S. mutans* may be more capable of maintaining the destructive process.

SALIVA: Saliva also has an important role in the maintenance of teeth and the development of caries. In addition to its functions in moistening and lubricating oral surfaces, saliva has a high buffering capacity that helps neutralize microbially produced acids in the mouth. In addition, saliva contains several potentially bacteriostatic factors, such as lysozyme, lactoferrin, the lactoperoxidase system, and secretory immunoglobulins. Removal of the major salivary glands in rats results in a 10-fold increase in caries. In humans, *xerostomia* (chronic dryness of the mouth from lack of saliva) results in rampant caries.

DIETARY FACTORS: There is a consensus that one of the most important factors in the development of caries is a high carbohydrate intake. Raw and unrefined foods contain a great deal of roughage that cleanses the teeth. Additionally, roughage necessitates more mastication, which further contributes to the cleansing of the teeth. By contrast, soft and refined foods tend to stick to the teeth and also require less chewing.

FLUORIDE: The presence of fluoride in the drinking water protects against dental caries. Fluoride is incorporated into the crystal lattice structure of enamel where it forms fluoroapatite, a less acid-soluble compound than the apatite of enamel. The fluoridation of drinking water in many communities has been followed by a dramatic reduction in the incidence of dental caries in children, whose teeth were formed while they drank fluoride-containing water.

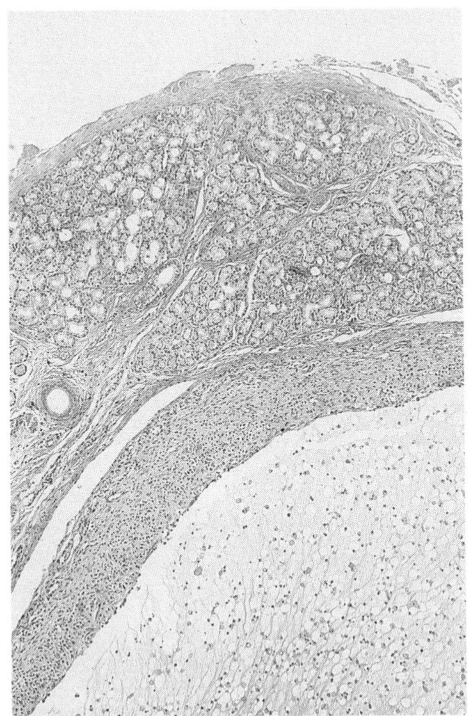

FIGURE 25-10
Mucocele of lower lip. This cystic lesion is associated with the minor salivary glands and is probably caused by trauma that permits escape of mucus. The cyst has a fibrous wall and is lined by granulation tissue. The lumen is filled with mucus that contains numerous macrophages.

☐ **Pathology:** Caries begins with the disintegration of the enamel prisms after decalcification of the interprismatic substance, events that lead to the accumulation of debris and microorganisms (Figs. 25-11 and 25-12). These changes produce a small pit or fissure in the enamel. When the process reaches the dentinoenamel junction, it spreads laterally and also penetrates the dentin along the dentinal tubules. A substantial cavity then forms in the dentin, leading to a flask-shaped lesion with a narrow orifice. Calcification of the dentinal tubules may seal them off, thereby barring further penetration by microorganisms. However, decalcification of dentin usually continues and leads to a focal coalescence of the destroyed dentinal tubules. Damage to dentin stimulates the odontoblasts that line the wall of the pulp chamber to form secondary dentin. Unfortunately, this reparative process usually does not prevent the microorganisms of the oral flora from reaching the dental pulp and causing pulpitis. Only when the vascular pulp of the tooth is invaded does an inflammatory reaction *(pulpitis)* appear, accompanied for the first time by pain.

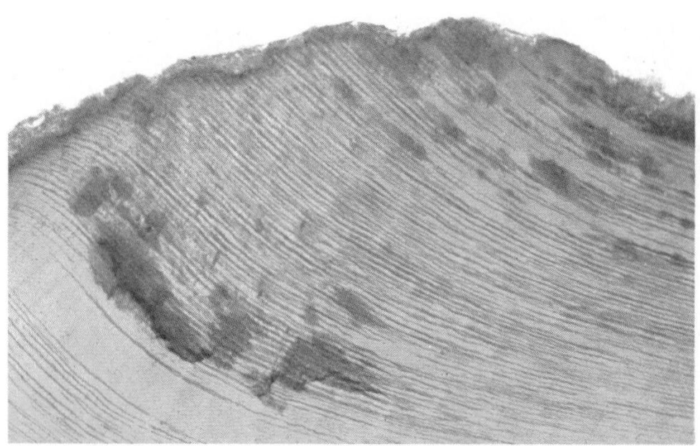

FIGURE *25-12*
Dental caries. Deposits of debris cover the surface. Bacterial colonies (dark purple) have extended into dentinal canals.

DISEASES OF THE PULP AND PERIAPICAL TISSUES

The dental pulp consists of delicate connective tissue enclosed within the calcified walls of dentin. The pulp chamber is lined by odontoblasts and has a minute apical foramen, through which blood vessels, lymphatics, and small nerves penetrate.

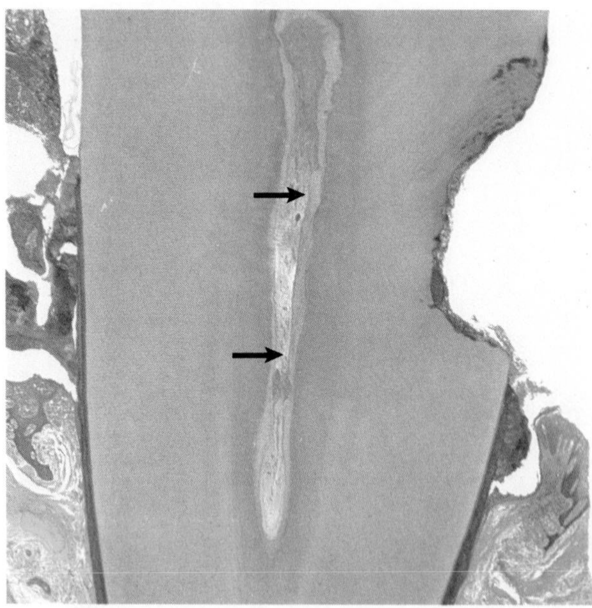

FIGURE *25-11*
Dental caries. A large cavity close to the gingival margin is illustrated. ***Arrows,*** **band of secondary dentin that lines the pulp chamber. This newly formed dentin is opposite the area of tooth destruction and was produced by the stimulated odontoblasts.**

PULPITIS: Inflammation of the dental pulp, known as pulpitis, results from invasion by the oral bacteria involved in dental caries. Pain in acute pulpitis reflects an increase in the pressure of the pulp chamber caused by edema and exudate. Increased pressure in the pulp chamber also facilitates the spread of inflammation. Acute pulpitis may be accompanied by the formation of a small pulp abscess, and several small abscesses may lead to necrosis of the entire pulp. Chronic pulpitis may be the outcome of a subsiding acute inflammation or may be a chronic inflammation from its onset.

Acute or chronic pulpitis, if untreated, ultimately results in complete necrosis of the dental pulp. The infection may spread through a root canal into the periapical region, thereby leading to more serious lesions.

APICAL (OR PERIAPICAL) GRANULOMA: The most common sequel of pulpitis is the formation of chronically inflamed periapical granulation tissue (Fig. 25-13). The inflammatory tissue gradually becomes surrounded by a fibrous capsule, and when the tooth is extracted, the encapsulated granuloma is found attached to the root. Histological examination of apical granulomas reveals the presence of stratified squamous epithelium, which may be derived from a periodontal pocket or from epithelial rests commonly attached to the root.

RADICULAR CYST (APICAL PERIODONTAL CYST): The squamous epithelium of an apical granuloma proliferates, forming a cavity, or cyst, lined by stratified squamous epithelium.

PERIAPICAL ABSCESS: As a result of pulpitis, an abscess may develop around the root of the tooth, either directly or after the formation of periapical granulomas and cysts.

OSTEOMYELITIS: A periapical abscess, if not contained, rapidly extends to the adjacent bone, where it produces osteomyelitis. Bacteriological cultures in all stages of pulpitis and periapical infections grow *Staphylococcus*

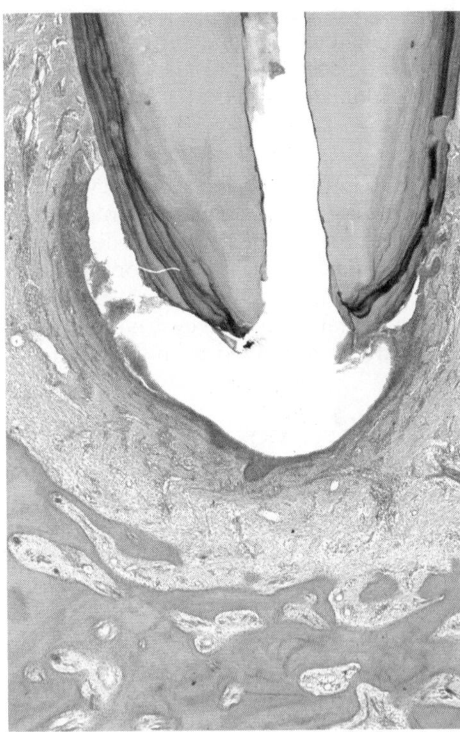

FIGURE 25-13
Advanced caries with periapical granuloma.

aureus, S. epidermidis, various streptococci, or mixed organisms.

Osteomyelitis of the mandible or maxilla is an uncommon complication of odontogenic disease, usually of periapical infection. Similar to osteomyelitis of other bones, it may become localized or propagate within the jawbones. The infection may break through the cortical bone and spread in various tissue spaces of the head and neck, causing cellulitis (*phlegmon*) or abscesses. The purulent exudate may discharge into the surface of the mucous membranes or skin and create fistulas. In advanced cases, the infection follows the line of gravity in the tissue planes and ultimately reaches the mediastinum. These grave complications of osteomyelitis caused by dental infection were often lethal in the preantibiotic era but are rare today.

PERIODONTAL DISEASE

Periodontal disease refers to acute and chronic disorders of the soft tissues surrounding the teeth, which eventually leads to the loss of supporting bone. The gingiva (gum) is the part of the oral mucosa that surrounds the teeth and ends in a thin edge (free gingiva) closely adherent to the teeth. The periodontal ligament is composed of collagen fibers that hold the tooth in position by suspending it in the socket (alveolus) of the jawbones. These structures form the periodontium.

Chronic periodontal disease typically occurs in adults, particularly in persons with poor oral hygiene. However, many persons with apparently impeccable habits, but with a strong family history of periodontal disease, manifest the disorder. Chronic periodontitis causes loss of more teeth in adults than does any other disease, including caries.

☐ **Pathogenesis and Pathology:** Periodontal disease is caused by the accumulation of bacteria under the gingiva in the periodontal pocket. As the mass of bacteria adhering to the surface of tooth (*dental plaque*) ages and mineralizes, it forms *calculus* (tartar). Of the more than 300 types of bacteria that may reside in the oral cavity, only a few are involved in the tissue destruction seen in periodontal disease. Adult periodontitis is associated very strongly with *Bacteroides gingivalis.* In addition, *B. intermedius, Actinomyces* species, *Haemophilus* species, and a few other microorganisms also may participate in active adult periodontitis.

The inflammation often starts as a marginal gingivitis (Fig. 25-14), which, if untreated, progresses to chronic periodontitis. Once initiated, periodontitis continues to progress in the absence of treatment. Chronic inflammation weakens and destroys the periodontium, causing loosening and eventual loss of teeth.

Special Forms of Periodontal Disease

Hematological disorders may affect the oral tissues. Agranulocytosis causes necrotizing ulcers anywhere in the oral and pharyngeal mucosa, but involvement of the gingiva is particularly common. Infectious mononucleosis often results in gingivitis and stomatitis, with exudate and ulceration. Acute and chronic leukemias of all types cause oral lesions. The most common involvement of oral tissues is seen in acute monocytic leukemia, in which 80% of the patients exhibit gingivitis, gingival hyperplasia, petechiae, and hemorrhage. Necrosis and ulceration of the

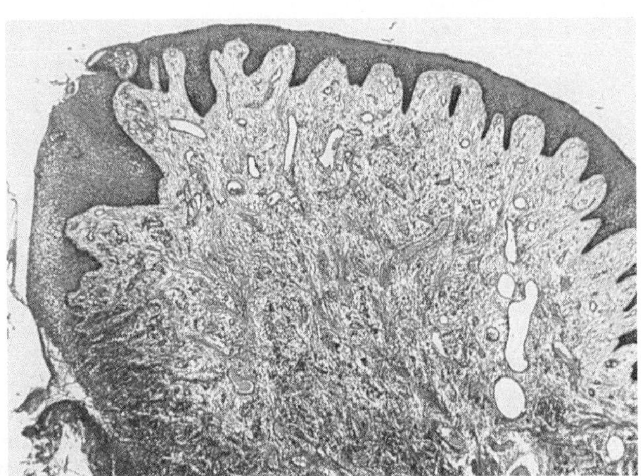

FIGURE 25-14
Hyperplastic chronic gingivitis. A section of gingiva shows a hyperplastic epithelium overlying chronically inflamed granulation tissue.

gingiva lead to severe superimposed infection, which may cause loss of teeth and alveolar bone. A hemorrhagic diathesis may be reflected in gingival hemorrhage.

Scurvy (vitamin C deficiency) is of historical interest, but in less dramatic forms is still encountered, particularly in poor, neglected, or ignorant persons. Scurvy tends to affect the marginal and interdental gingiva, which becomes swollen and bright red and readily bleeds and ulcerates. Hemorrhage into the periodontal membrane causes loosening and loss of teeth.

ODONTOGENIC CYSTS AND TUMORS

The mandible and maxilla, similar to other bones, are affected by both generalized and localized forms of skeletal diseases. However, they differ from other bones in that they provide an abode for the teeth. Besides the inflammatory processes of dental origin described earlier, a variety of odontogenic cysts and tumors arise in the jawbones and the adjacent soft tissues, the pathogenesis of which can be understood on the basis of dental histogenesis (Fig. 25-15).

ODONTOGENIC CYSTS: These cysts have been classified according to the stage of odontogenesis during which they originate. As mentioned earlier, the most common is the radicular, or apical, periodontal cyst, which involves the apex of an erupted tooth, usually after an infection of the dental pulp. The cyst is lined by stratified squamous epithelium derived from the epithelial rests of Malassez.

DENTIGEROUS CYSTS: These cysts are associated with the crown of an impacted, embedded, or unerupted tooth, most often involving the mandibular and maxillary third molars. The cyst forms after the crown of the tooth has completely developed, and fluid accumulates be-

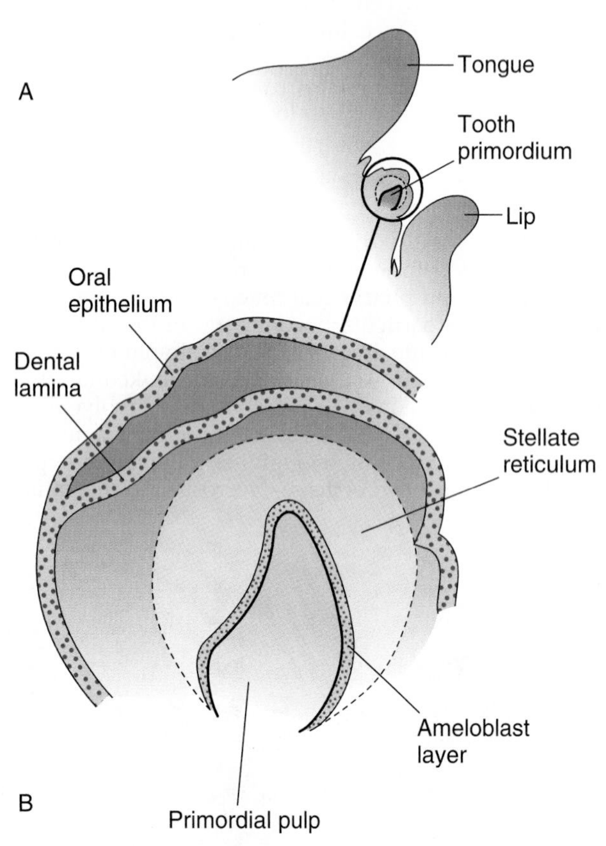

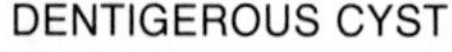

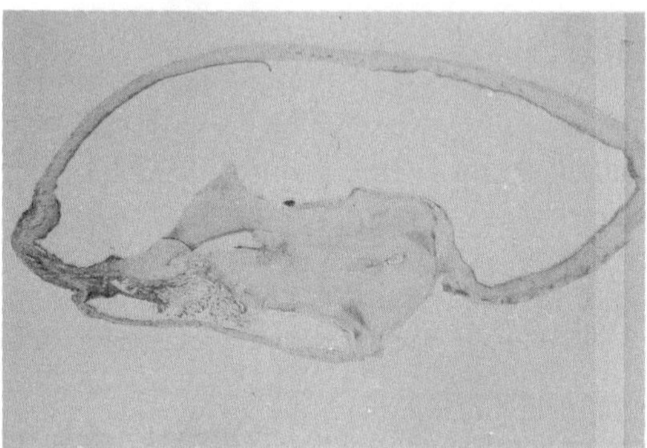

AMELOBLASTOMA

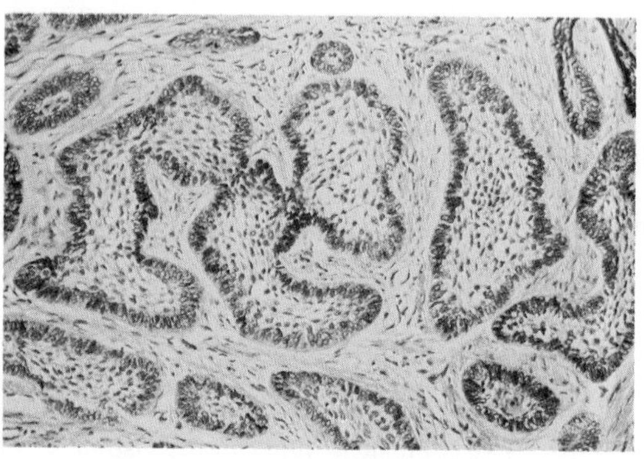

FIGURE 25-15
Development of teeth and odontogenic tumors. Diagrammatic representation of the normal development of a tooth and the mode of formation of a dentigerous cyst and ameloblastoma. (*A*) Sagittal section of the lower jaw of a human embryo at 14 weeks, through the primordium of the lower central incisor. (*B*) Higher-power representation of the circled area in *A*. The enamel organ at this stage is a double-walled sac, composed of an outer convex wall and an inner concave wall. Between the two are looser ectodermal cells (stellate reticulum). The stellate reticulum gives rise to dentigerous cysts, whereas the ameloblasts may form an ameloblastoma.

tween the crown and the overlying enamel epithelium (see Fig. 25-15). Dentigerous cysts tend to be unilocular and are lined by a thin layer of stratified squamous epithelium. Pressure by an enlarging cyst can cause marked resorption of bone and adjacent teeth. Among the potential complications of a dentigerous cyst are (1) recurrence after incomplete removal, (2) the development of an ameloblastoma from the cyst lining or from epithelial rests of Malassez, and (3) progression to squamous cell carcinoma.

AMELOBLASTOMA: *Ameloblastoma is a tumor of the jaws derived from odontogenic epithelium, most likely from cell rests of the enamel organ.* Rare cases have been reported in other sites, such as the long bones and sella turcica.

☐ **Pathology:** The large majority of ameloblastomas arise in the mandible, and most of these occur in the ramus or molar area. Ameloblastomas in the maxilla are most common in the molar area, but they can also involve the maxillary antrum or floor of the nasal cavity. The tumor tends to grow slowly as a central lesion of bone. Radiographs show a multilocular cyst-like appearance, with a smooth periphery, expansion of the bone, and thinning of the cortex.

Microscopically, ameloblastoma resembles the enamel organ in its various stages of differentiation, and a single tumor may show various histological patterns. Accordingly, the tumor cells resemble ameloblasts at the periphery of the epithelial nests or cords, where columnar cells are oriented perpendicular to the basement membrane (Fig. 25-16). The centers of these cell nests consist of loosely arranged, larger, polyhedral cells, which resemble the stellate reticulum of the developing tooth. Frequently, the complete breakdown of these looser areas results in the formation of microcysts.

The prognosis of ameloblastoma is favorable. Incompletely excised tumors recur, but malignant transformation does not occur.

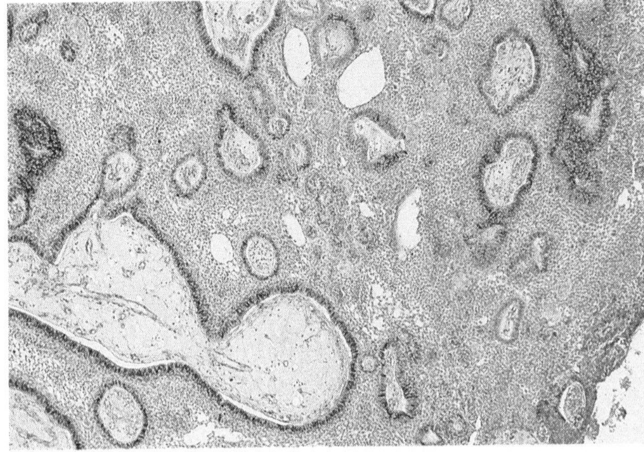

FIGURE *25-16*
Ameloblastoma. A common histological pattern is characterized by confluent islands of epithelium. The peripheral cells form bands that separate the tumor from the stroma.

Salivary Glands

The salivary glands, which develop as buds of the oral ectoderm, are tubuloalveolar structures that secrete saliva. The major salivary glands are paired organs. The parotid glands secrete serous saliva, whereas the submandibular and sublingual glands produce mixed serous and mucous saliva. The minor salivary glands are widespread, being present under the mucosa of the lips, cheeks, palate, and tongue.

XEROSTOMIA: *Xerostomia refers to chronic dryness of the mouth from the lack of saliva and has many causes.* Diseases that involve the major salivary glands and produce xerostomia include mumps, Sjögren syndrome, sarcoidosis, radiation-induced atrophy (Fig. 25-17), and drug sensitivity (antihistamines, tricyclic antidepressants, hypotensive drugs, phenothiazines).

SIALORRHEA: Increased salivary flow is associated with many conditions, for example, acute inflammation of the oral cavity, as in aphthous stomatitis, Parkinson disease, rabies, mental retardation, nausea, and pregnancy.

ENLARGEMENT: Unilateral enlargement of the major salivary glands is due to inflammation, cysts, or neoplasms. Bilateral enlargement is caused by inflammation

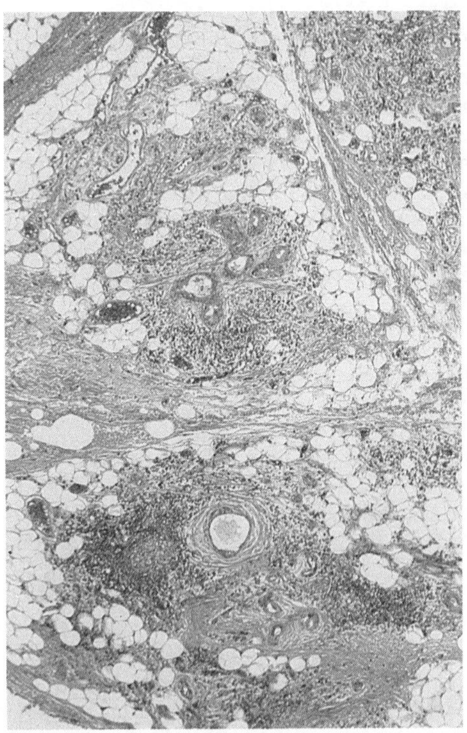

FIGURE *25-17*
Chronic sialadenitis. Severe chronic inflammation and marked atrophy of the submandibular gland are present after irradiation of an adjacent oral cancer. The atrophic acini have been replaced by fat.

(mumps, Sjögren syndrome), granulomatous disease (sarcoidosis), or diffuse neoplastic involvement (leukemia or malignant lymphoma).

SIALOLITHIASIS: Calcific stones occur in the ducts of salivary glands, most commonly in the submandibular gland. The etiology of sialolithiasis is unknown, although in some instances stones have been found around a foreign body. The most important consequence of stone formation is obstruction of the duct, often followed by inflammation distal to the occlusion.

PAROTITIS: Acute suppurative parotitis is caused by the ascent of bacteria, usually *S. aureus*, from the oral cavity when the salivary flow is reduced. It is most frequently seen in debilitated or postoperative patients. Acute and chronic parotitis is often associated with stricture of the salivary ducts or obstruction by stones. The stagnant secretions serve as a medium for retrograde bacterial invasion.

Epidemic parotitis (mumps) is an acute viral disease of the parotid glands, which spreads with infected saliva. The submandibular and sublingual salivary glands also may be involved. In addition to infection of the salivary glands in mumps, pancreatitis and orchitis are not uncommon. Microscopically, the salivary glands are densely infiltrated by lymphocytes and macrophages and exhibit degenerative changes and necrosis of the epithelial cells. Mumps is discussed in more detail in Chapter 9.

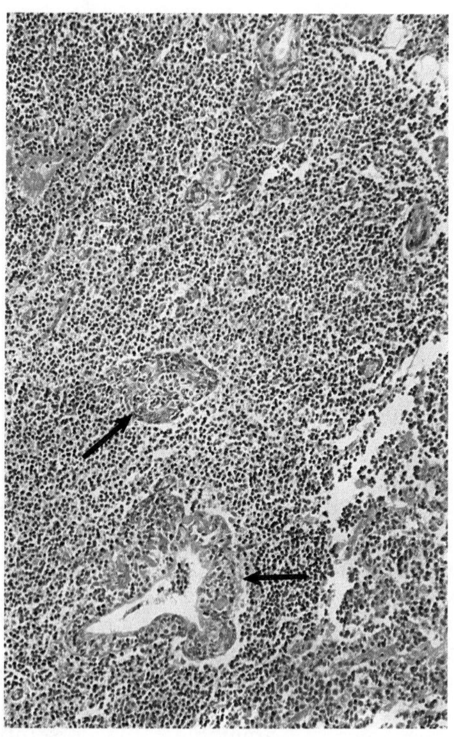

FIGURE *25-18*
Sjögren syndrome. A massive lymphoid infiltrate and epimyoepithelial islands (*arrows*) in the parotid gland are shown. Marked acinar atrophy caused xerostomia.

SJÖGREN SYNDROME

Sjögren syndrome is a chronic inflammatory disease of the salivary and lacrimal glands; it may be restricted to these sites or may be associated with a systemic collagen vascular disease. Involvement of the salivary glands leads to dry mouth (xerostomia), and disease of the lacrimal glands results in dry eyes (keratoconjunctivitis sicca). The pathogenesis and clinical features of Sjögren syndrome are discussed in Chapter 4; only the changes in the salivary glands are described here.

☐ **Pathology:** The parotid glands and sometimes the submandibular glands in Sjögren syndrome are unilaterally or bilaterally enlarged, but their lobular appearance is preserved. Contrast radiography of the salivary ducts reveals irregular dilatation of the ducts. Histologically, an initial periductal round cell infiltrate gradually extends to the acini, until the glands are completely replaced by a sea of polyclonal lymphocytes, immunoblasts, germinal centers, and plasma cells. Proliferating myoepithelial cells surround remnants of the damaged ducts and form so-called epimyoepithelial islands (Fig. 25-18). The term *benign lymphoepithelial lesion* has been introduced to describe these characteristic microscopic changes. Similar changes can be seen in the lacrimal glands and in the minor salivary glands. Focal lymphocytic sialadenitis can be demonstrated also in minor salivary glands obtained by labial biopsy in most patients with Sjögren syndrome (Fig. 25-19). Late in the course of the disease, the affected glands become atrophic, with fibrosis and fatty infiltration of the parenchyma.

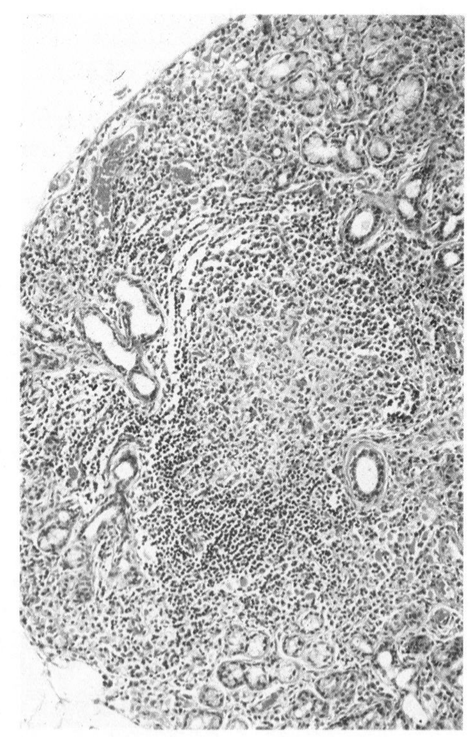

FIGURE *25-19*
Sjögren syndrome. A lip biopsy shows lobules of mucous glands infiltrated by lymphocytes and plasma cells. Slightly dilated ducts without acini indicate glandular atrophy.

Mikulicz syndrome *refers to a symmetric enlargement of the salivary and lacrimal glands due to a specific disease, such as leukemic infiltrates, malignant lymphoma, amyloidosis, tuberculosis, or sarcoidosis.* The use of this term in such situations is not warranted, because it is ambiguous.

PLEOMORPHIC ADENOMA (MIXED TUMOR)

Pleomorphic adenoma, the most common tumor of the salivary glands, is a benign neoplasm characterized by a biphasic appearance, which represents an admixture of epithelial and stromal elements. Two thirds of all tumors of the major salivary glands, and about half of those in the minor ones, are pleomorphic adenomas. The tumor is nine times more frequent in the parotid than in the submandibular gland and usually arises in the superficial lobe of the parotid. It occurs most frequently in middle-aged persons and shows a female preponderance.

☐ **Pathology:** Pleomorphic adenoma is seen as a slowly growing, painless, movable, firm mass, which has a smooth surface. Those tumors that arise deep in the parotid gland may grow between the ramus of the mandible and the styloid process and stylomandibular ligament into the parapharyngeal space, seen as a swelling of the lateral pharyngeal or tonsillar region.

Microscopically, pleomorphic adenoma shows a mixture of epithelial tissue intermingled with myxoid, mucoid, or chondroid areas (Fig. 25-20). The older term, mixed tumor, referred to this peculiar mixture of epithelial cells and mesenchymal ground substance. However, the neoplasm is now considered to be of epithelial origin: hence the label "adenoma."

The epithelial component of pleomorphic adenoma consists of two cell types, ductal and myoepithelial cells. The cells lining the ducts form tubules or small cystic structures and contain clear fluid or eosinophilic, periodic acid–Schiff (PAS)-positive material. Around the epithelial cells of the ducts are smaller myoepithelial cells, which constitute the main cellular component. The myoepithelial cells form well-defined sheaths, cords, or nests (Fig. 25-21), and often they are separated by a cellular ground substance, which resembles cartilaginous, myxoid, or mucoid material and appears to be the product of the myoepithelial cells.

☐ **Clinical Features:** Pleomorphic adenomas have a fibrous capsule, and as they grow, the surrounding fibrous tissue condenses around them. The tumors become larger and tend to protrude focally into the adjacent tissues, thereby becoming nodular (Fig. 25-22). At surgery, these tumor projections can be missed, if the tumor is not carefully dissected to leave an intact capsule and an adequate margin of surrounding glandular parenchyma. Tu-

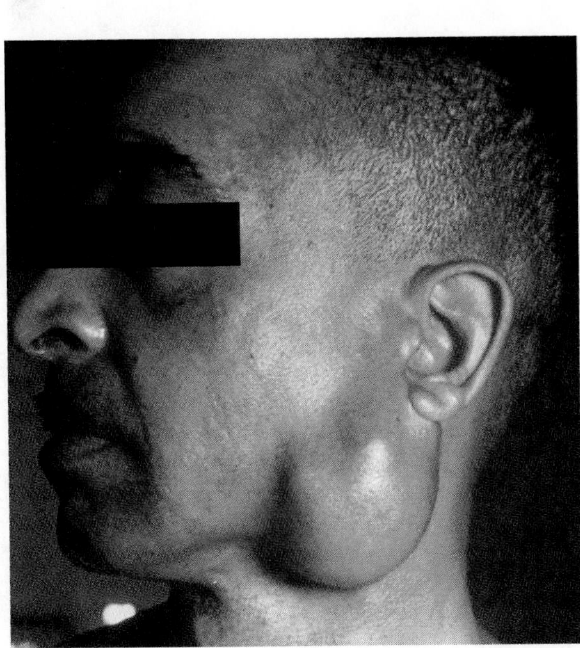

A

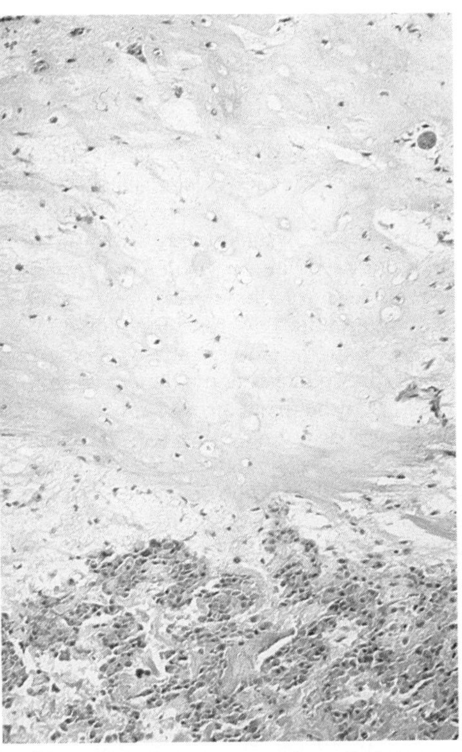

B

FIGURE *25-20*
Pleomorphic adenoma of the parotid. (*A*) A conspicuous tumor mass is seen at the angle of the jaw. (*B*) A microscopic view shows myoepithelial cells embedded in a myxoid stroma, which is adjacent to a chondroid area (*top*).

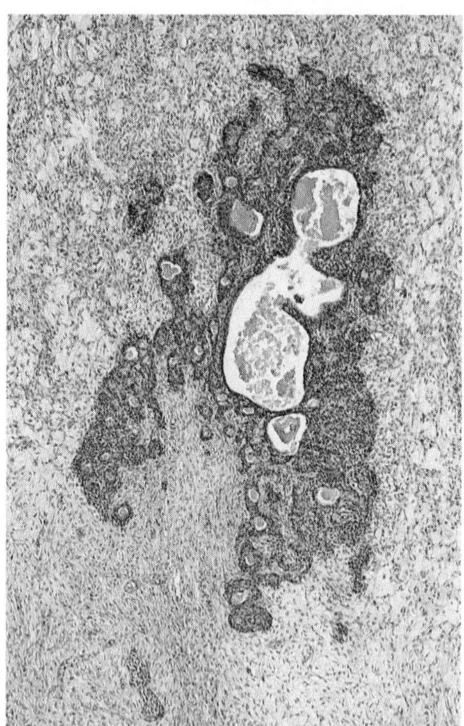

FIGURE 25-21
Pleomorphic adenoma of the parotid gland. Many myoepithelial cells have a fusiform appearance and are partly dispersed in a mucoid background. Nests of dark myoepithelial cells surround dilated ducts that contain eosinophilic material.

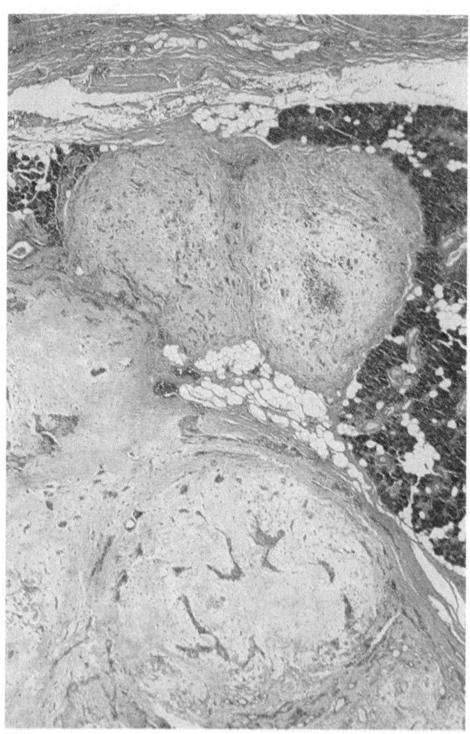

FIGURE 25-22
Pleomorphic adenoma of the parotid gland. The tumor contains characteristic myxoid and chondroid portions. The tumor is partly encapsulated, but a nodule protruding into the parotid gland lacks a capsule. If such nodules are not included in the resection, the tumor will recur.

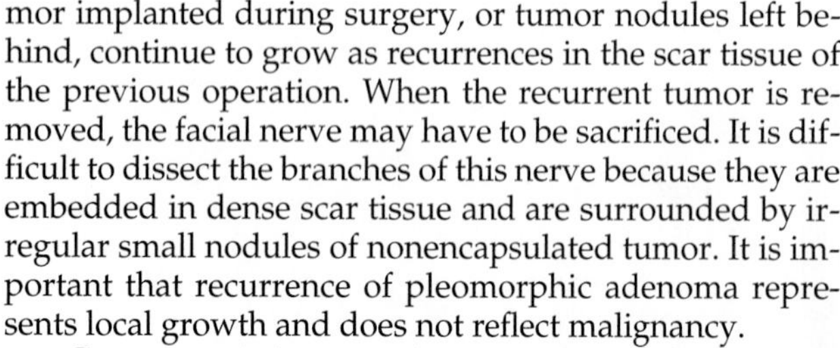

mor implanted during surgery, or tumor nodules left behind, continue to grow as recurrences in the scar tissue of the previous operation. When the recurrent tumor is removed, the facial nerve may have to be sacrificed. It is difficult to dissect the branches of this nerve because they are embedded in dense scar tissue and are surrounded by irregular small nodules of nonencapsulated tumor. It is important that recurrence of pleomorphic adenoma represents local growth and does not reflect malignancy.

On rare occasions, carcinomas arise in pleomorphic adenomas. A pleomorphic adenoma that has been present for many years may begin to grow rapidly or become painful. Histological examination reveals an unequivocal carcinoma in an otherwise benign pleomorphic adenoma. These tumors are usually adenocarcinomas, but mucoepidermoid or adenoid cystic carcinomas also may develop in pleomorphic adenomas.

MONOMORPHIC ADENOMA

A small proportion (5% to 10%) of benign epithelial tumors of the salivary glands consist of epithelium arranged in a regular, usually glandular, pattern without a mesenchyme-like component.

ADENOLYMPHOMA (WARTHIN TUMOR): *Warthin tumor is a benign neoplasm of the parotid gland composed of cystic glandular spaces embedded in dense lymphoid tissue.*

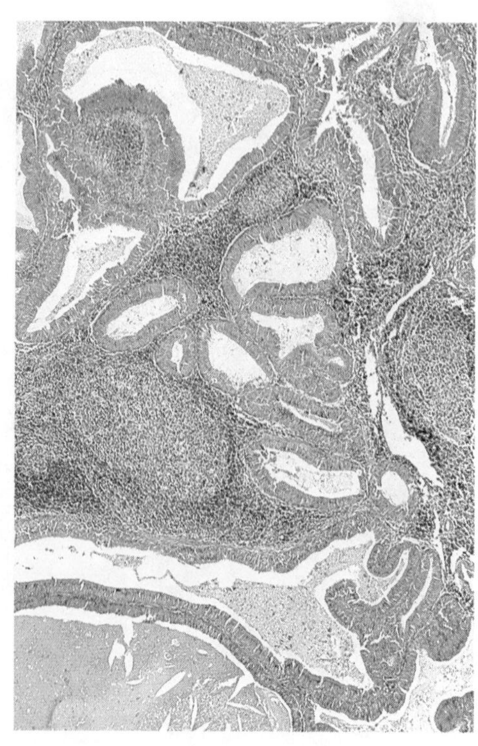

FIGURE 25-23
Adenolymphoma (Warthin tumor). Cystic spaces and duct-like structures are lined by oncocytes. Follicular lymphoid tissue is present.

This tumor is the most common monomorphic adenoma. Although the tumor is clearly benign, it can be bilateral (15% of cases) or multifocal within the same gland. Adenolymphoma is the only tumor of the salivary glands that is more common in men than in women. Adenolymphomas generally occur after the age of 30 years, with the majority arising after age 50 years.

The tumor is composed of glandular spaces, which tend to become cystic and show papillary projections. The cysts are lined by characteristic eosinophilic epithelial cells (oncocytes) and are embedded in dense lymphoid tissue with germinal centers (Fig. 25-23).

The histogenesis of this peculiar tumor has been much debated. Lymph nodes, which are normally found in the parotid gland and in its immediate vicinity, usually contain a few ducts or small islands of salivary gland tissue. It has been suggested that adenolymphomas arise from the proliferation of these salivary gland inclusions.

ONCOCYTOMA (OXYPHIL ADENOMA): These rare benign tumors are composed of nests or cords of oncocytes, most of which occur in the parotid glands of elderly persons. Oncocytes are benign epithelial cells that are swollen with mitochondria, which impart a granular appearance to the cytoplasm. They can be found scattered or in small clusters among the epithelial cells of various normal organs (e.g., the thyroid and parathyroid glands). For unknown reasons, oncocytes begin to appear in early adulthood, and their number increases with age. Their function is unknown.

MALIGNANT TUMORS

Mucoepidermoid Carcinoma

Mucoepidermoid carcinoma is a malignant salivary gland tumor composed of a mixture of neoplastic squamous cells, mucus-secreting cells, and epithelial cells of an intermediate type. Mucoepidermoid tumors probably originate from ductal epithelium, which has a considerable potential for metaplasia. They account for 5% to 10% of major salivary gland tumors and 10% of those in the minor salivary glands. Within the major salivary glands, more than half of mucoepidermoid carcinomas arise in the parotid gland. In the minor salivary glands, they develop most frequently in the palate. Although the tumor may occur in adolescents, most tumors are seen in adults and are more common in women.

□ **Pathology:** Mucoepidermoid carcinoma grows slowly and is seen as a firm painless mass. Microscopically, well-differentiated tumors form irregular duct-like and cystic spaces that are lined by squamous or mucus-secreting cells (Fig. 25-24). Poorly differentiated carcinomas contain few mucus-secreting cells and resemble squamous cell carcinomas.

Even well-differentiated mucoepidermoid carcinomas can metastasize, but the 5-year survival is better than 90%, regardless of the primary site. However, poorly differentiated mucoepidermoid carcinomas have a much lower survival rate (20% to 40%).

ADENOID CYSTIC CARCINOMA (CYLINDROMA)

Adenoid cystic carcinoma is a slowly growing malignant neoplasm of the salivary gland, which is notorious for its tendency to invade locally and to recur after surgical resection. Adenoid cystic carcinoma constitutes 5% of all tumors of the major salivary glands and 20% of those of the minor salivary glands. Of all adenoid cystic carcinomas, one third arise in the major salivary glands and two thirds in the minor ones. These tumors not only occur in the oral cavity but also arise in the lacrimal glands, nasopharynx, nasal cavity, paranasal sinuses, and lower respiratory tract. They are most common in persons between 40 and 60 years of age.

□ **Pathology:** Histologically, adenoid cystic carcinomas present varying patterns. The tumor cells are small, have scant cytoplasm, and grow in solid sheets or as small groups, strands, or columns. Within these structures, the tumor cells interconnect to enclose cystic spaces, resulting in a solid, tubular or cribriform (sieve-like) arrangement (Fig. 25-25). These two types are replicated in different combinations, resulting in various histological patterns. The tumor cells produce a homogeneous basement membrane material that gives them the characteristic cylindromatous appearance.

The tumors probably originate from cells that are differentiating toward intercalated ducts and toward

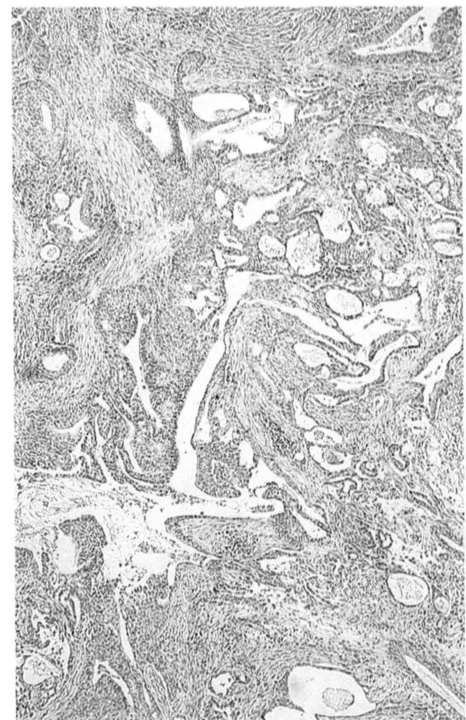

FIGURE **25-24**
Mucoepidermoid carcinoma of a minor salivary gland. This tumor invades the fibrous stroma and forms irregular duct-like and cystic spaces. The cysts, lined by squamous and mucus-secreting cells, contain mucus.

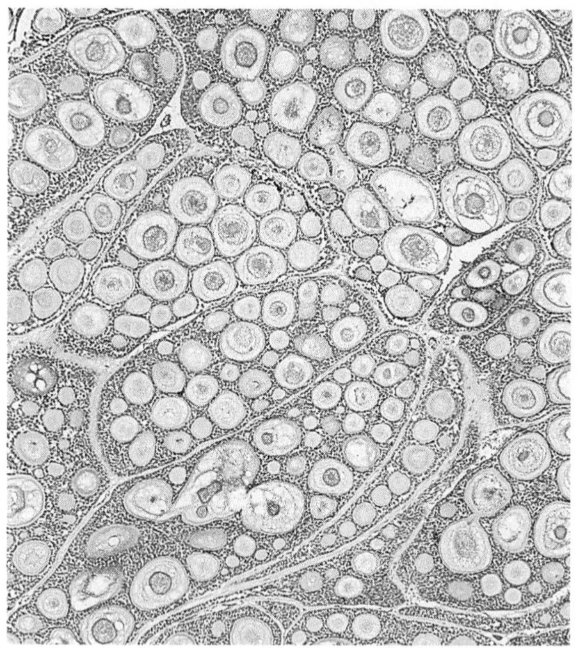

FIGURE 25-25
Adenoid cystic carcinoma of the palate. The tumor shows a cribriform arrangement, duct-like structures, and small groups of cells in a dense stroma.

myoepithelium. Adenoid cystic carcinoma tends to infiltrate the perineural spaces (Fig. 25-26) and is frequently painful. For these reasons, the tumors are often diagnosed in an advanced stage. Although most adenoid cystic carcinomas do not metastasize for many years, they are difficult to eradicate completely, and their long-term prognosis is poor.

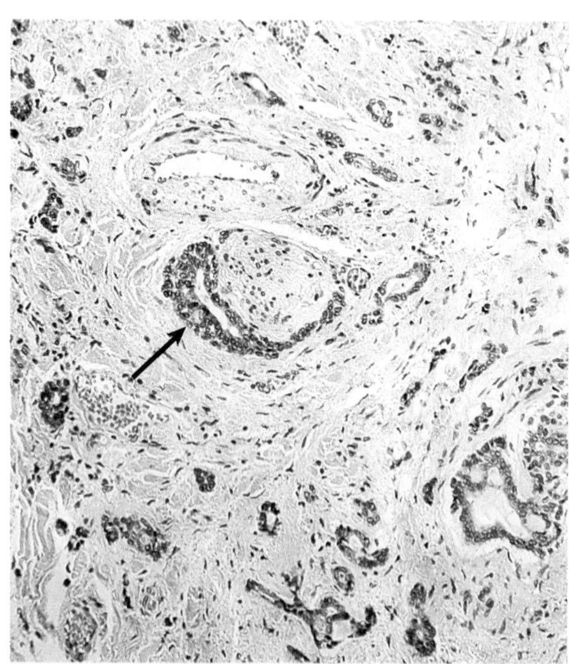

FIGURE 25-26
Adenoid cystic carcinoma. A photomicrograph shows perineural infiltration by the tumor (*arrow*).

ACINIC CELL CARCINOMA

Acinic cell carcinoma is an uncommon tumor of the parotid gland (1% to 3% of all salivary gland tumors), which arises from the epithelial secretory cells of the gland. It is occasionally encountered in the other salivary glands. The tumor occurs principally in young men between the ages of 20 and 30 years. It is seen as an encapsulated, round mass, usually smaller than 3 cm across, and is sometimes cystic. Microscopically, acinic cell carcinomas are composed of uniform cells with a small central nucleus and abundant basophilic cytoplasm, similar to the secretory (acinic) cells of the normal salivary glands. The tumor metastasizes to the regional lymph nodes.

After surgical resection of the tumor, the large majority (90%) of patients survive for 5 years, but local recurrence may be expected in one third of the patients, and only half survive for 20 years.

Intraparotid Lymph Nodes

Lymph nodes are normally embedded in the parotid gland. They drain the eyelids, the frontotemporal region, and the external ear canal. The intraparotid lymph nodes may be involved in a variety of inflammatory, reactive, or proliferative processes, including malignant lymphoma. They also may become enlarged by leukemic infiltrates. Rarely intraparotid lymph nodes harbor metastatic tumor, particularly malignant melanoma from primary sites in the face or scalp.

Nose and Paranasal Sinuses

ANATOMY

The apertures of the nostrils (anterior nares) lead into the nasal vestibule, a space lined by skin that contains hairs and sebaceous glands. Beyond the nares, the nasal cavity is divided by the median septum into two symmetric chambers, termed the nasal fossae. Each nasal fossa has an olfactory region, consisting of the superior nasal concha and the opposed part of the septum, and a respiratory region, which comprises the rest of the cavity. On the lateral wall are the inferior, middle, and superior nasal conchae (turbinates), overhanging the corresponding nasal passages or meatuses.

The paranasal sinuses are paired air spaces that communicate with the nasal cavity through ostia as follows:

- The nasolacrimal duct opens into the inferior meatus.
- The maxillary sinus, the frontal sinus, and the anterior ethmoid air cells open into the middle meatus.
- The sphenoid sinuses communicate with the sphenoethmoid recess or posterior ethmoid air cells.

The mucous membrane covering the respiratory portion of the nasal cavity has a ciliated, columnar epithelium

TABLE 25-1 **Pathological Processes in the Nose and Paranasal Sinuses and Their Relation to Adjacent Structures**

Nasopharynx ⇌ Nasal cavity	⇌ Maxillary sinus ⇌ Intraorbital, oral, and odontogenic disease
	⇌ Ethmoid sinuses ⇌ Intraorbital and intracranial disease
	⇌ Frontal sinus ⇌ Intraorbital and intracranial disease
	⇌ Sphenoid sinus ⇌ Cranial and intracranial disease

with interspersed goblet cells. The underlying lamina propria is rich in mucous glands and blood vessels. The paranasal sinuses are likewise lined by ciliated columnar epithelium, but their lamina propria lacks a rich vascular plexus. The ostia of the sinuses can be obstructed by mucosal swelling (e.g., edema caused by inflammation), tumor, or foreign body. The anatomical interrelations favor certain routes of spread of disease and therefore play an important role in the development of complications (Table 25-1; Fig. 25-27).

DISEASES OF THE EXTERNAL NOSE AND NASAL VESTIBULE

Virtually all diseases of the skin can occur on the external nose, including lesions due to solar damage (e.g., actinic keratosis, basal cell carcinoma, squamous cell carcinoma, and malignant melanoma). The numerous sebaceous glands of the nose are a frequent site of acne vulgaris.

Rhinophyma refers to a protuberant bulbous mass on the nose caused by marked hyperplasia of the sebaceous glands and chronic inflammation of the skin in acne rosacea.

Pyogenic granuloma is an inflammatory lesion often seen on the anterior nasal septum. It appears clinically to be an ulcerated capillary hemangioma but is actually exuberant granulation tissue secondary to trauma.

NOSEBLEED (EPISTAXIS): Trauma of the nose or to the nasal mucosa is the most common cause of nosebleed. Hypertension, a variety of hematological abnormalities, inflammatory conditions, and neoplastic diseases of the nasal mucosa may cause bleeding from the nose. Epistaxis frequently originates in a triangular area of the anterior nasal septum called Little's area. In this region, the epidermis is thin, and not infrequently numerous dilated blood vessels, or telangiectasias, are apparent. Little's area is also the location of ulcerations and perforations, which may be caused by various diseases or by trauma to the nasal septum (Table 25-2).

DISEASES OF THE NASAL CAVITY AND PARANASAL SINUSES

Rhinitis

Rhinitis is defined as inflammation of the mucous membranes of the nasal cavity and sinuses. The causes range from the com-

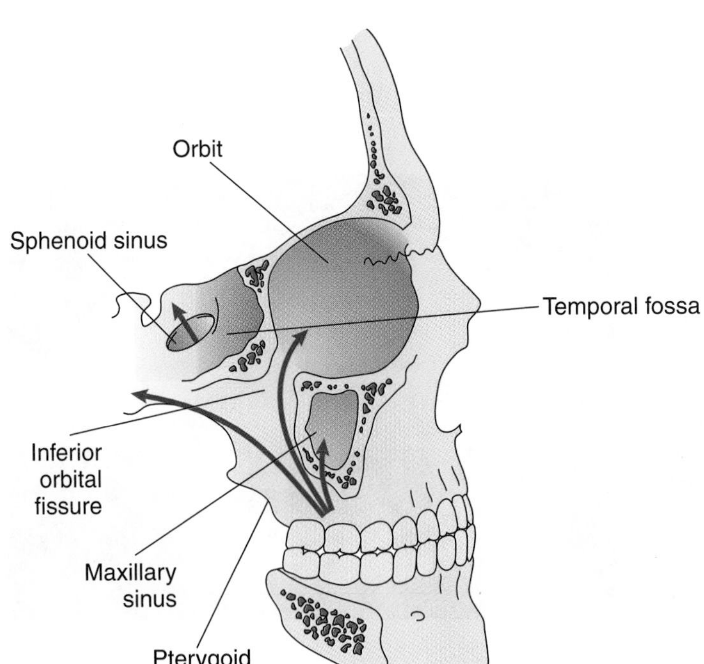

FIGURE 25-27
Pathways of infection to the intracranial cavity. Osseous pathways of infection from the jaws. *Arrows*, the direction of spread from the teeth to the maxillary sinus (1) and through the inferior orbital fissure to the orbit (2). A deeper route (3) is along the lateral pterygoid lamina up to the base of the skull, where, medial to the foramen ovale, a small aperture admits the vein of Vesalius. Through this small vein, the pterygoid plexus communicates with the cavernous sinus.

TABLE 25-2 **Causes of Perforation of the Nasal Septum**

Trauma
Specific infections (tuberculosis, syphilis, leprosy)
Wegener granulomatosis
Lupus erythematosus
Chronic exposure to dust (containing arsenic, chromium, copper, etc.)
Cocaine abuse
Malignant tumors

mon cold to unusual infections such as diphtheria, anthrax, and glanders.

VIRAL RHINITIS: The most common cause of acute rhinitis is viral infection, especially the common cold *(acute coryza)*. In viral rhinitis, the agent replicates in the epithelial cells, after which the degenerating epithelial cells are shed. The mucosa is edematous and engorged and is infiltrated by neutrophils and mononuclear cells. Clinically, mucosal swelling is manifested as nasal stuffiness. Abundant mucus secretion and increased vascular permeability lead to *rhinorrhea* (the free discharge of a thin nasal mucus).

Viral rhinitis is usually followed within a few days by secondary infections caused by the normal denizens of the nasal and pharyngeal mucus. The abundant serous discharge then becomes mucopurulent, after which the surface epithelium is shed. The epithelial cells regenerate rapidly after the inflammation subsides.

ALLERGIC RHINITIS: Numerous allergens are constantly present in our environment, and sensitivity to any one of them can cause allergic rhinitis. In this condition, airborne allergenic particles (e.g., pollens, molds, animal allergens) are deposited on the nasal mucosa. Often called *hay fever*, allergic rhinitis may be acute and seasonal or chronic and perennial.

The few plasma cells present in the nasal mucosa normally produce immunoglobulin E (IgE). Mast cells in the nasal mucosa or free in nasal secretions also bear specific IgE directed against allergens. On contact with an allergen, the mast cells release cytoplasmic granules containing a variety of chemical mediators and enzymes. Some mediators are preformed and thus rapidly acting (e.g., histamine); others are slowly eluted from the granule matrix (e.g., heparin or trypsin); and still others are newly synthesized (e.g., leukotrienes). Thus, an immediate, rapidly apparent reaction may give way to a prolonged inflammatory reaction as the various mediators exert their specific effects. The released mediators cause the signs and symptoms of allergic rhinitis, and many of the responses are attributable to histamine acting through its H_1 receptor.

The increased capillary permeability mediated by vasodilator substances results in edema of the nasal mucosa, especially of the inferior turbinates. Microscopic examination of the nasal secretions or mucosa reveals numerous eosinophils. The late phase of mast cell–mediated reactions is associated with persistent edema of the nasal mucosa and is seen clinically as nasal obstruction.

CHRONIC RHINITIS: Repeated bouts of acute rhinitis may lead to the development of chronic rhinitis. Often a deviated nasal septum is a contributory factor. Chronic rhinitis is characterized by thickening of the nasal mucosa because of persistent hyperemia, hyperplasia of the mucous glands, and infiltration by lymphocytes and plasma cells.

Nasal Polyps

Nasal polyps are focal inflammatory swellings of the mucosa of the nose or paranasal sinuses.

ALLERGIC POLYPS: Recurrent allergic reactions cause chronic mucosal edema and enlargement of the turbinates, eventually leading to localized bulgings of the mucosa and the formation of polyps. Allergic polyps of the nose are usually multiple and appear as smooth, pale, movable, rounded tumors (Fig. 25-28), which protrude into the airway and cause symptoms of nasal obstruction. They may be sessile or pedunculated, although the stalk is often not well seen. Microscopically, allergic polyps are lined externally by respiratory epithelium and contain mucous glands within a loose mucoid stroma, which is infiltrated by plasma cells, lymphocytes, and numerous eosinophils. Thickening of the basement membrane and goblet cell hyperplasia are usually prominent (Fig. 25-29).

NONALLERGIC POLYPS: These lesions arise in cases of chronic rhinitis and chronic sinusitis and are not related to allergic diseases of the nose. In most respects, they are morphologically similar to allergic polyps. There is a variable infiltrate of neutrophils, lymphocytes, and plasma cells in the superficial tissue, but eosinophils may be lacking.

Sinusitis

Sinusitis refers to an inflammation of the mucous membranes of the paranasal sinuses. Any condition (inflammation, neo-

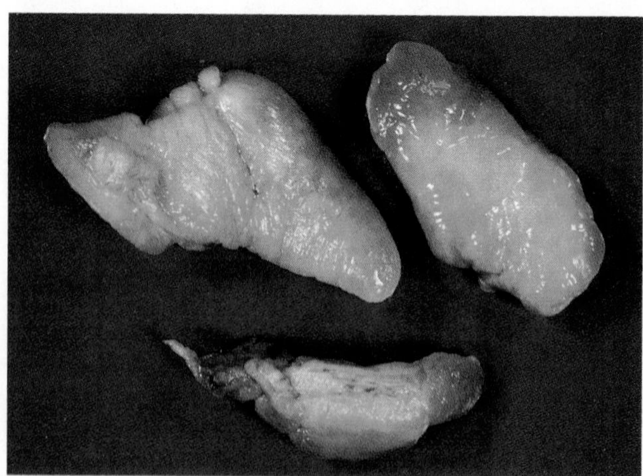

FIGURE 25-28
Nasal polyps. These smooth, pale, polypoid masses were removed from a patient with chronic rhinitis.

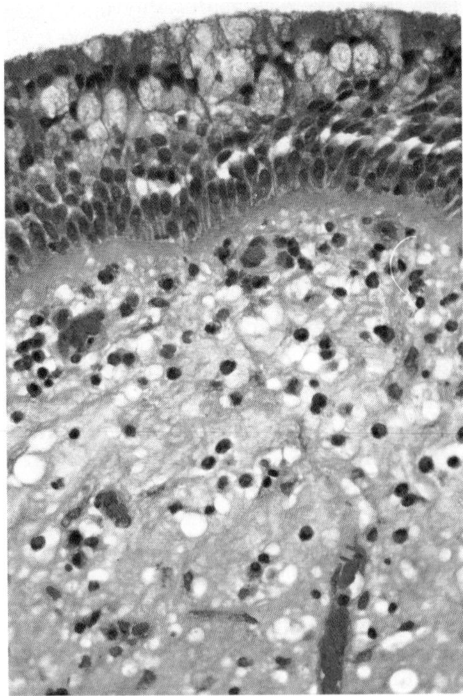

FIGURE 25-29
Nasal polyp. The ciliated respiratory epithelium has been replaced by goblet cells. The basement membrane is thickened, and the edematous stroma is infiltrated by many eosinophils.

plasm, foreign body) that interferes with drainage or aeration of a sinus renders it liable to infection. If the ostium of a sinus is blocked, the secretion or exudate accumulates behind the obstruction.

Acute sinusitis is a disorder of less than 3 weeks' duration, caused predominantly by the extension of infection from the nasal mucosa. In most cases, a rich bacterial flora is found, with *Haemophilus influenzae* and *Branhamella catarrhalis* most frequently present. Maxillary sinusitis may also be due to odontogenic infections, in which case, bacteria from the roots of the first and second molar teeth penetrate the thin bony plate that separates them from the floor of the maxillary sinus.

Chronic sinusitis is a sequel of acute inflammation, either as a result of incomplete resolution of the infection or because of recurrent acute complications. In contrast to acute sinusitis, the purulent exudate in chronic sinusitis almost always includes anaerobic bacteria. Acute or chronic sinusitis may be followed by a number of complications:

- **Mucocele:** *This term refers to the accumulation of mucous secretions in a nasal sinus.* Infection of a mucocele results in a sinus filled with mucopurulent exudate, termed *pyocele*. Purulent exudate in the sinus is termed *empyema* (Fig. 25-30). Mucoceles occur most often in the anterior compartments ("cells") of the ethmoid sinus and in the frontal sinus. The lesions develop slowly and by pressure cause resorption of bone (pressure atrophy). Mucoceles of the anterior ethmoid or frontal sinuses may be large enough to displace the contents of the orbit.
- **Osteomyelitis:** Bone infection results from the extension of a suppurative infection in the frontal sinus to the bone. Infection of the walls of a nasal sinus may spread through Volkmann canals to the periosteum, producing periostitis and a subperiosteal abscess. If these occur on the orbital side of the bone, orbital cellulitis or an orbital abscess forms. The skin overlying the infection is often markedly edematous, and subcutaneous cellulitis or a subcutaneous abscess also may develop. Osteomyelitis also may spread rapidly between the outer and inner tables of the skull.
- **Septic thrombophlebitis:** Infection in the sinuses may penetrate the bone and spread to the frontal and diploe venous systems. The spread of septic thrombophlebitis to the cavernous venous sinus through the superior ophthalmic veins is a life-threatening complication.
- **Intracranial infections:** Spread of infection to the cranial cavity also may complicate sinusitis. Lesions include epidural, subdural, and cerebral abscesses and purulent leptomeningitis. These consequences may develop without extensive destruction of the bone, because the infection can spread through the lymphatics or veins. Before the days of chemotherapy, these dreaded complications often led to death within a few days. With proper treatment, they are today uncommon.

Tuberculosis

Tuberculous infection of the nose is almost always the result of tuberculosis of the lungs, from which the tubercle

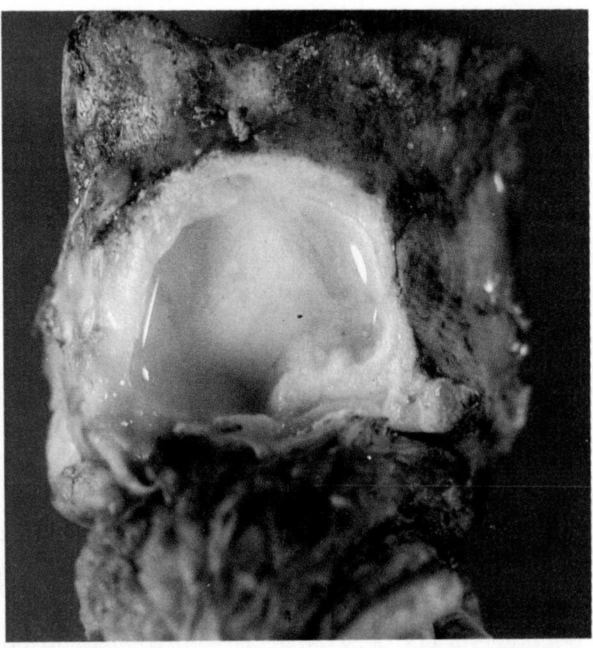

FIGURE 25-30
Empyema of the maxillary sinus (sagittal section). Infection followed chronic obstruction of the orifice caused by adenocarcinoma of the nasal mucosa.

bacilli spread by droplet infection. Tuberculosis of the facial skin, called *lupus vulgaris*, may spread to the nasal vestibule and then to the nasal mucosa. Granulomatous tuberculosis of the nasal mucosa usually originates on the anterior nasal septum. If the tuberculous lesion in the vestibule heals, scar formation and retraction may cause a deformity that narrows or even occludes the nostrils. Tuberculous infection may spread into the paranasal sinuses or along the nasolacrimal duct to cause tuberculous dacryocystitis and conjunctivitis. For more details, see Chapter 9.

Syphilis

Although a primary chancre in the nose is rare, the mucosal lesions of secondary syphilis are commonly observed in the nose and nasopharynx. In tertiary syphilis, the inflammatory process may involve large portions of the nasal mucosa, the underlying cartilage, and bone. Perichondrial or periosteal gummas may destroy nasal cartilage and bone. The ensuing collapse of the nasal bridge produces so-called saddle nose. Destruction of the bony walls of the nose may also lead to perforation of the nasal septum, hard palate, wall of the orbit, or maxillary sinus. For the full spectrum of syphilis, see Chapter 9.

Leprosy

Because *Mycobacterium leprae* multiplies more readily at a lower body temperature, it frequently infects cooler body sites, such as the nares and the anterior nasal mucosa. Indeed, nasal involvement is commonly the first manifestation of leprosy. The skin around the nares and the anterior nasal mucosa shows nodules, ulceration, or perforations. Nasal involvement is important because leprosy is spread through nasal secretions that teem with bacilli. Tuberculoid and intermediate forms of leprosy, which compose the majority of cases, are microscopically characterized by chronic granulomatous inflammation. Patients with deficient cellular immunity develop lepromatous leprosy, in which numerous foamy macrophages, so-called lepra cells, contain many phagocytosed mycobacteria. Leprosy is discussed in more detail in Chapter 9.

Scleroma

Originally named rhinoscleroma, scleroma is a chronic inflammatory process that usually begins in the nose and remains localized to that site, although it may extend slowly into the nasopharynx, larynx, and trachea. Rarely scleroma is seen in other locations, including the paranasal sinuses, orbital tissues, skin, lips, oral mucosa, gastrointestinal tract, and cervical lymph nodes. Cases of intracranial invasion also have been described.

Scleroma is endemic in some Mediterranean countries and in parts of Asia, Africa, and Latin America. Indigenous cases also have been recognized in the United States. The disease occurs in both sexes and at any age. Poor domestic and personal hygiene are common to most patients. Epidemiological evidence suggests that household relationships are the decisive factor in the development of this disorder.

Although the gram-negative diplobacillus, *Klebsiella rhinoscleromatis*, also known as *von Frisch bacillus*, was identified more than a century ago, Koch's postulates were fulfilled only in the 1970s. Experimental disease was produced by repeatedly injecting bacilli suspended in sterile mucin into the same site. The organisms are present in the throats of many healthy persons, but the mode of transmission is unknown.

The infected tissues appear firm, greatly thickened, irregularly nodular, and often ulcerated. Microscopically, the granulation tissue is strikingly rich in plasma cells, lymphocytes, and foamy macrophages (Fig. 25-31). The characteristic large macrophages, referred to as *Mikulicz cells*, contain masses of phagocytosed bacilli.

Serological tests are valuable in establishing the diagnosis of scleroma, because specific antibodies are present in many patients. The disease is successfully treated with various antibiotics.

Fungal Infections

Pathogenic fungi occasionally involve the nose and paranasal sinuses as part of a cutaneous or mucocutaneous infection, particularly in immunodeficient persons.

Candidiasis is the most common fungal infection of the nasal mucosa, usually accompanying oral and pharyngeal candidiasis (thrush).

Aspergillosis is uncommon and usually occurs in a paranasal sinus. Aspergillus organisms may disseminate to the venous sinuses, meninges, and brain. This rare form of infection, termed rhinocerebral aspergillosis, has a high mortality rate.

Rhinosporidiosis of the nose is produced by the enigmatic *Rhinosporidium seeberi*, an organism whose

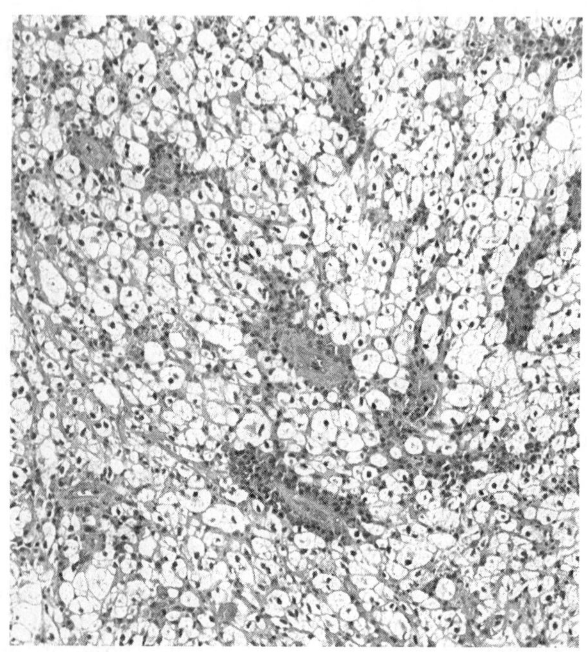

FIGURE *25-31*
Scleroma. Granulation tissue contains numerous foamy macrophages (Mikulicz cells).

source remains unknown. The microbe is classified among the fungi, although it has not been grown in culture and has not been transmitted experimentally. The disease is endemic in Sri Lanka and in parts of India, Central America, and South America.

The nasal mucosa afflicted with rhinosporidiosis contains vascular polyploid masses. Occasionally, similar lesions occur in the mucosa of other parts of the upper respiratory tract, the conjunctiva, the ear, or the skin. Microscopically, the polypoid masses show marked chronic inflammation and characteristic spherical sporangia. The sporangia, 50 to 350 μm in diameter, have a thick, homogeneous wall and contain clear cytoplasm and innumerable small endospores. The rupture of the sporangia evokes a foreign-body giant cell reaction. The treatment of choice is surgical removal of the lesions.

Leishmaniasis

The nose is a frequent site of the mucocutaneous form of leishmaniasis, caused by *Leishmania braziliensis* (see Chapter 9). The nasal disease, known as *espundia*, occurs in Central and South America. The initial lesion is a cutaneous sore, which heals within a few months. In some patients, mucocutaneous lesions develop in the nose or upper lip after an interval of months or years. The infection probably spreads by nasal contact with contaminated fingers.

The infected mucosa exhibits polypoid inflammatory lesions and superficial ulcers. In the earlier phases of the infection, many macrophages contain parasites. Later, a tuberculoid type of granulomatous response develops. Such lesions contain few recognizable parasites. Bacterial infection may supervene and lead to destruction of the soft tissues and collapse of the anterior cartilaginous nasal septum.

Wegener Granulomatosis

Wegener granulomatosis affects the upper airways (see Chapter 10). In its fully developed form, this uncommon disease involves the lungs, kidneys, and small arteries throughout the body. The disease is often first manifested as mucosal thickening and granulations in the nose. The resulting "runny nose," sinusitis, and nosebleeds may be accompanied by constitutional symptoms, such as fever, malaise, and weight loss. Microscopically, the nasal lesions reveal necrotizing granulomas with multinucleated giant cells.

Lethal Midline Granuloma (Polymorphic Reticulosis)

Lethal midline granuloma, also known as midline lethal reticulosis or polymorphic reticulosis, is a peripheral T-cell lymphoma that presents as necrotizing, ulcerating mucosal lesions of the upper respiratory tract (Fig. 25-32A). If untreated, the disease is invariably fatal. Although the designation "lethal

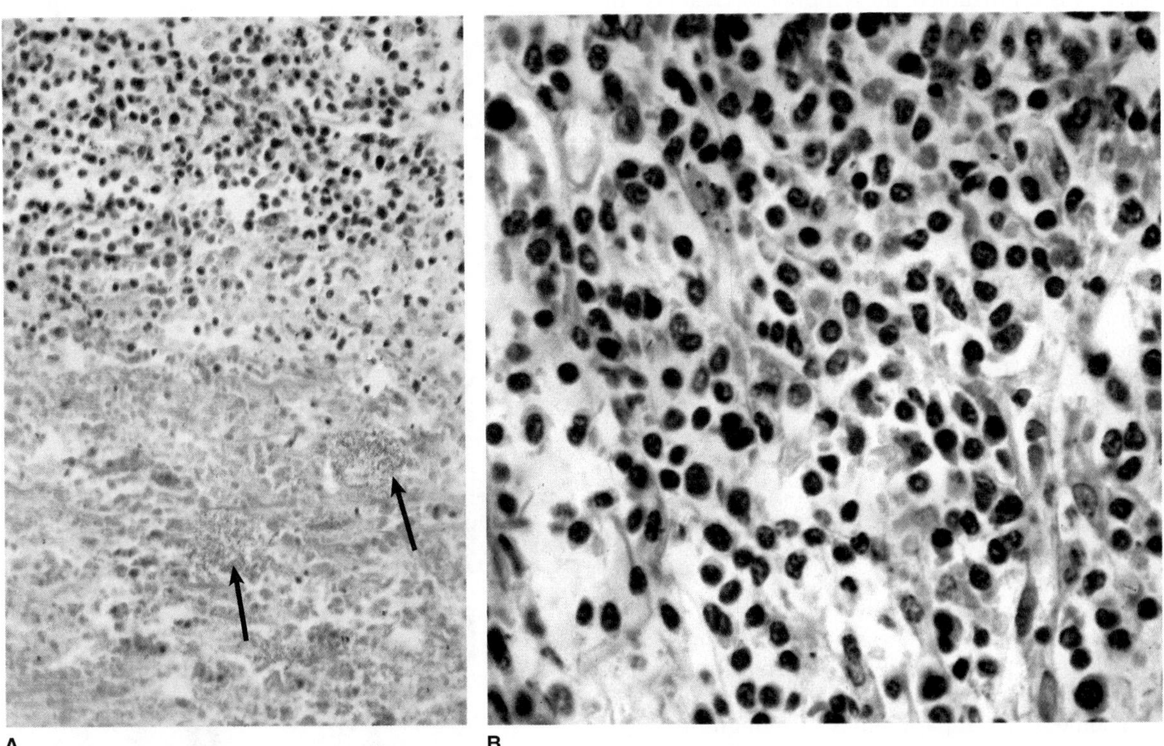

FIGURE 25-32
Lethal midline granuloma. (*A*) A cellular infiltrate of the nasal mucosa is covered by a crust of necrotic debris containing bacterial colonies (*arrows*). (*B*) A higher-power view of the cellular infiltrate in *A* demonstrates the polymorphism of the neoplastic lymphocytes.

midline granuloma" has occasionally been used in the literature to describe any clinical syndrome associated with destructive lesions of the nasal cavities, nasopharynx, palate, paranasal sinuses, or midface (e.g., Wegener granulomatosis, cocaine abuse, conventional malignant lymphoma), here we restrict the definition to an atypical peripheral T-cell lymphoma.

☐ **Pathology:** The polymorphism of the atypical T lymphocytes is a characteristic feature that distinguishes lethal midline granuloma from a conventional lymphoma (see Fig. 25-32B). Similar necrotizing infiltrates can also occur in the upper airways, lungs, and alimentary tract, but any organ may be involved, including the skin, lymph nodes, spleen, bone marrow, liver, kidneys, and central nervous system.

☐ **Clinical Features:** The clinical course of lethal midline granuloma is characterized by an insidious onset, with symptoms of nonspecific rhinitis or sinusitis. Gradually, the nasal mucosa becomes focally swollen and indurated and eventually ulcerated. The ulcers are covered by a black crust, under which the lesions progress to erode and destroy cartilage and bone. This destruction causes defects of the nasal septum, hard palate, and nasopharynx, with serious functional consequences. Frequently, the skin of the midface also becomes involved, hence the descriptive name. In half the patients, the disease remains localized, but an equal proportion exhibit widespread dissemination of the lymphoma. Death is due to secondary bacterial infection, aspiration pneumonia, or hemorrhage from an eroded large blood vessel.

The infiltrates of midline lethal granuloma are, at least initially, radiosensitive, and remission with cytotoxic agents also has been reported.

Benign Tumors

SQUAMOUS PAPILLOMA: The most frequent benign tumor of the nasal cavity is squamous papilloma, which almost always occurs in the nasal vestibule. The lesion is often clinically and microscopically indistinguishable from a wart (verruca vulgaris). For more details on human papillomavirus infection, see Chapter 9.

INVERTED PAPILLOMA: This tumor involves the lateral nasal wall and may spread into the paranasal uses. Inverted papillomas occur mainly in middle-aged persons. As the name implies, they show characteristic inversions of the surface epithelium into the underlying stroma (Fig. 25-33). Intranuclear bodies with the ultrastructural characteristics of human papillomavirus (HPV) particles and HPV type 11 DNA have been detected in some inverted papillomas. Although histologically benign, the tumors may erode bone by pressure. Unless surgical resection extends beyond the boundaries of the grossly visible lesion, they frequently recur. In 5% of the cases, inverted papillomas give rise to squamous cell carcinomas.

Malignant Tumors

Carcinomas of the Nasal Cavity and Paranasal Sinuses

More than half of these tumors originate in the antrum of the maxillary sinus, one third in the nasal cavity, 10% in the ethmoid sinus, and 1% in the sphenoid and frontal sinuses (Fig. 25-34). Most cancers of the nasal cavity and paranasal sinuses are squamous cell carcinomas. About 15% are adenocarcinomas, transitional cell carcinomas, or anaplastic carcinomas.

Several industrial chemicals have been implicated in the causation of the cancer of the nose and sinuses, including nickel, chromium, and aromatic hydrocarbons. Occupational settings that carry an increased risk for cancer of the nose and sinuses (but for which a specific chemical agent has not been identified) are woodworking in the furniture industry, the use of cutting oils, and employment in the leather textile industries.

Tumors in nickel workers are squamous cell carcinomas, which usually arise from the middle turbinate. The latency period varies from 2 to 32 years. The tumors related to other occupational exposures are predominantly adenocarcinomas and occur mostly in the maxillary and ethmoid sinuses. Because of the industrial setting in which many cancers of the nose and sinuses arise, they are much more common in men and occur after age 50 years.

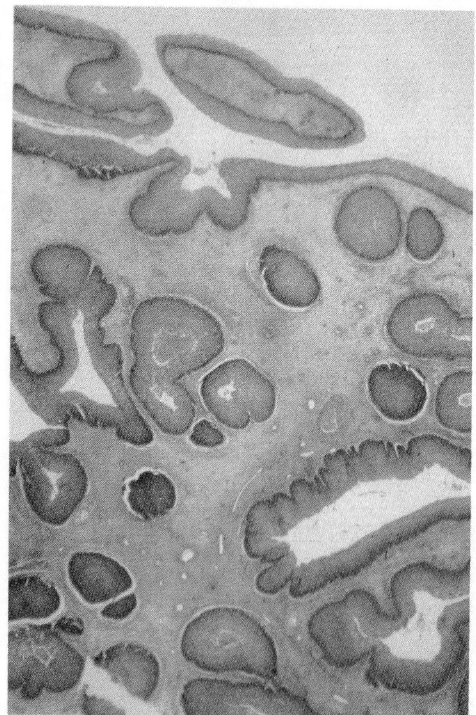

FIGURE *25-33*
Inverted papilloma. Stratified nonkeratinizing squamous epithelium covers the surface and inverts into the underlying stroma.

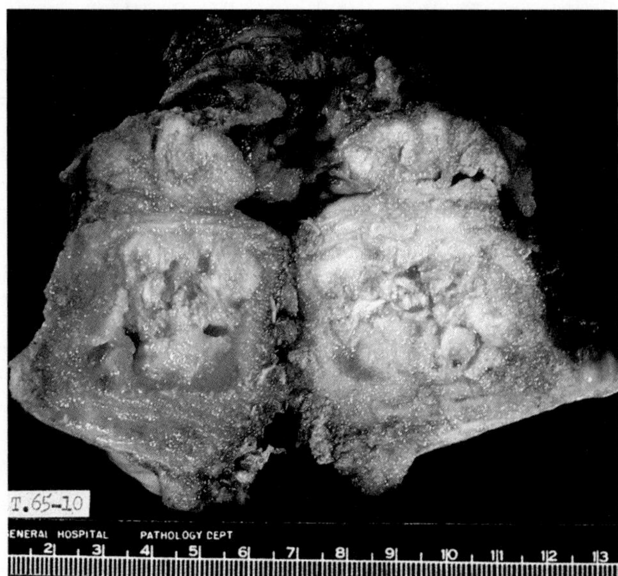

FIGURE 25-34
Squamous cell carcinoma of the maxillary sinus. In this sagittal section, the tumor has destroyed the nasal turbinates and the roof of the maxillary sinus. The tumor extends into the orbit (*top*).

The tumors grow relentlessly and invade adjacent structures but do not give rise to distant metastases. The usual survival is only a few years.

Olfactory Neuroblastoma

Olfactory neuroblastoma (esthesioneuroblastoma) is an unusual malignant tumor of the nose of neural crest origin. It arises from the olfactory mucosa that covers the superior third of the nasal septum, the cribriform plate, and the superior turbinate. Olfactory neuroblastoma is usually polypoid and highly vascular and displays diverse histological patterns, depending on the amount of intercellular neurofibrillary material (Fig. 25-35). The tumor cells are slightly larger than lymphocytes, exhibit round nuclei with an even distribution of chromatin, and have an inconspicuous cytoplasm. In some cases, the tumor cells form true rosettes (Fig. 25-36). By electron microscopy, olfactory neuroblastoma reveals intracytoplasmic secretory granules and cytoplasmic fibrils and microtubules, similar to those of neuroblastomas at other sites.

Olfactory neuroblastomas slowly invade and destroy

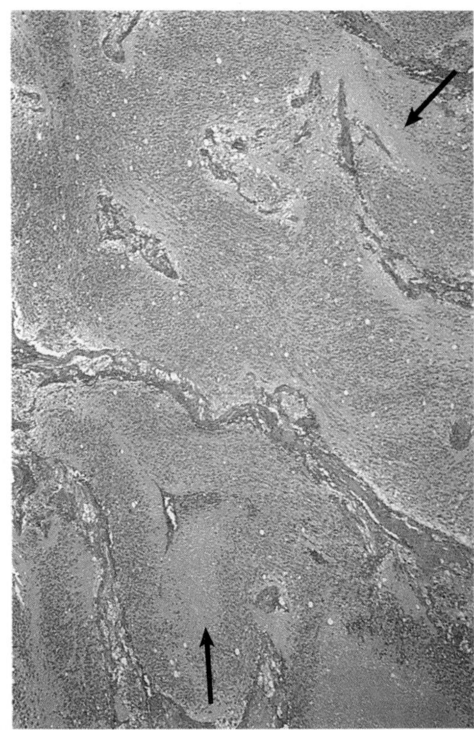

FIGURE 25-35
Olfactory neuroblastoma. The cellular tumor is divided by vascular septa and has an intercellular neurofibrillary matrix (*arrows*).

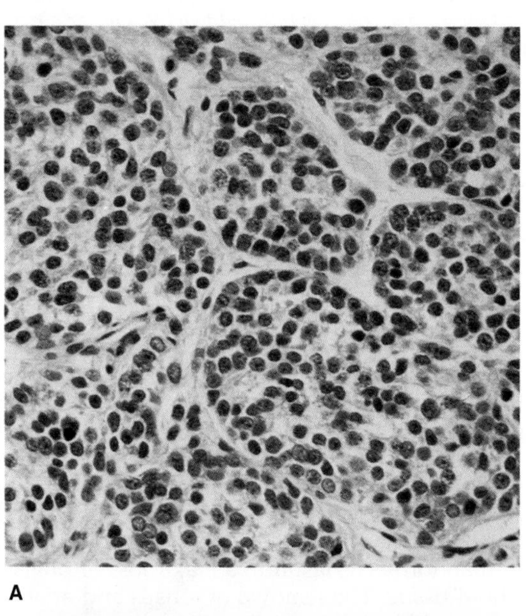

A

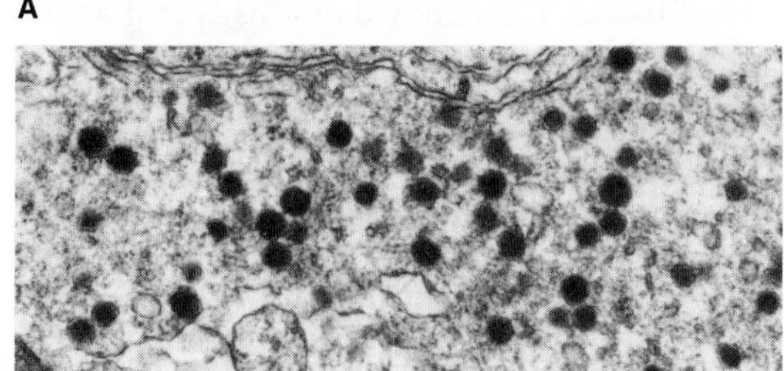

B

FIGURE 25-36
Olfactory neuroblastoma. (*A*) The tumor cells have round or oval nuclei, finely granular chromatin, and scanty cytoplasm. A rosette-like arrangement is seen in the center. (*B*) An electron micrograph shows intracytoplasmic, secretory-type, membrane-bound granules with dense cores.

bony structures and are readily spread through the lymphatics to involve regional and distant lymph nodes. Hematogenous metastases are less frequent. The 5-year survival rate is 50%, and death is usually due to invasion of the cranial cavity.

Nasopharynx

ANATOMY AND FUNCTION

The nasopharynx is continuous anteriorly with the nasal cavities; its roof is formed by the body of the sphenoid bone, and its posterior wall is formed by the cervical vertebrae. On the lateral walls of the nasopharynx are the openings of the eustachian tubes.

The nasopharynx of the newborn is covered by pseudostratified ciliated columnar epithelium. With advancing age, it is replaced by a stratified squamous epithelium over large areas (about 80%). The mucosa contains numerous mucous glands and abundant lymphoid tissue.

WALDEYER'S RING: *The circular band of lymphoid tissue located at the opening of the oropharynx into the respiratory and digestive tracts is referred to as Waldeyer's ring.* The lymphoid tissue on the superior posterior wall forms the nasopharyngeal tonsils, which, when hyperplastic, are better known as *adenoids*. The palatine tonsils, situated laterally where the pharynx connects with the oral cavity, are covered by stratified squamous epithelium, which dips into the lymphoid tissue and lines the infoldings (crypts). The crypts normally contain desquamated epithelium, lymphocytes, some neutrophils, and saprophytic organisms, including bacteria, *Candida*, and *Actinomyces*. Virulent pathogens may also be present in the pharynx of healthy persons (e.g., *C. diphtheriae*, meningococcus).

Waldeyer's ring is well developed in children and contains follicles with germinal centers. In fact, the largest collection of B lymphocytes in the normal child is found in the tonsils. The pharyngeal lymphoid tissue diminishes considerably on reaching adulthood, and with increasing age, it gradually involutes but does not totally disappear. Tonsillectomy and adenoidectomy, less widely practiced today than formerly, result in a major loss of pharyngeal lymphoid tissue. The removal of tonsils and adenoids is not followed by a decrease in serum immunoglobulins, nor does it alter the serological response to several human respiratory viruses. However, secretory IgA is decreased locally in the nasopharynx. In the time before immunization against poliomyelitis, patients after tonsillectomy had an increased incidence of bulbar poliomyelitis. Interestingly, tonsillectomy triples the risk of developing Hodgkin's disease later in life.

HYPOPLASIA AND HYPERPLASIA OF PHARYNGEAL LYMPHOID TISSUE

Bruton sex-linked agammaglobulinemia represents a congenital absence of pharyngeal lymphoid tissue (see Chapter 4). This familial disease affects only male offspring, who have minimal or no lymphoid tissue in their tonsils, pharynx, and intestines (Peyer's patches and appendix). On the other hand, they have a normally developed thymus.

Atrophy of pharyngeal lymphoid tissue is commonly seen in advanced states of AIDS and in chronically immunosuppressed patients. Local radiation therapy also results in marked loss of lymphoid tissue in Waldeyer's ring.

Hyperplasia of nasopharyngeal lymphoid tissue follows infections or chronic irritation of the pharynx by dust, smoke, and fumes. In some primary immunodeficiency syndromes (dysgammaglobulinemia type I or nodular lymphoid hyperplasia), the tonsils may be enlarged, presumably reflecting an adaptive response by the immune system.

INFLAMMATION

Pharyngitis and tonsillitis are among the most common diseases of the head and neck. Inflammation of the nasopharynx occurs predominantly in children, although it is also frequent in adolescence and in early adulthood. Viral or bacterial infections may be limited to the palatine tonsils, but the nasopharyngeal tonsils or adjacent pharyngeal mucosa may also be involved, often as part of a general upper respiratory tract infection. In the latter case, the initial infecting agent is most often a virus spread by droplet or by direct contact. Viral pharyngitis is usually caused by influenza, parainfluenza, adenovirus, respiratory syncytial virus, and rhinovirus.

Infectious mononucleosis is often accompanied by a sore throat. Unlike most other viral diseases, infectious mononucleosis typically produces an exudative pharyngitis.

Streptococcus pyogenes is the most important cause of pharyngitis and tonsillitis, because of the possibility of serious suppurative and nonsuppurative sequelae. Diphtheria is still an important cause of pharyngitis in some countries. These infections are characterized by an exudate, or in the case of diphtheria, a pseudomembrane, on the tonsils and pharynx.

Acute tonsillitis is a bacterial infection, usually with *S. pyogenes* (group A β-hemolytic streptococci). Follicular tonsillitis is characterized by pinpoint exudates that can be extruded from the crypts.

Pseudomembranous tonsillitis refers to a necrotic mucosa covered by a coat of exudate, for instance in diphtheria or in *Vincent angina*. The latter is caused by fusiform bacilli and spirochetes that are present in the normal bacterial flora of the mouth. These organisms become pathogenic when the local or systemic resistance is low (e.g., after mucosal injury or in malnutrition).

Recurrent or chronic tonsillitis is not so common as once believed, and enlarged tonsils in children do not necessarily mean chronic tonsillitis. However, repeated infections can cause enlargement of the tonsils and adenoids to a degree that may obstruct the air passages. In some persons, usually children, repeated bouts of streptococcal tonsillitis may be associated with rheumatic fever or glomerulonephritis; these persons may benefit from tonsillectomy.

Peritonsillar abscess (quinsy) is usually the sequel of

inappropriately treated acute bacterial tonsillitis. If it is not recognized and appropriately managed, it may lead to several life-threatening situations: (1) aided by gravity, it may dissect inferiorly to the pyriform sinus, with obstruction of or rupture into the airway; (2) a peritonsillar abscess may extend laterally into the parapharyngeal space (parapharyngeal abscess) and weaken the wall of the carotid artery; or (3) the abscess may penetrate along the carotid sheath inferiorly into the mediastinum or, superiorly, to the base of the skull or into the cranial cavity, with disastrous consequences.

Adenoids is a term that stems from the time when lymph nodes were called lymph "glands" and lymphoid tissue was thought to be "gland-like." Adenoids represent chronic inflammatory hyperplasia of the pharyngeal lymphoid tissue. This condition is often accompanied by chronic tonsillitis or rhinitis, almost always in children. Enlarged adenoids may cause partial or complete block of the eustachian tube, leading to serous or suppurative otitis media.

TUMORS

Juvenile Nasopharyngeal Angiofibroma

Juvenile angiofibroma is an uncommon, highly vascular neoplasm of the nasopharynx, which is histologically benign but locally aggressive. It occurs almost exclusively in adolescent boys. The tumor is rounded or nodular and has a sessile or pedunculated attachment to the upper posterior or lateral nasopharyngeal wall. Angiofibroma may grow into the fissures and foramina of the skull or may destroy bone and spread into adjacent structures, such as the nasal cavity, paranasal sinuses, orbit, middle cranial fossa, or pterygomaxillary fossa.

Histologically, the tumor has vascular and stromal components (Fig. 25-37). The blood vessels vary in size and shape. Their muscular walls display irregularly arranged smooth muscle, which may be absent focally. These defects in the vessel wall preclude vasoconstriction, thereby contributing to brisk bleeding after trauma. Biopsies are, therefore, dangerous and contraindicated. Although many surgeons still advocate a surgical approach, good results can be obtained with radiation therapy.

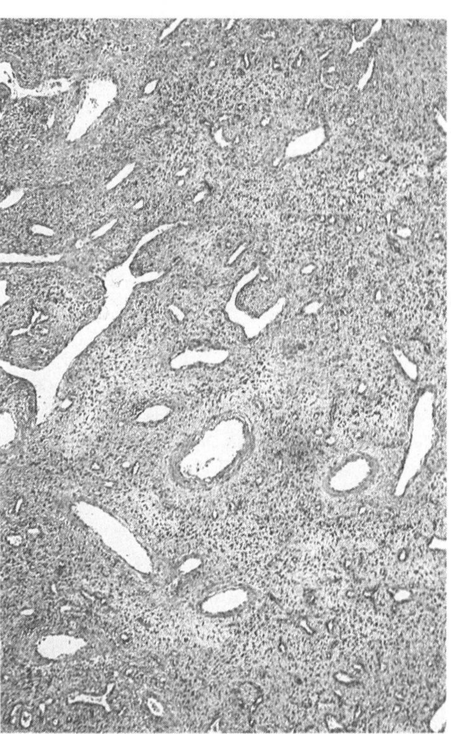

FIGURE 25-37
Juvenile angiofibroma. The tumor contains cellular fibrous tissue with numerous interspersed vascular channels of different caliber. The blood vessels have a varying configuration and a smooth muscle wall, which is often incomplete.

Squamous Cell Carcinoma

The oropharynx, including the tonsillar bed and the anterior and posterior faucial pillars, is a common site for squamous carcinomas. These tumors tend to be less differentiated and biologically more aggressive than squamous carcinomas of the anterior oral cavity. Squamous cell carcinomas of the oropharynx often metastasize early because of the rich lymphatic network in this region. The primary lymphatics drain into the superior deep jugular and submandibular lymph nodes and, to a somewhat lesser degree, into the retropharyngeal lymph nodes.

Nasopharyngeal Carcinoma

Nasopharyngeal carcinoma is an epithelial cancer, which is often related to infection with EBV and is particularly common in southeast Asia and parts of Africa. By far the most common cancer of the nasopharynx, nasopharyngeal carcinoma is the most frequent of all malignant tumors in the Chinese. In Hong Kong, nasopharyngeal carcinoma represents 18% of all cancers, compared with a worldwide prevalence of 0.25%. Chinese born in the United States have about a 20-fold greater mortality from carcinoma of the nasopharynx than do persons of other races. There is also a high incidence in Tunisia and East Africa.

☐ **Pathogenesis:** Various environmental risk factors for nasopharyngeal carcinoma (diet, inhalation of various substances, ethnic customs) have been sought, but no association has been positively demonstrated. Recent studies point to a possible combined role for environmental and genetic factors in the pathogenesis of nasopharyngeal carcinoma. There is an association with the A2/sin HLA profile in the Chinese, suggesting a genetic susceptibility.

Epstein–Barr virus is present in the tumor cells and B lymphocytes of patients with nasopharyngeal carcinoma. Moreover, 85% of patients also have antibodies to EBV and have anti-EBV IgA in the serum. Although a direct cause-and-effect relation between EBV and nasopharyngeal carcinoma remains to be proved, the presence of the virus is a useful tumor marker. For more details on the Epstein–Barr virus infection, see Chapters 5 and 9.

☐ **Pathology:** Nasopharyngeal carcinoma is seen as either keratinizing (squamous cell) tumors or nonkeratinizing ones. The keratinizing tumors occur in an older population and do not bear the same relation to EBV infection as do the nonkeratinizing types. The latter are classified as differentiated or undifferentiated. Differentiated nonkeratinizing nasopharyngeal carcinomas display a stratified appearance and distinct cell margins. By contrast, undifferentiated tumors exhibit clusters of poorly delimited or syncytial cells bearing large oval nuclei and scant eosinophilic cytoplasm (Fig. 25-38A). The undifferentiated variant often features a conspicuous lymphoid infiltrate, accounting for the obsolete (and misleading) term *lymphoepithelioma.*

Electron microscopy and immunohistochemical studies consistently demonstrate the presence of desmosomes and keratin (see Fig. 25-38B) and usually epithelial membrane antigen. On the basis of these features, it is thought that nasopharyngeal carcinoma derives from the basal layers of pseudostratified and stratified epithelia.

□ **Clinical Features:** Because of their location, most nasopharyngeal carcinomas remain asymptomatic for a long time. Palpable cervical lymph node metastases are the first sign of disease in about half of the cases, and even then, many patients have no complaints referable to the nasopharynx. The delay in diagnosis is mostly due to the growth pattern of nasopharyngeal carcinoma. The tumor does not form a large, space-occupying mass or extend into contiguous cavities. Rather it infiltrates neighboring regions, such as the parapharyngeal space, orbit, and cranial cavity. This locally aggressive growth results in various neurological symptoms and disturbances of hearing. Invasion of the base of the skull leads to involvement of the cranial nerves. Neoplasms growing in the fossa of Rosenmüller and in the lateral wall of the nasopharynx produce symptoms referable to the middle ear. Obstruction of the eustachian tube is common. The rich lymphatic network draining the nasopharynx is the route of frequent and early metastases to the cervical lymph nodes.

Nasopharyngeal carcinomas are radiosensitive, and more than half of the patients with tumor restricted to the nasopharynx survive 5 or more years. Metastasis to the cervical lymph nodes considerably reduces the survival rate, and cranial nerve involvement or distant metastasis carries a dismal prognosis.

Lymphomas of Waldeyer's Ring

Lymphomas constitute 5% of head and neck cancers. In this region, Waldeyer's ring is by far the most common site of origin of lymphoma. The palatine tonsils are the most common primary site of lymphoma, followed by the lymphoid tissue of the nasopharynx and the base of the tongue. Enlargement of a single tonsil in any age group, or bilateral painless tonsillar enlargement in adults, suggests the possibility of a lymphoma. In these cases, the cervical lymph nodes are most often involved by metastases.

Histologically, 90% of nasopharyngeal lymphomas

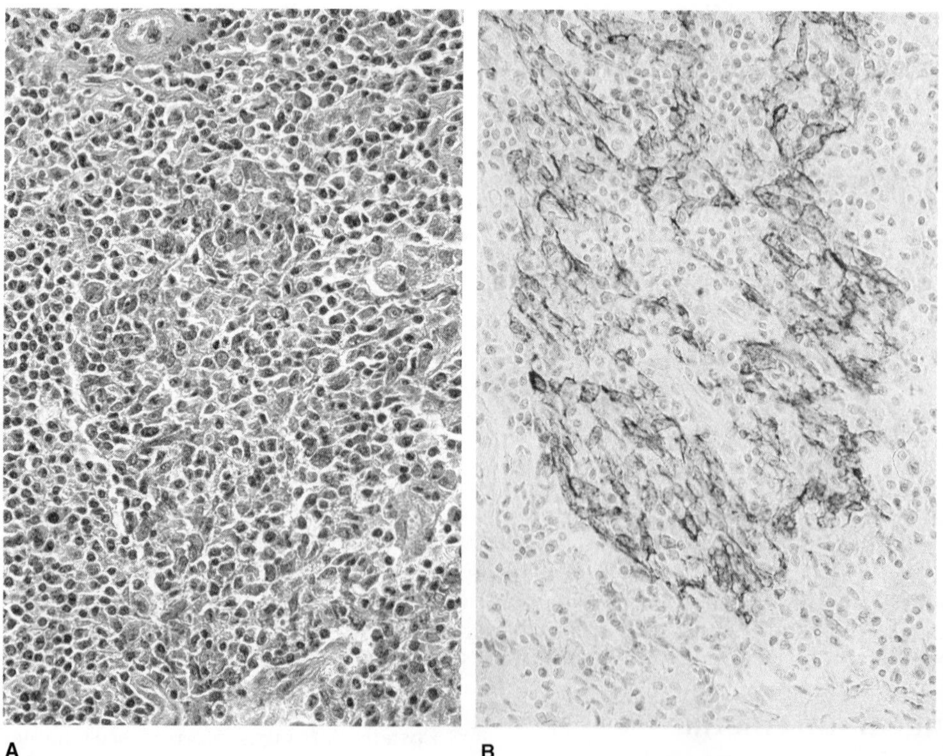

FIGURE *25-38*
Anaplastic carcinoma of the nasopharynx. (*A*) Poorly differentiated neoplastic cells are mingled with inflammatory mononuclear cells. (*B*) An immunohistochemical stain of *A* reveals that the tumor cells contain abundant keratin.

are diffuse, and more than half have been classified as large cell lymphomas. In the United States, the vast majority of lymphomas of Waldeyer's ring are of B-cell origin. In Japan, however, where T-cell lymphomas in general are far more common, nasopharyngeal lymphomas are predominantly of the T-cell type. Hodgkin's disease rarely is seen in Waldeyer's ring.

Plasmacytoma

Three fourths of all extramedullary plasmacytomas occur in the head and neck, with a strong predilection for the nasopharynx, nasal cavity, and paranasal sinuses. Similar to extramedullary plasmacytomas in other body sites, these tumors are best considered as part of a spectrum of plasma cell disorders. The tumors may remain localized or may evolve into systemic plasma cell myeloma.

Chordoma

Chordoma arises from the vestigial remnants of the embryonic notochord. In one third of the cases, the tumors extend into the nasopharynx. In the cranial region, chordomas originate from the area of the spheno-occipital synchondrosis. Histologically, they exhibit large vacuolated (*physaliferous*) cells surrounded by abundant intercellular matrix (Fig. 25-39). Chordomas usually grow slowly, but they infiltrate bone and are ordinarily not accessible to complete surgical removal. Few patients with chordomas of the cranial region survive longer than 5 years.

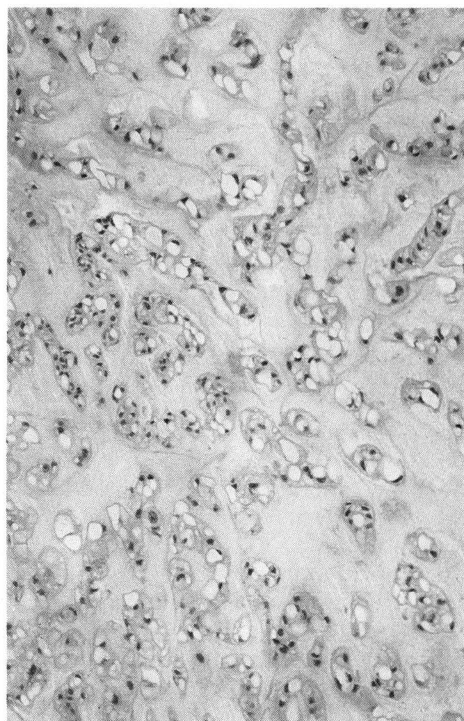

FIGURE *25-39*
Chordoma. Nests and cords of tumor cells are surrounded by abundant acellular ground substance. The tumor cell have a characteristic vacuolated, bubbly cytoplasm (physaliferous cells).

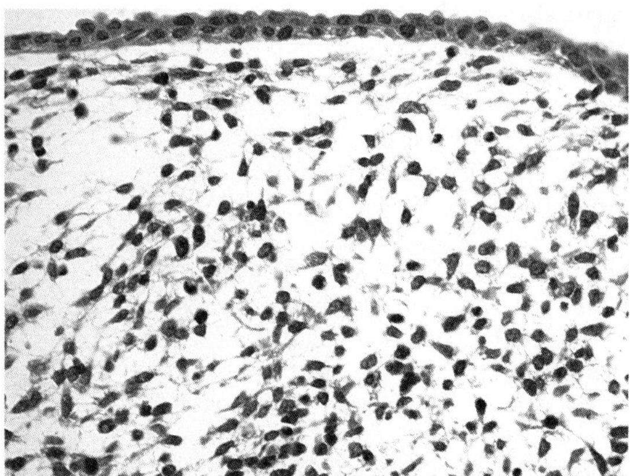

FIGURE *25-40*
Embryonal rhabdomyosarcoma from a 3-year-old girl. This highly malignant tumor arose in the parapharyngeal space and invaded the adjacent structures. The oval or tadpole-shaped tumor cells under the epithelium have hyperchromatic, eccentric nuclei and immunohistochemical and ultrastructural features of rhabdomyoblasts.

Other Malignant Tumors

Other malignant tumors of the nasopharynx are rare. They may arise from various components of the mucosa or adjacent supportive soft tissues and skeleton. *Embryonal rhabdomyosarcoma* (Fig. 25-40) arises in the pharyngeal tissues of young children. This highly malignant tumor invades contiguous structures and metastasizes by both the bloodstream and the lymphatics. In recent years, *Kaposi sarcoma* has been frequently seen in the nasopharyngeal mucosa of patients with AIDS.

The Ear

EXTERNAL EAR

The elastic cartilage of the auricle and that of the external ear canal are continuous and are covered by skin. The external auditory canal ends blindly at the tympanic membrane (eardrum), which separates the external ear from the middle ear. The outer surface of this airtight membrane is covered by squamous epithelium, which is continuous with the skin of the external ear canal. Its inner surface is lined by the cuboidal epithelium of the middle ear. Between these two epithelial covers of the tympanic membrane is a middle layer of dense fibrous tissue.

KELOIDS: These benign overgrowths of dermal scar tissue usually form within a year after trauma. Keloids frequently occur on the skin of the head and neck, shoulders, and upper chest, and back but are particularly common on the ear lobes after piercing for earrings or other trauma. They are much more frequent in blacks and Asians than in whites. The lesions can attain considerable size and tend to recur. Histologically, keloids are composed of thick, hyalinized bundles of collagen in the deep dermis (see Fig. 3-14).

CAULIFLOWER EARS: These deformities are particularly common in wrestlers and boxers and are the result of repeated mechanical trauma to the external ear. Blows to the ears cause subperichondrial hematomas, which organize and deform the ears.

RELAPSING POLYCHONDRITIS: *This rare, chronic disorder of unknown origin is characterized by intermittent inflammation that destroys the cartilaginous structures in the ears, nose, larynx, tracheobronchial tree, ribs, and joints.* It may involve hyaline cartilage, elastic cartilage, or fibrocartilage.

The cause of the cell damage is obscure, although immune mechanisms are suspected. Antibodies to cartilage, type II collagen, and chondroitin sulfate have been demonstrated in the serum of patients during acute attacks. The presence of immune complexes has been demonstrated in the involved cartilage. Relapsing polychondritis occurs alone or in association with one of the connective tissue diseases. Noncartilaginous tissues, such as the sclera and cardiac valves, also may be affected. Aortitis can cause fatal rupture of the aorta.

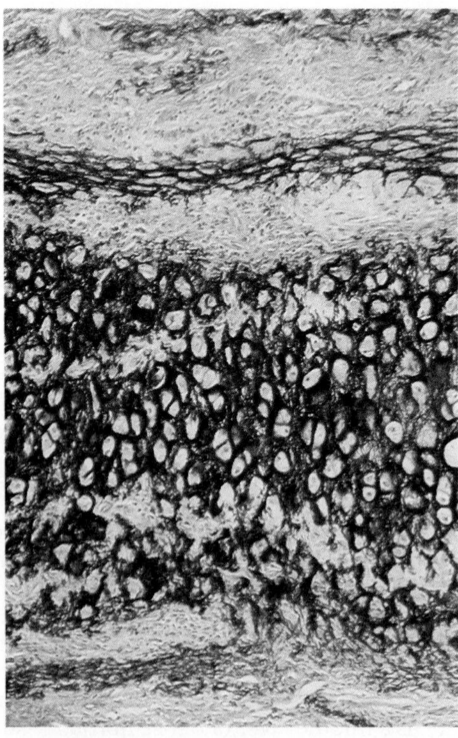

FIGURE *25-41*
Relapsing polychondritis. The perichondrium and elastic cartilage are infiltrated and partially destroyed by inflammatory cells and replaced by fibrosis.

Microscopically, the perichondrium is infiltrated with lymphocytes, plasma cells, and neutrophils, which also extend into the adjacent cartilage (Fig. 25-41). The chondrocytes die, and the cartilaginous matrix degenerates and fragments. Ultimately, the cartilage is destroyed and replaced by granulation tissue and fibrosis.

MALIGNANT OTITIS EXTERNA: This infection of the external auditory canal is caused by *Pseudomonas aeruginosa*. The infection may spread through the skin and cartilage to cause mastoiditis or osteomyelitis of the skull, thrombosis of the venous sinuses, meningitis, and death. Malignant otitis externa occurs primarily in elderly diabetics but has also been reported in patients with blood dyscrasias (e.g., leukemia, granulocytopenia).

AURAL POLYPS: These benign inflammatory lesions arise from within the external ear canal or extrude into the canal from the middle ear. Aural polyps are composed of ulcerated and inflamed granulation tissue, which readily bleeds. Polyps arising in the middle ear are the result of chronic otitis media.

MIDDLE EAR

Anatomy

The middle ear, or tympanic cavity, is an oblong space in the temporal bone lined by a mucous membrane (see Fig. 25-1). Together with the mastoid, it forms a closed mucosal compartment, also referred to as the middle ear cleft. The walls of the middle ear, except for the lateral wall, are bony. Most of the lateral wall consists of the tympanic membrane. Anteriorly, the eustachian tube connects the middle ear with the nasopharynx and provides an air passage to equalize air pressure on both sides of the tympanic membrane. The three auditory ossicles—the malleus, incus, and stapes—form a chain that connects the tympanic membrane with the oval window (on the medial wall of the tympanic cavity) and conducts sound across the middle ear space. The freedom of motion of the ossicles, particularly that of the stapes in the oval window, is more important for hearing than is an intact tympanic membrane.

The middle ear opens posteriorly into the mastoid antrum, a honeycomb of small, aerated, bony compartments (air cells) lined by a thin mucous membrane, which is continuous with that of the middle ear. The mastoid air cells are separated from the dura of the temporal lobe and from the cerebellum by thin cortical bone. Tracts of air cells in the temporal bone extend deep behind the internal ear and into the petrous portion of the temporal bone that houses the internal ear.

Otitis Media

Otitis media refers to inflammation of the middle ear cleft which is usually the result of an upper respiratory tract infection that extends from the nasopharynx. The infection almost invariably penetrates through the mastoid antrum into the mastoid cells. In the presence of an infection in the nasopharynx, microorganisms may reach the middle ear by ascending through the eustachian tube. Acute otitis media may be due to viral or bacterial infections or to obstruction of the eustachian tube without microorganisms. In the case of viral otitis media, the process may resolve without suppuration, or the middle ear may be secondarily invaded by pus-forming bacteria.

Obstruction of the eustachian tube is important in the production of middle ear effusion. When the pharyngeal end of the eustachian tube is swollen, air cannot enter the tube. If the tube is blocked, air in the middle ear is absorbed through the mucosa, and negative pressure develops. Over time, this negative pressure causes transudation of plasma, and occasionally bleeding, in the middle ear. Antibiotics usually cure or suppress the condition.

ACUTE SEROUS OTITIS MEDIA: Obstruction of the eustachian tube may result from sudden changes in atmospheric pressure, as may be encountered during flying in an aircraft or deep-sea diving. This effect is particularly severe in the presence of an upper respiratory tract infection, an acute allergic reaction, or viral or bacterial infection at the orifice of the eustachian tube. Inflammation may occur without bacterial invasion of the middle ear. More than half of the children in the United States have had at least one episode of serous otitis media before their third birthday. It has become increasingly evident that repeated bouts of otitis media in early childhood often contribute to unsuspected hearing loss, which is due to residual (usually sterile) fluid in the middle ear.

CHRONIC SEROUS OTITIS MEDIA: Recurrent or chronic serous effusion of the middle ear is due to the same conditions that cause acute obstruction of the eustachian tube. Inadequate antibiotic treatment of acute suppurative otitis media may also lead to recurrent serous otitis media. Carcinoma of the nasopharynx may be the cause of chronic serous otitis media in an adult and should always be suspected when a unilateral effusion occurs in the middle ear of an adult.

In chronic serous otitis media, the mucosal lining of the middle ear cleft undergoes changes that render it secretory, and mucus-producing (goblet) cells become preponderant. If the obstruction occurs acutely, there may be accompanying hemorrhage, for example, in the mastoid cells. Extravasation of blood and the degradation of erythrocytes liberate cholesterol. Cholesterol crystals stimulate a foreign-body reaction and the formation of granulation tissue, referred to as a cholesterol granuloma. Large cholesterol granulomas may destroy tissue in the mastoid or antrum. If the cholesterol granuloma is allowed to persist for many months, the granulation tissue may become fibrotic, a process that eventually results in complete obliteration of the middle ear and mastoid by fibrous tissue.

ACUTE SUPPURATIVE OTITIS MEDIA: One of the most common infections of childhood, acute suppurative otitis media, is caused by virulent pyogenic bacteria that invade the middle ear, usually through the eustachian tube. *Streptococcus pneumoniae* (pneumococcus) is the most common causative agent in all age groups (30% to 40%). *Haemophilus influenzae* causes about 20% of cases and is less frequent with increasing age. In about one fourth of cases, no bacteria can be cultured. If the purulent exudate in the middle ear accumulates, the eardrum ruptures, and the pus is then discharged. In most cases, the infection is self-limited, and even without therapy tends to heal. A few untreated persons continue to have suppuration and develop chronic otitis media.

ACUTE MASTOIDITIS: Infection of the mastoid bone was a common complication of acute otitis media before the advent of antibiotics, and it is still seen, albeit rarely, in cases of inadequately treated otitis media. Characteristically, the mastoid air cells are filled with pus, and the thin osseous intercellular walls become destroyed. The extension of the infection from the mastoid to contiguous structures causes complications.

ACUTE NECROTIZING OTITIS MEDIA: This rapidly progressive and destructive inflammation mainly affects children who are severely ill with infections (measles, scarlet fever, typhoid) or other systemic diseases, particularly those that are associated with impaired immunological resistance. Characteristically, the tympanic membrane and ossicles are destroyed, inevitably leading to chronic otitis media. Acute necrotizing otitis media is today uncommon in industrialized countries.

CHRONIC SUPPURATIVE OTITIS MEDIA AND MASTOIDITIS: Neglected or recurrent infection of the middle ear and mastoid process may eventually produce a chronic inflammation of the mucosa or destruction of the periosteum covering the ossicles (Fig. 25-42). However, recurrent episodes of acute middle ear infection are not considered to be chronic unless there is a permanent perforation of the tympanic membrane or destruction of the ossicles. Most organisms are aerobes; *S. pneumoniae, H. influenzae,* staphylococci, gram-negative bacilli, and diphtheroids are common. Chronic otitis media is much more common in persons who had ear disease in early childhood, which may have arrested normal development of the air cells in the mastoid. Most patients have a small, undeveloped mastoid process.

Chronic otitis media occurs in various forms, depending on the anatomical and functional characteristics of the middle ear, the type of pathogenic bacteria, and host resistance. The inflammatory process tends to be insidious, persistent, and destructive. By definition, the eardrum is always perforated in chronic otitis media. Painless discharge (otorrhea) and varying degrees of hearing loss are constant symptoms. Exuberant granulation tissue may form polyps, which can extend through the perforated eardrum into the external ear canal.

Cholesteatoma *is a mass of accumulated keratin that results from the growth of squamous epithelium from the external ear canal thorough the perforated eardrum into the middle ear.* In that location, it continues to produce keratin. Microscopically, cholesteatomas are identical to epidermal inclusion cysts and are surrounded by granulation tissue and fibrosis. The keratin mass frequently becomes infected and shields the bacteria from antibiotics. The principal dangers of cholesteatoma arise from erosion of bone, a process that may lead to the destruction of important contiguous structures (e.g., auditory ossicles, facial nerve, labyrinth).

COMPLICATIONS OF ACUTE AND CHRONIC OTITIS MEDIA: As a result of antibiotic treatment, complications of otitis media are now rare. However, a potential for serious, and even fatal, complications still exists with any suppurative inflammation of the middle ear cleft. Factors influencing the spread of infection beyond the middle ear space include the type and virulence of pathogenic organisms, the adequacy of treatment, and host resistance (e.g., diabetes, leukemia, immunosuppressive therapy).

Infection can extend from the middle ear cleft to other contiguous structures. The following cranial and intracranial complications may develop:

- Destruction of the facial nerve
- Deep cervical or subperiosteal abscess, when the cortical bone of the mastoid process is eroded
- Petrositis, when the infection spreads to the petrous portion of the temporal bone through the chain of air cells
- Suppurative labyrinthitis, as a result of infection of the internal ear
- Epidural, subdural, or cerebral abscess, after extension of the infection through the inner table of the mastoid bone
- Meningitis, when the infection extends to the meninges
- Thrombophlebitis of the sigmoid sinus, which occurs when the infection spreads through the dura to the posterior cranial fossa

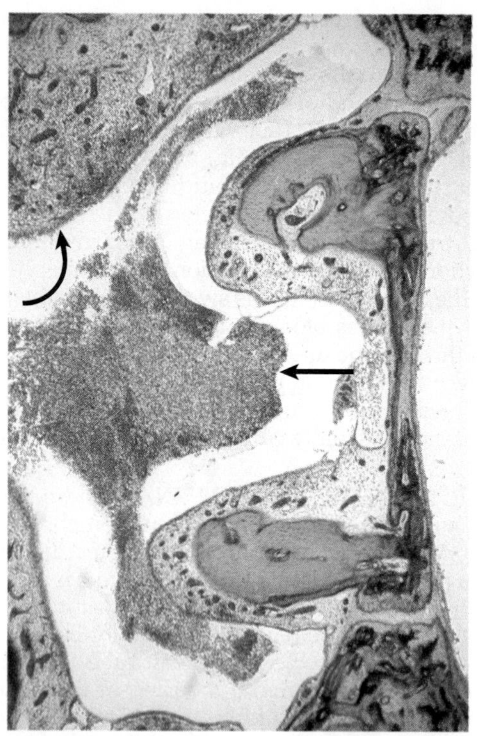

FIGURE 25-42
Chronic suppurative otitis media. A purulent exudate (*straight arrow*) is present in the middle ear cavity. The entire mucosa (*curved arrow*) is thickened by chronic inflammation and granulation tissue. The footplate and the crura of the stapes are at right.

Chemodectoma

Chemodectoma, also termed nonchromaffin paraganglioma, is the most frequent benign tumor of the middle ear and arises from the paraganglia of the middle ear (glomus jugulare or glomus tympanicum). Chemodectomas grow slowly but, over the years, cause extensive destruction of the middle ear and may extend into the internal ear and cranial cavity. Metastases are rare.

Histologically, chemodectomas of the middle ear are identical to those arising in other paraganglia and show characteristic lobules of cells embedded in a richly vascular connective tissue (Fig. 25-43). The glomus cells are of neural crest origin and contain varying amounts of catecholamines, mostly epinephrine and norepinephrine.

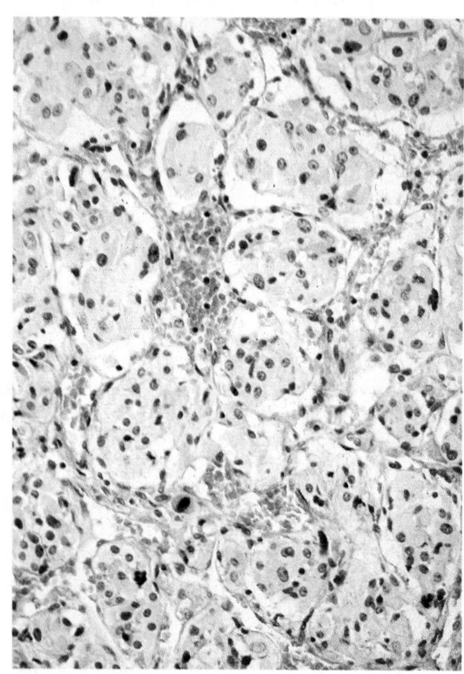

FIGURE 25-43
Chemodectoma (nonchromaffin paraganglioma) of glomus jugulare. Nests (lobules) of large cells with prominent nuclei and a vascular stroma are characteristic.

INTERNAL EAR

Anatomy

The petrous portion of the temporal bone contains the labyrinth that shelters the end organs for hearing (the cochlea) and equilibrium (the vestibular labyrinth; see Fig. 25-1). The complex cavities of the osseous labyrinth contain the membranous labyrinth, which forms a series of communicating membranous sacs and ducts. The membranous labyrinth is separated from the bony walls and is surrounded by a clear fluid, the perilymph. The perilymphatic system is continuous with the subarachnoid space through the cochlear aqueduct, which provides direct exchange with the cerebrospinal fluid. The membranous labyrinth contains a different fluid, the endolymph, which circulates in a closed system. Because of the lack of barriers between the cochlear and vestibular labyrinths, injury or disease of the inner ear frequently affects both hearing and equilibrium.

The cochlea is coiled upon itself like a snail shell and makes two and one-half turns. There are three compartments in the cochlea; two of these contain perilymph, whereas the third (the cochlear duct) contains endolymph. The cochlear duct encompasses the end organ for hearing, the organ of Corti, which rests on the basement membrane. The organ of Corti is arranged as a spiral, with three rows of outer hair cells and a row of inner hair cells. When the hairs of these neuroepithelial cells are bent or distorted by sonic vibration, the mechanical force is converted into electrochemical impulses and is interpreted in the temporal cortex as sound. High-pitched sounds stimulate the basal portion of the cochlea, and low-pitched ones, the apical end. The vestibular portion of the membranous labyrinth consists of the utricle, the saccule, and the semicircular canals. Each of these structures contains the specialized neuroepithelium that is the end organ for equilibrium.

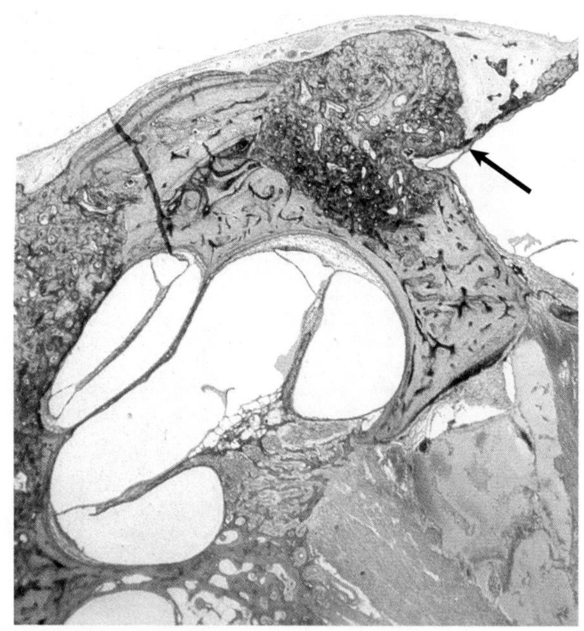

FIGURE *25-44*
Otosclerosis. Otosclerotic foci appear as dark purple areas in the bony labyrinth. At the anterior margin of the oval window (*arrow*), otosclerosis has immobilized the footplate of the stapes by bony ankylosis.

Otosclerosis

Otosclerosis refers to the formation of new spongy bone about the stapes and the oval window, which results in progressive deafness. Otosclerosis is an autosomal dominant hereditary defect and is the most common cause of conductive hearing loss in young and middle-aged adults in the United States. Ten percent of white and 1% of black adult Americans have some degree of otosclerosis, although 90% of cases are asymptomatic. The female-to-male ratio is 2:1, and both ears are usually affected. The pathogenesis of otosclerosis is obscure.

Although any part of the petrous bone may be affected, otosclerotic bone tends to form at particular points. The most frequent site (80% to 90%) is immediately anterior to the oval window. The focus of sclerotic bone extends posteriorly and may infiltrate and replace the stapes. This process progressively immobilizes the footplate of the stapes, and the developing bony ankylosis (Fig. 25-44) is functionally manifested as a slowly progressive conductive hearing loss.

Histologically, the initial lesion of otosclerosis is resorption of bone, with formation of highly cellular fibrous tissue, which contains wide vascular spaces and osteoclasts (Fig. 25-45). The focus of resorbed bone is later replaced by immature bone (Fig. 25-46). By repeated remodeling, this bone develops into more mature bone.

Otosclerosis is successfully treated by surgical mobilization of the auditory ossicles.

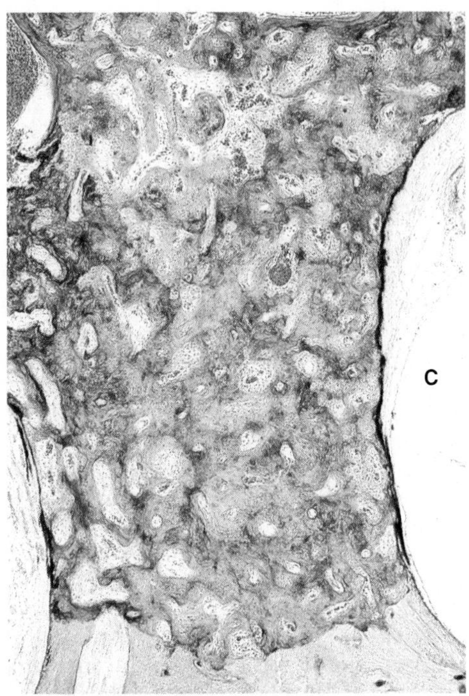

FIGURE *25-45*
Otosclerosis. In the lateral wall of the cochlea, the basophilic and more vascular bone is well demarcated. C, organ of Corti.

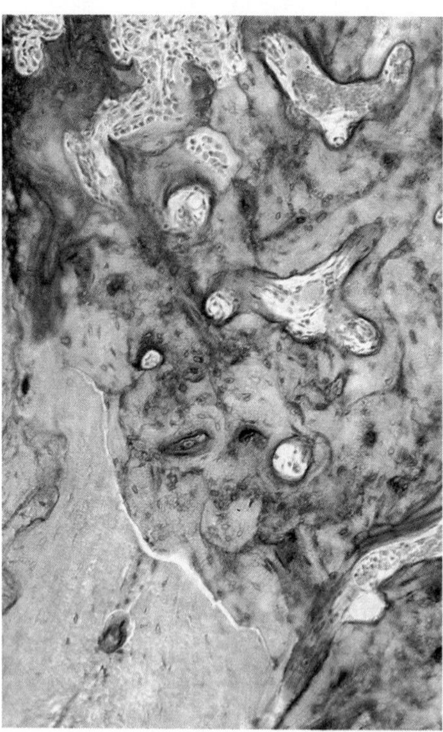

FIGURE 25-46
Otosclerosis. Otosclerotic bone (*top*) is less compact and more cellular than normal bone (*bottom*). The young otosclerotic bone contains widened interosseous spaces, which are cellular and contain small blood vessels.

Meniere Disease

Meniere disease is characterized by episodes of the triad of vertigo, sensorineural hearing loss, and tinnitus (ringing in the ears). A wide variety of etiological factors have been suggested, but the cause of Meniere disease remains uncertain. Its pathological correlate is hydropic distention of the endolymphatic system of the cochlea. Meniere disease is most common in the fourth and fifth decades and is bilateral in 15% of patients.

Microscopically, the earliest changes are dilatation of the cochlear duct and saccule. As the disease (*hydrops*) progresses, the entire endolymphatic system becomes dilated, and the membranous wall frequently tears (Fig. 25-47). Ruptures are sometimes followed by collapse of the membranous labyrinth, but atrophy of the sensory and neural structures is rare. It is thought that the symptoms of Meniere disease occur when endolymphatic hydrops causes rupture, and the endolymph escapes into the perilymph.

The attacks of vertigo, which are accompanied by nausea and vomiting and are often incapacitating, last less than 24 hours. Weeks or months go by before another episode, and in time, the remissions become longer. The hearing loss recovers between attacks but later becomes permanent. Meniere disease seems to be improved by a low-salt diet and the administration of diuretics.

Labyrinthine Toxicity

Drug-induced damage to the inner ear is the most frequent and serious cause of labyrinthine toxicity and is usually dose related. The best known drugs that produce ototoxic side effects are the aminoglycoside antibiotics, which cause irreversible damage to the vestibular or cochlear sensory cells. Other antibiotics, diuretics, antimalarial drugs, and salicylates may also cause transient or permanent sensorineural hearing loss. Among the antineoplastic agents, cisplatin frequently causes temporary or permanent hearing loss. Ototoxicity has been observed after a single therapeutic dose of cisplatin. Animal studies with cisplatin have documented loss of outer hair cells at the based of the cochlea, providing histological evidence of permanent high-frequency hearing loss. The labyrinth of the embryo is especially sensitive to some drugs (congenital deafness due to thalidomide, quinine, and chloroquine).

Viral Labyrinthitis

Viral infections are becoming increasingly recognized as the cause of several inner ear disorders, particularly deafness. Most cases represent invasion of the labyrinth by the virus. Cytomegalovirus and rubella are the best known prenatal viral infections that cause congenital deafness through maternal-to-fetal transmission. Cytomegalovirus antigen has been demonstrated in the cells of the organ of Corti and neurons of the spiral ganglia.

Mumps is the most common cause of deafness among the postnatal viral infections. The infection can cause a rapid hearing loss, which is unilateral in 80% of cases. By contrast, prenatal infection of the labyrinth with rubella is usually bilateral, with permanent loss of cochlear and vestibular function. A number of other viruses are suspected to cause labyrinthitis, including influenza and parainfluenza viruses, EBV (infectious mononucleosis),

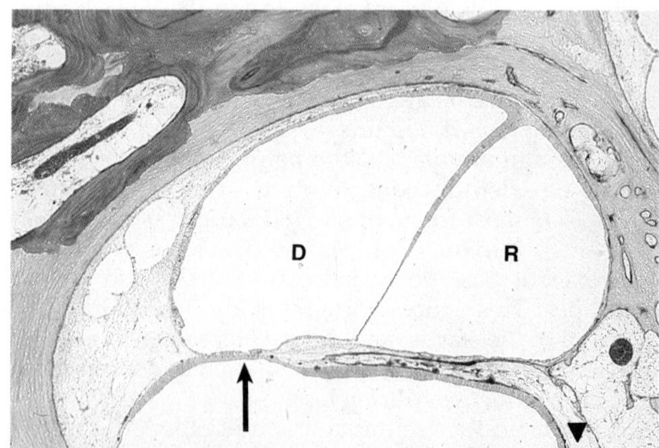

FIGURE 25-47
Meniere disease. The cochlear duct (D) is markedly distended, and Reissner membrane (R) is pushed back by endolymphatic hydrops. Neither the organ of Corti (*arrow*) nor the spiral ganglion (*arrowhead*) is seen in its usual location.

herpesviruses, and adenoviruses. Temporal bone specimens of such cases reveal severe damage to the organ of Corti, with almost total loss of both inner and outer hair cells.

Acoustic Trauma

Noise-induced hearing loss is a significant health problem in industrialized countries. Occupational or recreational exposure to loud tones or noises may cause temporary or permanent loss of hearing. The earliest damage occurs in the external hair cells of the organ of Corti. The loss of sensory hairs is followed by deformation, swelling, and disintegration of the hair cells. Progressive injury leads to damage of the supporting cells.

Tumors

SCHWANNOMA: Nearly all schwannomas in the internal auditory canal arise from the vestibular nerves. Vestibular schwannomas, which account for about 10% of all intracranial tumors, are slow growing and encapsulated. Larger tumors protrude from the internal auditory meatus into the cerebellopontine angle and may deform the brainstem and adjacent cerebellum (see Fig. 28-136). Schwannomas cause slowly progressive vestibular and auditory symptoms.

Neurofibromatosis, type 2, is characterized by a high incidence of bilateral vestibular schwannomas. Histologically, these tumors are indistinguishable from other vestibular schwannomas. For a more detailed discussion of acoustic neurinomas, see Chapter 28.

MENINGIOMA: Meningiomas of the cerebellopontine angle take origin from the meningothelial cells in the arachnoid villi. The favored sites for these tumors are the sphenoid ridge and the petrous pyramid. Meningiomas may extend into the adjacent temporal bone or dural sinuses.

SUGGESTED READING

BOOKS

Barnes L (ed): *Surgical pathology of the head and neck*, vols 1 and 2. New York: Marcel Dekker, 1985.

Michaels L (ed): Ear, nose and throat histopathology. New York: Springer-Verlag, 1987.

Neville BW, Damm DD, Allen CM, Bouquot JE: Oral and maxillofacial pathology. Philadelphia: WB Saunders, 1995.

Wenig BM: *Atlas of head and neck pathology*. Philadelphia: WB Saunders, 1993.

SPECIALIZED BOOKS AND REVIEW ARTICLES

ORAL CAVITY

Ellis GL, Auclair PL, Gnepp DR: *Surgical pathology of the salivary glands*. Philadelphia: WB Saunders, 1991.

Hooks JJ, Jordan GH: Viral infections in the oral cavity. New York: Elsevier-North Holland, 1982.

Kramer IRH, Lucas RB, Pindborg JJ, Sobin LH: Definition of leukoplakia and related lesions: An aid to studies on oral precancer. *Oral Surg* 46:518, 1978.

McCarthy PL, Shklar G: *Diseases of the oral mucosa*, 2nd ed. Philadelphia: Lea & Febiger, 1980.

Regezi JA, Sciubba J: *Oral pathology: Clinical-pathologic correlations*, 2nd ed. Philadelphia: WB Saunders, 1993.

Robertson PB, Greenspan JS: *Perspectives on oral manifestations of AIDS: Diagnosis and management of HIV-associated infections*. Littleton, MA: PSG Publishing, 1988.

Robinson HBG, Miller AS: *Colby, Kerr and Robinson's color atlas of oral pathology*, 5th ed., Philadelphia: JB Lippincott, 1990.

Shaw JH: Causes and control of dental caries. *N Engl J Med* 316:996–1004, 1987.

Tala H, Moutsopoulos HM, Kassan SG (eds): Sjögren's syndrome: *Clinical and immunological aspects*. New York: Springer-Verlag, 1987.

Williams RC: Periodontal disease. *N Engl J Med* 322: 373–382, 1990.

NOSE AND PARANASAL SINUSES

Batsakis JG, Luna MA: Midfacial necrotizing lesions. *Semin Diagn Pathol* 4:90–103, 1987.

Fienberg R, et al: Correlation of antineutrophil cytoplasmic antibodies with the extrarenal histopathology of Wegener's (pathergic) granulomatosis and related forms of vasculitis. *Hum Pathol* 24:160–168, 1993.

Lee NK, et al: Head and neck squamous cell carcinomas associated with human papillomaviruses and an increased incidence of cervical pathology. *Otolaryngol Head Neck Surg* 99:296–301, 1988.

Naclerio RM: Allergic rhinitis. *N Engl J Med* 325:860–869, 1991.

Vokes EE, Weichselbaum RR, Lippman SM, Hong WK: Head and neck cancer. *N Engl J Med* 328:184–186, 1993.

Wald ER: Sinusitis in children. *N Engl J Med* 326:319–323, 1992.

Wu TC, et al: Association of human papillomavirus with nasal neoplasia. *Lancet* 341:522–524, 1993

NASOPHARYNX

De The G, Ito Y (eds): *Nasopharyngeal carcinoma: Etiology and control*. Lyon: IARC Scientific Publications, No. 20, 1978.

Feinmesser R, Miyazaki I, Cheung R, Freeman JL, Noyek AM, Dosch HM: Diagnosis of nasopharyngeal carcinoma by DNA amplification of tissue obtained by fine-needle aspiration. *N Engl J Med* 326:17–21, 1992.

Grundmann E, Krueger GRF, Ablashi DV (eds): *Nasopharyngeal carcinoma*. Stuttgart: Gustav Fischer Verlag, 1981.

Saul SH, Kapadia SB: Primary lymphoma of Waldeyer's ring. *Cancer* 56:157, 1985.

EAR

Friedmann I, Arnold W: *Pathology of the ear*. Edinburgh: Churchill Livingstone, 1992.

Hawke M, Jahn AF (eds): *Disease of the ear: Clinical and pathological aspects*. Philadelphia: Lea & Febiger, 1986.

Konigsmark BW, Gorlin RJ: *Genetic and metabolic deafness.* Philadelphia: WB Saunders, 1976.

Melamed Y, Shupak A, Bitterman H: Medical problems associated with underwater diving. *N Engl J Med* 326:30–35, 1992.

Nadol JB: Hearing loss. *N Engl J Med* 329:1092–1102, 1993.

Nager GT: *Pathology of the ear and temporal bone.* Baltimore: Williams & Wilkins, 1993.

Schuknecht HF: *Pathology of the ear*. Cambridge, MA: Harvard University Press, 1974.

Swanson JA, Hoecker JL: Otitis media in young children. *Mayo Clin Proc* 71:179–183, 1996.

CHAPTER 26

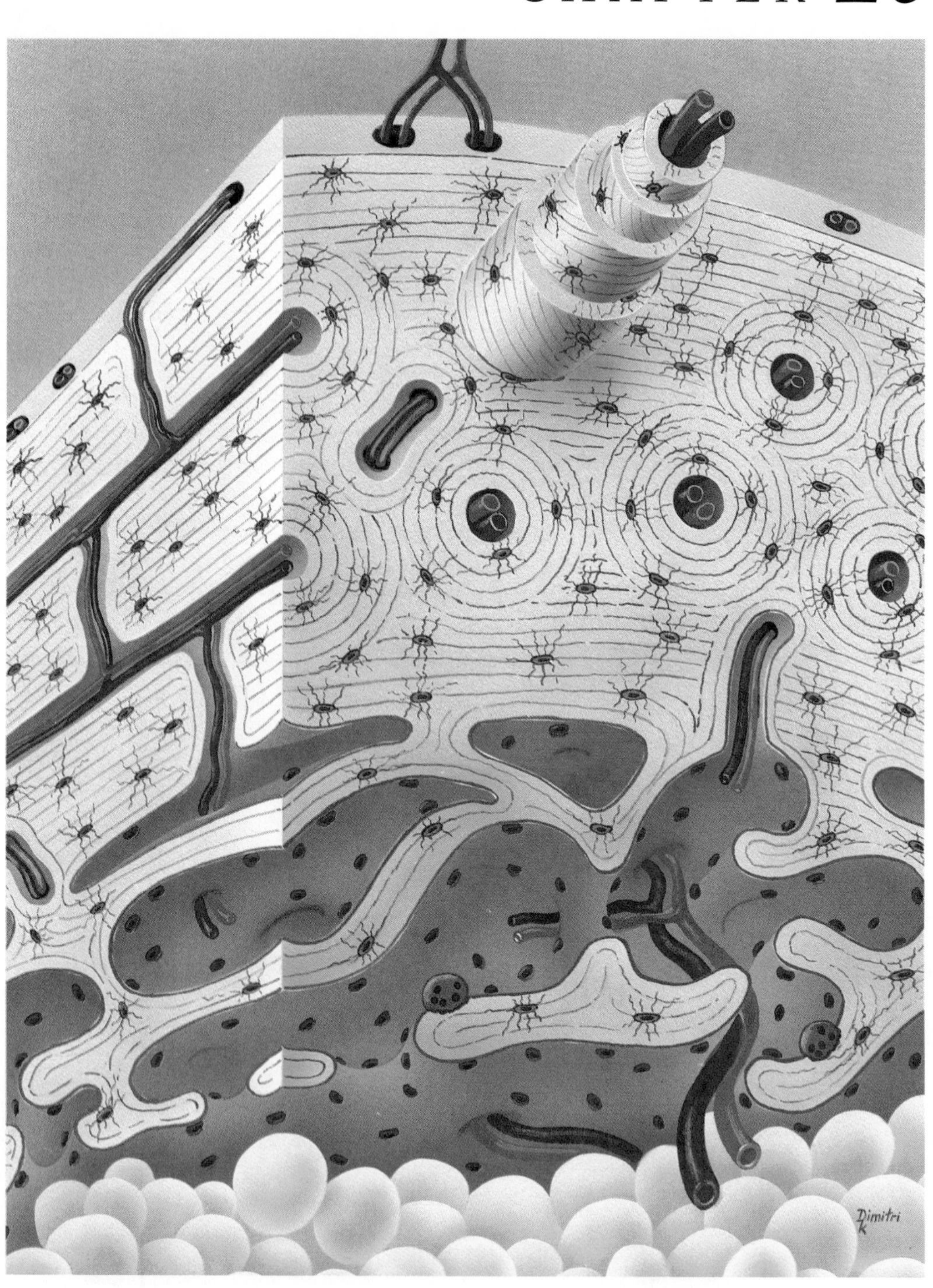

Bones and Joints

Alan L. Schiller
Steven L. Teitelbaum

FIGURE ***26-1*** ***(see opposite page)***
Anatomy of bone. A schematic representation of cortical and trabecular bone. The longitudinal section on the left shows the vasculature entering the periosteum via the periosteal perforating arteries and coursing through the bone perpendicular to the long axis in Volkmann's canals. The vessels that proceed longitudinally, or parallel to the long axis, are located in Haversian canals. Each artery is accompanied by a vein. Within the cortex, osteocytes reside in lacunae, and their cell processes extend into the canaliculi. The cross-sectional view *(right)* illustrates the various types of lamellar bone in the cortex. Circumferential lamellar bone is located adjacent to the periosteum and borders the marrow space. Concentric lamellar bone surrounds the central Haversian canals to form an osteon. Each layer of the concentric lamellar bone displays a change in the pitch of the collagen fibers, such that each layer has a different arrangement of collagen. The interstitial lamellar bone occupies the space between osteons. The marrow space is filled with fat, and its trabecular bone is contiguous with the cortex. Multinucleated osteoclasts are present, and palisaded osteoblasts surround the bone surfaces. The perforating arteries from the periosteum and the nutrient artery from the marrow space communicate within the cortex via Haversian and Volkmann's canals.

Bones

The functions of bone are classified as mechanical, mineral storage, and hemopoietic. The mechanical functions of bone include protection for the brain, spinal cord, and chest organs, rigid internal support for the limbs, and deployment as lever arms in the skeletal muscle. Bone is the principal reservoir for calcium and stores other ions, such as phosphate, sodium, and magnesium. The bones also serve as hosts for the hemopoietic bone marrow.

The mechanical properties of bone are related to its construction and internal architecture. Although extremely light, bone has a high tensile strength. This combination of strength and light weight is a result of its hollow tubular shape, the layering of bone tissue, and the internal buttressing of the matrix.

The term bone can refer to both an organ and a tissue. The "organ" is composed of bone tissue, cartilage, fat, marrow elements, vessels, nerves, and fibrous tissue. Bone "tissue" is described in microscopic terms and is defined by the relation of its collagen and mineral structure to the bone cells.

ANATOMY

Macroscopically two types of bone are recognized.

- **Cortical bone** is dense, compact bone, whose outer shell defines the shape of the bone. Cortical bone composes 80% of the skeleton, and because of its density, its functions are principally biomechanical.
- **Coarse cancellous bone** (also termed spongy, trabecular, or marrow bone) is generally found at the ends of long bones within the medullary canal. Cancellous bone has a high surface-to-volume ratio and as such, contains many more bone cells per unit volume than does cortical bone. Changes in the rate of bone turnover are manifested principally in cancellous bone.

All bones contain both cancellous and cortical elements (Fig. 26-1), but their proportions differ. The body, or shaft, of a long tubular bone, such as the femur, is composed of cortical bone, and its marrow is formed principally by fat. Toward the ends of the femur, the cortex becomes thin, and coarse cancellous bone becomes the predominant structure. By contrast, the skull is formed by outer and inner tables of compact bone, with only a small amount of cancellous bone within the marrow space, called the **diploë**.

The anatomical structures of bone are defined in relation to a transverse cartilage plate, which is present in the growing child. This structure is termed *the growth plate, the epiphyseal cartilage plate, or the physis* (Fig. 26-2). The terms epiphysis, metaphysis, and diaphysis are defined in relation to the growth plate.

- **The epiphysis** is the area of the bone that extends from the subarticular bone plate to the base of the growth plate.
- **The metaphysis** describes the region from the side of the growth plate facing away from the joint to the area where the bone develops its fluted or funnel shape. The metaphysis contains coarse cancellous bone.
- **The diaphysis** corresponds to the body or shaft of the bone and is the zone between the two metaphyses in a long tubular bone.

The metaphysis blends into the diaphysis and represents the area where the coarse cancellous bone dissipates. It is the area of bone that is particularly important in hematogenous infections, tumors, and malformations of the skeleton.

Two additional terms are essential to an understanding of the organization of bone:

- **Endochondral ossification** is the process by which bone tissue replaces cartilage.
- **Intramembranous ossification** refers to the mechanism by which bone tissue supplants membranous or fibrous tissue laid down by the periosteum.

All bones in the body are formed by at least some intramembranous ossification. Some bones, for instance, the calvaria of the skull, are forged purely by intramembranous ossification. Microscopically, it cannot be determined whether bone formation occurred as a result of replacement of cartilage or of fibrous tissue. Because bone tumors tend to recapitulate their embryological origins, it is not surprising that cartilaginous tumors of the frontal bone have not been seen, because the calvaria of the skull do not originate from cartilage.

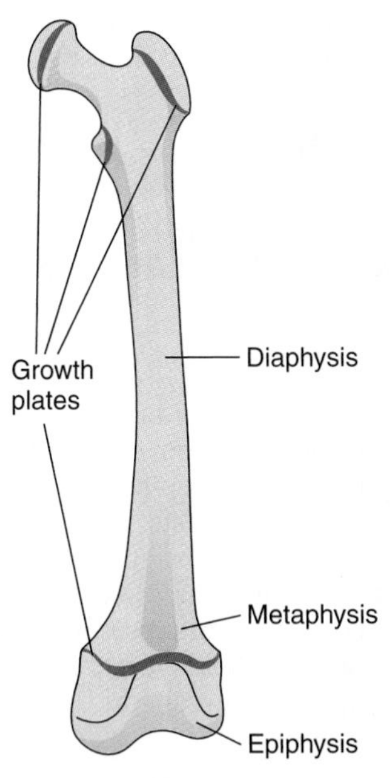

FIGURE 26-2
Anatomy of a long bone. (*A*) Diagram of the femur illustrates the various compartments. (*B*) Coronal section of the proximal femur illustrates the various anatomical parts of a long bone. The epiphyses of the femoral head and the greater trochanter are separated from the metaphysis by their respective epiphyseal plates. The cortex and medullary space are well visualized. (*C*) A section of the epiphysis with a zone of proliferating cartilage cells. Beneath this zone, the hypertrophic cartilage cells are arrayed in columns. At the bottom, the calcifying matrix is invaded by blood vessels. E, epiphysis; PC, proliferative cartilage; HC, hypertrophic cartilage; CC, calcified cartilage; V, vascular invasion.

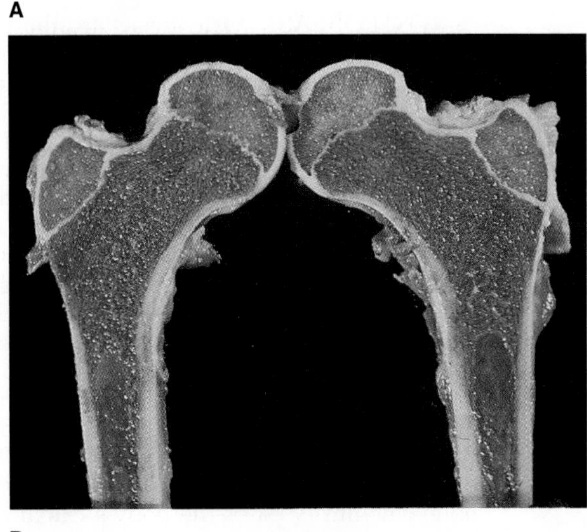

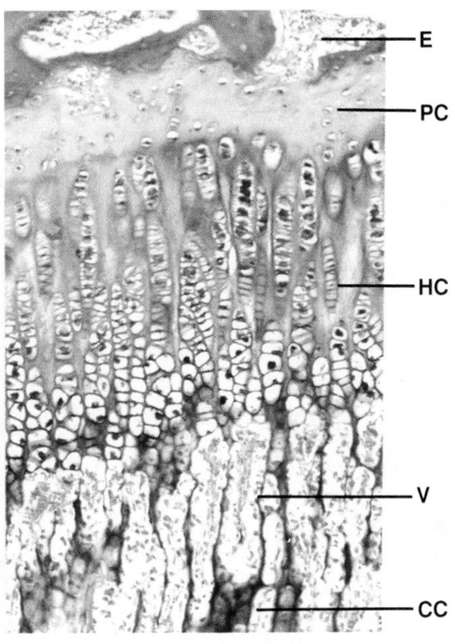

The Bone Marrow

The bone marrow resides in the space enclosed by the cortical bone, called the marrow space or medullary canal. It is supported by a delicate connective tissue framework that enmeshes the marrow cells and the blood vessels. Three types of marrow may be seen by the naked eye:

- **Red marrow** corresponds to hemopoietic tissue and is found in virtually all bones at the time of birth. At the time of adolescence, the red marrow is confined to the axial skeleton, which includes the skull, vertebrae, sternum, ribs, scapulae, clavicles, pelvis, and the proximal humerus and femur. Red marrow may also be pathological, depending on the age of the patient and the site of the marrow. For example, the presence of red marrow in the femoral diaphysis of a 55-year-old man is abnormal and may reflect underlying disease, such as leukemia.
- **Yellow marrow** appears microscopically as fat tissue and is found in the bones of the limbs. Yellow marrow in a normally hemopoietic area, such as a vertebral body, is abnormal at any age.
- **Gray or white marrow** is deficient in hemopoietic elements and is often fibrotic. **It is always a pathological tissue in a nongrowing adult bone or in areas distant from the growth plate in a child.**

The Blood Supply

The long tubular bones are provided with blood from two sources and contain canals to supply the tissues.

- **Nutrient arteries** enter the bone through a nutrient foramen and supply the marrow space and the internal one third to one half of the cortex.
- **Perforating arteries** are small straight vessels that ex-

tend inward from the periosteal arteries on the external surface of the periosteum (the fibrous capsule of the bone). The perforating arteries anastomose in the cortex with branches from the nutrient arteries coming from the marrow space.

- **Haversian canals** are spaces in the bone of the cortex that course parallel to the long axis of the bone for a short distance and then branch and communicate with other similar canals. Each canal contains one or two blood vessels, lymphatics, and some nerve fibers.
- **Volkmann's canals** are spaces within the cortex that run perpendicular to the long axis of the cortex to connect adjacent Haversian canals. Volkmann's canals also contain blood vessels.

Each artery has its paired vein and, perhaps, free nerve endings. Drainage of the veins proceeds either from the cortex outward to the periosteal veins or inward into the marrow space and out the nutrient veins.

Periosteum

The periosteum is a specialized connective tissue that covers all bones of the body and is capable of forming bone. The internal layer of the periosteum, termed the *cambium layer*, is applied to the surface of the bone and consists of loosely arranged collagenous bundles, with spindle-shaped connective tissue cells and a network of thin elastic fibers. The outer *fibrous layer* is contiguous with soft tissue planes and fascia. It is composed of a dense connective tissue containing blood vessels.

The Bone Matrix

Bone tissue is composed of cells (10% by weight), a mineralized phase (hydroxyapatite crystals, representing 60% of the total tissue), and an organic matrix (30%). Thus, with the exception of the cells, bone is a biphasic structure comprising an organic and an inorganic matrix.

The mineralized matrix consists of poorly crystalline hydroxyapatite, $Ca_{10}(PO_4)_6(OH)_2$. Because of its net negative charge, this material can neutralize substantial amounts of acid. Other important ions in bone are carbonate, citrate, fluoride, chloride, sodium, magnesium, potassium, and strontium.

The organic matrix consists of 88% type I collagen, 10% other proteins, and 1% to 2% lipids and glycosaminoglycans. **Thus, type I collagen essentially defines the organic matrix,** yet studies of the other proteins are of great interest, because they participate in bone morphogenesis and mineral crystallization. Examples of such proteins include the following:

- **Osteocalcin** is a protein produced by osteoblasts, and blood levels of this protein serve as a useful marker of bone formation. Interestingly, mice incapable of producing osteocalcin have increased bone mass, indicating that the protein inhibits bone resorption.
- **Osteopontin and sialoprotein** are bone matrix proteins containing the amino acid sequence *Arg-Gly-Asp*, which is recognized by the cell-attachment proteins termed *integrins*. Thus osteopontin and bone sialoprotein probably help anchor cells to the bone matrix.

The Cells of Bone

There are four types of cells in bone tissue, each of which has specific functions related to the formation, resorption, and remodeling of bone.

OSTEOPROGENITOR CELL: The osteoprogenitor cell, which ultimately differentiates into osteoblasts and osteocytes, is itself derived from a primitive stem cell. The stem cell is capable of developing into adipocytes, myoblasts, fibroblasts, or osteoblasts. The osteoprogenitor cell is found in the marrow, periosteum, and all the supporting structures within the marrow cavity. This cell is not readily recognized by light microscopy because it appears as a small, nonspecific, stellate or spindle-shaped cell. In response to an appropriate signal, the osteoprogenitor gives rise to an osteoblast.

OSTEOBLAST: Osteoblasts are the protein-synthesizing cells that produce and mineralize bone tissue. Precursor cells are turned into osteoblasts under the influence of the transcription factor CBFA-1. These large mononuclear and polygonal cells are arrayed in a line alone the bone surface (Fig. 26-3A). Underlying the layer of osteoblasts is a thin, eosinophilic zone of organic bone matrix that has not yet been mineralized, termed *osteoid*. The time from the deposition of osteoid to its mineralization is known as the *mineralization lag time*. Reflecting its protein synthetic capacity, the osteoblast has a complex cytoplasm, containing abundant endoplasmic reticulum, a prominent Golgi apparatus, and mitochondria with calcium-containing granules. Cytoplasmic processes that extend into the osteoid are in contact with cells embedded within the matrix, called osteocytes. The syncytium of osteocytes and osteoblasts probably serves to prevent bone calcium (99% of the body's calcium) from equilibrating with the general extracellular space. When the osteoblast is inactive, it flattens on the surface of bone tissue. The osteoblast contains alkaline phosphatase, manufactures osteocalcin, and has parathyroid hormone receptors. Collagenase secreted by the osteoblasts may also facilitate osteoclastic activity. Finally, a number of growth factors, including transforming growth factor-beta (TGF-β), insulin-like growth factor-1 (IGF-1), IGF-2, platelet-derived growth factor (PDGF), interleukin-1 (IL-1), fibroblast growth factor (FGF), and tumor necrosis factor-alpha (TNF-α), are produced by osteoblasts and play an important role in regulating growth and differentiation of bone.

OSTEOCYTE: The osteocyte is an osteoblast that is completely embedded in bone matrix and isolated in a lacuna (see Fig. 26-3B). Although osteocytes are responsible for depositing small quantities of bone around lacunae, with time this cell loses its capacity for protein synthesis, and the Golgi apparatus and endoplasmic reticulum become inconspicuous. The osteocyte has numerous processes that extend through bony canals, called *canaliculi*,

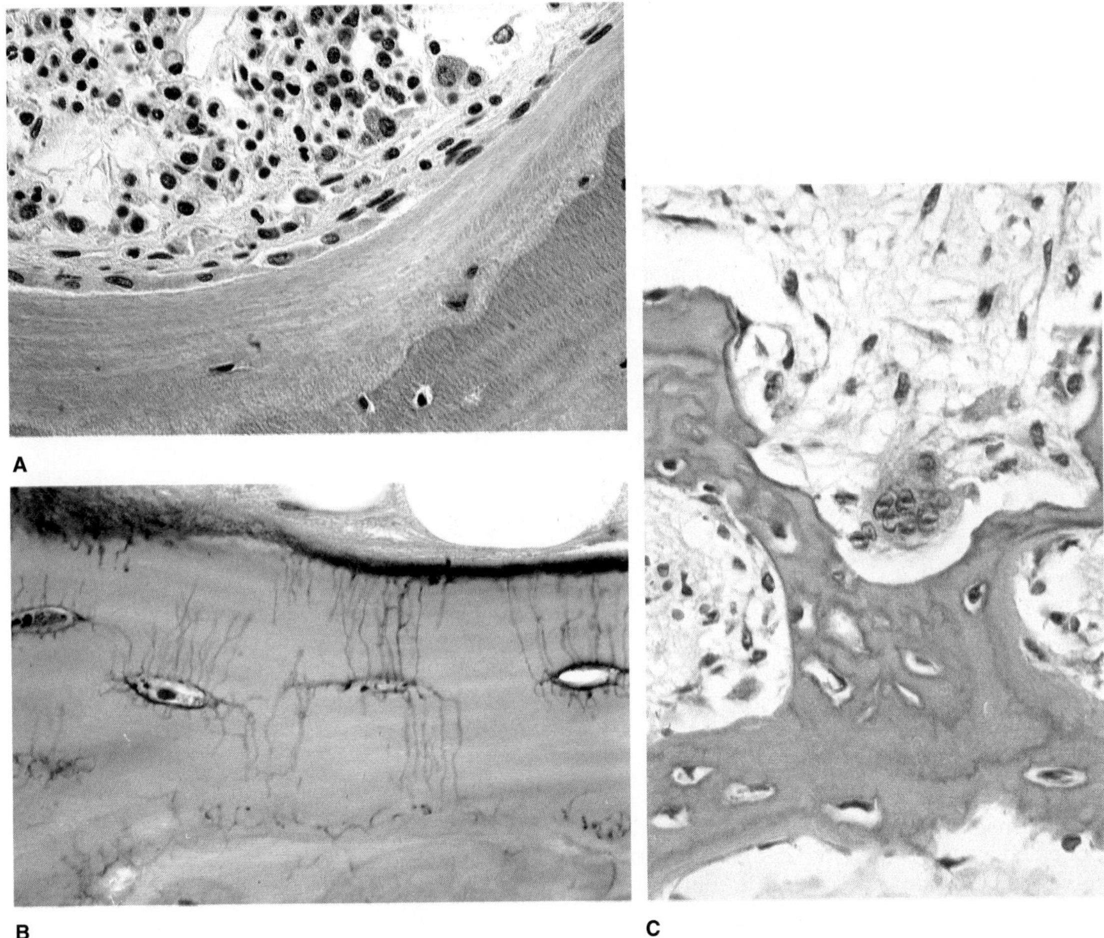

FIGURE 26-3
The cells of bones. (*A*) Osteoblast. A photomicrograph of bone reveals a layer of osteoblasts overlying an eosinophilic osteoid seam. Below the osteoid is mineralized bone. (*B*) Osteocyte. Osteocytes represent trapped osteoblasts embedded in a bony matrix. They are located in lacunae, and their cytoplasm extends into bony canals, called canaliculi. (*C*) Osteoclast. The osteoclast is a multinucleated cell found on the surface of bones in a small depression, termed a Howship's lacuna.

and communicate with those from other osteocytes. The cytoplasmic processes contain actin filaments and are separated from processes of other osteocytes by tight gap junctions. Recent evidence suggests the osteocyte may be the bone cell that recognizes and responds to mechanical forces.

OSTEOCLAST: The osteoclast, which is the exclusive bone-resorptive cell, is of hemopoietic origin and is a member of the monocyte/macrophage family. It is a multinucleated cell that contains many lysosomes and is rich in hydrolytic enzymes. Osteoclasts are found on the surfaces of bones in small depressions, termed *Howship's lacunae* (see Fig. 26-3C). Osteoclasts are highly polarized cells. The most strikingly polarized structure of the cell is its *ruffled membrane*, a complex infolding of plasmalemma, juxtaposed to the bone surface, which is visualized by electron microscopy (Fig. 26-4). The ruffled membrane is the osteoclast's resorptive organelle and forms only when the cell is in contact with and is actively degrading bone. Osteoclastic resorption is a multistep process that involves attachment of the cell to bone by integrins. A tight gasket-like seal isolates an extracellular compartment, which forms between bone and the osteoclast ruffled membrane. A proton pump then acidifies this compartment to a pH approximating 4.5, in effect creating a giant extracellular lysosome. This proton-rich environment mobilizes bone mineral, thereby exposing the organic matrix of bone to degradation by lysosomal enzymes. Degraded fragments of bone are transcytosed to the opposite side of the osteoclasts and then released to the extracellular space. Although the machinery of an osteoclast is superbly suited for bone resorption, it functions only if the matrix is mineralized. In fact, any bone that contains abundant osteoid or unmineralized cartilage is protected from osteoclastic activity. In rickets, the growth plate does not calcify normally; it therefore grows without osteoclastic resorption and becomes very thick.

The resorptive action of osteoclasts initiates the constant remolding of bone that is a normal part of skeletal maintenance (Fig. 26-5).

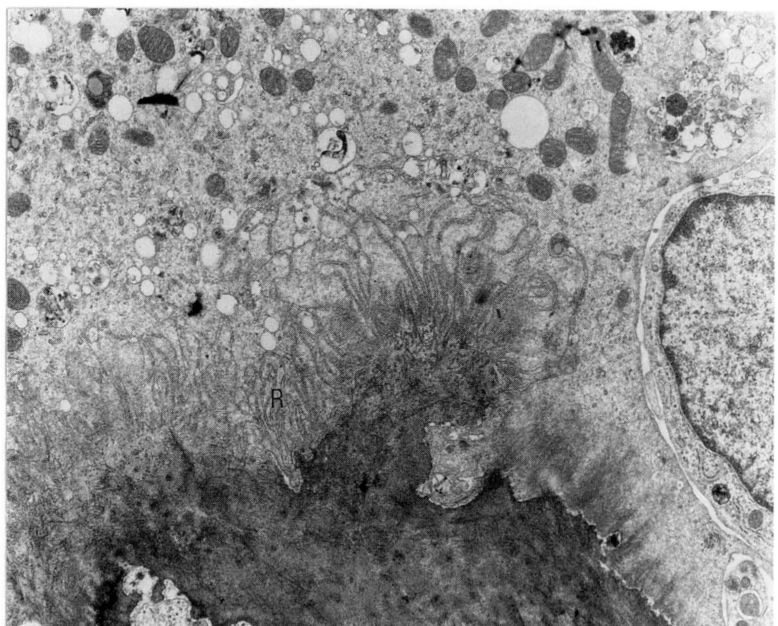

FIGURE 26-4
Osteoclast. An electron micrograph shows the ruffled membrane (R), which consists of a complex infolding of the plasma membrane juxtaposed to bone.

Microscopic Organization of Bone Tissue

Microscopic examination reveals two types of bone tissue: lamellar bone and woven bone (Fig. 26-6). Both varieties may be mineralized or unmineralized, the latter being termed *osteoid.*

Lamellar Bone

Lamellar bone is produced slowly and is highly organized. As the stronger bone tissue, it forms the adult skeleton. **Anything other than lamellar bone in the adult skeleton is abnormal.** Lamellar bone is defined by three characteristics: (1) a parallel arrangement of type I collagen fibers, (2) few osteocytes in the matrix, and (3) uniform osteocytes in lacunae parallel to the long axis of the collagen fibers. There are four types of lamellar bone.

- **Circumferential bone** forms the outer periosteal and inner endosteal lamellar envelopes of the cortex.
- **Concentric lamellar bone** is arranged around the Haversian canals. In two dimensions, concentric lamellar bone and its Haversian artery and vein constitute the *osteon* (see Fig. 26-1). In three dimensions, the osteons compose the Haversian system. These cylinders of bone around the Haversian canals run parallel to the long axis of the cortex and are the strongest bone made.
- **Interstitial lamellar bone** represents remnants of either circumferential or concentric lamellar bone, which have been remodeled and are wedged between the osteons.
- **Trabecular lamellar bone** forms the coarse cancellous bone of the medullary cavity. It exhibits plates of lamellar bone perforated by marrow spaces.

With the exception of trabecular bone, lamellar bone is found in the cortex (Fig. 26-7). The osteons form only if there

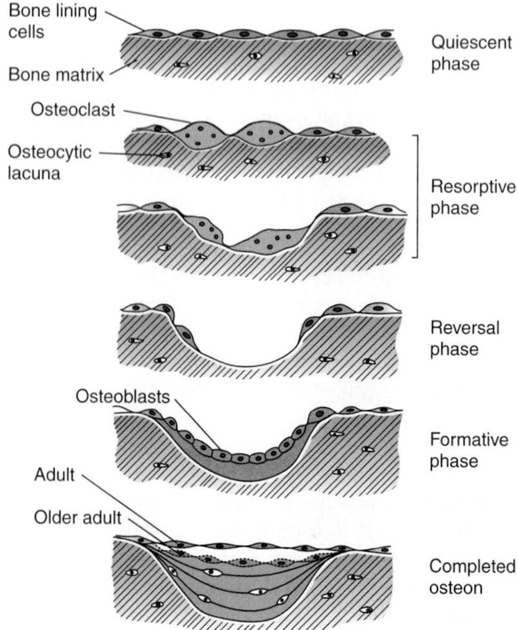

FIGURE 26-5
Bone-remodeling sequence. Bone remodeling is initiated by the appearance of osteoclasts on a bone surface previously lined by fusiform cells. After development of a resorption bay, osteoclasts are replaced by osteoblasts, which deposit new bone. The bone loss that attends aging (senile osteoporosis) is due to incomplete filling of resorption bays.

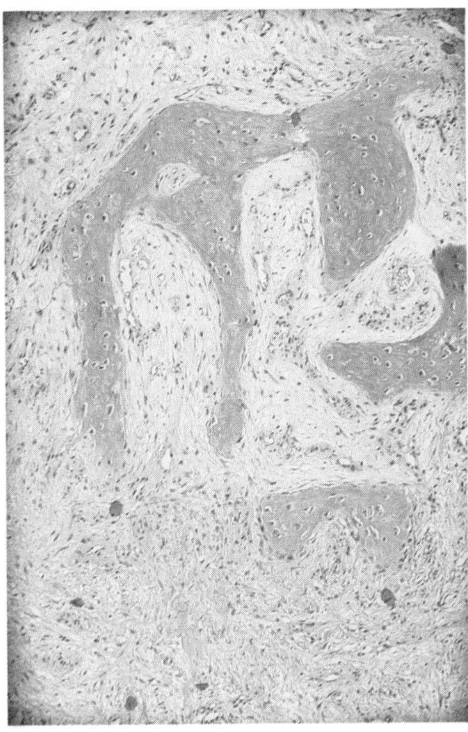

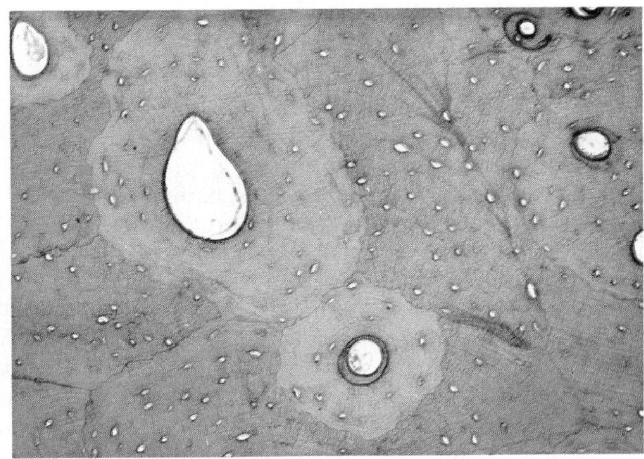

A B

FIGURE 26-6
Woven and lamellar bone. (*A*) Woven bone is characterized by a random distribution of collagen fibers, numerous osteocytes, and variation in the size of the osteocytes. (*B*) Lamellar bone shows a parallel and concentric arrangement of the collagen fibers and fewer osteocytes.

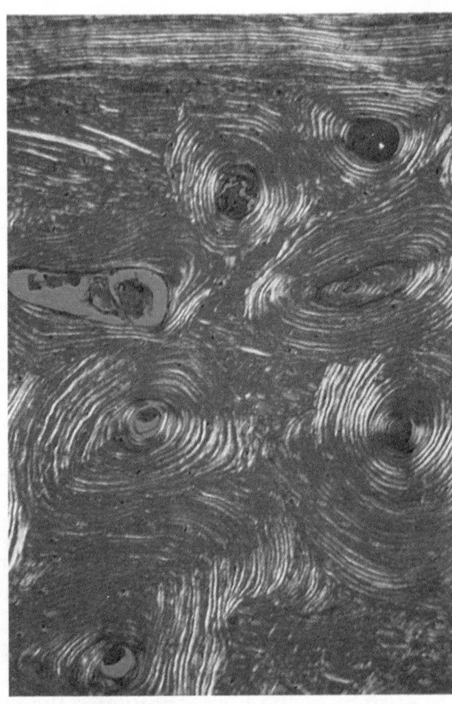

FIGURE 26-7
Cortical lamellar bone. Under polarized light, the concentric lamellar bone is arranged around the empty space where a Haversian canal traverses.

is appropriate stress. For example, a paralyzed limb in a child has a cortex composed exclusively of poorly formed Haversian systems and circumferential lamellar bone.

Woven Bone

Woven bone is identified by (1) an irregular arrangement of type I collagen fibers, hence the term woven; (2) numerous osteocytes in the matrix; and (3) variation in the size and shape of the osteocytes.

Woven bone is more rapidly deposited than lamellar bone. It is haphazardly arranged and of low tensile strength, serving as a temporary scaffolding for support. It is not surprising that woven bone is found in the developing fetus, in areas surrounding tumors and infections, and as part of a healing fracture. **The presence of woven bone in the adult skeleton always represents a pathological condition and indicates that reactive tissue has been produced in response to some stress in the bone.**

A few comparative points related to the presence of woven or lamellar bone deserve emphasis. Slowly manufactured bone tends to be lamellar, whereas rapidly deposited bone is woven. The presence of a fragment of Haversian bone and interstitial lamellar bone in a small biopsy specimen indicates the presence of cortical tissue. A persistent stress, such as that produced by a slowly growing tumor or an indolent infection, may actually be walled off by pathological lamellar bone, whereas a rapidly growing tumor or virulent infection may stimulate the formation of woven bone. Woven bone is the product of most bone-forming tumors. By contrast, lamellar bone is rarely found in bone-forming tumors.

Cartilage

In contrast to bone, cartilage does not contain blood vessels, nerves, or lymphatics. It may be focally calcified to provide some internal strength in the appropriate areas.

The Cartilage Matrix

Similar to bone, cartilage may be viewed as an organic and inorganic biphasic material. The inorganic phase is composed of calcium hydroxyapatite crystals, equivalent to those found in bone matrix. However, the organic matrix is quite different from that of bone. Essentially, cartilage is a hyperhydrated structure, with water forming some 80% of its weight. The remaining 20% is composed principally of two macromolecular substances, namely type II collagen and proteoglycans. Trace amounts of neutral lipids, phospholipids, lysozyme, and glycoproteins are also found. The water content is extremely important in the function of articular cartilage because it enhances the resilience and lubrication of the joint. The proteoglycans are complex macromolecules composed of a central linear protein core, to which are attached long side arms of polysaccharides called glycosaminoglycans. These molecules are polyanionic because of the regular presence of carboxyl groups and sulfates along the molecules. Cartilage glycosaminoglycans comprise three long-chain, unbranched, repeating, polydimeric saccharides: chondroitin-4-sulfate, chondroitin-6-sulfate, and keratan sulfate. The chondroitin sulfates are the most abundant, accounting for 55% to 90% of the cartilage matrix, depending on the age of the tissue.

Types of Cartilage

There are three types of cartilage:

- **Hyaline cartilage:** This is the prototypic cartilage, comprising the articular cartilage of the joints, the cartilaginous anlage of developing bones, the growth plates, the costochondral cartilages, the cartilages of the trachea, bronchi, and larynx, and the nasal cartilages. Hyaline cartilage is the most common cartilage in tumors, in fracture callus, and in areas of relative avascularity.
- **Fibrocartilage:** This tissue is essentially hyaline cartilage that contains numerous type I collagen fibers for tensile and structural strength. It is found in the annulus fibrosus of the intervertebral disk, tendinous and ligamentous insertions, menisci, the symphysis pubis, and insertions of joint capsules. Fibrocartilage may also occur in a fracture callus and in some cartilage-forming tumors.
- **Elastic cartilage:** Hyaline cartilage in specialized areas contains elastin. This yellow cartilage is found in the pinna of the ears, in the epiglottis, and in the arytenoid cartilages of the larynx.

Chondrocytes

Chondrocytes are derived from a primitive mesenchymal cell that is similar to the precursor of the bone cells. The chondroblast gives rise to the chondrocyte. The cell that destroys calcified cartilage is also the osteoclast.

BONE FORMATION AND GROWTH

Bone tissue grows only by appositional growth, defined as the deposition of new matrix on the surface by adjacent surface cells. By contrast, virtually all other tissues, especially cartilage, increase by interstitial cell proliferation within the matrix as well as by appositional growth. The development of bone in the fetus follows a stereotyped sequence.

Most of the skeleton (except the bones of the calvarium and the clavicles) develop from cartilage anlagen that are present during fetal development. Thus, bone is first represented by tissue cartilage, which is eventually resorbed and replaced by bone in a process termed endochondral ossification. The development of bone can be illustrated by using a limb as an example.

Primary Ossification

The process of primary ossification follows a temporal sequence:

1. **Cartilage anlage:** By 5 weeks of gestation, a thin layer of mesenchymal cells forms between the ectoderm and endoderm of the limb bud and condenses into a core of hyaline cartilage. This cartilaginous anlage becomes the precursor of the future long bone of that limb. The fibrous capsule of the cartilage anlage is called a *perichondrium*. The width of the cartilaginous anlage is increased by appositional growth of chondroblasts, which deposit cartilage matrix on the internal surface of the perichondrium. At the same time, the anlage increases in length by a combination of appositional and interstitial growth of the chondrocytes. At this stage, the long "bone" is actually composed of cartilage. Bone formation occurs at the perichondrium according to a predetermined program.
2. **The primary center of ossification:** The first true bone tissue is laid down on the fibrous surface of the cartilage anlage in the midportion of the future bone (diaphysis). At the perichondrium, the vascular bed increases, and the perichondrium begins to lay down woven bone on the surface of the cartilage core. This circumferential sleeve of woven bone is the primary center of ossification, because it is the first bone tissue to be formed. At this point, the perichondrium covers bone tissue and is thus termed *periosteum*.
3. **Cylinderization:** At the same time that the primary center of ossification forms, the increased vascularity on the surface of the bone stimulates the chondrocytes within the cartilaginous anlage to form proliferating columns of chondrocytes, which eventually undergo focal calcification. The calcification is the signal

for osteoclastic resorption and invasion of vessels into the cartilaginous mass. Thus, the earliest endochondral ossification occurs after the cartilage is hollowed out from the center of the anlage. This "cavitation" of the cartilaginous core forms the future marrow space. The progressive hollowing of the diaphysis is termed *cylinderization*.

4. **Primary spongiosum:** The swollen, hypertrophied chondrocytes within the central cartilage begin to die, and capillary invasion becomes more extensive. The surfaces of the calcified cartilage cores become enveloped by woven bone laid down by osteoblasts, which arrive through the pluripotential mesenchymal tissue that enters with the capillaries. This cartilaginous core, surrounded by woven bone, is called *primary spongiosum*, or *primary trabeculum*. It is the first bone formed after the replacement of cartilage in the process of endochondral ossification.

Cavitation continues along the future diaphysis toward each end of the bone. Meanwhile, the bone enlarges in width by appositional bone growth from the ever-increasing periosteal sleeve, which makes additional woven bone for the future cortex. The chondrocytes renew themselves by interstitial growth to keep pace with the enlarging cavitation of the future marrow cavity.

Secondary Ossification

Programmed events similar to those in the primary spongiosum take place in the cartilaginous ends of the future bone. Resting (reserve) cartilage is stimulated to become columns of proliferating cartilage, which then progress to hypertrophied chondrocytes and, eventually, calcified cartilage.

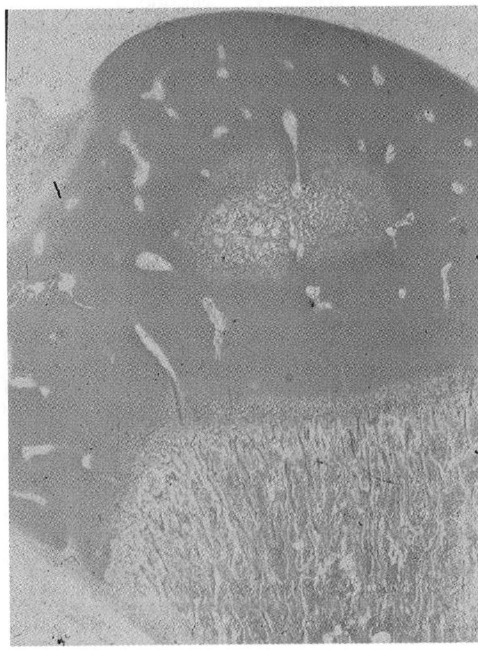

FIGURE *26-8*
Secondary center of ossification is present in the proximal femur.

1. **The secondary center of ossification** (Fig. 26-8): Also termed the *epiphyseal center of ossification*, this structure is formed at the ends of the bone when cartilage is resorbed. The centrifugal enlargement of the secondary ossification is called *hemispherization* and occurs simultaneously with the longitudinal development of the marrow cavity of the diaphysis.
2. **Formation of the growth plate:** Eventually, as the ends of the bone expand during hemispherization, and cylinderization occurs in the future diaphysis, a zone of cartilage is trapped between the end of the bone and the diaphysis. This cartilage is destined to be the *growth plate* (Fig. 26-9A). The growth plate is a layer of modified cartilage between the diaphysis and the epiphysis, and its structure is essentially unchanged from early fetal life to skeletal maturity. **The growth plate controls the longitudinal growth of bones and ultimately determines adult height.**
3. **Structure of the growth plate:** The chondrocytes of the growth plate are arranged in vertical rows, which, in three dimensions, are really helices. When viewed longitudinally, the growth plate, proceeding from the epiphysis to the metaphysis, is divided into zones (see Figs. 26-2B and 26-9).

The reserve (resting) zone is supplied by the epiphyseal arteries and has small chondrocytes and very little matrix. An additional peripheral zone, known as the *zone of Ranvier*, lies directly under the perichondrium.

The proliferative zone is the next deeper zone, in which active proliferation of chondrocytes occurs both longitudinally and transversely, although the main growth thrust is in the longitudinal direction. In a very active growth plate, the proliferative zones form more than half the thickness of the growth plate.

The hypertrophy zone is the next cartilaginous area and is characterized by a substantial increase in the size of the chondrocytes. The intercellular matrix is prominent, and chondrocytes are surrounded by a dense zone, called the *territorial matrix*.

The zone of calcification is the cartilaginous zone closest to the metaphysis, where the matrix becomes mineralized.

The zone of ossification is the area where a coating of bone is laid down on the surface of the calcified cartilage. Capillaries grow into the calcified cartilage and give access to osteoclasts, which resorb much of the calcified matrix. Residual vertical walls of calcified cartilage act as scaffolding for the deposition of bone.

The molecular mechanisms governing endochondral growth are beginning to be understood. For example, mutations of the FGF-3 receptor lead to either growth arrest or acceleration. Similarly, development of a normal growth plate depends on the expression of parathyroid hormone–related protein. Failure to produce this protein (initially isolated from malignant tumors that induce hypercalcemia) leads to severe growth retardation and distorted growth plates.

Formation of the Metaphysis

The formation of the metaphysis, which is called *funnelization*, occurs at the ring of LaCroix, a periosteal cuff of

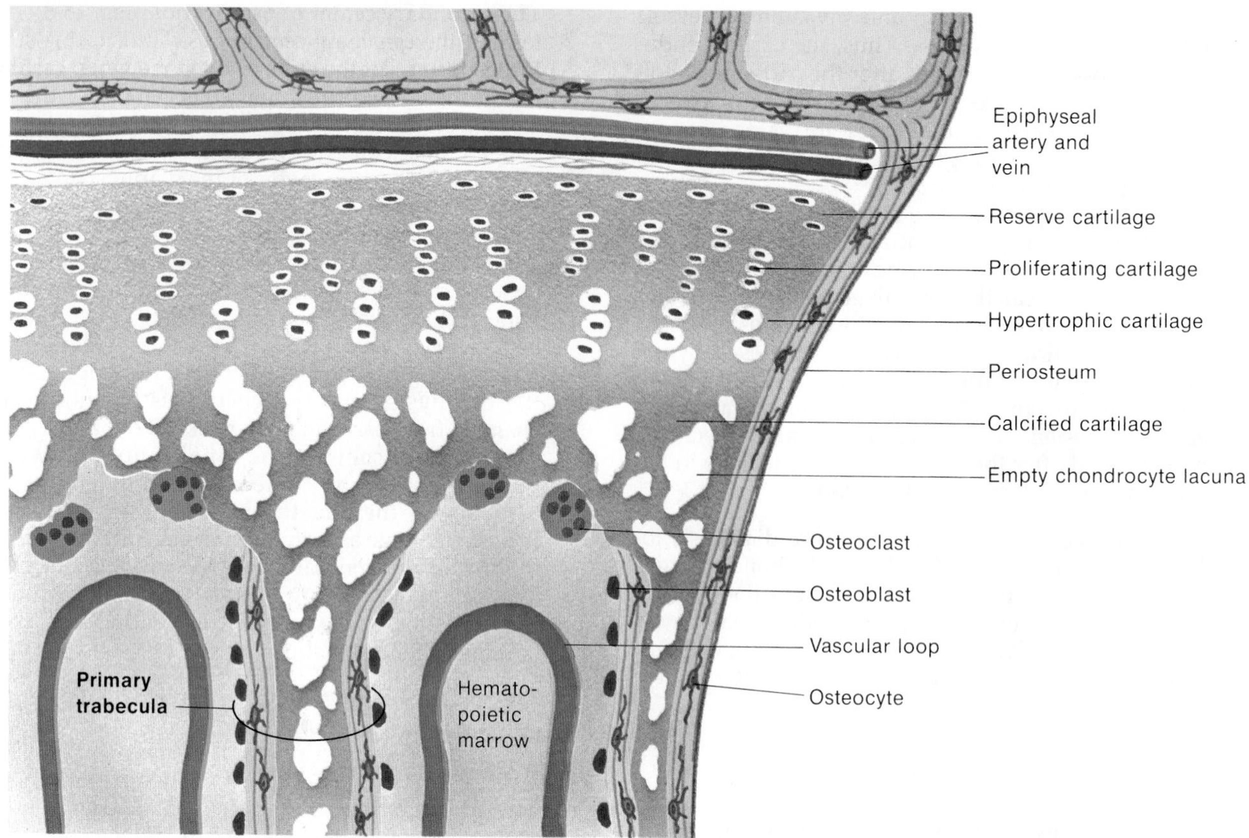

Epiphyseal artery and vein
Reserve cartilage
Proliferating cartilage
Hypertrophic cartilage
Periosteum
Calcified cartilage
Empty chondrocyte lacuna
Osteoclast
Osteoblast
Vascular loop
Osteocyte
Primary trabecula
Hemato-poietic marrow
A

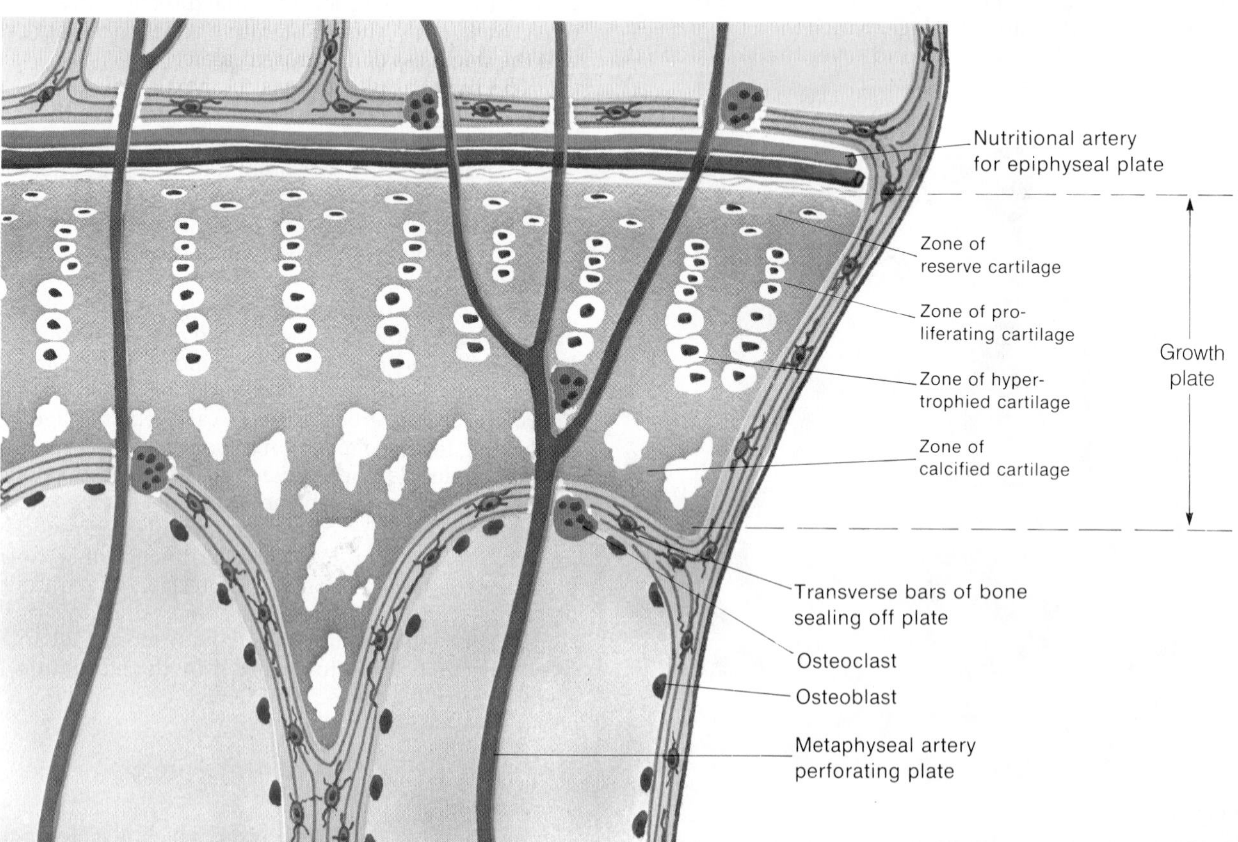

Nutritional artery for epiphyseal plate
Zone of reserve cartilage
Zone of pro-liferating cartilage
Zone of hyper-trophied cartilage
Zone of calcified cartilage
Growth plate
Transverse bars of bone sealing off plate
Osteoclast
Osteoblast
Metaphyseal artery perforating plate
B

FIGURE *26-9*

bone surrounding the epiphyseal cartilage. Here a wave of periosteal osteoclasts resorbs the cortex, so that a fluted or funnel shape begins to appear. At the same time, endosteal osteoblastic bone is deposited to keep pace with and to offset some of the osteoclastic resorption. The net result is the funnel or fluted shape of the bone.

Obliteration of the Growth Plate

The growth plate is normally obliterated at a specific age for each bone (see Fig. 26-9B). Closure of the growth plate is induced by sex hormones and occurs earlier in girls than in boys. The renewal of chondrocytes slows and ultimately ceases. The entire plate is eventually replaced by bone. In some persons, a transverse bony plate representing the site of closure can be seen radiologically.

DISORDERS OF THE GROWTH PLATE

Cretinism

Cretinism, the syndrome that results from maternal iodine deficiency (see Chapter 21), has profound effects on the skeleton. Linear growth is severely impaired, resulting in dwarfism, with the limbs disproportionately short in relation to the trunk. The delayed closure of the fontanelles of the skull causes an unusually large head. There is a delay in the closure of the epiphyses, as well as radiological stippling of these zones. Shedding of deciduous teeth and eruption of permanent teeth are retarded.

The skeletal deformities in cretinism are related to a defect in cartilage maturation. The chondrocytes do not follow the orderly progression of the endochondral sequence. Instead, the maturation of the hypertrophied zone is retarded, and the zone of proliferative cartilage is narrow. Endochondral ossification, therefore, does not proceed appropriately, and transverse bars of bone in the metaphysis seal off the growth plate. Although the growth plates may remain open, the failure of endochondral ossification produces severe dwarfism. The malshaped epiphyses seen on radiography reflect the incomplete penetration of the secondary centers of ossification of the epiphysis.

Morquio Syndrome

Many of the mucopolysaccharidoses (see Chapter 6) involve skeletal deformities, which can be attributed to the deposition of mucopolysaccharides (glycosaminoglycans) in the developing bones (Fig. 26-10). An example is Morquio syndrome (mucopolysaccharidosis type IV), which leads to a particularly severe form of dwarfism, in addition to dental defects, mental retardation, corneal opacities, and increased urinary excretion of keratan sulfate. Mucopolysaccharides accumulate in the chondrocytes, a process that ultimately interferes with the normal endochondral sequence. The result is a disorganized growth plate, which is also sealed off by transverse bars of bone.

Achondroplasia

Achondroplasia refers to a syndrome of short-limbed dwarfism and macrocephaly and represents a failure of normal epiphyseal cartilage formation. It is the most common genetic form of dwarfism (1:15,000 live births) and is inherited as an autosomal dominant trait. The large majority of cases represent new mutations. The mean adult height in achondroplasia is 131 cm (51 inches) in men and 125 cm (49 inches) in women. Achondroplastic dwarfs have normal mentation and an average life span. However, some patients develop severe kyphoscoliosis and its complications.

☐ **Pathogenesis:** Achondroplasia is caused by a mutation in the FGF-3 receptor on chromosome 4p16.3. When activated, this receptor suppresses physeal growth. The achondroplastic mutation constitutively activates the FGF-3 receptor, thereby arresting the development of the growth plate. Consistent with this observation, an inactivating FGF-3 mutation leads to accelerated longitudinal growth.

☐ **Pathology:** The growth plate in achondroplasia is greatly thinned, and the zone of proliferative cartilage is either absent or extensively attenuated (Fig. 26-11). The zone of provisional calcification, if present, undergoes endochondral ossification, but at a greatly reduced rate. A transverse bar of bone often seals off the growth plate, thereby preventing further bone formation and causing dwarfism. Interestingly, the secondary centers of ossification and the articular cartilage are normal. Because intramembranous ossification is undisturbed, the periosteum functions normally, and the bones become very short and thick. For the same reasons, the heads of affected patients appear unusually large, compared with the bones formed from the cartilage of the face. The spine is of normal length, but the limbs are abnormally short.

FIGURE *26-9*
Anatomy of the growth (epiphyseal) plate. (*A*) Normal growing epiphyseal plate. The epiphysis is separated from the epiphyseal plate by transverse plates of bone that seal the plate so that it grows only toward the metaphysis. The various zones of cartilage are illustrated. As the calcified cartilage migrates toward the metaphysis, the chondrocytes die, and the lacunae are empty. At the interface of the epiphyseal plate and the metaphysis, osteoclasts bore into the calcified cartilage, accompanied by a capillary loop from the metaphyseal vessels. Osteoblasts follow the osteoclasts and lay down osteoid on the cartilage core, thereby forming the primary spongiosum, or primary trabeculae. (*B*) Normal closure. The epiphyseal cartilage has ceased to grow, and metaphyseal vessels penetrate the cartilage plate. Transverse bars of bone separate the plate from the metaphysis.

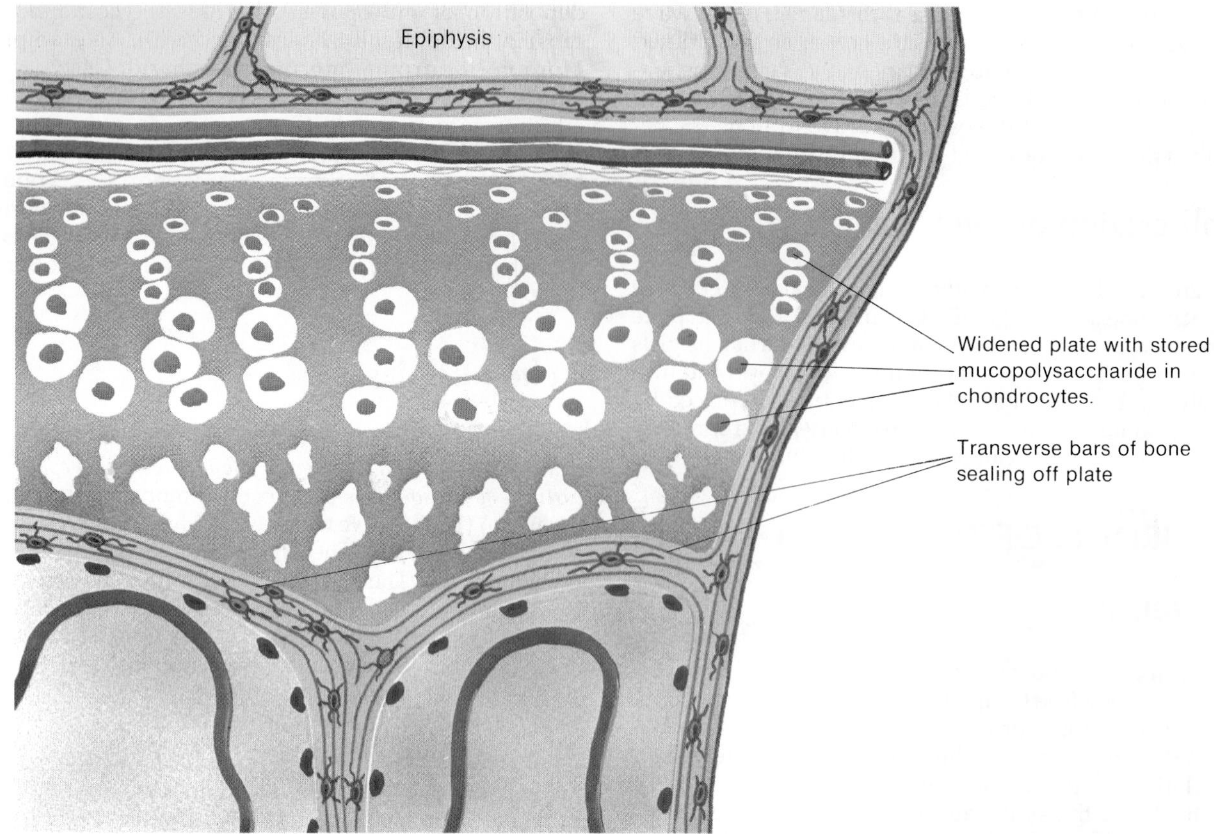

FIGURE 26-10
The growth (epiphyseal) plate in the mucopolysaccharidoses. These disorders are characterized by disorganized and abbreviated columns of swollen chondrocytes that are engorged with mucopolysaccharides. There is interference with the normal endochondral sequence, and the epiphyseal plate is sealed off by transverse bars of bone from the metaphysis. Dwarfism results from the lack of vascular penetration into the epiphyseal plate. Such penetration normally sustains new bone formation, thereby allowing continued lengthening of the bone.

Scurvy (Vitamin C Deficiency)

Scurvy, the clinical expression of vitamin C deficiency, is today a rare disease (see Chapter 8). Vitamin C is essential for the synthesis and proper structure of collagen. Wound healing and bone growth are, therefore, impaired in patients with scurvy. Furthermore, the basement membrane of capillaries is damaged by this condition, and widespread capillary bleeding is common.

□ **Pathology:** The skeletal changes of scurvy reflect the lack of osteoblastic function. Because the osteoblasts cannot produce and normally cross-link collagen, woven bone is not formed. At the growth plate, the chondrocytes continue to grow. The zone of calcified cartilage may actually become more prominent, because it is more heavily calcified. Osteoclasts resorb this zone, but the primary spongiosum does not form properly, and there is irregular vascular perforation of the cartilage plate (Fig. 26-12). Fractures and capillary bleeding occur, leading to further disorganization in the metaphysis—hence the German term *Trümmerfeld* ("field of ruin") for this area of the subepiphyseal plate. The subperiosteal bleeding may be so severe that is leads to diminution of the cortex, reduced appositional growth, and osteoporosis. Dislocation of the growth plate also may occur.

Children with scurvy have visible bone deformities, similar to those associated with rickets. In adults, bone deformities are not seen, but subperiosteal bleeding may occur, leading to joint and muscle pain.

Asymmetric Cartilage Growth

Asymmetric cartilage growth, such as occurs in patients with knock-knees and bowed legs, develops when one part of the growth plate, either medial or lateral, grows faster than the other. Most cases are hereditary, but mechanical forces, such as trauma near the growth plate, may stimulate one side to grow faster or in an asymmetric fashion.

To correct a severe condition in a child, the growth of this portion of the plate is retarded by surgically implanting a staple or a brace, thereby allowing the opposite side of the plate to grow. In an adult, because the growth plates have already closed, surgical osteotomy (fracture) is used. Aside from the cosmetic appearance, these conditions may require correction to prevent future incongruity, eventual loss of articular cartilage, and joint destruction.

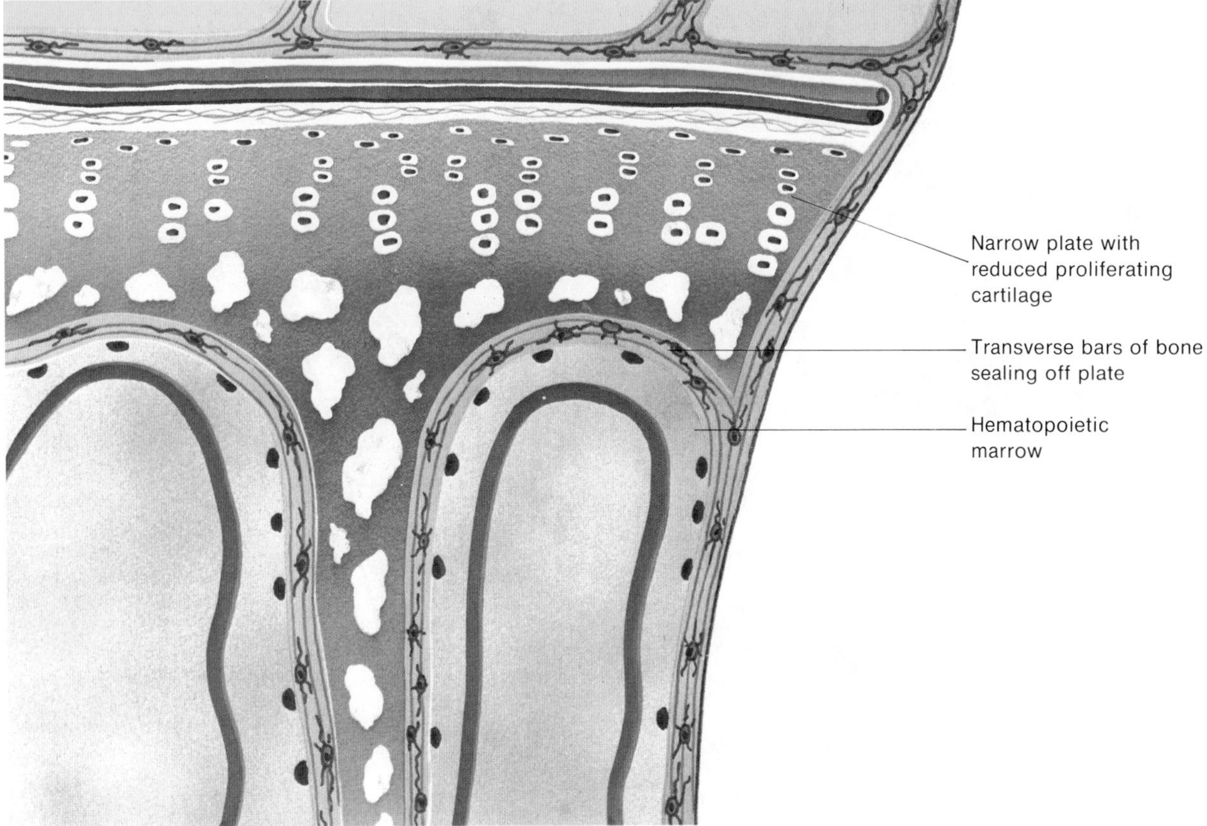

FIGURE *26-11*
The growth (epiphyseal) plate of an achondroplastic dwarf. In achondroplasia, the epiphyseal plate is reduced in thickness, and the zones of proliferating cartilage are attenuated. Osteoclastic activity is inconspicuous, and the interface between the plate and the metaphysis is often sealed by transverse bars of bone that prevent further endochondral ossification. As a result, the bones are shortened.

Scoliosis and Kyphosis

Scoliosis *is an abnormal lateral curvature of the spine, usually affecting adolescent girls.* ***Kyphosis*** *refers to an abnormal anteroposterior curvature.* When both conditions are present, the term ***kyphoscoliosis*** is used. A vertebral body grows in length (height) from the end plates of the vertebrae, which correspond to the growth plates of the long tubular bones. As in tubular bones, the vertebral bodies increase in width by appositional bone growth from the periosteum. In scoliosis, for unknown reasons, one portion of the end plate grows faster than the other, thereby producing a lateral curvature of the spine. The treatment is appropriate stress on the vertebral body, through the use of braces or internal fixation, to straighten the spine. If kyphoscoliosis is severe, the patient may eventually develop chronic pulmonary disease, cor pulmonale, and joint problems, particularly involving the hip.

Osteochondroma

Osteochondroma is a developmental defect (hamartoma) of the skeleton, which arises from a defect at the ring of Ranvier of the growth plate. Solitary osteochondroma is the most common form of the lesion. The tumor may have to be removed if it is cosmetically displeasing or presses on an artery or nerve.

☐ **Pathogenesis:** The ring of Ranvier guides the growth of the growth cartilage toward the metaphysis. If the ring of Ranvier is absent or defective, growth cartilage grows laterally into the soft tissue. Vessels originating in the marrow cavity of the bone extend into this cartilage mass. Continuation of this process results in a cartilage-capped, bony, stalked osteochondroma (Fig. 26-13), which is in direct continuity with the marrow cavity of the parent bone.

☐ **Pathology:** Osteochondromas tend to grow away from the joint. On radiograph, a cartilaginous mass is in direct continuity with the parent bone and is without an underlying cortex. On histological examination, a cartilage-capped, bony mass is surrounded by a surface fibrous membrane, which actually represents the perichondrium. Active endochondral ossification deep to the cartilage cap allows the bony protuberance to lengthen.

HEREDITARY MULTIPLE OSTEOCHONDROMATOSIS: This inherited, autosomal dominant disorder is characterized by numerous osteochondromas. Although not as common as solitary osteochondroma, the multiple form is not rare. It occurs predominantly in men and is primarily transmitted as a mendelian dominant

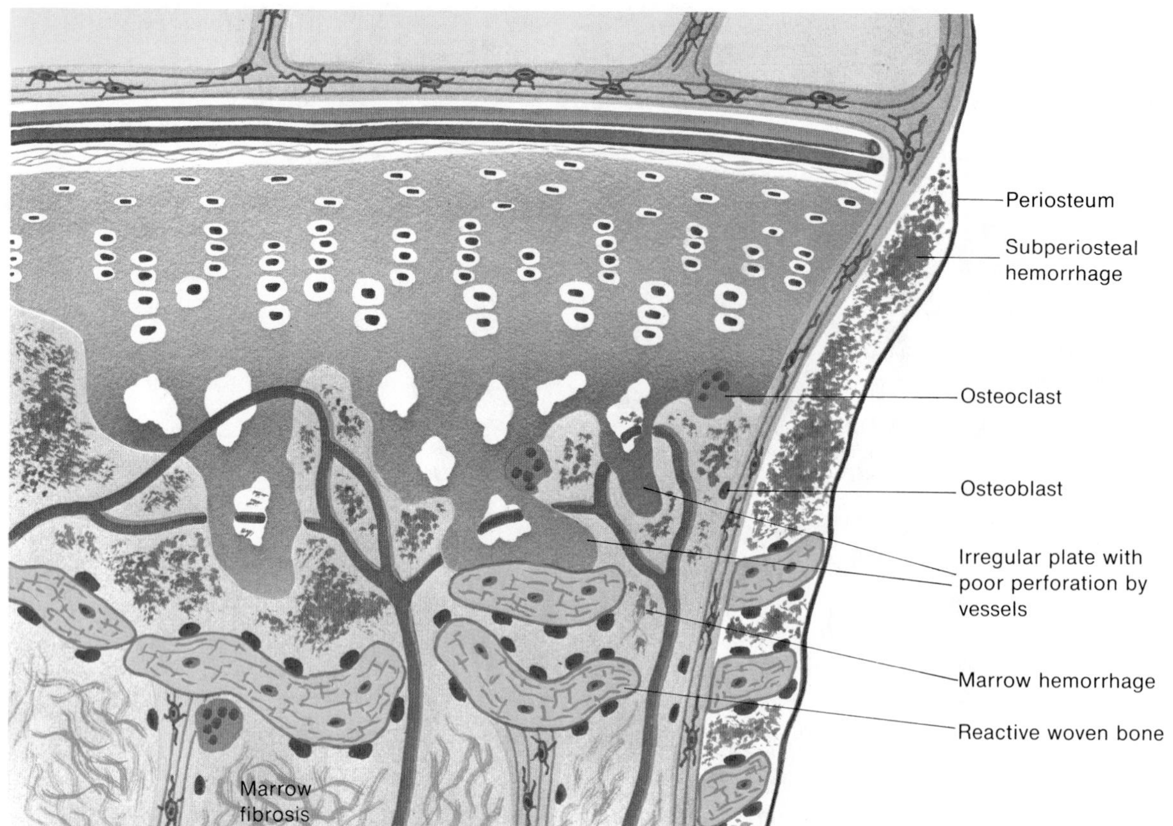

FIGURE *26-12*
The growth (epiphyseal) plate in scurvy. Defective collagen formation leads to capillary fragility and periosteal hemorrhage. Osteoclasts do not perforate the plate in a regular fashion. There is often extensive hemorrhage in this region. Microfractures cause secondary microcalluses; reactive bone is, therefore, seen in this region.

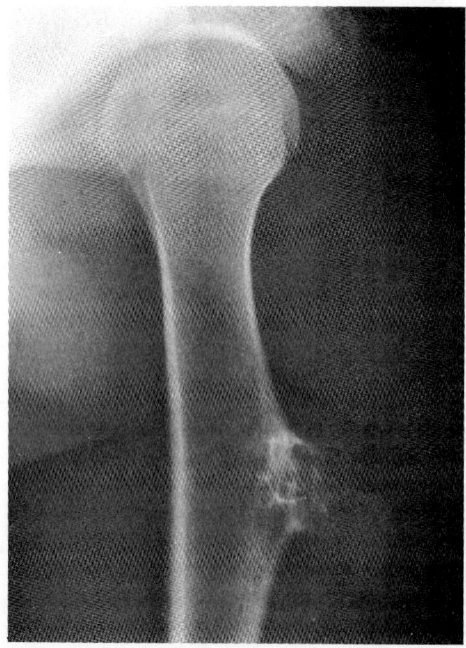
A

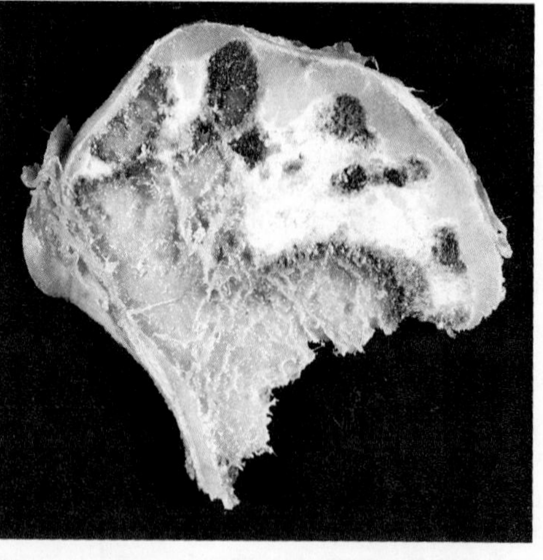
B

FIGURE *26-13*
Osteochondroma. (*A*) A radiograph of an osteochondroma of the humerus shows a legion that is directly contiguous with the marrow space. (*B*) The cross-sectional appearance of an osteochondroma shows the cap of calcified cartilage overlying poorly organized cancellous bone.

trait. However, an unaffected woman from an afflicted family also may transmit the disorder. In severe cases of hereditary osteochondromatosis, dwarfism may result because of the displacement of the longitudinal growth plate laterally by the osteochondroma. Metacarpals may be shortened, and fixed pronation or supination may develop if the lesions occur in the forearm and interfere with the function of the wrist. Further orthopedic difficulties may be caused by unequal leg length and joint function because of the encroaching osteochondromas.

The lesions of multiple osteochondromatosis are identical to those of solitary osteochondroma. Especially in multiple osteochondromatosis, there is a long-term increased risk of developing a chondrosarcoma in the cartilage cap, although this is a rare event. The enlargement of a known osteochondroma is worthy of investigation, although it may be attributable to adjacent trauma or to pregnancy and lactation.

Hemihypertrophy

Hemihypertrophy refers to a number of conditions that stimulate the growth plate in one limb to undergo rapid and prolonged endochondral ossification. As a consequence, the limb is much longer than the contralateral one. An infection in the metaphyseal area may stimulate the growth plate to grow rapidly. An arteriovenous malformation may also cause the growth plate to grow faster than its counterpart. Fractures and tumors near the growth plate may produce the same result. In some cases, hemihypertrophy is part of an inherited syndrome.

MODELING ABNORMALITIES

Osteopetrosis (Marble Bone Disease of Albers–Schönberg)

Osteopetrosis is a group of at least nine, rare, inherited disorders that are all characterized by abnormally dense bone. The most common, autosomal recessive form is a severe, sometimes fatal disease, affecting infants and children. Death of infants with this severe variant is attributable to marked anemia, cranial nerve entrapment, hydrocephalus, and infections. A more benign form, which is transmitted as an autosomal dominant trait and is seen in adulthood or adolescence, is associated with mild anemia or no symptoms at all.

☐ **Pathogenesis:** **The sclerotic skeleton of osteopetrosis is the result of failed osteoclastic bone resorption.** The disease is caused by mutations in genes that govern osteoclast formation or function. For example, mutation of genes coding proteins necessary for the generation of macrophages, which are osteoclast precursors, prompts one form of osteopetrosis distinguished by an absence of osteoclasts. Mutation of the oncogene c-*src*, which is necessary for osteoclast polarization, results in another type of osteopetrosis. In the latter form of the disease, abundant, yet ineffective, osteoclasts fail to polarize, as evidenced by the lack of a ruffled membrane.

Because osteoclast function is arrested, osteopetrosis is characterized by (1) the retention of the primary spongiosum with its cartilage cores, (2) lack of funnelization of the metaphysis, and (3) a thickened cortex. The result is short, block-like, radiodense bones, hence the term marble bone disease (Fig. 26-14). These bones are extremely radiopaque and weigh two to three times more than normal bone. However, they are basically weak because the bone structure is intrinsically disorganized, being unable to be remodeled along lines of stress. The mineralized cartilage is also weak and friable. As a result, the bones in osteopetrosis fracture easily.

☐ **Pathology and Clinical Features:** On gross examination, the bones in osteopetrosis are widened in the metaphysis and diaphysis, resulting in the characteristic "Erlenmeyer flask" deformity. Histologically, the bone tissue is extremely irregular, and almost all areas contain a cartilage core. Depending on the mutation, osteoclasts may be absent, present in normal numbers, or even abundant. In the case of osteopetrosis characterized by normal or increased numbers of osteoclasts, the molecular defect lies in a gene involved in the function of osteoclasts, rather in their formation.

The suppression of hemopoiesis in osteopetrosis is generally not due to encroachment of mineralized tissue on the marrow, but rather to its replacement by sheets of abnormal osteoclasts or extensive fibrosis. The magnitude of marrow suppression in patients with the malignant form of osteopetrosis is sufficient to cause severe anemia and even pancytopenia. To compensate for the encroachment on the marrow space, extramedullary hemopoiesis occurs in the liver, spleen, and lymph nodes, with result-

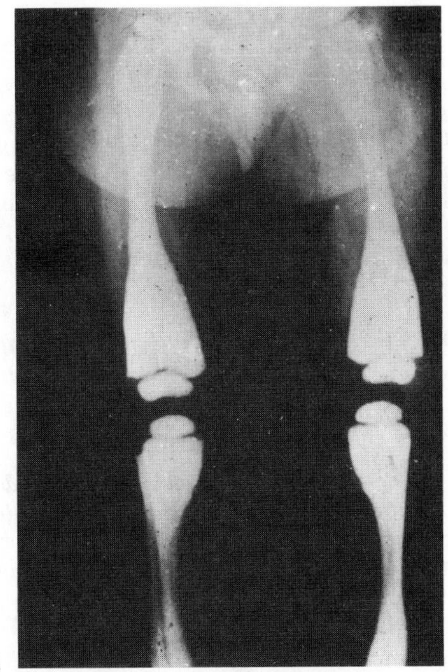

FIGURE 26-14
Osteopetrosis. (*A*) A radiograph of a child shows markedly misshapen and dense bones of the lower extremities, characteristic of "marble bone disease." *(figure continues)*

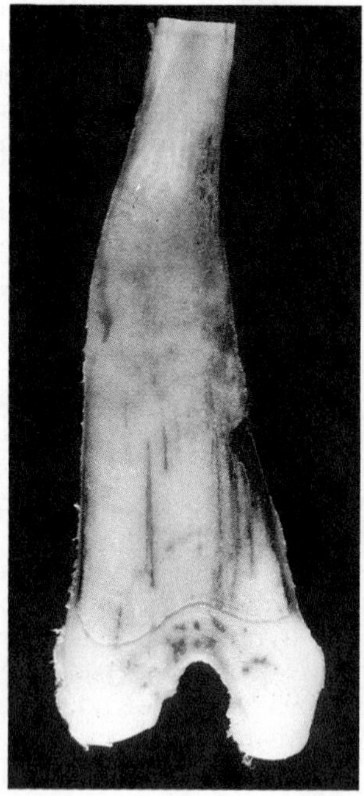
B

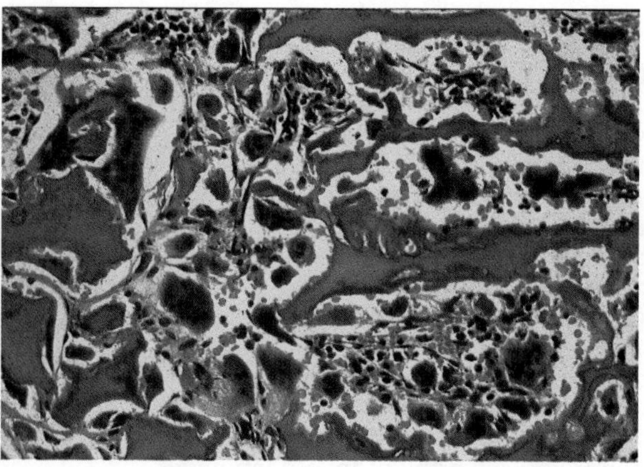
C

FIGURE *26-14 continued*
(*B*) A gross specimen of the femur shows obliteration of the marrow space by dense bone. (*C*) A photomicrograph of the bone of a child with osteopetrosis reveals a total disorganization of the bony trabeculae, most of which contain a core of calcified cartilage.

ing enlargement of these structures. Cranial nerve involvement is caused by the narrowing of neural foramina, and subsequent strangulation of nerves leads to blindness and deafness. The treatment currently used for osteopetrosis is bone marrow transplantation, which gives rise to a new clone of functional osteoclasts.

Progressive Diaphyseal Dysplasia (Camurati–Engelmann Disease)

Progressive diaphyseal dysplasia is an autosomal dominant disorder of children in which cylinderization does not proceed appropriately, resulting in a symmetric thickening in and an increased diameter of the diaphyses of long bones. The disease particularly affects the femur, tibia, fibula, radius, and ulna. Patients have pain over the affected areas, fatigue, muscle wasting, atrophy, and gait abnormalities.

DELAYED MATURATION OF BONE

Osteogenesis Imperfecta

Osteogenesis imperfecta refers to a group of autosomal dominant, heritable disorders of connective tissue, caused by mutations in the gene for type I collagen, which affect the skeleton, joints, ears, ligaments, teeth, sclerae, and skin (see Chapter 6). There are at least four types of osteogenesis imperfecta, each with a different mode of inheritance and clinical features.

Osteogenesis Imperfecta Type I

Osteogenesis imperfecta type I is characterized by multiple fractures after birth, blue sclerae, and hearing abnormalities. In some cases, abnormalities of the teeth are conspicuous. The initial fractures usually occur after the infant begins to sit and walk. There may be hundreds of fractures a year with minor movement or trauma. On radiological examination, the bones are extremely thin, delicate, and abnormally curved (Fig. 26-15). When a fracture occurs, the fracture callus may be so extensive as to resemble a tumor. As the child grows, the fractures tend to decrease in severity and frequency, and stature is generally unaffected.

The sclerae are very thin, with the blue color being attributable to the underlying choroid. The progressive hearing loss, which develops to total deafness in adulthood, results from fusion of the auditory ossicles. The joint laxity associated with the condition eventually leads to kyphoscoliosis and flat feet. Because of hypoplasia of the dentine and pulp, the teeth are misshapen and bluish yellow.

Osteogenesis Imperfecta Type II

Osteogenesis imperfecta type II is a lethal, perinatal disease. The affected infants are stillborn or die within a few days, in a sense being crushed to death. They exhibit markedly short stature and severe deformities of the limbs, and almost all of the bones sustain fractures during delivery or during uterine contractions in labor. As in osteogenesis imperfecta type I, the sclerae are blue.

Osteogenesis Imperfecta Type III

Osteogenesis imperfecta type III is the progressive, deforming type of disease and is characterized by many bone fractures, growth retardation, and severe skeletal deformities. Fractures are present at birth, but the bones are less fragile than in the type II form. These patients eventually develop severe shortening of their stature because of pro-

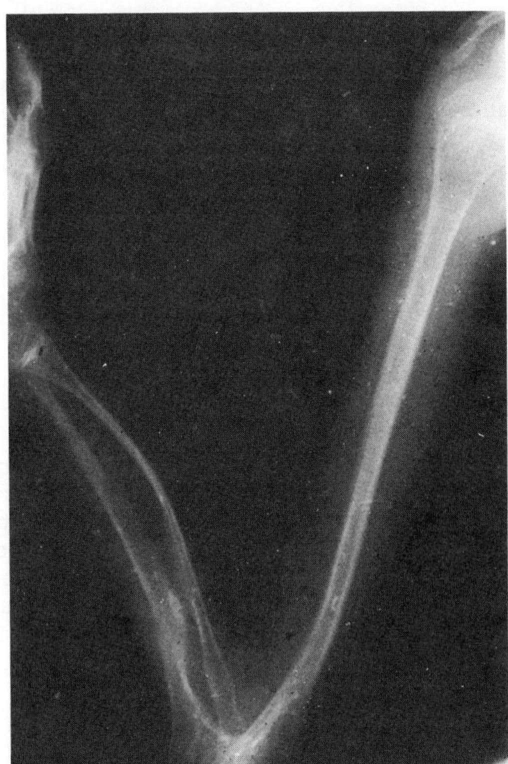

FIGURE 26-15
Osteogenesis imperfecta. A radiograph illustrates the markedly thin and attenuated humerus and bones of the forearm. There is a fracture callus in the proximal ulna.

gressive bone fractures and severe kyphoscoliosis. Although the sclerae may be blue at birth, they become white shortly thereafter. Abnormalities of the teeth are common.

Osteogenesis Imperfecta Type IV

Osteogenesis imperfecta type IV is similar to type I except that the sclerae are normal. The condition is heterogeneous in its presentation, and there may or may not be dental disease. In this disorder, abnormal cross-linkages of collagen result in thin, delicate, and weak collagen fibrils. This inappropriate collagen does not allow the bone cortex to mature, so that at birth, the cortex of the bone resembles that of a fetus. The cortex is composed of woven bone and small areas of lamellar bone. Over a period of years, the cortex matures, but this may not occur until adolescence or even later. In any event, the frequency of fractures tends to decrease over a long period. These patients are vigorously treated with orthopedic devices, including rods inserted into the medullary cavities, to prevent the dwarfing effect of multiple fractures.

Enchondromatosis (Ollier Disease)

Enchondromatosis is a bone disorder characterized by the development of multiple cartilaginous tumors, which lead to bony deformities. The condition is not strictly a disease of delayed maturation of bone, but one in which residual hyaline cartilage, anlage cartilage, or cartilage from the growth plate does not undergo endochondral ossification and remains in the bones. As a consequence, the bones show multiple, tumor-like masses of abnormally arranged hyaline cartilage (enchondromas), with zones of proliferative and hypertrophied cartilage (Fig. 26-16). These cartilaginous masses tend to be located in the metaphyses. As growth continues, the enchondromas settle in the diaphysis of adolescents and adults.

Enchondromatosis is asymmetric and may cause bone deformities. To some investigators, enchondromas represent true neoplasms. These cartilage nodules exhibit a strong tendency to undergo malignant change into chondrosarcomas in adult life. Therefore a patient with enchondromatosis who has increasing pain or an increasingly significant abnormality at one site should be evaluated to rule out an underlying sarcoma.

Maffucci syndrome *is characterized by multiple enchondromas and cavernous hemangiomas of the skin.* Chondrosarcoma develops in as many as half of all patients with Maffucci syndrome. There is also a solitary form of enchondroma that has the same histological features (perhaps less atypical) as the chondrocytes in Mafucci syndrome. This solitary form also principally affects the

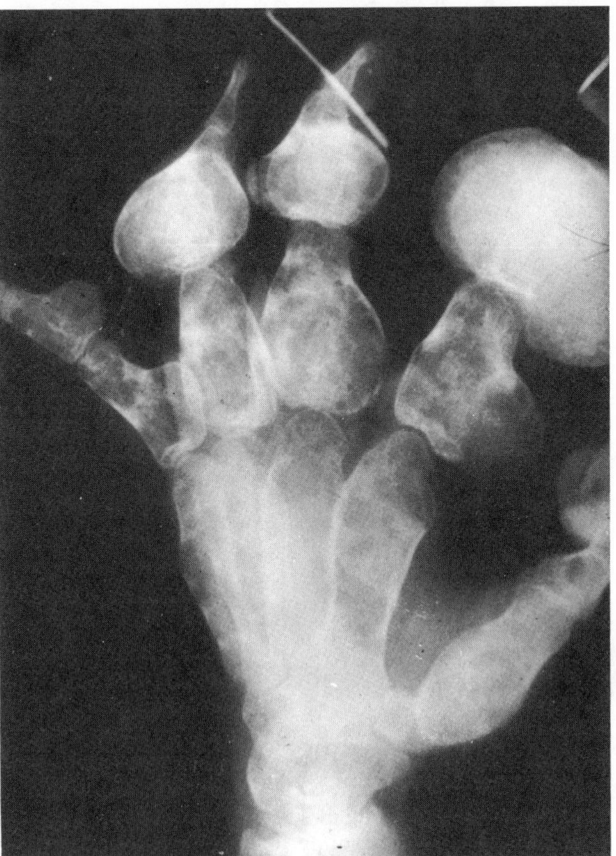

FIGURE 26-16
Multiple enchondromatosis (Ollier disease). A radiograph of the hand shows bulbous swellings that represent cartilage masses composed of hyaline cartilage, which is sometimes admixed with more primitive myxoid cartilage.

hands and feet, but is less likely to undergo malignant change. **It is noteworthy that all chondrosarcomas of the skeletal system probably arise from preexisting cartilage rests or enchondromas.**

FRACTURE

The most common bone lesion is a fracture, which is defined as a discontinuity of the bone. A force perpendicular to the long axis of the bone results in a transverse fracture. If the applied force is in the long axis of the bone, the resulting fracture is caused by compression. A torsional force results in a spiral fracture, and combined tension and compression shear forces cause angulation and displacement of the fractured ends.

A force powerful enough to fracture a bone also injures the adjacent soft tissues. In this situation, there is often (1) extensive muscle necrosis, (2) hemorrhage because of shearing of capillary beds and larger vessels of the soft tissues, (3) tearing of tendinous insertions and ligamentous attachments, and (4) even nerve damage, caused by stretching or direct tearing of the nerve.

Fracture Healing

In the repair of a bone fracture, anything other than the formation of bone tissue at the fracture site represents incomplete healing. The healing of a fracture is divided into three phases: the inflammatory phase, the reparative phase, and the remodeling phase (Fig. 26-17). The duration of each phase depends on the patient's age, the site of fracture, the patient's overall health and nutritional status, and the degree of soft tissue injury. Furthermore, local factors, such as vascular supply and mechanical forces at the site, also play a role in healing.

The Inflammatory Phase

In the first 1 to 2 days after a fracture, there is extensive tearing of the periosteum. The resultant rupture of blood vessels in the periosteum and adjacent soft tissue leads to extensive hemorrhage. In addition, muscle and other soft tissues may undergo necrosis and hemorrhage. There is also extensive necrosis of bone at the fracture site because of the disruption of large vessels in

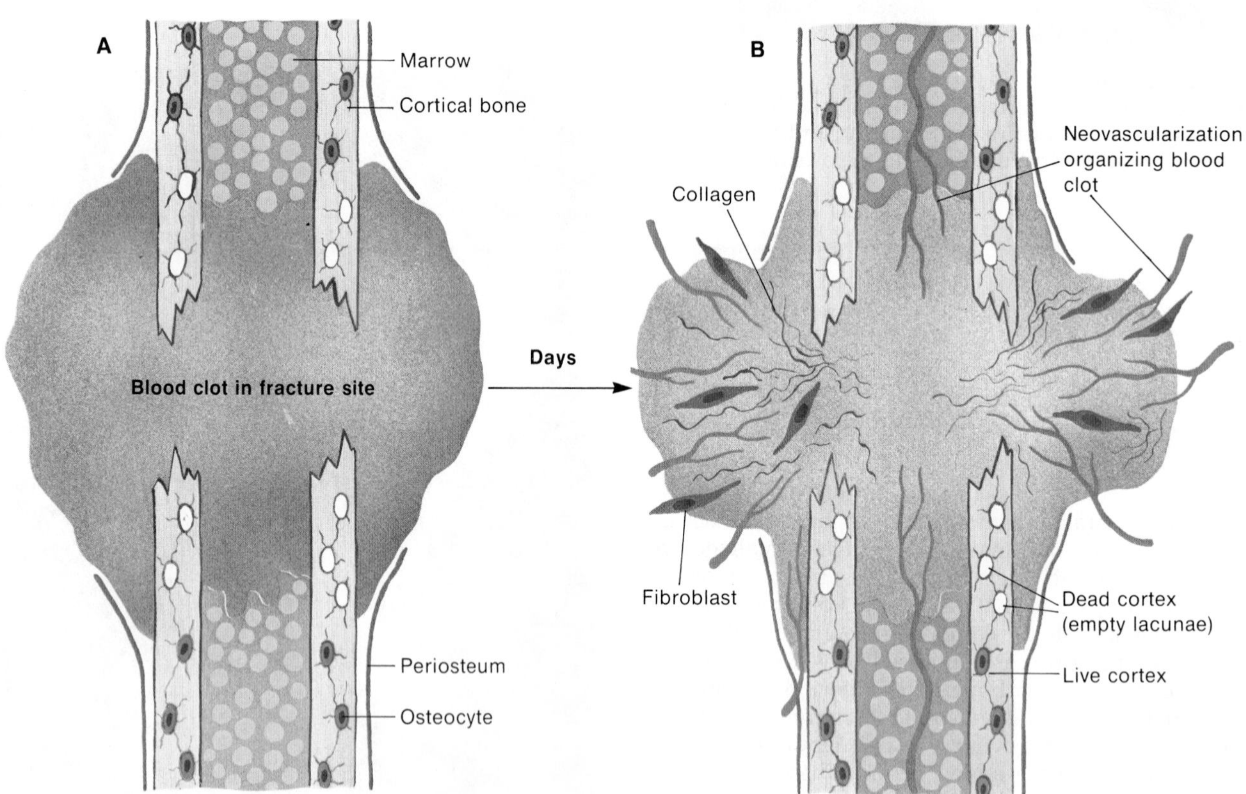

FIGURE 26-17
Healing of a fracture. (*A*) Soon after a fracture is sustained, an extensive blood clot forms in the subperiosteal and soft tissue, as well as in the marrow cavity. The bone at the fracture site is jagged. (*B*) The inflammatory phase of fracture healing is characterized by neovascularization and beginning organization of the blood clot. Because the osteocytes in the fracture site are dead, the lacunae are empty. The osteocytes of the cortex are necrotic well beyond the fracture site, owing to the traumatic interruption of the perforating arteries from the periosteum. (*figure continues*)

the bone and the interruption of the cortical vessels (i.e., the Volkmann and Haversian canals). **The hallmark of dead bone is the absence of osteocytes and empty bone lacunae.**

In 2 to 5 days, the hemorrhage forms a large clot, which must be resorbed so that the fracture can heal. Neovascularization begins to occur peripheral to this blood clot, which may extend deeply into the soft tissues and the medullary cavity. There is dilatation of adjacent vessels, transudation and exudation of fluids into the soft tissue and marrow, and the standard inflammatory response of polymorphonuclear leukocytes, macrophages, and mononuclear cells at the peripheral portion of the clot. By the end of the first week, most of the clot is organized by invasion of blood vessels and early fibrosis.

The earliest bone, which is invariably woven bone, also has formed after 7 days. **This corresponds to the "scar" of bone.** Because bone formation requires a good blood supply, the woven bone spicules begin to form at the periphery of the clot, where vascularization is greatest. Pluripotential mesenchymal cells from the soft tissue and within the bone marrow give rise to the osteoblasts that synthesize the woven bone. In most fractures, cartilage also is formed and is eventually resorbed by endochondral ossification. The granulation tissue containing bone or cartilage is termed a *callus*. Woven bone also forms inside the marrow cavity at the periphery of the blood clot because vascular tissue is also present in this location. At this time, the actual fracture site has not yet undergone remodeling.

The Reparative Phase

The reparative phase begins after the first week after the fracture and extends for months, depending on the degree of movement and the fixation of the fracture. By this time, the acute inflammatory cells have dissipated. The reparative process involves the differentiation of pluripotential cells into fibroblasts and osteoblasts. Repair proceeds from the periphery toward the center of the fracture site and accomplishes two objectives: (1) it organizes and resorbs the blood clot and, (2) more important, it furnishes neovascularization for the construction of the callus, which will eventually bridge the fracture site. The events leading to repair are as follows:

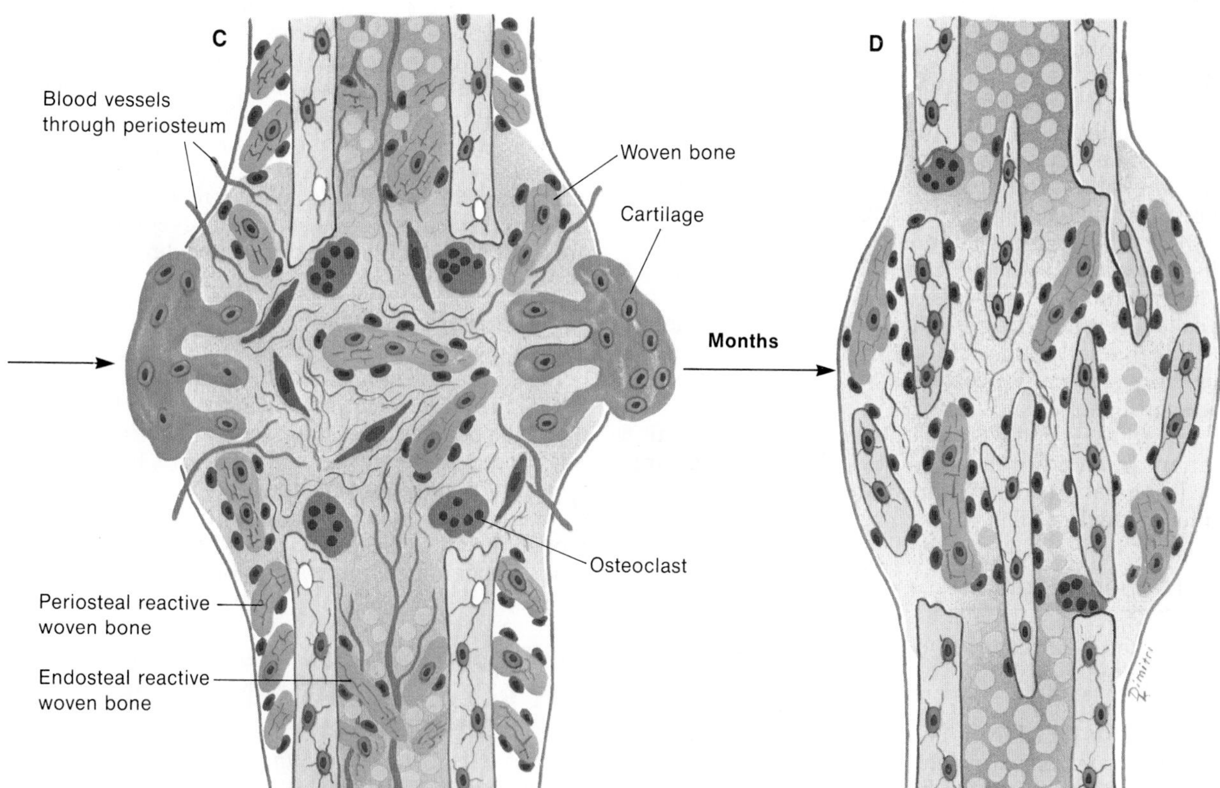

FIGURE *26-17 continued*
(*C*) The reparative phase of fracture healing is characterized by the formation of a callus of cartilage and woven bone near the fracture site. The jagged edges of the original cortex have been remodeled and eroded by osteoclasts. The marrow space has been revascularized and contains reactive woven bone, as does the periosteal area. (*D*) In the remodeling phase, during which the cortex is revitalized, the reactive bone may be lamellar or woven. The new bone is organized along stress lines and mechanical forces. Extensive osteoclastic and osteoblastic cellular activity is maintained.

1. Armies of osteoclasts within the Haversian canals form cutting cones that bore into the cortex toward the fracture site. A new vessel accompanies the cutting cone, supplying nutrients to these cells and providing more pluripotential cells for cell renewal.
2. At the same time, the external callus, which is found on the surface of the bone and is formed from the periosteum and the soft tissue mesenchymal cells, continues to grow toward the fracture site.
3. Simultaneously, an endosteal, or internal, callus forms within the medullary cavity and grows outward toward the fracture site.
4. The cortical cutting cones reach the fracture site, and the ends of the fractured bone begin to appear beveled and smooth, as the site is remodeled by osteoclasts.
5. The same is true of the endosteal surface of the cortex, as the internal callus works its way to the fracture site.
6. Where there are large areas of cartilage, new blood vessels invade the calcified cartilage, after which the endochondral sequence duplicates the normal formation of bone at the growth plate.

The Remodeling Phase

Several weeks after the fracture, the ingrowth of callus has sealed the bone ends, and remodeling begins. In the remodeling phase, the bone is reorganized, so that the original cortex is restored. Occasionally, the bone is strong enough to qualify as a clinically healed fracture, but biologically, the fracture may not be truly healed and may continue to undergo remodeling for years. For instance, the callus of rib fractures may remain throughout life because the continual respiratory movement of the ribs shears blood vessels and preserves extensive cartilage callus. In a child, in whom the growth plates are still open, the normal modeling process of growing bone overtakes the callus, so that a fracture may not be recognizable in later life. Similarly, in a child, the angulation of a bone at its fracture site may be corrected by a normal modeling process. If the fracture is near the growth plate, differential growth rates of the growth plate also correct the angulation. In an adult, however, because the plates are closed, angulation often requires correction with external or internal devices.

Special Considerations

There are unusual nuances to fracture healing that deserve mention.

PRIMARY HEALING: A fracture does not necessarily result in bone displacement and soft tissue injury. For example, a drill hole in the bone cortex or a controlled fracture, such as an osteotomy created with a fine saw during orthopedic surgery, does not displace bone. In this situation, there is almost no soft tissue reaction and callus formation because the bone is rigidly fixed. The fracture callus grows directly into the fracture site by a process called *primary healing*. This results in rapid reconstitution of the cortex, including restoration of the Haversian systems. Similarly, if a fracture site is held in rigid alignment by metal screws and plates, there is also little external callus. The cortical cutting cones will then be prominent and will heal the fracture site quickly.

NONUNION: If a fracture site does not heal, the condition is termed *nonunion*. Causes of nonunion include interposition of soft tissues at the fracture site, excessive motion, infection, poor blood supply, and other factors previously mentioned. Continued movement at the unhealed fracture site may also lead to *pseudoarthrosis*, a condition in which joint tissue is formed. Pluripotential tissue cells become synovial cells, secreting synovial fluid and forming a joint-like structure. In such cases, the fracture never heals, and the joint-like material must be removed surgically for the fracture to heal properly.

Stress Fractures (Fatigue or March Fractures)

Stress fracture refers to the accumulation of stress-induced microfractures, which eventually results in a true fracture through the bone cortex.

☐ **Pathogenesis:** A stress fracture occurs in bones in which the cortex has few osteons and forms only when stress is applied to the cortex. If the ill-prepared cortex (e.g., in the fifth metatarsal) undergoes repeated mechanical stress, such as from jogging, skiing, or ballet dancing, the bone produces cutting cones in an attempt to implant osteons. If the stress continues and microfractures accumulate, periosteal and endosteal calluses develop to strengthen the bone while active remodeling takes place. An actual fracture occurs as the last event, if the stresses are continually applied during remodeling.

☐ **Clinical Features:** Stress fractures are characterized clinically by pain and swelling over the affected bone. **At the site of a future stress fracture, callus forms before the fracture occurs.** When the actual fracture takes place, the pain becomes more severe. In the early stages of this condition, before the actual fracture, the radiological appearance may resemble that of a tumor. A biopsy will show that the cortex is riddled with cutting cones for remodeling, which is also the case with the reactive bone at the periphery of an invasive tumor.

OSTEONECROSIS (AVASCULAR NECROSIS, ASEPTIC NECROSIS)

Osteonecrosis refers to the death of bone and marrow in the absence of infection (Fig. 26-18). Causes of osteonecrosis are listed in Table 1.

It is important to recognize that necrotic bone heals differently in the cortex and in the underlying coarse cancellous bone.

Necrotic coarse cancellous bone heals by a process called "creeping substitution," in which the necrotic marrow is replaced by invading, or creeping, neovascular tissue that provides the pluripotential cells needed for bone

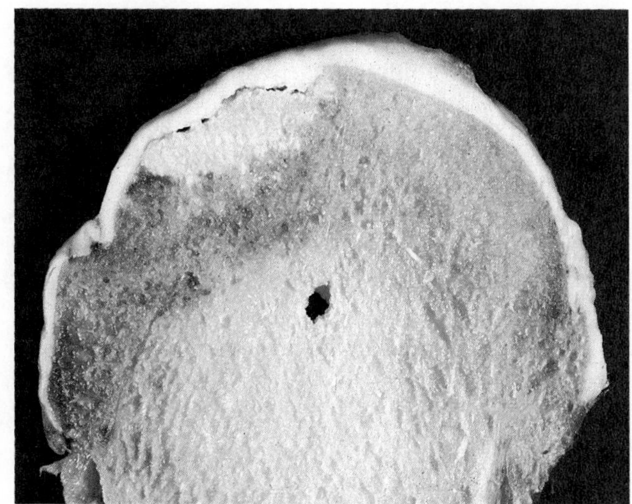

FIGURE *26-18*
Osteonecrosis of the head of the femur. Cross-section of the resected femoral head reveals a subchondral infarct, which is separated by a space from the articular cartilage.

remodeling. Although the necrotic bony trabeculae may be resorbed directly by osteoclastic activity, they are more commonly surrounded by new woven or lamellar bone generated by the osteoblastic activity of the granulation tissue. Eventually, the sandwich composed of necrotic bone in the center and the surrounding viable bone is remodeled by osteoclastic activity, and new bone is laid down through intramembranous bone formation.

Necrotic cortical bone is healed by a cutting cone. The cutting cone, as discussed earlier, forms by way of the preexisting vascular channels in the cortex. The appropriate signals reach this vascular channel and stimulate neovascularization by the surrounding pluripotential mesenchymal tissue. Osteoclasts make their way into the necrotic compact cortical bone, with osteoblasts trailing behind. As a result, tunnels bore their way into the necrotic cortex, thereby leading to new bone formation. This is a slow process, and the bone is often laid down *de novo* as lamellar bone.

TABLE *26-1* **Causes of Osteonecrosis**

Trauma, including fracture and surgery.
Emboli, producing focal bone infarction.
Systemic diseases, such as polycythemia, lupus erythematosus, Gaucher disease, sickle cell disease, and gout.
Radiation, either internal or external.
Corticosteroid administration.
Specific focal bone necrosis at various sites—for instance, in the head of the femur (Legg–Calvé–Perthes disease) or in the navicular bone (Köhler disease).
Organ transplantation, particularly renal, in patients with persistent hyperparathyroidism.
Osteochondritis dissecans, a condition of unknown etiology in which a piece of articular cartilage and subchondral bone breaks off into a joint. It is thought that a focal area of bone necrosis occurs and eventually detaches.
Autografts and allografts
Thrombosis of local vessels secondary to the pressure of adjacent tumors or other space-occupying lesions.
Idiopathic factors, as in the high incidence of osteonecrosis of the head and the femur in alcoholics. It is important to recognize that necrotic bone heals differently in the cortex and in the underlying coarse cancellous bone.

Legg–Calvé–Perthes disease involves the femoral head in children, and **idiopathic osteonecrosis** occurs in a similar location in adults. In both conditions, a collapse of the femoral head may lead to joint incongruity and eventual severe osteoarthritis. The collapse of the subchondral bone occurs as a result of several mechanisms:

- Necrotic bone may sustain stress fractures and compaction over a long period.
- The portion peripheral to the necrotic bone may undergo neovascularization. On radiological examination, there is a lucent area surrounding the necrotic zone.
- The rigid articular cartilage and subchondral bone may actually crack as the subchondral necrotic zone collapses, producing a fracture.

A radiograph of collapsed subchondral bone often shows the necrotic zone to be radiodense because of (1) the compaction of the preexisting dead bone, (2) the addition of new bone through creeping substitution, and (3) the formation of calcium soaps, which arise as a result of the necrosis of marrow fat. Because this necrotic zone tends to be wedge-shaped, focal vascular insufficiency may have occurred, although this has not been confirmed.

REACTIVE BONE FORMATION

Reactive bone is intramembranous bone that is formed in response to stress on bone or soft tissue. Conditions such as tumors, infections, trauma, or generalized or focal disease can stimulate bone formation. The periosteum may respond with a so-called *sunburst pattern* (Fig. 26-19), as seen with certain tumors, or a progressive layering of the periosteum, which produces an *onion-skin pattern* of the cortex. The endosteal or the marrow surface may produce new bone, so that on radiological studies, the cortex appears to be thickened, and the coarse cancellous bone appears to be more dense.

It is important that the reactive bone may be either woven or lamellar, depending on the rates of deposition of the reactive bone. For example, reactive bone around an indolent infection, such as a chronic osteomyelitis, may be laid down *de novo* as lamellar bone from the periosteum. In this case, the bone has time to respond to the persistent stress. Similarly, a benign tumor may stimulate a lamellar bone reaction. By contrast, a rapidly growing tumor is more likely to promote woven bone formation as a response to the rapid growth of the tumor cells. Invariably, reactive bone is of the intramembranous type, because it is derived from the periosteum or the endosteal tissue of the marrow.

Heterotopic Calcification

Reactive bone formation must be distinguished from heterotopic calcification, which is simply the deposition of acellular minerals in soft tissue. Reactive bone formation,

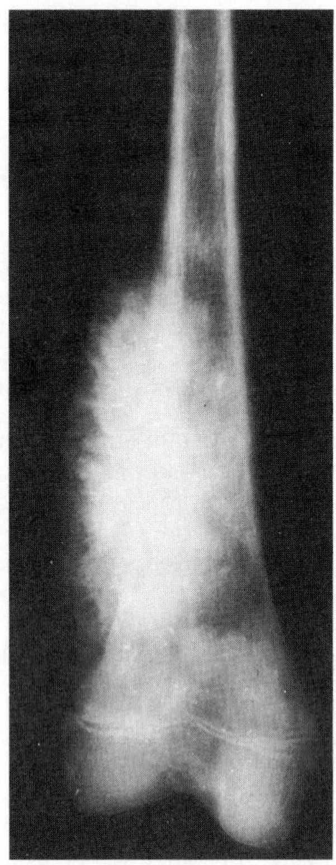

FIGURE *26-19*
Reactive bone formation. A radiograph of a resected femur bearing an osteosarcoma shows a sunburst pattern of hyperdense new bone in the distal diaphysis and metaphysis. This radiodensity is due to woven bone produced by the sarcoma and the periosteal reaction of the host bone. The epiphyseal plate is represented as a transverse lucent line that separates the metaphysis from the epiphysis. The radiating radiodense bone extends beyond the periosteum into the soft tissues, obscuring the underlying bone architecture.

or heterotopic bone formation, involves the production of woven or lamellar bone, which may or may not be mineralized. Radiologically, these entities are usually distinctive. Reactive bone often has a spicular or trabeculated pattern, whereas heterotopic calcification has an irregular, splotchy, and amorphous appearance. Heterotopic calcification tends to occur in necrotic soft tissue or in cartilage and is usually more dense than bone on radiography. Heterotopic calcification appears in two forms:

- **Metastatic calcification** occurs in conditions in which there is an increase in the calcium–phosphorus product. Thus, hypercalcemic states or hyperphosphatemic conditions predispose normal soft tissues to calcification.
- **Dystrophic calcification** is seen in abnormal soft tissues such as tumors, degenerative diseases such as arteriosclerosis, and areas subjected to trauma. In addition, loss of neurological function, as seen in quadriplegia and hemiplegia, predisposes the affected parts to soft tissue calcification.

Myositis Ossificans

Myositis ossificans refers to a condition in which there is formation of reactive bone in muscle as a result of injury. It affects young persons and, although it is entirely benign, often mimics a malignant neoplasm.

The lesion typically occurs as a result of blunt trauma to the muscle and soft tissues, usually of the lower limb. Peripheral neovascularization of the resulting hematoma leads in a short time to the formation of bone spicules in the soft tissue, because the local environment is similar to that of an initial hematoma in a healing fracture. Because myositis ossificans often occurs near a bone, such as the

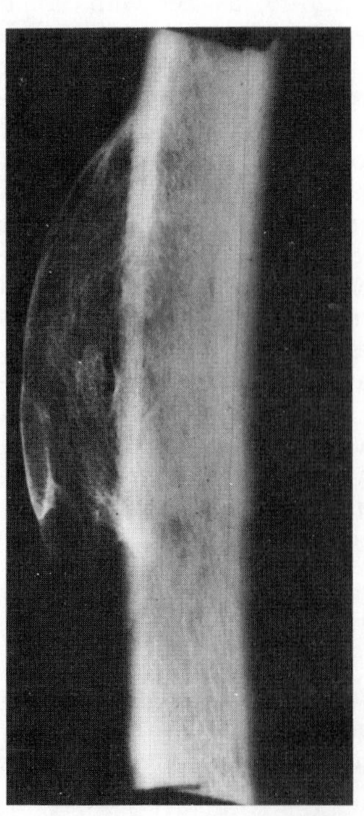

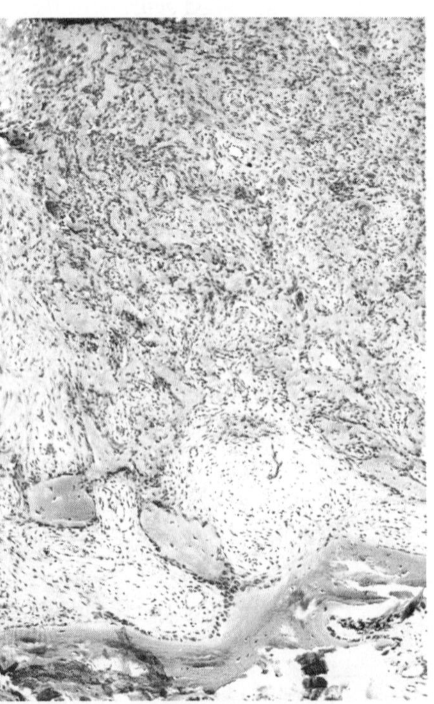

A B

FIGURE *26-20*
Myositis ossificans. (*A*) A radiograph of the mid-diaphyseal region of a long bone shows a surface excrescence of bone that represents long-standing myositis ossificans. The lesion is composed of distinct bony trabeculae and cortical bone. (*B*) A photomicrograph reveals mature bone (*bottom*) on the periphery of the lesion and immature bone in the center. The peripheral bone is lamellar, and the center contains woven bone surrounded by fibrous tissue.

femur or tibia, on radiography it may be misdiagnosed as a malignant bone-forming tumor.

☐ **Pathology:** Histologically, woven bone is formed within the granulation tissue (Fig. 26-20). In an early lesion of myositis ossificans, the cells of the woven bone and surrounding soft tissue are pleomorphic and show abundant mitoses, a histological appearance that also bears a resemblance to a malignant tumor. **The key feature that distinguishes myositis ossificans from a neoplasm is that the woven bone is well formed peripherally, whereas it is immature or not formed at all in the center of the lesion.** The phenomenon of peripheral maturity with central immaturity is called the *zonation effect* and clearly indicates a reactive process. A neoplasm has an opposite zonation effect, because the most mature tissue of the tumor is located centrally.

The growth pattern of myositis ossificans reflects the ingrowth of neovascular tissue from the peripheral portion into the center of the damaged area. The reason for this peripheral formation of bone is not understood, but it is well known that the closer the trauma is to the periosteum, the more likely it is that the healing tissue will contain reactive bone.

Myositis ossificans, especially in the late stages, may contain cartilage and even lamellar bone. Thus, in a well-developed lesion, it may mimic a sesamoid bone in the soft tissue. In this late stage, it is not difficult to distinguish this reactive lesion from a malignant tumor, which never forms such well-delineated bone.

INFECTIONS

Osteomyelitis

Osteomyelitis is an inflammation of bone caused by bacterial infection. Despite the common use of antibiotics, osteomyelitis is still a major diagnostic and therapeutic problem. The most common pathogens are *Staphylococcus* species, but other organisms, such as *Escherichia coli, Neisseria gonorrhoeae, Haemophilus influenzae,* and *Salmonella* species, are also seen. The organisms are introduced either through the hematogenous route or by direct introduction of the organisms into the bone.

Direct Penetration

Infection by direct penetration or extension of bacteria is now the most common cause of osteomyelitis in the United States. Bacterial organisms are introduced directly into the bone by penetrating wounds, fractures, or surgery. Staphylococci and streptococci are still commonly incriminated, but many other organisms produce such infections. *Staphylococcus aureus* is the most common organism involved after elective surgical procedures without preoperative antibiotics. When preoperative antibiotics are administered, *S. epidermidis* is the organism most frequently isolated, but in 25% of such postoperative infections, anaerobic organisms are detected. Rarely, a gram-negative organism may seed a hip after a urological or gastrointestinal surgical procedure.

Hematogenous Osteomyelitis

Infectious organisms may reach the bone from a focus elsewhere in the body through the bloodstream. Often the focus itself, for instance, a skin pustule or infected teeth and gums, poses little threat. Some suggest that even the mere brushing of teeth creates a temporary bacteremia, which may allow organisms to reach the bone.

The most common sites affected by hematogenous osteomyelitis are the ends of the long bones, such as the knee, ankle, and hip. The infection principally affects boys aged 5 to 15 years, but it is occasionally seen in older age groups as well. Drug addicts may develop hematogenous osteomyelitis from infected needles.

☐ **Pathogenesis and Pathology:** Hematogenous osteomyelitis primarily affects the metaphyseal area because of the unique vascular supply in this region (Fig. 26-21). Normally, arterioles enter the calcified portion of the growth plate, form a loop, and then drain into the medullary cavity without establishing a capillary bed. This loop system permits slowing and sludging of blood flow, thereby allowing bacteria time to penetrate the walls of the blood vessels and to establish an infective focus within the marrow. If the organism is virulent and continues to proliferate, it creates increased pressure on the adjacent thin-walled vessels because they lie in a closed space, the marrow cavity of bone. Such pressure further compromises the vascular supply in this region and produces bone necrosis. The necrotic areas coalesce into an avascular zone, thereby allowing further bacterial proliferation.

If the infection is not contained, pus and bacteria extend into the endosteal vascular channels that supply the cortex and spread throughout the Volkmann and Haversian canals of the cortex. Eventually, pus forms underneath the periosteum, shearing off the perforating arteries of the periosteum and further devitalizing the cortex. The pus flows between the periosteum and the cortex, isolating more bone from its blood supply, and may even invade the joint. Eventually, the pus penetrates the periosteum and the skin to form a draining sinus (Fig. 26-22). A sinus tract that extends from the cloaca to the skin may become epithelialized by epidermis that grows into the sinus tract. When this occurs, the sinus tract invariably remains open, continually draining pus, necrotic bone, and bacteria.

Periosteal new bone formation and reactive bone formation in the marrow tend to wall off the infection. At the same time, osteoclastic activity resorbs bone. If the infection is virulent, this attempt to contain it is overwhelmed, and the infection races through the bone, with virtually no bone formation but rather extensive bone necrosis. More commonly, pluripotential cells modulate into osteoblasts in an attempt to wall off the infection. Several lesions may develop:

- **Cloaca** is the hole formed in the bone during the formation of a draining sinus.
- **Sequestrum** is a fragment of necrotic bone that is embedded in the pus.
- **Brodie abscess** consists of reactive bone from the periosteum and the endosteum, which surrounds and contains the infection.

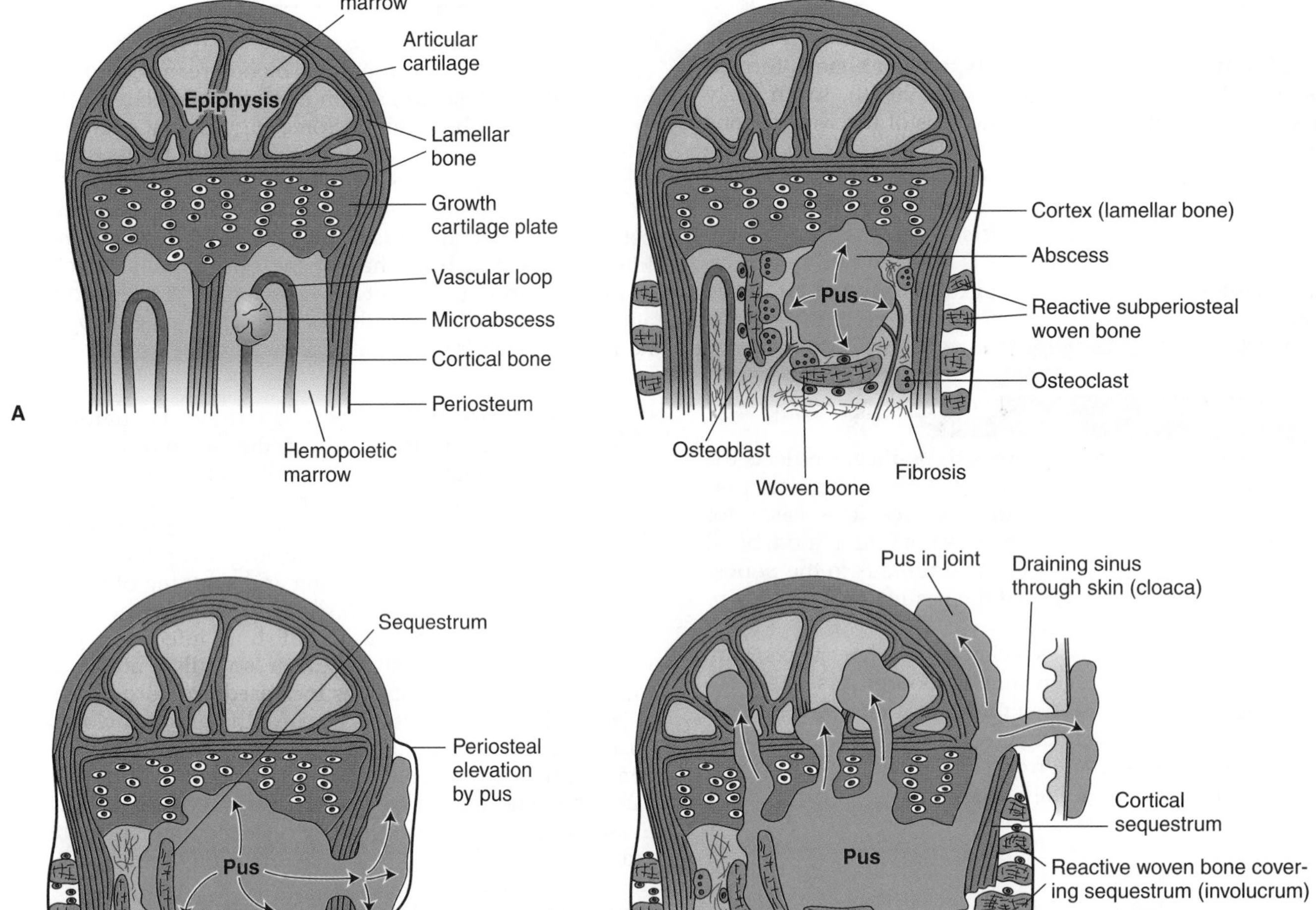

FIGURE 26-21
Pathogenesis of hematogenous osteomyelitis. (*A*) The epiphysis, metaphysis, and growth plate are normal. A small, septic microabscess is forming at the capillary loop. (*B*) The expansion of the septic focus stimulates resorption of adjacent bony trabeculae. Woven bone begins to surround this focus. The abscess expands into the cartilage and stimulates reactive bone formation by the periosteum. (*C*) The abscess, which continues to expand through the cortex into the subperiosteal tissue, shears off the perforating arteries that supply the cortex with blood, thereby leading to necrosis of the cortex. (*D*) The extension of this process into the joint space, the epiphysis, and the skin produces a draining sinus. The necrotic bone is called a sequestrum. The viable bone surrounding a sequestrum is termed the involucrum.

- **Involucrum** refers to a lesion in which periosteal new bone formation forms a sheath around the necrotic sequestrum. An involucrum that involves an entire bone may exist for several years before a patient seeks medical attention.

In very young children (1 year old or younger) afflicted with osteomyelitis, the adjacent joint is often involved because the periosteum is not firmly adherent to the cortex. From the age of 1 year to puberty, subperiosteal abscesses are common. Spread to adjacent joints may also occur in adults.

Vertebral Osteomyelitis

In adults, osteomyelitis frequently involves vertebral bodies (Fig. 26-23). The intervertebral disk is not a barrier for bacterial osteomyelitis, particularly for staphylococcal infection. Infections travel from one vertebra to the next by directly invading and traversing the intervertebral disk. Some investigators consider that the intervertebral disk is the primary source of infection, so-called *diskitis*. The disk expands with pus and is eventually destroyed as the pus bores into the adjacent vertebral bodies.

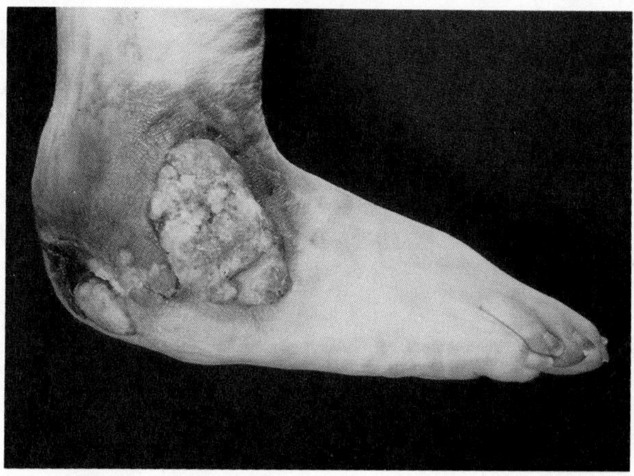

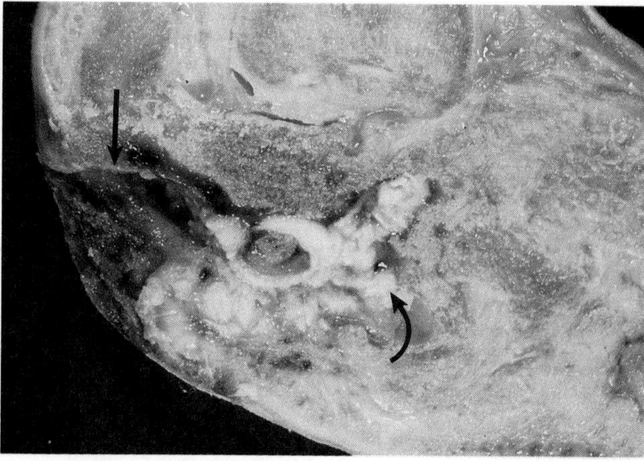

FIGURE 26-22
Chronic osteomyelitis. (*A*) In this patient with chronic osteomyelitis, the skin overlying the infected bone is ulcerated and a draining sinus *(dark area)* is evident over the heel. (*B*) After amputation of the foot, a sagittal section shows a draining sinus *(straight arrow)* that connects the infected bone with the surface of the ulcerated skin. The white tissue (*curved arrow)* is invasive squamous cell carcinoma, which arose in the skin.

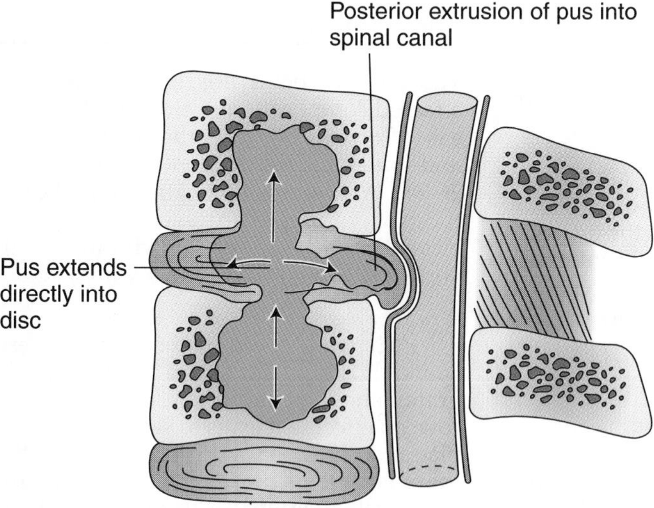

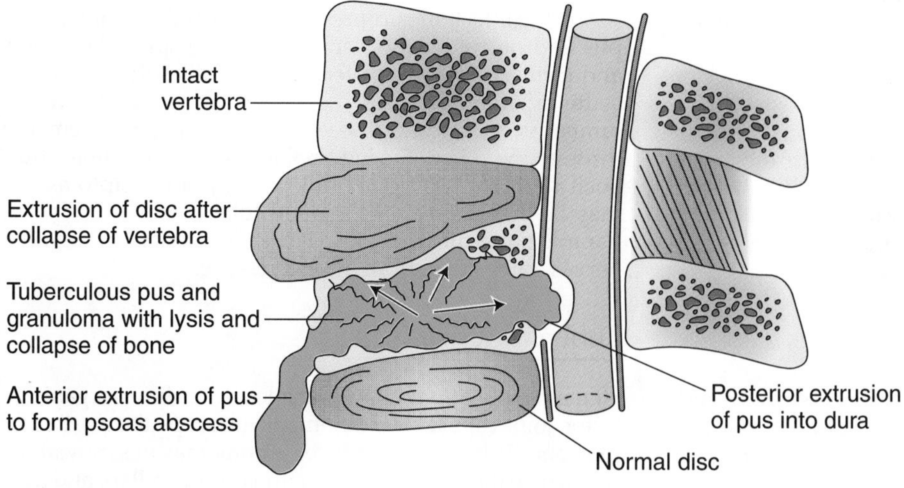

FIGURE 26-23
Osteomyelitis of the vertebral body. (*A*) Bacterial osteomyelitis expands from one vertebral body to the next by direct invasion of the intervertebral disc and may actually push posteriorly into the spinal canal. The sequence of events in the marrow cavity is similar to that in a long bone. (*B*) In tuberculous osteomyelitis, the bone is destroyed by resorption of bony trabeculae, which results in mechanical collapse of the vertebrae and extrusion of the intervertebral disc. Tuberculous organisms cannot penetrate the intervertebral disc directly; rather, they extend from one vertebra to the next after mechanical forces destroy and extrude the intervertebral disc.

Half or more of the cases of vertebral osteomyelitis are caused by *S. aureus*. Twenty percent represent infections with *E. coli* and other enteric organisms, many of which originate from the urinary tract. *Salmonella* species are also seen in the vertebral bodies, as are *Brucella* species. The predisposing factors are intravenous drug abuse, upper urinary tract infections, urological procedures, and hematogenous spread of organisms from other sites. Back pain, with point tenderness over the area of infection, is associated with low-grade fever and an increased sedimentation rate.

Occasionally, a paravertebral abscess draining the bone may "point" and emerge in the groin or elsewhere. Vertebral osteomyelitis may lead to (1) vertebral collapse with paravertebral abscesses, (2) spinal epidural abscesses, with cord compression from the abscess or from displaced fragments of the infected bone, and (3) compression fractures of the vertebral body, leading to neurological deficits.

Complications

The complications of osteomyelitis include the following:

- **Septicemia:** Dissemination of organisms through the bloodstream may occur as a result of bone infection. It is unusual for osteomyelitis to occur from septicemia.
- **Acute bacterial arthritis:** Joint infection arises as a result of osteomyelitis in children and in adults and represents a medical emergency. Direct digestion of cartilage by inflammatory cells destroys the articular cartilage and leads to osteoarthritis. Rapid intervention to prevent this complication is mandatory.
- **Pathological fractures:** Osteomyelitis may lead to fractures, which heal poorly and may require surgical drainage.
- **Squamous cell carcinoma:** This cancer develops in the bone or in the sinus tract of long-standing chronic osteomyelitis, often years after the initial infection. In such cases, squamous tissue arises from the epithelialization of the sinus tract and eventually undergoes malignant transformation (see Fig. 26-22).
- **Amyloidosis:** This systemic disease was a common complication of chronic osteomyelitis in the preantibiotic era, and patients often would die of cardiac and renal disease. Currently, it is rare in inhabitants of industrialized countries.
- **Chronic osteomyelitis:** Chronic infection of bone may follow acute osteomyelitis. Chronic osteomyelitis, especially that involving the entire bone, is incurable because necrotic bone or sequestra function as foreign bodies in avascular areas, and antibiotics do not reach the bacteria. Chronic osteomyelitis is therefore treated symptomatically with surgery or antibiotics for the duration of the patient's life.

Clinical Features

Hematogenous osteomyelitis in children is seen as a sudden illness, with fever and systemic toxicity, or as a subacute illness in which local manifestations predominate. Swelling, erythema, and tenderness over the involved bone are characteristic. The leukocyte count is often conspicuously increased, but it is normal in so many cases that absence of leukocytosis does not rule out the disease.

The treatment of osteomyelitis depends on the stage of the infection. Early osteomyelitis is treated with intravenous antibiotics for 6 or more weeks. Surgery is used to drain and decompress the infection within the bone or to drain abscesses that do not respond to antibiotic therapy. As already mentioned, in long-standing, chronic osteomyelitis, antibiotics alone are not curative, and extensive surgical debridement of necrotic bone is often required.

Tuberculosis

Tuberculosis of bone is invariably caused by a primary focus elsewhere in the body, usually the lungs or lymph nodes (see Chapter 9). When the bone infection is caused by the rare bovine type of tubercle bacillus, the initial focus is often the gut or tonsils. The mycobacteria spread to the bone hematogenously; only rarely is there direct spread into bone from a lung or lymph node.

Tuberculous Spondylitis (Pott Disease)

Tuberculous spondylitis, that is, infection of the spine, is a feared complication of childhood tuberculosis. The disease affects the bodies of the vertebrae, sparing the lamina and spines and the adjacent vertebrae (see Figs. 26-23 and 26-24). With antibiotic treatment, Pott disease is rare. The thoracic vertebrae are usually affected, especially the eleventh thoracic vertebra, with the lumbar and cervical vertebrae being less commonly involved.

☐ **Pathology:** The pathological process in tuberculous spondylitis is similar to that at other sites. The tuberculous granulomas first produce caseous necrosis of the bone marrow, an effect that leads to slow resorption of bony trabeculae and, occasionally, to cystic spaces in the bone. **Because there is little or no reactive bone formation, collapse of the affected vertebra is usual, after which kyphosis and scoliosis ensue.** The intervertebral disk is crushed and destroyed by the compression fracture, rather than by invasion of organisms. The typical hunchback of bygone days was often the victim of Pott disease.

If the infection ruptures into the soft tissue anteriorly, pus and necrotic debris drain along the spinal ligaments and form a *cold abscess*, a term that signifies the absence of acute inflammation. A *psoas abscess* forms near the lower lumbar vertebrae and dissects along the pelvis, to emerge through the skin of the inguinal region as a draining sinus. Such a process may occur without any prior symptoms and may be the first manifestation of tuberculous spondylitis. Paraplegia results from vascular insufficiency of the spinal nerves, rather than from direct pressure.

Tuberculous Arthritis

Hematogenous spread of tuberculosis may bring organisms to the joint capsule, synovium, or intracapsular portion of the bone. Tuberculosis induces granulomas in synovial tissue, which then becomes edematous and papillary and may

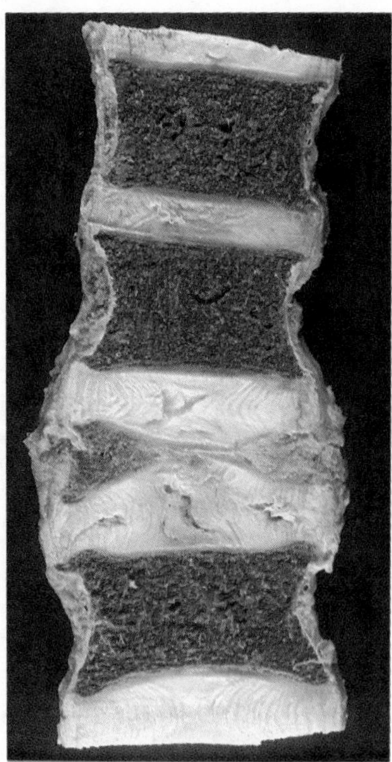

FIGURE *26-24*
Tuberculous spondylitis (Pott disease). A vertebral body is almost completely replaced by tuberculous tissue. Note the preservation of the intervertebral discs.

fill the entire joint space. Massive destruction of the articular cartilage results from undermining granulation tissue in the bone. The destroyed joint is replaced by bone, an effect that leads to an immovable joint *(bony ankylosis).*

Tuberculous Osteomyelitis of the Long Bones

Infection of the long bones is the least common bone manifestation of tuberculosis. Tuberculosis of a long bone occurs near the joint, where it also produces an arthritis. For unknown reasons, the greater trochanter of the femur is a common site for this disease.

Syphilis

Syphilis causes a slowly progressive, chronic, inflammatory disease of bone, which is characterized by granulomas, necrosis, and marked reactive bone formation. It may be acquired through sexual contact, or it may be passed through the placenta from mother to the fetus (see Chapter 9). The bone changes in syphilis depend on the age of the patient, the endosteal and periosteal changes, and the presence or absence of gummas.

Congenital Syphilis

Involvement of bone in congenital syphilis may appear as early as the fifth month of gestation and is fully developed at birth. The spirochetes are ubiquitous in the epiphysis and periosteum, where they produce osteochondritis (epiphysitis) and periostitis, respectively (Fig. 26-25). If the disease is severe, the epiphysis may become dislocated, leaving the child with a functionless limb (pseudoparalysis of Parrot).

The knee is most often affected by congenital syphilis. The growth plate is irregularly widened and displays a yellow discoloration. The zone of calcified cartilage is destroyed, and the marrow spaces are filled by a sea of lymphocytes, plasma cells, and spirochetes. Because the periosteum is stimulated to produce reactive new bone, the thickness of the cortex may actually be doubled. The inflammatory infiltrate permeates the cortex through the Volkmann and Haversian canals and settles in the elevated periosteum. Ultimately, the affected bones grow to become short and deformed.

Acquired Syphilis

Acquired syphilis in adults produces lesions of the bone early in the tertiary stage, 2 to 5 years after inoculation of the organisms. Periostitis is predominant because the growth plates have already closed. The bones most commonly affected are the tibia, nose, palate, and skull. The tibial lesions are marked by a periostitis, with deposition of new bone on the medial and anterior aspects of the shaft, a process that leads to the *saber shin* deformity. The skull is also increased in thickness because of periosteal stimulation.

The formation of gummas is most common during the tertiary stage of the disease. The bone adjacent to gummas is slowly replaced by fibrous marrow. Ultimately, perforations occur through the cortex. The markedly irregular, thickened periosteal surfaces, which are perforated by pits and serpiginous ulcerations, are characteristic of syphilis. Lysis and collapse of the nasal

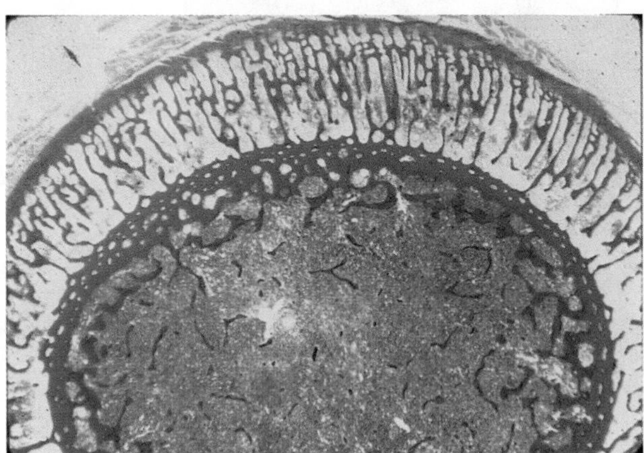

FIGURE *26-25*
Congenital syphilis of bone. A cross-section of a tubular bone infected by syphilis shows marked periosteal new bone formation. The medullary cavity is filled with a lymphoplasmocytic infiltrate that replaces the normal marrow fat. The cortex is irregularly destroyed by osteoclastic resorption, a process that stimulates periosteal new bone formation.

and palatal bones produce the classic *saddle nose:* perforation, destruction, and collapse of the nasal septum.

LANGERHANS CELL HISTIOCYTOSIS

Langerhans cell histiocytosis (LCH) is a generic term (previously referred to as histiocytosis X) for three entities characterized by the proliferation of Langerhans cells in various tissues: (1) eosinophilic granuloma, a localized form, (2) Hand–Schüller–Christian disease, a disseminated variant, and (3) Letterer–Siwe disease, a fulminant and often fatal generalized disease (see Chapter 20). The term *histiocyte* is synonymous with tissue macrophage, and the use of the label *histiocytosis* in LCH was originally based on the presumption that the proliferated cells were histiocytes.

☐ **Pathology:** The histological appearance of the bones in all three variants of LCH is identical and is characterized by collections of large, phagocytic cells with pale, eosinophilic, foamy cytoplasm and convoluted nuclei. By electron microscopy, these cells have the typical racquet-shaped, tubular structures (*Birbeck granules*) of the Langerhans cells of the skin. Numerous, scattered eosinophils are located throughout the lesions, occasionally forming collections called eosinophilic abscesses. Multinucleated giant cells of the foreign body (Touton) type are often seen in the lesion, as are chronic inflammatory cells.

The lesions of LCH may occur in any part of the body, including bones, skin, brain, lungs, lymph nodes, liver, and spleen. Although cholesterol deposition is prominent in the macrophages, there is no defined abnormality related to cholesterol metabolism, and these patients do not exhibit hypercholesterolemia.

The radiological findings in the bones in all three diseases are identical. The lesions may occur in the metaphysis or diaphysis of a long bone, or in a flat bone, especially in the skull. They are visualized as punched-out, lytic defects, with virtually no reactive bone. Such lesions may lead to fractures and periosteal callus formation.

Eosinophilic Granuloma

Eosinophilic granuloma, in either its solitary or multiple form, accounts for 70% of all cases of LCH. It is seen as a self-limited disease, usually in the first two decades of life, but occasionally in older persons. In eosinophilic granuloma, there are typically one or two lytic areas in bones of the axial or appendicular skeleton (Fig. 26-26) or the vertebrae. These lesions may cause mild pain or may be an incidental finding on a routine chest radiograph. Foci of disease in the lower thoracic or upper lumbar vertebrae may lead to collapse and pathological fractures.

Hand–Schüller–Christian Disease

Hand–Schüller–Christian disease occurs in younger children (aged 2 to 5 years) and is more widespread than eosinophilic granuloma. It represents some 20% of all cases of LCH. The disorder is characterized by lytic bony lesions, most frequently in the calvarium, ribs, pelvis, and scapulae. Involvement of the jaw bone results in the loss of teeth, evident radiologically as "floating teeth." A lesion may infiltrate the retro-orbital space, producing exophthalmos. Infiltration of the stalk of the hypothalamus

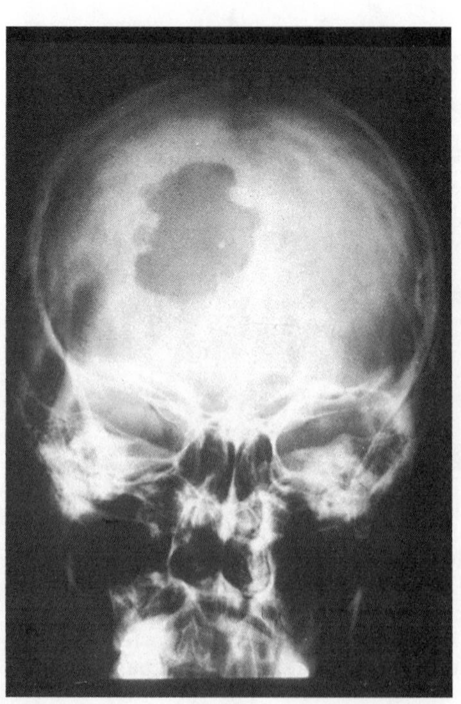
A

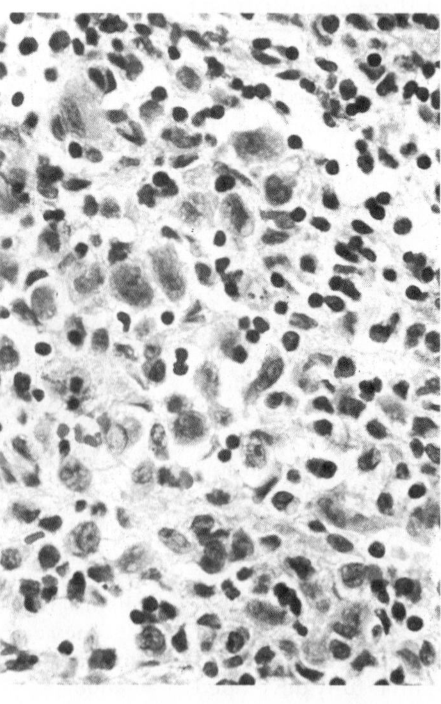
B

FIGURE *26-26*
Eosinophilic granuloma. (*A*) A radiograph of the skull shows a large, lytic lesion. (*B*) A photomicrograph of a lesion of eosinophilic granuloma reveals large histiocytes (Langerhans cells), eosinophils, and lymphoid cells.

by the proliferated Langerhans cells leads to diabetes insipidus. Twenty percent of patients have lymphadenopathy and lung infiltrates.

Crusty, red, and weepy skin lesions occur at the hairline and on the extensor surfaces of the extremities, the abdomen, and occasionally the soles of the feet. Deafness results from involvement of the external auditory canal and mastoid air cells. One third of affected patients demonstrate disease in the liver and spleen, and 40% have bone lesions, half of which involve the skull. Thus, the classic triad of Hand–Schüller–Christian disease, **lytic lesions of the skull, diabetes insipidus,** and **exophthalmos,** occurs in only one third of patients.

Letterer–Siwe Disease

Letterer–Siwe disease is an aggressive systemic malady that occurs in children younger than 2 years and accounts for 10% of cases of LCH. Affected children fail to thrive and become cachectic. Multiple organ involvement culminates in massive hepatosplenomegaly, lymphadenopathy, anemia, leukopenia, and thrombocytopenia. Widely scattered, seborrheic skin lesions, which are often hemorrhagic, are usual. The bone lesions are not prominent initially, but progressive marrow replacement and pulmonary infiltration occasionally cause death.

Treatment

Eosinophilic granuloma is a self-limited disease, and most of the lesions disappear if left alone. A lytic lesion in bone may have to be curetted and packed with bone chips. Sometimes the biopsy itself is enough to stimulate repair of the lytic lesion. A collapsed vertebra may actually reconstitute itself over time. Hand–Schüller–Christian disease may require radiation therapy for some bone and retro-orbital lesions. Diabetes insipidus seems to be irreversible, despite irradiation of the pituitary region. Drugs such as corticosteroids, cyclophosphamide, and tumoricidal agents may also be used to treat Hand–Schüller–Christian disease. Similarly aggressive therapy for Letterer–Siwe disease may improve the prognosis.

OSTEOPOROSIS

Osteoporosis is a metabolic bone disease characterized by diffuse skeletal lesions in which normally mineralized bone is decreased in mass to the point that it no longer provides adequate mechanical support. Whereas osteoporosis reflects a host of etiologies, it is always characterized by loss of skeletal mass. The remaining bone exhibits a normal ratio of mineralized to nonmineralized (i.e., osteoid) matrix. Although the severity of a metabolic bone disease may differ somewhat in various bones, its manifestations are extant throughout the skeleton. Thus evaluation of this family of skeletal disorders lends itself to random bone biopsy (Fig. 26-27).

☐ **Epidemiology:** In normal persons of both sexes, bone mass peaks between the ages of 25 and 35 years and begins to decline in the fifth or sixth decade. Bone loss with age occurs in all races, but because of higher peak bone mass, blacks are less prone to osteoporosis than are Asians and whites. At a certain point, this loss of bone is sufficient to justify the label osteoporosis and renders weight-bearing bones susceptible to fractures. The most common fractures occur in the neck and intertrochanteric region of the femur (hip fracture), the vertebral bodies (compression fracture; Fig. 26-28), and the distal radius (*Colles fracture*). In whites in the United States, 15% of persons have had a hip fracture by the age of 80 years, and by age 90 years, this figure increases to 25%. Women are at double the risk of hip fracture compared with men, although among blacks and some Asian populations, the incidence is equal among the sexes. The female sex predominance is particularly striking for vertebral fractures, in which the female-to-male ratio is 8:1. The propensity of men to sustain hip fractures as opposed to vertebral ones also reflects factors other than bone mass, such as loss of proprioception. A subset of women in the early postmenopausal years is at particular risk of vertebral fractures, which are rare in middle-aged men.

☐ **Pathogenesis:** **Regardless of the cause of osteoporosis, it always reflects enhanced bone resorption relative to formation.** Thus this family of diseases should be viewed in the context of the remodeling cycle. Persons younger than 35 or 40 years completely replace bone resorbed during the remodeling cycle. With age, less bone is replaced in resorption bays than is removed, leading to a small deficit at each remodeling site. Given the thousands of remodeling sites in the skeleton, the net bone loss, even in a short time, can be substantial.

Osteoporosis is classified as either primary or secondary. **Primary osteoporosis**, by far the more common variety, is of uncertain origin and occurs principally in postmenopausal women (type 1) and elderly persons of both sexes (type 2). **Secondary osteoporosis** is a disorder associated with a defined cause, including a variety of endocrine and genetic abnormalities.

Type 1 primary osteoporosis is due to an absolute increase in osteoclast activity. Given that osteoclasts initiate bone remodeling, the number of remodeling sites increases in this state of enhanced osteoclast formation, a phenomenon known as increased activation frequency.

The increased number of osteoclasts that appears in the early postmenopausal skeleton is the direct result of estrogen withdrawal. The effects of estrogen lack are not, however, targeted directly to the osteoclast, but rather to cells derived from marrow stroma, which secrete cytokines that recruit osteoclasts. These cytokines, which are believed to be estrogen sensitive, include IL-1 and IL-6, TNF, and macrophage colony-stimulating factor (MCSF).

Type 2 primary osteoporosis, also known as **senile osteoporosis**, has a more complex pathogenesis than does type 1. Type 2 osteoporosis generally appears after age 70 years and reflects attenuated osteoblast function. Thus, although osteoclast activity is no longer increased, the number of osteoblasts and the amount of bone produced per cell are insufficient to replace the bone removed during the resorptive phase of the remodeling cycle.

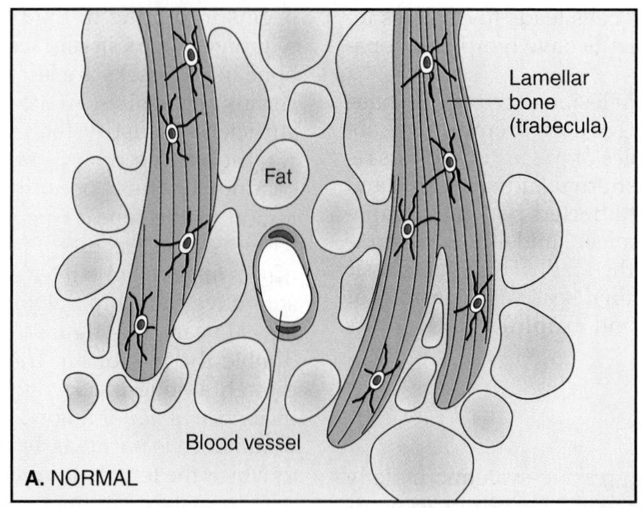
Lamellar
bone
(trabecula)
Fat
Blood vessel
A. NORMAL

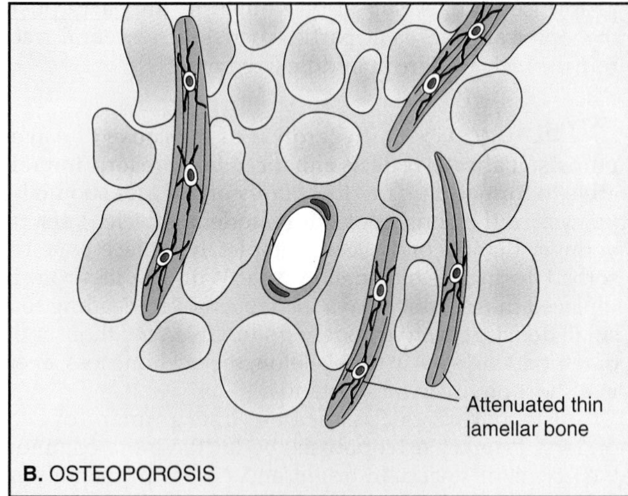
Attenuated thin
lamellar bone
B. OSTEOPOROSIS

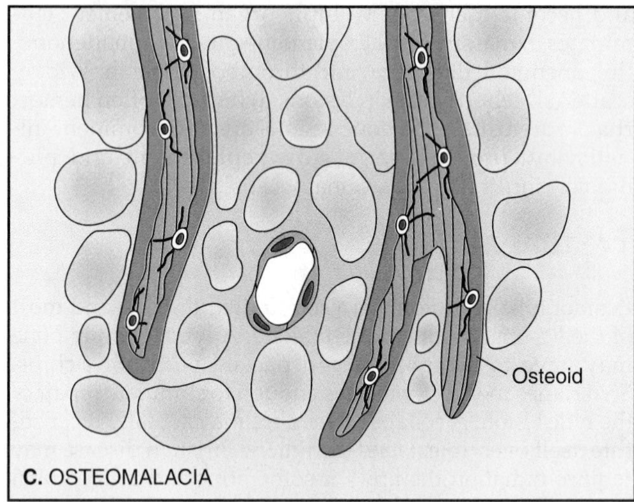
Osteoid
C. OSTEOMALACIA

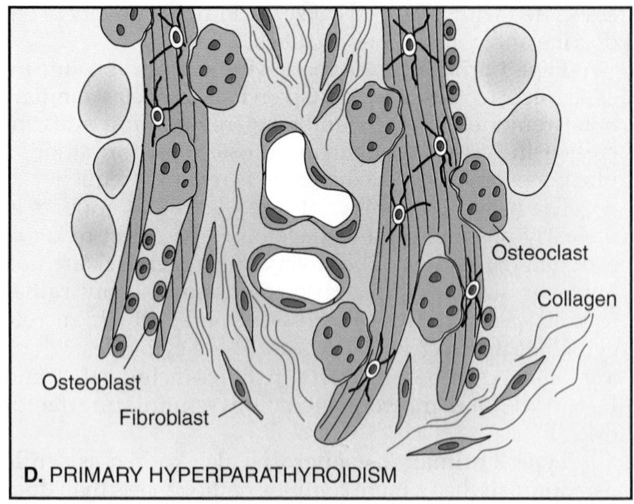
Osteoclast
Collagen
Osteoblast
Fibroblast
D. PRIMARY HYPERPARATHYROIDISM

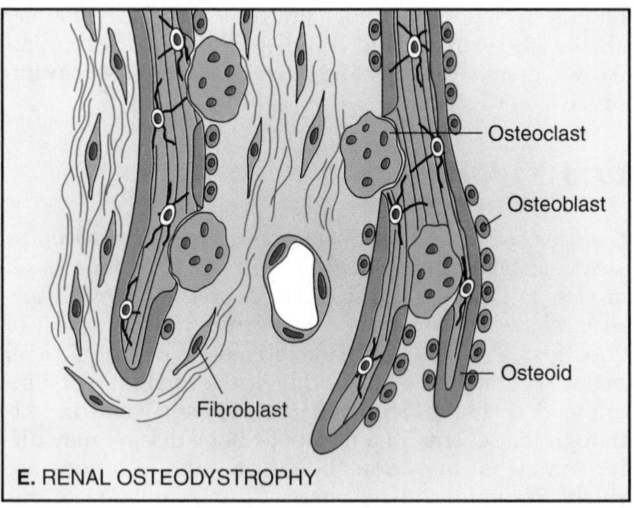
Osteoclast
Osteoblast
Osteoid
Fibroblast
E. RENAL OSTEODYSTROPHY

FIGURE *26-27*

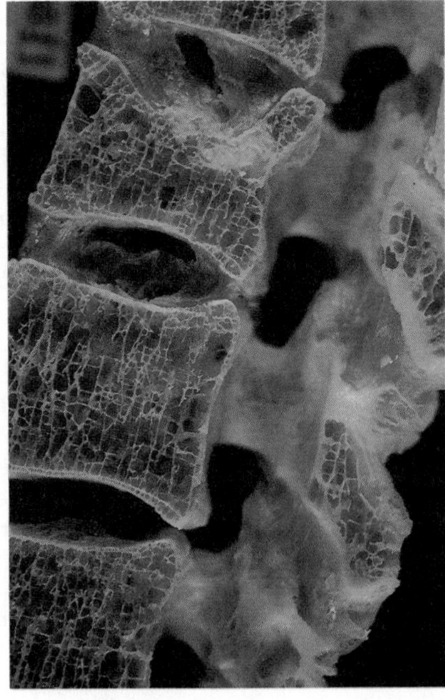
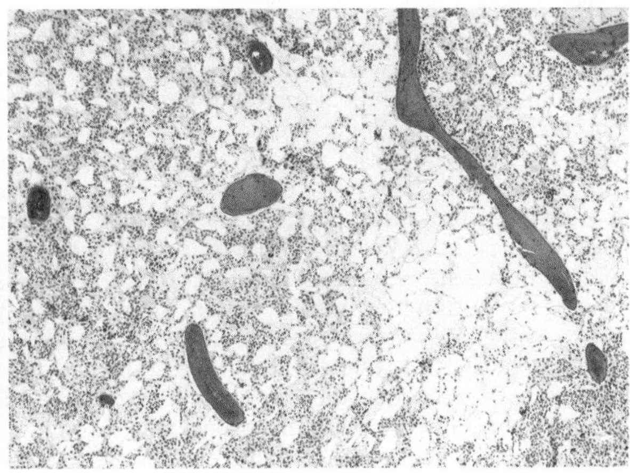

FIGURE 26-28
Osteoporosis. (*A*) A section of the vertebral column, in which the bone marrow has been washed out, demonstrates a loss of bone tissue and a compression fracture of a vertebral body (*top*). (*B*) A photomicrograph of a vertebral body shows very attenuated bony trabeculae.

Primary osteoporosis has been linked to a number of factors that influence peak bone mass and the rate of bone loss:

- **Genetic factors:** The development of clinically significant osteoporosis is related, in largest part, to the maximal amount of bone in a given person, referred to as *the peak bone mass*. The determinants of peak bone mass are to a large extent genetic. In general, peak bone mass is greater in men than in women and in blacks compared with whites or Asians. There is a higher concordance of peak bone mass in monozygotic as opposed to dizygotic twins. Women of reproductive age whose mothers have postmenopausal osteoporosis exhibit a lower bone mineral density than do women in the general population. The peak bone mass among blacks and whites is as follows: black men > white men > black women > white women.
- **Calcium intake:** The average calcium intake of postmenopausal women in the United States is below the recommended value of 800 mg/day. However, whether this seeming dietary deficiency contributes to the development of osteoporosis is controversial, in view of a number of studies to the contrary. Nevertheless, it has been recommended that the intake of calcium and vitamin D be increased by both premenopausal and postmenopausal women.
- **Calcium absorption and vitamin D:** Absorption of calcium in the intestine is known to decrease with age. Because calcium absorption is largely under the control of vitamin D, attention has been directed to the role of this steroid hormone in osteoporosis. Compared

FIGURE 26-27
Metabolic bone diseases. (*A*) Normal trabecular bone and fatty marrow. The trabecular bone is lamellar and contains evenly distributed osteocytes. (*B*) Osteoporosis. The lamellar bone exhibits discontinuous, thin trabeculae. (*C*) Osteomalacia. The trabeculae of the lamellar bone have abnormal amounts of nonmineralized bone (osteoid). These osteoid seams are thickened and cover a larger than normal area of the trabecular bone surface. (*D*) Primary hyperparathyroidism. The lamellar bone trabeculae are actively resorbed by numerous osteoclasts that bore into each trabecula. The appearance of osteoclasts dissecting into the trabeculae, a process termed dissecting osteitis, is diagnostic of hyperparathyroidism. Osteoblastic activity also is pronounced. The marrow is replaced by fibrous tissue adjacent to the trabeculae. (*E*) Renal osteodystrophy. The morphological appearance is similar to that of primary hyperparathyroidism, except that prominent osteoid covers the trabeculae. Osteoclasts do not resorb osteoid, and wherever an osteoid seam is lacking, osteoclasts bore into the trabeculae. Osteoblastic activity, in association with osteoclasts, is again prominent.

with controls, persons with osteoporosis evidence somewhat lower circulating levels of $1,25(OH)_2D$, although the difference is not large. This decrease has been attributed to an age-related decrease in the activity of 1α-hydroxylase in the kidney, the enzyme that catalyzes the formation of $1,25(OH)_2D$, the active form of vitamin D that promotes calcium absorption in the intestine. The decrease in 1α-hydroxylase activity has been attributed to decreased stimulation of the enzyme by parathyroid hormone, as well as an age-related decrease in the response of the renal tubule to parathyroid hormone (PTH). Interestingly, the administration of estrogens to postmenopausal women with osteoporosis increases both the circulating level of $1,25(OH)_2D$ and calcium absorption. It has been suggested that a decrease in 1α-hydroxylase activity in the kidney may stimulate the secretion of parathyroid hormone, thereby contributing to bone resorption.

- **Exercise:** Physical activity is necessary for the maintenance of bone mass, and athletes often have an increased bone mass. By contrast, the immobilization of a bone (e.g., prolonged bed rest, application of a cast) leads to accelerated bone loss. As a matter of current interest, the weightlessness of space flight results in severe bone loss (33% of trabecular bone mass in 25 weeks). Despite earlier expectations, there is no evidence that vigorous exercise substantially increases bone mass or helps prevent osteoporosis.
- **Environmental factors:** Cigarette smoking in women has been correlated with an increased incidence of osteoporosis. It is possible that the decreased level of active estrogens produced by smoking (see Chapter 8) is responsible for this effect.

In summary, the two major determinants of primary osteoporosis are estrogen deficiency in postmenopausal women and the aging process in both sexes. The possible mechanisms for these effects are summarized in Figure 26-29.

□ Pathology:

The ratio of osteoid to mineralized bone is normal in persons with osteoporosis. Newer densitometric and imaging techniques, such as computerized tomography, are sufficiently sensitive and precise to detect small deficiencies of bone. Although these noninvasive techniques visualize decrements in bone mass, they do not delineate the pathological mechanisms underlying the bone loss, which generally requires biochemical and occasionally, histological evaluation of the skeleton.

Because of the abundance of cancellous bone, osteoporotic changes are generally most dramatic in the spine. In vertebral body fractures caused by osteoporosis, the vertebra is deformed, with anterior wedging and collapse. If the vertebral body is not fractured, there is a general outline of both end plates, with a virtual absence of cancellous bone.

Histologically, osteoporosis is characterized by a decrease in the thickness of the cortex and a reduction in the number and size of trabeculae of the coarse cancellous bone. Whereas senile osteoporosis tends to feature reduced trabecular thickness, postmenopausal osteoporosis exhibits disrupted connections between trabeculae. The loss of trabecular connectivity, which is attended by diminished biomechanical strength and ultimately leads to fracture, is due to perforation of the trabeculae by resorbing osteoclasts in remodeling sites. In histological sections, the loss of connectivity results in the appearance of "isolated" islands of bone (see Fig. 26-27).

□ Clinical Features:

Postmenopausal osteoporosis usually becomes recognizable within 10 years after the onset of the menopause, whereas senile osteoporosis generally becomes symptomatic after age 70 years. Until recently, most patients were unaware of their disease until they had a fracture of a vertebra, hip, or other bone. However, the development of sensitive screening techniques now permits early diagnosis. Compression fractures of the vertebral bodies often occur after trivial trauma or may even follow lifting a heavy object. With each com-

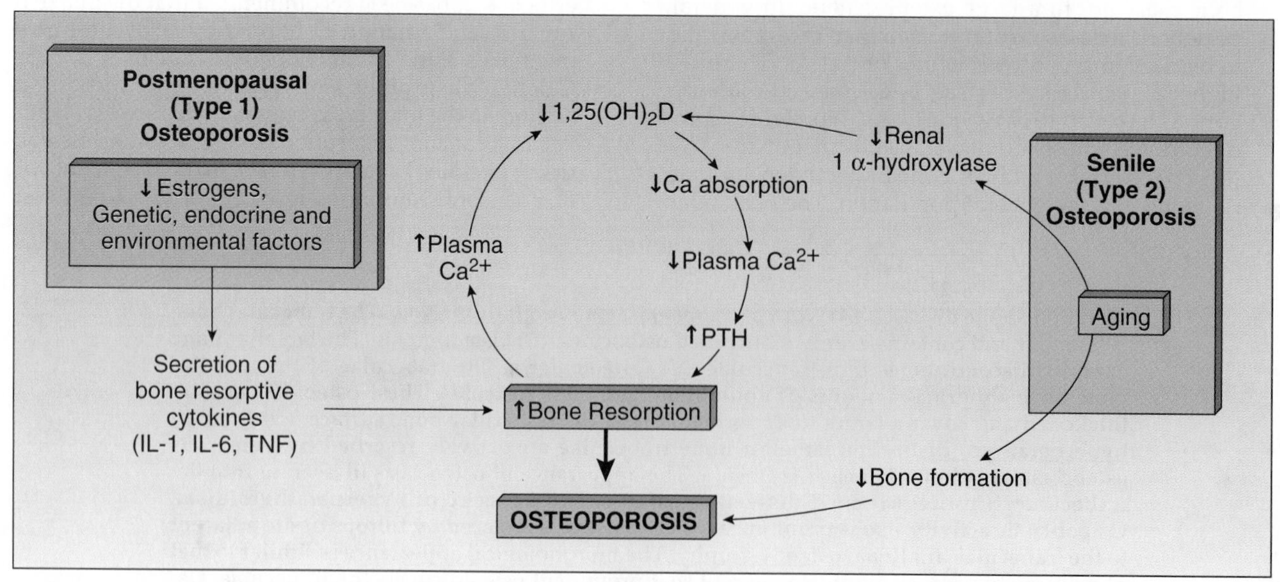

FIGURE 26-29
Pathogenesis of primary osteoporosis.

pression fracture, the patient becomes shorter and develops kyphosis ("dowager hump"). Serum calcium and phosphorus levels remain normal.

Estrogen therapy is an effective means of preventing postmenopausal osteoporosis. Because hormone treatment carries with it slightly increased risks of breast and endometrial cancers, other bone-specific antiosteoporotic drugs have been developed. A new class of inorganic compounds, known as *bisphosphonates*, appears particularly promising. All successful antiosteoporotic agents thus far developed block bone resorption but do not stimulate formation. Thus, the drugs may prevent progression of the disease but are incapable of curing the patient who already has osteoporosis. Dietary supplementation with calcium in elderly patients has been shown to reduce the risk of osteoporotic fractures by 30% to 70%.

Secondary Osteoporosis

Osteoporosis develops in association with a large number of other conditions (see Table 26-1).

- **Endocrine conditions:** Corticosteroid administration leads to the most common form of secondary osteoporosis. Bone loss may also result from an excess of endogenous glucocorticoids, as in Cushing disease. Corticosteroids inhibit osteoblastic activity, thereby reducing bone formation. They also impair vitamin D–dependent intestinal calcium absorption, an effect that leads to increased secretion of PTH and increased bone resorption.

  Hyperthyroidism causes accelerated turnover of bone and an increase in osteoclastic activity. Although thyrotoxicosis is associated with some degree of secondary osteoporosis, bone loss is limited.

  Hypogonadism in both men and women is accompanied by osteoporosis. In women with primary gonadal failure (Turner syndrome) or with secondary amenorrhea as a result of pituitary disease, estrogen deficiency is likely the cause. Hypogonadal men (e.g., Klinefelter syndrome, hemochromatosis) are at risk of osteoporosis because of a deficiency of anabolic androgens.
- **Hematological malignancies:** A variety of hematological cancers, particularly multiple myeloma, are accompanied by significant bone loss. The malignant plasma cells of multiple myeloma secrete osteoclast-activating factor, which is presumably responsible for secondary osteoporosis. Some leukemias and lymphomas are also associated with osteoporosis. The bone loss found in systemic mastocytosis has been attributed to the local release of heparin, which activates bone resorption. Even in the absence of skeletal metastases, some neoplasms are associated with severe hypercalcemia due to bone resorption. Osteoclastic activity is enhanced in these patients owing to secretion of PTH-related protein by the tumor.
- **Malabsorption:** Gastrointestinal and hepatic diseases that cause malabsorption often lead to osteoporosis, probably because of impaired absorption of calcium, phosphate, and vitamin D.
- **Alcoholism:** Chronic alcohol abuse also has been linked to the development of osteoporosis. Alcohol is a direct inhibitor of osteoblasts and may also inhibit calcium absorption.

OSTEOMALACIA AND RICKETS

Osteomalacia *(soft bones) is a disorder of adults characterized by inadequate mineralization of newly formed bone matrix.* ***Rickets*** *refers to a similar disorder in children, in whom the growth plates (physes) are open.* Thus children with rickets manifest defective mineralization not only of bone (osteomalacia) but also of the cartilaginous matrix of the growth plate. Diverse conditions associated with osteomalacia and rickets include abnormalities in vitamin D metabolism, phosphate deficiency states, and defects in the mineralization process itself.

Vitamin D Metabolism

An understanding of the pathogenesis of osteomalacia and rickets requires a brief discussion of the metabolism of vitamin D (Fig. 26-30). Vitamin D is ingested in food or synthesized in the skin from 7-dehydrocholesterol under the influence of the ultraviolet component of sunlight. The vitamin is first hydroxylated in the liver at carbon 25 to form its major circulating metabolite, 25-hydroxyvitamin D. It is then again hydroxylated in the proximal renal tubule at carbon 1 to produce the active hormone 1,25-dihydroxyvitamin D [$(1,25(OH)_2D)$]. Exposure to sunlight provides sufficient vitamin D for bone growth and mineralization, even in the face of an inadequate dietary source.

Receptors for $1,25(OH)_2D$ are present not only in classic targets, such as intestine, bone, and kidney, but are ubiquitous. This observation led to the realization that vitamin D targets many cells. This steroid hormone is a general inducer of differentiation, for example, influencing the maturation of hemopoietic and dermal cells, as well as a number of cancers. In the intestine, $1,25(OH)_2D$ stimulates the absorption of calcium and phosphate. It is also essential for osteoclast maturation. Although $1,25(OH)_2D$ enhances bone resorption *in vitro*, this effect does not occur *in vivo*, probably because of suppressed secretion of PTH. Regardless of the mechanism, $1,25(OH)_2D$ in concert with PTH serves to maintain the concentrations of calcium and phosphate in the blood that are required for proper mineralization of bone.

The principal determinant of the formation of $1,25(OH)_2D$ is the serum calcium concentration. A decrease in the level of blood calcium stimulates the release of PTH, which acts to augment the synthesis of $1,25(OH)_2D$ by the kidney.

Hypovitaminosis D can result from (1) inadequate exposure to sunlight, (2) deficient dietary intake, or (3) defective intestinal absorption. In addition there are hereditary and acquired disorders of vitamin D metabolism.

Dietary Deficiency of Vitamin D and Inadequate Exposure to Sunlight

Rickets plagued the children of the industrial cities of the United States and Europe from the 17th century through

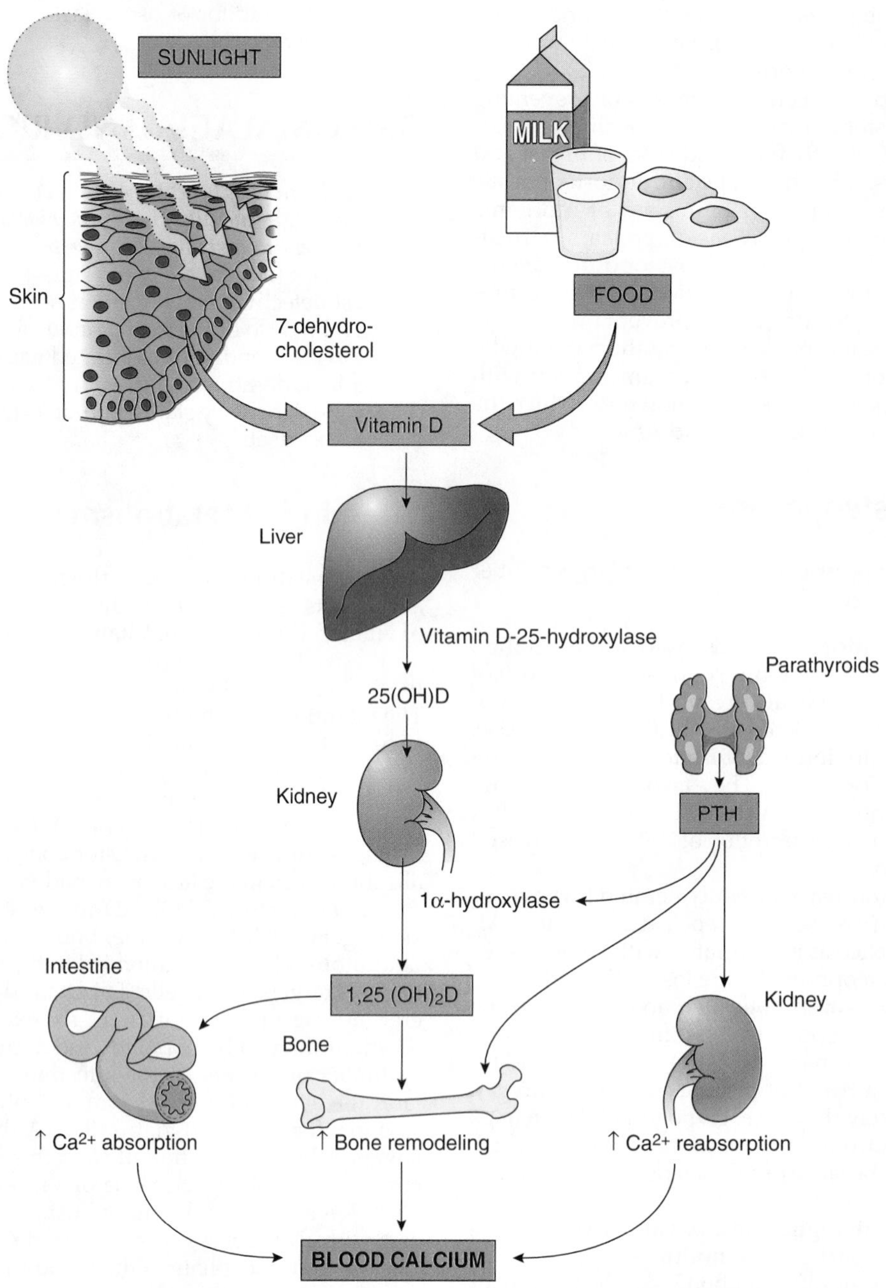

FIGURE *26-30*
Metabolism of vitamin D and the regulation of blood calcium.

the 19th century. Less than 100 years ago, 85% of the children in these regions had rickets. These children had insufficient sun exposure, and the dietary intake of vitamin D was inadequate to avert hypovitaminosis D. The administration of vitamin D–rich cod liver oil and later the fortification of milk and other foods with vitamin D effectively terminated the epidemic of rickets in Western countries. However, nutritional vitamin D deficiency remains a problem in some underdeveloped regions of the world, as well as in neglected elderly persons and food faddists.

Intestinal Malabsorption

In industrialized countries, osteomalacia is more often caused by diseases that are associated with intestinal malabsorption than by poor nutrition. **Diseases of the small intestine, cholestatic disorders of the liver, biliary obstruction, and chronic pancreatic insufficiency are the most frequent causes of osteomalacia in the United States.**

Malabsorption of vitamin D and calcium complicates a number of small intestinal diseases, including celiac disease, Crohn disease, scleroderma, and the post-surgical blind-loop syndrome. In obstructive jaundice, the lack of bile salts in the intestine impairs the absorption of lipids and lipid-soluble substances, among which is the fat-soluble vitamin D. Furthermore, with sufficient liver damage, the hydroxylation of vitamin D is reduced. Interestingly, the severe bone loss often attending biliary cirrhosis, a disease characterized by severe intestinal malabsorption leading to vitamin D deficiency, is osteoporosis rather than osteomalacia. This surprising finding indicates that vitamin D is essential not only for mineralization but also for the synthesis of bone collagen.

Disorders of Vitamin D Metabolism

There are hereditary and acquired disorders of vitamin D metabolism that involve either defective 1α-hydroxylation of vitamin D in the kidney or insensitivity of the target organ to 1,25$(OH)_2$D. Two autosomal recessive diseases associated with rickets are together known as vitamin D–dependent rickets.

Vitamin D–dependent rickets type I results from an inherited deficiency of renal 1α-hydroxylase activity. The clinical and biochemical changes of rickets appear during the first year of life, and these children exhibit hypocalcemia, hypophosphatemia, and high levels of serum PTH and alkaline phosphatase. The disease is controlled by the administration of 1,25$(OH)_2$D.

Vitamin D–dependent rickets type II represents inherited mutations of the vitamin D receptor, which render end organs insensitive to 1,25$(OH)_2$D. The manifestations of rickets usually become evident early in life but may appear at any time up to adolescence. The serum concentration of 1,25$(OH)_2$D is very high. The patients do not respond to 1,25$(OH)_2$D but are helped by repeated intravenous administration of calcium.

Acquired alterations in vitamin D metabolism also include defective renal 1α-hydroxylation and end-organ insensitivity. Some of the causes of impaired α-hydroxylation are hypoparathyroidism, tumor-induced osteomalacia, chronic renal diseases, and osteomalacia of old age. Osteomalacia occasionally complicates the treatment of epilepsy with anticonvulsant drugs, particularly phenobarbital and phenytoin. It is believed that these drugs block the action of 1,25$(OH)_2$D on target organs.

Renal Disorders of Phosphate Metabolism

Both rickets and osteomalacia may result from impaired reabsorption of phosphate by the proximal renal tubules, with resulting hypophosphatemia.

X-LINKED HYPOPHOSPHATEMIA: This condition, also termed *vitamin D–resistant rickets or phosphate diabetes*, is the most common type of hereditary rickets and is inherited as a dominant trait. The defective gene has been mapped to the short arm of the X chromosome (Xp22.31-p21.3) and has recently been cloned. Hypophosphatemia is caused by impaired transport of phosphate across the luminal membrane of proximal renal tubular cells, but the precise nature of the defect remains to be elucidated. Although renal phosphate wasting is central to the disease, osteoblast function is also impaired. In boys, florid rickets appears during childhood, whereas girls often have only hypophosphatemia. The disease is treated with life-long administration of phosphate and 1,25$(OH)_2$D. Pathologically, the bones of patients with X-linked hypophosphatemia show severe osteomalacia and contain wide osteoid seams. They also exhibit characteristic hypomineralized areas surrounding osteocytes, known as "halos." The presence of these structures indicates that osteocytes are responsible for the terminal mineralization of bone.

FANCONI SYNDROMES: *These inborn errors of metabolism are characterized by renal wastage of phosphate, glucose, bicarbonate, and amino acids.* They are all characterized by renal tubular acidosis and result in rickets and osteomalacia. Fanconi syndromes include Wilson disease, tyrosinemia, galactosemia, glycogen storage disease, and cystinosis. Renal tubular damage that leads to phosphate wastage may also be acquired, as in lead or mercury intoxication, amyloidosis, and Bence Jones proteinuria.

TUMOR-ASSOCIATED OSTEOMALACIA: This disorder is a phosphate-wasting syndrome that occurs with a number of benign and malignant tumors, including hemangiomas, nonossifying tumors of bone, prostate cancer, and neurofibromatosis. Such tumors presumably release substances that inhibit 1α-hydroxylase and impair the proximal tubular reabsorption of phosphate.

Defective Mineralization

Hypophosphatasia is a rare autosomal recessive disease in which a low activity of alkaline phosphatase in the blood and bones is associated with inadequate bone mineralization, resulting in rickets and osteomalacia. No effective treatment is available.

Some bisphosphonates, used in the treatment of Paget disease, and high doses of fluoride impair mineralization of newly forming bone matrix and may lead to osteomalacia.

□ Pathology

OSTEOMALACIA: Osteomalacia, like osteoporosis, is a cause of an osteopenic radiological pattern. The only findings may be compression fractures of the vertebrae and a decrease in bone thickness, as occur in osteoporosis. However, some specific findings may be seen in osteomalacia, including the pseudofractures of Milkman–Looser syndrome. These are radiolucent transverse defects, which are most common on the concave side of a long bone, the medial side of the neck of the femur, the ischial and pubic rami, the ribs, and the scapula.

Histologically, defective mineralization in osteomalacia results in an **exaggeration of the osteoid seams**, both in the thickness and in the proportion of trabecular surface covered (see Figs. 26-27 and 26-31). Osteoid seams reflect a time lag between the deposition of collagen and the appearance of the calcium salt. Adults add 1 μm of new matrix to the surfaces of bone every day, but it requires 10 days to mineralize this new bone. The normal thickness of osteoid seams, therefore, does not exceed 12 μm. Areas of pseudofracture display abundant osteoid and may function as stress points for true fractures. These areas do not evoke formation of callus and do not extend through the entire diameter of the bone.

RICKETS: Rickets is a disease of children and therefore results in extensive changes at the physeal plate (Fig. 26-32). This structure does not become adequately mineralized. The calcified cartilage and the zones of hypertrophy and proliferative cartilage continue to grow because osteoclastic activity does not resorb the cartilage growth plate. As a consequence, the growth plate is conspicuously thickened, irregular, and lobulated. Endochondral ossification proceeds very slowly and, preferentially, at the peripheral portions of the metaphysis. The result is a flared and cup-shaped epiphysis. The largest part of the primary spongiosum is composed of lamellar or woven bone, which importantly remains unmineralized.

On histological examination, the growth plate exhibits striking changes. Although the resting zone is normal, the zones of proliferating cartilage are greatly distorted. The ordered progression of helix-forming chondrocytes is lost and is replaced by a disorderly profusion of cells separated by small amounts of matrix. The resulting lobulated masses of proliferating and hypertrophied cartilage are associated with an increasing width of the growth plate, which may be 5 to 15 times the normal width. The zone of provisional calcification is poorly defined, and only a minimal amount of primary spongiosum is formed. Masses of proliferating cartilage extend into the metaphyseal region, without any apparent vascular invasion and with little osteoclastic activity.

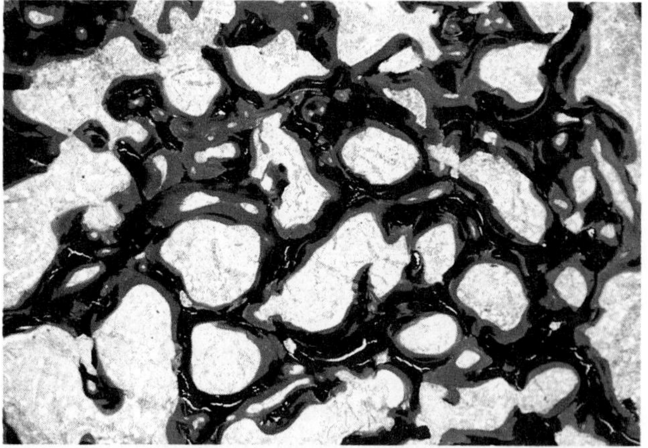

FIGURE *26-31*
Osteomalacia. The surfaces of the bony trabeculae (*black*) are covered by a thicker than normal layer of osteoid (*red*) with the von Kossa stain, which colors calcified tissue black.

□ Clinical Features

OSTEOMALACIA: The clinical diagnosis of osteomalacia is often difficult. Patients have nonspecific complaints, such as muscle weakness or diffuse aches and pains. In mild forms of the disease, only slowly progressive changes in bone are seen, and many patients are totally asymptomatic for years. In advanced cases, poorly localized bone pain and tenderness are common, especially in the spine, pelvis, and proximal parts of the extremities. In such cases, the diagnosis of osteomalacia may be made only after an acute fracture, the most common sites being the femoral neck, pubic ramus, spine, or ribs. Muscular weakness and hypotonia lead to a waddling gait in severe cases, and some patients are not be able to walk at all.

RICKETS: Children with rickets are apathetic and irritable and have a short attention span. They are content to be sedentary, assuming a Buddha-like posture. Rachitic children are short and exhibit characteristic changes of bones and teeth. Flattening of the skull, prominent frontal bones (frontal bossing), and conspicuous suture lines are typical. There is delayed dentition, with severe dental caries and enamel defects. The chest has the classic *rachitic rosary* (a grossly beaded appearance of the costochondral junctions that is produced by enlargement of the costal cartilages) and indentations of the lower ribs at the insertion of the diaphragm. *Pectus carinatum* ("pigeon breast") reflects an outward curvature of the sternum.

The overall musculature is weak, and abdominal weakness leads to a "potbelly." The limbs are shortened and deformed, with severe bowing of the arms and forearm and frequent fractures. The femoral head may dislocate from the growth plate (slipped capital femoral epiphysis).

PRIMARY HYPERPARATHYROIDISM

Primary hyperparathyroidism refers a metabolic bone disease characterized by generalized bone resorption caused by inappropriate secretion of PTH. Early in the century, bone disease in patients diagnosed with primary hyperparathyroidism was often advanced and crippling. Owing to screening of hospitalized patients for abnormalities of serum calcium, severe primary hyperparathyroidism is rarely encountered, and clinically significant bone disease is unusual. Thus, although bone biopsies of patients with primary hyperparathyroidism almost always exhibit evidence of the disease, there is generally no deficit in bone mass.

The histological changes of primary hyperparathyroidism are known as *osteitis fibrosa.* This term applies to all circumstances of markedly accelerated remodeling and may be seen in Paget disease, in hyperthyroidism, and even in some patients with postmenopausal osteoporosis. Almost all (90%) of the cases of primary hyperparathyroidism are caused by one or more parathyroid adenomas, whereas hyperplasia of all four glands ac-

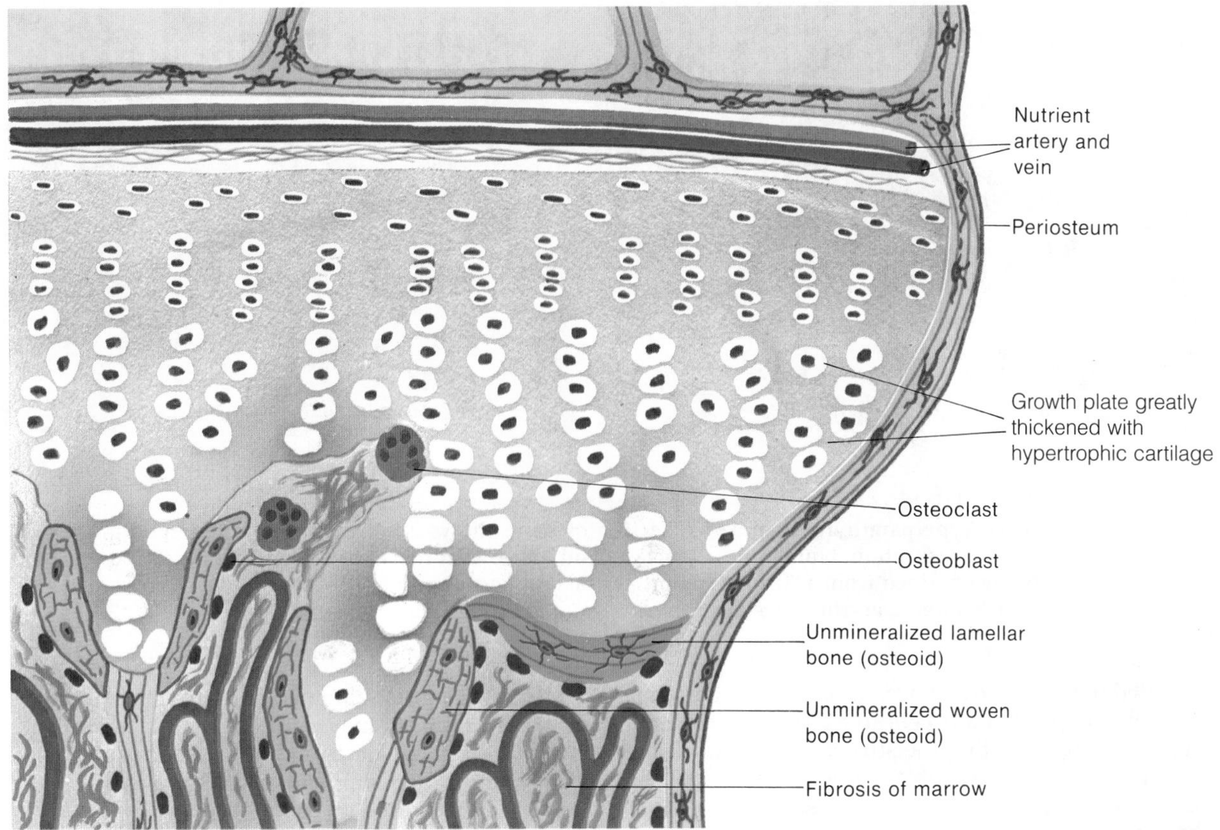

FIGURE *26-32*
The growth plate in rickets. The growth plate is thickened and disorganized, with a large zone of hypertrophic cartilage cells. There is irregular perforation of the cartilage plate by osteoclasts because there is little calcified cartilage. The woven bone on the surface of some of the primary trabeculae is unmineralized and therefore easily fractured. Such microfractures often lead to hemorrhage at the interface between the plate and the metaphysis.

counts for only 10%. Rarely, hyperparathyroidism complicates a parathyroid carcinoma. Because PTH promotes excretion of phosphate in the urine and stimulates osteoclastic bone resorption, low serum phosphate and high serum calcium levels are characteristic.

Actions of Parathyroid Hormone

The principal function of PTH is the regulation of the calcium concentration in the extracellular fluid. This task is accomplished by the effect of the hormone on the bone, kidney, and (indirectly) intestine.

BONE: PTH mobilizes calcium from bone, the major reservoir of calcium in the body. PTH increases the resorption of bone in the context of accelerated remodeling. Thus, enhanced bone formation is also a component of hyperparathyroidism. Depending on the relative increase in bone resorption and formation, respectively, the secretion of excess PTH may result in decreased, normal, or increased bone mass.

KIDNEY: PTH stimulates the reabsorption of calcium by the thick ascending and the granular portions of the distal renal tubules. It also enhances phosphate excretion in the proximal and distal convoluted tubules by directly inhibiting sodium-dependent phosphate transport. In addition, the hormone augments the activity of 1α-hydroxylase in the proximal tubules.

INTESTINE: PTH does not act directly on the intestine, but rather stimulates intestinal calcium absorption indirectly by increasing renal synthesis of $1,25(OH)_2D$.

☐ **Pathogenesis and Pathology:** The histogenesis of osteitis fibrosa cystica may be classified into three stages.

- **The early stage:** Initially osteoclasts are stimulated by the increased PTH levels to resorb bone. From the subperiosteal and endosteal surfaces, osteoclasts bore their way into the cortex as cutting cones. This process is termed *dissecting osteitis* because each trabecula is continually hollowed out by osteoclastic activity (see Figs. 26-27 and 26-33A). At the same time, collagen fibers are laid down in the endosteal marrow, and additional osteoclasts penetrate the bone. In contrast to myelofibrosis of hematological origin, in which fibrous tissue is randomly dis-

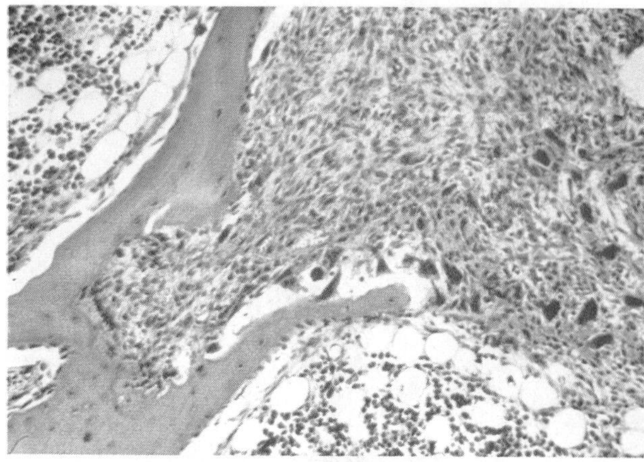

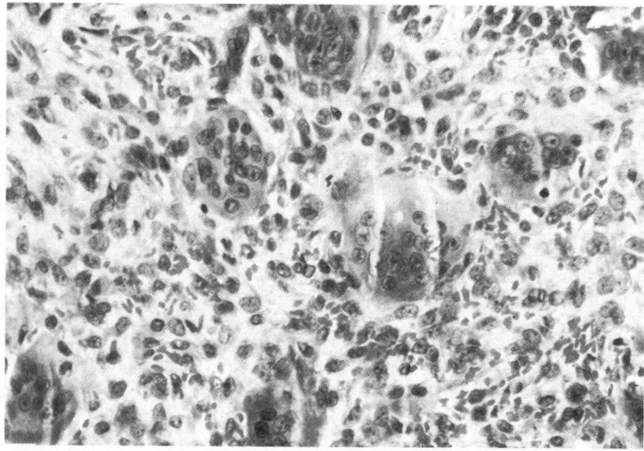

FIGURE 26-33
Primary hyperparathyroidism. (*A*) A section of bone shows a bony trabecula undergoing tunneling resorption. Numerous osteoclasts and marrow fibrosis are evident. (*B*) A section of tissue obtained from a "brown tumor" reveals numerous giant cells in a cellular, fibrous stroma. Scattered erythrocytes are present throughout the tissue.

tributed in the marrow space, the collagen of osteitis fibrosa is deposited adjacent to trabeculae. This observation suggests that the stromal cells depositing matrix material are osteoblast precursors.

- **Osteitis fibrosa:** In the second stage, the trabecular bone is resorbed and the marrow is replaced by loose fibrosis, hemosiderin-laden macrophages, areas of hemorrhage from microfractures, and reactive woven bone. This combination of features constitutes the "osteitis fibrosa" portion of the complex.
- **Osteitis fibrosa cystica:** As primary hyperparathyroidism progresses and hemorrhage continues, cystic degeneration ultimately occurs, leading to the final stage of the disease. The areas of fibrosis that contain reactive woven bone and hemosiderin-laden macrophages often display many giant cells, which are actually osteoclasts. Because of its macroscopic appearance, this lesion has been termed a *brown tumor* (see Fig. 26-33B). This is not a true tumor, but rather a repair reaction as an end stage of hyperparathyroidism.

The skeletal radiographs of most persons with primary hyperparathyroidism are normal. Some patients exhibit mottled bone cortex, with an irregular frayed surface in the outer table of the skull, the tufts of the terminal digits, and the shafts of the metacarpals (Fig. 26-34). A distinctive radiological peculiarity, referred to as *subperiosteal bone resorption*, is evident in the subperiosteal outer surface of the cortex and reflects dissecting osteitis. Resorption around the tooth sockets causes the lamina dura of the teeth to disappear.

A classic feature of **osteitis fibrosa cystica** is the presence of multiple, localized, lytic lesions, which represent hemorrhagic cysts or masses of fibrous tissue. These eccentric and well-demarcated lesions are separated from the soft tissue by a periosteal shell of bone. **The focal, tumor-like, lytic lesions always occur in the context of an abnormal skeleton produced by hyperparathyroidism.** If a single lesion is examined without considering the rest of the skeleton, it may be mistaken for a primary neoplasm of bone. The differential diagnosis of primary hyperparathyroidism includes other causes of hypercalcemia, such as osteolytic metastases, sarcoidosis, vitamin D intoxication, and, rarely, multiple myeloma.

□ **Clinical Features:** The symptoms of primary hyperparathyroidism are related to the abnormality of calcium homeostasis and have been summarized as "stones, bones, moans, and groans." The "stones" refer to kidney stones, and the "bones" to the skeletal changes. The "moans" describe psychiatric depression and other abnormalities associated with hypercalcemia, whereas

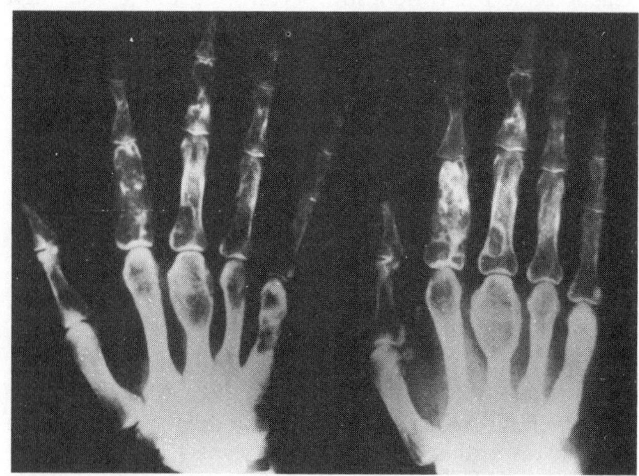

FIGURE 26-34
Primary hyperparathyroidism. A radiograph of the hands reveals bulbous swellings ("brown tumors") and numerous cavities, both representing bone resorption.

the "groans" characterize the gastrointestinal irregularities associated with a high serum calcium level.

Primary hyperparathyroidism is treated with surgical removal of the parathyroid adenomas. In cases in which parathyroid hyperplasia is the cause of the disease, three and a half glands are usually removed. The remaining fragment is sufficient to ensure that the patient does not develop hypocalcemia. After surgery, the histological appearance of the affected skeleton gradually normalizes.

RENAL OSTEODYSTROPHY

Renal osteodystrophy is a complex metabolic bone disease that occurs in the context of chronic renal failure. Severe renal osteodystrophy is most common in patients maintained on chronic dialysis, because they live long enough to develop conspicuous bone disease.

☐ **Pathogenesis:** The pathogenesis of renal osteodystrophy is similar to that of osteomalacia, with secondary hyperparathyroidism exerting its influence by way of osteoclastic resorption of bone (see Fig. 26-27). The sequence of events that leads to renal osteodystrophy may be summarized as follows:

1. In chronic renal disease, a reduced glomerular filtration rate leads to the retention of phosphate, thereby producing **hyperphosphatemia**.
2. Tubular injury causes a reduction in 1α-hydroxylase activity, with a resulting deficiency of 1,25$(OH)_2$D.
3. Intestinal calcium absorption is, in turn, decreased, thereby producing **hypocalcemia**.
4. Hypocalcemia stimulates the elaboration of parathyroid hormone. In fact, most patients with end-stage renal disease have substantial hyperparathyroidism. However, PTH does not effectively promote intestinal calcium absorption or renal tubular resorption of calcium because of failure to produce adequate 1,25$(OH)_2$D.
5. Perhaps because of hyperparathyroidism and hyperphosphatemia, a substantial proportion of patients with end-stage renal disease have increased bone mass. Renal osteosclerosis is particularly prominent in vertebrae where, owing to alternating bands of radiopaque and normally dense bone, the lesion is named "rugger jersey spine."

In some patients, defects in bone matrix mineralization (osteomalacia) also occur. Aluminum accumulation from dialysate contamination or the ingestion of aluminum-containing gels to prevent hyperphosphatemia has been a major factor in the induction of osteomalacia. Awareness of the detrimental effects of aluminum on the skeleton has greatly reduced the incidence of renal osteomalacia.

The adynamic variant of renal osteodystrophy is characterized by arrested bone remodeling. Few osteoclasts or osteoblasts are present, and no bone formation or resorption occurs. As a result, old bone accumulates, leading to structural compromise of the skeleton and a tendency to fractures. Affected patients tend to have mild hyperparathyroidism. Although this lesion, in the past,

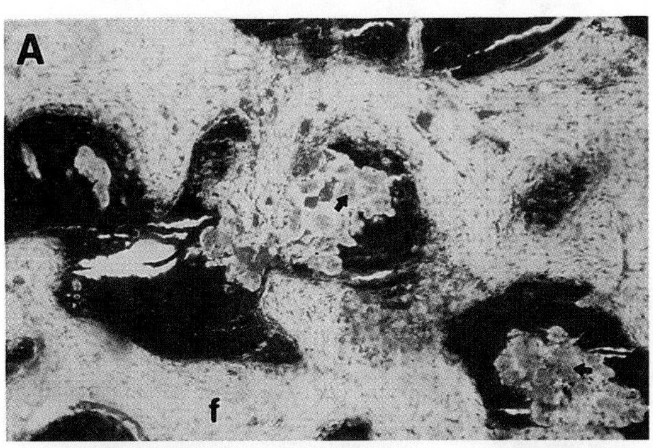

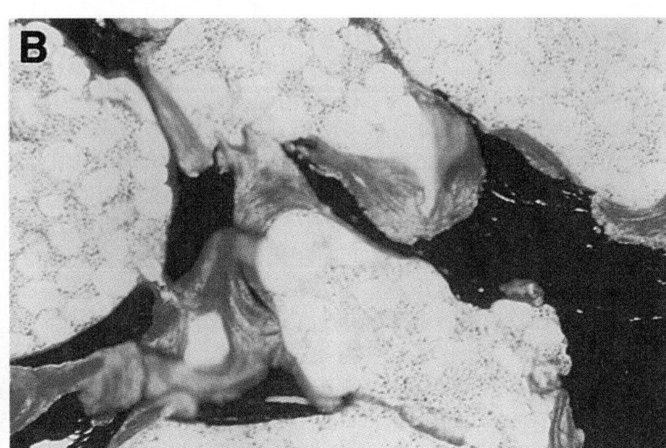

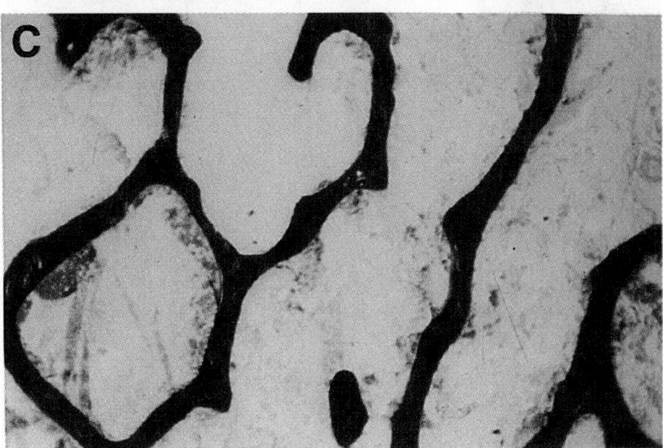

FIGURE 26-35
Renal osteodystrophy. (*A*) Osteitis fibrosa, with numerous osteoclasts (*arrows*), osteoblasts, and marrow fibrosis (*f*). (*B*) Osteomalacia, characterized by abundant osteoid (*red*), which is appreciated in specimens that have not been decalcified. (*C*) Adynamic bone disease in which remodeling is attenuated, with a paucity of osteoblasts, osteoclasts, and osteoid.

was generally associated with aluminum accumulation from the dialysis apparatus, such is no longer the case. Curiously, adynamic bone disease is now the most common form of renal osteodystrophy and is often disabling and difficult to manage.

☐ **Pathology and Clinical Features:** As a result of these effects of chronic renal failure, renal osteodystrophy is characterized by varying degrees of osteomalacia, osteitis fibrosa (Fig. 26-35A), osteomalacia (Fig. 26-35B), osteosclerosis, and adynamic bone disease (Fig. 26-35C). Combinations of osteitis fibrosa and osteomalacia are particularly common. Hyperphosphatemic patients with terminal chronic renal disease may display metastatic calcification at various sites, including the eyes, skin, muscular coats of arteries and arterioles, and periarticular soft tissues.

The management of renal osteodystrophy involves not only the treatment of renal failure but also the control of phosphate levels by appropriate drug therapy and infusions. Occasionally, parathyroidectomy is necessary to control hyperparathyroidism, and the administration of vitamin D may also be necessary.

PAGET DISEASE OF BONE

Paget disease is a chronic condition characterized by enlargement and lytic lesions of bone caused by disordered bone remodeling, in which excessive bone resorption initially results in lytic lesions, to be followed by disorganized and excessive bone formation.

☐ **Epidemiology:** Paget disease is common and generally affects men and women older than 60 years. In predisposed populations, 3% to 4% of elderly persons manifest the disease at autopsy or on radiographic examination. The disorder has an unusual worldwide distribution, afflicting populations of the British Isles and following their migrations throughout the world. Persons of English descent living in the United States, Australia, New Zealand, and Canada have a high incidence of the disease. Northern Europeans also have more Paget disease than Southern Europeans. It is striking that the disorder is almost nonexistent in Asia and in the indigenous populations of Africa and South America.

☐ **Pathogenesis:** Paget disease is of unknown origin. Interestingly, James Paget, who coined the term *osteitis deformans* for this disease more than a century ago, thought that it was likely an infection of bone. Since then, virtually every type of disease process, including neoplasia, has been proposed as the cause. A hereditary predisposition is suggested by the reports of almost 100 families in which Paget disease seems to be transmitted as an autosomal dominant trait.

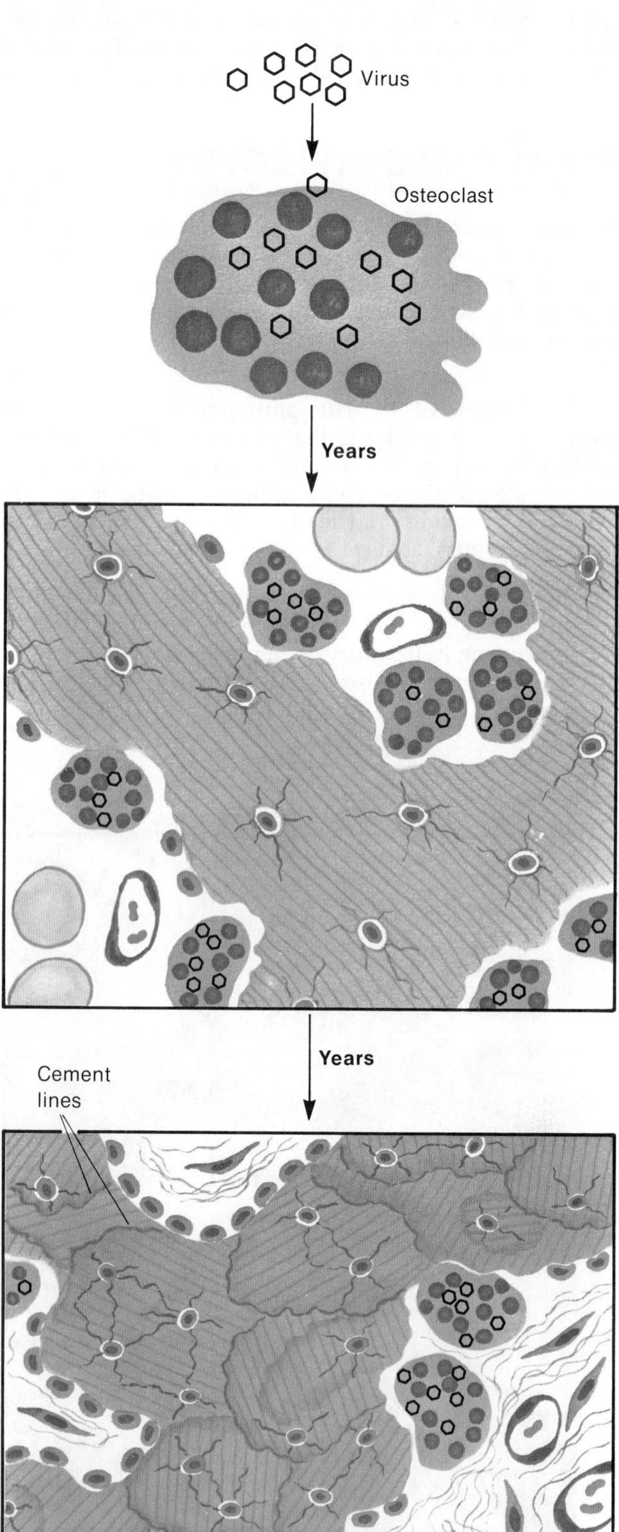

FIGURE *26-36*
Hypothetical viral etiology of Paget disease of bone. A virus infects osteoclastic progenitors or osteoclasts and stimulates osteoclastic activity, thereby leading to excessive resorption of bone. Over a period of years, the bone develops a characteristic mosaic pattern, produced by chaotically juxtaposed units of lamellar bone that form irregular cement lines. The adjacent marrow is often fibrotic, and there is a mixture of osteoclasts and osteoblasts on the surface of the bone.

An abundance of evidence indicates that Paget disease is of viral origin. Inclusions consistent with the structure of a virus have been demonstrated in the osteoclasts of Paget disease. Virtually all patients exhibit these inclusions, which are not found in any other skeletal disease other than giant cell tumors of bone. They consist of microfilaments in a paracrystalline array and have been compared with the inclusions in the brains of patients with subacute sclerosing encephalitis (see Chapter 29). This similarity has suggested the possibility that a slow virus may be involved (Fig. 26-36). Support for this hypothesis has come from the finding that the marrow of Paget disease patients contains viral transcripts.

□ **Pathology:** The lesions of Paget disease may be solitary or may occur at multiple sites. They tend to localize to the bones of the axial skeleton, including the spine, skull, and pelvis. The proximal femur and tibia may also be involved in the polyostotic form of the disease. Solitary Paget disease rarely involves the humerus, but in polyostotic disease, lesions involving this bone are common.

Paget disease is an example of bone remodeling gone awry. The disease is triphasic, as follows:

1. **"Hot" or osteoclastic resorptive stage:** Radiologically, there is a characteristic, sharply defined, flame-shaped or wedge-shaped lysis of the cortex, which may mimic a tumor.
2. **Mixed stage of osteoblastic and osteoclastic activity:** By radiograph, the bones are larger than normal. In fact, Paget disease is one of only two diseases that produce **larger than normal bones** (the other is fibrous dysplasia, discussed later). The cortex in the mixed phase is thickened, and the accentuation of the coarse cancellous bone makes the bone look heavy and enlarged (Fig. 26-37A,B). Involvement of vertebral bodies leads to a "picture frame" appearance (see Fig. 26-37C), as the cortices and end plates become greatly exaggerated in comparison with the coarse cancellous bone of the vertebral body. Although the bone is abnormal, the distorted, coarse cancellous bone and cortex still tend to align along stress lines. The pelvis is often thickened in the area of the acetabulum.
3. **"Cold" or burnt-out stage:** This period is characterized histologically by little cellular activity and radiologically by thickened and disordered bones.

The disease need not progress through all three stages, and in polyostotic disease, various foci may appear in different stages.

The osteoclast is the pathological cell of Paget disease and its appearance is characteristic. Whereas normal osteoclasts contain fewer than a dozen nuclei, those of Paget disease are huge and may encompass more than 100 (see Fig. 26-35B). Interestingly, osteoclasts generated *in*

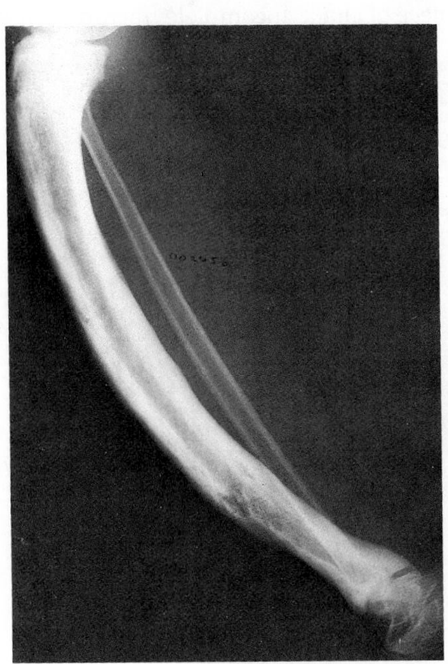

A

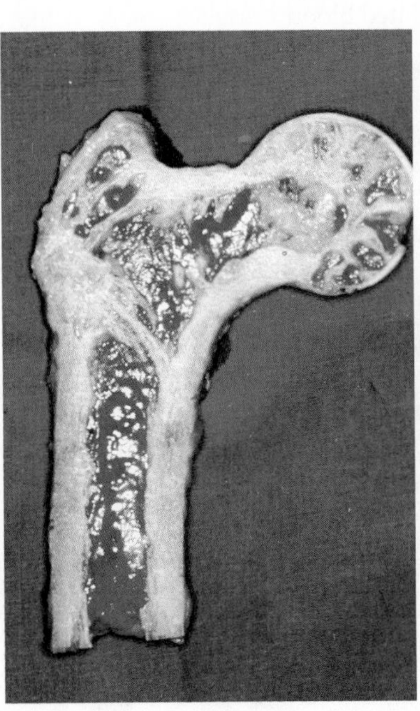

B

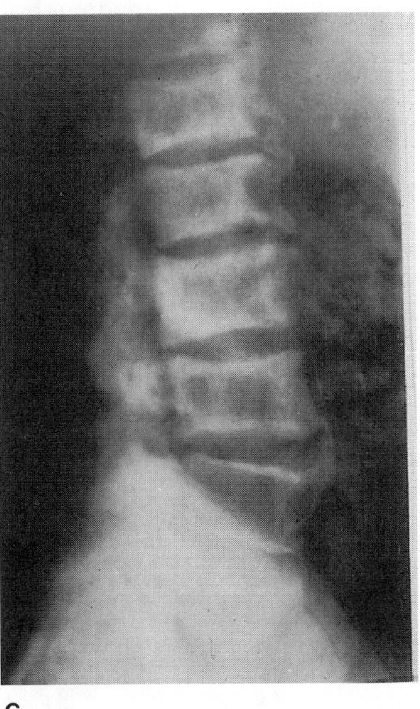

C

FIGURE *26-37*
Paget disease. (*A*) A radiograph of the leg shows marked involvement of the tibia by Paget disease with thickening and disorganization of the cortex. Note the normal appearance of the fibula. (*B*) The proximal end of a femur affected by Paget disease shows replacement of the normal cancellous architecture by coarse, thick bundles of trabecular bone. The cortical bone is irregularly thickened and exhibits a coarse, granular appearance instead of the normally smooth cortical bone. (*C*) A radiograph of the spine shows vertebrae affected by Paget disease. The vertebrae are shorter and wider than normal, and display the characteristic "picture frame" appearance.

vitro from the marrow of patients with Paget disease are also increased in number, size, and number of nuclei.

Because active Paget disease is a disorder of accelerated remodeling, its histological features are those of severe osteitis fibrosa. Numerous osteoclasts, large active osteoblasts, and peritrabecular marrow fibrosis are encountered. The rapid remodeling leads to disruption of trabecular architecture. Trabeculae are characteristically distorted and irregular, with a high surface-to-volume ratio. Bone collagen is often arranged in a woven rather than lamellar pattern.

With time, the lesions of Paget disease burn out and become inactive. The diagnostic hallmark of this stage is the abnormal arrangement of lamellar bone, in which islands of irregular bone formation, resembling pieces of a jigsaw puzzle, are separated by prominent *cement lines* (Fig. 26-38A). The result is a mosaic pattern in the bone, which can be seen particularly well under polarized light. In the cortex of an affected bone, the osteons tend to be destroyed, and concentric lamellae are incomplete. Although the changes in lamellar bone are diagnostic, it is not uncommon to see woven bone as part of the pathological process. In this situation, the woven bone is a reactive phenomenon, as in a microcallus, and represents a temporary bridge between islands of the mosaic bone of Paget disease.

□ **Clinical Features:** The most common focal symptom of Paget disease is pain, although its cause is not clear. The pain may be related to microfractures, to the stimulation of free nerve endings by dilated blood vessels adjacent to the bones, or to weight bearing in weaker bones.

SKULL INVOLVEMENT: Involvement of the skull is particularly common in Paget disease (see Fig. 26-37A). The skull exhibits localized lysis, generally in the frontal and parietal bones, which is termed *osteoporosis circumscripta*. Alternatively, there may be thickening of the outer and inner tables, which is most pronounced in the frontal and occipital bones (see Fig. 26-37B). The skull becomes very heavy and may collapse over the C1 vertebra, thereby compressing the brain and spinal cord. Hearing loss is caused by involvement of the ossicles and bony impingement on the eighth cranial nerve at the foramen. *Platybasia* (flattening of the base of the skull) impinges on the foramen magnum, thereby compressing the medulla and upper spinal cord.

The jaws may be grossly misshapen, and the teeth may fall out. Often, the facial bones increase in size, producing so-called *leontiasis ossea* (lion-like face). This deformity is particularly likely to result when the maxillary bones are affected.

PAGETIC STEAL: Occasionally, patients feel lightheaded, a symptom thought to be due to so-called pagetic steal, in which blood is shunted from the internal carotid system to the bones rather than directed to the brain.

FRACTURES AND ARTHRITIS: Bone fractures are common in Paget disease, the bones snapping transversely like a piece of chalk. Incomplete fractures without

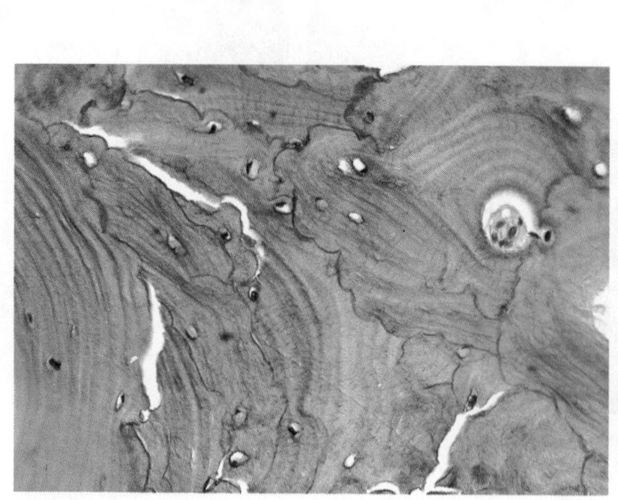
A

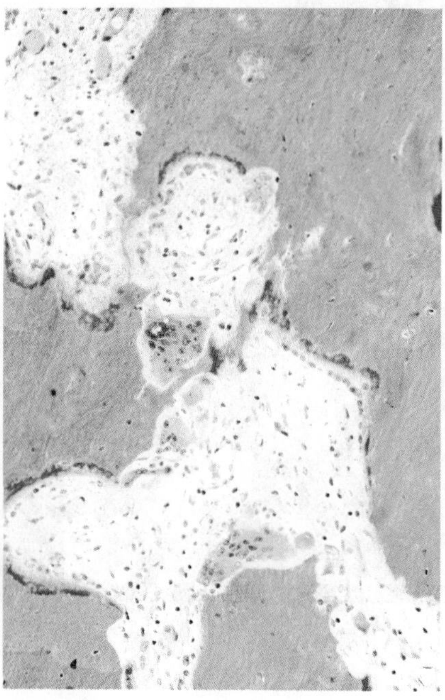
B

FIGURE 26-38
Paget disease. (*A*) A section of bone shows prominent basophilic cement lines with several microfractures. (*B*) With this Goldner stain, two osteoclasts are evident, each containing many more nuclei than normal. There are numerous osteoblasts, together with new, unmineralized osteoid (*red*) and marrow fibrosis.

displacement are called *infractions*. Involvement of the pelvis leads to hip problems. The loss of subchondral bone compliance causes secondary osteoarthritis and destruction of the articular cartilage.

HIGH-OUTPUT CARDIAC FAILURE: With extensive Paget disease, the blood flow to bone and subcutaneous tissue is remarkably increased, requiring an increase in cardiac output, which may be severe enough to result in cardiac failure.

SARCOMATOUS CHANGE: Neoplastic transformation may occur in a focus of Paget disease, usually in the femur, humerus, or pelvis. This complication occurs in less than 1% of all cases and usually arises in patients with severe Paget disease. Interestingly, the skull and vertebrae, which are the bones most commonly involved in Paget disease, rarely undergo sarcomatous change. The sarcoma is usually osteogenic but may be fibrosarcoma or chondrosarcoma.

GIANT CELL TUMOR: This lesion is not a neoplasm but rather a reactive phenomenon, similar to the "brown tumor" of hyperparathyroidism. Giant cell tumor is thought to represent an overshoot of osteoclastic activity and an associated fibroblastic response. Radiation therapy to the giant cell tumor is curative in many cases.

The serum calcium and phosphorus levels in Paget disease are normal, even though the turnover rate of bone is increased more than 20-fold. Although hypercalcemia is rare, it does occur if the patient is immobilized. The collagen structure of bone in Paget disease is entirely normal, but because of the accelerated bone turnover, levels of collagen breakdown products are increased in the serum and urine, especially hydroxyproline and hydroxylysine. Hydroxyproline excretion may reach 1,000 mg/day (normal, <40 mg). The serum alkaline phosphatase level serves as the most useful laboratory test in diagnosing Paget disease. It is enormously increased and correlates with osteoblastic activity. The alkaline phosphatase levels are disproportionately high with skull involvement, but tend to be low when only the pelvis is affected. A sudden increase in the activity of serum alkaline phosphatase may reflect sarcomatous change within a lesion.

Fortunately, most patients with Paget disease are asymptomatic and require no treatment. Fractures, osteoarthritis, and other orthopedic complications are treated symptomatically. Drugs directed at abnormal osteoclast function, including calcitonin, diphosphonates, and mithramycin, may be useful.

GAUCHER DISEASE

Gaucher disease is a hereditary storage disease that affects the bones, as well as other organs. The symptoms of the disorder relate to the accumulation within macrophages of large amounts of glucocerebroside (see Chapter 6 for a detailed discussion). Virtually all patients with Gaucher disease type I have some abnormality of the skeleton.

FAILURE OF REMODELING OF THE DISTAL FEMUR AND PROXIMAL TIBIA: This is the most common, although the least troublesome, skeletal abnormality in Gaucher disease. The defect is manifested as an absence of appropriate flaring, and, therefore, funnelization and cylinderization are abnormal (Fig. 26-39). The resulting bone has an Erlenmeyer flask shape, similar to that seen in other modeling deformities (e.g., osteopetrosis).

GAUCHER CRISIS: This event occurs in only a few patients with the disease, but it is intensely painful and disabling. The crisis seems to result from acute infarction of a large segment of bone, usually the spine, pelvis, or femoral head. The lesion may even be multifocal in one or several bones. In many cases, Gaucher crisis occurs after an acute viral illness. The patients have sudden, severe, and progressive pain, which is localized to an anatomical focus. Fever, tenderness in the area of the bone, and soft tissue swelling are characteristic. Gaucher crisis lasts for 2 or more weeks and then gradually improves.

LOCALIZED AND DIFFUSE BONE LOSS: Localized lytic lesions, cortical thinning, and loss of coarse cancellous bone are seen radiologically. Bone loss is usually most severe in the axial skeleton and the proximal appendicular skeleton. On histological examination, areas of decreased bone mass contain marrow packed with Gaucher cells. These patients are generally asymptomatic until a fracture or osteonecrosis occurs.

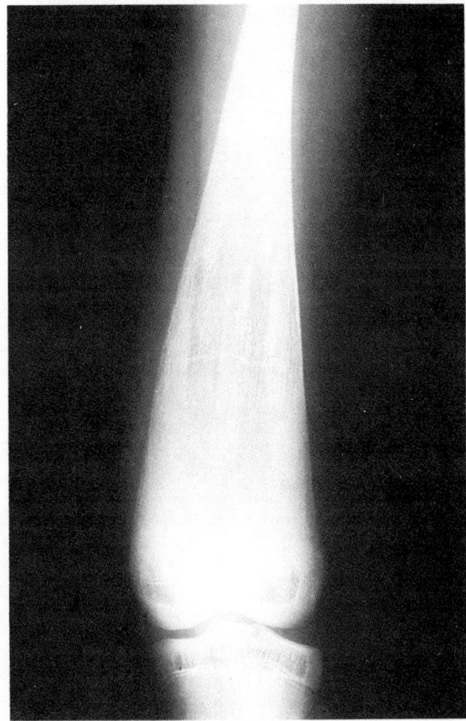

FIGURE *26-39*
Gaucher disease. A radiograph of the distal femur displays the characteristic flaring of the metaphysis and distal diaphysis.

OSTEOSCLEROTIC LESIONS: Increased bone formation occurs in the medullary cavity of the long bones and pelvis. Reactive new bone forms in areas that have undergone osteonecrosis, as evidenced by the presence in these zones of dead bone, fat necrosis, and calcification of fat. Occasionally, osteosclerotic lesions are present in the flat bones of the skull.

CORTICOMEDULLARY OSTEONECROSIS: This is the most disabling of the skeletal problems associated with Gaucher disease and occurs most commonly in young patients between the ages of 8 and 35 years. It affects the femoral head or proximal humerus or, less commonly, a femoral or tibial condyle, talus, or capitulum. Corticomedullary osteonecrosis may involve the shaft of long bones, as well. It is bilateral in more than half of the patients and is often multifocal. The pathogenesis of this lesion is not clear; one theory holds that it involves an occlusion of a vessel leading to the femoral or humeral head.

PATHOLOGICAL FRACTURES: The vertebrae, the long bones, and even the pelvis may have spontaneous fractures.

HEMATOGENOUS OSTEOMYELITIS AND SEPTIC ARTHRITIS: These infections are not uncommon in patients with Gaucher disease, and the incidence of postoperative wound infection also is high. The most common agents are coliform or anaerobic organisms. It may be that bacteria are deposited in areas of bone infarction, or perhaps the phagocytic cells filled with glucocerebroside are incompetent and cannot respond to the invading bacteria.

FIBROUS DYSPLASIA

Fibrous dysplasia is a peculiar developmental abnormality of the skeleton characterized by a disorganized mixture of fibrous and osseous elements in the interior of affected bones. It occurs in children or adults and may involve a single bone (monostotic) or many bones (polyostotic). In 5% of cases of fibrous dysplasia, the skeletal lesions are associated with skin pigmentation and endocrine dysfunction, in which case the term *McCune–Albright syndrome* is applied.

Recently activating mutations in the alpha subunit of the stimulatory guanine nucleotide binding protein ($G_s\alpha$), which is linked to adenylyl cyclase, has been described in bone cells from patients with fibrous dysplasia and McCune–Albright syndrome. The result would be constitutive activation of adenylyl cyclase and an increase in the levels of cyclic adenosine monophosphate (cAMP), thereby enhancing the function of the affected cells.

MONOSTOTIC FIBROUS DYSPLASIA: Monostotic fibrous dysplasia is the most common form of the disease and is most often seen in the second and third decades, without any predilection for either sex. The bones commonly involved are the proximal femur, tibia, ribs, and facial bones, although any bone may be involved. The disease may be asymptomatic, or it may lead to a pathological fracture.

POLYOSTOTIC FIBROUS DYSPLASIA: One fourth of patients with polyostotic fibrous dysplasia exhibit disease in more than half of the skeleton, including the facial bones. Symptoms usually are seen in childhood, and almost all patients have pathological fractures, limb defor-

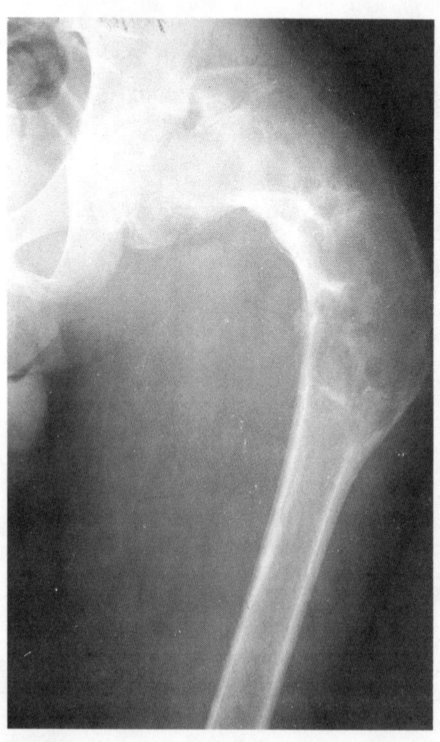
A

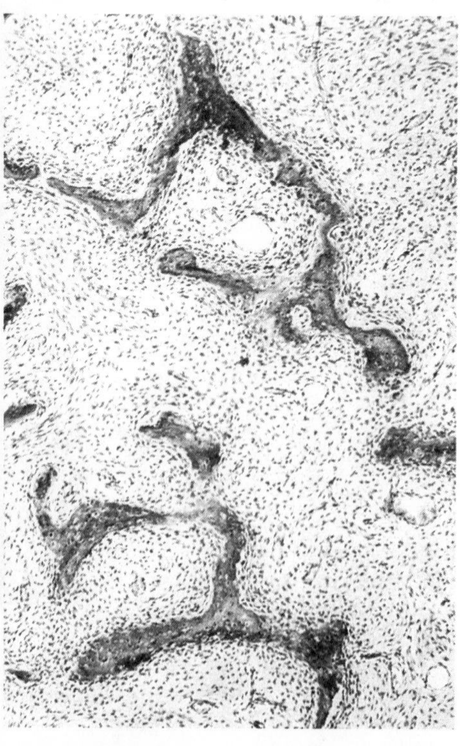
B

FIGURE *26-40*
Fibrous dysplasia. (*A*) A radiograph of the proximal femur shows a "shepherd's crook" deformity, caused by fractures sustained over the years. Irregular, marginated, ground-glass lucencies are surrounded by reactive bone. The shaft has an appearance that has been likened to a soap bubble. (*B*) A photomicrograph reveals whorled fibrous tissue surrounding irregularly shaped spicules of woven bone.

mities, or limb-length discrepancies. Polyostotic fibrous dysplasia is more common in females. Sometimes the disease becomes quiescent at puberty, whereas pregnancy may stimulate the growth of lesions.

McCUNE–ALBRIGHT SYNDROME: This condition is characterized by endocrine dysfunction, including acromegaly, Cushing syndrome, hyperthyroidism, and vitamin D–resistant rickets. The most common endocrine abnormality is precocious puberty in girls (boys rarely have McCune–Albright syndrome). As a result, premature closure of the growth plates may lead to an abnormally short stature. The most frequent extraskeletal manifestations of McCune–Albright syndrome are the characteristic skin lesions. These are pigmented macules ("café-au-lait" spots) with irregular ("coast of Maine") borders, which do not cross the midline of the body and are usually located over the buttocks, back, and sacrum. These macules have a tendency to overlie the skeletal lesions.

☐ **Pathology:** The radiographic features of fibrous dysplasia are distinctive. The bone lesion has a lucent ground-glass appearance with well-marginated borders and a thin cortex. The bone may be ballooned, deformed, or enlarged, and involvement may be focal, or it may encompass the entire bone (Fig. 26-40A).

All forms of fibrous dysplasia have an identical histological pattern (see Fig. 26-40B). Benign fibroblastic tissue is arranged in a loose, whorled pattern. Irregularly arranged, purposeless spicules of woven bone, which lack osteoblastic rimming, are embedded in the fibrous tissue. In 10% of cases, irregular islands of hyaline cartilage also are present. Occasionally, cystic degeneration occurs, with hemosiderin-laden macrophages, hemorrhage, and osteoclasts congregated about the cyst. Rarely (<1% of cases), malignant degeneration (osteosarcoma, chondrosarcoma, or fibrosarcoma) has been reported, but most of these cases involved previous irradiation. Treatment of fibrous dysplasia consists of curettage, repair of fractures, and prevention of deformities.

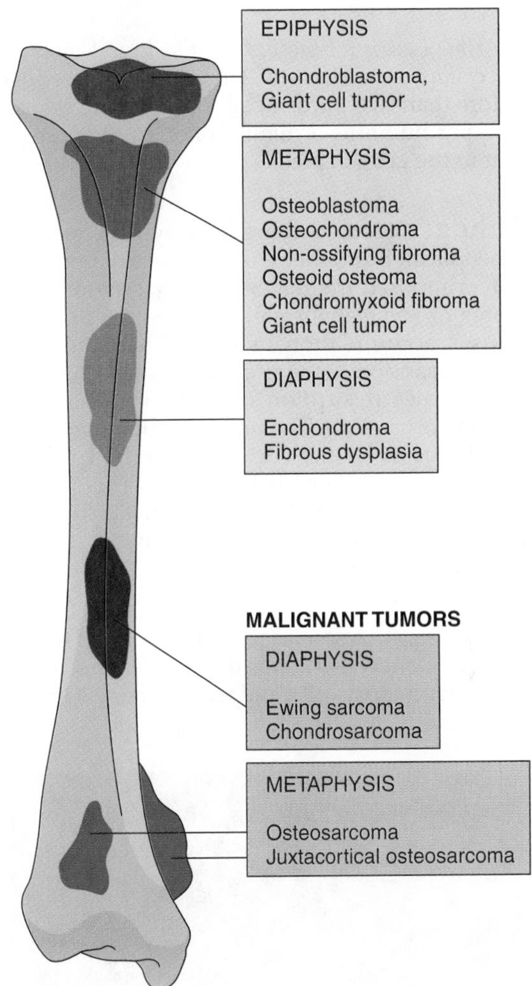

FIGURE *26-41*
Location of primary bone tumors in long tubular bones.

BENIGN TUMORS OF BONE

Bone tumors of all kinds are uncommon but are nevertheless important neoplasms, because many occur in children and young persons and are potentially lethal. A primary bone tumor may arise from any one of the cellular elements of bone. Most neoplasms of bone occur near the metaphyseal area, and more than 80% of primary tumors occur in either the distal femur or the proximal tibia (Fig. 26-41). In the growing child, these areas are characterized by conspicuous growth activity and are, therefore, more likely to develop a tumor.

Nonossifying Fibroma (Fibrous Cortical Defect)

Nonossifying fibroma is a benign, usually solitary lesion of childhood that occurs in the metaphysis of a long bone, most commonly the tibia or femur. The disorder is very common and may be present in as many as 25% of all children between ages 4 and 10 years, after which it characteristically regresses. The histogenesis is uncertain, and it remains controversial whether nonossifying fibroma is a neoplastic or developmental lesion. Most cases are asymptomatic, although pain or fracture through the thin cortex overlying the lesion occasionally calls attention to the condition.

☐ **Pathology:** Radiologically, nonossifying fibromas are identified by a cortical, eccentric position and by well-demarcated, central lucent zones surrounded by scalloped, sclerotic margins. On gross examination, the lesion is granular and dark red to brown. Microscopically, bland spindle cells are arranged in an interlacing, whorled pattern in which multinuclear giant cells and foamy macrophages may be seen. The rare, symptomatic, or expanded lesions are treated with curettage and bone grafting.

Solitary (Unicameral) Bone Cyst

Solitary bone cyst is a benign, fluid-filled, unilocular, lesion found in children or adolescents. There is a male predilection (3:1). More than two thirds of all solitary bone cysts occur in the upper humerus or femur, often in the metaphysis adjacent to the growth plate.

☐ **Pathogenesis:** Solitary bone cyst seems not to be a true neoplasm but rather a disturbance of bone growth with superimposed trauma. Secondary organization of a hematoma or some abnormality of the metaphyseal vessels causes accumulation of fluid. The "tumor" then grows by expansion of the fluid cavity, and the resulting pressure causes resorption of bone, mediated by the neighboring osteoclasts. The process is slow, so that as the endosteal surface of the cortex is resorbed, a thin periosteal shell of new bone is laid down. This process results in a thin, lytic bone lesion (Fig. 26-42) that is never greater in diameter than the growth plate and is particularly susceptible to pathological fracture.

☐ **Pathology:** A solitary bone cyst is lined by fibrous tissue, a few giant cells, hemosiderin-laden macrophages, chronic inflammatory cells, and reactive bone. Osteoclasts are present in the advancing front of the cyst and allow the expansion of the lesion. The cyst contains masses of amorphous proteinaceous material.

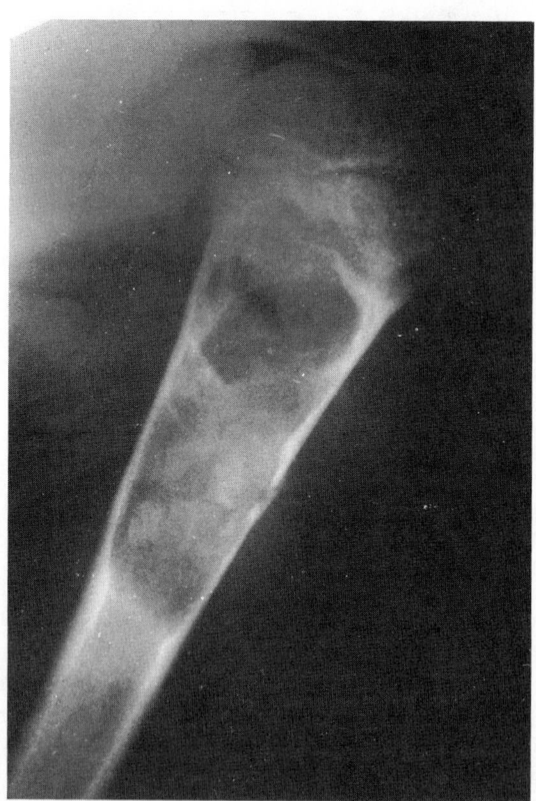

FIGURE 26-42
Solitary bone cyst. A radiograph of the proximal humerus of a child (note the epiphyseal plate) shows a large, well-demarcated, lytic epiphyseal and diaphyseal lesion. The cortex is thinned, but there is no cortical distortion or malformation of the shape of the bone.

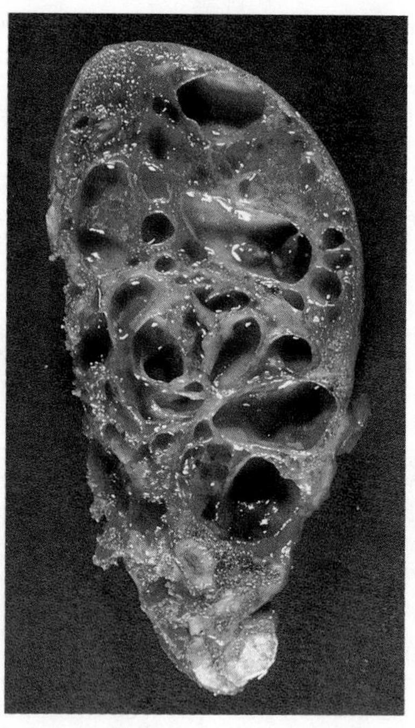

FIGURE 26-43
Aneurysmal bone cyst. In cross-section, the lesion consists of a spongy mass in which are seen multiple blood-filled cysts. Some of the septa between the cysts contain bony tissue.

☐ **Clinical Features:** Most solitary bone cysts are entirely asymptomatic until a pathological fracture calls attention to the lesion. Curettage and the deposition of bone chips are curative.

Aneurysmal Bone Cyst

Aneurysmal bone cyst is again not a true tumor, but rather an uncommon, expansive, hyperemic lesion arising from the surface of bone. It occurs in children and young adults, with a peak in the second decade. The lesion has been observed at every skeletal site but prefers the long bones and the vertebral column. The pathogenesis is obscure, but may represent cystic degeneration of an underlying lesion such as chondroblastoma, osteoblastoma, osteosarcoma, fibrous dysplasia, or giant cell tumor.

☐ **Pathology:** The periosteum around an aneurysmal bone cyst is ballooned but intact. At surgery, incision of the cyst results in brisk bleeding, which may be difficult to control. The cut surface of the lesion resembles a sponge permeated with blood and blood clots (Fig. 26-43). The walls and the septa of the aneurysmal cyst are composed of granulation tissue containing multinucleated giant cells, with occasional osteoid trabeculae.

☐ **Clinical Features:** Although some aneurysmal bone cysts tend to grow slowly, most expand rapidly and may reach an enormous size. The lesions usually are seen as pain and swelling, often in relation to trauma. The bone cyst may "blow out," that is, rupture and produce local hemorrhage. The treatment of choice is extraperiosteal excision and curettage. In sites such as the vertebral column or the pelvis, selective arterial embolization has been successful.

Osteoid Osteoma

Osteoid osteoma is a small, painful, benign lesion of bone composed of osseous tissue (the nidus) and surrounded by a halo of reactive bone formation. The tumor typically occurs in young persons, ranging in age from 5 to 25 years. Boys are affected more commonly than girls (3:1). Osteoid osteoma frequently arises in the cortex of the diaphysis of the tubular bones of the lower extremity.

☐ **Pathology:** Osteoid osteoma is a spherical, hyperemic tumor, about 1 cm in diameter, which is considerably softer than the surrounding bone (see Fig. 26-44) and easily enucleated at surgery. Microscopically, the tumor is composed of thin, irregular, trabeculae within a cellular granulation tissue containing osteoblasts and osteoclasts. The trabeculae are more mature in the center, which is often partially calcified. Reactive, sclerotic bone surrounds the nidus.

☐ **Clinical Features:** Pain, typically nocturnal, is out of proportion to the size of the lesion. It is often exacerbated by the intake of alcoholic beverages and promptly relieved by aspirin, possibly because of the high prostaglandin content of the tumor. Surgical excision or electrocautery is curative and leaves the patient very grateful to the surgeon.

Osteoblastoma

Osteoblastoma is an uncommon, benign neoplasm that is histologically similar to osteoid osteoma but is larger and not accompanied by the sharp pain of the latter. It stimulates less bone reaction and appears as a purely lytic lesion, with only a thin shell of surrounding bone. Osteoblastoma occurs in persons between the ages of 10 and 35 years, with no sex predilection, and mainly affects the spine and long bones. Curettage cures small osteoblastomas, but larger lesions may require wide resection.

Solitary Chondroma (Enchondroma)

Solitary chondroma is a benign, intraosseous tumor composed of well-differentiated cartilage. Although it has been debated whether it represents a true neoplasm or a hamartoma, recent cytogenetic analyses have implied a clonal origin for these lesions, suggesting that they are in fact neoplasms. The diagnosis is made at any age, because many cases are entirely asymptomatic. Most cases of solitary chondroma occur in the metacarpals and phalanges of the hands, the remainder being in almost any other tubular bone. The tumor is small and grows slowly. Radiologically, it appears as a well-delimited osteolytic area.

On gross examination, solitary chondroma has the semitranslucent appearance of hyaline cartilage, often with a few calcified areas. Microscopically, the cartilaginous tissue is well differentiated, with sparse chondrocytes.

Asymptomatic chondromas are best left untreated. When pain intervenes, curettage and bone grafting are the treatment of choice.

Chondroblastoma

Chondroblastoma is an uncommon, benign chondrogenic tumor, which occurs almost exclusively in the epiphyses of large bones, especially the upper femur, tibia, and humerus. It is more common in males than in females (2:1), and 90% of cases occur in young persons between the ages of 5 and 25 years.

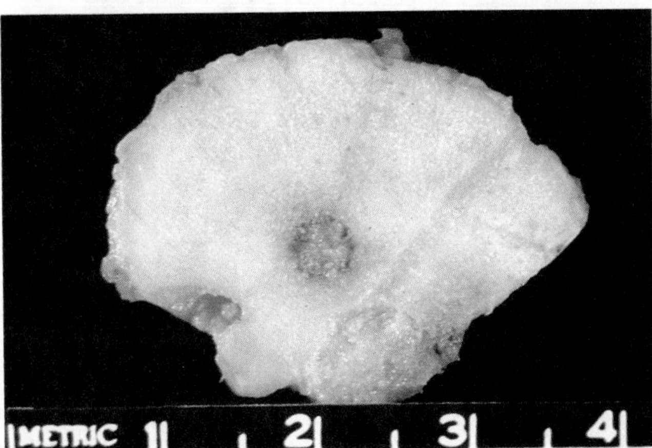

A

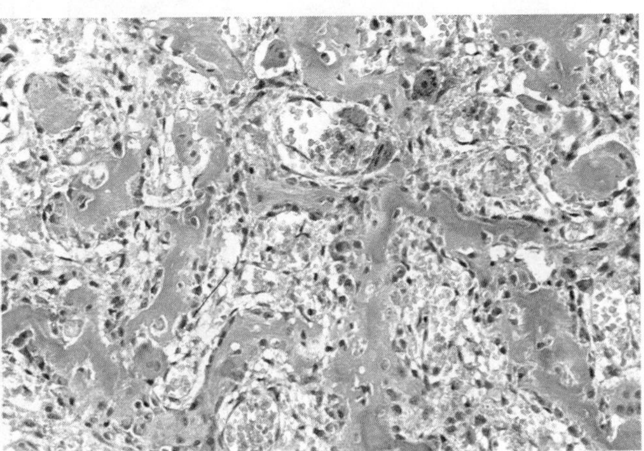

B

FIGURE 26-44
Osteoid osteoma. (*A*) A gross specimen of an osteoid osteoma shows the central nidus, which is embedded in dense bone. (*B*) A photomicrograph of the nidus reveals irregular trabeculae of woven bone surrounded by osteoblasts, osteoclasts, and fibrovascular marrow.

Pathology: Chondroblastoma grows slowly, and on radiological examination, displays an eccentric lytic appearance with sharply defined borders (Fig. 26-45). On gross examination, the tumor is soft and compact with scattered grayish white or hemorrhagic areas. Microscopically, primitive chondroblasts are arranged as sheets of round-to-polyhedral cells, which have well-defined cytoplasmic borders and large nuclei. The cartilage matrix appears primitive and is variably calcified, which accounts for the mottled pattern in radiographs. Chondroblastoma expands by stimulating osteoclastic resorption. In fact, these tumors may perforate the cortex, although they remain confined by the periosteum.

Clinical Features: Because of its para-articular location, the symptoms of chondroblastoma tend to be related to a joint, with moderate pain, mild swelling, and functional limitation of joint movement. If neglected, the tumor may on rare occasions attain a large size and destroy the epiphyseal area and invade the joint. Curettage is the treatment of choice, although in 10% of cases, the tumor recurs.

Chondromyxoid Fibroma

Chondromyxoid fibroma is a rare, benign cartilage-containing tumor of bone, which occurs in the femur or tibia of children and young adults. The tumor is also found occasionally in almost any bone.

Pathology: Radiologically, chondromyxoid fibroma is identified as an eccentric, lucent defect with a thin scalloped border of sclerotic bone. On gross examination, the tumor is a firm, lobulated, grayish white or tan mass, which replaces bone and thins the cortex. Microscopically, sparsely cellular lobules show spindle and stellate cells and multinucleated giant cells embedded within a chondroid or myxoid matrix. The lobules may be separated by bands of highly cellular tissue composed of similar cells. In some instances, the presence of large, pleomorphic cells in the chondroid matrix has led to an erroneous diagnosis of chondrosarcoma.

Chondromyxoid fibroma is best treated by surgical excision when possible, because the tumor tends to recur after simple curettage.

MALIGNANT TUMORS OF BONE

Osteosarcoma (Osteogenic Sarcoma)

Osteosarcoma is a highly malignant bone tumor characterized by the formation of neoplastic bone tissue. It is the most common primary malignant bone tumor, representing one fifth of all bone cancers. Osteosarcoma is most frequent in adolescents between the ages of 10 and 20 years, affecting boys more often than girls (2:1).

Pathogenesis: Almost two thirds of cases of osteosarcoma that have been studied exhibit mutations in the retinoblastoma (Rb) gene (see Chapter 5), and many tumors also contain mutations in the p53 gene. Thus, osteosarcoma takes its place among cancers related to the inactivation of tumor-suppressor genes. When the tumor arises in older persons, it is almost always a complication of Paget disease or radiation exposure. For example, radium watch dial painters who wetted their brushes with saliva developed osteosarcoma many years later as a result of the deposition of radium in their bones. Moreover, osteosarcoma has also developed in adults and children previously subjected to external, therapeutic radiation.

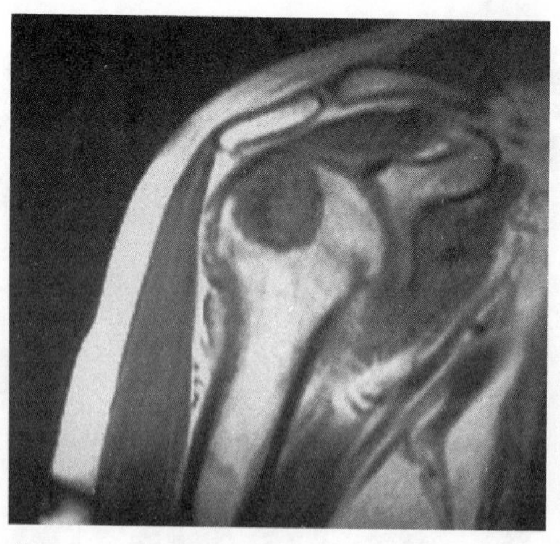
A

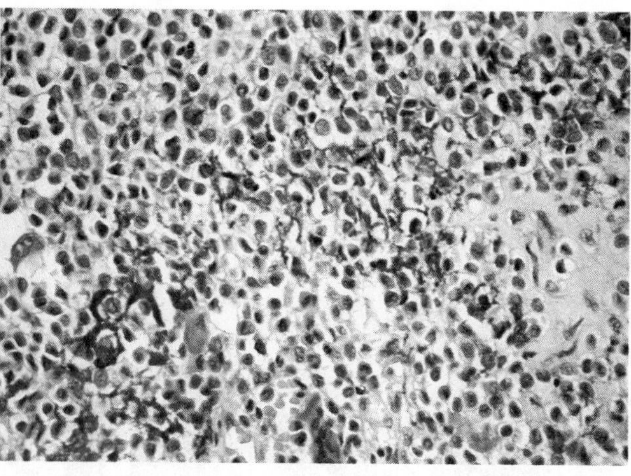
B

FIGURE *26-45*
Chondroblastoma. (*A*) A magnetic resonance image of the shoulder of a child shows a prominent lytic lesion of the head of the humerus, which involves the epiphysis and extends across the epiphyseal plate. (*B*) The histological appearance of a chondroblastoma is defined by plump, round cells (chondroblasts) surrounded by a mineralized matrix.

Several preexisting benign bone lesions are associated with an increased risk of later osteosarcoma, including fibrous dysplasia, bone infections, and bone marrow infarcts. It is important that, although trauma may call attention to an existing osteosarcoma, there is no evidence that it ever causes the tumor.

□ **Pathology:** Osteosarcoma often arises in the vicinity of the knee, that is, the lower femur (Fig. 26-46A), upper tibia, or fibula, although any metaphyseal area of a long bone may be affected. The proximal humerus is second to the knee area as a site of osteosarcoma, and 75% of all these tumors arise adjacent to the knee or shoulder. The hands, feet, skull, and jaw are less common sites for this disease, being affected more frequently in persons older than 25 years.

Radiological evidence of bone destruction and bone formation is characteristic, the latter representing neoplastic bone. Often, the periosteum is elevated by reactive bone adjacent to the tumor, a pattern that appears on radiographic studies as a triangular area between the cortex and the periosteal bone (Codman's triangle). A "sunburst" pattern is also often present (see Fig. 26-19).

In bones amputated for osteosarcoma, the gross appearance of the tumor is highly variable, depending on the relative amounts of bone, cartilage, stroma, and blood vessels. The cut surface may show any combination of hemorrhagic, cystic, soft, and bony hard areas. The neoplastic tissue may invade and break through the cortex, spread into the marrow cavity, elevate or perforate the periosteum, or grow into the epiphysis and even reach the joint space.

Histological examination reveals malignant osteoblasts, producing woven bone (see Fig. 26-46B). The malignant cells stain prominently for alkaline phosphatase and osteonectin. The tumorous bone is usually woven and is laid down haphazardly, and not aligned along stress lines. Often, foci of malignant cartilage cells or malignant giant cells are intermixed. In areas of bone lysis, non-neoplastic osteoclasts are found at the advancing front of the tumor.

Osteosarcoma spreads through the bloodstream to the lungs. In fact, almost all patients (98%) who die of this disease have lung metastases. Less commonly, the tumor metastasizes to other bones (35%), the pleura (33%), and the heart (20%).

□ **Clinical Features:** Osteosarcoma usually is seen as mild or intermittent pain around the knee or other involved areas. As the pain becomes more intense, the involved area swells, and palpation is painful. The movement of the adjacent joint is functionally limited. The serum alkaline phosphatase level is increased in half of the patients and may decrease after amputation, only to increase again with a recurrence or metastasis. Metastatic disease heralds a rapid clinical deterioration and death.

Traditionally, osteosarcoma was treated exclusively by amputation or disarticulation of the involved limb, but the prognosis for 5-year survival did not exceed 20%. More recent developments in chemotherapy and limb-sparing surgery have resulted in 5-year disease-free rates as high as 60%. Osteosarcoma is one of the few tumors in which the resection of isolated pulmonary metastases appears to prolong survival.

Juxtacortical osteosarcoma is a rare variant of osteosarcoma that occurs on the periosteal surface of the bone, especially the lower posterior metaphysis of the femur (72% of cases). Unlike classic osteosarcoma, most patients are older than 25 years, and the tumor is more common in women. Juxtacortical osteosarcoma spares the deep cortex and medulla of the bone and grows external to the shaft (Fig. 26-47). Usually, Codman's triangle is not evident radiologically. Surgical excision is the treatment of choice, and the prognosis is good, with a 5-year survival more than 80%.

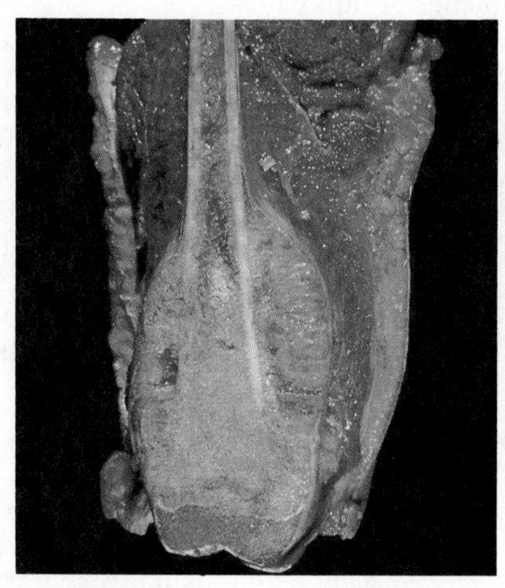

A

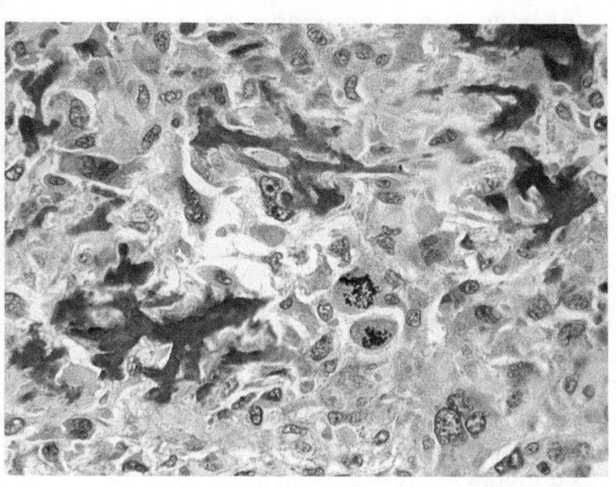

B

FIGURE *26-46*
Osteosarcoma. (*A*) The distal femur contains a dense osteoblastic malignant tumor that extends through the cortex into the soft tissue and the epiphysis. (*B*) A photomicrograph reveals pleomorphic malignant cells, tumor giant cells, and mitoses. The tumor produces woven bone that is focally calcified.

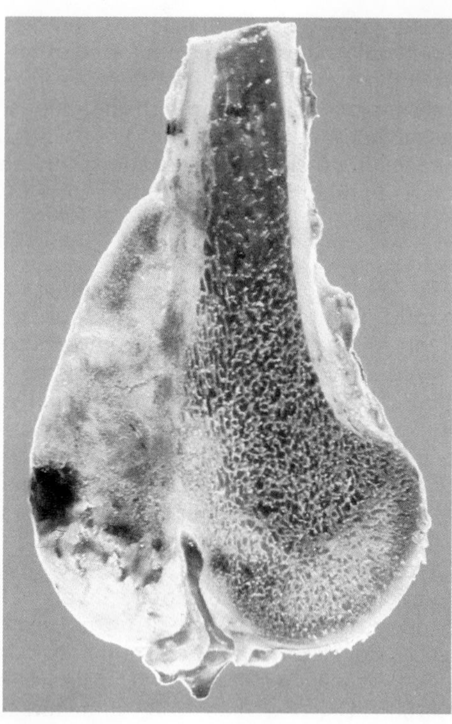

FIGURE *26-47*
Juxtacortical osteosarcoma. The lower femur contains a malignant tumor arising from the periosteal surface of the bone and sparing the medullary cavity.

Chondrosarcoma

Chondrosarcoma is a malignant tumor that originates from cartilage cells and maintains its cartilaginous nature throughout its evolution. Most cases arise from cartilage rests or endochondromas. A few have a history of a preexisting multiple osteochondromatosis or solitary osteochondroma. Chondrosarcoma is the second most common primary malignant bone tumor, occurring more commonly in men than in women (2:1). It is most frequently seen in the fourth to sixth decades (average age, 45 years).

☐ **Pathology:** Chondrosarcoma occurs in three variants, classified according to location.

CENTRAL CHONDROSARCOMA: This form arises in the medullary cavity of pelvic bones, ribs, and long bones, although any site may on occasion be affected. Radiologically, these tumors are characterized by poorly defined borders, a thickened shaft, and perforation of the cortex. Although they may penetrate the cortex, extension beyond the periosteum is uncommon. On gross examination, the neoplastic cartilaginous tissue is compressed inside the bone and exhibits areas of necrosis, cystic change, and hemorrhage. The cortex of the bone is infiltrated by the tumor.

Central chondrosarcoma begins with deep pain, which becomes more intense with time. In most cases, the tumor cannot be palpated, but in untreated cases, large masses may eventually form.

PERIPHERAL CHONDROSARCOMA: This variant is less common than the central variety of chrondrosarcoma and arises outside the bone, either *de novo* or in the cartilaginous cap of an osteochondroma. It occurs after the age of 20 years and never before puberty. The most frequent location of peripheral chondrosarcoma is the pelvis, followed by the femur, vertebrae, sacrum (Fig. 26-48A), humerus, and other long bones. It occurs only rarely distal to the knee or elbow. Radiologically, characteristic radiopacities representing calcification or ossification of the neoplastic cartilage are virtually pathognomonic for the lesion. Macroscopically, peripheral chondrosarcoma tends to be a large bosselated mass, which surrounds the base of an osteochondroma and invades the bone.

Peripheral chondrosarcoma usually is seen as a slowly growing mass. In a few cases, the affected person has a history of multiple osteochondromatosis, whereas in others, a solitary osteochondroma was known to the patient. The expansion of the mass causes pain and local symptoms. In the pelvis, the lumbosacral plexus may be compressed, and tumors in the vertebrae may cause paraplegia.

JUXTACORTICAL CHONDROSARCOMA: This is the least common variety of chondrosarcoma and is similar to central chondrosarcoma in its predilection for middle-aged men. It tends to be situated in the metaphysis of long bones, lying on the outer surface of the cortex. Thus it is probably of periosteal or parosteal origin. Radiologically, it may be entirely translucent or focally calcified. The symptoms of juxtacortical chondrosarcoma are dominated by swelling, with little accompanying pain.

Histologically, chondrosarcomas are composed of malignant cartilage cells in various stages of maturity (see Fig. 26-48B). Occasionally, a well-differentiated chondrosarcoma is difficult to distinguish from a benign tumor based on cytological grounds alone. Zones of calcification are often conspicuous and are seen on radiography as splotches or bulky masses.

Chondrosarcoma is one of the few tumors in which microscopic grading has a significant prognostic value. The 5-year survival rate for low-grade chondrosarcomas is 80%, for moderate-grade tumors about 50%, and for high-grade tumors only 20%.

Chondrosarcoma expands by stimulating osteoclastic resorption of bone and often breaks through the cortex. Most chondrosarcomas grow slowly, but hematogenous metastases to the lungs are common in poorly differentiated variants. Wide excision is often necessary.

Giant Cell Tumor

Giant cell tumor of bone is a locally aggressive, potentially malignant neoplasm characterized by the presence of osteoclastic, multinucleated, giant cells. It usually occurs in the third and fourth decades, with a slight predilection for women, and seems to be more common in Asia than in Western countries. Giant cell tumors in the elderly may be secondary to irradiation. Paget disease may produce a giant cell lesion that closely resembles a true giant cell tumor. The neo-

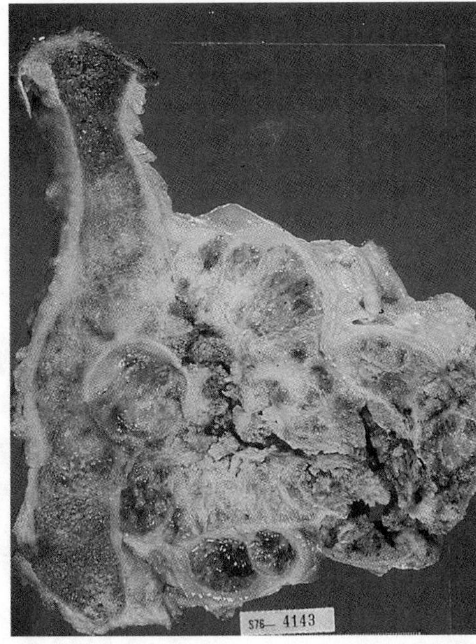

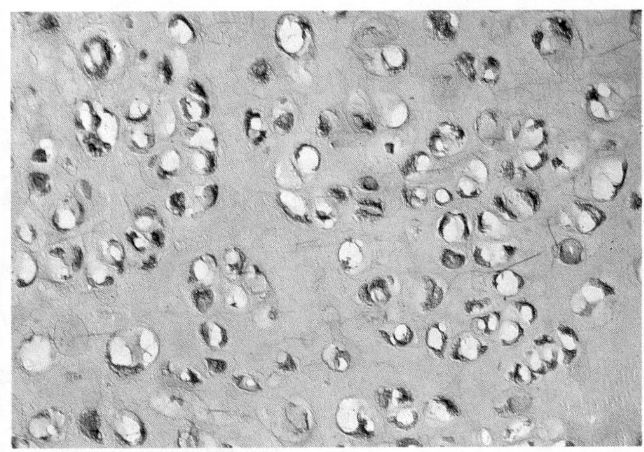

A B

FIGURE *26-48*
Chondrosarcoma. (*A*) A section through a chondrosarcoma of the pelvis shows a glistening surface with focal calcification and cyst formation. (*B*) A photomicrograph of a chondrosarcoma demonstrates malignant chondrocytes with pronounced atypia.

plasms are thought to arise from primitive stromal cells that have the capacity to modulate into osteoclasts.

□ **Pathology:** In the large majority of cases (90%), giant cell tumor of bone originates at the junction between the metaphysis and the epiphysis of a long bone, with more than half being situated in the knee area (distal femur and proximal tibia; Fig. 26-49A). The lower end of the radius, humerus, and fibula are also occasionally involved. The neoplasm is often a lytic lesion that grows slowly enough to allow a periosteal reaction. Thus, radiologically, the tumor tends to be surrounded by a thin, bony shell and expands the bone. Often, it has a multiloculated or "soap bubble" appearance, representing endosteal resorption of the bone.

On gross examination, giant cell tumor is clearly circumscribed, and the cut surface is soft and light brown, without bone or calcification. Numerous hemorrhagic areas result in the appearance of a sponge full of blood. In some cases, cystic cavities and necrotic areas are present. Giant cell tumor is often limited by the periosteum, although aggressive forms penetrate the cortex and the periosteum, even reaching the joint capsule and the synovial membrane.

Microscopically, giant cell tumor exhibits two types of cells (see Fig. 26-49B). The mononuclear ("stromal") cells are plump and oval, with large nuclei and scanty cytoplasm. Large osteoclastic giant cells, some with more than 100 nuclei, are scattered throughout the richly vascularized stroma. Diffuse interstitial hemorrhage is common.

Only the mononuclear cells are thought to be neoplastic and are the only components that proliferate. Indeed, the diagnosis of malignancy in a giant cell tumor depends on an analysis of the mononuclear cells rather than the multinucleated ones. All giant cell tumors must be viewed as potentially malignant, because as many as half recur locally after simple curettage. After this procedure, 5% to 10% metastasize to distant sites, particularly the lungs. Virtually all cases of metastases have occurred after an initial surgical intervention. Thus, some hold that recurrence of the tumor reflects inadequate resection and that distant metastases result from dislodgment of tumor fragments during surgery.

□ **Clinical Features:** Giant cell tumors commonly are seen with pain, often in the joint adjacent to the tumor. Microfractures and pathological fractures are frequent, owing to thinning of the cortex. The tumor is usually treated with thorough curettage and bone grafting, although more aggressive management, including *en bloc* resection or even amputation, may be necessary.

Ewing Sarcoma

Ewing sarcoma (EWS) is an uncommon malignant bone tumor composed of small, uniform, round cells, belonging to a family of primitive neuroectodermal tumors of childhood. EWS represents only 5% of all bone tumors and is found in children and adolescents, with two thirds of the cases occurring in patients younger than 20 years. Boys are affected more often than girls (2:1). It is very rare in blacks.

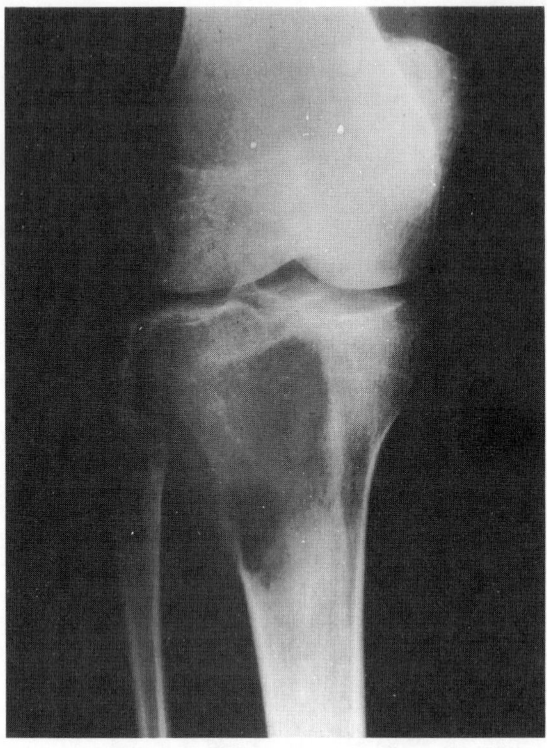
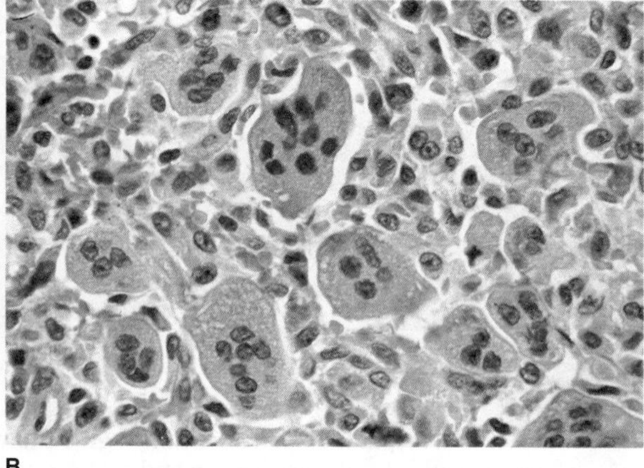

A B

FIGURE *26-49*
Giant cell tumor of bone. (*A*) A radiograph of the proximal tibia shows an eccentric lytic lesion, with virtually no new bone formation. The tumor extends to the subchondral bone plate and breaks through cortex into the soft tissue. (*B*) A photomicrograph shows osteoclast-type giant cells and plump, oval, mononuclear cells. The nuclei of both types of cells are identical.

Ewing sarcoma is believed to arise from primitive marrow elements or immature mesenchymal cells. Virtually all (90%) of these tumors have a reciprocal translocation between chromosomes 11 and 22 (t(11;22)p13;q12). This translocation results in the fusion of the amino-terminus region of the ubiquitously expressed EWS1 gene to the carboxy-terminus of a transcription factor termed the FLI-1 gene. The resulting chimeric gene product (fusion protein), EWS/FLI-1, is an aberrant transcription factor. Although EWS/FLI-1 is tumorigenic, the target genes are not yet identified. This chromosomal abnormality has been identified in primitive neuroectodermal tumors and has been used as evidence that Ewing sarcoma may belong to this family of neoplasms. Interestingly, another translocation that results in the fusion of the EWS1 gene with the Wilms tumor gene (WT1, see Chapter 16) has been identified in a related pediatric tumor (desmoplastic small round cell tumor).

□ **Pathology:** EWS is primarily a tumor of the long bones, especially the humerus, tibia, and femur, where it occurs as a midshaft or metaphyseal lesion. However, no bone is immune from involvement, and the tumor also occurs in the hands and feet and other bones.

The onion-skin pattern that is characteristically seen on radiological examination represents a circumferential layer of reactive periosteal bone, which is associated with a lytic lesion involving the medulla and endosteal surface of the cortex.

On gross examination, EWS is typically soft and grayish white, often studded by hemorrhagic foci and areas of necrosis. The tumor may infiltrate the medullary spaces without destroying the bony trabeculae. It may also diffusely infiltrate the cortical bone or form nodules in which the bone is completely resorbed. In many cases, the tumor mass penetrates the periosteum and extends into the soft tissues.

Microscopically, the tumor cells appear as sheets of closely packed, small, round cells with little cytoplasm, which are up to twice the size of a lymphocyte (Fig. 26-50). In some areas, the neoplastic cells tend to form rosettes, formed by tumor cells arranged about small areas of cell secretions of neurofilaments. An important diagnostic feature is the presence of substantial amounts of glycogen in the cytoplasm of the tumor cells, which is well visualized with the periodic acid–Schiff (PAS) stain. Fibrous strands separate the sheets of cells into irregular nests. There is little or no interstitial stroma, and mitoses are infrequent.

Ewing sarcoma metastasizes to many organs, including the lungs and brain. Other bones, especially the skull, are common sites for metastases (45% to 75% of cases).

□ **Clinical Features:** EWS is seen initially with pain, which becomes more intense and is followed by

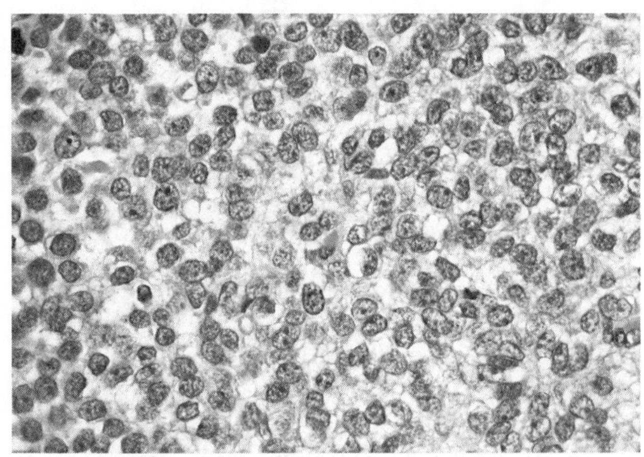

FIGURE 26-50
Ewing sarcoma. The tumor shows small, round cells, with glycogen-filled clear cytoplasm.

swelling of the affected area. Nonspecific symptoms, including fever and leukocytosis, commonly follow. In some cases, a soft tissue mass is encountered.

In the past, the prognosis of EWS was dismal, with 5-year survival rates of only 5% after surgery or radiation therapy. The use of chemotherapy, combined with irradiation and surgery, has now led to a 5-year disease-free survival of 75%.

Multiple Myeloma

Malignant tumors of plasma cells may be either local (plasmacytoma) or diffuse (multiple myeloma; see Chapter 20). Multiple myeloma occurs most often in older persons (average age, 65 years) and affects men twice as often as women. Because myeloma cells secrete cytokines that recruit osteoclasts, the lesions are unique in that they are almost exclusively lytic. The bones most frequently involved are the skull (Fig. 26-51), spine, ribs, pelvis, and femur. Pathological fractures are common. On microscopic examination, sheets of plasma cells show varying degrees of maturity. Amyloid deposits, in both skeletal and extraskeletal sites, are seen in 10% of patients.

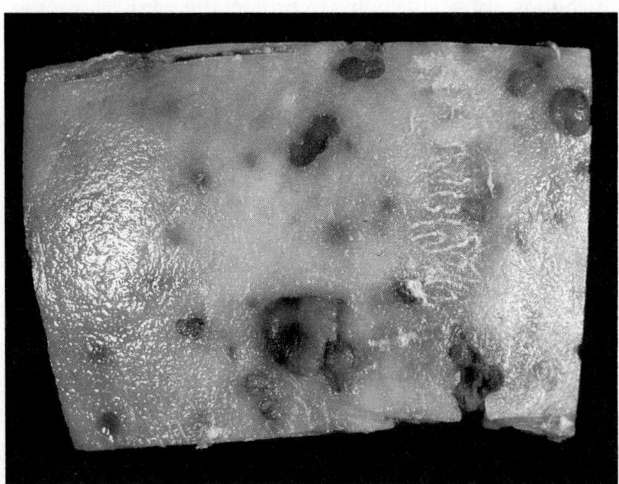

FIGURE 26-51
Multiple myeloma. A segment of the skull from a patient with multiple myeloma demonstrates numerous punched-out, lytic lesions.

Despite irradiation and chemotherapy, the prognosis is poor (the median survival time is 32 months). The cause of death is usually infection or kidney failure. Solitary plasmacytoma has a better prognosis, with a 60% 5-year survival.

Metastatic Tumors

The most common malignant tumor of bone is metastatic cancer. Carcinomas compose the large majority of metastatic lesions to bone, specifically tumors of the breast, prostate, lung, thyroid, and kidney. Tumor cells usually arrive in the bone by way of the bloodstream; in the case of spinal metastases, they are often transported by the vertebral veins. It is estimated that skeletal metastases are found in at least 85% of cancer cases that have run their full clinical course. The vertebral column is, by far, the most commonly affected bony structure.

Some tumors (cancers of the thyroid, gastrointestinal tract, and kidney and neuroblastoma) produce mostly lytic lesions by stimulating osteoclasts. A few neoplasms (prostate, breast, lung, and stomach cancers) stimulate osteoblastic components to make bone, creating dense foci on radiographs (Fig. 26-52). However, most deposits of

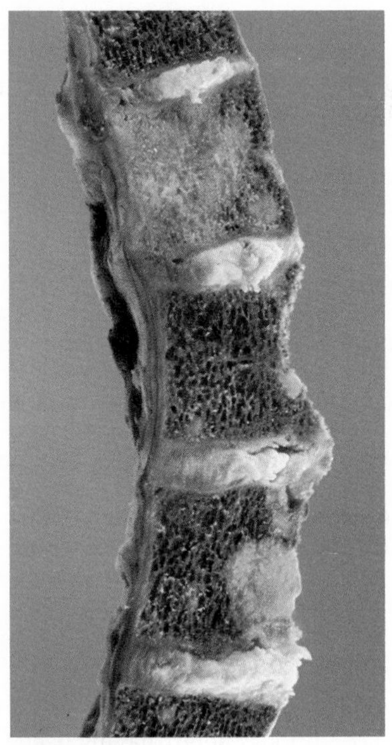

FIGURE 26-52
Metastatic carcinoma to bone. A section through the vertebral column reveals conspicuous nodules of metastatic tumor.

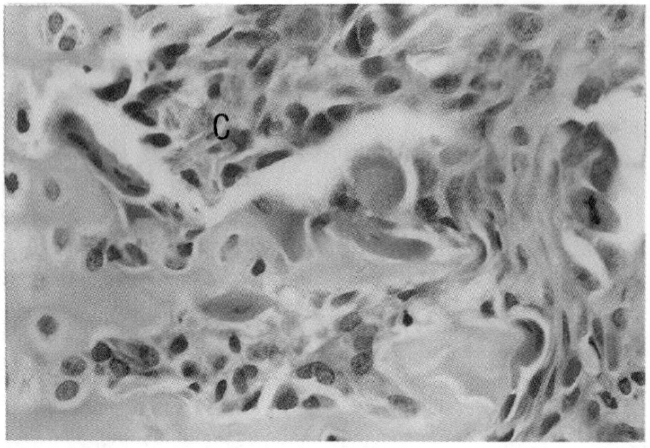

FIGURE 26-53
Tumor-induced osteolysis. Breast cancer (*C*) metastatic to bone recruits numerous osteoclasts (*red-staining cells*), which resorb bone and lead to osteolytic lesions.

metastatic cancer in the bones have mixtures of both lytic and blastic elements. The metastatic cancer itself does not resorb or make bone, but instead stimulates (by unknown mechanisms) the formation of osteoblasts and osteoclasts (Fig. 26-53).

Joints

A joint (or articulation) is a union between two or more bones, whose construction varies with the function of that joint. There are two types of joints: (1) **a synovial or diarthrodial joint**, which is a movable joint, such as the knee or elbow, that is lined by a synovial membrane; and (2) **a synarthrosis**, which is a joint that has little movement. Synarthroses are further divided into four subclassifications:

- **A symphysis** is an articulation joined by fibrocartilaginous tissue and firm ligaments that allows little movement. Examples are the symphysis pubis and the ends of vertebral joints.
- **A synchondrosis**, found at the articulated ends of bones, has articular cartilage, but no synovium or significant joint cavity. An example of such a joint is the sternal manubrial joint.
- **A syndesmosis** connects bones by fibrous tissue without any cartilaginous elements. The distal tibiofibular articulation and the cranial sutures are syndesmoses.
- **A synostosis** refers to a pathological bony bridge between bones, as occurs with ankylosis of the spine.

Diseases of diarthrodial joints are among the oldest pathological conditions known, having been found in the fossil bones of dinosaurs. Up to one third of the population of the United States older than 50 years develop some form of clinically significant joint disease.

CLASSIFICATION OF SYNOVIAL JOINTS AND THEIR MOVEMENTS

The synovial joints (or diarthrodial joints) are classified according to the type of movement they permit.

- **A uniaxial joint** allows movement around only one axis. In a hinge joint, such as the elbow, the axis is transverse across the articular surfaces, permitting both flexion and extension. In a pivot joint, such as the radioulnar joint, the axis is longitudinal along the shaft of the bone, and the motion is rotational.
- **A biaxial joint** allows movement around two axes. In the condyloid joint of the wrist, where the articular surfaces are oval, one axis is oriented in the long diameter and the other along the short diameter of the articular surfaces. This joint permits four-way movement: flexion, extension, abduction, and adduction. In a saddle joint, such as the carpometacarpal joint of the thumb, the joint surfaces allow movement as in a condyloid joint.
- **Polyaxial joints** permit movement in virtually any axis. In a ball-and-socket joint, such as is found in the shoulder and hip, all movements, including rotation, are possible.
- **A plane joint,** represented by the patella, allows the articular surfaces to glide over one another, the surfaces being essentially flat.

UNIT LOAD: The concept of unit load is the most important principle in the understanding of joint function. The unit load is the compressive force, expressed as kg/cm^3 of articular cartilage. The unit load is fairly constant over the hip, knee, and ankle (20 to 26 kg/cm^3 along the articular surfaces). Because the articular cartilage is injured if the load exceeds these values, a number of mechanisms protect the joint from exceeding the unit load.

The adjacent muscles are the major shock-absorbing structures that protect the joint. In addition, deformation, even to the extent of microscopic fractures of the coarse cancellous bone, also helps to protect the joint. Moreover, the deformation of the joint allows increasing the contact area with increasing load. In diarthrodial joints, there may be intra-articular structures, such as ligaments and menisci. The menisci hold distributed force along the articular surface and allow two planes of motion, such as flexion and rotation. However, 90% or more of the absorption of energy across the knee joint is by active muscle contraction, and only 10% or less is by secondary mechanisms, such as absorption of force by the coarse cancellous bone of the knee joint. **Thus, virtually any structure is sacrificed, even to the point of a bone fracture, to protect the articular cartilage from forces that exceed the critical unit load, thereby killing the irreplaceable articular cartilage.**

Development of Diarthrodial Joints

There are two basic principles that relate to the formation of diarthrodial joints: (1) The appendicular skeleton develops proximal to the distal skeleton (e.g., the shoulder joint develops before the elbow joint), and (2) development progresses in a cranial-to-caudal manner. This means that the upper limb develops 24 hours or more before the lower limb. Thus, it is unusual to find developmental abnormalities of the humerus and femur in the same patient, because injurious agents act during discrete time intervals.

The upper limb bud appears when the embryo is 26 days of age and is completely formed 4 weeks later. The limb bud is covered by ectodermal tissue, and by 31 days of gestation, the tip of the upper limb bud has a well-defined, ridge-like area called the apical ectodermal ridge. This structure is necessary for the sequential development of the limb elements; and it stimulates the underlying mesoderm to proceed in a proximal-to-distal direction. If the **apical ectodermal ridge** is removed, mesodermal proliferation ceases. The mesodermal tissue condenses to form a blastema soon after the limb bud appears. In the region of the future bone, the blastema differentiates to form cartilage. The space between two adjacent bones destined to become the future joint is termed the *interzone*.

The synovial tissue arises from the periphery of the interzone. Joint capsules, interarticular ligaments, menisci, tendons, and all other joint structures develop from this synovial mesenchyme. Vascular penetration takes place in this tissue, and the synovium soon becomes a rich capillary network, bringing to this area extra blastema cells, such as mast cells and macrophages. The macrophages, which secrete acid phosphatase and other esterases, play a major role in cavitation. *Cavitation* is a process by which vascular tissue is removed from the interzone region, thereby creating a future joint cavity. Administration of corticosteroids at this time arrests joint development. The joint becomes fused, leading to syndactyly of the hands. *Syndactyly*, which is a fused or web-shaped hand, occurs because the tissue between the digits is not removed.

Cleft palate results when the two palatine bones grow toward the midline, and the intervening tissue is not resorbed. Corticosteroids can also cause this condition.

Movement also plays a major role in the formation of a joint. A lack of movement retards joint development and may result in a rare but extremely crippling disease termed *arthrogryposis*, which is characterized by joint fusion. This condition may be produced experimentally by administering curare to chick embryos, thereby paralyzing movement.

Structures of the Synovial Joint

The Synovium

Synovial joints are partially lined on their internal aspects by the synovium. In a synovial joint, only the articular cartilage surfaces are devoid of synovium. The recesses and internal aspects of the capsule, as well as the areas around the intra-articular structures, such as the menisci and ligaments, all show synovial lining tissue. The synovial lining is not a true membrane, because there is no basement membrane separating the synovial lining cells from the subsynovial tissue.

The synovium is composed of one to three layers of synovial lining cells and is made up of two types of cells, distinguishable only by electron microscopy. **Type A cells** are macrophages that contain lysosomal enzymes and dense bodies. **Type B cells** secrete hyaluronic acid. The synovial cell membranes are disposed in villi and microvilli, an arrangement that creates an enormous surface area. It is estimated that, in the knee alone, there are 100 m^2 of synovial lining. The subsynovial tissue is a loose, vascularized areolar tissue. In some locations, the synovium is closely applied to the dense connective tissue of the joint capsule. On the other hand, if the synovial tissue lines a fat pad, for example, that of the knee, then the subsynovial tissue is composed mostly of adipose tissue.

The synovium controls a number of functions, including (1) diffusion in and out of the joint; (2) ingestion of debris; (3) secretion of hyaluronate, immunoglobulins, and lysosomal enzymes; and (4) lubrication of the joints by secretion of glycoproteins. The clear, sticky, viscid synovial fluid is present in small amounts not exceeding 1 to 4 mL. It is the chief source of nourishment for chondrocytes of the articular cartilage, which lacks a blood supply.

The synovial fluid is an ultrafiltrate that functions as a molecular sieve. It does not contain fibrinogen and therefore has no clotting capacity. It does not normally contain α_2-macroglobulin, although in disease states, this protein may accumulate. Hyaluronate is a very large molecule and has a great affinity for water because of its high number of negative charges. The function of hyaluronate may be disturbed if the charges are altered. For example, when a hemophiliac bleeds into a joint, the positively charged iron neutralizes the negative charges of hyaluronate. In ochronosis, homogentisic acid also cancels the negative charges of the hyaluronate. As a result, the synovium becomes a leaky sieve, and fibrinogen, α_2-macroglobulin, and other foreign substances gain entrance to the joint cavity.

Articular Cartilage

The hyaline cartilage that covers the articular ends of the bones does not participate in endochondral ossification and is well suited for its dual role in absorbing shocks and lubricating the surface of the movable joint. On gross examination, the articular cartilage is glistening, smooth, white, and semiridgid and is generally not thicker than 6 mm.

Histological Characteristics

Although the articular surface appears smooth on gross examination, scanning electron microscopy reveals gentle waves and pits that correspond to the underlying lacunae of the surface chondrocytes. There are five histological zones in the articular cartilage.

- **Tangential or gliding zone:** This is the region closest to the articular surface, where the chondrocytes are elongated, flattened, and parallel to the long axis of the surface. Within this zone, a condensation of type II collagen fibers forms the so-called skin of the articular cartilage.

- **Transitional zone:** The chondrocytes in this slightly deeper zone are larger, ovoid, and more randomly distributed than in the tangential zone. The standard hyaline cartilage matrix is present, and by electron microscopy, the collagen fibers are arranged transverse to the articular surface.
- **Radial zone:** The next deeper zone is the radial zone where the chondrocytes are small and are arranged in short columns, similar to those seen in the epiphyseal plate. In this area, the collagen fibers are large and are oriented perpendicular to the long axis of the articular surface.
- **Calcified zone:** The deepest region is characterized by small chondrocytes and a heavily calcified matrix.
- **Tide mark:** The calcified zone is separated from the radial zone by a transverse, undulating, heavily calcified "blue line" (evident on hematoxylin–eosin staining), called the *tide mark*. The tide mark is the interface between mineralized and unmineralized cartilage. It is also the division between the true articular cartilage and the calcified remnant of the cartilage anlage that participated in endochondral ossification. Furthermore, the tide mark divides the nutritional sources for the chondrocytes. Above the tide mark on the joint side, all of the cartilage receives its nutrition from the synovial fluid by diffusion. Deep to the tide mark, the calcified cartilage is nourished by epiphyseal blood vessels.

  The tide mark also is significant because it is the area where the cartilage cells are renewed. As a result of cell division, there is an upward migration of true articular chondrocytes toward the joint surface. Cell division below the tide mark occurs in the calcified cartilage, if there is appropriate stimulation. For example, in acromegaly, when the epiphyseal plates have already closed, the bones may grow in minute increments, because growth hormone stimulates the calcified cartilage remnant of the epiphyseal cartilage anlage. Because the joints in acromegaly do not keep pace, joint incongruity leads to severe osteoarthritis.
- **Subchondral bone plate:** Deep to the calcified cartilage, the transverse bony plate, termed the subchondral bone plate, supports the articular cartilage. It is directly contiguous with the coarse cancellous bone of the epiphysis.

Chemical Characteristics

The articular cartilage is a hyperhydrated structure, with water composing 70% to 80% of its weight. The remaining 20% to 30% is composed of type II collagen (70% of dry weight) and proteoglycans. The ash content is about 6%, and there are trace amounts of lipids, phospholipids, lysozyme, and, perhaps, glycoprotein.

- **Water content:** Water is crucial to the function of the articular cartilage. Both adult cartilage and immature hyaline cartilage contain large amounts of water, which may be bound to collagen and proteoglycan by hydrogen bonding.
- **Proteoglycans:** These elastic macromolecules form the intercellular matrix of hyaline cartilage and the nucleus pulposus of the intervertebral disk. The breakdown of proteoglycans in diseases such as osteoarthritis and rheumatoid arthritis leads to the loss of cartilage resistance to wear. Proteoglycans resemble a bottle brush, with the core of the molecule being a linear protein. Linked to the core and radiating outward are numerous glycosaminoglycan chains that extend stiffly into the matrix space because of repelling negative charges. The result is the creation of a molecular sieve.
- **Type II collagen:** This molecule forms 70% of the dry weight of articular cartilage. Type II collagen fibers are arranged in arcades (*Benninghoff arcades*), which extend up from the tide mark toward the articular surface and then curve down, returning to the tide mark. The collagen fibrils are not contiguous but tend to run in an "arcade" pattern. Surface cracks, or fibrillations, tend to run parallel to the surface, because that is generally the plane of the collagen within the articular cartilage. If the cracks extend deeper into the articular cartilage, they tend to be oriented perpendicular to the articular surface, because they follow the course of the collagen fibrils. Although articular cartilage is capable of synthesizing matrix and collagen over a lifetime, the rate of synthesis after injury is not sufficient to keep pace with needed repair.

Collagenases have been demonstrated in the articular cartilage of osteoarthritis, a finding that may explain the mechanism by which articular cartilage is degraded. Lysosomes that are present in normal tissue can release acid hydrolases in disease processes such as osteoarthritis or even a laceration of the articular cartilage. Cathepsin F has also been found in cartilage, although its role is unknown. Cell division and DNA synthesis, which are not usually seen in adult cartilage, may be initiated in response to injury.

OSTEOARTHRITIS

Osteoarthritis is a slowly progressive destruction of the articular cartilage that is manifested in the weight-bearing joints and fingers of older persons or the joints of younger persons subjected to trauma. **Osteoarthritis is the single most common form of joint disease.** The disorder is not a single nosological entity but rather a group of conditions that have in common the mechanical destruction of a joint. Osteoarthritis can be classified into primary and secondary types.

Primary osteoarthritis is a disease of unknown etiology in which the destruction of the joints is believed to result from an intrinsic defect of the joint cartilage. The prevalence and severity of primary osteoarthritis increases with age. Persons aged 18 to 24 years have a rate of 4%, whereas 85% of those who are aged 75 to 79 years are afflicted. Before the age of 45 years, the disease predominantly affects men. After age 55 years, however, osteoarthritis is more frequent in women. Many cases of primary osteoarthritis seem to exhibit a familial clustering, suggesting that hereditary factors may predispose to the disease.

Primary osteoarthritis has variously been called "wear and tear" arthritis and "degenerative joint disease." Progressive degradation of articular cartilage leads to joint narrowing, subchondral bone thickening, and eventually a nonfunctioning, painful joint. Although osteoarthritis is not primarily an inflammatory process, a mild inflammatory reaction may occur within the synovium.

Secondary osteoarthritis has a known underlying cause, including congenital or acquired incongruity of joints, trauma, crystal deposits, infection, metabolic diseases, endocrinopathies, inflammatory diseases, osteonecrosis, and hemarthrosis.

Chondromalacia is a term applied to a subcategory of osteoarthritis that affects the patellar surface of the femoral condyles of young persons and produces pain and stiffness of the knee.

☐ **Pathogenesis:** The factors that play a major role in the etiology of osteoarthritis include the following:

- Increased unit load on the chondrocyte
- Decreased resilience of the articular cartilage
- Increased stiffness of the coarse cancellous bone of the epiphysis
- Genetic influences

These factors lead to increased degradation of articular cartilage, with accompanying focally increased synthesis of cartilage matrix and even increased replication of chondrocytes. However, this attempt at repair does not keep pace with the continuing stress, and eventually the articular cartilage is degraded and disappears.

INCREASED UNIT LOAD: Abnormal force on the cartilage may result from a number of factors, but it is often attributable to pathological incongruities of the joint. For example, in congenital hip dysplasia, a fairly common abnormality, the socket of the acetabulum is shallow, covering only 30% to 40% of the femoral head (normal, 50%). As a result, there is less surface area covered by cartilage and an increased load on the articular cartilage. When the critical unit load is exceeded, the death of chondrocytes leads to degradation of the articular cartilage.

RESILIENCE OF THE ARTICULAR CARTILAGE: Because articular cartilage binds extensive amounts of water, it normally has a swelling pressure of at least 3 atmospheres. A disruption in the water bonding resulting from the events discussed earlier leads directly to decreased resilience.

STIFFNESS OF THE SUBCHONDRAL COARSE CANCELLOUS BONE: The structure of the bone adjacent to a joint is also an important factor in the maintenance of articular cartilage. The mechanical forces are not transferred to articular cartilage by normal stress, but rather are dissipated by microfractures of the coarse cancellous bone. Damage to the coarse cancellous bone results in an increased unit load on the cartilage because of an increase in the stiffness of subchondral bone, for example, in Paget disease. When endoprostheses and bone cement are used to repair injured bone, the transfer of mechanical forces to the articular cartilage eventually destroys it. Furthermore, the increased pressure also interferes with the lubricating function of the articular cartilage, which normally reduces friction to less than one third of that created when two blocks of ice slide across each other.

BIOCHEMICAL ABNORMALITIES: The biochemical changes of osteoarthritis primarily involve proteoglycans. There is a decrease in proteoglycan content and aggregation, as well as a reduction in the chain length of the glycosaminoglycans. Compared with the levels in normal articular cartilage, keratan sulfate is decreased, and chondroitin sulfate is increased. There is also a decline in the glucosamine concentration, but there is no change in the concentration of galactosamine. The collagen fibers are thicker than normal, and the arcades of Benninghoff are disrupted. The water content of osteoarthritic cartilage is increased. It is thought that the reduction in proteoglycans allows more water to be bound to the collagen fibers. Thus, osteoarthritic cartilage, or any cartilage that is fibrillated, tends to swell more than normal cartilage.

Although the synthesis of matrix by chondrocytes is augmented in the early stages of osteoarthritis, protein synthesis eventually tends to decrease, suggesting that the cells reach a point at which they fail to respond to reparative stimuli. Similarly, whereas chondrocytes in early osteoarthritic cartilage replicate, with advanced disease, cell replication diminishes. Acid cathepsin, which attacks the protein cores of the matrix macromolecules, is increased in osteoarthritic cartilage. Although collagenase is not present in normal cartilage, it is found in osteoarthritic cartilage.

GENETIC FACTORS: Studies of identical twins have demonstrated genetic contributions to the prevalence of osteoarthritis, which are estimated to account for half of the influences that determine the development of disease. In addition, genetic analysis of patients with a type of familial, early-onset osteoarthritis has disclosed a variety of mutations in the gene for type II collagen (COL2A1), the major collagen species of articular cartilage.

☐ **Pathology:** The joints commonly affected by osteoarthritis are the proximal and distal interphalangeal joints of the upper extremity, knees, and hips, and the cervical and lumbar segments of the spine. Radiologically, osteoarthritis is characterized by (1) narrowing of the joint space, which represents the loss of articular cartilage; (2) increased thickness of the subchondral bone; (3) subchondral bone cysts; and (4) large peripheral growths of bone and cartilage called *osteophytes*, which represent the bone's attempt to grow a new articular surface. The progressive pathological changes in osteoarthritis can be arbitrarily divided into a number of stages:

1. The earliest histological changes of osteoarthritis involve the loss of proteoglycans from the surface of the articular cartilage, manifested as a decrease in metachromatic staining. At the same time, empty lacunae in the articular cartilage indicate the death of chondrocytes (Fig. 26-54). The viable chondrocytes enlarge, aggregate into groups or clones, and become

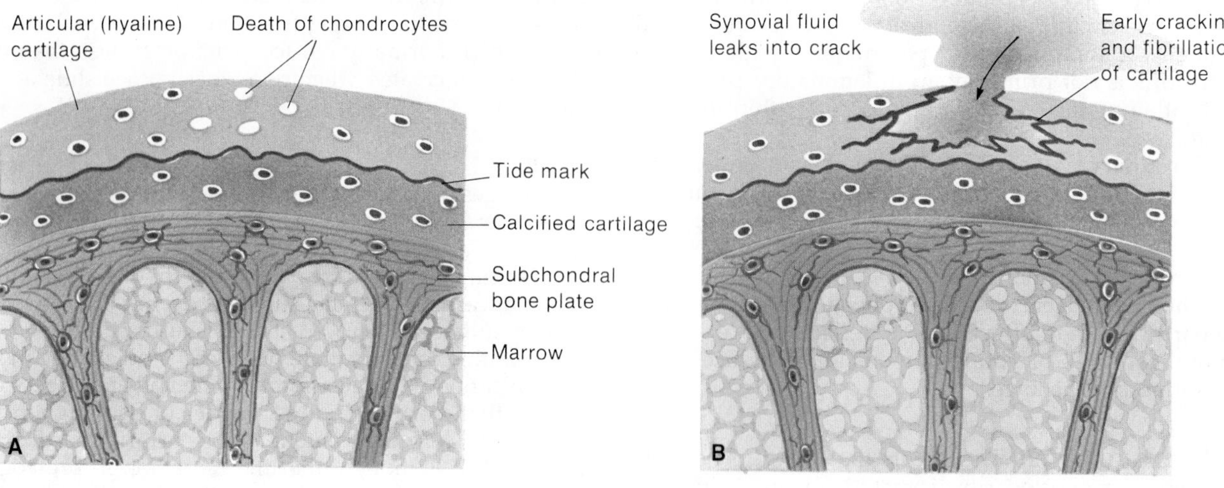
Articular (hyaline) cartilage
Death of chondrocytes
Tide mark
Calcified cartilage
Subchondral bone plate
Marrow
A
Synovial fluid leaks into crack
Early cracking and fibrillation of cartilage
B

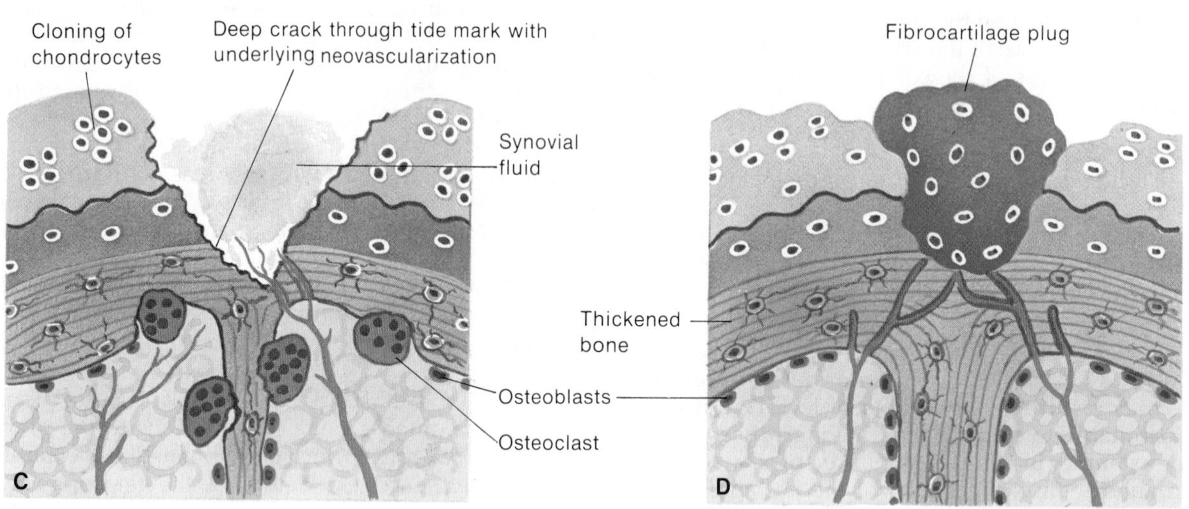
Cloning of chondrocytes
Deep crack through tide mark with underlying neovascularization
Synovial fluid
Osteoblasts
Osteoclast
C
Fibrocartilage plug
Thickened bone
D

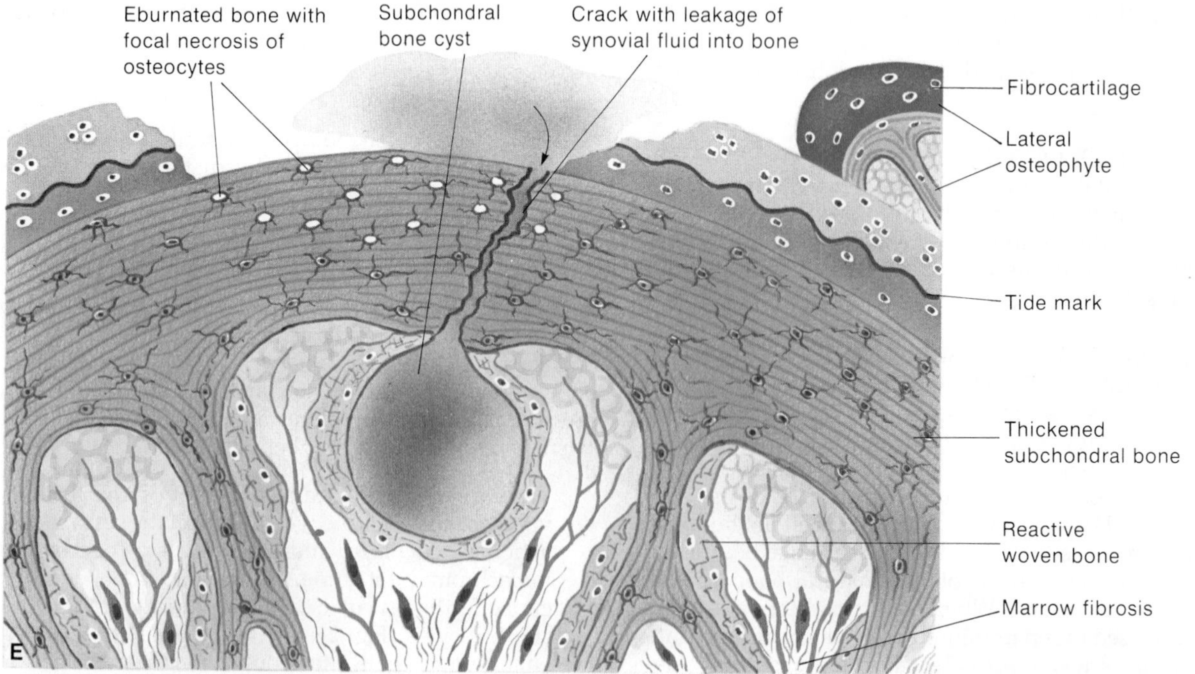
Eburnated bone with focal necrosis of osteocytes
Subchondral bone cyst
Crack with leakage of synovial fluid into bone
Fibrocartilage
Lateral osteophyte
Tide mark
Thickened subchondral bone
Reactive woven bone
Marrow fibrosis
E

FIGURE *26-54*

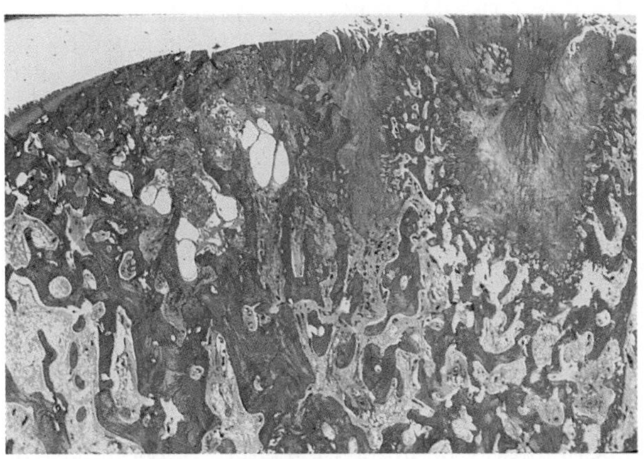

A

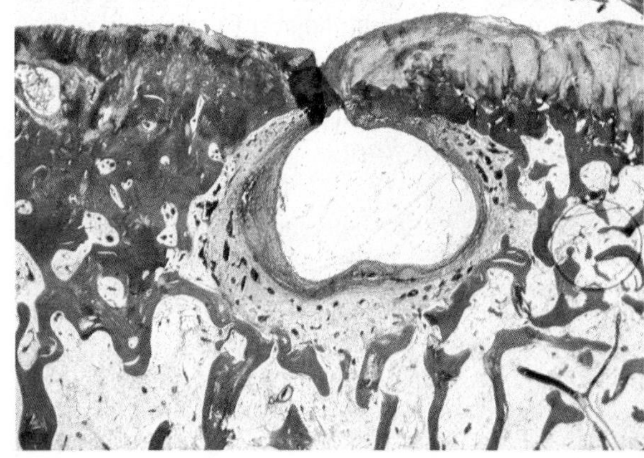

B

FIGURE *26-55*
Osteoarthritis. (*A*) A femoral head with osteoarthritis illustrating a fibrocartilaginous plug (*far right*) extending from the marrow onto the joint surface. Eburnated bone is present over the remaining surface. (*B*) A section through the articular surface of an osteoarthritic joint demonstrates focal absence of the articular cartilage, thickening of subchondral bone (*left*), and a subchondral bone cyst.

surrounded by basophilic staining matrix, called the *territorial matrix*.

2. Osteoarthritis may arrest at this stage for many years before it proceeds to the next stage, which is characterized by fibrillation (i.e., the development of surface cracks parallel to the long axis of the articular surface). These fibrillations also may persist for many years before further progression occurs.
3. As fibrillations propagate, synovial fluid begins to flow into the defects. The cracks are progressively oriented more vertically, tending to parallel the long axis of the collagen fibrils. Synovial fluid works its way deeper into the articular cartilage along the crack. Eventually, pieces of articular cartilage break off and lodge in the synovium, thereby inducing inflammation and a foreign-body giant cell reaction. The result is a hyperemic and hypertrophied synovium.
4. As the crack extends down toward the tide mark and eventually crosses it, neovascularization from the epiphysis and subchondral bone extends into the area of the crack, inducing subchondral osteoclastic bone resorption. Adjacent osteoblastic activity also occurs, and the result is a thickening of the subchondral bone plate in the area of the crack. As neovascularization progressively extends into the area of the crack, mesenchymal cells invade, and fibrocartilage forms as a poor substitute for the articular hyaline cartilage (Fig. 26-55A). These fibrocartilaginous plugs may persist, or they may be swept into the joint. The subchondral bone becomes exposed and burnished as it grinds against the opposite joint surface, which is undergoing the same process. These thick, shiny, and smooth areas of subchondral bone are referred to as *eburnated* (ivory-like) bone (see Figs. 26-54 and 26-55B).
5. In some areas, the eburnated bone eventually cracks, allowing synovial fluid to extend from the joint surface into the subchondral bone marrow, where it eventually leads to a *subchondral bone cyst* (see Fig. 26-55B). These cysts increase in size as synovial fluid is forced into the space but cannot exit. Eventually, there is bone resorption by osteoclasts and an attempt to wall off the area by osteoblastic activity. The result is a subchondral bone cyst filled with synovial fluid, with a well-marginated, reactive bone wall.
6. An osteophyte develops, usually in the lateral portions of the joint, when the mesenchymal tissue of the synovium modulates into osteoblasts and chondroblasts to form a mass of cartilage and bone. On gross examination, osteophytes are pearly, grayish bone nodules appearing on the peripheral portion of the joint surface. These osteophytes, or bony spurs, also

FIGURE *26-54*
Histogenesis of osteoarthritis. (*A, B*) The death of chondrocytes leads to a crack in the articular cartilage that is followed by an influx of synovial fluid and further loss and degeneration of cartilage. (*C*) As a result of this process, cartilage is gradually worn away. Below the tide mark, new vessels grow in from the epiphysis, and fibrocartilage (*D*) is deposited. (*E*) The fibrocartilage plug is not mechanically sufficient and may be worn away, thereby exposing the subchondral bone plate, which becomes thickened and eburnated. If there is a crack in this region, synovial fluid leaks into the marrow space and produces a subchondral bone cyst. Focal regrowth of the articular surface leads to the formation of osteophytes.

occur at the lateral portions of the intervertebral disks, extending from the adjacent vertebral bodies. They produce the "lipping" pattern seen on radiological studies as osteoarthritis of the spine. In the fingers, osteophytes at the distal interphalangeal joints are termed *Heberden nodes*.

☐ **Clinical Features:** The signs and symptoms of osteoarthritis are related to the location of the involved joints and the severity and duration of the joint deterioration. The physical findings are variable. The involved joints may be enlarged, tender, and boggy and may demonstrate crepitus. Deep, achy joint pain that follows activity and is relieved by rest is the clinical hallmark of osteoarthritis. Pain is usually a manifestation of significant joint destruction and arises in the periarticular structures, because articular cartilage lacks a nerve supply. Discomfort also is caused by short periods of stiffness, which is frequently experienced in the morning or after periods of minimal activity. Restriction of joint motion is a harbinger of severe disease and may result from joint or muscle contractures, intra-articular loose bodies, large osteophytes, and loss of congruity of the joint surfaces. There are no specific laboratory abnormalities in primary osteoarthritis.

At present there is no specific treatment to prevent or arrest osteoarthritis. Therapy is directed at specific orthopedic conditions and includes exercise, weight loss, and other supportive measures. In disabling osteoarthritis, joint replacement may be necessary.

RHEUMATOID ARTHRITIS

Rheumatoid arthritis (RA) is a systemic, chronic, inflammatory disease in which chronic polyarthritis involves diarthrodial joints bilaterally. The proximal interphalangeal and metacarpophalangeal joints, elbows, knees, ankles, and spine are commonly affected. The onset is usually in the third or fourth decade, but the prevalence increases with age until age 70 years. However, RA may occur at any age. The disease afflicts 1% to 2% of the adult population, and its incidence is greater in women than in men (3:1). The excess incidence of RA in women is firmly established before the menopause, after which the incidences for men and women increase uniformly. Commonly, the joints of the extremities are affected simultaneously and often in a symmetric pattern. The course of the disease is variable and is often punctuated by remissions and exacerbations. The broad spectrum of clinical manifestations ranges from barely discernible and mild signs and symptoms to severe, destructive, and mutilating disease.

It is now thought that classic RA probably comprises a heterogeneous group of disorders. Patients who are persistently seronegative for rheumatoid factor may have disease of a different etiology than do those who are seropositive. There are also rheumatoid-like diseases that are associated with underlying maladies, such as inflammatory bowel disease and cirrhosis.

☐ **Pathogenesis:** The cause of RA is unknown, but a number of factors have been implicated.

GENETIC FACTORS: A contribution of hereditary factors to the susceptibility to RA is suggested by the increased frequency of the disease in first-degree relatives of affected persons and by the concordance for the illness in monozygotic twins (30%). In addition, it is generally agreed that certain major histocompatibility (human leukocyte antigen; HLA) genes are expressed in a nonrandom manner in patients with RA. An important genetic locus that predisposes to RA is present in HLA II genes, and a specific set of HLA-DR alleles (DR4, DR1, DR10, DR14) is consistently increased in these patients. These alleles share a pentapeptide sequence motif (shared epitope) in a hypervariable segment of the **HLA-DRB1 gene**. This stretch of amino acids forms the rheumatoid pocket on the HLA molecule. It is likely that the binding properties of this pocket influence the type of peptides that can be bound by RA-associated HLA-DR molecules, thereby affecting the immune response to these peptides. Interestingly, seropositive (poor prognosis) RA (see later) is associated with a high frequency of an arginine in the shared epitope, whereas seronegative (good prognosis) disease commonly exhibits a lysine in the same position, further suggesting that the physical characteristics of the rheumatoid pocket influence the immune response in RA.

HUMORAL IMMUNITY: It is thought that immunological mechanisms play an important role in the pathogenesis of RA. Lymphocytes and plasma cells accumulate in the synovium, where they produce immunoglobulins, mainly of the IgG class. In addition, immune-complex deposits are present in the articular cartilage and the synovium. Increased serum levels of IgM, IgA, and IgG also may be found in patients with RA.

Some 80% of patients with classic RA are positive for **rheumatoid factor**. This factor actually represents multiple antibodies, principally IgM, but sometimes IgG or IgA, directed against the Fc fragment of IgG. Such antibodies are known as *anti-idiotype antibodies*. In rare cases, rheumatoid factor may be absent in the serum but is detectable in synovial fluid. Nevertheless, rheumatoid factor is not specifically diagnostic for RA. Significant titers of this factor are also found in patients with related collagen vascular diseases, such as systemic lupus erythematosus, progressive systemic sclerosis, and dermatomyositis. Rheumatoid factor also occurs in a wide variety of nonrheumatic disorders, including pulmonary fibrosis, cirrhosis, sarcoidosis, Waldenström macroglobulinemia, tuberculosis, kala-azar, lepromatous leprosy, and viral hepatitis. Even healthy elderly persons, particularly women, occasionally test positive for rheumatoid factor.

Although patients with classic RA may be seronegative, the presence of rheumatoid factor in high titer is frequently associated with severe and unremitting disease, many systemic complications, and a serious prognosis. The presence of IgG rheumatoid factor may be associated with the development of systemic complications, such as necrotizing vasculitis.

Immune complexes (IgG rheumatoid factor with IgG) and complement components are found in the synovium, synovial fluid, and extra-articular lesions of patients with RA. Furthermore, patients with seropositive RA have lower levels of complement in their synovial fluid than do patients who have the seronegative type.

CELLULAR IMMUNITY: It has also been postulated that cell-mediated immunity contributes to RA. Abundant T lymphocytes in the rheumatoid synovium are frequently Ia positive ("activated") and of the helper type. They are often in close contact with HLA-DR–positive cells, which are either macrophages or so-called dendritic Ia-positive cells; the latter do not demonstrate antigens of monocyte lineage.

T cells may directly or indirectly interact with macrophages through the production of cytokines that inhibit the migration and division of the latter. Such substances have been found in rheumatoid synovial fluid and in supernatants from rheumatoid tissue explants. These studies provide strong evidence that the joint destruction in RA reflects local production of cytokines, especially TNF and IL-1. Based on this information, future treatment of this disease is likely to target these inflammatory mediators. For example, IL-1 can stimulate the production of collagenase and prostaglandins in cultured synovial cells.

Patients with RA demonstrate a reactivity of T lymphocytes with collagen types I and III. In therapeutic trials, drainage of the thoracic duct, which primarily contains T cells, improved the condition of patients with RA. Furthermore, irradiation of lymphoid tissue has improved the clinical condition of some patients.

INFECTIOUS AGENTS: Neither infectious bacteria nor viruses have been detected in the joints of patients with RA, although in animal models, some bacterial wall fragments have produced a chronic synovitis.

Structures resembling viruses have been reported early in the course of the disease. It has been suggested that Epstein–Barr virus (EBV) may play a role in this disease, especially considering the high incidence of circulating antibodies to a variety of EBV antigens in patients with RA. Most patients with RA develop antibodies against a nuclear antigen in EBV-infected B cells. This antigen is termed RA-associated nuclear antigen (RANA) and is closely related to the nuclear antigen encoded by EBV (EBNA). Moreover, EBV is a polyclonal B-cell activator that stimulates the production of rheumatoid factor. Interestingly, the peripheral blood of many patients with RA contains an increased number of EBV-infected B cells.

LOCAL FACTORS: Synovial cells cultured from rheumatic joints exhibit a decreased response to glucocorticoids and an increased production of hyaluronate. These cells release a peptide (connective tissue-activating peptide) that may influence the function of other cells, producing increased amounts of prostaglandins, particularly prostaglandin E_2 (PGE_2).

A hypothetical scenario consistent with the evidence presented earlier might be constructed as follows:

1. In a genetically susceptible person, an unknown agent (possibly a virus, possibly EBV) infects a joint or some other tissue and stimulates the formation of antibodies.
2. These immunoglobulins act as new antigens, that is, they trigger the production of anti-idiotype antibodies (rheumatoid factor).
3. Immune complexes, which contain rheumatoid factor, are deposited in the synovium and activate the complement cascade. This results in increased vascular permeability and the uptake of immune complexes by leukocytes, which in turn release lysosomal enzymes, activated oxygen species, and other injurious products.
4. Activated macrophages in the synovium present unknown antigens to T cells, thereby stimulating the production of cytokines, which amplify inflammation, tissue injury, and the proliferation of synovial cells.

□ **Pathology:** The early synovial changes of RA are edema and the accumulation of plasma cells, lymphocytes, and macrophages (Fig. 26-56). There is a concomitant increase in vascularity and exudation of fibrin in the joint space, which may result in small fibrin nodules that float in the joint (*rice bodies*).

PANNUS FORMATION: The synovial lining cells, which are normally only one to three layers thick, undergo hyperplasia and form layers 8 to 10 cells deep. Multinucleated giant cells are often found among the synovial cells. **The result is a synovial lining thrown into numerous villi and frond-like folds that fill the peripheral recesses of the joint** (Fig. 26-57A).

As the synovium undergoes hyperplasia and hypertrophy, it creeps over the surface of the articular cartilage and adjacent structures. This inflammatory synovium, now containing mast cells, is termed a *pannus* (cloak). The pannus proceeds to cover the articular cartilage and isolate it from its nutritional synovial fluid. Lymphocytes aggregate into masses and eventually develop follicular centers (*Allison–Ghormley bodies;* see Fig. 26-57B).

The pannus erodes the articular cartilage and the adjacent bone, probably through the action of collagenase produced by the pannus (see Fig. 26-57C). The mechanisms for demineralization of bone adjacent to the pannus are unknown, but perhaps osteoclasts play a role. Because PGE_2 and IL-1 stimulate osteoclasts and are actively produced in the rheumatoid synovium, they may be mediators of bone erosion.

The characteristic bone loss of RA is juxta-articular, that is it is immediately adjacent to both sides of the joint. Because the remaining bone is normal, juxta-articular bone loss is probably related to a factor elaborated locally by the rheumatoid synovium.

The pannus invades the joint and subchondral bones as if it were a neoplasm. Eventually, the joint is destroyed and undergoes fibrous fusion, termed *ankylosis* (Fig. 26-58). Long-standing cases lead to a fused joint with bony bridging, called *bony ankylosis*.

An alternative route of joint destruction is cartilage loss, which leads to the changes already described for osteoarthritis. The synovial pannus may stimulate cartilage resorption, by depriving it of its nourishing synovial fluid. The pannus may also stimulate T lymphocytes to secrete a factor that incites chondrocytes to release lysosomal enzymes.

SYNOVIAL FLUID: Fluid in a joint inflamed by RA contains abundant polymorphonuclear leukocytes, although they are rarely present in the synovial tissue. Over

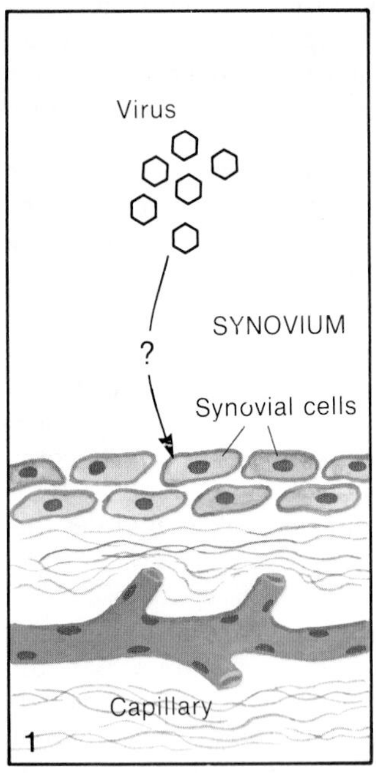

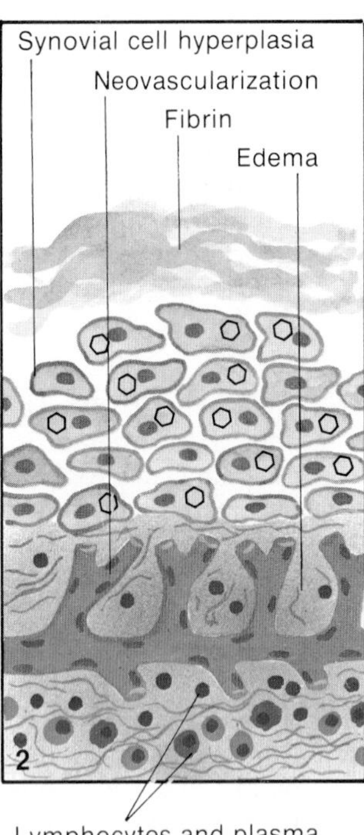

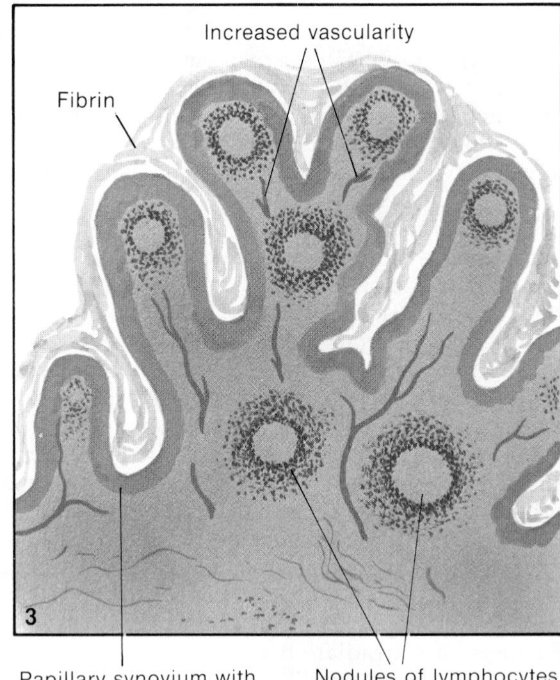

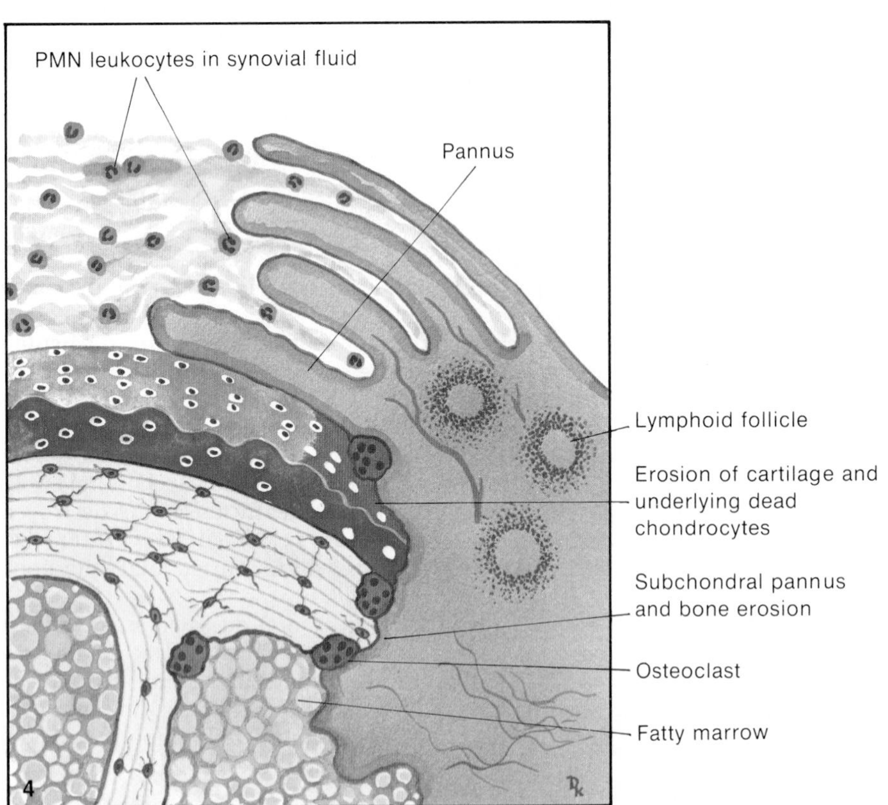

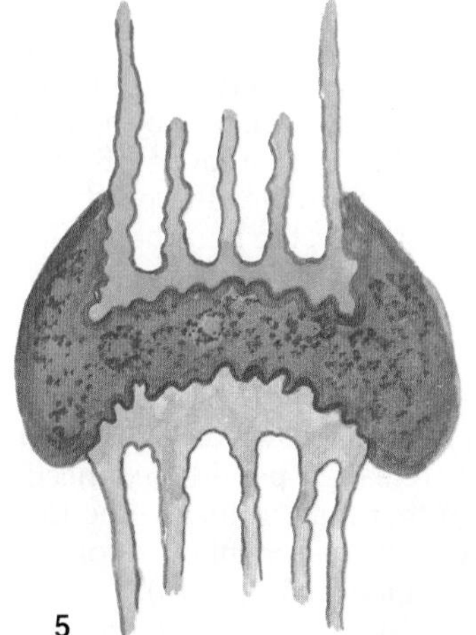

Destruction of joint by fibrosis and loss of articular cartilage, with periarticular bone loss

FIGURE **26-56**

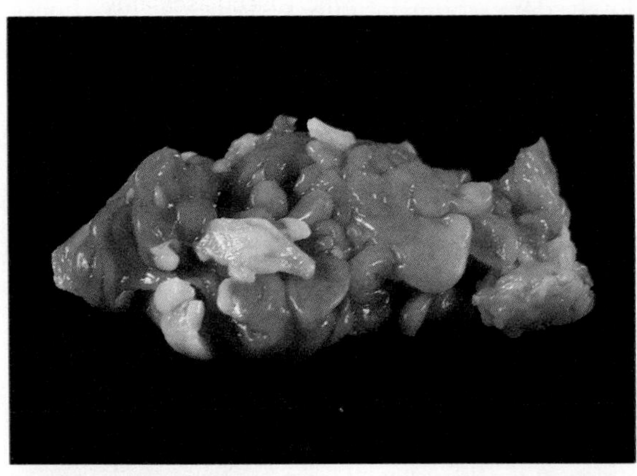

A

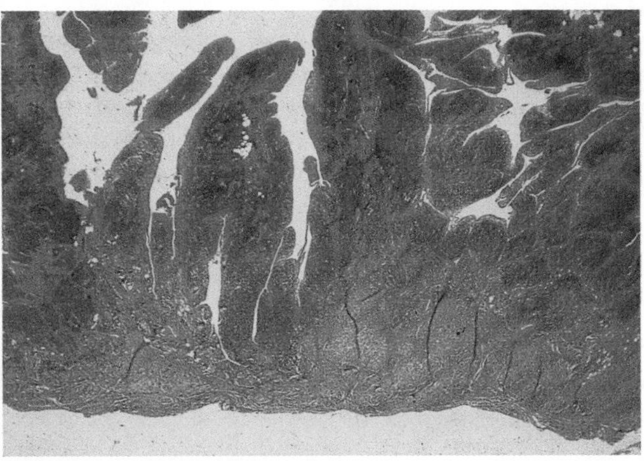

B

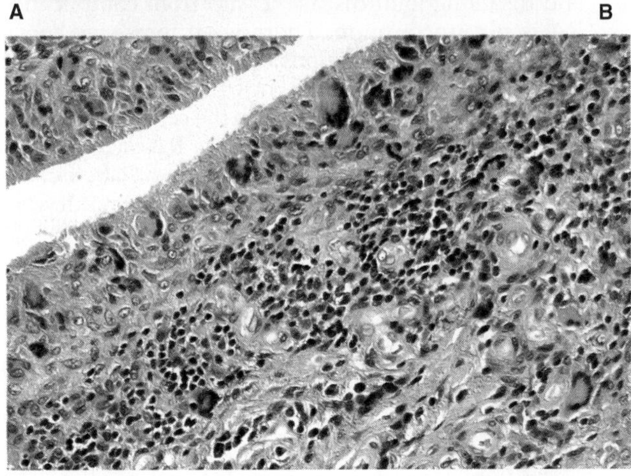

C

FIGURE 26-57
Rheumatoid arthritis. (*A*) The hyperplastic synovium from a patient with rheumatoid arthritis shows numerous finger-like projections, with focal pale areas of fibrin deposition. The brownish color of the synovium reflects hemosiderin accumulation derived from old hemorrhage. (*B*) A microscopic view reveals prominent lymphoid follicles (Allison–Ghormley bodies), synovial hyperplasia and hypertrophy, villous folds, and thickening of the synovial membrane by fibrosis and inflammation. (*C*) A higher-power view of the inflamed synovium demonstrates hyperplasia and hypertrophy of the lining cells. Numerous giant cells are noted on and below the surface. The stroma is chronically inflamed.

the years, as the disease waxes and wanes, the degree of acute inflammation also correlates with the varying activity of the rheumatoid process.

Changes in the synovial fluid include a massive increase in volume, increased turbidity, and decreased viscosity. The protein content of the fluid is increased, as well as the number of inflammatory cells. In some cases, the leukocyte count exceeds 50,000/μL, with 95% polymorphonuclear leukocytes.

Rheumatoid Nodules

Rheumatoid arthritis is a systemic disease that also involves tissues other than the joints and tendons. A characteristic lesion, termed the *rheumatoid nodule,* is found in other systemic locations. This structure has a centrally located core of fibrinoid necrosis, which is a mixture of fibrin and other proteins, such as degraded collagen (Fig. 26-59). A surrounding rim of macrophages is arranged in a radial, or palisading, fashion. Peripheral to the macrophages is an outer circle of lymphocytes, plasma cells, and other mononuclear cells. The overall appearance resembles a peculiar granuloma surrounding a core of fibrinoid necrosis. Rheumatoid nodules, which are usually found in areas of pressure (e.g., the skin of the elbows and legs), are movable, firm, rubbery, and occasionally tender. A large nodule may ulcerate. Recurrence after surgical removal is common.

Rheumatoid nodules may also be seen in lupus ery-

FIGURE 26-56
Histogenesis of rheumatoid arthritis. *1:* A virus or an unknown stress stimulates the synovial cells to proliferate. *2:* The influx of lymphocytes, plasma cells, and mast cells, together with neovascularization and edema, leads to hypertrophy and hyperplasia of the synovium. *3:* Lymphoid nodules are prominent. *4:* The proliferating synovium extends into the joint space, burrows into the bone beneath the articular cartilage and covers the cartilage as a pannus. The articular cartilage is eventually destroyed by direct resorption or deprivation of its nutrient synovial fluid. The synovial tissue continues to proliferate in the subchondral region, as well as in the joint. *5:* Eventually, the joint is destroyed and becomes fused, a condition termed ankylosis.

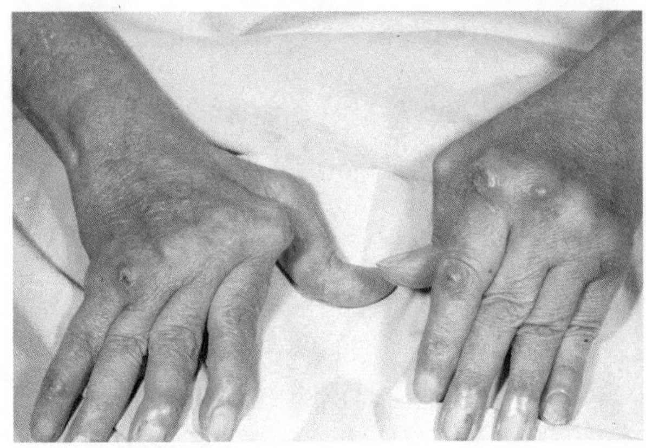

FIGURE 26-58
Rheumatoid arthritis. The hands of a patient with advanced arthritis show swelling of the metacarpal phalangeal joints and the classic ulnar deviation of the fingers.

thematous and rheumatic fever. They are sometimes found in visceral organs, such as the heart, lungs, and intestinal tract, and even the dura. Nodules in the bundle of His may cause cardiac arrhythmias, whereas in the lungs, they produce fibrosis and even respiratory failure (rheumatoid lung; see Chapter 12).

Rheumatoid arthritis also may be accompanied by acute necrotizing vasculitis, which can affect virtually any organ. Vasculitis may produce myocardial infarction, cerebrovascular occlusion, renal failure, mesenteric infarction, or gangrene of a digit.

□ Clinical Features:

The clinical diagnosis of RA is imprecise and is based on a number of criteria, such as the number and types of joints involved, the presence of rheumatoid nodules and rheumatoid factor, and radiographic features characteristic of the disease.

The onset of the disease may be acute, slowly progressing, or insidious. Most patients give a history of slowly developing fatigue, weight loss, weakness, and vague musculoskeletal discomfort, which eventually localizes to the involved joints. Diseased joints are frequently warm, swollen, and painful. The pain is heightened by motion and is most severe after periods of disuse. Unabated disease causes progressive destruction of the joint surfaces and periarticular structures. Eventually, the patients manifest severe flexion and extension deformities, associated with joint subluxation, which may terminate in joint ankylosis.

The natural history of RA is variable, and in most patients, the activity of the disease will wax and wane. One fourth of the patients seem to recover completely. Another fourth remain for many years with only slight functional impairment, whereas half have serious progressive and disabling joint disease. Death from complications of RA is not uncommon. There is an increased mortality from a variety of infections, gastrointestinal hemorrhage and perforation, vasculitis, heart and lung involvement, amyloidosis, and subluxation of the cervical spine. In fact, the survival of patients with active RA is comparable to that observed in Hodgkin's disease and diabetes.

The drugs used to suppress the inflammatory process of the synovium and to induce a remission are essentially of three classes:

- **Anti-inflammatory agents** include aspirin, nonsteroidal antiinflammatory drugs (such as indomethacin, naproxen, and ibuprofen), phenylbutazone, glucocorticoids, and even intra-articular corticosteroids administered by injection.
- **Remission-inducing drugs** used are gold salts, penicillamine, and antimalarial drugs, such as chloroquine.
- **Immunosuppressive drugs** are used in patients with severe progressive disease who do not respond to antiinflammatory or remission-inducing drugs. They include cyclophosphamide, azathioprine, 6-mercaptopurine, chlorambucil, and methotrexate.

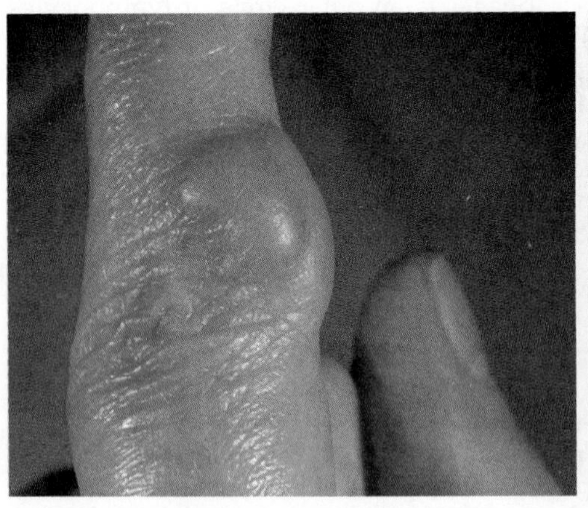

A

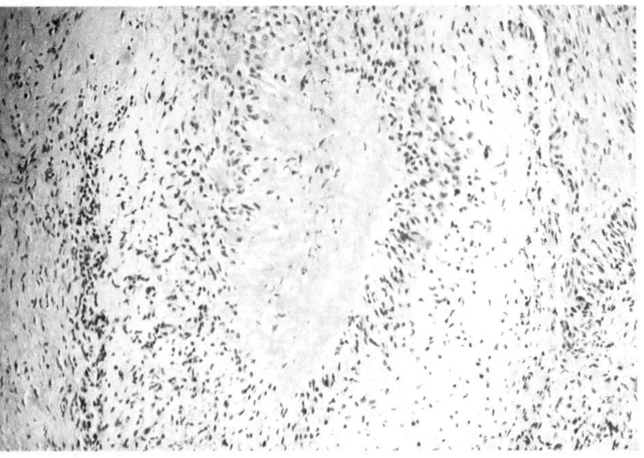

B

FIGURE 26-59
Rheumatoid nodule. (*A*) A patient with rheumatoid arthritis has a mass on a digit. (*B*) A microscopic view of a rheumatoid nodule shows a central area of necrosis surrounded by palisaded macrophages and a chronic inflammatory infiltrate.

Spondyloarthropathy

A number of clinical entities were formerly classified as variants of RA but are now recognized to be distinct disorders. These forms of arthritis are now termed *spondyloarthropathies* and include ankylosing spondylitis, Reiter syndrome, psoriatic arthritis, and arthritis associated with inflammatory bowel disease. These conditions have in common the following features:

- Seronegativity for rheumatoid factor and other serological markers of RA
- An association with class I histocompatibility antigens, particularly HLA-B27
- Preferential localization to the sacrum and vertebral column
- Asymmetric involvement of only few peripheral joints
- A tendency to inflammation of periarticular tendons and fascia
- Systemic involvement of other organs, especially uveitis, carditis, and aortitis
- Preferential onset in young men

Ankylosing Spondylitis

Ankylosing spondylitis is an inflammatory arthropathy of the vertebral column and sacroiliac joints. It may be accompanied by asymmetric, peripheral arthritis (30% of patients) and systemic manifestations. Ankylosing spondylitis is most common in young men, and the peak incidence is at about age 20 years. **More than 90% of patients are positive for HLA-B27 (normal, 4% to 8%), although the disorder affects only 1% of persons with this haplotype**.

☐ **Pathology:** Ankylosing spondylitis begins at the sacroiliac joints bilaterally and then ascends the spinal column by involving the small joints of the posterior elements of the spine. The result is ultimate destruction of these joints, after which the spine becomes fused posteriorly. The unburdened vertebral bodies become square and osteoporotic, because the main force of gravity is borne by the fused posterior elements. In such cases, the intervertebral disk undergoes ossification and may disappear. Eventually, bony fusion of the vertebral bodies ensues (Fig. 26-60).

Although a few patients with ankylosing spondylitis have an usually rapid development of crippling spinal disease, most are able to maintain their employment and live a normal life span. However, up to 5% of patients develop AA amyloidosis and uremia, and a few manifest severe cardiac involvement.

Reiter Syndrome

Reiter syndrome is a triad that includes (1) seronegative polyarthritis, (2) conjunctivitis, and (3) nonspecific urethritis. The disorder is almost exclusively encountered in men and usually follows venereal exposure or an episode of bacillary dysentery. As in ankylosing spondylitis, Reiter syndrome is associated with HLA-B27 antigen in up to 90% of patients. In fact, after an attack of dysentery, 20% of HLA-B27–positive men develop Reiter syndrome.

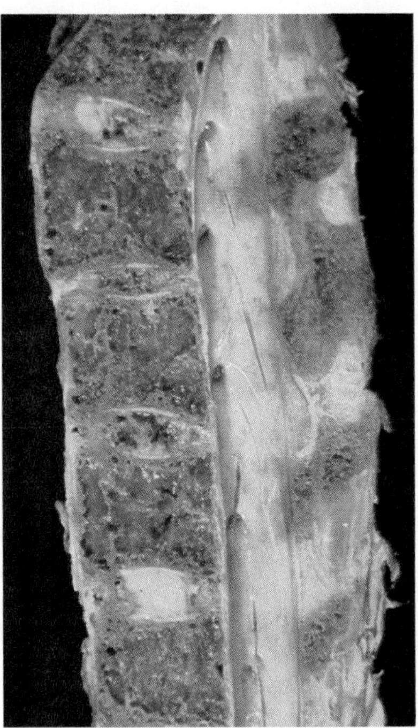

FIGURE *26-60*
Ankylosing spondylitis. The vertebrae have been cut longitudinally. The vertebral bodies are square and have lost most of their trabecular bone, owing to osteoporosis from disuse. Bone bridges fuse one vertebral body to the next across the intervertebral discs. Portions of the intervertebral disc are replaced by bone marrow. Bony bridges also fuse the posterior elements, a condition termed ankylosis.

The pathological features of Reiter arthritis are comparable to those of RA. More than half of the patients develop mucocutaneous lesions similar to those of pustular psoriasis, termed *keratoblennorrhagicum,* over the palms, soles, and trunk. In most patients, the disease remits within a year, but in 20%, progressive arthritis develops, including ankylosing spondylitis.

Psoriatic Arthritis

Of all patients with psoriasis, particularly in those with severe disease, 7% develop an inflammatory seronegative arthritis. HLA-B27 has been linked to psoriatic spondylitis and inflammation of the distal interphalangeal joints, and HLA-DR4 has been associated with a rheumatoid pattern of involvement. The joint disease is usually mild and only slowly progressive, although a mutilating form is occasionally encountered.

Enteropathic Arthritis

Ulcerative colitis and Crohn disease are accompanied by seronegative peripheral arthritis in 20% of the cases and spondylitis in 10%. This form of arthritis also is seen in patients with Whipple disease and after certain bacterial infections of the gut. No particular tissue type is associated with peripheral arthritis, but the majority of patients with ankylosing spondylitis are HLA-B27 positive. Although the mechanism by which HLA-B27 influences the occurrence of enteropathic arthritis (and other spondyloarthropathies) remains to be discovered, it has been proposed that HLA-B27 and proteins from enteric bacteria are structurally related in a manner that potentially affects antigen presentation to the T-cell receptor. Resection of the affected bowel in ulcerative colitis relieves the arthritis, but in Crohn disease, this complication often does not resolve.

Juvenile Arthritis (Still Disease)

Juvenile arthritis refers to a number of different chronic arthritic conditions in children. At one time, this term signified a variant of RA that was characterized by chronic synovitis and extra-articular symptoms. However, it is now recognized that in addition to RA, many children with juvenile arthritis eventually develop ankylosing spondylitis, psoriatic arthritis, and other connective tissue diseases. The term *juvenile arthritis* is now applied to any chronic inflammatory arthritis in children and can be classified as follows:

- **Seropositive arthritis:** Fewer than 10% of children with arthritis are positive for rheumatoid factor and have a polyarticular presentation. There is a female predominance (80%) among children with Still disease, and in most cases (75%), antinuclear antibodies are present. There is an association with HLA-D4, and more than half of the children eventually develop severe arthritis.
- **Polyarticular disease without systemic symptoms:** About one fourth of all cases of juvenile arthritis (90% girls) are seen as disease of several joints, are seronegative, and do not manifest systemic symptoms. Fewer than 15% of these patients eventually develop severe arthritis.
- **Polyarticular disease with systemic symptoms:** Roughly 20% of children with polyarticular juvenile arthritis have prominent systemic symptoms, which include high fever, rash, hepatosplenomegaly, lymphadenopathy, pleuritis, pericarditis, anemia, and leukocytosis. The majority (60%) of patients are boys who are negative for rheumatoid factor, and one fourth of these patients are left with severe arthritis.
- **Pauciarticular arthritis:** Children with involvement of only a few large joints, such as the knee, ankle, elbow, or hip girdle, account for about half of all cases juvenile arthritis, in two general groups. The larger group are mainly (80%) girls who are negative for rheumatoid factor but exhibit antinuclear antibodies and are positive for HLA-DR5, HLA-DRw6, or HLA-DRw8. Of these patients, one third have ocular disease characterized by chronic iridocyclitis (inflammation of the iris and ciliary body). Only a small minority of these children have residual polyarthritis or ocular damage.

The other group of children with a pauciarticular presentation are almost all boys, are negative for both rheumatoid factor and antinuclear bodies, and are positive for HLA-B27 (75%). A few have acute iridocyclitis, which resolves spontaneously. Some of these children subsequently develop ankylosing spondylitis.

GOUT

Gout is a heterogeneous group of diseases in which the common denominator is an increased serum uric acid level and the deposition of urate crystals in the joints and kidneys. Although all patients with gout display hyperuricemia, fewer than 15% of all persons with increased serum uric acid have gout.

Gout is characterized by acute and chronic arthritis. The varieties of gout are classified according to the etiology of the hyperuricemia into primary and secondary forms. Primary gout refers to hyperuricemia in the absence of any other disease, whereas secondary gout occurs in association with another illness that results in hyperuricemia. It has been estimated that of all cases of hyperuricemia, one third are primary and the remainder secondary.

Pathogenesis of Hyperuricemia

Uric acid results from the catabolism of purines, derived either from the diet or synthesized *de novo*. In most mammals, relatively insoluble uric acid is converted to highly soluble allantoin by urate oxidase. The loss of this enzyme during the course of human evolution imposed a narrow balance between uric acid production and the tissue deposition of urates. In humans, uric acid is eliminated from the body only in the urine. Thus, the level of uric acid in the blood (normal, <7.0 mg/dL in men and 6.0 mg/dL in women) reflects the difference between the amounts of purines ingested and synthesized and the extent of renal excretion. Gout can result from (1) overproduction of purines, (2) augmented catabolism of nucleic acids as a result of increased cell turnover, (3) decreased salvage of free purine bases, or (4) decreased urinary excretion of uric acid (Fig. 26-61). Increased dietary intake of purine-rich foods, particularly meat, in an otherwise normal person does not lead to hyperuricemia and gout.

Primary (Idiopathic) Gout

In the large majority of cases of primary gout, the specific biochemical defect responsible for the hyperuricemia is unknown. **Most cases (85%) of idiopathic gout result from an as-yet-unexplained impairment of uric acid excretion by the kidneys.** In the remainder, there is a primary overproduction of uric acid, but only in a minority of cases has the the underlying abnormality been identified.

In principle, a reduction in urate clearance in primary gout can result from (1) decreased glomerular filtration, (2) increased tubular reabsorption, or (3) decreased urate excretion by the renal tubules. Although none of these mechanisms has been conclusively demonstrated, current opinion favors decreased urate excretion.

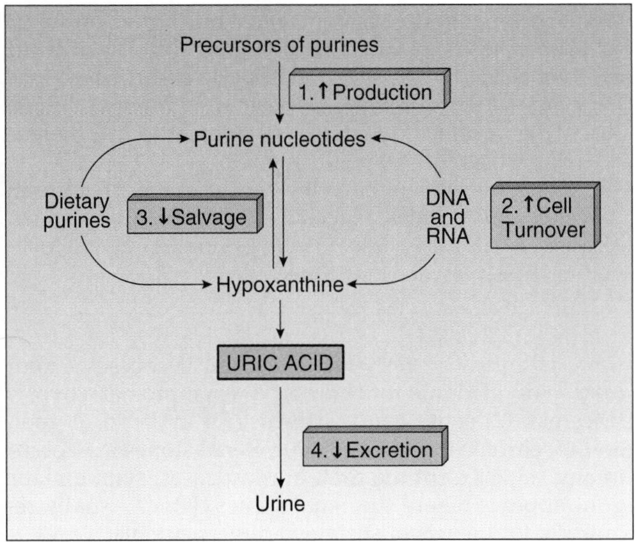

FIGURE *26-61*
Pathogenesis of hyperuricemia and gout. Purine nucleotides are synthesized *de novo* from nonpurine precursors or derived from preformed purines in the diet. Purine nucleotides are catabolized to hypoxanthine or incorporated into nucleic acids. The degradation of nucleic acids and of dietary urines also produces hypoxanthine. Hypoxanthine is converted to uric acid, which in turn is excreted into the urine. Hyperuricemia and gout result from (*1*) increased *de novo* purine synthesis, (2) increased cell turnover, (3) decreased salvage of dietary purines and hypoxanthine, and (4) decreased uric acid excretion by the kidneys.

GENETIC FACTORS: A familial tendency to gout has been recognized since the time of Galen. Hyperuricemia is common among the relatives of persons with gout. On the basis of familial studies, it has been proposed that primary hyperuricemia in some persons is inherited as an autosomal dominant trait with variable penetrance. However, large population studies have implicated X-linked transmission in some cases, whereas others have favored multifactorial inheritance. It is generally agreed that precocious gout exhibits a strong familial tendency, a feature that is consistent with the fact that the early onset of many diseases with multifactorial inheritance (e.g., atherosclerosis, diabetes) is likely to be associated with a clearly visible genetic component. The consensus today holds that the level of serum uric acid is controlled by multiple genes.

Gout Due to Inborn Errors of Metabolism

Whereas the specific cause of an abnormally high rate of urate production is not identifiable in most cases of primary gout, two inborn errors of metabolism that result in an elevated level of phosphoribosyl pyrophosphate (PP-ribose-P) are known. In this respect, the rate-limiting step in purine synthesis is the condensation of glutamine with PP-ribose-P to form phosphoribosyl amine. An increased intracellular concentration of PP-ribose-P accelerates the biosynthesis of purines. PP-ribose-P, through the activity of hypoxanthine phosphoribosyl transferase (HPRT), also condenses with and thereby salvages purine bases (hypoxanthine and guanine) derived from the catabolism of nucleic acids.

LESCH–NYHAN SYNDROME: This condition represents an inherited, X-linked (Xq26-q27) deficiency of HPRT, a defect that leads to the accumulation of PP-ribose-P and in turn to enhanced purine synthesis. Children with this syndrome are clinically normal at birth, but exhibit delays in development and neurological dysfunction within the first year. The large majority are afflicted by self-mutilation and are mentally retarded. The patients exhibit hyperuricemia and eventually develop gouty arthritis. In addition, obstructive nephropathy and hematological abnormalities are often present.

In another hereditary condition characterized by increased intracellular PP-ribose-P levels, an abnormally high activity of PP-ribose-P synthetase accelerates *de novo* purine synthesis.

Secondary Gout

A number of conditions result in hyperuricemia and secondary gout. As in primary gout, secondary hyperuricemia may reflect urate overproduction or decreased urinary excretion of uric acid. Increased production of uric acid is most commonly associated with increased turnover of nucleic acids, as seen in leukemias and lymphomas, and after chemotherapy for cancer. Accelerated ATP degradation may also lead to overproduction of uric acid and occurs in glycogen-storage diseases and tissue hypoxia. Ethanol intake is a cause of secondary hyperuricemia, in part owing to accelerated ATP catabolism and, to a lesser degree, decreased renal excretion of uric acid.

Similar to primary hyperuricemia, reduced urate excretion in secondary gout can result from decreased glomerular filtration, increased tubular reabsorption, and decreased tubular secretion. The most common causes of decreased urinary excretion of uric acid are chronic diseases that lead to a reduction in functional renal mass. In renal failure, the clearance of uric acid is decreased, and with a decrease in the rate of glomerular filtration, hyperuricemia ensues.

Dehydration and the administration of diuretic drugs increase tubular reabsorption of uric acid and lead to hyperuricemia. Impaired urate secretion by the renal tubules results from competitive inhibition by a variety of organic anions, including lactate (ethanol intake), β-hydroxybutyrate and acetoacetate (diabetes), and branched-chain ketoacids (maple-syrup urine disease). Other conditions that reduce renal urate excretion, but whose mechanisms are not clear, include lead nephropathy and the intake of certain drugs, such as salicylates, ethambutol, and nicotinic acid. In fact, drugs are implicated in as many as 20% of patients with hyperuricemia.

Saturnine gout was described in 18th century England, where this disease was prevalent among the upper classes who had lead plumbing in their houses (Saturn is the symbol for lead). It is now recognized that these patients were afflicted with lead nephropathy. The Romans had a similar problem, because they drank from vessels containing lead.

☐ **Epidemiology:** Primary gout is a disease of adult men, and only 5% of cases occur in women. It is rare in children before the age of puberty and in women during the reproductive period. The peak incidence is in the fifth decade. This sex distribution can be traced to the fact that at all ages, the mean serum urate concentration in women is lower than that in men, although the level in the former increases after the menopause. A family history is elicited in many patients with gout, but environmental factors also play an important role. Positive correlations exist between the prevalence of hyperuricemia in a population and the mean values for weight, protein intake, alcohol consumption, social class, and intelligence. Thus, gout is a disease that exemplifies the interplay between genetic predisposition and environmental influences.

☐ **Pathology:** When sodium urate crystals precipitate from supersaturated body fluids, they absorb fibronectin, complement, and a number of other proteins on their surface. On phagocytizing these protein-coated crystals, neutrophils release activated oxygen species and lysosomal enzymes, which mediate tissue injury. Moreover, neutrophils that have ingested urate crystals also secrete leukotriene B_4, kinins, collagenase, kallikrein, prostaglandins, and IL-1, all factors that promote the inflammatory response.

The presence of long, needle-shaped crystals that are negatively birefringent under polarized light is diagnostic of gout. Urate crystals may be found intracellularly in leukocytes of the synovial fluid. Extracellular soft-tissue deposits of these crystals (*tophi*) (Fig. 26-62A) are surrounded by foreign-body giant cells and an associated inflammatory response of mononuclear cells (see Fig. 26-62B). These granuloma-like areas are found in cartilage, in any of the soft tissues around joints, and even in the subchondral bone marrow adjacent to joints.

Macroscopically, any chalky, white deposit on the surfaces of intra-articular structures, including articular cartilage, is suggestive of gout, and a touch preparation of this substance is in order. Radiologically, gouty arthritis exhibits characteristic, punched-out, juxta-articular, lytic ("rat bite") lesions that are associated with only minimal reactive new bone (Fig. 26-63). In contrast to RA, there is no juxta-articular osteopenia in gout.

Urate deposits in the kidney occur in the interstitium between renal tubules, especially at the medullary apices. These deposits are grossly visible as small, shiny, golden-yellow, linear streaks in the medulla.

☐ **Clinical Features:** The clinical course of gout may be divided into four stages: (1) asymptomatic hyperuricemia, (2) acute gouty arthritis, (3) intercritical gout, and (4) chronic tophaceous gout. Renal stones may occur in any stage except the first. In most cases, symptomatic gout appears before the renal stones, which usually require 20 to 30 years of sustained hyperuricemia.

- **Asymptomatic hyperuricemia** often precedes clinically evident gout by many years.
- **Acute gouty arthritis** was well characterized by Thomas Sydenham, who described his own disease in the 1600s. It is a painful condition that usually involves one joint and is unaccompanied by constitutional symptoms. Later in the course of the disease, polyarticular involvement with fever is common. At least half of patients are first seen with a painful and red first metatarsophalangeal joint (great toe), designated *podagra*. Eventually, 90% of all patients have such an attack. Although the disease primarily affects the lower extremities, fingers, elbows, and wrists also become involved.

  Commonly, a gouty attack begins at night and is exquisitely painful, simulating an acute bacterial infection of the affected joint. An attack may be triggered by consuming a large meal or drinking alcoholic beverages, but other specific events, such as trauma, certain drugs, and surgery, also may be responsible. Even when untreated, an acute attack of gout is self-limited.

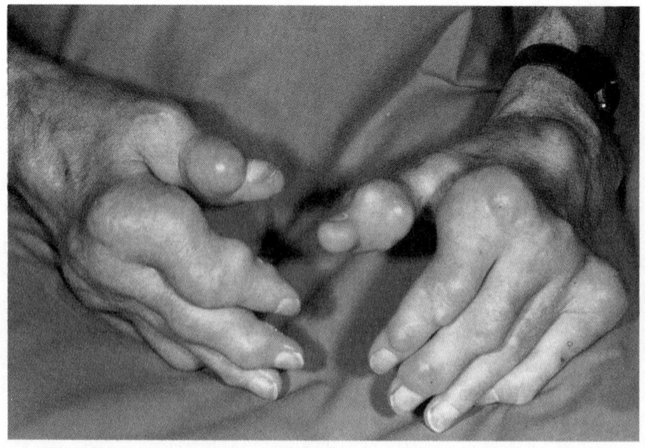
A

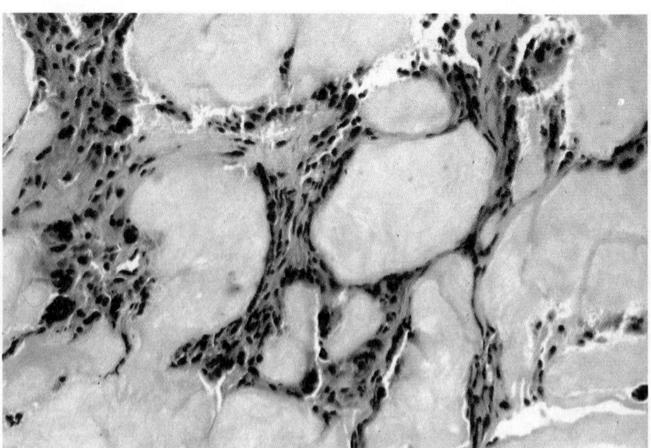
B

FIGURE 26-62
Gout. (*A*) Gouty tophi project from the fingers as rubbery nodules. (*B*) A section from a tophus shows extracellular masses of urate crystals with accompanying foreign-body giant cells.

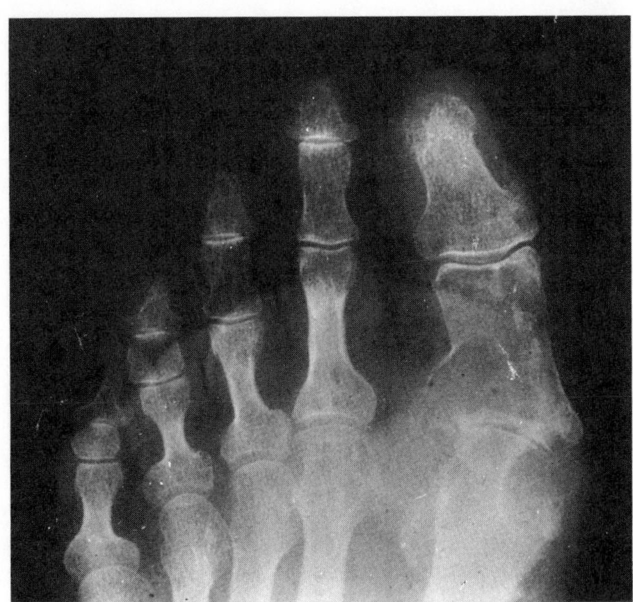

FIGURE 26-63
Gout. A radiograph of the first metatarsophalangeal joint shows a lytic lesion that destroys the joint space. There is an adjacent soft tissue tophus, as well as surrounding edema.

- **The intercritical period** is the asymptomatic interval between the initial acute attack and subsequent attacks. These periods may last up to 10 years, but later attacks tend to be increasingly severe and prolonged, polyarticular, and febrile.
- **Tophaceous gout** eventually appears in the untreated patient in the form of tophi in the cartilage, synovial membranes, tendons, and soft tissues. A tophus is a chalky, cheesy, yellow-white, pasty deposit of monosodium urate crystals. Classic locations of a tophus are the helix or the antihelix of the ear. They also occur on the hands (see Fig. 26-62A), in the olecranon bursa, and in the Achilles tendon. Tophi are rare in patients treated with antihyperuricemic drugs.

Renal failure is responsible for 10% of the deaths in patients with gout. However, the contribution of urate nephropathy to chronic renal dysfunction is unclear, and hypertension, preexisting kidney disease, and the intake of analgesic drugs may be more important. About one third of patients with gout have mild albuminuria, a reduced glomerular filtration rate, and a decreased renal concentrating ability. In patients with severe gout caused by inherited enzyme deficiencies and in those with a precocious presentation, urate nephropathy is a prominent feature of the clinical course.

Urate stones constitute 10% of all renal calculi in patients in the United States and up to 40% of all renal calculi in patients in Israel and Australia. The prevalence of stones correlates with the serum concentration of uric acid and is 1000 times greater in gout patients than in the general population, affecting up to 25% of the former. Gout patients also have an increased frequency of calcium-containing stones, in which case the uric acid may serve as a nidus for a calcium stone.

DISORDERS ASSOCIATED WITH GOUT: Hyperuricemia and gout are linked to a number of other chronic conditions, but the reasons for many of these associations are poorly understood. Hyperlipidemia is found in 80% of patients with gout, although there is no evidence for a genetic basis for this association. Half of gouty persons have hypertension, a relation that may reflect decreased renal blood flow and obesity. Indeed, one third of untreated hypertensive persons have hyperuricemia, and patients with gout have a mean body weight almost 20% greater than that of the normal population. As previously noted, ethanol intake can precipitate attacks of acute gouty arthritis, principally because of an increase in uric acid production.

TREATMENT: The treatment of gout is designed to (1) decrease the severity of acute attacks, (2) reduce the serum urate levels, (3) prevent future attacks, (4) promote the dissolution of urate deposits, and (5) alkalinize the urine to prevent stone formation. The principal drugs used to interrupt the inflammatory process, thereby preventing or controlling the acute attack, are indomethacin and other nonsteroidal anti-inflammatory agents. Colchicine has been used for hundreds of years and has been administered prophylactically during the intervals between gouty attacks to prevent recurrent episodes. However, colchicine has toxic side effects, including diarrhea, nausea, and vomiting, which limit its effectiveness. Occasionally, glucocorticoids, such as prednisone, are prescribed. The uricosuric drugs that interfere with urate resorption by the renal tubule include probenecid and sulfinpyrazone.

A drug worthy of special attention is **allopurinol**, a competitive inhibitor of xanthine oxidase, the enzyme that converts xanthine and hypoxanthine to uric acid. This drug causes a prompt decrease in uricosemia and uricosuria. It is used in patients who have renal insufficiency and in those who are resistant to other uricosuric drugs. It also may be administered to patients undergoing chemotherapy for hemopoietic proliferative disorders, in whom the rate of urate production is increased.

CALCIUM PYROPHOSPHATE DIHYDRATE–DEPOSITION DISEASE (CHONDROCALCINOSIS AND PSEUDOGOUT)

Calcium pyrophosphate dihydrate (CPPD)-deposition disease refers to the accumulation of this compound in synovial membranes (pseudogout), joint cartilage (chondrocalcinosis), ligaments, and tendons. The disease can be idiopathic, associated with trauma, linked to a number of metabolic disorders, or, in rare cases, hereditary.

CPPD-deposition disease is principally a condition of old age, with half of the population older than 85 years being afflicted. The large majority of cases in the elderly are without symptoms. Because fully two thirds of these patients manifest preexisting joint damage, it is believed that trauma and the aging process in cartilage promote nucleation of CPPD crystals. In asymptomatic cases, punctate or linear calcifications may be present in any fibrocartilage or hyaline cartilage surface. For example, radiography of the knee may disclose linear streaks that outline the menisci.

☐ Pathogenesis: **The major predisposing abnormality in patients with CPPD-deposition disease is an excessive level of inorganic pyrophosphate in the synovial fluid.** This material derives from the hydrolysis of nucleoside triphosphates in the chondrocytes of the joint. Increased pyrophosphate levels in the synovial fluid can result from either increased production or decreased catabolism.

Calcium pyrophosphate deposition is commonly found in the knees after trauma and after surgical removal of the meniscus. It is possible that released nucleotides after injury to the articular cartilage serve as a substrate for nucleotide triphosphate pyrophosphohydrolase (NTP), thereby increasing the production of pyrophosphate. A number of other disorders are associated with the deposition of calcium pyrophosphate crystals, including hyperparathyroidism, hypothyroidism, hemochromatosis, Wilson disease, and ochronosis. Iron and copper are presumed to inhibit pyrophosphatase, accounting for decreased degradation of pyrophosphate.

Hypophosphatasia is a heritable condition in which the activity of alkaline phosphatase (the enzyme that hydrolyzes pyrophosphate) in serum and tissue is deficient. As a result, pyrophosphate is not adequately metabolized and accumulates in the synovial fluid.

☐ Pathology and Clinical Features: The minority of cases of CPPD-deposition disease that are symptomatic are classified according to the nature of joint involvement.

- **Pseudogout** refers to self-limited attacks of acute arthritis lasting from 1 day to 4 weeks and involving one or two joints. About 25% of patients with CPPD-deposition disease have an acute onset of gout-like symptoms, presenting as inflammation and swelling of the knees, ankles, wrists, elbows, hips, or shoulders. Metatarsophalangeal joints, which are frequently affected in gout, are usually spared. The synovial fluid exhibits abundant leukocytes containing CPPD crystals.
- **Pseudorheumatoid arthritis** is a variant of CPPD-deposition disease in which multiple joints are chronically involved. The symptoms are mild and resemble those of RA.
- **Pseudo-osteoarthritis** has symptoms similar to those of osteoarthritis.
- **Pseudoneurotrophic disease** is characterized by joint destruction so severe as to resemble a neurotrophic joint.

On gross examination, calcium pyrophosphate deposits appear as chalky white areas on the cartilaginous surfaces (Fig. 26-64). Unlike needle-shaped urate crystals, they are stubby, short, and rhomboid ("coffin shaped") and are only weakly birefringent under polarized light. In contrast to urate crystals, CPPD crystals do not dissolve in water and are easily found in tissue sections. Only a few mononuclear cells and macrophages surround the foci of crystal deposition.

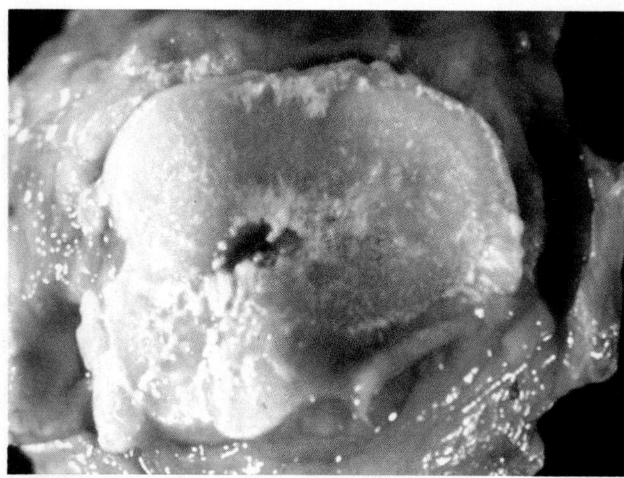

FIGURE *26-64*
Calcium pyrophosphate–deposition disease. A degenerated patella exhibits deposits of chalky-white calcific material on its surface.

Calcium Hydroxyapatite–Deposition Disease

Calcium hydroxyapatite–deposition disease is an acute or chronic arthritis characterized by hydroxyapatite crystals within leukocytes and mononuclear cells in joint tissue and synovial fluid. Calcium hydroxyapatite (HA) is the major mineral of bone and teeth and is the compound deposited in dystrophic and metastatic calcification. Hydroxyapatite crystals are frequently encountered in the synovial fluid of joints involved by osteoarthritis, but there is reason to believe that severe HA deposition is a distinct entity. The joints most frequently involved are the knee, shoulder, hip, and fingers. Attacks may last several days.

HEMOPHILIA, HEMOCHROMATOSIS, AND OCHRONOSIS

Hemophilia, hemochromatosis, and ochronosis (see Chapter 6) all produce joint disease with degradation of the matrix and destruction of the articular cartilage.

Hemophilia gives rise to severe forms of arthritis because of extensive bleeding into joints (hemarthrosis), particularly the knees, elbows, ankles, shoulders, and hips. In addition to the effects within the articular cartilage matrix, synovial proliferation also simulates RA.

Hemochromatosis is complicated by arthritis in half of affected patients. The hands, hips, and knees may be involved in recurrent attacks.

Ochronosis is a rare, autosomal recessive disease caused by a defect in homogentisic acid oxidase. The deposition of ochronotic pigment in the cartilage of the joints, including the intravertebral disks, eventually causes them to become brittle and to degenerate.

TUMORS AND TUMOR-LIKE LESIONS OF JOINTS

True neoplasms of the joints are rare. The most common malignant lesions of the synovium are metastatic carcinomas, particularly adenocarcinoma of the colon, breast, and lung. Lymphoproliferative diseases (e.g., leukemia) may also involve the synovium, mimicking other conditions, such as RA. It is unusual for primary malignant bone tumors to extend into the joint, although they may invade the joint capsule from the soft tissues.

Ganglion

A ganglion is a thin-walled, simple cyst containing clear mucinous fluid, which occurs most commonly on the extensor surfaces of the hands and feet, especially the wrist. The cyst arises either from the synovium or from areas of myxoid change in the connective tissue, possibly after trauma. If the lesion is painful, it can be readily removed surgically, although a ganglion on the dorsum of the wrist was traditionally treated by a blow with the family Bible.

Baker cyst refers to a herniation of the synovium of the knee joint into the popliteal space. It is most often seen in association with various forms of arthritis, in which the intra-articular pressure is increased.

Synovial Chondromatosis

Synovial chondromatosis is a benign, self-limited disease in which hyaline cartilage nodules, which form in the synovium, detach from that structure, and float in the synovial fluid, in a manner similar to grains of sand between gears. The chronic irritation produced by these foreign bodies stimulates the synovium to secrete large amounts of synovial fluid and also causes bleeding in the synovial membrane. Synovial chondromatosis involves the large diarthrodial joints of young and middle-aged men, affecting the knee in most cases, but also the hip, elbow, shoulder, and ankle. Patients have pain, stiffness, and locking of the joint, with associated bloody effusions.

Unlike the cartilage that detaches from the articular surface in osteoarthritis, in synovial chondromatosis, fragments of hyaline cartilage are formed *de novo* in the synovium. Therefore, they do not have a tide mark and thus differ from true articular cartilage. Occasionally, the cartilage nodules, while still residing in the synovium, undergo endochondral ossification, in which case, the disease is called *synovial osteochondromatosis*. If these nodules detach, the bony portions die, but the cartilage fragments remain viable and enlarge because they are nourished by synovial fluid. The condition is treated by evacuating the joint and performing a partial synovectomy.

Pigmented Villonodular Synovitis

Pigmented villonodular synovitis, despite its obsolete name, is a benign neoplasm of the synovial lining characterized by an exuberant proliferation of synovial lining cells with extension into the subsynovial tissue. This tumor involves a single joint, usually occurs in young adults, and is equally distributed between male and female subjects. The most common site (80%) is the knee, although pigmented villonodular synovitis also occurs in the hip, ankles, calcaneocuboid joint, elbow, and tendon sheaths of the fingers and toes.

The tumors arise on the synovium of tendon sheaths, bursae, and diarthrodial joints. The lesions of pigmented villonodular synovitis invade the joint and erode the bone. They may insinuate through joint capsules into soft tissue and encompass nerves and arteries, sometimes necessitating radical surgical excision. The synovium develops enlarged folds and nodular excres-

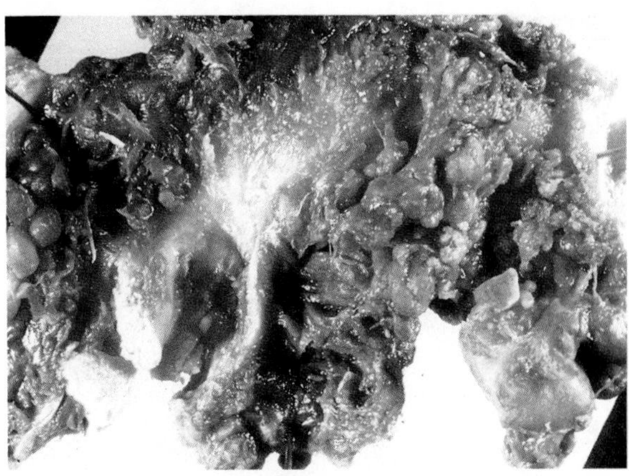

A

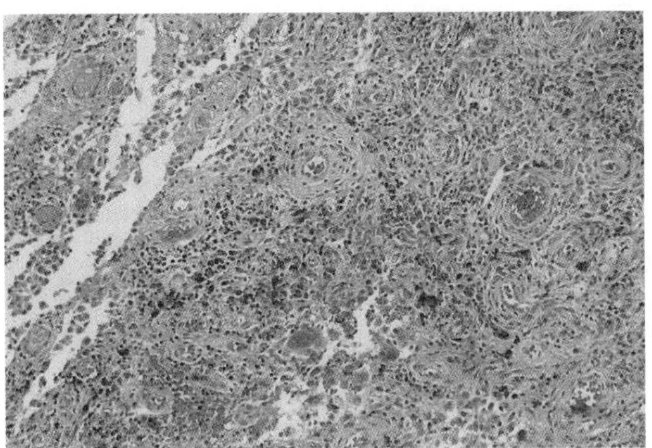

B

FIGURE *26-65*
Pigmented villonodular synovitis. (*A*) A specimen of synovium exhibits the characteristic pigmented, thickened, opaque, and nodular appearance. (*B*) A microscopic section reveals an infiltrate of mononuclear cells, many of which contain hemosiderin pigment, and a number of giant cells.

cences (Fig 26-65A). Microscopically, the tumor is composed of bland mononuclear cells with scattered multinucleated giant cells, in which the nuclei are arrayed peripherally. Hemosiderin-laden macrophages reflect previous hemorrhage (see Fig. 26-65B).

Localized nodular synovitis is a similar condition of the knee that involves only one portion of the synovium rather than the entire membrane. The symptoms are limited to pain, joint locking, and joint effusions.

Localized nodular tenosynovitis, also called **giant cell tumor of the tendon sheath**, involves the tendon sheaths of the hands and feet. **It is the most common soft tissue tumor of the hand.** The lesion occurs mostly in young and middle-aged women and involves the flexor surface of the middle or index finger.

The treatment for all forms of pigmented villonodular synovitis is surgical. Radiation therapy produces fibrosis of the proliferating synovial tissue, but amputation is occasionally necessary.

Soft Tissue Tumors

The term soft tissue tumor refers to neoplastic conditions that arise in certain extraskeletal mesodermal tissues of the body, including skeletal muscle, fat, fibrous tissue, blood, and lymphatic vessels. Tumors of peripheral nerves are included in the category of soft tissue tumors, despite their derivation from the neuroectoderm.

In the context of soft tissue tumors, the term benign is relative, because so-called benign tumors may have a limited capacity for invasive growth and may recur locally. By definition, a *benign* soft tissue tumor does not metastasize. Malignant soft tissue tumors are usually highly invasive and metastasize and are often associated with a poor prognosis. Soft tissue tumors are rare, accounting for less than 1% of all cancers in the United States. Benign soft tissue neoplasms are 100 times more common than malignant ones.

Trauma is occasionally ascribed a causative role in the pathogenesis of soft tissue tumors, usually in cases in which possible compensation is involved. However, there is no evidence to support such a correlation with trauma, and the injury simply draws attention to a preexisting tumor. Burns in childhood produce scars, which in rare instances lead to soft tissue fibroblastic tumors many years later. Radiation injury has been reported to be associated with the development of sarcomas years after exposure. A group of genetic disorders that are associated with soft tissue tumors includes neurofibromatosis type 1, tuberous sclerosis, Osler–Weber–Rendu disease, and mesenteric fibromatosis in Gardner syndrome.

A few important general principles relate to soft tissue tumors:

- Deep lesions tend to be malignant.
- The more superficial the location of the tumor, the more likely it is to be benign.
- Larger tumors tend to be malignant more often than small ones.
- A rapidly growing tumor is more likely to be malignant than one that develops slowly.
- Calcification may exist in both benign and malignant tumors.
- Benign tumors are relatively avascular, whereas most malignant ones are hypervascular.

The classification of soft tissue tumors is based primarily on the pattern of differentiation of the neoplastic cells. For example, a tumor that produces collagen may be called a benign fibroma or fibromatosis, whereas its malignant counterpart is called a fibrosarcoma. Similarly, a tumor of fat cells is either a benign lipoma or a liposarcoma.

TUMORS AND TUMOR-LIKE CONDITIONS OF FIBROUS ORIGIN

Nodular Fasciitis

Nodular fasciitis is a benign but rapidly growing reactive lesion, which is probably the result of trauma and commonly affects the forearm, trunk, and back (Fig. 26-66). Most cases occur in adults, and the rapid growth of this lesion usually prompts the patient to seek medical attention. Histologically, nodular fasciitis may be mistaken for a sarcoma, because it is hypercellular and has abundant mitoses and numerous, pleomorphic, spindle-shaped cells. Its true nature is defined when it is recognized that the entire "mass" is the counterpart of granulation tissue in response to trauma. The lesion is self-limited and is cured by surgical excision.

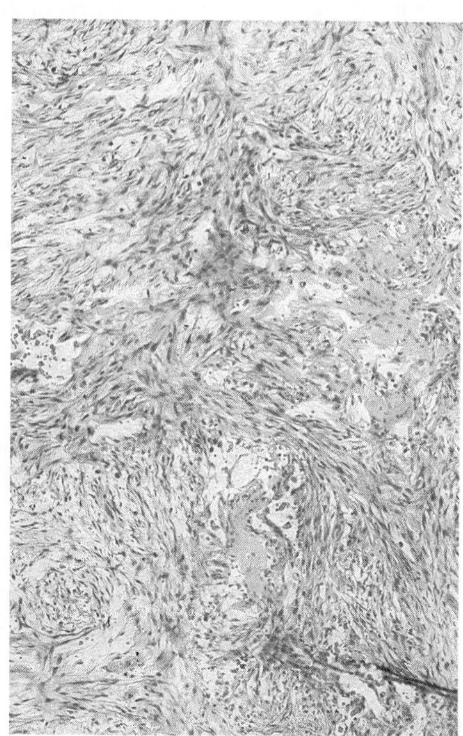

FIGURE *26-66*
Nodular fasciitis. Swirls of tightly woven spindle cells and collagen are admixed with a few lymphoid cells and vascular channels.

Fibromatosis

Fibromatosis, also known as "desmoid tumor," is a locally invasive, slowly growing, collagenous mass, which may occur virtually anywhere in the body. Although they do not metastasize, the lesions of fibromatosis are locally aggressive, and surgical resection is often followed by a local recurrence. An increased incidence of fibromatosis has been reported in diabetics, alcoholics, and epileptics. Therefore, this "tumor" may represent a reaction to repeated trauma at a specific site.

☐ **Pathology:** On gross examination, the lesions of fibromatosis tend to be large, firm, and whitish, with poorly demarcated borders and a whorled cut surface. They frequently originate in a muscular fascia. Microscopic examination reveals sheets and interdigitating fascicles of benign-appearing spindle cells (fibroblasts) with little mitotic activity. Because microscopic tongues of tumor extend between preexisting structures, surgical "shelling out" of the lesion is followed by recurrences in half of the cases. Complete surgical excision is curative.

Specific forms of fibromatosis are identified by their characteristic locations:

- **Palmar fibromatosis** (Dupuytren contracture) is the single most common form of fibromatosis, occurring in 1% to 2% of the general population, but in as many as 20% of persons older than 65 years. In half the cases, the lesion is bilateral, and in 10% of cases, it is associated with fibromatosis in other locations. Fibrous nodules and cord-like bands in the palmar fascia eventually lead to flexion contractures of the fingers, particularly the fourth and fifth digits.
- **Plantar fibromatosis** is similar to palmar fibromatosis, except that it is less frequent and involves the plantar aponeurosis.
- **Penile fibromatosis (Peyronie disease)** is the least common of the localized fibromatoses and is characterized by an induration of, or mass in, the shaft of the penis, causing it to curve toward the affected side (penile strabismus). The lesion leads to urethral obstruction and pain on erection.

Fibrosarcoma

Fibrosarcoma is a malignant tumor of fibroblasts, which is most commonly found in the thigh, particularly around the knee. This neoplasm typically occurs in adults, although it may be encountered in any age group and may even be congenital. Fibrosarcomas arise from connective tissue, such as fascia, scar tissue, periosteum, and tendons. Macroscopically, the tumors are sharply demarcated and frequently exhibit necrosis and hemorrhage. They are characterized histologically by pleomorphic fibroblasts (Fig. 26-67), which often form densely interlacing bundles and fascicles, producing a "herringbone" pattern. The prognosis for fibrosarcoma is at best guarded, the survival at 5 years being only 40% and that at 10 years 30%. Poorly differentiated fibrosarcomas have a worse prognosis than better differentiated ones.

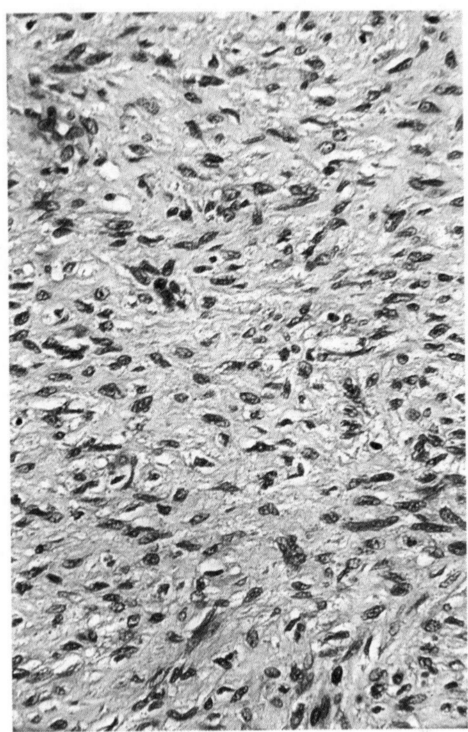

FIGURE *26-67*
Fibrosarcoma. A photomicrograph demonstrates irregularly arranged neoplastic fibroblasts.

Malignant Fibrous Histiocytoma

Malignant fibrous histiocytoma (MFH) is a soft tissue tumor that contains foci of histiocytic (macrophage) differentiation. It is the most common type of soft tissue sarcoma and is the most frequent sarcoma encountered after radiation therapy. MFH typically occurs in older adults, but cases have been recorded at all ages. In half of the cases, MFH arises in the deep fascia or within a skeletal muscle, and the tumor has been reported in association with surgical scars and foreign bodies.

☐ **Pathology:** Histologically, MFH displays a highly variable morphological pattern, with areas of spindle-shaped tumor cells arrayed in an irregularly whorled (storiform) pattern adjacent to pleomorphic fields (Fig. 26-68). The spindle cells tend to be well differentiated and resemble fibroblasts. There are occasional plump cells (histiocytes), abundant mitoses, a few xanthomatous (lipid-laden) cells, and a moderate chronic inflammatory reaction. Some tumors contain numerous tumor giant cells, which exhibit an intense eosinophilia. The extent of collagen deposition is variable, and sometimes dominates the microscopic pattern. A few tumors reveal a conspicuous myxoid stroma.

The prognosis of MFH depends on the degree of cytological atypia. Almost half of the patients develop a local recurrence after surgery, and a comparable proportion later manifest metastatic disease, particularly in the lungs.

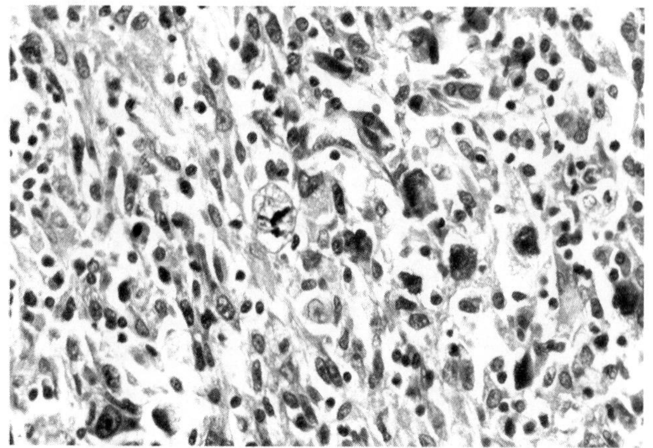

FIGURE *26-68*
Malignant fibrous histiocytoma. An anaplastic tumor exhibits spindle cells, plump lipid-laden histiocytes, tumor giant cells, an abnormal mitosis (*center*), and a mild chronic inflammatory infiltrate.

TUMORS OF ADIPOSE TISSUE

LIPOMA: This benign, circumscribed tumor is composed of well-differentiated adipocytes and is the most common soft tissue mass. The tumor can originate at any site in the body that contains adipose tissue, but most appear in the subcutaneous tissues of the upper half of the body, especially on the trunk and neck. Lipomas are encountered mainly in adults, and patients with multiple tumors often have relatives with a similar history.

☐ **Pathology:** On gross examination, lipomas are encapsulated, soft, yellow lesions, which vary in size and may become very large. Deeper tumors are often poorly circumscribed. Histologically, a lipoma is often indistinguishable from normal adipose tissue. Lipomas are adequately treated by simple local excision.

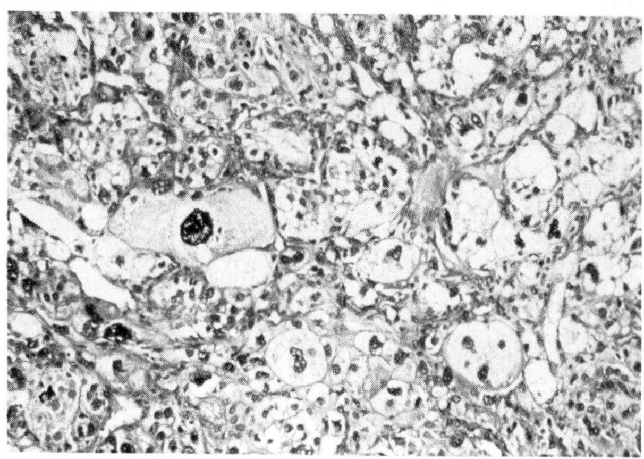

FIGURE *26-69*
Liposarcoma. Large pleomorphic cells with bizarre nuclei and vacuolated cytoplasm are evident.

ANGIOLIPOMA: This term refers to a small, well-circumscribed, subcutaneous lipoma that exhibits extensive vascular proliferation and usually appears shortly after puberty. Angiolipoma is often multiple and painful.

LIPOSARCOMA: The second most common sarcoma in adults, liposarcoma composes 20% of all malignant soft tissue tumors. The neoplasm arises after age 50 years and is most frequent in the deep thigh and retroperitoneum. Liposarcomas tend to grow slowly but may become extremely large.

The myxoid variant of liposarcoma (see later) is another example of the growing list of human cancers that are associated with specific chromosomal translocations that result in the synthesis of abnormal fusion protein. In the case of liposarcoma, most tumors exhibit a translocation between chromosomes 12 and 16, t(12;16)(q13;p11), in which the TLS/FUS gene on chromosome 16 is fused with the CHOP gene on chromosome 12. The TLS/FUS gene product is a novel RNA-binding protein with substantial homology to the EWS protein of Ewing sarcoma, whereas the CHOP protein is a transcriptional repressor.

On gross examination, the typical liposarcoma measures 5 to 10 cm in diameter, although examples measuring 40 cm in diameter and weighing is excess of 50 pounds have been encountered. On cut section, the appearance of the tumor is variable, depending on the proportions of adipose, mucinous, and fibrous tissue. Poorly differentiated liposarcomas grossly appear similar to brain tissue and display necrosis, hemorrhage, and cysts. Microscopically, the most common pattern is one of variably differentiated, "signet ring" lipoblasts embedded in a vascularized myxoid stroma (Fig. 26-69). Poorly differentiated liposarcomas show uniform round cells with vesicular nuclei, which may be difficult to distinguish from other small cell sarcomas. Well-differentiated liposarcomas can be confused with lipomas.

Local recurrence rates and metastases after surgery are high for round cell and pleomorphic liposarcomas, and the 5-year survival for these tumors is less than 20%. By contrast, the 5-year survival for patients with well-differentiated and myxoid tumors exceeds 70%.

RHABDOMYOSARCOMA

Rhabdomyosarcoma is a malignant tumor that displays features of striated muscle differentiation. It is uncommon in mature adults, but is the most frequent soft tissue sarcoma of children and young adults. The histogenesis of rhabdomyosarcoma is controversial, but it is probable that most of these tumors derive from primitive mesenchyme that has retained the capacity for skeletal muscle differentiation. Alternatively, rhabdomyosarcoma may arise from embryonal muscle tissue that is displaced into the soft tissues during embryogenesis.

☐ **Pathology:** Most cases of rhabdomyosarcoma can be classified according to four histological categories.

EMBRYONAL RHABDOMYOSARCOMA: This form is most common in children between the ages of 3 and 12 years and frequently involves the head and neck, genitourinary tract, and retroperitoneum. The morphological appearance varies from that of a highly differentiated tumor containing rhabdomyoblasts, with large eosinophilic cytoplasm and cross-striations (Fig. 26-70A), to that of a poorly differentiated neoplasm, which is difficult to classify.

BOTRYOID EMBRYONAL RHABDOMYOSARCOMA: This tumor, also known as *sarcoma botryoides*, is distinguished by the formation of polypoid, grape-like tumor masses. Microscopically, the malignant cells are scattered in an abundant myxoid stroma. Botryoid foci may occur in any type of embryonal rhabdomyosarcoma, but they are most common in tumors of hollow visceral organs, including the vagina (see Chapter 18) and the bladder.

ALVEOLAR RHABDOMYOSARCOMA: This neoplasm occurs less frequently than the embryonal type and principally affects young persons between ages 10 and 25 years. It is most common in the upper and lower extremities, but it can also be distributed in the same sites as the embryonal type. Typically, club-shaped tumor cells are arranged in clumps that are outlined by fibrous septa. The loose arrangement of the cells in the center of the clusters leads to the "alveolar" pattern (see Fig. 26-70B). The tumor cells exhibit an intense eosinophilia, and occasional multinucleated giant cells are identified. Malignant rhabdomyoblasts, recognizable by their cross-striations, occur less commonly in the alveolar variant than in embryonal rhabdomyosarcoma, being present in only 25% of cases.

PLEOMORPHIC RHABDOMYOSARCOMA: The least common form of rhabdomyosarcoma is found in the skeletal muscles of older persons, often in the thigh. This tumor differs from the other types of rhabdomyosarcoma in the pleomorphism of its irregularly arranged cells. Large, granular, and eosinophilic rhabdomyoblasts, together with multinucleated giant cells, are common. Cross-striations are virtually nonexistent.

The previously dismal prognosis associated with most rhabdomyosarcomas has improved in the past 2 decades as a result of the introduction of combined therapeutic modalities, including surgery, radiation therapy, and chemotherapy. Today, more than 80% of patients with localized or regional disease are cured.

SMOOTH MUSCLE TUMORS

LEIOMYOMA: This benign soft tissue tumor usually arises in the subcutaneous tissues or from the walls of blood vessels. Leiomyomas are painful lesions, which appear as firm, yellow, circumscribed nodules. Microscopically, intersecting fascicles of regular smooth cells are evident. Simple excision is curative.

LEIOMYOSARCOMA: This malignant soft tissue neoplasm is an uncommon tumor of adults, which typically arises in the extremities from the wall of blood vessels. Macroscopically, leiomyosarcomas tend to be well circumscribed, but they are larger and softer than leiomyomas and often exhibit necrosis, hemorrhage, and cystic degeneration. Histologically, the tumor cells are arranged in fascicles, often with palisaded nuclei. Well-differentiated tumor cells have elongated nuclei and eosinophilic cytoplasm, whereas poorly differentiated ones may show severe nuclear atypism. Leiomyosarcoma is differentiated from leiomyoma mainly by a high mitotic activity, which is also an indicator of prognosis. The majority of leiomyosarcomas eventually metastasize, although dissemination may be seen as late as 15 or more years after resection of the primary tumor.

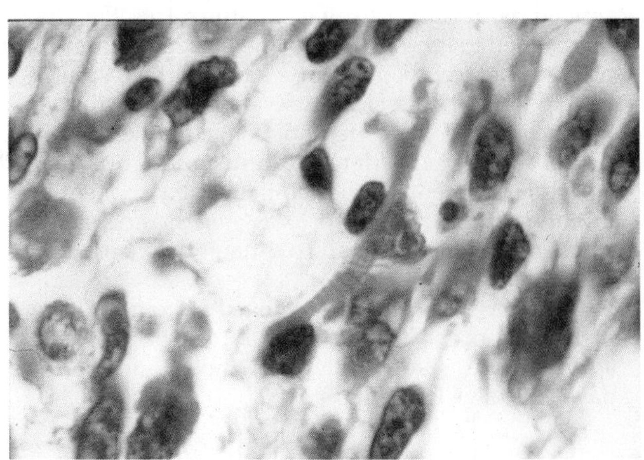

A

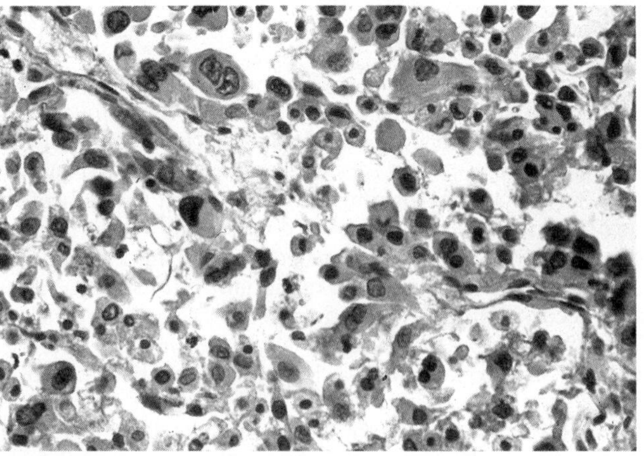

B

FIGURE *26-70*
Rhabdomyosarcoma. (*A*) Embryonal rhabdomyosarcoma. The center of the field shows a well-differentiated rhabdomyoblast with cross-striations. (*B*) Alveolar rhabdomyosarcoma. The neoplastic cells are arranged in clusters that display an alveolar pattern.

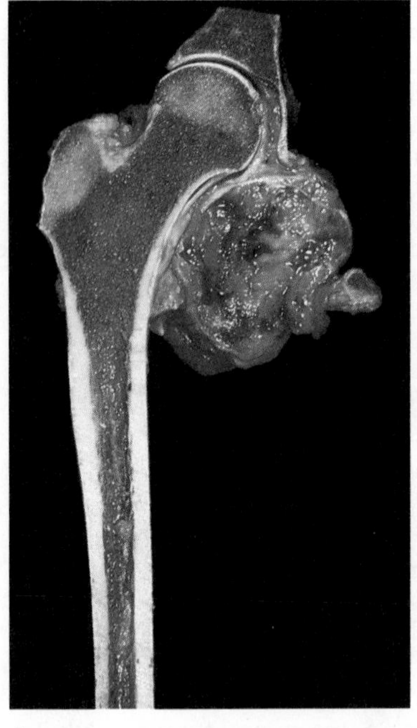

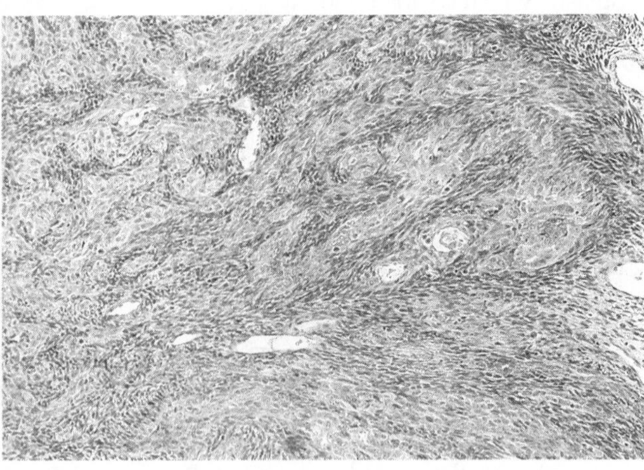

FIGURE *26-71*
Synovial sarcoma. (*A*) A section of the upper femur and acetabulum reveals a tumor adjacent to the hip joint and the neck of the femur. (*B*) A microscopic view demonstrates the biphasic appearance of a synovial sarcoma. Irregular spaces are lined by plump, synovial-like neoplastic cells. The intervening tissue contains cells with similar nuclei.

VASCULAR TUMORS

Benign vascular tumors (hemangiomas) are among the most common soft tissue tumors and are the most frequent neoplasms of infancy and childhood. By contrast, angiosarcomas are among the rarest of soft tissue tumors, accounting for fewer than 1% of all sarcomas. Vascular tumors are discussed in detail in Chapter 10.

SYNOVIAL SARCOMA

Synovial sarcoma is a highly malignant soft tissue tumor that arises in the region of a joint, usually in association with tendon sheaths, bursae, and joint capsules. Fewer than 10% of synovial sarcomas are intra-articular. Although the tumor bears a microscopic resemblance to the synovium, its origin from this tissue has not been established. Synovial sarcoma accounts for 10% of malignant soft tissue tumors and occurs principally in adolescents and young adults. The tumor typically is seen as a painful or tender mass, usually in the vicinity of a large joint, particularly the knee.

Synovial sarcomas contain a characteristic and specific, balanced chromosomal translocation involving chromosomes X and 18 [t(x;18)(p11.2;q11.2)]. This translocation results in the fusion of the SYT (synteny) gene on chromosome 18 to the SSX gene (a transcriptional repressor) on the X chromosome, leading to the production of a hybrid protein, SYT-SSX.

☐ **Pathology:** On gross examination, synovial sarcomas are usually circumscribed, round or multilobular masses attached to tendons, tendon sheaths, or the exterior wall of the joint capsule (Fig. 26-71A). The tumors tend to be surrounded by a glistening pseudocapsule and in many instances are cystic. They range from small nodules to masses of 15 cm or more in diameter, the average being 3 to 5 cm.

Microscopically, synovial sarcoma is classically described as having a **biphasic pattern** (see Fig. 26-71B). Fluid-filled glandular spaces lined by epithelium-like tumor cells are embedded in a sarcomatous, spindle cell background. These elements vary in proportion, distribution, and cellular differentiation, with the spindle cells usually being considerably more numerous than the glandular elements. If the "epithelial" component is lacking, the tumor is referred to as *monophasic synovial sarcoma* and may be difficult to differentiate from fibrosarcoma.

The recurrence rate of synovial sarcoma is high, and metastases occur in more than 60% of cases. The 5-year survival rate is about 50%, and those who die usually have extensive lung metastases.

SUGGESTED READING

BOOKS

Avioli LV, Krane SM (eds): *Metabolic diseases and clinically related disorders,* 3rd ed. Philadelphia: WB Saunders, 1997.

Collins DH: *Pathology of bone.* London: Butterworth, 1966.

Enzinger FM, Weiss SW: *Soft tissue tumors,* 2nd ed. St. Louis: CV Mosby, 1988.

Farvus M (ed): *Primer on the metabolic bone diseases and disorders of mineral metabolism.* : American Society for Bone and Mineral Research, 1990.

Kelley WN, Harris ED Jr, Ruddy S, Sledge CB: *Textbook of rheumatology,* 5th ed. Philadelphia: WB Saunders, 1997.

Marcus R, Feldman D, Kelsey J (eds): *Osteoporosis.* San Diego: Academic Press, 1996.

Rodman GP, Shumacher HR (eds): *Primer in the rheumatic diseases,* 8th ed. Atlanta: Arthritis Foundation, 1983.

Scriver CR, Beaudet AL, Sly SW, Valle D (eds): *The metabolic basis of inherited disease,* 6th ed. New York: McGraw-Hill, 1989.

Spjut HJ, Dorfman HD, Fechner RE, Ackerman LV: *Tumors of bone and cartilage,* fascicle 5. Washington, DC: Armed Forces Institute of Pathology, 1971.

REVIEW ARTICLES

Gallacher SJ: Paget disease of bone. *Curr Opin Rheumatol* 5:351–356, 1993.

Glimcher MJ: On the form and function of bone: From molecules to organs: Wolff's law revisited. In: Veis A (ed): *Chemistry and biology of mineralized connective tissue.* New York: Elsevier-North Holland, 1981.

Hruska KA, Teitelbaum SL: Renal osteodystrophy. *N Engl J Med* 333:166–174, 1995.

Inman RD, Scofield RH: Etiopathogenesis of ankylosing spondylitis and reactive arthritis. *Curr Opin Rheumatol* 6:360–370, 1994.

Manolagas AC, Jilka RL: Bone marrow, cytokines, and bone remodeling: Emerging insights into the pathophysiology of osteoporosis. *N Engl J Med* 332:305–311, 1995.

Marcus R: Normal and abnormal bone remodeling in man. *Annu Rev Med* 38:129–143, 1987.

Schiller AL: Diagnosis of borderline cartilage lesions of bone. *Semin Diagn Pathol* 2:42–61, 1985.

Sledge CB: Structure, development, and function of joints. *Orthop Clin North Am* 6:619–629, 1975.

CHAPTER 27

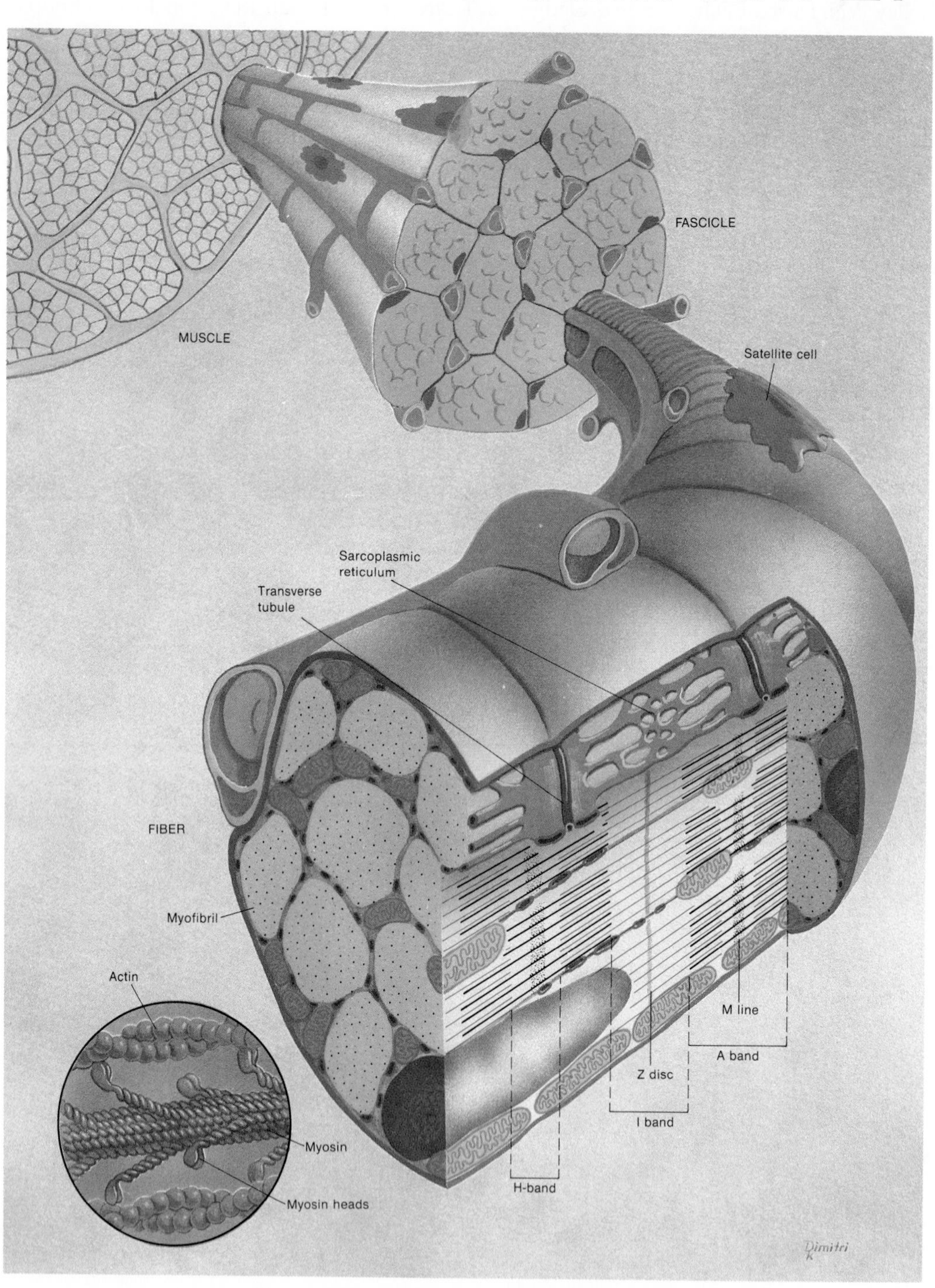

MUSCLE
FASCICLE
Satellite cell
Sarcoplasmic reticulum
Transverse tubule
FIBER
Myofibril
Actin
Myosin
Myosin heads
H-band
I band
Z disc
A band
M line
Dimitri K

Skeletal Muscle

Arthur P. Hays
Vernon W. Armbrustmacher

continued

FIGURE 27-1 *(see opposite page)*
Anatomy of skeletal muscle. The composite drawing demonstrates the morphological features of striated muscle from grossly visible to macromolecular levels. In the upper left, a portion of a muscle is contained by a distinct outer connective tissue layer, called the epimysium or fascia. Fascicles are groups of muscle fibers separated by connective tissue septa called perimysium. Within the fascicle, individual muscle fibers (myofibers) are closely packed and are surrounded by an intricate array of microvasculature and a barely perceptible network of connective tissue called the endomysium. The enlarged fascicle also shows scattered, flattened cells (*green*), called satellite cells, lying on the surface of the fiber. Each muscle fiber is covered by a basement membrane (*orange*) and packed with bundles of myofilaments called myofibrils. The endoplasmic reticulum (sarcoplasmic reticulum) forms an extensive, complex tubular network with periodic dilatations (cisternae) around each myofibril. The cisternae are closely apposed to the transverse tubules, which are derived from the cell membrane (sarcolemma) and form a transverse network, which resembles chicken wire, around each myofibril, giving extensive communication between the internal and external environments. The cross-striations of striated muscle are created by the arrangement of the myofilaments of the myofibril. The dark A-band results from the thick myosin filaments and the thinner, partially overlapping actin filaments. In the middle portion of the myosin filaments where the actin does not overlap, there is a lighter band called the H-zone or H-band. In the middle of the H-band, the center of each myosin filament thickens, forming intermolecular bridging with the adjacent myosin filament and giving rise to the M-line. The finer actin filaments are anchored on the dark Z-disc of the lighter I-band. With contraction, the myosin filaments pull the actin filaments, causing the H-zone to disappear, the A-band to widen, and the I-band to shrink. The mitochondria are scattered throughout the sarcoplasm among the myofibrils. In the final enlargement, the myosin filament is covered with myosin heads that attach to receptor sites on the surrounding actin filaments. The movement of these heads, with attachment and detachment, pulls the actin filaments, ratchet fashion, past the myosin filament.

Inherited Metabolic Diseases

Glycogen Storage Diseases (Glycogenoses)

Lipid Myopathies

Mitochondrial Diseases

Myoadenylate Deaminase Deficiency

Familial Periodic Paralysis

Rhabdomyolysis

Denervation

Spinal Muscular Atrophy

Type II Fiber Atrophy

EMBRYOLOGY AND ANATOMY

The myoblast is a primitive cell committed to developing into skeletal muscle. The myoblast develops the capacity to fuse with other myoblasts to form a multinucleated myotube. This structure soon assumes a cylindrical configuration, with its nuclei arranged centrally along the longitudinal axis. The periphery of the myotube rapidly accumulates myofibrils, composed of myosin and actin, among other proteins. Myosin and actin become arrayed in the cross-banded pattern characteristic of striated muscle (Fig. 27-1).

The myotube does not mature completely until it is innervated by the terminal axon of a lower motor neuron. Before innervation, the sarcolemma of the myotube contains diffusely distributed nicotinic receptors for acetylcholine on its surface membrane. When innervation occurs, these receptors (now designated *extrajunctional receptors*) disappear from the sarcolemma, except at the developing motor end plate, where they become highly concentrated. Although an individual muscle fiber is innervated by only a single nerve ending, a given motor neuron innervates numerous muscle fibers.

Structure of the Myofiber

Only after innervation has occurred does the muscle fiber progress to maturity. The nuclei of each fiber move from the center to arrange themselves in a regular pattern beneath the sarcolemma (see Fig. 27-3A). The myofiber has a distinctive architecture that is visualized by electron microscopy. Muscle contraction is produced by the sliding of the actin filaments past the myosin filaments (see Figs. 27-1 and 27-2). A few definitions are in order.

- **Sarcomere:** The functional unit of the myofibril is the sarcomere, which extends from one Z-band to the next.
- **Z-band:** This is a distinct electron-dense band that anchors the thin actin filaments.
- **I-band:** This zone consists of the actin filaments as they extend from the Z-band into the A-band.
- **A-band:** This structure is composed of the thick myosin filaments. The actin filaments overlap the myosin filaments to a variable extent, depending on the degree of muscle contraction. The thin filaments form a hexagonal array around each thick filament.
- **H-zone:** This is a pale region in the midportion of the A-band where the actin filaments end.
- **M-line:** At the midline of the A-band, a zone of intermolecular bridging and thickening of the myosin filaments forms a thin, slightly darker electron-dense band, designated the M-line.

During contraction, the sliding actin filaments advance farther into the A-band, producing a shorter sarcomere length. As a result, the lengths of the I-band and H-zone decrease, whereas that of the A-band remains nearly constant.

The sarcoplasmic reticulum surrounds each myofibril and forms an elaborate membranous network that has irregular dilatations (cisternae) juxtaposed to a transverse tubular network derived from the sarcolemma. The transverse tubular system (T-system) is arranged across the fiber-like chicken wire, each ring wrapping around an individual myofibril (see Fig. 27-1). This arrangement allows an electrical stimulus to proceed along the surface of the muscle fiber and to become diffusely and rapidly internalized by way of the transverse tubular system. The electrical signal is translated into a chemical signal between the transverse tubule and the cisternae of the sarcoplasmic reticulum. This process releases calcium from the sarcoplasmic reticulum into the vicinity of myofibrils, where the chemical signal triggers muscle contraction.

The lower motor neuron and the fibers that it innervates are referred to as the motor unit. The size of a motor unit varies. In limb muscles, a single motor unit can comprise as many as several hundred myofibers. By contrast, each motor unit of the extraocular muscles may have as few as 20 myofibers. The muscles of the eye are also exceptional because a single fiber may have more than one motor end plate.

Myofiber Types

After innervation, a characteristic metabolic profile develops for different muscle fibers. In lower mammals, some muscles have a deep red color (type I), whereas others are pale (type II).

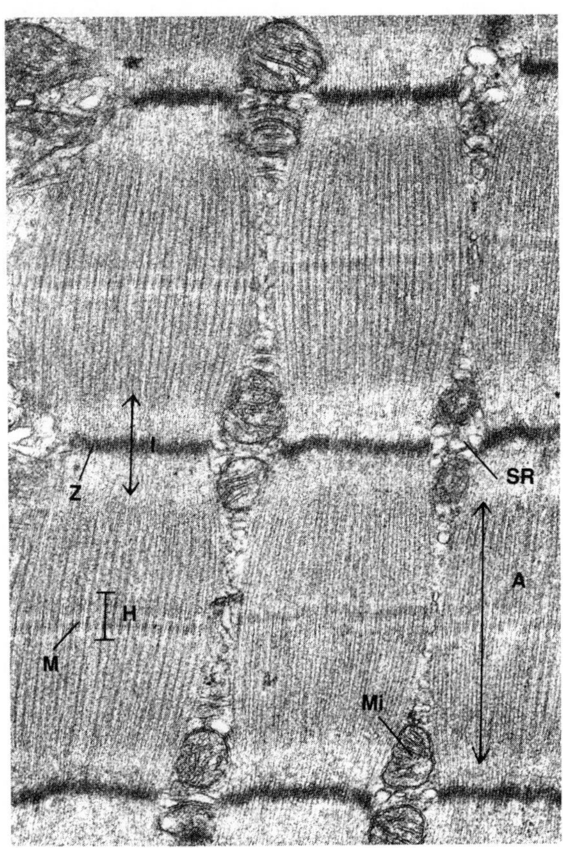

FIGURE 27-2
Normal muscle. This electron micrograph of the biceps muscle shows that each parallel bundle of filaments is a myofibril. The thin dark band, the Z-disc (*Z*), bisects the broad, pale I-band (*I*), a zone composed of the thin actin filaments. The broad, dark band, made up of the thick myosin filaments and overlapping actin filaments, is the A-band (*A*). The middle of the A-band consists of the pale H-zone (*H*), which in turn is bisected by a slightly darker M-line (*M*), representing a zone of intermolecular bridging of myosin. Small membrane-bound vesicles compose the sarcoplasmic reticulum (*SR*) and the transverse tubules. Pairs of mitochondria (*Mi*) tend to be located between myofibrils at the level of the I-bands.

TYPE I FIBERS (RED, SLOW TWITCH): If a nerve stimulates a dark (red) muscle, the resulting contraction is slower and more prolonged than when a nerve excites a pale (white) muscle. For this reason, red muscles have been classified as "slow twitch." Type I fibers tend to have more oxygen-storing red pigment (myoglobin) and more numerous mitochondria. The corresponding mitochondrial enzymes of the Krebs cycle and the carrier proteins of the electron-transport chain are all present in greater amounts in the red, slow-twitch muscle than in the white, fast-twitch muscle. The genes that encode myosin and other contractile proteins of type I fibers differ from those expressed in type II fibers. These differences provide the molecular basis for the alkaline histochemical reaction for myosin adenosine triphosphatase (ATPase), which gives a crisp distinction between the two fiber types. Type I fibers remain almost unstained (Fig. 27-3).

Functionally, type I muscles have a greater capacity for long, sustained contractions, and they resist fatigue. A training program to increase endurance produces little change in size of type I fibers, but conditioning of these fibers results in a proliferation of mitochondria and an expanded capacity for generating energy.

TYPE II FIBERS (WHITE, FAST TWITCH): Stimulation of type II fibers elicits a faster, shorter, and more powerful contraction than occurs in type I fibers. Glycogen, phosphorylase, and other enzymes in the Embden–Meyerhof pathway, which produce energy by anaerobic glycolysis, are present in higher concentrations in white muscle. Type II fibers stain darkly for ATPase.

Type II muscle fibers are suitable for rapid contractions of brief duration and react to training for strength with hypertrophy. Androgenic steroids induce hypertrophy of type II fibers, and disuse of the muscle results in their selective atrophy.

The lower motor neuron greatly influences fiber type. During embryonic development of mammals, the early muscle cells begin to express type-specific contractile proteins before muscle is innervated. Thus, the phenotype of a myofiber seems to be a genetically determined property of the cell, rather than one that is determined by the nerve supply. However, the innervation of muscle can alter the types of myofibers. For example, after denervation injury, the reinnervation of a slow-twitch muscle by the nerve from a fast-twitch muscle causes the newly in-

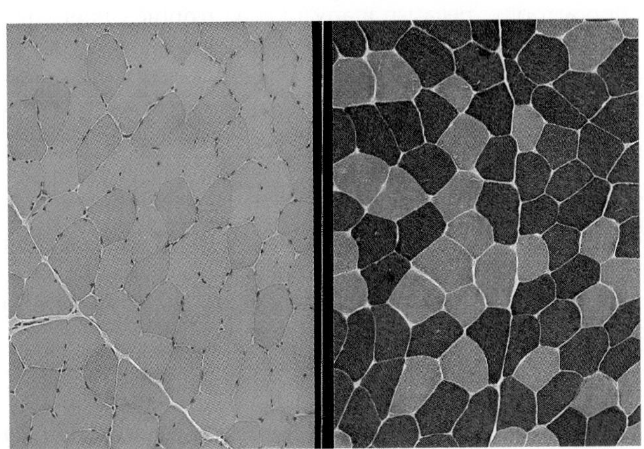

FIGURE 27-3
Normal muscle. (*A*) Hematoxylin and eosin stain. In this transverse frozen section of the vastus lateralis, the polygonal myofibers are separated from each other by an indistinct, thin layer of connective tissue, the endomysium. The thicker band of connective tissue, the perimysium, demarcates a bundle or fascicle of fibers. All of the nuclei in this field are located at the periphery of the cells. Occasional nuclei are contained within satellite cells but cannot be distinguished from those of the myofibers by light microscopy. (*B*) Myofibrillar (myosin) ATPase. Type I fibers are pale, whereas type II fibers are dark. Note the intermixture of fiber types.

nervated type I fibers to assume the staining characteristic of type II fibers. It is thought that the pattern or rate of discharge of the lower motor neuron plays an important role in this process. Because the lower motor neuron can determine the fiber type, it follows that all the muscle fibers in a given motor unit are of the same type. When looking at a cross-section of human muscle that has been stained with the alkaline ATPase reaction, one sees a random mixture of fiber types (see Fig. 27-3B), because the motor units interdigitate extensively with each other.

In humans, no muscles are composed exclusively of one fiber type. However, the proportion of fiber types does vary from muscle to muscle. For example, the soleus muscle is composed of predominantly type I fibers (80% or greater). The pattern of fiber types in a given muscle varies between persons, a difference that is apparently genetically determined. There is some evidence that changing the use of a muscle over a long period through intensive training may alter the pattern of muscle fiber types. Type I and type II fibers often maintain their properties even in the presence of advanced pathological alterations in disease.

ENZYME HISTOCHEMISTRY

Application of enzyme histochemical reactions is helpful in the interpretation of pathological changes in muscle biopsy specimens.

NONSPECIFIC ESTERASE: With this stain, type I fibers are slightly darker than type II fibers. The nonspecific esterase reaction is important in identifying denervation atrophy, because many of the atrophic denervated fibers are selectively stained, whether they are type I or type II (see Fig. 27-20). Macrophages also are intensively stained by the nonspecific esterase reaction, as are motor end plates, owing to their acetylcholine esterase activity.

NADH-TETRAZOLIUM REDUCTASE: The reaction product in the reduced nicotinamide adenine dinucleotide–tetrazolium reductase (NADH-TR) reaction is reduced tetrazolium (formazan), which appears as a dark precipitate. The staining reflects the enzyme activity of complex II of the electron transport chain. Nuclear DNA (nDNA) encodes some of the subunits of this complex, whereas mitochondrial DNA (mtDNA) specifies other subunits. Myofibrils are outlined as unstained areas. Because type I fibers have many mitochondria, they appear dark with this stain. The NADH-TR stain does not distinguish the two fiber types as clearly as with the ATPase reaction. In addition, the identity of the fiber type is often not maintained in pathological states. Abnormal collections of mitochondria are darkly stained in primary mitochondrial disorders. Also, excessive staining occurs in atrophic fibers as a result of denervation, whether they were originally type I or type II. Target fibers characteristic of denervation are best recognized with this stain (see Fig. 27-21).

SUCCINATE DEHYDROGENASE (SDH): The SDH reaction is based on complex II of the electron-transport chain. The protein reduces tetrazolium in the presence of the substrate, succinate, and the staining pattern closely resembles that of NADH-TR. The subunits of the SDH complex are entirely encoded by nDNA. It is the most sensitive histochemical index of mitochondrial proliferation caused by mutations of mtDNA, presumably because the genetic defect does not interfere with the electron carrier function (see Fig. 27-18B).

CYTOCHROME C OXIDASE: Cytochrome C oxidase is complex IV of the electron-transport chain. The protein transfers electrons from cytochrome c to molecular oxygen. Three of the 13 subunits are encoded by mtDNA, and one of them includes the active site of the enzyme. The histochemical reaction reduces diaminobenzidine in the presence of cytochrome c, producing a brownish color (see Fig. 27-18C).

ALKALINE PHOSPHATASE: Muscle fibers are normally unstained with the alkaline phosphatase reaction, but regenerating ones are selectively stained. Small blood vessels (probably arterioles) appear black. Cases of dermatomyositis often exhibit abnormal staining of the blood vessels in perifascicular and endomysial connective tissue, which can be a helpful sign of the inflammatory nature of the disease (see Fig. 27-15C).

FIGURE *27-4*
Segmental necrosis and regeneration of a muscle fiber. (*A*) A normal muscle fiber contains myofibrils and subsarcolemmal nuclei and is covered by a basement membrane. Scattered satellite cells are situated on the surface of the sarcolemma, inside the basement membrane. These cells are dormant myoblasts, capable of proliferating and fusing to form differentiated fibers. They constitute 3% to 5% of the nuclei, as observed in a cross-section of skeletal muscle. (*B*) In many muscle diseases (for example, Duchenne muscular dystrophy or polymyositis), injury to the muscle fiber causes segmental necrosis with disintegration of the sarcoplasm, leaving a preserved basement membrane and nerve supply (not shown). (*C*) The damaged segment attracts circulating macrophages, which penetrate the basement membrane and begin to digest and engulf the sarcoplasmic contents (myophagocytosis). Regenerative processes begin with the activation and proliferation of the satellite cells, forming myoblasts within the basement membrane. Macrophages gradually leave the site of injury with their load of debris. (*D*) At a later stage, the myoblasts are aligned in close proximity to each other in the center of the fiber and begin to fuse. (*E*) Regeneration of the fiber segment is prominent, as indicated by the large, pale, vesicular, centrally located nuclei. (*F*) The fiber is nearly normal except for a few persistent central nuclei. Eventually, the normal state (*A*) is restored.

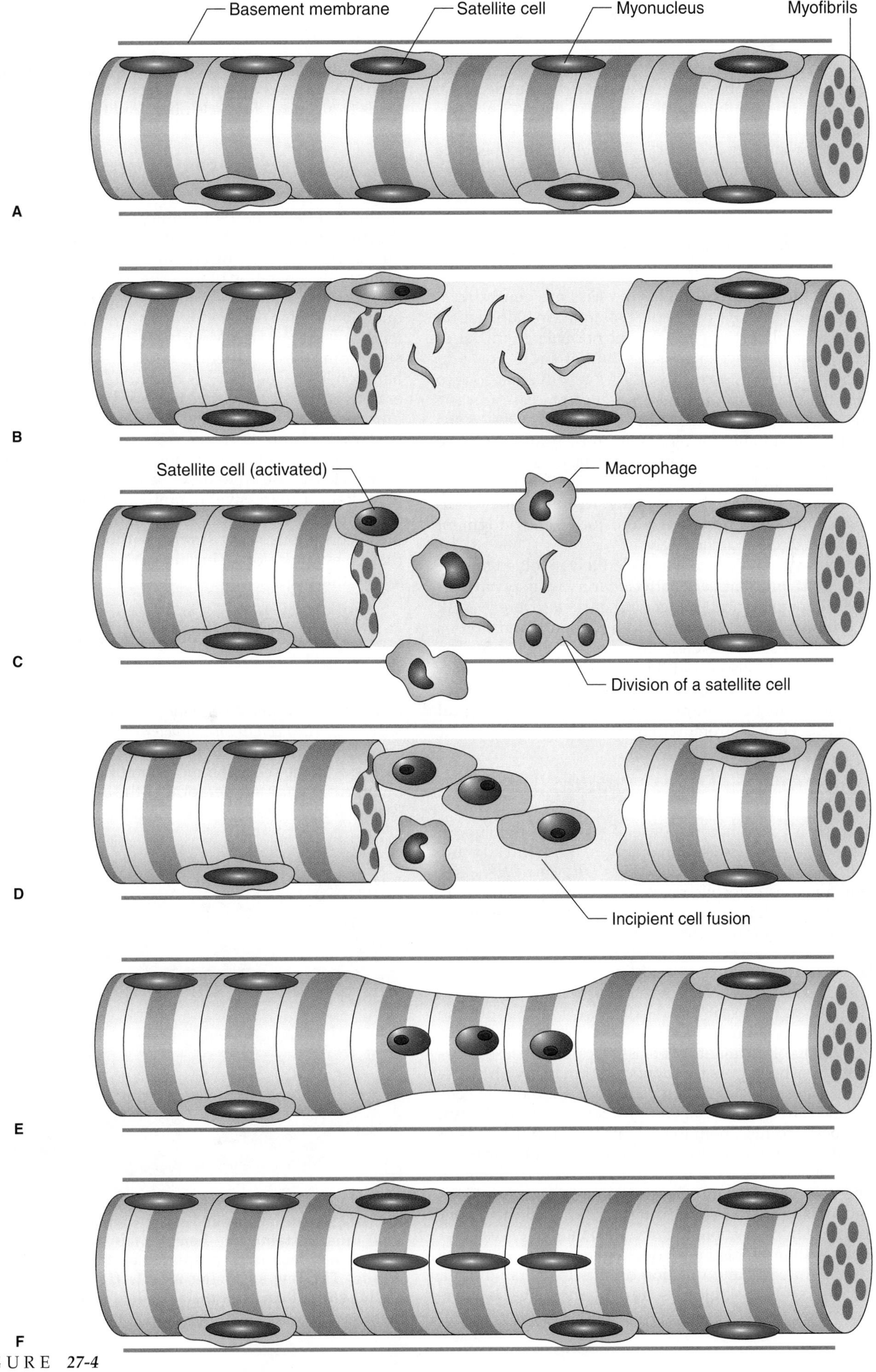
Basement membrane
Satellite cell
Myonucleus
Myofibrils
A
B
Satellite cell (activated)
Macrophage
C
Division of a satellite cell
D
Incipient cell fusion
E
F

FIGURE *27-4*

PERIODIC ACID–SCHIFF (PAS): The PAS reaction demonstrates the basement membrane of muscle fibers and capillaries. Within the fiber, most of the PAS-positive material is glycogen, a finely granular material distributed around the myofibrils throughout the fiber. The PAS stain is helpful in the diagnosis of glycogen-storage diseases.

MUSCLE BIOPSY

Because most neuromuscular diseases are generalized, pathological changes can be demonstrated in biopsy specimens from almost any muscle. The normal pattern varies considerably between muscles, but is more constant within a specific muscle. It is, therefore, advantageous to limit the biopsy to the same muscle from case to case. Samples from either the quadriceps femoris or the biceps brachii are suitable for biopsy in most primary muscle diseases (myopathies). Biopsy of the gastrocnemius muscle and the sural nerve is often performed in patients with a suspected peripheral neuropathy. However, some neuromuscular conditions are more focal, and judgment must be exercised accordingly.

Biopsy sampling from a moderately involved muscle is the most informative. Unaffected muscles may have little or no pathological changes, whereas a severely weak muscle may be largely replaced by adipose and fibrous connective tissue (see end-stage muscle, Fig. 27-5). The surgeon should also avoid the site of a tendon insertion, because the histological appearance of a normal myotendinous junction can mimic some of the pathological changes seen in neuromuscular diseases.

General Pathological Reactions

Necrosis is a common response of myofibers to injury in primary muscle diseases (myopathies). Widespread acute necrosis of skeletal muscle fibers (*rhabdomyolysis*, see later) releases cytosolic proteins, including myoglobin, into the circulation, an event that may result in myoglobinuria and acute renal failure. In many human myopathies, necrosis occurs in a segment along the length of the fiber, leaving two intact portions that flank the site of damage (Fig. 27-4). The injury quickly elicits two responses: an influx of blood-borne monocytes into the necrotic cytoplasm and activation of the satellite cells, a population of dormant myoblasts located in close proximity to each fiber. As the monocytes gradually phagocytose the necrotic debris and remove it, the satellite cells become active myoblasts and proliferate. Within 2 days, they begin to fuse, both to each other and to the ends of the intact fiber remnants, to form a joining multinucleated segment. This regenerating segment resembles the myotube of developing muscle during embryogenesis. This regenerating fiber is smaller in diameter than the parent fiber, and it has basophilic cytoplasm and large, vesicular nuclei with prominent nucleoli. **Regeneration** can restore normal structure and function of muscle fibers within a few weeks after a single episode of injury, as in the inherited disorder myophosphorylase deficiency (see later). With subacute or chronic disorders, fiber necrosis proceeds concurrent with fiber regeneration. This gradually leads to atrophy of muscle fibers and fibrosis.

MUSCULAR DYSTROPHY

In the middle of the 19th century, physicians discovered that progressive weakness of the voluntary muscles could be caused by either a disorder of the nervous system or a primary degeneration of muscles. *Muscular dystrophy was the name applied to primary muscular degeneration.* It was frequently found to be hereditary, or at least familial, and relentlessly progressive. Morphological study of muscle tissue from these patients, obtained with a "muscle harpoon," showed necrosis of muscle fibers, with regenerative activity, progressive fibrosis, and infiltration of the muscle with fatty tissue (Fig. 27-5). Little or no inflammation was recognized.

In subsequent years, numerous variants of this type of muscle disease were described, and a classification of hereditary, progressive, noninflammatory degenerative conditions of muscle has evolved. In general, many of these conditions show similar pathological alterations, that is, evidence of a chronic, active, noninflammatory myopathic process.

Duchenne and Becker Muscular Dystrophies

Duchenne muscular dystrophy is a severe, progressive, X-linked, inherited condition characterized by progressive degeneration of muscles, particularly those of the pelvic and shoulder girdles. It is the most common noninflammatory myopathy in children. A milder form of the disease is known as *Becker muscular dystrophy* (see Chapter 6 for the molecular

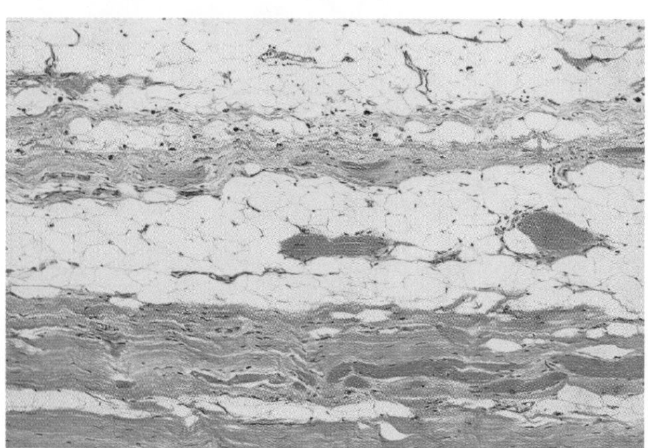

FIGURE 27-5
End-stage neuromuscular disease. In this section of the deltoid muscle stained by hematoxylin and eosin, skeletal muscle has been largely replaced by fibrofatty connective tissue. The few surviving muscle fibers have a deeper eosinophilia than does the abundant collagenous component.

genetics of both diseases). The serum creatine kinase activity is greatly increased in both conditions.

□ Pathogenesis:

Duchenne muscular dystrophy is caused by mutations of a large gene on the short arm of the X chromosome (Xp21). This gene codes for *dystrophin*, a 427-kDa protein localized on the inner surface of the sarcolemma. Dystrophin links the subsarcolemmal cytoskeleton to the exterior of the cell through a transmembrane complex of proteins and glycoproteins that binds to laminin. Dystrophin is absent or greatly reduced in amount, often as a result of deletions of the gene (Fig. 27-6). Dystrophin-deficient muscle fibers thus lack the normal interaction between the sarcolemma and the extracellular matrix. This disruption may be responsible for the observed increased osmotic fragility of dystrophic muscle, the excessive influx of calcium ions, and the release of soluble muscle enzymes, such as creatine kinase, into the serum. Further evidence to support this hypothesis is the fact that a breakdown of the sarcolemma precedes muscle cell necrosis, and the basal lamina seems to separate from the sarcolemma early in Duchenne muscular dystrophy.

The results of molecular genetic analysis of other forms of muscular dystrophy support these concepts. Becker muscular dystrophy is allelic to Duchenne dystrophy, and mutations of the genes produce an altered dystrophin, usually a truncated protein. This mutated protein is localized to the surface membrane of muscle fibers, but the immunocytochemical staining is often reduced in intensity or focally absent (see Fig. 27-6). The abnormal protein apparently retains sufficient function to result in a less severe phenotype. Other muscle diseases closely resemble Duchenne and Becker dystrophies, but are inherited in a recessive autosomal fashion. Some of these patients have mutations that affect the expression of transmembrane proteins or glycoproteins and interrupt the link between the cytoskeleton and extracellular matrix.

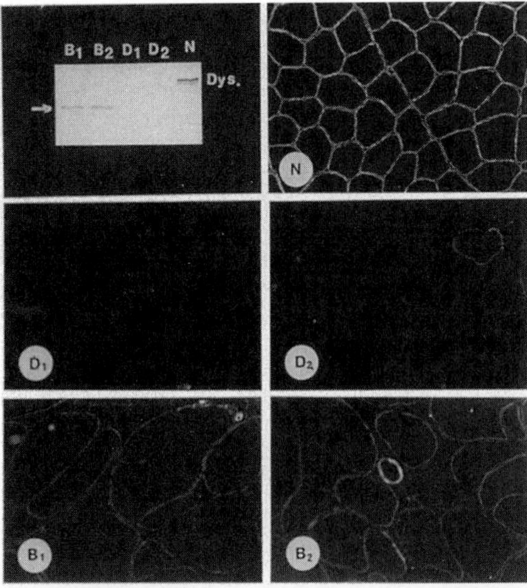

FIGURE 27-6
Dystrophin analysis in Duchenne and Becker muscular dystrophies. Immunofluorescence stain for dystrophin. The sections illustrate a normal subject (*N*), two patients with Duchenne dystrophy (*D*), and two with Becker dystrophy (*B*). Dystrophin is normally concentrated at the surface membrane of every muscle fiber, but in Duchenne dystrophy, the protein is absent or is only barely detected in a small proportion of muscle fibers. Becker dystrophy exhibits hypertrophic muscle fibers with reduced expression of dystrophin. The immunoblot (*upper left*) of normal muscle shows a band near the top of the gel corresponding to the 427-kDa protein, dystrophin. Dystrophin is undetectable in Duchenne dystrophy. In Becker dystrophy, a weaker band has migrated farther down the gel relative to the normal protein, and it corresponds to a smaller, truncated protein. The combined analysis (immunolocalization and immunoblot) of the dystrophin protein is diagnostic of this group of dystrophies (dystrophinopathies).

□ Pathology:

The disease process in Duchenne dystrophy consists of (1) a relentless necrosis of muscle fibers, (2) a continuous effort at repair and regeneration, and (3) progressive fibrosis. The degenerative process eventually outstrips the regenerative capacity of the muscle. As a consequence, there is a progressively decreasing number of muscle fibers and increasing amounts of fibrofatty connective tissue. The end stage is characterized by an almost complete loss of skeletal muscle fibers, but relative sparing of the muscle spindle fibers (see Fig. 27-5).

In the early stage of the disease, necrotic fibers and regenerating fibers tend to occur in small groups, together with scattered, large, hyalinized dark fibers. The latter are overly contracted and are thought to precede fiber necrosis (Figs. 27-7 and 27-8). Breakdown of the sarcolemma is one of the earliest ultrastructural changes. Macrophages invade necrotic fibers and reflect a scavenging function rather than an inflammatory process.

The diagnosis of Duchenne dystrophy can be established by polymerase chain reaction (PCR) analysis of genomic DNA derived from leukocytes in a blood sample. In practice, diagnosis by using this method is limited to large deletions of the gene. About 30% of the patients have small rearrangements or point mutations of the gene, and they can be evaluated by muscle biopsy, which shows little or no detectable dystrophin by immunoblot or immunocytochemical staining.

□ Clinical Features:

Boys with Duchenne muscular dystrophy have markedly increased serum creatine kinase levels from birth and morphologically abnormal muscle, even *in utero*. Clinical weakness is not detectable during the first year, but usually becomes so by the age of 3 or 4 years. The weakness is noted mainly around the pelvic and shoulder girdles (proximal muscle weakness) and is relentlessly progressive. "Pseudohypertrophy" of the calf muscles develops eventually. The patients are usually wheelchair-bound by the age of 10 years and bedridden by 15 years. The most common causes of death are complications of respiratory insufficiency caused by muscular weakness or cardiac arrhythmia owing to myocardial involvement.

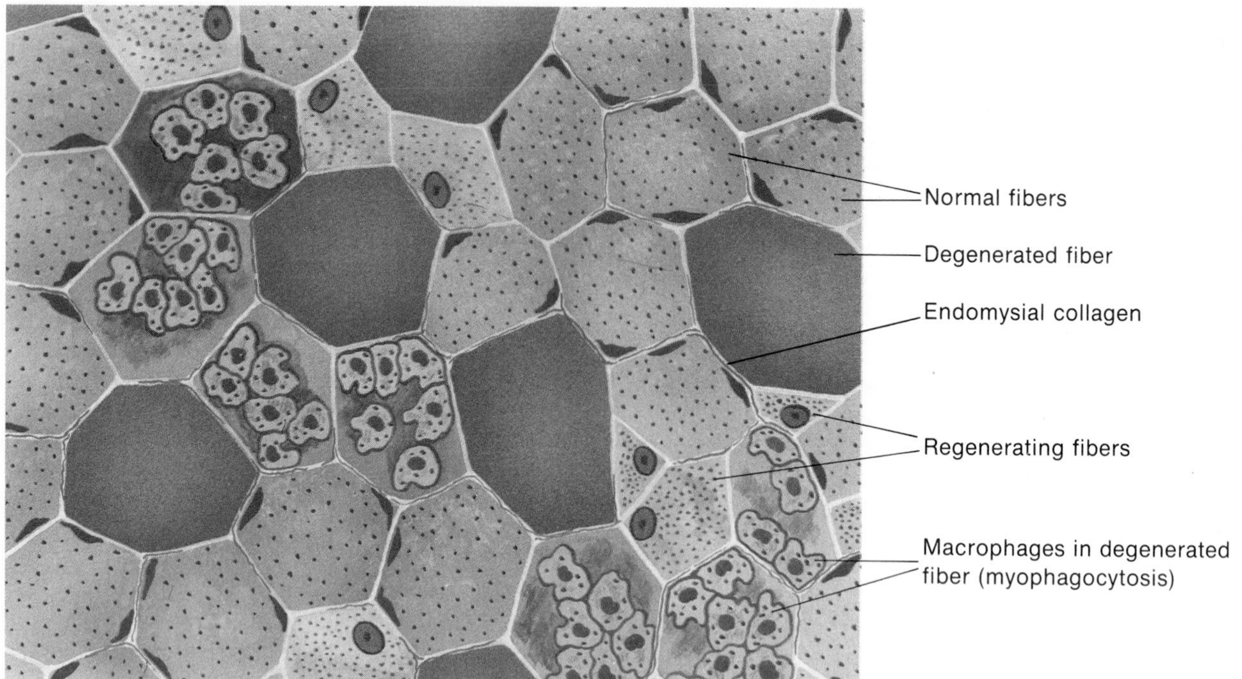

FIGURE 27-7
Duchenne muscular dystrophy. The pathological changes in skeletal muscle are illustrated by staining with the modified Gomori trichrome stain. Some fibers are slightly larger and darker than normal. These represent overcontracted segments of sarcoplasm situated between degenerated segments. Some fibers are packed with macrophages (myophagocytosis), which remove degenerated sarcoplasm. Some fibers are smaller than normal and have granular sarcoplasm. These fibers have enlarged, vesicular nuclei with prominent nucleoli and represent regenerating fibers. Developing endomysial fibrosis is represented by the deposition of collagen around individual muscle fibers. The changes are those of a chronic, active noninflammatory myopathy.

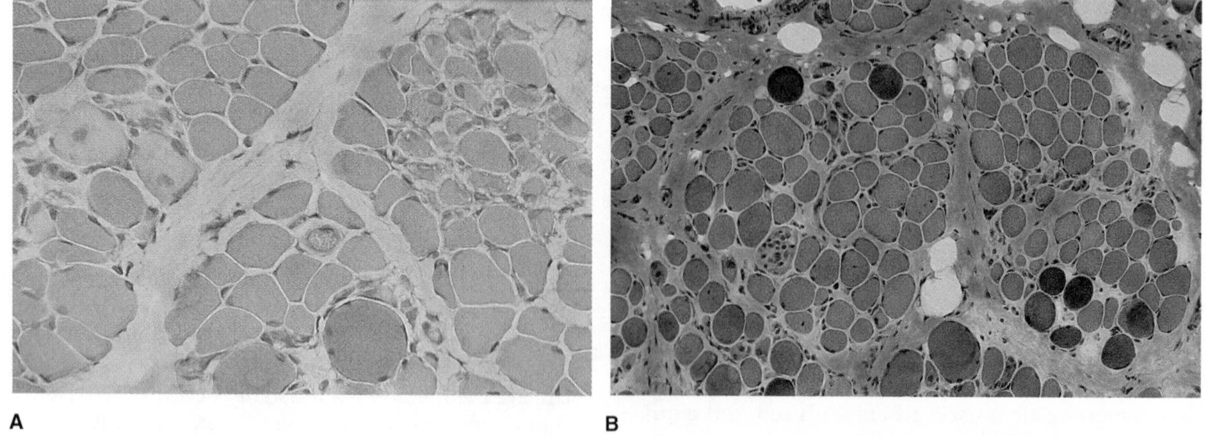

FIGURE 27-8
Duchenne muscular dystrophy. (*A*) Hematoxylin and eosin stain. A section of vastus lateralis muscle shows necrotic muscle fibers, some of them invaded by macrophages. The endomysial septa are thickened, indicating fibrosis. (*B*) Modified Gomori trichrome. A similar section demonstrates dark-staining enlarged fibers, which represent overly contracted fibers. Calcium influx across the defective surface membrane overwhelms mechanisms that maintain a low resting Ca^{2+} concentration and triggers excessive contraction. There is conspicuous perimysial and endomysial fibrosis.

Occasional cases that are indistinguishable from Duchenne muscular dystrophy occur in girls. These patients represent a genetically different disease or a nonrandom inactivation of the X chromosome.

CARRIER DETECTION: Because Duchenne muscular dystrophy is inherited as an X-linked recessive disease, the disease is passed from a mother who is a heterozygote carrier of the abnormal gene. Alternatively, the disease can stem from a spontaneous somatic mutation of the gene, which occurs at a high rate and accounts for 30% of cases. In these instances, there is no carrier. Until recently, the best method to detect carriers has been multiple determinations of serum creatine kinase levels, which are moderately increased in 75% of heterozygotes. There is considerable variability in the expression of the carrier state, probably because of variations in the random inactivation of the X chromosome. Some of the carriers can now be detected by dystrophin immunolocalization performed on a muscle biopsy. This procedure shows a characteristic mosaic pattern of deficient and normal myofibers. Molecular probes are able to detect more than two thirds of these individuals who carry large deletions.

Myotonic Dystrophy

Myotonic dystrophy, the most common form of adult muscular dystrophy, is an autosomal dominant disorder characterized by a slowing of muscle relaxation (myotonia) and progressive muscle weakness and wasting. The prevalence has been estimated to be as high as 14 per 100,000, although it may be higher because of the difficulty in detecting minimally affected persons. The age at onset and severity of symptoms show extreme variations. Myotonic dystrophy can be separated into two clinical groups: (1) adult onset, and (2) congenital.

☐ **Pathogenesis:** The gene for myotonic dystrophy has been localized to the long arm of chromosome 19 (19q13.3), and most cases seem to be descended from one original mutation. The mutation responsible for the disease is the expansion of a CTG repeat near the 3′ end of the gene. Normal persons have fewer than 30 copies of this trinucleotide repeat, whereas it is present in 50 copies or more in minimally affected patients with myotonic dystrophy. An interesting genetic characteristic of this disease is the phenomenon of anticipation, that is, an earlier age at onset and increasing severity of symptoms in successive generations. The number of trinucleotide repeats increases with successive generations, the size of the repeat sequence correlating with the severity of symptoms. Expansion of a trinucleotide repeat is a common mechanism in many human genetic diseases and has now been observed in fragile X syndrome, Kennedy disease, and Huntington disease, among others. The gene for myotonic dystrophy encodes a novel serine–threonine protein kinase. Apparently, abnormal phosphorylation of ion channels alters the excitability of the sarcolemma.

☐ **Pathology:** The pathological changes of adult myotonic dystrophy are highly variable, even in muscles from the same patient. Most cases display atrophy of type I fibers and hypertrophy of type II fibers. Internally situated nuclei are a constant feature. The ATPase reaction shows many ring fibers, in which there is a circumferential concentration of heavily stained sarcoplasm. Necrosis and regeneration, although occasionally present, are not prominent (as they are in Duchenne muscular dystrophy).

The muscle of congenital myotonic dystrophy shows myofiber atrophy, frequent central nuclei, and a failure of fiber differentiation. These pathological features closely resemble those of the X-linked recessive type of myotubular myopathy (see later).

☐ **Clinical Features:** In addition to skeletal muscle, myotonic dystrophy affects many systems, including the heart, smooth muscle, central nervous system, endocrine glands, and the eye. The diagnosis is based on the clinical features, the family history, and the characteristic electromyography, which exhibits myotonic discharges. DNA analysis showing an expanded trinucleotide repeat is predictive *in utero* and can be diagnostic in patients.

Adult myotonic dystrophy is seen most commonly with slowly progressive muscle weakness and stiffness, principally in the distal limbs. The facial and jaw muscles are virtually always affected, and ptosis can be severe. Extramuscular features of myotonic dystrophy are sometimes present and include cataracts, testicular atrophy with diminished fertility, and variable degrees of personality deterioration. A few patients exhibit involvement of smooth muscle, with disorders of the gastrointestinal tract, gallbladder, and uterus. Cardiac arrhythmias and, less commonly, cardiomyopathy have been reported.

Congenital myotonic dystrophy is seen only in the offspring of women who themselves exhibit symptoms of myotonic dystrophy. The infants are born with severe muscle weakness, but myotonia is inconspicuous or absent, although it appears in later childhood. A significant number of these patients have some degree of mental retardation.

CONGENITAL MYOPATHIES

Occasionally, a newborn manifests generalized hypotonia, with decreased deep tendon reflexes and muscle bulk. Many of these children have a difficult perinatal period because of weak respirations and consequent pulmonary complications. Some have "malignant" hypotonia, which is progressive and results in death within the first 12 months of life. *Werdnig–Hoffman disease* and infantile acid maltase deficiency (*Pompe disease*) are examples.

Other hypotonic patients have a "benign" course. Although the hypotonia persists throughout their lives, it shows little or no progression. The patients become ambulatory and live a normal life span, although sometimes complicated by secondary skeletal complications of the hypotonia. It is this group of patients that is subsumed in the category of "congenital myopathies."

Morphological study of the muscle of these patients rarely exhibits distinctive structural abnormalities of

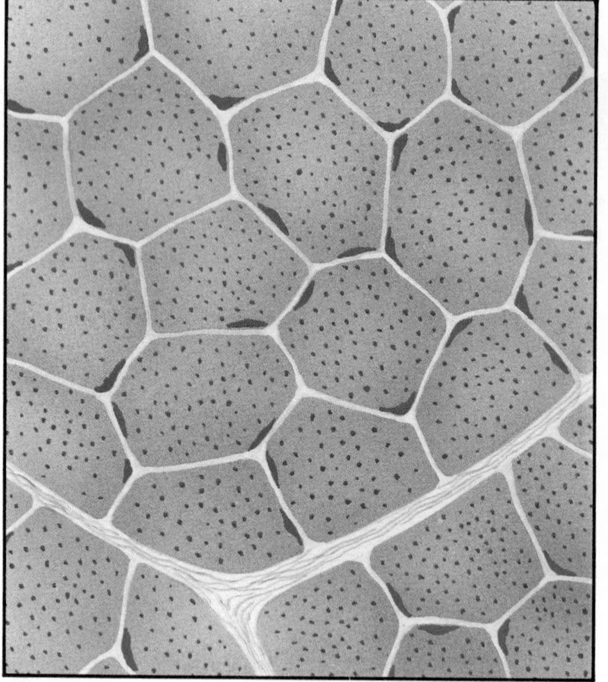

A. NORMAL

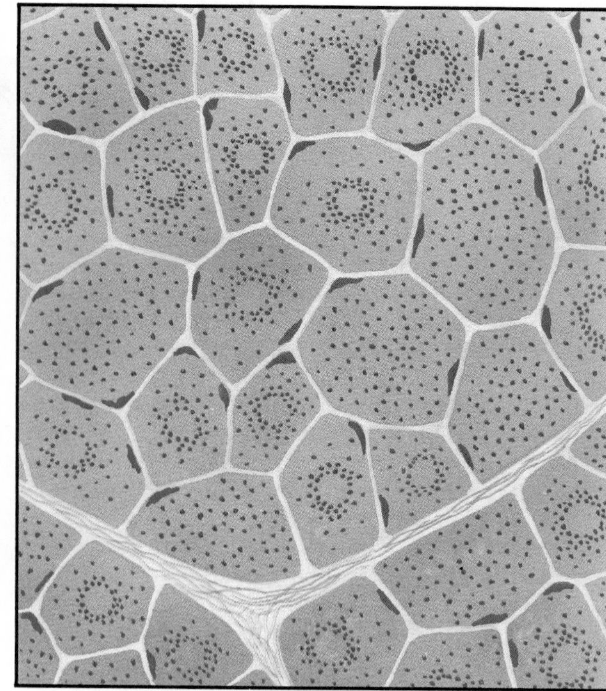

B. CENTRAL CORE DISEASE

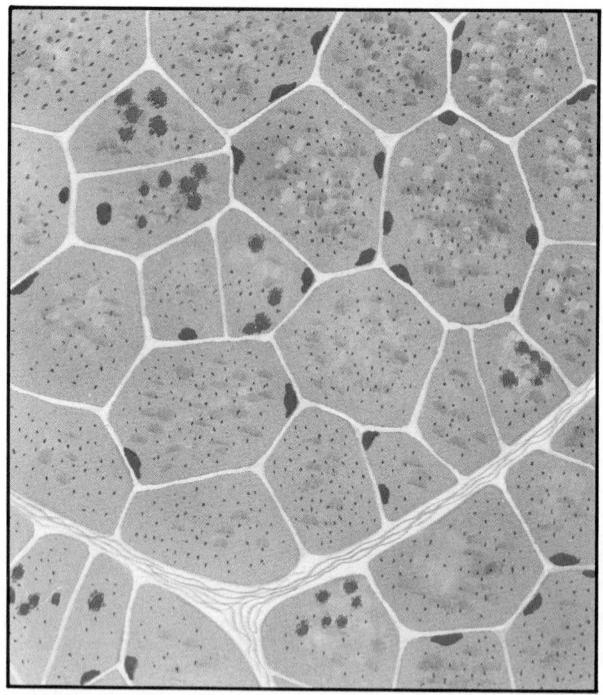

C. ROD MYOPATHY

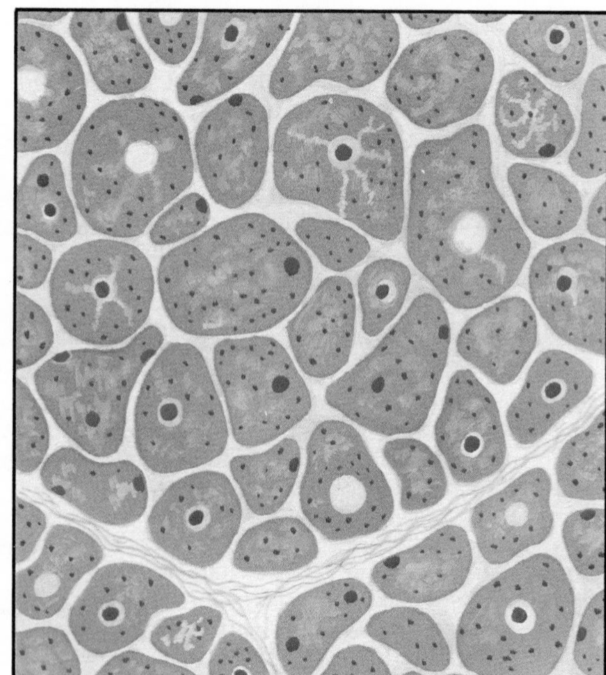

D. CENTRONUCLEAR MYOPATHY

FIGURE *27-9*

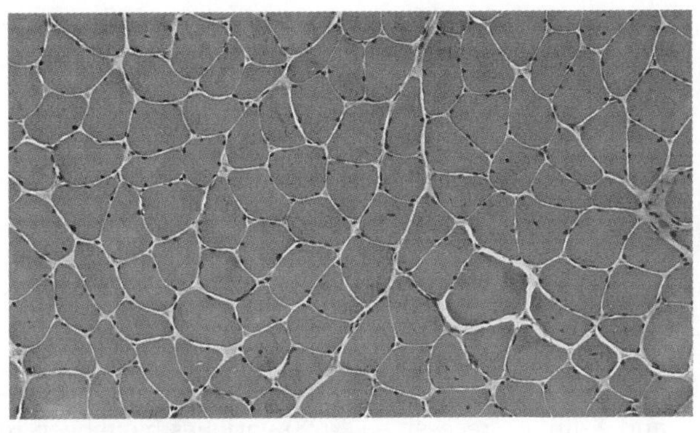

A

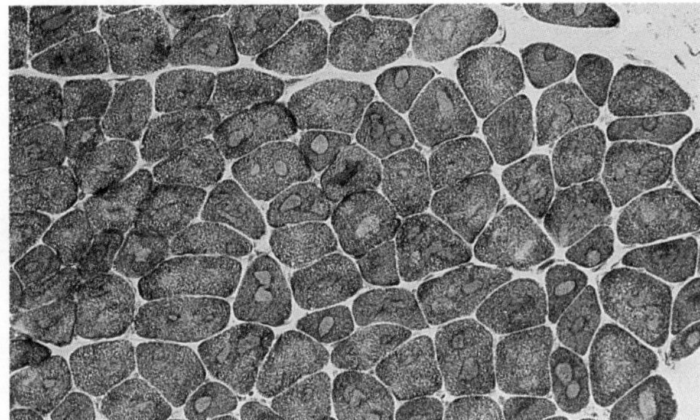

B

FIGURE 27-10
Central core disease. (*A*) Hematoxylin and eosin stain. A section of vastus lateralis muscle appears nearly normal. (*B*) Stained for NADH-tetrazolium reductase, the same muscle shows a distinct circular zone of pallor in the center of most muscle fibers. A thin zone of excessive staining surrounds the core lesion. All of the myofibers in this case were type I, as demonstrated by the myofibrillar ATPase stain (not shown). Note the close resemblance of the core lesions to the target formations found in the muscle fibers of neurogenic disorders (see Fig. 27-21).

myofibers. Three of the most common forms of congenital myopathies are central core disease, nemaline (rod) myopathy, and central nuclear myopathy (Fig. 27-9).

Some generalizations can be made about these three conditions. They all have congenital hypotonia, decreased deep tendon reflexes, decreased muscle bulk, and delayed motor milestones. In addition, the morphological abnormality expressed in the muscle biopsy in all three conditions is usually limited to type I (red) fibers. Furthermore, these patients often have an abnormal predominance of type I fibers or, perhaps or possibly, a failure of type II (white) fibers to develop. The skeletal muscle does not show signs of active myofiber necrosis or fibrosis, and the patients do not ordinarily have increased activity of serum creatine kinase.

Central Core Disease

Central core disease is an autosomal dominant condition characterized by congenital hypotonia, with proximal muscle weakness, decreased deep tendon reflexes, and delayed motor development. The disease has been traced to a mutation on the long arm of chromosome 19 (19q13.1), which codes for the ryanodine receptor, the calcium-release channel of the sarcoplasmic reticulum. Occasional cases are sporadic or show autosomal recessive inheritance. The typical patient becomes ambulatory, although muscle strength never develops to a normal level.

☐ **Pathology:** Muscle biopsy reveals a striking predominance of type I fibers. Many or all of these fibers display a central zone of degeneration, which exhibits a loss of staining in the NADH-TR reaction (Fig. 27-10B). This central core abnormality extends throughout the entire length of the fiber. The central core is difficult to see with the hematoxylin and eosin stain (see Fig. 27-10A) but can often be demonstrated with the PAS reaction. By electron microscopy, the central core is characterized by a loss of mitochondria and other membranous organelles, with or without disorganization of the myofibrils. Membranous organelles tend to condense around the margin of the central core. The structure of the periphery of the fiber is otherwise unremarkable.

FIGURE 27-9
Congenital myopathies. (*A*) Normal. A frozen section of normal skeletal muscle stained with modified Gomori trichrome is depicted. The nuclei are purple, the membranous organelles (mitochondria and sarcoplasmic reticulum) are red, myofibrils are light green, and perifascicular collagen is light green. The fibers are of uniform size and somewhat polygonal. (*B*) Central core myopathy. Many type I fibers are slightly smaller than normal and contain a round central core, which runs the length of the muscle fiber. The core is devoid of membranous organelles and is surrounded by a condensed ring. "Core fibers" resemble target fibers (see Fig. 27-21), although no neuropathic process has yet been demonstrated in central core disease. (*C*) Rod (nemaline) myopathy. Many type I fibers are slightly smaller than normal and contain reddish aggregates of rods. In transverse section, many of the rods appear as granules because they are oriented in parallel to the longitudinal axis of the fiber. (*D*) Central nuclear myopathy (myotubular myopathy). Many type I fibers are smaller and rounder than normal. Some contain a single, central nucleus, whereas others contain a round central pale zone, representing the zone between adjacent longitudinally arranged nuclei. These fibers resemble the myotube stage during embryonic development of skeletal muscle.

The central core anomaly bears a striking resemblance to the target fibers (see Fig. 27-21) seen in active denervating conditions. However, no evidence of active denervation is seen in patients with central core disease. The motor end plates are architecturally unremarkable, and no extrajunctional nicotinic acetylcholine receptors are present in the muscle membrane.

Mutations of the ryanodine receptor gene also cause one form of *malignant hyperthermia,* a potentially fatal disorder in patients triggered by the use of anesthesia for surgery. Both central core disease and this adverse response to anesthesia can coexist in some of these patients.

Rod (Nemaline) Myopathy

Rod myopathy includes a heterogeneous group of diseases that have in common the accumulation of rod-like inclusions within the sarcoplasm of skeletal muscle. The disease was initially named "nemaline" myopathy because the inclusions within the muscle fiber were interpreted as a tangled, thread-like mass. In reality, they are clusters of rod-shaped structures.

The classic congenital form of rod myopathy is characterized by congenital hypotonia and delayed motor milestones of variable clinical severity, with associated secondary skeletal changes, such as kyphoscoliosis. In some cases, there is severe involvement of muscles of the face, pharynx, and neck. Later-onset (childhood and adult) forms tend to be associated with some muscle degeneration, increases of serum creatine kinase levels, and a slowly progressive course. A few of the patients originally designated as having limb girdle muscular dystrophy have eventually been found to have rod myopathy. The cause of the condition is unknown. Inheritance seems to be either autosomal dominant or autosomal recessive. The genes responsible for rod myopathy are just beginning to be identified, and a mutation of the gene for α-tropomyosin was found in one family with an autosomal dominant disorder.

☐ **Pathology:** The findings on muscle biopsy consist of a variable predominance of type I fibers and the accumulation of rod-shaped structures within their sarcoplasm. The aggregates of these inclusions are often located in subsarcolemmal regions near nuclei. They are brilliant red to dark red when stained with the modified Gomori trichrome stain (see Figs. 27-9 and 27-11A) and may or may not be visible with hematoxylin and eosin. The rods are almost always positive with the phosphotungstic acid hematoxylin (PTAH) stain and are negative with the ATPase and NADH-TR reactions. Ultrastructural studies demonstrate that the inclusions are indeed rod-shaped and arise from the Z-band, which they resemble ultrastructurally (see Fig. 27-11B).

It should be pointed out that rods have been described in a variety of neuromuscular diseases, including denervation atrophy, muscular dystrophy, and inflammatory myopathies. Experimental tenotomy (cutting a tendon) induces formation of rods in the muscle when the nerve supply remains intact. In rod myopathy, however, the inclusions constitute the predominant pathological change.

Central Nuclear Myopathy (Myotubular Myopathy)

Central nuclear myopathy refers to a group of clinically and genetically heterogeneous inherited conditions, which have in common the presence of a centrally located nucleus in skeletal muscle cells. Autosomal recessive, autosomal dominant, and X-linked recessive (Xq28) varieties have been recognized. In X-linked inheritance, the newborn is strikingly weak and hypotonic and may die of respiratory insufficiency during the neonatal period. The autosomal dominant form tends to be of later onset and is associated with modestly increased serum creatine kinase levels. It has a slowly progressive course and, like rod myopathy, resembles the so-called limb girdle muscular dystrophy syndrome. In some patients, there is a striking involvement of the facial and extraocular musculature.

☐ **Pathology:** Biopsy specimens from patients with central nuclear myopathy are variable, but are characterized by type I fiber predominance (Fig. 27-12). Many of these fibers are small and round, with a single central nucleus (see Fig. 27-12), accounting for the name of the disease. In this respect, they resemble the myotubular stage in the embryogenesis of skeletal muscle. This apparent immature state suggests a possible defect in the nerve supply to the muscle fiber, because the lower motor neuron requires subsequent maturation of the fiber. However, studies of the lower motor neuron, including the motor end plate, have failed to demonstrate any abnormality in these patients. Mutations of a gene for a tyrosine phosphatase cause the X-linked form of myotubular myopathy.

The later-onset forms of myotubular myopathy are characterized morphologically by more mature muscle fibers, in which the fibers are larger, have more numerous myofibrils, and display single central nuclei that appear more mature.

INFLAMMATORY MYOPATHIES

The inflammatory myopathies represent a heterogeneous group of acquired disorders, all of which feature symmetrical proximal muscle weakness, increased serum levels of muscle-derived enzymes, and nonsuppurative inflammation of skeletal muscle. From a historical point of view, the two major inflammatory myopathies, *polymyositis* and *dermatomyositis*, were considered variants of the same entity. A third type of inflammatory myopathy, termed *inclusion-body myositis*, was recognized recently. All three diseases are distinct entities, with their own characteristic immunopathological, morphological, and clinical features.

Inflammatory myopathies are uncommon, the annual incidence being 1 in 100,000. Dermatomyositis af-

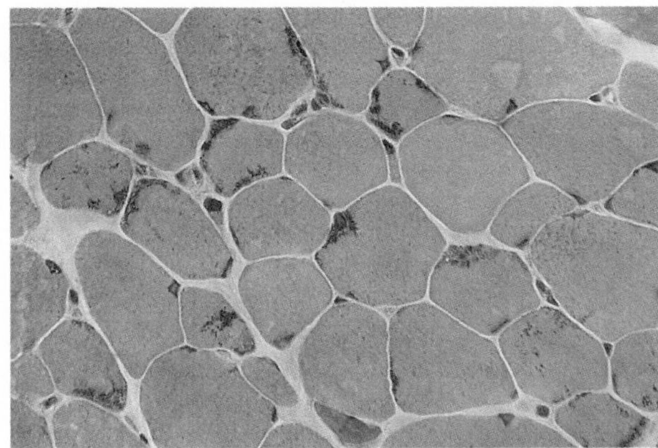

A

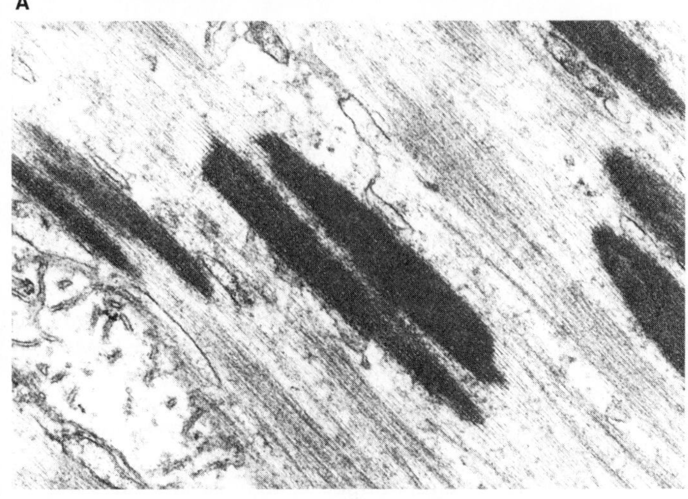

B

FIGURE 27-11
Rod (nemaline) myopathy. (*A*) Modified Gomori trichrome stain. Muscle fibers contain dark aggregates of rods and granules. These rods tend to be located at the fiber periphery near nuclei. All of the affected fibers are type I. (*B*) An electron micrograph of the same biopsy shows that the structures are rod-shaped and are derived from the Z-disc, having the same periodic substructure.

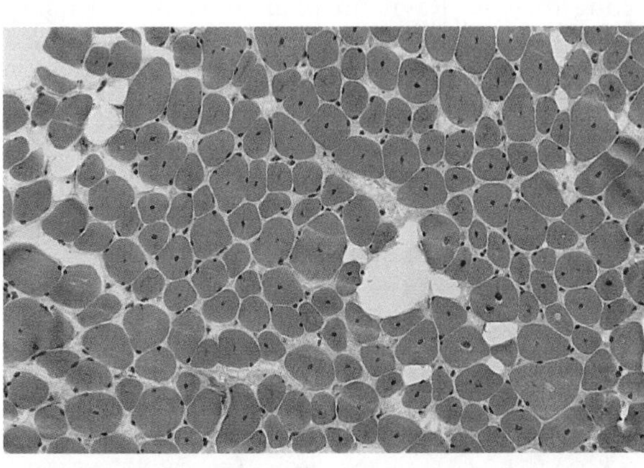

A

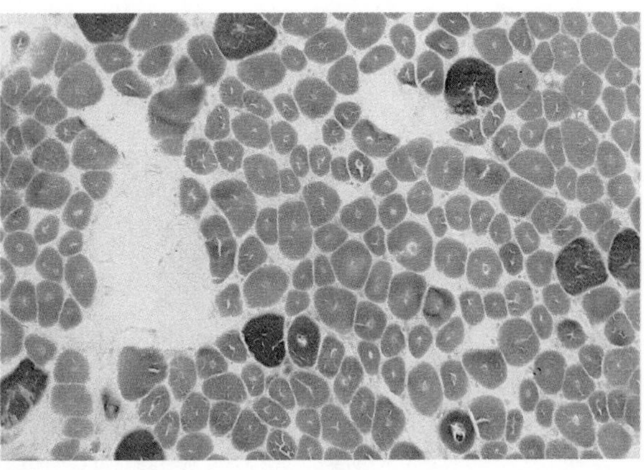

B

FIGURE 27-12
Central nuclear (myotubular) myopathy. (*A*) Hematoxylin and eosin stain. Many muscle fibers contain a single, central nucleus, and most of the affected muscle fibers are abnormally small. These fibers resemble the late myotube stage of fetal development of skeletal muscle. (*B*) Myofibrillar (myosin) ATPase. The section demonstrates a type I phenotype in the fibers with central nuclei. It also illustrates type I fiber predominance, which is a general feature of congenital myopathies.

flicts children and adults, whereas polymyositis almost always occurs after the age of 20 years. Both disorders occur more commonly in female than in male persons. The incidence of inclusion-body myositis is three times greater in men than in women, and the disorder usually occurs after age 50 years.

The inflammatory myopathies are thought to have an autoimmune origin because of (1) their association with other autoimmune and connective tissues diseases, (2) pathological evidence of autoimmune mechanisms of muscle cell injury, (3) detection of autoantibodies in serum, (4) a beneficial response to immunosuppressive agents in polymyositis and dermatomyositis (but not inclusion-body myositis), and (5) failure to isolate or detect an infectious agent in muscle. No specific target autoantigens in muscle or blood vessels have been identified.

The most prominent morphological characteristics that the inflammatory myopathies share are (1) the presence of inflammatory cells, (2) necrosis and phagocytosis of muscle fibers, (3) a mixture of regenerating and atrophic fibers, and (4) fibrosis.

☐ **Clinical Features:** All varieties of inflammatory myopathy discussed here are seen as insidious proximal and symmetric muscle weakness, gradually increasing over a period of weeks to months. The patients have problems with simple activities that require the use of proximal muscles, including lifting objects, climbing steps, or combing the hair. Dysphagia and difficulty in holding up the head reflect involvement of the pharyngeal and neck-flexor muscles. Some patients with inclusion-body myositis have distal muscle weakness of the limbs that equals or exceeds that of proximal muscles. In advanced cases, the respiratory muscles may be affected. The weakness progresses over weeks or months and leads to severe muscular wasting.

Dermatomyositis is distinguished from the other myopathies by the presence of a characteristic rash on the upper eyelids, face, trunk, and occasionally other body surfaces. It may occur alone or in association with scleroderma, mixed connective tissue disease, or other autoimmune conditions. When dermatomyositis occurs in a middle-aged man, it is associated with an increased risk of an epithelial cancer, most commonly carcinoma of the lung. By contrast, polymyositis and inclusion-body myositis have only a chance association with malignancy.

Patients with inflammatory myopathies have a moderate to markedly increased serum creatine kinase level and increases in other muscle enzyme levels. Antinuclear and anticytoplasmic antibodies exist in all of these diseases, with specificity to several different antigens. Treatment of polymyositis and dermatomyositis with corticosteroids is usually successful, but inclusion-body myositis is generally resistant to all therapy.

Polymyositis

☐ **Pathogenesis:** Polymyositis is thought to be related to direct muscle cell damage produced by cytotoxic T cells, and there is no evidence of a microangiopathy such as that found in dermatomyositis (see later). In these disorders, healthy muscle fibers are initially surrounded by CD8+ T lymphocytes (Fig. 27-13) and macrophages, after which the muscle fibers degenerate. In contrast to normal muscle tissue, the affected muscles in polymyositis express major histocompatibility complex-I (MHC-I) antigen on the sarcolemma. Because cytotoxic T cells attack antigenic targets in association with MHC-I molecules, these findings are taken as evidence for the immunopathological basis of these disorders.

The role of autoantibodies against nuclear antigens and cytoplasmic ribonucleoproteins in the pathogenesis of muscle injury is unknown. There is a frequent association between anti-Jo-1, an antibody against histidyl-tRNA synthetase, with the concomitant presence of interstitial lung disease, Raynaud phenomenon, and nonerosive arthritis.

Although viral infections may trigger these inflam-

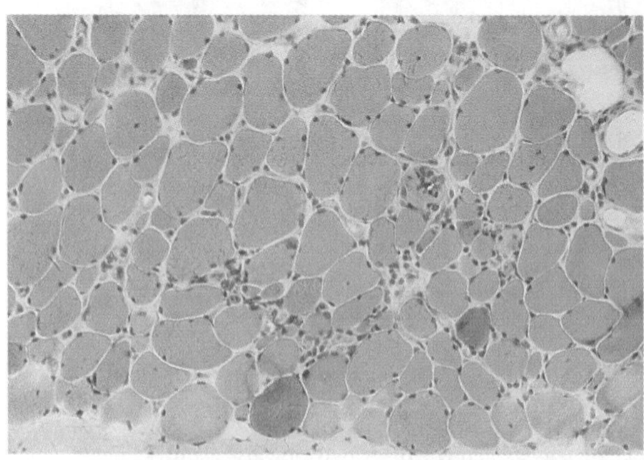
A

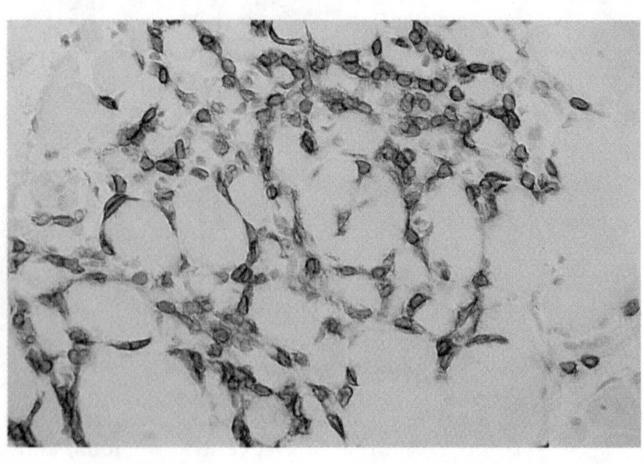
B

FIGURE *27-13*
Polymyositis. (*A*) Hematoxylin and eosin stain. A section of affected muscle shows an inflammatory myopathy. Mononuclear inflammatory cells infiltrate chiefly the endomysium. The field includes single-fiber necrosis. (*B*) An immunoperoxidase stain shows CD8+ cytotoxic T cells.

matory myopathies, muscle tissue has not yielded a virus on culture, despite many attempts to recover these agents. An inflammatory myopathy indistinguishable from polymyositis occurs in many cases of human immunodeficiency virus-1 (HIV-1), but the role of the retrovirus is unclear.

☐ **Pathology:** Inflammatory cells infiltrate connective tissue mostly within the fascicles (that is, endomysial inflammation) and invade apparently healthy muscle fibers (see Fig. 27-13A). Angiopathy is absent. Isolated degenerating or regenerating fibers are scattered throughout fascicles. Perifascicular atrophy is not present in polymyositis (see later).

Inclusion Body Myositis

The pathological features of inclusion body myositis resemble those of polymyositis and consist of single-fiber necrosis and regeneration with predominantly endomysial cytotoxic T cells. In addition, basophilic granular material is seen at the edge of slit-like vacuoles (rimmed vacuoles) within the muscle fibers. The fibers also contain small eosinophilic cytoplasmic inclusions, often located near the rimmed vacuoles (Fig. 27-14A). The inclusions are stained by Congo red and represent a form of intracellular amyloid (see Fig. 27-14B). The substance is immunoreactive for β-amyloid protein, the same type of amyloid present in the senile plaques of Alzheimer disease. The pathogenic significance of these inclusions is not understood. Small groups of angulated fibers are present. By electron microscopy, the granules of rimmed vacuoles contain membranous whorls. Distinctive filaments are found in the vicinity of the rimmed vacuoles (see Fig. 27-14C). The pathognomonic features of inclusion body myositis include the Congo red–positive inclusions and the characteristic filaments in the cytoplasm (or rarely in nuclei) of muscle fibers.

Dermatomyositis

☐ **Pathogenesis:** This myopathy is characterized by (1) immune complexes of immunoglobulin G (IgG), IgM, and complement components, including membrane attack complement (C5b-9; Fig 27-15B), in the walls of capillaries and other blood vessels; (2) microangiopathy with loss of capillaries; (3) signs of injury and atrophy of myofibers; and (4) perivascular infiltrates of B cells and T cells with a predominantly CD4-helper phenotype. These features suggest that muscle injury in dermatomyositis is produced primarily by complement-mediated cytotoxic antibodies directed against the microvasculature of skeletal muscle tissues. In fact, the presence of complement on the capillaries precedes inflammation or damage to the muscle fibers and is the most specific lesion of dermatomyositis. This microangiopathy is thought to lead to is-

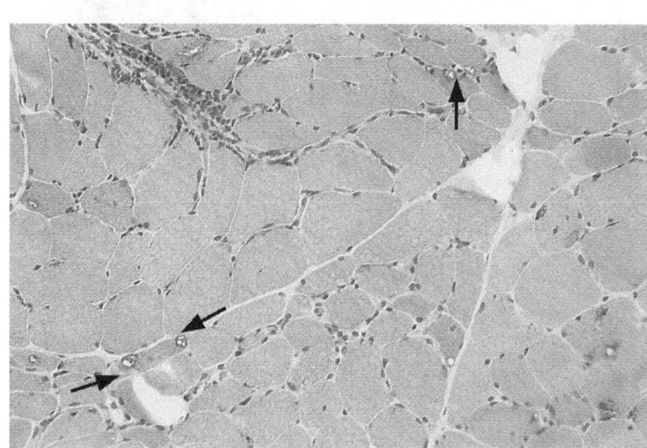

A

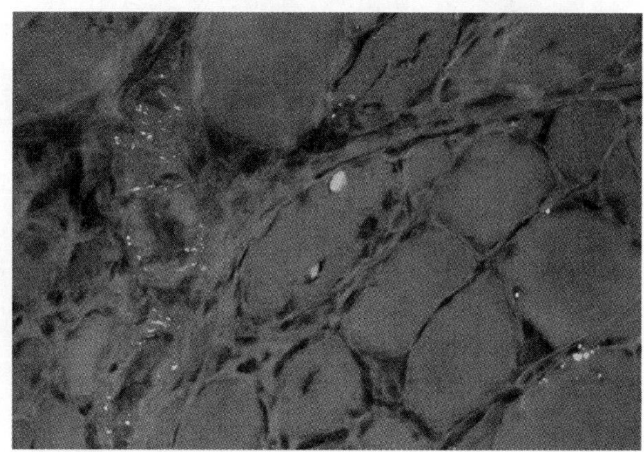

B

C

FIGURE 27-14
Inclusion body myositis (IBM). (*A*) Hematoxylin and eosin stain. The features in IBM resemble those of polymyositis, but the muscle fibers also exhibit rimmed vacuoles (*arrows*), corresponding to enlarged lysosomes. The hyaline inclusions are sparse and difficult to visualize with this stain. (*B*) Congo red stain. The inclusion has weak congophilia, but the color signal is strong because it has been enhanced by fluorescence excitation. (*C*) This electron micrograph demonstrates the characteristic filaments of the amyloid inclusions.

chemic injury of individual muscle fibers and eventually to fiber atrophy. True infarcts may result from the involvement of larger intramuscular arteries. The skin rash, which clinically distinguishes dermatomyositis from the other types of inflammatory myopathies, is presumably related to the same microangiopathy.

☐ **Pathology:** This disorder features lymphoid infiltrates around blood vessels and in connective tissue of chiefly the perimysium (see Fig. 27-15). The infiltrates are composed of B cells and T cells with a high ratio of helper cells (CD4+) to cytotoxic/suppressor (CD8+) T cells. Immune complexes in the walls of blood vessels (see Fig. 27-15B) are associated with microangiopathy. The intramuscular blood vessels exhibit endothelial hyperplasia, fibrin thrombi, and obliteration of capillaries. Perifascicular atrophy consists of one or more layers of atrophic fibers located at the periphery of the fascicles. The combination of perifascicular atrophy and immune complexes in capillary walls is virtually diagnostic of dermatomyositis, even in the absence of inflammation. The abnormal staining of the endomysial connective tissue with the alkaline phosphatase reaction reflects the damage to the blood vessels (see Fig. 27-15C).

MYASTHENIA GRAVIS

Myasthenia gravis is an acquired autoimmune disease characterized by abnormal muscular fatigability and caused by circulating antibodies to the acetylcholine (Ach) receptor at the myoneural junction. It occurs in all races and is twice as common in women as in men. The disease typically begins in young adults, but cases in children and the very old have also been described.

☐ **Pathogenesis:** Myasthenia gravis is mediated by an immunological attack on the Ach receptor of the motor end plate. Polyclonal antibodies attach to various epitopes of the receptor protein, and act by reducing the number of the receptors. A syndrome resembling human myasthenia can be induced in animals by injecting the Ach receptor together with Freund adjuvant.

In myasthenia gravis, the antigen–antibody complex binds complement components and produces shedding of the terminal portions of the junction folds of the neuromuscular junction, which are rich in Ach receptors. The IgG antibodies are bivalent, and they cross-link the receptor proteins remaining in the postsynaptic membrane. This effect increases the rate of endocytosis of the recep-

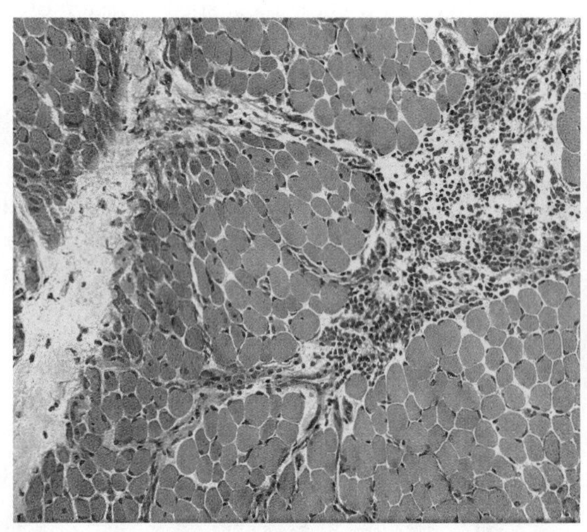

A

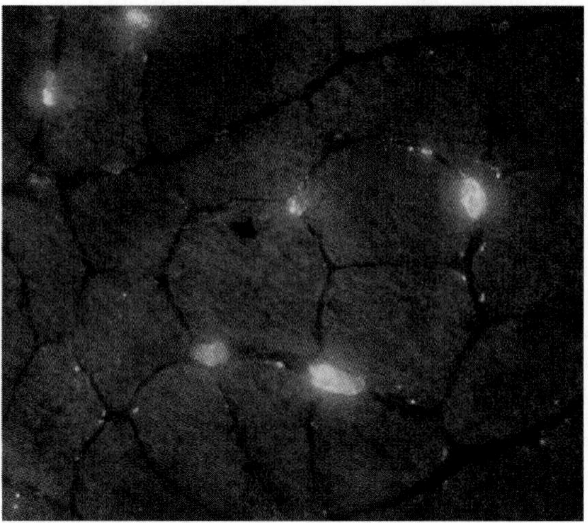

B

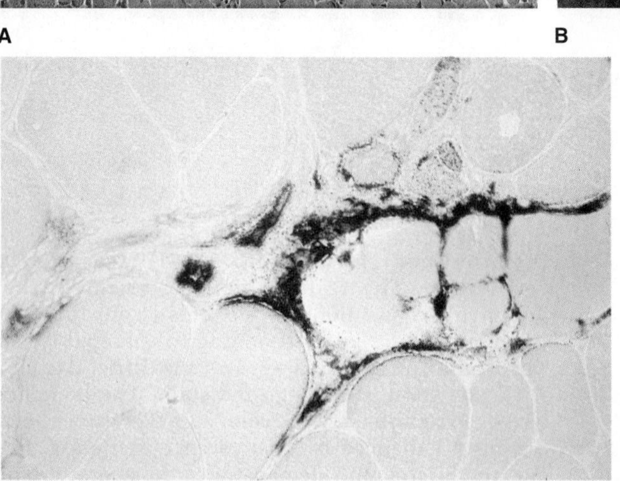

C

FIGURE 27-15
Dermatomyositis. *(A)* Hematoxylin and eosin stain. In dematomyositis, the inflammatory cells infiltrate predominantly the perimysium rather than the endomysium. In addition, narrow, peripheral zones of muscle fascicles disclose atrophic fibers, a pattern referred to as perifascicular atrophy. *(B)* In this immunofluorescence photograph, the walls of many capillaries display C5b-9 (membrane attack complex). *(C)* Alkaline phosphatase stain. The abnormal staining of the tissue is located largely in the blood vessels of the endomysium, reflecting the altered microvasculature typical of dermatomyositis. A few small regenerating fibers are also stained by this method.

tors, exceeding the muscle fiber's ability to replace them. The combination of a reduced area of the postsynaptic membrane, a decreased number of Ach receptors per unit area, and a widened synaptic space results in muscle weakness and abnormal fatigability. There is little evidence that the antireceptor antibodies directly block the action of Ach to prevent neuromuscular transmission.

The thymus clearly plays an important role in the pathogenesis of myasthenia gravis. Up to 40% of patients have an associated thymoma, and surgical removal is often curative. As many as 75% of the remaining patients have thymic hyperplasia, and in such cases, thymectomy is often an effective treatment. Ach receptors have been demonstrated on the surface of some thymic cells in both thymoma and thymic hyperplasia. Thus, there is evidence to suggest that in myasthenia gravis, thymic T lymphocytes activate B lymphocytes to produce antireceptor antibodies.

☐ **Pathology:** By light microscopy, the pathological changes in myasthenia gravis are not impressive. At best, a muscle biopsy may reveal atrophy of type II muscle fibers. Focal collections of lymphocytes may be present within the fascicles, particularly in autopsy tissue. By electron microscopy, most muscle endplates are abnormal, even in muscles that are not weakened. There is simplification of the sarcolemmal secondary folds, breakdown and loss of the crests of the folds, and widening of the clefts.

☐ **Clinical Features:** Patients with myasthenia gravis show considerable variation in the severity of the condition, and, similar to other autoimmune diseases, the symptoms tend to wax and wane. Weakness of the extraocular muscles is typically severe and causes ptosis and diplopia. In fact, myasthenia gravis may remain confined to these muscles. More frequently, the disease progresses to other muscles, such as those associated with swallowing, the trunk, and extremities. Patients with myasthenia gravis also have a high incidence of other autoimmune diseases.

The overall mortality of myasthenia gravis is about 10%, often owing to respiratory insufficiency because of muscle weakness. In addition to thymectomy, corticosteroid therapy, with or without methotrexate, and anticholinesterase drugs are used alone or in combination for treatment of these patients. Plasmapheresis acts to reduce the titers of anti-Ach receptor antibodies and can ameliorate symptoms, but the clinical effects are short-lived.

LAMBERT–EATON SYNDROME

Lambert-Eaton syndrome is a paraneoplastic disorder that presents as muscular weakness, wasting, and fatigability of the proximal limbs and trunk. Also termed *myasthenic–myopathic syndrome,* the disease is usually associated with small cell carcinoma of the lung, although it may also occur in patients with other malignant diseases and rarely in the absence of an underlying malignancy. There is neurophysiological evidence for a defect in the release of Ach at the nerve terminals. Similar to myasthenia gravis, the disease seems to have an autoimmune basis, because it can be transferred to mice by IgG from patients, and it responds to treatment with corticosteroids. The pathogenic IgG autoantibodies recognize voltage-sensitive calcium channels that are expressed both in motor nerve terminals and in the cells of the lung cancer. The calcium channels are necessary for release of Ach, and they are greatly reduced in the presynaptic membrane in these patients, thereby interfering with neuromuscular transmission. The Lambert–Eaton syndrome is one of several different paraneoplastic syndromes of the nervous system that are thought to be caused by pathogenic antibodies reactive to autoantigens of nerve cells.

INHERITED METABOLIC DISEASES

Skeletal muscle is dramatically affected by a variety of endocrine and metabolic diseases, such as Cushing syndrome, Addison disease, hypothyroidism, hyperthyroidism, and conditions associated with hepatic or renal failure. In the following discussion, however, a primary hereditary abnormality in the metabolism of skeletal muscle results in abnormal muscular function.

Glycogen Storage Diseases (Glycogenoses)

Glycogen storage diseases are autosomal recessive, inherited, metabolic disorders characterized by an inability to degrade glycogen (see Chapter 6). There are in excess of a dozen known glycogenoses caused by abnormalities of different enzymes involved in glycogen metabolism.

For the purpose of this discussion, we illustrate four conditions that significantly affect the function of skeletal muscle. When these disorders were initially described, they were often identified according to the person who first recognized the abnormality (e.g., Pompe disease, McArdle disease). Later, as the specific enzyme deficiency was identified, the disease was classified according to the deficient enzyme (e.g., acid maltase deficiency, myophosphorylase deficiency). However, we now know that different genetic mutations (genotypes) can affect the same enzyme and lead to different clinical phenotypes. For example, infantile acid maltase deficiency and adult-onset acid maltase deficiency represent distinct mutations. Another nomenclature attaches a Roman numeral to the enzyme deficiency. For instance, Pompe disease (acid maltase deficiency, infantile acid maltase deficiency) is also known as type II glycogenosis. Diagnoses of all four glycogenoses can be established by biochemical analysis of the deficient enzyme in skeletal muscle. The genes for these enzymes have been cloned and sequenced. Genomic DNA analysis of blood leukocytes or other cells can potentially provide *in utero* diagnosis or detect the heterozygote state.

Type II Glycogenosis (Acid Maltase Deficiency, α-1,4-Glucosidase Deficiency, Pompe Disease)

Various genetic mutations affect the acid maltase activity of muscle and lead to distinctly different clinical syndromes. Acid maltase is a lysosomal enzyme that is expressed in all cells and participates in the degradation of glycogen. When the enzyme is deficient, glycogen is not broken down, accumulates within lysosomes, and remains membrane bound (Fig. 27-16).

☐ **Pathology:** In all forms of glycogenosis due to acid maltase deficiency, the morphological changes are distinctive and almost pathognomonic. The muscle in Pompe disease displays massive accumulation of membrane-bound glycogen and disappearance of the myofilaments and other sarcoplasmic organelles. Surprisingly, there is very little regeneration, and apparently inactive satellite cells are present on the surface of muscle fibers that have been almost completely destroyed by the disease process.

The pathological features of late infantile, juvenile, and adult-onset forms of type II glycogenosis are milder. The morphological changes range from an overt vacuolar myopathy demonstrated by routine histology to very subtle accumulation of membrane-bound glycogen particles detectable only by electron microscopy. Vacuoles observed by light microscopy are empty or they contain PAS-positive granular material that is removed by diastase, indicating that it is composed of glycogen (see Fig. 27-16B).

☐ **Clinical Features:** The first acid maltase deficiency to be recognized, described by Pompe, is the most severe form and occurs in the neonatal or early infantile stage. These patients have severe hypotonia and areflexia and clinically resemble patients with Werdnig–Hoffmann disease (see later under Denervation). Sometimes the patients have an enlarged tongue and cardiomegaly. They die of cardiac failure, usually within the first 2 years of life. Many tissues are affected, but the most significant involvement is in skeletal and cardiac muscle, the central nervous system (CNS), and the liver. The serum creatine kinase level is only slightly to moderately increased.

Many patients with later-onset forms of the disease have a mild but relentlessly progressive myopathy. Glycogen accumulates in other organs, but clinical expression of the disorder is usually limited to muscle. In the past, it was often mistaken for muscular dystrophy affecting the girdle muscles.

Type III Glycogenosis (Debranching Enzyme Deficiency, Cori Disease, Limit Dextrinosis, Amylo-1,6-Glucosidase Deficiency)

Type III glycogenosis is a rare, autosomal recessive disease that affects children or adults. In these patients, phosphorylase is able to hydrolyze 1,4-glycosidic linkages of the terminal glucose chains of glycogen, but not beyond the 1,6-glycosidic linkage at the site of a branch point, owing to the absence of the debranching enzyme. Glycogen without surface glucose chains is referred to as "limit dextrin." Hepatomegaly and growth retardation are usual. The muscle involvement and symptoms are variable, and the most severe and consistent involvement is related to liver dysfunction in children. Liver dysfunction usually subsides or it may not ever be clinically manifest. Rarely, these patients appear in adulthood with a slowly progressive myopathy. Electron microscopy reveals large masses of glycogen granules free in the sarcoplasm.

Type V Glycogenosis (McArdle Disease, Myophosphorylase Deficiency)

Type V glycogenosis is a more common metabolic myopathy, which is usually not progressive or severely debilitating. The enzyme, myophosphorylase, is a tissue-specific protein of normal skeletal muscle. In the absence of enzyme activity, skeletal muscle glycogen cannot be cleaved at 1,4-glycosidic chains to produce glucose for energy pro-

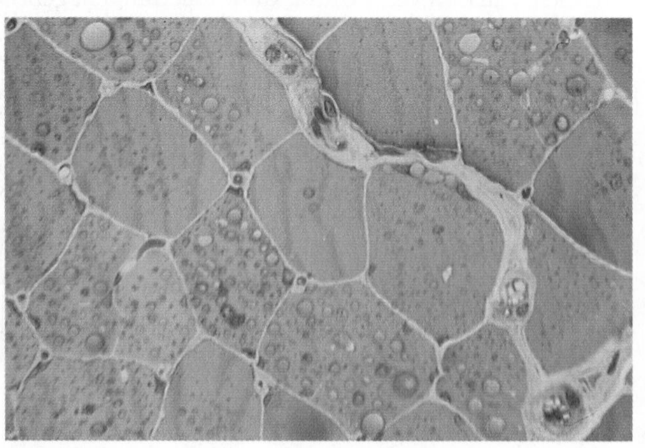

A

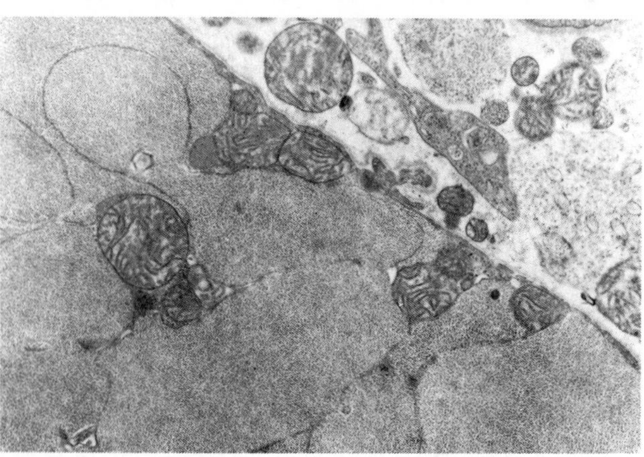

B

FIGURE *27-16*
Acid maltase deficiency—adult onset. (*A*) Semithin plastic section of muscle stained with toluidine blue. Vacuoles in muscle fibers contain metachromatic (slightly reddish) glycogen, which contrasts with the orthochromatic (bluish) staining of other structures. (*B*) An electron micrograph shows an accumulation of glycogen particles within lysosomes.

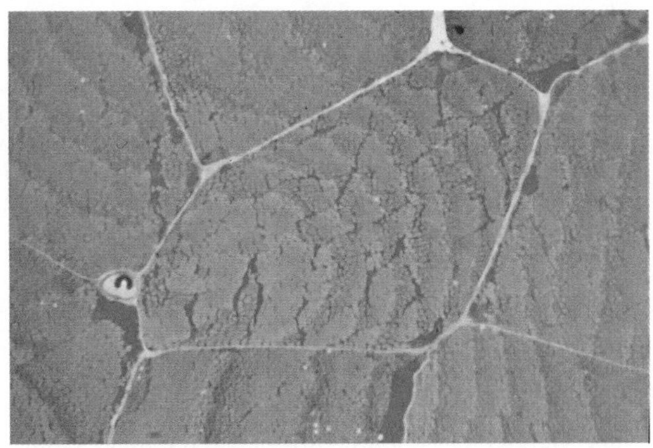
A

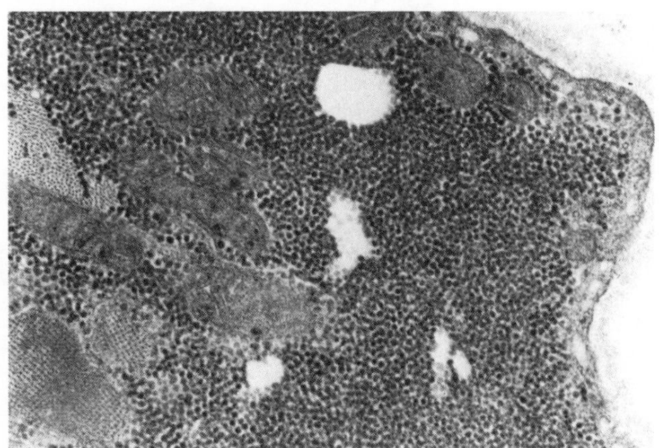
B

FIGURE 27-17
McArdle disease (myophosphorylase deficiency). (*A*) Transverse semithin plastic section of muscle stained by periodic acid–Schiff (PAS) and toluidine blue. PAS-positive glycogen accumulates predominantly in the subsarcolemmal region. (*B*) An electron micrograph demonstrates an abnormal mass of glycogen particles just beneath the sarcolemma. The glycogen is not surrounded by a membrane, in contrast to the lysosomal glycogen storage of acid maltase deficiency.

duction during periods of physical exertion. As a result, muscle cramps occur with exercise. The patient is also unable to produce lactate during ischemic exercise, a defect that is the basis for a metabolic test for the condition.

If the patient avoids strenuous exercise, the abnormality does not seriously interfere with his life. However, prolonged, vigorous exercise can lead to widespread necrosis of myofibers and release of soluble muscle proteins, such as creatine kinase and myoglobin, into the circulation. This event, in turn, can produce myoglobinuria and renal failure. The renal disorder must be treated immediately by giving life-saving intravenous fluids and osmotic agents to induce a diuresis.

Muscle biopsy should be performed several weeks after an episode of symptoms to allow regeneration of the muscle. The tissue may appear completely normal, except for the absence of phosphorylase activity. However, there is usually evidence of subtle abnormal accumulation of glycogen granules within the sarcoplasm, predominantly within the subsarcolemmal area (Fig. 27-17). The specific diagnosis can be made by the histochemical reaction for myophosphorylase, but it must be confirmed by biochemical assay of the muscle enzyme activity or by analysis of genomic DNA.

Type VII Glycogenosis (Phosphofructokinase Deficiency)

Phosphofructokinase (PFK) deficiency is less common than McArdle disease but causes an identical syndrome. PFK is a key enzyme in the Embden–Meyerhof pathway that catalyzes the conversion of fructose-6-phosphate to fructose-1,6-diphosphate. In muscle, this enzyme is composed of four identical subunits (M4), whereas in erythrocytes, the tetramer is assembled by two different subunits (the M and L subunits), each under separate genetic control. As a result, a genetic lack of the muscle subunit results in a complete absence of PFK activity in muscle, but only a 50% decrease in activity in erythrocytes. In the latter cells, the remaining active enzyme is made up of four normal L subunits.

Patients with type VII glycogenosis often have slight anemia or low-grade hemolysis. The morphological findings are similar to those in McArdle disease, except that the patients exhibit phosphorylase activity in the muscle. By contrast, a histochemical reaction for PFK shows little or no staining for the enzyme. The diagnosis is substantiated by biochemical analysis of the enzyme activity in muscle.

Lipid Myopathies

Occasionally, the muscle biopsy specimen from a patient with exercise intolerance or muscle weakness contains an excess amount of neutral lipids. Such conditions are caused by a variety of metabolic disorders affecting lipid metabolism, of which more than a dozen have been identified. In brief, lipid myopathies may involve (1) deficient transport of fatty acids into the mitochondria (carnitine deficiency syndromes and carnitine palmityl transferase deficiency), (2) defects in a variety of enzymes that mediate β-oxidation of fatty acids, (3) abnormalities in respiratory chain enzymes, and (4) defects in triglyceride utilization. Only disorders involving carnitine metabolism are discussed here.

Carnitine Deficiency

Carnitine, which is synthesized in the liver and is present in large quantities in skeletal muscle, is necessary for the transport of long-chain fatty acids into the mitochondria. Patients with muscle carnitine deficiency, an autosomal recessive condition, have progressive proximal muscle weakness and atrophy and often show signs of denervation and peripheral neuropathy. The absence of carnitine leads to massive accumulation of lipid droplets in the sarcoplasm outside the mitochondria, a change readily evident in a muscle biopsy. Sometimes oral carnitine therapy alleviates the symptoms. Carnitine deficiency in skeletal muscle also occurs as part of a systemic disorder that can affect the central nervous system, heart, and liver.

Carnitine Palmityl Transferase Deficiency

As in carnitine deficiency, persons with carnitine palmityl transferase deficiency are unable to metabolize long-chain fatty acids because of an inability to transport these lipids into the mitochondria, where they undergo β-oxidation. After prolonged exercise, these patients have muscular pain, which may progress to myoglobinuria. Prolonged fasting can produce the same symptoms. After such an episode, fibers regenerate and restore muscle structure. Biopsy specimens show no excess sarcoplasmic lipid or other microscopic abnormalities, and the diagnosis depends on the biochemical assay for carnitine palmityl transferase activity.

Mitochondrial Diseases

Inherited defects of mitochondrial metabolism are an uncommon but conceptually important group of disorders. Historically, diseases of muscle were recognized first and designated mitochondrial myopathies, but others affect the CNS as well as muscle and are known as the mitochondrial encephalomyopathies. The nervous system, skeletal muscle, heart, kidney, and other organs can be affected in different combinations as part of a multisystem disease.

The inherited diseases of mitochondria are classified genetically into two broad groups, defects of either nDNA or mtDNA. Point mutations, deletions, and duplications of mtDNA have been identified and linked to several syndromes of the mitochondrial encephalomyopathies. This group of syndromes is discussed here.

☐ **Pathogenesis:** The majority of mitochondrial proteins are encoded by nDNA, but 13 of the approximately 80 polypeptide subunits of the respiratory chain complexes are specified by mtDNA, and defects in these proteins compose the mitochondrial encephalomyopathies.

The diseases of mtDNA have a maternal form of inheritance, contrasting with the Mendelian pattern of nDNA mutations. MtDNA of the zygote is derived exclusively from the oocyte. The zygote and its daughter cells have many mitochondria, each of which contains several copies of the maternally derived mitochondrial genome. Mutations in copies of mtDNA are passed on randomly to subsequent generations of cells. During growth of the fetus or later, it is likely that some cells contain only mutant genomes (mutant homoplasmy), whereas others have only normal genomes (wild-type homoplasmy). Still others receive a mixed population of mutant and normal mtDNA (heteroplasmy). In turn, clinical expression of a disease produced by a given mutation of mtDNA depends on the total content of mitochondrial genomes and the proportion that is mutant. **The fraction of mutant mtDNA must exceed a critical value for a mitochondrial disease to become symptomatic.** This threshold varies in different organs and is presumably related to the energy requirements of the cells.

☐ **Pathology:** In skeletal muscle, the pathological signature of a defect of mtDNA is the accumulation of mitochondria. The excessive organelles are expressed as aggregates of reddish granular material in the sarcoplasm, as demonstrated by the modified Gomori trichrome stain (Fig. 27-18A). The abnormality has been termed a ragged red fiber because of the irregular contour of the reddish deposits at the fiber periphery. Pathogenic mutations of mtDNA in these diseases often impair the activity of complex IV (cytochrome oxidase). Three of the subunits are encoded by mtDNA, and they are required for function of the assembled electron transport carrier. Hence, histochemical stains for ragged red fibers are often deficient in cytochrome oxidase activity (see Fig. 27-18C). By contrast, the ragged red fibers stain intensely for succinate dehydrogenase (complex II), a complex that is exclusively encoded by nDNA (see Fig. 27-18B). The increased activity of succinic dehydrogenase presumably reflects the proliferation of mitochondria, and it is one of the many proteins synthesized in the cytoplasm and imported into the mitochondrion. The defects of mitochondria (see Fig. 27-18D) result in atrophy of myofibers and the accumulation of sarcoplasmic lipid and glycogen. Death of nerve cells and reactive astrocytosis occur in the CNS.

☐ **Clinical Features:** The clinical manifestations of the encephalomyopathies are extremely variable, but usually begin in childhood. Some of the patients begin with muscle weakness and later develop a brain disorder. Others begin with a neurological disease of the brain and may or may not have overt muscle weakness, even though the muscle biopsy indicates a mitochondrial disorder. Other organs, such as the heart, are often affected as part of a multisystem disorder.

Three neurological syndromes have been defined clinically and designated (1) *Kearns–Sayre syndrome* (progressive ophthalmoplegia, retinal pigmentary degeneration, cardiac arrhythmias, and other features), (2) *MELAS* (mitochondrial myopathy, encephalopathy, lactic acidosis, and stroke-like episodes), and (3) *MERRF* (myoclonic epilepsy and ragged red fibers). Most of the patients with Kearns–Sayre syndrome have large deletions of mtDNA and are not familial. MELAS and MERRF usually display point mutations of mitochondrial genes for certain transfer RNA and show a maternal pattern of inheritance.

Myoadenylate Deaminase Deficiency

Adenosine monophosphate deaminase (AMP-DA) is present in large quantities in skeletal muscle, particularly in type II fibers. AMP-DA is an important enzyme in the regulation of the purine nucleotide cycle that helps to main-

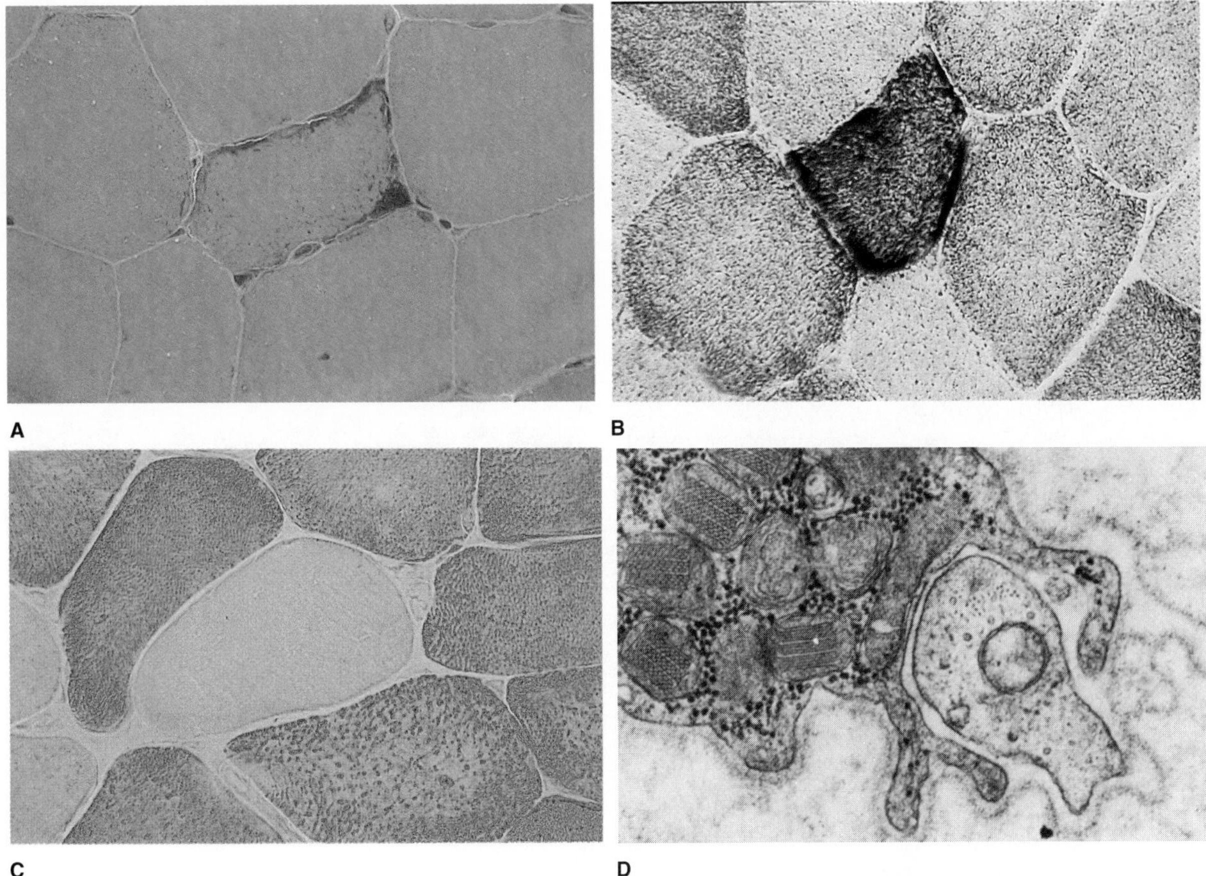

FIGURE 27-18
Mitochondrial myopathy caused by deletions of mitochondrial DNA (mtDNA). (*A*) Modified Gomori trichrome. A ragged red fiber shows prominent proliferation of reddish, granular mitochondria, located chiefly in a subsarcolemmal region. (*B*) Succinate dehydrogenase (SDH) stain. A ragged red fiber shows overexpression of SDH, an electron-transport carrier that is entirely encoded by nuclear DNA (nDNA). (*C*) Another ragged red fiber displays lack of histochemical staining for cytochrome oxidase. Three subunits of this electron-transport carrier are coded by mtDNA, and the mutations have interfered with function in this fiber. (*D*) An electron micrograph reveals mitochondria with ultrastructural abnormalities, including paracrystalline inclusions.

tain the ATP/ADP ratio during exercise. A group of patients with mild proximal muscle weakness and exercise intolerance exhibit complete absence of AMP-DA activity. It is a common, autosomal recessive condition, occurring in 1% to 2% of all muscle biopsy specimens. There is a question as to whether AMP-DA deficiency represents a separate disease entity or a malady that is unmasked by other neuromuscular diseases.

Familial Periodic Paralysis

Familial periodic paralysis refers to a group of autosomal dominant disorders characterized by episodes of muscular weakness or even complete paralysis, followed by a rapid recovery. The disorders are related to abnormalities in sodium and potassium fluxes into and out of muscle cells. During an attack, the surface of the muscle fibers does not propagate an action potential, although the delivery of calcium inside the muscle fiber results in contraction. Muscle biopsy specimens taken during the attack exhibit no detectable abnormalities of recent onset. Later, permanent mild myopathic features and sarcoplasmic vacuoles appear. The vacuoles correspond to dilated or remodeled sarcoplasmic reticulum and transverse tubules. In some cases, a distinct subpopulation of fibers (type IIB) contains large numbers of tubular aggregates, which are derived from the tubular network of the sarcoplasmic reticulum.

There are three clinically and genetically distinct syndromes—hypokalemic, hyperkalemic, and normokalemic periodic paralysis. The hypokalemic type has been linked to mutations of the gene that encodes a voltage-gated calcium channel of skeletal muscle, whereas the hyperkalemic and normokalemic forms reflect mutations in the SCN4A gene on chromosome 17q, which specifies the sodium channel.

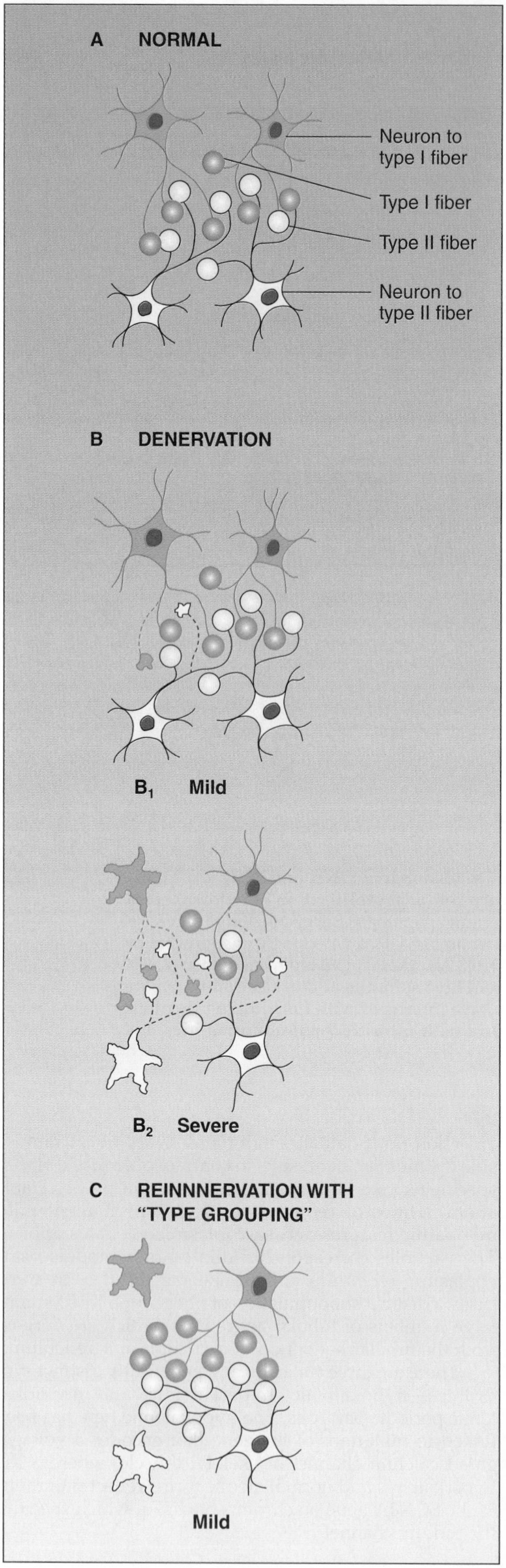

A NORMAL

Neuron to type I fiber

Type I fiber

Type II fiber

Neuron to type II fiber

B DENERVATION

B_1 Mild

B_2 Severe

C REINNNERVATION WITH "TYPE GROUPING"

Mild

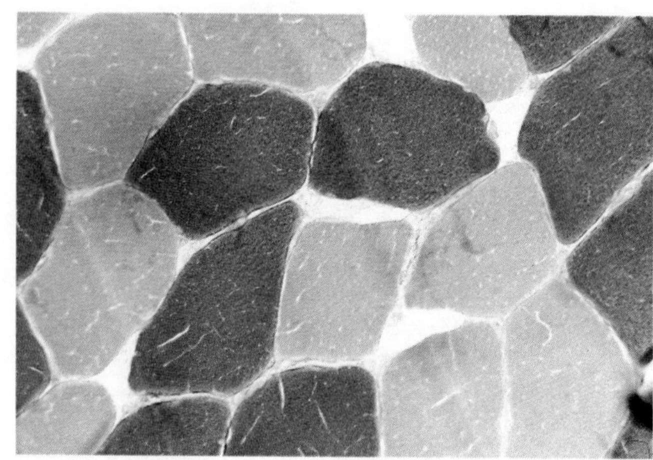

A

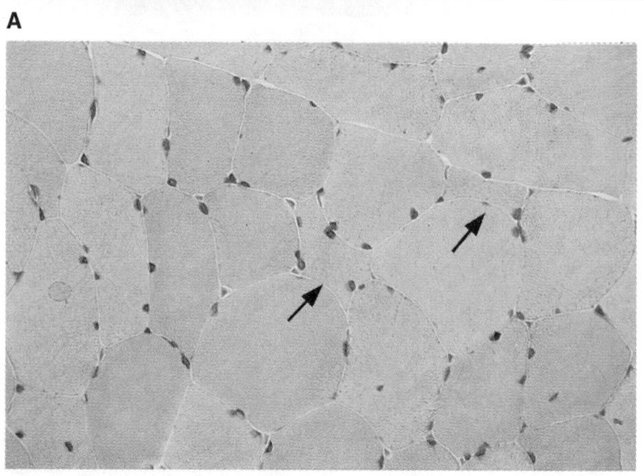

B_1

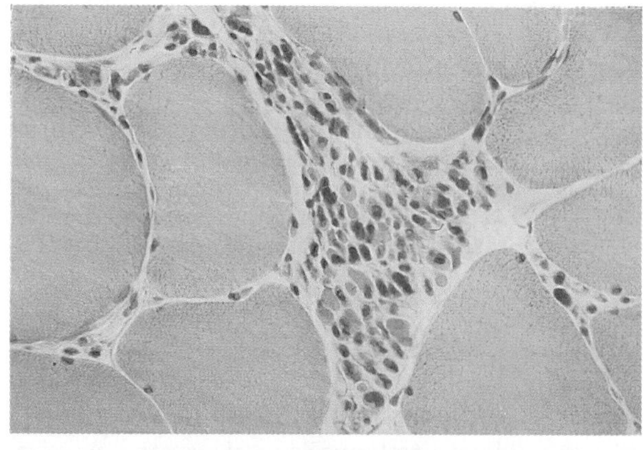

B_2

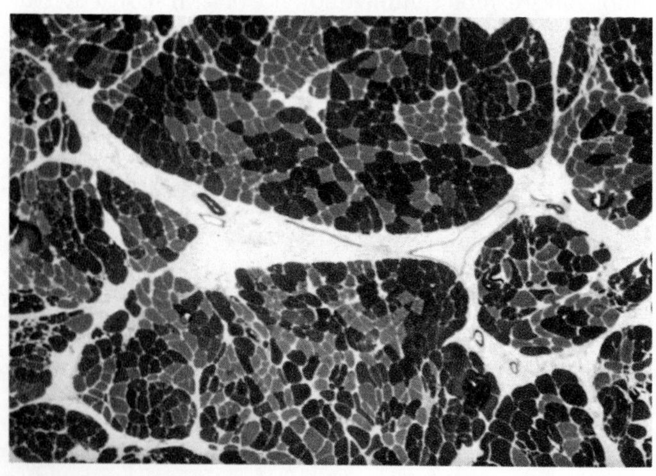

C

RHABDOMYOLYSIS

Rhabdomyolysis refers to the dissolution of skeletal muscle fibers and the release of myoglobin into the circulation, an event that may result in myoglobinuria and acute renal failure. The disorder may be acute, subacute, or chronic. During acute rhabdomyolysis, the muscles are swollen and tender and profoundly weak.

Occasionally, an episode of rhabdomyolysis may complicate or follow influenza. Some patients develop rhabdomyolysis with apparently mild exercise and probably have some form of metabolic myopathy. After recovery, a subsequent biopsy may reveal muscle that is morphologically normal. Rhabdomyolysis also may complicate heat stroke or malignant hyperthermia after the administration of an anesthetic such as halothane. Alcoholism is occasionally associated with either acute or chronic rhabdomyolysis.

The pathological changes in rhabdomyolysis correspond to an active, noninflammatory myopathy, with scattered necrosis of muscle fibers and varying degrees of degeneration and regeneration. Clusters of macrophages are seen in and around muscle fibers, but these are not accompanied by lymphocytes or inflammatory cells.

DENERVATION

The pathology of denervation reflects lesions of the lower motor neuron. Lesions of the upper motor neuron, as occur in multiple sclerosis or stroke, result in paralysis and atrophy. However, the lower motor neuron in these conditions remains intact, and the pathological changes reflect a nonspecific diffuse atrophy rather than denervation atrophy.

A muscle biopsy is a highly sensitive test for detecting a lesion of the lower motor neuron, but the pattern of denervation does not identify the cause of the lesion. For example, it does not distinguish between a disease such as amyotrophic lateral sclerosis, a disorder of motor neurons and a peripheral neuropathy due to diabetes mellitus. The morphological changes indicate whether the denervation is recent or chronic.

When a skeletal muscle fiber becomes separated from contact with its lower motor neuron, it invariably atrophies, owing to the progressive loss of myofibrils. On cross-section, the atrophic fiber has a characteristic angular configuration, seemingly compressed by surrounding normal muscle fibers (Fig. 27-19). If the fiber is not reinnervated, the atrophy proceeds to complete loss of myofibrils, and the nuclei condense into aggregates. In the end stage, the muscle fibers disappear and are replaced chiefly by adipose tissue.

The early phase of denervating disease is characterized by irregularly scattered angular atrophic fibers. As the disease progresses, these fibers are seen in groups, at first in small clusters of several fibers, and later in progressively larger groups (see Fig. 27-19B). Denervated, angular, atrophic fibers are excessively dark when stained for nonspecific esterase (Fig. 27-20) and NADH-TR reactions, in contrast to atrophy caused by disuse or wasting. With the ATPase reaction, the groups of dark-stained, angular, atrophic fibers are a mixture of type I and type II fibers. In virtually all of the known denervating conditions, there is no selective denervation of one type of motor neuron.

Another abnormality occasionally present in a denervating condition is the "target fiber" (Fig. 27-21), seen in 20% of cases. This change is apparently transient, occurring during or shortly after the process of denervation or reinnervation and indicating that the process is active. This lesion consists of a central pallor of the muscle fiber. This area is surrounded by a condensed zone, which in turn is surrounded by a normal zone of sarcoplasm. Target fibers are difficult to see with the hematoxylin and eosin stain but are clearly demonstrated by the NADH-TR stain, which shows a greatly reduced staining in the central zone (see Fig. 27-21). This alteration reflects a reduction or absence of mitochondria.

With every episode of denervation, there is an effort at reinnervation. In a slowly progressive denervating pro-

FIGURE *27-19*
Denervation/reinnervation. *(A)* As shown in the photomicrograph, the normal intermixed distribution of type I (*pale*) and type II (*dark*) muscle fibers is shown by staining for adenosine triphosphatase (ATPase). In the drawing, two neurons (*red*) innervate type I muscle fibers, and two neurons (*black*) supply type II fibers. *(B)* Denervation; hematoxylin and eosin stain. With early (mild) denervation (B_1), portions of the axonal tree degenerate, resulting in angular atrophy of scattered type I and II muscle fibers. With more advanced (severe) denervation (B_2), entire lower motor neurons or numerous axonal processes degenerate, causing small groups of angular atrophic fibers to appear as illustrated in the photomicrograph. *(C)* Reinnervation; myofibrillar ATPase. As neurons degenerate, surviving neurons sprout more nerve endings and reinnervate some of the denervated fibers. These reinnervated fibers become either type I or type II, according to the type of neuron that reinnervates them. This process results in fewer, but larger, motor units and the appearance of clusters of fibers of one type adjacent to clusters of the other type, a pattern called "type grouping." The photomicrograph demonstrates type grouping. (Compare with the normal pattern illustrated in Fig. 27-3B or 27-19A.) This field would appear normal except for a few atrophic fibers if it were stained with hematoxylin and eosin.

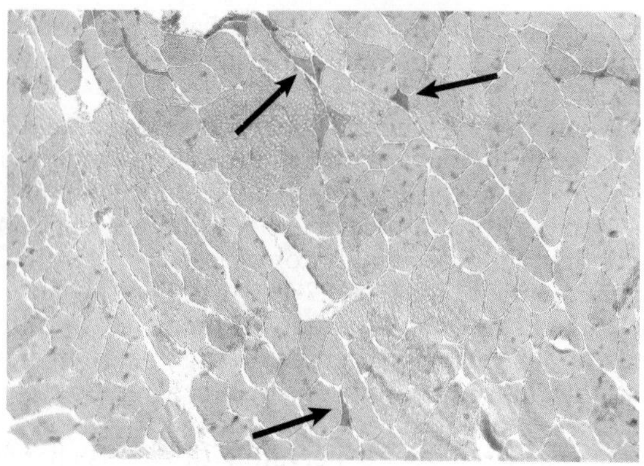

FIGURE 27-20
Denervation. In this frozen section of the biceps muscle subjected to the nonspecific esterase reaction, there are a few irregularly scattered, angular, atrophic fibers (*arrows*), which are excessively dark-stained. This pattern is highly characteristic of atrophy due to denervation.

cess, reinnervation may actually keep pace with denervation. New sprouting nerve endings make synaptic contact with the muscle fiber at the site of the previous motor end plate. Shortly after denervation, the muscle fiber becomes covered with the nicotinic Ach receptor (extrajunctional receptor), a situation similar to that in the myotubular phase of embryogenesis. This denervated state induces the sprouting of new nerve endings from adjacent surviving nerve. With reinnervation, the extrajunctional receptor again disappears from the sarcolemma, except at the point of synaptic contact.

In a chronic denervating condition, reinnervation of each surviving motor unit gradually becomes larger. As a lower motor neuron of a specific type takes over the innervation of a given field of fibers, fiber groups of one type are seen adjacent to groups of another type. This pattern is designated *type grouping* and is pathognomonic of denervation followed by reinnervation (see Figs. 27-19C and 27-22).

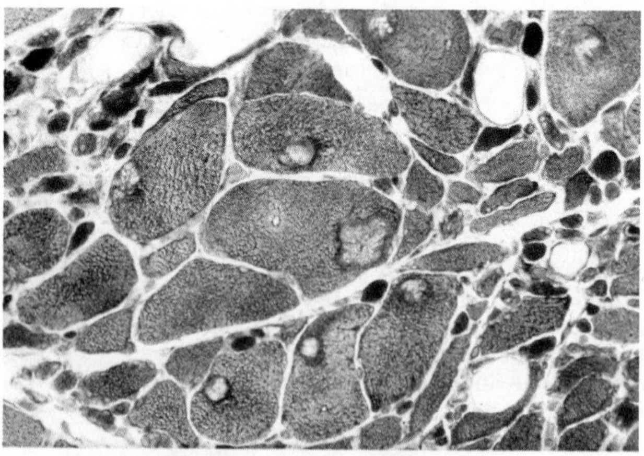

FIGURE 27-21
Target fiber. A cross-section of striated muscle treated with an reduced nicotinamide adenine dinucleotide (NADH)-TR stain demonstrates several "target fibers," a characteristic feature of some cases of denervation. Because the enzyme reaction creates a product (formazan) that selectively fixes to membranous organelles, the centers of the target areas appear devoid of mitochondria and sarcoplasmic reticulum. The myofibrils may or may not be intact.

Patients with striking type grouping often have symptoms of muscle cramping in addition to progressive muscular weakness. After a single episode of denervation, such as occurs with poliomyelitis, reinnervation often leads to a remarkable recovery of strength. Years later, a biopsy shows a conspicuous pattern of type grouping, with scattered pyknotic nuclear clumps (see Fig. 27-22B). In such cases, there are neither angular atrophic fibers nor target fibers.

Occasionally, a biopsy specimen reveals an abnormal prominence of one fiber type over the other. This situation is designated *type predominance* and may involve either type I or type II fibers. The explanation for this effect is often not clear, but there is frequently evidence of denervation. It could be that in type predominance, reinnervation favors one type of lower motor neuron over another.

It is not uncommon to see occasional muscle fibers undergoing necrosis or regeneration in neuropathic conditions. In these patients, a modest increase in serum creatine kinase levels reflects mild muscle degeneration. This finding is common in patients with slowly progressive forms of spinal muscular atrophy, as in Kugelberg–Welander disease and Kennedy disease.

Spinal Muscular Atrophy

The syndrome of spinal muscular atrophy (SMA) is characterized by degeneration of anterior horn cells of the spinal cord and represents the second most common, lethal, autosomal recessive disorder after cystic fibrosis. Childhood SMA is classified into type I (Werdnig–Hoffmann disease), type II (intermediate), and type III (Kugelberg–Welander disease). The survival motor neuron gene (5q11.2-13.3) is absent in virtually all (99%) cases of SMA.

WERDNIG–HOFFMANN DISEASE (INFANTILE SMA): *Werdnig–Hoffmann disease results in progressive and severe weakness in early infancy, and these infants seldom live beyond the first year of life.* The denervation seems to have begun *in utero* after the establishment of motor units. The histological pattern is virtually pathognomonic (Fig. 27-23). Groups of minute, rounded, atrophic fibers are still identifiable with the ATPase reaction as being either type I or type II. In addition, there are fascicles of normal muscle fibers and, almost invariably, striking clusters of markedly hypertrophied type I fibers. In addition to the absent survival motor neuron gene, a second gene (neuronal apoptosis inhibitory protein gene) has also been implicated in the pathogenesis of Werdnig–Hoffmann disease.

KUGELBERG–WELANDER DISEASE (JUVENILE SMA): *This variant is a later-onset form of SMA and is not necessarily progressive.* Previously, these patients were often designated as having limb-girdle muscular dystrophy. The electromyographic pattern of denervation helps to identify these patients. The muscle biopsy shows type grouping and other evidence of a neurogenic disorder, but can resemble a myopathy in a small sample because of coexisting necrotic fibers and regenerating fibers.

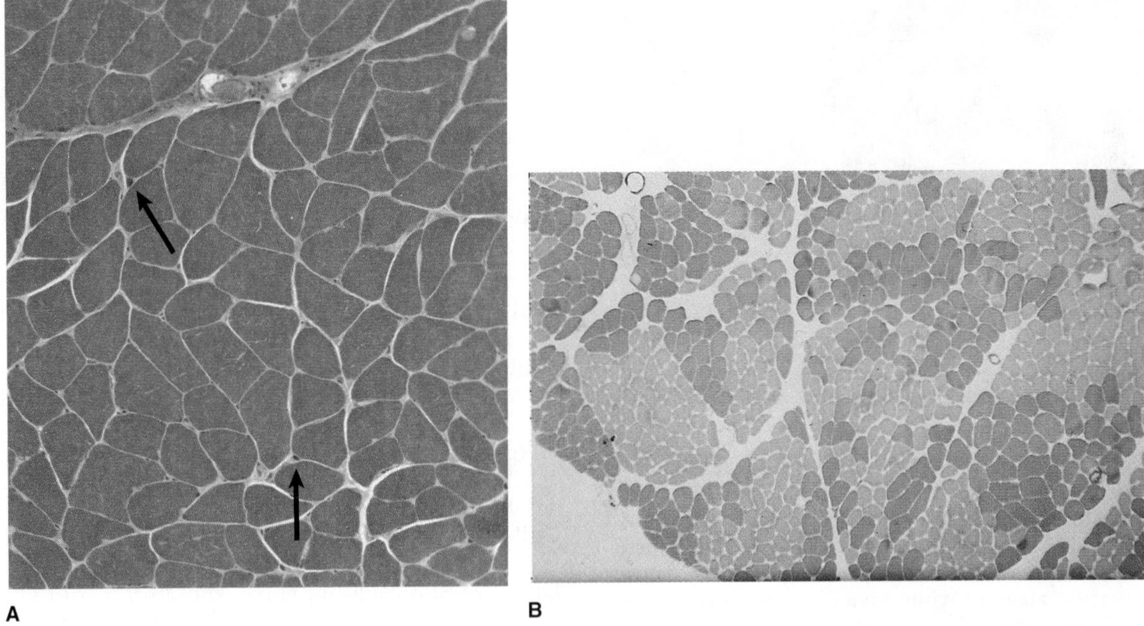

FIGURE 27-22
Type grouping. (*A*) This biopsy of the biceps was obtained from a 27-year-old woman who had contracted poliomyelitis at age 7 years. A section of the biceps stained with hematoxylin and eosin shows muscle fibers that vary slightly in size and shape. The scattered black "dots" (*arrows*) among some of the fibers are pyknotic nuclear clumps in extremely atrophic fibers that were not reinnervated. The fiber types cannot be distinguished with this stain. (*B*) A similar case stained for ATPase. Striking type grouping reflects reinnervation. Groups of type II fibers (*dark*) are adjacent to groups of type I fibers. As a result, there are fewer but larger motor units. The absence of angular atrophic fibers or target fibers suggests that there is no active denervation.

Type II Fiber Atrophy

A commonly misinterpreted pathological pattern in muscle biopsy specimens is atrophy resulting from disuse, wasting, upper motor neuron disease, and corticosteroid toxicity. This diffuse, nonspecific atrophy is manifested histologically by selective angular atrophy of type II fibers. With the hematoxylin and eosin stain, it is sometimes impossible to distinguish this pattern of atrophy from that of denervation. However, with the ATPase reaction, all of the angular atrophic fibers are type II (Fig. 27-24). Furthermore, these abnormal fibers do not stain heavily with the nonspecific esterase reaction or the NADH-TR reaction. Type II atrophy is a common condition, which is often an epiphenomenon related to a more chronic problem.

STEROID MYOPATHY: Corticosteroid therapy can produce muscle weakness, and the muscle biopsy is characterized histologically by type II atrophy. This pathological feature raises an important point clinically, because patients with polymyositis are often treated with large doses of corticosteroids. If the patient develops worsening weakness, the physician must decide whether the symptom represents a relapse of the polymyositis and requires an increase in the dose of corticosteroids. Alternatively, the weakness may represent steroid myopathy, in which case, a decrease in the dosage is indicated.

In weakness caused by corticosteroid toxicity, the patients do not demonstrate an increase in the serum creatine kinase level and histologically manifest a selective atrophy of type II fibers, in the absence of muscle fiber degeneration and inflammation. By contrast, fiber degeneration and inflammation would be expected in recurrent

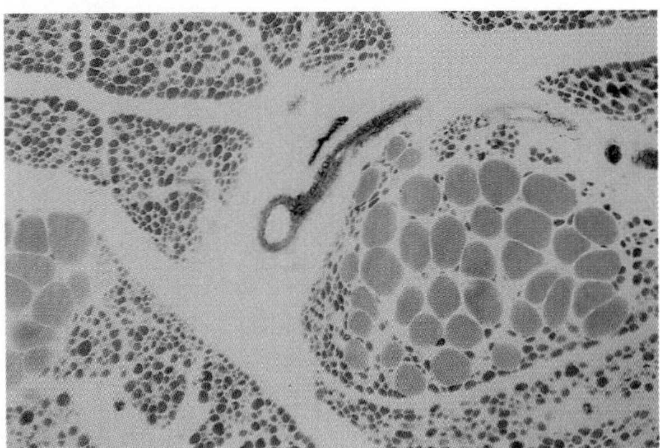

FIGURE 27-23
Werdnig–Hoffman disease (infantile spinal muscular atrophy). This cross-section of skeletal muscle stained for myofibrillar ATPase is derived from an infant with severe hypotonia. It shows groups of extremely atrophic, rounded type I and type II fibers and clusters of markedly hypertrophied type I fibers.

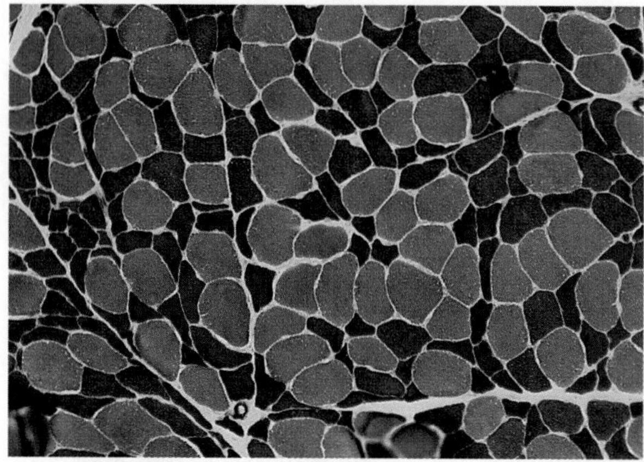

FIGURE 27-24
Type II fiber atrophy. This biopsy of the vastus lateralis muscle was taken from a 48 year-old man with proximal muscle weakness because of endogenous corticosteroid toxicity (Cushing syndrome). Virtually all of the angular atrophic fibers are type II. This form of atrophy closely mimics denervation atrophy when visualized with the hematoxylin and eosin stain.

polymyositis, a process that is reflected in an increase of the serum creatine kinase activity.

SUGGESTED READING

BOOKS

DiMauro S: Mitochondrial encephalomyopathies. In: Rosenberg RN (ed). *Molecular and genetic basis of neurological disease.* Stoneham: Butterworth, pp. 665–694, 1993.

Engel AG, Franzini-Armstrong C (eds): *Myology,* 2nd ed. New York: McGraw-Hill, 1994.

Emery AEH: *Duchenne muscular dystrophy,* revised ed. Oxford Monographs on Medical Genetics, vol 15. New York: Oxford University Press, 1988.

Mastaglia FL, Walton OF, Detchant L (eds): *Skeletal muscle pathology,* 2nd ed. Edinburgh: Churchill Livingstone, 1992.

Walton JA (ed): *Disorders of voluntary muscle,* 5th ed. London: Churchill Livingstone, 1988.

REVIEW ARTICLES

Ahn AH, Kunkel LM: The structural and functional diversity of dystrophin. *Nature Genet* 3:283–291, 1993.

Asbury AK, McKhann GM, McDonald WI (eds): Diseases of the central nervous system. *Clin Neurol* 1:11–15, 1992.

Beggs AH, Kunkel LM: Improved diagnosis of Duchenne/Becker muscular dystrophy. *J Clin Invest* 85:613–619, 1990.

Cullen MJ, Mastaglia FL: Morphological changes in dystrophic muscle. *Br Med Bull* 36:145–152, 1980.

DiMauro S, Bresolin E, Hays AP: Disorders of glycogen metabolism of muscle. *Crit Rev Clin Neurobiol* 1:83–116, 1984.

DiMauro S, Trevisan C, Hays A: Disorders of lipid metabolism in muscle. *Muscle Nerve* 3:369–388, 1980.

Mastaglia FL, Ojeda VJ: Inflammatory myopathies: Part 1. *Ann Neurol* 17:215–227, 1985.

Mastaglia FL, Ojeda VJ: Inflammatory myopathies: Part 2. *Ann Neurol* 17:317–323, 1985.

Plotz PH, Dalakas M, Leff RL, et al: Current concepts in the idiopathic inflammatory myopathies: Polymyositis, dermatomyositis and related disorders. *Ann Intern Med* 111:143–157, 1989.

Worton RG, Thompson MW: Genetics of Duchenne muscular dystrophy. *Annu Rev Genet* 22:601–629, 1988.

CHAPTER 28

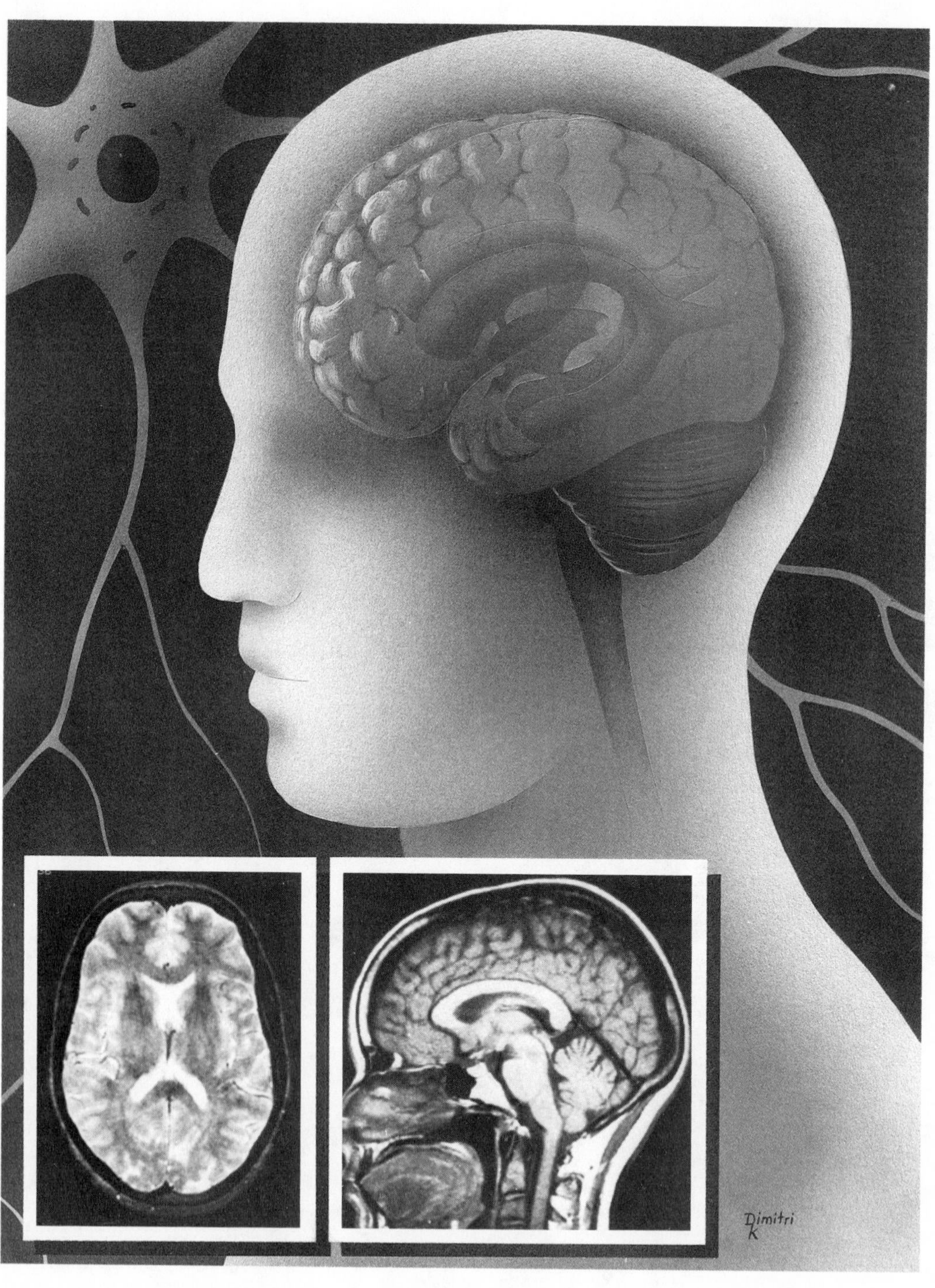

The Nervous System

F. Stephen Vogel
Gregory N. Fuller
Thomas W. Bouldin

FIGURE 28-1 *(see opposite page)*
The brain. The anatomical structures of the brain are well visualized by magnetic resonance imaging.

The Central Nervous System

Anatomically and functionally, the nervous system is the most complex structure in the body (Fig. 28-1). In some respects, the brain and the spinal cord can be viewed as consisting of many distinct organs, which are nevertheless intimately interconnected and are capable of exquisite and rapid communications. Thus, the sensory, motor, cognitive, memory, and autonomic functions of the nervous system have distinct anatomical correlates, although defects in one area may have significant effects on the functionality of other regions. Despite this intricate organization, the nervous system is governed by the same principles that control the function of cells in the rest of the body. The study of neuropathology emphasizes the unique character of the nervous system and, at the same time, the biological attributes that it shares with other tissues.

TOPOGRAPHY: The functional properties of the nervous system are topographically localized, and thus neurological diseases are also geographically distributed. The differential sensitivity of neurons to various types of degenerative and inflammatory disorders is remarkable. For example, Huntington disease is characterized by selective degeneration of neurons in the caudate nuclei, whereas Parkinson disease targets the substantia nigra, and amyotrophic lateral sclerosis singles out the motor neurons of the spinal cord, the brainstem, and the cerebrum. Similarly, infectious diseases have distinctive geographic distributions. Poliomyelitis involves the anterior horn cells of the spinal cord and the motor nuclei of the brainstem; herpes simplex localizes preferentially in the temporal lobes of the cerebrum; rabies seeks out the medulla. Vascular diseases and demyelinating conditions also display geographic preferences within the nervous system, and a degree of geographic predictability characterizes most brain tumors.

AGE: Neurological disorders assail the nervous system throughout life. Nevertheless, an individual disease commonly manifests a predilection for a selected age group. For example, inborn errors of metabolism, such as Tay–Sachs disease, the leukodystrophies, and several tumors, are encountered largely in childhood. Multiple sclerosis shows a strong preference for young adults, rarely having its onset before puberty or after the age of 40 years. Huntington disease typically strikes youthful and middle-aged adults. Parkinson disease is rarely evidenced before the later decades of life, and Alzheimer disease tends to be a malady of the aged brain.

THE CELLS OF THE NERVOUS SYSTEM

Neurons

Cognition, the supreme biological function of the brain, requires stability of structure. The human nervous system, seemingly by necessity, has relinquished certain cellular capabilities to achieve this unique function. Thus, mature neurons do not divide. A full quota exists at birth or shortly thereafter. The nervous system loses neurons as a part of the aging process. This neuronal loss is generalized, although not universally synchronous.

The need for stability of structure in the nervous system is further exemplified by the fact that neurons of the central nervous system (CNS) cannot effectively regenerate axons. Thus an infarct that transects the internal capsule creates a permanent motor deficit. Furthermore, neurons of the brain and spinal cord are not efficiently remyelinated after injury. Consequently, a plaque of multiple sclerosis establishes a lasting area of demyelination, which in turn creates a permanent functional deficit.

ANATOMY: Neurons have a variety of shapes and sizes, but certain features are common to all of them. Microscopically, the centrally located nuclei are round and, particularly in large neurons, contain a prominent nucleolus. The cytoplasm is abundant, and the ribosome-studded endoplasmic reticulum forms prominent basophilic granules known as Nissl bodies (Fig. 28-2). Some neurons, for example, those in the substantia nigra or locus ceruleus, normally contain cytoplasmic pigment (Fig. 28-3). The cytoplasm is also rich in neurofilaments, which are the counterparts of the intermediate filaments of other cells.

The surface of the neuronal cell body is disposed in numerous branching projections, termed *dendrites*; this results in an enormous expansion of the surface area of the

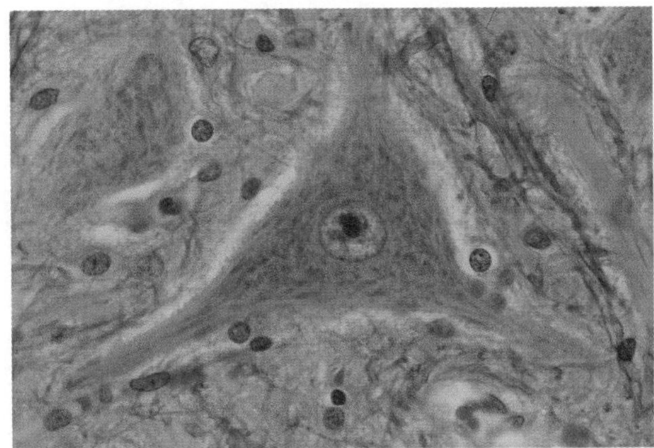

FIGURE 28-2
Neuron. The neuron is a pyramidal cell with a rounded nucleus and prominent nucleolus. The granularity of the cytoplasm is imparted by rough endoplasmic reticulum (Nissl substance).

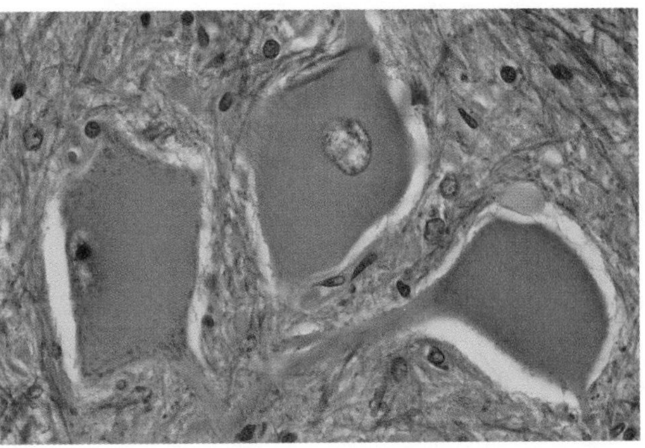

FIGURE 28-4
Chromatolysis. An injured neuron has imbibed fluid and appears swollen, with a pale cytoplasm and Nissl substance marginated toward the plasma membrane.

neuron. Dendrites are best demonstrated by silver impregnation. The cell body of a neuron leads into a single axon, which—depending on its location—may extend for more than a meter. Some axons are surrounded by a myelin sheath, whereas others are unmyelinated.

Neurons react to injury and, on occasion, they do so in very specific ways. Some of these reactions are reversible, whereas others forecast cell death.

CHROMATOLYSIS: As in other cells, injury to a neuron frequently causes it to swell. As the cytoplasm expands, the Nissl substance is displaced centrifugally and becomes marginated near the plasma membrane (Fig. 28-4). The nucleus assumes an eccentric position. This process, termed chromatolysis, may be a response to injury to, or transection of, an axon. In this setting, the process is reversible, except in those instances in which the transection closely approximates the cell body. Alternatively, chromatolysis may signal a serious metabolic disturbance, as occurs when a motor neuron grapples with the poliovirus. Less commonly, fluid accumulates as droplets in the cytosol (Fig. 28-5).

ATROPHY: The loss of neurons in the brain may be appreciated on gross examination as a reduction in brain weight or as a selective decrease in mass of a specific region (e.g., the caudate nucleus in Huntington disease). Atrophy may also refer to a single neuron, in which case, the cell shrivels and becomes hyperchromatic (Fig. 28-6). Such injured cells may ultimately disappear.

NEURONOPHAGIA: Injuries that kill neurons abruptly create cellular debris, which elicits phagocytosis. Some phagocytic cells are mononuclear macrophages, but most are polymorphonuclear leukocytes. The process of aggregation of inflammatory cells about a dead neuron, coupled with phagocytosis, is termed neuronophagia (Fig. 28-7).

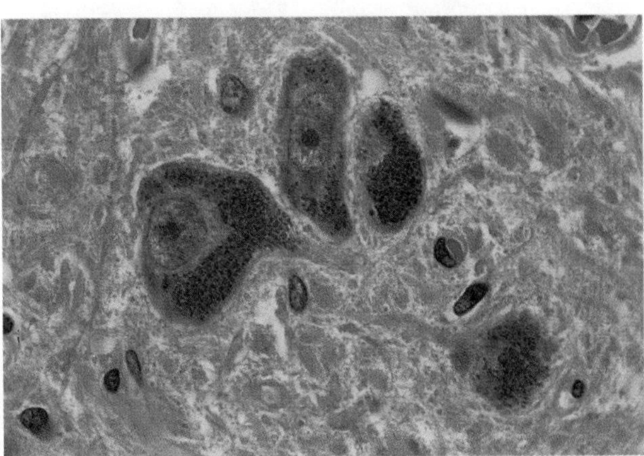

FIGURE 28-3
Pigmented neurons. Neurons of the substantia nigra and locus ceruleus are heavily pigmented with neuromelanin.

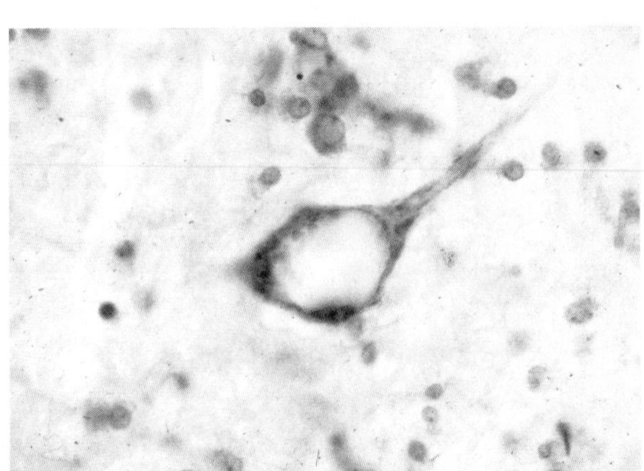

FIGURE 28-5
Hydropic degeneration. Fluid-filled vacuoles distend the cytoplasmic compartment and displace the nucleus.

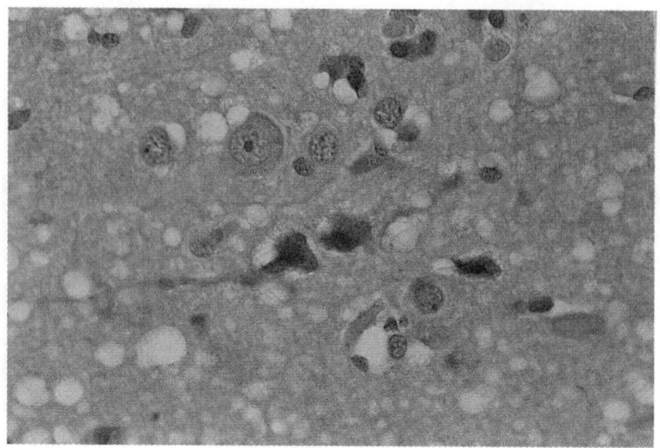

FIGURE *28-6*
Atrophy. In this case of Creutzfeldt–Jakob disease, several injured neurons are shriveled and hyperchromatic.

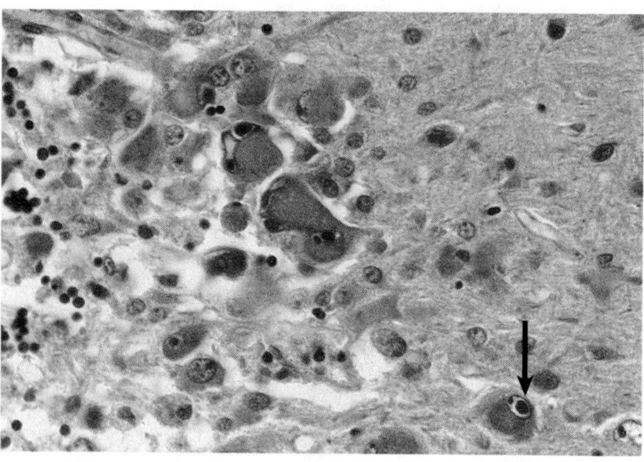

FIGURE *28-8*
Intranuclear inclusions. Cytomegalovirus induces intranuclear inclusions, made prominent by the presence of clear halos (*arrow*). These inclusions are demonstrated in the Purkinje cells of a patient with acquired immunodeficiency syndrome (AIDS).

INTRANEURONAL INCLUSIONS: A variety of nuclear and cytoplasmic inclusions appear in neurons, particularly in certain viral encephalitides and degenerative diseases. The characteristics of specific inclusions are described with the diseases they mark (Figs. 28-8 and 28-9).

Astrocytes

Astrocytes, as the name implies, are star-shaped cells distributed throughout the nervous system. Similar to neurons, they are of neuroectodermal origin. Although astrocytes clearly serve a supportive purpose, their precise functions have not been clearly defined. However, they do play a prominent role in the response of the nervous system to injury.

ANATOMY: Although many species of astrocytes are recognized by the characteristics of their cytoplasm and their geographic distribution in the brain, two varieties are worthy of attention. *Fibrillary astrocytes* are located in the white matter, and *protoplasmic astrocytes* reside in the gray matter. By light microscopy, both types of astrocytes display a rounded nucleus, 7 to 10 μm in diameter, with a homogeneous chromatin pattern. The cytoplasm of "resting" astrocytes is not clearly evident. With silver impregnation, delicate, sinuous cytoplasmic processes extend in all directions from the cell body (Fig. 28-10), often terminating in foot processes that rest on blood vessels. Protoplasmic astrocytes tend to have broad, branching processes, whereas those of fibrillary astrocytes are longer, thinner, and less branched. By electron microscopy, both types of astrocytes contain a meshwork of fine glial (intermediate) filaments.

REACTIONS: Astrocytes multiply in and about localized sites of tissue injury (astrogliosis, or simply glio-

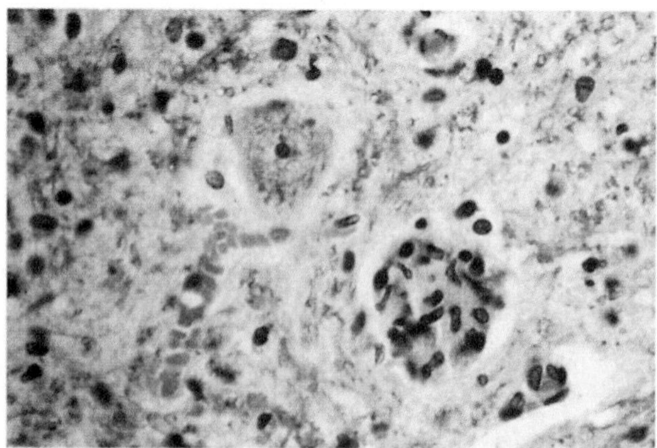

FIGURE *28-7*
Neuronophagia. Leukocytes may accumulate at sites of neuronal necrosis, as shown in this case of acute poliomyelitis.

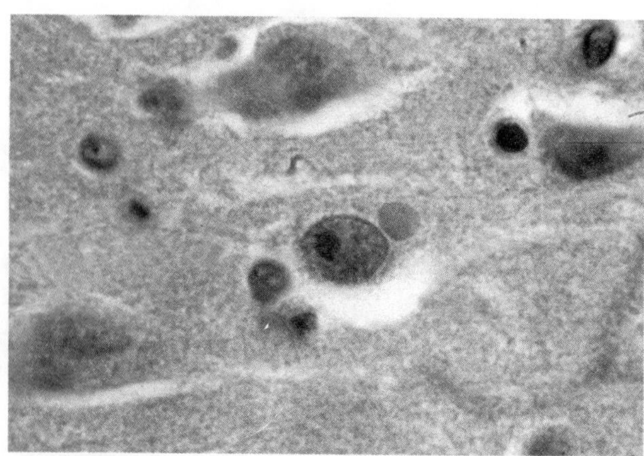

FIGURE *28-9*
Negri body. Rabies encephalitis is characterized by round, eosinophilic cytoplasmic inclusions that resemble an erythrocyte.

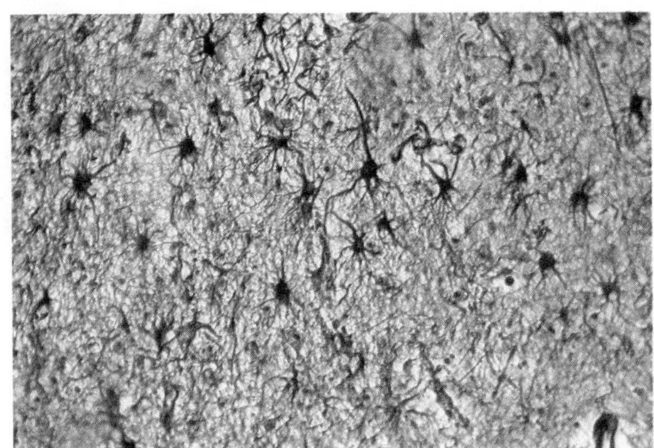

FIGURE 28-10
Astrocytes. Astrocytes have proliferated in the chronically injured brain of a patient with tertiary syphilis. The processes are well outlined with silver carbonate.

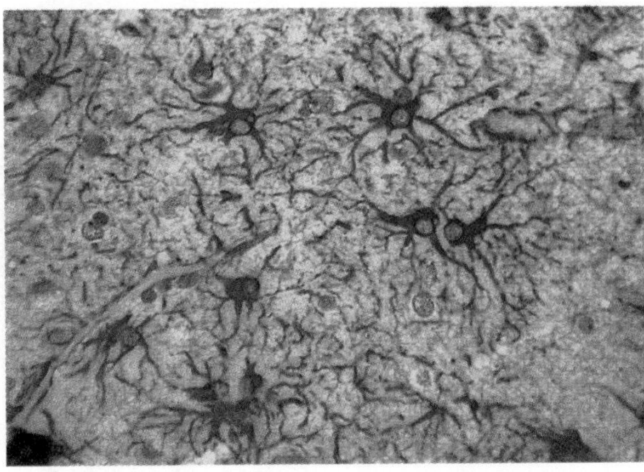

FIGURE 28-12
Reactive astrocytes. The glial processes of astrocytes stain intensely for glial fibrillary acidic protein (GFAP).

sis), for example, in contusions, penetrating wounds, abscesses, granulomas, metastatic tumors, infarcts, and cerebral hemorrhages (Fig. 28-11). Proliferation of fibrillary astrocytes is induced over a period of several days, and the persistence of the response is commensurate with the duration of the stimulus. There are some analogies between the proliferation of astrocytes and fibroblasts in the response to injury, but astrocytes form only a "glial scar" composed predominantly of cell processes rather than collagen (Fig. 28-12).

Astrogliosis also marks certain generalized disease states, while selectively sparing others. For instance, general paresis, a form of tertiary syphilis, and Pick disease are characterized by capricious gliosis. By contrast, the early course of spongiform degeneration of Creutzfeldt–Jakob disease and, to a remarkable degree, the entire course of Alzheimer disease, progress with little attention by astrocytes (see Fig. 28-10 through Fig. 28-12).

Fibrillary astrocytes are prone to neoplastic transformation and are responsible for the dominant family of gliomas. Protoplasmic astrocytomas are uncommon antecedents of cancer.

Corpora amylacea appear within the brains of all aged persons, with a predilection for the subpial and subependymal regions. They are spherical, 5- to 20-nm amorphous structures (Fig. 28-13), with basophilic and argentophilic staining affinities, which are composed of carbohydrate and protein. Although they appear extracellular by light microscopy, electron microscopy has disclosed their evolution within glial processes of astrocytes.

Oligodendroglia

Oligodendroglia are the myelin-producing cells of the CNS and are related to astrocytes insofar as they are both of neuroectodermal origin. In sections stained with hema-

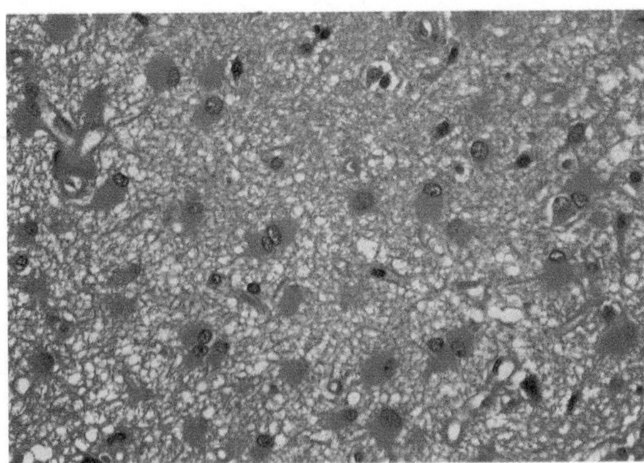

FIGURE 28-11
Astrocytes. In a section stained with hematoxylin and eosin, reactive astrocytes appear plump and display pink cytoplasm (gemistocytic astrocytes).

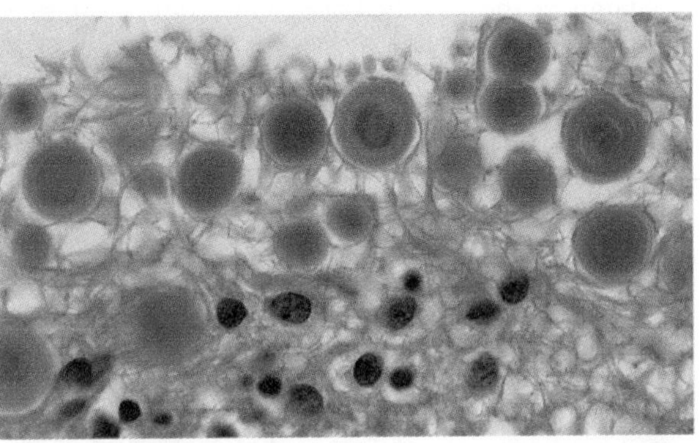

FIGURE 28-13
Corpora amylacea. These products of astrocytes are amorphous, slightly basophilic bodies that accumulate in the subependymal area of elderly persons. They also are found in sites of degeneration, notably the posterior columns in tabes dorsalis.

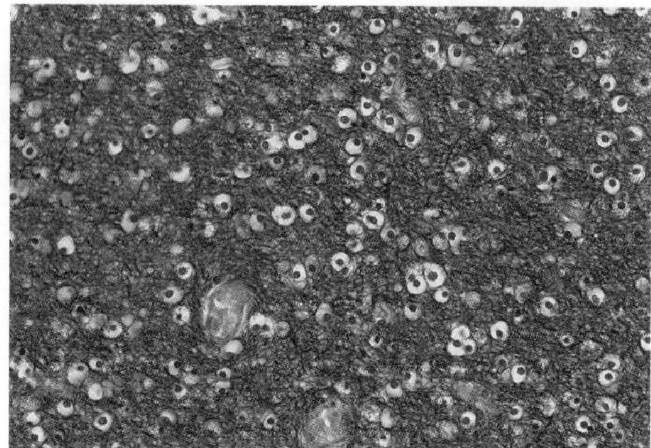

FIGURE 28-14
Normal white matter. In this section stained with luxol fast blue for myelin, the white matter is sparsely populated by oligodendroglia, which are aligned along the myelinated axons.

toxylin and eosin or luxol fast blue, oligodendroglia have dark, rounded nuclei, which resemble those of lymphocytes. A thin rim of cytoplasm surrounds the nucleus. In the gray matter, many oligodendroglia are satellites of neurons, residing in a small depression on the surface of the latter. In the white matter, oligodendroglia are arrayed longitudinally between myelinated fibers (Fig. 28-14).

Oligodendroglia synthesize myelin during the late gestational period and through the first two postnatal years. Subsequently, they serve to maintain these lipid membranes throughout life. Damage to oligodendroglia results in demyelination, as in progressive multifocal leukoencephalopathy. These glial cells can undergo neoplastic transformation, but compared with astrocytes, do so infrequently.

Ependyma

A single layer of ependymal cells lines the four ventricular chambers, the aqueduct of Sylvius, the central canal of the spinal cord, and the filum terminale. These cells vary from cuboidal to flat (Fig. 28-15) and modulate fluid transfer between the cerebrospinal fluid (CSF) and cells of the nervous system. During gestation, some viral infections target the ependymal cells, an event responsible in part for aqueductal stenosis and congenital hydrocephalus. Ependymomas, which result from the neoplastic transformation of ependymal cells, are exophytic masses protruding into a ventricle, particularly the fourth. Ependymomas also constitute a common intramedullary tumor of the spinal cord and filum terminale.

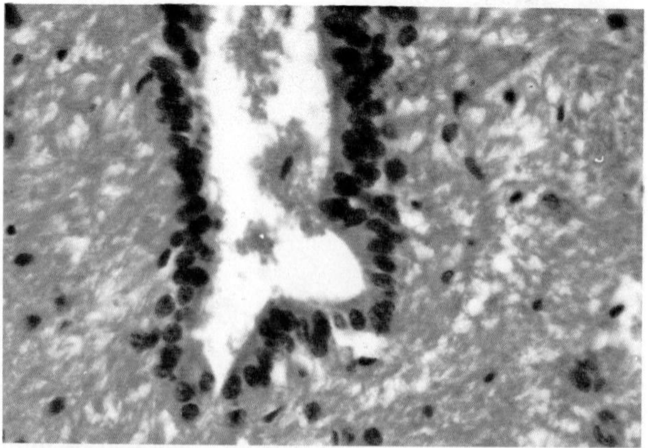

FIGURE 28-15
Ependyma. The central canal of the spinal cord is lined by a single layer of closely aligned cuboidal to columnar cells.

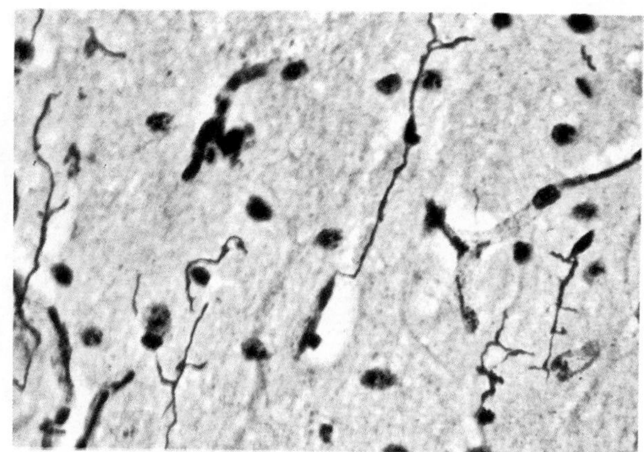

FIGURE 28-16
Microglia. The native macrophages of the central nervous system, termed microglia, are elongated when resting and exhibit few "glial" processes. Silver carbonate stain.

Microglia

Microglia are phagocytic elements of the CNS, accounting for 5% of all glial cells.

ANATOMY: Resting microglia are identified in tissues stained with hematoxylin and eosin by their hyperchromatic, elongated nuclei, which are surrounded by

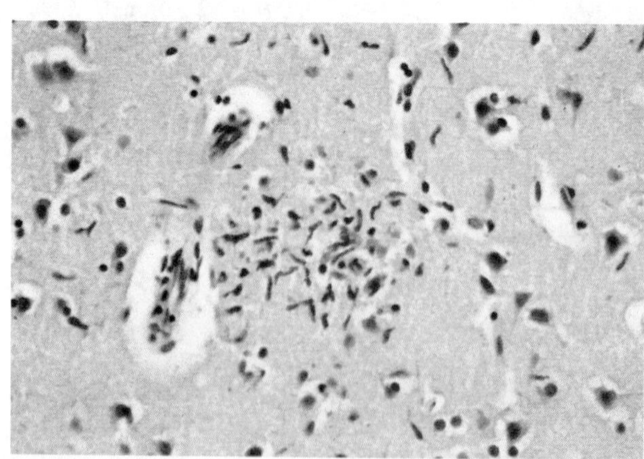

FIGURE 28-17
Glial nodule. Microglia and astrocytes create cellular nodules in response to viral, protozoan, or rickettsial infections.

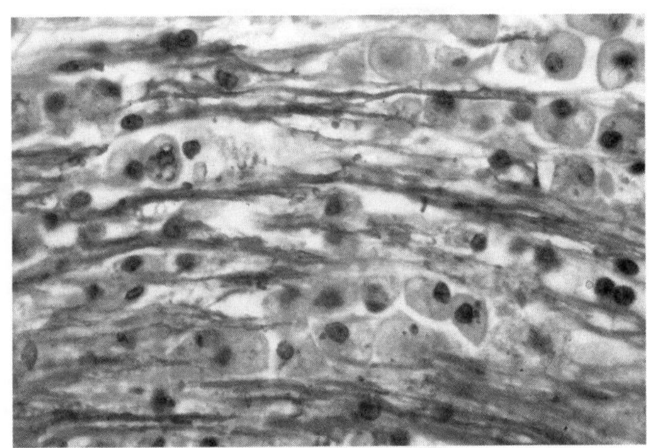

FIGURE 28-18
Macrophages. In this section from a patient with central pontine myelinolysis, macrophages, activated microglia, and other cells derived from the circulation have accumulated at sites of tissue destruction.

only a thin rim of cytoplasm. When stained with silver, their linear form appears with fine lateral projections (Fig. 28-16). Microglia often contain lipofuscin, dense bodies, and multivesicular bodies. In the gray matter, microglia may appear as isolated cells or as neuronal or vascular satellites. In the white matter, they are predominantly perivascular.

REACTIONS: Microglia proliferate and show reactive changes in areas of injury. Two patterns are recognized, focal microglial nodules and diffuse microgliosis. *Microglial nodules* are formed of microglia and astrocytes (Fig. 28-17), and characterize viral, rickettsial, and protozoal infections. Reactive microglia may exhibit a prominent elongated nucleus and are referred to as *rod cells.* As befits their phagocytic nature, in response to tissue necrosis, they become distended by lipid droplets and other cellular debris and are then designated *gitter cells* (Fig. 28-18).

The origin of microglia is still debated. There is general agreement that some resting microglia do not bear monocyte/macrophage surface markers. Whether this fact is firm evidence for a glial origin of these cells, or whether blood-borne monocytes take up residence in the brain as resting microglia that do not express surface markers until activated, remains to be determined. In this respect, it is important to note that most of the phagocytic cells in inflammatory reactions of the CNS are clearly monocyte/macrophages derived from the circulation.

CONGENITAL MALFORMATIONS

The development of the CNS proceeds according to a precise schedule, and each morphological event is the cornerstone for those that follow. For example, myelination is initiated late in embryonic development only after the neurons and oligodendroglia have achieved complex differentiation and migration. If either of the latter processes is flawed, myelination does not occur or becomes disordered. **In this context, a congenital anomaly is the result of an interruption in the proper completion of a single developmental sequence.**

Because the developmental schedule is rigid, the characteristics of a congenital malformation are defined more by the time of the insult than by the nature of the injury itself. Accordingly, a specific congenital malformation may have many causes, all sharing a common time-related target. For instance, either anoxia or ionizing radiation administered to pregnant rats early in the eighth day induces anencephaly in the pups. The same agents applied only a few hours later fail to induce anencephaly but rather result in cleft palate.

Neural Tube Defects (Dysraphic States)

Neural tube defect (NTD) refers to the defective closure of the dorsal aspect of the vertebral column.

Spina Bifida

Spina bifida is an NTD that is most common in the lumbosacral region (Fig. 28-19), *the terminology being determined by the extent of the defect.*

- **Spina bifida occulta:** This defect is restricted to the vertebral arches. It is usually asymptomatic, and its presence is frequently marked externally only by a dimple or small tuft of hair.
- **Meningocele:** This is a condition in which a more extensive bony and soft tissue defect permits protrusion

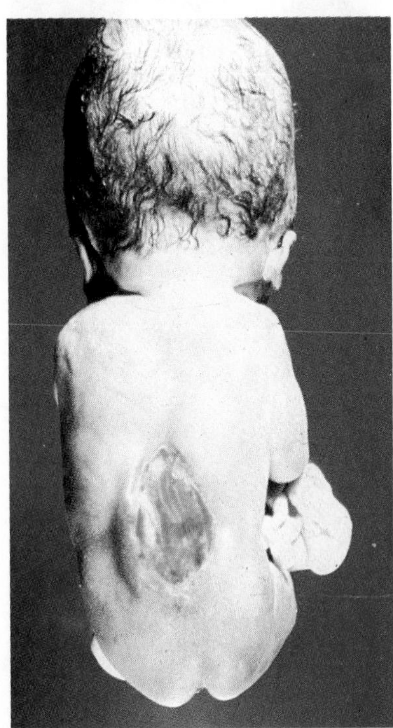

FIGURE 28-19
Spina bifida with meningomyelocele. The deformity is evident at birth as an elliptical, cutaneous defect over the lumbar spine.

of the meninges as a fluid-filled sac. The lateral aspects of the sac are characteristically covered by skin, whereas the apex is usually ulcerated.

- **Meningomyelocele:** This term refers to a more extensive defect that exposes the spinal canal and causes the nerve roots, particularly those of the cauda equina, to be entrapped in subcutaneous scar tissue (Fig. 28-20). Characteristically, the spinal cord appears as a flattened, ribbon-like structure.
- **Rachischisis:** In the extreme defect, the spinal column is converted into a gaping canal, often without a recognizable spinal cord (Fig. 28-21).

☐ **Pathogenesis:** Spina bifida is induced readily in rats and chicks by chemicals, such as trypan blue, or by hypervitaminosis A. The critical interval is the eighth to the ninth gestational day. A favored concept holds that spina bifida results from failure of closure of the neural tube. However, because spina bifida occulta involves only the bone, the validity of this concept has been questioned. Maternal folic acid deficiency has been associated with an increased incidence of NTDs, including spina bifida. As a result, folic acid has been approved for inclusion as a food supplement in commercial flour.

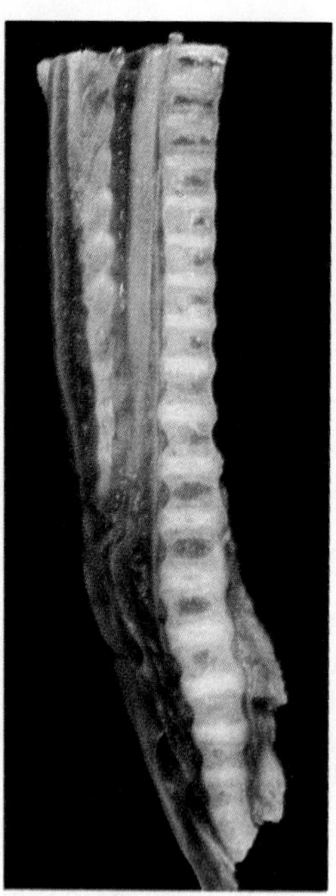

FIGURE *28-21*
Rachischisis. A sagittal section of the vertebral column shows a bony and cutaneous defect, with segmental absence of the spinal cord.

☐ **Clinical Features:** The spectrum of neurological deficits ranges from an absence of symptoms in spina bifida occulta to lower limb paresis or paralysis, sensory loss, and rectal and vesicle incontinence with meningomyelocele. The clinical consequences of such a lesion must also take into account the possibility of other malformations. In the case of a meningomyelocele, this potential includes the Arnold–Chiari malformation, hydrocephalus, polymicrogyria, and hydromyelia segmental dilatation of the central canal of the spinal cord (Fig. 28-22).

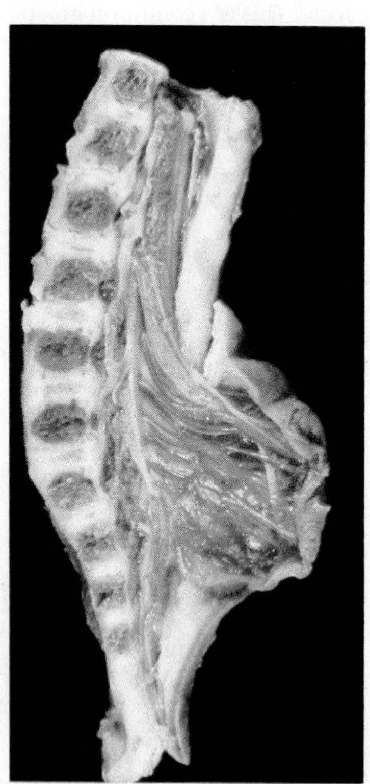

FIGURE *28-20*
Meningomyelocele. A sagittal section of the vertebral column discloses nerve roots arching through the saccular defect.

Anencephaly

Anencephaly refers to the congenital absence of all or part of the brain (Fig. 28-23). Among lethal malformations of the CNS, the incidence of anencephaly is second only to that of spina bifida. It occurs in 0.5 to 2.0 per 1000 births, with a modest female predominance. Anencephalic fetuses are either stillborn or die within the first few days of life.

☐ **Pathogenesis:** There are many theories regarding the pathogenesis of anencephaly. One involves closure of the anterior neuropore; another incriminates disturbed angiogenesis. The concurrence of anencephaly with other NTDs, such as spina bifida, suggests a shared pathogenetic mechanism in which failure of closure of the anterior neuropore is the primary event. This concept is supported by the occurrence of anterior NTDs among very young aborted human embryos.

Certain features, however, are not consistent with the theory that anencephaly results simply from the failure of the neuropore to close.

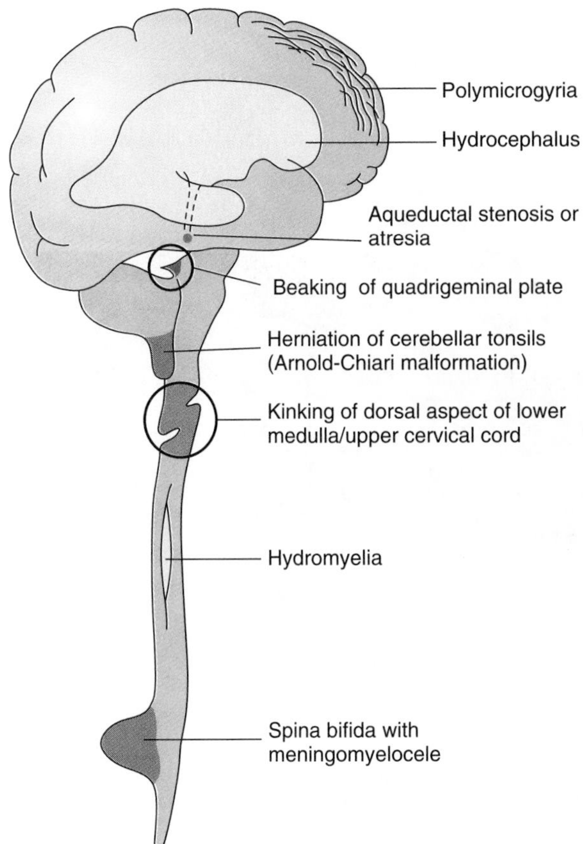

FIGURE 28-22
Arnold–Chiari malformation and associated lesions.

- The presence of well-formed eyes attests to the prior existence of properly formed optic cups. These structures normally arise from the lateral wall of the diencephalon after closure of the neural tube in the fourth week.
- The preservation of the retina affirms the absence of significant intrinsic deficiencies in the neuroectodermal potential for differentiation.
- The presence of the choroid plexus in the "cranial" mass, the "cerebrovasculosa," indicates that the pia has been brought into physical contact with the ependyma through infolding of the neural tube, an event that also follows the closure of the anterior neuropore and dates the cerebral injury to about the sixth week of gestation.

Many events occur in the 2-week interval before the sixth week of gestation, including the incorporation of the cerebrum into the systemic circulation. By the sixth to seventh week of fetal development, the carotid and vertebral arteries have united to form the circle of Willis. This structure becomes the hub for vessels that establish union with the intrinsic parenchymal vasculature, thereby integrating the developing cerebrum into the systemic circulation. The intrinsic blood pressure of a vessel is the determinant for smooth muscle proliferation. Thus, the scant muscularis in the vessels of the cerebrovasculosa in anencephaly suggests that these channels represent the "unused" parenchymal vascular bed, which failed to unite with the systemic circulation. The eyes have avoided dependency on the internal carotid circulation, having acquired an alternate supply from the external carotid vessels.

□ **Pathology:** The cranial vault in anencephaly is absent, and the cerebral hemispheres are represented by a discoid mass of highly vascularized, poorly differentiated neural tissue, the so-called *cerebrovasculosa*. This diminutive mass lies on the flattened base of the skull, behind two well-formed and normally positioned eyes, which mark the anterior margin of disturbed organogenesis. A well-differentiated retina attests to the preservation of this selected neuroectoderm, and short segments of the optic nerve extend posteriorly. The posterior aspect of the malformation is a transitional zone, which varies from case to case. On occasion, the midbrain structures are recognized, but most often the entire brainstem and cerebellum are rudimentary. The upper spinal cord tends to be hypoplastic and deformed. A dysraphic bony defect of the posterior spinal column (rachischisis) may involve the cervical area. Vertebral arteries and an atretic basilar artery are usually identifiable in a tangle of meningeal vessels (Fig. 28-24A).

The cerebrovasculosa represents a residuum of the underdeveloped cerebral hemispheres and typically contains discrete islands of immature neural and glial tissue (see Fig. 28-24B). It also encloses cavities that are partially lined by ependyma and occasionally contain choroid plexus. However, the mass is composed predominantly of vascular channels that vary considerably in size. These channels are lined by endothelium but are largely devoid of muscularis. Beneath the cerebrovasculosa, but sharing a common origin with the brain, are cranial nerves and intraosseous ganglia.

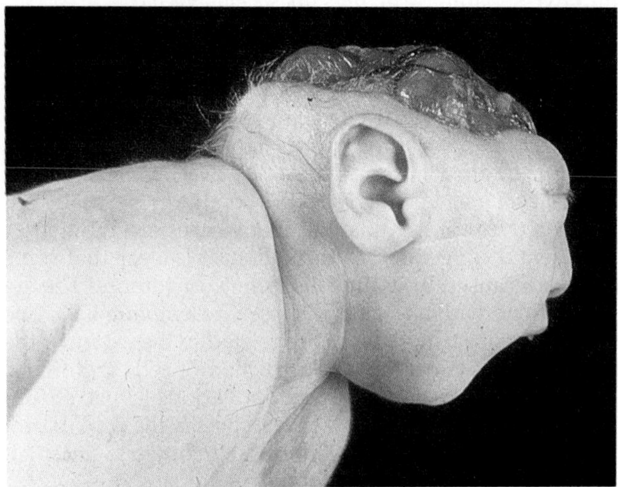

FIGURE 28-23
Anencephaly. The absence of a calvarium has exposed a discoid mass of highly vascularized tissue (cerebrovasculosa), in which there are rudimentary neuroectodermal structures. The lesion is bounded anteriorly by normally formed eyes and posteriorly by the brainstem.

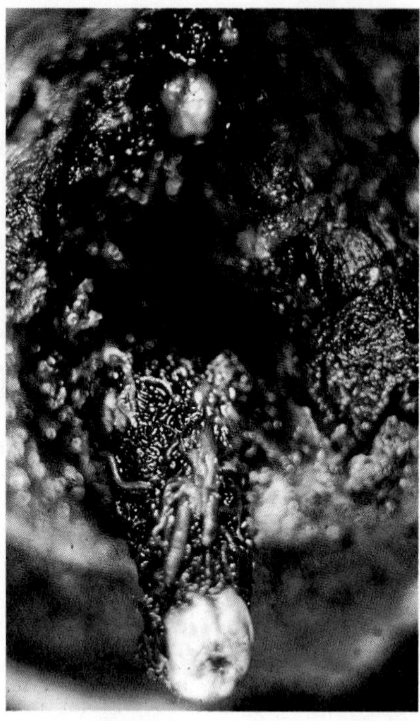

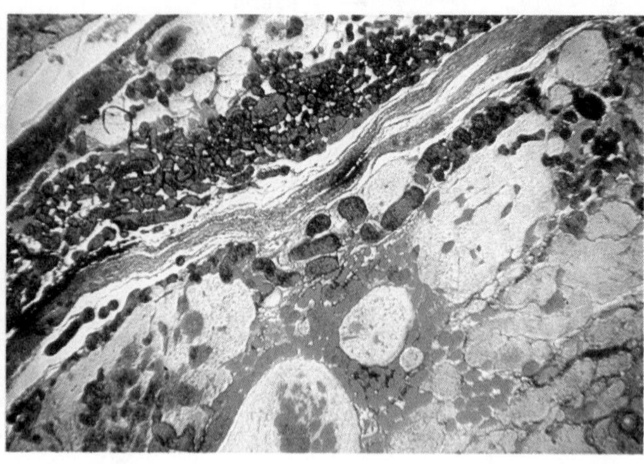

A B

FIGURE 28-24
Anencephaly. (*A*) An inferior view of the discoid mass (cerebrovasculosa) that replaces the brain in anencephaly shows a well-formed medulla encircled by a plexus of abnormal blood vessels. (*B*) A microscopic section shows that the cerebrovasculosa contains islands of neural tissue and an abundance of thin-walled blood vessels.

Malformations of the Spinal Cord

The spinal cord on occasion harbors congenital malformations that are less apparent at birth than are neural tube defects. Rare duplications occur, ranging from complete duplication (*dimyelia*) to lateral bifurcation of the spinal cord into two separate structures (*diastematomyelia*).

Hydromyelia refers to dilatation of the central canal of the spinal cord (see Fig. 28-22).

SYRINGOMYELIA: *In this congenital malformation, a tubular cavitation (syrinx) extends for variable distances along the entire length of the spinal cord, which may or may not communicate with the central canal.* The condition is usually encountered in adults, although many cases are thought to represent a congenital malformation. It is clear that some cases are caused by trauma, ischemia, or tumors. The syrinx is filled with a clear fluid closely resembling CSF. The symptoms of syringomyelia are related to the extent of the syrinx and its concomitant destruction of cells and fibers. Motor and sensory deficits occur at various levels, reflecting the anatomical location of the lesions in the spinal cord.

Syringobulbia is a variant of syringomyelia in which slit-like cavities are located in the medulla.

Arnold–Chiari Malformation

Arnold–Chiari malformation is a condition in which the brainstem and cerebellum are compacted into a shallow, bowl-shaped posterior fossa with a low-positioned tentorium. It is usually associated with a lumbosacral meningomyelocele (see Fig. 28-22).

☐ **Pathogenesis:** One theory of the origin of the Arnold–Chiari malformation holds that the meningomyelocele serves to anchor the lower end of the spinal cord and that the downward growth of the vertebral column creates traction on the medulla (see Fig. 28-22). However, the curvature of the medulla and the beaking of the quadrigeminal plate in the Arnold–Chiari malformation are not readily explained by this mechanism.

Another theory proposes that the downward thrust is initiated by the increased intracranial pressure of hydrocephalus. Still another focuses on the restricted size of the posterior fossa and views the bony defect of the skull as the primary event, with consequent extrusion of the cerebellar tissue through the foramen magnum.

☐ **Pathology:** In Arnold–Chiari malformation, the caudal aspect of the cerebellar vermis is herniated through an enlarged foramen magnum (Fig. 28-25) and protrudes as a tongue on the dorsal aspect of the cervical cord, often reaching the level of C3 to C5. The herniated tissue is bound in position by thickened meninges and shows pressure atrophy, with depletion of Purkinje and granular cells. The brainstem also is displaced caudally. Typically, the displacement is more exaggerated dorsally than ventrally, and thus landmarks such as the obex of the fourth ventricle are appreciably more caudal than are ventral structures such as the inferior olive. As viewed

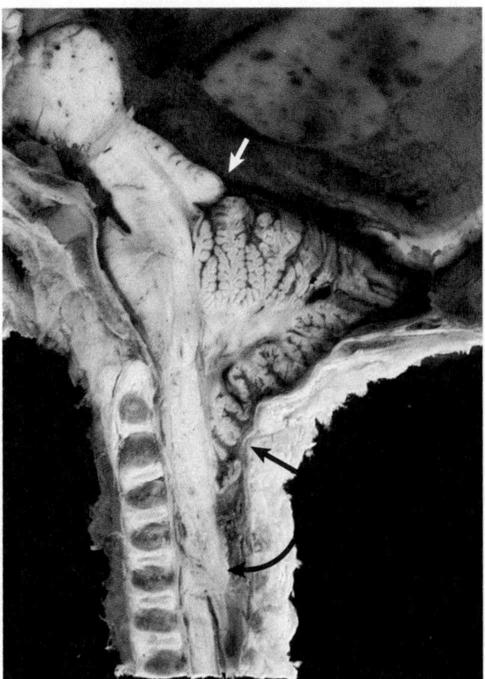

FIGURE 28-25
Arnold–Chiari malformation. The cerebellar vermis is herniated below the level of the foramen magnum (*straight arrow*). The downward displacement of the dorsal portion of the cord causes the obex of the fourth ventricle to occupy a position below the foramen magnum. The beaking of the inferior colliculus of the quadrigeminal plate (*white arrow*) and the S-shaped angulation of the upper cervical cord are seen (*curved arrow*).

from a lateral aspect, the lower medulla is sharply angulated in its midsegment, thereby creating a dorsal protrusion (Fig. 28-26). The foramina of Magendie and Luschka are compressed by the bony ridge of the foramen magnum. The cerebellum is flattened and has a discoid, rather than an ovoid, contour, similar to a clam. Frequently, the quadrigeminal plate is also deformed by a "beak-shaped" dorsal protrusion of the inferior colliculi. The Arnold–Chiari malformation also causes hydrocephalus, through obstruction of the foramina of Magendie and Luschka.

Congenital Hydrocephalus

Hydrocephalus refers to an excessive amount of CSF. The fluid accumulations are in varied locations and have many causes, as discussed later in the section entitled Cerebrospinal Fluid.

Congenital atresia of the aqueduct of Sylvius is the most common cause of congenital hydrocephalus (Fig. 28-27). It occurs with an incidence of 1 in 1000 live births. Histological examination of the midbrain may disclose multiple atretic channels (Fig. 28-28) or an aqueduct stenosed by periaqueductal gliosis (Fig. 28-29). The latter has been attributed to the transplacental transmission of one of the many viruses known to induce ependymitis.

Disorders of Cerebral Gyri

Abnormalities of the cerebral gyri are frequently associated with mental retardation. These deviations provide a spectrum of entities, among which are the following:

- ***Polymicrogyria*** *refers to the presence of small and excessive gyri* (Fig. 28-30).
- ***Pachygyria*** *is a condition in which the gyri are reduced in number and unusually broad* (Fig. 28-31).
- ***Lissencephaly*** *is a congenital disorder in which the cortical surface of the cerebral hemispheres is smooth or only lightly furrowed.* Almost all patients with lissencephaly (92%) show deletions in the region of the *LIS1* gene on chromosome 17p13.3.

  Gyral malformations arise from disturbances in neuronal migration, a highly patterned event of the first trimester of embryonic development. The primitive neurons move centrifugally from the germinal mantle to populate the cortex. The number of neurons and their positions in the cortex are determining factors in the redundancy of the cortical mantle, which, in turn, initiates the infolding that creates sulci.
- ***Heterotopia*** represents a focal disturbance in neuronal migration that leads to nodular collections of ectopic neurons, usually in the white matter. Heterotopia is often associated with mental retardation and seizures. Migrational disturbances of neurons have been associated with maternal alcoholism.

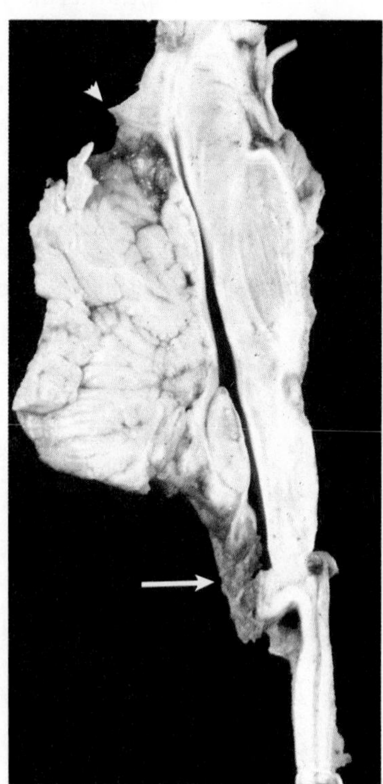

FIGURE 28-26
Arnold–Chiari malformation. A sagittal section of the brainstem illustrates the features enumerated in Fig. 28-22. A tongue of cerebellar vermis extends downward over the dorsum of the cervical cord (*arrow*). Note the sharp beak of the inferior colliculus (*arrowhead*).

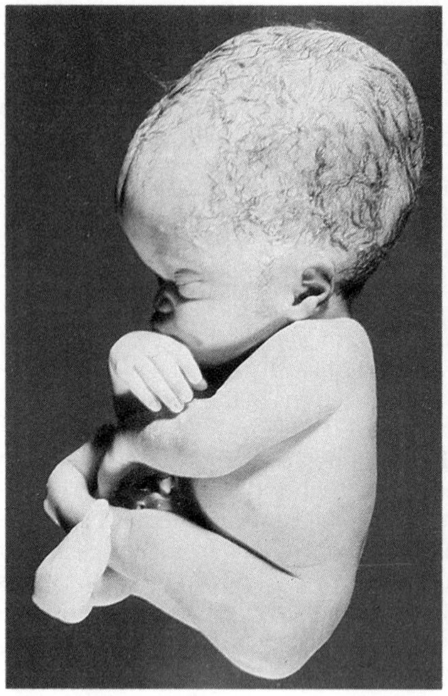

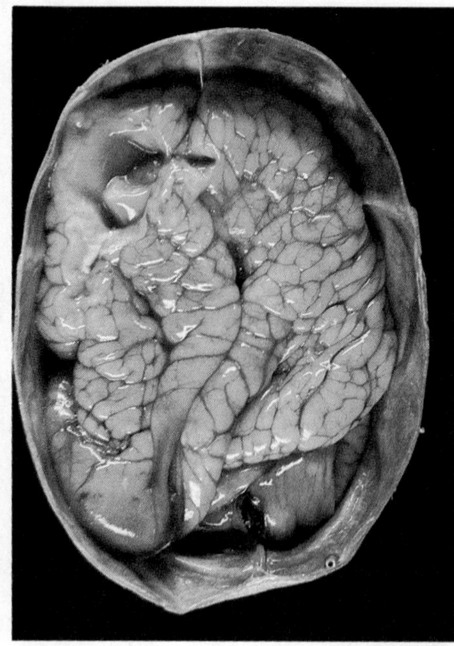

A B

FIGURE *28-27*
Congenital hydrocephalus. (*A*) Hydrocephalus occurring before the fusion of the cranial sutures causes pronounced enlargement of the head. (*B*) Removal of the calvarium demonstrates an atrophic and collapsed cerebral cortex.

Congenital Defects Associated with Chromosomal Abnormalities

Derangements of the larger autosomes, 1 through 12, are incompatible with sustained intrauterine life, and affected fetuses are aborted. Structural and functional abnormalities attributable to gross chromosomal derangements are best exemplified by trisomies of chromosomes 13-15 and chromosome 21 (Down syndrome).

Down Syndrome

Down syndrome is a chromosomal disorder caused by trisomy 21, which is characterized by mental retardation, distinctive facial features, and a variety of other anomalies. Although most cases reflect trisomy 21, a few are the result of translocations or mosaicism. Down syndrome is discussed in detail in Chapter 6, and here we deal only with the pathology in the brain.

The weight of the brain is moderately reduced, and the organ is shortened in its anteroposterior dimension. There is a simple gyral pattern, with disproportionately slender superior temporal gyri (Fig. 28-32). On histological examination, the cytoarchitecture of the cortex in Down syndrome so closely approximates the normal as to be indistinguishable from it. Of interest is the propensity for the precocious development of the histological features of Alzheimer disease. Typically, the lesions of Alzheimer disease (see later) occur before the midportion of the fourth decade of life.

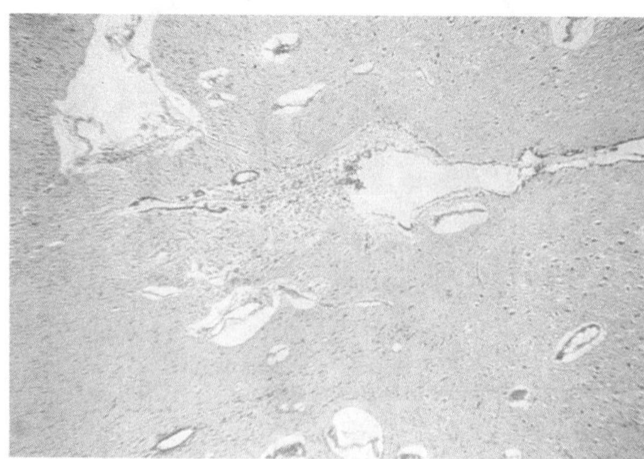

FIGURE *28-28*
Neonatal hydrocephalus. Multiple atretic canals replace the normal single aqueduct of Sylvius.

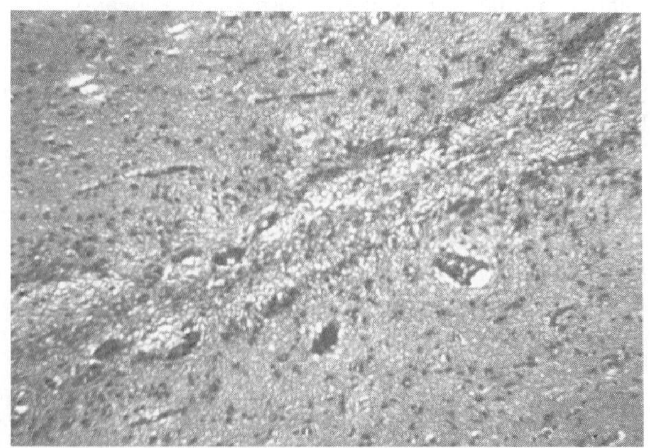

FIGURE *28-29*
Neonatal hydrocephalus. The aqueduct of Sylvius is occluded by astroglial tissue, a response that may represent an intrauterine viral infection.

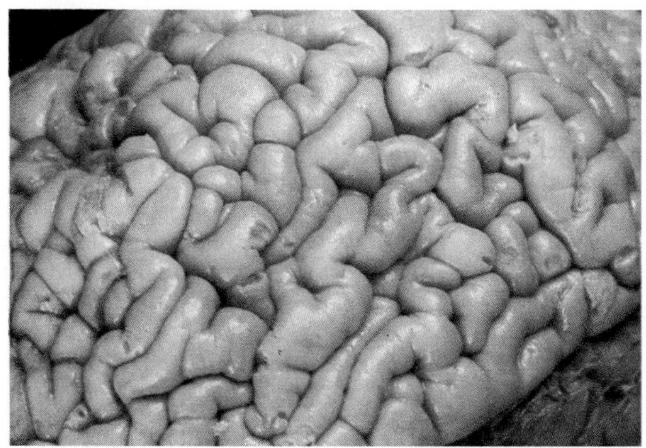

FIGURE 28-30
Polymicrogyria. The surface of the brain exhibits an excessive number of small, irregularly sized, randomly distributed gyral folds.

Trisomy 13-15

Trisomy 13-15 has an incidence of 1 per 5000 births, with a modest female predominance. The congenital deformities involve the brain, facial features, and extremities. The complex is dominated by holoprosencephaly, arrhinencephaly, microphthalmia, cyclopia, low-set ears, harelip, and cleft palate. The extremities exhibit polydactyly and "rocker bottom" feet.

HOLOPROSENCEPHALY: *This term refers to a microcephalic brain that features an absence of the interhemispheric fissure.* The horseshoe-shaped cerebral hemispheres have an uncleaved frontal pole, across which the gyri show an irregular horizontal orientation (Fig. 28-33). Behind this lens-shaped cortex is a common ventricular chamber created by the lateral displacement of the posterior portions of the cerebral hemispheres. The base of the ventricular chamber is formed by the bilobed structures of the caudate nuclei and thalami. Holoprosencephaly is rarely compatible with life beyond a few weeks or months.

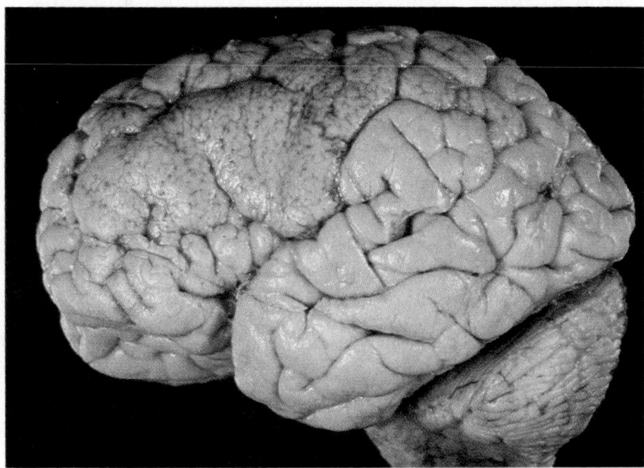

FIGURE 28-31
Pachygyria. The occurrence of broad gyri marks a deformity of embryonic development.

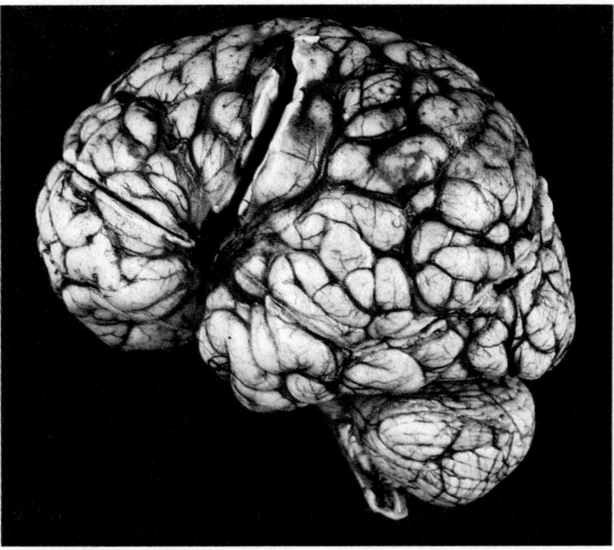

FIGURE 28-32
Down syndrome. Mild microcephaly and underdevelopment of the superior temporal gyri are noted.

ARRHINENCEPHALY: *The absence of the olfactory tracts and bulbs (rhinencephalon) is associated with holoprosencephaly or occurs as a solitary malformation* (Fig. 28-34).

ABSENCE OF THE CORPUS CALLOSUM: This anomaly is a regular feature of holoprosencephaly, al-

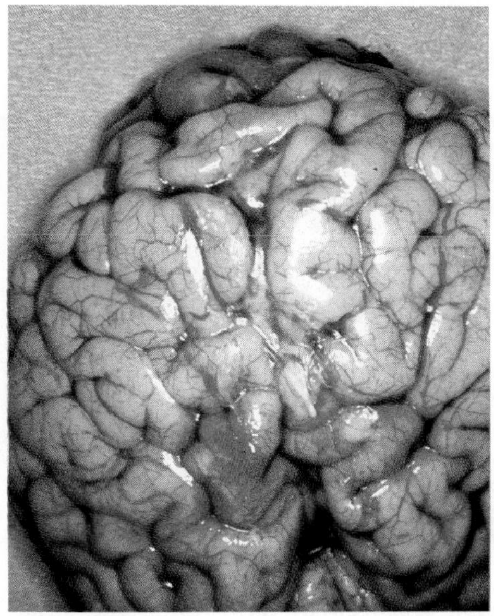

FIGURE 28-33
Holoprosencephaly. A view from the superior aspect of the brain shows the absence of the anterior interhemispheric fissure.

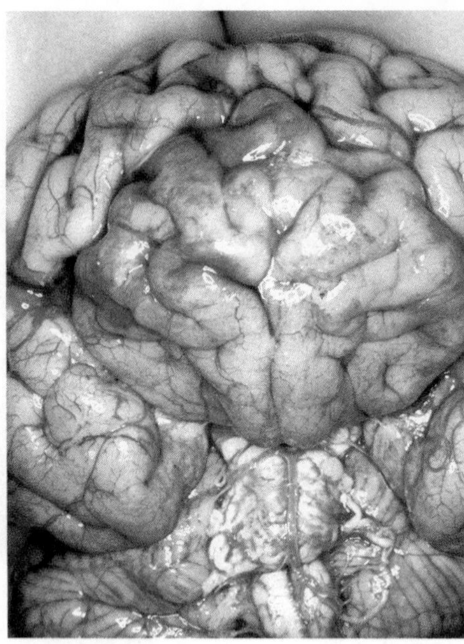

FIGURE 28-34
Arrhinencephaly. An absence of the olfactory system frequently accompanies holoprosencephaly.

though it can also be a solitary lesion. Remarkably, the absence of the corpus callosum occurs without any significant impairment of interhemispheric functional coordination. On the other hand, it is occasionally associated with seizures. The corpus callosum physically tethers the hemispheres, and its absence permits the lateral ventricles to drift outward and upward (Fig. 28-35), a position that is radiographically diagnostic.

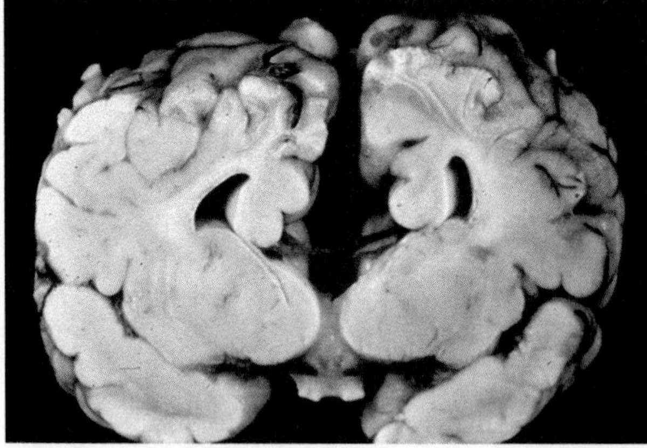

FIGURE 28-35
Congenital absence of the corpus callosum. The lateral ventricles have assumed a more lateral position, whereas the cingulate gyri have rolled downward to occupy the position of the absent corpus callosum.

Epilepsy

The term epilepsy (Gk., "overcome or seized") refers to paroxysmal, transient disturbances (seizures) in brain function that are expressed as impairment in or loss of consciousness, abnormal motor activity, or sensory or mental disturbances. Epilepsy is not uncommon, the prevalence being 6 per 1000. Newborns and infants are particularly vulnerable, as are the elderly. The majority of seizures (75%) occur without a demonstrable organic lesion and are classed as idiopathic epilepsy. Most of these cases are sporadic, although hereditary forms are recognized.

☐ **Pathology:** Careful studies of the brains of patients who had idiopathic epilepsy have described neuronal loss and reactive gliosis. The affected areas include the hippocampus, cerebellum, thalamus, and cerebral neocortex. Whether these changes are the cause of idiopathic epilepsy or result from the anoxia that occurs with generalized seizures is still debated.

A lesser number of cases of epilepsy are initiated by a defined entity, for instance, an intracranial tumor, an arteriovenous malformation, or a brain scar from a penetrating wound. The incidence of acquired seizures is defined by (1) the proximity of the lesion to the motor cortex, (2) the nearness to the surface of the brain, and (3) the duration of the lesion.

TRAUMA

Epidural Hematoma

Epidural hematoma refers to the accumulation of blood between the calvarium and the dura. This lesion is usually the result of a blow to the side of the head that fractures the temporal bone. Unless treated promptly, an epidural hematoma is generally fatal.

☐ **Pathogenesis:** The intracranial dura is securely bound to the inner aspect of the calvarium and thus is analogous to the periosteum. The middle meningeal arteries occupy the theoretical space between the dura and the calvarium. They are grooved into the inner table of the bone, and their branches splay across the temporal–parietal area, generally as three major vessels. The temporal bone is one of the thinnest bones of the skull and, therefore, particularly vulnerable to fracture. Even trauma that seems inconsequential may be sufficient to fracture the temporal–parietal bone and thereby cause transection of branches of the middle meningeal artery. The result is life-threatening epidural hemorrhage (Figs. 28-36).

☐ **Pathology and Clinical Course:** Transection of the middle meningeal artery permits the escape of arterial blood into the epidural space. This bleeding slowly, but inevitably, separates the dura from the calvarium, and the hematoma enlarges relentlessly (Fig. 28-37). During

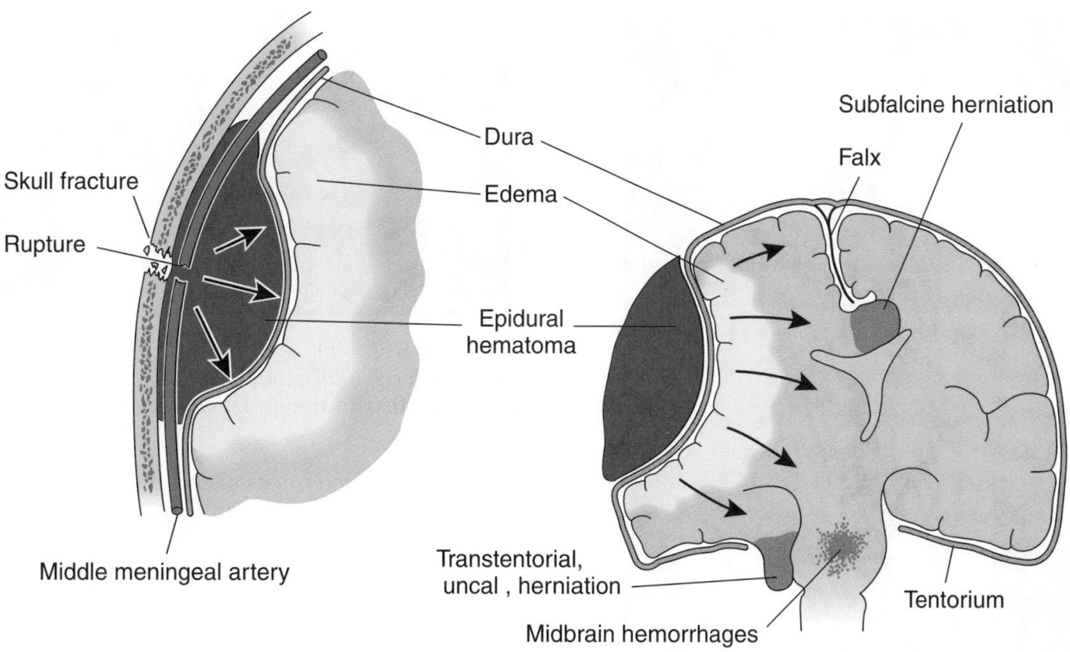

FIGURE 28-36
Development of an epidural hematoma. Transection of a branch of the middle meningeal artery by the sharp edge of a fracture initiates bleeding under arterial pressure. This bleeding slowly dissects the dura from the calvarium and produces an expanding hematoma. After an asymptomatic interval of several hours, transtentorial herniation becomes life-threatening.

the initial 4 to 8 hours, the intracranial events are largely asymptomatic. Symptoms, which become evident when the hematoma has attained a volume of 30 to 50 mL, reflect a space-occupying lesion. Because the supratentorial compartment has a fixed volume, the introduction of a space-occupying mass necessitates the displacement of an equal volume from this compartment. During the asymptomatic interval, the earliest volumetric adjustment is accomplished by the downward displacement of CSF through the aperture in the tentorium.

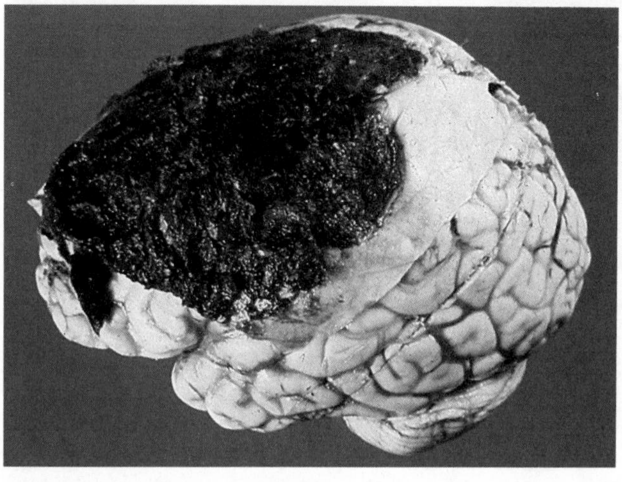

Bleeding continues, and the hematoma enlarges progressively. When the increased intracranial pressure exceeds the venous pressure, the large venous sinuses are compressed. This collapse of the venous conduits creates circulatory stagnation, thereby causing cerebral ischemia and hypoxia. During this interval of global cerebral hypoxia, the patient manifests diffuse cortical impairment, evidenced as confusion and disorientation.

The Cushing reflex is a protective response that augments cerebral circulation and increases cerebral oxygenation. The heart rate slows to increase ventricular filling, and myocardial contraction becomes more forceful. The blood pressure, particularly systolic pressure, is increased.

Bleeding continues into the hematoma, which has now attained a size of approximately 60 mL within 6 to 10 hours. Compensatory mechanisms have been exhausted, and the brain is shifted laterally away from the side of the lesion. The medial aspect of the temporal lobe on the side of the hematoma is compressed against the midbrain and displaced downward through the horseshoe-shaped opening of the tentorium, an event termed transtentorial herniation (Fig. 28-38). This herniation compresses the tissues of the uncus of the hippocampus against the midbrain and also against contiguous structures, such as the third nerve. Thus, the oculomotor nerve is compressed against the edge of the tentorium, causing third-nerve palsy. The pupil, generally on the side of the lesion, becomes fixed and dilated.

FIGURE 28-37
Epidural hematoma. A discoid mass of fresh hemorrhage overlies the frontal–parietal cortex.

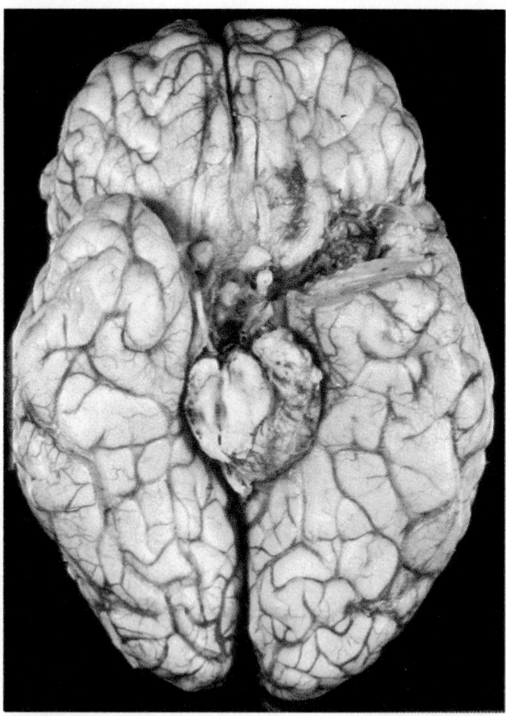

FIGURE 28-38
Transtentorial herniation. The uncus of the hippocampus is herniated downward and displaces the midbrain, which is the site of secondary ("Duret") hemorrhages.

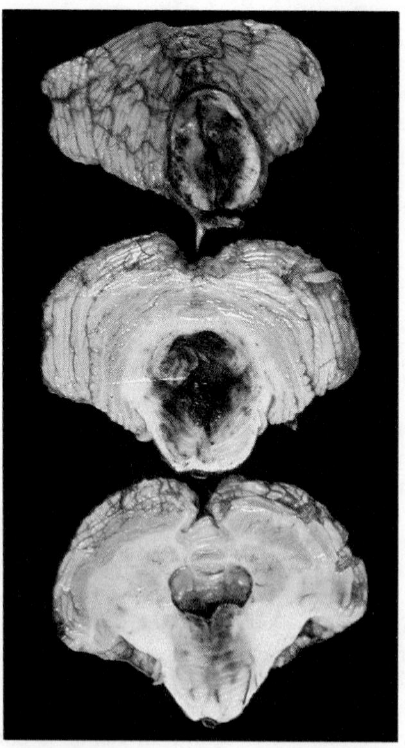

FIGURE 28-39
Transtentorial herniation. Duret hemorrhages in a case of transtentorial herniation tend to be midline and to occupy the brainstem from the upper midbrain to midpons.

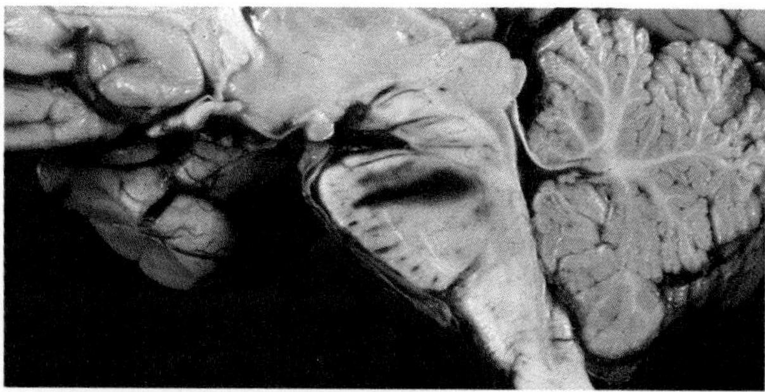

FIGURE 28-40
Transtentorial herniation. A sagittal section reveals the longitudinal distribution of Duret hemorrhages.

The herniated uncus also compresses the vasculature of the midbrain, most important, the paired mesencephalic veins (great veins of Rosenthal). Venous stagnation in the midbrain causes further hypoxia and impairs neuronal function. Damage to the reticular formation is expressed clinically as a decline in the level of consciousness. Shortly thereafter, hemorrhage (Figs. 28-38 through 28-40) and necrosis appear, after which the regional injury to the reticular formation becomes irreversible (Fig. 28-41). Death is imminent, or if the supratentorial pressure is relieved, unconsciousness is permanent. **Epidural hematomas are invariably progressive and, when not recognized and evacuated, are fatal in 24 to 48 hours.**

The blow to the head that causes an epidural hematoma does not necessarily have to produce a concussion, defined as the transient loss of consciousness due to trauma. Consciousness is a positive neurological activity that is dependent on the function of specific neurons,

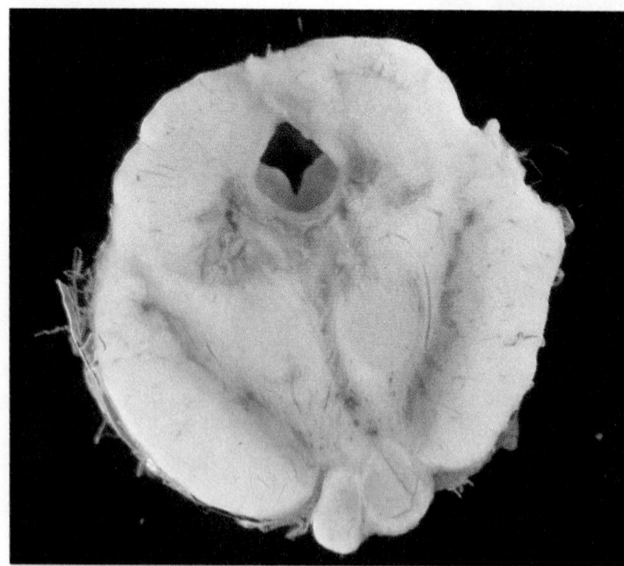

FIGURE 28-41
Transtentorial herniation. This is a cross-section of the midbrain of a patient who survived transtentorial herniation but remained unconscious for several months. Hemosiderin-stained areas of necrosis mark the sites of previous Duret hemorrhages.

those of the reticular formation of the brainstem. Concussion is exemplified in the boxing ring, generally as the consequence of a blow that deflects the head upward and posteriorly, often with a rotatory component. These motions impart a quick torque on the brainstem and cause functional paralysis of the neurons of the reticular formation.

A blow to the temporal–parietal area sufficiently vigorous to cause a skull fracture does not generally cause a concussion, because lateral movement of the cerebral hemispheres is prevented by the falx. Therefore, the absence of a loss of consciousness in a patient under consideration for an epidural hematoma has no clinical relevance.

Subdural Hematoma

Subdural hematoma is an accumulation of blood in the subdural space as a consequence of bleeding from torn bridging veins. This lesion is a significant cause of death after head injuries from falls, assaults, vehicular accidents, and sporting mishaps. Victims of child abuse commonly have subdural hematomas.

☐ **Pathogenesis:** The cerebral hemispheres are immersed in CSF. They are tethered loosely by blood vessels and cranial nerves and are free to float in an anteroposterior direction. The venous drainage from the cerebral hemispheres flows upward through veins in the pia. As these veins reach the parasagittal region, they cross the subarachnoid space and the arachnoid and traverse the theoretical subdural space. After breaching the dura, they then enter the dural sinus.

Significantly, the arachnoid is intimately applied to the undersurface of the dura. Recent ultrastructural studies have demonstrated that the innermost layer of the dura, referred to as the dural border cell (DBC) layer, and the outermost layer of the arachnoid (the arachnoid barrier cell [ABC] layer) are joined together by intercellular junctions. In actuality, they constitute a single continuous membrane. There is no evidence that an actual or potential true space exists between the dura and arachnoid. However, the intercellular attachments that unite the cells of the DBC layer are sparse, and this layer is the weakest structural plane of the meninges. The arachnoid is firmly bound to the underlying pia and subjacent cerebral hemisphere by the arachnoid trabeculae, and the dura is tightly adherent to the overlying inner table of the calvarium by its periosteal layer. Thus, pathological fluid accumulations, such as hematomas and hygromas, tend to separate the meninges along the path of least resistance (i.e., within the DBC layer). Nevertheless, the terms subdural space and subdural hematoma are firmly ingrained and have been retained by most authors.

When the frontal or occipital portion of the moving head strikes a fixed object, or when the stationary head is struck by a blunt object, the cerebral hemispheres are displaced in an anteroposterior direction. The cerebral hemispheres hit forcefully against the inner aspect of the occipital or frontal bone. The soft cerebral tissues become compact and then recoil, a response that initiates a rippled movement in the cerebral parenchyma. Because the dura is adherent to the skull, and the arachnoid is attached to the cerebrum, the disparate movement of these membranes produces a shearing effect localized to the DBC layer ("subdural space"). As a result, the cortical veins are torn where they pass across this structurally weak plane (Fig. 28-42). The motions of the skull and the brain are thereafter in opposite directions. The subdural space is readily expansible, unlike the restricted epidural space. Fortunately, the bleeding, being venous in origin, usually stops spontaneously, after an accumulation of 25 to 50 mL. The compression of the severed bridging veins by the hematoma initiates thrombosis. Because the brain is symmetric and a force applied in the sagittal plane similarly affects both hemispheres, it is not surprising that subdural hematomas are frequently bilateral.

☐ **Pathology:** A subdural hematoma that is stationary in size and too small to cause symptoms nevertheless induces important tissue responses. The contact between the hematoma and the inferior aspect of the dura is a site of irritation. Granulation tissue, rich in capillaries and fibroblasts, forms over the subsequent several weeks, creating a layer above the hematoma, termed the *outer membrane* (Fig. 28-43). From this membrane, migratory fibroblasts invade the subjacent hematoma, where they percolate downward and knit a fibrous membrane across the deep, or inner, aspect of the blood clot. Approximately 2 weeks pass before this *inner membrane* is grossly visible (Fig. 28-44). Unlike the outer membrane, the delicate encapsulating inner membrane lacks blood vessels.

A subdural hematoma, static in size and generally asymptomatic, has the potential for three routes of evolution:

- The hematoma may be reabsorbed, as occurs regularly when blood is introduced experimentally into the subdural space of a laboratory animal.
- The hematoma may remain static, with the potential for calcification.
- The hematoma may enlarge.

Expansion of the hematoma and the onset of symptoms is most often the result of rebleeding from the outer membrane, usually within 6 months. The granulation tissue is analogous to a wet scab, which is vulnerable to even minor trauma, perhaps no greater than the mild pressure from the underlying cerebral hemisphere that has been set in motion by shaking the head. Rebleeding creates a new hematoma, which lies immediately subjacent to the original outer membrane. With time, the new hematoma becomes compartmentalized from the initial hematoma by the development of a second inner membrane.

Such episodes of sporadic rebleeding expand the lesion periodically and at unpredictable intervals. Alternatively, it has been postulated that lysis of the original hematoma creates a hyperosmotic state, which attracts fluid across the inner membrane, thereby enlarging the lesion. This process is of lesser consequence than rebleeding, because a subdural hematoma at surgery or postmortem examination resembles dense clotted blood, undiluted by clear fluid.

Remarkably, during the genesis of a subdural hematoma, the severance of the cortical bridging veins is

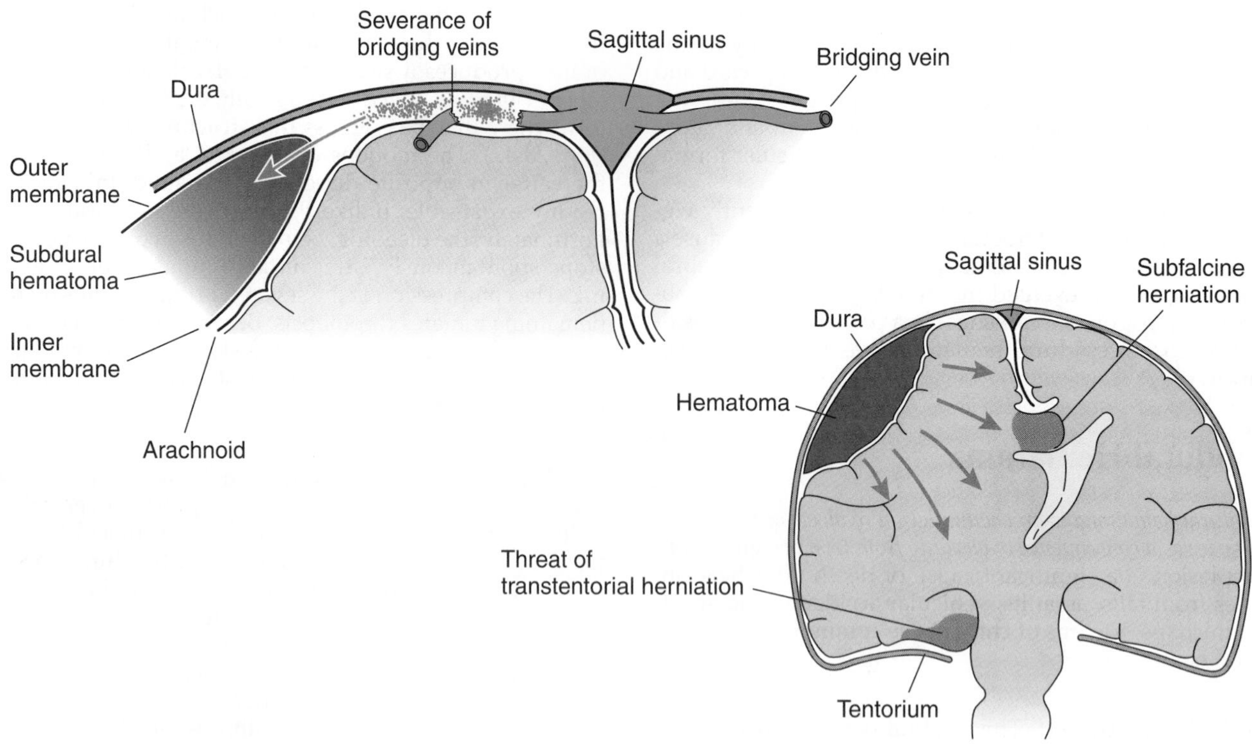

FIGURE 28-42
Development of a subdural hematoma. With head trauma, the dura moves with the skull, and the arachnoid moves with the cerebrum. As a result, the bridging veins are sheared as they cross between the dura and the arachnoid. Venous bleeding creates a hematoma in the expansile subdural space. Subsequent transtentorial herniation is life-threatening.

so precisely localized to the subdural space as to compartmentalize blood away from the CSF. Throughout the evolution of a subdural hematoma, the continuity and integrity of the diaphanous arachnoid are preserved. The arachnoid is not incorporated into the inner membrane nor, for unexplained reasons, does it participate in this contiguous fibroblastic proliferation. **Thus, the absence of blood in the CSF does not negate the presence of a subdural hematoma.**

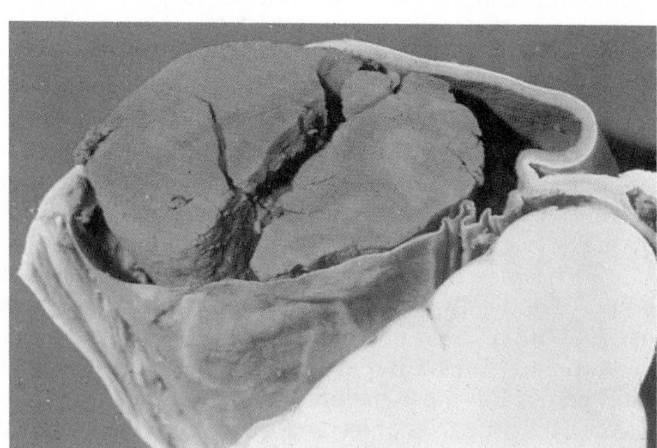

FIGURE 28-43
Subdural hematoma. A chronic subdural hematoma is encapsulated by an outer membrane, evidenced as a narrow brown layer beneath the white dura.

☐ **Clinical Features:** The symptoms of a subdural hematoma are protean. Stretching of the meninges causes headaches. Pressure on the motor cortex produces contralateral weakness, and focal irritation of the cortex may initiate seizures. Diffuse, often bilateral, subdural hematomas may impair cognitive function and lead to de-

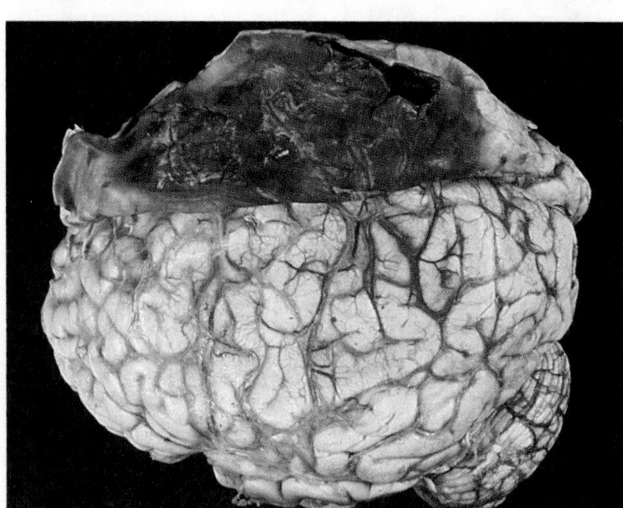

FIGURE 28-44
Subdural hematoma. The left leaf of the dura has been deflected upward to disclose a subdural hematoma that is thinly encapsulated by an inner membrane.

mentia, which invites the mistaken diagnosis of senility. One or several episodes of rebleeding may enlarge the mass and initiate a lethal transtentorial herniation.

Subarachnoid Hemorrhage

Subarachnoid hemorrhage refers to bleeding into the subarachnoid space of any cause. This type of hemorrhage may be seen in association with traumatic head injuries (e.g., cerebral contusion or laceration). However, subarachnoid hemorrhage is rarely an isolated finding with trauma and usually complicates hemorrhage in other parts of the brain. **Two thirds of cases of subarachnoid hemorrhages reflect the rupture of a preexisting arterial aneurysm.** In 10% of the cases, an arteriovenous malformation is demonstrated. The remaining cases result from a variety of conditions, including blood dyscrasias, infections, vasculitis, and tumors. Subarachnoid hemorrhage and cerebral aneurysms are discussed more fully later in this chapter.

Cerebral Contusion

A cerebral contusion is a bruise of the cortical surface of the brain as a result of head trauma.

☐ **Pathogenesis:** Similar to subdural hematomas, cerebral contusions are generally the result of energetic anteroposterior displacement, when the moving head strikes a fixed object. The flotation of the cerebral hemispheres in the anteroposterior direction and the soft gelatinous quality of the cerebral tissues create a vulnerability to bruising or laceration of the cortex by forces applied to the head, particularly those in the midsagittal plane. The magnitude of the contusion parallels the velocity of the motion and the abruptness of the deceleration.

When the cerebral contusion occurs at the point of impact, the lesion is referred to as a *coup* (Fr., "blow") contusion (Fig. 28-45). When the occipital area strikes the ground in a backward fall, the resulting abrasions are prone to occur on the contralateral side of the brain opposite the point of contact, that is, in the frontal or temporal cortex. Such lesions are designated *contrecoup* contusions (see Fig. 28-45).

The distant location of contracoup lesions underscores the anatomical features that determine the nature of the injury: (1) The occipital bone against which the cerebrum first hits has a broad, smooth contour that does not favor injury; (2) the gelatinous quality of the cerebral tissues causes recoil and permits disparate motion between the cerebrum and the skull; and (3) the frontal and temporal poles hit against the irregular, cobbled surface of the frontal and middle fossae.

☐ **Pathology:** If the force is minimal, the contusion is limited to the gray cortex and is restricted to the apex of the gyri (Fig. 28-46A). Greater forces destroy larger expanses of the cortex, creating deeper cavitary lesions that extend into the white matter or that lacerate the cortex

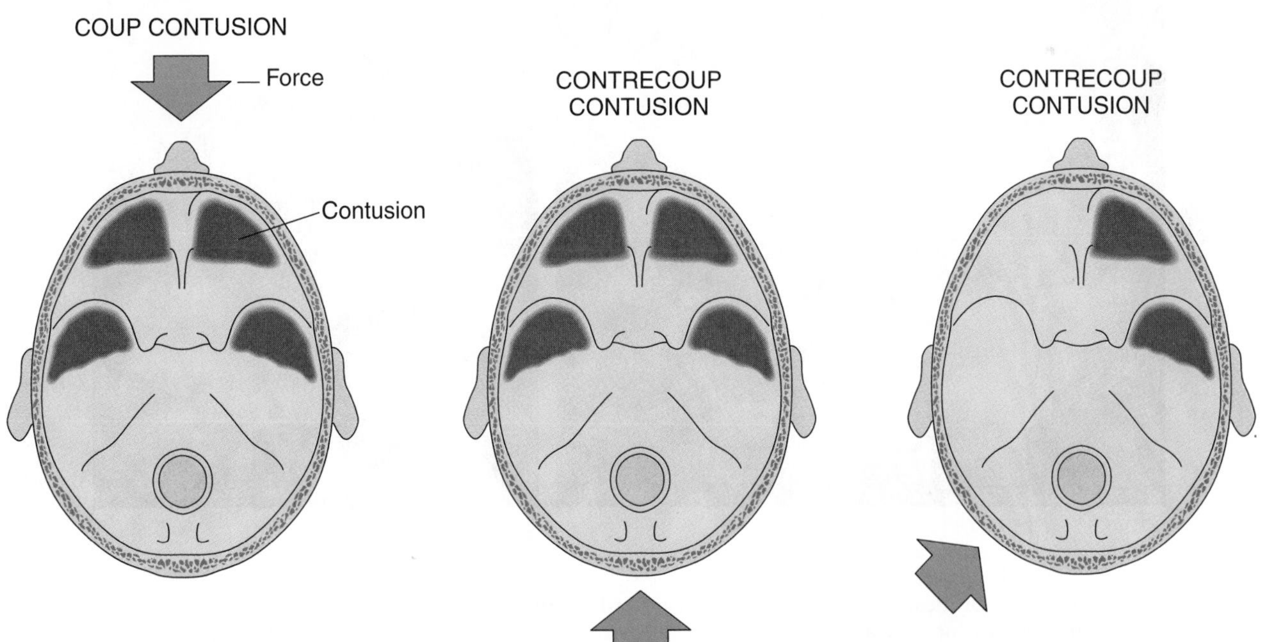

FIGURE *28-45*
Mechanisms of cerebral contusion. The cerebral hemispheres float in the cerebrospinal fluid. Rapid deceleration or, less commonly, acceleration of the skull causes the cortex to impact forcefully into the anterior and middle fossae. The position of a contusion is determined by the direction of the force and the intracranial anatomy.

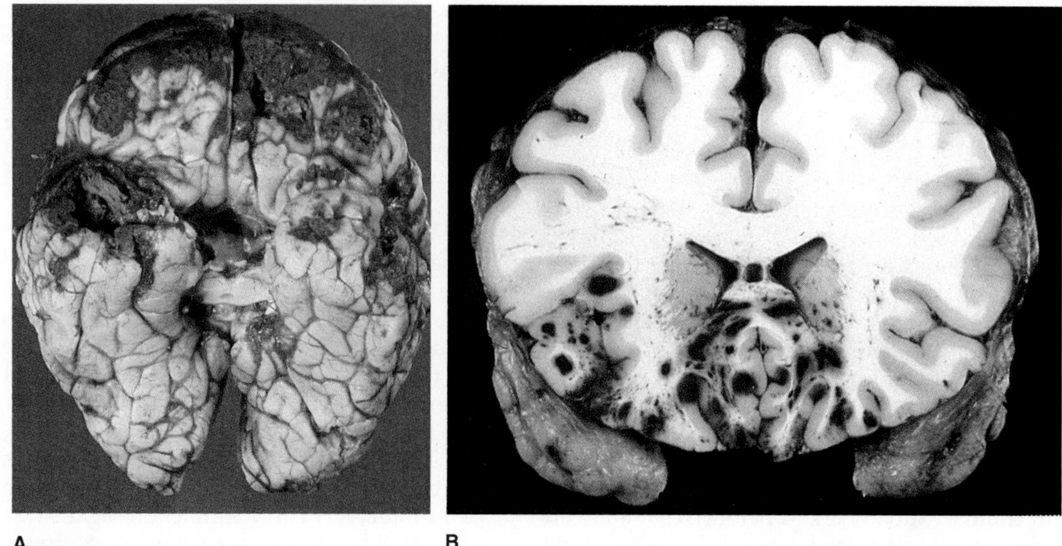

FIGURE 28-46
Recent cerebral contusions. (*A*) Multiple areas of hemorrhage mark the poles of the frontal and temporal lobes. (*B*) A coronal section of *A* shows underlying parenchymal hemorrhages.

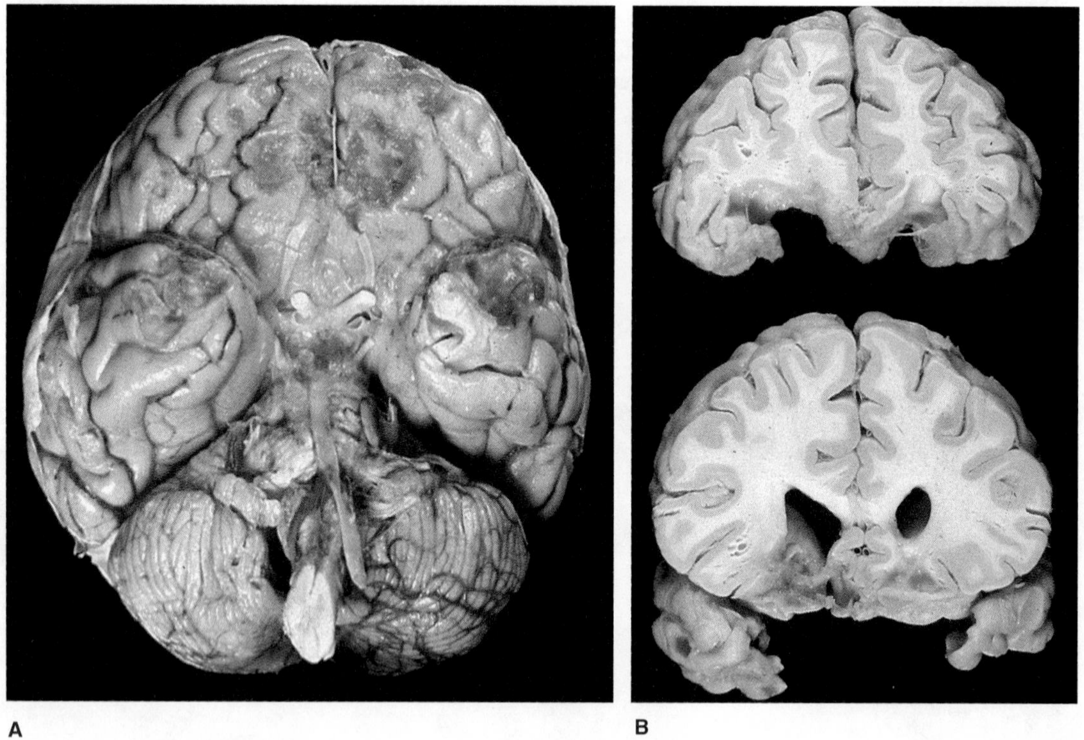

FIGURE 28-47
Remote cerebral contusion. (*A*) Previous cerebral contusions are evidenced by a ragged appearance and focal excavation of the injured parenchyma. (*B*) Coronal section through the sites of old cerebral contusions discloses cystic areas that mark previous hemorrhages.

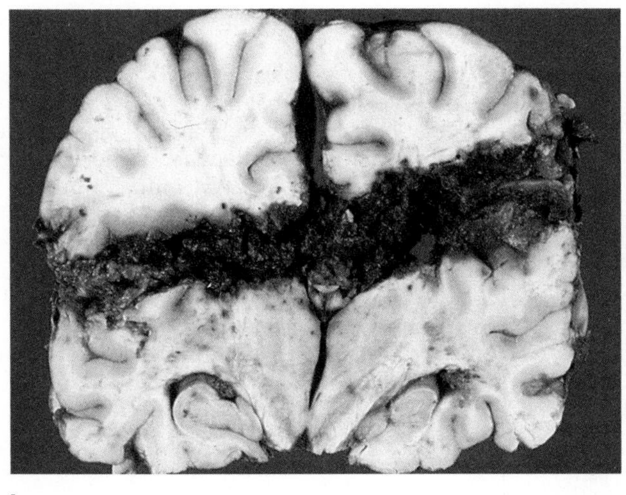

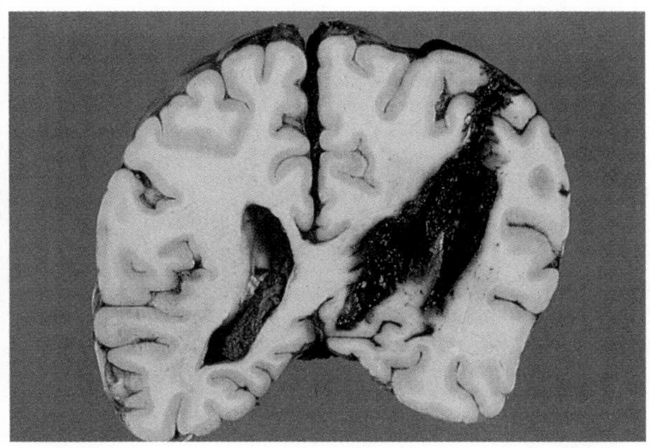

FIGURE 28-48
Penetrating wound. (*A*) A .32-caliber bullet created a hemorrhagic tract through the cerebrum. (*B*) A butcher knife was plunged deep into the brain, causing lethal hemorrhage.

and initiate cortical or subcortical hemorrhages (see Fig. 28-46B). The hemorrhage and edema associated with large contusions create a mass lesion, which threatens life by transtentorial herniation.

Contusions are permanent. The bruised, necrotic tissue is promptly phagocytized by macrophages and is ultimately transported in large part into the bloodstream. Mild astrocytic proliferation forms a local scar, and the lesion persists as a telltale crater (Fig. 28-47).

Contusional injury to the cerebrum may be internal and apparent only on microscopic examination. The parasagittal cortex is anchored by its attachment to the arachnoid villi (*pacchionian granulations*), whereas the lateral aspects of the cerebral hemispheres have greater freedom of motion. This discrepancy permits laminar planes of shearing forces, which lead to axonal injury, particularly in vehicular accidents. When axons are broken, owing to this shearing phenomenon that occurs during forceful rotatory acceleration and deceleration, they retract into "spheroids," and their myelin is lost. These changes are typically present in the parasagittal white matter and are accompanied acutely by multiple small hemorrhages. In such instances, the patient is typically rendered comatose, and the computed tomographic scan

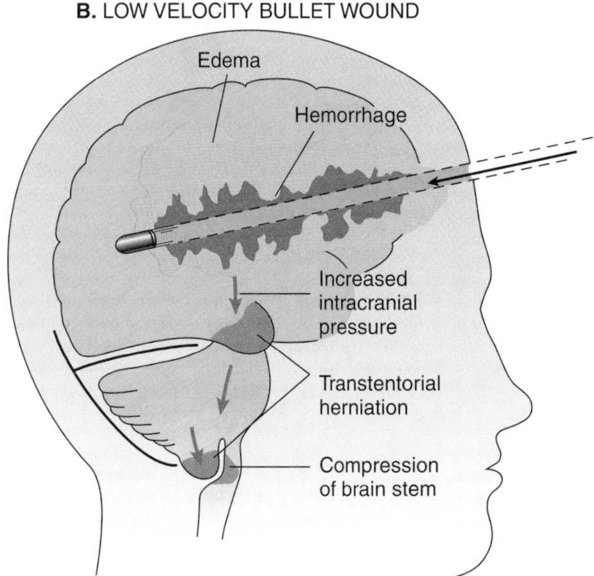

FIGURE 28-49
Consequences of high- and low-velocity bullet wounds. (*A*) The "blast effect" of a high-velocity projectile causes an immediate increase in supratentorial pressure and results in death because of impaction of the cerebellum and medulla into the foramen magnum. (*B*) A low-velocity projectile increases the pressure at a more gradual rate through hemorrhage and edema.

may disclose cerebral edema without hemorrhage. Magnetic resonance imaging often reveals small hemorrhages and foci of edema.

Penetrating Wounds

Penetrating objects such as bullets and knives enter the cranium and traverse the brain with variable velocities. In the absence of direct injury to the vital medullary centers, the immediate threat to life is hemorrhage (Fig. 28-48). Bleeding creates a space-occupying mass, the presence of which threatens transtentorial herniation. When the hemorrhage occurs in the cerebellum, the immediate threat is herniation of the cerebellar tonsils into the foramen magnum. This compresses the medulla and often paralyzes the cardiac and respiratory centers.

Velocity contributes a blast effect to a projectile (Fig. 28-49). As a high-velocity bullet traverses the brain, it disrupts tissues, not only by its own mass but also by a centrifugal blast that enlarges the diameter of the cylinder of disruption. Thus, a high-velocity (military) bullet can cause immediate death through an explosive increase in intracranial pressure. This pressure forcefully herniates the cerebellar tonsils into the foramen magnum and compresses the medulla, thereby causing immediate cardiac or respiratory paralysis.

Seizures are a threat in healed penetrating wounds, usually manifested 6 to 12 months after the trauma. Collagenous tissue is displaced into the brain from the scalp

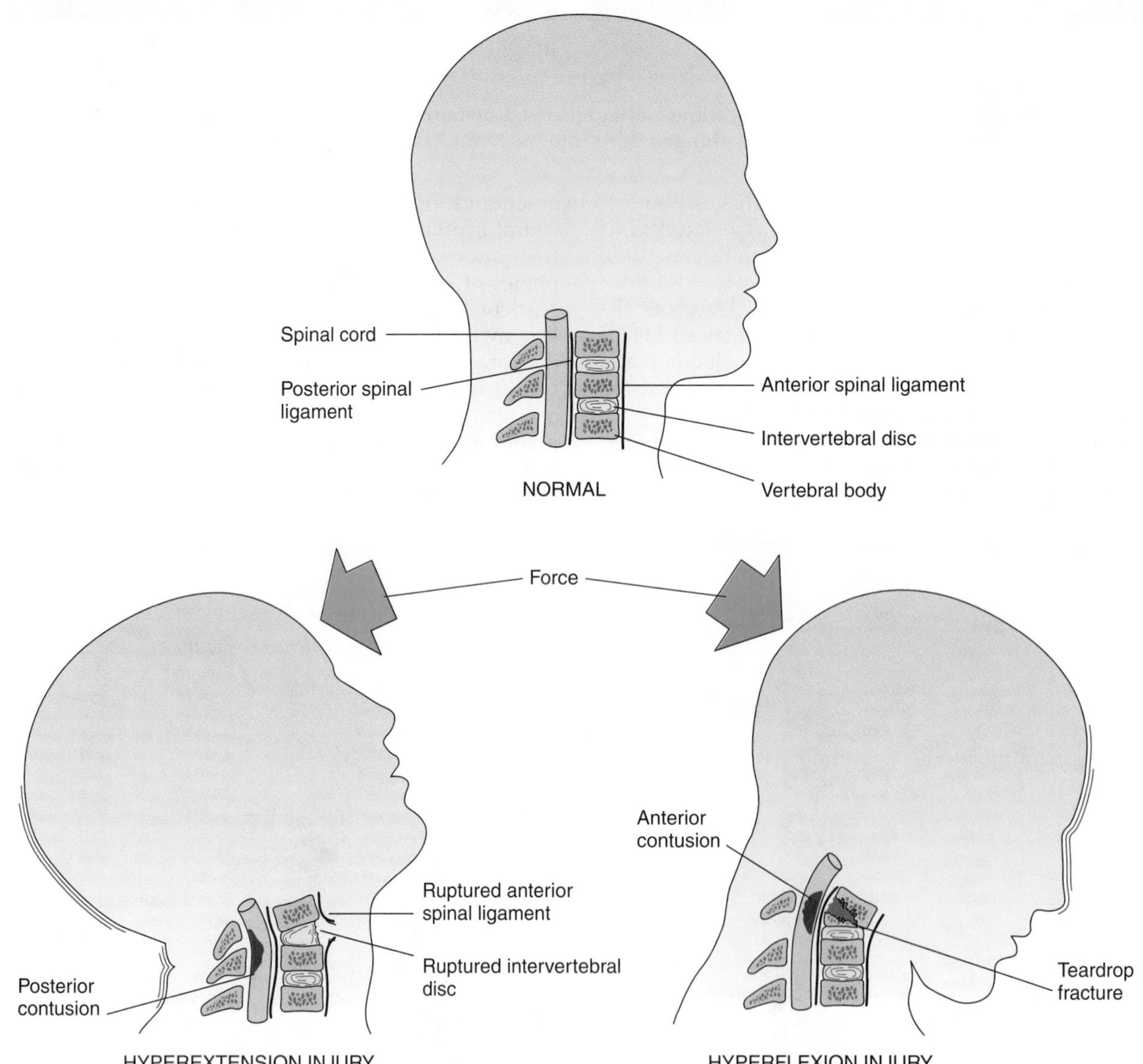

FIGURE *28-50*
Spinal injury. Numerous angles of force can be applied to the highly vulnerable cervical spine. Posterior (hyperextension) and anterior (hyperflexion) injuries are the most common. Hyperextension injury causes rupture of the anterior spinal ligament and permits excessive posterior angulation. Hyperflexion injury causes compression, frequently associated with a "teardrop" fracture of a vertebral body, and produces excessive forward angulation of the cord.

or dura, and fibroblasts subsequently proliferate to form a dense scar. The precise mechanism by which a scar activates neurons and leads to seizures remains obscure.

Spinal Cord Injuries

Trauma to the spinal cord is a significant cause of morbidity, often leading to paraplegia or quadriplegia, depending on the location and extent of the injury. Traumatic lesions may result from direct injury to the cord by penetrating wounds (stab wounds, bullets) or indirect injury as a consequence of vertebral fractures, fracture–dislocations, or subluxation of the spine. The spinal cord may be contused not only at the site of injury but also above and below the point of trauma. Traumatic injury may be complicated by compromise of the arterial supply to the cord, with resulting infarction.

The bodies of the vertebrae are separated by intravertebral disks and are stabilized in normal alignment by two longitudinal ligaments, as well as by the posterior bony processes. The anterior spinal ligament adheres to the ventral surface of the vertebral bodies, whereas the posterior spinal ligament is affixed to the posterior vertebral column. As a result of extreme flexion or extension (Fig. 28-50), the angulation of the bony vertebral column brings the spinal cord forcefully into contact with bone, or alternatively, interferes with the regional circulation.

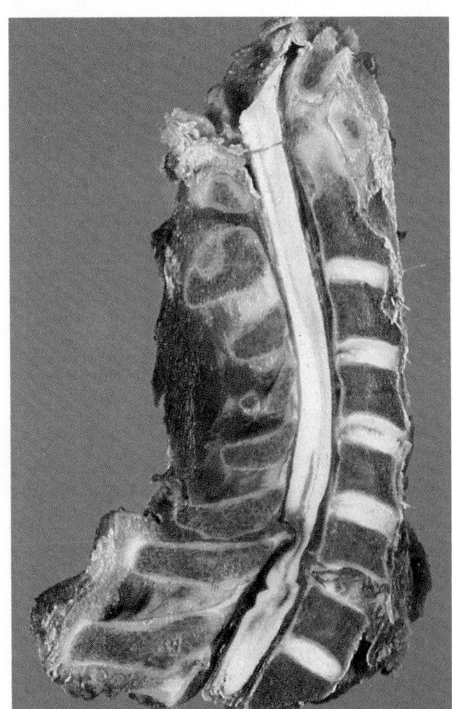

FIGURE *28-51*
Cervical contusion. A hyperextension injury of cervical cord from a blow to the forehead resulted in posterior angulation. The anterior spinal ligament ruptured, the intervertebral disc fragmented, and the cord was brought forcibly against the posterior process of the underlying fixed vertebral body.

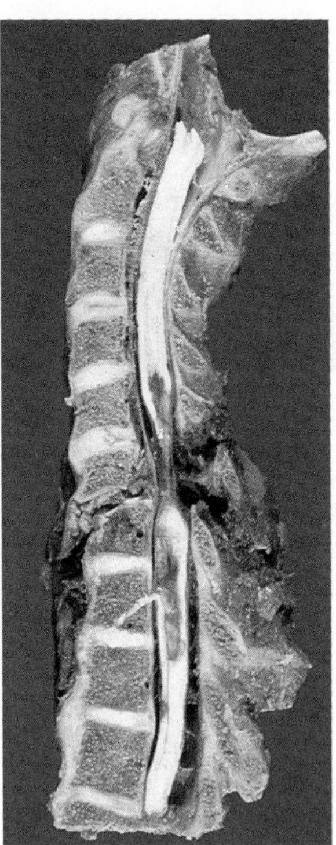

FIGURE *28-52*
Cervical contusion. Hyperflexion injury caused forward angulation of the cervical cord, with fracture of the anterior lip of the underlying vertebral body. The cord is angulated over the superior–posterior ridge of the fixed underlying cervical body.

HYPEREXTENSION INJURY: When the forehead is struck and driven posteriorly, as during a diving impact in shallow water, the posterior displacement of the head (hyperextension) tears the anterior spinal ligament, thereby permitting a sharp posterior angulation of the spinal canal. At the point of angulation, the posterior aspect of the spinal cord is brought into forceful and damaging contact with the posterior process of the stationary vertebral body, which lies immediately caudal to the angulation (Fig. 28-51).

HYPERFLEXION INJURY: When the head or shoulders are struck from behind by an object of considerable weight, or when this region of a falling human body (generally in a flexed position) strikes a stationary object, the head is driven forcefully forward and downward (hyperflexion). The impact forces one vertebral body down upon the underlying one. The anterior lip of the underlying vertebral body is fractured, with forward slippage and downward displacement of the overlying vertebra. This disfigurement of the spinal canal results in sharp forward angulation of the spinal cord. The anterior surface of the angulated cord forcefully contacts the posterior superior edge of the stable underlying vertebral body (Fig. 28-52).

The consequences of a spinal cord injury vary with the severity of the trauma.

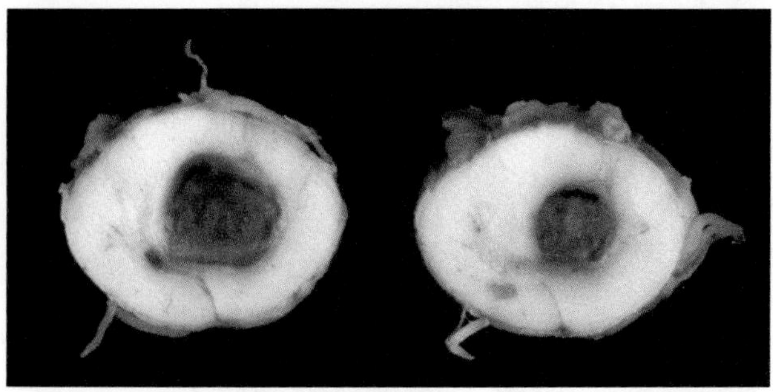

FIGURE 28-53
Cervical contusion. A cross-section of a contused spinal cord shows central hemorrhage, termed "hematomyelia with myelomalacia."

- **Concussion of the spinal cord** is the mildest injury and represents a transient and reversible disturbance of spinal cord function.
- **Contusion of the spinal cord** is the result of more severe trauma, ranging from a minor transient bruise to hemorrhagic necrosis of nervous tissue. The edema and softening of the cord that follow a severe contusion are referred to as *myelomalacia*. A collection of blood within the substance of the spinal cord is termed *hematomyelia* (Fig. 28-53).
- **Lacerations and transections of the spinal cord**, usually produced by penetrating wounds, are ordinarily irreversible and result in complete loss of function, the nature of which depends on the location and extent of the injury.

CIRCULATORY DISORDERS

Vascular Malformations

There are four major categories of vascular anomalies:

- **Arteriovenous malformation** (Fig. 28-54): This is the most common congenital vascular malformation and of the greatest clinical significance. Seizure disorders and intracranial hemorrhages, usually subarachnoid or intracerebral, supervene in the second or third decades. The lesion evolves during embryonic development as a result of a focal absence of a capillary bed, which permits direct communication between cerebral arteries and veins. The resultant conglomeration of abnormal vessels is located in a region of cerebral cortex and the contiguous underlying white matter. The area of involvement enlarges as a result of the gradual recruitment of tributary vessels.
- **Cavernous angioma:** This congenital anomaly is considerably less common than arteriovenous malformation. It is similar in structure to a cavernous angioma of the liver, being formed by large vascular spaces compartmentalized by prominent fibrous walls. Most cavernous angiomas remain asymptomatic. However, a significant minority of patients have intracranial bleeding, epilepsy, or focal neurological disturbances.
- **Telangiectasia:** This focal aggregate of uniformly small vessels, with intervening neural parenchyma, may initiate seizures but rarely ruptures.
- **Venous angioma:** This structure consists of a focus of a few enlarged veins distributed randomly in the spinal cord or brain. The lesion is generally asymptomatic.

Aneurysms

Intravascular pressure exploits weakness in arterial walls and causes aneurysms. Among the many causes of aneurysms are the following:

- **Developmental defects**, which give rise to berry (saccular, medial defect) aneurysms (Fig. 28-55)
- **Atherosclerosis** (Fig. 28-56)
- **Hypertension**, which is associated with lipohyalinosis of cerebral arterioles and induces Charcot–Bouchard aneurysms (Fig. 28-57)
- **Bacterial infections**, leading to mycotic aneurysms
- **Trauma**, which on rare occasions causes dissecting aneurysms

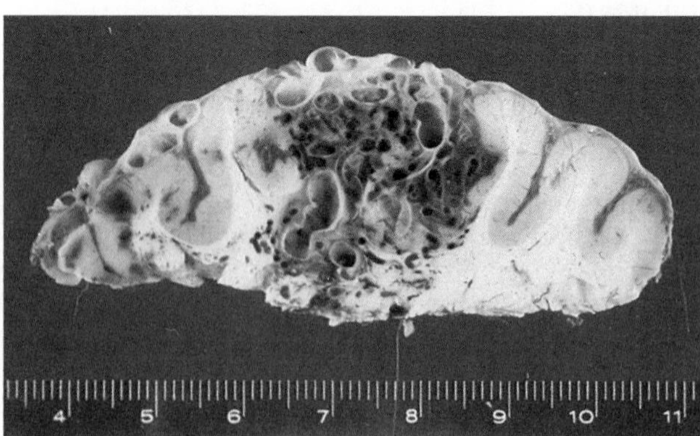

FIGURE 28-54
Arteriovenous malformation. Abnormal blood vessels replace the cortical gray matter and extend deeply into the underlying white matter.

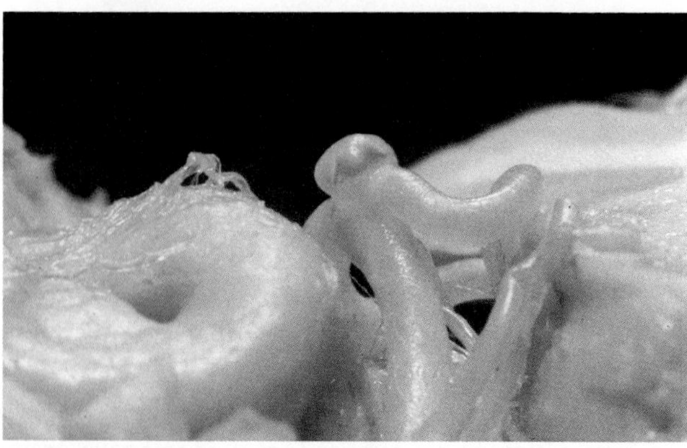

FIGURE 28-55
Berry aneurysm. A thin-walled aneurysm protrudes from an arterial bifurcation in the circle of Willis.

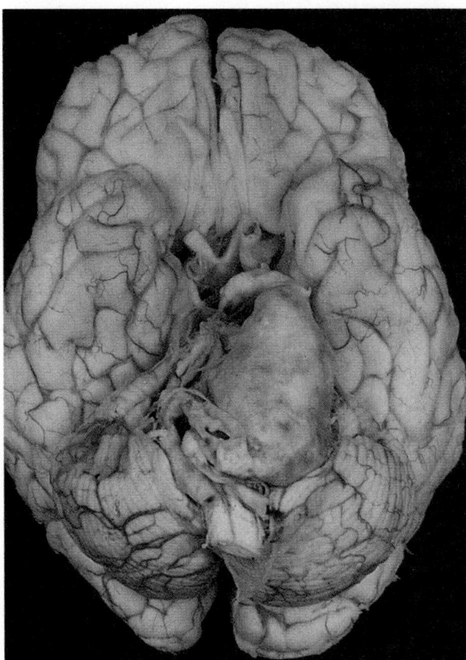

FIGURE *28-56*
Atherosclerotic aneurysm. A fusiform dilatation of the basilar and internal carotid arteries has resulted from severe atherosclerosis.

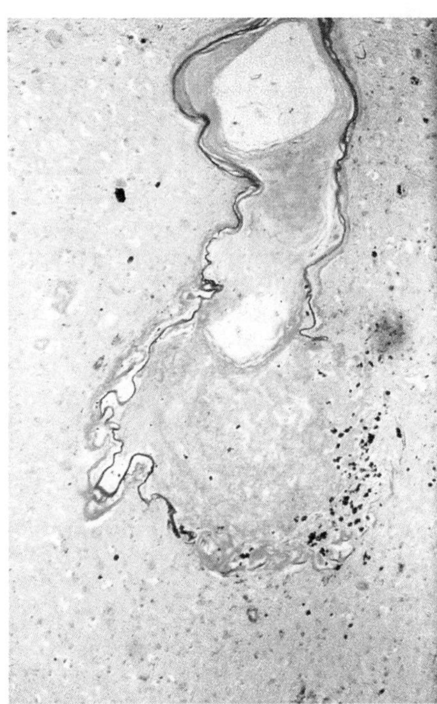

FIGURE *28-57*
Charcot–Bouchard aneurysm. Chronic hypertension initiated the deposition of lipid in and the hyalinization of the arterial wall. A microaneurysm arises from the damaged wall of the arteriole. The hemosiderin-laden macrophages attest to previous hemorrhage.

Berry Aneurysms

☐ **Pathogenesis and Pathology:** Berry aneurysms are the consequence of arterial defects that originate during embryonic development, when the bifurcation of an artery creates a Y-shaped configuration (Fig. 28-58). The circumferential muscular layer of the parent vessel, and that of two branches, are separate and may fail to interdigitate adequately across the notch of the Y. This creates a point of congenital muscular weakness, bridged only by endothelium, the internal elastic membrane, and a slender coating of adventitia. The bloodstream from the parent vessel exerts relentless pressure at the notch of the Y, and time and trauma then exploit the congenital defect. Eventually, the internal elastic membrane degenerates and fragments, after which the endothelium yields. A saccular aneurysm evolves, its wall being formed precariously only of adventitia.

More than 90% of saccular aneurysms occur at branch points in the carotid system. They are about equally distributed at the unions of (1) the anterior cerebral and the anterior communicating arteries, (2) the complex of the internal carotid–posterior communicating–anterior cerebral–anterior choroidal arteries, and (3) the trifurcation of the middle cerebral artery. In 20% of the cases, multiple berry aneurysms are present. Careful autopsies have revealed that undetected berry aneurysms are found in as many as 25% of persons older than 55 years.

☐ **Clinical Features:** **Rupture of a berry aneurysm results in life-threatening subarachnoid hemorrhage, with a 35% mortality during the initial hemorrhage.** Rupture produces intracerebral or intraventricular hemorrhage in up to one third of the patients. A sudden severe headache characteristically heralds the onset of subarachnoid hemorrhage and may be followed by coma. Patients who survive for 3 to 4 days often manifest a progressive decline in consciousness, an effect that has been attributed to arterial spasm and consequent cerebral ischemia and infarction. Survivors of the initial episode may rebleed, in which case the prognosis is worse.

The enlargement of a saccular aneurysm may form a mass large enough to compress cranial nerves and produce palsies or to impinge on parenchymal structures and induce neurological symptoms. A "giant" saccular aneurysm of the internal carotid complex produces palsies of the third, fourth, and sixth cranial nerves and seizures initiated by the compression of the medial aspect of the temporal lobe.

Atherosclerotic Aneurysms

Aneurysms caused by atherosclerosis are preferentially localized in the major cerebral vessels (vertebral, basilar, and internal carotid arteries), the favored sites of atherosclerosis. Fibrous replacement of the media and destruction of the internal elastic membrane weaken the arterial wall and permit aneurysmal dilatation (Fig. 28-59). Atherosclerotic aneurysms are characteristically fusiform, and as they enlarge, the vessel elongates. Thus, an atherosclerotic aneurysm of the basilar artery is prone to

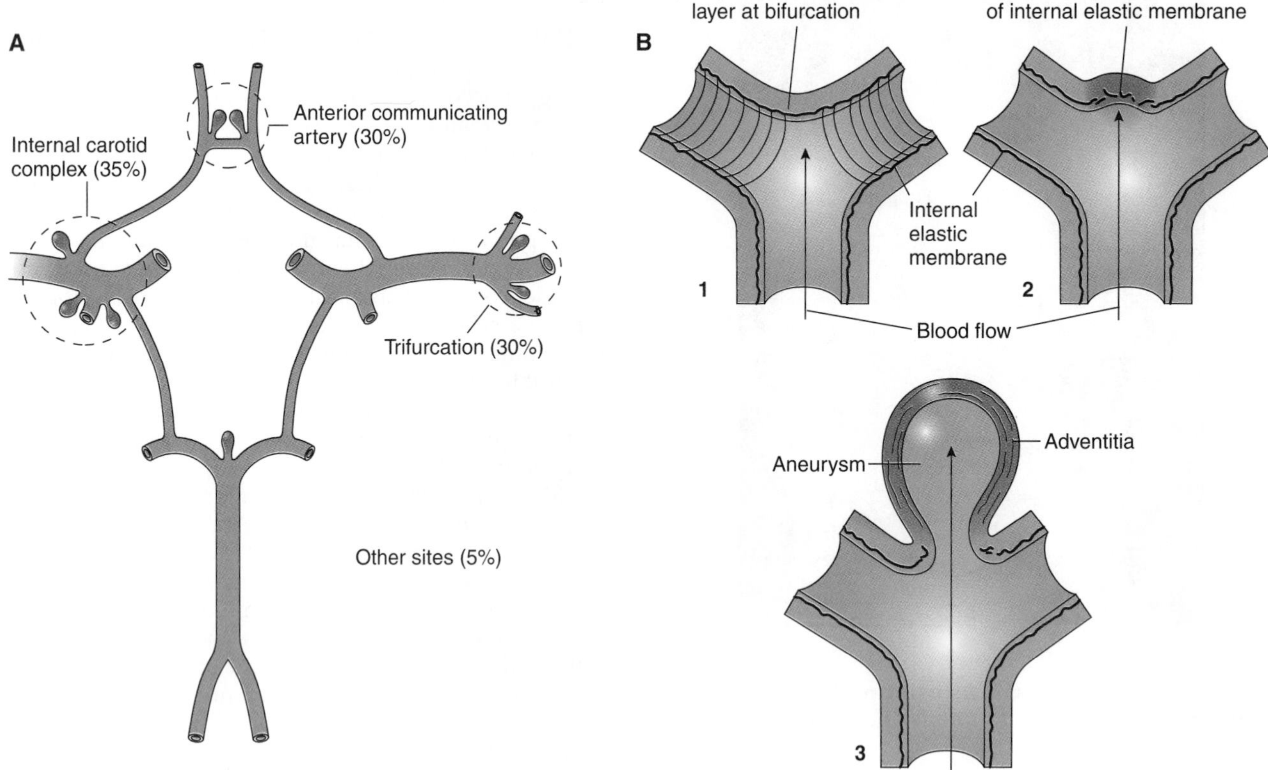

FIGURE *28-58*
Saccular aneurysm. (*A*) The incidence of saccular aneurysms (berry aneurysms), which preferentially involve the carotid tributaries, is depicted. (*B*) Their pathogenesis is illustrated. The lesion evolves as a result of blood acting on an early embryonic defect.

move laterally into the cerebellopontine angle, where it forms a mass that compresses cranial nerves and produces neurological deficits (see Fig. 28-56). Atherosclerotic aneurysms rarely rupture, and the major complication is thrombosis. Pontine infarctions are often the sequelae of atherosclerotic aneurysms of the basilar artery.

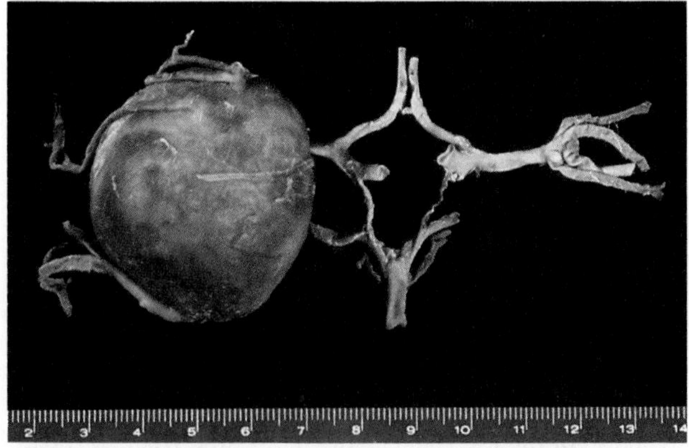

FIGURE *28-59*
Giant saccular aneurysm. A large aneurysm of the middle cerebral artery created a mass lesion, which produced symptoms clinically mistaken for those of a tumor.

Mycotic Aneurysms

Infections of arterial walls result from septic emboli, usually with origins in an infected cardiac valve. The embolus flows through the carotid circulation and typically lodges in a branch of the middle cerebral artery, commonly at the origin of a short penetrating carotid vessel. The bacteria proliferate, induce inflammation, and destroy the integrity of the arterial wall. The compromised vessel yields to an aneurysm, which may rupture and be seen as an intracerebral or subarachnoid hemorrhage. Alternatively, microorganisms may be released and produce a cerebral abscess or suppurative meningitis.

Cerebral Hemorrhage

Cerebral hemorrhages that occur without trauma are referred to as "spontaneous," although most are caused by a vascular anomaly (see earlier) or are the consequence of long-standing hypertension. Such events have been traditionally referred to as "strokes" or "apoplexy," terms that also include occlusive cerebrovascular lesions (infarcts).

Hypertensive intracerebral hemorrhage occurs at preferential sites, which are in order of frequency: (1) the basal ganglia–thalamus (65%; Fig. 28-60), (2) the pons (15%; Fig. 28-61), and (3) the cerebellum (8%; Fig. 28-62).

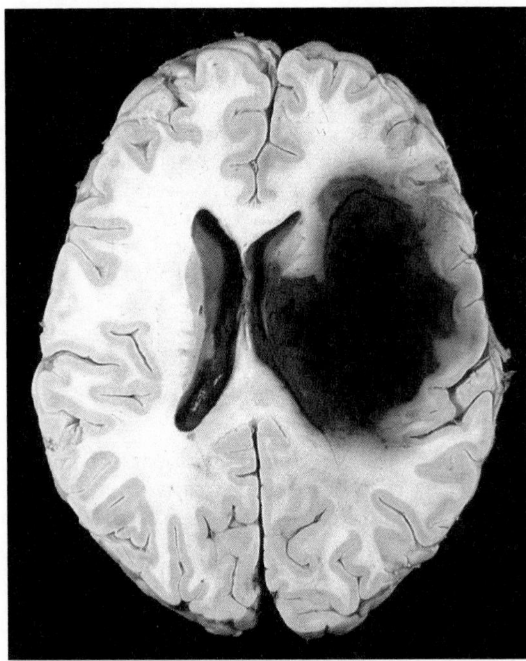

FIGURE *28-60*
Cerebral hemorrhage. A spontaneous cerebral hemorrhage began near the external capsule and produced a hematoma that threatened rupture into a lateral ventricle.

Interestingly, although the frequency of cerebral hemorrhage is notably increased by the presence of hypertension, the topographic pattern is not altered by the absence of this major risk factor.

The integrity of cerebral arterioles is compromised by hypertension through the deposition of lipid and hyaline material in their walls, an alteration referred to as *lipohyalinosis* (see Fig. 28-57). The resulting weakening of the wall leads to the formation of *Charcot–Bouchard* aneurysms. These small fusiform aneurysms are located on the trunk of a vessel rather than at a bifurcation and are disposed to rupture and hemorrhage. The fact that Charcot–Bouchard aneurysms and lipohyalinosis associated with long-standing hypertension occur in a geographic distribution that closely corresponds to the pattern of spontaneous cerebral hemorrhage argues strongly for a relation between them.

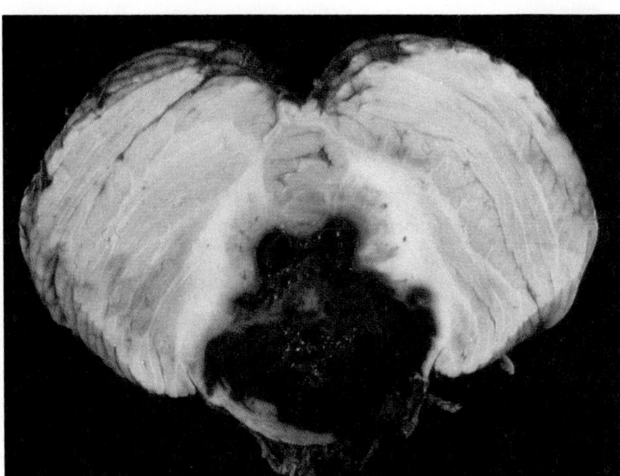

FIGURE *28-61*
Pontine hemorrhage. A spontaneous hemorrhage is present in the midpons.

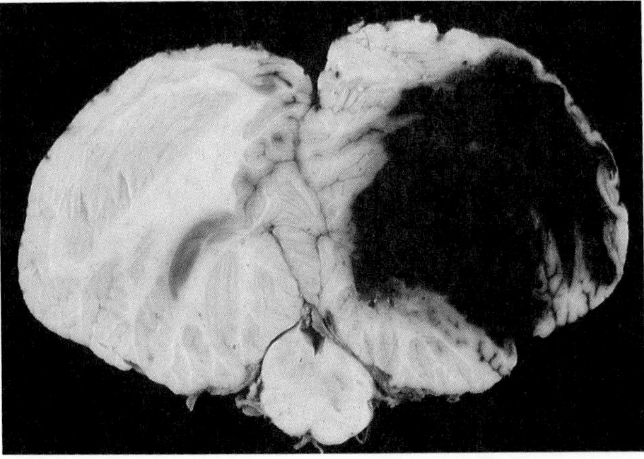

FIGURE *28-62*
Cerebellar hemorrhage. A spontaneous hemorrhage has destroyed a lateral lobe of the cerebellum.

The onset of symptoms in the case of a hypertensive cerebral hemorrhage (hemorrhagic stroke) is abrupt, and weakness usually dominates. When hemorrhage is progressive, and it usually is, death occurs within a period of hours or several days. As the hematoma enlarges, it may cause death by transtentorial herniation, or it may rupture into a lateral ventricle and initiate massive intraventricular hemorrhage (Fig. 28-63).

INTRAVENTRICULAR HEMORRHAGE: Rupture of a vessel into a ventricle rapidly distends the entire ventricular system with blood. The forward edge of this col-

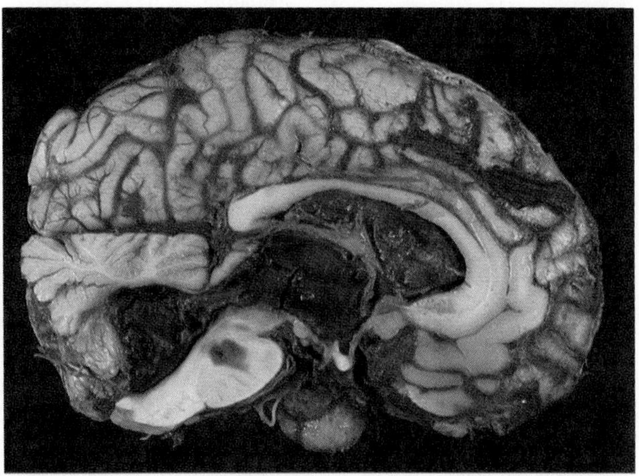

FIGURE *28-63*
Intraventricular hemorrhage. A sagittal section of the brain shows ventricular chambers filled with blood. The patient died rapidly, owing to compression of the brainstem by blood in the fourth ventricle.

umn of blood expands the fourth ventricle but rarely emerges from the foramina of Magendie and Luschka. The rush of blood through the ventricular system seemingly causes death by distention of the fourth ventricle and the compression of vital centers in the medulla.

PONTINE HEMORRHAGE: In this catastrophic event, the loss of consciousness reflects damage to the reticular formation, an injury that overshadows all other specific cranial nerve deficits. The initial focus of hemorrhage is generally in the midpons and, thus, is more caudal than hemorrhage induced by transtentorial herniation. With minimal enlargement, pontine hemorrhage encroaches on the vital medullary centers. Patients rarely survive, and death usually occurs before arrival at the hospital.

CEREBELLAR HEMORRHAGE: Bleeding into the cerebellum causes abrupt ataxia, usually accompanied by a severe occipital headache and vomiting. The expanding hematoma threatens life acutely through compression of the medulla, either directly or as a consequence of the herniation of the cerebellar tonsils into the foramen magnum. The lack of localized functional representation in the cerebellum generally permits surgical evacuation of the lesion without serious neurological deficits. This contrasts favorably with the universally disappointing surgical results when cerebral hematomas are drained.

Spontaneous cerebral hemorrhages have causes other than hypertension, including the following:

- Leakage from an arteriovenous malformation
- Erosion of vessels by a primary or secondary neoplasm
- A bleeding diathesis, as exemplified by thrombocytopenic purpura
- Endothelial injury by microorganisms, notably rickettsiae
- Embolic infarction, with consequent hemorrhage into the area of necrosis

Ischemia and Infarction

Inadequate perfusion of the brain may result from generalized low blood flow resulting from extracerebral events, such as shock or cardiac arrest, or from occlusive disease of the cerebral circulation. In the case of a generalized decrease in cerebral blood flow, the resultant ischemia is global, whereas vascular obstruction produces regional ischemia and often a localized infarct. The lesions that follow global ischemia can also be produced by hypoxia (e.g., near-drowning, carbon monoxide poisoning, or entrapment in a burning building).

Global Ischemia

The pattern of injury produced by global ischemia (or hypoxia) reflects the anatomical arrangement of cerebral blood vessels and the sensitivity of individual neurons to oxygen deprivation (Fig. 28-64). The topography of the cerebral vasculature is primarily responsible for two lesions, watershed infarcts and laminar necrosis.

WATERSHED INFARCTS: These ischemic lesions reflect the fact that the major cerebral vessels, notably the anterior, middle, and posterior cerebral arteries, provide overlapping circulations (Fig. 28-65). For example, although the anterior cerebral arteries principally supply the cortex on the medial aspects of both cerebral hemispheres, they also interface with the distribution of the middle cerebral arteries in the parasagittal cortex. However, the overlapping zone in the parasagittal cortex is not so richly vascularized as are the regions supplied by the primary distributions of the anterior and middle cerebral arteries. A precipitate decline in cerebral blood flow abruptly diminishes the circulation in the overlapping branches of both the anterior and middle cerebral arteries. This inflicts a dual ischemic insult to the intervening circulatory zones, and watershed infarcts result.

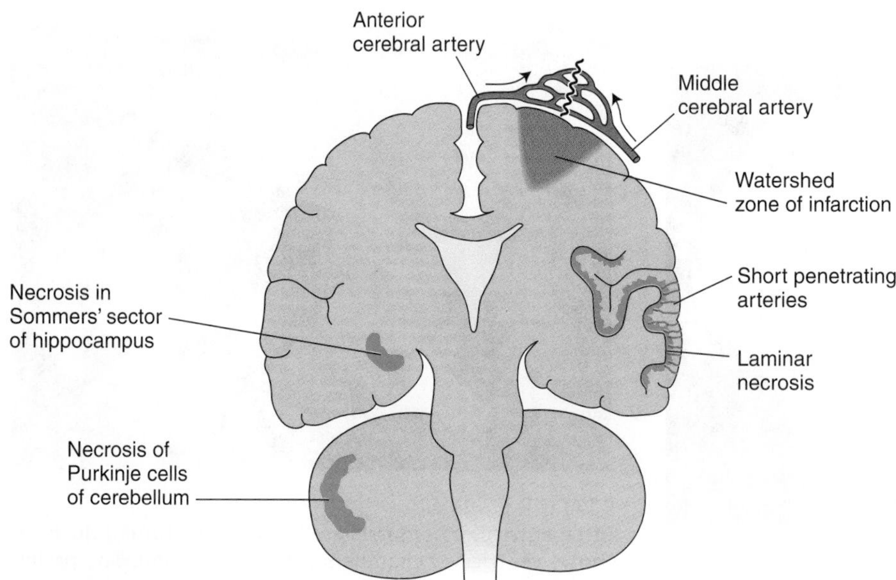

FIGURE *28-64*
Consequences of global ischemia. A global insult induces lesions that reflect the vascular architecture (watershed infarcts, laminar necrosis) and the sensitivity of individual neuronal systems (pyramidal cells of Sommer sector, Purkinje cells).

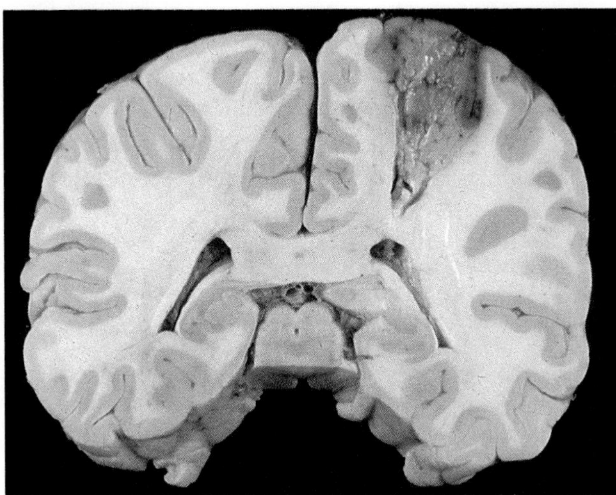

FIGURE *28-65*
Watershed infarct. A coronal section of the brain shows a recent infarct between the distributions of the anterior and middle cerebral arteries.

LAMINAR NECROSIS: This localized lesion similarly portrays an injury patterned by the topography of the normal cerebral vasculature (Figs. 28-66 and 28-67). The cerebral gray matter receives its major blood supply through the "short penetrators," which take origin at right angles from larger vessels in the pia and then form a cascade as they penetrate into the gray matter. In that location, they branch frequently, finally constructing a rich plexus of capillaries deep in the gray matter, notably in the fourth to sixth neuronal cell layers. An abrupt loss of circulatory pressure selectively diminishes flow through this terminal capillary plexus. The necrotic zone is laminar, and the necrosis is understandably most severe in the deeper layers of the gray cortex.

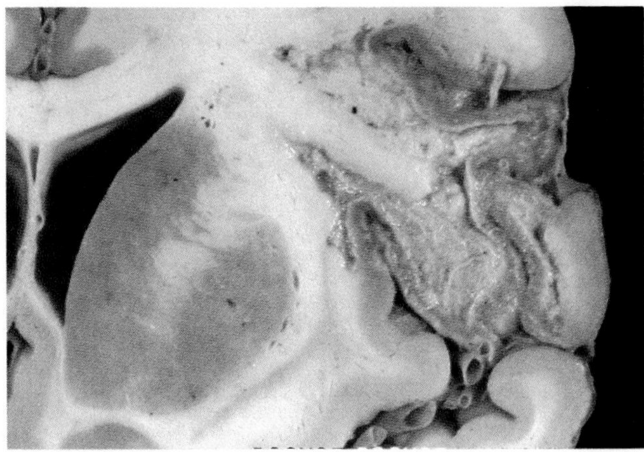

FIGURE *28-66*
Laminar necrosis. A narrow zone of infarction is seen within the cerebral cortex.

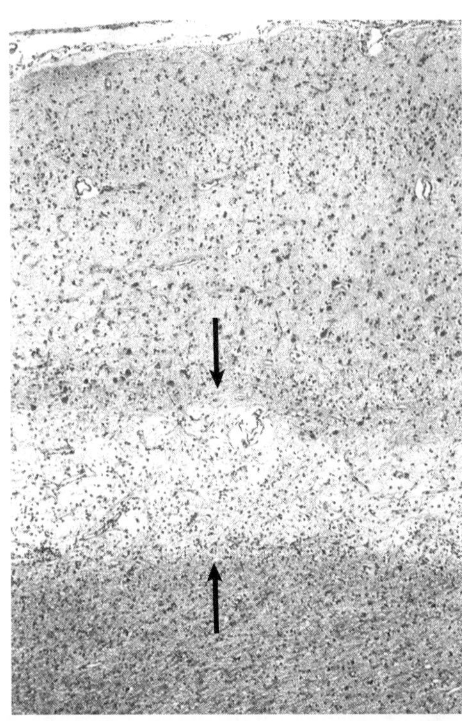

FIGURE *28-67*
Laminar necrosis. A microscopic view of Fig. 28-66 shows that the zone of infarction (*arrows*) selectively involves the fourth to the sixth cortical layers.

Selective neuronal sensitivity to a lack of oxygen is expressed most dramatically in the Purkinje cells of the cerebellum and the pyramidal neurons of Sommer sector in the hippocampus. Presumably, these neurons have unusual metabolic requirements for oxygen or inordinate sensitivity to lactic acid. Thus, in global ischemia, selective, neuronal sensitivity may lead to localized areas of necrosis.

Regional Ischemia and Cerebral Infarction

The prevalence and progressive nature of atherosclerosis are reflected in the fact that cerebrovascular occlusive disease remains a major cause of morbidity and mortality. Atherosclerosis predisposes to vascular thrombosis and embolic events, both of which result in localized ischemia and subsequent cerebral infarction (Fig. 28-68).

☐ **Pathology:** Cerebral infarcts are traditionally designated "hemorrhagic" or "bland." These descriptors are overly simplistic and admit of only two extreme possibilities. Yet in general, infarcts that are caused by embolization are the sites of hemorrhage, whereas those initiated by thrombotic occlusion *in situ* are largely ischemic and therefore bland. These differences are accounted for by the tempo of evolution. An embolus occludes vascular flow abruptly, after which the ischemic region undergoes necrosis. The blood vessels that traverse the area of in-

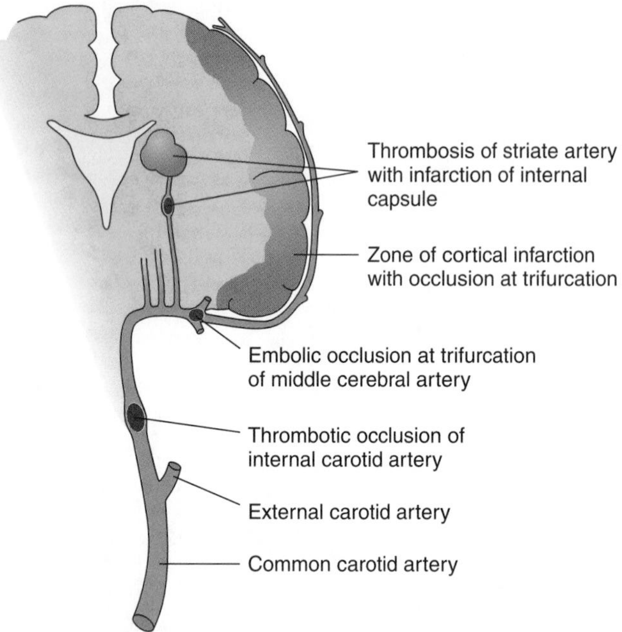

FIGURE 28-68
Distribution of cerebral infarcts. The normal geographic distribution of the cerebral vasculature defines the pattern and size of infarcts, and consequently, their symptoms. Occlusion at the trifurcation initiates cortical infarction, with motor and sensory loss, and often, aphasia. Occlusion of a striate branch transects the internal capsule and causes a motor deficit.

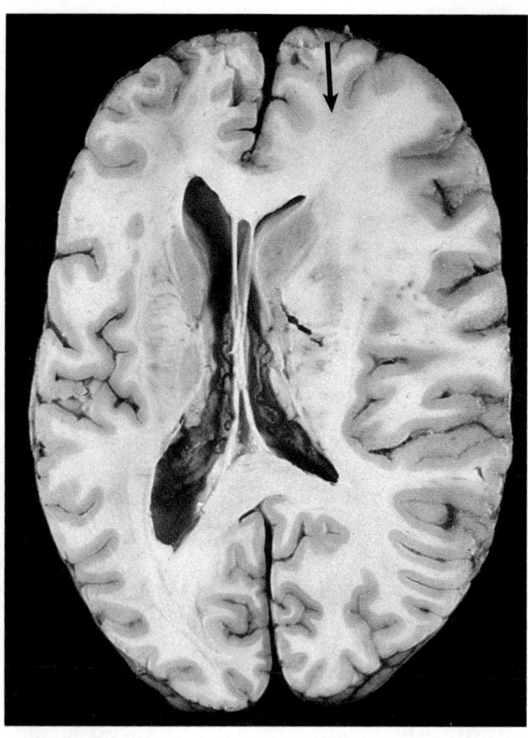

FIGURE 28-69
Recent cerebral infarct. A horizontal section of the brain shows expansion and softening in the distribution of the right middle cerebral artery (*arrow*).

farction also become necrotic and leak blood into that region. Because thrombosis *in situ* progresses more slowly, the collateral vessels also thrombose, thereby guarding against secondary hemorrhage.

A recent infarct of the brain transforms the cerebral tissue into necrotic, putty-like debris (Fig. 28-69), which is ultimately phagocytized by macrophages (Fig. 28-70). Unlike infarcts of the heart and kidneys, cerebral infarcts are not repaired by fibroblasts. As an early response, capillaries proliferate at the margin of the lesion and become numerous by the fifth day. Within months, in proportion to the size of the lesion, the necrotic area is excavated by phagocytosis, and a permanent cyst is formed. At the same time, neovascularity regresses. If the initial area of the infarction is large, the residual cyst is bridged by a cobweb of atretic blood vessels (Fig. 28-71). Although fluid-filled, cerebral infarcts have been referred to as examples of liquefactive necrosis, the fluid is derived from seepage and is not the end-product of necrosis. Thus, it is more accurate to speak of a cerebral infarct as an example of coagulative necrosis rather than of liquefactive necrosis.

☐ **Clinical Features:** Localized neurological deficits are produced by the occlusion of different cerebral vessels. For example, the lengthy and slender striate arteries, which take origin from the proximal middle cerebral artery, are commonly occluded by atherosclerosis and thrombosis. The resultant infarct often transects the internal capsule and produces hemiparesis or hemiplegia (Fig. 28-72). Similarly, the trifurcation of the middle cerebral artery, a point of major step-down in vascular caliber, is a favored site not only for the lodgement of emboli but also for atherosclerosis, which promotes thrombosis *in situ*. Occlusion of the middle cerebral artery at the trifurcation deprives the parietal cortex of circulation and produces motor and sensory deficits, as well as aphasias, when the dominant hemisphere is involved.

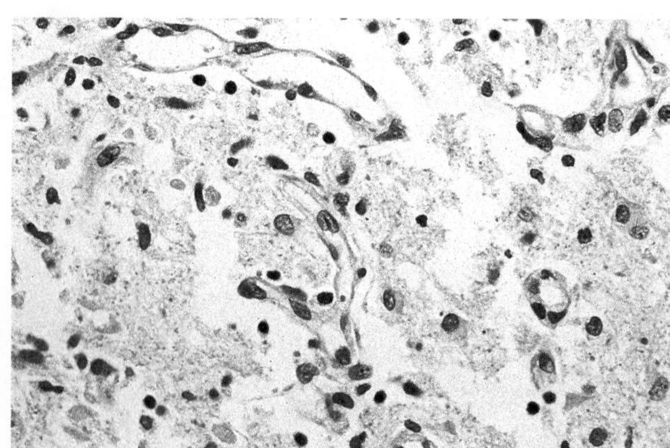

FIGURE 28-70
Recent cerebral infarct. A microscopic view of Fig. 28-69 shows destruction of the parenchymal architecture, numerous debris-laden macrophages, and proliferated capillaries.

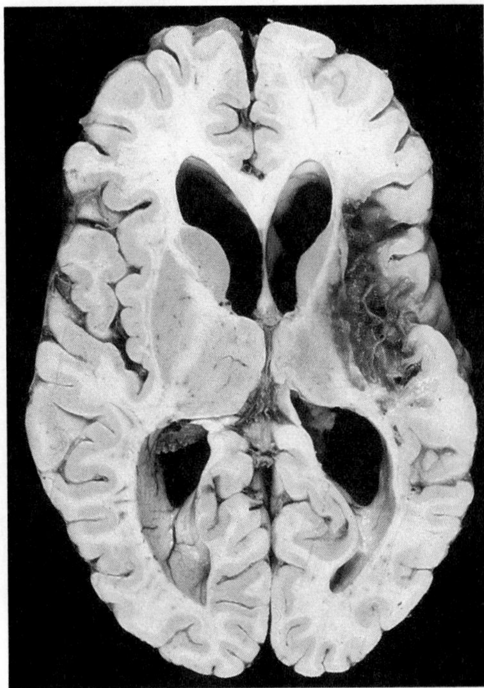

FIGURE 28-71
Remote cerebral infarct. A horizontal section of the brain demonstrates that the end stage of a cerebral infarct is a cyst traversed by atretic vessels.

Localized ischemia is associated with three distinct clinical syndromes:

- **Transient ischemic attack (TIA)** refers to focal cerebral dysfunction that lasts less than 24 hours and is often of only a few minutes' duration. Although it is followed by complete neurological recovery, a TIA signifies an increased risk of a cerebral infarct.
- **Stroke in evolution** describes the progression of neurological symptoms while the patient is under observation. This syndrome is uncommon and usually reflects the propagation of a thrombus in the carotid or basilar arteries.
- **Completed stroke** is the term for a stable neurological deficit resulting from a cerebral infarct.

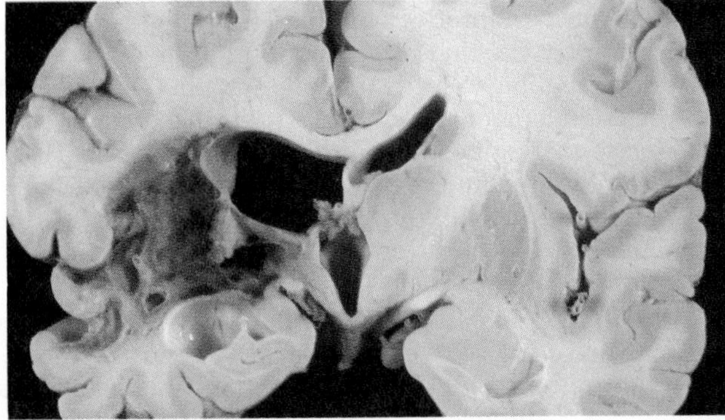

FIGURE 28-72
Remote cerebral infarction. Occlusion of the striate vessels resulted in an infarct in the region of the internal capsule and basal ganglia. Resorption of destroyed tissue led to cyst formation, with dilatation of the adjacent ventricle.

Regional Occlusive Cerebrovascular Disease

The various occlusive cerebrovascular diseases, which lead to cerebral infarcts, may be classified into five categories, in accord with the caliber and nature of the involved vessel:

- Large extracranial and intracranial vessels, such as the carotid, vertebral, and basilar arteries
- Arteries of the circle of Willis and their immediate branches
- Parenchymal arteries and arterioles
- Capillaries
- Large veins and dural sinuses

THE LARGE EXTRACRANIAL AND INTRACRANIAL ARTERIES: These arteries are frequent sites of atherosclerosis (Fig. 28-73). The most notable example is the common carotid artery, in which atherosclerotic plaques are particularly prominent where the artery bifurcates to form the external and internal branches. Occlusion or severe stenosis of an internal carotid artery affects the hemisphere on that side proportional to the

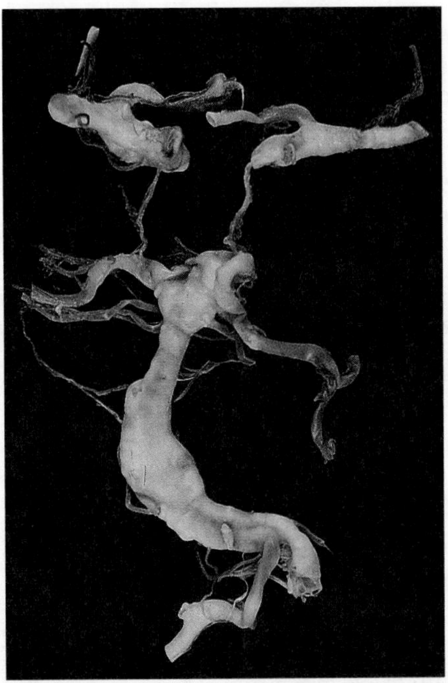

FIGURE 28-73
Atherosclerosis of the cerebral vasculature. In this dissected specimen, the large vessels (the vertebral, basilar, internal carotid, and middle cerebral arteries) show significant atherosclerosis, whereas the smaller vessels are less involved.

degree of collateral circulation through the anterior and posterior communicating arteries. Most often, occlusion of a carotid artery initiates infarction in the distribution of the middle cerebral artery, often with a less intense insult to the frontal lobe on the same side (see Fig. 28-68).

THE CIRCLE OF WILLIS: The various branches of this structure may be occluded, but the consequences are dependent on the configuration of the circle. Thus, if the anterior communicating artery is large, it can provide collateral circulation to a frontal lobe whose arterial supply has been compromised by occlusion of the internal carotid artery. Among the branches of the circle of Willis, the middle cerebral artery is most often occluded by thrombosis complicating atherosclerosis. Because the trifurcation of the middle cerebral artery represents a major step-down in vascular caliber, it is the predominant site of occlusion by emboli from a mural thrombus in the heart. Such emboli, which typically have diameters of 5 mm or greater, fit snugly behind the trifurcation or enter and occlude a branch of the middle cerebral artery (Fig. 28-74).

THE PARENCHYMAL ARTERIES AND ARTERIOLES: These vessels are not disposed to atherosclerosis, but they are damaged by hypertension and become stenotic because of arteriosclerosis. The narrowing of these vessels initiates small ischemic lesions, referred to as lacunar infarcts. When multiple, these minute infarcts can impair cognition and create the entity termed multiple infarct dementia.

Hypertensive encephalopathy refers to the CNS manifestations of malignant hypertension (see Chapter 10). As in other organs assailed by malignant hypertension, fibrinoid necrosis of small arteries and arterioles and minute hemorrhages (petechiae) are conspicuous. Cerebral edema, and resulting papilledema, may complicate the vascular pathology. Clinically, hypertensive encephalopathy usually is seen as headache and vomiting and progresses to lethargy, coma, and death. With modern antihypertensive therapy, malignant hypertension and its complications are no longer common.

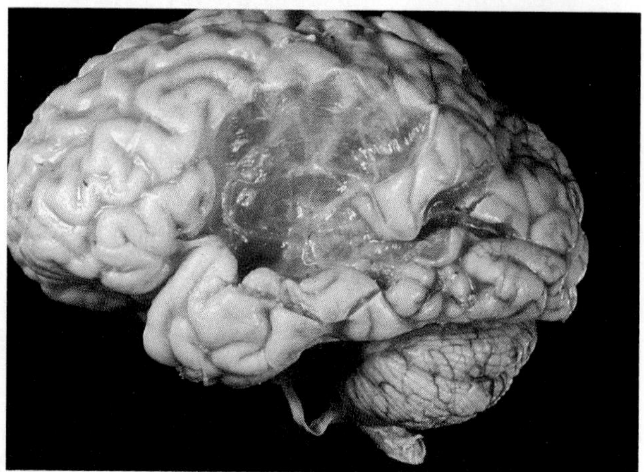

FIGURE *28-74*
Remote cerebral infarction. Occlusion of the middle cerebral artery at the trifurcation resulted in a large infarct, which has become cystic.

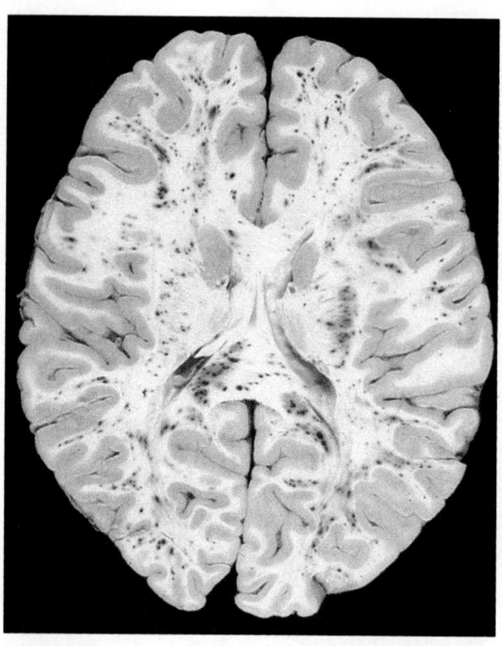

FIGURE *28-75*
Fat embolization. A horizontal section of the brain from a patient who had massive trauma exhibits numerous petechiae throughout the white matter.

THE CAPILLARY BED: Small emboli, notably those composed of fat or air, occlude capillaries (Fig. 28-75).

Fat emboli are carried downstream through the cerebral vessels until the caliber of the embolus exceeds that of the tributaries. When they lodge, their semifluid consistency creates a major, but not absolute, barrier to blood flow. The distal capillary endothelium becomes hypoxic and permeable, and petechiae develop. Typically, the petechiae are restricted to the white matter, because the greater density of capillaries in the gray cortex provides regional oxygenation, and the endothelial integrity of an embolized vessel is adequately preserved.

Air emboli introduced into the cerebrovascular system liberate a multitude of bubbles. Each divides as it encounters a constricting bifurcation, until the surface tension of the bubble exceeds the forces applied by vascular flow. On lodgement, a bubble of air acts in a manner comparable to that of a droplet of fat and deprives the distal capillary endothelium of oxygen. This again results in the formation of petechiae, which are less restricted to the white matter than in the case of fat embolization.

THE CEREBRAL VEINS: Unlike veins in other locations, the cerebral veins empty into large conduits, the venous sinuses. Among these, the sagittal sinus occupies a prominent position, because it accommodates the venous drainage from the superior portions of the cerebral hemispheres (Fig. 28-76). Blood flows sluggishly in these aqueducts, and the walls are irregularly contoured with estuaries. Venous sinus thrombosis in the brain is a serious complication of the following:

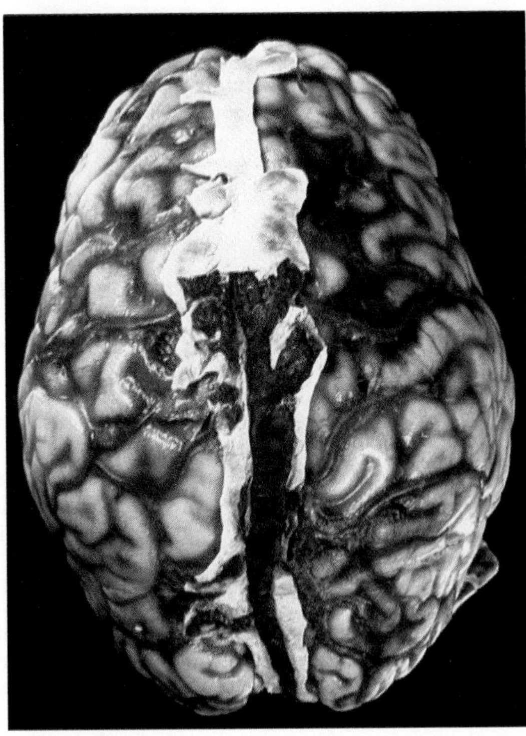

FIGURE *28-76*
Sagittal sinus thrombosis. Removal of the dura reveals the sagittal sinus to be filled with clotted blood. Secondary thrombosis of the veins in the cerebral cortex has led to bilateral hemorrhagic infarcts.

- Systemic dehydration, as occurs in an infant with gastrointestinal fluid loss
- Phlebitis, caused for example by mastoiditis or bacteremia
- Obstruction by a neoplasm, notably a meningioma
- Sickle cell disease

Because venous obstruction causes stagnation upstream, abrupt thrombosis of the sagittal sinus results in bilateral hemorrhagic infarctions of the frontal regions of the cerebral hemispheres. A more indolent occlusion of the sinus, such as invasion by a meningioma, permits the recruitment of collateral circulation through the inferior sagittal sinus, a small channel that lies at the lower edge of the falx and empties into the straight sinus.

CEREBROSPINAL FLUID

The cerebrospinal fluid (CSF) constitutes an "accessory circulatory system," which is adapted to the needs of the brain and spinal cord. This fluid flows in a leisurely fashion from its intraventricular origin to its sites of reabsorption, principally through the arachnoid villi and into the dural sinuses. The flow of CSF transports metabolites, which are provided to the ependymal membrane and to the subpial cortex. The CSF also serves as a sump for metabolic waste. Most important, its fluid properties create a protective jacket for the brain and spinal cord.

Cerebrospinal fluid is present in a volume of 120 to 150 mL. It is formed principally by the choroid plexus, at a rate of 500 mL/day and reabsorbed by the arachnoid villi. A small volume of fluid also is formed near the surface of the brain and reaches the subarachnoid compartment through the Virchow–Robin spaces. Although age disfigures the delicate anatomy of the choroid plexus by the deposition of fibrous tissue, cholesterol, and calcium, its filtrative capacity is maintained, and no disease state is characterized by a lack of CSF.

The choroid plexus stretches as a cord along the roof of the third ventricle. After bifurcating and passing through the foramina of Monro, each cord then angles sharply posteriorly to lie on the floor of the lateral ventricle. It then curves gently downward into the temporal horns of the ventricular chambers, where it expands to form a bulbous mass, the glomus. Thus, the choroid plexus is not present in the frontal or occipital poles of the lateral ventricles, nor does it enter the aqueduct of Sylvius.

During embryonic development, the cerebellum rotates on its transverse axis, and the pia is carried onto the posterior surface of the fourth ventricle, where it contacts the ependyma. In this way, the tela choroidea is formed from the pia, and the cuboidal "epithelium" of the choroid is contributed by the ependyma. Thus, the posterior aspect of the fourth ventricle is covered by choroid plexus, which extends laterally through the foramen of Luschka into the immediate subarachnoid space of the cerebellopontine angle. Analogously, the inward rotation of the cerebral hemispheres contributes pia to the formation of the choroid plexus of the third ventricle and the lateral ventricles.

Hydrocephalus

Obstruction to the flow of CSF in the brain results in hydrocephalus, a condition marked by dilatation of the cerebral ventricles by accumulated CSF. When the obstruction is within the ventricular chambers, the hydrocephalus is designated *noncommunicating* (Fig. 28-77). *Communicating* hydrocephalus refers to the situation in which there is no obstruction in the ventricular system, but the reabsorption of CSF by the arachnoid villi is impaired.

NONCOMMUNICATING HYDROCEPHALUS: Flow through a ventricular chamber or a foramen may be obstructed by (1) a congenital malformation, (2) a neoplasm, (3) inflammation, or (4) hemorrhage. As discussed earlier, the aqueduct of Sylvius is the most common location of an obstructive congenital malformation. Some tumors, notably papillomas or carcinomas of the choroid plexus and ependymomas, arise within a ventricular chamber. In that location, they can obstruct the flow of CSF and produce hydrocephalus. In addition to physical obstruction, neoplasms of the choroid plexus form excessive volumes of CSF. Parenchymal tumors, notably gliomas, compress the aqueduct or a ventricular chamber and cause hydrocephalus behind the point of stenosis. The ependyma is sensitive to viral infections, particularly during embryonic development; thus ependymitis is believed to be a cause of congenital aqueductal stenosis (see Fig. 28-29).

COMMUNICATING HYDROCEPHALUS: An impairment of reabsorption of CSF with resultant communi-

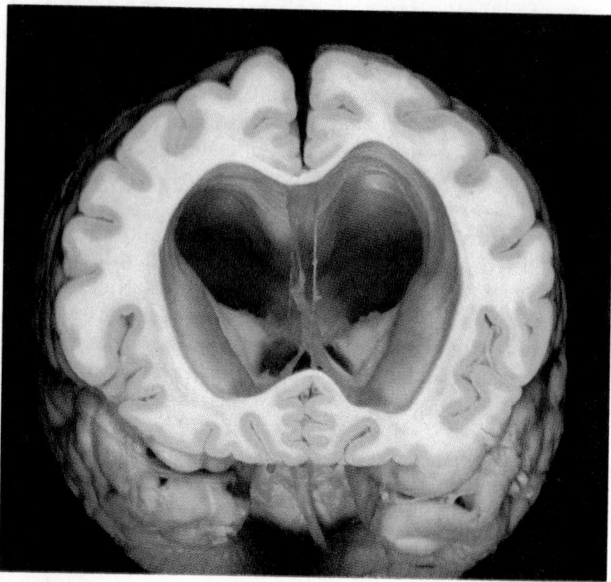

FIGURE 28-77
Hydrocephalus. A coronal section of the brain from a patient who died of a brain tumor that obstructed the aqueduct of Sylvius shows marked dilatation of the lateral ventricles.

cating hydrocephalus can complicate subarachnoid hemorrhage, meningitis, and the spread of tumor within the subarachnoid space.

☐ **Pathology:** Similar pathological changes occur in hydrocephalus of all etiologies. The cerebral hemispheres are enlarged, and the ventricular system is dilated behind the point of obstruction. The external pattern of the gyri tends to be less prominent as sulci are compressed. The white matter is reduced in volume, and the basal ganglia and thalamus are attenuated (see Figs. 28-77 and 28-78).

When hydrocephalus develops *in utero* or in early life, usually because of obstruction at the aqueduct of Sylvius, the ventricles expand behind the point of obstruction, the cranial sutures separate, the head enlarges, and the cerebral cortex becomes attenuated. Histological examination of the region of the obstructed aqueduct reveals multiple small, irregular, ependyma-lined canals (see Fig. 28-28). In some cases, the single aqueduct, or the clustered aborted canals, are surrounded by astrogliosis, in which case, the condition is thought to represent an inflammatory ependymitis, probably due to an interuterine viral infection (see Fig. 28-29). Without surgical drainage of the CSF from the ventricles, the hydrocephalus is slowly progressive, and the head may attain a huge size.

☐ **Clinical Features:** The infantile cranium expands easily, and the symptoms of increased intracranial pressure are generally absent. Convulsions are common, and in severe cases, optic atrophy leads to blindness. Weakness and incoordination are common. Interestingly, intelligence may be unimpaired even in the face of severe ventricular dilatation, although dementia may ultimately supervene. The insertion of shunts that link the ventricles to the venous system has been successful in controlling hydrocephalus in some children.

In adults, the onset of hydrocephalus is usually marked by symptoms of increased intracranial pressure, including headache and vomiting and, shortly thereafter, papilledema. If the obstruction is not relieved, mental deterioration eventually appears. The pressure of the CSF is not always increased, and a syndrome of low-pressure hydrocephalus is recognized.

Hydrocephalus ex vacuo refers to the enlargement of the ventricular system that represents a compensatory re-

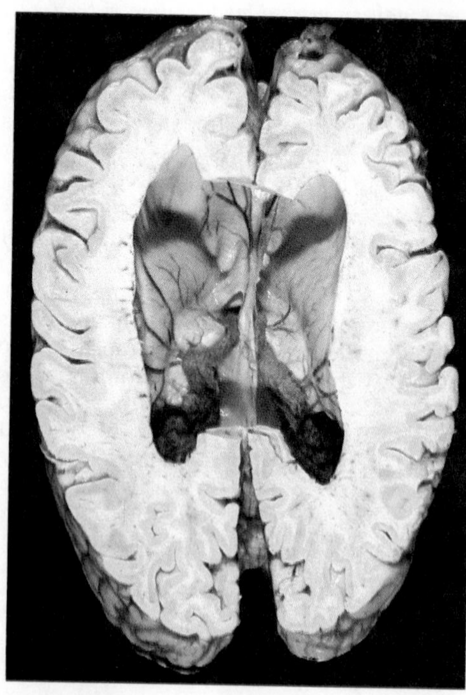

FIGURE 28-78
Hydrocephalus. A horizontal section of the brain from a patient with obstructive hydrocephalus caused by a neoplasm emphasizes the enlargement of the lateral ventricles.

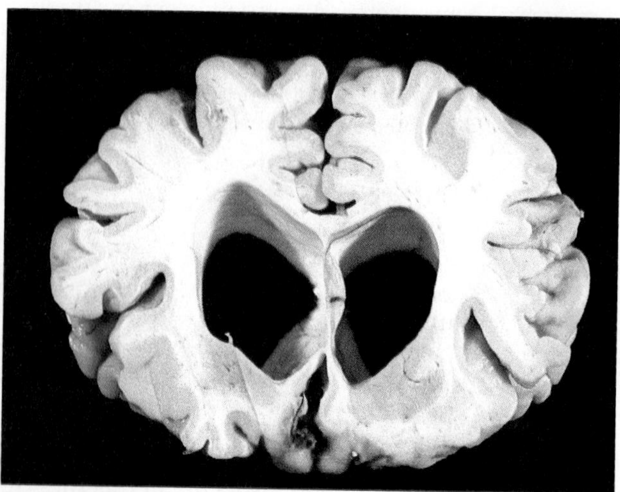

FIGURE 28-79
Hydrocephalus *ex vacuo*. Atrophy of the cerebral cortex in an aged, demented person is associated with enlargement of the ventricles.

sponse to severe cortical atrophy and is not related to obstruction (Fig. 28-79). By itself, it has no functional significance.

INFECTIOUS DISEASES

The list of organisms that infect the CNS is long and includes virtually all types of microorganisms that infect the rest of the body. Most species of organisms localize in preferred intracranial and intraspinal sites. For example, poliovirus selects the motor neurons of the spinal cord and bulbar area, herpes simplex virus localizes to the temporal lobes, and progressive multifocal leukoencephalopathy (JC virus) preferentially involves the parasagittal white matter. Bacteria generally localize in the leptomeninges and produce meningitis. However, the same organism can, on occasion, lodge in the parenchyma and initiate a cerebritis, which often progresses to abscess formation. On rare occasions, bacteria enter the subdural compartment and clandestinely induce subdural empyema.

Fungi such as *Cryptococcus neoformans* grow indolently in the leptomeninges. Others, such as *Aspergillus fumigatus*, aggressively induce cerebral abscesses and occasionally initiate leptomeningitis. *Treponema pallidum*, the cause of syphilis, gains access to the nervous system through the bloodstream and assumes a prolonged residency in neural tissues. Here the organisms propagate and induce highly distinctive clinical disorders, among which dementia paralytica and tabes dorsalis are of greatest historical interest. On other occasions, the spirochete selects the meninges, where it initiates fibrosis and an obliterative endarteritis, thereby creating meningovascular syphilis.

Rickettsial infections, such as Rocky Mountain spotted fever, target endothelial cells. In the brain, endothelial injury produces petechiae and cerebral edema, and the global nature of this process induces a serious encephalopathy. *Toxoplasma gondii* pits its low virulence against the natural resistance of the human adult and generally is unable to induce an active infection. Yet through transplacental transmission, it gains access to the fetal brain, where it produces paraventricular necrosis and calcification, mostly in the basal ganglia and thalamus. This protozoan also takes advantage of the susceptibility of the immunocompromised adult and constitutes a significant source of infection in patients with acquired immunodeficiency syndrome (AIDS). Clearly, the anatomical localization, the character of the tissue response, and the age and immunological status of the patient are all cardinal in an understanding and recognition of intracranial infections.

Meningitis

Leptomeningitis *denotes an inflammatory process that is localized to the interfacing surfaces of the pia and arachnoid* (Fig. 28-80A). This compartment houses the CSF, an excellent culture medium for most microorganisms. The changes in the CSF vary with the nature and the extent of the infection. These include its cellular constituents, protein and sugar contents, electrolyte composition, and serological reactivities (see Fig. 28-80B).

Pachymeningitis *refers to inflammation of the dura. It is usually the consequence of contiguous infection, such as chronic sinusitis or mastoiditis.* The dura is a substantial bar-

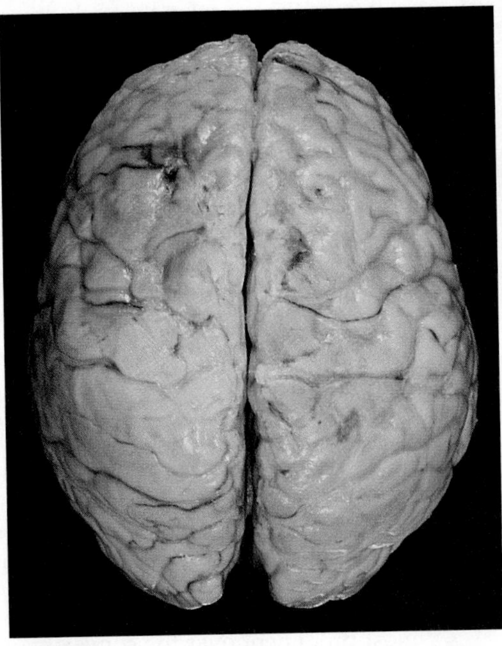

A

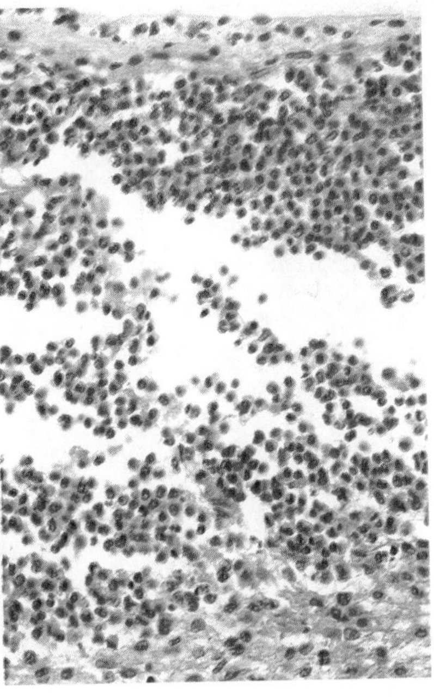

B

FIGURE 28-80
Purulent meningitis. (*A*) A creamy exudate opacifies the leptomeninges. (*B*) A microscopic section shows the accumulation of numerous neutrophils in the subarachnoid space.

rier to infection, and inflammation is usually restricted to its outer surface.

Bacterial Meningitis

With few exceptions, all forms of meningitis are initiated by microorganisms, bacteria being the principal offenders. Among these, suppurative organisms predominate.

Suppurative Meningitis

- ***Escherichia coli:*** In the newborn, in whom resistance to gram-negative bacteria has not yet fully developed, *E. coli* is the prime cause of meningitis. The cross-placental transfer of maternal immunoglobulin G (IgG) imparts protection to the newborn against many bacteria. However, *E. coli* and similar gram-negative organisms require IgM for neutralization, a protein that does not cross the placental barrier. Consequently, gram-negative organisms quickly produce a purulent meningitis, with a high mortality during infancy (Fig. 28-81).
- ***Haemophilus influenzae:*** Environmental exposure to *H. influenzae*, also a gram-negative organism, is somewhat delayed, and the incidence of meningitis is maximal between 3 months and 3 years (Fig. 28-82).
- ***Streptococcus pneumoniae:*** The pneumococcus predominates as a cause of meningitis later in life. In patients with a history of basilar skull fracture, there is an unusually high incidence of pneumococcal meningitis, which often recurs after treatment.

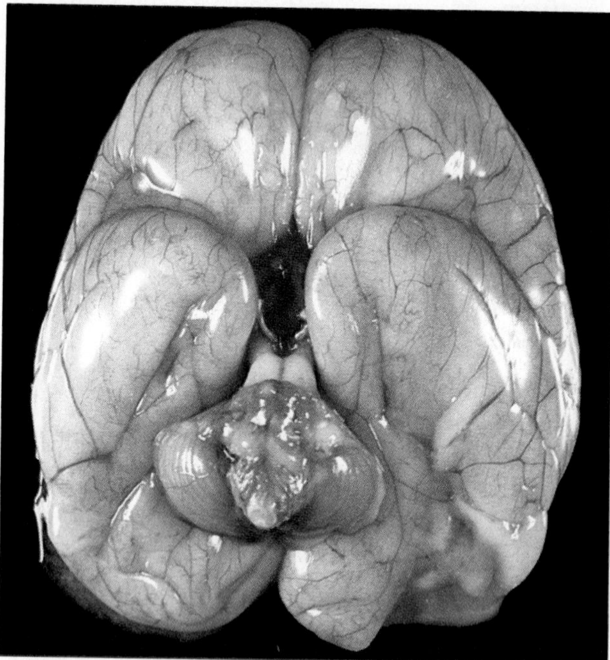

FIGURE 28-81
***Escherichia coli* meningitis. The brain of an infant who died of *E. coli* meningitis shows a purulent exudate in the leptomeninges at the base of the brain.**

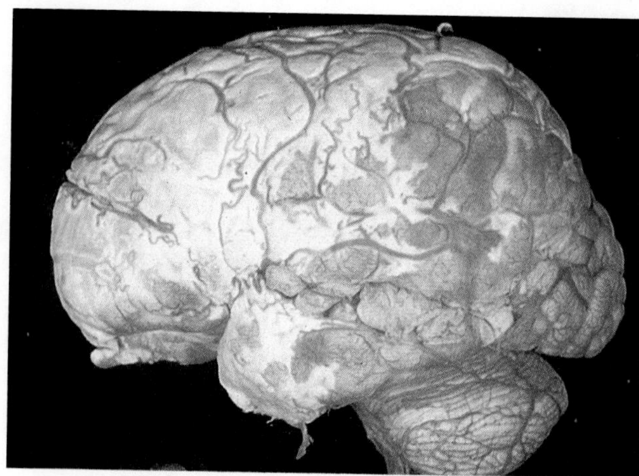

FIGURE 28-82
***Hemophilus influenzae* meningitis. A loculated fibrinous exudate involves the meninges.**

- ***Neisseria meningitidis:*** The meningococcus frequents the human nasopharynx, and airborne transmission in crowded environments causes "epidemic meningitis," a serious event in military barracks. The initial phase of the infection is a bacteremia, manifested by fever, malaise, and a petechial rash. An intravascular coagulopathy may be associated with lethal adrenal hemorrhages (*Waterhouse–Friderichsen syndrome*). Untreated meningococcal bacteremia is prone to initiate an acute fulminant meningitis.

Although organisms reach the intracranial compartment by way of the bloodstream, it is not clear how they exit from the vascular channels. It is possible that blood-borne bacteria lodge in the pial blood vessels, from which they escape into the CSF. Alternatively, they may gain entry to the CSF by way of the choroid plexus (Fig. 28-83).

Because most organisms initiate a purulent or suppurative response, the presence of polymorphonuclear leukocytes in the CSF is the most definitive index of meningitis (see Fig. 28-80B). Yet lymphocytes are the hallmark of tuberculosis and the viral meningitides, as well as of some chronic infections, such as those due to *Cryptococcus neoformans*.

☐ **Pathology:** Gross examination of the brain discloses an exudate of leukocytes and fibrin, which opacifies the arachnoid. When the meningitis is marked, this membrane acquires a creamy appearance. The intensity of the exudate may be so slight as to be equivocal to the naked eye. At other times, it is sufficiently prominent to form white cords along the vessels that traverse the sulci, particularly those in the parasagittal areas and those in proximity to the sylvian fissure. A purulent exudate is most prominent over the convexity of the cerebral hemispheres (see Fig. 28-80A), but it also extends along the base of the brain, where the interpeduncular fossa constitutes a reservoir of infection. Because the intracranial and

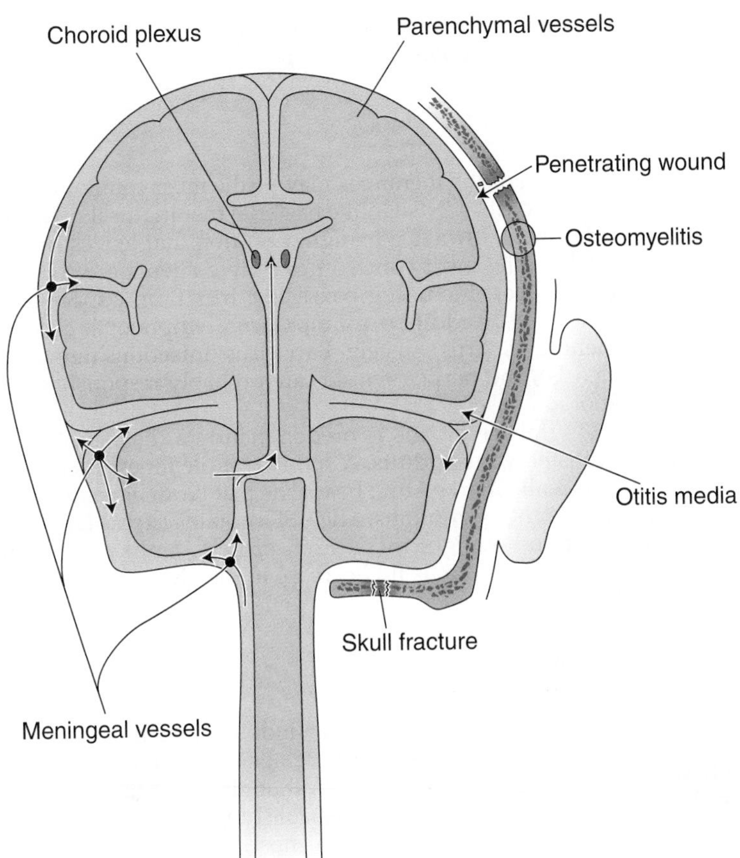

FIGURE 28-83
Routes of entry of infectious organisms into the cranial cavity.

intraspinal subarachnoid spaces are in continuity, the exudate passes freely between these conjoined compartments.

Although delicate and diaphanous, the pia is a remarkably efficient barrier against the spread of infection, and it generally prevents involvement of the underlying brain. Thus cerebral abscesses are rarely a complication of meningitis. The pia forms conical sleeves about the blood vessels as they penetrate through the surface of the brain. These slender perivascular compartments, termed the *Virchow–Robin spaces*, are in direct continuity with the subarachnoid space. They may harbor leukocytes and microorganisms, but they rarely provide a portal of entry for infection of the parenchyma.

Haemophilus influenzae elicits a dense leukocytic exudate, which is rich in fibrin. As a result, the exudate becomes loculated, creating a barrier to antibiotics (see Fig. 28-82).

□ **Clinical Features:** All forms of suppurative meningitis share a number of symptoms, although the onset ranges from fulminant to insidious. Headache, vomiting, and fever are particularly common. Convulsions frequently occur in children. The classic signs of meningeal infection include cervical rigidity, head retraction, pain in the knee when the hip is flexed (Kernig sign), and spontaneous flexion of the knees and hips when the neck is flexed (Brudzinski sign). In untreated cases, delirium often gives way to stupor, coma, and eventually death.

Tuberculous Meningitis and Tuberculomas

Tuberculous granulomas in the meninges are analogous to those in visceral sites (Fig. 28-84). Epithelioid cells, Langhans giant cells, and lymphocytes surround areas of caseous necrosis. Inadequately treated tuberculous meningitis results in meningeal fibrosis, which is responsible for communicating hydrocephalus. Arteritis in tuberculous meningitis may also lead to parenchymal infarcts. Because tuberculous meningitis has a strong predilection for the base of the brain, particularly for the sylvian fissure, such infarcts are most often in the distribution of the striate arteries. Untreated tuberculous meningitis is uniformly fatal in 4 to 6 weeks.

Parenchymal involvement of the brain by tuberculosis produces a *tuberculoma*, which is a solitary spherical mass with a central area of caseous necrosis surrounded by granulomatous tissue (Fig. 28-85). In the early era of neurosurgery, tuberculomas accounted for about 10% of intracranial "tumors."

The mechanism by which the tubercle bacillus gains access to the brain is not entirely clear, although most cases appear to represent hematogenous dissemination. In end-stage tuberculous meningitis, granulomas are frequently encountered in the choroid plexus. Tubercle bacilli may lodge in parenchymal capillaries, in a manner similar to that of pyogenic organisms that produce abscesses. The tubercle bacilli might then initiate a tuberculoma, which secondarily erodes into the subarachnoid space. Perhaps all of the potential portals (pial blood ves-

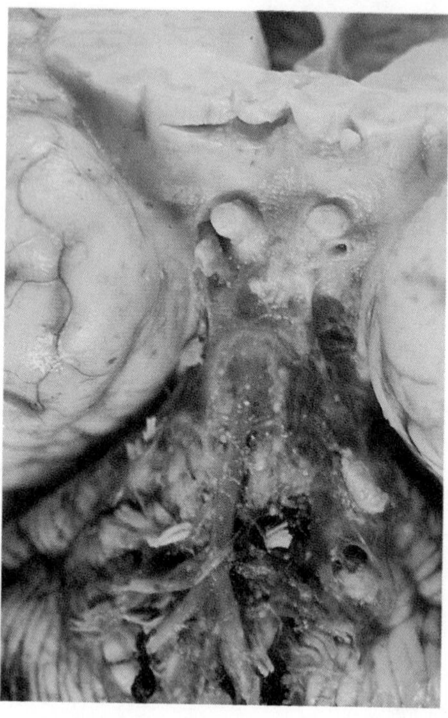

FIGURE 28-84
Tuberculous meningitis. The meninges covering the base of the brain, particularly about the optic chiasm and interpeduncular fossa, are opacified. Note the minute tubercles overlying the basilar artery.

sels, the choroid plexus, and the parenchymal capillaries) may be used as avenues of entry for the tubercle bacillus.

Tuberculosis of the spinal column (*Pott disease*) produces an epidural mass of granulomatous tissue and frequently causes destruction and angulation of the spine, with the threat of spinal cord compression (Fig. 28-86). The marked spinal deformity of Pott disease was formerly responsible for many so-called "hunchbacks," a condition that is rare today.

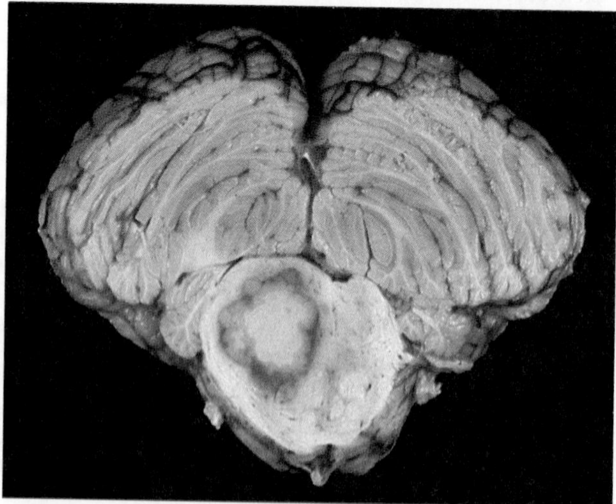

FIGURE 28-85
Tuberculoma. A spherical mass is present in the tegmentum of the pons. The center is caseous and is encapsulated by a rim of darker granulomatous tissue.

Viral Meningitis

Infection of the meninges may be the most common viral disease of the CNS. Unlike bacterial meningitis, however, it is almost always a benign condition that leaves no sequelae. The most common causative agents are the enteroviruses, including coxsackievirus B and species of echovirus. In addition, mumps virus, lymphocytic choriomeningitis virus, Epstein–Barr virus (infectious mononucleosis), and herpes simplex are probably responsible for sporadic cases.

Viral meningitis is predominantly a disease of children and young adults. A sudden febrile illness is characteristically marked by a headache that is out of proportion to the other symptoms. The CSF contains excess lymphocytes and a slight increase in protein. Unlike bacterial meningitis, there is no decrease in the glucose content of the CSF.

Cryptococcal Meningitis

Cryptococcal meningitis is an indolent infection in which the virulence of the causative agent marginally exceeds the resistance of the host. Although the organism is on rare occasions capable of establishing a meningitis in an immunologically competent host, in most instances, it acts opportunistically in immunocompromised persons.

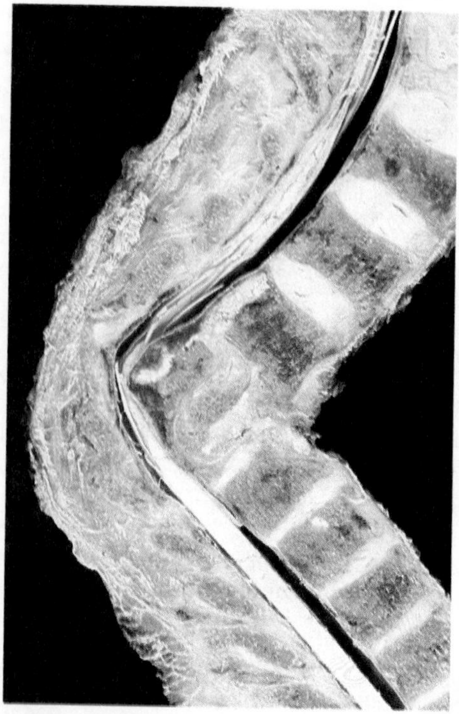

FIGURE 28-86
Pott disease. Tuberculosis of the spine has initiated a destructive spondylitis, with resulting kyphosis and compression of the spinal cord.

In this situation, the disease usually evolves over a period of months. *Cryptococcus neoformans* customarily enters the human host by the inhalation of contaminated particulates. Birds are a major reservoir, and their inhaled excreta initiate a pneumonitis, after which the fungi enter the bloodstream and attain the intracranial compartment.

□ **Pathology:** The tissue response in the meninges to *C. neoformans* is typically sparse. The lesions are widely disseminated in the meninges, ependyma, and choroid plexus. To the naked eye, they appear as discrete white nodules, a millimeter or so in diameter. Organisms may abound, particularly in the Virchow–Robin spaces. The tissue response features an occasional multinucleated giant cell, sometimes with phagocytized organisms, accompanied by scant epithelioid cells and a scattering of lymphocytes.

Cryptococcal organisms are encapsulated spheres, 5 to 15 μm in diameter. They have an external gelatinous capsule and reproduce by budding (Fig. 28-87). When a drop of contaminated CSF is mixed with India ink, microscopic examination shows a clear halo about the encapsulated organism. This capsule sheds specific antigens that can be detected in the CSF by the latex cryptococcal antigen test.

Cryptococcus neoformans usually causes only a meningitis, with organisms occupying the subarachnoid space and sometimes extending into the Virchow–Robin spaces around cerebral blood vessels. Rare cases of infection with this fungus, however, show collections of organisms within the brain parenchyma, forming gelatinous pseudocysts (Fig. 28-88).

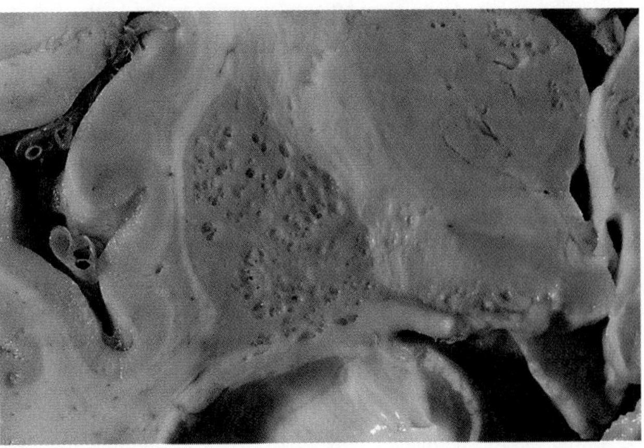

FIGURE *28-88*
Cryptococcal infection. The historic term for cryptococcus, "Torula histolytica," referred to the propensity of this organism to create a lytic, spongy lesion in the parenchyma, shown here in the basal ganglia from a patient who died of acquired immunodeficiency syndrome (AIDS).

Amoebic Meningoencephalitis

Two genera of amoebae, *Naegleria* and *Acanthamoeba*, gain entry into the intracranial compartment by way of the cribriform plate, via the olfactory nerves, after a person is exposed to contaminated water while swimming. The more common infection by *Naegleria* produces a fulminant and rapidly fatal leptomeningitis, with death usually occurring in less than a week. In tissue sections, the trophozoites of *Naegleria* are of a size and appearance similar to those of macrophages. Infection by *Acanthamoeba*, the trophozoites of which resemble those of *Naegleria* (Fig. 28-89), is equally fatal, but generally after a more protracted course. In addition to meningitis, the latter organism produces parenchymal abscesses and a granulomatous tissue reaction. *Acanthamoeba* has a distinctive double, serrated cell wall.

Syphilitic (Luetic) Meningitis and Related Lesions

The spirochete of syphilis, *Treponema pallidum*, enters the bloodstream from the primary lesion, the chancre. The

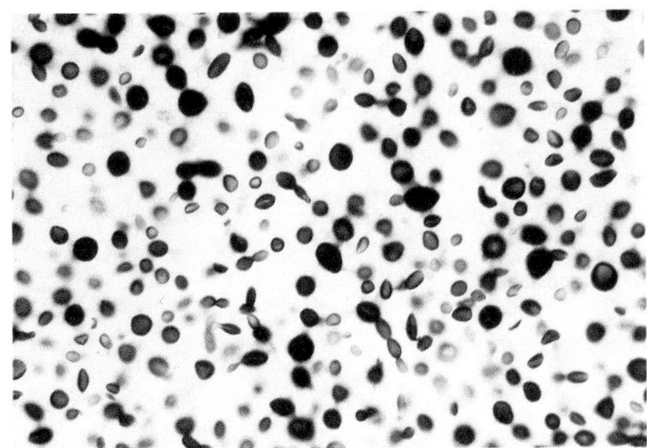

FIGURE *28-87*
Cryptococcal meningitis. The cryptococcal organisms vary in size, with diameters between 5 and 15 μm. They reproduce by budding.

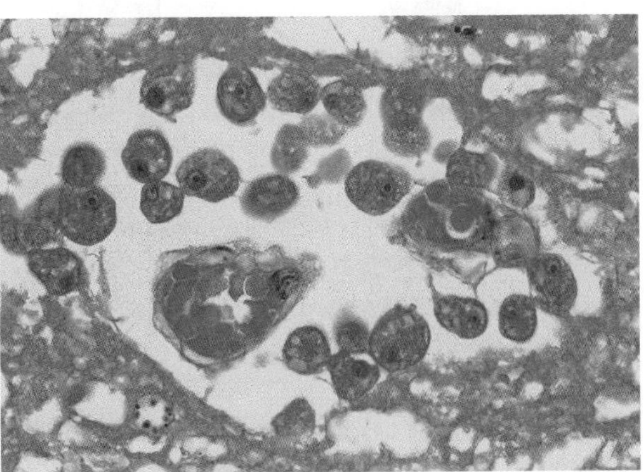

FIGURE *28-89*
***Acanthamoeba* infection. The protozoa bear a close resemblance to macrophages.**

onset of secondary syphilis is marked externally by the appearance of a maculopapular rash on the skin and mucous membranes and internally by a few lymphocytes and plasma cells and increased protein in the CSF. This is presumably the period when the blood-borne spirochetes lodge, at least transiently, in the meninges. The organisms do not survive for long and cannot be demonstrated histologically in cases of meningovascular syphilis. The CSF serology characteristically reverts to negative.

On occasion, the transient spirochete initiates a fibroblastic response in the meninges, accompanied by a proliferative, obliterative endarteritis (Fig. 28-90). Vascular obstruction induces multiple small infarcts in the cerebral cortex. Plasma cells, the hallmark of syphilis, surround the arterioles of the cerebral cortex in luetic meningovascular syphilis.

TABES DORSALIS: Although this condition is commonly ascribed to a degeneration of the posterior fasciculi of the spinal cord, the initial lesion is actually a variant of chronic meningitis. The dorsal nerve roots that approach the spinal cord, proximal to the dorsal root ganglia, are met by a conical sleeve of arachnoid. This sheath, with its estuary filled with CSF, can be the site of syphilitic inflammation.

The inflammatory response generates fibrous tissue, which constricts the nerve roots and causes wallerian degeneration of the axons. The axons that course cephalad in the posterior fasciculus have not synapsed with intramedullary neurons, as do all other ascending pathways in the cord. They are rather direct extensions of axons from the posterior roots, and the wallerian degeneration that is initiated in the dorsal spinal nerve roots extends directly into the posterior fasciculi. This is the most readily visualized morphological lesion of tabes dorsalis and accounts for the loss of position and proprioceptive sense in the lower extremities. The serological reaction of the CSF generally reverts to negative before the onset of tabetic symptoms.

LUETIC DEMENTIA: *Treponema pallidum* also may lodge in the brain and be clinically latent for decades. In that location, the spirochetes replicate sluggishly but escape eradication, being shielded from the immune system by the blood–brain barrier. Their presence can be demonstrated in histological sections several decades later. The

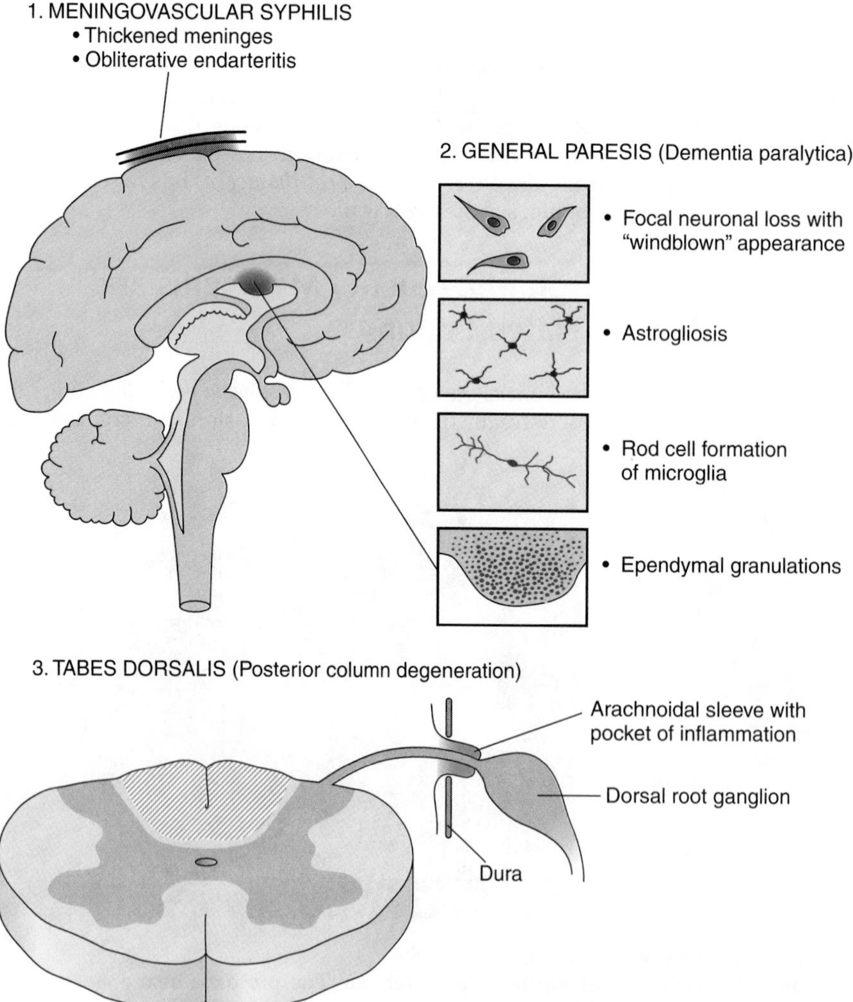

FIGURE *28-90*
Involvement of the central nervous system in syphilis.

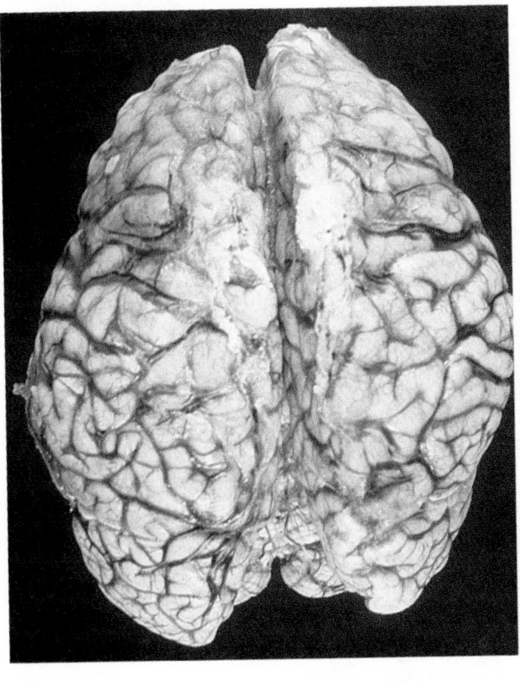

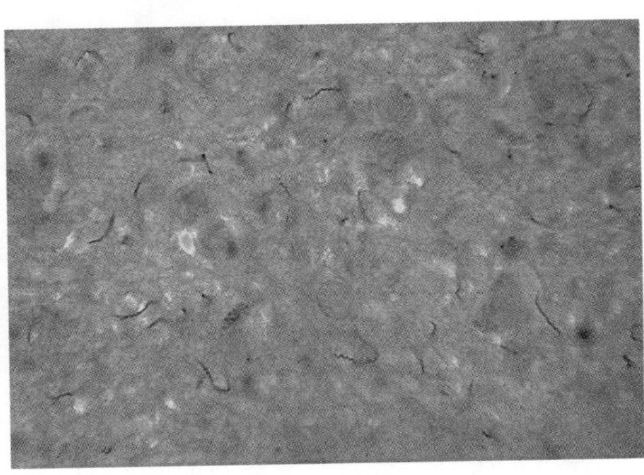

A B

FIGURE 28-91
Tertiary syphilis (general paresis). (*A*) The brain shows cortical atrophy, most marked in the frontal lobes. (*B*) Spirochetes are evident with a silver stain.

morphological features of luetic dementia include the following:

- Focal loss of cortical neurons (Fig. 28-91)
- Disfigurement of the topography of the residual nerve cells ("wind-blown appearance")
- Marked gliosis
- Conversion of microglia into elongated forms encrusted with iron ("rod cells") and
- Nodular ependymitis

These morphological alterations are accompanied by a marked decrement in cognitive function, referred to as *dementia paralytica*.

Cerebral Abscess

The cerebral cortex and the subjacent white matter contain the richest capillary bed in the brain. It is not surprising, therefore, that microorganisms carried by the bloodstream lodge preferentially in this location. Here they replicate and elicit an acute inflammatory reaction and regional edema termed *cerebritis* (Fig. 28-92). Within several days, liquefaction necrosis converts the lesion to an expanding abscess (Figs. 28-93 and 28-94), which threatens life by transtentorial herniation or by rupture into a ventricle.

Although astrocytes are ordinarily the predominant cell in cerebral repair, in this situation they yield the role of containment to fibroblasts, which knit a capsule around the abscess. Astrocytes multiply at the margin of the abscess outside the fibrous capsule, but their contribution to encapsulation is minimal.

If the abscess is not excised or drained or if the infection is not restrained by antibiotic therapy, pressure builds within the abscess cavity. Edema is prone to develop in the underlying white matter, which is already vulnerable because of the normal paucity of blood vessels.

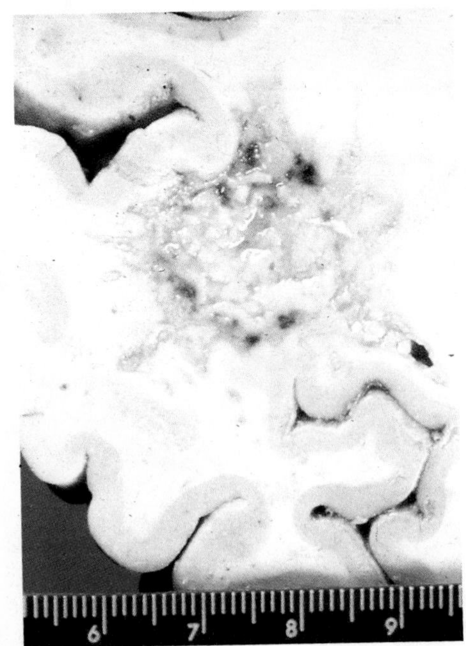

FIGURE 28-92
Cerebritis. An irregular, soft, gelatinous area in the white matter is the prodromal phase of a cerebral abscess.

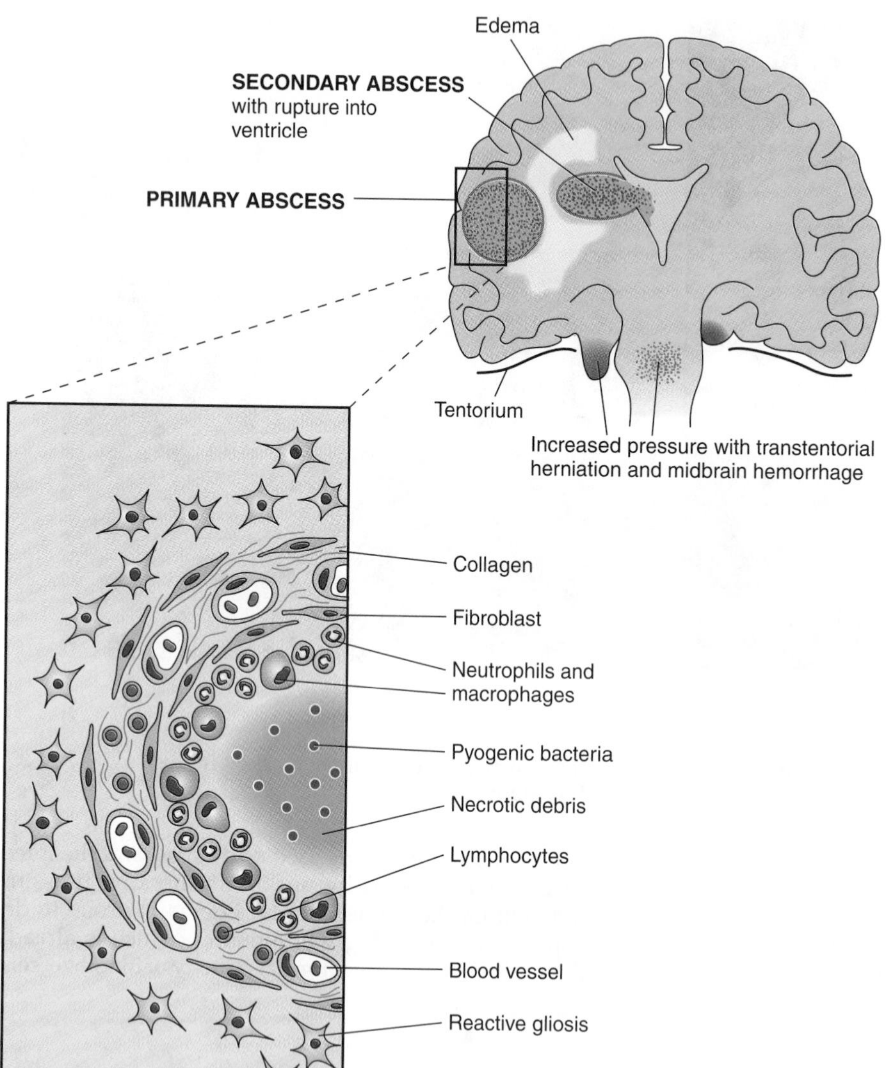

FIGURE 28-93
Brain abscess and its complications. A cerebral abscess may cause death through the production of secondary abscesses with intraventricular rupture; alternatively, death may result from transtentorial herniation.

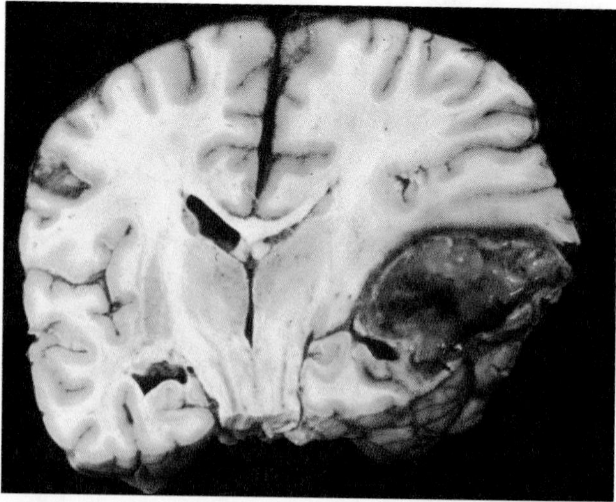

FIGURE 28-94
Cerebral abscess. A young man with chronic otitis media developed an abscess in the temporal lobe, which then ruptured into the temporal horn of the lateral ventricle.

This region is further disposed to ischemia by the overlying position of the abscess, which compresses circulation through the deep penetrating vessels that course perpendicularly from the pia into the depths of the white matter. Thus, the region below an abscess is susceptible to the growth of microorganisms that escape from the "mother" abscess. Frequently, a "daughter" abscess forms beneath the primary lesion and, through one or several generations of contiguous abscesses, carries the inflammatory process inward to threaten intraventricular rupture. Purulent material liberated into the ventricle passes through the chambers across the absorptive ependymal surfaces, through the foramina of Magendi and Luschka, and onto the meninges. Such an event is promptly fatal, presumably because of the absorption of toxic products.

Viral Encephalomyelitis

The manifestations of viral infections of the parenchyma of the CNS are heterogeneous. The attribute that permits recognition of viral infections, both clinically and pathologically, is their propensity for localization in specific areas of the nervous system (Fig. 28-95). Thus, poliomyelitis selects the motor neurons of the spinal cord and bulbar area. Rabies assails the brainstem. Herpes simplex targets the temporal lobes. Subacute sclerosing panencephalitis and progressive multifocal leukoencephalopathy afflict the cerebral hemispheres, the former generally in childhood and the latter in immunocompromised patients.

The mechanisms of viral tropism are largely obscure. There are specific binding sites on the plasma membranes of motor neurons for the poliovirus. Thus, the experimental injection of poliovirus into the occipital lobes of a monkey fails to destroy the neurons at the injection site. Rather the virus "seeks out" the motor neurons of the spinal cord. It is not clear why other viruses elicit regional inflammation. For example, why does the herpes simplex virus preferentially involve the temporal lobes? Because this virus may reside latently in the gasserian ganglion, it is considered that the proximity of this ganglion to the temporal lobe may be responsible for the geographic distribution of herpetic encephalitis.

The transmission of viruses within neural tissues, and specifically within axons, is clearly exemplified in the pathogenesis of the herpetic "cold sore." It is also dramatically evident from studies of rabies. Intra-axonal transmission of rabies virus has been demonstrated in peripheral nerves, from the site of the bite to the spinal cord or brainstem. Transmission also occurs centrifugally from cranial nerves to the salivary glands, after which the contaminated saliva transmits the disease through a subsequent bite.

☐ **Pathology:** The classic, although not universal, hallmark of viral infections in the CNS is the presence of **perivascular cuffs of lymphocytes** involving small arteries and arterioles (Fig. 28-96). A complementary and more diagnostic feature of viral infections of the brain is the formation of inclusion bodies (Fig. 28-97). However, they are by no means a constant feature. For example, inclusion bodies are not present in some classic infections, such as poliomyelitis.

The characteristics of the most common inclusions are as follows:

- **Herpes simplex and herpes zoster infection:** The inclusions are small, intranuclear, and eosinophilic and cannot be distinguished by their morphological appearance (see Fig. 28-101).
- **Rabies:** The cytoplasmic Negri body is unequivocal evidence of rabies encephalitis (see Fig. 28-9).
- **Progressive multifocal leukoencephalopathy:** The intranuclear inclusions that characterize this disease reflect the presence of a papovavirus (JC virus) and are found within oligodendroglia. They are associated with mild enlargement of the nucleus and exhibit a "ground glass" appearance. The inclusion enlarges the nucleus and alters the appearance of its chromatin without forming a discrete "body" (see Fig. 28-104).
- **Subacute sclerosing panencephalitis:** The discrete intranuclear inclusions found in this condition are basophilic and are associated with a prominent halo.
- **Cytomegalovirus infection:** Eosinophilic inclusions are present in both the nucleus and cytoplasm of astrocytes and neurons. They are most conspicuous in the enlarged nucleus, where they are sharply defined and surrounded by a halo (see Fig. 28-8 and Fig. 28-103).

As a further adjunct to diagnosis, viral particles may be visualized by electron microscopy. Intranuclear viral particles abound in progressive multifocal leukoencephalopathy, and they can be readily visualized in her-

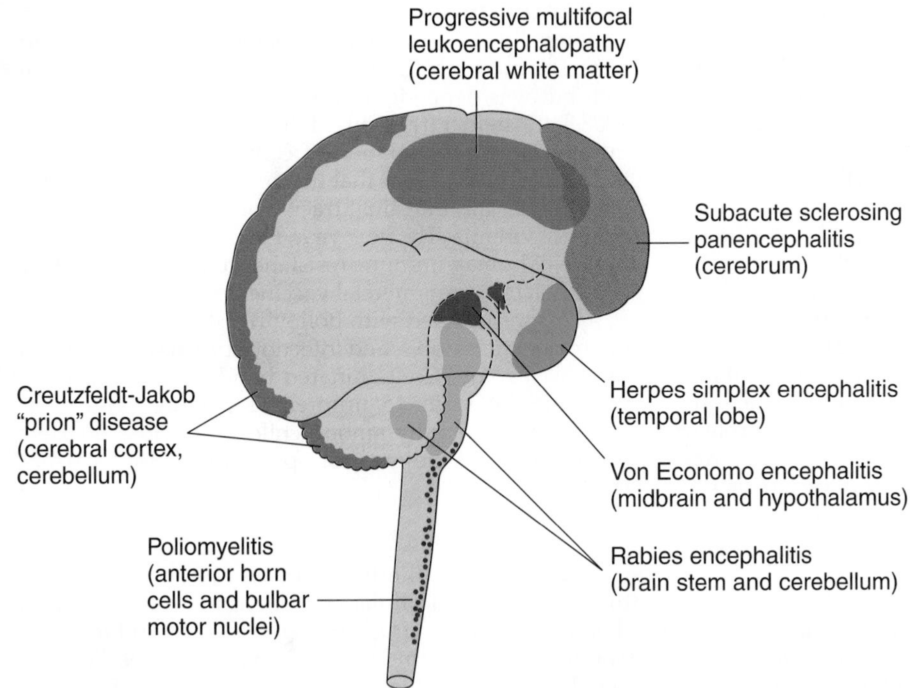

FIGURE 28-95
Distribution of the lesions of viral encephalitides.

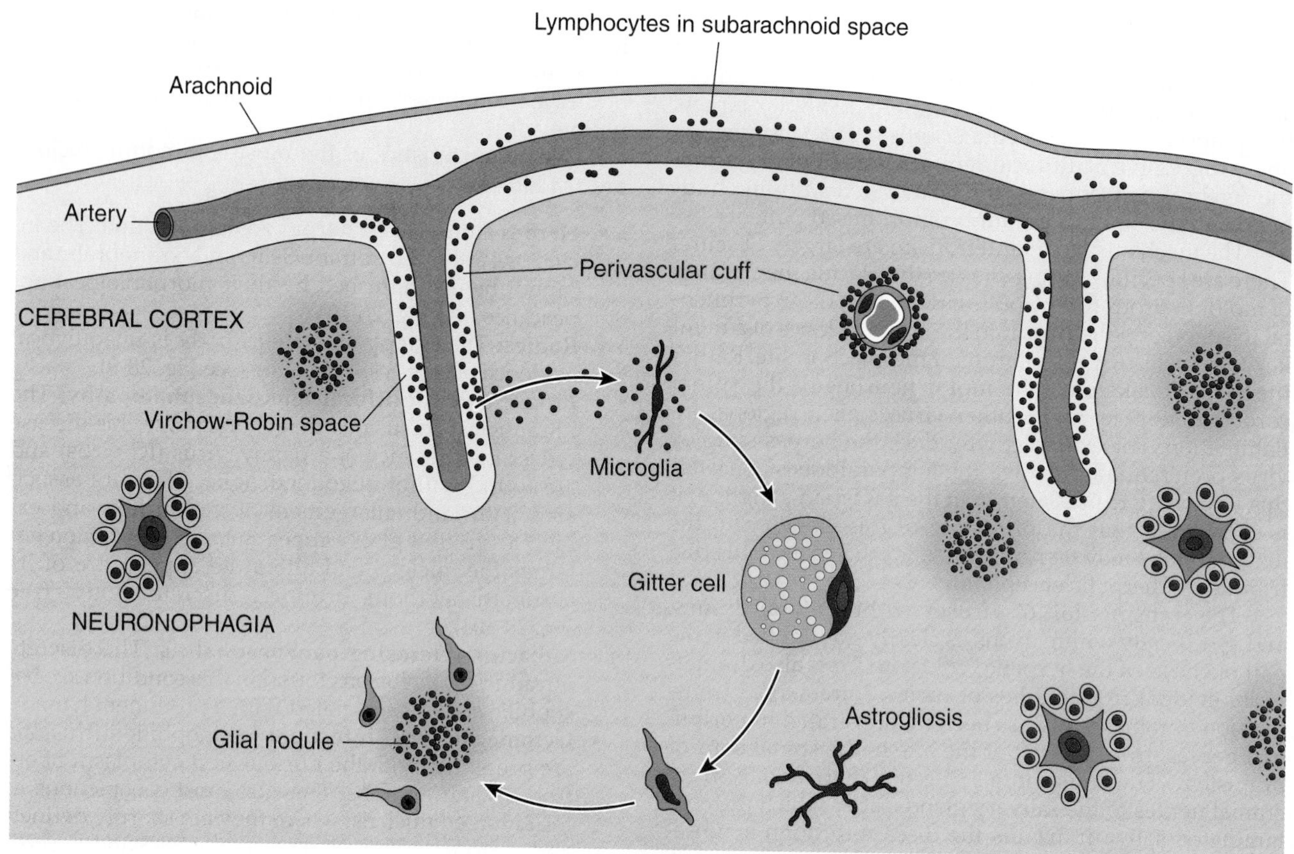

FIGURE 28-96
The lesions of viral encephalitis.

pes simplex. The use of immunohistochemical methods is also an important technique for recognition of viral infections (see Fig. 28-103).

☐ **Clinical Features:** The onset of most viral encephalitides is abrupt. The more specific neurological deficits, for example, the paralysis of poliomyelitis or the difficulty in swallowing (hydrophobia) in rabies, reflect the geographic localization of the lesions. Although most encephalitides run a brief course, the tempo can unquestionably be variable. For example, the clinical course of subacute sclerosing panencephalitis may extend over many years. It is likely that the same would be true for progressive multifocal leukoencephalopathy were this infection not present in a host whose life expectancy is already limited by a major illness. The herpes simplex virus, as mentioned earlier, resides latently in the gasserian ganglion for decades, and there is suggestive evidence that it can do the same in the brain. For this and other reasons, there are unresolved concerns about the potential role of viral infections in the genesis of a variety of chronic cerebral disorders, such as epilepsy and multiple sclerosis.

Poliomyelitis

The term poliomyelitis refers to any inflammation of the gray matter of the spinal cord, but in common usage, it implies an infection with one of three strains of poliovirus (Brunhilde, Lancing, Leon). The organism is one of the enteroviruses, which are all small, nonenveloped, single-stranded, RNA viruses.

☐ **Epidemiology:** Historical evidence suggests that poliomyelitis has occurred in epidemic form since antiquity. The medical triumph over this disease has been recent but was dependent on many prior observations. In 1908, Landsteiner transmitted the infection to monkeys by intraperitoneal inoculation of contaminated CSF. Three years later, he reported that the virus replicates in the human tonsils and intestinal tract, from which it spreads to produce viremia. The next year, Flexner characterized the nature of human immune resistance to poliovirus. A half-century later, a commercial vaccine became available.

Persons infected with poliovirus shed large amounts of virus in their stools, and infection spreads by way of the fecal–oral route. Contaminated hands, food, and water transmit the virus to uninfected persons. The agent spreads most rapidly among children in close quarters, where there are the greatest opportunities for fecal–oral contact.

☐ **Pathology:** Binding sites on motor neurons, and the favorable intracellular conditions for viral replication therein, permit the virus to enter these cells and replicate. The infected cells undergo chromatolysis (see Fig. 28-4 and Fig. 28-98), after which they are phagocytized by

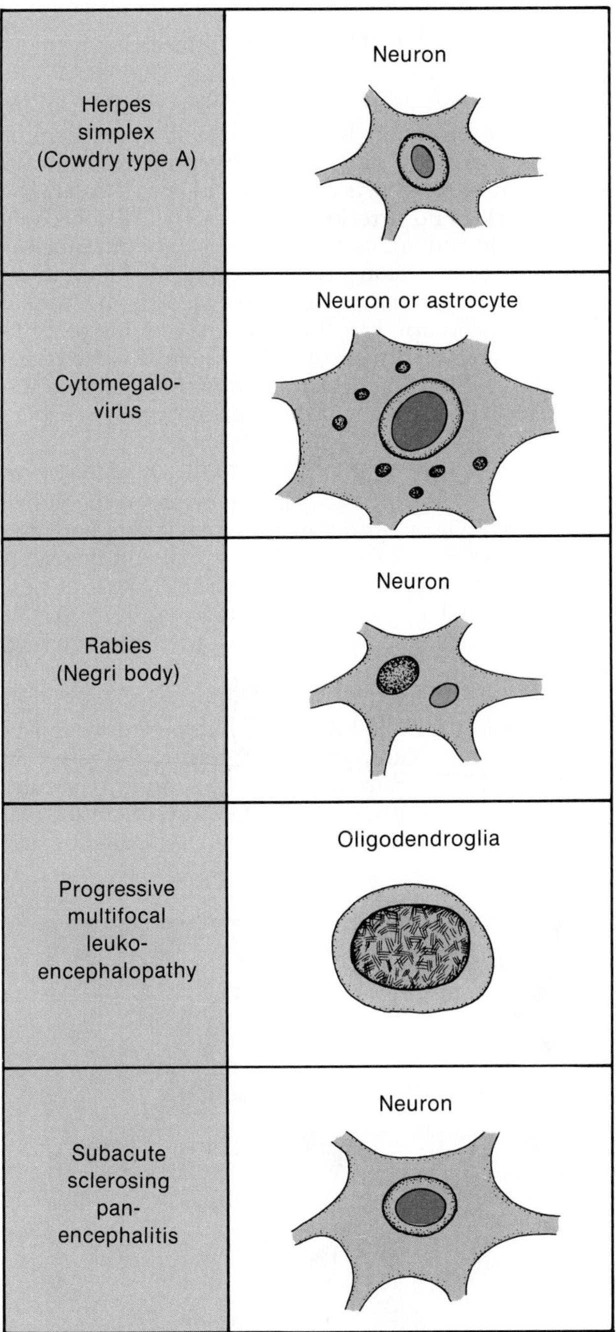

FIGURE 28-97
Inclusion bodies in viral encephalitides.

macrophages (neuronophagia; see Fig. 28-7). The initial inflammatory response transiently features polymorphonuclear leukocytes, but they soon yield to lymphocytes. The latter surround blood vessels in the anterior horns of the spinal cord and the medulla and may extend in lesser degrees into the meninges. The motor cortex usually lacks frank inflammation but may contain "glial nodules," which are focal collections of microglia and lymphocytes (see Fig. 28-17). The immunological response of the host to poliovirus sterilizes the tissues within several weeks. This limits the duration of the inflammation and halts the progression of clinical disease. Sections of spinal cord in cases of healed poliomyelitis show a paucity of neurons in the anterior horns of the affected regions, with secondary degeneration of the corresponding ventral roots and peripheral nerves.

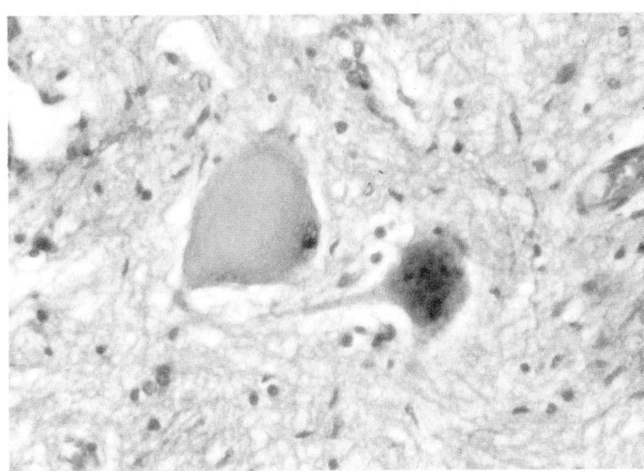

FIGURE 28-98
Poliomyelitis. Chromatolysis and neuronal necrosis are seen in the anterior horn of the spinal cord.

☐ **Clinical Features:** After infection with poliovirus, nonspecific symptoms, such as fever, malaise, and headache, are followed in several days by signs of meningitis and shortly thereafter by paralysis. In severe cases, the muscles of the neck, trunk, and all four limbs may be powerless, and paralysis of the respiratory muscles may become life threatening. Milder cases exhibit an asymmetric and patchy paralysis, most prominently in the lower limbs.

Improvement begins in about a week, and only some of the muscles affected at the outset remain permanently paralyzed. The mortality varies from 5% to 25%, with death usually resulting from respiratory failure. The development in the 1950s of effective vaccines against poliovirus has largely eliminated the disease, and sporadic cases occur only in nonimmunized children and young adults.

Rabies

Rabies is an encephalitis caused by rabies virus, an enveloped, single-stranded RNA virus of the rhabdovirus group. Rabies has been recognized throughout recorded history. Lower animals serve as a reservoir of this zoonosis and transmit the lethal encephalitis to humans. Carnivores, notably dogs, wolves, foxes, and skunks, are the principal reservoirs, but the infection also extends to bats and domestic animals, including cattle, goats, and swine. The infectious agent is transmitted to humans through contaminated saliva introduced by a bite. In the United States, where dogs are routinely vaccinated against rabies, the few human rabies infections (one to five per year) usually result from exposure to rabid wild animals. By contrast, in areas of Asia, Africa, and South America, where rabies is endemic in dogs, most human infections result from dog bites. In these areas of the world, rabies kills more than 50,000 persons annually.

☐ **Pathogenesis:** The virus enters a peripheral nerve and is transported by centripetal axoplasmic flow to the spinal cord and brain. The latent interval varies in proportion to the distance of transport, being as short as 10 days or as long as 3 months. Centrifugal, intra-axonal transmission of the virus contaminates visceral organs, importantly, the salivary glands, where the saliva becomes infectious.

☐ **Pathology:** Lymphocytes aggregate about small arteries and veins in the brainstem. Scattered neurons show chromatolysis and neuronophagia, and glial nodules attest to the infectious nature of the process. The inflammation is centered in the brainstem and spills into the cerebellum and hypothalamus. The presence of Negri bodies (see Fig. 28-9) in the hippocampus, brainstem, and Purkinje cells of the cerebellum confirms the diagnosis of rabies.

☐ **Clinical Features:** Destruction of neurons in the brainstem by rabies virus initiates painful spasms of the throat, difficulty in swallowing, and a consequent tendency to aspirate fluids. These symptoms prompted the original designation "hydrophobia." The clinical symptoms also reflect a general encephalopathy, characterized by irritability, agitation, seizures, and delirium. The CSF is altered in accord with the "typical viral response" showing (1) a modest increase in the number of lymphocytes, (2) a moderate increase in protein content, and (3) unaltered glucose levels and CSF pressure. The illness progresses to death in an interval of 1 to several weeks.

Specific treatment of rabies is not available. Dating from the time of Pasteur, postexposure prophylaxis is accomplished by a series of vaccine injections and is usually effective.

Herpes Simplex Encephalitis and Related Infections

Herpesviruses include herpes simplex (types 1 and 2), varicella-zoster virus, cytomegalovirus, Epstein–Barr virus, and simian B virus.

HERPES SIMPLEX VIRUS TYPE 1 (HSV-1): Herpes simplex virus type 1 is largely responsible for the "cold sore." The region of the vesicular lesion on the lip is innervated from the gasserian ganglion through its mandibular nerve trunk. HSV-1 may reside latently within the gasserian ganglion, where it proliferates during periods of stress and is transmitted centrifugally through the nerve trunk to the lip.

Herpes encephalitis is a major viral infection of the human nervous system. In adults, the encephalitis is caused principally by HSV-1 and curiously is localized predominantly in one or both temporal lobes. The reason for this localization is uncertain but, as mentioned previously, it is considered to result from intra-axonal spread of the virions from the gasserian ganglion to the overlying brain through meningeal nerve fibers. This explanation is weakened, however, by the occurrence of encephalitis in persons who lack a history of cold sores and by the frequency of bilateral temporal lobe involvement.

☐ **Pathology:** Herpes encephalitis is a fulminant infection. The temporal lobes become swollen, hemorrhagic, and necrotic (Fig. 28-99). The inflammatory exudate is predominantly lymphocytic and perivascular. The small arteries and arterioles characteristically become hemorrhagic and edematous (Fig. 28-100). Intranuclear inclusions occur in neurons but also may be found in astrocytes and oligodendrocytes. The inclusions are weakly eosinophilic, occupy less than half the volume of a nucleus, and are usually surrounded by an inconspicuous halo (Fig. 28-101). The detection of viral proteins by immunohistochemical techniques is diagnostically reliable.

HERPES SIMPLEX VIRUS TYPE 2 (HSV-2): In women, HSV-2 initiates a vesicular lesion on the vulva, coupled with a latent infection in the pelvic ganglia. Newborns acquire HSV-2 from the birth canal and thereafter have an encephalitis. At this age, the neural tissues are extremely vulnerable, and the infection promptly causes extensive liquefaction in the cerebrum and cerebellum (Fig. 28-102).

VARICELLA-ZOSTER VIRUS: Herpes zoster causes a disease that is anatomically analogous to the gasserian ganglion–cold sore complex of herpes simplex. The cutaneous vesicular eruption of "shingles" occurs in the distribution of a dermatome whose dorsal root ganglion har-

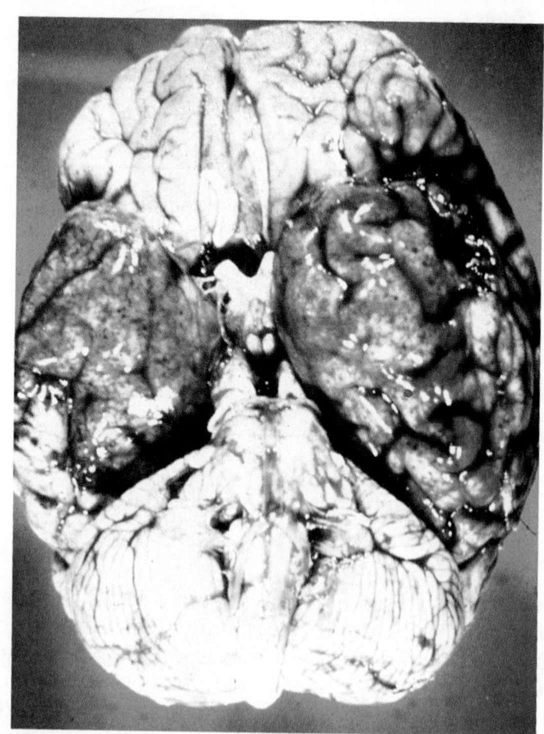

FIGURE 28-99
Herpes simplex encephalitis. The temporal lobes are preferentially involved by a hemorrhagic, necrotizing inflammation.

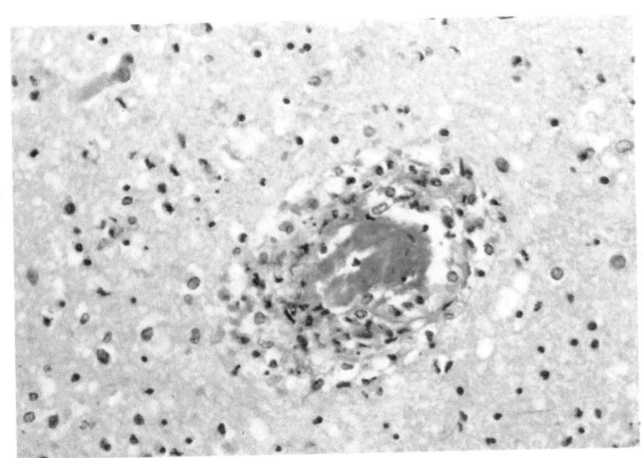

FIGURE 28-100
Herpes simplex encephalitis. A microscopic view of Fig. 28-99 shows a necrotizing arteritis in a temporal lobe.

bors the varicella-zoster virus. The infection elicits only mild inflammation, and it rarely spreads to the CNS.

CYTOMEGALOVIRUS: This agent crosses the placenta to induce encephalitis *in utero*. The lesions in the embryonic nervous system predominate in the periventricular areas and are characterized by necrosis and calcification. Because of the proximity of these lesions to the third ventricle and the aqueduct, they are prone to induce hydrocephalus. Cytomegalovirus is one of the agents of the so-called toxoplasmosis, other (congenital syphilis and viruses), rubella, cytomegalovirus, and herpes simplex virus (TORCH) complex of newborns (see Chapter 6). In adults, cytomegalovirus initiates encephalitis in immunocompromised hosts (see Fig. 28-8 and Fig. 28-103).

SIMIAN B VIRUS: This virus contaminates the saliva of lower primates and is transmitted to humans through a bite, causing fulminant encephalitis and myelitis.

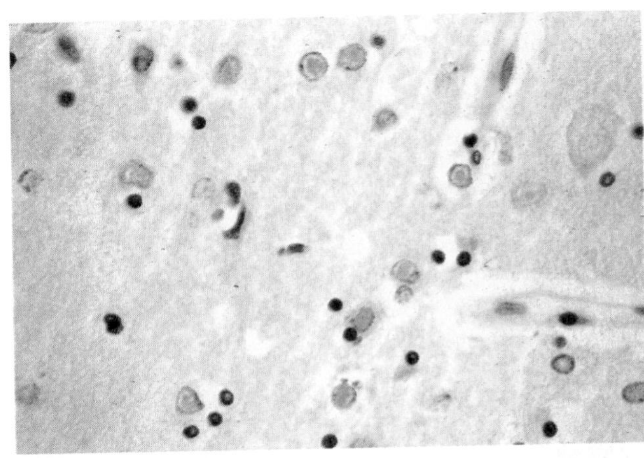

FIGURE 28-101
Herpes simplex encephalitis. The infected neurons display small, intranuclear, eosinophilic inclusions that lack halos.

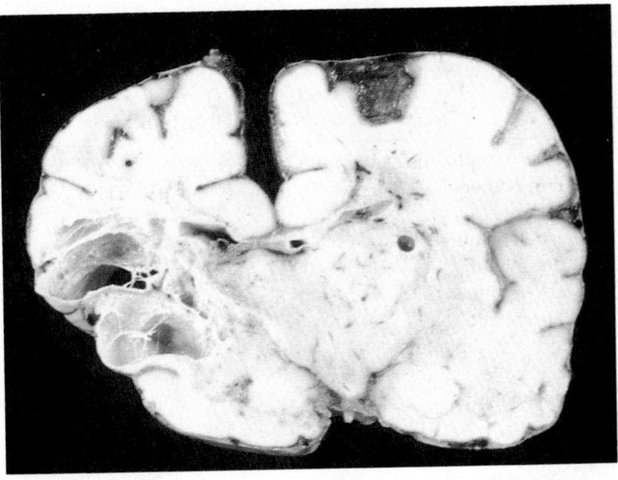

FIGURE 28-102
Herpes simplex type 2 encephalitis. The brain of an infant born to a mother with genital herpes shows conspicuous cavitary lesions.

Arthropod-Borne Viral Encephalitis

Arthropod-borne viruses, often termed arboviruses, comprise a heterogeneous group of agents transmitted between vertebrates by blood-sucking vectors, such as mosquitoes and ticks. The Togaviridae and Bunyaviridae contain most of the arboviruses that cause human encephalitis. Arbovirus infections are zoonoses of wild and domestic animals, and humans become accidentally infected if bitten by an infected arthropod. Human infection is a dead end and does not contribute to continued viral propagation for the virus.

The various encephalitides caused by arboviruses have been named principally for the geographic regions where they were first noted (Table 28-1). These diseases include Eastern, Western, and Venezuelan equine en-

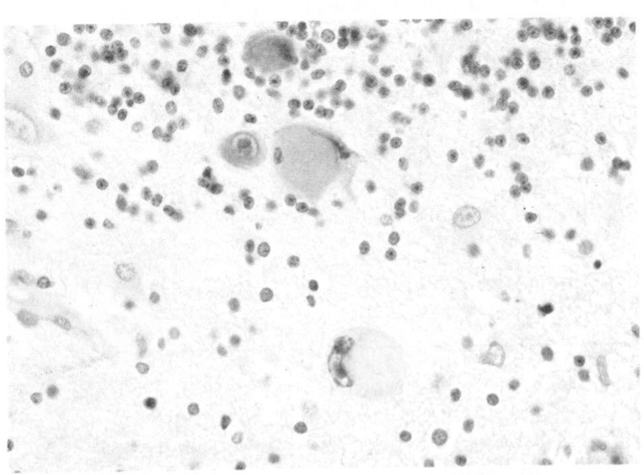

FIGURE 28-103
Cytomegalovirus (CMV) encephalitis. Immunohistochemical localization of CMV antigens demonstrates intranuclear and intracytoplasmic inclusions within Purkinje cells of the cerebellum.

TABLE 28-1 Insect-Borne Viral Encephalitis

Virus	Insect Vector	Distribution
St. Louis encephalitis	Mosquito	North and South America
Western equine encephalitis	Mosquito	North and South America
Venezuelan equine encephalitis	Mosquito	North and South America
Eastern equine encephalitis	Mosquito	North America
California encephalitis	Mosquito	North America
Murray Valley encephalitis	Mosquito	Australia, Papua New Guinea
Japanese B encephalitis	Mosquito	Eastern and southeastern Asia
Tick-borne encephalitis	Tick	Eastern Europe, Scandinavia

cephalitis, St. Louis encephalitis, Japanese B encephalitis, and California encephalitis.

☐ **Pathology:** The lesions in the brain do not differentiate among the various arboviruses that cause encephalitis. The lesions vary from a mild meningitis with scattered lymphocytes, to severe inflammation of the gray matter, to prominent necrosis. No inclusion bodies are present in the infected neurons. Perivascular lymphoid infiltrates are conspicuous, and in severe cases, thrombosis of small vessels occurs. In necrotic foci, neuronophagia is evident. In cases in which survival has been prolonged, areas of demyelination and gliosis may be apparent.

☐ **Clinical Features:** The arthropod-borne encephalitides share many features, but each type has a different course. For example, Eastern equine encephalitis is commonly a fulminant disease that kills in a few days, whereas Venezuelan equine encephalitis tends to be benign. Mild cases of arbovirus encephalitis may be manifested by no more than an influenza-like syndrome and are not diagnosed as encephalitis. In severe cases, the onset is abrupt, with high fever, headache, vomiting, and meningeal signs. Shortly thereafter, lethargy and coma supervene, with most victims dying within 5 days. Young children often survive but may be left with mental retardation, epilepsy, and other neurological sequelae.

Encephalitis Lethargica (von Economo Encephalitis)

Beginning in the winter of 1916 with the pandemic of influenza and lasting for about 5 years, the agent of encephalitis lethargica induced a single, severe epidemic of encephalitis. Although the infectious agent was neither isolated nor identified, the characteristic perivascular cuffs of lymphocytes in the midbrain and hypothalamus testified to its viral nature. As the name implies, the dominant symptom was somnolence, which on occasion persisted unabated for weeks. The regression of this symptom in an occasional patient disclosed the presence of parkinsonism (see later). Other victims of von Economo encephalitis developed Parkinson disease ("postencephalitis parkinsonism") a decade or so later. This occurrence suggests that subclinical injury to the neurons of the substantia nigra compromised the longevity of these cells.

Subacute Sclerosing Panencephalitis

Subacute sclerosing panencephalitis (SSPE) is a chronic, lethal, viral infection of the brain caused by the measles virus. The disease was first recognized in 1933 and was descriptively named "subacute inclusion-body encephalitis." A decade later, its features were defined as (1) an encephalitis of insidious onset that predominates in childhood, (2) a protracted course, and (3) inflammation, principally in the cerebral gray matter. It is now recognized that occasional cases occur in adults and may follow a more rapid course.

☐ **Pathogenesis:** The etiology of subacute sclerosing panencephalitis remained uncertain until 1969, when it was demonstrated that an agent having the general properties of measles virus proliferated in cells maintained in co-culture with infected tissue of the host. Moreover, most patients with SSPE give a history of measles, usually before several years of age. The consistent association of SSPE with a measles-like virus argues strongly for an etiological role for this agent.

Two different mechanisms have been proposed to account for the protracted course of the infection in the brain, which is characterized by the persistence of the virus within infected cells. Antimeasles antibody has been shown to transform an otherwise acute encephalitis into a persistent one, presumably by interacting with viral antigens on the surface of infected cells and inhibiting viral budding. It has also been demonstrated in SSPE that virus isolated from the brain is always defective. A viral protein necessary for viral budding (M protein) is unusually sensitive to proteases of the host cell, thereby presumably preventing the release of nascent virus from the cell.

☐ **Pathology and Clinical Features:** In tissue sections, the inflammation is highlighted by (1) the presence of prominent haloed intranuclear inclusions within neurons and oligodendroglial cells, (2) marked astrogliosis in damaged areas in both the gray and white matter (accounting for the term *sclerosing*), (3) patchy loss of myelin, and (4) ubiquitous perivascular cuffs of lymphocytes and macrophages.

The classic, protracted disease insidiously creates cognitive deficits, alters personality and behavior, inflicts motor and sensory deficits, and ultimately causes stupor and death, all over a period of several years. The CSF is minimally altered but typically contains an increased titer against the measles virus.

Progressive Multifocal Leukoencephalopathy

Progressive multifocal leukoencephalopathy (PML) is a relentless and destructive focal disease caused by JC virus, which principally affects the white matter in all areas of the nervous system. PML is seen insidiously as dementia, weakness,

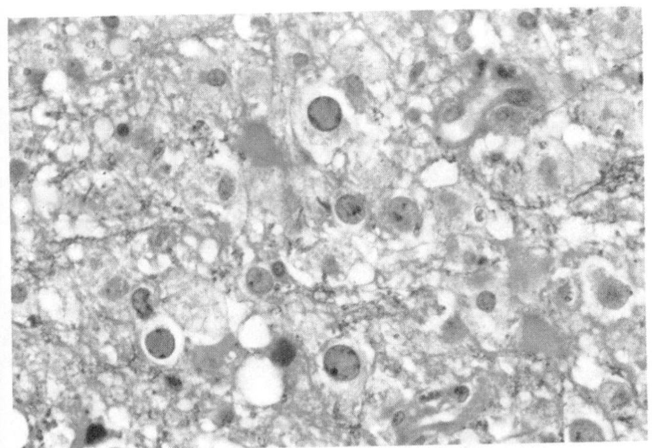

FIGURE 28-104
Progressive multifocal leukoencephalopathy. The oligodendroglia are enlarged and exhibit intranuclear inclusions.

visual loss, and ataxia, and most patients die within 6 months. The malady exemplifies many of the fundamental characteristics of neurotropic viruses: (1) opportunism, (2) selectivity for an individual cell species, notably oligodendroglia (Fig. 28-104), (3) the capacity to induce demyelination by damaging oligodendrocytes (Fig. 28-105), and (4) oncogenicity (Fig. 28-106).

JC virus, a papovavirus closely analogous to simian virus 40 (SV40 virus), is the causative agent of PML. With few exceptions, the encephalitis is a terminal complication in immunosuppressed patients, for example, persons treated for cancer or lupus erythematosus, patients receiving organ transplants, and particularly persons with AIDS. In fact, PML is no longer a rare disease: it occurs in 1% to 3% of patients with AIDS in the United States and in an even higher proportion in studies from Europe.

☐ **Pathology:** The typical lesions of PML appear as widely disseminated discrete foci of demyelination near the gray–white junction in the cerebral hemispheres and the brainstem (see Fig. 28-105). The characteristic lesion of PML exhibits the following morphological features:

- It is spherical, measuring several millimeters in diameter.
- A central area is largely devoid of myelin.
- Axons are retained.
- Few oligodendrocytes are seen.
- The lesion is infiltrated by macrophages, without necrosis.
- Pleomorphic astrocytes are present (see Fig. 28-106).

A pathognomonic feature of PML is a peripheral area of demyelination that contains enlarged oligodendrocytes, with homogeneously dense, hyperchromatic, intranuclear inclusions, which lack a halo and have a ground-glass appearance (see Fig. 28-104). Electron microscopy discloses intranuclear, crystalline arrays of spherical virions, 35 to 40 nm in diameter.

The pleomorphic astrocytes appear anaplastic. Their nuclei are often multiple and irregular in contour and display dense chromatin material. Astrocytomas have developed in several patients with PML.

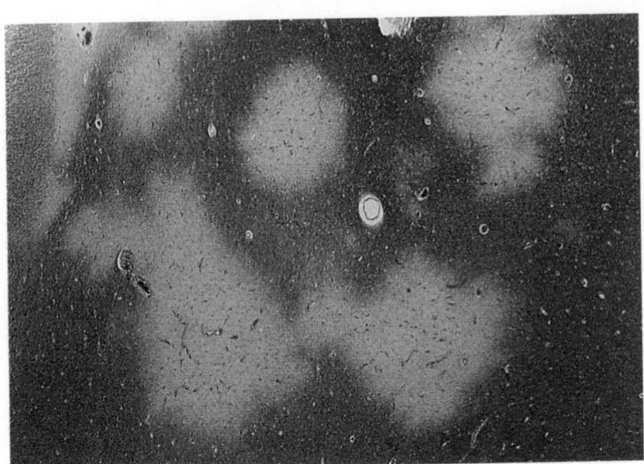

FIGURE 28-105
Progressive multifocal leukoencephalopathy. A luxol fast blue stain of the brain demonstrates conspicuous demyelination.

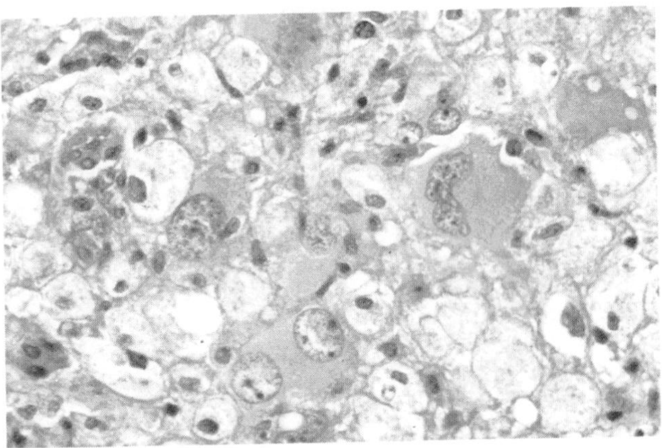

FIGURE 28-106
Progressive multifocal leukoencephalopathy. The astroglia display marked nuclear pleomorphism.

AIDS Encephalopathy

Among patients with AIDS, half manifest a clinical encephalopathy, and an even larger proportion demonstrate morphological lesions in the CNS at autopsy. Some patients have an opportunistic infection in the brain (e.g., toxoplasmosis, cytomegalovirus [see Fig. 28-8], herpes simplex, progressive multifocal leukoencephalopathy, or a primary lymphoma). However, the majority of AIDS patients with encephalopathy have a disease that is attributable to an active infection of the CNS by the retrovirus itself. **Dementia is the most common clinical manifestation of AIDS encephalopathy, also termed *AIDS dementia complex*.** The symptoms range from loss of memory and concentration to severe cognitive impairment with paralysis and loss of sensory functions.

☐ **Pathogenesis:** Macrophages and microglial cells in the CNS are productively infected by human immunodeficiency virus-1 (HIV-1) in AIDS encephalopathy and are considered to play a key pathogenetic role. Although other cells, including neurons and astrocytes, also may interact with the virus, they do not seem to be productively infected in AIDS encephalopathy but are believed to be injured indirectly. A number of indirect mechanisms have been invoked to explain the loss of neurons and demyelination found in AIDS encephalopathy. These include (1) the release of toxic cytokines (e.g., TNF-α, IL-1, and IL-6) by infected macrophages and microglia, (2) the secretion of other neurotoxic agents from these same cells, (3) excessive concentrations of abnormal neurotransmitters, and (4) disruption of the cerebral microvasculature.

□ **Pathology:** On gross examination, AIDS encephalopathy is characterized by mild cerebral atrophy, with dilatation of the lateral ventricles and slight prominence of the gyri and sulci. The diminution in brain weight rarely exceeds 200 g. The histological changes are usually most intense in the subcortical gray and white matter, whereas few changes are seen in the cerebral cortex. **The hallmark of AIDS encephalopathy is the presence of multinucleated giant cells of the monocyte/macrophage lineage associated with microglial nodules** (Fig. 28-107). In addition, myelin pallor (Fig. 28-108), reflecting diffuse demyelination, and an intense astrogliosis are commonly found.

Vacuolar myopathy is a second distinct neurological lesion attributed to HIV infection, although it is considerably less frequent than encephalopathy. It occurs alone or concurrent with AIDS encephalopathy and is characterized by marked vacuolation of the posterior and lateral columns, principally at the thoracic level of the spinal cord. Ataxia and spastic paraparesis dominate the clinical presentation.

Congenital HIV encephalopathy and myelopathy differ from the adult disease more in their intensity than in their specific attributes. Calcification of the basal ganglia and thalamus are more common in the childhood infections and can be visualized radiographically.

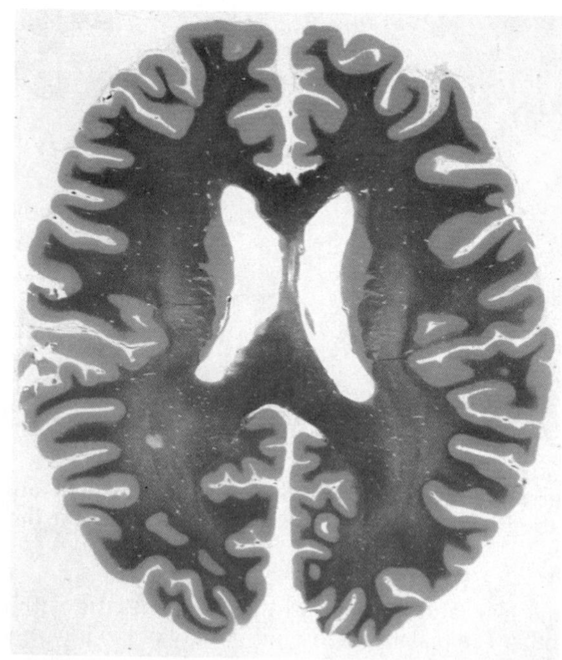

FIGURE *28-108*
Acquired immunodeficiency syndrome (AIDS) encephalopathy. A horizontal section of the brain stained for myelin demonstrates a symmetric pallor, predominantly in the corona radiata, indicating demyelination.

PRION DISEASES (SPONGIFORM ENCEPHALOPATHIES)

Prion diseases comprise a group of neurodegenerative conditions characterized clinically by slowly progressive ataxia and dementia and pathologically by a peculiar vacuolization termed ***spongiform degeneration*** (Fig. 28-109). The spongiform encephalopathies include four human diseases: kuru, Creutzfeldt–Jakob disease (CJD), Gerstmann–Straussler–Scheinker syndrome, and fatal familial insomnia (Table 28-2). In addition, similar diseases occur in ani-

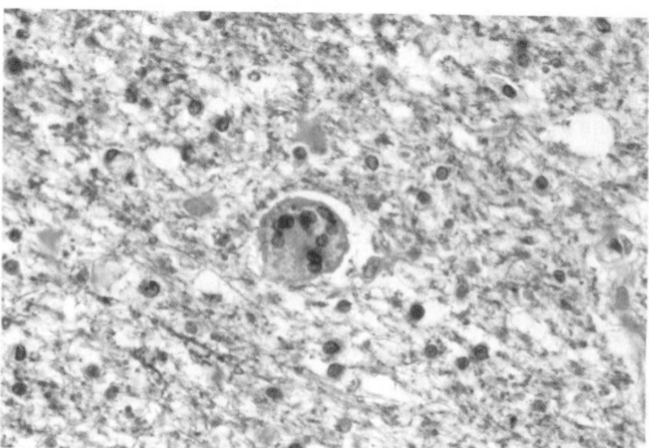

FIGURE *28-107*
Acquired immunodeficiency syndrome (AIDS) encephalopathy. This higher-power view of Fig. 28-108 shows a multinucleated macrophage and diffuse astrogliosis.

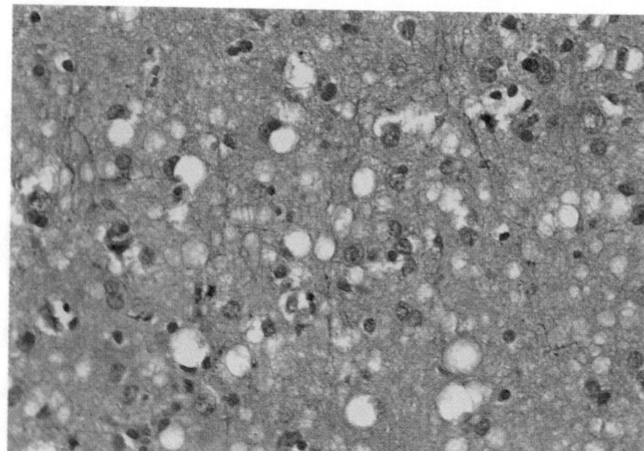

FIGURE *28-109*
Creutzfeldt–Jakob disease. Spongiform degeneration of the gray matter is characterized by individual and clustered vacuoles, without evidence of inflammation.

mals, including scrapie in sheep and goats, bovine spongiform encephalopathy (BSE; mad cow disease), transmissible mink encephalopathy, and chronic wasting disease in mule deer and elk.

Prion diseases encompass infectious and familial (inherited prion gene mutation) forms, but cases predominate in which the mode of acquisition is uncertain. In addition to their many singular clinical and molecular pathological features, prion diseases are currently under intense scrutiny because of recent data that indicate a link between BSE ("mad cow disease") and a new variant of human CJD, namely vCJD.

☐ **Pathogenesis:** It is now known that all the spongiform encephalopathies are transmissible diseases. The initial demonstration of the transmissibility of these diseases was accomplished in sheep with scrapie, when transmission of spongiform encephalopathy to other animals was produced by the inoculation of infected nervous tissue. Subsequently, Gajdusek et al. in 1966 produced similar lesions in chimpanzees by the intracerebral injection of homogenized brain tissue from patients with kuru. Two years later, the same investigators successfully passed CJD by the same technique. Unfortunately, inadvertent human transmission of CJD has also been observed as a consequence of the administration of contaminated human pituitary growth hormone, corneal transplantation from a diseased donor, insufficiently sterilized neurosurgical instruments, and the surgical implantation of contaminated dura.

Studies of the infectious agent of the spongiform encephalopathies were greatly facilitated by the development of infectious models in mice and hamsters. On partial purification of infectious particles from these models, it was apparent that the putative "slow virus" of scrapie was not a virus at all, but rather an unprecedented protein that was not associated with nucleic acid. The term *prion* was introduced by Prusiner in 1982 to differentiate these *proteinaceous infectious particles* from viruses.

The human prion gene (termed *PRNP*) is located on the short arm of chromosome 20, and the open reading frame consists of a single exon encoding 254 amino acid residues. The normal prion gene product, prion protein (PrP), is a constitutively expressed cell-surface glycoprotein, which is bound to the plasmalemma by a glycolipid anchor. The highest levels of PrP messenger RNA (mRNA) are found in CNS neurons, but the function of the protein is unknown. Remarkably, the normal cellular prion protein, termed cellular PrP or PrP^{C}, and the pathogenic (infectious) prion protein, known as scrapie PrP or PrP^{SC}, do not differ in primary structure (amino acid sequence). Rather they have very different three-dimensional conformations and patterns of glycosylation. Specifically, PrP^{C} is rich in the α-helix configuration, with four putative domains. Conversely, it exhibits little β-pleated sheet configuration. By contrast, the content of β-pleated sheets in PrP^{SC} is greatly increased. It is thought that this difference in conformation underlies the greater resistance of PrP^{SC} to proteinase digestion compared with PrP^{C}. The posttranslational conversion of α-helices to β-pleated sheets is hypothesized to underlie the prion-propagation mechanism, whereby normal host PrP^{C} is converted to PrP^{SC}. The newly converted proteins then change other PrP^{C} proteins into pathogenic PrP^{SC}. The result is an autocatalytic, exponentially expanding accrual of abnormal PrP^{SC}. The intraneuronal accumulation of PrP^{SC} occurs before the characteristic microcystic change can be appreciated histologically. Thus, the toxic accumulation of PrP^{SC} eventually compromises cell function and ultimately results in neuronal loss and neuropil vacuolation.

TABLE *28-2* **Prion Diseases**

I. Human
  A. Creutzfeldt–Jakob disease (CJD)
    1. Sporadic (85% of all CJD cases; incidence 1 per million worldwide)
    2. Inherited mutation of the prion gene, autosomal dominant transmission (15% of all CJD cases)
    3. Iatrogenic
      a. Hormone injection
        Human growth hormone (55 cases)
        Human pituitary gonadotropin (5 cases)
      b. Tissue grafts
        Dura mater (11 cases)
        Cornea (1 case)
        Pericardium (1 case)
      c. Medical devices (inadequate sterilization)
        Depth electrodes (2 cases)
        Surgical instruments (not definitely proven)
    4. New variant CJD (vCJD)
  B. Gerstmann–Staussler–Scheinker disease (GSS; inherited prion gene mutation, autosomal dominant transmission)
  C. Fatal familial insomnia (FFI; inherited prion gene mutation, autosomal dominant transmission)
  D. Kuru (confined to the Fore people of Papua New Guinea; formerly transmitted by cannibalistic ritual)
II. Animal
  A. Scrapie (sheep and goats)
  B. Bovine spongiform encephalopathy (BSE; "mad cow disease")
  C. Transmissible mink encephalopathy
  D. Feline spongiform encephalopathy
  E. Captive exotic ungulate spongiform encephalopathy (nyala, gemsbok, eland, arabian oryx, greater kudu)
  F. Chronic wasting disease of deer and elk
  G. Experimental transmission to many species, including primates and transgenic mice

☐ **Pathology:** The cardinal morphological feature of the prion diseases is spongiform degeneration, that is, the presence of small aggregates of microcysts (see Fig. 28-109). These are most prevalent in the cortical gray matter but also involve the deeper nuclei of the basal ganglia and hypothalamus and, importantly, the cerebellum. Within the areas of spongiform degeneration, neurons disappear, and astrogliosis becomes prominent. The cortical spinal pathways degenerate.

The various human prion diseases have distinctive features.

KURU: In 1956, a medical officer in New Guinea provided an account of kuru, a progressive, fatal neurological disorder, in members of an isolated cannibalistic tribe.

The disease takes its name from the word "trembling" in the language of the Fore tribe. The transmission of kuru in New Guinea was linked to ritualistic cannibalism, wherein women and children consumed human brain. The initial incidence of the disease is dated to the entry of Europeans to New Guinea in 1920. The incidence of kuru has sharply abated with the elimination of cannibalism.

Kuru was the first human prion disease shown to be transmissible. The disease formerly reached epidemic proportions in the Fore people of New Guinea but has been virtually eliminated after the cessation of ritualistic cannibalism by which the Fore honored their dead. The initial and most prominent clinical features of kuru are limb and truncal ataxia, which reflect severe involvement of the cerebellum. In 70% of kuru cases, prion protein accumulates extracellularly as amyloid plaques ("kuru-type plaques"), and spongiform change is present in both the cerebral hemispheres and cerebellum. Dementia is also seen in some patients, but occurs late in the clinical course. As with all of the prion diseases, kuru is lethal; death typically supervenes a year after the onset of ataxia.

CREUTZFELDT–JAKOB DISEASE: This rare, subacute encephalopathy was first fully described by Jakob in 1921. The disease has a worldwide annual incidence of 1 per million. Symptoms begin insidiously, but within 6 months, the patient exhibits severe dementia and is usually dead within a year. The involvement of the cerebellum adds ataxia to the predominant symptom of dementia and distinguishes CJD clinically from Alzheimer disease.

Creutzfeldt–Jakob disease is by far the most common form of human prion disease and can be classified into four types based on etiology:

- **Sporadic CJD:** The sporadic form occurs worldwide, with an incidence of 1 per million, and accounts for 75% of all cases of CJD. The mode of acquisition is unknown; patients do not exhibit the mutations associated with the inherited forms of CJD or other prion diseases, and there is no history of iatrogenic exposure. A normal polymorphism, which codes either for methionine (M) or valine (V), occurs at codon 129 of the prion gene. Susceptibility to all forms of CJD, including the sporadic type, appears to be influenced by this polymorphism, with a disproportionate number of patents being homozygous at this locus. The frequencies for the white population are as follows: 51% M/V, 37% M/M, and 12% V/V.

  Sporadic CJD exhibits prototypical histological features of the spongiform encephalopathies: microcystic neuropil vacuolation (Fig. 28-109), astrogliosis, and neuronal loss. As in all other prion diseases, no host inflammatory response is seen.

  Clinically, sporadic CJD is characterized by the classic triad of dementia, myoclonus, and periodic spike–wave complexes on electroencephalogram (EEG). The dementia is rapidly progressive, with death occurring within 4 to 12 months. However, longer courses of 2 to 5 years are well documented. Some 15% of cases are first seen with ataxia similar to that of kuru, with dementia following later.
- **Inherited CJD:** Familial CJD composes 15% of prion diseases, with an incidence of 1 per 10 million. Several different mutations of the prion gene have been documented in various kindreds. The mutated PrP in familial CJD, fatal familial insomnia, and Gerstmann–Straussler–Scheinker disease, is designated δPrP.
- **Iatrogenic CJD:** As listed in Table 28-2, a number of iatrogenic cases of CJD have also been documented; however, most of the causes have now been eliminated. For example, recombinant human growth hormone is now available and has supplanted human pituitary–derived preparations.
- **New variant CJD:** New variant CJD (vCJD) was recently identified by a surveillance program established in the United Kingdom in response to the BSE epidemic that devastated the cattle industry. A group of patients was identified that differed from other patients with sporadic CJD in several important characteristics, the most striking of which is age. The mean age at onset of symptoms for sporadic CJD is 65 years, whereas it is 26 years for vCJD patients. Other significant differences include a longer duration of illness for vCJD (median, 12 months vs. 4 months) and an atypical clinical presentation. Instead of the typical memory impairment, vCJD patients had various behavioral changes or sensory disturbances (dysesthesias) and lacked the characteristic EEG findings seen in sporadic CJD. At autopsy, vCJD is characterized by prominent spongiform change in the basal ganglia and thalamus and extensive PrP plaques in the cerebrum and cerebellum. The plaques are distinctive in that they are surrounded by a zone of spongiform change, a feature that is not found in sporadic CJD but is seen in scrapie. Finally, the amount of PrP present in vCJD brains is much greater that that in sporadic CJD. Subsequent physicochemical analysis revealed that the vCJD PrP^{SC} exhibits strain characteristics that are distinct from other types of CJD PrP^{SC} but resemble those of BSE transmitted to mice and primates. These data indicate that BSE is the source of the new CJD variant.

GERSTMANN–STRAUSSLER–SCHEINKER SYNDROME (GSS): This disorder was initially described in 1936 as a familial syndrome of spinocerebellar ataxia combined with dementia. Patients are seen with limb and truncal ataxia, which is slowly progressive over 2 to 10 years. At autopsy, prominent prion protein amyloid plaques ("kuru-type") and spongiform change are found in the cerebellum, cerebrum, and brainstem. Dementia is a late feature of the disease.

FATAL FAMILIAL INSOMNIA: This disease is the most recent addition to the list of human prion diseases. Patients have a profound disturbance of sleep–wake cycles, which is manifested as intractable insomnia. Dysautonomia, abnormal endocrine function, and signs of pyramidal and cerebellar dysfunction are common. Although cognitive function usually remains intact, dementia may supervene. Neuropathological findings at autopsy are limited primarily to atrophy of specific thalamic nuclei. The insomnia has been described in several Italian families, in which afflicted patients have a point mutation in codon 178 of the *PRNP* gene. The mutation consists of the substitution of aspartic acid by asparagine. Interestingly, the same mutation is found in another prion disorder, a subtype of inherited CJD termed CJD^{178} or CJD (D178N). The two disorders differ in that fatal insomnia contains a codon for methionine at the polymorphic locus 178, whereas the CJD (D178N) allele at this locus codes for valine.

DEMYELINATING DISEASES

The category of demyelinating disease is restricted to those disorders in which myelin is lost selectively, whereas other neural structures are preserved. In this context, the leukodystrophies, multiple sclerosis, central pontine myelinolysis, and perhaps PML are appropriately viewed as demyelinating states. By contrast, the coagulative necrosis of a cerebral infarct, the liquefactive necrosis of an abscess, the traumatic injury of a contusion, and the secondary demyelination of wallerian degeneration serve only as reminders that myelin is vulnerable to many injuries.

Leukodystrophies

The leukodystrophies are a heterogeneous group of inherited diseases characterized by profound disturbances in the formation and preservation of myelin.

Metachromatic Leukodystrophy

Metachromatic leukodystrophy (MLD), the most common type of leukodystrophy, is an autosomal recessive disorder of myelin metabolism that is characterized by the accumulation of a cerebroside (galactosyl sulfatide) in the white matter of the brain and peripheral nerves. MLD predominates in infancy, but rare "juvenile" or "adult" cases have been described. The disorder is lethal within several years.

☐ **Pathogenesis:** MLD is caused by a deficiency in the activity of arylsulfatase A, a lysosomal enzyme involved in the degradation of myelin. As a result of the inability of the mutant enzyme to hydrolyze sulfatides, there is a progressive accumulation of sulfatides within the lysosomes of Schwann cells and oligodendrocytes, the cells responsible for the maintenance of myelin.

☐ **Pathology:** Metachromasia refers to a change in the color of a dye when it reacts with tissue. In MLD, the accumulated sulfatides form cytoplasmic spherical granules, 15 to 20 μm in diameter, which stain metachromatically with a variety of dyes, including acidified cresyl violet and toluidine blue.

At autopsy, the cerebral hemispheres and cerebellum feature a diffuse loss of myelin, with (1) the accumulation of metachromatic material, principally in the white matter, (2) prominent astrogliosis, and (3) preservation of the subcortical arcuate fibers. Demyelination of peripheral nerves is less severe.

Krabbe Disease

Krabbe disease is a rapidly progressive, invariably fatal, autosomal recessive neurological disorder caused by a deficiency of galactocerebroside β-galactosidase. The condition appears in young infants and is defined by the presence of perivascular aggregates of mononuclear and multinucleated "globoid cells" in the white matter, hence the alternative name *globoid cell leukodystrophy*. The globoid cells are macrophages that contain undigested galactocerebroside (galactosylceramide).

☐ **Pathogenesis:** Krabbe disease features an almost complete loss of oligodendroglia and myelin in the brain. It is difficult to relate the inability to catabolize galactocerebroside to the selective destruction of oligodendroglia. It has been hypothesized that a highly toxic, alternative metabolite, psychosin, is also a substrate for galactocerebroside β-galactosidase and is generated within oligodendroglia. The accumulation of psychosin is thought to destroy oligodendroglia, thereby producing demyelination.

☐ **Pathology:** At autopsy, the brain is small, and the loss of myelin is diffuse, but the cerebral cortex is normal. Marbled areas of partial and total demyelination are present. Astrogliosis is typically severe.

As demyelination proceeds, clusters of globoid cells are found around blood vessels. These cells measure up to 50 μm in diameter and contain as many as 20 peripherally located nuclei. In the end stage of Krabbe disease, the number of globoid cells decreases, and in areas of severe myelin loss, only scattered globoid cells remain. By electron microscopy, the globoid cells contain inclusions with straight or tubular profiles, which appear crystalloid in cross section.

Krabbe disease appears in the early months of life and progresses to death within 1 to 2 years. Severe motor, sensory, and cognitive impairment reflects the diffuse involvement of the nervous system.

Adrenoleukodystrophy

Adrenoleukodystrophy (ALD) refers to an X-linked (Xq28), inherited disorder in which dysfunction of the adrenal cortex and demyelination of the nervous system are associated with unusually high levels of saturated very-long-chain fatty acids (VLCFAs) in tissue and body fluids. ALD occurs in children between the ages of 3 and 10 years, and neurological symptoms precede the signs of adrenal insufficiency. The disease progresses rapidly, and the body is quickly reduced to a vegetative state, which may persist for several years before death supervenes.

☐ **Pathogenesis:** The cause of ALD involves an enzyme defect that impairs the capacity to degrade VLCFAs. A defect in the peroxisomal membrane prevents the normal activation of free VLCFAs by the addition of coenzyme A (CoA). As a result of the inability to degrade VLCFAs, fatty acids of C24 or C30 or more accumulate as cholesterol esters in gangliosides and in myelin. The pathogenesis of the adrenal atrophy is considered to relate to the accumulation of abnormal cholesterol esters in that gland. In the nervous system, VLCFAs may be directly toxic, although immunological responses to abnormal lipids have also been invoked.

□ **Pathology:** The tissue alterations of ALD are dominated by confluent and often bilaterally symmetric demyelination. The most severe lesions are in the subcortical white matter of the parietooccipital region, which with time extend in a rostral direction. The cerebral cortex is spared. Histologically, a severe loss of myelinated axons and oligodendrocytes is noted in the affected areas, together with astrogliosis. A conspicuous perivascular infiltrate of mononuclear cells, mostly lymphocytes, is common. Scattered macrophages contain periodic acid–Schiff (PAS)-positive and sudanophilic material. The peripheral nerves are also depleted of myelin, but to a lesser degree than the brain.

The adrenals are characteristically atrophic, and electron microscopy reveals pathognomonic cytoplasmic, membrane-bound, curvilinear inclusions or clefts (lamellae) in the cortical cells. These lamellae contain VLCFAs, probably in the form of cholesterol esters. Similar inclusions have been observed in Schwann cells and macrophages in the nervous system lesions.

Alexander Disease

Alexander disease is a rare neurological disorder of infants and children characterized pathologically by a loss of myelin in the brain and a striking accumulation of irregular, extracellular fibers (Rosenthal fibers; Fig. 28-110). Clinically, these children have psychomotor retardation, progressive dementia, and paralysis and eventually die.

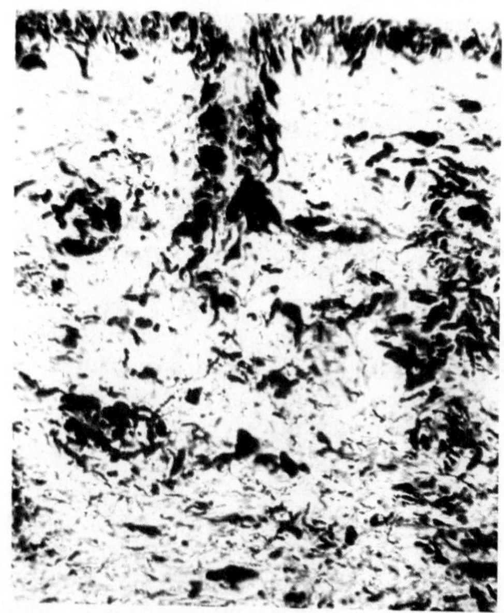

FIGURE *28-110*
Alexander disease. Rosenthal fibers are aggregated beneath the pia and about blood vessels.

□ **Pathogenesis:** The basis for demyelination and the genesis of the Rosenthal fibers is not clear. The degeneration of myelin, and in this instance, its lack of formation suggest an inborn error of metabolism. The primitive glial cells take origin in the germinal mantle and migrate centrifugally into the hemispheres, where they align along axons for the purpose of myelination. It has been suggested that in Alexander disease, the primitive glial cells fail to establish this critical structural alignment. As a consequence, they continue to migrate outward until they encounter a barrier, such as a blood vessel or the pia. It is presumed that in this ectopic position, these glial cells elaborate proteolipids that have the staining characteristics of myelin but not the normal membranous configuration that is acquired through an anatomic relation with an axon.

□ **Pathology:** The histological appearance of the CNS in Alexander disease is strikingly abnormal, because of the presence of innumerable Rosenthal fibers. These irregular, beaded formations of proteolipids are deposited in the subpial mantle of the cerebrum, in the molecular cortex of the cerebellum, in the periphery of the spinal cord, and in the outer margins of the optic and olfactory nerves. Less intense depositions surround the blood vessels (see Fig. 28-110). Small Rosenthal fibers are present in glial processes. Larger Rosenthal fibers appear as irregular elongated or spiral extracellular accumulations. The content of myelin in the white matter is strikingly deficient. Interestingly, in Alexander disease, myelin is well preserved in the peripheral nerves.

Multiple Sclerosis

Multiple sclerosis (MS) is a chronic demyelinating disease of the CNS in which there are numerous patches of demyelination throughout the white matter. MS is the single most common chronic disease of the CNS of young adults in the United States, with a prevalence approaching 1 in 1000. The disorder affects sensory and motor functions, and in most cases, is characterized by exacerbations and remissions over a period of many years.

□ **Epidemiology:** MS is principally a disease of temperate climates, being rare in the tropics and increasing in frequency with distance from the equator. Persons who emigrate before age 15 years from areas with a low prevalence of MS to endemic areas acquire an increased risk of developing the disease, suggesting the involvement of an environmental factor acting early in life. MS is acquired at a mean age of 30 years; an onset in children younger than 14 years and in adults after age 60 years is distinctly unusual. Women are afflicted almost twice as often as men.

□ **Pathogenesis:** The precise etiology of MS remains obscure. However, experimental and clinical studies have pointed to a genetic predisposition to MS and an immune pathogenesis. In addition, the epidemiological data discussed earlier suggest the possibility that an infection, presumably viral, acquired before age 15 years might also play a role.

GENETIC FACTORS: A genetic predisposition to MS is suggested by studies showing a familial aggregation of the disease, with an increased risk in second- and third-degree relatives of patients with MS. Moreover, monozygotic twins show a 25% concordance for MS, whereas only 2% of dizygotic twins are both afflicted. Susceptibility also is associated with a number of major histocompatibility complex (MHC) alleles, particularly HLA-DR2. This association suggests that immune mechanisms are involved in the pathogenesis. Indeed, studies of siblings, both of whom had MS, revealed a striking concordance for the same T-cell receptor haplotype.

IMMUNE FACTORS: The evidence supporting a role for immune mechanisms in MS comes from the histological appearance of the lesions and from the experimental production of demyelination by sensitization to myelin-derived antigens.

The chronic lesions of MS demonstrate perivascular lymphocytes and macrophages, and at the margins, numerous CD4+ (helper-inducer subset) and CD8+ T cells accumulate. Whereas rearrangements of the T-cell receptor gene are not present in peripheral lymphocytes of patients with MS, the CD4+ T cells isolated from the CSF appear to be oligoclonal. Although the target antigen of this oligoclonal population has not been identified, the data suggest an immune response to a specific protein of the CNS.

Further support for immune mechanisms in the pathogenesis of MS comes from the experimental production of an antigen-specific, T cell–mediated autoimmune demyelinating disease, termed *experimental allergic encephalitis* (*EAE*). The injection of myelin basic protein into a variety of experimental animals, including nonhuman primates, results in relapsing or progressive paralysis and demyelinating lesions in the CNS, which exhibit perivascular lymphocytic infiltrates. As in MS, EAE is linked to class II immune response genes.

INFECTIOUS AGENTS: A wide variety of viruses have been implicated in the etiology of MS at one time or another, including vaccinia, mumps, rubella, herpes simplex, and measles. However to date, no direct evidence exists for the involvement of any infectious agent. More recently, a possible role for JC virus, the etiological agent of progressive multifocal leukoencephalopathy, has been proposed but requires further study. This agent can selectively initiate demyelination in the CNS, presumably because the virus replicates in oligodendrocytes, where it may interfere with the support of myelin metabolism.

☐ **Pathology: The plaque is the hallmark of MS** (Fig. 28-111A). Characteristically, plaques of variable size, rarely more than 2 cm in diameter, accumulate in great numbers in the brain and spinal cord. They are remarkably discrete and frequently possess smoothly rounded contours. Usually situated in the white matter, the plaques occasionally breach the gray–white junction, but only rarely are they seated entirely in the gray cortex. The lesion exhibits a preference for the optic nerves and chiasm and uniformly localizes to the paraventricular white

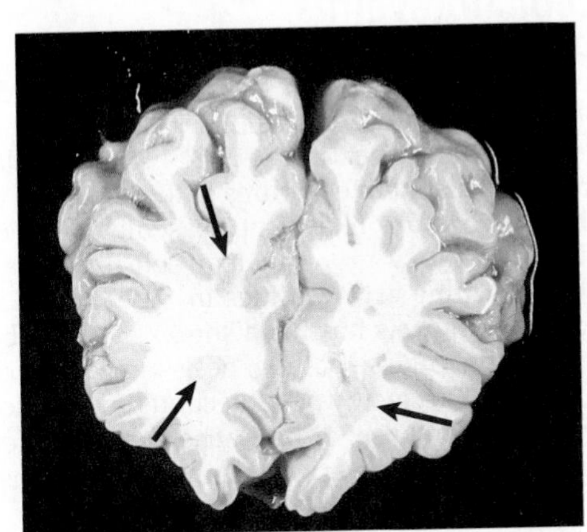

A

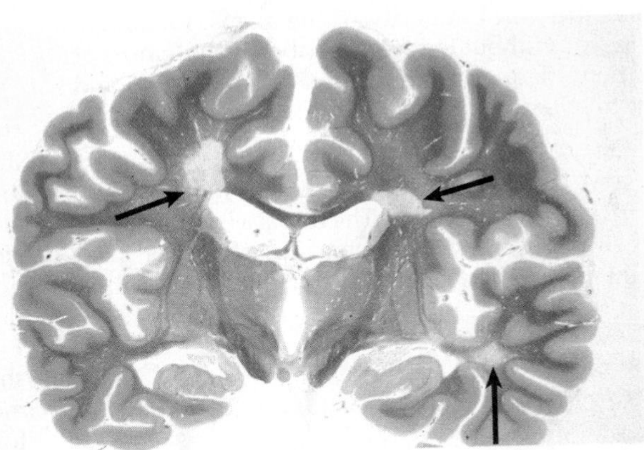

B

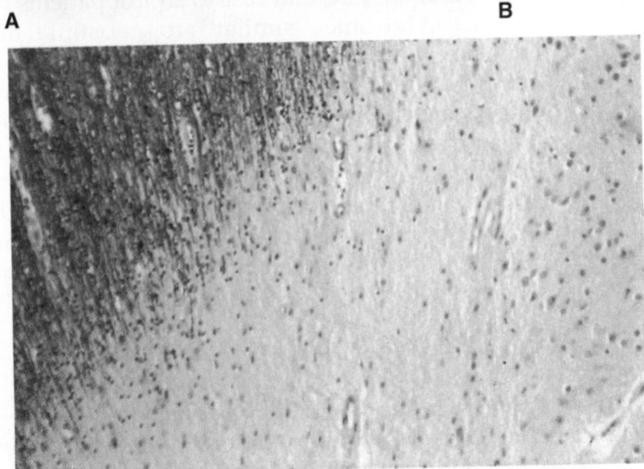

C

FIGURE *28-111*
Multiple sclerosis. (*A*) In this unfixed brain, the plaques of multiple sclerosis in the white matter (*arrows*) assume the darker color of the cerebral cortex. (*B*) A coronal section of the brain from a patient with long-standing multiple sclerosis, which has been stained for myelin, shows discrete areas of demyelination (*arrows*), with characteristic involvement of the superior angles of the lateral ventricles. (*C*) A higher magnification of *B* shows the edge of a plaque and emphasizes the regional character of the lesion. Both motor and sensory fibers lose their myelin but retain axonal continuity as they traverse the lesion.

matter of the corona radiata (see Fig. 28-111B). Otherwise, the distribution of plaques is highly random, and they indiscriminately involve the cerebrum, cerebellum, brainstem, and spinal cord.

The evolving plaque is marked by the following morphological hallmarks:

- Selective loss of myelin in a region of axonal preservation (see Fig. 28-111C)
- A few lymphocytes that cluster about small veins and arteries (Fig. 28-112)
- An influx of macrophages
- Considerable edema

When neurons are encompassed by the boundaries of a plaque, the neuronal cell bodies are remarkably spared. The number of oligodendrocytes is moderately diminished, although they show no distinctive structural alterations. As the plaque ages, it becomes more discrete, and edema regresses. This serves to emphasize the focal nature of the tissue injury, its selectivity for myelin, and its severity, because demyelination is total within the area of the plaque. A rare plaque that is traversed by a few myelinated fibers is referred to as a "shadow plaque."

Characteristically, an axon that approaches the area of tissue injury loses its myelin sheath abruptly, in precisely the same physical relation to the plaque as that of all other neighboring axons, although some may be motor and others sensory. The denuded axons traverse the plaque, and in unison again acquire myelin on the opposite edge of the lesion (see Fig. 28-111C).

The aging plaque acquires astrocytes, and with time the tissue becomes dense with glial processes. This "scar" impairs the structural integrity of the axons. Oligodendroglia are lost without evidence of abortive attempts at remyelination. Plaques rarely exhibit frank necrosis and are not cystic.

☐ **Clinical Features:** MS usually has its onset during the third or fourth decades. The disease is punctuated thereafter by abrupt and brief episodes of clinical progression interspersed with periods of relative stability.

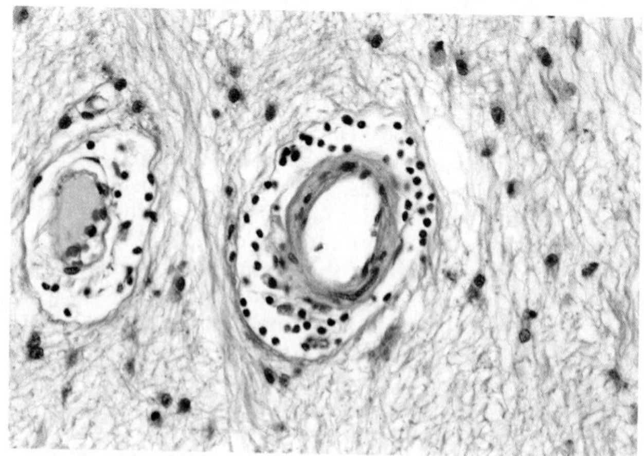

FIGURE *28-112*
Multiple sclerosis. An end-stage lesion features astrogliosis, thick-walled blood vessels, moderate perivascular inflammation, and a secondary loss of axons.

However, some patients with MS exhibit a relentless course without any remissions. Each exacerbation is the expression of the formation of additional plaques of demyelination. The visual system and the paraventricular areas are particularly vulnerable to the disease, whereas the peripheral nerves are uniformly spared.

Multiple sclerosis typically begins with symptoms relating to lesions in the optic nerves, brainstem, or spinal cord. Blurred vision, or the loss of vision in one eye, is often the presenting complaint. When the initial lesion is in the brainstem, the most troubling early symptoms are double vision and vertigo. Plaques within the spinal cord are reflected in weakness of one or both legs and sensory symptoms in the form of numbness in the lower extremities. Many of the initial symptoms are partially reversible within a few months.

Unfortunately, in most patients with MS, the disease recurs and thereafter follows a chronic relapsing and remitting course, with the development of permanent lesions. In established cases, the degree of functional impairment is highly variable, ranging from minor disability to severe incapacity, with widespread paralysis, dysarthria, severe visual defects, incontinence, and dementia. The patients usually die of respiratory paralysis or urinary tract infections in terminal coma. Most patients with MS survive 20 to 30 years after the onset of symptoms. In some people with MS, treatment with interferon beta has been reported to be helpful.

Postinfectious and Postvaccinal Encephalomyelitis

A number of viral exanthems (e.g., measles, varicella, and rubella) are on rare occasions followed by an encephalomyelitis, appearing between 3 and 21 days after the rash. The distinctive features of the lesions in the brain and spinal cord are foci of perivascular demyelination and a conspicuous mononuclear cell infiltrate around small to medium-sized venules in the white matter. An immunological basis for this disorder has long been suspected, but the precise pathogenesis remains unclear.

Children affected by postinfectious encephalomyelitis show the sudden onset of headache, vomiting, fever, and meningeal signs. In severe cases, these symptoms may be followed by paraplegia, incontinence, and stupor. The disease is often severe, and 15% to 20% of patients die.

A syndrome similar to postinfectious encephalomyelitis may follow immunization against several infectious agents, notably smallpox (historically) and rabies, and is termed *postvaccinal encephalomyelitis*. Postrabies immunization encephalomyelitis occurred for many years after using a vaccine made from rabbit spinal cord and contaminated with neural antigens. With the development of rabies vaccines prepared from human cells in culture, this complication has virtually disappeared.

Central Pontine Myelinolysis

Central pontine myelinolysis is a rare demyelinating disorder that affects the pons of malnourished persons, principally alcoholics. Discrete areas of selective demyelination occur as

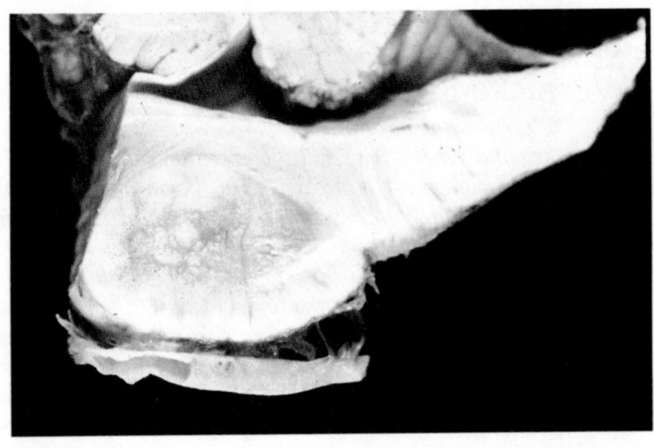

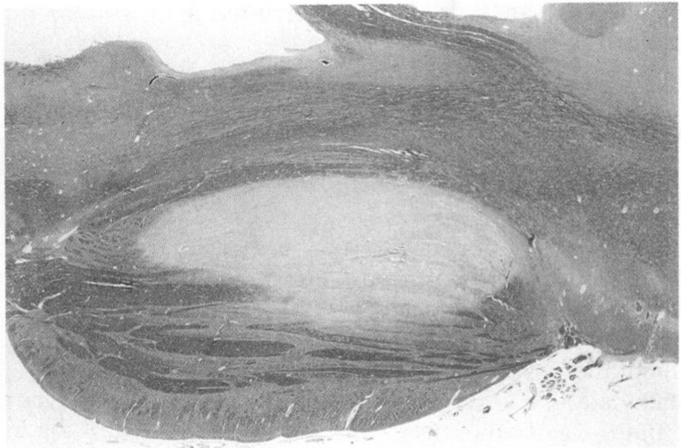

FIGURE *28-113*
Central pontine myelinolysis. (*A*) A sagittal section of the brainstem shows a soft lesion in the tegmentum of the pons. (*B*) A section of *A* stained for myelin reveals a sharply demarcated loss of myelin.

solitary lesions in the pons (Fig. 28-113). In many cases, the lesions are too small to have clinical manifestations and are discovered only at autopsy. In a few patients, quadriparesis, pseudobulbar palsy, or a severe depression of consciousness ("pseudocoma") may occur. The precise etiology of central pontine myelinolysis has not been established, but it is thought to relate to disturbances associated with the rapid therapeutic correction of hyponatremia.

NEURONAL STORAGE DISEASES

Neuronal storage diseases are all the result of the accumulation of normal metabolic products within lysosomes owing to an inherited deficiency in specific catabolic enzymes. They are discussed in detail in Chapter 6, and only the highlights of the neurological manifestations are presented here.

Tay–Sachs Disease

Tay–Sachs disease (amaurotic familial idiocy) is a lethal, autosomal recessive disorder caused by an inborn deficiency of hexosaminidase A, which permits the accumulation of a ganglioside within the neurons of the CNS. The disease is fatal in infancy and early childhood. Retinal involvement increases macular transparency and is responsible for a *cherry-red spot* in the position of the macula.

The brain is the major site of storage of gangliosides, and this organ progressively enlarges during infancy. On histological examination, lipid droplets are seen within the cytoplasm of distended nerve cells, both in the central and peripheral nervous systems. Electron microscopy reveals the lipid to be largely present within lysosomes in the form of whorled "myelin figures." The neural tissues respond with a diffuse astrogliosis.

An affected infant appears normal at birth but shows a delay in motor development by age 6 months. Thereafter, progressive deterioration leads to a state of flaccid weakness, blindness, and severe mental impairment. Death usually supervenes before the end of the second year.

Hurler Syndrome

Hurler syndrome is an autosomal recessive disturbance in glycosaminoglycan metabolism that results in the intraneuronal accumulation of mucopolysaccharides. The clinical variants of this syndrome are distinguished by variable involvement of visceral organs and the nervous system. The disease is typically expressed in infancy or early childhood as dwarfism, corneal opacities, skeletal deformities, and hepatosplenomegaly. The intraneuronal storage distends the cytoplasmic compartment and is accompanied by astrogliosis.

Gaucher Disease

Gaucher disease is an autosomal recessive genetic disorder characterized by a deficiency of glucocerebrosidase and the accumulation of glucocerebroside, principally in macrophages. The CNS is most severely involved in the infantile type (type II) of Gaucher disease. Although intraneuronal accumulation of glucocerebroside is not conspicuous, neuronal loss is severe and is accompanied by diffuse astrogliosis. These infants fail to thrive and die at an early age.

Niemann–Pick Disease

Niemann–Pick disease is an autosomal recessive disorder in which intraneuronal storage of sphingomyelin results from a deficiency of sphingomyelinase. The clinical symptoms occur early, and the disease is marked by failure of the infant to develop and thrive. The mononuclear phagocyte system is targeted for storage, but the nervous system may predominate symptomatically during infancy. The brain becomes atrophic and shows marked astrogliosis. Retinal degeneration may produce a cherry-red spot, similar to that in Tay–Sachs disease.

METABOLIC NEURONAL DISEASES

Phenylketonuria

Phenylketonuria (PKU) is an autosomal recessive disorder that reflects a deficiency in phenylalanine hydroxylase (see Chapter 6). Phenylalanine accumulates in the blood and tissues, owing to a block in the conversion of phenylalanine to tyrosine. The condition becomes apparent in the early months of life and leads to mental retardation, seizures, and impaired physical development. Untreated patients rarely obtain an IQ above 50. Although cognitive functions are seriously disturbed, there is no consistent alteration in neuronal cytoarchitecture. In a few cases, the brain has been found to be underweight and deficient in myelination.

Cretinism

Severe hypothyroidism in infancy, termed cretinism, alters the functional capacity of the CNS. The disorder is reversible by the early administration of thyroxine, but when the deficiency persists beyond a few months, the disease becomes unalterable. Even in the dysfunctional state, the brain acquires a near-normal weight, has appropriate neuronal cytoarchitecture, and is well myelinated. However, the patient is typically stunted in growth and severely handicapped intellectually.

Wilson Disease

This autosomal recessive disease is an inherited disorder of copper metabolism, which affects the brain and the liver, thus the synonym "hepatolenticular degeneration" (see Chapter 14). Although the pathogenesis of Wilson disease is still debated, there is a consensus that defective biliary excretion of copper is involved. The total circulating copper in Wilson disease is decreased, but free copper (i.e., not bound to ceruloplasmin) is increased, a situation that may favor the deposition of copper in the brain. The cerebral intoxication generally appears clinically in the second decade and is evidenced in athetoid movements. Before, during, or after the appearance of neurological symptoms, an insidiously developing cirrhosis of the liver may be seen as hepatic failure. The deposition of copper in the limbus of the cornea produces a visible golden-brown band, the *Kayser–Fleischer ring* (see Chapter 29).

On gross examination of the brain, the lenticulate nuclei may show a light golden discoloration. In one fourth of the cases, small cysts or clefts are evident macroscopically either in the putamen or in the lower margins of the cortical gray mantle. Histologically a scant loss of neurons and a mild gliosis in the lenticulate nuclei understate the severe chorioathetoid movement disorder that characterizes the disease.

VITAMIN DEFICIENCIES

Wernicke Syndrome

Wernicke syndrome is the result of thiamine (vitamin B_1) deficiency, characterized clinically as a disturbance in thermal regulation, altered consciousness, ophthalmoplegia, and nystagmus and pathologically by lesions in the hypothalamus and mamillary bodies, the periaqueductal regions of the midbrain, and the tegmentum of the pons (Fig. 28-114). The syndrome arises most commonly in association with chronic alcoholism, but it may appear in patients whose nutrition is sustained by infusions that lack thiamine. Typically, the onset of symptoms is precipitate.

Wernicke syndrome may progress rapidly to death, but in most cases, it is promptly reversible on the administration of thiamine. In fatal cases, petechiae about small capillaries are conspicuous in the mamillary bodies, the hypothalamus, the periaqueductal gray matter, and the floor of the fourth ventricle. The prior occurrence of lesions is permanently marked by the presence of brown hemosiderin. Interestingly, neurons and myelin are spared in Wernicke encephalopathy. However, the mamillary bodies become atrophic.

Wernicke–Korsakoff syndrome is a clinical term that refers to a state of disordered memory for recent events, often compensated for by confabulation, in chronic alcoholism. The histological changes, when present, are distinguished from those of Wernicke syndrome by chromatolysis and degeneration of neurons in the medial–dorsal nucleus of the thalamus. Thus, Wernicke syndrome and Korsakoff psychosis occur concurrently in the setting of chronic alcoholism, but their causes may (or may not) be different.

Alcoholism

The problems associated with alcoholism embrace both nutrition and intoxication. Four cerebral lesions warrant consideration (Fig. 28-115):

- Cortical atrophy
- Atrophy of the superior aspect of the vermis of the cerebellum (Fig. 28-116)
- Wernicke syndrome (see Fig. 28-114)
- Central pontine myelinolysis (see Fig. 28-113)

Many chronic alcoholics display cerebral atrophy, but the cause of this association is still not entirely clear. The relative roles of direct alcohol toxicity, malnutrition, and perhaps other factors remain to be defined. The same lack of precise causation prevails with regard to the atrophy of the Purkinje and granular cells of the cerebellum. This alteration is the most common corollary of chronic alcoholism and is ostensibly the cause of truncal ataxia, which persists during periods of sobriety. As previously noted, the lesions of Wernicke syndrome are intimately related to thiamine deficiency, and central pontine myelinolysis is presumably an iatrogenic complication caused by the rapid correction of hyponatremia.

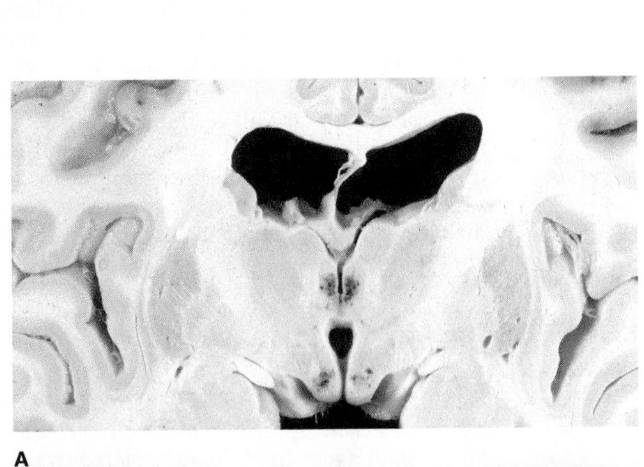

A

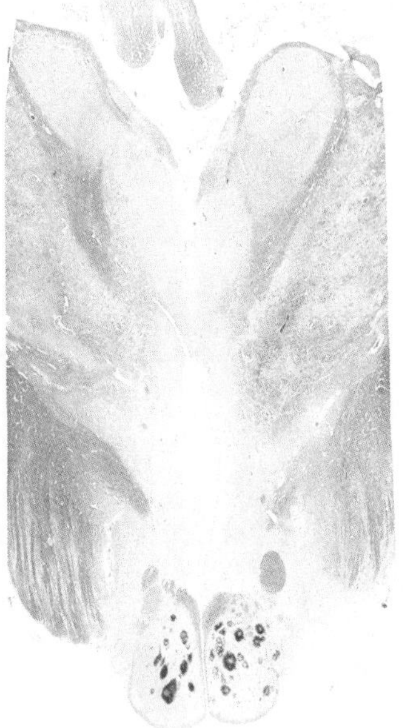

B

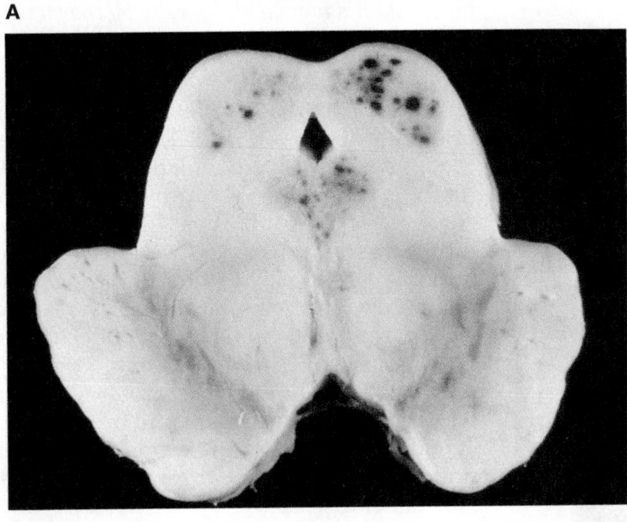

C

FIGURE *28-114*
Wernicke encephalopathy. (*A*) The mamillary bodies and the paraventricular regions exhibit petechiae. (*B*) A histological section of *A*, stained with luxol fast blue, emphasizes the selectivity for the mamillary bodies. (*C*) The quadrigeminal plate and periaqueductal regions display conspicuous petechiae.

Hepatic Encephalopathy

Hepatic encephalopathy is a common clinical expression of severe liver failure, manifested as delirium, seizures, and coma (see Chapter 14). In general, the clinical symptoms greatly exceed their morphological corollaries. The latter are restricted to the appearance of altered astroglia, termed Alzheimer type II astrocytes. In these cells, the nuclei are enlarged, and the chromatin material is marginated. These changes are generally more prominent in the thalamus.

Subacute Combined Degeneration of the Spinal Cord

Subacute combined degeneration of the spinal cord is a result of a deficiency of vitamin B_{12} (pernicious anemia) and features lesions in the posterolateral portions of the spinal cord (see Chapters 14 and 20). The initial lesion is a symmetrical loss of myelin and axons at the thoracic level of the spinal cord (see Fig. 28-121). Although astrogliosis is typically mild in the acute lesion, with time the area of degeneration loses its spongiform appearance, and the cord becomes atrophic and scarred by astrocytes. When progressive, the lesions extend both caudad and cephalad, producing an edematous, spongiform appearance in the posterolateral areas of the cord.

A burning sensation in the soles of the feet, along with other paresthesias, ushers in a rapidly progressive, only partially reversible, neurological deficit. Weakness is usually present in all four limbs. Eventually, defective postural sensibility leads to incoordination of the lower limbs and ataxia.

In addition to pernicious anemia, subacute combined degeneration may complicate a rare case of extensive gastric resection and other malabsorption syn-

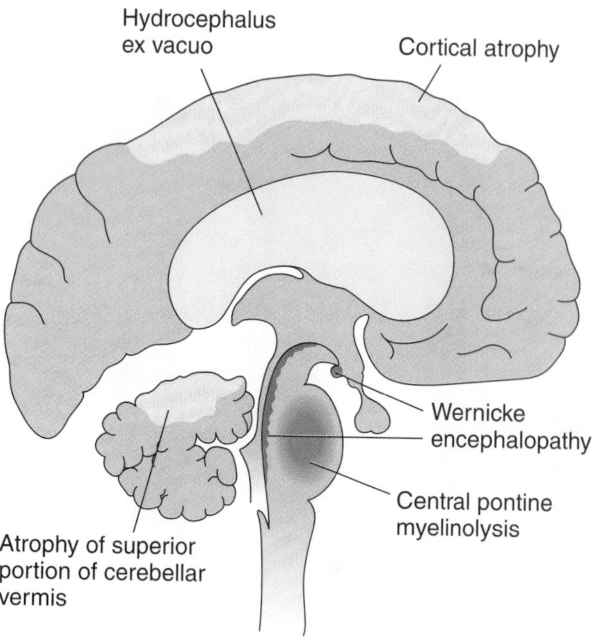

FIGURE 28-115
Lesions of the brain associated with chronic alcoholism.

dromes. Because vitamin B_{12} is not found in plants, some extreme vegetarians who eschew all animal products, even milk and eggs, have developed subacute combined degeneration after many years on the restricted diet.

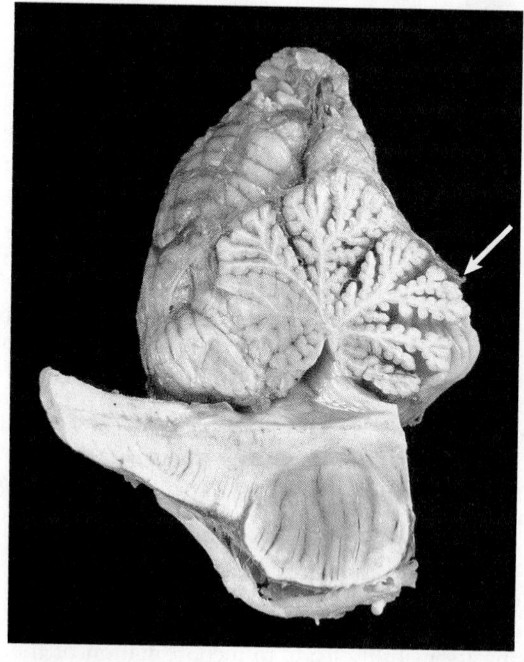

FIGURE 28-116
Chronic alcoholism. The superior and anterior portions of the vermis of the cerebellum (*arrow*) are atrophic.

DEGENERATIVE DISEASES

This heterogeneous group of disorders includes Parkinson disease, amyotrophic lateral sclerosis, Huntington disease, the spinocerebellar ataxias, and Alzheimer disease (Fig. 28-117). Some of these maladies involve primarily a single neuronal species (Parkinson disease), whereas others affect specific neuroanatomic systems or regions (Huntington disease) or the nervous system diffusely (Alzheimer disease). Until recently, the etiology and pathophysiology of all of these disorders has been frustratingly idiopathic. Modern investigative techniques, however, are now providing exciting insights, as exemplified by the discovery of trinucleotide repeat expansion mutations as the genetic basis for a number of neurodegenerative diseases.

Parkinson Disease

First described in 1817, Parkinson disease (PD) is a neurological disorder characterized pathologically by the loss of neurons in the substantia nigra and clinically by tremors at rest, muscular rigidity, expressionless countenance, and emotional lability.

☐ **Epidemiology:** PD typically appears in the sixth to eighth decades of life. The disease is common, and more than 2% of the population in North America eventually develop PD. The prevalence has remained unchanged for at least the past 40 years, and no sex or racial differences are apparent. Genetic factors do not seem to be important, especially in view of the low concordance rate in monozygotic twins. However, a rare, autosomal dominant, early-onset, familial form of PD has been identified. This variant is characterized by a point mutation in the α-synuclein gene on the long arm of chromosome 4, which codes for a prosynaptic protein. Interestingly, α-synuclein is the source of a small peptide that forms the nonamyloid component of the amyloid plaques in Alzheimer disease.

☐ **Pathogenesis:** The vast majority of cases of PD are idiopathic, but the disease has been recorded after viral encephalitis (von Economo encephalitis) and after the intake of a toxic chemical (1-methyl-4-phenyl-1,2,3,6-tetrahydropyridine; MPTP). The substantia nigra is a component of the extrapyramidal system that relays information to the basal ganglia through dopaminergic synapses. Normal aging is associated with a loss of neurons in the substantia nigra and a reduction in the dopamine content of that region. It has been suggested that PD is simply an acceleration of normal age-related changes. Yet this explanation does not account for the declining incidence of the disease after the age of 80 years.

One theory advanced to explain the loss of neurons in the substantia nigra holds that oxidative stress produced by the autooxidation of catecholamines during melanin formation injures these cells. There is accumulating evidence that the pathogenesis of PD may be related to both oxidative stress and a reduced ability to deal with it.

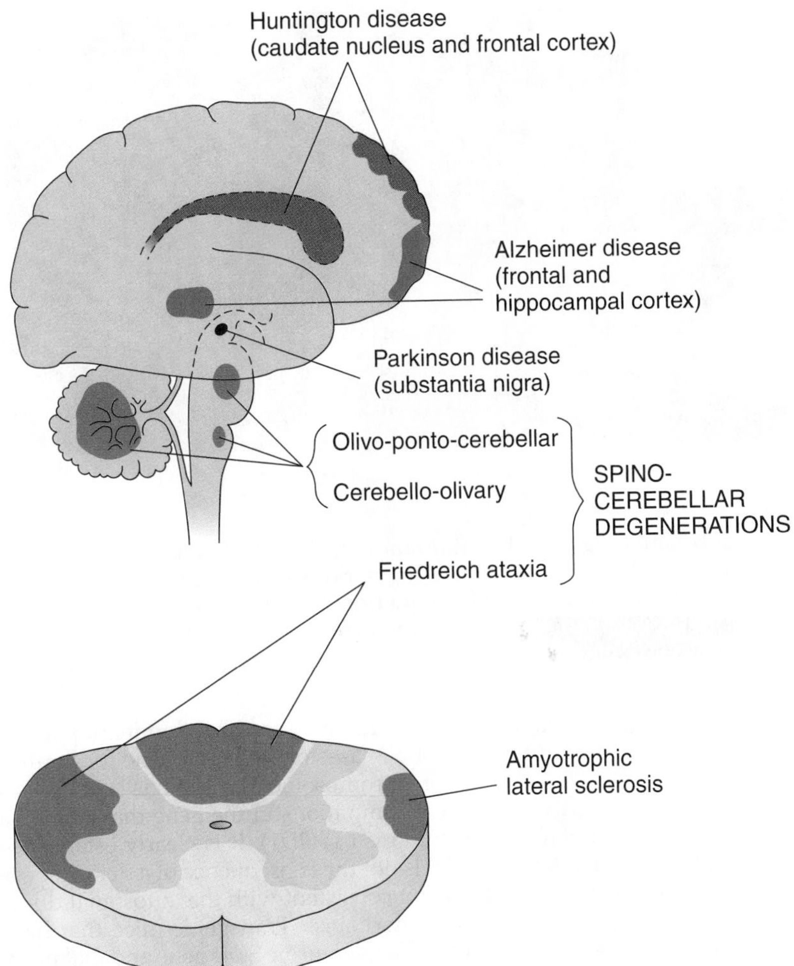

FIGURE *28-117*
Distribution of degenerative diseases of the central nervous system.

Defects in mitochondrial electron transport have been described in patients with PD. Mitochondrial defects in the presence of oxidative stress could be lethal to the dopaminergic neurons of the substantia nigra. In this respect, it is noteworthy that a by-product of the illicit synthesis of meperidine analogues, MPTP, induced a PD-like syndrome in intravenous drug users. MPTP is an inhibitor of mitochondrial electron transport and thus may produce parkinsonism by a mechanism similar to that of naturally occurring PD.

Historically, von Economo encephalitis (encephalitis lethargica) during the influenza epidemic of 1916 to 1920 resulted in injury to the substantia nigra. Depending on the extent of neuronal destruction, the consequent clinical expressions of postencephalitic parkinsonism were immediate or delayed. Although postmortem examination disclosed a gross loss of pigmentation in the substantia nigra and locus ceruleus, the neuropathology of postencephalitic parkinsonism differs from that of idiopathic PD. Whereas PD is characterized by Lewy bodies (see later), these neuronal inclusions were rare in postencephalitic parkinsonism. Moreover, the latter displayed neurofibrillary tangles, which are uncommon in idiopathic PD.

☐ **Pathology:** Gross examination of the brain reveals a loss of pigmentation in the substantia nigra and locus ceruleus (Fig. 28-118A). On microscopic examination, pigmented neurons are scarce, and there are small extracellular deposits of melanin, derived from necrotic neurons. Some residual nerve cells are atrophic, and a few contain spherical, eosinophilic cytoplasmic inclusions, termed *Lewy bodies* (Fig. 28-118B). As viewed by electron microscopy, these are dense accumulations of filamentous and granular debris.

With the passage of time, the neuronal degeneration of PD extends beyond the substantia nigra to involve the dopaminergic nigrostriatal pathways. Secondary degenerative changes are present in the striatum, particularly the putamen.

☐ **Clinical Features:** PD is characterized by a slowness of all voluntary movements and a muscular rigidity throughout the entire range of movement. Most patients have a coarse tremor of the distal extremities, which is present at rest and disappears with voluntary movement. The face is expressionless (mask-like), and a reduced rate of swallowing leads to drooling. There is an

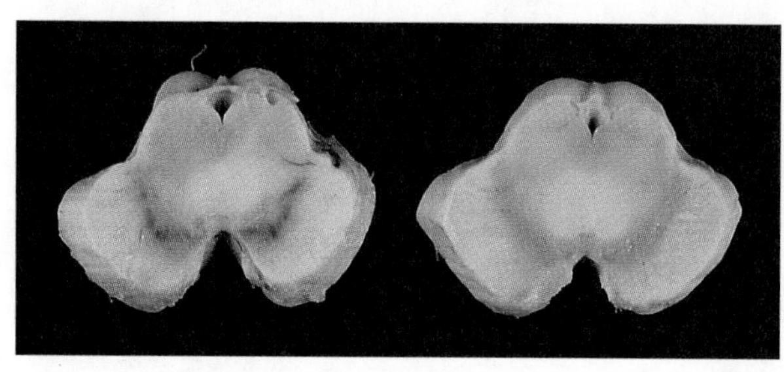

A

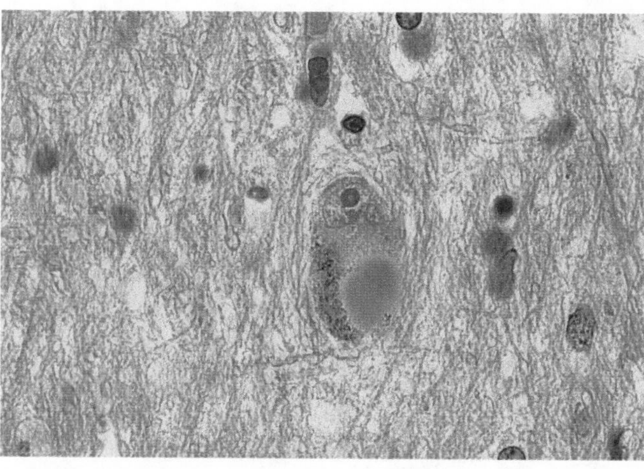

B

FIGURE 28-118
Parkinson disease. (*A*) The normal substantia nigra of the midbrain (*left*) is heavily pigmented, whereas the same region from a patient with long-standing parkinsonism (*right*) has lost the pigment. (*B*) A microscopic section of the substantia nigra from the patient with parkinsonism shows a spherical eosinophilic inclusion within the cytoplasm of a pigmented dopaminergic neuron, termed a "Lewy body."

increased incidence of depression and dementia. In early parkinsonism, substitution therapy with levodopa is beneficial. However, this therapy does not rectify the underlying disorder and with the passage of several years becomes ineffective.

Striatonigral degeneration is a rare disorder that mimics PD so closely that it is rarely diagnosed during life. At autopsy, the corpus striatum (caudate and putamen) is visibly atrophied, and microscopic examination shows severe loss of neurons in these loci. Less severe changes occur in the substantia nigra and locus ceruleus.

Progressive supranuclear palsy is another unusual neurological disorder that is clinically similar to PD but adds a progressive paralysis of vertical eye movements. The course of the disease is relentless, with death within 5 to 10 years. The pathological changes in the brain are more widespread than those of PD, with loss of neurons in the globus pallidus, subthalamic nucleus, red nucleus, tectum, periaqueductal gray matter, and dentate nuclei.

Amyotrophic Lateral Sclerosis

Amyotrophic lateral sclerosis (ALS) is a degenerative disease of motor neurons of the brain and spinal cord, which results in progressive weakness and wasting of the extremities and eventually impairment of the respiratory muscles.

☐ **Epidemiology and Pathogenesis:** ALS is a worldwide disease with an incidence of 1 in 100,000. The frequency of the disease peaks in the fifth decade of life, and it is rare in persons younger than 35 years. There is a 1.5- to 2.0-fold excess of ALS in men. Restricted geographic areas with a particularly high incidence of ALS exist in Guam and parts of Japan and Papua New Guinea, but there is some question whether these cases are the same disorder as in the rest of the world.

Familial cases, with an autosomal dominant pattern, account for 5% of all cases of ALS. The gene for familial ALS is located on chromosome 21q and has been associated with missense mutations in the gene that codes for superoxide dismutase 1 (*SOD1*). It is clearly established that familial ALS is not the consequence of a deficiency of SOD activity, a fact consistent with the autosomal dominant pattern of inheritance. Transgenic mice that have two normal copies of the murine SOD gene and that in addition express the human mutant SOD1 protein develop a syndrome that closely resembles ALS. Thus, the mutant gene in ALS seems to act through a gain of function, which has been hypothesized to represent an exaggerated peroxidase activity of *SOD1*. It is suspected that oxidative reactions catalyzed by mutant *SOD1* may initiate the neurodegenerative lesions of familial ALS.

☐ **Pathology:** ALS affects motor neurons in three locations: (1) the anterior horn cells of the spinal cord; (2) the motor nuclei of the brainstem, particularly the hypoglossal nuclei; and (2) the upper motor neurons of the cerebral cortex. The injury to the motor neurons leads to degeneration of their axons, visualized in striking alterations of the lateral pyramidal pathways in the spinal cord.

The defining histological change in ALS is a loss of large motor neurons accompanied by mild gliosis (Fig. 28-119A). This change is most evident in the anterior horns of the lumbar cord and cervical enlargements of the spinal cord and in the hypoglossal nuclei. There is also a loss of the giant pyramidal Betz cells in the motor cortex of the cerebrum. The most striking secondary change in the spinal cord is a loss of myelinated fibers in the lateral corticospinal tracts (see Fig. 28-121), which imparts a pallor to these areas when they are viewed with myelin stains. The anterior nerve roots are atrophic (Fig. 28-119B), and the affected muscles are pale and shrunken.

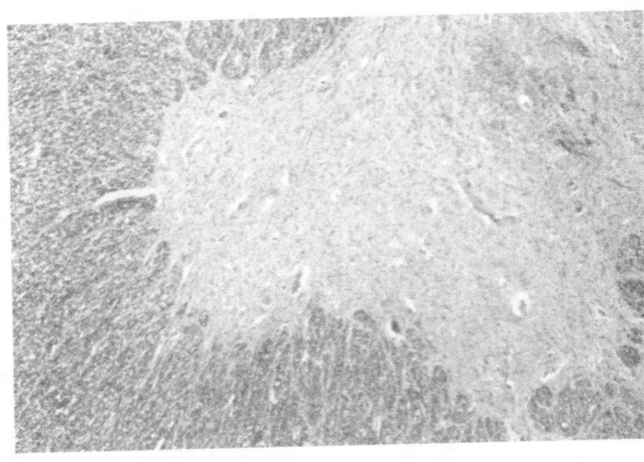
A

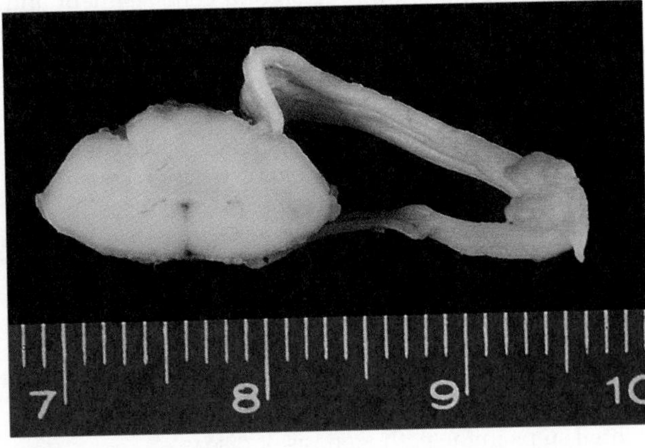

B

FIGURE 28-119
Amyotrophic lateral sclerosis. (*A*) A photomicrograph of the anterior horn of the spinal cord reveals a severe loss of motor neurons, without evidence of inflammation. (*B*) The ventral root is grossly atrophic as a result of neuronal depletion in the anterior horn.

☐ **Clinical Features:** ALS generally is seen as weakness and wasting of the muscles of a hand, often accompanied by painful cramps of the muscles of the arm. Irregular rapid contractions of the muscles that do not move the limb (fasciculations) are characteristic. The disease is inexorably progressive, with increasing weakness of the limbs leading to total disability. Speech may become unintelligible, and respiratory weakness supervenes. Despite the dramatic wasting of the body, intellectual capacity is preserved to the end. The clinical course generally extends beyond a decade.

Trinucleotide Repeat Expansion Syndromes

The striking progress seen in elucidation of the genetic basis for many medical disorders over the past decade is reflected in the investigation of the central nervous system degenerative diseases. In particular, a large group of neurological diseases can now be classified on a genetic basis as trinucleotide repeat expansion syndromes (Table 28-3). The first such disorder to be identified was Fragile X syndrome in 1991, followed by spinal and bulbar muscular atrophy and myotonic dystrophy. The triplet repeat mutation disorders now include Huntington disease and Friedreich ataxia.

As seen in Table 28-3, trinucleotide repeats are a normal feature of many genes, and the expansion of the number of triplet repeats confers pathogenicity. Some triplet repeat diseases feature only a narrow gap between the normal and disease distributions (e.g., Huntington disease), whereas in others, the separation is large (e.g., Fragile X syndrome and Friedreich ataxia). This class of mutation encompasses examples of all forms of inheritance, including X-linked, autosomal dominant, and autosomal recessive. In some of these disorders, the expansion muta-

TABLE 28-3 **Trinucleotide Repeat Expansion Syndromes**

Disease (year triplet identified)	Inheritance Pattern	Chromosome Locus/Protein	Trinucleotide	Normal Repeat Range	Disease Repeat Range
Fragile X syndrome (1991)	X-linked	Xq27.3	CGG	5–54	230–4000
Spinal and bulbar muscular atrophy (1991)	X-linked	Xq11-12/androgen receptor	CAG	12–34	40–62
Myotonic dystrophy (1992)	AD	19q13.2/cAMP-dependent serine-threonine protein kinase	CTG	5–37	44–3000
Huntington disease (1993)	AD	4p16.3/huntingtin	CAG	11–30	36–121
Olivopontocerevellar atrophy (Spinocerebellar atrophy type 1) (1993)	AD	6p22-23/ataxin	CAG	19–36	40–81
Dentato-rubro-pallido-luysian atrophy (DRPLA) (1994)	AD	12p12-ter/atrophin	CAG	8–35	54–79
Machado–Joseph disease (Spinocerebellar atrophy type 3) (1994)	AD	14q24.3–32	CAG	12–37	61–84
Friedreich ataxia (1996)	AR	9q13.3–21.1/frataxin	GAA	7–22	120–1700

AD, autosomal dominant; AR, autosomal recessive; cAMP, cyclic adenosine monophosphate.

tion lies within the coding region of a gene segment and results in the production of an abnormal ("toxic") protein, as appears to be the case for most of the autosomal dominant CAG expansion disorders. In others, the expansion occurs in a noncoding region of the gene and presumably interferes with transcription or message processing. The resulting decreased level of protein production constitutes a loss-of-function mutation (as appears to be the case with the GAA expansion of Friedreich ataxia). The identification of the specific chromosomal locus, gene, and mutation in these disorders is only the first step in understanding the pathophysiology of the disease. For most of the triplet expansion disorders, our knowledge is embryonic, and much work remains to be done, including characterization of the normal protein function and elucidation of the sequential steps in the pathogenesis of disease.

Huntington Disease

Huntington disease (HD) is an autosomal dominant genetic disorder characterized by involuntary movements of all parts of the body, deterioration of cognitive functions, and often severe emotional disturbance. First described by a medical student (George Huntington) in 1872, the disorder principally affects whites of northwestern European ancestry, among whom the incidence is 1 in 12,000 to 1 in 20,000. Genealogical studies indicate that all cases of HD derive from the spread of an original focus in northern Europe, and the malady is notably rare in Asia and Africa.

☐ **Pathogenesis:** The HD gene is located on chromosome 4 (4p16.3) and codes for a novel protein, *huntingtin*. In 1993, it was discovered that the genetic alteration at this locus consists of a trinucleotide (CAG) repeat expansion (Table 28-3). The repeat is located within the coding region of the gene and results in production of an altered protein, which contains a polyglutamine tract near the N terminus. In agreement with the dominant mode of inheritance, the triplet expansion likely results in a toxic gain of function. In most autosomal dominant diseases, heterozygotes tend to be less severely affected than homozygotes. **By contrast, HD is one of the purest examples of a true autosomal dominant disorder (i.e., heterozygotes do no differ clinically from homozygotes); the abnormal allele exhibits complete dominance.**

The huntingtin gene product is widely expressed in tissues throughout the body and in all regions of the nervous system, by both neurons and glia. However, its function is unknown. By what mechanism altered huntingtin produces the specific neuroanatomical damage seen in HD is also unknown. A likely possibility is the presence of additional proteins that interact specifically with the expanded polyglutamine tract and are expressed only by the affected cell populations. Recently, a protein (HAP-1) that binds to huntingtin was identified. This protein is particularly expressed in the brain, and its binding to huntingtin is enhanced by expanded polyglutamine repeats.

As with other CAG repeat expansion diseases, a strong inverse correlation is seen between the magnitude of the expansion and the age of clinical onset. Accordingly, the most numerous repeats are seen in juvenile-onset cases. The huntingtin CAG repeat length is unstable in gametes, especially among sperm. Accordingly, the CAG length is more unstable and tends to be longer when inherited from the father, compared with maternal transmission. As a result, HD transmitted from the father results in clinical disease some 3 years earlier than when it is passed from the mother. Moreover, the ratio of children with juvenile-onset HD who inherit the expanded CAG allele from their father compared with their mother is 10:1.

Sporadic (new mutation) cases of HD have until now been thought to be rare. However, testing for huntingtin CAG expression is now revealing increasing numbers of these patients. Most new mutations arise from unstable transmission of triplet repeats from an asymptomatic parent whose alleles exhibit repeat lengths in the zone between the normal (<30) and HD (>36) ranges (referred to as "intermediate alleles").

☐ **Pathology:** On gross examination of the brain from patients who died of HD, the frontal cortex is symmetrically and moderately atrophic, whereas the lateral ventricles appear disproportionately enlarged, owing to the loss of the normal convex curvature of the caudate nuclei (Fig. 28-120). There is symmetric atrophy of the caudate nuclei, with lesser involvement of the putamen. Microscopically, the neuronal population of the caudate and putamen, particularly the small neurons, is greatly

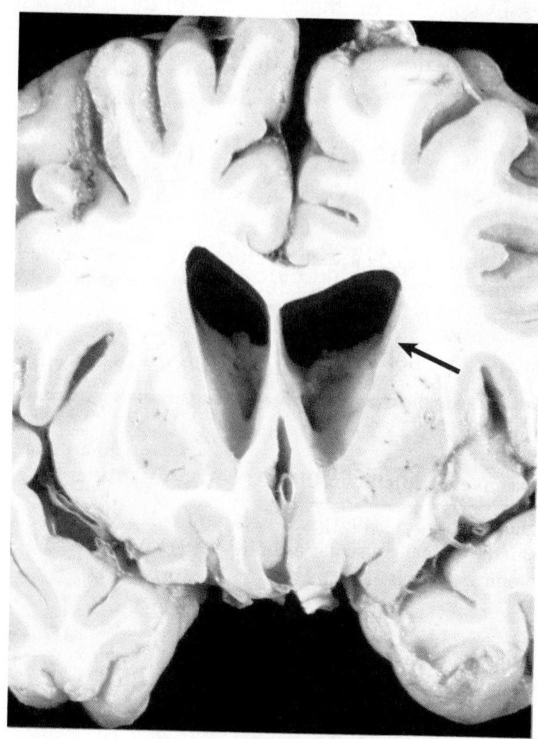

FIGURE *28-120*
Huntington disease. The caudate nuclei (*arrow*) are markedly atrophic, thereby imparting a concave rather than a normal convex curvature to the lateral walls of the ventricles.

depleted, and there is an accompanying moderate astrogliosis. The cortical neurons are similarly, but less severely, depleted. Biochemical assays at the termination of the disease show a marked decrease in γ-aminobutyric acid (GABA) and glutamic acid decarboxylase.

□ **Clinical Features:** The symptoms of HD usually are first seen at about age 40 years, but 5% of persons with the disorder develop neurological signs before age 20 years, and a comparable proportion develop manifestations after age 60 years. Cognitive and emotional disturbances precede, sometimes by many years, the development of abnormal movements in more than half of the patients. Because of the prominent involvement of the extrapyramidal system, the symptoms inevitably feature a choreoathetoid movement disorder, which progresses to total incapacitation. Subsequent involvement of the cortex leads to a severe loss of cognitive function and intellectual deterioration, often accompanied by paranoia and delusions. The interval from the onset of symptoms to death averages 15 years.

The Inherited Spinocerebellar Ataxias

The spinocerebellar ataxias represent a heterogeneous category of disease that features (1) a broad but system-based topography, (2) a genetic contribution, and (3) a precocious loss of neurons and neural tracts in the cerebellum, brainstem, and spinal cord. The symptoms reflects the topography of the lesions. Thus, ataxia and intention tremor suggest involvement of the cerebellum; rigidity and tremor reflect degeneration of the brainstem; and losses of deep tendon reflexes, vibration sense, and pain sensation are caused by disease of the spinal cord.

Because there is a greater anatomical and clinical uniformity among cases from a particular family than among random cases from different families, case reports have generally focused on specific families, and the original authors' names have been appended to the different syndromes. For example, an inherited form of cerebello-olivary degeneration is designated "cerebello-olivary degeneration of Holmes"; this is distinguished from the sporadic "cerebello-olivary degeneration of Marie." In turn, these cases share many anatomical features with "olivopontocerebellar degeneration of Menzel." A similar complexity pertains to the nosology of spinal cord degeneration, although in this location, Friedreich ataxia is of major importance.

This complex nosology is now being clarified, owing to the identification of the precise genetic defects in many of these disorders. As seen in Table 28-3, several inherited ataxias, including olivopontocerebellar atrophy, Machado–Joseph disease, and Friedreich ataxia, have recently been shown to be disorders of triplet repeat expansion mutations.

Friedreich Ataxia

Friedreich ataxia is the most common inherited ataxia, with a prevalence in European populations of approximately 1 in 50,000. Although the inheritance pattern is autosomal recessive, many cases arise sporadically as new mutations and thus lack a family history. The onset of symptoms is usually before age 25 years, followed by an unremitting and progressive course of up to 30 years before death. The hallmark of Friedreich ataxia is a combined ataxia of both the upper and lower limbs. Dysarthria, lower-limb areflexia, extensor plantar reflexes, and sensory loss also occur in most patients. Frequently associated systemic abnormalities include deformities of the skeletal system, notable scoliosis and pes cavus, and hypertrophic cardiomyopathy, which is a common cause of death. An increased frequency of glucose intolerance and diabetes mellitus also is seen.

□ **Pathogenesis:** The genetic defect in Friedreich ataxia was mapped to chromosome 9 in 1988. The candidate gene (*X25*), located on chromosome 9, codes for a mitochondrial protein (*frataxin*) of 210 amino acid residues, which is probably involved in iron transport into mitochondria. In 1996, a mutation consisting of an unstable expansion of a trinucleotide (GAA) repeat was shown to be present in the first intron of the frataxin gene (9q13.3-21.1). The recessive pattern of inheritance suggests that this expansion results in a loss of function. Support for this hypothesis is provided by the absence or extremely low levels of frataxin mRNA transcripts in cases of Friedreich ataxia, which suggests that the expansion mutation interferes with transcription or RNA processing. In normal persons, the highest levels of frataxin gene expression are found in the heart and spinal cord. It is, therefore, likely that a lack of frataxin is responsible for both the neuropathological manifestations of Friedreich ataxia and the cardiomyopathy. There is a strong correlation between the size of the triplet expansion and the age at which symptoms appear, as well as the rate of clinical progression. Moreover, the frequency of hypertrophic cardiomyopathy also increases with increasing size of the GAA expansion.

The clinical spectrum of Friedreich ataxia is broader than previously thought. Many patients have sporadic ataxia, in which the typical clinical features of Friedreich ataxia are not fully expressed or in which atypical signs or symptoms are present. In such cases, identification of a GAA repeat expansion in the frataxin gene confirms the diagnosis of Friedreich ataxia. In one study, a significant proportion of patients (14%) with proven GAA expansion of the frataxin gene had an onset at older than 25 years (26 to 51), and 12% had retained lower-limb reflexes.

□ **Pathology:** The most prominent postmortem findings in Friedreich ataxia are seen in the spinal cord. The classic lesion consists of degeneration of three major pathways: the posterior columns, corticospinal pathways, and the spinocerebellar tracts (Fig. 28-121). Posterior column degeneration accounts for the sensory loss experienced by patients with Friedreich ataxia and occurs as a result of loss of the parent neuronal cell bodies, which are located in the dorsal root ganglia (see Fig. 28-121). In advanced cases, this degeneration can be appreciated grossly as shrinkage of the dorsal spinal roots and posterior funiculi. Similarly, atrophy of the spinocerebellar tracts, with attendant ataxia, follows neuronal degenera-

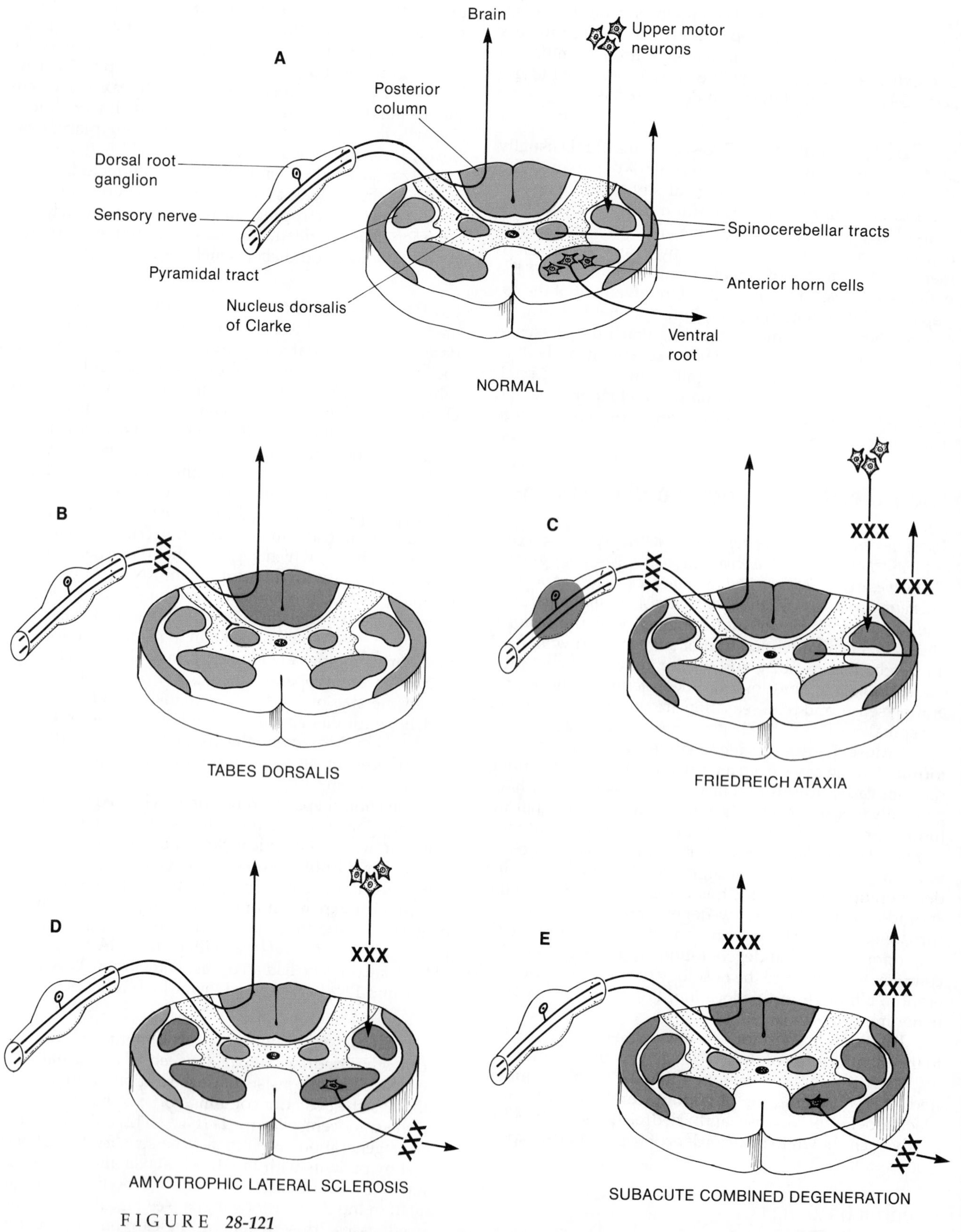

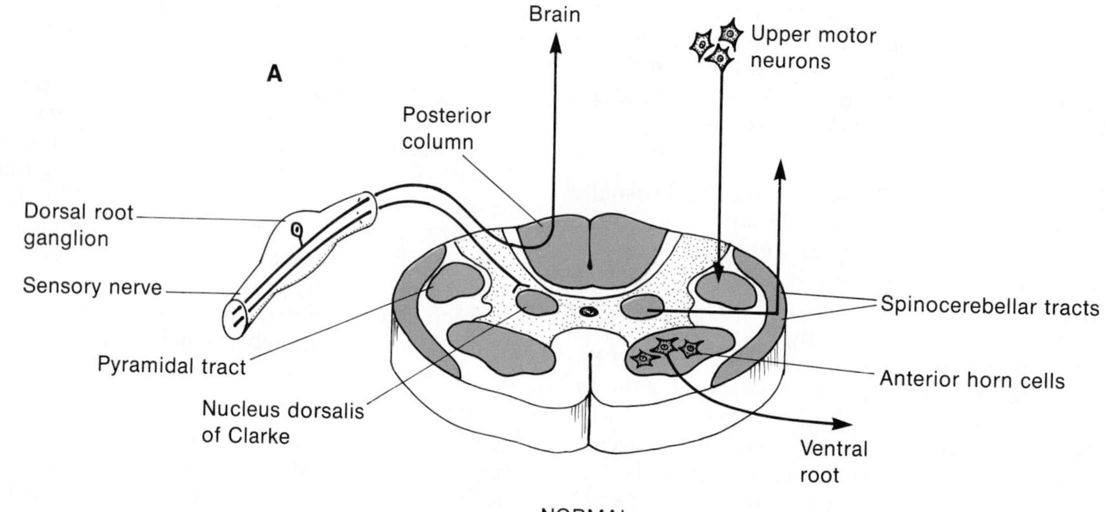

A
Brain
Upper motor neurons
Posterior column
Dorsal root ganglion
Sensory nerve
Spinocerebellar tracts
Pyramidal tract
Anterior horn cells
Nucleus dorsalis of Clarke
Ventral root
NORMAL
B
XXX
TABES DORSALIS
C
XXX
XXX
XXX
FRIEDREICH ATAXIA
D
XXX
XXX
AMYOTROPHIC LATERAL SCLEROSIS
E
XXX
XXX
XXX
SUBACUTE COMBINED DEGENERATION

FIGURE *28-121*
Degenerative disorders of the spinal cord. Many ascending (*blue*) and descending (*green*) pathways traverse the spinal cord. The four diseases illustrated produce differing patterns of disruption (*red*) of these pathways, depending on the location of the primary pathological process.

tion in the dorsal nucleus of Clarke. The corticospinal tracts show the most pronounced degeneration more distally in the cord, with gradually less pronounced atrophy as the cord is followed proximally toward the brainstem. This process is referred to as a "dying back" phenomenon.

CEREBELLO-OLIVARY DEGENERATION OF HOLMES: This autosomal inherited disorder is most commonly expressed during the second and third decades of life. Progressive cerebellar ataxia predominates, although dysphagia and nystagmus often reflect brainstem involvement. A loss of Purkinje cells and neurons of the inferior olives is characteristic.

Alzheimer Disease

Alzheimer disease (AD) is an insidious and progressive neurological disorder characterized clinically by loss of memory, cognitive impairment, and eventual dementia, and pathologically by amyloid-containing neuritic plaques and neurofibrillary tangles. The term Alzheimer disease was originally restricted to patients younger than 65 years in whom dementia was associated with characteristic neuropathological alterations. Thus, the designation "presenile dementia" was synonymous with this disorder of middle age, in contrast to an analogous clinical and morphological state in the later decades of life, which was termed "senile dementia." Currently, the term Alzheimer disease is used generically for all ages and identifies a specific morphological corollary of dementia.

☐ **Epidemiology:** Although AD is a worldwide disease, its distribution has been best studied in Western countries. **It is the most common cause of dementia in the elderly, accounting for more than half of all the cases.** The prevalence of the condition is closely related to age. Before age 65 years, the prevalence of AD is at most 1% to 2%, whereas it is 10% or greater after age 85 years. Women are affected twice as often as men. The large majority of cases of Alzheimer disease are sporadic, but a familial variant is recognized.

☐ **Pathogenesis:** Although the cause of AD has not been fully elucidated, there have been significant advances in our understanding of the origin of both AD-associated amyloid in the neuritic plaques and the neurofibrillary tangles in the cytoplasm of neurons.

AMYLOID β-PROTEIN (Aβ): Increasing evidence points to the importance of the deposition of Aβ in the neuritic plaques of AD. These plaques are located in areas of the cerebral cortex that are linked to intellectual function and are a constant feature of AD. The core of these plaques contains a distinct form of Aβ, which is 42 amino acids in length. Aβ is derived by proteolysis from a much larger (695 amino acids) membrane-spanning amyloid precursor protein (APP). Full-length APP exhibits an extracellular region, a transmembrane sequence, and a cytoplasmic domain. The region comprising Aβ serves to anchor the amino-terminal portion of APP to the membrane. The physiological function of APP is unknown, but it appears that the cytoplasmic portion of the molecule is associated with the cytoskeleton and is modulated by phosphorylation. Cytoskeleton-associated APP has also been demonstrated in the cytosol-free region of the surface membrane, but the relation between APPs in these two sites is not clear.

Normally, the degradation of APP involves a proteolytic cleavage in the middle of the Aβ domain, with the release of a fragment extending from the middle of the Aβ domain to the amino-terminal of APP. This fragment is lost to the extracellular fluid. By contrast, in AD, for reasons still to be determined, the APP molecule is cut at both ends of the Aβ domain, thereby releasing an intact Aβ molecule, which accumulates in neuritic plaques as amyloid fibrils.

The centrality of the deposition of Aβ in the pathogenesis of AD is suggested by several observations:

- Patients with **Down syndrome** (trisomy 21) develop the clinical and histopathological features of AD, including amyloid deposition in neuritic plaques, generally by age 40 years. The gene for APP is located on chromosome 21, and it is thought that the additional dose of the gene product in trisomy 21 predisposes to the precocious accumulation of Aβ.
- Some patients with the familial form of AD carry mutant APP genes. In this case, mutant APP is presumably more likely to be processed at either end of the Aβ domain than the normal protein, thereby releasing the intact, amyloidogenic fragment.
- A transgenic mouse expressing a mutant human APP gene develops lesions in the brain that are very similar to those of AD, although neurofibrillary tangles have not been observed.

The cell of origin of APP is not known, although it is suspected that the most likely candidates are circulating blood cells and endothelial cells. Neurons and glial cells may also be sites of APP synthesis. The demonstration of Aβ in the walls of cerebral blood vessels raises the possibility that the amyloid protein deposited in the brain may originate in the bloodstream (Fig. 28-122).

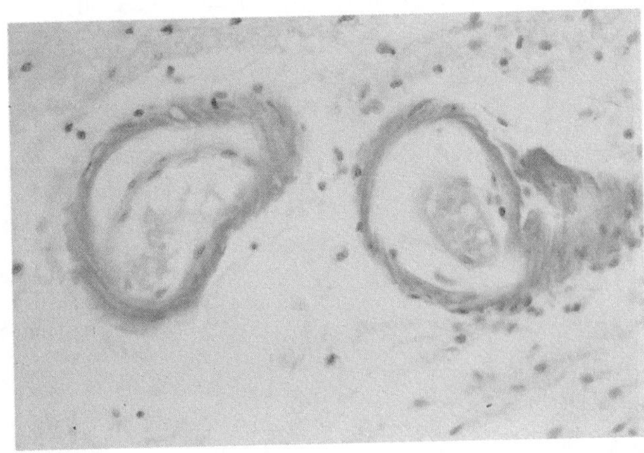

FIGURE *28-122*
Congophilic angiopathy. The cerebral blood vessels stain with Congo red, indicating the presence of amyloid.

NEUROFIBRILLARY TANGLES: Neurofibrillary tangles are composed of paired helical filaments that consist of an abnormal form of a normally occurring microtubule-associated protein (MAP), termed *tau*. It is thought that tau serves to stabilize neuronal microtubules, a function that may be necessary for proper axonal transport. In AD, the phosphorylation of tau at aberrant sites results in a protein that does not associate with microtubules but instead aggregates in the form of paired helical filaments. Current research is directed at the study of the kinases and phosphatases that presumably play a role in the aberrant phosphorylation of tau. Whatever the mechanism, the destabilization of microtubules might initiate a cascade of secondary perturbations, the culmination of which could be axonal degeneration.

Important questions remain to be answered. The relation between the number and size of amyloid-containing neuritic plaques, neuronal loss, and the degree of dementia in AD needs further definition. Whether neuronal injury, including neurofibrillary tangles, results from the plaque itself or from a direct action of β-amyloid peptide (BAP), or both, also requires further study. Cortical neurons in AD have been shown to accumulate aluminum, but this seems to be an effect of neuronal injury, rather than the cause of AD.

GENETIC FACTORS: Significant progress toward elucidations of the complex genetics of AD has recently been made, yielding insights into the inherited subtypes, as well as the much more common sporadic variant. As mentioned earlier, mutations of the *APP* gene have been associated with certain early-onset familial variants of AD. Additional genetic associations (Table 28-4) involve the apolipoprotein E (apoE) genotype and two recently discovered genes, presenilin 1 and presenilin 2.

APOLIPOPROTEIN E: ApoE has long been known for its role in cholesterol metabolism. Its relevance to dementia was uncovered in 1993, when it was reported that specific apoE alleles are susceptibility factors for sporadic and late-onset familial subtypes of AD. The human apoE gene is found on chromosome 19 (19q13.2). The three common alleles, $\epsilon 2$, $\epsilon 3$, and $\epsilon 4$, occur in North American apoE genotypes with the following frequencies: $\epsilon 3/\epsilon 3$, 60%; $\epsilon 3/\epsilon 4$, 23%; $\epsilon 2/\epsilon 3$, 13%; $\epsilon 2/\epsilon 4$, 2%; $\epsilon 2/\epsilon 2$, 1%; and $\epsilon 4/\epsilon 4$, 2%. An increased risk of late-onset familial and sporadic AD is associated with inheritance of the $\epsilon 4$ allele, particularly the homozygous $\epsilon 4/\epsilon 4$ genotype. Conversely, the $\epsilon 2$ allele may confer some protection. The age at which symptoms appear in late-onset AD also correlates with the $\epsilon 4$ allele; $\epsilon 4/\epsilon 4$ homozygotes exhibit the earliest age at onset (<70 years), whereas patients with the $\epsilon 2$ allele experience the latest onset (>90 years). The presence of the $\epsilon 4$ allele has also been correlated with an increased number of plaques in AD patients. It should be noted, however, that the apoE genotype is by no means an absolute determinant of AD. Not all persons with an $\epsilon 4$ allele develop AD, and, conversely, AD occurs in some persons who lack an $\epsilon 4$ allele.

Current data suggest several mechanisms by which apoE may influence the development of AD. *In vitro*, apoE binds amyloid β-peptide, and apoE-$\epsilon 4$ specifically promotes amyloid fibril formation more effectively than apoE-$\epsilon 3$. With respect to tau, apoE-$\epsilon 3$ binds to nonphosphorylated tau with higher affinity than apoE-$\epsilon 4$. It has, therefore, been suggested that apoE-$\epsilon 3$ might protect tau from phosphorylation and subsequent polymerization into neurofibrillary tangles.

TABLE 28-4 Genetic Factors in Alzheimer Disease (AD)

Gene	Chromosome	Disease Association
Amyloid precursor protein (*APP*)	21	Mutations of the *APP* gene are associated with early-onset familial AD
Presenilin 1 (*PS1*)	14	Mutations of the *PS1* gene are associated with early-onset familial AD
Presenilin 2 (*PS2*)	1	Mutations of the *PS2* gene are associated with Volga German familial AD
Apolipoprotein E (*apoE*)	19	Presence of the $\epsilon 4$ allele is associated with increased risk and younger age of onset of both inherited and sporadic forms of late-onset AD

PRESENILIN: Two genes with significant homology are associated with different kindreds of familial AD. Mutations of the gene presenilin 1 (*PS1*), located on chromosome 14, are associated with the most common form of autosomal dominant early-onset AD. The presenilin 2 gene (*PS2*) resides on chromosome 1 and is associated with AD in Volga German pedigrees. Importantly, presenilin mutations occur in half of all inherited AD, compared with only a few percent for mutant *APP* genes. Both presenilin genes code for proteins characterized by multiple transmembrane domains. There is some evidence to suggest that PS1 and PS2 mutant proteins alter the processing of the β-APP, thereby favoring increased production and deposition of amyloid β-peptides. Cellular processing of APP releases Aβ fragments of varying lengths, but the Aβ42 variant (see earlier) appears to be particularly dangerous. It is precisely the Aβ molecule whose production is enhanced by mutant *PS1*. It is thought that mutant PS1 allows misfolded APP to accumulate in cells, whereas the wild-type protein does not. In turn, the misfolded protein is more susceptible to enzymatic cleavage at the Aβ42 site.

☐ **Pathology:** The pathology of AD (Fig. 28-123) is dominated by the presence of (1) neuritic plaques, (2) neurofibrillary tangles, and (3) granulovacuolar degeneration. Identical morphological alterations also are present in lesser intensity in the cerebrum of a large proportion of elderly persons with symptoms as minor as forgetfulness. Indeed, the "disease process" is seemingly as inescapable in the aging human brain as is systemic atherosclerosis.

During the course of AD, neurons and neuritic processes are lost. The gyri narrow, the sulci widen, and cor-

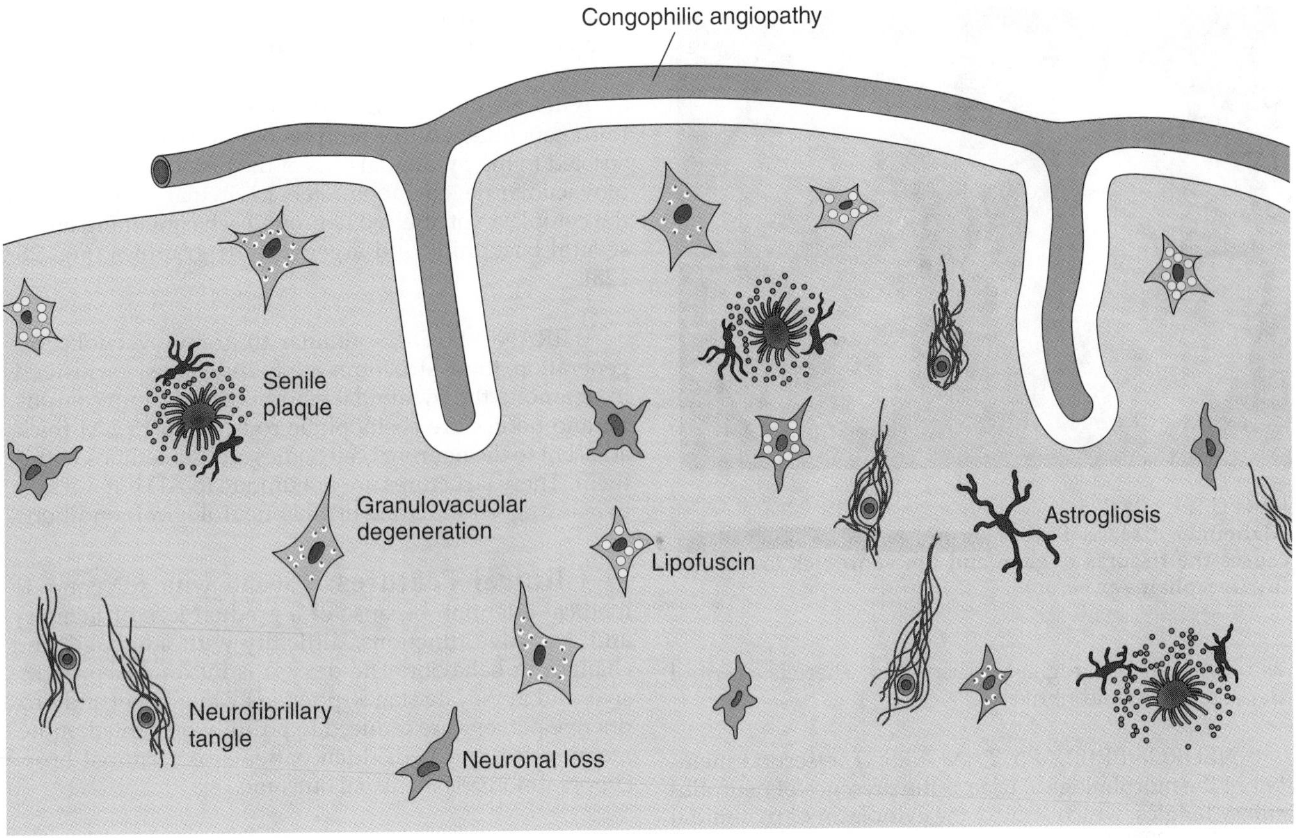

FIGURE *28-123*
Microscopic lesions of Alzheimer disease.

tical atrophy becomes apparent. The brain loses approximately 200 g in an interval of 3 to 8 years (Fig. 28-124). The atrophy is bilateral and symmetric and targets the frontal and hippocampal cortex (Fig. 28-125).

NEURITIC PLAQUES: The most conspicuous histological lesion, the neuritic plaque, is a discrete spherical area, several hundred μM in diameter, which in severe cases may occupy as much as one half of the volume of the gray matter of the cerebral cortex (Fig. 28-126). The neuritic plaque is argentophilic and contains abundant glial processes, as well as deposits that stain positively for amyloid. By electron microscopy, the plaques are composed of innumerable neuritic processes, among which

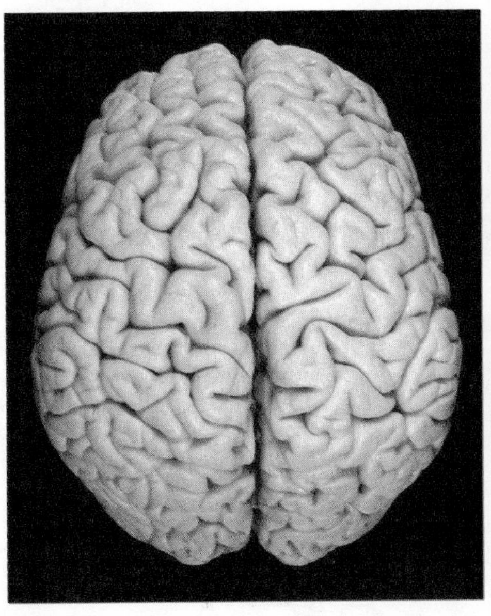
A

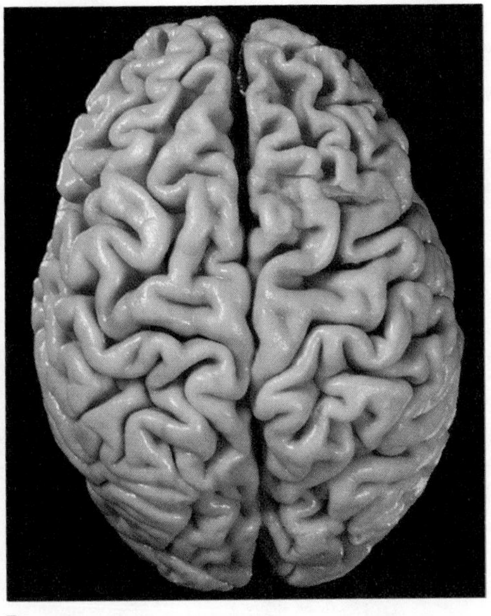
B

FIGURE *28-124*
Alzheimer disease. (*A*) Normal brain. (*B*) The brain of a patient with Alzheimer disease shows cortical atrophy characterized by slender gyri and prominent sulci.

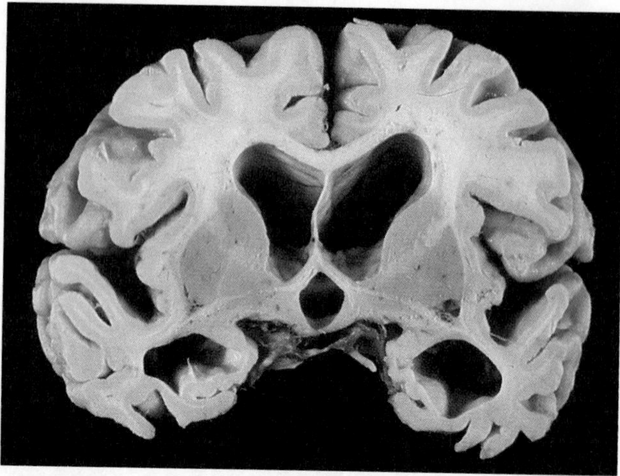

FIGURE 28-125
Alzheimer disease. Severe atrophy of the hippocampus causes the fissures to gape and the ventricles to enlarge (hydrocephalus *ex vacuo*).

astrocytes and microglia are dispersed. There is a central deposit of amyloid fibrils.

NEUROFIBRILLARY TANGLES: The second member of the morphological triad is the presence of neurofibrillary tangles, which occupy the cytoplasm of pyramidal cells (Fig. 28-127). By light microscopy, neurofibrillary tangles are composed of argentophilic fibers arranged in irregular bundles, knots, and curves. Electron microscopy reveals the tangles to be composed of paired helical filaments, each filament being 10 nm in width.

It deserves mention that neurofibrillary tangles are not pathognomonic of AD, because they also mark the neurons of some boxers (*dementia pugilistica*) and are seen in the substantia nigra in postencephalitic parkinsonism.

GRANULOVACUOLAR DEGENERATION: The third constituent of the morphological triad is largely restricted to the pyramidal cells of the hippocampus. Granulovacuolar degeneration refers to circular clear zones in the cytoplasm of affected neurons, each containing one or several basophilic and argentophilic granules (Fig. 28-128).

HIRANO BODIES: Similar to granulovacuolar degeneration, these structures are found almost exclusively in or among the pyramidal neurons of the hippocampus. Hirano bodies are eosinophilic rods, 10 to 15 μM thick, adjacent to the neuronal cell bodies and sometimes within them. These structures are not unique to AD but are seen in many aged brains and in other neurological conditions.

☐ **Clinical Features:** Patients with AD come to medical attention because of a gradual loss of memory and cognitive functions, difficulty with language, and changes in behavior. The disease is inexorably progressive, and in the late stages, previously intelligent and productive persons are reduced to pitifully demented, mute, incontinent, and bedridden patients. A terminal bronchopneumonia is the usual outcome.

Pick Disease

Pick disease (*lobar sclerosis*) is expressed clinically as a dementia that is indistinguishable from that of AD. This disorder, among the rarest of the cortical dementias (Fig. 28-129), becomes symptomatic in midadult life and progresses

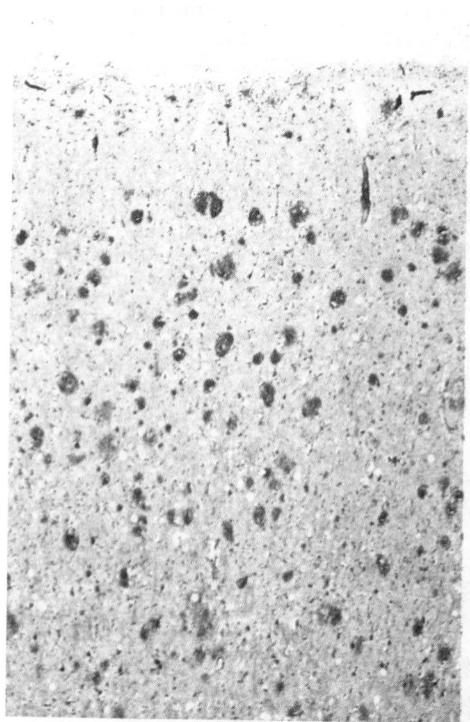

A

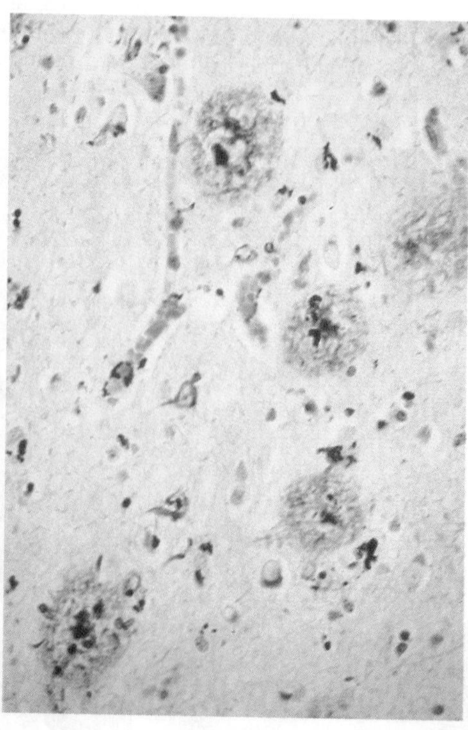

B

FIGURE 28-126
Alzheimer disease. (*A*) A section of the cerebral cortex impregnated with silver reveals the presence of neuritic plaques. (*B*) A higher-magnification view of A shows the uniform size and spherical shape of the neuritic plaque, which contains a dense core of amyloid.

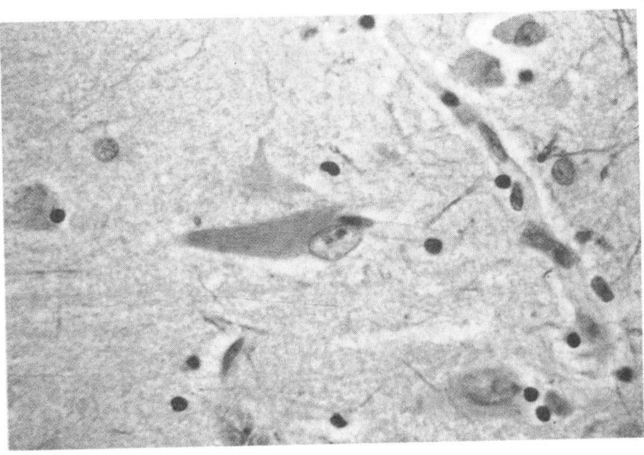
A

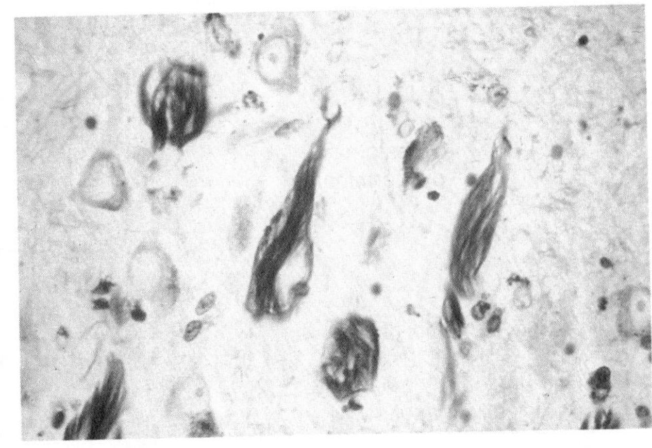
B

FIGURE 28-127
Alzheimer disease. (*A*) The cytoplasm of a neuron is distended by neurofibrillary tangles. (*B*) A silver stain of *A* demonstrates the fibrillary character of the cytoplasmic inclusions.

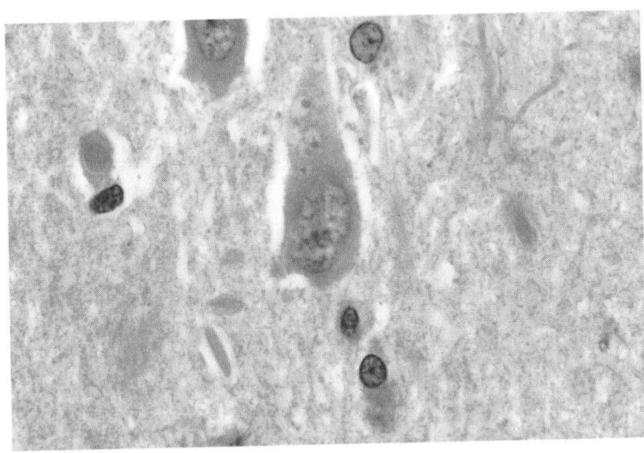

FIGURE 28-128
Alzheimer disease. A section of the hippocampus shows granulovacuolar degeneration of a pyramidal neuron, evidenced as clear cytoplasmic vacuoles containing granules.

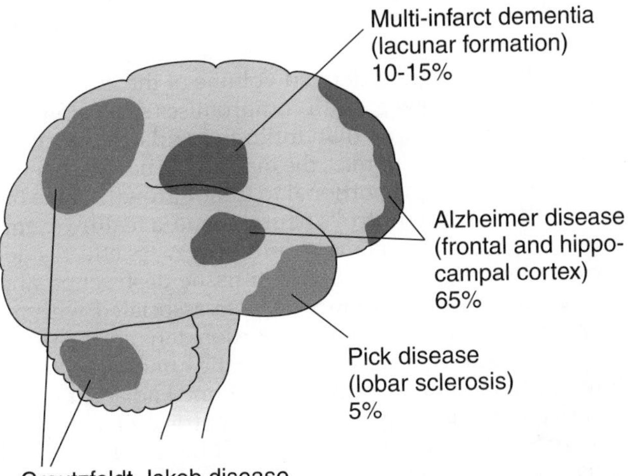

FIGURE 28-129
Diseases associated with dementia.

relentlessly to death over a period of 3 to 10 years. Some examples of Pick disease cluster in a single family, but the case distributions do not conform to a hereditary pattern. Women are involved more often than men.

Unlike AD, cortical atrophy in Pick disease is often unilateral and is usually localized in a frontal or a temporal lobe. The atrophy may attain extreme proportions, so that the affected gyri are reduced to a thin edge (*knife-blade atrophy*). Histologically, the involved cortex is markedly depleted of neurons, and their place is taken by conspicuous astrogliosis. Many residual neurons have a ballooned cytoplasm, occasionally containing one or several eosinophilic and intensely argentophilic cytoplasmic inclusions termed Pick bodies. By electron microscopy, these structures are formed by densely aggregated neurofilaments.

NEOPLASIA

Tumors within the intracranial compartment can be classified according to five cytological origins:

- **Neuroectoderm**, principally gliomas
- **Mesenchymal structures**, notably meningiomas and schwannomas
- **Ectopic tissues**, such as those that have been displaced intracranially during embryonic development, including craniopharyngiomas, dermoid and epidermoid cysts, lipomas, and dysgerminomas
- **Retained embryonal structures** (e.g., paraphyseal cysts)
- **Metastases**

Intracranial tumors constitute only 2% of all "aggressive" neoplasms, but their frequency in childhood imparts a greater clinical significance. Gliomas account for 60% of primary intracranial neoplasms, meningiomas for 20%, and all others for 20% (Fig. 28-130).

Tumors of neuroectodermal origin are predominantly glial. They are derived from astrocytes (astrocytomas), oligodendroglia (oligodendrogliomas), or ependyma (ependymomas). Each of these tumors exhibits varying

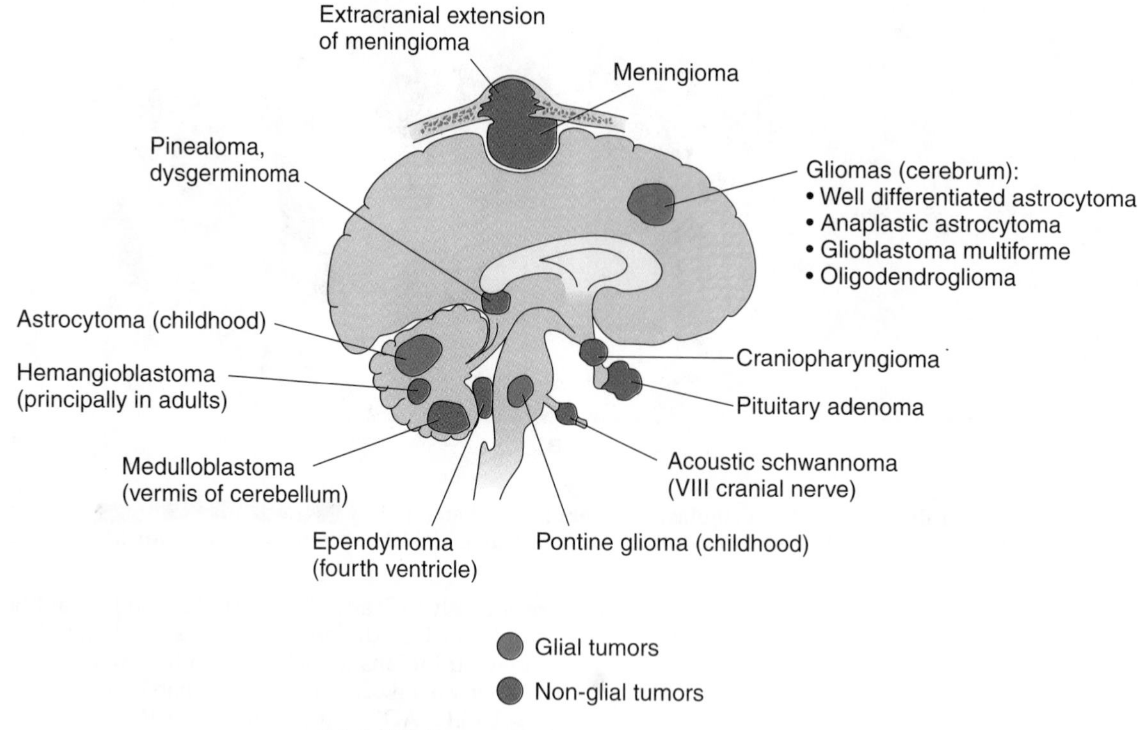

FIGURE *28-130*
The distribution of common intracranial tumors.

degrees of anaplasia, from well-differentiated tumors that are difficult to distinguish from normal tissue to anaplastic tumors that do not resemble nervous tissue at all.

BENIGN VERSUS MALIGNANT: The descriptive terms benign and malignant require qualification when used in reference to the gliomas. For example, even a very well-differentiated astrocytoma infiltrates freely through the surrounding brain tissue and has a poorly defined margin. The term benign may be applied to this lesion, because its growth is indolent and permits survival for 5 to 10 years. Nevertheless, unlike "benign" neoplasms elsewhere, many astrocytomas are eventually fatal. Conventionally, the less-differentiated tumors, anaplastic astrocytoma and glioblastoma multiforme, are designated "malignant." These cancers grow more rapidly, infiltrate without restraint, and are fatal in a short time. Yet, unlike malignant tumors elsewhere, even the most anaplastic glioma rarely metastasizes outside the CNS.

AGE OF THE PATIENT AND LOCATION OF THE TUMOR: The location of the lesion is particularly relevant in the diagnosis of a suspected neoplasm. Most tumors in the intracranial or intraspinal compartment have predictable geographic localizations. Thus, tumors of the astrocytic series occur predominantly in the cerebral hemispheres in middle life and old age, in the cerebellum and pons in childhood, and in the spinal cord in young adults. Oligodendrogliomas predominantly involve the cerebrum in adults. Ependymomas have their highest incidence in the fourth ventricle, followed by intramedullary lesions that are derived from the lining of the spinal canal and from the filum terminale.

Totally without logic, the lowest incidence of ependymomas is found in the largest ependymal surface, that of the lateral ventricles. Some tumors, such as the craniopharyngiomas, medulloblastomas, and germinomas, have highly specific sites of origin. A few tumors, notably the third ventricular cyst, are rigidly restricted to a single position in the septum pellucidum, where the lesion regularly abuts against the foramen of Monro, lifts the fornix, and compresses the medial aspects of the internal capsules. Thus, the symptoms of intracranial pressure (hydrocephalus), personality changes, bilateral leg weakness, and urinary incontinence relate to the position of this expansible mass. Meningiomas arise from widely distributed arachnoid villi but display preferred sites of origin (see later).

Within the rigidly defined volume of the intracranial compartment, a new growth compromises space. If it displaces the brain, rather than infiltrates and destroys it, as in the case of meningiomas, the mass of the neoplasm may "consume" space proportional to tumor growth. If the tumor infiltrates and destroys neural tissue, a feature exemplified by glioblastoma multiforme, the mass effect is determined by the balance between tissue destruction and tumor growth. Most tumors are also associated with regional edema, which is disproportionately abundant in the immediate environs of a metastatic tumor and constitutes additional mass. Tumors positioned adjacent to the ventricles, particularly the fourth ventricle or the aqueduct of Sylvius, are prone to obstruct these conduits and cause hydrocephalus.

NEURONAL TUMORS: Infrequently, the neuroectoderm gives rise to a neoplasm of neuronal heritage.

These tumors occur most often in childhood, and their cellular composition is usually primitive. An important example is the medulloblastoma, which arises in the cerebellum, generally in the first decade of life. This entity is usually situated in the vermis; its growth is rapid, and regional infiltration is extensive.

It has been emphasized that the neuroectodermal tumors, even though highly anaplastic, rarely metastasize outside the cranial cavity. However, certain tumors, notably medulloblastoma and less commonly ependymoma and pineal parenchymal tumor, have a marked propensity to disseminate or "seed" by way of the CSF. The implants generally involve the subarachnoid compartment over the spinal cord and cauda equina. In conformity with the principle that a cell must be capable of replication to undergo neoplastic transformation, medulloblastomas and the better differentiated ganglionic tumors typically are seen symptomatically during infancy or childhood. In fact, many tumors have their origin during embryonic development. An interesting exception is esthesioneuroblastoma of the olfactory mucosa, which occurs in adults. This seems to be puzzling until one recalls that the olfactory epithelium is a neural structure that retains a proliferative potential.

SYMPTOMS OF INTRACRANIAL TUMORS: An infiltrative neoplasm that destroys functional neural tissue creates a neurological deficit, which may be sensory or motor or both. Cognitive functions are not infrequently impaired. Alternatively, a neoplasm that "irritates" a functional area may initiate an involuntary release of neuronal activity, and its presence is then manifested as a seizure. Seizures may originate from many neuronal systems; thus, there are (1) motor seizures, (2) subtle visual and olfactory seizures ("uncinate fits"), and (3) seizure disorders that stem from vegetative centers of the brain. Among the neoplasms, meningiomas and the well-differentiated gliomas, such as astrocytomas, oligodendrogliomas, and gangliomas, are most likely to be associated with seizures.

The mass of a neoplasm, combined with edema or hydrocephalus, causes increased intracranial pressure, which leads to headaches and vomiting. A mass effect, if progressive, ultimately causes various herniations of neural tissue:

- **Transtentorial herniation:** The medial aspect of the hippocampus (uncus) herniates into the aperture of the tentorium (see Fig. 28-38). Transtentorial herniation interferes with the circulatory dynamics of the midbrain and causes a decline in the level of consciousness as a result of impaired function of the reticular formation. It frequently compresses the third nerve against the edge of the tentorium and causes third nerve palsy, evidenced as a fixed dilated pupil. Shortly thereafter, irreversible midbrain necrosis and hemorrhage lead to permanent loss of consciousness and then to death (see Fig. 28-39).
- **Foramen magnum herniation:** As a result of increased pressure in the posterior fossa, cerebellar tonsils herniate into the foramen magnum. This compresses the cardiac and respiratory centers, in which case, death follows promptly.
- **Subfalcine herniation:** The cingulate gyrus herniates beneath the falx, which on rare occasions may result in infarction in the territories supplied by the pericallosal vessels, with weakness or sensory loss in the legs.

Tumors Derived from Astrocytes

Neoplasms derived from astrocytes show a wide spectrum of differentiation, ranging from tumors whose histological structure is remarkably similar to normal brain tissue to highly aggressive growths that are hardly recognizable as of glial origin. These tumors have been assigned three grades in order of increasing anaplasia, the first two being astrocytoma (grade I) and anaplastic astrocytoma (grade II). The least differentiated tumor derived from astrocytes (grade III) is referred to as glioblastoma multiforme.

Astrocytoma

Astrocytoma is a glioma composed of well-differentiated astrocytes. It composes approximately 20% of primary intracranial neoplasms. It frequents (1) the cerebral hemispheres in adults (Fig. 28-131); (2) the optic nerve, walls of the third ventricle, midbrain, pons, and cerebellum in the first two decades of life (Fig. 28-132); and (3) the spinal cord, predominantly in the thoracic and cervical segments, in young adults.

☐ **Pathology:** On gross examination, astrocytoma is poorly demarcated and infiltrates the brain with an indistinct margin. Childhood astrocytomas of the cerebellar hemispheres are frequently cystic. Astrocytomas of the cerebrum often contain microcysts. An occasional astrocytoma contains sufficient calcospherites to be visible radiographically. Microscopically, astrocytoma is distinguished by a matrix of slender glial cytoplasmic processes, in which the nuclei are dispersed randomly (Fig. 28-133). There are several well-recognized morphological variations of astrocytoma:

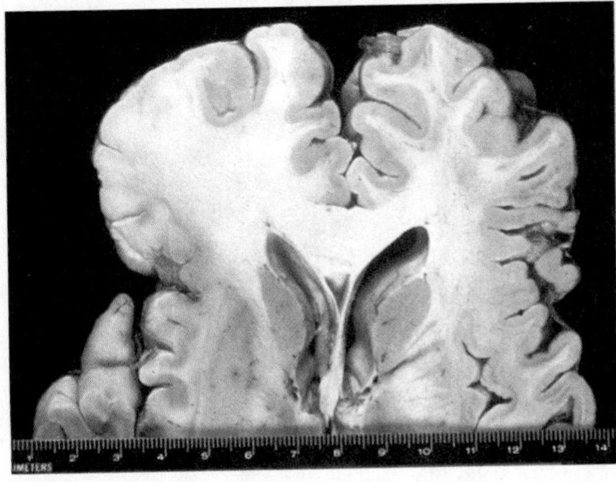

FIGURE *28-131*
Astrocytoma. A poorly demarcated, expansile mass occupies the left frontal lobe.

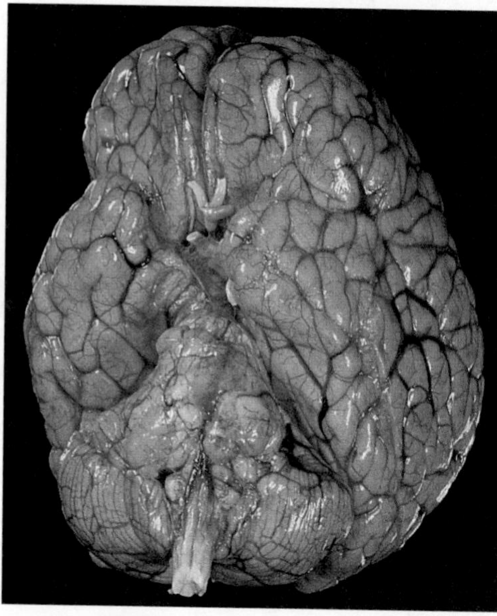

FIGURE *28-132*
Astrocytoma. During childhood, the brainstem is a common site of astrocytomas. Note the entrapment of the basilar artery.

- **Fibrillary astrocytoma:** Most astrocytomas, particularly those in the cerebral hemispheres of adults, have intermediately dense glial processes.
- **Gemistocytic astrocytoma:** Abundant eosinophilic cytoplasm encases the tumor cell nuclei.
- **Juvenile pilocytic astrocytoma:** This tumor occurs in children, is characterized by abundant, hair-like glial processes, and typically contains Rosenthal fibers.

The life expectancy of patients with astrocytoma is widely variable, but approximates 5 years. Transformation to a higher degree of anaplasia, often to glioblastoma multiforme, occurs in 10% of cases and shortens life expectancy.

Anaplastic Astrocytoma

Anaplastic astrocytoma is distinguished from the other astrocytomas by (1) greater cellularity, (2) cellular pleomorphism, and (3) anaplasia (Fig. 28-134). The topographic distribution parallels that of astrocytoma. The growth of the tumor is rapid, and life expectancy averages 3 years.

Glioblastoma Multiforme

Glioblastoma multiforme is the extreme expression of anaplasia among the glial neoplasms and accounts for 40% of all primary intracranial tumors. Most glioblastomas have constituent cells with recognizable astrocytic properties, but they display (1) marked pleomorphism, (2) frequent mitoses, (3) regional zones of necrosis, and (4) endothelial proliferation. The last feature is a manifestation of cellular hyperplasia induced by angiogenic growth factors. A similar hyperplasia of fibroblasts also is initiated by the presence of glioblastoma multiforme near the dura or vascular adventitia. Hyperplasia of fibroblasts may actually attain malignant proportions, in which case, the sarcomatous growth intermingles fibrosarcoma with the glioma, resulting in a *gliosarcoma*.

Glioblastoma typically infiltrates extensively, frequently crossing the corpus callosum and producing a bilateral lesion likened to a butterfly in its gross configuration and in its mottled red and yellow coloration (Fig. 28-135). These colors are imparted by multiple areas of recent (red) and remote (yellow) hemorrhage. The cardinal histological features of glioblastoma multiform are as follows:

- **Marked cellularity**, with variable degrees of cellular pleomorphism and multinucleated cells (Fig. 28-136)
- **Serpentine areas of necrosis** surrounded by zones of crowded tumor cells ("palisading"; Fig. 28-137)
- **Endothelial cell proliferation**, which creates clusters of small vessels, referred to as "glomeruloid" formations (Fig. 28-138)

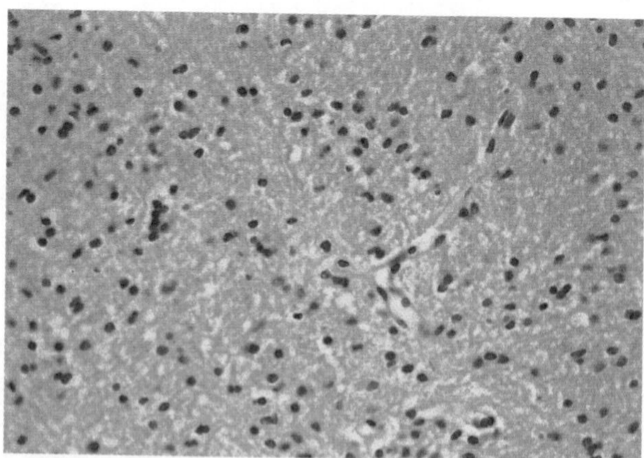

FIGURE *28-133*
Astrocytoma. A microscopic section shows a moderately cellular, well-differentiated astrocytoma, which displays minimal pleomorphism.

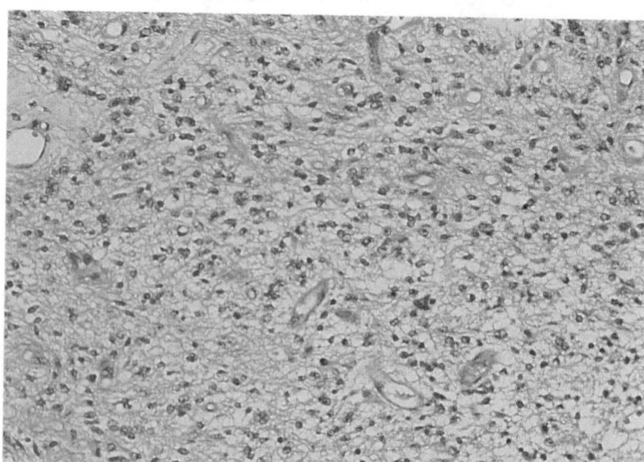

FIGURE *28-134*
Anaplastic astrocytoma. Anaplasia introduces hypercellularity, nuclear pleomorphism, and increased vascularity, but retains a glial fibrillary background.

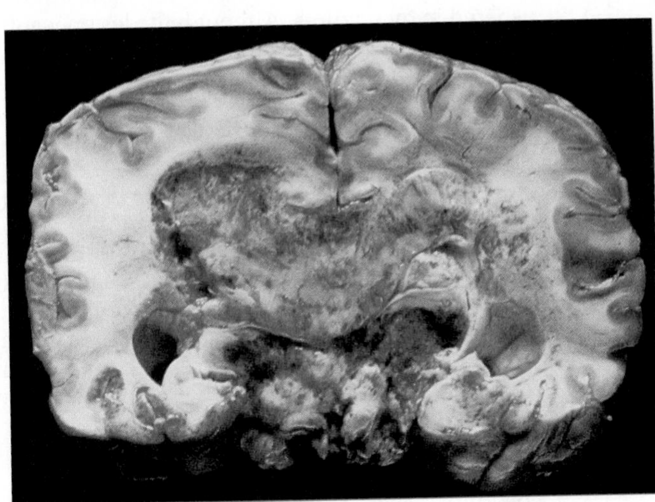

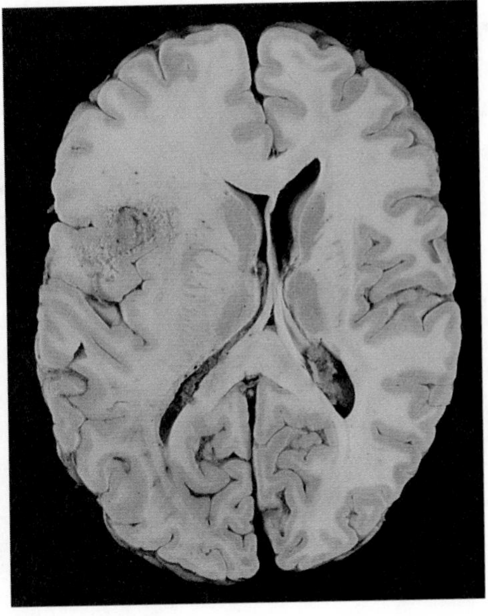

FIGURE 28-135
Glioblastoma multiforme. (*A*) The tumor occupies the splenium of the corpus callosum with bilateral extension into the white matter, where it imparts variegated shades of red and yellow ("butterfly tumor"). (*B*) A horizontal section of the brain from another patient with a glioblastoma multiforme reveals a partially necrotic and edematous mass in the left insula.

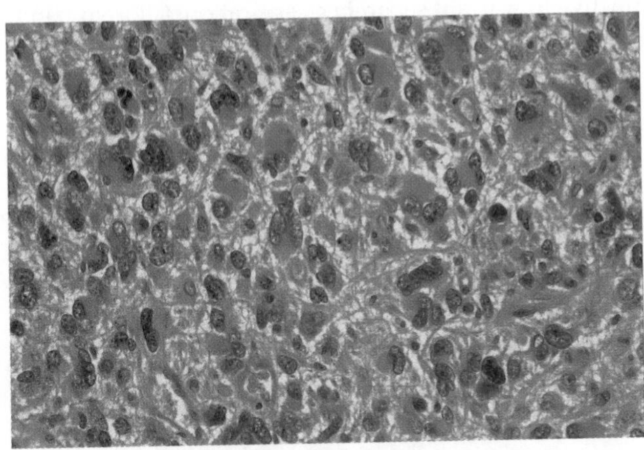

FIGURE 28-136
Glioblastoma multiforme. A malignant glioma features marked nuclear pleomorphism and bizarre multinucleated cells. The eosinophilic cytoplasm flows into coarse glial processes.

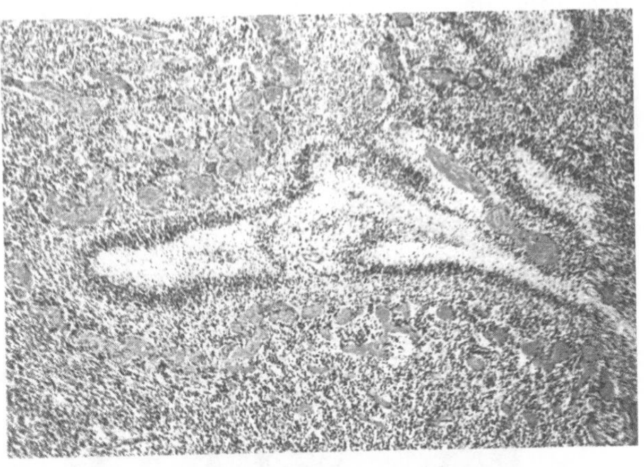

FIGURE 28-137
Glioblastoma multiforme. A photomicrograph demonstrates a highly vascularized tumor with serpentine areas of necrosis, bordered by hypercellular zones (palisading).

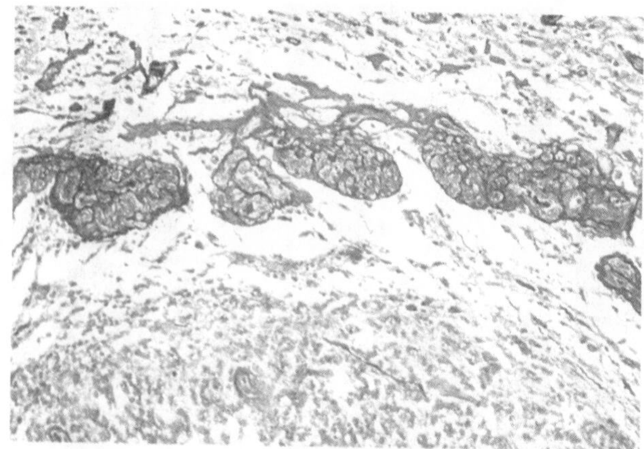

FIGURE 28-138
Glioblastoma multiforme. A silver stain shows aggregates of proliferated endothelial cells, which grow as glomeruloid structures from the arcuate vessels toward the tumor.

- The clinical course of glioblastoma multiforme rarely exceeds 18 months. The tumor predominates in the later decades of life and occurs twice as frequently as astrocytoma.

Oligodendroglioma

Oligodendroglioma, in accord with its cell of origin, arises in the white matter, predominantly in the cerebral hemispheres of adults. The histological composition of oligodendroglioma recreates the small rounded nuclei of oligodendrocytes but introduces variable densities in cell population and cellular pleomorphism. Calcospherites, which on occasion are visualized radiographically, appear as grains of sand scattered randomly throughout the lesion. The slow growth is reflected in an absence of mitotic figures and necrosis.

The symptoms of oligodendroglioma are frequently ushered in by seizures. Although the lesion is infiltrative, its slow growth permits survival for 5 to 10 years.

Ependymoma

Ependymoma is most common in the fourth ventricle (Fig. 28-139A), *producing obstruction and resulting in hydrocephalus.* Ependymoma is also second only to astrocytoma as an intramedullary tumor of the spinal cord. In that location, it arises from the lining of the central canal or the filum terminale, most often seen at the lumbosacral level. This is at variance with the location of intramedullary astrocytoma, which usually appears at a cervical–thoracic level.

The cells of an ependymoma characteristically have an "epithelial" appearance, similar to that of normal ependymal cells. They possess ovoid nuclei, with coarse chromatin material and well-defined plasma membranes. The cells of an ependymoma form clefts or may arrange around blood vessels, creating an anuclear mantle of glial processes about the adventitia (see Fig. 28-139B). The tumor generally grows slowly, but it can seed the subarachnoid space.

CHOROID PLEXUS PAPILLOMA: This benign tumor is a variant of ependymoma, but it is sufficiently distinctive to warrant separate classification. Choroid papilloma occurs most commonly in young boys and usually arises in a lateral ventricle. Hydrocephalus is the major complication. On gross examination, choroid papilloma appears as an intraventricular papillary mass. Microscopically, it duplicates the structure of the normal choroid plexus. Excision is curative.

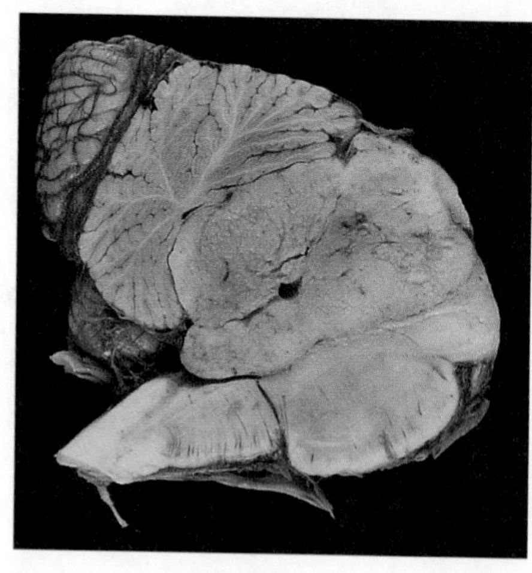

A

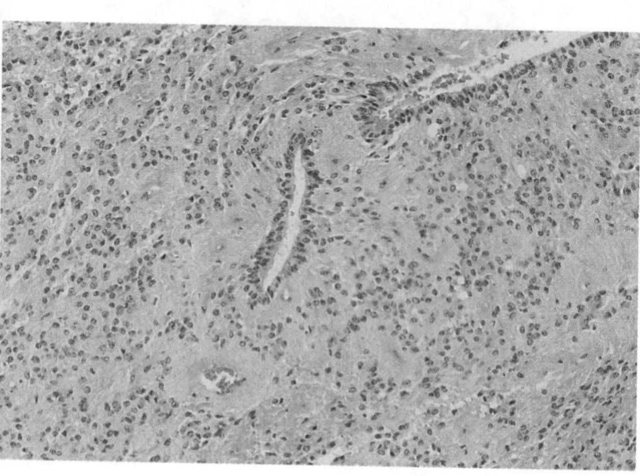

B

FIGURE 28-139
Ependymoma. (*A*) The fourth ventricle is greatly distended by a well-demarcated mass that flattens the pons and elevates the cerebellum. (*B*) A microscopic section of the tumor in *A* shows randomly arranged cells, a fibrillary matrix, and clefts lined by tumor cells.

Medulloblastoma

Medulloblastoma, the most common intracranial neuroblastic lesion, is derived from the transient cerebellar external granular cell layer of neurons. It arises exclusively in the cerebellum and has its highest frequency toward the end of the first decade. The tumor infiltrates aggressively and frequently disseminates through the CSF.

Medulloblastoma features hyperchromatic, round-to-oval nuclei and scant cytoplasm. The cells crowd together with no structural pattern. The neuroblastic character of the cells is occasionally expressed in rosette formation, a distinctive feature of embryonic and neoplastic neuroblasts

Children with medulloblastoma are first seen with cerebellar dysfunction or hydrocephalus. Similar to embryonic neuroblasts, the tumor is highly sensitive to ionizing radiation, but unfortunately, subarachnoid dissemination is frequent. The 10-year survival rate is only 50%.

Ganglioglioma

Ganglioglioma is a rare brain tumor composed of mature and immature neurons in a stroma of glia. It commonly expresses its presence in seizures during the first two decades of life. The neuronal constituents are represented by (1) small rounded nuclei of neuroblasts, (2) intermediate forms, and (3) large nuclei with prominent nucleoli and the well-defined cytoplasm of ganglionic cells. The matrix of ganglioglioma is contributed by astrocytes. The lesion typically grows indolently.

Neoplasms of Mesenchymal Origin

Meningioma

Meningiomas are intracranial tumors that arise from the arachnoid villi and produce symptoms by compressing adjacent brain tissue. They account for almost 20% of all primary intracranial neoplasms. The peak frequency is in the fourth to fifth decades, but there is a significant incidence in youthful adults. These tumors produce a globoid or discoid (meningioma *en plaque*) mass (Fig. 28-140). Although meningiomas may occur at almost any intracranial site, they are most common in parasagittal areas, convexities of the cerebral hemispheres, the olfactory groove, and the lateral wing of the sphenoid. Meningiomas occur with a 60:40 female-to-male incidence, but in the spinal canal, this ratio approaches 10:1. The tumor has a propensity to erode contiguous bone (Fig. 28-141). The superficial position of meningiomas, coupled with neural displacement rather than infiltration, invites total surgical excision. However, particularly with lesions at the base of the brain, invasion of the skull often limits complete resection and recurrence is common.

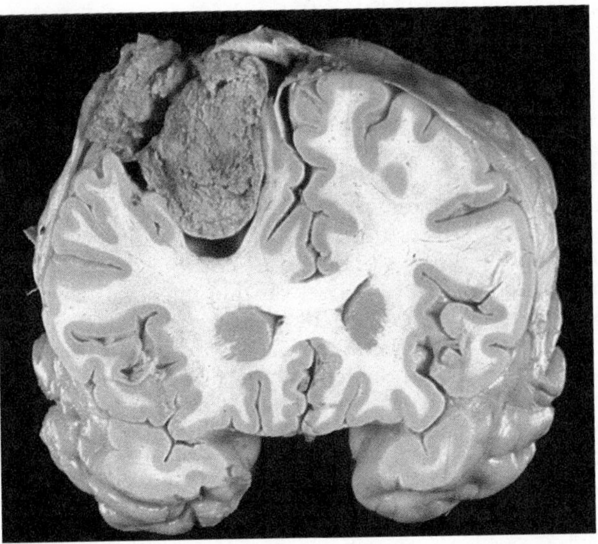

FIGURE *28-140*
Meningioma. A tumor that arises from the arachnoid indents the underlying cortex.

☐ **Pathogenesis:** Meningiomas typically arise in one of three settings:

- Sporadic cases (most common)
- Iatrogenic cases caused by prior radiation therapy to the cranium
- In association with a genetic disorder, especially neurofibromatosis type 2

The majority of meningiomas arise sporadically. Significantly, many sporadic meningiomas exhibit loss, partial deletion, or mutation of chromosome 22, involving the *NF2* locus (22q12). Similar cytogenetic observations have also been found with sporadic schwannomas (see later). These findings suggest that inactivations of the putative *NF2* tumor-suppressor gene is involved in the genesis of many meningiomas and schwannomas arising

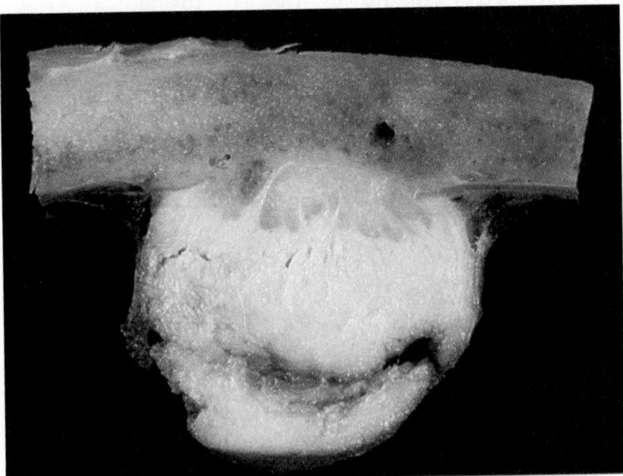

FIGURE *28-141*
Meningioma. The calvarium is infiltrated by a locally aggressive meningioma.

sporadically, in addition to those occurring in patients with NF2.

The induction of meningiomas by radiation therapy involves a latent period of a decade or more and is directly related to the radiation dosage. Low-dose scalp irradiation for tinea capitis was widely used from 1909 until the introduction of the antifungal drug griseofulvin in 1960. For these patients, the average interval between the treatment and the detection of a meningioma was 35 years. With higher radiation doses, such as would be administered for head and neck cancers, intervals as short as 5 years have been reported. Meningiomas also occur in conjunction with several genetic syndromes, most important with neurofibromatosis type 2 (NF2). An association has also been reported with basal cell nevus syndrome (Gorlin syndrome), and rare, familial, multiple meningioma syndromes have been documented.

☐ **Pathology:** On gross examination, most meningiomas appear as well-circumscribed, firm, bosselated masses of variable size. The cut surface presents a gray, binder-twine pattern similar to that of uterine leiomyomas. The histological hallmark of meningiomas is a whorled pattern of "meningothelial" cells (Fig. 28-142), in association with psammoma bodies (laminated, spherical calcospherites). Although this morphological appearance is distinctive, in many meningiomas, it is obscured by a predominantly fibroblastic proliferation. Some meningiomas are dominated by blood vessels (*angiomatous meningioma*); others have a papillary appearance (*papillary meningiomas*); a rare lesion features microcystic formations (*microcystic meningioma*). The different subtypes of meningioma do not differ significantly in their biological behavior, and the historic separation into many histological categories does not serve a useful purpose.

☐ **Clinical Features:** The indolent growth of meningiomas creates a symptomatic interval that often spans years. Well-differentiated lesions displace the brain but do not infiltrate it. Thus, seizures rather than neurological deficits frequently characterize the clinical presentation. This is particularly true of meningiomas positioned in parasagittal sites and of those situated over the convexity of the hemispheres. In other locations, meningiomas compress functional structures. Tumors of the olfactory groove produce anosmia; those in the suprasellar region lead to visual deficits; meningiomas in the cerebellopontine angle create cranial nerve palsies; and those in the spinal column result in dysfunction of the spinal nerve roots and spinal cord.

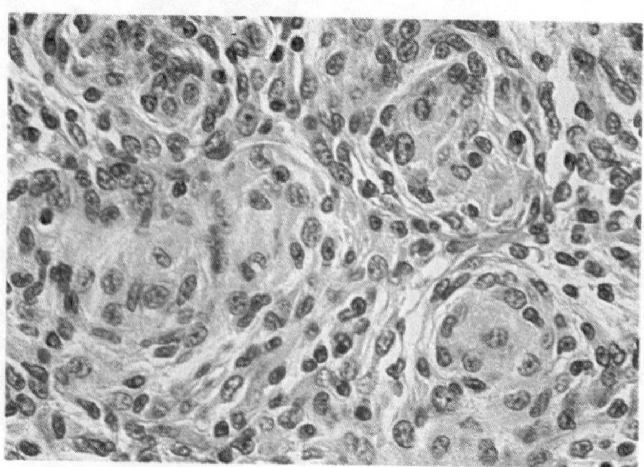

FIGURE 28-142
Meningioma. A microscopic section shows whorled meningothelial cells.

Because meningiomas are intimately related to the meninges, which are innervated by pain fibers, headaches are common. Penetration of the calvarium may create a tumor mass on the external table of the skull, historically recognized as a "brain tumor" by barbers. Meningiomas that are not completely excised tend to recur. Although the symptom-free interval after surgery is variable, a typical meningioma doubles in size approximately every 2 years.

Schwannoma

Schwannoma is a tumor derived from Schwann cells, a cell species that produces collagen as well as myelin. This tumor is also known as neurilemmoma, perineural fibroblastoma, and neurinoma. Histologically, schwannomas feature fascicles of spindle cells. Occasionally, parallel, picketed, and regimented patterns of cells are noted at the ends of a fibrillar bundle, an arrangement referred to as a Verocay body. Fortunately, Schwann cell tumors are rarely malignant. Nuclear pleomorphism, particularly when limited to an occasional cell, does not predict accelerated growth.

Acoustic neuromas are intracranial schwannomas that are restricted to the eighth nerve (Fig. 28-143). Interestingly, the tumor invariably begins where the stromal matrix undergoes transition from oligodendroglial to Schwann cell origin. This junction corresponds anatomically to the position of the internal auditory meatus. Thus, the occurrence of the lesion not only initiates tinnitus and deafness but also expands the bony meatus, an effect that is useful for radiographic diagnosis. The growth of an acoustic neurinoma causes it to protrude into the cerebellopontine angle, where other nerves are compressed.

Schwannomas also arise on spinal nerve roots. On occasion, they are entirely within the spinal canal, although at other times, they span a bony foramen, with a "dumb-bell" configuration. Together with meningiomas, schwannomas compose most intradural–extramedullary neoplasms. Tumors of Schwann cells also occur on peripheral nerves as schwannomas and neurofibromas. As mentioned with regard to sporadic meningiomas, a significant proportion of sporadic schwannomas also exhibit deletions or mutations of chromosome 22 involving the region of the *NF2* gene.

Neoplasms Derived from Ectopic Tissues

Craniopharyngioma

Craniopharyngiomas are solid and cystic lesions that arise from the epithelium of Rathke's pouch, a part of the embryonic nasopharynx that migrates cephalad and gives origin to the anterior lobe of the hypophysis. Derivations of this epithelium as-

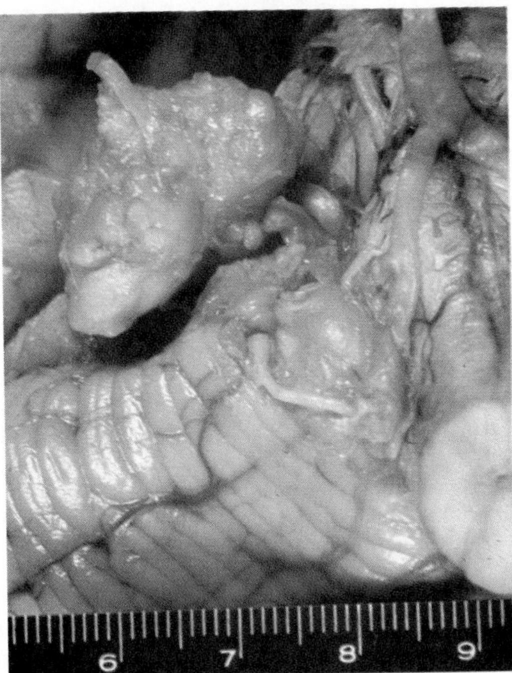

FIGURE *28-143*
Acoustic neuroma. A tumor in the cerebellar pontine angle arises from the eighth cranial nerve.

sume positions above the sella turcica (Fig. 28-144A). Some cystic lesions are lined by squamous epithelium, whereas others, referred to as *adamantinomas*, are solid and resemble lesions of dentigerous origin (see Fig. 28-144B). Craniopharyngiomas generally become symptomatic in the first two decades of life, creating visual deficits and headaches. They may cause anterior pituitary failure or involve the posterior pituitary to produce diabetes insipidus.

Dermoid and Epidermoid Cysts

Dermoid and epidermoid cysts stem from misdirected events of embryonic development. The term dermoid refers to cysts whose walls contain not only squamous epithelium but also skin appendages and hair. These cystic analogues of cutaneous structures are displaced into the bone of the skull and occasionally into the intracranial compartment. The displaced squamous cells proliferate and develop into a cyst, whose inwardly oriented epithelium desquamates keratotic debris, which resembles "mother of pearl." The intracranial lesions tend to occur in the posterior fossa or about the sella turcica. Although these cysts are not true neoplasms, their symptoms are related to the presence of an expanding intracranial mass.

Lipoma

Lipomas arise from rudiments of adipose tissue that were carried inward as the brain infolded embryologically. Thus lipomas are positioned (1) along the superior aspect of the corpus callosum (Fig. 28-145), (2) across the dorsum of the quadrigeminal plate, and (3) down the dorsal sagittal plane of the spinal cord to the level of the cauda equina. They enlarge slowly, if at all, but may enmesh cranial or spinal nerves and interfere with nerve conduction. Most lipomas of the CNS are encountered incidentally at postmortem examination and histologically mimic normal fat cells.

Tumors of Germ Cell Origin

Neoplasms that are thought to originate from misplaced germ cells occur within the cranial cavity and, less commonly, in the spinal cord. Such tumors are almost invariably located in midline structures, especially in the area of the pineal gland, but also at sites immediately adjacent to this gland, in the cerebellopontine angle, and around the

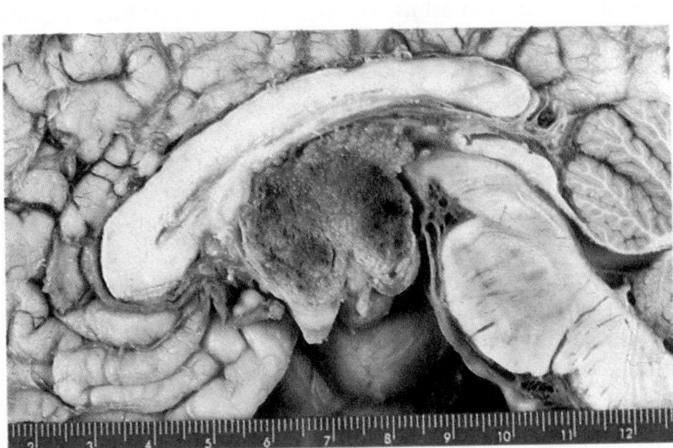

A

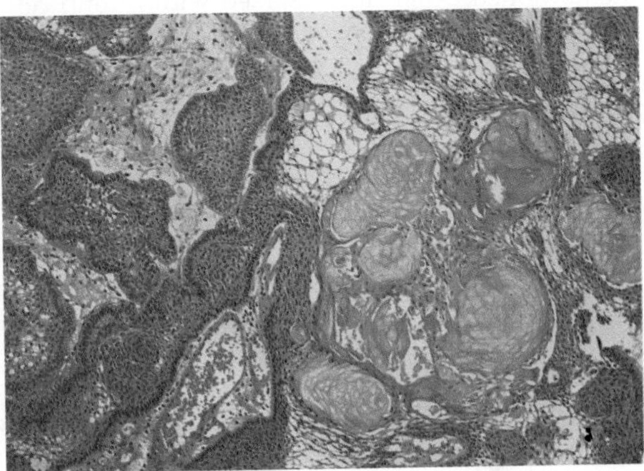

B

FIGURE *28-144*
Craniopharyngioma. (*A*) The tumor arises above the sella turcica, producing a spherical mass that impinges on the optic chiasm, hypothalamus, and third ventricle. (*B*) A microscopic section shows cords of epithelial cells interspersed with keratotic debris, resembling a lesion of dentigerous origin (see Fig. 25-16).

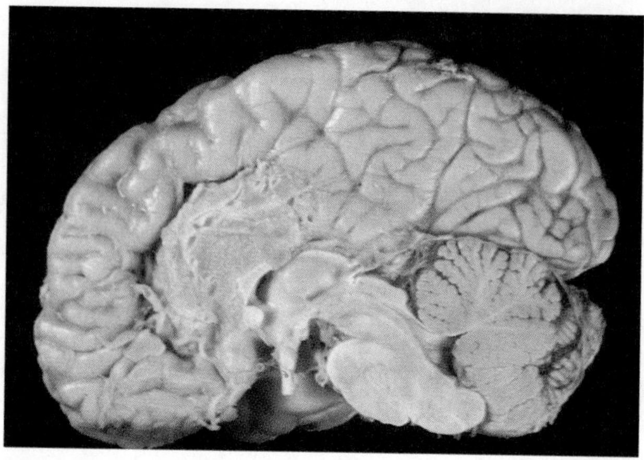

FIGURE 28-145
Lipoma. A soft yellow mass is seen in the dorsal, midsagittal axis of the brain.

sella turcica. Intracranial germ cell tumors display a number of phenotypes that parallel gonadal neoplasms, including seminoma, choriocarcinoma, embryonal carcinoma, endodermal sinus tumor, and teratoma.

Intracranial germ cell tumors are seen primarily in young adult men, and the symptoms depend on the location of the expanding mass. Destruction of the pineal gland by a germ cell tumor may produce precocious puberty, particularly in boys. When the tumor occurs in the pineal area, it may compress the superior colliculus and restrict ocular motion. Compression of the aqueduct of Sylvius leads to hydrocephalus.

Hemangioblastoma

Hemangioblastoma is a highly vascularized tumor that originates predominantly in the cerebellum. Although its name suggests that it arises from endothelial cells, the true cell of origin is still debated. Hemangioblastoma features endothelium-lined canals interspersed with plump cells (Fig. 28-146) that do not generate factor VIII and, therefore, cannot be identified as of endothelial origin. **In 20% of cases, these cells secrete erythropoietin and induce polycythemia.** A rare hemangioblastoma arises in the spinal cord, and on occasion they originate above the tentorium. Hemangioblastoma usually becomes clinically apparent between the ages of 20 and 40 years.

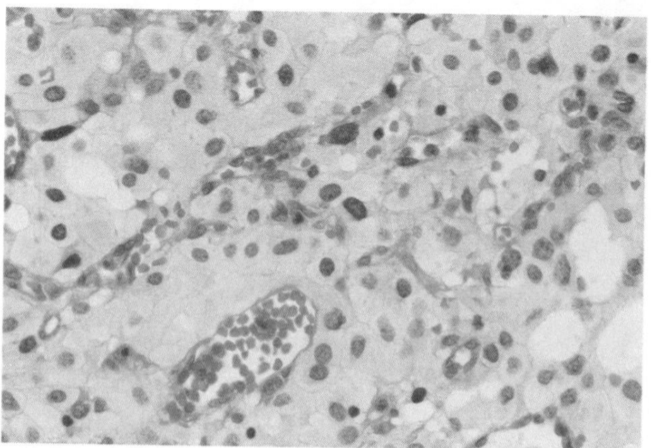

FIGURE 28-146
Hemangioblastoma. The tumor is composed of cells that display abundant pink cytoplasm and is traversed by thin-walled vascular channels.

Lindau syndrome refers to the hereditary occurrence of a cerebellar hemangioblastoma that is not associated with other lesions.

Von Hippel–Lindau syndrome is a hereditary variant in which cerebellar hemangioblastoma is associated with retinal hemangiomas.

Lymphoma

Lymphoma originates as a primary lesion in the brain in a manner analogous to its occurrence in the stomach, small bowel, or testis. In the brain, the tumor often arises deep in the cerebral hemispheres, commonly in bilateral periventricular positions (Fig. 28-147A,B). A mixture of small and large lymphocytes portray strong angiocentricity (see Fig. 28-147C). The constituent cells are generally identified by surface markers as B lymphocytes. The lesion has a close, but not absolute, relation with immunosuppression and is a well-recognized complication of AIDS. The Epstein–Barr virus coexists in a very high proportion of primary lymphomas and is viewed as causative by many investigators.

Extracranial lymphomas may secondarily involve the CNS, usually late in the course of the disease. The meninges, epidural space, and nerve roots are most commonly affected.

Metastatic Tumors

Metastatic tumors reach the intracranial compartment through the bloodstream, generally in patients with advanced cancer. Tumors of different organs vary in their incidence of intracranial metastases. For example, a patient with disseminated melanoma has a greater than 50% likelihood of acquiring intracranial metastases, whereas the incidence of such metastases for carcinoma of the breast and lung is approximately 35%, and that for cancer of the kidney or colon is only 5%. Certain carcinomas, such as those of the prostate, liver, and adrenals, and sarcomas of all types rarely establish intracranial metastases. Most metastatic lesions seed to the gray–white junction, reflecting the rich capillary bed in this area. Carcinomas may seed the calvarium and extend into the intracranial compartment.

A metastasis contrasts with a primary glioma in its discrete appearance, globoid shape, and prominent halo of edema (Fig. 28-148). Metastases to the leptomeninges permit tumor cells to grow in the CSF, suspended as if they were in tissue culture.

Colloid Cyst

Colloid cysts (paraphyseal cyst, third ventricular cyst) are distinctive for their anterior, midline location in the tegmental portion of the third ventricle (Fig. 28-149). In

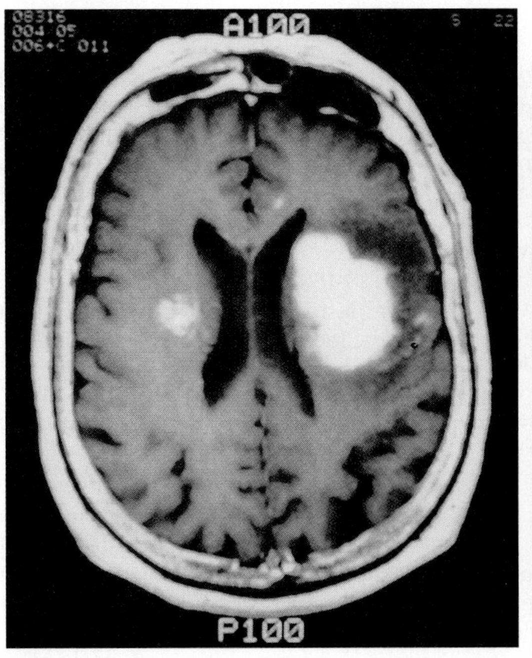

A

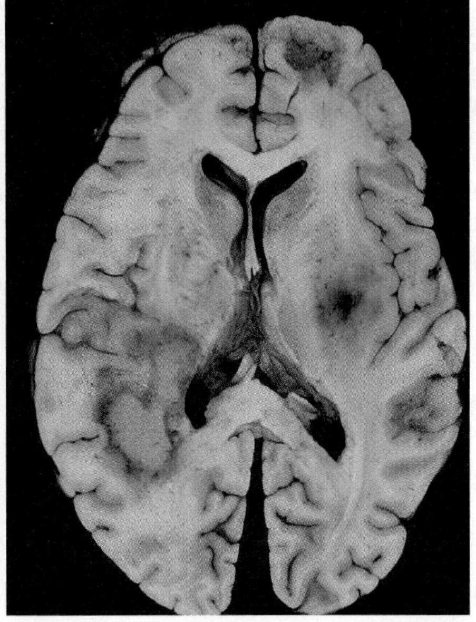

B

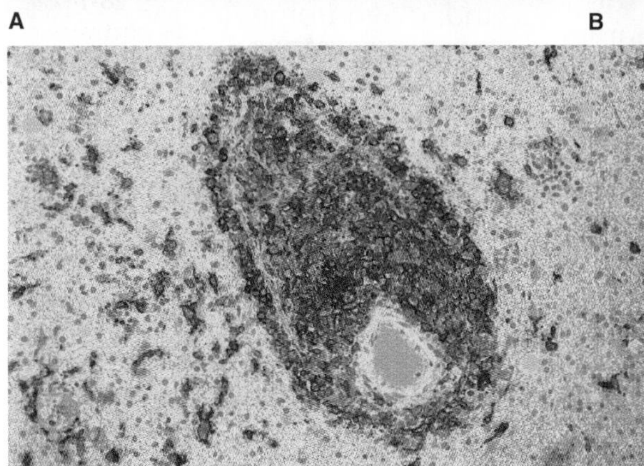

C

FIGURE *28-147*
Primary lymphoma of the brain. (*A*) Magnetic resonance imaging shows a multicentric primary lymphoma, with a predilection for localization near the ventricles. (*B*) A multiplicity of lesions is distributed through both hemispheres in a patient with acquired immunodeficiency syndrome (AIDS). (*C*) A microscopic section of the tumor reveals an angiocentric distribution of small and large neoplastic lymphocytes, which are stained for a B-cell antigen.

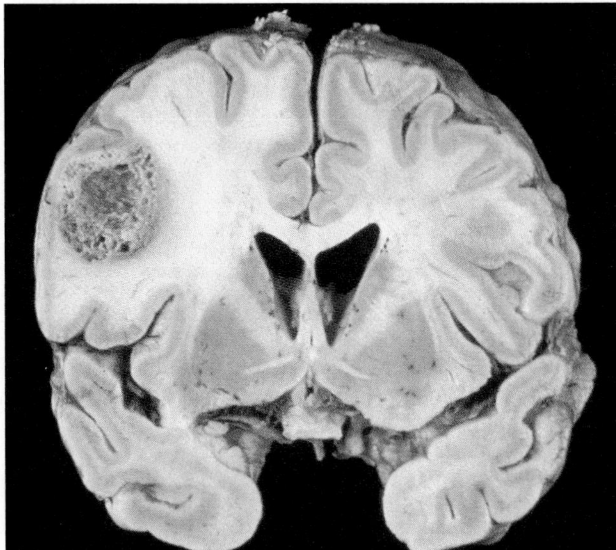

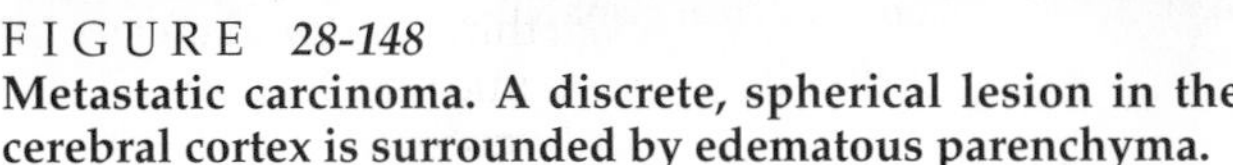

FIGURE *28-148*
Metastatic carcinoma. A discrete, spherical lesion in the cerebral cortex is surrounded by edematous parenchyma.

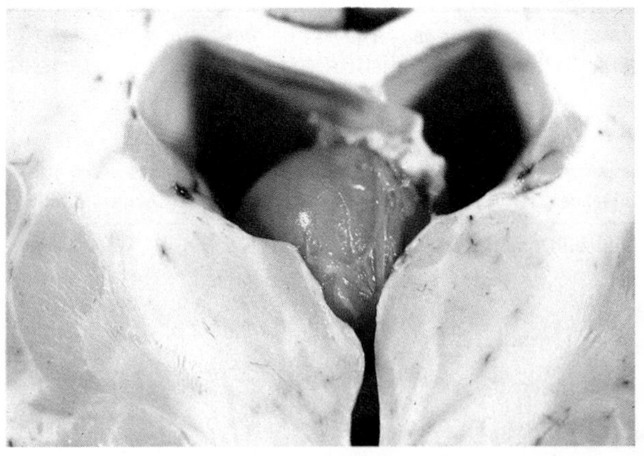

FIGURE *28-149*
Colloid cyst. The lesion arises in the roof of the third ventricle, disfigures the fornix, and impinges on the foramen of Monro to produce hydrocephalus.

this location, they (1) occlude the foramina of Monro, (2) elevate and compress the fornix, and (3) press on the lateral wall of the third ventricle. These effects result in hydrocephalus, alterations in personality, weakness of the lower legs, and loss of bladder control. The pyramidal fibers to the legs and the pathway that originates in the cingulate gyrus to control the bladder pass medially in the internal capsule subjacent to the ependyma.

Colloid cysts are lined by ciliated cuboidal epithelium. The lesions enlarge slowly, usually over decades, by the accumulation of desquamated and secretory products. The origin of a colloid cyst remains in doubt, but it is conjectured to arise from the paraphysis, a sense organ of lower vertebrates that may remain as a vestigial structure in humans.

Hereditary Intracranial Neoplasms

A number of hereditary disorders are associated with tumors of the brain and spinal cord. The major syndromes and principal nervous system tumors are listed in Table 28-5 and include the neurofibromatoses, tuberous sclerosis, and von Hippel–Lindau syndrome. In addition, many other inherited diseases in which neoplasms of systemic organs figure prominently may include variable expression of nervous system tumors, such as malignant gliomas arising in patients with Li–Fraumeni syndrome and medulloblastomas associated with Turcot syndrome.

Neurofibromatosis (von Recklinghausen Disease)

Neurofibromatosis occurs in two distinct forms, both of which are inherited as autosomal dominant traits (see Chapter 6). Type 2 neurofibromatosis is usually characterized by bilateral acoustic neuromas. However, the disease can be diagnosed in patients with a unilateral eighth nerve tumor if two of the following are present: neurofibroma, meningioma, glioma, or schwannoma.

Tuberous Sclerosis (Bourneville Disease)

Tuberous sclerosis is an autosomal dominant disease characterized by hamartomas (tubers) of the brain, retina, and viscera. In this entity, disordered migration and arrested maturation of the neuroectoderm result in the appearance of "tubers" of the cerebral cortex and of subependymal astrocytic nodules (Fig. 28-150A). The tubers are discrete, firm, cortical areas composed of bizarre cells that possess both neuronal and glial features. The subependymal nodules have been likened to "candle drippings" and provide the substrate for gemistocytic astrocytomas (see Fig. 28-150B). In addition to the intracranial neuroectodermal lesions, the syndrome includes (1) angiofibromas of the face (adenoma sebaceum), (2) rhabdomyomas of the heart, and (3) mixed mesenchymal tumors of the kidney (angiomyolipomas). Almost all patients with tuberous sclerosis have seizures, and the majority are mentally retarded.

Mutations in two genes have been linked to tuberous sclerosis. *TSC1* (9q34) codes for a 130-kDa protein, termed *hamartin*. *TSC2* (16p13) encodes *tuberin*, a protein with homology to a GTPase-activating protein. Both genes seem to act as tumor suppressors.

Lindau Syndrome

As was mentioned previously, some hemangioblastomas of the cerebellum assume a hereditary pattern (Lindau syndrome). An identical tumor may occur in the retina (von Hippel–Lindau syndrome). In the latter syndrome, cysts may also occur in the kidneys and pancreas.

Sturge–Weber Syndrome (Encephalofacial Angiomatosis)

Sturge–Weber syndrome is a rare, nonfamilial congenital disorder characterized by angiomas of the brain and face. The facial lesion is usually unilateral and is termed a port wine stain (*nevus flammeus*). The leptomeninges exhibit large angiomas, which in severe cases may occupy an entire hemisphere. Cerebral calcification and atrophy often underlie the intracranial angiomas. The link between angiomas of the face and the brain has been attributed to the continuity of the embryological vascular supply of the telencephalon, the eye, and the overlying skin. In most instances, Sturge–Weber syndrome is associated with mental deficiency.

TABLE *28-5* **Hereditary Syndromes Associated with Intracranial Tumors**

Disease	Chromosome Locus	Gene (Protein)	Nervous System Tumor(s)
Neurofibromatosis 1	17q11	*NF1* (neurofibromin)	Neurofibroma Neurofibrosarcoma Juvenile pilocytic astrocytoma of the optic nerves ("optic glioma")
Neurofibromatosis 2	22q12	*NF2* (schwannomin/merlin)	Schwannoma Meningioma Ependymoma (spinal cord)
Tuberous sclerosis	9q34 16p13.3	*TSC1* (hamartin) *TSC2* (tuberin)	Subependymal giant cell Astrocytoma
von Hippel–Lindau syndrome	3p25	*VHL*	Hemangioblastoma

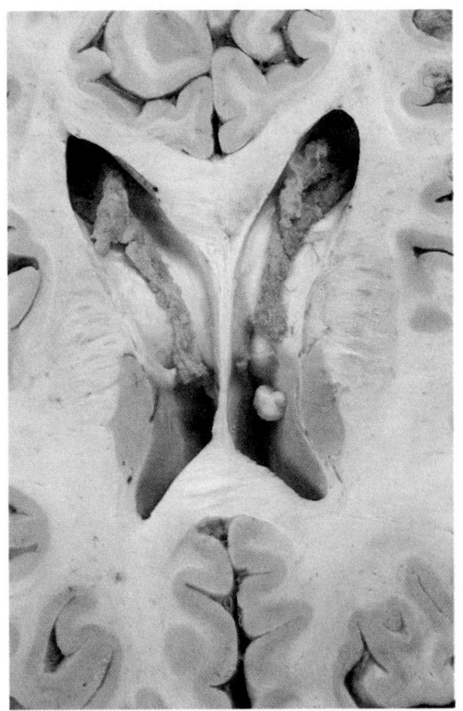

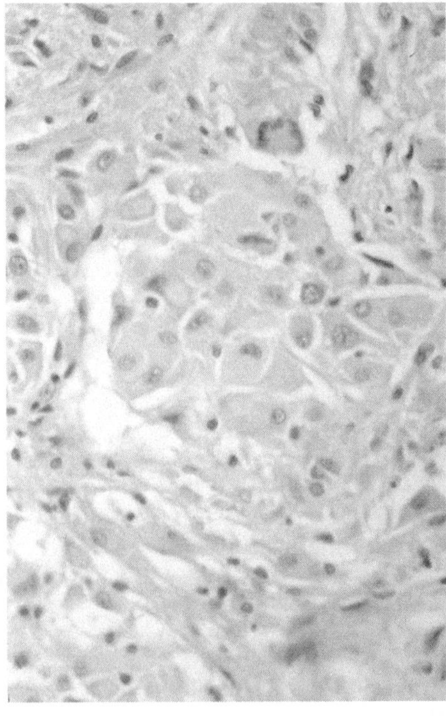

A B

FIGURE 28-150
Tuberous sclerosis. (*A*) A horizontal section of the brain shows subependymal astrocytic nodules in the lateral ventricles ("candle drippings"). (*B*) A giant cell astrocytoma has developed from one of the subependymal hamartomas.

The Peripheral Nervous System

ANATOMY

The peripheral nervous system is external to the brain and spinal cord and includes cranial nerves, dorsal and ventral spinal roots, spinal nerves and their continuations, and ganglia. Peripheral nerves carry somatic motor, somatic sensory, visceral sensory, and autonomic fibers.

The somatic motor and preganglionic autonomic fibers arise from neuronal cell bodies within the CNS. The sensory and postganglionic autonomic fibers originate from neuronal cell bodies within ganglia located on cranial nerves, dorsal roots, and autonomic nerves. The neurons and satellite cells of the ganglia and all of the Schwann cells are derived from the neural crest.

The peripheral nerves, but not their ganglia, have a blood–nerve barrier analogous to the blood–brain barrier. Endoneurial connective tissue surrounds the individual nerve fibers, which are bundled into fascicles by the perineurial connective tissue. Epineurial connective tissue binds the fascicles together and contains the nutrient arteries.

Peripheral nerve fibers are either myelinated or unmyelinated (Fig. 28-151). Myelinated fibers range from 1 to 20 μm in diameter, whereas unmyelinated ones are considerably smaller, measuring 0.4 to 2.4 μm. Myelin is an elaboration of the Schwann cell plasmalemma and is necessary for saltatory nerve conduction. Schwann cells ensheath both the myelinated and the unmyelinated fibers. The axon determines whether the ensheathing Schwann cell differentiates into a myelin-forming cell.

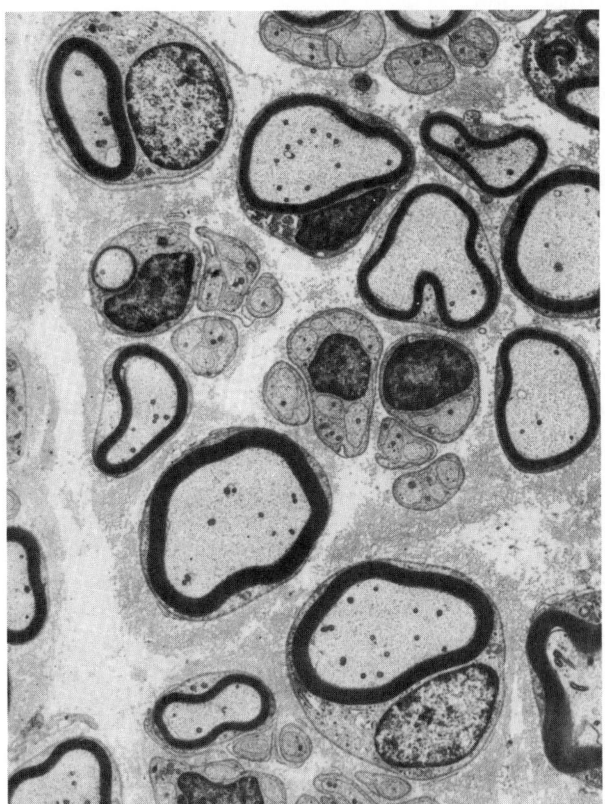

FIGURE 28-151
Structure of peripheral nerve. An electron micrograph of a peripheral nerve shows myelinated fibers interspersed with groups of unmyelinated fibers. Note that in contrast to myelinated axons, several unmyelinated axons may share a Schwann cell.

Myelin-sheath thickness, internodal length (i.e., the distance between two nodes of Ranvier), and conduction velocity are proportional to the axonal diameter.

REACTIONS TO INJURY

Peripheral nerve fibers display only a limited number of reactions to injury. The major types of nerve fiber damage are axonal degeneration and segmental demyelination. The peripheral nervous system differs from the CNS in having the capacity for functionally significant axonal regeneration and remyelination.

Axonal Degeneration

Degeneration (necrosis) of the axon occurs in many neuropathies and reflects significant injury of the neuronal cell body or its axon. Axonal degeneration is quickly followed by breakdown of the myelin sheath and Schwann cell proliferation. Myelin degradation is initiated by Schwann cells and completed by macrophages, which infiltrate the nerve within 3 days after axonal degeneration. If the degeneration is restricted to the distal axon, regenerating axons may sprout within 1 week from the intact, proximal axonal stump. There are several types of axonal degeneration.

DISTAL AXONOPATHY: In many neuropathies, axonal degeneration is initially restricted to the distal ends of the larger, longer fibers (Fig. 28-152). Peripheral neuropathies characterized by the selective degeneration of distal axons are known as *dying-back neuropathies* (distal axonopathies) and typically are seen as distal ("glove-and-stocking") neuropathies. The basis for the selective vulnerability of the distal axon in these neuropathies is unknown.

In distal axonopathy, the neuronal cell body and proximal axon remain intact. Therefore, axonal regeneration and return of nerve function may be possible if the cause of the distal axonal degeneration can be identified and removed. This must occur before the dying-back degeneration extends sufficiently centripetally to involve the proximal axon and cell body. Recovery is also limited in some dying-back neuropathies, because the distal axonal degeneration involves not only the peripherally directed axon of the dorsal root-ganglion neuron, but also its centrally directed axon traveling in the dorsal columns of the spinal cord. These centrally directed axons, like other axons within the CNS, have little capacity for regeneration.

NEURONOPATHY: Axonal degeneration may also be the result of degeneration of the neuronal cell body, as occurs in poliomyelitis. Neuropathies showing selective degeneration of the neuronal cell body are referred to as neuronopathies and are much less common than distal axonopathies. There is little potential for recovery of function in neuronopathy because degeneration of the neuronal cell body precludes axonal regeneration.

A. INTACT MYELINATED FIBER

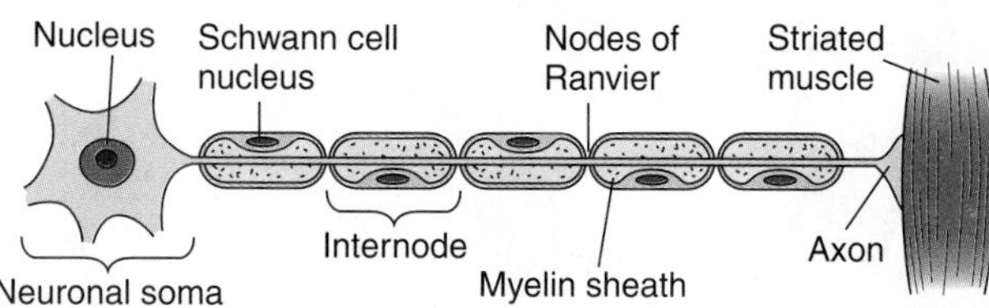

B. DISTAL AXONAL DEGENERATION

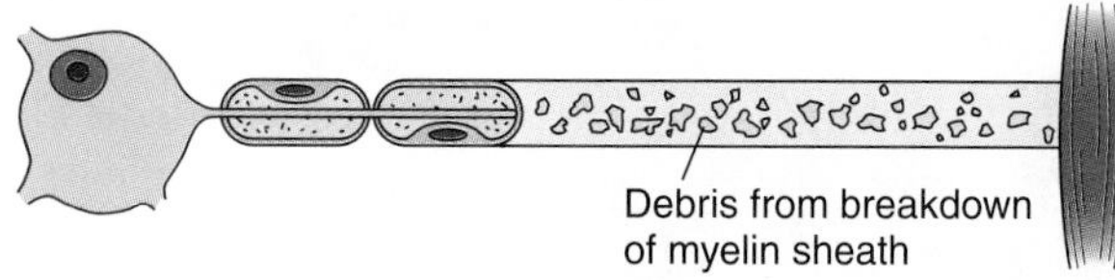

C. DEGENERATION OF CELL BODY AND AXON

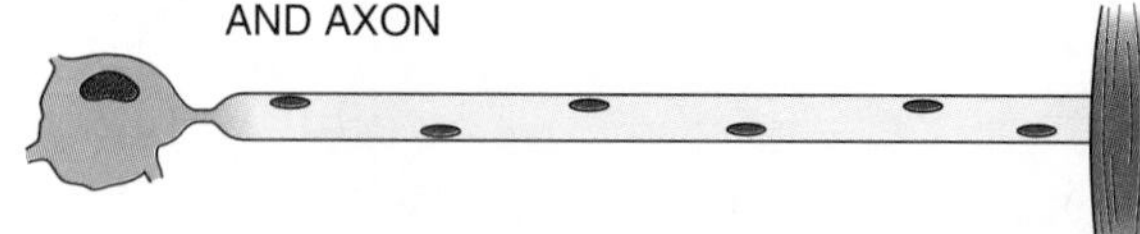

D. SEGMENTAL DEMYELINATION

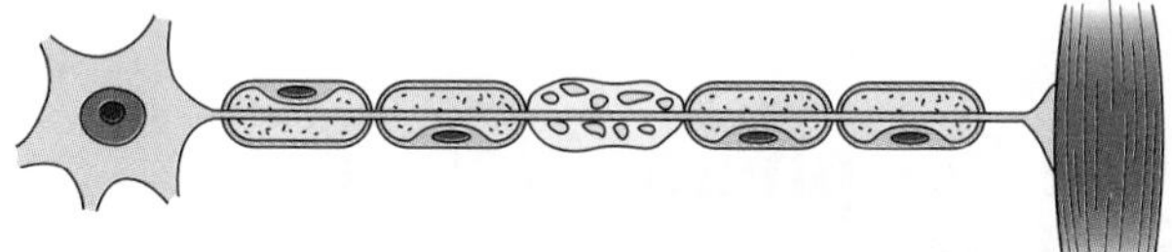

E. REMYELINATION

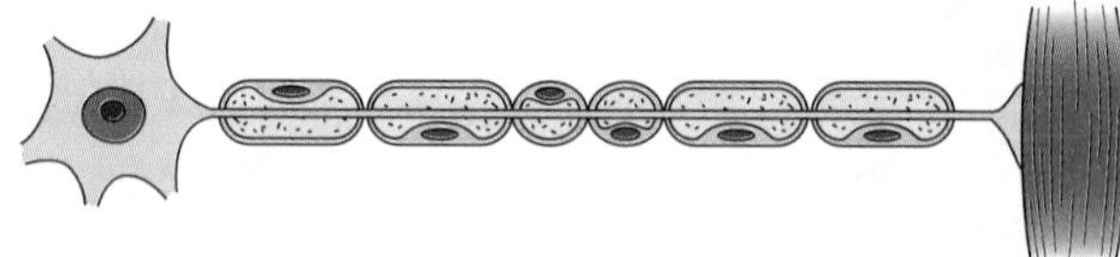

F. REGENERATING AXON

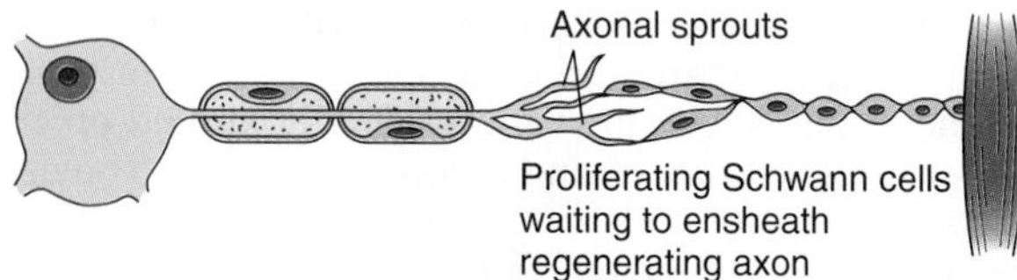

G. REGENERATED NERVE FIBER

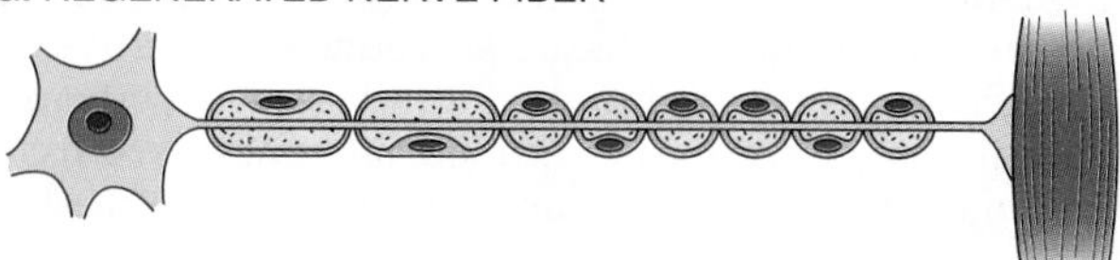

FIGURE *28-152*
Basic responses of peripheral nerve fibers to injury.

WALLERIAN DEGENERATION: This term refers to the axonal degeneration that occurs in a nerve distal to a transection or crush of the nerve.

Segmental Demyelination

The loss of myelin from one or more internodes (segments) along a myelinated fiber is common in many neuropathies and reflects Schwann cell dysfunction (see Fig. 28-152). This dysfunction may be caused by direct injury of the Schwann cell–myelin sheath (*primary demyelination*), or it may be the result of underlying axonal abnormalities (*secondary demyelination*).

The degeneration of the myelin sheath is unaccompanied by degeneration of the underlying axon. Macrophages infiltrate the nerve and clear the myelin debris. Degeneration of the internodal myelin sheath is followed sequentially by (1) Schwann cell proliferation, (2) remyelination of the demyelinated segments, and (3) recovery of function. The remyelinated internodes have shortened internodal lengths. Repeated episodes of segmental demyelination and remyelination of peripheral nerves, as occurs in chronic demyelinating neuropathies, lead to the accumulation of supernumerary Schwann cells around axons (*onion-bulbs*) and clinically apparent nerve enlargement (*hypertrophic neuropathy*; Fig. 28-153).

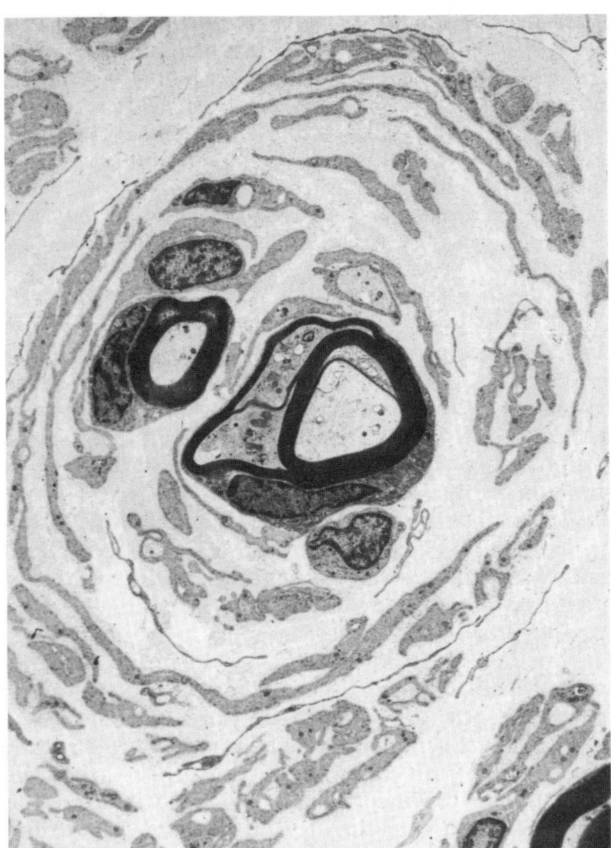

FIGURE *28-153*
Onion-bulb formation in peripheral nerve. An electron micrograph shows multiple layers of flattened Schwann cell processes encircling two myelinated axons. Onion-bulb formations are common in the demyelinating form of Charcot–Marie–Tooth disease.

PERIPHERAL NEUROPATHIES

Peripheral neuropathy is a process that affects the function of one or more peripheral nerves. The disease may be restricted to the peripheral nervous system, involve both the peripheral and central nervous systems, or affect multiple organ systems. Peripheral neuropathies are encountered in all age groups and may be hereditary or acquired.

The causes of peripheral neuropathy are diverse (Table 28-6). Charcot–Marie–Tooth disease (CMT) is the most common hereditary peripheral neuropathy. Diabetic neuropathy is the most common acquired neuropathy in the United States. Pathologically, the involved nerves may show mainly axonal degeneration (*axonal neuropathy*), segmental demyelination (*demyelinating neuropathy*), or a mixture of both. Most neuropathies are axonal. The demyelinating form of CMT and inflammatory demyelinating neuropathy are the common demyelinating neuropathies.

☐ **Clinical Features:** The major clinical manifestations of peripheral neuropathy are muscle weakness, muscle atrophy, alterations of sensation, and autonomic dysfunction. Motor, sensory, and autonomic functions may be equally or preferentially affected. Sensory abnormalities may reflect predominant involvement of large-diameter fibers (position and vibration sense) or small-

TABLE *28-6* **Etiological Classification of Neuropathy**

Autoimmune	Toxic neuropathy
Acute inflammatory demyelinating neuropathy	Paraneoplastic neuropathy
Chronic inflammatory demyelinating neuropathy	Amyloid neuropathy
Acute motor axonal neuropathy	Paraproteinemic neuropathy
Multifocal motor neuropathy	Inherited neuropathy
Dorsal root ganglionitis	Neuropathy associated with infections
Metabolic	Cytomegalovirus
Diabetic polyneuropathy	Diphtheria (toxin)
Uremic neuropathy	Herpes zoster
Hypothyroid neuropathy	Human immunodeficiency virus
Critical-illness polyneuropathy	Leprosy
Nutritional	Lyme disease
Alcoholic neuropathy	Sarcoid neuropathy
Vitamin B_1–deficiency neuropathy	Radiation neuropathy
Vitamin B_6–deficiency neuropathy	Traumatic neuropathy
Vitamin B_{12}–deficiency neuropathy	Cryptogenic neuropathy
Vitamin E–deficiency neuropathy	
Ischemic	
Vasculitic neuropathy	
Neuropathy of peripheral vascular disease	
Diabetic mononeuropathies	

diameter fibers (pain and temperature). The tempo of the neuropathy may be acute (days to weeks), subacute (weeks to months), or chronic (months to years). The disease may be localized to one nerve (*mononeuropathy*) or several nerves (*mononeuropathy multiplex*), or it may be diffuse and symmetric (*polyneuropathy*). Electrophysiological studies are often helpful in differentiating between axonal and demyelinating neuropathies. Nerve-conduction velocity is typically near normal in axonal neuropathies but greatly decreased in demyelinating neuropathies.

Inflammatory Demyelinating Neuropathy

Inflammatory demyelinating neuropathy is an acquired neuropathy that (1) may be sporadic; (2) may follow immunization, surgery, or viral and mycoplasmal infections; or (3) may complicate cancer. There is also an increased incidence of inflammatory demyelinating neuropathy in persons with HIV infection. The pathogenesis of demyelination in the inflammatory neuropathies is unknown, but current evidence suggests that it may be immunologically mediated.

☐ **Pathology:** An inflammatory demyelinating neuropathy may involve all levels of the peripheral nervous system, including spinal roots, ganglia, craniospinal nerves, and autonomic nerves. The distribution of the lesions varies from case to case. The involved regions show endoneurial infiltrates of lymphocytes and macrophages, segmental demyelination, and relative sparing of axons. The lymphoid infiltrates are often perivascular, but there is no true vasculitis. Macrophages are frequently found adjacent to degenerating myelin sheaths and have been observed to strip off and phagocytose the superficial myelin lamellae. Such macrophage-mediated demyelination is rarely observed in other neuropathies. When the neuropathy has a chronic course, there may be numerous onion bulbs, owing to recurring episodes of demyelination, Schwann cell proliferation, and remyelination.

☐ **Clinical Features:** Inflammatory demyelinating neuropathy usually is seen as an acutely evolving, predominantly motor polyneuropathy (*acute inflammatory demyelinating polyneuropathy, Guillain–Barré syndrome*). Sensory or autonomic disturbances predominate in some cases. Some 5% of cases are seen with ophthalmoplegia, ataxia, and areflexia (*Fisher syndrome*). The muscular paralysis may cause respiratory embarrassment, and the autonomic involvement may result in cardiac arrhythmias, hypotension, or hypertension. Resolution of acute inflammatory demyelinating neuropathy begins 2 to 4 weeks after onset, and most patients make a good recovery. Less frequently, inflammatory demyelinating neuropathy has a chronic course, characterized by multiple relapses or a slow continuous progression (*chronic inflammatory polyneuropathy*). Lumbar puncture characteristically reveals an increase in the protein level of the CSF, but only slight pleocytosis. The increased protein level is attributable to the inflammation of the spinal roots. Plasmapheresis and intravenously administered gamma globulin have proven beneficial in both acute and chronic forms of the disease. Corticosteroids are effective only in the chronic form of inflammatory demyelinating neuropathy.

Acute motor axonal neuropathy is a polyneuropathy that is seen clinically like acute inflammatory demyelinating neuropathy. This axonal form of the Guillain–Barré syndrome is often associated with evidence of prior *Campylobacter jejuni* infection. The disease is presumed to have an immune-mediated pathogenesis.

Multifocal motor neuropathy is a chronic asymmetric neuropathy that may be mistaken clinically for motor neuron disease. The neuropathy is characterized pathologically by chronic inflammation and demyelination, suggesting that it is related to chronic inflammatory demyelinating neuropathy. There is often an associated increased titer of anti-GM_1 antibodies, but the role of these antibodies in the pathogenesis of the disorder is unknown.

Dorsal Root Ganglionitis (Sensory Ganglionitis)

Dorsal root ganglionitis is a sensory neuronopathy that may occur independently, as a remote effect of cancer (paraneoplastic neuropathy), or in association with Sjögren syndrome. The neuronopathy typically is seen as a subacute or chronic sensory polyneuropathy with sensory ataxia. The pathogenesis of the ganglionitis is unknown, but an immune mechanism is likely. The dorsal root ganglia show infiltration by lymphocytes and loss of sensory neurons.

Diabetic Neuropathy

Peripheral neuropathy is a common complication of diabetes mellitus. The neuropathy may manifest as a distal sensory or sensorimotor polyneuropathy, autonomic neuropathy, mononeuropathy, or mononeuropathy multiplex. **Distal, predominantly sensory, polyneuropathy is the most common form of diabetic neuropathy.**

The pathogenesis of the nerve fiber injury in diabetes is unknown. It has long been held that the metabolic alterations of diabetes are responsible for the distal symmetric polyneuropathy and that nerve ischemia caused by the small-vessel disease is responsible for the mononeuropathies. There is some evidence, however, to suggest that local nerve ischemia may also play a role in the pathogenesis of the symmetric polyneuropathy.

The distal symmetric polyneuropathy of diabetes is characterized pathologically by a mixture of axonal degeneration and segmental demyelination, with axonal degeneration predominating. The axonal loss involves fibers of all sizes, but occasionally preferentially affects the large myelinated fibers (*large-fiber neuropathy*) or the small myelinated fibers and unmyelinated fibers (*small-fiber neuropathy*). There may also be loss of neurons in the dorsal root ganglia and anterior horns, but this appears to be a consequence of centripetal progression of dying-back axonal degeneration rather than a neuropathy.

Uremic Neuropathy

Uremic neuropathy is a distal sensorimotor axonal polyneuropathy that may complicate chronic renal failure. The pathogenesis of the nerve fiber damage is not known, but the disease usually stabilizes or improves with chronic dialysis. Uremic neuropathy is characterized pathologically by both distal axonal degeneration and segmental demyelination, with axonal degeneration predominating and preferentially involving large-diameter fibers. The neuropathy resolves after renal transplantation.

Critical-Illness Polyneuropathy

Critical-illness polyneuropathy is a distal axonal neuropathy that develops in patients with sepsis and multiorgan failure. The pathogenesis of the condition is obscure. The acute, predominantly motor, neuropathy may first become apparent when the patient cannot be weaned from ventilatory support.

Alcoholic Neuropathy

Alcoholic neuropathy is a distal sensorimotor axonal polyneuropathy that is generally attributed to nutritional deficiencies, rather than to a direct toxic effect of ethanol on the peripheral nervous system. Peripheral nerves show loss of nerve fibers from axonal degeneration of the dying-back type. Axonal neuropathy is also associated with a lack of vitamins B_1, B_6, B_{12}, or E, but is much less common in the United States than alcoholic neuropathy. The axonal neuropathy associated with isoniazid therapy for tuberculosis is due to the drug's interference with the metabolism of vitamin B_6.

Vasculitic Neuropathy

Vasculitis may involve the nutrient arteries of nerves and produce ischemic nerve injury (*ischemic neuropathy*). Vasculitis-induced ischemic neuropathy may complicate polyarteritis nodosa and other systemic vasculitidies, rheumatoid arthritis, other collagen-vascular diseases, cryoglobulinemia, and HIV infection. A "nonsystemic" vasculitic neuropathy, in which the vasculitis is primarily limited to the peripheral nervous system, also has been recognized. Vasculitic neuropathy is characterized pathologically by axonal degeneration and typically is seen as a mononeuropathy or mononeuropathy multiplex (Fig. 28-154).

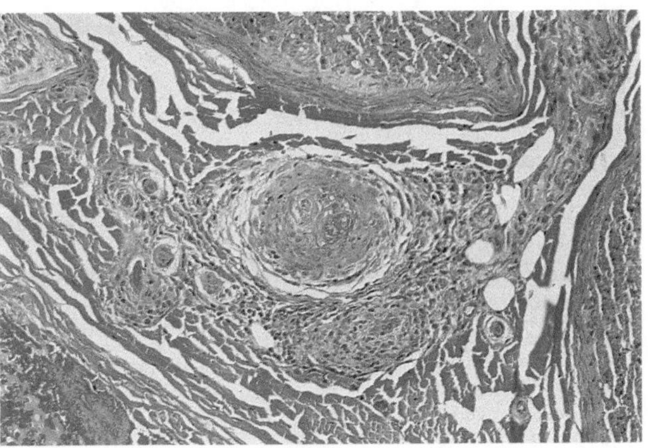

FIGURE *28-154*
Vasculitic neuropathy in a patient with polyarteritis nodosa. A photomicrograph from a cross-section of a sural nerve reveals an inflamed epineurial artery, with a disorganized wall and thrombosis in its lumen.

Toxic Neuropathy

A wide variety of drugs, environmental agents, and industrial compounds cause peripheral neuropathy (Table 28-7). The majority of toxic neuropathies are iatrogenic (i.e., they are caused by drugs). Most toxic neuropathies are characterized by axonal degeneration, usually of the dying-back type. Amiodarone, buckthorn toxin, and diphtheria toxin are notable for producing demyelinating neuropathies. Because diphtheria toxin does not cross the blood–nerve barrier, the demyelination in diphtheritic neuropathy is limited to the barrier-deficient ganglia and contiguous regions of the spinal roots and nerves.

Paraneoplastic Neuropathy

Paraneoplastic neuropathy is a disease of peripheral nerves that occurs as a remote effect of cancer. Other paraneoplastic diseases of the nervous system include chronic encephalomyelitis, necrotizing myelopathy, cerebellar degeneration, and the Eaton–Lambert syndrome. It is not uncommon for a paraneoplastic disorder to precede the

TABLE *28-7* **Agents Associated with Toxic Neuropathy**

Drugs	Environmental and Industrial Agents
Amiodarone	Acrylamide
Chloramphenicol	Allyl chloride
Colchicine	Arsenic
Dapsone	Buckthorn toxin
Dideoxycytidine	Carbon disulfide
Disulfiram	Chlordecone
Ethambutol	Dimethylaminopropionitrile
Gold	Diphtheria toxin
Isoniazid	Ethylene oxide
Metronidazole	*n*-Hexane
Misonidazole	Methyl *n*-butyl ketone
Nitrofurantoin	Lead
Perhexiline	Mercury
Phenytoin	Methyl bromide
Platinum	Organophosphates
Pyridoxine (vitamin B_6)	Polychlorinated biphenyls
Suramin	Thallium
Thalidomide	Trichloroethylene
Vincristine	Vacor

recognition of the underlying cancer. Several different clinicopathological types of paraneoplastic peripheral neuropathy have been defined, although the pathogenetic mechanisms responsible for these diseases are unknown.

- **Chronic axonal polyneuropathy:** This distal sensorimotor polyneuropathy is characterized by axonal degeneration and demyelination, with axonal loss predominating.
- **Dorsal root ganglionitis (subacute sensory polyneuropathy, sensory ganglionitis):** Much less commonly, paraneoplastic neuropathy is seen as a subacute sensory neuronopathy. The dorsal root ganglionitis may be be accompanied by similar histological changes in the CNS (*paraneoplastic encephalomyelitis*).
- **Subacute motor polyneuropathy:** This rare paraneoplastic syndrome is due to a loss of neurons in the anterior horns of the spinal cord and typically occurs in the context of Hodgkin disease.
- **Inflammatory demyelinating neuropathy:** Acute and chronic versions of this disorder also have been associated with cancer.

Not all neuropathies associated with cancer result from remote effects of neoplasia on the nervous system. Cancer may also cause neuropathy by direct compression or infiltration of nerves or nerve roots.

Amyloid Neuropathy

Amyloid infiltration of the peripheral nervous system typically produces a distal sensorimotor axonal polyneuropathy, often with prominent autonomic dysfunction. Although amyloid neuropathy may be hereditary, it usually complicates the acquired form of systemic amyloidosis that is associated with plasma cell dyscrasias and the deposition of immunoglobulin light-chain (AL) amyloid. A point mutation in the transthyretin (prealbumin) gene is responsible for dominantly inherited, familial, amyloid polyneuropathy. Pathologically, amyloid neuropathy is characterized by the deposition of amyloid in peripheral nerves, dorsal root ganglia, and autonomic ganglia. The interstitial amyloid deposits are both endoneurial and epineurial and frequently involve the walls of blood vessels. The deposition of amyloid is accompanied by loss of myelinated and unmyelinated fibers. Postulated mechanisms for the nerve-fiber damage include direct mechanical injury of nerve fibers and ganglion cells by the amyloid deposits and nerve ischemia caused by amyloid infiltration of the vasa nervorum.

Carpal tunnel syndrome is a chronic entrapment neuropathy of the median nerve at the wrist and represents another complication of systemic amyloidosis. The nerve entrapment is the result of amyloid infiltration of the flexor retinaculum.

Paraproteinemic (Dysproteinemic) Neuropathy

Monoclonal gammopathy may be associated with amyloid neuropathy, cryoglobulinemia-associated vasculitic neuropathy, a chronic axonal polyneuropathy of unknown pathogenesis, or a chronic demyelinating polyneuropathy. ***Chronic demyelinating polyneuropathy*** occurs in the context of IgM monoclonal gammopathy of unknown significance or Waldenstrom macroglobulinemia. It is characterized pathologically by extensive segmental demyelination, a variable number of onion bulbs, axonal loss, and a distinctive widening of the myelin lamellae (Fig. 28-155). The IgM paraprotein binds to myelin-associated glycoprotein (MAG), suggesting that the paraprotein is involved in the pathogenesis of the demyelination.

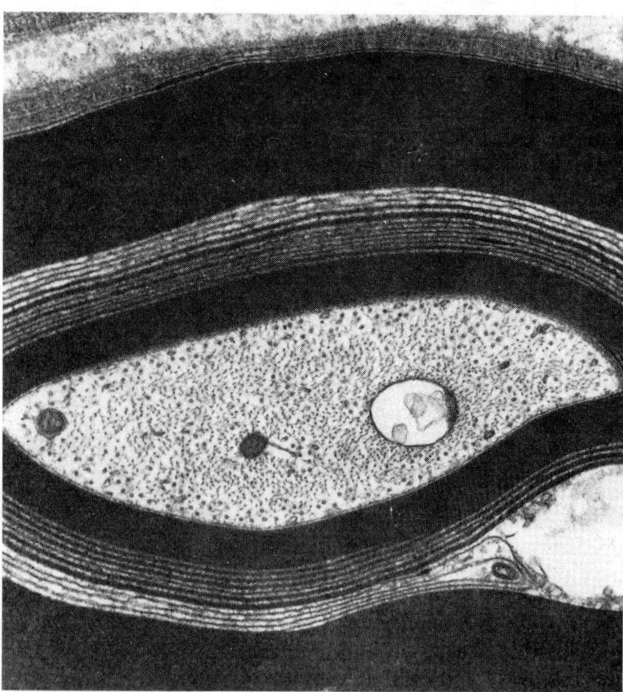

FIGURE *28-155*
Paraproteinemic neuropathy. An electron micrograph shows a myelinated fiber with multiple abnormally widely spaced myelin lamellae from a patient with an immunoglobulin M (IgM) monoclonal gammopathy of unknown significance and a chronic demyelinating neuropathy.

Hereditary Neuropathy

Peripheral neuropathy is a manifestation of a variety of inherited diseases (Table 28-8). Hereditary neuropathy is the most common form of chronic neuropathy in children and an often unrecognized cause in adults.

CHARCOT–MARIE–TOOTH DISEASE: CMT is a slowly progressive form of hereditary motor and sensory neuropathy (HMSN), which is seen in late childhood or adolescence as a distal sensorimotor polyneuropathy. ***CMT1 (HMSN I)*** features decreased nerve-conduction velocity and is characterized pathologically by chronic demyelination, onion bulbs, nerve hypertrophy, and distal axonal degeneration. ***CMT2 (HMSN II)*** has near-normal

TABLE *28-8* **Inherited Diseases Associated with Neuropathy**

Abetalipoproteinemia
Fabry disease (α-galactosidase deficiency)
Familial amyloid polyneuropathies
  Apolipoprotein A_1-related
  Gelsolin-related
  Transthyretin-related
Friedreich ataxia
Giant axonal neuropathy
Hereditary motor and sensory neuropathies
Hereditary motor neuropathies (spinal muscular atrophies)
Hereditary sensory neuropathies
Leukodystrophies
  Adrenoleukomyeloneuropathy
  Globoid cell leukodystrophy
  Metachromatic leukodystrophy
Porphyria
Refsum disease (phytanic acid storage disease)
Tangier disease

nerve-conduction velocity and microscopically shows distal axon degeneration. CMT is genetically heterogeneous, with subtypes defined by their specific genetic defects (Table 28-9).

***Dejerine–Sottas syndrome* (*HMSN III*)** is a much more severe form of HMSN that is seen at birth or early infancy with extremely decreased nerve-conduction velocities. Peripheral nerves show a severe, chronic demyelinating neuropathy, with onion bulbs and distal axonal degeneration.

Neuropathy Associated with AIDS

Human immunodeficiency virus infection may be associated clinically with acute or chronic inflammatory demyelinating neuropathy, distal predominantly sensory polyneuropathy, mononeuropathy, polyradiculopathy, and toxic neuropathy.

- **Chronic axonal polyneuropathy** is the most common type of neuropathy associated with HIV infection. This distal, predominantly sensory, polyneuropathy is characterized by distal axonal degeneration and usually occurs during the later stages of AIDS. The pathogenesis of the axonal degeneration is obscure, and there is no effective therapy.
- **Inflammatory demyelinating neuropathy** associated with AIDS may be acute or chronic and is pathologically similar to the inflammatory demyelinating neuropathy associated with the Guillain–Barré syndrome. The disorder is thought to be immunologically mediated. The neuropathy typically occurs early in the course of HIV infection, before the full onset of AIDS. The inflammatory demyelinating neuropathy often responds to plasmapheresis, intravenous gamma globulin, or corticosteroids.
- **Cytomegalovirus infection** of the peripheral nervous system has been responsible for some of the mononeuropathies and polyradiculopathies associated with AIDS.
- **Vasculitic neuropathy** is the cause of mononeuropathy and mononeuropathy multiplex in some AIDS patients.
- **Toxic neuropathy** is caused by several drugs used in the therapy of AIDS.

TABLE *28-9* **Charcot–Marie–Tooth Disease (CMT) and Related Hereditary Motor and Sensory Neuropathies (HMSN)**

Disease	Inheritance	Linkage	Candidate Gene	Pathology
CMT1A (HMSN IA)	Dominant	Chromosome 17	Peripheral myelin protein-22 (PMP22)	Chronic demyelinating polyneuropathy with numerous onion bulbs and nerve hypertrophy; distal axonal degeneration also is present
CMT1B (HMSN IB)	Dominant	Chromosome 1	Myelin protein zero (P_0) (a protein of PNS myelin)	
CMTX1	Dominant	Chromosome X	Connexin-32 (a gap junction protein)	
CMT2 (HMSN II)	Dominant	Chromosome 1	Unknown	Distal axonal degeneration
Dejerine–Sottas syndrome (HMSN III)	Recessive or dominant	Chromosome 17 or 1	PMP22 or P_0	Chronic demyelinating neuropathy with onion bulbs and nerve hypertrophy; distal axonal degeneration also is present
Hereditary liability to pressure palsies	Dominant	Chromosome 17	PMP22	Chronic demyelinating neuropathy with focally thickened myelin sheaths (tomacula) and axonal degeneration

Cryptogenic Neuropathy

In at least 10% of patients who have peripheral neuropathy, no etiology is apparent, despite careful and extensive investigations. These cryptogenic neuropathies are usually axonal and are seen as a chronic, distal, sensorimotor polyneuropathy.

NERVE TRAUMA

Traumatic Neuroma

Traumatic neuroma is a mass of regenerating axons and scar tissue that forms at the end of the proximal stump of a nerve that has been disrupted physically. After the transection of a peripheral nerve, regenerating axonal sprouts arise within 1 week from the distal ends of the intact axons in the proximal nerve stump. If the severed ends of the proximal and distal nerve stumps are closely approximated, the regenerating axonal sprouts may find and reinnervate the distal stump. The regenerating axons advance in the distal stump at a rate of about 1 mm/day. However, in many instances, the severed ends of the nerve are not closely approximated, and there is considerable scar tissue between the proximal and distal stumps. This scar tissue and the wide gap between the proximal and distal stumps prevent the regenerating sprouts from successfully reinnervating the distal stump. In this situation, the Schwann cell–ensheathed regenerating axons grow haphazardly into the scar tissue at the end of the proximal stump to form a painful swelling known as a traumatic or amputation neuroma.

Plantar Neuroma (Morton Neuroma)

Plantar neuroma is a painful, sausage-shaped swelling of the plantar digital nerve between the second and third or third and fourth metatarsal bones. It is probably caused by repeated nerve compression. The swelling is not a true neuroma, because it is the result of endoneurial, perineurial, and epineurial fibrosis rather than of a mass of regenerating axons. The fibrotic nerve also shows nerve fiber loss and areas of myxoid degeneration.

TUMORS

Primary tumors of the peripheral nervous system are of neuronal or nerve sheath origin. The neuronal tumors (e.g., neuroblastoma and ganglioneuroma) usually arise from the adrenal medulla or sympathetic ganglia. The common nerve sheath tumors are schwannoma and neurofibroma.

Schwannoma (Neurilemmoma)

Schwannoma is a benign, slowly growing neoplasm of Schwann cells that may arise in any nerve, including cranial nerves, spinal roots, or peripheral nerves. These tumors usually are seen in adults.

ACOUSTIC SCHWANNOMA (ACOUSTIC NEURINOMA): Intracranial schwannomas account for 8% of all intracranial tumors. With few exceptions, the intracranial schwannomas arise from the eighth cranial nerve (usually the superior or inferior vestibular branch, rarely the cochlear branch) within the internal auditory canal or at the meatus and cause unilateral, sensorineural hearing loss and tinnitus. The slowly growing tumor enlarges the meatus, extends medially into the subarachnoid space of the cerebellopontine angle (*cerebellopontine angle tumor*) (see Fig. 28-143), and compresses the fifth and seventh cranial nerves, brainstem, and cerebellum. The posterior fossa mass may also lead to increased intracranial pressure, hydrocephalus, and tonsillar herniation. Most vestibular schwannomas are unilateral and are unassociated with neurofibromatosis. Bilateral vestibular schwannomas are a defining feature of NF2.

INTRASPINAL AND PERIPHERAL SCHWANNOMAS: These tumors arise most often from the dorsal (sensory) spinal roots. They typically are seen as intradural, extramedullary tumors, producing radicular (root) pain and spinal cord compression. More peripheral schwannomas most commonly arise on nerves of the head, neck, and extremities

☐ **Pathology:** Schwannomas tend to be oval and well demarcated and vary in diameter from a few millimeters to several centimeters. The nerve of origin, if sufficiently large, may be identifiable. The cut surface is firm,

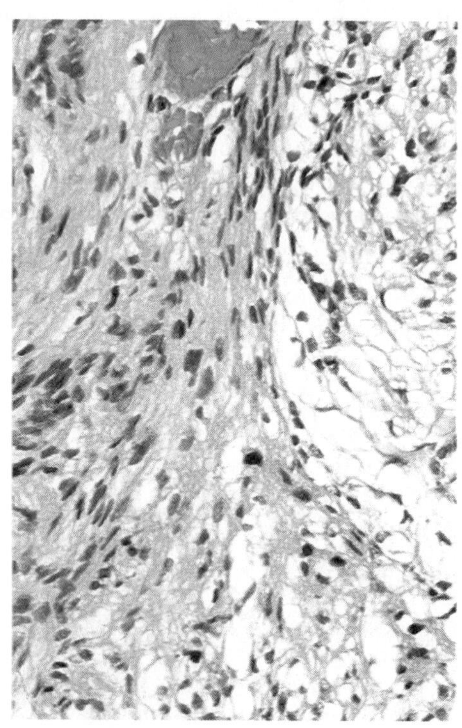

FIGURE *28-156*
Schwannoma. A photomicrograph shows the characteristically abrupt transition between the compact Antoni type A histological pattern (*left*) and the spongy Antoni type B histological pattern (*right*).

tan to gray, and often shows foci of hemorrhage, necrosis, xanthomatous change, and cystic degeneration. Microscopically, the proliferating Schwann cells form two distinctive histological patterns (Fig. 28-156).

Antoni type A pattern is characterized by interwoven fascicles of spindle cells with elongated nuclei, eosinophilic cytoplasm, and indistinct cytoplasmic borders. The nuclei may palisade in areas to form structures known as *Verocay bodies*.

Antoni type B pattern features spindle or oval cells with indistinct cytoplasm in a loose, vacuolated background.

Degenerative changes in schwannomas are common and include collections of foam cells, recent or old hemorrhage, foci of fibrosis, and hyalinized blood vessels. Scattered atypical nuclei are frequently encountered in schwannomas, but mitotic figures are uncommon.

Neurofibroma

Neurofibroma is a benign, slowly growing tumor of peripheral nerve composed principally of Schwann cells. The tumor may be more hamartomatous than neoplastic. A distinction between neurofibroma and schwannoma is warranted because of the close association of neurofibroma with neurofibromatosis type 1 (NF1; von Recklinghausen disease) and its potential for sarcomatous degeneration.

Neurofibromas may be solitary or multiple and may arise on any nerve. They are found in both children and adults. Most commonly, neurofibromas involve the skin, major nerve plexuses, large deep nerve trunks, retroperitoneum, and gastrointestinal tract. The large majority of *solitary cutaneous neurofibromas* occur outside the context of neurofibromatosis and do not have the potential for sarcomatous degeneration. The presence of multiple neurofibromas or one large plexiform neurofibroma strongly suggests the diagnosis of NF1 and should prompt a careful search for other stigmata of the disease.

☐ **Pathology:** On gross examination, a neurofibroma arising in a large nerve appears as a poorly circumscribed, fusiform enlargement. The diffuse, intrafascicular growth of the tumor within multiple nerve fascicles may so enlarge the nerve's fascicles that they appear grossly as the cords of a nerve plexus (*plexiform neurofibroma*). The neurofibroma may involve long segments of the nerve, making complete surgical excision impossible. When neurofibromas arise from small nerves, the nerve of origin may not be apparent. Cutaneous neurofibromas originate from dermal nerves and are seen as soft, nodular, or pedunculated skin tumors.

The cut surface of a neurofibroma is soft and light gray, and the enlarged nerve fascicles of the plexiform neurofibroma may be prominent. Microscopically, neurofibroma arising in a large nerve is characterized by an endoneurial proliferation of spindle cells with elongated nuclei, eosinophilic cytoplasm, and indistinct cell borders. The spindle cells often aggregate to form tiny strands coursing haphazardly through the tumor (Fig. 28-157). Interspersed among the spindle cells are wavy bands of collagen, an extracellular myxoid matrix, and residual nerve fibers. The coursing of nerve fibers through the neurofibroma contrasts with the pattern in schwannoma, in which nerve fibers are pushed peripherally into the tumor capsule. When arising from a small nerve, neurofibroma usually extends beyond the nerve and diffusely infiltrates the surrounding tissue.

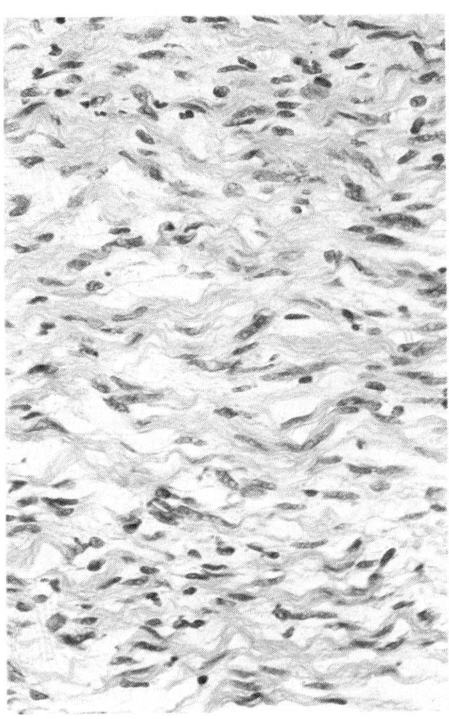

FIGURE *28-157*
Neurofibroma. A photomicrograph shows that the proliferating spindle-shaped Schwann cells form small strands that course haphazardly through a myxoid matrix.

Some 5% of NF1-associated neurofibromas exhibit sarcomatous transformation, with foci of malignant peripheral nerve-sheath tumor. The presence of increased cellularity and mitotic figures heralds malignant transformation.

Malignant Peripheral Nerve-Sheath Tumor (Malignant Schwannoma, Neurofibrosarcoma)

Malignant peripheral nerve-sheath tumor is a poorly differentiated, spindle cell sarcoma of peripheral nerve of uncertain histogenesis. The tumor may arise *de novo* or from malignant transformation of a neurofibroma. Malignant peripheral nerve sheath tumor is most common in adults. **About half of these sarcomas occur in patients with neurofibromatosis.** There is an increased incidence of malignant peripheral nerve-sheath tumors at sites of previous irradiation.

Malignant peripheral nerve-sheath tumor presents grossly as an unencapsulated, fusiform enlargement of a nerve. Microscopically, the neoplasm resembles fibrosarcoma. The tumor is prone to local recurrence and bloodborne metastases.

SUGGESTED READING

BOOKS

Adams JH, Duchen LW (eds): *Greenfield's neuropathology*, 6th ed. New York: Oxford University Press, 1997.

Asbury AK, Thomas PK (eds): *Peripheral nerve disorders 2*. Oxford: Butterworth-Heinemann, 1995.

Davis RL, Robertson DM: *Textbook of neuropathology*, 3rd ed. Baltimore: Williams & Wilkins, 1997.

Dyck PJ, Thomas PK, Griffin JW, et al (eds): *Peripheral neuropathy*, 3rd ed. Philadelphia: WB Saunders, 1993.

Enzinger FM, Weiss SW: *Soft tissue tumors*, 3rd ed. St. Louis: Mosby-Year Book, 1995.

Midroni G, Bilbao JM: *Biopsy diagnosis of peripheral neuropathies*. Boston: Butterworth-Heinemann, 1995.

Ouvrier RA: Peripheral neuropathies. In: Berg BO (ed): *Principles of child neurology*. New York: McGraw-Hill, pp. 1607–1655, 1996.

Schaumburg HH, Berger AR, Thomas PK: *Disorders of peripheral nerves*, 2nd ed. Philadelphia: FA Davis, 1992.

REVIEW ARTICLES

DeArmond SJ, Prusiner SB: Etiology and pathogenesis of prion diseases. *Am J Pathol* 146:785–811, 1995.

Fuller GN: Central nervous system tumors. In: Parham DM (ed): *Pediatric neoplasia: morphology and biology*. New York: Lippincott–Raven, pp. 153–204, 1996.

Fuller GN, Burger PC: Central nervous system. In: Stemberg SS (ed): *Histology for pathologists*, 2nd ed. New York: Lippincott–Raven, pp. 243–282, 1997.

Haines DE: On the question of a subdural space. *Anat Rec* 230:3–21, 1991.

Haines DE, Harkey HL, Al-Mefty O: The subdural space: a new look at an outdated concept. *Neurosurgery* 32:111–120, 1993.

Harding AE: From the syndrome of Charcot, Marie and Tooth to disorders of peripheral myelin proteins. *Brain* 118:809–818, 1995.

Martin R, McFarland HF, McFarlin DE: Immunological aspects of demyelinating diseases. *Annu Rev Immunol* 10:153–188, 1992.

Parry GJ: Peripheral neuropathies associated with human immunodeficiency virus infection. *Ann Neurol* 23(suppl):S49–S53, 1988.

Prusiner SB: The prion diseases. *Sci Am* 272:48–57, 1995.

Rose LM, Richards TL, Petersen R, et al: Remitting-relapsing EAE in nonhuman primates: a valid model of multiple sclerosis. *Clin Immunol Immunopathol* 59:1–15, 1991.

Suter U, Snipes GJ: Biology and genetics of hereditary motor and sensory neuropathies. *Annu Rev Neurosci* 18:45–75, 1995.

Yankner BA: Mechanisms of neuronal degeneration in Alzheimer's disease. *Neuron* 16:921–932, 1996.

Youdim BH, Riederer P: Understanding Parkinson's disease. *Sci Am* 276:52–59, 1997.

CHAPTER 29

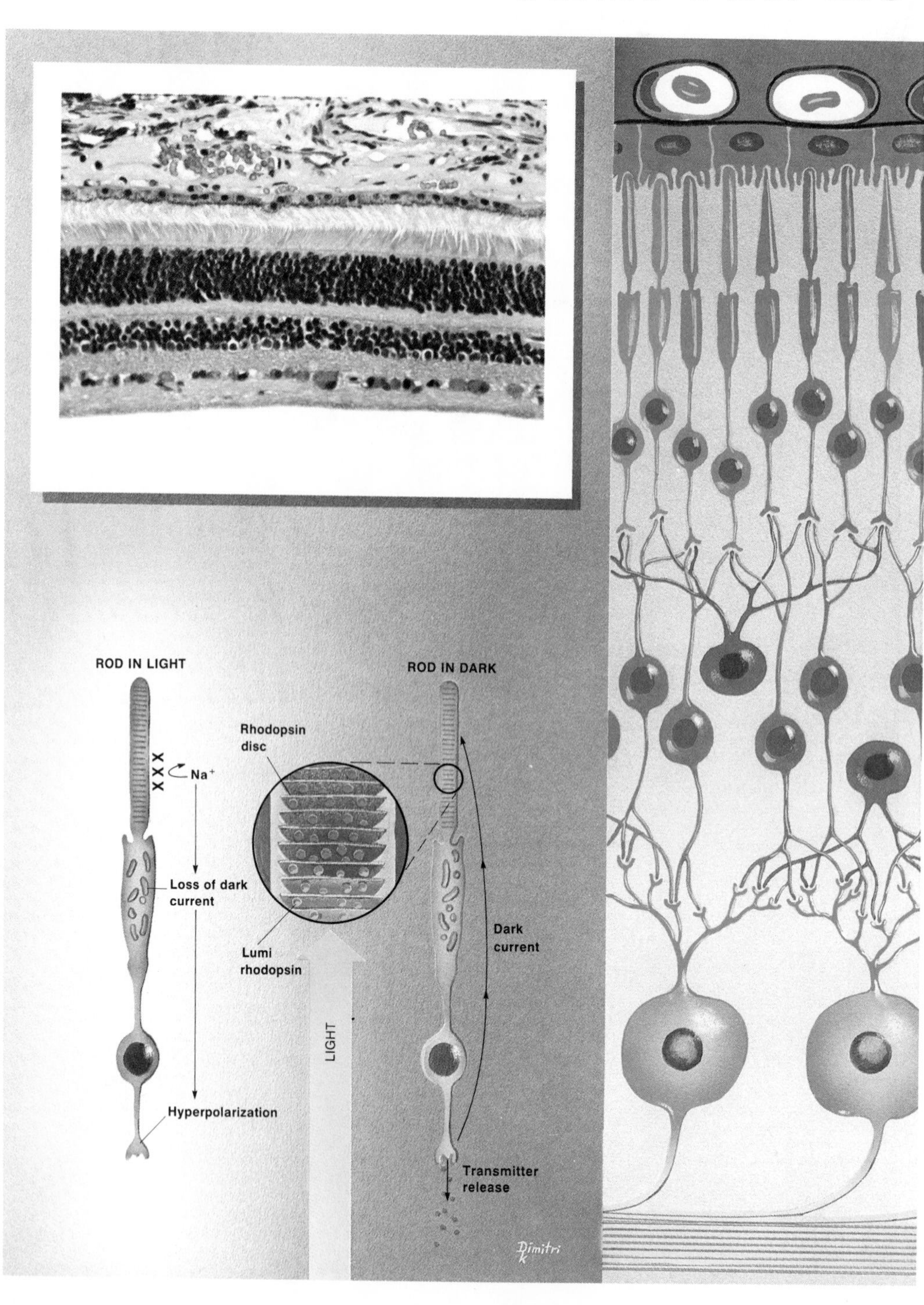

ROD IN LIGHT
ROD IN DARK
Rhodopsin disc
Na⁺
Loss of dark current
Lumi rhodopsin
LIGHT
Dark current
Hyperpolarization
Transmitter release
Dimitri

The Eye

Gordon K. Klintworth

FIGURE **29-1** *(see opposite page)*
The retinal basis of vision. The retina, the specialized tissue that responds to light, contains neurons arranged in distinct layers. In the vertebrate retina, light passes through the entire eye before reaching the photoreceptors (rods and cones). The outer segment of each photoreceptor is its light-sensitive region. The rod outer segment contains a dense stack of disc membranes in which the photoprotein, rhodopsin, is embedded. The biochemical transduction of light into neural impulses is dependent on ion fluxes.

Disorders of the eye are common, and many of its afflictions result in blindness. The eye is exposed to myriad microorganisms, antigens, and toxic chemicals, as well as to solar radiation and adverse climatic conditions. The unprotected position of the eye makes it vulnerable to a host of injuries. The eye is also involved in numerous systemic diseases (Table 29-1), and the recognition of ocular abnormalities aids in the diagnosis of many conditions.

DEVELOPMENTAL ANOMALIES AND GENETIC DISORDERS

Anomalous development of the eye results in a variety of malformations that involve the entire globe or specific parts of it. The causes of many of these developmental anomalies are unknown, but some are genetically determined or are due to chromosomal abnormalities, viruses, or drugs. Numerous genetically determined diseases of the eye are X-linked, including ocular albinism, retinitis pigmentosa, retinoschisis, some congenital cataracts, choroideremia, Norrie disease, X-linked coloboma, and red–green color blindness (protanopia or deuteranopia). The genes that specify the protein moieties (opsins) of the three different color-sensitive pigments in the human retina have been isolated and characterized. The mutant genes responsible for numerous ocular disorders, including color blindness, Norrie disease, and retinitis pigmentosa, have been sequenced and cloned. The Pax 6 gene plays an important role in normal ocular development, and mutations in it cause a variety of ocular developmental anomalies, especially of the anterior segment.

PHYSICAL AND CHEMICAL INJURIES

Physical trauma to the eye commonly causes ecchymosis of the highly vascular eyelids (black eye); when this occurs, other parts of the eye also may be injured. Superficial disruptions of the corneal epithelium follow traumatic abrasions, prolonged wearing of a contact lens, foreign bodies on the eye, exposure to ultraviolet light, and exposure to caustic chemicals. Blunt trauma increases the intraorbital pressure momentarily, causing the bones in the floor of the orbit to fracture into the maxillary sinus (blowout fracture). The inferior rectus muscle may become entrapped in the fracture, thereby causing the eye to sink into the orbit (enophthalmos).

An almost infinite variety of foreign materials are capable of injuring the eye. Whereas small particles often lodge in the superficial ocular tissues, some penetrate into or through the eye. The patient may not even be aware of the intraocular foreign body if it reaches the eye at high velocity, as occurs in accidents with industrial machinery. A foreign particle may damage the eye during entry or because of secondary infection after the introduction of microorganisms. Some foreign bodies provoke a prominent acute inflammatory or granulomatous reaction. Others, such as those containing iron, cause retinal degeneration and even discoloration of the ocular tissues (siderosis bulbi), effects that may not be evident for several years. Other complications of ocular injuries include cataracts, retinal detachment, and glaucoma.

The eye is commonly injured by a variety of household and industrial chemicals that enter it accidentally or as a result of a malicious act. The damage created depends on the nature of the chemical.

THE EYELIDS

The more important conditions that affect the eyelids include the following:

Blepharitis is a common inflammation of the eyelids, which sometimes is seen as an acute, red, tender, inflammatory mass.

Hordeolum (or sty) refers to an acute, inflammatory, focal lesion of the eyelid. Acute inflammation involving the meibomian glands is termed an *internal hordeolum,* whereas acute folliculitis of the glands of Zeis is an *external hordeolum.*

Chalazion is a granulomatous inflammation centered around the meibomian glands or the glands of Zeis. It is thought to represent a reaction to extruded lipid secretions. A chalazion usually produces a painless swelling in the eyelid.

Inflammatory pseudotumor of the orbit describes an idiopathic chronic inflammatory reaction associated with a variable degree of fibrosis. It is a common cause of proptosis and partial immobility of the eyeball.

Xanthelasma refers to a yellow plaque of lipid-containing macrophages, usually involving the nasal aspect of the eyelids. It is often seen in older persons and patients

TABLE 29-1 Systemic Disease with Ocular Involvement

Ocular Tissue	Ocular Abnormalities	Disease
Choroid	Hemangioma	Sturge-Weber syndrome
conjunctiva	Bitot spot	Vitamin A deficiency
	Crystals	Cystinosis
	Dry eyes	Avitaminosis A
		Benign mucous membrane pemphigoid
		Familial dysautonomia (Riley-Day syndrome)
		Polyarteritis nodosa
		Psoriatic arthritis
		Rheumatoid arthritis
		Sjögren syndrome
		Systemic lupus erythematosus
		Systemic sclerosis
		Stevens-Johnson syndrome
	Granulomatous inflammation	Sarcoidosis
	Telangiectasia	Ataxia telangiectasia (Louis-Bar syndrome)
Cornea	Amyloid deposits	Inherited amyloid neuropathy type IV (Meretoja)
	Arcus lipoides (arcus senilis)	Hyperlipoproteinemia type II
		Hyperlipoproteinemia type III (occasionally)
		Hyperlipoproteinemia type IV
	Band keratopathy	Hyperparathyroidism
		Marie-Strümpell disease
		Sarcoidosis
		Severe renal disease
		Still disease
		Vitamin D toxicity
	Clouding/opacification	Familial lecithin cholesterol acyltransferase deficiency
		Familial high-density lipoprotein deficiency (Tangier disease)
		Metachromatic leukodystrophy variant
		Mucolipidosis type III
		Mucopolysaccharidoses (some types)
	Crystals	Benign monoclonal gammopathies
		Cystinosis
		Multiple myeloma
	Dry cornea	(See under conjunctiva, dry eyes)
	Kayser-Fleischer ring	Hepatolenticular degeneration (Wilson disease)
	Thick corneal nerves	Multiple endocrine neoplasia syndrome type IIB
	Ulcers (dendritic)	Tyrosinemia
	Verticillate lines	Fabry disease
Eyelid	Epicanthic folds	de Lange syndrome
		Deletion of short arm of chromosome 5 (5p−)
		Deletion of long arm of chromosome 13 (13q−)
		Deletion of short arm of chromosome 18 (18p−)
		Down syndrome
		Ehlers-Danlos syndrome
		Klinefelter syndrome (45X and mosaic variants)
		Marinesco-Sjögren syndrome
		Rubinstein-Taybi syndrome
		Turner syndrome
	Xanthomas/xanthelasmas	Hyperlipoproteinemia type I, II, and V
		Hyperlipoproteinemia type III (occasionally)
Iris	Aniridia	Nephroblastoma (Wilms tumor)
	Blue color	Various forms of oculocutaneous albinism
	Heterochromia iridis	Waardenburg-Klein syndrome
	Neovascularization	Carotid cavernous fistula
		Carotid ischemia
		Diabetes mellitus
Lacrimal gland	Granulomatous inflammation	Sarcoidosis

(continued)

TABLE **29-1** *(continued)*

Ocular Tissue	Ocular Abnormalities	Disease
Lens	Cataract	Alport syndrome
		Cretinism
		Diabetes mellitus
		Down syndrome
		Fabry disease
		Galactosemia
		Sturge-Weber syndrome
		Hidrotic ectodermal dysplasia (Marshall type)
		Hypocalcemia
		Incontinentia pigmenti
		Laurence-Moon-Biedl syndrome
		Mannosidosis
		Marinesco-Sjögren syndrome
		Myotonic dystrophy
		Norrie disease
		Pierre Robin syndrome
		Rothmund-Thomson syndrome
		Rubella (congenital)
		Trisomy 13
	Dislocated/subluxation	Ehlers-Danlos syndrome
		Homocystinuria
		Marfan syndrome
Miscellaneous	Glaucoma	Lowe oculocerebrorenal syndrome
		Sturge-Weber syndrome
	Photophobia	Chédiak-Higashi syndrome
		Oculocutaneous albinism (various types)
	Progressive myopia	Stickler progressive arthro-ophthalmopathy
Muscles	Strabismus	Gaucher disease type II (infantile, acute neuronopathic)
Optic nerve	Optic atrophy	Globoid cell leukodystrophy (Krabbe disease)
		GM_2 gangliosidosis type III
		Neuronal ceroid lipofuscinosis type I (infantile, Hagberg-Haltia-Santavuori)
Orbit	Proptosis	Hyperthyroidism
Retina	Angioid streaks	Paget disease of bone
		Pseudoxanthoma elasticum
	Astrocytic hamartomas	Tuberous sclerosis
	Cherry-red spot at macula	GM_1 gangliosidosis type I
		GM_2 gangliosidosis type II variant B (Tay-Sachs)
		GM_2 gangliosidosis type II variant O (Sandhoff)
		Mucolipidosis type I
		Niemann-Pick disease
	Cotton-wool spots	Collagen diseases
		Diabetes mellitus
		Malignant hypertension
		Pernicious anemia
	Degeneration	Farber disease
		Hyperornithinemia (chorioretinal gyrate atrophy)
		Neuronal ceroid-lipofuscinosis type I (infantile, Hagberg-Haltia-Santavuori)
		Niemann-Pick disease
		Sulfatide lipidosis (metachromatic leukodystrophy)
		X-linked copper malabsorption syndrome (Menke disease)
		(See also pigmentary retinopathy, next page)
	Emboli	Atrial myxoma
		Bacterial endocarditis
		Calcified cardiac valves
		Cardiac mural thrombi
		Ulcerated atheromatous plaques
	Fat	Fractures of long bones
	Air	Sudden barometric decompression
	Air	Surgical procedures or accidental injuries to neck or thorax
	Talc	Intravenous drug addiction
	Hemangioblastoma	Von Hippel-Lindau disease

(continued)

TABLE **29-1** *(continued)*

Ocular Tissue	Ocular Abnormalities	Disease
	Lipemia retinalis	Hyperlipoproteinemia types I and V
		Young diabetes with marked acidosis
	Microaneurysms	Aortic arch syndrome
		Diabetes mellitus
		Macroglobulinemia
	Neovascularization	Diabetes mellitus
		Retinopathy of prematurity
		Sickle cell disease
	Occlusovascular disease	Aortic arch syndrome (Takayasu disease, pulseless disease)
		Atherosclerosis
		Diabetes mellitus
		Disseminated intravascular coagulation
		Giant cell arteritis
		Sickle cell disease
	Pigmentary retinopathy	Cystinosis
		Abetalipoproteinemia (Bassen-Kornzweig syndrome)
		Neuronal ceroid lipofuscinosis
		Type II late infantile (Jansky-Bielschowsky)
		Type III juvenile (Spielmeyer-Sjögren-Batten)
		Niemann-Pick disease
		Phytanic acid storage disease (Refsum syndrome)
		Cockayne syndrome
		Congenital ichthyosis
		Drugs
		Chloroquine
		Quinacrine hydrochloride (Atabrine)
		Chlorpromazine
		Hallervorden-Spatz syndrome
		Hallgren syndrome
		Kearns-Sayre syndrome
		Laurence-Moon-Biedl syndrome
		Pelizaeus-Merzbacher syndrome
		Usher syndrome
		Vitamin A deficiency
		Mucopolysaccharidoses
		Type I-H (Hurler)
		Type I-S (Scheie)
		Type II (Hunter)
		Types IIIA and IIIB (Sanfilippo)
		Postinflammatory and degenerative conditions
		Behçet disease
		Cytomegalovirus
		Measles
		Onchocerciasis
		Rubella
		Smallpox vaccination
		Syphilis
		Toxoplasmosis
		Typhoid fever
	Retinal detachment	Norrie disease
	Retinopathy	Diabetes mellitus
		Hypertension
		Sickle cell hemoglobin C disease
Sclera	Pigmentation	
	Brown/black	Alkaptonuria (ochronosis)
	Blue	de Lange syndrome
	Blue	Ehlers-Danlos syndrome
	Blue	Osteogenesis imperfecta
	Yellow	Jaundice
	Yellow	Liver disease
Vitreous body	Amyloid deposits	Transthyretin amyloidosis

with disorders of lipid metabolism (e.g., familial hypercholesterolemia, primary biliary cirrhosis).

THE ORBIT

Exophthalmos *or* **proptosis** *is an abnormal forward protrusion of the eyeball.* The term exophthalmos is used mainly when the condition is bilateral; proptosis refers to a unilateral protrusion of the eye. Numerous conditions cause a forward protrusion of the eye. The most common cause is thyroid disease, followed by orbital dermoid cysts and hemangiomas. Other orbital conditions can cause proptosis: various inflammatory lesions, lymphomas, developmental anomalies, vascular problems, and neoplasms all contribute cases. Proptosis also results from lesions of the paranasal sinuses and intracranial cavity.

Exophthalmos of Hyperthyroidism

Exophthalmos due to Graves disease may precede or follow other manifestations of thyroid dysfunction. Exophthalmos resulting from thyroid disease usually occurs in early adult life, especially in women (female-to-male ratio, 4:1). It may be severe and progressive, particularly in middle life, when exophthalmos no longer correlates well with the state of the thyroid function. Dysthyroid exophthalmos may be associated with edema of the eyelids, chemosis (edema of the conjunctiva), and limited ocular motion.

☐ **Pathogenesis:** Exophthalmos results from an increase in the volume of orbital tissue, produced largely by (1) an increase in orbital water, as a result of the osmotic pressure of glycosaminoglycans; and (2) enlarged extraocular muscles that are infiltrated with lymphocytes and other mononuclear cells.

The pathogenesis of dysthyroid exophthalmos remains uncertain, but it has been suggested that exophthalmos may be an organ-specific autoimmune condition distinct from Graves disease but closely linked to it. The serum of patients with hyperthyroidism and exophthalmos often contain antibodies to the extraocular muscles, whereas the blood of those without eye disease does not. There is also a familial predisposition to this autoimmune disorder. The responsible antigen remains elusive; those that have been considered as possible triggers for the immune response include a 64-kDa protein of unknown function, thyrotropin or fragments of it, thyroglobulin, acetyl cholinesterase, and bacteria. The ocular disorder may precede, accompany, or follow hyperthyroidism, but the large majority of patients with exophthalmos will develop Graves disease at some time.

☐ **Clinical Features:** Although it is usually bilateral, one eye may be involved earlier or more extensively than the other. Other ocular manifestations of hyperthyroidism include retraction of the upper eyelid (owing to increased sympathetic tone) and a characteristic stare or apparent proptosis as a result of exposure of the conjunctiva above the corneoscleral limbus.

Complications of severe exophthalmos include several potentially blinding complications: corneal exposure with subsequent ulceration and optic nerve compression. Paradoxically, thyroidectomy may increase the incidence and severity of exophthalmos associated with hyperthyroidism.

THE CONJUNCTIVA

Hyperemia

Hyperemic conjunctival blood vessels (called conjunctival injection by ophthalmologists) occur in conjunctivitis, certain corneal disease, iridocyclitis, and glaucoma. In conjunctivitis, irrespective of the cause, the conjunctival vessels become diffusely congested, with the engorged vessels tapering toward the corneoscleral limbus. Another variety of conjunctival hyperemia (ciliary flush) is associated with iritis and corneal defects. In this condition, finer vessels radiate for a short distance from the limbus.

Hemorrhage

Conjunctival hemorrhage follows blunt trauma, anoxia, or severe bouts of coughing. It also occurs spontaneously, often first noted on arising after sleep. Conjunctival hemorrhages do not extend into the cornea because of the barrier imposed by the close apposition of the corneal epithelium to the underlying substantia propria.

Conjunctivitis

Microorganisms lodging on the surface of the eye frequently cause conjunctivitis, keratitis (corneal inflammation), or a corneal ulcer. The eye may also become infected by hematogenous spread from a focus of infection elsewhere. Iatrogenic infections of the eye are always a distinct possibility in ophthalmic surgical procedures, such as cataract extractions, corneal grafts, and the intraocular instillation of prosthetic lenses. Adenoviruses and other pathogens may be introduced into the eye by a physician using infected eyedrops or a contaminated tonometer (an instrument used to measure intraocular pressure).

At some stage in life, virtually everyone has viral or bacterial conjunctivitis. This most common of eye diseases is characterized by hyperemic conjunctival blood vessels (pink eye). The inflammatory exudate that accumulates in the conjunctival sac commonly crusts, causing the eyelids to stick together in the morning. The conjunctival discharge may be purulent, fibrinous, serous, or hemorrhagic and contains inflammatory cells that vary with the etiological agent. In keeping with the seasonal nature of many allergens, allergic conjunctivitis sometimes occurs only during a particular time of the year.

Trachoma

Trachoma is a chronic, contagious conjunctivitis caused by Chlamydia trachomatis. Different serotypes of *C. trachomatis* cause ocular, genital, and systemic infections (trachoma, inclusion conjunctivitis, and lymphogranuloma venereum) in millions of people (see Chapter 9).

☐ **Epidemiology:** About 500 million people are afflicted by trachoma, an acute, infectious, cicatrizing keratoconjunctivitis caused by *C. trachomatis* (serotypes A, B, and C). **This infection is the most common cause of blindness in the world and is especially prevalent in Asia, the Middle East, and parts of Africa.** Trachoma is not very contagious, but overcrowding and poor hygienic conditions favor its transmission by fingers, fomites, and flies. Spontaneous healing is common in children, but in adults, the disease progresses more rapidly and rarely heals in the absence of treatment.

☐ **Pathology:** Trachoma is virtually always bilateral and involves the upper half of the conjunctiva more extensively than the lower (Fig. 29-2). The cellular infiltrate is predominantly lymphocytic, and conjunctival lymph follicles with necrotic germinal centers are characteristic. Eventually lymphocytes and blood vessels invade the superior portion of the cornea between the epithelium and Bowman's zone (trachomatous pannus). Scarring of the conjunctiva and eyelids distorts the eyelids. On microscopic examination, the desquamated conjunctival epithelium exhibits glycogen-rich intracytoplasmic inclusion bodies and large macrophages containing nuclear fragments (*Leber cells*). Secondary bacterial infection is a common complication.

Other Chlamydial Infections

Chlamydia is responsible for a purulent conjunctivitis (inclusion blennorrhea) that develops in the newborn, who becomes infected during passage through the birth canal. The infection is also acquired by swimming in nonchlorinated pools (swimming pool conjunctivitis) or from discharges of lesions of the conjunctiva, urethra, or cervix uteri.

In adults and older children, *Chlamydia* causes a chronic follicular conjunctivitis with focal lymphoid hyperplasia (inclusion conjunctivitis) and intracytoplasmic inclusion bodies indistinguishable from those of trachoma. In contrast to trachoma, however, the lower tarsal conjunctiva is involved. Scarring and necrosis do not develop, and keratitis is rare and mild.

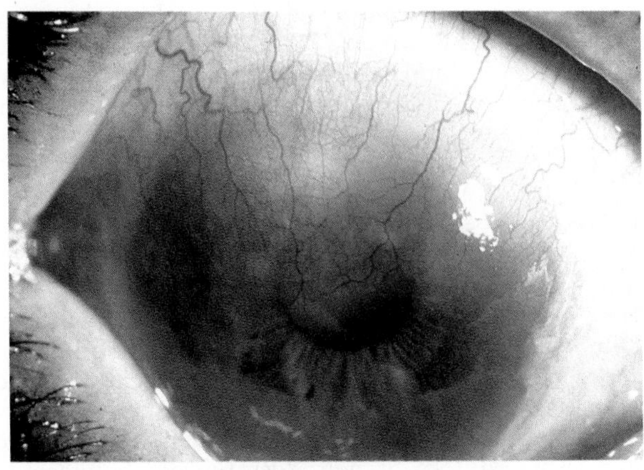

FIGURE 29-2
Trachoma. A clinical photograph of the cornea of a patient with severe trachoma shows an extensive fibrovascular opacity (pannus) in the superior cornea.

Ophthalmia Neonatorum

Ophthalmia neonatorum is a severe, acute conjunctivitis with a copious purulent discharge, especially in the newborn, caused by Neisseria gonorrhoeae. The infection, a common cause of blindness in some parts of the world, is complicated by corneal ulceration, perforation and scarring, and panophthalmitis. The infant usually becomes infected while passing through the birth canal of an infected mother. Aside from gonorrhea, ophthalmia neonatorum has other causes, including other pyogenic bacteria and *C. trachomatis* (serotypes D to K, also known as *Chlamydia oculogenitalis*). Even the silver nitrate previously administered to the conjunctiva of newborns to prevent gonococcal infection can itself provoke a conjunctivitis. Accordingly, today newborns are routinely treated with penicillin eyedrops.

Dry-Eye Syndrome

Basal tear production is diminished in certain ocular and systemic diseases (see Table 29-1). It may also be decreased for no apparent reason, especially in older women, and sometimes occurs during the menopause. Dry-eye syndrome associated with Sjögren disease (keratoconjunctivitis sicca) usually affects middle-aged women and results from inflammation and atrophy of the lacrimal glands (see Chapter 4).

Pinguecula and Pterygium

***Pinguecula** is a yellowish conjunctival lump usually located nasal to the corneoscleral limbus.* It is the most common conjunctival lump. Despite its yellowish appearance, the lesion does not contain fat; rather, it consists of sun-damaged connective tissue identical to that in similarly injured skin (actinic elastosis).

***Pterygium** is a fold of vascularized conjunctiva that grows horizontally onto the cornea in the shape of an insect wing (hence the name).* It is often associated with a pinguecula and frequently recurs after excision.

THE CORNEA

Herpes Simplex

Herpesvirus (HSV) has a predilection for the corneal epithelium, where it causes keratitis, but it can invade the corneal stroma and occasionally other ocular tissues.

PRIMARY INFECTION BY HSV TYPE 1: Subclinical or undiagnosed localized ocular lesions are caused by HSV type 1 in childhood. These infections are accompanied by regional lymphadenopathy, systemic infection, and fever. HSV type 2 rarely causes ocular infection, but when it does, it can produce widespread lesions of the cornea and retina. An exception occurs in the newborn, who becomes infected during passage through the birth canal of a mother who harbors genital herpes. Most corneal lesions due to HSV are asymptomatic plaques of diseased epithelial cells that contain replicating virus. These usually heal without ulceration, but an acute unilateral follicular conjunctivitis may occur. Corneal ulcers appear after the serum antibody levels become increased.

REACTIVATION OF HSV INFECTION: Latent in the trigeminal ganglion, HSV may pass down the nerves and reactivate the infection. In contrast to primary infection by the virus, reactivation disease is characterized by ulceration of the cornea and a more severe inflammatory reaction. On the other hand, fever and lymphadenopathy are not evident.

Recurrence of corneal ulcers due to HSV may be precipitated by ultraviolet light, trauma, menstruation, emotional and physical stress, exposure to light or sunlight, vaccination, and other factors. These recurrences occur despite high titers of circulating anti-HSV antibodies and specific cell-mediated immunity.

□ Pathology: HSV causes multiple, minute, discrete, intraepithelial corneal ulcers (superficial punctate keratopathy). Although some of these lesions heal, others enlarge and eventually coalesce to form linear or branching fissures (dendritic ulcers, from Gk., *dendron*, "tree"). The epithelium between the fissures desquamates, causing sharply demarcated, irregular geographic ulcers. The corneal ulcers are readily seen in the patient after the cornea has been stained with fluorescein. The affected epithelial cells, which may become multinucleated, contain eosinophilic, intranuclear inclusion bodies (*Lipschutz bodies*).

The lesions of the corneal stroma vary in reactivated HSV infection. Typically, a central disc-shaped corneal opacity develops beneath the epithelium, owing to edema and a minimal inflammatory cell infiltrate (*disciform keratitis*). The corneal stroma may become markedly thinned, and Descemet's membrane may bulge into it (*descemetocele*). Corneal perforation can also occur.

Onchocerciasis

The nematode *Onchocerca volvulus*, which is transmitted by bites of infected blackflies, is by far the most important helminthic infection of the eye (see Chapter 9). **This parasite accounts for blindness in at least half a million people in regions of Africa and Latin America in which it is endemic.** Microfilaria released from fertilized adult female worms migrate into the superficial cornea, bulbar conjunctiva, aqueous humor, and other ocular tissues. After the demise of the intracorneal microfilaria, an inflammatory response causes corneal opacification and visual impairment (*river blindness*). Less frequently, endophthalmitis, retinal lesions, and optic atrophy occur.

Arcus Lipoides (Arcus Senilis)

Arcus lipoides (formerly called arcus senilis because of its frequency in the elderly) is a white arc due to lipid deposition in the peripheral cornea. It may also form an entire ring, in which case the term *annulus lipoides* is more appropriate. Although not necessarily associated with increased serum lipid levels, arcus lipoides accompanies certain disorders of lipid metabolism (see Table 29-1), and its presence alerts the perceptive clinician to the systemic disorder.

Band Keratopathy

Band keratopathy refers to an opaque horizontal band across the superficial central cornea. The opacification may contain calcium phosphate (calcific band keratopathy) or noncalcified protein (chronic actinic keratopathy, noncalcific band keratopathy, climatic droplet keratopathy).

In calcific band keratopathy, calcium phosphate deposits in a horizontal band across the superficial central cornea in conditions associated with hypercalcemia. However, the disorder most often occurs in the absence of an increased serum calcium concentration, as in chronic uveitis and other ocular disorders.

Chronic actinic keratopathy occurs worldwide, but is most severe in regions in which people spend a considerable amount of time outdoors. Their unprotected eyes are exposed to excessive ultraviolet light, such as that reflected from desert, water, or snow.

Corneal Dystrophies

The corneal dystrophies encompass a heterogeneous group of hereditary, noninflammatory diseases of the cornea. Although literally indicating corneal disorders with defective nutrition, keratopathies due to nutritional deficiencies have traditionally not been included under the umbrella of corneal dystrophy. Most corneal dytrophies are autosomal dominant or recessive, but rare cases are X-linked recessive. The corneal dystrophies have traditionally been classified according to the primary layer that is involved: (1) the outer layer composed of epithelium, basement membrane, and Bowman's layer, (2) the stroma, and (3) the endothelium and Descemet's membrane. A shortcoming of such a classification is its artificiality, because many of the conditions involve more than one layer.

EPITHELIAL DYSTROPHIES: The different epithelial dystrophies are characterized by a variety of distinct abnormalities, which include (1) microcysts or accumulations of anomalous material within the cytoplasm of the corneal epithelium, (2) defects in the epithelial basement membrane, and (3) the deposition of a finely fibrillar substance in Bowman's layer. In some epithelial dystrophies, faulty desmosomes may permit the separation of adjacent epithelial cells, leading to the accumulation of fluid-filled microcysts. A loss of hemidesmosomes between the epithelium and Bowman's layer leads to painful, recurrent erosions that begin in early childhood. Although there may be a slow decrease in visual acuity, epithelial dystrophies do not ordinarily cause blindness.

STROMAL DYSTROPHIES: The stromal dystrophies are clear-cut entities in which different substances, including amyloid, glycosaminoglycans, unidentified proteins, and a variety of lipids, accumulate within the corneal stroma because of an inherited metabolic disorder. Each stromal dystrophy causes a characteristic form of corneal opacification. The age of onset and the rate of progression vary with the particular disorder. Although the clinical manifestations may be limited to the cornea, other tissues are involved in some of these dystrophies.

ENDOTHELIAL DYSTROPHIES: Several different endothelial dystrophies are recognized, usually accompanied by abnormalities in Descemet's membrane, the basement membrane of the corneal endothelium. In one dystrophy of the corneal endothelium (*Fuchs dystrophy*), wart-like excrescences form on Descemet's membrane, and progressive visual loss follows corneal edema and the degeneration of the endothelial cells.

THE LENS

Cataracts

A cataract is an opacification in the crystalline lens (Fig. 29-3). Some ophthalmologists restrict the term cataract to those opacifications within the lens that affect vision. Cataracts are a major cause of visual impairment and blindness throughout the world and are the outcome of numerous conditions. They can be caused by disorders of carbohydrate metabolism that result in monosaccharide excesses (diabetes) or by deficiencies in riboflavin or tryptophan. A variety of cataracts result from genetic disorders. Others are related to the actions of toxins, drugs, or physical agents. Examples of substances that may cause cataracts include dinitrophenol, naphthalene, ergot, phospholine iodide (topical), corticosteroids, and phenothiazines. Physical agents that cause cataracts are heat, ultraviolet light, trauma, intraocular surgery, and ultrasound.

Ocular diseases that may be complicated by cataracts include uveitis, intraocular neoplasms, glaucoma, retinitis pigmentosa, and retinal detachment. Cataracts also are associated with congenital rubella virus infection, aging, some skin diseases (atopic dermatitis, scleroderma), and various systemic diseases (see Table 29-1).

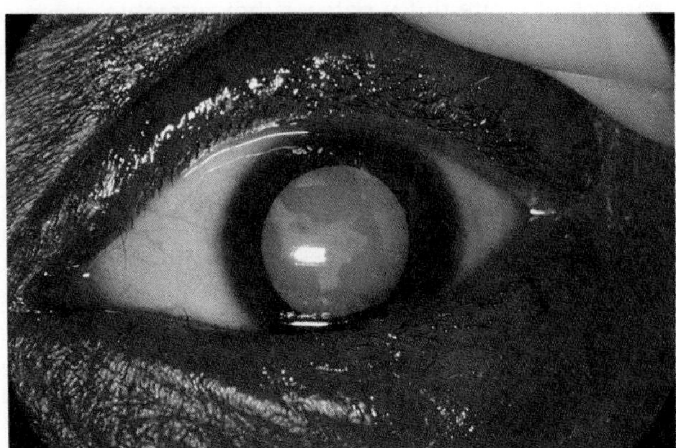

FIGURE 29-3
Cataract. The white appearance of the pupil in this eye is due to complete opacification of the lens ("mature cataract").

☐ **Pathology:** The most common cataract in the United States is associated with aging (age-related cataract). Clefts appear between the lens fibers, and degenerated lens material accumulates in these spaces (morgagnian corpuscles, incipient cataract). The degenerated lens material exerts an osmotic pressure, causing the damaged lens to increase in volume by imbibing water. Such a swollen lens may obstruct the pupil and cause glaucoma (*phakomorphic glaucoma*).

After the entire lens degenerates (mature cataract), its volume diminishes because lenticular debris escapes into the aqueous humor through a degenerated lens capsule (hypermature cataract). After becoming engulfed by macrophages, the extruded lenticular material may obstruct the aqueous outflow and produce glaucoma (*phakolytic glaucoma*). The compressed lens fibers in the center of the lens normally harden with aging (simple nuclear sclerotic cataract) and may become brown or black. If the peripheral portion of the lens, or lens cortex, becomes liquefied (*morgagnian cataract*), the sclerotic nucleus may sink within the lens by gravity.

Fortunately, cataractous lenses can be surgically removed, and optical devices can be provided to permit the focusing of light on the retina (spectacles, contact lenses, implantation of prosthetic lenses).

Presbyopia

Presbyopia is an impairment of vision associated with aging, in which the near point of distinct vision becomes located farther from the eye. At the equator of the crystalline lens, the cuboidal subcapsular cells differentiate into elongated lens fibers throughout life. Once formed, these lens fibers persist indefinitely. Older fibers become displaced into the center of the lens, causing it to enlarge with age. After this process has occurred for many years, the lens loses it elasticity, an effect that interferes with its normal tendency to become spherical, thereby diminishing the power of accommodation. As a result, most persons after age 40 years begin to have difficulty reading and require spectacles for near vision.

Phacoanaphylactic Endophthalmitis

Phacoanaphylactic endophthalmitis is an immunologically evoked, granulomatous response to lens proteins. The inflammatory lesion occurs around or within the lens (or its remains) in an eye with a traumatized or cataractous lens or after the surgical removal of a cataractous lens. A similar reaction may occur spontaneously in the contralateral eye months or years later. This autoimmune reaction to unique lens proteins, which are normally sequestered from the immune system, can be provoked experimentally by immunization with autologous lens material.

THE UVEA

A variety of inflammatory conditions affect the uveal tract. Inflammation of the uvea (*uveitis*) also encompasses inflammation of the iris (*iritis*), the ciliary body (*cyclitis*), and the iris plus the ciliary body (*iridocyclitis*). Inflammation of the iris and ciliary body typically causes a red eye, photophobia, moderate pain, blurred vision, a pericorneal halo, ciliary flush, and slight miosis. A flare is common in the anterior chamber on slit-lamp biomicroscopy, and keratic precipitates or a *hypopyon* also develop.

Posterior synechiae are adhesions that develop between the iris and the lens.

Peripheral anterior synechiae are adhesions between the peripheral iris and the anterior chamber angle. Both types of synechiae are complications of iritis and can cause glaucoma.

Sympathetic Ophthalmitis

Sympathetic ophthalmitis is an autoimmune uveitis in which the entire uvea develops granulomatous inflammation after a latent period in response to an injury in the other eye. Perforating ocular injury and prolapse of uveal tissue often lead to a progressive, bilateral, diffuse, granulomatous inflammation of the uvea. This uveitis develops in the originally injured eye (exciting eye) after a latent period of 4 to 8 weeks. The latent period may, however, be as short as 10 days or as long as many years. The uninjured eye (sympathizing eye) becomes affected at the same time as the injured eye or shortly thereafter. Vitiligo and graying of the eyelashes sometimes accompanies the uveitis. Nodules containing reactive retinal pigment epithelium, macrophages, and epithelioid cells commonly appear between Bruch's membrane and the retinal pigment epithelium (*Dalen–Fuchs nodules*).

It is widely believed that sympathetic ophthalmitis is an autoimmune reaction to sensitization by uveal antigens. Because melanin granules are frequently found within macrophages in sympathetic ophthalmia, they were once suspected of containing the offending antigen, but evidence for this is weak. In recent years, experimental studies have suggested that the antigen responsible for sympathetic ophthalmitis resides in the photoreceptors of the retina (arrestin).

Sarcoidosis

Ocular involvement occurs in one fourth to one third of patients with sarcoidosis and is frequently the initial clinical manifestation. Although any of the ocular and orbital tissues may be involved, this granulomatous disease has a predilection for the anterior segment of the eye. Ocular involvement is usually bilateral and most often takes the form of a granulomatous uveitis. Other ocular manifestations of sarcoidosis include calcific band keratopathy, cataracts, retinal vascularization, vitreous hemorrhage, and bilateral enlargement of the lacrimal and salivary glands (*Mikulicz syndrome*).

THE RETINA

Retinal Hemorrhage

Retinal hemorrhages are a feature of many disorders, including hypertension, diabetes mellitus, and central retinal vein occlusion. The appearance varies with the location. Hemorrhage in the nerve fiber layer spreads between axons and causes a flame-shaped appearance on funduscopy, whereas deep retinal hemorrhages tend to be round. When located between the retinal pigment epithelium and Bruch's membrane, blood appears as a dark mass and clinically resembles a melanoma.

After accidental or surgical perforation of the globe, choroidal hemorrhages may detach the choroid and displace the retina, vitreous body, and lens through the wound.

Retinal Occlusive Vascular Disease

Vascular occlusion results from thrombosis, embolism, stenosis (as in atherosclerosis), vascular compression, intravascular sludging or coagulation, or vasoconstriction (for instance, in hypertensive retinopathy or migraine). Thrombosis of the ocular vessels may accompany primary disease of these vessels, as in giant cell arteritis.

Certain disorders of the heart and of major vessels, such as the carotid arteries, predispose to emboli that lodge in the retina (see Table 29-1) and are evident on funduscopic examination at points of vascular bifurcation. Within the optic nerve, emboli in the central retinal artery frequently lodge in the vessel where it passes though the scleral perforations in the scleral (lamina cribrosa). In this location, the arterial lumen is narrower than in the orbital portion of the artery.

☐ **Pathology:** The effect of vascular occlusion depends on the size of the vessel involved, the degree of resultant ischemia, and the nature of the embolus. Small emboli often do not interfere with retinal function, whereas septic emboli may cause foci of ocular infection. Retinal ischemia of any cause frequently results in the appearance of white fluffy patches that resemble cotton on ophthalmoscopic examination (*cotton-wool patches*). These round spots, which are seldom wider than the optic disc, consist of aggregates of swollen axons in the nerve-fiber layer of the retina. The affected axons contain numerous degenerated mitochondria and dense bodies related to the lysosomal system, which accumulate because of impaired axoplasmic flow. Histologically, in cross-section, the individual swollen axons resemble cells (*cytoid bodies*). Cotton-wool spots are reversible if the circulation is restored in time.

Central Retinal Artery Occlusion

Like the neurons in rest of the nervous system, those in the retina (Fig. 29-4), similar to those in the rest of the nervous system, are extremely susceptible to hypoxia. Central retinal artery occlusion (Figs. 29-5 and 29-6) may fol-

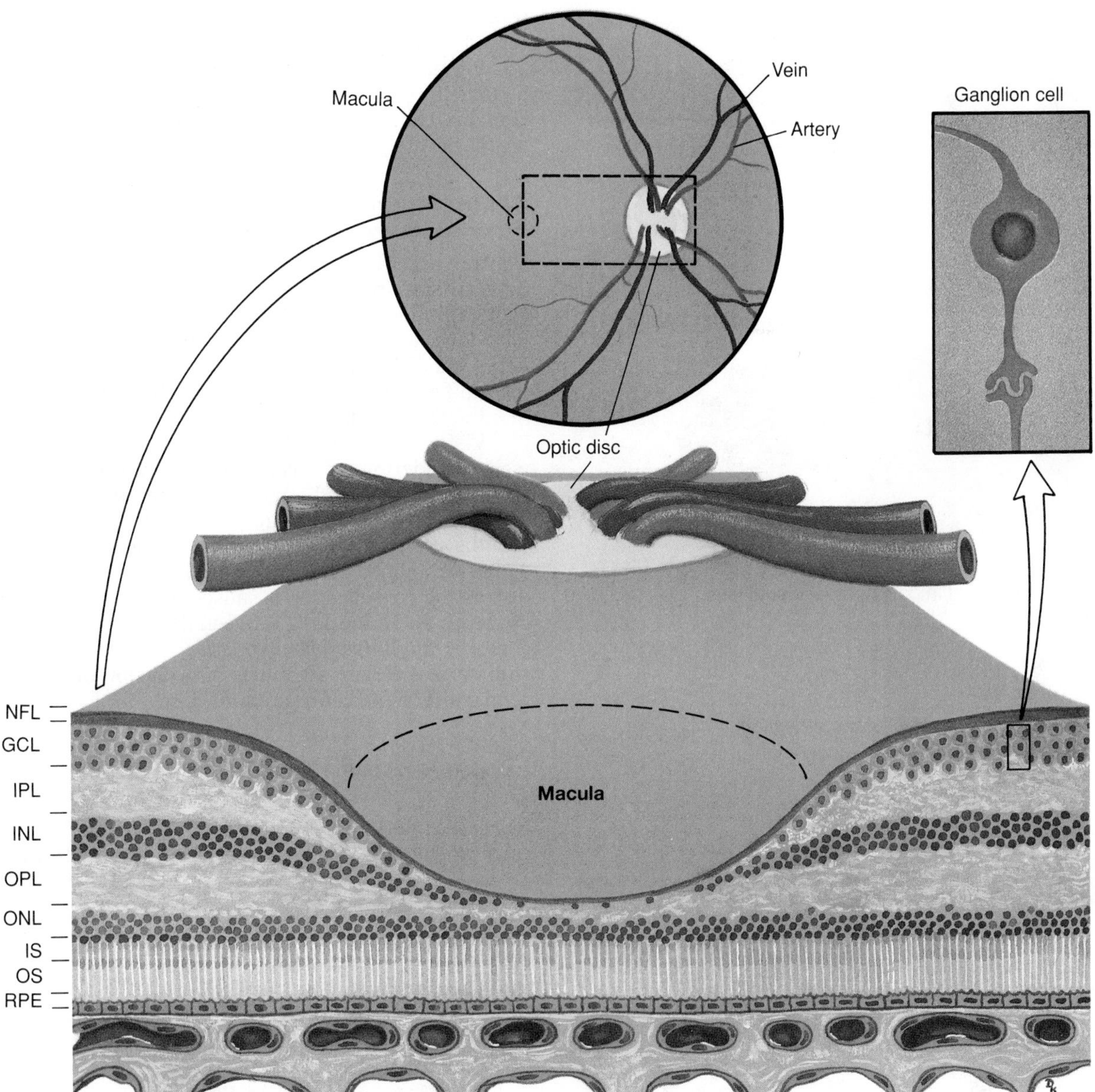

FIGURE *29-4*
The normal retina. The constituents of the normal retina are arranged in distinct layers. These include the nerve fiber layer (*NFL*), ganglion cell layer (*GCL*), inner plexiform layer (*IPL*), inner nuclear layer (*INL*), outer plexiform layer (*OPL*), outer nuclear layer (*ONL*), inner segments (*IS*) and outer segments (*OS*) of the photoreceptors, and the retinal pigment epithelium (*RPE*). The axons from the ganglion cells enter the nerve fiber layer and converge toward the optic disc. The inner retina contains arteries and veins. The retina is thinnest at the center of the macula, where bare photoreceptors rest on the retinal pigment epithelium. Only one cell thick in most of the retina, the ganglion cell layer is multilayered at the macula.

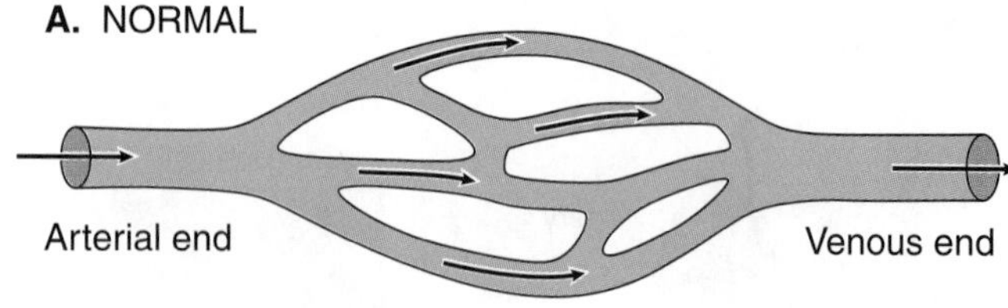

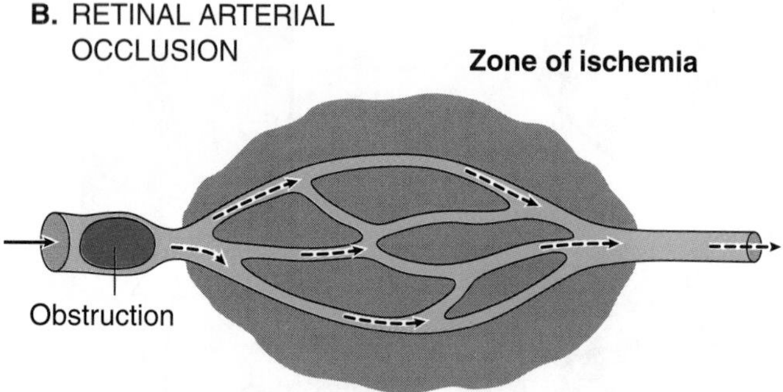

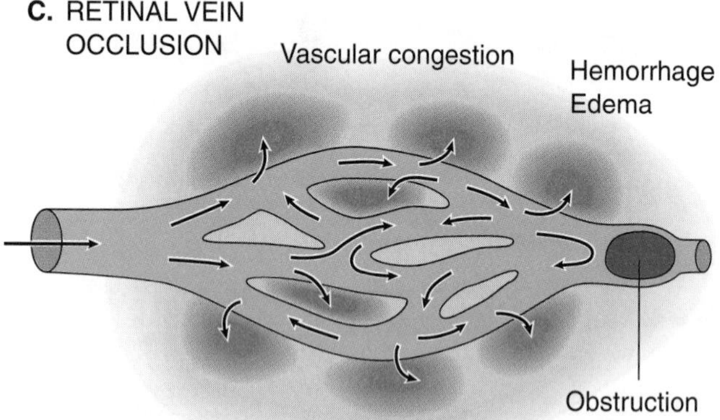

FIGURE *29-5*
Occlusion of the retinal artery and vein. (*A*) In the retina, as in other parts of the body, blood normally flows through a capillary network. When the retinal arteries become occluded, as with an embolus, a zone of retinal ischemia ensues. This is accompanied by impaired neuronal function and visual loss, and the ischemic retina becomes pale (*B*). Because the intravascular pressure within the ischemic tissue is low, hemorrhage is inconspicuous. On the other hand, with retinal vein occlusion (*C*), vascular congestion, hemorrhage, and edema are prominent, whereas ischemia is mild and neuronal function remains intact.

low thrombosis of the retinal artery, as in atherosclerosis or giant cell arteritis, or embolization to that vessel. Intracellular edema, manifested by retinal pallor, is prominent, especially in the macula, where the ganglion cells are most numerous. The foveola, that is, the vascularized choroid beneath the center of the macula, stands out in sharp contrast as a prominent *cherry-red spot*. The lack of retinal circulation reduces the retinal arterioles to delicate threads (see Fig. 29-6).

Permanent blindness follows central retinal artery obstruction, unless the ischemia is of short duration. Unilateral blurred vision, lasting a few minutes (*amaurosis fugax*), occurs with small retinal emboli.

Central Retinal Vein Occlusion

Central retinal vein occlusion results in flame-shaped hemorrhages in the nerve-fiber layer of the retina, especially around the optic disc. The hemorrhages reflect the high intravascular pressure that dilates and ruptures the veins and collateral vessels (Fig. 29-7). Edema of the optic disc and retina occurs because of an impaired absorption of interstitial fluid.

Vision is disturbed but may recover surprisingly well, considering the severity of the funduscopic changes. An intractable closed-angle glaucoma, with severe pain and repeated hemorrhages, commonly ensues 2 to 3 months after central retinal vein occlusion (100-day glaucoma, thrombotic glaucoma, neovascular glaucoma). This distressing complication is caused by neovascularization of the iris and adhesions between the iris and the anterior chamber angle (*peripheral anterior synechiae*). Table 29-2 summarizes certain attributes of occlusion of the central retinal artery and central retinal vein.

Hypertensive Retinopathy

Increased blood pressure commonly affects the retina, causing changes that can readily be seen with the oph-

TABLE *29-2* **Comparison Between Occlusions of the Central Retinal Vein and Central Retinal Artery**

	Central Retinal Vein Occlusion	Central Retinal Artery Occlusion
Incidence	More common	Less common
Intravascular pressure	High	Low
Metabolites	Impaired drainage	
Funduscopic features		
Hemorrhage	Marked Flame shaped	Not a feature
Cherry-red spot	Absent	Present
Cotton-wool spot	Occasionally	Uncommon[a]
Veins	Engorged and tortuous	Collapsed
Retinal arterioles	Prominent	Delicate threads
Vision	Poor	Poor
Recovery	Good	Poor
Onset	Gradual	Sudden
Ischemia	Less prominent	Prominent
Sequelae		
Glaucoma	Common	Uncommon
Iris neovascularization	Common	Uncommon

[a] Sometimes seen in patients with ischemia (e.g., carotid artery stenosis) preceding central retinal artery occlusion.

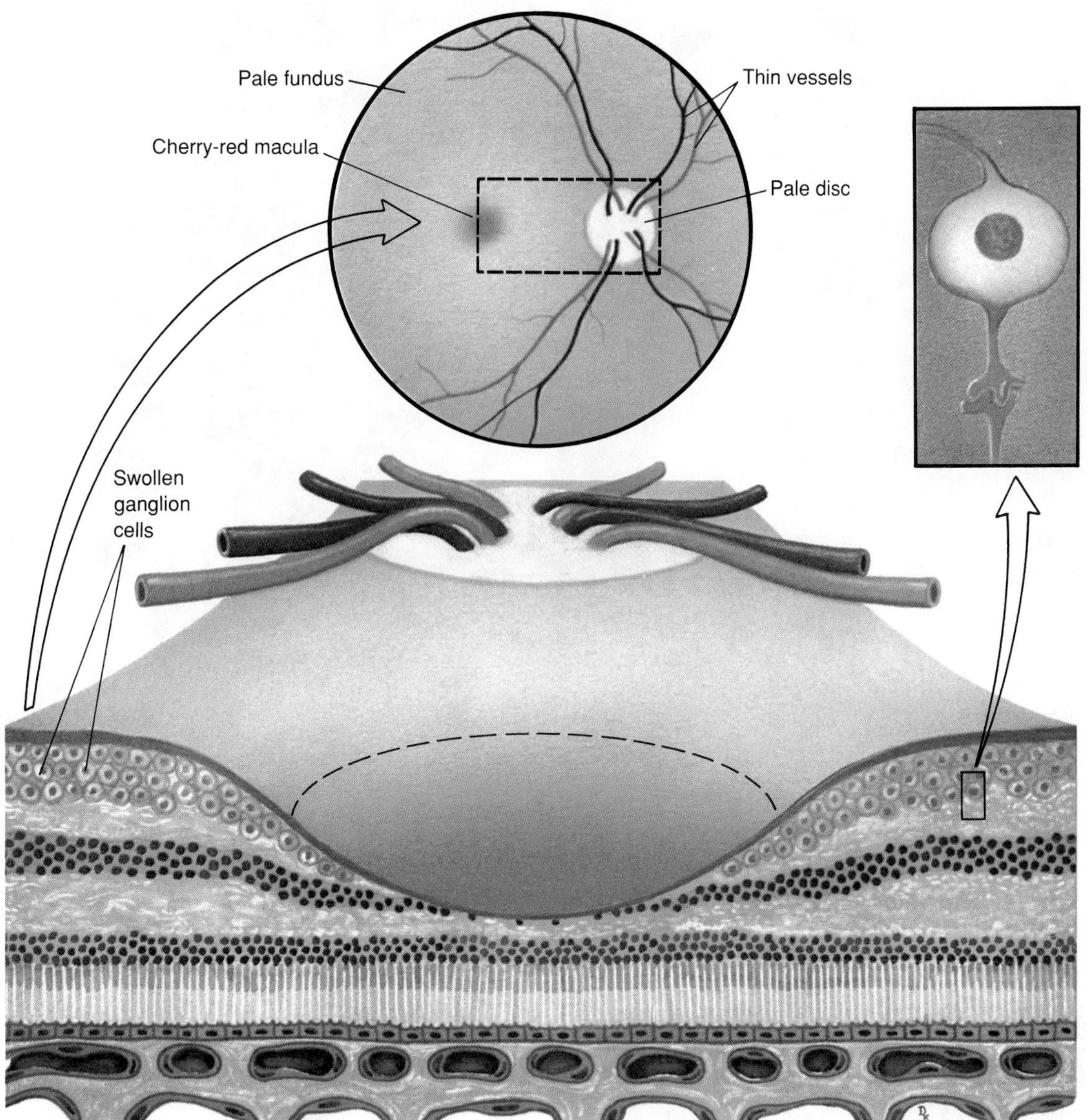

FIGURE *29-6*
Central retinal artery occlusion. When the central retinal artery becomes occluded, as with an embolus, the entire retina becomes edematous and pale. The decreased blood flow makes the retinal vessels less visible on funduscopic examination. The macula becomes cherry-red in color, owing to the prominent, but normal, underlying vasculature of the choroid.

thalmoscope and that relate to the severity of the hypertension (Figs. 29-8 and 29-9).

☐ **Pathology:** Features of hypertensive retinopathy include the following:

- Arteriolar narrowing
- Hemorrhages in the retinal nerve fiber layer (flame-shaped hemorrhages)
- Exudates, including some that radiate from the center of the macula (macular star)
- Fluffy white bodies in the superficial retina (cotton-wool spots)
- Microaneurysms

In the eye, arteriolosclerosis accompanies long-standing hypertension and commonly affects the retinal and choroidal vessels. The lumina of the thickened retinal arterioles become narrowed, increasingly tortuous, and of irregular caliber. At sites where the arterioles cross veins, the latter appear kinked (*arteriovenous nicking*). However, the venous diameter before the site of compression is not wider than that after it. Thus, the kinked appearance of the vein is not due to compression by a taut sclerotic artery. Rather, it reflects sclerosis within the venous walls because the retinal arteries and veins share a common adventitia at sites of arteriovenous crossings.

By funduscopy, abnormal retinal arterioles appear as parallel white lines at sites of vascular crossings (*arterial*

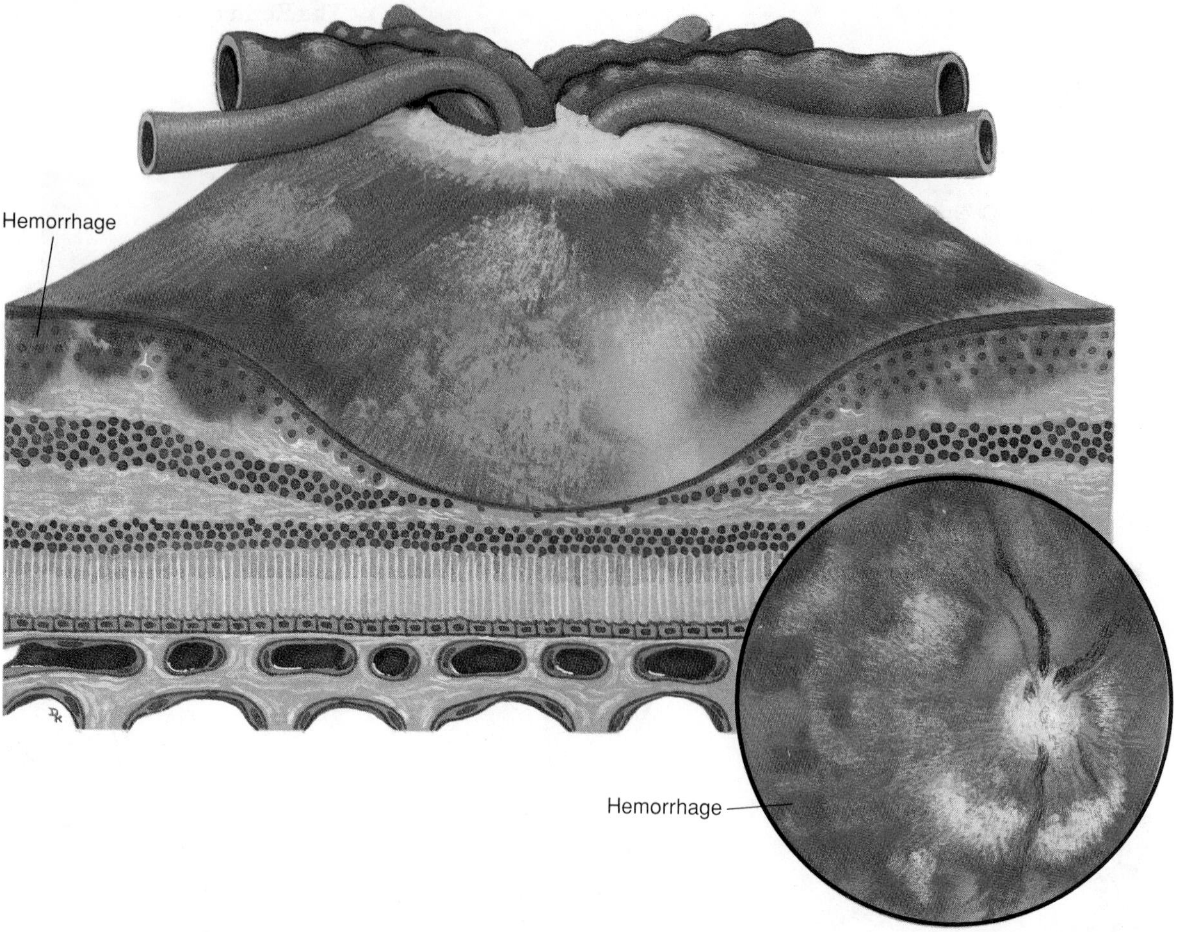

Hemorrhage

Hemorrhage

FIGURE *29-7*
Central retinal vein occlusion. In contrast to central retinal artery occlusion, central retinal vein occlusion produces considerable vascular engorgement and retinal hemorrhage as a consequence of the increased intravascular pressure.

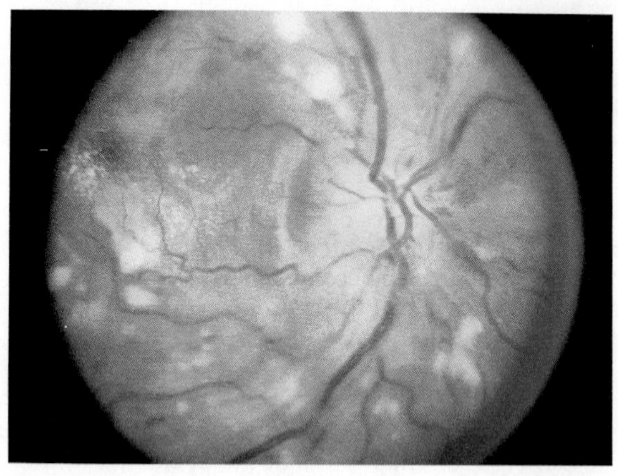

FIGURE *29-8*
Hypertensive retinopathy. A photograph of the ocular fundus in a patient with extensive retinopathy. The optic nerve head is edematous; the retina contains numerous exudates and "cotton-wool" spots.

FIGURE *29-9*
Hypertensive retinopathy. Various abnormalities develop within the retina in hypertension. The commonly associated arteriolosclerosis affects the appearance of the retinal microvasculature. Light reflected from the thickened arteriolar walls mimics silver or copper wire. Blood flow through the retinal venules is not well visualized at the sites of arteriolar–venular crossings. This effect is due to a thickening of the venular wall rather than to an impediment to blood flow caused by compression; the column of blood proximal to the compression is not wider than the part distal to the crossing. Impaired axoplasmic flow within the nerve fiber layer, caused by ischemia, results in swollen axons with cytoplasmic bodies. Such structures resemble cotton on funduscopy ("cotton-wool spots"). Hemorrhages are common in the retina, and exudates frequently form a star around the macula.

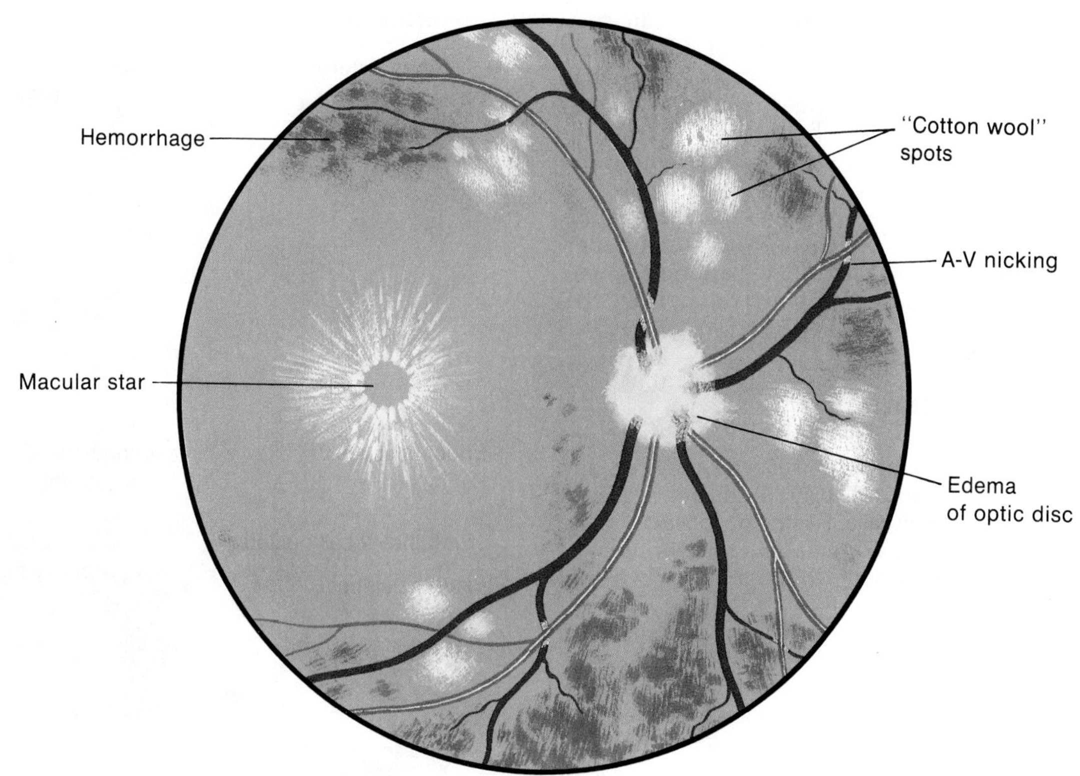
Hemorrhage
"Cotton wool" spots
A-V nicking
Macular star
Edema of optic disc

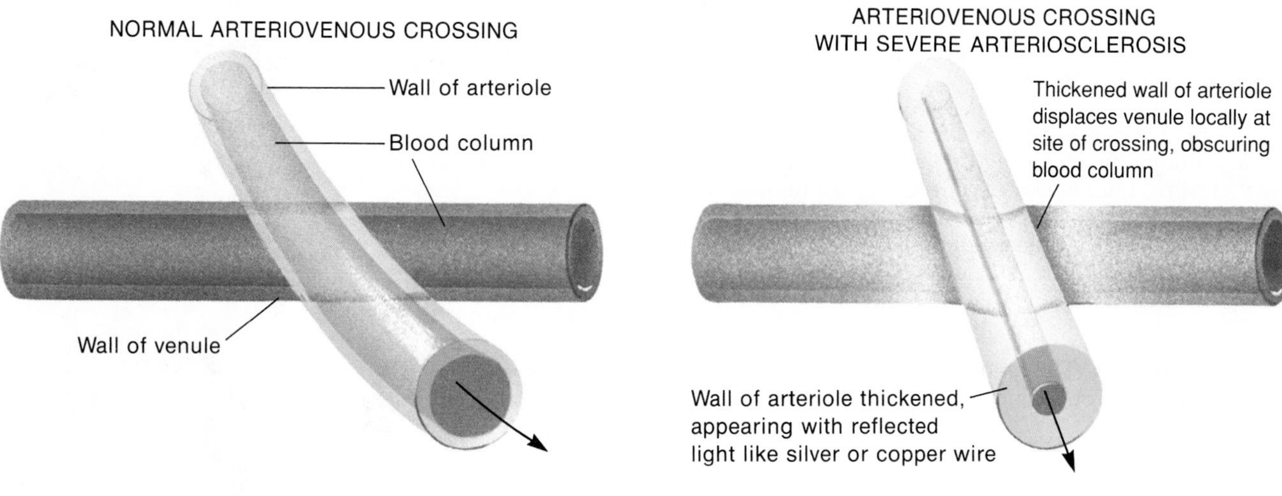
NORMAL ARTERIOVENOUS CROSSING
Wall of arteriole
Blood column
Wall of venule
ARTERIOVENOUS CROSSING WITH SEVERE ARTERIOSCLEROSIS
Thickened wall of arteriole displaces venule locally at site of crossing, obscuring blood column
Wall of arteriole thickened, appearing with reflected light like silver or copper wire

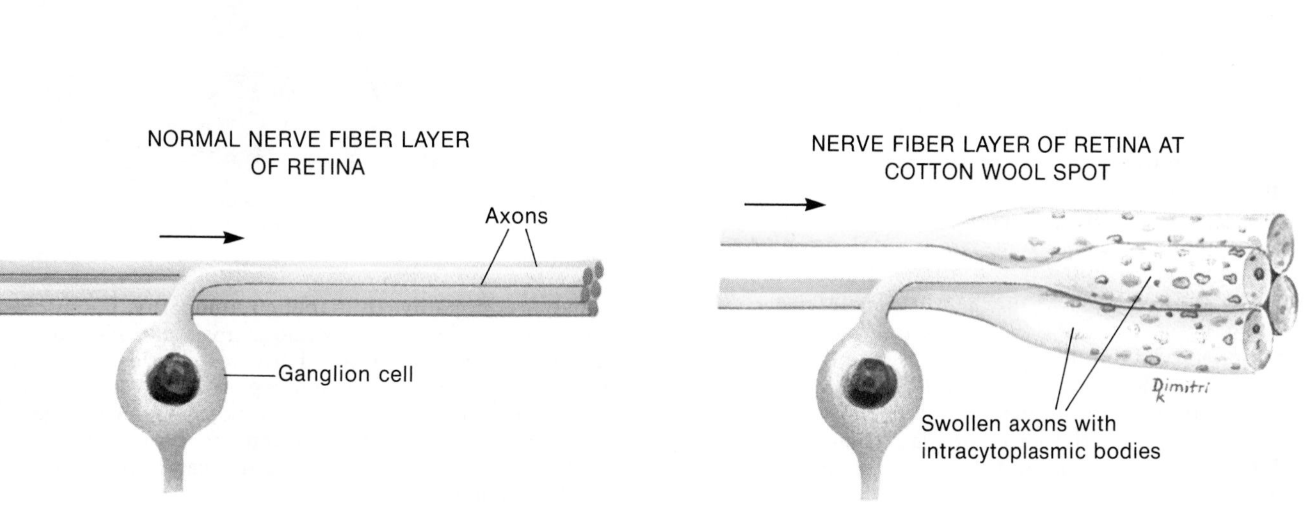
NORMAL NERVE FIBER LAYER OF RETINA
Axons
Ganglion cell
NERVE FIBER LAYER OF RETINA AT COTTON WOOL SPOT
Swollen axons with intracytoplasmic bodies

sheathing). Initially, the narrowed lumen of the retinal vessels decreases the visibility of the blood column and makes it appear orange on ophthalmoscopic examination (*copper wiring*). However, as the blood column eventually becomes completely obscured, light reflected from the sclerotic vessels appears as threads of silver wire (*silver wiring*).

Small superficial or deep retinal hemorrhages often accompany retinal arteriolosclerosis. **Malignant hypertension** is characterized by a necrotizing arteriolitis, with fibrinoid necrosis and thrombosis of the precapillary retinal arterioles.

Diabetic Retinopathy

The eye is frequently involved in diabetes mellitus, and ocular symptoms occur in 20% to 40% of diabetics even at the clinical onset of the disease. For the purposes of a unified discussion, the various ophthalmic complications of diabetes are all described here, although they do not all primarily affect the retina.

Virtually all patients with type 1 (insulin-dependent) diabetes and many of those with type 2 (non–insulin-dependent) diabetes develop some degree of background retinopathy (see later) within 5 to 15 years of the onset of diabetes (Figs. 29-10 to 29-12). The more dangerous proliferative retinopathy does not appear until at least 10 years of diabetes, after which the incidence increases rapidly and remains high for many years. **The frequency of proliferative retinopathy correlates with the degree of glycemic control; the better the control, the lower the rate of retinopathy.**

Retinal ischemia can account for most features of diabetic retinopathy, including the cotton-wool spots, capillary closure, microaneurysms, and retinal neovascularization. Ischemia results from narrowing or occlusion of retinal arterioles (as from arteriolosclerosis or platelet and lipid thrombi) or from atherosclerosis of the central retinal or ophthalmic arteries.

☐ **Pathology:** The retinopathy of diabetes is characterized by background and proliferative stages.

BACKGROUND (NONPROLIFERATIVE) DIABETIC RETINOPATHY: This stage exhibits venous engorgement, small hemorrhages (*dot and blot hemorrhages*), capillary microaneurysms, and exudates. These lesions usually do not impair vision, unless associated with macular edema. The retinopathy begins at the posterior pole but eventually may involve the entire retina.

On funduscopy, the first discernible clinical abnormality in background diabetic retinopathy is engorged retinal veins, with localized sausage-shaped distentions, coils, and loops. This is followed by small hemorrhages in the same areas, mostly in the inner nuclear and outer plexiform layers. With time, "waxy" exudates accumulate, chiefly in the vicinity of the microaneurysms. The retinopathy of the elderly diabetic frequently displays numerous exudates (*exudative diabetic retinopathy*), whereas this is not a feature in diabetics with type 1 disease. Because of the hyperlipoproteinemia of diabetics, the exudates are rich in lipid and thus appear yellowish (*waxy exudates*).

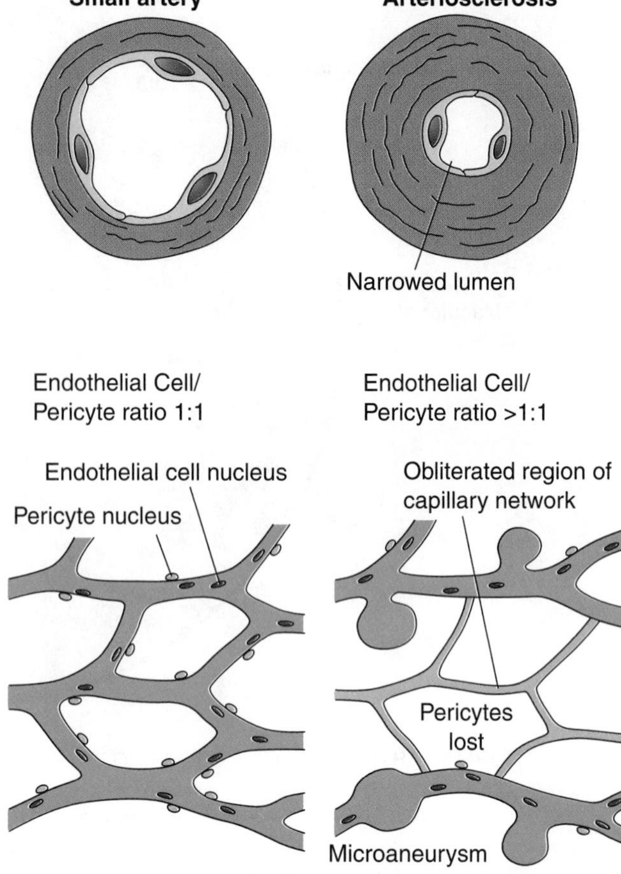

FIGURE 29-10
Diabetic retinopathy. In diabetic retinopathy, the microvasculature is abnormal. Arteriosclerosis narrows the lumen of the small arteries. Pericytes are lost and the endothelial cell-to-pericyte ratio is greater than 1. Capillary microaneurysms are prominent, and portions of the capillary network become acellular and show no blood flow. The basement membrane of the retinal capillaries is thickened and vacuolated.

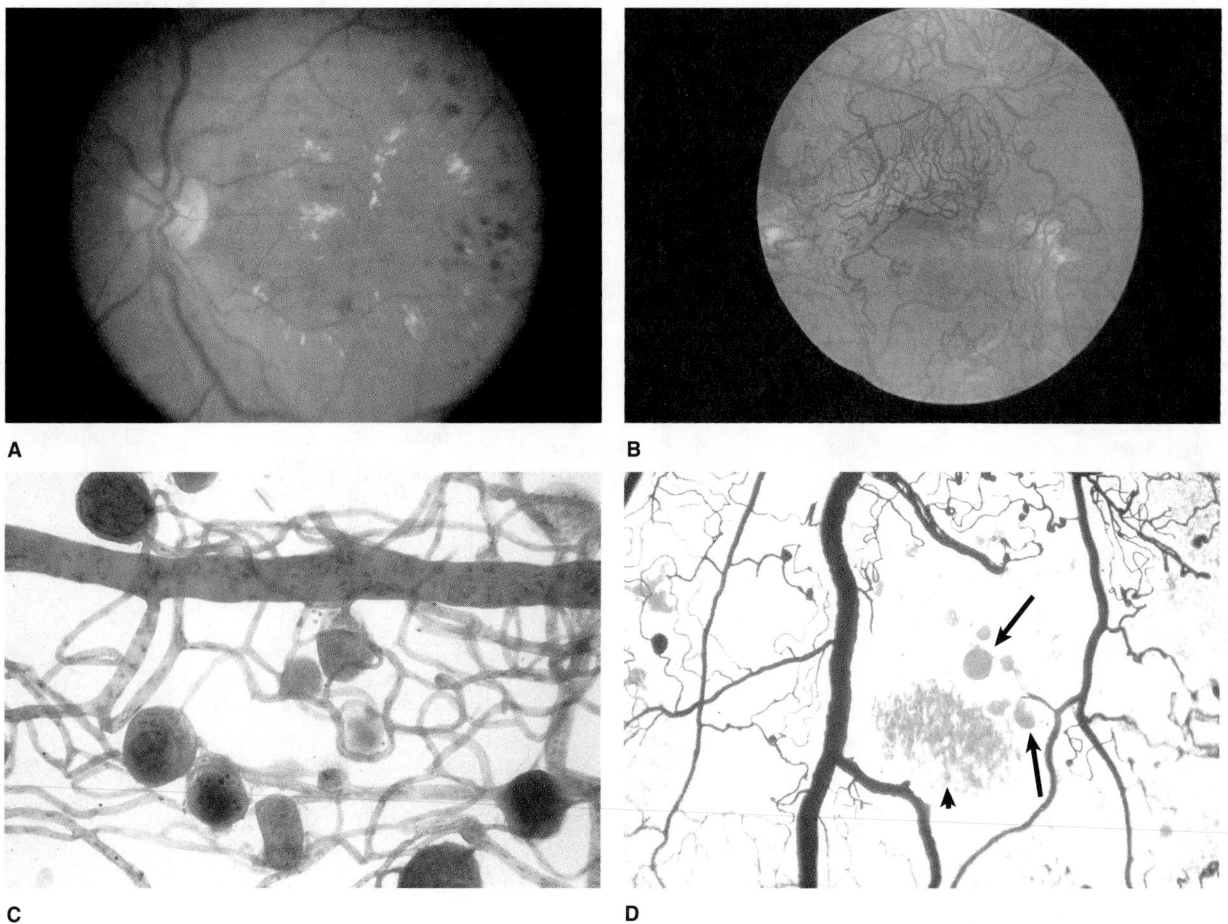

FIGURE 29-11
Diabetic retinopathy. (*A*) View of the ocular fundus in a patient with background diabetic retinopathy. Several yellowish "hard" exudates, which are rich in lipids, are evident, together with several relatively small retinal hemorrhages. (*B*) A vascular frond has extended anterior to the retina in the eye with proliferative diabetic retinopathy. (*C*) Numerous microaneurysms are present in this flat preparation of a diabetic retina. (*D*) This flat preparation from a diabetic was stained with periodic acid–Schiff (PAS) after the retinal vessels had been perfused with India ink. Microaneurysms (*arrows*) and an exudate (*arrowhead*) are evident in a region of retinal nonperfusion.

PROLIFERATIVE RETINOPATHY: After many years, diabetic retinopathy becomes proliferative. Delicate new blood vessels grow along with fibrous and glial tissue toward the vitreous body. Neovascularization of the retina is a prominent feature of diabetic retinopathy and of other conditions caused by retinal ischemia. Tortuous new vessels first appear on the surface of the retina and optic nerve head and then grow into the vitreous cavity. The newly formed friable vessels bleed easily, and the resultant vitreal hemorrhages obscure vision. Neovascularization is associated with the proliferation and migration of astrocytes, which grow around the new vessels to form delicate white veils (gliosis). The proliferating fibrovascular and glial tissue contracts, often causing retinal detachment and blindness. Frequently, features of hypertensive and arteriolosclerotic retinopathy are associated with diabetic retinopathy.

Diabetic retinopathy and glaucoma are the leading causes of irreversible blindness in the United States. Blindness in diabetic retinopathy results when the macula is involved, but it also follows vitreous hemorrhage, retinal detachment, and glaucoma. Once blindness ensues, it heralds an ominous future for the patient, because death from ischemic heart disease or renal failure often follows. In fact, the mean life expectancy in such cases is less than 6 years, and only one fifth of blind diabetics survive 10 years. Laser phototherapy early in the course of proliferative retinopathy has proved effective in controlling this complication.

Diabetic Iridopathy

In diabetics with severe retinopathy, a fibrovascular layer frequently grows along the anterior surface of the iris and in the anterior chamber angle. Because such iris neovascularization (*rubeosis iridis*) is a feature of several conditions associated with retinal ischemia, it is believed to be

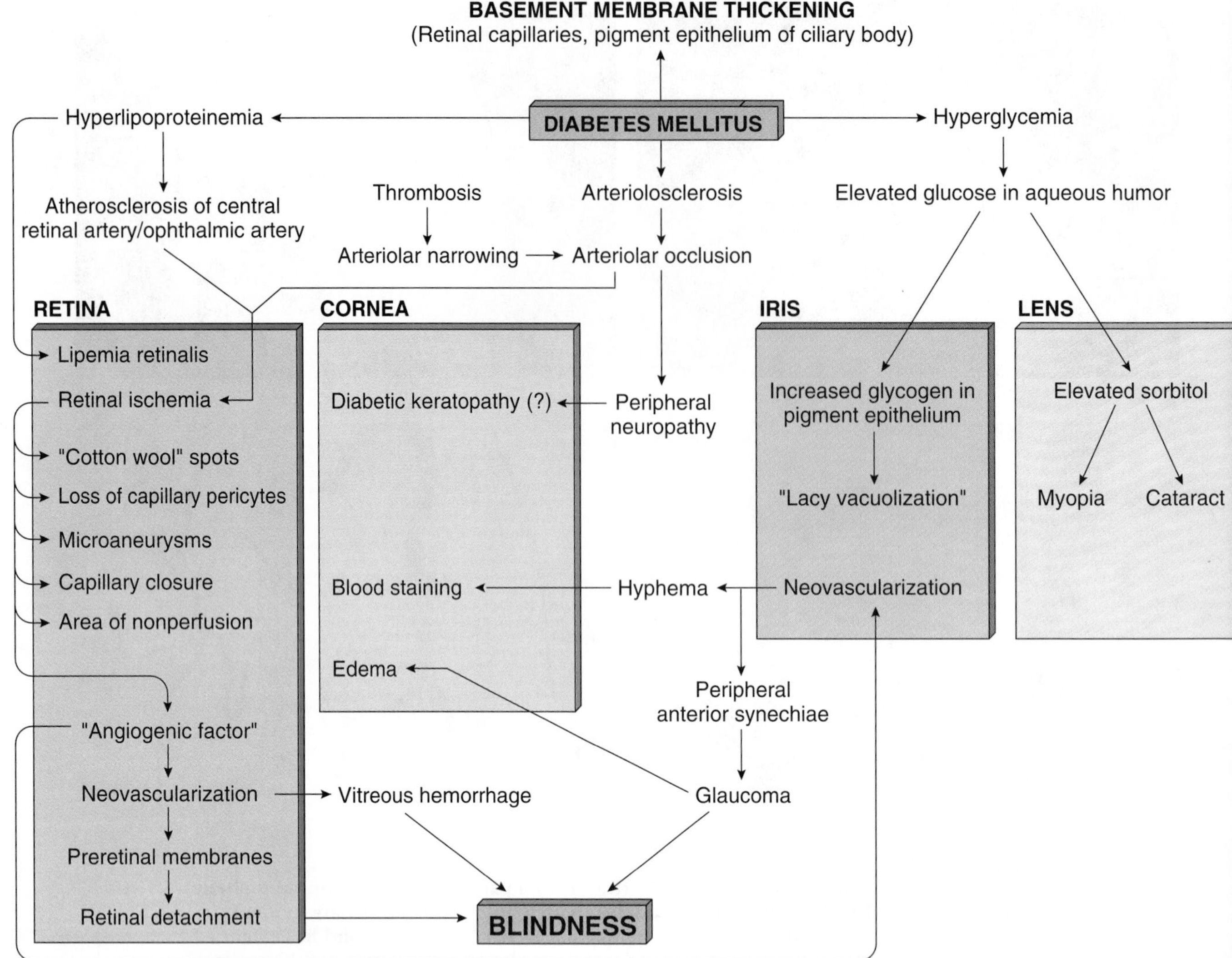

FIGURE 29-12
The effect of diabetes on the eye.

due to an angiogenic factor produced by the ischemic retina.

☐ **Pathology:** A fibrovascular membrane leads to adhesions between the iris and the cornea (*peripheral anterior synechiae*) and between the iris and lens (*posterior synechiae*), while traction by the fibrovascular membrane pulls the iris pigment epithelium around the pupillary margin (*ectropion uveae*). The friable new vessels on the iris bleed easily and cause *hyphema* (hemorrhage within the anterior chamber of the eye). Neovascularization of the iris is clinically important because it frequently culminates in a blind, painful eye, owing to secondary glaucoma (*neovascular glaucoma*).

Hyperglycemia leads to glycogen storage in the pigmented epithelium of the iris, a phenomenon analogous to that produced in the renal tubules by glycosuria (*Armanni–Ebstein phenomenon*). When tissue sections of diabetic eyes are processed in the usual manner, the pigment epithelium of the iris sometimes contains numerous vacuoles, which imparts a lacy appearance. The vacuoles result from the loss of glycogen in the preparation of tissue sections. Glycogen storage within the pigment epithelium of the iris is thought to account for the scattering of the iris pigment observed clinically in diabetic patients.

Diabetic Cataracts

Patients with type 1 diabetes often develop bilateral "snowflake" cataracts. These consist of a blanket of white needle-shaped opacities in the lens immediately beneath the anterior and posterior lens capsule. The opacities coalesce within a few weeks in adolescents, and within days in children, until the whole lens becomes opaque. Snowflake cataracts can be produced experimentally in young animals and result from an osmotic effect caused by the accumulation of sorbitol, the alcohol derived from glucose (see Chapter 22). The increased sorbitol content of the lens causes imbibition of water and an enlargement of the lens.

Age-related cataracts occur in diabetics at an earlier age than in the general population and progress more rapidly to maturity. A sudden temporary myopia, caused by an increase in the refractive power of the lens, may be the presenting manifestation of diabetes.

Other Ophthalmic Manifestations of Diabetes

Diabetics are at increased risk for inflammation of the anterior segment of the eye, phycomycosis (mucormycosis) of the orbit, and primary open-angle glaucoma. They are also prone to the *Argyll Robertson pupil* (unequal and irregularly shaped pupils that react to accommodation but not to light). Cranial nerve palsies occur, especially of the oculomotor nerve. Some patients with long-standing diabetes develop recurrent corneal erosions, which are thought to be due to impaired innervation of the cornea.

Retinal Detachment

Retinal detachment refers to the separation of the sensory retina from the retinal pigment epithelium. During fetal development, the space between the sensory retina and the retinal pigment epithelium is obliterated when these two layers become apposed. However, the sensory retina readily separates from the retinal pigment epithelium when fluid (liquid vitreous, hemorrhage, or exudate) accumulates within the potential space between these structures. Such a separation is a common cause of blindness.

Factors predisposing to retinal detachment include retinal defects (due to trauma or certain retinal degenerations), vitreous traction, diminished pressure on the retina (as after vitreous loss), and weakening of the fixation of the retina. The photoreceptors and retinal pigment epithelium normally function as a unit. After they separate in a retinal detachment, oxygen and nutrients that normally reach the outer retina from the choroid need to diffuse across a greater distance. This situation causes the photoreceptors to degenerate, after which cyst-like extracellular spaces appear within the retina. Three varieties of retinal detachment are recognized—rhegmatogenous, tractional, and exudative.

RHEGMATOGENOUS RETINAL DETACHMENT: This condition is associated with a retinal tear and often with degenerative changes in the vitreous body or peripheral retina. Full-thickness holes in the retina are not complicated by retinal detachment, unless liquid vitreous gains access to the potential space between the retina and the retinal pigment epithelium. Even then some vitreoretinal traction seems to be necessary for retinal detachment to occur. Retinal detachment follows intraocular hemorrhage (as after trauma) and is a potential complication of cataract extractions and several other ocular operations.

TRACTIONAL RETINAL DETACHMENT: In some instances, the retina is detached by being pulled toward the center of the eye by adherent vitreoretinal adhesions, as occurs in proliferative diabetic retinopathy and retinopathy of prematurity, and after intraocular infection.

EXUDATIVE RETINAL DETACHMENT: An accumulation of fluid in the potential space between the sensory retina and the retinal pigment epithelium causes a detached retina in disorders such as choroiditis, choroidal hemangioma, and choroidal melanoma.

Retinitis Pigmentosa (Pigmentary Retinopathy)

Retinitis pigmentosa is a generic term that refers to a variety of bilateral, progressive, degenerative retinopathies characterized clinically by night blindness and constriction of peripheral visual fields and pathologically by the loss of retinal photoreceptors (rods and cones) and pigment accumulation within the retina.

☐ **Pathogenesis:** Multiple genetic disorders result in retinitis pigmentosa. Some are isolated ocular disorders, with autosomal dominant, autosomal recessive, or X-linked recessive inheritance; in others, the pigmentary retinopathies are associated with neurological and systemic disorders (see Table 29-1). To date, at least seven loci are known for autosomal dominant retinitis pigmentosa, and three loci for autosomal recessive retinitis pigmentosa are known. Retinitis pigmentosa has also been mapped to two distinct loci on the X chromosome. Almost 12% of autosomal dominant cases of retinitis pigmentosa have a mutation in the rhodopsin genes. Currently, more than 70 different rhodopsin mutations have been identified, usually point mutations or small deletions. Other cases of retinitis pigmentosa have mutations in the genes for the photoreceptor proteins peripherin and ROM-1, and the genes for the β subunit of guanosine triphosphate (GTP) phosphodiesterase or the α subunit of a rod cyclic guanosine monophosphate (cGMP)–gated channel.

Because multiple different mutations result in retinitis pigmentosa, a single defective protein cannot explain the death of photoreceptor cells that is characteristic of the condition. Presumably the abnormal metabolic pathways that result from all mutations ultimately converge at a final common point. Studies in experimental models of retinitis pigmentosa, including some with transgenic mice, indicate that programmed cell death (apoptosis) is involved.

☐ **Pathology:** In retinitis pigmentosa, the destruction of rods, and later cones, is followed by the migration of retinal pigment epithelial cells into the sensory retina (Fig. 29-13). Melanin appears within slender processes of spidery cells and accumulates mainly around small branching retinal blood vessels (especially in the equatorial portion of the retina), like spicules of bone. A gradual attenuation of the retinal blood vessels ensues, and the optic nerve head acquires a characteristic waxy pallor.

☐ **Clinical Features:** The clinical manifestations of retinitis pigmentosa, as well as the appearance and distribution of the retinal pigmentation, vary with the causes of the retinopathy. Half of all patients with retinitis pigmentosa have a family history of the disease. Patients with autosomal recessive and X-linked disease are more

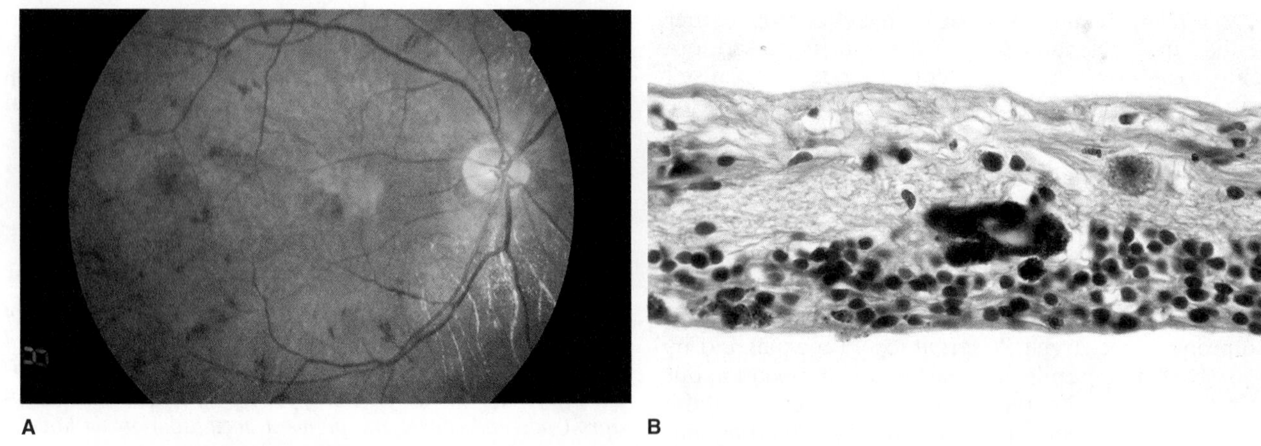

FIGURE 29-13
(*A*) Fundus photograph of the retina of a patient with pigmentary retinopathy (retinitis pigmentosa) showing attenuated retinal vessels and foci of retinal pigmentation. (*B*) Microscopic appearance of a severely degenerated retina in pigmentary retinopathy. Note the focal accumulations of pigmented cells (derived from retinal pigmented epithelium) within the retina.

severely affected and usually are seen in childhood with night blindness and peripheral field defects. Autosomal dominant forms of retinitis pigmentosa tend to be less severe, and symptoms begin later in life. As the condition progresses, contraction of the visual fields eventually leads to tunnel vision. Central vision is usually preserved until late in the course of the disease. In a few cases, the macula becomes involved, and blindness ensues.

Macular Degeneration

The center of the macula, the foveola, is the point of greatest visual acuity. In this area, there is a high concentration of cones resting on the retinal pigment epithelium. Surrounding the macula, the retina has a multilayered concentration of ganglion cells. With aging, in certain drug toxicities (e.g., chloroquine), and in several inherited disorders, the macula degenerates, and central vision is impaired. **Perhaps the most common cause of reduced vision in the United States is age-related maculopathy.** This condition is sometimes associated with a subretinal fibrovascular tissue and sometimes bleeding into the subretinal space (hemorrhagic macular degeneration). Interestingly, in one series of patients with age-related macular degeneration, mutations in the *ABCR* gene (ATP–binding cassette transporter–retina) were found. *ABCR* codes for a rod cell protein (rim protein), which is thought to be a transporter involved in molecular recycling. Mutations in this gene may allow degraded material to accumulate and interfere with retinal function.

Cherry-Red Spot at the Macula

Cherry-red spot at the macula describes a condition in which the central foveola appears bright red in comparison with the surrounding retina. In lysosomal storage diseases (see Table 29-1), including the gangliosidoses, myriad intracytoplasmic lysosomal inclusions within the multilayered ganglion cell layer of the macula impart a striking pallor to the affected retina. As a result, the central foveola appears bright red because of the underlying choroidal vasculature (Fig. 29-14). A cherry-red spot also occurs at the macula after central retinal artery occlusion, but for a different reason. Edema causes the entire retina to appear pale, a situation that highlights the subfoveolar vascular choroid.

Angioid Streaks

Angioid streaks refer to the vessel-like appearance of fractures in Bruch's membrane when the posterior segment of the eye is examined clinically. In a variety of systemic conditions (see Table 29-1), Bruch's membrane fractures spontaneously, thereby causing characteristic irregular lines that radiate beneath the retina from the optic nerve head (angioid streaks).

Retinopathy of Prematurity (Retrolental Fibroplasia)

Retinopathy of prematurity is a bilateral, iatrogenic, retinal disorder that occurs predominantly in premature infants who have been treated after birth with oxygen. The entity was originally called retrolental fibroplasia because of a mass of scarred tissue behind the lens in advanced cases. In the United States and in some other countries some 50 years ago, retinopathy of prematurity (Fig. 29-15) was the leading cause of blindness in infants. This bilateral, iatrogenic ocular disorder is almost restricted to premature infants administered high concentrations of oxygen.

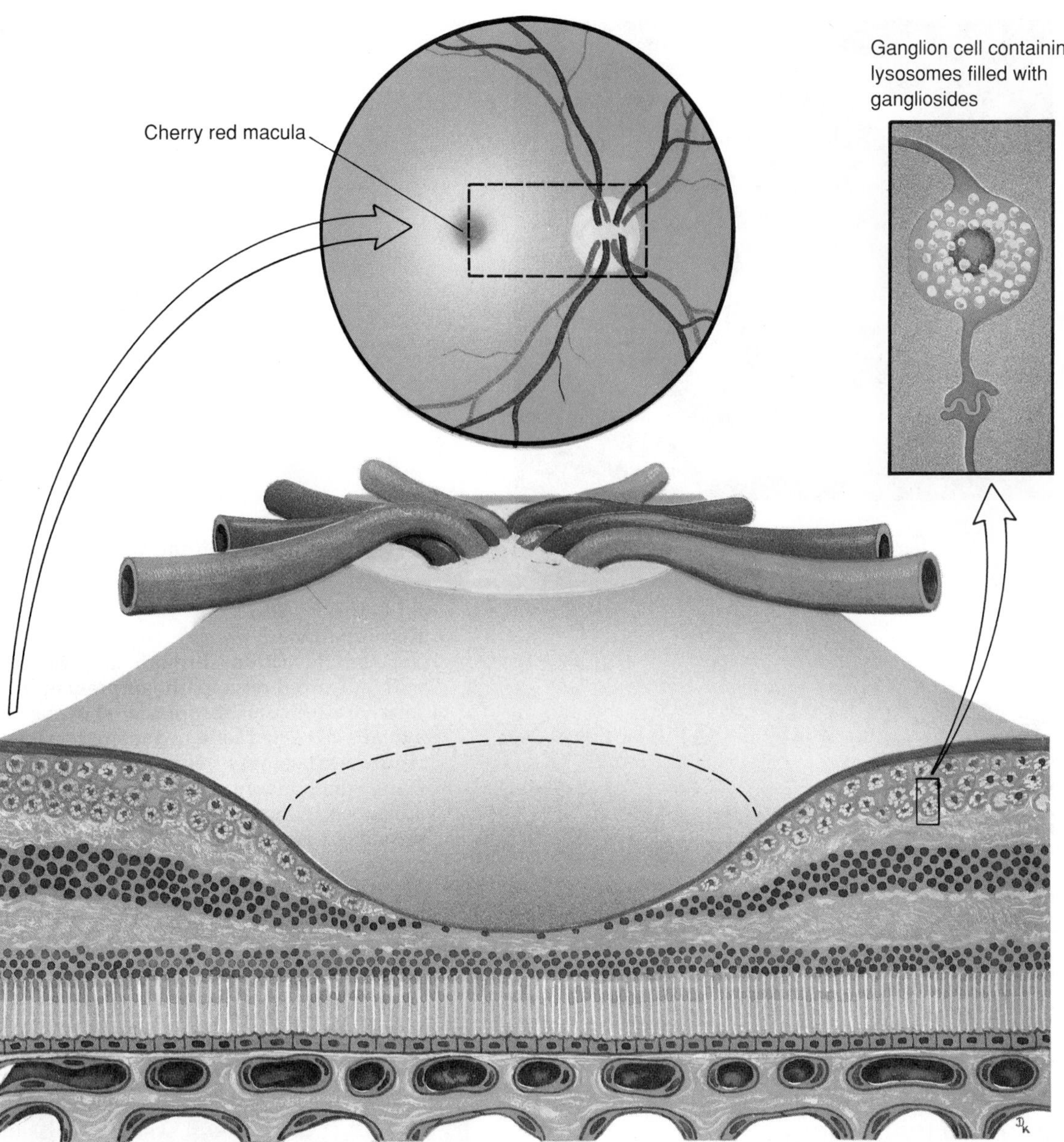

FIGURE *29-14*
Cherry-red macula. A cherry-red spot appears at the macula in several lysosomal storage diseases that are characterized by intracytoplasmic accumulations within the retinal ganglion cells, such as granulocyte–macrophage-2 (GM_2) gangliosidosis type II (Tay–Sachs disease). The macula develops this appearance because the pallor created by the deposits within the multilayered ganglion cells enhances the visibility of the underlying normal choroidal vasculature.

When a premature infant is exposed to excessive amounts of oxygen, as in an incubator, the developing retinal blood vessels become obliterated, and the peripheral retina, which is normally avascular until the end of fetal life, does not vascularize. The more mature the retina, the less the vaso-obliterative effect of hyperoxia. When the infant eventually returns to ambient air, an intense proliferation of vascular endothelium and glial cells begins at the junction of the avascular and vascularized portions of the retina. This becomes apparent 5 to 10 weeks after removal of the infant from the incubator and, as in diabetic retinopathy, it is thought to result from the liberation of an angiogenic factor produced by the avascular and ischemic peripheral retina. This angiogenic factor is also believed to account for the neovascularization of the iris that sometimes accompanies the retinopathy of prematurity. In 25% of cases, retinopathy progresses to a cicatricial phase, characterized by retinal detachment, a fibrovascular mass behind the lens (retrolental), and blindness.

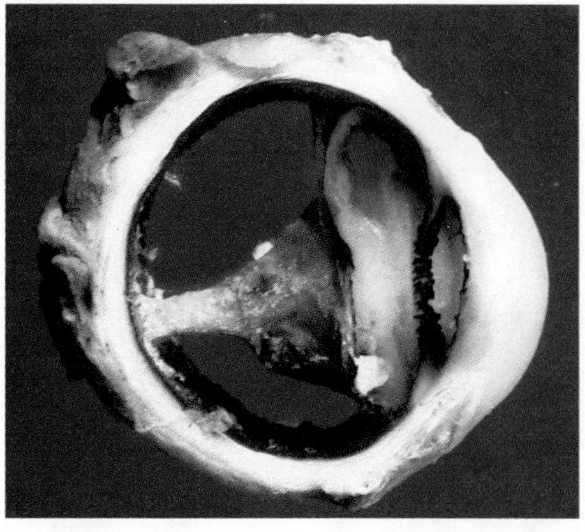
A

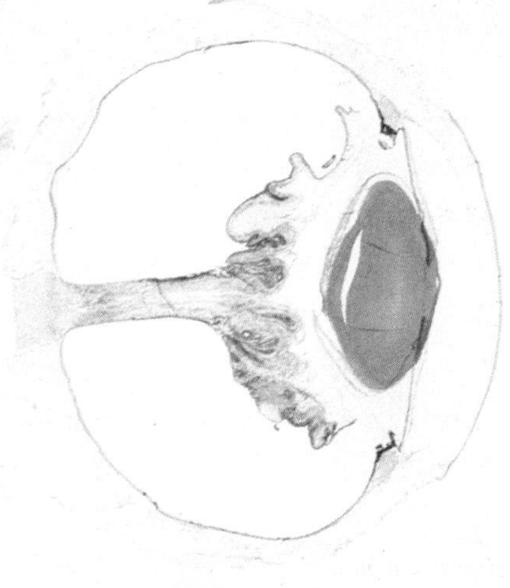
B

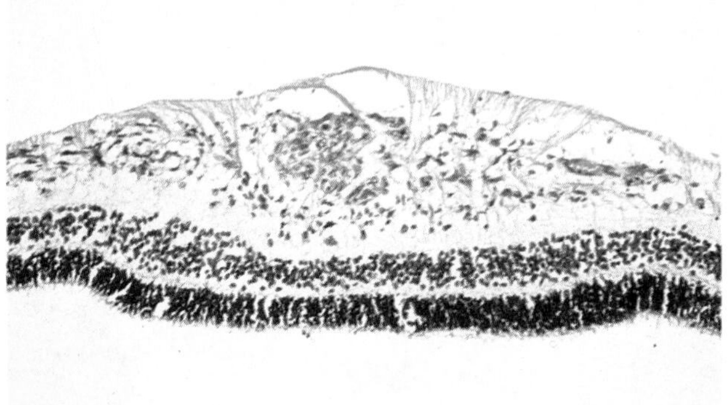
C

FIGURE 29-15
Retinopathy of prematurity. (*A*) A horizontal section through an eye with advanced retinopathy of prematurity (retrolental fibroplasia) shows a totally detached retina adherent to a fibrovascular mass behind the lens. (*B*) A whole mount of an eye with an advanced retinopathy of prematurity provides a view corresponding to the macroscopic eye illustrated in *A*. (*C*) Light-microscopic view of an early angiogenic focus in the retina with retinopathy of prematurity.

THE OPTIC NERVE

Optic Nerve Head Edema

Optic nerve head (optic disc) edema refers to a swelling of the optic nerve head where it enters the globe. The condition is also known by the misnomer *papilledema*, which is imprecise because an optic papilla does not exist. Optic nerve head edema can result from various causes, the most important of which is **increased intracranial pressure**. The term papilledema is still widely used in that context. Other important causes of optic nerve head edema are (1) obstruction to the venous drainage of the eye, such as may occur with compressive lesions of the orbit, (2) an infarct of the optic nerve (ischemic optic neuropathy), (3) inflammation of the optic nerve close to the eyeball (optic neuritis, papillitis), and (4) multiple sclerosis.

Edema of the optic nerve head is characterized clinically by a swollen optic disc, which displays blurred margins and dilated vessels (Fig. 29-16). Frequently, hemorrhages (Fig. 29-17), exudates, and cotton-wool spots are seen, and concentric folds of the choroid and retina may

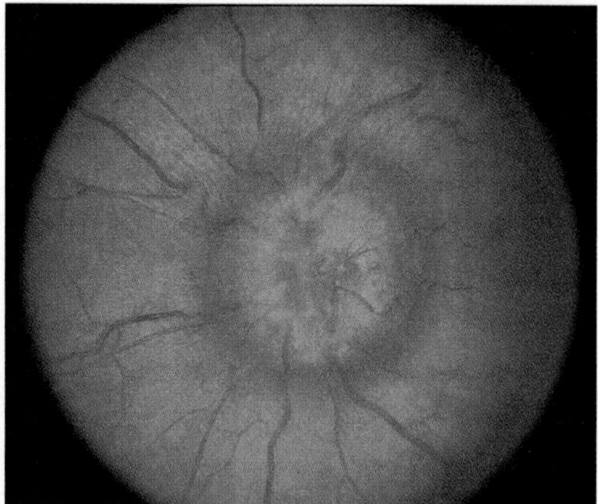

FIGURE 29-16
Chronic papilledema. The optic nerve head is congested and protrudes anteriorly toward the interior of the eye. It has blurred margins, and the vessels within it are poorly seen. In contrast to acute papilledema, the veins are not so congested, and hemorrhage is not a feature.

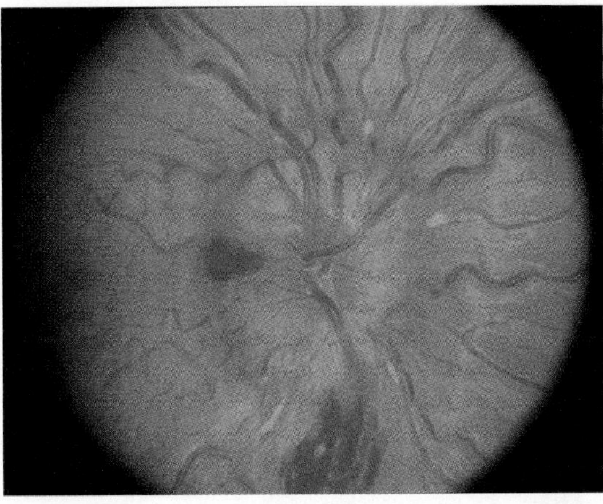

FIGURE 29-17
The optic nerve head is markedly congested, with dilated veins and a blurred margin. A small hemorrhage is evident within the optic nerve head at its junction with the retina. Several small "cotton-wool" spots are present within the adjacent retina.

surround the nerve head. Acutely, optic nerve head edema results in few if any visual symptoms. As the condition becomes established, swelling of the optic nerve head enlarges the normal blind spot. After many months, atrophic changes lead to a loss of visual acuity.

Optic Atrophy

Optic atrophy is a thinning of the optic nerve caused by a loss of axons within its substance. The nerve axons within the optic nerve are lost in many conditions. Possible causes include (1) long-standing edema of the optic nerve head, (2) optic neuritis, (3) optic nerve compression, (4) glaucoma, and (5) retinal degeneration. Optic atrophy also can be caused by some drugs, such as ethambutol and isoniazid. The optic nerve head is usually flat and pale in optic atrophy (Fig. 29-18), but when this disorder follows glaucoma, the disc is excavated (*glaucomatous cupping*).

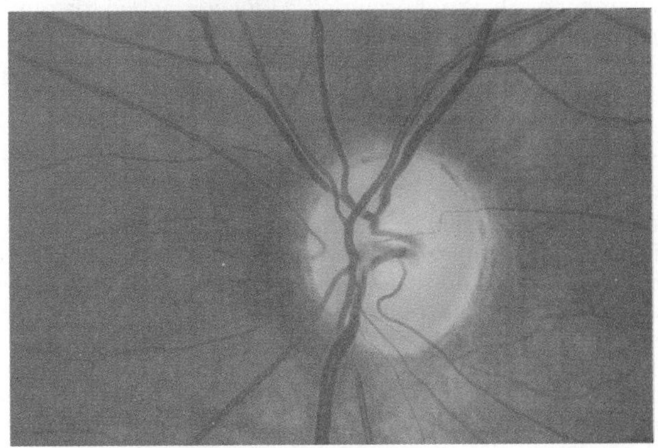

FIGURE 29-18
Optic atrophy. The margin of the optic nerve head is sharply demarcated from the adjacent retina. Because the myelinated axons in the optic nerve are markedly diminished, the optic nerve head appears much whiter than normal.

GLAUCOMA

Glaucoma refers to a collection of disorders that feature an optic neuropathy accompanied by a characteristic excavation of the optic nerve head and a progressive loss of visual field sensitivity. In most cases, glaucoma is produced by increased intraocular pressure (*ocular hypertension*). It deserves emphasis that an increased intraocular pressure does not necessarily cause glaucoma.

After being produced by the ciliary body, the aqueous humor enters the posterior chamber (the space between the iris and the zonules) before passing through the pupil to the anterior chamber (between the iris and the cornea). From that site, it drains into veins by way of the trabecular meshwork and Schlemm canal (Fig. 29-19). A delicate balance between the production and drainage of the aqueous humor maintains intraocular pressure within its physiological range (10 to 20 mm Hg). In certain pathological states, aqueous humor accumulates within the eye, and the intraocular pressure becomes increased. Temporary or permanent impairment of vision results from pressure-induced degenerative changes in the retina and optic nerve head (Fig. 29-20) and from corneal edema and opacification.

Glaucoma almost always follows a congenital or acquired lesion of the anterior segment of the eye that mechanically obstructs the aqueous drainage. The obstruction may be located between the iris and lens, in the angle of the anterior chamber, in the trabecular meshwork, in Schlemm's canal, or in the venous drainage of the eye.

Types of Glaucoma

Congenital Glaucoma (Infantile Glaucoma, Buphthalmos)

Congenital glaucoma refers to glaucoma caused by an obstruction to the aqueous drainage by developmental anomalies. The disorder develops even though the intraocular pressure may not become increased until early infancy or childhood. Most cases of congenital glaucoma occur in boys (65%), and an X-linked recessive mode of inheritance is common. The developmental anomaly usually involves both eyes and, although often limited to the angle of the anterior chamber, may be accompanied by a variety of other ocular malformations. Congenital glaucoma is associated with a deep anterior chamber, corneal cloudiness, sensitivity to bright lights (*photophobia*), excessive tearing, and buphthalmos. The term *buphthalmos* (Gk. *bous*, "ox"; *ophthalmos*, "eye") designates the enlarged eyes of congenital glaucoma that result from an expansion caused by increased intraocular pressure beneath a pliable sclera.

Primary Open-Angle Glaucoma

Primary glaucoma develops in a person with no apparent underlying eye disease. The disorder is subdivided into *open-angle glaucoma*, in which the anterior chamber angle is open and appears normal, and *closed-angle glaucoma*, in which the anterior chamber is shallower than normal, and the angle is abnormally narrow. **Primary open-angle glaucoma is the most frequent type of glaucoma and a major cause of blindness in the United States.** It affects 1% to 3% of the population older than 40 years and occurs principally in the sixth decade. The intraocular pressure becomes increased insidiously and asymptomatically, and although almost always bilateral, one eye may be affected more severely than the other. With time, damage to the retina and optic nerve causes an irreversible loss of peripheral vision.

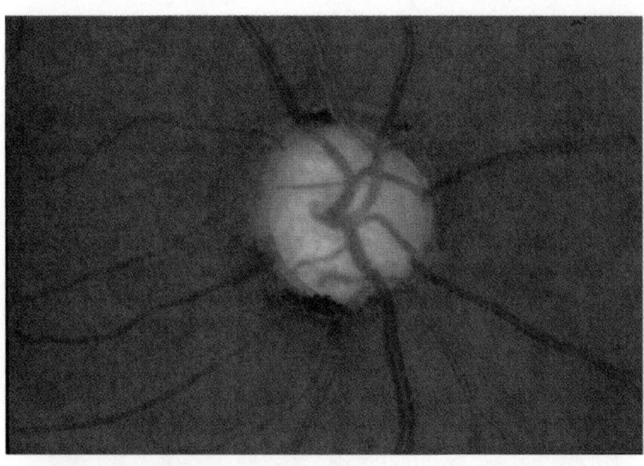

FIGURE *29-20*
Optic nerve head in glaucoma. The anterior part of the optic nerve is depressed ("optic cupping"), and the blood vessels crossing the margin of the optic nerve head are displaced nasally. The fundus appears dark because this eye from a black patient contains numerous pigmented melanocytes in the choroid.

The angle of the anterior chamber is open and appears normal, but an increased resistance to the outflow of the aqueous humor is present within the vicinity of Schlemm's canal. Persons with diabetes mellitus and myopia have an increased risk of primary open-angle glaucoma.

Primary Closed-Angle Glaucoma

Primary closed-angle glaucoma occurs after age 40 years. It afflicts persons whose peripheral iris is displaced anteriorly toward the trabecular meshwork, thereby creating an abnormally narrow angle. When the pupil is constricted (*miotic*), the iris remains stretched, so that the chamber angle is not occluded. However, when the pupil dilates (*mydriasis*), the iris obstructs the anterior chamber angle, thereby impairing aqueous drainage and resulting in sudden episodes of intraocular hypertension. This is

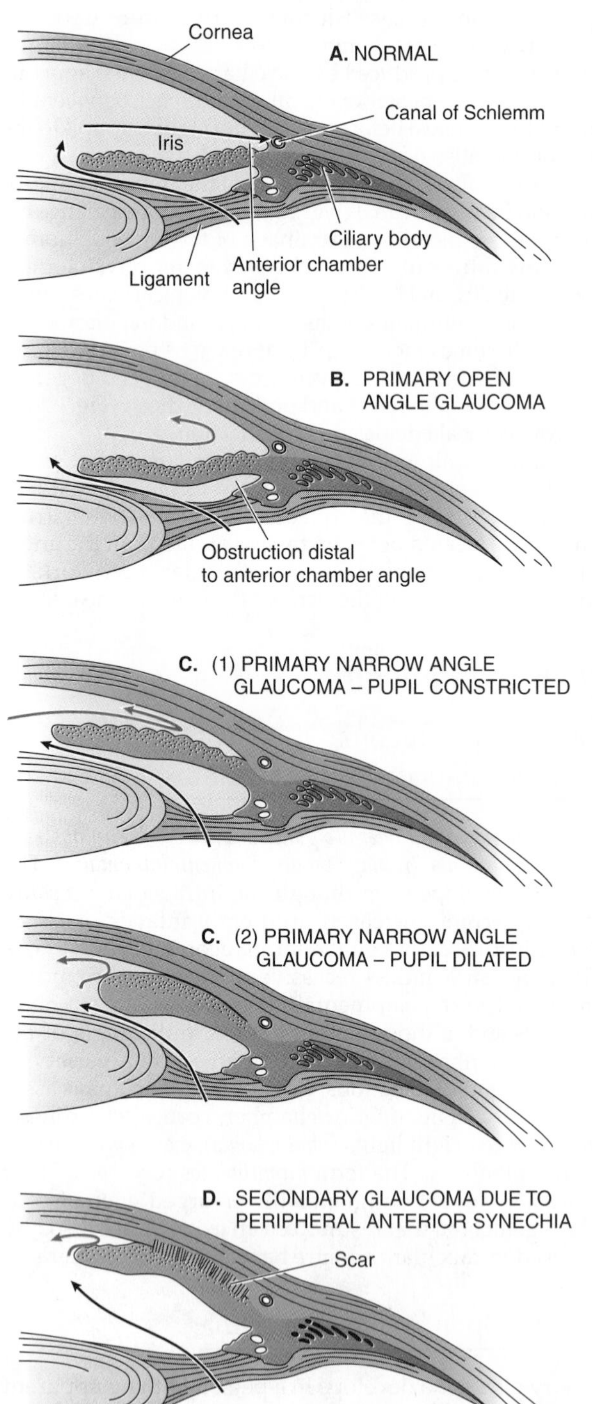

FIGURE *29-19*
Pathogenesis of glaucoma. The anterior segment of the eye is affected differently in various forms of glaucoma. (*A*) Structure of the normal eye. In primary open-angle glaucoma (*B*), the obstruction to the aqueous outflow is distal to the anterior chamber angle, and the anterior segment resembles that of the normal eye. In primary narrow-angle glaucoma (*C*), the anterior chamber angle is open, but narrower than normal when the pupil is constricted (*C1*). When the pupil becomes dilated in such an eye, the thickened iris obstructs the anterior chamber angle (*C2*), thereby causing an increase in intraocular pressure. The anterior chamber angle can become obstructed by a variety of pathological processes, including an adhesion between the iris and the posterior surface of the cornea (peripheral anterior synechia) (*D*).

accompanied by ocular pain, and halos or rings are seen around lights. In such persons, the intraocular pressure may also become increased if the pupil becomes blocked (e.g., by a swollen lens) and aqueous humor accumulates in the posterior chamber. **Acute closed-angle glaucoma is an ocular emergency, and it is essential to start ocular hypotensive treatment within the first 24 to 48 hours if vision is to be maintained.**

Primary closed-angle glaucoma affects both eyes, but it may become apparent in one eye 2 to 5 years before it is noted in the other. The intraocular pressure is normal between attacks, but after many episodes, adhesions form between the iris and the trabecular meshwork and cornea (peripheral anterior synechiae) and accentuate the block to the outflow of the aqueous humor.

Secondary Glaucoma

The causes of secondary glaucoma are many and include inflammation, hemorrhage, neovascularization of the iris, and adhesions. In secondary glaucoma, the anterior chamber angles may be open or closed. Because the underlying disorder is usually limited to one eye, secondary glaucoma tends to be unilateral.

Low-Tension Glaucoma

Low-tension glaucoma refers to an entity in which the characteristic visual-field defect and all of the ophthalmoscopic features of chronic open-angle glaucoma occur without an increase in intraocular pressure. The characteristic visual-field defect and all of the ophthalmoscopic features of chronic simple (open-angle) glaucoma often occur in the elderly without an increase in intraocular pressure. Although some eyes may be hypersensitive to normal intraocular pressure, most cases of low-tension glaucoma probably represent an infarction of the optic nerve head.

Effects of Increased Intraocular Pressure

Prolonged ocular hypertension has several effects on the eye:

- In adults, increased intraocular pressure leads to a characteristic cupped excavation of the optic nerve head (glaucomatous cupping), accompanied by a nasal displacement of the retinal blood vessels. In infants, cupping of the optic disc tends to be less prominent.
- The cornea or sclera bulges at weak points, such as sites of scars in the outer coat of the eye.
- Optic atrophy, with a loss of axons, gliosis, and thickening of the pial septa, follows the retinal degeneration and damage to the nerve fibers at the optic disc.
- The ganglion cell layer of the retina degenerates, thereby impairing vision. The outer retina, which derives its nutrition from the underlying choroid, remains intact.
- When the intraocular pressure is increased before age 3 years, the pliable eye sometimes enlarges extensively (*buphthalmos*). After the first few years of life, a rigid sclera prevents glaucomatous eyes from enlarging under the increased pressure.

MYOPIA

Myopia is a refractive ocular abnormality in which light from the visualized object focuses at a point in front of the retina because of a longer than usual anteroposterior diameter of the eye. Myopia affects more then 70 million people in the United States, requiring correction with glasses or contact lenses. Highly controversial procedures for correcting myopia include the creation of radial incisions into the cornea (radial keratopathy) and more recently other forms of refractive surgery by using an excimer laser. Myopia usually begins in young people and varies in severity. A mild form (*stationary or simple myopia*) is generally nonprogressive after the cessation of body growth, whereas a genetically determined "progressive myopia" is more severe.

PHTHISIS BULBI

Phthisis bulbi refers to a nonspecific, end-stage eye that is disorganized and atrophic. This condition (Fig. 29-21) is most common after trauma to or inflammation of the eye. The eye is small and soft, and the choroid and ciliary body are separated from the sclera. The sclera is thickened, wrinkled, and indented owing to the loss of intraocular pressure. The cornea is flattened, shrunken, and opaque. The intraocular contents are disorganized by diffuse scarring, and detachment of the sensory retina is invariably encountered. The lens is displaced and often calcified. A typical finding in phthisis bulbi is intraocular bone for-

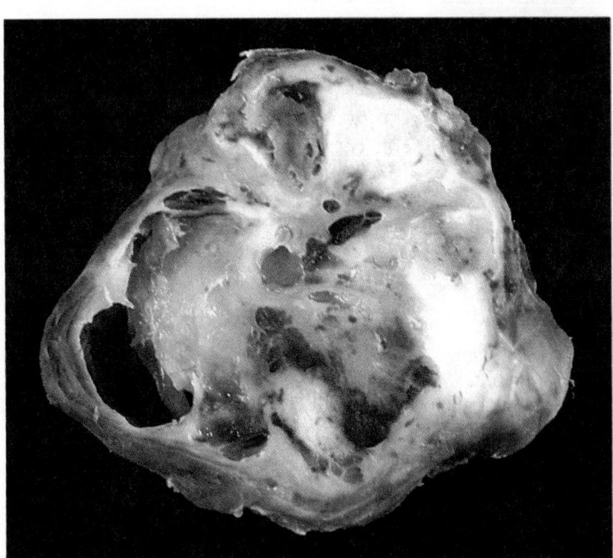

FIGURE *29-21*
Section through an eye with phthisis bulbi, exemplifying the markedly disorganized nature of the intraocular contents of such atrophic disordered globes.

mation, which seems to be derived from the hyperplastic pigment epithelium.

Eyes afflicted with phthisis bulbi are often enucleated.

NEOPLASMS

The eye and adjacent structures contain a wide variety of cell types, and, as one might expect, benign and malignant neoplasms arise from them (Table 29-3). **Intraocular neoplasms arise mostly from immature retinal neurons (retinoblastoma) and uveal melanocytes (melanoma).** Although the retinal pigment epithelium often undergoes reactive proliferation, it seldom becomes neoplastic.

Malignant Melanoma

Uveal melanoma is a malignant neoplasm that arises from melanocytes or nevi in the uvea. Malignant melanoma is the most common primary intraocular malignancy. It may arise from melanocytes in any part of the eye, the choroid being the most common site.

□ **Pathology:** Choroidal melanomas are mostly circumscribed and invade Bruch's membrane, causing a collar stud–shaped or mushroom-shaped mass (Fig. 29-22). By contrast, some tumors are flat (diffuse melanoma) and cause a gradual deterioration of vision over many years. Some do not become apparent until extraocular dissemination has occurred. Orange lipofuscin pigment is evident over the surface of some choroidal melanomas.

Microscopically, uveal melanomas may be composed mainly of variable amounts of spindle-shaped cells without nucleoli (spindle A cells), spindle-shaped cells with prominent nucleoli (spindle B cells), and polygonal cells with distinct cell borders and prominent nucleoli (epithelioid cells). The cells vary in their amount of pigmentation, and some cells may contain abundant cytoplasmic lipid ("balloon cell degeneration"). Variable amounts of necrosis are common in uveal melanomas.

Melanomas of the ciliary body and iris may extend circumferentially around the globe (ring melanoma). In the iris, melanomas are seen clinically 1 to 2 decades ear-

TABLE *29-3* **Primary Neoplasms of the Eye and its Adnexa**

Intraocular Neoplasms
Retinoblastoma
Medulloepithelioma
Teratoid medulloepithelioma
Glioneuroma
Adenomas and adenocarcinomas of ciliary epithelium
Melanoma
Leiomyoma
Neurofibroma
Schwannoma
Lymphoma
Neoplasms of the Eyelid and Lacrimal Drainage Apparatus
Benign
Squamous papilloma
Seborrheic keratosis
Inverted folliculoma (inverted follicular keratosis)
Adenoma of sebaceous glands (Meibomian glands)
Adenoma of Krause's accessory lacrimal gland
Adenoma of sweat glands and apocrine glands (Moll's glands)
Keratoacanthoma
Papilloma of lacrimal sac
Leiomyoma
Pilomatrixoma
Trichoepithelioma
Neurofibroma
Schwannoma
Malignant
Basal cell carcinoma
Squamous cell carcinoma
Sebaceous carcinoma (Meibomian gland carcinoma)
Malignant melanoma
Lymphoma
Adenocarcinoma of sweat gland
Extramammary Paget disease
Adenoacanthoma

Neoplasms of Conjunctiva	
Dysplasia	Primary acquired melanosis
Intraepithelial carcinoma (carcinoma *in situ*)	Melanoma
Squamous cell carcinoma	Oncocytoma
Lymphoma	Neurofibroma
Neoplasms of Orbit	
Neoplasms of lacrimal gland:	Mucoepidermoid carcinoma
Mixed tumors	Oncocytoma
Adenocystic carcinoma	
Neoplasms of optic nerve:	
Meningioma	Astrocytoma
Other Orbital Tumors	
Benign	
Hemangiopericytoma	Chondroma
Fibrous histiocytoma	Leiomyoma
Schwannoma	Aneurysmal bone cyst
Lipoma	Fibrous dysplasia
Osteoma	Fibrous xanthoma
Fibroma	Myxoma
Hemangioendothelioma	
Malignant	
Rhabdomyosarcoma	Malignant hemangioendothelioma
Malignant lymphomas	Malignant hemangiopericytoma
Plasma cell myeloma	Malignant fibrous histiocytoma
Neurofibrosarcoma	Chondrosarcoma
Liposarcoma	Kaposi sarcoma
Osteogenic sarcoma	

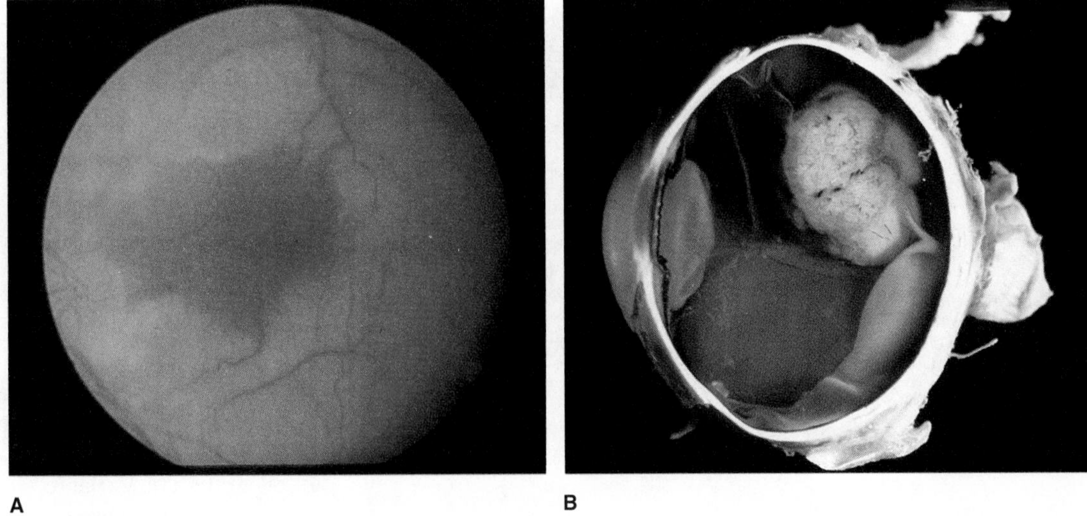

FIGURE 29-22
Malignant melanoma. (*A*) A malignant melanoma of the choroid is apparent as a dark mass visible beneath the retinal blood vessels. (*B*) A mushroom-shaped melanoma of the choroid is present in this eye. Choroidal melanomas commonly invade through Bruch's membrane and result in this appearance.

lier than those in the choroid and ciliary body, perhaps because they are more easily seen.

Aside from hematogenous spread, uveal melanomas disseminate by traversing the sclera to enter the orbital tissues, usually at sites where blood vessels and nerves pass through the sclera. Unlike melanomas of the skin, those of the uvea do not spread by lymphatics because the eye lacks these structures. Intraocular melanomas sometimes cause cataract, glaucoma, retinal detachment, inflammation, and even hemorrhage.

The usual treatment for most uveal melanomas is enucleation of the eye, but some are treated with other methods, such as radiotherapy or local excision. More than half of patients with uveal melanomas survive for 15 years after enucleation. Deaths have been reported within 5 years from spindle A melanomas, but tumors composed purely of epithelioid cells have the worst prognosis. Anecdotally, the diagnosis of metastatic ocular melanoma has been made intuitively by astute clinicians who discovered an enlarged liver in a patient with a "glass eye."

***Primary acquired melanosis of the conjunctiva* refers to irregular areas of pigmentation that appear spontaneously in the conjunctiva of one eye.** It is analogous to cutaneous lentigo maligna melanoma. Primary acquired melanosis of the conjunctiva develops in a nonpigmented portion of the conjunctiva of one eye at about age 40 to 50 years. This condition may regress spontaneously or evolve into a more aggressive tumor. Other malignant melanomas of the conjunctiva are preceded by a nevus or have no overt antecedent lesion. Still others represent an extension of an intraocular melanoma.

Retinoblastoma

Retinoblastoma is a malignant neoplasm that arises from immature neurons in the retina. It the most common intraocular malignant neoplasm of childhood (Fig. 29-23) affecting 1:20,000 to 1:34,000 children. The tumor most frequently is seen within the first 2 years of life, and sometimes even at birth. The presenting signs include a white pupil (leukocoria), squint (strabismus), poor vision, spontaneous hyphema, or a red, painful eye. Secondary glaucoma is a frequent complication. Light entering the eye commonly reflects a yellowish color similar to that from the tapetum of a cat (cat's eye reflex). Most retinoblastomas occur sporadically and are unilateral. Some 6% to 8% of retinoblastomas are inherited. Up to 25% of the sporadic retinoblastomas, and most inherited retinoblastomas are bilateral.

Retinoblastomas are related to inherited or acquired deletions of or mutations in the retinoblastoma (Rb) tumor-suppressor gene, located on the long arm of chromosome 13 (13q14) (see Chapter 5).

☐ **Pathology:** Some retinoblastomas grow toward the vitreous body and can be seen with an ophthalmoscope (endophytic retinoblastoma). Others grow between the sensory retina and the retinal pigment epithelium, thereby detaching the retina (exophytic retinoblastoma). A few retinoblastomas are both endophytic and exophytic. The retina often contains several distinct foci of tumor in the same eye, some of which represent multifocal origin, whereas others reflect tumor implantations from dissemination through the vitreous body.

Retinoblastoma is a cream-colored tumor that contains scattered, chalky white, calcified flecks within yellow necrotic zones, which may be detected radiologically. The tumors are intensely cellular and display several morphological patterns. In some instances, densely packed, round neoplastic cells with hyperchromatic nuclei, scant cytoplasm, and abundant mitoses are randomly distributed. In other retinoblastomas, the cells are arranged radially around a central cavity (Flexner–Wintersteiner rosettes), as they differentiate toward photoreceptors. In some cases,

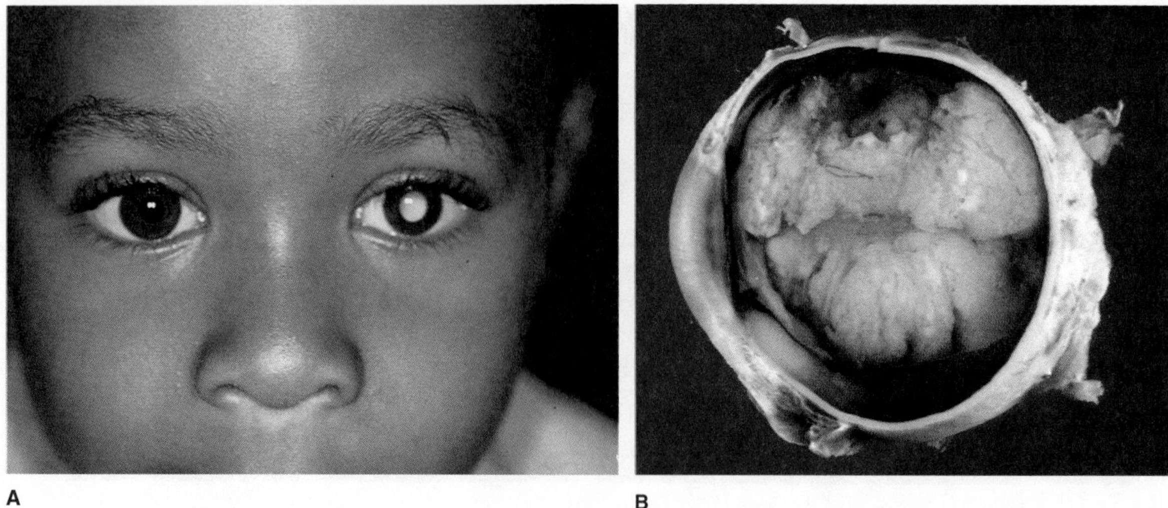

FIGURE *29-23*
Retinoblastoma. (*A*) The white pupil (leukocoria) in the left eye is the result of an intraocular retinoblastoma. (*B*) This surgically excised eye is almost filled by a cream-colored intraocular retinoblastoma with calcified flecks.

the cellular arrangement resembles the *fleur-de-lis* (fleurette). Viable tumor cells align themselves around blood vessels, and necrotic areas with calcification are seen a short distance from the vascularized regions.

Retinoblastomas disseminate by several routes. They commonly extend into the optic nerve, from where they spread intracranially. They also invade blood vessels, especially in the highly vascular choroid, before metastasizing hematogenously throughout the body. The bone marrow is a common site of blood-borne metastases, but surprisingly, the lung is rarely involved.

Retinoblastomas are almost always fatal if left untreated. However, with early diagnosis and modern therapy, survival is high (about 90%). Rarely, spontaneous regression occurs for reasons that remain unknown. Patients with inherited retinoblastomas, presumably as a consequence of the loss of *Rb* gene function, have an increased susceptibility to other malignant tumors, includ-

TABLE *29-4* **Comparison Between Melanoma and Retinoblastoma**

	Melanoma	**Retinoblastoma**
Inheritance	Very rare	5% to 8%
Cell of origin	Melanocytes and related precursors	Retinal neurons
Age	Most after 50 years Rare before puberty	Infancy
Location	Choroid (most) Ciliary body Iris Conjunctiva Eyelid (rare)	Retina
Race	Mostly whites Uncommon in blacks Rare in Asians	No predisposition
Sex	No sex predisposition	No sex predisposition
Bilaterality	Rare	Common (30%)
Color	Variable Gray to black	Creamy with chalky white flecks
Spread		
Hematogenous	Yes	Yes
Via optic nerve	Rare and only in blind glaucomatous eye	Common
Transcleral	Common	Uncommon

ing osteogenic sarcoma, Ewing sarcoma, and pinealoblastoma.

Features of retinoblastomas are compared with similar attributes of melanomas in Table 29-4.

Metastatic Intraocular and Orbital Neoplasms

Metastatic neoplasms in the eye are more common than those that arise within the ocular tissues. Sometimes an ocular metastasis is the initial clinical manifestation of the cancer, but most cases are diagnosed only after death. Leukemias and cancers of the breast and lung account for most cases of intraocular metastases, usually to the posterior choroid. Neuroblastoma frequently metastasizes to the orbit in infancy and childhood. The orbit may be invaded by malignant neoplasms of the eyelid, conjunctiva, paranasal sinuses, nose, nasopharynx, and intracranial cavity.

SUGGESTED READING

Garner A, Klintworth GK (eds): *Pathobiology of ocular disease: A dynamic approach,* 2nd ed. New York: Marcel Dekker, 1994.

Klintworth GK, Eagle RC, Jr: Eye and ocular adnexa. In: Damjanov I, Linder J (eds). *Anderson's pathology,* 10th ed. St. Louis: Mosby, pp. 2832–2875, 1996.

Klintworth GK, Hitchcock MG: The eye. In: Craighead JE (ed). *Pathology of environmental and occupational disease.* St. Louis, Mosby, pp. 601–631, 1995.

Scroggs MW, Klintworth GK: The eye and ocular adnexa. In: Sternberg SS (ed): *Diagnostic surgical pathology,* 2nd ed. New York: Raven Press, pp. 949–980, 1994.

Spencer WH (ed): *Ophthalmic pathology: An atlas and textbook,* 4th ed, 3 vols. Philadelphia: WB Saunders, 1996.

Yanoff M, Fine BS: *Ocular pathology: A text and atlas,* 3rd ed. St. Louis: Mosby-Year Book, 1997.

CHAPTER 30

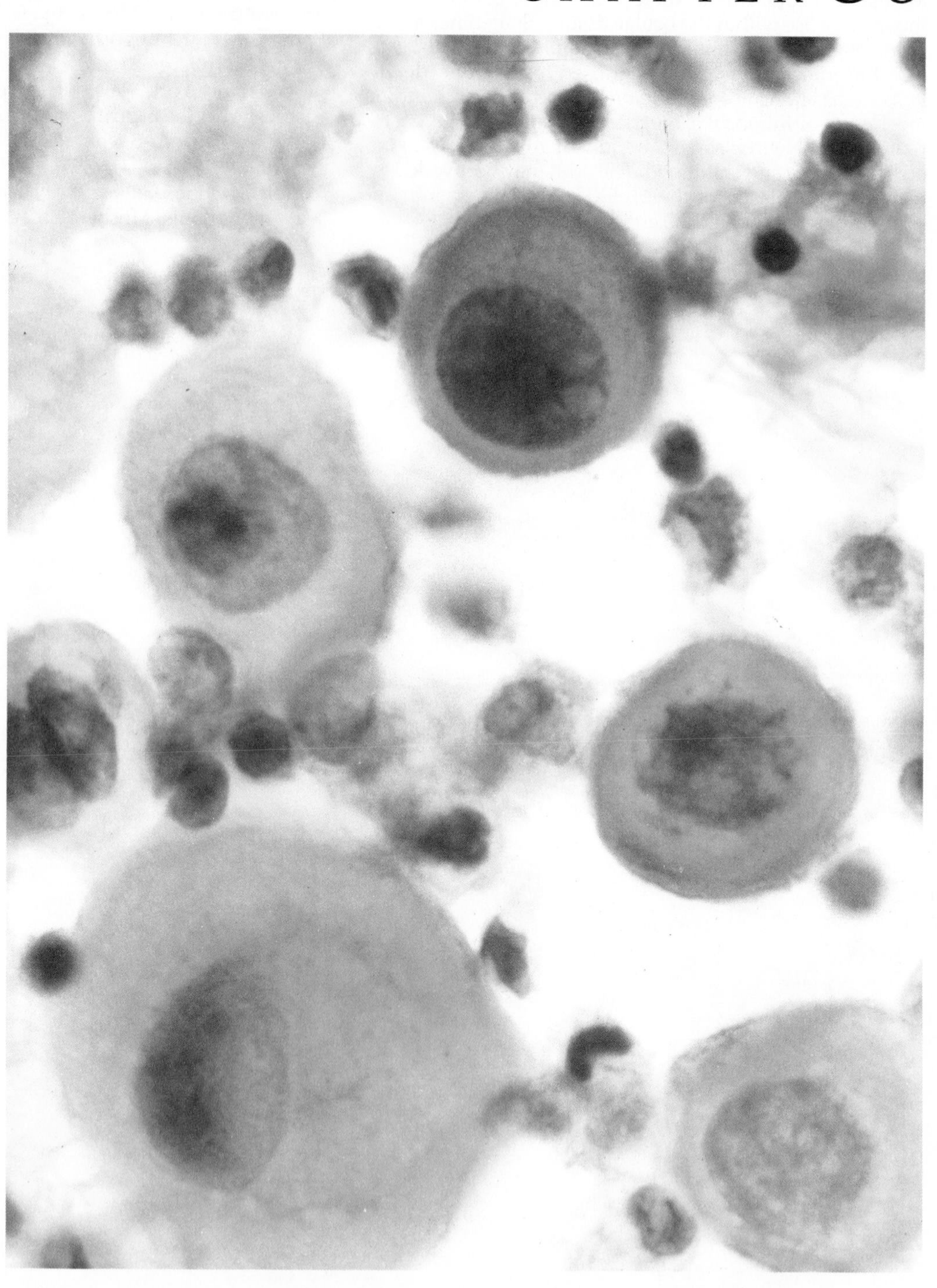

Cytopathology

Hormoz Ehya

FIGURE *30-1* *(see opposite page)*
Cytological preparation of pleural fluid from a patient with mesothelioma.

Cytopathology refers to diagnostic techniques that are used to examine cells from various body sites to determine the cause or nature of disease. Cytological methods date to the mid-19th century, when investigators detected abnormal cells in body fluids, such as urine, sputum, effusions, and gastric secretions. George Papanicolaou in New York City initiated the modern era of diagnostic cytology in 1928, when he delivered a paper entitled "New Cancer Diagnosis." While studying the hormonal effects of the menstrual cycle on squamous cells exfoliated from human uterine cervix, Papanicolaou discovered cellular abnormalities that were associated with uterine cancer. In the same year, Aureli Babes of Bucharest independently reported similar findings. Despite initial skepticism, cytological examination, popularly termed the **"Pap" test**, has been widely accepted as the most reliable screening test for the early detection of cancer and precancerous conditions of the uterine cervix.

In addition to its impact on saving human life, routine cytological testing has helped us to understand carcinogenesis in the uterine cervix. The past several decades have witnessed a tremendous surge in the application of cytology to numerous human organs and tissues, so that it is now considered a routine modality in the diagnosis and surveillance of cancer.

APPLICATIONS OF CYTOPATHOLOGY

Screening for the Early Detection of Asymptomatic Cancer

The most important application of cytopathology in the area of cancer prevention is the examination of scrapings from the cervix. Widespread screening of the female population by Pap smears has resulted in a conspicuous reduction in the incidence of cervical cancer in the United States and many other countries. The rate of the decline varies from one country to another, depending on the proportion of the population screened. In Iceland, which has one of the most intensive screening programs in the world, an 80% decline in mortality from cervical cancer has been achieved. Similarly, in one Canadian study, the incidence of cervical cancer was reported to be 4.5 cases per 100,000 in screened populations, compared with 29 cases in unscreened ones.

The bladder, lung, and endometrium are other organs in which cytopathology is useful in the detection of cancers in their early stages. However, economic considerations preclude mass screening of the general public for such tumors. Instead, specific populations at high risk for the development of certain cancers are screened by cytological methods. Examples of such surveys include sputum cytology in uranium mine workers who have a high incidence of lung cancer; urine cytology in industrial workers exposed to chemical carcinogens who are at high risk for bladder cancer; and colonic lavage for the detection of colon cancer in patients with ulcerative colitis.

In China, where the incidence of esophageal cancer is very high, cytological screening has achieved a 90% accuracy in detecting this tumor. For sampling, a deflated balloon attached to a catheter is swallowed. The balloon is then inflated and pulled out, scraping the surface of the esophageal mucosa. Smears are made from the surface of the balloon and examined microscopically. Whereas the vast majority of esophageal cancers in the United States are at an advanced stage at the time of discovery, 75% of the neoplasms detected through mass surveys in China have been *in situ* or minimally invasive.

Diagnosis of Symptomatic Cancer

Cytology may be used alone or in conjunction with other modalities to diagnose tumors revealed by physical or radiological examinations. Cytological sampling by needle aspiration is generally more convenient and less complicated than an open biopsy. Diseases that are commonly diagnosed by cytology are listed in Table 30-1. Diagnosis by cytological tests is particularly important in malignant tumors of an advanced stage, which are not amenable to surgical treatment. Examples of such neoplasms include pancreatic carcinoma with metastases, hepatocellular carcinoma, and small cell carcinoma of the lung. A definitive diagnosis in such instances precludes the dangers of surgical intervention.

In endoscopic evaluation of the respiratory system, alimentary canal, and upper urinary tract, cytological samples are obtained concurrent with biopsy samples. Combining the two methods increases the diagnostic

TABLE *30-1* **Entities Commonly Diagnosed by Cytological Methods**

Procedure	Entity
Uterine Cervix and Vagina	
Scraping	Hormonal status
Brushing	Inflammation
	Reparative changes
	Infection
	Viral (herpes simplex virus, human papillomavirus)
	Bacterial (*Gardnerella, Actinomyces, Chlamydia*)
	Fungal (*Candida*)
	Protozoal (*Trichomonas vaginalis*)
	Helminthic (*Enterobius vermicularis,* microfilaria)
	Vaginal adenosis
	Cervical intraepithelial neoplasia (squamous dysplasia, *in situ* carcinoma)
	Malignant neoplasms
	Squamous cell carcinoma
	Endocervical adenocarcinoma
	Endometrial adenocarcinoma
	Mixed mesodermal tumor
	Extrauterine neoplasms (particularly ovarian)
	Metastatic tumors
Respiratory Tract	
Sputum	Extracellular substances
Bronchial washing	Curschmann's spirals
Bronchial brushing	Charcot–Leyden crystals
Bronchoalveolar lavage	Ferruginous bodies
Fine-needle aspiration	Inflammation
	Abscess
	Granuloma
	Infection
	Bacterial (*Mycobacterium, Actinomyces*)
	Viral (herpes simplex virus, cytomegalovirus)
	Fungal (*Candida, Aspergillus, Cryptococcus, Histoplasma, Blastomyces, Coccidioides, Phycomycetes*)
	Pneumocytis carinii
	Reactive changes
	Bronchial epithelial atypia
	Goblet cell hyperplasia
	Reserve cell hyperplasia
	Squamous metaplasia
	Radiation and chemotherapy effect
	Benign neoplasms
	Pulmonary hamartoma
	Pleural fibroma
	Malignant neoplasms
	Squamous cell carcinoma
	Adenocarcinoma
	Small cell carcinoma
	Undifferentiated large cell carcinoma
	Carcinoid tumor
	Metastatic tumors
Serous Cavities (Pericardium, Pleura, Peritoneum)	
Paracentesis	Inflammation (acute, chronic, granulomatous)
	Eosinophilic pleuritis
	Rheumatoid pleuritis
	Infection
	Viral
	Fungal
	Parasitic
	Malignant mesothelioma
	Metastatic neoplasms
Urinary Tract	
Urine	Renal casts and crystals
Washing	Inflammation
Brushing	Malakoplakia
	Infection
	Viral (cytomegalovirus, herpes simplex virus, polyomavirus)
	Fungal (*Candida*)
	Protozoal (ameba, schistosoma)
	Drug-induced acute intestitial nephritis (presence of eosinophils)
	Neoplasms
	Transitional cell carcinoma
	Squamous carcinoma
	Adenocarcinoma
	Metastatic tumors
Kidney	
Fine-needle aspiration	Cysts
	Abscess
	Granuloma
	Neoplasms
	Angiomyolipoma
	Oncocytoma
	Renal cell carcinoma
	Transitional cell carcinoma
	Nephroblastoma (Wilms tumor)
	Metastatic tumors
Alimentary Tract	
Brushing	Inflammation
Washing	Benign ulcer
Balloon scraping	Infection
	Bacterial (*Helicobacter pylori*)
	Viral (herpes simplex virus, cytomegalovirus)
	Fungal (*Candida*)
	Protozoal (ameba, *Giardia*)
	Barrett esophagus
	Neoplastic polyps (adenomas)
	Malignant neoplasms
	Squamous carcinoma
	Adenocarcinoma
	Carcinoid tumor
	Leiomyosarcoma
	Malignant lymphoma

(continued)

TABLE **30-1** *(continued)*

Procedure	Entity
Central Nervous System	
Cerebrospinal fluid	Cerebral hemorrhage (presence of erythrocytes and hemosiderin-laden macrophages)
Fine-needle aspiration	Inflammation (acute, chronic, granulomatous)
	Infection
	Fungal (*Cryptococcus*)
	Primary neoplasms
	Meningioma
	Astrocytoma
	Glioblastoma multiforme
	Ependymoma
	Oligodendroglioma
	Medulloblastoma
	Malignant lymphoma
	Metastatic neoplasms
Breast	
Nipple discharge	Inflammation
Fine-needle aspiration	Abscess
	Granuloma
	Fat necrosis
	Fibrocystic disease
	Benign neoplasms
	Fibroadenoma
	Lactating adenoma
	Granular cell tumor
	Malignant neoplasms
	Ductal carcinoma
	Medullary carcinoma
	Colloid carcinoma
	Lobular carcinoma
	Phyllodes tumor
	Metastatic tumors
Thyroid	
Fine-needle aspiration	Thyroiditis
	Acute
	Granulomatous
	Lymphocytic
	Hashimoto
	Benign cysts
	Nodular goiter
	Neoplasms
	Follicular neoplasm
	Hurthle cell tumor
	Papillary carcinoma
	Medullary carcinoma
	Anaplastic carcinoma
	Malignant lymphoma
	Metastatic tumors
Lymph Nodes	
Fine-needle aspiration	Lymphadenitis
	Hyperplasia
	Neoplasms
	Malignant lymphoma
	Hodgkin's disease
	Metastatic tumors
Salivary Gland	
Fine-needle aspiration	Inflammation (acute, chronic, granulomatous)
	Mucocele
	Benign lymphoepithelial lesion (Mikulicz disease)
	Benign neoplasms
	Pleomorphic adenoma
	Monomorphic adenoma
	Oncocytoma
	Warthin tumor
	Malignant neoplasms
	Adenoid cystic carcinoma
	Mucoepidermoid carcinoma
	Acinic cell carcinoma
	Malignant mixed tumor
	Malignant lymphoma
	Metastatic tumors
Liver	
Fine-needle aspiration	Cysts (simple, hydatid)
	Inflammation
	Abscess
	Granuloma
	Neoplasms
	Hepatocellular carcinoma
	Cholangiocarcinoma
	Angiosarcoma
	Metastatic tumors
Pancreas	
Fine-needle aspiration	Cysts and pseudocysts
	Abscess
	Neoplasms
	Cystadenomas (serous, mucinous)
	Adenocarcinoma
	Giant cell carcinoma
	Islet cell tumor
	Papillary–cystic neoplasm
	Metastatic tumors
Adrenal	
Fine-needle aspiration	Neoplasms
	Cortical adenoma
	Cortical carcinoma
	Pheochromocytoma
	Neuroblastoma
	Metastatic tumors
Prostate	
Fine-needle aspiration	Cysts
	Inflammation
	Abscess
	Granuloma
	Hyperplasia
	Adenocarcinoma

(continued)

TABLE **30-1** *(continued)*

Procedure	Entity
Ovary	
Fine-needle aspiration	Non-neoplastic cysts
	Abscess
	Endometriosis
	Neoplasms
	Benign cystic neoplasms
	Adenocarcinoma
	Granulosa cell tumor
	Germ cell tumors
Eye and Orbit	
Fine-needle aspiration	Orbital cysts and pseudotumor
Vitrectomy	Uveitis (acute, chronic, granulomatous)
	Infection (viral, fungal, parasitic)
	Non-neoplastic intraocular lesions
	Hemorrhage
	Phacoanaphylactic endophthalmitis
	Asteroid hyalosis
	Amyloidosis
	Coats disease
	Intraocular neoplasms
	Malignant melanoma
	Retinoblastoma
	Medulloepithelioma
	Malignant lymphoma/leukemia
	Metastatic tumors
	Orbital neoplasms
	Mixed tumor
	Meningioma
	Glioma
	Lacrimal gland carcinoma
	Rhabdomyosarcoma
	Malignant lymphoma/leukemia
	Metastatic tumors
Skin, Conjunctiva, Oral Mucosa	
Scraping	Infection
Fine-needle aspiration	Viral (herpes simplex virus, molluscum contagiosum)
	Fungal
	Parasitic
	Pemphigus vulgaris
	Neoplasms
	Squamous carcinoma
	Basal cell carcinoma
	Malignant melanoma
	Metastatic tumors
Bone	
Fine-needle aspiration	Non-neoplastic lesions
	Osteomyelitis
	Cysts
	Eosinophilic granuloma
	Neoplasms
	Osteosarcoma
	Chondrosarcoma
	Giant cell tumor
	Ewing sarcoma
	Plasma cell myeloma
	Ameloblastoma
	Chordoma
	Metastatic tumors
Soft Tissue	
Fine-needle aspiration	Non-neoplastic lesions
	Abscess
	Hematoma
	Neoplasms
	Liposarcoma
	Fibrosarcoma
	Rhabdomyosarcoma
	Leiomyosarcoma
	Synovial sarcoma
	Malignant fibrous histiocytoma
	Malignant schwannoma
	Metastatic tumors

yield and often averts repeated endoscopy when either alone misses the lesion. In fact, the diagnostic accuracy of esophageal, gastric, and colonic endoscopy is improved from about 75% to well over 90% when cytology is used in addition to biopsy.

Surveillance of Patients Treated for Cancer

For some types of cancers, cytology is the most feasible method of surveillance to detect recurrence. The best example is periodic urine cytology, usually at 3-month intervals, to monitor the recurrence of cancer of the urinary tract. In patients with ovarian carcinoma, after the initial surgery and completion of chemotherapy, an exploratory laparotomy is performed to assess the response of the tumor to treatment ("second-look" operation). Even in the absence of grossly visible residual or recurrent tumor, smears made from peritoneal washings are examined to assess the presence of malignant cells.

Cytology is valuable in documenting the development of metastases. Cytological methods are readily used in the evaluation of patients previously treated for cancer who develop an effusion, neurological symptoms, lymphadenopathy, or nodules in the skin, lung, or liver.

Cytology also is helpful in the diagnosis of cysts, benign neoplasms, inflammatory conditions, and infections of various organs. The most common disorders are listed in Table 30-1.

CYTOLOGICAL METHODS

Exfoliative Cytology

Exfoliative cytology refers to the examination of cells that are shed spontaneously into body fluids or secretions. Examples include sputum, cerebrospinal fluid, urine, effusions in body cavities (pleura, pericardium, peritoneum), nipple discharge, and vitreous and aqueous humors. The number of cells in such specimens is usually not sufficient to allow an adequate assessment by direct smearing of the fluid on a glass slide. Therefore, cytology laboratories use various cell-concentration techniques, such as centrifugation or membrane filtration, to prepare smears. Subsequently, the smears are stained by one or more of several methods, the most popular of which is the Papanicolaou stain.

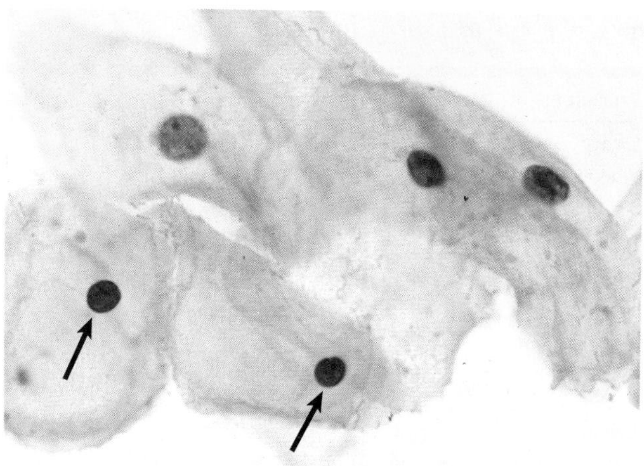

FIGURE *30-2*
Normal cervical Papanicolaou (Pap) smear. Large squamous cells from the superficial, and intermediate layers of the epithelium are illustrated. The cells have abundant cytoplasm, which varies in staining from pink to blue. The nuclei are small, and the nuclear–cytoplasmic ratio is low. The most superficial cells have pyknotic nuclei (*arrows*).

Abrasive Cytology

Abrasive cytology encompasses methods by which cells are dislodged by various tools from body surfaces (skin, mucous membranes, serous membranes). A classic example is the preparation of cervical smears with a spatula or a small brush. By contrast, a smear made from vaginal secretions, which contain spontaneously shed cells, is considered an exfoliative cytological specimen. Other abrasive methods include the endoscopic brushing of the mucosal surfaces of the gastrointestinal, respiratory, and urinary tracts; the balloon technique for obtaining cells from the esophagus; and the scraping of cutaneous, oral, vaginal, or conjunctival lesions to detect herpesvirus inclusions. Washing (or lavage) of mucosal or serosal surfaces during endoscopy or open surgery may be considered a combined exfoliative and abrasive method, because it samples both cells that are shed spontaneously and those dislodged mechanically.

Cells obtained by scraping or brushing are directly smeared on glass slides and fixed immediately in 95% ethanol or with a spray fixative before staining. Lavage specimens are sent to the laboratory for cell concentration, as described in Exfoliative Cytology (above).

Fine-Needle Aspiration Cytology

Aspiration cytology is a technique that uses cells obtained by aspiration under negative pressure through a thin-gauge needle. Although sporadic attempts to collect diagnostic samples from tumors by means of a needle were documented as early as the mid-19th century, it was not until the 1920s that this method was used systematically. Despite remarkable success with this technique, needle aspiration did not become popular for several decades. Today we use a modified version of aspiration biopsy, with a 22-gauge or a smaller size needle, known as fine-needle aspiration.

Virtually any organ or tissue can be sampled by fine-needle aspiration. Superficial organs (e.g., thyroid, breast, lymph nodes, prostate, skin, and soft tissues) are easily targeted. Deep organs, such as the lung, mediastinum, liver, pancreas, kidney, adrenal gland, and retroperitoneum, are aspirated with guidance by fluoroscopy, computed tomography, or ultrasound.

To obtain optimal results, several points deserve emphasis:

- In aspirating solid masses, one need not see material entering the syringe. In fact, aspiration is stopped as soon as blood appears in the hub of the needle, because it dilutes the cells. The small amount of material in the lumen of the needle is smeared on glass slides and stained.
- If the lesion is cystic, the fluid is aspirated into the syringe and sent to the cytology laboratory for processing.
- Sometimes aspiration must be repeated several times to obtain adequate diagnostic material.

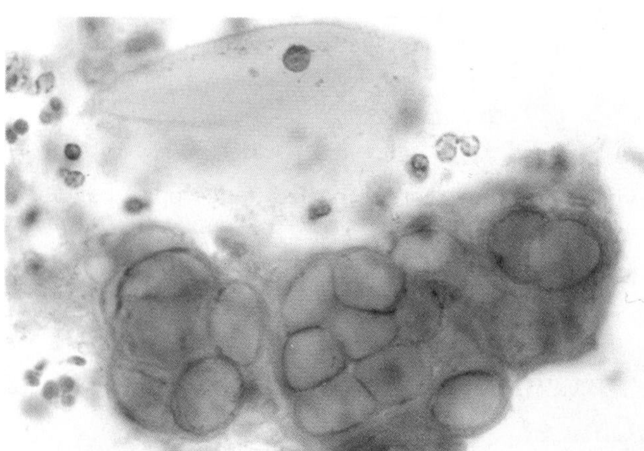

FIGURE *30-3*
Herpes simplex virus infection in a cervical smear. Note multinucleation of squamous cells, nuclear molding, margination of the chromatin, and "ground glass" appearance of the nuclei. A normal superficial squamous cell serves for comparison.

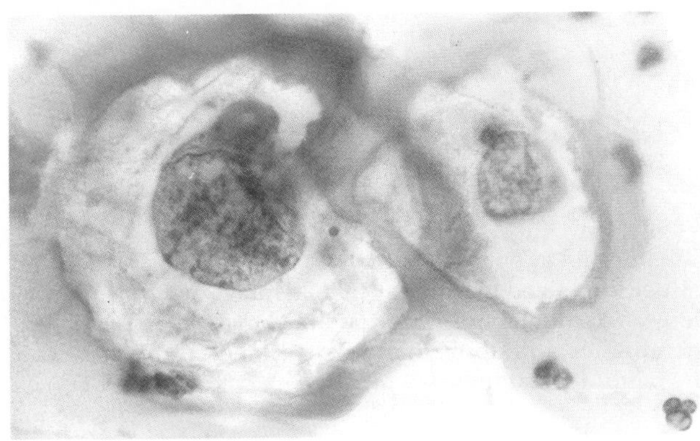

FIGURE 30-4
Papillomavirus infection in a cervical smear. Two superficial squamous cells exhibit "koilocytotic atypia," a term that denotes the presence of sharply demarcated, large perinuclear vacuoles, combined with alterations in the chromatin pattern.

- When aspirating large masses, it should be kept in mind that the center of the tumor may be necrotic. Thus, the needle should be placed in the periphery of the mass to obtain viable tumor cells.
- Whereas some European cytopathologists prefer air-dried, Romanowsky-stained smears, most Americans favor alcohol-fixed smears stained by the Papanicolaou method or with hematoxylin and eosin.

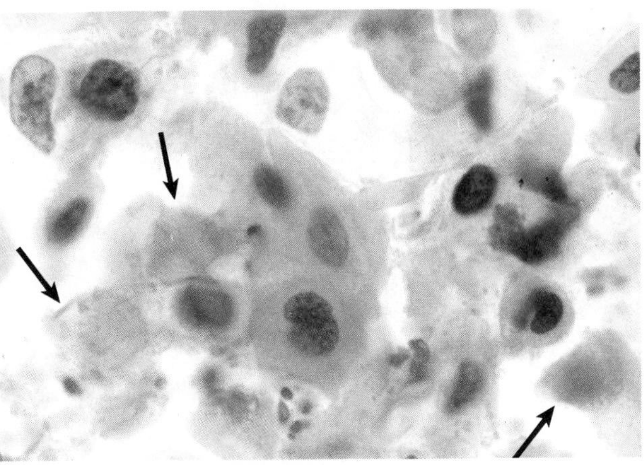

FIGURE 30-6
Invasive squamous cell carcinoma of the cervix. Pleomorphic squamous cells, with enlarged, irregular, and hyperchromatic nuclei, are present. Note the abnormalities of the chromatin and the irregularity of the nuclear membrane. The presence of necrotic cells in the background (*arrows*) is a helpful criterion to distinguish this invasive carcinoma from carcinoma *in situ*.

Some examples of exfoliative, abrasive, and aspiration cytology of various organs are illustrated in Figs. 30-1 through 30-14.

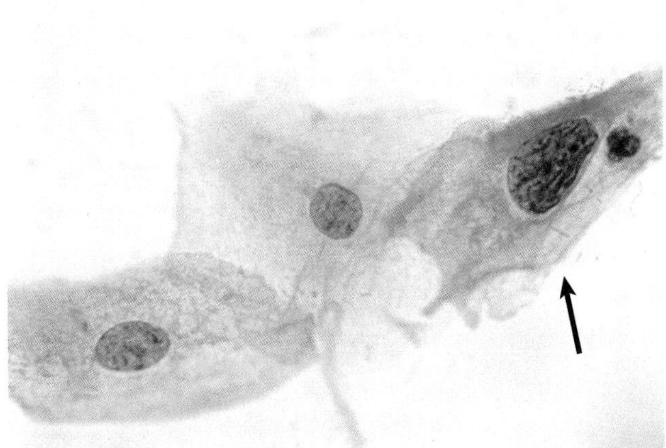

A

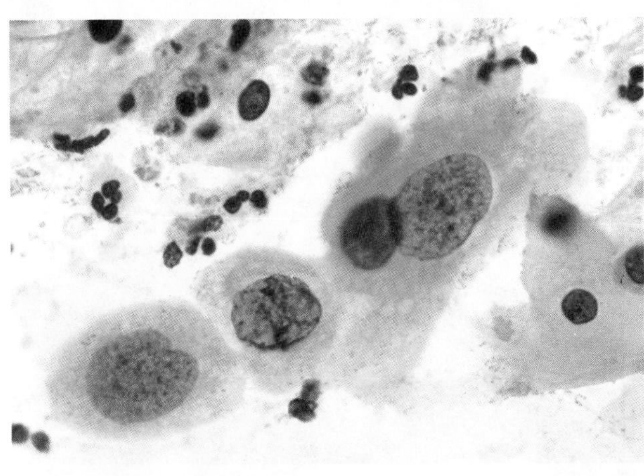

B

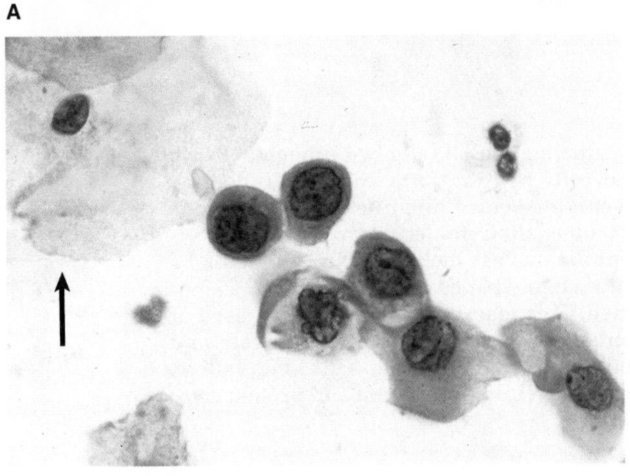

C

FIGURE 30-5
Spectrum of cervical intraepithelial neoplasia (CIN) in cervical smears. (*A*) CIN grade I (mild dysplasia). The dysplastic cell (*arrow*) has abundant cytoplasm. The nucleus is enlarged and hyperchromatic. The chromatin is evenly dispersed, and a nucleolus is not evident. Compare this cell with the other two normal squamous cells. (*B*) CIN grade II (moderate dysplasia). The dysplastic cells (center) are more numerous and have a higher nuclear-to-cytoplasmic ratio than do mildly dysplastic cells. (*C*) CIN grade III (severe dysplasia/carcinoma *in situ*). Multiple dysplastic squamous cells with scant cytoplasm and very high nuclear–cytoplasmic ratios are seen. Note the normal superficial squamous cell (*arrow*).

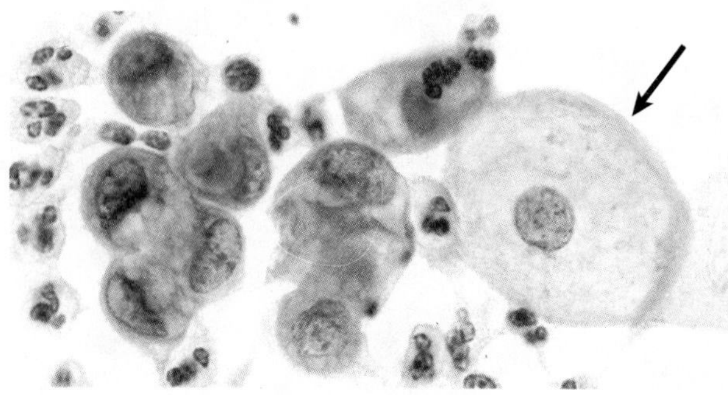

FIGURE *30-7*
Endometrial adenocarcinoma in a cervical smear. A cluster of medium-sized malignant cells displays cytoplasmic vacuoles. The nuclei are eccentric and have irregular nuclear membranes and abnormally distributed chromatin. Note the benign squamous cell (*arrow*).

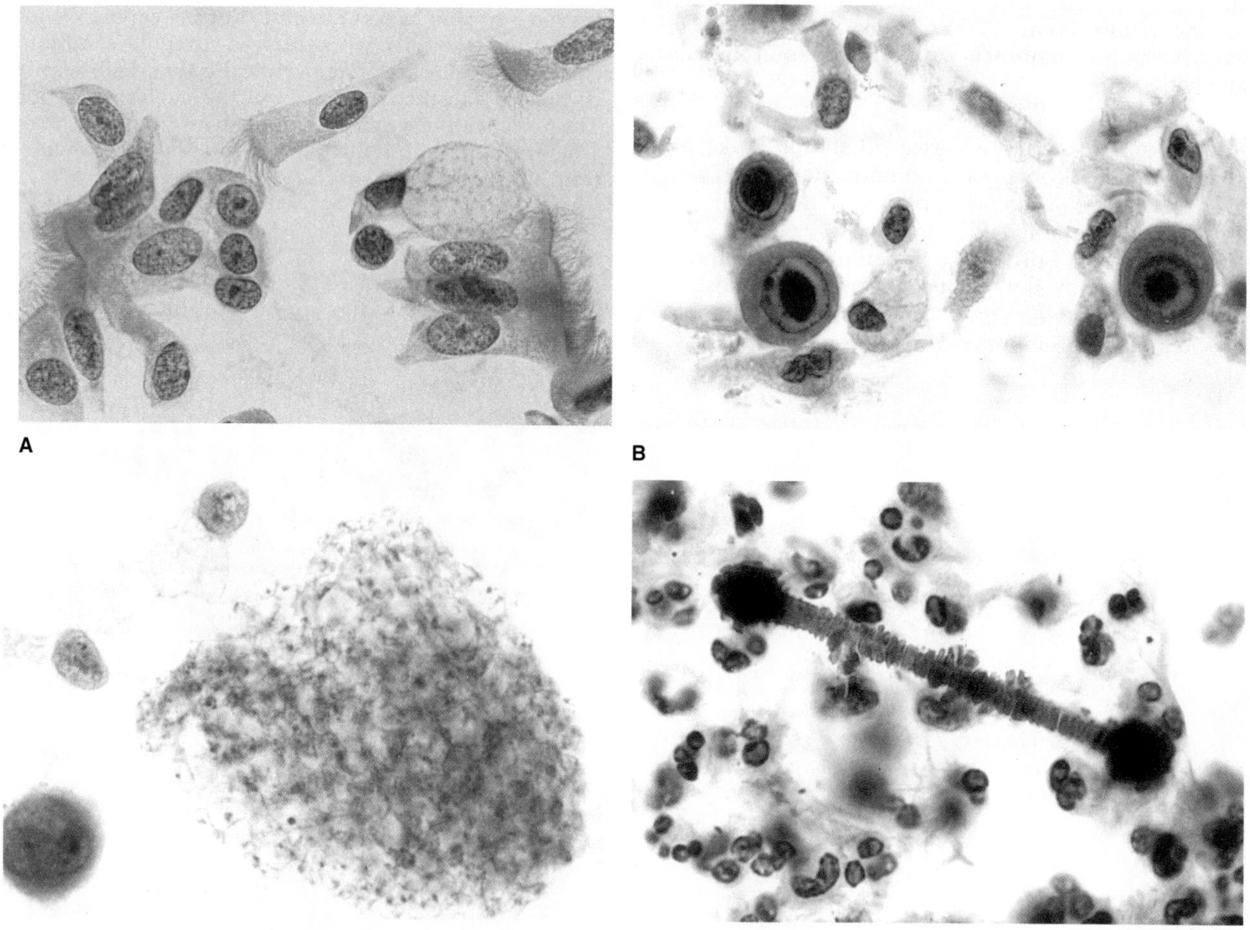

A

B

C

D

FIGURE *30-8*
Cytology of the respiratory tract. (*A*) Normal bronchial epithelial cells in a bronchial brush specimen are shown. Note the ciliated columnar cells with uniform and basally located nuclei. The chromatin is finely granular and evenly dispersed, the nuclear membrane is smooth and regular, and the nucleoli are inconspicuous. (*B*) Cytomegalovirus (CMV) infection in bronchial washings. Note the large basophilic nuclear inclusions surrounded by a halo and marginated chromatin, forming the typical target-shaped appearance. (*C*) *Pneumocystis carinii* in a bronchoalveolar lavage specimen. This foamy alveolar cast composed of small cysts, each with an eccentric dot, is characteristic of *P. carinii*. Two bronchial cells and an alveolar macrophage are evident. (*D*) Ferruginous body in the sputum. This long, yellow, beaded structure with clubbed ends is formed by the precipitation of iron and protein complexes on asbestos fibers.

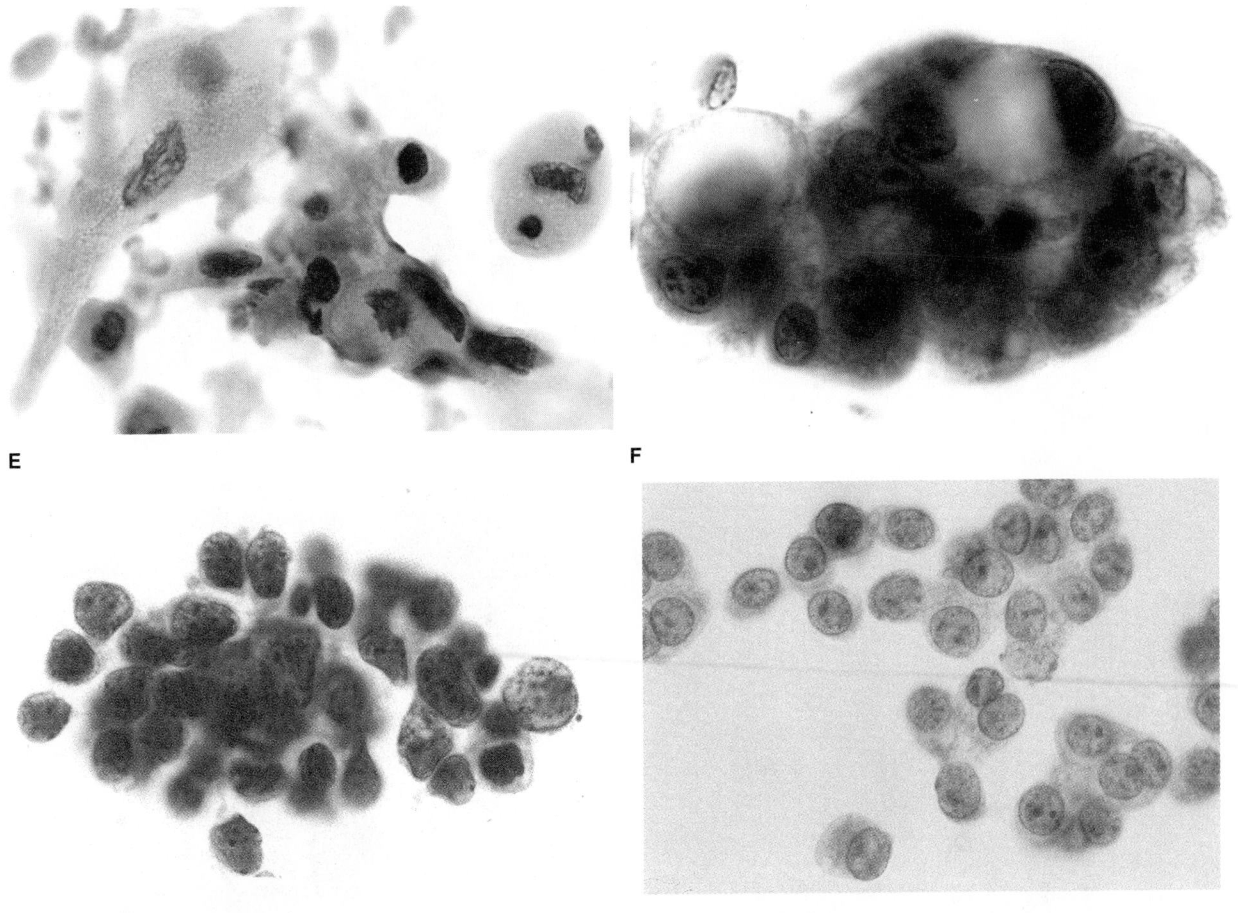

FIGURE 30-8 *continued*
(*E*) Squamous cell carcinoma in a bronchial brush specimen. Note the highly atypical squamous cells with marked variation in size and shape. The nuclei are hyperchromatic and irregular. The orange color in some of the cells is imparted by the presence of keratin. (*F*) Adenocarcinoma cells in the sputum. A cluster of epithelial cells with highly atypical nuclei, prominent nucleoli, and cytoplasmic vacuoles is seen. (*G*) Small cell carcinoma in a bronchial brush specimen. The cells are small, the cytoplasm is scanty, and the nuclei are molded where they abut adjacent ones. (*H*) Carcinoid tumor in a fine-needle aspirate of the lung. These medium-sized cells are arranged in loosely cohesive sheets. The cells possess granular cytoplasm and uniform, round nuclei. The chromatin is evenly dispersed and the nucleoli are indistinct.

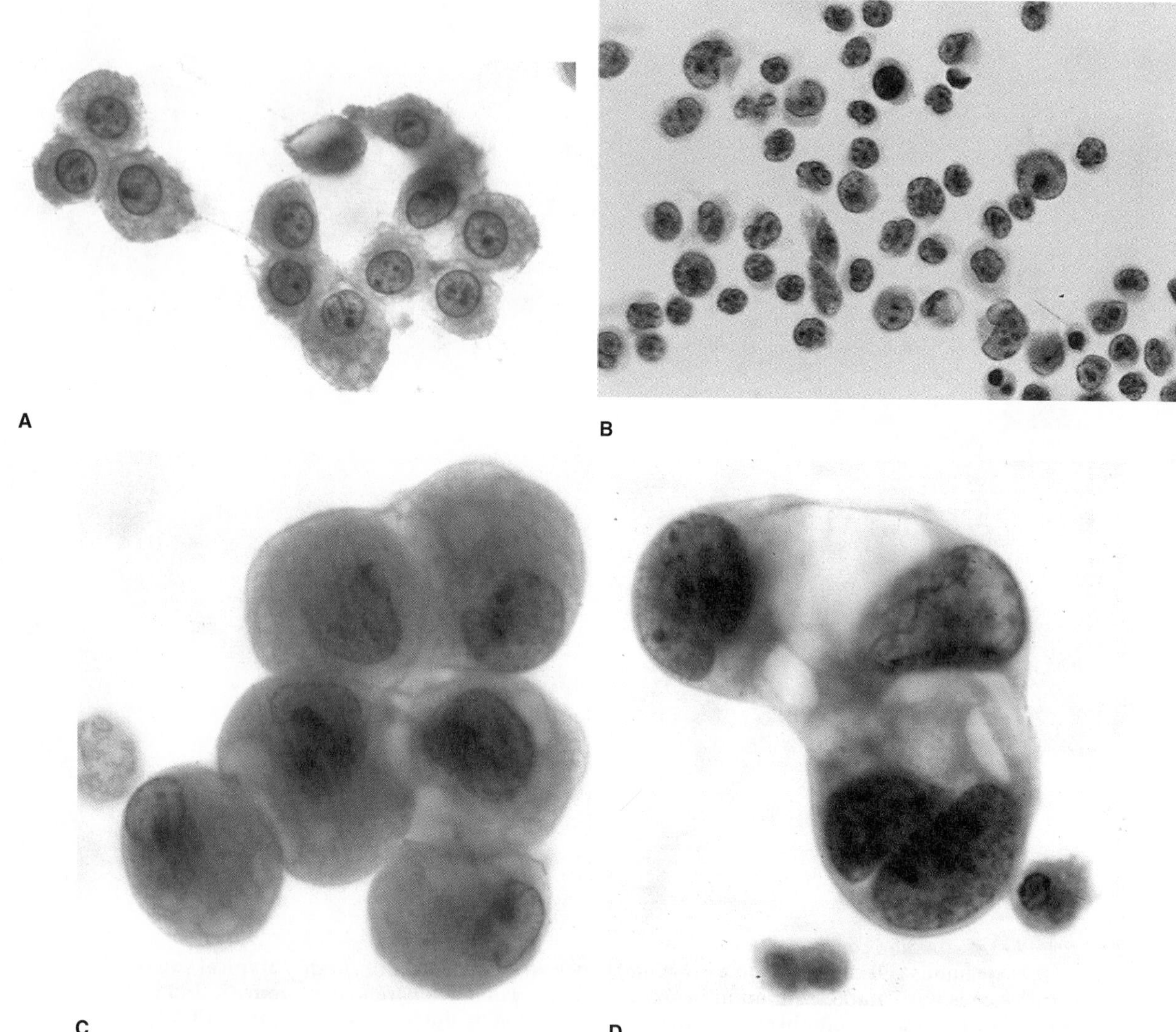

FIGURE 30-9
Cytology of effusions. (*A*) Benign mesothelial cells in a pleural fluid. The nuclei are small, round, and uniform. The nuclear membrane is smooth, and the nucleoli are small. (*B*) Malignant lymphoma in a pleural fluid. There are single small atypical cells with high nuclear–cytoplasmic ratio, coarse chromatin, and irregular nuclear membrane. (*C*) Cells of a malignant mesothelioma in a pleural fluid. The cytoplasm resembles that of normal mesothelial cells, but the nuclei are large, hyperchromatic, and irregular. The chromatin is abnormally distributed; the nucleoli are prominent, and the nuclear membrane has irregular indentations. (*D*) Metastatic ovarian adenocarcinoma in an ascitic fluid. The nuclei exhibit malignant criteria, and the cytoplasm contains secretory vacuoles.

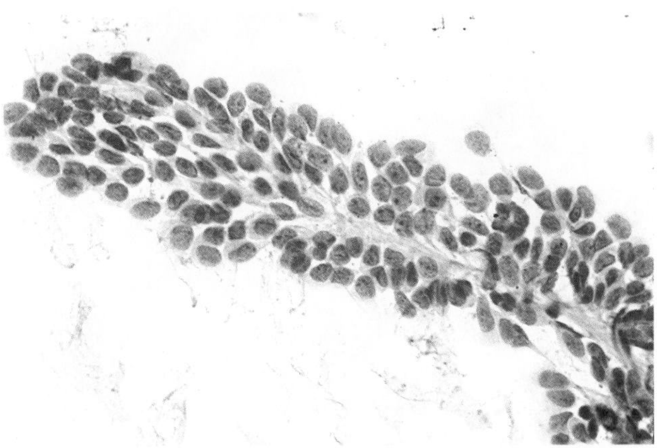
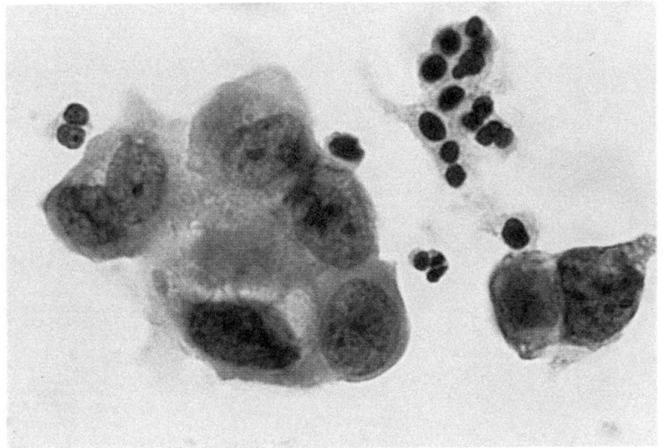

A B

FIGURE *30-10*
Cytology of the urinary tract. (*A*) Low-grade papillary urothelial neoplasm in an endoscopic brush specimen from the renal pelvis. The cells are uniform and resemble normal urothelial cells. Architecturally, however, the cells form a papillary structure with a central core, which facilitates the diagnosis of a papillary neoplasm. (*B*) High-grade urothelial carcinoma in the urine. Highly pleomorphic cells with varying sized, hyperchromatic, and irregular nuclei are evident. The nucleoli are prominent in some cells.

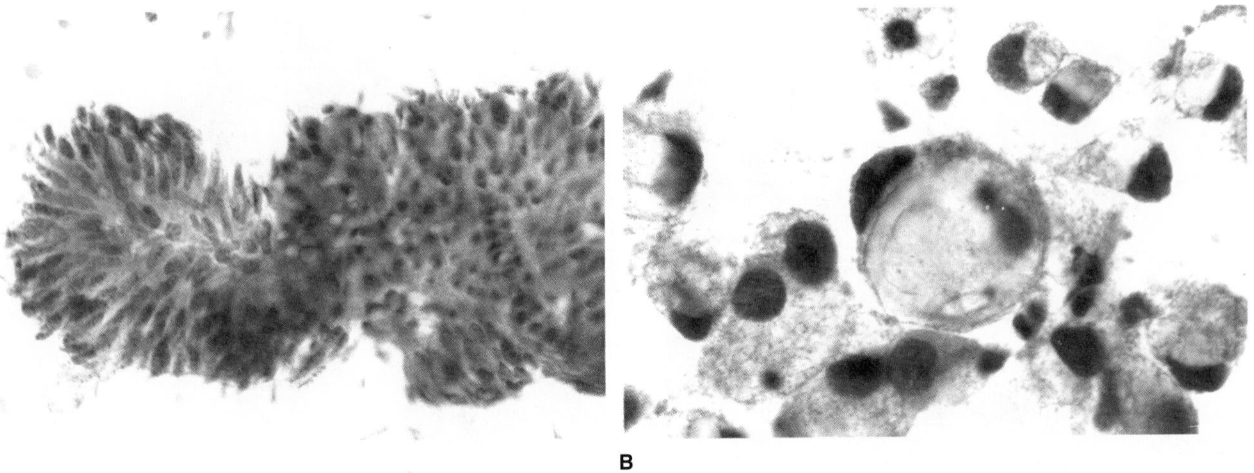

A B

FIGURE *30-11*
Cytology of the alimentary tract. (*A*) Benign colonic adenoma in a colonoscopic brushing specimen. This cohesive cluster of columnar cells exhibits crowding and elongation of the nuclei, but without significant variations in size or shape. (*B*) Signet ring cell adenocarcinoma in a gastric brushing specimen. There is a lack of cohesiveness among the tumor cells. The nuclei appear malignant and are displaced by large amounts of cytoplasmic mucin.

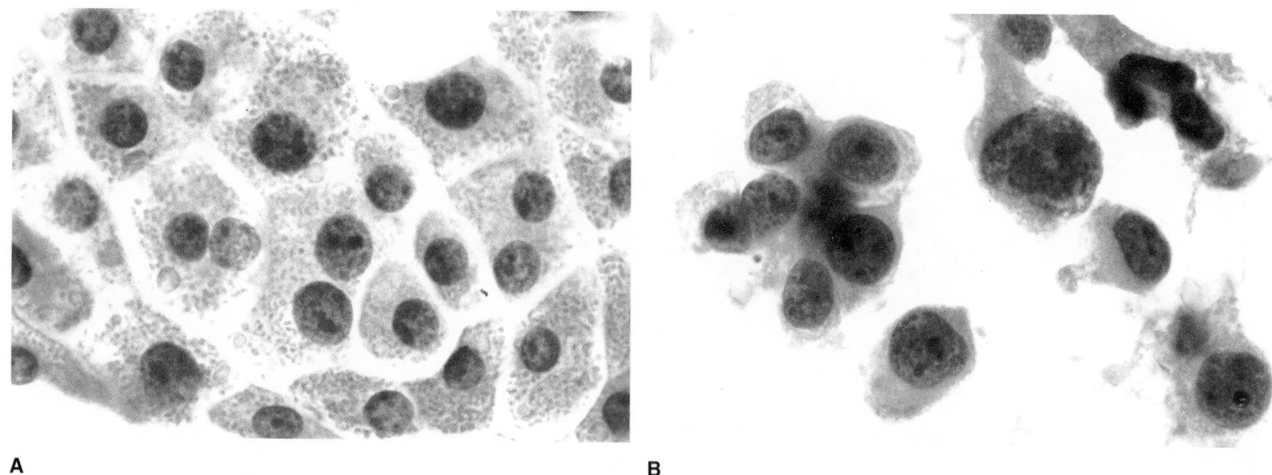

FIGURE *30-12*
Fine-needle aspiration (FNA) cytology of the breast. (*A*) Apocrine metaplasia. These benign cells form a monolayer sheet. The cytoplasm is abundant and granular. The nuclei are round and uniform and possess small nucleoli. (*B*) Mammary duct carcinoma. The cells vary in size and shape and are poorly cohesive. The nuclei are hyperchromatic, with clumping of the chromatin. The nucleoli are prominent.

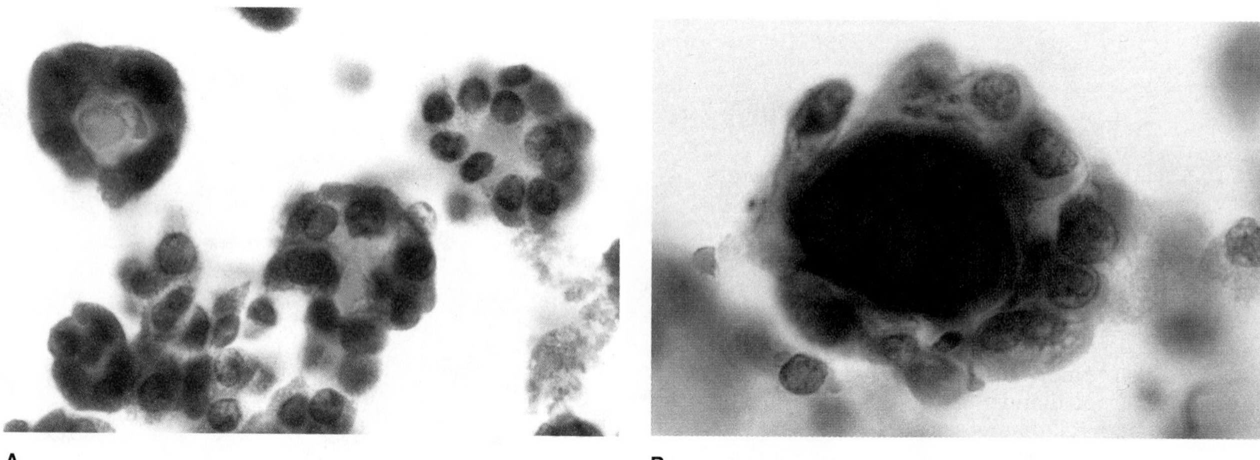

FIGURE *30-13*
Fine-needle aspiration (FNA) cytology of the thyroid. (*A*) Follicular neoplasm. The tumor cells form small follicles with scant colloid. There is a mild degree of nuclear atypia. (*B*) Papillary carcinoma. There is a psammoma body surrounded by atypical epithelial cells. The nuclei exhibit clearing of the chromatin, folding of the nuclear membrane (nuclear grooves), and an occasional intranuclear cytoplasmic invagination (pseudoinclusion).

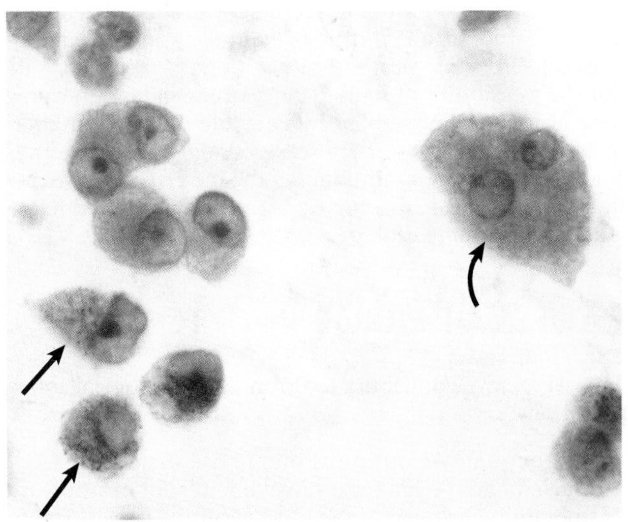

FIGURE 30-14
Metastatic malignant melanoma in a fine-needle aspirate of the liver. Poorly cohesive tumor cells with eccentric nuclei and prominent nucleoli are present. The cytoplasm contains fine melanin granules (*straight arrows*). A benign binucleated hepatocyte is evident (*curved arrow*).

ADVANTAGES OF CYTOPATHOLOGY

Cytology has both advantages and limitations compared with the examination of histological samples (biopsy). The following are the most important advantages.

Less trauma is produced by cytological techniques than by biopsy. Thus, there are fewer complications, such as hemorrhage or perforation. For example, aspirating pleural fluid with a thin needle is much less traumatic than obtaining a piece of the pleura by open biopsy or with a large needle. Similarly, brushing the surface of an endobronchial tumor or a colonic lesion is less likely to cause hemorrhage than is removing a piece of the tissue. Because of the small diameter of the needle used for fine-needle aspiration, the risk of hemorrhage, infection, or tumor spread is negligible compared with that associated with large-core needle biopsy or punch biopsy. Acute pancreatitis, a serious complication of large-core needle biopsy or open biopsy of the pancreas, is vanishingly rare with fine-needle aspiration. The complications of anesthesia are of no concern, because collection of cytological samples usually does not require general or local anesthesia.

A larger sampling surface is available for cytological methods. This is particularly important in endoscopic procedures and in the assessment of the intraperitoneal spread of cancer cells during laparotomy. In peritoneal washings, a very large area of the peritoneum is sampled, whereas biopsy samples are limited to a few, small, grossly visible foci. A focus of flat *in situ* carcinoma of the bladder that is not evident by cystoscopy is more likely to be discovered by cytological examination of the urine or bladder washings than by a few random biopsy samples.

Tumors that are difficult to access by biopsy may be sampled by cytological methods. Examples include cerebrospinal fluid cytology to diagnose meningeal carcinomatosis; brushing or washing of a gastrointestinal tract stricture that does not permit passage of the biopsy instrument; and fine-needle aspiration of a peripheral carcinoma of the lung that is beyond the reach of a bronchoscope.

A rapid diagnosis is one of the major advantages of cytological methods. Direct smears and fine-needle aspirates can be read within a few minutes of the collection. Fluids that need laboratory preparation can be processed, if necessary, in less than an hour.

Greater convenience is afforded by the collection of cytological specimens compared with biopsy. In most instances, no prior preparation of the patient is necessary, and the sampling is done as an office procedure. For endoscopically collected specimens, no preparations are needed beyond those required routinely for visualization.

An increased detection rate of malignancy in endoscopic procedures is achieved by combining cytological sampling (washing or brushing) with biopsy. In turn, this reduces the possibility that a repeated diagnostic procedure will be required.

A greater cost-effectiveness of cytology as a method of cancer detection has been amply demonstrated. Often, it eliminates needless tests, procedures, and surgical operations.

The following case histories illustrate the advantages of cytology:

- A 45-year-old woman visited a physician after noticing a "lump" in her neck. The physician discovered a thyroid nodule, and during the same visit, performed a fine-needle aspiration. Within hours, the cytopathologist diagnosed papillary carcinoma of the thyroid. The patient was referred to a surgeon for thyroidectomy without the need for further confirmatory tests. An alternative course of action might have been tests of thyroid function, radionuclide scanning of the thyroid, ultrasonography, and a trial of thyroid hormone–suppression therapy for several months.
- A pregnant woman discovered a rapidly enlarging mass in her breast. Her physician performed fine-needle aspiration of the nodule, which was diagnosed as a benign fibroadenoma. Surgery was delayed until after delivery to avoid possible complications of surgery or anesthesia during pregnancy. The alternative might have been an immediate surgical excision of the mass for fear of breast cancer, which may grow more rapidly during pregnancy.

LIMITATIONS OF CYTOPATHOLOGY

The classification of the type of tumor is generally more difficult with cytological samples than with the biopsy specimens because of the small size of cytological samples and the loss of tissue pattern. Cytological interpretation relies heavily on morphological alterations of individual cells, and to a lesser degree on the relation between the cells (e.g., formation of acini or squamous pearls, molding of cells, papillary arrangement). The patterns of tumor infiltration and invasion of the adjacent structures and vascular channels are important histological parameters in the determination of malignancy but cannot be evaluated by cytology. For example, the differential diagnosis between follicular adenoma and well-differentiated follicular carcinoma of the thyroid depends on the absence or presence of capsular and vascular invasion, rather than the appearance of the tumor cells. Because such invasion cannot be determined by aspiration of the lesion, a diagnosis of "follicular neoplasm" is rendered by the cytopathologist; further classification of the tumor requires histological examination of the excised tumor.

The small size of the specimen may preclude accurate classification of some neoplasms with mixed elements, such as adenosquamous carcinoma, carcinosarcoma, or synovial sarcoma, if only one component of the tumor is sampled. In exfoliative cytology, carcinomas are more readily diagnosed than sarcomas, because epithelial neoplasms have a higher tendency to shed tumor cells. For the same reason, malignant mixed mesodermal tumor of the female genital tract is frequently diagnosed as adenocarcinoma on examination of the peritoneal fluid or cervicovaginal smears.

The extent and depth of invasion cannot be assessed by cytological examination. For example, it is not possible to distinguish with certainty between *in situ* and invasive transitional cell carcinoma of the bladder by cytological examination of the urine, between microinvasive and deeply invasive squamous carcinoma of the cervix with cervical smears, or between intraductal carcinoma and invasive duct carcinoma of the breast by needle aspiration.

ACCURACY OF CYTOLOGICAL METHODS

The accuracy of cytological diagnosis depends on several factors, including the experience of the collector of the specimen, the sampling method, the target organ, and the expertise of the examiner. False-positive diagnoses are rarely made by experienced cytopathologists; thus, the specificity of a malignant diagnosis approaches 100%. The sensitivity of the test, however, is in the range of 80% to 90% for most specimen types.

A higher sensitivity has been achieved by some endoscopic brushing methods, particularly for alimentary tract malignancies, whereas for some specimen types, the sensitivity is lower. For example, cytological examination of cerebrospinal fluid detects only one third of primary neoplasms of the central nervous system and only one half of metastatic cancers, because only tumors that communicate with the ventricles or meninges can shed cells. For urinary tract cancers, the sensitivity of cytology depends on the type and grade of the tumor. Low-grade transitional cell carcinomas, which by definition have little or no nuclear atypia, are difficult to detect, whereas high-grade neoplasms are usually diagnosed correctly.

The sensitivity of fine-needle aspiration has been reported to be about 90% in large series. The existence of false-negative results indicates that the absence of malignant cells in cytological samples does not completely rule out the possibility of malignancy. Unless a benign cause for a lesion can be established by cytological examination (e.g., fibroadenoma of the breast, benign cyst of the thyroid, liver abscess, granuloma of the lung), further investigation, including histological biopsy, is warranted to exclude a malignant etiology.

CAUSES OF ERROR IN CYTOLOGY

Several factors contribute to erroneous cytological interpretations:

- **Inadequate sampling** is one of the major causes of false-negative diagnoses in cytology. For example, in obtaining a smear of the uterine cervix, it is critical to sample the transformation zone, because most precancerous lesions of the cervix arise in this area. Thus, an adequate cervical smear should contain squamous cells as well as endocervical material (columnar cells, mucus, and metaplastic squamous cells). The adequacy of a sputum specimen is assessed by the presence of pulmonary macrophages, which indicates a deep cough sample. Examples of inadequate cytological samples include (1) a peritoneal washing specimen that lacks mesothelial cells, (2) a smear of a cutaneous vesicle, which is obtained to search for viral changes, but which lacks squamous cells, and (3) a gastric brushing specimen, which contains blood and inflammatory cells but no epithelial cells.
- **Poor fixation of the smears or inadequate preservation of a fluid** is another preventable cause of error in cytology. For the Papanicolaou staining method, cells must be fixed in 95% ethanol or by a spray fixative immediately after smearing on the slide. A few seconds of delay in fixation can cause air-drying artifacts, which create substantial difficulties in interpretation.

  Cells in body fluids undergo degeneration, the rate of which varies according to the type of fluid. Generally, cells are better protected in fluids with a high protein concentration, such as effusions, than in those that contain little protein (e.g., urine or cerebrospinal fluid). To prevent cell degeneration, fluids must be transported to the laboratory and processed rapidly. Refrigeration slows cell degeneration and bacterial growth for a few hours or a day, but if delay is inevitable, a preservative should be used. Addition of an equal volume of 50% ethanol is a good method for preservation of fluids. Formaldehyde, a commonly used fixative for histological samples, is not appropriate for cytological preparations.
- **Suboptimal laboratory preparation and staining** can cause considerable difficulty in the interpretation of cytological smears. Examples include (1) inadequate cell concentration or poor adhesion to the glass slide, (2) thick smears containing multiple layers of cells, (3) poor fixation, and (4) inadequate or excessive exposure of the cells to various staining reagents.

MORPHOLOGICAL PARAMETERS USED IN CYTOLOGICAL EVALUATION

Cellularity of the Specimen

Several factors influence the cellularity of a cytological sample, including the sampling method and device, the expertise of the collector, and the type of the tissue being sampled. In general, abrasive methods produce more cells than spontaneously exfoliated samples. For example, samples of a lung neoplasm obtained by bronchial washing or brushing are more likely to have a large number of tumor cells than is a sputum specimen.

In fine-needle aspiration, larger size needles produce more cellular samples than very thin ones. The cellularity of abrasive and fine-needle aspiration specimens is also dependent on the expertise of the physician who performs the procedure. The placement of the needle or brush in the proper position, application of optimal pressure or suction, adequate movement of the device within the target tissue, and avoidance of dilution of cells with excessive blood are all important factors in obtaining adequately cellular samples.

The type of tissue being sampled greatly influences the cellularity of the specimen. Epithelial cells are generally detached with greater ease than stromal cells or fibrous tissue. Malignant cells have a lower degree of cohesiveness than their benign counterparts; thus they are more likely to exfoliate spontaneously or mechanically. Malignant neoplasms that have little connective tissue support (e.g., small cell carcinoma of the lung, lymphoma, malignant melanoma) produce more cellular samples than those with a generous fibrous stroma (e.g., scirrhous carcinoma of the breast). In general, carcinomas have a higher tendency to exfoliate cells than do sarcomas.

Cell Arrangement

The tissue pattern is lost in cytological preparations, particularly in exfoliative cytology. However, the relation between cells is a helpful criterion for cytological diagnosis. Cells may appear singly, in small groups, in monolayer sheets, or in three-dimensional clusters. Several cells may fuse, forming a large multinucleated cell termed a *syncytium*. Cell clusters may form (1) papillary configurations with fibrovascular cores (papillary transitional cell carcinoma, papillary adenocarcinoma, malignant mesothelioma); (2) glandular or tubular structures (adenocarcinoma); (3) follicles (follicular adenoma of the thyroid); (4) rosettes (neuroblastoma); or (5) pearls (squamous cell carcinoma).

Cell Size and Shape

The size of tumor cells varies greatly depending on the type of neoplasm. Small cell carcinoma of the lung, some types of lymphoma, and many childhood tumors are composed of small regular cells. By contrast, squamous cell carcinoma, giant cell carcinoma, pleomorphic sarcomas, some endocrine carcinomas, and choriocarcinoma display very large cells. Malignant neoplasms tend to have a greater variability in cell size than do benign tumors, a feature termed *anisocytosis*. However, this rule does not apply to all neoplasms. Well-differentiated adenocarcinomas and low-grade transitional cell carcinomas, for example, have little anisocytosis. Conversely, marked anisocytosis may be seen in some benign conditions, such as lymph node hyperplasia or radiation effects.

Cell shape may vary widely from one tissue to another, but cells of the same type in normal tissues and in benign neoplasms are generally uniform (monomorphic). By contrast, most malignant tumors exhibit marked variation in cell shape (pleomorphic).

Cytoplasm

The cytoplasm is evaluated for color, texture, presence of inclusions, vacuoles, pigments, and other cell products. With the Papanicolaou method, the cytoplasm assumes various shades of pink to blue; keratin is characterized by an orange color. The cytoplasm may vary in texture from homogeneous to granular or foamy. The presence of pigments, including melanin, hemosiderin, bile, lipofuscin, and carbon particles, is helpful in identifying the cell type. Single or multiple vacuoles in the cytoplasm indicate degenerative changes, secretory activity, or phagocytosis. Viral and chlamydial infections may form inclusions in the cytoplasm. Squamous cells infected by human papillomavirus show characteristic changes called *koilocytotic atypia*, which consists of a large perinuclear halo and nuclear abnormalities. The accumulation of immunoglobulin in the cytoplasm of reactive or neoplastic plasma cells forms an eosinophilic globule termed the *Russell body*. Small cytoplasmic concretions called *Michaelis–Gutmann bodies* are seen in malakoplakia.

Nucleus

The size and shape of the nucleus, alterations of nuclear membrane and chromatin, prominence of the nucleolus, and mitotic activity are important parameters in cytological evaluation. The nuclei of normal cells show little variation in size and shape. Modest nuclear enlargement occurs in normal cells during the S phase of the cell cycle and in reactive or regenerating cells. Malignant cells usually exhibit significant nuclear enlargement, which is frequently disproportionate to the enlargement of the cell and results in an increased nuclear-to-cytoplasmic ratio. In addition, significant variations in nuclear size (*anisokaryosis*) and nuclear shape are common in malignant neoplasms. The nuclei of most cancer cells, with the exception of some well-differentiated tumors, are abnormally shaped and have an irregular contour, with protrusions, indentations, and grooves. Molding of the nuclei against one another is seen in some tumors (classically in small cell carcinomas), probably owing to a rapid growth rate and a scanty cytoplasm.

The nuclei of cancer cells are usually darker (*hyperchromatic*) than those of normal cells, and the chromatin tends to be coarser and unevenly distributed. Multinucleation *per se* is not helpful in the diagnosis of malignancy, because this feature may be seen in (1) normal cells (e.g., superficial urothelial cells, osteoclasts, syncytiotrophoblasts), (2) inflammatory conditions (e.g., multinucleated giant cells in granulomas), (3) benign neoplasms (e.g., giant cell tumor of the tendon sheath), or (4) malignant neoplasms (e.g., giant cell carcinoma, malignant fibrous histiocytoma, choriocarcinoma).

The nucleoli of cancer cells, particularly in poorly differentiated tumors, are often larger and more numerous than those in their benign counterparts. However, prominent nucleoli also can be seen in metabolically active benign cells. Furthermore, in some types of cancer (e.g., small cell carcinoma of the lung), tumor cells lack conspicuous nucleoli. Cytoplasmic invagination into the nucleus, which is seen in cross-section as a pale intranuclear inclusion, may occur in some benign and malignant neoplasms and may be helpful in their classification. For example, the presence of such cytoplasmic "inclusions" in a thyroid aspirate is a strong indication of papillary carcinoma.

Mitoses

Whereas increased mitotic activity can occur in both benign and malignant tumors, cancer cells in general have a higher rate of mitosis. Additionally, the presence of abnormal mitoses (abnormal distribution of chromosomes or presence of more than two mitotic poles) is a reliable criterion for the diagnosis of malignancy.

Extracellular Material and Cellular Background

The background of the smear is evaluated for the presence of inflammation, blood, various extracellular substances, cell products, necrotic debris, and microorganisms. The type of inflammation (acute, chronic, granulomatous) and some varieties of microorganisms, including bacteria, fungi, protozoa, and helminths, can be identified. Cell necrosis may occur in a variety of benign conditions (for example, in infections, trauma, ischemia, and irradiation). Cell necrosis may also be a prominent feature of many malignant neoplasms. Thus, in the absence of recognizable intact cells, a definitive diagnosis cannot be made on a sample composed entirely of necrotic debris. However, when present in association with malignant cells, necrosis is generally an indication of an invasive cancer. In this way, necrosis may help to distinguish an invasive squamous cell carcinoma of the uterine cervix from carcinoma *in situ*. This criterion, however, cannot be generalized to all types of cancers. For instance, carcinoma *in situ* of the breast may also contain foci of necrosis (comedocarcinoma). Common entities found in the smear background are listed in Table 30-2.

TABLE *30-2* Smear Background in Cytological Specimens

Inflammation (acute, chronic, granulomatous)
Microorganisms
Bacteria
Fungi
Helminths
Protozoa (*Trichomonas vaginalis, Pneumocystis carinii,* amebae)
Necrotic debris
Blood, hemosiderin
Mucin
Amyloid
Colloid
Psammoma bodies
Ferruginous bodies
Curschmann's spirals
Charcot–Leyden crystals
Renal casts
Urinary crystals

REPORTING SYSTEMS

Various methods have been used for reporting the results of cytological tests. Papanicolaou devised a numerical classification system, which ranged from class I for the absence of abnormal cells to class V for conclusive evidence of cancer. In the early years of cytopathology, this classification was widely adopted, but it proved inadequate as the field expanded. Most laboratories have replaced the Papanicolaou classification with narrative reports, similar to the terminology used in histopathological reporting.

In 1988, a group of pathologists and gynecologists met in Bethesda, Maryland, in an attempt to standardize gynecological cytology reports. The group concluded that the Papanicolaou classification was unacceptable in the modern practice of cytopathology and proposed a new reporting classification, which has since become known as the **Bethesda system**. This reporting system has been adopted by most laboratories in the United States. A second Bethesda workshop in 1991 revised the original classification. Each cytology report should include the following elements:

- A statement regarding the adequacy of the specimen for diagnostic evaluation
- A general categorization of the diagnosis (as "within normal limits," "benign cellular changes," or "epithelial cell abnormality")
- A descriptive diagnosis

One of the most important accomplishments of the Bethesda system is a mandate for a statement on adequacy of the specimen. The following elements must be present to deem a cervical smear satisfactory for evaluation: (1) Technical interpretability (optimal smearing, proper fixation, lack of excessive blood or inflammation, etc.), and (2) adequate sampling of the transformation zone (presence of ectocervical squamous cells and endocervical columnar or metaplastic squamous cells).

The Bethesda system also introduced a new classification for cervical precancerous lesions, which consists of two categories: (1) low-grade squamous intraepithelial lesion (human papillomavirus infection and mild dysplasia), and (2) high-grade squamous intraepithelial lesion (moderate dysplasia, severe dysplasia, carcinoma *in situ*).

SUGGESTED READING

BOOKS

Atkinson BF (ed): *Atlas of diagnostic cytopathology.* Philadelphia: WB Saunders, 1992.

Bibbo M (ed): *Comprehensive cytopathology.* 2nd ed. Philadelphia: WB Saunders, 1997.

DeMay RM: *The art and science of cytopathology.* Chicago: ASCP Press, 1996.

Koss LG: *Diagnostic cytology and its histopathologic bases,* 4th ed. Philadelphia: JB Lippincott, 1997.

Koss LG, Woyke S, Olszewski W: *Aspiration biopsy: Cytologic interpretation and histologic bases,* 2nd ed. Tokyo: Igaku-Shoin, 1992.

Kurman RJ, Solomon D. *The Bethesda System for reporting cervical/vaginal cytologic diagnoses: Definitions, criteria, and explanatory notes for terminology and specimen adequacy.* New York: Springer-Verlag, 1994.

REVIEW ARTICLES

Bigner SH, Johnston WW: The cytopathology of cerebrospinal fluid: II. Metastatic cancer, meningeal carcinomatosis and primary central nervous system neoplasms. *Acta Cytol* 25:461–479, 1981.

Christopherson WM: Cytologic detection and diagnosis of cancer: Its contributions and limitations. *Cancer* 51:1201–1208, 1983.

Ehya H: Effusion cytology: The value and limitations of cytologic examination. *Clin Lab Med* 11:443–467, 1991.

Frable WJ: Needle aspiration biopsy: Past, present, and future. *Hum Pathol* 20:504–517, 1989.

Gharib H, Goellner JR. Fine needle aspiration biopsy of the thyroid: An appraisal. *Ann Intern Med* 118:282–289, 1993.

Hajdu SI: Cytology from antiquity to Papanicolaou. *Acta Cytol* 21:668–676, 1977.

Hajdu SI, Ehya H, Frable WJ, et al: The value and limitations of aspiration cytology in the diagnosis of primary tumors: A symposium. *Acta Cytol* 33:741–790, 1989.

Hajdu SI, Melamed MR: Limitations of aspiration cytology in the diagnosis of primary neoplasms. *Acta Cytol* 28:337–345, 1984.

Johnston WW, Frable WJ: Cytopathology of the respiratory tract: A review. *Am J Pathol* 84:372–424, 1976.

Kline TS: Survey of aspiration biopsy cytology of the breast. *Diagn Cytopathol* 7:98–105, 1991.

Koss LG: Cytology: Accuracy of diagnosis. *Cancer* 64(suppl):249–252, 1989.

Koss LG: The Papanicolaou test for cervical cancer detection: A triumph and a tragedy. *JAMA* 261:737–743, 1989.

Zakowski MF: Fine needle aspiration cytology of tumors: Diagnostic accuracy and potential pitfalls. *Cancer Invest* 12:505–515, 1994.

Acknowledgments

Specific acknowledgment is made for permission to use the following material:

Chapter 1, Figure 7. Okazaki H, Scheithauer BW: Atlas of Neuropathology. New York, Gower Medical Publishing, 1988. By permission of Mayo Foundation.

Chapter 3, Figure 18. Okazaki H, Scheithauer BW: Atlas of Neuropathology. New York, Gower Medical Publishing, 1988. By permission of Mayo Foundation.

Chapter 5, Figure 6. Bullough PG, Vigorita VJ: Atlas of Orthopaedic Pathology. New York, Gower Medical Publishing, 1984.

Chapter 5, Figure 18. Bullough PG, Boachie-Adjei O: Atlas of Spinal Diseases. New York, Gower Medical Publishing, 1988.

Chapter 6, Figure 30. Bullough PG, Vigorita VJ: Atlas of Orthopaedic Pathology. New York, Gower Medical Publishing, 1988.

Chapter 8, Figure 14. Okazaki H, Scheithauer BW: Atlas of Neuropathology. New York, Gower Medical Publishing, 1988. By permission of Mayo Foundation.

Chapter 8, Figure 16. McKee PH: Pathology of the Skin. London, Gower Medical Publishing, 1989.

Chapter 9, Figures 21A, 21B, 28, 54A, 71, 83, 89, 90, 98A, and 98B. Farrar WE, Wood MJ, Innes JA, Tubbs H: Infectious Diseases Text and Color Atlas, 2nd ed. New York, Gower Medical Publishing, 1992.

Chapter 12, Figure 58. Courtesy of the Armed Forces Institute of Pathology.

Chapter 12. The authors would like to gratefully acknowledge Dr. Bruce Wenig for the contribution of Figure 5 and Dr. Anthony Gal for the contribution of Figure 73.

Chapter 13, Figures 6A, 6B, 9, 11, 14, 15, 23, 25, 27, 43, 45, 47, 50, 53A, 55, 61, and 62. Mitros FA: Atlas of Gastrointestinal Pathology. New York, Gower Medical Publishing, 1988.

Chapter 13, Figure 12. Courtesy of Dr. Cecilia M. Fenoglio-Preiser.

Chapter 14, Figure 43. Yanoff M: Ocular Pathology: A Color Atlas. New York, Gower Medical Publishing, 1988.

Chapter 14, Figure 63. Thung SN, Gerber MA: Histopathology of liver transplantation. In Fabry TL, Klion FM (eds): Guide to Liver Transplantation. New York, Igaku-Shoin Medical Publishers, 1992.

Chapter 17, Figures 4A and 10. Weiss MA, Mills SE: Atlas of Genitourinary Tract Diseases. New York, Gower Medical Publishers, 1988.

Chapter 18, Figures 59A and 59B. Woodruff JD, Parmley TH: Atlas of Gynecologic Pathology. New York, Gower Medical Publishing, 1988.

Chapter 21, Figure 13. Sandoz Pharmaceutical Corporation.

Chapter 26, Figures 22A, 22B, 43, 55B, 60, and 71A. Bullough PG: Atlas of Orthopaedic Pathology, 2nd ed. New York, Gower Medical Publishing, 1992.

Chapter 28, Figures 57 and 135A. Okazaki H, Scheithauer BW: Atlas of Neuropathology. New York, Gower Medical Publishing, 1988. By permission of Mayo Foundation.

Index

Note: Page numbers followed by *t* and *f* indicate tables and figures, respectively.

E

I

T